DAVIS'S DRUG GUIDE for NURSES®

TWENTIETH EDITION

Cynthia A. Sanoski, PharmD, BCPS, FCCP
Associate Dean of Student Affairs, Office of Professional Education
Professor of Instruction, Department of Pharmacy Practice & Science
University of Iowa College of Pharmacy
Iowa City, Iowa

F.A. DAVIS
Philadelphia

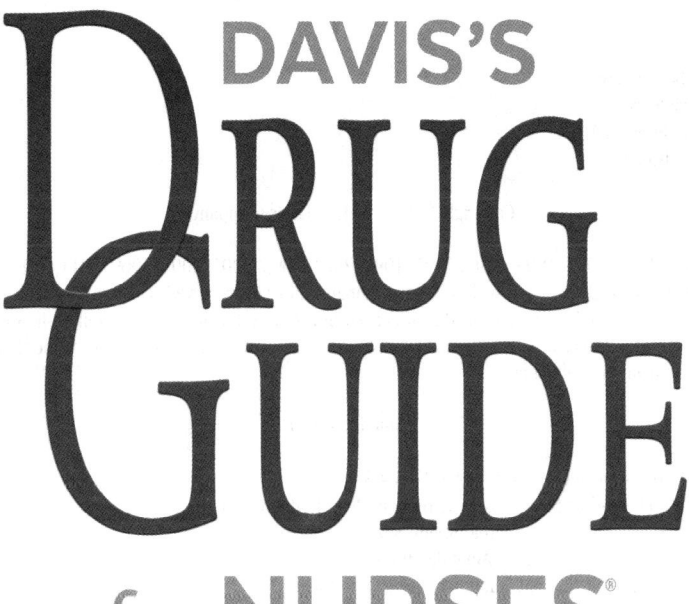

F. A. Davis Company
1915 Arch Street
Philadelphia, PA 19103
www.fadavis.com

Printed in China

Last digit indicates print number 10 9 8 7 6 5 4 3 2 1
Editor-in-Chief, Product Strategy & Development: Jean Rodenberger
Publisher, Product Strategy & Development: Suzanne Czehut Toppy
Senior Content Project Manager: Amanda Minutola
Senior Project Editor, Content Solutions: Megan Schindele
Manager, Content Architecture: Robert Allen

NOTE: As new scientific information becomes available through basic and clinical research, recommended treatments and drug therapies undergo changes. The authors and publisher have done everything possible to make this book accurate, up to date, and in accord with accepted standards at the time of publication. However, the reader is advised always to check product information (package inserts) for changes and new information regarding dose and contraindications before administering any drug. Caution is especially urged when using new or infrequently ordered drugs.

Library of Congress Control Number: 2025949810

IN MEMORIAM—APRIL HAZARD VALLERAND, PHD, RN, FAAN (1957–2024)

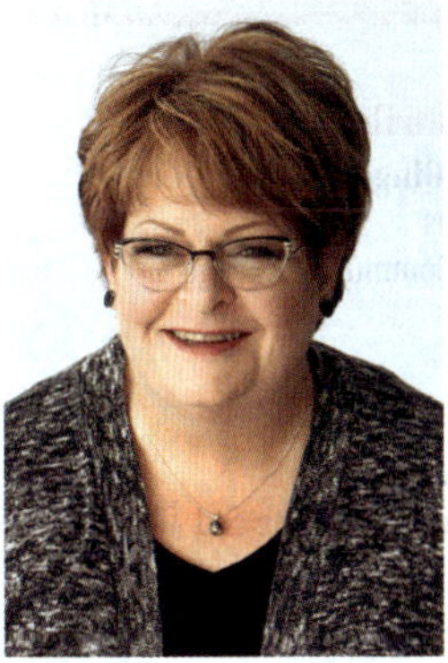

With profound respect and enduring gratitude, we dedicate this 20th edition of *Davis's Drug Guide for Nurses* to the memory of Dr. April Hazard Vallerand—a visionary nursing educator, esteemed researcher, and tireless advocate for patient-centered care.

Dr. Vallerand was a nationally recognized nurse educator, scholar, and clinician whose passion for pharmacology and commitment to improving pain management transformed nursing education and practice. As a lead author for *Davis's Drug Guide for Nurses* for more than 35 years, she was devoted to equipping nurses and nursing students with the most current evidence-based information on the safe and effective use of medications. As an Endowed Professor and Director of the PhD Program at Wayne State University College of Nursing, April mentored countless students and colleagues, always with grace, rigor, and generosity. Her legacy lives on in the countless lives she touched. We honor Dr. Vallerand by continuing the work she championed—empowering nurses with the knowledge and confidence to deliver safe, effective, and empathetic care.

April will be remembered not only for her remarkable professional contributions but also for her warmth, generosity, wit, and the inspiration she brought to all who had the privilege of knowing and working with her.

The Editorial Team of *Davis's Drug Guide*

DEDICATION

In loving memory of my mother, Geraldine, whose unwavering love, wisdom, and support graced every chapter of my life for 91 extraordinary years. Her presence was my constant source of strength and inspiration, guiding me through every personal and professional pursuit. The memories we shared are a lasting blessing—etched into my heart and spirit. I love you deeply, Momma.

Cindy

ACKNOWLEDGMENTS

I offer my thanks to the students and nurses who have used this book for more than 35 years. I hope this book provides you with the current knowledge of pharmacotherapeutics you need to continue to give quality care in our rapidly changing health care environment.

Cindy

Contributors

Monograph Contributors

Marlene Jones, DNP, MS, RN
Nursing Instructor
St. Elizabeth College of Nursing
Utica, New York

Sally Villaseñor, DNP, MSN, ACNP-BC, CNE
Assistant Professor (Clinical)
Wayne State University College of Nursing
Detroit, Michigan

Rachel Elizabeth Woolley, MSN, APRN
Family Nurse Practitioner
McMinnville, Oregon
Assistant Professor
Oregon Health & Science University
Monmouth, Oregon

Additional Contributors

Margaret Mary Gingrich, RN, MSN, CRNP
Professor Emeritus
Harrisburg Area Community College
Hospice CRNP
Homeland Hospice
Harrisburg, Pennsylvania

Gladdi Tomlinson, RN, MSN
Professor (Adjunct) of Nursing and Allied Health
Harrisburg Area Community College
Harrisburg, Pennsylvania

Erin Ziegler, PhD, NP-PHC
Associate Professor
Toronto Metropolitan University
Toronto, Ontario

Contents

How to Use *Davis's Drug Guide for Nurses*

Davis's Drug Guide for Nurses provides comprehensive, current drug information in well-organized nursing-focused monographs. It also includes extensive supplemental material in 14 appendices, addresses the issue of safe medication administration, and educates the reader about 40 different therapeutic classes of drugs. In this 20th edition, we continue to focus on safe medication administration by including **Medication Safety Tools** and even more information about health care's most vulnerable patients: children, older adults, pregnant patients, and breastfeeding (sometimes referred to as chest feeding) patients. Look for more Pedi, Geri, OB, Lactation, and Rep headings in the monographs. For Canadian students and nurses, we include an appendix comparing Canadian and U.S. pharmaceutical practices, more Canada-only combination drugs in the Combination Drugs appendix, and additional Canadian brand names in the drug monographs. The following sections describe the organization of *Davis's Drug Guide for Nurses*.

Safe Medication Use Articles

This book includes several articles that describe the medication safety issues that confront clinicians and patients. "Medication Errors: Improving Practices and Patient Safety" familiarizes you with the systems issues and clinical situations repeatedly implicated in medication errors and suggests means to avoid them. It also teaches you about *high alert* medications that have a greater potential to cause patient harm than other medications. "Detecting and Managing Adverse Drug Reactions" explains and provides guidance on identifying and managing adverse drug reactions. "Risk Evaluation and Mitigation Strategies (REMS)" explains strategies developed by the pharmaceutical industry and required by the Food and Drug Administration (FDA) to minimize adverse drug reactions from potentially dangerous drugs. "Special Dosing Considerations" identifies the patient populations (e.g., neonates, patients with renal or hepatic impairment, older adults) who require careful dose adjustments to ensure optimal therapeutic outcomes. "Educating Patients About Medication Use" reviews the most important teaching points for nurses to discuss with their patients and their families. Other critical safety information is highlighted in red in each drug monograph. In addition to these articles, please refer to the Medication Safety Tools in the back of the book for the BEERS criteria drug list, proper dosing for pediatric intravenous medications, confused drug names, FDA-approved tall man letters, and more.

Classifications

Medications in the same therapeutic class often share similar mechanisms of action, assessment guidelines, precautions, and interactions. The Classifications section provides summaries of the major therapeutic classifications we cover and commonly prescribed drugs in that class. It also provides patient teaching information common to all agents within the class. A list of drugs within each class can also be found in the Comprehensive Index.

Drug Monographs

Drug monographs are organized in the following manner:

High Alert Status: Some medications, such as chemotherapeutic agents, anticoagulants, and insulins, have a greater potential for harm than others. These medications are identified by the *Institute for Safe Medication Practices* as **high alert drugs**. *Davis's Drug Guide for Nurses* includes a HIGH ALERT label in the upper right corner of the monograph header in appropriate medications to alert the nurse to the medication's risk. The term "high alert" is used in other parts of the monograph to help the nurse administer these medications safely.

BEERS Criteria: A BEERS label appears at the top of applicable drug monographs for those medications listed in the most recent Beers Criteria developed by the American Geriatrics Society.

These medications are potentially inappropriate for use in older adults because they are associated with more risk than benefit in this patient population.

REMS status: We highlight the drugs that currently have approved REMS programs associated with their use by adding a REMS label at the top of applicable drug monographs.

Generic/Brand Name: The generic name appears first, with a pronunciation key, followed by an alphabetical list of trade names. Canadian trade names are preceded by a maple leaf (🍁). Many brand names have been discontinued by the manufacturer, requiring nurses to know the generic names of drugs. Brand names that have been discontinued have a slash through them (~~Decadron~~). A vesicant icon (V) will appear here and elsewhere in the text if the drug is considered a vesicant, which can cause severe tissue damage to the patient if not administered correctly. A double helix icon (🧬) may also appear here and elsewhere in the text to indicate pharmacogenomic implications, which can impact how a patient may respond to a drug based on their unique genetic makeup.

Classification: The therapeutic classification, which categorizes drugs by the disease state they are used to treat, appears first, followed by the pharmacologic classification, which is based on the drug's mechanism of action.

Controlled Substance Schedule: All drugs regulated by federal law are placed into one of five schedules, based on the drug's medicinal value, harmfulness, and potential for abuse or addiction. Schedule I drugs, the most dangerous and having no medicinal value, are not included in *Davis's Drug Guide for Nurses*. (See Appendix H for Controlled Substances Schedules.)

Pregnancy Category: The FDA discontinued the Pregnancy Category system (A, B, C, D, and X) because this categorization may not appropriately communicate the risk that a drug may have during pregnancy or breastfeeding. Therefore, Pregnancy Categories have been removed from all drug monographs and replaced with *Rep*, *OB*, and *Lactation* tags in drug prescribing information and Patient/Family Teaching sections. Here you will find information on the potential risk of using the drug in women and men of reproductive potential as well as during pregnancy and breastfeeding and contraception suggestions.

Special Note About Boxed Warnings: *The FDA requires* Boxed Warnings *to be included in the manufacturer's package insert for certain drugs that have serious or life-threatening adverse effects. We have highlighted this information throughout the drug monographs as applicable to promote safe administration and use of these drugs.*

Indications: Medications are approved by the FDA for specific disease states. This section identifies the diseases or conditions for which the drug is approved and includes significant unlabeled uses as well.

Action: This section contains a concise description of how the drug produces the desired therapeutic effect.

Pharmacokinetics: This section provides information on how the body processes a medication by absorption, distribution, metabolism, and excretion and includes information on the drug's half-life.

Absorption: Absorption is the process that follows drug administration and its subsequent delivery to systemic circulation. If only a small fraction is absorbed following oral administration (diminished bioavailability), then the oral dose must be much greater than the parenteral dose. Absorption into systemic circulation also follows other routes of administration, such as topical, transdermal, intramuscular, subcutaneous, rectal, and ophthalmic routes. Drugs administered intravenously are 100% bioavailable.

Distribution: This section comments on the drug's distribution in body tissues and fluids. Distribution becomes important in choosing one drug over another, as in selecting an antibiotic that will penetrate the central nervous system to treat meningitis or that will penetrate into the urine to treat a urinary tract infection. Information on protein binding is included for drugs that are >90% bound to plasma proteins, which has implications for drug-drug interactions.

Metabolism and Excretion: Drugs are primarily eliminated from the body either by hepatic metabolism to active or inactive compounds and subsequent excretion by the kidneys or by renal elimination of unchanged drug. Therefore, drug metabolism and excretion information is important in determining dose regimens and intervals for patients with renal or hepatic impairment. The creatinine clearance (CCr) helps quantify renal function and guides dose adjustments. Formulas to estimate CCr are included in Appendix E.

Half-Life: The half-life of a drug is the amount of time it takes for the drug concentration to decrease by 50%. It takes approximately 4–5 half-lives for a drug to achieve steady-state concentrations upon initiation or for the drug to be eliminated from the body upon discontinuation. Half-lives are given for drugs assuming the patient has normal renal or hepatic function. Conditions that alter the half-life are noted.

Time/Action Profile: The time/action profile table provides the drug's onset of action, peak effect, and duration of activity for each route. This information can aid in planning administration schedules and allows the reader to appreciate differences in choosing one route over another.

Contraindications and Precautions: Situations in which drug use should be avoided are listed as contraindications. In general, most drugs are contraindicated in pregnancy or lactation, unless the potential benefits outweigh the possible risks to the mother or baby (e.g., anticonvulsants, antihypertensives, and antiretrovirals). Contraindications may be absolute (i.e., the drug in question should be avoided completely) or relative, in which certain clinical situations may allow cautious use of the drug. The precautions portion includes disease states or clinical situations in which drug use involves risks or in which dose modification may be necessary. Extreme cautions are noted separately to draw attention to conditions under which use of the drug results in serious, potentially life-threatening consequences.

Adverse Reactions/Side Effects: It is not possible to list all reported reactions, but major side effects for all drugs are included. Life-threatening adverse reactions or side effects are **CAPITALIZED**, and the most frequent side effects are underlined. Those underlined generally have an incidence of >10%. Those not underlined occur in <10% but >1% of patients. Although life-threatening reactions may be rare (<1%), they are included because of their significance. For each body system, the most frequent adverse reactions are listed first alphabetically (including life-threatening); then all other reactions are subsequently listed alphabetically (including life-threatening). The following abbreviations are used for body systems:

CV: cardiovascular
Derm: dermatologic
EENT: eye, ear, nose, and throat
Endo: endocrinologic
F and E: fluid and electrolyte
GI: gastrointestinal
GU: genitourinary
Hemat: hematologic
Local: local
Metab: metabolic
MS: musculoskeletal
Neuro: neurologic
Resp: respiratory
Misc: miscellaneous

Interactions: Drug interactions are a significant risk for patients. As the number of medications a patient receives increases, so does the likelihood of drug-drug interactions. This section provides the most important drug-drug interactions and their physiological effects. Significant drug-food and drug-natural product interactions are also noted, as are recommendations for avoiding or minimizing these interactions.

Route/Dosage: This section includes recommended doses for adults, children, and other more specific age groups by route. Dose units are expressed in the terms in which they are usually prescribed. For example, the penicillin G dose is given in units rather than in milligrams. Dosing intervals are also provided in the way they are frequently ordered. If a specific clinical situation (indication) requires a different dose or interval, this is listed separately for clarity. Specific dosing regimens for hepatic or renal impairment are also included. Dosing recommendations for significant drug interactions are also included in this section.

Availability: This section lists the strengths and concentrations of available dose forms, which is useful in planning more convenient regimens (fewer tablets/capsules, less injection volume) and in determining whether certain dose forms are available. Flavors of oral liquids and chewable tablets have been included to improve compliance and adherence in pediatric patients. This section will also indicate whether a drug is available as a generic product.

Nursing Implications: This section helps the nurse apply the nursing process to pharmacotherapeutics. The subsections provide a guide to clinical assessment, implementation (drug administration), and evaluation of the outcomes of pharmacologic therapy.

Assessment: This section includes guidelines for assessing patient history and physical data before, during, and following drug therapy. Assessments specific to the drug's various indications are also included. **Lab Test Considerations** provides information regarding which laboratory tests to monitor and how the results may be affected by the medication. This section also includes dose modifications required for changes in lab values. **Toxicity and Overdose** identifies therapeutic serum drug concentrations that must be monitored as well as signs and symptoms of toxicity. The antidote and treatment for toxicity or overdose are also included.

Implementation: This section provides guidelines for administering medication. **High Alert** information relates to preventing medication errors with inherently dangerous drugs. Sound-alike, look-alike name confusion alerts are also included here. Other headings in this section provide data regarding routes of administration. Dose modifications for side effects are included for drugs that provide this information. **PO** describes when and how to administer an oral drug, whether tablets may be crushed or capsules opened, and when to administer the medication in relation to food. The Do Not Crush (DNC) tag identifies drugs that should be swallowed whole. In the **IV Administration** section, bold blue headings are included to highlight the recommended **reconstitution**, **dilution**, and **concentrations**. These headings complement the rate heading and make this critical information easy to find. **IV Push** refers to administering medications from a syringe directly into a saline lock, Y-site of IV tubing, or a 3-way stopcock; **Intermittent** and **Continuous Infusion** specifies standard dilution solutions and amounts, stability information, and rates. In addition, a quick reference for information about dilution amounts in neonates and infants, who are extremely sensitive to excess fluids, is contained in the **Medication Safety Tools** section. **Y-Site Compatibility/Incompatibility** identifies medications compatible or incompatible with each drug when administered via Y-site injection or 3-way stopcock in IV tubing. Information for drugs not included in these lists is conflicting or unavailable. Compatibility information is compiled from *Lexidrug*. Vesicant information and guidance on managing cases of IV drug extravasation are also included in this section.

Patient/Family Teaching: This section includes information that should be taught to patients and/or families of patients. Side effects that should be reported, information on minimizing and managing side effects, details on administration, and follow-up requirements are presented. The nurse also should refer to the **Implementation** section for specific information to teach to the patient and family about taking the medication. The Rep tag identifies information on contraception, breastfeeding, monitoring parameters for infants exposed to the drug, and fertility data. **Home Care Issues** discusses aspects to be considered for medications taken in the home setting.

Evaluation/Desired Outcomes: Outcome criteria for determination of the effectiveness of the medication are provided.

Additional Resources

Readers may create an account on fadavis.com to access free additional resources available. These include:

- Pronunciation library of 1,600+ drug names
- Tutorials on psychotropic drugs and preventing medication errors
- Online calculators for body mass index, metric conversions, IV drip rates, dosage/kg, and Fahrenheit/Celsius conversions
- Interactive case studies
- Medication administration videos
- Appendices M-P:
  - M: Natural/Herbal Products
  - N: Combination Drugs
  - O: Routine Pediatric and Adult Immunizations
  - P: Bibliography

Web and Mobile Options

Prefer online or app access? Choose the option that fits your needs. Trial offers are available, and access fee or subscription rates apply.

Davis Nursing Consult: Print purchasers: Check out the inside front cover for a 30-day free trial to our comprehensive reference resource, including *Davis's Drug Guide For Nurses, Davis's Comprehensive Manual of Laboratory and Diagnostic Tests,* and *Taber's Cyclopedic Medical Dictionary*. Davis Nursing Consult can also be purchased on fadavis.com. Web and mobile access included.

Drugguide.com: Access the full *Davis's Drug Guide for Nurses* online from Unbound Medicine—easy to search and always up to date.

App Stores: Stay current with the *Davis's Drug Guide for Nurses* app. Start your free trial for quick, on-the-go access.

Evidence-Based Practice and Pharmacotherapeutics

The purpose of evidence-based practice (EBP) is to use the best available evidence to make informed patient-care decisions that ultimately improve the treatment outcomes and safety of treatment for patients. How pharmacologic agents affect patients is often the subject of research; such research is required by the Food and Drug Administration (FDA) before and after drug approval. Any medication can be the subject of an evidence-based clinical review. But what does "evidence-based" mean, and how does it relate to nursing?

Evidence-based nursing practice can be viewed as a foundation of professional practice. It is an approach to making decisions, providing nursing care, and improving clinical practice based upon clinical expertise in combination with the most current and relevant research evidence. Still subject to debate are questions about the sufficiency and quality of evidence. For example, what kind of evidence is needed? How much evidence is necessary to support, modify, or change clinical practice? And were the studies reviewed of "good" quality, and are their results valid?

Clinicians use a **hierarchy of evidence** to rank types of research reports from the most valuable and scientifically rigorous to the least useful. The hierarchy makes clear that some level of evidence about the effect of a particular treatment or condition exists, even if the evidence is considered weak. Figure 1 illustrates a hierarchy of evidence pyramid with widely accepted rankings: the most scientifically rigorous at the top, the least scientifically rigorous at the bottom. Clinicians should look for the highest level of available evidence to answer their clinical questions. It is important that clinicians also apply the second fundamental principle of EBP, which is that evidence alone is not sufficient to make clinical decisions. Decision makers must always trade off the benefits and risks, as well as the costs associated with alternative treatment options, and consider the patient's values and preferences.

Evidence-Based Practice and Its Importance in Pharmacology

Evidence-based practices in pharmacology generally are derived from well-designed randomized controlled trials (RCTs) or other experimental designs that investigate a drug's therapeutic and nontherapeutic effects. FDA-approved pharmacologic agents have undergone rigorous testing through RCTs, but nurses have the responsibility to evaluate the findings for the best scientific

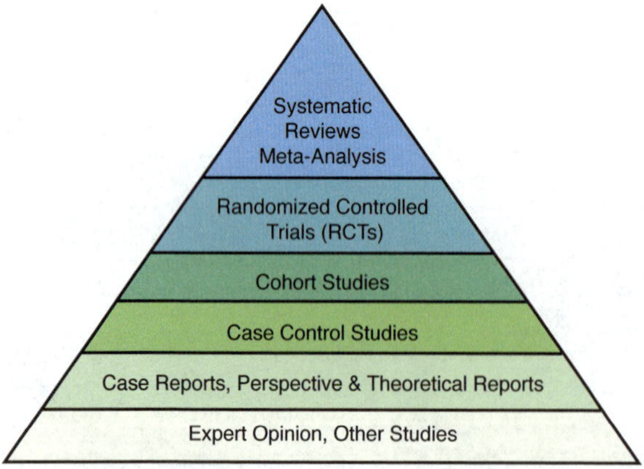

Figure 1: Hierarchy of Scientific Evidence Pyramid

evidence available and to recognize the most appropriate, safest, and efficacious drugs for their patients.

One valuable and quickly accessible resource for evaluating the current highest level of pharmacologic evidence is the Cochrane Database of Systematic Reviews. The Cochrane library and databases provide full text of high-quality, regularly updated systematic reviews, protocols, and clinical trials.

AHRQ's Evidence-Based Practice Centers (EPCs) provide evidence reports and technology assessments that can assist nurses in their efforts to provide the highest quality and safest pharmacologic health care available. The EPCs systematically review the relevant scientific literature, conduct additional analyses (when appropriate) prior to developing their reports and assessments, and provide guideline comparisons.

Evidence-based systematic guidelines provide nurses with access to the most current knowledge, enabling them to critically appraise the scientific evidence and its appropriateness to their patient population. This is especially important given the need for nurses to keep abreast of the rapidly changing pharmacologic agents in use. New drugs are approved each month, compelling nurses to know these drugs' intended uses, therapeutic effects, interactions, and adverse effects.

Evidence-based practice requires a shift from the traditional paradigm of clinical practice—grounded in intuition, clinical experience, and pathophysiologic rationale—to a paradigm in which nurses must combine clinical expertise, patient values and preferences, and clinical circumstances with the integration of the best scientific evidence to make conscientious, well-informed, research-based decisions that affect nursing patient care.

***

Sally Villasenor, DNP, RN, ACNP-BC
Nurse Practitioner and Assistant Professor
Wayne State University College of Nursing
Detroit, Michigan

RESOURCES

1. Curtis, K., Fry, M., Shaban, R. Z., & Considine, J. (2017). Translating research findings to clinical nursing practice. *Journal of Clinical Nursing*, 26(5–6), 862–872. https://doi.org/10.1111/jocn.13586
2. Melnyk, B. M., & Fineout-Overholt, E. (2019). *Evidence-based practice in nursing and healthcare: A guide to best practice*. (4th ed). Wolters Kluwer.
3. Polit, D. F., & Beck, C. T. (2021). *Essentials of nursing research: Appraising evidence for nursing practice*. (10th ed). Wolters Kluwer Health.

Pharmacogenomics

Introduction

Multiple variables influence the selection and optimization of drug therapy for each individual patient. Pharmacogenomics, the study of the influence of individual genetic variations on drug response in patients, may yield additional information to further enhance safe and effective medication use. Originally the field focused on the effects of specific variants within individual genes on drug response (i.e., pharmaco *genetics*); however, more recent research has focused on the role of multiple variants across the genome (i.e., pharmaco *genomics*) and their combined potential to modify and alter drug therapy outcomes.

The understanding of pharmacogenomics has increased considerably. Most emerging research has fallen into one of three domains:

- Gene variants that influence the function of drug transporter proteins (how efficiently drugs are delivered to their site(s) of activity)
- Gene variants that cause differences in the function of drug-metabolizing enzymes (how quickly or slowly drugs are used and broken down in the body)
- Gene variants that alter a drug's "target" proteins (variations in the genes coding for a target protein may alter the protein's three-dimensional shape, changing the binding affinity for drugs to that protein)

As the biological relevance of specific genetic variants has increased, it is understood that multiple variations across the genome can contribute to significant yet *relatively predictable* treatment outcomes. Virtually every therapeutic area involving medication use includes a drug for which documented genetic variability has the potential to affect drug response. Some of this information is included in the Food and Drug Administration–approved package insert prescribing information. For some agents, the suitability of a specific drug or the determination of an appropriate initial dose for an individual patient based on pharmacogenetic information has been incorporated into dosing algorithms and patient care. As such, it is essential that health care providers be able to interpret and utilize this information to facilitate safer and more effective use of medications for individual patients.

Genetic Variation Within the Human Genome

The human genome is comprised of approximately 3 billion nucleotide base pair sequences that encode for molecular DNA with each individual having their own unique human genome sequence (except for identical twins). Four nucleotide bases (adenine, guanine, cytosine, and thymine) form the sequence of each single strand of DNA. Variations in nucleotide sequences can occur and contribute to alterations in the expression and activities of certain genes as well as their protein products. The location of these variations within a DNA sequence on a particular chromosome can have a profound impact on the biological activity of that gene; however, it should also be understood that some gene variants may lead to little or no discernible change to biologic activity at all. As new gene variants are discovered, the process of understanding the *degree of impact* becomes a focus for investigators.

Proteins are involved in most enzymatic, structural, and biologic functions associated with drug disposition and effects. The processes involved in DNA replication, RNA transcription, and translation to synthesized proteins are complex. Each of these processes is potentially susceptible to consequences of DNA sequence variations.

Genetic variations can take many forms, but most fall into three general categories:

- Single nucleotide base substitutions (e.g., a cytosine substituted for an adenine)
- Insertions or deletions of a nucleotide base within a sequence

- Deletions or extra copies of entire DNA sequences (e.g., trisomy 21, in which an extra copy of *all* genes on the 21st chromosome are present)

Variations in DNA that occur at a frequency of greater than 1% in the population are called polymorphisms. The most common gene varients in humans are single nucleotide polymorphisms (SNPs, pronounced as the word "snips" in dialogue). SNPs result from the substitution of one nucleotide base for another. The location of a SNP within a gene is important, as the location may or may not elicit a downstream effect on protein made from the gene. It is helpful to recall the importance of introns and exons for mRNA manufacturing when considering how SNPs can impact protein function. An important point to keep in mind is that *any* gene variant may have a spectrum-like impact on protein manufacture, ranging from zero clinical consequences (no discernible effect on proteins) to complete lack of functional proteins associated with significant alterations in drug response. Also, pharmacogenomic clinical effects must always be considered within the larger sphere of environmental influences on drugs and drug responses. Finally, due to the commonality of polymorphisms, multiple gene variants may be present within one patient, making prediction of drug response particularly challenging.

Clinical Significance of Genetic Polymorphisms

SNPs and other genetic variations influence drug response at different levels through alterations in the activities of enzymes or proteins involved in drug absorption, transport, metabolism, elimination, or at the drug target receptor (site of drug action). Clinically relevant polymorphisms have been identified for genes that encode for most of the common enzymes involved in drug metabolism. Most enzymes are localized intracellularly throughout a wide variety of tissues in the body, including the enterocytes that line the intestine and within hepatocytes. Variants that cause diminished or absent enzyme activity decrease drug metabolism processes. In this case, if the drug is metabolized to an inactive product, then the prolonged persistence of the parent drug in the body could result in excessive pharmacologic effects, and potential toxicities may occur. If the drug requires enzymatic conversion to a pharmacologically active metabolite, drug response may be reduced or absent. In contrast, if the variation is due to extra copies of a gene that results in increased enzymatic activity, opposite effects on drug metabolism and response can occur.

Similar outcomes can be associated with polymorphisms in genes that encode for membrane transporter proteins that are responsible for drug transport into cells (influx) as well as proteins that participate in energy-dependent processes that export drugs out of cells (efflux transporters). Polymorphisms in drug transport proteins can influence drug response by altering drug gastrointestinal absorption, uptake and distribution in tissues, exposure to intracellular drug-metabolizing enzymes, and elimination via the bile or urine. Finally, some genes that encode for certain drug receptors are highly polymorphic, resulting in attenuated or exaggerated drug responses. The number of polymorphic genes responsible for variations in drug response at drug receptors is relatively small compared to those associated with drug-metabolizing enzymes or transport proteins; however, this area has undergone the least amount of study to date.

Incorporating Pharmacogenomic Information into Clinical Practice

Most drugs are initiated in individual patients based on knowledge about their safety and effectiveness within the general population. Information regarding patient characteristics (e.g., age, ethnicity, renal/hepatic function, concurrent disease, etc.) known to contribute to variability in drug response, when available, is considered at this time. It is becoming more and more common, however, to consider gene variants as well when initiating drugs, as interindividual gene factors are thought to contribute to drug response variability in 15–30% of patients. Currently, there are more than 100 drugs with pharmacogenomic information included in the package insert. For selected agents, dosing recommendations based on an individual's genetic information (i.e., genotype) for specific drugs and drug classes are also considered. Genomic biomarkers can play an important role in identifying responders and nonresponders, avoiding drug toxicity, and adjusting the dose of drugs to optimize their efficacy and safety. However, the typical strategy for most drug therapy is to monitor the patient's response to treatment and modify regimens as necessary. Patients who develop exaggerated pharmacologic responses or elicit no pharmacologic effect may be expressing a phenotype suggestive of altered drug disposition or target receptor effect that could be associated with an underlying genetic polymorphism. As we continue to learn more about these associations and can incorporate pharmacogenomic information into decisions regarding drug therapy for individual patients, the ultimate goal is to improve therapeutic outcomes by limiting drug exposure to patients that are most likely to derive no therapeutic benefit and/or experience toxic drug effects.

For example, some genetic variants are associated with hypersensitivity reactions to a specific drug. A prescriber who is contemplating initiating that drug for a patient may need to determine whether the patient possesses that variant in their DNA. If that specific variant is present, the prescriber might select an alternate agent, thereby avoiding a potentially life-threatening hypersensitivity reaction. In another example, patients who are determined to have a genetic variant that results in an inactive metabolizing enzyme would not be appropriate candidates for an analgesic drug that requires that enzyme to convert the drug to the active analgesia-producing form. On the other hand, if that metabolizing enzyme is responsible for conversion of an active parent drug to an inactive metabolite, the starting dose of the drug may be reduced or perhaps an alternative drug might be selected.

Several Clinical Laboratory Improvement Amendment–approved laboratories offer pharmacogenetic testing to identify relevant genetic polymorphisms that predict drug response and can be used to initiate appropriate drugs and dosing regimens for individual patients. Some of these tests, while recommended in drug prescribing information, are costly and may not be covered by insurance. Patients may not fully understand the utility of undergoing genetic testing and providing a specimen for DNA analysis, which is typically performed on blood, saliva, buccal swab, or other tissue collection. On the other hand, patients who are engaged in their medical care may be familiar with the concept of "personalized medicine" and seek information about available tests to individualize their own drug therapy. Many drugs are now required to have pharmacogenetic testing performed before they are prescribed. Other drugs have labeling that includes "test recommended" or "for information only." Health care professionals will need to be familiar with pharmacogenetic tests that are recommended for specific drug therapies, how to interpret the results of those tests, and how to incorporate pharmacogenetic data with other clinical information to optimize patient drug therapy and health care outcomes.

RESOURCES

1. Benjeddou, M., & Peiró, A. M. (2021). Pharmacogenomics and prescription opioid use. *Pharmacogenomics*, 22(4), 235–245. https://doi.org/10.2217/pgs-2020-0032
2. Carr, D. F., Turner, R. M., & Pirmohamed, M. (2021). Pharmacogenomics of anticancer drugs: Personalising the choice and dose to manage drug response. *British Journal of Clinical Pharmacology*, 87(2), 237–255. https://doi.org/10.1111/bcp.14407
3. Cheek, D. J., & Walker, T. (2025). Pharmacogenomics for nurses. *Nursing Clinics of North America*, 60(2), 283–292. https://doi.org/10.1016/j.cnur.2025.01.006
4. Genetics Primer. (2012). *Alcohol Research: Current Reviews*, 34(3), 270–271. https://pmc.ncbi.nlm.nih.gov/articles/PMC3860415/
5. Nicholson, W. T., Formea, C. M., Matey, E. T., Wright, J. A., Giri, J., & Moyer, A. M. (2021). Considerations when applying pharmacogenomics to your practice. *Mayo Clinic Proceedings*, 96(1), 218–230. https://doi.org/10.1016/j.mayocp.2020.03.011

Medication Errors: Improving Practices and Patient Safety

It is widely acknowledged that medication errors result in thousands of adverse drug events, preventable reactions, and deaths per year. Nurses, physicians, pharmacists, patient safety organizations, the Food and Drug Administration, the pharmaceutical industry, Health Canada, and other parties share in the responsibility for determining how medication errors occur and designing strategies to reduce error.

One impediment to understanding the scope and nature of the problem has been the reactive "blaming, shaming, training" culture that singled out one individual as the cause of the error. Also historically, medication errors that did not result in patient harm—near-miss situations in which an error could have but didn't happen—or errors that did not result in serious harm were not reported. In contrast, serious errors often instigated a powerful punitive response in which one or a few persons were deemed to be at fault and, as a result, lost their jobs and sometimes their licenses.

In 1999, the Institute of Medicine (IOM) published *To Err Is Human: Building a Safer Health System*, which drew attention to the problem of medication errors. It pointed out that excellent health care providers do make medication errors, that many of the traditional processes involved in the medication-use system were error-prone, and that other factors, notably drug labeling and packaging, contributed to error. Furthermore, the IOM report, in conjunction with other groups such as the United States Pharmacopeia and the Institute for Safe Medication Practices (ISMP), called for the redesign of error-prone systems to include processes that anticipated the fallibility of humans working within the system. This initiative is helping shift the way the health care industry addresses medication errors from a single person/bad apple cause to a systems issue.

The National Coordinating Council for Medication Error Reporting and Prevention developed the definition of a medication error that reflects this shift and captures the scope and breadth of the issue:

> "A medication error is any preventable event that may cause or lead to inappropriate medication use or patient harm while the medication is in the control of the health care provider, patient, or consumer. Such events may be related to professional practice, health care products, procedures, and systems, including prescribing; order communication; product labeling, packaging, and nomenclature; compounding; dispensing; distribution; administration; education; monitoring; and use."

Inherent in this definition's mention of related factors are the human factors that are part of the medication use system. For example, a nurse or pharmacist may automatically reach into the bin where dobutamine is usually kept, see "do" and "amine," and select dopamine instead of dobutamine. Working amid distractions, working long hours or shorthanded, and working in a culture where perfection is expected and questioning is discouraged are other examples of the human factors and environmental conditions that contribute to error.

The goal for the design of any individual or hospital-wide medication use system is to determine where systems are likely to fail and to build in safeguards that minimize the potential for error. One way to begin that process is to become familiar with medications or practices that have historically been shown to be involved in serious errors.

High-Alert Medications

Some medications, because of a narrow therapeutic range or inherent toxic nature, have a high risk of causing devastating injury or death if improperly ordered, prepared, stocked, dispensed, administered, or monitored. Although these medications may not be involved in more errors, they require special attention due to the potential for serious, possibly fatal consequences. These have been termed **high-alert medications**, to communicate the need for extra care and safeguards. Many of these drugs are used commonly in the general population or are used frequently in urgent clinical situations. The Joint Commission monitors the use of frequently prescribed high-alert medications, which include insulin, opioids, injectable potassium chloride (or phosphate) concentrate, antithrombotics, sodium chloride solutions with a concentration greater than 0.9%, and others. Visit the Institute for Safe Medication Practices at www.ismp.org for a complete list of High-Alert Drugs.

Causes of Medication Errors

Many contributing factors and discrete causes of error have been identified, including failed communication, poor pharmaceutical supply chain distribution practices, dose miscalculations, drug packaging and drug-device related problems, incorrect drug administration, and lack of patient education.

Failed Communication: Failed communication covers many of the errors made in the ordering phase, and although ordering is performed by the prescriber, the nurse, the clerk, and the pharmacist who interpret that order are also involved in the communication process.

- ***Poorly handwritten or verbal orders.*** Handwriting is a major source of error and has led to inaccurate interpretations of the drug intended, the route of administration, the frequency, and dose. Telephone and verbal orders are likewise prone to misinterpretation. The current use of electronic drug order entry within hospitals and electronic prescribing to pharmacies contributes to increased legibility and consistency of medication orders and prescriptions.
- ***Drugs with similar-sounding or similar-looking names.*** Similar sounding names, or names that look similar when handwritten, are frequently confused. Doxorubicin hydrochloride and doxorubicin liposomal, or Lunesta® and Neulasta® are two examples. Mix-ups are more likely when each drug has similar dose ranges and frequencies.

Several of the sound-alike/look-alike drugs were targeted for labeling intervention by the FDA, which requested manufacturers with look-alike names to voluntarily revise the appearance of the established names. The revision visually differentiates the drug names by using "tall man" letters (capitals) to highlight distinguishing syllables (e.g., buPROPrion versus busPIRone or ceFAZolin versus cefTAZidime. See the TALL MAN Lettering table in the **Medication Safety Tools** section for the list of the pairs of drugs that are commonly confused, often with serious consequences.

- ***Misuse of zeroes in decimal numbers.*** Massive, tenfold overdoses are traceable to not using a leading zero (.2 mg instead of 0.2 mg) or adding an unnecessary trailing zero (2.0 mg instead of 2 mg) in decimal expressions of dose. Similar overdoses are found in decimal expressions in which the decimal point is obscured by poor handwriting, stray marks, or lined orders sheets (e.g., reading 3.1 grams as 31 grams). Underdosing also may occur by the same mechanism and prevent a desired, perhaps life-saving effect.
- ***Misinterpreted abbreviations.*** Abbreviations can be misinterpreted or, when used in the dose part of the order, can result in incorrect dose of the correct medication. For example, lower- or uppercase "U" for units has been read as a zero, making 10 u of insulin look like 100 units when handwritten. The Latin abbreviation "QOD" for every other day has been misinterpreted as QID (4 times per day). Current widespread use of electronic drug ordering and prescriptions increases legibility; frequency choices are often in plain language such as "every other day" instead of "QOD." See Table 1 for a list of confusing abbreviations and safer alternatives.
- ***Ambiguous or incomplete orders.*** Orders that do not clearly specify dose, route, frequency, or indication do not communicate complete information and are open to misinterpretation.

Poor Distribution Practices: Poor distribution includes error-prone storing practices such as keeping similar-looking products next to each other. Dispensing multidose floor stock vials of potentially dangerous drugs instead of unit (single) dose vials is also associated with error, as is allowing nonpharmacists to dispense medications in the absence of the pharmacist.

Dose Miscalculations: Dose miscalculations are a prime source of medication error. Also, many medications need to be dose-adjusted for renal or hepatic impairment, age, height and weight, and body composition (i.e., correct for obesity). Complicated dosing formulas provide many opportunities to introduce error. Often vulnerable populations, such as premature infants, children, older adults, and those with serious underlying illnesses, are at greatest risk.

Drug Packaging: Similar packaging or poorly designed packaging encourages error. Drug companies may use the same design for different formulations or fail to highlight information about concentration or strength. Lettering, type size, color, and packaging methods can either help or hinder drug identification.

Drug Delivery Systems: Drug delivery systems include infusion pumps and drip rate controllers. Some models do not prevent free flow of medication, leading to sudden high dose infusion of potent and dangerous medications. The lack of safeguards preventing free flow and programming errors are among the problems encountered with infusion control devices. Newer models, which are integrated with the medication administration record (MAR) via scanned barcodes to match the patient with drug, dose, and timing, contribute to increased dosing safety; however, it is a nursing responsibility to verify the dose and determine that the infusion pump is delivering properly at the point of drug administration.

Incorrect Drug Administration: Incorrect drug administration covers many problems. Misidentification of a patient, incorrect route of administration, missed doses, or improper drug preparation are types of errors that occur during the administration phase. Barcode scanning to identify the patient and correlate with the correct MAR decreases the likelihood of incorrect drug administration.

Lack of Patient Education: Safe medication use is enhanced in the hospital and the home when the patient is well informed. The knowledgeable patient can recognize when something has changed in their medication regimen and can question the health care provider. At the same time, many issues related to medication errors, such as ambiguous directions, unfamiliarity with a drug, and confusing packaging, affect the patient as well as the health care provider, underscoring the need for careful education. Patient education also enhances adherence, which is a factor in proper medication use.

Prevention Strategies

Since medication use systems are complex and involve many steps and people, they are error-prone. On an individual basis, nurses can help reduce the incidence of error by implementing the following strategies:

- Clarify any order that is not obviously and clearly legible. Ask the prescriber to print orders using block style letters if handwritten.
- Do not accept orders with the abbreviation "u" or "IU" for units. Clarify the dosage and ask the prescriber to write out the word units.
- Clarify any abbreviated drug name or the abbreviated dosing frequencies q.d. QD, q.o.d. QOD, and q.i.d or QID. To minimize any confusion associated with drug names, abbreviation of drugs names should ALWAYS be avoided. Suggest abandoning Latin abbreviations in favor of spelling out dosing frequency.
- Decimal point errors can be hard to see. Suspect a missed decimal point and clarify any order if the dose requires more than 3 dosing units.
- If dose ordered requires use of multiple dosage units or very small fractions of a dose unit, review the dose, have another health care provider check the original order and recalculate formulas, and confirm the dose with the prescriber.
- If taking a verbal order, ask prescriber to spell out the drug name and dosage to avoid sound-alike confusion (e.g., hearing Cerebyx for Celebrex, or fifty for fifteen). Read back the order

to the prescriber after you have written it in the chart. Confirm and document the indication to further enhance accurate communication.

- Clarify any order that does not include metric weight, dosing frequency, or route of administration.
- Weigh each patient as soon as possible on admission and during each outpatient or emergency department encounter. Avoid the use of a stated, estimated, or historical weight.
- Do not start a patient on new medication by borrowing medications from another patient. This action bypasses the double-check provided by the pharmacist's review of the order.
- Always check the patient's name band before administering medications. Verbally addressing a patient by name does not provide sufficient identification. If available, use of barcode scanning per institutional policy recommended.
- Use the facility's standard drug administration times to reduce the chance of an omission error.
- Be sure to fully understand any drug administration device before using it. This includes infusion pumps, inhalers, and transdermal patches.
- Have a second practitioner independently check original order, dose calculations, and infusion pump settings for high-alert medications.
- Realize that the printing on packaging boxes, vials, ampules, prefilled syringes, or any container in which a medication is stored can be misleading. Be sure to differentiate clearly the medication and the number of milligrams per milliliter versus the total number of milligrams contained within. Massive overdoses have been administered by assuming that the number of milligrams per milliliter is all that is contained within the vial or ampule. Read the label when obtaining the medication, before preparing or pouring the medication, and after preparing or pouring the medication.
- Educate patients about the medications they take. Provide verbal and written instructions and ask the patient to restate important points.

RESOURCES

1. Billstein-Leber, M., Carrillo, C., Cassano, A. T., Moline, K., & Robertson, J. (2018). ASHP guidelines on preventing medication errors in hospitals. *American Journal of Health-System Pharmacy*, 75(19), 1493–1517. https://doi.org/10.2146/ajhp170811
2. Wang, H., Tao, D., & Yan, M. (2021). Effects of text enhancement on reduction of look-alike drug name confusion: A systematic review and meta-analysis. *Quality Management in Health Care*, 30(4), 233–243. https://doi.org/10.1097/qmh.0000000000000303
3. Institute for Safe Medication Practices. (2024). *Targeted medication safety best practices for hospitals*. https://www.ismp.org/guidelines/best-practices-hospitals
4. Kohn, L. T., Corrigan, J. M., & Donaldson, M. S. (Eds.). (1999). *To err is human: Building a safer health system*. National Academy Press.
5. Manias, E., Kusljic, S., & Wu, A. (2020). Interventions to reduce medication errors in adult medical and surgical settings: A systematic review. *Therapeutic Advances in Drug Safety*, 11, 2042098620968309. https://doi.org/10.1177/2042098620968309
6. National Coordinating Council for Medication Error Reporting and Prevention. (2025). *About medication errors: What is a medication error?* https://www.nccmerp.org/about-medication-errors
7. Hutton, K., Ding, Q., & Wellman, G. (2021). The effect of bar-coding technology on medication errors: A systematic literature review. *Journal of Patient Safety*, 17(3), e192–e206. https://doi.org/10.1097/pts.0000000000000366

Table 1: Abbreviations and Symbols Associated with Medication Errors

ABBREVIATION/SYMBOL	INTENDED MEANING	MISTAKEN FOR	RECOMMENDATION
APAP	acetaminophen	not recognized as acetaminophen	Use full drug name
AT II	angiotensin II	antithrombin III	Use full drug name
AT III	antithrombin III	angiotensin II	Use full drug name
AZT	zidovudine	azithromycin, azathioprine, aztreonam	Use full drug name
Coined names for compounded products (e.g., magic mouthwash, banana bag, GI cocktail, pink lady)	specific ingredients compounded together	mistaken ingredients	Use complete drug/product names for all ingredients
CPZ	Compazine (prochlorperazine)	chlorpromazine	Use full drug name
DOR	doravirine	Dovato (dolutegravir/ lamivudine)	Use full drug name
HCT	hydrocortisone	hydrochlorothiazide	Use full drug name
HCTZ	hydrochlorothiazide	hydrocortisone	Use full drug name
IV vanc	intravenous vancomycin	Invanz (ertapenem)	Use full drug name
"Levo"	levofloxacin	Levophed (norepinephrine)	Use full drug name
$MgSO_4$*	magnesium sulfate	morphine sulfate	Use full drug name
MS or MSO_4*	morphine sulfate	magnesium sulfate	Use full drug name
MTX	methotrexate	mitoxantrone	Use full drug name
Na at the beginning of a drug name (e.g., Na bicarbonate)	sodium bicarbonate	no bicarbonate	Use full drug name
Neo	Neo-Synephrine (phenylephrine)	neostigmine	Use full drug name
"Nitro" drip	nitroglycerin infusion	nitroprusside infusion	Use full drug name
NoAC	novel/new oral anticoagulant	no anticoagulant	Use full drug name
Number embedded in drug name (e.g., 5-fluorouracil, 6-mercaptopurine)	fluorouracil or mercaptopurine	embedded number mistaken as the dose or number of tablets/capsules to be administered	Use full drug name without an embedded number
OXY	oxytocin	oxycodone, Oxycontin	Use full drug name
PCA	procainamide	patient controlled analgesia	Use full drug name
PIT	Pitocin (oxytocin)	Pitressin (vasopressin)	Use full drug name
PNV	prenatal vitamins	penicillin VK	Use full drug name
PTU	propylthiouracil	Purinethol (mercaptopurine)	Use full drug name
T3	Tylenol with codeine No. 3	Liothyronine	Use full drug name
TAC or tac	triamcinolone or tacrolimus	one mistaken for the other or as tetracaine, Adrenalin, cocaine, Taxotere, Adriamycin, or cyclophosphamide	Use full drug name
TAF	tenofovir alafenamide	tenofovir disoproxil fumarate	Use full drug name
TDF	tenofovir disoproxil fumarate	tenofovir alafenamide	Use full drug name
TNK	TNKase	TPA	Use full drug name
TPA or tPA	tissue plasminogen activator, Activase (alteplase)	TNK or TNKase (tenecteplase), TXA (tranexamic acid), Retevase (reteplase)	Use full drug name
TXA	tranexamic acid	TPA	Use full drug name
$ZnSO_4$	zinc sulfate	morphine sulfate	Use full drug name
µg	microgram	mg (milligram)	Use "mcg"
AD, AS, or AU	right ear, left ear, each ear	right eye, left eye, each eye	Spell out "right ear," "left ear," or "each ear"
BIW or biw	2 times a week	2 times a day	Spell out "2 times weekly"
cc	cubic centimeters	u (units)	Use "mL"
D/C	Discharge or discontinue	One mistaken for the other	Spell out "discharge" or "discontinue"
gr	grain(s)	gram	Use the metric system (e.g., mcg, g)
HS or hs	half strength or hours of sleep (at bedtime)	one mistaken for the other	Spell out "half strength" or use "HS" for at bedtime
IN	intranasal	IM or IV	Spell out "intranasal"

Table 1: Abbreviations and Symbols Associated with Medication Errors—cont'd

ABBREVIATION/SYMBOL	INTENDED MEANING	MISTAKEN FOR	RECOMMENDATION
IT	intrathecal	Intratracheal, intratumor, intratympanic, inhalation therapy	Spell out "intrathecal"
IU*	international units	IV or 10	Spell out "units"
l	liter	1 (one)	Use uppercase "L"
M or K	thousand	million	Spell out "thousand"
ml	milliliter	1 (one)	Use "mL" (with lowercase "m" and uppercase "L")
MM or M	million	thousand	Spell out "million"
Ng or ng	nanogram	mg (milligram) or nasogastric	Spell out "nanogram"
OD, OS, or OU	right eye, left eye, each eye	right ear, left ear, each ear	Spell out "right eye," "left eye," or "each eye"
o.d. or OD	once daily	right eye	Spell out "daily"
OJ	orange juice	OD (right eye), OS (left eye)	Spell out "orange juice"
oz	ounce(s)	zero or O2	Use the metric system (e.g., mL)
q.d. qd, Q.D. or QD*	every day	qid (4 times per day)	Spell out "daily"
q1d	daily	qid (4 times per day)	Spell out "daily"
q6PM, etc.	every evening at 6 PM	every 6 hours	Spell out "daily at 6 PM" or "6 PM daily"
Qhs	nightly at bedtime	qhr (every hour)	Use "QHS" or "qhs"
q.o.d. qod, Q.O.D, or QOD*	every other day	qid (4 times per day) or qd (daily)	Spell out "every other day"
SC, SQ, sq, or sub q	subcutaneously	SC mistaken as SL (sublingual); SQ mistaken as "5 every"; q in sub q mistaken as "every"	Use "SUBQ" or spell out "subcutaneously"
SSRI or SSI	sliding scale regular insulin, sliding scale insulin	selective serotonin reuptake inhibitor or strong solution of iodine (Lugol's)	Spell out "sliding scale insulin"
tbsp or Tbsp	tablespoon(s)	teaspoon(s)	Use the metric system (e.g., mL)
TIW or tiw	3 times a week	3 times a day or twice a week	Spell out "3 times weekly"
tsp	teaspoon(s)	tablespoon(s)	Use the metric system (e.g., mL)
u or U*	units	0 (zero), 4 (four) or cc	Spell out "units"
UD	as directed (ut dictum)	unit dose	Spell out "use as directed"
/ (slash mark)	separates two doses	1 (one)	Spell out "and" between drug doses
+	plus or and	4 (four)	Spell out "plus," "and," or "in addition to"
1/2 tablet	half tablet	1 or 2 tablets	Spell out "half tablet"; avoid using fractions or decimals
Doses expressed as Roman numerals (e.g., V)	5	designated letter (e.g., the letter "V") or the wrong numeral (e.g., 10 instead of 5)	Use only Arabic numbers (e.g., 1, 2, 3) to express doses
Zero **after** a decimal point (e.g., 1.0 mg)*	1 mg	10 mg	DO NOT USE zero after a decimal point for doses expressed as a whole number
No zero **before** a decimal point (e.g., .1 mg)*	0.1 mg	1 mg	ALWAYS USE zero before a decimal point when the number is less than 1
Ratio expression of a concentration of a SINGLE-ENTITY injectable drug product (e.g., epinephrine 1:1,000; 1:10,000; 1:100,000) (note: combination local anesthetics are an exception [e.g., lidocaine 1% and epinephrine 1:100,000])	1:1,000 (contains 1 mg/mL); 1:10,000 (contains 0.1 mg/mL); 1:100,000 (contains 0.01 mg/mL)	wrong strength	Express the concentration in terms of quantity per total volume (e.g., 1 mg per 10 mL)
@	at	2 (two)	Spell out "at"

Table 1: Abbreviations and Symbols Associated with Medication Errors—cont'd

ABBREVIATION/SYMBOL	INTENDED MEANING	MISTAKEN FOR	RECOMMENDATION
x1	administer once	administer for 1 day	Spell out "for 1 dose"
>	greater than	<	Spell out "greater than"
<	less than	4 or >	Spell out "less than"
&	and	2 (two)	Spell out "and"
°	hour	zero	Spell out "hr," "h," or "hour"
Ø or Ⓘ	zero or null sign	4 (four), 6 (six), 8 (eight) or 9 (nine)	Use "0" or "zero" or describe intent using whole words
#	pound(s)	Number sign	Use the metric system (kg or g) rather than pounds or use "lb" if referring to "pounds"
Drug name and dose run together (e.g., propranolol 20 mg; Tegretol 300 mg)	propranolol 20 mg; Tegretol 300 mg	propranolol 120 mg or Tegretol 1300 mg	Place space between drug name, dose, and unit of measure
Numerical dose and unit of measure run together (e.g., 10 mg; 10 units)	10 mg; 10 units	m in "mg" and u in "units" mistaken for one or two zeroes	Place space between drug dose and unit of measure
Large doses without properly placed commas (e.g., 100000 units; 1000000 units)	100,000 units; 1,000,000 units	100000 mistaken as 10,000 or 1,000,000; 1,000,000 mistaken as 100,000	Use commas for drug doses at or above 1,000 or spell out ("100 thousand" or "1 million")

*Appears on The Joint Commission's "Do Not Use" list of abbreviations.

Modified from ISMP's List of Error-Prone Abbreviations, Symbols, and Dose Designations, 2024.

Detecting and Managing Adverse Drug Reactions

An *adverse drug reaction* (ADR) is any unexpected, undesired, or excessive response to a medication that results in:

- temporary or permanent serious harm or disability;
- admission to a hospital, transfer to a higher level of care, or prolonged stay;
- death.

Adverse drug reactions are distinguished from adverse drug events, in which causality is uncertain, and side effects, which may be bothersome to the patient and necessitate a change in therapy but are not considered serious. Although some ADRs are the result of medication errors, many are not.

Types of ADRs

The Food and Drug Administration (FDA) classifies ADRs into two broad categories: type A and type B. Type A reactions are predictable reactions based on the primary or secondary pharmacologic effect of the drug. Dose-related reactions and drug-drug interactions are examples of type A reactions. Type B reactions are unpredictable, are not related to dose, and are not the result of the drug's primary or secondary pharmacologic effect. Idiosyncratic and hypersensitivity reactions are examples of type B reactions.

Dose-Related Reactions (Toxic Reactions): In dose-related reactions, the dose prescribed for the patient is excessive. Although a variety of mechanisms may interact, reasons for this type of reaction include:

- renal or hepatic impairment;
- extremes in age (neonates and frail older adults);
- drug-drug or drug-food interactions;
- underlying illness.

Dose-related reactions are often the result of preventable errors in prescribing in which physiologic factors such as age, renal impairment, and weight were not considered sufficiently or in inadequate therapeutic monitoring. Medications with narrow therapeutic ranges (digoxin, aminoglycosides, antiepileptic drugs) and those that require careful monitoring or laboratory testing (anticoagulants, nephrotoxic drugs) are most frequently implicated in dose-related reactions. Dose-related reactions usually are managed successfully by temporarily discontinuing the drug and then reducing the dose or increasing the dosing interval. In some instances, the toxic effects need to be treated with another agent (e.g., Digibind for digoxin toxicity or protamine for heparin toxicity). Appropriately timed therapeutic drug level monitoring, review of new drugs added to an existing regimen that may affect the drug level, and frequent assessment of relevant laboratory values are critical to safe medical management and prevention of dose-related reactions.

Drug-Drug Interactions: Drug-drug interactions occur when the pharmacokinetic or pharmacodynamic properties of an individual drug affect another drug. Pharmacokinetics refers to the way the body processes a medication (absorption, distribution, metabolism, and elimination). In a drug-drug interaction, the pharmacokinetic properties of one drug can cause a change in drug concentration of another drug and an altered response. For example, one drug may block enzymes that metabolize a second drug. The concentration of the second drug is then increased and may become toxic or cause adverse reactions. Pharmacodynamic drug-drug interactions involve the known effects and side effects of the drugs. For example, two drugs with similar therapeutic effects may act together in a synergistic way. The increased antithrombotic effects that occur when warfarin and aspirin are taken together or the increased central nervous system (CNS) depression that results when two drugs with CNS depressant effects potentiate each other are examples of pharmacodynamic drug-drug interactions. Certain classes of drugs are more likely to result in serious drug-drug interactions, and patients receiving these agents should be monitored carefully. These medication classes include anticoagulants, oral hypoglycemic agents, nonsteroidal anti-inflammatory drugs, antihypertensives, antibiotics, antiseizure agents, antiretrovirals, antidepressants, and antipsychotic agents.

Idiosyncratic Reactions: Idiosyncratic reactions occur without relation to dose and are unpredictable and sporadic. Reactions of this type may manifest in many different ways, including fever, blood dyscrasias, cardiovascular effects, or mental status changes. The time frame between the occurrence of a problem and initiation of therapy is sometimes the only clue linking drug to symptom. Some idiosyncratic reactions may be explained by genetic differences in drug-metabolizing enzymes.

Hypersensitivity Reactions: Hypersensitivity reactions are usually allergic responses. Manifestations of hypersensitivity reactions range from mild rashes to nephritis, pneumonitis, hemolytic anemia, and anaphylaxis. Protein drugs (vaccines, enzymes) are frequently associated with hypersensitivity reactions. In most instances, antibody formation is involved in the process, and therefore cross-sensitivity may occur. An example of this type of reaction is a hypersensitivity to penicillin and cross-sensitivity with other penicillins and/or cephalosporins. Documenting drugs to which the patient is allergic and the specific hypersensitivity reaction is very important. If the reaction to an agent is anaphylaxis, the nurse should monitor the patient during administration of a cross-hypersensitive agent, especially during the initial dose, and ensure ready access to emergency resuscitative equipment.

Recognizing an ADR

Adverse drug reactions should be suspected whenever there is a negative change in a patient's condition, particularly when a new drug has been introduced. Strategies that can enhance recognition include knowing the side effect/adverse reaction profile of medications. Nurses should be familiar with a drug's most commonly encountered side effects and adverse reactions before administering it. In *Davis's Drug Guide for Nurses*, most frequent ADRs are underlined, and life-threatening ADRs are CAPITALIZED and appear in red in the **Adverse Reactions and Side Effects** section. Within each organ system in this section, ADRs occurring at a frequency of ≥10% are underlined and are listed first (in alphabetical order). Adverse drug reactions occurring at a frequency of <10% will not be underlined and will be listed (in alphabetical order) after the underlined ADRs. As always, monitoring the patient's response to a medication and ongoing assessment are key nursing actions. Learn to recognize patient findings that suggest an ADR has occurred. These include:

- rash;
- change in respiratory rate, HR, BP, or mental state;
- seizure;
- anaphylaxis;
- diarrhea;
- fever.

Any of these findings can suggest an ADR and should be reported and documented promptly so that appropriate interventions, including discontinuation of suspect medications, can occur. Prompt intervention can prevent a mild adverse reaction from escalating into a serious health problem. Other steps taken by the health care team when identifying and treating an ADR include:

- Determining that the drug ordered was the drug given and intended.
- Determining that the drug was given in the correct dosage and by the correct route.
- Establishing the chronology of events: time drug was taken and onset of symptoms.
- Stopping the drug and monitoring patient status for improvement (dechallenge).
- Restarting the drug, if appropriate, and monitoring closely for adverse reactions (rechallenge).

Prevention

Health care organizations have responded to consumer, regulator, and insurer pressures by developing programs that aim to eliminate preventable ADRs. In the inpatient setting, computer systems can display the patient's age, height, weight, and CCr (or estimated glomerular filtratration rate) and send an alert to the clinician if a prescribed dose is out of range for any of the displayed parameters. Allergy alerts and drug-drug interaction alerts can be presented to the clinician at the time an order is entered.

In the outpatient setting, strategies that increase the patient's knowledge base and access to pharmacists and nurses may help prevent adverse reactions. Outpatient pharmacy computer systems that are linked within a chain of pharmacies may allow the pharmacist to view the patient's profile if the patient is filling a prescription in a pharmacy other than the usual one. Many pharmacy computers have dose limits and drug-drug interaction verification to assist pharmacists filling orders.

Such strategies are a valuable auxiliary to but cannot replace conscientious history taking, careful patient assessment, and ongoing monitoring. A thorough medication history, including all prescription and nonprescription drugs, all side effects and adverse reactions encountered, allergies, and all pertinent physical data should be available to the prescriber. The prescriber is responsible for reviewing this data, along with current medications, laboratory values, and any other variable that affects drug response.

It is not expected that practitioners will remember all relevant information when prescribing. In fact, reliance on memory is error-fraught, and clinicians need to use available resources to verify drug interactions whenever adding a new drug to the regimen. Setting expectations that clinicians use evidence-based information rather than their memories when prescribing, dispensing, administering, or monitoring patients has the potential to reduce the incidence of preventable ADRs.

Reporting ADRs in the United States:

FDA MedWatch Program: To monitor and assess the incidence of adverse reactions, the FDA sponsors MedWatch, a program that allows health care practitioners and consumers the opportunity to report serious adverse reactions or product defects encountered from medications, medical devices, special nutritional products, or other FDA-regulated items. The FDA considers serious those reactions that result in death, life-threatening illness or injury, hospitalization, disability, or congenital anomaly or those that require medical/surgical intervention.

In addition to reporting serious ADRs, health care providers should also report problems related to suspected contamination, questionable stability, defective components, or poor packaging/labeling. Reports should be submitted even if there is some uncertainty about the cause-effect relationship or if some details are missing. This reporting form may be accessed at https://www.fda.gov/safety/medwatch-fda-safety-information-and-adverse-event-reporting-program. Reactions to vaccines should be reported to the Vaccine Adverse Event Reporting System (VAERS; https://vaers.hhs.gov/). Nurses share with other health care providers an obligation to report adverse reactions to the MedWatch program so that all significant data can be analyzed for opportunities to improve patient care.

Reporting ADRs in Canada:

The Marketed Health Products Directorate of Health Canada coordinates ADR reporting activities and analyzes reports submitted from regional centers in each province. MedEffect Canada encourages health providers, patients, and regulatory authorities to report adverse reactions as they occur, either by email, mail, or the Health Canada website. Health care providers reporting ADRs are required to supply information regarding patient characteristics, details about the reaction(s), current treatment, and outcomes. Information identifying the patient or health care provider remains confidential.

Adverse drug reaction reports are analyzed to investigate any associations with the health product. Based on the outcome, regulatory bodies decide on a course of action, which may include performing additional postmarketing studies, reassessment of the risk versus benefit of the product, packaging modification, addition of warnings in patient information leaflets, or issuing public alerts or market withdrawals. Updates regarding adverse reactions are published in the Health Product InfoWatch every month.

Access the following link for the Side Effect Reporting Form for consumers and health providers: https://www.canada.ca/en/health-canada/services/drugs-health-products/medeffect-canada/adverse-reaction-reporting.html.

RESOURCES

1. Zazzara, M. B., Palmer, K., Vetrano, D. L., Carfi, A., & Onder, G. (2021). Adverse drug reactions in older adults: A narrative review of the literature. *European Geriatric Medicine*, 12(3), 463–473. https://doi.org/10.1007/s41999-021-00481-9
2. Schiavo, G., Forgerini, M., Lucchetta, R. C., Silva, G. O., & Mastroianni, P. D. C. (2022). Cost of adverse drug events related to potentially inappropriate medication use: A systematic review. *Journal of the American Pharmacists Association*, 62(5), 1463–1476. https://doi.org/10.1016/j.japh.2022.04.008
3. MedEffect Canada. (2017). *Adverse Reaction Information*. Government of Canada. https://www.canada.ca/en/health-canada/services/drugs-health-products/medeffect-canada/adverse-reaction-information.html

Overview of Risk Evaluation and Mitigation Systems (REMS)

Over the past several decades, the Food and Drug Administration (FDA) has employed a number of risk management programs designed to detect, evaluate, prevent, and mitigate drug adverse events for drugs with the potential for serious adverse drug reactions. Some of the risk management plans used by the FDA over the years have included the use of patient package inserts, medication guides, restricted access programs, and classification of drugs as controlled substances. These programs were acknowledged by the FDA as Risk Minimization Action Plans in 2005. With these programs, the FDA only had the authority to mandate postmarketing commitments from drug manufacturers before the drug was approved; however, these requirements could not be enforced after the drug was approved.

The Food and Drug Administration Amendments Act of 2007 gave the FDA the authority to subject drugs to new risk identification and communication strategies in the postmarketing period. These new strategies, called Risk Evaluation and Mitigation Strategies (REMS), can be required for any drug or drug class that is associated with serious risks. The FDA can require a REMS if it believes that this program is necessary to ensure that the benefits outweigh the potential risks of the drug. The FDA can require a REMS either as part of the drug approval process or during the postmarketing period if new information becomes available regarding potentially harmful effects that are associated with the use of the drug.

Components of the REMS may include a medication guide, a patient package insert, and/or a communication plan. A REMS for New Drug Applications or Biologics License Applications requires a timetable for submission of assessment of the REMS. A variety of elements to ensure safe use of drugs can be required as part of the REMS if it is believed that a medication guide, patient package insert, or communication plan are not adequate to mitigate the serious risks associated with a particular drug. These elements may include the following:

- Health care providers who prescribe the drug are specifically trained and/or certified.
- Pharmacies, practitioners, or health care settings that dispense the drug are specifically trained and/or certified.
- The drug is dispensed to patients only in certain health care settings, such as hospitals.
- The drug is dispensed only to patients with evidence or other documentation of safe-use conditions, such as laboratory test results.
- Patients using the drug are subject to certain monitoring.
- Patients using the drug are enrolled in a registry.

The FDA maintains an updated list of these REMS programs at https://www.accessdata.fda.gov/scripts/cder/rems/index.cfm. A REMS tag has been added at the top of and within the monographs of drugs associated with these programs.

Special Dosing Considerations

For many patients the average dose range for a given drug can be toxic. The purpose of this section is to describe vulnerable patient populations for which special dosing considerations must be made to protect the patient and improve clinical outcomes.

The Pediatric Patient

Most drugs prescribed to children are not approved by the Food and Drug Administration (FDA) for use in pediatric populations. This does not mean it is wrong to prescribe these drugs to children; rather, it means that the medications were not tested in children. The lack of pediatric drug information can result in patient harm or death, such as what occurred with the drug chloramphenicol. When given to very young children, chloramphenicol caused toxicity and multiple deaths. Referred to as "gray baby syndrome," this toxic reaction was eventually found to be dose dependent. The FDA now requires that new drugs that may be used in children include information for safe pediatric use.

The main reason for adjusting doses in pediatric patients is body size, which is measured by body weight or body surface area (BSA). Weight-based pediatric drug doses are expressed in number of milligrams per kilogram of body weight (mg/kg) while doses calculated on BSA are expressed in number of milligrams per meter squared (mg/m^2). BSA is determined using a BSA nomogram or calculated by using formulas (see Appendix E).

The neonate and the premature infant require additional adjustments secondary to immature function of body systems. For example, absorption may be incomplete or altered due to differences in gastric pH or motility. Distribution may be altered because of varying amounts of total body water, and metabolism and excretion can be delayed due to immature liver and kidney function. Furthermore, rapid weight changes and progressive maturation of hepatic and renal function require frequent monitoring and careful dose adjustments. Gestational age, as well as weight, may be needed to properly dose some drugs in the neonate.

The Older Adult Patient

Absorption, distribution, metabolism, and excretion are altered in adults over 65 years of age, putting the older patient at risk for toxic reactions. Pharmacokinetic properties in older adults are affected by (1) diminished GI motility and blood flow, which delays absorption; (2) changes in ratios of percentage of body fat, lean muscle mass, and total body water, which alter distribution; (3) decreased plasma proteins, especially in the malnourished patient, which alters distribution by allowing a larger proportion of free or unbound drug to circulate and exert effects; (4) diminished hepatic function, which slows metabolism; and (5) diminished renal function, which delays excretion.

Older adults should be prescribed the lowest effective dose at the initiation of therapy, followed by careful titration of doses. Monitor carefully for signs and symptoms of adverse drug reactions.

Another concern is that many older adult patients are prescribed multiple drugs and are at risk for polypharmacy. As the number of medications a patient takes increases, so does the risk for an adverse drug reaction. One drug may negate or potentiate the effects of another drug (drug-drug interaction). This situation is compounded by concurrent use of nonprescription or over-the-counter drugs, herbal supplements, and vitamins. In general, doses of most medications (especially digoxin, sedative/hypnotics, anticoagulants, nonsteroidal anti-inflammatory agents, antibiotics, and antihypertensives) should be decreased in the older adult population. The Beers List/Criteria, which appears in the *Medication Safety Tools* section, is a list of drugs to be used with caution in older adults.

Women of Reproductive Potential

Generally, pregnant women should avoid medications, except when necessary. Both the mother and the fetus must be considered. The placenta is a membrane that allows rapid and complete diffusion of lipid soluble drugs and protects the fetus only from extremely large molecules. The fetus is particularly vulnerable during the first and the last trimesters of pregnancy. During the first trimester, vital organs are forming, and ingestion of teratogenic drugs may lead to fetal malformation or miscarriage. Unfortunately, this is the time when a woman is least likely to know that she is pregnant. In the third trimester, drugs administered to the mother and transferred to the fetus may not be safely metabolized and excreted by the fetus. This is especially true of drugs administered near term. After the infant is delivered, they no longer have the placenta to help with drug excretion, and drugs administered before delivery may result in toxicity.

Of course, many conditions, such as asthma, diabetes, gastrointestinal disorders, and mental illness, affect pregnant women and require long-term medication use. When the medications are used, whether over-the-counter or prescription, prescribing the lowest effective dose for the shortest period of time necessary is the rule. The Centers for Disease Control and Prevention has a variety of resources and treatment guidelines called Treating for Two: Medicine and Pregnancy, found online at https://www.cdc.gov/pregnancy/meds/treatingfortwo/.

The possibility of a medication altering sperm quality and quantity in a potential father is also an area of concern. Male patients should be informed of this risk when taking any medications known to have this potential.

Renal Impairment

The kidneys are the major organ of drug elimination. Failure to account for decreased renal function is a preventable source of adverse drug reactions. Renal function is measured by the creatinine clearance, which can be approximated in the absence of a 24-hour urine collection (see Appendix E). In addition, doses in patients with renal impairment can be optimized by measuring blood levels of certain drugs (e.g., digoxin, aminoglycosides).

Patients with underlying renal impairment, premature infants with immature renal function, and older adults with an age-related decrease in renal function require careful dose adjustments. Renal function may fluctuate over time and should be reassessed periodically.

Hepatic Impairment

The liver is the major organ of drug metabolism. The cytochrome P-450 (CYP450) system changes a drug from a relatively fat-soluble compound to a more water-soluble substance, which means that the drug can then be excreted by the kidneys. Liver function is not as easily quantified as renal function, and it therefore is difficult to predict the correct dose for a patient with hepatic impairment based on laboratory tests.

A patient who is severely jaundiced or who has very low serum proteins (particularly albumin) can be expected to have some problems metabolizing drugs. In advanced liver disease, portal vascular congestion also impairs drug absorption. Examples of drugs that should be carefully dosed in patients with hepatic impairment include theophylline, diuretics, phenytoin, and sedatives. Some drugs (e.g., enalapril, carisoprodol) must be activated in the liver to exert their effect and are known as prodrugs. In patients with hepatic impairment, these drugs may not be converted to the active component, thereby resulting in decreased efficacy.

Heart Failure

Heart failure results in passive congestion of blood vessels in the gastrointestinal tract, which impairs drug absorption. Heart failure also slows drug delivery to the liver, delaying metabolism. Renal function is frequently compromised, adding to delayed elimination and prolonged drug action. Doses of drugs metabolized mainly by the liver or excreted mainly by the kidneys should be decreased in patients with chronic heart failure.

Body Size

Drug dosing is often based on total body weight. However, some drugs selectively penetrate fatty tissues. If the drug does not penetrate fatty tissues (e.g., digoxin, gentamicin), doses for the obese patient should be determined by ideal body weight or estimated lean body mass. Ideal body weight may be determined from tables of optimal weights or may be estimated using formulas for lean body mass when the patient's height and weight are known (see Appendix E). If such adjustments are not made, considerable toxicity can result.

Body size is also a factor in patients who are grossly underweight. Older adults, chronic alcoholics, patients with acquired immune deficiency, and patients who are terminally ill from cancer or other debilitating illnesses need careful attention to dosing. Patients who have had a limb amputated also need to have this change in body size considered.

Drug Interactions

Use of multiple drugs, especially those known to interact with other drugs, may necessitate dose adjustments. Drugs highly bound to plasma proteins, such as warfarin and phenytoin, may be displaced by other highly protein-bound drugs. When this phenomenon occurs, the drug that has been displaced exhibits an increase in its activity because the free or unbound drug is thus available to be active.

Some drugs decrease the liver's ability to metabolize other drugs by inhibiting the CYP450 system. Drugs capable of doing this include ketoconazole and itraconazole. Coadministered drugs that are also highly metabolized by the liver may need to be administered in decreased doses. Other agents, such as phenobarbital, rifampin, phenytoin, and carbamazepine, can stimulate the liver to metabolize drugs more rapidly by inducing the CYP450 system, requiring larger doses to be administered. Coadministered drugs that are also highly metabolized by the liver may need to be administered in higher doses.

Drugs that significantly alter urine pH can affect excretion of drugs for which the excretory process is pH dependent. Alkalinizing the urine will hasten the excretion of acidic drugs. An example of this is administering sodium bicarbonate in cases of aspirin overdose to promote the renal excretion of aspirin. Alkalinizing the urine will increase reabsorption of alkaline drugs, which prolongs and enhances drug action. Acidification of the urine will hasten the excretion of alkaline drugs. Acidification of the urine will also enhance reabsorption of acidic drugs, prolonging and enhancing drug action.

Some drugs compete for enzyme systems with other drugs. Allopurinol inhibits the enzyme involved in uric acid production, but it also inhibits metabolism (inactivation) of 6-mercaptopurine, greatly increasing its toxicity. The dose of mercaptopurine needs to be significantly reduced when coadministered with allopurinol.

The same potential for interactions exists for some foods. Dietary calcium, found in high concentrations in dairy products, combines with tetracycline or fluoroquinolones and prevents their absorption. Foods high in pyridoxine (vitamin B_6) can negate the antiparkinsonian effect of levodopa. Grapefruit juice inhibits the enzyme that breaks down some drugs, and concurrent ingestion may significantly increase drug levels and the risk for toxicity.

Many commonly taken natural products interact with pharmaceutical drugs. St. John's wort, garlic, ephedra, and other natural products can interact with medications and cause known or unpredictable reactions.

Nurses and prescribers should consult drug references and remember that the average dosing range for drugs is intended for an average patient. Every patient is an individual with specific drug-handling capabilities. Taking these special dosing considerations into account allows for an individualized drug regimen that promotes the desired therapeutic outcome and minimizes the risk of toxicity.

RESOURCES

1. Burchum, J., & Rosenthal, L. (2021). *Lehne's pharmacology for nursing care* (11th ed.). Elsevier.
2. Ziend, C. S., & Carvalho, M. D. (2023). *Applied therapeutics: The clinical use of drugs* (12th ed.). Lippincott Williams & Wilkins.

The Cytochrome P450 System: What Is It and Why Should I Care?

Looking beyond the obvious takes time, energy, insight, and fortitude, yet this is what we are called to do. We are nurses—tireless care providers. Yet when the subject of the liver's enzyme system, also called the cytochrome P450 system, is discussed, we feel the urge to run the other way—or better yet, to just ignore the conversation. But can we do this as the tireless care provider? The answer to this question is clear and simple: no, we cannot. This is because numerous medications, nutrients, and herbal therapies are metabolized through the cytochrome P450 (CYP450) enzyme system. This system can be inhibited or induced by drugs and, once altered, can be clinically significant in the development of drug-drug interactions that may cause unanticipated adverse reactions or therapeutic failures. This article will review the basic concepts of the CYP450 system and relate these concepts to clinically significant altered responses.

The CYP450 enzymes are essential for the production of numerous agents, including cholesterol and steroids. Additionally, these enzymes are necessary for the detoxification of foreign chemicals and the metabolism of drugs. CYP450 enzymes are so named because they are bound to membranes within a cell (cyto) and contain a heme pigment (chrome and P) that absorbs light at a wavelength of 450 nm when exposed to carbon monoxide. There are more than 50 CYP450 enzymes, but the CYP1A2, CYP2C19, CYP2D6, CYP1A2, CYP3A4, and CYP3A5 enzymes are responsible for metabolizing 45% of drug metabolism. The CYP2D6 (20–30%), the CYP2C9 (10%), and the CYP2E1 and CYP1A2 (5%) complete this enzyme system.

Drugs that cause CYP450 drug interactions are referred to as either inhibitors or inducers. An inducing agent can increase the rate of another drug's metabolism by as much as two- to threefold, developing over a period of a week. When an inducing agent is prescribed with another medication, the dose of the other medication may need to be adjusted because the rate of metabolism is increased and the effect of the medication reduced. This can lead to a therapeutic failure of the medication. Conversely, if a medication is taken with an agent that inhibits its metabolism, then the drug level can rise and possibly result in a harmful or adverse effect. Information regarding a drug's CYP450 metabolism and its potential for inhibition or induction can be found on the drug label and accessed through the U.S. Food and Drug Administration or manufacturer's websites.

When we assess our patients and provide management modalities, these are implemented within a framework of the patient's heritage, race, and culture. This is also true in pharmacology as well (i.e., pharmacogenetics). This concept is important to examine because we know that there exists genetic variability that may influence a patient's response to commonly prescribed drug classes. This genetic variability can be defined as polymorphism. Seven percent of White patients and 2–7% of Black patients are poor metabolizers of drugs dependent on CYP2D6, which metabolizes many beta blockers, antidepressants, and opioids. This is because the drug's metabolism via CYP450 enzymes exhibits genetic variability.

Recently, researchers have studied the genetic variability in metabolism among women who were prescribed tamoxifen and medications that inhibit the CYP2D6 enzyme. To review, tamoxifen is biotransformed to the potent antiestrogen endoxifen by this enzyme. CYP2D6 genetic variation (individuals considered extensive metabolizers versus poor metabolizers) and inhibitors of the enzyme markedly reduce endoxifen plasma concentrations in tamoxifen-treated patients.

The researchers concluded that CYP2D6 metabolism is an "independent predictor of breast cancer outcome in postmenopausal women receiving tamoxifen for early breast cancer. Determination of CYP2D6 genotype may be of value in selecting adjuvant hormonal therapy and it appears CYP2D6 inhibitors should be avoided in tamoxifen-treated women." Do oncology patients come to us with only their cancer and its treatment? No, they come with multifaceted dimensions and comorbid conditions such as hypertension, dyslipidemia, depression, seizure disorders, and so forth. For example, several antidepressants (paroxetine and fluoxetine) are inhibitors of metabolism when given with drugs metabolized through the CYP2D6 enzyme, such as haloperidol, metoprolol, and hydrocodone. Thus, the therapeutic response can be accentuated. Medications that inhibit the CYP3A4 enzyme, such as amiodarone and antifungals, can affect the therapeutic response of fentanyl, alprazolam, and numerous statins; as a result, the effect of these drugs can be enhanced, leading to potential toxic levels.

At times, these CYP450 inducers and inhibitors are commonly ingested items such as grapefruit juice and tobacco. There are numerous medications known to interact with grapefruit juice, including statins, antiarrhythmic agents, immunosuppressive agents, and calcium channel blockers. Furthermore, the inhibition of the enzyme system seems to be dose dependent; thus, the more a patient drinks, the more the inhibition that occurs. Additionally, the effects can last for several days if grapefruit juice is consumed on a regular basis. Luckily, the effect of this is not seen with other citrus juices.

Hopefully, this brief review has opened the door to your inquisitive nature on how the liver's enzyme system is affected by numerous medications and why some patients experience clinically significant unanticipated adverse reactions or therapeutic failures.

CYP1A2

SENSITIVE SUBSTRATES	MODERATE OR STRONG INHIBITORS	MODERATE OR STRONG INDUCERS
alosetron, caffeine, duloxetine, melatonin, pirfenidone ramelteon tasimelteon theophylline, tizanidine	ciprofloxacin, fluvoxamine, mexiletine, vemurafenib	cigarette smoke, phenytoin, rifampin, teriflunomide

CYP2C9

SENSITIVE SUBSTRATES	STRONG OR MODERATE INHIBITORS	STRONG OR MODERATE INDUCERS
celecoxib, glimepiride, phenytoin, (S)-warfarin	amiodarone, fluconazole, miconazole	enzalutamide, rifampin

CYP2C19

SENSITIVE SUBSTRATES	STRONG OR MODERATE INHIBITORS	STRONG OR MODERATE INDUCERS
diazepam, lansoprazole, omeprazole, rabeprazole, voriconazole	cenobamate, felbamate, fluconazole, fluoxetine, fluvoxamine, voriconazole	apalutamide, efavirenz, enzalutamide, phenytoin, rifampin

CYP2D6

SENSITIVE SUBSTRATES	STRONG OR MODERATE INHIBITORS	STRONG OR MODERATE INDUCERS
atomoxetine, desipramine, dextromethorphan, eliglustat, imipramine, metoprolol, nebivolol, nortriptyline, perphenazine, propafenone, propranolol, tramadol, tolterodine, venlafaxine	abiraterone, bupropion, cinacalcet, duloxetine, fluoxetine, lorcaserin, mirabegron, paroxetine, quinidine, rolapitant, terbinafine	None

CYP3A

SENSITIVE SUBSTRATES	STRONG OR MODERATE INHIBITORS	STRONG OR MODERATE INDUCERS
alprazolam, aprepitant, atorvastatin, avanafil budesonide, buspirone, colchicine, conivaptan, darifenacin, darunavir, dasatinib, dronedarone, eletriptan, eliglustat, eplerenone, everolimus, felodipine, ibrutinib, isavuconazonium, ivabradine, lemborexant, lomitapide, lovastatin, lurasidone, maraviroc, midazolam, mobocertinib, naloxegol, nisoldipine, pimozide, quetiapine, rilpivirine, rivaroxaban, sildenafil, simvastatin, sirolimus, tacrolimus, tadalafil, ticagrelor, tipranavir, tolvaptan, triazolam, vardenafil, venetoclax	aprepitant, ceritinib, ciprofloxacin, clarithromycin, cobicistat, conivaptan, crizotinib, diltiazem, dronedarone, erythromycin, fluconazole, grapefruit juice, idelalisib, imatinib, isavuconazonium, itraconazole, ketoconazole, nefazodone, nelfinavir, posaconazole, ritonavir, verapamil, voriconazole	apalutamide, bosentan, carbamazepine, cenobamate, dabrafenib, efavirenz, enzalutamide, etravirine, ivosidenib, lorlatinib, lumacaftor/ivacaftor, mitotane, pexidartinib, phenobarbital, phenytoin, primidone, rifampin, sotorasib, St. John's wort

RESOURCES

1. U.S. Food and Drug Administration. (2025, June 27). *FDA's examples of drugs that interact with CYP enzymes and transporter systems*. https://www.fda.gov/drugs/drug-interactions-labeling/healthcare-professionals-fdas-examples-drugs-interact-cyp-enzymes-and-transporter-systems
2. Krau, S. D. (2013). Cytochrome p450, part 1: What nurses really need to know. *Nursing Clinics of North America*, 48(4), 671–680. https://doi.org/10.1016/j.cnur.2013.09.002
3. Krau, S. D. (2013). Cytochrome p450, part 2: What nurses need to know about the cytochrome p450 family systems. *Nursing Clinics of North America*, 48(4), 681–696. https://doi.org/10.1016/j.cnur.2013.09.003
4. Krau, S. D. (2013). Cytochrome p450, part 3: Drug interactions: Essential concepts and considerations. *Nursing Clinics of North America*, 48(4), 697–706. https://doi.org/10.1016/j.cnur.2013.09.004

Educating Patients About Safe Medication Use

Research has shown that patients need information about several medication-related topics, no matter what the medication is. A well-informed patient and/or family can help prevent medication errors by hospital staff and is less likely to make medication errors at home. Adherence to the medication regimen is another goal achieved through patient education.

Before beginning any teaching, however, always assess the patient's current knowledge by asking if they are familiar with the medication, how it is taken at home, what precautions or follow-up care is required, and other questions specific to each drug. Based on the patient's current knowledge level and taking into consideration factors such as readiness to learn, environmental and social barriers to learning or adherence, and cultural factors, discuss the following:

- **Generic and brand names of the medication.** Patients should know both the brand and generic names of each medication for two reasons. It helps them identify their medications when a generic equivalent is substituted for a brand name version, and it prevents patients or health care providers from making sound-alike confusion errors when giving or documenting a medication history. An example of this is saying Celebrex but meaning or hearing Cerebyx.
- **Purpose of the medication.** Patients have a right to know what the therapeutic benefit of the medication will be but also should be told the consequences of not taking the prescribed medication. This may enhance adherence. For example, a patient may be more likely to take blood pressure medication if told lowering high blood pressure will prevent heart attack, kidney disease, or stroke rather than hearing only that it will lower blood pressure.
- **Dose and how to take the medication.** To derive benefit and avoid adverse reactions or other poor outcomes, the patient must know how much of the medication to take and when to take it. Refer to doses in metric weight (e.g., milligram, gram) rather than dosage unit (tablet) or volume (1 teaspoon). The patient must also be informed of the best time to take the medication—for example, on an empty or a full stomach, before bedtime, or with or without other medications. If possible, help the patient fit the medication schedule into their own schedule so that taking the medication is not difficult or forgotten.
- **What to do if a dose is missed.** Always explain to patients what to do if a dose is missed. Patients have reported taking a double dose of medication when a missed dose occurs, putting themselves at risk for side effects and adverse reactions.
- **Duration of therapy.** It is not uncommon for patients to stop taking a medication when they feel better or to discontinue a medication when they cannot perceive a benefit. For very long-term and even lifelong therapy, the patient may need to be reminded that the medication helps maintain the current level of wellness. Patients may need to be reminded to finish short-term courses of medications (such as antibiotics) even though they frequently will feel much better before the prescription runs out. Some medications cannot be discontinued abruptly, and patients should be warned to consult a health care provider before discontinuing such agents. Patients will need to know to refill prescriptions several days before running out or to take extra medication if traveling.
- **Minor side effects and what to do if they occur.** Inform the patient that all medications have potential side effects. Explain the most common side effects associated with the medication and how to avoid or manage them if they occur. An informed patient is less likely to stop taking a medication because of a minor and potentially avoidable side effect.
- **Serious side effects and what to do if they occur.** Inform the patient of the possibility of serious side effects. Describe signs and symptoms associated with serious side effects, and tell the patient to immediately inform a health care provider should they occur. Tell the patient to call before the next dose of the medication is scheduled and to not assume that the medication is the source of the symptom and prematurely discontinue it.

- **Medications to avoid.** Drug-drug interactions can dampen drug effects, enhance drug effects, or cause life-threatening adverse events such as cardiac arrhythmias, liver injury, renal failure, or internal bleeding. The patient and family need to know which other medications, including over-the-counter medications, to avoid.
- **Foods to avoid and other precautions.** Food-drug interactions are not uncommon and can have effects similar to drug-drug interactions. Excessive sun exposure resulting in severe dermal reactions is not uncommon and represents an environmental-drug interaction. Likewise, the patient should be informed of what activities to avoid, in case the medication affects alertness or coordination, for example.
- **How to store the medication.** Medications must be stored properly to maintain potency. Most medications should not be stored in the bathroom medicine cabinet because of excess heat and humidity. In addition, thoughtful storage practices, such as separating two family members' medications, can prevent mix-ups and inadvertent accessibility by children (or pets). Some medications, such as those with potential for abuse, must be kept in a safe/locked container away from children or others. Review storage with patients and ask about current methods for storing medications.
- **Follow-up care.** Anyone taking medication requires ongoing care to assess effectiveness and appropriateness of medications. Many medications require testing to monitor blood levels; effects on hematopoietic, hepatic, or renal function; or other effects on other body systems. Ongoing medical evaluation may result in dosage adjustments, change in medication, or discontinuation of medication.
- **What not to take.** Inform patients not to take expired medications or someone else's medication. Warn them not to self-medicate with older, no-longer-used prescriptions, even if the remaining supply is not expired. Tell patients to keep a current record of all medications taken and to ask health care providers if new medications are meant to replace a current medication.

As you teach, encourage the patient and the family to ask questions. Providing feedback about medication questions will increase their understanding and help you identify areas that need reinforcement. Also, ask patients to repeat what you have said and return to demonstrate application or administration techniques.

Stress the importance of concurrent therapies. Medications often are only a part of a recommended therapy. Review with the patient and family other measures that will enhance or maintain health. Always consider the cultural context in which health information is provided and plan accordingly. This might include obtaining a same-gender translator or adjusting dosing times to avoid conflict with traditional rituals.

Finally, provide written instructions in a simple and easy-to-read format. Keep in mind that most health care information is written at a 10th-grade reading level, while many patients read at a 5th-grade level. Tell patients to keep the written instructions so that they can be reviewed at home, when stress levels are lower and practical difficulties in maintaining the medication plan are known.

Classifications

ANTI-ALZHEIMER'S AGENTS

Commonly Prescribed Drugs

See Mechanism of Action of Select Anti-Alzheimer Drugs table.

Pharmacologic Profile

General Use

Alzheimer dementia.

General Action and Information

MECHANISM OF ACTION OF SELECT ANTI-ALZHEIMER DRUGS

DRUG	MECHANISM
Donanemab and lecanemab	Monoclonal antibody directed against amyloid beta
Donepezil, galantamine, and rivastigmine	Acetylcholinesterase inhibitors
Memantine	N-methyl-D-aspartate (NMDA) receptor antagonist

Contraindications

Hypersensitivity.

Precautions

Acetylcholinesterase inhibitors should be used cautiously in patients with a history of sick sinus syndrome or other supraventricular cardiac conduction abnormalities (may cause bradycardia). Cholinergic effects may result in adverse GI effects (nausea, vomiting, diarrhea, weight loss) and may also ↑ gastric acid secretion resulting in GI bleeding, especially during concurrent NSAID therapy. Other cholinergic effects may include urinary tract obstruction, seizures, or bronchospasm. Neuropsychiatric side effects, including confusion, dizziness, headache, and sedation, are frequently reported with use of memantine. Lecanemab and donanemab should be used with caution in patients who are apolipoprotein E ∊4 homozygotes because of the risk of amyloid-related imaging abnormalities (ARIA), which can be life-threatening. These drugs may also cause infusion-related reactions.

Interactions

Acetylcholinesterase inhibitors may have additive effects with other drugs having cholinergic properties, exaggerate the effects of succinylcholine-type muscle relaxation during anesthesia, and ↓ therapeutic effects of anticholinergics. Lecanemab and donanemab should be used cautiously in patients receiving anticoagulant medications because of an ↑ risk of bleeding.

Nursing Implications

Assessment

- Assess cognitive function (memory, attention, reasoning, language, ability to perform simple tasks) throughout therapy.
- Acetylcholinesterase inhibitors: Monitor HR periodically during therapy. May cause bradycardia.
- Donanemab and lecanemab: Perform brain MRI at baseline and periodically during therapy (each drug has specific recommendations). Enhanced clinical vigilance for ARIA is recommended during the 1st 14 wk of therapy. Also, monitor for infusion-related reactions (fever and flu-like symptoms [chills, generalized aches, feeling shaky, joint pain], nausea, vomiting, hypotension, hypertension, oxygen desaturation).

C L A S S I F I C A T I O N S

Implementation

- Donanemab and lecanemab are administered as IV infusions.
- **Donepezil:** Can be administered PO or via transdermal patch. Administer oral donepezil in the evening just before going to bed. Apply transdermal patch once weekly.
- **Rivastigmine:** Can be administered PO or via transdermal patch. Apply transdermal patch every 24 hr.

Patient/Family Teaching

- Instruct patient and caregiver that medication should be taken as directed.
- Advise patient and caregiver to notify health care provider if nausea, vomiting, diarrhea, or changes in color of stool occur or if new symptoms occur or previously noted symptoms ↑ in severity.

Evaluation/Desired Outcomes

- Improvement in cognitive function (memory, attention, reasoning, language, ability to perform simple tasks) in patients with Alzheimer disease.

ANTIANEMICS

Commonly Prescribed Drugs

See Mechanism of Action of Select Antianemics table.

Pharmacologic Profile

General Use

Prevention and treatment of anemias.

General Action and Information

MECHANISM OF ACTION OF SELECT ANTIANEMICS

DRUG	MECHANISM
Ferrous sulfate and iron sucrose	Required for production of hemoglobin
Darbepoetin and epoetin alfa	Erythropoiesis stimulating agents
Cyanocobalamin and folic acid	Water-soluble vitamin required for hematopoiesis

Contraindications

Undiagnosed anemias. Hemochromatosis, hemosiderosis, hemolytic anemia (iron). Uncontrolled hypertension (darbepoetin and epoetin alfa).

Precautions

Use parenteral iron (iron sucrose) cautiously in patients with a history of allergy or hypersensitivity reactions.

Interactions

Oral iron can ↓ the absorption of tetracyclines, fluoroquinolones, bisphosphonates, mycophenolate mofetil, levothyroxine, or penicillamine. Concurrent use of proton pump inhibitors, H_2 antagonists, or antacids may ↓ absorption of oral iron. Phenytoin and other anticonvulsants may ↓ the absorption of folic acid.

Nursing Implications

Assessment

- Assess patient's nutritional status and dietary history to determine possible causes for anemia and need for patient teaching.

Implementation

- When administering parenteral iron, assess for hypersensitivity reactions and anaphylaxis (rash, dyspnea, loss of consciousness, hypotension, collapse, convulsions) for ≥30 min following injection. Equipment for resuscitation should be readily available.

- Monitor hemoglobin, hematocrit, serum ferritin, and transferrin saturation prior to and periodically during therapy.

Patient/Family Teaching

- Encourage patients to comply with diet recommendations of health care provider. Explain that the best source of vitamins and minerals is a well-balanced diet with foods from the four basic food groups.
- Patients self-medicating with vitamin and mineral supplements should be cautioned not to exceed RDA. The effectiveness of megadoses for treatment of various medical conditions is unproven and may cause side effects.

Evaluation/Desired Outcomes

- Resolution of anemia.

ANTIANGINALS

Commonly Prescribed Drugs

See Mechanism of Action of Select Antianginals table.

Pharmacologic Profile

General Use

Nitrates are used to treat and prevent attacks of angina. Only nitrates (sublingual, translingual spray, transdermal ointment, or intravenous) may be used in the acute treatment of attacks of angina pectoris. Nitrates, calcium channel blockers (CCBs), beta blockers, and ranolazine are used prophylactically in long-term management of angina.

General Action and Information

MECHANISM OF ACTION OF SELECT ANTIANGINALS

DRUG	MECHANISM
Atenolol, metoprolol, nadolol, propranolol, and timolol	Beta blockers (selective: atenolol and metoprolol; nonselective: nadolol, propranolol, and timolol): ↓ HR, contractility and wall tension → ↓ myocardial oxygen demand
Amlodipine, nicardipine, and nifedipine	Dihydropyridine CCBs: dilate coronary arteries (↑ myocardial oxygen supply); ↓ contractility and wall tension (↓ myocardial oxygen demand)
Diltiazem and verapamil	Nondihydropyridine CCBs: dilate coronary arteries (↑ myocardial oxygen supply); ↓ HR, contractility, and wall tension (↓ myocardial oxygen demand)
Isosorbide dinitrate/mononitrate and nitroglycerin	Nitrates: dilate coronary arteries (↑ myocardial oxygen supply); ↓ myocardial wall tension (↓ myocardial oxygen demand)
Ranolazine	↓ wall tension and myocardial oxygen consumption (↓ myocardial oxygen demand)

Contraindications

Hypersensitivity. Avoid use of beta blockers and nondihydropyridine CCBs in sick sinus syndrome or 2nd/3rd-degree heart block, cardiogenic shock, or decompensated HF. Avoid nitrates in ↑ intracranial pressure and during concurrent use of phosphodiesterase (PDE)-5 inhibitors (avanafil, sildenafil, tadalafil, vardenafil) or riociguat.

Precautions

Beta blockers should be used cautiously in patients with diabetes mellitus or pulmonary disease.

Interactions

Nitrates, CCBs, and beta blockers may cause hypotension with other antihypertensives or acute ingestion of alcohol. Nitrates may also cause significant hypotension with PDE-5 inhibitors or riociguat. Verapamil, diltiazem, and beta blockers may ↑ risk of bradycardia when used with digoxin, ivabradine, or clonidine. Verapamil, diltiazem, and ranolazine have a number of other significant drug-drug interactions.

Nursing Implications

Assessment

- Assess location, duration, intensity, and precipitating factors of patient's anginal pain.
- Monitor BP and HR periodically throughout therapy.

Implementation

- Available in various dose forms. See specific drugs for information on administration.

Patient/Family Teaching

- Instruct patient on concurrent nitrate therapy and prophylactic antianginals to continue taking both medications as ordered and to use sublingual/translingual nitroglycerin as needed for anginal attacks.
- Advise patient to contact health care provider immediately if chest pain does not improve; worsens after therapy; is accompanied by diaphoresis or shortness of breath; or if severe, persistent headache occurs.
- Inform patient that headache is a common side effect of nitrates that should ↓ with continuing therapy. Aspirin or acetaminophen may be ordered to treat headache.
- Caution patient to make position changes slowly to minimize orthostatic hypotension.
- Advise patient to avoid concurrent use of alcohol with these medications.

Evaluation/Desired Outcomes

- Decrease in frequency and severity of anginal attacks.
- Increase in activity tolerance.

ANTIANXIETY AGENTS

Commonly Prescribed Drugs

See Mechanism of Action of Select Antianxiety Agents table.

Pharmacologic Profile

General Use

Antianxiety agents are used in the management of various forms of anxiety, including generalized anxiety disorder. Some agents are more suitable for intermittent or short-term use (benzodiazepines), while others are more useful long term (buspirone, paroxetine, venlafaxine).

General Action and Information

MECHANISM OF ACTION OF SELECT ANTIANXIETY AGENTS

DRUG	MECHANISM
Alprazolam, chlordiazepoxide, diazepam, lorazepam, and oxazepam	Benzodiazepines
Paroxetine	Selective serotonin reuptake inhibitor
Venlafaxine	Selective serotonin/norepinephrine reuptake inhibitor
Buspirone	Binds to serotonin and dopamine receptors in brain
Hydroxyzine	Has activity at muscarinic, serotonin, and dopamine receptors in brain

Contraindications

Hypersensitivity. Should not be used in comatose patients or in those with pre-existing CNS depression. Should not be used in patients with uncontrolled severe pain. Avoid use during pregnancy or lactation.

Precautions

Use cautiously in patients with hepatic impairment, severe renal impairment, or severe underlying pulmonary disease (benzodiazepines only). Use with caution in patients who may be suicidal or who may have had previous drug addictions. Patients may be more sensitive to CNS depressant effects; dosage ↓ may be required.

Interactions

Mainly for benzodiazepines; additive CNS depression with alcohol, antihistamines, some antidepressants, opioid analgesics, or phenothiazines may occur. Most agents should not be used with MAO inhibitors.

Nursing Implications

Assessment

- Monitor BP, HR, and respiratory status frequently throughout IV administration.
- Prolonged high-dose therapy may lead to psychological or physical dependence. Restrict the amount of drug available to patient, especially if patient is depressed, suicidal, or has a history of addiction.
- Assess degree of anxiety and level of sedation (ataxia, dizziness, slurred speech) before and periodically throughout therapy.

Implementation

- Patients changing to buspirone from other antianxiety agents should receive gradually ↓ doses. Buspirone will not prevent withdrawal symptoms.

Patient/Family Teaching

- May cause daytime drowsiness. Caution patient to avoid driving and other activities requiring alertness until response to medication is known.
- Advise patient to avoid the use of alcohol and other CNS depressants concurrently with these medications.
- Advise patient to inform health care provider if pregnancy is planned or suspected.

Evaluation/Desired Outcomes

- Decrease in anxiety level.

ANTIARRHYTHMICS

Commonly Prescribed Drugs

See Mechanism of Action of Select Antiarrhythmics table.

Pharmacologic Profile

General Use

Suppression of cardiac arrhythmias.

General Action and Information

MECHANISM OF ACTION OF SELECT ANTIARRHYTHMICS

DRUG	MECHANISM
Lidocaine	Class Ib (Na channel blocker)
Esmolol, metoprolol, and propranolol	Class II (beta blockers: ↓ AV nodal conduction and ↓ automaticity)
Amiodarone	Class III (K channel blocker; also has Na channel, beta receptor, and Ca channel blocking properties)
Diltiazem and verapamil	Class IV (nondihydropyridine calcium channel blockers: ↓ AV nodal conduction)
Adenosine	Restores sinus rhythm by slowing conduction and interrupting re-entrant pathways in the AV node
Atropine	Inhibits the action of acetylcholine at postganglionic sites located in the heart → ↑ HR
Digoxin	↓ SA and AV nodal conduction

* AV = atrioventricular; Ca = calcium; K = potassium; Na = sodium; SA = sinoatrial.

Contraindications

Differ greatly among various agents. See individual drugs.

Precautions
Differ greatly among agents used. Appropriate dosage adjustments should be made in older adults and those with renal or hepatic impairment, depending on agent chosen. Correctable causes of arrhythmias (electrolyte abnormalities, drug toxicity) should be evaluated. See individual drugs.

Interactions
Differ greatly among agents used. See individual drugs.

Nursing Implications

Assessment
- Monitor ECG, HR, and BP continuously throughout IV administration and periodically throughout oral administration.

Implementation
- Take HR before administration of oral doses. Withhold dose and notify physician or other health care provider if HR <50 bpm.

Patient/Family Teaching
- Instruct patient to take oral doses around the clock, as directed, even if feeling better.
- Instruct patient or family member on how to take pulse. Advise patient to report changes in pulse rate or rhythm to health care provider.
- Caution patient to avoid taking OTC medications without consulting health care provider.
- Advise patient to carry identification describing disease process and medication regimen at all times.
- Emphasize the importance of follow-up exams to monitor progress.

Evaluation/Desired Outcomes
- Resolution of cardiac arrhythmias without detrimental side effects.

ANTIASTHMATICS

Commonly Prescribed Drugs
See Mechanism of Action of Select Antiasthmatics table.

Pharmacologic Profile

General Use
Management of acute and chronic episodes of reversible bronchoconstriction. Goal of therapy is to treat acute attacks (short-term control) and to ↓ incidence and intensity of future attacks (long-term control). The choice of modalities depends on the continued requirement for short-term control agents.

General Action and Information

MECHANISM OF ACTION OF SELECT ANTIASTHMATICS

DRUG	MECHANISM
Beclomethasone, budesonide, ciclesonide, fluticasone, methylprednisolone, mometasone, prednisolone, and prednisone	Corticosteroids: ↓ airway inflammation
Albuterol, levalbuterol, and salmeterol	Beta$_2$ agonists: ↑ levels of cyclic-3', 5'-adenosine monophosphate (cAMP) → Bronchodilation
Benralizumab, dupilumab, and mepolizumab	Interleukin antagonists
Montelukast	Leukotriene receptor antagonist
Omalizumab	Inhibits binding of IgE to receptors on mast cells and eosinophils, preventing the release of inflammatory mediators
Tiotropium	Anticholinergic: Inhibits the action of acetylcholine at muscarinic receptors in bronchial smooth muscle → Bronchodilation

Contraindications
Only short-acting adrenergic bronchodilators should be used during acute attacks of asthma.

Precautions
Adrenergic bronchodilators and anticholinergics should be used cautiously in patients with cardiovascular disease. Chronic use of systemic corticosteroids should be avoided in children or during pregnancy or lactation. Patients with diabetes may experience loss of glycemic control during corticosteroid therapy. Corticosteroids should never be abruptly discontinued.

Interactions
Adrenergic bronchodilators and phosphodiesterase inhibitors may have additive CNS and cardiovascular effects with other adrenergic agents. Corticosteroids may ↓ the effectiveness of antidiabetics. Corticosteroids may cause hypokalemia, which may be additive with potassium-losing diuretics and may also ↑ the risk of digoxin toxicity.

Nursing Implications

Assessment
- Assess lung sounds and respiratory function prior to and periodically throughout therapy.
- Assess cardiovascular status of patients taking adrenergic bronchodilators or anticholinergics. Monitor for ECG changes and chest pain.

Implementation
- **Inhaln:** Shake inhaler well, and allow ≥1 min between inhalations of aerosol medication. Prime the inhaler before first use. Use of spacer recommended for children.

Patient/Family Teaching
- Instruct patient to take antiasthmatics as directed. Do not take more than prescribed or discontinue without discussing with health care provider.
- Advise patient to avoid smoking and other respiratory irritants.
- Instruct patient in correct use of metered-dose inhaler or other administration devices (see Appendix C).
- Advise patient to contact health care provider promptly if the usual dose of medication fails to produce the desired results, if symptoms worsen after treatment, or if toxic effects occur.
- Patients using inhalation medications and bronchodilators should be advised to use the bronchodilator first and allow 5 min to elapse before administering other medications, unless otherwise directed by health care provider.

Evaluation/Desired Outcomes
- Prevention of and reduction in symptoms of asthma.

ANTICHOLINERGICS

Commonly Prescribed Drugs
Atropine, benztropine, darifenacin, dicyclomine, fesoterodine, glycopyrrolate, ipratropium, oxybutynin, scopolamine, solifenacin, tiotropium, tolterodine, umeclidinium

Pharmacologic Profile

General Use
Atropine: Bradyarrhythmias; also used as ophthalmic mydriatic. **Ipratropium:** Bronchospasm (inhalation) and rhinorrhea (intranasal). **Scopolamine:** Nausea and vomiting related to motion sickness and vertigo. **Glycopyrrolate:** Inhibits salivation and excessive respiratory secretions. **Benztropine:** Parkinson disease; also used to manage drug-induced extrapyramidal effects. **Umeclidinium:** Chronic obstructive pulmonary disease. **Tiotropium:** Chronic obstructive pulmonary disease and asthma. **Darifenacin, fesoterodine, oxybutynin, solifenacin, and tolterodine:** Overactive bladder.

CLASSIFICATIONS

General Action and Information
Competitively inhibit the action of acetylcholine. In addition, atropine, glycopyrrolate, and scopolamine are antimuscarinic in that they inhibit the action of acetylcholine at sites innervated by postganglionic cholinergic nerves.

Contraindications
Hypersensitivity, narrow-angle glaucoma, severe hemorrhage, tachycardia (due to thyrotoxicosis or cardiac insufficiency), or myasthenia gravis.

Precautions
Older adults and pediatric patients are more susceptible to adverse effects. Use cautiously in patients with urinary tract pathology; those at risk for GI obstruction; and those with chronic renal, hepatic, pulmonary, or cardiac disease.

Interactions
Additive anticholinergic effects (dry mouth, dry eyes, blurred vision, constipation) with other agents possessing anticholinergic activity, including antihistamines, antidepressants, quinidine, and disopyramide. May alter GI absorption of other drugs by inhibiting GI motility and ↑ transit time. Antacids may ↓ absorption of orally administered anticholinergics.

Nursing Implications

Assessment
- Assess vital signs and ECG frequently during IV drug therapy. Report any significant changes in HR or BP promptly.
- Assess respiratory status (rate, breath sounds, degree of dyspnea) before administration and at peak of medication effect for inhalers.
- Monitor intake and output in older adults or surgical patients; may cause urinary retention.
- Assess patient regularly for abdominal distention and auscultate for bowel sounds. Constipation may become a problem. Increasing fluids and adding bulk to the diet may help alleviate constipation.

Implementation
- **PO:** Administer oral doses of glycopyrrolate 1 hr before or 2 hr after meals.
- Scopolamine transdermal patch should be applied ≥4 hr before travel.
- Tiotropium capsules are for inhalation only and must not be swallowed.

Patient/Family Teaching
- Instruct patient that frequent rinses, sugarless gum or candy, and good oral hygiene may help relieve dry mouth.
- May cause drowsiness. Caution patient to avoid driving or other activities requiring alertness until response to medication is known.
- Advise patient that tiotropium and umeclidinium are not to be used for acute bronchospasm attacks but may be continued during an acute exacerbation.
- **Ophth:** Advise patients that ophthalmic preparations may temporarily blur vision and impair ability to judge distances. Dark glasses may be needed to protect eyes from bright light.

Evaluation/Desired Outcomes
- Increase in heart rate.
- Decrease in nausea and vomiting related to motion sickness or vertigo.
- Dryness of mouth.
- Dilation of pupils.
- Decrease in GI motility.
- Resolution of signs and symptoms of Parkinson disease.
- Decreased urinary frequency, urgency, and urge incontinence.

ANTICOAGULANTS

Commonly Prescribed Drugs

See Mechanism of Action of Select Anticoagulants table.

Pharmacologic Profile

General Use

Prevention and treatment of thromboembolic disorders, including deep vein thrombosis (DVT), pulmonary embolism (PE), and atrial fibrillation (AF)-induced stroke and systemic thromboembolism. Also used in the management of myocardial infarction (MI) sequentially or in combination with thrombolytics and/or antiplatelet agents.

General Action and Information

MECHANISM OF ACTION OF SELECT ANTICOAGULANTS

DRUG	MECHANISM
Oral	
Apixaban, edoxaban, and rivaroxaban	Factor Xa inhibitors; direct oral anticoagulants (DOACs)
Dabigatran	Direct thrombin inhibitor; DOAC
Warfarin	Vitamin K antagonist
Parenteral	
Argatroban and bivalirudin	Direct thrombin inhibitors
Dalteparin and enoxaparin	Low molecular weight heparins: potentiate the inhibitory effect of antithrombin on factor Xa and thrombin (factor IIa)
Fondaparinux	Factor Xa inhibitor
Heparin	Potentiates the inhibitory effect of antithrombin on factor Xa and thrombin (factor IIa)

Contraindications

Underlying coagulation disorders, ulcer disease, malignancy, recent surgery, or active bleeding.

Precautions

Anticoagulation should be undertaken cautiously in any patient with a potential site for bleeding. Pregnant or lactating patients should not receive warfarin or dabigatran. Heparin does not cross the placenta. All anticoagulants should be used cautiously in patients receiving epidural analgesia.

Interactions

Warfarin is highly protein bound and may displace or be displaced by other highly protein-bound drugs. The resultant interactions depend on which drug is displaced. Bleeding may be potentiated by aspirin or large doses of penicillins or penicillin-like drugs, cefotetan, valproic acid, or NSAIDs. Apixaban, dabigatran, edoxaban, and rivaroxaban have a number of other significant drug-drug interactions. See individual drugs.

Nursing Implications

Assessment

- Assess patient taking anticoagulants for signs of bleeding and hemorrhage (bleeding gums; nosebleed; unusual bruising; tarry, black stools; hematuria; ↓ hematocrit or BP; guaiac-positive stools; urine; nasogastric aspirate).
- Assess patient for evidence of thrombosis. Symptoms will depend on area of involvement.
- **Lab Test Considerations:** Monitor prothrombin time (PT) or international normalized ratio (INR) with warfarin therapy, activated partial thromboplastin time (aPTT) with full-dose heparin therapy, and hematocrit frequently during therapy.
- **Toxicity and Overdose:** If overdose occurs or anticoagulation needs to be immediately reversed, the antidote for heparins is protamine sulfate; for warfarin, the antidote is vitamin K (phytonadione); for dabigatran, the antidote is idarucizumab; for rivaroxaban and apixaban, the antidote is andexanet alfa. Administration of fresh frozen plasma or prothrombin complex

concentrate may also be required in severe bleeding due to warfarin, oral direct thrombin inhibitors, or oral factor Xa inhibitors.

Implementation

- Inform all health care providers caring for patient of anticoagulant therapy. Venipunctures and injection sites require application of pressure to prevent bleeding or hematoma formation.
- If apixaban, dabigatran, edoxaban, or rivaroxaban must be discontinued for reasons other than bleeding, consider replacing with another anticoagulant; discontinuation ↑ risk of thrombotic events.
- Use an infusion pump with continuous infusions to ensure accurate dosage.

Patient/Family Teaching

- Caution patient to avoid activities leading to injury, to use a soft toothbrush and electric razor, and to report any symptoms of unusual bleeding or bruising to health care provider immediately.
- Instruct patient not to take OTC medications, especially those containing aspirin, NSAIDs, or alcohol, without advice of health care provider.
- Review foods high in vitamin K (see Appendix J) with patients on warfarin. Patient should have consistent limited intake of these foods, as vitamin K is the antidote for warfarin and greatly alternating intake of these foods will cause the INR to fluctuate.
- Emphasize the importance of frequent lab tests to monitor the degree of anticoagulation with unfractionated heparin or warfarin.
- Instruct patient to carry identification describing medication regimen at all times and to inform all health care providers caring for patient of anticoagulant therapy before laboratory tests, treatment, or surgery.

Evaluation/Desired Outcomes

- Prevention of undesired clotting and its sequelae without signs of hemorrhage. Prevention of stroke, MI, and death in patients at risk.

ANTICONVULSANTS

Commonly Prescribed Drugs

See Mechanism of Action of Select Anticonvulsants table.

Pharmacologic Profile

General Use

Anticonvulsants are used to ↓ the incidence and severity of seizures due to various etiologies. Some anticonvulsants are used parenterally in the immediate treatment of seizures. It is not uncommon for patients to require more than one anticonvulsant to control seizures on a long-term basis. Several anticonvulsants are evaluated with serum level monitoring. Several anticonvulsants also are used to treat neuropathic pain.

General Action and Information

MECHANISM OF ACTION OF SELECT ANTICONVULSANTS

DRUG	MECHANISM
Brivaracetam and levetiracetam	Bind to synaptic vesicle protein 2A, modulating neurotransmitter release
Carbamazepine, fosphenytoin, lacosamide, lamotrigine, phenytoin, and oxcarbazepine	Inhibit voltage-gated sodium channels to ↓ neuronal excitability
Diazepam, clonazepam, midazolam, phenobarbital, and valproates	Potentiate the effects of GABA (an inhibitory neurotransmitter)
Gabapentin and pregabalin	Inhibit voltage-gated calcium channels to ↓ neuronal excitability
Topiramate	Inhibits voltage-gated sodium channels; potentiates effects of GABA; glutamate antagonist; carbonic anhydrase inhibitor

Contraindications

Previous hypersensitivity.

Precautions

Use cautiously in patients with severe hepatic or renal impairment; dose adjustment may be required. Choose agents carefully in pregnant and lactating women. Fetal hydantoin syndrome may occur in offspring of patients who receive phenytoin during pregnancy.

Interactions

Barbiturates, carbamazepine, and phenytoin stimulate the metabolism of other drugs that are metabolized by the liver, ↓ their effectiveness. Phenytoin is highly protein-bound and may displace or be displaced by other highly protein-bound drugs. Lamotrigine, tiagabine, and topiramate are capable of interacting with several other anticonvulsants. Many drugs are capable of lowering seizure threshold and may ↓ the effectiveness of anticonvulsants, including tricyclic antidepressants and phenothiazines. For more specific interactions, see individual drugs.

Nursing Implications

Assessment

- Assess location, duration, and characteristics of seizure activity.
- **Toxicity and Overdose:** Monitor serum drug levels routinely throughout anticonvulsant therapy, especially when adding or discontinuing other medications.

Implementation

- Administer anticonvulsants around the clock. Abrupt discontinuation may precipitate status epilepticus.
- Implement seizure precautions.

Patient/Family Teaching

- Instruct patient to take medication every day, exactly as directed.
- May cause drowsiness. Caution patient to avoid driving or other activities requiring alertness until response to medication is known. Do not resume driving until physician gives clearance based on control of seizures.
- Advise patient to avoid taking alcohol or other CNS depressants concurrently with these medications.
- Advise patient to carry identification describing disease process and medication regimen at all times.

Evaluation/Desired Outcomes

- Decrease or cessation of seizures without excessive sedation.
- Decreased neuropathic pain.

ANTIDEPRESSANTS

Commonly Prescribed Drugs

See Mechanism of Action of Select Antidepressants table.

Pharmacologic Profile

General Use

Used in the treatment of various forms of endogenous depression, often in conjunction with psychotherapy.

CLASSIFICATIONS

General Action and Information

MECHANISM OF ACTION OF SELECT ANTIDEPRESSANTS

DRUG	MECHANISM
Amitriptyline, desipramine, imipramine, and nortriptyline	Tricyclic antidepressants (TCAs)
Citalopram, escitalopram, fluoxetine, fluvoxamine, paroxetine, sertraline, vilazodone, and vortioxetine	Selective serotonin reuptake inhibitors (SSRIs)
Desvenlafaxine, duloxetine, and venlafaxine	Serotonin/norepinephrine reuptake inhibitors (SNRIs)
Phenelzine and selegiline	Monoamine oxidase (MAO) inhibitors
Brexpiprazole	Serotonin/dopamine activity modulator
Bupropion	Dopamine/norepinephrine reuptake inhibitor
Esketamine	N-methyl-D-aspartate (NMDA) receptor antagonist
Mirtazapine	Tetracyclic antidepressant
Zuranolone	GABA A receptor positive modulator

Contraindications
Hypersensitivity. Should not be used in narrow-angle glaucoma, pregnancy/lactation, or immediately after MI.

Precautions
Use cautiously in older adults and those with pre-existing cardiovascular disease. Men with prostatic enlargement may be more susceptible to urinary retention. Anticholinergic side effects of TCAs (dry eyes, dry mouth, blurred vision, constipation) may require dosage modification or drug discontinuation. Dosage requires slow titration; onset of therapeutic response may be 2–4 wk. May ↓ seizure threshold, especially bupropion.

Interactions
TCAs: May cause hypertension, tachycardia, and seizures when used with MAO inhibitors or MAO-inhibitor-like drugs. May prevent therapeutic response to some antihypertensives. Additive CNS depression with other CNS depressants. Sympathomimetic activity may be enhanced when used with other sympathomimetics. Additive anticholinergic effects with other drugs possessing anticholinergic properties. **SSRIs/SNRIs:** May cause hypertension, tachycardia, and seizures when used with MAO inhibitors or MAO-inhibitor-like drugs. May ↑ risk of serotonin syndrome when used with other drugs with serotonergic properties. These drugs have a number of other significant drug-drug interactions. See individual drugs.

Nursing Implications

Assessment
- Monitor mental status and affect. Assess for suicidal tendencies, especially during early therapy. Restrict amount of drug available to patient.

Implementation
- Administer drugs that are sedating at bedtime to avoid excessive drowsiness during waking hours, and administer drugs that cause insomnia in the morning.

Patient/Family Teaching
- Caution patient to avoid alcohol and other CNS depressants.
- Inform patient that dizziness or drowsiness may occur. Caution patient to avoid driving and other activities requiring alertness until response to the drug is known.
- Caution patient to make position changes slowly to minimize orthostatic hypotension.
- Advise patient to notify health care provider if dry mouth, urinary retention, or constipation occurs. Frequent rinses, good oral hygiene, and sugarless candy or gum may diminish dry mouth. An ↑ in fluid intake, fiber, and exercise may prevent constipation.
- Advise patient to notify health care provider of medication regimen and any herbal alternative therapies before treatment or surgery.

- Emphasize the importance of participation in psychotherapy and follow-up exams to evaluate progress.

Evaluation/Desired Outcomes

- Resolution of depression.

ANTIDIABETICS

Commonly Prescribed Drugs

See Mechanism of Action of Select Antidiabetics table.

Pharmacologic Profile

General Use

Insulin is used in the management of type 1 diabetes mellitus (DM). It may also be used in type 2 DM when diet and/or oral medications fail to adequately control blood sugar. The choice of insulin preparation (rapid-acting, intermediate-acting, long-acting) depends on the degree of control desired, daily blood glucose fluctuations, and history of previous reactions. Oral agents and noninsulin injectable agents are used primarily in type 2 DM. Oral agents are used when diet therapy alone fails to control blood glucose or symptoms or when patients are not amenable to using insulin or another injectable agent. Some oral agents may be used with insulin.

General Action and Information

MECHANISM OF ACTION OF SELECT ANTIDIABETICS

DRUG	MECHANISM
Dapagliflozin and empagliflozin	Sodium-glucose co-transporter 2 (SGLT2) inhibitors: Inhibit SGLT2 in proximal renal tubules → ↓ reabsorption of glucose → ↑ excretion of glucose in urine
Dulaglutide, liraglutide, and semaglutide	Glucagon-like peptide-1 (GLP-1) receptor agonists: ↑ glucose-dependent insulin secretion; ↓ inappropriate glucagon secretion; slows gastric emptying
Glimepiride, glipizide, and glyburide	Sulfonylureas: stimulate endogenous insulin secretion by beta cells of the pancreas and ↑ insulin sensitivity
Linagliptin and sitagliptin	Dipeptidyl peptidase-4 (DPP-4) inhibitors: Slow inactivation of incretin hormones → ↑ insulin secretion and ↓ glucagon
Insulin	↑ transport of glucose into cells and promotes the conversion of glucose to glycogen
Metformin	↓ hepatic glucose production and intestinal absorption of glucose; ↑ insulin sensitivity
Pioglitazone	Thiazolidinedione: ↑ insulin sensitivity
Tirzepatide	Glucose-dependent insulinotropic polypeptide (GIP) receptor and GLP-1 receptor agonist: ↑ glucose-dependent insulin secretion; ↓ inappropriate glucagon secretion; slows gastric emptying

Contraindications

Insulin: Hypoglycemia. **Oral hypoglycemic agents:** Hypersensitivity (cross-sensitivity with other sulfonylureas and sulfonamides may exist). Hypoglycemia. Type 1 DM. Avoid use in patients with severe kidney, liver, thyroid, and other endocrine dysfunction. Should not be used in pregnancy or lactation. **DPP-4 inhibitors:** Type 1 DM. **GLP-1 agonists:** Personal or family history of medullary thyroid carcinoma. Multiple Endocrine Neoplasia syndrome type 2. Type 1 DM. **SGLT2 inhibitors:** Severe renal impairment. Type 1 DM. Diabetic ketoacidosis.

Precautions

Insulin: Infection, stress, or changes in diet may alter requirements. **Oral hypoglycemic agents:** Use cautiously in older adults; dose ↓ may be necessary. Infection, stress, or changes in diet may alter requirements. Use sulfonylureas with caution in patients with a history of cardiovascular disease. Metformin may cause lactic acidosis. **DPP-4 inhibitors:** Use cautiously in patients with renal impairment, history of pancreatitis, or history of angioedema to another DPP-4 inhibitor. **GLP-1 agonists:** Use cautiously in patients with a history of pancreatitis, diabetic retinopathy, history of angioedema to another GLP-1 agonist, or undergoing elective surgery or procedure requiring general anesthesia or deep sedation. **SGLT2 inhibitors:** Moderate renal impairment or use of loop diuretics may ↑ risk of hypotension and hypovolemia. History of pancreatitis, pancreatic surgery, reduced caloric intake due to illness or surgery, surgical procedures, or alcohol abuse may ↑ risk of ketoacidosis. Peripheral arterial disease, diabetic foot infection, or osteomyelitis may ↑ risk of lower limb amputation.

Interactions

Insulin: Additive hypoglycemic effects with oral hypoglycemic agents. **Oral hypoglycemic agents:** Ingestion of alcohol with sulfonylureas may result in disulfiram-like reaction with some agents. Alcohol, corticosteroids, rifampin, glucagon, and thiazide and loop diuretics may ↓ effectiveness. Anabolic steroids, chloramphenicol, MAO inhibitors, most NSAIDs, salicylates, sulfonamides, and warfarin may ↑ hypoglycemic effect. Beta blockers may produce hypoglycemia and mask signs and symptoms of hypoglycemia. **DPP-4 inhibitors and GLP-1 agonists:** Use with insulin or sulfonylureas may ↑ hypoglycemic effect. **SGLT2 inhibitors:** Use with insulin or sulfonylureas may ↑ hypoglycemic effect. NSAIDs, diuretics, ACE inhibitors, or ARBs may ↑ risk of acute kidney injury.

Nursing Implications

Assessment

- Observe patient for signs and symptoms of hypoglycemic reactions.
- Metformin and pioglitazone do not cause hypoglycemia when taken alone but may ↑ the hypoglycemic effect of other hypoglycemic agents.
- Patients who have been well controlled on metformin but develop illness or laboratory abnormalities should be assessed for ketoacidosis or lactic acidosis. Assess serum electrolytes, renal function, ketones, glucose, and, if indicated, blood pH and lactate and pyruvate levels. If either form of acidosis is present, discontinue metformin immediately and treat acidosis.
- For SGLT2 inhibitors, monitor for signs and symptoms of volume depletion (dizziness, feeling faint, weakness, orthostatic hypotension) after initiating therapy, especially in older adults and patients with renal impairment, low systolic BP, or on diuretics. Monitor for signs/symptoms of urinary tract infection during therapy. Monitor for ketoacidosis, especially during prolonged fasting for illness or surgery.
- **Lab Test Considerations:** Serum glucose and A1c should be monitored periodically throughout therapy to evaluate effectiveness of treatment.

Implementation

- Patients stabilized on a treatment regimen who are exposed to stress, fever, trauma, infection, or surgery may require sliding scale insulin. Withhold oral hypoglycemic agents and reinstitute after resolution of acute illness.
- Discontinue SGLT2 inhibitors ≥3 days before surgery; therapy can be resumed once patient is clinically stable following surgery and has resumed oral intake.
- **Insulin:** Available in different types and strengths and from different species. Check type, species, source, dose, and expiration date with another licensed nurse. Do not interchange insulins without physician's order. Use only insulin syringes to draw up dose. Use only U100 syringes to draw up insulin lispro dose.

Patient/Family Teaching

- Explain to patient that medication controls hyperglycemia but does not cure diabetes. Therapy is long term.
- Review signs of hypoglycemia and hyperglycemia with patient. If hypoglycemia occurs, advise patient to take a glass of orange juice or 2–3 teaspoons of sugar, honey, or corn syrup dissolved in water, and notify health care provider.
- Encourage patient to follow prescribed diet, medication, and exercise regimen to prevent hypoglycemic or hyperglycemic episodes.
- Instruct patient in proper testing of serum glucose and ketones.

- Advise patient to notify health care provider if nausea, vomiting, or fever develops; if unable to eat usual diet; or if blood glucose levels are not controlled.
- Advise patient to carry sugar or a form of glucose and identification describing medication regimen at all times.
- Insulin is the recommended method of controlling blood glucose during pregnancy.
- **Insulin:** Instruct patient on proper technique for administration; include type of insulin, equipment (syringe and cartridge pens), storage, and syringe disposal. Discuss the importance of not changing brands of insulin or syringes, selection and rotation of injection sites, and compliance with therapeutic regimen.
- **Metformin:** Explain to patient the risk of lactic acidosis and the potential need for discontinuation of metformin therapy if a severe infection, dehydration, or severe or continuing diarrhea occurs or if medical tests or surgery is required.
- **SGLT2 inhibitors:** Advise patient to notify health care provider immediately if new pain or tenderness, sores or ulcers, or infections involving the leg or foot occur and to immediately seek care if pain or tenderness, redness, or swelling of the genitals or area from the genitals back to the rectum, along with a fever above 100.4°F or malaise, occur.

Evaluation/Desired Outcomes

- Control of blood glucose levels without the appearance of hypoglycemic or hyperglycemic episodes.

ANTIDIARRHEALS

Commonly Prescribed Drugs

Loperamide and octreotide

Pharmacologic Profile

General Use

For the control and symptomatic relief of acute and chronic nonspecific diarrhea.

General Action and Information

Loperamide slows intestinal motility and propulsion. Octreotide is used specifically for diarrhea associated with GI endocrine tumors.

Contraindications

Previous hypersensitivity. Severe abdominal pain of unknown cause, especially when associated with fever. Diarrhea associated with *Clostridioides difficile*-associated diarrhea.

Precautions

Use cautiously in patients with severe liver disease or inflammatory bowel disease. Safety in pregnancy and lactation not established (loperamide). Octreotide may aggravate gallbladder disease.

Interactions

Octreotide may alter the response to insulin or oral hypoglycemic agents.

Nursing Implications

Assessment

- Assess the frequency and consistency of stools and bowel sounds before and throughout therapy.
- Assess patient's fluid and electrolyte status and skin turgor for dehydration.

Implementation

- Shake liquid preparations before administration.

Patient/Family Teaching

- Instruct patient to notify health care provider if diarrhea persists or if fever, abdominal pain, or palpitations occur.

C L A S S I F I C A T I O N S

Evaluation/Desired Outcomes

- Decrease in diarrhea.

ANTIEMETICS

Commonly Prescribed Drugs

See Mechanism of Action of Select Antiemetics table.

Pharmacologic Profile

General Use

Phenothiazines, granisetron, metoclopramide, ondansetron, and palonosetron are used to manage nausea and vomiting of many causes, including surgery, anesthesia, and antineoplastic and radiation therapy. Aprepitant, fosnetupitant, and netupitant are used specifically with emetogenic chemotherapy. Scopolamine and meclizine are used almost exclusively to prevent motion sickness. Doxylamine/pyridoxine is used exclusively for the treatment of nausea and vomiting during pregnancy that has not responded to conservative management.

General Action and Information

MECHANISM OF ACTION OF SELECT ANTIEMETICS

DRUG	MECHANISM
Aprepitant, netupitant, and fosnetupitant	Substance P/neurokinin-1 receptor antagonist
Chlorpromazine, prochlorperazine, and promethazine	Phenothiazines: depress the chemoreceptor trigger zone in the CNS
Granisetron, ondansetron, and palonosetron	Serotonin (5-HT_3) receptor antagonists
Doxylamine/pyridoxine	Doxylamine has antihistaminic effects
Meclizine	Antihistaminic and anticholinergic effects
Metoclopramide	Blocks dopamine receptors in chemoreceptor trigger zone in the CNS
Scopolamine	Anticholinergic effects

Contraindications

Previous hypersensitivity.

Precautions

Use phenothiazines cautiously in children who may have viral illnesses. Use granisetron, palonosetron, and ondansetron with caution in patients with QT interval prolongation.

Interactions

Additive CNS depression with other CNS depressants including antidepressants, antihistamines, opioid analgesics, and sedative/hypnotics. Phenothiazines may produce hypotension when used with antihypertensives, nitrates, or acute ingestion of alcohol. Granisetron, palonosetron, and ondansetron may ↑ the risk of serotonin syndrome when used with other serotonergic agents. Aprepitant, fosnetupitant, and netupitant have numerous drug interactions with CYP450 agents. See individual drugs.

Nursing Implications

Assessment

- Assess nausea, vomiting, bowel sounds, and abdominal pain before and following administration.
- Monitor hydration status and intake and output. Patients with severe nausea and vomiting may require IV fluids in addition to antiemetics.

Implementation

- For prophylactic administration, follow directions for specific drugs so that peak effect corresponds to time of anticipated nausea.

Patient/Family Teaching

- Advise patient and family to use general measures to ↓ nausea (begin with sips of liquids and small, nongreasy meals; provide oral hygiene; remove noxious stimuli from environment).
- May cause drowsiness. Advise patient to call for assistance when ambulating and to avoid driving or other activities requiring alertness until response to medication is known.
- Advise patient to make position changes slowly to minimize orthostatic hypotension.

Evaluation/Desired Outcomes

- Prevention of, or reduction in, nausea and vomiting.

ANTIFUNGALS

Commonly Prescribed Drugs

See Mechanism of Action of Select Antifungals table.

Pharmacologic Profile

General Use

Treatment of fungal infections. Infections of skin or mucous membranes may be treated with topical or vaginal preparations. Deep-seated or systemic infections require oral or parenteral therapy.

General Action and Information

MECHANISM OF ACTION OF SELECT ANTIFUNGALS

DRUG	MECHANISM
Anidulafungin, caspofungin, and micafungin	Echinocandins: inhibit β-1,3-glucan synthase → weakens fungal cell wall
Butenafine, naftifine, and terbinafine	Inhibit squalene epoxidase → disrupts ergosterol synthesis → ↓ fungal cell membrane synthesis
Butoconazole, clotrimazole, econazole, efinaconazole, isavuconazonium, ketoconazole, luliconazole, miconazole, oxiconazole, posaconazole, sertaconazole, sulconazole, terconazole, tioconazole, and voriconazole	Azole antifungals: inhibits fungal cytochrome P450 → disrupts ergosterol synthesis → ↓ fungal cell membrane synthesis
Ciclopirox	Inhibits transport of essential elements in fungal cell, disrupting synthesis of DNA, RNA, and protein
Nystatin	Binds to ergosterol in fungal membranes → leakage of cell contents → changes fungal cell membrane permeability
Tavaborole	Inhibits fungal protein synthesis
Tolnaftate	Distorts the hyphae and stunts mycelial growth in fungi

Contraindications

Previous hypersensitivity.

Precautions

Because most systemic antifungals may have adverse effects on bone marrow function, use cautiously in patients with depressed bone marrow reserve. Fluconazole requires dosage adjustment in the presence of renal impairment. Adverse reactions to fluconazole may be more severe in HIV-positive patients. The IV formulation of voriconazole should be avoided in patients with renal impairment.

Interactions

Differ greatly among various agents. See individual drugs.

Nursing Implications

Assessment

- Assess patient for signs of infection and assess involved areas of skin and mucous membranes before and throughout therapy. Increased skin irritation may indicate need to discontinue medication.

CLASSIFICATIONS

Implementation

- Available in various dosage forms. Refer to specific drugs for directions for administration.
- **Topical:** Consult physician or other health care provider for cleansing technique before applying medication. Wear gloves during application. Do not use occlusive dressings unless specified by physician or other health care provider.

Patient/Family Teaching

- Instruct patient on proper use of medication form.
- Instruct patient to continue medication as directed for full course of therapy, even if feeling better.
- Advise patient to report ↑ skin irritation or lack of therapeutic response to health care provider.

Evaluation/Desired Outcomes

- Resolution of signs and symptoms of infection. Length of time for complete resolution depends on organism and site of infection. Deep-seated fungal infections may require prolonged therapy (weeks–months). Recurrent fungal infections may be a sign of serious systemic illness.

ANTIHISTAMINES

Commonly Prescribed Drugs

Azelastine, cetirizine, diphenhydramine, fexofenadine, hydroxyzine, levocetirizine, loratadine, meclizine, and promethazine

Pharmacologic Profile

General Use

Relief of symptoms associated with allergies, including rhinitis, urticaria, and angioedema, and as adjunctive therapy in anaphylactic reactions. Some antihistamines are used to treat motion sickness (dimenhydrinate and meclizine), insomnia (diphenhydramine), and other nonallergic conditions.

General Action and Information

Antihistamines block the effects of histamine at the H_1 receptor. They do not block histamine release, antibody production, or antigen-antibody reactions. The 1st-generation antihistamines (diphenhydramine) have anticholinergic properties and may cause constipation, dry eyes, dry mouth, and blurred vision; in addition, these antihistamines cause sedation (because they cross the blood-brain barrier). The 2nd-generation antihistamines (cetirizine, fexofenadine, levocetirizine, loratadine) do not cross the blood-brain barrier and are much less likely to cause sedation.

Contraindications

Hypersensitivity and angle-closure glaucoma. Should not be used in premature or newborn infants.

Precautions

Older adults may be more susceptible to adverse anticholinergic effects of antihistamines. Use cautiously in patients with pyloric obstruction, prostatic hypertrophy, hyperthyroidism, cardiovascular disease, or severe liver disease. Use cautiously in pregnancy and lactation.

Interactions

Additive sedation when used with other CNS depressants, including alcohol, antidepressants, opioid analgesics, and sedative/hypnotics. MAO inhibitors prolong and intensify the anticholinergic properties of antihistamines.

Nursing Implications

Assessment

- Assess allergy symptoms (rhinitis, conjunctivitis, hives) before and periodically throughout therapy.
- Assess lung sounds and character of bronchial secretions. Maintain fluid intake of 1500–2000 mL/day to ↓ viscosity of secretions.

CLASSIFICATIONS

- **Nausea and Vomiting:** Assess degree of nausea and frequency and amount of emesis when administering for nausea and vomiting.
- **Pruritus:** Observe the character, location, and size of affected area when administering for pruritic skin conditions.

Implementation

- When used for prophylaxis of motion sickness, administer ≥30 min and preferably 1–2 hr before exposure to conditions that may precipitate motion sickness.

Patient/Family Teaching

- Inform patient that drowsiness may occur. Avoid driving or other activities requiring alertness until response to drug is known.
- Caution patient to avoid using concurrent alcohol or CNS depressants.
- Advise patient that good oral hygiene, frequent rinsing of mouth with water, and sugarless gum or candy may help relieve dryness of mouth.
- Instruct patient to contact health care professional if symptoms persist.

Evaluation/Desired Outcomes

- Decrease in allergic symptoms.
- Prevention or decreased severity of nausea and vomiting.
- Relief of pruritus.
- Sedation when used as a hypnotic.

ANTIHYPERTENSIVES

Commonly Prescribed Drugs

See Mechanism of Action of Select Antihypertensives table.

Pharmacologic Profile

General Use

Treatment of hypertension. Parenteral products are used in the treatment of hypertensive emergencies. Oral treatment should be initiated as soon as possible and individualized to ensure adherence and compliance for long-term therapy.

General Action and Information

MECHANISM OF ACTION OF SELECT ANTIHYPERTENSIVES

DRUG	MECHANISM
Acebutolol, atenolol, betaxolol, bisoprolol, carvedilol, labetalol, metoprolol, nadolol, nebivolol, pindolol, propranolol, and timolol	Beta blockers (selective: acebutolol, atenolol, betaxolol, bisoprolol, metoprolol, and nebivolol; nonselective: carvedilol, labetalol, nadolol, pindolol, propranolol, and timolol)
Amlodipine, diltiazem, felodipine, isradipine, nicardipine, nifedipine, nisoldipine, and verapamil	Calcium channel blockers (dihydropyridine: amlodipine, felodipine, isradipine, nicardipine, nifedipine, and nisoldipine; nondihydropyridine: diltiazem and verapamil)
Azilsartan, candesartan, irbesartan, losartan, olmesartan, telmisartan, and valsartan	Angiotensin II receptor blockers (ARBs)
Benazepril, captopril, enalapril/enalaprilat, fosinopril, lisinopril, moexipril, perindopril, quinapril, ramipril, and trandolapril	Angiotensin-converting enzyme (ACE) inhibitors
Chlorothiazide, chlorthalidone, hydrochlorothiazide, and metolazone	Thiazide diuretics
Doxazosin, prazosin, and terazosin	Alpha$_1$ receptor antagonists
Eplerenone and spironolactone	Mineralocorticoid receptor antagonists
Hydralazine and nitroprusside	Direct-acting vasodilators
Aprocitentan	Endothelin receptor antagonist
Clonidine	Centrally acting alpha$_2$ receptor agonist

Contraindications

Hypersensitivity to individual agents.

Precautions

Choose agents carefully in pregnancy and during lactation. ACE inhibitors and ARBs should be avoided during pregnancy. Clonidine and beta blockers should be used only in patients who are compliant with their medications because abrupt discontinuation of these agents may result in rapid and excessive ↑ in BP (rebound phenomenon). Thiazide and loop diuretics may ↑ the risk of hyperglycemia and hyperuricemia. Hydralazine may cause tachycardia if used alone and are commonly used in combination with beta blockers; it may also cause sodium and water retention and is usually combined with a diuretic.

Interactions

Many drugs can negate the therapeutic effectiveness of antihypertensives, including NSAIDs, sympathomimetics, decongestants, appetite suppressants, SNRIs, and MAO inhibitors. Hypokalemia from diuretics may ↑ the risk of digoxin toxicity. Potassium supplements and potassium-sparing diuretics may cause hyperkalemia when used with ACE inhibitors or ARBs. ACE inhibitors, ARBs, and diuretics may ↑ the risk of lithium toxicity. Digoxin, ivabradine, and clonidine may ↑ the risk of bradycardia when used with beta blockers, verapamil, or diltiazem.

Nursing Implications

Assessment

- Monitor BP and HR frequently during dosage adjustment and periodically throughout therapy.
- Monitor intake and output and daily weight with use of diuretics.

Implementation

- Many antihypertensives are available as combination products to enhance compliance (see Appendix N).

Patient/Family Teaching

- Instruct patient to continue taking medication, even if feeling well. Abrupt withdrawal may cause rebound hypertension. Medication controls but does not cure hypertension.
- Encourage patient to comply with additional interventions for hypertension (weight ↓, low-sodium diet, regular exercise, discontinuation of smoking, moderation of alcohol consumption, stress management).
- Instruct patient and family on proper technique for monitoring BP. Advise them to check BP weekly and report significant changes.
- Caution patient to make position changes slowly to minimize orthostatic hypotension. Advise patient that exercise or hot weather may enhance hypotensive effects.
- Advise patient to consult health care provider before taking any OTC medications, especially cold remedies.
- Advise patient to inform health care provider of medication regimen before treatment or surgery.
- Patients taking ACE inhibitors or ARBs should notify health care provider if pregnancy is planned or suspected.
- Emphasize the importance of follow-up exams to monitor progress.

Evaluation/Desired Outcomes

- Decrease in BP.

ANTI-INFECTIVES

Commonly Prescribed Drugs

See Mechanism of Action of Select Anti-infectives table.

Pharmacologic Profile

General Use

Treatment and prophylaxis of various bacterial infections. See specific drugs for spectrum and indications. Some infections may require additional surgical intervention and supportive therapy.

General Action and Information

MECHANISM OF ACTION OF SELECT ANTI-INFECTIVES

DRUG CLASS	DRUG(S)	MECHANISM
Aminoglycosides	Amikacin, gentamicin, neomycin, streptomycin, and tobramycin	Inhibit protein synthesis by binding to 30S ribosomal subunit
Beta-lactams		
β-lactamase inhibitor	Sulbactam/durlobactam	Inhibit bacterial cell wall synthesis by binding to penicillin-binding proteins
Carbapenems	Ertapenem, imipenem/cilastatin, and meropenem	
Cephalosporins	1st generation: Cefadroxil, cefazolin, and cephalexin 2nd generation: Cefaclor, cefotetan, cefoxitin, cefprozil, and cefuroxime 3rd generation: Cefdinir, cefixime, cefotaxime, cefpodoxime, ceftazidime, and ceftriaxone 4th generation: Cefepime 5th generation: Ceftaroline and ceftobiprole	
Monobactam	Aztreonam and aztreonam/avibactam	
Penem	Sulopenem etzadroxil/probenecid	
Penicillins	Amoxicillin, ampicillin, penicillin G, and penicillin V	
Penicillins, Penicillinase-Resistant	Dicloxacillin, nafcillin, and oxacillin	
Cyclic lipopeptide	Daptomycin	Causes rapid depolarization of cell membrane → inhibits protein, DNA, and RNA synthesis
Fluoroquinolones	Ciprofloxacin, delafloxacin, levofloxacin, moxifloxacin, and ofloxacin	Inhibit DNA gyrase and topoisomerase IV → inhibit DNA synthesis
Glycopeptides	Dalbavancin, oritavancin, telavancin, and vancomycin	Inhibits bacterial cell wall synthesis by blocking glycopeptide polymerization
Glycylcycline	Tigecycline	Inhibit protein synthesis by binding to 30S ribosomal subunit
Lincosamide	Clindamycin	Inhibits protein synthesis by binding to 50S ribosomal subunit
Macrolides	Azithromycin, erythromycin, and fidaxomicin	Inhibit protein synthesis by binding to 50S ribosomal subunit
Nitroimidazole	Metronidazole and secnidazole	Cause DNA strand breakage
Oxazolidinone	Linezolid and tedizolid	Inhibits protein synthesis by binding to the 23S ribosome of the 50S subunit
Tetracyclines	Doxycycline	Inhibit protein synthesis by binding to 30S ribosomal subunit
Triazaacenaphthylene	Gepotidacin	Inhibits DNA gyrase and topoisomerase IV inhibits DNA synthesis

Contraindications

Known hypersensitivity to individual agents. Cross-sensitivity among related agents may occur.

Precautions

Culture and susceptibility testing are desirable to optimize therapy. Dosage modification may be required in patients with hepatic or renal impairment. Use cautiously in pregnant and lactating women. Prolonged inappropriate use of broad spectrum anti-infective agents may lead to superinfection with fungi or resistant bacteria.

Interactions

Penicillins and aminoglycosides chemically inactivate each other and should not be physically admixed. Erythromycin may ↓ hepatic metabolism of other drugs. Probenecid ↑ serum levels of penicillins and related compounds. Fluoroquinolone and tetracycline absorption may be ↓ by antacids, bismuth subsalicylate, calcium, iron salts, sucralfate, and zinc salts.

Nursing Implications

Assessment

- Assess patient for signs and symptoms of infection prior to and throughout therapy.
- Determine previous hypersensitivities in patients receiving penicillins or cephalosporins.
- Obtain specimens for culture and sensitivity prior to initiating therapy. First dose may be given before receiving results.
- Monitor bowel function. Diarrhea, abdominal cramping, fever, and bloody stools should be reported to health care provider promptly as a sign of *Clostridioides difficile*-associated diarrhea.

Implementation

- Most anti-infectives should be administered around the clock to maintain therapeutic serum drug levels.

Patient/Family Teaching

- Instruct patient to continue taking medication around the clock until finished completely, even if feeling better.
- Advise patient to report the signs of superinfection (black, furry overgrowth on the tongue; vaginal itching or discharge; loose or foul-smelling stools) and allergy to health care provider.
- Instruct patient to notify health care provider if fever and diarrhea develop, especially if stool contains pus, blood, or mucus. Advise patient not to treat diarrhea without consulting health care provider.
- Instruct patient to notify health care provider if symptoms do not improve.

Evaluation/Desired Outcomes

- Resolution of the signs and symptoms of infection. Length of time for complete resolution depends on organism and site of infection.

ANTINEOPLASTICS

Commonly Prescribed Drugs

See Traditional Chemotherapy Drugs and Targeted Cancer Therapies tables.

Pharmacologic Profile

General Use

Used in the treatment of various solid tumors, lymphomas, and leukemias. Also used in some autoimmune disorders such as rheumatoid arthritis (methotrexate). Often used in combinations to minimize individual toxicities and ↑ response. Chemotherapy may be combined with other treatment modalities such as surgery and radiation therapy. Dosages vary greatly, depending on extent of disease, other agents used, and patient's condition.

General Action and Information

TRADITIONAL CHEMOTHERAPY DRUGS

DRUG CLASS	DRUG(S)
Alkylating agent	Busulfan, cyclophosphamide, dacarbazine, ifosfamide, and melphalan
Anthracyclines	Daunorubicin and doxorubicin
Antiandrogens	Abiraterone, apalutamide, bicalutamide, darolutamide, and enzalutamide

DRUG CLASS	DRUG(S)
Antimetabolite	Fluorouracil, gemcitabine, methotrexate, and pemetrexed
Antitumor antibiotic	Bleomycin and cytarabine
Aromatase inhibitor	Anastrozole, exemestane, and letrozole
Estrogen receptor antagonist	Tamoxifen
Hormones	Goserelin, leuprolide, and megestrol
Platinum compounds	Carboplatin, cisplatin, and oxaliplatin
Taxane derivatives	Cabazitaxel, docetaxel, paclitaxel, and paclitaxel protein-bound particles
Topoisomerase inhibitors	Irinotecan, mitoxantrone, and topotecan
Vinca alkaloids	Vinblastine, vincristine, and vinorelbine

TARGETED CANCER THERAPIES

TARGET	DRUG(S)
AKT	Capivasertib
Anaplastic lymphoma kinase (ALK)	Alectinib
BRAF	Dabrafenib and encorafenib
CD20	Rituximab
CD30	Brentuximab vedotin
CD38	Daratumumab
CD79b	Polatuzumab vedotin
Cyclin-dependent kinase (CDK)	Abemaciclib, palbociclib, and ribociclib
Cytotoxic T-lymphocyte associated antigen-4 (CTLA-4)	Ipilimumab
Epidermal growth factor receptor (EGFR)	Cetuximab, erlotinib, lazertinib, osimertinib, and panitumumab
HER2	Ado-trastuzumab, fam-trastuzumab deruxtecan, pertuzumab, and trastuzumab
Immunomodulatory	Lenalidomide, pomalidomide, and thalidomide
Mitogen-activated extracellular kinase (MEK)	Binimetinib and trametinib
mTOR	Everolimus
Nectin-4	Enfortumab vedotin
PD-1	Nivolumab and pembrolizumab
PD-L1	Atezolizumab and durvalumab
Phosphatidylinositol 3-kinase alpha (PIK3CA)	Alpelisib and inavolisib
Poly (ADP-ribose) polymerase (PARP)	Olaparib
Proteasome	Carfilzomib
Tyrosine kinases	Cabozantinib, imatinib, lapatinib, lenvatinib, and nilotinib
Vascular endothelial growth factor (VEGF)	Axitinib and bevacizumab

Contraindications

Previous bone marrow depression or hypersensitivity. Contraindicated in pregnancy and lactation.

Precautions

Use cautiously in patients with active infections, ↓ bone marrow reserve, radiation therapy, or other debilitating illnesses. Use cautiously in women of reproductive potential.

Interactions

Allopurinol ↓ metabolism of mercaptopurine. Toxicity from methotrexate may be ↑ by other nephrotoxic drugs or larger doses of aspirin or NSAIDs. Bone marrow depression is additive. See individual drugs.

Nursing Implications

Assessment

- Monitor for bone marrow depression. Assess for bleeding (bleeding gums; bruising; petechiae; guaiac stools, urine, and emesis) and avoid IM injections and rectal temperatures if platelet count is low. Apply pressure to venipuncture sites for 10 min. Assess for signs of infection during neutropenia. Anemia may occur. Monitor for ↑ fatigue, dyspnea, and orthostatic hypotension.
- Monitor intake and output ratios, appetite, and nutritional intake. Prophylactic antiemetics may be used. Adjusting diet as tolerated may help maintain fluid and electrolyte balance and nutritional status.

- Monitor IV site carefully and ensure patency. Discontinue infusion immediately if discomfort, erythema along vein, or infiltration occurs. Tissue ulceration and necrosis may result from infiltration.
- Monitor for symptoms of gout (↑ uric acid, joint pain, edema). Encourage patient to drink ≥2 L of fluid each day. Allopurinol may be given to ↓ uric acid levels. Alkalinization of urine may be ordered to ↑ excretion of uric acid.

Implementation

- Solutions for injection should be prepared in a biologic cabinet. Wear gloves, gown, and mask while handling medication. Discard equipment in designated containers.
- Check dose carefully. Fatalities have resulted from dosing errors.

Patient/Family Teaching

- Caution patient to avoid crowds and persons with known infections. Health care provider should be informed immediately if symptoms of infection occur.
- Instruct patient to report unusual bleeding. Advise patient of thrombocytopenia precautions.
- These drugs may cause gonadal suppression; however, patient should still use birth control, as most antineoplastics are teratogenic. Advise patient to inform health care provider immediately if pregnancy is suspected.
- Discuss with patient the possibility of hair loss. Explore methods of coping.
- Instruct patient to inspect oral mucosa for erythema and ulceration. If ulceration occurs, advise patient to use sponge brush and to rinse mouth with water after eating and drinking. Topical agents may be used if mouth pain interferes with eating. Stomatitis pain may require treatment with opioid analgesics.
- Instruct patient not to receive any vaccinations without advice of health care provider. Antineoplastics may ↓ antibody response and ↑ risk of adverse reactions.
- Advise patient of need for medical follow-up and frequent lab tests.

Evaluation/Desired Outcomes

- Decrease in size and spread of tumor.
- Improvement in hematologic status in patients with leukemia.

ANTIPARKINSON AGENTS

Commonly Prescribed Drugs

See Mechanism of Action of Select Antiparkinson Agents table.

Pharmacologic Profile

General Use

Parkinson disease.

General Action and Information

MECHANISM OF ACTION OF SELECT ANTIPARKINSON AGENTS

DRUG	MECHANISM
Carbidopa/levodopa, pramipexole, and ropinirole	Dopamine agonists
Rasagiline, safinamide, and selegiline	Monoamine oxidase (MAO)-B inhibitors → ↑ dopamine
Benztropine	Anticholinergic
Entacapone	Catechol-O-methyltransferase (COMT) inhibitor → ↑ levodopa

Contraindications

Anticholinergics should be avoided in patients with angle-closure glaucoma. MAO-B inhibitors should not be used with other MAO inhibitors.

Precautions

Use cautiously in patients with severe cardiac disease, pyloric obstruction, or prostatic enlargement.

Interactions
Pyridoxine, MAO inhibitors, benzodiazepines, phenytoin, phenothiazines, and haloperidol may antagonize the effects of levodopa. Agents that antagonize dopamine (phenothiazines, metoclopramide) may ↓ effectiveness of dopamine agonists.

Nursing Implications
Assessment
- Assess parkinsonian and extrapyramidal symptoms (akinesia, rigidity, tremors, pill rolling, mask facies, shuffling gait, muscle spasms, twisting motions, drooling) before and throughout course of therapy. On-off phenomenon may cause symptoms to appear or improve suddenly.
- Monitor BP frequently during therapy. Instruct patient to remain supine during and for several hours after 1st dose of bromocriptine, as severe hypotension may occur.

Implementation
- In the carbidopa/levodopa combination, the number following the drug name represents the milligram of each respective drug.

Patient/Family Teaching
- May cause drowsiness or dizziness. Advise patient to avoid driving or other activities that require alertness until response to medication is known.
- Caution patient to make position changes slowly to minimize orthostatic hypotension.
- Instruct patient that frequent rinsing of mouth, good oral hygiene, and sugarless gum or candy may ↓ dry mouth. Patient should notify health care provider if dryness persists (saliva substitutes may be used). Also notify the dentist if dryness interferes with use of dentures.
- Advise patient to confer with health care provider before taking OTC medications, especially cold remedies, or drinking alcoholic beverages. Patients receiving levodopa should avoid multivitamins because vitamin B_6 (pyridoxine) may interfere with levodopa's action.
- Caution patient that ↓ perspiration may occur. Overheating may occur during hot weather. Patients should remain indoors in an air-conditioned environment during hot weather.
- Advise patient to ↑ activity, bulk, and fluid in diet to minimize constipating effects of medication.
- Advise patient to notify health care provider if confusion, rash, urinary retention, severe constipation, visual changes, or worsening of parkinsonian symptoms occur.

Evaluation/Desired Outcomes
- Resolution of parkinsonian signs and symptoms.
- Resolution of drug-induced extrapyramidal symptoms.

ANTIPLATELET AGENTS
Commonly Prescribed Drugs
See Mechanism of Action of Select Antiplatelet Agents table.

Pharmacologic Profile
General Use
To treat and prevent thromboembolic events such as stroke and MI.

General Action and Information

MECHANISM OF ACTION OF SELECT ANTIPLATELET AGENTS

DRUG	MECHANISM
Clopidogrel and ticagrelor	Inhibits P2Y12 receptor on platelets → Inhibits ADP-mediated platelet activation
Aspirin	Inhibits cyclooxygenase-1 → ↓ thromboxane A2
Eptifibatide	Glycoprotein IIb/IIIa receptor inhibitor

C L A S S I F I C A T I O N S

Contraindications
Hypersensitivity, ulcer disease, active bleeding, and recent surgery.

Precautions
Use cautiously in patients at risk for bleeding (trauma, surgery) or a history of GI bleeding or ulcer disease.

Interactions
Concurrent use with NSAIDs, heparin, thrombolytics, warfarin, dabigatran, rivaroxaban, apixaban, or edoxaban may ↑ the risk of bleeding. All proton pump inhibitors, except pantoprazole, may ↓ the antiplatelet effects of clopidogrel. Opioids may ↓ effectiveness of clopidogrel and ticagrelor.

Nursing Implications

Assessment
- Assess patient taking antiplatelet agents for signs/symptoms of stroke, peripheral arterial disease, or MI periodically throughout therapy.
- Monitor for signs/symptoms of bleeding (pallor of skin and conjunctiva, fatigue, weakness, easy bruising, nosebleeds, bleeding gums, hematuria), including GI bleeding (hematochezia, melena, coffee ground emesis).

Implementation
- Use an infusion pump with continuous infusions to ensure accurate dosage.

Patient/Family Teaching
- Instruct patient to notify health care provider immediately if any bleeding is noted.
- Inform patient that ticagrelor may cause shortness of breath, which usually resolves during therapy.

Evaluation/Desired Outcomes
- Prevention of stroke, MI, and vascular death in patients at risk.

ANTIPSYCHOTICS

Commonly Prescribed Drugs
Typical: chlorpromazine, haloperidol, and prochlorperazine; *Atypical:* aripiprazole, brexpiprazole, cariprazine, clozapine, iloperidone, lurasidone, olanzapine, paliperidone, pimavanserin, quetiapine, risperiDONE, xanomelene/trospium, and ziprasidone

Pharmacologic Profile

General Use
Treatment of schizophrenia. Use of clozapine is limited to schizophrenia unresponsive to conventional therapy. Selected agents are also used for acute treatment of manic and mixed episodes associated with bipolar I disorder, maintenance treatment of bipolar I disorder, and as adjunctive treatment of depression.

General Action and Information
Block dopamine receptors in the brain; also alter dopamine release and turnover. Peripheral effects include anticholinergic properties and alpha-adrenergic blockade. Atypical antipsychotics may have fewer adverse reactions compared to the typical antipsychotics.

Contraindications
Hypersensitivity. Cross-sensitivity may exist among phenothiazines. Should not be used in angle-closure glaucoma. Should not be used in patients who have CNS depression.

Precautions
Use cautiously in patients with symptomatic cardiac disease. Avoid exposure to extremes in temperature. Use cautiously in severely ill or debilitated patients and patients with respiratory insufficiency,

diabetes, prostatic hypertrophy, or intestinal obstruction. May ↓ seizure threshold. Clozapine may cause agranulocytosis. Most agents are capable of causing neuroleptic malignant syndrome. Should not be used routinely for anxiety or agitation not related to psychoses.

Interactions

Additive hypotension with acute ingestion of alcohol, antihypertensives, or nitrates. Phenobarbital may ↓ effectiveness. Additive CNS depression with other CNS depressants, including alcohol, antihistamines, antidepressants, opioid analgesics, or sedative/hypnotics. Lithium may ↓ levels and effectiveness of phenothiazines. May ↓ the therapeutic response to levodopa. May ↑ the risk of agranulocytosis with antithyroid agents. Many of the atypical antipsychotics have CYP450 interactions. See individual agents.

Nursing Implications

Assessment

- Assess patient's mental status (orientation, mood, behavior) before and periodically throughout therapy.
- Monitor BP (sitting, standing, lying), HR, and respiratory rate before and frequently during the period of dosage adjustment.
- Observe patient carefully when administering medication to ensure medication is actually taken and not hoarded.
- Monitor patient for onset of *akathisia*—restlessness or desire to keep moving—and extrapyramidal side effects; *parkinsonian effects*—difficulty speaking or swallowing, loss of balance control, pill rolling, masklike face, shuffling gait, rigidity, tremors; and *dystonia*—muscle spasms, twisting motions, twitching, inability to move eyes, weakness of arms or legs—every 2 mo during therapy and 8–12 wk after therapy has been discontinued. Parkinsonian effects are more common in older adults, and dystonias are more common in younger patients. Notify health care provider if these symptoms occur, as ↓ in dosage or discontinuation of medication may be necessary. Trihexyphenidyl or benztropine may be used to control these symptoms.
- Monitor for *tardive dyskinesia*—uncontrolled rhythmic movement of mouth, face, and extremities; lip smacking or puckering; puffing of cheeks; uncontrolled chewing; rapid or wormlike movements of tongue. Notify health care provider immediately if these symptoms occur; these side effects may be irreversible.
- Monitor for development of *neuroleptic malignant syndrome*—fever, respiratory distress, tachycardia, convulsions, diaphoresis, hypertension or hypotension, pallor, tiredness, severe muscle stiffness, loss of bladder control. Notify health care provider immediately if these symptoms occur.

Implementation

- Keep patient recumbent for ≥30 min following parenteral administration to minimize hypotensive effects.
- **PO:** Administer with **food**, **milk**, or a full glass of **water** to minimize gastric irritation.

Patient/Family Teaching

- Advise patient to take medication exactly as directed and not to skip doses or double up on missed doses. Abrupt withdrawal may lead to gastritis, nausea, vomiting, dizziness, headache, tachycardia, and insomnia.
- Advise patient to make position changes slowly to minimize orthostatic hypotension.
- Medication may cause drowsiness. Caution patient to avoid driving or other activities requiring alertness until response to the medication is known.
- Caution patient to avoid taking alcohol or other CNS depressants concurrently with this medication.

- Advise patient to use sunscreen and protective clothing when exposed to the sun to prevent photosensitivity reactions. Extremes of temperature should also be avoided, as these drugs impair body temperature regulation.
- Advise patient that ↑ activity, bulk, and fluids in the diet helps minimize the constipating effects of this medication.
- Instruct patient to use frequent mouth rinses, good oral hygiene, and sugarless gum or candy to minimize dry mouth.
- Advise patient to notify health care provider of medication regimen before treatment or surgery.
- Emphasize the importance of routine follow-up exams and continued participation in psychotherapy as indicated.

Evaluation/Desired Outcomes

- Decrease in excitable, paranoic, or withdrawn behavior. Decrease in incidence of mood swings in patients with bipolar disorders. Increase in sense of well-being in patients with depression.

ANTIRETROVIRALS

Commonly Prescribed Drugs

See Mechanism of Action of Select Antiretrovirals table.

Pharmacologic Profile

General Use

The goal of antiretroviral therapy in the management of HIV infection is to improve CD4 cell counts and ↓ viral load. If accomplished, this generally results in slowed progression of the disease, improved quality of life, and ↓ opportunistic infections. Perinatal use of agents also prevents transmission of the virus to the fetus. Postexposure and pre-exposure prophylaxis with certain antiretrovirals is also recommended.

General Action and Information

MECHANISM OF ACTION OF SELECT ANTIRETROVIRALS

DRUG	MECHANISM
Lamivudine, tenofovir alafenamide, and zidovudine	Nucleoside reverse transcriptase inhibitors (NRTIs)
Cabotegravir and dolutegravir	Integrase strand transfer inhibitors (INSTIs)
Darunavir and ritonavir	Protease inhibitors
Lencapavir	Capsid inhibitor
Rilpivirine	Non-nucleoside reverse transcriptase inhibitor (NNRTI)

Contraindications

Hypersensitivity. Because of highly varying toxicities among agents, see individual monographs for more specific information.

Precautions

Many agents require modification for renal impairment. Protease inhibitors may cause hyperglycemia and hyperlipidemia and should be used cautiously in patients with diabetes and patients at increased risk for cardiovascular disease. Hemophiliacs may also be at risk of bleeding when taking protease inhibitors. See individual monographs for specific information.

Interactions

There are many significant and potentially serious drug-drug interactions among the antiretrovirals. Many of these interactions involve the cytochrome P450 system. See individual agents.

Nursing Implications

Assessment

- Assess patient for change in severity of symptoms of HIV and for symptoms of opportunistic infections throughout therapy.

- **Lab Test Considerations:** Monitor viral load and CD4 counts prior to and periodically during therapy.

Implementation

- Administer doses around the clock.

Patient/Family Teaching

- Instruct patient to take medication exactly as directed. Emphasize the importance of complying with therapy, not taking more than prescribed amount, and not discontinuing without consulting health care provider. Missed doses should be taken as soon as remembered unless almost time for next dose; patient should not double doses.
- Inform patient that antiretroviral therapy does not cure HIV and does not ↓ the risk of transmission of HIV to others through sexual contact or blood contamination. Caution patient to use a condom during sexual contact and to avoid sharing needles or donating blood to prevent spreading the HIV virus to others.
- Advise patient to avoid taking any Rx, OTC, or herbal products without consulting health care provider.
- Emphasize the importance of regular follow-up exams and blood counts to determine progress and to monitor for side effects.

Evaluation/Desired Outcomes

- Decrease in viral load and increase in CD4 counts in patients with HIV.

ANTIRHEUMATICS

Commonly Prescribed Drugs

See Mechanism of Action of Select Antirheumatics table.

Pharmacologic Profile

General Use

Antirheumatics are used to manage symptoms of rheumatoid arthritis (pain, swelling) and in more severe cases to slow down joint destruction and preserve joint function. NSAIDs, aspirin, and other salicylates are used to manage symptoms such as pain and swelling, allowing continued motility and improved quality of life. Corticosteroids are reserved for more advanced swelling and discomfort, primarily because of their ↑ side effects, especially with chronic use. They can be used to control acute flares of disease. Neither NSAIDs nor corticosteroids prevent disease progression or joint destruction. Disease-modifying antirheumatics drugs (DMARDs) slow the progression of rheumatoid arthritis and delay joint destruction. Several months of therapy may be required before benefit is noted and maintained.

General Action and Information

MECHANISM OF ACTION OF SELECT ANTIRHEUMATICS

DRUG	MECHANISM
Adalimumab, certolizumab, etanercept, golimumab, and infliximab	Tumor necrosis factor (TNF)-α inhibitors
Diclofenac, ibuprofen, indomethacin, and naproxen	NSAIDs
Cyclophosphamide, hydroxychloroquine, leflunomide, methotrexate, and sulfasalazine	DMARDs
Baricitinib, tofacitinib, and upadacitinib	Janus kinase (JAK) inhibitors
Sarilumab and tocilizumab	Interleukin-6 inhibitors
Abatacept	Inhibits T-cell activation
Apremilast	Phosphodiesterase–4 inhibitor
Celecoxib	Cyclo-oxygenase-2 (COX-2) inhibitor
Cyclosporine	Interleukin-2 inhibitor

Contraindications
Hypersensitivity. Patients who are allergic to aspirin should not receive other NSAIDs. Corticosteroids should not be used in patients with active untreated infections. Many DMARDs have immunosuppressive properties and should be avoided in patients for whom immunosuppression poses a serious risk, including patients with active infections, underlying malignancy, and transplant recipients.

Precautions
NSAIDs and corticosteroids should be used cautiously in patients with a history of GI bleeding. Corticosteroids should be used with caution in patients with diabetes.

Interactions
NSAIDs may diminish the response to diuretics and other antihypertensives. Corticosteroids may augment hypokalemia from other medications and ↑ the risk of digoxin toxicity. DMARDs ↑ the risk of serious immunosuppression with other immunosuppressants. Live vaccines should not be given concurrently with DMARDs.

Nursing Implications

Assessment
- Assess patient monthly for pain, swelling, and range of motion.

Implementation
- Most agents require regular administration to obtain maximum effects.

Patient/Family Teaching
- Instruct patient to contact health care provider if no improvement is noticed within a few days.
- Instruct patient to contact health care provider promptly if signs or symptoms of infection develop.

Evaluation/Desired Outcomes
- Improvement in signs and symptoms of rheumatoid arthritis.

ANTITUBERCULARS

Commonly Prescribed Drugs
Ethambutol, isoniazid, pyrazinamide, and rifampin.

Pharmacologic Profile

General Use
To treat and prevent tuberculosis. Combinations are used in the treatment of active tuberculosis to rapidly ↓ the infectious state and delay or prevent the emergence of resistant strains. In selected situations, intermittent (twice weekly) regimens may be employed. Rifampin is also used in the prevention of meningococcal meningitis and *Haemophilus influenzae* type B and in treatment of S. aureus infections (in combination with other antimicrobial agents).

General Action and Information
Kill or inhibit the growth of mycobacteria responsible for causing tuberculosis. Combination therapy with ≥2 agents is required, unless used as prophylaxis (isoniazid alone).

Contraindications
Hypersensitivity. Severe liver disease.

Precautions
Use cautiously in patients with a history of liver disease or in older adults. Ethambutol requires ophthalmologic follow-up. Compliance is required for optimal response.

Interactions
Isoniazid inhibits the metabolism of phenytoin. Rifampin significantly ↓ levels of many drugs.

Nursing Implications

Assessment

- Mycobacterial studies and susceptibility tests should be performed prior to and periodically throughout therapy to detect possible resistance.
- Assess lung sounds and character and amount of sputum periodically throughout therapy.

Implementation

- Most medications can be administered with food if GI irritation occurs.

Patient/Family Teaching

- Advise patient of the importance of continuing therapy even after symptoms have subsided.
- Emphasize the importance of regular follow-up exams to monitor progress and check for side effects.
- Inform patients taking rifampin that saliva, sputum, sweat, tears, urine, and feces may become red-orange to red-brown and that soft contact lenses may become permanently discolored.

Evaluation/Desired Outcomes

- Resolution of the signs and symptoms of tuberculosis. Negative sputum cultures.

ANTIULCER AGENTS

Commonly Prescribed Drugs

See Mechanism of Action of Select Antiulcer Agents table.

Pharmacologic Profile

General Use

Treatment and prophylaxis of peptic ulcer and gastric hypersecretory conditions such as Zollinger-Ellison syndrome. H_2-receptor antagonists and proton pump inhibitors (PPIs) are also used in the management of gastroesophageal reflux disease.

General Action and Information

MECHANISM OF ACTION OF SELECT ANTIULCER AGENTS

DRUG	MECHANISM
Dexlansoprazole, esomeprazole, lansoprazole, omeprazole, pantoprazole, and rabeprazole	PPIs
Famotidine	H_2 receptor antagonist
Misoprostol	Prostaglandin E_1 analog
Sucralfate	Gastroduodenal protective agent
Vonoprazan	Potassium-competitive acid blocker

Contraindications

Hypersensitivity.

Precautions

Most H_2 antagonists require dose ↓ in renal impairment and in older adults. Magnesium-containing antacids should be used cautiously in patients with renal impairment. Misoprostol should be used cautiously in women of reproductive potential. Long-term therapy (>1 yr) with PPIs may be associated with an ↑ risk of hip, wrist, or spine fractures; fundic gland polyps; and vitamin B_{12} deficiency.

Interactions

Calcium- and magnesium-containing antacids ↓ the absorption of tetracycline and fluoroquinolones. Omeprazole ↓ metabolism of phenytoin, diazepam, and warfarin. All agents that ↑ gastric pH will ↓ the absorption of itraconazole, ketoconazole, iron salts, erlotinib, nilotinib, atazanavir, nelfinavir, rilpivirine, and mycophenolate mofetil. All PPIs, except pantoprazole, may ↓ the antiplatelet effects of clopidogrel.

CLASSIFICATIONS

Nursing Implications

Assessment

- Assess patient routinely for epigastric or abdominal pain and frank or occult blood in the stool, emesis, or gastric aspirate.
- **H_2 Receptor Antagonists:** Assess older adults and severely ill patients for confusion routinely. Notify health care provider promptly should this occur.
- **Misoprostol:** Assess women of reproductive potential for pregnancy. Medication is usually begun on 2nd or 3rd day of menstrual period following a negative serum pregnancy test within 2 wk of beginning therapy.

Implementation

- **Misoprostol:** Administer with meals and at bedtime to ↓ the severity of diarrhea.
- **PPIs:** Administer before meals, preferably in the morning. Capsules should be swallowed whole; do not open, crush, or chew.
- May be administered concurrently with antacids.
- **Sucralfate:** Administer on an empty stomach 1 hr before meals and at bedtime. Do not crush or chew tablets. Shake suspension well prior to administration. If nasogastric administration is required, consult pharmacist, as protein-binding properties of sucralfate have resulted in formation of a bezoar when administered with enteral feedings and other medications.

Patient/Family Teaching

- Instruct patient to take medication as directed for the full course of therapy, even if feeling better. If a dose is missed, it should be taken as soon as remembered but not if almost time for next dose. Do not double doses.
- Advise patient to avoid alcohol, products containing aspirin, NSAIDs, and foods that may cause an ↑ in GI irritation.
- Advise patient to report onset of black, tarry stools to health care provider promptly.
- Inform patient that cessation of smoking may help prevent the recurrence of duodenal ulcers.
- **Misoprostol:** Inform patient that misoprostol may cause spontaneous abortion. Women of reproductive potential must be informed of this effect through verbal and written information and must use contraception throughout therapy. If pregnancy is suspected, the woman should stop taking misoprostol and immediately notify her health care provider.
- **Sucralfate:** Advise patient that an ↑ in fluid intake, dietary bulk, and exercise may prevent drug-induced constipation.

Evaluation/Desired Outcomes

- Decrease in GI pain and irritation.
- Prevention of gastric irritation and bleeding.
- Decreased symptoms of GERD.
- Prevention of gastric ulcers in patients receiving chronic NSAID therapy (misoprostol only).

ANTIVIRALS

Commonly Prescribed Drugs

Acyclovir, entecavir, famciclovir, foscarnet, ganciclovir, lamivudine, molnupiravir, nirmatrelvir/ritonavir, oseltamivir, remdesivir, valacyclovir, and valganciclovir

Pharmacologic Profile

General Use

Acyclovir, famciclovir, and valacyclovir are used in the management of herpes virus infections. Acyclovir and valacyclovir are also used in the management of chickenpox. Oseltamivir is used primarily in the prevention and/or treatment of influenza infection. Foscarnet, ganciclovir, and valganciclovir are used in the prevention and/or treatment of cytomegalovirus (CMV) infection. Entecavir and lamivudine are used for the treatment of hepatitis B infection. Molnupiravir, nirmatrelvir/ritonavir, and remdesivir are used in the treatment of COVID-19 infection.

General Action and Information
Most agents inhibit viral replication.

Contraindications
Previous hypersensitivity.

Precautions
Many antiviral agents require dose adjustment in renal impairment. Acyclovir may cause renal impairment. Acyclovir may cause CNS toxicity. Foscarnet ↑ risk of seizures.

Interactions
Acyclovir may have additive CNS and nephrotoxicity with drugs causing similar adverse reactions. Nirmatrelvir/ritonavir has numerous drug interactions involving the cytochrome P450 system.

Nursing Implications

Assessment
- Assess patient for signs and symptoms of infection before and throughout therapy.
- **Ophth:** Assess eye lesions before and daily during therapy.
- **Topical:** Assess lesions before and daily during therapy.

Implementation
- Most systemic antiviral agents should be administered around the clock to maintain therapeutic serum drug levels.

Patient/Family Teaching
- Instruct patient to continue taking medication around the clock for full course of therapy, even if feeling better.
- Advise patient that antivirals do not prevent transmission to others. Precautions should be taken to prevent spread of virus.
- Instruct patient in correct technique for topical or ophthalmic preparations.
- Instruct patient to notify health care provider if symptoms do not improve.

Evaluation/Desired Outcomes
- Prevention or resolution of the signs and symptoms of viral infection. Length of time for complete resolution depends on organism and site of infection.

BONE RESORPTION INHIBITORS

Commonly Prescribed Drugs
See Mechanism of Action of Select Bone Resorption Inhibitors table.

Pharmacologic Profile

General Use
Bone resorption inhibitors are primarily used to treat and prevent osteoporosis in postmenopausal women. Other uses include treatment of osteoporosis due to other causes, including corticosteroid therapy, treatment of Paget disease of the bone, and management of hypercalcemia.

General Action and Information

MECHANISM OF ACTION OF SELECT BONE RESORPTION INHIBITORS

DRUG	MECHANISM
Alendronate, ibandronate, pamidronate, risedronate, and zoledronic acid	Bisphosphonates
Denosumab	Receptor activator of nuclear factor kappa-B-ligand (RANKL) inhibitor
Raloxifene	Selective estrogen receptor modulator (SERM)
Romosozumab	Sclerostin inhibitor

Contraindications

Hypersensitivity. Bisphosphonates and denosumab should not be used in patients with hypocalcemia. Bisphosphonates should not be used in patients with abnormalities of the esophagus that delay esophageal emptying. Raloxifene should not be used in women of reproductive potential or a history of thromboembolic disease. Romosozumab should not be used in patients who have experienced an MI or stroke in the past year.

Precautions

Use bisphosphonates cautiously in patients with renal impairment; some agents should be avoided in moderate to severe renal impairment. Invasive dental procedures, cancer, chemotherapy, corticosteroids, angiogenesis inhibitors, poor oral hygiene, diabetes, gingival infections, periodontal disease, dental disease, anemia, coagulopathy, infection, or poorly fitting dentures may ↑ risk of jaw osteonecrosis in patients receiving bisphosphonates, denosumab, or romosozumab. Patients with hypoparathyroidism, previous thyroid/parathyroid surgery, malabsorption syndromes, history of small intestinal excision, concurrent use of calcium-lowering medications, or severe renal impairment/hemodialysis are at ↑ risk of hypocalcemia with denosumab.

Interactions

Calcium supplements ↓ absorption of bisphosphonates. Aspirin and NSAIDs may ↑ GI adverse reactions with bisphosphonates.

Nursing Implications

Assessment

- Assess patients for low bone density before and periodically during therapy.
- Assess for symptoms of Paget disease (bone pain, headache, decreased visual and auditory acuity, ↑ skull size).
- For patients receiving denosumab, monitor for signs/ symptoms of hypersensitivity reactions (hypotension, dyspnea, upper airway edema, lip swelling, rash, pruritus, urticaria) after administration. Treat symptomatically and discontinue medication if symptoms occur.
- **Lab Test Considerations:** Monitor serum calcium in patients with osteoporosis. Monitor alkaline phosphatase in patients with Paget disease.

Implementation

- Denosumab and romosozumab are administered SUBQ.
- Duration of therapy with romosozumab is limited to 1 yr due to ↓ effectiveness. If continued therapy is needed, continue therapy with an antiresorptive agent.

Patient/Family Teaching

- Instruct patient to take medication exactly as directed.
- Emphasize the importance of follow-up tests for bone mineral density.
- Discuss the importance of other treatments for osteoporosis (supplemental calcium and/or vitamin D, weight-bearing exercise, modification of behavioral factors such as smoking and/or alcohol consumption).

- Advise patient to take good care of teeth and gums (brush and floss regularly) and to inform health care provider of therapy prior to dental surgery.
- Inform patient of ↑ risk of fractures upon discontinuation of denosumab. If denosumab is discontinued, consider another bone resorption inhibitor.

Evaluation/Desired Outcomes

- Prevention of, or decrease in, the progression of osteoporosis with a reduction in fractures.
- Decrease in the progression of Paget disease.

BRONCHODILATORS

Commonly Prescribed Drugs

See Mechanism of Action of Select Bronchodilators table.

Pharmacologic Profile

General Use

Used in the treatment of reversible airway obstruction due to asthma or chronic obstructive pulmonary disease. Rapid-acting inhaled beta-agonist bronchodilators (albuterol or levalbuterol) should be reserved as acute relievers of bronchospasm; repeated or chronic use indicates the need for additional long-term control agents, including inhaled corticosteroids, mast cell stabilizers, long-acting bronchodilators (oral theophylline, $beta_2$ agonists, or anticholinergics), and leukotriene modifiers (montelukast, zafirlukast).

General Action and Information

MECHANISM OF ACTION OF SELECT BRONCHODILATORS

DRUG	MECHANISM
Albuterol, epinephrine, formoterol, levalbuterol, terbutaline, and vilanterol	$Beta_2$ receptor agonists
Ipratropium and tiotropium	Anticholinergics

Contraindications

Hypersensitivity to agents or preservatives (bisulfites) used in their formulation. Avoid use in uncontrolled cardiac arrhythmias.

Precautions

Use $beta_2$ agonists cautiously in patients with diabetes, cardiovascular disease, or hyperthyroidism. Use anticholinergic agents cautiously in narrow-angle glaucoma, prostatic hyperplasia, or bladder-neck obstruction.

Interactions

Therapeutic effectiveness of $beta_2$ agonists may be antagonized by concurrent use of beta blockers. $Beta_2$ agonists may have additive sympathomimetic effects with other adrenergic drugs, including vasopressors and decongestants. Use of anticholinergic agents with other agents with anticholinergic activity may result in additive anticholinergic effects (dry mouth, dry eyes, blurred vision, constipation).

Nursing Implications

Assessment

- Assess BP, HR, respiratory rate, lung sounds, and character of secretions before and throughout therapy.
- Patients with a history of cardiovascular problems should be monitored for ECG changes and chest pain with use of $beta_2$ agonists.

Implementation

- Administer around the clock to maintain therapeutic plasma levels.

CLASSIFICATIONS

Patient/Family Teaching
- Emphasize the importance of taking only the prescribed dose at the prescribed time intervals.
- Encourage the patient to drink adequate liquids (2000 mL/day minimum) to ↓ the viscosity of the airway secretions.
- Advise patient to avoid OTC cough, cold, or breathing preparations without consulting health care provider and to minimize intake of xanthine-containing foods or beverages (colas, coffee, and chocolate), as these may ↑ side effects of theophylline.
- Caution patient to avoid smoking and other respiratory irritants.
- Instruct patient on proper use of metered-dose inhaler (see Appendix C).
- Advise patient to contact health care provider promptly if the usual dose of medication fails to produce the desired results, symptoms worsen after treatment, or toxic effects occur.
- Patients using other inhalation medications and bronchodilators should be advised to use bronchodilator 1st and allow 5 min to elapse before administering the other medication, unless otherwise directed by health care provider.

Evaluation/Desired Outcomes
- Decreased bronchospasm.
- Increased ease of breathing.

CENTRAL NERVOUS SYSTEM STIMULANTS

Commonly Prescribed Drugs
Amphetamine mixtures, dexmethylphenidate, lisdexamfetamine, methylphenidate, modafinil, and solriamfetol.

Pharmacologic Profile

General Use
Amphetamine mixtures, dexmethylphenidate, lisdexamfetamine, and methylphenidate are used in the treatment of narcolepsy and as adjunctive treatment in the management of attention-deficit hyperactivity disorder (ADHD). Modafinil and solriamfetol are used for the treatment of excessive daytime drowsiness due to narcolepsy or obstructive sleep apnea.

General Action and Information
Produce CNS stimulation by ↑ levels of neurotransmitters in the CNS. Produce CNS and respiratory stimulation, dilated pupils, ↑ motor activity and mental alertness, and a diminished sense of fatigue.

Contraindications
Hypersensitivity. Should not be used in pregnant or lactating women. Should not be used in hyperexcitable states, patients with psychotic personalities or suicidal/homicidal tendencies, glaucoma, or severe cardiovascular disease.

Precautions
Use cautiously in patients with a history of cardiovascular disease, hypertension, diabetes mellitus, substance use disorder, or in older adults.

Interactions
Additive sympathomimetic (adrenergic) effects. Use with MAO inhibitors can result in hypertensive crises. Alkalinizing the urine (sodium bicarbonate, acetazolamide) ↓ excretion and enhances effects of amphetamines. Acidification of the urine (ammonium chloride, large doses of ascorbic acid) ↓ effect of amphetamines.

Nursing Implications

Assessment
- Monitor BP, HR, and respiratory rate before administering and periodically during therapy.
- Monitor weight biweekly and inform health care provider of significant weight loss.

- Monitor height periodically in children; inform health care provider if growth inhibition occurs.
- May produce false sense of euphoria and well-being. Provide frequent rest periods and observe patient for rebound depression after the effects of the medication have worn off.
- **ADHD:** Assess attention span, impulse control, and interactions with others. Therapy may be interrupted at intervals to determine if symptoms are sufficient to warrant continued therapy.
- **Narcolepsy:** Observe and document frequency of episodes.

Implementation
- Follow administration directions associated with individual formulations.

Patient/Family Teaching
- Instruct patient not to alter dose without consulting health care provider. Abrupt cessation with high doses may cause extreme fatigue and mental depression.
- Advise patient to avoid intake of large amounts of caffeine.
- Advise patient that many of these medications have known abuse potential. Caution patient to protect the medications from theft, and never give them to anyone other than the individual for whom it was prescribed. Store the medications out of sight and reach of children, and in a location not accessible by others.
- Advise patient to notify health care provider if nervousness, insomnia, palpitations, vomiting, skin rash, fever, painful and prolonged erections, or circulation problems (fingers or toes feel numb, cool, or painful; fingers or toes change color from pale to blue to red) occur.
- Medication may impair judgment. Caution patient to avoid driving or other activities requiring judgment until response to medication is known.
- Inform patient that periodic holidays from the drug may be used to assess progress and decrease dependence.

Evaluation/Desired Outcomes
- Decreased frequency of narcoleptic episodes.
- Improved attention span and social interactions.

CORTICOSTEROIDS

Commonly Prescribed Drugs
Alclometasone, amcinonide, beclomethasone, betamethasone, budesonide, ciclesonide, clobetasol, clocortolone, desonide, desoximetasone, dexamethasone, diflorasone, fludrocortisone, fluocinolone, fluocinonide, flurandrenolide, fluticasone, halcinonide, halobetasol, hydrocortisone, methylprednisolone, mometasone, prednisolone, prednisone, and triamcinolone.

Pharmacologic Profile

General Use
Used in replacement doses (20 mg of hydrocortisone or equivalent) systemically to treat adrenocortical insufficiency. Larger doses are usually used for their anti-inflammatory, immunosuppressive, or antineoplastic activity. Used adjunctively in many other situations, including autoimmune diseases. Topical corticosteroids are used in a variety of inflammatory and allergic conditions. Inhaled corticosteroids are used in the chronic management of asthma or chronic obstructive pulmonary disease; intranasal and ophthalmic corticosteroids are used in the management of chronic allergic and inflammatory conditions.

General Action and Information
Produce profound and varied metabolic effects, in addition to modifying the normal immune response and suppressing inflammation. Available in a variety of dosage forms, including oral, injectable, topical, ophthalmic, intranasal, and inhalation. Prolonged use of large amounts of topical, ophthalmic, intranasal, or inhaled agent may result in systemic absorption and/or adrenal suppression.

Contraindications
Serious infections (except for certain forms of meningitis). Do not administer live vaccines to patients on larger doses.

Precautions
Prolonged treatment will result in adrenal suppression. Use lowest dose possible for shortest time possible. Do not discontinue abruptly. Additional doses may be needed during stress (surgery and infection). Long-term use in children will result in ↓ growth. May mask signs of infection.

Interactions
Additive hypokalemia with amphotericin B and potassium-losing diuretics. Hypokalemia may ↑ the risk of digoxin toxicity. May ↑ requirements for oral or injectable hypoglycemic agents. Phenytoin, phenobarbital, and rifampin may ↓ effectiveness. Oral contraceptives may block metabolism of corticosteroids.

Nursing Implications

Assessment
- These drugs are indicated for many conditions. Assess involved systems prior to and periodically throughout course of therapy.
- Assess patient for signs of adrenal insufficiency (hypotension, weight loss, weakness, nausea, vomiting, anorexia, lethargy, confusion, restlessness) prior to and periodically throughout course of therapy.
- Children should have periodic evaluations of growth during chronic therapy.

Implementation
- If dose is ordered daily or every other day, administer in the morning to coincide with the body's normal secretion of cortisol.
- **PO:** Administer with meals to minimize gastric irritation.

Patient/Family Teaching
- Emphasize need to take medication exactly as directed. Review symptoms of adrenal insufficiency that may occur when stopping the medication and that may be life-threatening.
- These drugs cause immunosuppression and may mask symptoms of infection. Instruct patient to avoid people with known contagious illnesses and to report possible infections. Advise patient to consult health care provider before receiving any vaccinations.
- Advise patient to carry identification in the event of an emergency in which patient cannot relate medical history.

Evaluation/Desired Outcomes
- Suppression of the inflammatory and immune responses in autoimmune disorders, allergic reactions, and organ transplants.
- Replacement therapy in adrenal insufficiency.
- Resolution of skin inflammation, pruritus, or other dermatologic conditions.

HORMONES

Commonly Prescribed Drugs
See General Uses of Select Hormones table.

Pharmacologic Profile

General Use

GENERAL USES OF SELECT HORMONES

DRUG	MECHANISM
Estradiol and estrogens	Amenorrhea; contraception; postmenopausal osteoporosis (prevention); vasomotor symptoms associated with menopause; vulvar/vaginal atrophy associated with menopause
Desmopressin	Diabetes insipidus; hemophilia A; nocturia; nocturnal enuresis; von Wildebrand disease
Glucagon	Hypoglycemia
Goserelin	Breast cancer; endometriosis; prostate cancer; uterine bleeding
Insulin	Type 1 and 2 diabetes
Levothyroxine	Hypothyroidism
Megestrol	Anorexia/cachexia; breast cancer; endometrial cancer
Nafarelin	Central precocious puberty; endometriosis
Octreotide	Acromegaly; carcinoid syndrome; variceal bleeding
Ospemifene	Vulvar/vaginal atrophy associated with menopause
Oxytocin	Labor induction
Progesterone	Amenorrhea; contraception; uterine bleeding
Testosterone	Delayed puberty (males); hypogonadism (males)
Vasopressin	Hypotension (associated with septic shock)

General Action and Information

Natural or synthetic substances that have a specific effect on target tissue. Differ greatly in their effects, depending on individual agent and function of target tissue.

Contraindications

Differ greatly among individual agents; see individual entries.

Precautions

Differ greatly among individual agents; see individual entries.

Interactions

Differ greatly among individual agents; see individual entries.

Nursing Implications

Assessment

- Monitor patient for symptoms of hormonal excess or insufficiency.
- **Sex Hormones:** BP and liver function tests should be monitored periodically throughout therapy.

Implementation

- **Sex Hormones:** During hospitalization, continue to administer according to schedule followed prior to hospitalization.

Patient/Family Teaching

- Explain dose schedule (and withdrawal bleeding with female sex hormones).
- Emphasize the importance of follow-up exams to monitor effectiveness of therapy and to ensure proper development of children and early detection of possible side effects.
- **Female Sex Hormones:** Advise patient to report signs and symptoms of fluid retention, thromboembolic disorders, mental depression, or hepatic dysfunction to health care professional.

Evaluation/Desired Outcomes

- Resolution of clinical symptoms of hormone imbalance including menopause symptoms and contraception.
- Correction of fluid and electrolyte imbalances.
- Control of the spread of advanced metastatic breast or prostate cancer.
- Slowed progression of postmenopausal osteoporosis.

IMMUNOSUPPRESSANTS

Commonly Prescribed Drugs

Azathioprine, belimumab, cyclosporine, everolimus, mycophenolate, pimecrolimus, sirolimus, and tacrolimus.

Pharmacologic Profile

General Use

Azathioprine, cyclosporine, everolimus, mycophenolate, sirolimus, and tacrolimus are used with corticosteroids in the prevention of transplantation rejection reactions. Azathioprine and cyclosporine are also used in the management of selected autoimmune diseases (nephrotic syndrome of childhood and severe rheumatoid arthritis). Belimumab is used for the treatment of lupus nephritis and systemic lupus erythematosus. Pimecrolimus is used in the treatment of atopic dermatitis.

General Action and Information

Inhibit cell-mediated immune responses by different mechanisms. In addition to azathioprine and cyclosporine, which are used primarily for their immunomodulating properties, cyclophosphamide and methotrexate are used to suppress the immune responses in certain disease states (nephrotic syndrome of childhood and severe rheumatoid arthritis).

Contraindications

Hypersensitivity to drug or vehicle.

Precautions

Use cautiously in patients with infections.

Interactions

Allopurinol inhibits the metabolism of azathioprine. Drugs that alter liver-metabolizing processes may change the effect of cyclosporine, tacrolimus, or sirolimus. The risk of toxicity with methotrexate may be ↑ by other nephrotoxic drugs, large doses of aspirin, or NSAIDs.

Nursing Implications

Assessment

- Monitor for infection (vital signs, sputum, urine, stool, WBC). Notify physician or other health care provider immediately if symptoms occur.
- Assess for symptoms of organ rejection throughout therapy.
- **Lab Test Consideration:** Monitor CBC and differential throughout therapy.

Implementation

- Protect transplant patients from staff and visitors who may carry infection.
- Maintain protective isolation as indicated.

Patient/Family Teaching

- Reinforce the need for lifelong therapy to prevent transplant rejection. Review symptoms of rejection for transplanted organ and stress the need for patient to notify health care provider immediately if they occur.
- Advise patient to avoid contact with contagious persons. Patients should not receive vaccinations without first consulting with health care provider.
- Emphasize the importance of follow-up exams and lab tests.

Evaluation/Desired Outcomes

- Prevention or reversal of rejection of organ transplants.
- Decrease in symptoms of autoimmune disorders.

LAXATIVES

Commonly Prescribed Drugs

Bisacodyl, docusate, lactulose, magnesium citrate/hydroxide/oxide, methylnaltrexone, naloxegol, plecanatide, polyethylene glycol 3350, and senna.

Pharmacologic Profile

General Use

To treat or prevent constipation or to prepare the bowel for radiologic or endoscopic procedures.

General Action and Information

Induce one or more bowel movements per day. Groups include stimulants (bisacodyl, senna), saline laxatives (magnesium salts), stool softeners (docusate), and osmotic cathartics (lactulose, polyethylene glycol). Methylnaltrexone and naloxegol are used to specifically manage opioid-induced constipation. Plecanatide is used to manage chronic constipation that is idiopathic in nature or due to irritable bowel syndrome. ↑ fluid intake, exercising, and adding more dietary fiber are also useful in the management of chronic constipation.

Contraindications

Hypersensitivity. Contraindicated in persistent abdominal pain, nausea, or vomiting of unknown cause, especially if accompanied by fever or other signs of an acute abdomen.

Precautions

Excessive or prolonged use may lead to dependence. Should not be used in children unless advised by a physician or other health care provider.

Interactions

Theoretically may ↓ the absorption of other orally administered drugs by ↓ transit time.

Nursing Implications

Assessment

- Assess patient for abdominal distention, presence of bowel sounds, and usual pattern of bowel function.
- Assess color, consistency, and amount of stool produced.

Implementation

- May be administered at bedtime for morning results.
- Taking oral doses on an empty stomach will usually produce more rapid results.
- Do not crush or chew enteric-coated tablets. Take with a full glass of water or juice.
- Stool softeners may take several days for results.

Patient/Family Teaching

- Advise patients, other than those with spinal cord injuries, that laxatives should be used only for short-term therapy. Long-term therapy may cause electrolyte imbalance and dependence.
- Encourage patients to use other forms of bowel regulation: ↑ bulk in the diet, ↑ fluid intake, and ↑ mobility. Normal bowel habits are individualized and may vary from 3 times/day to 3 times/wk.
- Instruct patients with cardiac disease to avoid straining during bowel movements (Valsalva maneuver).
- Advise patient that laxatives should not be used when constipation is accompanied by abdominal pain, fever, nausea, or vomiting.

Evaluation/Desired Outcomes

- A soft, formed bowel movement.
- Evacuation of the colon.

LIPID-LOWERING AGENTS

Commonly Prescribed Drugs

See Mechanism of Action of Select Lipid-Lowering Agents table.

Pharmacologic Profile

General Use

Used as a part of a total plan including diet and exercise to ↓ blood lipids in an effort to ↓ the morbidity and mortality of atherosclerotic cardiovascular disease and its sequelae.

General Action and Information

MECHANISM OF ACTION OF SELECT LIPID-LOWERING AGENTS

DRUG	MECHANISM
Atorvastatin, fluvastatin, lovastatin, pitavastatin, pravastatin, rosuvastatin, and simvastatin	HMG-CoA reductase inhibitors
Evolocumab	Proprotein convertase subtilisin kexin type 9 (PCSK9) inhibitor
Ezetimibe	Cholesterol absorption inhibitor
Fenofibrate	Peroxisome proliferator-activated receptor-α (PPAR-α) agonist
Omega-3-acid ethyl esters	↓ hepatic production of TG-rich very low-density lipoproteins

Contraindications

Hypersensitivity. HMG-CoA reductase inhibitors are contraindicated in pregnancy.

Precautions

Differ greatly among individual agents; see individual entries.

Interactions

HMG-CoA reductase inhibitors have numerous drug interactions involving cytochrome P450 system.

Nursing Implications

Assessment

- Obtain a diet history, especially in regard to **fat** and alcohol consumption.
- **Lab Test Considerations:** Serum cholesterol, LDL-C, HDL-C, and TG levels should be evaluated before initiating and periodically throughout therapy.
- Liver function tests should be assessed before and periodically throughout therapy with HMG Co-A reductase inhibitors, niacin, and fibric acid derivatives.

Implementation

- See specific medications to determine timing of doses in relation to meals.
- PCSK9 inhibitors are administered SUBQ.

Patient/Family Teaching

- Advise patient that these medications should be used in conjunction with diet restrictions (**fat**, **cholesterol**, **carbohydrates**, and alcohol), exercise, and cessation of smoking.

Evaluation/Desired Outcomes

- Decreased serum cholesterol, TG, and LDL-C levels and improved HDL-C levels.

OPIOID ANALGESICS

Commonly Prescribed Drugs

Buprenorphine, codeine, fentanyl, hydrocodone, hydromorphone, meperidine, methadone, morphine, nalbuphine, oxycodone, tapentadol, and tramadol.

Pharmacologic Profile

General Use

Moderate to severe pain. Fentanyl is also used as a general anesthetic adjunct.

General Action and Information

Opioids bind to opiate receptors in the CNS, where they act as agonists of endogenously occurring opioid peptides (eukephalins and endorphins). The result is alteration to the perception of and response to pain.

Contraindications

Hypersensitivity to individual agents.

Precautions

Use cautiously in patients with undiagnosed abdominal pain, head trauma or pathology, liver disease, or history of addiction to opioids. Use smaller doses initially in older adults and those with respiratory diseases. Prolonged use may result in tolerance and the need for larger doses to relieve pain. Psychological or physical dependence may occur.

Interactions

↑ the CNS depressant properties of other drugs, including alcohol, antihistamines, antidepressants, sedative/hypnotics, phenothiazines, and MAO inhibitors. Use of partial-antagonist opioid analgesics (buprenorphine, butorphanol, nalbuphine) may precipitate opioid withdrawal in physically dependent patients. Use with MAO inhibitors or procarbazine may result in severe paradoxical reactions (especially with meperidine). Methadone may ↑ the risk of QT interval prolongation when use with other QT interval prolonging medications.

Nursing Implications

Assessment

- Assess type, location, and intensity of pain prior to and at peak following administration. When titrating opioid doses, ↑ of 25–50% should be administered until there is either a 50% ↓ in the patient's pain rating on a numerical or visual analogue scale or the patient reports satisfactory pain relief. A repeat dose can be safely administered at the time of the peak if previous dose is ineffective and side effects are minimal.
- Opioid agonist-antagonists are not recommended for prolonged use or as first-line therapy for acute or cancer pain.
- An equianalgesic chart (see Appendix I) should be used when changing routes or when changing from one opioid to another.
- Assess BP, HR, and respiratory rate before and periodically during administration. If respiratory rate <10/min, assess level of sedation. Physical stimulation may be sufficient to prevent significant hypoventilation. Dose may need to be ↓ by 25–50%. Initial drowsiness will diminish with continued use.
- Assess prior analgesic history. Antagonistic properties of agonist-antagonists may induce withdrawal symptoms (vomiting, restlessness, abdominal cramps, ↑ BP and temperature) in patients physically dependent on opioids.
- Prolonged use may lead to physical and psychological dependence and tolerance. This should not prevent patient from receiving adequate analgesia. Most patients who receive opioid analgesics for pain do not develop psychological dependence. Progressively higher doses may be required to relieve pain with chronic therapy.

- Assess bowel function routinely. Prevention of constipation should be instituted with ↑ intake of fluids and bulk, stool softeners, and laxatives to minimize constipating effects. Stimulant laxatives should be administered routinely if opioid use >2–3 days, unless contraindicated.
- Monitor intake and output. If significant discrepancies occur, assess for urinary retention and inform physician or other health care provider.
- **Toxicity and Overdose:** If an opioid antagonist is required to reverse respiratory depression or coma, naloxone is the antidote. Dilute the 0.4-mg ampule of naloxone in 10 mL of 0.9% NaCl and administer 0.5 mL (0.02 mg) by IV push every 2 min. For children and patients weighing <40 kg, dilute 0.1 mg of naloxone in 10 mL of 0.9% NaCl for a concentration of 10 mcg/mL and administer 0.5 mcg/kg every 1–2 min. Naloxone may also be administered intranasally to reverse opioid-induced respiratory depression or coma. Administer 1 spray (2 mg or 4 mg) in one nostril; may repeat dose every 2–3 min (with each subsequent dose being administered in alternate nostril). Titrate dose to avoid withdrawal, seizures, and severe pain.

Implementation

- Explain therapeutic value of medication before administration to enhance the analgesic effect.
- Regularly administered doses may be more effective than prn (as needed) administration. Analgesic is more effective if given before pain becomes severe.
- Coadministration with nonopioid analgesics may have additive analgesic effects and may permit lower doses.
- Medication should be discontinued gradually after long-term use to prevent withdrawal symptoms.

Patient/Family Teaching

- Instruct patient on how and when to ask for pain medication.
- Advise patient that opioid analgesics have known abuse potential. Advise the patient to protect these medications from theft, and never give them to anyone other than the individual for whom it was prescribed. Store out of sight and reach of children and in a location not accessible by others.
- Medication may cause drowsiness or dizziness. Caution patient to call for assistance when ambulating or smoking and to avoid driving or other activities requiring alertness until response to medication is known.
- Advise patient to make position changes slowly to minimize orthostatic hypotension.
- Caution patient to avoid concurrent use of alcohol or other CNS depressants with this medication.
- Encourage patient to turn, cough, and breathe deeply every 2 hr to prevent atelectasis.

Evaluation/Desired Outcomes

- Decreased severity of pain without a significant alteration in level of consciousness or respiratory status.

SEDATIVE/HYPNOTICS

Commonly Prescribed Drugs

See Mechanism of Action of Select Sedative Hypnotics table.

Pharmacologic Profile

General Use

Sedatives are used to provide sedation, usually prior to procedures. Hypnotics are used to manage insomnia. Selected agents are useful as anticonvulsants (diazepam, phenobarbital), skeletal muscle relaxants (diazepam), adjuncts in the management of alcohol withdrawal syndrome (chlordiazepoxide, diazepam, oxazepam), or as amnestics (midazolam, diazepam).

General Action and Information

MECHANISM OF ACTION OF SELECT SEDATIVE HYPNOTICS

DRUG	MECHANISM
Chlordiazepoxide, diazepam, lorazepam, midazolam, oxazepam, and temazepam	Benzodiazepines: potentiates the effect of GABA (an inhibitory neurotransmitter)
Eszopiclone, phenobarbital, zaleplon, and zolpidem	Potentiates the effects of GABA
Daridorexant, suvorexant	Orexin receptor antagonist
Dexmedetomidine	Alpha-2 receptor agonist
Hydroxyzine	Antihistamine
Promethazine	Phenothiazine

Contraindications

Hypersensitivity. Should not be used in comatose patients or in those with pre-existing CNS depression. Should not be used in patients with uncontrolled severe pain. Avoid use during pregnancy or lactation.

Precautions

Use cautiously in patients with hepatic impairment, severe renal impairment, or severe underlying pulmonary disease. Use with caution in patients who may be suicidal or who may have had previous drug addictions. Hypnotic use should be short-term. Older adults may be more sensitive to CNS depressant effects; dosage ↓ may be required.

Interactions

Additive CNS depression with alcohol, antihistamines, some antidepressants, opioid analgesics, or phenothiazines. Should not be used with MAO inhibitors.

Nursing Implications

Assessment

- Monitor BP, HR, and respiratory rate frequently throughout IV administration.
- Prolonged high-dose therapy may lead to psychological or physical dependence. Restrict the amount of drug available to patient, especially if patient is depressed, suicidal, or has a history of addiction.
- **Insomnia:** Assess sleep patterns before and periodically throughout course of therapy.
- **Seizures:** Observe and record intensity, duration, and characteristics of seizure activity. Institute seizure precautions.
- **Muscle Spasms:** Assess muscle spasms, associated pain, and limitation of movement before and throughout therapy.
- **Alcohol Withdrawal:** Assess patient experiencing alcohol withdrawal for tremors, agitation, delirium, and hallucinations. Protect patient from injury.

Implementation

- Supervise ambulation and transfer of patients following administration of hypnotic doses. Side rails should be raised and call bell within reach at all times. Keep bed in low position.

Patient/Family Teaching

- Discuss the importance of preparing the environment for sleep (dark room, quiet, avoidance of nicotine and caffeine). If less effective after a few weeks, consult health care provider; do not ↑ dose. Gradual withdrawal may be required to prevent reactions following prolonged therapy.
- May cause daytime drowsiness. Caution patient to avoid driving and other activities requiring alertness until response to medication is known.
- Advise patient to avoid the use of alcohol and other CNS depressants concurrently with these medications.
- Advise patient to inform health care provider if pregnancy is planned or suspected.

Evaluation/Desired Outcomes

- Improvement in sleep patterns.
- Control of seizures.
- Decrease in muscle spasms.
- More rational ideation when used for alcohol withdrawal.

SKELETAL MUSCLE RELAXANTS

Commonly Prescribed Drugs

Baclofen, cyclobenzaprine, diazepam, methocarbamol, orphenadrine, and tizanidine.

Pharmacologic Profile

General Use

Two major uses are spasticity associated with spinal cord diseases or lesions (baclofen) or adjunctive therapy in the symptomatic relief of acute painful musculoskeletal conditions (cyclobenzaprine, diazepam, and methocarbamol).

General Action and Information

Act centrally (baclofen, cyclobenzaprine, diazepam, methocarbamol, and tizanidine).

Contraindications

Baclofen should not be used in patients in whom spasticity is used to maintain posture and balance.

Precautions

Use cautiously in patients with a history of liver disease.

Interactions

Additive CNS depression with other CNS depressants, including alcohol, antihistamines, antidepressants, opioid analgesics, and sedative/hypnotics.

Nursing Implications

Assessment

- Assess patient for pain, muscle stiffness, and range of motion before and periodically throughout therapy.

Implementation

- Provide safety measures as indicated. Supervise ambulation and transfer of patients.

Patient/Family Teaching

- Encourage patient to comply with additional therapies prescribed for muscle spasm (rest, physical therapy, heat).
- Medication may cause drowsiness. Caution patient to avoid driving or other activities requiring alertness until response to drug is known.
- Advise patient to avoid concurrent use of alcohol or other CNS depressants with these medications.

Evaluation/Desired Outcomes

- Decreased musculoskeletal pain.
- Decreased muscle spasticity.
- Increased range of motion.

THROMBOLYTICS

Commonly Prescribed Drugs

Alteplase and tenecteplase.

Pharmacologic Profile

General Use

Acute ST-segment-elevation MI and acute ischemic stroke. Alteplase is also used in the management of acute pulmonary embolism and for occluded central venous access devices.

General Action and Information

Directly convert plasminogen to plasmin, which then degrades fibrin in clots, resulting in lysis of the clot.

Contraindications

Hypersensitivity. Active internal bleeding, history of cerebrovascular accident, recent CNS trauma or surgery, neoplasm, arteriovenous malformation, severe uncontrolled hypertension, or known bleeding tendencies.

Precautions

Recent (within 10 days) major surgery, trauma, or GI or GU bleeding. Severe hepatic or renal disease. Subacute bacterial endocarditis or acute pericarditis. Use cautiously in older adults.

Interactions

Concurrent use with antiplatelet agents, NSAIDs, warfarin, dabigatran, rivaroxaban, apixaban, edoxaban, or heparins may ↑ the risk of bleeding, although these agents are frequently used together or in sequence. Risk of bleeding may also be ↑ by concurrent use with cefotetan and valproic acid.

Nursing Implications

Assessment

- Begin therapy as soon as possible after the onset of symptoms.
- Monitor vital signs continuously for coronary thrombosis and at least every 4 hr during therapy for other indications. Do not use lower extremities to monitor BP.
- Assess patient carefully for bleeding every 15 min during the 1st hr of therapy, every 15–30 min during the next 8 hr, and at least every 4 hr for the duration of therapy. Frank bleeding may occur from sites of invasive procedures or from body orifices. Internal bleeding may also occur (↓ neurologic status; abdominal pain with coffee-ground emesis or black, tarry stools; hematuria; joint pain). If uncontrolled bleeding occurs, stop medication and notify physician immediately.
- Assess neurologic status throughout therapy.
- Altered sensorium or neurologic changes may be indicative of intracranial bleeding.
- **Acute ST-segment elevation MI:** Monitor BP, HR, and ECG continuously. Notify physician if significant arrhythmias occur. Cardiac enzymes should be monitored. Coronary angiography may be ordered following therapy.
- Monitor heart sounds and breath sounds frequently. Inform physician if signs of HF occur (rales/crackles, dyspnea, S3 heart sound, jugular venous distention).
- **Acute Ischemic Stroke:** Assess neurologic status. Determine time of onset of stroke symptoms. Must be administered within 3–4.5 hr of onset (within 3 hr in patients >80 yr, those taking oral anticoagulants, those with a baseline National Institutes of Health Stroke Scale score >25, or those with both a history of stroke and diabetes).
- **Pulmonary Embolism:** Monitor BP, HR, hemodynamics, and respiratory status (rate, degree of dyspnea, arterial blood gases).
- **Cannula/Catheter Occlusion:** Monitor ability to aspirate blood as indicator of patency. Ensure that patient exhales and holds breath when connecting and disconnecting IV syringe to prevent air embolism.

- **Lab Test Considerations:** Hematocrit, hemoglobin, platelet count, fibrin/fibrin degradation product titer, fibrinogen concentration, PT, and aPTT may be evaluated prior to and frequently throughout therapy. Bleeding time may be assessed prior to therapy if patient has received platelet aggregation inhibitors. Obtain type and crossmatch and have blood available at all times in case of hemorrhage. Stools should be tested for occult blood loss and urine for hematuria periodically during therapy.
- **Toxicity and Overdose:** If local bleeding occurs, apply pressure to site. If severe or internal bleeding occurs, discontinue infusion. Clotting factors and/or blood volume may be restored through infusions of whole blood, packed RBCs, fresh frozen plasma, or cryoprecipitate. Do not administer dextran, as it has antiplatelet activity. Aminocaproic acid may be used as an antidote.

Implementation

- Starting two IV lines prior to therapy is recommended: one for the thrombolytic agent, the other for any additional infusions.
- Avoid invasive procedures, such as IM injections or arterial punctures, with this therapy. If such procedures must be performed, apply pressure to all arterial and venous puncture sites for ≥30 min. Avoid venipunctures at noncompressible sites (jugular vein, subclavian site).
- Systemic anticoagulation with heparin is usually begun several hours after the completion of thrombolytic therapy.

Patient/Family Teaching

- Explain purpose of medication and the need for close monitoring to patient and family. Instruct patient to report hypersensitivity reactions (rash, dyspnea) and bleeding or bruising.
- Explain need for bedrest and minimal handling during therapy to avoid injury. Avoid all unnecessary procedures such as shaving and vigorous tooth brushing.

Evaluation/Desired Outcomes

- Lysis of thrombi and restoration of blood flow.
- Prevention of neurologic sequelae in acute ischemic stroke.
- Cannula or catheter patency.

VASCULAR HEADACHE SUPPRESSANTS

Commonly Prescribed Drugs

See Mechanism of Action of Select Vascular Headache Suppressants table.

Pharmacologic Profile

General Use

Used for acute treatment of vascular headaches (migraine, cluster headaches, migraine variants). Other agents such as some beta blockers and some calcium channel blockers are used for suppression of frequently occurring vascular headaches. The (5-HT_1) agonists and some of the calcitonin gene-related peptide (CGRP) inhibitors (rimegepant, ubrogepant, zavegepant) are used for the acute treatment of migraine headaches. Some CGRP inhibitors (atogepant, erenumab, fremanezumab, galcanezumab, rimegepant) are used for migraine prevention.

General Action and Information

MECHANISM OF ACTION OF SELECT VASCULAR HEADACHE SUPPRESSANTS

DRUG	MECHANISM
Atogepant, erenumab, fremanezumab, galcanezumab, rimegepant, ubrogepant, and zavegepant	CGRP receptor inhibitors
Rizatriptan, sumatriptan, and zolmitriptan	5-HT_1 agonists

Contraindications

Use of 5-HT_1 agonists should be avoided in patients with ischemic cardiovascular disease.

Precautions
Use 5-HT_1 agonists cautiously in patients who are at risk for cardiovascular disease. ↑ risk of serotonin syndrome with 5-HT_1 agonists when used with serotonergic agents.

Interactions
Many of the CGRP antagonists have interactions involving the cytochrome P450 system.

Nursing Implications

Assessment
- Assess pain location, intensity, duration, and associated symptoms (photophobia, phonophobia, nausea, vomiting) during migraine attack and frequency of attacks.

Implementation
- Medications used for acute treatment of headache should be administered at the first sign of a headache.

Patient/Family Teaching
- Advise patient that lying down in a darkened room following medication administration may further help relieve headache.
- May cause dizziness or drowsiness. Caution patient to avoid driving or other activities requiring alertness until response to medication is known.
- Advise patient to avoid alcohol, which aggravates headaches.

Evaluation/Desired Outcomes
- Relief of migraine attack.

WEIGHT CONTROL AGENTS

Commonly Prescribed Drugs
Bupropion/naltrexone, phentermine, phentermine/topiramate, semaglutide, and tirzepatide.

Pharmacologic Profile

General Use
These agents are used in the management of exogenous obesity as part of a regimen including a reduced-calorie diet. They are especially useful in the presence of other risk factors, including hypertension, diabetes, or dyslipidemias.

General Action and Information
Phentermine is an anorexiant designed to ↓ appetite via its action in the CNS. Semaglutide and tirzepatide are glucagon-like peptide-1 (GLP-1) receptor agonists.

Contraindications
None of these agents should be used during pregnancy or lactation. Phentermine should not be used in patients with severe hepatic or renal disease, uncontrolled hypertension, known HF, or cardiovascular disease. Bupropion/naltrexone should not be used in patients with uncontrolled hypertension, anorexia/bulimia, or a history of seizure disorders. Semaglutide and tirzepatide should not be used in patients with a personal or family history of medullary thyroid carcinoma, multiple endocrine neoplasia syndrome type 2, or type 1 DM.

Precautions
Phentermine should be used cautiously in patients with a history of seizures or angle-closure glaucoma and in geriatric patients. Semaglutide and tirzepatide should be used with caution in patients with a history of pancreatitis, diabetic retinopathy, history of angioedema to another GLP-1 agonist, or undergoing elective surgery or procedure requiring general anesthesia or deep sedation.

Interactions

Phentermine may have additive adverse effects with CNS stimulants, some vascular headache suppressants, MAO inhibitors, and some opioids (concurrent use should be avoided). Concurrent use of bupropion/naltrexone with MAO inhibitors should be avoided.

Nursing Implications

Assessment

- Monitor weight and dietary intake prior to and periodically during therapy. Adjust concurrent medications (antihypertensives, antidiabetics, lipid-lowering agents) as needed.

Implementation

- Do not administer bupropion/naltrexone with a high-fat meal; may ↑ risk of seizures.
- Discontinue opioids prior to starting bupropion/naltrexone. Patients should be opioid-free for ≥7–10 days in those receiving short-acting opioids and up to 14 days in those receiving buprenorphine or methadone.
- Administer phentermine or phentermine/topiramate in the morning; avoid dosing in the evening because they may cause insomnia.
- Bupoprion/naltrexone, phentermine, and phentermine/topiramate are administered orally. Semaglutide can be administered either orally or SUBQ. Tirzepatide is administered SUBQ.

Patient/Family Teaching

- Advise patient that regular physical activity, approved by health care provider, should be used in conjunction with medication and diet.

Evaluation/Desired Outcomes

- Slow, consistent weight loss when combined with a reduced-calorie diet.

abatacept (a-bat-a-cept)

Orencia

Classification

Therapeutic: antirheumatics (DMARDs)

Pharmacologic: fusion proteins

Indications

Moderate to severely active rheumatoid arthritis in adults (as monotherapy or in combination with other disease modifying antirheumatic drugs, other than tumor-necrosis factor (TNF) inhibitors. Moderate to severely active polyarticular juvenile idiopathic arthritis (as monotherapy or in combination with methotrexate). Active psoriatic arthritis. Prophylaxis of acute graft versus host disease in patients undergoing hematopoietic stem cell transplantation from a matched or 1 allele-mismatched unrelated-donor (in combination with a calcineurin inhibitor and methotrexate).

Action

Inhibits T-cell activation (and the inflammatory process) by binding to specific receptors. **Therapeutic Effects:** Decreased progression of rheumatoid arthritis, juvenile idiopathic arthritis, and psoriatic arthritis. Improved survival and graft versus host disease-free survival in patients undergoing hematopoietic stem cell transplantation.

Pharmacokinetics

Absorption: IV administration results in complete bioavailability.

Distribution: Unknown.

Metabolism and Excretion: Unknown.

Half-life: 13 days.

TIME/ACTION PROFILE (improvement in symptoms)

ROUTE	ONSET	PEAK	DURATION
IV	within 15 days–3 mo	6–12 mo	3 yr (maintenance of response)

Contraindications/Precautions

Contraindicated in: Hypersensitivity; Concurrent use of TNF inhibitors or anakinra.

Use Cautiously in: Chronic obstructive pulmonary disease (↑ risk of exacerbations and other adverse events); OB: Safety not established in pregnancy; Lactation: Safety not established in breastfeeding; Pedi: Safety and effectiveness not established in children <18 yr (rheumatoid arthritis) or 2 yr (all other indications); Geri: ↑ risk of adverse reactions in older adults.

Adverse Reactions/Side Effects

Neuro: headache, dizziness. **Misc:** INFECTION (INCLUDING CYTOMEGALOVIRUS AND EPSTEIN-BARR VIRUS REACTIVATION), HYPERSENSITIVITY REACTIONS (INCLUDING ANAPHYLAXIS), infusion-related events, MALIGNANCY.

Interactions

Drug-Drug: Concurrent use with **TNF antagonists** may ↑ risk and severity of infections. May ↑ risk of adverse reactions and ↓ effectiveness of **live-virus vaccines**.

Route/Dosage

Rheumatoid Arthritis

IV (Adults >100 kg): 1000 mg initially; repeat dose at 2 wk and 4 wk after initial dose, then every 4 wk thereafter.

IV (Adults 60–100 kg): 750 mg initially; repeat dose at 2 wk and 4 wk after initial dose, then every 4 wk thereafter.

IV (Adults <60 kg): 500 mg initially; repeat dose at 2 wk and 4 wk after initial dose, then every 4 wk thereafter.

SUBQ (Adults): Treatment may be initiated with or without a single IV dose (according to weight-based dosing guidelines above); then give 125 mg SUBQ within 1 day; then give 125 mg SUBQ once weekly; if patient does not receive IV dose, initiate once weekly SUBQ injections; if transitioning from IV therapy, administer next scheduled dose as SUBQ injection.

Juvenile Idiopathic Arthritis

IV (Children ≥6 yr and >100 kg): 1000 mg initially; repeat dose at 2 wk and 4 wk after initial dose, then every 4 wk thereafter.

IV (Children ≥6 yr and 75–100 kg): 750 mg initially; repeat dose at 2 wk and 4 wk after initial dose, then every 4 wk thereafter.

IV (Children ≥6 yr and <75 kg): 10 mg/kg initially; repeat dose at 2 wk and 4 wk after initial dose, then every 4 wk thereafter.

SUBQ (Children ≥2 yr and ≥50 kg): 125 mg once weekly.

SUBQ (Children ≥2 yr and 25–<50 kg): 87.5 mg once weekly.

SUBQ (Children ≥2 yr and 10–<25 kg): 50 mg once weekly.

Psoriatic Arthritis

IV (Adults >100 kg): 1000 mg initially; repeat dose at 2 wk and 4 wk after initial dose, then every 4 wk thereafter.

IV (Adults 60–100 kg): 750 mg initially; repeat dose at 2 wk and 4 wk after initial dose, then every 4 wk thereafter.

IV (Adults <60 kg): 500 mg initially; repeat dose at 2 wk and 4 wk after initial dose, then every 4 wk thereafter.

SUBQ (Adults): 125 mg once weekly.

SUBQ (Children ≥2 yr and ≥50 kg): 125 mg once weekly.

SUBQ (Children ≥2 yr and 25–<50 kg): 87.5 mg once weekly.
SUBQ (Children ≥2 yr and 10–<25 kg): 50 mg once weekly.

Prophylaxis of Acute Graft Versus Host Disease

IV (Adults and Children ≥6 yr): 10 mg/kg (max dose = 1000 mg) on the day before transplantation; repeat dose on Days 5, 14, and 28 after transplantation.
IV (Children 2–<6 yr): 15 mg/kg on the day before transplantation, then 12 mg/kg on Days 5, 14, and 28 after transplantation.

Availability

Lyophilized powder for IV administration: 250 mg/vial. **Solution for SUBQ administration (prefilled syringes):** 50 mg/0.4 mL, 87.5 mg/0.7 mL, 125 mg/mL. **Solution for SUBQ administration (prefilled ClickJect autoinjector):** 125 mg/mL.

NURSING IMPLICATIONS

Assessment

- Assess range of motion, degree of swelling, and pain in affected joints before and periodically during therapy.
- Assess for infusion-related reaction (dizziness, headache, hypertension) and signs of allergic reaction (hypotension, urticaria, dyspnea). Infusion-related reactions usually occur within 1 hr of start of infusion. Keep epinephrine, an antihistamine, and resuscitation equipment close by in case of an anaphylactic reaction.
- Assess for latent tuberculosis with a tuberculin skin test. If positive, tuberculosis should be treated prior to abatacept therapy.
- Assess health status at each session. Monitor patients who develop a new infection while taking abatacept closely. Discontinue therapy in patients who develop a serious infection or sepsis. Do not initiate therapy in patients with active infections.
- Monitor for signs and symptoms of hypersensitivity reactions (angioedema) during therapy. Make sure oxygen and supportive measures are available. If reactions occur, discontinue abatacept permanently.

Lab Test Considerations

- Prescreen patient for viral hepatitis prior to therapy; may reactivate hepatitis. If test is positive, do not start abatacept.
- Patients receiving IV abatacept may record false positive blood glucose due to maltose in injection; discuss with health care professional.
- Monitor patient for Epstein-Barr virus and cytomegalovirus infection or reactivation for 6 mo post-transplant. Consider prophylaxis for 6 mo post-transplant.

Implementation

- Do not confuse Orencia with Oracea.
- **Prophylaxis of Acute Graft Versus Host Disease:** Before administering abatacept, administer recommended antiviral prophylactic treatment for Epstein-Barr virus reactivation; continue for 6 mo following hematopoietic stem cell transplantation. Consider prophylactic antivirals for cytomegalovirus infection/reactivation during treatment and for 6 mo following hematopoietic stem cell transplantation.
- **SUBQ**: Remove prefilled syringe from refrigerator and allow to reach room temperature for 30–60 min; do not use other methods to warm solution. Leave needle cover on during warming. Inspect solution; do not administer solutions that are discolored, contain particulate matter, are expired, or do not have the correct amount of fluid in syringe. Front of thigh is the preferred site; abdomen (except for 2 inches from navel) or upper arm, if administered by caregiver, may also be used. Pinch skin and inject at a 45° angle. Do not rub injection site. Rotate each injection at least 1 inch from last injection; avoid areas where skin is tender, bruised, red, or hard or contains scars or stretch marks. *ClickJect autoinjector* should not be used with children <18 yr.

IV Administration

- **Intermittent Infusion: Reconstitution:** Reconstitute each vial with 10 mL of sterile water for injection, using ONLY SILICONE-FREE DISPOSABLE SYRINGE PROVIDED WITH EACH VIAL and an 18–21-gauge needle for a concentration of 25 mg/mL. Discard solutions prepared using siliconized syringes. Additional silicone-free syringes are available from manufacturer. Direct stream of sterile water to side of vial. Rotate vial by gently swirling to minimize foaming. Do not shake. Upon dissolution, vent vial to dissipate foam. Solution should be clear and colorless to pale yellow. Do not use solutions that are discolored or contain particulate matter. **Dilution:** Further dilute solution to 100 mL of 0.9% NaCl by withdrawing volume of abatacept solution from 100 mL infusion bag or bottle. Slowly add reconstituted solution using the same SILICONE-FREE DISPOSABLE SYRINGE PROVIDED WITH EACH VIAL. Mix gently. **Concentration:** 5, 7.5, or 10 mg/mL depending on whether 2, 3, or 4 vials were used. Discard unused portion of vial. Infusion must be completed within 24 hr of reconstitution. Diluted solution may be stored at room temperature or refrigerated before use. **Rate:** Administer over 30 min with a sterile nonpyrogenic, low-protein-binding filter with a 0.2–1.2-micron pore size.
- For prophylaxis of acute graft versus host disease: Administer over 60 min with a sterile nonpyrogenic, low-protein-binding filter with a 0.2–1.2 micron pore size.
- **Y-Site Incompatibility:** Do not infuse in same infusion line as other agents.

Patient/Family Teaching

- Instruct patient on purpose of abatacept. Advise patient to read the *Orencia Patient Information* leaflet prior to each session. Provide an opportunity for patient to ask questions. If a dose is missed, ask health care professional when to schedule next dose.
- Advise patient not to receive live vaccines during or 3 mo following therapy. Advise patients and parents that adults and children should complete immunizations to date before initiation of abatacept.
- Advise patient that methotrexate, analgesics, NSAIDs, corticosteroids, and salicylates may be continued during therapy.
- Instruct patient that abatacept should not be taken with TNF antagonists; may increase risk for infections.
- Instruct patient to notify health care professional if signs and symptoms of upper respiratory or other infections or hypersensitivity reactions occur. Therapy may need to be discontinued if serious infection occurs.
- Inform patient of increased risk of malignancies, including skin cancer. Advise patient to examine skin regularly for new or changes in lesions. Notify health care professional if changes in skin are seen.
- Rep: Advise patient to notify health care professional if pregnancy is planned or suspected. Caution patient to avoid breastfeeding during therapy.

Evaluation/Desired Outcomes

- Reduction in symptoms of rheumatoid arthritis, juvenile idiopathic arthritis, and psoriatic arthritis.
- Improved survival and acute graft versus host disease-free survival in patients undergoing hematopoietic stem cell transplantation.

HIGH ALERT

abemaciclib (a-bem-a-**sye**-klib)

Verzenio

Classification

Therapeutic: antineoplastics

Pharmacologic: kinase inhibitors

Indications

Adjuvant treatment of hormone receptor (HR)-positive, human epidermal growth factor 2 (HER2)-negative, node-positive early breast cancer at high risk of recurrence (in combination with tamoxifen or an aromatase inhibitor). Advanced or metastatic HR-positive, HER2-negative breast cancer in patients with disease progression following endocrine therapy (in combination with fulvestrant). HR-positive, HER2-negative advanced or metastatic breast cancer in patients with disease progression following endocrine therapy and prior chemotherapy in the metastatic setting (as monotherapy). HR-positive, HER2-negative advanced or metastatic breast cancer (as initial endocrine-based therapy in combination with an aromatase inhibitor).

Action

Inhibits kinases (cyclin-dependent kinases 4 and 6) that are part of the signaling pathway for cell proliferation. **Therapeutic Effects:** Improved survival and decreased spread of breast cancer.

Pharmacokinetics

Absorption: 45% absorbed following oral administration.

Distribution: Extensively distributed to tissues.

Protein Binding: 96%.

Metabolism and Excretion: Primarily metabolized in the liver by CYP3A4 to several active metabolites; 81% excreted in feces, 3% in urine.

Half-life: 18.3 hr.

TIME/ACTION PROFILE (plasma concentrations)

ROUTE	ONSET	PEAK	DURATION
PO	unknown	8 hr	24 hr

Contraindications/Precautions

Contraindicated in: OB: Pregnancy; Lactation: Lactation.

Use Cautiously in: Severe renal impairment (CCr <30 mL/min); Severe hepatic impairment (↓ dose); History of venous thromboembolism; Rep: Women of reproductive potential; Pedi: Safety and effectiveness not established in children.

Adverse Reactions/Side Effects

CV: peripheral edema, DEEP VEIN THROMBOSIS (DVT). **Derm:** alopecia, pruritus, rash. **GI:** ↑ liver enzymes, abdominal pain, constipation, diarrhea, dry mouth, nausea, stomatitis, vomiting, HEPATOTOXICITY. **GU:** ↑ serum creatinine, ↓ fertility (men). **Hemat:** ANEMIA, LEUKOPENIA, NEUTROPENIA, THROMBOCYTOPENIA. **Metab:** ↓ appetite, weight loss. **MS:** arthralgia. **Neuro:** dizziness, dysgeusia, fatigue, headache. **Resp:** cough, INTERSTITIAL LUNG DISEASE/PNEUMONITIS, PULMONARY EMBOLISM (PE). **Misc:** fever, INFECTION.

Interactions

Drug-Drug: Strong CYP3A inhibitors, including **itraconazole** or **ketoconazole**, may ↑ levels and risk of toxicity; avoid concurrent use with ketoconazole; ↓ abemaciclib dose when using other strong CYP3A4 inhibitors (resume original dose after 3–5 half-lives of offending drug have passed following discontinuation). **Strong CYP3A inducers**, including **rifampin**, may ↓ levels and effectiveness; avoid concurrent use.

Route/Dosage

PO (Adults): *With fulvestrant, tamoxifen, or an aromatase inhibitor:* 150 mg twice daily; for early breast cancer, continue for 2 yr or until disease progression or unacceptable toxicity; for advanced or metastatic breast cancer, continue until disease progression or unacceptable toxicity. *As monotherapy:* 200 mg twice daily; continue until disease progression or unacceptable toxicity. *Concurrent use of strong CYP3A inhibitor (other then ketoconazole):* 100 mg twice daily (with fulvestrant, tamoxifen, an aromatase inhibitor, or as monotherapy); if dose already at 100 mg twice daily due to adverse reactions, ↓ dose to 50 mg twice daily; for early breast cancer, continue for 2 yr or until disease progression or unacceptable toxicity; for advanced or metastatic breast cancer, continue until disease progression or unacceptable toxicity.

Hepatic Impairment

PO (Adults): *Severe hepatic impairment:* With fulvestrant, tamoxifen, or an aromatase inhibitor: 150 mg once daily; for early breast cancer, continue for 2 yr or until disease progression or unacceptable toxicity; for advanced or metastatic breast cancer, continue until disease progression or unacceptable toxicity. As monotherapy: 200 mg once daily; continue until disease progression or unacceptable toxicity. Concurrent use of strong CYP3A inhibitor (other than ketoconazole): 100 mg once daily (with fulvestrant, tamoxifen, an aromatase inhibitor, or as monotherapy); if dose already at 100 mg once daily due to adverse reactions, ↓ dose to 50 mg once daily; for early breast cancer, continue for 2 yr or until disease progression or unacceptable toxicity; for advanced or metastatic breast cancer, continue until disease progression or unacceptable toxicity.

Availability

Tablets: 50 mg, 100 mg, 150 mg, 200 mg.

NURSING IMPLICATIONS

Assessment

- Monitor for diarrhea; may result in dehydration and infection. *If Grade 1 diarrhea,* no dose ↓ required. *If Grade 2 diarrhea,* if diarrhea resolves in 24 hr to Grade ≤1, hold therapy until resolution. No dose ↓ required. *If Grade 2 diarrhea that persists or recurs after resuming same dose despite maximum supportive measures,* hold dose until diarrhea resolves to Grade ≤1. Resume at next lower dose. *If Grade 3 or 4 diarrhea or diarrhea that requires hospitalization,* hold therapy until diarrhea resolves to Grade ≤1; then resume at next lower dose.
- Monitor for signs and symptoms of DVT and PE and treat as needed.
- Monitor weight throughout therapy, and for ↓ in appetite.

Lab Test Considerations

- Verify negative pregnancy test before starting therapy.
- Monitor CBC with differential before starting, every 2 wk for 1st 2 mo, monthly for next 2 mo, and as clinically indicated. *If Grade 1 or 2 neutropenia,* no dose ↓ required. *If Grade 3 neutropenia,* hold dose until resolves to Grade ≤2. *If Grade 3 recurrent or Grade 4 neutropenia,* hold therapy until resolved to Grade ≤2. Resume at next lower dose.
- Monitor ALT, AST, and serum bilirubin prior to starting therapy, every 2 wk for 1st 2 mo, monthly for next 2 mo, and as clinically indicated. *If Grade 1 (AST and/or ALT > upper limit of normal [ULN] to 3 times ULN), Grade 2 (AST and/or ALT >3–5 times ULN, without ↑ in total bilirubin >2 times ULN),* no dose ↓ required. *If persistent or recurrent Grade 2 AST and/or ALT ↑, or Grade 3 (AST and/or ALT >5–20 times ULN), without ↑ in total bilirubin above 2 times ULN,* hold therapy until toxicity resolves to Grade ≤1. Resume at next lower dose. *If AST and/or ALT >3 times ULN with total bilirubin >2 times ULN, in the absence of cholestasis or Grade 4 (AST and/or ALT >20 times ULN),* permanently discontinue abemaciclib.
- May ↑ serum creatinine without glomerular function being affected. Monitor BUN, cystatin C, or calculated glomerular filtration rate to determine impaired renal function.

Implementation

- **Dose Reduction Recommendations:** *1st dose reduction:* 100 twice daily for combination therapy OR 150 mg twice daily for monotherapy. *2nd dose reduction:* 50 mg twice daily for combination therapy OR 100 mg twice daily for monotherapy. *3rd dose reduction:* Discontinue combination therapy OR 50 mg twice daily for monotherapy.
- **PO:** Administer twice daily, at the same times each day, without regard to food. ***DNC:*** Swallow tablets whole; do not crush, break, or chew.

Patient/Family Teaching

- Explain purpose and side effects of medication to patient. Advise patient to read *Patient Information* before starting therapy and with each Rx refill in case of changes. Instruct patient to take at the same time each day as directed. If patient vomits or misses a dose, omit dose and take next dose as scheduled. Do not ingest tablets that are broken, cracked, or not intact.
- Instruct patient to notify health care professional of all Rx or OTC medications, vitamins, or herbal products being taken and to consult with health care professional before taking other medications.
- Advise patient that at first sign of diarrhea, start antidiarrheal therapy (loperamide), ↑ oral fluids, and notify health care professional.
- Advise patient to notify health care professional if signs and symptoms of infection (fever, chills), liver problems (feeling very tired, pain on upper right side of abdomen, loss of appetite, weight loss, unusual bleeding or bruising), or venous

thromboembolism (pain or swelling in arms or legs, shortness of breath, chest pain, rapid breathing, rapid heart rate) occur.

- Rep: May cause fetal harm. Advise women of reproductive potential to use effective contraception and avoid breastfeeding during therapy and for >3 wk after last dose. Inform health care professional if pregnancy is planned or suspected. May impair male fertility.

Evaluation/Desired Outcomes

- Improved survival and decreased spread of breast cancer.

HIGH ALERT

abiraterone (a-bi-ra-te-rone)

Yonsa, Zytiga

Classification

Therapeutic: antineoplastics

Pharmacologic: enzyme inhibitors

Indications

Zytiga: Treatment of the following conditions: Metastatic castration-resistant prostate cancer (in combination with prednisone). Metastatic high-risk castration-sensitive prostate cancer (in combination with prednisone). **Yonsa:** Metastatic castration-resistant prostate cancer (in combination with methylprednisolone).

Action

Inhibits the enzyme 17α-hydroxylase/C17,20-lyase (CYP17), which is required for androgen production. May also result in increased mineralocortocoid production. **Therapeutic Effects:** Decreased androgen production with decreased spread of androgen-sensitive prostate cancer.

Pharmacokinetics

Absorption: Hydrolyzed to its active compound following oral administration.
Distribution: Widely distributed to tissues.
Protein Binding: >99%.
Metabolism and Excretion: Metabolized by esterases to inactive compounds; eliminated primarily in feces as unchanged drug and metabolites; 5% excreted in urine.
Half-life: 12 hr.

TIME/ACTION PROFILE (plasma concentrations)

ROUTE	ONSET	PEAK	DURATION
PO	unknown	2 hr	12 hr

Contraindications/Precautions

Contraindicated in: Severe hepatic impairment; Concurrent use of radium Ra 223 dichloride (↑ risk of fractures and mortality).

Use Cautiously in: HF, recent MI, other cardiovascular disease, or ventricular arrhythmias; Electrolyte abnormalities or hypertension (correct/treat prior to initiation); Stress, infection, trauma, or acute disease process (may result in adrenocortical insufficiency requiring additional corticosteroids); Moderate hepatic impairment; Rep: Men with female partners of reproductive potential.

Adverse Reactions/Side Effects

CV: hypertension, arrhythmia, edema, QT interval prolongation (in presence of hypokalemia), TORSADES DE POINTES (IN PRESENCE OF HYPOKALEMIA). **Derm:** hot flushing. **Endo:** adrenocortical insufficiency (due to concurrent corticosteroid), hypoglycemia. **F and E** hypokalemia. **GI:** diarrhea, dyspepsia, HEPATOTOXICITY. **GU:** ↓ fertility, nocturia, urinary frequency. **MS:** fracture, joint pain/discomfort. **Resp:** cough.

Interactions

Drug-Drug: May ↑ levels of and risk of toxicity from **CYP2D6 substrates**, including **thioridazine** and **dextromethorphan**; if concurrent use necessary, ↓ dose of CYP2D6 substrate. May ↑ levels of and risk of toxicity from **CYP2C8 substrates**, including **pioglitazone**; if concurrent use necessary, ↓ dose of CYP2C8 substrate may be required. **Strong CYP3A4 inducers**, including **carbamazepine**, **phenobarbital**, **phenytoin**, **rifabutin**, **rifapentine**, or **rifampin**, may ↓ levels and effectiveness; avoid concurrent use. May ↑ risk of hypoglycemia when used with **pioglitazone** or **repaglinide**.

Route/Dosage

Zytiga and Yonsa are not interchangeable.

Zytiga

PO (Adults): 1000 mg once daily; *Concurrent use with strong CYP3A4 inducer:* 1000 mg twice daily.

Hepatic Impairment

PO (Adults): *Moderate hepatic impairment:* 250 mg once daily.

Yonsa

PO (Adults): 500 mg once daily; *Concurrent use with strong CYP3A4 inducer:* 500 mg twice daily.

Hepatic Impairment

PO (Adults): *Moderate hepatic impairment:* 125 mg once daily.

Availability

Tablets (Zytiga): 250 mg, 500 mg. **Tablets (Yonsa):** 125 mg.

NURSING IMPLICATIONS

Assessment

- Monitor BP and assess for fluid retention monthly. Control hypertension during therapy.
- Monitor for signs and symptoms of adrenocortical insufficiency (hypotension, weight loss, weakness, nausea, vomiting, anorexia, lethargy, confusion, restlessness), especially in patients under stress or who are withdrawn from or have ↓ prednisone dose. Symptoms may be masked by abiraterone.

Lab Test Considerations

- Monitor AST, ALT, and bilirubin before starting therapy, every 2 wk for 3 mo, and monthly thereafter. Administer ↓ dose to patients with baseline moderate hepatic impairment and monitor AST, ALT, and bilirubin before starting therapy, every wk for first mo, every 2 wk for 2 mo, and monthly thereafter. If clinical signs of hepatic toxicity occur, measure serum bilirubin, AST, and ALT promptly; monitor frequently if ↑ levels. *If AST and/or ALT ↑ >5 times upper limit of normal (ULN) or bilirubin ↑ >3 times ULN in patients with baseline moderate hepatic impairment,* hold therapy. Following return of liver function to baseline or AST and ALT ↑>2.5 times ULN or bilirubin ↑ >1.5 times ULN, may restart at ↓ dose of 750 mg once daily. Monitor AST, ALT, and bilirubin every 2 wk for 3 mo and monthly thereafter. If hepatotoxicity recurs, may restart at 500 mg once daily following return to baseline or AST and ALT ↑>2.5 times ULN or bilirubin ↑ >1.5 times ULN. If hepatotoxicity recurs at 500 mg once daily dose, permanently discontinue abiraterone. *If concurrent ↑ ALT >3 times ULN and total bilirubin ↑>2 times ULN without biliary obstruction or other causes,* permanently discontinue abiraterone.
- Monitor serum potassium and sodium at least monthly during therapy. May cause hypokalemia correct prior to starting and during therapy.
- May ↑ triglycerides and ↓ phosphorous.

Implementation

- Patients should receive a gonadotropin-releasing hormone analog concurrently or should have had bilateral orchiectomy.
- ***DNC:*** Swallow tablets whole with water; do not crush, break, or chew.
- **Zytiga:** *For castration-resistant prostate cancer:* Administer once daily with prednisone 5 mg twice daily on an empty stomach >1 hr before or 2 hr after meals; food ↑ absorption and adverse reactions. *For castration-sensitive prostate cancer:* Administer once daily with prednisone 5 mg once daily on an empty stomach >1 hr before or 2 hr after meals; food ↑ absorption.
- **Yonsa:** Administer orally once daily in combination with methylprednisolone 4 mg orally twice daily. Administer without regard to meals.

Patient/Family Teaching

- Explain purpose and side effects of medication to patient. Advise to read *Patient Information* before starting therapy. Instruct patient to take medications as directed and not to stop abiraterone, prednisone, methylprednisolone, or gonadotropin-releasing hormone analog without consulting health care professional. If a dose is missed, take the following day. If >1 dose is missed, consult health care professional. Explain need for continued follow-up exams and lab tests to assess possible side effects.
- Advise parents to notify health care professional of all Rx or OTC medications, vitamins, or herbal products being taken and to consult with health care professional before taking other medications.
- Advise patient to notify health care professional if signs and symptoms of high BP, low potassium, and fluid retention (dizziness, fast heartbeat, feeling faint or light-headed, headache, confusion, muscle weakness, pain in legs, swelling in legs or feet); adrenal insufficiency; or hepatotoxicity (yellowing of skin and eyes, dark urine, pain in upper right quadrant, severe nausea or vomiting, difficulty concentrating, disorientation, confusion) occur or of side effects that are bothersome or persistent.
- Rep: Advise patients to use effective contraception methods during sex, throughout therapy, and for 3 wk after therapy. Individuals who are pregnant or of reproductive potential should not touch tablets without wearing gloves. May impair reproductive function and fertility in men of reproductive potential.

Evaluation/Desired Outcomes

- Decreased androgen production with decreased spread of androgen-sensitive prostate cancer.

abrocitinib

(a-broe-**sye**-ti-nib)

Cibinqo

Classification

Therapeutic: anti-inflammatories

Pharmacologic: kinase inhibitors

Indications

Refractory moderate to severe atopic dermatitis in patients whose disease is not adequately controlled with other systemic drug products, including biologics, or when use of those therapies are not recommended (not to be used with other JAK inhibitors, biologic immunomodulators, or other immunosuppressants).

A

Action

Inhibits JAK enzymes, which prevents the signaling of interleukin-4, interleukin-13, and other cytokines involved in the pathogenesis of atopic dermatitis.
Therapeutic Effects: Improvement in clinical and symptomatic parameters of atopic dermatitis.

Pharmacokinetics

Absorption: Well absorbed following oral administration.
Distribution: Extensively distributed to tissues.
Metabolism and Excretion: Primarily metabolized by the liver via the CYP2C19, CYP2C9, CYP3A4, and CYP2B6 isoenzymes into two active metabolites (M1 and M2). 2% of White people, 4% of Black people, and 14% of Asian people have CYP2C19 genotype that results in ↓ metabolism of abrocitinib. Primarily excreted in urine (<1% as unchanged drug).
Half-life: 3–5 hr.

TIME/ACTION PROFILE (plasma concentrations)

ROUTE	ONSET	PEAK	DURATION
PO	rapid	<1 hr	unknown

Contraindications/Precautions

Contraindicated in: Concurrent use of antiplatelet therapies (excluding low-dose aspirin [≤81 mg/day]) for the 1st 3 mo of treatment; Active infection; Platelet count <150,000/mm³, lymphocyte count <500 cells/mm³, ANC <1000 cells/mm³, or hemoglobin level <8 g/dL; ↑ risk for thrombosis; Severe renal impairment or end-stage renal disease; Severe hepatic impairment; Lactation: Lactation.
Use Cautiously in: Patients who are >50 yr old and have ≥1 cardiovascular risk factor (↑ risk of all-cause mortality, cardiovascular death, MI, stroke, and thrombosis); Chronic or recurrent infection; Previously exposed to tuberculosis (TB); History of serious or opportunistic infection; Resided or traveled in areas of endemic tuberculosis or endemic mycoses; Underlying conditions that predispose to infection; Malignancy (other than successfully treated nonmelanoma skin cancer); Current or previous smoker (↑ risk of malignancy); Known or suspected CYP2C19 poor metabolizers (↓ dose); Moderate renal impairment (↓ dose); OB: Other agents for atopic dermatitis preferred in pregnancy; Pedi: Children <12 yr (safety and effectiveness not established); Geri: Older adults may have ↑ risk of lymphopenia, thrombocytopenia, and herpes infection.

Adverse Reactions/Side Effects

CV: CARDIOVASCULAR DEATH, DEEP VEIN THROMBOSIS (DVT), hypertension, MI. **Derm:** acne, contact dermatitis, impetigo. **EENT:** nasopharyngitis, retinal detachment. **GI:** nausea, abdominal pain, oropharyngeal pain, vomiting. **Hemat:** lymphopenia, thrombocytopenia. **Metab:** hyperlipidemia. **MS:** ↑ CK. **Neuro:** dizziness, fatigue, headache, STROKE. **Resp:** PULMONARY EMBOLISM (PE). **Misc:** INFECTION (INCLUDING SERIOUS BACTERIAL, FUNGAL, VIRAL, OR OPPORTUNISTIC INFECTIONS, INCLUDING TB), MALIGNANCY (INCLUDING NONMELANOMA SKIN CANCER).

Interactions

Drug-Drug: May ↑ risk of bleeding and thrombocytopenia when used with **antiplatelet drugs**, excluding low-dose **aspirin** (≤81 mg/day); concurrent use during 1st 3 mo of abrocitinib contraindicated. **Moderate to strong inhibitors of both CYP2C9 and CYP2C19**, including **fluconazole**, significantly ↑ levels and risk of toxicity; avoid concurrent use. **Strong CYP2C9 inducers** and **strong CYP2C19 inducers**, including **rifampin**, ↓ levels and effectiveness; avoid concurrent use. **Strong CYP2C19 inhibitors**, including **fluvoxamine**, may ↑ levels and risk of toxicity; ↓ abrocitinib dose. May ↑ levels and risk of toxicity of **P-glycoprotein substrates**, including **dabigatran**; closely monitor. May ↑ risk of adverse reactions and ↓ antibody response to **live vaccines**; avoid concurrent use.

Route/Dosage

PO (Adults and Children ≥12 yr): 100 mg once daily initially; if adequate response not achieved after 12 wk, may ↑ to 200 mg once daily. Discontinue therapy if inadequate response after dose ↑ to 200 mg once daily. *CYP2C19 poor metabolizers or concurrent use of strong CYP2C19 inhibitors:* 50 mg once daily initially; if adequate response not achieved after 12 wk, may ↑ to 100 mg once daily. Discontinue therapy if inadequate response after dose ↑ to 100 mg once daily.

Renal Impairment

PO (Adults and Children ≥12 yr): *CCr 30–59 mL/min:* 50 mg once daily initially; if adequate response not achieved after 12 wk, may ↑ to 100 mg once daily. Discontinue therapy if inadequate response after dose ↑ to 100 mg once daily.

Availability

Tablets: 50 mg, 100 mg, 200 mg.

NURSING IMPLICATIONS

Assessment

- Assess involved area of skin before starting and periodically during therapy.
- Determine TB infection status. For patients with latent TB or those with a negative latent TB test who are at high risk for TB, start preventive therapy for latent TB before starting abrocitinib. Monitor all patients for active TB during treatment, even patients with initial negative latent TB test.

- Conduct viral hepatitis screening in accordance with clinical guidelines. Starting abrocitinib is not recommended in patients with active hepatitis B or hepatitis C.
- Monitor for development of signs and symptoms of infection, including TB, during and after therapy. If a serious or opportunistic infection, discontinue therapy. Begin diagnostic testing and antimicrobial therapy. Consider risks and benefits of therapy before reinitiating therapy.
- Monitor for signs and symptoms of major adverse cardiac events. Patients who are current or past smokers and patients with other cardiovascular risk factors are at greatest risk.
- Monitor for thrombosis, including DVT, PE, and arterial thrombosis. If symptoms of thrombosis occur, discontinue therapy and evaluate and treat patients.

Lab Test Considerations

- Monitor CBC with differential at baseline, 4 wk after starting therapy, and 4 wk after ↑ dose. *If platelet count <50,000/mm³*, permanently discontinue abrocitinib and follow with CBC until >100,000/mm³. *If ALC <500/mm³*, temporarily discontinue abrocitinib; may be restarted once ALC returns above this value. *If ANC <1000/mm³*, temporarily discontinue abrocitinib; may be restarted once ANC returns above this value. *If Hgb <8 g/dL*, temporarily discontinue abrocitinib; may be restarted once Hgb returns above this value.
- May ↑ lipids. Monitor lipid levels after 4 wk of therapy and periodically thereafter.

Implementation

- Complete any necessary immunizations, including herpes zoster vaccinations, in agreement with current immunization guidelines prior to starting therapy.
- Can be used with or without topical corticosteroids.
- **PO:** Administer without regard to food, at the same time each day. ***DNC:*** Swallow tablets whole with water; do not crush, split, or chew.

Patient/Family Teaching

- Explain purpose and side effects of medication to patient. Advise patient to read *Patient Information* before starting therapy. Instruct patient to take as directed. Take missed dose as soon as possible unless <12 hr before next dose. If <12 hr before next dose, omit dose and resume dosing at the regular scheduled time.
- Instruct patient to notify health care professional of all Rx or OTC medications, vitamins, or herbal products being taken and to consult with health care professional before taking other medications.
- Advise patient to notify health care professional if signs and symptoms of infection (fever, sweating, or chills; blood in phlegm; diarrhea or stomach pain; muscle aches; weight loss; burning during urination or urinating more often than usual; cough or shortness of breath; warm, red, or painful skin or sores on body; feeling very tired) occur.
- Caution patients with signs and symptoms of a heart attack or stroke (discomfort in the center of chest that lasts for more than a few minutes or that goes away and comes back; severe tightness, pain, pressure, or heaviness in chest, throat, neck, or jaw; pain or discomfort in arms, back, neck, jaw, or stomach; weakness in one part or on one side of the body; slurred speech; shortness of breath with or without chest discomfort; breaking out in a cold sweat; nausea or vomiting; light-headedness) to notify health care professional immediately.
- Inform patient of ↑ risk of DVT and pulmonary embolism. If signs and symptoms (swelling, pain, or tenderness in one or both legs; sudden, unexplained chest or upper back pain; shortness of breath or difficulty breathing) occur, stop therapy and get immediate medical care. Advise patient to notify health care professional if they have had blood clots in the legs or lungs in the past.
- May ↑ risk of cancer. Advise patient to have skin checked for skin cancer during therapy. Limit amount of time spent in sunlight. Avoid using tanning beds or sunlamps. Wear protective clothing and use sunscreen with a high protection factor (SPF 30 and above); especially important for patients with very fair skin or with a family history of skin cancer. Instruct patient to notify health care professional if they have ever had any type of cancer.
- Rep: Advise women of reproductive potential to notify health care professional if pregnancy is planned or suspected. Advise to avoid breastfeeding during and for one day after last dose. May impair female fertility; may be reversible. There is a pregnancy exposure registry that monitors pregnancy outcomes in women exposed to abrocitinib during pregnancy. Pregnant women exposed to abrocitinib and health care providers are encouraged to call 1-877-311-3770 or visit www.cibinqopregnancyregistry.com.

Evaluation/Desired Outcomes

- Improvement in clinical and symptomatic parameters of atopic dermatitis.

acebutolol, See BETA BLOCKERS (selective).

acetaminophen

(a-seet-a-**min**-oh-fen)

✱ Abenol, ✱ Acet, ✱ Children Feverhalt, ✱ Fortolin, Infant's Feverall, ~~Ofirmev,~~ ✱ Pediaphen, ✱ Pediatrix, ✱ Taminol, ✱ Tempra, Tylenol

Classification

Therapeutic: antipyretics, nonopioid analgesics

Indications

PO, Rect Treatment of: Mild pain, Fever. **IV:** Treatment of: Mild to moderate pain, Moderate to severe pain with opioid analgesics, Fever.

Action

Inhibits synthesis of prostaglandins that may serve as mediators of pain and fever, primarily in the CNS. Has no significant anti-inflammatory properties or GI toxicity. **Therapeutic Effects:** Analgesia. Antipyresis.

Pharmacokinetics

Absorption: Well absorbed following oral administration. Rectal absorption is variable. Intravenous administration results in complete bioavailability.
Distribution: Widely distributed. Crosses the placenta; enters breast milk in low concentrations.
Metabolism and Excretion: 85–95% metabolized by the liver (CYP2E1 enzyme system). Metabolites may be toxic in overdose situation. Metabolites excreted by the kidneys.
Half-life: *Neonates:* 7 hr; *Infants and Children:* 3–4 hr; *Adults:* 1–3 hr.

TIME/ACTION PROFILE (analgesia and antipyresis)

ROUTE	ONSET	PEAK	DURATION
PO	0.5–1 hr	1–3 hr	3–8 hr†
Rect	0.5–1 hr	1–3 hr	3–4 hr
IV‡	within 30 min	30 min	4–6 hr

† Depends on dose.
‡ Antipyretic effects.

Contraindications/Precautions

Contraindicated in: Previous hypersensitivity; Products containing alcohol, aspartame, saccharin, sugar, or tartrazine (FDC yellow dye #5) should be avoided in patients who have hypersensitivity or intolerance to these compounds; Severe hepatic impairment/active liver disease.
Use Cautiously in: Hepatic disease/renal disease (lower chronic doses recommended); Alcoholism, chronic malnutrition, severe hypovolemia, or severe renal impairment (CCr <30 mL/min, ↑ dosing interval and ↓ daily dose may be necessary); Chronic alcohol use/abuse; Malnutrition; OB: Use in pregnancy only if clearly needed (for IV); Lactation: Use cautiously (for IV).

Adverse Reactions/Side Effects

CV: hypertension (IV), hypotension (IV). **Derm:** ACUTE GENERALIZED EXANTHEMATOUS PUSTULOSIS, rash, STEVENS-JOHNSON SYNDROME (SJS), TOXIC EPIDERMAL NECROLYSIS, urticaria. **F and E:** hypokalemia (IV). **GI:** ↑ liver enzymes, constipation (↑ in children) (IV), HEPATOTOXICITY (WITH HIGHER DOSES), nausea (IV), vomiting (IV). **GU:** renal failure (high doses/chronic use). **Hemat:** neutropenia, pancytopenia. **MS:** muscle spasms (IV), trismus (IV). **Neuro:** agitation (↑ in children) (IV), anxiety (IV), fatigue (IV), headache (IV), insomnia (IV). **Resp:** atelectasis (↑ in children) (IV), dyspnea (IV).

Interactions

Drug-Drug: Chronic high-dose acetaminophen (>2 g/day) may ↑ risk of bleeding with **warfarin** (INR should not exceed 4). Hepatotoxicity is additive with other **hepatotoxic substances**, including **alcohol**. Concurrent use of **isoniazid**, **rifampin**, **rifabutin**, **phenytoin**, **barbiturates**, and **carbamazepine** may ↑ the risk of acetaminophen-induced liver damage (limit self-medication); these agents will also ↓ therapeutic effects of acetaminophen. Concurrent use of **NSAIDs** may ↑ the risk of adverse renal effects (avoid chronic concurrent use). **Propranolol** ↓ metabolism and may ↑ effects. May ↓ effects of **lamotrigine** and **zidovudine**.

Route/Dosage

Children ≤12 yr should not receive >5 PO or rectal doses/24 hr without notifying physician or other health care professional. No dose adjustment needed when converting between IV and PO acetaminophen in adults and children ≥50 kg
PO (Adults and Children >12 yr): 325–650 mg every 6 hr or 1 g 3–4 times daily or 1300 mg every 8 hr (not to exceed 3 g or 2 g/24 hr in patients with hepatic/renal impairment).
PO (Children 1–12 yr): 10–15 mg/kg/dose every 6 hr as needed (not to exceed 5 doses/24 hr).
PO (Infants): 10–15 mg/kg/dose every 6 hr as needed (not to exceed 5 doses/24 hr).
PO (Neonates): 10–15 mg/kg/dose every 6–8 hr as needed.
IV (Adults and Children ≥13 yr and ≥50 kg): 1000 mg every 6 hr or 650 mg every 4 hr (not to exceed 1000 mg/dose, 4 g/day [by all routes], and less than 4 hr dosing interval).
IV (Adults and Children ≥13 yr and <50 kg): 15 mg/kg every 6 hr or 12.5 mg/kg every 4 hr (not to exceed 15 mg/kg/dose [up to 750 mg/dose], 75 mg/kg/day [up to 3750 mg/day] [by all routes], and less than 4 hr dosing interval).
IV (Children 2–12 yr): 15 mg/kg every 6 hr or 12.5 mg/kg every 4 hr (not to exceed 15 mg/kg/dose [up to 750 mg/dose], 75 mg/kg/day [up to 3750 mg/day] [by all routes], and less than 4 hr dosing interval).
IV (Infants 29 days–2 yr): 15 mg/kg every 6 hr (not to exceed 60 mg/kg/day [by all routes]).
IV (Neonates Birth–28 days): 12.5 mg/kg every 6 hr (not to exceed 50 mg/kg [by all routes]).
Rect (Adults and Children >12 yr): 325–650 mg every 4–6 hr as needed or 1 g 3–4 times/day (not to exceed 4 g/24 hr).

Rect (Children 1–12 yr): 10–20 mg/kg/dose every 4–6 hr as needed.
Rect (Infants): 10–20 mg/kg/dose every 4–6 hr as needed.
Rect (Neonates): 10–15 mg/kg/dose every 6–8 hr as needed.

Availability

Chewable tablets (fruit, bubblegum, or grape flavor): 80 mg[OTC], 160 mg[OTC]. **Tablets:** 160 mg[OTC], 325 mg[OTC]. **Caplets:** 325 mg[OTC]. **Solution (berry, fruit, and grape flavor):** 100 mg/mL[OTC]. **Liquid (mint):** 160 mg/5 mL[OTC]. **Elixir (grape and cherry flavor):** 160 mg/5 mL[OTC]. **Drops:** 160 mg/ 5 mL [OTC]. **Suspension:** 🍁 100 mg/mL[OTC]🍁 160 mg/5 mL[OTC]. **Syrup:** 160 mg/5 mL[OTC]. **Suppositories:** 80 mg[OTC], 120 mg[OTC], 325 mg[OTC]. **Solution for injection:** 10 mg/mL. ***In combination with:*** many other medications. See Appendix N.

NURSING IMPLICATIONS

Assessment

- Assess overall health status and alcohol usage before administering acetaminophen. Patients who are malnourished or chronically abuse alcohol are at higher risk of developing hepatotoxicity with chronic use of usual doses of this drug.
- Assess amount, frequency, and type of drugs taken in patients self-medicating, especially with OTC drugs. Prolonged use of acetaminophen ↑ risk of adverse hepatic and renal effects. Do not exceed maximum daily dose of acetaminophen when considering all routes of administration and all combination products containing acetaminophen.
- Assess for rash periodically during therapy. May cause SJS. Discontinue therapy if rash (reddening of skin, blisters, and detachment of upper surface of skin peeling) or if accompanied with fever, general malaise, fatigue, muscle or joint aches, blisters, oral lesions, conjunctivitis, hepatitis, or eosinophilia.
- **Pain:** Assess type, location, and intensity prior to and 30–60 min following administration.
- **Fever:** Assess fever; note presence of associated signs (diaphoresis, tachycardia, and malaise).

Lab Test Considerations

- Evaluate hepatic, hematologic, and renal function periodically during prolonged high-dose therapy.
- May alter results of blood glucose monitoring. May cause falsely ↓ values when measured with glucose oxidase/peroxidase method, but probably not with hexokinase/G6PD method. May also cause falsely ↑ values with certain instruments; see manufacturer's instruction manual.
- ↑ serum bilirubin, LDH, AST, ALT, and prothrombin time may indicate hepatotoxicity.

Toxicity and Overdose

- If overdose occurs, **N-acetylcysteine** is the antidote.

Implementation

- Do not confuse Tylenol with Tylenol PM. Do not confuse acetaminophen with acetazolamide.
- To prevent fatal medication errors with IV dosing, ensure dose in milligrams (mg) and milliliters (mL) is not confused, dosing is based on weight for patients under 50 kg, infusion pump is programmed for accuracy, and total daily dose of acetaminophen from all sources does not exceed maximum daily limits.
- When combined with opioids, do not exceed the maximum recommended daily dose of acetaminophen.
- **PO:** Administer with a full glass of water.
- May be taken with food or on an empty stomach.

IV Administration

- **Intermittent Infusion:** *For 1000 mg dose*, insert vented IV set through septum of 100 mL vial; may be administered without further dilution. *For doses <1000 mg*, withdraw appropriate dose from vial and place in a separate empty, sterile container for IV infusion. Place small volume pediatric doses up to 60 mL in a syringe and administer via syringe pump. Solution is clear and colorless; do not administer solutions that are discolored or contain particulate matter. Administer within 6 hr of breaking vial seal. **Rate:** Infuse over 15 min. Monitor end of infusion in order to prevent air embolism, especially if acetaminophen is primary infusion.
- **Y-Site Compatibility:** buprenorphine, butorphanol, caffeine citrate, cefazolin, cefoxitin, ceftriaxone, clindamycin, D5W, defibrotide, dexamethasone, dexmedetomidine, D10W, D5/LR, D5/0.9% NaCl, diphenhydramine, droperidol, esmolol, gentamicin, granisetron, haloperidol, heparin, hydrocortisone, hydromorphone, hydroxyzine, ketamine, LR, labetalol, lidocaine, lorazepam, magnesium sulfate, mannitol, meperidine, methylprednisolone, metoclopramide, metoprolol, midazolam, morphine, nalbuphine, 0.9% NaCl, ondansetron, oxytocin, piperacillin/tazobactam, potassium chloride, prochlorperazine, protamine, remimazolam, rocuronium, sildenafil, sufentanil, vancomycin.
- **Y-Site Incompatibility:** acyclovir, blinatumomab, chlorpromazine, diazepam, metronidazole, phenobarbital, phenytoin, posaconazole, propofol.

Patient/Family Teaching

- Advise patient to take medication exactly as directed and not to take more than the recommended amount. Chronic excessive use of >4 g/day (2 g in chronic alcoholics) may lead to hepatotoxicity, renal, or cardiac damage. Adults should not take acetaminophen longer than 10 days and children not longer than 5 days unless directed by health care professional. Short-term doses of acetaminophen with salicylates or NSAIDs should not exceed recommended daily dose of either drug alone.

- Advise patient to avoid alcohol (3 or more glasses per day increase the risk of liver damage) if taking more than an occasional 1–2 doses and to avoid taking concurrently with salicylates or NSAIDs for more than a few days, unless directed by health care professional.
- Advise patient to discontinue acetaminophen and notify health care professional if rash occurs.
- Inform patients with diabetes that acetaminophen may alter results of blood glucose monitoring. Advise patient to notify health care professional if changes are noted.
- Caution patient to check labels on all OTC products. Advise patients to avoid taking more than one product containing acetaminophen at a time to prevent toxicity.
- Advise patient to consult health care professional if discomfort or fever is not relieved by routine doses of this drug or if fever is greater than 39.5°C (103°F) or lasts longer than 3 days.
- Pedi: Advise parents or caregivers to check concentrations of liquid preparations. All OTC single ingredient acetaminophen liquid products now come in a single concentration of 160 mg/5 mL. Errors have resulted in serious liver damage. Have parents or caregivers determine the correct formulation and dose for their child (based on the child's age/weight), and demonstrate how to measure it using an appropriate measuring device.

Evaluation/Desired Outcomes

- Relief of mild to moderate pain.
- Reduction of fever.

acetaZOLAMIDE

(a-seet-a-**zole**-a-mide)

~~Diamox, Diamox Sequels~~

Classification

Therapeutic: anticonvulsants, antiglaucoma agents, diuretics, ocular hypotensive agent

Pharmacologic: carbonic anhydrase inhibitors

Indications

Elevated intraocular pressure associated with acute angle-closure glaucoma (as adjunctive therapy). Prevention or treatment of acute altitude sickness. Edema.

Action

Inhibition of carbonic anhydrase in the eye results in decreased secretion of aqueous humor. Inhibition of renal carbonic anhydrase, resulting in self-limiting urinary excretion of sodium, potassium, bicarbonate, and water. **Therapeutic Effects:** Lowering of intraocular pressure. Prevention and treatment of acute altitude sickness. Diuresis and subsequent mobilization of excess fluid.

Pharmacokinetics

Absorption: Dose dependent; erratic with doses >10 mg/kg/day.

Distribution: Crosses the blood-brain barrier.

Protein Binding: 95%.

Metabolism and Excretion: Excreted mostly unchanged in urine.

Half-life: 2.4–5.8 hr.

TIME/ACTION PROFILE (↓ intraocular pressure)

ROUTE	ONSET	PEAK	DURATION
PO	1–1.5 hr	2–4 hr	8–12 hr
PO-ER	2 hr	8–18 hr	18–24 hr
IV	2 min	15 min	4–5 hr

Contraindications/Precautions

Contraindicated in: Hypersensitivity or cross-sensitivity with sulfonamides may occur; Hepatic impairment; Concurrent use with ophthalmic carbonic anhydrase inhibitors (brinzolamide, dorzolamide) is not recommended; OB: Avoid use during 1st trimester of pregnancy.

Use Cautiously in: Chronic respiratory disease; Electrolyte abnormalities; Gout; Renal disease (↓ dose for CCr <50 mL/min); Diabetes mellitus; OB: Use with caution during 2nd or 3rd trimester of pregnancy; Lactation: Safety not established during breastfeeding.

Adverse Reactions/Side Effects

Derm: rash, STEVENS-JOHNSON SYNDROME. **EENT:** transient nearsightedness. **Endo:** hyperglycemia. **F and E:** hyperchloremic acidosis, growth retardation (in children receiving chronic therapy), hypokalemia. **GI:** anorexia, weight loss, melena, nausea, vomiting. **GU:** crystalluria, renal calculi. **Hemat:** APLASTIC ANEMIA, HEMOLYTIC ANEMIA, LEUKOPENIA. **Metab:** hyperuricemia. **Neuro:** depression, dysgeusia, fatigue, paresthesias, weakness, drowsiness. **Misc:** HYPERSENSITIVITY REACTIONS (INCLUDING ANAPHYLAXIS).

Interactions

Drug-Drug: May ↓ levels and effectiveness of **barbiturates**, **aspirin**, and **lithium**. May ↑ levels and risk of toxicity of **amphetamine**, **cyclosporine**, **quinidine**, **procainamide**, and possibly **tricyclic antidepressants**.

Route/Dosage

Acute Angle-Closure Glaucoma

PO IV (Adults): 500 mg as single dose (to be used when there is a ≥1-hr delay to ophthalmologist evaluation, as an adjunct to topical therapy).

PO (Children): 10–30 mg/kg/day in 2–4 divided doses (max dose = 1000 mg/day) (immediate release).

PO (Children ≥12 yr): 500 mg twice daily (extended release).

Acute Altitude Sickness

PO (Adults): *Prevention:* 125 mg twice daily (immediate release); start 24–48 hr before ascent and discontinue after staying at the target elevation for 2–4 days or when descent initiated for individuals who ascended to target elevation and immediately descend. *Treatment:* 250 mg twice daily (immediate release). Continue until descent or 24 hr after resolution of symptoms.

PO (Children): *Prevention:* 1.25 mg/kg every 12 hr (max dose = 125 mg/dose) (immediate release); start either the day before or on the day of ascent and discontinue after staying at the target elevation for 2–4 days or when descent initiated for individuals who ascended to target elevation and immediately descend. *Treatment:* 2.5 mg/kg every 12 hr (max dose = 250 mg/dose) (immediate release).

Edema

PO IV (Adults): 250–500 mg once daily or every other day (immediate release for oral).

PO IV (Children): 5 mg/kg once daily or every other day (immediate release for oral).

Availability

Extended-release capsules: 500 mg. **Powder for injection:** 500 mg/vial. **Tablets:** 125 mg, 250 mg.

NURSING IMPLICATIONS

Assessment

- Assess for hypersensitivity reactions and anaphylaxis (rash; hives; wheezing; trouble breathing, swallowing, or talking). Implement supportive measures (epinephrine) if indicated.
- Observe for signs of hypokalemia (muscle weakness, malaise, fatigue, ECG changes, vomiting).
- Assess for allergies to sulfonamides.
- **Intraocular Pressure:** Assess for eye discomfort or decrease in visual acuity.
- **Seizures:** Monitor neurologic status in patients receiving acetazolamide for seizures. Initiate seizure precautions.
- **Altitude Sickness:** Monitor for ↓ in severity of symptoms (headache, nausea, vomiting, fatigue, dizziness, drowsiness, shortness of breath). Notify health care provider immediately if neurologic symptoms worsen or if patient becomes more dyspneic and rales or crackles develop.
- **Edema:** Monitor intake and output and daily weight during therapy.

Lab Test Considerations

- Serum electrolytes, complete blood counts, and platelet counts should be evaluated initially and periodically during prolonged therapy. May ↓ potassium, bicarbonate, WBCs, and RBCs. May ↑ chloride.
- May ↑ serum and urine glucose; monitor serum and urine glucose carefully in patients with diabetes.
- May cause false-positive results for urine protein and 17-hydroxysteroid tests.
- May ↑ ammonia, bilirubin, uric acid, calcium, and urine urobilinogen. May ↓ urine citrate.

Implementation

- Do not confuse acetazolamide with acetaminophen.
- Encourage fluid intake up to 2000–3000 mL/day, unless contraindicated, to prevent crystalluria and stone formation.
- A potassium supplement without chloride should be administered concurrently with acetazolamide.
- **PO:** Give with food to minimize GI irritation. Tablets may be crushed and mixed with fruit-flavored syrup to minimize bitter taste for patients with difficulty swallowing. ***DNC:*** Extended-release capsules may be opened and sprinkled on soft food. Do not crush, chew, or swallow contents dry. Extended-release capsules are only indicated for glaucoma and altitude sickness; do not use for seizure disorders or diuresis.

IV Administration

- **IV Push: Reconstitution:** Reconstitute 500 mg in ≥5 mL of sterile water for injection. Use reconstituted solution within 24 hr. **Concentration:** 100 mg/mL. **Rate:** Not to exceed 500 mg/min.
- **Intermittent Infusion: Reconstitution:** Reconstitute 500 mg in ≥5 mL of sterile water for injection. Use reconstituted solution within 24 hr. **Dilution:** Further dilute reconstituted solution in 50–100 mL of D5W, D10W, 0.45% NaCl, 0.9% NaCl, LR, or combinations of dextrose and saline or dextrose and LR solution. **Concentration:** 5–10 mg/mL. **Rate:** Infuse over 15–30 min.
- **Y-Site Compatibility:** pantoprazole.
- **Y-Site Incompatibility:** multiple vitamins.

Patient/Family Teaching

- Explain purpose and side effects of medication to patient. Advise patient to read *Patient Information* before starting therapy. Instruct patient to take as directed. Take missed doses as soon as possible unless almost time for next dose. Do not double doses. Patients on anticonvulsant therapy may need to gradually withdraw medication.
- Advise patient to notify health care provider of all Rx or OTC medications, vitamins, or herbal products being taken and to consult with health care provider before taking other medications.
- Advise patient to report numbness or tingling of extremities, weakness, rash, sore throat, unusual bleeding or bruising, fever, or signs/symptoms of a sulfonamide adverse reaction (Stevens-Johnson syndrome [flu-like symptoms, spreading red rash, skin/mucous membrane blistering], toxic epidermal necrolysis [widespread peeling/blistering of skin]) to health care provider. If hematopoietic reactions, fever, rash, hepatic, or renal problems occur, acetazolamide should be discontinued.

A

- May occasionally cause drowsiness. Caution patient to avoid driving and other activities that require alertness until response to the drug is known.
- Caution patient to use sunscreen and wear protective clothing to prevent photosensitivity reactions.
- **Intraocular Pressure:** Advise patient of the need for periodic ophthalmologic exams; loss of vision may be gradual and painless.
- Rep: Advise women of reproductive potential to notify health care provider if pregnancy is planned or suspected or if breastfeeding.

Evaluation/Desired Outcomes

- Lowering of intraocular pressure.
- Prevention and treatment of acute altitude sickness.
- Diuresis and subsequent mobilization of excess fluid.

acetylcysteine
(a-se-teel-**sis**-teen)

Acetadote, ~~Mucomyst~~

Classification

Therapeutic: antidotes (for acetaminophen toxicity), mucolytic

Indications

PO IV: Antidote for the management of potentially hepatotoxic overdose of acetaminophen. **Inhaln:** Mucolytic in the management of conditions associated with thick viscid mucous secretions. **Unlabeled Use: PO:** Prevention of radiocontrast-induced renal impairment.

Action

PO IV: Decreases the buildup of a hepatotoxic metabolite in acetaminophen overdosage. **Inhaln:** Degrades mucus, allowing easier mobilization and expectoration. **Therapeutic Effects: PO:** Prevention or lessening of liver damage following acetaminophen overdose. **Inhaln:** Lowers the viscosity of mucus.

Pharmacokinetics

Absorption: Absorbed from the GI tract following oral administration. Action is local following inhalation; remainder may be absorbed from pulmonary epithelium. IV administration results in complete bioavailability.
Distribution: Well distributed to tissues.
Metabolism and Excretion: Partially metabolized by the liver, 22% excreted renally.
Half-life: *Adults:* 5.6 hr (↑ in hepatic impairment) *Newborns:* 11 hr.

ROUTE	ONSET	PEAK	DURATION
PO (antidote)	unknown	30–60 min	4 hr
IV (antidote)	unknown	unknown	unknown
Inhaln (mucolytic)	1 min	5–10 min	short

Contraindications/Precautions

Contraindicated in: Hypersensitivity.
Use Cautiously in: Severe respiratory insufficiency, asthma, or history of bronchospasm; History of GI bleeding (oral only); OB: Use during pregnancy only if potential maternal benefit justifies potential fetal risk; Lactation: Safety not established in breastfeeding.

Adverse Reactions/Side Effects

CV: hypotension, tachycardia. **Derm:** rash, clamminess, pruritus, urticaria. **EENT:** rhinorrhea. **F and E:** fluid overload. **GI:** nausea, vomiting, stomatitis. **Neuro:** drowsiness. **Resp:** bronchospasm, ↑ secretions, bronchial/tracheal irritation, chest tightness. **Misc:** chills, fever, HYPERSENSITIVITY REACTIONS (INCLUDING ANAPHYLAXIS AND ANGIOEDEMA) (PRIMARILY WITH IV).

Interactions

Drug-Drug: Activated charcoal may adsorb orally administered acetylcysteine and ↓ its effectiveness as an antidote.

Route/Dosage

Acetaminophen Overdose

PO (Adults and Children): 140 mg/kg initially, followed by 70 mg/kg every 4 hr for 17 additional doses.
IV (Adults and Children): *Loading dose:* 150 mg/kg (maximum: 15 g) over 60 min initially, followed by *First maintenance dose:* 50 mg/kg (maximum: 5 g) over 4 hr. *Second maintenance dose:* 100 mg/kg (maximum: 10 g) over 16 hr.

Mucolytic

Inhaln: (Adults and Children 1–12 yr): *Nebulization via face mask:* 3–5 mL of 20% solution or 6–10 mL of the 10% solution 3–4 times daily; *Nebulization via tent or croupette:* volume of 10–20% solution required to maintain heavy mist; *Direct instillation:* 1–2 mL of 10–20% solution every 1–4 hr; *Intratracheal instillation via tracheostomy:* 1–2 mL of 10–20% solution every 1–4 hr (up to 2–5 mL of 20% solution via tracheal catheter into particular segments of the bronchopulmonary tree).
Inhaln: (Infants): *Nebulization:* 1–2 mL of 20% solution or 2–4 mL of 10% solution 3–4 times daily.

Prevention of Radiocontrast-Induced Renal Impairment

PO (Adults): 600 mg twice daily for 2 days, beginning the day before the procedure.

Availability

Solution for inhalation: 10% (100 mg/mL), 20% (200 mg/mL). **Solution for injection:** 200 mg/mL.

NURSING IMPLICATIONS

Assessment

- **Antidote in Acetaminophen Overdose:** Assess type, amount, and time of acetaminophen ingestion. Assess plasma acetaminophen levels. Initial levels are drawn at least 4 hr after ingestion of acetaminophen. Plasma level determinations may be difficult to interpret following ingestion of extended-release preparations. Do not wait for results to administer dose.
- *IV:* Assess for anaphylaxis. Erythema and flushing are common, usually occurring 30–60 min after initiating infusion, and may resolve with continued administration. If rash, hypotension, wheezing, or dyspnea occur, initiate treatment for anaphylaxis (antihistamine and epinephrine). Interrupt acetylcysteine infusion until symptoms resolve and restart carefully. If anaphylaxis recurs, discontinue acetylcysteine and use alternative form of treatment.
- Assess patient for nausea, vomiting, and urticaria. Notify health care professional if these occur. Monitor for signs and symptoms of fluid overload (dyspnea, edema, increased BP) during therapy. Adjust volume of diluent as needed. May result in hyponatremia, seizures, and death.
- **Mucolytic:** Assess respiratory function (lung sounds, dyspnea) and color, amount, and consistency of secretions before and immediately following treatment to determine effectiveness of therapy.

Lab Test Considerations

- Monitor AST, ALT, and bilirubin levels along with INR every 24 hr for 96 hr in patients with plasma acetaminophen levels indicating potential hepatotoxicity.
- Monitor cardiac and renal function (serum creatinine, BUN), serum glucose, hemoglobin, hematocrit, and electrolytes. Maintain fluid and electrolyte balance; correct hypoglycemia.

Implementation

- After opening, solution for inhalation may turn light purple; does not alter potency. Refrigerate open vials and discard after 96 hr.
- Drug reacts with rubber and metals (iron, nickel, copper); avoid contact.
- **PO:** Prepare oral solution by diluting 20% acetylcysteine solution with diet cola or other diet soft drink to a final concentration of 5% (add 3 mL of diluent for each 1 mL of 20% acetylcysteine solution; do not decrease the proportion of diluent). Water may be used as diluent if administered via gastric tube or Miller-Abbott tube. Dilution should be freshly prepared and administered within 1 hr. Undiluted solutions are stable for 96 hr if refrigerated.
- **Acetaminophen Overdose:** Empty stomach contents by inducing emesis or lavage prior to administration.

IV Administration

- **Intermittent Infusion:** Most effective if administered within 8 hr of acetaminophen ingestion. **Dilution:** Dilute in sterile water for injection, D5W/0.45% NaCl, or D5W. Solution is colorless to slight pink or purple; do not administer solutions that are cloudy, discolored, or contain particulate matter. Stable for 24 hr at room temperature. **Concentration:** **For loading dose:** *For patients 5–20 kg:* Dilute 150 mg in 3 mL/kg of diluent. *For patients 21–40 kg:* Dilute 150 mg/kg in 100 mL of diluent. *For patients 41–100 kg:* Dilute 150 mg/kg in 200 mL of diluent. **For Second Dose:** *For patients 5–20 kg:* Dilute 50 mg/kg in 7 mL/kg of diluent. *For patients 21–40 kg:* Dilute 50 mg/kg in 250 mL of diluent. *For patients 41–100 kg:* Dilute 50 mg/kg in 500 mL of diluent. **For Third Dose:** *For patients 5–20 kg:* Dilute 100 mg/kg in 14 mL/kg of diluent. *For patients 21–40 kg:* Dilute 100 mg/kg in 500 mL of diluent. *For patients 41–100 kg:* Dilute 100 mg/kg in 1000 mL of diluent. Adjust fluid volume for patients requiring fluid resuscitation. Vials are single-use. Discard after using. Reconstituted solution is stable for 24 hr at room temperature. **Rate:** Administer **Loading Dose** over 1 hr.
- Administer **Second Dose** over 4 hr.
- Administer **Third Dose** over 16 hr.
- **Y-Site Compatibility:** heparin, meropenem, naloxone, tigecycline, vancomycin.
- **Y-Site Incompatibility:** cefepime, ceftazidime.
- **Inhaln: Mucolytic:** Encourage adequate fluid intake (2000–3000 mL/day) to decrease viscosity of secretions.
- For nebulization, 20% solution may be diluted with 0.9% NaCl for injection or inhalation or sterile water for injection or inhalation. May use 10% solution undiluted. May be administered by nebulization, or 1–2 mL may be instilled directly into airway. During administration, when 25% of medication remains in nebulizer, dilute with equal amount of 0.9% NaCl or sterile water.
- An increased volume of liquefied bronchial secretions may occur following administration. Have suction equipment available for patients unable to effectively clear airways.
- If bronchospasm occurs during treatment, discontinue and consult health care professional regarding possible addition of bronchodilator to therapy. Patients with asthma or hyperactive airway disease should be given a bronchodilator prior to acetylcysteine to prevent bronchospasm.
- Rinse patient's mouth and wash face following treatment, as drug leaves a sticky residue.

Patient/Family Teaching

- Advise patient to notify health care professional if symptoms of hypersensitivity reaction or fluid overload occur.

- Rep: Advise females of reproductive potential to notify health care professional if pregnancy is planned or suspected and to avoid breastfeeding for 30 hr after administration.
- **Acetaminophen Overdose:** Explain purpose of medication to patient.
- **Inhaln:** Instruct patient to clear airway by coughing deeply before taking aerosol treatment.
- Inform patient that unpleasant odor of this drug becomes less noticeable as treatment progresses and medicine dissipates.

Evaluation/Desired Outcomes

- Decreased acetaminophen levels.
- No further increase in hepatic damage during acetaminophen overdose therapy.
- Decreased dyspnea and clearing of lung sounds when used as a mucolytic.
- Prevention of radiocontrast-induced renal impairment.

V acyclovir (ay-sye-kloe-veer)

Zovirax

Classification

Therapeutic: antivirals

Pharmacologic: purine analogues

Indications

PO: Treatment of: Recurrent genital herpes infections, Localized cutaneous herpes zoster infections (shingles) and chickenpox (varicella). **IV:** Treatment of: Severe initial episodes of genital herpes in nonimmunosuppressed patients, Mucosal or cutaneous herpes simplex infections or herpes zoster infections (shingles) in immunosuppressed patients, Herpes simplex encephalitis, Neonatal herpes simplex infections. **Topical:** *Cream:* Recurrent herpes labialis (cold sores). *Ointment:* Treatment of limited non-life-threatening herpes simplex infections in immunocompromised patients (systemic treatment is preferred).

Action

Interferes with viral DNA synthesis. **Therapeutic Effects:** Inhibition of viral replication, decreased viral shedding, and reduced time for healing of lesions.

Pharmacokinetics

Absorption: Despite poor absorption (15–30%), therapeutic plasma concentrations are achieved.
Distribution: Widely distributed. CSF concentrations are 50% of plasma.
Metabolism and Excretion: >90% eliminated unchanged by kidneys; remainder metabolized by liver.
Half-life: *Neonates:* 4 hr; *Children (1–12 yr):* 2–3 hr; *Adults:* 2–3.5 hr (↑ in renal failure).

TIME/ACTION PROFILE (plasma concentrations)

ROUTE	ONSET	PEAK	DURATION
PO	unknown	1.5–2.5 hr	4 hr
IV	prompt	end of infusion	8 hr

† Salivary concentrations

Contraindications/Precautions

Contraindicated in: Hypersensitivity to acyclovir or valacyclovir.
Use Cautiously in: Pre-existing serious neurologic, hepatic, pulmonary, or fluid and electrolyte abnormalities; Renal impairment (dose alteration recommended if CCr <50 mL/min); Obese patients (dose should be based on ideal body weight); Patients with hypoxia; OB: Use during pregnancy only if potential maternal benefit justifies potential fetal risk; systemic exposure minimal following buccal or topical administration; Lactation: Use while breastfeeding only if potential maternal benefit justifies potential risk to infant; systemic exposure minimal following buccal or topical administration; Geri: May need to ↓ dose in older adults due to age-related ↓ in renal function.

Adverse Reactions/Side Effects

Derm: acne, hives, rash, STEVENS-JOHNSON SYNDROME, unusual sweating. **Endo:** changes in menstrual cycle. **F and E:** polydipsia. **GI:** diarrhea, nausea, vomiting, ↑ liver enzymes, abdominal pain, anorexia, hyperbilirubinemia. **GU:** crystalluria, hematuria, RENAL FAILURE, renal pain. **Hemat:** THROMBOTIC THROMBOCYTOPENIC PURPURA/HEMOLYTIC UREMIC SYNDROME (HIGH DOSES IN IMMUNOSUPPRESSED PATIENTS). **Local:** pain, phlebitis, local irritation. **MS:** joint pain. **Neuro:** dizziness, headache, hallucinations, SEIZURES, trembling.

Interactions

Drug-Drug: Probenecid and **theophylline** may ↑ levels and risk of toxicity. **Valproic acid** or **phenytoin** may ↓ levels and effectiveness. Concurrent use of other **nephrotoxic drugs** may ↑ risk nephrotoxicity. **Zidovudine** and intrathecal **methotrexate** may ↑ risk of CNS side effects.

Route/Dosage

Initial Genital Herpes

PO (Adults and Children): 200 mg every 4 hr while awake (5 times/day) for 7–10 days or 400 mg every 8 hr for 7–10 days; maximum dose in children: 80 mg/kg/day in 3–5 divided doses.
IV (Adults and Children ≥12 yr): 5 mg/kg every 8 hr for 5 days.

Chronic Suppressive Therapy for Recurrent Genital Herpes

PO (Adults and Children): 400 mg twice daily or 200 mg 3–5 times/day for up to 12 mo. Maximum dose in children: 80 mg/kg/day in 2–5 divided doses.

Intermittent Therapy for Recurrent Genital Herpes

PO (Adults and Children): 200 mg every 4 hr while awake (5 times/day) or 400 mg every 8 hr or 800 mg every 12 hr for 5 days; start at first sign of symptoms. Maximum dose in children: 80 mg/kg/day in 2–5 divided doses.

Acute Treatment of Herpes Zoster in Immunosuppressed Patients

PO (Adults): 800 mg every 4 hr while awake (5 times/day) for 7–10 days. *Prophylaxis:* 400 mg 5 times/day.
PO (Children): 250–600 mg/m²/dose 4–5 times/day.

Herpes Zoster in Immunocompetent Patients

PO (Adults and Children): 4000 mg/day in 5 divided doses for 5–7 days. Maximum dose in children: 80 mg/kg/day in 5 divided doses.

Chickenpox

PO (Adults and Children): 20 mg/kg (not to exceed 800 mg/dose) 4 times daily for 5 days. Start within 24 hr of rash onset.

Mucosal and Cutaneous Herpes Simplex Infections in Immunosuppressed Patients

IV (Adults and Children >12 yr): 5 mg/kg every 8 hr for 7 days.
IV (Children 3 mo–12 yr): 10 mg/kg every 8 hr for 7 days.
Topical: (Adults): ½-inch ribbon of 5% *ointment* for every 4-square-inch area every 3 hr (6 times/day) for 7 days.

Herpes Simplex Encephalitis

IV (Adults and Children ≥12 yr): 10 mg/kg every 8 hr for 10 days.
IV (Children 3 mo–12 yr): 20 mg/kg every 8 hr for 10 days.
IV (Children birth–3 mo): 20 mg/kg every 8 hr for 14–21 days.
IV (Neonates, premature): 10 mg/kg every 12 hr for 14–21 days.

Neonatal Herpes Simplex Infections

IV (Children postmenstrual age of ≥34 wk): 20 mg/kg every 8 hr for 21 days.
IV (Children postmenstrual age of <34 wk): 20 mg/kg every 12 hr for 21 days.

Varicella Zoster Infections in Immunosuppressed Patients

IV (Adults and Children ≥12 yr): 10 mg/kg every 8 hr for 7 days.
IV (Children <12 yr): 20 mg/kg every 8 hr for 7 days.

Renal Impairment

PO IV (Adults and Children >3 mo): *CCr 25.1–50 mL/min/1.73 m²:* Normal dose every 12 hr; *CCr 10.1–25 mL/min/1.73 m²:* Normal dose every 24 hr; *CCr ≤10 mL/min/1.73 m²:* 50% of dose every 24 hr.

Herpes Labialis

Topical: (Adults and Children >12 yr): Apply 5 times/day for 4 days; start at first symptoms.

Availability (generic available)

Tablets: 🍁 200 mg, 400 mg, 800 mg. **Capsules:** 200 mg. **Oral suspension (banana flavor):** 200 mg/5 mL. **Solution for injection:** 🍁 25 mg/mL, 50 mg/mL. **Cream:** 5%. **Ointment:** 5%. ***In combination with:*** hydrocortisone (Xerese). See Appendix N.

NURSING IMPLICATIONS

Assessment

- Assess lesions before and daily during therapy.
- Monitor frequency of recurrences.
- Monitor neurologic status in patients with herpes encephalitis or for encephalopathic changes such as lethargy, obtundation, tremors, confusion, hallucinations, agitation, or seizures. Initiate seizure precautions as indicated.

Lab Test Considerations

- Monitor BUN, serum creatinine, and CCr before and during therapy. May ↑ BUN and serum creatinine or ↓ CCr, which may indicate renal failure.

Implementation

- Do not confuse Zovirax with Zyvox or Zostrix.
- Start acyclovir treatment as soon as possible after herpes simplex symptoms appear and within 24 hr of a herpes zoster outbreak.
- **PO:** Acyclovir may be administered with food or on an empty stomach, with a full glass of water.
- Shake oral suspension well before administration.
- **Topical:** Apply to skin lesions only; do not use in the eye.

IV Administration

- **IV:** Maintain adequate hydration (2000–3000 mL/day), especially during first 2 hr after IV infusion, to prevent crystalluria.
- **V** IV acyclovir is a vesicant. Concentration <7 mg/mL preferred for peripheral IV administration. Can also be infused through a midline catheter or PICC. If extravasation occurs, immediately stop infusion. Leave needle/cannula in place temporarily but do not flush the line. Gently aspirate extravasated solution; then remove needle/cannula. Elevate patient's extremity and apply dry warm compresses. Initiate hyaluronidase antidote for refractory cases in addition to supportive management. For hyaluronidase, inject a total of 1 mL (15 units/mL) intradermally or SUBQ as five separate 0.2-mL injections (using a tuberculin syringe) around the site of extravasation; if IV catheter remains in place, administer IV through the infiltrated catheter; may repeat in 30–60 min if no resolution.
- Do not administer acyclovir injectable topically, IM, SUBQ, PO, or in the eye.
- **Intermittent Infusion:** Reconstitute 500-mg or 1-g vial with 10 mL or 20 mL, respectively, of

sterile water for injection. Do not reconstitute with bacteriostatic water with benzyl alcohol or parabens. Shake well to dissolve completely. **Dilution:** Further dilute solution in ≥100 mL of D5W, 0.9% NaCl, dextrose/saline combinations, or LR. **Concentration:** 7 mg/mL. Patients requiring fluid restriction: 10 mg/mL. Use reconstituted solution within 12 hr. Once diluted for infusion, use solution within 24 hr. Refrigeration results in precipitation, which dissolves at room temperature. **Rate:** Administer via infusion pump over 1 hr to minimize renal tubular damage.

- **Y-Site Compatibility:** alemtuzumab, allopurinol, amikacin, aminophylline, amphotericin B deoxycholate, amphotericin B liposomal, ampicillin, anidulafungin, argatroban, arsenic trioxide, atracurium, azithromycin, bivalirudin, bleomycin, bumetanide, buprenorphine, busulfan, butorphanol, calcium chloride, calcium gluconate, carboplatin, carmustine, cefazolin, cefotaxime, cefotetan, cefoxitin, ceftaroline, ceftazidime, ceftriaxone, cefuroxime, cisplatin, clindamycin, cyclophosphamide, cytarabine, dactinomycin, dantrolene, defibrotide, dexamethasone, dexmedetomidine, digoxin, dimenhydrinate, docetaxel, doxorubicin liposomal, doxycycline, enalaprilat, ephedrine, ertapenem, erythromycin, etoposide, etoposide phosphate, famotidine, fentanyl, filgrastim, fluconazole, fluorouracil, fosphenytoin, furosemide, glycopyrrolate, heparin, hydrocortisone, hydromorphone, ifosfamide, imipenem/cilastatin, insulin, regular, isoproterenol, leucovorin, linezolid, lorazepam, magnesium sulfate, mannitol, melphalan, methohexital, methotrexate, methylprednisolone, metoprolol, metronidazole, milrinone, mitoxantrone, multivitamins, nafcillin, nitroglycerin, octreotide, oxacillin, oxytocin, paclitaxel, pamidronate, pemetrexed, penicillin G potassium, pentobarbital, phenobarbital, potassium acetate, potassium chloride, propofol, propranolol, remifentanil, rituximab, rocuronium, sodium acetate, sodium bicarbonate, succinylcholine, sufentanil, theophylline, thiotepa, tigecycline, tirofiban, tobramycin, trastuzumab, trimethoprim/sulfamethoxazole, vancomycin, vasopressin, vinblastine, vincristine, voriconazole, zidovudine, zoledronic acid.
- **Y-Site Incompatibility:** acetaminophen, aminocaproic acid, amiodarone, ampicillin/sulbactam, aztreonam, cefepime, chlorpromazine, ciprofloxacin, dacarbazine, daptomycin, daunorubicin, dexrazoxane, diazepam, dobutamine, dopamine, doxorubicin hydrochloride, epinephrine, epirubicin, eptifibatide, esmolol, fludarabine, foscarnet, gemcitabine, gemtuzumab ozogamicin, haloperidol, hydralazine, idarubicin, irinotecan, ketamine, ketorolac, labetalol, levofloxacin, lidocaine, mesna, methadone, midazolam, mitomycin, mycophenolate, nicardipine, nitroprusside, ondansetron, palonosetron, pentamidine, phenylephrine, phenytoin, piperacillin/tazobactam, potassium phosphates, procainamide, prochlorperazine, promethazine, sargramostim, sodium phosphates, tacrolimus, topotecan, vecuronium, verapamil, vinorelbine.

Patient/Family Teaching

- Explain the purpose and side effects of acyclovir. Instruct patient to take medication as directed for the full course of therapy. Take missed doses as soon as possible but not just before next dose is due; do not double doses. Acyclovir should not be used more frequently or longer than prescribed. Advise patient to read *Patient Information* before starting and with each Rx refill in case of changes.
- Advise patients that the additional use of OTC creams, lotions, and ointments may delay healing and may cause spreading of lesions.
- Inform patient that acyclovir is not a cure; the virus lies dormant in the ganglia. Acyclovir will not prevent the spread of infection to others.
- Instruct patient to consult health care provider if symptoms are not relieved after 7 days of topical therapy or if oral acyclovir does not decrease the frequency and severity of recurrences. Immunocompromised patients may require a longer time, usually 2 wk, for crusting over of lesions.
- Instruct women with genital herpes to have yearly Papanicolaou smears because they may be more likely to develop cervical cancer.
- **Topical:** Instruct patient to apply ointment in sufficient quantity to cover all lesions every 3 hr, 6 times/day, for 7 days. A ½-inch ribbon of ointment covers approximately 4 square inches. Use a finger cot or glove when applying to prevent inoculation of other areas or spread to other people. Keep affected areas clean and dry. Loose-fitting clothing should be worn to prevent irritation.
- Avoid drug contact in or around eyes. Report any unexplained eye symptoms to health care provider immediately; ocular herpetic infection can lead to blindness.
- Rep: Advise women of reproductive potential to notify health care provider if pregnancy is planned or suspected or if breastfeeding. Advise patient that condoms should be used during sexual contact and to avoid sexual contact while lesions are present.

Evaluation/Desired Outcomes

- Crusting over and healing of skin lesions.
- Decrease in frequency and severity of recurrences.
- Acceleration of complete healing and cessation of pain in herpes zoster.
- Decrease in intensity of chickenpox.

adalimumab

(a-da-li-**mu**-mab)

Abrilada, ✤ Amgevita, Amjevita, ~~Cyltezo~~, Hadlima, Hulio, Humira, Hyrimoz, Idacio, Simlandi, Yuflyma, Yusimry

Classification

Therapeutic: antirheumatics

Pharmacologic: DMARDs, monoclonal antibodies

Indications

- **Abrilada, Amjevita, Hadlima, Hulio, Humira, Idacio, Hyrimoz, Simlandi, Yuflyma, and Yusimry:** Treatment of the following conditions: Moderately to severely active rheumatoid arthritis (may be used alone or with methotrexate or other non-biologic disease-modifying antirheumatic drugs [DMARDs]); Psoriatic arthritis (may be used alone or with other non-biologic DMARDs); Active ankylosing spondylitis; Moderately to severely active Crohn disease in patients who have responded inadequately to conventional therapy; Moderately to severely active ulcerative colitis in patients who have responded inadequately to immunosuppressants such as corticosteroids, azathioprine, or 6-mercaptopurine; Moderately to severely active polyarticular juvenile idiopathic arthritis (as monotherapy or with methotrexate); Moderate to severe chronic plaque psoriasis in patients who are candidates for systemic therapy or phototherapy and when other systemic therapies are deemed inappropriate; Non-infectious intermediate, posterior, and panuveitis. **Abrilada, Amjevita, Hadlima, Humira, Hyrimoz, Idacio, Simlandi, Yuflyma, and Yusimry only:** Treatment of the following condition: Moderate to severe hidradenitis suppurativa.

Action

Neutralizes and prevents the action of tumor necrosis factor (TNF), resulting in anti-inflammatory and antiproliferative activity. **Therapeutic Effects:** Decreased pain and swelling with decreased rate of joint destruction in patients with rheumatoid arthritis, psoriatic arthritis, juvenile idiopathic arthritis, and ankylosing spondylitis. Reduced signs and symptoms and maintenance of clinical remission of Crohn disease. Induction and maintenance of clinical remission of ulcerative colitis. Reduced severity of plaques. Reduced number of abscesses and inflammatory nodules. Decreased progression of uveitis.

Pharmacokinetics

Absorption: 64% absorbed after SUBQ administration.

Distribution: Synovial fluid concentrations are 31–96% of serum.

Metabolism and Excretion: Unknown.

Half-life: 14 days (range 10–20 days).

TIME/ACTION PROFILE (improvement)

ROUTE	ONSET	PEAK	DURATION
SUBQ	8–26 wk	131 hr*	2 wk†

* Plasma concentration.

† Following discontinuation.

Contraindications/Precautions

Contraindicated in: Hypersensitivity; Concurrent use of anakinra or abatacept; Active infection (including localized).

Use Cautiously in: History of chronic or recurrent infection or underlying illness/treatment predisposing to infection; History of exposure to tuberculosis; History of opportunistic infection; Patients residing or who have resided where tuberculosis, histoplasmosis, coccidioidomycoses, or blastomycosis is endemic; Pre-existing or recent-onset CNS demyelinating disorders; History of lymphoma; OB: Use during pregnancy only if potential maternal benefit justifies potential fetal risk; Lactation: Use while breastfeeding only if potential maternal benefit justifies potential risk to infant; Pedi: Children <2 yr (safety not established); ↑ risk of lymphoma (including hepatosplenic T-cell lymphoma [HSTCL] in patients with Crohn disease or ulcerative colitis), leukemia, and other malignancies in children; Geri: ↑ risk of infection/malignancy in older adults.

Adverse Reactions/Side Effects

CV: hypertension. **Derm:** rash, psoriasis. **EENT:** optic neuritis. **GI:** abdominal pain, nausea. **GU:** hematuria. **Hemat:** neutropenia, thrombocytopenia. **Local:** injection site reactions. **Metab:** hyperlipidemia. **MS:** back pain. **Neuro:** headache, Guillain-Barré syndrome, multiple sclerosis. **Misc:** fever, HYPERSENSITIVITY REACTIONS (INCLUDING ANAPHYLAXIS AND ANGIOEDEMA), INFECTION (INCLUDING REACTIVATION TUBERCULOSIS [TB] AND OTHER OPPORTUNISTIC INFECTIONS DUE TO BACTERIAL, INVASIVE FUNGAL, VIRAL, MYCOBACTERIAL, AND PARASITIC PATHOGENS), MALIGNANCY (INCLUDING LYMPHOMA, HSTCL, LEUKEMIA, AND SKIN CANCER).

Interactions

Drug-Drug: Concurrent use with **anakinra**, **abatacept**, or other **TNF-blocking agents** ↑ risk of serious infections; concurrent use contraindicated. Concurrent use with **azathioprine** and/or **methotrexate** may ↑ risk of HSTCL. **Live vaccinations** should not be given concurrently. Risks and benefits should be considered before using live vaccinations in an infant exposed to adalimumab therapy in utero.

Route/Dosage

Rheumatoid Arthritis, Ankylosing Spondylitis, and Psoriatic Arthritis

SUBQ (Adults): 40 mg every other wk. Methotrexate, non-biologic DMARDs, corticosteroids, and/or analgesics may be continued during therapy. Patients not receiving concurrent methotrexate may receive additional benefit by ↑ dose to 40 mg once weekly *or* 80 mg every other wk.

Crohn Disease

SUBQ (Adults): 160 mg initially on Day 1 (given in one day or over two consecutive days), followed by 80 mg 2 wk later on Day 15. Two wk later (Day 29), begin maintenance dose of 40 mg every other wk. Aminosalicylates, corticosteroids, and/or immunomodulatory agents (e.g. azathioprine, 6-mercaptopurine, methotrexate) may be continued during therapy.

SUBQ (Children ≥6 yr and ≥40 kg): *Abrilada, Amjevita, Hadlima, Hulio, Humira, Hyrimoz, Idacio, and Simlandi only:* 160 mg initially on Day 1 (given in one day or over two consecutive days), followed by 80 mg 2 wk later on Day 15. Two wk later (Day 29), begin maintenance dose of 40 mg every other wk. Aminosalicylates, corticosteroids, and/or immunomodulatory agents (e.g. azathioprine, 6-mercaptopurine, methotrexate) may be continued during therapy.

SUBQ (Children ≥6 yr and 17–<40 kg): *Abrilada, Amjevita, Hadlima, Hulio, and Humira only:* 80 mg initially on Day 1, followed by 40 mg 2 wk later on Day 15. Two wk later (Day 29), begin maintenance dose of 20 mg every other wk. Aminosalicylates, corticosteroids, and/or immunomodulatory agents (e.g. azathioprine, 6-mercaptopurine, methotrexate) may be continued during therapy.

Ulcerative Colitis

SUBQ (Adults): 160 mg initially on Day 1 (given in one day or over two consecutive days), followed by 80 mg 2 wk later on Day 15. Two wk later (Day 29), begin maintenance dose of 40 mg every other wk. Aminosalicylates, corticosteroids, and/or immunomodulatory agents (e.g. azathioprine, 6-mercaptopurine, methotrexate) may be continued during therapy. Should be continued only if patients have evidence of clinical remission by wk 8 of therapy.

SUBQ (Children ≥5 yr and ≥40 kg): *Humira only:* 160 mg initially on Day 1 (given in one day or over two consecutive days), followed by 80 mg 1 wk later on Day 8, and then followed by 80 mg 1 wk later on Day 15. Two wk later (Day 29), begin maintenance dose of either 80 mg every other wk *or* 40 mg every wk. Aminosalicylates, corticosteroids, and/or immunomodulatory agents (e.g. azathioprine, 6-mercaptopurine, methotrexate) may be continued during therapy.

SUBQ (Children ≥5 yr and 20–<40 kg): *Humira only:* 80 mg initially on Day 1, followed by 40 mg 1 wk later on Day 8, and then followed by 40 mg 1 wk later on Day 15. Two wk later (Day 29), begin maintenance dose of either 40 mg every other wk *or* 20 mg every wk. Aminosalicylates, corticosteroids, and/or immunomodulatory agents (e.g. azathioprine, 6-mercaptopurine, methotrexate) may be continued during therapy.

Juvenile Idiopathic Arthritis

SUBQ (Children 2–17 yr (Abrilada, Amjevita, Hadlima, Hulio, Humira, Hyrimoz, Idacio, and Simlandi)): *10–<15 kg (Abrilada, Hadlima, Humira, and Hyrimoz only):* 10 mg every other wk; *15–<30 kg (Abrilada, Amjeveta, Hadlima, Hulio, and Humira only):* 20 mg every other wk; *≥30 kg:* 40 mg every other wk.

Plaque Psoriasis

SUBQ (Adults): 80 mg initially; then in 1 wk, begin regimen of 40 mg every other wk.

Uveitis

SUBQ (Adults): 80 mg initially; then in 1 wk, begin regimen of 40 mg every other wk.

SUBQ (Children ≥2 yr and ≥30 kg): *Humira only:* 40 mg every other wk.

SUBQ (Children ≥2 yr and 15–<30 kg): *Humira only:* 20 mg every other wk.

SUBQ (Children ≥2 yr and 10–<15 kg): *Humira only:* 10 mg every other wk.

Hidradenitis Suppurativa

SUBQ (Adults): *Abrilada, Amjevita, Hadlima, Humira, Hyrimoz, Idacio, Simlandi, Yuflyma, or Yusimry:* 160 mg initially (given in one day or over two consecutive days), followed by 80 mg 2 wk later on Day 15. Two wk later (Day 29), begin maintenance dose of 40 mg every wk *or* 80 mg every other wk.

SUBQ (Children ≥12 yr and ≥60 kg): *Humira only:* 160 mg initially (given in one day or over two consecutive days), followed by 80 mg 2 wk later on Day 15. Two wk later (Day 29), begin maintenance dose of 40 mg every wk *or* 80 mg every other wk.

SUBQ (Children ≥12 yr and 30–59 kg): *Humira only:* 80 mg initially on Day 1, followed by 40 mg 1 wk later on Day 8. Two wk later (Day 22), begin maintenance dose of 40 mg every other wk.

Availability

Solution for injection (prefilled syringes): 10 mg/0.1 mL, 10 mg/0.2 mL, 20 mg/0.2 mL, 20 mg/0.4 mL, 40 mg/0.4 mL, 40 mg/0.8 mL, 80 mg/0.8 mL. **Solution for injection (vials):** 40 mg/0.8 mL. **Solution for injection (prefilled pens):** 40 mg/0.4 mL, 40 mg/0.8 mL, 80 mg/0.8 mL.

NURSING IMPLICATIONS

Assessment

- Assess for signs of infection (fever, dyspnea, flu-like symptoms, frequent or painful urination, redness or swelling at the site of a wound), including tuberculosis and hepatitis B virus (HBV), prior to, during, and after therapy. *If serious infection occurs,* discontinue adalimumab and initiate treatment as indicated. Monitor new infections closely.

- Assess for latex allergy. Needle cover of syringe contains latex and should not be handled by persons sensitive to latex.
- Monitor for signs of anaphylaxis (urticaria, dyspnea, facial edema) following injection. *If severe allergic reaction occurs,* discontinue adalimumab immediately. Resuscitation medications and equipment should be readily available.
- Assess for signs and symptoms of systemic fungal infection (fever, malaise, weight loss, sweats, cough, dyspnea, pulmonary infiltrates, serious systemic illness). *If serious systemic illness occurs and the patient has lived or traveled where mycoses are endemic,* consider empiric antifungal treatment until pathogen identified.
- Monitor for signs of autoimmunity during therapy. *If a lupus-like syndrome occurs,* discontinue adalimumab.
- **Arthritis:** Assess pain and range of motion before and periodically during therapy.
- **Crohn Disease or Ulcerative Colitis:** Monitor frequency and consistency of bowel movements periodically during therapy.
- **Plaque Psoriasis:** Assess skin lesions periodically during therapy.
- **Hidradenitis Suppurativa:** Monitor skin lesions (abscesses, inflammatory nodules, draining fistulas) during therapy.
- **Uveitis:** Monitor signs and symptoms of uveitis (red eye with or without pain, photosensitivity, blurry vision, suddenly seeing "floaters") during therapy.

Lab Test Considerations

- Complete tuberculin skin test prior to initiation of therapy. *For induration ≥5 mm,* consult with TB specialist and start treatment of latent TB before therapy initiation with adalimumab. Monitor CBC with differential periodically during therapy. May cause leukopenia, neutropenia, thrombocytopenia, and pancytopenia. *If signs or symptoms of blood dyscrasias (persistent fever, bruising, bleeding, pallor) occur,* consider discontinuing adalimumab.
- Monitor HBV blood tests before initiation and for several months after therapy is complete. *If active or reactivated HBV occurs,* stop adalimumab and treat as indicated. Use caution when considering resumption of therapy.
- Antigen and antibody testing for histoplasmosis and TB skin test may be negative with active infection during adalimumab therapy.

Implementation

- Update age-appropriate vaccines according to guidelines prior to initiation of therapy.
- Administer initial injection under health care professional supervision.
- Vial is for single use and institutional use only.
- **SUBQ**: Solution may be left at room temperature for 15–30 min before injecting. *For vial,* draw up adequate volume for dose and *for either the prepared or prefilled syringe,* administer SUBQ at 45° angle. *For pen,* point cap down to make sure solution reaches fill line. Remove gray cap, pinch skin, place pen against skin at 90° angle, and press button until a click is heard. Hold pen in place until all solution is injected (10 sec) and yellow marker is visible in window. Administer in upper thigh or abdomen, avoiding 2 inches around navel. Rotate injection sites; avoid areas that are tender, bruised, hard, or red.
- Solution is clear to slightly opalescent, colorless to pale brownish-yellow; do not administer solution that is cloudy, discolored, or contains particulates.

Patient/Family Teaching

- Explain purpose and side effects of medication. Advise patient to read *Patient Information* before starting therapy.
- Instruct patient on the appropriate steps for administration technique and disposal of equipment, if self-administration is appropriate.
- Advise patient, if dose missed, to administer as soon as possible; then take next dose according to regular schedule.
- Inform patient of risk for injection site reaction (redness and/or itching, rash, hemorrhage, bruising, pain, swelling); rash usually disappears in a few days.
- Caution patient to notify health care professional immediately if signs of infection, HBV (muscle aches, clay-colored stools, fatigue, fever, dark urine, chills, yellow skin or eyes, stomach pain, ↓ appetite, skin rash, vomiting), severe rash, swollen face, or difficulty breathing occurs or if nervous system problems (numbness or tingling, visual changes, weakness in arms or legs, dizziness) occur.
- Inform patient of ↑ risk of cancer.
- Advise patient to notify health care professional of all Rx or OTC medications, vitamins, or herbal products being taken and to consult with health care professional before taking other medications.
- Instruct patient to notify health care professional of medication regimen prior to treatment or surgery.
- Advise patient to avoid live vaccines during therapy.
- Rep: Advise women of reproductive potential to notify health care professional if pregnancy is planned or suspected or if breastfeeding.

Evaluation/Desired Outcomes

- Decreased pain and swelling with decreased rate of joint destruction in patients with rheumatoid arthritis.

A

- Decreased signs and symptoms, slowed progression of joint destruction, and improved physical function in patients with psoriatic arthritis.
- Reduced signs and symptoms of ankylosing spondylitis.
- Decreased signs and symptoms and maintenance of remission in patients with Crohn disease or ulcerative colitis.
- Reduced pain and swelling in patients moderate to severe polyarticular juvenile idiopathic arthritis in children 2 yr of age and older.
- Reduced severity of plaques in patients with severe chronic plaque psoriasis.
- Improvement in skin lesions in patients with hidradenitis suppurativa.
- Decreased progression of uveitis.

adenosine (a-den-oh-seen)

~~Adenocard, Adenoscan~~

Classification

Therapeutic: antiarrhythmics

Indications

Conversion of paroxysmal supraventricular tachycardia to normal sinus rhythm when vagal maneuvers are unsuccessful. As a diagnostic agent (with noninvasive techniques) to assess myocardial perfusion defects occurring as a consequence of coronary artery disease.

Action

Restores sinus rhythm by interrupting re-entrant pathways in the AV node. Slows conduction time through the AV node. Produces coronary artery vasodilation. **Therapeutic Effects:** Restoration of sinus rhythm.

Pharmacokinetics

Absorption: IV administration results in complete bioavailability.

Distribution: Taken up by erythrocytes and vascular endothelium.

Metabolism and Excretion: Rapidly converted to inosine and adenosine monophosphate.

Half-life: <10 sec.

TIME/ACTION PROFILE (antiarrhythmic effect)

ROUTE	ONSET	PEAK	DURATION
IV	immediate	unknown	1–2 min

Contraindications/Precautions

Contraindicated in: Hypersensitivity; 2nd- or 3rd-degree AV block or sick sinus syndrome, unless a functional artificial pacemaker is present; Myocardial ischemia/infarction (only when used as diagnostic agent); Lactation: Lactation.

Use Cautiously in: Asthma (may induce bronchospasm); Unstable angina; OB: Safety not established in pregnancy.

Adverse Reactions/Side Effects

CV: <u>arrhythmias</u>, chest pain, hypotension, MI, palpitations, VENTRICULAR TACHYCARDIA. **Derm:** <u>facial flushing</u>, burning sensation, sweating. **EENT:** blurred vision, throat tightness. **GI:** metallic taste, nausea. **MS:** neck and back pain. **Neuro:** apprehension, dizziness, head pressure, headache, light-headedness. numbness, SEIZURES (ONLY WHEN USED FOR DIAGNOSTIC USE), STROKE (ONLY WHEN USED FOR DIAGNOSTIC USE), tingling. **Resp:** <u>shortness of breath</u>, chest pressure, hyperventilation. **Misc:** heaviness in arms, HYPERSENSITIVITY REACTIONS, pressure sensation in groin.

Interactions

Drug-Drug: Carbamazepine may ↑ risk of progressive heart block. **Dipyridamole** ↑ effects of adenosine; ↓ adenosine dose. Effects of adenosine ↓ by **theophylline** or **caffeine**; may need to ↑ adenosine dose. Concurrent use with **digoxin** may ↑ risk of ventricular fibrillation.

Route/Dosage

IV (Adults and Children >50 kg): *Antiarrhythmic:* 6 mg by rapid IV bolus; if no results, repeat 1–2 min later as 12-mg rapid bolus. This dose may be repeated (single dose not to exceed 12 mg). *Diagnostic use:* 140 mcg/kg/min for 6 min (0.84 mg/kg total).

IV (Children <50 kg): *Antiarrhythmic:* 0.05–0.1 mg/kg as a rapid bolus; may repeat in 1–2 min; if response is inadequate, may ↑ by 0.05–0.1 mg/kg until sinus rhythm is established or maximum dose of 0.3 mg/kg is used.

Availability (generic available)

Solution for injection: 3 mg/mL.

NURSING IMPLICATIONS

Assessment

- Monitor HR frequently (every 15–30 sec) and ECG continuously during therapy. A short, transient period of 1st-, 2nd-, or 3rd-degree heart block or asystole may occur following injection; usually resolves quickly due to short duration of adenosine. Once conversion to sinus rhythm is achieved, transient arrhythmias (premature ventricular contractions, atrial premature contractions, sinus tachycardia, sinus bradycardia, skipped beats, AV nodal block) may occur, but generally last a few sec.
- Monitor BP during therapy.
- Assess respiratory status following administration. Dyspnea may occur; condition is usually self-limiting. Patients with history of asthma may experience bronchospasm.

Implementation

IV Administration

- **IV:** Crystals may occur if adenosine is refrigerated. Warm to room temperature to dissolve crystals. Solution must be clear before use. Do not administer solutions that are discolored or contain particulate matter. Discard unused portions.
  IV Push: Dilution: Administer undiluted. **Concentration:** 3 mg/mL. **Rate:** Administer over 1–2 sec via peripheral IV as proximal as possible to trunk. Slow administration may cause ↑ HR in response to vasodilation. Follow each dose with 20-mL rapid saline flush to ensure injection reaches systemic circulation. **Intermittent Infusion:** (for use in diagnostic testing) **Dilution:** Administer 30-mL vial undiluted. **Concentration:** 3 mg/mL. **Rate:** Administer at a rate of 140 mcg/kg/min over 6 min for a total dose of 0.84 mg/kg. Thallium-201 should be injected as close to the venous access as possible at the midpoint (after 3 min) of the infusion.

Patient/Family Teaching

- Explain the purpose and side effects of adenosine; side effects may include chest, throat, neck, jaw, or GI discomfort.
- Caution patient to change positions slowly to minimize orthostatic hypotension. Doses >12 mg ↓ BP by ↓ peripheral vascular resistance.
- Instruct patient to report facial flushing, shortness of breath, or dizziness.
- Advise patient to avoid products containing methylxanthines (caffeinated coffee, tea, carbonated drinks, energy drinks, or drugs such as aminophylline or theophylline) prior to myocardial perfusion imaging study.
- Rep: Advise women of reproductive potential to notify health care professional if pregnancy is suspected or if breastfeeding.

Evaluation/Desired Outcomes

- Conversion of supraventricular tachycardia to sinus rhythm.
- Diagnosis of myocardial perfusion defects.

HIGH ALERT

ado-trastuzumab

(ado tras-**too**-zoo-mab)

Kadcyla

Classification

Therapeutic: antineoplastics

Pharmacologic: drug-antibody conjugates

Indications

HER2-positive metastatic breast cancer in patients previously treated with trastuzumab and a taxane who have either received prior therapy for metastatic disease or developed disease recurrence during or within 6 mo of completing adjuvant therapy. Adjuvant treatment of HER2-positive early breast cancer in patients who have residual invasive disease after neoadjuvant taxane and trastuzumab-based therapy.

Action

A HER2-targeted antibody and microtubule inhibitor conjugate. Trastuzumab, the antibody, attaches to receptors and is taken into the cell, where the microtubule inhibitor DM1 causes cell cycle arrest and death. **Therapeutic Effects:** Decreased spread of metastatic breast cancer, with improved progression-free survival.

Pharmacokinetics

Absorption: IV administration results in complete bioavailability.

Distribution: Unknown.

Metabolism and Excretion: DM1 is metabolized by CYP3A4/5.

Half-life: 4 days.

TIME/ACTION PROFILE (comparative improvement in progression-free survival)

ROUTE	ONSET	PEAK	DURATION
IV	4–6 mo	10–12 mo	2 yr

Contraindications/Precautions

Contraindicated in: Interstitial lung disease or pneumonitis; OB: Pregnancy; Lactation: Lactation.

Use Cautiously in: Underlying cardiovascular or pulmonary disease, including dyspnea at rest; Rep: Women of reproductive potential and men with female partners of reproductive potential should use effective contraception; Pedi: Safety and effectiveness not established in children.

Adverse Reactions/Side Effects

CV: HF, hypertension, peripheral edema. **Derm:** pruritus, rash. **EENT:** ↑ lacrimation, blurred vision, conjunctivitis, dry eyes. **F and E:** hypokalemia. **GI:** ↑ liver enzymes, constipation, nausea, altered taste, diarrhea, dry mouth, dyspepsia, HEPATOTOXICITY, stomatitis, vomiting. **GU:** ↓ fertility. **Hemat:** anemia, HEMORRHAGE, neutropenia, THROMBOCYTOPENIA. **MS:** musculoskeletal pain, arthralgia, myalgia. **Neuro:** fatigue, headache, peripheral neuropathy, dizziness, insomnia, weakness. **Resp:** cough, INTERSTITIAL LUNG DISEASE (ILD)/PNEUMONITIS. **Misc:** chills, fever, HYPERSENSITIVITY REACTIONS, infusion-related reactions.

Interactions

Drug-Drug: Strong CYP3A4 inhibitors, including **atazanavir, clarithromycin, itraconazole, ketoconazole, nefazodone, nelfinavir, ritonavir,** and **voriconazole**, may ↑ levels and risk of toxicity; avoid concurrent use. Concurrent use of **anticoagulants** or **antiplatelet agents**, especially during the first cycle, may ↑ risk of bleeding.

Route/Dosage

Should not be used interchangeably with trastuzumab.

Metastatic Breast Cancer

IV (Adults): 3.6 mg/kg every 3 wk until disease progression or unacceptable toxicity.

Early Breast Cancer

IV (Adults): 3.6 mg/kg every 3 wk (21-day cycle) for a total of 14 cycles unless there is disease progression or unacceptable toxicity.

Availability

Lyophilized powder for injection: 100 mg/vial, 160 mg/vial.

NURSING IMPLICATIONS

Assessment

- Evaluate left ventricular function in all patients prior to and every 3 mo during therapy. **For patients with metastatic disease:** *If symptomatic HF:* Permanently discontinue ado-trastuzumab. *If left ventricular ejection fraction (LVEF) <40%:* Hold dose. Repeat LVEF assessment within 3 wk. If LVEF <40% is confirmed, permanently discontinue ado-trastuzumab. *If LVEF 40–≤45% and ↓ is ≥10% points from baseline:* Hold dose. Repeat LVEF within 3 wk. If LVEF has not recovered to within 10% points from baseline, permanently discontinue ado-trastuzumab. *If LVEF 40–≤45% and ↓ is <10% points from baseline:* Continue therapy. Repeat LVEF within 3 wk. *If LVEF >45%:* Continue therapy. **For patients with early breast cancer:** *If LVEF <45%:* Hold dose. Repeat LVEF within 3 wk. If LVEF <45% is confirmed, permanently discontinue ado-trastuzumab. *If LVEF 45–< 50% and ↓ is ≥10% points from baseline:* Hold dose. Repeat LVEF within 3 wk. *If LVEF <50% and not recovered to <10% points from baseline:* Permanently discontinue ado-trastuzumab. *If LVEF 45–<50% and ↓ is <10% points from baseline:* Continue therapy. Repeat LVEF within 3 wk. *If LVEF ≥50%:* Continue therapy. *If symptomatic HF, Grade 3–4 left ventricular systolic dysfunction, Grade 3–4 HF, or Grade 2 HF accompanied by LVEF <45%:* Permanently discontinue ado-trastuzumab.
- Assess for signs and symptoms of infusion reactions (fever, chills, flushing, dyspnea, hypotension, wheezing, bronchospasm, tachycardia). Slow or interrupt therapy if symptoms are severe. Observe closely during first infusion. Permanently discontinue for life-threatening reactions.
- Monitor neurologic status before and during treatment. Assess for paresthesia, loss of deep tendon reflexes (Achilles reflex is usually first involved), weakness (wrist drop or footdrop, gait disturbances), cranial nerve palsies (jaw pain, hoarseness, ptosis, visual changes), arthralgia, myalgia, muscle spasm, autonomic dysfunction (ileus, difficulty voiding, orthostatic hypotension, impaired sweating), and CNS dysfunction (↓ level of consciousness, agitation, hallucinations). *If Grade 3 or 4 peripheral neuropathy (severe symptoms; limiting self-care activities of daily living [ADL]) occurs:* Temporarily discontinue therapy until resolution to Grade ≤2 (moderate symptoms; limiting instrumental ADL) neuropathy.
- Monitor for signs and symptoms of pulmonary toxicity (dyspnea, cough, fatigue, pulmonary infiltrates). Permanently discontinue ado-trastuzumab if ILD or pneumonitis develops.
- Monitor for hemorrhage during therapy, especially in patients receiving anticoagulants or antiplatelet therapy or who have thrombocytopenia.

Lab Test Considerations

- HER2-protein overexpression is used to determine whether treatment with ado-trastuzumab is indicated and should be determined by labs with proficiency in specific technology used. Information on approved tests is available at http://www.fda.gov/CompanionDiagnostics.
- Verify negative pregnancy status before starting therapy.
- Monitor serum AST, ALT, and bilirubin prior to starting therapy and before each dose. **For patients with metastatic disease:** *If AST/ALT >2.5–≤5 times upper limit of normal (ULN):* Treat at same dose. *If AST/ALT >5–≤20 times ULN:* Hold dose until AST/ALT recovers to Grade ≤2; then ↓ by one dose level. *If AST/ALT >20 times ULN:* Permanently discontinue ado-trastuzumab. *If serum bilirubin >1.5–≤3 times ULN:* Hold dose until bilirubin recovers to Grade ≤1; then treat at same dose level. *If bilirubin >3–≤10 times ULN:* Hold dose until bilirubin recovers to Grade ≤1; then ↓ by one dose level. *If bilirubin >10 times ULN:* Permanently discontinue ado-trastuzumab. *If AST/ALT >3 times ULN and concurrent total bilirubin >2 times ULN:* Permanently discontinue ado-trastuzumab. **For patients with early breast cancer:** *If ALT >3–≤20 times ULN on day of scheduled treatment:* Hold dose until ALT recovers to Grade ≤1; then ↓ by one dose level. *If ALT >20 times ULN at any time:* Permanently discontinue ado-trastuzumab. *If AST >3–≤5 times ULN on day of scheduled treatment:* Hold dose until AST recovers to Grade ≤1; then treat with same dose. *If AST >5–≤20 times ULN on day of scheduled treatment:* Hold dose until AST recovers to Grade ≤1; then ↓ by one dose level. *If AST >20 times ULN at any time:* Permanently discontinue ado-trastuzumab. *If total bilirubin >1–≤2 times ULN on day of scheduled treatment:*

Hold dose until total bilirubin ≤1 times ULN; then ↓ by one dose level. *If total bilirubin >2 times ULN at any time:* Permanently discontinue ado-trastuzumab.

- Monitor platelet count prior to starting therapy and before each dose. Nadir of thrombocytopenia occurs by Day 8 and generally improves to Grade 0 or 1 by next scheduled dose. **For patients with metastatic disease:** *If platelets 25,000–<50,000/mm³:* Hold dose until platelet count recovers to ≥75,000/mm³; then treat at same dose level. *If platelets <25,000/mm³:* Hold dose until platelet count recovers to ≥75,000/mm³; then ↓ by one dose level. **For patients with early breast cancer:** *If platelets 25,000–<75,000/mm³:* Hold dose until platelet count recovers to ≥75,000/mm³); then treat at same dose level. If two delays required due to thrombocytopenia, ↓ by one dose level. *If platelets <25,000/mm³:* Hold dose until platelet count recovers to ≥75,000/mm³; then ↓ by one dose level.
- May ↓ hemoglobin, neutrophils, and serum potassium.

Implementation

- ***High Alert:*** Do not confuse ado-trastuzumab with trastuzumab. Trade name of administered product should be clearly recorded in patient file to improve traceability.
- ***High Alert:*** Fatalities have occurred with chemotherapeutic agents. Before administering, clarify all ambiguous orders; double-check single, daily, and course-of-therapy dose limits; have second practitioner independently double-check original order, dose calculations, and infusion pump settings.
- Dose reduction schedule: *1st dose reduction:* 3 mg/kg; *2nd dose reduction:* 2.4 mg/kg; *Need for further dose reduction:* Permanently discontinue ado-trastuzumab.
- Solution should be prepared in a biologic cabinet. Wear gloves, gown, and mask while handling medication. Discard IV equipment in specially designated containers.

IV Administration

- Ado-trastuzumab is an irritant. If extravasation occurs, immediately stop infusion. Leave needle/cannula in place temporarily but do not flush the line. Gently aspirate extravasated solution; then remove needle/cannula. Elevate patient's extremity.
- **Intermittent Infusion: Reconstitution:** Slowly inject 5 or 8 mL of sterile water for injection into 100 or 160 mg vial of ado-trastuzumab respectively. Swirl gently until dissolved; do not shake. Solution is clear, colorless to pale brown, and slightly opalescent; do not administer solutions that are discolored or contain particulates. Use reconstituted vials immediately or store in refrigerator up to 4 hr; then discard. Do not freeze. **Concentration:** 20 mg/mL. **Dilution:** Withdraw required dose from vial and add to infusion bag containing 250 mL of 0.9% NaCl; do not use dextrose solutions. Gently invert bag to mix without foaming. Use diluted solution immediately; may be stored in refrigerator up to 24 hr prior to use; then discard; do not freeze or shake. **Rate:** Infuse through a 0.2- or 0.22-micron in-line non-protein-adsorptive polyethersulfone filter. Do not administer as IV push or bolus. *1st infusion:* Infuse over 90 min; observe for infusion-related reaction. *Subsequent infusions:* Infuse over 30 min if prior infusions were well tolerated. Observe patient during and for ≥90 min after infusion.
- **Y-Site Incompatibility:** Do not administer other drugs through same IV line.

Patient/Family Teaching

- Explain purpose of medication to patient. If dose is missed, administer as soon as possible; do not wait until next scheduled dose. Adjust schedule to maintain 3-wk interval between doses.
- Advise patient to notify health care provider immediately if signs and symptoms of liver injury (nausea, vomiting, abdominal pain, jaundice, dark urine, pruritus, anorexia) or HF (new onset or worsening shortness of breath, cough, swelling of ankles/legs, palpitations, weight gain of >5 lbs in 24 hr, dizziness, loss of consciousness) occur.
- Advise patient to notify health care provider if signs of peripheral neuropathy (burning, numbness, pain in hands and feet/legs) occur.
- Rep: May cause fetal harm. Advise women of reproductive potential to use a highly effective method of contraception during therapy and for ≥7 mo after last dose. Advise men with a female partner of reproductive potential to use a highly effective method of contraception during therapy and for ≥4 mo after last dose. Notify health care provider promptly if pregnancy is suspected and avoid breastfeeding for ≥7 mo after last dose. Encourage women who have been exposed to ado-trastuzumab during pregnancy, either directly or through seminal fluid to immediately report exposure to Genentech Adverse Event Line at 1-888-835-2555. May impair fertility in all patients.

Evaluation/Desired Outcomes

- Decreased spread of metastatic breast cancer.

albuterol (al-**byoo**-ter-ole)

~~Accuneb,~~ ✱ Airomir, Proair Respiclick, Proventil HFA, ✱ Salbutamol, Ventolin HFA, ✱ Ventolin Diskus, ~~VoSpire ER~~

Classification

Therapeutic: bronchodilators
Pharmacologic: adrenergics

Indications
Treatment or prevention of bronchospasm in asthma or chronic obstructive pulmonary disease (COPD). **Inhaln:** Prevention of exercise-induced bronchospasm. **PO:** Treatment of bronchospasm in asthma or COPD.

Action
Binds to $beta_2$-adrenergic receptors in airway smooth muscle, leading to activation of adenyl cyclase and increased levels of cyclic-3′, 5′-adenosine monophosphate (cAMP). Increases in cAMP activate kinases, which inhibit the phosphorylation of myosin and decrease intracellular calcium. Decreased intracellular calcium relaxes smooth muscle airways. Relaxation of airway smooth muscle with subsequent bronchodilation. Relatively selective for $beta_2$ (pulmonary) receptors. **Therapeutic Effects:** Bronchodilation.

Pharmacokinetics
Absorption: Well absorbed after oral administration but rapidly undergoes extensive metabolism.
Distribution: Small amounts appear in breast milk.
Metabolism and Excretion: Extensively metabolized by the liver and other tissues.
Half-life: Oral 2.7–5 hr; Inhalation: 3.8 hr.

TIME/ACTION PROFILE (bronchodilation)

ROUTE	ONSET	PEAK	DURATION
PO	15–30 min	2–3 hr	4–6 hr or more
Inhaln	5–15 min	60–90 min	3–6 hr

Contraindications/Precautions
Contraindicated in: Hypersensitivity to adrenergic amines.
Use Cautiously in: Cardiac disease; Hypertension; Hyperthyroidism; Diabetes; Glaucoma; Seizure disorders; Excess inhaler use may lead to tolerance and paradoxical bronchospasm; OB: Use during pregnancy only if potential maternal benefit justifies potential fetal risk; Lactation: Use while breastfeeding only if potential maternal benefit justifies potential risk to infant; Pedi: Children <2 yr (safety and effectiveness not established); Geri: ↑ risk of adverse reactions in older adults; may require dose ↓.

Adverse Reactions/Side Effects
CV: chest pain, palpitations, angina, arrhythmias, hypertension. **Endo:** hyperglycemia. **F and E:** hypokalemia. **GI:** nausea, vomiting. **Neuro:** nervousness, restlessness, tremor, headache, hyperactivity (children), insomnia. **Resp:** PARADOXICAL BRONCHOSPASM (EXCESSIVE USE OF INHALERS).

Interactions
Drug-Drug: Concurrent use with other **adrenergic agents** will have ↑ adrenergic side effects. Use with **MAO inhibitors** may lead to hypertensive crisis. **Beta blockers** may negate therapeutic effect. May ↓ serum **digoxin** levels. Cardiovascular effects are potentiated in patients receiving **tricyclic antidepressants**. Risk of hypokalemia ↑ concurrent use of **potassium-losing diuretics**. Hypokalemia ↑ the risk of **digoxin** toxicity.
Drug-Natural Products: Use with caffeine-containing herbs (**cola nut**, **guarana**, **tea**, **coffee**) ↑ stimulant effect.

Route/Dosage
PO (Adults and Children ≥12 yr): 2–4 mg 3–4 times daily (not to exceed 32 mg/day).
PO (Geriatric Patients): Initial dose should not exceed 2 mg 3–4 times daily; may be ↑ carefully (up to 32 mg/day).
PO (Children 6–12 yr): 2 mg 3–4 times daily; may be carefully ↑ as needed (not to exceed 8 mg/day).
PO (Children 2–6 yr): 0.1 mg/kg 3 times daily (not to exceed 2 mg 3 times daily initially); may be carefully ↑ to 0.2 mg/kg 3 times daily (not to exceed 4 mg 3 times daily).
Inhaln: (Adults and Children ≥4 yr): *Via metered-dose inhaler or dry powder inhaler:* 2 inhalations every 4–6 hr (some patients may respond to 1 inhalation) or 2 inhalations 15 min before exercise; *NIH Guidelines for acute asthma exacerbation: Children:* 4–8 puffs every 20 min for 3 doses then every 1–4 hr; *Adults:* 4–8 puffs every 20 min for up to 4 hr then every 1–4 hr as needed.
Inhaln: (Adults and Children >12 yr): *NIH Guidelines for acute asthma exacerbation via nebulization or IPPB:* 2.5–5 mg every 20 min for 3 doses then 2.5–10 mg every 1–4 hr as needed; *Continuous nebulization:* 10–15 mg/hr.
Inhaln: (Children 2–12 yr): *NIH Guidelines for acute asthma exacerbation via nebulization or IPPB:* 0.15 mg/kg/dose (minimum dose 2.5 mg) every 20 min for 3 doses; then 0.15–0.3 mg/kg (not to exceed 10 mg) every 1–4 hr as needed *or* 1.25 mg 3–4 times daily for children 10–15 kg *or* 2.5 mg 3–4 times daily for children >15 kg; *Continuous nebulization:* 0.5–3 mg/kg/hr.
Inhaln: (Neonates): 1.25 mg/dose every 8 hr via nebulization or 1–2 puffs via MDI into the ventilator circuit every 6 hr.

Availability (generic available)
Immediate-release tablets: 2 mg, 4 mg. **Oral syrup (strawberry flavored):** 2 mg/5 mL. **Inhalation solution:** 0.63 mg/3 mL (0.021%), 1.25 mg/3 mL (0.042%), 2.5 mg/3 mL (0.083%)🍁 1 mg/mL🍁 2 mg/mL, 5 mg/mL (0.5%). **Metered-dose aerosol:** 90 mcg/inhalation in 6.7-g, 8-g, 8.5-g, and 18-g canisters (200 metered inhalations)🍁 100 mcg/spray. **Powder**

for inhalation (Proair Respiclick): 90 mcg/inhalation (200 metered inhalations). **Powder for inhalation (Ventolin Diskus):** 🍁 200 mcg. ***In combination with:*** budesonide (Airsupra); ipratropium (Combivent Respimat). See Appendix N.

NURSING IMPLICATIONS

Assessment

- Assess lung sounds, pulse, and BP before administration and during peak of medication. Note amount, color, and character of sputum produced.
- Monitor pulmonary function tests before initiating therapy and periodically during therapy.
- Observe for paradoxical bronchospasm (wheezing). If condition occurs, withhold medication and notify health care professional immediately.

Lab Test Considerations

- May cause transient ↓ in serum potassium concentrations with nebulization or higher-than-recommended doses.

Implementation

- **PO:** Administer oral medication with meals to minimize gastric irritation.
- **Inhaln:** Shake inhaler well, and allow at least 1 min between inhalations of aerosol medication. Prime the inhaler before first use by releasing 4 test sprays into the air away from the face. *Proair Respiclick* does not require priming. Pedi: Use spacer for children <8 yr of age.
- For nebulization or IPPB, the 0.5-, 0.83-, 1-, and 2-mg/mL solutions do not require dilution before administration. The 5 mg/mL (0.5%) solution must be diluted with 1–2.5 mL of 0.9% NaCl for inhalation. Diluted solutions are stable for 24 hr at room temperature or 48 hr if refrigerated.
- For nebulizer, compressed air or oxygen flow should be 6–10 L/min; a single treatment of 3 mL lasts about 10 min.
- IPPB usually lasts 5–20 min.

Patient/Family Teaching

- Instruct patient to take albuterol as directed. If on a scheduled dosing regimen, take missed dose as soon as remembered, spacing remaining doses at regular intervals. Do not double doses or increase the dose or frequency of doses. Caution patient not to exceed recommended dose; may cause adverse effects, paradoxical bronchospasm (more likely with first dose from new canister), or loss of effectiveness of medication.
- Instruct patient to contact health care professional immediately if shortness of breath is not relieved by medication or is accompanied by diaphoresis, dizziness, palpitations, or chest pain.
- Instruct patient to prime unit with 4 sprays before using and to discard canister after 200 sprays. Actuators should not be changed among products.
- Inform patient that these products contain hydrofluoroalkane (HFA) and the propellant and are described as non-CFC or CFC-free (contain no chlorofluorocarbons).
- Instruct patient to notify health care professional of all Rx or OTC medications, vitamins, or herbal products being taken and to consult health care professional before taking any OTC medications or alcoholic beverages concurrently with this therapy. Caution patient also to avoid smoking and other respiratory irritants.
- Inform patient that albuterol may cause an unusual or bad taste.
- Rep: Advise females of reproductive potential to notify health care professional if pregnancy is planned or suspected or if breastfeeding. Encourage patients who become pregnant during therapy to enroll in the pregnancy registry that monitors pregnancy outcomes in women exposed to asthma medications during pregnancy. For more information, contact the MothersToBaby Pregnancy Studies conducted by the Organization of Teratology Information Specialists at 1-877-311-8972 or visit http://mothertobaby.org/pregnancy-studies/.
- **Inhaln:** Instruct patient in the proper use of the metered-dose inhaler or nebulizer (see Appendix C).
- Advise patients to use albuterol first if using other inhalation medications and allow 5 min to elapse before administering other inhalant medications unless otherwise directed.
- Advise patient to rinse mouth with water after each inhalation dose to minimize dry mouth and clean the mouthpiece with water at least once a wk.
- Instruct patient to notify health care professional if there is no response to the usual dose or if contents of one canister are used in less than 2 wk. Asthma and treatment regimen should be re-evaluated and corticosteroids should be considered. Need for increased use to treat symptoms indicates decrease in asthma control and need to re-evaluate patient's therapy.

Evaluation/Desired Outcomes

- Prevention or relief of bronchospasm.

alclometasone, See CORTICOSTEROIDS (TOPICAL)

HIGH ALERT

alectinib (al-ekti-nib)

Alecensa, 🍁 Alecensaro

Classification

Therapeutic: antineoplastics

Pharmacologic: kinase inhibitors

Indications

Patients with anaplastic lymphoma kinase (ALK)-positive metastatic non-small cell lung cancer (NSCLC).

Adjuvant treatment following tumor resection of ALK-positive NSCLC (tumors ≥ 4 cm or node positive).

Action

Inhibits tyrosine kinase receptors targeting ALK and RET. **Therapeutic Effects:** Decreased spread of NSCLC and improved disease-free survival.

Pharmacokinetics

Absorption: 37% absorbed following oral administration; high-fat, high-calorie meals ↑ absorption.
Distribution: Extensively distributed to tissues.
Protein Binding: 99%.
Metabolism and Excretion: Primarily metabolized by the liver via the CYP3A4 isoenzyme to its active metabolite, M4 (also metabolized by CYP3A4). 84% excreted in feces unchanged; minimal excretion in urine.
Half-life: *Alectinib:* 33 hr; *M4 active metabolite:* 31 hr.

TIME/ACTION PROFILE (plasma concentrations)

ROUTE	ONSET	PEAK	DURATION
PO	unknown	4 hr	unknown

Contraindications/Precautions

Contraindicated in: OB: Pregnancy; Lactation: Lactation.
Use Cautiously in: Severe renal impairment or end-stage renal disease; Severe hepatic impairment (↓ dose); Rep: Women of reproductive potential; Pedi: Safety and effectiveness not established in children.

Adverse Reactions/Side Effects

CV: bradycardia, edema. **Derm:** photosensitivity, rash. **EENT:** blurred vision, diplopia. **Endo:** hyperglycemia. **F and E:** hypocalcemia, hypokalemia, hyponatremia, hypophosphatemia. **GI:** constipation, diarrhea, HEPATOTOXICITY, hyperbilirubinemia, nausea, vomiting. **GU:** renal impairment. **Hemat:** anemia, lymphopenia, BLEEDING, hemolytic anemia. **Metab:** ↑ weight. **MS:** ↑ creatine kinase, back pain, myalgia. **Neuro:** fatigue, headache. **Resp:** cough, dyspnea, INTERSTITIAL LUNG DISEASE (ILD)/PNEUMONITIS, PULMONARY EMBOLISM.

Interactions

Drug-Drug: None reported.

Route/Dosage

Metastatic Non-Small Cell Lung Cancer

PO (Adults): 600 mg twice daily; continue until disease progression or unacceptable toxicity.

Hepatic Impairment

PO (Adults): *Severe hepatic impairment:* 450 mg twice daily; continue until disease progression or unacceptable toxicity.

Adjuvant Treatment of Resected Non-Small Cell Lung Cancer

PO (Adults): 600 mg twice daily; continue for a total of 2 yr or until disease recurrence or unacceptable toxicity.

Hepatic Impairment

PO (Adults): *Severe hepatic impairment:* 450 mg twice daily; continue for a total of 2 yr or until disease recurrence or unacceptable toxicity.

Availability

Capsules: 150 mg.

NURSING IMPLICATIONS

Assessment

- Monitor for signs and symptoms of ILD/pneumonitis (worsening of respiratory symptoms, dyspnea, cough, fever). Withhold therapy if symptoms occur and permanently discontinue if no other potential causes are identified.
- Monitor heart rate and BP regularly during therapy. *If symptomatic bradycardia occurs*, withhold therapy until asymptomatic or heart rate ≥60 bpm. If concomitant medication identified as contributing and is discontinued, or its dose adjusted, resume alectinib at previous dose upon recovery to asymptomatic bradycardia or to heart rate ≥60 bpm. If no contributing medication identified, or if contributing medications are not discontinued or dose modified, resume alectinib at reduced dose upon recovery to asymptomatic bradycardia or to heart rate of ≥60 bpm. *If life-threatening bradycardia occurs*, permanently discontinue alectinib if no contributing medication is identified. If contributing medication is identified and discontinued, or its dose is adjusted, resume alectinib at reduced dose upon recovery to asymptomatic bradycardia or to heart rate of ≥60 bpm, with frequent monitoring as clinically indicated. Permanently discontinue alectinib in case of recurrence.
- Assess for myalgia periodically during therapy.

Lab Test Considerations

- Verify negative pregnancy test before starting therapy. For patient selection, determine presence of ALK positivity in tumor tissue or plasma specimens using FDA approved test. Information on FDA-approved tests for the detection of ALK rearrangements in NSCLC is available at http://www.fda.gov/CompanionDiagnostics. Dose reduction schedule: 1st dose reduction: 450 mg twice daily, 2nd dose reduction 300 mg twice daily. Discontinue if unable to tolerate 300 mg twice daily.
- Monitor liver function tests every 2 wk during first 3 mo of therapy, and then monthly and as clinically indicated during treatment. *If ALT or AST ↑ >5*

times upper limit of normal (ULN) with total bilirubin ≤2 times ULN, temporarily withhold until recovery to baseline or ≤3 times ULN; then resume at reduced dose. *If ALT or AST ↑ >3 times ULN with total bilirubin ↑>2 times ULN in absence of cholestasis or hemolysis*, permanently discontinue alectinib. *If total bilirubin ↑ >3 times ULN*, temporarily withhold until recovery to baseline or to ≤1.5 times ULN; then resume at reduced dose.

- Assess CK every 2 wk during 1st mo of therapy and in patients reporting unexplained muscle pain, tenderness, or weakness. *If ↑ CK >5 times ULN*, temporarily withhold until recovery to baseline or ≤2.5 times ULN; then resume at same dose. *If ↑ CK >10 times ULN or 2nd occurrence of ↑ CK >5 times ULN*, temporarily withhold until recovery to baseline or ≤2.5 times ULN; then resume at reduced dose.
- Monitor serum creatinine periodically during therapy. *If Grade 3 renal impairment occurs*, hold doses until serum creatinine ≤ 1.5 times ULN; then resume at reduced dose. *If Grade 4 renal impairment occurs*, discontinue alectinib permanently.
- May cause hyperglycemia, hypocalcemia, hypokalemia, hypophosphatemia, and hyponatremia.
- May cause anemia and lymphopenia.

Implementation

- **PO:** Administer twice daily with food. ***DNC:*** Swallow capsules whole; do not open or dissolve capsule contents.

Patient/Family Teaching

- Instruct patient to take alectinib as directed. If a dose is missed or vomiting occurs after taking, omit dose and take next dose at scheduled time. Advise patient to read *Patient Information* before starting therapy and with each Rx refill in case of changes.
- Advise patient to use sunscreen and lip balm (SPF ≥50) and to wear protective clothing to prevent photosensitivity reaction.
- Advise patient to notify health care professional if signs and symptoms of liver problems (feeling tired, itchy skin, feeling less hungry than usual, nausea or vomiting, yellowing of skin or whites of eyes, pain on right side of stomach, dark urine, bleeding or bruising more easily than normal), respiratory problems (trouble breathing, shortness of breath, cough, fever), bradycardia (dizziness, light-headedness, syncope), or myalgia (unexplained muscle pain, tenderness, or weakness) occur.
- Instruct patient to notify health care professional of all Rx or OTC medications, vitamins, or herbal products being taken and consult health care professional before taking any new medications.
- Rep: May cause fetal harm. Advise females of reproductive potential to use effective contraception and avoid breastfeeding during and for at least 1 wk following therapy. Advise males with female partners of reproductive potential to use effective contraception during and for 3 mo after last dose.

Evaluation/Desired Outcomes

- Decreased spread of NSCLC and improved disease-free survival.

alendronate

(a-**len**-drone-ate)

Binosto, Fosamax

Classification

Therapeutic: bone resorption inhibitors

Pharmacologic: bisphosphonates

Indications

Treatment and prevention of postmenopausal osteoporosis. Treatment of osteoporosis in men. Treatment of Paget disease of the bone. Treatment of corticosteroid-induced osteoporosis in patients (men and women) who are receiving ≥7.5 mg of prednisone/day (or equivalent) with evidence of decreased bone mineral density.

Action

Inhibits resorption of bone by inhibiting osteoclast activity. **Therapeutic Effects:** Reversal of the progression of osteoporosis with decreased fractures. Decreased progression of Paget disease.

Pharmacokinetics

Absorption: Poorly absorbed (0.6–0.8%) after oral administration.

Distribution: Transiently distributes to soft tissue; then distributes to bone.

Metabolism and Excretion: Excreted in urine.

Half-life: 10 yr (reflects release of drug from skeleton).

TIME/ACTION PROFILE (inhibition of bone resorption)

ROUTE	ONSET	PEAK	DURATION
PO	1 mo	3–6 mo	3 wk–7 mo†

† After discontinuation of alendronate.

Contraindications/Precautions

Contraindicated in: Abnormalities of the esophagus that delay esophageal emptying (e.g. strictures, achalasia); Inability to stand/sit upright for at least 30 min; Renal impairment (CCr <35 mL/min); OB: Pregnancy.

Use Cautiously in: History of upper GI disorders; Pre-existing hypocalcemia or vitamin D deficiency; Invasive dental procedures; cancer; receiving chemotherapy, corticosteroids, or angiogenesis inhibitors; poor oral hygiene; periodontal disease; dental disease; anemia; coagulopathy; infection; or poorly fitting dentures (may ↑ risk of jaw osteonecrosis); HF or hypertension (effervescent tablet only); Lactation:

Safety not established in breastfeeding; Pedi: Safety and effectiveness not established in children.

Adverse Reactions/Side Effects

CV: atrial fibrillation. **Derm:** erythema, photosensitivity, rash. **EENT:** blurred vision, conjunctivitis, eye pain/inflammation. **GI:** abdominal distention, abdominal pain, acid regurgitation, constipation, diarrhea, dyspepsia, dysphagia, esophageal cancer, esophageal ulcer, esophagitis, flatulence, gastritis, nausea, taste perversion, vomiting. **MS:** musculoskeletal pain, femur fractures, osteonecrosis (primarily of jaw). **Neuro:** headache. **Resp:** asthma exacerbation.

Interactions

Drug-Drug: Calcium supplements, antacids, and **levothyroxine** may ↓ absorption. Doses >10 mg/day ↑ risk of adverse GI events when used with **NSAIDs**.
Drug-Food: Food significantly ↓ absorption. **Caffeine (coffee, tea, cola), mineral water,** and **orange juice** also ↓ absorption.

Route/Dosage

Treatment of Osteoporosis

PO (Adults): 10 mg once daily or 70 mg once weekly.

Prevention of Osteoporosis

PO (Adults): 5 mg once daily or 35 mg once weekly.

Paget Disease

PO (Adults): 40 mg once daily for 6 mo. Retreatment may be considered for patients who relapse.

Treatment of Corticosteroid-Induced Osteoporosis in Men and Women

PO (Adults): *Men and premenopausal women:* 5 mg once daily. *Postmenopausal women not receiving estrogen:* 10 mg once daily.

Availability (generic available)

Tablets: 5 mg, 10 mg, 35 mg, 40 mg, 70 mg. **Effervescent tablets (strawberry flavor) (contains 603 mg of sodium/tablet) (Binosto):** 70 mg. **Oral solution (raspberry flavor):** 70 mg/75 mL. ***In combination with:*** cholecalciferol (Fosamax plus D). See Appendix N.

NURSING IMPLICATIONS

Assessment

- **Osteoporosis:** Assess for low bone mass before and periodically during therapy.
- **Paget Disease:** Assess for symptoms of Paget disease (bone pain, headache, ↓ visual and auditory acuity, ↑ skull size).
- Assess for upper GI adverse effects (dysphagia, odynophagia, upper abdominal pain, retrosternal pain, new or worsening heartburn). *If these GI adverse effects occur,* discontinue alendronate and evaluate for gastric or duodenal ulcers.
- Monitor for fractures; temporary discontinuation may be necessary especially with atypical femur fractures.
- Assess for signs and symptoms of osteonecrosis of the jaw (halitosis, jaw pain, jaw swelling, exposed bone, loose teeth, dental pain); discontinuation may be necessary.
- Assess pain levels; if severe musculoskeletal pain develops, notify provider for evaluation; discontinuation may be necessary.

Lab Test Considerations

- *Osteoporosis:* Assess serum calcium, phosphate, and vitamin D levels before and periodically during therapy. Correct hypocalcemia and vitamin D deficiency before initiating alendronate therapy. May cause mild, transient ↑ of calcium and phosphate.
- **Paget Disease:** Monitor alkaline phosphatase before and periodically during therapy. Alendronate is indicated for patients with alkaline phosphatase twice the upper limit of normal.

Implementation

- **PO:** Administer 1st thing in the morning with 6–8 ounces of plain water 30 min before other medications, beverages, or food. Oral solution should be followed by ≥2 ounces of water. ***DNC:*** Swallow tablets whole; do not crush, break, or chew.
- For *effervescent tablets,* dissolve one tablet in half a glass (4 ounces) of plain room temperature water (not mineral water or flavored water). Wait ≥5 min after the effervescence stops, stir the solution for approximately 10 sec, and drink contents.

Patient/Family Teaching

- Explain the purpose and side effects of alendronate to patient. Instruct on the importance of taking exactly as directed, 1st thing in the morning, 30 min before other medications, beverages, or food. Waiting >30 min will improve absorption. Take alendronate with 6–8 ounces of plain water (mineral water, orange juice, coffee, and other beverages ↓ absorption). If a dose is missed, skip dose and resume the next morning; do not double doses or take later in the day. If a weekly dose is missed, take the morning after remembered and resume the following wk on the chosen day. Do not take two tablets on the same day. Do not discontinue without consulting health care professional. Advise patient to read *Medication Guide* before starting therapy and with each Rx refill in case of changes.
- Caution patient to remain upright for 30 min following dose to facilitate passage to stomach and ↓ risk of esophageal irritation. Advise patient to discontinue alendronate and notify health care provider if pain or difficulty swallowing, retrosternal pain, or new/worsening heartburn occur.

- Caution patient not to swallow, chew, or allow undissolved effervescent tablet to dissolve in their mouth; may cause oropharyngeal irritation.
- Counsel patient on sodium-restricted diet that the effervescent tablet contains 603 mg sodium.
- Advise patient to eat a balanced diet and consult health care professional about the need for supplemental calcium and vitamin D.
- Encourage patient to participate in regular exercise and to modify behaviors that ↑ the risk of osteoporosis (stop smoking, ↓ alcohol consumption).
- Advise parents to notify health care professional of all Rx or OTC medications, vitamins, or herbal products being taken and to consult with health care professional before taking other medications.
- Advise patient to inform health care professional of alendronate therapy prior to dental surgery.
- Caution patient to use sunscreen and protective clothing to prevent photosensitivity reactions.
- Advise patient to notify health care professional if blurred vision, eye pain, or inflammation occur.
- Rep: May cause fetal harm. Advise women of reproductive potential to notify health care professional if pregnancy is planned or suspected or if breastfeeding during therapy. If pregnancy is detected, discontinue alendronate as soon as possible.

Evaluation/Desired Outcomes
- Prevention of or decrease in the progression of osteoporosis in postmenopausal women. Reassess need for medication periodically. Consider discontinuation of alendronate after 3–5 yr in patients with low risk of fractures. If discontinued, reassess fracture risk periodically.
- Treatment of osteoporosis in men.
- Decrease in the progression of Paget disease.
- Treatment of corticosteroid-induced osteoporosis.

alfuzosin (al-fyoo-zo-sin)
Uroxatral, ✱ Xatral

Classification
Therapeutic: urinary tract antispasmodics
Pharmacologic: peripherally acting antiadrenergics

Indications
Symptomatic benign prostatic hyperplasia (BPH).

Action
Selectively blocks $alpha_1$-adrenergic receptors in the lower urinary tract to relax smooth muscle in the bladder neck and prostate. **Therapeutic Effects:** Increased urine flow and decreased symptoms of BPH.

Pharmacokinetics
Absorption: 49% absorbed following oral administration; food ↑ absorption.
Distribution: Unknown.
Metabolism and Excretion: Mostly metabolized by the liver via the CYP3A4 isoenzyme system; 11% excreted unchanged in urine.
Half-life: 10 hr.

TIME/ACTION PROFILE

ROUTE	ONSET	PEAK	DURATION
PO-ER	within hr	8 hr	24 hr

Contraindications/Precautions
Contraindicated in: Hypersensitivity; Moderate to severe hepatic impairment; Concurrent use of strong CYP3A4 inhibitors; Severe renal impairment.
Use Cautiously in: Congenital or acquired QTc interval prolongation or concurrent use of other drugs known to prolong QTc interval; Mild hepatic impairment; Symptomatic hypotension; Concurrent use of antihypertensive agents, phosphodiesterase type 5 inhibitors, or nitrates (↑ risk of postural hypotension); Previous hypotensive episode with other medications; Geri: Consider age-related changes in body mass and cardiac, renal, and hepatic function when prescribing in older adults.

Adverse Reactions/Side Effects
CV: postural hypotension. **Derm:** TOXIC EPIDERMAL NECROLYSIS. **EENT:** intraoperative floppy iris syndrome. **GI:** abdominal pain, constipation, dyspepsia, nausea. **GU:** erectile dysfunction, priapism. **Hemat:** thrombocytopenia. **Neuro:** dizziness, fatigue, headache. **Resp:** bronchitis, pharyngitis, sinusitis.

Interactions
Drug-Drug: Strong CYP3A4 inhibitors, including **ketoconazole**, **itraconazole**, and **ritonavir**, may significantly ↑ levels and risk of toxicity; concurrent use contraindicated. Other **alpha adrenergic antagonists**, including **doxazosin**, **prazosin**, or **terazosin**, may ↑ risk of hypotension; avoid concurrent use. **Cimetidine**, **atenolol**, and **diltiazem** may ↑ levels and risk of toxicity. May ↑ levels and risk of toxicity of **atenolol** and **diltiazem**; monitor BP and heart rate. ↑ risk of hypotension with **antihypertensives**, **nitrates**, **phosphodiesterase type 5 inhibitors** (including **sildenafil**, **tadalafil**, and **vardenafil**) and acute ingestion of **alcohol**. **QT interval prolonging medications** may ↑ risk of QT interval prolongation.

Route/Dosage
PO (Adults): 10 mg once daily.

Availability
Extended-release tablets: 10 mg.

NURSING IMPLICATIONS
Assessment
- Assess for symptoms of BPH (urinary hesitancy, feeling of incomplete bladder emptying, interruption of urinary stream, impairment of size and

force of urinary stream, terminal urinary dribbling, straining to start flow, dysuria, urgency) before and periodically during therapy.

- Rule out prostatic carcinoma before therapy; symptoms are similar.
- Assess for postural hypotension. Monitor orthostatic BP and HR frequently during initial dose adjustment and periodically thereafter. May occur within a few hr after initial doses and occasionally thereafter.

Implementation

- **PO:** Administer with food at the same meal each day. ***DNC:*** Tablets must be swallowed whole; do not crush, break, or chew.

Patient/Family Teaching

- Instruct patient to take medication with the same meal each day. Take missed doses as soon as remembered. If not remembered until next day, omit; do not double doses.
- May cause dizziness or drowsiness. Advise patient to avoid driving or other activities requiring alertness until response to the medication is known.
- Caution patient to avoid sudden changes in position to ↓ orthostatic hypotension.
- Advise patient to consult health care professional before taking any cough, cold, or allergy remedies.
- Instruct patient to notify health care professional of medication regimen before any surgery, especially cataract surgery.
- Advise patient to notify health care professional immediately if priapism (persistent painful penile erection), angina (chest pain), frequent dizziness, rash, or fainting occurs.
- Emphasize the importance of follow-up exams to evaluate effectiveness of medication.
- Geri: Assess risk for falls; implement fall prevention program and instruct patient and family in preventing falls at home.

Evaluation/Desired Outcomes

- Decreased symptoms of BPH.

allopurinol

(al-oh-**pure**-i-nole)

Aloprim, Zyloprim

Classification

Therapeutic: antigout agents, antihyperuricemics

Pharmacologic: xanthine oxidase inhibitors

Indications

PO: Prevention of attack of gouty arthritis and nephropathy. **PO IV:** Treatment of secondary hyperuricemia, which may occur during treatment of tumors or leukemias.

Action

Inhibits the production of uric acid by inhibiting the action of xanthine oxidase. **Therapeutic Effects:** Lowering of serum uric acid levels.

Pharmacokinetics

Absorption: Well absorbed (80%) following oral administration.

Distribution: Widely distributed to tissues.

Protein Binding: <1%.

Metabolism and Excretion: Metabolized to oxypurinol, an active compound with a long half-life. 12% excreted unchanged; 76% excreted as oxypurinol.

Half-life: 1–3 hr (oxypurinol 18–30 hr).

TIME/ACTION PROFILE (hypouricemic effect)

ROUTE	ONSET	PEAK	DURATION
PO, IV	1–2 days	1–2 wk	1–3 wk†

† Duration after discontinuation of allopurinol.

Contraindications/Precautions

Contraindicated in: Hypersensitivity; Presence of HLA-B*58:01 allele (↑ risk of hypersensitivity reactions); Lactation: Lactation.

Use Cautiously in: Acute attacks of gout; Renal impairment (dose ↓ required if CCr <20 mL/min); Dehydration (adequate hydration necessary); OB: Safety not established in pregnancy; Geri: Begin at lower end of dosage range in older adults.

Adverse Reactions/Side Effects

CV: bradycardia, flushing, HF (reported with IV administration), hypertension, hypotension. **Derm:** rash (discontinue drug at first sign of rash), DRUG REACTION WITH EOSINOPHILIA AND SYSTEMIC SYMPTOMS (DRESS), STEVENS-JOHNSON SYNDROME, TOXIC EPIDERMAL NECROLYSIS, urticaria. **GI:** diarrhea, hepatitis, nausea, vomiting. **GU:** hematuria, renal failure. **Hemat:** bone marrow depression. **Neuro:** drowsiness. **Misc:** HYPERSENSITIVITY REACTIONS.

Interactions

Drug-Drug: Mercaptopurine and **azathioprine** ↑ bone marrow depressant properties; doses of these drugs should be ↓. **Ampicillin** or **amoxicillin** ↑ risk of rash. May ↑ effects of **oral hypoglycemic agents** and **warfarin**. **Thiazide diuretics** or **ACE inhibitors** may ↑ risk of hypersensitivity reactions. Large doses of allopurinol may ↑ risk of **theophylline** toxicity. May ↑ levels and risk of toxicity of **cyclosporine**.

Route/Dosage

Gout

PO (Adults and Children >10 yr): *Initially:* 100 mg/day; ↑ at weekly intervals based on serum uric acid (not to exceed 800 mg/day). Doses

>300 mg/day should be given in divided doses; *Maintenance dose:* 100–200 mg 2–3 times daily. Doses of ≤300 mg may be given as a single daily dose.

Renal Impairment

(Adults and Children): *CCr 10–50 mL/min:* ↓ dose to 50% of recommended; *CCr <10 mL/min:* ↓ dose to 30% of recommended.

Secondary Hyperuricemia

PO (Adults and Children >10 yr): 600–800 mg/day in 2–3 divided doses starting 1–2 days before chemotherapy or radiation.
PO (Children 6–10 yr): 10 mg/kg/day in 2–3 divided doses (maximum 800 mg/day) or 300 mg/day in 2–3 divided doses.
PO (Children <6 yr): 10 mg/kg/day in 2–3 divided doses (maximum 800 mg/day) or 150 mg/day in 3 divided doses.
IV (Adults and Children >10 yr): 200–400 mg/m^2/day (up to 600 mg/day) as a single daily dose or in divided doses every 8–24 hr.
IV (Children <10 yr): 200 mg/m^2/day initially as a single daily dose or in divided doses every 8–24 hr (maximum dose 600 mg/day).

Renal Impairment

(Adults and Children): *CCr 10–50 mL/min:* ↓ dose to 50% of recommended; *CCr <10 mL/min:* ↓ dose to 30% of recommended.

Availability

Tablets: 100 mg, 200 mg, 300 mg. **Powder for injection:** 500 mg/vial.

NURSING IMPLICATIONS

Assessment

- Monitor intake and output. Renal impairment can cause drug accumulation and toxic effects. Ensure adequate fluid intake, sufficient to yield 2 liters per day of urine output in adults and 2 liters/m^2/day in pediatrics to ↓ risk of kidney stone formation.
- Consider testing for HLA-B*58:01 allele in patients of African, Asian, and Native Hawaiian/Pacific Islander ancestry prior to using allopurinol; use not recommended if allele present.
- Assess for hypersensitivity reactions, including rash. *At first sign of rash or other hypersensitivity,* discontinue allopurinol immediately and provide appropriate medical attention.
- Monitor for signs and symptoms of DRESS (fever, rash, lymphadenopathy, and/or facial swelling, associated with involvement of other organ systems [hepatitis, nephritis, hematologic abnormalities, myocarditis, myositis]) during therapy. May resemble an acute viral infection. Eosinophilia is often present. Discontinue therapy if signs occur.
- **Gout:** Monitor for joint pain and swelling. Addition of colchicine or NSAIDs may be necessary for acute attacks. Prophylactic doses of colchicine or an NSAID should be administered concurrently during first 3–6 mo of therapy because of ↑ risk of gout flares during first few mo of allopurinol therapy.

Lab Test Considerations

- Prior to therapy initiation for gout, assess serum uric acid, CBC, comprehensive metabolic panel, and liver and kidney function tests.
- Monitor serum creatinine at least daily during early therapy. *If uric acid concentration ↑, associated with ↓ urate clearance,* ↓ dose based on renal impairment dosage guidelines.
- Monitor serum alkaline phosphatase and AST/ALT in patients who develop anorexia, weight loss, or pruritus during therapy. *If ↑ liver enzymes occur,* permanently discontinue allopurinol.
- Monitor blood glucose in patients receiving oral hypoglycemic agents.
- Monitor blood counts periodically during therapy. *If unexplained cytopenias occur,* permanently discontinue allopurinol.

Implementation

- Do not confuse Zyloprim with zolpidem.
- **PO:** May be administered after milk or meals to ↓ gastric irritation; give with plenty of fluid. May be crushed and given with liquid or food if swallowing tablet is difficult.

IV Administration

- **Intermittent Infusion: Reconstitution:** Reconstitute each 500 mg vial with 25 mL of sterile water for injection. Solution is clear and almost colorless with slight opalescence. **Dilution:** Dilute with 0.9% NaCl or D5W. Administer within 10 hr of reconstitution; do not refrigerate. Do not administer solution if discolored, cloudy or contains particulates. **Concentration:** <6 mg/mL. **Rate:** Infusion should be initiated 24–48 hr before start of chemotherapy known to cause tumor cell lysis. Rate of infusion depends on volume of infusate (100–300 mg doses may be infused over 30 min). Administered as a single infusion or equally divided infusions at 6-, 8-, or 12-hr intervals.
- **Y-Site Compatibility:** acyclovir, aminophylline, anidulafungin, argatroban, arsenic trioxide, aztreonam, bivalirudin, bleomycin, bumetanide, buprenorphine, butorphanol, calcium gluconate, carboplatin, caspofungin, cefazolin, cefotetan, ceftazidime, ceftriaxone, cefuroxime, cisplatin, cyclophosphamide, dactinomycin, dexamethasone, dexmedetomidine, docetaxel, doxorubicin liposomal, enalaprilat, etoposide, famotidine, filgrastim, fluconazole, fludarabine, fluorouracil, fosphenytoin, furosemide, ganciclovir, gemcitabine, gemtuzumab ozogamicin, granisetron, heparin, hetastarch, hydrocortisone, hydromorphone, ifosfamide, leucovorin calcium, linezolid, lorazepam, mannitol, mesna, methotrexate, metronidazole, milrinone, mitoxantrone, morphine, octreotide, oxaliplatin,

oxytocin, paclitaxel, pamidronate, pantoprazole, pemetrexed, piperacillin/tazobactam, potassium chloride, sodium acetate, thiotepa, tigecycline, tirofiban, trimethoprim/sulfamethoxazole, vancomycin, vasopressin, vinblastine, vincristine, voriconazole, zidovudine, zoledronic acid.

- **Y-Site Incompatibility:** alemtuzumab, amikacin, amiodarone, amphotericin B deoxycholate, carmustine, cefotaxime, chlorpromazine, clindamycin, cytarabine, dacarbazine, daptomycin, daunorubicin, dexrazoxane, diltiazem, diphenhydramine, doxorubicin hydrochloride, doxycycline, droperidol, epirubicin, ertapenem, etoposide phosphate, floxuridine, foscarnet, gentamicin, haloperidol, hydroxyzine, idarubicin, imipenem/cilastatin, irinotecan, meperidine, methadone, methylprednisolone, metoprolol, minocycline, mitomycin, moxifloxacin, mycophenolate, nalbuphine, ondansetron, palonosetron, potassium acetate, prochlorperazine, promethazine, sodium bicarbonate, tacrolimus, tobramycin, topotecan, vecuronium, vinorelbine.

Patient/Family Teaching

- Instruct patient to take allopurinol as directed. Take missed doses as soon as remembered. If dosing schedule is once daily, do not take if remembered the next day. If dosing schedule is more than once a day, take up to 300 mg for next dose.
- Instruct patient to continue taking allopurinol along with an NSAID or colchicine and plenty of fluids during an acute gout flare.
- Alkaline diet may be ordered. Urinary acidification with large doses of vitamin C or other acids may ↑ kidney stone formation (see Appendix J). Advise patient of need for ↑ fluid intake.
- May occasionally cause drowsiness. Caution patient to avoid driving or other activities requiring alertness until response to drug is known.
- Instruct patient to report skin rash, blood in urine, influenza symptoms (chills, fever, muscle aches and pains, nausea, vomiting), or symptoms of DRESS to health care professional immediately; skin rash may indicate hypersensitivity.
- Advise patient that large amounts of alcohol ↑ uric acid concentrations and may ↓ effectiveness of allopurinol.
- Rep: Advise women of reproductive potential to notify health care professional if pregnancy is planned or suspected and to avoid breastfeeding during therapy and for 1 wk after last dose.
- Emphasize importance of follow-up exams to monitor effectiveness and side effects.

Evaluation/Desired Outcomes

- Decreased serum and urinary uric acid levels. May take 2–6 wk to observe clinical improvement in patients treated for gout.

HIGH ALERT

⧖ alpelisib (al-pe-lisib)

Piqray, Vijoice

Classification

Therapeutic: antineoplastics

Pharmacologic: kinase inhibitors

Indications

Piqray: ⧖ Hormone receptor-positive, human epidermal growth factor receptor 2-negative, PIK3CA-mutated, advanced, or metastatic breast cancer (in combination with fulvestrant). **Vijoice:** ⧖ Severe manifestations of PIK3CA-related overgrowth spectrum in patients who require systemic therapy.

Action

⧖ Acts as an inhibitor of phosphatidylinositol 3-kinase (PI3K). Mutations in the gene encoding the catalytic α-subunit of PI3K (PI3KCA) lead to activation of PI3Kα and Akt-signaling, cellular transformation, and tumor generation. Alpelisib inhibits phosphorylation of PI3K downstream targets (including Akt) and demonstrated activity in cell lines harboring a PIK3CA mutation. Activating mutations in PIK3CA may induce overgrowths and malformations in PIK3CA-related overgrowth spectrum. **Therapeutic Effects:** Decreased progression of breast cancer. Reduction in lesion volume in PIK3CA-related overgrowth spectrum.

Pharmacokinetics

Absorption: Well absorbed following oral administration.

Distribution: Widely distributed to tissues.

Metabolism and Excretion: Primarily metabolized via hydrolysis; also metabolized to a lesser extent by the CYP3A4 isoenzyme. Excreted in feces (36% as unchanged drug; 32% as metabolites) and urine (2% as unchanged drug; 7% as metabolites).

Half-life: 8–9 hr.

TIME/ACTION PROFILE (plasma concentrations)

ROUTE	ONSET	PEAK	DURATION
PO	unknown	2–4 hr	24 hr

Contraindications/Precautions

Contraindicated in: History of serious hypersensitivity reactions including anaphylaxis, Stevens-Johnson syndrome, erythema multiforme, or toxic epidermal necrolysis; OB: Pregnancy; Lactation: Lactation.

Use Cautiously in: Diabetes or risk factors for hyperglycemia (obesity, elevated fasting plasma glucose, elevated A1c, concurrent use of systemic corticosteroids, or age ≥75 yr); Severe renal impairment (Piqray only); Rep: Women of reproductive potential and men with female partners of reproductive potential; Pedi: Safety and effectiveness not established in children <18 yr (breast cancer) or <2 yr (PIK3CA-related overgrowth spectrum); Geri: Older adults may be more sensitive to drug effects.

Adverse Reactions/Side Effects

CV: peripheral edema. **Derm:** alopecia, DRUG REACTION WITH EOSINOPHILIA AND SYSTEMIC SYMPTOMS (DRESS), dry skin, ERYTHEMA MULTIFORM (EM), pruritus, rash, STEVENS-JOHNSON SYNDROME (SJS), TOXIC EPIDERMAL NECROLYSIS (TEN), cellulitis, eczema. **Endo:** hyperglycemia, hypoglycemia, hyperglycemic hyperosmolar nonketotic syndrome, KETOACIDOSIS. **F and E:** hyperkalemia, hypocalcemia, hypokalemia, hypomagnesemia, hyponatremia, hypophosphatemia. **GI:** ↑ lipase, ↑ liver enzymes, abdominal pain, DIARRHEA, hyperbilirubinemia, metallic taste, nausea, stomatitis, vomiting, colitis, hypoalbuminemia. **GU:** ↑ serum creatinine, ↓ fertility, acute kidney injury. **Hemat:** anemia, lymphopenia, thrombocytopenia. **Metab:** ↓ appetite, hypercholesterolemia, hypertriglyceridemia, weight loss. **Neuro:** fatigue, headache, insomnia. **Resp:** cough, PNEUMONITIS. **Misc:** fever, INFECTION, HYPERSENSITIVITY REACTIONS (INCLUDING ANAPHYLAXIS AND ANGIOEDEMA).

Interactions

Drug-Drug: Strong CYP3A4 inducers may ↓ levels and effectiveness; avoid concurrent use. **Breast cancer resistance protein inhibitors** may ↑ levels and risk of toxicity; avoid concurrent use. May ↓ levels of **CYP2C9 substrates**, including **warfarin**.

Route/Dosage

Breast Cancer

PO (Adults): *Piqray:* 300 mg once daily until disease progression or unacceptable toxicity.

PIK3CA-Related Overgrowth Spectrum

PO (Adults): *Vijoice tablets:* 250 mg once daily until disease progression or unacceptable toxicity.

PO (Children 6–<18 yr): *Vijoice:* 50 mg once daily (as oral tablets or granules) until disease progression or unacceptable toxicity. After 24 wk, may ↑ to 125 mg once daily (as oral tablets only) to optimize clinical/radiological response; continue until disease progression or unacceptable toxicity. Once patient becomes 18 yr old, gradually ↑ to 250 mg once daily (as oral tablets only).

PO (Children 2–<6 yr): *Vijoice:* 50 mg once daily until disease progression or unacceptable toxicity.

Availability

Tablets (Piqray): 50 mg, 150 mg, 200 mg. **Tablets (Vijoice):** 50 mg, 125 mg, 200 mg. **Oral granules (Vijoice):** 50 mg/pkt.

NURSING IMPLICATIONS

Assessment

- Monitor for signs and symptoms of hypersensitivity reactions (dyspnea, flushing, rash, fever, tachycardia) during therapy. If symptoms occur, permanently discontinue alpelisib.
- Assess for severe cutaneous adverse reactions including SJS, EM, TEN, and DRESS (prodrome of fever, flu-like symptoms, mucosal lesions, progressive skin rash) during therapy. *If rash is Grade 1 (< 10% body surface area [BSA] with active skin toxicity),* no dose adjustment needed. Initiate topical corticosteroid treatment. Consider adding oral antihistamine to manage symptoms. If rash is not improved within 28 days of treatment, add a low-dose systemic corticosteroid. If the cause is SJS, EM, TEN, or DRESS, permanently discontinue alpelisib. *If Grade 2 (10–30% BSA with active skin toxicity),* no dose adjustment necessary. Initiate or intensify topical corticosteroid and oral antihistamines. Consider low-dose systemic corticosteroid treatment. If rash improves to Grade ≤ 1 within 10 days, systemic corticosteroid may be discontinued. If the cause is SJS, EM, TEN, or DRESS, permanently discontinue alpelisib. *If Grade 3 (severe rash not responsive to medical management and >30% BSA with active skin toxicity),* hold alpelisib. Initiate or intensify topical/systemic corticosteroid and oral antihistamines. If the cause is SJS, EM, TEN, or DRESS, permanently discontinue alpelisib. If the etiology is not SJS, EM, TEN, or DRESS, hold dose until improvement to Grade ≤ 1; then resume alpelisib at next lower dose. *If Grade 4 (severe bullous, blistering, or exfoliating skin conditions and any % BSA associated with extensive superinfection, with IV antibiotics indicated; life-threatening),* permanently discontinue alpelisib.
- Monitor for signs and symptoms of pneumonitis (hypoxia, cough, dyspnea, interstitial infiltrates) during therapy. If pneumonitis is confirmed, discontinue alpelisib permanently.
- Monitor for signs and symptoms of diarrhea and colitis (abdominal pain, mucus or blood in stool) during therapy. *If Grade 1 diarrhea occurs,* do not adjust alpelisib dose. Start antidiarrheal therapy and monitor symptoms. *If Grade 2 diarrhea occurs,* start or intensify antidiarrheal therapy and monitor symptoms. May add enteric-acting and/or systemic steroids to therapy for Grade 2 or Grade 3 colitis. Hold alpelisib until recovery to Grade ≤1; then resume at same dose. *If Grade 3 diarrhea occurs,* start or intensify antidiarrheal therapy and monitor symptoms. Hold alpelisib until recovery to Grade ≤1; then resume at the next lower dose. *If Grade 4 diarrhea occurs,* permanently discontinue alpelisib.

Lab Test Considerations

- Verify negative pregnancy test before starting therapy.

Information on FDA approved tests for the detection of PIK3CA mutations in breast cancer is available at: http://www.fda.gov/CompanionDiagnostics.

- May cause hyperglycemia. Consider premedication with metformin prior to the initiation of *Piqray* in combination with fulvestrant based on patient risk factors for hyperglycemia, GI tolerability, and clinical situation. Before starting alpelisib therapy, test fasting blood glucose (FBG) and A1c; optimize blood glucose. After starting therapy, monitor blood glucose at least weekly for first 2 wk, then at least once every 4 wk, and as indicated. Monitor A1c every 3 mo and as indicated. If hyperglycemia develops, monitor FBG at least twice weekly until FBG decreases to normal. During treatment with antihyperglycemic agents, continue monitoring FBG at least weekly for 8 wk, then once every 2 wk, and as needed clinically. *If Grade 1 FBG >upper limit of normal (ULN)–160 mg/dL,* no dose adjustment needed. Begin or intensify antihyperglycemic treatment. *If Grade 2 FBG >160–250 mg/dL:* no dose adjustment needed. Begin or further intensify antihyperglycemic therapy. If FBG does not decrease to ≤ 160 mg/dL within 21 days, reduce alpelisib dose by one dose level and follow FBG value recommendations. *If Grade 3 FBG >250–500 mg/dL,* hold alpelisib. Begin or intensify oral antihyperglycemic therapy and consider additional antihyperglycemic agents for 1–2 days until hyperglycemia improves. Administer IV hydration and consider added intervention for electrolyte/ketoacidosis/hyperosmolar disturbances. If FBG decreases to ≤160 mg/dL within 3–5 days under appropriate antihyperglycemic therapy, resume alpelisib at one lower dose level. If FBG does not decrease to ≤160 mg/dL within 3–5 days under appropriate antihyperglycemic therapy, consult with a specialist in the treatment of hyperglycemia. If FBG does not decrease to ≤160 mg/dL within 21 days following appropriate antihyperglycemic therapy, permanently discontinue alpelisib. *If Grade 4 FBG >500 mg/dL,* hold alpelisib. Begin or intensify appropriate antihyperglycemic therapy (administer IV hydration and consider appropriate intervention for electrolyte/ketoacidosis/hyperosmolar disturbances); recheck FBG within 24 hr and as indicated. If FBG decreases to ≤500 mg/dL, follow FBG recommendations for Grade 3. If FBG is confirmed at >500 mg/dL, discontinue alpelisib permanently.

Implementation

- When starting at *Piqray* at 300 mg once daily (two 150 mg tablets), dose adjustments for adverse reactions include: *First dose reduction:* 250 mg once daily (one 200 mg tablet and one 50 mg tablet). *Second dose reduction:* 200 mg tablet once daily.
- Dose reductions for *Vijoice* include: *First dose reduction:* 125 mg once daily. *Second dose reduction:* 50 mg once daily. If adult or pediatric patients cannot tolerate 50 mg, discontinue alpelisib.
- **PO:** Administer with food once daily at same time of day. ***DNC:*** Swallow tablets whole; do not crush, break, or chew. For patients with difficulty swallowing, administer *Vijoice* as an oral suspension with food. Place *Vijoice* tablets in 2–4 ounces of water and let stand for 5 min. Make suspension with water only. Crush tablets with a spoon and stir until an oral suspension is obtained. Administer immediately after preparation. Discard oral suspension if not administered within 60 min after preparation. After administration, add 2–3 tablespoons of water to same glass. Stir with same spoon to resuspend any remaining particles and administer entire contents. Repeat if particles remain.
- Only use *Vijoice* oral granules when the dose is 50 mg once daily. Do not use multiple or partial packets of the oral granules to obtain a dose of 125 mg or 250 mg. Do not combine *Vijoice* tablets and oral granule packets to obtain a specific dose. Administer *Vijoice* oral granules using either of the following methods: 1) Pour the contents of one oral granule packet directly onto the patient's tongue and have patient swallow with approximately 2–4 ounces of water. Have patient rinse their mouth with additional water and swallow to ensure no particles remain in the mouth. 2) Pour the contents of one oral granule packet into a cup. Add 1–3 teaspoons of water, milk, apple juice, applesauce, or yogurt and administer the mixture immediately. Rinse the cup with up to 2 ounces of water, milk, or apple juice and administer the mixture immediately. If particles remain in the cup, repeat until the full dose is administered. Discard the mixture if not administered within 2 hr after preparation.

Patient/Family Teaching

- Instruct patient to take alpelisib as directed. Take missed doses with food within 9 hr of time usually taken. If >9 hr, omit dose and take next dose next day at usual time. If patient vomits after dose, skip dose and take next dose next day. Advise patient to read *Patient Information* before starting and with each Rx refill in case of changes.
- Advise patients to notify health care professional if the signs and symptoms of hypersensitivity reactions, skin reactions, hyperglycemia (excessive thirst, urinating more often than usual or higher amount of urine than usual, or increased appetite with weight loss), and lung problems occur. Advise patients to immediately report new or worsening respiratory symptoms.
- If diarrhea occurs, advise patient to start antidiarrheal treatment, increase oral fluids, and notify health care professional.

- Advise patient to notify health care professional of all Rx or OTC medications, vitamins, or herbal products being taken and to consult health care professional before taking any new medications.
- Rep: May cause fetal harm. Advise females of reproductive potential and males with female partners of reproductive potential to use effective contraception during and for 1 wk after last dose. Advise patient to avoid breastfeeding during and for 1 wk after last dose. May impair fertility in male and female patients.

Evaluation/Desired Outcomes

- Decreased progression of breast cancer.
- Reduction in lesion volume in PIK3CA-related overgrowth spectrum.

BEERS

ALPRAZolam

(al-**pray**-zoe-lam)

Xanax, Xanax XR

Classification

Therapeutic: antianxiety agents

Pharmacologic: benzodiazepines

Schedule IV

Indications

Generalized anxiety disorder. Panic disorder. Anxiety associated with depression.

Action

Acts at many levels in the CNS to produce anxiolytic effect. May produce CNS depression. Effects may be mediated by GABA, an inhibitory neurotransmitter. **Therapeutic Effects:** Relief of anxiety.

Pharmacokinetics

Absorption: Well absorbed (90%) from the GI tract; absorption is slower with extended-release tablets.
Distribution: Widely distributed; crosses blood-brain barrier. Accumulation is minimal.
Metabolism and Excretion: Metabolized by the liver by the CYP3A4 isoenzyme to an active compound that is subsequently rapidly metabolized.
Half-life: 12–15 hr.

TIME/ACTION PROFILE (sedation)

ROUTE	ONSET	PEAK	DURATION
PO	1–2 hr	1–2 hr	up to 24 hr

Contraindications/Precautions

Contraindicated in: Hypersensitivity; Cross-sensitivity with other benzodiazepines may exist; Pre-existing CNS depression; Severe uncontrolled pain; Angle-closure glaucoma; Obstructive sleep apnea or pulmonary disease; Concurrent use with itraconazole or ketoconazole; Lactation: Lactation.

Use Cautiously in: Renal impairment (↓ dose); Hepatic impairment (↓ dose); History of suicide attempt or alcohol/drug dependence, debilitated patients (↓ dose); OB: Use late in pregnancy can result in sedation (respiratory depression, lethargy, hypotonia) and/or withdrawal symptoms (hyperreflexia, irritability, restlessness, tremors, inconsolable crying, feeding difficulties) in neonates; Pedi: Safety and effectiveness not established in children; Geri: Appears on Beers list. ↑ risk of cognitive impairment, delirium, falls, fractures, and motor vehicle accidents in older adults. If possible, avoid use in older adults.

Adverse Reactions/Side Effects

Derm: rash. **EENT:** blurred vision. **GI:** constipation, diarrhea, nausea, vomiting, weight gain. **Neuro:** dizziness, drowsiness, lethargy, confusion, depression, hangover, headache, paradoxical excitation. **Misc:** physical dependence, psychological dependence, tolerance.

Interactions

Drug-Drug: Use with **opioids** or other **CNS depressants**, including other **benzodiazepines**, **nonbenzodiazepine sedative/hypnotics**, **anxiolytics**, **general anesthetics**, **muscle relaxants**, **antipsychotics**, and **alcohol**, may cause profound sedation, respiratory depression, coma, and death; reserve concurrent use for when alternative treatment options are inadequate. **Hormonal contraceptives**, **disulfiram**, **fluoxetine**, **isoniazid**, **metoprolol**, **propranolol**, **valproic acid**, and **CYP3A4 inhibitors** (**erythromycin**, **ketoconazole**, **itraconazole**, **fluvoxamine**, **cimetidine**, **nefazodone**) ↑ levels and effects; dose adjustments may be necessary; concurrent use with ketoconazole and itraconazole contraindicated. May ↓ efficacy of **levodopa**. **CYP3A4 inducers**, including **rifampin**, **carbamazepine**, or **barbiturates**, may ↓ levels and effectiveness. Sedative effects may be ↓ by **theophylline**. **Cigarette smoking** may ↓ levels and effectiveness.
Drug-Natural Products: **Kava-kava**, **valerian**, or **chamomile** can ↑ risk of CNS depression. **St. John's wort** may ↓ levels and effectiveness.
Drug-Food: **Grapefruit juice** may ↑ levels and risk of toxicity.

Route/Dosage

Anxiety

PO (Adults): 0.25–0.5 mg 2–3 times daily (not to exceed 4 mg/day).
PO (Geriatric Patients): Begin with 0.25 mg 2–3 times daily.

Panic Attacks

PO (Adults): 0.5 mg 3 times daily; may ↑ by ≤1 mg every 3–4 days as needed (not to exceed 10 mg/day). *Extended-release tablets:* 0.5–1 mg once daily in the morning; may ↑ every 3–4 days by not more than 1 mg/day; up to 10 mg/day (usual range 3–6 mg/day).

Availability (generic available)

Tablets: 0.25 mg, 0.5 mg, 1 mg, 2 mg. **Extended-release tablets:** 0.5 mg, 1 mg, 2 mg, 3 mg. **Orally disintegrating tablets (orange flavor):** 0.25 mg, 0.5 mg, 1 mg, 2 mg. **Oral solution (concentrate):** 1 mg/mL.

NURSING IMPLICATIONS

Assessment

- Assess degree and manifestations of anxiety and mental status (orientation, mood, behavior) prior to and periodically during therapy.
- Assess for drowsiness, light-headedness, and dizziness. These symptoms usually disappear as therapy progresses. Dose should be ↓ if these symptoms persist.
- Geri: Assess CNS effects and risk of falls. Institute falls prevention strategies.
- Assess risk for addiction, abuse, or misuse before administration and periodically during therapy.
- Prolonged high-dose therapy may lead to psychological or physical dependence. Risk is greater in patients taking >4 mg/day. Restrict the amount of drug available to patient. Assess regularly for continued need for treatment.

Lab Test Considerations

- Monitor CBC and liver and renal function periodically during long-term therapy. May ↓ hematocrit and cause neutropenia.

Toxicity and Overdose

- Flumazenil is the antidote for alprazolam toxicity or overdose. Flumazenil may induce seizures in patients with a history of seizures disorder or who are taking tricyclic antidepressants.

Implementation

- Do not confuse Xanax with Fanapt.
- Do not confuse alprazolam with clonazepam or lorazepam.
- If early-morning anxiety or anxiety between doses occurs, same total daily dose should be divided into more frequent intervals.
- **PO:** May be administered with food if GI upset occurs. Administer greatest dose at bedtime to avoid daytime sedation.
- Tablets may be crushed and taken with food or fluids if patient has difficulty swallowing. ***DNC:*** Do not crush, break, or chew extended-release tablets.
- Taper by 0.5 mg every 3 days to prevent withdrawal; may require even more gradual taper if withdrawal symptoms (heightened sensory perception, impaired concentration, dysosmia, clouded sensorium, paresthesias, muscle cramps, muscle twitch, diarrhea, blurred vision, ↓ appetite, weight loss) occur. Some patients may require longer tapering period (wks to >12 mo).
- For *orally disintegrating tablets:* Remove tablet from bottle with dry hands just before taking medication. Place tablet on tongue. Tablet will dissolve with saliva; may also be taken with water. Remove cotton from bottle and reseal tightly to prevent moisture from entering bottle. If only ½ tablet taken, discard unused portion immediately; may not remain stable.

Patient/Family Teaching

- Explain purpose and side effects of medication to patient. Advise to read *Patient Information* before starting therapy. Instruct patient to take medication as directed; do not skip or double up on missed doses. If a dose is missed, take within 1 hr; otherwise, skip the dose and return to regular schedule. If medication is less effective after a few wk, check with health care provider; do not ↑ dose.
- Caution patient not to stop taking alprazolam without consulting health care provider. Abrupt withdrawal may cause sweating, vomiting, muscle cramps, tremors, and seizures; may be life-threatening.
- Advise patient to avoid the use of alcohol or other CNS depressants, including opioids, concurrently with alprazolam; may cause respiratory depression and overdose. Instruct patient to consult health care provider before taking Rx, OTC, or herbal products concurrently with this medication, especially St. John's wort.
- Advise patient to avoid drinking grapefruit juice during therapy. May ↑ levels and risk of toxicity.
- Advise patient to not take more than prescribed or share medication with anyone.
- Advise patient that alprazolam is a drug with known abuse potential. Protect it from theft, and never give to anyone other than the individual for whom it was prescribed. Store out of sight and reach of children, and in a location not accessible by others.
- May cause drowsiness or dizziness. Caution patient to avoid driving and other activities requiring alertness until response to the medication is known. Geri: Instruct patient and family how to reduce falls risk at home.
- Inform patient that benzodiazepines are usually prescribed for short-term use and do not cure underlying problems.
- Rep: May cause fetal harm. Advise patient to notify health care provider if pregnancy is planned or suspected or if breastfeeding. Monitor neonates exposed to benzodiazepines during pregnancy (especially during 3rd trimester) and labor for signs of sedation (respiratory depression, lethargy, hypotonia) and/or withdrawal symptoms

(hyperreflexia, irritability, restlessness, tremors, inconsolable crying, and feeding difficulties) in the neonate. Monitor neonates and infants exposed to alprazolam during breastfeeding for sedation and withdrawal symptoms. Inform women who take alprazolam during pregnancy about the National Pregnancy Registry for Other Psychiatric Medications to monitor pregnancy outcomes in women exposed to alprazolam during pregnancy. Enroll patient by calling 1-866-961-2388 or visiting online at https://womensmentalhealth.org/research/pregnancyregistry/.

Evaluation/Desired Outcomes

- Relief of anxiety.

alteplase, See THROMBOLYTIC AGENTS.

amcinonide, See CORTICOSTEROIDS (TOPICAL).

amikacin, See AMINOGLYCOSIDES.

AMINOGLYCOSIDES

amikacin (am-i-**kay**-sin)
~~Amikin~~, Arikayce

gentamicin (jen-ta-**mye**-sin)
~~Garamycin~~

neomycin (neo-oh-**mye**-sin)

streptomycin (strep-toe-**mye**-sin)

tobramycin (toe-bra-**mye**-sin)
Bethkis, Kitabis Pak, TOBI, TOBI Podhaler

Classification
Therapeutic: anti-infectives
Pharmacologic: aminoglycosides
See Appendix B for ophthalmic use

Indications

Amikacin, gentamicin, and tobramycin: Treatment of serious gram-negative bacterial infections and infections caused by staphylococci when penicillins or other less toxic drugs are contraindicated. **Streptomycin:** In combination with other agents in the management of active tuberculosis. **Neomycin:** Used orally to prepare the GI tract for surgery, to decrease the number of ammonia-producing bacteria in the gut as part of the management of hepatic encephalopathy, and to treat diarrhea caused by *Escherichia coli*. **Amikacin by inhalation:** Treatment of *Mycobacterium avium* complex (MAC) lung disease in patients who have limited or no other treatment options and who do not achieve negative sputum cultures after ≥6 consecutive mo of a multidrug treatment regimen (in combination with other antibacterial drugs). **Tobramycin by inhalation:** Management of *Pseudomonas aeruginosa* in cystic fibrosis patients. **Gentamicin, streptomycin:** In combination with other agents in the management of serious enterococcal infections. **Gentamicin IV:** Prevention of infective endocarditis. **Gentamicin (topical):** Treatment of localized infections caused by susceptible organisms. **Unlabeled Use: Amikacin:** In combination with other agents in the management of *Mycobacterium avium* complex infections.

Action

Inhibits protein synthesis in bacteria at level of 30S ribosome. **Therapeutic Effects:** Bactericidal action. **Spectrum:** Most aminoglycosides notable for activity against: *P. aeruginosa, Klebsiella pneumoniae, E.coli, Proteus, Serratia, Acinetobacter, Staphylococcus aureus*. In treatment of enterococcal infections, synergy with a penicillin is required. Streptomycin and amikacin also active against *Mycobacterium*.

Pharmacokinetics

Absorption: Well absorbed after IM administration. IV administration results in complete bioavailability. Some absorption follows administration by other routes. Minimal systemic absorption with neomycin (may accumulate in patients with renal failure).
Distribution: Widely distributed throughout extracellular fluid. Poor penetration into CSF (↑ when meninges are inflamed).
Metabolism and Excretion: Excretion is >90% renal.
Half-life: 2–4 hr (↑ in renal impairment).

TIME/ACTION PROFILE (plasma concentrations*)

ROUTE	ONSET	PEAK	DURATION
PO (neomycin)	rapid	1–4 hr	N/A
IM	rapid	30–90 min	6–24 hr
IV	rapid	15–30 min†	6–24 hr

* All parenterally administered aminoglycosides.
† Postdistribution peak occurs 30 min after the end of a 30-min infusion and 15 min after the end of a 1-hr infusion.

Contraindications/Precautions

Contraindicated in: Hypersensitivity to aminoglycosides; Most parenteral products contain bisulfites and should be avoided in patients with known intolerance; Intestinal obstruction (neomycin only); OB: Pregnancy; Pedi: Products containing benzyl alcohol should be avoided in neonates.
Use Cautiously in: Renal or auditory impairment (dose adjustments necessary; plasma concentration monitoring useful in preventing ototoxicity and nephrotoxicity); Mitochondrial DNA variants in

A

the 12S rRNA gene (*MTRNR1*) or maternal history of ototoxicity (↑ risk of ototoxicity); Neuromuscular diseases such as myasthenia gravis; Obesity (dose should be based on ideal body weight); COPD or asthma (amikacin inhalation may worsen condition); OB: Minimal systemic absorption anticipated (inhalation formulations); Lactation: Safety not established in breastfeeding; Pedi: Neonates have ↑ risk of neuromuscular blockade; difficulty in assessing auditory and vestibular function and immature renal function; safety and effectiveness of amikacin inhalation not established in children; Geri: Older adults due to age-related renal impairment; may be difficult to assess vestibular and auditory function in older adults.

Adverse Reactions/Side Effects

Derm: rash (amikacin inhalation). **EENT:** ototoxicity (vestibular and cochlear), voice alteration (amikacin inhalation), epistaxis (amikacin inhalation), oral candidiasis (amikacin inhalation). **F and E:** hypomagnesemia. **GI:** diarrhea (amikacin inhalation), nausea (amikacin inhalation), diarrhea (neomycin), dry mouth (amikacin inhalation), nausea (neomycin), vomiting (amikacin inhalation and neomycin), weight loss(amikacin inhalation). **GU:** nephrotoxicity. **MS:** muscle paralysis (high parenteral doses). **Neuro:** ataxia, headache (amikacin inhalation), anxiety (amikacin inhalation), dysgeusia (amikacin inhalation), enhanced neuromuscular blockade, vertigo. **Resp:** bronchospasm (amikacin inhalation), cough (amikacin inhalation), hemoptysis (amikacin inhalation), apnea, bronchospasm (tobramycin inhalation), hypersensitivity pneumonitis (amikacin inhalation), wheezing (tobramycin inhalation). **Misc:** hypersensitivity reactions.

Interactions

Drug-Drug: Inactivated by **penicillins** and **cephalosporins** when coadministered to patients with renal insufficiency. May potentiate effects of **inhalation anesthetics** or **neuromuscular blockers**. ↑ incidence of ototoxicity with **loop diuretics**. ↑ incidence of nephrotoxicity with other **nephrotoxic drugs**, such as **amphotericin**, **vancomycin**, **acyclovir**, **cisplatin**, or **cephalosporins**. Neomycin may ↑ anticoagulant effects of **warfarin**. Neomycin may ↓ absorption of **digoxin** and **methotrexate**.

Route/Dosage

Amikacin

IM IV (Adults and Children): 5 mg/kg every 8 hr or 7.5 mg/kg every 12 hr (not to exceed 1.5 g/day). *Mycobacterium avium complex:* 7.5–15 mg/kg/day divided every 12–24 hr.
IM IV (Neonates): *Loading dose:* 10 mg/kg; *Maintenance dose:* 7.5 mg/kg every 12 hr.
Inhaln: (Adults): 590 mg once daily.

Renal Impairment

IM IV (Adults): *Loading dose:* 7.5 mg/kg; further dosing based on blood level monitoring and renal function assessment.

Gentamicin

IM IV (Adults): 1–2 mg/kg every 8 hr (up to 6 mg/kg/day in 3 divided doses); *Once-daily dosing (unlabeled):* 4–7 mg/kg every 24 hr.
IM IV (Children >5 yr): 2–2.5 mg/kg every 8 hr; *Once daily:* 5–7.5 mg/kg every 24 hr; *Cystic fibrosis:* 2.5–3.3 mg/kg every 6–8 hr; *Hemodialysis:* 1.25–1.75 mg/kg postdialysis.
IM IV (Children 1 mo–5 yr): 2.5 mg/kg every 8 hr; *Once daily:* 5–7.5 mg/kg every 24 hr; *Cystic fibrosis:* 2.5–3.3 mg/kg every 6–8 hr; *Hemodialysis:* 1.25–1.75 mg/kg postdialysis.
IM IV (Neonates full term and/or >1 wk): *Weight <1200 g:* 2.5 mg/kg every 18–24 hr; *Weight 1200–2000 g:* 2.5 mg/kg every 8–12 hr; *Weight >2000 g:* 2.5 mg/kg every 8 hr; *ECMO:* 2.5 mg/kg every 18 hr; subsequent doses based on serum concentrations; *Once daily:* 3.5–5 mg/kg every 24 hr.
IM IV (Neonates premature and/or ≤1 wk): *Weight <1000 g:* 3.5 mg/kg every 24 hr; *Weight 1000–1200 g:* 2.5 mg/kg every 18–24 hr; *Weight >1200 g:* 2.5 mg/kg every 12 hr; *Once daily:* 3.5–4 mg/kg every 24 hr.
IT: (Adults): 4–8 mg/day.
IT: (Infants >3 mo and Children): 1–2 mg/day.
IT: (Neonates): 1 mg/day.
Topical: (Adults and Children >1 mo): Apply cream or ointment 3–4 times daily.

Renal Impairment

IM IV (Adults): Initial dose of 2 mg/kg. Subsequent doses/intervals based on blood level monitoring and renal function assessment.

Neomycin

PO (Adults): *Preoperative intestinal antisepsis:* 1 g every hr for 4 doses, then 1 g every 4 hr for 5 doses *or* 1 g at 1 PM, 2 PM, and 11 PM on day before surgery; *Hepatic encephalopathy:* 1–3 g every 6 hr for 5–6 days; may be followed by 4 g/day chronically.
PO (Children): *Preoperative intestinal antisepsis:* 15 mg/kg every 4 hr for 2 days *or* 25 mg/kg at 1 PM, 2 PM, and 11 PM on day before surgery; *Hepatic encephalopathy:* 12.5–25 mg/kg every 6 hr for 5–6 days (maximum dose = 12 g/day).

Streptomycin

IM (Adults): *Tuberculosis:* 1 g/day initially; ↓ to 1 g 2–3 times weekly; *Other infections:* 250 mg–1 g every 6 hr *or* 500 mg–2 g every 12 hr.

IM (Children): *Tuberculosis:* 20 mg/kg/day (not to exceed 1 g/day); *Other infections:* 5–10 mg/kg every 6 hr *or* 10–20 mg/kg every 12 hr.

Renal Impairment

IM (Adults): 1 g initially; further dosing determined by blood level monitoring and assessment of renal function.

Tobramycin

IM IV (Adults): 1–2 mg/kg every 8 hr *or* 4–6.6 mg/kg/day every 24 hr.
IM IV (Adults): 3–6 mg/kg/day in 3 divided doses, or 4–6.6 mg/kg once daily.
IM IV (Children >5 yr): 6–7.5 mg/kg/day divided every 8 hr, up to 13 mg/kg/day divided every 6–8 hr in cystic fibrosis patients (dosing interval may vary from every 6 hr–every 24 hr, depending on clinical situation).
IM IV (Children 1 mo–5 yr): 7.5 mg/kg/day divided every 8 hr, up to 13 mg/kg/day divided every 6–8 hr in cystic fibrosis.
IM IV (Neonates): *Preterm <1000 g:* 3.5 mg/kg every 24 hr; *0–4 weeks, <1200 g:* 2.5 mg/kg every 18 hr; *Postnatal age <7 days:* 2.5 mg/kg every 12 hr; *Postnatal age ≥8 days, 1200–2000 g:* 2.5 mg/kg every 8–12 hr; *Postnatal age ≥8 days, >2000 g:* 2.5 mg/kg every 8 hr.
Inhaln: (Adults and Children ≥6 yr): *Nebulizer solution:* 300 mg twice daily for 28 days; then off for 28 days; then repeat cycle; *Powder for inhalation:* Inhale contents of four 28-mg capsules twice daily for 28 days; then off for 28 days; then repeat cycle.

Renal Impairment

IM IV (Adults): 1 mg/kg initially; further dosing determined by blood level monitoring and assessment of renal function.

Availability

Amikacin (generic available)

Solution for injection: 250 mg/mL. **Suspension for oral inhalation:** 590 mg/8.4 mL.

Gentamicin (generic available)

Premixed infusion: 60 mg/50 mL, 80 mg/50 mL, 80 mg/100 mL, 100 mg/50 mL, 100 mg/100 mL, 120 mg/100 mL. **Solution for injection:** 10 mg/mL, 40 mg/mL. **Topical cream:** 0.1%. **Topical ointment:** 0.1%.

Neomycin (generic available)

Tablets: 500 mg. ***In combination with:*** other topical antibiotics or anti-inflammatory agents for skin, ear, and eye infections. See Appendix N.

Streptomycin (generic available)

Lyophilized powder for injection: 1 g/vial.

Tobramycin (generic available)

Lyophilized powder for injection: 1200 mg/vial. **Nebulizer solution (Bethkis):** 300 mg/4 mL. **Nebulizer solution (TOBI, Kitabis Pak):** 300 mg/5 mL. **Powder for inhalation (TOBI Podhaler):** 28 mg/capsule. **Solution for injection:** 10 mg/mL, 40 mg/mL.

NURSING IMPLICATIONS

Assessment

- Assess for infection (vital signs, wound appearance, sputum, urine, stool, WBC) at beginning of and throughout therapy.
- Obtain specimens for culture and sensitivity before starting therapy. 1st dose may be given before receiving results.
- Evaluate 8th cranial nerve function by audiometry before and throughout therapy. Hearing loss is usually in the high-frequency range and irreversible. Prompt recognition and intervention are essential in preventing permanent damage. Also monitor for vestibular dysfunction (vertigo, ataxia, nausea, vomiting, numbness, skin tingling, muscle twitching, seizures). 8th cranial nerve dysfunction is associated with persistently elevated peak or trough aminoglycoside concentrations. Aminoglycosides should be discontinued if tinnitus or subjective hearing loss occurs.
- Monitor intake and output and daily weight to assess hydration status and renal function.
- Assess for signs of superinfection (fever, upper respiratory infection, vaginal itching or discharge, increasing malaise, diarrhea).
- **Inhaln:** Assess for hypersensitivity pneumonitis with inhaled amikacin (e.g. allergic alveolitis, pneumonitis, interstitial lung disease, allergic reaction). *If hypersensitivity pneumonitis occurs,* discontinue inhaled amikacin and treat as appropriate.
- Monitor for hemoptysis, bronchospasm, or exacerbation of underlying pulmonary disease.
- **Hepatic Encephalopathy:** Monitor neurologic status. Before administering oral medication, assess patient's ability to swallow.

Lab Test Considerations

- Monitor renal function by urinalysis, specific gravity, BUN, serum creatinine, and CCr before and during therapy. May ↑ BUN and serum creatinine.
- May ↑ AST, ALT, serum alkaline phosphatase, bilirubin, and LDH concentrations.
- May ↓ serum calcium, magnesium, potassium, and sodium concentrations (streptomycin and tobramycin).

Toxicity and Overdose

- Monitor plasma concentrations periodically during oral, IM, and IV therapy; not needed for inhalation therapy. Timing of plasma concentrations is important in interpreting results. Draw blood for peak concentrations 1 hr after IM injection and 30 min after a 30-min IV infusion is completed. Draw trough concentrations just before next dose. Peak concentration for **amikacin** is 20–30 mcg/mL; trough concentration should be <10 mcg/mL. Peak concentration for **gentamicin** and **tobramycin** should not exceed 10 mcg/mL; trough concentrations should not exceed 2 mcg/mL. Peak concentration for **streptomycin** should not exceed 25 mcg/mL.

Implementation

- Do not confuse gentamicin with gentian violet.
- Patients treated with parenteral aminoglycosides should be under close clinical observation because of the potential ototoxicity and nephrotoxicity associated with its use. Safety has not been established for using parenteral aminoglycosides for >14 days.
- Keep patient well hydrated (1500–2000 mL/day) during therapy.
- **Preoperative Bowel Prep:** Neomycin is usually used in conjunction with erythromycin, a low-residue diet, and a cathartic or enema.
- **PO:** Neomycin may be administered without regard to meals.
- **IM:** IM administration should be deep into a well-developed muscle. Alternate injection sites.
- **IV:** If aminoglycosides and penicillins or cephalosporins must be administered concurrently, administer in separate sites, >1 hr apart.

Amikacin

IV Administration

- **Intermittent Infusion: Dilution:** Dilute with D5W, D10W, 0.9% NaCl, dextrose/saline combinations, or LR. Solution may be pale yellow without ↓ potency. Stable for 24 hr at room temperature. **Concentration:** 10 mg/mL. **Rate:** Infuse over 30–60 min for adults and children and over 1–2 hr in infants.
- **Y-Site Compatibility:** acyclovir, aldesleukin, alemtuzumab, aminocaproic acid, aminophylline, amiodarone, anidulafungin, argatroban, arsenic trioxide, ascorbic acid, atracurium, atropine, aztreonam, benztropine, bivalirudin, bleomycin, bumetanide, buprenorphine, butorphanol, calcium chloride, calcium gluconate, cangrelor, carboplatin, carmustine, caspofungin, cefazolin, cefepime, cefotaxime, cefotetan, cefoxitin, ceftaroline, ceftazidime, ceftolozane/tazobactam, ceftriaxone, cefuroxime, chloramphenicol, chlorpromazine, cisatracurium, cisplatin, clindamycin, cyanocobalamin, cyclophosphamide, cyclosporine, cytarabine, dactinomycin, daptomycin, daunorubicin, dexamethasone, dexmedetomidine, dexrazoxane, digoxin, diltiazem, diphenhydramine, dobutamine, docetaxel, dopamine, doxorubicin hydrochloride, doxorubicin liposomal, doxycycline, enalaprilat, ephedrine, epinephrine, epirubicin, epoetin alfa, eptifibatide, ertapenem, erythromycin, esmolol, etoposide, etoposide phosphate, famotidine, fentanyl, filgrastim, fluconazole, fludarabine, fluorouracil, foscarnet, fosphenytoin, furosemide, gemcitabine, gentamicin, glycopyrrolate, granisetron, hydrocortisone, hydromorphone, idarubicin, ifosfamide, imipenem/cilastatin, imipenem/cilastatin/relebactam, irinotecan, isavuconazonium, isoproterenol, ketamine, ketorolac, labetalol, leucovorin, levofloxacin, lidocaine, linezolid, lorazepam, magnesium sulfate, mannitol, melphalan, meperidine, meropenem, meropenem/vaborbactam, mesna, methadone, methotrexate, methylprednisolone, metoclopramide, metoprolol, metronidazole, midazolam, milrinone, minocycline, mitoxantrone, morphine, multivitamins, mycophenolate, nafcillin, nalbuphine, naloxone, nicardipine, nitroglycerin, nitroprusside, norepinephrine, octreotide, ondansetron, oxaliplatin, oxytocin, paclitaxel, palonosetron, pamidronate, pemetrexed, papaverine, penicillin G, phenobarbital, phentolamine, phenylephrine, phytonadione, piperacillin/tazobactam, posaconazole, potassium acetate, potassium chloride, procainamide, prochlorperazine, promethazine, propranolol, protamine, pyridoxine, remifentanil, rituximab, rocuronium, sargramostim, sodium acetate, sodium bicarbonate, succinylcholine, sufentanil, sulbactam/durlobactam, tacrolimus, tedizolid, theophylline, thiamine, thiotepa, tigecycline, tirofiban, tobramycin, topotecan, vancomycin, vasopressin, vecuronium, verapamil, vinblastine, vincristine, vinorelbine, voriconazole, zidovudine, zoledronic acid.
- **Y-Site Incompatibility:** allopurinol, amphotericin B deoxycholate, amphotericin B liposomal, azathioprine, dacarbazine, dantrolene, defibrotide, diazepam, diazoxide, folic acid, ganciclovir, gemtuzumab ozogamicin, ibuprofen lysine, indomethacin, mitomycin, pentamidine, pentobarbital, phenytoin, propofol, trastuzumab, trimethoprim/sulfamethoxazole, **Inhaln:** If using a bronchodilator or with known hyperreactive airway disease, chronic obstructive pulmonary disease, asthma, or bronchospasm, pretreat with short-acting selective beta-2 agonists.
- Allow to come to room temperature before administering with *Lamira™ Nebulizer System* only. Shake vial well for 10–15 sec. until contents appear uniform and well mixed. Flip up plastic top of vial and pull down on metal ring to open. Remove metal ring and rubber stopper carefully. Pour contents of vial into medication reservoir of the nebulizer handset.

Gentamicin

IV Administration

- **Intermittent Infusion: Dilution:** Dilute each dose with D5W, 0.9% NaCl, or LR. Do not use solutions that are discolored or that contain a precipitate. **Concentration:** 10 mg/mL. **Rate:** Infuse slowly over 30 min–2 hr.

- **Y-Site Compatibility:** acetaminophen, aldesleukin, alemtuzumab, alprostadil, amikacin, aminocaproic acid, aminophylline, amiodarone, anidulafungin, argatroban, arsenic trioxide, ascorbic acid, atropine, aztreonam, benztropine, bivalirudin, bleomycin, bumetanide, buprenorphine, butorphanol, caffeine citrate, calcium chloride, calcium gluconate, carboplatin, carmustine, caspofungin, cefazolin, cefepime, cefotaxime, cefoxitin, ceftaroline, ceftazidime, ceftazidime/avibactam, ceftolozane/avibactam, ceftriaxone, cefuroxime, chlorothiazide, chlorpromazine, ciprofloxacin, cisatracurium, cisplatin, clindamycin, cyanocobalamin, cyclophosphamide, cyclosporine, cytarabine, dactinomycin, daptomycin, daunorubicin, dexmedetomidine, dexrazoxane, digoxin, diltiazem, dimenhydrinate, diphenhydramine, dobutamine, docetaxel, dopamine, doxorubicin hydrochloride, doxorubicin liposomal, doxycycline, edetate calcium disodium, enalaprilat, ephedrine, epinephrine, epirubicin, epoetin alfa, eptifibatide, eravacycline, ertapenem, erythromycin, esmolol, etoposide, etoposide phosphate, famotidine, fentanyl, fluconazole, fludarabine, fluorouracil, foscarnet, fosphenytoin, gemcitabine, glycopyrrolate, granisetron, hydromorphone, ifosfamide, imipenem/cilastatin, imipenem/cilastatin/relebactam, irinotecan, isavuconazonium, isoproterenol, ketamine, ketorolac, labetalol, leucovorin, levofloxacin, lidocaine, linezolid, lorazepam, magnesium sulfate, mannitol, melphalan, meperidine, meropenem, meropenem/vaborbactam, mesna, methadone, methylprednisolone, metoclopramide, metoprolol, metronidazole, midazolam, milrinone, minocycline, mitoxantrone, morphine, multivitamins, mycophenolate, nafcillin, nalbuphine, naloxone, nicardipine, nitroglycerin, nitroprusside, norepinephrine, octreotide, ondansetron, oxaliplatin, oxytocin, paclitaxel, palonosetron, pamidronate, papaverine, penicillin G, phenobarbital, phentolamine, phenylephrine, phytonadione, posaconazole, potassium acetate, potassium chloride, procainamide, prochlorperazine, promethazine, propranolol, protamine, pyridoxine, remifentanil, rituximab, rocuronium, sargramostim, sildenafil, sodium acetate, sodium bicarbonate, succinylcholine, sufentanil, sulbactam/durlobactam, tacrolimus, telavancin, theophylline, thiamine, thiotepa, tigecycline, tirofiban, tobramycin, topotecan, trastuzumab, vancomycin, vasopressin, vecuronium, verapamil, vinblastine, vincristine, vinorelbine, voriconazole, zidovudine, zoledronic acid.
- **Y-Site Incompatibility:** allopurinol, amphotericin B deoxycholate, amphotericin B liposomal, azathioprine, cangrelor, cefotetan, dacarbazine, dantrolene, diazepam, diazoxide, folic acid, ganciclovir, gemtuzumab ozogamicin, idarubicin, indomethacin, letermovir, methotrexate, mitomycin, oxacillin, pemetrexed, pentamidine, pentobarbital, phenytoin, propofol, trimethoprim/sulfamethoxazole, tedizolid.

Tobramycin

IV Administration

- **Intermittent Infusion: Dilution:** Dilute each dose of tobramycin in 50–100 mL of D5W, D10W, D5/0.9% NaCl, 0.9% NaCl, Ringer's, or lactated Ringer's solution. **Concentration:** Not >10 mg/mL. Pediatric doses may be diluted in proportionately smaller amounts. Stable for 24 hr at room temperature, 96 hr if refrigerated. **Rate:** Infuse slowly over 30–60 min in both adult and pediatric patients.
- **Y-Site Compatibility:** acyclovir, aldesleukin, alemtuzumab, alprostadil, alteplase, amikacin, aminocaproic acid, aminophylline, amiodarone, anidulafungin, argatroban, arsenic trioxide, ascorbic acid, atropine, aztreonam, benztropine, bivalirudin, bleomycin, bumetanide, buprenorphine, butorphanol, calcium chloride, calcium gluconate, carboplatin, carmustine, caspofungin, cefepime, cefotaxime, cefoxitin, ceftaroline, ceftazidime, ceftazidime/avibactam, ceftolozane/avibactam, cefuroxime, chloramphenicol, chlorpromazine, ciprofloxacin, cisatracurium, cisplatin, clindamycin, cyanocobalamin, cyclophosphamide, cyclosporine, cytarabine, dactinomycin, daptomycin, daunorubicin, dexmedetomidine, dexrazoxane, digoxin, diltiazem, dimenhydrinate, diphenhydramine, dobutamine, docetaxel, dopamine, doxorubicin hydrochloride, doxorubicin liposomal, doxycycline, enalaprilat, ephedrine, epinephrine, epirubicin, epoetin alfa, eravacycline, ertapenem, erythromycin, esmolol, etoposide, etoposide phosphate, famotidine, fentanyl, filgrastim, fluconazole, fludarabine, fluorouracil, foscarnet, fosphenytoin, furosemide, gemcitabine, gentamicin, glycopyrrolate, granisetron, hydromorphone, idarubicin, ifosfamide, imipenem/cilastatin, imipenem/cilastatin/relebactam, irinotecan, isavuconazonium, isoproterenol, ketamine, ketorolac, labetalol, leucovorin, levofloxacin, lidocaine, linezolid, lorazepam, magnesium sulfate, mannitol, melphalan, meperidine, meropenem, meropenem/vaborbactam, mesna, methadone, methotrexate, methylprednisolone, metoclopramide, metoprolol, metronidazole, midazolam, milrinone, minocycline, mitomycin, mitoxantrone, morphine, multivitamins, mycophenolate, nafcillin, nalbuphine, naloxone, nicardipine, nitroglycerin, nitroprusside, norepinephrine, octreotide, ondansetron, oritavancin, oxaliplatin, oxytocin, paclitaxel, palonosetron, pamidronate, papaverine, penicillin G, phenobarbital, phentolamine, phenylephrine, phytonadione, potassium acetate, potassium chloride, procainamide, prochlorperazine, promethazine, propranolol, protamine, pyridoxine, remifentanil, rituximab, rocuronium, sodium

acetate, sodium bicarbonate, succinylcholine, sufentanil, sulbactam/durlobactam, tacrolimus, telavancin, theophylline, thiamine, thiotepa, tigecycline, tirofiban, topotecan, trastuzumab, vancomycin, vasopressin, vecuronium, verapamil, vinblastine, vincristine, vinorelbine, voriconazole, zidovudine, zoledronic acid.

- **Y-Site Incompatibility:** allopurinol, amphotericin B deoxycholate, amphotericin B liposomal, azathioprine, cangrelor, cefazolin, cefiderocol, cefotetan, ceftobiprole, ceftriaxone, dacarbazine, dantrolene, defibrotide, dexamethasone, diazepam, diazoxide, folic acid, ganciclovir, gemtuzumab ozogamicin, indomethacin, oxacillin, pemetrexed, pentamidine, pentobarbital, phenytoin, piperacillin/tazobactam, propofol, sargramostim, tedizolid, trimethoprim/sulfamethoxazole. **Topical:** Cleanse skin before application. Wear gloves during application.
- **Inhaln:** Do not mix *TOBI* with dornase alpha in nebulizer.
- *TOBI Podhaler* capsules are not for oral use. Store capsules in blister until immediately before use. Use new Podhaler device provided with each weekly packet. Check to see capsule is empty after inhaling. If powder remains in capsule, repeat inhalation until capsule is empty.

Patient/Family Teaching

- Explain purpose and side effects of medication to patient. Advise patient to read *Patient Information* before starting therapy.
- Advise patient to notify health care provider of all Rx or OTC medications, vitamins, or herbal products being taken and to consult with health care provider before taking other medications.
- Advise patient to report signs of hypersensitivity, tinnitus, vertigo, hearing loss, rash, dizziness, or difficulty urinating.
- Advise patient of the importance of drinking plenty of liquids.
- Advise patient with a history of rheumatic heart disease or valve replacement the importance of using antimicrobial prophylaxis before invasive medical or dental procedures.
- **PO:** Advise patient to take neomycin as directed for full course of therapy. Take missed doses as soon as possible if not almost time for next dose; do not take double doses.
- Caution patient that neomycin may cause nausea, vomiting, or diarrhea.
- **Topical:** Advise patient to wash affected skin gently and pat dry. Apply a thin film of ointment. Apply occlusive dressing only if directed by health care provider. Patient should assess skin and inform health care provider if skin irritation develops or infection worsens.
- **Inhaln: Amikacin:** Advise patient to omit missed doses and administer next dose next day; do not double doses. Instruct patient to read *Medication Guide* before starting and with each Rx refill in case of changes.
- Advise patient to notify health care provider if signs and symptoms of allergic inflammation of lungs (fever, wheezing, coughing, shortness of breath, fast breathing), hemoptysis (coughing up blood), bronchospasm (shortness of breath, difficult or labored breathing, wheezing, coughing, chest tightness), or worsening of COPD occur.
- **Tobramycin:** Advise patient to take inhalation twice daily as close to 12 hr apart as possible and not <6 hr apart. Solution is colorless to pale yellow and may darken with age without affecting quality. Administer over 15-min period using a handheld PARI LC PLUS reusable nebulizer with a *PARI VIOS (for Bethkis) or DeVibiss Pulmo Aide (for TOBI)* compressor. Instruct patient on multiple therapies to take others first and use *tobramycin* last. Tobramycin-induced bronchospasm may be reduced if tobramycin is administered after bronchodilators. Instruct patient to sit or stand upright during inhalation and breathe normally through mouthpiece of nebulizer. Nose clips may help patient breath through mouth. Store at room temperature for up to 28 days. Advise patient to disinfect the nebulizer parts (except tubing) by boiling them in water for a full 10 min every other treatment day.
- Advise patient in correct technique for use of *TOBI Podhaler*. Wipe mouthpiece with clean, dry cloth after use; do not wash with water.
- Rep: May cause fetal harm. Advise women of reproductive potential to notify health care provider if pregnancy is planned or suspected or if breastfeeding. May cause irreversible deafness in infants.

Evaluation/Desired Outcomes

- Bactericidal action.

BEERS HIGH ALERT

V amiodarone
(am-ee-**oh**-da-rone)

Nexterone, Pacerone

Classification

Therapeutic: antiarrhythmics (class III)

Indications

Life-threatening ventricular arrhythmias unresponsive to less toxic agents. **Unlabeled Use: PO:**

Supraventricular tachyarrhythmias. **IV:** As part of the Advanced Cardiac Life Support (ACLS) and Pediatric Advanced Life Support (PALS) guidelines for the management of ventricular fibrillation (VF)/pulseless ventricular tachycardia (VT) after cardiopulmonary resuscitation and defibrillation have failed; also for other life-threatening tachyarrhythmias.

Action

Prolongs action potential and refractory period. Inhibits adrenergic stimulation. Slows the sinus rate, increases PR and QT intervals, and decreases peripheral vascular resistance (vasodilation). **Therapeutic Effects:** Suppression of arrhythmias.

Pharmacokinetics

Absorption: Slowly and variably absorbed from the GI tract (35–65%). IV administration results in complete bioavailability.
Distribution: Distributed to and accumulates slowly in body tissues. Reaches high levels in fat, muscle, liver, lungs, and spleen.
Protein Binding: 96%.
Metabolism and Excretion: Metabolized by the liver; excreted into bile. Minimal renal excretion. One metabolite has antiarrhythmic activity.
Half-life: 13–107 days.

TIME/ACTION PROFILE (suppression of ventricular arrhythmias)

ROUTE	ONSET	PEAK	DURATION
PO	2–3 days (up to 2–3 mo)	3–7 hr	wk–mos
IV	2 hr	3–7 hr	unknown

Contraindications/Precautions

Contraindicated in: Cardiogenic shock; Severe sinus node dysfunction; 2nd- or 3rd-degree AV block; Bradycardia (unless a pacemaker is in place); Hypersensitivity to amiodarone or iodine; Lactation: Lactation.
Use Cautiously in: Thyroid disorders; Corneal refractive laser surgery; Severe pulmonary or liver disease; OB: Should only be used during pregnancy when arrhythmias are refractory to other treatments or when other treatments are contraindicated; Pedi: Safety and effectiveness not established in children; Geri: Appears on Beers list. Avoid use as first-line therapy for rhythm control in atrial fibrillation in older adults unless HF or significant left ventricular hypertrophy present.

Adverse Reactions/Side Effects

CV: bradycardia, hypotension, HF, QT interval prolongation, WORSENING VENTRICULAR ARRHYTHMIAS. **Derm:** photosensitivity, blue discoloration. **EENT:** corneal microdeposits, abnormal sense of smell, dry eyes, optic neuritis, optic neuropathy, photophobia. **Endo:** hypothyroidism, hyperthyroidism. **GI:** anorexia, constipation, nausea, vomiting, ↑ liver enzymes, abdominal pain, abnormal sense of taste, HEPATOTOXICITY. **GU:** ↓ libido, epididymitis. **Neuro:** ataxia, dizziness, fatigue, involuntary movement, malaise, paresthesia, peripheral neuropathy, poor coordination, tremor, confusional states, disorientation, hallucinations, headache, insomnia. **Resp:** ACUTE RESPIRATORY DISTRESS SYNDROME, PULMONARY FIBROSIS.

Interactions

Drug-Drug: ↑ risk of QT interval prolongation with **fluoroquinolones**, **macrolides**, and **azole antifungals**. ↑ levels and risk of toxicity of **digoxin**; ↓ digoxin dose by 50%. ↑ levels and risk of toxicity of **cyclosporine**, **dextromethorphan**, **methotrexate**, **phenytoin**, **carvedilol**, and **theophylline**. **Phenytoin** may ↓ levels and effectiveness. ↑ levels and risk of bleeding of **warfarin**; ↓ warfarin dose by 30%. ↑ risk of bradyarrhythmias, sinus arrest, or heart block with **beta blockers**, **verapamil**, **diltiazem**, **digoxin**, **ivabradine**, or **clonidine**. ↑ risk of bradycardia when used with **sofosbuvir**, **ledipasvir/sofosbuvir**, **sofosbuvir/velpatasvir**, or **sofosbuvir/velpatasvir/voxilaprevir**; concurrent use not recommended. **Cholestyramine** may ↓ levels and effectiveness. **Cimetidine** and **ritonavir** may ↑ levels and risk of toxicity. Risk of myocardial depression is ↑ by **volatile anesthetics**. ↑ risk of myopathy with **lovastatin** and **simvastatin**; do not exceed 40 mg/day of lovastatin or 20 mg/day of simvastatin.
Drug-Natural Products: St. John's wort may ↓ levels and effectiveness; avoid concurrent use.
Drug-Food: Grapefruit juice may ↑ levels and risk of toxicity; avoid concurrent use.

Route/Dosage

Ventricular Arrhythmias

PO (Adults): 800–1600 mg/day in 1–2 doses for 1–3 wk; then 600–800 mg/day in 1–2 doses for 1 mo; then 400 mg/day maintenance dose.
PO (Children): 10 mg/kg/day (800 mg/1.72 m^2/day) for 10 days or until response or adverse reaction occurs; then 5 mg/kg/day (400 mg/1.72 m^2/day) for several wk; then ↓ to 2.5 mg/kg/day (200 mg/1.72 m^2/day) or lowest effective maintenance dose.
IV (Adults): 150 mg over 10 min, followed by 360 mg over the next 6 hr and then 540 mg over the next 18 hr. Continue infusion at 0.5 mg/min until oral therapy is initiated. If arrhythmia recurs, a small loading infusion of 150 mg over 10 min should be given; in addition, the rate of the maintenance infusion may be ↑. *Conversion to initial oral therapy:* If duration of IV infusion was <1 wk, oral dose should be 800–1600 mg/day; if IV infusion was 1–3 wk, oral dose should be 600–800 mg/day; if IV infusion was >3 wk, oral dose should be 400 mg/day. *ACLS guidelines for pulseless VF/VT:* 300 mg IV push; may repeat once after 3–5 min with 150 mg IV push (maximum cumulative dose 2.2 g/24 hr; unlabeled).

A

IV: Intraosseous: (Children and infants): *PALS guidelines for pulseless VF/VT:* 5 mg/kg as a bolus; *Perfusion tachycardia:* 5 mg/kg loading dose over 20–60 min (maximum of 15 mg/kg/day; unlabeled).

Supraventricular Tachycardia

PO (Adults): 600–800 mg/day for 1 wk or until desired response occurs or side effects develop; then ↓ to 400 mg/day for 3 wk; then maintenance dose of 200–400 mg/day.

PO (Children): 10 mg/kg/day (800 mg/1.72 m^2/day) for 10 days or until response or side effects occur; then 5 mg/kg/day (400 mg/1.72 m^2/day) for several wk; then ↓ to 2.5 mg/kg/day (200 mg/1.72 m^2/day) or lowest effective maintenance dose.

Availability (generic available)

Premixed infusion (Nexterone): 150 mg/100 mL D5W (does not contain polysorbate 80 or benzyl alcohol), 360 mg/200 mL D5W (does not contain polysorbate 80 or benzyl alcohol). **Solution for injection:** 50 mg/mL. **Tablets:** 100 mg, 200 mg, 400 mg.

NURSING IMPLICATIONS

Assessment

- Monitor ECG continuously during IV therapy or initiation of oral therapy. Monitor HR and rhythm throughout therapy; PR prolongation, slight QRS widening, and T-wave amplitude reduction with T-wave widening and bifurcation may occur. QT interval prolongation may be associated with worsening of arrhythmias; monitor closely during IV therapy. Report bradycardia or ↑ in arrhythmias promptly; patients receiving IV therapy may require slowing infusion rate, discontinuing infusion, or inserting a temporary pacemaker.
- Assess pacing and defibrillation threshold in patients with pacemakers and implanted defibrillators at beginning and periodically during therapy.
- Assess for signs of pulmonary toxicity (rales/crackles, ↓ breath sounds, pleuritic friction rub, fatigue, dyspnea, cough, wheezing, pleuritic pain, fever, hemoptysis, hypoxia). Chest x-ray and pulmonary function tests are recommended before therapy. Monitor chest x-ray yearly during therapy to detect diffuse interstitial changes or alveolar infiltrates. Bronchoscopy or gallium radionuclide scan may also be used for diagnosis. Usually reversible after withdrawal, but fatalities have occurred.
- **IV:** Assess for signs and symptoms of ARDS during therapy. Report dyspnea, tachypnea, or rales/crackles promptly. Bilateral, diffuse pulmonary infiltrates are seen on chest x-ray.
- Monitor BP frequently. Hypotension usually occurs during first several hr of therapy and is related to rate of infusion. If hypotension occurs, slow rate.
- **PO:** Assess for neurotoxicity (ataxia, proximal muscle weakness, tingling or numbness in fingers or toes, uncontrolled movements, tremors); common during initial therapy, but may occur within 1 wk to several mo of initiation of therapy and may persist for >1 yr after withdrawal. Dose ↓ is recommended. Assist patient during ambulation to prevent falls.
- Ophthalmic exams should be performed before and regularly during therapy and whenever visual changes (photophobia, halos around lights, ↓ acuity) occur. May cause permanent loss of vision.
- Assess for signs of thyroid dysfunction, especially during initial therapy. Lethargy; weight gain; edema of the hands, feet, and periorbital region; and cool, pale skin suggest hypothyroidism and may require ↓ in dose or discontinuation of therapy and thyroid supplementation. Tachycardia; weight loss; nervousness; sensitivity to heat; insomnia; and warm, flushed, moist skin suggest hyperthyroidism and may require discontinuation of therapy and treatment with antithyroid agents.

Lab Test Considerations

- Monitor thyroid function tests before starting therapy and every 6 mo during therapy.
- Monitor AST and ALT before starting therapy and every 6 mo during therapy. *If liver function studies are 3 times the upper limit of normal or double in patients with elevated baseline levels or if hepatomegaly occurs,* ↓ dose.
- Monitor serum potassium, calcium, and magnesium levels before starting therapy and periodically during therapy. Hypokalemia, hypocalcemia, and/or hypomagnesemia may cause additional arrhythmias; correct levels before beginning therapy.

Implementation

- ***High Alert:*** IV vasoactive medications are inherently dangerous; fatalities have occurred from medication errors involving amiodarone. Before administering, have second practitioner check original order, dose calculations, and infusion pump settings. Patients should be hospitalized and monitored closely during IV therapy and initiation of oral therapy. IV therapy should be administered only by clinicians experienced in treating life-threatening arrhythmias.
- Do not confuse amiodarone with amantadine.
- **PO:** May be administered with meals and in divided doses if GI intolerance occurs or if daily dose ≥1000 mg.

IV Administration

- V IV amiodarone is a vesicant. If extravasation occurs, immediately stop infusion. Leave needle/cannula in place temporarily but do not flush the line. Gently aspirate extravasated solution; then remove needle/cannula. Elevate patient's extremity and apply dry warm compresses. Initiate hyaluronidase antidote for refractory cases in addition to supportive management. For hyaluronidase, inject a total of 1 mL (15 units/mL) intradermally or SUBQ as five separate 0.2 mL injections (using a tuberculin syringe) around the site of extravasation; if IV catheter remains in place, administer IV through the infiltrated catheter; may repeat in 30–60 min if no resolution.

- **IV:** Administer via volumetric pump; drop size may be ↓, causing altered dosing with drop counter infusion sets.
- Administer through an in-line filter.
- Infusions exceeding 2 hr must be administered in glass or polyolefin bottles to prevent adsorption. However, polyvinyl chloride (PVC) tubing must be used during administration because concentrations and infusion rate recommendations have been based on PVC tubing.
- **IV Push: Dilution:** Used for treatment of pulseless VT/VF. Administer undiluted. May also be diluted in 20–30 mL of D5W or 0.9% NaCl. **Concentration:** 50 mg/mL. **Rate:** Administer IV push.
- **Intermittent Infusion: Dilution:** Dilute 150 mg of amiodarone in 100 mL of D5W. Infusion stable for 2 hr in PVC bag, or use premixed bags. **Concentration:** 1.5 mg/mL. **Rate:** Infuse over 10 min. Do not administer IV push.
- **Continuous Infusion: Dilution:** Dilute 900 mg of amiodarone in 500 mL of D5W. Infusion stable for 24 hr in glass or polyolefin bottle. **Concentration:** 1.8 mg/mL. Concentration may range from 1–6 mg/mL (concentrations >2 mg/mL must be administered via central venous catheter).
- **Rate:** Infuse at a rate of 1 mg/min for the first 6 hr; then ↓ infusion rate to 0.5 mg/min and continue until oral therapy initiated.
- **Y-Site Compatibility:** alemtuzumab, alprostadil, amikacin, anidulafungin, arsenic trioxide, atracurium, atropine, bleomycin, buprenorphine, busulfan, butorphanol, calcium chloride, cangrelor, carboplatin, carmustine, caspofungin, cefepime, ceftaroline, ceftolozane/tazobactam, chlorpromazine, ciprofloxacin, cisatracurium, cisplatin, clindamycin, cyclophosphamide, cyclosporine, dacarbazine, dactinomycin, daptomycin, daunorubicin, dexmedetomidine, dexrazoxane, diltiazem, diphenhydramine, docetaxel, dopamine, doxycycline, droperidol, enalaprilat, ephedrine, epinephrine, erythromycin lactobionate, esmolol, etoposide, etoposide phosphate, famotidine, fluconazole, gemcitabine, gentamicin, glycopyrrolate, granisetron, haloperidol, hetastarch, hydralazine, hydromorphone, idarubicin, ifosfamide, irinotecan, isavuconazonium, isoproterenol, ketamine, labetalol, lidocaine, linezolid, lorazepam, mannitol, meperidine, mesna, methadone, metoclopramide, metoprolol, metronidazole, midazolam, milrinone, mitoxantrone, morphine, moxifloxacin, mycophenolate, nafcillin, nalbuphine, naloxone, nicardipine, nitroglycerin, octreotide, ondansetron, oxaliplatin, palonosetron, pemetrexed, penicillin G potassium, pentamidine, phentolamine, phenylephrine, procainamide, prochlorperazine, promethazine, propranolol, remifentanil, rifampin, rocuronium, succinylcholine, sufentanil, tacrolimus, tedizolid, theophylline, tirofiban, tobramycin, topotecan, vancomycin, vasopressin, vecuronium, vinblastine, vincristine, vinorelbine, voriconazole, zidovudine, zoledronic acid.
- **Y-Site Incompatibility:** acyclovir, allopurinol, aminocaproic acid, aminophylline, ampicillin, ampicillin/sulbactam, azithromycin, bivalirudin, cefiderocol, cefotaxime, cefotetan, ceftazidime, chloramphenicol, clevidipine, cytarabine, dantrolene, dexamethasone, diazepam, digoxin, doxorubicin hydrochloride, doxorubicin liposomal, eravacycline, ertapenem, fludarabine, fluorouracil, foscarnet, fosphenytoin, ganciclovir, gemtuzumab ozogamicin, heparin, hydrocortisone, imipenem/cilastatin, ketorolac, LR, letermovir, leucovorin, levofloxacin, melphalan, meropenem, meropenem/vaborbactam, methotrexate, micafungin, mitomycin, paclitaxel, pentobarbital, phenobarbital, phenytoin, piperacillin/tazobactam, plazomicin, potassium acetate, potassium phosphates, sodium acetate, sodium bicarbonate, sodium phosphates, sulbactam/durlobactam, thiotepa, tigecycline, trimethoprim/sulfamethoxazole, verapamil.

Patient/Family Teaching

- Explain purpose and side effects of medication to patient. Advise patient to read *Patient Information* before starting therapy. Instruct patient to take as directed. If a dose is missed, do not take at all. Consult health care provider if >2 doses are missed.
- Advise patient to notify health care provider of all Rx or OTC medications, vitamins, or herbal products being taken and to consult with health care provider before taking other medications, especially St. John's wort.
- Advise patient to avoid drinking grapefruit juice during therapy.
- Inform patient that side effects may not appear until several days, wks, or yr after initiation of therapy and may persist for several mo after withdrawal.
- Teach patients to monitor HR daily and report abnormalities.
- Advise patients that photosensitivity reactions may occur through window glass, thin clothing, and sunscreens. Protective clothing and sunblock are recommended during and for 4 mo after therapy. If photosensitivity occurs, dose ↓ may be useful.

- Inform patients that bluish discoloration of the face, neck, and arms is a possible side effect of this drug after prolonged use. This is usually reversible and will fade over several mo. Notify health care provider if this occurs.
- Instruct male patients to notify health care provider if signs and symptoms of epididymitis (pain and swelling in scrotum) occur. May require ↓ in dose.
- Instruct patient to notify health care provider of medication regimen before treatment or surgery.
- Advise patient to notify health care provider if signs and symptoms of thyroid dysfunction occur.
- Emphasize the importance of follow-up exams, including chest x-ray once yearly and liver and thyroid function tests every 6 mo.
- Rep: May cause fetal harm. Advise women of reproductive potential to use effective contraception and to avoid breastfeeding during therapy. May cause neonatal bradycardia, QT prolongation, periodic ventricular extrasystoles; neonatal hypothyroidism (with or without goiter) detected antenatally or in the newborn and reported even after a few days of exposure; neonatal hyperthyroxinemia; neurodevelopmental abnormalities independent of thyroid function, including speech delay and difficulties with written language and arithmetic, delayed motor development, and ataxia; jerk nystagmus with synchronous head titubation; fetal growth retardation; and premature birth. Advise patient to notify health care provider if pregnancy is planned or suspected.

Evaluation/Desired Outcomes

- Suppression of arrhythmias.

BEERS

amitriptyline

(a-mee-**trip**-ti-leen)

Elavil

Classification

Therapeutic: antidepressants

Pharmacologic: tricyclic antidepressants

Indications

Depression. **Unlabeled Use:** Anxiety. Insomnia. Chronic pain syndromes (e.g. fibromyalgia, neuropathic pain/chronic pain, headache, low back pain).

Action

Potentiates the effect of serotonin and norepinephrine in the CNS. Has significant anticholinergic properties. **Therapeutic Effects:** Antidepressant action.

Pharmacokinetics

Absorption: Well absorbed from the GI tract.

Distribution: Widely distributed.

Protein Binding: 95%.

Metabolism and Excretion: Extensively metabolized by the liver, primarily by the CYP2D6 isoenzyme; the CYP2D6 enzyme system exhibits genetic polymorphism (7% of population may be poor metabolizers and may have significantly ↑ amitriptyline concentrations and an ↑ risk of adverse effects). Some metabolites have antidepressant activity. Undergoes enterohepatic recirculation and secretion into gastric juices.

Half-life: 10–50 hr.

TIME/ACTION PROFILE (antidepressant effect)

ROUTE	ONSET	PEAK	DURATION
PO	2–3 wk (up to 30 days)	2–6 wk	days–wk

Contraindications/Precautions

Contraindicated in: Angle-closure glaucoma; History of QTc interval prolongation, recent MI, or HF; Lactation: Lactation.

Use Cautiously in: May ↑ risk of suicide attempt/ideation especially during early treatment or dose adjustment; risk may be greater in children or adolescents; Patients with pre-existing cardiovascular disease; Prostatic hyperplasia (↑ risk of urinary retention); History of seizures (threshold may be ↓); Hypovolemia or dehydration (↑ risk of syndrome of inappropriate antidiuretic hormone secretion [SIADH]); OB: Use during pregnancy only if potential maternal benefit justifies potential fetal risk; Pedi: Children <12 yr (safety and effectiveness not established); Geri: Appears on Beers list. ↑ risk of adverse reactions in older adults, including falls secondary to sedative and anticholinergic effects, orthostatic hypotension, and SIADH. Avoid use in older adults.

Adverse Reactions/Side Effects

CV: hypotension, ARRHYTHMIAS, QT interval prolongation, TORSADES DE POINTES. **Derm:** photosensitivity. **EENT:** blurred vision, dry eyes, dry mouth. **Endo:** changes in blood glucose, gynecomastia. **F and E:** hyponatremia, SIADH. **GI:** constipation, hepatitis, paralytic ileus. **GU:** ↓ libido, urinary retention. **Hemat:** blood dyscrasias. **Metab:** ↑ appetite, weight gain. **Neuro:** lethargy, sedation, SUICIDAL THOUGHTS/BEHAVIORS.

Interactions

Drug-Drug: Amitriptyline is metabolized in the liver by the cytochrome P450 2D6 enzyme, and its action may be affected by drugs that compete for metabolism by this enzyme, including other **antidepressants, phenothiazines, carbamazepine, propafenone,** and **flecainide**; when these drugs are used concurrently with amitriptyline, may need to ↓ dose of one or the other or both. Concurrent use of other drugs that inhibit the activity of the enzyme, including **cimetidine**, **quinidine**, **amiodarone**, and **ritonavir**, may ↑ levels and risk of toxicity of amitriptyline. May cause hypotension, tachycardia, and potentially fatal reactions when used with **MAO inhibitors**; avoid concurrent use; discontinue 2 wk before starting amitriptyline. Concurrent use with **SSRIs** may result in ↑ toxicity and should be avoided; **fluoxetine** should be stopped 5 wk before starting amitriptyline. **Clonidine** may result in hypertensive crisis and should be avoided. **Levodopa** may result in delayed or ↓ absorption of levodopa or hypertension. **Rifampin**, **rifapentine**, and **rifabutin** may ↓ levels and effectiveness. **Moxifloxacin** may ↑ risk of adverse cardiovascular reactions. ↑ risk of CNS depression with other **CNS depressants**, including **alcohol**, **antihistamines**, **clonidine**, **opioids**, and **sedative/hypnotics**. **Barbiturates** may ↓ levels and effectiveness. **Adrenergic** and **anticholinergic** side effects may be ↑ with other agents having **anticholinergic** properties. **Phenothiazines** or **oral contraceptives** may ↑ levels and risk of toxicity. **Nicotine** may ↓ levels and effectiveness. **Diuretics** may ↑ risk of SIADH.

Drug-Natural Products: St. John's wort may ↓ levels and effectiveness. **Kava-kava**, **valerian**, or **chamomile** can ↑ risk of CNS depression. ↑ anticholinergic effects with **jimson weed** and **scopolia**.

Route/Dosage

PO (Adults): 75 mg/day in divided doses; may ↑ up to 150 mg/day *or* 50–100 mg at bedtime; may ↑ by 25–50 mg up to 150 mg (in hospitalized patients, may initiate with 100 mg/day and ↑ total daily dose up to 300 mg).

PO (Geriatric Patients): 10–25 mg at bedtime; may ↑ by 10–25 mg weekly if tolerated (usual dose range = 25–150 mg/day).

Availability (generic available)

Tablets: 10 mg, 25 mg, 50 mg, 75 mg, 100 mg, 150 mg.

NURSING IMPLICATIONS

Assessment

- Obtain weight and body mass index initially and periodically during treatment.
- Assess fasting glucose and cholesterol levels in overweight/obese individuals.
- Monitor BP and HR before and during initial therapy. Notify health care provider of ↓ in BP (10–20 mm Hg) or sudden ↑ in HR. Monitor ECG before and periodically during therapy in patients taking high doses or with a history of cardiovascular disease.
- Assess for signs and symptoms of SIADH (hyponatremia, headache, muscle cramps or weakness, tremors).
- **Depression:** Monitor mental status (orientation, mood behavior) frequently. Assess for suicidal tendencies, especially during early therapy. Restrict amount of drug available to patient. Risk may be ↑ in children, adolescents, and adults ≤24 yr. After starting therapy, children, adolescents, and young adults should be seen by health care provider at least weekly for 4 wk, every 3 wk for next 4 wk, and on advice of health care provider thereafter.
- **Pain:** Assess intensity, quality, and location of pain periodically during therapy. May require several weeks for effects to be seen. Use pain scale to monitor effectiveness of medication. Assess for sexual dysfunction (↓ libido; erectile dysfunction). Geri: Older adults started on amitriptyline may be at ↑ risk for falls; start with low dose and monitor closely. Assess for anticholinergic effects (weakness and sedation).

Lab Test Considerations

- Assess CBC, sodium, liver function, and serum glucose before and periodically during therapy. May ↓ sodium. Serum glucose may be ↑ or ↓. May ↑ serum bilirubin and alkaline phosphatase. May cause bone marrow depression.

Implementation

- Dose ↑ should be made at bedtime due to sedation. Dose titration is a slow process; may take weeks to months to become effective. May give entire dose at bedtime. Sedative effect may be apparent before antidepressant effect is noted. May require tapering to avoid withdrawal effects.
- **PO:** Administer medication with or immediately after a meal to minimize gastric upset. Tablet may be crushed and given with food or fluids.

Patient/Family Teaching

- Explain purpose and side effects of medication to patient. Advise to read *Patient Information* before starting therapy. Instruct patient to take medication as directed. If a dose is missed, take as soon as possible unless almost time for next dose; if regimen is a single dose at bedtime, do not take in the morning because of side effects. Advise patient that drug effects may not be noticed for >2 wk. Abrupt discontinuation may cause nausea, vomiting, diarrhea, headache, trouble sleeping with vivid dreams, and irritability.
- Advise patient to notify health care provider of all Rx or OTC medications, vitamins, or herbal products being taken and to consult health care provider before taking other medications.
- May cause drowsiness and blurred vision. Caution patient to avoid driving and other activities requiring alertness until response to drug is known.
- Orthostatic hypotension, SIADH, sedation, and confusion are common during early therapy, especially in older adults. Protect patient from falls and advise

patient to make position changes slowly. Institute fall precautions. Advise patient to make position changes slowly. Refer as appropriate for nutrition/weight management and medical management.

- Advise patient to avoid alcohol or other CNS depressant drugs during and for 3–7 days after therapy has been discontinued.
- Advise patient, family, and caregivers to look for suicidality, especially during early therapy or dose changes. Notify health care provider immediately if thoughts about suicide or dying, attempts to commit suicide, new or worse depression or anxiety, agitation or restlessness, panic attacks, insomnia, new or worse irritability, aggressiveness, acting on dangerous impulses, mania, or other changes in mood or behavior occur.
- Instruct patient to notify health care provider if urinary retention, dry mouth, or constipation persists. Sugarless candy or gum may diminish dry mouth, and an ↑ in fluid intake or fiber may prevent constipation. If symptoms persist, dose ↓ or discontinuation may be necessary. Consult health care provider if dry mouth persists for >2 wk.
- Caution patient to use sunscreen and protective clothing to prevent photosensitivity reactions.
- Alert patient that medication may turn urine blue-green in color.
- Inform patient of need to monitor dietary intake. ↑ in appetite may lead to undesired weight gain.
- Advise patient to notify health care provider of medication regimen before treatment or surgery. Medication should be discontinued as long as possible before surgery.
- Rep: May cause fetal harm. Advise women of reproductive potential to notify health care provider if pregnancy is planned or suspected and to avoid breastfeeding. Assess neonates of women taking amitriptyline during pregnancy for irritability, jitteriness, ↑ crying, constipation, problems with urinating, respiratory distress, nausea, and convulsions. Patients exposed to antidepressants during pregnancy are encouraged to enroll in the National Pregnancy Registry for Antidepressants. Patients or their health care providers may contact the registry by calling 1-866-961-2388 or https://womensmentalhealth.org/research/pregnancyregistry/antidepressants.

Evaluation/Desired Outcomes

- Antidepressant action.

amLODIPine, See CALCIUM CHANNEL BLOCKERS.

amoxicillin (a-mox-i-sill-in)

~~Amoxil~~, ✦ Novamoxin, ~~Trimox~~

Classification

Therapeutic: anti-infectives, antiulcer agents

Pharmacologic: aminopenicillins

Indications

Treatment of: Skin and skin structure infections, Otitis media, Sinusitis, Respiratory infections, Genitourinary infections. Endocarditis prophylaxis. Postexposure inhalational anthrax prophylaxis. Management of ulcer disease due to *Helicobacter pylori*.

Action

Inhibits bacterial cell wall synthesis. **Therapeutic Effects:** Bactericidal action; spectrum is broader than penicillins. **Spectrum:** Active against: Streptococci, Pneumococci, Enterococci, *Haemophilus influenzae*, *Escherichia coli*, *Proteus mirabilis*, *Neisseria meningitidis*, *Neisseria gonorrhoeae*, *Shigella*, *Chlamydia trachomatis*, *Salmonella*, *Borrelia burgdorferi*, *H. pylori*.

Pharmacokinetics

Absorption: Well absorbed from duodenum (75–90%). More resistant to acid inactivation than other penicillins.

Distribution: Diffuses readily into most body tissues and fluids. CSF penetration ↑ when meninges are inflamed.

Metabolism and Excretion: 30% metabolized by the liver; 70% excreted unchanged in the urine.

Half-life: *Neonates:* 3.7 hr; *Infants and Children:* 1–2 hr; *Adults:* 0.7–1.4 hr.

TIME/ACTION PROFILE (plasma concentrations)

ROUTE	ONSET	PEAK	DURATION
PO	30 min	1–2 hr	8–12 hr

Contraindications/Precautions

Contraindicated in: Hypersensitivity to penicillins (cross-sensitivity exists to cephalosporins and other beta-lactams).

Use Cautiously in: Severe renal impairment; Infectious mononucleosis, acute lymphocytic leukemia, or cytomegalovirus infection (↑ risk of rash).

Adverse Reactions/Side Effects

Derm: <u>rash</u>, ACUTE GENERALIZED EXANTHEMATOUS PUSTULOSIS, DRUG REACTION WITH EOSINOPHILIA AND SYSTEMIC SYMPTOMS, STEVENS-JOHNSON SYNDROME (SJS), TOXIC EPIDERMAL NECROLYSIS, urticaria. **GI:** <u>diarrhea</u>, ↑ liver enzymes, CLOSTRIDIOIDES DIFFICILE-ASSOCIATED DIARRHEA (CDAD), nausea, vomiting. **Hemat:** blood dyscrasias.

Neuro: SEIZURES (HIGH DOSES). **Misc:** HYPERSENSITIVITY REACTIONS (INCLUDING ANAPHYLAXIS), SERUM SICKNESS, superinfection.

Interactions

Drug-Drug: Probenecid ↓ renal excretion and ↑ levels; therapy may be combined for this purpose. May ↑risk of bleeding with **warfarin**. May ↓ effectiveness of **oral contraceptives**. **Allopurinol** may ↑ frequency of rash.

Route/Dosage

Most Infections

PO (Adults): 250–500 mg every 8 hr *or* 500–875 mg every 12 hr (not to exceed 2–3 g/day).
PO (Children >3 mo): 25–50 mg/kg/day in divided doses every 8 hr *or* 25–50 mg/kg/day in divided doses every 12 hr; *Acute otitis media due to highly resistant strains of S. pneumoniae:* 80–90 mg/kg/day in divided doses every 12 hr; *Postexposure inhalational anthrax prophylaxis:* <40 kg: 45 mg/kg/day in divided doses every 8 hr; >40 kg: 500 mg every 8 hr.
PO (Infants ≤3 mo and neonates): 20–30 mg/kg/day in divided doses every 12 hr.

Renal Impairment

PO (Adults): *CCr 10–30 mL/min:* 250–500 mg every 12 hr; *CCr <10 mL/min:* 250–500 mg every 24 hr.

Helicobacter pylori

PO (Adults): *Triple therapy:* 1000 mg amoxicillin twice daily with lansoprazole 30 mg twice daily and clarithromycin 500 mg twice daily for 14 days *or* 1000 mg amoxicillin twice daily with omeprazole 20 mg twice daily and clarithromycin 500 mg twice daily for 14 days *or* amoxicillin 1000 mg twice daily with esomeprazole 40 mg daily and clarithromycin 500 mg twice daily for 10 days. *Dual therapy:* 1000 mg amoxicillin three times daily with lansoprazole 30 mg three times daily for 14 days.

Endocarditis Prophylaxis

PO (Adults): 2 g 1 hr prior to procedure.
PO (Children): 50 mg/kg 1 hr prior to procedure (not to exceed adult dose).

Gonorrhea

PO (Adults and Children ≥40 kg): 3 g as a single dose.
PO (Children >2 yr and <40 kg): 50 mg/kg with probenecid 25 mg/kg as a single dose.

Availability

Capsules: 250 mg, 500 mg. **Tablets:** 500 mg, 875 mg. **Chewable tablets (cherry, banana, peppermint flavors):** 125 mg, 250 mg. **Powder for oral suspension (strawberry [125 mg/5 mL] and bubblegum [200 mg/5 mL, 250 mg/5 mL, 400 mg/5 mL] flavors):** 125 mg/5 mL, 200 mg/5 mL, 250 mg/5 mL, 400 mg/5 mL. ***In combination with:*** clarithromycin and lansoprazole in a compliance package; omeprazole and clarithromycin (Omeclamox-Pak); omeprazole and rifabutin (Talicia); clarithromycin and vonoprazan in a compliance package (Voquenza Triple Pak); vonoprazan in a compliance package (Voquenza Dual Pak). See Appendix N.

NURSING IMPLICATIONS

Assessment

- Assess for infection (vital signs; appearance of wound, sputum, urine, and stool; WBC) at beginning of and throughout therapy.
- Obtain a history before initiating therapy to determine previous use of and reactions to penicillins or cephalosporins. Persons with a negative history of penicillin sensitivity may still have an allergic response.
- Monitor for signs and symptoms of anaphylaxis (rash, urticaria, pruritus, angioedema, hoarseness, dyspnea, wheezing). Notify health care professional immediately if these occur.
- Assess for rash or signs and symptoms of SJS periodically during therapy (fever, general malaise, fatigue, muscle or joint aches, blisters, oral lesions, conjunctivitis). Discontinue therapy and provide supportive care.
- Obtain specimens for culture and sensitivity prior to therapy. First dose may be given before receiving results.
- Monitor bowel function. Diarrhea, abdominal cramping, fever, and bloody stools should be reported to health care professional promptly as a sign of CDAD. May begin up to several wk following cessation of therapy.

Lab Test Considerations

- May cause ↑ serum alkaline phosphatase, LDH, AST, and ALT concentrations.
- Consider CBC to monitor for therapeutic response.
- May cause false-positive direct Coombs test result.
- May cause false positive readings on urine glucose tests.

Implementation

- **PO:** Administer around the clock. May be given without regard to meals or with meals to ↓ GI side effects. Capsule contents may be emptied and swallowed with liquids.
- Shake oral suspension before administering. Suspension may be given straight or mixed in formula, milk, fruit juice, water, or ginger ale. Administer immediately after mixing. Discard refrigerated reconstituted suspension after 10 days.

Patient/Family Teaching

- Educate patient on reason and side effects of amoxicillin. Instruct patients to take medication around the clock and to finish the drug completely as directed, even if feeling better. Advise patient that sharing of this medication may be dangerous.

Advise patient to read *Patient Information* before starting therapy.

- Pedi: Teach parents or caregivers to calculate and measure doses accurately. Reinforce importance of using measuring device supplied by pharmacy or with product, not household items.
- Instruct the patient to notify health care professional if symptoms do not improve.
- Advise patient to report the signs of superinfection (furry overgrowth on the tongue, vaginal itching or discharge, loose or foul-smelling stools) and allergy.
- Instruct patient to notify health care professional immediately if diarrhea, abdominal cramping, fever, or bloody stools occur and not to treat with antidiarrheals without consulting health care professional.
- Teach patients with a history of rheumatic heart disease or valve replacement the importance of using antimicrobial prophylaxis before invasive medical or dental procedures.
- Rep: Caution women of reproductive potential taking oral contraceptives to use an alternate or additional nonhormonal method of contraception during therapy with amoxicillin and until next menstrual period.

Evaluation/Desired Outcomes

- Resolution of the signs and symptoms of infection. Length of time for complete resolution depends on the organism and site of infection.
- Endocarditis prophylaxis.
- Eradication of *H. pylori* with resolution of ulcer symptoms.
- Prevention of inhalational anthrax (postexposure).

amoxicillin/clavulanate

(a-mox-i-**sill**-in/klav-yoo-**lan**-ate)

Augmentin, Augmentin ES,
Clavulin

Classification

Therapeutic: anti-infectives

Pharmacologic: aminopenicillins/beta-lactamase inhibitors

Indications

Treatment of a variety of infections, including: Skin and skin structure infections, Otitis media, Sinusitis, Respiratory tract infections, Genitourinary tract infections.

Action

Inhibits bacterial cell wall synthesis; spectrum of amoxicillin is broader than penicillin. Clavulanate resists action of beta-lactamase, an enzyme produced by bacteria that is capable of inactivating some penicillins. **Therapeutic Effects:** Bactericidal action against susceptible bacteria. **Spectrum:** Active against: Streptococci, Pneumococci, Enterococci, *Haemophilus influenzae*, *Escherichia coli*, *Proteus mirabilis*, *Neisseria meningitidis*, *Neisseria gonorrhoeae*, *Staphylococcus aureus*, *Klebsiella pneumoniae*, *Shigella*, *Salmonella*, *Moraxella catarrhalis*.

Pharmacokinetics

Absorption: Well absorbed from the duodenum (75–90%). More resistant to acid inactivation than other penicillins.

Distribution: Diffuses readily into most body tissues and fluids. Does not readily enter brain/CSF; CSF penetration is ↑ in the presence of inflamed meninges.

Metabolism and Excretion: 30% metabolized by the liver; 70% excreted unchanged in the urine.

Half-life: 1–1.3 hr.

TIME/ACTION PROFILE (plasma concentrations)

ROUTE	ONSET	PEAK	DURATION
PO	30 min	1–2 hr	8–12 hr

Contraindications/Precautions

Contraindicated in: Hypersensitivity to penicillins or clavulanate; Suspension and chewable tablets contain aspartame and should be avoided in phenylketonurics; History of amoxicillin/clavulanate-associated cholestatic jaundice.

Use Cautiously in: Severe renal impairment; Hepatic impairment; Infectious mononucleosis (↑ risk of rash).

Adverse Reactions/Side Effects

Derm: rash, ACUTE GENERALIZED EXANTHEMATOUS PUSTULOSIS, DRUG REACTION WITH EOSINOPHILIA AND SYSTEMIC SYMPTOMS, STEVENS-JOHNSON SYNDROME (SJS), TOXIC EPIDERMAL NECROLYSIS, urticaria. **GI:** diarrhea, CLOSTRIDIOIDES DIFFICILE-ASSOCIATED DIARRHEA (CDAD), hepatic impairment, nausea, vomiting. **GU:** vaginal candidiasis. **Hemat:** blood dyscrasias. **Neuro:** SEIZURES (HIGH DOSES). **Misc:** ALLERGIC REACTIONS (INCLUDING ANAPHYLAXIS AND SERUM SICKNESS), superinfection.

Interactions

Drug-Drug: Probenecid ↓ renal excretion and ↑ levels; therapy may be combined for this purpose. May ↑ risk of bleeding of **warfarin**. Concurrent **allopurinol** therapy ↑ risk of rash. May ↓ effectiveness of **hormonal contraceptives**.

Drug-Food: Clavulanate absorption is ↓ by a **high-fat** meal.

Route/Dosage

Most Infections (Dosing based on amoxicillin component)

PO (Adults and Children >40 kg): 250 mg every 8 hr *or* 500 mg every 12 hr.

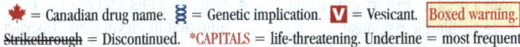

Serious Infections and Respiratory Tract Infections

PO (Adults and Children >40 kg): 875 mg every 12 hr *or* 500 mg every 8 hr; *Acute bacterial sinusitis:* 2000 mg every 12 hr for 10 days (extended release); *Community-acquired pneumonia:* 2000 mg every 12 hr for 7–10 days (extended release).

Recurrent/Persistent Acute Otitis Media Due to Multidrug-Resistant *Streptococcus pneumoniae, H. influenzae,* or *M. catarrhalis*

PO (Children <40 kg): 80–90 mg/kg/day in divided doses every 12 hr for 10 days (ES formulation only).

Renal Impairment

PO (Adults): *CCr 10–30 mL/min:* 250–500 mg every 12 hr; *CCr <10 mL/min:* 250–500 mg every 24 hr.

Otitis Media, Sinusitis, Lower Respiratory Tract Infections, Serious Infections

PO (Children ≥3 mo): *200 mg/5 mL or 400 mg/5 mL suspension:* 45 mg/kg/day divided every 12 hr; *125 mg/5 mL or 250 mg/5 mL suspension:* 40 mg/kg/day divided every 8 hr.

Less Serious Infections

PO (Children ≥3 mo): *200 mg/5 mL or 400 mg/5 mL suspension:* 25 mg/kg/day divided every 12 hr; *125 mg/5 mL or 250 mg/5 mL suspension:* 20 mg/kg/day divided every 8 hr.
PO (Children <3 mo): *125 mg/5 mL suspension:* 15 mg/kg every 12 hr.

Availability (generic available)

Immediate-release tablets: 250 mg amoxicillin with 125 mg clavulanate, 500 mg amoxicillin with 125 mg clavulanate, 875 mg amoxicillin with 125 mg clavulanate. **Chewable tablets (cherry-banana flavor):** 200 mg amoxicillin with 28.5 mg clavulanate, 400 mg amoxicillin with 57 mg clavulanate. **Extended-release tablets (scored):** 1000 mg amoxicillin with 62.5 mg clavulanate. **Powder for oral suspension (200 mg/5 mL is fruit flavor; 250 mg/5 mL is orange flavor; 400 mg/5 mL is fruit flavor; 600 mg/5 mL is orange or strawberry-creme flavor):** 200 mg amoxicillin with 28.5 mg clavulanate/5 mL, 250 mg amoxicillin with 62.5 mg clavulanate/5 mL, 400 mg amoxicillin with 57 mg clavulanate/5 mL, 600 mg amoxicillin with 42.9 mg clavulanate/5 mL (ES formulation).

NURSING IMPLICATIONS

Assessment

- Assess for infection (vital signs; appearance of wound, sputum, urine, and stool; WBC) at beginning of and during therapy.
- Obtain a history before initiating therapy to determine previous use of and reactions to penicillins or cephalosporins. Persons with a negative history of penicillin sensitivity may still have an allergic response.
- Observe for signs and symptoms of anaphylaxis (rash, urticaria, pruritus, angioedema, hoarseness, dyspnea, wheezing). Notify health care professional immediately if these occur.
- Assess for rash or signs and symptoms of SJS periodically during therapy (fever, general malaise, fatigue, muscle or joint aches, blisters, oral lesions, conjunctivitis). Discontinue therapy and provide supportive care.
- Obtain specimens for culture and sensitivity prior to therapy. First dose may be given before receiving results.
- Monitor bowel function. Diarrhea, abdominal cramping, fever, and bloody stools should be reported to health care professional promptly as a sign of CDAD. May begin up to several wk following cessation of therapy.

Lab Test Considerations

- May cause ↑ serum alkaline phosphatase, LDH, AST, and ALT concentrations. Elderly men and patients receiving prolonged treatment are at ↑ risk for hepatic impairment.
- Consider CBC to monitor for therapeutic response.
- May cause false-positive direct Coombs test result.
- May cause false positive readings on urine glucose tests.

Implementation

- **PO:** Administer around the clock. Administer at the start of a meal to enhance absorption and to ↓ GI side effects. Do not administer with high-fat meals; clavulanate absorption is ↓. Extended-release tablet is scored and can be broken for ease of administration; ***DNC:*** however, do not crush extended-release tablet. Capsule contents may be emptied and swallowed with liquids. Chewable tablets should be crushed or chewed before swallowing with liquids. Shake oral suspension before administering. Refrigerated reconstituted suspension should be discarded after 10 days.
- Two 250-mg tablets are not bioequivalent to one 500-mg tablet; 250-mg tablets and 250-mg chewable tablets are also not interchangeable. Two 500-mg tablets are not interchangeable with one 1000-mg extended release tablet; amounts of clavulanic acid and durations of action are different. Augmentin ES 600 (600 mg/5 mL) does not contain the same amount of clavulanic acid as any of the other Augmentin suspensions. Suspensions are not interchangeable.
- Pedi: Do not administer 250-mg chewable tablets to children <40 kg due to clavulanate content. Children <3 mo should receive the 125-mg/5 mL oral solution.

Patient/Family Teaching

- Educate patient on reason and side effects of amoxicillin/clavulanate. Instruct patients to take medication around the clock and to finish the drug completely as directed, even if feeling better. Advise patients that sharing of this medication may be dangerous. Advise patient to read *Patient Information* before starting therapy.

- Pedi: Teach parents or caregivers to calculate and measure doses accurately. Reinforce importance of using measuring device supplied by pharmacy or with product, not household items.
- Advise patient to report the signs of superinfection (furry overgrowth on the tongue, vaginal itching or discharge, loose or foul-smelling stools) and allergy.
- Instruct patient to notify health care professional immediately if diarrhea, abdominal cramping, fever, or bloody stools occur and not to treat with antidiarrheals without consulting health care professionals.
- Instruct the patient to notify health care professional if symptoms do not improve or if nausea or diarrhea persists when drug is administered with food.
- Rep: Instruct women of reproductive potential taking oral contraceptives to use an alternate or additional method of contraception during therapy and until next menstrual period; may ↓ effectiveness of hormonal contraceptives. Advise patient to notify health care professional if pregnancy is planned or suspected or if breastfeeding.

Evaluation/Desired Outcomes

- Resolution of the signs and symptoms of infection. Length of time for complete resolution depends on the organism and site of infection.

amphetamine mixtures

(am-**fet**-a-meen)

Adderall, Adderall XR, Mydayis

Classification

Therapeutic: central nervous system stimulants

Schedule II

Indications

Attention-deficit hyperactivity disorder (ADHD). Narcolepsy.

Action

Causes release of norepinephrine from nerve endings. Pharmacologic effects are: CNS and respiratory stimulation, Vasoconstriction, Mydriasis (pupillary dilation). **Therapeutic Effects:** Increased motor activity, mental alertness, and decreased fatigue in narcoleptic patients. Increased attention span in ADHD.

Pharmacokinetics

Absorption: Well absorbed after oral administration.

Distribution: Widely distributed in body tissues, with high concentrations in the brain and CSF.

Metabolism and Excretion: Some metabolism by the liver. Urinary excretion is pH-dependent. Alkaline urine promotes reabsorption and prolongs action.

Half-life: *Children 6–12 yr:* 9–11 hr; *Adults:* 10–13 hr (depends on urine pH).

TIME/ACTION PROFILE (CNS stimulation)

ROUTE	ONSET	PEAK	DURATION
PO	tablet: 0.5–1 hr	tablet: 3 hr capsule: 7 hr	4–6 hr

Contraindications/Precautions

Contraindicated in: Hypersensitivity; Hyperexcitable states including hyperthyroidism; Psychotic personalities; Concurrent use or use within 14 days of MAO inhibitors or MAO-like drugs (linezolid or methylene blue); Suicidal or homicidal tendencies; Chemical dependence; Glaucoma; Serious structural cardiac abnormalities, cardiomyopathy, serious cardiac arrhythmia, coronary artery disease, or other serious cardiac disease (may ↑ risk of sudden death); End-stage renal disease; Lactation: Lactation.

Use Cautiously in: History of substance abuse; Continual use (may produce psychological dependence or physical addiction); Hypertension; Diabetes mellitus; Tics or family history/diagnosis of Tourette syndrome (may worsen condition); Severe renal impairment (↓ dose); OB: Use during pregnancy only if potential maternal benefit justifies potential fetal risk; may lead to premature delivery and low birth weight infants; Geri: Older adults may be more susceptible to side effects.

Adverse Reactions/Side Effects

CV: palpitations, tachycardia, cardiomyopathy (↑ with prolonged use or high doses), hypertension, hypotension, peripheral vasculopathy, SUDDEN DEATH. **Derm:** alopecia, urticaria. **EENT:** blurred vision, ↑ intraocular pressure, mydriasis. **Endo:** growth inhibition (with long term use in children). **GI:** anorexia, constipation, cramps, diarrhea, dry mouth, intestinal ischemia, nausea, vomiting. **GU:** libido changes, erectile dysfunction, priapism. **MS:** RHABDOMYOLYSIS. **Neuro:** hyperactivity, insomnia, restlessness, tremor, aggression, anger, behavioral disturbances, dizziness, dysgeusia, hallucinations, headache, irritability, mania, paresthesia, skin picking, talkativeness, thought disorder, tics, Tourette syndrome. **Misc:** HYPERSENSITIVITY REACTIONS (INCLUDING ANAPHYLAXIS AND ANGIOEDEMA), physical dependence, psychological dependence.

Interactions

Drug-Drug: Concurrent use with **MAO inhibitors** or **MAO-inhibitor-like drugs**, such as **linezolid** or **methylene blue**, may result in serious, potentially fatal reactions; wait at least 14 days following discontinuation of MAO inhibitor before initiation of amphetamine mixtures. Drugs that affect serotonergic neurotransmitter systems, including **MAO inhibitors, tricyclic antidepressants, SSRIs, SNRIs, fentanyl, buspirone, tramadol, lithium**, and **triptans**, may ↑ risk of serotonin syndrome. ↑ adrenergic effects with other **adrenergics** or **thyroid preparations. Drugs that alkalinize urine**, including **sodium bicarbonate** or **acetazolamide**, may ↓ excretion and ↑ risk of toxicity. **Drugs that acidify urine**, including large doses of **ascorbic acid**, may ↑ excretion and ↓ effectiveness. ↑ risk of hypertension and bradycardia with **beta blockers.** ↑ risk of arrhythmias with **digoxin. Tricyclic antidepressants** may ↑ risk of arrhythmias, hypertension, or hyperpyrexia. **Proton pump inhibitors** may ↑ risk of toxicity.

Drug-Natural Products: Use with **St. John's wort** may ↑ risk of serotonin syndrome.

Drug-Food: Foods that alkalinize the urine (fruit juices) can ↑ effect of amphetamine.

Route/Dosage

Dose is expressed in total amphetamine content (amphetamine + dextroamphetamine).

Attention-Deficit Hyperactivity Disorder

PO (Adults): *Immediate-release tablets:* 5 mg 1–2 times daily; may ↑ daily dose in 5-mg increments at weekly intervals; usual dose range = 5–40 mg/day in 1–3 divided doses. *Extended-release capsules (Adderall XR):* 20 mg once daily; *Extended-release capsules (Mydayis):* 12.5–25 mg once daily in the morning upon awakening; may ↑ daily dose in 12.5-mg increments at weekly intervals (maximum dose = 50 mg/day).

PO (Children ≥13 yr): *Immediate-release tablets:* 5 mg 1–2 times daily; may ↑ daily dose in 5-mg increments at weekly intervals; usual dose range = 5–40 mg/day in 1–3 divided doses. *Extended-release capsules (Adderall XR):* 10 mg once daily in the morning; may ↑ to 20 mg once daily in the morning after 1 wk; *Extended-release capsules (Mydayis):* 12.5 mg once daily in the morning upon awakening; may ↑ daily dose in 12.5-mg increments at weekly intervals (maximum dose = 25 mg/day).

PO (Children 6–12 yr): *Immediate-release tablets:* 5 mg 1–2 times daily; may ↑ daily dose in 5-mg increments at weekly intervals; usual dose range = 5–40 mg/day in 1–3 divided doses. *Extended-release capsules (Adderall XR):* 5–10 mg once daily in the morning; may ↑ daily dose in 5–10-mg increments at weekly intervals (maximum dose = 30 mg/day).

PO (Children 3–5 yr): *Immediate-release tablets:* 2.5 mg once daily in the morning; may ↑ daily dose in 2.5-mg increments at weekly intervals; usual dose range = 2.5–40 mg/day in 1–3 divided doses.

Renal Impairment

PO (Adults): *GFR 15–29 mL/min/1.73 m²:* Extended-release capsules (Adderall XR): 15 mg once daily in the morning; Extended-release capsules (Mydayis): 12.5 mg once daily in the morning upon awakening; may ↑ daily dose in 12.5-mg increments at weekly intervals (maximum dose = 25 mg/day).

Renal Impairment

(Children ≥13 yr): *GFR 15–29 mL/min/1.73 m²:* Extended-release capsules (Mydayis): 12.5 mg once daily in the morning upon awakening (maximum dose = 12.5 mg/day).

Renal Impairment

(Children ≥6 yr): *GFR 15–29 mL/min/1.73 m²:* Extended-release capsules (Adderall XR): 5 mg once daily in the morning (maximum dose = 20 mg/day in children 6–12 yr).

Narcolepsy

PO (Adults and Children ≥13 yr): *Immediate-release tablets:* 10 mg once daily in the morning; may ↑ daily dose in 10-mg increments at weekly intervals; usual dosage range = 5–60 mg/day in 1–3 divided doses.

PO (Children 6–12 yr): *Immediate-release tablets:* 5 mg once daily; may ↑ daily dose in 5-mg increments at weekly intervals; usual dose range = 5–60 mg/day in 1–3 divided doses.

Availability (generic available)

Amount is expressed in total amphetamine content (amphetamine + dextroamphetamine).

Immediate-release tablets: 5 mg, 7.5 mg, 10 mg, 12.5 mg, 15 mg, 20 mg, 30 mg. **Extended-release capsules (Adderall XR):** 5 mg, 10 mg, 15 mg, 20 mg, 25 mg, 30 mg. **Extended-release capsules (Mydayis):** 12.5 mg, 25 mg, 37.5 mg, 50 mg.

NURSING IMPLICATIONS

Assessment

- Monitor BP, HR, and respiratory rate before and periodically during therapy. Obtain a history (including assessment of family history of sudden death, ventricular arrhythmia, tics, or Tourette syndrome), physical exam to assess for cardiac disease, and further evaluation (ECG and echocardiogram), if indicated. If exertional chest pain, unexplained syncope, or other cardiac symptoms occur, evaluate promptly.
- May produce a false sense of euphoria and well-being. Provide frequent rest periods and observe patient for rebound depression after the effects of the medication have worn off.
- Monitor closely for behavior change during therapy.
- Assess for risk of abuse, misuse, or addiction prior to starting therapy and during therapy. Has high dependence and abuse or misuse potential. Misuse and abuse of CNS stimulants can result in overdose and death; this risk is ↑ with higher doses or

unapproved methods of administration, such as snorting or injection. Tolerance to medication occurs rapidly; do not ↑ dose.

- Assess infants born to mothers taking amphetamines for symptoms of withdrawal (feeding difficulties, irritability, agitation, excessive drowsiness).
- **ADHD:** Monitor weight biweekly and inform health care provider of significant loss. Pedi: Monitor height periodically in children; report growth inhibition. Growth suppression may occur in children with long-term use.
- Assess child's attention span, impulse control, and interactions with others. Therapy may be interrupted at intervals to determine whether symptoms are sufficient to continue therapy.
- **Narcolepsy:** Observe and document frequency of narcoleptic episodes.

Lab Test Considerations

- May interfere with urinary steroid determinations.
- May cause ↑ plasma corticosteroid concentrations; greatest in evening.

Implementation

- ***High Alert:*** Do not confuse Adderall with Adderall XR.
- **PO:** Administer in the morning to prevent insomnia. May be taken without regard to food. Individualize dose to therapeutic needs and response of patient. Use the lowest effective dose.
- Administer short acting doses 4–6 hr apart.
- ***DNC:*** Extended-release capsules may be swallowed whole or opened and sprinkled on applesauce; swallow contents without chewing. Applesauce should be swallowed immediately; do not store. Do not divide contents of capsule; entire contents of capsule should be taken.
- **ADHD:** Pedi: When symptoms are controlled, dose ↓ or interruption of therapy may be possible during summer months or may be given on each of the five school days, with medication-free weekends and holidays.

Patient/Family Teaching

- Instruct patient to take medication once in the early morning as directed. With extended release capsule, avoid afternoon doses to prevent insomnia. Omit missed doses and resume schedule next day. Do not double doses. Discuss safe use, risks, and proper storage and disposal of amphetamines with patients and caregivers with each Rx. Advise patient and parents to read the *Medication Guide* prior to starting therapy and with each Rx refill in case of changes. Instruct patient not to alter dose without consulting health care provider. Abrupt cessation of high doses may cause extreme fatigue and mental depression.
- Advise patient that amphetamine mixtures is a drug with known potential for abuse, misuse, and/or addiction. Store in safe place, protect it from theft, and never give to anyone other than the individual for whom it was prescribed.
- Inform patient that the effects of drug-induced dry mouth can be minimized by rinsing frequently with water or chewing sugarless gum or candies.
- Advise patient to limit intake of foods that alkalinize the urine (fruit juices).
- May impair judgment. Advise patient to use caution when driving or during other activities requiring alertness until response to medication is known.
- Advise patient to notify health care provider of all Rx or OTC medications, vitamins, or herbal products being taken and to consult with health care provider before taking other medications, especially St. John's wort.
- Inform patient that periodic holidays from the drug may be used to assess progress and decrease dependence. Pedi: Children should be given a drug-free holiday each yr to reassess symptoms and treatment. Doses will change as children age due to pharmacokinetic changes such as slower hepatic metabolism. If reduced appetite and weight loss occur, advise parents to provide high-calorie meals when drug levels are low (at breakfast and or bedtime).
- Advise patient and/or parents to notify health care provider of behavioral changes (new or worse behavior and thought problems, bipolar illness, or aggressive behavior or hostility; new psychotic symptoms such as hearing voices, believing things that are not true, suspicion, or new manic symptoms).
- Advise patient to notify health care provider if symptoms of heart problems (chest pain, shortness of breath, fainting), nervousness, restlessness, insomnia, dizziness, anorexia, or dry mouth becomes severe.
- Inform patients of risk of peripheral vasculopathy. Instruct patients to notify health care provider of any new numbness, pain, skin color change from pale to blue to red, or coolness or sensitivity to temperature in fingers or toes, and call if unexplained wounds appear on fingers or toes.
- Rep: May cause fetal harm. Advise women of reproductive potential to notify health care provider if pregnancy is planned or suspected or and to avoid breastfeeding during therapy. May ↑ risk or premature birth and low birth weight. Monitor infants born to mothers taking amphetamines for symptoms of withdrawal (feeding difficulties, irritability, agitation, excessive drowsiness). Encourage patients exposed to amphetamines during pregnancy to join the registry. Health care providers may call the National Pregnancy Registry

for Psychiatric Medications at 1-866-961-2388 or online at https://womensmentalhealth.org/clinical-and-research-programs/pregnancyregistry/othermedications/ to register patients.

- Emphasize the importance of routine follow-up exams to monitor progress.
- **Home Care Issues:** Advise parents to notify school nurse of medication regimen.

Evaluation/Desired Outcomes

- Improved attention span in patients with ADHD.
- Increased motor activity, mental alertness, and decreased fatigue in patients with narcolepsy.

ampicillin (am-pi-**sil**-in)

Classification
Therapeutic: anti-infectives
Pharmacologic: aminopenicillins

Indications

Treatment of the following infections: Skin and skin structure infections, Soft-tissue infections, Otitis media, Sinusitis, Respiratory infections, Genitourinary infections, Meningitis, Septicemia. Endocarditis prophylaxis. **Unlabeled Use:** Prevention of infection in certain high-risk patients undergoing cesarean section.

Action

Inhibits bacterial cell wall synthesis. **Therapeutic Effects:** Bactericidal action; spectrum is broader than penicillin. **Spectrum:** Active against: Streptococci, nonpenicillinase-producing staphylococci, *Listeria*, Pneumococci, Enterococci, *Haemophilus influenzae*, *Escherichia coli*, *Enterobacter*, *Klebsiella*, *Proteus mirabilis*, *Neisseria meningitidis*, *N. gonorrhoeae*, *Shigella*, *Salmonella*.

Pharmacokinetics

Absorption: Moderately absorbed from the duodenum (30–50%).
Distribution: Diffuses readily into body tissues and fluids. CSF penetration is ↑ in the presence of inflamed meninges.
Metabolism and Excretion: Variably metabolized by the liver (12–50%). Renal excretion is variable (25–60% after oral dosing; 50–85% after IM administration).
Half-life: *Neonates:* 1.7–4 hr; *Children and Adults:* 1–1.5 hr (↑ in renal impairment).

TIME/ACTION PROFILE (blood levels)

ROUTE	ONSET	PEAK	DURATION
PO	rapid	1.5–2 hr	4–6 hr
IM	rapid	1 hr	4–6 hr
IV	rapid	end of infusion	4–6 hr

Contraindications/Precautions

Contraindicated in: Hypersensitivity to penicillins (cross sensitivity to cephalosporins and other beta-lactams may exist).
Use Cautiously in: Severe renal impairment (↓ dose if CCr <10 mL/min); Infectious mononucleosis, acute lymphocytic leukemia or cytomegalovirus infection (↑ incidence of rash).

Adverse Reactions/Side Effects

Derm: rash, urticaria. **GI:** diarrhea, CLOSTRIDIOIDES DIFFICILE-ASSOCIATED DIARRHEA (CDAD), nausea, vomiting. **Hemat:** blood dyscrasias. **Neuro:** SEIZURES (HIGH DOSES). **Misc:** HYPERSENSITIVITY REACTIONS (INCLUDING ANAPHYLAXIS AND SERUM SICKNESS), superinfection.

Interactions

Drug-Drug: Probenecid ↑ levels and effects; therapy may be combined for this purpose. Large doses may ↑ risk of bleeding with **warfarin**. ↑ risk of hypersensitivity reactions with **allopurinol** therapy. May ↓ effectiveness of oral **hormonal contraceptives**.

Route/Dosage

Respiratory and Soft-Tissue Infections

PO (Adults and Children ≥20 kg): 250–500 mg every 6 hr.
PO (Children <20 kg): 50–100 mg/kg/day in 3–4 divided doses (not to exceed 2–3 g/day).
IM IV (Adults and Children ≥40 kg): 500 mg–3 g every 6 hr (not to exceed 14 g/day).
IM IV (Children <40 kg): 100–200 mg/kg/day in 3–4 divided doses (not to exceed 12 g/day).

Bacterial Meningitis Caused by *H. influenzae*, *Streptococcus pneumoniae*, Group B streptococcus, or *N. meningitidis*; Septicemia

IM IV (Adults): 500 mg–3 g every 6 hr (not to exceed 14 g/day).
IM IV (Children >1 mo): 200–400 mg/kg/day in 4 divided doses (not to exceed 12 g/day).
IM IV (Neonates ≤7 days): 200 mg/kg/day in 3 divided doses.
IM IV (Neonates >7 days): 300 mg/kg/day in 4 divided doses.

GI/GU Infections other than *N. gonorrhoeae*

PO (Adults and Children >20 kg): 250–500 mg every 6 hr (larger doses for more serious/chronic infections).
PO (Children ≤20 kg): 50–100 mg/kg/day in 4 divided doses.

N. gonorrhoeae

PO (Adults): 3 g as single dose with 1 g probenecid.
IM IV (Adults and Children ≥40 kg): 500 mg every 6 hr.
IM IV (Children <40 kg): 100–200 mg/kg/day in 3–4 divided doses.

Urethritis Caused by *N. gonorrhoeae* in Men

IM IV (Adults and Children ≥40 kg): 500 mg, repeated 8–12 hr later; additional doses may be necessary for more complicated infections (prostatitis, epididymitis).

Prevention of Bacterial Endocarditis

IM IV (Adults): 2 g 30 min before procedure (gentamicin may be added for high-risk patients); additional 1 g may be given 6 hr later for high-risk patients.
IM IV (Children): 50 mg/kg (not to exceed 2 g) 30 min before procedure (gentamicin may be added for high-risk patients); additional 25 mg/kg may be given 6 hr later for high-risk patients.

Renal Impairment

(Adults and Children): *CCr ≤10 mL/min:* ↑ dosing interval to every 12 hr.

Availability (generic available)

Capsules: 500 mg. **Powder for injection:** 250 mg/vial, 500 mg/vial, 1 g/vial, 2 g/vial, 10 g/vial.

NURSING IMPLICATIONS

Assessment

- Assess for signs and symptoms of therapeutic response to treatment based on resolving infection (vital signs; appearance of wound, sputum, urine, and stool; WBC) throughout therapy.
- Obtain a history before initiating therapy to determine previous use and reactions to penicillins, cephalosporins, or other beta-lactam antibiotics. Persons with a negative history of penicillin sensitivity may still have an allergic response.
- Obtain specimens for culture and sensitivity before therapy. 1st dose may be given before receiving results.
- Observe patient for signs and symptoms of anaphylaxis (rash, pruritus, laryngeal edema, wheezing). Discontinue the drug and notify health care provider immediately if these occur. Keep epinephrine, an antihistamine, and resuscitation equipment close by in the event of an anaphylactic reaction.
- Monitor for signs and symptoms of CDAD, including watery diarrhea with mucus, fever, abdominal pain or cramping, anorexia, nausea, and in severe cases, dehydration, colitis, and blood or pus in the stool. May begin up to several weeks following cessation of therapy.
- Assess skin for "ampicillin rash," a nonallergic, dull red, macular or maculopapular, mildly pruritic rash.

Lab Test Considerations

- Monitor CBC with differential for therapeutic response.
- Monitor hepatic and renal function periodically during prolonged therapy. May ↑ AST and ALT.
- May cause transient ↓ estradiol, total conjugated estriol, estriol-glucuronide, or conjugated estrone in pregnant women.
- May cause a false-positive direct Coombs test result.
- May cause a false-positive urinary glucose.

Implementation

- Reserve IM or IV route for moderately severe or severe infections or patients unable to take oral medication. Change to PO as soon as possible.
- **PO:** Administer around the clock on an empty stomach ≥1 hr before or 2 hr after meals with a full glass of water. Capsules may be opened and mixed with water. Reconstituted oral suspensions retain potency for 7 days at room temperature and 14 days if refrigerated. Ampicillin has ↓ absorption in the presence of food, so it is recommended that enteral feedings be interrupted for 1 hr before and 2 hr after administration.
- **IM: Reconstitution:** Add sterile water for injection: 0.9–1.2 mL to the 125-mg vial, 1 mL to the 250-mg vial, 1.8 mL to the 500-mg vial, 3.5 mL to the 1-g vial, and 6.8 mL to the 2-g vial. Should be used within 1 hr of reconstitution.

IV Administration

- **IV Push:** Add sterile water for injection: 5 mL to each 125-, 250-, or 500-mg vial; 7.4 mL to each 1-g vial; or 14.8 mL to each 2-g vial. Should be used within 1 hr of reconstitution. **Rate:** Doses of 125–500 mg may be given over 3–5 min (not to exceed 100 mg/min). Rapid administration may cause seizures.
- **Intermittent Infusion: Dilution:** Reconstitute vials as per the directions above. Further dilute in 50 mL or more of 0.9% NaCl, D5W, D5/0.45% NaCl, or LR. Administer within 4 hr (more stable in NaCl). **Concentration:** Not to exceed 30 mg/mL. **Rate:** Infuse over 10–15 min.
- **Y-Site Compatibility:** acyclovir, alemtuzumab, alprostadil, aminocaproic acid, anidulafungin, argatroban, arsenic, azithromycin, bivalirudin, bleomycin, caffeine citrate, cangrelor, carboplatin, carmustine, cisplatin, cytarabine, dactinomycin, daptomycin, dexmedetomidine, dexrazoxane, dimenhydrinate, docetaxel, doxorubicin liposomal, eptifibatide, etoposide, etoposide phosphate, filgrastim, fludarabine, fluorouracil, foscarnet, fosphenytoin, gemcitabine, gemtuzumab ozogamicin, granisetron, hetastarch, ifosfamide, irinotecan, letermovir, leucovorin, levofloxacin, linezolid, mannitol, melphalan, meropenem, mesna, methadone, methotrexate, metronidazole, milrinone, mitomycin, nafcillin, octreotide, oxaliplatin, paclitaxel, palonosetron, pamidronate, pantoprazole, pemetrexed, perphenazine, potassium acetate, propofol,

remifentanil, rituximab, rocuronium, sodium acetate, thiotepa, tigecycline, tirofiban, trastuzumab, vecuronium, vinblastine, vincristine, vitamin B complex with C, voriconazole, zoledronic acid.

- **Y-Site Incompatibility:** If aminoglycosides and penicillins must be administered concurrently, administer in separate sites ≥1 hr apart acetaminophen, aminophylline, amiodarone, amphotericin B deoxycholate, amphotericin B liposomal, buprenorphine, caspofungin, chlorpromazine, dacarbazine, dantrolene, daunorubicin, diazepam, diazoxide, diphenhydramine, dobutamine, dopamine, doxorubicin hydrochloride, doxycycline, epirubicin, fluconazole, ganciclovir, haloperidol, hydroxyzine, idarubicin, ketamine, lorazepam, midazolam, mitoxantrone, mycophenolate, nicardipine, nitroprusside, ondansetron, papaverine, penicillin G potassium, pentamidine, phenytoin, prochlorperazine, promethazine, protamine, sargramostim, sodium bicarbonate, topotecan, tranexamic acid, trimethoprim/sulfamethoxazole, verapamil, vinorelbine.

Patient/Family Teaching

- Explain the purpose and side effects of ampicillin to patient. Do not stop receiving drug without consulting health care provider. If an appointment is missed, contact health care provider as soon as possible to reschedule. Advise patient to read *Medication Guide* before starting and periodically during therapy in case of changes.
- Instruct patient to take medication around the clock and to finish the drug completely as directed, even if feeling better. Advise patients that sharing of this medication can be dangerous.
- Explain need for continued medical follow-up to monitor progress and assess effectiveness and possible side effects of medication. Instruct patient to notify health care provider if symptoms do not improve.
- Advise patient to report the signs of superinfection (furry overgrowth on the tongue, vaginal itching or discharge, loose or foul-smelling stools) and allergy.
- Caution patient to notify health care provider if fever and diarrhea occur, especially if stool contains blood, pus, or mucus. Advise patient not to treat diarrhea without consulting health care provider. May occur up to several weeks after discontinuation of medication.
- Patients with a history of rheumatic heart disease or valve replacement need to be taught the importance of using antimicrobial prophylaxis before invasive medical or dental procedures.
- Advise patient to notify health care provider of all Rx or OTC medications, vitamins, or herbal products being taken and to consult with health care provider before taking other medications.
- Rep: Advise women of reproductive potential to notify health care provider if pregnancy is planned or suspected or if breastfeeding. Advise patients taking oral contraceptives to use an alternate or additional nonhormonal method of contraception while taking ampicillin and until next menstrual period.

Evaluation/Desired Outcomes

- Resolution of the signs and symptoms of infection. Length of time for complete resolution depends on the organism and site of infection.
- Endocarditis prophylaxis.

ampicillin/sulbactam

(am-pi-**sil**-in/sul-**bak**-tam)

Unasyn

Classification

Therapeutic: anti-infectives

Pharmacologic: aminopenicillins/beta-lactamase inhibitors

Indications

Treatment of the following infections: Skin and skin structure infections, Soft-tissue infections, Otitis media, Intra-abdominal infections, Sinusitis, Respiratory infections, Genitourinary infections, Meningitis, Septicemia.

Action

Inhibits bacterial cell wall synthesis; spectrum is broader than that of penicillin. Addition of sulbactam increases resistance to beta-lactamases, enzymes produced by bacteria that may inactivate ampicillin. **Therapeutic Effects:** Bactericidal action. **Spectrum:** Active against: Streptococci, Pneumococci, Enterococci, *Haemophilus influenzae*, *Escherichia coli*, *Proteus mirabilis*, *Neisseria meningitidis*, *Neisseria gonorrhoeae*, *Shigella*, *Salmonella*, *Bacteroides fragilis*, *Moraxella catarrhalis*. Use should be reserved for infections caused by beta-lactamase–producing strains.

Pharmacokinetics

Absorption: Well absorbed from IM sites.

Distribution: Ampicillin diffuses readily into bile, blister, and tissue fluids. Poor CSF penetration unless meninges are inflamed.

Metabolism and Excretion: Ampicillin is variably metabolized by the liver (12–50%). Renal excretion is also variable. Sulbactam is eliminated unchanged in urine.

Protein Binding: *Ampicillin:* 28%; *sulbactam:* 38%. **Half-life:** *Ampicillin:* 1–1.8 hr; *sulbactam:* 1–1.3 hr.

TIME/ACTION PROFILE (plasma concentrations)

ROUTE	ONSET	PEAK	DURATION
IM	rapid	1 hr	6–8 hr
IV	immediate	end of infusion	6–8 hr

Contraindications/Precautions

Contraindicated in: Hypersensitivity to penicillins or sulbactam; History of cholestatic jaundice or hepatic impairment with ampicillin/sulbactam.

Use Cautiously in: Severe renal impairment; Epstein-Barr virus infection, acute lymphocytic leukemia, or cytomegalovirus infection (↑ risk of rash); OB: Safety not established in pregnancy; Lactation: Use while breastfeeding only if potential maternal benefit justifies potential risk to infant.

Adverse Reactions/Side Effects

Derm: rash, ACUTE GENERALIZED EXANTHEMATOUS PUSTULOSIS (AGEP), DRUG REACTION WITH EOSINOPHILIA AND SYSTEMIC SYMPTOMS (DRESS), ERYTHEMA MULTIFORME (EM), STEVENS-JOHNSON SYNDROME (SJS), TOXIC EPIDERMAL NECROLYSIS (TEN), urticaria. **GI:** diarrhea, cholestasis, CLOSTRIDIOIDES DIFFICILE-ASSOCIATED DIARRHEA (CDAD), HEPATOTOXICITY, nausea, vomiting. **Hemat:** blood dyscrasias. **Local:** pain at injection site, phlebitis. **Neuro:** SEIZURES (HIGH DOSES). **Misc:** HYPERSENSITIVITY REACTIONS (INCLUDING ANAPHYLAXIS AND MYOCARDIAL ISCHEMIA [WITH OR WITHOUT MI]), superinfection.

Interactions

Drug-Drug: **Probenecid** ↓ renal excretion and ↑ levels; therapy may be combined for this purpose. May ↑ risk of bleeding of **warfarin**. **Allopurinol** may ↑ risk of rash. May ↓ levels and effectiveness of **hormonal contraceptives**.

Route/Dosage

Dosage based on ampicillin component. Contains 5 mEq (115 mg) sodium/1.5 g of ampicillin/sulbactam.

IM IV (Adults and Children ≥40 kg): 1–2 g ampicillin every 6–8 hr (not to exceed 12 g ampicillin/day).

IM IV (Children ≥1 yr): 100–200 mg ampicillin/kg/day divided every 6 hr; *Meningitis:* 200–400 mg ampicillin/kg/day divided every 6 hr; maximum dose: 8 g ampicillin/day.

IM IV (Infants >1 mo): 100–150 mg ampicillin/kg/day divided every 6 hr.

Renal Impairment

IM IV (Adults, Children, and Infants): *CCr 15–29 mL/min:* Administer every 12 hr; *CCr 5–14:* Administer every 24 hr.

Availability (generic available)

Powder for injection: 1.5 g/vial (1 g ampicillin with 500 mg sulbactam), 3 g/vial (2 g ampicillin with 1 g sulbactam), 15 g/vial (10 g ampicillin with 5 g sulbactam).

NURSING IMPLICATIONS

Assessment

- Assess patient for infection (vital signs, wound appearance, sputum, urine, stool, WBCs) at beginning and throughout therapy.
- Obtain a history before initiating therapy to determine previous use of and reactions to penicillins or cephalosporins. Persons with a negative history of penicillin sensitivity may still have an allergic response.
- Obtain specimens for culture and sensitivity before therapy. First dose may be given before receiving results.
- Monitor for signs and symptoms of hypersensitivity reactions (rash, urticaria, pruritus, flushing, dizziness, vomiting, abdominal pain) and angioedema (swelling of throat, lips, tongue, or face; dyspnea; wheezing; hoarseness). Discontinue drug immediately and provide supportive care. Keep epinephrine, an antihistamine, and resuscitation equipment close by in the event of an anaphylactic reaction.
- Monitor patients for development of severe cutaneous adverse reactions, including AGEP, DRESS, EM, SJS, and TEN. Advise patients of signs and symptoms of these reactions (prodrome of fever, flu-like symptoms, muscle or joint aches, mucosal lesions, progressive skin rash, blisters, lymphadenopathy, conjunctivitis). *If a severe cutaneous adverse reaction is suspected,* interrupt therapy until etiology of reaction is determined. Consultation with a dermatologist is recommended. *If a severe cutaneous adverse reaction is confirmed, or for other Grade 4 skin reactions,* permanently discontinue ampicillin/sulbactam.
- Monitor bowel function. Diarrhea, abdominal cramping, fever, and bloody stools should be reported to health care professional promptly as a sign of CDAD. May begin up to several mo following cessation of therapy

Lab Test Considerations

- Monitor hepatic and renal function periodically during therapy. May ↑ AST, ALT, LDH, bilirubin, alkaline phosphatase, BUN, and serum creatinine.
- May ↓ hemoglobin, hematocrit, RBC, WBC, neutrophils, and lymphocytes.
- May cause transient ↓ estradiol, total conjugated estriol, estriol-glucuronide, or conjugated estrone in pregnant women.
- May cause a false-positive Coombs test result.

Implementation

- **IM** Reconstitute for IM use by adding 3.2 mL of sterile water or 0.5% or 2% lidocaine to the 1.5-g vial or 6.4 mL to the 3-g vial. Administer within 1 hr of preparation, deep IM into well-developed muscle.

IV Administration

- **IV Push: Reconstitution:** Reconstitute 1.5-g vial with 3.2 mL of sterile water for injection and the 3-g vial with 6.4 mL. **Concentration:** 375 mg ampicillin/sulbactam per mL. **Rate:** Administer over at least 10–15 min within 1 hr of reconstitution. More rapid administration may cause seizures.

- **Intermittent Infusion: Reconstitution:** Reconstitute vials as per directions for IV push above. **Dilution:** Further dilute in 50–100 mL of 0.9% NaCl, D5W, D5/0.45% NaCl, or LR. Stability of solution varies from 2–8 hr at room temperature or 3–72 hr if refrigerated, depending on concentration and diluent. **Concentration:** 3–45 mg of ampicillin/sulbactam per mL. **Rate:** Infuse over 15–30 min.
- **Y-Site Compatibility:** alemtuzumab, aminocaproic acid, anidulafungin, argatroban, azithromycin, bivalirudin, bleomycin, cangrelor, carboplatin, carmustine, cefepime, ceftolozane/tazobactam, cisplatin, cyclophosphamide, cytarabine, dactinomycin, daptomycin, dexmedetomidine, dexrazoxane, docetaxel, doxorubicin liposomal, eptifibatide, etoposide, etoposide phosphate, filgrastim, fludarabine, fluorouracil, foscarnet, fosphenytoin, gemcitabine, gemtuzumab, granisetron, hydromorphone, ifosfamide, irinotecan, letermovir, leucovorin, levofloxacin, linezolid, meropenem/vaborbactam, mesna, methadone, methotrexate, metronidazole, milrinone, mitomycin, octreotide, oxaliplatin, paclitaxel, palonosetron, pamidronate, pantoprazole, pemetrexed, plazomicin, potassium acetate, remifentanil, rituximab, rocuronium, sodium acetate, tedizolid, telavancin, thiotepa, tigecycline, tirofiban, trastuzumab, vecuronium, vinblastine, vincristine, voriconazole, zoledronic acid.
- **Y-Site Incompatibility:** acyclovir, amiodarone, amphotericin B deoxycholate, amphotericin B liposomal, azathioprine, caspofungin, chlorpromazine, ciprofloxacin, dacarbazine, dantrolene, daunorubicin, diazepam, diazoxide, dobutamine, doxorubicin hydrochloride, doxycycline, epirubicin, ganciclovir, haloperidol, hydralazine, hydrocortisone, hydroxyzine, idarubicin, isavuconazonium, lorazepam, methylprednisolone, midazolam, mitoxantrone, mycophenolate, nicardipine, ondansetron, papaverine, pentamidine, phenytoin, prochlorperazine, promethazine, protamine, sargramostim, topotecan, tranexamic acid, trimethoprim/sulfamethoxazole, verapamil, vinorelbine, If aminoglycosides and penicillins must be given concurrently, administer in separate sites at least 1 hr apart.

Patient/Family Teaching

- Educate patient on reason and side effects of ampicillin/sulbactam. Instruct patients to take medication around the clock and to finish the drug completely as directed, even if feeling better. Advise patients that sharing of this medication may be dangerous. Advise patient to read *Patient Information* before starting therapy.
- Instruct the patient to notify health care professional if symptoms do not improve.
- Advise patient to report rash, signs of superinfection (furry overgrowth on the tongue, vaginal itching or discharge, loose or foul-smelling stools) and allergy.
- Instruct patient to notify health care professional if any rash (particularly with fever, flu-like symptoms, swollen lymph nodes) develops within the 1–2 wk of therapy.
- Caution patient to notify health care professional if fever and diarrhea occur, especially if stool contains blood, pus, or mucus. Advise patient not to treat diarrhea without consulting health care professional. May occur up to several wk after discontinuation of medication.
- Rep: Instruct women of reproductive potential taking oral contraceptives to use an alternate or additional method of contraception during therapy and until next menstrual period; may ↓ effectiveness of hormonal contraceptives. Advise patient to notify health care professional if pregnancy is planned or suspected or if breastfeeding.

Evaluation/Desired Outcomes

- Resolution of signs and symptoms of infection. Length of time for complete resolution depends on the organism and site of infection.

HIGH ALERT

anastrozole (a-nass-troe-zole)

Arimidex

Classification

Therapeutic: antineoplastics

Pharmacologic: aromatase inhibitors

Indications

Adjuvant treatment of postmenopausal hormone receptor-positive early breast cancer. Initial therapy in women with postmenopausal hormone receptor-positive or hormone receptor unknown, locally advanced, or metastatic breast cancer. Advanced postmenopausal breast cancer in women with disease progression despite tamoxifen therapy.

Action

Inhibits the enzyme aromatase, which is partially responsible for conversion of precursors to estrogen. **Therapeutic Effects:** Lowers levels of circulating estrogen, which may halt progression of estrogen-sensitive breast cancer.

Pharmacokinetics

Absorption: 83–85% absorbed following oral administration.
Distribution: Unknown.
Metabolism and Excretion: 85% metabolized by the liver; 11% excreted renally.
Half-life: 50 hr.

A

TIME/ACTION PROFILE (lowering of serum estradiol)

ROUTE	ONSET	PEAK	DURATION
PO	within 24 hr	14 days	6 days†

† Following cessation of therapy.

Contraindications/Precautions

Contraindicated in: OB: Pregnancy; Lactation: Lactation.

Use Cautiously in: Ischemic heart disease; Rep: Women of reproductive potential; Pedi: Safety and effectiveness not established in children.

Adverse Reactions/Side Effects

CV: angina, MI, peripheral edema. **Derm:** hot flashes, rash, sweating. **EENT:** pharyngitis. **F and E:** hypercalcemia. **GI:** nausea, abdominal pain, anorexia, constipation, diarrhea, dry mouth, vomiting. **GU:** ↓ fertility (women), pelvic pain, vaginal bleeding, vaginal dryness. **Metab:** hypercholesterolemia, weight gain. **MS:** back pain, arthritis, bone pain, carpal tunnel syndrome, fracture, myalgia. **Neuro:** headache, weakness, dizziness, paresthesia. **Resp:** cough, dyspnea. **Misc:** pain, HYPERSENSITIVITY REACTIONS (INCLUDING ANAPHYLAXIS AND ANGIOEDEMA).

Interactions

Drug-Drug: None reported.

Route/Dosage

PO (Adults): 1 mg once daily.

Availability (generic available)

Tablets: 1 mg.

NURSING IMPLICATIONS

Assessment

- Assess for pain (muscle, joint, bone, pelvic, chest, neck, head) periodically during therapy.

Lab Test Considerations

- Verify negative pregnancy test before starting therapy.
- May cause ↑ GGT, AST, ALT, alkaline phosphatase, total cholesterol, and LDL-C levels.
- Monitor bone mineral density at baseline and periodically during therapy.

Implementation

- **PO:** Take medication consistently with regard to food.

Patient/Family Teaching

- Instruct patient to take medication as directed. Take missed doses as soon as remembered unless it is almost time for next dose. Do not double doses. Advise patient to read *Patient Information* before starting and with each Rx refill; changes may occur.
- Inform patient of potential for adverse reactions and to notify health care professional immediately if allergic reactions (swelling of the face, lips, tongue, or throat; difficulty in swallowing and/or breathing), liver problems (general feeling of not being well, yellowing of skin or whites of eyes, pain on the right side of abdomen), skin reactions (lesions, ulcers, blisters), or chest pain occurs.
- Advise patient that vaginal bleeding may occur during first few wk after changing over from other hormonal therapy. Continued bleeding should be evaluated.
- Advise patient to report ↑ pain so treatment can be initiated.
- Rep: May cause fetal harm. Advise women of reproductive potential to use effective contraception during and for ≥3 wk after last dose of therapy and to avoid breastfeeding for ≥2 wk after last dose. Advise patient to notify health care professional immediately if pregnancy is planned or suspected. May impair female fertility.

Evaluation/Desired Outcomes

- Slowing of disease progression in women with advanced breast cancer.

ANGIOTENSIN-CONVERTING ENZYME (ACE) INHIBITORS

benazepril (ben-**aye**-ze-pril)
Lotensin

captopril (**kap**-toe-pril)
~~Capoten~~

enalapril/enalaprilat
(e-**nal**-a-pril/e-**nal**-a-pril-at)
Epaned, Vasotec, ✱ Vasotec IV

fosinopril (foe-**sin**-oh-pril)
~~Monopril~~

lisinopril (lyse-**in**-oh-pril)
~~Prinivil~~, Qbrelis, Zestril

moexipril (moe-**eks**-i-pril)
~~Univase~~

perindopril (pe-**rin**-do-pril)
~~Aceon,~~ ✱ Coversyl

quinapril (**kwin**-a-pril)
Accupril

ramipril (ra-**mi**-pril)
Altace

trandolapril (tran-**doe**-la-pril)
✱ Mavik

Classification
Therapeutic: antihypertensives
Pharmacologic: ACE inhibitors

Indications

Hypertension (as monotherapy or in combination with other antihypertensives). **Captopril, enalapril, fosinopril, lisinopril, quinapril, ramipril, trandolapril:** HF. **Captopril, lisinopril, ramipril, trandolapril:** Reduction of risk of death or development of HF following MI. **Enalapril:** Slowed progression of left ventricular dysfunction into overt HF. **Ramipril:** Reduction of the risk of MI, stroke, and death from cardiovascular disease in patients at risk (>55 yr old with a history of CAD, stroke, peripheral vascular disease, or diabetes with another cardiovascular risk factor). **Captopril:** ↓ progression of diabetic nephropathy. **Perindopril:** Reduction of risk of death from cardiovascular causes or nonfatal MI in patients with stable CAD.

Action

ACE inhibitors block the conversion of angiotensin I to the vasoconstrictor angiotensin II. ACE inhibitors also prevent the degradation of bradykinin and other vasodilatory prostaglandins. ACE inhibitors also ↑ plasma renin levels and ↓ aldosterone levels. Net result is systemic vasodilation. **Therapeutic Effects:** Lowering of BP in hypertensive patients. Improved symptoms in patients with HF (selected agents only). ↓ development of overt heart failure (enalapril only). Improved survival and ↓ development of overt HF after MI (selected agents only). ↓ risk of death from cardiovascular causes or MI in patients with stable CAD (perindopril only). ↓ risk of MI, stroke, or death from cardiovascular causes in high-risk patients (ramipril only). ↓ progression of diabetic nephropathy (captopril only).

Pharmacokinetics

Absorption: *Benazepril:* 37% absorbed after oral administration. *Captopril:* 60–75% absorbed after oral administration (↓ by food). *Enalapril:* 55–75% absorbed after oral administration. *Enalaprilat:* IV administration results in complete bioavailability. *Fosinopril:* 36% absorbed after oral administration. *Lisinopril:* 25% absorbed after oral administration (much variability). *Moexipril:* 13% bioavailability as moexiprilat after oral administration (↓ by food). *Perindopril:* 25% bioavailability as perindoprilat after oral administration. *Quinapril:* 60% absorbed after oral administration (high-fat meal may ↓ absorption). *Ramipril:* 50–60% absorbed after oral administration. *Trandolapril:* 70% bioavailability as trandolapril at after oral administration.

Distribution: All well distributed to tissues

Protein Binding: *Benazepril:* 95%, *Fosinopril:* 99.4%, *Moexipril:* 90%, *Quinapril:* 97%.

Metabolism and Excretion: *Benazepril:* Converted by the liver to benazeprilat, the active metabolite. 20% excreted by kidneys; 11–12% nonrenal (biliary elimination). *Captopril:* 50% metabolized by the liver to inactive compounds, 50% excreted unchanged by the kidneys. *Enalapril, enalaprilat:* Enalapril is converted by the liver to enalaprilat, the active metabolite; primarily eliminated by the kidneys. *Fosinopril:* Converted by the liver and GI mucosa to fosinoprilat, the active metabolite; 50% excreted in urine; 50% in feces. *Lisinopril:* 100% eliminated by the kidneys. *Moexipril:* Converted by liver and GI mucosa to moexiprilat, the active metabolite; 13% excreted in urine, 53% in feces. *Perindopril:* Converted by the liver to perindoprilat, the active metabolite; primarily excreted in urine. *Quinapril:* Converted by the liver, GI mucosa, and tissue to quinaprilat, the active metabolite: 96% eliminated by the kidneys. *Ramipril:* Converted by the liver to ramiprilat, the active metabolite; 60% excreted in urine, 40% in feces. *Trandolapril:* Converted by the liver to trandolaprilat, the active metabolite; 33% excreted in urine, 66% in feces.

Half-life: *Benazeprilat:* 10–11 hr. *Captopril:* 2 hr (↑ in renal impairment). *Enalapril:* 2 hr (↑ in renal impairment). *Enalaprilat:* 35–38 hr (↑ in renal impairment). *Fosinoprilat:* 12 hr. *Lisinopril:* 12 hr (↑ in renal impairment). *Moexiprilat:* 2–9 hr (↑ in renal impairment). *Perindoprilat:* 3–10 hr (↑ in renal impairment). *Quinaprilat:* 3 hr (↑ in renal impairment). *Ramiprilat:* 13–17 hr (↑ in renal impairment). *Trandolaprilat:* 22.5 hr (↑ in renal impairment).

TIME/ACTION PROFILE (effect on BP: single dose†)

ROUTE	ONSET	PEAK	DURATION
Benazepril	within 1 hr	2–4 hr	24 hr
Captopril	15–60 min	60–90 min	6–12 hr
Enalapril PO	1 hr	4–8 hr	12–24 hr
Enalapril IV	15 min	1–4 hr	4–6 hr
Fosinopril	within 1 hr	2–6 hr	24 hr
Lisinopril	1 hr	6 hr	24 hr
Moexipril	within 1 hr	3–6 hr	up to 24 hr
Perindoprilat	within 1–2 hr	3–7 hr	up to 24 hr
Quinapril	within 1 hr	2–4 hr	up to 24 hr
Ramipril	within 1–2 hr	3–6 hr	24 hr
Trandolapril	within 1–2 hr	4–10 hr	up to 24 hr

† Full effects may not be noted for several weeks.

Contraindications/Precautions

Contraindicated in: Hypersensitivity; History of angioedema with previous use of ACE inhibitors (also in absence of previous use of ACE inhibitors for benazepril); Concurrent use with aliskiren in patients with diabetes or moderate to severe renal impairment (CCr <60 mL/min); Concurrent use with sacubitril/valsartan; must be a 36-hr washout period after switching to/from sacubitril/valsartan; OB: Pregnancy; Lactation: Lactation.

Use Cautiously in: Renal impairment, hepatic impairment, hypovolemia, hyponatremia, or concurrent diuretic therapy; Black patients with hypertension (monotherapy less effective; may require additional therapy; ↑ risk of angioedema); Surgery/

anesthesia (hypotension may be exaggerated); Rep: Women of reproductive potential; Pedi: Safety and effectiveness not established in children <18 yr (moexipril, perindopril, quinapril ramipril, trandolapril) or <6 yr (benazepril, fosinopril, lisinopril); Geri: Initial dose ↓ recommended for most agents in older adults due to age-related ↓ in renal function.
Exercise Extreme Caution in: Family history of angioedema.

Adverse Reactions/Side Effects

CV: hypotension, chest pain, edema, tachycardia. **Derm:** flushing, pruritus, rashes. **F and E:** hyperkalemia. **GI:** abdominal pain, anorexia, constipation, diarrhea, nausea, vomiting. **GU:** erectile dysfunction, proteinuria, renal impairment. **Hemat:** AGRANULOCYTOSIS, neutropenia (captopril only). **Metab:** hyperuricemia. **MS:** back pain, muscle cramps, myalgia. **Neuro:** dysgeusia, dizziness, drowsiness, fatigue, headache, insomnia, vertigo, weakness. **Resp:** cough, dyspnea. **Misc:** ANGIOEDEMA, fever.

Interactions

Drug-Drug: Sacubitril ↑ risk of angioedema; concurrent use contraindicated; do not administer within 36 hr of switching to/from **sacubitril/valsartan**. Excessive hypotension may occur with **diuretics** and other **antihypertensives**. ↑ risk of hyperkalemia with **potassium supplements**, **potassium-sparing diuretics**, or **potassium-containing salt substitutes**. ↑ risk of hyperkalemia, renal dysfunction, hypotension, and syncope with **angiotensin II receptor blockers** or **aliskiren**; avoid concurrent use with aliskiren in patients with diabetes or CCr <60 mL/min; avoid concurrent use with angiotensin II receptor blockers. **NSAIDs** and selective **COX-2 inhibitors** may blunt the antihypertensive effect and ↑ risk of renal impairment. Absorption of fosinopril may be ↓ by **antacids** (separate administration by 1–2 hr). May ↑ levels and risk of toxicity of **lithium**. Quinapril may ↓ absorption of **tetracycline**, **doxycycline**, and **fluoroquinolones** (because of magnesium in tablets). ↑ risk of angioedema with **temsirolimus**, **sirolimus**, or **everolimus**.
Drug-Food: Food significantly ↓ absorption of captopril and moexipril; administer drugs 1 hr before meals.

Route/Dosage

Benazepril

PO (Adults): 10 mg once daily; ↑ gradually to maintenance dose of 20–40 mg/day in 1–2 divided doses (begin with 5 mg/day in patients receiving diuretics).
PO (Children ≥6 yr): 0.2 mg/kg once daily; may titrate up to 0.6 mg/kg/day (or 40 mg/day).

Renal Impairment

PO (Adults): *CCr <30 mL/min:* Initiate therapy with 5 mg once daily.

Renal Impairment

PO (Children ≥6 yr): *CCr <30 mL/min:* Contraindicated.

Captopril

PO (Adults): *Hypertension:* 12.5–25 mg 2–3 times daily; may ↑ at 1–2 wk intervals up to 150 mg 3 times daily (begin with 6.25–12.5 mg 2–3 times daily in patients receiving diuretics) (maximum dose = 450 mg/day); *HF:* 25 mg 3 times daily (6.25–12.5 mg 3 times daily in patients who have been vigorously diuresed); titrate up to target dose of 50 mg 3 times daily; *Post-MI:* 6.25-mg test dose, followed by 12.5 mg 3 times daily; may ↑ up to 50 mg 3 times daily; *Diabetic nephropathy:* 25 mg 3 times daily.
PO (Children): *HF:* 0.3–0.5 mg/kg/dose 3 times daily; titrate up to a maximum of 6 mg/kg/day in 2–4 divided doses; *Older Children:* 6.25–12.5 mg/dose every 12–24 hr; titrate up to a maximum of 6 mg/kg/day in 2–4 divided doses.
PO (Infants): *HF:* 0.15–0.3 mg/kg/dose; titrate up to a maximum of 6 mg/kg/day in 1–4 divided doses.
PO (Neonates): *HF:* 0.05–0.1 mg/kg/dose every 8–24 hr; may ↑ as needed up to 0.5 mg/kg every 6–24 hr; *Premature neonates:* 0.01 mg/kg/dose every 8–12 hr.

Renal Impairment

PO (Adults): *CCr 10–50 mL/min:* Administer 75% of dose; *CCr <10 mL/min:* Administer 50% of dose.

Enalapril/Enalaprilat

PO (Adults): *Hypertension:* 2.5–5 mg once daily; ↑ as required up to 40 mg/day in 1–2 divided doses (initiate therapy at 2.5 mg once daily in patients receiving diuretics); *HF:* 2.5 mg 1–2 times daily; titrate up to target dose of 10 mg twice daily; begin with 2.5 mg once daily in patients with hyponatremia (serum sodium <130 mEq/L); *Asymptomatic left ventricular dysfunction:* 2.5 mg twice daily; titrate up to a target dose of 10 mg twice daily.
PO (Children >1 mo): *Hypertension:* 0.08 mg/kg once daily; may slowly titrate up to a maximum of 0.58 mg/kg/day.
IV (Adults): *Hypertension:* 0.625–1.25 mg (0.625 mg if receiving diuretics) every 6 hr; can titrate up to 5 mg every 6 hr.
IV (Children >1 mo): *Hypertension:* 5–10 mcg/kg/dose given every 8–24 hr.

Renal Impairment

PO IV (Adults): *Hypertension CCr 10–50 mL/min:* Administer 75% of dose; *CCr <10 mL/min:* Administer 50% of dose.

Renal Impairment

PO IV (Children >1 mo): *CCr <30 mL/min:* Contraindicated.

Fosinopril

PO (Adults): *Hypertension:* 10 mg once daily; may ↑ as required up to 80 mg/day. *HF:* 10 mg once daily (5 mg once daily in patients who have been vigorously diuresed); may ↑ over several weeks up to 40 mg/day.
PO (Children ≥6 yr and >50 kg): *Hypertension:* 5–10 mg once daily.

Lisinopril

PO (Adults): *Hypertension:* 10 mg once daily; can ↑ up to 20–40 mg/day (initiate therapy at 5 mg/day in patients receiving diuretics); *HF:* 5 mg once daily; may titrate every 2 wk up to 40 mg/day; begin with 2.5 mg once daily in patients with hyponatremia (serum sodium <130 mEq/L); *Post-MI:* 5 mg once daily for 2 days, then 10 mg daily.
PO (Children ≥6 yr): *Hypertension:* 0.07 mg/kg once daily (up to 5 mg/day); may titrate every 1–2 wk up to 0.6 mg/kg/day (or 40 mg/day).

Renal Impairment

PO (Adults): *CCr 10–30 mL/min:* Begin with 5 mg once daily; may slowly titrate up to 40 mg/day; *CCr <10 mL/min:* Begin with 2.5 mg once daily; may slowly titrate up to 40 mg/day.

Renal Impairment

(Children ≥6 yr): *CCr <30 mL/min:* Contraindicated.

Moexipril

PO (Adults): 7.5 mg once daily; may ↑ up to 30 mg/day in 1–2 divided doses (begin with 3.75 mg/day in patients receiving diuretics).

Renal Impairment

PO (Adults): *CCr ≤40 mL/min:* Initiate therapy at 3.75 mg once daily; may titrated upward carefully to 15 mg/day.

Perindopril

PO (Adults): *Hypertension:* 4 mg once daily; may slowly titrate up to 16 mg/day in 1–2 divided doses (should not exceed 8 mg/day in older adults) (begin with 2–4 mg/day in 1–2 divided doses in patients receiving diuretics); *Stable CAD:* 4 mg once daily for 2 wk; may ↑, if tolerated, to 8 mg once daily; for older adults, begin with 2 mg once daily for 1 wk (may ↑, if tolerated, to 4 mg once daily for 1 wk; then ↑ as tolerated to 8 mg once daily).

Renal Impairment

PO (Adults): *CCr 30–60 mL/min:* 2 mg/day initially; may slowly titrate up to 8 mg/day in 1–2 divided doses.

Quinapril

PO (Adults): *Hypertension:* 10–20 mg once daily initially; may titrated every 2 wk up to 80 mg/day in 1–2 divided doses (initiate therapy at 5 mg/day in patients receiving diuretics); *HF:* 5 mg twice daily initially; may titrate at weekly intervals up to 20 mg twice daily.

Renal Impairment

PO (Adults): *CCr >60 mL/min:* Initiate therapy at 10 mg/day; *CCr 30–60 mL/min:* Initiate therapy at 5 mg/day; *CCr 10–30 mL/min:* Initiate therapy at 2.5 mg/day.

Ramipril

PO (Adults): *Hypertension:* 2.5 mg once daily; may ↑ slowly up to 20 mg/day in 1–2 divided doses (initiate therapy at 1.25 mg/day in patients receiving diuretics). *HF post-MI:* 1.25–2.5 mg twice daily initially; may ↑ slowly up to 5 mg twice daily. *Reduction in risk of MI, stroke, and death from cardiovascular causes:* 2.5 mg once daily for 1 wk, then 5 mg once daily for 3 wk; then ↑ as tolerated to 10 mg once daily (can also be given in 2 divided doses).

Renal Impairment

PO (Adults): *CCr <40 mL/min:* Initiate therapy at 1.25 mg once daily; may slowly titrate up to 5 mg/day in 1–2 divided doses.

Trandolapril

PO (Adults): *Hypertension:* 1 mg once daily (2 mg once daily in Black patients); *HF post-MI:* Initiate therapy at 1 mg once daily; titrate up to 4 mg once daily if possible.

Renal Impairment

PO (Adults): *CCr <30 mL/min:* Initiate therapy at 0.5 mg once daily; may slowly titrate upward (maximum dose = 4 mg/day).

Hepatic Impairment

PO (Adults): Initiate therapy at 0.5 mg once daily; may slowly titrated upward (maximum dose = 4 mg/day).

Availability

Benazepril (generic available)

Tablets: 5 mg, 10 mg, 20 mg, 40 mg. ***In combination with:*** amlodipine (Lotrel) and hydrochlorothiazide (Lotensin HCT). See Appendix N.

Captopril (generic available)

Tablets: 12.5 mg, 25 mg, 50 mg, 100 mg. ***In combination with:*** hydrochlorothiazide.

Enalapril (generic available)

Tablets: 2.5 mg, 5 mg, 10 mg, 20 mg. **Oral solution (mixed berry flavor):** 1 mg/mL. ***In combination with:*** hydrochlorothiazide (Vaseretic). See Appendix N.

Enalaprilat (generic available)

Solution for injection: 1.25 mg/mL.

Fosinopril (generic available)

Tablets: 10 mg, 20 mg, 40 mg. ***In combination with:*** hydrochlorothiazide.

Lisinopril (generic available)

Tablets: 2.5 mg, 5 mg, 10 mg, 20 mg, 30 mg, 40 mg. **Oral solution:** 1 mg/mL. ***In combination with:*** hydrochlorothiazide (Zestoretic). See Appendix N.

Moexipril (generic available)

Tablets: 7.5 mg, 15 mg.

Perindopril (generic available)

Tablets: 2 mg, 4 mg, 8 mg.

Quinapril (generic available)

Tablets: 5 mg, 10 mg, 20 mg, 40 mg. ***In combination with:*** hydrochlorothiazide.

Ramipril (generic available)

Capsules: 1.25 mg, 2.5 mg, 5 mg, 10 mg ✱ 15 mg.

Trandolapril (generic available)

Tablets: ✱ 0.5 mg, 1 mg, 2 mg, 4 mg. ***In combination with:*** verapamil.

NURSING IMPLICATIONS

Assessment

- **Hypertension:** Monitor BP and HR frequently during initial dose adjustment and periodically during therapy. Notify health care provider of significant changes.
- Monitor frequency of prescription refills to determine adherence.
- Assess for signs of angioedema (swelling of face, extremities, eyes, lips, or tongue; difficulty in swallowing or breathing); may occur at any time during therapy. Discontinue medication and provide supportive care. **HF:** Monitor weight and assess patient routinely for resolution of fluid overload (peripheral edema, rales/crackles, dyspnea, weight gain, jugular venous distention).

Lab Test Considerations

- Monitor BUN, serum creatinine, and electrolytes periodically. May ↑ serum potassium, BUN and creatinine. May ↓ sodium. If ↑ BUN or serum creatinine concentrations occur, dose ↓ or withdrawal may be required.
- Monitor CBC periodically during therapy. Certain drugs may rarely cause slight ↓ in hemoglobin and hematocrit, leukopenia, and eosinophilia.
- May ↑ AST, ALT, alkaline phosphatase, serum bilirubin, uric acid, and glucose.
- Assess urine protein before and periodically during therapy for up to 1 yr in patients with renal impairment or those receiving >150 mg/day of captopril. If excessive or ↑ proteinuria occurs, re-evaluate ACE inhibitor therapy.
- *Captopril:* May cause positive ANA titer.
- *Captopril:* May cause false-positive test results for urine acetone.
- *Captopril:* Monitor CBC with differential before initiation of therapy, every 2 wk for 1st 3 mo, and periodically for up to 1 yr in patients at risk for neutropenia (patients with renal impairment or collagen-vascular disease) or at 1st sign of infection. Discontinue therapy if neutrophil count <1000/mm^3.

Implementation

- Do not confuse Accupril with Aciphex. Do not confuse benazepril with Benadryl. Do not confuse captopril with carvedilol. Do not confuse Zestril with Zegerid, Zetia, or Zyprexa.
- Correct volume depletion, if possible, before initiation of therapy.
- **PO:** Precipitous drop in BP during 1st 1–3 hr after 1st dose may require volume expansion with normal saline but is not usually considered an indication for stopping therapy. Discontinuing diuretic therapy or cautiously ↑ salt intake 2–3 days before initiation may ↓ risk of hypotension. Monitor closely for >1 hr after BP has stabilized. Resume diuretics if BP not controlled.

Benazepril

- **PO:** If difficulty swallowing tablets, pharmacist may compound oral suspension; stable for 30 days if refrigerated. Shake suspension before each use.

Captopril

- **PO:** Administer 1 hr before or 2 hr after meals. May be crushed if patient has difficulty swallowing. Tablets may have a sulfurous odor.
- An oral solution may be prepared by crushing a 25-mg tablet and dissolving it in 25–100 mL of water. Shake for >5 min and administer within 30 min.

Enalapril

- **PO:** For patients with difficulty swallowing tablets, oral solution is available ready to use. Shake solution before each use. Solution is stable at controlled room temperature for 60 days.

Enalaprilat

IV Administration

- **IV Push:** **Dilution:** May be administered undiluted. **Concentration:** 1.25 mg/mL. **Rate:** Administer over ≥5 min.
- **Intermittent Infusion:** **Dilution:** Dilute in up to 50 mL of D5W, 0.9% NaCl, D5/0.9% NaCl, or D5/LR. Diluted solution is stable for 24 hr. **Rate:** Infuse slowly over ≥5 min.
- **Y-Site Compatibility:** acyclovir, alemtuzumab, allopurinol, amikacin, aminocaproic acid, aminophylline, amiodarone, amphotericin B liposomal, anidulafungin, argatroban, arsenic trioxide, ascorbic acid, atracurium, atropine, azathioprine,

azithromycin, aztreonam, benztropine, bivalirudin, bleomycin, bumetanide, buprenorphine, butorphanol, calcium chloride, calcium gluconate, cangrelor, carboplatin, carmustine, cefazolin, cefotaxime, cefotetan, cefoxitin, ceftaroline, ceftazidime, ceftobiprole, ceftriaxone, cefuroxime, chloramphenicol, chlorpromazine, cisatracurium, cisplatin, cladribine, clindamycin, cyanocobalamin, cyclophosphamide, cyclosporine, cytarabine, dacarbazine, dactinomycin, daptomycin, daunorubicin, dexamethasone, dexmedetomidine, dexrazoxane, digoxin, diltiazem, diphenhydramine, dobutamine, docetaxel, dopamine, doxorubicin hydrochloride, doxorubicin liposomal, doxycycline, ephedrine, epinephrine, epirubicin, epoetin alfa, eptifibatide, ertapenem, erythromycin, esmolol, etoposide, etoposide phosphate, famotidine, fentanyl, filgrastim, fluconazole, fludarabine, fluorouracil, folic acid, foscarnet, fosphenytoin, furosemide, ganciclovir, gemcitabine, gentamicin, glycopyrrolate, granisetron, heparin, hydrocortisone, hydromorphone, idarubicin, ifosfamide, imipenem/cilastatin, imipenem/cilastatin/relebactam, indomethacin, insulin, regular, irinotecan, isoproterenol, ketorolac, labetalol, leucovorin, levofloxacin, lidocaine, linezolid, lorazepam, magnesium sulfate, mannitol, melphalan, meperidine, meropenem, mesna, methadone, methotrexate, methylprednisolone, metoclopramide, metoprolol, metronidazole, midazolam, milrinone, mitomycin, mitoxantrone, morphine, moxifloxacin, multivitamins, mycophenolate, nafcillin, nalbuphine, naloxone, nicardipine, nitroglycerin, nitroprusside, norepinephrine, octreotide, ondansetron, oxacillin, oxaliplatin, oxytocin, paclitaxel, palonosetron, pamidronate, papaverine, pemetrexed, penicillin G, pentamidine, pentobarbital, phenobarbital, phentolamine, phenylephrine, phytonadione, piperacillin/tazobactam, potassium acetate, potassium chloride, potassium phosphates, procainamide, prochlorperazine, promethazine, propofol, propranolol, protamine, pyridoxine, remifentanil, rituximab, rocuronium, sodium acetate, sodium bicarbonate, succinylcholine, sufentanil, tacrolimus, theophylline, thiamine, thiotepa, tigecycline, tirofiban, tobramycin, topotecan, trastuzumab, vancomycin, vasopressin, vecuronium, verapamil, vinblastine, vincristine, vinorelbine, voriconazole, zoledronic acid.

- **Y-Site Incompatibility:** amphotericin B deoxycholate, caspofungin, cefepime, dantrolene, diazepam, diazoxide, gemtuzumab ozogamicin, phenytoin.

Lisinopril

- **PO:** Oral solution is clear to slightly opalescent. Administer without dilution.

Moexipril

- **PO:** Administer moexipril on an empty stomach, 1 hr before a meal.

Ramipril

- **PO:** Capsules may be opened and sprinkled on applesauce or dissolved in 4 ounces water or apple juice for patients with difficulty swallowing. Effectiveness is same as capsule. Prepared mixtures can be stored for up to 24 hr at room temperature or up to 48 hr if refrigerated.

Trandolapril

- **PO:** May be taken with or without food.

Patient/Family Teaching

- Explain purpose and side effects of medication to patient. Advise patient to read *Patient Information* before starting therapy. Advise to take medication as directed at the same time each day, even if feeling well. Take missed doses as soon as possible but not if almost time for next dose. Do not double doses. Advise not to discontinue therapy unless directed by health care provider.
- Advise patient to notify health care provider of all Rx or OTC medications, vitamins, or herbal products being taken and to consult with health care provider before taking other medications, especially cough, cold, or allergy remedies.
- Advise patient to avoid salt substitutes or foods containing high levels of potassium or sodium unless directed by health care provider (see Appendix J).
- Advise patient to change positions slowly to minimize hypotension. Use of alcohol, standing for long periods, exercising, and hot weather may ↑ risk of orthostatic hypotension.
- May cause dizziness. Advise patient to avoid driving and other activities requiring alertness until response to medication is known.
- Advise patient to inform health care provider of medication regimen before treatment or surgery.
- Advise patient that medication may cause impairment of taste that generally resolves within 8–12 wk, even with continued therapy.
- Advise patient to notify health care provider immediately if rash; mouth sores; sore throat; fever; swelling of hands or feet; irregular heartbeat; chest pain; dry cough; hoarseness; swelling of face, eyes, lips, or tongue; or difficulty swallowing or breathing occur; or if taste impairment or skin rash persists. Persistent dry cough may occur and may not subside until medication is discontinued. Consult health care provider if cough becomes bothersome. Also notify health care provider if nausea, vomiting, or diarrhea occurs and continues.
- Advise patient with diabetes to monitor blood glucose closely, especially during 1st month of therapy; may cause hypoglycemia.
- **Hypertension:** Encourage patient to comply with additional interventions for hypertension (weight reduction, low sodium diet, discontinuation of smoking, moderation of alcohol consumption, regular exercise, stress management). Medication controls but does not cure hypertension.

A

- Advise patient and family/caregiver on correct technique for monitoring BP. Advise them to check BP at least weekly and to report significant changes to health care provider.
- Rep: May cause fetal harm. Advise women of reproductive potential to use effective contraception during therapy and notify health care provider if pregnancy is planned or suspected. If pregnancy is detected, discontinue medication as soon as possible. Closely observe infants with histories of in utero exposure to ACE inhibitors for hypotension, oliguria, and hyperkalemia. If oliguria or hypotension occur, support blood pressure and renal perfusion. Exchange transfusions or dialysis may be required as a means of reversing hypotension and substituting for disordered renal function. Advise patient to avoid breastfeeding during therapy.

Evaluation/Desired Outcomes

- Lowering of BP in hypertensive patients.
- Improved symptoms in patients with HF (selected agents only).
- ↓ development of overt heart failure (enalapril only).
- Improved survival and ↓ development of overt HF after MI (selected agents only).
- ↓ risk of death from cardiovascular causes or MI in patients with stable CAD (perindopril only).
- ↓ risk of MI, stroke or death from cardiovascular causes in high-risk patients (ramipril only).
- ↓ progression of diabetic nephropathy (captopril only).

ANGIOTENSIN II RECEPTOR ANTAGONISTS

azilsartan (a-zill-**sar**-tan)
Edarbi

candesartan (can-de-**sar**-tan)
Atacand

irbesartan (ir-be-**sar**-tan)
Avapro

losartan (loe-**sar**-tan)
Cozaar

olmesartan (ole-me-**sar**-tan)
Benicar, Olmetec

telmisartan (tel-mi-**sar**-tan)
~~Micardis~~

valsartan (val-**sar**-tan)
Diovan

Classification
Therapeutic: antihypertensives
Pharmacologic: angiotensin II receptor antagonists

Indications

Hypertension (as monotherapy or in combination with other antihypertensives). Diabetic nephropathy in patients with type 2 diabetes and hypertension (irbesartan and losartan only). HF (New York Heart Association class II–IV) in patients who cannot tolerate ACE inhibitors (candesartan and valsartan only) or in combination with an ACE inhibitor and beta blocker (candesartan only). Prevention of stroke in patients with hypertension and left ventricular hypertrophy (losartan only). Reduction of risk of death from cardiovascular causes in patients with left ventricular systolic dysfunction after MI (valsartan only). Reduction of risk of MI, stroke, or cardiovascular death in patients ≥55 yr who are at high risk for cardiovascular events and are unable to take ACE inhibitors (telmisartan only).

Action

Blocks vasoconstrictor and aldosterone-producing effects of angiotensin II at receptor sites, including vascular smooth muscle and the adrenal glands. **Therapeutic Effects:** Lowering of BP. Slowed progression of diabetic nephropathy (irbesartan and losartan only). Reduced cardiovascular death and hospitalizations due to HF in patients with HF (candesartan and valsartan only). Decreased risk of cardiovascular death in patients with left ventricular systolic dysfunction who are post-MI (valsartan only). Decreased risk of stroke in patients with hypertension and left ventricular hypertrophy (effect may be less in black patients) (losartan only).

Pharmacokinetics

Absorption: *Azilsartan:* Azilsartan medoxomil is converted to azilsartan, the active component. 60% absorbed; *Candesartan:* Candesartan cilexetil is converted to candesartan, the active component; 15% bioavailability of candesartan; *Irbesartan:* 60–80% absorbed after oral administration; *Losartan:* Well absorbed, with extensive first-pass hepatic metabolism, resulting in 33% bioavailability; *Olmesartan:* Olmesartan medoxomil is converted to olmesartan, the active component; 26% bioavailability of olmesartan; *Telmisartan:* 42–58% absorbed following oral administration (bioavailability ↑ in patients with hepatic impairment); *Valsartan:* 10–35% absorbed following oral administration; systemic exposure 60% higher with the oral solution compared to tablets.
Distribution: All are well distributed to tissues.
Protein Binding: All >90%.
Metabolism and Excretion: *Azilsartan:* 50% metabolized by the liver, primarily by the CYP2C9 enzyme system. 55% eliminated in feces, 42% in urine (15% as unchanged drug); *Candesartan:*

Minor metabolism by the liver; 33% excreted in urine, 67% in feces (via bile); *Irbesartan:* Some hepatic metabolism; 20% excreted in urine, 80% in feces; *Losartan:* Undergoes extensive first-pass hepatic metabolism; 14% is converted to an active metabolite. 4% excreted unchanged in urine; 6% excreted in urine as active metabolite; some biliary elimination; *Olmesartan:* 30–50% excreted unchanged in urine; remainder eliminated in feces via bile; *Telmisartan:* Excreted mostly unchanged in feces via biliary excretion; *Valsartan:* Minor metabolism by the liver; 13% excreted in urine, 83% in feces.

Half-life: *Azilsartan:* 11 hr; *Candesartan:* 9 hr; *Irbesartan:* 11–15 hr; *Losartan:* 2 hr (6–9 hr for metabolite); *Olmesartan:* 13 hr; *Telmisartan:* 24 hr; *Valsartan:* 6 hr.

TIME/ACTION PROFILE (antihypertensive effect with chronic dosing)

DRUG	ONSET	PEAK	DURATION
Azilsartan	within 2 hr	18 hr	24 hr
Candesartan	2–4 hr	4 wk	24 hr
Irbesartan	within 2 hr	2 wk	24 hr
Losartan	6 hr	3–6 wk	24 hr
Olmesartan	within 1 wk	2 wk	24 hr
Telmisartan	within 3 hr	4 wk	24 hr
Valsartan	within 2 hr	4 wk	24 hr

Contraindications/Precautions

Contraindicated in: Hypersensitivity; Concurrent use with aliskiren in patients with diabetes or moderate to severe renal impairment (CCr <60 mL/min); Severe hepatic impairment (candesartan); OB: Pregnancy; Lactation: Lactation.

Use Cautiously in: HF (may result in azotemia, oliguria, acute renal failure, and/or death); Volume- or salt-depleted patients or patients receiving high doses of diuretics (correct deficits before initiating therapy or initiate at lower doses); Black patients (may not be effective); Impaired renal function due to primary renal disease or HF (may worsen renal function); Obstructive biliary disorders (telmisartan) or hepatic impairment (losartan, telmisartan); Severe renal impairment (valsartan); Rep: Women of reproductive potential; Pedi: Safety and effectiveness not established in children <18 yr (azilsartan, candesartan, irbesartan, telmisartan), <6 yr (losartan, olmesartan), and <1 yr (valsartan).

Adverse Reactions/Side Effects

CV: hypotension, chest pain, edema, tachycardia. **Derm:** rash. **EENT:** nasal congestion, pharyngitis, rhinitis, sinusitis. **F and E:** hyperkalemia. **GI:** abdominal pain, diarrhea, drug-induced hepatitis, dyspepsia, nausea, vomiting. **GU:** renal impairment. **MS:** arthralgia, back pain, myalgia. **Neuro:** dizziness, anxiety, depression, fatigue, headache, insomnia, weakness. **Misc:** ANGIOEDEMA.

Interactions

Drug-Drug: NSAIDs and selective **COX-2 inhibitors** may blunt the antihypertensive effect and ↑ risk of renal dysfunction. ↑ antihypertensive effects with other **antihypertensives** and **diuretics**. Telmisartan may ↑ levels and risk of toxicity of **digoxin**. **Potassium-sparing diuretics**, **potassium-containing salt substitutes**, or **potassium supplements** may ↑ risk of hyperkalemia. ↑ risk of hyperkalemia, renal impairment, hypotension, and syncope with concurrent use of **ACE inhibitors** or **aliskiren**; avoid concurrent use with aliskiren in patients with diabetes or CCr <60 mL/min; avoid concurrent use with ACE inhibitors. Candesartan, valsartan, and irbesartan may ↑ levels and risk of toxicity of **lithium**. Irbesartan and losartan may ↑ levels and risk of toxicity of **amiodarone**, **fluoxetine**, **glimepiride**, **glipizide**, **phenytoin**, and **warfarin**. **Rifampin** may ↓ levels and effectiveness of losartan. Telmisartan may ↑ risk of renal impairment when used with **ramipril**; concurrent use not recommended. **Colesevelam** may ↓ levels and effectiveness of olmesartan; administer olmesartan ≥4 hr before colesevelam.

Route/Dosage

Azilsartan

PO (Adults): 80 mg once daily; may ↓ initial dose to 40 mg once daily if high doses of diuretics are used concurrently.

Candesartan

PO (Adults): *Hypertension:* 16 mg once daily; may ↑ up to 32 mg/day in 1–2 divided doses (begin therapy at a lower dose in patients who are receiving diuretics or are volume depleted). *HF:* 4 mg once daily initially; may double dose every 2 wk up to target dose of 32 mg once daily.

PO (Children 6–16 yr and >50 kg): 8–16 mg/day (in 1–2 divided doses); may ↑ up to 32 mg/day (in 1–2 divided doses).

PO (Children 6–16 yr and <50 kg): 4–8 mg/day (in 1–2 divided doses); may ↑ up to 16 mg/day (in 1–2 divided doses).

PO (Children 1–5 yr): 0.20 mg/kg/day (in 1–2 divided doses); may ↑ up to 0.4 mg/kg/day (in 1–2 divided doses).

Hepatic Impairment

PO (Adults): *Moderate hepatic impairment:* Initiate at 8 mg once daily.

Irbesartan

PO (Adults): *Hypertension:* 150 mg once daily; may ↑ to 300 mg once daily. Initiate therapy at 75 mg once daily in patients who are receiving diuretics or are volume depleted. *Type 2 diabetic nephropathy:* 300 mg once daily.

Losartan

PO (Adults): *Hypertension:* 50 mg once daily initially (range 25–100 mg/day as a single daily dose or 2 divided doses) (initiate therapy at 25 mg once daily in patients who are receiving diuretics or are volume depleted). *Prevention of stroke in patients with hypertension and left ventricular hypertrophy:* 50 mg once daily initially; hydrochlorothiazide 12.5 mg once daily should be added and/or dose of losartan ↑ to 100 mg once daily followed by ↑ in hydrochlorothiazide to 25 mg once daily based on BP response. *Type 2 diabetic nephropathy:* 50 mg once daily; may ↑ to 100 mg once daily depending on BP response.

Hepatic Impairment

PO (Adults): 25 mg once daily initially; may ↑ as tolerated.

PO (Children >6 yr): *Hypertension:* 0.7 mg/kg once daily (up to 50 mg/day); may titrate up to 1.4 mg/kg/day (or 100 mg/day).

Renal Impairment

PO (Children >6 yr): *CCr <30 mL/min:* Contraindicated.

Olmesartan

PO (Adults): 20 mg once daily; may ↑ up to 40 mg once daily (patients who are receiving diuretics or are volume-depleted should be started on lower doses).

PO (Children 6–16 yr): *≥35 kg:* 20 mg once daily; may ↑ after 2 wk up to 40 mg once daily; *20–34.9 kg:* 10 mg once daily; may ↑ after 2 wk up to 20 mg once daily.

Telmisartan

PO (Adults): *Hypertension:* 40 mg once daily (volume-depleted patients should start with 20 mg once daily); may titrate up to 80 mg/day; *Cardiovascular risk reduction:* 80 mg once daily.

Valsartan

Oral tablets and solution are NOT interchangeable on a mg-per-mg basis. These dosage forms should not be combined to arrive at a particular dose.

PO (Adults): *Hypertension:* 80 mg or 160 mg once daily initially in patients who are not volume-depleted; may ↑ to 320 mg once daily; *HF:* 40 mg twice daily; may titrate up to target dose of 160 mg twice daily as tolerated; *Post-MI:* 20 mg twice daily (may initiate ≥ 12 hr after MI); may titrate up to target dose of 160 mg twice daily, as tolerated.

PO (Children 1–16 yr): *Hypertension:* 1 mg/kg once daily (maximum dose = 40 mg/day) (may consider using starting dose of 2 mg/kg once daily if greater BP ↓ needed); may ↑ up to 4 mg/kg once daily (maximum dose = 160 mg/day).

Availability

Azilsartan (generic available)

Tablets: 40 mg, 80 mg. ***In combination with:*** chlorthalidone (Edarbyclor); see Appendix N.

Candesartan (generic available)

Tablets: 4 mg, 8 mg, 16 mg, 32 mg. ***In combination with:*** hydrochlorothiazide (Atacand HCT); see Appendix N.

Irbesartan (generic available)

Tablets: 75 mg, 150 mg, 300 mg. ***In combination with:*** hydrochlorothiazide (Avalide); see Appendix N.

Losartan (generic available)

Tablets: 25 mg, 50 mg, 100 mg. ***In combination with:*** hydrochlorothiazide (Hyzaar); see Appendix N.

Olmesartan (generic available)

Tablets: 5 mg, 20 mg, 40 mg. ***In combination with:*** hydrochlorothiazide (Benicar HCT); amlodipine (Azor); amlodipine and hydrochlorothiazide (Tribenzor); see Appendix N.

Telmisartan (generic available)

Tablets: 20 mg, 40 mg, 80 mg. ***In combination with:*** hydrochlorothiazide (Micardis HCT); amlodipine; amlodipine and indapamide (Widaplik); see Appendix N.

Valsartan (generic available)

Tablets: 40 mg, 80 mg, 160 mg, 320 mg.

Oral solution (grape flavor): 4 mg/mL. ***In combination with:*** amlodipine (Exforge); hydrochlorothiazide (Diovan HCT); amlodipine and hydrochlorothiazide (Exforge HCT); see Appendix N.

NURSING IMPLICATIONS

Assessment

- Assess BP (lying, sitting, standing) and HR periodically during therapy. Notify health care provider of significant changes.
- Assess for signs of angioedema (dyspnea, facial swelling). May rarely cause angioedema.
- **HF:** Monitor daily weight and assess routinely for resolution of fluid overload (peripheral edema, rales/crackles, dyspnea, weight gain, JVD).

Lab Test Considerations

- Monitor renal function and electrolyte levels periodically. May ↑ potassium, BUN, and serum creatinine.
- May ↑ AST, ALT, and bilirubin (candesartan and olmesartan only).
- May ↑ uric acid, and ↓ hemoglobin and hematocrit. May cause neutropenia, and thrombocytopenia.

Implementation

- Do not confuse Atacand with antacid. Do not confuse Cozaar with Colace or Zocor.

- Correct volume depletion, if possible, before starting therapy.
- **PO:** Administer without regard to meals.

Losartan

- **PO:** *If difficulty swallowing tablets,* pharmacist can compound oral suspension; stable for 4 wk if refrigerated. Shake suspension before each use.

Valsartan

- For pediatric patients unable to swallow tablets, solution can be prepared by pharmacist. Tablets and suspension are not interchangeable. Do not combine tablets and suspension. Solution should be used for pediatric patients aged 1–5 yr, for patients >5 yr of age who cannot swallow tablets, and for pediatric patients for whom the calculated dose (mg/kg) does not correspond to the available tablet strengths of valsartan.

Patient/Family Teaching

- Explain purpose and side effects of medication to patient. Advise patient to read *Patient Information* before starting therapy. Advise to take as medication directed, even if feeling well. Take missed doses as soon as remembered if not almost time for next dose; do not double doses. Advise patient to take medication at the same time each day and not to discontinue therapy unless directed by health care provider.
- Advise patient to notify health care provider of all Rx or OTC medications, vitamins, or herbal products being taken and to consult with health care provider before taking other medications, especially NSAIDs and cough, cold, or allergy remedies.
- Advise patient to avoid salt substitutes containing potassium or food containing high levels of potassium or sodium unless directed by health care provider. See Appendix J.
- Advise patient to avoid sudden changes in position. Use of alcohol, standing for long periods, exercising, and hot weather may ↑ risk of orthostatic hypotension.
- May cause dizziness. Advise patient to avoid driving or other activities requiring alertness until response to medication is known.
- Advise patient to notify health care provider of medication regimen before treatment or surgery.
- Advise patient to notify health care provider immediately if swelling of face, eyes, lips, or tongue occurs or if difficulty swallowing or breathing occurs.
- **Hypertension:** Encourage patient to comply with additional interventions for hypertension (weight reduction, low-sodium diet, discontinuation of smoking, moderation of alcohol consumption, regular exercise, stress management). Medication controls but dose not cure hypertension.
- Instruct patient and family/caregiver on proper technique for monitoring BP. Advise to check BP at least weekly and to report significant changes.
- Rep: May cause fetal harm. Advise women of reproductive potential to use contraception and notify health care provider if pregnancy is planned or suspected or if breastfeeding. If pregnancy is detected, discontinue medication as soon as possible. In patients taking during pregnancy, perform serial ultrasound examinations to assess the intra-amniotic environment. Fetal testing may be appropriate, based on the week of gestation. Patients should be aware, however, that oligohydramnios may not appear until after the fetus has sustained irreversible injury. If oligohydramnios is observed, consider alternative drug treatment. Closely observe neonates with histories of in utero exposure to valsartan for hypotension, oliguria, and hyperkalemia. In neonates with a history of in utero exposure to valsartan, if oliguria or hypotension occurs, support blood pressure and renal perfusion. Exchange transfusions or dialysis may be required as a means of reversing hypotension and replacing renal function.

Evaluation/Desired Outcomes

- Lowering of BP.
- Slowed progression of diabetic nephropathy (irbesartan and losartan only).
- Reduced cardiovascular death and hospitalizations due to HF in patients with HF (candesartan and valsartan only).
- Decreased risk of cardiovascular death in patients with left ventricular systolic dysfunction who are post-MI (valsartan only).
- Decreased risk of stroke in patients with hypertension and left ventricular hypertrophy (effect may be less in black patients) (losartan only).

anidulafungin

(a-**ni**-du-la-fun-gin)

Eraxis

Classification

Therapeutic: antifungals

Pharmacologic: echinocandins

Indications

Candidemia and other serious candidal infections, including intra-abdominal abscess, peritonitis. Esophageal candidiasis.

Action

Inhibits the synthesis of fungal cell wall. **Therapeutic Effects:** Death of susceptible fungi. **Spectrum:** Active against *Candida albicans*, *Candida glabrata*, *Candida parapsilosis*, and *Candida tropicalis*.

Pharmacokinetics

Absorption: IV administration results in complete bioavailability.

Distribution: Widely distributed to tissues.

A

Metabolism and Excretion: Undergoes chemical degradation without hepatic metabolism; <1% excreted in urine.
Half-life: 40–50 hr.

TIME/ACTION PROFILE (plasma concentrations)

ROUTE	ONSET	PEAK	DURATION
IV	rapid	end of infusion	24 hr

Contraindications/Precautions

Contraindicated in: Hypersensitivity; Known or suspected hereditary fructose intolerance.
Use Cautiously in: Underlying liver disease (may worsen); OB: Safety not established in pregnancy; other antifungal agents preferred in pregnancy for infections caused by *Candida*; Lactation: Use while breastfeeding only if potential maternal benefit justifies potential risk to infant; Pedi: Safety and effectiveness not established in children <1 mo (candidemia and intra-abdominal abscess and peritonitis caused by *Candida*) or <18 yr (esophageal candidiasis); may lead to polysorbate toxicity in low-birth weight infants.

Adverse Reactions/Side Effects

CV: hypotension. **Derm:** flushing, rash, urticaria. **F and E:** hypokalemia. **GI:** ↑ liver enzymes, diarrhea. **Resp:** bronchospasm, dyspnea. **Misc:** ANAPHYLAXIS, infusion reactions.

Interactions

Drug-Drug: None reported.

Route/Dosage

Candidemia and Intra-abdominal Abscess or Peritonitis Caused by *Candida*

IV (Adults): 200 mg loading dose on Day 1; then 100 mg once daily. Continue therapy for ≥14 days after last positive culture.
IV (Children ≥1 mo): 3 mg/kg (max = 200 mg) loading dose on Day 1; then 1.5 mg/kg (max = 100 mg) once daily. Continue therapy for ≥14 days after last positive culture.

Esophageal Candidiasis

IV (Adults): 100 mg loading dose on Day 1; then 50 mg once daily. Continue therapy for a minimum of 14 days and for ≥7 days following resolution of symptoms.

Availability

Lyophilized powder for injection (contains fructose and polysorbate 80): 50 mg/vial, 100 mg/vial.

NURSING IMPLICATIONS

Assessment

- Assess infected area at baseline and periodically during therapy to monitor effectiveness of therapy.
- Monitor for anaphylaxis (rash, urticaria, flushing, pruritus, bronchospasm, dyspnea, hypotension); usually related to histamine release. *If symptoms occur,* stop therapy and provide appropriate treatment. ↓ risk by not exceeding recommended infusion rate.

Lab Test Considerations

- Obtain culture specimens before starting therapy. Therapy may be started before results are obtained.
- May cause ↑ ALT, AST, alkaline phosphatase, and hepatic enzymes. *If liver function abnormality occurs,* monitor closely and consider discontinuing anidulafungin.
- May cause hypokalemia.
- May cause neutropenia and leukopenia.

Implementation

IV Administration

- **Adults: Intermittent Infusion: Reconstitution:** Reconstitute each 50 mg vial with 15 mL or the 100 mg vial with 30 mL of sterile water for injection. Stable at room temperature for 24 hr. **Concentration:** 3.33 mg/mL. **Dilution:** *For 50 mg dose,* dilute contents of reconstituted vial with 50 mL of D5W or 0.9% NaCl for an infusion volume of 65 mL. *For 100-mg dose,* dilute contents of reconstituted vial with 100 mL of D5W or 0.9% NaCl for an infusion volume of 130 mL. *For 200-mg dose,*d ilute contents of two reconstituted 100-mg vials with 200 mL of D5W or 0.9% NaCl for an infusion volume of 260 mL. **Concentration:** 0.77 mg/mL. Do not administer solutions that are discolored or contain particulates. Stable for 48 hr at room temperature. Do not freeze. **Rate:** Do not exceed 1.1 mg/min. Infuse 50 mg dose over ≥45 min, 100 mg dose over 90 min, or 200 mg dose over 180 min.
- **Children: Intermittent Infusion: Reconstitution:** Reconstitute each 50 mg vial with 15 mL or the 100 mg vial with 30 mL of sterile water for injection. Stable at room temperature for 24 hr. **Concentration:** 3.33 mg/mL. **Dilution:** Dilute with 0.9% NaCl or D5W. **Concentration:** 0.77 mg/mL. Prepare in infusion syringe or IV infusion bag. Do not administer solutions that are discolored or contain particulates. Stable for 48 hr at room temperature. Do not freeze. **Rate:** Do not exceed 1.1 mg/min.
- **Y-Site Compatibility:** acyclovir, alemtuzumab, allopurinol, amikacin, aminocaproic acid, aminophylline, amiodarone, amphotericin B liposomal, ampicillin, ampicillin/sulbactam, argatroban, arsenic trioxide, atracurium, azithromycin, aztreonam, bivalirudin, bleomycin, bumetanide, buprenorphine, busulfan, butorphanol, calcium chloride, calcium gluconate, cangrelor, carboplatin, carmustine, caspofungin, cefazolin, cefepime, cefotaxime, cefotetan, cefoxitin, ceftazidime, ceftolozane/

tazobactam, ceftriaxone, cefuroxime, chlorpromazine, ciprofloxacin, cisatracurium, cisplatin, clindamycin, cyclophosphamide, cyclosporine, cytarabine, dacarbazine, dactinomycin, daunorubicin, dexamethasone, dexmedetomidine, dexrazoxane, digoxin, diltiazem, diphenhydramine, dobutamine, docetaxel, dopamine, doxorubicin hydrochloride, doxorubicin liposomal, doxycycline, droperidol, enalaprilat, ephedrine, epinephrine, epirubicin, eptifibatide, erythromycin, esmolol, etoposide, etoposide phosphate, famotidine, fentanyl, fluconazole, fludarabine, fluorouracil, foscarnet, fosphenytoin, furosemide, ganciclovir, gemcitabine, gentamicin, glycopyrrolate, granisetron, haloperidol, heparin, hydralazine, hydrocortisone, hydromorphone, hydroxyzine, idarubicin, ifosfamide, imipenem/cilastatin, insulin, regular, irinotecan, isavuconazonium, isoproterenol, ketorolac, labetalol, letermovir, leucovorin calcium, levofloxacin, lidocaine, linezolid, lorazepam, mannitol, melphalan, meperidine, meropenem, mesna, methadone, methotrexate, methylprednisolone, metoclopramide, metoprolol, metronidazole, midazolam, milrinone, mitomycin, mitoxantrone, morphine, moxifloxacin, mycophenolate, nafcillin, naloxone, nicardipine, nitroglycerin, nitroprusside, norepinephrine, octreotide, ondansetron, oxaliplatin, oxytocin, paclitaxel, palonosetron, pamidronate, pantoprazole, pentamidine, pentobarbital, phenobarbital, phentolamine, phenylephrine, piperacillin/tazobactam, potassium acetate, potassium chloride, procainamide, prochlorperazine, promethazine, propranolol, remifentanil, rocuronium, sodium acetate, succinylcholine, sufentanil, sulbactam/durlobactam, tacrolimus, tedizolid, theophylline, thiotepa, tirofiban, tobramycin, topotecan, trimethoprim/sulfamethoxazole, vancomycin, vasopressin, vecuronium, verapamil, vinblastine, vincristine, vinorelbine, voriconazole, zidovudine, zoledronic acid.

- **Y-Site Incompatibility:** amphotericin B deoxycholate, dantrolene, diazepam, ertapenem, gemtuzumab ozogamicin, magnesium sulfate, meropenem/vaborbactam, nalbuphine, pemetrexed, phenytoin, plazomicin, potassium phosphates, sodium bicarbonate, sodium phosphates.

Patient/Family Teaching

- Explain purpose and side effects of medication. Advise patient to read *Patient Information* before starting therapy.
- Instruct patient to notify health care professional immediately if signs and symptoms of anaphylaxis occur or if diarrhea becomes pronounced.
- Inform patient that anidulafungin contains fructose. May be life-threatening when administered to patients with hereditary fructose intolerance.
- Rep: Advise women of reproductive potential to notify health care professional if pregnancy is planned or suspected or if breastfeeding.

Evaluation/Desired Outcomes

- Resolution of clinical and laboratory indication of fungal infection.

ANTIFUNGALS (TOPICAL)

butenafine (byoo-**ten**-a-feen)
Lotrimin Ultra

ciclopirox (sye-kloe-**peer**-ox)
Ciclodan, ✱ Loprox

clotrimazole (kloe-**trye**-ma-zole)
Alevazol, ✱ Canesten, ✱ Clotrimaderm

econazole (ee-**kon**-a-zole)
Ecoza

efinaconazole (eff-in-a-**kon**-a-zole)
Jublia

ketoconazole (kee-toe-**koe**-na-zole)
Ketodan, ✱ Ketoderm

luliconazole (loo-li-**kon**-a-zole)
Luzu

miconazole (mye-**kon**-a-zole)
Fungoid, Lotrimin AF, Micatin, ✱ Micozole, Zeasorb-AF

naftifine (**naff**-ti-feen)
Naftin

nystatin (nye-**stat**-in)
Klayesta, ~~Mycostatin~~, Nyamyc, ✱ Nyaderm, Nystop

oxiconazole (ox-i-**kon**-a-zole)
Oxistat

sertaconazole (ser-ta-**kon**-a-zole)
Ertaczo

sulconazole (sul-**kon**-a-zole)
Exelderm

tavaborole (ta-va-**bor**-ole)
~~Kerydin~~

terbinafine (ter-**bin**-a-feen)
✱ Lamisil, Lamisil AT

tolnaftate (tol-**naff**-tate)
Tinactin

Classification
Therapeutic: antifungals (topical)

Indications

Treatment of a variety of cutaneous fungal infections, including cutaneous candidiasis, tinea pedis (athlete's foot), tinea cruris (jock itch), tinea corporis (ringworm), tinea versicolor, seborrheic dermatitis, dandruff, and onychomycosis of fingernails and toenails.

A

Action
Butenafine, nystatin, clotrimazole, econazole, efinaconazole, ketoconazole, luliconazole, miconazole, naftifine, oxiconazole, sertaconazole, sulconazole, and terbinafine affect the synthesis of the fungal cell wall, allowing leakage of cellular contents. Tolnaftate distorts the hyphae and stunts mycelial growth in fungi. Ciclopirox inhibits the transport of essential elements in the fungal cell, disrupting the synthesis of DNA, RNA, and protein. Tavaborole inhibits fungal protein synthesis via inhibition of aminoacyl-transfer ribonucleic acid (tRNA) synthetase. **Therapeutic Effects:** Decrease in symptoms of fungal infection.

Pharmacokinetics
Absorption: Absorption through intact skin is minimal.
Distribution: Distribution after topical administration is primarily local.
Metabolism and Excretion: Metabolism and excretion not known following local application.
Half-life: *Butenafine:* 35 hr; *Ciclopirox:* 5.5 hr (gel); *Efinaconazole:* 29.9 hr; *Terbinafine:* 21 hr.

TIME/ACTION PROFILE (resolution of symptoms/lesions†)

ROUTE	ONSET	PEAK	DURATION
Butenafine	unknown	up to 4 wk	unknown
Luliconazole	unknown	3–4 wk	unknown
Tolnaftate	24–72 hr	unknown	unknown

† Only the drugs with known information included in this table.

Contraindications/Precautions
Contraindicated in: Hypersensitivity to active ingredients, additives, preservatives, or bases; Some products contain alcohol or bisulfites and should be avoided in patients with known intolerance.
Use Cautiously in: Nail and scalp infections (may require additional systemic therapy); OB: Safety not established in pregnancy; Lactation: Safety not established in breastfeeding.

Adverse Reactions/Side Effects
Local: burning, itching, local hypersensitivity reactions, redness, stinging.

Interactions
Drug-Drug: Econazole may ↑ levels of and risk of bleeding from **warfarin**.

Route/Dosage
Butenafine
Topical: (Adults and Children >12 yr): Apply once daily for 2 wk for tinea corporis, tinea cruris, or tinea versicolor. Apply once daily for 4 wk or once daily for 7 days for tinea pedis.

Ciclopirox
Topical: (Adults and Children >10 yr): *Cream/lotion:* Apply twice daily for 2–4 wk; *Topical solution (nail lacquer):* Apply to nails at bedtime or 8 hr prior to bathing for up to 48 wk. Each daily application should be made over the previous coat and then removed with alcohol every 7 days; *Gel:* Apply twice daily for 4 wk; *Shampoo:* 5–10 mL applied to scalp; lather and leave on for 3 min; rinse; repeat twice weekly for 4 wk (≥3 days between applications).

Clotrimazole
Topical: (Adults and Children >3 yr): Apply twice daily for 1–4 wk.

Econazole
Topical: (Adults and Children): Apply once daily for tinea pedis (for 4 wk), tinea cruris (for 2 wk), tinea corporis (for 2 wk), or tinea versicolor (for 2 wk). Apply twice daily for cutaneous candidiasis (for 2 wk).

Efinaconazole
Topical: (Adults and Children ≥6 yr): Apply to affected toenails once daily for 48 wk.

Ketoconazole
Topical: (Adults): Apply cream once daily for cutaneous candidiasis (for 2 wk), tinea corporis (for 2 wk), tinea cruris (for 2 wk), tinea pedis (for 6 wk), or tinea versicolor (for 2 wk). Apply cream twice daily for seborrheic dermatitis (for 4 wk). For dandruff, use shampoo twice weekly (wait 3–4 days between treatments) for 4 wk and then intermittently.

Luliconazole
Topical: (Adults and Children ≥12 yr): *Interdigital tinea pedis:* Apply to affected and surrounding areas once daily for 2 wk; *Tinea cruris:* Apply to affected and surrounding areas once daily for 1 wk.
Topical: (Adults and Children ≥2 yr): *Tinea corporis:* Apply to affected and surrounding areas once daily for 1 wk.
Topical: (Adults): *Interdigital tinea pedis:* Apply to affected and surrounding areas once daily for 2 wk; *Tinea cruris and tinea corporis:* Apply to affected and surrounding areas once daily for 1 wk.

Miconazole
Topical: (Adults and Children >2 yr): Apply twice daily. Treat tinea cruris for 2 wk and tinea pedis or tinea corporis for 4 wk.

Naftifine

Topical: (Adults): *Interdigital tinea pedis:* Apply cream or gel once daily for 2 wk; *Tinea cruris or tinea corporis:* apply cream once daily for 2 wk.
Topical: (Children ≥12 yr): *Interdigital tinea pedis:* Apply cream or gel once daily for 2 wk.
Topical: (Children ≥2 yr): *Tinea corporis:* Apply cream once daily for 2 wk.

Nystatin

Topical: (Adults and Children): Apply 2–3 times daily until healing is complete.

Oxiconazole

Topical: (Adults and Children): Apply cream or lotion 1–2 times daily for tinea pedis (for 4 wk), tinea corporis (for 2 wk), or tinea cruris (for 2 wk). Apply cream once daily for tinea versicolor (for 2 wk).

Sertaconazole

Topical: (Adults and Children >12 yr): Apply twice daily for 4 wk.

Sulconazole

Topical: (Adults): Apply 1–2 times daily (twice daily for tinea pedis). Treat tinea corporis, tinea cruris, or tinea versicolor for 3 wk, and tinea pedis for 4 wk.

Tavaborole

Topical: (Adults and Children ≥6 yr): Apply to affected nail once daily for 48 wk.

Terbinafine

Topical: (Adults): Apply twice daily for tinea pedis (for 1 wk) or daily for tinea cruris or tinea corporis for 1 wk.

Tolnaftate

Topical: (Adults): Apply twice daily for tinea cruris (for 2 wk), tinea pedis (for 4 wk), or tinea corporis (for 4 wk).

Availability

Butenafine (generic available)

Cream: 1%$^{\text{Rx, OTC}}$.

Ciclopirox (generic available)

Cream: 0.77%. **Gel:** 0.77%. **Lotion:** 🍁 1%. **Nail lacquer:** 8%. **Shampoo:** 1%. **Suspension:** 0.77%.

Clotrimazole (generic available)

Cream: 1%^{OTC}. **Ointment:** 1%^{OTC}. **Solution:** 1%^{OTC}. ***In combination with:*** betamethasone.

Econazole (generic available)

Cream: 1%. **Foam:** 1%.

Efinaconazole (generic available)

Solution: 10%.

Ketoconazole (generic available)

Cream: 2%. **Foam:** 2%. **Shampoo:** 2%.

Luliconazole (generic available)

Cream: 1%.

Miconazole (generic available)

Cream: 2%$^{\text{Rx, OTC}}$. **Ointment:** 2%^{OTC}. **Powder:** 2%^{OTC}. **Solution:** 2%^{OTC}. **Spray powder:** 2%^{OTC}. ***In combination with:*** zinc oxide (Vusion). See Appendix N.

Naftifine

Cream: 1%, 2%. **Gel:** 2%.

Nystatin (generic available)

Cream: 100,000 units/g$^{\text{Rx, OTC}}$. **Ointment:** 100,000 units/g$^{\text{Rx, OTC}}$. **Powder:** 100,000 units/g$^{\text{Rx, OTC}}$. ***In combination with:*** triamcinolone.

Oxiconazole (generic available)

Cream: 1%. **Lotion:** 1%.

Sertaconazole

Cream: 2%.

Sulconazole (generic available)

Cream: 1%. **Solution:** 1%.

Tavaborole (generic available)

Solution: 5%.

Terbinafine (generic available)

Cream: 1%^{OTC}.

Tolnaftate (generic available)

Cream: 1%^{OTC}. **Powder:** 1%^{OTC}. **Solution:** 1%^{OTC}. **Spray powder:** 1%^{OTC}.

NURSING IMPLICATIONS

Assessment

- Assess involved areas of skin and mucous membranes before and frequently during therapy. ↑ skin irritation may indicate need to discontinue medication.

Implementation

- Consult health care provider for proper cleansing technique before applying medication.
- Choice of vehicle is based on use. Ointments, creams, and liquids are used as primary therapy. Lotion is usually preferred in intertriginous areas; if cream is used, apply sparingly to avoid maceration. Powders are usually used as adjunctive therapy but may be used as primary therapy for mild conditions (especially for moist lesions).
- **Topical:** Apply small amount to cover affected area completely. Avoid use of occlusive wrappings or dressings unless directed by health care provider.
- **Nail lacquer:** Avoid contact with skin other than skin immediately surrounding treated nail. Avoid contact with eyes or mucous membranes. Removal of unattached, infected nail, as frequently as monthly, by health care provider is needed with use of this medication. Up to 48 wk of daily application and provider removal may be required to achieve

clear or almost clear nail. 6 mo of treatment may be required before results are noticed.

- **Ciclopirox or ketoconazole shampoo:** Moisten hair and scalp thoroughly with water. Apply sufficient shampoo to produce enough lather to wash scalp and hair and gently massage it over the entire scalp area for approximately 1 min. Rinse hair thoroughly with warm water. Repeat process, leaving shampoo on hair for an additional 3 min. After the 2nd shampoo, rinse and dry hair with towel or warm air flow. Shampoo twice a week for 4 wk with >3 days between each shampooing and then intermittently as needed to maintain control.
- **Ketoconazole or econazole foam:** Hold container upright and dispense foam into cap of can or other smooth surface; dispensing directly on to hand is not recommended as the foam begins to melt immediately on contact with warm skin. Pick up small amounts with fingertips and gently massage into affected areas until absorbed. Move hair to allow direct application to skin.

Patient/Family Teaching

- Explain purpose and side effects of medication to patient. Advise patient to read *Patient Information* before starting therapy. Instruct patient to apply medication as directed for full course of therapy, even if feeling better. Emphasize the importance of avoiding the eyes.
- Advise patient to notify health care provider of all Rx or OTC medications, vitamins, or herbal products being taken and to consult with health care provider before taking other medications.
- Advise patient that some products may stain fabric, skin, or hair. Check label information. Fabrics stained from cream or lotion can usually be cleaned by handwashing with soap and warm water; stains from ointments can usually be removed with standard cleaning fluids.
- Patients with athlete's foot should be taught to wear well-fitting, ventilated shoes; to wash affected areas thoroughly; and to change shoes and socks at least once a day.
- Advise patient to report ↑ skin irritation or lack of response to therapy to health care provider.
- **Nail lacquer:** File away loose nail and trim nails every 7 days after solution is removed with alcohol. Do not use nail polish on treated nails. Inform health care provider if patient has diabetes mellitus before using.
- Rep: Advise women of reproductive potential to notify health care provider if pregnancy is planned or suspected or breastfeeding.

Evaluation/Desired Outcomes

- Decrease in symptoms of fungal infection.

ANTIFUNGALS (VAGINAL)

butoconazole
(byoo-toe-**kon**-a-zole)
Gynazole-1
clotrimazole (kloe-**trye**-ma-zole)
✦Canesten, ✦Clotrimaderm
miconazole (mye-**kon**-a-zole)
terconazole (ter-**kon**-a-zole)
tioconazole (tye-oh-**kon**-a-zole)
Monistat-1Day

Classification
Therapeutic: antifungals (vaginal)

Indications

Vulvovaginal candidiasis.

Action

Affects the permeability of the fungal cell wall, allowing leakage of cellular contents. Not active against bacteria. **Therapeutic Effects:** Inhibited growth and death of susceptible *Candida*, with decrease in accompanying symptoms of vulvovaginitis (vaginal burning, itching, discharge).

Pharmacokinetics

Absorption: Absorption through intact skin is minimal.
Distribution: Unknown. Action is primarily local.
Metabolism and Excretion: Negligible with local application.
Half-life: Not applicable.

ROUTE	ONSET	PEAK	DURATION
All agents	rapid	unknown	24 hr

Contraindications/Precautions

Contraindicated in: Hypersensitivity to active ingredients, additives, or preservatives; OB: Safety not established in pregnancy; Lactation: Safety not established in breastfeeding.
Use Cautiously in: None noted.

Adverse Reactions/Side Effects

Derm: terconazole: TOXIC EPIDERMAL NECROLYSIS. **GU:** itching, pelvic pain, vulvovaginal burning. **Misc: terconazole:** ANAPHYLAXIS.

Interactions

Drug-Drug: Concurrent use of vaginal miconazole with **warfarin** ↑ risk of bleeding/bruising; appropriate monitoring recommended.

Route/Dosage

Butoconazole

Vag (Adults and Children ≥12 yr): One applicatorful as a single dose.

Clotrimazole
Vag (Adults and Children >12 yr): One applicatorful (5 g) of 1% cream at bedtime for 7 days *or* one applicatorful (5 g) of 2% cream at bedtime for 3 days.

Miconazole
Vag (Adults and Children ≥12 yr): *Vaginal suppositories:* One 100-mg suppository at bedtime for 7 days *or* one 200-mg suppository at bedtime for 3 days *or* one 1200-mg suppository as a single dose. *Vaginal cream:* One applicatorful of 2% cream at bedtime for 7 days *or* one applicatorful of 4% cream at bedtime for 3 days. *Combination packages:* Contain a cream or suppositories as well as an external vaginal cream (may be used twice daily for up to 7 days, as needed, for symptomatic management of itching).

Terconazole
Vag (Adults): *Vaginal cream:* One applicatorful (5 g) of 0.4% cream at bedtime for 7 days *or* one applicatorful (5 g) of 0.8% cream at bedtime for 3 days. *Vaginal suppositories:* one suppository (80 mg) at bedtime for 3 days.

Tioconazole
Vag (Adults and Children ≥12 yr): One applicatorful (4.6 g) at bedtime as a single dose.

Availability
Butoconazole
Vaginal cream: 2%[Rx, OTC].

Clotrimazole (generic available)
Vaginal cream: 1%[OTC]2%[OTC].

Miconazole (generic available)
Vaginal cream: 2%[OTC]. **Vaginal suppositories:** 100 mg[OTC], 200 mg[Rx, OTC]. ***In combination with:*** combination package of three 200-mg suppositories and 2% external cream[OTC]; one 1200-mg suppository and 2% external cream[OTC]; 4% vaginal cream and 2% external cream[OTC]; seven 100-mg suppositories and 2% external cream[OTC]; 2% vaginal cream and 2% external cream[OTC].

Terconazole (generic available)
Vaginal cream: 0.4%, 0.8%. **Vaginal suppositories:** 80 mg.

Tioconazole
Vaginal ointment: 6.5%[OTC].

NURSING IMPLICATIONS
Assessment
- Assess involved areas of skin and mucous membranes before and frequently during therapy. ↑ skin irritation may indicate need to discontinue medication.

Implementation
- Consult health care provider for proper cleansing technique before applying medication.
- **Vag:** Applicators are supplied for vaginal administration.

Patient/Family Teaching
- Explain purpose and side effects of medication to patient. Advise to read *Patient Information* before starting therapy. Advise patient to apply medication as directed for full course of therapy, even if feeling better. Therapy should be continued during menstrual period.
- Advise patient to notify health care provider of all Rx or OTC medications, vitamins, or herbal products being taken and to consult health care provider before taking other medications, especially cold preparations.
- Advise patient on proper use of vaginal applicator. Medication should be inserted high into the vagina at bedtime. Instruct patient to remain recumbent for >30 min after insertion. Advise use of sanitary napkins to prevent staining of clothing or bedding.
- Advise patient to avoid using tampons while using this product.
- Advise patient to consult health care provider regarding intercourse during therapy. Vaginal medication may cause minor skin irritation in sexual partner. Advise patient to refrain from sexual contact during therapy or have male partner wear a condom. Some products may weaken latex contraceptive devices. Another method of contraception should be used during treatment.
- Advise patient to report to health care provider ↑ skin irritation or lack of response to therapy. A 2nd course may be necessary if symptoms persist.
- Advise patient to stop using medication and notify health care provider immediately if rash or signs and symptoms of anaphylaxis (wheezing, rash, hives, shortness of breath) occur.
- Advise patient to dispose of applicator after each use (except for terconazole).
- Rep: Advise women of reproductive potential to notify health care provider if pregnancy is planned or suspected or if breastfeeding.

Evaluation/Desired Outcomes
- Inhibited growth and death of susceptible *Candida*, with decrease in accompanying symptoms of vulvovaginitis (vaginal burning, itching, discharge).

HIGH ALERT

apalutamide
(a-pa-**loo**-ta-mide)

Erleada

Classification

Therapeutic: antineoplastics

Pharmacologic: androgen receptor inhibitors

A

Indications
Nonmetastatic castration-resistant prostate cancer. Metastatic castration-sensitive prostate cancer.

Action
Acts as an androgen receptor inhibitor, preventing the binding of androgen; also inhibits androgen nuclear translocation and DNA interaction. Decreases proliferation and induces cell death of prostate cancer cells.
Therapeutic Effects: Decreased growth and spread of prostate cancer.

Pharmacokinetics
Absorption: Completely absorbed following oral administration.
Distribution: Extensively distributed to tissues.
Protein Binding: *Apalutamide:* 96%; *N-desmethyl apalutamide:* 95%.
Metabolism and Excretion: Metabolized by the CYP2C8 and CYP3A4 isoenzymes in the liver to an active metabolite (N-desmethyl apalutamide). Primarily excreted in urine (65%) and 24% excreted in feces, with only minimal amounts being excreted as unchanged drug.
Half-life: 3 days.

TIME/ACTION PROFILE (plasma concentrations)

ROUTE	ONSET	PEAK	DURATION
PO	unknown	2 hr	unknown

Contraindications/Precautions
Contraindicated in: None.
Use Cautiously in: History of seizures, underlying brain pathology, cerebrovascular accident, TIA, brain metastases, or brain arteriovenous malformation (may ↑ risk of seizures); Ischemic heart disease, HF, stroke, or TIA; Rep: Men with female partners of reproductive potential; Pedi: Safety and effectiveness not established in children.

Adverse Reactions/Side Effects
CV: hypertension, peripheral edema, MI, unstable angina. **Derm:** hot flushing, rash, DRUG REACTION WITH EOSINOPHILIA AND SYSTEMIC SYMPTOMS (DRESS), pruritus, STEVENS-JOHNSON SYNDROME (SJS), TOXIC EPIDERMAL NECROLYSIS (TEN). **Endo:** hyperglycemia, hypothyroidism. **F and E:** hyperkalemia. **GI:** diarrhea, nausea. **GU:** ↓ fertility (males). **Hemat:** anemia, leukopenia, lymphopenia. **Metab:** ↓ appetite, hypercholesterolemia, hypertriglyceridemia, weight loss. **MS:** arthralgia, fracture. **Neuro:** falls, fatigue, SEIZURES. **Resp:** INTERSTITIAL LUNG DISEASE/PNEUMONITIS.

Interactions
Drug-Drug: Strong CYP2C8 and CYP3A4 inhibitors, including **gemfibrozil**, may ↑ levels and risk of toxicity; may need to ↓ apalutamide dose. May ↓ levels and effectiveness of **CYP3A4, CYP2C9, and CYP2C19 substrates**; avoid concurrent use when possible. May ↓ levels and effectiveness of **fexofenadine** and **rosuvastatin. Drugs that ↓ seizure threshold** may ↑ risk of seizures.

Route/Dosage
PO (Adults): 240 mg once daily.

Availability
Tablets: 60 mg, 240 mg.

NURSING IMPLICATIONS
Assessment
- Monitor for seizures. Implement seizure precautions. If a seizure occurs during therapy, permanently discontinue apalutamide therapy.
- Monitor for signs of ILD/pneumonitis (dyspnea, cough, hypoxia, fever). CT scan or chest x-ray should be done prior to and periodically during therapy to monitor lung status. *If clinically significant symptoms occur,* discontinuation of therapy and/or treatment with corticosteroids and/or antibiotics may be required.
- Assess for falls risk. Institute prevention if indicated. Monitor and manage patients at risk for fractures.
- Monitor patients for development of severe cutaneous adverse reactions, including DRESS, SJS, and TEN. Advise patients of signs and symptoms of these reactions (prodrome of fever, flu-like symptoms, mucosal lesions, progressive skin rash, lymphadenopathy). *If a severe cutaneous adverse reaction is suspected,* interrupt therapy until etiology of reaction is determined. Consultation with a dermatologist is recommended. *If a severe cutaneous adverse reaction is confirmed or for other Grade 4 skin reactions,* permanently discontinue therapy.

Lab Test Considerations
- May cause ↑ TSH levels.

Implementation
- Patients should also receive a gonadotropin-releasing hormone analog concurrently or should have had a bilateral orchiectomy.
- **PO:** Administer four of the 60-mg tablets or one of the 240-mg tablets once daily without regard to food. ***DNC:*** Swallow tablets whole; do not crush, break, dissolve, or chew.
- *For patients with difficulty swallowing:* Tablets can be dispersed in noncarbonated water and then administered with orange juice, applesauce, or additional water. Place tablets in cup. Do not crush or split tablets. Add about 2 teaspoons (10 mL) (for 240-mg tablet) or 4 teaspoons (20 mL) (for 60-mg tablets) of noncarbonated water to make sure tablets

are completely immersed in water. Wait 2 min until tablets are broken up and spread out; then stir mixture. Add 2 tablespoons (30 mL) of orange juice, applesauce, or additional water and stir mixture. Swallow mixture immediately. Rinse cup with enough water to make sure whole dose is taken and drink it immediately; do not save for later. *To administer via feeding tube:* Place one 240-mg tablet in the barrel of syringe (use at least a 20-mL syringe) and draw up 10 mL of noncarbonated water into the syringe. For 60-mg tablets, place all the needed tablets in the barrel of syringe (use at least a 50-mL syringe) and draw up 20 mL of noncarbonated water into the syringe. For the 240-mg or 60-mg tablets, wait 10 min and then shake vigorously to disperse contents completely. Administer immediately through feeding tube. Refill syringe with noncarbonated water and administer. Repeat until no tablet residue is left in syringe or feeding tube.

- *If ≥Grade 3 toxicity or intolerable side effects occur,* withhold dose until symptoms improve to ≤Grade 1; then resume at same or ↓ dose (180 mg or 120 mg). *For Grade 3 or 4 cerebrovascular and ischemic cardiovascular events,* consider permanent discontinuation. *For confirmed severe cutaneous adverse reactions or other Grade 4 skin reactions,* permanently discontinue therapy.

Patient/Family Teaching

- Explain purpose and side effects of apalutamide to patient. Instruct patient to take apalutamide as directed at the same time each day. Take missed doses as soon as remembered within the same day. If a whole day is missed, omit dose and take next day's scheduled dose; do not double doses. Advise patient not to interrupt, modify dose, or stop taking apalutamide without consulting health care professional. Advise patient to read *Patient Information* before starting therapy and with each Rx refill in case of changes.
- Instruct patient to notify health care professional of all Rx or OTC medications, vitamins, or herbal products being taken and to consult health care professional before taking other Rx, OTC, or herbal products.
- May cause seizures, falls, and fractures. Caution patient to avoid driving and other activities requiring alertness until response to medication is known. Notify health care professional immediately if seizure occurs.
- Advise patient to notify health care professional immediately of symptoms of lung problems (e.g. shortness of breath, cough, fever).
- Advise patient to notify health care professional if rash occurs.
- Advise patient to notify health care professional and go to nearest emergency room if signs and symptoms of cardiac problems (chest pain or discomfort at rest or with activity, shortness of breath) occur.
- Rep: May cause fetal harm. Caution patients that apalutamide is not approved for use by females. Advise male patients with female partners of reproductive potential to use effective contraception during and for 3 mo after last dose of therapy. May impair fertility in males of reproductive potential.

Evaluation/Desired Outcomes

- Decreased growth and spread of prostate cancer.

HIGH ALERT

apixaban (a-pix-a-ban)

Eliquis, Eliquis Sprinkle

Classification

Therapeutic: anticoagulants

Pharmacologic: factor Xa inhibitors

Indications

Reduction in risk of stroke/systemic embolism associated with nonvalvular atrial fibrillation. Prevention of deep vein thrombosis (DVT) that may lead to pulmonary embolism (PE) following knee or hip replacement surgery. Treatment of and reduction in risk of recurrence of DVT or PE.

Action

Acts as a selective, reversible site inhibitor of factor Xa, inhibiting both free and bound factor. Does not affect platelet aggregation directly but does inhibit thrombin-induced platelet aggregation. Decreases thrombin generation and thrombus development. **Therapeutic Effects:** Treatment and prevention of thromboembolic events.

Pharmacokinetics

Absorption: 50% absorbed following oral administration.

Distribution: Unknown.

Metabolism and Excretion: Primarily metabolized by the liver by the CYP3A4 isoenzyme; excreted in urine and feces. Biliary and direct intestinal excretion account for fecal elimination.

Half-life: 6 hr (12 hr after repeated dosing due to prolonged absorption).

TIME/ACTION PROFILE (effect on hemostasis)

ROUTE	ONSET	PEAK	DURATION
PO	unknown	3–4 hr†	24 hr

† Blood levels.

Contraindications/Precautions

Contraindicated in: Previous severe hypersensitivity reactions; Active pathological bleeding; Severe hepatic impairment; Prosthetic heart valves; PE with hemodynamic instability or requiring thrombolysis or pulmonary embolectomy; Triple-positive antiphospholipid syndrome (↑ risk of thrombosis); Lactation: Lactation.

Use Cautiously in: Neuroaxial spinal anesthesia or spinal puncture, especially if concurrent with an indwelling epidural catheter; drugs affecting hemostasis; or history of traumatic/repeated spinal puncture or spinal deformity (↑ risk of epidural or spinal hematoma); Surgery; Renal impairment (dose ↓ may be required); Moderate hepatic impairment (↑ risk of bleeding); Rep: Women of reproductive potential; OB: Use during pregnancy only if potential maternal benefit justifies potential fetal risk.

Adverse Reactions/Side Effects

Hemat: BLEEDING. **Misc:** HYPERSENSITIVITY REACTIONS (INCLUDING ANAPHYLAXIS).

Interactions

Drug-Drug: ↑ risk of bleeding with other **anticoagulants**, **aspirin**, **clopidogrel**, **ticagrelor**, **prasugrel**, **fibrinolytics**, **NSAIDs**, **SNRIs**, or **SSRIs**. **Strong CYP3A4 and P-glycoprotein (P-gp) inhibitors**, including **itraconazole**, **ketoconazole**, and **ritonavir**, ↑ levels and risk of bleeding; may need to ↓ apixaban dose or avoid concurrent use. **Strong CYP3A4 and P-gp inducers**, including **carbamazepine**, **phenytoin**, and **rifampin**, may ↓ levels and ↑ risk of thromboses; avoid concurrent use.
Drug-Natural Products: St. John's wort may ↓ levels and ↑ risk of thromboses; avoid concurrent use.

Route/Dosage

Reduction in Risk of Stroke/Systemic Embolism in Nonvalvular Atrial Fibrillation

PO (Adults): 5 mg twice daily; *Any 2 of the following: age ≥80 yr, weight ≤60 kg, serum creatinine ≥1.5 mg/dL:* 2.5 mg twice daily; *Concurrent use of strong CYP3A4 and P-gp inhibitors:* 2.5 mg twice daily; if patient already taking 2.5 mg twice daily, avoid concurrent use.

Renal Impairment

PO (Adults): *Hemodialysis:* 5 mg twice daily; *Hemodialysis and either age ≥80 yr or weight ≤60 kg:* 2.5 mg twice daily.

Prevention of Deep Vein Thrombosis Following Knee or Hip Replacement Surgery

PO (Adults): 2.5 mg twice daily, initiated 12–24 hr postoperatively (when hemostasis is achieved); continued for 35 days after hip replacement or 12 days after knee replacement; *Concurrent use of strong CYP3A4 and P-gp inhibitors:* Avoid concurrent use.

Treatment of Deep Vein Thrombosis or Pulmonary Embolism

PO (Adults): 10 mg twice daily for 7 days; then 5 mg twice daily; *Concurrent use of strong CYP3A4 and P-gp inhibitors:* 2.5 mg twice daily
PO (Children ≥35 kg): 10 mg twice daily for 7 days; then 5 mg twice daily.
PO (Children 25–<35 kg): 8 mg twice daily for 7 days; then 4 mg twice daily.
PO (Children 18–<25 kg): 6 mg twice daily for 7 days; then 3 mg twice daily.
PO (Children 12–<18 kg): 4 mg twice daily for 7 days; then 2 mg twice daily.
PO (Children 9–<12 kg): 3 mg twice daily for 7 days; then 1.5 mg twice daily.
PO (Children 6–<9 kg): 2 mg twice daily for 7 days; then 1 mg twice daily.
PO (Children 4–<6 kg): 1 mg twice daily for 7 days; then 0.5 mg twice daily.
PO (Children 2.6–<4 kg): 0.3 mg twice daily for 7 days; then 0.15 mg twice daily.

Reduction in Risk of Recurrence of Deep Vein Thrombosis or Pulmonary Embolism

PO (Adults): 2.5 mg twice daily after ≥6 mo of treatment of DVT or PE; *Concurrent use of strong CYP3A4 and P-gp inhibitors:* Avoid concurrent use.

Availability

Tablets: 2.5 mg, 5 mg. **Tablets for oral suspension:** 0.5 mg. **Sprinkle capsules:** 0.15 mg.

NURSING IMPLICATIONS

Assessment

- Assess patient for symptoms of stroke, DVT, PE, bleeding, or peripheral vascular disease periodically during therapy. *If pathological hemorrhage occurs,* discontinue apixaban and provide appropriate treatment.
- Monitor frequently for signs and symptoms of neurological impairment in patients with indwelling epidural or intrathecal catheters and after removal. *If neurological compromise occurs,* treat immediately.

Toxicity and Overdose

- Antidote is andexanet alfa, indicated for adults only. Effects persist for ≥24 hr after last dose. Oral activated charcoal also ↓ apixaban plasma concentrations. Other agents and hemodialysis do not have a significant effect.

Implementation

- ***High Alert:*** Do not confuse apixaban with axitinib.
- If apixaban is discontinued for a reason other than bleeding or completion of a course of therapy, consider coverage with another anticoagulant because of ↑ risk of thromboembolism when apixaban is prematurely discontinued.
- When *converting from warfarin,* discontinue warfarin and start apixaban when INR <2.0.

- When *converting from apixaban to warfarin*, apixaban affects INR, so INR measurements may not be useful for determining appropriate dose of warfarin. If continuous anticoagulation is necessary, discontinue apixaban and begin both a parenteral anticoagulant and warfarin at time of next dose of apixaban. Discontinue parenteral anticoagulant when INR reaches acceptable range.
- When *switching between apixaban and anticoagulants other than warfarin*, discontinue one being taken and begin the other at the next scheduled dose.
- *For surgery*, discontinue apixaban ≥48 hr before invasive or surgical procedures with a moderate or high risk of unacceptable or clinically significant bleeding or ≥24 hr prior to procedures with a low risk of bleeding or where the bleeding would be noncritical and easily controlled.
- *For indwelling epidural or intrathecal catheters*, do not remove within 24 hr after the last dose of apixaban; do not administer next dose <5 hr after catheter removal. *If traumatic or repeated puncture occurs,* delay dose for 48 hr.
- **PO:** Administer twice daily without regard to food.
- **For adults and children weighing ≥35 kg who cannot swallow a tablet,** 5 mg and 2.5 mg tablets can be crushed; suspended in water, D5W, or apple juice; or mixed with applesauce and administered immediately orally. May also be suspended in 60 mL of water or D5W and promptly administered through a 12 French nasogastric tube.
- **For children weighing <35 kg,** *capsules* must be opened and entire contents sprinkled in water or infant formula, mixed as described in Instructions for Use (IFU). Administer within 2 hr. Do not swallow capsule. For 0.5 mg *tablet for oral suspension,* mix with water, infant formula, apple juice, or applesauce as described in IFU. Administer mixture within 2 hr or immediately when mixed in applesauce. Each packet is for single use only. Liquid mixtures may be delivered through a 5–12 French nasogastric or gastrostomy tube.

Patient/Family Teaching

- Explain purpose and side effects of medication. Advise patient to read *Patient Information* before starting therapy and to take missed dose as soon as remembered on the same day; then resume twice daily; do not double doses. Do not discontinue without consulting health care provider.
- Advise patient to store apixaban at room temperature.
- Advise patient to notify health care provider immediately if signs of bleeding (easy bruising, discolored urine, red or tarry stools, coughing or vomiting blood, pain or swelling of joints, headache, dizziness, weakness, recurring nosebleed, bleeding from gums, ↑ menstrual bleeding, dyspepsia, abdominal pain, epigastric pain) occur or if injury occurs, especially head injury.
- Caution patient to notify health care provider if skin rash or signs of severe allergic reaction (chest pain or tightness, swelling of face or tongue, trouble breathing or wheezing, feeling dizzy or faint) occur.
- Advise patient to notify health care provider of medication regimen prior to treatment or surgery.
- Instruct patient to notify health care provider of all Rx or OTC medications, vitamins, or herbal products being taken and consult health care provider before taking any new medications, especially St. John's wort. Risk of bleeding is ↑ with aspirin, NSAIDs, warfarin, heparin, SSRIs, or SNRIs.
- Inform patient having had neuraxial anesthesia or spinal puncture to watch for signs and symptoms of spinal or epidural hematoma (numbness or weakness of legs, bowel or bladder dysfunction). Notify health care provider immediately if symptoms occur.
- Rep: Advise women of reproductive potential to notify health care provider if pregnancy is planned or suspected and to avoid breastfeeding during therapy. May ↑ risk of uterine bleeding in pregnant women, fetus, and neonate; advise patient to notify health care provider if significant uterine bleeding occurs.

Evaluation/Desired Outcomes

- Reduction in the risk and treatment of stroke and systemic embolism.

apremilast (a-pre-mil-ast)

Otezla

Classification

Therapeutic: antirheumatics, antipsoriatics
Pharmacologic: phosphodiesterase type 4 inhibitors

Indications

Active psoriatic arthritis. Plaque psoriasis in adults who are candidates for phototherapy or systemic therapy. Moderate to severe plaque psoriasis in children who are candidates for phototherapy or systemic therapy. Oral ulcers associated with Behçet's disease.

Action

Acts as an inhibitor of phosphodiesterase type 4 (PDE4). Inhibition of PDE4 results in ↑ intracellular levels of cyclic adenosine monophosphate. **Therapeutic Effects:** Reduction in severity of psoriatic arthritis with improved joint function. Reduction in severity of plaques. Reduction in number of and pain associated with oral ulcers.

Pharmacokinetics

Absorption: 73% absorbed following oral administration.
Distribution: Unknown.
Metabolism and Excretion: Extensively metabolized (mostly by CYP3A4); metabolites are not pharmacologically active. Excreted in urine (58%)

and feces (39%) as inactive metabolites; 3% excreted unchanged in urine, 7% in feces.
Half-life: 6–9 hr.

TIME/ACTION PROFILE (plasma concentrations†)

ROUTE	ONSET	PEAK	DURATION
PO	unknown	2.5 hr	12–24 hr

† Improvement in joint symptoms make take up to 4 mo.

Contraindications/Precautions

Contraindicated in: Hypersensitivity; Concurrent use of CYP450 enzyme inducers.
Use Cautiously in: History of depression or suicidal ideation; Severe renal impairment (dose ↓ required for CCr <30 mL/min); Taking diuretics or antihypertensive medications (may be at higher risk of complications from severe nausea, vomiting, and diarrhea); OB: Use during pregnancy only if potential maternal benefits justify potential fetal risks; Lactation: Use while breastfeeding only if potential maternal benefits justify potential risks to infant; Pedi: Safety and effectiveness not established in children <18 yr (psoriatic arthritis or Behçet's disease) or <6 yr (plaque psoriasis); Geri: Older adults may be at ↑ risk of complications from severe nausea, vomiting, and diarrhea.

Adverse Reactions/Side Effects

GI: diarrhea, nausea, upper abdominal pain, vomiting. **Metab:** weight loss. **Neuro:** depression, headache. **Misc:** HYPERSENSITIVITY REACTIONS (INCLUDING ANAPHYLAXIS AND ANGIOEDEMA).

Interactions

Drug-Drug: Concurrent use of CYP450 inducers, including **carbamazepine**, **phenobarbital**, **phenytoin** and **rifampin**, may ↓ blood levels and effectiveness; concurrent use should be avoided.

Route/Dosage

Adult Patients with Psoriatic Arthritis, Plaque Psoriasis, or Behçet's Disease

PO (Adults): *Day 1:* 10 mg in the morning; *Day 2:* 10 mg in the morning and 10 mg in the evening; *Day 3:* 10 mg in the morning and 20 mg in the evening; *Day 4:* 20 mg in the morning and 20 mg in the evening; *Day 5:* 20 mg in the morning and 30 mg in the evening; *Day 6 and thereafter:* 30 mg in the morning and 30 mg in the evening.

Renal Impairment

PO (Adults): *CCr <30 mL/min:* Days 1–3: 10 mg in the morning; Days 4–5: 20 mg in the morning; Day 6 and afterward: 30 mg in the morning.

Children with Moderate to Severe Plaque Psoriasis

PO (Children ≥6 yr and ≥50 kg): *Day 1:* 10 mg in the morning; *Day 2:* 10 mg in the morning and 10 mg in the evening; *Day 3:* 10 mg in the morning and 20 mg in the evening; *Day 4:* 20 mg in the morning and 20 mg in the evening; *Day 5:* 20 mg in the morning and 30 mg in the evening; *Day 6 and thereafter:* 30 mg in the morning and 30 mg in the evening.
PO (Children ≥6 yr and 20–<50 kg): *Day 1:* 10 mg in the morning; *Day 2:* 10 mg in the morning and 10 mg in the evening; *Day 3:* 10 mg in the morning and 20 mg in the evening; *Day 4:* 20 mg in the morning and 20 mg in the evening; *Day 5:* 20 mg in the morning and 20 mg in the evening; *Day 6 and thereafter:* 20 mg in the morning and 20 mg in the evening.

Renal Impairment

PO (Children ≥6 yr and ≥50 kg): *CCr <30 mL/min:* Days 1–3: 10 mg in the morning; Days 4–5: 20 mg in the morning; Day 6 and afterward: 30 mg in the morning.

Renal Impairment

PO (Children ≥6 yr and 20–<50 kg): *CCr <30 mL/min:* Days 1–3: 10 mg in the morning; Day 4 and afterward: 20 mg in the morning.

Availability (generic available)

Tablets: 10 mg, 20 mg, 30 mg.

NURSING IMPLICATIONS

Assessment

- Assess pain and range of motion before and periodically during therapy.
- Monitor mental status for signs and symptoms of depression (orientation, mood behavior) frequently. Assess for suicidal tendencies, especially during early therapy.
- Obtain weight and BMI initially and periodically during treatment in adults. Closely monitor height and weight in children. If clinically significant weight loss occurs, evaluate weight loss and consider discontinuation of therapy. Treatment may need to be interrupted if children are not growing or gaining weight as expected.

Implementation

- Follow titration guidelines when beginning therapy to minimize GI side effects.
- **PO:** Administer without regard for meals. ***DNC:*** Swallow tablet whole; do not crush, break, or chew.

Patient/Family Teaching

- Instruct patient to take apremilast as directed.
- Advise patient, family and caregivers to look for suicidality, especially during early therapy or dose

changes. Notify health care professional immediately if thoughts about suicide or dying, attempts to commit suicide, new or worse depression or anxiety, agitation or restlessness, panic attacks, insomnia, new or worse irritability, aggressiveness, acting on dangerous impulses, mania, or other changes in mood or behavior occur.
- Inform patient of risk of nausea, vomiting, and diarrhea. Instruct patient to notify health care professional if severe nausea, vomiting, or diarrhea occur; may need to consider dose reduction or interruption of therapy.
- Inform patient of need to monitor weight regularly. Notify health care professional if unexplained or clinically significant weight loss occurs; may need to discontinue therapy.
- Advise patient to notify health care professional of all Rx or OTC medications, vitamins, or herbal products being taken and to consult with health care professional before taking other medications.
- Rep: Advise patient to notify health care professional if pregnancy is planned or suspected or if breastfeeding.

Evaluation/Desired Outcomes
- Improvement in pain and function in patients with psoriatic arthritis.
- Increased healing of lesions in plaque psoriasis.
- Improvement in oral ulcers associated with Behçet's disease.

aprepitant (a-prep-i-tant)
Aponvie, Cinvanti, Emend

Classification
Therapeutic: antiemetics
Pharmacologic: neurokinin antagonists

Indications
IV, PO: Prevention of: Acute and delayed nausea and vomiting associated with initial and repeat courses of highly emetogenic chemotherapy (in combination with other antiemetic agents) (Cinvanti and Emend); Nausea and vomiting associated with initial and repeat courses of moderately emetogenic chemotherapy (in combination with other antiemetic agents) (Cinvanti and Emend). **IV:** Prevention of delayed nausea and vomiting associated with initial and repeat courses of moderately emetogenic chemotherapy (in combination with other antiemetic agents) (Cinvanti). **IV:** Prevention of postoperative nausea and vomiting (Aponvie).

Action
Acts as a selective antagonist at substance P/neurokinin 1 (NK_1) receptors in the brain. **Therapeutic Effects:** Decreased nausea and vomiting associated with chemotherapy or surgical procedures. Augments the antiemetic effects of dexamethasone and 5-HT_3 antagonists in patients receiving chemotherapy.

Pharmacokinetics
Absorption: 60–65% absorbed following oral administration. IV administration results in complete bioavailability.
Distribution: Crosses the blood-brain barrier; remainder of distribution unknown.
Protein Binding: 95–99%.
Metabolism and Excretion: Mostly metabolized by the liver via the CYP3A4 isoenzyme.
Half-life: 9–13 hr.

TIME/ACTION PROFILE (antiemetic effect)

ROUTE	ONSET	PEAK	DURATION
PO	1 hr	4 hr*	24 hr
IV	rapid	end of infusion*	24 hr

* Plasma concentration.

Contraindications/Precautions
Contraindicated in: Hypersensitivity; Concurrent use with pimozide; OB: Pregnancy (IV only; contains alcohol).
Use Cautiously in: OB: Safety not established in pregnancy (PO only); Rep: Women of reproductive potential; Lactation: Safety not established in breastfeeding; Pedi: Safety and effectiveness not established in children <18 yr (IV) or <6 mo (PO).

Adverse Reactions/Side Effects
CV: dizziness, fatigue, weakness. **Derm:** STEVENS-JOHNSON SYNDROME (SJS). **GI:** diarrhea. **Neuro:** headache. **Misc:** hiccups, HYPERSENSITIVITY REACTIONS (INCLUDING ANAPHYLAXIS).

Interactions
Drug-Drug: May significantly ↑ levels of **pimozide**, which can ↑ risk of torsades de pointes; concurrent use contraindicated. May ↑ levels and risk of toxicity of **CYP3A4 substrates**, including **docetaxel**, **paclitaxel**, **etoposide**, **irinotecan**, **ifosfamide**, **imatinib**, **vinorelbine**, **vinblastine**, **vincristine**, **midazolam**, **triazolam**, and **alprazolam**; concurrent use should be undertaken with caution. **Moderate or strong CYP3A4 inhibitors**, including **ketoconazole**, **itraconazole**, **nefazodone**, **clarithromycin**, **ritonavir**, **nelfinavir**, and **diltiazem**, may ↑ levels and risk of toxicity. **Strong CYP3A4 inducers**, including **rifampin**, **carbamazepine**, and **phenytoin**, may ↓ levels and effectiveness. May ↑ levels and risk of toxicity of **dexamethasone**; regimen reflects a 50% dose ↓. A similar effect occurs with **methylprednisolone**; ↓ IV dose by 25%; ↓ PO dose by 50% when used concurrently. May ↓ the effects of **warfarin** (carefully monitor INR for 2 wk), **oral contraceptives** (use alternate method), and **phenytoin**.

Route/Dosage

Prevention of Acute and Delayed Nausea and Vomiting Associated With Highly Emetogenic Chemotherapy

PO (Adults and Children ≥12 yr): *Capsules:* 125 mg given 1 hr prior to chemotherapy (Day 1); then 80 mg once daily for 2 days (Days 2 and 3). *Suspension (if unable to swallow capsules):* 3 mg/kg (max dose = 125 mg) given 1 hr prior to chemotherapy (Day 1); then 2 mg/kg (max dose = 80 mg) once daily for 2 days (Days 2 and 3).

IV (Adults): *Cinvanti:* 130 mg given 30 min prior to chemotherapy on Day 1 only.

PO (Children 6 mo–<12 yr and >6 kg): *Suspension:* 3 mg/kg (max dose = 125 mg) given 1 hr prior to chemotherapy (Day 1); then 2 mg/kg (max dose = 80 mg) once daily for 2 days (Days 2 and 3).

Prevention of Nausea and Vomiting Associated With Moderately Emetogenic Chemotherapy

PO (Adults and Children ≥12 yr): *Capsules:* 125 mg given 1 hr prior to chemotherapy (Day 1); then 80 mg once daily for 2 days (Days 2 and 3). *Suspension (if unable to swallow capsules):* 3 mg/kg (max dose = 125 mg) given 1 hr prior to chemotherapy (Day 1); then 2 mg/kg (max dose = 80 mg) once daily for 2 days (Days 2 and 3).

IV (Adults): *Cinvanti (single-dose regimen for delayed nausea/vomiting):* 130 mg given 30 min prior to chemotherapy on Day 1 (with dexamethasone 12 mg PO given 30 min prior to chemotherapy and a 5-HT_3 antagonist prior to chemotherapy). *Cinvanti (3-day regimen):* 100 mg given 30 min prior to chemotherapy on Day 1 (with dexamethasone 12 mg PO given 30 min prior to chemotherapy and a 5-HT_3 antagonist prior to chemotherapy). Continue aprepitant 80 mg PO on Days 2 and 3.

PO (Children 6 mo–<12 yr and >6 kg): *Suspension:* 3 mg/kg (max dose = 125 mg) given 1 hr prior to chemotherapy (Day 1); then 2 mg/kg (max dose = 80 mg) once daily for 2 days (Days 2 and 3).

Prevention of Postoperative Nausea and Vomiting

IV (Adults): *Aponvie:* 32 mg as a single dose administered prior to induction of anesthesia.

Availability (generic available)

Capsules (Emend): 40 mg, 80 mg, 125 mg. **Powder for oral suspension (Emend):** 125 mg/pouch. **Emulsion for injection (Aponvie, Cinvanti) (contains alcohol):** 7.2 mg/mL.

NURSING IMPLICATIONS

Assessment

- Assess nausea, vomiting, appetite, bowel sounds, and abdominal pain before and following administration.
- Monitor hydration, nutritional status, and intake and output. Patients with severe nausea and vomiting may require IV fluids in addition to antiemetics.
- Assess for rash periodically during therapy. May cause SJS. Discontinue therapy if severe rash or if accompanied by fever, general malaise, fatigue, muscle or joint aches, blisters, skin peeling, sores, oral lesions, conjunctivitis, hepatitis, or eosinophilia.
- Monitor for signs and symptoms of infusion site reaction (erythema, edema, pain, thrombophlebitis). Treat symptomatically. Avoid infusion into small veins or through a butterfly catheter.
- Monitor for signs and symptoms of hypersensitivity reactions (flushing, erythema, dyspnea, hypotension, syncope) periodically during therapy. If symptoms occur, discontinue therapy and treat symptoms; do not reinitiate therapy if symptoms occur with first use.

Lab Test Considerations

- Monitor INR closely during the 2-wk period, especially at 7–10 days, following aprepitant therapy in patients on chronic warfarin therapy.
- May cause mild, transient ↑ in alkaline phosphatase, AST, ALT, and BUN.
- May cause proteinuria, erythrocyturia, leukocyturia, hyperglycemia, hyponatremia, and ↑ leukocytes.
- May ↓ hemoglobin and WBC.

Implementation

- For chemotherapy, aprepitant is given as part of a regimen that includes a corticosteroid and a 5-HT_3 antagonist (see Route/Dosage).
- **PO:** Administer daily for 3 days. *Day 1:* Administer 1 hr before chemotherapy. *Days 2 and 3:* Administer once in the morning. May be administered without regard to food. ***DNC:*** Swallow capsules whole; do not open, crush, or chew.
- Oral suspension may be used for pediatric patients or those with difficulty swallowing. Follow manufacturer's instructions for preparing suspension. Refrigerate suspension; may be stored at room temperature for up to 3 hr before use. To administer, take cap off, and place dispenser in patient's mouth along inner cheek. Dispense slowly. Discard after 72 hr.

IV Administration

Cinvanti

- Complete injection or infusion 30 min before chemotherapy.
- **IV Push:** Withdraw 18 mL for the 130-mg dose or 14 mL for the 100-mg dose from the vial. Do not dilute. **Rate:** Inject over 2 min. Flush line with 0.9% NaCl before and after injection.
- **Intermittent Infusion:** *For 130-mg dose,* withdraw 18 mL from the injection vial and transfer into

diluent. *For 100-mg dose,* withdraw 14 mL from the aprepitant injection vial and transfer into diluent. **Dilution:** 100 mL of 0.9% NaCl or D5W. Mix by gently inverting bag 4–5 times. Solution is an opaque, off-white emulsion. Do not administer solutions that are discolored or contain particulate matter. May be stored at room temperature for 6 hr if mixed with 0.9% NaCl or 12 hr if mixed with D5W or in refrigerator for up to 72 hr. **Rate:** Infuse over 30 min.

- **Y-Site Incompatibility:** LR, Solutions containing divalent cations (calcium, magnesium).

Emend

- Complete injection or infusion 30 min prior to chemotherapy.
- **Intermittent Infusion: Reconstitution:** Inject 5 mL of 0.9% NaCl into vial along the vial wall to prevent foaming. Swirl vial gently. Avoid shaking and jetting 0.9% NaCl into the vial. **Dilution:** Withdraw entire volume from vial and transfer to infusion bag containing 145 mL of 0.9% NaCl for a volume of 150 mL. **Concentration:** Final concentration of 1 mg/mL. Gently invert bag 2–3 times. Solution is stable for 24 hr at room temperature. Discard unused portion. **Rate:** Infuse over 20–30 min for adults, over 30 min for children 12–17 yr, or over 60 min for children 6 mo to <12 yr. **For children, may also be given as a 3-day regimen via central venous catheter:** *For children 12–17 yr,* Day 1: infuse 115 mg over 30 min; Days 2 and 3: infuse 80 mg over 30 min. *For children 6 mo to <12 yr,* Day 1: infuse 3 mg/kg up to 115 mg over 60 min; Days 2 and 3: infuse 2 mg/kg up to 80 mg over 60 min.
- **Y-Site Incompatibility:** LR, Solutions containing divalent cations (calcium, magnesium).

Aponvie

- **IV Push:** Withdraw 4.4 mL from vial. Solution is opaque and off-white to amber. Do not administer solutions that are discolored or contain particulate matter. Do not dilute. Flush the infusion line with 0.9% NaCl before and after administration. **Rate:** Administer over 30 sec before induction of anesthesia.
- **Y-Site Incompatibility:** D5W, LR, Solutions containing divalent cations (calcium, magnesium).

Patient/Family Teaching

- Explain purpose and side effects of medication to patient. Advise patient to read *Patient Information* before starting therapy. Instruct patient to take as directed.
- Instruct patient to notify health care professional of all Rx or OTC medications, vitamins, or herbal products being taken and consult health care professional before taking any new medications.
- Instruct patient to notify health care professional if nausea and vomiting occur prior to administration.
- Advise patient to notify health care professional immediately if symptoms of hypersensitivity reaction (hives, rash, itching, redness of the face/skin, difficulty in breathing or swallowing) occur.
- Advise patient/caregiver to use general measures to ↓ nausea (begin with sips of liquids and small, nongreasy meals; provide oral hygiene; remove noxious stimuli from environment).
- Rep: Caution women of reproductive potential that aprepitant may ↓ efficacy of oral contraceptives. Advise patient to use effective alternate nonhormonal methods of contraception during and for 1 mo following treatment. Advise women of reproductive potential that *Cinvanti* contains alcohol and may cause fetal harm including central nervous system abnormalities, behavioral disorders, and impaired intellectual development. Avoid use of *Cinvanti* during pregnancy. Advise patient to notify health care professional if pregnancy is planned or suspected or if breastfeeding.

Evaluation/Desired Outcomes

- Decreased nausea and vomiting associated with chemotherapy or surgery.
- Augmentation of antiemetic effects of dexamethasone and 5-HT_3 antagonists in patients receiving chemotherapy.

aprocitentan
(a-proe-sye-**ten**-tan)

Tryvio

Classification

Therapeutic: antihypertensives

Pharmacologic: endothelin receptor antagonists

Indications

Hypertension (in combination with other antihypertensive agents).

Action

Acts as an endothelin receptor antagonist, inhibiting the binding of endothelin-1 to endothelin A and B receptors. **Therapeutic Effects:** Reduction in BP.

Pharmacokinetics

Absorption: Extent of absorption unknown.
Distribution: Well distributed to tissues.
Protein Binding: >99%.
Metabolism and Excretion: Primarily metabolized by the liver via UGT1A1 and UGT2B7. 52% excreted in urine (<1% as unchanged drug); 25% excreted in feces (7% as unchanged drug).
Half-life: 41 hr.

TIME/ACTION PROFILE (plasma concentrations)

ROUTE	ONSET	PEAK	DURATION
PO	unknown	4–5 hr	24 hr

A

Contraindications/Precautions

Contraindicated in: Hypersensitivity; New York Heart Association class III–IV HF; Unstable cardiac disease; NT-pro-BNP ≥500 pg/mL; Severe anemia; End-stage renal disease or hemodialysis; Moderate to severe hepatic impairment or AST/ALT >3 times upper limit of normal; OB: Pregnancy; Lactation: Lactation.
Use Cautiously in: Chronic kidney disease (↑ risk of edema); Rep: Women of reproductive potential; Pedi: Safety and effectiveness not established in children; Geri: Older adults may be at ↑ risk of edema.

Adverse Reactions/Side Effects

CV: edema. **GI:** ↑ liver enzymes. **GU:** ↓ fertility (men). **Hemat:** anemia. **Misc:** hypersensitivity reactions.

Interactions

Drug-Drug: None reported.

Route/Dosage

PO (Adults): 12.5 mg once daily

Availability

Tablets: 12.5 mg.

NURSING IMPLICATIONS

Assessment

- Assess BP and HR before and during treatment. Monitor for hypotension or insufficient BP control.
- Assess for signs and symptoms of fluid retention, weight gain, and worsening HF. If clinically significant fluid retention develops, treat appropriately, and consider discontinuation.

Lab Test Considerations

- Verify negative pregnancy test before starting therapy, monthly during treatment, and 1 mo after discontinuation. If positive pregnancy test, discontinue therapy.
- May cause hepatotoxicity. Measure AST/ALT and total bilirubin before starting treatment and repeat periodically during treatment and as clinically indicated.
- Monitor BUN, serum creatinine, and eGFR periodically during treatment.
- Monitor potassium levels and correct imbalances.
- May ↓ hemoglobin and hematocrit.

Implementation

- **PO:** Administer daily with or without food. Swallow tablets whole.

Patient/Family Teaching

- Explain purpose and side effects of medication. Advise patient to read *Patient Information* before starting therapy. Advise to take as directed. If a dose is missed, skip the missed dose and take the next dose at the regular time. Do not take two doses on the same day.
- Advise patient to notify health care provider of all Rx or OTC medications, vitamins, or herbal products being taken and to consult health care provider before taking other medications.
- Advise patient with symptoms of hepatotoxicity (nausea, vomiting, right upper quadrant pain, fatigue, anorexia, jaundice, dark urine, fever, itching) to immediately stop treatment and notify health care provider.
- Educate patient on signs of fluid retention and to weigh themselves daily. Advise patient to contact health care provider if ↑ weight or swelling of the ankles or legs.
- Educate patient on how to properly measure BP, symptoms of hypotension (dizziness, fainting) and hypertension (headache, visual disturbances).
- Rep: May cause fetal harm. Advise women who can become pregnant to avoid pregnancy and use acceptable contraception before starting treatment, monthly during treatment, and for 1 mo after last dose. Acceptable forms of contraception include an IUD, contraceptive implant, tubal sterilization, a combination of a hormone method plus a barrier method, or two barrier methods. When a hormone method is chosen, a barrier method must also be used. If the patient's partner has had a vasectomy, a hormone or barrier method must also be used. Health care providers should counsel patients on use of emergency contraception. May impair fertility in men. Health care providers should enroll any patient exposed to aprocitentan during pregnancy in the Pregnancy Safety Study by calling 1-866-429-8964.

Evaluation/Desired Outcomes

- Reduction in BP.

HIGH ALERT

argatroban (ar-gat-tro-ban)

Classification
Therapeutic: anticoagulants
Pharmacologic: thrombin inhibitors

Indications

Prophylaxis or treatment of thrombosis in patients with heparin-induced thrombocytopenia (HIT). As an anticoagulant in patients with or at risk for HIT who are undergoing percutaneous coronary intervention (PCI).

Action

Inhibits thrombin by binding to its receptor sites. Inhibition of thrombin prevents activation of factors V, VIII, and XII; the conversion of fibrinogen to fibrin; platelet adhesion and aggregation. **Therapeutic Effects:** Decreased thrombus formation and extension with decreased sequelae of thrombosis (emboli, postphlebitic syndromes).

Pharmacokinetics

Absorption: IV administration results in complete bioavailability.

Distribution: Unknown.

Metabolism and Excretion: Mostly metabolized by the liver; excreted primarily in feces via biliary excretion. 16% excreted unchanged in urine; 14% excreted unchanged in feces.

Half-life: 39–51 min (↑ in hepatic impairment).

TIME/ACTION PROFILE (anticoagulant effect)

ROUTE	ONSET	PEAK	DURATION
IV	immediate	1–3 hr	2–4 hr

Contraindications/Precautions

Contraindicated in: Major bleeding; Hypersensitivity.

Use Cautiously in: Hepatic impairment (↓ initial infusion rate); OB: Use during pregnancy only if potential maternal benefit justifies potential fetal risk; Lactation: Use while breastfeeding only if potential maternal benefit justifies potential risk to infant; Pedi: Safety and effectiveness not established in children.

Adverse Reactions/Side Effects

CV: hypotension. **GI:** diarrhea, nausea, vomiting. **Hemat:** BLEEDING. **Misc:** fever, HYPERSENSITIVITY REACTIONS (INCLUDING ANAPHYLAXIS).

Interactions

Drug-Drug: Risk of bleeding may be ↑ by **antiplatelet agents**, **thrombolytic agents**, or **other anticoagulants**.

Drug-Natural Products: ↑ bleeding risk with **anise, arnica, chamomile, clove, feverfew, garlic, ginger, ginkgo, Panax ginseng**, and others.

Route/Dosage

IV (Adults): 2 mcg/kg/min as a continuous infusion; adjust infusion rate on the basis of activated partial thromboplastin time (aPTT). *Patients undergoing PCI:* 350 mcg/kg bolus followed by infusion at 25 mcg/kg/min, activated clotting time (ACT) should be assessed 5–10 min later. If ACT is 300–450 sec, procedure may be started. If ACT <300 sec, give additional bolus of 150 mcg/kg and ↑ infusion rate to 30 mcg/kg/min. If ACT is >450 sec, infusion rate should be ↓ to 15 mcg/kg/min and ACT rechecked after 5–10 min. If thrombotic complications occur or ACT drops to <300 sec, an additional bolus of 150 mcg/kg may be given and the infusion rate ↑ to 40 mcg/kg/min followed by ACT monitoring. If anticoagulation is required after surgery, lower infusion rates should be used.

Hepatic Impairment

IV (Adults): 0.5 mcg/kg/min as a continuous infusion; adjust infusion rate on the basis of aPTT.

Availability

Premixed infusion: 50 mg/50 mL. **Solution for injection:** 100 mg/mL.

NURSING IMPLICATIONS

Assessment

- Monitor vital signs periodically during therapy. Unexplained ↓ in BP may indicate hemorrhage. Assess patient for bleeding. Minimize arterial and venous punctures, IM injections, and use of urinary catheters, nasotracheal intubation, and nasogastric tubes. Avoid noncompressible sites for IV access. Monitor for blood in urine, lower back pain, or pain or burning on urination. If bleeding cannot be controlled with pressure, ↓ dose or discontinue argatroban immediately.
- Monitor for signs and symptoms of anaphylaxis (rash, coughing, dyspnea) during therapy. Implement medical management (epinephrine) if necessary.

Lab Test Considerations

- Monitor aPTT before initiation of continuous infusion, 2 hr after initiation of therapy, and periodically during therapy to confirm aPTT is within desired therapeutic range.
- For patients undergoing PCI, monitor ACT as described in Route and Dose section.
- Assess hemoglobin, hematocrit, and platelet count before and periodically during argatroban therapy. May ↓ hemoglobin and hematocrit. Unexplained ↓ hematocrit may indicate hemorrhage.
- Use of argatroban concurrently with multiple doses of warfarin will result in more prolonged prothrombin time and INR (although there is not an ↑ in vitamin K–dependent factor Xa activity). Monitor INR daily during concomitant therapy. Repeat INR 4–6 hr after argatroban is discontinued. If repeat value is below desired therapeutic value for warfarin alone, restart argatroban therapy and continue until desired therapeutic range for warfarin alone is reached. To obtain the INR for warfarin alone when dose of argatroban is >2 mcg/kg/min, temporarily ↓ argatroban dose to 2 mcg/kg/min; INR for combined therapy may then be obtained 4–6 hr after argatroban dose was ↓.

Toxicity and Overdose

- There is no specific antidote for argatroban. If overdose occurs, discontinue argatroban. Anticoagulation parameters usually return to baseline with 2–4 hr after discontinuation.

Implementation

- Do not confuse argatroban with Aggrastat.
- Discontinue all parenteral anticoagulants before argatroban therapy is started. Oral anticoagulation may be initiated with maintenance dose of warfarin; do not administer loading dose. Discontinue argatroban therapy when INR for combined therapy is >4.

IV Administration

- **IV:** Do not administer solutions that are cloudy or contain particulate matter. Discard unused portion.
- **IV Push: Dilution:** Bolus dose of 350 mcg/kg should be given prior to continuous infusion in patients undergoing PCI. For diluent information, see Continuous Infusion section below. **Rate:** Administer bolus over 3–5 min.
- **Continuous Infusion: Dilution:** Dilute 250 mg in 250 mL of 0.9% NaCl, D5W, or LR. **Concentration:** 1 mg/mL. Mix by repeated inversion for 1 min. Diluted solution is slightly viscous, clear, and colorless to pale yellow; may show a slight haziness that disappears upon mixing; solution must be clear before use. Solution is stable at controlled room temperature and ambient light for 24 hr, or for 96 hr at controlled room temperature or refrigerated and protected from light; do not expose to direct sunlight. Premixed solutions are clear, colorless, and ready to be infused (no further dilution needed). Store at room temperature; do not refrigerate or freeze.
- **Rate:** Based on patient's weight (see Route/Dosage section). Dose adjustment may be made 2 hr after starting infusion or changing dose until steady-state aPTT is 1.5–3 times the initial baseline value (not to exceed 100 sec).
- **Y-Site Compatibility:** acyclovir, alemtuzumab, allopurinol, amikacin, aminocaproic acid, aminophylline, amphotericin B liposomal, ampicillin, ampicillin/sulbactam, anidulafungin, arsenic trioxide, atracurium, atropine, azithromycin, aztreonam, bivalirudin, bleomycin, bumetanide, buprenorphine, busulfan, butorphanol, calcium acetate, calcium chloride, calcium gluconate, carboplatin, carmustine, caspofungin, cefazolin, cefotaxime, cefotetan, cefoxitin, ceftazidime, ceftriaxone, cefuroxime, chloramphenicol, chlorpromazine, ciprofloxacin, cisatracurium, cisplatin, clindamycin, cyclophosphamide, cyclosporine, cytarabine, dacarbazine, dactinomycin, daptomycin, daptomycin, daunorubicin, dexamethasone, dexmedetomidine, dexrazoxane, digoxin, diltiazem, diphenhydramine, dobutamine, docetaxel, dopamine, doxorubicin hydrochloride, doxorubicin liposomal, doxycycline, droperidol, enalaprilat, ephedrine, epinephrine, epirubicin, eptifibatide, ertapenem, erythromycin, esmolol, etoposide, etoposide phosphate, famotidine, fentanyl, fluconazole, fludarabine, fluorouracil, foscarnet, fosphenytoin, furosemide, ganciclovir, gemcitabine, gemtuzumab ozogamicin, gentamicin, glycopyrrolate, granisetron, haloperidol, heparin, hydralazine, hydrocortisone, hydromorphone, ibutilide, idarubicin, ifosfamide, imipenem/cilastatin, insulin, regular, irinotecan, isoproterenol, ketorolac, labetalol, leucovorin, levofloxacin, lidocaine, linezolid, lorazepam, magnesium sulfate, mannitol, melphalan, meperidine, meropenem, mesna, methadone, methotrexate, methylprednisolone, metoclopramide, metoprolol, midazolam, milrinone, mitomycin, mitoxantrone, morphine, moxifloxacin, mycophenolate, nafcillin, nalbuphine, naloxone, nicardipine, nitroglycerin, nitroprusside, norepinephrine, octreotide, ondansetron, oxaliplatin, oxytocin, paclitaxel, palonosetron, pamidronate, pantoprazole, pentamidine, pentobarbital, phenobarbital, phentolamine, phenylephrine, phenytoin, piperacillin/tazobactam, potassium acetate, potassium chloride, potassium phosphate, procainamide, prochlorperazine, promethazine, propranolol, remifentanil, rocuronium, sodium acetate, sodium bicarbonate, sodium phosphate, succinylcholine, sufentanil, tacrolimus, theophylline, thiotepa, tigecycline, tirofiban, tobramycin, topotecan, trimethoprim/sulfamethoxazole, vancomycin, vasopressin, vecuronium, verapamil, vinblastine, vincristine, vinorelbine, voriconazole, zidovudine, zoledronic acid.
- **Y-Site Incompatibility:** cefepime, dantrolene, diazepam, phenytoin.

Patient/Family Teaching

- Explain the purpose and side effects of the medication to patient.
- Advise patient to avoid other products known to affect bleeding.
- Instruct patient to notify health care professional immediately if any bleeding or signs and symptoms of allergic reaction is noted.
- Rep: Advise women of reproductive potential to notify health care professional if pregnancy is planned or suspected or if breastfeeding.

Evaluation/Desired Outcomes

- Decreased thrombus formation and extension with decreased sequelae of thrombosis (emboli, postphlebitic syndromes).

BEERS

ARIPiprazole

(a-ri-**pip**-ra-zole)

Abilify, Abilify Asimtufii, Abilify Maintena, Aristada, Aristada Initio, Opipza

Classification

Therapeutic: antipsychotics, mood stabilizers

Pharmacologic: serotonin-dopamine activity modulators (SDAM)

Indications

Abilify, Abilify Asimtufii, Abilify Maintena, Aristada, and Opipza: Schizophrenia. **Abilify:**

Treatment of the following conditions: Acute treatment of manic and mixed episodes associated with bipolar I disorder (as monotherapy or with lithium or valproate). Agitation associated with schizophrenia or bipolar disorder. **Abilify Asimtufii and Abilify Maintena:** Maintenance treatment of bipolar I disorder (as monotherapy). **Abilify and Opipza:** Treatment of the following conditions: Adjunctive treatment of depression. Irritability associated with autistic disorder. Tourette disorder.

Action

Psychotropic activity may be due to agonist activity at dopamine D_2 and serotonin 5-HT_{1A} receptors and antagonist activity at the 5-HT_{2A} receptor. Also has $alpha_1$-adrenergic blocking activity. **Therapeutic Effects:** Decreased manifestations of schizophrenia. Decreased mania in bipolar patients. Decreased symptoms of depression. Decreased agitation associated with schizophrenia or bipolar disorder. Decreased emotional and behavioral symptoms of irritability. Decreased incidence of tics.

Pharmacokinetics

Absorption: Well absorbed (87%) following oral administration; 100% following IM injection.
Distribution: Extensively distributed to tissues.
Protein Binding: >99%.
Metabolism and Excretion: Mostly metabolized by the liver by the CYP3A4 and CYP2D6 isoenzymes; the CYP2D6 enzyme system exhibits genetic polymorphism; 7% of population may be poor metabolizers (PMs) and may have significantly ↑ aripiprazole concentrations and an ↑ risk of adverse effects (↓ dose by 50% in PMs); one metabolite (dehydro-aripiprazole) has antipsychotic activity. 18% excreted unchanged in feces; <1% excreted unchanged in urine.
Half-life: *Aripiprazole:* 75 hr; *dehydro-aripiprazole: 94 hr*; ER injectable suspension: 30–46 days (Abilify Maintena); 29–35 days (Aristada).

TIME/ACTION PROFILE (antipsychotic effect)

ROUTE	ONSET	PEAK	DURATION
PO	unknown	2 wk	unknown
ER-IM	unknown	unknown	unknown

Contraindications/Precautions

Contraindicated in: Hypersensitivity; CYP2D6 PMs or concurrent use of strong CYP3A4 inhibitors, strong CYP2D6 inhibitors, or strong CYP3A4 inducers (Aristada Initio only).
Use Cautiously in: May ↑ risk of suicide attempt/ideation, especially during early treatment or dose adjustment; this risk appears to be greater in adolescents or children; Known cardiovascular or cerebrovascular disease; CYP2D6 PMs (↓ dose); Conditions that cause hypotension (dehydration, treatment with antihypertensives or diuretics); Diabetes (may ↑ risk of hyperglycemia); Seizure disorders; Patients at risk for aspiration pneumonia or falls; OB: Use during pregnancy only if potential maternal benefit justifies potential fetal risk; neonates at ↑ risk for extrapyramidal symptoms and withdrawal after delivery when exposed during the 3rd trimester; Lactation: Use while breastfeeding only if potential maternal benefit justifies potential risk to infant; Pedi: Safety and effectiveness not established in children; Geri: Appears on Beers list. ↑ risk of stroke, cognitive decline, and mortality in older adults with dementia. Avoid use in older adults, except for schizophrenia, bipolar disorder, or adjunctive treatment of major depressive disorder.

Adverse Reactions/Side Effects

CV: bradycardia, chest pain, edema, hypertension, orthostatic hypotension, tachycardia. **Derm:** DRUG REACTION WITH EOSINOPHILIA AND SYSTEMIC SYMPTOMS (DRESS), dry skin, ecchymosis, skin ulcer, sweating. **EENT:** blurred vision, conjunctivitis, ear pain. **Endo:** ↓ prolactin, hyperglycemia. **GI:** constipation, ↑ salivation, anorexia, nausea, vomiting, weight loss. **GU:** urinary incontinence. **Hemat:** AGRANULOCYTOSIS, anemia, leukopenia, neutropenia. **Local:** injection site reactions. **Metab:** dyslipidemia, weight gain. **MS:** muscle cramps, neck pain. **Neuro:** drowsiness, extrapyramidal reactions, tremor, abnormal gait, akathisia, confusion, depression, fatigue, hostility, impaired cognitive function, impaired motor function, impulse control disorders (eating/binge eating, gambling, sexual, shopping), insomnia, light-headedness, manic reactions, nervousness, restlessness, sedation, SEIZURES, SUICIDAL THOUGHTS, tardive dyskinesia. **Resp:** dyspnea. **Misc:** ↓ heat regulation, HYPERSENSITIVITY REACTIONS, NEUROLEPTIC MALIGNANT SYNDROME.

Interactions

Drug-Drug: Strong CYP3A4 inhibitors, including **ketoconazole** and **clarithromycin**, may ↑ levels and risk of toxicity; ↓ aripiprazole dose by 50%. **Strong CYP2D6 inhibitors**, including **quinidine**, **fluoxetine**, or **paroxetine**, may ↑ levels and risk of toxicity; ↓ aripiprazole dose by ≥50%. **CYP3A4 inducers** may ↓ levels and effectiveness; double aripiprazole dose.

Route/Dosage

If used concurrently with combination of strong, moderate, or weak CYP3A4 and CYP2D6 inhibitors, ↓ oral aripiprazole dose by 75%. Aripiprazole dose should be ↓ by 75% in CYP2D6 PMs who are concurrently receiving a strong CYP3A4 inhibitor. Do NOT substitute Aristada Initio for Aristada.

Schizophrenia

PO (Adults): 10 or 15 mg once daily; doses up to 30 mg/day have been used; increments in dosing should not be made before 2 wk at a given dose. *CYP2D6 PMs:* ↓ dose by 50%. *CYP2D6 PMs concurrently using CYP3A4 inhibitor:* ↓ dose by 75%. *Concurrent use of strong CYP2D6 or CYP3A4 inhibitor:* ↓ dose by 50%. *Concurrent use of strong CYP2D6 and CYP3A4 inhibitor:* ↓ dose by 75%. *Concurrent use of strong CYP3A4 inducer:* Double usual dose over 1–2 wk.

PO (Children 13–17 yr): 2 mg once daily; ↑ to 5 mg once daily after 2 days, and then to target dose of 10 mg once daily after another 2 days; may further ↑ dose in 5-mg increments if needed (max: 30 mg/day). *CYP2D6 PMs:* ↓ dose by 50%. *CYP2D6 PMs concurrently using CYP3A4 inhibitor:* ↓ dose by 75%. *Concurrent use of strong CYP2D6 or CYP3A4 inhibitor:* ↓ dose by 50%. *Concurrent use of strong CYP2D6 and CYP3A4 inhibitor:* ↓ dose by 75%. *Concurrent use of strong CYP3A4 inducer:* Double usual dose over 1–2 wk.

Abilify Maintena (1-day initiation)

IM (Adults): Administer two injections of 400 mg (total of 800 mg) in two different injection sites and one dose of oral aripiprazole 20 mg on the 1st day of treatment with Abilify Maintena; then continue with 400 mg once monthly. If no adverse reactions to 400 mg once monthly dose, may ↓ dose to 300 mg once monthly. *CYP2D6 PMs:* Administer two injections of 300 mg (total of 600 mg) in two different injection sites and one dose of oral aripiprazole 20 mg on the 1st day of treatment with Abilify Maintena; then continue with 300 mg once monthly. *CYP2D6 PMs concurrently using CYP3A4 inhibitor:* Avoid use; *Concurrent use of strong CYP2D6 or CYP3A4 inhibitor:* Administer two injections of 300 mg (total of 600 mg) in two different injection sites and one dose of oral aripiprazole 20 mg on the 1st day of treatment with Abilify Maintena; then continue with 300 mg once monthly. *Concurrent use of CYP2D6 and CYP3A4 inhibitor:* Avoid use; *Concurrent use of CYP3A4 inducer:* Avoid use.

Abilify Maintena (14-day initiation)

IM (Adults): 400 mg once monthly; after 1st injection, if previously receiving oral aripiprazole, continue treatment with oral aripiprazole (10–20 mg/day) for 14 days. If previously stable on another oral antipsychotic (but known to tolerate aripiprazole), after 1st injection, continue treatment with oral antipsychotic for 14 days. If no adverse reactions to 400 mg once monthly dose, may ↓ dose to 300 mg once monthly. *CYP2D6 PMs:* ↓ dose to 300 mg once monthly; *CYP2D6 PMs concurrently using CYP3A4 inhibitor:* ↓ dose to 200 mg once monthly; *Concurrent use of strong CYP2D6 or CYP3A4 inhibitor:* ↓ dose to 300 mg once monthly (if originally receiving 400 mg once monthly) or 200 mg once monthly (if originally receiving 300 mg once monthly); *Concurrent use of CYP2D6 and CYP3A4 inhibitor:* ↓ dose to 200 mg once monthly (if originally receiving 400 mg once monthly) or 160 mg once monthly (if originally receiving 300 mg once monthly); *Concurrent use of CYP3A4 inducer:* Avoid use.

Abilify Asimtufii (1-day initiation)

IM (Adults): *Receiving oral antipsychotics:* Administer one injection of Abilify Asimtufii 960 mg in the gluteal muscle, one injection of Abilify Maintena 400 mg in a separate gluteal or deltoid muscle, and one dose of oral aripiprazole 20 mg on the first day of treatment with Abilify Asimtufii; then continue with Abilify Asimtufii 960 mg every 2 mo. *CYP2D6 PMs:* Administer one injection of Abilify Asimtufii 720 mg in the gluteal muscle, one injection of Abilify Maintena 300 mg in a separate gluteal or deltoid muscle, and one dose of oral aripiprazole 20 mg on the first day of treatment with Abilify Asimtufii; then continue with Abilify Asimtufii 720 mg every 2 mo; *CYP2D6 PMs concurrently using CYP3A4 inhibitor:* Avoid use; *Concurrent use of strong CYP2D6 or CYP3A4 inhibitor:* Administer one injection of Abilify Asimtufii 720 mg in the gluteal muscle, one injection of Abilify Maintena 300 mg in a separate gluteal or deltoid muscle, and one dose of oral aripiprazole 20 mg on the first day of treatment with Abilify Asimtufii; then continue with Abilify Asimtufii 720 mg every 2 mo; *Concurrent use of strong CYP2D6 and strong CYP3A4 inhibitor:* Avoid use; *Concurrent use of CYP3A4 inducer:* Avoid use.

Abilify Asimtufii (14-day initiation)

IM (Adults): *Receiving oral antipsychotics:* 960 mg every 2 mo (56 days after previous injection); after 1st injection, if previously receiving oral aripiprazole, continue treatment with oral aripiprazole (10–20 mg/day) for 14 days. If previously stable on another oral antipsychotic (but known to tolerate aripiprazole), after 1st injection, continue treatment with oral antipsychotic for 14 days. *Previously receiving Abilify Maintena:* 960 mg every 2 mo in place of the next scheduled Abilify Maintena injection; the 1st injection may be administered in place of the 2nd or later injection of Abilify Maintena; *CYP2D6 PMs:* ↓ dose to 720 mg every 2 mo; *CYP2D6 PMs concurrently using CYP3A4 inhibitor:* Avoid use; *Concurrent use of strong CYP2D6 or CYP3A4 inhibitor:* ↓ dose to 720 mg every 2 mo; *Concurrent use of strong CYP2D6 and strong CYP3A4 inhibitor:* Avoid use; *Concurrent use of CYP3A4 inducer:* Avoid use.

Aristada

IM (Adults): *With Aristada Initio:* Administer 675-mg injection of Aristada Initio **with** first injection of Aristada (dose is based on total daily dose of oral aripiprazole; if patient receiving 10 mg/day of oral aripiprazole, administer 441 mg once monthly; if patient receiving 15 mg/day of oral aripiprazole, administer 662 mg once monthly, 882 mg every 6 wk, or 1064 mg every 2 mo; if patient receiving ≥20 mg/day of oral aripiprazole, administer 882 mg once monthly) (initial Aristada dose can be given on same day as or within 10 days of Aristada Initio) **AND** one dose of oral aripiprazole 30 mg; *Without Aristada Initio:* Dose is based on total daily dose of oral aripiprazole; if patient receiving 10 mg/day of oral aripiprazole, administer 441 mg once monthly; if patient receiving 15 mg/day of oral aripiprazole, administer 662 mg once monthly, 882 mg every 6 wk, or 1064 mg every 2 mo; if patient receiving ≥20 mg/day of oral aripiprazole, administer 882 mg once monthly; after 1st injection; continue treatment with oral aripiprazole for 21 days; *Concurrent use of strong CYP2D6 or CYP3A4 inhibitor for >2 wk:* ↓ dose of Aristada to 441 mg once monthly (if originally receiving 662 mg once monthly) or 662 mg once monthly (if originally receiving 882 mg once monthly); no dose adjustment necessary if originally receiving 441 mg once monthly; avoid use of Aristada Initio; *CYP2D6 PMs concurrently using strong CYP3A4 inhibitor for >2 wk:* ↓ dose of Aristada to 441 mg once monthly (if originally receiving 662 mg or 882 mg once monthly); no dose adjustment necessary if originally receiving 441 mg once monthly; avoid use of Aristada Initio; *Concurrent use of strong CYP2D6 and CYP3A4 inhibitor:* Avoid use of Aristada in patients requiring 662 mg or 882 mg once monthly dose; no dose adjustment of Aristada necessary if originally receiving 441 mg once monthly; avoid use of Aristada Initio; *Concurrent use of CYP3A4 inducer:* ↑ dose of Aristada to 662 mg once monthly (if originally receiving 441 mg once monthly); no dose adjustment if Aristada necessary if originally receiving 662 mg or 882 mg once monthly; avoid use of Aristada Initio.

Acute Manic or Mixed Episodes Associated With Bipolar I Disorder

PO (Adults): 15 mg once daily as monotherapy or 10–15 mg once daily with lithium or valproate; target dose is 15 mg once daily; may ↑ to 30 mg once daily, if needed. *CYP2D6 PMs:* ↓ dose by 50%. *CYP2D6 PMs concurrently using CYP3A4 inhibitor:* ↓ dose by 75%. *Concurrent use of strong CYP2D6 or CYP3A4 inhibitor:* ↓ dose by 50%. *Concurrent use of strong CYP2D6 and CYP3A4 inhibitor:* ↓ dose by 75%. *Concurrent use of strong CYP3A4 inducer:* Double usual dose over 1–2 wk.

PO (Children 10–17 yr): 2 mg once daily; ↑ to 5 mg once daily after 2 days, and then to target dose of 10 mg once daily after another 2 days; may further ↑ dose in 5-mg increments if needed (max: 30 mg/day). *CYP2D6 PMs:* ↓ dose by 50%. *CYP2D6 PMs concurrently using CYP3A4 inhibitor:* ↓ dose by 75%. *Concurrent use of strong CYP2D6 or CYP3A4 inhibitor:* ↓ dose by 50%. *Concurrent use of strong CYP2D6 and CYP3A4 inhibitor:* ↓ dose by 75%. *Concurrent use of strong CYP3A4 inducer:* Double usual dose over 1–2 wk.

Maintenance Treatment of Bipolar I Disorder

Abilify Maintena (1-day initiation)

IM (Adults): Administer two injections of 400 mg (total of 800 mg) in two different injection sites and one dose of oral aripiprazole 20 mg on the 1st day of treatment with Abilify Maintena; then continue with 400 mg once monthly. If no adverse reactions to 400 mg once monthly dose, may ↓ dose to 300 mg once monthly. *CYP2D6 PMs:* Administer two injections of 300 mg (total of 600 mg) in two different injection sites and one dose of oral aripiprazole 20 mg on the 1st day of treatment with Abilify Maintena; then continue with 300 mg once monthly. *CYP2D6 PMs concurrently using CYP3A4 inhibitor:* Avoid use; *Concurrent use of strong CYP2D6 or CYP3A4 inhibitor:* Administer two injections of 300 mg (total of 600 mg) in two different injection sites and one dose of oral aripiprazole 20 mg on the 1st day of treatment with Abilify Maintena; then continue with 300 mg once monthly. *Concurrent use of CYP2D6 and CYP3A4 inhibitor:* Avoid use; *Concurrent use of CYP3A4 inducer:* Avoid use.

Abilify Maintena (14-day initiation)

IM (Adults): 400 mg once monthly; after 1st injection, if previously receiving oral aripiprazole, continue treatment with oral aripiprazole (10–20 mg/day) for 14 days. If previously stable on another oral antipsychotic (but known to tolerate aripiprazole), after 1st injection, continue treatment with oral antipsychotic for 14 days. If no adverse reactions to 400 mg once monthly dose, may ↓ dose to 300 mg once monthly. *CYP2D6 PMs:* ↓ dose to 300 mg once monthly; *CYP2D6 PMs concurrently using CYP3A4 inhibitor:* ↓ dose to 200 mg once monthly; *Concurrent use of strong CYP2D6 or CYP3A4 inhibitor:* ↓ dose to 300 mg once monthly (if originally receiving 400 mg once monthly) or 200 mg once monthly (if originally receiving 300 mg once monthly); *Concurrent use of CYP2D6 and CYP3A4 inhibitor:* ↓ dose to 200 mg once monthly (if originally receiving 400 mg once monthly) or 160 mg once monthly (if originally receiving 300 mg once monthly); *Concurrent use of CYP3A4 inducer:* Avoid use.

Abilify Asimtufii

IM (Adults): *Receiving oral antipsychotics:* 960 mg every 2 mo (56 days after previous injection); after 1st injection, if previously receiving oral aripiprazole, continue treatment with oral aripiprazole (10–20 mg/day) for 14 days. If previously stable on another oral antipsychotic (but known to tolerate aripiprazole), after 1st injection, continue treatment with oral antipsychotic for 14 days. *Previously receiving Abilify Maintena:* 960 mg every 2 mo in place of the next scheduled Abilify Maintena injection; the 1st injection may be administered in place of the 2nd or later injection of Abilify Maintena; *CYP2D6 PMs:* ↓ dose to 720 mg every 2 mo; *CYP2D6 PMs concurrently using* *strong CYP3A4 inhibitor:* Avoid use; *Concurrent use of strong CYP2D6 or CYP3A4 inhibitor:* ↓ dose to 720 mg every 2 mo; *Concurrent use of strong CYP2D6 and CYP3A4 inhibitor:* Avoid use; *Concurrent use of CYP3A4 inducer:* Avoid use.

Depression

PO (Adults): 2–5 mg once daily; may titrate upward at 1-wk intervals to 5–10 mg once daily (max: 15 mg/day). *CYP2D6 PMs:* ↓ dose by 50%. *CYP2D6 PMs concurrently using CYP3A4 inhibitor:* ↓ dose by 75%. *Concurrent use of strong CYP2D6 or CYP3A4 inhibitor:* ↓ dose by 50%. *Concurrent use of strong CYP2D6 and CYP3A4 inhibitor:* ↓ dose by 75%. *Concurrent use of strong CYP3A4 inducer:* Double usual dose over 1–2 wk.

Irritability Associated with Autistic Disorder

PO (Children 6–17 yr): 2 mg once daily; ↑ to 5 mg once daily after at least 1 wk; may further ↑ dose in 5-mg increments if needed at ≥1-wk intervals (max: 15 mg/day). *CYP2D6 PMs:* ↓ dose by 50%. *CYP2D6 PMs concurrently using CYP3A4 inhibitor:* ↓ dose by 75%. *Concurrent use of strong CYP2D6 or CYP3A4 inhibitor:* ↓ dose by 50%. *Concurrent use of strong CYP2D6 and CYP3A4 inhibitor:* ↓ dose by 75%. *Concurrent use of strong CYP3A4 inducer:* Double usual dose over 1–2 wk.

Tourette Disorder

PO (Children 6–18 yr and ≥50 kg): 2 mg once daily; ↑ to target dose of 5 mg once daily after 2 days; may further ↑ dose if needed at ≥1-wk intervals (max: 10 mg/day). *CYP2D6 PMs:* ↓ dose by 50%. *CYP2D6 PMs concurrently using CYP3A4 inhibitor:* ↓ dose by 75%. *Concurrent use of strong CYP2D6 or CYP3A4 inhibitor:* ↓ dose by 50%. *Concurrent use of strong CYP2D6 and CYP3A4 inhibitor:* ↓ dose by 75%. *Concurrent use of strong CYP3A4 inducer:* Double usual dose over 1–2 wk.

PO (Children 6–18 yr and <50 kg): 2 mg once daily; ↑ to 5 mg once daily after 2 days, and then to target dose of 10 mg once daily after 5 days; may further ↑ dose in 5-mg increments if needed at ≥1-wk intervals (max: 20 mg/day). *CYP2D6 PMs:* ↓ dose by 50%. *CYP2D6 PMs concurrently using CYP3A4 inhibitor:* ↓ dose by 75%. *Concurrent use of strong CYP2D6 or CYP3A4 inhibitor:* ↓ dose by 50%. *Concurrent use of strong CYP2D6 and CYP3A4 inhibitor:* ↓ dose by 75%. *Concurrent use of strong CYP3A4 inducer:* Double usual dose over 1–2 wk.

Availability (generic available)

Immediate-release tablets: 2 mg, 5 mg, 10 mg, 15 mg, 20 mg, 30 mg. **Orally disintegrating tablets (vanilla flavor):** 10 mg, 15 mg. **Oral film (Opipza):** 2 mg, 5 mg, 10 mg. **Oral solution (orange cream):** 1 mg/mL. **Extended-release suspension for injection (Abilify Maintena) (prefilled syringes or vials):** 300 mg, 400 mg. **Extended-release suspension for injection (Aristada) (prefilled syringes):** 441 mg/1.6 mL, 662 mg/2.4 mL, 882 mg/3.2 mL, 1064 mg/3.9 mL. **Extended-release suspension for injection (Aristada Initio) (prefilled syringes):** 675 mg/2.4 mL. **Extended-release suspension for injection (Abilify Asimtufii) (prefilled syringes):** 720 mg/2.4 mL, 960 mg/3.2 mL.

NURSING IMPLICATIONS

Assessment

- Assess mental status (orientation, mood, behavior) before and periodically during therapy.
- Assess for suicidal tendencies, especially during early therapy. Restrict amount of drug available to patient. Risk may be ↑ in adults ≤24 yr. After starting therapy, young adults should be seen by health care provider at least weekly for 4 wk, every 3 wk for next 4 wk, and on advice of health care provider thereafter.
- Assess weight and body mass index initially and during therapy. Compare weight of children and adolescents with that expected during normal growth.
- Monitor BP (sitting, standing, lying), HR, and respiratory rate before and periodically during therapy.
- Observe patient carefully when administering medication to ensure that medication is actually taken and not hoarded or cheeked.
- Monitor patient for onset of akathisia (restlessness or desire to keep moving) and extrapyramidal side effects (*parkinsonian:* difficulty speaking or swallowing, loss of balance control, pill rolling of hands, masklike face, shuffling gait, rigidity, tremors; and *dystonic:* muscle spasms, twisting motions, twitching, inability to move eyes, weakness of arms or legs) periodically during therapy. Report these symptoms.
- Monitor for tardive dyskinesia (uncontrolled rhythmic movement of mouth, face, and extremities; lip smacking or puckering; puffing of cheeks; uncontrolled chewing; rapid or worm-like movements of tongue). Notify health care provider immediately if these symptoms occur, as these side effects may be irreversible.
- Monitor for development of neuroleptic malignant syndrome (fever, muscle rigidity, altered mental status, respiratory distress, tachycardia, seizures, diaphoresis, hypertension or hypotension, pallor, tiredness, loss of bladder control). Notify health care provider immediately if these symptoms occur.
- Assess for falls risk. Drowsiness, orthostatic hypotension, and motor and sensory instability ↑ risk. Institute prevention as indicated.

- Assess for injection site reactions (pain at site, redness, irritation).

Lab Test Considerations

- May ↑ CK.
- Monitor CBC frequently during initial months of therapy in patients with pre-existing or history of low WBC. May cause leukopenia, neutropenia, or agranulocytosis. Discontinue therapy if this occurs.
- Monitor blood glucose and cholesterol levels before starting and periodically during therapy. Patients with diabetes or risk factors for diabetes mellitus (obesity, family history of diabetes) who are starting treatment with atypical antipsychotics should undergo fasting blood glucose testing at beginning and periodically during therapy.

Implementation

- Do not confuse aripiprazole with rabeprazole or proton pump inhibitors.
- *Aristada Initio* is only used as a one-time dose to initiate *Aristada* therapy or if doses of *Aristada* are missed. Administer missed doses as soon as possible; may supplement next *Aristada* injection with *Aristada Initio.* **If last Aristada injection 441 mg** *and time since last injection ≤6 wk,* do not supplement; *if >6 wk but ≤7 wk since last dose,* supplement with single dose of *Aristada Initio*; *if >7 wk since last dose,* reinitiate with a single dose of *Aristada Initio* and a single dose of oral aripiprazole 30 mg. **If last Aristada injection 662 mg or 882 mg** *and time since last injection ≤8 wk,* do not supplement; *if >8 wk but ≤12 wk since last dose,* supplement with single dose of *Aristada Initio*; *if ≥12 wk since last dose,* reinitiate with a single dose of *Aristada Initio* and a single dose of oral aripiprazole 30 mg. **If last Aristada injection 1064 mg** *and time since last injection ≤10 wk,* do not supplement; *if >8 wk but ≤12 wk since last dose,* supplement with single dose of *Aristada Initio*; *if ≥12 wk since last dose,* reinitiate with a single dose of *Aristada Initio* and a single dose of oral aripiprazole 30 mg.
- **PO:** Administer once daily without regard to meals.
- *Orally disintegrating tablets:* Do not open blister until ready to administer. For single tablet removal, open package and peel back foil on blister to expose tablet. Do not push tablet through foil; may damage tablet. Immediately upon opening blister, using dry hands, remove tablet and place entire oral disintegrating tablet on tongue. Tablet disintegration occurs rapidly in saliva. Take tablet without liquid, but if needed, it can be taken with liquid. Do not attempt to split tablet.
- **Extended-Release IM:** *Abilify Maintena* is available in vials or dual chamber prefilled syringes. *For vials,* reconstitute 300-mg vial with 1.5 mL and 400-mg vial with 1.9 mL of sterile water for injection; discard extra sterile water. Withdraw air to equalize pressure in vial. Shake vial vigorously for 30 sec until suspension is uniform; suspension is opaque and milky white. If injection is not given immediately, shake vial vigorously to resuspend prior to injection. Do not store suspension in syringe. Determine volume needed for dose: from 400-mg vial: 400 mg = 2 mL, 300 mg = 1.5 mL, 200 mg = 1.0, and 160 mg = 0.8 mL. From 300-mg vial: 300 mg = 1.5 mL, 200 mg = 1 mL, and 160 mg = 0.8 mL. *For prefilled syringes,* push plunger rod slightly to engage threads. Rotate plunger rod until rod stops rotating to release diluent; middle stopper will be at indicator line. Vertically shake syringe vigorously for 20 sec until drug is uniformly milky-white. *For deltoid site,* use 23-gauge needle, 1 inch in length, for nonobese patients and 22-gauge, 1½ inches, for obese patients. *For gluteal site,* use 22-gauge needle, 1½ inches in length, for nonobese patients and 22-gauge, 2 inches, for obese patients. Inject deep into deltoid or gluteal site; do not massage. Continue oral dosing of aripiprazole for 2 wk after 1st dose of *Abilify Maintena*. *Abilify Maintena* should be administered no sooner than 26 days after the previous injection.
- If 2nd or 3rd doses of *Abilify Maintena* are missed and >4 wk but <5 wk since last injection, administer injection as soon as possible. Resume monthly injections no sooner than 26 days later. If >5 wk since last injection, reinitiate treatment with single or double injection start. If 4th or subsequent doses are missed and >4 wk but <6 wk since last injection, administer injection as soon as possible. Resume monthly injections no sooner than 26 days later. If >6 wk since last injection, reinitiate treatment with single or double injection start.
- *Aristada* comes in a kit with several needle sizes. Tap syringe ≥10 times to dislodge settled material, and shake syringe vigorously for ≥30 sec to ensure suspension is uniform. Shake again if syringe not used within 15 min. Select needle and injection site. Deltoid may be used for 441 mg dose only. May use gluteal site for all doses. Remove air from syringe. Inject entire contents rapidly and continuously over <10 sec.
- *Abilify Asimtufii* must be administered as an IM gluteal injection by a health care provider. Do not administer by any other route. For patients who have never taken aripiprazole, establish tolerability with oral aripiprazole prior to initiating treatment with *Abilify Asimtufii*. Due to the half-life of oral aripiprazole, it may take up to 2 wk to fully assess tolerability. The suspension should appear to be a uniform, homogeneous suspension that is opaque and milky-white in color. Do not use *Abilify Asimtufii* prefilled syringe if the suspension is discolored or contains particulate matter. Tap syringe on your hand ≥10 times. After tapping, shake syringe vigorously for ≥10 sec until medication is uniform. For nonobese patients use a 22-gauge, 1½-inch needle; for

obese patients use a 21-gauge, 2-inch needle. Slowly inject the entire contents of prefilled syringe IM into gluteal muscle of patient; do not massage injection site. *Abilify Asimtufii* should be administered no sooner than 56 days after previous injection.

- If dose of *Abilify Asimtufii* is missed >8 wk but <14 wk since last injection, administer dose as soon as possible. Resume regular maintenance injections no sooner than 2 mo later. If >14 wk since last injection, reinitiate treatment with single or double injection start.
- ***Opipza:*** Administer orally with or without food. Apply on top of the tongue to dissolve in saliva. Can be swallowed without liquid. Administer only one film at a time. If additional film is needed, administer after the previous film has completely dissolved. Refrain from chewing or swallowing undissolved film. Do not cut or split film.

Patient/Family Teaching

- Explain purpose and side effects of medication. Advise patient to read *Patient Information* before starting therapy. Advise patient to take medication as directed and not to skip doses or double up on missed doses. Explain what the following steps would be if an injection dose is missed.
- Instruct patient to notify health care provider of all Rx or OTC medications, vitamins, or herbal products being taken and to consult health care provider before taking any new medications. Caution patient to avoid taking alcohol or other CNS depressants concurrently with this medication.
- Inform patient of possibility of extrapyramidal symptoms and tardive dyskinesia. Instruct patient to report these symptoms immediately.
- Advise patient to make position changes slowly to minimize orthostatic hypotension.
- Medication may cause drowsiness and light-headedness. Caution patient to avoid driving or other activities requiring alertness until response to medication is known.
- Advise patient, family, and caregivers to look for suicidality, especially during early therapy or dose changes. Notify health care provider immediately if thoughts about suicide or dying, attempts to commit suicide, new or worse depression or anxiety, agitation or restlessness, panic attacks, insomnia, new or worse irritability, aggressiveness, acting on dangerous impulses, mania, or other changes in mood or behavior occur.
- Inform patient that aripiprazole may cause weight gain. Advise patient to monitor weight periodically. Notify health care provider of significant weight gain.
- Advise patient that extremes in temperature should be avoided, because this drug impairs body temperature regulation.
- Advise patient to notify health care provider if new or ↑ eating/binge eating, gambling, sexual, shopping, or other impulse control disorders occur.
- Advise patient to notify health care provider of medication regimen prior to treatment or surgery.
- Emphasize the importance of routine follow-up exams and continued participation in psychotherapy as indicated.
- Rep: Advise women of reproductive potential to notify health care provider if pregnancy is planned or suspected or if breastfeeding. Extrapyramidal and/or withdrawal symptoms (agitation, hypertonia, hypotonia, tremor, somnolence, respiratory distress, feeding disorder) have been reported in neonates who were exposed to antipsychotic drugs during the 3rd trimester of pregnancy. Monitor neonates closely. Encourage pregnant patients to enroll in pregnancy exposure registry by contacting National Pregnancy Registry for Atypical Antipsychotics at 1-866-961-2388 or visit http://womensmentalhealth.org/clinical-and-research-programs/pregnancyregistry/.

Evaluation/Desired Outcomes

- Decreased manifestations of schizophrenia.
- Decreased mania in bipolar patients.
- Decreased symptoms of depression.
- Decreased agitation associated with schizophrenia or bipolar disorder.
- Decreased emotional and behavioral symptoms of irritability.
- Decreased incidence of tics.

BEERS

aspirin (as-pir-in)

Acuprin, ✱ Asaphen, Aspergum, Aspir-Low, Aspirtab, Bayer Aspirin, Bayer Timed-Release Arthritic Pain Formula, Easprin, Ecotrin, 8-Hour Bayer Timed-Release, Empirin, ✱ Entrophen, Halfprin, Healthprin, ✱ Lowprin, Norwich Aspirin, ✱ Novasen, ✱ Rivasa, Sloprin, St. Joseph Adult Chewable Aspirin, Therapy Bayer, Vazalore, ZORprin

Classification

Therapeutic: antiplatelet agents, antipyretics, nonopioid analgesics

Pharmacologic: salicylates, nonsteroidal anti-inflammatory drugs (NSAIDs)

Indications

Inflammatory disorders, including: Rheumatoid arthritis, Osteoarthritis. Mild to moderate pain. Fever.

Prophylaxis of transient ischemic attacks and MI. **Unlabeled Use:** Adjunctive treatment of Kawasaki disease.

Action

Produce analgesia and reduce inflammation and fever by inhibiting the production of prostaglandins. Decreases platelet aggregation. **Therapeutic Effects:** Analgesia. Reduction of inflammation. Reduction of fever. Decreased incidence of transient ischemic attacks and MI.

Pharmacokinetics

Absorption: Well absorbed from the upper small intestine; absorption from enteric-coated preparations may be unreliable; rectal absorption is slow and variable.
Distribution: Rapidly and widely distributed; crosses the placenta and enters breast milk.
Metabolism and Excretion: Extensively metabolized by the liver; inactive metabolites excreted by the kidneys. Amount excreted unchanged by the kidneys depends on urine pH; as pH ↑, amount excreted unchanged ↑ from 2–3% up to 80%.
Half-life: 2–3 hr for low doses; up to 15–30 hr with larger doses because of saturation of liver metabolism.

TIME/ACTION PROFILE (analgesia/↓ fever)

ROUTE	ONSET	PEAK	DURATION
PO	5–30 min	1–3 hr	3–6 hr

Contraindications/Precautions

Contraindicated in: Hypersensitivity to aspirin or other salicylates; Cross-sensitivity with other NSAIDs may exist (less with nonaspirin salicylates); Bleeding disorders or thrombocytopenia; OB: Avoid use after 30 wk gestation; Pedi: May ↑ risk of Reye syndrome in children or adolescents with viral infections.
Use Cautiously in: History of GI bleeding or ulcer disease; Chronic alcohol use/abuse; Severe renal impairment; Severe hepatic impairment; OB: Use at or after 20 wk gestation may cause fetal or neonatal renal impairment; if NSAID treatment is necessary between 20 wk and 30 wk gestation, limit use to the lowest effective dose and shortest duration possible; Lactation: Safety not established in breastfeeding; Geri: Appears on Beers list. ↑ risk of major bleeding in older adults. Avoid use for primary prevention of cardiovascular disease in older adults. Avoid chronic use for pain (at doses >325 mg/day) in older adults unless other alternatives are not effective and the patient can take a gastroprotective agent; avoid short-term use for pain (at doses >325 mg/day) in older adults in combination with oral or parenteral corticosteroids, anticoagulants, or antiplatelet agents unless other alternatives are not effective and the patient can take a gastroprotective agent.

Adverse Reactions/Side Effects

Derm: DRUG REACTION WITH EOSINOPHILIA AND SYSTEMIC SYMPTOMS (DRESS), EXFOLIATIVE DERMATITIS, GENERALIZED BULLOUS FIXED DRUG ERUPTION, rash, STEVENS-JOHNSON SYNDROME (SJS), TOXIC EPIDERMAL NECROLYSIS (TEN), urticaria. **EENT:** tinnitus. **GI:** dyspepsia, epigastric distress, nausea, abdominal pain, anorexia, GI BLEEDING, hepatotoxicity, vomiting. **Hemat:** anemia, hemolysis. **Misc:** HYPERSENSITIVITY REACTIONS (INCLUDING ANAPHYLAXIS, LARYNGEAL EDEMA, AND SERIOUS SKIN REACTIONS).

Interactions

Drug-Drug: May ↑ the risk of bleeding with **warfarin**, **heparin**, **heparin-like agents**, **thrombolytic agents**, **dipyridamole**, **clopidogrel**, **tirofiban**, or **eptifibatide**, although these agents are frequently used safely in combination and in sequence. **Ibuprofen:** may negate the cardioprotective antiplatelet effects of low-dose aspirin. May ↑ risk of bleeding with **cefotetan** and **valproic acid**. May ↑ activity of **penicillins**, **phenytoin**, **methotrexate**, **valproic acid**, **oral hypoglycemic agents**, and **sulfonamides**. **Urinary acidification** ↑ reabsorption and may ↑ serum salicylate levels. **Alkalinization of the urine** or the ingestion of large amounts of **antacids** ↑ excretion and ↓ serum salicylate levels. May blunt the therapeutic response to **diuretics** and **ACE inhibitors**. ↑ risk of GI irritation with **NSAIDs**.
Drug-Natural Products: ↑ anticoagulant effect and bleeding risk with **arnica**, **chamomile**, **clove**, **feverfew**, **garlic**, **ginger**, **ginkgo**, **Panax ginseng**, and others.
Drug-Food: Foods capable of acidifying the urine (see Appendix J) may ↑ serum salicylate levels.

Route/Dosage

Pain/Fever

PO, Rect (Adults): 325–1000 mg every 4–6 hr (not to exceed 4 g/day). *Extended-release tablets:* 650 mg every 8 hr or 800 mg every 12 hr.
PO, Rect (Children 2–11 yr): 10–15 mg/kg/dose every 4–6 hr; maximum dose: 4 g/day.

Inflammation

PO (Adults): 2.4 g/day initially; ↑ to maintenance dose of 3.6–5.4 g/day in divided doses (up to 7.8 g/day for acute rheumatic fever).
PO (Children): 60–100 mg/kg/day in divided doses (up to 130 mg/kg/day for acute rheumatic fever).

Prevention of Transient Ischemic Attacks

PO (Adults): 50–325 mg once daily.

Prevention of Myocardial Infarction/Antiplatelet Effects

PO (Adults): 80–325 mg once daily. *Suspected acute MI:* 160 mg as soon as MI is suspected.
PO (Children): 3–10 mg/kg/day given once daily (round dose to a convenient amount).

Kawasaki Disease

PO (Children): 80–100 mg/kg/day in 4 divided doses until fever resolves; may be followed by maintenance dose of 3–5 mg/kg/day as a single dose for up to 8 wk.

Availability (generic available)

Immediate-release tablets: 81 mg^{OTC}, 162.5 mg^{OTC}, 325 mg^{OTC}, 500 mg^{OTC}, 650 mg^{OTC}, ✱ 975 mg^{OTC}. **Immediate-release capsules:** 325 mg^{OTC}. **Extended-release tablets:** ✱ 325 mg^{OTC}, 650 mg^{OTC}, 800 mg. **Enteric-coated (delayed-release) tablets:** 80 mg^{OTC}, 165 mg^{OTC}, ✱ 300 mg^{OTC}, 325 mg^{OTC}, 500 mg^{OTC}, ✱ 600 mg^{OTC}, 650 mg^{OTC}, 975 mg^{OTC}. **Delayed-release capsules:** ✱ 325 mg^{OTC}, ✱ 500 mg^{OTC}. **Chewable tablets:** ✱ 80 mg^{OTC}, 81 mg^{OTC}.
Dispersible tablets: 325 mg^{OTC}, 500 mg^{OTC}.
Suppositories: 60 mg^{OTC}, 120 mg^{OTC}, 125 mg^{OTC}, 130 mg^{OTC}, ✱ 150 mg^{OTC}, ✱ 160 mg^{OTC}, 195 mg^{OTC}, 200 mg^{OTC}, 300 mg^{OTC}, ✱ 320 mg^{OTC}, 325 mg^{OTC}, 600 mg^{OTC}, ✱ 640 mg^{OTC}, 650 mg^{OTC}, 1.2 g^{OTC}. ***In combination with:*** antihistamines, decongestants, cough suppressants^{OTC}, and opioids. See Appendix N.

NURSING IMPLICATIONS

Assessment

- Patients who have asthma, allergies, and nasal polyps or who are allergic to tartrazine are at an ↑ risk for developing hypersensitivity reactions.
- Monitor for signs and symptoms of DRESS (fever, rash, lymphadenopathy, facial swelling), exfoliative dermatitis, generalized bullous fixed drug eruption, SJS, or TEN periodically during therapy. Discontinue therapy if symptoms occur.
- **Pain:** Assess pain and limitation of movement; note type, location, and intensity before and 60 min after administration.
- **Fever:** Assess fever and note associated signs (diaphoresis, tachycardia, malaise, chills).

Lab Test Considerations

- Monitor hepatic function before antirheumatic therapy and if symptoms of hepatotoxicity occur; more likely in patients, especially children, with rheumatic fever, systemic lupus erythematosus, juvenile arthritis, or pre-existing hepatic disease. May cause ↑ serum AST, ALT, and alkaline phosphatase, especially when plasma concentrations exceed 25 mg/100 mL. May return to normal despite continued use or dose ↓. If severe abnormalities or active liver disease occurs, discontinue aspirin.
- Monitor serum salicylate levels periodically with prolonged high-dose therapy to determine dose, safety, and efficacy, especially in children with Kawasaki disease.
- May alter results of serum uric acid, urine vanillylmandelic acid, protirelin-induced TSH, urine hydroxyindoleacetic acid determinations, and radionuclide thyroid imaging.
- Prolongs bleeding time for 4–7 days, and in large doses, may cause prolonged prothrombin time. Monitor hematocrit periodically in prolonged high-dose therapy to assess for GI blood loss.

Toxicity and Overdose

- Monitor for the onset of tinnitus, headache, hyperventilation, agitation, mental confusion, lethargy, diarrhea, and sweating. If these symptoms appear, withhold medication and notify health care professional immediately.

Implementation

- Use lowest effective dose for shortest period of time.
- **PO:** Administer after meals or with food or an antacid to minimize gastric irritation. Food slows but does not alter the total amount absorbed.
- *DNC:* Do not crush or chew enteric-coated tablets. Do not take antacids within 1–2 hr of enteric-coated tablets. Chewable tablets may be chewed, dissolved in liquid, or swallowed whole. Some extended-release tablets may be broken or crumbled but must not be ground up before swallowing. See manufacturer's prescribing information for individual products.

Patient/Family Teaching

- Explain purpose and side effects of medication to patient. Advise patient to read *Patient Information* before starting therapy. Instruct patient to take aspirin with a full glass of water and to remain in an upright position for 15–30 min after administration. Advise patient to notify health care professional of all Rx or OTC medications, vitamins, or herbal products being taken and to consult health care professional before taking other medications.
- Advise patient to report tinnitus; unusual bleeding of gums; bruising; black, tarry stools; or fever lasting >3 days.
- Caution patient to avoid concurrent use of alcohol with this medication to minimize possible gastric irritation; ≥3 glasses of alcohol per day may ↑ risk of GI bleeding. Caution patient to avoid taking concurrently with acetaminophen or NSAIDs for more than a few days, unless directed by health care professional to prevent analgesic nephropathy.
- Instruct patients on a sodium-restricted diet to avoid effervescent tablets or buffered-aspirin preparations.
- Tablets with an acetic (vinegar-like) odor should be discarded.
- Advise patients on long-term therapy to inform health care professional of medication regimen before surgery. Aspirin may need to be withheld for 1 wk before surgery.

- Advise patient about signs and symptoms of DRESS, exfoliative dermatitis, generalized bullous fixed drug eruption, SJS, or TEN and to notify health care professional if any occur.
- Rep: May cause fetal harm. Advise women of reproductive potential to notify health care professional if pregnancy is planned or suspected or if breastfeeding. Advise women to avoid aspirin in the 3rd trimester of pregnancy (after 29 wk); may cause premature closure of the fetal ductus arteriosus. Use of aspirin after 20 wk may cause fetal renal dysfunction leading to oligohydramnios. May cause reversible infertility in women attempting to conceive; may consider discontinuing aspirin.
- Pedi: Centers for Disease Control and Prevention warns against giving aspirin to children or adolescents with varicella (chickenpox) or influenza-like or viral illnesses because of a possible association with Reye syndrome.
- **Transient Ischemic Attacks or MI:** Advise patients receiving aspirin prophylactically to take only prescribed dose. ↑ dose has not been found to provide additional benefits.

Evaluation/Desired Outcomes

- Analgesia.
- Reduction of inflammation.
- Reduction of fever.
- Prevention of transient ischemic attacks and MI.

atenolol, See BETA BLOCKERS (selective).

HIGH ALERT

atezolizumab

(a-te-zoe-**liz**-ue-mab)

Tecentriq

Classification

Therapeutic: antineoplastics

Pharmacologic: monoclonal antibodies programmed death ligand 1 (PD-L1) inhibitors

Indications

First-line treatment of metastatic non-small cell lung cancer (NSCLC) in patients whose tumors have high PD-L1 expression (PD-L1 stained ≥50% of tumor cells or PD-L1 stained tumor-infiltrating immune cells covering ≥ 10% of the tumor area) and have no epidermal growth factor receptor (EGFR) or anaplastic lymphoma kinase (ALK) genomic tumor aberrations (as monotherapy). Metastatic NSCLC in patients who have disease progression during or following platinum-containing chemotherapy (as monotherapy). Patients with EGFR or ALK genomic tumor aberrations should have disease progression on FDA-approved therapy for these aberrations prior to receiving atezolizumab. Stage II to IIIA NSCLC as adjuvant treatment following resection and platinum-based chemotherapy in patients whose tumors have PD-L1 expression on ≥ 1% of tumor cells (as monotherapy). Metastatic non-squamous, NSCLC as first-line therapy in patients whose tumors have no EGFR or ALK genomic tumor aberrations (in combination with bevacizumab, paclitaxel, and carboplatin). Metastatic nonsquamous NSCLC as first-line therapy in patients whose tumors have no EGFR or ALK genomic tumor aberrations (in combination with paclitaxel protein bound and carboplatin). Extensive-stage small cell lung cancer as first-line therapy (in combination with carboplatin and etoposide). Unresectable or metastatic hepatocellular carcinoma in patients who have not previously received systemic therapy (in combination with bevacizumab). BRAF V600 mutation-positive unresectable or metastatic melanoma (in combination with cobimetinib and vemurafenib). Unresectable or metastatic alveolar soft part sarcoma (as monotherapy).

Action

Binds to (PD-L1) to prevent its interaction with the programmed cell death-1 (PD-1) and B7.1 (or CD80) receptors, which activates the antitumor immune response. **Therapeutic Effects:** Decreased spread of NSCLC, small cell lung cancer, hepatocellular carcinoma, and melanoma with increased survival. Decreased spread of alveolar soft part sarcoma.

Pharmacokinetics

Absorption: IV administration results in complete bioavailability.

Distribution: Minimally distributed to tissues.

Metabolism and Excretion: Unknown.

Half-life: 27 days.

TIME/ACTION PROFILE (plasma concentrations)

ROUTE	ONSET	PEAK	DURATION
IV	unknown	unknown	unknown

Contraindications/Precautions

Contraindicated in: OB: Pregnancy; Lactation: Lactation.

Use Cautiously in: Allogeneic hematopoietic stem cell transplant recipients (↑ risk of transplantation complications); Solid organ transplant recipients (↑ risk of rejection); Rep: Women of reproductive potential; Pedi: Children <2 yr (alveolar soft part sarcoma) or <18 yr (all other indications) (safety and effectiveness not established).

Adverse Reactions/Side Effects

CV: peripheral edema, myocarditis, pericarditis. **Derm:** pruritus, rash, DRUG REACTION WITH EOSINOPHILIA AND SYSTEMIC SYMPTOMS (DRESS), STEVENS-JOHNSON SYNDROME (SJS), TOXIC EPIDERMAL NECROLYSIS (TEN). **Endo:** hypothyroidism, ADRENAL INSUFFICIENCY, hyperglycemia, hyperthyroidism, hypophysitis, type 1 diabetes mellitus. **F and E:** hyponatremia, dehydration. **GI:** ↓ appetite, COLITIS/DIARRHEA, constipation, HEPATOTOXICITY, nausea, vomiting, ↑ liver enzymes, abdominal pain, PANCREATITIS. **GU:** hematuria, ↓ fertility (females), ↑ serum creatinine, acute kidney injury, nephritis, urinary obstruction. **Hemat:** lymphopenia, anemia. **Metab:** hypoalbuminemia. **MS:** arthralgia. **Neuro:** Guillain-Barré syndrome, ENCEPHALITIS, MENINGITIS, MYASTHENIA GRAVIS, myelitis, nerve paresis. **Resp:** cough, dyspnea, INTERSTITIAL LUNG DISEASE. **Misc:** fatigue, fever, INFECTION (INCLUDING HERPES ENCEPHALITIS AND TUBERCULOSIS), INFUSION-RELATED REACTIONS.

Interactions

Drug-Drug: None reported.

Route/Dosage

Non-Small Cell Lung Cancer

IV (Adults): *As monotherapy (metastatic NSCLC):* 840 mg every 2 wk until disease progression or unacceptable toxicity *or* 1200 mg every 3 wk until disease progression or unacceptable toxicity *or* 1680 mg every 4 wk until disease progression or unacceptable toxicity. *As monotherapy (adjuvant treatment):* 840 mg every 2 wk for up to 1 yr unless there is disease recurrence or unacceptable toxicity *or* 1200 mg every 3 wk for up to 1 yr unless there is disease recurrence or unacceptable toxicity *or* 1680 mg every 4 wk for up to 1 yr unless there is disease recurrence or unacceptable toxicity. *Combination therapy:* 840 mg every 2 wk until disease progression or unacceptable toxicity *or* 1200 mg every 3 wk until disease progression or unacceptable toxicity *or* 1680 mg every 4 wk until disease progression or unacceptable toxicity. Administer prior to bevacizumab and chemotherapy when given on same day.

Small Cell Lung Cancer

IV (Adults): 840 mg every 2 wk until disease progression or unacceptable toxicity *or* 1200 mg every 3 wk until disease progression or unacceptable toxicity *or* 1680 mg every 4 wk until disease progression or unacceptable toxicity. Administer prior to carboplatin and etoposide when given on same day.

Hepatocellular Carcinoma

IV (Adults): 840 mg every 2 wk until disease progression or unacceptable toxicity *or* 1200 mg every 3 wk until disease progression or unacceptable toxicity *or* 1680 mg every 4 wk until disease progression or unacceptable toxicity. Administer prior to bevacizumab when given on same day.

Melanoma

IV (Adults): 840 mg every 2 wk until disease progression or unacceptable toxicity *or* 1200 mg every 3 wk until disease progression or unacceptable toxicity *or* 1680 mg every 4 wk until disease progression or unacceptable toxicity. A 28-day treatment cycle of cobimetinib and vemurafenib should be administered prior to starting atezolizumab therapy.

Alveolar Soft Part Sarcoma

IV (Adults): 840 mg every 2 wk until disease progression or unacceptable toxicity *or* 1200 mg every 3 wk until disease progression or unacceptable toxicity *or* 1680 mg every 4 wk until disease progression or unacceptable toxicity.

IV (Children ≥2 yr): 15 mg/kg (max dose = 1200 mg) every 3 wk until disease progression or unacceptable toxicity.

Availability

Solution for injection: 60 mg/mL.

NURSING IMPLICATIONS

Assessment

- Monitor for signs and symptoms of pneumonitis (new or worsening cough, dyspnea, chest pain) during therapy. Monitor with x-rays as needed. *For ≥Grade 2 pneumonitis,* hold atezolizumab and administer corticosteroids at a dose of 1–2 mg/kg/day prednisolone equivalents followed by a taper. Resume after taper corticosteroid if Grade 0–1. If no complete or partial resolution within 12 wk of starting corticosteroids or inability to reduce prednisone to ≤10 mg per day within 12 wk of starting steroids, permanently discontinue atezolizumab. *For Grade 3 or 4 pneumonitis,* permanently discontinue atezolizumab.
- Monitor for signs and symptoms of hepatitis (jaundice, severe nausea or vomiting, pain on right side of abdomen, lethargy, dark urine, unusual bleeding or bruising, anorexia) periodically during therapy.
- Monitor for signs and symptoms of diarrhea or colitis (blood in stools, dark tarry stools, abdominal pain or tenderness) periodically during therapy. *For Grade 2 or 3,* hold atezolizumab until Grade 1 or resolved and corticosteroid dose ≤prednisone 10 mg per day (or equivalent). *For Grade 4,* permanently discontinue atezolizumab.
- Monitor for signs and symptoms of adrenal insufficiency (extreme tiredness, dizziness or fainting, frequent urination, nausea or vomiting, changes in mood or behavior, ↓ sex drive, irritability, forgetfulness), hypophysitis (unusual headaches, persistent headaches, vision problems), hyperthyroidism, and type 1 diabetes periodically during therapy. *If Grades 2, 3, or 4 occur,* hold dose until Grade 1 or resolved and clinically stable on hormone replacement therapy.
- Monitor for signs and symptoms of immune-mediated skin reactions (rash, pruritus, blistering, painful sores in mouth, nose, throat, genital area) periodically during therapy. Topical emollients

and/or topical corticosteroids may treat mild to moderate nonexfoliative rashes. May cause exfoliative dermatitis (SJS, TEN, DRESS). *If SJS, TEN, or DRESS is suspected,* hold atezolizumab. *If SJS, TEN, or DRESS are confirmed,* permanently discontinue atezolizumab.

- Monitor for signs and symptoms of meningitis or encephalitis (fever, confusion, changes in mood or behavior, extreme sensitivity to light, neck stiffness) during therapy. If symptoms occur, permanently discontinue atezolizumab. Administer 1–2 mg/kg/day methylprednisolone or equivalent. Convert to oral prednisone 60 mg/day or equivalent once improved. When symptoms improve to ≤ Grade 1, taper steroids over ≥1 mo.
- Monitor for signs and symptoms of motor or sensory neuropathy (severe muscle weakness, numbness or tingling in hands or feet) periodically during therapy. For Grade 2 neurological toxicities, hold atezolizumab and administer corticosteroids at a dose of 1–2 mg/kg/day prednisolone equivalents followed by a taper. Resume after taper corticosteroid if Grade 0–1. If no complete or partial resolution within 12 wk of starting corticosteroids or inability to reduce prednisone to ≤10 mg per day within 12 wk of starting steroids, permanently discontinue atezolizumab. *If Grades 3 or 4 or symptoms of myasthenic syndrome/myasthenia gravis or Guillain-Barré syndrome occur,* permanently discontinue atezolizumab. Institute treatment as needed.
- Monitor for signs and symptoms of pancreatitis (abdominal pain) during therapy. *If Grade 2 or 3 pancreatitis occurs,* hold atezolizumab. Treat with methylprednisolone IV 1–2 mg/kg/day or equivalent. Once symptoms improve, follow with 1–2 mg/kg/day of oral prednisone or equivalent. Resume atezolizumab if symptoms of pancreatitis resolved and corticosteroid reduced to ≤10 mg/day oral prednisone or equivalent. *For Grade 4 or recurrent pancreatitis,* permanently discontinue atezolizumab.
- Monitor for signs and symptoms of infection (fever, cough, frequent urination, flu-like symptoms, painful urination) periodically during therapy. Treat suspected or confirmed infections with antibiotics. *For ≥Grade 3 or 4 infections,* withhold atezolizumab until Grade 1 or resolved.
- Monitor for signs and symptoms of infusion-related reactions (chills or shaking, itching or rash, flushing, dyspnea, wheezing, dizziness, fever, feeling faint, back or neck pain, facial swelling) during therapy. *For Grade 1 or 2,* interrupt or slow infusion. *For Grade 3 or 4 infusion reactions,* permanently discontinue atezolizumab.
- Monitor for signs and symptoms of myocarditis (chest pain, irregular heartbeat, shortness of breath, swelling of ankles) during therapy. *If Grade 2, 3, or 4 myocarditis occurs,* discontinue atezolizumab permanently.

Lab Test Considerations

- Verify a negative pregnancy test before starting therapy. Confirm PD-L1 expression in melanoma via tests and BRAF V600 in unresectable or metastatic melanoma at http://www.fda.gov/CompanionDiagnostics. An FDA-approved test for the detection of other BRAF V600 mutations for this use is not currently available.
- For patients with hepatitis with no tumor involvement of the liver, monitor AST, ALT, and serum bilirubin prior to and periodically during therapy. *If AST or ALT >3 and ≤ 8 times upper limit of normal (ULN) or total bilirubin >1.5 and ≤ 3 times ULN* hold dose until Grade 1 or resolved and corticosteroid dose ≤prednisone 10 mg per day (or equivalent). *If AST or ALT >8 times ULN or total bilirubin >3 times ULN,* permanently discontinue atezolizumab. For patients with hepatitis with tumor involvement of the liver, *If baseline AST or ALT >1 and ≤3 times ULN and increases to >5 and ≤10 times ULN or baseline AST or ALT >3 and ≤5 times ULN and increases to >8 and ≤10 times ULN,* hold atezolizumab and administer corticosteroids at a dose of 1–2 mg/kg/day prednisolone equivalents followed by a taper. Resume after taper corticosteroid if Grade 0–1. If no complete or partial resolution within 12 wk of starting corticosteroids or inability to reduce prednisone to ≤10 mg per day within 12 wk of starting steroids, permanently discontinue atezolizumab. *If AST or ALT increases to >10 times ULN or total bilirubin increases to >3 times ULN,* permanently discontinue atezolizumab.
- Monitor thyroid function prior to and periodically during therapy. *If asymptomatic,* continue therapy. *For symptomatic hypothyroidism (extreme tiredness, weight gain, constipation, feeling cold, hair loss, deepening voice),* withhold atezolizumab and begin thyroid replacement therapy as needed without corticosteroids. *For symptomatic hyperthyroidism (hunger, irritability, mood swings, weight loss),* hold atezolizumab until Grade 1 or resolved and clinically stable on hormone replacement therapy. Resume therapy when symptoms of hyper- or hypothyroidism are controlled and thyroid function is improving.
- Monitor blood glucose periodically during therapy. For type 1 diabetes, begin treatment with insulin. For ≥Grade 2, 3, or 4 hyperglycemia (fasting glucose >250–500 mg/dL), hold atezolizumab until Grade 1 or resolved and control is achieved on insulin replacement therapy.
- Monitor serum amylase or lipase in patients with symptoms of pancreatitis. If serum amylase or lipase levels ≥Grade 3 (>2 times ULN), withhold atezolizumab. Treat with methylprednisolone IV 1–2 mg/kg/day or equivalent. Once symptoms improve, follow with 1–2 mg/kg/day of oral prednisone or equivalent. Resume atezolizumab if

symptoms of pancreatitis resolved and corticosteroid ↓ to ≤10 mg/day oral prednisone or equivalent.

- Monitor renal function prior to and periodically during therapy. *If serum creatinine increases to Grades 2 or 3,* hold atezolizumab and administer corticosteroids at a dose of 1–2 mg/kg/day prednisolone equivalents followed by a taper. Resume after taper corticosteroid if Grade 0–1. If no complete or partial resolution within 12 wk of starting corticosteroids or inability to reduce prednisone to ≤10 mg per day within 12 wk of starting steroids, permanently discontinue atezolizumab. *If serum creatinine increases to Grade 4,* permanently discontinue atezolizumab.
- May cause lymphopenia, hyponatremia, anemia, ↑ alkaline phosphatase, ↑ serum creatinine, and hypoalbuminemia.

Implementation

IV Administration

- **Intermittent Infusion: Dilution:** Dilute with 0.9% NaCl in a polyvinyl chloride, polyethylene, or polyolefin infusion bag. **Concentration:** 3.2 mg/mL to 16.8 mg/mL. Gently invert to dilute; do not shake. Solution is clear and colorless to slightly yellow. Do not administer solutions that are discolored or contain particulate matter. Administer immediately once prepared or store for ≤6 hr at room temperature (including infusion time) or ≤24 hr if refrigerated. Do not freeze.
- Administer atezolizumab before chemotherapy or other antineoplastic drugs when given on same day. **Rate:** Administer over 60 min with or without a sterile, nonpyrogenic, low-protein-binding in-line filter (0.2–0.22 micron); do not administer via IV push or bolus. If first infusion is tolerated, subsequent infusions may be infused over 30 min.
- **Y-Site Incompatibility:** Do not administer other drugs through same IV line.

Patient/Family Teaching

- Explain purpose of atezolizumab to patient. Advise patient to read the *Medication Guide* before starting and periodically during therapy in case of changes.
- Advise patient to notify health care professional immediately if symptoms of pneumonitis, hepatitis, colitis, endocrine problems, meningitis, nervous system problems, ocular inflammatory toxicity (blurry or double vision, eye pain or redness), pancreatitis, infection, infusion-related reactions, or rash occur.
- Advise patient to notify health care professional of all Rx or OTC medications, vitamins, or herbal products being taken and to consult with health care professional before taking other medications.
- Rep: May cause fetal harm. Advise females of reproductive potential to use effective contraception and to avoid breastfeeding during and for at least 5 mo after last dose. Inform females that atezolizumab may impair fertility during therapy.

Evaluation/Desired Outcomes

- Decreased spread of NSCLC, small cell lung cancer, hepatocellular carcinoma, and melanoma with increased survival.
- Decreased spread of alveolar soft part sarcoma.

atogepant (a-toe-je-pant)

Qulipta

Classification

Therapeutic: vascular headache suppressants

Pharmacologic: calcitonin gene related peptide receptor antagonists

Indications

Preventive treatment of migraines.

Action

Binds to and inhibits the calcitonin gene-related peptide (CGRP) receptor, which reduces the neuroinflammatory and vasodilatory effects of CGRP. **Therapeutic Effects:** Reduction in number of monthly migraine days.

Pharmacokinetics

Absorption: Well absorbed following oral administration.

Distribution: Well distributed to tissues.

Metabolism and Excretion: Primarily metabolized in the liver via the CYP3A4 isoenzyme. Primarily excreted as unchanged drug in feces (42%) and urine (5%).

Half-life: 11 hr.

TIME/ACTION PROFILE (plasma concentrations)

ROUTE	ONSET	PEAK	DURATION
PO	rapid	1–2 hr	unknown

Contraindications/Precautions

Contraindicated in: Hypersensitivity; Severe renal impairment or end-stage renal disease (for chronic migraine prevention); Severe hepatic impairment.

Use Cautiously in: Hypertension; Raynaud phenomenon; Severe renal impairment or end-stage renal disease (for episodic migraine prevention); OB: Oral CGRP antagonists not currently recommended for prevention of migraine during pregnancy; Lactation: Oral CGRP antagonists not currently recommended for prevention of migraine while breastfeeding; Pedi: Safety and effectiveness not established in children.

Adverse Reactions/Side Effects

CV: hypertension, Raynaud phenomenon. **GI:** constipation, nausea. **Metab:** ↓ appetite, weight loss. **Neuro:** dizziness, fatigue, sedation. **Misc:** HYPERSENSITIVITY REACTIONS (INCLUDING ANAPHYLAXIS).

Interactions

Drug-Drug: Strong CYP3A4 inhibitors, including **itraconazole**, may ↑ levels and risk of toxicity; ↓ dose. **Strong CYP3A4 inducers**, including **rifampin**; **moderate CYP3A4 inducers**; or **weak CYP3A4 inducers**, including **topiramate**, may ↓ levels and effectiveness; ↑ atogepant dose for episodic migraine prevention; avoid concurrent use for chronic migraine prevention. **OATP inhibitors**, including **rifampin**, may ↑ levels and risk of toxicity; ↓ atogepant dose for episodic or chronic migraine prevention. **St. John's wort** may ↓ levels and effectiveness; avoid concurrent use. **Drug-Food: Grapefruit juice** may ↑ levels and risk of toxicity; avoid concurrent use.

Route/Dosage

Episodic Migraine

PO (Adults): 10 mg, 30 mg, or 60 mg once daily. *Concurrent use of strong CYP3A4 inhibitors:* 10 mg once daily. *Concurrent use of strong, moderate, or weak CYP3A4 inducers:* 30 mg or 60 mg once daily. *Concurrent use of OATP inhibitors:* 10 mg or 30 mg once daily.

Renal Impairment

PO (Adults): *CCr <30 mL/min:* 10 mg once daily.

Chronic Migraine

PO (Adults): 60 mg once daily. *Concurrent use of strong CYP3A4 inhibitors:* 10 mg once daily. *Concurrent use of strong, moderate, or weak CYP3A4 inducers:* Avoid concurrent use. *Concurrent use of OATP inhibitors:* 30 mg once daily.

Renal Impairment

PO (Adults): *CCr <30 mL/min:* Avoid use.

Availability

Tablets: 10 mg, 30 mg, 60 mg.

NURSING IMPLICATIONS

Assessment

- Assess pain location, character, intensity, duration, and associated symptoms (photophobia, phonophobia, nausea, vomiting) of migraine pain.
- Monitor frequency of migraine headaches.
- Monitor BP periodically and more frequently in patients with pre-existing HTN.
- Monitor for signs and symptoms of hypersensitivity reactions (rash, urticaria, pruritus, flushing, dizziness, vomiting, abdominal pain) and angioedema (swelling of throat, lips, tongue, or face; dyspnea; wheezing; hoarseness). Hypersensitivity reactions can occur days after administration. If a hypersensitivity reaction occurs, discontinue atogepant and begin supportive therapy as needed.

Implementation

- Doses for episodic and chronic migraines are different.
- **PO:** Administer without regard to food.

Patient/Family Teaching

- Explain the purpose and side effects of atogepant. Instruct patient to take as directed. Advise patient to read *Patient Information* before starting and with each Rx refill in case of changes.
- Advise patient that use of triptans, ergotamine derivatives, NSAIDs, acetaminophen, and opioids for headache treatment while taking atogepant is acceptable.
- Advise patient to avoid alcohol, which aggravates headaches, during atogepant use.
- Advise patient that lying down in a darkened room following atogepant administration may further help relieve headache.
- Inform patients of potential for hypersensitivity reaction and that these reactions can occur days after administration of atogepant. Advise patients to call 911 and immediately seek treatment for signs and symptoms of hypersensitivity reactions (difficulty breathing; chest tightness; hives; rash; light-headedness; itching; swelling of the face, lips, tongue, or throat). *If hypersensitivity reaction occurs,* discontinue atogepant.
- Advise patient to avoid grapefruit juice during therapy.
- Advise patient to report symptoms of ↑ BP or worsening pre-existing HTN.
- Advise patient to notify health care provider of all Rx or OTC medications, vitamins, or herbal products being taken and to consult with health care provider before taking other medications. Avoid St. John's wort during treatment.
- Rep: Advise women of reproductive potential to notify health care provider if pregnancy is planned or suspected or if breastfeeding. Inform patient of the pregnancy exposure registry that monitors pregnancy outcomes in women exposed to *Qulipta*. For more information, health care providers or patients are encouraged to contact: 1-833-277-0206 or visit http://empresspregnancyregistry.com.

Evaluation/Desired Outcomes

- Decrease in number of migraines/month.

atomoxetine

(a-to-**mox**-e-teen)

Strattera

Classification

Therapeutic: agents for attention deficit hyperactivity disorder (ADHD)

Pharmacologic: selective norepinephrine reuptake inhibitors

Indications
Attention-deficit/hyperactivity disorder (ADHD).

Action
Selectively inhibits the presynaptic transporter of norepinephrine. **Therapeutic Effects:** Increased attention span.

Pharmacokinetics
Absorption: Well absorbed following oral administration.
Distribution: Unknown.
Protein Binding: 98%.
Metabolism and Excretion: Mostly metabolized by the liver via the CYP2D6 isoenzyme pathway; the CYP2D6 enzyme system exhibits genetic polymorphism (7% of population may be poor metabolizers and may have significantly ↑ atomoxetine concentrations and an ↑ risk of adverse effects).
Half-life: 5 hr.

ROUTE	ONSET	PEAK	DURATION
PO	unknown	1–2 hr	12–24 hr

Contraindications/Precautions
Contraindicated in: Hypersensitivity; Concurrent or within 2 wk of therapy with MAO inhibitors; Angle-closure glaucoma; Pheochromocytoma; Hypertension, tachycardia, cardiovascular, or cerebrovascular disease.
Use Cautiously in: Personal or family history of bipolar disorder, mania, or hypomania; Concurrent albuterol or vasopressors (↑ risk of adverse cardiovascular reactions); CYP2D6 poor metabolizers (↓ dose); OB: Use during pregnancy only if potential maternal benefit justifies potential fetal risk; Lactation: Safety not established in breastfeeding; Pedi: May ↑ risk of suicide attempt/ideation especially during dose early treatment or dose adjustment; risk may be greater in children or adolescents; Pedi: Children <6 yr (safety and effectiveness not established).

Adverse Reactions/Side Effects
CV: hypertension, orthostatic hypotension, QT interval prolongation, syncope, tachycardia. **Derm:** ↑ sweating, rash, urticaria. **GI:** nausea, vomiting, dyspepsia, HEPATOTOXICITY **Adults:** constipation, dry mouth. **GU: Adults:** dysmenorrhea, ejaculatory problems, erectile dysfunction, libido changes, priapism, urinary hesitation, urinary retention. **Metab:** ↓ appetite, ↓ growth, weight loss. **MS:** RHABDOMYOLYSIS. **Neuro:** dizziness, fatigue, insomnia, mood swings, aggression, behavioral disturbances, delusions, hallucinations, hostility, mania, paresthesia, SUICIDAL THOUGHTS, thought disorder. **Misc:** HYPERSENSITIVITY REACTIONS (INCLUDING ANAPHYLAXIS AND ANGIOEDEMA).

Interactions
Drug-Drug: Concurrent use with **MAO inhibitors** may result in serious, potentially fatal reactions; concurrent use within 2 wk of each other contraindicated. ↑ risk of cardiovascular effects with **albuterol** or **vasopressors**; use cautiously. **CYP2D6 inhibitors**, including **quinidine**, **fluoxetine**, or **paroxetine**, may ↑ levels and risk of toxicity; dose ↓ recommended.

Route/Dosage
PO (Adults and Children ≥6 yr and >70 kg): 40 mg/day initially; may ↑ every 3 days to a daily target dose of 80 mg/day given as a single dose in the morning or evenly divided doses in the morning and late afternoon/early evening; may further ↑ after 2–4 wk up to 100 mg/day. *Concurrent use of CYP2D6 inhibitor (quinidine, fluoxetine, paroxetine):* 40 mg/day initially; may ↑ if needed to 80 mg/day after 4 wk.
PO (Children ≥6 yr and ≤70 kg): 0.5 mg/kg/day initially; may ↑ every 3 days to a daily target dose of 1.2 mg/kg, given as a single dose in the morning or evenly divided doses in the morning and late afternoon/early evening (not to exceed 1.4 mg/kg/day or 100 mg/day, whichever is less). *Concurrent use of CYP2D6 inhibitor (quinidine, fluoxetine, paroxetine) or CYP2D6 poor metabolizer:* 0.5 mg/kg/day initially; may ↑ if needed to 1.2 mg/kg/day after 4 wk.

Hepatic Impairment
PO (Adults and Children): *Moderate hepatic impairment:* ↓ initial and target dose by 50%; *Severe hepatic impairment:* ↓ initial and target dose to 25% of normal.

Availability (generic available)
Capsules: 10 mg, 18 mg, 25 mg, 40 mg, 60 mg, 80 mg, 100 mg.

NURSING IMPLICATIONS
Assessment
- Assess attention span, impulse control, and interactions with others.
- Assess for bipolar disorder (screen patients for a personal or family history of bipolar disorder, mania, or hypomania) before starting therapy.
- Monitor BP and HR periodically during therapy. Obtain a history (including assessment of family history of sudden death or ventricular arrhythmia), physical exam to assess for cardiac disease, and further evaluation (ECG and echocardiogram), if indicated. If exertional chest pain, unexplained syncope, or other cardiac symptoms occur, evaluate promptly.
- Monitor growth, body height, and weight in children.

- Assess for signs of liver injury (pruritus, dark urine, jaundice, right upper quadrant tenderness, unexplained flu-like symptoms) during therapy. Discontinue and do not restart atomoxetine in patients with jaundice or laboratory evidence of liver injury.
- Monitor closely for notable changes in behavior that could indicate the emergence or worsening of suicidal thoughts or behavior or depression. Psychotic or manic symptoms (hallucinations, delusional thinking, mania) in patients without a history of psychotic illness or mania can be caused by atomoxetine at usual doses. If symptoms occur, consider discontinuing therapy.

Lab Test Considerations

- Monitor liver enzymes (at signs/symptoms of liver dysfunction and for several wk after discontinuation).
- In normal, intermediate, and ultrarapid CYP2D6 metabolizers or in patients with unknown CYP2D6 metabolizer status, draw peak plasma concentrations 1–2 hr after dose. In intermediate CYP2D6 metabolizers, consider drawing peak plasma concentrations 2–4 hr after dose in patients with lower enzyme activity or if the *10 allele is present. For poor CYP2D6 metabolizers, draw peak plasma concentrations 4 hr after dose. *Therapeutic reference range:* 200–1000 ng/mL. *Laboratory alert level:* 2000 ng/mL.

Implementation

- Do not confuse atomoxetine with atorvastatin.
- **PO:** Administer without regard to food. Doses may be discontinued without tapering. ***DNC:*** Swallow capsules whole; do not open, crush, or chew.

Patient/Family Teaching

- Explain purpose and side effects of medication to patient. Advise patient/caregiver to read *Patient Information* before starting therapy. Instruct patient to take medication as directed. Take missed doses as soon as possible, but should not take more than the total daily amount in any 24-hr period.
- Instruct patient to notify health care provider of all Rx or OTC medications, vitamins, or herbal products being taken and consult health care provider before taking any new medications.
- Inform patient that sharing this medication may be dangerous.
- Advise patient and/or caregiver to notify health care provider if thoughts about suicide or dying, attempts to commit suicide, new or worse depression, new or worse anxiety, feeling very agitated or restless, panic attacks, trouble sleeping, new or worse irritability, acting aggressive or hostile, being angry or violent, acting on dangerous impulses, an extreme ↑ in activity and talking, or other unusual changes in behavior or mood occur or if signs and symptoms of severe liver injury (pruritus, dark urine, jaundice, right upper quadrant tenderness, unexplained flu-like symptoms) occur.
- May cause dizziness. Caution patient to avoid driving or other activities requiring alertness until response to medication is known.
- Rep: Advise women of reproductive potential to notify health care provider if pregnancy is planned or suspected or if breastfeeding. Register patients who took atomoxetine during pregnancy in Pregnancy Exposure Registry to monitor pregnancy outcomes by calling the National Pregnancy Registry for ADHD Medications at 1-866-961-2388 or visiting https://womensmentalhealth.org/adhd-medications/.

Evaluation/Desired Outcomes

- Increased attention span.

atorvastatin, See HMG-CoA REDUCTASE INHIBITORS (statins).

BEERS

atropine (at-ro-peen)

Classification

Therapeutic: antiarrhythmics

Pharmacologic: anticholinergics, antimuscarinics

See Appendix B for ophthalmic use

Indications

IV: Given preoperatively to decrease oral and respiratory secretions. **IV:** Sinus bradycardia and heart block. **IV:** Reversal of adverse muscarinic effects of anticholinesterase agents (neostigmine or pyridostigmine). **IV:** Anticholinesterase (organophosphate pesticide) poisoning. **Inhaln:** Exercise-induced bronchospasm.

Action

Inhibits the action of acetylcholine at postganglionic sites located in: Smooth muscle, Secretory glands, CNS (antimuscarinic activity). Low doses decrease: Sweating, Salivation, Respiratory secretions. Intermediate doses result in: Mydriasis (pupillary dilation), Cycloplegia (loss of visual accommodation), Increased heart rate. GI and GU tract motility are decreased at larger doses. **Therapeutic Effects:** Increased heart rate. Decreased GI and respiratory secretions. Reversal of muscarinic effects. May have a spasmolytic action on the biliary and genitourinary tracts.

Pharmacokinetics

Absorption: Well absorbed following SUBQ administration. IV administration results in complete bioavailability.

Distribution: Readily crosses the blood-brain barrier. Crosses the placenta and enters breast milk.

Metabolism and Excretion: Mostly metabolized by the liver; 30–50% excreted unchanged by the kidneys.

Half-life: Children <2 yr: 4–10 hr; Children >2 yr: 1.5–3.5 hr; Adults: 4–5 hr.

TIME/ACTION PROFILE (inhibition of salivation)

ROUTE	ONSET	PEAK	DURATION
SUBQ	rapid	15–50 min	4–6 hr
IV	immediate	2–4 min	4–6 hr

Contraindications/Precautions

Contraindicated in: Hypersensitivity; Angle-closure glaucoma; Acute hemorrhage; Tachycardia secondary to cardiac insufficiency or thyrotoxicosis; Obstructive disease of the GI tract.

Use Cautiously in: Intra-abdominal infections; Prostatic hyperplasia; Chronic renal, hepatic, pulmonary, or cardiac disease; OB: Safety not established in pregnancy; Lactation: Use while breastfeeding only if potential maternal benefit justifies potential risk to infant; Pedi: Infants with Down syndrome have ↑ sensitivity to cardiac effects and mydriasis. Children may have ↑ susceptibility to adverse reactions. Exercise care when prescribing to children with spastic paralysis or brain damage; Geri: Appears on Beers list. ↑ risk of adverse reactions in older adults due to anticholinergic effects. Avoid use of all formulations in older adults except for ophthalmic formulations.

Adverse Reactions/Side Effects

CV: tachycardia, arrhythmias, palpitations. **Derm:** ↓ sweating, flushing. **EENT:** blurred vision, cycloplegia, dry eyes, mydriasis, photophobia. **GI:** dry mouth, constipation, impaired GI motility. **GU:** urinary hesitancy, impotency, retention. **Neuro:** drowsiness, confusion. **Resp:** pulmonary edema, tachypnea.

Interactions

Drug-Drug: ↑ anticholinergic effects with other **anticholinergics**, including **antihistamines**, **tricyclic antidepressants**, **quinidine**, and **disopyramide**. Anticholinergics may alter the absorption of other **orally administered drugs** by slowing motility of the GI tract. **Antacids** ↓ absorption of **anticholinergics**. May ↑ GI mucosal lesions in patients taking oral **potassium chloride** tablets. May alter response to **beta-blockers**.

Route/Dosage

Preanesthesia (To Decrease Salivation/Secretions)

IV: SUBQ (Adults): 0.4–0.6 mg 30–60 min preop.
IV: SUBQ (Children >5 kg): 0.01–0.02 mg/kg/dose 30–60 min preop to a maximum of 0.4 mg/dose; minimum: 0.1 mg/dose.
IV: SUBQ (Children <5 kg): 0.02 mg/kg/dose 30–60 min preop then every 4–6 hr as needed.

Bradycardia

IV (Adults): 0.5–1 mg; may repeat as needed every 5 min, not to exceed a total of 2 mg (every 3–5 min in Advanced Cardiac Life Support guidelines) or 0.04 mg/kg (total vagolytic dose).
IV (Children): 0.02 mg/kg (maximum single dose is 0.5 mg in children and 1 mg in adolescents); may repeat every 5 min up to a total dose of 1 mg in children (2 mg in adolescents).
Endotracheal: (Children): use the IV dose and dilute before administration.

Reversal of Adverse Muscarinic Effects of Anticholinesterases

IV (Adults): 0.6–12 mg for each 0.5–2.5 mg of neostigmine or 10–20 mg of pyridostigmine concurrently with anticholinesterase.

Organophosphate Poisoning

IV (Adults): 1–2 mg/dose every 10–20 min until atropinic effects observed then every 1–4 hr for 24 hr; up to 50 mg in first 24 hr and 2 g over several days may be given in severe intoxication.
IV (Children): 0.02–0.05 mg/kg every 10–20 min until atropinic effects observed then every 1–4 hr for 24 hr.

Bronchospasm

Inhaln: (Adults): 0.025–0.05 mg/kg/dose every 4–6 hr as needed; maximum 2.5 mg/dose.
Inhaln: (Children): 0.03–0.05 mg/kg/dose 3–4 times/day; maximum 2.5 mg/dose.

Availability (generic available)

Solution for injection: 0.05 mg/mL, 0.1 mg/mL, 0.4 mg/mL, 1 mg/mL.

NURSING IMPLICATIONS

Assessment

- Assess vital signs and ECG tracings frequently during IV drug therapy. Report any significant changes in heart rate or BP, or increased ventricular ectopy or angina to health care professional promptly.
- Monitor intake and output ratios in elderly or surgical patients because atropine may cause urinary retention.
- Assess patients routinely for abdominal distention and auscultate for bowel sounds. If constipation becomes a problem, increasing fluids and adding bulk to the diet may help alleviate constipation.

Implementation

IV Administration

- **IV Push: Dilution:** Administer undiluted.
- **Rate:** Administer over 1 min; more rapid administration may be used during cardiac resuscitation (follow with 20 mL saline flush). Slow administration

(over >1 min) may cause a paradoxical bradycardia (usually resolved in approximately 2 min).

- **Y-Site Compatibility:** amikacin, aminophylline, amiodarone, argatroban, ascorbic acid, azathioprine, aztreonam, benztropine, bivalirudin, bumetanide, buprenorphine, butorphanol, calcium chloride, calcium gluconate, cangrelor, cefazolin, cefotaxime, cefotetan, cefoxitin, ceftazidime, ceftriaxone, cefuroxime, chloramphenicol, chlorpromazine, clindamycin, cyanocobalamin, cyclosporine, dexamethasone, dexmedetomidine, digoxin, diphenhydramine, dobutamine, dopamine, doxycycline, enalaprilat, ephedrine, epinephrine, epoetin alfa, eptifibatide, erythromycin, esmolol, etomidate, famotidine, fentanyl, fluconazole, folic acid, furosemide, ganciclovir, gentamicin, glycopyrrolate, heparin, hydrocortisone, hydromorphone, imipenem/cilastatin, indomethacin, insulin, regular, isoproterenol, ketamine, ketorolac, labetalol, LR, lidocaine, magnesium sulfate, mannitol, meperidine, meropenem, methadone, methylprednisolone, metoclopramide, metoprolol, midazolam, morphine, multivitamins, nafcillin, nalbuphine, naloxone, nitroglycerin, nitroprusside, norepinephrine, ondansetron, oxacillin, oxytocin, palonosetron, papaverine, penicillin G, pentamidine, pentobarbital, phenobarbital, phentolamine, phenylephrine, phytonadione, potassium chloride, procainamide, prochlorperazine, promethazine, propranolol, protamine, pyridoxine, sodium bicarbonate, succinylcholine, sufentanil, theophylline, thiamine, tirofiban, tobramycin, vancomycin, vasopressin, verapamil.
- **Y-Site Incompatibility:** acetaminophen, dantrolene, diazepam, pantoprazole, phenytoin, trimethoprim/sulfamethoxazole. **Endotracheal:** Dilute with 5–10 mL of 0.9% NaCl.
- Rate: Inject directly into the endotracheal tube followed by several positive pressure ventilations.

Patient/Family Teaching

- Explain purpose of atropine to patient.
- May cause drowsiness. Caution patients to avoid driving or other activities requiring alertness until response to medication is known.
- Instruct patient that oral rinses, sugarless gum or candy, and frequent oral hygiene may help relieve dry mouth.
- Caution patients that atropine impairs heat regulation. Strenuous activity in a hot environment may cause heat stroke.
- Advise patient to notify health care professional of all Rx or OTC medications, vitamins, or herbal products being taken and to consult with health care professional before taking other medications.
- Rep: Advise patient to notify health care professional if pregnancy is planned or suspected or if breastfeeding.
- Pedi: Instruct parents or caregivers that medication may cause fever and to notify health care professional before administering to a febrile child.
- Geri: Inform male patients with benign prostatic hyperplasia that atropine may cause urinary hesitancy and retention. Changes in urinary stream should be reported to health care professional.

Evaluation/Desired Outcomes

- Increase in heart rate.
- Dryness of mouth.
- Reversal of muscarinic effects.

HIGH ALERT

axitinib (ax-i-ti-nib)

Inlyta

Classification

Therapeutic: antineoplastics

Pharmacologic: kinase inhibitors

Indications

First-line treatment of advanced renal cell carcinoma (in combination with avelumab or pembrolizumab). Advanced renal cell carcinoma following failure of one other systemic therapy.

Action

Inhibits tyrosine kinases on various receptors, including vascular endothelial growth factor receptors that may be involved in tumor angiogenesis/growth and cancer progression. **Therapeutic Effects:** Inhibited tumor growth with decreased disease progression.

Pharmacokinetics

Absorption: Well absorbed (58%) following oral administration.

Distribution: Unknown.

Protein Binding: >99%.

Metabolism and Excretion: Mostly metabolized by the CYP3A4/5 isoenzymes, with some metabolism by CYP2C19 and UGT1A1 systems. 41% eliminated in feces (12% as unchanged drug); 23% eliminated in urine as metabolites.

Half-life: 2.5–6.1 hr.

TIME/ACTION PROFILE (plasma concentrations)

ROUTE	ONSET	PEAK	DURATION†
PO	unknown	2.5–4.1 hr	12 hr

† ↓ progression of disease may last up to 18 mo.

Contraindications/Precautions

Contraindicated in: Untreated brain metastases; Recent active GI bleeding; OB: Pregnancy; Lactation: Lactation.

Use Cautiously in: Hypertension (must be well controlled prior to/during therapy); Moderate hepatic impairment (↓ dose); Surgery (discontinue 24 hr prior if possible); End-stage renal disease (CCr <15 mL/min); Rep: Woman of reproductive potential and men with female partners of reproductive

A

potential; Pedi: Safety and effectiveness not established in children.

Adverse Reactions/Side Effects

CV: HYPERTENSION, AORTIC ANEURYSM, ARTERIAL/VENOUS THROMBOEMBOLIC EVENTS, CARDIAC DEATH (WITH AVELUMAB), MI (WITH AVELUMAB), HF. **Derm:** dry skin, rash, palmar-plantar erythrodysesthesia (hand-foot syndrome), alopecia, erythema, wound healing impairment, pruritus. **EENT:** dysphonia. **Endo:** hypothyroidism. **F and E:** ↓ bicarbonate, hyperglycemia, hyperkalemia, hypernatremia, hypoalbuminemia, hypocalcemia, hypoglycemia, hyponatremia, hypophosphatemia, hypercalcemia. **GI:** ↑ liver enzymes, abdominal pain, altered taste, constipation, diarrhea, HEPATOTOXICITY, nausea, stomatitis, burning mouth, GI PERFORATION/FISTULA. **GU:** ↑ serum creatinine, proteinuria. **Hemat:** anemia, neutropenia, thrombocytopenia, BLEEDING. **Metab:** ↓ appetite, weight loss. **MS:** arthralgia, extremity pain. **Neuro:** dysphoria, fatigue, headache, REVERSIBLE POSTERIOR LEUKOENCEPHALOPATHY SYNDROME (RPLS). **Resp:** cough.

Interactions

Drug-Drug: Strong CYP3A4/5 inhibitors, including **atazanavir**, **clarithromycin**, **itraconazole**, **ketoconazole**, **nefazodone**, **nelfinavir**, **ritonavir**, and **voriconazole**, may ↑ levels and risk of toxicity; avoid concurrent use, if possible; if concurrent use unavoidable, select alternative agent. If none is acceptable, ↓ axitinib dose by 50%. **Strong CYP3A4/5 inducers**, including **carbamazepine**, **dexamethasone**, **phenobarbital**, **phenytoin**, **rifabutin**, **rifampin**, and **rifapentin**, as well as **moderate CYP3A4/5 inducers**, including **bosentan**, **efavirenz**, **etravirine**, **modafanil**, and **nafcillin**, may ↓ levels and effectiveness; avoid concurrent use, if possible.

Drug-Natural Products: St. John's wort may ↓ levels and effectiveness; avoid concurrent use.

Drug-Food: Grapefruit/grapefruit juice may ↑ levels and risk of toxicity; avoid concurrent used.

Route/Dosage

First-Line Treatment of Advanced Renal Cell Carcinoma

PO (Adults): *In combination with avelumab:* 5 mg twice daily, approximately 12 hr apart initially; after tolerating therapy for ≥2 consecutive wk (i.e. no adverse reactions Grade >2, remaining normotensive, and not receiving antihypertensive medications), may ↑ to 7 mg twice daily; after tolerating adjusted dose for ≥2 consecutive wk (using same criteria), may ↑ to 10 mg twice daily. Continue treatment until unacceptable toxicity or disease progression. *In combination with pembrolizumab:* 5 mg twice daily, approximately 12 hr apart initially; after tolerating therapy for ≥6 wk (i.e. no adverse reactions Grade >2, remaining normotensive, and not receiving antihypertensive medications), may ↑ to 7 mg twice daily; after tolerating adjusted dose for ≥6 consecutive wk (using same criteria), may ↑ to 10 mg twice daily. Continue treatment until unacceptable toxicity or disease progression. *Concurrent use of strong CYP3A4/5 inhibitors:* ↓ dose by 50%.

Hepatic Impairment

PO (Adults): *Moderate hepatic impairment:* ↓ dose by 50%.

Second-Line Treatment of Advanced Renal Cell Carcinoma

PO (Adults): 5 mg twice daily, approximately 12 hr apart initially; after tolerating therapy for ≥2 consecutive wk (i.e. no adverse reactions Grade >2, remaining normotensive, and not receiving antihypertensive medications), may ↑ to 7 mg twice daily; after tolerating adjusted dose for ≥2 consecutive wk (using same criteria), may ↑ to 10 mg twice daily. Continue treatment until unacceptable toxicity or disease progression. *Concurrent use of strong CYP3A4/5 inhibitors:* ↓ dose by approximately 50%.

Hepatic Impairment

PO (Adults): *Moderate hepatic impairment:* ↓ dose by 50%.

Availability

Tablets: 1 mg, 5 mg.

NURSING IMPLICATIONS

Assessment

- Ensure BP is well controlled before starting therapy. Monitor BP periodically during therapy. *If SBP >150 mm Hg or DBP >100 mm Hg despite antihypertensive treatment,* ↓ dose by one level. *If SBP >160 mm Hg or DBP >105 mm Hg,* hold until BP <150/100 mm Hg. Resume at ↓ dose. *If Grade 4 or hypertensive crisis occurs,* permanently discontinue axitinib.
- Monitor for bleeding during therapy. *If Grade 3 or 4 hemorrhage occurs,* hold until Grade 0 or 1 or baseline. Either resume at ↓ dose or discontinue based on severity and persistence of adverse reaction.
- Monitor for signs or symptoms of cardiac failure during therapy. *If asymptomatic cardiomyopathy (left ventricular ejection fraction >20% but <50% below baseline or below the lower limit of normal if baseline not obtained),* hold until resolution to Grade 0 or 1 or baseline. Resume at ↓ dose. *If HF with clinical signs and symptoms occurs,* permanently discontinue axitinib.

- Axitinib in combination with avelumab may cause severe and fatal cardiovascular events. Monitor for signs and symptoms of severe cardiovascular events. Consider baseline and periodic evaluation of left ventricular ejection fraction. Manage cardiovascular risk factors (hypertension, diabetes, dyslipidemia). *If Grade 3 or 4 cardiovascular events occur,* permanently discontinue axitinib and avelumab.
- May cause diarrhea when in combination with avelumab or pembrolizumab. *If Grade 1–2 diarrhea occurs,* start antidiarrheal medications. *If Grade 3 diarrhea occurs,* hold axitinib. If diarrhea is controlled with antidiarrheals, resume at same dose or ↓ dose by one level. *If Grade 4 diarrhea occurs,* hold axitinib until Grade <2; then resume with ↓ dose by one level.

Lab Test Considerations

- Verify negative pregnancy test before starting therapy. Monitor thyroid function tests before and periodically during therapy. May cause hypothyroidism or hyperthyroidism. Monitor for proteinuria before and periodically during therapy. *If ≥ 2 g proteinuria/24 hr occurs,* hold axitinib until resolution to <2 g/24 hr. Resume at ↓ dose.
- Monitor liver function tests prior to and periodically during therapy. May ↑ ALT, AST and bilirubin. **In combination with avelumab or pembrolizumab:** *If ALT or AST ≥3 times upper limit of normal (ULN) but <10 times ULN without concurrent total bilirubin ≥2 times ULN,* hold both axitinib and avelumab or pembrolizumab until resolution to Grades 0–1. Consider rechallenge with axitinib and/or avelumab or pembrolizumab. *If ALT or AST >3 times ULN with concurrent total bilirubin ≥2 times ULN or ALT or AST ≥10 times ULN,* discontinue both axitinib and avelumab or pembrolizumab permanently.
- May ↑ serum creatinine, alkaline phosphatase, blood sugar, lipase, amylase, sodium, or potassium and ↓ hemoglobin, absolute lymphocytes, platelets, bicarbonate, serum calcium, albumin, blood sugar, sodium, or phosphate.

Implementation

- Do not confuse axitinib with apixaban.
- **Dose Modification Guidelines: *Dose Increase:*** May ↑ dose in patients who have no adverse reactions Grade >2, are normotensive, and are not receiving antihypertensive medication for ≥2 consecutive wk. ***Starting dose:*** 5 mg twice daily. *1st dose ↑:* 7 mg twice daily. *2nd dose ↑:* 10 mg twice daily. ***Dose Reduction:*** *1st dose ↓:* 3 mg twice daily. *2nd dose ↓:* 2 mg twice daily.
- May impair wound healing. Hold therapy for ≥2 days prior to elective surgery. Do not administer for ≥2 wk following major surgery and until adequate wound healing. Resume at ↓ dose or discontinue based on severity and persistence of impaired wound healing.
- **PO:** Administer twice daily with doses 12 hr apart. May be administered without regard to food. ***DNC:*** Swallow tablets whole followed by a full glass of water.

Patient/Family Teaching

- Explain purpose and side effects of medication. Instruct patient that if a dose is vomited or missed, omit dose and take next dose at regular time; do not double doses. Advise patient to read *Patient Information* before starting therapy.
- Advise patient to avoid drinking grapefruit juice or eating grapefruit during axitinib therapy.
- Advise patient to notify health care professional of therapy prior to treatment, dental procedure, or surgery.
- Advise patient to notify health care professional immediately if unexpected bleeding; bleeding of gums; heavier than normal menses; severe or uncontrollable bleeding; pink or brown urine; red or black stools; bloody or dark coffee-ground looking vomit; unexpected pain, swelling, or joint pain; headaches; feeling dizzy; or weakness occur.
- Advise patient to notify health care professional immediately with signs and symptoms of venous or arterial clots (chest pain or pressure; pain in arms, back, neck, or jaw; shortness of breath; numbness or weakness on one side of body; confusion; difficulty talking; headache; or vision changes) occur.
- May cause stomach or intestinal wall perforation. Caution patient to notify health care professional if severe abdominal pain, vomiting blood, or red or black stools occur.
- Advise patient to notify health care professional promptly if signs and symptoms of RPLS (headache, seizures, weakness, confusion, high BP, blindness or change in vision, problems thinking), thyroid problems (worsening or persistent tiredness, feeling hot or cold, voice deepening, weight gain or loss, hair loss, muscle cramps and aches), or HF (tiredness, swelling abdomen, legs or ankles, shortness of breath, protruding neck veins) occur.
- Instruct patient to notify health care professional of all Rx or OTC medications, vitamins, or herbal products being taken and consult health care professional before taking any new medications, especially St. John's wort.
- Rep: May cause fetal harm. Advise women of reproductive potential and men with female partners of reproductive potential to use effective contraception during therapy and for 1 wk after last dose. Advise female patients to avoid breastfeeding during therapy and for 2 wk after last dose. May impair fertility in male and female patients.

Evaluation/Desired Outcomes

- Decreased growth and spread of advanced renal cell carcinoma.

☒ azaTHIOprine
(ay-za-**thye**-oh-preen)
Azasan, Imuran
Classification
Therapeutic: immunosuppressants
Pharmacologic: purine antagonists

Indications

Prevention of renal transplant rejection (in combination with corticosteroids, local radiation, or other cytotoxic agents). Severe, active, erosive rheumatoid arthritis unresponsive to more conventional therapy. **Unlabeled Use:** Crohn disease or ulcerative colitis.

Action

Antagonizes purine metabolism with subsequent inhibition of DNA and RNA synthesis. **Therapeutic Effects:** Suppression of cell-mediated immunity and altered antibody formation.

Pharmacokinetics

Absorption: Readily absorbed after oral administration. IV administration results in complete bioavailability. **Distribution:** Unknown
Metabolism and Excretion: Metabolized to 6-mercaptopurine, which is further metabolized ☒ (one route is by thiopurine methyltransferase [TPMT] to form an inactive metabolite; nucleotide diphosphatase [NUDT15] is also involved in inactivation process). Minimal renal excretion of unchanged drug.
Half-life: 3 hr.

TIME/ACTION PROFILE

ROUTE	ONSET	PEAK	DURATION
PO (anti-inflammatory)	6–8 wk	12 wk	unknown

Contraindications/Precautions

Contraindicated in: Hypersensitivity; OB: Pregnancy; Lactation: Lactation.
Use Cautiously in: Infection; Malignancies; ↓ bone marrow reserve; Previous or concurrent radiation therapy; Severe renal impairment/oliguria; ☒ TPMT or NUDT15 enzyme deficiency (alternative therapy or substantial dose ↓ are required to avoid hematologic adverse events); Rep: Women of reproductive potential; Pedi: ↑ risk of hepatosplenic T-cell lymphoma (HSTCL) in children with inflammatory bowel disease.

Adverse Reactions/Side Effects

CV: Raynaud phenomenon. **Derm:** alopecia, rash. **EENT:** retinopathy. **GI:** <u>anorexia</u>, <u>hepatotoxicity</u>,

nausea, <u>vomiting</u>, diarrhea, mucositis, pancreatitis. **Hemat:** <u>anemia</u>, <u>leukopenia</u>, pancytopenia, <u>thrombocytopenia</u>. **MS:** arthralgia. **Neuro:** PROGRESSIVE MULTIFOCAL LEUKOENCEPHALOPATHY (PML). **Resp:** pulmonary edema. **Misc:** <u>chills</u>, <u>fever</u>, MALIGNANCY (INCLUDING POST-TRANSPLANT LYMPHOMA, HSTCL, AND SKIN CANCER), SERUM SICKNESS.

Interactions

Drug-Drug: **Febuxostat** may ↑ levels and risk of toxicity; concurrent use not recommended. Additive myelosuppression with **antineoplastics**, **cyclosporine**, and **myelosuppressive agents**. **Allopurinol** may ↑ levels and risk of toxicity; ↓ azathioprine dose to 25–33% of the usual dose. May ↓ antibody response to **live-virus vaccines** and ↑ the risk of adverse reactions.
Drug-Natural Products: **Echinacea** and **melatonin** may interfere with immunosuppression.

Route/Dosage
Renal Allograft Rejection Prevention
PO IV (Adults and Children): 3–5 mg/kg/day initially; maintenance dose 1–3 mg/kg/day.

Rheumatoid Arthritis
PO IV (Adults and Children): 1 mg/kg/day for 6–8 wk; ↑ by 0.5 mg/kg/day every 4 wk until response or up to 2.5 mg/kg/day; then ↓ by 0.5 mg/kg/day every 4–8 wk to minimal effective dose.

Inflammatory Bowel Disease (Crohn Disease or Ulcerative Colitis) (unlabeled use)
PO (Adults and Children): 50 mg once daily; may ↑ by 25 mg/day every 1–2 wk as tolerated to target dose of 2–3 mg/kg/day.

Availability (generic available)
Tablets: 50 mg, 75 mg, 100 mg. **Powder for injection:** 100 mg/vial.

NURSING IMPLICATIONS
Assessment

- Assess for infection (vital signs, sputum, urine, stool, WBC) during therapy.
- Monitor intake and output and daily weight. ↓ urine output may lead to toxicity with this medication.
- Monitor for signs of malignancy (splenomegaly, hepatomegaly, abdominal pain, persistent fever, night sweats, and weight loss).
- Monitor for signs of PML (confusion, depression, trouble with memory, behavioral changes, changes in strength on one side, difficulty speaking, change in balance or vision).
- **Rheumatoid Arthritis:** Assess range of motion; degree of swelling, pain, and strength in affected

☘ = Canadian drug name. ☒ = Genetic implication. **V** = Vesicant. Boxed warning.
~~Strikethrough~~ = Discontinued. *CAPITALS = life-threatening. <u>Underline</u> = most frequent.

joints; and ability to perform activities of daily living before and periodically during therapy.

Lab Test Considerations

- Monitor renal, hepatic, and hematologic functions before beginning therapy, weekly during the 1st mo, bimonthly for the next 2–3 mo, and monthly thereafter.
- Leukocyte count of <3000/mm³ or platelet count of <100,000/mm³ may necessitate a ↓ in dose or temporary discontinuation.
- ↓ in hemoglobin may indicate bone marrow suppression.
- Hepatotoxicity may be manifested by ↑ alkaline phosphatase, bilirubin, AST, ALT, and amylase concentrations. Usually occurs within 6 mo of transplant, rarely with rheumatoid arthritis, and is reversible on discontinuation of azathioprine.
- May ↓ serum and urine uric acid and plasma albumin.

Implementation

- Do not confuse azathioprine with azacitidine.
- Protect transplant patients from staff members and visitors who may carry infection. Maintain protective isolation as indicated.
- **PO:** May be administered with or after meals or in divided doses to minimize nausea.

IV Administration

- **Intermittent Infusion: Reconstitution:** Add 10 mL of sterile water for injection, and swirl until a clear solution results. Reconstituted solution should be used within 24 hr. **Dilution:** Further dilute with 0.9% NaCl or D5W; final volume depends on time for the infusion. Inspect solution for particulate matter and discoloration prior to administration.
- **Y-Site Compatibility:** atracurium, atropine, benztropine, calcium gluconate, cyanocobalamin, cyclosporine, digoxin, enalaprilat, epoetin alfa, erythromycin, fentanyl, fluconazole, folic acid, furosemide, glycopyrrolate, heparin, insulin, regular, mannitol, metoclopramide, metoprolol, naloxone, nitroglycerin, oxytocin, pentobarbital, phenobarbital, penicillin G, phytonadione, potassium chloride, propranolol, protamine, sufentanil, vasopressin.
- **Y-Site Incompatibility:** amikacin, aminophylline, ampicillin/sulbactam, ascorbic acid, aztreonam, bumetanide, buprenorphine, butorphanol, calcium chloride, cefazolin, cefotaxime, cefotetan, cefoxitin, ceftazidime, ceftriaxone, cefuroxime, chloramphenicol, chlorpromazine, clindamycin, dantrolene, diazepam, diazoxide, diphenhydramine, dobutamine, dopamine, doxycycline, ephedrine, epinephrine, esmolol, famotidine, ganciclovir, gentamicin, haloperidol, hydralazine, hydrocortisone, imipenem/cilastatin, isoproterenol, ketorolac, labetalol, lidocaine, magnesium sulfate, meperidine, midazolam, minocycline, morphine, multivitamins, nafcillin, nalbuphine, nitroprusside, norepinephrine, ondansetron, pentamidine, phenylephrine, phenytoin, procainamide, prochlorperazine, promethazine, pyridoxine, rocuronium, sodium bicarbonate, succinylcholine, tacrolimus, theophylline, thiamine, tobramycin, trimethoprim/sulfamethoxazole, vancomycin, verapamil. **Rate:** Infuse over 30–60 min; 5 min to 8 hr have been used.

Patient/Family Teaching

- Instruct patient to take azathioprine as directed. If a dose is missed on a once-daily regimen, omit dose; if a dose is missed on several-times-a-day dosing, take as soon as possible or double next dose. Consult health care professional if more than one dose is missed or if vomiting occurs shortly after dose is taken. Do not discontinue without consulting health care professional.
- Advise patient to report unusual tiredness or weakness; cough or hoarseness; fever or chills; lower back or side pain; painful or difficult urination; severe diarrhea; black, tarry stools; blood in urine; or transplant rejection to health care professional immediately.
- Reinforce the need for lifelong therapy to prevent transplant rejection.
- Inform patient of ↑ risk of malignancy. For patients with ↑ risk for skin cancer, exposure to sunlight and ultraviolet light should be limited by wearing protective clothing and using a sunscreen with a high protection factor.
- Instruct patient to notify health care professional of all Rx or OTC medications, vitamins, or herbal products being taken and consult health care professional before taking any new medications or receiving any vaccinations while taking this medication.
- Advise patient to avoid contact with persons with contagious diseases and persons who have recently taken oral poliovirus vaccine or other live viruses.
- Rep: May cause fetal harm. Advise patient to use contraception during and for ≥4 mo after therapy is completed and to avoid breastfeeding during therapy. May also cause intrahepatic cholestasis of pregnancy.
- Emphasize the importance of follow-up exams and lab tests.
- **Rheumatoid Arthritis:** Concurrent therapy with salicylates, NSAIDs, or corticosteroids may be necessary. Patient should continue physical therapy and adequate rest. Explain that joint damage will not be reversed; goal is to slow or stop disease process.

Evaluation/Desired Outcomes

- Prevention of transplant rejection.
- Decreased stiffness, pain, and swelling in affected joints in 6–8 wk in rheumatoid arthritis. Therapy is discontinued if no improvement in 12 wk.

azelastine (a-zel-as-teen)
Astepro Allergy

Classification
Therapeutic: allergy, cold, cough remedies, antihistamines

See Appendix B for ophthalmic use

Indications
Temporary relief of nasal congestion, runny nose, sneezing, and itchy nose due to hay fever or other upper respiratory allergies.

Action
Locally antagonizes the effects of histamine at H_1-receptor sites; does not bind to or inactivate histamine. **Therapeutic Effects:** Decreased sneezing, nasal rhinitis, pruritus and postnasal drip.

Pharmacokinetics
Absorption: 40% absorbed after intranasal administration.
Distribution: Widely distributed to tissues.
Metabolism and Excretion: Most of absorbed azelastine is metabolized by the liver (converted to an active metabolite.
Half-life: 22–25 hr.

TIME/ACTION PROFILE (relief of symptoms)

ROUTE	ONSET	PEAK	DURATION
Intranasal	rapid	2–3 hr†	12 hr

† Plasma concentration.

Contraindications/Precautions
Contraindicated in: Hypersensitivity.
Use Cautiously in: OB: Safety not established in pregnancy; Lactation: Safety not established in breastfeeding; Pedi: Safety not established in children <6 yr.

Adverse Reactions/Side Effects
EENT: epistaxis, nasal burning, pharyngitis, sinusitis, sneezing. **GI:** bitter taste, dry mouth, nausea. **Metab:** ↑ weight. **MS:** myalgia. **Neuro:** drowsiness, dizziness, dysesthesia, fatigue, headache.

Interactions
Drug-Drug: Additive CNS depression with **CNS depressants**, including **alcohol**, **sedative/hypnotics**, and **opioid analgesics**. Concurrent use of **cimetidine** ↑ blood levels.
Drug-Natural Products: Concomitant use of **kava**, **valerian**, **skullcap**, **chamomile**, or **hops** can ↑ CNS depression.

Route/Dosage
Intranasal (Adults and Children ≥12 yr): 2 sprays/nostril once daily *or* 1–2 sprays/nostril twice daily.
Intranasal (Children 6–11 yr): 1 spray/nostril twice daily.

Availability (generic available)
Nasal spray: 205.5 mcg/spray (60–200 sprays/bottle) OTC. ***In combination with:*** fluticasone (Dymista); see Appendix N.

NURSING IMPLICATIONS
Assessment
- Assess allergy symptoms (rhinitis, sneezing, conjunctivitis, hives) before and periodically during therapy.
- Assess lung sounds and character of bronchial secretions. Maintain fluid intake of 1500–2000 mL/day to decrease viscosity of secretions.

Lab Test Considerations
- May cause false-negative allergy skin testing. Discontinue antihistamines at least 72 hr before testing.

Implementation
- **Intranasal** Before initial use, remove the safety clip on the bottle and prime the delivery system with 6 sprays or until a fine mist appears. When ≥3 days have elapsed since last use, reprime the unit with 2 sprays or until a fine mist appears.

Patient/Family Teaching
- Instruct patient in the proper technique for administration of azelastine. Keep head tilted downward toward toes during instillation of intranasal spray to decrease bitter taste.
- May cause drowsiness. Caution patient to avoid driving or other activities requiring alertness until effects of the medication are known.
- Advise patient to avoid taking alcohol or other CNS depressants concurrently with this drug.
- Advise patient that good oral hygiene, frequent rinsing of the mouth, and sugarless gum or candy may help relieve dry mouth. Patient should notify dentist if dry mouth persists >2 wk.
- Instruct patient to notify health care professional of all Rx or OTC medications, vitamins, or herbal products being taken and consult health care professional before taking any new medications.
- Rep: Advise females of reproductive potential to notify health care professional if pregnancy is planned or suspected or if breastfeeding.
- Instruct patient to contact health care professional if symptoms persist.

Evaluation/Desired Outcomes

- Decreased sneezing, nasal rhinitis, pruritus and postnasal drip.

azilsartan, See ANGIOTENSIN II RECEPTOR ANTAGONISTS.

V azithromycin (aye-zith-roe-mye-sin)

~~Zithromax, Zmax~~

Classification

Therapeutic: agents for atypical mycobacterium anti-infectives

Pharmacologic: macrolides

Indications

Acute bacterial exacerbations of chronic bronchitis. Acute bacterial sinusitis. Community-acquired pneumonia. Pharyngitis/tonsillitis (as alternative in patients who cannot use 1st line therapy). Acute otitis media. Uncomplicated skin/skin structure infections. Urethritis/cervicitis. Pelvic inflammatory disease. Genital ulcer disease in men with chancroid. **Unlabeled Use:** Prevention of disseminated *Mycobacterium avium* complex (MAC) infection in patients with advanced HIV infection.

Action

Inhibits protein synthesis at the level of the 50S bacterial ribosome. **Therapeutic Effects:** Bacteriostatic action against susceptible bacteria. **Spectrum:** Active against the following gram-positive aerobic bacteria: *Staphylococcus aureus*, *Streptococcus pneumoniae*, *S. pyogenes* (group A strep). Active against these gram-negative aerobic bacteria: *Haemophilus influenzae*, *Moraxella catarrhalis*, *Neisseria gonorrhoeae*. Also active against: *Bordetella pertussis*, *Mycoplasma*, *Legionella*, *Chlamydia pneumoniae*, *Ureaplasma urealyticum*, *Borrelia burgdorferi*, *M. avium*. Not active against methicillin-resistant *S. aureus*.

Pharmacokinetics

Absorption: Rapidly absorbed (40%) after oral administration. IV administration results in complete bioavailability.

Distribution: Widely distributed to body tissues and fluids. Intracellular and tissue levels exceed those in serum; low CSF levels.

Protein Binding: 7–51%.

Metabolism and Excretion: Mostly excreted unchanged in bile; 4.5% excreted unchanged in urine.

Half-life: 11–14 hr after single dose; 2–4 days after several doses.

TIME/ACTION PROFILE (plasma concentrations)

ROUTE	ONSET	PEAK	DURATION
PO	rapid	2.5–3.2 hr	24 hr
IV	rapid	end of infusion	24 hr

Contraindications/Precautions

Contraindicated in: Hypersensitivity to azithromycin, erythromycin, or other macrolide anti-infectives; History of cholestatic jaundice or hepatic dysfunction with prior use of azithromycin; QT interval prolongation, hypokalemia, hypomagnesemia, or bradycardia.
Use Cautiously in: Severe hepatic impairment (dose adjustment may be required); Severe renal impairment (CCr <10 mL/min); Myasthenia gravis (may worsen symptoms); OB: Use during pregnancy only if potential maternal benefit justifies potential fetal risk; Lactation: Use while breastfeeding only if potential maternal benefit justifies potential risk to infant; Pedi: Neonates (↑ risk of infantile hypertrophic pyloric stenosis at up to 42 days of life); Geri: Older adults may have ↑ risk of QT interval prolongation.

Adverse Reactions/Side Effects

CV: CARDIOVASCULAR DEATH, chest pain, hypotension, palpitations, QT interval prolongation, TORSADES DE POINTES. **Derm:** ACUTE GENERALIZED EXANTHEMATOUS PUSTULOSIS, DRUG REACTION WITH EOSINOPHILIA AND SYSTEMIC SYMPTOMS (DRESS), photosensitivity, rash, STEVENS-JOHNSON SYNDROME (SJS), TOXIC EPIDERMAL NECROLYSIS (TEN). **EENT:** ototoxicity. **F and E:** hyperkalemia. **GI:** abdominal pain, diarrhea, nausea, ↑ liver enzymes, cholestatic jaundice, CLOSTRIDIOIDES DIFFICILE-ASSOCIATED DIARRHEA (CDAD), dyspepsia, flatulence, HEPATOTOXICITY, melena, oral candidiasis, pyloric stenosis. **GU:** nephritis, vaginitis. **Hemat:** anemia, leukopenia, thrombocytopenia. **Neuro:** dizziness, drowsiness, fatigue, headache, seizures. **Misc:** HYPERSENSITIVITY REACTIONS (INCLUDING ANAPHYLAXIS AND ANGIOEDEMA).

Interactions

Drug-Drug: Quinidine, **procainamide**, **dofetilide**, **sotalol**, and **amiodarone** may ↑ risk of QT interval prolongation; avoid concurrent use. **Aluminum-** and **magnesium-containing antacids** ↓ may levels and effectiveness. **Nelfinavir** may ↑ levels and risk of toxicity; azithromycin also ↓ nelfinavir levels and effectiveness. **Efavirenz** may ↑ levels and risk of toxicity. May ↑ the effects and risk of toxicity of **warfarin** and **zidovudine**. Other macrolide anti-infectives have been known to ↑ levels and risk of toxicity of **digoxin**, **theophylline**, **ergotamine**, **dihydroergotamine**, **triazolam**, **carbamazepine**, **cyclosporine**, **tacrolimus**, and **phenytoin**.

Route/Dosage

Acute Bacterial Exacerbations of Chronic Bronchitis

PO (Adults): 500 mg on 1st day; then 250 mg once daily for 4 more days (total dose of 1.5 g) *or* 500 mg once daily for 3 days.

Acute Bacterial Sinusitis

PO (Adults): 500 mg once daily for 3 days.
PO (Children >6 mo): 10 mg/kg once daily for 3 days (not to exceed 500 mg/dose).

Community-Acquired Pneumonia

IV: PO (Adults): *More severe:* 500 mg IV every 24 hr for at least 2 doses; then 500 mg PO every 24 hr for a total of 7–10 days; *Less severe:* 500 mg PO; then 250 mg/day PO for 4 more days.
PO (Children >6 mo): 10 mg/kg on 1st day; then 5 mg/kg once daily for 4 more days (not to exceed 500 mg/dose).

Pharyngitis/Tonsillitis

PO (Adults): 500 mg on 1st day; then 250 mg/day for 4 more days.
PO (Children ≥2 yr): 12 mg/kg once daily for 5 days (not to exceed 500 mg/dose);

Acute Otitis Media

PO (Children ≥6 mo): 30 mg/kg single dose (not to exceed 1500 mg/dose) *or* 10 mg/kg once daily (not to exceed 500 mg/dose) for 3 days *or* 10 mg/kg (not to exceed 500 mg/dose) on 1st day; then 5 mg/kg once daily (not to exceed 250 mg/dose) for 4 more days.

Uncomplicated Skin/Skin Structure Infection

PO (Adults): 500 mg on 1st day; then 250 mg/day for 4 more days.

Urethritis/Cervicitis

PO (Adults): *Nongonococcal:* Single 1-g dose. *Gonococcal:* Single 2-g dose.

Pelvic Inflammatory Disease

IV: PO (Adults): 500 mg IV every 24 hr for 1–2 days; then 250 mg PO every 24 hr for a total of 7 days.

Genital Ulcer Disease in Men with Chancroid

PO (Adults): Single 1-g dose.

Prevention of Disseminated MAC Infection

PO (Adults): 1.2 g once weekly (as monotherapy or in combination with rifabutin).
PO (Children): 5 mg/kg once daily (not >250 mg/dose) or 20 mg/kg (not >1200 mg/dose) once weekly (as monotherapy or in combination with rifabutin).

Availability (generic available)

Tablets: 250 mg, 500 mg, 600 mg. **Powder for oral suspension (cherry and banana flavor):** 1 g/pkt. **Powder for oral suspension (cherry, creme de vanilla, and banana flavor):** 100 mg/5 mL, 200 mg/5 mL. **Powder for injection:** 500 mg/vial.

NURSING IMPLICATIONS

Assessment

- Assess for infection (vital signs; appearance of wound, sputum, urine, and stool; WBC) at beginning of and throughout therapy.
- Obtain specimens for culture and sensitivity before initiating therapy. 1st dose may be given before receiving results.
- Observe for signs and symptoms of anaphylaxis (rash, pruritus, laryngeal edema, wheezing). Notify health care professional immediately if these occur.
- Assess for skin rash frequently during therapy. Discontinue azithromycin at first sign of rash; may be life-threatening. SJS or TEN may develop. Treat symptomatically; may recur once treatment is stopped.
- Assess cardiac history and ECG at baseline; optimally avoid use in patients with long QT syndrome or cardiac arrhythmias associated with prolonged QT interval or those on concurrent medications that can prolong the QT interval;

Lab Test Considerations

- May ↑ serum bilirubin, AST, ALT, LDH, and alkaline phosphatase concentrations.
- May ↑ CK, potassium, PT, BUN, serum creatinine, and blood glucose.
- May occasionally cause ↓ WBC and platelet count.

Implementation

- **PO:** Administer 1 hr before or 2 hr after meals. Do not give simultaneously with aluminum- or magnesium-containing antacids.
- For administration of single 1-g packet, thoroughly mix entire contents of packet with 2 ounces (60 mL) of water. Drink entire contents immediately; add an additional 2 ounces of water, mix, and drink to assure complete consumption of dose. Do not use the single packet to administer doses other than 1000 mg of azithromycin. Pedi: 1-g packet is not for pediatric use.

IV Administration

- V IV azithromycin is a vesicant. Can be administered through peripheral IV, midline catheter, or PICC. If extravasation occurs, immediately stop infusion. Leave needle/cannula in place temporarily, but do not flush the line. Gently aspirate extravasated solution; then remove needle/cannula. Elevate patient's extremity and apply warm dry compresses.

- **Intermittent Infusion: Reconstitution:** Reconstitute each 500-mg vial with 4.8 mL of sterile water for injection. Reconstituted solution is stable for 24 hr at room temperature. **Concentration:** 100 mg/mL. **Dilution:** Further dilute the 500-mg dose in 250 mL or 500 mL of 0.9% NaCl, 0.45% NaCl, D5W, LR, D5/0.45% NaCl, or D5/LR. Infusion is stable for 24 hr at room temperature or for 7 days if refrigerated. **Concentration:** 1–2 mg/mL. **Rate:** Infuse over 3 hr (1 mg/mL solution) or 1 hr (2 mg/mL solution). Do not administer as an IV bolus.
- **Y-Site Compatibility:** acyclovir, alemtuzumab, aminocaproic acid, aminophylline, amphotericin B liposomal, ampicillin, ampicillin/sulbactam, anidulafungin, argatroban, arsenic trioxide, atracurium, bivalirudin, bleomycin, bumetanide, buprenorphine, butorphanol, calcium chloride, calcium gluconate, cangrelor, carboplatin, carmustine, cefazolin, cefepime, cefotetan, cefoxitin, ceftaroline, ceftazidime, ceftolozane/tazobactam, cisatracurium, cisplatin, cyclophosphamide, cyclosporine, cytarabine, dacarbazine, daptomycin, dexamethasone, dexmedetomidine, dexrazoxane, digoxin, diltiazem, diphenhydramine, dobutamine, docetaxel, dopamine, doxorubicin liposomal, doxycycline, droperidol, enalaprilat, ephedrine, epinephrine, eptifibatide, ertapenem, esmolol, etoposide, etoposide phosphate, fluconazole, fluorouracil, foscarnet, fosphenytoin, ganciclovir, gemcitabine, granisetron, haloperidol, heparin, hetastarch, hydrocortisone, hydromorphone, idarubicin, ifosfamide, irinotecan, isoproterenol, labetalol, LR, leucovorin, lidocaine, linezolid, lorazepam, magnesium sulfate, mannitol, meperidine, meropenem, meropenem/vaborbactam, mesna, methadone, methohexital, methotrexate, methylprednisolone, metoclopramide, milrinone, nalbuphine, naloxone, nitroglycerin, nitroprusside, octreotide, ondansetron, oxaliplatin, oxytocin, paclitaxel, palonosetron, pamidronate, pantoprazole, pemetrexed, pentobarbital, phenobarbital, phenylephrine, plazomicin, potassium acetate, potassium phosphates, procainamide, prochlorperazine, promethazine, propranolol, remifentanil, rocuronium, sodium acetate, sodium bicarbonate, sodium phosphates, succinylcholine, sufentanil, tacrolimus, telavancin, thiotepa, tigecycline, tirofiban, trimethoprim/sulfamethoxazole, vancomycin, vasopressin, vecuronium, verapamil, vincristine, voriconazole, zidovudine, zoledronic acid.
- **Y-Site Incompatibility:** amiodarone, amphotericin B deoxycholate, chlorpromazine, diazepam, doxorubicin hydrochloride, epirubicin, gemtuzumab ozogamicin, midazolam, mitoxantrone, mycophenolate, nicardipine, pentamidine, phenytoin.

Patient/Family Teaching

- Educate patient on reason for azithromycin and side effects. Instruct patients to take medication as directed and to finish the drug completely, even if they are feeling better. Take missed doses as soon as possible unless almost time for next dose; do not double doses. Advise patients that sharing of this medication may be dangerous, even if others have similar symptoms. Advise patient to read *Patient Information* before starting.
- Instruct patient not to take azithromycin with food or antacids.
- May cause drowsiness and dizziness. Caution patient to avoid driving or other activities requiring alertness until response to medication is known.
- Advise patient to use sunscreen and protective clothing to prevent photosensitivity reactions.
- Advise patient to report symptoms of chest pain, palpitations, yellowing of skin or eyes, or signs of superinfection (black, furry overgrowth on the tongue; vaginal itching or discharge; loose or foul-smelling stools) or rash.
- Instruct patient to notify health care professional if fever and diarrhea develop, especially if stool contains blood, pus, or mucus. Advise patient not to treat diarrhea without advice of health care professional.
- Advise patients being treated for nongonococcal urethritis or cervicitis that sexual partners should also be treated.
- Instruct parents, caregivers, or patient to notify health care professional if symptoms do not improve.
- Rep: Advise women of reproductive potential to notify health care professional if pregnancy is planned or suspected or if breastfeeding. Advise parents to monitor breastfed infant for diarrhea, vomiting, or rash.

Evaluation/Desired Outcomes

- Resolution of the signs and symptoms of infection. Length of time for complete resolution depends on the organism and site of infection.

aztreonam (az-**tree**-oh-nam)

Azactam, Cayston

Classification

Therapeutic: anti-infectives

Pharmacologic: monobactams

Indications

IM IV: Treatment of serious gram-negative infections, including: Septicemia, Skin and skin structure infections, Intra-abdominal infections, Gynecologic infections, Respiratory tract infections, Urinary tract infections. Useful for treatment of multiresistant strains of some bacteria including aerobic gram-negative pathogens. **Inhaln:** To improve respiratory symptoms in patients with cystic fibrosis (CF) with *Pseudomonas aeruginosa*.

Action

Inhibits bacterial cell wall synthesis. **Therapeutic Effects:** Bactericidal action against susceptible bacteria. **Spectrum:** Displays significant activity against gram-negative aerobic organisms only: *Escherichia coli, Serratia, Klebsiella oxytoca or pneumoniae, Citrobacter, Proteus mirabilis, Pseudomonas aeruginosa, Enterobacter, Haemophilus influenzae*. Not active against: *Staphylococcus aureus, Enterococcus, Bacteroides fragilis, Streptococci*.

Pharmacokinetics

Absorption: Well absorbed following IM administration. IV administration results in complete bioavailability. Low absorption follows administration by oral inhalation.

Distribution: Widely distributed to tissues. High concentrations achieved in sputum with inhalation.

Metabolism and Excretion: 60–70% excreted unchanged by the kidneys. 10% of inhaled dose excreted unchanged in urine. Small amounts metabolized by the liver.

Half-life: *Adults:* 1.5–2 hr; *Children:* 1.7 hr; *Neonates:* 2.4–9 hr (↑ in renal impairment).

TIME/ACTION PROFILE (plasma concentrations)

ROUTE	ONSET	PEAK	DURATION
IM	rapid	60 min	6–8 hr
IV	rapid	end of infusion	6–8 hr
Inhaln	rapid	unknown	Several hr

Contraindications/Precautions

Contraindicated in: Hypersensitivity; Lactation: Lactation (IV/IM formulation).

Use Cautiously in: Severe renal impairment; Cross-sensitivity with penicillins or cephalosporins may occur rarely; has been used safely in patients with a history of penicillin or cephalosporin allergy; Patients with FEV_1 <25% or >75% predicted, or patients colonized with *Burkholderia cepacia* (safety and effectiveness not established); OB: Safety of IV/IM formulation not established in pregnancy; systemic absorption of oral inhalation expected to be minimal; Lactation: Systemic absorption of oral inhalation expected to be minimal; Pedi: Children <7 yr (oral inhalation) (safety and effectiveness not established); Geri: Consider age-related ↓ in renal function in older adults.

Adverse Reactions/Side Effects

CV: chest discomfort (oral inhalation). **Derm:** rash. **EENT:** nasal congestion (oral inhalation), nasopharyngeal pain (oral inhalation). **GI:** abdominal pain (oral inhalation), altered taste, CLOSTRIDIOIDES DIFFICILE-ASSOCIATED DIARRHEA (CDAD), diarrhea, nausea, vomiting. **Local:** pain at IM site, phlebitis at IV site. **Neuro:** SEIZURES. **Resp:** cough (oral inhalation), wheezing (oral inhalation), bronchospasm (oral inhalation). **Misc:** fever (inhalation), HYPERSENSITIVITY REACTIONS (INCLUDING ANAPHYLAXIS), superinfection.

Interactions

Drug-Drug: Levels may be ↑ by **furosemide** or **probenecid**.

Route/Dosage

IM IV (Adults): *Moderately severe infections:* 1–2 g every 8–12 hr; *severe or life-threatening infections (including those due to Pseudomonas aeruginosa):* 2 g every 6–8 hr; *urinary tract infections:* 0.5–1 g every 8–12 hr.

IV (Children 1 mo–16 yr): *Mild to moderate infections:* 30 mg/kg every 8 hr; *moderate to severe infections:* 30 mg/kg every 6–8 hr; *cystic fibrosis:* 50 mg/kg every 6–8 hr.

IV (Neonates >2 kg): 30 mg/kg every 6–8 hr.

IV (Neonates ≤2 kg): 30 mg/kg every 8–12 hr.

Inhaln: (Adults and Children >7 yr): 75 mg three times daily for 28 days.

Renal Impairment

IV (Adults): *CCr 10–30 mL/min:* 1–2 g initially; then 50% of usual dosage at usual interval; *CCr <10 mL/min:* 500 mg–2 g initially; then 25% of usual dosage at usual interval (of initial dose should also be given after each hemodialysis session).

Availability (generic available)

Powder for injection: 1 g/vial, 2 g/vial. **Lyophilized powder for use with diluent provided in Altera Nebulizer System only (Cayston):** 75 mg/vial with 1 mL ampule of diluent (0.17% NaCl).

NURSING IMPLICATIONS

Assessment

- Assess infection at baseline and monitor for effectiveness of aztreonam throughout therapy.
- Assess history of previous use and reaction to penicillins and cephalosporins prior to initiating therapy. Aztreonam can often still be used in patients allergic to these drugs.
- Assess respiratory status prior to and following inhalation therapy.
- Observe for signs and symptoms of anaphylaxis (rash, pruritus, laryngeal edema, wheezing). Notify the health care professional immediately if these occur.
- Monitor for diarrhea, abdominal cramping, fever, and bloody stools during and up to 8 wk

after cessation of therapy. *If CDAD suspected or confirmed,* discontinue antibiotics not directed at *Clostridium difficile* and treat as clinically indicated.

Lab Test Considerations

- Obtain specimens for culture and sensitivity before initiating therapy. First dose may be given before receiving results.
- May ↑ in AST, ALT, alkaline phosphatase, LDH, and serum creatinine. May ↑ prothrombin and partial thromboplastin times, and positive Coombs test.

Implementation

- After adding diluent to vial, shake immediately and vigorously. Solution is colorless to light straw yellow to slightly pink. Do not administer if discolored, cloudy, or contains particulates. Not for multidose use; discard unused solution. IV route is recommended if single dose >1 g or for severe or life-threatening infection.
- **IM Reconstitution:** Add at least 3 mL 0.9% NaCl or sterile or bacteriostatic water for injection to each gram of aztreonam. Stable at room temperature for 48 hr or 7 days if refrigerated.
- Administer into large, well-developed muscle.

IV Administration

- **IV Push: Reconstitution:** Add 6–10 mL of sterile water for injection into each vial. **Rate:** Administer slowly over 3–5 min by direct injection or into tubing of a compatible solution.
- **Intermittent Infusion: Reconstitution:** Add 3 mL of sterile water for injection into each vial. **Dilution:** Dilute further with 0.9% NaCl, Ringer's or LR, D5W, D10W, D5/0.9% NaCl, D5/0.45% NaCl, D5/0.2% NaCl, D5/LR, or sodium lactate. **Concentration:** Do not exceed 50 mg/mL. Solution is stable for 48 hr at room temperature and 7 days refrigerated. **Rate:** Infuse over 20–60 min.
- **Y-Site Compatibility:** alemtuzumab, allopurinol, amikacin, aminocaproic acid, aminophylline, anidulafungin, argatroban, arsenic trioxide, ascorbic acid, atracurium, atropine, benztropine, bivalirudin, bleomycin, bumetanide, buprenorphine, butorphanol, calcium chloride, calcium gluconate, cangrelor, carboplatin, carmustine, caspofungin, cefazolin, cefepime, cefotaxime, cefotetan, cefoxitin, ceftazidime, ceftolozane/tazobactam, ceftriaxone, cefuroxime, ciprofloxacin, cisatracurium, cisplatin, clindamycin, cyanocobalamin, cyclophosphamide, cyclosporine, cytarabine, dacarbazine, dactinomycin, daptomycin, dexamethasone, dexmedetomidine, dexrazoxane, digoxin, diltiazem, dobutamine, docetaxel, dopamine, doxorubicin hydrochloride, doxorubicin liposomal, doxycycline, droperidol, enalaprilat, ephedrine, epinephrine, epirubicin, epoetin alfa, eptifibatide, eravacycline, ertapenem, esmolol, etoposide, etoposide phosphate, famotidine, fentanyl, filgrastim, floxuridine, fluconazole, fludarabine, fluorouracil, folic acid, foscarnet, fosphenytoin, furosemide, gemcitabine, gentamicin, glycopyrrolate, granisetron, heparin, hetastarch, hydrocortisone, hydromorphone, idarubicin, ifosfamide, insulin, regular, irinotecan, isavuconazonium, isoproterenol, ketorolac, labetalol, leucovorin calcium, levofloxacin, lidocaine, linezolid, magnesium sulfate, mannitol, melphalan, meperidine, meropenem, meropenem/vaborbactam, mesna, methadone, methotrexate, methylprednisolone, metoclopramide, metoprolol, midazolam, milrinone, morphine, multivitamin, nafcillin, nalbuphine, naloxone, nicardipine, nitroglycerin, nitroprusside, norepinephrine, octreotide, ondansetron, oxacillin, oxaliplatin, oxytocin, paclitaxel, palonosetron, pamidronate, pemetrexed, penicillin G, phenobarbital, phentolamine, phenylephrine, phytonadione, piperacillin/tazobactam, plazomicin, plicamycin, potassium acetate, potassium chloride, procainamide, propofol, propranolol, protamine, pyridoxine, remifentanil, rituximab, rocuronium, sargramostim, sodium acetate, sodium bicarbonate, succinylcholine, sufentanil, sulbactam/durlobactam, tacrolimus, tedizolid, theophylline, thiamine, thiotepa, tigecycline, tirofiban, tobramycin, topotecan, vasopressin, vecuronium, verapamil, vinblastine, vincristine, vinorelbine, voriconazole, zidovudine, zoledronic acid.
- **Y-Site Incompatibility:** acyclovir, amphotericin B deoxycholate, amphotericin B liposomal, azathioprine, azithromycin, chlorpromazine, dantrolene, daunorubicin, diazepam, diazoxide, erythromycin, ganciclovir, gemtuzumab ozogamicin, indomethacin, letermovir, lorazepam, metronidazole, mitomycin, mitoxantrone, mycophenolate, oritavancin, pantoprazole, papaverine, pentamidine, pentobarbital, phenytoin, prochlorperazine, trastuzumab.
- **Inhaln: Reconstitution:** Open glass vial; remove metal ring, pull tab, and remove gray stopper. Twist tip of included diluent ampule and squeeze contents into glass vial. Replace stopper and swirl gently until contents are completely dissolved. Administer immediately after reconstitution using *Altera Nebulizer System*. Pour reconstituted solution into handset of nebulizer. Turn unit on. Place mouthpiece into mouth and breathe normally only through mouth. Administration takes 2–3 min. Do not use other nebulizers or mix with other medications. Refrigerate aztreonam and diluent; may be stored at room temperature for up to 28 days. Protect from light.
- Administer short-acting bronchodilator between 15 min and 4 hr or long-acting bronchodilator

between 30 min and 12 hr prior to treatment. If taking multiple inhaled therapies, administer in the following order: bronchodilator, mucolytic, and lastly aztreonam.

Patient/Family Teaching

- Advise patient to report signs of superinfection (furry overgrowth on the tongue, vaginal itching or discharge, loose or foul-smelling stools) and allergy.
- Instruct patient to notify health care professional if fever and diarrhea develop, especially if stool contains blood, pus, or mucus. Advise patient not to self-treat diarrhea.
- Advise patient to notify health care professional of new or worsening symptoms of infection or if anaphylaxis occurs.
- Rep: Advise women of reproductive potential to notify health care professional if pregnancy is planned or suspected or if breastfeeding. Patients receiving IV aztreonam should consider temporarily discontinuing breastfeeding during therapy.
- **Inhaln:** Instruct patient to use aztreonam as directed for the full 28-day course, even if feeling better. If a dose is missed, take all three daily doses, as long as doses are ≥4 hr apart. Skipping doses or not completing full course of therapy may ↓ effectiveness and ↑ likelihood of bacterial resistance. Inform patient of the importance of using a bronchodilator prior to treatment and in use and cleaning of nebulizer. Advise patient to read *Patient Information* before starting therapy.

Evaluation/Desired Outcomes

- Resolution of signs and symptoms of infection.
- Improvement in respiratory symptoms in patients with CF.

aztreonam/avibactam

(az-tree-oh-nam/a-vi-**bak**-tam)

Emblaveo

Classification

Therapeutic: anti-infectives

Pharmacologic: monobactams, beta-lactamase inhibitors

Indications

Complicated intra-abdominal infections in patients who have limited or no treatment options (in combination with metronidazole).

Action

Aztreonam: Inhibits bacterial cell wall synthesis. *Avibactam:* Inhibits beta-lactamase, an enzyme that destroys penicillins and cephalosporins. **Therapeutic Effects:** Death of susceptible bacteria with resolution of infection. **Spectrum:** Active against *Escherichia coli*, *Klebsiella pneumoniae*, *Enterobacter cloacae*, *Klebsiella oxytoca*, *Citrobacter freundii*, and *Serratia marcescens*.

Pharmacokinetics

Aztreonam

Absorption: IV administration results in complete bioavailability.

Distribution: Widely distributed to tissues.

Metabolism and Excretion: 60–70% excreted unchanged by the kidneys. Small amounts metabolized by the liver.

Half-life: 2 hr.

Avibactam

Absorption: IV administration results in complete bioavailability.

Distribution: Widely distributed to tissues.

Metabolism and Excretion: Minimally metabolized; mainly excreted unchanged in urine.

Half-life: 2 hr.

TIME/ACTION PROFILE (plasma concentrations)

ROUTE	ONSET	PEAK	DURATION
IV	rapid	end of infusion	unknown

Contraindications/Precautions

Contraindicated in: Hypersensitivity.

Use Cautiously in: Renal impairment (CCr <50 mL/min); Hepatic impairment; OB: Safety not established in pregnancy; Lactation: Safety not established in breastfeeding; Pedi: Safety and effectiveness not established in children; Geri: Consider age-related impairment of renal function in older adults.

Adverse Reactions/Side Effects

CV: hypotension. **Derm:** flushing, rash, TOXIC EPIDERMAL NECROLYSIS (TEN). **F and E:** hypokalemia. **GI:** ↑ liver enzymes, abdominal pain, CLOSTRIDIOIDES DIFFICILE-ASSOCIATED DIARRHEA (CDAD), constipation, diarrhea, nausea, vomiting. **Hemat:** anemia, eosinophilia, leukocytosis, thrombocytopenia, thrombocytosis. **Local:** phlebitis. **Neuro:** ageusia, dizziness, headache, insomnia, mental status changes. **Misc:** fever, hypersensitivity reactions.

Interactions

Drug-Drug: Concurrent use with **probenecid** not recommended.

Route/Dosage

IV (Adults): 2.67 g (2 g aztreonam/0.67 g avibactam) initially as loading dose, then 2 g (1.5 g aztreonam/0.5 g avibactam) every 6 hr for 5–14 days.

Renal Impairment

IV (Adults): *CCr 30–<50 mL/min:* 2.67 g (2 g aztreonam/0.67 g avibactam) initially as loading dose, then 1 g (0.75 g aztreonam/0.25 g avibactam) every 6 hr for 5–14 days. *CCr 15–<30 mL/min:* 1.8 g (1.35 g aztreonam/0.45 g avibactam) initially as loading dose, then 0.9 g (0.675 g aztreonam/0.225 g avibactam) every 8 hr for 5–14 days. *CCr <15 mL/min or Hemodialysis:* 1.33 g (1 g aztreonam/0.33 g avibactam) initially as loading dose, then 0.9 g (0.675 g aztreonam/0.225 g avibactam) every 12 hr for 5–14 days.

Availability

Powder for injection: aztreonam 1.5 g/avibactam 0.5 g/vial.

NURSING IMPLICATIONS

Assessment

- Monitor body temperature. May cause fever.
- Assess for hypersensitivity reactions (rash, flushing, and bronchospasm). *If hypersensitivity reaction occurs,* discontinue aztreonam/avibactam and start appropriate medications and/or supportive care.
- Assess for skin reactions such as TEN (sore throat, painful erosions in the mouth, eyes, or genitalia, red/purple blistering rash). *If a serious skin reaction occurs,* discontinue aztreonam/avibactam.
- Monitor for diarrhea, abdominal cramping, fever, and bloody stools during and up to 8 wk after cessation of therapy. *If CDAD suspected or confirmed,* discontinue aztreonam/avibactam and treat as clinically indicated.

Lab Test Considerations

- Obtain specimens for culture and sensitivity before initiating therapy. First dose may be given before receiving results.
- May ↑ ALT and AST.
- May ↓ potassium and hemoglobin.

Implementation

- Administer after hemodialysis if applicable.

IV Administration

- **Intermittent Infusion:**
- **Reconstitution:** Reconstitute vial with 10 mL of sterile water for injection. Mix gently until contents dissolve completely. Solution may be stored for up to 60 min under ambient light before further dilution. **Dilution:** Further dilute appropriate volume of reconstituted solution to 50–250 mL in 0.9% NaCl, D5W, or LR. Diluted solution may be refrigerated for up to 24 hr followed by 4 hr (solution diluted in D5W) or 12 hr (solution diluted in 0.9% NaCl or LR) at room temperature under ambient light. **Concentration:** 2.7–40 mg/mL (aztreonam); 0.9–13.3 mg/mL (avibactam). **Rate:** Infuse over 3 hr
- **Y-Site Incompatibility:** Do not administer other drugs through same IV line.

Patient/Family Teaching

- Explain purpose and side effects of medication to patient. Advise patient to read *Patient Information* before starting therapy. Emphasize on the importance of completing the full course of therapy.
- Advise patient to notify health care professional of all Rx or OTC medications, vitamins, or herbal products being taken and to consult health care professional before taking other medications.
- Advise patient about the hypersensitivity reactions that can occur and to notify health care professional or seek immediate medical attention.
- Advise patient to notify health care professional if signs/symptoms of a severe rash, blistering or peeling skin with or without a fever or joint pain occur.
- Advise patient to notify health care professional if severe watery or bloody diarrhea develops.
- Rep: Advise women of reproductive potential to notify health care professional if pregnancy is planned or suspected or if breastfeeding.

Evaluation/Desired Outcomes

- Death of susceptible bacteria with resolution of infection.

B

baclofen (bak-loe-fen)

Fleqsuvy, Gablofen, Lioresal, Ozobax DS

Classification

Therapeutic: antispasticity agents, skeletal muscle relaxants (centrally acting)

Indications

PO: Reversible spasticity due to multiple sclerosis or spinal cord lesions. **IT:** Severe spasticity of cerebral or spinal origin (should be reserved for patients who do not respond or are intolerant to oral baclofen) (should wait at least one yr in patients with traumatic brain injury before considering therapy). **Unlabeled Use:** Pain in trigeminal neuralgia.

Action

Inhibits reflexes at the spinal level. **Therapeutic Effects:** Decreased muscle spasticity; bowel and bladder function may also be improved.

Pharmacokinetics

Absorption: Well absorbed after oral administration.
Distribution: Widely distributed to tissues.
Metabolism and Excretion: 70–80% eliminated unchanged by the kidneys.
Half-life: 2.5–4 hr.

TIME/ACTION PROFILE (effects on spasticity)

ROUTE	ONSET	PEAK	DURATION
PO	hr–wk	unknown	unknown
IT	0.5–1 hr	4 hr	4–8 hr

Contraindications/Precautions

Contraindicated in: Hypersensitivity.
Use Cautiously in: Patients in whom spasticity maintains posture and balance; Seizure disorders (may ↓ seizure threshold); Renal impairment (↓ dose may be required); OB: Safety not established in pregnancy; Lactation: Use while breastfeeding only if potential maternal benefit justifies potential risk to infant; Pedi: Children <4 yr (intrathecal) (safety and effectiveness not established); Geri: ↑ risk of CNS side effects in older adults.

Adverse Reactions/Side Effects

CV: edema, hypotension. **Derm:** pruritus, rash. **EENT:** nasal congestion, tinnitus. **GI:** <u>nausea</u>, constipation. **GU:** frequency. **Metab:** ↑ weight, hyperglycemia. **Neuro:** <u>dizziness</u>, <u>drowsiness</u>, <u>fatigue</u>, <u>weakness</u>, ataxia, confusion, depression, headache, insomnia, SEIZURES (IT). **Misc:** hypersensitivity reactions, sweating.

Interactions

Drug-Drug: ↑ CNS depression with other **CNS depressants**, including **alcohol**, **antihistamines**, **opioid analgesics**, and **sedative/hypnotics**. Use with **MAO inhibitors** may lead to ↑ CNS depression or hypotension.
Drug-Natural Products: Kava-kava, **valerian**, or **chamomile** can ↑ CNS depression.

Route/Dosage

PO (Adults): 5 mg 3 times daily. May ↑ every 3 days by 5 mg/dose up to 80 mg/day (some patients may have a better response to 4 divided doses).
PO (Children ≥8 yr): 30–40 mg/day divided every 8 hr; titrate to a maximum of 120 mg/day.
PO (Children 2–7 yr): 20–30 mg/day divided every 8 hr; titrate to a maximum of 60 mg/day.
PO (Children <2 yr): 10–20 mg/day divided every 8 hr; titrate to a maximum of 40 mg/day.
IT: (Adults): 100–800 mcg/day infusion; dose is determined by response during screening phase.
IT: (Children ≥4 yr): 25–1200 mcg/day infusion (average 275 mcg/day); dose is determined by response during screening phase.

Availability (generic available)

Tablets: 5 mg, 10 mg, 15 mg, 20 mg. **Oral solution (grape flavor):** 1 mg/mL, 2 mg/mL. **Oral suspension (grape flavor):** 5 mg/mL. **Solution for intrathecal injection:** 50 mcg/mL, 500 mcg/mL, 1000 mcg/mL, 2000 mcg/mL.

NURSING IMPLICATIONS

Assessment

- Assess muscle spasticity before and periodically during therapy.
- Observe patient for drowsiness, dizziness, or ataxia. May be alleviated by a change in dose.
- **IT:** Monitor patient closely during test dose and titration. Have resuscitative equipment immediately available for life-threatening or intolerable side effects.

Lab Test Considerations

- May ↑ serum glucose, alkaline phosphatase, AST, and ALT.

Implementation

- **PO:** Administer with milk or food to ↓ GI irritation.
- **Oral suspension:** Shake oral suspension well before use. Use a calibrated measuring device to measure and deliver dose accurately; a household teaspoon or tablespoon is not an adequate measuring device. Discard unused portion 2 mo after first opening.
- **IT:** For *screening phase:* **Dilution:** dilute for a concentration of 50 mcg/mL with sterile

preservative-free NaCl for injection. Test dose should be administered over ≥1 min. Observe patient for a significant ↓ in muscle tone or frequency or severity of spasm. If response is inadequate, two additional test doses, each 24 hr apart, 75 mcg/1.5 mL and 100 mcg/2 mL respectively, may be administered. Patients with an inadequate response should not receive chronic IT therapy. Avoid use of prefilled syringes for filling reservoir of pump; prefilled syringes are not sterile.
- Dose titration for implantable IT pumps is based on patient response. If no substantive response after dose ↑, check pump function and catheter patency.

Patient/Family Teaching

- Instruct patient to take baclofen as directed. Take a missed dose within 1 hr; do not double doses. Caution patient to avoid abrupt withdrawal of this medication; may precipitate an acute withdrawal reaction (hallucinations, increased spasticity, seizures, mental changes, restlessness). Discontinue baclofen gradually over 2 wk or more.
- May cause dizziness and drowsiness. Advise patient to avoid driving or other activities requiring alertness until response to drug is known.
- Instruct patient to change positions slowly to minimize orthostatic hypotension.
- Advise patient to avoid concurrent use of alcohol or other CNS depressants while taking this medication.
- Instruct patient to notify health care provider if frequent urge to urinate or painful urination, constipation, nausea, headache, insomnia, tinnitus, depression, or confusion persists.
- Advise patient to report signs and symptoms of hypersensitivity (rash, itching) promptly.
- Rep: Advise women of reproductive potential to notify health care provider if pregnancy is planned or suspected or if breastfeeding. Inform patient that use during pregnancy or breastfeeding may cause withdrawal symptoms (↑ muscle tone, tremor, jitteriness, seizures) in infants starting hours to days after delivery.
- **IT:** Caution patient and caregiver not to discontinue IT therapy abruptly. May result in fever, mental status changes, exaggerated rebound spasticity, and muscle rigidity. Advise patient not to miss scheduled refill appointments and to notify health care provider promptly if signs of withdrawal occur.

Evaluation/Desired Outcomes

- Decrease in muscle spasticity and associated musculoskeletal pain with an increased ability to perform activities of daily living.
- Decreased pain in patients with trigeminal neuralgia. May take wk to obtain optimal effect.

baricitinib (bar-i-sye-ti-nib)

Olumiant

Classification

Therapeutic: antirheumatics

Pharmacologic: kinase inhibitors

Indications

Moderately to severely active rheumatoid arthritis (RA) in patients who have had an inadequate response/intolerance to ≥1 tumor necrosis factor inhibitor therapies (as monotherapy or in combination with methotrexate or other non-biologic disease-modifying antirheumatic drugs [DMARDs]) (not to be used with other Janus kinase [JAK] inhibitors, biologic DMARDs, or potent immunosuppressants, including azathioprine and cyclosporine). Coronavirus disease 2019 (COVID-19) in hospitalized patients requiring supplemental oxygen, noninvasive or invasive mechanical ventilation, or extracorporeal membrane oxygenation (ECMO). Severe alopecia areata (not to be used with other JAK inhibitors, biologic immunomodulates, cyclosporine, or other potent immunosuppressants).

Action

Acts as a JAK inhibitor, which prevents the activation of signal transducers and activators of transcription, resulting in a reduction in immunoglobulins and C-reactive protein. **Therapeutic Effects:** Improvement in clinical and symptomatic parameters of RA. Shortened time to recovery and reduction in death from COVID-19. Improvement in scalp hair coverage in alopecia areata.

Pharmacokinetics

Absorption: Well absorbed following oral administration (80%).
Distribution: Widely distributed into tissues.
Metabolism and Excretion: Metabolized by the liver by CYP3A4; primarily excreted in the urine (69% as unchanged drug); 15% excreted in feces as unchanged drug.
Half-life: 12 hr.

TIME/ACTION PROFILE (clinical improvement)

ROUTE	ONSET	PEAK	DURATION
PO	1 wk	3 mo	unknown

Contraindications/Precautions

Contraindicated in: Active infection; Severe renal impairment (for RA); Patients with end-stage renal disease (ESRD), acute kidney injury, or receiving dialysis (for COVID-19); Severe hepatic impairment (for RA or alopecia areata); ↑ risk for thrombosis; Absolute lymphocyte count (ALC) <500 cells/mm^3, ANC <1000 cells/mm^3, or hemoglobin <8 g/dL; Lactation: Lactation.

B

Use Cautiously in: Patients who are >50 yr old and have ≥1 cardiovascular risk factor (↑ risk of all-cause mortality, cardiovascular death, MI, stroke, and thrombosis); Current or past history of smoking (↑ risk of malignancy, cardiovascular death, MI, or stroke); Malignancy (other than successfully treated nonmelanoma skin cancer); Chronic or recurrent infection; Previously exposed to tuberculosis (TB); History of serious or opportunistic infection; Resided or traveled in areas of endemic tuberculosis or endemic mycoses; Underlying conditions that predispose to infection; Severe hepatic impairment (use for treatment of COVID-19 only if potential benefit outweighs potential risk); Diverticulitis (↑ risk of GI perforation); OB: Use during pregnancy only if potential maternal benefit justifies potential fetal risk; Pedi: Safety and effectiveness not established in children; Geri: Infection risk may be ↑ in older adults.

Adverse Reactions/Side Effects

CV: CARDIOVASCULAR DEATH, DEEP VEIN THROMBOSIS (DVT), MI. **GI:** ↑ liver enzymes, GI PERFORATION, nausea. **GU:** ↑ serum creatinine. **Hemat:** anemia, lymphopenia, neutropenia, thrombocytosis. **Metab:** ↑ lipids. **MS:** ↑ CK. **Neuro:** STROKE. **Resp:** PULMONARY EMBOLISM (PE). **Misc:** HYPERSENSITIVITY REACTIONS (INCLUDING ANGIOEDEMA), INFECTION (INCLUDING SERIOUS BACTERIAL, FUNGAL, VIRAL, OR OPPORTUNISTIC INFECTIONS, INCLUDING TB), MALIGNANCY (INCLUDING NONMELANOMA SKIN CANCER).

Interactions

Drug-Drug: Organic anion transporter 3 (OAT3) inhibitors, including **probenecid**, may ↑ levels and risk of toxicity; avoid concurrent use.

Route/Dosage

Rheumatoid Arthritis

PO (Adults): 2 mg once daily. *Concurrent use of OAT3 inhibitors (if recommended baricitinib dose is 2 mg once daily):* 1 mg once daily. *Concurrent use of OAT3 inhibitors (if recommended baricitinib dose is 1 mg once daily):* Consider discontinuing OAT3 inhibitor. *Concurrent use of OAT3 inhibitors:* 1 mg once daily.

Renal Impairment

PO (Adults): *eGFR 30–<60 mL/min/m²:* 1 mg once daily. *eGFR <30 mL/min/m²:* Not recommended.

COVID-19

PO (Adults): 4 mg once daily for 14 days or until hospital discharge, whichever occurs first. *Concurrent use of OAT3 inhibitors (if recommended baricitinib dose is 4 mg once daily):* 2 mg once daily. *Concurrent use of OAT3 inhibitors (if recommended baricitinib dose is 2 mg once daily):* 1 mg once daily. *Concurrent use of OAT3 inhibitors (if recommended baricitinib dose is 1 mg once daily):* Consider discontinuing OAT3 inhibitor.

Renal Impairment

PO (Adults): *eGFR 30–<60 mL/min/m²:* 2 mg once daily. *eGFR 15–<30 mL/min/m²:* 1 mg once daily. *eGFR <15 mL/min/m²:* Not recommended.

Alopecia Areata

PO (Adults): 2 mg once daily; may ↑ to 4 mg once daily if response inadequate. For patients with nearly complete or complete scalp hair loss, with or without substantial eyelash or eyebrow hair loss, consider starting treatment with 4 mg once daily. In patients receiving 4 mg once daily (as initial therapy or after a dose ↑), ↓ to 2 mg once daily once adequate response achieved. *Concurrent use of OAT3 inhibitors (if recommended baricitinib dose is 4 mg once daily):* 2 mg once daily. *Concurrent use of OAT3 inhibitors (if recommended baricitinib dose is 2 mg once daily):* 1 mg once daily. *Concurrent use of OAT3 inhibitors (if recommended baricitinib dose is 1 mg once daily):* Consider discontinuing OAT3 inhibitor.

Renal Impairment

PO (Adults): *eGFR 30–<60 mL/min/m² (if recommended baricitinib dose is 4 mg once daily):* 2 mg once daily. *eGFR 30–<60 mL/min/m² (if recommended baricitinib dose is 2 mg once daily):* 1 mg once daily. *eGFR <30 mL/min/m²:* Not recommended.

Availability (generic available)

Film-coated tablets: 1 mg, 2 mg, 4 mg.

NURSING IMPLICATIONS

Assessment

- Assess pain and range of motion before and periodically during therapy.
- Determine TB infection status. For patients with latent TB or those with a negative latent TB test who are at high risk for TB, start preventive therapy for latent TB before starting baricitinib. Monitor all patients for active TB during treatment, even patients with initial negative latent TB test.
- Assess for signs of infection (fever, dyspnea, flu-like symptoms, frequent or painful urination, redness or swelling at the site of a wound), including tuberculosis and hepatitis B virus, prior to and periodically during therapy. New infections should be monitored closely (upper respiratory tract infections, bronchitis, urinary tract infections). Infections may be fatal, especially in patients taking immunosuppressive therapy.

- Monitor for signs and symptoms of major adverse cardiac events. Patients who are current or past smokers and patients with other cardiovascular risk factors are at greatest risk.
- Monitor for thrombosis, including DVT, PE, and arterial thrombosis. If symptoms of thrombosis occur, discontinue therapy and evaluate and treat patients.
- Monitor for signs and symptoms of hypersensitivity reactions (hives; rash; pruritus; swelling of lips, face, or tongue; dyspnea) during therapy. Discontinue if symptoms occur.

Lab Test Considerations

- May cause neutropenia. Monitor ANC at baseline and periodically during therapy. *Patients with RA or alopecia areata: If ANC ≥1000 cells/mm³*, maintain dose. *If ANC <1000 cells/mm³*, hold therapy until ANC ≥1000 cells/mm³. *Patients with COVID-19:* Do not start therapy if ANC <500 cells/mm³.
- May cause lymphopenia. *Patients with RA or alopecia areata:* Monitor ALC at baseline and periodically during therapy. *If ALC ≥500 cells/mm³*, maintain dose. *If ALC <500 cells/mm³*, hold therapy until ALC ≥500 cells/mm³. Do not start therapy if ALC <500 cells/mm³. *Patients with COVID-19:* Do not start therapy if ALC <200 cells/mm³.
- May cause anemia. *Patients with RA or alopecia areata:* Monitor hemoglobin at baseline and periodically during therapy. *If hemoglobin ≥8 g/dL*, maintain dose. *If hemoglobin <8 g/dL*, hold therapy until hemoglobin ≥8 g/dL. Do not start therapy if hemoglobin <8 g/dL.
- Monitor liver enzymes at baseline and periodically during therapy. If ↑ in AST or ALT and liver injury are suspected, hold therapy until cause determined.
- May cause elevations in serum lipids. Monitor total cholesterol, low-density lipoprotein cholesterol, and high-density lipoprotein cholesterol 12 wk after starting therapy.
- Monitor renal function at baseline and periodically during therapy.

Implementation

- Administer a tuberculin skin test before starting therapy. Patients with active latent TB should be treated for TB prior to therapy.
- Immunizations for patients with RA and alopecia areata should be current prior to initiating therapy. Patients may receive concurrent vaccinations, except for live vaccines.
- **PO:** Administer once daily without regard to food.
- For patients unable to swallow tablets, tablets may be dispersed in water. Place tablets in a container with 10 mL (5 mL minimum) of room temperature water, disperse by gently swirling the tablet(s), and administer immediately orally. Rinse container with 10 mL (5 mL minimum) of water and swallow entire contents.
- *Administration via G tube:* Place tablet(s) in a container with approximately 15 mL (10 mL minimum) of room temperature water and disperse with gentle swirling. Ensure tablet(s) are sufficiently dispersed to allow free passage through tip of syringe. Withdraw entire contents into an appropriate syringe and immediately administer through gastric feeding tube. Rinse container with approximately 15 mL (10 mL minimum) of room temperature water, withdraw contents into syringe, and administer through the tube.
- *Administration via NG or OG tube:* Place tablet(s) into a container with approximately 30 mL of room temperature water and disperse with gentle swirling. Ensure tablet(s) are sufficiently dispersed to allow free passage through tip of syringe. Withdraw entire contents into an appropriate syringe and immediately administer through enteral feeding tube. To avoid clogging of small diameter tubes (smaller than 12 Fr), syringe can be held horizontally and shaken during administration. Rinse container with at least 15 mL of room temperature water, withdraw contents into syringe, and administer through the tube.

Patient/Family Teaching

- Explain purpose and side effects of medication to patient. Advise patient to read *Patient Information* before starting therapy. Instruct patient to take baricitinib as directed.
- Advise patient to notify health care provider of all Rx or OTC medications, vitamins, or herbal products being taken and to consult with health care provider before taking other medications.
- Advise patient to notify health care provider if signs and symptoms of infection (fever, sweating, or chills; blood in phlegm; diarrhea or stomach pain; muscle aches; weight loss; burning during urination or urinating more often than usual; cough or shortness of breath; warm, red, or painful skin or sores on body; feeling very tired) occur.
- Caution patients with signs and symptoms of a heart attack or stroke (discomfort in the center of chest that lasts for more than a few min or that goes away and comes back; severe tightness, pain, pressure, or heaviness in chest, throat, neck, or jaw; pain or discomfort in arms, back, neck, jaw, or stomach; weakness in one part or on one side of the body; slurred speech; shortness of breath with or without chest discomfort; breaking out in a cold sweat; nausea or vomiting; light-headedness) to notify health care provider immediately.
- Inform patient of ↑ risk of DVT and PE. If signs and symptoms (swelling, pain, or tenderness in one or both legs; sudden, unexplained chest or upper back pain; shortness of breath or difficulty breathing) occur, stop therapy and get immediate medical care. Advise patient to notify health care

B

provider if they have had blood clots in the legs or lungs in the past.

- May ↑ risk of cancer. Advise patient to have skin checked for skin cancer during therapy. Limit amount of time spent in sunlight. Avoid using tanning beds or sunlamps. Wear protective clothing and use sunscreen with a high protection factor (SPF 30 and above); especially important for patients with very fair skin or with a family history of skin cancer. Instruct patient to notify health care provider if they have ever had any type of cancer.
- Educate patient on smoking cessation. Those who are current or past smokers are at ↑ risk for major adverse cardiovascular events.
- Advise patient to avoid live vaccines during therapy.
- Rep: May cause fetal harm. Advise women of reproductive potential to notify health care provider if pregnancy is planned or suspected and to avoid breastfeeding during and for 4 days after last dose of therapy.

Evaluation/Desired Outcomes

- Decreased pain and swelling with decreased rate of joint destruction in patients with RA.
- Shortened time to recovery and reduction in death from COVID-19.
- Improvement in scalp hair coverage in alopecia areata.

beclomethasone, See CORTICOSTEROIDS (INHALATION).

beclomethasone, See CORTICOSTEROIDS (NASAL).

belimumab (be-li-moo-mab)

Benlysta

Classification

Therapeutic: immunosuppressants

Pharmacologic: monoclonal antibodies

Indications

Active autoantibody-positive systemic lupus erythematosus in patients currently receiving standard therapy. Active lupus nephritis in patients currently receiving standard therapy.

Action

A monoclonal antibody produced by recombinant DNA technique that specifically binds to B-lymphocyte stimulator protein, thereby inactivating it. **Therapeutic Effects:** ↓ survival of B cells, including autoreactive ones and ↓ differentiation into immunoglobulin-producing plasma cells. Result is ↓ disease activity with lessened damage/improvement in mucocutaneous, musculoskeletal, and immunologic manifestations of systemic lupus erythematosus. Improvement in or stabilization of renal function in lupus nephritis.

Pharmacokinetics

Absorption: 74% absorbed after SUBQ administration; IV administration results in complete bioavailability.

Distribution: Unknown.

Metabolism and Excretion: Unknown.

Half-life: 19.4 days.

TIME/ACTION PROFILE (↓ in activated B cells)

ROUTE	ONSET	PEAK	DURATION
IV or SUBQ	8 wk	unknown	52 wk†

† With continuous treatment.

Contraindications/Precautions

Contraindicated in: Hypersensitivity; Receiving therapy for chronic infection.

Use Cautiously in: Infections (consider temporary withdrawal for acute infections, treat aggressively); Concurrent use of immunosuppressant therapy or impaired immune function (↑ risk of progressive multifocal leukoencephalopathy [PML]); Previous history of depression or suicidal ideation (may worsen); OB: Use during pregnancy only if potential maternal benefit justifies potential fetal risk; Lactation: Safety not established in breastfeeding; Rep: Women of reproductive potential; Pedi: Children <5 yr (safety and effectiveness not established); Geri: Older adults may be more sensitive to drug effects.

Adverse Reactions/Side Effects

Derm: rash. **GI:** diarrhea, nausea. **GU:** cystitis. **Hemat:** leukopenia. **MS:** extremity pain, myalgia. **Neuro:** depression, insomnia, migraine, anxiety, fatigue, PML, SUICIDAL IDEATION/BEHAVIOR. **Misc:** fever, infusion reactions, ANAPHYLAXIS, facial edema, INFECTION.

Interactions

Drug-Drug: ↑ risk of adverse reactions and ↓ immune response to **live vaccines**; should not be given concurrently. ↑ risk of serious infections and postinjection systemic reactions when used with **rituximab**.

Route/Dosage

Systemic Lupus Erythematosus

IV (Adults and Children ≥5 yr): 10 mg/kg every 2 wk for 3 doses; then 10 mg/kg every 4 wk.

SUBQ (Adults and Children ≥5 yr and ≥40 kg): 200 mg once weekly; if transitioning from IV therapy, give 1st SUBQ dose 1–4 wk after last IV dose.
SUBQ (Children ≥5 yr and 15–<40 kg): 200 mg every 2 wk; if transitioning from IV therapy, give 1st SUBQ dose 1–4 wk after last IV dose.

Lupus Nephritis

IV (Adults and Children ≥5 yr): 10 mg/kg every 2 wk for 3 doses; then 10 mg/kg every 4 wk.
SUBQ (Adults and Children ≥5 yr and ≥40 kg): 400 mg (given as two 200-mg injections) once weekly for 4 wk; then 200 mg once weekly. May transition from IV therapy after completing 1st two IV doses; give 1st 200 mg SUBQ dose 1–2 wk after last IV dose.
SUBQ (Children ≥5 yr and 15–<40 kg): 200 mg once weekly for 4 wk; then 200 mg every 2 wk; if transitioning from IV therapy, give 1st SUBQ dose 1–2 wk after last IV dose; then continue with 200 mg every 2 wk.

Availability

Lyophilized powder for IV injection: 120 mg/vial, 400 mg/vial. **Solution for SUBQ injection (prefilled syringes and autoinjectors):** 200 mg/mL.

NURSING IMPLICATIONS

Assessment

- Monitor for signs of anaphylaxis (hypotension, angioedema, urticaria, rash, pruritus, wheezing, dyspnea, facial edema) during and following injection. Medications (antihistamines, corticosteroids, epinephrine) and equipment should be readily available. *If anaphylaxis or other severe allergic reaction occurs,* discontinue belimumab immediately.
- Monitor for infusion reactions (headache, nausea, skin reactions, bradycardia, myalgia, rash, urticaria, hypotension). *If infusion reaction occurs,* infusion rate may be slowed or interrupted.
- Assess for signs of infection, including tuberculosis, prior to injection. *If active infection is present,* do not initiate belimumab. *If serious infection occurs during therapy,* monitor, treat as indicated, and consider holding belimumab until infection controlled.
- Assess for signs of PML (hemiparesis, apathy, confusion, cognitive deficiencies, ataxia) periodically during therapy.

Implementation

- Consider premedication for prophylaxis against infusion and hypersensitivity reaction.
- **SUBQ**: Allow autoinjector or prefilled syringe to sit at room temperature for 30 min prior to injection. Solution is clear to opalescent and colorless to pale yellow; do not use if discolored or contains particulates. Inject into abdomen or thigh; rotate sites each week. Avoid areas of tenderness, bruising, redness, or induration. Do not freeze or shake. Avoid exposure to heat. May store at room temperature for ≤12 hr if protected from sunlight.

IV Administration

- **Intermittent Infusion:** Allow to stand 10–15 min at room temperature. **Reconstitution:** Using a 21–25-gauge needle, reconstitute 120-mg vial with 1.5 mL and 400-mg vial with 4.8 mL of sterile water for injection by directing stream toward side of vial to minimize foaming. Swirl gently for 60 sec. Allow vial to sit at room temperature during reconstitution, swirling gently for 60 sec every 5 min until powder is dissolved. Do not shake. Reconstitution usually takes 10–15 min but may take up to 30 min. Protect from sunlight. Solution is opalescent and colorless to pale yellow and without particles. Small bubbles are expected and acceptable. **Concentration:** 80 mg/mL. **Dilution:** 0.9% NaCl, 0.45% NaCl or LR. Remove volume of patient's dose from a 250-mL infusion bag and discard. Replace with required amount of reconstituted solution. Gently invert bag to mix. Do not administer if discolored or contains particulates. Discard unused solution in vial. If not used immediately, refrigerate or store at room temperature and protect from light. Total time from reconstitution to completion of infusion should not exceed 8 hr. **Rate:** Infuse over 1 hr; may slow or interrupt rate if infusion reaction occurs.
- **Y-Site Incompatibility:** Do not administer other drugs through same IV line.

Patient/Family Teaching

- Explain purpose and side effects of medication. Advise patient to read *Patient Information* before starting therapy.
- Instruct patient or caregiver in correct technique for SUBQ injection, care, and disposal of equipment. Inject on the same day each week. Inject missed dose as soon as remembered; then resume on usual day or start a new weekly schedule from the day missed dose was administered. Do not inject two doses on same day.
- Caution patient to notify health care provider immediately if signs of infection (fever; sweating; chills; muscle aches; cough; shortness of breath; blood in phlegm; weight loss; warm, red, or painful skin or sores; diarrhea or stomach pain; burning on urination; urinary frequency; feeling tired), PML, severe rash, or swollen face occurs.
- Advise patient and caregiver to notify health care provider immediately for signs of suicidality, attempts to die by suicide, new or worse depression or anxiety, agitation or restlessness, panic attacks, insomnia, new or worse irritability, aggressiveness, acting on dangerous impulses, mania, other changes in mood or behavior, or symptoms of serotonin syndrome.

- Caution patient to avoid receiving live vaccines for 30 days before and during belimumab therapy.
- Advise patient to notify health care provider of all Rx or OTC medications, vitamins, or herbal products being taken and to consult health care provider before taking other medications.
- Rep: Advise women of reproductive potential to use effective contraception during and for ≥4 mo after final dose and to notify health care provider if breastfeeding. Encourage pregnant patients to enroll in pregnancy registry by calling 1-877-311-8972 or visiting https://mothertobaby.org/ongoing-study/benlysta-belimumab/.

Evaluation/Desired Outcomes

- Improvement in mucocutaneous, musculoskeletal, and immunologic disease activity in patients with systemic lupus erythematosus.
- Improvement in or stabilization of renal function in lupus nephritis.

benazepril, See ANGIOTENSIN-CONVERTING ENZYME (ACE) INHIBITORS.

benralizumab

(ben-ra-**liz**-ue-mab)

Fasenra

Classification

Therapeutic: antiasthmatics

Pharmacologic: monoclonal antibodies, interleukin antagonists

Indications

Add-on maintenance treatment of severe asthma that is of an eosinophilic phenotype. Eosinophilic granulomatosis with polyangiitis.

Action

Interleukin-5 (IL-5) antagonist that inhibits binding of IL-5 to the surface of the eosinophil, which reduces the production and survival of eosinophils. **Therapeutic Effects:** Decreased incidence of asthma exacerbations. Reduction in use of maintenance oral corticosteroid therapy in patients with asthma. Induction of remission in eosinophilic granulomatosis with polyangiitis.

Pharmacokinetics

Absorption: 58% absorbed following SUBQ administration.

Distribution: Minimally distributed to tissues.

Metabolism and Excretion: Degraded by proteolytic enzymes located throughout the body.

Half-life: 15 days

TIME/ACTION PROFILE (plasma concentrations)

ROUTE	ONSET	PEAK	DURATION
SUBQ	unknown	unknown	unknown

Contraindications/Precautions

Contraindicated in: Hypersensitivity; Acute bronchospasm or status asthmaticus.

Use Cautiously in: Pre-existing helminth infections; OB: Use during pregnancy only if potential maternal benefit outweighs potential fetal risk; Lactation: Safety not established in breastfeeding; Pedi: Children <6 yr (safety and effectiveness not established).

Adverse Reactions/Side Effects

EENT: pharyngitis. **Neuro:** headache. **Misc:** fever, HYPERSENSITIVITY REACTIONS (INCLUDING ANAPHYLAXIS, ANGIOEDEMA, URTICARIA, AND RASH), injection site reactions.

Interactions

Drug-Drug: None reported.

Route/Dosage

Asthma

SUBQ (Adults and Children ≥12 yr): 30 mg every 4 wk for first three doses, then 30 mg every 8 wk thereafter.

SUBQ (Children 6–11 yr and ≥35 kg): 30 mg every 4 wk for first three doses, then 30 mg every 8 wk thereafter.

SUBQ (Children 6–11 yr and <35 kg): 10 mg every 4 wk for first three doses, then 10 mg every 8 wk thereafter.

Eosinophilic Granulomatosis with Polyangiitis

SUBQ (Adults): 30 mg every 4 wk.

Availability

Solution for injection (prefilled syringes or autoinjectors): 10 mg/0.5 mL, 30 mg/mL.

NURSING IMPLICATIONS

Assessment

- Assess lung sounds, BP, and HR periodically during therapy. Note amount, color, and character of sputum produced.
- Monitor for signs and symptoms of hypersensitivity reactions (rash, pruritus, hives, swelling of face and neck, dyspnea, fainting, dizziness, light-headedness) periodically during therapy; usually occur within hrs, but may occur days after injection. Discontinue medication and provide supportive care if reaction occurs.

Implementation

- Treat pre-existing helminth infections before starting therapy.
- Prefilled syringe is for administration by a health care professional. Autoinjector can be administered by patient or caregiver with training. Autoinjector should be administered by health care professional or caregiver for children aged 6–11 yr weighing ≥35 kg.
- **SUBQ**: ***Asthma:*** Administer every 4 wk for the 1st three doses and every 8 wk thereafter in upper arm, thigh, or abdomen. ***Eosinophilic Granulomatosis with Polyangiitis:*** Administer every 4 wk in upper arm, thigh, or abdomen.
- Store in refrigerator; protect from light. Do not freeze or shake. Leave carton at room temperature for 30 min before administration. Solution is clear to opalescent, colorless to slightly yellow; may contain a few translucent or white to off-white particles. Do not administer if liquid is cloudy, discolored, or contains large particles or foreign particulate matter. Do not expel the air bubble prior to administration. Pinch skin to inject medication.

Patient/Family Teaching

- Explain the purpose and side effects of benralizumab to patient. Instruct patient in correct technique for injection, care, and disposal of equipment. Advise patient to read *Patient Information* before starting therapy and with each Rx refill in case of changes.
- Advise patient that benralizumab should not be used to treat an acute asthma attack. Patient should continue asthma medications, including corticosteroids, unless otherwise instructed by health care professional.
- Advise patient to stop using medication and notify health care professional immediately if signs and symptoms of hypersensitivity reactions occur.
- Instruct patient to notify health care professional of all Rx or OTC medications, vitamins, or herbal products being taken and to consult health care professional before taking any OTC medications or alcoholic beverages concurrently with this therapy. Caution patient also to avoid smoking and other respiratory irritants.
- Instruct patient whose systemic corticosteroids have been recently reduced or withdrawn to carry a warning card indicating the need for supplemental systemic corticosteroids in the event of stress or severe asthma attack unresponsive to bronchodilators.
- Advise patient to have helminth infections treated before starting benralizumab therapy.
- Rep: Advise women of reproductive potential to notify health care professional if pregnancy is planned or suspected or if breastfeeding. Encourage health care professional or pregnant patients to enroll in pregnancy registry to monitor outcomes of women exposed to benralizumab during pregnancy by calling 1-877-311-8972 or visiting mothertobaby.org/Fasenra.

Evaluation/Desired Outcomes

- Decreased incidence of asthma exacerbations. Reduction in use of maintenance oral corticosteroid therapy.
- Induction of remission in eosinophilic granulomatosis with polyangiitis.

benzonatate (ben-zoe-na-tate)

~~Tessalon Perles~~

Classification

Therapeutic: allergy, cold, and cough remedies, antitussives (local anesthetic)

Indications

Relief of nonproductive cough due to minor throat or bronchial irritation from inhaled irritants or colds.

Action

Anesthetizes cough or stretch receptors in vagal nerve afferent fibers found in lungs, pleura, and respiratory passages. May also decrease transmission of the cough reflex centrally. **Therapeutic Effects:** Reduction in cough.

Pharmacokinetics

Absorption: Unknown.
Distribution: Unknown.
Metabolism and Excretion: Unknown.
Half-life: Unknown.

TIME/ACTION PROFILE (antitussive effect)

ROUTE	ONSET	PEAK	DURATION
PO	15–20 min	unknown	3–8 hr

Contraindications/Precautions

Contraindicated in: Hypersensitivity to benzonatate. Cross-sensitivity with other ester-type local anesthetics (tetracaine, procaine, and others) may occur.
Use Cautiously in: OB: Safety not established in pregnancy; Lactation: Safety not established in breastfeeding; Pedi: Children <10 yr (safety and effectiveness not established).

Adverse Reactions/Side Effects

Derm: pruritus, skin eruptions. **EENT:** burning sensation in eyes, nasal congestion. **GI:** GI upset, constipation, nausea. **Neuro:** dizziness, headache, sedation. **Misc:** chest numbness, chilly sensation, hypersensitivity reactions.

Interactions

Drug-Drug: Additive CNS depression may occur with **antihistamines**, **alcohol**, **opioids**, and **sedative/hypnotics**.

Route/Dosage

PO (Adults and Children ≥10 yr): 100 mg 3 times daily (up to 600 mg/day).

Availability (generic available)

Capsules: 100 mg, 150 mg, 200 mg.

NURSING IMPLICATIONS

Assessment

- Assess frequency and nature of cough, lung sounds, and amount and type of sputum produced. Unless contraindicated, maintain fluid intake of 1500–2000 mL to ↓ viscosity of bronchial secretions.
- Assess for psychiatric effects such as mental confusion and visual hallucinations.
- Monitor for hypersensitivity reactions (bronchospasm, cardiovascular collapse, laryngospasm). Implement medical support if needed.

Implementation

- ***DNC:*** Swallow capsule whole. Do not chew or dissolve in mouth; release of benzonatate from capsules may cause local anesthetic effect and choking.
- If numbness or tingling of the tongue, mouth, throat, or face occurs, avoid oral ingestion of food or liquid until numbness has resolved.

Patient/Family Teaching

- Explain purpose and side effects of medication to patient. Advise to read *Patient Information* before starting therapy. Instruct to take exactly as directed. If a dose is missed, take as soon as possible unless almost time for next dose. Do not double doses.
- Advise patient to notify health care professional of all Rx or OTC medications, vitamins, or herbal products being taken and to consult health care professional before taking other medications.
- ***DNC:*** Caution patient not to chew capsules.
- Advise parents to keep benzonatate in a child-resistant container and store it out of reach of children. Overdose with benzonatate in children <2 yr has been reported following accidental ingestion of as few as one or two capsules. If a child accidentally ingests benzonatate, seek medical attention immediately.
- May occasionally cause dizziness or drowsiness. Caution patient to avoid driving or other activities requiring alertness until response to the medication is known.
- Instruct patient to cough effectively. Sit upright and take several deep breaths before attempting to cough.
- Advise patient to minimize cough by avoiding irritants, such as cigarette smoke, fumes, and dust. Humidification of environmental air, frequent sips of water, and sugarless hard candy may also ↓ the frequency of dry, irritating cough.
- Caution patient to avoid taking alcohol or other CNS depressants, including opioids and cannabinoids, concurrently with this medication.
- Advise patient that any cough lasting >1 wk or accompanied by fever, chest pain, persistent headache, or skin rash warrants medical attention.
- Advise patient to notify health care professional if symptoms of overdose (seizures, restlessness, trembling) occur.
- Rep: Advise women of reproductive potential to notify health care professional if pregnancy is planned or suspected or if breastfeeding.

Evaluation/Desired Outcomes

- Reduction in cough.

BEERS

benztropine (benz-troe-peen)

~~Cogentin~~

Classification

Therapeutic: antiparkinson agents

Pharmacologic: anticholinergics

Indications

Adjunctive treatment of all forms of Parkinson disease, including drug-induced extrapyramidal effects and acute dystonic reactions.

Action

Blocks cholinergic activity in the CNS, which is partially responsible for the symptoms of Parkinson disease. Restores the natural balance of neurotransmitters in the CNS. **Therapeutic Effects:** Reduction of rigidity and tremors.

Pharmacokinetics

Absorption: Well absorbed following PO and IM administration. IV administration results in complete bioavailability.

Distribution: Unknown.

Metabolism and Excretion: Unknown.

Half-life: Unknown.

TIME/ACTION PROFILE (antidyskinetic activity)

ROUTE	ONSET	PEAK	DURATION
PO	1–2 hr	several days	24 hr
IM, IV	within min	unknown	24 hr

Contraindications/Precautions

Contraindicated in: Hypersensitivity; Angle-closure glaucoma; Tardive dyskinesia; Pedi: Children <3 yr.
Use Cautiously in: Prostatic hyperplasia; Seizure disorders; Cardiac arrhythmias; OB: Safety not established in pregnancy; Lactation: Safety not established in pregnancy; Geri: Appears on Beers list. Not recommended for prevention or treatment of extrapyramidal symptoms due to antipsychotics in older adults; more effective agents available for treatment of Parkinson disease. Avoid use of oral formulation in older adults.

Adverse Reactions/Side Effects

CV: arrhythmias, hypotension, palpitations, tachycardia. **Derm:** ↓ sweating. **EENT:** blurred vision, dry eyes, mydriasis. **GI:** constipation, dry mouth, ileus, nausea. **GU:** hesitancy, urinary retention. **Neuro:** confusion, depression, dizziness, hallucinations, headache, sedation, weakness.

Interactions

Drug-Drug: Additive anticholinergic effects with **drugs sharing anticholinergic properties**, such as **antihistamines**, **phenothiazines**, **quinidine**, **disopyramide**, and **tricyclic antidepressants**. Counteracts the cholinergic effects of **bethanechol**. **Antacids** and **antidiarrheals** may ↓ absorption.
Drug-Natural Products: ↑ anticholinergic effect with **angel's trumpet**, **jimson weed**, and **scopolia**.

Route/Dosage

Parkinsonism

PO (Adults): 1–2 mg/day in 1–2 divided doses (range 0.5–6 mg/day).

Acute Dystonic Reactions

IM, IV (Adults): 1–2 mg initially; then 1–2 mg PO twice daily.

Drug-Induced Extrapyramidal Reactions

PO, IM, IV (Adults): 1–4 mg given once or twice daily (1–2 mg 2–3 times daily may also be used PO).

Availability (generic available)

Tablets: 0.5 mg, 1 mg, 2 mg. **Solution for injection:** 1 mg/mL.

NURSING IMPLICATIONS

Assessment

- Assess parkinsonian and extrapyramidal symptoms (restlessness or desire to keep moving, rigidity, tremors, pill rolling, masklike face, shuffling gait, muscle spasms, twisting motions, difficulty speaking or swallowing, loss of balance control) before and during therapy.
- Assess bowel function daily. Monitor for constipation, abdominal pain, distention, or absence of bowel sounds.
- Monitor intake and output ratios and assess patient for urinary retention (dysuria, distended abdomen, infrequent voiding of small amounts, overflow incontinence).
- Patients with mental illness are at risk of developing exaggerated symptoms of their disorder during early therapy with benztropine. Hold benztropine and notify health care professional if significant behavioral changes occur.
- **IM/IV:** Monitor BP and HR closely and maintain bedrest for 1 hr after administration. Advise patients to change positions slowly to minimize orthostatic hypotension.

Implementation

- **PO:** Administer with food or immediately after meals to minimize gastric irritation. May be crushed and administered with food if patient has difficulty swallowing.
- **IM:** Parenteral route is used only for dystonic reactions.
- Geri: Start with dose selection at the low end of the recommended dosage range and ↑ dosage only as needed while monitoring for adverse effects.

IV Administration

- **IV Push:** IV route is rarely used because onset is same as with IM route. **Rate:** Administer at a rate of 1 mg over 1 min.
- **Y-Site Compatibility:** amikacin, aminophylline, ascorbic acid, atracurium, atropine, azathioprine, aztreonam, bumetanide, buprenorphine, butorphanol, calcium chloride, calcium gluconate, cefazolin, cefotaxime, cefotetan, cefoxitin, ceftazidime, ceftriaxone, cefuroxime, chlorpromazine, clindamycin, cyanocobalamin, cyclosporine, dexamethasone, digoxin, diphenhydramine, dobutamine, dopamine, doxycycline, enalaprilat, ephedrine, epinephrine, epoetin alfa, erythromycin, esmolol, famotidine, fentanyl, fluconazole, folic acid, gentamicin, glycopyrrolate, heparin, hydrocortisone, hydroxyzine, imipenem/cilastatin, insulin, regular, isoproterenol, ketorolac, labetalol, LR, lidocaine, magnesium sulfate, mannitol, meperidine, meropenem, methylprednisolone, metoclopramide, metoprolol, midazolam, morphine, multivitamins, nafcillin, nalbuphine, naloxone, nitroglycerin, nitroprusside, norepinephrine, ondansetron, oxacillin, oxytocin, papaverine, penicillin G, pentamidine, phenobarbital, phentolamine, phenylephrine, phytonadione, potassium chloride, procainamide, prochlorperazine, promethazine, propranolol, protamine, pyridoxine, sodium bicarbonate, succinylcholine, sufentanil, tacrolimus, theophylline, thiamine, tobramycin, vancomycin, vasopressin, verapamil.

- **Y-Site Incompatibility:** amphotericin B deoxycholate, chloramphenicol, dantrolene, diazepam, diazoxide, furosemide, ganciclovir, indomethacin, pentobarbital, phenytoin, sulfamethoxazole/trimethoprim.

Patient/Family Teaching

- Explain the purpose and side effects of benztropine. Encourage patient to take as directed. Take missed doses as soon as possible, up to 2 hr before the next dose. Taper gradually when discontinuing or a withdrawal reaction may occur (anxiety, tachycardia, insomnia, return of parkinsonian or extrapyramidal symptoms). Advise patient to read *Patient Information* before starting and with each Rx refill in case of changes.
- May cause drowsiness or dizziness. Advise patient to avoid driving or other activities that require alertness until response to the drug is known.
- Instruct patient that frequent rinsing of mouth, good oral hygiene, and sugarless gum or candy may ↓ dry mouth. Patient should notify health care professional if dryness persists (saliva substitutes may be used). Also, notify the dentist if dryness interferes with use of dentures.
- Caution patient to change positions slowly to minimize orthostatic hypotension.
- Instruct patient to notify health care professional if difficulty with urination, constipation, abdominal discomfort, rapid or pounding heartbeat, confusion, eye pain, or rash occur.
- Advise patient to notify health care professional of all Rx or OTC medications, vitamins, or herbal products being taken and to consult with health care professional before taking other medications, especially cold remedies, or drinking alcoholic beverages.
- Caution patient that this medication ↓ perspiration. Overheating may occur during hot weather. Patient should notify health care professional if unable to remain indoors in an air-conditioned environment during hot weather.
- Advise patient to avoid taking antacids or antidiarrheals within 1–2 hr of this medication.
- Emphasize the importance of routine follow-up exams.
- Rep: Advise women of reproductive potential to notify health care professional if pregnancy is planned or suspected or if breastfeeding.

Evaluation/Desired Outcomes

- Decrease in tremors and rigidity and an improvement in gait and balance. Therapeutic effects are usually seen 2–3 days after the initiation of therapy.

BETA BLOCKERS (nonselective)

carvedilol (kar-**ve**-di-lole)
Coreg, ~~Coreg CR~~

labetalol (la-**bet**-oh-lole)
🍁 Trandate

nadolol (**nay**-doe-lole)
~~Corgard~~

pindolol (**pin**-doe-lole)
🍁 Visken

propranolol (proe-**pran**-oh-lole)
Hemangeol, ~~Inderal~~, Inderal LA, Inderal XL, Innopran XL

timolol (**tim**-oh-lole)
~~Blocadren~~

Classification
Therapeutic: antianginals, antiarrhythmics, antihypertensives
Pharmacologic: beta-blockers (nonselective)

Indications

Hypertension. **Carvedilol:** HF (ischemic or cardiomyopathic) with other agents, left ventricular dysfunction after MI. **Nadolol, propranolol:** Management of angina. **Propranolol:** Management of arrhythmias. **Propranolol, timolol:** Prevention/management of myocardial infarction (MI). **Propranolol:** Management of hypertension, angina, arrhythmias, hypertrophic cardiomyopathy, thyrotoxicosis, essential tremors, or pheochromocytoma (all but Hemangeol); Also used in the prevention and management of MI, and the prevention of vascular headaches (all but Hemangeol); Proliferating infantile hemangioma requiring systemic therapy (Hemangeol only). **Timolol:** Prevention of vascular headaches.

Action

Block stimulation of beta$_1$-adrenergic (myocardial) and beta$_2$-adrenergic (pulmonary vascular and uterine) receptor sites. Labetalol and carvedilol have alpha$_1$-adrenergic blocking activity, which may result in more orthostatic hypotension. Pindolol has intrinsic sympathomimetic activity (ISA), which may produce less bradycardia. Propranolol's mechanism for the treatment of infantile hemangiomas is unknown. **Therapeutic Effects:** Decreased heart rate and BP. Suppression of arrhythmias. Increased cardiac output, decreased risk of death from HF, slowed progression of HF (carvedilol only). Prevention of MI. Hemangioma resolution (propranolol only)

Pharmacokinetics

Absorption: *Carvedilol:* Well absorbed but rapidly undergoes extensive first-pass hepatic metabolism, resulting in 25–35% bioavailability; *nadolol:* Variably (30%) absorbed after oral administration; *labetalol:* Well absorbed but rapidly undergoes extensive first-pass hepatic metabolism, resulting in 25% bioavailability; *pindolol* and *timolol:* Well absorbed after oral administration; *propranolol:* Well absorbed but undergoes extensive first-pass hepatic metabolism.

Distribution: *Carvedilol:* Unknown; *nadolol:* Minimal penetration of the CNS; *labetalol:* Some CNS penetration.

Metabolism and Excretion: *Carvedilol:* Extensively metabolized, excreted in feces via bile, <2% excreted unchanged in urine; *labetalol:* Extensively metabolized by the liver; *nadolol:* 70% excreted unchanged by the kidneys; *pindolol:* Partially metabolized by the liver, 50% excreted unchanged by the kidneys; *propranolol* and *timolol:* Extensively metabolized by the liver.

Half-life: *Carvedilol:* 7–10 hr; *labetalol:* 3–8 hr; *nadolol:* 10–24 hr (↑ in renal impairment); *pindolol:* 3–4 hr; *propranolol:* 3.4–6 hr; *timolol:* 3–4 hr.

TIME/ACTION PROFILE (cardiovascular effects)

ROUTE	ONSET	PEAK	DURATION
Carvedilol–PO	within 1 hr	1–2 hr	12 hr
Labetalol–PO	20 min–2 hr	1–4 hr	8–12 hr
Labetalol–IV	2–5 min	5–15 min	2–4 hr (up to 24 hr)
Nadolol–PO	up to 5 days	6–9 days	24 hr
Pindolol–PO	7 days	2 wk	8–24 hr
Propranolol–PO	30 min	60–90 min	6–12 hr
Propranolol–PO-ER	unknown	6 hr	24 hr
Propranolol–IV	immediate	1 min	4–6 hr
Timolol–PO	unknown	1–2 hr*	12–24 hr

* After single dose, full effect not seen until several wk of therapy.

Contraindications/Precautions

Contraindicated in: Hypersensitivity; Uncompensated HF; Pulmonary edema; Cardiogenic shock; Bradycardia, sick sinus syndrome, or heart block (unless pacemaker present); Severe hepatic impairment; Bronchial asthma/bronchospasm; Premature infants with corrected age <5 wk (Hemangeol only); Asthma or history of bronchospasm (Hemangeol only); BP <50/30 mmHg (Hemangeol only); Pheochromocytoma (Hemangeol only); Pedi: Infants <2 kg (Hemangeol only).

Use Cautiously in: HF (condition may deteriorate after initial therapy); Diabetes mellitus (may mask signs of hypoglycemia); Thyrotoxicosis (may mask symptoms); Peripheral vascular disease; History of severe allergic reactions (intensity of reactions may be ↑); Skeletal muscle disease (with propranolol) (may exacerbate myopathy); Renal impairment; Hepatic impairment; OB: Lactation: All agents cross the placenta and may cause fetal/neonatal bradycardia, hypotension, hypoglycemia, or respiratory depression; Pedi: Safety and effectiveness not established in children; Geri: Older adults may have ↑ sensitivity; use lower initial dose; consider age-related ↓ in body mass and renal/hepatic/cardiac function.

Adverse Reactions/Side Effects

CV: ARRHYTHMIAS, BRADYCARDIA, HF, orthostatic hypotension (with carvedilol and labetalol), peripheral vasoconstriction. **Derm:** ERYTHEMA MULTIFORME (WITH PROPRANOLOL), EXFOLIATIVE DERMATITIS (WITH PROPRANOLOL), itching, rash, STEVENS-JOHNSON SYNDROME (SJS), TOXIC EPIDERMAL NECROLYSIS (TEN). **EENT:** blurred vision, dry eyes, intraoperative floppy iris syndrome (with carvedilol and labetalol), nasal stuffiness. **Endo:** hyperglycemia, hypoglycemia. **GI:** constipation, diarrhea, nausea. **GU:** erectile dysfunction, ↓ libido. **MS:** arthralgia, back pain, muscle cramps, myopathy (with propranolol). **Neuro:** fatigue, weakness, anxiety, depression, dizziness, drowsiness, insomnia (with propranolol), memory loss, mental status changes, nightmares, paresthesia. **Resp:** bronchospasm, PULMONARY EDEMA, wheezing. **Misc:** drug-induced lupus syndrome.

Interactions

Drug-Drug: General anesthetics, **IV phenytoin**, **diltiazem**, and **verapamil** ↑ risk of myocardial depression. **Verapamil**, **diltiazem**, **digoxinclonidine**, and **ivabradine** may ↑ risk of bradycardia. ↑ risk of hypotension may occur with **other antihypertensives**, acute ingestion of **alcohol**, or **nitrates**. **Amphetamines**, **cocaine**, **ephedrine**, **epinephrine**, **norepinephrine**, **phenylephrine**, or **pseudoephedrine** may result in unopposed alpha-adrenergic stimulation (excessive hypertension, bradycardia). Chronic **alcohol** use may ↓ levels and effectiveness. May alter the effectiveness of **insulin** or **oral hypoglycemic agents**; dose adjustments may be necessary. May ↓ effectiveness of **theophylline**. May ↓ beneficial beta$_1$ cardiovascular effects of **dopamine** or **dobutamine**. Use cautiously within 14 days of **MAO inhibitor** therapy; concurrent use may result in hypertension. **Cimetidine** may ↑ toxicity from carvedilol, labetalol, timolol, or propranolol. **NSAIDs** may ↓ antihypertensive action. **Rifampin** may ↓ levels and effectiveness of carvedilol. Carvedilol may ↑ levels and risk of toxicity of **digoxin**. **Amiodarone** or **fluconazole** may ↑ levels and risk of toxicity of carvedilol. Propranolol may ↑ levels and risk of toxicity of **lidocaine** and **bupivacaine**.

Route/Dosage

Carvedilol

PO (Adults): *Hypertension:* Immediate release: 6.25 mg twice daily; may ↑ every 7–14 days up to 25 mg twice daily. Extended release: 20 mg once daily; may double dose every 7–14 days up to 80 mg once daily; *HF:* Immediate release: 3.125 mg twice daily for 2 wk; may ↑ to 6.25 mg twice daily. May double dose every 2 wk as tolerated (not to exceed 25 mg twice daily in patients <85 kg or 50 mg twice daily in patients >85 kg. Extended release: 10 mg once daily; may double dose every 2 wk as tolerated up to 80 mg once daily; *Left ventricular dysfunction after MI:* Immediate release: 6.25 mg twice daily; ↑ after 3–10 days to 12.5 twice daily then to target dose of 25 mg twice daily; some patients may require lower initial doses and slower titration. Extended release: 20 mg once daily; may double dose every 3–10 days up to 80 mg once daily.

Labetalol

PO (Adults): 100 mg twice daily; may ↑ by 100 mg twice daily every 2–3 days as needed (usual range 400–800 mg/day in 2–3 divided doses; doses up to 1.2–2.4 g/day have been used).
IV (Adults): 20 mg; additional doses of 40–80 mg may be given every 10 min as needed (not to exceed 300-mg total dose) or 0.5–2 mg/min infusion; may be titrated up to 10 mg/min.

Nadolol

PO (Adults): 40 mg once daily initially; may ↑ by 40–80 mg/day every 3–7 days as needed (up to 240–320 mg/day).

Pindolol

PO (Adults): 5 mg twice daily initially; may ↑ by 10 mg/day every 2–3 wk as needed (up to 45–60 mg/day).

Propranolol

PO (Adults): *Angina:* 80–320 mg/day in 2–4 divided doses or once daily as extended/sustained-release capsules. *Hypertension:* Immediate release: 40 mg twice daily initially; may ↑ as needed (usual range 120–240 mg/day; doses up to 1 g/day have been used). Extended release: 80 mg once daily; ↑ as needed up to 120 mg once daily (Innopran XL should be given once daily at bedtime). *Arrhythmias:* 10–30 mg 3–4 times daily. *Prevention of MI:* 180–240 mg/day in divided doses. *Hypertrophic cardiomyopathy:* 20–40 mg 3–4 times daily. *Adjunct therapy of pheochromocytoma:* 20 mg 3 times daily to 40 mg 3–4 times daily concurrently with alpha-blocking therapy, started 3 days before surgery is planned. *Vascular headache prevention:* Immediate release: 20 mg 4 times daily. Extended release: 80 mg/day; may ↑ as needed up to 240 mg/day. *Tremor:* 40 mg twice daily; may ↑ up to 120 mg/day (up to 320 mg have been used).
PO (Children): *Hypertension/arrhythmias:* 0.5–1 mg/kg/day in 2–4 divided doses; may ↑ as needed (usual range for maintenance dose is 2–4 mg/kg/day in 2 divided doses).
PO (Children 5 wk–5 mo): *Infantile hemangioma:* 0.6 mg/kg twice daily (≥9 hr apart); after 1 wk, ↑ to 1.1 mg/kg twice daily; after another wk, ↑ to 1.7 mg/kg twice daily and maintain for 6 mo.
IV (Adults): *Arrhythmias:* 1–3 mg; may repeat after 2 min, and again in 4 hr if needed.
IV (Children): *Arrhythmias:* 10–100 mcg (0.01–0.1 mg)/kg (up to 1 mg/dose); may repeat every 6–8 hr if needed.

Timolol

PO (Adults): *Hypertension:* 10 mg twice daily; may ↑ every 7 days (usual maintenance dose is 10–20 mg twice daily; up to 60 mg/day); *Prevention of MI:* 10 mg twice daily, starting 1–4 wk after MI; *Prevention of vascular headache:* 10 mg twice daily; may give as a single daily dose; may ↑ up to 10 mg in the morning and 20 mg in the evening.

Availability

Carvedilol (generic available)

Extended-release capsules: 10 mg, 20 mg, 40 mg, 80 mg. **Tablets:** 3.125 mg, 6.25 mg, 12.5 mg, 25 mg.

Labetalol (generic available)

Tablets: 100 mg, 200 mg, 300 mg, 400 mg. **Premixed infusion:** 100 mg/100 mL 0.72% NaCl, 200 mg/200 mL D5W, 200 mg/200 mL 0.72% NaCl, 300 mg/300 mL 0.72% NaCl. **Solution for injection:** 5 mg/mL.

Nadolol (generic available)

Tablets: 20 mg, 40 mg, 80 mg, ✱ 160 mg.

Pindolol (generic available)

Tablets: 5 mg, 10 mg, ✱ 15 mg.

Propranolol (generic available)

Immediate-release tablets: 10 mg, 20 mg, 40 mg, 60 mg, 80 mg. **Extended-release capsules:** 60 mg, 80 mg, 120 mg, 160 mg. **Oral solution:** 20 mg/5 mL, 40 mg/5 mL. **Oral solution (Hemangeol):** 4.28 mg/mL. **Solution for injection:** 1 mg/mL. ***In combination with:*** hydrochlorothiazide (generic only).

Timolol (generic available)

Tablets: 5 mg, 10 mg, 20 mg.

NURSING IMPLICATIONS

Assessment

- Monitor BP and HR frequently during dose adjustment and periodically during therapy. Assess for bradycardia and orthostatic hypotension when assisting patient up from supine position.

- Patients receiving *labetalol IV* must be supine during and for 3 hr after administration. Monitor vital signs every 5–15 min during and for several hours after administration. Check BP at 5 and 10 min after each IV push injection, until the target BP is achieved.
- Patients receiving *propranolol IV* must have continuous ECG monitoring and may have pulmonary capillary wedge pressure or central venous pressure monitoring during and for several hr after administration.
- Consider that patients taking *propranolol* for noncardiac indications may have undiagnosed cardiac disease. Abrupt discontinuation or withdrawal over too short a period of time (<9 days) should be avoided, as it may precipitate life-threatening arrhythmias, hypertension, or myocardial ischemia. Assess patient carefully during tapering (optimally over 2 wk) and after medication is discontinued.
- Monitor intake and output and daily weight. Assess patient routinely for evidence of fluid overload (peripheral edema, dyspnea, rales/crackles, fatigue, weight gain, jugular venous distention). Patients with HF may have worsening of symptoms during therapy initiation.
- Monitor patients for development of severe cutaneous adverse reactions during therapy with *carvedilol* or *propranolol*, including SJS and TEN (prodrome of fever, malaise, mucosal lesions, progressive skin rash, blisters, lymphadenopathy, conjunctivitis, myalgias, hepatitis, eosinophilia). *If a severe cutaneous adverse reaction is suspected,* interrupt therapy until etiology of reaction is determined. Consultation with a dermatologist is recommended. *If a severe cutaneous adverse reaction is confirmed or for other Grade 4 skin reactions,* permanently discontinue therapy.
- Monitor for signs and symptoms of hypersensitivity reactions with *carvedilol* and *propranolol* (rash, urticaria, pruritus, flushing, dizziness, vomiting, abdominal pain) and anaphylaxis/angioedema with *timolol* (swelling of throat, lips, tongue, or face; dyspnea; wheezing; hoarseness). Immediately discontinue medication and provide supportive care.
- **Angina:** Assess frequency and characteristics of angina periodically during therapy.
- **Vascular Headache Prophylaxis:** Assess frequency, severity, characteristics, and location of vascular headache periodically during therapy.
- **Infantile Hemangioma:** Monitor BP and HR for 2 hr after propranolol initiation or dose ↑. May worsen bradycardia or hypotension. Discontinue if symptomatic bradycardia (<80 bpm) or hypotension (systolic BP <50 mmHg) occurs.

Lab Test Considerations

- May ↑ BUN, potassium, triglycerides, and uric acid.
- May ↑ ANA titers.
- May ↑ blood glucose.
- *Labetalol* and *carvedilol* may ↑ serum alkaline phosphatase, LDH, AST, and ALT. Liver function should be evaluated at baseline and periodically. *If jaundice or laboratory signs of hepatic impairment occurs,* permanently discontinue therapy.
- *Propranolol (Hemangeol)* may cause hypoglycemia in children, especially if not feeding, vomiting, or taking corticosteroids.

Toxicity and Overdose

- Monitor patients receiving beta blockers for signs of overdose (bradycardia, severe dizziness or fainting, severe drowsiness, dyspnea, bluish fingernails or palms, seizures). Notify health care provider immediately if these signs/symptoms occur.
- Unless contraindicated, hypotension may be treated with modified Trendelenburg position and IV fluids, and bradycardia with atropine. Glucagon has been used to treat bradycardia and hypotension unresponsive to IV fluids.

Implementation

- Do not confuse carvedilol with captopril. Do not confuse Inderal (propranolol) with Adderall (amphetamine/dextroamphetamine).
- ***High Alert:*** Patient harm or fatalities have occurred when switching from oral to IV propranolol. Oral and IV doses of *propranolol* are not interchangeable. Check dose carefully. IV dose is the oral dose and may be a temporary alternative if patient is NPO. Change to oral therapy as soon as possible.
- Discontinuation of concurrent clonidine should be done gradually with beta blocker discontinued 1st over 1–2 wk. Then, after several days, discontinue clonidine to ↓ risk of rebound hypertension.
- **PO:** Take HR before administering. If <50 bpm or if arrhythmia occurs, withhold medication and notify health care provider.
- Most beta blockers may be administered with food or on an empty stomach. Administer *carvedilol, labetalol,* and *propranolol* with meals or directly after eating to enhance absorption and minimize orthostatic hypotension.
- ***DNC:*** Swallow extended release tablets whole; do not crush, break, or chew. *Nadolol, pindolol, propranolol tablets,* and *timolol* may be crushed and mixed with food. *Carvedilol* extended-release capsules may be opened and sprinkled on cold applesauce and taken immediately; do not store mixture.
- Mix *propranolol oral solution* with liquid or semisolid food (water, juices, soda, applesauce,

puddings). Rinse glass with more liquid to ensure that all medication is taken. Do not store after mixing.

- Administer *propranolol (Hemangeol)* during or right after a feeding to prevent hypoglycemia. Skip dose if child is not eating or vomiting. Administer using oral syringe provided; if necessary may be diluted in small amount of milk or fruit juice and given in babys bottle.
- To convert from immediate-release to extended-release *carvedilol*, convert 3.125 mg twice daily (immediate release) to 10 mg once daily (extended release); convert 6.25 mg twice daily (immediate release) to 20 mg once daily (extended release); convert 12.5 mg twice daily (immediate release) to 40 mg once daily (extended release); convert 25 mg twice daily (immediate release) to 80 mg once daily (extended release).

IV Administration

- ***High Alert:*** IV vasoactive medications are inherently dangerous. Before administering IV, have 2nd practitioner independently check original order, dosage calculations, and infusion pump settings.

Labetalol

- **IV Push: Dilution:** Administer undiluted. **Concentration:** 5 mg/mL. **Rate:** Administer slowly over 2 min.
- **Continuous Infusion: Dilution:** Add 200 mg of labetalol to 160 mL or 250 mL of 0.9% NaCl, 0.45% NaCl, D5W, LR, D5/0.25% NaCl, D5/0.9% NaCl, D5/LR, or 5% dextrose. Do not dilute in 5% sodium bicarbonate. **Concentration:** 0.67–1 mg/mL. **Rate:** See Route/Dosage section.
- **Y-Site Compatibility:** acetaminophen, alemtuzumab, amikacin, aminocaproic acid, aminophylline, amiodarone, anidulafungin, argatroban, arsenic trioxide, ascorbic acid, atracurium, atropine, azithromycin, aztreonam, benztropine, bleomycin, bumetanide, buprenorphine, butorphanol, calcium chloride, calcium gluconate, carboplatin, carmustine, caspofungin, ceftazidime, ceftolozane/tazobactam, chlorpromazine, ciprofloxacin, cisplatin, cyanocobalamin, cyclophosphamide, cyclosporine, dacarbazine, dactinomycin, daptomycin, daunorubicin, dexmedetomidine, dexrazoxane, digoxin, diltiazem, diphenhydramine, dobutamine, docetaxel, dopamine, doxorubicin hydrochloride, doxorubicin liposomal, doxycycline, enalaprilat, ephedrine, epinephrine, epirubicin, epoetin alfa, eptifibatide, ertapenem, erythromycin, esmolol, etoposide, etoposide phosphate, famotidine, fentanyl, fluconazole, fludarabine, fluorouracil, folic acid, fosphenytoin, ganciclovir, gemcitabine, gentamicin, glycopyrrolate, granisetron, hetastarch, hydromorphone, idarubicin, ifosfamide, imipenem/cilastatin, imipenem/cilastatin/relebactam, irinotecan, isavuconazonium, isoproterenol, leucovorin, levofloxacin, levothyroxine, lidocaine, linezolid, lorazepam, magnesium sulfate, mannitol, meperidine, meropenem, meropenem/vaborbactam, mesna, methylprednisolone, metoclopramide, metoprolol, metronidazole, midazolam, milrinone, minocycline, mitoxantrone, morphine, moxifloxacin, multivitamins, mycophenolate, nalbuphine, naloxone, nicardipine, nitroglycerin, nitroprusside, norepinephrine, octreotide, ondansetron, oxacillin, oxaliplatin, oxytocin, palonosetron, pamidronate, papaverine, pemetrexed, pentamidine, pentobarbital, phenobarbital, phentolamine, phenylephrine, phytonadione, plazomicin, potassium acetate, potassium chloride, potassium phosphates, procainamide, prochlorperazine, promethazine, propofol, propranolol, protamine, pyridoxine, rocuronium, sodium acetate, sodium bicarbonate, succinylcholine, sufentanil, sulbactam/durlobactam, tacrolimus, tedizolid, telavancin, theophylline, thiamine, thiotepa, tigecycline, tirofiban, tobramycin, topotecan, vancomycin, vasopressin, vecuronium, verapamil, vinblastine, vincristine, vinorelbine, voriconazole, zoledronic acid.
- **Y-Site Incompatibility:** acyclovir, albumin, amphotericin B deoxycholate, amphotericin B liposomal, azathioprine, cangrelor, cefepime, cefiderocol, cefotaxime, cefotetan, cefoxitin, ceftaroline, ceftobiprole, ceftriaxone, cefuroxime, dantrolene, dexamethasone, diazepam, diazoxide, foscarnet, gemtuzumab ozogamicin, hydrocortisone, ibuprofen (Caldolor), indomethacin, ketorolac, micafungin, mitomycin, paclitaxel, pantoprazole, penicillin G sodium, phenytoin, piperacillin/tazobactam.

Propranolol

- **IV Push: Dilution:** Administer undiluted or dilute each 1 mg in 10 mL of D5W. **Concentration:** 0.1–1 mg/mL. **Rate:** Administer at a rate not to exceed 1 mg/min. **Intermittent Infusion: Dilution:** May be diluted in 50 mL of 0.9% NaCl, D5W, D5/0.45% NaCl, D5/0.9% NaCl, or LR. **Concentration:** 0.02 mg/mL. **Rate:** Infuse over 10–15 min.
- **Y-Site Compatibility:** acyclovir, alemtuzumab, alteplase, amikacin, aminocaproic acid, aminophylline, amiodarone, anidulafungin, argatroban, arsenic trioxide, ascorbic acid, atracurium, atropine, azathioprine, aztreonam, benztropine, bivalirudin, bleomycin, bumetanide, buprenorphine, butorphanol, calcium chloride, calcium gluconate, carboplatin, carmustine, caspofungin, cefazolin, cefotaxime, cefotetan, cefoxitin, ceftazidime, ceftriaxone, cefuroxime, chloramphenicol, chlorothiazide, chlorpromazine, cisplatin, clindamycin, cyanocobalamin, cyclophosphamide, cyclosporine, cytarabine, dacarbazine, dactinomycin,

daptomycin, daunorubicin, dexamethasone, dexmedetomidine, dexrazoxane, digoxin, diltiazem, diphenhydramine, dobutamine, docetaxel, dopamine, doxorubicin hydrochloride, doxorubicin liposomal, doxycycline, edetate calcium disodium, enalaprilat, ephedrine, epinephrine, epirubicin, epoetin alfa, eptifibatide, ertapenem, erythromycin, esmolol, etoposide, etoposide phosphate, famotidine, fentanyl, fluconazole, fludarabine, fluorouracil, folic acid, foscarnet, fosphenytoin, furosemide, ganciclovir, gemcitabine, gemtuzumab ozogamicin, gentamicin, glycopyrrolate, granisetron, heparin, hetastarch, hydrocortisone, hydromorphone, idarubicin, ifosfamide, imipenem/cilastatin, irinotecan, isoproterenol, ketorolac, labetalol, leucovorin, levofloxacin, lidocaine, linezolid, lorazepam, magnesium sulfate, mannitol, meperidine, meropenem, mesna, methadone, methohexital, methotrexate, methylprednisolone, metoclopramide, metoprolol, metronidazole, midazolam, milrinone, minocycline, mitoxantrone, morphine, moxifloxacin, multivitamins, mycophenolate, nafcillin, nalbuphine, naloxone, nicardipine, nitroglycerin, nitroprusside, norepinephrine, octreotide, ondansetron, oxacillin, oxaliplatin, oxytocin, palonosetron, pamidronate, papaverine, pemetrexed, penicillin G, pentamidine, pentobarbital, phenobarbital, phentolamine, phenylephrine, phytonadione, potassium acetate, potassium chloride, procainamide, prochlorperazine, promethazine, propofol, protamine, pyridoxine, rocuronium, sodium acetate, sodium bicarbonate, succinylcholine, sufentanil, tacrolimus, theophylline, thiamine, thiotepa, tigecycline, tirofiban, tobramycin, topotecan, vancomycin, vasopressin, vecuronium, verapamil, vinblastine, vincristine, vinorelbine, voriconazole, zoledronic acid.

- **Y-Site Incompatibility:** amphotericin B deoxycholate, amphotericin B liposomal, clevidipine, dantrolene, diazepam, diazoxide, indomethacin, insulin regular, mitomycin, paclitaxel, pantoprazole, phenytoin, piperacillin/tazobactam, trimethoprim/sulfamethoxazole.

Patient/Family Teaching

- Explain the purpose and side effects of the medication. Instruct patient to take medication as directed, at the same time each day, even if feeling well; do not skip or double up on missed doses. Take missed doses as soon as possible up to 4 hr before next dose (8 hr with *labetalol, nadolol, or extended-release propranolol*). Instruct parent or caregiver on proper use of dosing syringe with *propranolol oral solution*. Keep out of children's reach. Advise patient to read *Patient Information* before starting and with each Rx refill in case of changes.
- Advise patient that abrupt withdrawal may precipitate life-threatening arrhythmias, hypertension, or myocardial ischemia. Discontinue beta blockers slowly over 1–2 wk as directed by a health care provider.
- Advise patient to ensure that enough medication is available for weekends, holidays, and vacations. An electronic prescription refill may be available for emergency use.
- Teach patient and family how to check pulse and BP. Instruct them to check pulse daily and BP biweekly. Advise patient to hold dose and contact health care provider if pulse is <50 bpm or BP changes significantly.
- May cause drowsiness or dizziness. Caution patients to avoid driving or other activities that require alertness until response to the drug is known. Caution patients receiving *labetalol IV* or *propranolol IV* to call for assistance during ambulation or transfer.
- Advise patients to change positions slowly to minimize orthostatic hypotension, especially during initiation of therapy or with dose ↑. Patients taking *oral labetalol* should be especially cautious when drinking alcohol, standing for long periods, exercising, and during hot weather, as orthostatic hypotension is enhanced.
- Caution patient that this medication may ↑ sensitivity to cold.
- Instruct patient to notify health care provider of all Rx or OTC medications, vitamins, or herbal products being taken and to consult health care provider before taking other Rx, OTC, or herbal products, especially NSAIDs and cold preparations, concurrently with this medication.
- Advise patients with diabetes to closely monitor blood sugar, especially if weakness, malaise, irritability, or fatigue occurs. Medication may mask some signs of hypoglycemia, but dizziness and sweating may still occur. Acute hypertension may occur following insulin-induced hypoglycemia in patients receiving propranolol. Instruct parents/caregivers of children receiving *propranolol (Hemangeol)* how to recognize signs of hypoglycemia, to notify health care provider, and to take child to nearest emergency department if hypoglycemia is suspected.
- Advise patient to notify health care provider if slow pulse, difficulty breathing, wheezing, cold hands and feet, dizziness, confusion, depression, rash, fever, sore throat, unusual bleeding, or bruising occurs.
- Instruct patient to inform health care provider of medication regimen before treatment or surgery.
- Advise patient to carry identification describing disease process and medication regimen at all times.
- **Hypertension:** Reinforce the need to continue additional therapies for hypertension (weight loss, sodium restriction, stress reduction, regular exercise, moderation of alcohol consumption, smoking cessation). Medication controls but does not cure hypertension.
- **Angina:** Caution patient to avoid overexertion with decrease in chest pain.

B

- **Vascular Headache Prophylaxis:** Caution patient that sharing this medication may be dangerous.
- Rep: May cause fetal harm. Advise women of reproductive potential to notify health care provider if pregnancy is planned or suspected or if breastfeeding. Beta blockers are generally considered drugs of choice (with *labetalol* having the most evidence) for managing mild hypertension in pregnancy. If a beta blocker is taken during 3rd trimester, monitor fetal growth and for bradycardia, hypotension, and hypoglycemia; the newborn should be monitored for bradycardia, hypotension, hypoglycemia, and respiratory depression for 48 hr after delivery.

Evaluation/Desired Outcomes

- Decrease in HR and BP. Full effects of lower doses may not be seen for 4–6 wk. Hypotensive effects of *pindolol* may begin within 7 days, but maximum effect is reached in approximately 2 wk.
- Control of arrhythmias without appearance of detrimental side effects.
- Reduction in frequency of angina.
- Increase in activity tolerance; *nadolol* may require up to 5 days before therapeutic effects are seen.
- Improved cardiac output and ↓ progression of HF.
- Prevention of MI.
- Prevention of vascular headaches (propranolol and timolol).
- Management of thyrotoxicosis.
- Management of pheochromocytoma.
- Decrease in tremors.
- Management of hypertrophic cardiomyopathy.
- Resolution of infantile hemangioma (propranolol only).

BETA BLOCKERS (selective)

acebutolol (a-se-**byoo**-toe-lol)
~~Sectral~~

atenolol (a-**ten**-oh-lol)
Tenormin

betaxolol (be-**tax**-oh-lol)
~~Kerlone~~

bisoprolol (bis-**oh**-proe-lol)
~~Zebeta~~

metoprolol (me-**toe**-proe-lol)
Kaspargo Sprinkle, Lopressor, Toprol XL

nebivolol (ne-**bi**-vi-lole)
Bystolic

Classification
Therapeutic: antianginals, antiarrhythmics, antihypertensives
Pharmacologic: beta-blockers (selective)

Indications

Hypertension. Angina pectoris (atenolol and metoprolol). Prevention of MI (atenolol and metoprolol). Stable symptomatic HF due to ischemic heart disease, hypertension, or cardiomyopathy (Toprol XL only). **unlabeled Use:** Prevention of migraine headaches. Tremors.

Action

Block stimulation of $beta_1$ (myocardial)-adrenergic receptors, usually without affecting $beta_2$ (pulmonary, vascular, uterine)-receptor sites. Acebutolol has mild intrinsic sympathomimetic activity (ISA), which may result in less bradycardia. **Therapeutic Effects:** Decreased BP and HR. Decreased frequency of attacks of angina pectoris. Improved performance/survival in HF.

Pharmacokinetics

Absorption: *Acebutolol*, *betaxolol*, *metoprolol*, and *nebivolol:* Well absorbed after oral administration. *Atenolol:* 50–60% absorbed after oral administration. *Bisoprolol:* Well absorbed after oral administration, but 20% undergoes first-pass hepatic metabolism. IV administration of *metoprolol* results in complete bioavailability.
Distribution: *Acebutolol* and *atenolol:* Minimal penetration of CNS. *Betaxolol* and *nebivolol:* Widely distributed. *Metoprolol:* Crosses the blood-brain barrier.
Metabolism and Excretion: *Acebutolol:* Mostly converted by the liver to diacetolol, which is also a beta blocker. *Atenolol:* 40–50% excreted unchanged by the kidneys; remainder excreted in feces as unabsorbed drug. *Betaxolol:* Mostly metabolized by the liver; 20% excreted unchanged by the kidneys. *Bisoprolol:* 50% excreted unchanged by the kidneys; remainder renally excreted as metabolites; 2% excreted in feces. *Metoprolol:* Mostly metabolized by the liver. *Nebivolol:* Mostly metabolized by the liver; some metabolites have antihypertensive action; minimal excretion of unchanged drug.
Half-life: *Acebutolol:* 3–4 hr (8–13 hr for diacetolol); *Atenolol:* 6–9 hr; *Betaxolol:* 15–20 hr; *Bisoprolol:* 9–12 hr; *Metoprolol:* 3–7 hr; *Nebivolol:* 12 hr.

TIME/ACTION PROFILE (cardiovascular effects)

ROUTE	ONSET	PEAK	DURATION
Acebutolol PO (antihypertensive effect)	1–1.5 hr	2–8 hr	12–24 hr
Acebutolol PO (antiarrhythmic effect)	1 hr	4–6 hr	Up to 10 hr
Atenolol PO	1 hr	2–4 hr	24 hr

Continued

ROUTE	ONSET	PEAK	DURATION
Betaxolol PO	3–4 hr	7–14 days*	24 hr
Bisoprolol PO	unknown	1–4 hr	24 hr
Metoprolol PO†	15 min	unknown	6–12 hr
Metoprolol PO–ER	unknown	6–12 hr	24 hr
Metoprolol IV	immediate	20 min	5–8 hr
Nebivolol PO	unknown	unknown	unknown

* With multiple dosing.
† Maximal effects on BP (chronic therapy) may not occur for 1 wk. Hypotensive effects may persist for up to 4 wk after discontinuation.

Contraindications/Precautions

Contraindicated in: Decompensated HF; Compensated HF with reduced ejection fraction (acebutolol, atenolol, betaxolol, metoprolol immediate release, and nebivolol) (only metoprolol extended release and bisoprolol should be used); Pulmonary edema; Cardiogenic shock; Bradycardia, heart block, or sick sinus syndrome (in absence of a pacemaker); Severe hepatic impairment (nebivolol); Bronchospastic disease (nebivolol); Lactation: Lactation (nebivolol).
Use Cautiously in: Renal impairment (↓ dose of *acebutolol* if CCr <50 mL/min; ↓ dose of *bisoprolol* if CCr <40 mL/min; ↓ dose of *atenolol* if CCr <35 mL/min; ↓ dose of *betaxolol* and *nebivolol* if CCr <30 mL/min); Hepatic impairment (↓ dose of *bisoprolol*); Pulmonary disease (including asthma; $beta_1$ selectivity may be lost at higher doses; avoid use if possible); Diabetes mellitus (may mask signs of hypoglycemia); Thyrotoxicosis (may mask symptoms); History of severe allergic reactions (intensity of reactions may be ↑); Major surgery (anesthesia may augment myocardial depression); Untreated pheochromocytoma (initiate only after alpha blocker therapy started); OB: ↑ risk of fetal hypotension, bradycardia, hypoglycemia, and respiratory depression when used during third trimester; use in pregnancy only if potential maternal benefit outweighs potential fetal risk; Lactation: Safety not established; Pedi: Safety and effectiveness not established in children <18 yr (all agents, except metoprolol extended-release capsules) or <6 yr (metoprolol extended-release capsules); Geri: Older adults may have ↑ sensitivity; ↓ initial dose.

Adverse Reactions/Side Effects

CV: BRADYCARDIA, HF, hypotension, peripheral vasoconstriction, PULMONARY EDEMA. **Derm:** rash. **EENT:** blurred vision, stuffy nose. **Endo:** hyperglycemia, hypoglycemia. **GI:** ↑ liver enzymes, constipation, diarrhea, nausea, vomiting. **GU:** erectile dysfunction, ↓ libido, urinary frequency. **Hemat:** thrombocytopenia (betaxolol). **MS:** arthralgia, back pain, joint pain. **Neuro:** fatigue, weakness, anxiety, depression, dizziness, drowsiness, insomnia, memory loss, mental status changes, nervousness, nightmares. **Resp:** bronchospasm, wheezing. **Misc:** drug-induced lupus syndrome.

Interactions

Drug-Drug: General anesthesia, IV phenytoin, and **verapamil** may cause ↑ myocardial depression. ↑ risk of bradycardia when used with **digoxin, verapamil, diltiazem, clonidine,** or **ivabradine**. ↑ risk hypotension with other **antihypertensives**, acute ingestion of **alcohol**, or **nitrates**. **Amphetamines, cocaine, ephedrine, epinephrine, norepinephrine, phenylephrine,** or **pseudoephedrine** may result in unopposed alpha-adrenergic stimulation (excessive hypertension, bradycardia). May alter the effectiveness of **insulin** or **oral hypoglycemic agents**; dosage adjustments may be necessary. May ↓ the effectiveness of **theophylline**. May ↓ the beneficial $beta_1$-cardiovascular effects of **dopamine** or **dobutamine**. Use cautiously within 14 days of **monoamine oxidase (MAO) inhibitor** therapy; may result in hypertension.

Route/Dosage

Acebutolol

PO (Adults): *Arrhythmias:* 200 mg twice daily; may ↑ as needed (range 600–1200 mg/day). *Hypertension:* 400 mg/day, as a single dose or in 2 divided doses; may ↑ as needed (range 400–800 mg/day).

Atenolol

PO (Adults): *Angina:* 50 mg once daily initially; may ↑ after 1 wk to 100 mg/day; may then ↑ as needed (up to 200 mg/day). *Hypertension:* 25–50 mg once daily initially; may ↑ after 2 wk to 50–100 mg once daily. *MI:* 50 mg (given 10 min after last IV dose), then 50 mg 12 hr later, then 100 mg/day as a single dose or in 2 divided doses for 6–9 days or until hospital discharge.

Betaxolol

PO (Adults): 10 mg once daily; may ↑ to 20 mg after 7 days; start with 5 mg in older adults or patients with renal impairment.

Bisoprolol

PO (Adults): 5 mg once daily initially; may ↑ to 10 mg once daily (range 2.5–20 mg/day); start with 2.5 mg/day in patients with bronchospasm.

Metoprolol

PO (Adults): *Hypertension/angina:* 25–100 mg/day initially as a single dose or in 2 divided doses; may ↑ every 7 days as needed up to 450 mg/day (immediate release) or 400 mg/day (extended release) (for angina, give in divided doses). Extended-release products are given once daily. *MI:* 25–50 mg (starting 15 min after last IV dose) every 6 hr for 48 hr, then 100 mg twice daily. *Migraine prevention:* 50–100 mg 2–4 times daily (unlabeled). *HF:* 12.5–25 mg once daily (of extended release); may double dose every 2 wk up to 200 mg/day.

IV (Adults): *MI:* 5 mg every 2 min for 3 doses, followed by oral dosing.
PO (Children ≥6 yr): *Hypertension:* 1 mg/kg once daily (extended-release capsules); may titrate, as needed (not to exceed 50 mg/day).

Nebivolol
PO (Adults): 5 mg once daily initially; may ↑ at 2 wk intervals up to 40 mg/day.

Availability (generic available)
Acebutolol
Capsules: 200 mg, 400 mg.
Tablets: ✱ 100 mg ✱ 200 mg ✱ 400 mg.

Atenolol
Tablets: 25 mg, 50 mg, 100 mg. **In combination with:** chlorthalidone (Tenoretic). See Appendix N. Betaxolol
Tablets: 10 mg, 20 mg.

Bisoprolol
Tablets: ✱ 1.25 mg, 2.5 mg, 5 mg, 10 mg. **In combination with:** hydrochlorothiazide (Ziac). See Appendix N.

Metoprolol
Immediate-release tablets (tartrate): 25 mg, 37.5 mg, 50 mg, 75 mg, 100 mg. **Extended-release capsules (succinate; Kapspargo Sprinkle):** 25 mg, 50 mg, 100 mg, 200 mg. **Extended-release tablets (succinate; Toprol XL):** 25 mg, 50 mg, 100 mg, 200 mg. **Oral solution:** 10 mg/mL. **Solution for injection:** 1 mg/mL. **In combination with:** hydrochlorothiazide (Lopressor HCT). See Appendix N.

Nebivolol
Tablets: 2.5, 5 mg, 10 mg, 20 mg.

NURSING IMPLICATIONS
Assessment
- Monitor BP, HR, and ECG frequently during dose adjustment and periodically throughout therapy.
- Monitor intake and output and daily weights. Assess routinely for signs and symptoms of HF (dyspnea, rales/crackles, weight gain, peripheral edema, jugular venous distention).
- **Angina:** Assess frequency and characteristics of anginal attacks periodically during therapy.
- **Metoprolol:** Monitor vital signs and ECG every 5–15 min during and for several hours after parenteral administration. If HR <40 bpm, administer atropine 0.25–0.5 mg IV.

Lab Test Considerations
- May ↑ glucose and triglycerides.
- Acebutolol and metoprolol may ↑ serum alkaline phosphatase, LDH, AST, and ALT levels.

Toxicity and Overdose
- Monitor patients receiving beta-adrenergic blocking agents for signs of overdose (bradycardia, severe dizziness, or fainting, severe drowsiness, dyspnea, bluish fingernails or palms, seizures). Notify health care provider immediately if these signs occur.

Implementation
- Do not confuse Toprol-XL (metoprolol) with Topamax (topiramate). Do not confuse Lopressor (metoprolol) with Lyrica (pregabalin). Do not confuse metoprolol tartrate with metoprolol succinate.
- **PO:** Take apical pulse before administering. If <50 bpm or if arrhythmia occurs, withhold medication and notify health care provider.
- Most selective beta blockers may be administered with food or on an empty stomach. Administer metoprolol with meals or directly after eating. ***DNC:*** Extended-release tablets should be swallowed whole; do not crush, break, or chew.
- Swallow *Kapspargo Sprinkle* whole. If unable to swallow capsule, capsule may be opened and contents sprinkled over soft food (applesauce, pudding, yogurt). Swallow contents of capsule along with a small amount (teaspoon) of soft food. Swallow drug/food mixture within 60 min; do not store for future use. May also be administered via NG tube by opening and adding capsule contents to an all plastic oral tip syringe and adding 15 mL of water. Gently shake syringe for about 10 sec. Promptly administer through a 12 French or larger NG tube. Rinse with additional water to ensure no granules are left in syringe.

IV Administration
Metoprolol
- **IV Push: Dilution:** May be administered undiluted. **Concentration:** 1 mg/mL. **Rate:** May be administered by injecting 5 mg rapidly at 2-min intervals for 3 doses. Oral therapy should begin 15 min after last IV dose.
- **Y-Site Compatibility:** acetaminophen, acyclovir, albumin, human, alemtuzumab, amikacin, aminocaproic acid, aminophylline, amiodarone, amphotericin B liposomal, anidulafungin, argatroban, arsenic trioxide, ascorbic acid, atropine, aztreonam, benztropine, bivalirudin, bleomycin, bumetanide, buprenorphine, butorphanol, calcium chloride, calcium gluconate, cangrelor, carboplatin, carmustine, caspofungin, cefazolin, cefepime, cefotaxime, cefotetan, cefoxitin, ceftaroline, ceftazidime, ceftriaxone, cefuroxime, chloramphenicol, chlorpromazine, ciprofloxacin, cisplatin, clindamycin, cyanocobalamin, cyclophosphamide, cyclosporine, cytarabine, dacarbazine, dactinomycin, daptomycin, daunorubicin

hydrochloride, dexamethasone, dexmedetomidine, dexrazoxane, digoxin, diltiazem, diphenhydramine, dobutamine, docetaxel, dopamine, doxorubicin hydrochloride, doxorubicin liposomal, doxycycline, enalaprilat, ephedrine, epinephrine, epirubicin, epoetin alfa, eptifibatide, erythromycin, esmolol, esomeprazole, etoposide, etoposide phosphate, famotidine, fentanyl, fluconazole, fludarabine, fluorouracil, folic acid, foscarnet, fosphenytoin, furosemide, ganciclovir, gemcitabine, gentamicin, glycopyrrolate, granisetron, heparin, hetastarch, hydrocortisone, hydromorphone, ibuprofen, idarubicin, ifosfamide, imipenem/cilastatin, indomethacin, insulin regular, irinotecan, isoproterenol, ketorolac, labetalol, LR, leucovorin, levofloxacin, levothyroxine, linezolid, lorazepam, magnesium sulfate, mannitol, meperidine, meropenem, mesna, methadone, methotrexate, methylprednisolone, metoclopramide, metronidazole, midazolam, milrinone, mitomycin, mitoxantrone, morphine, moxifloxacin, multivitamins, mycophenolate, nafcillin, nalbuphine, naloxone, nicardipine, nitroprusside, norepinephrine, 0.9% NaCl, octreotide, ondansetron, oxacillin, oxaliplatin, oxytocin, paclitaxel, palonosetron, pamidronate, papaverine, pemetrexed, penicillin G, pentamidine, pentobarbital, phenobarbital, phentolamine, phenylephrine, phytonadione, piperacillin/tazobactam, potassium acetate, potassium chloride, procainamide, prochlorperazine, promethazine, propranolol, protamine, pyridoxine, rocuronium, sodium bicarbonate, succinylcholine, sufentanil, tacrolimus, theophylline, thiamine, thiotepa, tigecycline, tirofiban, tobramycin, topotecan, vancomycin, vasopressin, vecuronium, verapamil, vinblastine, vincristine, vinorelbine, voriconazole, zoledronic acid.

- **Y-Site Incompatibility:** allopurinol, amphotericin B deoxycholate, dantrolene, diazepam, gemtuzumab ozogamicin, pantoprazole, phenytoin, trimethoprim/sulfamethoxazole.

Patient/Family Teaching

- Instruct patient to take medication as directed, at the same time each day, even if feeling well; do not skip or double up on missed doses. Take missed doses as soon as possible up to 4 hr before next dose (8 hr with atenolol, betaxolol, or metoprolol). Abrupt withdrawal may precipitate life-threatening arrhythmias, hypertension, or myocardial ischemia.
- Teach patient and family how to check pulse and BP. Instruct them to check pulse daily and BP biweekly and to report significant changes to health care provider.
- May cause drowsiness. Caution patients to avoid driving or other activities that require alertness until response to the drug is known.
- Advise patients to change positions slowly to minimize orthostatic hypotension.
- Caution patient that this medication may ↑ sensitivity to cold.
- Instruct patient to notify health care provider of all Rx or OTC medications, vitamins, or herbal products being taken and to consult health care provider before taking any Rx, OTC, or herbal products, especially cold preparations. Patients on antihypertensive therapy should also avoid excessive amounts of coffee, tea, and cola.
- Patients with diabetes should closely monitor blood sugar, especially if weakness, malaise, irritability, or fatigue occurs. Medication does not block dizziness or sweating as signs of hypoglycemia.
- Advise patient to notify health care provider if slow pulse, difficulty breathing, wheezing, cold hands and feet, dizziness, light-headedness, confusion, depression, rash, fever, sore throat, unusual bleeding, or bruising occurs.
- Instruct patient to inform health care provider of medication regimen before treatment or surgery.
- Rep: Advise women of reproductive potential to notify health care provider if pregnancy is planned or suspected or if breastfeeding. Monitor neonates of women taking metoprolol for symptoms of hypotension, bradycardia, hypoglycemia, and respiratory depression and manage accordingly. Monitor breastfed infants for bradycardia, dry mouth, skin or eyes, and diarrhea or constipation.
- Advise patient to carry identification describing disease process and medication regimen at all times.
- **Hypertension:** Reinforce the need to continue additional therapies for hypertension (weight loss, sodium restriction, stress reduction, regular exercise, moderation of alcohol consumption, smoking cessation). Medication controls but does not cure hypertension.

Evaluation/Desired Outcomes

- Decrease in BP.
- Control of arrhythmias without appearance of detrimental side effects.
- Reduction in frequency of anginal attacks.
- Increase in activity tolerance.
- Prevention of MI.
- Management of stable, symptomatic heart failure (Toprol XL 25 mg only).

betamethasone, See CORTICOSTEROIDS (SYSTEMIC).

betamethasone, See CORTICOSTEROIDS (TOPICAL).

betaxolol, See BETA BLOCKERS (selective).

B

bethanechol (be-than-e-kole)

✱ Duvoid, ~~Urecholine~~

Classification

Therapeutic: urinary tract stimulant

Pharmacologic: cholinergics

Indications

Postpartum and postoperative nonobstructive urinary retention. Neurogenic atony of the urinary bladder with retention.

Action

Stimulates cholinergic receptors. Effects include: Contraction of the urinary bladder, Decreased bladder capacity, Increased frequency of ureteral peristaltic waves, **Therapeutic Effects:** Bladder emptying.

Pharmacokinetics

Absorption: Poorly absorbed after oral administration.
Distribution: Does not cross the blood-brain barrier.
Metabolism and Excretion: Unknown.
Half-life: Unknown.

TIME/ACTION PROFILE (response on bladder muscle)

ROUTE	ONSET	PEAK	DURATION
PO	30–90 min	1 hr	6 hr

Contraindications/Precautions

Contraindicated in: Hypersensitivity; Mechanical obstruction of the GI or GU tract; Lactation: Lactation.
Use Cautiously in: History of asthma; Ulcer disease; Cardiovascular disease; Seizure disorders; Hyperthyroidism; Sensitivity to cholinergic agents or effects; OB: Safety not established in pregnancy; Pedi: Safety and effectiveness not established in children.

Adverse Reactions/Side Effects

CV: bradycardia, HEART BLOCK, hypotension, SYNCOPE/CARDIAC ARREST. **Derm:** flushing, sweating. **EENT:** lacrimation, miosis. **GI:** abdominal discomfort, diarrhea, nausea, salivation, vomiting. **GU:** urgency. **Neuro:** headache, malaise. **Resp:** bronchospasm. **Misc:** hypothermia.

Interactions

Drug-Drug: Quinidine and **procainamide** may antagonize cholinergic effects. Additive cholinergic effects with **cholinesterase inhibitors**. Use with **ganglionic blocking agents** may result in severe hypotension. Effectiveness will be ↓ by **anticholinergics**.
Drug-Natural Products: Cholinergic effects may be antagonized by **angel's trumpet**, **jimson weed**, or **scopolia**.

Route/Dosage

PO (Adults): 25–50 mg 3 times daily. Dose may be determined by administering 5–10 mg every 1–2 hr until response is obtained or total of 50 mg administered *or* by starting with 10 mg, giving 25 mg 6 hr later, and then, if needed, 50 mg 6 hr later.
PO (Children): 0.2 mg/kg 3 times daily or 0.15 mg/kg 4 times daily.

Availability (generic available)

Tablets: 5 mg, 10 mg, 25 mg, 50 mg.

NURSING IMPLICATIONS

Assessment

- Monitor BP, HR, and respiratory rate before administering.
- Monitor intake and output. Palpate abdomen for bladder distention. Notify health care provider if drug fails to relieve condition for which it was prescribed. Catheterization may be ordered to assess postvoid residual.

Lab Test Considerations

- May ↑ AST, amylase, and lipase.

Toxicity and Overdose

- Observe for drug toxicity (sweating, flushing, abdominal cramps, nausea, salivation). If overdose occurs, treatment includes atropine sulfate (specific antidote).

Implementation

- A test dose is usually employed before maintenance to determine minimum effective dose.
- **PO:** Administer on an empty stomach, 1 hr before or 2 hr after meals, to prevent nausea and vomiting.

Patient/Family Teaching

- Explain purpose and side effects of medication. Advise patient to read *Patient Information* before starting therapy. Instruct to take medication exactly as directed. Missed doses should be taken as soon as possible within 2 hr; otherwise, return to regular dosing schedule. Do not double doses.
- Advise patient to notify health care provider of all Rx or OTC medications, vitamins, or herbal products being taken and to consult with health care provider before taking other medications.
- Caution patient to change positions slowly to minimize orthostatic hypotension.
- Advise patient to report abdominal discomfort, salivation, sweating, or flushing to health care provider.
- Rep: Advise women of reproductive potential to notify health care provider if pregnancy is planned or suspected or if breastfeeding.

Evaluation/Desired Outcomes

- Bladder emptying.

HIGH ALERT

bevacizumab (be-va-**siz**-uh-mab)
✱ Abevmy, Alymsys, Avastin, Avzivi, ✱ Aybintio, ✱ Bambevi, Jobevne, Mvasi, Vegzelma, Zirabev

Classification
Therapeutic: antineoplastics
Pharmacologic: monoclonal antibodies

Indications

Alymsys, Avastin, Avzivi, Jobevne, Mvasi, Vegzelma, and Zirabev: Treatment of the following conditions: First- or second-line treatment of metastatic colorectal cancer (in combination with IV 5-fluorouracil-based chemotherapy); Second-line treatment of metastatic colorectal cancer in patients who have progressed on a first-line regimen containing bevacizumab (in combination with fluoropyrimidine-irinotecan- or fluoropyrimidine-oxaliplatin-based chemotherapy); First-line treatment of patients with unresectable, locally advanced, recurrent, or metastatic nonsquamous non-small cell lung cancer (in combination with carboplatin and paclitaxel); Recurrent glioblastoma (as monotherapy); Metastatic renal cell carcinoma (in combination with interferon alfa); Persistent, recurrent, or metastatic cervical cancer (in combination with paclitaxel and cisplatin or paclitaxel and topotecan); Platinum-resistant recurrent epithelial ovarian, fallopian tube, or primary peritoneal cancer in patients who have received ≤2 previous chemotherapy regimens (in combination with paclitaxel, pegylated liposomal doxorubicin, or topotecan). **Avastin, Jobevne, Mvasi, Vegzelma, and Zirabev:** Treatment of the following conditions: Platinum-sensitive recurrent epithelial ovarian, fallopian tube, or primary peritoneal cancer (in combination with carboplatin and paclitaxel or with carboplatin and gemcitabine followed by bevacizumab as a single agent); Stage III or IV epithelial ovarian, fallopian tube, or primary peritoneal cancer following initial surgical resection (in combination with carboplatin and paclitaxel followed by bevacizumab as a single agent). **Avastin only:** Unresectable or metastatic hepatocellular carcinoma in patients who have not previously received systemic therapy (in combination with atezolizumab).

Action

A monoclonal antibody that binds to vascular endothelial growth factor, preventing its attachment to binding sites on vascular endothelium, thereby inhibiting growth of new blood vessels (angiogenesis). **Therapeutic Effects:** Decreased metastatic disease progression and microvascular growth.

Pharmacokinetics

Absorption: IV administration results in complete bioavailability.
Distribution: Unknown.
Metabolism and Excretion: Unknown.
Half-life: 20 days (range 11–50 days).

ROUTE	ONSET	PEAK	DURATION
IV	rapid	end of infusion	14 days

Contraindications/Precautions

Contraindicated in: Hypersensitivity; Recent hemoptysis or other serious recent bleeding episode; First 28 days after major surgery; OB: Pregnancy; Lactation: Lactation.
Use Cautiously in: Cardiovascular disease; Diabetes (↑ risk of arterial thromboembolic events); Previous use of anthracyclines (↑ risk of HF); Esophageal varices (in patients with hepatocellular carcinoma); Rep: Women of reproductive potential; Pedi: Safety and effectiveness not established in children; cases of nonmandibular osteonecrosis reported; Geri: ↑ risk of serious adverse reactions including arterial thromboembolic events in older adults.

Adverse Reactions/Side Effects

CV: angina, DEEP VEIN THROMBOSIS (DVT), HF, hypertension, hypotension, MI. **Derm:** impaired wound healing, NECROTIZING FASCIITIS, WOUND DEHISCENCE. **EENT:** nasal septum perforation. **GI:** GI PERFORATION. **GU:** ↑ serum creatinine, nephrotic syndrome, ovarian failure, proteinuria. **Hemat:** BLEEDING. **Neuro:** POSTERIOR REVERSIBLE ENCEPHALOPATHY SYNDROME (PRES), STROKE, transient ischemic attack. **Resp:** HEMOPTYSIS, PULMONARY EMBOLISM (PE). **Misc:** INFUSION REACTIONS.

Interactions

Drug-Drug: ↑ blood levels of SN 38 (the active metabolite of **irinotecan**); significance is not known. ↑ risk of microangiopathic hemolytic anemia when used with **sunitinib**; concurrent use should be avoided.

Route/Dosage

Colorectal Cancer

IV (Adults): *Alymsys, Avastin, Avzivi, Jobevne, Mvasi, Vegzelma, or Zirabev:* 5 mg/kg every 14 days when given with bolus-IFL chemotherapy regimen *or* 10 mg/kg every 14 days when given with FOLFOX4 chemotherapy regimen *or* 5 mg/kg every 14 days or 7.5 mg/kg every 21 days when given with a fluoropyrimidine-irinotecan or fluoropyrimidine-oxaliplatin based chemotherapy regimen.

Lung Cancer or Cervical Cancer

IV (Adults): *Alymsys, Avastin, Avzivi, Jobevne, Mvasi, Vegzelma, or Zirabev:* 15 mg/kg every 3 wk.

B

Glioblastoma or Renal Cell Carcinoma

IV (Adults): *Alymsys, Avastin, Avzivi, Jobevne, Mvasi, Vegzelma, or Zirabev:* 10 mg/kg every 2 wk.

Platinum-Resistant Epithelial Ovarian, Fallopian Tube, or Primary Peritoneal Cancer

IV (Adults): *Alymsys, Avastin, Avzivi, Jobevne, Mvasi, Vegzelma, or Zirabev:* 10 mg/kg every 2 wk when given with paclitaxel, pegylated liposomal doxorubicin, or topotecan *or* 15 mg/kg every 3 wk when given with topotecan.

Platinum-Sensitive Epithelial Ovarian, Fallopian Tube, or Primary Peritoneal Cancer

IV (Adults): *Avastin, Jobevne, Mvasi, Vegzelma, or Zirabev:* 15 mg/kg every 3 wk when given with carboplatin and paclitaxel for 6–8 cycles, followed by 15 mg/kg every 3 wk as monotherapy *or* 15 mg/kg every 3 wk when given with carboplatin and gemcitabine for 6–10 cycles, followed by 15 mg/kg every 3 wk as monotherapy.

Stage III or IV Epithelial Ovarian, Fallopian Tube, or Primary Peritoneal Cancer Following Surgical Resection

IV (Adults): *Avastin, Jobevne, Mvasi, Vegzelma, or Zirabev:* 15 mg/kg every 3 wk when given with carboplatin and paclitaxel for up to 6 cycles, followed by 15 mg/kg every 3 wk as monotherapy for a total up to 22 cycles or until disease progression, whichever occurs earlier.

Hepatocellular Carcinoma

IV (Adults): *Avastin:* 15 mg/kg every 3 wk (administer after atezolizumab on same day) until disease progression or unacceptable toxicity.

Availability

Solution for injection: 25 mg/mL.

NURSING IMPLICATIONS

Assessment

- Assess for signs of GI perforation (abdominal pain associated with constipation, fever, nausea, and vomiting), fistula formation, and wound dehiscence during therapy. *If GI perforation occurs,* discontinue therapy.
- Assess for signs of hemorrhage (epistaxis, hemoptysis, bleeding) and thromboembolic events (stroke, MI, DVT, PE) during therapy. *If Grade 3 or 4 hemorrhage, severe arterial thromboembolism, or Grade 4 venous thromboembolism occurs,* discontinue therapy. Hold bevacizumab for patients with recent history of hemoptysis of ≥½ teaspoon (2.5 mL) of red blood.
- Monitor BP every 2–3 wk during therapy. *If severe hypertension occurs that is not controlled with medical management,* temporarily suspend therapy. *If hypertensive crisis or encephalopathy occurs,* permanently discontinue bevacizumab.
- Assess for infusion reactions (stridor, wheezing, hypertension, oxygen desaturation, chest pain, headache, rigors, diaphoresis) during therapy. May require epinephrine, corticosteroids, IV antihistamines, bronchodilators, and/or oxygen. *If clinically significant reaction occurs,* hold therapy until resolved and resume at ↓ infusion rate. *If severe reaction occurs,* permanently discontinue bevacizumab.
- Assess for signs of HF (dyspnea, peripheral edema, rales/crackles, jugular venous distension) during therapy. *If symptoms occur,* permanently discontinue bevacizumab.
- Monitor for signs of PRES (headache, seizure, lethargy, confusion, blindness). Hypertension may or may not be present. May occur within 16 hr–1 yr of initiation of therapy. *If PRES suspected,* treat hypertension, if present, and discontinue bevacizumab therapy. Symptoms usually resolve within days.
- Monitor wound healing. *If wound healing complications occur,* hold bevacizumab until adequate wound healing. *If necrotizing fasciitis occurs,* permanently discontinue bevacizumab.

Lab Test Considerations

- Monitor serial urinalysis for proteinuria during therapy. Patients with a ≥2+ urine dipstick require further testing with a 24-hr urine collection. Hold therapy for ≥2 g of proteinuria/24 hr and resume when proteinuria <2 g/24 hr. *If nephrotic syndrome occurs,* permanently discontinue bevacizumab.
- May cause leukopenia, thrombocytopenia, hypokalemia, and hyperbilirubinemia.
- May ↑ serum creatinine.

Implementation

- Avoid administration for ≥28 days before elective surgery and following major surgery; surgical incision should be fully healed due to potential for impaired wound healing.

IV Administration

- **Intermittent Infusion: Dilution:** Dilute prescribed dose in 100 mL of 0.9% NaCl. Do not shake. Discard unused portions. Solution is colorless to pale yellow or brown; do not administer solution that is discolored or contains particulate matter. Stable if refrigerated for up to 4 hr (*Alymsys*), 8 hr (*Avastin, Jobevne, Mvasi*), 24 hr (*Vegzelma*), 16 days (*Zirabev*), or at room temperature up to 4 hr (*Vegzelma*). **Rate:** Administer initial dose over 90 min. If well tolerated, 2nd infusion may be administered over 60 min. If well tolerated, all subsequent infusions may be administered over 30 min. **Do not administer as an IV push or bolus.**

- **Y-Site Incompatibility:** Do not administer other drugs through same IV line.

Patient/Family Teaching

- Explain the purpose and side effects of bevacizumab to patient. Do not stop receiving drug without consulting health care provider. If an appointment is missed, contact health care provider as soon as possible to reschedule. Advise patient to read *Medication Guide* before starting and periodically during therapy in case of changes.
- Explain need for continued medical follow-up to assess effectiveness and possible side effects of medication. Periodic lab tests and may be needed.
- Advise patient of the need for monitoring BP periodically during therapy; notify health care provider if BP is elevated.
- Advise patient to report any signs of unusual bleeding, high fever, rigors, sudden onset of worsening neurological function, persistent or severe abdominal pain, severe constipation, or vomiting immediately to health care provider.
- Inform patient of ↑ risk of wound healing complications and arterial thromboembolic events.
- Rep: May cause fetal harm. Advise women of reproductive potential to use effective contraception and avoid breastfeeding during therapy and for 6 mo after last dose. Inform women of reproductive potential of risk of ovarian failure that may lead to sterility following therapy.

Evaluation/Desired Outcomes

- Decreased metastatic disease progression and microvascular growth.

HIGH ALERT

bicalutamide (bye-ka-**loot**-a-mide)

Casodex

Classification

Therapeutic: antineoplastics

Pharmacologic: antiandrogens

Indications

Metastatic prostate cancer (in combination with a luteinizing hormone-releasing hormone [LHRH] analog).

Action

Antagonizes the effects of androgen at the cellular level. **Therapeutic Effects:** Decreased spread of prostate cancer.

Pharmacokinetics

Absorption: Well absorbed following oral administration.

Distribution: Unknown.

Protein Binding: 96%.

Metabolism and Excretion: Mostly metabolized by the liver. Excreted in the urine and feces.

Half-life: 5.8 days.

TIME/ACTION PROFILE (plasma concentrations)

ROUTE	ONSET	PEAK	DURATION
PO	unknown	31.3 hr	unknown

Contraindications/Precautions

Contraindicated in: Hypersensitivity.

Use Cautiously in: Moderate to severe hepatic impairment; Rep: Men with female partners of reproductive potential.

Adverse Reactions/Side Effects

CV: chest pain, hypertension, peripheral edema. **Derm:** hot flashes, alopecia, photosensitivity, rash, sweating. **Endo:** breast pain, gynecomastia, hyperglycemia. **GI:** constipation, diarrhea, nausea, ↑ liver enzymes, abdominal pain, HEPATOTOXICITY, vomiting. **GU:** ↓ fertility, erectile dysfunction, hematuria, incontinence, nocturia, urinary tract infections. **Hemat:** anemia. **Metab:** weight loss. **MS:** pain. **Neuro:** weakness, dizziness, headache, insomnia, paresthesia. **Resp:** dyspnea. **Misc:** flu-like syndrome, infection.

Interactions

Drug-Drug: May ↑ the effect of **warfarin.**

Route/Dosage

PO (Adults): 50 mg once daily.

Availability (generic available)

Tablets: 50 mg.

NURSING IMPLICATIONS

Assessment

- Assess patient for adverse GI effects. Diarrhea is the most common cause of discontinuation of therapy.

Lab Test Considerations

- Monitor serum prostate-specific antigen periodically to determine response to therapy. If levels ↑, assess patient for disease progression. May require periodic LHRH analog administration without bicalutamide.
- Monitor serum transaminases before therapy, monthly during first 4 mo of therapy, and periodically thereafter. May ↑ serum alkaline phosphatase, AST, ALT, and bilirubin concentrations. *If patient is jaundiced or if transaminases ↑ >2 times upper limit of normal,* discontinue bicalutamide; levels usually return to normal after discontinuation.

- May ↑ BUN and serum creatinine and ↓ hemoglobin and WBCs.
- May ↓ glucose tolerance in patients taking LHRH agonists concurrently; monitor blood glucose in patients receiving bicalutamide in combination with LHRH analog.
- Monitor PT/INR closely in patients taking warfarin. May lead to severe bleeding.

Implementation
- Start treatment with bicalutamide at the same time as LHRH analog.
- Handle intact tablets or capsules with single gloves; use double gloves, respiratory protection, and a protective gown in the preparation of tablets or capsules, including cutting, crushing, manipulating, or handling uncoated tablets; optimally prepare in a ventilated control device. During administration, wear single gloves, and wear eye/face protection if the patient may resist, vomit, spit up, or experience difficulty swallowing.
- **PO:** May be administered in the morning or evening, without regard to food.

Patient/Family Teaching
- Explain the purpose and side effects. Instruct patient to take bicalutamide along with the LHRH analog as directed at the same time each day. If a dose is missed, omit and take the next dose at regular time; do not double doses. Do not discontinue without consulting health care professional. Advise patient to read *Patient Information* prior to starting and with each Rx refill in case of changes.
- Emphasize the importance of regular follow-up exams and blood tests to determine progress; monitor for side effects.
- May cause dizziness. Caution patient to avoid driving or other activities requiring alertness until response to medication is known.
- Advise patient to stop taking bicalutamide and notify health care professional immediately of symptoms of liver dysfunction (nausea, vomiting, abdominal pain, fatigue, anorexia, flu-like symptoms, dark urine, jaundice, right upper quadrant tenderness) or interstitial lung disease (trouble breathing with or without a cough or fever).
- Advise patient to notify health care professional of all Rx or OTC medications, vitamins, or herbal products being taken and to consult health care professional before taking any new medications.
- Instruct patient to report severe or persistent diarrhea.
- Discuss with patient the possibility of hair loss, breast enlargement, and breast pain. Explore methods of coping.
- Advise patient to use sunscreen, avoid sunlight or sunlamps and tanning beds, and wear protective clothing to prevent photosensitivity reactions.
- Rep: Advise men with female partners of reproductive potential to use effective contraception during and for 130 days after last dose of therapy. Advise patients that bicalutamide may impair fertility.

Evaluation/Desired Outcomes
- Decreased spread of prostate cancer.

bictegravir/emtricitabine/tenofovir alafenamide (bik-**teg**-ra-vir/em-trye-**sye**-ta-been/ten-**of**-oh-veer al-a-**fen**-a-mide)

Biktarvy

Classification

Therapeutic: antiretrovirals

Pharmacologic: nucleoside reverse transcriptase inhibitors, integrase strand transfer inhibitors (INSTI)

Indications
HIV infection in patients who have no antiretroviral treatment history or in those on a stable antiretroviral regimen who are virologically suppressed (with HIV-1 RNA <50 copies/mL) and no history of treatment failure or no known substitutions associated with resistance to bictegravir or tenofovir (to replace their current antiretroviral regimen).

Action
Bictegravir: Inhibits HIV-1 integrase, which is required for viral replication; *Emtricitabine:* Phosphorylated intracellularly, where it inhibits HIV reverse transcriptase, resulting in viral DNA chain termination; *Tenofovir:* Phosphorylated intracellularly, where it inhibits HIV reverse transcriptase, resulting in disruption of DNA synthesis. **Therapeutic Effects:** Slowed progression of HIV infection and decreased occurrence of sequelae.

Pharmacokinetics
Bictegravir

Absorption: Extent of absorption following oral administration unknown.

Distribution: Unknown.

Protein Binding: >99%.

Metabolism and Excretion: Primarily metabolized by the CYP3A4 isoenzyme and UGT1A1 in the liver; 60% excreted in feces; 35% excreted in urine.

Half-life: 17.3 hr.

Emtricitabine

Absorption: Well absorbed (93%) following oral administration.
Distribution: Unknown.
Metabolism and Excretion: Undergoes some metabolism; 70% excreted in urine; 14% excreted in feces.
Half-life: 10.4 hr.

Tenofovir Alafenamide

Absorption: Tenofovir alafenamide is a prodrug, which is hydrolyzed into tenofovir, the active component; absorption enhanced by high-fat meals.
Distribution: Unknown.
Metabolism and Excretion: Tenofovir is phosphorylated to tenofovir diphosphate (active metabolite); 32% excreted in feces; <1% excreted in urine.
Half-life: *Tenofovir alafenamide:* 0.51 hr; *Tenofovir diphosphate:* 150–180 hr.

TIME/ACTION PROFILE (plasma concentrations)

ROUTE	ONSET	PEAK	DURATION
bictegravir PO	unknown	2–4 hr	24 hr
emtricitabine PO	unknown	1.5–2 hr	24 hr
tenofovir PO	unknown	0.5–2 hr	24 hr

Contraindications/Precautions

Contraindicated in: Concurrent use of dofetilide or rifampin; Severe renal impairment or end-stage renal disease not receiving hemodialysis; Patients with no antiretroviral treatment history and end-stage renal disease who are receiving chronic hemodialysis; Severe hepatic impairment.
Use Cautiously in: Hepatitis B virus (HBV) coinfection; History of suicidal ideation or depression (↑ risk of suicidal thoughts); Renal impairment or receiving nephrotoxic medications (↑ risk of renal impairment); OB: Recommended in pregnant individuals who are virologically suppressed on a stable antiretroviral regimen with no known substitutions associated with resistance to bictegravir, emtricitabine, or tenofovir alafenamide; Lactation: Safety of bictegravir not established in breastfeeding; breastfeeding should be supported in people with HIV who are taking antiretroviral therapy as prescribed and are maintaining an undetectable amount of virus in the body; Pedi: Children weighing <14 kg (safety and effectiveness not established).

Adverse Reactions/Side Effects

GI: ↑ amylase, ↑ liver enzymes, ACUTE EXACERBATION OF HBV, diarrhea, LACTIC ACIDOSIS/HEPATOMEGALY WITH STEATOSIS, nausea. **GU:** ACUTE RENAL FAILURE/FANCONI SYNDROME. **Hemat:** neutropenia. **Metab:** hyperlipidemia. **MS:** ↑ CK. **Neuro:** abnormal dreams, dizziness, fatigue, headache, insomnia. **Misc:** immune reconstitution syndrome.

Interactions

Drug-Drug: Bictegravir may ↑ **dofetilide** levels and the risk of torsades de pointes; concurrent use contraindicated. **Rifampin** may ↓ levels and effectiveness of bictegravir; concurrent use contraindicated. Medications that compete for active tubular secretion, including **acyclovir**, **cidofovir**, **ganciclovir**, **valacyclovir**, **valganciclovir**, or **aminoglycosides**, may ↑ levels and risk of toxicity of emtricitabine and tenofovir. Nephrotoxic agents, including **NSAIDs**, ↑ risk of nephrotoxicity of tenofovir; avoid concurrent use. **Carbamazepine**, **oxcarbazepine**, **phenobarbital**, **phenytoin**, **rifabutin**, and **rifapentine** may ↓ levels and effectiveness of bictegravir and tenofovir; avoid concurrent use. Administration with **antacids** containing **magnesium** or **aluminum** ↓ absorption of bictegravir; take ≥2 hr before or ≥6 hr after magnesium- or aluminum-containing antacids. Administration with supplements or antacids containing **calcium** or **iron** ↓ absorption of bictegravir; take at the same time as calcium or iron supplements with food (and not on an empty stomach). May ↑ levels and risk of toxicity of **metformin**.
Drug-Natural Products: St. John's wort may ↓ levels and effectiveness of bictegravir and tenofovir; avoid concurrent use.

Route/Dosage

PO (Adults and Children ≥25 kg): One tablet (bictegravir 50 mg/emtricitabine 200 mg/tenofovir alafenamide 25 mg) once daily
PO (Children 14–24 kg): One tablet (bictegravir 30 mg/emtricitabine 120 mg/tenofovir alafenamide 15 mg) once daily.

Renal Impairment

PO (Adults): *Virologically suppressed with CCr <15 mL/min and receiving chronic hemodialysis:* One tablet (bictegravir 50 mg/emtricitabine 200 mg/tenofovir alafenamide 25 mg) once daily (on days of hemodialysis, give dose after hemodialysis session).

Availability

Tablets: bictegravir 30 mg/emtricitabine 120 mg/tenofovir alafenamide 15 mg, bictegravir 50 mg/emtricitabine 200 mg/tenofovir alafenamide 25 mg.

NURSING IMPLICATIONS

Assessment

- Assess patient for change in severity of HIV symptoms and for symptoms of opportunistic infections during therapy.
- May cause lactic acidosis and severe hepatomegaly with steatosis. Monitor patient for signs (↑ serum lactate, ↑ liver enzymes, liver enlargement on palpation). Suspend therapy if clinical or laboratory signs occur.

B

Lab Test Considerations

- Monitor viral load and CD4 cell count regularly during therapy.
- Test patients for chronic HBV before initiating therapy. Medication is not indicated for treatment of HBV. Exacerbations of HBV have occurred upon discontinuation of therapy.
- Assess serum creatinine, estimated CCr, urine glucose, and urine protein prior to and periodically during therapy. Also monitor serum phosphorous in patients with chronic kidney disease. Discontinue therapy in patients who develop clinically significant ↓ renal function or evidence of Fanconi syndrome.
- Monitor liver function tests in patients coinfected with HIV and HBV who discontinue *Biktarvy*. May cause an exacerbation of HBV. May ↑ AST, ALT, bilirubin, CK, serum amylase, serum lipase, and triglycerides.
- May ↓ neutrophil count.
- May ↑ LDL cholesterol.

Implementation

- **PO:** Administer once daily without regard to food.
- Administer medication ≥2 hr before or 6 hr after antacids containing aluminum or magnesium. Medication may be taken with food at same time as supplements or antacids containing iron or calcium.

Patient/Family Teaching

- Emphasize the importance of taking medication as directed. Do not take more than prescribed amount, and do not stop taking without consulting health care provider. Take missed doses as soon as remembered, but not if almost time for next dose; do not double doses. Advise patient to read *Patient Information* before starting therapy and with each Rx refill in case of changes.
- Instruct patient that medication should not be shared with others.
- Inform patient that medication does not cure HIV or prevent associated or opportunistic infections. Therapy may ↓ the risk of transmission of HIV to others through sexual contact or blood contamination. Caution patient to use a condom and to avoid sharing needles or donating blood to prevent spreading HIV to others.
- Instruct patient to notify health care provider immediately if signs/symptoms of lactic acidosis (tiredness or weakness, unusual muscle pain, trouble breathing, stomach pain with nausea and vomiting, cold especially in arms or legs, dizziness, fast or irregular heartbeat) or signs/symptoms of hepatotoxicity (yellow skin or whites of eyes, dark urine, light-colored stools, lack of appetite for several days or longer, nausea, abdominal pain) occur.
- Instruct patient to notify health care provider of all Rx or OTC medications, vitamins, or herbal products being taken and consult health care provider before taking any new medications, especially St. John's wort.
- Advise patient to notify health care provider if signs and symptoms of immune reconstitution syndrome (signs and symptoms of an infection) occur.
- Rep: Advise women of reproductive potential to notify health care provider if pregnancy is planned or suspected or if breastfeeding is planned. Enroll pregnant patients in the Antiretroviral Pregnancy Registry by calling 1-800-258-4263.
- Emphasize the importance of regular follow-up exams and blood counts to determine progress and monitor for side effects.

Evaluation/Desired Outcomes

- Delayed progression of HIV and decreased opportunistic infections in patients with HIV.
- Decrease in viral load and increase in CD4 cell counts.

HIGH ALERT

binimetinib (bin-i-me-ti-nib)

Mektovi

Classification

Therapeutic: antineoplastics

Pharmacologic: kinase inhibitors

Indications

Metastatic/unresectable melanoma in patients with the BRAF V600E or V600K mutation (in combination with encorafenib). Metastatic non-small cell lung cancer (NSCLC) in patients with the BRAF V600E mutation (in combination with encorafenib).

Action

Inhibits the activity of mitogen-activated extracellular kinase 1 and 2, which are enzymes that normally promote cellular proliferation. **Therapeutic Effects:** Decreased progression of melanoma and improved survival. Decreased progression of NSCLC.

Pharmacokinetics

Absorption: At least 50% absorbed following oral administration.

Distribution: Extensively distributed to tissues.

Protein Binding: 97%.

Metabolism and Excretion: Mostly metabolized by the liver via glucuronidation. 62% excreted in feces (32% as unchanged drug); 31% excreted in urine (6.5% as unchanged drug).

Half-life: 3.5 hr.

TIME/ACTION PROFILE (plasma concentrations)

ROUTE	ONSET	PEAK	DURATION
PO	unknown	1.6 hr	unknown

Contraindications/Precautions

Contraindicated in: OB: Pregnancy; Lactation: Lactation.

Use Cautiously in: Left ventricular ejection fraction (LVEF) <50%; History of retinal vein occlusion; Uncontrolled glaucoma or history of hypercoagulability (↑ risk of retinal vein occlusion); Moderate or severe hepatic impairment (↓ dose); Rep: Women of reproductive potential; Pedi: Safety and effectiveness not established in children.

Adverse Reactions/Side Effects

CV: CARDIOMYOPATHY, hypertension, peripheral edema, DEEP VENOUS THROMBOSIS (DVT). **Derm:** rash, photosensitivity. **EENT:** retinopathy, visual impairment, macular edema, retinal detachment, retinal vein occlusion (RVO), uveitis. **F and E:** hyponatremia. **GI:** ↑ liver enzymes, abdominal pain, constipation, diarrhea, nausea, vomiting, colitis, HEPATOTOXICITY. **GU:** ↑ serum creatinine. **Hemat:** anemia, HEMORRHAGE, leukopenia, lymphopenia, neutropenia. **MS:** ↑ CK, RHABDOMYOLYSIS. **Neuro:** dizziness, fatigue. **Resp:** INTERSTITIAL LUNG DISEASE (ILD), PULMONARY EMBOLISM (PE). **Misc:** fever, MALIGNANCY.

Interactions

Drug-Drug: None reported.

Route/Dosage

PO (Adults): 45 mg twice daily; continue until disease progression or unacceptable toxicity.

Hepatic Impairment

PO (Adults): *Moderate or severe hepatic impairment:* 30 mg twice daily; continue until disease progression or unacceptable toxicity.

Availability

Tablets: 15 mg.

NURSING IMPLICATIONS

Assessment

- Monitor LVEF by echocardiogram or multigated acquisition scan before starting therapy with binimetinib, 1 mo after initiation, and then at 2–3-mo intervals during therapy. *If asymptomatic, absolute ↓ in LVEF >10% from baseline that is also below lower limit of normal (LLN) occurs,* hold binimetinib for up to 4 wk and evaluate LVEF every 2 wk. Resume binimetinib at ↓ dose if present LVEF ≥ LLN, absolute ↓ from baseline is ≤10%, and patient is asymptomatic. If LVEF does not recover within 4 wk, permanently discontinue binimetinib. *If symptomatic HF occurs with absolute ↓ in LVEF >20% from baseline that is also below LLN,* discontinue binimetinib permanently.
- Monitor for signs and symptoms of venous thromboembolism (shortness of breath, chest pain, arm or leg swelling, cool or pale arm or leg) during therapy. *If uncomplicated DVT or PE occurs,* hold binimetinib. If improves to Grade 0–1, resume at ↓ dose. If not improved, permanently discontinue binimetinib. *If life-threatening PE occurs,* permanently discontinue binimetinib.
- Assess for visual symptoms at each visit. Perform regular ophthalmic exam. Monitor for signs and symptoms of ocular toxicities (blurred vision, loss of vision, other vision changes, seeing colored dots, halo around objects, swelling, redness, photophobia, eye pain). *If symptomatic retinopathy/retinal pigment epithelial detachments occur,* hold binimetinib for up to 10 days. If improves and becomes asymptomatic, resume at same dose. If not improved, resume at a ↓ dose or permanently discontinue binimetinib. *If any grade RVO occurs,* permanently discontinue binimetinib. *If Grade 1 or 2 uveitis does not respond to ocular therapy, or if Grade 3 uveitis occurs,* withhold binimetinib for up to 6 wk. If improved, resume at same or ↓ dose. If not improved, permanently discontinue binimetinib. *If Grade 4 uveitis occurs,* permanently discontinue binimetinib.
- Monitor for signs and symptoms of ILD or pneumonitis (cough, dyspnea, hypoxia, pleural effusion, infiltrates) during therapy. *If Grade 2 ILD occurs,* hold binimetinib for up to 4 wk. If improved to Grade 0–1, resume at ↓ dose. If not resolved within 4 wk, permanently discontinue binimetinib. *If Grade 3 or 4 ILD occurs,* permanently discontinue binimetinib.
- Assess for bleeding (headaches, dizziness, feeling weak, coughing up blood or blood clots, vomiting blood or vomit looks like coffee grounds, red or black tarry stools) during therapy. *If recurrent Grade 2 or 1st occurrence of Grade 3 hemorrhagic event occurs,* hold binimetinib for up to 4 wk. If improves to Grade 0–1 or baseline levels, resume at ↓ dose. If no improvement, permanently discontinue binimetinib. *If 1st occurrence of Grade 4 hemorrhagic event occurs,* permanently discontinue binimetinib, or hold for up to 4 wk. If improves to Grade 0–1 or to baseline levels, resume at ↓ dose. If no improvement, permanently discontinue binimetinib. *If recurrent Grade 3 hemorrhagic event occurs,* consider discontinuing binimetinib permanently. *If recurrent Grade 4 hemorrhagic event occurs,* permanently discontinue binimetinib.
- Monitor patients for new malignancies prior to initiation as well as during and after discontinuation of therapy.

B

Lab Test Considerations
- Verify negative pregnancy test prior to starting therapy.
- Confirm presence of BRAF V600E or V600K mutation in tumor specimens before starting therapy. Information on FDA-approved tests for the detection of BRAF V600 mutations in melanoma is available at: http://www.fda.gov/CompanionDiagnostics.
- Monitor liver function tests before starting therapy, monthly during therapy, and as indicated. *If Grade 2 ↑ AST or ALT occurs,* continue dose. If no improvement within 2 wk, hold binimetinib until improved to Grade 0–1 or to baseline levels and resume at same dose. *If Grade 3 or 4 ↑ AST or ALT occurs,* consider permanently discontinuing binimetinib.
- May cause rhabdomyolysis. Monitor CK and serum creatinine levels prior to starting therapy, periodically during therapy, and as indicated. *If Grade 4 asymptomatic CK ↑ or any Grade CK ↑ with symptoms or with renal impairment occurs,* hold dose for up to 4 wk. If improved to Grade 0–1, resume at ↓ dose. If not resolved within 4 wk, permanently discontinue binimetinib.

Implementation
- Dose adjustments for adverse reactions include: *First dose reduction:* 30 mg twice daily. *If patient unable to tolerate 30 mg twice daily,* discontinue binimetinib.
- **PO:** Administer without regard to food. Usually taken with encorafenib.

Patient/Family Teaching
- Explain purpose and side effects of medication to patient. Advise to read *Patient Information* before starting therapy.
- Instruct patient to take missed dose as soon as remembered, but no closer than 6 hr to next dose. If patient vomits after dose, omit and take next scheduled dose.
- Advise patient to notify health care professional promptly if signs and symptoms of HF, venous thromboembolism (sudden onset of difficulty breathing, leg pain, swelling), changes in vision, ILD (new or worsening cough or dyspnea), hepatotoxicity (jaundice, dark urine, nausea, vomiting, loss of appetite, fatigue, bruising, bleeding), rhabdomyolysis (unusual or new onset weakness, myalgia, darkened urine), hemorrhage, or abnormal skin changes (mole color/shape changes, new wart, unhealed skin sores) occur.
- Advise patient to notify health care professional of all Rx or OTC medications, vitamins, or herbal products being taken and to consult health care professional before taking other medications.
- Rep: May cause fetal harm. Advise women of reproductive potential to use effective contraception during and for ≥30 days after last dose and to avoid breastfeeding for 3 days after last dose. Advise patient to notify health care professional if pregnancy is planned or suspected.

Evaluation/Desired Outcomes
- Decreased progression of melanoma and improved survival.
- Decreased progression of NSCLC.

bisacodyl (bis-a-**koe**-dill)
Dulcolax, Ex-Lax Ultra

Classification
Therapeutic: laxatives
Pharmacologic: stimulant laxatives

Indications
Constipation. Evacuation of the bowel before radiologic studies or surgery. Part of a bowel regimen in spinal cord injury patients.

Action
Stimulates peristalsis. Alters fluid and electrolyte transport, producing fluid accumulation in the colon.
Therapeutic Effects: Evacuation of the colon.

Pharmacokinetics
Absorption: Variable absorption follows oral administration; rectal absorption is minimal; action is local in the colon.
Distribution: Unknown.
Metabolism and Excretion: Small amounts absorbed are metabolized by the liver.
Half-life: Unknown.

TIME/ACTION PROFILE (evacuation of bowel)

ROUTE	ONSET	PEAK	DURATION
PO	6–12 hr	unknown	unknown
Rectal	15–60 min	unknown	unknown

Contraindications/Precautions
Contraindicated in: Hypersensitivity; Abdominal pain; Obstruction; Nausea or vomiting (especially with fever or other signs of an acute abdomen).
Use Cautiously in: Severe cardiovascular disease; Anal or rectal fissures; Excess or prolonged use (may result in dependence).

Adverse Reactions/Side Effects
F and E: hypokalemia (with chronic use). **GI:** abdominal cramps, nausea, diarrhea, rectal burning. **MS:** muscle weakness (with chronic use). **Misc:** protein-losing enteropathy, tetany (with chronic use).

Interactions

Drug-Drug: Antacids, histamine H_2-receptor antagonists, and **proton pump inhibitors** may remove enteric coating of tablets, resulting in gastric irritation/dyspepsia. May ↓ the absorption of other **orally administered drugs** because of ↑ motility and ↓ transit time.
Drug-Food: Milk may remove enteric coating of tablets, resulting in gastric irritation/dyspepsia.

Route/Dosage

PO (Adults and Children ≥12 yr): 5–15 mg/day (up to 30 mg/day) as a single dose.
PO (Children 3–11 yr): 5–10 mg/day (0.3 mg/kg) as a single dose.
Rect (Adults and Children ≥12 yr): 10 mg/day single dose.
Rect (Children 2–11 yr): 5–10 mg/day single dose.
Rect (Children <2 yr): 5 mg/day single dose.

Availability (generic available)

Enteric-coated tablets: 5 mg^{OTC}. **Rectal suppositories:** 10 mg^{OTC}. **Rectal enema:** 10 mg/30 mL^{OTC}.

NURSING IMPLICATIONS

Assessment

- Assess for abdominal distention, presence of bowel sounds, and pattern of bowel function.
- Monitor amount of stool produced during therapy. *If nausea, vomiting, or change in bowel habits last >2 wk,* discontinue bisacodyl.

Implementation

- Do not confuse Dulcolax (bisacodyl) with Dulcolax (docusate sodium).
- May be administered at bedtime for morning results.
- **PO:** Taking on an empty stomach will produce more rapid results.
- ***DNC:*** Do not crush or chew enteric-coated tablets. Take with a full glass of water or juice.
- Do not administer oral doses within 1 hr of milk or antacids; this may lead to premature dissolution of tablet and gastric or duodenal irritation.
- **Rect** Rectal suppository or enema can be given at the time a bowel movement is desired. Lubricate suppositories with water or water-soluble lubricant before insertion. Encourage patient to retain the suppository or enema 15–30 min before expelling.

Patient/Family Teaching

- Advise patients, other than those with spinal cord injuries, that laxatives should be used only for short-term therapy. Prolonged therapy may cause electrolyte imbalance and dependence.
- Explain purpose and side effects of medication. Advise patient to read *Patient Information* before starting therapy.
- Advise patient to ↑ fluid intake to ≥1500–2000 mL/day during therapy to prevent dehydration.
- Encourage patients to use other forms of bowel regulation (↑ oral intake of bulk-forming fiber, ↑ fluid intake, ↑ mobility as able). Normal bowel habits vary from 3 times/day to 3 times/wk.
- Instruct patients with cardiac disease to avoid straining during bowel movements.
- Advise patient to stop bisacodyl and notify health care professional if significant abdominal pain, fever, nausea, vomiting, or rectal bleeding occur or if no bowel movement occurs after using bisacodyl ≥1 wk.
- Advise patient to notify health care professional of all Rx or OTC medications, vitamins, or herbal products being taken and to consult health care professional before taking other medications.
- Rep: Advise women of reproductive potential to notify health care professional if pregnancy is planned or suspected or if breastfeeding.

Evaluation/Desired Outcomes

- Soft, formed bowel movement when used for constipation.
- Evacuation of colon before surgery or radiologic studies or for patients with spinal cord injuries.

bisoprolol, See BETA BLOCKERS (selective).

HIGH ALERT

bivalirudin (bi-val-i-roo-din)

Angiomax

Classification
Therapeutic: anticoagulants
Pharmacologic: thrombin inhibitors

Indications

Patients undergoing percutaneous coronary intervention (PCI), including those with heparin-induced thrombocytopenia (HIT) or heparin-induced thrombocytopenia and thrombosis syndrome (HITTS).

Action

Specifically and reversibly inhibits thrombin by binding to its receptor sites. Inhibition of thrombin prevents activation of factors V, VIII, and XII; the conversion of fibrinogen to fibrin; and platelet adhesion and aggregation. **Therapeutic Effects:** Decreased acute ischemic complications in patients with unstable angina (death, MI, or the urgent need for revascularization procedures).

Pharmacokinetics

Absorption: IV administration results in complete bioavailability.

B

Distribution: Unknown.
Metabolism and Excretion: Cleared from plasma by a combination of renal mechanisms and proteolytic breakdown.
Half-life: 25 min (↑ in renal impairment).

TIME/ACTION PROFILE (anticoagulant effect)

ROUTE	ONSET	PEAK	DURATION
IV	immediate	unknown	1–2 hr

Contraindications/Precautions

Contraindicated in: Active major bleeding; Hypersensitivity.
Use Cautiously in: Any disease state associated with an ↑ risk of bleeding; HIT or HITTS; Patients with unstable angina not undergoing PCI; Patients with other acute coronary syndromes; Severe renal impairment; OB: Safety not established in pregnancy; Lactation: Use while breastfeeding only if potential maternal benefit justifies potential risk to infant; Pedi: Safety and effectiveness not established in children.

Adverse Reactions/Side Effects

CV: hypotension, ACUTE STENT THROMBOSIS (ESPECIALLY IN PATIENTS WITH ST-SEGMENT ELEVATION MI UNDERGOING PCI), bradycardia, hypertension. **GI:** nausea, abdominal pain, dyspepsia, vomiting. **Hemat:** BLEEDING. **Local:** injection site pain. **MS:** pain. **Neuro:** headache, anxiety, insomnia, nervousness. **Misc:** fever.

Interactions

Drug-Drug: ↑ risk of bleeding with **heparin, low molecular weight heparins, clopidogrel, thrombolytics**, or any other **drugs that inhibit coagulation**.
Drug-Natural Products: ↑ risk of bleeding with **arnica, chamomile, clove, dong quai, feverfew, garlic, ginger, gingko, Panax ginseng**, and others.

Route/Dosage

IV (Adults): 0.75 mg/kg as a bolus injection, followed by an infusion at a rate of 1.75 mg/kg/hr for the duration of the PCI procedure. An activated clotting time (ACT) should be performed 5 min after bolus dose and an additional bolus dose of 0.3 mg/kg may be administered if needed. Continuation of the infusion (at a rate of 1.75 mg/kg/hr) for up to 4 hr postprocedure is optional (should be considered in patients with ST-segment elevation MI). Therapy should be initiated prior to the procedure and given in conjunction with aspirin.

Renal Impairment

IV (Adults): No ↓ in the bolus dose is needed in any patient with renal impairment. *CCr <30 mL/min:* ↓ infusion rate to 1 mg/kg/hr; *Hemodialysis:* ↓ infusion rate to 0.25 mg/kg/hr.

Availability (generic available)

Lyophilized powder for injection: 250 mg/vial.
Premixed infusion: 250 mg/50 mL.

NURSING IMPLICATIONS

Assessment

- Assess for bleeding; most common is oozing from the arterial access site for cardiac catheterization. Minimize use of arterial and venous punctures; IM injections; and use of urinary catheters, nasotracheal intubation, and nasogastric tubes. *If bleeding cannot be controlled with pressure to site,* discontinue bivalirudin immediately.
- Monitor vital signs. May cause bradycardia, hypertension, or hypotension. An unexplained ↓ in BP may indicate hemorrhage.
- Monitor patients with ST-segment elevation MI undergoing primary PCI with bivalirudin for acute stent thrombosis for ≥24 hr in a facility capable of managing ischemic complications.

Lab Test Considerations

- Assess hemoglobin, hematocrit, and platelets at baseline and periodically during therapy. An unexplained ↓ in hematocrit may indicate hemorrhage.
- Bivalirudin interferes with INR measurements; INR may not be useful in determining appropriate dose of warfarin.
- Monitor ACT periodically in patients with renal impairment.

Implementation

- Administer IV just prior to PCI, in conjunction with aspirin 300–325 mg/day. Do not administer IM.

IV Administration

- **IV Push:** (for bolus dose) **Reconstitution:** Reconstitute each 250-mg vial with 5 mL of sterile water for injection. Reconstituted vials are stable for 24 hr if refrigerated. **Dilution:** Further dilute in 50 mL of D5W or 0.9% NaCl. Withdraw bolus dose out of bag. Infusion is stable for 24 hr at room temperature. **Concentration:** Final concentration of infusion is 5 mg/mL. **Rate:** Administer as a bolus injection. **Intermittent Infusion: Reconstitution:** Reconstitute each 250-mg vial as per the above directions. **Dilution:** Further dilute in 50 mL of D5W or 0.9% NaCl. If infusion will be continued after 4 hr (at a rate of 0.2 mg/kg/hr), reconstituted vial should be diluted in 500 mL of D5W or 0.9% NaCl. Infusion is stable for 24 hr at room temperature. Premixed infusion is stable for 24 hr at room temperature or 14 days if refrigerated. **Concentration:** 5 mg/mL (infusion rate: 1.75 mg/kg/hr); 0.5 mg/mL (infusion rate: 0.2 mg/kg/hr). **Rate:** Based on patient's weight (see Route/Dosage section).

- **Y-Site Compatibility:** acyclovir, allopurinol, amikacin, aminocaproic acid, aminophylline, amphotericin B liposomal, ampicillin, ampicillin/sulbactam, anidulafungin, argatroban, arsenic trioxide, atropine, azithromycin, aztreonam, bleomycin, bumetanide, buprenorphine, busulfan, butorphanol, calcium chloride, calcium gluconate, cangrelor, carboplatin, carmustine, cefazolin, cefepime, cefotaxime, cefotetan, cefoxitin, ceftazidime, ceftriaxone, cefuroxime, chloramphenicol, ciprofloxacin, cisatracurium, cisplatin, clindamycin, cyclophosphamide, cyclosporine, cytarabine, dacarbazine, dactinomycin, daptomycin, daunorubicin, dexamethasone, dexmedetomidine, dexrazoxane, digoxin, diltiazem, diphenhydramine, docetaxel, dopamine, doxorubicin hydrochloride, doxorubicin liposomal, doxycycline, droperidol, enalaprilat, ephedrine, epinephrine, epirubicin, epoprostenol, eptifibatide, ertapenem, erythromycin, esmolol, etoposide, etoposide phosphate, fentanyl, fluconazole, fludarabine, fluorouracil, foscarnet, fosphenytoin, furosemide, ganciclovir, gemcitabine, gentamicin, glycopyrrolate, granisetron, heparin, hydralazine, hydrocortisone, hydromorphone, hydroxyzine, idarubicin, ifosfamide, imipenem/cilastatin, insulin, regular, irinotecan, isoproterenol, ketorolac, leucovorin calcium, levofloxacin, lidocaine, linezolid, magnesium sulfate, mannitol, melphalan, meperidine, meropenem, mesna, methohexital, methotrexate, methylprednisolone, metoclopramide, metoprolol, metronidazole, midazolam, milrinone, mitomycin, mitoxantrone, morphine, moxifloxacin, mycophenolate, nafcillin, nalbuphine, naloxone, nicardipine, nitroglycerin, nitroprusside, norepinephrine, octreotide, ondansetron, oxaliplatin, oxytocin, paclitaxel, palonosetron, pamidronate, pemetrexed, pentobarbital, phenobarbital, phenylephrine, piperacillin/tazobactam, potassium acetate, potassium chloride, potassium phosphate, procainamide, propranolol, remifentanil, rocuronium, sodium acetate, sodium bicarbonate, sodium phosphate, succinylcholine, sufentanil, tacrolimus, theophylline, thiotepa, tigecycline, tirofiban, tobramycin, topotecan, trimethoprim/sulfamethoxazole, vasopressin, vecuronium, verapamil, vinblastine, vincristine, vinorelbine, voriconazole, warfarin, zidovudine, zoledronic acid.
- **Y-Site Incompatibility:** alteplase, amiodarone, amphotericin B deoxycholate, caspofungin, chlorpromazine, dantrolene, diazepam, dobutamine, pentamidine, phenytoin, prochlorperazine, vancomycin.

Patient/Family Teaching

- Explain purpose and side effects of medication. Advise patient to read *Patient Information* before starting therapy.
- Instruct patient to notify health care professional immediately if any bleeding or bruising is noted.
- Instruct patient to notify health care professional of all Rx or OTC medications, vitamins, or herbal products being taken and consult health care professional before taking any new medications.
- Rep: Advise women of reproductive potential to notify health care professional if pregnancy is planned or suspected or if breastfeeding.

Evaluation/Desired Outcomes

- ↓ acute ischemic complications in patients with unstable angina (death, MI, or the urgent need for revascularization procedures).

HIGH ALERT

bleomycin (blee-oh-**mye**-sin)

Classification

Therapeutic: antineoplastics

Pharmacologic: antitumor antibiotics

Indications

Treatment of: Lymphomas, Squamous cell carcinoma, Testicular embryonal cell carcinoma, Choriocarcinoma, Teratocarcinoma. Intrapleural administration to prevent the reaccumulation of malignant effusions.

Action

Inhibits DNA and RNA synthesis. **Therapeutic Effects:** Death of rapidly replicating cells, particularly malignant ones.

Pharmacokinetics

Absorption: IV administration results in complete bioavailability. Well absorbed from IM and SUBQ sites. Absorption follows intrapleural and intraperitoneal administration.

Distribution: Widely distributed; concentrates in skin, lungs, peritoneum, kidneys, and lymphatics.

Metabolism and Excretion: 60–70% excreted unchanged by the kidneys.

Half-life: 2 hr (↑ in renal impairment).

TIME/ACTION PROFILE (tumor response)

ROUTE	ONSET	PEAK	DURATION
IV, IM, SUBQ	2–3 wk	unknown	unknown

Contraindications/Precautions

Contraindicated in: Hypersensitivity; OB: Pregnancy; Lactation: Lactation.

Use Cautiously in: Renal impairment (dose ↓ required if CCr <35 mL/min); Pulmonary disease; Rep: Women of reproductive potential; Geri: ↑ risk of pulmonary toxicity and renal impairment in older adults.

Adverse Reactions/Side Effects

CV: hypotension, peripheral vasoconstriction. **Derm:** hyperpigmentation, mucocutaneous toxicity, alopecia, erythema, rash, urticaria, vesiculation. **GI:** anorexia, nausea, stomatitis, vomiting. **Hemat:** anemia, leukopenia, thrombocytopenia. **Local:** pain at tumor site, phlebitis at IV site. **Metab:** weight loss. **Neuro:** aggressive behavior, disorientation, weakness. **Resp:** pneumonitis, PULMONARY FIBROSIS. **Misc:** chills, fever, ANAPHYLACTOID REACTIONS.

Interactions

Drug-Drug: Hematologic toxicity ↑ with **radiation therapy** and other **antineoplastics**. **Cisplatin** may ↑ risk of toxicity. ↑ risk of pulmonary toxicity with other **antineoplastics**, thoracic **radiation therapy**, or **general anesthesia**. ↑ risk of Raynaud phenomenon when used with **vinblastine**.

Route/Dosage

Patients with lymphoma should receive initial test doses of ≤2 units for the first two doses.

IV: IM SUBQ (Adults and Children): 0.25–0.5 unit/kg (10–20 units/m²) weekly or twice weekly initially. If favorable response, ↓ maintenance doses to 1 unit/day or 5 units/wk IM or IV. May also be given as continuous IV infusion at 0.25 unit/kg or 15 units/m²/day for 4–5 days.

Intrapleural: (Adults): 15–20 units instilled for 4 hr; then removed.

Availability (generic available)

Powder for injection: 15 units/vial, 30 units/vial.

NURSING IMPLICATIONS

Assessment

- Monitor vital signs before and frequently during therapy.
- Assess for fever and chills. May occur 3–6 hr after administration and last for 4–12 hr.
- Monitor for anaphylactic (fever, chills, hypotension, wheezing) and idiosyncratic (confusion, hypotension, fever, chills, wheezing) reactions. Keep resuscitation equipment and medications nearby. Patients with lymphoma are at particular risk for idiosyncratic reactions that may occur immediately or several hr after therapy, usually after the 1st or 2nd dose.
- Assess for dyspnea and fine rales, the earliest sign and symptom of pulmonary toxicity. Monitor chest x-ray every 1–2 wk during therapy. *If pulmonary changes occur*, hold bleomycin to determine if causal. Consider monitoring pulmonary diffusion capacity (DL_{co}) at baseline and monthly during therapy. *If DL_{co} <30–35% of baseline value*, permanently discontinue bleomycin.
- Assess nausea, vomiting, and appetite. Weigh weekly. Modify diet as tolerated. Antiemetics may be given before administration.

Lab Test Considerations

- Verify negative pregnancy status before starting therapy. Monitor CBC before and periodically during therapy. May cause thrombocytopenia and leukopenia (nadir occurs in 12 days and usually returns to pretreatment levels by day 17).
- Monitor baseline and periodic renal and hepatic function.

Implementation

- ***High Alert:*** Fatalities have occurred with chemotherapeutic agents. Before administering, clarify all ambiguous orders; double-check single, daily, and course-of-therapy dose limits; have second practitioner independently double-check original order and dose calculations.
- ***High Alert:*** Bleomycin should be administered in a monitored setting under the supervision of a physician experienced in cancer chemotherapy.
- Prepare solution in a biologic cabinet. Wear gloves, gown, and mask while handling medication. Discard equipment in specially designated containers.
- Patients with lymphoma should receive a 1- or 2-unit test dose 2–4 hr before initiation of therapy. Monitor closely for anaphylactic reaction. May not detect reactors.
- Premedication with acetaminophen, corticosteroids, and diphenhydramine may ↓ drug fever and risk of anaphylaxis.
- **IM SUBQ**: **Reconstitution:** Inject 1–5 mL or 2–10 mL of sterile or bacteriostatic water for injection or 0.9% NaCl into 15 unit or 30 unit vials, respectively.

IV Administration

- Bleomycin is an irritant. If extravasation occurs, immediately stop infusion. Leave needle/cannula in place temporarily but do not flush the line. Gently aspirate extravasated solution; then remove needle/cannula. Elevate patient's extremity. **Intermittent Infusion: Reconstitution:** Inject 5 mL or 10 mL of 0.9% NaCl into 15 unit or 30 unit vials, respectively. Reconstituted solution is stable for 24 hr at room temperature and for 14 days if refrigerated. Do not administer solution if discolored or contains particulates. **Concentration:** 3 units/mL. **Rate:** Administer slowly over 10 min.
- **Y-Site Compatibility:** acyclovir, allopurinol, amikacin, aminocaproic acid, aminophylline, amiodarone, ampicillin, ampicillin/sulbactam, anidulafungin, argatroban, atracurium, azithromycin, aztreonam, bivalirudin, bumetanide, buprenorphine, busulfan, butorphanol, calcium chloride, calcium gluconate, carboplatin, carmustine, caspofungin, cefazolin, cefepime, cefotaxime, cefotetan,

cefoxitin, ceftazidime, ceftriaxone, cefuroxime, chloramphenicol, chlorpromazine, ciprofloxacin, cisatracurium, cisplatin, clindamycin, cyclophosphamide, cyclosporine, cytarabine, dacarbazine, dactinomycin, daptomycin, daunorubicin, dexamethasone, dexmedetomidine, dexrazoxane, digoxin, diltiazem, diphenhydramine, dobutamine, docetaxel, dopamine, doxorubicin hydrochloride, doxorubicin liposomal, doxycycline, droperidol, enalaprilat, ephedrine, epinephrine, epirubicin, ertapenem, erythromycin, esmolol, etoposide, etoposide phosphate, famotidine, fentanyl, filgrastim, fluconazole, fludarabine, fluorouracil, foscarnet, fosphenytoin, furosemide, ganciclovir, gemcitabine, gentamicin, glycopyrrolate, granisetron, haloperidol, heparin, hetastarch, hydralazine, hydrocortisone, hydromorphone, idarubicin, ifosfamide, imipenem/cilastatin, insulin, regular, irinotecan, isoproterenol, ketorolac, labetalol, leucovorin, levofloxacin, lidocaine, linezolid, lorazepam, magnesium sulfate, mannitol, melphalan, meperidine, meropenem, mesna, methadone, methohexital, methotrexate, methylprednisolone, metoclopramide, metoprolol, metronidazole, midazolam, milrinone, minocycline, mitomycin, mitoxantrone, morphine, moxifloxacin, nafcillin, nalbuphine, naloxone, nicardipine, nitroglycerin, nitroprusside, norepinephrine, octreotide, ondansetron, oxaliplatin, paclitaxel, palonosetron, pamidronate, pantoprazole, pemetrexed, pentamidine, pentobarbital, phenobarbital, phentolamine, phenylephrine, piperacillin/tazobactam, potassium acetate, potassium chloride, potassium phosphates, procainamide, prochlorperazine, promethazine, propranolol, remifentanil, rituximab, rocuronium, sargramostim, sodium acetate, sodium bicarbonate, sodium phosphates, succinylcholine, sufentanil, tacrolimus, theophylline, thiotepa, tirofiban, tobramycin, topotecan, trastuzumab, trimethoprim/sulfamethoxazole, vancomycin, vasopressin, vecuronium, verapamil, vinblastine, vincristine, vinorelbine, voriconazole, zidovudine, zoledronic acid.

- **Y-Site Incompatibility:** amphotericin B deoxycholate, amphotericin B liposomal, dantrolene, diazepam, phenytoin, tigecycline.
- **Intrapleural:** Dissolve 60 units in 50–100 mL of 0.9% NaCl.
- Administer through thoracotomy tube. Position patient from supine to left and right lateral several times over the next 4 hr; then unclamp tube and re-establish suction as directed.

Patient/Family Teaching

- Explain purpose and side effects of medication. Advise patient to read *Patient Information* before starting therapy.
- Instruct patient to notify health care provider if fever, chills, wheezing, faintness, diaphoresis, shortness of breath, prolonged nausea and vomiting, anorexia, weight loss, or mouth sores occur.
- Encourage patient not to smoke due to risk of worsen pulmonary toxicity.
- Explain that skin toxicity may manifest itself as skin sensitivity, hyperpigmentation (especially at skin folds and points of skin irritation), and skin rashes and thickening.
- Advise patient to notify health care provider prior to surgery so pulmonary toxicity prevention measures may be provided (FIO_2 at 25%, fluid replacement with colloid versus crystalloid).
- Instruct patient to inspect oral mucosa for erythema and ulceration. If ulceration occurs, advise patient to use sponge brush and rinse mouth with water after eating and drinking. Opioid analgesics may be required if pain interferes with eating.
- Discuss with patient the possibility of hair loss. Explore coping strategies.
- Instruct patient not to receive vaccinations without advice of health care provider.
- Advise patient to notify health care provider of all Rx or OTC medications, vitamins, or herbal products being taken and to consult health care provider before taking other medications.
- Rep: May cause fetal harm. Advise women of reproductive potential to avoid pregnancy and use effective contraception during therapy. Advise patient to notify health care provider if pregnancy is planned or suspected or if breastfeeding.

Evaluation/Desired Outcomes

- Decreased tumor size without evidence of hypersensitivity or pulmonary toxicity.

HIGH ALERT

brentuximab vedotin

(bren-**tux**-i-mab)

Adcetris

Classification

Therapeutic: antineoplastics

Pharmacologic: drug-antibody conjugates

Indications

Classical Hodgkin lymphoma in patients who have failed autologous hematopoietic stem cell transplant or who have failed ≥2 prior multiagent chemotherapies and are not candidates for autologous hematopoietic stem cell transplant. Previously untreated, high-risk classical Hodgkin lymphoma (in combination with doxorubicin, vincristine, etoposide, prednisone, and cyclophosphamide). Classical Hodgkin lymphoma in patients who are at high risk of relapse or progression as autologous hematopoietic stem cell transplant consolidation.

Previously untreated stage III or IV classical Hodgkin lymphoma (in combination with doxorubicin, vinblastine, and dacarbazine). Systemic anaplastic large cell lymphoma after failure of ≥1 multiagent chemotherapy regimen. Primary cutaneous anaplastic large cell lymphoma or CD30-expressing mycosis fungoides in patients who have received prior systemic therapy. Previously untreated systemic anaplastic large cell lymphoma or other CD30-expressing peripheral T-cell lymphoma (in combination with cyclophosphamide, doxorubicin, and prednisone). Relapsed or refractory large B-cell lymphoma, including diffuse large B-cell lymphoma not otherwise specified, diffuse large B-lymphoma arising from indolent lymphoma, or high-grade B-cell lymphoma, after ≥2 lines of systemic therapy in patients who are not eligible for autologous hematopoietic stem cell transplant or chimeric antigen receptor T-cell therapy (in combination with lenalidomide and rituximab).

Action

An antibody-drug conjugate (ADC) made up of three parts: an antibody specific for human CD30 (cAC10, a cell membrane protein of the tumor necrosis factor receptor), a microtubule disrupting agent monomethyl auristatin (MMAE), and a protease-cleavable linker that attaches MMAE covalently to cAC10. The combination disrupts the intracellular microtubule network causing cell-cycle arrest and apoptotic cellular death. **Therapeutic Effects:** Decreased spread of lymphoma.

Pharmacokinetics

Absorption: IV administration results in complete bioavailability.

Distribution: Unknown.

Metabolism and Excretion: Small amounts of MMAE that are released are metabolized by the liver and eliminated mostly by the kidneys.

Half-life: *ADC:* 4–6 days.

TIME/ACTION PROFILE (plasma concentrations)

ROUTE	ONSET	PEAK	DURATION
IV (ADC)	unknown	end of infusion	3 wk
IV (MMAE)	unknown	1–3 days	3 wk

Contraindications/Precautions

Contraindicated in: Concurrent use of bleomycin (↑ risk of pulmonary toxicity); Severe renal impairment; Moderate or severe hepatic impairment; OB: Pregnancy; Lactation: Lactation.

Use Cautiously in: Preexisting GI involvement (↑ risk of GI perforation); High body mass index (BMI) or diabetes (↑ risk of hyperglycemia); Rep: Women of reproductive potential and men with female partners of reproductive potential; Pedi: Children <2 yr (safety and effectiveness not established).

Adverse Reactions/Side Effects

CV: peripheral edema. **Derm:** alopecia, night sweats, pruritus, rash, STEVENS-JOHNSON SYNDROME (SJS), TOXIC EPIDERMAL NECROLYSIS (TEN), dry skin. **EENT:** oropharyngeal pain. **Endo:** hyperglycemia. **F and E:** KETOACIDOSIS. **GI:** ↓ appetite, abdominal pain, BOWEL OBSTRUCTION, constipation, diarrhea, GI HEMORRHAGE, GI PERFORATION, GI ULCER, HEPATOTOXICITY, ILEUS, nausea, PANCREATITIS, vomiting, weight loss, ENTEROCOLITIS, NEUTROPENIC COLITIS, ulcer. **GU:** ↓ fertility. **Hemat:** anemia, NEUTROPENIA, THROMBOCYTOPENIA. **MS:** arthralgia, back pain, extremity pain, myalgia, muscle spasm. **Neuro:** anxiety, dizziness, fatigue, headache, insomnia, peripheral neuropathy, PROGRESSIVE MULTIFOCAL LEUKOENCEPHALOPATHY (PML). **Resp:** ACUTE RESPIRATORY DISTRESS SYNDROME, cough, dyspnea, INTERSTITIAL LUNG DISEASE. **Misc:** fever, lymphadenopathy, chills, INFUSION REACTIONS (INCLUDING ANAPHYLAXIS), TUMOR LYSIS SYNDROME.

Interactions

Drug-Drug: **Bleomycin** may ↑ risk of pulmonary toxicity; concurrent use contraindicated. **Strong CYP3A4 inhibitors**, including **ketoconazole**, may ↑ levels and risk of toxicity. **Strong CYP3A4 inducers**, including **rifampin**, may ↓ levels and effectiveness.

Route/Dosage

Relapsed Classical Hodgkin Lymphoma or Relapsed Systemic Anaplastic Large Cell Lymphoma

IV (Adults): 1.8 mg/kg (max dose = 180 mg) every 3 wk until disease progression or unacceptable toxicity.

Renal Impairment

IV (Adults): *CCr <30 mL/min:* Avoid use.

Hepatic Impairment

IV (Adults): *Mild hepatic impairment:* 1.2 mg/kg (max dose = 120 mg) every 3 wk until disease progression or unacceptable toxicity; *Moderate or severe hepatic impairment:* Avoid use.

Previously Untreated, High-Risk Classical Hodgkin Lymphoma

IV (Children ≥2 yr): 1.8 mg/kg (max dose = 180 mg) every 3 wk until a maximum of 5 doses completed.

Renal Impairment

IV (Children ≥2 yr): *CCr <30 mL/min:* Avoid use.

Hepatic Impairment

IV (Children ≥2 yr): *Mild hepatic impairment:* 1.2 mg/kg (max dose = 120 mg) every 3 wk until a maximum of 5 doses completed; *Moderate or severe hepatic impairment:* Avoid use.

Classical Hodgkin Lymphoma Consolidation

IV (Adults): 1.8 mg/kg (max dose = 180 mg) every 3 wk until a maximum of 16 cycles completed, disease progression, or unacceptable toxicity. Initiate therapy within 4–6 wk postautologous hematopoietic stem cell transplant or upon recovery of autologous hematopoietic stem cell transplant.

Renal Impairment

IV (Adults): *CCr <30 mL/min:* Avoid use.

Hepatic Impairment

IV (Adults): *Mild hepatic impairment:* 1.2 mg/kg (max dose = 120 mg) every 3 wk until a maximum of 16 cycles completed, disease progression, or unacceptable toxicity; *Moderate or severe hepatic impairment:* Avoid use.

Previously Untreated Stage III or IV Classical Hodgkin Lymphoma

IV (Adults): 1.2 mg/kg (max dose = 120 mg) every 2 wk until a maximum of 12 doses completed, disease progression, or unacceptable toxicity.

Renal Impairment

IV (Adults): *CCr <30 mL/min:* Avoid use.

Hepatic Impairment

IV (Adults): *Mild hepatic impairment:* 0.9 mg/kg (max dose = 90 mg) every 2 wk until a maximum of 12 doses completed, disease progression, or unacceptable toxicity; *Moderate or severe hepatic impairment:* Avoid use.

Relapsed Primary Cutaneous Anaplastic Large Cell Lymphoma or CD30-Expressing Mycosis Fungoides

IV (Adults): 1.8 mg/kg (max dose = 180 mg) every 3 wk until a maximum of 16 cycles completed, disease progression, or unacceptable toxicity.

Renal Impairment

IV (Adults): *CCr <30 mL/min:* Avoid use.

Hepatic Impairment

IV (Adults): *Mild hepatic impairment:* 1.2 mg/kg (max dose = 120 mg) every 3 wk until a maximum of 16 cycles completed, disease progression, or unacceptable toxicity; *Moderate or severe hepatic impairment:* Avoid use.

Previously Untreated Systemic Anaplastic Large Cell Lymphoma or Other CD30-Expressing Peripheral T-Cell Lymphomas

IV (Adults): 1.8 mg/kg (max dose = 180 mg) every 3 wk with each cycle of chemotherapy for 6–8 doses.

Renal Impairment

IV (Adults): *CCr <30 mL/min:* Avoid use.

Hepatic Impairment

IV (Adults): *Mild hepatic impairment:* 1.2 mg/kg (max dose = 120 mg) every 3 wk with each cycle of chemotherapy for 6–8 doses; *Moderate or severe hepatic impairment:* Avoid use.

Relapsed or Refractory Large B-Cell Lymphoma

IV (Adults): 1.2 mg/kg (max dose = 120 mg) every 3 wk until disease progression or unacceptable toxicity.

Renal Impairment

IV (Adults): *CCr <30 mL/min:* Avoid use.

Hepatic Impairment

IV (Adults): *Mild hepatic impairment:* 0.9 mg/kg (max dose = 90 mg) every 3 wk until disease progression or unacceptable toxicity; *Moderate or severe hepatic impairment:* Avoid use.

Availability

Lyophilized powder for injection: 50 mg/vial.

NURSING IMPLICATIONS

Assessment

- Monitor for signs and symptoms of peripheral neuropathy (hypoesthesia, hyperesthesia, paresthesia, discomfort, burning, neuropathic pain, weakness). *If new or worsening Grade 2 peripheral neuropathy occurs,* ↓ dose of vincristine per prescribing information. Continue dosing with brentuximab. If neuropathy improves to Grade ≤1 by day 8 of next cycle, resume vincristine at full dose. *If Grade 3 peripheral neuropathy occurs,* discontinue vincristine. For 1st occurrence, delay next dose of brentuximab until neuropathy improves to Grade ≤1; then restart at 1.2 mg/kg (max dose = 120 mg). For 2nd occurrence, hold brentuximab until improvement to Grade ≤2; then restart at 0.8 mg/kg (max dose = 80 mg). For 3rd occurrence, discontinue brentuximab. *If Grade 4 peripheral neuropathy occurs,* discontinue brentuximab and vincristine.
- Monitor temperature periodically during therapy, especially if neutropenic.
- Assess for signs and symptoms of infusion-related reactions, including anaphylaxis (rash, pruritus, dyspnea, swelling of face and neck). *If anaphylaxis occurs,* discontinue infusion immediately; do not restart. Treat other infusion-related reactions by stopping and treating symptoms. Premedicate patients who have experienced a prior infusion-related reaction with acetaminophen, an antihistamine, and a corticosteroid prior to subsequent infusions.
- Monitor for tumor lysis syndrome due to rapid ↓ in tumor volume (acute renal failure, hyperkalemia, hypocalcemia, hyperuricemia,

hypophosphatemia). Risks are higher in patients with greater tumor burden and rapidly proliferating tumors; may be fatal. Correct electrolyte abnormalities, monitor renal function and fluid balance, and administer supportive care, including dialysis, as indicated.

- Assess for skin rash frequently during therapy. Discontinue at 1st sign of rash; may be life-threatening. SJS or TEN may develop. Treat symptomatically; may recur once treatment is stopped.
- Assess for any new signs or symptoms that may be suggestive of PML, an opportunistic infection of the brain caused by the JC virus that leads to death or severe disability; withhold dose and notify health care provider promptly. PML symptoms may begin gradually but usually worsen rapidly. Symptoms vary depending on which part of brain is infected (mental function declines rapidly and progressively, causing dementia; speaking becomes increasingly difficult; partial blindness; difficulty walking; rarely, headaches and seizures occur). Diagnosis is usually made via gadolinium-enhanced MRI and CSF analysis. Risk of PML ↑ with the number of infusions. Withhold brentuximab at 1st sign of PML.
- Monitor for signs and symptoms of pulmonary toxicity (cough, dyspnea) during therapy. *If new or worsening pulmonary symptoms occur,* hold brentuximab during assessment and until symptoms improve.
- Monitor for severe abdominal pain during therapy; may cause pancreatitis.

Lab Test Considerations

- Verify negative pregnancy status before starting therapy.
- Monitor CBC before each dose and more frequently in patients with Grade 3 or 4 neutropenia. Prolonged (≥1 wk) severe neutropenia may occur. *If Grade 3 or 4 neutropenia occurs,* hold dose of brentuximab until resolution to Grade ≤2. Consider growth factor support for subsequent cycles for patients who developed Grade 3 or 4 neutropenia. *If recurrent Grade 4 neutropenia occurs despite use of growth factors,* discontinue brentuximab or ↓ dose to 1.2 mg/kg (max dose = 120 mg).
- Monitor liver enzymes and bilirubin periodically during therapy. Signs of new, worsening, or recurrent hepatotoxicity may require ↓ in dose or interruption or discontinuation of therapy.
- Monitor blood glucose frequently during therapy; hyperglycemia may occur more frequently in patients with high BMI or diabetes. If hyperglycemia develops, administer antihyperglycemic agents as clinically indicated.

Implementation

IV Administration

- Premedicate patients with previously untreated stage III or IV classical Hodgkin lymphoma, peripheral T-cell lymphoma, or relapsed or refractory large B-cell lymphoma who are treated with brentuximab in combination with chemotherapy with G-CSF beginning with Cycle 1.
- **Intermittent Infusion:** Calculate dose and number of brentuximab vials needed. Calculate for 100 kg for patients weighing >100 kg. **Reconstitution:** Reconstitute each 50 mg vial with 10.5 mL of sterile water for injection. Direct stream to side of vial. Swirl gently; do not shake. Solution should be clear to slightly opalescent and colorless. Do not administer solutions that are discolored or contain a precipitate. Dilute immediately into infusion bag or store solution in refrigerator; use within 24 hr of reconstitution. **Concentration:** 5 mg/mL. **Dilution:** Withdraw volume of brentuximab dose from infusion bag of >100 mL. Dilute appropriate volume of reconstituted drug in 0.9% NaCl, D5W, or LR. **Concentration:** 0.4–1.8 mg/mL. Invert bag gently to mix. Do not freeze. Infuse the diluted solution immediately or store solution in refrigerator; use within 24 hr of reconstitution. **Rate:** Infuse over 30 min. Do not administer as IV push or bolus.
- **Y-Site Incompatibility:** Do not administer other drugs through same IV line.

Patient/Family Teaching

- Explain purpose and side effects of medication to patient. Advise to read *Patient Information* before starting therapy.
- Advise patient to notify health care provider of all Rx or OTC medications, vitamins, or herbal products being taken and to consult health care provider before taking other medications.
- Instruct patient to notify health care provider of any numbness or tingling of hands or feet or any muscle weakness.
- Advise patient to notify health care provider immediately if signs and symptoms of infection (fever of ≥100.5°F, chills, cough, pain on urination), hepatotoxicity (fatigue, anorexia, right upper abdominal discomfort, dark urine, jaundice), PML (changes in mood or usual behavior; confusion; thinking problems; loss of memory; changes in vision, speech, or walking; ↓ strength or weakness on one side of body), pulmonary toxicity, GI complications or pancreatitis (abdominal pain, nausea, vomiting, diarrhea, rash), or infusion reactions (fever, chills, rash, breathing problems within 24 hr of infusion) occur.

- Educate patient about signs and symptoms of hyperglycemia (blurred vision; drowsiness; dry mouth; flushed, dry skin; fruit-like breath odor; ↑ urination; ketones in urine; loss of appetite; stomachache; nausea or vomiting; tiredness; rapid, deep breathing; unusual thirst; unconsciousness). Advise patient to notify health care provider if symptoms occur.
- Rep: May cause fetal harm. Advise women of reproductive potential and men with female partners of reproductive potential to use effective contraception during therapy and for >6 mo after last dose and to avoid breastfeeding during therapy. If pregnancy is suspected, notify health care provider promptly. Inform men that therapy may impair fertility.

Evaluation/Desired Outcomes

- Decreased spread of lymphoma.

BEERS

brexpiprazole (brex-pip-ra-zole)

Rexulti

Classification

Therapeutic: antipsychotics, antidepressants
Pharmacologic: serotonin-dopamine activity modulators (SDAM)

Indications

Schizophrenia. Adjunctive treatment of major depressive disorder. Agitation associated with dementia due to Alzheimer disease.

Action

Psychotropic activity may be due to partial agonist activity at dopamine D_2 and serotonin 5-HT_{1A} receptors and antagonist activity at the 5-HT_{2A} receptor. **Therapeutic Effects:** Decreased manifestations of schizophrenia, including excitable, paranoic, or withdrawn behavior. Improvement in symptoms of depression with increased sense of well-being. Decreased agitation associated with dementia due to Alzheimer disease.

Pharmacokinetics

Absorption: Well absorbed (95%) following oral administration.
Distribution: Well distributed to tissues.
Protein Binding: >99%.
Metabolism and Excretion: Primarily metabolized by the liver via the CYP3A4 and CYP2D6 isoenzymes; the CYP2D6 enzyme system exhibits genetic polymorphism (7% of population may be poor metabolizers and may have significantly ↑ brexpiprazole concentrations and an ↑ risk of adverse effects). 25% excreted in urine (<1% unchanged); 46% in feces (14% unchanged).
Half-life: 91 hr.

TIME/ACTION PROFILE (improvement in symptoms)

ROUTE	ONSET	PEAK	DURATION
PO (schizophrenia)	within 1–2 wk	4–6 wk	unknown
PO (depression)	within 1 wk	5 wk	unknown

Contraindications/Precautions

Contraindicated in: Hypersensitivity.
Use Cautiously in: History of seizures or concurrent use of medications that may ↓ seizure threshold; Pre-existing cardiovascular disease, dehydration, hypotension, concurrent antihypertensives, diuretics, electrolyte imbalance (↑ risk of orthostatic hypotension, correct deficits before treatment); Pre-existing low WBC (may ↑ risk of leukopenia/neutropenia); History of diabetes, metabolic syndrome, or dyslipidemia (may exacerbate); May ↑ risk of suicide attempt/ideation especially during early treatment or dose adjustment; risk may be greater in children or adolescents; Patients at risk for falls; Poor CYP2D6 metabolizers (↓ dose); OB: Use during 3rd trimester may result in extrapyramidal/withdrawal symptoms in infant; use during pregnancy only if potential maternal benefit justifies potential fetal risk; Lactation: Safety not established during breastfeeding; Pedi: Safety and effectiveness not established in children <18 yr (major depressive disorder) or <13 yr (schizophrenia); Geri: Appears on Beers list. ↑ risk of stroke, cognitive decline, and mortality in older adults with dementia. Avoid use in older adults, except for schizophrenia, adjunctive treatment of major depressive disorder, or agitation associated with dementia due to Alzheimer disease (not indicated for dementia-related psychosis without agitation).

Adverse Reactions/Side Effects

CV: cerebrovascular adverse reactions (↑ in older adults with dementia-related psychoses), orthostatic hypotension/syncope. **EENT:** blurred vision. **Endo:** hyperglycemia/diabetes. **GI:** abdominal pain, constipation, diarrhea, dry mouth, dysphagia, excess salivation, flatulence. **Hemat:** agranulocytosis, leukopenia, neutropenia. **Metab:** weight gain, ↑ appetite, dyslipidemia. **Neuro:** akathisia, abnormal dreams, cognitive impairment, dizziness, drowsiness, dystonia, extrapyramidal symptoms, headache, NEUROLEPTIC MALIGNANT SYNDROME, restlessness, sedation, SEIZURES, SUICIDAL THOUGHTS/BEHAVIORS, tardive dyskinesia, tremor, urges (eating, gambling, sexual, shopping). **Misc:** body temperature dysregulation, HYPERSENSITIVITY REACTIONS (INCLUDING ANAPHYLAXIS).

Interactions

Drug-Drug: Strong CYP3A4 inhibitors, including **clarithromycin, itraconazole** or **ketoconazole**, may ↑ levels and risk of toxicity; ↓ dose. **Strong CYP2D6 inhibitors**, including **fluoxetine, paroxetine**, or **quinidine**,

B

may ↑ levels and risk of toxicity; ↓ dose. Combined use of **strong or moderate CYP3A4 inhibitors with strong or moderate CYP2D6 inhibitors** in addition to brexpiprazole, including the following combinations: **itraconazole + quinidine**, **fluconazole + paroxetine**, **itraconazole + duloxetine** or **fluconazole + duloxetine**: may ↑ levels and risk of toxicity; ↓ dose. **Strong CYP3A4 inducers**, including **rifampin**, may ↓ levels and effectiveness; ↑ dose. **Antihypertensives** or **diuretics** may ↑ the risk of hypotension. **Medications that may ↓ seizure threshold** may ↑ the risk of seizures.
Drug-Natural Products: St. John's wort may ↓ levels and effectiveness; ↑ dose.

Route/Dosage

Schizophrenia

PO (Adults): 1 mg once daily on Days 1–4; then ↑ to 2 mg once daily on Days 5–7; then ↑ to 4 mg once daily on Day 8 (not to exceed 4 mg once daily). *Known CYP2D6 poor metabolizers:* Use 50% of the usual dose. *Concurrent use of strong CYP2D6 inhibitors (schizophrenia only) or CYP3A4 inhibitors:* Use 50% of the usual dose; *Concurrent use of strong/moderate CYP2D6 inhibitors AND strong/moderate CYP3A4 inhibitors:* Use 25% of the usual dose; *Known CYP2D6 poor metabolizer taking concurrent strong/moderate CYP3A4 inhibitors:* Use 25% of the usual dose; *Concurrent use of strong CYP3A4 inducers:* Double usual dose over 1–2 wk; titrate by clinical response.
PO (Children 13–17 yr): 0.5 mg once daily on Days 1–4; then ↑ to 1 mg once daily on Days 5–7; then ↑ to 2 mg once daily on Day 8. May ↑ dose by 1 mg/day on weekly basis (not to exceed 4 mg once daily). *Known CYP2D6 poor metabolizers:* Use 50% of the usual dose. *Concurrent use of strong CYP2D6 inhibitors (schizophrenia only) or CYP3A4 inhibitors:* Use 50% of the usual dose; *Concurrent use of strong/moderate CYP2D6 inhibitors AND strong/moderate CYP3A4 inhibitors:* Use 25% of the usual dose; *Known CYP2D6 poor metabolizer taking concurrent strong/moderate CYP3A4 inhibitors:* Use 25% of the usual dose; *Concurrent use of strong CYP3A4 inducers:* Double usual dose over 1–2 wk; titrate by clinical response.

Renal Impairment

PO (Adults and Children 13–17 yr): *CCr <60 mL/min:* Maximum daily dose should not exceed 3 mg.

Hepatic Impairment

(Adults and Children 13–17 yr): *Moderate to severe hepatic impairment:* Maximum daily dose should not exceed 3 mg.

Major Depressive Disorder

PO (Adults): 0.5 or 1 mg once daily initially; may be ↑ to 2 mg once daily (not to exceed 3 mg once daily); *Known CYP2D6 poor metabolizers:* Use 50% of the usual dose. *Concurrent use of strong CYP2D6 inhibitors (schizophrenia only) or CYP3A4 inhibitors:* Use 50% of the usual dose; *Concurrent use of strong/moderate CYP2D6 inhibitors AND strong/moderate CYP3A4 inhibitors:* Use 25% of the usual dose; *Known CYP2D6 poor metabolizer taking concurrent strong/moderate CYP3A4 inhibitors:* Use 25% of the usual dose; *Concurrent use of strong CYP3A4 inducers:* Double usual dose over 1–2 wk; titrate by clinical response.

Renal Impairment

PO (Adults): *CCr <60 mL/min:* Maximum daily dose should not exceed 2 mg.

Hepatic Impairment

PO (Adults): *Moderate to severe hepatic impairment:* Maximum daily dose should not exceed 2 mg.

Agitation Associated With Dementia Due to Alzheimer Disease

PO (Adults): 0.5 mg once daily on Days 1–7; then ↑ to 1 mg once daily on Days 8–14; then ↑ to 2 mg once daily on Day 15. May ↑ to 3 mg once daily after ≥14 days based on clinical response and tolerability. *Known CYP2D6 poor metabolizers:* Use 50% of the usual dose. *Concurrent use of strong CYP2D6 inhibitors (schizophrenia only) or CYP3A4 inhibitors:* Use 50% of the usual dose; *Concurrent use of strong/moderate CYP2D6 inhibitors AND strong/moderate CYP3A4 inhibitors:* Use 25% of the usual dose; *Known CYP2D6 poor metabolizer taking concurrent strong/moderate CYP3A4 inhibitors:* Use 25% of the usual dose; *Concurrent use of strong CYP3A4 inducers:* Double usual dose over 1–2 wk; titrate by clinical response.

Renal Impairment

PO (Adults): *CCr <60 mL/min:* Maximum daily dose should not exceed 2 mg.

Hepatic Impairment

PO (Adults): *Moderate to severe hepatic impairment:* Maximum daily dose should not exceed 2 mg.

Availability (generic available)

Tablets: 0.25 mg, 0.5 mg, 1 mg, 2 mg, 3 mg, 4 mg.

NURSING IMPLICATIONS

Assessment

- Assess mental status (orientation, mood, behavior) before and periodically during therapy. Assess for suicidal tendencies, especially during early therapy for depression. Restrict amount of drug available to patient. Risk may be ↑ in children, adolescents, and adults ≤24 yr.
- Assess weight and BMI initially and throughout therapy.
- Monitor BP (sitting, standing, lying), HR, and respiratory rate before and periodically during therapy.

- Observe patient carefully when administering medication to ensure that medication is actually taken and not hoarded or cheeked.
- Monitor patient for onset of akathisia (restlessness or desire to keep moving) and extrapyramidal side effects (*parkinsonian:* difficulty speaking or swallowing, loss of balance control, pill rolling of hands, masklike face, shuffling gait, rigidity, tremors; and *dystonic:* muscle spasms, twisting motions, twitching, inability to move eyes, weakness of arms or legs) periodically during therapy. Report these symptoms.
- Monitor for tardive dyskinesia (uncontrolled rhythmic movement of mouth, face, and extremities; lip smacking or puckering; puffing of cheeks; uncontrolled chewing; rapid or worm-like movements of tongue). Notify health care provider immediately if these symptoms occur; symptoms may partially or completely resolve but may be irreversible.
- Monitor for development of neuroleptic malignant syndrome (fever, muscle rigidity, altered mental status, respiratory distress, tachycardia, seizures, diaphoresis, hypertension or hypotension, pallor, tiredness, loss of bladder control, ↑ CK, myoglobinuria/rhabdomyolysis, acute renal failure). Notify health care provider immediately if these symptoms occur.
- Assess for fall risk. Drowsiness, orthostatic hypotension, and motor and sensory instability ↑ risk. Institute prevention if indicated.

Lab Test Considerations

- Monitor CBC frequently during initial mo of therapy in patients with pre-existing or history of low WBC. May cause leukopenia, neutropenia, or agranulocytosis. Discontinue therapy if severe neutropenia (ANC <1000 mm^3 occurs). Monitor blood glucose and cholesterol levels initially and periodically during therapy.

Implementation

- Not indicated as an as-needed ("prn") treatment for agitation associated with dementia due to Alzheimer disease.
- **PO:** Administer once daily without regard to meals.

Patient/Family Teaching

- Advise patient to take medication as directed and not to skip doses or double up on missed doses. Take missed doses as soon as remembered unless almost time for the next dose. Do not stop taking brexpiprazole without consulting health care provider. Advise patient to read *Medication Guide* before starting and with each Rx refill in case of changes.
- Inform patient of possibility of extrapyramidal symptoms and tardive dyskinesia. Instruct patient to report these symptoms immediately.
- Advise patient to make position changes slowly to minimize orthostatic hypotension. Protect from falls.
- Medication may cause drowsiness and light-headedness. Caution patient to avoid driving or other activities requiring alertness until response to medication is known.
- Advise patient, family, and caregivers to look for suicidality, especially during early therapy or dose changes. Notify health care provider immediately if thoughts about suicide or dying, attempts to commit suicide, new or worse depression or anxiety, agitation or restlessness, panic attacks, insomnia, new or worse irritability, aggressiveness, acting on dangerous impulses, mania, or other changes in mood or behavior occur.
- Advise patient and family to notify health care provider if signs and symptoms of high blood sugar (feel very thirsty, urinating more than usual, feel very hungry, feel weak or tired, nausea, confusion, breath smells fruity) occur.
- Inform patient that brexpiprazole may cause weight gain. Advise patient to monitor weight periodically. Notify health care provider of significant weight gain.
- Instruct patient to notify health care provider of all Rx or OTC medications, vitamins, or herbal products being taken and to consult health care provider before taking any new medications. Caution patient to avoid taking alcohol or other CNS depressants concurrently with this medication.
- Advise patient that extremes in temperature should be avoided because this drug impairs body temperature regulation.
- Advise patient to notify health care provider if new or ↑ eating/binge eating or gambling, sexual, shopping, or other impulse control disorders occur.
- Advise patient to notify health care provider of medication regimen prior to treatment or surgery.
- Rep: May cause fetal harm. Advise women of reproductive potential to notify health care provider if pregnancy is planned or suspected and to avoid breastfeeding during therapy. May cause extrapyramidal and/or withdrawal symptoms (agitation, hypertonia, hypotonia, tremor, somnolence, respiratory distress, feeding disorder) in neonates whose mothers were exposed to antipsychotic drugs during 3rd trimester of pregnancy. Symptoms vary in severity. Some neonates recover within hours or days without specific treatment; others require prolonged hospitalization. Monitor neonates for extrapyramidal and/or withdrawal symptoms and manage symptoms appropriately. Encourage pregnant patients to enroll in registry by contacting National Pregnancy Registry for Atypical Antipsychotics at 1-866-961-2388 or visit http://womensmentalhealth.org/clinical-and-research-programs/pregnancyregistry/.
- Emphasize the importance of routine follow-up exams and continued participation in psychotherapy as indicated.

Evaluation/Desired Outcomes

- Decrease in excitable, paranoic, or withdrawn behavior.

- Increased sense of wellbeing in patients with depression.
- Decreased agitation associated with dementia due to Alzheimer disease.

brivaracetam (briv-a-ra-se-tam)

Briviact, Brivlera

Classification

Therapeutic: anticonvulsants

Schedule V

Indications

Partial-onset seizures.

Action

Displays a high and selective affinity for synaptic vesicle protein 2A in the brain, which may contribute to its anticonvulsant effect. **Therapeutic Effects:** Decreased incidence of seizures.

Pharmacokinetics

Absorption: Rapidly and completely absorbed following oral administration. IV administration results in complete bioavailability.

Distribution: Widely distributed to tissues.

Metabolism and Excretion: Hepatic and extrahepatic amidase-mediated hydrolysis of the amide moiety to form carboxylic acid metabolite (primary route) and hydroxylation primarily by the CYP2C19 isoenzyme to form the hydroxy metabolite (secondary route) (all metabolites inactive). The CYP2C19 isoenzyme exhibits genetic polymorphism (2% of White people, 4% of Black people, and 14% of Asian people may be poor metabolizers and may have significantly ↑ brivaracetam concentrations and an ↑ risk of adverse effects). >95% excreted by the kidneys (<10% excreted unchanged).

Half-life: 9 hr.

TIME/ACTION PROFILE (plasma concentrations)

ROUTE	ONSET	PEAK	DURATION
PO	unknown	1–4hr†	unknown
IV	unknown	end of infusion	unknown

† 1 hr in fasting state; 4 hr with high-fat meal.

Contraindications/Precautions

Contraindicated in: Hypersensitivity; End-stage renal disease.

Use Cautiously in: All patients (may ↑ risk of suicidal thoughts/behaviors); Known or suspected poor CYP2C19 metabolizers (may require dose ↓); Hepatic impairment (dose ↓ recommended); OB: Safety not established in pregnancy; Lactation: Safety not established in breastfeeding; Pedi: Children <1 mo (safety and effectiveness not established); Geri: Dose adjustment may be needed because of ↓ renal and hepatic function in older adults.

Adverse Reactions/Side Effects

EENT: nystagmus. **GI:** constipation, nausea, vomiting. **Hemat:** leukopenia. **Local:** infusion site pain. **Neuro:** aggression, agitation, anger, anxiety, apathy, belligerence, depression, dizziness, drowsiness, hallucinations, irritability, mood swings, paranoia, psychosis, restlessness, SUICIDAL THOUGHTS/BEHAVIOR, tearfulness, vertigo, ataxia, balance disorder, coordination difficulties, dysgeusia, euphoria, fatigue. **Misc:** HYPERSENSITIVITY REACTIONS (INCLUDING BRONCHOSPASM AND ANGIOEDEMA).

Interactions

Drug-Drug: CYP2C19 inducers, including **rifampin**, may ↓ levels and effectiveness; ↑ brivaracetam dose by up to 100%. Concurrent use with **carbamazepine** may ↑ levels of carbamazepine-epoxide (active metabolite); consider ↓ dose of carbamazepine if tolerability issues occur. May ↑ levels and risk of toxicity of **phenytoin**.

Route/Dosage

IV route should only be used when oral therapy is not feasible.

PO IV (Adults and Children ≥16 yr): 50 mg twice daily; may titrate down to 25 mg twice daily or up to 100 mg twice daily based on tolerability and effectiveness.

PO IV (Children ≥1 mo and ≥50 kg): 25–50 mg twice daily; may titrate up to 100 mg twice daily based on tolerability and effectiveness.

PO IV (Children ≥1 mo and 20–<50 kg): 0.5–1 mg/kg twice daily; may titrate up to 2 mg/kg twice daily based on tolerability and effectiveness.

PO IV (Children ≥1 mo and 11–<20 kg): 0.5–1.25 mg/kg twice daily; may titrate up to 2.5 mg/kg twice daily based on tolerability and effectiveness.

PO IV (Children ≥1 mo and <11 kg): 0.75–1.5 mg/kg twice daily; may titrate up to 3 mg/kg twice daily based on tolerability and effectiveness.

Hepatic Impairment

PO IV (Adults and Children ≥16 yr): 25 mg twice daily; may titrate up to 75 mg twice daily based on tolerability and effectiveness.

Hepatic Impairment

PO IV (Children ≥1 mo and ≥50 kg): 25 mg twice daily; may titrate up to 75 mg twice daily based on tolerability and effectiveness.

Hepatic Impairment

PO IV (Children ≥1 mo and 20–<50 kg): 0.5 mg/kg twice daily; may titrate up to 1.5 mg/kg twice daily based on tolerability and effectiveness.

Hepatic Impairment

PO IV (Children ≥1 mo and 11–<20 kg): 0.5 mg/kg twice daily; may titrate up to 2 mg/kg twice daily based on tolerability and effectiveness.

Hepatic Impairment

PO IV (Children ≥1 mo and <11 kg): 0.75 mg/kg twice daily; may titrate up to 2.25 mg/kg twice daily based on tolerability and effectiveness.

Availability (generic available)

Tablets: 10 mg, 25 mg, 50 mg, 75 mg, 100 mg.
Oral solution (raspberry flavored): 10 mg/mL.
Solution for injection: 10 mg/mL.

NURSING IMPLICATIONS

Assessment

- Assess mental status (orientation, mood, behavior) before and periodically during therapy. Monitor closely for notable changes in behavior that could indicate the emergence or worsening of suicidal thoughts or behavior or depression.
- Monitor for signs and symptoms of bronchospasm (wheezing, dyspnea) and angioedema (rash, pruritus, perioral swelling) during therapy. If signs of hypersensitivity occur, discontinue brivaracetam.

Lab Test Considerations

- May ↓ WBC and neutrophil counts. Monitor liver function tests as clinically indicated, especially if pre-existing liver condition.

Implementation

- ***High Alert:*** Do not confuse Briviact with Brilinta.
- Initiate therapy with oral or IV administration. IV administration may be used when oral dose is not feasible; administer at same dose and frequency as oral doses.
- **PO:** Administer twice daily without regard to food. ***DNC:*** Swallow tablets whole with liquid; do not crush or chew.
- Use a calibrated measuring device for accuracy with oral solution. **Dilution** is not necessary. May be administered via nasogastric or gastrostomy tube. Oral solution is stable for 5 mo after opening.

IV Administration

- **Intermittent Infusion: Dilution:** May be administered undiluted or diluted with 0.9% NaCl, LR, or D5W. Solution is clear and colorless; do not administer solutions that are discolored or contain particulate matter. Solution is stable for up to 4 hr at room temperature; may be stored in polyvinyl chloride bags. **Rate:** Administer over 2–15 min.

Patient/Family Teaching

- Explain purpose and side effects of medication to patient. Advise patient to read *Patient Information* before starting therapy. Instruct patient to take as directed. ↓ dose gradually; do not stop abruptly to minimize risk of ↑ seizure frequency and status epilepticus.
- Advise patient to notify health care professional of all Rx or OTC medications, vitamins, or herbal products being taken and to consult with health care professional before taking other medications.
- May cause drowsiness, fatigue, dizziness, and balance problems. Caution patient to avoid driving or other activities requiring alertness until response to medication is known. Do not resume driving until provider gives clearance based on control of seizure disorder.
- Advise patient to avoid alcohol or CNS depressants. These can worsen side effects like sedation or dizziness.
- Advise patient and caregiver to notify health care professional if behavioral changes, thoughts about suicide or dying, attempts to commit suicide, new or worse depression, new or worse anxiety, feeling very agitated or restless, panic attacks, trouble sleeping, new or worse irritability, acting aggressive, being angry or violent, acting on dangerous impulses, an extreme ↑ in activity and talking, or other unusual changes in behavior or mood occur.
- Rep: Advise women of reproductive potential to notify health care professional if pregnancy is planned or suspected or if breastfeeding. Encourage patients who become pregnant to enroll in the North American Antiepileptic Drug Pregnancy Registry by calling 1-888-233-2334 or on the web at www.aedpregnancyregistry.org.

Evaluation/Desired Outcomes

- Decreased incidence of seizures.

budesonide, See CORTICOSTEROIDS (INHALATION).

budesonide, See CORTICOSTEROIDS (NASAL).

budesonide, See CORTICOSTEROIDS (SYSTEMIC).

budesonide/formoterol/glycopyrrolate (byoo-**des**-oh-nide/for-**moe**-te-rol/glye-koe-**pye**-roe-late)

Breztri Aerosphere

Classification

Therapeutic: anti-inflammatories (steroidal), bronchodilators

Pharmacologic: corticosteroids, long-acting $beta_2$-adrenergic agonists (LABAs), anticholinergics

Indications

Maintenance treatment of COPD.

Action

Budesonide: Potent, locally acting anti-inflammatory; *formoterol:* a $beta_2$-adrenergic agonist that stimulates adenyl cyclase, resulting in accumulation of cyclic adenosine monophosphate at $beta_2$-adrenergic receptors resulting in bronchodilation; *glycopyrrolate:* acts as an anticholinergic by inhibiting M3 muscarinic receptors in bronchial smooth muscle resulting in bronchodilation. **Therapeutic Effects:** Bronchodilation with decreased airflow obstruction.

Pharmacokinetics

Budesonide

Absorption: Unknown.
Distribution: Extensively distributed to extravascular tissues.
Metabolism and Excretion: Primarily metabolized by the liver by the CYP3A4 isoenzyme into inactive metabolites; primarily excreted in urine and feces as metabolites.
Half-life: 5 hr.

Formoterol

Absorption: Unknown.
Distribution: Extensively distributed to extravascular tissues.
Metabolism and Excretion: Primarily metabolized by the liver by glucuronidation and O-demethylation to inactive metabolites; 62% of drug excreted in urine; 24% excreted in feces.
Half-life: 10 hr.

Glycopyrrolate

Absorption: Unknown.
Distribution: Extensively distributed to extravascular tissues.
Metabolism and Excretion: Primarily metabolized by the liver, with the CYP2D6 isoenzyme playing a minor role in elimination; 85% excreted in urine.
Half-life: 15 hr.

TIME/ACTION PROFILE (improvement in FEV_1)

ROUTE	ONSET	PEAK	DURATION
Inhalation	within 5 min	4 wk	unknown

Contraindications/Precautions

Contraindicated in: Hypersensitivity; Asthma; Acutely deteriorating COPD or acute respiratory symptoms.
Use Cautiously in: Systemic corticosteroid therapy (should not be abruptly discontinued when inhaled therapy is started; additional corticosteroids needed during stress or trauma); Prolonged immobilization, family history of osteoporosis, postmenopausal status, cigarette smoking, advanced age, or poor nutrition (↑ risk of osteoporosis); Narrow-angle glaucoma; Seizure disorders; Thyrotoxicosis; Urinary retention, prostatic hyperplasia, bladder-neck obstruction; Diabetes; Severe hepatic impairment; Severe renal impairment or end-stage renal disease requiring dialysis (use only if expected benefit exceeds potential risk); OB: Safety not established in pregnancy; Lactation: Use while breastfeeding only if potential maternal benefit justifies potential risk to infant; Pedi: Safety and effectiveness not established in children.
Exercise Extreme Caution in: Concurrent use of MAO inhibitors, tricyclic antidepressants, or drugs that prolong the QTc interval.

Adverse Reactions/Side Effects

CV: arrhythmias, hypertension, tachycardia. **EENT:** cataracts, glaucoma, sinusitis. **Endo:** adrenal suppression (high dose, long-term therapy only), hyperglycemia. **F and E:** hypokalemia. **GI:** diarrhea, oropharyngeal candidiasis. **MS:** ↓ bone density, muscle spasms. **Resp:** bronchospasm, cough, pneumonia. **Misc:** HYPERSENSITIVITY REACTIONS (INCLUDING ANGIOEDEMA, URTICARIA, OR RASH).

Interactions

Drug-Drug: Strong **CYP3A4 inhibitors**, including **atazanavir**, **clarithromycin**, **itraconazole**, **ketoconazole**, **nefazodone**, **nelfinavir**, and **ritonavir**, may ↑ levels and risk of toxicity. **Anticonvulsants**, **oral corticosteroids**, and **proton pump inhibitors** may ↑ risk of osteoporosis. Concurrent use with other **adrenergics** may ↑ adrenergic adverse reactions of formoterol (↑ heart rate, ↑ BP, jitteriness). **Xanthine derivatives**, **corticosteroids**, and **diuretics** may ↑ risk of hypokalemia or ECG changes with formoterol. ↑ risk of serious adverse cardiovascular effects with **MAO inhibitors**, **tricyclic antidepressants**, and **QT interval prolonging drugs**; use with extreme caution. Effectiveness of formoterol may be ↓ by **beta blockers**; use cautiously and only when necessary. ↑ risk of anticholinergic adverse reactions with glycopyrrolate when used concurrently with other **anticholinergics**; avoid concurrent use.

Route/Dosage

Inhaln: (Adults): 2 inhalations twice daily.

Availability

Inhalation aerosol: budesonide 160 mcg/glycopyrrolate 9 mcg/formoterol 4.8 mcg per inhalation in 10.7-g canister (120 inhalations).

NURSING IMPLICATIONS

Assessment

- Assess lung sounds, pulse, and BP before administration and during peak of medication. Note amount, color, and character of sputum produced.
- Observe for paradoxical bronchospasm (wheezing, dyspnea, tightness in chest) and hypersensitivity reaction (rash; urticaria; swelling of the face, lips, or eyelids). If condition occurs, withhold medication and notify health care professional immediately.
- Monitor patient for signs of hypersensitivity reactions (difficulties in breathing or swallowing; swelling of tongue, lips, and face; urticaria; skin rash) during therapy. Discontinue therapy and consider alternative if reaction occurs.

Lab Test Considerations

- May ↑ serum glucose and ↓ serum potassium.

Implementation

- **Inhaln:** Administer as 2 inhalations twice daily, morning and evening. Shake well before use. Prime by releasing 4 sprays into air away from face before 1st use and by releasing 2 sprays if unused for >7 days. After inhalation, rinse mouth with water without swallowing. See Appendix C for use of metered-dose inhalers.

Patient/Family Teaching

- Explain purpose and side effects of medication to patient. Advise patient to read *Patient Information* before starting therapy. Instruct to use as directed. Do not discontinue therapy without discussing with health care professional, even if feeling better. If a dose is missed, skip dose and take next dose at regularly scheduled time. Do not double doses. Use a rapid-acting bronchodilator if symptoms occur before next dose is due. Caution patient not to use >2 times a day; may cause adverse effects, paradoxical bronchospasm, or loss of effectiveness of medication.
- Advise patient to consult health care professional before taking any Rx, OTC, or herbal products or alcohol concurrently with this therapy. Caution patient also to avoid smoking and other respiratory irritants.
- Advise patient that inhaler should be discarded when display window indicates zero or 3 mo (120-inhalation canister) or 3 wk (28-inhalation canister) after removal of canister from pouch, whichever comes first. Never immerse the canister into water to determine the amount remaining in the canister ("float test").
- Caution patient not to use medication to treat acute symptoms. A rapid-acting inhaled beta-adrenergic bronchodilator should be used for relief of acute asthma attacks. Notify health care professional immediately if symptoms get worse or more inhalations than usual are needed from rescue inhaler.
- Advise patient to rinse the mouth with water without swallowing after inhalation to help ↓ the risk of getting a fungus infection (thrush) in the mouth and throat.
- Instruct patient to contact health care professional immediately if shortness of breath is not relieved by medication or if nausea; vomiting; shakiness; headache; fast or irregular heartbeat; sleeplessness; or signs and symptoms of narrow-angle glaucoma (eye pain or discomfort, blurred vision, visual halos or colored images, red eyes), urinary retention (difficulty passing urine, painful urination), or pneumonia (increase in mucus [sputum] production, change in mucus color, fever, chills, ↑ cough, ↑ breathing problems) occur.
- Rep: Advise women of reproductive potential to notify health care professional if pregnancy is planned or suspected or if breastfeeding.

Evaluation/Desired Outcomes

- Bronchodilation with decreased airflow obstruction.

bumetanide, See DIURETICS (LOOP).

REMS HIGH ALERT

buprenorphine

(byoo-pre-**nor**-feen)

Belbuca, Brixadi, ~~Buprenex~~, Butrans, Sublocade, ~~Subutex~~

Classification

Therapeutic: opioid analgesics

Pharmacologic: opioid agonists/antagonists

Schedule III

Indications

IM IV: Moderate to severe acute pain. **Buccal:** transdermal Pain that is severe enough to require daily, around-the-clock long-term opioid treatment and for which alternative treatment options (e.g. nonopioid analgesics or immediate-release opioids) are inadequate. **sublingual** Opioid use disorder (preferred for induction only); suppresses withdrawal symptoms in opioid detoxification. **SUBQ**: Moderate to severe opioid use disorder in patients who have initiated treatment with a buprenorphine-containing product for ≥7 days (Sublocade). **SUBQ**: Moderate to severe opioid use disorder in patients who have initiated treatment with a single dose of a transmucosal buprenorphine product or who are already being treated with buprenorphine (Brixadi).

Action

Binds to opiate receptors in the CNS. Alters the perception of and response to painful stimuli while producing generalized CNS depression. Has partial antagonist properties that may result in opioid withdrawal in physically dependent patients when used as an analgesic. **Therapeutic Effects: IM IV:** transdermal Decreased severity of pain. **sublingual** Suppression of withdrawal symptoms during detoxification and maintenance from heroin or other opioids. Produces a relatively mild withdrawal compared to other agents. **SUBQ**: Continued cessation of opioid use.

Pharmacokinetics

Absorption: Well absorbed after IM and SL use; 46–65% absorbed with buccal use; 15% of transdermal dose absorbed through skin; IV administration results in complete bioavailability.
Distribution: Extensively distributed to tissues; CNS concentration is 15–25% of plasma.
Protein Binding: 96%.
Metabolism and Excretion: Mostly metabolized by the liver mostly via the CYP3A4 isoenzyme; one metabolite is active; 70% excreted in feces; 27% excreted in urine.
Half-life: *IV:* 2–3 hr; *Buccal:* 27 hr; *Transdermal:* 26 hr; *SL:* 37 hr; *Subdermal:* 24–48 hr; *SUBQ:* 43–60 days.

TIME/ACTION PROFILE (analgesia)

ROUTE	ONSET	PEAK	DURATION
IM	15 min	60 min	6 hr†
IV	rapid	less than 60 min	6 hr†
SL	unknown	unknown	unknown
Transdermal	unknown	unknown	7 days
Buccal	unknown	unknown	unknown
SUBQ	unknown	unknown	unknown

† 4–5 hr in children.

Contraindications/Precautions

Contraindicated in: Hypersensitivity; Significant respiratory depression (transdermal, buccal); Acute or severe bronchial asthma (transdermal, buccal); Paralytic ileus (transdermal, buccal); Acute, mild, intermittent, or postoperative pain (transdermal); Long QT syndrome; Lactation: Lactation.
Use Cautiously in: Personal or family history of substance use disorder or mental illness (for pain management); ↑ intracranial pressure; Compromised respiratory function including COPD, cor pulmonale, diminished respiratory reserve, hypoxia, hypercapnia, or respiratory depression of other causes; Severe renal impairment; Moderate or severe hepatic impairment (dose ↓ needed for severe impairment); Hypothyroidism; Seizure disorders; Adrenal insufficiency; Biliary tract disease; Acute pancreatitis; Debilitated patients (dose ↓ required); Oral mucositis (dose ↓ required) (buccal); Undiagnosed abdominal pain; Hypokalemia, hypomagnesemia, unstable atrial fibrillation, symptomatic bradycardia, unstable HF, QT interval prolongation, or myocardial ischemia; Prostatic hyperplasia; OB: Safety not established in pregnancy; prolonged use of buccal, transdermal, or SL buprenorphine during pregnancy can result in neonatal opioid withdrawal syndrome; Pedi: Safety and effectiveness not established in children <18 yr (SL and transdermal) or <2 yr (parenteral); Geri: ↑ risk of respiratory depression in older adults (dose ↓ required).

Adverse Reactions/Side Effects

CV: hypertension, hypotension, palpitations, QT interval prolongation. **Derm:** sweating, clammy feeling, erythema, pruritus, rash. **EENT:** blurred vision, diplopia, miosis (high doses). **Endo:** adrenal insufficiency. **GI:** nausea, constipation, dry mouth, HEPATOTOXICITY, ileus, vomiting. **GU:** urinary retention. **Local:** injection site reactions. **Neuro:** confusion, dysphoria, hallucinations, sedation, dizziness, euphoria, floating feeling, headache, unusual dreams. **Resp:** RESPIRATORY DEPRESSION (INCLUDING CENTRAL SLEEP APNEA AND SLEEP-RELATED HYPOXEMIA). **Misc:** allodynia, HYPERSENSITIVITY REACTIONS (INCLUDING ANAPHYLAXIS, ANGIOEDEMA, AND BRONCHOSPASM), opioid-induced hyperalgesia, physical dependence, psychological dependence, tolerance.

Interactions

Drug-Drug: Concurrent use with **class Ia antiarrhythmics**, **class III antiarrhythmics**, or other **QT interval prolonging medications** may ↑ risk of QT interval prolongation; avoid concurrent use. Use with **benzodiazepines** or other **CNS depressants**, including other **opioids**, **nonbenzodiazepine sedative/hypnotics**, **anxiolytics**, **general anesthetics**, **muscle relaxants**, **antipsychotics**, and **alcohol**, may cause profound sedation, respiratory depression, coma, and death; reserve concurrent use for when alternative treatment options are inadequate. Use with extreme caution in patients receiving **MAO inhibitors**; ↑ CNS and respiratory depression and hypotension; ↓ buprenorphine dose by 50%; may need to ↓ **MAO inhibitor** dose; do not use transdermal formulation within 14 days of **MAO inhibitor**. May ↓ effectiveness of other **opioid analgesics**. **CYP3A4 inhibitors**, including **itraconazole**, **ketoconazole**, **erythromycin**, **ritonavir**, **atazanavir**, or **fosamprenavir**, may ↑ levels and risk of toxicity; may need to ↓ dose. **CYP3A4 inducers**, including **carbamazepine**, **rifampin**, or **phenytoin**, may ↓ levels and effectiveness; dose modification may be necessary during concurrent use. Drugs that affect serotonergic neurotransmitter systems, including **tricyclic antidepressants**, **SSRIs**, **SNRIs**, **MAO inhibitors**, **TCAs**, **tramadol**, **trazodone**, **mirtazapine**, **5-HT_3 receptor antagonists**, **linezolid**, **methylene blue**, and **triptans**, may ↑ risk of serotonin syndrome.

Drug-Natural Products: Kava-kava, valerian, chamomile, or **hops** can ↑ CNS depression.

Route/Dosage

Analgesia

IM IV (Adults): 0.3 mg every 4–6 hr as needed. May repeat initial dose after 30 min (up to 0.3 mg every 4 hr or 0.6 mg every 6 hr); 0.6-mg doses should be given only IM.

IM IV (Children 2–12 yr): 2–6 mcg (0.002–0.006 mg)/kg every 4–6 hr.

Transdermal (Adults): *Opioid-naive:* Transdermal system delivering 5–20 mcg/hr applied every 7 days. Initiate with 5 mcg/hr system; each dose titration may occur after 72 hr; do not exceed dose of 20 mcg/hr; *Previously taking <30 mg/day of morphine or equivalent:* Initiate with 5 mcg/hr system; each dose titration may occur after 72 hr; do not exceed dose of 20 mcg/hr; apply patch every 7 days; *Previously taking 30–80 mg/day of morphine or equivalent:* Initiate with 10 mcg/hr system; each dose titration may occur after 72 hr; do not exceed dose of 20 mcg/hr; apply patch every 7 days; *Previously taking >80 mg/day of morphine or equivalent:* Consider use of alternate analgesic.

Buccal (Adults): *Opioid-naive:* Initiate therapy with 75 mcg once daily or every 12 hr for ≥4 days; then ↑ dose to 150 mcg every 12 hr; may then titrate dose in increments of 150 mcg every 12 hr no more frequently than every 4 days; do not exceed dose of 450 mcg every 12 hr (based on clinical studies); *Previously taking <30 mg/day of morphine or equivalent:* Initiate therapy with 75 mcg once daily or every 12 hr for ≥4 days; then ↑ dose to 150 mcg every 12 hr; may then titrate dose in increments of 150 mcg every 12 hr no more frequently than every 4 days; do not exceed dose of 900 mcg every 12 hr; *Previously taking 30–89 mg/day of morphine or equivalent:* Initiate therapy with 150 mcg every 12 hr for ≥4 days; may then titrate dose in increments of 150 mcg every 12 hr no more frequently than every 4 days; do not exceed dose of 900 mcg every 12 hr; *Previously taking 90–160 mg/day of morphine or equivalent:* Initiate therapy with 300 mcg every 12 hr for ≥4 days; may then titrate dose in increments of 150 mcg every 12 hr no more frequently than every 4 days; do not exceed dose of 900 mcg every 12 hr; *Previously taking >160 mg/day of morphine or equivalent:* Consider use of alternate analgesic; *Patients with oral mucositis:* ↓ initial dose by 50% then titrate dose in increments of 75 mcg every 12 hr no more frequently than every 4 days.

Hepatic Impairment

Transdermal (Adults): *Mild to moderate hepatic impairment:* Initiate with 5 mcg/hr system.

Hepatic Impairment

Buccal: (Adults): *Severe hepatic impairment:* ↓ initial dose by 50%; then titrate dose in increments of 75 mcg every 12 hr no more frequently than every 4 days.

Treatment of Opioid Use Disorder

sublingual (Adults): *Induction:* 8 mg once daily on Day 1; then 16 mg once daily on Day 2–4; *Maintenance:* Patients should preferably be transitioned to buprenorphine/naloxone; if patient cannot tolerate naloxone, then can use buprenorphine (usual dosage range = 4–24 mg/day); recommended target dose = 16 mg/day; dose can be ↑ or ↓ by 2–4 mg, as needed to prevent signs/symptoms of opioid withdrawal.

SUBQ (Adults): *Sublocade:* 300 mg once monthly for 2 mo; then 100 mg once monthly; may ↑ maintenance dose to 300 mg once monthly if patient reports illicit opioid use or has positive urine drug screen for illicit opioid use.

SUBQ (Adults): *Patients not currently receiving buprenorphine treatment (Brixadi [weekly formulation] only):* To avoid precipitating an opioid withdrawal syndrome, a single 4-mg test dose of transmucosal buprenorphine-containing product should be administered prior to administration of Brixadi weekly injection. If the test dose is tolerated without precipitating withdrawal, administer 16 mg (weekly formulation) initially, followed by an additional 8 mg (weekly formulation) within 3 days of the initial dose for a total recommended weekly dose of 24 mg. If needed, during the 1st wk of treatment, may administer an additional 8 mg (weekly formulation) after ≥24 hr after the previous dose, for a total weekly dose of 32 mg. Administer subsequent injections (weekly formulation) once weekly based on the total weekly dose that was established during Wk 1 (16–32 mg). Dose adjustments can be made at weekly intervals (max dose = 32 mg once weekly). *Patients currently receiving buprenorphine treatment (Brixadi [weekly formulation]):* If daily dose of SL buprenorphine ≤6 mg, administer 8 mg once weekly (weekly formulation). If daily dose of SL buprenorphine 8–10 mg, administer 16 mg once weekly (weekly formulation). If daily dose of SL buprenorphine 12–16 mg, administer 24 mg once weekly (weekly formulation). If daily dose of SL buprenorphine 18–24 mg, administer 32 mg once weekly (weekly formulation). *Patients currently receiving buprenorphine treatment (Brixadi [monthly formulation]):* If daily dose of SL buprenorphine 8–10 mg, administer 64 mg once monthly (monthly formulation). If daily dose of SL buprenorphine 12–16 mg, administer 96 mg once monthly (monthly formulation). If daily dose of SL buprenorphine 18–24 mg, administer 128 mg once monthly (monthly formulation). *Transitioning between Brixadi (monthly formulation) and Brixadi (monthly formulation):* If dose of weekly formulation 16 mg once weekly, convert to 64 mg once monthly (monthly formulation). If dose of weekly formulation

24 mg once weekly, convert to 96 mg once monthly (monthly formulation). If dose of weekly formulation 32 mg once weekly, convert to 128 mg once monthly (monthly formulation).

Hepatic Impairment

sublingual (Adults): *Severe hepatic impairment:* ↓ initial dose and adjustment dose by 50%.

Availability (generic available)

Buccal film (Belbuca): 75 mcg, 150 mcg, 300 mcg, 450 mcg, 600 mcg, 750 mcg, 900 mcg. **Extended-release solution for SUBQ injection (prefilled syringes) (Sublocade):** 100 mg/0.5 mL, 300 mg/1.5 mL. **Extended-release solution for SUBQ injection (prefilled syringes) (Brixadi [weekly]):** 8 mg/0.16 mL, 16 mg/0.32 mL, 24 mg/0.48 mL, 32 mg/0.64 mL. **Extended-release solution for SUBQ injection (prefilled syringes) (Brixadi [monthly]):** 64 mg/0.18 mL, 96 mg/0.27 mL, 128 mg/0.36 mL. **Solution for injection:** 0.3 mg/mL. **Sublingual tablets:** 2 mg, 8 mg. **Transdermal systems (Butrans):** 5 mcg/hr, 7.5 mcg/hr, 10 mcg/hr, 15 mcg/hr, 20 mcg/hr. ***In combination with:*** naloxone (Suboxone, Zubsolv). See Appendix N.

NURSING IMPLICATIONS

Assessment

- Monitor for signs and symptoms of adrenal insufficiency (nausea, vomiting, anorexia, fatigue, weakness, dizziness, low BP) during therapy. *If adrenal insufficiency suspected,* confirm with diagnostic testing. If confirmed, treat with physiologic doses of replacement corticosteroids. Wean patient off opioid to allow adrenal recovery and continue corticosteroids until adrenal function recovers. Other opioids may be tried.
- **Pain:** Assess type, location, and intensity of pain before and 1 hr after IM and 5 min (peak) after IV administration. When titrating opioid doses, ↑ of 25–50% should be administered until there is either a 50% ↓ in the patient's pain rating on a numerical or visual analogue scale or the patient reports satisfactory pain relief. A repeat dose can be safely administered at the time of the peak if previous dose is ineffective and side effects are minimal. Single doses of 600 mcg (0.6 mg) should be administered IM. Patients requiring doses >600 mcg (0.6 mg) should be converted to an opioid agonist. Buprenorphine is not recommended for prolonged use (except buccal or transdermal) or as first-line therapy for acute or cancer pain. SL formulations should not be used to relieve pain.
- An equianalgesic chart (see Appendix I) should be used when changing routes or when changing from one opioid to another.
- Monitor patients for opioid-induced hyperalgesia occurs when an opioid paradoxically causes an ↑ in pain or an ↑ in sensitivity to pain. Opioid-induced hyperalgesia differs from tolerance, which is the need for ↑ doses of opioids to maintain a defined effect. Symptoms of opioid-induced hyperalgesia include ↑ levels of pain upon opioid dosage ↑, ↓ levels of pain upon opioid dosage ↓, or pain from ordinarily nonpainful stimuli. If opioid-induced hyperalgesia suspected, consider ↓ buprenorphine dose.
- Assess level of consciousness, BP, HR, and respiratory rate before and periodically during administration, especially within first 24–72 hr of buccal therapy. If respiratory rate <10/min, assess level of sedation. Dose may need to be ↓ by 25–50%. Buprenorphine 0.3–0.4 mg has approximately equal analgesic and respiratory depressant effects to morphine 10 mg. Monitor for respiratory depression, especially during initiation or following dose ↑; serious, life-threatening, or fatal respiratory depression may occur. May cause sleep-related breathing disorders (central sleep apnea, sleep-related hypoxemia).
- Assess previous analgesic history. Antagonistic properties may induce withdrawal symptoms (vomiting, restlessness, abdominal cramps, ↑ BP and temperature) in patients who are physically dependent on opioid agonists. Symptoms may occur up to 15 days after discontinuation and persist for 1–2 wk.
- Buprenorphine has a lower potential for dependence than other opioids; however, prolonged use may lead to physical and psychological dependence and tolerance. This should not prevent patient from receiving adequate analgesia. Most patients receiving buprenorphine for pain rarely develop psychological dependence. If tolerance develops, changing to an opioid agonist may be required to relieve pain.
- Assess bowel function routinely. Prevent constipation with ↑ intake of fluids and bulk, and laxatives to minimize constipating effects. Administer stimulant laxatives routinely if opioid use >2–3 days, unless contraindicated. Consider drugs for opioid-induced constipation.
- **Transdermal:** Assess risk for opioid addiction, abuse, or misuse prior to administration. Monitor for respiratory depression, especially during initiation or following dose ↑; serious, life-threatening, or fatal respiratory depression may occur. Misuse or abuse of *Butrans* by chewing, swallowing, snorting, or injecting buprenorphine extracted from transdermal system will result in the uncontrolled delivery of buprenorphine and risk of overdose and death.

- Maintain frequent contact during periods of changing analgesic requirements, including initial titration, between the prescriber, other members of the health care team, the patient, and the caregiver/family.
- **Treatment of Opioid Dependence:** Assess patient for signs and symptoms of opioid withdrawal before and during therapy.

Lab Test Considerations

- May ↑ serum amylase and lipase.
- Monitor liver function tests before and periodically during opioid dependence therapy.

Toxicity and Overdose

- If an opioid antagonist is required to reverse respiratory depression or coma, naloxone is the antidote. Dilute the 0.4-mg ampule of naloxone in 10 mL of 0.9% NaCl and administer 0.5 mL (0.02 mg) by IV push every 2 min. For children and patients weighing <40 kg, dilute 0.1 mg of naloxone in 10 mL of 0.9% NaCl for a concentration of 10 mcg/mL and administer 0.5 mcg/kg every 1–2 min. Titrate dose to avoid withdrawal, seizures, and severe pain. Naloxone may not completely reverse respiratory depressant effects of buprenorphine; may require mechanical ventilation, oxygen, IV fluids, and vasopressors.

Implementation

- Do not confuse buprenorphine with hydromorphone.
- **Pain:** Explain therapeutic value of medication before administration to enhance the analgesic effect.
- Regularly administered doses may be more effective than prn administration. Analgesic is more effective if given before pain becomes severe.
- Coadministration with nonopioid analgesics has additive effects and may permit lower opioid doses.
- For patients taking forms of long-acting buprenorphine, if acute pain management or anesthesia is needed, treat with a nonopioid analgesic, if possible. Patients requiring opioid therapy for analgesia may be treated with a high-affinity full opioid analgesic under the supervision of a physician, with particular attention to respiratory function. Higher doses may be required for analgesic effect. Monitor patient closely.
- ***REMS:*** FDA strongly encourages health care providers to complete a REMS-compliant education program that includes all the elements of the FDA Education *Blueprint for Health Care Providers Involved in the Management or Support of Patients with Pain,* available at www.fda.gov/OpioidAnalgesicREMSBlueprint. Information on programs can be found at 1-800-503-0784 or www.opioidanalgesicrems.com.
- Discuss availability of naloxone for emergency treatment of opioid overdose with the patient and caregiver and assess the potential need for access to naloxone, both when initiating and renewing therapy, especially if patient has household members (including children) or other close contacts at risk for accidental exposure or overdose. Consider prescribing naloxone, based on the patient's risk factors for overdose, such as concurrent use of CNS depressants, a history of opioid use disorder, or prior opioid overdose. However, the presence of risk factors for overdose should not prevent the proper management of pain in any patient.
- **Buccal:** Have patient wet inside of cheek with tongue or rinse mouth with water. Apply film immediately after removal from package. Place yellow side of film against inside of cheek. Hold film in place with dry fingers for 5 sec; then leave in place on inside of cheek until fully dissolved. If chewed or swallowed, may result in lower peak concentrations and lower bioavailability. Do not administer if package seal is broken or film is cut, damaged, or changed. Avoid applying to areas of mouth with sores or lesions. To dispose of unused film, remove from foil package, drop into toilet, and flush.
- **IM** Administer IM injections deep into well-developed muscle. Rotate sites of injections.

IV Administration

- **IV Push:** May give IV undiluted. ***High Alert:*** Administer slowly. Rapid administration may cause respiratory depression, hypotension, and cardiac arrest. **Rate:** Give over ≥2 min
- **Y-Site Compatibility:** acetaminophen, acyclovir, allopurinol, amikacin, aminocaproic acid, amiodarone, amphotericin B liposomal, anidulafungin, argatroban, arsenic trioxide, ascorbic acid, atracurium, atropine, azithromycin, aztreonam, benztropine, bivalirudin, bleomycin, bumetanide, butorphanol, calcium chloride, calcium gluconate, carboplatin, carmustine, cefazolin, cefepime, cefotaxime, cefotetan, cefoxitin, ceftazidime, ceftriaxone, cefuroxime, chloramphenicol, chlorpromazine, cisatracurium, cisplatin, cladribine, clindamycin, cyanocobalamin, cyclophosphamide, cyclosporine, cytarabine, dacarbazine, dactinomycin, daptomycin, daunorubicin, dexamethasone, dexmedetomidine, dexrazoxane, digoxin, diltiazem, diphenhydramine, dobutamine, docetaxel, dopamine, doxorubicin hydrochloride, doxycycline, enalaprilat, ephedrine, epinephrine, epirubicin, epoetin alfa, eptifibatide, ertapenem, erythromycin, esmolol, etoposide, etoposide phosphate, famotidine, fentanyl, filgrastim, fluconazole, fludarabine, foscarnet, fosphenytoin, gemcitabine, gentamicin, glycopyrrolate, granisetron, heparin, hetastarch, hydrocortisone, idarubicin, ifosfamide, imipenem/

cilastatin, insulin, regular, irinotecan, isoproterenol, ketorolac, labetalol, leucovorin, levofloxacin, lidocaine, linezolid, lorazepam, magnesium sulfate, mannitol, melphalan, meperidine, mesna, methotrexate, methylprednisolone, metoclopramide, metoprolol, metronidazole, midazolam, milrinone, minocycline, mitomycin, mitoxantrone, morphine, multivitamins, mycophenolate, nafcillin, nalbuphine, naloxone, nicardipine, nitroglycerin, nitroprusside, norepinephrine, octreotide, ondansetron, oxacillin, oxaliplatin, oxytocin, paclitaxel, palonosetron, pamidronate, papaverine, pemetrexed, penicillin G, pentamidine, phentolamine, phenylephrine, phytonadione, piperacillin/tazobactam, potassium acetate, potassium chloride, procainamide, prochlorperazine, promethazine, propofol, propranolol, protamine, pyridoxine, remifentanil, rituximab, rocuronium, sodium acetate, succinylcholine, sufentanil, tacrolimus, theophylline, thiamine, thiotepa, tigecycline, tirofiban, tobramycin, topotecan, trastuzumab, vancomycin, vasopressin, vecuronium, verapamil, vinblastine, vincristine, vinorelbine, voriconazole, zoledronic acid.

- **Y-Site Incompatibility:** alemtuzumab, aminophylline, ampicillin, azathioprine, dantrolene, diazepam, diazoxide, doxorubicin liposomal, fluorouracil, gemtuzumab ozogamicin, indomethacin, pantoprazole, pentobarbital, phenobarbital, phenytoin, sodium bicarbonate, trimethoprim/sulfamethoxazole.
- **Transdermal:** Buprenorphine may cause withdrawal in patients who are already taking opioids. For conversion from other opioids to buprenorphine transdermal, taper current around-the-clock opioids for up to 7 days to no more than 30 mg of morphine or equivalent per day before beginning treatment with buprenorphine transdermal. May use short-acting analgesics as needed until analgesic efficacy with buprenorphine transdermal is attained. Buprenorphine transdermal may not provide adequate analgesia for patients requiring >80 mg/day oral morphine equivalents.
- Apply system to flat, hairless, nonirritated, and nonirradiated site on the upper outer arm, upper chest, upper back, or side of the chest. If skin preparation is necessary, use clear water and clip hair (do not shave). Allow skin to dry completely before application. Apply immediately after removing from package. Do not alter the system (i.e. cut) in any way before application. Remove liner from adhesive layer and press firmly in place with palm of hand for 30 sec, especially around the edges, to make sure contact is complete. Remove used system and fold so that adhesive edges are together. Flush system down toilet immediately on removal or follow the institutional policy. Apply new system to a different site. After removal, wait ≥3 wk before applying to the same site. If patch falls off during 7-day dosing interval, dispose of patch and place a new patch on at a different site.
- May be titrated no less than every 72 hr. Dose adjustments in 5 mcg/hr, 7.5 mcg/hr, or 10 mcg/hr increments may be used by using no more than two patches.
- To discontinue, taper dose gradually to prevent signs and symptoms of withdrawal; consider introduction of immediate-release opioid medication. For patients taking buprenorphine regularly for a wk or more, initiate taper by a small enough increment (no more than 10%–25% of the total daily dose) to avoid withdrawal symptoms, and proceed with dose-lowering at an interval of every 2–4 wk or longer. Provision of lower dose strengths may be necessary for a successful taper. Monitor for withdrawal symptoms (restlessness; lacrimation; rhinorrhea; yawning; perspiration; chills; myalgia; mydriasis; irritability; anxiety; backache; joint pain; weakness; abdominal cramps; insomnia; nausea; anorexia; vomiting; diarrhea; ↑ BP, respiratory rate, or HR) during taper. If withdrawal symptoms occur, it may be necessary to pause the taper for a period of time or raise the dose of the opioid analgesic to the previous dose and then proceed with a slower taper. Monitor for changes in mood, emergence of suicidal thoughts, or use of other substances.
- **Treatment of Opioid Use Disorder:** Must be prescribed by health care provider with special training.
- **sublingual:** Induction is usually started with buprenorphine SL over 3–4 days. Initial dose should be administered ≥4 hr after last opioid dose and preferably when early signs of opioid withdrawal appear. Once patient is on a stable dose, maintenance therapy with buprenorphine/naloxone (Suboxone) is preferred for continued, unsupervised treatment.
- Administer sublingually. Usually takes 2–10 min for tablets to dissolve. If more than one tablet is prescribed, place multiple tablets under the tongue or two at a time until all tablets are dissolved. Do not chew or swallow; ↓ amount of medication absorbed. Not used for analgesia; may cause death in opioid-naive patients.
- **SUBQ**: *Sublocade* is for patients who have initiated treatment with a transmucosal buprenorphine product followed by dose adjustment for ≥7 days. Prepare and administer only by health care

provider monthly with a minimum of 26 days between doses. Use syringe and needle provided by manufacturer. Remove from refrigerator ≥15 min before injection to allow to reach room temperature. Do not open foil pouch until patient has arrived. Discard if left at room temperature for >12 wk. Do not administer solutions that are discolored or contain particulate matter. Pinch injection site and administer into abdomen; do not rub. May cause a lump that will ↓ over several wk. Do not administer IV or IM. If discontinued, withdrawal effects will be delayed (2–5 mo) due to long half-life. Monitor patients discontinuing for withdrawal signs and symptoms. May use transmucosal buprenorphine to treat withdrawal. In patients taking *Sublocade* for ≥4–6 mo, plasma and urine levels of buprenorphine may be detectable for ≥12 mo following discontinuation. Administer missed doses as soon as possible with following dose given ≥26 days later. For patients with regular therapy of 100 mg monthly, a 2-mo dosing interval may be used on occasion (e.g. extended travel); a single 300-mg dose may be given to cover a 2-mo period, and then resume 100 mg monthly regimen. Caution patient that 300-mg dose may cause sedation.

- *REMS:* *Brixandi* is only available through a restricted program called the *Brixandi REMS.* Health care settings and pharmacies that order and dispense *Brixandi* must be certified in this program and comply with REMS requirements.
- **Treatment of Opioid Use Disorder:** There are two formulations of *Brixandi*; one lasting 7 days and one lasting 1 mo. Doses of *Brixandi* (weekly) cannot be combined to yield a monthly dose.
- Only health care providers should prepare and administer *Brixandi*. Administer *Brixandi* as a single injection. Do not divide.
- For patients not currently receiving buprenorphine, begin with a test dose of 4 mg transmucosal buprenorphine to establish that buprenorphine is tolerated without precipitated withdrawal, and then transition to *Brixandi* (weekly).
- *Brixandi* is only for SUBQ injection; do not administer IV, IM, or intradermally.
- **SUBQ**: Inject slowly at a 90° angle into SUBQ tissue of the buttock, thigh, abdomen, or upper arm. Hold safety syringe in place for an additional 2 seconds keeping plunger pressed down fully. Rotate injection sites. In patients not currently receiving buprenorphine, for *Brixandi* (weekly), use the upper arm site only after steady state has been achieved (4 consecutive doses). Injection in the arm site was associated with approximately 10% lower plasma levels than other sites.
- Needle cap is synthetically derived from natural rubber latex; may cause allergic reactions in latex-sensitive individuals.
- If a dose of *Brixandi* (weekly) is missed, administer next dose as soon as possible. *Brixandi* (weekly) should be administered in 7-day intervals and *Brixandi* monthly should be administered every 28 days.

Patient/Family Teaching

- *REMS:* Instruct patient on risk of addiction, abuse, and misuse, which could lead to death. Discuss safe use, risks, and proper storage and disposal of opioid analgesics with patients and caregivers with each Rx. *The Patient Counseling Guide* is available at www.fda.gov/OpioidAnalgesicREMSPCG. Advise patient not to share buprenorphine with others and to protect from theft or misuse. Advise patient to avoid abrupt discontinuation; may lead to withdrawal symptoms.
- Educate patients and caregivers on how to recognize respiratory depression and emphasize the importance of calling 911 or getting emergency medical help right away in the event of a known or suspected overdose. Inform patients and caregivers about various ways to obtain naloxone as permitted by individual state naloxone dispensing and prescribing requirements or guidelines (by prescription, directly from a pharmacist, or as part of a community-based program).
- Medication may cause drowsiness or dizziness. Advise patient to call for assistance when ambulating and to avoid driving or other activities requiring alertness until response to medication is known, especially within 24–48 hr after subdermal implant insertion.
- Advise patient to avoid concurrent use of alcohol or other CNS depressants.
- Instruct patient to notify health care provider of all Rx or OTC medications, vitamins, or herbal products being taken and to consult health care provider before taking any Rx, OTC, or herbal products, especially CNS depressants.
- Advise patient and family members to inform health care providers of physical dependence on an opioid and of buprenorphine therapy.
- Rep: Advise patient to notify health care provider if pregnancy is planned or suspected and to avoid breastfeeding during therapy. Inform patient of potential for neonatal opioid withdrawal syndrome with prolonged use during pregnancy. Monitor infant for signs and symptoms of neonatal opioid withdrawal syndrome (irritability, hyperactivity and abnormal sleep pattern, high-pitched cry, tremor, vomiting, diarrhea, and/or failure to gain weight); usually occur in the first days after birth. Chronic use may impair fertility.
- **Pain:** Instruct patient on how and when to ask for pain medication.
- Encourage patients on bedrest to turn, cough, and breathe deeply every 2 hr to prevent atelectasis.

B

- Instruct patient to change positions slowly to minimize orthostatic hypotension.
- Advise patient that good oral hygiene, frequent mouth rinses, and sugarless gum or candy may decrease dry mouth.
- **Buccal:** Instruct patient on proper technique of buccal film and to avoid eating or drinking until film dissolves. Apply at same time each day. Avoid touching or moving buccal film with tongue or fingers. After product has completely dissolved, take a sip of water, swish gently around teeth and gums, and swallow. Wait for ≥1 hr after taking *Belbuca* before brushing teeth. Do not stop using buprenorphine without consulting health care provider. Advise patient to read *Instructions for Use* prior to starting therapy and with each Rx refill in case of changes.
- Advise patient to notify health care provider if the dose does not control pain.
- **Transdermal:** Instruct patient in correct method for application, removal, storage, and disposal of transdermal system. Wear patches for 7 days. May be worn while bathing, showering, or swimming. Do not discontinue or change dose without consulting health care provider. Instruct patient to read the *Medication Guide* prior to starting and with each Rx refill.
- Advise patients and caregivers/family members of the potential side effects. Instruct patient to notify health care provider if pain is not controlled or if bothersome side effects occur. Contact immediately if difficulty or changes in breathing; unusual deep "sighing" breathing; slow or shallow breathing; new or unusual snoring; slow heartbeat; severe sleepiness; cold, clammy skin; feeling faint, dizzy, or confused; having difficulty thinking, walking, or talking normally; or swelling or blistering around patch occur.
- Advise patient that fever, electric blankets, heating pads, saunas, hot tubs, and heated water beds increase release of buprenorphine from patch.
- Advise patient referred for MRI test to discuss patch with referring health care provider and MRI facility to determine if removal of patch is necessary prior to test and for directions for replacing patch.
- **Opioid Use Disorder:** Explain techniques for use to patient.
- Caution patient that buprenorphine may be a target for people who abuse drugs; store medications in a safe place to protect them from theft. Selling or giving this medication to others is against the law.
- Caution patient that injection of *Suboxone* can lead to severe withdrawal symptoms.
- Advise patient if admitted to the emergency department to inform treating health care provider and emergency room staff of physical dependence on opioids and of treatment regimen.
- Advise patient to notify health care provider promptly if faintness, dizziness, confusion, slowed breathing, skin or whites of eyes turning yellow, urine turning dark, light-colored stools, ↓ appetite, nausea, or abdominal pain occur.
- **SL:** Instruct patient in correct use of medication; directions for use must be followed exactly. Medication must be used regularly, not occasionally. Take missed doses as soon as remembered; if almost time for next dose, skip missed dose and return to regular dosing schedule. Do not take two doses at once unless directed by health care provider. Do not discontinue use without consulting health care provider; abrupt discontinuation may cause withdrawal symptoms. If medication is discontinued, flush unused tablets down the toilet if a drug take-back option is not readily available.
- **SUBQ:** ***REMS:*** Inform patient *Sublocade* and *Brixandi* are only available through a restricted program, *Sublocade* or *Brixandi* REMS program. *Sublocade* can only be dispensed to directly to a health care provider. *Brixandi* can only be administered by a health care provider.

Evaluation/Desired Outcomes

- Decrease in severity of pain without a significant alteration in level of consciousness or respiratory status.
- Suppression of withdrawal symptoms during detoxification and maintenance from heroin or other opioids.
- Continued cessation of opioid use.

REMS HIGH ALERT

buprenorphine/naloxone

(byoo-pre-**nor**-feen/na-**lox**-one)

~~Bunavail~~, Suboxone, Zubsolv

Classification

Therapeutic: opioid addiction agents

Pharmacologic: opioid agonists/antagonists, opioid antagonists

Schedule III

Indications

Treatment of opioid dependence as part of a comprehensive program including counseling and psychological support (Suboxone sublingual films and Zubsolv indicated for induction therapy for patients dependent on short-acting opioid products and maintenance treatment; Suboxone sublingual tablets indicated for maintenance treatment only).

Action

Buprenorphine: Binds to opiate receptors in the CNS. *Sublingual naloxone:* has no pharmacological effect; it is present in the formulation to discourage injection of the product by opioid-dependent patients.
Therapeutic Effects: Suppression of withdrawal symptoms during detoxification and maintenance from opioids.

Pharmacokinetics

Absorption: *Buprenorphine:* Well absorbed following SL administration; *naloxone:* Negligible absorption follows SL administration.
Distribution: *Buprenorphine:* Crosses the placenta; enters breast milk. CNS concentration is 15–25% of plasma.
Protein Binding: *Buprenorphine:* 96%.
Metabolism and Excretion: *Buprenorphine:* Mostly metabolized by the liver mostly via the CYP3A4 enzyme system; one metabolite is active; 70% excreted in feces; 27% excreted in urine.
Half-life: *Buprenorphine:* 33 hr; *Naloxone:* 60–90 min (up to 3 hr in neonates).

TIME/ACTION PROFILE

ROUTE	ONSET	PEAK†	DURATION
SL	Unknown	1.5–1.7 hr	24 hr

† Blood level.

Contraindications/Precautions

Contraindicated in: Hypersensitivity to buprenorphine or naloxone; Severe hepatic impairment (induction or maintenance therapy); Moderate hepatic impairment (induction therapy).
Use Cautiously in: Compromised respiratory function including COPD, cor pulmonale, diminished respiratory reserve, hypoxia, hypercapnia, or respiratory depression of other causes; Moderate hepatic impairment (maintenance therapy); Hypokalemia, hypomagnesemia, unstable atrial fibrillation, symptomatic bradycardia, unstable HF, QT interval prolongation, or myocardial ischemia; OB: Use during pregnancy only if potential maternal benefit justifies potential fetal risk; Lactation: Use while breastfeeding only if potential maternal benefit justifies potential risk to infant; Pedi: Safety and effectiveness not established in children; Geri: Older adults may be more sensitive to drug effects.

Adverse Reactions/Side Effects

CV: QT interval prolongation, orthostatic hypotension. **Derm:** ↑ sweating. **Endo:** ADRENAL INSUFFICIENCY. **F and E:** peripheral edema. **GI:** constipation, nausea, oral hypoesthesia, oral mucosal erythema, vomiting, glossodynia, hepatitis. **Neuro:** headache, insomnia. **Resp:** RESPIRATORY DEPRESSION (INCLUDING CENTRAL SLEEP APNEA AND SLEEP-RELATED HYPOXEMIA). **Misc:** HYPERSENSITIVITY REACTIONS (INCLUDING ANAPHYLAXIS), physical dependence, psychological dependence, tolerance, withdrawal phenomenon.

Interactions

Drug-Drug: Use with extreme caution in patients receiving **MAO inhibitors** (↑ CNS and respiratory depression and hypotension: ↓ buprenorphine dose by 50%; may need to ↓ **MAO inhibitor** dose). Concurrent use with **class Ia antiarrhythmics**, **class III antiarrhythmics**, or other **QT interval prolonging medications** may ↑ risk of QT interval prolongation; avoid concurrent use. Concurrent use of **CYP3A4 inhibitors**, including **ritonavir**, **ketoconazole**, **itraconazole**, **fluconazole**, **clarithromycin**, **erythromycin**, **nefazodone**, **diltiazem**, **verapamil**, **nelfinavir**, and **fosamprenavir**, ↑ levels and risk of opioid toxicity; careful monitoring during initiation, dose changes, or discontinuation of the inhibitor is recommended. Concurrent use with **CYP3A4 inducers**, including **barbiturates**, **carbamazepine**, **efavirenz**, **corticosteroids**, **modafinil**, **nevirapine**, **oxcarbazepine**, **phenobarbital**, **phenytoin**, **rifabutin**, or **rifampin**, may ↓ fentanyl levels and analgesia; if inducers are discontinued or dose ↓, patients should be monitored for signs of opioid toxicity and necessary dose adjustments should be made. Use with **benzodiazepines** or other **CNS depressants**, including other **opioids**, **nonbenzodiazepine sedative/hypnotics**, **anxiolytics**, **general anesthetics**, **muscle relaxants**, **antipsychotics**, and **alcohol**, may cause profound sedation, respiratory depression, coma, and death; reserve concurrent use for when alternative treatment options are inadequate. Drugs that affect serotonergic neurotransmitter systems, including **tricyclic antidepressants**, **SSRIs**, **SNRIs**, **MAO inhibitors**, **TCAs**, **tramadol**, **trazodone**, **mirtazapine**, **5-HT$_3$ receptor antagonists**, **linezolid**, **methylene blue**, and **triptans**, ↑ risk of serotonin syndrome.
Drug-Natural Products: Concomitant use of **kava-kava**, **valerian**, **chamomile**, or **hops** can ↑ CNS depression.

Route/Dosage

A Zubsolv 1.4/0.36 tablet is equivalent in terms of buprenorphine content to a Suboxone 2/0.5 tablet. A Zubsolv 5.7/1.4 tablet is equivalent in terms of buprenorphine content to a Suboxone 8/2 tablet.

Induction

SL (Adults): *Suboxone film:* Initiate therapy on Day 1 with buprenorphine 2 mg/naloxone 0.5 mg or buprenorphine 4 mg/naloxone 1 mg; then titrate up in increments of buprenorphine 2–4 mg every 2 hr until achieve dose of buprenorphine 8 mg/naloxone 2 mg based on control of acute withdrawal symptoms.

On Day 2, a single daily dose of up to buprenorphine 16 mg/naloxone 4 mg is recommended. *Zubsolv:* Induction: Initiate therapy on Day 1 with buprenorphine 1.4 mg/naloxone 0.36 mg; then follow with up to buprenorphine 4.2 mg/naloxone 1.08 mg given as 1–2 tablets of buprenorphine 1.4 mg/naloxone 0.36 mg every 1.5–2 hr on Day 1 (not to exceed 3 tablets). On Day 2, a single daily dose of up to buprenorphine 11.4 mg/naloxone 2.9 mg is recommended.

Maintenance

Buccal: SL (Adults): *Suboxone film:* Dose taken once daily. Progressively ↑/adjust in increments of buprenorphine 2 mg/naloxone 0.5 mg or buprenorphine 4 mg/naloxone 1 mg. Titrate to keep patient engaged in treatment while suppressing opioid withdrawal; usual target dose is buprenorphine 16 mg/naloxone 4 mg once daily;

SL (Adults): *Tablets (generic):* Dose taken once daily. Progressively ↑/adjust in increments of buprenorphine 2 mg/naloxone 0.5 mg or buprenorphine 4 mg/naloxone 1 mg. Titrate to keep patient engaged in treatment while suppressing opioid withdrawal; usual target dose is buprenorphine 16 mg/naloxone 4 mg once daily. *Zubsolv tablets:* Dose taken once daily. Progressively ↑/adjust in increments of buprenorphine 1.4 mg/naloxone 0.36 mg or buprenorphine 2.8 mg/naloxone 0.72 mg. Titrate to keep patient engaged in treatment while suppressing opioid withdrawal; usual target dose is buprenorphine 11.4 mg/naloxone 2.8 mg once daily.

Availability (generic available)

Sublingual film (Suboxone) (lime flavored): buprenorphine 2 mg/naloxone 0.5 mg, buprenorphine 4 mg/naloxone 1 mg, buprenorphine 8 mg/naloxone 2 mg, buprenorphine 12 mg/naloxone 3 mg ✱ buprenorphine 16 mg/naloxone 4 mg. **Sublingual tablets:** buprenorphine 2 mg/naloxone 0.5 mg, buprenorphine 8 mg/naloxone 2 mg. **Sublingual tablets (Zubsolv):** buprenorphine 0.7 mg/naloxone 0.18 mg, buprenorphine 1.4 mg/naloxone 0.36 mg, buprenorphine 2.9 mg/naloxone 0.71 mg, buprenorphine 5.7 mg/naloxone 1.4 mg, buprenorphine 8.6 mg/naloxone 2.1 mg, buprenorphine 11.4 mg/naloxone 2.9 mg.

NURSING IMPLICATIONS

Assessment

- During initial therapy, assess patient at least weekly during first mo and frequently thereafter for compliance, effectiveness of treatment plan, and overall patient progress. Once a stable dose is achieved, monthly assessment may be used. Determine absence of medication toxicity, medical, or behavioral adverse effect; responsible handling of medications by patient; compliance with treatment plan, including recovery-oriented activities and psychotherapy or other modalities; abstinence from illicit drug use.
- Monitor for signs and symptoms of adrenal insufficiency (nausea, vomiting, anorexia, fatigue, weakness, dizziness, low blood pressure) during therapy. If adrenal insufficiency is suspected, confirm with diagnostic testing. If confirmed, treat with physiologic doses of replacement corticosteroids. Wean patient off opioid to allow adrenal recovery and continue corticosteroids until adrenal function recovers. Other opioids may be tried.

Lab Test Considerations

- Monitor liver function test prior to beginning therapy and periodically during treatment.

Implementation

- Buprenorphine/naloxone sublingual film and sublingual tablets are not appropriate as an analgesic.
- *REMS:* Can only be prescribed by clinicians who meet qualifying requirements, and who have notified the Secretary of Health and Human Services of their intent to prescribe this product for the treatment of opioid dependence and have been assigned a unique identification number that must be included on every prescription.
- Induction of therapy begins with patient being in a moderate state of opioid withdrawal and receiving buprenorphine or buprenorphine/naloxone, not <6 hr after patient last used opioids. Once the induction phase is completed, maintenance begins with buprenorphine/naloxone titration.
- Patients receiving buprenorphine/naloxone sublingual film may be switched to sublingual tablets of same dose. Due to the greater bioavailability of sublingual film, monitor patients switched from tablets to film for overdose and patients switched from film to tablets for withdrawal symptoms. Dose adjustments may be required.
- Discuss availability of naloxone for emergency treatment of opioid overdose with the patient and caregiver and assess the potential need for access to naloxone, both when initiating and renewing therapy, especially if patient has household members (including children) or other close contacts at risk for accidental exposure or overdose. Consider prescribing naloxone, based on the patient's risk factors for overdose, such as concomitant use of CNS depressants, a history of opioid use disorder, or prior opioid overdose. However, the presence of risk factors for overdose should not prevent the proper management of pain in any patient.

- **SL:** *Film:* Place film under tongue. If additional film is required for dose, place on opposite side of tongue from first film, minimizing overlap. Keep film under tongue until dissolved (5–7 min); do not chew, swallow, or move film after placement. Film may also be used buccally.
- *Tablets:* Place under tongue until dissolves, about 5 min. Do not cut, chew, or swallow. Do not eat or drink anything until tablet is dissolved.
- **Buccal:** Have patient wet inside of cheek with tongue or rinse mouth with water. Apply film immediately after removal from package. Place yellow side of film against inside of cheek. Hold film in place with dry fingers for 5 sec; then leave in place on inside of cheek until fully dissolved. If chewed or swallowed, may result in lower peak concentrations and lower bioavailability. Do not administer if package seal if broken or film is cut, damaged, or changed. Avoid applying to areas of mouth with sores or lesions. To dispose of unused film, remove from foil package, drop into toilet, and flush.

Patient/Family Teaching

- Instruct patient to take medication as directed. Take missed doses as soon as remembered unless almost time for next dose; do not double doses. Do not take more often than prescribed or take other forms of buprenorphine/naloxone and consult health care professional before stopping; gradually discontinue dose to prevent withdrawal syndrome. Instruct patient to read *Medication Guide* before starting therapy and with each Rx refill in case of changes. Advise patient to keep medication in a safe place, out of reach of children, and protected from being stolen, and do not share with others, even if they have the same symptoms. Explain that buprenorphine/naloxone sublingual film may be fatal to children and individuals not tolerant to opioids. Advise patient that selling or giving medication away is against the law.
- To dispose of unused films, remove from foil pouch and drop each film into toilet and flush.
- Educate patients and caregivers on how to recognize respiratory depression and emphasize the importance of calling 911 or getting emergency medical help right away in the event of a known or suspected overdose. Inform patients and caregivers about various ways to obtain naloxone as permitted by individual state naloxone dispensing and prescribing requirements or guidelines (by prescription, directly from a pharmacist, or as part of a community-based program).
- Caution patient of the danger of taking nonprescribed benzodiazepines or other CNS depressants, including alcohol, during therapy. Combination may be fatal.
- May cause dizziness. Caution patient to avoid driving and other activities requiring alertness until response to medication is known.
- Advise patient to make position changes slowly to prevent orthostatic hypotension.
- Instruct patient to notify health care professional of all Rx or OTC medications, vitamins, or herbal products being taken and consult health care professional before taking any new medications.
- Advise patient to notify health care professional if signs and symptoms of adrenal insufficiency occur.
- Rep: Advise females of reproductive potential to notify health care professional if pregnancy is planned or suspected or if breastfeeding. Inform patient of potential for neonatal opioid withdrawal syndrome with prolonged use during pregnancy. Monitor neonate for signs and symptoms of withdrawal symptoms (irritability, hyperactivity and abnormal sleep pattern, high-pitched cry, tremor, vomiting, diarrhea, and/or failure to gain weight); usually occur the first days after birth. Advise breastfeeding women taking buprenorphine/naloxone to monitor infants for increased drowsiness and breathing difficulties. Chronic opioid use may cause impaired fertility in females and males of reproductive potential.
- Instruct patient to inform family that, in the event of an emergency, treating health care professionals should be informed that patient is physically dependent on an opioid and being treated with buprenorphine/naloxone sublingual film.

Evaluation/Desired Outcomes

- Suppression of withdrawal symptoms during detoxification and maintenance from opioids.

buPROPion (byoo-**proe**-pee-on)

Aplenzin, ~~Wellbutrin~~, Wellbutrin SR, Wellbutrin XL, Zyban

Classification

Therapeutic: antidepressants, smoking deterrents

Pharmacologic: aminoketones

Indications

Major depressive disorder. Depression with seasonal affective disorder. Smoking cessation.

Action

Decreases neuronal reuptake of dopamine in the CNS. Diminished neuronal uptake of serotonin and norepinephrine (less than tricyclic antidepressants). **Therapeutic Effects:** Diminished depression. Decreased craving for cigarettes.

B

Pharmacokinetics

Absorption: Although well absorbed, rapidly and extensively metabolized by the liver.
Distribution: Unknown.
Metabolism and Excretion: Extensively metabolized by the liver into 3 active metabolites (CYP2B6 isoenzyme involved in formation of one of the active metabolites).
Half-life: 14 hr (active metabolites may have longer half-lives).

TIME/ACTION PROFILE (antidepressant effect)

ROUTE	ONSET	PEAK	DURATION
PO	1–3 wk	unknown	unknown

Contraindications/Precautions

Contraindicated in: Hypersensitivity; Concurrent use of MAO inhibitors or MAO-like drugs (linezolid or methylene blue); Seizure disorders; Arteriovenous malformation; severe head injury; CNS tumor; CNS infection; severe stroke; anorexia nervosa; bulimia; or abrupt discontinuation of alcohol, benzodiazepines, barbiturates, or antiepileptic drugs (↑ risk of seizures).
Use Cautiously in: Renal/hepatic impairment (↓ dose recommended); Recent history of MI; History of suicide attempt; Unstable cardiovascular status; May ↑ risk of suicide attempt/ideation especially during early treatment or dose adjustment; this risk appears to be greater in adolescents or children; Psychiatric illness; Angle-closure glaucoma; OB: Use during pregnancy only if potential maternal benefit justifies potential fetal risk; Lactation: Use while breastfeeding only if potential maternal benefit justifies potential risk to infant; Pedi: Safety and effectiveness not established in children; Geri: ↑ risk of drug accumulation and ↑ sensitivity to effects in older adults.

Adverse Reactions/Side Effects

CV: hypertension. **Derm:** photosensitivity. **Endo:** hyperglycemia, hypoglycemia, syndrome of inappropriate antidiuretic hormone secretion. **GI:** dry mouth, nausea, vomiting. **Metab:** change in appetite, weight gain, weight loss. **Neuro:** agitation, headache, tremor, aggression, anxiety, delusions, depression, hallucinations, HOMICIDAL THOUGHTS/BEHAVIOR, hostility, insomnia, mania, panic, paranoia, psychoses, SEIZURES, SUICIDAL THOUGHTS/BEHAVIOR.

Interactions

Drug-Drug: **MAO inhibitors** may ↑ risk of hypertensive reactions; concurrent use contraindicated; ≥14 days should elapse between discontinuation of MAO inhibitor and initiation of bupropion (or vice versa). **MAO-inhibitor-like drugs**, such as **linezolid** or **methylene blue**, may ↑ risk of hypertensive reactions; concurrent use contraindicated; do not start therapy in patients receiving **linezolid** or **methylene blue**; if **linezolid** or **methylene blue** need to be started in a patient receiving bupropion, immediately discontinue bupropion and monitor for 2 wk or until 24 hr after last dose of linezolid or methylene blue, whichever comes first (may resume bupropion therapy 24 hr after last dose of linezolid or methylene blue). ↑ risk of adverse reactions when used with **amantadine** or **levodopa**. ↑ risk of seizures with **phenothiazines**, **antidepressants**, **theophylline**, **corticosteroids**, **OTC stimulants/anorectics**, or cessation of **alcohol** or **benzodiazepines**; avoid or minimize alcohol use. **Ritonavir**, **lopinavir/ritonavir**, and **efavirenz** may ↓ levels and effectiveness; may need to ↑ dose. May ↑ levels and risk of toxicity of **citalopram**. **Carbamazepine** may ↓ levels and effectiveness. **Nicotine** replacement may cause hypertension. ↑ risk of bleeding with **warfarin**. May ↑ levels and risk of toxicity of **SSRIs**, **tricyclic antidepressants**, **haloperidol**, **risperidone**, **thioridazine**, **beta blockers**, **flecainide**, and **propafenone**. May ↓ levels and effectiveness of **tamoxifen**. May ↓ levels and effectiveness of **digoxin**.

Route/Dosage

Depression

PO (Adults): *Immediate release:* 100 mg twice daily initially; after 3 days, may ↑ to 100 mg 3 times daily; after at least 4 wk of therapy, may ↑ up to 450 mg/day in divided doses (not to exceed 150 mg/dose; wait at least 6 hr between doses at the 300 mg/day dose or at least 4 hr between doses at the 450-mg/day dose). *12-hr sustained release:* 150 mg once daily in the morning; after 3 days, may ↑ to 150 mg twice daily with at least 8 hr between doses; after at least 4 wk of therapy, may ↑ to a maximum daily dose of 400 mg given as 200 mg twice daily. *24-hr extended release (Wellbutrin XL):* 150 mg once daily in the morning; may be ↑ after 4 days to 300 mg once daily; some patients may require up to 450 mg/day as a single daily dose. *24-hr extended release (Aplenzin):* 174 mg once daily in the morning; may be ↑ after 4 days to 348 mg once daily; some patients may require up to 522 mg/day as a single daily dose. *24-hr extended release (generic):* 450 mg once daily (should NOT be used as initial therapy; should only be used in patients who have been receiving 300 mg/day of another bupropion formulation for at least 2 wk and require titration up to 450 mg/day or in those patients receiving 450 mg/day of another bupropion formulation).

Hepatic Impairment

PO (Adults): *Moderate to severe hepatic impairment (Aplenzin):* Max dose: 174 mg every other day.

Seasonal Affective Disorder

PO (Adults): *24-hr extended release (Wellbutrin XL):* 150 mg/day in the morning; if dose is well tolerated, ↑ to 300 mg/day in one wk. Doses should be tapered to 150 mg/day for 2 wk before discontinuing; *24-hr extended release (Aplenzin):* 174 mg once daily in the morning; may be ↑ after 7 days to 348 mg once daily.

Hepatic Impairment

PO (Adults): *Moderate to severe hepatic impairment (Aplenzin):* Max dose: 174 mg every other day.

Smoking cessation

PO (Adults): *12-hr sustained release:* 150 mg once daily for 3 days; then 150 mg twice daily for 7–12 wk (doses should be at least 8 hr apart).

Availability (generic available)

Immediate-release tablets: 75 mg, 100 mg. **12-hr sustained-release tablets:** 100 mg, 150 mg, 200 mg. **24-hr extended-release tablets (Wellbutrin XL):** 150 mg, 300 mg. **24-hr extended-release tablets (Aplenzin):** 174 mg, 348 mg, 522 mg. **24-hr extended-release tablets (generic):** 450 mg.
In combination with: dexamethasone (Auvelity); naltrexone (Contrave). See Appendix N.

NURSING IMPLICATIONS

Assessment

- Monitor mood changes and level of anxiety during therapy.
- Assess for suicidal tendencies, especially during early therapy. Restrict amount of drug available to patient. Risk may be ↑ in children, adolescents, and adults ≤24 yr. After starting therapy, children, adolescents, and young adults should be seen by health care provider face-to-face at least weekly for 4 wk, then every other wk for next 4 wk, then at 12 wk, and then on advice of health care provider thereafter.
- Monitor BP and HR at baseline and regularly for hypertension during therapy, especially during the initial 3 mo; ↑ risk in patients with concurrent use of other drugs that ↑ dopaminergic or noradrenergic activity.
- Monitor for signs and symptoms of seizure activity with higher doses, patient factors, clinical situations, and concurrent medications that ↓ the seizure threshold; ↑ dose gradually and discontinue use if a seizure occurs.
- Monitor for signs and symptoms of anaphylactic reactions (pruritus, urticaria, hives, angioedema, dyspnea). Discontinue therapy and treat symptomatically.

Lab Test Considerations

- Monitor hepatic and renal function closely in patients with renal or hepatic impairment.
- May cause false-positive urine test for amphetamines.

Implementation

- Do not confuse bupropion with buspirone. Do not confuse Wellbutrin SR with Wellbutrin XL.
- Administer doses in equally spaced time increments during the day to minimize the risk of seizures. Risk of seizures ↑ 4-fold in doses >450 mg/day.
- Insomnia may be ↓ by avoiding bedtime doses. May require treatment during 1st wk of therapy.
- Nicotine patches, gum, inhalers, and spray may be used concurrently with bupropion.
- When converting from other brands of bupropion to *Aplenzin*, 522 mg/day of *Aplenzin* is equivalent to 450 mg/day bupropion hydrochloride, 348 mg/day of *Aplenzin* is equivalent to 300 mg/day bupropion hydrochloride, and 174 mg/day of *Aplenzin* is equivalent to 150 mg/day bupropion hydrochloride.
- **PO:** ***DNC:*** Swallow sustained-release or extended-release tablets whole; do not break, crush, or chew.
- May be administered with food to lessen GI irritation.
- **Seasonal Affective Disorder:** Begin administration in autumn prior to the onset of depressive symptoms. Continue therapy through winter and begin to taper and discontinue in early spring.

Patient/Family Teaching

- Educate patient on purpose and side effects of bupropion. Instruct patient to take as directed at the same time each day. Missed doses should be omitted. Do not double doses or take more than prescribed. May require ≥4 wk for full effects. Do not discontinue without consulting health care provider. May require gradual dose ↓ before discontinuation. Advise patient to read *Medication Guide* before starting and with each Rx refill in case of changes.
- Emphasize the importance of follow-up exams to monitor progress.
- May impair judgment or motor and cognitive skills. Caution patient to avoid driving and other activities requiring alertness until response to medication is known.
- Advise patient and caregivers to look for suicidality, especially during early therapy or dose changes. Notify health care provider immediately if thoughts about suicide or dying, attempts to commit suicide, new or worse depression or anxiety, agitation or restlessness, panic attacks, insomnia, new or worse irritability, aggressiveness, acting on dangerous impulses, mania, or other changes in mood or behavior occur.
- Instruct patient to notify health care provider of all Rx or OTC medications, vitamins, or herbal products being taken; to avoid alcohol during therapy; and to consult with health care provider before taking other medications with bupropion.
- Inform patient that frequent mouth rinses, good oral hygiene, and sugarless gum or candy may minimize

dry mouth. If dry mouth persists for >2 wk, consult health care provider regarding use of saliva substitute.

- Advise patient to notify health care provider if rash or other troublesome side effects occur.
- Inform patient that unused shell of XL tablets may appear in stool; this is normal.
- Advise patient to use sunscreen and protective clothing to prevent photosensitivity reactions.
- Advise patient to notify health care provider of medication regimen before treatment or surgery.
- **Smoking Cessation:** Smoking should be stopped during the 2nd wk of therapy to allow for the onset of bupropion and to maximize the chances of quitting.
- Rep: Instruct women of reproductive potential to inform health care provider if pregnancy is planned or suspected or if breastfeeding. Inform patient about pregnancy exposure registry to monitor pregnancy outcomes in women exposed to antidepressants during pregnancy. Register patients by calling the National Pregnancy Registry for Antidepressants at 1-844-405-6185 or visiting online at https://womensmentalhealth.org/clinical-and-researchprograms/pregnancyregistry/antidepressants/.

Evaluation/Desired Outcomes

- Increased sense of well-being.
- Renewed interest in surroundings. Acute episodes of depression may require several months of treatment.
- Cessation of smoking.

bupropion/naltrexone

(byoo-**proe**-pee-on nal-**trex**-one)

Contrave

Classification

Therapeutic: weight control agents

Pharmacologic: aminoketones, opioid antagonists

Indications

Adjunct to calorie-reduced diet and increased physical activity for chronic weight management in obese patients (BMI ≥30 kg/m^2) or overweight patients (BMI ≥27 kg/m^2) with at least one other comorbidity (hypertension, type 2 diabetes, or dyslipidemia).

Action

Bupropion: Antidepressant that acts as a weak inhibitor of neuronal reuptake of dopamine and norepinephrine. *Naltrexone:* Acts as an opioid antagonist. In combination they affect two different brain areas involved in food intake: the hypothalamic appetite regulatory center and mesolimbic dopamine circuit reward system. **Therapeutic Effects:** Decreased appetite with associated weight loss.

Pharmacokinetics

Bupropion

Absorption: Well absorbed but rapidly metabolized by the liver. Absorption is enhanced by a high-fat meal.
Distribution: Unknown.
Metabolism and Excretion: Extensively metabolized; three metabolites are pharmacologically active. Excretion is mostly renal as metabolites; minimal renal excretion of unchanged drug.
Half-life: 21 hr (longer for some metabolites).

Naltrexone

Absorption: Well absorbed orally; undergoes extensive first-pass hepatic metabolism, resulting in 5–40% bioavailability. Absorption is enhanced by a high-fat meal.
Distribution: Parent drug and metabolites enter breast milk.
Metabolism and Excretion: Metabolized to 6-beta-naltrexol. Both parent drug and metabolite are pharmacologically active. Excretion is mostly renal as metabolite; less than 2% as unchanged drug.
Half-life: *naltrexone:* 5 hr; *6-beta-naltrexol:* 13 hr.

TIME/ACTION PROFILE (weight loss)

ROUTE	ONSET	PEAK	DURATION
PO	within 4 wk	6 mo	unknown

Contraindications/Precautions

Contraindicated in: Known hypersensitivity to bupropion or naltrexone; Uncontrolled hypertension; End-stage renal disease; Severe hepatic impairment; Seizure disorders; Anorexia or bulimia; During withdrawal from or discontinuation of alcohol, benzodiazepines, barbiturates, or antiepileptics; Chronic opioid/opiate agonist or partial agonist use or acute opiate withdrawal; During/within 14 days of MAO inhibitors; Concurrent use of other bupropion-containing medications; OB: Pregnancy; Pedi: Not recommended for use in children.

Use Cautiously in: History of suicidal behavior/ideation; History of seizure risk (avoid administration with a high-fat meal, adhere to recommended dose); Cardiac/cerebrovascular disease; Angle-closure glaucoma; Diabetes mellitus (weight loss may result in hypoglycemia if treatment is not adjusted); Moderate or severe renal impairment (use lower dose); Moderate hepatic impairment (↓ dose); Lactation: Use while breastfeeding only if potential maternal benefit justifies potential risk to infant; Geri: Older adults may have ↑ sensitivity to adverse CNS reactions.

Adverse Reactions/Side Effects

CV: hypertension, tachycardia. **Derm:** hot flush, sweating. **EENT:** angle-closure glaucoma (bupropion), tinnitus. **GI:** <u>constipation</u>, <u>nausea</u>, <u>vomiting</u>, abdominal pain, diarrhea, dry mouth, hepatotoxicity (naltrexone).

Neuro: headache, aggression, agitation, anxiety, delusions, depression, dizziness, dysgeusia, hallucinations, HOMICIDAL THOUGHTS/BEHAVIOR, hostility, insomnia, mania, panic, paranoia, psychosis, SEIZURES, SUICIDAL THOUGHTS/BEHAVIOR, tremor. **Misc:** HYPERSENSITIVITY REACTIONS (INCLUDING ANAPHYLAXIS AND ANAPHYLACTOID REACTIONS).

Interactions

Drug-Drug: Concurrent use with **MAO inhibitors** may ↑ risk of hypertensive reactions; concurrent use contraindicated; at least 14 days should elapse between discontinuation of MAO inhibitor and initiation of bupropion (or vice versa). Concurrent use with **MAO-inhibitor-like drugs**, such as **linezolid** or **methylene blue**, may ↑ risk of hypertensive reactions; concurrent use contraindicated; do not start therapy in patients receiving **linezolid** or **methylene blue**; if **linezolid** or **methylene blue** need to be started in a patient receiving bupropion, immediately discontinue bupropion and monitor for 2 wk or until 24 hr after last dose of linezolid or methylene blue, whichever comes first (may resume bupropion therapy 24 hr after last dose of linezolid or methylene blue). May ↑ levels and risk of toxicity of **CYP2D6 substrates**, including **SSRIs**, **tricyclic antidepressants**, **haloperidol**, **risperidone**, **thioridazine**, **metoprolol**, **flecainide**, and **propafenone**. **CYP2B6 inducers**, including **carbamazepine**, **efavirenz**, **ritonavir**, **lopinavir**, **phenobarbital**, and **phenytoin**, may ↓ levels and effectiveness; avoid concurrent use. **CYP2B6 inhibitors**, including **clopidogrel**, may ↑ levels and risk of toxicity; do not exceed one tablet twice daily. Concurrent use of **drugs that ↓ seizure threshold** may ↑ risk of seizures. **Dopaminergic drugs**, including **amantadine** and **levodopa**, may ↑ risk of CNS toxicity. Concurrent ingestion of **alcohol** may ↑ risk of neuropsychiatric reactions (reduce or avoid consumption). May ↓ renal excretion of and ↑ levels/risk of toxicity from **amantadine**, **amiloride**, **cimetidine**, **dopamine**, **famotidine**, **memantine**, **metformin**, **pindolol**, **procainamide**, **varenicline**, and **oxaliplatin**. May ↓ analgesic effects of **opioids**.

Route/Dosage

PO (Adults): *Week 1:* One tablet in the morning; *Week 2:* One tablet in the morning and one tablet in the evening; *Week 3:* Two tablets in the morning and one tablet in the evening; *Week 4 and onward:* Two tablets in the morning and two tablets in the evening. *Concurrent use of CYP2B6 inhibitors:* Dose should not exceed one tablet twice daily.

Renal Impairment

PO (Adults): *Moderate or severe renal impairment:* Dose should not exceed one tablet in the morning and one tablet in the evening.

Hepatic Impairment

PO (Adults): *Moderate hepatic impairment:* Dose should not exceed one tablet in the morning and one tablet in the evening.

Availability

Extended-release tablets: 90 mg bupropion/8 mg naltrexone.

NURSING IMPLICATIONS

Assessment

- Monitor for weight loss and adjust concurrent medications (antihypertensives, antidiabetics, lipid-lowering agents) as needed. Discontinue if ≥5% ↓ in baseline body weight is not achieved after 12 wk at maintenance dosage.
- Assess mental status and mood changes, especially during initial few months of therapy. Risk may be ↑ in children, adolescents, and adults ≤24 yr. Inform health care professional if patient demonstrates significant ↑ in signs of depression (depressed mood, loss of interest in usual activities, insomnia or hypersomnia, psychomotor agitation or retardation, ↑ fatigue, feelings of guilt or worthlessness, slowed thinking or impaired concentration, irritability, hostility, suicide or homicide attempt, suicidal ideation). Restrict amount of drug available to patient.
- Monitor for signs and symptoms of opioid withdrawal (tachycardia, diaphoresis, nausea, vomiting, anxiety, tremor, excessive yawning) in opioid-dependent patients.
- Monitor BP and HR at baseline and regularly for hypertension during therapy, especially during the initial 3 mo; ↑ risk in patients with concurrent use of other drugs that ↑ dopaminergic or noradrenergic activity.
- Monitor for signs and symptoms of seizure activity with higher doses, patient factors, clinical situations, and concurrent medications that lower the seizure threshold; ↑ dose gradually and discontinue use if a seizure occurs.
- Monitor for signs and symptoms of anaphylactic reactions (pruritus, urticaria, hives, angioedema, dyspnea). Discontinue therapy and treat symptomatically.

Lab Test Considerations

- Monitor blood glucose prior to and during therapy in patients with type 2 diabetes; may cause hypoglycemia.
- May cause false-positive urine test for amphetamines.

Implementation

- **PO:** Administer in the morning and evening according to dose escalation schedule. ***DNC:*** Swallow tablets whole; do not break, crush, or chew.
- Do not administer with a high-fat meal; may ↑ risk of seizures.
- Discontinue opioids prior to starting extended-release naltrexone/bupropion. Patients should be opioid-free for a minimum of 7–10 days in those receiving short-acting opioids and up to 14 days in those receiving buprenorphine or methadone.

Patient/Family Teaching

- Explain the purpose and side effects to patient. Instruct patient to take medication as directed, following the dose escalation schedule. If a dose is missed, omit and wait until next scheduled dose; do not double doses. Advise patient to read *Medication Guide* before starting therapy and with each Rx refill in case of changes.

- Instruct patient to adhere to a reduced-calorie diet and ↑ physical activity.
- Advise patient, family, and caregivers to look for suicidality, especially during early therapy. Notify health care professional immediately if thoughts about suicide, homicide, or dying; attempts to commit suicide; new or worse depression or anxiety, agitation, or restlessness; panic attacks; insomnia; new or worse irritability; aggression; hostility; acting on dangerous impulses; mania; or other changes in mood or behavior occur.
- Advise patient to notify health care professional if signs and symptoms of liver damage (stomach pain lasting more than a few days, dark urine, yellowing of skin and whites of eyes, tiredness) occurs.
- Advise patients they may be less sensitive to opioids during therapy. Advise patients to notify health care professional of bupropion/naltrexone therapy.
- Advise patient to notify health care professional of all Rx or OTC medications, vitamins, or herbal products being taken; to consult with health care professional before taking other medications; and to minimize or avoid alcohol during therapy.
- Rep: Instruct women of reproductive potential to notify health care professional if pregnancy is planned or suspected and to avoid breastfeeding during therapy. Advise pregnant patients to discontinue medication, as appropriate weight gain based on prepregnancy weight is recommended for all pregnant patients, including those who are overweight or obese, due to the weight gain that occurs in maternal tissues during pregnancy.

Evaluation/Desired Outcomes

- Decreased appetite with associated weight loss. Evaluate therapy after 12 wk at maintenance dose. If patient has not lost 5% of baseline body weight discontinue medication; clinically meaningful weight loss is unlikely.

busPIRone (byoo-**spye**-rone)

~~BuSpar~~

Classification

Therapeutic: antianxiety agents

Indications

Anxiety.

Action

Binds to serotonin and dopamine receptors in the brain. Increases norepinephrine metabolism in the brain. **Therapeutic Effects:** Relief of anxiety.

Pharmacokinetics

Absorption: Rapidly absorbed.

Distribution: Widely distributed to tissues.

Protein Binding: 95%.

Metabolism and Excretion: Extensively metabolized by the liver via the CYP3A4 isoenzyme; 20–40% excreted in feces.

Half-life: 2–3 hr.

TIME/ACTION PROFILE (relief of anxiety)

ROUTE	ONSET	PEAK	DURATION
PO	7–10 days	3–4 wk	unknown

Contraindications/Precautions

Contraindicated in: Hypersensitivity; Severe renal impairment; Severe hepatic impairment; Concurrent use of MAO inhibitors; Lactation: Lactation.

Use Cautiously in: Concurrent use of other antianxiety agents (other agents should be slowly withdrawn to prevent withdrawal or rebound phenomenon); Patients receiving other psychotropics; OB: Safety not established in pregnancy; Pedi: Children <6 yr (safety and effectiveness not established).

Adverse Reactions/Side Effects

CV: <u>chest pain</u>, <u>palpitations</u>, <u>tachycardia</u>, hypertension, hypotension, syncope. **Derm:** <u>rash</u>, <u>sweating</u>, alopecia, blisters, bruising, dry skin, edema, flushing, pruritus. **EENT:** <u>blurred vision</u>, <u>nasal congestion</u>, <u>sore throat</u>, <u>tinnitus</u>, altered taste or smell, conjunctivitis. **Endo:** irregular menses. **GI:** <u>nausea</u>, abdominal pain, constipation, diarrhea, dry mouth, vomiting. **GU:** changes in libido, dysuria, urinary frequency, urinary hesitancy. **MS:** <u>myalgia</u>. **Neuro:** <u>dizziness</u>, <u>drowsiness</u>, <u>excitement</u>, <u>fatigue</u>, <u>headache</u>, <u>incoordination</u>, <u>insomnia</u>, <u>nervousness</u>, <u>numbness</u>, <u>paresthesia</u>, <u>weakness</u>, personality changes, tremor. **Resp:** chest congestion, hyperventilation, shortness of breath. **Misc:** <u>clamminess</u>, fever.

Interactions

Drug-Drug: Concurrent use with **MAO inhibitors** may ↑ risk of hypertensive reactions; concurrent use contraindicated; at least 14 days should elapse between discontinuation of MAO inhibitor and initiation of buspirone (or vice versa). **CYP3A4 inhibitors**, including **erythromycin**, **nefazodone**, **ketoconazole**, **itraconazole**, and **ritonavir**, may ↑ levels and risk of toxicity; ↓ dose to 2.5 mg twice daily with erythromycin; ↓ dose to 2.5 mg once daily with nefazodone. **CYP3A4 inducers**, including **rifampin**,

dexamethasone, **phenytoin**, **phenobarbital**, and **carbamazepine**, may ↓ levels and effectiveness. Avoid concurrent use with **alcohol**.
Drug-Natural Products: Concurrent use of **kava-kava**, **valerian**, or **chamomile** can ↑ CNS depression.
Drug-Food: Grapefruit juice ↑ levels and risk of toxicity; ingestion of large amounts of grapefruit juice is not recommended.

Route/Dosage

PO (Adults): 7.5 mg twice daily; may ↑ by 5 mg/day every 2–4 days as needed (not to exceed 60 mg/day). Usual dose is 10–15 mg twice daily.
PO (Children ≥6 yr): 5 mg once daily; may ↑ by 5 mg/day every 2–7 days as needed. Usual dose is 7.5–30 mg twice daily

Availability (generic available)

Tablets: 5 mg, 7.5 mg, 10 mg, 15 mg, 30 mg.

NURSING IMPLICATIONS

Assessment

- Assess degree and manifestations of anxiety before and periodically during therapy.
- Buspirone does not appear to cause physical or psychological dependence or tolerance. However, patients with a history of substance use disorder should be assessed for tolerance or impaired control. Restrict amount of drug available to these patients.

Implementation

- Do not confuse buspirone with bupropion.
- Patients changing from other antianxiety agents should receive gradually ↓ doses. Buspirone will not prevent withdrawal symptoms.
- CNS depressant drugs should be withdrawn gradually before initiating buspirone.
- **PO:** May be administered with food to minimize gastric irritation. Food slows but does not alter extent of absorption.

Patient/Family Teaching

- Explain the purpose and side effects of buspirone. Instruct patient to take exactly as directed. Take missed doses as soon as possible if not just before next dose; do not double doses. Do not take more than amount prescribed. Advise patient to read *Patient Information* before starting and with each Rx refill in case of changes.
- May cause dizziness or drowsiness. Caution patient to avoid driving or other activities requiring alertness until response to the medication is known.
- Advise patient to avoid concurrent use of alcohol or other CNS depressants.
- Instruct patient to avoid large amounts of grapefruit juice while taking this drug.
- Instruct patient to notify health care professional of all Rx or OTC medications, vitamins, or herbal products being taken and to consult health care professional before taking any Rx, OTC, or herbal products.
- Instruct patient to notify health care professional if any chronic abnormal movements occur (dystonia, motor restlessness, involuntary movements of facial or cervical muscles).
- Emphasize the importance of follow-up exams to determine effectiveness of medication.
- Rep: Advise women of reproductive potential to notify health care professional if pregnancy is planned or suspected or if breastfeeding.

Evaluation/Desired Outcomes

- Increase in sense of well-being.
- Decrease in subjective feelings of anxiety. Some improvement may be seen in 7–10 days. Optimal results take 3–4 wk of therapy. Buspirone is usually used for short-term therapy (3–4 wk). If prescribed for long-term therapy, efficacy should be periodically assessed.

HIGH ALERT

busulfan (byoo-sul-fan)

Busulfex, Myleran

Classification
Therapeutic: antineoplastics
Pharmacologic: alkylating agents

Indications

PO: Chronic myelogenous leukemia (CML) and bone marrow disorders. **IV:** Conditioning regimen before allogenic hematopoietic progenitor cell transplantation for CML (in combination with cyclophosphamide).

Action

Disrupts nucleic acid function and protein synthesis (cell-cycle phase-nonspecific). **Therapeutic Effects:** Death of rapidly growing cells, especially malignant ones.

Pharmacokinetics

Absorption: Rapidly absorbed from the GI tract following oral administration. IV administration results in complete bioavailability.
Distribution: Unknown.
Metabolism and Excretion: Extensively metabolized by the liver.
Half-life: 2.5 hr.

TIME/ACTION PROFILE (effect on blood counts)

ROUTE	ONSET	PEAK	DURATION
PO	1–2 wk	wk	up to 1 mo†
IV	unknown	unknown	13 days‡

† Complete recovery may take up to 20 mo.
‡ After administration of last dose.

Contraindications/Precautions

Contraindicated in: Hypersensitivity; Failure to respond to previous courses; OB: Pregnancy; Lactation: Lactation.

Use Cautiously in: Active infection; ↓ bone marrow reserve; Obese patients (base dose on ideal body weight); Other chronic debilitating diseases; Rep: Women of reproductive potential and men with female partners of reproductive potential; Geri: Begin therapy at lower end of dose range in older adults due to ↑ frequency of impaired cardiac, hepatic, or renal function.

Adverse Reactions/Side Effects

Incidence and severity of adverse reactions and side effects are increased with IV use

CV: PO: CARDIAC TAMPONADE (WITH HIGH-DOSE CYCLOPHOSPHAMIDE) **IV:** chest pain, hypotension, tachycardia, thrombosis, arrhythmias, atrial fibrillation, cardiomegaly, ECG changes, edema, heart block, HF, hypertension, pericardial effusion, ventricular extrasystoles. **Derm: PO:** itching, rash, acne, alopecia, erythema nodosum, exfoliative dermatitis, hyperpigmentation. **EENT: PO:** cataracts **IV:** epistaxis, pharyngitis, ear disorders. **Endo: PO and IV:** hyperuricemia **IV:** hyperglycemia **PO:** sterility, gynecomastia. **F and E:** hypokalemia, hypomagnesemia, hypophosphatemia. **GI: PO:** drug-induced hepatitis, nausea, vomiting **IV:** abdominal enlargement, anorexia, constipation, diarrhea, dry mouth, hematemesis, nausea, rectal discomfort, vomiting, abdominal pain, dyspepsia, hepatic veno-occlusive disease (↑ in allogenic transplantation), hepatomegaly, pancreatitis, stomatitis. **GU:** oliguria, ↓ fertility, dysuria, hematuria. **Hemat:** MYELOSUPPRESSION. **Local:** inflammation/pain at injection site. **MS:** arthralgia, myalgia, back pain. **Neuro: IV:** anxiety, confusion, depression, dizziness, headache, weakness, CEREBRAL HEMORRHAGE/COMA, encephalopathy, mental status changes, SEIZURES. **Resp: PO:** PULMONARY FIBROSIS **IV:** alveolar hemorrhage, asthma, atelectasis, cough, hemoptysis, hypoxia, pleural effusion, pneumonia, rhinitis, sinusitis. **Misc:** allergic reactions, chills, fever, infection.

Interactions

Drug-Drug: Concurrent or previous (within 72 hr) use of **acetaminophen** may ↑ levels and risk of toxicity. Concurrent use with high-dose **cyclophosphamide** in patients with thalassemia may result in cardiac tamponade. **Itraconazole**, **metronidazole**, or **deferasirox** may ↑ levels and risk of toxicity. **Phenytoin** may ↓ levels and effectiveness. Long-term continuous therapy with **thioguanine** may ↑ risk of hepatic toxicity. ↑ bone marrow suppression with other **antineoplastics** or **radiation therapy**. May ↓ the antibody response to and ↑ risk of adverse reactions from **live-virus vaccines**.

Route/Dosage

PO (Adults): *Induction:* 1.8 mg/m²/day or 0.06 mg/kg/day until WBCs <15,000/mm³. Usual dose is 4–8 mg/day (range 1–12 mg/day). *Maintenance:* 1–3 mg/day.
PO (Children): 0.06–0.12 mg/kg/day or 1.8–4.6 mg/m²/day initially. Titrate dose to maintain WBC of approximately 20,000/mm³.
IV (Adults): 0.8 mg/kg every 6 hr (dose based on ideal body weight or actual weight, whichever is less; in obese patients, dosage should be based on adjusted ideal body weight) for 4 days (total of 16 doses); given in combination with cyclophosphamide.

Availability (generic available)

Tablets: 2 mg. **Solution for injection:** 6 mg/mL.

NURSING IMPLICATIONS

Assessment

- ***High Alert:*** Monitor for myelosuppression. Assess for bleeding (bleeding gums; bruising; petechiae; guaiac stools, urine, or emesis) and avoid IM injections and taking rectal temperatures. Apply pressure to venipuncture sites for ≥10 min. Assess for signs of infection (fever, chills, sore throat, cough, hoarseness, lower back or side pain, difficult or painful urination) during neutropenia. Anemia may occur. Monitor for fatigue, dyspnea, and orthostatic hypotension. Notify health care provider if these symptoms occur.
- Monitor for significant changes in intake/output and daily weights.
- Monitor for symptoms of gout (↑ uric acid, joint pain, lower back or side pain, swelling of feet or lower legs). Encourage patient to drink ≥2 L of fluid each day. Allopurinol may be given to ↓ uric acid levels. Alkalinization of urine may be ordered to ↑ excretion of uric acid.
- Assess for pulmonary fibrosis (fever, cough, shortness of breath) periodically during and after therapy. Discontinue therapy at the first sign of pulmonary fibrosis. Usually occurs 8 mo–10 yr (average 4 yr) after initiation of therapy.

Lab Test Considerations

- Monitor CBC with differential before and weekly during therapy. The nadir of leukopenia occurs within 10–15 days and the nadir of WBC at 11–30 days. Recovery usually occurs within 12–20 wk. *If WBC <15,000/mm³ or if a precipitous drop occurs,* treat as per guidelines. *If platelet count <150,000/mm³,* institute thrombocytopenia precautions. Myelosuppression may be severe and progressive, with recovery taking 1 mo–2 yr after discontinuation of therapy.
- Monitor serum ALT, bilirubin, alkaline phosphatase, and uric acid before and periodically during therapy. May ↑ uric acid levels.

- May cause false-positive cytology results of breast, bladder, cervix, and lung tissues.

Implementation

- ***High Alert:*** Fatalities have occurred with chemotherapeutic agents. Before administering, clarify all ambiguous orders; double-check single, daily, and course-of-therapy dose limits; have second practitioner independently double-check original order, calculations, and infusion pump settings.
- ***High Alert:*** Do not confuse Myleran with Alkeran or Leukeran.
- **IV:** Premedicate patient with phenytoin before IV administration to minimize seizure risk.
- Administer antiemetics before and on a fixed schedule during IV administration.
- **PO:** Administer at the same time each day on an empty stomach to ↓ nausea and vomiting.

IV Administration

- **IV:** Prepare solution in a biologic cabinet. Wear gloves, gown, and mask while handling IV medication. Discard IV equipment in specially designated containers.
- Busulfan is an irritant. If extravasation occurs, immediately stop infusion. Leave needle/cannula in place temporarily but do not flush the line. Gently aspirate extravasated solution; then remove needle/cannula. Elevate patient's extremity.
- **Intermittent Infusion: Dilution:** Use needle with 5-micron nylon filter provided to remove calculated volume of busulfan from vial; remove and replace needle, and inject busulfan into diluent. Do not use polycarbonate syringe. Add 9.3 mL busulfan to 93 mL 0.9% NaCl or D5W. Mix by inverting several times. Solution diluted with 0.9% NaCl or D5W is stable for 8 hr at room temperature, and solution diluted with 0.9% NaCl is stable for 12 hr if refrigerated. Administration must be completed during this time. Solution is clear and colorless; do not administer solution if discolored or contains precipitates. **Concentration:** ≥0.5 mg/mL. **Rate:** Administer via central venous catheter over 2 hr every 6 hr for 4 days for a total of 16 doses. Before and after infusion, flush catheter with 5 mL 0.9% NaCl or D5W.
- **Y-Site Compatibility:** acyclovir, amiodarone, amphotericin B liposomal, anidulafungin, argatroban, arsenic trioxide, bivalirudin, bleomycin, caspofungin, dacarbazine, daptomycin, dexmedetomidine, dexrazoxane, diltiazem, docetaxel, ertapenem, foscarnet, fosphenytoin, granisetron, hetastarch, hydromorphone, leucovorin, levofloxacin, linezolid, lorazepam, meperidine, mesna, methadone, metronidazole, milrinone, moxifloxacin, octreotide, ondansetron, paclitaxel, palonosetron, piperacillin/tazobactam, potassium acetate, rituximab, sodium acetate, tacrolimus, tigecycline, tirofiban, trastuzumab, vasopressin, vinblastine, zoledronic acid.
- **Y-Site Incompatibility:** idarubicin, thiotepa, vecuronium, voriconazole.

Patient/Family Teaching

- Instruct patient to take medication as directed, at the same time each day. Consult health care provider if vomiting occurs shortly after dose is taken. If dose is missed, omit; do not double doses.
- Advise patient to notify health care provider if fever; sore throat; signs of infection; lower back or side pain; difficult or painful urination; sores in mouth or on lips; chills; dyspnea; persistent cough; bleeding gums; easy bleeding, bruising; petechiae; or blood in urine, stool, or emesis occurs. Instruct patient to use soft toothbrush and electric razor. Caution patient not to drink alcoholic beverages or take products containing aspirin or NSAIDs.
- Caution patient to avoid crowds and persons with known infections. Health care provider should be informed immediately if symptoms of infection occur.
- Discuss with patient the possibility of hair loss. Explore methods of coping.
- Instruct patient not to receive any vaccinations without advice of health care provider.
- Advise patients on long-term therapy to notify health care provider immediately if cough, shortness of breath, fever, or joint pain occur or if darkening of skin, diarrhea, dizziness, fatigue, anorexia, confusion, or nausea and vomiting become pronounced.
- Inform patient of ↑ risk of a second malignancy with busulfan.
- Rep: May cause fetal harm. Advise women of reproductive potential to use effective contraception during therapy and for 6 mo after last dose and to avoid breastfeeding during therapy. Advise men with female partners of reproductive potential to use effective contraception during and for 3 mo after last dose of therapy. May impair fertility.
- Advise patient of the importance of periodic blood counts.

Evaluation/Desired Outcomes

- Decrease in leukocyte count to within normal limits.
- Decreased night sweats. Increase in appetite. Increased sense of well-being. Therapy is resumed when leukocyte count reaches 50,000/mm³.

butenafine, See ANTIFUNGALS (TOPICAL).

butoconazole, See ANTIFUNGALS (VAGINAL).

HIGH ALERT

cabazitaxel (ka-ba-zi-tax-el)

Jevtana

Classification

Therapeutic: antineoplastics

Pharmacologic: taxoids

Indications

Hormone-refractory metastatic prostate cancer previously treated with a regimen including docetaxel (in combination with prednisone).

Action

Binds to intracellular tubulin and promotes its assembly into microtubules while inhibiting disassembly. Result is inhibition of mitosis and interphase. **Therapeutic Effects:** Death of rapidly replicating cells, particularly malignant ones, with ↓ spread of metastatic prostate cancer.

Pharmacokinetics

Absorption: IV administration results in complete bioavailability.

Distribution: Extensively distributed to tissues.

Metabolism and Excretion: Extensively (>95%) metabolized by the liver, 80–90% by the CYP3A4/5 isoenzymes. Metabolites are excreted in urine and feces. Minimal renal excretion.

Half-life: 95 hr.

TIME/ACTION PROFILE (plasma concentrations)

ROUTE	ONSET	PEAK	DURATION
IV	rapid	end of infusion	unknown

Contraindications/Precautions

Contraindicated in: Severe hypersensitivity to cabazitaxel or polysorbate 80; Neutrophil count ≤1500/mm³; Hepatic impairment (total bilirubin ≥3 times upper limit of normal [ULN]).

Use Cautiously in: Neutropenia or a history of pelvic radiation, adhesions, ulceration, or GI bleeding (↑ risk of GI and urinary adverse reactions); Concurrent use of steroids, NSAIDs, or antithrombotics (↑ risk of GI adverse reactions); Severe renal impairment or end-stage renal disease; Hemoglobin <10 g/dL; Lung disease (↑ risk of pulmonary toxicity); Mild or moderate hepatic impairment (↓ dose); Poor performance status, previous episodes of febrile neutropenia, extensive prior radiation ports, or poor nutritional status (↑ risk of complications from prolonged neutropenia); Rep: Men with female partners of reproductive potential; Pedi: Safety and effectiveness not established in children; Geri: ↑ risk of adverse reactions in older adults (especially prolonged neutropenia and febrile neutropenia).

Adverse Reactions/Side Effects

CV: arrhythmias, hypotension. **Derm:** alopecia. **F and E:** electrolyte imbalance. **GI:** abdominal pain, abnormal taste, anorexia, constipation, DIARRHEA, GI BLEED, GI PERFORATION, nausea, vomiting, dyspepsia, ENTEROCOLITIS, ILEUS. **GU:** hematuria, cystitis, RENAL FAILURE. **Hemat:** anemia, leukopenia, NEUTROPENIA, THROMBOCYTOPENIA. **MS:** arthralgia, back pain, muscle spasms. **Neuro:** peripheral neuropathy, weakness, fatigue. **Resp:** dyspnea, ACUTE RESPIRATORY DISTRESS SYNDROME, INTERSTITIAL LUNG DISEASE. **Misc:** fever, HYPERSENSITIVITY REACTIONS (INCLUDING ANAPHYLAXIS).

Interactions

Drug-Drug: Strong CYP3A inhibitors, including **ketoconazole**, **itraconazole**, **clarithromycin**, **atazanavir**, **nefazodone**, **nelfinavir**, **ritonavir**, and **voriconazole**, may ↑ levels and risk of toxicity; concurrent use contraindicated. **Strong CYP3A inducers**, including **phenytoin**, **carbamazepine**, **rifampin**, **rifabutin**, **rifapentin**, and **phenobarbital**, may ↓ levels and effectiveness; concurrent use contraindicated.

Drug-Natural Products: St. John's wort may ↓ levels and effectiveness; concurrent use contraindicated.

Route/Dosage

IV (Adults): 20 mg/m² every 3 wk (with prednisone 10 mg PO daily). A dose of 25 mg/m² may be considered in select patients.

Hepatic Impairment

IV (Adults): *Mild hepatic impairment (total bilirubin >1–≤1.5 times ULN or AST >1.5 times ULN):* 20 mg/m² every 3 wk (with prednisone 10 mg PO daily); *Moderate hepatic impairment (total bilirubin >1.5–≤3 times ULN):* 15 mg/m² every 3 wk (with prednisone 10 mg PO daily); *Severe hepatic impairment (total bilirubin >3 times ULN):* Contraindicated.

Availability (generic available)

Viscous solution for injection: 40 mg/mL (contains polysorbate 80); comes with diluent (5.7 mL of 13% [w/w] ethanol in water for injection). **Solution for injection:** 10 mg/mL.

C

NURSING IMPLICATIONS

Assessment

- Assess for hypersensitivity reactions (generalized rash/erythema, hypotension, bronchospasm, swelling of face). May occur within minutes following initiation of infusion. *If severe reaction occurs,* discontinue infusion immediately and provide supportive therapy.
- Assess for signs and symptoms of GI toxicity (abdominal pain and tenderness, fever, persistent constipation, nausea, vomiting, severe diarrhea); resulting electrolyte imbalances may result in death. Premedication is recommended. Treat with rehydration, antidiarrheal, or antiemetic therapy as needed. *If Grade ≥3 or persisting diarrhea occurs despite appropriate medication and fluid and electrolyte replacement,* hold cabazitaxel until improvement or resolution; then ↓ by one dose level.
- Assess for signs and symptoms of peripheral neuropathy (pain, burning, or numbness in hands, feet, or legs) during therapy. *If Grade 2 peripheral neuropathy occurs,* withhold until improvement or resolution; then ↓ by one dose level. *If Grade ≥3 peripheral neuropathy occurs,* permanently discontinue cabazitaxel.
- Monitor for signs and symptoms of respiratory compromise (trouble breathing, dyspnea, chest pain, cough, fever) during therapy; hold for new or worsening symptoms and consider discontinuation.

Lab Test Considerations

- Monitor CBC with differential weekly during Cycle 1 and before each cycle thereafter. *If prolonged grade 3 neutropenia (>1 wk) despite appropriate treatment, including filgrastim, occurs,* hold cabazitaxel until neutrophils $>1500/mm^3$; then ↓ by one dose level. *If febrile neutropenia occurs,* hold cabazitaxel until improvement or resolution and neutrophils $>1500/mm^3$; then ↓ by one dose level. Use filgrastim for secondary prophylaxis.
- May cause hematuria.
- May ↑ AST, ALT, and bilirubin.

Implementation

- ***High Alert:*** Fatalities have occurred with chemotherapeutic agents. Before administering, clarify all ambiguous orders; double-check single, daily, and course-of-therapy dose limits; have second practitioner independently double-check original order and dose calculations.
- Prepare solution in a biologic cabinet. Wear gloves, gown, and mask while handling medication. Discard equipment in specially designated containers. If solution comes in contact with skin or mucosa, wash with soap and water immediately.
- Premedicate ≥30 min before each dose with antihistamine (diphenhydramine 25 mg or equivalent), corticosteroid (dexamethasone 8 mg or equivalent), and H_2 antagonist (famotidine 20 mg or equivalent). Antiemetic prophylaxis, PO or IV, is recommended.
- Primary prophylaxis with G-CSF (filgrastim) recommended in older adults, poor performance status, previous episodes of febrile neutropenia, extensive prior radiation ports, poor nutritional status, and in all patients receiving a dose of 25 mg/m^2 to minimize complications due to prolonged neutropenia.

IV Administration

- Two dilutions are required. Do not use PVC infusion containers or polyurethane infusion sets for preparation or infusion.
- **First Dilution: Reconstitution:** Mix vial with entire contents of supplied diluent. Direct needle to inside wall of vial and inject slowly to avoid foaming. Mix gently by repeated inversions for at least 45 sec; do not shake. Let stand for a few minutes to allow foam to dissipate. **Concentration:** 10 mg/mL.
- **Second Dilution: Dilution:** Withdraw recommended dose from cabazitaxel solution and dilute further into a sterile 250 mL PVC-free container of 0.9% NaCl or D5W. If dose >65 mg is required, use a larger volume of infusion vehicle so concentration does not exceed 0.26 mg/mL. Gently invert container to mix. **Concentration:** 0.10–0.26 mg/mL. Stable for 8 hr (including 1 hr infusion) at room temperature or 24 hr if refrigerated. May crystallize over time. Do not use if crystallized, discolored, or contains particulates.
  Rate: Infuse over 1 hr at room temperature through a 0.22 micrometer nominal pore size filter.
- **Y-Site Incompatibility:** Do not administer other drugs through same IV line.

Patient/Family Teaching

- Instruct patient to take oral prednisone as prescribed and to notify health care professional if a dose is missed or not taken in time.
- Explain purpose and side effects of medication. Advise patient to read *Patient Information* before starting therapy.
- Advise patient to notify health care professional immediately if signs or symptoms of hypersensitivity reactions; fever; sore throat; signs of infection; lower back or side pain; difficult or painful urination; sores on mouth or lips; bleeding gums; bruising; petechiae; blood in urine, stool, or emesis; unusual swelling; shortness of breath; trouble breathing; chest pain; or cough occur. Caution patient to avoid crowds and persons with known infections. Instruct patient to use soft toothbrush and electric razor and to avoid falls. Patient should also be cautioned not to drink alcoholic beverages or to take products containing aspirin or NSAIDs; may precipitate GI hemorrhage.

C

- May cause dizziness. Caution patient to avoid driving or other activities requiring alertness until response to medication is known.
- Instruct patient to notify health care professional of all Rx or OTC medications, vitamins, or herbal products being taken and consult health care professional before taking any new medications, especially St. John's wort.
- Instruct patient not to receive any vaccinations without advice of health care professional.
- Rep: Advise men with female partners of reproductive potential to use effective contraception during therapy and for ≥4 mo after last dose of cabazitaxel. May impair male fertility.
- Emphasize need for periodic lab tests to monitor for side effects. Advise patient to monitor temperature frequently.

Evaluation/Desired Outcomes

- ↓ in size and spread of metastatic prostate cancer.

cabotegravir (ka-boe-teg-ra-vir)

Apretude, Vocabria

Classification

Therapeutic: antiretrovirals

Pharmacologic: integrase strand transfer. inhibitors instis

Indications

PO: Short-term treatment of HIV-1 infection in patients who are virologically suppressed (HIV-1 RNA <50 copies/mL) on a stable antiretroviral regimen with no history of treatment failure and with no known or suspected resistance to either cabotegravir or rilpivirine (in combination with rilpivirine). To be used in one of the following situations: (1) As an oral lead-in therapy to assess the tolerability of cabotegravir prior to administration of cabotegravir/rilpivirine extended-release injection (Cabenuva); or (2) As oral therapy for patients who will miss planned dosing with the cabotegravir/rilpivirine extended-release injection (Cabenuva). **PO IM** Pre-exposure prophylaxis (PrEP) to reduce the risk of sexually acquired HIV-1 infection in at-risk individuals. To be used in one of the following situations: (1) As an oral lead-in therapy to assess the tolerability of cabotegravir prior to administration of cabotegravir extended-release injection (Apretude); or (2) As oral PrEP for patients who will miss planned dosing with the cabotegravir extended-release injection (Apretude).

Action

Inhibits HIV-1 integrase, which is required for viral replication. **Therapeutic Effects:** Evidence of decreased viral replication and reduced viral load with slowed progression of HIV and its sequelae. Reduction in risk of sexually acquired HIV infection in at-risk individuals.

Pharmacokinetics

Absorption: ↑ with high-fat meals after oral administration.

Distribution: Widely distributed to extravascular tissues.

Protein Binding: >99%.

Metabolism and Excretion: Primarily metabolized by the uridine diphosphate glucuronosyltransferase (UGT) 1A1 enzyme system, with some involvement of UGT1A9. Primarily excreted in feces as unchanged drug (47%), with 27% excreted in urine as metabolites.

Half-life: *PO:* 41 hr; *IM:* 5.6–11.5 wk.

TIME/ACTION PROFILE (plasma concentrations)

ROUTE	ONSET	PEAK	DURATION
PO	unknown	3 hr	24 hr
IM	unknown	7 days	2 mo

Contraindications/Precautions

Contraindicated in: Hypersensitivity; Concurrent use of carbamazepine, oxcarbazepine, phenobarbital, phenytoin, rifampin, or rifapentine; Unknown or positive HIV-1 status (for HIV-1 PrEP only); Lactation: Breastfeeding not recommended in patients with HIV.

Use Cautiously in: Severe hepatic impairment; End-stage renal disease; Severe renal impairment (injection only); OB: Safety not established in pregnancy; Lactation: Use while breastfeeding in HIV-uninfected mothers only if potential maternal benefit outweighs potential risk to infant; Pedi: Safety and effectiveness not established in children <12 yr; Geri: Use with caution in older adults, considering concurrent disease states, drug therapy, and age-related ↓ in hepatic and renal function.

Adverse Reactions/Side Effects

Derm: STEVENS-JOHNSON SYNDROME, TOXIC EPIDERMAL NECROLYSIS. **GI:** diarrhea, HEPATOTOXICITY, nausea. **Local:** injection site reactions. **MS:** ↑ CK (injection). **Neuro:** abnormal dreams, anxiety, depression, dizziness, fatigue, headache, insomnia, mood disturbances, SUICIDAL THOUGHTS/BEHAVIOR. **Misc:** fever, HYPERSENSITIVITY REACTIONS (INCLUDING ANGIOEDEMA).

Interactions

Drug-Drug: Strong UGT1A1 inducers, including **carbamazepine**, **oxcarbazepine**, **phenobarbital**, **phenytoin**, **rifampin**, and **rifapentine**, may significantly ↓ levels and effectiveness; concurrent use contraindicated. **Antacids** containing polyvalent cations, including **aluminum hydroxide**, **calcium carbonate**, or **magnesium hydroxide**, may ↓ absorption and effectiveness of cabotegravir; administer antacids ≥2 hr before or ≥4 hr after cabotegravir. May ↓ levels and effectiveness of **methadone**.

Route/Dosage

HIV-1 Treatment

Oral Lead-in Dosing to Assess Tolerability of Cabotegravir

PO (Adults and Children ≥12 yr and ≥35 kg): 30 mg once daily (taken with rilpivirine 25 mg once daily). Continue for ≥28 days to assess tolerability prior to initiating cabotegravir/rilpivirine extended-release injection (Cabenuva) therapy. The last dose of oral cabotegravir should be taken on the same day that cabotegravir/rilpivirine extended-release injection (Cabenuva) therapy is initiated.

Oral Dosing to Replace Planned Missed Doses of Cabotegravir/Rilpivirine Extended-Release Injection (Cabenuva)

PO (Adults and Children ≥12 yr and ≥35 kg): *To replace planned missed cabotegravir/rilpivirine extended-release injections (Cabenuva) for patients on monthly dosing schedule (if patient plans to miss scheduled monthly injection by >7 days):* 30 mg once daily (with rilpivirine 25 mg once daily) initiated at the same time as missed injection of cabotegravir/rilpivirine and then continued until day the cabotegravir/rilpivirine extended-release injection (Cabenuva) is restarted (oral replacement therapy can be continued for up to 2 mo). *To replace planned missed cabotegravir/rilpivirine extended-release injections (Cabenuva) for patients on every-2-mo dosing schedule (if patient plans to miss scheduled every-2-mo injection by >7 days):* 30 mg once daily (with rilpivirine 25 mg once daily) initiated the same time as missed injection of cabotegravir/rilpivirine and then continued until day the cabotegravir/rilpivirine extended-release injection (Cabenuva) is restarted (oral replacement therapy can be continued for up to 2 mo).

HIV-1 Pre-exposure Prophylaxis

May initiate with cabotegravir oral lead-in therapy (to assess tolerability of cabotegravir) prior to cabotegravir IM injections or may precede directly to cabotegravir IM injections without oral lead-in.

Oral Lead-in Therapy

PO (Adults and Children ≥12 yr and ≥35 kg): 30 mg once daily. Continue for ≥28 days to assess tolerability prior to initiating IM therapy (see Initiation Injections section below).

Initiation Injections

IM (Adults and Children ≥12 yr and ≥35 kg): *With oral lead-in therapy:* 600 mg once monthly for 2 consecutive mo (2nd initiation injection may be administered up to 7 days before or after the date the individual is scheduled to receive the injection); then proceed with continuation injections. 1st initiation injection should be given on the last day of oral cabotegravir lead-in therapy or within 3 days of the last dose of oral cabotegravir lead-in therapy (see Oral Lead-in Therapy section above to assess tolerability of cabotegravir). *Without oral lead-in therapy:* 600 mg once monthly for 2 consecutive mo (2nd initiation injection may be administered up to 7 days before or after the date the individual is scheduled to receive the injection); then proceed with continuation injections.

Continuation Injections

IM (Adults and Children ≥12 yr and ≥35 kg): 600 mg every 2 mo starting 2 mo after the last initiation injection (injection may be administered up to 7 days before or after the date the individual is scheduled to receive the injection).

Missed Doses of Injection

PO (Adults and Children ≥12 yr and ≥35 kg): *Planned missed injections:* If a patient plans to miss a scheduled every-2-mo dose of cabotegravir extended-release injection (Apretude) by >7 days, use cabotegravir 30 mg once daily to replace one every-2-mo injection. The 1st dose of oral therapy should be taken approximately 2 mo after the last dose of cabotegravir extended-release injection (Apretude) and continued until the day that injection dosing is restarted or within 3 days of injection dosing being restarted. For oral PrEP durations >2 mo, use an alternative oral regimen for PrEP. *Unplanned missed injections:* If a scheduled injection visit is missed or delayed by >7 days and oral dosing has not been taken in the interim, clinically reassess to determine if injection therapy remains appropriate.

Availability

Tablets (Vocabria): 30 mg. **Extended-release suspension for injection (Apretude):** 200 mg/mL.

NURSING IMPLICATIONS

Assessment

- Assess patient for change in severity of HIV symptoms and for symptoms of opportunistic infections during therapy.
- Observe patient for 10 min following injection for postinjection reactions (dyspnea, agitation, abdominal cramping, flushing, sweating, oral numbness, changes in BP).
- Monitor mental status, mood changes, and affect. Monitor for anxiety, depression (especially in patients with a history of psychiatric illness), suicidal ideation, and paranoia during therapy.
- Monitor for development of severe cutaneous adverse reactions (SJS and TEN), including signs and symptoms of prodrome of fever, malaise,

mucosal lesions, progressive skin rash, blisters, lymphadenopathy, conjunctivitis, myalgias, hepatitis, and/or eosinophilia. *If a severe cutaneous adverse reaction is suspected,* interrupt therapy until etiology of reaction is determined. Consultation with a dermatologist is recommended. *If a severe cutaneous adverse reaction is confirmed,* permanently discontinue cabotegravir.

- Monitor for signs and symptoms of hypersensitivity reactions (rash, urticaria, pruritus, flushing, dizziness, vomiting, abdominal pain) and angioedema (swelling of throat, lips, tongue, face, dyspnea, wheezing, hoarseness). *If hypersensitivity reaction occurs,* immediately discontinue cabotegravir and provide supportive care.
- Monitor for signs and symptoms of hepatotoxicity (fatigue, nausea, upper abdominal pain, jaundice, scleral icterus, dark urine, clay-colored stools). *If hepatotoxicity suspected,* discontinue cabotegravir.

Lab Test Considerations

- Perform HIV-1 test in patients before starting *Apretude* or *Vocabria* and before each subsequent injection of *Apretude*. Do not initiate *Apretude* for HIV-1 PrEP unless negative HIV status is confirmed.
- Monitor liver function tests periodically during therapy.

Implementation

- Oral lead-in is used for ≥28 days concurrently with rilpivirine to assess the tolerability of cabotegravir prior to the initiation of cabotegravir/rilpivirine. Administer last oral dose on same day injections with cabotegravir/rilpivirine are started.
- If taking to replace a missed scheduled injection of cabotegravir/rilpivirine, take 1st dose of oral therapy approximately 1 mo after last injection dose and continue until the day injection dosing is restarted.
- **PO:** Administer once daily with a meal at the same time each day.
- **IM** *Apretude*: Before starting *Apretude* for HIV-1 PrEP, ask seronegative individuals about recent (<1 mo) potential exposure events (condomless sex or condom breaking during sex with a partner of unknown HIV-1 status or unknown viremic status, a recent sexually transmitted infection [STI]), and evaluate for current or recent signs or symptoms consistent with acute HIV-1 infection (fever, fatigue, myalgia, skin rash). If recent (<1 mo) exposures to HIV-1 are suspected or symptoms consistent with acute HIV-1 infection are present, use an FDA-approved test as an aid in diagnosis of acute or primary HIV-1 infection. When using *Apretude* for HIV-1 PrEP, test for HIV-1 before each injection and upon diagnosis of any other STIs. If an individual has confirmed HIV-1 infection, transition individual to a complete HIV-1 treatment regimen.
- *Apretude* may be initiated with oral cabotegravir prior to IM injections, or patient may proceed directly to injection of *Apretude* without an oral lead-in.
- Prior to starting *Apretude*, carefully select individuals who agree to the required injection dosing and testing schedule and counsel individuals about the importance of adherence to scheduled dosing visits to help ↓ the risk of acquiring HIV-1 infection and development of resistance.
- Bring to room temperature prior to administration. Administer undiluted in the ventrogluteal or dorsogluteal site using the Z-track method; do not administer by any other route or anatomical site. Consider the body mass index (BMI) of the individual to ensure that the needle length is sufficient to reach the gluteus muscle. Longer needle lengths may be required for individuals with higher BMI (>30 kg/m²) to ensure injection is administered IM and not SUBQ. Solution is white to light pink; do not administer solutions that are discolored or contain particulate matter. Do not freeze. Do not mix with any other product or diluent. Administer dose as soon as possible; may remain in the syringe for up to 2 hr.

Patient/Family Teaching

- Explain the purpose and side effects of cabotegravir. Instruct patient to take as directed. Take missed doses as soon as remembered. Do not stop taking cabotegravir without consulting health care provider. Instruct patient to read *Patient Information* before starting cabotegravir and with each Rx refill in case of changes.
- **IM** Tell patient to contact their health care provider if they miss or plan to miss a scheduled monthly injection.
- Advise patient to take antacid products ≥2 hr before or 4 hr after taking this drug.
- Advise patient to notify health care provider if signs and symptoms of allergic reaction (fever; general ill feeling; tiredness; muscle or joint aches; trouble breathing; blisters or sores in mouth; blisters; redness or swelling of eyes; swelling of mouth, face, lips, or tongue), liver problems (yellow skin or white part of eyes; dark or tea-colored urine; light-colored stools; nausea or vomiting; loss of appetite; pain, aching, or tenderness on the right side of stomach area; itching) or depression

(feeling sad or hopeless, feeling anxious or restless, have thoughts of hurting yourself [suicide], have tried to hurt yourself) occur.

- Apretude is not always effective in preventing HIV-1. Encourage consistent and correct condom use; communication of HIV-1 status to partner(s); knowledge of partner(s)' HIV-1 status, including viral suppression status; and regular testing for STIs that can facilitate HIV-1 transmission.
- Instruct patient to notify health care provider of all Rx or OTC medications, vitamins, or herbal products being taken and consult health care provider before taking any new medications.
- Rep: May cause fetal harm. Advise women of reproductive potential to use effective contraception during therapy. Advise women with HIV to avoid breastfeeding. Cabotegravir is detected in systemic circulation for ≥12 mo after discontinuing *Apretude*. Inform patient of pregnancy exposure registry that monitors pregnancy outcomes in women exposed to cabotegravir during pregnancy. Register patients by calling the Antiretroviral Pregnancy Registry at 1-800-258-4263.

Evaluation/Desired Outcomes

- Decrease in viral load and improvement in CD4 cell counts.
- Delayed progression of HIV and decreased opportunistic infections in patients with HIV.

cabotegravir/rilpivirine (ka-boe-teg-ra-vir/ril-pi-vir-een)

Cabenuva

Classification

Therapeutic: antiretrovirals

Pharmacologic: integrase strand transfer inhibitors (INSTIs), non-nucleoside reverse transcriptase inhibitors

Indications

HIV-1 infection to replace the current antiretroviral regimen in patients who are virologically suppressed (HIV-1 RNA <50 copies/mL) on a stable antiretroviral regimen with no history of treatment failure and with no known or suspected resistance to either cabotegravir or rilpivirine.

Action

Cabotegravir: Inhibits HIV-1 integrase, which is required for viral replication; *Rilpivirine:* Inhibits HIV-replication by noncompetitively inhibiting HIV reverse transcriptase. **Therapeutic Effects:** Evidence of decreased viral replication and reduced viral load with slowed progression of HIV and its sequelae.

Pharmacokinetics

Cabotegravir

Absorption: Increased with high-fat meals.
Distribution: Distributed to extravascular tissues.
Protein Binding: >99%.
Metabolism and Excretion: Primarily metabolized by the uridine diphosphate glucuronosyltransferase (UGT) 1A1 enzyme system, with some involvement of UGT1A9. Primarily excreted in feces as unchanged drug (47%), with 27% excreted in urine as metabolites.
Half-life: 41 hr.

Rilpivirine

Absorption: Well absorbed following oral administration.
Distribution: Unknown.
Protein Binding: 99.7%.
Metabolism and Excretion: Primarily metabolized by the liver via the CYP3A isoenzyme; 25% excreted unchanged in feces; <1% excreted unchanged in urine.
Half-life: 50 hr

TIME/ACTION PROFILE (plasma concentrations)

ROUTE	ONSET	PEAK	DURATION
cabotegravir IM	unknown	7 days	unknown
rilpivirine IM	unknown	3–4 days	unknown

Contraindications/Precautions

Contraindicated in: Hypersensitivity to cabotegravir or rilpivirine; Concurrent use of carbamazepine, dexamethasone (more than a single dose), oxcarbazepine, phenobarbital, phenytoin, rifabutin, rifampin, rifapentine, or St. John's wort; OB: Pregnancy; Lactation: Breastfeeding not recommended in patients with HIV.

Use Cautiously in: History of depression or suicide attempt; Hepatic impairment; Severe renal impairment or end-stage renal disease; Pedi: Children <12 yr (safety and effectiveness not established); Geri: Use with caution in older adults, considering concurrent disease states, drug therapy, and age-related ↓ in hepatic and renal function.

Adverse Reactions/Side Effects

CV: QT interval prolongation. **Derm:** DRUG REACTION WITH EOSINOPHILIA AND SYSTEMIC SYMPTOMS (DRESS), rash, STEVENS-JOHNSON SYNDROME, TOXIC EPIDERMAL NECROLYSIS. **GI:** ↑ lipase, HEPATOTOXICITY, nausea. **Local:** injection site reactions. **Metab:** weight gain. **MS:** ↑ CK, pain. **Neuro:** depression, dizziness, fatigue, headache, insomnia, mood disturbances, somnolence, SUICIDAL THOUGHTS/BEHAVIORS. **Misc:** fever, HYPERSENSITIVITY REACTIONS (INCLUDING ANGIOEDEMA).

Interactions

Drug-Drug: **Strong UGT1A1 inducers** or **CYP3A inducers**, including **carbamazepine**, **oxcarbazepine**, **phenobarbital**, **phenytoin**, **rifabutin**, **rifampin**, or **rifapentine**, may significantly ↓ cabotegravir and rilpivirine levels and effectiveness; concurrent use contraindicated. Use of more than a single dose of **dexamethasone** may significantly ↓ rilpivirine levels and effectiveness; concurrent use contraindicated. **Macrolide antibiotics**, including **azithromycin**, **clarithromycin**, and **erythromycin**, may ↑ rilpivirine levels and risk of toxicity, including QT interval prolongation; use alternative antibiotic therapy. **QT interval prolonging drugs** may ↑ risk of QT interval prolongation and torsades de pointes. May ↓ levels and effectiveness of **methadone**.
Drug-Natural Products: **St. John's wort** may significantly ↓ rilpivirine levels and effectiveness; concurrent use contraindicated.

Route/Dosage

Lead-in therapy with oral cabotegravir and oral rilpivirine must be used for ≥28 days to assess tolerability to both cabotegravir and rilpivirine prior to initiating cabotegravir/rilpivirine extended-release injection therapy.

Monthly Dosing

IM (Adults and Children ≥12 yr and ≥35 kg): *Initiation injections:* Cabotegravir 600 mg as a single injection and rilpivirine 900 mg as a single injection, both administered on the final day of lead-in therapy with oral cabotegravir and oral rilpivirine. *Continuation injections:* Cabotegravir 400-mg injection and rilpvirine 600-mg injection once monthly (administer both injections during same visit). Start continuation injections 1 mo following initiation injections. Monthly injections may be given within 7 days of originally scheduled date of injection. *Switching to every-2-mo injection dosing:* Administer cabotegravir 600-mg injection and rilpivirine 900-mg injection 1 mo after the last monthly continuation injection and then every 2 mo thereafter. *Planned missed injections:* If patient plans to miss a scheduled injection visit by >7 days, give oral cabotegravir 30 mg once daily and oral rilpivirine 25 mg once daily initiated at the same time as missed injection of cabotegravir/rilpivirine and then continue until day the cabotegravir/rilpivirine extended-release injection is restarted (oral replacement therapy can be continued for up to 2 mo). If time since last injection ≤2 mo, resume injection with cabotegravir 400-mg injection and rilpivirine 600-mg injection once monthly. If time since last injection >2 mo, resume injection with initiation of cabotegravir 600-mg single injection and rilpivirine 900-mg single injection followed in 1 mo by continuation injections of cabotegravir 400-mg injection and rilpivirine 600-mg injection once monthly (start continuation injections 1 mo following initiation injections). *Unplanned missed injections:* If monthly injections are missed or delayed by >7 days and oral cabotegravir and oral rilpivirine therapy have not been taken in the interim, reassess patient to determine if resumption of injection dosing remains appropriate.

Every-2-Month Dosing

IM (Adults and Children ≥12 yr and ≥35 kg): *Initiation injections:* Cabotegravir 600-mg injection and rilpivirine 900-mg injection once monthly for 2 consecutive mo, with the 1st set of injections being administered on the final day of lead-in therapy with oral cabotegravir and oral rilpivirine. 2nd initiation injection may be given within 7 days of originally scheduled date of injection. *Continuation injections:* Cabotegravir 600-mg injection and rilpvirine 900-mg injection every 2 mo (administer both injections during same visit). Start continuation injections 2 mo following 2nd initiation injection. Every-2-mo injections may be given within 7 days of originally scheduled date of injection. *Switching to monthly injection dosing:* Administer cabotegravir 400-mg injection and rilpivirine 600-mg injection 2 mo after the last monthly continuation injection and then once monthly thereafter. *Planned missed injections:* If patient plans to miss a scheduled injection visit by >7 days, give oral cabotegravir 30 mg once daily and oral rilpivirine 25 mg once daily initiated at the same time as missed injection of cabotegravir/rilpivirine and then continue until day the cabotegravir/rilpivirine extended-release injection is restarted (oral replacement therapy can be continued for up to 2 mo). If time since 2nd initiation injection ≤2 mo, resume initiation injection with cabotegravir 600-mg injection and rilpivirine 900-mg injection, followed by continuation injections every 2 mo (starting 2 mo following 2nd initiation injection). If time since 2nd initiation injection >2 mo, restart the two initiation injections (see above) given once monthly for 2 consecutive mo, followed by the continuation injections (see above) given every 2 mo. If patient misses a continuation injection by ≤3 mo, resume injection with cabotegravir 600-mg injection and rilpivirine 900-mg injection every 2 mo. If time since last injection >3 mo, restart the two initiation injections (see above) given once monthly for 2 consecutive mo followed by the continuation injections (see above) given every 2 mo. *Unplanned missed injections:* If monthly injections are missed or delayed by >7 days and oral cabotegravir and oral rilpivirine therapy have not been taken in the interim, reassess patient to determine if resumption of injection dosing remains appropriate.

Availability

Extended-release suspension for injection: 400-mg/600-mg kit (200 mg/mL vial of cabotegravir and 300 mg/mL vial of rilpivirine), 600-mg/900-mg kit (200 mg/mL vial of cabotegravir and 300 mg/mL vial of rilpivirine).

NURSING IMPLICATIONS

Assessment

- Assess patient for change in severity of HIV symptoms and for symptoms of opportunistic infections during therapy.
- Observe patient for 10 min following injections for postinjection reactions (dyspnea, agitation, abdominal cramping, flushing, sweating, oral numbness, changes in BP).
- Monitor mental status, mood changes, and affect. Monitor for anxiety, depression (especially in patients with a history of psychiatric illness), suicidal ideation, and paranoia during therapy.
- Monitor for development of severe cutaneous adverse reactions, (DRESS, SJS, TEN), including signs and symptoms of prodrome of fever, malaise, mucosal lesions, progressive skin rash, blisters, lymphadenopathy, conjunctivitis, myalgias, hepatitis, and/or eosinophilia. *If a severe cutaneous adverse reaction is suspected,* interrupt therapy until etiology of reaction is determined. Consultation with a dermatologist is recommended. *If a severe cutaneous adverse reaction is confirmed,* permanently discontinue cabotegravir/rilpivirine.
- Monitor for signs and symptoms of hypersensitivity reactions (rash, urticaria, pruritus, flushing, dizziness, vomiting, abdominal pain) and angioedema (swelling of throat, lips, tongue, or face; dyspnea; wheezing; hoarseness). *If hypersensitivity reaction occurs,* immediately discontinue cabotegravir/rilpivirine and provide supportive care.
- Monitor for signs and symptoms of hepatotoxicity (fatigue, nausea, upper abdominal pain, jaundice, scleral icterus, dark urine, clay-colored stools). *If hepatotoxicity suspected,* discontinue cabotegravir/rilpivirine.

Lab Test Considerations

- Monitor liver function tests periodically during therapy.

Implementation

- Lead-in therapy with oral cabotegravir and oral rilpivirine must be used for ≥28 days to assess tolerability to both cabotegravir and rilpivirine prior to initiating cabotegravir/rilpivirine extended-release injection therapy. Start injections of cabotegravir/rilpivirine on last day of PO lead-in therapy.
- Injection must be administered by health care provider.
- **IM** Administer cabotegravir and rilpivirine at separate gluteal (preferably ventrogluteal) injection sites (on opposite sides or 2 cm apart) during the same visit. Use needles long enough for IM injection. Allow suspensions to come to room temperature for 15 min before administration. Stable at room temperature for up to 6 hr. Shake suspensions vigorously to mix. Do not administer solutions that contain particulate matter. Administer within 2 hr of drawing into syringe; if >2 hr, discard injection. Do not refrigerate syringes. Start continuation injections 1 mo after the initiation injections. Injections may be given 7 days before or after the date to receive the injection.

Patient/Family Teaching

- Explain the purpose and side effects of cabotegravir/rilpivirine. Instruct patient in the importance of adhering to monthly schedule of injections. *Planned Missed Injections:* If a scheduled injection visit by >7 days, take daily PO therapy to replace up to 2 consecutive monthly injection visits. Take 1st dose of PO therapy approximately 1 mo after the last injection dose and continue until the day injection dosing is restarted. *Unplanned Missed Injections:* If monthly injections are missed or delayed by >7 days and PO therapy has not been taken in the interim, health care provider will reassess patient to determine if resumption of injection dosing remains appropriate. Instruct patient to read *Patient Information* before starting cabotegravir/rilpivirine therapy and with each injection in case of changes.
- Counsel patients that adherence to scheduled dosing visits helps maintain viral suppression and ↓ risk of viral rebound and potential development of resistance with missed doses.
- Advise patient to notify health care provider if signs and symptoms of allergic reaction (fever; generally ill feeling; tiredness; muscle or joint aches; trouble breathing; blisters or sores in mouth; blisters; redness or swelling of eyes; swelling of mouth, face, lips, or tongue), postinjection reactions (trouble breathing, stomach cramps, sweating, numbness of mouth, feeling anxious, feeling warm, feeling light-headed or faint, blood pressure changes), liver problems (yellow skin or white part of eyes; dark or tea-colored urine; light-colored stools; nausea or vomiting; loss of appetite; pain, aching, or tenderness on the right side of stomach area; itching), or depression (feeling sad or hopeless, feeling anxious or restless, have thoughts of hurting yourself [suicide], or have tried to hurt yourself) occur.
- Encourage consistent and correct condom use; communication of HIV-1 status to partner(s);

knowledge of partner(s)' HIV-1 status, including viral suppression status; and regular testing for sexually transmitted infections that can facilitate HIV-1 transmission.

- Instruct patient to notify health care provider of all Rx or OTC medications, vitamins, or herbal products being taken and consult health care provider before taking any new medications, especially St. John's wort.
- Rep: May cause fetal harm. Advise women of reproductive potential to use effective contraception during therapy and to avoid breastfeeding. Cabotegravir is detected in systemic circulation for ≥12 mo after discontinuing cabotegravir/rilpivirine. Inform patient of pregnancy exposure registry that monitors pregnancy outcomes in women exposed to cabotegravir. Register patients by calling the Antiretroviral Pregnancy Registry at 1-800-258-4263.

Evaluation/Desired Outcomes

- Decrease in viral load and improvement in CD4 cell counts.
- Delayed progression of HIV and decreased opportunistic infections in patients with HIV.

HIGH ALERT

cabozantinib (ka-boe-**zan**-ti-nib)

Cabometyx, Cometriq

Classification

Therapeutic: antineoplastics

Pharmacologic: kinase inhibitors

Indications

Cabometyx: Advanced renal cell carcinoma. First-line treatment of advanced renal cell carcinoma (in combination with nivolumab). Hepatocellular carcinoma in patients previously treated with sorafenib. Locally advanced or metastatic differentiated thyroid cancer that has progressed following prior vascular endothelial growth factor receptor-targeted therapy in patients who are refractory to or ineligible to receive radioactive iodine. Previously treated, unresectable, locally advanced or metastatic, well-differentiated pancreatic neuroendocrine tumors. Previously treated, unresectable, locally advanced or metastatic, well-differentiated extra-pancreatic neuroendocrine tumors. **Cometriq:** Progressive, metastatic medullary thyroid cancer.

Action

Inhibits tyrosine kinase, resulting in disruption of cellular function including tumor formation and progression. **Therapeutic Effects:** Improved survival with renal cell carcinoma and hepatocellular carcinoma. Decreased spread of medullary thyroid cancer. Improved progression-free survival with differentiated thyroid cancer and neuroendocrine tumors.

Pharmacokinetics

Absorption: Well absorbed following oral administration; food significantly enhances absorption.
Distribution: Extensively distributed to tissues.
Protein Binding: >99.7%.
Metabolism and Excretion: Highly metabolized by the liver, mostly by the CYP3A4 isoenzyme. 54% excreted in feces, 27% in urine (as metabolites).
Half-life: *Cometriq:* 55 hr; *Cabometyx:* 99 hr.

TIME/ACTION PROFILE (improved survival)

ROUTE	ONSET	PEAK	DURATION
PO	within 2 mo	unknown	14.7–21.4 mo

Contraindications/Precautions

Contraindicated in: Severe hepatic impairment; OB: Pregnancy; Lactation: Lactation.
Use Cautiously in: Elective surgical procedures (discontinue 28 days prior, if possible); Hypertension (control prior to treatment); Severe renal impairment; Moderate hepatic impairment (Cabometyx); Rep: Women of reproductive potential; Pedi: Safety and effectiveness not established in children <12 yr (differentiated thyroid cancer) or children <18 yr (all other indications).

Adverse Reactions/Side Effects

CV: hypertension, DEEP VEIN THROMBOSIS, MI. **Derm:** dry skin, hair color changes, palmar-plantar erythrodysesthesia (PPE), rash, impaired wound healing. **Endo:** hypothyroidism, ADRENAL INSUFFICIENCY (IN COMBINATION WITH NIVOLUMAB). **F and E:** hypocalcemia, hypophosphatemia, hypokalemia, hypomagnesemia, hyponatremia. **GI:** ↓ appetite, ↑ liver enzymes, abdominal pain, constipation, diarrhea, dyspepsia, HEPATOTOXICITY (IN COMBINATION WITH NIVOLUMAB), nausea, oral pain, stomatitis, vomiting, weight loss, GI PERFORATION/FISTULA. **GU:** proteinuria, infertility, nephrotic syndrome. **Hemat:** lymphopenia, neutropenia, thrombocytopenia, anemia, BLEEDING. **MS:** arthralgia, muscle spasms, osteonecrosis of the jaw. **Neuro:** dizziness, dysgeusia, fatigue, headache, POSTERIOR REVERSIBLE ENCEPHALOPATHY SYNDROME (PRES), STROKE. **Resp:** cough, dyspnea, PULMONARY EMBOLISM.

Interactions

Drug-Drug: Strong CYP3A4 inhibitors, including **atazanavir, clarithromycin, conivaptan, itraconazole, ketoconazole, lopinavir/ritonavir, nefazodone, nelfinavir, posaconazole, ritonavir,** and **voriconazole,** may ↑ levels and risk of toxicity;

avoid concurrent use, if possible. If concurrent use necessary, ↓ cabozantinib dose. **Strong CYP3A4 inducers**, including **carbamazepine**, **dexamethasone**, **phenobarbital**, **phenytoin**, **rifabutin**, **rifampin**, and **rifapentine**, may ↓ levels and effectiveness; avoid concurrent use, if possible. If concurrent use necessary, ↓ cabozantinib dose. **MRP2 inhibitors**, including **abacavir**, **adefovir**, **cidofovir**, **furosemide**, **lamivudine**, **nevirapine**, **ritonavir**, **probenecid**, and **tenofovir**, may ↑ levels and risk of toxicity.
Drug-Natural Products: St. John's wort may ↓ levels and effectiveness; avoid concurrent use.
Drug-Food: Grapefruit juice may ↑ levels and risk of toxicity; avoid concurrent use.

Route/Dosage

Capsules and tablets are not interchangeable.

Cabometyx

Advanced Renal Cell Carcinoma

PO (Adults): *As monotherapy:* 60 mg once daily until disease progression or unacceptable toxicity. *With nivolumab:* 40 mg once daily until disease progression or unacceptable toxicity. *Concurrent use of strong CYP3A4 inhibitor (as monotherapy):* 40 mg once daily until disease progression or unacceptable toxicity (resume full dose 2–3 days after discontinuing inhibitor). *Concurrent use of strong CYP3A4 inhibitor (with nivolumab):* 20 mg once daily until disease progression or unacceptable toxicity (resume full dose 2–3 days after discontinuing inhibitor). *Concurrent use of strong CYP3A4 inducer (as monotherapy):* 80 mg once daily until disease progression or unacceptable toxicity (resume full dose 2–3 days after discontinuing inducer). *Concurrent use of strong CYP3A4 inducer (with nivolumab):* 60 mg once daily until disease progression or unacceptable toxicity (resume full dose 2–3 days after discontinuing inducer).

Hepatic Impairment

PO (Adults): *Moderate hepatic impairment:* 40 mg once daily until disease progression or unacceptable toxicity.

Hepatocellular Carcinoma

PO (Adults): 60 mg once daily until disease progression or unacceptable toxicity. *Concurrent use of strong CYP3A4 inhibitor:* 40 mg once daily until disease progression or unacceptable toxicity (resume full dose 2–3 days after discontinuing inhibitor). *Concurrent use of strong CYP3A4 inducer:* 80 mg once daily until disease progression or unacceptable toxicity (resume full dose 2–3 days after discontinuing inducer).

Hepatic Impairment

PO (Adults): *Moderate hepatic impairment:* 40 mg once daily until disease progression or unacceptable toxicity.

Differentiated Thyroid Cancer and Neuroendocrine Tumors

PO (Adults and Children ≥12 yr and ≥40 kg): 60 mg once daily until disease progression or unacceptable toxicity. *Concurrent use of strong CYP3A4 inhibitor:* 40 mg once daily until disease progression or unacceptable toxicity (resume full dose 2–3 days after discontinuing inhibitor). *Concurrent use of strong CYP3A4 inducer:* 80 mg once daily until disease progression or unacceptable toxicity (resume full dose 2–3 days after discontinuing inducer).
PO (Adults and Children ≥12 yr and <40 kg): 40 mg once daily until disease progression or unacceptable toxicity. *Concurrent use of strong CYP3A4 inhibitor:* 20 mg once daily until disease progression or unacceptable toxicity (resume full dose 2–3 days after discontinuing inhibitor). *Concurrent use of strong CYP3A4 inducer:* 60 mg once daily until disease progression or unacceptable toxicity (resume full dose 2–3 days after discontinuing inducer).

Hepatic Impairment

PO (Adults and Children ≥12 yr and BSA ≥1.2 m^2): 40 mg once daily until disease progression or unacceptable toxicity.

Hepatic Impairment

PO (Adults and Children ≥12 yr and BSA <1.2 m^2): 20 mg once daily until disease progression or unacceptable toxicity.

Cometriq

PO (Adults): 140 mg once daily until disease progression or unacceptable toxicity. *Concurrent use of strong CYP3A4 inhibitor:* 100 mg once daily until disease progression or unacceptable toxicity (resume full dose 4 days after discontinuing inhibitor). *Concurrent use of strong CYP3A4 inducer:* 180 mg once daily until disease progression or unacceptable toxicity (resume full dose 2–3 days after discontinuing inducer).

Hepatic Impairment

PO (Adults): *Mild or moderate hepatic impairment:* 80 mg once daily.

Availability (generic available)

Capsules (Cometriq): 20 mg, 80 mg. **Tablets (Cabometyx):** 20 mg, 40 mg, 60 mg.

NURSING IMPLICATIONS

Assessment

- Monitor BP prior to and periodically during therapy. *If hypertension occurs,* do not initiate, or hold therapy and manage medically; once BP controlled, resume cabozantinib at ↓ dose. *If uncontrollable, severe hypertension or hypertensive crisis occurs,* permanently discontinue cabozantinib.

C

- Monitor for symptoms of perforations and fistulas, including abscess (severe abdominal pain, coughing, gagging, choking especially when eating or drinking, abscess, sepsis). *If symptoms occur,* permanently discontinue cabozantinib.
- Monitor for diarrhea. *If intolerable Grade 2, Grade 3 not managed with treatment, or Grade 4 diarrhea occur,* hold cabozantinib until Grade 1; then resume at ↓ dose.
- Monitor for signs and symptoms of PPE. *If intolerable Grade 2 or Grade 3 PPE occurs,* hold cabozantinib until Grade 1; then resume at ↓ dose.
- Perform an oral examination for inflammation, infection, or ulceration prior to and periodically during therapy.
- Evaluate patients with seizures, headache, visual disturbances, confusion, or altered mental status for PRES via MRI. *If PRES confirmed,* permanently discontinue cabozantinib.
- Monitor for signs and symptoms of adrenal insufficiency. *If Grade ≥2 adrenal insufficiency occurs,* begin symptomatic treatment and hormone replacement therapy. May require holding cabozantinib.
- Pedi: Physeal and longitudinal growth monitoring is recommended in children with open growth plates.

Lab Test Considerations

- Verify negative pregnancy test before starting therapy.
- Monitor urine protein periodically during therapy. *If nephrotic syndrome occurs,* discontinue cabozantinib.
- Monitor CBC with differential periodically during therapy. May ↓ WBC, ANC, hemoglobin, lymphocytes, and platelets.
- Monitor liver enzymes prior to and periodically during therapy and more frequently when used in combination with other drugs. May ↑ AST, ALT, and alkaline phosphatase. **When used with nivolumab:** *If ALT or AST >3 times upper limit of normal (ULN) but ≤10 times ULN with concurrent total bilirubin <2 times ULN,* hold cabozantinib and nivolumab until recovery to Grade ≤1. *If ALT or AST >10 times ULN or >3 times ULN with concurrent total bilirubin ≥2 times ULN,* permanently discontinue both cabozantinib and nivolumab.
- May cause hypophosphatemia, hyperbilirubinemia, hypomagnesemia, hypokalemia, hyponatremia, lymphopenia, neutropenia, and thrombocytopenia.
- Monitor thyroid function periodically during therapy and manage dysfunction as needed.
- Monitor calcium levels and replace calcium as necessary during treatment. Hold; then resume at ↓ dose upon recovery or permanently discontinue cabozantinib depending on severity.

Implementation

- Do not confuse Cometriq with coenzyme Q10.
- Do not interchange tablets and capsules.
- Stop treatment ≥21 days before scheduled surgery, including dental surgery. Do not resume therapy for ≥14 days after major surgery and until the wound is adequately healed. Hold doses in patients with dehiscence or wound-healing complications.
- Permanently discontinue cabozantinib if severe hemorrhage, serious arterial thrombotic event (MI, cerebral infarction), or osteonecrosis of the jaw occur.
- **PO:** *Cometriq*: Administer 140 mg dose as one 80-mg and three 20-mg capsules on an empty stomach ≥1 hr before or 2 hr after meals. ***DNC:*** Swallow capsules whole; do not open, crush, or chew.
- **Dose Reduction Schedule (Cometriq):** Upon resolution of adverse reactions to Grade ≤1: hold cabozantinib; resume at ↓ dose once Grade ≤1. *If previous dose was 140 mg once daily*, resume at 100 mg once daily. *If previous dose was 100 mg once daily*, resume at 60 mg once daily. *If previous dose was 60 mg once daily*, resume at 60 mg once daily as tolerated or discontinue.
- **PO:** *Cabometyx*: Administer tablet on an empty stomach with ≥8 ounces of water ≥1 hr before or 2 hr after meals. ***DNC:*** Swallow tablet whole; do not break, crush, or chew.
- **Dose Reduction Schedule (Cabometyx):** Upon resolution of adverse reactions to Grade ≤1: *If previous dose was 60 mg once daily,* ↓ to 40 mg once daily. 2nd dose reduction: ↓ to 20 mg once daily. *If previous dose was 40 mg once daily,* ↓ to 20 mg once daily. 2nd dose reduction: ↓ to 20 mg every other day. *If previous dose was 40 mg once daily (with nivolumab)*, ↓ to 20 mg every other day.

Patient/Family Teaching

- Explain purpose and side effects of medication. Advise patient to read *Patient Information* before starting therapy. Take missed doses as soon as remembered if within 12 hr of dose; then take next dose at regularly scheduled time. If >12 hr, omit dose and take next dose at normal time; do not double doses.
- Advise patient to avoid grapefruit, grapefruit juice, and any foods or supplements that contain grapefruit during therapy.
- Caution patient to notify health care provider immediately if signs and symptoms of hemorrhage

(coughing up blood or blood clots, vomiting blood or coffee-ground-like vomit, red or black tarry stools, menstrual bleeding heavier than usual, any unusual or heavy bleeding); perforation or fistula (abdominal pain or tenderness); stroke or heart attack (swelling or pain in hands, arms, feet, or legs; shortness of breath; unusual sweating; numbness or weakness of face, arm, or leg, especially on one side of body; sudden confusion or trouble speaking or understanding; sudden trouble seeing in one or both eyes; sudden trouble walking; dizziness; loss of balance or coordination; sudden severe headache); diarrhea; PPE (rash, redness, pain, swelling, or blisters on palms or soles of feet); swelling in hands, arms, legs, or feet; jaw pain; toothache or sores on gums; or PRES occur.

- Instruct patient to notify health care provider if signs and symptoms of hand-foot skin reactions (progressive or intolerable rash, redness, pain, swelling, blisters on hands or soles of feet); severe diarrhea; mouth sores; oral pain; changes in taste; severe nausea or vomiting, preventing eating or drinking; or weight loss occur.
- Advise patient to notify health care provider of all Rx or OTC medications, vitamins, or herbal products being taken and to consult with health care provider before taking other medications, especially St. John's wort.
- Instruct patient to maintain good oral hygiene and regular dentist exams during therapy. If jaw pain, toothache, or sores on gums occur, notify health care provider.
- Advise patient to notify health care provider of medication regimen prior to treatment or surgery. Therapy must be stopped 28 days before planned surgery, including dental procedures.
- Rep: May cause fetal harm. Advise women of reproductive potential and men with female partners of reproductive potential to use effective contraception during therapy and for ≥4 mo after completion of therapy and to avoid breastfeeding during therapy and for 4 mo following last dose. May impair fertility in men and women.

Evaluation/Desired Outcomes

- ↓ spread of metastatic medullary thyroid cancer.
- Improved survival with renal cell carcinoma and hepatocellular carcinoma.
- Improved progression-free survival with differentiated thyroid cancer and neuroendocrine tumors.

calcifediol, See VITAMIN D COMPOUNDS.

calcitriol, See VITAMIN D COMPOUNDS.

CALCIUM CHANNEL BLOCKERS

amLODIPine (am-**loe**-di-peen)
Katerzia, Norliqva, Norvasc

diltiazem (dil-**tye**-a-zem)
Cardizem, Cardizem CD, Cardizem LA, Cartia XT, ~~Taztia XT~~, Tiazac, 🍁 Tiazac XC

felodipine (fe-**loe**-di-peen)
🍁 Plendil

isradipine (is-**ra**-di-peen)
~~DynaCirc~~

niCARdipine (nye-**kar**-di-peen)
Cardene IV

NIFEdipine (nye-**fed**-i-peen)
~~Adalat CC~~, 🍁 Adalat XL, ~~Afeditab CR~~, Procardia, Procardia XL

niMODipine (nye-**moe**-di-peen)
🍁 Nimotop, Nymalize

nisoldipine (nye-**sole**-di-peen)
Sular

verapamil (ver-**ap**-a-mil)
~~Calan, Calan SR, Verelan~~, Verelan PM

Classification
Therapeutic: antianginals, antiarrhythmics, antihypertensives

Indications

Hypertension. Angina pectoris. Vasospastic (Prinzmetal) angina. **Nimodipine:** Subarachnoid hemorrhage

Action

Inhibits the transport of calcium into myocardial and vascular smooth muscle cells, resulting in inhibition of excitation-contraction coupling and subsequent contraction. **Diltiazem, verapamil:** Decrease SA and AV conduction and prolong AV node refractory period in conduction tissue. **Therapeutic Effects:** Systemic vasodilation resulting in decreased BP. Coronary vasodilation resulting in decreased frequency and severity of attacks of angina. **Nimodipine:** Prevention of vascular spasm after subarachnoid hemorrhage, resulting in decreased neurologic impairment. **Diltiazem, verapamil:** Reduction of ventricular rate during atrial fibrillation or flutter.

Pharmacokinetics

Absorption: *Amlodipine:* Well absorbed after oral administration (64–90%); *Diltiazem* and *verapamil:* Well absorbed after oral administration but rapidly metabolized; *Felodipine*, *isradipine*, *nicardipine*, *nimodipine*, and *nisoldipine:* Well absorbed after oral administration but extensively metabolized, resulting in ↓ bioavailability; *Nifedipine:* Well absorbed after oral administration but rapidly metabolized, resulting in ↓ bioavailability (45–70%); bioavailability is ↑ (80%) with extended-release forms.

Distribution: *Amlodipine, diltiazem, isradipine, nicardipine, verapamil:* Well distributed to tissues; *nimodipine:* Crosses the blood-brain barrier.

Metabolism and Excretion: All agents are mostly metabolized by the liver; ≤10% excreted unchanged by kidneys.

Half-life: *Amlodipine:* 30–50 hr; *diltiazem:* 3.5–9 hr; *felodipine:* 11–16 hr; *isradipine:* 8 hr; *nicardipine:* 2–4 hr; *nifedipine:* 2–5 hr; *nimodipine:* 1–2 hr; *verapamil:* 4.5–12 hr.

TIME/ACTION PROFILE (cardiovascular effects)

ROUTE	ONSET	PEAK	DURATION
Amlodipine PO	unknown	6–9	24 hr
Diltiazem PO	30 min	2–3 hr	6–8 hr
Diltiazem PO-CD	unknown	14 days†	24 hr
Diltiazem PO-XR	unknown	14 days†	24 hr
Diltiazem IV	2–5 min	unknown	unknown
Felodipine PO	1 hr	2–4 hr	up to 24 hr
Isradipine PO	<2 hr	2–3 hr	12 hr
Nicardipine PO	20 min	1–2 hr	8 hr
Nicardipine IV	within min	45 min	50 hr‡
Nifedipine PO	20 min	unknown	6–8 hr
Nifedipine PO-ER	unknown	unknown	24 hr
Nimodipine PO	unknown	1 hr	unknown
Nisoldipine	unknown	6–12 hr	24 hr
Verapamil PO	1–2 hr	30–90 min	3–7 hr
Verapamil PO-ER	unknown	5–7 hr	24 hr
Verapamil IV	1–5 min	3–5 min	2 hr

† Maximum antihypertensive effect with chronic therapy.
‡ After discontinuation.
Single dose; effects from multiple doses may not be evident for 24–48 hr.
Antiarrhythmic effects; hemodynamic effects begin 3–5 min after injection and persist for 10–20 min.

Contraindications/Precautions

Contraindicated in: Hypersensitivity (cross-sensitivity may occur); Sick sinus syndrome; 2nd- or 3rd-degree heart block (unless artificial pacemaker is in place); BP <90 mmHg (especially with diltiazem and verapamil); Recent MI or pulmonary congestion (diltiazem only); HF, severe ventricular dysfunction, or cardiogenic shock, unless associated with supraventricular tachyarrhythmias (diltiazem and verapamil only); Concurrent use of IV beta blocker (IV diltiazem and verapamil only); Advanced aortic stenosis (nicardipine only); Concurrent use of strong CYP3A4 inhibitors (nimodipine only); Concurrent use of strong CYP3A4 inducers (nifedipine and nimodipine only).

Use Cautiously in: Severe hepatic impairment (dose ↓ recommended for most agents); Severe renal impairment (dose ↓ of nicardipine may be necessary); History of serious ventricular arrhythmias or HF; History of porphyria (nifedipine); OB: Use during pregnancy only if potential maternal benefit justifies potential fetal risk; extended-release nifedipine preferred during pregnancy; Lactation: Use while breastfeeding only if potential maternal benefit justifies potential risk to infant; Pedi: Safety and effectiveness not established in children <18 yr (diltiazem, felodipine, nicardipine, nifedipine, nimodipine, nisoldipine), <6 yr (amlodipine); Geri: Dose ↓/slower IV infusion rates recommended for most agents in older adults; ↑ risk of hypotension; consider age-related ↓ in body mass, ↓ hepatic/renal/cardiac function, concurrent drug therapy and other disease states in older adults.

Adverse Reactions/Side Effects

CV: peripheral edema (with amlodipine, felodipine, nifedipine), ARRHYTHMIAS, HF, bradycardia, chest pain, hypotension, palpitations, syncope, tachycardia. **Derm:** ↑ sweating, dermatitis, erythema multiforme, flushing (with nifedipine, nicardipine), photosensitivity, pruritus/urticaria, rash, STEVENS-JOHNSON SYNDROME (SJS). **EENT:** blurred vision, disturbed equilibrium, epistaxis, tinnitus. **Endo:** gynecomastia, hyperglycemia. **GI:** ↑ liver enzymes, anorexia, constipation, diarrhea, dry mouth, dyspepsia, GI obstruction (with nifedipine), gingival hyperplasia, nausea, ulcer (with nifedipine), vomiting. **GU:** dysuria, nocturia, polyuria, sexual dysfunction, urinary frequency. **Hemat:** anemia, leukopenia, thrombocytopenia. **Metab:** weight gain. **MS:** joint stiffness, muscle cramps. **Neuro:** abnormal dreams, anxiety, confusion, dizziness, drowsiness, dysgeusia, headache (with nifedipine, isradipine, felodipine), nervousness, paresthesia, psychiatric disturbances, tremor, weakness. **Resp:** cough, dyspnea.

Interactions

Drug-Drug: **Strong CYP3A4 inhibitors**, including **clarithromycin**, **nelfinavir**, **ritonavir**, **ketoconazole**, **itraconazole**, **posaconazole**, **voriconazole**, **conivaptan**, and **nefazodone**, may ↑ levels and risk of toxicity; avoid concurrent use with nimodipine. **Strong CYP3A4 inducers**, including **carbamazepine**, **phenobarbital**, **phenytoin**, and **rifampin**, may ↓ levels and effectiveness; avoid concurrent use with nifedipine and nimodipine. Additive hypotension may occur with acute ingestion of **alcohol**, **quinidine**, **fentanyl**, **nitrates**, or other **antihypertensives**. Antihypertensive effects may be ↓

by **NSAIDs**. Diltiazem, nifedipine, and verapamil may ↑ levels and risk of toxicity of **digoxin**. Concurrent use of diltiazem or verapamil with **beta blockers**, **digoxin**, **clonidine**, or **ivabradine** may ↑ risk of bradycardia. Amlodipine, diltiazem, and verapamil may ↑ risk of myopathy with **simvastatin** and **lovastatin**; do not exceed simvastatin dose of 20 mg/day (with amlodipine) or 10 mg/day (with diltiazem or verapamil); do not exceed lovastatin dose of 20 mg/day (with diltiazem or verapamil). **Phenobarbital** and **phenytoin** may ↓ levels and effectiveness of diltiazem. **Cimetidine** and **propranolol** may ↑ levels and risk of toxicity of diltiazem, felodipine, nicardipine, or nifedipine. Amlodipine, diltiazem, nicardipine, nifedipine, and verapamil may ↑ levels and risk of toxicity of **carbamazepine**, **cyclosporine**, **tacrolimus**, **prazosin**, or **quinidine**. Verapamil may ↑ muscle-paralyzing effects of **nondepolarizing neuromuscular blocking agents**. Effectiveness of verapamil may be ↓ by coadministration with **vitamin D** and calcium. Verapamil may alter **lithium** levels. Concurrent use of verapamil with **erythromycin** or **clarithromycin** may ↑ risk of hypotension and bradycardia. Verapamil may ↑ levels and risk of toxicity of **doxorubicin** and **paclitaxel**. Concurrent use of verapamil with **aspirin** may ↑ risk of bleeding. ↑ risk of GI obstruction when nifedipine used concurrently with **H_2 blockers**, **opioids**, **NSAIDs**, **laxatives**, **anticholinergic drugs**, **levothyroxine**, or **neuromuscular blockers**. Concurrent use of verapamil with **sirolimus**, **temsirolimus**, or **everolimus** may ↑ levels of sirolimus, temsirolimus, everolimus, and verapamil; consider ↓ dose of sirolimus, temsirolimus, everolimus, and verapamil.

Drug-Natural Products: Verapamil ↑ caffeine levels with caffeine-containing herbs (cola nut, guarana, mate, tea, coffee). **St. John's wort** may significantly ↓ levels and effectiveness; concurrent use is contraindicated.

Drug-Food: Grapefruit juice may ↑ levels and risk of toxicity of **felodipine**, **nifedipine**, **nimodipine**, **nicardipine**, **nisoldipine**, and **verapamil**; avoid concurrent use with nifedipine and nimodipine.

Route/Dosage

Amlodipine

PO (Adults): 5–10 mg once daily; *Fragile or small patients or patients already receiving other antihypertensives:* Initiate at 2.5 mg/day; ↑ as required/tolerated (up to 10 mg/day) as an antihypertensive therapy with 2.5 mg/day in patients with hepatic impairment.

PO (Geriatric Patients): *Hypertension:* Initiate therapy at 2.5 mg/day; ↑ as required/tolerated (up to 10 mg/day); *Angina:* Initiate therapy at 5 mg/day; ↑ as required/tolerated (up to 10 mg/day).

PO (Children 6–17 yr): 2.5–5 mg once daily.

Hepatic Impairment

PO (Adults): *Hypertension:* Initiate therapy at 2.5 mg/day; ↑ as required/tolerated (up to 10 mg/day); *Angina:* Initiate therapy at 5 mg/day; ↑ as required/tolerated (up to 10 mg/day).

Diltiazem

PO (Adults): Immediate release: 30–120 mg 3–4 times daily. Extended release: 120–240 mg once daily (up to 360 mg/day); *Concurrent use of simvastatin:* Diltiazem dose should not exceed 240 mg/day, and simvastatin dose should not exceed 10 mg/day.

IV (Adults): 0.25 mg/kg; may repeat in 15 min with a dose of 0.35 mg/kg. May follow with continuous infusion at 10 mg/hr (range 5–15 mg/hr) for up to 24 hr.

Felodipine

PO (Adults): 5 mg/day initially (2.5 mg/day in older adults). May ↑ every 2 wk. Usual daily dose is 5–10 mg (not to exceed 20 mg/day).

Isradipine

PO (Adults): 2.5 mg twice daily; may ↑ every 2–4 wk by 5 mg/day (not to exceed 20 mg/day).

Nicardipine

PO (Adults): *Immediate release:* 20 mg 3 times daily; may ↑ every 3 days (range 20–40 mg 3 times daily). *Extended release:* 30 mg twice daily (up to 60 mg twice daily).

IV (Adults): *Substitute for PO nicardipine:* If PO dose is 20 mg every 8 hr, then infusion rate is 0.5 mg/hr; if PO dose is 30 mg every 8 hr, then infusion rate is 1.2 mg/hr; if PO dose is 40 mg every 8 hr, then infusion rate is 2.2 mg/hr. *Patients not receiving PO nicardipine:* Initiate therapy at 5 mg/hr; may ↑ by 2.5 mg every 5–15 min as needed (up to 15 mg/hr).

Nifedipine

PO (Adults): *Immediate release:* 10–30 mg 3 times daily (not to exceed 180 mg/day); *Extended release:* 30–90 mg once daily (not to exceed 90–120 mg/day).

Nimodipine

PO (Adults): 60 mg every 4 hr for 21 days; therapy should be started within 96 hr of subarachnoid hemorrhage.

Nisoldipine

PO (Adults): 20 mg once daily; may ↑ by 10 mg/day every 7 days (range 20–40 mg/day; not to exceed 60 mg/day).

Verapamil

PO (Adults): 80–120 mg 3 times daily; ↑ as needed. *Patients with poor ventricular function or hepatic impairment, or older adults:* Immediate release: 40 mg 3 times daily initially. Extended release:

120–240 mg once daily; may ↑ as needed (range 240–480 mg/day).
PO (Geriatric Patients): *Immediate release:* 40 mg 3 times daily initially.
PO (Children <15 yr): 4–8 mg/kg/day in divided doses.
IV (Adults): 5–10 mg (75–150 mcg/kg); may repeat with 10 mg after 30 min.
IV (Children 1–15 yr): 100–300 mcg/kg; may repeat after 30 min (initial dose not to exceed 5 mg; repeat dose not to exceed 10 mg).
IV (Children <1 yr): 100–200 mcg/kg.

Availability

Amlodipine (generic available)
Tablets: 2.5 mg, 5 mg, 10 mg. **Oral solution (Norliqva) (peppermint flavor):** 1 mg/mL. **Oral suspension (Katerzia):** 1 mg/mL. ***In combination with***: aliskiren/hydrochlorothiazide (Amturnide), atorvastatin (Caduet), benazepril (Lotrel), olmesartan (Azor), olmesartan/hydrochlorothiazide (Tribenzor), telmisartan, telmisartan/indapamide (Widaplik), valsartan (Exforge), and valsartan/hydrochlorothiazide (Exforge HCT). See Appendix N.

Diltiazem (generic available)
Tablets: 30 mg, 60 mg, 90 mg, 120 mg. **Extended-release capsules (Cardizem CD, Tiazac, Cartia XT):** 120 mg, 180 mg, 240 mg, 300 mg, 360 mg, 420 mg. **Extended-release tablets (Cardizem LA):** 120 mg, 180 mg, 240 mg, 300 mg, 360 mg, 420 mg. **Solution for injection:** 5 mg/mL.

Felodipine (generic available)
Extended-release tablets: 2.5 mg, 5 mg, 10 mg.

Isradipine (generic available)
Capsules: 2.5 mg, 5 mg.

Nicardipine (generic available)
Capsules: 20 mg, 30 mg. **Premixed infusion:** 20 mg/200 mL dextrose 4.8% in water or 0.86% NaCl, 40 mg/200 mL 0.83% NaCl. **Solution for injection:** 2.5 mg/mL.

Nifedipine (generic available)
Capsules: 🍁 5 mg, 10 mg, 20 mg. **Tablets:** 🍁 10 mg. **Extended-release tablets (Nifedical XL, Procardia XL):** 🍁 10 mg, 🍁 20 mg, 30 mg, 60 mg, 90 mg.

Nimodipine (generic available)
Capsules: 30 mg. **Oral solution:** 6 mg/mL.

Nisoldipine (generic available)
Extended-release tablets: 20 mg, 30 mg, 40 mg. **Geomatrix extended-release tablets:** 8.5 mg, 17 mg, 25.5 mg, 34 mg.

Verapamil (generic available)
Immediate-release tablets: 40 mg, 80 mg, 120 mg. **Extended-release capsules:** 120 mg, 180 mg, 240 mg, 360 mg. **Extended-release capsules (Verelan PM):** 100 mg, 200 mg, 300 mg. **Extended-release tablets:** 120 mg, 180 mg, 240 mg. **Solution for injection:** 2.5 mg/mL. ***In combination with***: trandolapril (Tarka); see Appendix N.

NURSING IMPLICATIONS

Assessment
- Monitor BP and HR before therapy, during dose titration, and periodically during therapy. Monitor ECG at baseline and then periodically during prolonged therapy.
- Monitor intake and output and daily weight. Assess for signs of HF (peripheral edema, rales/crackles, dyspnea, weight gain, jugular venous distention).
- Assess for rash or signs and symptoms of SJS periodically during therapy (fever, general malaise, fatigue, muscle or joint aches, blisters, oral lesions, conjunctivitis, hepatitis, eosinophilia). *If SJS occurs,* discontinue therapy and provide supportive care.
- **Angina:** Assess location, duration, intensity, and precipitating factors of patient's anginal pain.
- **Hypertension:** BP should be checked monthly when initiating or adjusting therapy and then every 3–6 mo once BP goals have been met.
- **Arrhythmias:** Monitor ECG continuously during administration. Report bradycardia or prolonged hypotension promptly. Emergency equipment and medication should be available.
- **Nimodipine:** Assess patient's neurologic status (level of consciousness, movement) before and periodically after administration.
- Patients receiving digoxin concurrently with diltiazem, nifedipine, or verapamil should have routine serum digoxin level and be monitored for signs and symptoms of digoxin toxicity.

Lab Test Considerations
- Total serum calcium concentrations are not affected by calcium channel blockers.
- Monitor serum potassium periodically. Hypokalemia ↑ risk of arrhythmias; should be corrected.
- Monitor renal and hepatic functions periodically during long-term therapy. Several days of therapy may cause ↑ in liver enzymes, which return to normal on discontinuation of therapy.
- Nifedipine may cause positive antinuclear antibody (ANA) and direct Coombs test results.
- Nimodipine may occasionally cause ↓ platelet count.

Implementation

- Do not confuse amlodipine with amiloride. Do not confuse diltiazem with diazepam. Do not confuse nicardipine with nifedipine or nimodipine. Do not confuse Cardizem with Cardene. Do not confuse Tiazac with Ziac.
- **PO:** May be administered without regard to meals. Administer with meals if GI irritation becomes a problem. Administer *verapamil* with meals or milk to minimize gastric irritation. *Cardizem and felodipine* should be taken on empty stomach or with a light meal. Administer *nisoldipine* on an empty stomach 2 hr after or 1 hr before meals.
- *DNC:* Do not open, crush, break, or chew sustained-release capsules or tablets. Empty tablets that appear in stool are not significant.
- Crush and mix diltiazem tablets with food or fluids for patients having difficulty swallowing.
- *Tiazac* capsules may be opened and contents sprinkled on a spoonful of applesauce. Swallow immediately without chewing and follow with full glass of water; do not store mixture or subdivide capsule contents.
- *Norliqva* is a pale straw-colored solution stored at room temperature. *Katerzia* is a white to off-white liquid suspension that should be refrigerated. Shake before using.

Nifedipine

- Sublingual use is not recommended due to serious adverse drug reactions.

Nimodipine

- Administer by PO route ONLY; administration via IV or parenterally may cause serious adverse events, including death.
- **PO:** If patient is unable to swallow capsule, make a hole in both ends of the capsule with a sterile 18-gauge needle and extract the contents into a syringe that cannot accept a needle and is labeled "Not for IV Use." Empty contents into water or nasogastric (NG) tube and flush with 30-mL normal saline.
- Administer oral solution 1 hr before or 2 hr after meals. For administration via NG or gastric tube, administer via syringe included; then refill syringe with 20 mL of 0.9% saline water solution; flush remaining contents from NG or gastric tube into stomach.

IV Administration

Diltiazem

- **IV Push: Dilution:** Administer bolus dose undiluted. **Concentration:** 5 mg/mL. **Rate:** Administer over 2 min.
- **Continuous Infusion: Dilution:** Dilute 125 mg in 100 mL, 250 mg in 250 mL, or 250 mg in 500 mL of 0.9% NaCl, D5W, or D5/0.45% NaCl. **Concentration:** 0.45–1 mg/mL. Stable for 24 hr at room temperature or if refrigerated.
- **Rate:** See Route/Dosage section. Titrate to patient's HR and BP response.
- **Y-Site Compatibility:** albumin, alemtuzumab, amikacin, aminocaproic acid, amiodarone, amphotericin B deoxycholate, anidulafungin, argatroban, arsenic trioxide, atracurium, azithromycin, aztreonam, bivalirudin, bleomycin, bumetanide, buprenorphine, busulfan, butorphanol, calcium chloride, calcium gluconate, cangrelor, carboplatin, carmustine, caspofungin, cefazolin, cefotaxime, cefotetan, cefoxitin, ceftaroline, ceftazidime, ceftolozane/tazobactam, ceftriaxone, cefuroxime, chlorpromazine, ciprofloxacin, cisatracurium, cisplatin, clindamycin, cyclophosphamide, cyclosporine, cytarabine, dacarbazine, dactinomycin, daptomycin, daunorubicin, dexamethasone, dexmedetomidine, dexrazoxane, digoxin, diphenhydramine, dobutamine, docetaxel, dopamine, doxorubicin, doxycycline, droperidol, enalaprilat, ephedrine, epinephrine, epirubicin, eptifibatide, ertapenem, erythromycin, esmolol, etoposide, etoposide phosphate, famotidine, fentanyl, fluconazole, fludarabine, foscarnet, fosphenytoin, gemcitabine, gentamicin, glycopyrrolate, granisetron, haloperidol, hetastarch, hydralazine, hydromorphone, idarubicin, ifosfamide, imipenem/cilastatin, imipenem/cilastatin/relebactam, irinotecan, isoproterenol, labetalol, leucovorin, levofloxacin, lidocaine, linezolid, lorazepam, magnesium sulfate, mannitol, melphalan, meperidine, meropenem, meropenem/vaborbactam, mesna, methadone, metoclopramide, metoprolol, metronidazole, midazolam, milrinone, mitoxantrone, morphine, moxifloxacin, multivitamins, mycophenolate, nalbuphine, naloxone, nicardipine, nitroglycerin, nitroprusside, norepinephrine, octreotide, ondansetron, oxacillin, oxaliplatin, oxytocin, paclitaxel, palonosetron, pamidronate, pemetrexed, penicillin G potassium, pentamidine, phentolamine, phenylephrine, potassium acetate, potassium chloride, potassium phosphate, prochlorperazine, promethazine, propranolol, remifentanil, rocuronium, sodium acetate, succinylcholine, sufentanil, sulbactam/durlobactam, tacrolimus, telavancin, theophylline, thiotepa, tigecycline, tirofiban, tobramycin, topotecan, trimethoprim/sulfamethoxazole, vancomycin, vasopressin, vecuronium, verapamil, vinblastine, vincristine, vinorelbine, voriconazole, zidovudine, zoledronic acid.
- **Y-Site Incompatibility:** allopurinol, amphotericin B liposomal, cefepime, ceftobiprole, chloramphenicol, dantrolene, diazepam, doxorubicin liposomal, fluorouracil, furosemide, ganciclovir, gemtuzumab ozogamicin, ketorolac, letermovir, methotrexate, micafungin, mitomycin,

pantoprazole, pentobarbital, phenobarbital, phenytoin, piperacillin/tazobactam, rifampin.

Nicardipine

- To transfer from IV nicardipine infusion to oral therapy with other antihypertensive, start oral therapy simultaneously with discontinuation of nicardipine infusion. If transferring to oral nicardipine therapy, administer 1st dose of a 3-times-a-day regimen 1 hr before discontinuation of infusion.
- **Continuous Infusion: Dilution:** Dilute each 25-mg ampule/vial with 240 mL of D5W, D5/0.45% NaCl, D5/0.9% NaCl, D5/potassium chloride 40 mEq, 0.45% NaCl, or 0.9% NaCl. **Concentration:** 0.1 mg/mL. Stable for 24 hr at room temperature.
- **Rate:** See Route/Dosage section. Titrate rate according to BP response. Administer through large peripheral veins or central veins to ↓ risk of venous thrombosis, phlebitis, local irritation, swelling, extravasation, and vascular impairment. Change infusion site every 12 hr to minimize risk of peripheral venous irritation.
- **Y-Site Compatibility:** alemtuzumab, amikacin, amiodarone, anidulafungin, argatroban, arsenic trioxide, atracurium, aztreonam, bivalirudin, bleomycin, bumetanide, buprenorphine, butorphanol, calcium chloride, calcium gluconate, carboplatin, carmustine, caspofungin, cefazolin, cefiderocol, cefotaxime, cefotetan, cefoxitin, ceftriaxone, chloramphenicol, chlorpromazine, ciprofloxacin, cisatracurium, cisplatin, clevidipine, cyclophosphamide, cyclosporine, cytarabine, dacarbazine, daptomycin, dexmedetomidine, dexrazoxane, digoxin, diltiazem, diphenhydramine, dobutamine, docetaxel, dopamine, doxorubicin hydrochloride, doxorubicin liposomal, doxycycline, droperidol, enalaprilat, ephedrine, epinephrine, epirubicin, eptifibatide, eravacycline, erythromycin, esmolol, etoposide, etoposide phosphate, famotidine, fentanyl, fluconazole, gemcitabine, gentamicin, granisetron, haloperidol, hetastarch, hydromorphone, idarubicin, ifosfamide, irinotecan, isavuconazonium, isoproterenol, labetalol, leucovorin, levofloxacin, lidocaine, linezolid, magnesium sulfate, mannitol, meperidine, methadone, metoclopramide, metoprolol, metronidazole, midazolam, milrinone, mitoxantrone, morphine, moxifloxacin, mycophenolate, nafcillin, nalbuphine, naloxone, nitroglycerin, nitroprusside, norepinephrine, octreotide, ondansetron, oxaliplatin, oxytocin, paclitaxel, palonosetron, pamidronate, penicillin G potassium, pentamidine, phenylephrine, plazomicin, potassium chloride, procainamide, prochlorperazine, promethazine, propranolol, remifentanil, rocuronium, sodium phosphates, succinylcholine, sufentanil, sulbactam/durlobactam, tacrolimus, theophylline, tirofiban, tobramycin, vancomycin, vasopressin, vecuronium, vincristine, voriconazole, zidovudine, zoledronic acid.
- **Y-Site Incompatibility:** acyclovir, aminocaproic acid, amphotericin B deoxycholate, amphotericin B liposomal, ampicillin, ampicillin/sulbactam, azithromycin, ceftazidime, ceftolozane/tazobactam, cefuroxime, defibrotide, dexamethasone, diazepam, ertapenem, fludarabine, fluorouracil, foscarnet, fosphenytoin, furosemide, ganciclovir, gemtuzumab ozogamicin, hydrocortisone, imipenem/cilastatin, ketorolac, meropenem, meropenem/vaborbactam, mesna, methohexital, methotrexate, micafungin, pantoprazole, pemetrexed, pentobarbital, phenobarbital, phenytoin, piperacillin/tazobactam, potassium acetate, sodium bicarbonate, tedizolid, thiotepa, tigecycline.

Verapamil

- **IV:** Patients should remain recumbent for ≥1 hr after IV administration to minimize hypotensive effects.
- **IV Push: Dilution:** Administer undiluted. **Concentration:** 2.5 mg/mL **Rate:** Administer over 2 min. Geri: Administer over 3 min.
- **Y-Site Compatibility:** alemtuzumab, amikacin, aminocaproic acid, anidulafungin, argatroban, arsenic trioxide, ascorbic acid, atracurium, atropine, azithromycin, aztreonam, benztropine, bivalirudin, bleomycin, bumetanide, buprenorphine, butorphanol, calcium chloride, calcium gluconate, cangrelor, carboplatin, carmustine, caspofungin, cefazolin, cefotaxime, cefotetan, cefoxitin, ceftriaxone, cefuroxime, chlorpromazine, ciprofloxacin, cisplatin, clindamycin, cyanocobalamin, cyclophosphamide, cyclosporine, cytarabine, dacarbazine, dactinomycin, daptomycin, daunorubicin, dexamethasone, dexmedetomidine, dexrazoxane, digoxin, diltiazem, diphenhydramine, dobutamine, docetaxel, dopamine, doxorubicin hydrochloride, doxorubicin liposomal, doxycycline, enalaprilat, ephedrine, epinephrine, epirubicin, epoetin alfa, eptifibatide, erythromycin, esmolol, etoposide, etoposide phosphate, famotidine, fentanyl, fluconazole, fludarabine, gemcitabine, gemtuzumab ozogamicin, gentamicin, glycopyrrolate, granisetron, heparin, hetastarch, hydrocortisone, hydromorphone, idarubicin, ifosfamide, imipenem/cilastatin, insulin, regular, irinotecan, isoproterenol, ketorolac, labetalol, leucovorin, levofloxacin, lidocaine, linezolid, lorazepam,

magnesium sulfate, mannitol, meperidine, mesna, methadone, methotrexate, methylprednisolone, metoclopramide, metoprolol, metronidazole, midazolam, milrinone, minocycline, mitomycin, mitoxantrone, morphine, moxifloxacin, multivitamins, mycophenolate, nalbuphine, naloxone, nitroglycerin, nitroprusside, norepinephrine, octreotide, ondansetron, oxaliplatin, oxytocin, paclitaxel, palonosetron, pamidronate, papaverine, pemetrexed, penicillin G, pentamidine, phentolamine, phenylephrine, phytonadione, potassium acetate, potassium chloride, procainamide, prochlorperazine, promethazine, propranolol, protamine, pyridoxine, rocuronium, sodium acetate, succinylcholine, sufentanil, tacrolimus, theophylline, thiamine, tirofiban, tobramycin, topotecan, vancomycin, vasopressin, vecuronium, vinblastine, vincristine, vinorelbine, voriconazole, zoledronic acid.
- **Y-Site Incompatibility:** acyclovir, albumin, aminophylline, amiodarone, amphotericin B deoxycholate, amphotericin B liposomal, ampicillin, ampicillin/sulbactam, azathioprine, ceftazidime, chloramphenicol, dantrolene, diazepam, diazoxide, ertapenem, fluorouracil, folic acid, foscarnet, fosphenytoin, furosemide, ganciclovir, indomethacin, pantoprazole, pentobarbital, phenobarbital, phenytoin, piperacillin/tazobactam, propofol, sodium bicarbonate, suggamadex, thiotepa, tigecycline, trimethoprim/sulfamethoxazole.

Patient/Family Teaching

- Explain purpose and side effects of the medication. Instruct patient to take medication as directed, even if feeling well. Take missed doses as soon as possible unless almost time for next dose; do not double doses. May need to be discontinued gradually. Advise patient to read *Patient Information* before starting and with each Rx refill in case of changes.
- Advise patients taking *felodipine, nifedipine, nimodipine, nisoldipine, nicardipine, and verapamil* to avoid drinking grapefruit juice during therapy.
- Instruct patient on technique for monitoring pulse. Instruct patient to contact health care provider if HR <50 bpm.
- Caution patient to change positions slowly to minimize orthostatic hypotension.
- Advise patient to notify health care provider if rash, irregular heartbeat, dyspnea, swelling of hands and feet, pronounced dizziness, nausea, constipation, or hypotension occurs or if headache is severe or persistent.
- May cause drowsiness or dizziness. Advise patient to avoid driving or other activities requiring alertness until response to the medication is known.
- Geri: Teach patient and family about risk for falls and how to ↓ risk in the home.
- Instruct patient on importance of maintaining good dental hygiene and seeing dentist frequently for teeth cleaning to prevent tenderness, bleeding, and gingival hyperplasia (gum enlargement).
- Instruct patient to notify health care provider of all Rx or OTC medications, vitamins, or herbal products being taken and to avoid concurrent use of alcohol or OTC medications and herbal products, especially NSAIDs and cold preparations, without consulting health care provider.
- Caution patient to wear protective clothing and use sunscreen to prevent photosensitivity reactions.
- **Angina:** Instruct patient on concurrent nitrate or beta blocker therapy to continue taking both medications as directed and use SL nitroglycerin as needed for anginal attacks.
- Inform patient taking *isradipine or nifedipine* that anginal attacks may occur 30 min after administration as a result of reflex tachycardia. This is usually temporary and is not an indication for discontinuation.
- Advise patient to contact health care provider if chest pain does not improve, worsens after therapy, or occurs with diaphoresis or if shortness of breath or persistent headache occurs.
- Caution patient to discuss exercise restrictions with health care provider before exertion.
- **Hypertension:** Encourage patient to comply with other interventions for hypertension (weight reduction, low-sodium diet, smoking cessation, moderation of alcohol consumption, regular exercise, stress management). Medication controls but does not cure hypertension.
- Instruct patient and family in proper technique for monitoring BP. Advise patient to take BP weekly and to report significant changes to health care provider.
- Rep: Advise women of reproductive potential to notify health care provider if pregnancy is planned or suspected or if breastfeeding.

Evaluation/Desired Outcomes

- Decrease in BP.
- Decrease in frequency and severity of anginal attacks.
- Decrease in need for nitrate therapy.
- Increase in activity tolerance and sense of well-being.
- Suppression and prevention of atrial tachyarrhythmias.
- Improvement in neurologic deficits caused by vasospasm after subarachnoid hemorrhage.

REMS

calcium oxybate/magnesium oxybate/potassium oxybate/sodium oxybate (kal-see-um ox-ee-bate/mag-nee-zhum ox-ee-bate/po-tas-e-um ox-ee-bate/soe-dee-um ox-ee-bate)

Xywav

Classification

Therapeutic: anticataplectic

Pharmacologic: hydroxybutyrate

Schedule III

Indications

Cataplexy or excessive daytime sleepiness in patients with narcolepsy (generally with concurrent stimulant therapy).

Action

Oxybate, a CNS depressant, is also known as gamma hydroxybutyrate, a metabolite of GABA. Its mechanism of action as an anticataplectic is not known. **Therapeutic Effects:** Decreased incidence of cataplexy episodes in patients with narcolepsy.

Pharmacokinetics

Absorption: Rapidly absorbed; extent of absorption ↓ by a high-fat meal.

Distribution: Extensively distributed to extravascular tissues.

Metabolism and Excretion: Almost entirely biotransformed to carbon dioxide, which is eliminated by expiration; <5% excreted unchanged in urine.

Half-life: 40 min.

TIME/ACTION PROFILE (plasma concentrations)

ROUTE	ONSET	PEAK	DURATION
PO	rapid	1.3 hr	unknown

Contraindications/Precautions

Contraindicated in: Concurrent alcohol, CNS depressant, or sedative/hypnotic therapy; Succinic semialdehyde dehydrogenase deficiency.

Use Cautiously in: Hepatic impairment (↓ starting dose by 50%); History of depression or suicidal attempt; Obstructive sleep apnea; OB: Safety not established in pregnancy; Lactation: Use while breastfeeding only if potential maternal benefit justifies potential risk to infant; Pedi: Children < 7 yr or <20 kg (safety and effectiveness not established); Geri: ↑ sensitivity of drug's effects in older adults; dose ↓ may be required.

Adverse Reactions/Side Effects

Derm: ↑ sweating. **GI:** nausea, vomiting, diarrhea, dry mouth. **GU:** enuresis. **Metab:** ↓ appetite, weight loss. **MS:** muscle spasm. **Neuro:** dizziness, headache, aggression, agitation, anxiety, confusion, depression, hallucinations, irritability, paranoia, paresthesia, psychosis, sedation, SEIZURES, sleep walking, SUICIDAL THOUGHTS/BEHAVIORS, tremor. **Resp:** RESPIRATORY DEPRESSION. **Misc:** fatigue, physical dependence.

Interactions

Drug-Drug: ↑ risk of respiratory depression, hypotension, CNS depression, syncope, and death when used with other **CNS depressants**, including **alcohol, antidepressants, antipsychotics, benzodiazepines, muscle relaxants, opioids**, or **sedative/hypnotics**; concurrent use contraindicated. **Valproic acid** may ↑ levels and risk of toxicity; ↓ dose by ≥20% when starting valproic acid; use lower starting dose when initiating therapy in patient already receiving valproic acid.

Route/Dosage

PO (Adults and Children ≥7 yr and ≥45 kg): 2.25 g at bedtime and 2.25 g 2.5–4 hr later (total nightly dose = 4.5 g); may be ↑ at weekly intervals by 1.5 g/night (0.75 g/dose) (max dose = 9 g/night [4.5 g/dose]).

PO (Children ≥7 yr and 30–44.9 kg): 1.5 g at bedtime and 1.5 g 2.5–4 hr later (total nightly dose = 3 g); may be ↑ at weekly intervals by 1 g/night (0.5 g/dose) (max dose = 7.5 g/night [3.75 g/dose]).

PO (Children ≥7 yr and 20–29.9 kg): 1 g at bedtime and 1 g 2.5–4 hr later (total nightly dose = 2 g); may be ↑ at weekly intervals by 1 g/night (0.5 g/dose) (max dose = 6 g/night [3 g/dose]).

Hepatic Impairment

PO (Adults and Children ≥7 yr and ≥45 kg): ↓ starting dose by 50% (1.12 g at bedtime and 1.12 g 2.5–4 hr later) (total nightly dose = 2.25 g); dose increments should be titrated to desired effect with close monitoring.

Hepatic Impairment

PO (Children ≥7 yr and 30–44.9 kg): ↓ starting dose by 50% (0.75 g at bedtime and 0.75 g 2.5–4 hr later) (total nightly dose = 1.5 g); dose increments should be titrated to desired effect with close monitoring.

Hepatic Impairment

PO (Children ≥7 yr and 20–29.9 kg): ↓ starting dose by 50% (0.5 g at bedtime and 0.5 g 2.5–4 hr later) (total nightly dose = 1 g); dose increments should be titrated to desired effect with close monitoring.

Availability
Oral solution: 500 mg/mL.

NURSING IMPLICATIONS
Assessment
- Monitor for CNS depression (respiratory depression, hypotension, profound sedation, syncope) and ↑ apnea (sleep-related apnea). Implement immediate medical interventions if symptoms occur.
- Monitor for emergent or ↑ depression (depressed mood), suicidal ideation, and suicidal tendencies.
- Assess for seizure activity (myoclonus and tonic-clonic).
- Assess for confusion, agitation, anxiety, confusion, irritability, panic attack, tension, visual hallucinations, aggression, paranoia, and psychosis. Implement safety precautions.
- Evaluate for episodes of sleepwalking. May cause parasomnias (abnormal dreams, night terrors, sleep paralysis, sleep talking, somnambulism).
- Monitor patients closely with history of drug abuse for signs of misuse or abuse (↑ in size or frequency of dosing, drug-seeking behavior, feigned cataplexy).

Implementation
- ***REMS:*** Xywav is available only through a restricted distribution program called the *Xywav and XYREM REMS* because of the risks of CNS depression, abuse, and misuse. Health care providers are specially certified to prescribe *Xywav*, and it can only be dispensed by the central pharmacy that is specially certified. *Xywav* will be dispensed and shipped only to patients who are enrolled in the *XYWAV and XYREM REMS* with documentation of safe use. Further information is available at www.XYWAVXYREMREMS.com or 1-866-997-3688.
- **PO:** Administer without food and >2 hr after eating, while sitting up in bed. After taking dose, lie down and do not get out of bed. If dosing twice nightly, set an alarm to awaken for the 2nd dose; take ≥2.5–4 hr after 1st dose. Prepare both doses before bedtime.
- Dilute required amount of oral solution in cup (60 mL) of water in pharmacy-provided container. Consume prepared solution within 24 hr at room temperature.

Patient/Family Teaching
- Explain purpose and side effects of medication to patient. Advise patient to read *Patient Information* before starting therapy. If the second dose is missed, that dose should be skipped and should not be taken again until the next night. Two doses should never be taken at one time. If the nightly dose requires multiple administrations, inform patient on how to prepare each dose and to administer while in bed.
- Advise patient to notify health care provider of all Rx or OTC medications, vitamins, or herbal products being taken and to consult health care provider before taking other medications.
- Advise patients they will often fall asleep within 5–15 min of taking the medication, depending on the individual; may vary from night to night.
- Instruct patients and/or caregivers to contact a health care provider immediately if the patient develops depressed mood, markedly diminished interest or pleasure in usual activities, significant change in weight and/or appetite, psychomotor agitation or retardation, ↑ fatigue, feelings of guilt or worthlessness, slowed thinking, impaired concentration, or suicidal ideation.
- Advise patients not to engage in hazardous occupations or activities requiring complete mental alertness or motor coordination, such as operating machinery or a motor vehicle or flying an airplane, for ≥6 hr after dose.
- Inform patients and/or caregiver about sleepwalking and behavioral or psychiatric adverse reactions, including confusion, anxiety, and psychosis. Notify their health care provider if any of these types of symptoms occur.
- Advise patient to avoid alcohol and sedative hypnotics.
- **REMS:** Instruct the patient and/or caregiver about the risk of CNS depression, abuse, and misuse. Educate on how to take safely and effectively. *Xywav* is available only by prescription and filled through the central pharmacy certified in the *XYWAV and XYREM REMS*. Instruct the patient they must be enrolled in the *XYWAV and XYREM REMS* to receive *Xywav*.
- Rep: Advise women of reproductive potential to notify health care provider if pregnancy is planned or suspected or if breastfeeding.

Evaluation/Desired Outcomes
- Decrease incidence of cataplexy episodes in patients with narcolepsy.

HIGH ALERT

IV CALCIUM SALTS
calcium acetate (25% Ca or 12.6 mEq/g)
(**kal**-see-um **ass**-e-tate)
~~PhosLo~~

calcium carbonate (40% Ca or 20 mEq/g)
(**kal**-see-um **kar**-bo-nate)
~~Caltrate~~, Maalox, Titralac, Tums, Tums E-X

C

calcium chloride (27% Ca or 13.6 mEq/g)
(**kal**-see-um **kloh**-ride)
Calciject
calcium citrate (21% Ca or 12 mEq/g)
(**kal**-see-um **si**-trate)
Cal-Citrate
calcium gluconate (9% Ca or 4.5 mEq/g)
(**kal**-see-um **gloo**-koh-nate)
calcium lactate (13% Ca or 6.5 mEq/g)
(**kal**-see-um **lak**-tate)

Classification
Therapeutic: mineral and electrolyte replacements/supplements
Pharmacologic: antacids

Indications

PO IV: Treatment and prevention of hypocalcemia. **PO:** Adjunct in the prevention of postmenopausal osteoporosis. **IV:** Emergency treatment of hyperkalemia and hypermagnesemia and adjunct in cardiac arrest or calcium channel blocking agent toxicity (calcium chloride, calcium gluconate). **Calcium carbonate:** May be used as an antacid. **Calcium acetate:** Control of hyperphosphatemia in end-stage renal disease.

Action

Essential for nervous, muscular, and skeletal systems. Maintain cell membrane and capillary permeability. Act as an activator in the transmission of nerve impulses and contraction of cardiac, skeletal, and smooth muscle. Essential for bone formation and blood coagulation. Binds to dietary phosphate to form an insoluble calcium phosphate complex, which is excreted in the feces, resulting in decreased serum phosphorus concentrations (calcium acetate). **Therapeutic Effects:** Replacement of calcium in deficiency states. Control of hyperphosphatemia in end-stage renal disease without promoting aluminum absorption (calcium acetate).

Pharmacokinetics

Absorption: Absorption from the GI tract requires vitamin D. IV administration results in complete bioavailability.
Distribution: Readily enters extracellular fluid.
Metabolism and Excretion: Excreted mostly in the feces; 20% eliminated by the kidneys.
Half-life: Unknown.

TIME/ACTION PROFILE (effects on serum calcium)

ROUTE	ONSET	PEAK	DURATION
PO	unknown	unknown	unknown
IV	immediate	immediate	0.5–2 hr

Contraindications/Precautions

Contraindicated in: Hypercalcemia; Renal calculi; Ventricular fibrillation; Concurrent use of calcium supplements (calcium acetate).
Use Cautiously in: Severe respiratory insufficiency; Renal impairment; Cardiac disease; OB: Hypercalcemia may ↑ risk of maternal and fetal complications.

Adverse Reactions/Side Effects

CV: arrhythmias, bradycardia, CARDIAC ARREST (IV ONLY). **F and E:** hypercalcemia. **GI:** constipation, diarrhea (oral solution only), nausea, vomiting. **GU:** calculi, hypercalciuria. **Local:** phlebitis (IV only). **Neuro:** syncope (IV only), tingling.

Interactions

Drug-Drug: Hypercalcemia ↑ risk of **digoxin** toxicity. Chronic use with **antacids** in renal impairment may lead to milk-alkali syndrome. **Calcium supplements**, including calcium-containing antacids, may ↑ risk of hypercalcemia; avoid concurrent use. Ingestion by mouth ↓ the absorption of orally administered **phenytoin** and **iron salts**; take 1 hr before or 3 hr after oral calcium supplements. Excessive amounts may ↓ effectiveness of **calcium channel blockers**. Calcium acetate may ↓ absorption of orally administered **tetracyclines**; take ≥1 hr before calcium acetate Calcium acetate may ↓ absorption of orally administered **fluoroquinolones**; take ≥2 hr before or 6 hr after calcium acetate. Calcium acetate may ↓ absorption of orally administered **levothyroxine**; take ≥4 hr before or 4 hr after calcium acetate. ↓ absorption of **risedronate**; do not take within 2 hr of calcium supplements. **Thiazide diuretics** may result in hypercalcemia. May ↓ the ability of **sodium polystyrene sulfonate** to ↓ serum potassium.
Drug-Food: Cereals, **spinach**, or **rhubarb** may ↓ absorption of calcium supplements.

Route/Dosage

Doses are expressed in mg, g, or mEq of calcium.
PO (Adults): *Prevention of hypocalcemia, treatment of depletion, osteoporosis:* 1–2 g/day. *Antacid:* 0.5–1.5 g as needed (calcium carbonate only). *Hyperphosphatemia in end-stage renal disease (calcium acetate only):* 1334 mg with each meal; may ↑ gradually (in absence of hypercalcemia) to

achieve target serum phosphate levels (usual dose = 2001–2668 mg with each meal).
PO (Children): *Supplementation:* 45–65 mg/kg/day.
PO (Infants): *Neonatal hypocalcemia:* 50–150 mg/kg (not to exceed 1 g).
IV (Adults): *Emergency treatment of hypocalcemia, cardiac standstill:* 7–14 mEq. *Hypocalcemic tetany:* 4.5–16 mEq; repeat until symptoms are controlled. *Hyperkalemia with cardiac toxicity:* 2.25–14 mEq; may repeat in 1–2 min. *Hypermagnesemia:* 7 mEq.
IV (Children): *Emergency treatment of hypocalcemia:* 1–7 mEq. *Hypocalcemic tetany:* 0.5–0.7 mEq/kg 3–4 times daily.
IV (Infants): *Emergency treatment of hypocalcemia:* <1 mEq. *Hypocalcemic tetany:* 2.4 mEq/kg/day in divided doses.

Availability (generic available)

Calcium Acetate
Tablets: 667 mg (169 mg elemental Ca). **Gelcaps:** 667 mg (169 mg elemental Ca).

Calcium Carbonate
Tablets: 600 mg (240 mg Ca)^{OTC}, 650 mg (260 mg Ca)^{OTC}, 1.25 g (500 mg Ca)^{OTC}, 1.5 g (600 mg Ca)^{OTC}. **Chewable tablets:** 420 mg (168 mg Ca)^{OTC}, 500 mg (200 mg Ca)^{OTC}, 750 mg (300 mg Ca)^{OTC}, 1 g (400 mg Ca)^{OTC}, 1.25 g (500 mg Ca)^{OTC}. **Oral suspension:** 1.25 g (500 mg Ca)/5 mL^{OTC}. **Powder:** 6.5 g (2400 mg Ca)/packet^{OTC}.

Calcium Chloride
Solution for injection: 10% (1.36 mEq/mL).

Calcium Citrate
Tablets: 200 mg^{OTC}, 250 mg^{OTC}. **Capsules:** 150 mg.

Calcium Gluconate
Tablets: 500 mg (45 mg Ca)^{OTC}. **Premixed infusion (in sodium chloride):** 1 g/50 mL (4.65 mEq/50 mL), 2 g/100 mL (9.3 mEq/100 mL). **Solution for injection:** 10% (0.45 mEq/mL).

Calcium Lactate
Tablets: 100 mg ^{OTC}.

NURSING IMPLICATIONS

Assessment
- **Calcium Supplement/Replacement:** Assess closely for symptoms of hypocalcemia (paresthesia, muscle twitching, laryngospasm, colic, cardiac arrhythmias, Chvostek or Trousseau sign). Notify health care provider if these occur. Protect symptomatic patients by elevating and padding siderails and keeping bed in low position.
- Monitor BP, HR, and ECG frequently during parenteral therapy. May cause vasodilation with resulting hypotension, bradycardia, arrhythmias, and cardiac arrest. Transient ↑ in BP may occur during IV administration, especially in older adults or in patients with hypertension.
- Assess IV site for patency. Extravasation may cause cellulitis, necrosis, and sloughing.
- Monitor patient on digoxin for signs of toxicity.

Antacid: When used as an antacid, assess for heartburn, indigestion, and abdominal pain. Inspect abdomen; auscultate bowel sounds.

Lab Test Considerations
- Monitor serum calcium or ionized calcium, chloride, sodium, potassium, magnesium, albumin, and parathyroid hormone (PTH) concentrations before and periodically during therapy for treatment of hypocalcemia. *For patients with hyperphosphatemia:* Monitor serum calcium twice weekly during adjustment phase. If serum calcium level >12 mg/dL, discontinue therapy and start hemodialysis as needed; ↓ dose or temporarily stop therapy for calcium level between 10.5 and 11.9 mg/dL.
- May ↓ serum phosphate concentrations with excessive and prolonged use. When used to treat hyperphosphatemia in patients with renal failure, monitor phosphate levels.

Toxicity and Overdose
- Assess for nausea, vomiting, anorexia, thirst, severe constipation, paralytic ileus, and bradycardia. Contact health care provider immediately if these signs of hypercalcemia occur.

Implementation
- ***High Alert:*** Errors with IV calcium gluconate and calcium chloride have occurred secondary to confusion over which salt is ordered. Clarify incomplete orders. Confusion has occurred with milligram doses of calcium chloride and calcium gluconate, which are not equal. Chloride and gluconate forms are routinely available on most hospital crash carts; specify form of calcium desired.
- Do not confuse Os-Cal with Asacol.
- In cardiac arrest situations, the use of calcium chloride should be limited to patients with hyperkalemia, hypocalcemia, and calcium channel blocker toxicity.
- **PO:** Administer calcium carbonate 1–1.5 hr after meals and at bedtime. Chewable tablets should be well chewed before swallowing. Follow oral doses with a 8 ounces of water, except when using calcium carbonate as a phosphate binder in renal dialysis. Administer on an empty stomach before meals to optimize effectiveness in patients with hyperphosphatemia.
- **IM** IM administration of calcium salts can cause severe necrosis and tissue sloughing. Do not administer IM.

C

IV Administration

- **IV:** IV solution should be warmed to body temperature and given through a small-bore needle in a large vein to minimize phlebitis. May cause cutaneous burning sensation, peripheral vasodilation, and ↓ BP. Patient should remain recumbent for 30–60 min after IV administration.
- IV calcium chloride and calcium gluconate are vesicants. Should be administered via a central or deep vein; do not use small hand or foot veins for administration. If extravasation occurs, immediately stop infusion. Leave needle/cannula in place temporarily but do not flush the line. Gently aspirate extravasated solution; then remove needle/cannula. Elevate patient's extremity and apply dry warm compresses. Initiate hyaluronidase antidote for refractory cases in addition to supportive management. For hyaluronidase, inject a total of 1 mL (15 units/mL) intradermally or SUBQ as five separate 0.2-mL injections (using a tuberculin syringe) around the site of extravasation; if IV catheter remains in place, administer IV through the infiltrated catheter; may repeat in 30–60 min if no resolution.
- Administer slowly. High concentrations may cause cardiac arrest. Rapid administration may cause tingling, sensation of warmth, and a metallic taste. Stop infusion if these symptoms occur, and resume infusion at a slower rate when they subside.
- Do not administer solutions that are not clear or that contain a precipitate.

Calcium Chloride

IV Administration

- **IV Push:** May be administered undiluted by IV push.
- **Intermittent/Continuous Infusion: Dilution:** May be diluted with D5W, D10W, 0.9% NaCl, D5/0.25% NaCl, D5/0.45% NaCl, D5/0.9% NaCl, or D5/LR. **Rate:** Maximum rate for adults is 0.7–1.4 mEq/min; for children, 0.5 mL/min.
- **Y-Site Compatibility:** acyclovir, alemtuzumab, amikacin, aminocaproic acid, aminophylline, amiodarone, anidulafungin, argatroban, arsenic trioxide, ascorbic acid, atracurium, atropine, azithromycin, aztreonam, benztropine, bivalirudin, bleomycin, buprenorphine, butorphanol, carboplatin, carmustine, caspofungin, cefotaxime, cefotetan, cefoxitin, ceftaroline, ceftolozane/tazobactam, chloramphenicol, chlorothiazide, chlorpromazine, cisplatin, clindamycin, cyanocobalamin, cyclophosphamide, cyclosporine, cytarabine, dacarbazine, dactinomycin, daptomycin, daunorubicin, dexmedetomidine, dexrazoxane, digoxin, diltiazem, diphenhydramine, dobutamine, docetaxel, dopamine, doxapram, doxorubicin hydrochloride, doxycycline, edetate calcium disodium, enalaprilat, ephedrine, epinephrine, epirubicin, epoetin alfa, eptifibatide, eravacycline, ertapenem, erythromycin, esmolol, etoposide, etoposide phosphate, famotidine, fentanyl, fluconazole, fludarabine, furosemide, ganciclovir, gemcitabine, gentamicin, glycopyrrolate, granisetron, heparin, hetastarch, hydromorphone, idarubicin, ifosfamide, imipenem/cilastatin/relebactam, insulin, regular, irinotecan, isavuconazonium, isoproterenol, labetalol, LR, leucovorin, lidocaine, linezolid, lorazepam, mannitol, meperidine, meropenem, mesna, methadone, methohexital, methotrexate, metoclopramide, metoprolol, metronidazole, micafungin, midazolam, milrinone, minocycline, mitomycin, mitoxantrone, morphine, moxifloxacin, multivitamins, mycophenolate, nafcillin, nalbuphine, naloxone, nicardipine, nitroglycerin, nitroprusside, norepinephrine, octreotide, ondansetron, oxytocin, paclitaxel, palonosetron, papaverine, penicillin G, pentobarbital, phenobarbital, phentolamine, phenylephrine, phytonadione, piperacillin/tazobactam, potassium acetate, potassium chloride, procainamide, prochlorperazine, promethazine, propranolol, protamine, pyridoxine, rocuronium, succinylcholine, sufentanil, sulbactam/durlobactam, tacrolimus, theophylline, thiamine, thiotepa, tigecycline, tirofiban, tobramycin, topotecan, vancomycin, vasopressin, vecuronium, verapamil, vinblastine, vincristine, vinorelbine, voriconazole.
- **Y-Site Incompatibility:** amphotericin B deoxycholate, amphotericin B liposomal, azathioprine, cefazolin, ceftazidime, ceftobiprole, ceftriaxone, cefuroxime, dantrolene, diazepam, diazoxide, doxorubicin liposomal, fluorouracil, folic acid, foscarnet, fosphenytoin, gemtuzumab ozogamicin, haloperidol, indomethacin, ketorolac, magnesium sulfate, meropenem/vaborbactam, methylprednisolone, minocycline, oxacillin, oxaliplatin, pantoprazole, pemetrexed, phenytoin, plazomicin, potassium phosphates, prochlorperazine, propofol, sodium bicarbonate, sodium phosphates, tedizolid, trimethoprim/sulfamethoxazole.

Calcium Gluconate

IV Administration

- **IV Push: Rate:** Administer slowly by IV push. Maximum administration rate for adults is 1.5–2 mL/min.
- **Continuous Infusion: Dilution:** May be further diluted in 1000 mL of D5W, D10W, D20W, D5/0.9% NaCl, 0.9% NaCl, D5/LR, or LR. **Rate:** Administer at a rate not to exceed 200 mg/min over 12–24 hr.

- **Y-Site Compatibility:** acyclovir, aldesleukin, alemtuzumab, allopurinol, alprostadil, amikacin, aminocaproic acid, aminophylline, anidulafungin, argatroban, arsenic trioxide, ascorbic acid, atropine, azathioprine, azithromycin, aztreonam, benztropine, bivalirudin, bleomycin, bumetanide, buprenorphine, butorphanol, caffeine citrate, carboplatin, carmustine, caspofungin, cefazolin, cefepime, cefiderocol, cefotaxime, cefotetan, cefoxitin, ceftaroline, ceftazidime, ceftolozane/tazobactam, cefuroxime, chloramphenicol, chlorothiazide, chlorpromazine, ciprofloxacin, cisatracurium, cisplatin, cladribine, clevidipine, clindamycin, cyanocobalamin, cyclophosphamide, cyclosporine, cytarabine, dacarbazine, dactinomycin, daptomycin, daunorubicin hydrochloride, daunorubicin liposomal, dexmedetomidine, dexrazoxane, digoxin, diltiazem, dimenhydrinate, diphenhydramine, dobutamine, docetaxel, dopamine, doxapram, doxorubicin hydrochloride, doxorubicin liposomal, doxycycline, edetate calcium disodium, enalaprilat, ephedrine, epinephrine, epirubicin, epoetin alfa, eptifibatide, eravacycline, ertapenem, erythromycin, esmolol, etoposide, etoposide phosphate, famotidine, fentanyl, filgrastim, fludarabine, fluorouracil, folic acid, furosemide, ganciclovir, gemcitabine, gentamicin, glycopyrrolate, granisetron, hetastarch, hydromorphone, idarubicin, ifosfamide, imipenem/cilastatin/relebactam, insulin regular, irinotecan, isavuconazonium, isoproterenol, ketamine, labetalol, LR, leucovorin, levofloxacin, lidocaine, linezolid, lorazepam, magnesium sulfate, mannitol, melphalan, meperidine, meropenem/vaborbactam, mesna, methadone, methohexital, methotrexate, metoclopramide, metoprolol, metronidazole, micafungin, midazolam, milrinone, mitomycin, mitoxantrone, morphine, moxifloxacin, multivitamins, nafcillin, nalbuphine, naloxone, nicardipine, nitroglycerin, nitroprusside, norepinephrine, octreotide, ondansetron, oritavancin, oxaliplatin, oxytocin, paclitaxel, palonosetron, papaverine, penicillin G, pentamidine, pentobarbital, phenobarbital, phentolamine, phenylephrine, phytonadione, piperacillin/tazobactam, plazomicin, potassium acetate, potassium chloride, procainamide, prochlorperazine, promethazine, propofol, propranolol, protamine, pyridoxine, remifentanil, rituximab, rocuronium, sargramostim, sodium acetate, succinylcholine, sufentanil, sulbactam/durlobactam, tacrolimus, telavancin, theophylline, thiamine, thiotepa, tigecycline, tirofiban, tobramycin, trastuzumab, vancomycin, vasopressin, vecuronium, verapamil, vinblastine, vincristine, vinorelbine, voriconazole.
- **Y-Site Incompatibility:** amphotericin B deoxycholate, amphotericin B liposomal, cangrelor, ceftobiprole, ceftriaxone, dantrolene, diazepam, foscarnet, fosphenytoin, gemtuzumab ozogamicin, indomethacin, methylprednisolone, minocycline, mycophenolate, oxacillin, pemetrexed, phenytoin, potassium phosphates, remimazolam, sodium bicarbonate, sodium phosphates, tedizolid, topotecan, trimethoprim/sulfamethoxazole.

Patient/Family Teaching

- Explain purpose and side effects of medication to patient. Advise to read *Patient Information* before starting therapy. Instruct to take medication as directed. Instruct patients on a regular schedule to take missed doses as soon as possible; then go back to regular schedule.
- Advise patient to notify health care provider of all Rx or OTC medications, vitamins, or herbal products being taken and to consult health care provider before taking other medications, especially cold preparations.
- Instruct patient not to take enteric-coated tablets within 1 hr of calcium carbonate; this will result in premature dissolution of the tablets.
- Do not administer concurrently with foods containing large amounts of oxalic acid (spinach, rhubarb), phytic acid (brans, cereals), or phosphorus (milk or dairy products). Administration with milk products may lead to milk-alkali syndrome (nausea, vomiting, confusion, headache). Do not take within 1–2 hr of other medications if possible.
- Advise patient that calcium carbonate may cause constipation. Review methods of preventing constipation (↑ fiber in diet, fluid intake, and mobility) and using laxatives. Severe constipation may indicate toxicity.
- Advise patient to avoid excessive use of tobacco or beverages containing alcohol or caffeine.
- **Calcium Supplement:** Encourage patients to maintain a diet adequate in vitamin D (see Appendix J).
- **Osteoporosis:** Advise patient that exercise has been found to arrest and reverse bone loss. Patient should discuss any exercise limitations with health care provider before beginning program.
- **Hyperphosphatemia:** Advise patient to notify health care provider promptly if signs and symptoms of hypercalcemia (constipation, anorexia, nausea, vomiting, confusion, stupor) occur.
- Advise patient to avoid taking calcium-containing supplements, including calcium-based antacids, during therapy.
- Rep: Advise women of reproductive potential to notify health care provider if pregnancy is planned or suspected or if breastfeeding. Monitor infants born to mothers with hypocalcemia for signs of hypocalcemia or hypercalcemia (neuromuscular irritability, apnea, cyanosis, cardiac rhythm disorders).

Evaluation/Desired Outcomes

- Replacement of calcium in deficiency states.
- Control of hyperphosphatemia in end-stage renal disease without promoting aluminum absorption (calcium acetate).

canakinumab
(kan-a-**kin**-ue-mab)
Ilaris

Classification
Therapeutic: none assigned
Pharmacologic: interleukin antagonists

Indications
Cryopyrin-associated periodic syndromes including familial cold autoinflammatory syndrome and Muckle-Wells syndrome. Tumor necrosis factor receptor associated periodic syndrome. Hyperimmunoglobulin D syndrome/mevalonate kinase deficiency. Familial Mediterranean fever. Active Still disease, including adult-onset Still disease and systemic juvenile idiopathic arthritis. Gout flares when NSAIDs and colchicine are contraindicated, are not tolerated, or do not provide an adequate response, and when repeated courses of corticosteroids are not appropriate.

Action
Binds and neutralizes the activity of interleukin (IL)-1β by blocking its interaction with IL-1 receptors. **Therapeutic Effects:** Decreased flares of disease symptoms. Reduction in pain associated with gout flares and in risk of new gout flares.

Pharmacokinetics
Absorption: 70% absorbed following SUBQ administration.
Distribution: Unknown.
Metabolism and Excretion: Unknown.
Half-life: 26 days.

TIME/ACTION PROFILE

ROUTE	ONSET	PEAK	DURATION
SUBQ	within 8 days†	7 days‡	8 wk

† Noted as normalization of markers of inflammation.
‡ Blood levels.

Contraindications/Precautions
Contraindicated in: None.
Use Cautiously in: Active untreated infection, history of recurrent infections, or conditions increasing the propensity of infections; OB: Use during pregnancy only if clearly needed; Lactation: Use while breastfeeding only if potential maternal benefit justifies potential risk to infant; Pedi: Children <2 yr (safety and effectiveness not established).

Adverse Reactions/Side Effects
Derm: DRUG REACTION WITH EOSINOPHILIA AND SYSTEMIC SYMPTOMS (DRESS). **EENT:** nasopharyngitis. **GI:** diarrhea, nausea, gastroenteritis. **Local:** injection site reactions. **Metab:** weight gain. **MS:** musculoskeletal pain. **Neuro:** headache, vertigo. **Resp:** bronchitis. **Misc:** influenza, hypersensitivity reactions, INFECTION, MACROPHAGE ACTIVATION SYNDROME.

Interactions
Drug-Drug: Avoid concurrent use of **live vaccines**; all vaccinations should be completed prior to treatment. Concurrent use with **tumor necrosis factor inhibitors** may ↑ risk of serious infections. May alter activity of **CYP450 substrates**, including **warfarin**; careful monitoring of such drugs with narrow therapeutic indices should be undertaken.

Route/Dosage
Cryopyrin-Associated Periodic Syndromes
SUBQ (Adults >40 kg): 150 mg every 8 wk.
SUBQ (Adults and Children 15–40 kg): 2 mg/kg every 8 wk; may be ↑ to 3 mg/kg every 8 wk if response inadequate.

Tumor Necrosis Factor Receptor Associated Periodic Syndrome, Hyperimmunoglobulin D Syndrome/Mevalonate Kinase Deficiency, and Familial Mediterranean Fever
SUBQ (Adults >40 kg): 150 mg every 4 wk; may be ↑ to 300 mg every 4 wk if inadequate response.
SUBQ (Adults and Children ≤40 kg): 2 mg/kg every 4 wk; may be ↑ to 4 mg/kg every 4 wk if inadequate response.

Still Disease (Adult-Onset Still Disease and Systemic Juvenile Idiopathic Arthritis
SUBQ (Adults and Children ≥2 yr and ≥7.5 kg): 4 mg/kg (max dose = 300 mg) every 4 wk.

Gout Flares
SUBQ (Adults): 150 mg as single dose. If retreatment necessary, wait ≥12 wk before administering another dose.

Availability
Solution for injection: 150 mg/mL.

NURSING IMPLICATIONS
Assessment
- Assess for symptoms of cryopyrin-associated periodic syndromes (fever, headache, urticaria-like rash, arthralgia, myalgia, fatigue, conjunctivitis) prior to and periodically during therapy.
- Assess for signs and symptoms of infection (fever, sore throat, chills, cough, dyspnea, pain on

urination) before starting and periodically during therapy. Discontinue canakinumab if serious infection occurs.

- Assess for DRESS. *If serious skin eruptions or other severe hypersensitivity occur,* immediately discontinue canakinumab; treat promptly and monitor until resolved.
- Assess site and pain intensity in patients with gout.

Implementation

- Do not confuse Ilaris with Ilumya.
- Test for latent tuberculosis before initiating therapy. If positive, treat tuberculosis prior to therapy.
- Bring all recommended vaccinations up to date prior to therapy, including pneumococcal and inactivated influenza vaccines.
- **SUBQ**: Injection should be performed by health care professional. Administer undiluted. Solution is clear to opalescent, colorless to slightly brownish-yellow tint; if solution is brown, highly opalescent, or contains particulates, do not use. Refrigerate unopened vials and protect from light; do not freeze.
- Inject SUBQ using a 27-gauge 0.5-inch needle. Avoid injection into scar tissue.

Patient/Family Teaching

- Instruct patient to read *Medication Guide* prior to starting therapy.
- May cause vertigo. Caution patient to avoid driving and other activities requiring alertness until response to canakinumab is known.
- Advise patient to notify health care professional immediately if signs of infection (fever, sore throat, dyspnea) or macrophage activation syndrome (fever lasting >3 days, persistent cough, redness in one part of body, warm feeling or swelling of skin) occur.
- Inform patient to avoid receiving live vaccines during therapy.
- May cause injection site reactions (pain, erythema, swelling, pruritus, bruising, mass, inflammation, dermatitis, edema, urticaria, vesicles, warmth, hemorrhage). Notify health care professional if reaction is persistent.
- Advise patient to notify health care professional if signs and symptoms of hypersensitivity reactions (difficulty breathing or swallowing, nausea, dizziness, skin rash, itching, hives, palpitations, low BP) occur.
- Advise patient to notify health care professional of all Rx or OTC medications, vitamins, or herbal products being taken and to consult with health care professional before taking other medications.
- Rep: Advise women of reproductive potential to notify health care professional if pregnancy is planned or suspected or if breastfeeding. May interfere with immune response; consider risks and benefits before administering live vaccines to infants exposed to canakinumab in utero for ≥4–12 mo after mother's last dose.

Evaluation/Desired Outcomes

- Decreased flares of disease symptoms.
- Reduction in pain associated with gout flares and risk of new gout flares.

candesartan, See ANGIOTENSIN II RECEPTOR ANTAGONISTS.

cannabidiol (kan-a-bi-**dye**-ol)

Epidiolex

Classification

Therapeutic: anticonvulsants

Pharmacologic: cannabinoids

Schedule V

Indications

Seizures associated with Lennox-Gastaut syndrome, Dravet syndrome, or tuberous sclerosis complex.

Action

Cannabidiol is a cannabinoid that naturally occurs in the *Cannabis sativa* plant. Mechanism of anticonvulsant effect unknown; does not work by interacting with cannabinoid receptors. **Therapeutic Effects:** Reduction in frequency of atonic, tonic, clonic, and tonic-clonic seizures.

Pharmacokinetics

Absorption: Extent of absorption unknown. High-fat/high-calorie meals increase extent of absorption.
Distribution: Extensively distributed to tissues.
Protein Binding: >94%.
Metabolism and Excretion: Primarily metabolized in the liver by the CYP2C9 and CYP3A4 isoenzymes to an active metabolite (7-OH-CBD). Primarily excreted in feces.
Half-life: 56–61 hr.

TIME/ACTION PROFILE (plasma concentrations)

ROUTE	ONSET	PEAK	DURATION
PO	unknown	2.5–5 hr	unknown

Contraindications/Precautions

Contraindicated in: Hypersensitivity to cannabidiol or sesame oil.
Use Cautiously in: Elevated liver enzymes (at baseline); Moderate to severe hepatic impairment; OB: Use during pregnancy only if the potential maternal benefit justifies the potential fetal risk; Lactation: Use while breastfeeding only if the potential maternal

benefit justifies the potential risk to the infant; Pedi: Children <2 yr (safety and effectiveness not established); Geri: Choose dose carefully in older adults, considering concurrent disease states, drug therapy, and age-related ↓ in hepatic and renal function.

Adverse Reactions/Side Effects

Derm: rash. **EENT:** dry mouth. **GI:** ↓ appetite, ↑ liver enzymes, diarrhea, abdominal pain, HEPATOTOXICITY, weight loss. **GU:** ↑ serum creatinine. **Hemat:** anemia. **Neuro:** fatigue, insomnia, sedation, aggressive behavior, agitation, ataxia, SUICIDAL THOUGHTS/BEHAVIORS. **Misc:** HYPERSENSITIVITY REACTIONS (INCLUDING ANGIOEDEMA), infection, physical dependence, psychological dependence (high doses or prolonged therapy).

Interactions

Drug-Drug: Strong CYP2C9 inducers or **strong CYP3A4 inducers** may ↓ levels and effectiveness; consider ↑ cannabidiol dose. May ↑ levels and risk of toxicity of **CYP1A2 substrates**, including **theophylline** and **tizanidine**; consider ↓ dose of CYP1A2 substrate. May ↑ levels and risk of toxicity of **CYP2B6 substrates**, including **bupropion** and **efavirenz**. May ↑ levels and risk of toxicity of **CYP2C8 substrates** and **CYP2C9 substrates**; consider ↓ dose of CYP2C8 or CYP2C9 substrate. May ↑ levels and risk of toxicity of **UGT1A9 substrates**, including **propofol** and **fenofibrate**; consider ↓ dose of UGT1A9 substrate. May ↑ levels and risk of toxicity of **UGT2B7 substrates**, including **gemfibrozil**, **lamotrigine**, **morphine**, and **lorazepam**; consider ↓ dose of UGT2B7 substrate. May ↑ levels and risk of toxicity of **CYP2C19 substrates**, including **diazepam**; consider ↓ dose of CYP2C19 substrate. May ↑ risk of toxicity of **clobazam**. May ↑ levels and risk of toxicity of **P-glycoprotein substrates**, including **everolimus**, **sirolimus**, **tacrolimus**, and **digoxin**. May ↑ levels and risk of toxicity of **stiripentol**. Additive CNS depression with **alcohol**, **antihistamines**, **barbiturates**, **benzodiazepines**, **muscle relaxants**, **opioid analgesics**, **tricyclic antidepressants**, and **sedative/hypnotics**. **Valproic acid** may ↑ risk of hepatotoxicity; consider discontinuation of or adjustment of dose of cannabidiol and/or valproic acid if ↑ liver enzymes occur.

Route/Dosage

Seizures Associated With Lennox-Gastaut Syndrome or Dravet Syndrome

PO (Adults and Children ≥1 yr): 2.5 mg/kg twice daily; can ↑ to 5 mg/kg twice daily in 1 wk. If further ↓ in seizure frequency needed, may continue to ↑ dose on weekly basis (every other day if more rapid titration warranted) in increments of 2.5 mg/kg twice daily (max dose = 10 mg/kg twice daily).

Hepatic Impairment

PO (Adults and Children ≥1 yr): *Moderate hepatic impairment:* 1.25 mg/kg twice daily; can ↑ to 2.5 mg/kg twice daily in 1 wk. If further ↓ in seizure frequency needed, may continue to ↑ dose on weekly basis (every other day if more rapid titration warranted) in increments of 1.25 mg/kg twice daily (max dose = 5 mg/kg twice daily); *Severe hepatic impairment:* 0.5 mg/kg twice daily; can ↑ to 1 mg/kg twice daily in 1 wk. If further ↓ in seizure frequency needed, may continue to ↑ dose on weekly basis (every other day if more rapid titration warranted) in increments of 0.5 mg/kg twice daily (max dose = 2 mg/kg twice daily).

Seizures Associated with Tuberous Sclerosis Complex

PO (Adults and Children ≥1 yr): 2.5 mg/kg twice daily; can ↑ on weekly basis (every other day if more rapid titration warranted) in increments of 2.5 mg/kg twice daily to recommended maintenance dosage of 12.5 mg/kg twice daily.

Hepatic Impairment

PO (Adults and Children ≥1 yr): *Moderate hepatic impairment:* 1.25 mg/kg twice daily; can ↑ on weekly basis (every other day if more rapid titration warranted) in increments of 1.25 mg/kg twice daily to recommended maintenance dosage of 6.25 mg/kg twice daily; *Severe hepatic impairment:* 0.5 mg/kg twice daily; can ↑ on weekly basis (every other day if more rapid titration warranted) in increments of 0.5 mg/kg twice daily to recommended maintenance dosage of 2.5 mg/kg twice daily.

Availability

Oral solution (strawberry flavor): 100 mg/mL.

NURSING IMPLICATIONS

Assessment

- Assess location, duration, and characteristics of seizure activity. Institute seizure precautions.
- Monitor closely for suicidal behavior and ideation as soon as 1 wk following initiation of therapy. *If suicidal behavior occurs,* consider if symptoms may be related to the illness being treated.
- Monitor for signs and symptoms of hepatotoxicity. *If signs and symptoms occur,* promptly measure serum transaminases and total bilirubin and interrupt or discontinue cannabidiol therapy.
- Monitor for signs and symptoms of hypersensitivity reactions (pruritus, erythema, angioedema) during therapy. *If hypersensitivity reaction occurs,* discontinue cannabidiol.

Lab Test Considerations

- Obtain serum transaminases (ALT, AST) and total bilirubin levels before initiation; then at 1, 3, and

6 mo; within 1 mo following dose change; and as needed thereafter. *If ALT or AST >3 times upper limit of normal (ULN) and bilirubin >2 times ULN,* discontinue cannabidiol. *If ALT or AST persistently >5 times ULN,* discontinue cannabidiol.

Implementation

- **PO:** Administer with consistency in regard to food. Use included calibrated measuring device to ensure accurate dosing. Store solution at room temperature; do not refrigerate or freeze. Discard 12 wk after bottle is first opened.
- May be administered enterally via silicone nasogastric or gastrostomy tube. After each dose, flush the tube with approximately 5 times the priming volume of the tube with room-temperature drinking water. Volume may need to be modified for fluid restrictions. Do not use with tubes made of polyvinyl chloride or polyurethane and avoid use of silicone nasogastric tubes <50 cm in length and <5 FR in diameter.

Patient/Family Teaching

- Explain purpose and side effects of medication. Advise patient to read *Patient Information* before starting therapy.
- Advise patient not to stop cannabidiol without consulting health care provider; must be gradually discontinued to prevent seizures or discontinued rapidly under direct health care provider supervision.
- Caution patient to avoid driving or other activities requiring alertness and not to resume driving until health care provider gives clearance based on control of seizure disorder and response to medication is known.
- Advise patient to notify health care provider if signs and symptoms of hepatotoxicity (nausea, vomiting, right upper quadrant pain, fatigue, anorexia, jaundice, dark urine) occur.
- Instruct patient to notify health care provider of all Rx or OTC medications, vitamins, or herbal products being taken; consult health care provider before taking any new medications; and avoid alcohol during therapy.
- Inform patient and caregiver of risk of suicidal thoughts and behavior, and to notify health care provider immediately if behavioral or mood changes, worsening signs and symptoms of depression, or suicidal thoughts occur.
- Inform patients of potential for positive cannabis drug screens.
- Rep: Advise women of reproductive potential to notify health care provider if pregnancy is planned or suspected or if breastfeeding. Encourage patients who become pregnant to enroll in both of the following registries: North American Antiepileptic Drug (NAAED) Pregnancy Registry (1-888-233-2334; www.aedpregnancyregistry.org); and *Epidiolex* Pregnancy Surveillance Program (1-855-272-7158; www.epidiolexpregnancystudy.com). Enrollment must be done by patient.

Evaluation/Desired Outcomes

- Decreased frequency and intensity of seizure activity.

HIGH ALERT

capivasertib (kap-eye-va-ser-tib)

Truqap

Classification

Therapeutic: antineoplastics

Pharmacologic: kinase inhibitors

Indications

Hormone receptor-positive, human epidermal growth factor receptor 2 (HER2)-negative locally advanced or metastatic breast cancer with ≥1 *PIK3CA/AKT1/PTEN*-alteration following progression on ≥1 endocrine-based regimen in the metastatic setting or recurrence on or within 12 mo of completing adjuvant therapy (in combination with fulvestrant).

Action

Acts as an inhibitor of all three isoforms of serine/threonine kinase AKT (AKT1, AKT2, and AKT3) and inhibits phosphorylation of downstream AKT substrates. **Therapeutic Effects:** Improved progression-free survival and decreased spread of breast cancer.

Pharmacokinetics

Absorption: 29% absorbed following oral administration.

Distribution: Extensively distributed to extravascular tissues.

Metabolism and Excretion: Primarily metabolized in the liver via the CYP3A4 and UGT2B7. 45% excreted in the urine; 50% in the feces.

Half-life: 8.3 hr.

TIME/ACTION PROFILE (plasma concentrations)

ROUTE	ONSET	PEAK	DURATION
PO	unknown	1–2 hr	12 hr

Contraindications/Precautions

Contraindicated in: Hypersensitivity; Severe renal impairment; Severe hepatic impairment; OB: Pregnancy; Lactation: Lactation.

Use Cautiously in: Insulin-dependent diabetes; Diabetes, obesity, elevated fasting glucose (>160 mg/dL), elevated A1c, concurrent use of corticosteroids, or infection; Moderate hepatic impairment; Rep:

Women of reproductive potential and men with female partners of reproductive potential; Pedi: Safety and effectiveness not established in children.

Adverse Reactions/Side Effects

Derm: dermatitis, dry skin, eczema, pruritus, rash, skin discoloration, urticaria, DRUG REACTION WITH EOSINOPHILIA AND SYSTEMIC SYMPTOMS (DRESS), ERYTHEMA MULTIFORME, palmar-plantar erythrodysesthesia. **Endo:** HYPERGLYCEMIA, DIABETIC KETOACIDOSIS. **F and E:** hypocalcemia, hypokalemia, dehydration. **GI:** ↓ appetite, ↑ liver enzymes, DIARRHEA, nausea, stomatitis, vomiting. **GU:** ↑ serum creatinine, urinary tract infection. **Hemat:** anemia, leukopenia, lymphopenia, neutropenia, thrombocytopenia. **Metab:** hypertriglyceridemia. **Neuro:** fatigue, headache.

Interactions

Drug-Drug: Strong CYP3A4 inhibitors, including **itraconazole**, may ↑ levels and risk of toxicity; avoid concurrent use. If concurrent use necessary, ↓ capivasertib dose. **Moderate CYP3A4 inhibitors**, including **erythromycin** and **verapamil**, may ↑ levels and risk of toxicity; ↓ capivasertib dose. **Strong CYP3A4 inducers**, including **rifampin**, and **moderate CYP3A4 inducers**, including **efavirenz**, may ↓ levels and effectiveness; avoid concurrent use.

Route/Dosage

PO (Adults): 400 mg twice daily for 4 days, followed by 3 days off; continue until disease progression or unacceptable toxicity. *Concurrent use with strong or moderate CYP3A4 inhibitor:* 320 mg twice daily for 4 days, followed by 3 days off; continue until disease progression or unacceptable toxicity.

Availability

Tablets: 160 mg, 200 mg.

NURSING IMPLICATIONS

Assessment

- Monitor for signs and symptoms of diarrhea and dehydration. *At 1st signs of diarrhea,* advise patient to ↑ oral fluids and start antidiarrheal therapy. *If Grade 2 or 3 diarrhea occurs,* hold therapy until recovery to Grade ≤1. If recovery occurs in ≤28 days, resume at same or one lower dose as clinically indicated. If recovery occurs in >28 days or recurrence occurs, resume at one lower dose for Grade 2 or permanently discontinue for Grade 3. *If Grade 4 diarrhea occurs,* permanently discontinue capivasertib.
- Monitor skin for erythema, rash, and urticaria. *If Grade 2 skin reactions occur,* hold therapy until recovery to Grade ≤1; then resume at same dose. If symptoms persist or recur, resume at one lower dose. *If Grade 3 skin reactions occur,* hold therapy until recovery to Grade ≤1. If recovery occurs in ≤28 days, resume at same dose. If recovery occurs in >28 days, resume at one lower dose. *For recurrent Grade 3 or Grade 4 skin reactions,* permanently discontinue capivasertib.

Lab Test Considerations

- Verify negative pregnancy test before starting therapy.
- Monitor CBC with differential, triglycerides, and serum creatinine periodically during therapy.
- Evaluate fasting plasma glucose (FPG) and A1c and optimize FPG prior to initiating therapy. Monitor FPG on Day 3 or 4 of the dosing week during Weeks 1, 2, 4, 6, and 8; then monthly; and as clinically indicated. Monitor A1c every 3 mo and as clinically indicated. *If hyperglycemia occurs,* monitor FPG at least twice weekly until ↓ to baseline. Consider consultation with health care provider experienced in treating hyperglycemia for therapy with antihyperglycemics and monitor FPG at least once weekly for 2 mo, followed by once every 2 wk or as clinically indicated. *If FPG >upper limit of normal (ULN)–160 mg/dL or A1c >7%,* consider initiation or intensification of oral diabetic therapy. *If FPG 161–250 mg/dL,* hold therapy until ≤160 mg/dL. If recovery occurs in ≤28 days, resume at same dose. If recovery occurs in >28 days, resume at one lower dose. *If FPG 251–500 mg/dL,* hold therapy until ≤160 mg/dL. If recovery occurs in ≤28 days, resume at one lower dose. If recovery occurs in >28 days, permanently discontinue capivasertib. *If FPG >500 mg/dL,* hold therapy. If FPG ↓ to ≤500 mg/dL within 24 hr, follow guidance for the relevant grade. If FPG remains >500 mg/dL for >24 hr, or if ketoacidosis or life-threatening sequelae occur at any FPG level, permanently discontinue capivasertib.

Implementation

- **Dose reduction schedule:** *1st dose reduction:* 320 mg twice daily for 4 days followed by 3 days off. *2nd dose reduction:* 200 mg twice daily for 4 days followed by 3 days off. *If patient unable to tolerate 200 mg twice daily,* permanently discontinue capivasertib.
- Take with or without food. ***DNC:*** Swallow tablets whole. Do not chew, crush, or split tablets prior to swallowing. Do not take tablets that are broken or otherwise not intact.
- If a dose is missed, take within 4 hr of scheduled time; otherwise, omit and take at the next scheduled time. If a patient vomits a dose, instruct not to take an additional dose; take the next dose at its usual time.

- Administer a luteinizing hormone-releasing hormone (LHRH) agonist for premenopausal and perimenopausal women, and consider administration of LHRH agonist to men, according to current clinical practice standards.

Patient/Family Teaching

- Explain purpose and side effects of medication to patient. Advise patient to read *Patient Information* before starting therapy.
- Advise patient to notify health care provider of all Rx or OTC medications, vitamins, or herbal products being taken and to consult health care provider before taking other medications.
- Advise patient to immediately contact health care provider if symptoms of hyperglycemia (↑ thirst, ↑ hunger with weight loss, ↑ urination), diarrhea, dehydration, or skin changes occur.
- Rep: May cause fetal harm. Advise women of reproductive potential and male partners of women of reproductive potential to use effective contraception during therapy and for 1 mo (women) and 4 mo (female partners) after last dose. Advise patient to notify health care provider of known or suspected pregnancy and to avoid breastfeeding.

Evaluation/Desired Outcomes

- Improved progression-free survival and decreased spread of breast cancer.

captopril, See ANGIOTENSIN-CONVERTING ENZYME (ACE) INHIBITORS.

BEERS

carBAMazepine

(kar-ba-**maz**-e-peen)

Carbatrol, Equetro, TEGretol,
TEGretol CR, TEGretol XR

Classification

Therapeutic: anticonvulsants, mood stabilizers

Indications

Tonic-clonic, mixed, and complex-partial seizures. Pain in trigeminal neuralgia. **Equetro only:** Acute manic or mixed episodes associated with bipolar I disorder.

Action

Decreases synaptic transmission in the CNS by affecting sodium channels in neurons. **Therapeutic Effects:** Prevention of seizures. Relief of pain in trigeminal neuralgia. Decreased mania.

Pharmacokinetics

Absorption: Absorption is slow but complete. Suspension produces earlier, higher peak, and lower trough levels.

Distribution: Widely distributed to tissues. Crosses the blood-brain barrier.

Protein Binding: 75–90%.

Metabolism and Excretion: Extensively metabolized in the liver by the CYP3A4 isoenzyme to active epoxide metabolite; epoxide metabolite has anticonvulsant and antineuralgic activity.

Half-life: *Children:* 8–14 hr; *Adults:* 12–17 hr.

TIME/ACTION PROFILE (anticonvulsant activity)

ROUTE	ONSET	PEAK	DURATION
PO	up to 1 mo†	4–5 hr‡	6–12 hr
PO-ER	up to 1 mo†	2–12 hr‡	12 hr

† Onset of antineuralgic activity is 8–72 hr.
‡ Listed for tablets; peak level occurs 1.5 hr after a chronic dose of suspension.

Contraindications/Precautions

Contraindicated in: Hypersensitivity to carbamazepine or tricyclic antidepressants; Bone marrow suppression; Concurrent use or use within 14 days of MAO inhibitors; Concurrent use of nefazodone or NNRTIs that are CYP3A4 substrates; Lactation: Lactation.

Use Cautiously in: All patients (may ↑ risk of suicidal thoughts/behaviors); Cardiac or hepatic disease; Renal failure (adjust dose for CCr <10 mL/min); ↑ intraocular pressure; OB: Use during pregnancy only if potential maternal benefits outweigh potential fetal risks; additional vitamin K during last week of pregnancy has been recommended; Geri: Appears on Beers list. May worsen or cause syndrome of inappropriate antidiuretic hormone (SIADH) secretion in older adults. Use with caution in older adults and closely monitor sodium concentrations when starting therapy or ↑ dose.

Exercise Extreme Caution in: Patients positive for HLA-B*1502 or HLA-A*3101 alleles (unless benefits clearly outweigh the risks) (↑ risk of serious skin reactions).

Adverse Reactions/Side Effects

CV: edema, heart block, HF, hypertension, hypotension, syncope. **Derm:** DRUG REACTION WITH EOSINOPHILIA AND SYSTEMIC SYMPTOMS (DRESS), nail shedding, photosensitivity, rash, STEVENS-JOHNSON SYNDROME (SJS), TOXIC EPIDERMAL NECROLYSIS (TEN), urticaria. **EENT:** blurred vision, corneal opacities, nystagmus. **Endo:** SIADH. **F and E:** hyponatremia. **GI:** ↑ liver enzymes, HEPATOTOXICITY, PANCREATITIS. **GU:** urinary hesitancy, urinary retention. **Hemat:** AGRANULOCYTOSIS, APLASTIC ANEMIA, eosinophilia, leukopenia, lymphadenopathy,

THROMBOCYTOPENIA. **Metab:** weight gain. **Neuro:** ataxia, drowsiness, fatigue, psychosis, sedation, SUICIDAL THOUGHTS, vertigo. **Resp:** pneumonitis. **Misc:** chills, fever.

Interactions

Drug-Drug: May significantly ↓ levels and effectiveness of **nefazodone** or **NNRTIs** that are CYP3A4 substrates; concurrent use contraindicated. Concurrent or recent (within 2 wk) use of **MAO inhibitors** may result in hyperpyrexia, hypertension, seizures, and death; concurrent use contraindicated. May ↓ levels and effectiveness of **acetaminophen**, **alprazolam**, **aprepitant**, **buprenorphine**, **bupropion**, **calcium channel blockers**, **citalopram**, **clonazepam**, **corticosteroids**, **cyclosporine**, **doxycycline**, **estrogen-containing contraceptives**, **everolimus**, **haloperidol**, **imatinib**, **itraconazole**, **lamotrigine**, **levothyroxine**, **methadone**, **midazolam**, **olanzapine**, **paliperidone**, **phenytoin**, **protease inhibitors**, **risperidone**, **sertraline**, **sirolimus**, **tacrolimus**, **tadalafil**, **theophylline**, **tiagabine**, **topiramate**, **tramadol**, **trazodone**, **tricyclic antidepressants**, **valproic acid**, **warfarin**, **ziprasidone**, and **zonisamide**. May ↓ levels and effectiveness of **aripiprazole**; double aripiprazole dose. May ↓ levels and effectiveness of **temsirolimus** and **lapatinib**; avoid concurrent use. May ↓ levels and effectiveness of **apixaban**, **dabigatran**, **edoxaban**, and **rivaroxaban**; avoid concurrent use. **Aprepitant**, **brivaracetam**, **cimetidine**, **ciprofloxacin**, **clarithromycin**, **danazol**, **dantrolene**, **diltiazem**, **erythromycin**, **fluconazole**, **fluoxetine**, **fluvoxamine**, **ibuprofen**, **isoniazid**, **itraconazole**, **ketoconazole**, **loratadine**, **olanzapine**, **omeprazole**, **oxybutynin**, **protease inhibitors**, **trazodone**, **voriconazole**, and **verapamil** may ↑ levels and risk of toxicity. **Rifampin**, **phenobarbital**, and **phenytoin** may ↓ levels and effectiveness. May ↑ risk of hepatotoxicity from **isoniazid**. May ↑ risk of CNS toxicity from **lithium**. May ↓ levels and effectiveness of **nondepolarizing neuromuscular blocking agents**. May ↑ risk of toxicity of **cyclophosphamide**.

Drug-Natural Products: St. John's wort may ↓ levels and effectiveness.

Drug-Food: Grapefruit juice may ↑ levels and risk of toxicity.

Route/Dosage

When converting from immediate-release (IR) to extended-release (ER) formulation, administer same total daily dose (in 2 divided doses).

Seizures

PO (Adults and Children >12 yr): 200 mg twice daily (IR tablets and ER tablets/capsules) or 100 mg 4 times daily (suspension); ↑ by up to 200 mg/day in divided doses (every 12 hr for ER tablets; every 6–8 hr for IR tablets and suspension) every 7 days until therapeutic levels are achieved (usual range = 600–1200 mg/day); not to exceed 1000 mg/day in children 12–15 yr old or 1200 mg/day in children 15–18 yr old or 1600 mg/day in adults.

PO (Children 6–12 yr): 100 mg twice daily (IR tablets or ER tablets/capsules) or 50 mg 4 times daily (suspension). ↑ by up to 100 mg/day in divided doses (every 12 hr for ER tablets; every 6–8 hr for IR tablets and suspension) every 7 days until therapeutic levels are achieved (usual range = 400–800 mg/day); not to exceed 1000 mg/day.

PO (Children <6 yr): 10–20 mg/kg/day in 2 3 divided doses (IR tablets) or in 4 divided doses (suspension); may ↑ at weekly intervals until optimal response and therapeutic levels are achieved; not to exceed 35 mg/kg/day.

Trigeminal Neuralgia

PO (Adults): 100 mg twice daily (IR or ER tablets), 200 mg once daily (ER capsules), or 50 mg 4 times daily (suspension); ↑ by up to 200 mg/day in divided doses (every 12 hr for IR tablets or ER tablets/capsules; every 6 hr for suspension) as needed until pain is relieved (usual range = 400–800 mg/day); not to exceed 1200 mg/day.

Acute Manic or Mixed Episodes Associated With Bipolar I Disorder

PO (Adults): *Equetro:* 200 mg twice daily; ↑ by 200 mg/day until optimal response is achieved; not to exceed 1600 mg/day.

Availability (generic available)

Immediate-release tablets: 200 mg. **Chewable tablets:** 100 mg 🍁 200 mg. **Extended-release capsules (Carbatrol, Equetro):** 100 mg, 200 mg, 300 mg. **Extended-release tablets (Tegretol XR):** 100 mg200 mg, 400 mg. **Oral suspension (citrus-vanilla flavor):** 100 mg/5 mL.

NURSING IMPLICATIONS

Assessment

- Monitor closely for changes in behavior that could indicate the emergence or worsening of suicidal thoughts or behavior or depression.
- Monitor for changes in skin condition in early therapy. SJS and TEN are significantly more common in patients with a particular human leukocyte antigen (HLA) allele, HLA-B*1502 (occurs almost exclusively in patients with Asian ancestry, including South

🍁 = Canadian drug name. = Genetic implication. V = Vesicant. Boxed warning. ~~Strikethrough~~ = Discontinued. *CAPITALS = life-threatening. Underline = most frequent.

Asian Indians). Screen patients of Asian ancestry for the HLA-B*1502 allele before starting treatment with carbamazepine. If positive, carbamazepine should not be started unless the expected benefit outweighs ↑ risk of serious skin reactions. Patients who have been taking carbamazepine for more than a few months without developing skin reactions are at low risk of these events ever developing.

- Monitor for signs and symptoms of DRESS (fever, rash, and/or lymphadenopathy with organ system involvement [hepatitis, nephritis, hematologic abnormalities, myocarditis, myositis]) resembling an acute viral infection with eosinophilia. *If DRESS suspected,* discontinue carbamazepine if other cause not determined.
- Monitor for signs and symptoms of pancreatitis or hepatotoxicity (fatigue, severe nausea, vomiting, upper abdominal pain, jaundice, scleral icterus, dark urine, clay-colored stools).
- Assess height and weight or waist circumference at baseline, and follow weight after 6 mo and then annually.
- Perform baseline and periodic eye examinations, including slit-lamp, fundoscopy, and tonometry. Assess intraocular pressure (IOP) in patients with a history of ↑ IOP prior to treatment and periodically thereafter.
- **Seizures:** Assess frequency, location, duration, and characteristics of seizure activity. Implement seizure precautions as indicated.
- **Trigeminal Neuralgia:** Assess for facial pain (location, intensity, duration). Ask patient to identify stimuli that may precipitate facial pain (hot or cold foods, bedclothes, touching face).
- **Bipolar Disorder:** Assess mental status (mood, orientation, behavior) and cognitive abilities before and periodically during therapy.

Lab Test Considerations

- Monitor CBC, reticulocyte count, and serum iron at baseline, weekly during the 1st 2 mo, and yearly thereafter. Discontinue therapy if myelosuppression occurs.
- Perform genetic testing for the HLA-B*1502 allele in patients of Asian ancestry prior to beginning therapy.
- Perform liver function tests, urinalysis, electrolytes, BUN, and serum creatinine at baseline, monthly for the 1st 3 mo, and then annually. May ↑ AST, ALT, serum alkaline phosphatase, bilirubin, BUN, urine protein, and urine glucose levels.
- Monitor electrolytes at baseline, monthly for the 1st 3 mo, and then annually. May cause hyponatremia.
- Measure fasting lipid profile and glucose at baseline. May occasionally ↑ serum cholesterol, HDL-C, and triglyceride concentrations.
- May cause false-negative pregnancy test results with tests that determine human chorionic gonadotropin.

Toxicity and Overdose

- Plasma concentrations should be routinely monitored during therapy. Therapeutic levels range from 4–12 mcg/mL.

Implementation

- Do not confuse carbamazepine with oxcarbazepine. Do not confuse Tegretol with Tegretol XR.
- **PO:** Administer medication with food to ↓ GI irritation. May take at bedtime to ↓ daytime sedation. ***DNC:*** Do not crush or chew extended-release tablets. Extended-release capsules may be opened and the contents sprinkled on applesauce or other similar foods.
- Do not administer suspension simultaneously with other liquid medications or diluents; mixture produces an orange rubbery mass.

Patient/Family Teaching

- Explain the purpose and side effects of carbamazepine. Instruct patient to take around the clock, as directed. Take missed doses as soon as possible but not just before next dose; do not double doses. Notify health care provider if more than one dose is missed. Discontinue gradually to prevent seizures. Instruct patient to read the *Medication Guide* before starting and with each Rx refill in case of changes.
- Explain need for continued medical follow-up to assess effectiveness and possible side effects of medication. Periodic lab tests and eye exams may be needed.
- Advise patient to avoid grapefruit and grapefruit juice during therapy.
- May cause dizziness and drowsiness. Caution patient to avoid driving or other activities requiring alertness until response to medication is known.
- Inform patient that coating of *Tegretol XR* is not absorbed but is excreted in feces and may be visible in stool.
- Inform patient that frequent mouth rinses, good oral hygiene, and sugarless gum or candy may help ↓ dry mouth. Saliva substitute may be used. Consult dentist if dry mouth persists >2 wk.
- Instruct patients and caregivers to monitor for emergence of suicidal thoughts and behaviors. Notify health care provider immediately if suicidal thoughts, new or worsening depression, anxiety, changes in behavior or mood, thoughts of suicide, dying, or hurting self, or acting on dangerous impulses occur. Instruct patient to carry wallet card and to call the National Suicide Prevention Lifeline at 1-800-273-8255 or visit www.988lifeline.org if they experience suicidal thoughts.
- Advise patient and family to notify health care provider if new or worse depression, new or worse anxiety, feeling very agitated or restless, panic attacks, trouble sleeping, new or worse irritability,

acting aggressive, being angry or violent, acting on dangerous impulses, an extreme increase in activity and talking, or other unusual changes in behavior or mood occur.
- Instruct patient to report skin rash, fever, sore throat, mouth ulcers, easy bruising, petechiae, unusual bleeding, abdominal pain, chills, rash, pale stools, dark urine, or jaundice to health care provider immediately.
- Caution patients to use sunscreen and protective clothing to prevent photosensitivity reactions.
- Advise patient to notify health care provider of all Rx or OTC medications, vitamins, or herbal products being taken and to consult with health care provider before taking other medications. Advise patient not to take alcohol or other CNS depressants concurrently with this medication.
- Instruct patient to notify health care provider of medication regimen before treatment or surgery.
- **Seizures:** Medical ID describing disease process and medication regimen should be worn at all times in case of emergencies.
- Rep: May cause fetal harm. Advise women of reproductive potential to use a nonhormonal form of contraception while taking carbamazepine, to avoid breastfeeding during therapy, and to notify health care provider if pregnancy is planned or suspected or if breastfeeding. May ↓ effectiveness of estrogen-containing contraceptives. Encourage patients who become pregnant to enroll in the North American Antiepileptic Drug Pregnancy Registry by calling 1-888-233-2334 or on the web at www.aedpregnancyregistry.org.

Evaluation/Desired Outcomes

- Absence or reduction of seizure activity.
- Decrease in trigeminal neuralgia pain. Patients with trigeminal neuralgia who are pain-free should be re-evaluated every 3 mo to determine minimum effective dose.
- Decreased mania and depressive symptoms in bipolar I disorder.

carbidopa/levodopa

(**kar**-bi-doe-pa/**lee**-voe-doe-pa)

Crexont, Dhivy, Duopa, ✱ Duodopa, Rytary, Sinemet, ~~Sinemet CR~~

Classification

Therapeutic: antiparkinson agents

Pharmacologic: dopamine agonists

Indications

Parkinson's disease, postencephalitic parkinsonism, and symptomatic parkinsonism that may follow carbon monoxide intoxication or manganese intoxication.

Action

Levodopa is converted to dopamine in the CNS, where it serves as a neurotransmitter. Carbidopa, a decarboxylase inhibitor, prevents peripheral destruction of levodopa. **Therapeutic Effects:** Relief of tremor and rigidity in Parkinson's syndrome.

Pharmacokinetics

Absorption: Well absorbed following oral administration.

Distribution: Widely distributed. *Levodopa:* enters the CNS in small concentrations. *Carbidopa:* does not cross the blood-brain barrier but does cross the placenta.

Metabolism and Excretion: *Levodopa:* mostly metabolized by the GI tract and liver. *Carbidopa:* 30% excreted unchanged by the kidneys.

Half-life: *Levodopa:* 1 hr; *carbidopa:* 1–2 hr.

TIME/ACTION PROFILE (antiparkinson effects)

ROUTE	ONSET	PEAK	DURATION
Carbidopa	unknown	unknown	5–24 hr
Levodopa	10–15 min	unknown	5–24 hr or more
Carbidopa/levodopa extended release	unknown	2 hr	12 hr

Contraindications/Precautions

Contraindicated in: Hypersensitivity; Angle-closure glaucoma; Nonselective MAO inhibitor therapy; Malignant melanoma; Undiagnosed skin lesions; Some products contain tartrazine, phenylalanine, or aspartame and should be avoided in patients with known hypersensitivity.

Use Cautiously in: History of cardiac, psychiatric, or ulcer disease; OB: Safety not established in pregnancy; Lactation: May ↓ serum prolactin; levodopa enters breast milk; use while breastfeeding only if potential maternal benefit justifies potential risk to infant; Pedi: Safety and effectiveness not established in children.

Adverse Reactions/Side Effects

CV: orthostatic hypotension. **Derm:** melanoma. **EENT:** blurred vision, mydriasis. **GI:** constipation, nausea, vomiting, anorexia, bezoar (enteral suspension), dry mouth, GI HEMORRHAGE (ENTERAL SUSPENSION), GI ISCHEMIA (ENTERAL SUSPENSION), GI OBSTRUCTION

(ENTERAL SUSPENSION), GI PERFORATION (ENTERAL SUSPENSION), HEPATOTOXICITY, INTUSSUSCEPTION (ENTERAL SUSPENSION), PANCREATITIS (ENTERAL SUSPENSION), PERITONITIS (ENTERAL SUSPENSION). **Hemat:** hemolytic anemia, leukopenia. **MS:** dyskinesias. **Neuro:** depression, involuntary movements, anxiety, confusion, dizziness, drowsiness, hallucinations, memory loss, neuropathy, psychiatric problems, sudden sleep onset, urges (gambling, sexual). **Resp:** aspiration pneumonia (enteral suspension). **Misc:** darkening of urine or sweat, MELANOMA, SEPSIS (ENTERAL SUSPENSION).

Interactions

Drug-Drug: Use with **nonselective MAO inhibitors** may result in hypertensive reactions; concurrent use contraindicated (MAO inhibitor must be discontinued ≥2 wk before initiating carbidopa/levodopa). ↑ risk of arrhythmias with **inhalation hydrocarbon anesthetics**, especially **halothane**; if possible, discontinue 6–8 hr before anesthesia. **Phenothiazines**, **haloperidol**, **papaverine**, and **phenytoin** may ↓ effect of levodopa. Large doses of **pyridoxine** may ↓ beneficial effects of levodopa. ↑ hypotension may result with concurrent **antihypertensives**. **Anticholinergics** may ↓ absorption of levodopa. ↑ risk of adverse reactions with **selegiline** or **cocaine**.
Drug-Natural Products: Kava-kava may ↓ levodopa effectiveness.
Drug-Food: Ingestion of foods containing large amounts of **pyridoxine** may ↓ effect of levodopa.

Route/Dosage

Carbidopa/Levodopa

PO (Adults): *Immediate-release (IR) or orally disintegrating tablets:* 25 mg carbidopa/100 mg levodopa 3 times daily; may be ↑ every 1–2 days until desired effect is achieved (max = 8 tablets of 25 mg carbidopa/100 mg levodopa/day).
Enteral: (Adults): Patients must be converted to and be on stable dose of PO IR carbidopa/levodopa tablets before initiation of enteral suspension therapy. *Morning dose for Day 1 (mL) (to be administered over 10–30 min)* = (Amount of levodopa [in mg] in first dose of IR carbidopa/levodopa taken by patient on previous day * 0.8); *Continuous dose for Day 1 (mL) (to be administered over 16 hr)* = Determine amount of levodopa (in mg) patient received from IR carbidopa/levodopa doses throughout 16 waking hr of previous day (do not include doses of IR carbidopa/levodopa taken at night when calculating the levodopa amount). Then, subtract amount of first levodopa dose (in mg) taken by patient on previous day. Divide result by 20 to obtain the # of mL to be administered over 16 hr. Do not exceed dose of 2000 mg. At end of daily 16-hr infusion, patients will disconnect the pump from feeding tube and take their nighttime dose of oral IR carbidopa/levodopa tablets. Total daily dose can be titrated after Day 1 based on patient response and tolerability.

Carbidopa/Levodopa Extended-Release (ER) (doses of all other dosage forms of carbidopa/levodopa and Rytary are not interchangeable)

PO (Adults): *Patients not currently receiving levodopa (Sinemet CR):* 50 mg carbidopa/200 mg levodopa twice daily (minimum of 6 hr apart) initially. *Patients not currently receiving levodopa (Rytary):* 23.75 mg carbidopa/95 mg levodopa 3 times daily for 3 days; then 36.25 mg carbidopa/145 mg levodopa 3 times daily. May continue to ↑ dose as needed (max dose = 97.5 mg carbidopa/390 mg levodopa 3 times daily). May also ↑ frequency of administration up to 5 times daily (max dose = 612.5 mg carbidopa/2450 mg levodopa/day). *Patients not currently receiving levodopa (Crexont):* 35 mg carbidopa/140 mg levodopa twice daily for 3 days. May then gradually ↑ dose as needed to max dose of 525 mg carbidopa/2100 mg levodopa/day in up to 4 divided doses. *Conversion from IR carbidopa/levodopa to Sinemet CR:* Initiate therapy with at least 10% more levodopa content/day (may need up to 30% more) given at 4–8 hr intervals while awake. Allow 3 days between dosage changes; some patients may require larger doses and shorter dosing intervals. *Conversion from IR carbidopa/levodopa to Rytary:* If taking 400–549 mg/day of IR levodopa, give 3 capsules of Rytary 23.75 mg carbidopa/95 mg levodopa 3 times daily. If taking 550–749 mg/day of IR levodopa, give 4 capsules of Rytary 23.75 mg carbidopa/95 mg levodopa 3 times daily. If taking 750–949 mg/day of IR levodopa, give 3 capsules of Rytary 36.25 mg carbidopa/145 mg levodopa 3 times daily. If taking 950–1249 mg/day of IR levodopa, give 3 capsules of Rytary 48.75 mg carbidopa/195 mg levodopa 3 times daily. If taking ≥1250 mg/day of IR levodopa, give 4 capsules of Rytary 48.75 mg carbidopa/195 mg levodopa 3 times daily or 3 capsules of Rytary 61.25 mg carbidopa/245 mg levodopa 3 times daily; may then titrate as needed (max daily dose = 612.5 mg carbidopa/2450 mg levodopa). *Conversion from IR carbidopa/levodopa to Crexont:* If taking <500 mg/day of IR levodopa and most frequent single dose of IR levodopa is 100 mg, give Crexont 70 mg carbidopa/280 mg levodopa twice daily. If taking <500 mg/day of IR levodopa and most frequent single dose of IR levodopa is 150 mg, give 2 capsules of Crexont 52.5 mg carbidopa/210 mg levodopa twice daily. If taking <500 mg/day of IR levodopa and most frequent single dose of IR levodopa is 200 mg, give 2 capsules of Crexont 70 mg carbidopa/280 mg levodopa twice daily. If taking ≥500 mg/day of IR levodopa and most frequent single dose of IR levodopa is 100 mg, give Crexont 70 mg carbidopa/280 mg levodopa 3 times daily. If taking ≥500 mg/day of IR levodopa and most frequent single dose of IR levodopa is 150 mg, give 2 capsules of Crexont 52.5 mg carbidopa/210 mg levodopa 3 times daily. If taking ≥500 mg/day of IR levodopa and most frequent single dose of IR levodopa is 200 mg, give 2 capsules of Crexont 70 mg carbidopa/280 mg levodopa 3 times daily. If taking ≥500 mg/day of IR levodopa and most frequent single dose of IR levodopa is >200 mg, give 2 capsules of Crexont 87.5 mg carbidopa/350 mg levodopa 3 times daily. *Conversion from Rytary to Crexont:* Initiate Crexont on an approximately 1:1 mg basis using the levodopa component for conversion.

Availability (generic available)

Immediate-release tablets: carbidopa 10 mg/levodopa 100 mg, carbidopa 25 mg/levodopa 100 mg, carbidopa 25 mg/levodopa 250 mg. **Orally disintegrating tablet:** carbidopa 10 mg/levodopa 100 mg, carbidopa 25 mg/levodopa 100 mg, carbidopa 25 mg/levodopa 250 mg. **Extended-release capsules (Crexont):** carbidopa 35 mg/levodopa 140 mg, carbidopa 52.5 mg/levodopa 210 mg, carbidopa 70 mg/levodopa 280 mg, carbidopa 87.5 mg/levodopa 350 mg. **Extended-release capsules (Rytary):** carbidopa 23.75 mg/levodopa 95 mg, carbidopa 36.25 mg/levodopa 145 mg, carbidopa 48.75 mg/levodopa 195 mg, carbidopa 61.25 mg/levodopa 245 mg. **Extended-release tablets:** carbidopa 25 mg/levodopa 100 mg, carbidopa 50 mg/levodopa 200 mg. **Enteral suspension (Duopa):** carbidopa 4.63 mg/levodopa 20 mg/mL. ✱ carbidopa 5 mg/levodopa 20 mg/mL. ***In combination with:*** entacapone (Stalevo); see Appendix N.

NURSING IMPLICATIONS

Assessment

- Assess parkinsonian symptoms (akinesia, rigidity, tremors, pill rolling, shuffling gait, mask-like face, twisting motions, drooling) during therapy. On-off phenomenon may cause symptoms to appear or improve suddenly.
- Assess BP and HR frequently during period of dose adjustment.
- Duopa: Monitor for signs and symptoms of GI complications (abdominal pain, prolonged constipation, nausea, vomiting, fever, melanotic stool) during therapy.

Lab Test Considerations

- May cause false-positive test results in Coombs' test.
- May ↑ serum glucose. Dipstick for urine ketones may reveal false-positive results.
- Monitor hepatic and renal function and CBC periodically in patients on long-term therapy. May ↑ AST, ALT, bilirubin, alkaline phosphatase, LDH, and serum protein-bound iodine concentrations.
- May ↓ hemoglobin, ↓ hematocrit, and ↑ WBC.
- May cause agranulocytosis, hemolytic and nonhemolytic anemia, thrombocytopenia, and leukopenia.

Toxicity and Overdose

- Assess for signs of toxicity (involuntary muscle twitching, facial grimacing, spasmodic eye winking, exaggerated protrusion of tongue, behavioral changes). Consult health care professional if symptoms occur.

Implementation

- Do not confuse Sinemet with Janumet.
- In preoperative patients or patients who are NPO, confer with health care professional about continuing medication administration using oral disintegrating tablets.
- **PO:** Administer on a regular schedule. Hospitalized patients should be continued on same schedule as at home. Administer while awake, not around the clock, to improve sleep and prevent side effects.
- ***DNC:*** Controlled-release tablets may be administered as whole or half tablets. Do not crush or chew.
- Each *Dhivy* tablet is scored in three segments with each segment containing 6.25 mg of carbidopa and 25 mg of levodopa to help with titration.
- *For enteral administration,* administer *Duopa* into the jejunum through a percutaneous endoscopic gastrostomy with jejunal tube (PEG-J) with CADD-Legacy 1400 portable infusion pump. Take suspension out of refrigerator 20 min prior to use; must be at room temperature for use. Administer over 16 hr. If extra dose is needed, set function at 1 mL (20 mg of levodopa) when starting; may be adjusted in 0.2 mL increments. Limit to one extra dose every 2 hr. Frequent extra doses may cause or worsen dyskinesias. Discontinue gradually; do not stop abruptly.
- *For ER capsules,* administer without regard to food. ***DNC:*** Swallow capsules whole; do not chew, divide, or crush. For patients with difficulty swallowing, open capsule and sprinkle entire contents on 1–2 tablespoons of applesauce; consume immediately. Do not store mixture for future use. Inform patients that first dose of day may be taken 1–2 hr before eating, as a high-fat, high-calorie meal may delay the absorption of levodopa and onset of action by 2–3 hr. Discontinue gradually; do not stop abruptly. When adjusting dose of ER capsules, keep dose of other Parkinson's medications stable; dose may need to be ↑ in patients taking COMT inhibitor. ER capsules may be administered 3–5 times daily if more frequent dosing is needed and tolerated.

Patient/Family Teaching

- Explain purpose and side effects of medication to patient. Advise patient to read *Patient Information* before starting therapy.
- Instruct patient to take medication at regular intervals as directed. Do not change dose regimen or take additional antiparkinson drugs, including more carbidopa/levodopa, without consulting health care professional. Take missed doses as soon as remembered, unless next scheduled dose is within 2 hr; do not double doses. Advise patient therapeutic effects usually become evident after 2–3 wk of therapy but may require up to 6 mo. Patients who take this medication for several yr may experience a ↓ in the drug's effectiveness.
- Advise patient to notify health care professional of all Rx or OTC medications, vitamins, or herbal products being taken and to consult with health care professional before taking other medications, especially cold remedies. Large amounts of vitamin B_6 (pyridoxine) and iron may interfere with the action of levodopa.
- Explain that gastric irritation may be ↓ by eating food shortly after taking medications but that high-protein meals may impair levodopa's effects. Dividing daily protein intake among all the meals may help ensure adequate protein intake and drug effectiveness. Do not drastically alter diet during therapy without consulting health care professional.
- May cause sudden onset of sleep, drowsiness, or dizziness. Advise patient to avoid driving and other activities that require alertness until response to drug is known.
- Caution patient to change positions slowly to minimize orthostatic hypotension. Notify health care professional if orthostatic hypotension occurs.
- Instruct patient that frequent rinsing of mouth, good oral hygiene, and sugarless gum or candy may ↓ dry mouth.
- Caution patient to monitor skin lesions for any changes. Notify health care professional promptly because of the risk for malignant melanoma.
- Inform patient that harmless darkening of saliva, urine, or sweat may occur.
- Advise patient to notify health care professional if signs and symptoms of GI complications; palpitations; urinary retention; involuntary movements; behavioral changes; severe nausea and vomiting; new skin lesions; or new or ↑ gambling, sexual, binge or compulsive eating, or other intense urges occur. Dose ↓ may be required.
- Inform patient that sometimes a wearing-off effect may occur at end of dosing interval. Notify health care professional if this poses a problem to lifestyle.
- Rep: Advise female patients to notify health care professional if pregnancy is planned or suspected or if breastfeeding. May inhibit lactation.

Evaluation/Desired Outcomes

- Relief of tremors and rigidity in Parkinson's syndrome.

HIGH ALERT

CARBOplatin (kar-boe-**pla**-tin)

Paraplatin

Classification

Therapeutic: antineoplastics

Pharmacologic: alkylating agents

Indications

Advanced ovarian carcinoma (in combination with other agents). Palliative treatment of ovarian carcinoma unresponsive to other modalities.

Action

Inhibits DNA synthesis by producing cross-linking of parent DNA strands (cell-cycle phase-nonspecific). **Therapeutic Effects:** Death of rapidly replicating cells, particularly malignant ones.

Pharmacokinetics

Absorption: IV administration results in complete bioavailability.

Distribution: Well distributed to tissues.

Protein Binding: Platinum is irreversibly bound to plasma proteins.

Metabolism and Excretion: Excreted mostly by the kidneys.

Half-life: *Carboplatin:* 2.6–5.9 hr (↑ in renal impairment); *platinum:* 5 days.

TIME/ACTION PROFILE (effects on blood counts)

ROUTE	ONSET	PEAK	DURATION
IV	unknown	21 days	28 days

Contraindications/Precautions

Contraindicated in: Hypersensitivity to carboplatin, cisplatin, or mannitol; OB: Pregnancy; Lactation: Lactation.

Use Cautiously in: Hearing loss; Electrolyte abnormalities; Renal impairment (↓ dose); Active infection; Diminished bone marrow reserve (↓ dose); Rep: Women of reproductive potential; Pedi: Safety and effectiveness not established in children; Geri: ↑ risk of thrombocytopenia in older adults; consider renal function in dose determination.

Adverse Reactions/Side Effects

Derm: alopecia, rash. **EENT:** ototoxicity. **F and E** hypocalcemia, hypokalemia, hypomagnesemia, hyponatremia. **GI:** abdominal pain, nausea, vomiting, constipation, diarrhea, hepatitis, stomatitis. **GU:** gonadal suppression, nephrotoxicity. **Hemat:** ANEMIA, LEUKOPENIA, THROMBOCYTOPENIA. **Metab:** hyperuricemia.

Neuro: peripheral neuropathy, weakness. **Misc:** HYPERSENSITIVITY REACTIONS (INCLUDING ANAPHYLAXIS).

Interactions

Drug-Drug: ↑ risk of nephrotoxicity and ototoxicity with **aminoglycosides** and **loop diuretics**. ↑ bone marrow depression with other **bone marrow–depressing drugs** or **radiation therapy**. May ↓ antibody response to **live-virus vaccines** and ↑ risk of adverse reactions.

Route/Dosage

IV (Adults): *Initial treatment:* 300 mg/m² with cyclophosphamide at 4-wk intervals. *Treatment of refractory tumors:* 360 mg/m² as a single dose; may be repeated at 4-wk intervals, depending on response.

Renal Impairment

IV (Adults): *CCr 41–59 mL/min:* Initial dose 250 mg/m²; *CCr 16–40 mL/min:* Initial dose 200 mg/m².

Availability (generic available)

Solution for injection: 10 mg/mL.

NURSING IMPLICATIONS

Assessment

- Assess for nausea and vomiting; often occur 6–12 hr after therapy and may persist for 24 hr. Prophylactic antiemetics may be used. Adjust diet as tolerated to maintain fluid and electrolyte balance and ensure adequate nutritional intake. May require discontinuation of therapy.
- Monitor for bone marrow suppression. Assess for bleeding (bleeding gums; bruising; petechiae; guaiac stools, urine, and emesis), and avoid IM injections and rectal temperatures if platelet count is low. Apply pressure to venipuncture sites for 10 min. Assess for signs of infection during neutropenia. Anemia may occur and may be cumulative; transfusions are frequently required. Monitor for ↑ fatigue, dyspnea, and orthostatic hypotension.
- Monitor for signs of anaphylaxis (rash, urticaria, pruritus, facial swelling, wheezing, tachycardia, hypotension). Discontinue medication immediately and notify physician if these occur. Epinephrine and resuscitation equipment should be readily available.
- Audiometry is recommended before initiation of therapy and subsequent doses. Ototoxicity manifests as tinnitus and unilateral or bilateral hearing loss in high frequencies and becomes more frequent and severe with repeated doses. Ototoxicity is more pronounced in children.

Lab Test Considerations

- Monitor CBC with differential before and weekly during therapy. The nadirs of thrombocytopenia and leukopenia occur after 21 days and recover by 30 days after a dose. Nadir of WBC counts usually occurs after 21–28 days and recovers by day 35. Withhold subsequent doses until neutrophil count >2000/mm³ and platelet count >100,000/mm³.
- Monitor renal function and serum electrolytes before initiation of therapy and before each course of carboplatin.
- Monitor hepatic function before and periodically during therapy. May ↑ serum bilirubin, alkaline phosphatase, and AST concentrations.

Implementation

- ***High Alert:*** Fatalities have occurred with chemotherapeutic agents. Before administering, clarify all ambiguous orders; double-check single, daily, and course-of-therapy dose limits; have second practitioner independently double-check original order, calculations, and infusion pump settings.
- ***High Alert:*** Do not confuse carboplatin with cisplatin.
- ***High Alert:*** Carboplatin should be administered in a monitored setting under the supervision of a physician experienced in cancer chemotherapy.

IV Administration

- Solution should be prepared in a biologic cabinet. Wear gloves, gown, and mask while handling medication. Discard equipment in specially designated containers.
- Do not use aluminum needles or equipment during preparation or administration; aluminum reacts with the drug.
- Carboplatin is an irritant. If extravasation occurs, immediately stop infusion. Leave needle/cannula in place temporarily but do not flush the line. Gently aspirate extravasated solution; then remove needle/cannula. Elevate patient's extremity and apply dry cold compresses for 20 min 4 times day for 1–2 days.
- **Intermittent Infusion: Dilution:** Dilute appropriate volume of drug solution in 100 mL or 250 mL bag of 0.9% NaCl or D5W. **Concentration:** 0.5 mg/mL. Stable for 8 hr at room temperature. **Rate:** Infuse over 15–60 min.
- **Y-Site Compatibility:** acyclovir, alemtuzumab, allopurinol, amikacin, aminocaproic acid, aminophylline, amiodarone, amphotericin B liposomal, ampicillin, ampicillin/sulbactam, anidulafungin, argatroban, atracurium, azithromycin, aztreonam, bivalirudin, bleomycin, bumetanide, buprenorphine, butorphanol, calcium chloride, calcium gluconate, caspofungin, cefazolin, cefepime, cefotaxime, cefotetan, cefoxitin, ceftazidime,

ceftriaxone, cefuroxime, ciprofloxacin, cisatracurium, cisplatin, cladribine, clindamycin, cyclophosphamide, cyclosporine, cytarabine, dacarbazine, daptomycin, daunorubicin, dexamethasone, dexmedetomidine, dexrazoxane, digoxin, diltiazem, diphenhydramine, dobutamine, docetaxel, dopamine, doxorubicin hydrochloride, doxorubicin liposomal, doxycycline, droperidol, enalaprilat, ephedrine, epinephrine, epirubicin, ertapenem, erythromycin, esmolol, etoposide, etoposide phosphate, famotidine, fentanyl, filgrastim, fluconazole, fludarabine, fluorouracil, foscarnet, fosphenytoin, furosemide, ganciclovir, gemcitabine, gemtuzumab ozogamicin, gentamicin, glycopyrrolate, granisetron, haloperidol, heparin, hetastarch, hydrocortisone, hydromorphone, idarubicin, ifosfamide, imipenem/cilastatin, insulin, regular, isoproterenol, ketorolac, labetalol, levofloxacin, lidocaine, linezolid, lorazepam, magnesium sulfate, mannitol, melphalan, meperidine, meropenem, mesna, methadone, methotrexate, methylprednisolone, metoclopramide, metoprolol, metronidazole, micafungin, midazolam, milrinone, minocycline, mitomycin, mitoxantrone, morphine, moxifloxacin, nafcillin, nalbuphine, naloxone, nicardipine, nitroglycerin, nitroprusside, norepinephrine, octreotide, ondansetron, oxaliplatin, paclitaxel, palonosetron, pamidronate, pantoprazole, pemetrexed, pentamidine, pentobarbital, phenobarbital, phenylephrine, piperacillin/tazobactam, potassium acetate, potassium chloride, potassium phosphates, prochlorperazine, promethazine, propofol, propranolol, remifentanil, rituximab, rocuronium, sargramostim, sodium acetate, sodium bicarbonate, sodium phosphates, succinylcholine, sufentanil, tacrolimus, theophylline, thiotepa, tigecycline, tirofiban, tobramycin, trastuzumab, trimethoprim/sulfamethoxazole, vancomycin, vasopressin, vecuronium, verapamil, vinblastine, vincristine, vinorelbine, voriconazole, zidovudine, zoledronic acid.

- **Y-Site Incompatibility:** amphotericin B deoxycholate, chlorpromazine, diazepam, leucovorin, phenytoin, procainamide.

Patient/Family Teaching

- Explain purpose and side effects of medication to patient. Advise patient to read *Patient Information* before starting therapy. Emphasize the need for periodic lab tests to monitor for side effects.
- Advise patient to notify health care provider of all Rx or OTC medications, vitamins, or herbal products being taken and to consult health care provider before taking other medications.
- Instruct patient to notify health care provider promptly if fever; chills; sore throat; signs of infection; lower back or side pain; difficult or painful urination; bleeding gums; bruising; pinpoint red spots on skin; blood in stools, urine, or emesis; ↑ fatigue, dyspnea, or orthostatic hypotension occurs.
- Caution patient to avoid crowds and persons with known infections. Instruct patient to use soft toothbrush and electric razor and to avoid falls. Caution patients not to drink alcoholic beverages or take medication containing aspirin or NSAIDs because they may precipitate gastric bleeding.
- Instruct patient to promptly report any numbness or tingling in extremities or face, ↓ coordination, difficulty with hearing or ringing in the ears, unusual swelling, or weight gain to health care provider.
- Instruct patient not to receive any vaccinations without advice of health care provider and to avoid contact with persons who have received oral polio vaccine within the past several months.
- Instruct patient to inspect oral mucosa for erythema and ulceration. If ulceration occurs, advise patient to notify health care provider, rinse mouth with water after eating, and use sponge brush. Mouth pain may require treatment with opioids.
- Discuss with patient the possibility of hair loss. Explore methods of coping.
- Rep: Advise women of reproductive potential to notify health care provider if pregnancy is planned or suspected or if breastfeeding. Advise patient of the need for contraception during therapy.

Evaluation/Desired Outcomes

- Death of rapidly replicating cells, particularly malignant ones.

carboprost (kar-bo-prost)

Hemabate

Classification

Therapeutic: abortifacients

Pharmacologic: oxytocics, prostaglandins

Indications

Induction of midtrimester abortion. Postpartum hemorrhage that has not responded to conventional therapy.

Action

Causes uterine contractions by directly stimulating the myometrium. **Therapeutic Effects:** Expulsion of fetus. Control of postpartum bleeding.

Pharmacokinetics

Absorption: Well absorbed following IM administration.

Distribution: Unknown.

Metabolism and Excretion: Unknown.

Half-life: Unknown.

TIME/ACTION PROFILE (peak noted as mean abortion time)

ROUTE	ONSET	PEAK	DURATION
IM	unknown	16 hr	unknown

Contraindications/Precautions

Contraindicated in: Hypersensitivity; Acute pelvic inflammatory disease; Active pulmonary, renal, or hepatic disease.
Use Cautiously in: Uterine scarring; Asthma; Hypotension; Hypertension; Cardiac disease; Adrenal disease; Anemia; Jaundice; Diabetes mellitus; Seizure disorders.

Adverse Reactions/Side Effects

Derm: flushing. **GI:** diarrhea, nausea, vomiting, abdominal pain, cramps. **GU:** UTERINE RUPTURE. **Neuro:** dizziness, headache. **Resp:** wheezing. **Misc:** fever, chills, HYPERSENSITIVITY REACTIONS (INCLUDING ANAPHYLAXIS AND ANGIOEDEMA), shivering.

Interactions

Drug-Drug: Augments the effects of other **oxytocic agents**.

Route/Dosage

Test Dose

IM (Adults): 100 mcg.

Abortifacient

IM (Adults): 250 mcg every 1.5–3.5 hr depending upon uterine response; may be ↑ to 500 mcg if several doses of 250 mcg produce inadequate response (not to exceed 2 days of continuous therapy or total dose of 12 mg).

Refractory Postpartum Uterine Bleeding

IM (Adults): 250 mcg; may be repeated every 15–90 min (total dose not to exceed 2 mg).

Availability (generic available)

Solution for injection: 250 mcg/mL.

NURSING IMPLICATIONS

Assessment

- Monitor frequency, duration, and force of contractions and uterine resting tone. Notify health care provider if contractions are absent or last >1 min.
- Monitor temperature, BP, and HR periodically throughout course of therapy. Large dose may cause hypertension. Temperature elevation beginning 1–16 hr after initiation of therapy and lasting for several hours is not unusual.
- Monitor for signs and symptoms of anaphylaxis (wheezing; chest tightness; dyspnea; rash; pruritus; swelling of face, lips, or throat). Provide supportive care if symptoms occur.
- Assess for nausea, vomiting, and diarrhea. Vomiting and diarrhea occur in approximately two-thirds of patients. Premedication with antiemetic and antidiarrheal is recommended.
- Monitor amount and type of vaginal discharge. Notify health care provider immediately if symptoms of hemorrhage (increased bleeding, hypotension, pallor, tachycardia) occur.

Implementation

- Carboprost should be used only with strict adherence to recommended dosages. It should be used by medically trained personnel in a hospital that can provide immediate intensive care and acute surgical facilities.
- Avoid contact with skin. Thoroughly wash skin immediately after spillage.
- Opioid analgesic may be given for uterine cramping.
- Store in refrigerator.
- **IM:** Administer deep IM. Dose may be repeated every 1.5–3.5 hr. Rotate sites.

Patient/Family Teaching

- Explain purpose of vaginal examinations (to assess for trauma to cervix).
- Instruct patient to notify health care provider immediately if fever and chills, foul-smelling vaginal discharge, lower abdominal pain, or increased bleeding occurs.

Evaluation/Desired Outcomes

- Complete abortion.
- Control of postpartum or postabortal hemorrhage.

HIGH ALERT

carfilzomib (car- fil-zoe- mib)

Kyprolis

Classification
Therapeutic: antineoplastics
Pharmacologic: proteasome inhibitors

Indications

Multiple myeloma in patients whose disease has relapsed or is refractory despite receiving ≥1 previous drug therapies (as monotherapy). Multiple myeloma in patients whose disease has relapsed or is refractory despite receiving 1–3 previous drug therapies (in combination with dexamethasone, or lenalidomide + dexamethasone, or daratumumab + dexamethasone, or daratumumab/hyaluronidase + dexamethasone, or isatuximab + dexamethasone).

Action

Acts as a proteasome inhibitor by binding to sites on the 20s proteasome. Has antiproliferative and proapoptotic activity. **Therapeutic Effects:** Delayed progression of multiple myeloma.

Pharmacokinetics

Absorption: IV administration results in complete bioavailability.
Distribution: Unknown.
Metabolism and Excretion: Rapidly and extensively metabolized by extrahepatic enzymes. Metabolites have no antineoplastic activity.
Half-life: Unknown.

TIME/ACTION PROFILE (proteasome inhibition)

ROUTE	ONSET	PEAK	DURATION
IV	within 1 hr	unknown	>48 hr

Contraindications/Precautions

Contraindicated in: Severe hepatic impairment; Concurrent use with melphalan and prednisone in newly diagnosed patients ineligible for transplant (↑ risk of serious/fatal adverse reactions); OB: Pregnancy; Lactation: Lactation.
Use Cautiously in: History of cardiovascular disease (may ↑ risk of adverse cardiovascular reactions; safe and effective use in patients with New York Heart Association Class III and IV HF, recent MI, or conduction abnormalities has not been established); Large tumor load (↑ risk of tumor lysis syndrome); Dehydration, diarrhea, or electrolyte abnormalities (correct prior to treatment); Mild or moderate hepatic impairment (↓ dose); Renal impairment (↑ risk of acute renal failure); Prior or current use of immunosuppressants (↑ risk of progressive multifocal leukoencephalopathy); Rep: Women of reproductive potential and men with female sexual partners of reproductive potential; Pedi: Safety and effectiveness not established in children; Geri: ↑ risk of cardiovascular events in older adults.

Adverse Reactions/Side Effects

CV: hypertension, peripheral edema, DEEP VEIN THROMBOSIS, HF, MYOCARDIAL ISCHEMIA/INFARCTION, SUDDEN CARDIAC DEATH. **Endo:** hypoglycemia, atrial fibrillation. **F and E** hypercalcemia, hypokalemia, hypomagnesemia, hyponatremia, hypophosphatemia. **GI:** anorexia, constipation, diarrhea, HEPATIC FAILURE, hepatotoxicity, nausea. **GU:** ACUTE RENAL FAILURE. **Hemat:** anemia, leukopenia, THROMBOCYTOPENIA, THROMBOTIC THROMBOCYTOPENIC PURPURA (TTP)/HEMOLYTIC UREMIC SYNDROME (HUS), lymphopenia. **MS:** back pain, chest wall pain, muscle spasms. **Neuro:** dizziness, fatigue, headache, hypoesthesia, insomnia, POSTERIOR REVERSIBLE ENCEPHALOPATHY SYNDROME (PRES), weakness, peripheral neuropathy, PROGRESSIVE MULTIFOCAL LEUKOENCEPHALOPATHY (PML). **Resp:** cough, dyspnea, ACUTE RESPIRATORY DISTRESS SYNDROME, INTERSTITIAL LUNG DISEASE, PNEUMONITIS, pulmonary edema, PULMONARY EMBOLISM, pulmonary hypertension. **Misc:** fever/chills, INFUSION REACTIONS (INCLUDING FACIAL AND LARYNGEAL EDEMA), TUMOR LYSIS SYNDROME.

Interactions

Drug-Drug: None reported.

Route/Dosage

Combination Therapy with Lenalidomide + Dexamethasone

IV (Adults): *Cycle 1:* 20 mg/m² daily for 2 days (Days 1 and 2); if tolerated, ↑ dose to 27 mg/m² on Days 8, 9, 15, and 16 of a 28-day treatment cycle. *Cycles 2–12:* 27 mg/m² on Days 1, 2, 8, 9, 15, and 16 of a 28-day treatment cycle; *Cycles 13–18:* 27 mg/m² on Days 1, 2, 15, and 16 of a 28-day treatment cycle. *Cycles 19 and subsequent cycles:* Continue lenalidomide and dexamethasone (without carfilzomib) until unacceptable toxicity or disease progression.

Combination Therapy with Daratumumab + Dexamethasone or Daratumumab/Hyaluronidase + Dexamethasone

Twice Weekly Regimen

IV (Adults): *Cycle 1:* 20 mg/m² daily for 2 days (Days 1 and 2); if tolerated, ↑ dose to 56 mg/m² on Days 8, 9, 15, and 16 of a 28-day treatment cycle. *Cycle 2 and subsequent cycles:* 56 mg/m² on Days 1, 2, 8, 9, 15, and 16 of a 28-day treatment cycle. Continue carfilzomib, daratumumab (or daratumumab/hyaluronidase), and dexamethasone until unacceptable toxicity or disease progression.

Once Weekly Regimen

IV (Adults): *Cycle 1:* 20 mg/m² on Day 1; if tolerated, ↑ dose to 70 mg/m² on Days 8 and 15 of a 28-day treatment cycle. *Cycle 2 and subsequent cycles:* 70 mg/m² on Days 1, 8, and 15 of a 28-day treatment cycle. Continue carfilzomib, daratumumab (or daratumumab/hyaluronidase), and dexamethasone until unacceptable toxicity or disease progression.

Combination Therapy with Isatuximab + Dexamethasone

Twice Weekly Regimen

IV (Adults): *Cycle 1:* 20 mg/m² daily for 2 days (Days 1 and 2); if tolerated, ↑ dose to 56 mg/m² on Days 8, 9, 15, and 16 of a 28-day treatment cycle. *Cycle 2 and subsequent cycles:* 56 mg/m² on Days 1, 2, 8, 9, 15, and 16 of a 28-day treatment cycle. Continue carfilzomib, isatuximab, and dexamethasone until unacceptable toxicity or disease progression.

Combination Therapy with Dexamethasone

Twice Weekly Regimen

IV (Adults): *Cycle 1:* 20 mg/m² daily for 2 days (Days 1 and 2); if tolerated, ↑ dose to 56 mg/m² on Days 8, 9, 15, and 16 of a 28-day treatment cycle.

Cycle 2 and subsequent cycles: 56 mg/m^2 on Days 1, 2, 8, 9, 15, and 16 of a 28-day treatment cycle. Continue both carfilzomib and dexamethasone until unacceptable toxicity or disease progression.

Once Weekly Regimen

IV (Adults): *Cycle 1:* 20 mg/m^2 on Day 1; if tolerated, ↑ dose to 70 mg/m^{2}on Days 8 and 15 of a 28-day treatment cycle. *Cycle 2 and subsequent cycles:* 70 mg/m^2 on Days 1, 8, and 15 of a 28-day treatment cycle. Continue both carfilzomib and dexamethasone until unacceptable toxicity or disease progression.

Monotherapy

20/27 mg/m^2 Regimen

IV (Adults): *Cycle 1:* 20 mg/m^2 daily for 2 days (Days 1 and 2); if tolerated, ↑ dose to 27 mg/m^2 on Days 8, 9, 15, and 16 of a 28-day treatment cycle. *Cycles 2–12:* 27 mg/m^2 on Days 1, 2, 8, 9, 15, and 16 of a 28-day treatment cycle; *Cycle 13 and subsequent cycles:* 27 mg/m^2 on Days 1, 2, 15, and 16 of a 28-day treatment cycle. Continue carfilzomib until unacceptable toxicity or disease progression.

20/56 mg/m^2 Regimen

IV (Adults): *Cycle 1:* 20 mg/m^2 daily for 2 days (Days 1 and 2); if tolerated, ↑ dose to 56 mg/m^2 on Days 8, 9, 15, and 16 of a 28-day treatment cycle. *Cycles 2–12:* 56 mg/m^2 on Days 1, 2, 8, 9, 15, and 16 of a 28-day treatment cycle; *Cycle 13 and subsequent cycles:* 56 mg/m^2 on Days 1, 2, 15, and 16 of a 28-day treatment cycle. Continue carfilzomib until unacceptable toxicity or disease progression.

Renal Impairment

IV (Adults): *Hemodialysis:* Administer dose after hemodialysis.

Hepatic Impairment

IV (Adults): *Mild or moderate hepatic impairment:* ↓ dose by 25%.

Availability (generic available)

Lyophilized powder for injection: 10 mg/vial, 30 mg/vial, 60 mg/vial.

NURSING IMPLICATIONS

Assessment

- Maintain hydration status during therapy. Monitor for dehydration and fluid overload, especially in patients with or at risk for HF.
- Monitor for cardiac complications (BP, new or worsening HF, decreased left ventricular function, myocardial ischemia). Hold dose for Grade 3 or 4 cardiac events until recovery. Consider restarting at a reduced dose. If tolerated, may escalate to previous dose.
- Monitor BP before starting and periodically during therapy. Treat hypertension before starting therapy. Assess risks/benefits if hypertension cannot be adequately controlled.
- Assess for pulmonary hypertension with cardiac imaging. Hold dose until resolved or returned to baseline. Consider restarting based on risk/benefit ratio. May use a reduced dose and escalate as tolerated.
- Monitor for dyspnea frequently during therapy. Interrupt therapy until symptoms resolved; consider restarting with one dose level reduction and ↑ as tolerated. If drug-induced pulmonary toxicity occurs, discontinue carfilzomib.
- Assess for sensory and motor peripheral neuropathy periodically during therapy. If Grade 3 or 4 occurs, hold dose until resolved or returned to baseline. Restart with prior or reduced dose, may escalate if tolerated.
- Monitor for signs and symptoms of tumor lysis syndrome (hyperuricemia, hyperkalemia, hyperphosphatemia, hypocalcemia) during therapy. Consider uric acid–lowering drugs in patients at risk. Manage promptly; may require discontinuation.
- Monitor for signs/symptoms of infusion reactions (fever, chills, arthralgia, myalgia, facial flushing, facial edema, laryngeal edema, vomiting, weakness, shortness of breath, hypotension, syncope, chest tightness). May occur immediately or up to 24 hr after administration. Premedicate with dexamethasone prophylactically.
- Assess for signs and symptoms of TTP/HUS (weakness, confusion or coma, abdominal pain, nausea, vomiting, diarrhea, arrhythmias). Discontinue therapy if symptoms occur.
- Monitor for signs and symptoms of PRES (seizure, headache, lethargy, confusion, blindness, altered consciousness, other visual and neurological disturbances, hypertension). Determined with MRI. Discontinue if symptoms occur.
- Assess for any new signs or symptoms that may be suggestive of PML, an opportunistic infection of the brain caused by the JC virus that leads to death or severe disability; withhold dose and notify health care professional promptly. PML symptoms may begin gradually but usually worsen rapidly. Symptoms vary depending on which part of brain is infected (mental function declines rapidly and progressively, causing dementia; speaking becomes increasingly difficult; partial blindness; difficulty walking; rarely, headaches and seizures occur). Diagnosis is usually made via gadolinium-enhanced MRI and CSF analysis. Risk of PML ↑ with the number of infusions. Hold carfilzomib at first sign of PML.

Lab Test Considerations

- Verify negative pregnancy test before starting therapy.
- Monitor CBC and platelet count frequently during therapy. Nadir of thrombocytopenia occurs around Day 8 of 28-day cycle and recovery to baseline by start of next 28-day cycle. *If ANC <0.5 × 10^9/L,* hold dose. If recovered to ≥0.5 × 10^9/L, continue at same dose. For subsequent drops to <0.5 × 10^9/L, follow recommendations above and consider 1 dose level reduction when restarting carfilzomib. *If ANC <0.5 × 10^9/L and an oral temperature >38.5°C. or two consecutive readings of >38.0° for more than 2 hr,* hold dose. If ANC returns to baseline and fever resolves, resume therapy at same dose. *If platelets <10 × 10^9/L or evidence of bleeding with thrombocytopenia,* hold dose. If recovered to ≥10 × 10^9/L and/or bleeding is controlled, continue at same dose. For subsequent drops to <10 × 10^9/L, follow recommendations above and consider one dose level reduction when restarting carfilzomib.
- Monitor liver enzymes frequently during therapy. May cause ↑ serum transaminases and bilirubin. If Grade 3 or 4 ↑ of transaminases, bilirubin, or other liver abnormalities, hold dose until resolved or return to baseline. May be restarted at a reduced dose with frequently liver function monitoring; may escalate dose if tolerated.
- Monitor renal function frequently during therapy. *If serum creatinine ≥2 times baseline or CCr <15 mL/min, or CCr ↓ ≤50% of baseline, or need for dialysis,* hold dose and continue monitoring. If ↓ renal function due to carfilzomib, resume when renal function has recovered to within 25% of baseline; start at 1 dose level reduction. If not due to carfilzomib, dosing may be resumed at discretion of physician. For patients on dialysis receiving carfilzomib, administer dose after dialysis procedure.
- Monitor serum potassium periodically during therapy. May cause hyperglycemia, hypercalcemia, hypophosphatemia, and hyponatremia.

Implementation

- Hydrate patient to reduce risk of renal toxicity and tumor lysis syndrome. At least 48 hr before Cycle 1, Day 1, administer oral fluids (30 mL per kg) and IV fluids (250 mL to 500 mL of IV fluid prior to each dose in Cycle 1). Give an additional 250–500 mL of IV fluids following administration, if needed. Continue oral and/or IV hydration, as needed, in subsequent cycles. Monitor for fluid overload and adjust hydration to patient needs.
- *For monotherapy or combination therapy,* premedicate with dexamethasone 4 mg PO or IV at least 30 min but not >4 hr prior to all doses during Cycle 1 to reduce the incidence and severity of infusion reactions. If symptoms of infusion reaction occur during subsequent cycles, reinstate dexamethasone premedication. *For combination with other therapies,* premedicate with dexamethasone 40 mg PO or IV at least 30 min but not >4 hr before doses on Days 1, 8, 15, and 22 during each cycle to reduce incidence and severity of infusion reactions. Continue hydration as needed during subsequent cycles.
- Institute thromboprophylaxis regimen with combination therapy of carfilzomib with dexamethasone and other therapies.
- Use antiviral prophylaxis to decrease risk of herpes zoster reactivation.

IV Administration

- **Intermittent Infusion: Reconstitution:** Using a 21-gauge needle, reconstitute each 10 mg vial by injecting 5 mL, each 30 mg vial by injecting 15 mL, or each 60 mg vial by injecting 29 mL sterile water for injection respectively, directed onto inside wall of vial to minimize foaming. Swirl gently or invert slowly for 1 min or until complete dissolution of powder; do not shake. If foaming occurs, allow solution to rest for 2–5 min until foaming subsides. Solution should be clear and colorless; do not administer solutions that are discolored or contain particulate matter. **Dilution:** Withdraw calculated dose from vial and dilute in 50 or 100 mL D5W. Vial may exceed required dose; calculate dose carefully to prevent overdosing. Reconstituted solution is stable at room temperature for 4 hr and 24 hr if refrigerated. Discard unused portion.
- **Rate:** *For carfilzomib in combination with lenalidomide and dexamethasone,* infuse over 10 min. *For carfilzomib in combination with dexamethasone or daratumumab and dexamethasone,* infuse over 30 min. *For monotherapy with 20/27 mg/m² regimen,* infuse over 10 min. *For monotherapy with 20/27 mg/m² regimen,* infuse over 30 min. Do not administer as a bolus. Flush line with 0.9% NaCl or D5W immediately prior to and following administration.
- **Y-Site Incompatibility:** Do not mix with or infuse with other medications.

Patient/Family Teaching

- Explain purpose of medication to patient.
- Advise patient to notify health care professional immediately if signs and symptoms of infusion reactions (fever, chills, rigors, arthralgia, myalgia, facial flushing, facial edema, vomiting, weakness, shortness of breath, hypotension, syncope, chest tightness, chest pain, cough, swelling of feet or legs), venous thrombosis, bleeding, hepatitis (worsening fatigue, yellow discoloration of skin or eyes), or dyspnea occur.

- May cause fatigue, dizziness, fainting, and drop in BP. Caution patient to avoid driving or other activities requiring alertness until response to medication is known.
- Advise patient to maintain hydration status during therapy; may cause vomiting and/or diarrhea.
- Advise patient to notify health care professional of all Rx or OTC medications, vitamins, or herbal products being taken and to consult with health care professional before taking other medications.
- Rep: May cause fetal harm. Advise females of reproductive potential to use effective contraception during therapy and for 6 mo following last dose of therapy and to avoid breastfeeding during and for 2 wk after last dose. Avoid hormonal contraceptives during combination therapy to prevent ↑ risk of thrombosis. Advise males with female partners of reproductive potential to use effective contraception during and for 3 mo after last dose. May impair fertility in male and female patients.

Evaluation/Desired Outcomes

- Slowed progression of multiple myeloma.

BEERS

cariprazine (kar-ip-ra-zeen)

Vraylar

Classification

Therapeutic: antipsychotics

Indications

Schizophrenia. Acute treatment of mania/mixed episodes associated with bipolar I disorder. Depressive episodes associated with bipolar I disorder. Adjunctive treatment of major depressive disorder (in combination with antidepressants).

Action

Acts as a partial agonist at dopamine D_2 receptors in the CNS and serotonin 5-HT_{1A}; also acts an antagonist at 5-HT_{2A} receptors. **Therapeutic Effects:** Decreased incidence and severity of symptoms of schizophrenia. Decreased occurrence and severity of mania associated with bipolar I disorder. Antidepressant action.

Pharmacokinetics

Absorption: Well absorbed following oral administration.

Distribution: Unknown.

Protein Binding: 91–97%.

Metabolism and Excretion: Two metabolites, desmethyl cariprazine (DCAR) and didesmethyl cariprazine (DDCAR), have antipsychotic activity. Metabolism occurs mostly via the CYP3A4 isoenzyme, with further metabolism resulting in inactive metabolites; 21% excreted urine, 1.2% as unchanged drug.

Half-life: Cariprazine: 2–4 days; *DDCAR:* 1–3 wk.

TIME/ACTION PROFILE (improvement in symptoms)

ROUTE	ONSET	PEAK	DURATION
PO (schizophrenia)	within 1–2 wk	4–6 wk	2 wk†
PO (mania due to bipolar I disorder)	within 5–7 days	2–3 wk	2 wk†

† Plasma concentrations of drug and active metabolites following discontinuation.

Contraindications/Precautions

Contraindicated in: Hypersensitivity.

Use Cautiously in: Known cerebrovascular/cardiovascular disease, dehydration, concurrent use of diuretics/antihypertensives or syncope (↑ risk of orthostatic hypotension); May ↑ risk of suicide attempt/ideation, especially during early treatment or dose adjustment; risk may be greater in children or adolescents; Pre-existing ↓ WBC or ANC or history of drug-induced leukopenia/neutropenia; At risk of aspiration or falls; OB: Neonates exposed in the 3rd trimester may experience extrapyramidal symptoms/withdrawal; Lactation: Use while breastfeeding only if potential maternal benefit justifies potential risk to infant; Pedi: Safety and effectiveness not established; Geri: Appears on Beers list. ↑ risk of stroke, cognitive decline, and mortality in older adults with dementia. Avoid use in older adults, except for schizophrenia, bipolar disorder, or adjunctive treatment of major depressive disorder (not indicated for dementia-related psychosis).

Adverse Reactions/Side Effects

CV: hypertension, orthostatic hypotension, tachycardia. **Derm:** rash, STEVENS-JOHNSON SYNDROME (SJS). **EENT:** blurred vision. **Endo:** hyperglycemia/diabetes mellitus. **GI:** dyspepsia, nausea, ↑ liver enzymes, constipation, diarrhea, dry mouth, dysphagia (↑ aspiration risk), vomiting. **Hemat:** AGRANULOCYTOSIS, leukopenia, neutropenia. **Metab:** ↓ appetite, dyslipidemia, weight gain. **MS:** arthralgia, back pain, extremity pain. **Neuro:** akathisia, drowsiness, extrapyramidal symptoms, headache, agitation, dizziness, fatigue, insomnia, NEUROLEPTIC MALIGNANT SYNDROME (NMS), restlessness, SUICIDAL THOUGHTS/BEHAVIORS, tardive dyskinesia. **Resp:** cough. **Misc:** body temperature dysregulation.

Interactions

Drug-Drug: **Strong CYP3A4 inhibitors**, including **itraconazole** and **ketoconazole**, and **moderate CYP3A4 inhibitors**, including **erythromycin** and **fluconazole**, may ↑ levels and risk of toxicity; ↓ cariprazine dose. Levels and effectiveness may be ↓ by concurrent use of **strong CYP3A4 inducers**, including **carbamazepine** and **rifampin**; concurrent use not recommended. Concurrent use of **diuretics** or **antihypertensives** may ↑ risk of orthostatic hypotension/syncope.

Route/Dosage

Schizophrenia or Acute Treatment of Mania/Mixed Episodes Associated With Bipolar I Disorder

PO (Adults): 1.5 mg once daily; may ↑ to 3 mg once daily on Day 2; further dosage adjustments can be made in increments of 1.5 mg or 3 mg depending on response/tolerability (max dose = 6 mg once daily). *Initiation of strong CYP3A4 inhibitor while on stable dose of cariprazine:* If current dose 1.5–3 mg once daily: Change to 1.5 mg every 3 days. If current dose 4.5–6 mg once daily: Change to 1.5 mg every other day. *Initiation of moderate CYP3A4 inhibitor while on stable dose of cariprazine:* If current dose 1.5–3 mg once daily: Change to 1.5 mg every other day. If current dose 4.5–6 mg once daily: Change to 1.5 mg once daily. *Initiation of cariprazine while on stable dose of strong CYP3A4 inhibitor:* 1.5 mg every 3 days; may ↑ to 1.5 mg every other day if needed. *Initiation of cariprazine while on stable dose of moderate CYP3A4 inhibitor:* 1.5 mg every other day; may ↑ to 1.5 mg once daily, if needed.

Depressive Episodes Associated With Bipolar I Disorder or Adjunctive Treatment of Major Depressive Disorder

PO (Adults): 1.5 mg once daily; may ↑ to 3 mg once daily on Day 15 depending on response/tolerability (max dose = 3 mg once daily); *Initiation of strong CYP3A4 inhibitor while on stable dose of cariprazine:* If current dose 1.5–3 mg once daily: Change to 1.5 mg every 3 days. If current dose 4.5–6 mg once daily: Change to 1.5 mg every other day. *Initiation of moderate CYP3A4 inhibitor while on stable dose of cariprazine:* If current dose 1.5–3 mg once daily: Change to 1.5 mg every other day. If current dose 4.5–6 mg once daily: Change to 1.5 mg once daily. *Initiation of cariprazine while on stable dose of strong CYP3A4 inhibitor:* 1.5 mg every 3 days. *Initiation of cariprazine while on stable dose of moderate CYP3A4 inhibitor:* 1.5 mg every other day.

Availability

Capsules: 1.5 mg, 3 mg, 4.5 mg, 6 mg.

NURSING IMPLICATIONS

Assessment

- Assess mental status (orientation, mood, behavior) before and periodically during therapy. Assess for suicidal tendencies, especially during early therapy for depression. Restrict amount of drug available to patient. Risk may be ↑ in children, adolescents, and adults ≤24 yr.
- Assess waist circumference, weight, and BMI before treatment, at Wk 4, at Wk 8, at Wk 12, following initiation or change in therapy, and quarterly thereafter; Pedi: Evaluate weight gain against expected normal growth in children.
- Monitor BP (sitting, standing, lying), HR, and respiratory rate at baseline, at Wk 12, and annually thereafter; more frequently in patients with risk factors for hypertension.
- Observe patient carefully when administering medication to ensure that medication is actually taken and not hoarded or cheeked.
- Monitor for adverse reactions and patient response for several weeks after starting therapy and after each dose ↑. Due to long action, may not occur for several weeks. Consider ↓ dose or discontinuing drug if severe adverse reactions occur.
- Monitor patient for onset of akathisia (restlessness or desire to keep moving) and extrapyramidal side effects (*parkinsonian:* difficulty speaking or swallowing, loss of balance control, pill rolling of hands, masklike face, shuffling gait, rigidity, tremors; and *dystonic:* muscle spasms, twisting motions, twitching, inability to move eyes, weakness of arms or legs) periodically throughout therapy. Report these symptoms.
- Monitor for tardive dyskinesia (uncontrolled rhythmic movement of mouth, face, and extremities; lip smacking or puckering; puffing of cheeks; uncontrolled chewing; rapid or worm-like movements of tongue). Notify health care professional immediately if these symptoms occur, as these side effects may be irreversible.
- Monitor for development of NMS, such as hyperpyrexia, muscle rigidity, seizures, altered mental status, or evidence of autonomic instability (irregular HR or BP, tachycardia, diaphoresis, cardiac arrhythmia). *If NMS suspected,* discontinue cariprazine and institute seizure precautions as indicated.
- Assess for rash or signs and symptoms of SJS periodically during therapy (fever, general malaise, fatigue, muscle or joint aches, blisters, oral lesions, conjunctivitis). *If SJS confirmed,* discontinue cariprazine and provide supportive care.
- Assess for falls risk. Drowsiness, orthostatic hypotension, and motor and sensory instability ↑ risk. Institute prevention if indicated.

Lab Test Considerations

- Monitor CBC with differential frequently during therapy in patients with pre-existing or history of low WBC. May cause leukopenia, neutropenia, or agranulocytosis. *If ANC <1000/mm³,* discontinue cariprazine.
- Obtain fasting blood glucose, lipid profile, and cholesterol levels at baseline, Wk 12, and annually during therapy. Patients with diabetes should be closely monitored for worsening glycemic control.

Implementation

- **PO:** Administer once daily without regard to food.

Patient/Family Teaching

- Explain the purpose and side effects of cariprazine. Advise patient to take medication as directed and not to skip doses or double up on missed doses. Take missed doses as soon as remembered unless almost time for the next dose. Do not stop taking cariprazine without consulting health care professional. Advise patient to read *Patient Information* before starting and with each Rx refill in case of changes.
- Emphasize the importance of routine follow-up exams and continued participation in psychotherapy as indicated.
- Inform patient of possibility of extrapyramidal symptoms and tardive dyskinesia. Instruct patient to report these symptoms immediately.
- Advise patient to make position changes slowly to minimize orthostatic hypotension. Protect from falls.
- Medication may cause drowsiness. Caution patient to avoid driving or other activities requiring alertness until response to medication is known.
- Advise patient, family, and caregivers to look for suicidality, especially during early therapy or dose changes. Notify health care professional immediately if thoughts about suicide or dying, attempts to commit suicide, new or worse depression or anxiety, agitation or restlessness, panic attacks, insomnia, new or worse irritability, aggressiveness, acting on dangerous impulses, mania, or other changes in mood or behavior occur.
- Inform patient that cariprazine may cause weight gain. Advise patient to monitor weight periodically. Notify health care professional of significant weight gain.
- Instruct patient to notify health care professional of all Rx or OTC medications, vitamins, or herbal products being taken and to consult health care professional before taking any new medications. Caution patient to avoid taking alcohol or other CNS depressants concurrently with this medication.
- Advise patient that extremes in temperature should be avoided because this drug impairs body temperature regulation.
- Advise patient to notify health care professional of medication regimen prior to treatment or surgery.
- Advise patients with diabetes to report worsening of glucose control due to potential for hyperglycemia.
- Rep: May cause fetal harm. Advise women of reproductive potential to notify health care professional if pregnancy is planned or suspected during therapy or if breastfeeding. Encourage pregnant patients to enroll in registry by contacting National Pregnancy Registry for Atypical Antipsychotics at 1-866-961-2388 or visit http://womensmentalhealth.org/clinical-and-research-programs/pregnancyregistry/. May cause extrapyramidal and/or withdrawal symptoms (agitation, hypertonia, hypotonia, tremor, somnolence, respiratory distress, feeding disorder) in neonates whose mothers were exposed to antipsychotic drugs during 3rd trimester of pregnancy. Symptoms vary in severity. Some neonates recover within hours or days without specific treatment; others required prolonged hospitalization. Monitor neonates of women pregnant while taking cariprazine for extrapyramidal and/or withdrawal symptoms and manage symptoms appropriately.

Evaluation/Desired Outcomes

- Decrease in excitable, paranoid, or withdrawn behavior.
- Decreased occurrence and severity of mania associated with bipolar I disorder.
- Increased sense of well-being.
- Renewed interest in surroundings.

carvedilol, See BETA BLOCKERS (nonselective).

caspofungin (kas-po-**fun**-gin)

~~Cancidas~~

Classification

Therapeutic: antifungals

Pharmacologic: echinocandins

Indications

Invasive aspergillosis refractory to, or intolerant of, other therapies. Candidemia and associated serious infections (intra-abdominal abscesses, peritonitis, pleural space infections). Esophageal candidiasis. Suspected fungal infections in febrile neutropenic patients.

Action

Inhibits the synthesis of (1, 3)-D-glucan, a necessary component of the fungal cell wall. **Therapeutic Effects:** Death of susceptible fungi.

Pharmacokinetics

Absorption: IV administration results in complete bioavailability.
Distribution: Widely distributed to tissues.
Protein Binding: 97%.
Metabolism and Excretion: Slowly and extensively metabolized; <1.5% excreted unchanged in urine.
Half-life: Polyphasic: *phase:* 9–11 hr; *phase:* 40–50 hr.

TIME/ACTION PROFILE

ROUTE	ONSET	PEAK	DURATION
IV	unknown	end of infusion	24 hr

Contraindications/Precautions

Contraindicated in: Hypersensitivity; OB: Pregnancy.
Use Cautiously in: Moderate hepatic impairment (↓ maintenance dose recommended); Lactation: Use while breastfeeding only if potential maternal benefit justifies potential risk to infant.

Adverse Reactions/Side Effects

Derm: flushing, pruritus, rash, STEVENS-JOHNSON SYNDROME (SJS), TOXIC EPIDERMAL NECROLYSIS (TEN). **GI:** ↑ liver enzymes, diarrhea, nausea, vomiting. **GU:** ↑ serum creatinine. **Local:** venous irritation at injection site. **Neuro:** headache. **Resp:** bronchospasm. **Misc:** chills, fever, HYPERSENSITIVITY REACTIONS (INCLUDING ANAPHYLAXIS AND ANGIOEDEMA).

Interactions

Drug-Drug: ↑ risk of hepatotoxicity with **Cyclosporine**; closely monitor liver enzymes during concurrent therapy. May ↓ levels and effectiveness of **tacrolimus**. **Rifampin** may ↓ levels and effectiveness; maintenance dose should be ↑ to 70 mg/day (in patients with normal hepatic function). **Efavirenz**, **nelfinavir**, **nevirapine**, **phenytoin**, **dexamethasone**, or **carbamazepine** may ↓ levels and effectiveness; consider ↑ maintenance dose to 70 mg/day in patients who are not clinically responding.

Route/Dosage

IV (Adults): 70 mg initially, followed by 50 mg once daily; duration determined by clinical situation and response; *Esophageal candidiasis:* 50 mg once daily; duration determined by clinical situation and response.
IV (Children ≥3 mo): 70 mg/m^2 (max = 70 mg) initially, followed by 50 mg/m^2 once daily (max = 70 mg/day); duration determined by clinical situation and response.
IV (Infants 1 to <3 mo and Neonates): 25 mg/m^2 once daily.

Hepatic Impairment

IV (Adults): *Moderate hepatic impairment:* 70 mg initially, followed by 35 mg once daily; duration determined by clinical situation and response.

Availability (generic available)

Powder for injection: 50 mg/vial, 70 mg/vial.

NURSING IMPLICATIONS

Assessment

- Assess patient for signs and symptoms of fungal infections before and periodically during therapy.
- Assess for skin rash frequently during therapy. Discontinue at first sign of rash; may be life-threatening. SJS and TEN may develop. Treat symptomatically; may recur once treatment is stopped.
- Monitor for signs and symptoms of hypersensitivity reactions, including anaphylaxis (rash, dyspnea, stridor, facial swelling, angioedema, pruritus, sensation of warmth, bronchospasm) during therapy. *If hypersensitivity reaction occurs,* stop infusion and implement supportive medical management as needed.

Lab Test Considerations

- May ↑ serum alkaline phosphatase, serum creatinine, AST, ALT, eosinophils, and urine protein and RBCs. May ↓ serum potassium, hemoglobin, hematocrit, and WBC count.

Implementation

IV Administration

- **Intermittent Infusion:** Allow refrigerated vial to reach room temperature. **Reconstitution:** Reconstitute vials with 10.8 mL of 0.9% NaCl, sterile water for injection, bacteriostatic water for injection with methylparaben and propylparaben, or bacteriostatic water for injection with 0.9% benzyl alcohol. Use preservative-free diluents for neonates. Do not dilute with dextrose solutions. White cake should dissolve completely. Mix gently until a clear solution is obtained. Do not use a solution that is cloudy, discolored, or contains precipitates. Reconstituted solution is stable for 1 hr at room temperature. **Concentration:** 5 mg/mL (50 mg vial); 7 mg/mL (70 mg vial). **Dilution:** Further dilute appropriate volume of reconstituted solution with 0.9% NaCl, 0.45% NaCl, 0.225% NaCl, or LR. Infusion is stable for 24 hr at room temperature or 48 hr if refrigerated. **Concentration:** Not to exceed 0.5 mg/mL. **Rate:** Infuse over 1 hr.
- **Y-Site Compatibility:** alemtuzumab, allopurinol, amikacin, aminophylline, amiodarone, anidulafungin, argatroban, arsenic trioxide, atracurium, aztreonam, bleomycin, bumetanide, busulfan, butorphanol, calcium acetate, calcium chloride,

calcium gluconate, carboplatin, carmustine, chlorpromazine, ciprofloxacin, cisatracurium, cisplatin, cyclophosphamide, cyclosporine, dacarbazine, dactinomycin, daptomycin, daunorubicin, dexmedetomidine, dexrazoxane, diltiazem, diphenhydramine, dobutamine, docetaxel, dopamine, doxorubicin hydrochloride, doxorubicin liposomal, doxycycline, droperidol, epinephrine, epirubicin, erythromycin, esmolol, etoposide, etoposide phosphate, famotidine, fentanyl, fluconazole, fludarabine, ganciclovir, gemcitabine, gentamicin, glycopyrrolate, granisetron, haloperidol, hydrocortisone, hydromorphone, idarubicin, ifosfamide, imipenem/cilastatin, insulin, regular, irinotecan, isoproterenol, labetalol, leucovorin, levofloxacin, linezolid, magnesium sulfate, mannitol, melphalan, meperidine, meropenem, mesna, metoclopramide, metoprolol, midazolam, milrinone, mitomycin, mitoxantrone, morphine, moxifloxacin, mycophenolate, nalbuphine, naloxone, nicardipine, nitroglycerin, norepinephrine, octreotide, ondansetron, oxaliplatin, oxytocin, paclitaxel, palonosetron, pentamidine, phentolamine, phenylephrine, posaconazole, potassium acetate, potassium chloride, procainamide, prochlorperazine, promethazine, propranolol, remifentanil, rocuronium, succinylcholine, sufentanil, tacrolimus, telavancin, theophylline, thiotepa, tigecycline, tirofiban, tobramycin, topotecan, vancomycin, vasopressin, vecuronium, verapamil, vinblastine, vincristine, vinorelbine, voriconazole, zidovudine, zoledronic acid.

- **Y-Site Incompatibility:** aminocaproic acid, amphotericin B liposomal, ampicillin, ampicillin/sulbactam, bivalirudin, blinatumomab, cefazolin, cefepime, cefotaxime, cefotetan, cefoxitin, ceftaroline, ceftazidime, ceftriaxone, cefuroxime, chloramphenicol, clindamycin, dantrolene, dexamethasone, diazepam, digoxin, enalaprilat, ephedrine, ertapenem, fluorouracil, foscarnet, fosphenytoin, furosemide, heparin, ketorolac, lidocaine, methotrexate, methylprednisolone, nafcillin, nitroprusside, pamidronate, pemetrexed, pentobarbital, phenobarbital, phenytoin, piperacillin/tazobactam, potassium phosphates, sodium acetate, sodium bicarbonate, sodium phosphates, trimethoprim/sulfamethoxazole.
- Solutions containing dextrose

Patient/Family Teaching

- Explain purpose and side effects of medication to patient. Advise patient to read *Patient Information* before starting therapy. Inform patient about the need for routine lab monitoring during therapy.
- Advise patient to notify health care professional of all Rx or OTC medications, vitamins, or herbal products being taken and to consult health care professional before taking other medications.
- Advise patient to notify health care professional immediately if symptoms of allergic reactions (rash, facial swelling, pruritus, sensation of warmth, difficulty breathing) occur.
- Rep: Advise women of reproductive potential to notify health care professional if pregnancy is planned or suspected or if breastfeeding.

Evaluation/Desired Outcomes

- Death of susceptible fungi.

cefaclor, See CEPHALOSPORINS—SECOND GENERATION.

cefadroxil, See CEPHALOSPORINS—FIRST GENERATION.

ceFAZolin, See CEPHALOSPORINS—FIRST GENERATION.

cefdinir, See CEPHALOSPORINS—THIRD GENERATION.

cefepime (seff-e-peem)

~~Maxipime~~

Classification

Therapeutic: anti-infectives

Pharmacologic: fourth-generation cephalosporins

Indications

Treatment of the following infections caused by susceptible organisms: Uncomplicated skin and skin structure infections, Bone and joint infections, Uncomplicated and complicated urinary tract infections, Respiratory tract infections, Complicated intra-abdominal infections (with metronidazole), Septicemia. Empiric treatment of febrile neutropenic patients.

Action

Inhibits bacterial cell wall synthesis. **Therapeutic Effects:** Bactericidal action against susceptible bacteria. **Spectrum:** Similar to that of 2nd- and 3rd-generation cephalosporins, but activity against staphylococci is less, whereas activity against gram-negative pathogens is greater, even for organisms resistant to 1st-, 2nd-, and 3rd-generation cephalosporins. Notable is increased action against: *Enterobacter*, *Haemophilus influenzae* (including β-lactamase-producing strains), *Escherichia coli*, *Klebsiella pneumoniae*, *Neisseria*, *Proteus*, *Providencia*, *Pseudomonas aeruginosa*, *Serratia*, *Moraxella catarrhalis* (including β-lactamase-producing strains). Not active against methicillin-resistant staphylococci or enterococci.

Pharmacokinetics

Absorption: Well absorbed after IM administration; IV administration results in complete bioavailability.
Distribution: Widely distributed. Some CSF penetration.
Metabolism and Excretion: 85% excreted unchanged in urine.
Half-life: *Adults:* 2 hr (↑ in renal impairment); *Children 2 mo–6 yr:* 1.7–1.9 hr.

TIME/ACTION PROFILE (plasma concentrations)

ROUTE	ONSET	PEAK	DURATION
IM	rapid	1–2 hr	12 hr
IV	rapid	end of infusion	12 hr

Contraindications/Precautions

Contraindicated in: Hypersensitivity to cephalosporins; Serious hypersensitivity to penicillins.
Use Cautiously in: History of GI disease, especially colitis; Renal impairment (↓ dose/↑ dosing interval recommended if CCr ≤60 mL/min); Hepatic impairment or poor nutritional status (may be at ↑ risk of bleeding); OB: Safety not established in pregnancy; Lactation: Safety not established in breastfeeding; Geri: Dose adjustment due to age-related ↓ in renal function may be necessary in older adults.

Adverse Reactions/Side Effects

Derm: rash, pruritus, urticaria. **GI:** CLOSTRIDIOIDES DIFFICILE-ASSOCIATED DIARRHEA (CDAD), diarrhea, nausea, vomiting. **Hemat:** bleeding, eosinophilia, hemolytic anemia, neutropenia, thrombocytopenia. **Local:** pain at IM site, phlebitis at IV site. **Neuro:** aphasia, ENCEPHALOPATHY, headache, SEIZURES (↑ RISK IN RENAL IMPAIRMENT). **Misc:** fever, HYPERSENSITIVITY REACTIONS (INCLUDING ANAPHYLAXIS), superinfection.

Interactions

Drug-Drug: Probenecid ↓ excretion and ↑ levels. Concurrent use of **loop diuretics** or **aminoglycosides** may ↑ risk of nephrotoxicity.

Route/Dosage

IM (Adults): *Mild to moderate uncomplicated or complicated urinary tract infections due to Escherichia coli:* 0.5–1 g every 12 hr.
IV (Adults): *Moderate to severe pneumonia:* 1–2 g every 12 hr. *Mild to moderate uncomplicated or complicated urinary tract infections:* 0.5–1 g every 12 hr. *Severe uncomplicated or complicated urinary tract infections, moderate to severe uncomplicated skin and skin structure infections, complicated intra-abdominal infections:* 2 g every 12 hr. *Empiric treatment of febrile neutropenia:* 2 g every 8 hr.
IV (Children 1 mo–16 yr): *Uncomplicated and complicated urinary tract infections, uncomplicated skin and skin structure infections, pneumonia:* 50 mg/kg every 12 hr (not to exceed 2 g/dose). *Febrile neutropenia:* 50 mg/kg every 8 hr (not to exceed 2 g/dose).
IV (Neonates postnatal age ≥14 days): 50 mg/kg every 12 hr.
IV (Neonates postnatal age <14 days): 30 mg/kg every 12 hr; consider 50 mg/kg every 12 hr for *Pseudomonas* infections.

Renal Impairment

IM, IV (Adults): (See manufacturer's specific recommendations) *CCr 30–60 mL/min:* 0.5–1 g every 24 hr or 2 g every 12–24 hr; *CCr 11–29 mL/min:* 0.5–2 g every 24 hr; *CCr <11 mL/min:* 250 mg–1 g every 24 hr.

Availability (generic available)

Powder for injection: 1 g, 2 g. **Premixed infusion:** 1 g/50 mL D5W, 2 g/100 mL D5W.

NURSING IMPLICATIONS

Assessment

- Assess for infection (vital signs; appearance of wound, sputum, urine, and stool; WBC) at beginning of and throughout therapy.
- Before initiating therapy, obtain a history to determine previous use of and reactions to penicillins or cephalosporins. Persons with a negative history of penicillin sensitivity may still have an allergic response.
- Obtain specimens for culture and sensitivity before initiating therapy. 1st dose may be given before receiving results.
- Observe for signs and symptoms of anaphylaxis (rash, pruritus, laryngeal edema, wheezing). Discontinue the drug and notify health care professional immediately if these symptoms occur. Keep epinephrine, an antihistamine, and resuscitation equipment close by in the event of an anaphylactic reaction.
- Monitor bowel function. Diarrhea, abdominal cramping, fever, and bloody stools should be reported to health care professional promptly as a sign of CDAD. May begin up to several wk following cessation of therapy.
- Monitor for neurotoxic events, including encephalopathy, myoclonus, aphasia, seizures, and nonconvulsive status epilepticus, especially in patients

C

with renal impairment and the elderly; dosage adjustment or discontinuation may be necessary. Institute seizure precautions as indicated.

Lab Test Considerations

- May cause positive results for Coombs test in patients receiving high doses or in neonates whose mothers were given cephalosporins before delivery.
- May ↑ AST, ALT, bilirubin, BUN, and serum creatinine.
- May rarely cause leukopenia, neutropenia, thrombocytopenia, and eosinophilia.

Implementation

- **IM: Reconstitution:** Reconstitute IM doses with sterile or bacteriostatic water for injection, 0.9% NaCl, or D5W. May be diluted with lidocaine to minimize injection discomfort.
- Inject deep into a well-developed muscle mass; massage well.
- IM route should only be used for treatment of mild to moderate uncomplicated or complicated urinary tract infections due to *Escherichia coli*.

IV Administration

- **IV:** Monitor injection site frequently for phlebitis (pain, redness, swelling). Change sites every 48–72 hr to prevent phlebitis.
- If aminoglycosides are administered concurrently, administer in separate sites, if possible, ≥1 hr apart. If 2nd site is unavailable, flush lines between medications.
- **Intermittent Infusion: Reconstitution:** Reconstitute each 1 g or 2 g vial with 10 mL of sterile water for injection, 0.9% NaCl, or D5W. **Dilution:** Dilute further in 50–100 mL of D5W, 0.9% NaCl, D10W, D5/0.9% NaCl, or D5/LR. Solution is stable for 24 hr at room temperature and 7 days if refrigerated. Reconstituted solution color may darken depending on storage conditions; however, this does not affect potency. **Concentration:** Not to exceed 40 mg/mL. **Rate:** Infuse over 20–30 min.
- **Y-Site Compatibility:** amikacin, aminocaproic acid, amiodarone, ampicillin/sulbactam, anidulafungin, arsenic trioxide, azithromycin, aztreonam, bivalirudin, bleomycin, bumetanide, buprenorphine, butorphanol, calcium gluconate, carboplatin, carmustine, ceftolozane/tazobactam, cyclophosphamide, cytarabine, dactinomycin, daptomycin, dexamethasone, dexmedetomidine, docetaxel, doxorubicin liposomal, eptifibatide, eravacycline, esmolol, fluconazole, fludarabine, fluorouracil, foscarnet, fosphenytoin, furosemide, gentamicin, granisetron, hetastarch, hydrocortisone, hydromorphone, imipenem/cilastatin, insulin, regular, ketamine, LR, leucovorin calcium, levofloxacin, linezolid, lorazepam, melphalan, meropenem/vaborbactam, mesna, methadone, methotrexate, methylprednisolone, metoprolol, metronidazole, milrinone, octreotide, oxytocin, paclitaxel, palonosetron, pamidronate, piperacillin/tazobactam, plazomicin, potassium acetate, remifentanil, rocuronium, sargramostim, sodium acetate, sodium bicarbonate, sufentanil, sulbactam/durlobactam, tedizolid, telavancin, thiotepa, tigecycline, tirofiban, tobramycin, trimethoprim/sulfamethoxazole, valproate sodium, vasopressin, zidovudine, zoledronic acid.
- **Y-Site Incompatibility:** acetylcysteine, acyclovir, alemtuzumab, amphotericin B deoxycholate, amphotericin B liposomal, argatroban, caspofungin, chlorpromazine, ciprofloxacin, cisplatin, dacarbazine, daunorubicin, dexrazoxane, diazepam, diltiazem, diphenhydramine, doxorubicin hydrochloride, droperidol, enalaprilat, epirubicin, erythromycin, etoposide, etoposide phosphate, famotidine, filgrastim, floxuridine, ganciclovir, gemcitabine, gemtuzumab ozogamicin, haloperidol, hydroxyzine, idarubicin, ifosfamide, irinotecan, isavuconazonium, labetalol, letermovir, magnesium sulfate, mannitol, meperidine, metoclopramide, midazolam, mitomycin, mitoxantrone, nalbuphine, ondansetron, oxaliplatin, pantoprazole, pemetrexed, phenytoin, prochlorperazine, promethazine, tacrolimus, theophylline, topotecan, vecuronium, vinblastine, vincristine, vinorelbine, voriconazole.

Patient/Family Teaching

- Explain the purpose and side effects to patient. Inform patient of the importance of receiving the full course of therapy even if feeling better. Advise patient to read *Medication Guide* before starting and periodically during therapy in case of changes.
- Advise patient to report immediately any signs/symptoms of encephalopathy (confusion, hallucinations, stupor, coma), stiffness, or seizures.
- Advise patient to report signs and symptoms of superinfection (furry overgrowth on the tongue, vaginal itching or discharge, loose or foul-smelling stools) and allergy.
- Instruct patient to notify health care professional if fever and diarrhea develop, especially if stool contains blood, pus, or mucus. Advise patient not to treat diarrhea without consulting health care professional.
- Advise patient to notify health care professional of all Rx or OTC medications, vitamins, or herbal products being taken and to consult with health care professional before taking other medications. There are multiple significant possible drug-drug interactions.

- Rep: Advise women of reproductive potential to notify health care professional if pregnancy is planned or suspected or if breastfeeding.

Evaluation/Desired Outcomes

- Resolution of the signs and symptoms of infection. Length of time for complete resolution depends on the organism and site of infection.

cefixime, See CEPHALOSPORINS—THIRD GENERATION.

cefotaxime, See CEPHALOSPORINS—THIRD GENERATION.

cefoTEtan, See CEPHALOSPORINS—SECOND GENERATION.

cefOXitin, See CEPHALOSPORINS—SECOND GENERATION.

cefpodoxime, See CEPHALOSPORINS—THIRD GENERATION.

cefprozil, See CEPHALOSPORINS—SECOND GENERATION.

ceftaroline (sef-tar-oh-leen)

Teflaro

Classification

Therapeutic: anti-infectives

Pharmacologic: cephalosporin derivatives

Indications

Acute bacterial skin/skin structure infections. Community-acquired pneumonia.

Action

Inhibits bacterial cell wall synthesis. **Therapeutic Effects:** Bactericidal action against susceptible bacteria. **Spectrum:** Active against: *Staphylococcus aureus* (including methicillin-susceptible and -resistant strains), *Streptococcus pneumoniae*, *Streptococcus pyogenes*, *Streptococcus agalactiae*, *Escherichia coli*, *Haemophilus influenzae*, *Klebsiella pneumoniae*, and *Klebsiella oxytoca*.

Pharmacokinetics

Absorption: IV administration results in complete bioavailability of parent drug.

Distribution: Well distributed to tissues.

Metabolism and Excretion: Ceftaroline fosamil is rapidly converted by plasma phosphatases to ceftaroline, the active metabolite; 88% excreted in urine, 6% in feces.

Half-life: 2.6 hr (after multiple doses).

TIME/ACTION PROFILE (plasma concentrations)

ROUTE	ONSET	PEAK	DURATION
IV	rapid	end of infusion	12 hr

Contraindications/Precautions

Contraindicated in: Known serious hypersensitivity to cephalosporins.

Use Cautiously in: Known hypersensitivity to other beta-lactams; Renal impairment (↓dose); OB: Safety not established in pregnancy; Lactation: Use while breastfeeding only if potential maternal benefit justifies potential risk to infant; Pedi: Neonates <34 wk (gestational age) or <12 days (postnatal age) (acute bacterial skin/skin structure infections) and infants <2 mo (community-acquired pneumonia) (safety and effectiveness not established); Geri: Dose adjustment may be necessary in older adults for age-related ↓ in renal function.

Adverse Reactions/Side Effects

Derm: rash. **GI:** CLOSTRIDIOIDES DIFFICILE-ASSOCIATED DIARRHEA (CDAD), diarrhea, nausea. **Hemat:** hemolytic anemia. **Local:** phlebitis. **Neuro:** ENCEPHALOPATHY, SEIZURES. **Misc:** HYPERSENSITIVITY REACTIONS (INCLUDING ANAPHYLAXIS).

Interactions

Drug-Drug: None reported.

Route/Dosage

Acute Bacterial Skin/Skin Structure Infections

IV (Adults): 600 mg every 12 hr for 5–14 days.

IV (Children 2–17 yr and >33 kg): 400 mg every 8 hr for 5–14 days *or* 600 mg every 12 hr for 5–14 days.

IV (Children 2–17 yr and ≤33 kg): 12 mg/kg every 8 hr for 5–14 days.

IV (Children 2 mo–<2 yr): 8 mg/kg every 8 hr for 5–14 days.

IV (Neonates 0–<2 mo): 6 mg/kg every 8 hr for 5–14 days.

Renal Impairment

IV (Adults): *CCr >30 to ≤50 mL/min:* 400 mg every 12 hr; *CCr ≥15 to ≤30 mL/min:* 300 mg every 12 hr; *CCr <15 mL/min including hemodialysis:* 200 mg every 12 hr.

Community-Acquired Pneumonia

IV (Adults): 600 mg every 12 hr for 5–7 days.

IV (Children 2–17 yr and >33 kg): 400 mg every 8 hr for 5–14 days *or* 600 mg every 12 hr for 5–14 days.
IV (Children 2–17 yr and ≤33 kg): 12 mg/kg every 8 hr for 5–14 days.
IV (Children 2 mo–<2 yr): 8 mg/kg every 8 hr for 5–14 days.

Renal Impairment

IV (Adults): *CCr 31–50 mL/min:* 400 mg every 12 hr; *CCr 15–30 mL/min:* 300 mg every 12 hr; *CCr <15 mL/min including hemodialysis:* 200 mg every 12 hr.

Availability (generic available)

Powder for injection: 400 mg/vial, 600 mg/vial.

NURSING IMPLICATIONS

Assessment

- Assess for infection (vital signs; appearance of wound, sputum, urine, and stool; WBC) at beginning of and throughout therapy.
- Before initiating therapy, obtain a history to determine previous use of and reactions to penicillins, cephalosporins, or carbapenems. Persons with a negative history of sensitivity may still have an allergic response.
- Observe patient for signs and symptoms of anaphylaxis (rash, pruritus, laryngeal edema, wheezing). Discontinue the drug and notify health care provider immediately if these symptoms occur. Keep epinephrine, an antihistamine, and resuscitation equipment close by in the event of an anaphylactic reaction.
- Monitor bowel function. Diarrhea, abdominal cramping, fever, and bloody stools should be reported to health care provider promptly as a sign of CDAD. May begin up to several months following cessation of therapy.
- Monitor for neurotoxic events, including encephalopathy, myoclonus, aphasia, seizures, and nonconvulsive status epilepticus, especially in patients with renal impairment; dosage adjustment or discontinuation may be necessary. Institute seizure precautions as indicated.

Lab Test Considerations

- Obtain specimens for culture and sensitivity before initiating therapy. 1st dose may be given before receiving results. May cause seroconversion from a negative to a positive direct Coombs test. If anemia develops during or after therapy, perform a direct Coombs test. If drug-induced hemolytic anemia is suspected, discontinue ceftaroline and provide supportive care.

Implementation

IV Administration

- **Intermittent Infusion: Reconstitution:** Reconstitute with 20 mL of sterile water for injection, 0.9% NaCl, D5W, or LR. **Dilution:** Dilute further with 50–250 mL of same diluent unless reconstituted with sterile water for injection; then use 0.9% NaCl, D5W, D2.5W, 0.45% NaCl, or LR. Mix gently to dissolve. Solution is clear to light or dark yellow; do not administer solutions that are discolored or contain particulate matter. Solution is stable for 6 hr at room temperature or 24 hr if refrigerated. **Rate:** Infuse over 5–60 min.
- **Y-Site Compatibility:** acyclovir, amikacin, aminophylline, amiodarone, azithromycin, bumetanide, calcium chloride, calcium gluconate, cefiderocol, ceftolozane/tazobactam, ciprofloxacin, cisatracurium, clindamycin, cyclosporine, dexamethasone, digoxin, diltiazem, diphenhydramine, dopamine, enalaprilat, esomeprazole, famotidine, fentanyl, fluconazole, furosemide, gentamicin, granisetron, haloperidol, heparin, hydrocortisone, hydromorphone, insulin, regular, insulin lispro, letermovir, levofloxacin, lidocaine, lorazepam, mannitol, meperidine, methylprednisolone, metoclopramide, metoprolol, metronidazole, midazolam, milrinone, morphine, moxifloxacin, multivitamins, norepinephrine, ondansetron, pantoprazole, plazomicin, potassium chloride, promethazine, propofol, remifentanil, sodium bicarbonate, tobramycin, trimethoprim/sulfamethoxazole, vasopressin, voriconazole.
- **Y-Site Incompatibility:** amphotericin B deoxycholate, caspofungin, diazepam, eravacycline, filgrastim, isavuconazonium, labetalol, meropenem/vaborbactam, potassium phosphates, sodium phosphates, sulbactam/durlobactam, tedizolid.

Patient/Family Teaching

- Explain the purpose and side effects to patient.
- Advise patient to report immediately any signs/symptoms of encephalopathy (confusion, hallucinations, stupor, coma), stiffness, and seizures.
- Advise patient to report signs of superinfection (furry overgrowth on the tongue, vaginal itching or discharge, loose or foul-smelling stools) and allergy.
- Instruct patient to notify health care provider if fever and diarrhea develop, especially if stool contains blood, pus, or mucus. Advise patient not to treat diarrhea without consulting health care provider.
- Advise patient to notify health care provider of all Rx or OTC medications, vitamins, or herbal

products being taken and to consult with health care provider before taking other medications.

- Rep: Advise women of reproductive potential to notify health care provider if pregnancy is planned or suspected or if breastfeeding.

Evaluation/Desired Outcomes

- Resolution of the signs and symptoms of infection. Length of time for complete resolution depends on the organism and site of infection.

cefTAZidime, See CEPHALOSPORINS—THIRD GENERATION.

ceftobiprole (sef-toe-bye-prole)

Zevtera

Classification

Therapeutic: anti-infectives

Pharmacologic: cephalosporin derivatives

Indications

Bacteremia (including right-sided infective endocarditis). Acute bacterial skin/skin structure infections. Community-acquired pneumonia.

Action

Inhibits bacterial cell wall synthesis. **Therapeutic Effects:** Bactericidal action against susceptible bacteria. **Spectrum:** Active against: *Staphylococcus aureus* (including methicillin-susceptible and -resistant strains), *Streptococcus pneumoniae*, *Streptococcus pyogenes*, *Escherichia coli*, *Haemophilus influenzae*, *Haemophilus influenzae*, *Haemophilus parainfluenzae*, and *Klebsiella pneumoniae*.

Pharmacokinetics

Absorption: IV administration results in complete bioavailability.

Distribution: Well distributed to tissues.

Metabolism and Excretion: Minimally metabolized. Primarily excreted as unchanged drug in urine.

Half-life: 3.3 hr.

TIME/ACTION PROFILE (plasma concentrations)

ROUTE	ONSET	PEAK	DURATION
IV	rapid	end of infusion	6–8 hr

Contraindications/Precautions

Contraindicated in: Known serious hypersensitivity to cephalosporins.

Use Cautiously in: Ventilator-associated bacterial pneumonia (↑ risk of mortality); Seizure disorders; Renal impairment (↓ dose if CCr <50 mL/min); Augmented renal clearance (↑ dosing frequency if CCr >150 mL/min); OB: Safety not established in pregnancy; Lactation: Safety not established in breastfeeding; Pedi: Safety and effectiveness not established in children <18 yr (bacteremia or acute bacterial skin/skin structure infections) or <3 mo (community-acquired pneumonia). Geri: Dose adjustment may be necessary in older adults for age-related ↓ in renal function.

Adverse Reactions/Side Effects

CV: hypertension. **Derm:** rash. **F and E:** hypokalemia, hyponatremia. **GI:** ↑ liver enzymes, nausea, abdominal pain, CLOSTRIDIOIDES DIFFICILE-ASSOCIATED DIARRHEA (CDAD), diarrhea, vomiting. **GU:** ↑ serum creatinine. **Hemat:** anemia, leukopenia. **Local:** phlebitis. **Neuro:** dizziness, dysgeusia, headache, insomnia, SEIZURES. **Resp:** dyspnea. **Misc:** fever, fungal infection, HYPERSENSITIVITY REACTIONS (INCLUDING ANAPHYLAXIS).

Interactions

Drug-Drug: May ↑ levels and risk of toxicity of **organic anion transporting polypeptide (OATP) 1B1 substrates** and **OATP 1B3 substrates**.

Route/Dosage

Bacteremia

IV (Adults): *Days 1–8:* 667 mg every 6 hr; *Day 9 and thereafter:* 667 mg every 8 hr. Treatment duration is up to 42 days.

Renal Impairment

IV (Adults): *CCr >150 mL/min:* 667 mg every 6 hr for up to 42 days. *CCr 30–<50 mL/min:* Days 1–8: 667 mg every 8 hr; Day 9 and thereafter: 667 mg every 12 hr. Treatment duration is up to 42 days. *CCr 15–<30 mL/min:* Days 1–8: 333 mg every 8 hr; Day 9 and thereafter: 333 mg every 12 hr. Treatment duration is up to 42 days. *CCr <15 mL/min and Hemodialysis:* 333 mg every 24 hr for up to 42 days. Administer dose after hemodialysis on hemodialysis days.

Acute Bacterial Skin/Skin Structure Infections

IV (Adults): 667 mg every 8 hr for 5–14 days.

Renal Impairment

IV (Adults): *CCr >150 mL/min:* 667 mg every 6 hr for 5–14 days. *CCr 30–<50 mL/min:* 667 mg every 12 hr for 5–14 days. *CCr 15–<30 mL/min:* 333 mg every 12 hr for 5–14 days. *CCr <15 mL/min and Hemodialysis:* 333 mg every 24 hr for 5–14 days. Administer dose after hemodialysis on hemodialysis days.

Community-Acquired Pneumonia

IV (Adults): 667 mg every 8 hr for 5–14 days.

IV (Children 12–<18 yr): 13.3 mg/kg (max = 667 mg) every 8 hr for 7–14 days.
IV (Children 3 mo-<12 yr): 20 mg/kg (max = 667 mg) every 8 hr for 7–14 days.

Renal Impairment
IV (Adults): *CCr >150 mL/min:* 667 mg every 6 hr for 5–14 days. *CCr 30–<50 mL/min:* 667 mg every 12 hr for 5–14 days. *CCr 15–<30 mL/min:* 333 mg every 12 hr for 5–14 days. *CCr <15 mL/min and Hemodialysis:* 333 mg every 24 hr for 5–14 days. Administer dose after hemodialysis on hemodialysis days.

Renal Impairment
(Children 12–<18 yr): *CCr 30–<50 mL/min:* 10 mg/kg (max = 667 mg) every 12 hr for 7–14 days. *CCr 15–<30 mL/min:* 10 mg/kg (max = 333 mg) every 12 hr for 7–14 days.

Renal Impairment
(Children 6–<12 yr): *CCr 30–<50 mL/min:* 10 mg/kg (max = 667 mg) every 12 hr for 7–14 days. *CCr 15–<30 mL/min:* 10 mg/kg (max = 333 mg) every 24 hr for 7–14 days.

Renal Impairment
(Children 2–<6 yr): *CCr 30–<50 mL/min:* 13.3 mg/kg (max = 667 mg) every 12 hr for 7–14 days. *CCr 15–<30 mL/min:* 13.3 mg/kg (max = 333 mg) every 24 hr for 7–14 days.

Availability
Powder for injection: 667 mg/vial.

NURSING IMPLICATIONS
Assessment
- Assess for infection (vital signs; appearance of wound, sputum, urine, and stool; WBC) at beginning of and throughout therapy.
- Before initiating therapy, obtain a history to determine previous use of and reactions to penicillins or cephalosporins. Persons with a negative history of cephalosporin sensitivity may still have an allergic response.
- Observe patient for signs/symptoms of hypersensitivity reactions (rash, pruritus, laryngeal edema, wheezing). *If hypersensitivity reaction occurs,* discontinue ceftobiprole. Keep epinephrine, an antihistamine, and resuscitation equipment close by in the event of an anaphylactic reaction.
- Monitor for seizure activity especially in patients with renal impairment and implement seizure precautions if indicated.
- Monitor for diarrhea, abdominal cramping, fever, and bloody stools during and for several weeks after therapy. *If CDAD is suspected or confirmed,* discontinue ceftobiprole and treat as clinically indicated.

Lab Test Considerations
- Obtain specimens for culture and sensitivity before initiating therapy. 1st dose may be given before receiving results.
- Monitor CBC with differential. May cause neutropenia and thrombocytopenia.
- Monitor BUN and serum creatinine especially in those with renal impairment.
- May ↑ AST and ALT.

Implementation
IV Administration
- **Intermittent Infusion: Reconstitution:** *For adult and pediatric patients >12 yr,* reconstitute vial with 10 mL of sterile water for injection or D5W. *For pediatric patients aged 3 mo-<12 yr,* reconstitute vial with 10 mL of D5W. Shake vial vigorously (10 min). Solution may be stored in refrigerator for 24 hr or 1 hr at room temperature. **Dilution:** Withdraw dose from vial and add to 250 mL bag of 0.9% NaCl or D5W (125 mL for adults with CCr <30 mL/min). **Concentration:** 2.67– 5.33 mg/mL. **Rate:** Infuse over 2 hr.
- **Y-Site Compatibility:** aminophylline, azithromycin, bumetanide, clindamycin, cyclosporine, dexamethasone, digoxin, enalaprilat, fentanyl, fluconazole, furosemide, granisetron, heparin, hydrocortisone, lorazepam, mannitol, methylprednisolone, metoprolol, metronidazole, multivitamins, norepinephrine, potassium chloride, propofol, sodium bicarbonate, trimethoprim/sulfamethoxazole, vasopressin, voriconazole.
- **Y-Site Incompatibility:** amikacin, amiodarone, amphotericin B deoxycholate, calcium chloride, calcium gluconate, caspofungin, ciprofloxacin, cisatracurium, diazepam, diltiazem, diphenhydramine, dobutamine, dopamine, famotidine, filgrastim, gentamicin, haloperidol, hydromorphone, insulin regular, labetalol, levofloxacin, lidocaine, magnesium sulfate, meperidine, metoclopramide, midazolam, morphine, moxifloxacin, ondansetron, potassium phosphates, promethazine, tobramycin.

Patient/Family Teaching
- Explain purpose and side effects of medication to patient. Advise patient to read *Patient Information* before starting therapy. Advise to take the full course of treatment, even if symptoms improve.
- Advise patient to notify health care professional of all Rx or OTC medications, vitamins, or herbal products being taken and to consult health care professional before taking other medications.

- Advise patient that hypersensitivity reactions can occur and to notify health care professional or seek immediate medical attention if needed.
- Advise patient that seizures and other adverse CNS reactions can occur and to notify health care professional if any are experienced.
- Caution patient to notify health care provider if fever and diarrhea occur, especially if stool contains blood, pus, or mucus. Advise patient not to treat diarrhea without consulting health care provider. May occur up to several weeks after discontinuation of medication.
- Rep: Advise women of reproductive potential to notify health care professional if pregnancy is planned or suspected or breastfeeding.

Evaluation/Desired Outcomes

- Bactericidal action against susceptible bacteria.

cefTRIAXone, See CEPHALOSPORINS—THIRD GENERATION.

cefuroxime, See CEPHALOSPORINS—SECOND GENERATION.

celecoxib (sel-e-kox-ib)

CeleBREX, Elyxyb

Classification

Therapeutic: antirheumatics

Pharmacologic: COX-2 inhibitors

Indications

Osteoarthritis. Rheumatoid arthritis. Ankylosing spondylitis. Juvenile rheumatoid arthritis. Acute pain. Primary dysmenorrhea. Acute treatment of migraine (with or without aura) (oral solution only).

Action

Inhibits the enzyme COX-2. This enzyme is required for the synthesis of prostaglandins. Has analgesic, anti-inflammatory, and antipyretic properties. **Therapeutic Effects:** Decreased pain and inflammation caused by osteoarthritis, rheumatoid arthritis, ankylosing spondylitis, or juvenile rheumatoid arthritis. Decreased acute pain.

Pharmacokinetics

Absorption: Bioavailability unknown.

Distribution: Extensively distributed to tissues.

Protein Binding: 97%.

Metabolism and Excretion: Mostly metabolized by the liver via the CYP2C9 isoenzyme; the CYP2C9 isoenzyme exhibits genetic polymorphism; poor metabolizers may have significantly ↑ celecoxib concentrations and an ↑ risk of adverse effects; <3% excreted unchanged in urine and feces.

Half-life: 11 hr.

TIME/ACTION PROFILE (pain reduction)

ROUTE	ONSET	PEAK	DURATION
PO	24–48 hr	unknown	12–24 hr†

† After discontinuation.

Contraindications/Precautions

Contraindicated in: Hypersensitivity; Cross-sensitivity may exist with other NSAIDs, including aspirin; History of allergic-type reactions to sulfonamides; History of allergic-type reactions to aspirin or other NSAIDs, including the aspirin triad (asthma, nasal polyps, severe hypersensitivity reactions to aspirin); Advanced renal disease; Severe hepatic impairment; Coronary artery bypass graft surgery; Recent MI; HF; OB: Avoid use after 30 wk gestation.

Use Cautiously in: Cardiovascular disease or risk factors for cardiovascular disease (may ↑ risk of serious cardiovascular thrombotic events, MI, and stroke, especially with prolonged use or use of higher doses); Renal impairment; hepatic impairment; dehydration; or concurrent diuretic, ACE inhibitor, or angiotensin receptor blocker therapy (↑ risk of renal impairment); History of long duration of NSAID use, smoking, alcohol use, advanced liver disease, coagulopathy, or poor general health (↑ risk of GI bleeding); Hypertension or fluid retention; Asthma; Patients who are known or suspected to be poor CYP2C9 metabolizers (↓ initial dose by 50%; in patients with juvenile rheumatoid arthritis, use alternative treatment); OB: Use at or after 20 wk gestation may cause fetal or neonatal renal impairment; if treatment is necessary between 20 wk and 30 wk gestation, limit use to the lowest effective dose and shortest duration possible; Pedi: Safety not established in children <2 yr or for longer than 6 mo; Geri: ↑ risk of GI bleeding and renal impairment in older adults.

Exercise Extreme Caution in: History of peptic ulcer disease or GI bleeding.

Adverse Reactions/Side Effects

CV: edema, HF, hypertension, MI, THROMBOSIS. **Derm:** ACUTE GENERALIZED EXANTHEMATOUS PUSTULOSIS (AGEP), DRUG REACTION WITH EOSINOPHILIA AND SYSTEMIC SYMPTOMS (DRESS), EXFOLIATIVE DERMATITIS, GENERALIZED BULLOUS FIXED DRUG ERUPTION, rash, STEVENS-JOHNSON SYNDROME (SJS), TOXIC EPIDERMAL NECROLYSIS (TEN). **F and E:** hyperkalemia. **GI:** abdominal pain, diarrhea, dyspepsia, flatulence, GI BLEEDING, GI PERFORATION, GI ULCERATION, nausea. **GU:** renal impairment. **Hemat:** anemia. **Neuro:** dizziness, headache, insomnia, STROKE. **Misc:** HYPERSENSITIVITY REACTIONS (INCLUDING ANAPHYLAXIS AND SERIOUS SKIN REACTIONS).

C

Interactions

Drug-Drug: CYP2C9 inhibitors may ↑ levels and risk of toxicity. May ↓ effectiveness of **ACE inhibitors**, **thiazide diuretics**, and **furosemide**. **Fluconazole** may ↑ levels and risk of toxicity; use lowest recommended dosage. ↑ risk of GI bleeding with **anticoagulants, aspirin, clopidogrel, ticagrelor, prasugrel, corticosteroids, fibrinolytics, SNRIs, or SSRIs**. May ↑ levels and risk of toxicity of **lithium** and **methotrexate**. May ↑ risk of nephrotoxicity associated with **cyclosporine**. May ↑ risk of myelosuppression and renal and GI toxicity associated with **pemetrexed**.

Route/Dosage

Osteoarthritis

PO (Adults): 200 mg once daily *or* 100 mg twice daily. *CYP2C9 poor metabolizers:* ↓ dose by 50%.

Hepatic Impairment

PO (Adults): *Moderate hepatic impairment:* ↓ dose by 50%.

Rheumatoid Arthritis

PO (Adults): 100–200 mg twice daily (capsules). *CYP2C9 poor metabolizers:* ↓ dose by 50%.

Hepatic Impairment

PO (Adults): *Moderate hepatic impairment:* ↓ dose by 50%.

Ankylosing Spondylitis

PO (Adults): 200 mg once daily (capsules) *or* 100 mg twice daily (capsules); may ↑ dose after 6 wk to 400 mg/day. *CYP2C9 poor metabolizers:* ↓ dose by 50%.

Hepatic Impairment

PO (Adults): *Moderate hepatic impairment:* ↓ dose by 50%.

Juvenile Rheumatoid Arthritis

PO (Children ≥2 yr, 10–25 kg): 50 mg twice daily (capsules).

PO (Children ≥2 yr, ≥25 kg): 100 mg twice daily (capsules).

Hepatic Impairment

PO (Children ≥2 yr): *Moderate hepatic impairment:* ↓ dose by 50%.

Acute Pain or Primary Dysmenorrhea

PO (Adults): 400 mg initially; then a 200-mg dose if needed on the first day; then 200 mg twice daily as needed (capsules). *CYP2C9 poor metabolizers:* ↓ dose by 50%.

Hepatic Impairment

PO (Adults): *Moderate hepatic impairment:* ↓ dose by 50%.

Acute Treatment of Migraine

PO (Adults): *Oral solution:* 120 mg as a single dose (not to exceed 120 mg/24 hr). *CYP2C9 poor metabolizers:* Oral solution: 60 mg as a single dose (not to exceed 60 mg/24 hr).

Hepatic Impairment

PO (Adults): *Moderate hepatic impairment:* 60 mg as a single dose (not to exceed 60 mg/24 hr).

Availability (generic available)

Capsules: 50 mg, 100 mg, 200 mg, 400 mg. **Oral solution (peppermint flavor):** 25 mg/mL.

NURSING IMPLICATIONS

Assessment

- Assess range of motion, degree of swelling, and pain in affected joints before and periodically during therapy.
- Assess for allergy to sulfonamides, aspirin, or NSAIDs. Patients with these allergies should not receive celecoxib.
- Monitor for signs and symptoms of hypersensitivity reactions (anaphylaxis). *If hypersensitivity reaction occurs,* implement medical interventions (epinephrine) and treat as indicated.
- Assess for skin rash frequently during therapy. AGEP, exfoliative dermatitis, generalized bullous fixed drug eruption, SJS, or TEN may develop. *If rash, blisters, or erosions occur,* discontinue celecoxib. Treat symptomatically; may recur once treatment is stopped.
- Monitor for signs and symptoms of DRESS (fever, rash, lymphadenopathy, facial swelling) periodically during therapy. *If DRESS symptoms occur,* discontinue celecoxib.
- **Migraines:** Assess intensity and frequency of migraine pain.

Lab Test Considerations

- May ↑ AST and ALT.
- May cause hypophosphatemia, hyperkalemia, and ↑ BUN.

Implementation

- Do not confuse Celebrex with Celexa or Cerebyx.
- Use lowest effective dose for shortest period of time.
- **PO:** May be administered without regard to meals. Capsules may be opened and sprinkled on applesauce and ingested immediately with water. Mixture may be stored in the refrigerator for up to 6 hr.
- Oral solution is clear and colorless.
- Limit oral solution use to ≤10 days per month to avoid medication-overuse headache.

Patient/Family Teaching

- Explain purpose and side effects of medication to patient. Advise patient to read *Patient Information* before starting therapy. Instruct patient to take as directed. Do not take more than prescribed dose. ↑ doses does not appear to ↑ effectiveness.
- Advise patient to notify health care provider of all Rx or OTC medications, vitamins, or herbal products being taken and to consult health care provider before taking other medications.
- Caution patient to avoid use of more than one NSAID or aspirin at a time; ↑ risk of GI toxicity. ↑ dose or adding an NSAID or aspirin does not provide ↑ pain relief but may ↑ incidence of side effects.
- Advise patient to notify health care provider promptly if signs or symptoms of GI toxicity (abdominal pain, black stools), skin rash, unexplained weight gain, or edema occur.
- Advise patients to discontinue celecoxib and notify health care provider if signs and symptoms of hepatotoxicity (nausea, fatigue, lethargy, pruritus, jaundice, upper right quadrant tenderness, flu-like symptoms) occur.
- May cause hypertension. Instruct patient in correct technique for monitoring BP and to notify health care provider if significant changes occur.
- Inform patient of ↑ risk of MI and stroke. Use lowest effective dose for shortest time. Advise patient to notify health care provider immediately if signs and symptoms (shortness of breath or trouble breathing, chest pain, weakness in one part or side of body, slurred speech, swelling of the face or throat) occur.
- Inform patient of signs and symptoms of anaphylactic reactions (difficulty breathing, swelling of face/throat) and to seek immediate emergency help if these occur.
- Advise patient to stop celecoxib immediately if any type of skin rash/blister or fever occurs and to notify health care provider.
- Rep: May cause fetal harm. Advise women of reproductive potential to notify health care provider if pregnancy is planned or suspected or if breastfeeding. Advise patients to avoid celecoxib in the 3rd trimester of pregnancy (after 29 wk); may cause premature closure of the fetal ductus arteriosus. Use of celecoxib after 20 wk may cause fetal renal impairment, leading to oligohydramnios. May cause reversible infertility in women attempting to conceive; may consider discontinuing celecoxib.

Evaluation/Desired Outcomes

- Decreased pain and inflammation caused by osteoarthritis, rheumatoid arthritis, ankylosing spondylitis, or juvenile rheumatoid arthritis.
- Decreased acute pain.

cephalexin, See CEPHALOSPORINS—FIRST GENERATION.

CEPHALOSPORINS—FIRST GENERATION

cefadroxil (sef-a-**drox**-ill)
~~Duricef~~

ceFAZolin (sef-**a**-zoe-lin)
~~Ancef~~

cephalexin (sef-a-**lex**-in)
~~Keflex~~

Classification
Therapeutic: anti-infectives
Pharmacologic: first-generation cephalosporins

Indications

Treatment of the following infections caused by susceptible organisms: Skin and skin-structure infections (including burn wounds), Pneumonia, Urinary tract infections, Bone and joint infections, Septicemia. Not suitable for the treatment of meningitis. **Cefadroxil:** Pharyngitis and/or tonsillitis. **Cefazolin:** Perioperative prophylaxis, biliary tract infections, genital infections, bacterial endocarditis prophylaxis for dental and upper respiratory tract procedures. **Cephalexin:** Otitis media.

Action

Inhibits bacterial cell wall synthesis. **Therapeutic Effects:** Bactericidal action against susceptible bacteria. **Spectrum:** Active against many gram-positive cocci, including: *Streptococcus pneumoniae*, Group A beta-hemolytic streptococci, Penicillinase-producing staphylococci. Not active against: Methicillin-resistant staphylococci, *Bacteroides fragilis*, *Enterococcus*. Active against some gram-negative rods, including: *Klebsiella pneumoniae*, *Proteus mirabilis*, *Escherichia coli*.

Pharmacokinetics

Absorption: *Cefadroxil* and *cephalexin* are well absorbed following oral administration. *Cefazolin* is well absorbed following IM administration.
Distribution: Widely distributed. Cefazolin penetrates bone and synovial fluid well. Minimal CSF penetration.
Metabolism and Excretion: Excreted almost entirely unchanged by the kidneys.
Half-life: *Cefadroxil:* 60–120 min; *cefazolin:* 90–150 min; *cephalexin:* 50–80 min (all are ↑ in renal impairment).

C

TIME/ACTION PROFILE (blood levels)

ROUTE	ONSET	PEAK	DURATION
Cefadroxil PO	rapid	1.5–2 hr	12–24 hr
Cefazolin IM	rapid	0.5–2 hr	6–12 hr
Cefazolin IV	rapid	5 min	6–12 hr
Cephalexin PO	rapid	1 hr	6–12 hr

Contraindications/Precautions

Contraindicated in: Hypersensitivity to cephalosporins; Serious hypersensitivity to penicillins.

Use Cautiously in: Renal impairment (dosage ↓ and/or ↑ dosing interval recommended for: *cefadroxil* and *cephalexin*, if CCr ≤50 mL/min, and *cefazolin* if CCr <55 mL/min (adults) or <70 mL/min (children); History of GI disease, especially colitis; Renal or hepatic impairment, poor nutritional state, extended antibiotic therapy, or previously stabilized on anticoagulant therapy (may be at ↑ risk of bleeding) (cefazolin); OB: Lactation: Half-life is shorter and blood levels lower during pregnancy; have been used safely; Geri: Dose adjustment due to age-related ↓ in renal function may be necessary in older adults.

Adverse Reactions/Side Effects

Derm: rash, pruritus, STEVENS-JOHNSON SYNDROME (SJS), urticaria. **GI:** diarrhea, nausea, vomiting, CLOSTRIDIOIDES DIFFICILE-ASSOCIATED DIARRHEA (CDAD), cramps. **Hemat:** agranulocytosis, eosinophilia, hemolytic anemia, neutropenia, thrombocytopenia. **Local:** pain at IM site, phlebitis at IV site. **Neuro:** SEIZURES (HIGH DOSES). **Misc:** HYPERSENSITIVITY REACTIONS (INCLUDING ANAPHYLAXIS AND SERUM SICKNESS), superinfection.

Interactions

Drug-Drug: Probenecid ↓ excretion and ↑ levels and effects of renally excreted cephalosporins. **Loop diuretics** or **aminoglycosides** may ↑ risk of renal toxicity. Cefazolin may potentiate the effects of **anticoagulants** and ↑ the risk of bleeding.

Route/Dosage

Cefadroxil

PO (Adults): *Pharyngitis and tonsillitis:* 500 mg every 12 hr or 1 g every 24 hr for 10 days. *Skin and soft-tissue infections:* 500 mg every 12 hr or 1 g every 24 hr. *Urinary tract infections:* 500 mg–1 g every 12 hr or 1–2 g every 24 hr.

PO (Children): *Pharyngitis, tonsillitis, or impetigo:* 15 mg/kg every 12 hr or 30 mg/kg every 24 hr for 10 days. *Skin and soft-tissue infections:* 15 mg/kg every 12 hr. *Urinary tract infections:* 15 mg/kg every 12 hr.

Renal Impairment

PO (Adults): *CCr 25–50 mL/min:* 500 mg every 12 hr; *CCr 10–25 mL/min:* 500 mg every 24 hr; *CCr <10 mL/min:* 500 mg every 36 hr.

Cefazolin

IM, IV (Adults): *Moderate to severe infections:* 500 mg–1 g every 6–8 hr. *Mild infections with gram-positive cocci:* 250–500 mg every 8 hr. *Uncomplicated urinary tract infection:* 1 g every 12 hr. *Pneumococcal pneumonia:* 500 mg every 12 hr. *Severe, life-threatening infections (e.g. infective endocarditis or septicemia):* 1–1.5 g every 6 hr.

IV (Adults ≥120 kg): *Perioperative prophylaxis:* 3 g within 30–60 min prior to incision (an additional 500 mg–1 g should be given for surgeries ≥ 2 hr). 500 mg–1 g should then be given for all surgeries every 6–8 hr for 24 hr following the surgery.

IV (Adults <120 kg): *Perioperative prophylaxis:* 1–2 g within 30–60 min prior to incision (an additional 500 mg–1 g should be given for surgeries ≥ 2 hr). 500 mg–1 g should then be given for all surgeries every 6–8 hr for 24 hr following the surgery.

IV (Children ≥10 yr and ≥50 kg): *Perioperative prophylaxis:* 2 g within 30–60 min prior to incision (an additional 500 mg–1 g should be given for surgeries ≥2 hr). 500 mg–1 g should then be given for all surgeries every 6–8 hr for 24 hr following the surgery.

IV (Children ≥10 yr and <50 kg): *Perioperative prophylaxis:* 1 g within 30–60 min prior to incision (an additional 500 mg–1 g should be given for surgeries ≥2 hr). 500 mg–1 g should then be given for all surgeries every 6–8 hr for 24 hr following the surgery.

IV (Children): *Mild to moderate infections:* 25–50 mg/kg/day divided into 3 or 4 equal doses. *Severe infections:* 100 mg/kg/day divided into 3 or 4 equal doses.

Renal Impairment

IV (Adults): *CCr 35–54 mL/min:* 1–2 g every 8–12 hr; *CCr 11–34 mL/min:* 1 g every 12 hr; *CCr ≤10 mL/min:* 500 mg–1 g every 24 hr. *Hemodialysis:* 500 mg–1 g every 24 hr (on hemodialysis days, give dose after dialysis). *Peritoneal dialysis:* 500 mg every 12 hr *or* 1 g every 24 hr.

Renal Impairment

(Children): *CCr 40–70 mL/min:* Give 60% of normal daily dose in 2 divided doses (every 12 hr). *CCr 20–40 mL/min:* Give 25% of normal daily dose in 2 divided doses (every 12 hr). *CCr 5–20 mL/min:* Give 10% of normal daily dose every 24 hr.

Cephalexin

PO (Adults): *Most infections:* 250–500 mg every 6 hr. *Uncomplicated cystitis, skin and soft-tissue infections, streptococcal pharyngitis:* 500 mg every 12 hr.

PO (Children): *Most infections:* 25–50 mg/kg/day divided every 6–8 hr (can be administered every 12 hr in skin/skin structure infections or streptococcal pharyngitis). *Otitis media:* 18.75–25 mg/kg every 6 hr (maximum = 4 g/day).

Renal Impairment

PO (Adults): *CCr 10–50 mL/min:* 500 mg every 8–12 hr; *CCr <10 mL/min:* 250–500 mg every 12–24 hr.

Availability

Cefadroxil (generic available)

Capsules: 500 mg. **Tablets:** 1 g. **Oral suspension (orange-pineapple flavor):** 250 mg/5 mL, 500 mg/5 mL.

Cefazolin (generic available)

Powder for injection: 500 mg/vial, 1 g/vial, 2 g/vial, 3 g/vial, 10 g/vial, 20 g/vial, 100 g/vial, 300 g/vial. **Premixed containers:** 1 g/50 mL 4% dextrose in water, 2 g/50 mL 3% dextrose in water, 3 g/50 mL 2% dextrose in water.

Cephalexin (generic available)

Capsules: 250 mg, 500 mg, 750 mg. **Tablets:** 250 mg, 500 mg. **Oral suspension:** 125 mg/5 mL, 250 mg/5 mL.

NURSING IMPLICATIONS

Assessment

- Assess for resolving infection (WBC and vital signs trends; appearance of wound, sputum, urine, and stool) at beginning and during therapy.
- Before initiating therapy, obtain a history to determine previous use of and reactions to other beta-lactam antibiotics, including penicillins or cephalosporins. Persons with a negative history may still have an allergic response.
- Obtain specimens for culture and sensitivity before initiating therapy. First dose may be given before receiving results.
- Observe for signs and symptoms of hypersensitivity reactions (rash, urticaria, pruritus, flushing, dizziness, vomiting, abdominal pain) and angioedema (swelling of throat, lips, tongue, or face; dyspnea; wheezing; hoarseness). Discontinue drug immediately and provide supportive care. Keep epinephrine, an antihistamine, and resuscitation equipment close by in case of an anaphylactic reaction.
- Monitor for signs and symptoms of CDAD, including watery diarrhea with mucus, fever, abdominal pain or cramping, anorexia, nausea, and, in severe cases, dehydration and blood or pus in the stool. May begin up to several weeks after therapy. Report promptly to health care provider.
- Assess for rash or signs and symptoms of SJS frequently during therapy (fever, general malaise, fatigue, muscle or joint aches, blisters, oral lesions, conjunctivitis, hepatitis, eosinophilia). Discontinue cephalosporins at 1st sign of rash and provide supportive care; may be life-threatening. May recur once treatment is stopped.
- Monitor for seizure activity, particularly in patients with renal impairment; discontinue therapy if seizure occurs and treat as clinically indicated. Institute seizure precautions.
- Assess for signs and symptoms of superinfection such as oral thrush (white or yellow patches) or genital mycotic infections (pruritus and yeasty discharge). Treat infection promptly.

Lab Test Considerations

- May cause positive results for Coombs test in patients receiving high doses or in neonates whose mothers were given cephalosporins before delivery.
- May ↑ AST, ALT, alkaline phosphatase, bilirubin, LDH, BUN, and serum creatinine.
- May rarely cause leukopenia, neutropenia, agranulocytosis, thrombocytopenia, or eosinophilia.

Implementation

- Do not confuse cefazolin with cefotetan, cefoxitin, ceftazidime, or ceftriaxone.
- **PO:** Administer around the clock. May be administered on full or empty stomach. Administration with food may minimize GI irritation. Shake oral suspension well before administering. Use calibrated measuring device with liquid preparations. Refrigerate oral suspensions up to 14 days.

Cefazolin

- **Reconstitution:** For IM, IV push, and IV intermittent infusion, reconstitute 500-mg vial with 2 mL; 1-g vial with 2.5 mL; 2-g and 3-g vials with 15 mL; and 10-g vial with 45 mL sterile water for injection **Concentration:** 225 mg/mL (500-mg vial); 330 mg/mL (1-g vial); 136 mg/mL (2-g vial); 196 mg/mL (3-g vial); 1 g/5 mL (10-g vial), respectively. Shake well until dissolved. Stable for 24 hr at room temperature or for 10 days if refrigerated.
- **IM** Inject deep into a well-developed muscle mass; massage well.

IV Administration

- **IV:** Monitor site frequently for thrombophlebitis (pain, redness, swelling). Change sites every 48–72 hr to prevent phlebitis.
- Do not use solutions that are cloudy or contain a precipitate.
- If aminoglycosides are administered concurrently, administer in separate sites, if possible, >1 hr

apart. If 2nd site is unavailable, flush line between medications.

- **IV Push: Dilution:** Reconstituted solution may be further diluted with 0.9% NaCl, D5W, D10W, dextrose/saline combinations, or D5/LR. Do not use preparations containing benzyl alcohol for neonates. **Concentration:** 100–138 mg/mL. **Rate:** Administer slowly over 3–5 min.
- **Intermittent Infusion: Dilution:** Reconstituted solution may be further diluted with 0.9% NaCl, D5W, D10W, D5/0.25% NaCl, D5/0.45% NaCl, D5/0.9% NaCl, D5/LR, or LR solution. Solution is stable for 24 hr at room temperature and 10 days if refrigerated.
- **Concentration:** ≤20 mg/mL.
- **Rate:** Administer over 30–60 min.
- **Y-Site Compatibility:** acetaminophen, acyclovir, allopurinol, alprostadil, amikacin, aminocaproic acid, aminophylline, amphotericin B liposomal, anidulafungin, argatroban, arsenic trioxide, ascorbic acid, atracurium, atropine, azithromycin, aztreonam, benztropine, bivalirudin, bleomycin, bumetanide, buprenorphine, butorphanol, calcium gluconate, cangrelor, carboplatin, carmustine, cefiderocol, cefotetan, cefoxitin, ceftazidime, ceftolozane/tazobactam, ceftriaxone, cefuroxime, chloramphenicol, cisplatin, clindamycin, cyanocobalamin, cyclophosphamide, cyclosporine, cytarabine, dactinomycin, daptomycin, dexamethasone, dexmedetomidine, dexrazoxane, digoxin, diltiazem, docetaxel, doxorubicin liposomal, enalaprilat, ephedrine, epinephrine, epirubicin, epoetin alfa, eptifibatide, esmolol, etoposide, etoposide phosphate, fentanyl, filgrastim, fluconazole, fludarabine, fluorouracil, folic acid, foscarnet, fosphenytoin, furosemide, gemcitabine, gentamicin, glycopyrrolate, granisetron, heparin, hetastarch, hydrocortisone, ifosfamide, imipenem/cilastatin, indomethacin, insulin, regular, irinotecan, isoproterenol, ketamine, ketorolac, letermovir, leucovorin, levetiracetam, lidocaine, linezolid, lorazepam, mannitol, melphalan, meperidine, meropenem, meropenem/vaborbactam, mesna, methadone, methotrexate, methylprednisolone, metoclopramide, metoprolol, metronidazole, midazolam, milrinone, morphine, multivitamins, nafcillin, nalbuphine, nicardipine, nitroglycerin, nitroprusside, norepinephrine, octreotide, ondansetron, oxacillin, oxaliplatin, oxytocin, paclitaxel, palonosetron, pamidronate, penicillin G, phenobarbital, phenylephrine, phytonadione, plazomicin, potassium acetate, potassium chloride, procainamide, propofol, propranolol, remifentanil, remimazolam, rituximab, sargramostim, sodium acetate, sodium bicarbonate, succinylcholine, sufentanil, sulbactam/durlobactam, tacrolimus, tedizolid, theophylline, thiamine, thiotepa, tigecycline, tirofiban, topotecan, trastuzumab, vasopressin, vecuronium, verapamil, vinblastine, vincristine, voriconazole, zoledronic acid.
- **Y-Site Incompatibility:** alemtuzumab, azathioprine, calcium chloride, caspofungin, cefotaxime, chlorpromazine, dacarbazine, dantrolene, daunorubicin, diazepam, diazoxide, diphenhydramine, dobutamine, dopamine, doxorubicin hydrochloride, doxycycline, erythromycin, ganciclovir, gemtuzumab ozogamicin, haloperidol, hydralazine, idarubicin, isavuconazonium, minocycline, mitomycin, mitoxantrone, mycophenolate, papaverine, pemetrexed, pentamidine, pentobarbital, phentolamine, phenytoin, prochlorperazine, protamine, pyridoxine, tobramycin, trimethoprim/sulfamethoxazole, vinorelbine.

C

Patient/Family Teaching

- Explain the purpose and side effects of the medication. Instruct patient to take medication around the clock at evenly spaced times and to finish the medication completely as directed, even if feeling better. Take missed doses as soon as possible unless almost time for next dose; do not double doses. Pedi: Instruct parents or caregivers to use calibrated measuring device with liquid preparations. Advise patient that sharing this medication may be dangerous. Advise patient to read *Patient Information* before starting and with each Rx refill in case of changes.
- Advise patients and family to call 911 and seek urgent treatment for signs and symptoms of hypersensitivity reactions (difficulty breathing; chest tightness; hives; rash; feeling light-headed; itching; swelling of the face, lips, tongue, or throat).
- Advise patient to report signs of superinfection (furry overgrowth on the tongue, white patches in mouth, vaginal itching or discharge, loose or foul-smelling stools).
- Instruct patient to notify health care provider if rash or fever and diarrhea develop, especially if diarrhea contains blood, mucus, or pus. Advise patient not to treat diarrhea without consulting health care provider.
- Advise patient to notify health care provider of all Rx or OTC medications, vitamins, or herbal products being taken and to consult with health care provider before taking other medications.
- Rep: Advise women of reproductive potential to notify health care provider if pregnancy is planned or suspected or if breastfeeding.

Evaluation/Desired Outcomes

- Bactericidal action against susceptible bacteria.
- Resolution of signs and symptoms of infection. Length of time for complete resolution depends on the organism and site of infection.
- Decreased incidence of infection when used for prophylaxis.

CEPHALOSPORINS—SECOND GENERATION

cefaclor (**sef**-a-klor)

cefoTEtan (sef-oh-**tee**-tan)
Cefotan

cefOXitin (se-**fox**-i-tin)
~~Mefoxin~~

cefprozil (sef-**proe**-zil)

cefuroxime (se-fyoor-**ox**-eem)
Ceftin, ~~Zinacef~~

Classification
Therapeutic: anti-infectives
Pharmacologic: second-generation cephalosporins

Indications

Treatment of the following infections caused by susceptible organisms: Respiratory tract infections, Skin and skin structure infections, Bone and joint infections (not cefaclor or cefprozil), Urinary tract infections (not cefprozil). **Cefotetan and cefoxitin:** Intra-abdominal and gynecologic infections. **Cefuroxime:** Meningitis, gynecologic infections, and Lyme disease. **Cefaclor, cefprozil, cefuroxime:** Otitis media. **Cefoxitin and cefuroxime:** Septicemia. **Cefotetan, cefoxitin, cefuroxime:** Perioperative prophylaxis.

Action

Inhibits bacterial cell wall synthesis. **Therapeutic Effects:** Bactericidal action against susceptible bacteria. **Spectrum:** Similar to that of first-generation cephalosporins but have ↑ activity against several other gram-negative pathogens, including: *Haemophilus influenzae*, *Escherichia coli*, *Klebsiella pneumoniae*, *Morganella morganii*, *Neisseria gonorrhoeae* (including penicillinase-producing strains), *Proteus*, *Providencia*, *Serratia marcescens*, *Moraxella catarrhalis*. Not active against methicillin-resistant staphylococci or enterococci. **Cefuroxime:** Active against *Borrelia burgdorferi*. **Cefotetan and cefoxitin:** Active against *Bacteroides fragilis*.

Pharmacokinetics

Absorption: *Cefotetan, cefoxitin,* and *cefuroxime:* Well absorbed following IM administration. *Cefaclor, cefprozil,* and *cefuroxime:* Well absorbed following oral administration.
Distribution: Widely distributed. Penetration into CSF is poor, but adequate for cefuroxime (IV) to be used in treating meningitis.
Metabolism and Excretion: Excreted primarily unchanged by the kidneys.
Half-life: *Cefaclor:* 30–60 min; *cefotetan:* 3–4.6 hr; *cefoxitin:* 40–60 min; *cefprozil:* 90 min; *cefuroxime:* 60–120 min (all are ↑ in renal impairment).

ROUTE	ONSET	PEAK	DURATION
Cefaclor PO	rapid	30–60 min	6–12 hr
Cefaclor PO-CD	unknown	unknown	12 hr
Cefotetan IM	rapid	1–3 hr	12 hr
Cefotetan IV	rapid	end of infusion	12 hr
Cefoxitin IM	rapid	30 min	4–8 hr
Cefoxitin IV	rapid	end of infusion	4–8 hr
Cefprozil PO	unknown	1–2 hr	12–24 hr
Cefuroxime PO	unknown	2–3 hr	8–12 hr
Cefuroxime IM	rapid	15–60 min	6–12 hr
Cefuroxime IV	rapid	end of infusion	6–12 hr

Contraindications/Precautions

Contraindicated in: Hypersensitivity to cephalosporins; Serious hypersensitivity to penicillins.
Use Cautiously in: Renal impairment (↓ dose/↑ dosing interval for: *cefotetan* if CCr ≤30 mL/min, *cefoxitin* if CCr ≤50 mL/min, *cefprozil* if CCr <30 mL/min, *cefuroxime* if CCr <30 mL/min); Patients with hepatic dysfunction, poor nutritional state, or cancer (↑ risk for bleeding); History of GI disease, especially colitis; *Cefprozil (oral suspension)* contains aspartame and should be avoided in patients with phenylketonuria; Geri: Dose adjustment due to age-related ↓ in renal function may be necessary in older adults; may also be at ↑ risk for bleeding with *cefotetan* or *cefoxitin*.

Adverse Reactions/Side Effects

Derm: rash, urticaria. **GI:** diarrhea, CLOSTRIDIOIDES DIFFICILE-ASSOCIATED DIARRHEA (CDAD), cramps, nausea, vomiting. **Hemat:** agranulocytosis, bleeding (↑ with cefotetan and cefoxitin), eosinophilia, hemolytic anemia, neutropenia, thrombocytopenia. **Local:** pain (at IM site), phlebitis. **Neuro:** SEIZURES (HIGH DOSES). **Misc:** HYPERSENSITIVITY REACTIONS (INCLUDING ANAPHYLAXIS AND SERUM SICKNESS), superinfection.

Interactions

Drug-Drug: Probenecid ↓ excretion and ↑ levels. If **alcohol** is ingested within 48–72 hr of cefotetan, a disulfiram-like reaction may occur. Cefotetan may ↑ risk of bleeding with **anticoagulants, antiplatelet agents, thrombolytics,** and **NSAIDs. Antacids** ↓

absorption of cefaclor. **Aminoglycosides** or **loop diuretics** may ↑ risk of nephrotoxicity.

Route/Dosage

Cefaclor

PO (Adults): *Immediate release:* 250–500 mg every 8 hr; *Extended release:* 500 mg every 12 hr.

PO (Children >1 mo): 6.7–13.4 mg/kg every 8 hr or 10–20 mg/kg every 12 hr (up to 1 g/day).

Cefotetan

IM, IV (Adults): *Most infections:* 1–2 g every 12 hr. *Severe/life-threatening infections:* 2–3 g every 12 hr. *Urinary tract infections:* 500 mg–2 g every 12 hr *or* 1–2 g every 24 hr. *Perioperative prophylaxis:* 1–2 g 30–60 min before initial incision as a single dose).

Renal Impairment

IM, IV (Adults): *CCr 10–30 mL/min:* Give usual adult dose every 24 hr *or* 50% of usual adult dose every 12 hr; *CCr <10 mL/min:* Give usual adult dose every 48 hr *or* 25% of usual adult dose every 12 hr.

Cefoxitin

IM, IV (Adults): *Most infections:* 1 g every 6–8 hr. *Severe infections:* 1 g every 4 hr *or* 2 g every 6–8 hr. *Life-threatening infections:* 2 g every 4 hr *or* 3 g every 6 hr. *Perioperative prophylaxis:* 2 g 30–60 min before initial incision, then 2 g every 6 hr for up to 24 hr.

IM, IV (Children >3 mo): *Most infections:* 13.3–26.7 mg/kg every 4 hr *or* 20–40 mg/kg every 6 hr. *Perioperative prophylaxis:* 30–40 mg/kg within 60 min of initial incision, then 30–40 mg/kg every 6 hr for up to 24 hr.

Renal Impairment

IM, IV (Adults): *CCr 30–50 mL/min:* 1–2 g every 8–12 hr; *CCr 10–29 mL/min:* 1–2 g every 12–24 hr; *CCr 5–9 mL/min:* 0.5–1 g every 12–24 hr; *CCr <5 mL/min:* 0.5–1 g every 24–48 hr.

Cefprozil

PO (Adults): *Most infections:* 250–500 mg every 12 hr *or* 500 mg every 24 hr.

PO (Children 6 mo–12 yr): *Otitis media:* 15 mg/kg every 12 hr. *Acute sinusitis:* 7.5–15 mg/kg every 12 hr (higher dose should be used for moderate to severe infections).

PO (Children 2–12 yr): *Pharyngitis/tonsillitis:* 7.5 mg/kg every 12 hr. *Skin/skin structure infections:* 20 mg/kg every 24 hr.

Renal Impairment

PO (Adults and Children ≥6 mo): *CCr <30 mL/min:* Give 50% of usual dose at normal dosing interval.

Cefuroxime

PO (Adults and Children >12 yr): *Pharyngitis/tonsillitis, maxillary sinusitis, uncomplicated UTIs:* 250 mg every 12 hr. *Bronchitis, uncomplicated skin/skin structure infections:* 250–500 mg every 12 hr. *Gonorrhea:* 1 g as a single dose. *Lyme disease:* 500 mg every 12 hr for 20 days.

PO (Children 3 mo–12 yr): *Otitis media, acute bacterial maxillary sinusitis, impetigo:* 250 mg every 12 hr.

IM, IV (Adults): *Uncomplicated urinary tract infections, skin/skin structure infections, disseminated gonococcal infections, uncomplicated pneumonia:* 750 mg every 8 hr. *Bone/joint infections, severe or complicated infections:* 1.5 g every 8 hr. *Life-threatening infections:* 1.5 g every 6 hr. *Meningitis:* 3 g every 8 hr. *Perioperative prophylaxis:* 1.5 g IV 30–60 min before initial incision; 750 mg IM/IV every 8 hr can be given when procedure prolonged. *Prophylaxis during open-heart surgery:* 1.5 g IV at induction of anesthesia and then every 12 hr for 3 additional doses. *Gonorrhea:* 1.5 g IM (750 mg in two sites) with 1 g probenecid PO.

IM, IV (Children >3 mo): *Most infections:* 12.5–25 mg/kg every 6 hr *or* 16.7–33.3 mg/kg every 8 hr (max dose = 6 g/day). *Bone and joint infections:* 50 mg/kg every 8 hr (max dose = 6 g/day). *Bacterial meningitis:* 50–60 mg/kg every 6 hr *or* 66.7–80 mg/kg every 8 hr.

Renal Impairment

IM, IV (Adults): *CCr 10–29 mL/min:* Give standard dose every 24 hr; *CCr <10 mL/min (no hemodialysis):* Give standard dose every 48 hr; *Hemodialysis:* Give an additional dose at end of each dialysis session.

Availability

Cefaclor (generic available)

Capsules: 250 mg, 500 mg. **Extended-release tablets:** 500 mg. **Oral suspension (strawberry):** 250 mg/5 mL.

Cefotetan (generic available)

Powder for injection: 1 g/vial, 2 g/vial.

Cefoxitin (generic available)

Powder for injection: 1 g/vial, 2 g/vial, 10 g/vial.

Cefprozil (generic available)

Oral suspension (bubblegum flavor): 125 mg/5 mL, 250 mg/5 mL. **Tablets:** 250 mg, 500 mg.

Cefuroxime (generic available)

Tablets: 250 mg, 500 mg. **Powder for oral suspension (tutti frutti flavor):** 🍁 125 mg/5 mL. **Powder for injection:** 750 mg/vial, 1.5 g/vial.

NURSING IMPLICATIONS

Assessment

- Assess for infection (vital signs; appearance of wound, sputum, urine, and stool; WBC) at beginning and during therapy.
- Before initiating therapy, obtain a history to determine previous use of and reactions to penicillins or cephalosporins. Persons with a negative history of penicillin sensitivity may still have an allergic response.
- Obtain specimens for culture and sensitivity before initiating therapy. First dose may be given before receiving results.
- Assess for signs and symptoms of anaphylaxis (rash, pruritus, laryngeal edema, wheezing). *If anaphylaxis occurs,* immediately discontinue the drug. Keep epinephrine, an antihistamine, and resuscitation equipment close by in the event of an anaphylactic reaction.
- Monitor bowel function. Diarrhea, abdominal cramping, fever, and bloody stools should be reported to health care provider promptly as a sign of CDAD. May begin up to several weeks following cessation of therapy.

Lab Test Considerations

- May cause positive results for Coombs test in patients receiving high doses or in neonates whose mothers were given cephalosporins before delivery. *Cefotetan:* Monitor prothrombin time and assess patient for bleeding (guaiac stools; check for hematuria, bleeding gums, or ecchymosis) daily in high-risk patients; may cause hypoprothrombinemia.
- May ↑ AST, ALT, alkaline phosphatase, bilirubin, LDH, BUN, and serum creatinine.
- *Cefoxitin* may falsely ↑ test results for serum and urine creatinine; do not obtain serum samples within 2 hr of administration.
- Rarely causes leukopenia, neutropenia, agranulocytosis, thrombocytopenia, and eosinophilia.

Implementation

- Do not confuse cefotetan with cefazolin, cefoxitin, ceftazidime, or ceftriaxone. Do not confuse cefoxitin with cefazolin, cefotetan, ceftazidime, or cetriaxone. Do not confuse cefuroxime with sulfasalazine.
- **PO:** Administer as prescribed. May be administered on full or empty stomach. Administration with food may minimize GI irritation. Shake oral suspension well before administering.
- Administer cefaclor extended-release tablets with food; ***DNC:*** Swallow tablets whole. Do not crush, break, or chew.
- Do not administer *cefaclor* within 1 hr of antacids.
- *Cefuroxime:* ***DNC:*** Swallow tablets whole, do not crush; crushed tablets have a strong, persistent bitter taste. Tablets may be taken without regard to meals.
- **IM:** **Reconstitution:** Reconstitute IM doses with sterile or bacteriostatic water for injection or 0.9% NaCl for injection. May be diluted with lidocaine to minimize injection discomfort.
- Inject deep into a well-developed muscle mass; massage well.

IV Administration

- **IV:** Change sites every 48–72 hr to prevent phlebitis. Monitor site frequently for thrombophlebitis (pain, redness, swelling).
- If aminoglycosides are administered concurrently, administer in separate sites if possible, >1 hr apart. If 2nd site is unavailable, flush IV line between medications.

Cefotetan

- **IV Push:** **Reconstitution:** Reconstitute each gram with ≥10 mL of sterile or bacteriostatic water for injection, 0.9% NaCl, or D5W. Do not use preparations containing benzyl alcohol for neonates. **Concentration:** 95 mg/mL. **Rate:** Administer slowly over 3–5 min.
- **Intermittent Infusion:** **Dilution:** Further dilute reconstituted solution in 50–100 mL of D5W or 0.9% NaCl. Solution may be colorless or yellow. Solution is stable for 24 hr at room temperature or 96 hr if refrigerated. **Concentration:** 10–40 mg/mL. **Rate:** Administer over 20–30 min.
- **Y-Site Compatibility:** acyclovir, allopurinol, amikacin, aminocaproic acid, aminophylline, anidulafungin, argatroban, arsenic trioxide, ascorbic acid, atropine, azithromycin, aztreonam, benztropine, bivalirudin, bleomycin, bumetanide, buprenorphine, butorphanol, calcium chloride, calcium gluconate, carboplatin, carmustine, cefazolin, cefotaxime, cefoxitin, ceftazidime, ceftriaxone, cefuroxime, chloramphenicol, cisplatin, clindamycin, cyanocobalamin, cyclophosphamide, cyclosporine, cytarabine, dacarbazine, dactinomycin, daptomycin, dexamethasone, dexmedetomidine, dexrazoxane, digoxin, diltiazem, docetaxel, dopamine, doxorubicin liposomal, enalaprilat, ephedrine, epinephrine, epoetin alfa, eptifibatide, etoposide, etoposide phosphate, fentanyl, filgrastim, fluconazole, fludarabine, fluorouracil, folic acid, foscarnet, fosphenytoin, furosemide, gemcitabine, glycopyrrolate, granisetron, heparin, hydrocortisone, hydromorphone, ifosfamide, imipenem/cilastatin, irinotecan, isoproterenol, ketorolac, leucovorin, levofloxacin, lidocaine, linezolid, lorazepam, magnesium sulfate, mannitol, melphalan, mesna, methadone, methotrexate, methylprednisolone, metoclopramide, metoprolol, metronidazole, milrinone, mitoxantrone, morphine, multivitamins, nafcillin, nalbuphine,

naloxone, nicardipine, nitroglycerin, nitroprusside, norepinephrine, octreotide, oxacillin, oxaliplatin, oxytocin, paclitaxel, palonosetron, pamidronate, penicillin G, phenylephrine, phytonadione, potassium acetate, potassium chloride, procainamide, propofol, propranolol, pyridoxine, remifentanil, rituximab, rocuronium, sargramostim, sodium acetate, succinylcholine, sufentanil, sulbactam/durlobactam, tacrolimus, theophylline, thiamine, thiotepa, tigecycline, tirofiban, topotecan, vasopressin, vecuronium, verapamil, vinblastine, vincristine, voriconazole, zoledronic acid.

- **Y-Site Incompatibility:** alemtuzumab, amiodarone, amphotericin B deoxycholate, amphotericin B liposomal, azathioprine, caspofungin, chlorpromazine, dantrolene, daunorubicin, diazepam, diazoxide, diphenhydramine, dobutamine, doxorubicin hydrochloride, doxycycline, epirubicin, erythromycin, esmolol, ganciclovir, gemtuzumab ozogamicin, gentamicin, haloperidol, hydralazine, idarubicin, indomethacin, labetalol, minocycline, mitomycin, mycophenolate, pantoprazole, papaverine, pemetrexed, pentamidine, pentobarbital, phenobarbital, phentolamine, phenytoin, prochlorperazine, promethazine, protamine, sodium bicarbonate, tobramycin, trastuzumab, trimethoprim/sulfamethoxazole, vinorelbine.

Cefoxitin

- **IV Push:** Reconstitution: Reconstitute each gram with ≥10 mL of sterile or bacteriostatic water for injection, 0.9% NaCl, or D5W. Do not use preparations containing benzyl alcohol for neonates. Concentration: 200 mg/mL. Rate: Administer slowly over 3–5 min.
- **Intermittent Infusion:** Dilution: Further dilute reconstituted solution in 50–100 mL of D5W, D10W, 0.9% NaCl, dextrose/saline combinations, D5/LR, Ringer's, or LR. Stable for 24 hr at room temperature and 1 wk if refrigerated. Darkening of powder does not alter potency. Concentration: 40 mg/mL. Rate: Administer over 30–60 min.
- **Continuous Infusion:** May be diluted in 500–1000 mL for continuous infusion.
- **Y-Site Compatibility:** acetaminophen, acyclovir, amikacin, aminocaproic acid, aminophylline, amphotericin B deoxycholate, amphotericin B liposomal, anidulafungin, argatroban, arsenic trioxide, ascorbic acid, atropine, azithromycin, aztreonam, benztropine, bivalirudin, bleomycin, bumetanide, buprenorphine, butorphanol, calcium chloride, calcium gluconate, cangrelor, carboplatin, carmustine, cefazolin, cefotaxime, cefotetan, ceftazidime, ceftriaxone, cefuroxime, chloramphenicol, cisplatin, clindamycin, cyanocobalamin, cyclophosphamide, cyclosporine, cytarabine, dacarbazine, dactinomycin, daptomycin, dexamethasone, dexmedetomidine, dexrazoxane, digoxin, diltiazem, docetaxel, dopamine, doxorubicin liposomal, enalaprilat, ephedrine, epinephrine, epoetin alfa, eptifibatide, esmolol, etoposide, etoposide phosphate, fentanyl, fluconazole, fludarabine, fluorouracil, folic acid, foscarnet, fosphenytoin, furosemide, gemcitabine, glycopyrrolate, granisetron, heparin, hydrocortisone, hydromorphone, ifosfamide, imipenem/cilastatin, indomethacin, irinotecan, isoproterenol, ketorolac, leucovorin, lidocaine, linezolid, lorazepam, magnesium sulfate, mannitol, meperidine, meropenem, mesna, methotrexate, metoclopramide, metoprolol, metronidazole, midazolam, milrinone, mitomycin, morphine, multivitamins, nafcillin, nalbuphine, naloxone, nicardipine, nitroglycerin, nitroprusside, norepinephrine, octreotide, ondansetron, oxacillin, oxaliplatin, oxytocin, paclitaxel, palonosetron, pamidronate, penicillin G, phenylephrine, phytonadione, potassium acetate, potassium chloride, procainamide, propofol, propranolol, pyridoxine, remifentanil, rituximab, rocuronium, sodium acetate, succinylcholine, sulbactam/durlobactam, sufentanil, tacrolimus, theophylline, thiamine, thiotepa, tigecycline, tirofiban, topotecan, vasopressin, vecuronium, verapamil, vinblastine, vincristine, voriconazole, zoledronic acid.
- **Y-Site Incompatibility:** alemtuzumab, azathioprine, caspofungin, chlorpromazine, dantrolene, daunorubicin hydrochloride, diazepam, diazoxide, diphenhydramine, dobutamine, doxorubicin hydrochloride, doxycycline, epirubicin, erythromycin, filgrastim, ganciclovir, gemtuzumab ozogamicin, haloperidol, hydralazine, idarubicin, insulin, regular, labetalol, levofloxacin, methylprednisolone, minocycline, mitoxantrone, mycophenolate, papaverine, pemetrexed, pentamidine, pentobarbital, phenobarbital, phentolamine, phenytoin, prochlorperazine, promethazine, protamine, sodium bicarbonate, trastuzumab, trimethoprim/sulfamethoxazole, vinorelbine.

Cefuroxime

- **IV Push:** Reconstitution: Reconstitute 750-mg vial with 8.3 mL and 1.5-g vial with 16 mL of sterile water for injection, respectively. Do not use preparations containing benzyl alcohol for neonates. Rate: Administer slowly over 3–5 min.
- **Intermittent Infusion:** Dilution: Further dilute reconstituted solution in 50–100 mL of 0.9% NaCl, D5W, or 0.45% NaCl. Stable for 24 hr

at room temperature and 7 days if refrigerated. **Concentration:** 10–40 mg/mL. **Rate:** Administer over 15–60 min.

- **Continuous Infusion:** May also be diluted in 500–1000 mL 0.9% NaCl, D5W, D10W, D5/0.9% NaCl, D5/0.45% NaCl, or 1/6 M sodium lactate injection for continuous infusion.
- **Y-Site Compatibility:** acyclovir, allopurinol, aminocaproic acid, aminophylline, amphotericin B liposomal, anidulafungin, argatroban, arsenic trioxide, ascorbic acid, atracurium, atropine, aztreonam, benztropine, bivalirudin, bleomycin, bumetanide, buprenorphine, butorphanol, calcium gluconate, cangrelor, carboplatin, carmustine, cefazolin, cefotaxime, cefotetan, cefoxitin, ceftazidime, ceftolozane/tazobactam, ceftriaxone, chloramphenicol, cisplatin, clindamycin, cyclophosphamide, cyanocobalamin, cyclophosphamide, cyclosporine, cytarabine, dacarbazine, dactinomycin, daptomycin, dexmedetomidine, dexrazoxane, digoxin, diltiazem, docetaxel, dopamine, doxorubicin liposomal, enalaprilat, ephedrine, epinephrine, epoetin alfa, eptifibatide, erythromycin, esmolol, etoposide, etoposide phosphate, famotidine, fentanyl, fludarabine, fluorouracil, folic acid, foscarnet, fosphenytoin, furosemide, gemcitabine, gemtuzumab ozogamicin, glycopyrrolate, granisetron, heparin, hydrocortisone, hydromorphone, ifosfamide, imipenem/cilastatin, indomethacin, insulin, regular, irinotecan, isoproterenol, ketamine, ketorolac, leucovorin, levofloxacin, lidocaine, linezolid, lorazepam, mannitol, melphalan, meperidine, meropenem, meropenem/vaborbactam, mesna, methadone, methotrexate, methylprednisolone, metoclopramide, metoprolol, milrinone, morphine, multivitamins, nafcillin, nalbuphine, naloxone, nitroglycerin, nitroprusside, norepinephrine, octreotide, ondansetron, oxacillin, oxaliplatin, oxytocin, paclitaxel, palonosetron, pamidronate, pemetrexed, penicillin G, phenylephrine, phytonadione, plazomicin, potassium acetate, potassium chloride, procainamide, propofol, propranolol, pyridoxine, remifentanil, rituximab, rocuronium, sargramostim, sodium acetate, succinylcholine, sufentanil, sulbactam/durlobactam, tacrolimus, tedizolid, theophylline, thiamine, thiotepa, tigecycline, tirofiban, topotecan, trastuzumab, vasopressin, vecuronium, verapamil, vinblastine, vincristine, voriconazole, zoledronic acid.
- **Y-Site Incompatibility:** alemtuzumab, azathioprine, calcium chloride, caspofungin, chlorpromazine, dantrolene, daunorubicin, dexamethasone, diazepam, diazoxide, diphenhydramine, dobutamine, doxorubicin hydrochloride, doxycycline, epirubicin, filgrastim, ganciclovir, haloperidol, hydralazine, idarubicin, isavuconazonium, labetalol, magnesium sulfate, midazolam, minocycline, mitomycin, mitoxantrone, mycophenolate, nicardipine, papaverine, pentamidine, pentobarbital, phenobarbital, phentolamine, phenytoin, prochlorperazine, promethazine, protamine, sodium bicarbonate, trimethoprim/sulfamethoxazole, vinorelbine.

Patient/Family Teaching

- Explain purpose and side effects of medication to patient. Advise patient to read *Patient Information* before starting therapy. Instruct patient to take medication around the clock at evenly spaced times and to finish the medication completely, even if feeling better. Take missed doses as soon as possible unless almost time for next dose; do not double doses. Use calibrated measuring device with liquid preparations. Advise patient that sharing of this medication may be dangerous.
- Advise patient to notify health care provider of all Rx or OTC medications, vitamins, or herbal products being taken and to consult with health care provider before taking other medications.
- Advise patient to report signs of superinfection (furry overgrowth on the tongue, vaginal itching or discharge, loose or foul-smelling stools) and allergy.
- Caution patients that concurrent use of alcohol with *cefotetan* may cause a disulfiram-like reaction (abdominal cramps, nausea, vomiting, headache, hypotension, palpitations, dyspnea, tachycardia, sweating, flushing). Alcohol and alcohol-containing medications should be avoided during and for several days after therapy.
- Instruct patient to notify health care provider if fever and diarrhea develop, especially if stool contains blood, pus, or mucus. Advise patient not to treat diarrhea without consulting health care provider.
- Rep: Advise women of reproductive potential to notify health care provider if pregnancy is planned or suspected or if breastfeeding.

Evaluation/Desired Outcomes

- Bactericidal action against susceptible bacteria.

CEPHALOSPORINS—THIRD GENERATION

cefdinir (**sef**-di-nir)
~~Omnicef~~

cefixime (sef-**ik**-seem)
Suprax

cefotaxime (sef-oh-**taks**-eem)
~~Claforan~~

cefpodoxime (sef-poe-**dox**-eem)
~~Vantin~~

cefTAZidime (sef-**tay**-zi-deem)
~~Fortaz~~, Tazicef
cefTRIAXone (sef-try-**ax**-one)
~~Rocephin~~

Classification
Therapeutic: anti-infectives
Pharmacologic: third-generation cephalosporins

Indications
Treatment of the following infections caused by susceptible organisms: Skin and skin structure infections (not cefixime), Urinary and gynecologic infections (not cefdinir), Respiratory tract infections (not cefdinir). **Cefotaxime, ceftazidime, ceftriaxone:** Meningitis and bone/joint infections. **Cefotaxime, ceftazidime, ceftriaxone:** Intra-abdominal infections and septicemia. **Cefdinir, cefixime, cefpodoxime, ceftriaxone:** Otitis media. **Cefotaxime, ceftriaxone:** Perioperative prophylaxis. **Ceftazidime:** Febrile neutropenia. **Cefotaxime, ceftriaxone:** Lyme disease.

Action
Inhibits bacterial cell wall synthesis. **Therapeutic Effects:** Bactericidal action against susceptible bacteria. **Spectrum:** Similar to that of second-generation cephalosporins, but activity against staphylococci is less, whereas activity against gram-negative pathogens is greater, even for organisms resistant to first- and second-generation agents. Notable is increased action against: *Enterobacter*, *Haemophilus influenzae*, *Escherichia coli*, *Klebsiella pneumoniae*, *Neisseria gonorrhoeae*, *Citrobacter*, *Morganella*, *Proteus*, *Providencia*, *Serratia*, *Moraxella catarrhalis*, *Borrelia burgdorferi*. Some agents have activity against *N. meningitidis* (cefotaxime, ceftazidime, ceftriaxone). Some agents have enhanced activity against *Pseudomonas aeruginosa* (ceftazidime). Not active against methicillin-resistant staphylococci or enterococci. Some agents have activity against anaerobes, including *Bacteroides fragilis* (cefotaxime, ceftriaxone).

Pharmacokinetics
Absorption: *Cefotaxime, ceftazidime,* and *ceftriaxone* are well absorbed after IM administration. *Cefixime* 40–50% absorbed after oral administration (oral suspension); *cefdinir* 16–25% absorbed after oral administration. *Cefpodoxime proxetil* is a prodrug that is converted to its active component in GI tract during absorption (50% absorbed).
Distribution: Widely distributed. CSF penetration better than with first- and second-generation agents.
Protein Binding: *Ceftriaxone* ≥90%.
Metabolism and Excretion: *Cefdinir* and *ceftazidime*>85% excreted in urine. *Cefpodoxime:* 30% excreted in urine. *Ceftriaxone* and *cefotaxime:* partly metabolized and partly excreted in the urine. *Cefixime:* 50% excreted unchanged in urine, ≥10% in bile.
Half-life: *Cefdinir:* 1.7 hr; *cefixime:* 3–4 hr; *cefotaxime:* 1–1.5 hr; *cefpodoxime:* 2–3 hr; *ceftazidime:* 2 hr; *ceftriaxone:* 6–9 hr (all except *ceftriaxone* are ↑ in renal impairment).

ROUTE	ONSET	PEAK	DURATION
Cefdinir PO	rapid	2–4 hr	12–24 hr
Cefixime PO	rapid	2–6 hr	24 hr
Cefotaxime IM	rapid	0.5 hr	4–12 hr
Cefotaxime IV	rapid	end of infusion	4–12 hr
Cefpodoxime PO	unknown	2–3 hr	12 hr
Ceftazidime IM	rapid	1 hr	6–12 hr
Ceftazidime IV	rapid	end of infusion	6–12 hr
Ceftriaxone IM	rapid	1–2 hr	12–24 hr
Ceftriaxone IV	rapid	end of infusion	12–24 hr

Contraindications/Precautions
Contraindicated in: Hypersensitivity to cephalosporins; Serious hypersensitivity to penicillins; Pedi: Premature neonates up to a postmenstrual age of 41 wk (ceftriaxone only); Pedi: Hyperbilirubinemic neonates (may lead to bilirubin encephalopathy); Pedi: Neonates ≤28 days requiring calcium-containing IV solutions (↑ risk of precipitation formation).
Use Cautiously in: Renal impairment (↓ dosing/↑ dosing interval recommended for: *cefdinir* if CCr <30 mL/min, *cefixime* if CCr ≤60 mL/min, *cefotaxime* if CCr <20 mL/min, *cefpodoxime* if CCr <30 mL/min, *ceftazidime* if CCr ≤50 mL/min); Combined severe hepatic and renal impairment (↑ risk of neurological adverse reactions with *ceftriaxone*; dose ↓/↑ dosing interval recommended); Diabetes (*cefdinir* suspension contains sucrose); Phenylketonuria (*cefixime* chewable tablets contain aspartame); History of GI disease, especially colitis; Pedi: ↑ risk of urolithiasis and acute renal failure (ceftriaxone only); Geri: Dose adjustment due to age-related ↓ in renal function may be necessary.

Adverse Reactions/Side Effects
Derm: rash, STEVENS-JOHNSON SYNDROME (SJS), urticaria. **GI:** diarrhea, nausea, vomiting, cholelithiasis (ceftriaxone), CLOSTRIDIOIDES DIFFICILE ASSOCIATED DIARRHEA (CDAD), cramps, pancreatitis (ceftriaxone). **GU:** acute renal failure (ceftriaxone), hematuria, urolithiasis (ceftriaxone), vaginal moniliasis. **Hemat:** agranulocytosis, bleeding, eosinophilia, hemolytic anemia, lymphocytosis, neutropenia, thrombocytopenia, thrombocytosis. **Local:** pain at IM site, phlebitis at IV site. **Neuro:** encephalopathy, headache, SEIZURES (HIGH

C

DOSES). **Misc:** HYPERSENSITIVITY REACTIONS (INCLUDING ANAPHYLAXIS AND SERUM SICKNESS), superinfection.

Interactions

Drug-Drug: Probenecid ↓ excretion and ↑ serum levels (cefdinir, cefixime, cefotaxime, cefpodoxime, ceftriaxone). Concurrent use of **loop diuretics, aminoglycosides**, or **NSAIDs** may ↑ risk of nephrotoxicity. **Antacids** ↓ absorption of cefdinir and cefpodoxime. **Iron supplements** ↓ absorption of cefdinir. **H_2-receptor antagonists** ↓ absorption of cefpodoxime. Cefixime may ↑ **carbamazepine** levels. Ceftriaxone should not be administered concomitantly with any calcium-containing solutions. Ceftriaxone may ↑ risk of bleeding with **warfarin**.

Route/Dosage

Cefdinir

PO (Adults ≥13 yr): 300 mg every 12 hr *or* 600 mg every 24 hr (use every 12 hr dosing only for community-acquired pneumonia or skin and skin structure infections).

PO (Children 6 mo–12 yr): 7 mg/kg every 12 hr (use only for skin/skin structure infections) *or* 14 mg/kg every 24 hr; dose should not exceed 600 mg/day.

Renal Impairment

PO (Adults and Children ≥13 yr): *CCr <30 mL/min:* 300 mg every 24 hr.

Renal Impairment

PO (Children 6 mo–12 yr): *CCr <30 mL/min:* 7 mg/kg every 24 hr.

Cefixime

PO (Adults and Children >12 yr or >45 kg): *Most infections:* 400 mg once daily; *Gonorrhea:* 400 mg single dose.

PO (Children 6 mo–12 yr): 8 mg/kg once daily *or* 4 mg/kg every 12 h.

Renal Impairment

PO (Adults): *CCr 21–60 mL/min:* 75% of standard dose once daily; *CCr ≤20 mL/min:* 50% of standard dose once daily.

Cefotaxime

IM, IV (Adults and Children >12 yr): *Most uncomplicated infections:* 1 g every 12 hr. *Moderate or severe infections:* 1–2 g every 6–8 hr. *Life-threatening infections:* 2 g every 4 hr (maximum dose = 12 g/day). *Gonococcal urethritis/cervicitis or rectal gonorrhea in females:* 500 mg IM (single dose). *Rectal gonorrhea in males:* 1 g IM (single dose). *Perioperative prophylaxis:* 1 g 30–90 min before initial incision (one-time dose).

IM, IV (Children 1 mo–12 yr): *<50 kg:* 100–200 mg/kg/day divided every 6–8 hr. *Meningitis:* 200 mg/kg/day divided every 6 hr. *Invasive pneumococcal meningitis:* 225–300 mg/kg/day divided every 6–8 hr. *≥50 kg:* see adult dosing.

IV (Neonates 1–4 wk): 50 mg/kg every 6–8 hr.

IV (Neonates ≤1 wk): 50 mg/kg every 8–12 hr.

Renal Impairment

(Adults): *CCr <20 mL/min:* ↓ dose by 50%.

Cefpodoxime

PO (Adults): *Most infections:* 200 mg every 12 hr. *Skin and skin structure infections:* 400 mg every 12 hr. *Urinary tract infections/pharyngitis:* 100 mg every 12 hr. *Gonorrhea:* 200 mg single dose.

PO (Children 2 mo–12 yr): *Pharyngitis/tonsillitis/otitis media/acute maxillary sinusitis:* 5 mg/kg every 12 hr (not to exceed 200 mg/dose).

Renal Impairment

PO (Adults): *CCr <30 mL/min:* ↑ dosing interval to every 24 hr.

Ceftazidime

IM, IV (Adults and Children ≥12 yr): *Pneumonia and skin/skin structure infections:* 500 mg–1 g every 8 hr. *Bone and joint infections:* 2 g every 12 hr. *Severe and life-threatening infections:* 2 g every 8 hr. *Complicated urinary tract infections:* 500 mg every 8–12 hr. *Uncomplicated urinary tract infections:* 250 mg every 12 hr. *Cystic fibrosis lung infection caused by* P. aeruginosa: 30–50 mg/kg every 8 hr (maximum dose = 6 g/day).

IM, IV (Children 1 mo–12 yr): 33.3–50 mg/kg every 8 hr (maximum dose = 6 g/day).

IM, IV (Neonates ≤4 wk): 50 mg/kg every 8–12 hr.

Renal Impairment

IM, IV (Adults): *CCr 31–50 mL/min:* 1 g every 12 hr; *CCr 16–30 mL/min:* 1 g every 24 hr; *CCr 6–15 mL/min:* 500 mg every 24 hr; *CCr <5 mL/min:* 500 mg every 48 hr.

Ceftriaxone

IM, IV (Adults): *Most infections:* 1–2 g every 12–24 hr. *Gonorrhea:* 250 mg IM (single dose). *Meningitis:* 2 g every 12 hr. *Perioperative prophylaxis:* 1 g 30–120 min before initial incision (single dose).

IM, IV (Children): *Most infections:* 25–37.5 mg/kg every 12 hr *or* 50–75 mg/kg every 24 hr; dose should not exceed 2 g/day. *Meningitis:* 100 mg/kg every 24 hr *or* 50 mg/kg every 12 hr; dose should not exceed 4 g/day. *Acute otitis media:* 50 mg/kg IM single dose; dose should not exceed 1 g. *Uncomplicated gonorrhea:* 125 mg IM (single dose).

Hepatic/Renal Impairment

IM, IV (Adults): *Hepatic impairment with significant renal impairment:* Not to exceed 2 g/day.

Availability

Cefdinir (generic available)

Capsules: 300 mg. **Oral suspension(strawberry):** 125 mg/5 mL, 250 mg/5 mL.

Cefixime (generic available)

Capsules: 400 mg. **Chewable tablets (contain aspartame):** 100 mg, 150 mg, 200 mg. **Oral suspension(strawberry):** 100 mg/5 mL, 200 mg/5 mL, 500 mg/5 mL. **Tablets:** 400 mg.

Cefotaxime (generic available)

Powder for injection: 500 mg/vial, 1 g/vial, 2 g/vial, 10 g/vial.

Cefpodoxime (generic available)

Oral suspension (lemon creme): 50 mg/5 mL, 100 mg/5 mL. **Tablets:** 100 mg, 200 mg.

Ceftazidime (generic available)

Powder for injection: 1 g/vial, 2 g/vial, 6 g/vial. **Premixed infusion:** 1 g/50 mL, 2 g/50 mL.

Ceftriaxone (generic available)

Powder for injection: 250 mg/vial, 500 mg/vial, 1 g/vial, 2 g/vial, 10 g/vial, 100 g/vial. **Premixed infusion:** 1 g/50 mL, 2 g/50 mL.

NURSING IMPLICATIONS

Assessment

- Assess for infection (vital signs; appearance of wound, sputum, urine, and stool; WBC) at beginning of and throughout therapy.
- Before initiating therapy, obtain a history to determine previous use of and reactions to penicillins or cephalosporins. Persons with a negative history of penicillin sensitivity may still have an allergic response.
- Obtain specimens for culture and sensitivity before initiating therapy. First dose may be given before receiving results.
- Observe for signs and symptoms of anaphylaxis (rash, pruritus, laryngeal edema, wheezing). Discontinue drug and notify health care professional immediately if these symptoms occur. Keep epinephrine, an antihistamine, and resuscitation equipment close by in the event of an anaphylactic reaction.
- Monitor bowel function. Diarrhea, abdominal cramping, fever, and bloody stools should be reported to health care professional promptly as a sign of CDAD. May begin up to several wk following cessation of therapy.
- Assess patient for skin rash frequently during therapy. Discontinue at first sign of rash; may be life-threatening. SJS may develop. Treat symptomatically; may recur once treatment is stopped.
- Pedi: Assess newborns for jaundice and hyperbilirubinemia before making decision to use ceftriaxone (should not be used in jaundiced or hyperbilirubinemic neonates).

Lab Test Considerations

- May cause positive results for Coombs' test in patients receiving high doses or in neonates whose mothers were given cephalosporins before delivery.
- May cause ↑ AST, ALT, alkaline phosphatase, bilirubin, LDH, BUN, and serum creatinine.
- May rarely cause leukopenia, neutropenia, agranulocytosis, thrombocytopenia, eosinophilia, lymphocytosis, and thrombocytosis.

Implementation

- Do not confuse ceftazidime with cefazolin, cefoxitin, cefotetan, or ceftriaxone. Do not confuse ceftriaxone with cefazolin, cefotetan, cefoxitin, or ceftazidime.
- **PO:** Administer around the clock. May be administered on full or empty stomach. Administration with food may minimize GI irritation. Shake oral suspension well before administering. Administer *cefpodoxime tablets* with meals to enhance absorption (suspension may be administered without regard to meals.
- *Cefixime oral suspension* should be used to treat otitis media (results in higher peak concentrations than tablets).
- Do not administer *cefdinir* or *cefpodoxime* within 2 hr before or after an antacid. Do not administer *cefpodoxime* within 2 hr before or after an H_2 receptor antagonist. Do not administer *cefdinir* within 2 hr before or after iron supplements.
- **IM: Reconstitution:** Reconstitute IM doses with sterile or bacteriostatic water for injection or 0.9% NaCl for injection. May be diluted with lidocaine to minimize injection discomfort. Do not administer lidocaine-containing ceftriaxone IV.
- Inject deep into a well-developed muscle mass; massage well.

IV Administration

- **IV:** Monitor injection site frequently for phlebitis (pain, redness, swelling). Change sites every 48–72 hr to prevent phlebitis.
- If aminoglycosides are administered concurrently, administer in separate sites, if possible, at least 1 hr apart. If second site is unavailable, flush lines between medications.

Cefotaxime

- **IV Push: Reconstitution:** Reconstitute 500-mg, 1-g and 2-g vials in at least 10 mL of sterile water for injection. **Concentration:** 50 mg/mL (500 mg), 95 mg/mL (1 g), and 180 mg/mL (2 g). Do not use preparations containing benzyl alcohol for neonates. **Rate:** Administer slowly over 3–5 min.

- **Intermittent Infusion:** **Dilution:** Reconstituted solution may be further diluted in D5W, D10W, lactated Ringer's solution, D5/0.25% NaCl, D5/0.45% NaCl, D5/0.9% NaCl, or 0.9% NaCl. **Concentration:** 20–60 mg/mL. Solution may appear light yellow to amber. Solution is stable for 24 hr at room temperature and 5 days if refrigerated. **Rate:** Administer over 20–30 min.
- **Y-Site Compatibility:** acetaminophen, acyclovir, alprostadil, amikacin, aminocaproic acid, aminophylline, anidulafungin, argatroban, arsenic trioxide, ascorbic acid, atracurium, atropine, aztreonam, benztropine, bivalirudin, bleomycin, bumetanide, buprenorphine, butorphanol, calcium chloride, calcium gluconate, cangrelor, carboplatin, carmustine, cefotetan, cefoxitin, ceftriaxone, cefuroxime, cisplatin, clindamycin, cyanocobalamin, cyclophosphamide, cyclosporine, cytarabine, dactinomycin, daptomycin, dexamethasone, dexmedetomidine, dexrazoxane, digoxin, diltiazem, dimenhydrinate, docetaxel, dopamine, doxorubicin liposomal, doxycycline, enalaprilat, ephedrine, epinephrine, epirubicin, epoetin alfa, eptifibatide, erythromycin, esmolol, etoposide, etoposide phosphate, famotidine, fentanyl, fludarabine, fluorouracil, folic acid, foscarnet, fosphenytoin, furosemide, glycopyrrolate, granisetron, heparin, hetastarch, hydrocortisone, ifosfamide, imipenem/cilastatin, indomethacin, insulin, regular, isoproterenol, ketamine, ketorolac, LR, leucovorin calcium, lidocaine, linezolid, lorazepam, magnesium sulfate, mannitol, melphalan, meperidine, meropenem, mesna, methadone, methotrexate, metoclopramide, metoprolol, midazolam, milrinone, morphine, multivitamins, nafcillin, nalbuphine, naloxone, nicardipine, nitroglycerin, nitroprusside, norepinephrine, octreotide, ondansetron, oxacillin, oxaliplatin, oxytocin, paclitaxel, palonosetron, pamidronate, penicillin G, phenylephrine, phytonadione, potassium acetate, potassium chloride, procainamide, propofol, propranolol, pyridoxine, remifentanil, rituximab, rocuronium, sargramostim, sodium acetate, succinylcholine, sufentanil, tacrolimus, theophylline, thiamine, thiotepa, tigecycline, tirofiban, tobramycin, topotecan, vasopressin, verapamil, vinblastine, vinorelbine, voriconazole, zoledronic acid.
- **Y-Site Incompatibility:** alemtuzumab, allopurinol, amiodarone, amphotericin B liposomal, azathioprine, caspofungin, cefazolin, ceftazidime, chloramphenicol, chlorpromazine, dacarbazine, dantrolene, daunorubicin hydrochloride, diazepam, diphenhydramine, dobutamine, doxorubicin hydrochloride, filgrastim, ganciclovir, gemcitabine, gemtuzumab ozogamicin, haloperidol, hetastarch, hydralazine, hydroxyzine, idarubicin, irinotecan, labetalol, methylprednisolone, minocycline, mitomycin, mitoxantrone, mycophenolate, pantoprazole, papaverine, pemetrexed, pentamidine, pentobarbital, phenobarbital, phenytoin, prochlorperazine, promethazine, protamine, sodium bicarbonate, trastuzumab, trimethoprim/sulfamethoxazole, vecuronium.

Ceftazidime

- **IV Push:** **Reconstitution:** Reconstitute 500-mg, 1-g and 2-g vials with 5.3 mL, 10 mL or 10 mL, respectively, of sterile water for injection. **Concentration:** 100 mg/mL (500 mg), 100 mg/mL (1 g), and 170 mg/mL (2 g). Do not use preparations containing benzyl alcohol for neonates. **Rate:** Administer slowly over 3–5 min.
- **Intermittent Infusion:** **Dilution:** Reconstituted solution may be further diluted in at least 1 g/10 mL of 0.9% NaCl, D5W, D10W, dextrose/saline combinations, or LR. Dilution causes CO_2 to form inside vial, resulting in positive pressure; vial may require venting after dissolution to preserve sterility of vial. Solution may appear yellow to amber; darkening does not alter potency. Solution is stable for 18 hr at room temperature and 7 days if refrigerated. **Concentration:** 40 mg/mL. **Rate:** Administer over 15–30 min.
- **Y-Site Compatibility:** acetaminophen, acyclovir, allopurinol, aminocaproic acid, aminophylline, anakinra, anidulafungin, argatroban, arsenic trioxide, atropine, aztreonam, benztropine, bivalirudin, bleomycin, bumetanide, buprenorphine, butorphanol, calcium gluconate, cangrelor, carboplatin, carmustine, cefazolin, cefotetan, cefoxitin, ceftolozane/tazobactam, ceftriaxone, cefuroxime, ciprofloxacin, cisplatin, clindamycin, cyanocobalamin, cyclophosphamide, cyclosporine, cytarabine, dacarbazine, dactinomycin, daptomycin, dexamethasone, dexmedetomidine, dexrazoxane, digoxin, diltiazem, dimenhydrinate, docetaxel, dopamine, enalaprilat, ephedrine, epinephrine, epoetin alfa, eptifibatide, eravacycline, esmolol, etoposide, etoposide phosphate, famotidine, fentanyl, filgrastim, fludarabine, fluorouracil, folic acid, foscarnet, fosphenytoin, furosemide, gemcitabine, glycopyrrolate, granisetron, heparin, hetastarch, hydrocortisone, hydromorphone, ibuprofen lysine, ifosfamide, imipenem/cilastatin, indomethacin, insulin, regular, irinotecan, isoproterenol, ketamine, ketorolac, labetalol, LR, leucovorin calcium, levofloxacin, lidocaine, linezolid, lorazepam, magnesium sulfate, mannitol, melphalan, meperidine, meropenem, meropenem/vaborbactam, mesna, methadone, methotrexate, methylprednisolone, metoclopramide, metoprolol, metronidazole, milrinone, mitomycin, morphine, multivitamins, nafcillin, nalbuphine, naloxone, nitroglycerin, norepinephrine, octreotide, oxacillin, oxaliplatin, oxytocin, paclitaxel, palonosetron,

pamidronate, penicillin G, phenobarbital, phentolamine, phenylephrine, phytonadione, plazomicin, potassium acetate, potassium chloride, procainamide, propranolol, pyridoxine, remifentanil, rituximab, rocuronium, sodium acetate, sodium bicarbonate, succinylcholine, sufentanil, tacrolimus, tedizolid, telavancin, thiotepa, tigecycline, tirofiban, trastuzumab, vasopressin, vecuronium, vinblastine, vincristine, vinorelbine, voriconazole, zidovudine, zoledronic acid.

- **Y-Site Incompatibility:** acetylcysteine, alemtuzumab, amiodarone, amphotericin B deoxycholate, amphotericin B liposomal, ascorbic acid, azathioprine, blinatumomab, calcium chloride, caspofungin, cefotaxime, chloramphenicol, chlorpromazine, dantrolene, daunorubicin hydrochloride, diazepam, diphenhydramine, doxorubicin hydrochloride, doxorubicin liposomal, doxycycline, epirubicin, ganciclovir, gemtuzumab ozogamicin, haloperidol, hydralazine, hydroxyzine, idarubicin, isavuconazonium, midazolam, minocycline, mitoxantrone, mycophenolate, nitroprusside, papaverine, pemetrexed, pentamidine, phenytoin, prochlorperazine, promethazine, protamine, thiamine, topotecan, trimethoprim/sulfamethoxazole, verapamil.

Ceftriaxone

- **Intermittent Infusion: Reconstitution:** Reconstitute each 250-mg vial with 2.4 mL, each 500-mg vial with 4.8 mL, each 1-g vial with 9.6 mL, and each 2-g vial with 19.2 mL of sterile water for injection, 0.9% NaCl, or D5W for a concentration of 100 mg/mL. **Dilution:** Solution should be further diluted in 50–100 mL of 0.9% NaCl, D5W, D10W, D5/0.45% NaCl, or D5/0.9% NaCl. Solution may appear light yellow to amber. Solution is stable for 3 days at room temperature. **Concentration:** 40 mg/mL.
- **Rate:** Infuse over 30 min.
- **Y-Site Compatibility:** acetaminophen, acyclovir, allopurinol, aminocaproic acid, aminophylline, amphotericin B liposomal, anidulafungin, argatroban, arsenic trioxide, atropine, aztreonam, benztropine, bivalirudin, bleomycin, bumetanide, buprenorphine, butorphanol, cangrelor, carboplatin, carmustine, cefazolin, cefotaxime, cefotetan, cefoxitin, ceftazidime, ceftolozane/tazobactam, cefuroxime, cisatracurium, cisplatin, cyanocobalamin, cyclophosphamide, cyclosporine, cytarabine, dactinomycin, daptomycin, dexamethasone, dexmedetomidine, dexrazoxane, digoxin, diltiazem, docetaxel, dopamine, doxorubicin liposomal, doxycycline, enalaprilat, ephedrine, epinephrine, epoetin alfa, eptifibatide, erythromycin, esmolol, etoposide, etoposide phosphate, fentanyl, fludarabine, fluorouracil, folic acid, foscarnet, fosphenytoin, furosemide, gemcitabine, glycopyrrolate, granisetron, heparin, hydrocortisone, hydromorphone, ifosfamide, indomethacin, insulin, regular, isoproterenol, ketorolac, levofloxacin, lidocaine, linezolid, lorazepam, mannitol, melphalan, meperidine, meropenem, meropenem/vaborbactam, mesna, methadone, methotrexate, methylprednisolone, metoclopramide, metoprolol, metronidazole, midazolam, milrinone, mitomycin, morphine, multivitamins, nafcillin, nalbuphine, naloxone, nicardipine, nitroglycerin, nitroprusside, norepinephrine, octreotide, oxacillin, oxaliplatin, oxytocin, paclitaxel, palonosetron, pamidronate, pantoprazole, pemetrexed, penicillin G, phenobarbital, phentolamine, phenylephrine, phytonadione, plazomicin, potassium acetate, potassium chloride, procainamide, propranolol, pyridoxine, remifentanil, rituxumab, rocuronium, sargramostim, sodium acetate, sodium bicarbonate, succinylcholine, sufentanil, tacrolimus, tedizolid, telavancin, theophylline, thiamine, thiotepa, tigecycline, tirofiban, topotecan, trastuzumab, vasopressin, vecuronium, verapamil, vinblastine, vincristine, voriconazole, zidovudine, zoledronic acid.
- **Y-Site Incompatibility:** alemtuzumab, amphotericin B deoxycholate, ascorbic acid, azathioprine, blinatumomab, calcium chloride, calcium gluconate, caspofungin, chloramphenicol, chlorpromazine, clindamycin, dacarbazine, dantrolene, daunorubicin hydrochloride, diazepam, diphenhydramine, dobutamine, doxorubicin hydrochloride, epirubicin, filgrastim, ganciclovir, gemtuzumab ozogamicin, haloperidol, hetastarch, hydralazine, hydroxyzine, idarubicin, imipenem/cilastatin, irinotecan, isavuconazonium, labetalol, leucovorin calcium, minocycline, mitoxantrone, mycophenolate, papaverine, pentamidine, pentobarbital, phenytoin, prochlorperazine, promethazine, protamine, tobramycin, trimethoprim/sulfamethoxazole, vinorelbine, Calcium-containing solutions, including parenteral nutrition, should not be mixed or co-administered, even via different infusion lines at different sites in patients <28 days old. In older patients, flush line thoroughly between infusions.

Patient/Family Teaching

- Instruct patient to take medication around the clock and to finish the medication completely, even if feeling better. Take missed doses as soon as possible unless almost time for next dose; do not double doses. Advise patient that sharing of this medication may be dangerous.

- Pedi: Instruct parents or caregivers to use calibrated measuring device with liquid preparations.
- Advise patient to report signs of superinfection (furry overgrowth on the tongue, vaginal itching or discharge, loose or foul-smelling stools) and allergy.
- Instruct patient to notify health care professional if rash, fever, and diarrhea develop, especially if stool contains blood, pus, or mucus. Advise patient not to treat diarrhea without consulting health care professional.
- Rep: Advise females of reproductive potential to notify health care professional if pregnancy is planned or suspected, or if breastfeeding.

Evaluation/Desired Outcomes

- Resolution of the signs and symptoms of infection. Length of time for complete resolution depends on the organism and site of infection.
- Decreased incidence of infection when used for prophylaxis.

certolizumab

(ser-toe-**liz**-ue-mab)

Cimzia

Classification

Therapeutic: gastrointestinal anti-inflammatories, antirheumatics

Pharmacologic: tumor necrosis factor blockers, DMARDs, monoclonal antibodies

Indications

Moderately to severely active Crohn's disease when response to conventional therapy has been inadequate. Moderately to severely active rheumatoid arthritis. Active psoriatic arthritis. Active ankylosing spondylitis. Active polyarticular juvenile idiopathic arthritis. Moderate to severe plaque psoriasis in patients who are not candidates for systemic therapy or phototherapy. Active non-radiographic axial spondyloarthritis with objective signs of inflammation.

Action

Neutralizes tumor necrosis factor, a prime mediator of inflammation; pegylation provides a long duration of action. **Therapeutic Effects:** Decreased signs/symptoms of Crohn's disease. Decreased pain and swelling, decreased rate of joint destruction, and improved physical function in rheumatoid arthritis and polyarticular juvenile idiopathic arthritis. Decreased joint swelling and pain in psoriatic arthritis. Decreased spinal pain and inflammation in ankylosing spondylitis. Reduced severity of plaques. Decreased pain and swelling, reduced C-reactive protein levels, and improved physical function in axial spondyloarthritis.

Pharmacokinetics

Absorption: 80% absorbed following SUBQ administration.

Distribution: Minimally distributed to tissues.

Metabolism and Excretion: Unknown.

Half-life: 14 days.

TIME/ACTION PROFILE (plasma concentrations)

ROUTE	ONSET	PEAK	DURATION
SUBQ	unknown	50–120 hr	2–4 wk

Contraindications/Precautions

Contraindicated in: Hypersensitivity; Active infection (including localized); Concurrent use of anakinra.

Use Cautiously in: History of chronic or recurrent infection or underlying illness/treatment predisposing to infection; History of exposure to tuberculosis (TB); History of opportunistic infection; Patients residing, or who have resided, where TB, histoplasmosis, coccidioidomycoses, or blastomycosis is endemic; History of demyelinating disorders (may exacerbate); History of HF; OB: Use during pregnancy only if potential maternal benefits justify potential fetal risk; Lactation: Use while breastfeeding only if potential maternal benefits justify potential risk to infant; Pedi: Safety and effectiveness not established in children; Geri: May ↑ risk of infection in older adults.

Adverse Reactions/Side Effects

Derm: psoriasis, skin reactions (rarely severe). **Hemat:** hematologic reactions. **MS:** arthralgia. **Misc:** INFECTION (INCLUDING REACTIVATION TB, HEPATITIS B VIRUS [HBV] REACTIVATION, AND OTHER OPPORTUNISTIC INFECTIONS DUE TO BACTERIAL, INVASIVE FUNGAL, VIRAL, MYCOBACTERIAL, AND PARASITIC PATHOGENS), HYPERSENSITIVITY REACTIONS (INCLUDING ANAPHYLAXIS, ANGIOEDEMA, SERUM SICKNESS, AND URTICARIA), lupus-like syndrome, MALIGNANCY (INCLUDING LYMPHOMA, HEPATOSPLENIC T-CELL LYMPHOMA [HSTCL], LEUKEMIA, AND SKIN CANCER).

Interactions

Drug-Drug: Anakinra ↑ risk of serious infections; concurrent use contraindicated. Concurrent use with **azathioprine** and/or **methotrexate** may ↑ risk of HSTCL. May ↓ antibody response to or ↑ risk of adverse reactions to **live vaccines**; avoid concurrent use.

Route/Dosage

Crohn's Disease

SUBQ (Adults): 400 mg (given as two 200-mg injections) initially; then repeat 2 and 4 wk later; may be followed by maintenance dose of 400 mg (given as two 200-mg injections) every 4 wk.

Rheumatoid Arthritis or Psoriatic Arthritis

SUBQ (Adults): 400 mg (given as two 200-mg injections) initially; then repeat 2 and 4 wk later; then maintenance dose of 200 mg every 2 wk (400 mg [given as two 200-mg injections] every 4 wk may be used alternatively).

Ankylosing Spondylitis or Non-Radiographic Axial Spondyloarthritis

SUBQ (Adults): 400 mg (given as two 200-mg injections) initially; then repeat 2 and 4 wk later; then maintenance dose of 200 mg every 2 wk or 400 mg (given as two 200-mg injections) every 4 wk.

Polyarticular Juvenile Idiopathic Arthritis

SUBQ (Children ≥2 yr and ≥40 kg): 400 mg (given as two 200-mg injections) initially; then repeat 2 and 4 wk later; then maintenance dose of 200 mg every 2 wk (starting at Wk 6).

SUBQ (Children ≥2 yr and 20–<40 kg): 200 mg initially; then repeat 2 and 4 wk later; then maintenance dose of 100 mg every 2 wk (starting at Wk 6).

SUBQ (Children ≥2 yr and 10–<20 kg): 100 mg initially; then repeat 2 and 4 wk later; then maintenance dose of 50 mg every 2 wk (starting at Wk 6).

Plaque Psoriasis

SUBQ (Adults): 400 mg (given as two 200-mg injections) every 2 wk; *Patients ≤90 kg:* may consider giving 400 mg (given as two 200-mg injections) initially; then repeat 2 and 4 wk later; then maintenance dose of 200 mg every 2 wk.

Availability

Lyophilized powder for injection: 200 mg/vial. **Solution for injection (prefilled syringes):** 200 mg/mL.

NURSING IMPLICATIONS

Assessment

- Assess for signs and symptoms of improvement or progression of disease process being treated.
- Assess for signs of infection prior to and during therapy. Monitor all patients for active TB (persistent cough, wasting, weight loss, low-grade fever) during therapy, even if initial test was negative. Do not begin certolizumab during an active infection. If new infection develops, monitor closely and discontinue certolizumab if infection becomes serious.
- Monitor for signs of hypersensitivity reactions (angioedema, dyspnea, hypotension, rash, serum sickness, urticaria). If reactions occur, discontinue certolizumab and treat symptomatically.
- Assess for signs and symptoms of systemic fungal infection. Consider empiric antifungal treatment for patients at risk of histoplasmosis and other invasive fungal infections until pathogen identified. Consult with infectious diseases specialist. Consider stopping certolizumab until infection resolved.
- Monitor for signs and symptoms of lupus-like syndrome. If symptoms occur discontinue certolizumab.

Lab Test Considerations

- May cause anemia, leukopenia, pancytopenia, and thrombocytopenia.
- Monitor CBC with differential periodically during therapy. May cause anemia, leukopenia, pancytopenia, and thrombocytopenia. Consider discontinuing certolizumab if significant hematologic dyscrasias occur.
- Test for HBV infection before initiating therapy. Monitor carriers closely for clinical and lab signs of active infection during therapy and for several mo following last dose. If HBV reactivation occurs, discontinue certolizumab and initiate antiviral therapy.
- Perform test for latent TB. If positive for latent TB, active TB in whom an adequate course of treatment cannot be confirmed, and for patients with a negative test for TB who have risk factors for tuberculosis infection, begin treatment for TB prior to starting certolizumab therapy. Monitor for TB throughout therapy, even if latent TB test is negative.
- May ↑ liver enzymes.
- May erroneously ↑ aPTT.

Implementation

- Update immunizations according to current guidelines prior to therapy.
- Assess for latex allergy if using prefilled syringe. Removal cap contains natural latex derivative.
- **Lyophilized powder for injection: Reconstitution:** Bring vial to room temperature for 30 min prior to reconstitution. Do not use other warming methods. Using the provided 20-gauge needle, add 1 mL sterile water for injection to vial. Gently swirl for 1 min; do not shake. Swirl every 5 min for up to 30 min until fully reconstituted. Solution is clear to opalescent, colorless to yellow, and free from particulates. Administer within 2 hr or refrigerate up to 24 hr prior to injection. Do not freeze. **Concentration:** 200 mg/mL. Using a new 20-gauge needle for each vial, withdraw reconstituted solution into two separate syringes, each containing 1 mL of certolizumab. Switch each 20-gauge needle to a 23-gauge needle prior to injection. Give 400-mg dose as two injections of 200 mg each.

- **SUBQ**: Bring reconstituted solution and prefilled syringes to room temperature for 30 min and no longer than 2 hr prior to injection. Inject full contents of syringe subcutaneously into separate sides of the abdomen or thigh. Avoid areas of skin tenderness, bruising, induration, scars, or stretch marks.

Patient/Family Teaching

- Advise patient of potential benefits and risks of certolizumab. Instruct patient in correct technique for injection, and care and disposal of equipment. Advise patient to read the *Medication Guide* prior to starting therapy.
- Advise patient to avoid live vaccines during or immediately prior to initiating therapy.
- Inform patient of risk of infection. Advise patient to notify health care professional if symptoms of infection (fever, cough, flu-like symptoms, open cuts or sores), including TB or reactivation of HBV infection, occur.
- Counsel patient about possible risk of lymphoma and other malignancies while receiving certolizumab. Advise patient to obtain periodic skin examinations during therapy.
- Advise patient to notify health care professional if signs of hypersensitivity reactions (rash, swollen face, difficulty breathing) or new or worsening medical conditions, such as heart or neurological disease or autoimmune disorders, occur and to report signs of bone marrow depression (bruising, bleeding, or persistent fever).
- Advise patient to notify health care professional of all Rx or OTC medications, vitamins, or herbal products being taken and to consult with health care professional before taking other medications.
- Rep: Advise patient to notify health care professional if pregnancy is planned or suspected or if breastfeeding.

Evaluation/Desired Outcomes

- Reduction in signs and symptoms of Crohn's disease.
- Decreased pain and swelling with decreased rate of joint destruction in patients with rheumatoid arthritis.
- Decreased joint swelling and pain in psoriatic arthritis.
- Decreased spinal pain and inflammation in ankylosing spondylitis.
- Decreased severity of plaques.
- Decreased pain and swelling, decreased C-reactive protein levels, and improved physical function in axial spondyloarthritis.

cetirizine (se-ti-ra-zeen)

Quzyttir, ✱ Reactine, ZyrTEC

Classification

Therapeutic: allergy, cold, and cough remedies, antihistamines

Pharmacologic: piperazines (peripherally selective)

Indications

PO: Relief of allergic symptoms caused by histamine release including: Seasonal and perennial allergic rhinitis, Chronic urticaria. **IV:** Acute urticaria.

Action

Antagonizes the effects of histamine at H_1-receptor sites; does not bind to or inactivate histamine. Anticholinergic effects are minimal, and sedation is dose related. **Therapeutic Effects:** Decreased symptoms of histamine excess (sneezing, rhinorrhea, ocular tearing and redness, pruritus).

Pharmacokinetics

Absorption: Well absorbed following oral administration. IV administration results in complete bioavailability.
Distribution: Unknown.
Protein Binding: 93%.
Metabolism and Excretion: Excreted primarily unchanged by the kidneys.
Half-life: 7.4–9 hr (↓ in children to 6.2 hr, ↑ in renal impairment up to 19–21 hr).

TIME/ACTION PROFILE (antihistaminic effects)

ROUTE	ONSET	PEAK	DURATION
PO	30 min	4–8 hr	24 hr
IV	unknown	unknown	unknown

Contraindications/Precautions

Contraindicated in: Hypersensitivity to cetirizine, levocetirizine, hydroxyzine, or any component; Pedi: Children <6 yr with renal or hepatic impairment.
Use Cautiously in: Patients with hepatic or renal impairment (dose ↓ recommended if CCr ≤31 mL/min or hepatic function is impaired); OB: Use during pregnancy only if potential maternal benefit justifies potential fetal risk; Lactation: Use while breastfeeding only if potential maternal benefit justifies potential risk to infant; Pedi: Children <6 mo (safety and effectiveness not established); Geri: Initiate at lower doses in older adults.

Adverse Reactions/Side Effects

Derm: acute generalized exanthematous pustulosis. **EENT:** pharyngitis. **GI:** dry mouth. **Neuro:** dizziness, drowsiness (significant with oral doses >10 mg/day), fatigue.

Interactions

Drug-Drug: Additive CNS depression may occur with **alcohol**, **opioid analgesics**, or **sedative/ hypnotics**. **Theophylline** may ↓ clearance and ↑ toxicity.

Route/Dosage

PO (Adults and Children ≥6 yr): 5–10 mg given once or divided twice daily.

PO (Children 2–5 yr): 2.5 mg once daily initially, may be ↑ to 5 mg once daily or 2.5 mg every 12 hr.

PO (Children 1–2 yr): 2.5 mg once daily initially; may be ↑ to 2.5 mg every 12 hr.

PO (Children 6–12 mo): 2.5 mg once daily.

IV (Adults and Children ≥12 yr): 10 mg every 24 hr as needed.

IV (Children 6–11 yr): 5–10 mg every 24 hr as needed.

IV (Children 6 mo–5 yr): 2.5 mg every 24 hr as needed.

Hepatic/Renal Impairment

PO (Adults and Children ≥12 yr): *CCr ≤31 mL/ min, hepatic impairment or hemodialysis:* 5 mg once daily.

Hepatic/Renal Impairment

PO (Children 6–11 yr): start therapy at <2.5 mg/ day.

Availability (generic available)

Capsules: 10 mg[OTC]. **Chewable tablets:** 5 mg[OTC], 10 mg[OTC]. **Orally disintegrating tablets:** 10 mg. **Syrup(banana-grape and bubblegum flavors):** 1 mg/mL[OTC]. **Tablets:** 5 mg[OTC], 10 mg[OTC] 🍁 20 mg. **Solution for injection:** 10 mg/mL. ***In combination with:*** pseudoephedrine (Zyrtec-D 12 hr) (See Appendix N).

NURSING IMPLICATIONS

Assessment

- Assess allergy symptoms (rhinitis, conjunctivitis, hives) before and periodically during therapy.
- Assess lung sounds and character of bronchial secretions. Maintain fluid intake of 1500–2000 mL/ day to decrease viscosity of secretions.
- Assess severity of urticaria before and periodically after injection.

Lab Test Considerations

- May cause false-negative result in allergy skin testing.

Implementation

- Do not confuse cetirizine with sertraline. Do not confuse Zyrtec with Lipitor, Zocor, Zyprexa, or Zyrtec-D.
- **PO:** Administer once daily without regard to food.

IV Administration

- **IV Push:** Administer undiluted. Solution is clear and colorless; do not administer solutions that are cloudy, discolored, or contain precipitate matter.
- **Rate:** Administer IV push over 1–2 min.

Patient/Family Teaching

- Instruct patient to take medication as directed.
- May cause dizziness and drowsiness. Caution patient to avoid driving or other activities requiring alertness until response to medication is known.
- Advise patient to avoid taking alcohol or other CNS depressants, including opioids, concurrently with this drug.
- Advise patient that good oral hygiene, frequent rinsing of mouth with water, and sugarless gum or candy may minimize dry mouth. Patient should notify dentist if dry mouth persists >2 wk.
- Instruct patient to contact health care professional if rash or dizziness occurs or if symptoms persist.
- **Rep:** Advise females of reproductive potential to notify health care professional if pregnancy is planned or suspected or if breastfeeding.

Evaluation/Desired Outcomes

- Decrease in allergic symptoms.

HIGH ALERT

🧬 cetuximab (se-**tux**-i-mab)

Erbitux

Classification

Therapeutic: antineoplastics

Pharmacologic: monoclonal antibodies

Indications

Locally or regionally advanced squamous cell carcinoma of the head and neck (in combination with radiation therapy). Recurrent or metastatic squamous cell carcinoma of the head and neck progressing after platinum-based therapy. Recurrent or metastatic squamous cell carcinoma of the head and neck (in combination with platinum-based therapy with 5-fluorouracil). 🧬 K-Ras wild-type, epidermal growth factor receptor (EGFR)-expressing metastatic colorectal cancer in patients who have not responded to irinotecan and oxaliplatin or are intolerant to irinotecan. 🧬 K-Ras wild-type, EGFR-expressing metastatic colorectal cancer in patients who have not responded to irinotecan alone (in combination with irinotecan). 🧬 First-line treatment of K-Ras wild-type, EGFR-expressing metastatic colorectal cancer (in combination with irinotecan, 5-fluorouracil, and leucovorin [FOLFIRI]). 🧬 Metastatic colorectal cancer with a BRAF V600E mutation (in combination with encorafenib).

Action

Binds specifically to EGFR, thereby preventing the binding of endogenous epidermal growth factor. This prevents cell growth and differentiation processes.
Therapeutic Effects: Decreased tumor growth and spread.

Pharmacokinetics

Absorption: IV administration results in complete bioavailability.
Distribution: Minimally distributed to tissues.
Metabolism and Excretion: Unknown.
Half-life: 97–114 hr.

ROUTE	ONSET	PEAK	DURATION
IV	unknown	unknown	unknown

Contraindications/Precautions

Contraindicated in: Hypersensitivity to cetuximab or murine (mouse) proteins; RAS-mutant metastatic colorectal cancer or unknown RAS mutation status (↑ mortality and tumor progression); OB: Pregnancy; Lactation: Lactation.
Use Cautiously in: Exposure to sunlight (may exacerbate dermatologic toxicity); History of tick bites, red meat allergy, or in presence of IgE antibodies directed against galactose-α-1,3-galactose (alpha-gal) (↑ risk of anaphylaxis); Rep: Women of reproductive potential; Pedi: Safety and effectiveness not established in children.

Adverse Reactions/Side Effects

Most adverse reactions reflect combination therapy with irinotecan.

CV: CARDIOPULMONARY ARREST, peripheral edema, SUDDEN CARDIAC DEATH. **Derm:** acneform dermatitis, hypertrichosis, nail disorder, pruritus, skin desquamation, skin infection, STEVENS-JOHNSON SYNDROME (SJS), TOXIC EPIDERMAL NECROLYSIS (TEN). **EENT:** conjunctivitis, ulcerative keratitis. **F and E** dehydration, hypomagnesemia. **GI:** abdominal pain, constipation, diarrhea, nausea, vomiting, ↓ weight, anorexia, stomatitis. **GU:** ↓ fertility (women), renal failure. **Hemat:** anemia, leukopenia. **MS:** back pain. **Neuro:** malaise, depression, headache, insomnia. **Resp:** cough, dyspnea, INTERSTITIAL LUNG DISEASE (ILD), PULMONARY EMBOLISM. **Misc:** fever, INFUSION REACTIONS (INCLUDING ANAPHYLAXIS).

Interactions

Drug-Drug: None reported.

Route/Dosage

Head and Neck Cancer With Radiation

IV (Adults): 400 mg/m² administered 1 wk prior to initiation of radiation therapy, followed by 250 mg/m² once weekly for the duration of radiation therapy or until disease progression or unacceptable toxicity (complete infusion 1 hr prior to radiation therapy).

Head and Neck Cancer Monotherapy or in Combination With Platinum-Based Therapy and 5-Fluorouracil

IV (Adults): *Monotherapy (weekly regimen):* 400 mg/m² initially, followed by 250 mg/m² once weekly until disease progression or unacceptable toxicity. *Monotherapy (biweekly regimen):* 500 mg/m² every 2 wk until disease progression or unacceptable toxicity. *Combination therapy with platinum-based therapy and 5-fluorouracil (weekly regimen):* 400 mg/m² initially, followed by 250 mg/m² once weekly until disease progression or unacceptable toxicity (complete infusion 1 hr to prior to administering platinum-based therapy with 5-fluorouracil). *Combination therapy with platinum-based therapy and 5-fluorouracil (biweekly regimen):* 500 mg/m² every 2 wk until disease progression or unacceptable toxicity (complete infusion 1 hr prior to administering platinum-based therapy with 5-fluorouracil).

Colorectal Cancer

IV (Adults): *Monotherapy (weekly regimen):* 400 mg/m² initially, followed by 250 mg/m² once weekly until disease progression or unacceptable toxicity. *Monotherapy (biweekly regimen):* 500 mg/m² every 2 wk until disease progression or unacceptable toxicity. *Combination therapy with irinotecan or FOLFIRI (weekly regimen):* 400 mg/m² initially, followed by 250 mg/m² once weekly until disease progression or unacceptable toxicity (complete infusion 1 hr prior to administering irinotecan or FOLFIRI). *Combination therapy with irinotecan or FOLFIRI (biweekly regimen):* 500 mg/m² every 2 wk until disease progression or unacceptable toxicity (complete infusion 1 hr prior to administering irinotecan or FOLFIRI). *Combination therapy with encorafenib:* 400 mg/m² initially, followed by 250 mg/m² once weekly until disease progression or unacceptable toxicity.

Availability

Solution for injection: 2 mg/mL.

NURSING IMPLICATIONS

Assessment

- Assess for infusion reactions (bronchospasm, stridor, hoarseness, urticaria, hypotension, loss of consciousness, MI, cardiopulmonary arrest) for ≥1 hr following infusion. ↑ risk of anaphylaxis in patients with a history of tick bites or red meat allergy or the presence of IgE antibodies against galactose- -1, 3-galactose (alpha-gal). Most reactions occur during 1st dose, but may occur later. *For Grade 1 or 2 infusion reactions,* ↓ infusion rate by 50%. *For Grade 3 or 4 infusion reactions,* immediately discontinue cetuximab. Keep epinephrine, corticosteroid, antihistamine, bronchodilator, and oxygen nearby during infusion.

- Assess for pulmonary toxicity. *If acute onset or worsening of symptoms occur,* delay infusion 1–2 wk; when resolved, continue at previous dose. *If no improvement in 2 wk or ILD confirmed,* permanently discontinue cetuximab.
- Assess for dermatologic toxicity (acneform rash, inflammation, infection). Treat symptomatically. Acneform rash usually occurs in initial 2 wk of therapy and may continue up to 28 days following therapy. *If 1st occurrence of Grade 3 or 4 dermatologic toxicities,* delay infusion 1–2 wk; when improved, continue at 250 mg/m^2. *If 2nd occurrence of Grade 3 or 4 dermatologic toxicities,* delay infusion 1–2 wk; when improved, ↓ dose to 200 mg/m^2. *If 3rd occurrence of Grade 3 or 4 dermatologic toxicities,* delay infusion 1–2 wk; when improved, ↓ dose to 150 mg/m^2. *If 4th occurrence of Grade 3 or 4 dermatologic toxicities or no improvement at any occurrence,* permanently discontinue cetuximab.

Lab Test Considerations

- Verify negative pregnancy test before starting therapy.
- Determine RAS mutation and EGFR-expression status using FDA-approved tests before initiating treatment. Only patients whose tumors are K-Ras wild-type should receive cetuximab. Determine BRAF V600E mutation before use for metastatic colon cancer. Information on FDA-approved tests for the detection of K-Ras or BRAF V600E mutations for metastatic colorectal cancer is available at http://www.fda.gov/CompanionDiagnostics.
- Consider testing patients for alpha-gal IgE antibodies using FDA-cleared method before starting therapy. Negative results for alpha-gal antibodies do not rule out the risk of severe infusion reactions.
- May cause anemia and leukopenia.
- Monitor serum electrolytes, especially magnesium, potassium, and calcium, during and periodically for ≥8 wk following infusion. May cause hypomagnesemia, hypocalcemia, and hypokalemia; may occur from days to months after initiation of therapy. May lead to cardiopulmonary arrest and sudden death.

Implementation

- Premedicate with histamine$_1$ antagonist (diphenhydramine 50 mg) 30–60 min prior to first dose; base subsequent administration on presence and severity of infusion reaction.

IV Administration

- Administer through a low protein binding 0.22-micrometer in-line filter placed as proximal to patient as possible. Solution should be clear and colorless and may contain a small amount of white amorphous particles. Do not shake.
- Can be administered via infusion pump or syringe pump. Piggyback cetuximab into infusion line.
- Observe patient for 1 hr following infusion.
- **Intermittent Infusion:** *For administration via infusion pump:* Remove cetuximab from vial(s) using vented spike needle. Transfer to sterile evacuated container or bag. Repeat with new needle for each vial. Affix infusion line and prime with cetuximab before starting infusion.
- *For administration via syringe pump:* Remove cetuximab from vial(s) using vented spike needle. Place syringe into driver of a syringe pump and set rate. Connect infusion line and prime with cetuximab. Use a new needle and filter for each vial. **Concentration:** 2 mg/mL. **Rate:** Infuse over 2 hr at a rate not to exceed 10 mg/min. Use 0.9% NaCl to flush line at end of infusion.
- Cetuximab infusion must be completed 1 hr prior to FOLFIRI (irinotecan, 5-fluorouracil, leucovorin) regimen. May infuse subsequent weekly infusions over 1 hr.

Patient/Family Teaching

- Explain purpose of cetuximab and potential side effects to patient.
- Advise patient to notify health care professional promptly of dermatologic changes (itchy, dry, scaly, or cracking skin; inflammation, infection, or swelling at base of nails; loss of nails), conjunctivitis, blepharitis, ↓ vision, and signs and symptoms of pulmonary toxicity (new or worsening cough, chest pain, shortness of breath) or infusion reactions (fever, chills, breathing problems). ↑ risk for infusion reactions in patients who have had a tick bite or red meat allergy.
- Caution patient to wear sunscreen and hats and limit sun exposure during therapy and for 2 mo following last dose of cetuximab.
- Rep: May cause fetal harm. Advise women of reproductive potential to use effective contraception during therapy and for 2 mo after last dose and to avoid breastfeeding during therapy and for 2 mo after last dose. May impair female fertility.

Evaluation/Desired Outcomes

- Decreased tumor growth and spread.

BEERS

chlordiazePOXIDE
(klor-dye-az-e-**pox**-ide)

~~Libritabs, Librium~~

Classification

Therapeutic: antianxiety agents, sedative/hypnotics

Pharmacologic: benzodiazepines

Schedule IV

Indications
Anxiety disorders. Alcohol withdrawal. Adjunct management of preoperative apprehension or anxiety.

Action
Acts at many levels of the CNS to produce anxiolytic effect. Depresses the CNS, probably by potentiating GABA, an inhibitory neurotransmitter. **Therapeutic Effects:** Sedation. Relief of anxiety.

Pharmacokinetics
Absorption: Well absorbed from the GI tract.

Distribution: Widely distributed. Crosses the blood-brain barrier.

Metabolism and Excretion: Highly metabolized by the liver. Some products of metabolism are active as CNS depressants.

Half-life: 5–30 hr.

TIME/ACTION PROFILE (sedation)

ROUTE	ONSET	PEAK	DURATION
PO	1–2 hr	0.5–4 hr	up to 24 hr

Contraindications/Precautions
Contraindicated in: Hypersensitivity; Some products contain tartrazine and should be avoided in patients with known intolerance; Cross-sensitivity with other benzodiazepines may occur; Comatose patients or those with pre-existing CNS depression; Uncontrolled severe pain; Pulmonary disease; Angle-closure glaucoma; Porphyria; Lactation: Lactation.

Use Cautiously in: Hepatic impairment; Severe renal impairment; History of suicide attempt or substance abuse; OB: Use late in pregnancy can result in sedation (respiratory depression, lethargy, hypotonia) and/or withdrawal symptoms (hyperreflexia, irritability, restlessness, tremors, inconsolable crying, feeding difficulties) in neonates; Pedi: Children <6 yr (safety and effectiveness not established); Geri: Appears on Beers list. ↑ risk of cognitive impairment, delirium, falls, fractures, and motor vehicle accidents. If possible, avoid use in older adults.

Adverse Reactions/Side Effects
Derm: rash. **EENT:** blurred vision. **GI:** constipation, diarrhea, nausea, vomiting. **Metab:** weight gain. **Neuro:** dizziness, drowsiness, depression, hangover, headache, paradoxical excitation, sedation. **Misc:** physical dependence, psychological dependence, tolerance.

Interactions
Drug-Drug: Use with **opioids** or other **CNS depressants**, including other **benzodiazepines**, **nonbenzodiazepine sedative/hypnotics**, **anxiolytics**, **general anesthetics**, **muscle relaxants**, **antipsychotics**, and **alcohol**, may cause profound sedation, respiratory depression, coma, and death; reserve concurrent use for when alternative treatment options are inadequate. **Cimetidine**, **oral contraceptives**, **disulfiram**, **fluoxetine**, **isoniazid**, **ketoconazole**, **metoprolol**, **propranolol**, or **valproic acid** may enhance effects. May ↓ efficacy of **levodopa**. Effectiveness may be ↓ by **rifampin** or **barbiturates**. Sedative effects may be ↓ by **theophylline**.

Drug-Natural Products: Kava-kava, **valerian**, **chamomile**, or **hops** can ↑ risk of CNS depression.

Route/Dosage
Alcohol Withdrawal
PO (Adults): 50–100 mg, repeated until agitation is controlled (up to 400 mg/day).

Anxiety
PO (Adults): 5–25 mg 3–4 times daily.

PO (Geriatric Patients): 5 mg 2–4 times daily initially; ↑ as needed.

PO (Children >6 yr): 5 mg 2–4 times daily, up to 10 mg 2–3 times daily.

Availability (generic available)
Capsules: 5 mg, 10 mg, 25 mg. ***In combination with:*** amitriptyline (generic only); clidinium (Librax). See Appendix N.

NURSING IMPLICATIONS
Assessment
- Assess for anxiety and level of sedation (ataxia, dizziness, slurred speech) periodically during therapy.
- Assess degree and manifestations of anxiety and mental status (orientation, mood, behavior) prior to and periodically during therapy.
- Assess risk for addiction, abuse, or misuse prior to administration and periodically during therapy.
- Prolonged high-dose therapy may lead to psychological or physical dependence. Restrict the amount of drug available to patient. Assess regularly for continued need for treatment.
- Geri: Assess risk of falls and institute fall prevention strategies. **Alcohol Withdrawal:** Assess for tremors, agitation, delirium, and hallucinations. Protect patient from injury. Institute seizure precautions.

Lab Test Considerations

- Patients on prolonged therapy should have CBC and liver function tests evaluated periodically. May ↑ AST, ALT, and serum bilirubin.
- May alter results of urine 17-ketosteroids and 17-ketogenic steroids. May cause ↓ response on metyrapone tests and decreased thyroidal uptake of ^{123}I and ^{131}I.

Toxicity and Overdose

- Flumazenil reverses sedation caused by chlordiazepoxide toxicity or overdose. Flumazenil may induce seizures in patients with a history of seizure disorder or who are on tricyclic antidepressants.

Implementation

- Do not confuse chlordiazepoxide with chlorpromazine.
- **PO:** Administer after meals or with milk to ↓ GI irritation. Tablets may be crushed and taken with food or fluids if patient has difficulty swallowing. Administer greater dose at bedtime to avoid daytime sedation.
- Do not discontinue abruptly; taper by 10 mg every 3 days to ↓ risk of withdrawal symptoms (depressed mood, trouble sleeping). Some patients may require longer taper period (months). Monitor patients closely with seizure disorder as abrupt withdrawal may precipitate seizures.

Patient/Family Teaching

- Instruct patient to take chlordiazepoxide as directed. If medication is less effective after a few weeks, check with health care provider; do not ↑ dose.
- Advise patient not to share medication with others; may be dangerous.
- Caution patient not to stop taking chlordiazepoxide without consulting health care provider. Abrupt withdrawal may cause sweating, vomiting, muscle cramps, tremors, and seizures; may be life-threatening.
- Advise patient that chlordiazepoxide is a drug with known abuse potential. Protect it from theft, and never give to anyone other than the individual for whom it was prescribed. Store out of sight and reach of children and in a location not accessible by others.
- May cause drowsiness or dizziness. Caution patient to avoid driving or other activities requiring alertness until response to medication is known.
- Advise patient to avoid the use of alcohol or other CNS depressants, including opioids, concurrently with alprazolam; may cause respiratory depression and overdose. Instruct patient to consult health care provider before taking Rx, OTC, or herbal products concurrently with this medication, especially St. John's wort.
- Rep: May cause fetal harm. Advise patient to notify health care provider if pregnancy is planned or suspected or if breastfeeding. Monitor neonates exposed to benzodiazepines during pregnancy (especially during 3rd trimester) and labor for signs of sedation (respiratory depression, lethargy, hypotonia) and/or withdrawal symptoms (hyperreflexia, irritability, restlessness, tremors, inconsolable crying, feeding difficulties) in the neonate. Monitor neonates and infants exposed to chlordiazepoxide during breastfeeding for sedation and withdrawal symptoms. Inform women who take chlordiazepoxide during pregnancy about the National Pregnancy Registry for Other Psychiatric Medications to monitor pregnancy outcomes in women exposed to alprazolam during pregnancy. Enroll patient by calling 1-866-961-2388 or visiting online at https://womensmentalhealth.org/research/pregnancyregistry/.

Evaluation/Desired Outcomes

- Decreased sense of anxiety.
- Increased ability to cope.
- Decreased delirium tremens and more rational ideation when used for alcohol withdrawal.

chlorothiazide, See DIURETICS (THIAZIDE).

BEERS

chlorproMAZINE

(klor-**proe**-ma-zeen)

~~Thorazine~~

Classification

Therapeutic: antiemetics, antipsychotics

Pharmacologic: phenothiazines

Indications

Second-line treatment for schizophrenia and psychoses after failure with atypical antipsychotics. Hyperexcitable, combative behavior in children. Bipolar disorder. Nausea and vomiting. Intractable hiccups. Preoperative sedation. Acute intermittent porphyria.

Action

Alters the effects of dopamine in the CNS. Has significant anticholinergic/alpha-adrenergic blocking activity. **Therapeutic Effects:** Diminished signs/symptoms of psychosis and bipolar disorder. Relief of nausea/vomiting/intractable hiccups. Decreased symptoms of porphyria.

Pharmacokinetics

Absorption: Variable absorption from tablets. Well absorbed following IM administration.
Distribution: Widely distributed; high CNS concentrations.
Protein Binding: ≥90%.
Metabolism and Excretion: Highly metabolized by the liver and GI mucosa. Some metabolites are active.
Half-life: 30 hr.

TIME/ACTION PROFILE (antipsychotic activity, antiemetic activity, sedation)

ROUTE	ONSET	PEAK	DURATION
PO	30–60 min	unknown	4–6 hr
IM	unknown	unknown	4–8 hr
IV	rapid	unknown	unknown

Contraindications/Precautions

Contraindicated in: Hypersensitivity; Hypersensitivity to sulfites (injectable); Cross-sensitivity with other phenothiazines may occur; Angle-closure glaucoma; Bone marrow depression; Severe liver/cardiovascular disease; Concurrent use of pimozide; Lactation: Lactation.
Use Cautiously in: Diabetes; Respiratory disease; Prostatic hyperplasia; CNS tumors; Epilepsy; Intestinal obstruction; OB: Neonates at ↑ risk for extrapyramidal symptoms and withdrawal after delivery when exposed during the 3rd trimester; use during pregnancy only if potential maternal benefit outweighs potential fetal risk; Pedi: Children with acute illnesses, infections, gastroenteritis, or dehydration (↑ risk of extrapyramidal reactions); Geri: Appears on Beers list. ↑ risk of stroke, cognitive decline, and mortality in older adults with dementia. Avoid use in older adults, except for schizophrenia, bipolar disorder, or for short-term use as an antiemetic (not indicated for dementia-related psychosis).

Adverse Reactions/Side Effects

CV: hypotension (↑ with IM, IV), tachycardia. **Derm:** photosensitivity, pigment changes, rash. **EENT:** blurred vision, dry eyes, lens opacities. **Endo:** amenorrhea, galactorrhea. **GI:** constipation, dry mouth, anorexia, hepatitis, ileus, priapism. **GU:** urinary retention. **Hemat:** AGRANULOCYTOSIS, leukopenia. **Metab:** hyperthermia. **Neuro:** sedation, extrapyramidal reactions, NEUROLEPTIC MALIGNANT SYNDROME, tardive dyskinesia. **Misc:** allergic reactions.

Interactions

Drug-Drug: Pimozide ↑ the risk of potentially serious cardiovascular reactions; concurrent use contraindicated. May alter serum **phenytoin** levels. ↓ pressor effect of **norepinephrine** and eliminates bradycardia. Antagonizes peripheral vasoconstriction from **epinephrine** and may reverse some of its actions. May ↑ levels and risk of toxicity of **valproic acid** and **tricyclic antidepressants**. May ↓ the pharmacologic effects of **amphetamine** and **related compounds**. May ↓ the effectiveness of **bromocriptine**. **Antacids** or **adsorbent antidiarrheals** may ↓ adsorption; administer 1 hr before or 2 hr after chlorpromazine. ↑ risk of anticholinergic effects with **antihistamines**, **tricyclic antidepressants**, **quinidine**, or **disopyramide**. Premedication with chlorpromazine ↑ the risk of neuromuscular excitation and hypotension when followed by **barbiturate** anesthesia. **Barbiturates** may ↓ levels and effectiveness. May ↓ levels and effectiveness of **barbiturates**. Additive hypotension with **antihypertensives**. Additive CNS depression with **alcohol**, **antidepressants**, **antihistamines**, **MAO inhibitors**, **opioid analgesics**, **sedative/hypnotics**, or **general anesthetics**. Concurrent use with **lithium** may produce disorientation, unconsciousness, or extrapyramidal symptoms. Concurrent use with **meperidine** may produce excessive sedation and hypotension. Concurrent use with **propranolol** ↑ blood levels of both drugs.
Drug-Natural Products: Kava-kava, **valerian**, **chamomile**, or **hops** can ↑ risk of CNS depression. ↑ anticholinergic effects with **angel's trumpet**, **jimson weed**, and **scopolia**.

Route/Dosage

PO (Adults): *Psychoses:* 10–25 mg 2–4 times daily; may ↑ by 20–50 mg every 3–4 days (usual dose is 200 mg/day; up to 1 g/day). *Bipolar disorder:* 10–25 mg 2–4 times daily; may ↑ by 20–50 mg every 3–4 days (usual dose range is 400–800 mg/day). *Nausea and vomiting:* 10–25 mg every 4 hr as needed. *Preoperative sedation:* 25–50 mg 2–3 hr before surgery. *Hiccups/porphyria:* 25–50 mg 3–4 times daily.
PO (Children): *Psychoses/nausea and vomiting:* 0.55 mg/kg (15 mg/m²) every 4–6 hr as needed. *Preoperative sedation:* 0.55 mg/kg (15 mg/m²) 2–3 hr before surgery.
IV (Adults): *Nausea/vomiting during surgery:* up to 25 mg. *Hiccups/tetanus:* 25–50 mg. *Porphyria:* 25 mg every 8 hr.
IV (Children): *Nausea/vomiting during surgery:* 0.275 mg/kg. *Tetanus:* 0.55 mg/kg.
IM (Adults): *Severe psychoses:* 25–50 mg initially; may be repeated in 1 hr; ↑ to maximum of 400 mg every 3–12 hr if needed (up to 1 g/day). *Nausea/vomiting:* 25 mg initially; may repeat with 25–50 mg every 3–4 hr as needed. *Nausea/vomiting during surgery:* 12.5 mg; may be repeated in 30 min as needed. *Preoperative sedation:* 12.5–25 mg 1–2 hr prior to surgery. *Hiccups/tetanus:* 25–50 mg 3–4 times daily. *Porphyria:* 25 mg every 6–8 hr until patient can take PO.

IM (Children ≥6 mo): *Psychoses/nausea and vomiting:* 0.55 mg/kg (15 mg/m²) every 6–8 hr (not to exceed 40 mg/day in children 6 mo–5 yr, or 75 mg/day in children 5–12 yr). *Nausea/vomiting during surgery:* 0.275 mg/kg; may repeat in 30 min as needed. *Preoperative sedation:* 0.55 mg/kg 1–2 hr prior to surgery. *Tetanus:* 0.55 mg/kg every 6–8 hr.

Availability (generic available)

Tablets: 10 mg, 25 mg, 50 mg, 100 mg, 200 mg. **Oral solution:** 30 mg/mL, 100 mg/mL. **Solution for injection:** 25 mg/mL.

NURSING IMPLICATIONS

Assessment

- Assess mental status (orientation, mood, behavior) before and periodically during therapy.
- Assess weight and BMI initially and throughout therapy. Refer as appropriate for nutritional/weight and medical management.
- Assess positive (hallucinations, delusions, agitation) and negative (social withdrawal) symptoms of schizophrenia.
- Monitor BP (sitting, standing, lying), HR, and respiratory rate before and frequently during the period of dose adjustment.
- Observe carefully when administering medication to ensure medication is actually taken and not hoarded.
- Assess fluid intake and bowel function. ↑ bulk and fluids in the diet may help ↓ constipation.
- Monitor patient for onset of akathisia (restlessness or desire to keep moving) and extrapyramidal side effects (*parkinsonian:* difficulty speaking or swallowing, loss of balance control, pill rolling of hands, masklike face, shuffling gait, rigidity, tremors; and *dystonic:* muscle spasms, twisting motions, twitching, inability to move eyes, weakness of arms or legs) every 2 mo during therapy and 8–12 wk after therapy has been discontinued. Notify health care provider if these symptoms occur; reduction in dose or discontinuation may be necessary. Trihexyphenidyl, diphenhydramine, or benztropine may be used to control these symptoms. Benzodiazepines may alleviate symptoms of akathisia.
- Monitor for tardive dyskinesia (uncontrolled rhythmic movement of mouth, face, and extremities; lip smacking or puckering; puffing of cheeks; uncontrolled chewing; rapid or worm-like movements of tongue; excessive eye blinking). Report these symptoms immediately; may be irreversible.
- Monitor for development of neuroleptic malignant syndrome (fever, respiratory distress, tachycardia, convulsions, diaphoresis, hypertension or hypotension, pallor, tiredness, severe muscle stiffness, loss of bladder control). Report these symptoms immediately.
- Monitor for symptoms related to hyperprolactinemia (menstrual abnormalities, galactorrhea, sexual dysfunction).
- Assess for falls risk. Drowsiness, orthostatic hypotension, and motor and sensory instability ↑ risk. Institute prevention if indicated.
- **Preoperative Sedation:** Assess level of anxiety before and following administration.

Lab Test Considerations

- Monitor CBC, liver function tests, and ocular exam periodically during therapy. May ↓ hematocrit, hemoglobin, leukocytes, granulocytes, and platelets. May ↑ bilirubin, AST, ALT, and alkaline phosphatase. Agranulocytosis may occur 4–10 wk after initiation of therapy, with recovery 1–2 wk following discontinuation. May recur if medication is restarted. Liver function abnormalities may require discontinuation of therapy. May cause false-positive or false-negative pregnancy tests and false-positive urine bilirubin test results.
- Assess fasting blood glucose and cholesterol levels initially and periodically throughout therapy.
- May ↑ serum prolactin levels.

Implementation

- Do not confuse chlorpromazine with chlordiazepoxide.
- Keep patient recumbent for ≥30 min following parenteral administration to minimize hypotensive effects.
- **Hiccups:** Initial treatment is with oral doses. If hiccups persist 2–3 days, IM injection may be used, followed by IV infusion.
- **PO:** Administer oral doses with food, milk, or a full glass of water to ↓ GI irritation. Tablets may be crushed.
- Mix oral solution with ≥60 mL of a carbonated beverage, coffee, fruit or tomato juice, milk, orange syrup, simple syrup, tea, or water; may also add to semisolid food (pudding, soup).
- **IM:** Do not inject SUBQ. Inject slowly into deep, well-developed muscle. May be diluted with 0.9% NaCl or 2% procaine. Lemon-yellow color does not alter potency of solution. Do not administer solution that is markedly discolored or contains a precipitate.

IV Administration

- **IV Push: Dilution:** Dilute with 0.9% NaCl. **Concentration:** Do not exceed 1 mg/mL. **Rate:** Inject slowly at a rate of no more than 1 mg/min for adults and 0.5 mg/min for children.

- **Continuous Infusion: Dilution:** May further dilute 25–50 mg in 500–1000 mL of D5W, D10W, 0.45% NaCl, 0.9% NaCl, Ringer's or lactated Ringer's injection, dextrose/Ringer's or dextrose/lactated Ringer's combinations. **Rate:** 1 mg/min.
- **Y-Site Compatibility:** alemtuzumab, amikacin, amiodarone, anidulafungin, argatroban, arsenic trioxide, ascorbic acid, atracurium, atropine, benztropine, bleomycin, buprenorphine, butorphanol, calcium chloride, calcium gluconate, carmustine, caspofungin, cisatracurium, cisplatin, cladribine, cyanocobalamin, cyclophosphamide, cyclosporine, cytarabine, dacarbazine, dactinomycin, daptomycin, daunorubicin, dexmedetomidine, dexrazoxane, digoxin, diltiazem, diphenhydramine, dobutamine, docetaxel, dopamine, doxorubicin hydrochloride, doxorubicin liposomal, doxycycline, edetate calcium disodium, enalaprilat, ephedrine, epinephrine, epirubicin, erythromycin, esmolol, etoposide, famotidine, fentanyl, filgrastim, fluconazole, gemcitabine, gentamicin, glycopyrrolate, granisetron, hetastarch, hydrocortisone, hydromorphone, idarubicin, ifosfamide, isoproterenol, ketamine, labetalol, LR, levofloxacin, lidocaine, lorazepam, magnesium sulfate, mannitol, meperidine, mesna, methadone, methylprednisolone, metoclopramide, metoprolol, metronidazole, midazolam, milrinone, minocycline, mitomycin, mitoxantrone, morphine, moxifloxacin, multivitamins, mycophenolate, nafcillin, nalbuphine, naloxone, nicardipine, nitroglycerin, norepinephrine, octreotide, ondansetron, oxacillin, oxaliplatin, palonosetron, pamidronate, papaverine, penicillin G potassium, pentamidine, phentolamine, phytonadione, potassium acetate, potassium chloride, procainamide, prochlorperazine, promethazine, propofol, propranolol, protamine, pyridoxine, rituximab, rocuronium, sodium acetate, succinylcholine, sufentanil, tacrolimus, theophylline, thiamine, thiotepa, tirofiban, tobramycin, topotecan, vancomycin, vasopressin, vecuronium, verapamil, vinblastine, vincristine, vinorelbine, voriconazole, zoledronic acid.
- **Y-Site Incompatibility:** acetaminophen, acyclovir, allopurinol, aminocaproic acid, aminophylline, amphotericin B deoxycholate, amphotericin B liposomal, ampicillin, ampicillin/sulbactam, azathioprine, azithromycin, aztreonam, bivalirudin, bumetanide, cangrelor, carboplatin, cefazolin, cefepime, cefotaxime, cefotetan, cefoxitin, ceftazidime, ceftriaxone, cefuroxime, chloramphenicol, chlorothiazide, clindamycin, dantrolene, diazepam, diazoxide, epoetin alfa, eptifibatide, ertapenem, etoposide phosphate, fludarabine, fluorouracil, folic acid, foscarnet, fosphenytoin, ganciclovir, gemtuzumab ozogamicin, imipenem/cilastatin, indomethacin, insulin, regular, irinotecan, ketorolac, leucovorin, linezolid, melphalan, methohexital, methotrexate, nitroprusside, paclitaxel, pantoprazole, pemetrexed, pentobarbital, phenobarbital, phenytoin, piperacillin/tazobactam, sargramostim, sodium bicarbonate, tigecycline, trastuzumab, trimethoprim/sulfamethoxazole.

Patient/Family Teaching

- Advise patient to take medication as directed and not to skip doses or double up on missed doses. If a dose is missed, take within 1 hr or omit dose and return to regular schedule. Abrupt withdrawal may lead to gastritis, nausea, vomiting, dizziness, headache, tachycardia, and insomnia.
- Inform patient of possibility of extrapyramidal symptoms and tardive dyskinesia. Instruct patient to report these symptoms immediately to health care provider.
- Advise patient to change positions slowly to minimize orthostatic hypotension. Protect from falls.
- May cause drowsiness. Caution patient to avoid driving or other activities requiring alertness until response to the medication is known.
- Caution patient to avoid taking alcohol or other CNS depressants concurrently with this medication.
- Advise patient to use sunscreen and protective clothing when exposed to the sun. Exposed surfaces may develop a temporary pigment change (ranging from yellow-brown to grayish purple). Extremes of temperature (exercise, hot weather, hot baths, or showers) should also be avoided, because this drug impairs body temperature regulation.
- Instruct patient to use frequent mouth rinses, good oral hygiene, and sugarless gum or candy to minimize dry mouth. Consult health care provider if dry mouth continues for 2 wk.
- Advise patient not to take within 2 hr of antacids or antidiarrheal medication.
- Inform patient that this medication may turn urine a pink-to-reddish-brown color.
- Advise patient to notify health care provider of medication regimen prior to treatment or surgery.
- Instruct patient to notify health care provider promptly if sore throat, fever, unusual bleeding or bruising, rash, weakness, tremors, visual disturbances, dark-colored urine, or clay-colored stools occur.
- Rep: Advise women of reproductive potential to notify health care provider if pregnancy is planned or suspected or if breastfeeding.
- Emphasize the importance of routine follow-up exams to monitor response to medication and detect side effects. Encourage continued participation in psychotherapy as indicated.

Evaluation/Desired Outcomes

- Decrease in excitable, manic behavior. Therapeutic effects may not be seen for 7–8 wk.

- Relief of nausea and vomiting.
- Relief of hiccups.
- Preoperative sedation.
- Management of porphyria.
- Decrease in positive (hallucinations, delusions, agitation) symptoms of schizophrenia.

chlorthalidone (thiazide-like), See DIURETICS (THIAZIDE).

cholecalciferol, See VITAMIN D COMPOUNDS.

ciclesonide (inhalation), See CORTICOSTEROIDS (INHALATION).

ciclesonide, See CORTICOSTEROIDS (NASAL).

ciclopirox, See ANTIFUNGALS (TOPICAL).

cinacalcet (sin-a-**kal**-set)

Sensipar

Classification

Therapeutic: hypocalcemics

Pharmacologic: calcimimetic agents

Indications

Secondary hyperparathyroidism in patients with chronic kidney disease on dialysis. Hypercalcemia caused by parathyroid carcinoma. Severe hypercalcemia in patients with primary hyperparathyroidism who are unable to undergo parathyroidectomy.

Action

Increases sensitivity of calcium-sensing receptors located on the surface of chief cells of parathyroid gland to levels of extracellular calcium. This decreases parathyroid hormone (PTH) production with resultant decrease in serum calcium. **Therapeutic Effects:** Decreased bone turnover and fibrosis. Decreased serum calcium.

Pharmacokinetics

Absorption: Well absorbed following oral administration; absorption is enhanced by food and further enhanced by a high-fat meal.

Distribution: Extensively distributed to tissues.

Protein Binding: 93–97%.

Metabolism and Excretion: Primarily metabolized by the liver via the CYP3A4, CYP2D6, and CYP1A2 isoenzymes; 80% excreted in urine as metabolites, 15% in feces.

Half-life: 30–40 hr.

TIME/ACTION PROFILE (effect on PTH concentrations)

ROUTE	ONSET	PEAK	DURATION
PO	rapid	2–6 hr	6–12 hr

Contraindications/Precautions

Contraindicated in: Hypersensitivity; Hypocalcemia.

Use Cautiously in: History of seizure disorder (↑ risk of seizures with hypocalcemia); Chronic kidney disease patients who are not being dialyzed (↑ risk of hypocalcemia); Intact parathyroid hormone (iPTH) level <150 pg/mL (dose ↓ or discontinuation may be warranted); Moderate or severe hepatic impairment; Congenital long QT syndrome, QT interval prolongation, family history of long QT syndrome or sudden cardiac death, or concurrent use of QT interval prolonging medications; OB: Safety not established in pregnancy; Lactation: Use while breastfeeding only if potential maternal benefit justifies potential risk to infant; Pedi: Safety and effectiveness not established in children.

Adverse Reactions/Side Effects

CV: ARRHYTHMIA, HF exacerbation, hypotension, QT interval prolongation, TORSADES DE POINTES. **F and E:** HYPOCALCEMIA. **GI:** nausea, vomiting. **Metab:** adynamic bone disease. **Neuro:** SEIZURES.

Interactions

Drug-Drug: QT interval prolonging medications may ↑ risk of QT interval prolongation and/or torsades de pointes, especially in patients with hypocalcemia. May ↑ levels and risk of toxicity of **CYP2D6 substrates**, including **flecainide**, **vinblastine**, **thioridazine**, **metoprolol**, **carvedilol**, and most **tricyclic antidepressants**; dose adjustments may be necessary. **Strong CYP3A4 inhibitors**, including **ketoconazole**, **itraconazole**, and **erythromycin**, may ↑ levels and risk of toxicity; monitoring and dose adjustment may be necessary.

Route/Dosage

Secondary Hyperparathyroidism in Patients with Chronic Kidney Disease on Dialysis

PO (Adults): 30 mg once daily; may ↑ every 2–4 wk (dose range 30–180 mg once daily) based on iPTH levels. *Switching from etecalcetide:* Discontinue etecalcetide for ≥4 wk and ensure corrected serum calcium is at or above lower limit of normal prior to starting cinacalcet.

Parathyroid Carcinoma or Primary Hyperparathyroidism

PO (Adults): 30 mg twice daily; may ↑ every 2–4 wk up to 90 mg 3–4 times daily based on serum calcium levels.

Availability (generic available)

Tablets: 30 mg, 60 mg, 90 mg.

NURSING IMPLICATIONS

Assessment

- Monitor for signs and symptoms of hypocalcemia, which may prolong QT interval, ↓ seizure threshold, cause hypotension, and worsen HF and arrhythmias.
- Monitor ECG for prolonged QT interval periodically during therapy.
- Monitor for signs and symptoms of GI bleed. Promptly evaluate and treat if suspected.

Lab Test Considerations

- Monitor serum calcium and phosphorus levels ≤1 wk after initiation or dose adjustment, monthly for patients with hyperparathyroidism, or every 2 mo for patients with parathyroid carcinoma once maintenance dose has been established, especially in patients with history of seizures. *If serum calcium <8.4 mg/dL,* do not initiate cinacalcet. *If serum calcium of 7.5–8.4 mg/dL or if symptomatic,* use calcium-containing phosphate binders and/or vitamin D sterols to ↑ serum calcium level. *If serum calcium <7.5 mg/dL or if symptoms persist and vitamin D cannot be* ↑, hold cinacalcet until serum calcium levels 8.0 mg/dL and/or symptoms resolve. Reinitiate therapy using next ↓ dose of cinacalcet.
- Monitor serum iPTH levels 1–4 wk after initiation of therapy or dose adjustment and every 1–3 mo after maintenance dose has been established. If iPTH levels < target range of 150–300 pg/mL, ↓ dose or discontinue cinacalcet. Assess iPTH levels ≥12 hr after dose.
- Monitor liver function tests in patients with moderate to severe hepatic impairment during therapy.

Implementation

- Cinacalcet may be used alone or in combination with vitamin D and/or phosphate binders.
- **PO:** Administer with food or shortly after meal. ***DNC:*** Take tablets whole; do not crush, break, or chew.

Patient/Family Teaching

- Explain purpose and side effects of medication. Advise patient to read *Patient Information* before starting therapy.
- Advise patient to notify health care professional for signs and symptoms of hypocalcemia (paresthesias, myalgias, cramping, tetany, seizures) or GI bleeding (black tarry stools, abdominal pain, nausea, vomiting).
- Advise patient to notify health care professional for worsening HF symptoms.
- Inform patient that cinacalcet may cause adynamic bone disease.
- Rep: Advise women of reproductive potential to notify health care professional if pregnancy is planned or suspected or if breastfeeding.
- Emphasize importance of follow-up lab tests to monitor safety and efficacy.

Evaluation/Desired Outcomes

- Decreased serum calcium levels.

ciprofloxacin, See FLUOROQUINOLONES.

HIGH ALERT

V CISplatin (sis-pla-tin)

~~Platinol~~

Classification

Therapeutic: antineoplastics

Pharmacologic: alkylating agents

Indications

Metastatic testicular and ovarian carcinoma. Advanced bladder cancer. Head and neck cancer. Cervical cancer. Lung cancer.

Action

Inhibits DNA synthesis by producing cross-linking of parent DNA strands (cell-cycle phase-nonspecific). **Therapeutic Effects:** Death of rapidly replicating cells, particularly malignant ones.

Pharmacokinetics

Absorption: IV administration results in complete bioavailability.

Distribution: Widely distributed; accumulates for months.

Metabolism and Excretion: Excreted mainly by the kidneys.

Half-life: 30–100 hr.

TIME/ACTION PROFILE (effects on blood counts)

ROUTE	ONSET	PEAK	DURATION
IV	unknown	18–23 days	39 days

Contraindications/Precautions

Contraindicated in: Hypersensitivity; OB: Pregnancy; Lactation: Lactation.

C

Use Cautiously in: Hearing loss; Renal impairment (↓ dose); HF; Electrolyte abnormalities; Active infection; Bone marrow depression; Rep: Women of reproductive potential; Geri: ↑ risk of nephrotoxicity and peripheral neuropathy in older adults.

Adverse Reactions/Side Effects

Derm: alopecia. **EENT:** ototoxicity, tinnitus. **F and E** hypocalcemia, hypokalemia, hypomagnesemia. **GI:** nausea, vomiting, diarrhea, HEPATOTOXICITY. **GU:** nephrotoxicity, sterility. **Hemat:** anemia, LEUKOPENIA, THROMBOCYTOPENIA. **Local:** phlebitis at IV site. **Metab:** hyperuricemia. **Neuro:** malaise, peripheral neuropathy, REVERSIBLE POSTERIOR LEUKOENCEPHALOPATHY SYNDROME (RPLS), SEIZURES, weakness. **Misc:** ANAPHYLAXIS.

Interactions

Drug-Drug: ↑ risk of nephrotoxicity and ototoxicity with other **aminoglycosides** and **loop diuretics**. ↑ risk of hypokalemia and hypomagnesemia with **loop diuretics** and **amphotericin B.** May ↓ **phenytoin** levels and effectiveness. ↑ risk of bone marrow depression with other **antineoplastics** or **radiation therapy**. May ↓ antibody response to **live-virus vaccines** and ↑ risk of adverse reactions.

Route/Dosage

IV (Adults): *Metastatic testicular tumors:* 20 mg/m² daily for 5 days; repeat every 3–4 wk. *Metastatic ovarian cancer:* 75–100 mg/m²; repeat every 4 wk in combination with cyclophosphamide *or* 100 mg/m² every 3 wk if used as a single agent. *Advanced bladder cancer:* 50–70 mg/m² every 3–4 wk as a single agent.

Availability (generic available)

Solution for injection: 1 mg/mL.

NURSING IMPLICATIONS

Assessment

- Monitor vital signs frequently during administration. Report significant changes.
- Monitor intake and output and specific gravity frequently during therapy. To ↓ risk of nephrotoxicity, maintain urinary output of >100 mL/hr for 4 hr before initiating and for >24 hr after administration.
- Encourage patient to drink 2000–3000 mL/day of water to promote excretion of uric acid. Allopurinol and alkalinization of urine may be used to help prevent uric acid nephropathy.
- Severe and protracted nausea and vomiting usually occur 1–4 hr after a dose; vomiting may last for 24 hr. Administer parenteral antiemetic agents 30–45 min before therapy and routinely around the clock for the next 24 hr. Monitor amount of emesis and notify health care provider if emesis exceeds guidelines to prevent dehydration. Nausea and anorexia may persist for up to 1 wk.
- Monitor for bone marrow depression. Assess for bleeding (bleeding gums; bruising; petechiae; blood in stools, urine, and emesis) and avoid IM injections and taking rectal temperatures if platelet count is low. Apply pressure to venipuncture sites for 10 min. Assess for signs of infection during neutropenia. Anemia may occur. Monitor for ↑ fatigue, dyspnea, and orthostatic hypotension.
- Monitor for signs of anaphylaxis (facial edema, wheezing, dizziness, fainting, tachycardia, hypotension). Discontinue medication immediately and report symptoms. Epinephrine and resuscitation equipment should be readily available.
- Medication may cause ototoxicity and neurotoxicity. Assess patient frequently for dizziness, tinnitus, hearing loss, loss of coordination, loss of taste, or numbness and tingling of extremities; may be irreversible. Notify health care provider promptly if these occur. Audiometry should be performed before initiation of therapy and before subsequent doses. Hearing loss is more frequent with children, usually occurs first with high frequencies, and may be unilateral or bilateral.
- Monitor for inadvertent cisplatin overdose. Doses >100 mg/m²/cycle once every 3–4 wk are rarely used. Differentiate daily doses from total dose/cycle. Symptoms of high cumulative doses include muscle cramps (localized, painful involuntary skeletal muscle contractions of sudden onset and short duration) and are usually associated with advanced stages of peripheral neuropathy.
- Monitor for signs of RPLS (headache, seizure, lethargy, confusion, blindness). Hypertension may or may not be present. May occur within 16 hr–1 yr of initiation of therapy. Treat hypertension if present and discontinue cisplatin therapy. Symptoms usually resolve within days.

Lab Test Considerations

- Monitor CBC with differential before and routinely throughout therapy. The nadir of leukopenia, thrombocytopenia, and anemia occurs within 18–23 days, and recovery occurs within 39 days after a dose. Withhold further doses until WBC >4000/mm³ and platelet count >100,000/mm³.
- Monitor BUN, serum creatinine, and CCr before initiation of therapy and before each course of cisplatin to detect nephrotoxicity. May ↑ BUN and serum creatinine and ↓ calcium, magnesium, phosphate, sodium, and potassium, usually occurring 2nd wk after a dose. Do not administer additional doses until BUN <25 mg/dL and serum

creatinine <1.5 mg/dL. May ↑ uric acid level, which usually peaks 3–5 days after a dose.

- May transiently ↑ serum bilirubin and AST concentrations.
- May cause positive Coombs test result.

Implementation

- ***High Alert:*** Fatalities have occurred with chemotherapeutic agents. Before administering, clarify all ambiguous orders; double-check single, daily, and course-of-therapy dose limits; have second practitioner independently double-check original order, calculations, and infusion pump settings. Clarify dose to ensure cumulative dose is not confused with daily dose; errors may be fatal.
- ***High Alert:*** Do not confuse cisplatin with carboplatin. To prevent confusion, orders should include generic and brand names. Administer under supervision of a physician experienced in use of cancer chemotherapeutic agents.
- Solution should be prepared in a biologic cabinet. Wear gloves, gown, and mask while handling medication. If powder or solution comes in contact with skin or mucosa, wash thoroughly with soap and water. Discard equipment in specially designated containers.
- Hydrate patient with >1–2 L of IV fluid 8–12 hr before initiating therapy with cisplatin.
- Do not use aluminum needles or equipment during preparation or administration. Aluminum reacts with this drug, forms a black or brown precipitate, and renders the drug ineffective.

IV Administration

- V Cisplatin is a vesicant. If extravasation occurs, immediately stop infusion. Leave needle/cannula in place temporarily but do not flush the line. Gently aspirate extravasated solution; then remove needle/cannula. Elevate patient's extremity and apply dry cold compresses for 20 min 4 times day for 1–2 days. Initiate antidote (sodium thiosulfate). Inject 2 mL of a □ molar sodium thiosulfate solution into existing IV line for each 100 mg of cisplatin extravasated; then consider also injecting a total of 1 mL as 0.1-mL SUBQ injections (total of 10 injections) around the area of extravasation in a clockwise manner; may repeat SUBQ injections several times over the next 3–4 hr. Topical dimethyl sulfoxide may also be considered. Apply dimethyl sulfoxide by saturating a gauze pad and painting on an area twice the size of the extravasation. Allow site to air-dry and repeat application every 8 hr for 7 days. Do not cover the area with dressing.
- **Intermittent Infusion:** Solution should be clear and colorless; discard if turbid or if it contains precipitates.
- **Dilution:** Dilute in 2 L of 5% dextrose in 0.3% or 0.45% NaCl containing 37.5 g of mannitol. **Concentration:** Keep under 0.5 mg/mL to prevent tissue necrosis. **Rate:** Administer over 6–8 hr. Maximum rate 1 mg/min.
- **Continuous Infusion:** Has been administered as continuous infusion over 24 hr–5 days with resultant ↓ in nausea and vomiting.
- **Y-Site Compatibility:** acyclovir, allopurinol, amikacin, aminophylline, amiodarone, ampicillin, ampicillin/sulbactam, anidulafungin, argatroban, atracurium, azithromycin, aztreonam, bivalirudin, bleomycin, bumetanide, buprenorphine, butorphanol, calcium chloride, calcium gluconate, carmustine, caspofungin, cefazolin, cefotaxime, cefotetan, cefoxitin, ceftazidime, ceftriaxone, cefuroxime, chlorpromazine, ciprofloxacin, cisatracurium, cladribine, clindamycin, cyclophosphamide, cyclosporine, cytarabine, dacarbazine, dactinomycin, daptomycin, daunorubicin, dexamethasone, dexmedetomidine, dexrazoxane, digoxin, diltiazem, diphenhydramine, dobutamine, docetaxel, dopamine, doxorubicin hydrochloride, doxorubicin liposomal, doxycycline, droperidol, enalaprilat, ephedrine, epinephrine, epirubicin, ertapenem, erythromycin, esmolol, etoposide, etoposide phosphate, famotidine, fentanyl, filgrastim, fluconazole, fludarabine, fluorouracil, foscarnet, fosphenytoin, furosemide, ganciclovir, gemcitabine, gentamicin, glycopyrrolate, granisetron, haloperidol, heparin, hetastarch, hydrocortisone, hydromorphone, idarubicin, ifosfamide, imipenem/cilastatin, indomethacin, irinotecan, isoproterenol, ketorolac, labetalol, leucovorin, levofloxacin, lidocaine, linezolid, lorazepam, magnesium sulfate, mannitol, melphalan, meperidine, meropenem, methadone, methohexital, methotrexate, methylprednisolone, metoclopramide, metoprolol, metronidazole, midazolam, milrinone, mitomycin, mitoxantrone, moxifloxacin, nafcillin, naloxone, nicardipine, nitroglycerin, nitroprusside, norepinephrine, octreotide, ondansetron, oxaliplatin, paclitaxel, palonosetron, pamidronate, pemetrexed, pentamidine, pentobarbital, phenobarbital, phenylephrine, phenytoin, potassium acetate, potassium chloride, potassium phosphates, procainamide, prochlorperazine, promethazine, propofol, propranolol, remifentanil, rituximab, sargramostim, sodium acetate, sodium bicarbonate, sodium phosphates, succinylcholine, sufentanil, tacrolimus, theophylline, tigecycline, tirofiban, tobramycin, topotecan, trastuzumab, trimethoprim/sulfamethoxazole, vancomycin, vasopressin, vecuronium, verapamil, vinblastine, vincristine, vinorelbine, voriconazole, zidovudine, zoledronic acid.
- **Y-Site Incompatibility:** amphotericin B deoxycholate, amphotericin B liposomal, cefepime, dantrolene, diazepam, insulin, regular, pantoprazole, piperacillin/tazobactam, thiotepa.

C

Patient/Family Teaching

- Explain purpose and side effects of medication to patient. Advise patient to read *Patient Information* before starting therapy.
- Advise patient to notify health care provider of all Rx or OTC medications, vitamins, or herbal products being taken and to consult health care provider before taking other medications.
- Instruct patient to report pain at injection site immediately.
- Instruct patient to report difficulty with hearing or tinnitus immediately.
- Instruct patient to notify health care provider promptly if fever; chills; cough; hoarseness; sore throat; signs of infection; lower back or side pain; painful or difficult urination; bleeding gums; bruising; petechiae; blood in stools, urine, or emesis; ↑ fatigue; dyspnea; or orthostatic hypotension occurs. Caution patient to avoid crowds and persons with known infections. Instruct patient to use soft toothbrush and electric razor and to avoid falls. Caution patient not to drink alcoholic beverages or take medication containing aspirin or NSAIDs; may precipitate gastric bleeding.
- Instruct patient to report promptly any numbness or tingling in extremities or face, unusual swelling, or joint pain.
- Instruct patient not to receive any vaccinations without advice of health care provider.
- Emphasize the need for periodic lab tests to monitor for side effects.
- Rep: May cause fetal harm. Advise women of reproductive potential to notify health care provider if pregnancy is planned or suspected and to avoid breastfeeding. Advise patient of the need for contraception. May cause infertility.

Evaluation/Desired Outcomes

- Death of rapidly replicating cells, particularly malignant ones.

BEERS

citalopram (si-**tal**-oh-pram)

CeleXA

Classification

Therapeutic: antidepressants

Pharmacologic: selective serotonin reuptake inhibitors (SSRIs)

Indications

Depression. **Unlabeled Use:** Premenstrual dysphoric disorder. Obsessive-compulsive disorder. Panic disorder. Generalized anxiety disorder. Post-traumatic stress disorder. Social anxiety disorder (social phobia).

Action

Selectively inhibits the reuptake of serotonin in the CNS. **Therapeutic Effects:** Antidepressant action.

Pharmacokinetics

Absorption: 80% absorbed after oral administration.

Distribution: Enters breast milk.

Metabolism and Excretion: Mostly metabolized by the liver (10% by the CYP3A4 and CYP2C19 isoenzymes); the CYP2C19 isoenzyme exhibits genetic polymorphism (2% of White patients, 4% of Black patients, and 14% of Asian patients may be poor metabolizers and may have significantly ↑ citalopram concentrations and an ↑ risk of adverse effects). Excreted unchanged in the urine.

Half-life: 35 hr.

TIME/ACTION PROFILE (antidepressant effect)

ROUTE	ONSET	PEAK	DURATION
PO	1–4 wk	unknown	unknown

Contraindications/Precautions

Contraindicated in: Hypersensitivity; Concurrent use of MAO inhibitors or MAO-like drugs (linezolid or methylene blue); Concurrent use of pimozide; Congenital long QT syndrome, bradycardia, hypokalemia, hypomagnesemia, recent myocardial infarction, or decompensated heart failure (↑ risk of QT interval prolongation); Concurrent use of QT interval prolonging drugs.

Use Cautiously in: History of mania; May ↑ risk of suicide attempt/ideation especially during early treatment or dose adjustment; this risk appears to be greater in adolescents or children; History of seizure disorder; Illnesses or conditions that are likely to result in altered metabolism or hemodynamic responses; Severe renal or hepatic impairment (maximum dose of 20 mg/day in patients with hepatic impairment); Poor CYP2C19 metabolizers (↑ risk of QT interval prolongation) (maximum dose of 20 mg/day); Concurrent use of CYP2C19 inhibitors (↑ risk of QT interval prolongation) (maximum dose of 20 mg/day); Angle-closure glaucoma; OB: Use during pregnancy only if potential maternal benefit justifies potential fetal risk; Lactation: Use while breastfeeding only if potential maternal benefit justifies potential risk to infant; Pedi: Safety and effectiveness not established in children; Geri: Appears on Beers list. May worsen or cause syndrome of inappropriate antidiuretic hormone (SIADH) secretion and/or hyponatremia in older adults. Use with caution in older adults and closely monitor sodium concentrations when starting therapy or ↑ dose. Maximum dose of 20 mg/day in patients >60 yr.

Adverse Reactions/Side Effects

CV: QT interval prolongation, postural hypotension, tachycardia, TORSADES DE POINTES. **Derm:** sweating, photosensitivity, pruritus, rash. **EENT:** abnormal accommodation. **Endo:** SIADH. **F and E** hyponatremia. **GI:** ↑ salivation, abdominal pain, anorexia, diarrhea, dry mouth, dyspepsia, flatulence, nausea, altered taste, vomiting. **GU:** ↓ libido, amenorrhea, delayed/absent orgasm, dysmenorrhea, ejaculatory delay/failure, erectile dysfunction, polyuria. **Hemat:** BLEEDING. **Metab:** ↑ appetite, weight gain, weight loss. **MS:** arthralgia, myalgia. **Neuro:** apathy, confusion, drowsiness, insomnia, tremor, weakness, ↓ libido, ↑ depression, agitation, amnesia, anxiety, dizziness, fatigue, impaired concentration, migraine headache, NEUROLEPTIC MALIGNANT SYNDROME, paresthesia, SUICIDAL THOUGHTS/BEHAVIORS. **Resp:** cough. **Misc:** fever, SEROTONIN SYNDROME, yawning.

Interactions

Drug-Drug: May cause serious, potentially fatal reactions when used with **MAO inhibitors**; concurrent use contraindicated; allow ≥14 days between citalopram and **MAO inhibitors**. Concurrent use with **MAO-inhibitor like drugs**, such as **linezolid** or **methylene blue**, may ↑ risk of serotonin syndrome; concurrent use contraindicated; do not start therapy in patients receiving **linezolid** or **methylene blue**; if **linezolid** or **methylene blue** need to be started in a patient receiving citalopram, immediately discontinue citalopram and monitor for signs/symptoms of serotonin syndrome for 2 wk or until 24 hr after last dose of linezolid or methylene blue, whichever comes first (may resume citalopram therapy 24 hr after last dose of linezolid or methylene blue). **Pimozide** may ↑ risk of QT interval prolongation and torsades de pointes; concurrent use contraindicated. **QT interval prolonging drugs** may ↑ the risk of QT interval prolongation and torsades de pointes; avoid concurrent use. **CYP2C19 inhibitors**, including **cimetidine**, may ↑ levels and risk of toxicity (maximum dose = 20 mg/day). Drugs that affect serotonergic neurotransmitter systems, including **tricyclic antidepressants**, **SNRIs**, **fentanyl**, **lithium**, **buspirone**, **tramadol**, **meperidine**, **methadone**, **amphetamines**, and **triptans**, may ↑ risk of serotonin syndrome. Use cautiously with other **centrally acting drugs**, including **alcohol**, **antihistamines**, **opioid analgesics**, and **sedative/hypnotics**; concurrent use with **alcohol** is not recommended. Serotonergic effects may be ↑ by **lithium**; concurrent use should be carefully monitored. **Ketoconazole**, **itraconazole**, **erythromycin**, and **omeprazole** may ↑ levels and risk of toxicity. **Carbamazepine** may ↓ levels and effectiveness. May ↑ levels and risk of toxicity of **metoprolol**. ↑ risk of bleeding with **NSAIDs**, **aspirin**, **clopidogrel**, **prasugrel**, **ticagrelor**, **dabigatran**, **apixaban**, **edoxaban**, **rivaroxaban**, or **warfarin**.
Drug-Natural Products: ↑ risk of serotonergic side effects, including serotonin syndrome, with **St. John's wort** and **SAMe**.

Route/Dosage

PO (Adults): 20 mg once daily initially; may ↑ in 1 wk to 40 mg/day (maximum dose); *CYP2C19 poor metabolizers or concurrent use of CYP2C19 inhibitor:* Do not exceed 20 mg/day.
PO (Geriatric Patients): 20 mg once daily initially (do not exceed 20 mg/day in patients >60 yr).

Hepatic Impairment

PO (Adults): 20 mg once daily (do not exceed 20 mg/day).

Availability (generic available)

Capsules: 30 mg. **Tablets:** 10 mg, 20 mg, 30 mg, 40 mg. **Oral solution (peppermint flavor):** 10 mg/5 mL.

NURSING IMPLICATIONS

Assessment

- Screen patient for a personal or family history of bipolar disorder, mania, or hypomania before starting therapy; may precipitate a mixed/manic episode.
- Monitor mood changes during therapy.
- Assess for suicidal tendencies, especially during early therapy and dose changes. Restrict amount of drug available to patient. Risk may be ↑ in children, adolescents, and adults ≤24 yr. After starting therapy, young adults should be seen by health care provider at least weekly for 4 wk, every 3 wk for the next 4 wk, and on advice of health care provider thereafter.
- Assess sexual function before starting citalopram. Assess for changes in sexual function during treatment, including timing of onset; patient may not report.
- Assess for serotonin syndrome (mental changes [agitation, hallucinations, coma], autonomic instability [tachycardia, labile BP, hyperthermia], neuromuscular aberrations [hyperreflexia, incoordination], GI symptoms [nausea, vomiting, diarrhea]), especially in patients taking other serotonergic drugs (SSRIs, SNRIs, triptans).

Lab Test Considerations

- Monitor electrolytes (potassium and magnesium) in patients at risk for electrolyte imbalances prior to and periodically during therapy.

Implementation

- Do not confuse Celexa with Celebrex, Cerebyx, or Zyprexa. Do not confuse citalopram with escitalopram.
- **PO:** Administer as a single dose in the morning or evening without regard to food.

Patient/Family Teaching

- Instruct patient to take citalopram as directed. Take missed doses as soon as remembered unless almost time for next dose; do not double doses. Do not stop abruptly; may cause anxiety, irritability, high or low mood, feeling restless or changes in sleep habits, headache, sweating, nausea, dizziness, electric shock–like sensations, shaking, and confusion. Advise patient to read the *Medication Guide* prior to starting therapy and with each refill in case of changes.
- May cause drowsiness, dizziness, impaired concentration, and blurred vision. Caution patient to avoid driving and other activities requiring alertness until response to the drug is known.
- Instruct patient to notify health care provider of all Rx or OTC medications, vitamins, or herbal products being taken and to consult health care provider before taking any other Rx, OTC, or herbal products, especially alcohol or other CNS depressants, including opioids and St. John's wort.
- Caution patient to change positions slowly to minimize dizziness.
- Advise patient, family, and caregivers to look for suicidality, especially during early therapy or dose changes. Notify health care provider immediately if thoughts about suicide or dying, attempts to commit suicide, new or worse depression or anxiety, agitation or restlessness, panic attacks, insomnia, new or worse irritability, aggressiveness, acting on dangerous impulses, mania, or other changes in mood or behavior.
- Advise patient and caregivers to immediately notify health care provider if symptoms of serotonin syndrome occur.
- Advise patient to use sunscreen and wear protective clothing to prevent photosensitivity reactions.
- Inform patient that frequent mouth rinses, good oral hygiene, and sugarless gum or candy may minimize dry mouth. If dry mouth persists for >2 wk, consult health care provider regarding use of saliva substitute.
- Inform patient that citalopram may cause symptoms of sexual dysfunction. In men, ejaculatory delay or failure, ↓ libido, and erectile dysfunction may occur. In women, may result in ↓ libido and delayed or absent orgasm. Advise patient to notify health care provider if symptoms occur.
- Rep: Instruct women of reproductive potential to notify health care provider if pregnancy is planned or suspected or if breastfeeding. If used during pregnancy, should be tapered during 3rd trimester to avoid neonatal serotonin syndrome and ↑ risk of maternal postpartum hemorrhage. Monitor infants exposed to citalopram for excess sedation, restlessness, agitation, poor feeding, poor weight gain, or respiratory distress; may ↑ risk of persistent pulmonary hypertension of the newborn. Inform patient of pregnancy exposure registry that monitors pregnancy outcomes in women exposed to antidepressants during pregnancy. Encourage pregnant patients to enroll in pregnancy exposure registry that monitors outcomes of women exposed to antidepressants during pregnancy by contacting National Pregnancy Registry for Antidepressants at 1-866-961-2388 or visiting online at https://womensmentalhealth.org/research/pregnancyregistry/antidepressants/.
- Emphasize the importance of follow-up exams to monitor progress.

Evaluation/Desired Outcomes

- Increased sense of well-being.
- Renewed interest in surroundings. May require 1–4 wk of therapy to obtain antidepressant effects.

clindamycin (klin-da-**mye**-sin)

Cleocin, Cleocin T, Clinda-Derm, ✱ Clinda-T, Clindagel, Clindesse, ~~Clindets~~, ✱ Dalacin C, ✱ Dalacin Vaginal, Xaciato

Classification

Therapeutic: anti-infectives

Indications

PO, IM, IV: Treatment of: Skin and skin structure infections, Respiratory tract infections, Septicemia, Intra-abdominal infections, Gynecologic infections, Osteomyelitis, Endocarditis prophylaxis. **Topical:** Severe acne. **Vag:** Bacterial vaginosis. **Unlabeled Use: PO, IM, IV:** Treatment of *Pneumocystis jiroveci* pneumonia, CNS toxoplasmosis, and babesiosis.

Action

Inhibits protein synthesis in susceptible bacteria at the level of the 50S ribosome. **Therapeutic Effects:** Bactericidal or bacteriostatic, depending on susceptibility and concentration. **Spectrum:** Active against most gram-positive aerobic cocci, including: Staphylococci, *Streptococcus pneumoniae*, other streptococci, but not enterococci. Has good activity against those anaerobic bacteria that cause bacterial vaginosis, including *Bacteroides fragilis*, *Gardnerella vaginalis*, *Mobiluncus* spp., *Mycoplasma hominis*, and *Corynebacterium*. Also active against *Pneumocystis jirovecii*, *Propionibacterium acnes*, and *Toxoplasma gondii*.

Pharmacokinetics

Absorption: Well absorbed following PO/IM administration. Minimal absorption following topical/vaginal use.

Distribution: Widely distributed. Does not significantly cross blood-brain barrier.

Protein Binding: 94%.

Metabolism and Excretion: Mostly metabolized by the liver by the CYP3A4 isoenzyme.

Half-life: *Neonates:* 3.6–8.7 hr; *Infants up to 1 yr:* 3 hr; *Children and adults:* 2–3 hr.

TIME/ACTION PROFILE (plasma concentrations)

ROUTE	ONSET	PEAK	DURATION
PO	rapid	60 min	6–8 hr
IM	rapid	1–3 hr	6–8 hr
IV	rapid	end of infusion	6–8 hr

Contraindications/Precautions

Contraindicated in: Hypersensitivity; Regional enteritis or ulcerative colitis (topical foam); Previous *Clostridioides difficile*-associated diarrhea (CDAD); Severe hepatic impairment; Diarrhea; Known alcohol intolerance (topical solution, suspension).

Use Cautiously in: Rep: Women and men of reproductive potential (some vaginal products may contain mineral oil, which may weaken condoms or vaginal diaphragms); OB: Safety not established in pregnancy for topical or vaginal administration; systemic administration during 2nd and 3rd trimesters not associated with ↑ risk of congenital abnormalities; injection contains benzyl alcohol, which can cross placenta; Lactation: Use while breastfeeding only if potential maternal benefit justifies potential risk to infant; Pedi: Injection contains benzyl alcohol, which can cause gasping syndrome in infants and neonates.

Adverse Reactions/Side Effects

CV: arrhythmias, hypotension. **Derm:** DRUG REACTION WITH EOSINOPHILIA AND SYSTEMIC SYMPTOMS (DRESS), ERYTHEMA MULTIFORME, rash, STEVENS-JOHNSON SYNDROME, TOXIC EPIDERMAL NECROLYSIS, urticaria. **GI:** diarrhea, CDAD, bitter or metallic taste, esophagitis, esophageal ulcer, nausea, vomiting. **Local:** local irritation (topical products), phlebitis at IV site. **Neuro:** dizziness, headache, vertigo. **Misc:** HYPERSENSITIVITY REACTIONS (INCLUDING ANAPHYLAXIS).

Interactions

Drug-Drug: May enhance the neuromuscular blocking action of other **neuromuscular blocking agents**. **CYP3A4 inhibitors** may ↑ levels and risk of toxicity. **CYP3A4 inducers**, including **rifampin**, may ↓ levels and effectiveness. **Topical:** Concurrent use with **irritants**, **abrasives**, or **desquamating agents** may result in additive irritation.

Route/Dosage

PO (Adults): *Most infections:* 150–450 mg every 6 hr. *Pneumocystis jiroveci pneumonia:* 1200–1800 mg/day in divided doses with 15–30 mg primaquine/day (unlabeled). *CNS toxoplasmosis:* 1200–2400 mg/day in divided doses with pyrimethamine 50–100 mg/day (unlabeled); *Bacterial endocarditis prophylaxis:* 600 mg 1 hr before procedure.

PO (Children >1 mo): 10–30 mg/kg/day divided every 6–8 hr; maximum dose 1.8 g/day. *Bacterial endocarditis prophylaxis:* 20 mg/kg 1 hr before procedure.

IM, IV (Adults): *Most infections:* 300–600 mg every 6–8 hr *or* 900 mg every 8 hr (up to 4.8 g/day IV has been used; single IM doses of >600 mg are not recommended). *Pneumocystis jiroveci pneumonia:* 2400–2700 mg/day in divided doses with primaquine (unlabeled). *Toxoplasmosis:* 1200–4800 mg/day in divided doses with pyrimethamine. *Bacterial endocarditis prophylaxis:* 600 mg 30 min before procedure.

IM, IV (Children >1 mo): 20–40 mg/kg/day (based on total body weight) divided every 6–8 hr; maximum dose: 4.8 g/day. *Bacterial endocarditis prophylaxis:* 20 mg/kg 30 min before procedure; maximum dose: 600 mg.

Vag (Adults and Adolescents): *Cleocin, Clindamax:* 1 applicatorful (5 g) at bedtime for 3 or 7 days (7 days in pregnant patients); *Clindesse:* one applicatorful (5 g) single dose; *or* 1 suppository (100 mg) at bedtime for 3 nights. *Xaciato:* one applicatorful (5 g) single dose.

Topical (Adults and Adolescents): *Solution:* 1% solution/suspension applied twice daily (range 1–4 times daily). *Foam, gel:* 1% foam or gel applied once daily.

Availability (generic available)

Capsules: 75 mg, 150 mg, 300 mg. **Oral solution:** 75 mg/5 mL. **Solution for injection:** 150 mg/mL. **Premixed infusion:** 300 mg/50 mL 0.9% NaCl, 600 mg/50 mL 0.9% NaCl, 900 mg/50 mL 0.9% NaCl. **Topical:** 1% lotion, gel, foam, solution, suspension, single-use applicators. **Vaginal cream:** 2%. **Vaginal gel:** 2%. **Vaginal suppositories (ovules):** 100 mg. ***In combination with:*** benzoyl peroxide (Acanya, Onexton), tretinoin (Veltin, Ziana) (see Appendix N).

C

NURSING IMPLICATIONS

Assessment

- Assess for infection (vital signs; appearance of wound, sputum, urine, and stool; WBC) at beginning of and during therapy.
- Obtain specimens for culture and sensitivity before initiating therapy. First dose may be given before receiving results.
- Monitor bowel elimination. Report diarrhea, abdominal cramping, fever, and bloody stools to health care provider promptly as a sign of CDAD. May begin up to several weeks following the cessation of therapy.
- Assess patient for hypersensitivity reactions (skin rash, urticaria).

Lab Test Considerations

- Monitor CBC; may ↓ leukocytes, eosinophils, and platelets.
- May ↑ alkaline phosphatase, bilirubin, CK, AST, and ALT.

Implementation

- **PO:** Administer with 6–8 ounces of water. May cause esophageal irritation; patient should be in an upright (60–90°) position during and for 30–60 min after administration. May be given with or without meals. Shake liquid preparations well. Do not refrigerate. Stable for 14 days at room temperature. Avoid administering before bed.
- **Gastric tubes (NG, G-tube, J-tube):** Open and disperse contents of each capsule in 10–15 mL of purified water; draw up mixture into enteral dosing syringe and administer via feeding tube. Flush feeding tube with an appropriate volume of purified water before and after administration.
- **IM:** Inject undiluted. Do not administer >600 mg in a single IM injection.

IV Administration

- **Intermittent Infusion:** **Dilution:** Dilute a dose of 300 mg or 600 mg in 50 mL and a dose of 900 mg or 1200 mg in 100 mL. Compatible diluents include D5W, 0.9% NaCl, D5/0.9% NaCl, D5/0.45% NaCl, or LR. Admixed solution stable for 16 days at room temperature. Premixed infusion is already diluted and ready to use. **Concentration:** Not to exceed 18 mg/mL. **Rate:** Infuse over 10–60 min. Not to exceed 30 mg/min. Hypotension and cardiopulmonary arrest have been reported following rapid IV administration.
- **Y-Site Compatibility:** acetaminophen, acyclovir, alemtuzumab, amikacin, aminocaproic acid, aminophylline, amiodarone, amphotericin B liposomal, anidulafungin, argatroban, arsenic trioxide, ascorbic acid, atracurium, atropine, aztreonam, benztropine, bivalirudin, bleomycin, bumetanide, buprenorphine, butorphanol, calcium chloride, calcium gluconate, cangrelor, carboplatin, carmustine, cefazolin, cefiderocol, cefotaxime, cefotetan, cefoxitin, ceftaroline, ceftazidime, ceftobiprole, cefuroxime, chloramphenicol, cisatracurium, cisplatin, cyanocobalamin, cyclophosphamide, cyclosporine, cytarabine, dacarbazine, dactinomycin, daptomycin, dexamethasone, dexmedetomidine, dexrazoxane, digoxin, diltiazem, dimenhydrinate, diphenhydramine, dobutamine, docetaxel, dopamine, doxorubicin hydrochloride, doxorubicin liposomal, doxycycline, enalaprilat, ephedrine, epinephrine, epirubicin, epoetin alfa, eptifibatide, esmolol, etoposide, etoposide phosphate, famotidine, fentanyl, fludarabine, fluorouracil, folic acid, foscarnet, fosphenytoin, furosemide, gemcitabine, gemtuzumab ozogamicin, gentamicin, glycopyrrolate, granisetron, heparin, hetastarch, hydrocortisone, hydromorphone, ifosfamide, imipenem/cilastatin, imipenem/cilastatin/relebactam, indomethacin, insulin, regular, irinotecan, isoproterenol, ketamine, ketorolac, LR, leucovorin, levofloxacin, lidocaine, linezolid, lorazepam, magnesium sulfate, mannitol, melphalan, meperidine, meropenem, mesna, methadone, methotrexate, methylprednisolone, metoclopramide, metoprolol, metronidazole, milrinone, morphine, multivitamins, nafcillin, nalbuphine, naloxone, nitroglycerin, nitroprusside, norepinephrine, octreotide, ondansetron, oxacillin, oxaliplatin, oxytocin, paclitaxel, palonosetron, pamidronate, pemetrexed, penicillin G, phenobarbital, phenylephrine, phytonadione, piperacillin/tazobactam, potassium acetate, potassium chloride, procainamide, propofol, propranolol, protamine, pyridoxine, remifentanil, rituximab, rocuronium, sargramostim, sodium acetate, sodium bicarbonate, succinylcholine, sufentanil, tacrolimus, theophylline, thiamine, thiotepa, tigecycline, tirofiban, tobramycin, vancomycin, vasopressin, vecuronium, verapamil, vinblastine, vincristine, vinorelbine, voriconazole, zidovudine, zoledronic acid,.
- **Y-Site Incompatibility:** allopurinol, amphotericin B deoxycholate azathioprine, caspofungin, ceftriaxone, chlorpromazine, dantrolene, daunorubicin hydrochloride, diazepam, diazoxide, filgrastim, ganciclovir, haloperidol, idarubicin, minocycline, mitomycin, mitoxantrone, mycophenolate, oritavancin, papaverine, pentamidine, pentobarbital, phentolamine, phenytoin, prochlorperazine, promethazine, topotecan, trastuzumab, trimethoprim/sulfamethoxazole.
- **Vag:** Applicators are supplied for vaginal administration. When treating bacterial vaginosis,

concurrent treatment of male partner is not usually necessary.

- **Topical:** Contact with eyes, mucous membranes, and open cuts should be avoided during topical application. If accidental contact occurs, rinse with copious amounts of cool water.
- Wash affected areas with warm water and soap; rinse and pat dry before application. Apply to entire affected area.

Patient/Family Teaching

- Explain purpose and side effects of medication to patient. Advise patient to read *Patient Information* before starting therapy. Instruct patient to take as directed. Take missed doses as soon as possible unless almost time for next dose. Do not double doses. Advise patient that sharing of this medication may be dangerous.
- Advise patient to notify health care provider of all Rx or OTC medications, vitamins, or herbal products being taken and to consult health care provider before taking other medications.
- Instruct patient to notify health care provider immediately if diarrhea, abdominal cramping, fever, or bloody stools occur and not to treat with antidiarrheals without consulting health care provider.
- Advise patient to report signs of superinfection (furry overgrowth on the tongue, vaginal or anal itching or discharge).
- Notify health care provider if no improvement within a few days.
- Patients with a history of rheumatic heart disease or valve replacement need to be taught the importance of antimicrobial prophylaxis before invasive medical or dental procedures.
- Rep: Advise women of reproductive potential to notify health care provider if pregnancy is planned or suspected or if breastfeeding. Use with caution during 1st trimester. If breastfeeding, alternate drugs are preferred. If continued during breastfeeding, monitor infant for diarrhea, thrush, and diaper rash.
- **IV:** Inform patient that bitter or metallic taste occurring with IV administration is not clinically significant.
- **Vag:** Instruct patient on proper use of vaginal applicator. Insert high into vagina at bedtime. Instruct patient to remain recumbent for ≥30 min following insertion. Advise patient to use sanitary napkin to prevent staining of clothing or bedding. Continue therapy during menstrual period.
- Advise patient to refrain from vaginal sexual intercourse during treatment.
- Caution patient that mineral oil in clindamycin cream may weaken latex or rubber contraceptive devices. Such products should not be used within 72 hr of vaginal cream.
- **Topical:** Caution patient applying topical clindamycin that solution is flammable (vehicle is isopropyl alcohol). Avoid application while smoking or near heat or flame.
- Advise patient to notify health care provider if excessive drying of skin occurs.
- Advise patient to wait 30 min after washing or shaving area before applying.

Evaluation/Desired Outcomes

- Bactericidal or bacteriostatic, depending on susceptibility and concentration.

clobetasol, See CORTICOSTEROIDS (TOPICAL).

clocortolone, See CORTICOSTEROIDS (TOPICAL).

BEERS

clonazePAM (kloe-na-ze-pam)

KlonoPIN, Rivotril

Classification

Therapeutic: anticonvulsants

Pharmacologic: benzodiazepines

Schedule IV

Indications

Lennox-Gastaut, akinetic, or myoclonic seizures. Panic disorder with or without agoraphobia. **Unlabeled Use:** Uncontrolled leg movements during sleep. Neuralgias. Infantile spasms. Sedation. Adjunct management of acute mania, acute psychosis, or insomnia.

Action

Anticonvulsant effects may be due to presynaptic inhibition. Produces sedative effects in the CNS, probably by stimulating inhibitory GABA receptors. **Therapeutic Effects:** Prevention of seizures. Decreased manifestations of panic disorder.

Pharmacokinetics

Absorption: Well absorbed from the GI tract.

Distribution: Probably crosses the blood-brain barrier.

Metabolism and Excretion: Mostly metabolized by the liver.

Half-life: 18–50 hr.

TIME/ACTION PROFILE (anticonvulsant activity)

ROUTE	ONSET	PEAK	DURATION
PO	20–60 min	1–2 hr	6–12 hr

C

Contraindications/Precautions

Contraindicated in: Hypersensitivity to clonazepam or other benzodiazepines; Severe hepatic impairment.

Use Cautiously in: All patients (may ↑ risk of suicidal thoughts/behaviors); Angle-closure glaucoma; Obstructive sleep apnea; Chronic respiratory disease; History of porphyria; OB: Use late in pregnancy can result in sedation (respiratory depression, lethargy, hypotonia) and/or withdrawal symptoms (hyperreflexia, irritability, restlessness, tremors, inconsolable crying, feeding difficulties) in neonates; Lactation: Use while breastfeeding only if potential maternal benefit justifies potential risk to infant; Pedi: Safety and effectiveness not established in children for panic disorder; Geri: Appears on Beers list. ↑ risk of cognitive impairment, delirium, falls, fractures, and motor vehicle accidents. If possible, avoid use in older adults.

Adverse Reactions/Side Effects

CV: palpitations. **Derm:** rash. **EENT:** diplopia, nystagmus. **GI:** constipation, diarrhea, hepatitis. **GU:** dysuria, nocturia, urinary retention. **Hemat:** anemia, eosinophilia, leukopenia, thrombocytopenia. **Metab:** weight gain. **Neuro:** ataxia, behavioral changes, drowsiness, fatigue, hypotonia, sedation, slurred speech, SUICIDAL THOUGHTS. **Resp:** ↑ secretions. **Misc:** fever, physical dependence, psychological dependence, tolerance.

Interactions

Drug-Drug: Use with **opioids** or other **CNS depressants**, including other **benzodiazepines**, **nonbenzodiazepine sedative/hypnotics**, **anxiolytics**, **general anesthetics**, **muscle relaxants**, **antipsychotics**, and **alcohol**, may cause profound sedation, respiratory depression, coma, and death; reserve concurrent use for when alternative treatment options are inadequate. **Cimetidine**, **hormonal contraceptives**, **disulfiram**, **fluoxetine**, **isoniazid**, **ketoconazole**, **metoprolol**, **propranolol**, or **valproic acid** may ↑ levels and risk of toxicity. May ↓ efficacy of **levodopa**. **Rifampin**, **barbiturates**, or **phenytoin** may ↓ levels and effectiveness. Sedative effects may be ↓ by **theophylline**. May ↑ levels and risk of toxicity of **phenytoin**.

Drug-Natural Products: Kava-kava, **valerian**, or **chamomile** can ↑ risk of CNS depression.

Route/Dosage

PO (Adults): 0.5 mg 3 times daily; may ↑ by 0.5–1 mg every 3 days. Total daily maintenance dose not to exceed 20 mg. *Panic disorder:* 0.125 mg twice daily; may ↑ after 3 days toward target dose of 1 mg/day (some patients may require up to 4 mg/day).

PO (Children ≤10 yr or ≤30 kg): 0.01–0.03 mg/kg/day (not to exceed 0.05 mg/kg/day) given in 2–3 equally divided doses; ↑ by no more than 0.25–0.5 mg every 3 days until therapeutic blood levels are reached (not to exceed 0.2 mg/kg/day).

Availability (generic available)

Tablets: ✱ 0.25 mg, 0.5 mg, 1 mg, 2 mg. **Orally disintegrating tablets:** 0.125 mg, 0.25 mg, 0.5 mg, 1 mg, 2 mg.

NURSING IMPLICATIONS

Assessment

- Observe and record intensity, duration, and location of seizure activity.
- Assess degree and manifestations of anxiety and mental status (orientation, mood, behavior) prior to and periodically during therapy.
- Assess need for continued treatment regularly.
- Assess for drowsiness, unsteadiness, and clumsiness. These symptoms are dose related and most severe during initial therapy; may ↓ in severity or disappear with continued or long-term therapy.
- Monitor closely for notable changes in behavior that could indicate the emergence or worsening of suicidal thoughts or behavior or depression.
- Assess risk for addiction, abuse, or misuse before administration and periodically during therapy.
- Prolonged high-dose therapy may lead to psychological or physical dependence. Restrict the amount of drug available to patient. Assess regularly for continued need for treatment.

Lab Test Considerations

- Patients on prolonged therapy should have CBC and liver function test results evaluated periodically. May ↑ serum bilirubin, AST, and ALT.
- May ↓ thyroidal uptake of ^{123}I and ^{131}I.

Toxicity and Overdose

- Therapeutic serum concentrations are 20–80 mg/mL. Flumazenil antagonizes clonazepam toxicity or overdose (may induce seizures in patients with history of seizure disorder or who are on tricyclic antidepressants).

Implementation

- Do not confuse clonazepam with alprazolam, clonidine, clozapine, clobazam, or lorazepam. Do not confuse Klonopin with clonidine.
- Institute seizure precautions for patients on initial therapy or undergoing dose manipulations.
- **PO:** Administer with food to ↓ GI irritation. Tablets may be crushed if patient has difficulty swallowing. Administer largest dose at bedtime to avoid daytime sedation.

- Orally disintegrating tablets should be left in the package until use. Remove from the blister pouch. Do not push tablet through the blister; peel open the blister pack with dry hands and place tablet on tongue. Tablet will dissolve rapidly and be swallowed with saliva. No liquid is needed to take the orally disintegrating tablet.
- Gradually taper to discontinue or ↓ the dose to ↓ risk of withdrawal reactions, ↑ seizure frequency, and status epilepticus. Taper by 0.25 mg every 3 days to ↓ signs and symptoms of withdrawal. If patient develops withdrawal symptoms, pause taper or ↑ dose to previous tapered dose level; ↓ dose more slowly. Some patients may require longer tapering period (weeks–>12 mo).

Patient/Family Teaching

- Explain purpose and side effects of medication to patient. Advise patient to read *Patient Information* before starting therapy. Instruct patient to take exactly as directed. Take missed doses within 1 hr or omit; do not double doses.
- Caution patient not to stop taking clonazepam without consulting health care provider. Abrupt withdrawal may cause sweating, vomiting, muscle cramps, tremors, and seizures; may be life-threatening.
- Advise patient to avoid the use of alcohol or other CNS depressants, including opioids, concurrently with clonazepam; may cause respiratory depression and overdose. Instruct patient to consult health care provider before taking Rx, OTC, or herbal products concurrently with this medication.
- Advise patient that clonazepam is usually prescribed for short-term use.
- Advise patient that clonazepam is a drug with known abuse potential. Protect it from theft, and never give to anyone other than the individual for whom it was prescribed. Store out of sight and reach of children and in a location not accessible by others.
- Advise patient to not share medication with others.
- May cause drowsiness or dizziness. Advise patient to avoid driving or other activities requiring alertness until response to drug is known.
- Advise patient to notify health care provider of medication regimen prior to treatment or surgery.
- Instruct patient and family to notify health care provider of unusual tiredness, bleeding, sore throat, fever, clay-colored stools, yellowing of skin, or behavioral changes. Advise patient and family to notify health care provider if thoughts about suicide or dying, attempts to commit suicide, new or worse depression, new or worse anxiety, feeling very agitated or restless, panic attacks, trouble sleeping, new or worse irritability, acting aggressive, being angry or violent, acting on dangerous impulses, an extreme ↑ in activity and talking, or other unusual changes in behavior or mood occur.
- Rep: Advise women of reproductive potential to notify health care provider if pregnancy is planned or suspected or if breastfeeding. Monitor infants exposed to clonazepam during 2nd and 3rd trimester or immediately before or during childbirth for ↓ fetal movement and/or fetal heart rate variability, floppy infant syndrome, dependence, sedation (respiratory depression, lethargy, hypotonia), and symptoms of withdrawal (hypertonia, hyperreflexia, hypoventilation, irritability, tremors, diarrhea, vomiting, restlessness, inconsolable crying, feeding difficulties); may occur shortly after delivery to up to 3 wk after birth. Monitor breastfed infants for sedation, poor sucking, poor feeding, and poor weight gain. Encourage pregnant patients to enroll in North American Antiepileptic Drug Pregnancy Registry to collect information about safety of antiepileptic drugs during pregnancy. To enroll, patients can call 1-888-233-2334 or visit http://www.aedpregnancyregistry.org/.
- Patient on anticonvulsant therapy should carry identification at all times describing disease process and medication regimen.
- Emphasize the importance of follow-up exams to determine effectiveness of the medication.

Evaluation/Desired Outcomes

- Prevention of seizures.
- Decreased manifestations of panic disorder.

BEERS

cloNIDine (klon-i-deen)

~~Catapres~~, Catapres-TTS, Duraclon, ~~Kapvay~~, Nexiclon XR, Onyda XR

Classification

Therapeutic: antihypertensives

Pharmacologic: adrenergics (centrally acting)

Indications

PO transdermal Hypertension. **PO:** Attention-deficit hyperactivity disorder (ADHD) (as monotherapy or as adjunctive to stimulants). epidural Cancer pain unresponsive to opioids alone. **Unlabeled Use:** Opioid withdrawal.

Action

Stimulates alpha-adrenergic receptors in the CNS, which results in decreased sympathetic outflow, inhibiting cardioacceleration and vasoconstriction centers. Prevents pain signal transmission to the CNS by stimulating alpha-adrenergic receptors in the spinal cord. **Therapeutic Effects:** Decreased BP. Decreased pain. Improved ADHD symptoms.

C

Pharmacokinetics

Absorption: Well absorbed from the GI tract and skin. Enters systemic circulation following epidural use.
Distribution: Widely distributed; enters CNS.
Metabolism and Excretion: Mostly metabolized by the liver; 40–60% eliminated unchanged in urine.
Half-life: *Neonates:* 44–72 hr; *Children:* 8–12 hr; *Adults: Plasma:* 12–16 hr (↑ in renal impairment); *CNS:* 1.3 hr.

TIME/ACTION PROFILE (PO, TD = antihypertensive effect; epidural = analgesia)

ROUTE	ONSET	PEAK	DURATION
PO	30–60 min	1–3 hr	8–12 hr
Transdermal	2–3 days	unknown	7 days†
Epidural	unknown	unknown	unknown

† 8 hr following removal of patch.

Contraindications/Precautions

Contraindicated in: Hypersensitivity; Injection site infection, anticoagulant therapy, or bleeding problems (epidural only); Obstetrical, postpartum, or postoperative pain (↑ risk of hypotension and bradycardia) (epidural only).
Use Cautiously in: Serious cardiac or cerebrovascular disease; Renal impairment; OB: Use during pregnancy only if potential maternal benefit justifies potential fetal risk; Lactation: Use while breastfeeding only if potential maternal benefit justifies potential risk to infant; Pedi: Safety and efficacy not established in children <6 yr (ADHD); evaluation for cardiac disease should precede initiation of therapy for ADHD in children; Geri: Appears on Beers list. ↑ risk of CNS effects, orthostatic hypotension, and bradycardia in older adults. Avoid use as first-line treatment of hypertension in older adults.

Adverse Reactions/Side Effects

CV: bradycardia, heart block, hypotension (↑ with epidural), palpitations. **Derm:** rash, sweating. **EENT:** dry eyes. **GI:** dry mouth, constipation, nausea, vomiting. **GU:** ↓ fertility, erectile dysfunction. **Metab:** weight gain. **Neuro:** drowsiness, depression, dizziness, hallucinations, nervousness, nightmares, paresthesia.

Interactions

Drug-Drug: Additive sedation with **CNS depressants**, including **alcohol**, **antihistamines**, **opioid analgesics**, and **sedative/hypnotics**. Additive hypotension with other **antihypertensives** and **nitrates**. Additive bradycardia with **beta blockers**, **diltiazem**, **ivabradine**, **verapamil**, or **digoxin**. **MAO inhibitors**, **amphetamines**, or **tricyclic antidepressants** may ↓ antihypertensive effect. Withdrawal phenomenon may be ↑ by discontinuation of **beta blockers**. Epidural clonidine prolongs the effects of epidurally administered **local anesthetics**. May ↓ effectiveness of **levodopa**.

Route/Dosage

Do NOT substitute between clonidine products on a mg-per-mg basis.

Hypertension

PO (Adults): *Immediate release:* 0.1 mg twice daily; ↑ by 0.1–0.2 mg/day every 2–4 days until BP is controlled; usual maintenance dose is 0.2–0.6 mg/day in 2–3 divided doses (up to 2.4 mg/day). *Extended release:* 0.17 mg once daily; ↑ by 0.09 mg/day at weekly intervals until BP is controlled; usual maintenance dose is 0.17–0.52 mg/day. *Urgent treatment of hypertension (immediate release):* 0.2 mg loading dose; then 0.1 mg every hr until BP is controlled or 0.8 mg total has been administered; follow with maintenance dosing.
PO (Geriatric Patients): *Immediate release:* 0.1 mg at bedtime initially; ↑ as needed.
Transdermal **(Adults):** 0.1 mg/24 hr patch applied once every 7 days; ↑ by 0.1 mg every 1–2 wk (usual dose range: 0.1–0.3 mg/24-hr patch applied once every 7 days).

Attention-Deficit Hyperactivity Disorder

PO (Children ≥6 yr and >45 kg): *Immediate release:* 0.1 mg at bedtime; then ↑ every 2–3 days to 0.1 mg twice daily; then 0.1 mg 3 times daily; then 0.1 mg 4 times daily (max dose = 0.4 mg/day).
PO (Children ≥6 yr and 40.6–45 kg): *Immediate release:* 0.05 mg at bedtime; then ↑ every 2–3 days to 0.05 mg twice daily; then 0.05 mg 3 times daily; then 0.05 mg 4 times daily (max dose = 0.3 mg/day).
PO (Children ≥6 yr and 27–40.5 kg): *Immediate release:* 0.05 mg at bedtime; then ↑ every 2–3 days to 0.05 mg twice daily; then 0.05 mg 3 times daily; then 0.05 mg 4 times daily (max dose = 0.2 mg/day).
PO (Children ≥6 yr): *Extended release (generic):* 0.1 mg at bedtime; after 1 wk, ↑ dose to 0.1 mg in am and at bedtime; after 1 wk, ↑ dose to 0.1 mg in am and 0.2 mg at bedtime; after 1 wk, ↑ dose to 0.2 mg in am and at bedtime (max dose = 0.4 mg/day). *Extended release (Onyda XR):* 0.1 mg at bedtime; titrate dose by 0.1 mg/day at weekly intervals (max dose = 0.4 mg/day).

Cancer Pain

Epidural (Adults): 30 mcg/hr initially; titrated according to need.
Epidural (Children): 0.5 mcg/kg/hr initially; titrated according to need up to 2 mcg/kg/hr.

Opioid Withdrawal

PO (Adults): *Immediate release:* 0.3–1.2 mg/day; may ↓ by 50% per day for 3 days; then discontinued or ↓ by 0.1–0.2 mg/day.

Availability (generic available)

Immediate-release tablets: 🍁 0.025 mg, 0.1 mg, 0.2 mg, 0.3 mg. **Extended-release tablets:** 0.1 mg. **Extended-release tablets (Nexiclon XR):** 0.17 mg, 0.26 mg. **Extended-release oral suspension (orange flavor) (Onyda XR):** 0.1 mg/mL. **Solution for epidural injection (Duraclon):** 100 mcg/mL, 500 mcg/mL. **Transdermal patch:** 0.1 mg/24 hr, 0.2 mg/24 hr, 0.3 mg/24 hr.

NURSING IMPLICATIONS

Assessment

- **Hypertension:** Monitor intake and output and daily weight, and assess for edema daily, especially at beginning of therapy.
- Monitor BP and HR before starting, frequently during initial dose adjustment and dose ↑ and periodically during therapy. Titrate slowly in patients with cardiac conditions or those taking other sympatholytic drugs. Report significant changes.
- **Pain:** Assess location, character, and intensity of pain before therapy, frequently during first few days, and routinely during administration.
- Monitor for fever as potential sign of catheter infection. **Opioid Withdrawal:** Monitor patient for signs and symptoms of opioid withdrawal (tachycardia, fever, runny nose, diarrhea, sweating, nausea, vomiting, irritability, stomach cramps, shivering, unusually large pupils, weakness, difficulty sleeping, gooseflesh).
- **ADHD:** Assess attention span, impulse control, and interactions with others.

Lab Test Considerations

- May cause transient ↑ in blood glucose levels.
- May ↓ urinary catecholamine and vanillylmandelic acid concentrations; these may ↑ on abrupt withdrawal.
- May cause weakly positive Coombs test result.

Implementation

- Do not confuse clonidine with clonazepam (Klonopin) or clozapine.
- Do not substitute between clonidine products on a mg-per-mg basis because of differing pharmacokinetic profiles.
- In the perioperative setting, continue clonidine up to 4 hr before surgery and resume as soon as possible thereafter. Do not interrupt *transdermal clonidine* during surgery. Monitor BP carefully.
- **PO:** Administer last dose of the day at bedtime. May be taken with or without food.
- *DNC:* Extended-release tablets (Nexiclon XR) are scored and may be split in half; do not crush or chew.
- For extended-release oral suspension, insert bottle adapter into bottle; do not remove this adapter once it has been inserted. Shake suspension gently for 10 sec before administering. Use oral dosing syringe to obtain accurate dose; tip of syringe should be inserted into bottle adapter to obtain dose. Discard any unused suspension that remains in bottle after 60 days of opening the bottle.

Transdermal: Transdermal system should be applied once every 7 days. May be applied to any hairless site; avoid cuts or calluses. Absorption is greater when placed on chest or upper arm and decreased when placed on thigh. Rotate sites weekly. Wash area with soap and water; dry thoroughly before application. Apply firm pressure over patch to ensure contact with skin, especially around edges. Remove old system and discard. System includes a protective adhesive overlay to be applied over medication patch to ensure adhesion, should medication patch loosen.

Epidural: Dilute 500 mcg/mL with 0.9% NaCl for a concentration of 100 mcg/mL. Do not administer solutions that are discolored or contain a precipitate. Discard unused portion.

Patient/Family Teaching

- Instruct patient to take clonidine at the same time each day, even if feeling well. Take missed dose as soon as remembered. If dose of extended-release product is missed, omit dose and take next dose as scheduled. Do not take more than the prescribed daily dose in any 24 hr. If more than one oral dose in a row is missed or if transdermal system is late in being changed by ≥3 days, consult health care provider. All routes of clonidine should be gradually discontinued over 2–4 days to prevent rebound hypertension. Advise patients taking oral and transdermal forms to read *Patient Information* before starting and with each Rx refill in case of changes.
- Advise patient to make sure enough medication is available for weekends, holidays, and vacations. A written prescription may be kept in wallet in case of emergency.
- May cause drowsiness, which usually diminishes with continued use. Advise patient to avoid driving or other activities requiring alertness until response to medication is known.
- Caution patient to avoid sudden changes in position to ↓ orthostatic hypotension. Use of alcohol, standing for long periods, exercising, and hot weather may ↑ orthostatic hypotension.
- If dry mouth occurs, frequent mouth rinses, good oral hygiene, and sugarless gum or candy may ↓

effect. If dry mouth continues for >2 wk, consult health care provider.

- Caution patients with contact lenses that clonidine may cause dryness of eyes.
- Caution patient to avoid concurrent use of alcohol, marijuana or other forms of cannabis, and other CNS depressants, including opioids, with this medication.
- Instruct patient to notify health care provider of all Rx or OTC medications, vitamins, or herbal products being taken and to consult health care provider before taking any other Rx, OTC, or herbal products, especially cough, cold, or allergy remedies.
- Advise patient to notify health care provider of medication regimen prior to treatment or surgery.
- Advise patient to notify health care provider if itching or redness of skin (with transdermal patch), mental depression, swelling of feet and lower legs, paleness or cold feeling in fingertips or toes, or vivid dreams or nightmares occur. May require discontinuation of therapy, especially with depression.
- **Hypertension:** Encourage patient to comply with additional interventions for hypertension (weight ↓, low-sodium diet, discontinuation of smoking, moderation of alcohol consumption, regular exercise, stress management). Medication helps control but does not cure hypertension.
- Instruct patient and family on proper technique for BP monitoring. Advise them to check BP at least weekly and report significant changes. **Transdermal:** Instruct patient on proper application of transdermal system. Do not cut or trim unit. Transdermal system can remain in place during bathing or swimming.
- Advise patient referred for MRI test to discuss patch with referring health care provider and MRI facility to determine if removal of patch is necessary prior to test and for directions for replacing patch.
- Pedi: Advise parents to notify school nurse of medication regimen.
- Rep: Advise women of reproductive potential to notify health care provider if pregnancy is planned or suspected or if breastfeeding. Monitor breastfeeding infants exposed to *Kapvay* through breast milk for symptoms of hypotension and/or bradycardia, such as sedation, lethargy, tachypnea, and poor feeding. May impair female and male fertility. There is a pregnancy exposure registry that monitors pregnancy outcomes in women exposed to ADHD medications during pregnancy. Register patients by calling the National Pregnancy Registry for ADHD Medications at 1-866961-2388 or visiting https://womensmentalhealth.org/adhd-medications/.

Evaluation/Desired Outcomes

- Decrease in BP.
- Decrease in severity of pain.
- Decrease in the signs and symptoms of opioid withdrawal.
- Improved attention span and social interactions in ADHD.

clopidogrel (kloh-pid-oh-grel)

Plavix

Classification

Therapeutic: antiplatelet agents

Pharmacologic: platelet aggregation inhibitors

Indications

Acute coronary syndrome (ST-segment elevation MI, non-ST-segment elevation MI, or unstable angina). Patients with established peripheral arterial disease, recent MI, or recent stroke.

Action

Inhibits platelet aggregation by irreversibly inhibiting the binding of ATP to platelet receptors. **Therapeutic Effects:** Reduction in risk of MI and stroke.

Pharmacokinetics

Absorption: Well absorbed following oral administration; prodrug that is rapidly metabolized to an active antiplatelet compound. Parent drug has no antiplatelet activity.

Distribution: Unknown.

Protein Binding: *Clopidogrel:* 98%; *active metabolite:* 94%.

Metabolism and Excretion: Rapidly and extensively converted by the liver via the CYP2C19 isoenzyme to its active metabolite, which is then eliminated 50% in urine and 45% in feces; 2% of White people, 4% of Black people, and 14% of Asian people have CYP2C19 genotype, which results in reduced metabolism of clopidogrel (poor metabolizers) into its active metabolite (may result in ↓ antiplatelet effects).

Half-life: 6 hr (active metabolite 30 min).

TIME/ACTION PROFILE (effects on platelet function)

ROUTE	ONSET	PEAK	DURATION
PO	within 24 hr	3–7 days	5 days†

† Following discontinuation.

Contraindications/Precautions

Contraindicated in: Hypersensitivity to clopidogrel or prasugrel; Pathologic bleeding (peptic ulcer, intracranial hemorrhage); CYP2C19 poor metabolizers.

Use Cautiously in: Patients at risk for bleeding (trauma, surgery, or other pathologic conditions); History of GI bleeding/ulcer disease; Severe hepatic impairment; Hypersensitivity to another thienopyridine (prasugrel); OB: Use should not be withheld if needed for emergent treatment of stroke or MI during pregnancy. Discontinue use 5–7 days prior to labor, delivery, or neuraxial blockade, if possible, due to ↑ risk of maternal bleeding and hemorrhage; Lactation: Use while breastfeeding only if potential maternal benefit justifies potential risk to infant; Pedi: Safety and effectiveness not established in children.

Adverse Reactions/Side Effects

CV: chest pain, edema, hypertension. **Derm:** ACUTE GENERALIZED EXANTHEMATOUS PUSTULOSIS, DRUG RASH WITH EOSINOPHILIA AND SYSTEMIC SYMPTOMS, pruritus, purpura, rash, STEVENS-JOHNSON SYNDROME (SJS), TOXIC EPIDERMAL NECROLYSIS (TEN). **EENT:** epistaxis. **GI:** abdominal pain, diarrhea, dyspepsia, gastritis, GI BLEEDING. **Hemat:** BLEEDING, NEUTROPENIA, THROMBOTIC THROMBOCYTOPENIC PURPURA. **Metab:** hypercholesterolemia. **MS:** arthralgia, back pain. **Neuro:** depression, dizziness, fatigue, headache. **Resp:** cough, dyspnea, eosinophilic pneumonia. **Misc:** fever, HYPERSENSITIVITY REACTIONS (INCLUDING ANAPHYLAXIS).

Interactions

Drug-Drug: Eptifibatide, tirofiban, aspirin, dipyridamole, NSAIDs, heparin, LMWHs, thrombolytic agents, SSRIs, SNRIs, or **warfarin** may ↑ risk of bleeding. **Strong CYP2C19 inducers,** including **rifampin,** may ↑ risk of bleeding; avoid concurrent use. May ↑ levels and risk of toxicity of **phenytoin, repaglinide, tamoxifen, torsemide, fluvastatin,** and many **NSAIDs**; avoid concurrent use with **repaglinide. CYP2C19 inhibitors,** including **omeprazole,** or **esomeprazole,** may ↓ antiplatelet effects; avoid concurrent use; may consider using **H_2 antagonist** or **pantoprazole. Opioids** may ↓ absorption of clopidogrel and its active metabolite and ↓ its antiplatelet effects; consider using parenteral antiplatelet in patients with acute coronary syndrome if concurrent use of opioids needed.

Drug-Natural Products: ↑ bleeding risk with **anise, arnica, chamomile, clove, fenugreek, feverfew, garlic, ginger, ginkgo, Panax ginseng,** and others.

Route/Dosage

Acute Coronary Syndrome

PO (Adults): 300 mg initially; then 75 mg once daily; aspirin 75–325 mg once daily should be given concurrently.

Recent MI, Stroke, or Peripheral Arterial Disease

PO (Adults): 75 mg once daily.

Availability (generic available)

Tablets: 75 mg, 300 mg.

NURSING IMPLICATIONS

Assessment

- Assess for signs and symptoms of emerging cardiovascular disease such as MI (chest pain, dyspnea, diaphoresis, dizziness, nausea), stroke (weakness, slurred speech, confusion, dizziness), and peripheral arterial disease periodically during therapy.
- Monitor for signs and symptoms of bleeding (pallor of skin and conjunctiva, fatigue, weakness, easy bruising, nosebleeds, bleeding gums, hematuria), including GI bleeding (hematochezia, melena, coffee ground emesis).
- Monitor for signs and symptoms of thrombotic thrombocytopenic purpura (thrombocytopenia, microangiopathic hemolytic anemia, neurologic findings, renal impairment, fever). May rarely occur, even after short exposure (<2 wk). Requires prompt treatment.
- Monitor for development of severe cutaneous adverse reactions, including SJS and TEN. If a severe cutaneous adverse reaction is suspected, interrupt therapy.
- Monitor for signs and symptoms of exanthematous pustulosis (itching; burning; fever; nonfollicular pustular rash on a red base in the armpits or groin, behind the knees, on the inner elbows, or on the face, which then spreads to other areas), which can occur within 1–2 days of taking the medication but can take up to 2 wk; if suspected, discontinue clopidogrel.

Lab Test Considerations

- Monitor CBC with differential periodically during therapy. Neutropenia and thrombocytopenia may rarely occur.
- May ↑ serum bilirubin, hepatic enzymes, total cholesterol, nonprotein nitrogen, and uric acid concentrations.

Implementation

- Do not confuse Plavix with Paxil or Pradaxa.
- Antiplatelet effectiveness depends on activation by the CYP450 system, primarily CYP2C19. Patients homozygous for nonfunctional CYP2C19 alleles produce less active metabolite, reducing efficacy of clopidogrel; prevalence is higher in Asian patients. Testing can identify poor metabolizers, and alternative P2Y12 inhibitors should be considered for these patients.
- Discontinue clopidogrel 5–7 days before planned surgical procedures. If clopidogrel must be temporarily discontinued, restart as soon as possible.

Premature discontinuation of therapy may increase risk of cardiovascular events.

- **PO:** Administer once daily without regard to food.
- Nasogastric administration in critically ill patients after CPR ↑ risk of ↓ bioavailability.

Patient/Family Teaching

- Explain the purpose and side effects of clopidogrel to patient. Instruct patient to take medication exactly as directed. Take missed doses as soon as possible unless almost time for next dose; do not double doses. Do not discontinue clopidogrel without consulting health care provider; may ↑ risk of cardiovascular events. Advise patient to read the *Medication Guide* before starting clopidogrel and with each Rx refill in case of changes.
- Advise patient to notify health care provider promptly if signs and symptoms of bleeding (unexpected bleeding or bleeding that lasts a long time; blood in urine [pink, red, or brown urine], red or black tarry stools, bruises without known cause or that get larger; coughing up blood or blood clots; vomiting blood or vomit looks like coffee grounds); fever, weakness, chills, sore throat, rash, unusual bleeding or bruising, extreme skin paleness, purple skin patches, yellowing of skin or eyes, or neurological changes occur.
- Advise patients of signs and symptoms of skin reactions (fever, flu-like symptoms, mucosal lesions, progressive skin rash, swollen lymph nodes).
- Advise patient to notify health care provider of medication regimen prior to treatment or surgery.
- Caution patient to avoid taking omeprazole or esomeprazole during therapy. Consult health care provider for other options.
- Instruct patient to notify health care provider of all Rx or OTC medications, vitamins, or herbal products being taken and to consult health care provider before taking any other Rx, OTC, or herbal products, especially those containing aspirin or NSAIDs or proton pump inhibitors.
- Rep: Advise women of reproductive potential to notify health care provider if pregnancy is planned or suspected or if breastfeeding. Therapy should not be withheld because of potential concerns regarding effects of clopidogrel on the fetus. Use during labor or delivery ↑ risk of maternal bleeding and hemorrhage. Avoid neuraxial blockade during clopidogrel use due to risk of spinal hematoma. When possible, discontinue clopidogrel 5–7 days prior to labor, delivery, or neuraxial blockade.

Evaluation/Desired Outcomes

- Prevention of stroke, MI, and vascular death in patients at risk.

clotrimazole, See ANTIFUNGALS (TOPICAL).

clotrimazole, See ANTIFUNGALS (VAGINAL).

BEERS

cloZAPine (kloe-za-peen)

Clozaril, ~~FazaClo~~, Versacloz

Classification
Therapeutic: antipsychotics

Indications

Schizophrenia unresponsive to or intolerant of standard therapy with other antipsychotics (treatment refractory). To reduce recurrent suicidal behavior in schizophrenic patients.

Action

Binds to dopamine receptors in the CNS. Also has anticholinergic and alpha-adrenergic blocking activity. Produces fewer extrapyramidal reactions and less tardive dyskinesia than standard antipsychotics but carries high risk of hematologic abnormalities. **Therapeutic Effects:** Diminished schizophrenic behavior. Diminished suicidal behavior.

Pharmacokinetics

Absorption: Well absorbed after oral administration.
Distribution: Rapid and extensive distribution; crosses blood-brain barrier.
Protein Binding: 95%.
Metabolism and Excretion: Mostly metabolized through the liver by the CYP1A2, CYP2D6, and CYP3A4 isoenzymes; the CYP2D6 isoenzyme exhibits genetic polymorphism; ~7% of population may be poor metabolizers and may have significantly ↑ clozapine concentrations and an ↑ risk of adverse effects.
Half-life: 8–12 hr.

TIME/ACTION PROFILE (antipsychotic effect)

ROUTE	ONSET	PEAK	DURATION
PO	unknown	wk	4–12 hr

Contraindications/Precautions

Contraindicated in: Hypersensitivity; Bone marrow depression; Severe CNS depression/coma; Baseline ANC <1500 cells/mm^3 (or <1000 cells/mm^3 for patients with benign ethnic neutropenia [BEN]); Lactation: Lactation.

Use Cautiously in: Long QT syndrome; Risk factors for QT interval prolongation or ventricular arrhythmias (e.g., recent MI, HF, arrhythmias); Hypokalemia or hypomagnesemia; Presence/history of constipation, urinary retention, or prostatic hypertrophy; Angle-closure glaucoma; Malnourished or dehydrated patients; patients with cardiovascular, cerebrovascular, hepatic, or renal disease; or patients on antihypertensives (↑ risk of orthostatic hypotension, bradycardia, and syncope; use lower initial dose, titrate more slowly); Risk factors for stroke (↑ risk of stroke in patients with dementia); Diabetes; Seizure disorder; Patients at risk for falls; Clozapine-associated myocarditis or cardiomyopathy; CYP2D6 poor metabolizer (consider ↓ dose); OB: Use during pregnancy only if potential maternal benefit justifies potential fetal risk; neonates at ↑ risk for extrapyramidal symptoms and withdrawal after delivery when exposed during the 3rd trimester; Pedi: Children <16 yr (safety and effectiveness not established); Geri: Appears on Beers list. ↑ risk of stroke, cognitive decline, and mortality in older adults with dementia. Avoid use in older adults, except for schizophrenia, bipolar disorder, or psychosis in Parkinson disease.

Adverse Reactions/Side Effects

CV: hypotension, tachycardia, bradycardia, CARDIAC ARREST, DEEP VEIN THROMBOSIS (DVT), HF, hypertension, MITRAL VALVE INCOMPETENCE, MYOCARDITIS, PERICARDITIS, QT interval prolongation, syncope, TORSADES DE POINTES, VENTRICULAR ARRHYTHMIAS. **Derm:** rash, sweating. **EENT:** visual disturbances. **Endo:** hyperglycemia. **GI:** constipation, ↑ salivation, abdominal discomfort, dry mouth, GI ISCHEMIA/INFARCTION/NECROSIS, GI OBSTRUCTION, GI PERFORATION, HEPATOTOXICITY, nausea, ulceration, vomiting. **GU:** nocturnal enuresis. **Hemat:** AGRANULOCYTOSIS, NEUTROPENIA. **Metab:** hyperlipidemia, weight gain. **Neuro:** dizziness, sedation, extrapyramidal reactions, NEUROLEPTIC MALIGNANT SYNDROME (NMS), SEIZURES. **Resp:** PULMONARY EMBOLISM (PE). **Misc:** fever.

Interactions

Drug-Drug: ↑ anticholinergic effects with other **anticholinergic drugs**, including **antihistamines**, **quinidine**, **disopyramide**, and **antidepressants**; avoid concurrent use. **Strong CYP1A2 inhibitors**, including **fluvoxamine** or **ciprofloxacin**, may ↑ levels and risk of toxicity; ↓ clozapine dose to ⅓ of the original dose during concurrent use. **Moderate CYP1A2 inhibitors** or **weak CYP1A2 inhibitors**, including **oral contraceptives** or **caffeine**, may ↑ levels and risk of toxicity; consider ↓ clozapine dose. **CYP2D6 inhibitors** or **CYP3A4 inhibitors**, including **cimetidine**, **escitalopram**, **erythromycin**, **paroxetine**, **bupropion**, **fluoxetine**, **quinidine**, **duloxetine**, **terbinafine**, or **sertraline**, may ↑ levels and risk of toxicity; consider ↓ clozapine dose. **Strong CYP3A4 inducers**, including **carbamazepine**, **phenytoin**, or **rifampin**, may ↓ levels and effectiveness; concurrent use not recommended; if concurrent use necessary, ↑ clozapine dose. **Moderate CYP1A2 inducers** or **weak CYP1A2 inducers** may ↓ levels and effectiveness; consider ↑ clozapine dose. **Moderate CYP3A4 inducers** or **weak CYP3A4 inducers** may ↓ levels and effectiveness; consider ↑ clozapine dose. ↑ risk of CNS depression with **alcohol**, **antidepressants**, **antihistamines**, **opioid analgesics**, or **sedative/hypnotics**. ↑ risk of hypotension with **nitrates**, acute ingestion of **alcohol**, or **antihypertensives**. ↑ risk of bone marrow suppression with **antineoplastics** or **radiation therapy**. **Lithium** ↑ risk of adverse CNS reactions, including seizures. ↑ risk of QT interval prolongation with other **QT interval prolonging agents**.

Drug-Natural Products: Caffeine-containing herbs (**cola nut, tea, coffee**) may ↑ levels and risk of toxicity. **St. John's wort** may ↓ levels and effectiveness.

Route/Dosage

PO (Adults): 12.5 mg 1–2 times daily initially; ↑ by 25–50 mg/day over a period of 2 wk up to target dose of 300–450 mg/day. May then be ↑ by up to 100 mg/day once or twice weekly (not to exceed 900 mg/day). Treatment should be continued for ≥2 yr in patients with suicidal behavior.

Availability (generic available)

Tablets (Clozaril): 25 mg, 100 mg. **Orally disintegrating tablets (mint):** 12.5 mg, 25 mg, 100 mg, 150 mg, 200 mg. **Oral suspension (Versacloz):** 50 mg/mL.

NURSING IMPLICATIONS

Assessment

- Monitor mental status (orientation, mood, behavior) before and periodically during therapy.
- Assess orthostatic vitals (HR and BP lying, sitting, standing) frequently during initial dosage adjustment and periodically throughout therapy. Titrate slowly and monitor closely; may cause orthostatic hypotension, bradycardia, syncope, and cardiac arrest.
- Assess weight and body mass index initially and periodically during therapy. Refer as appropriate for nutritional/weight management and medical management.
- Observe patient carefully when administering medication to ensure that medication is actually taken and not hoarded or cheeked.
- Monitor for signs and symptoms of myocarditis (unexplained fatigue, dyspnea, tachypnea, fever, chest pain, palpitations), pericarditis (pericardial friction rub, chest pain relieved by leaning forward), or HF (dyspnea, peripheral edema,

rales/crackles, jugular venous distension, fluid weight gain). Monitor ECG changes (ST-T wave abnormalities, arrhythmias, or tachycardia during 1st months of therapy). If these occur, permanently discontinue clozapine.

- Monitor for onset of akathisia (restlessness or desire to keep moving) and extrapyramidal side effects (*parkinsonian:* difficulty speaking or swallowing, loss of balance control, pill-rolling motion of hands, masklike face, shuffling gait, rigidity, tremors and dystonic muscle spasms, twisting motions, twitching, inability to move eyes, weakness of arms or legs) every 2 mo during therapy and 8–12 wk after therapy has been discontinued. Notify health care provider if these symptoms occur; ↓ in dose or discontinuation of medication may be necessary. Trihexyphenidyl or benztropine may be used to control these symptoms.
- Monitor for possible tardive dyskinesia (uncontrolled rhythmic movement of mouth, face, and extremities; lip smacking or puckering; puffing of cheeks; uncontrolled chewing; rapid or worm-like movements of tongue). Report these symptoms immediately; may be irreversible.
- Monitor frequency and consistency of bowel movements and assess for symptoms of hypomotility (nausea, vomiting, abdominal distension, abdominal pain). Symptoms range from constipation to paralytic ileus; ↑ risk with use of other anticholinergic medications. ↑ fiber and fluids in the diet and laxatives may help to minimize constipation. Prophylactic laxatives may be used for high-risk patients.
- Clozapine ↓ the seizure threshold. Institute seizure precautions for patients with history of seizure disorder.
- Transient fevers may occur, especially during 1st 3 wk of therapy. Fever is usually self-limiting but may require discontinuation of medication. Monitor for signs and symptoms of NMS (hyperpyrexia, muscle rigidity, seizures, altered mental status, evidence of autonomic instability [irregular HR or BP, tachycardia, diaphoresis, cardiac arrhythmia]). Notify health care provider immediately if these symptoms occur.
- Assess respiratory status during therapy. Monitor for signs and symptoms of venous thromboembolism such as PE (chest pain, dyspnea, tachycardia) or DVT (calf pain or tenderness, lower extremity edema, localized warmth or erythema).
- Assess for falls risk. Drowsiness, orthostatic hypotension, and motor and sensory instability ↑ risk. Institute prevention if indicated.
- Monitor for signs and symptoms of hepatotoxicity (fatigue, malaise, anorexia, nausea, jaundice, hyperbilirubinemia, coagulopathy, hepatic encephalopathy). May require permanent discontinuation if combined with ↑ transaminases.

Lab Test Considerations

- Verify negative pregnancy status before starting theory. Monitor CBC with differential before starting therapy. **For the general population (patients without BEN),** ANC must be ≥1500 cells/mm^3 to begin therapy. Monitor ANC once weekly for the 1st 6 mo; then biweekly for the next 6 mo; then, if maintained within acceptable parameters, monthly after 12 mo. *If mild neutropenia (ANC 1000–1499 cells/mm^3) occurs,* continue therapy and monitor ANC 3 times/wk until ANC ≥1500 cells/mm^3; then return to patient's last ANC monitoring interval. *If moderate neutropenia (ANC 500–999 cells/mm^3) occurs,* hold clozapine and obtain hematology consultation. Resume therapy once ANC ≥1000 cells/mm^3. Monitor ANC daily until ANC ≥1000 cells/mm^3, and then 3 times/wk until ANC ≥1500 cells/mm^3. Once ANC ≥1500 cells/mm^3, check ANC once weekly for 4 wk; then return to patient's last ANC monitoring interval. *If severe neutropenia (<500 cells/mm^3) occurs,* discontinue clozapine and obtain hematology consultation. Monitor ANC daily until ANC ≥1000 cells/mm^3 and then 3 times/wk until ANC ≥1500 cells/mm^3. If benefits of treatment outweigh risks, resume clozapine and monitor ANC as if newly initiating therapy. **For patients with BEN,** obtain ≥2 baseline ANC levels before starting therapy. ANC must be ≥1000 cells/mm^3 to begin therapy. Monitor ANC once weekly for the 1st 6 mo; then biweekly for the next 6 mo; then, if maintained within acceptable parameters, monthly after 12 mo. *If neutropenia (ANC 500–999 cells/mm^3) occurs,* obtain hematology consultation and continue therapy. Monitor ANC 3 times/wk until ANC ≥1000 cells/mm^3 and at least at patient's known baseline. Once ANC ≥1000 cells/mm^3, check ANC once weekly for 4 wk; then return to patient's last ANC monitoring interval. *If severe neutropenia (<500/mm^3) occurs,* discontinue clozapine and obtain hematology consultation. Monitor ANC daily until ANC ≥500 cells/mm^3 and then 3 times/wk until ANC ≥1000 cells/mm^3 and at least at patient's known baseline. If benefits of treatment outweigh risks, resume clozapine and monitor ANC as if newly initiating therapy.
- Assess renal function, serum electrolytes, and magnesium prior to initiating and periodically during therapy.
- Assess fasting lipid profile at baseline, Wk 12, and every 5 yr thereafter.

- Monitor fasting blood glucose at baseline, Wk 12, and annually; patients with diabetes should be monitored more frequently.
- Monitor liver function tests periodically during therapy or if clinical signs of hepatotoxicity occur.

Implementation

- Do not confuse clozapine with clonazepam or clonidine. Do not confuse Clozaril with Colazal.
- If clozapine needs to be stopped, discontinue therapy over 1–2 wk. For abrupt discontinuation unrelated to neutropenia, continue ANC monitoring for general population patients until ANC ≥1500/mm^3 and for patients with BEN until their ANC ≥1000/mm^3 or above their baseline. Monitor for recurrence of psychotic symptoms and symptoms related to cholinergic rebound (profuse sweating, headache, nausea, vomiting, diarrhea).
- When restarting clozapine in patients after even a brief interruption in therapy, dose must be ↓ to minimize risk of hypotension, bradycardia, and syncope. If one day's dosing has been missed, resume treatment at 40–50% of the established dose. If 2 days dosing has been missed, resume dose at approximately 25% of established dosage. For longer interruptions, reinitiate with a dose of 12.5 mg once daily or twice daily. If these doses are well tolerated, the dose may be ↑ to previous dose more quickly than recommended for initial treatment.
- **PO:** Administer capsules with food or milk to ↓ gastric irritation.
- Leave orally disintegrating tablet in blister until time of use. Do not push tablet through foil. Just before use, peel foil and gently remove disintegrating tablet. Immediately place tablet in mouth and allow to disintegrate and swallow with saliva. If ½ tablet dose used, destroy other half of tablet.
- Oral solution may be taken without regard to food. Shake bottle for suspension for 10 sec before withdrawing. Use oral syringes and oral adaptor provided for accurate dosing. Do not store dose in syringe; wash between doses.

Patient/Family Teaching

- Explain purpose and side effects of clozapine. Instruct patient to take as directed. If clozapine is stopped for >2 days, do not restart medication; notify health care provider for new dosing instructions. Patients on long-term therapy may need to discontinue gradually over 1–2 wk. Advise patient of need for continued medical follow-up for psychotherapy, eye exams, and laboratory tests. Advise patient to read *Patient Information* before starting and with each Rx refill in case of changes.
- Instruct patient to notify health care provider of all Rx or OTC medications, vitamins, or herbal products being taken and to consult health care provider before taking any other medications. Caution patient to avoid concurrent use of alcohol and other CNS depressants.
- Inform patient of possibility of extrapyramidal symptoms. Instruct patient to report these symptoms immediately.
- Inform patient that cigarette smoking can ↓ levels and effectiveness of clozapine. Risk for relapse ↑ if patient begins or ↑ smoking.
- Advise patient to change positions slowly to minimize orthostatic hypotension. Protect from falls.
- May cause seizures and drowsiness. Caution patient to avoid driving or other activities requiring alertness while taking clozapine.
- Instruct patient to use frequent mouth rinses, good oral hygiene, and sugarless gum or candy to minimize dry mouth.
- Advise patient to notify health care provider of medication regimen before treatment or surgery.
- Instruct patient to notify health care provider promptly if unexplained fatigue, dyspnea, tachypnea, chest pain, palpitations, sore throat, fever, lethargy, weakness, malaise, constipation, or flu-like symptoms occur.
- Rep: May cause fetal harm. Advise women of reproductive potential to notify health care provider if pregnancy is planned or suspected or if breastfeeding. Consider early screening for gestational diabetes if used during pregnancy. Neonates exposed to antipsychotic drugs during 3rd trimester are at risk for extrapyramidal and/or withdrawal symptoms following delivery. Monitor neonates for symptoms of agitation, hypertonia, hypotonia, tremor, somnolence, respiratory distress, excessive sedation, and feeding difficulties. Monitor infants exposed to clozapine through breast milk for excessive sedation. Health care providers are encouraged to advise pregnant patients to enroll in registry that monitors outcomes in women exposed to atypical antipsychotics by calling the National Pregnancy Registry for Atypical Antipsychotics at 1-866-961-2388 or visiting https://womensmentalhealth.org/clinical-and-research-programs/pregnancyregistry/.

Evaluation/Desired Outcomes

- Diminished schizophrenic behavior.
- Diminished suicidal behavior.

REMS HIGH ALERT

codeine (koe-deen)

Classification

Therapeutic: allergy, cold, and cough remedies, antitussives, opioid analgesics

Pharmacologic: opioid agonists

Schedule II III IV V (depends on content)

C

Indications
Mild to moderate pain. Antitussive (in smaller doses).

Action
Binds to opiate receptors in the CNS. Alters the perception of and response to painful stimuli while producing generalized CNS depression. Decreases cough reflex. Decreases GI motility. **Therapeutic Effects:** Decreased severity of pain. Suppression of the cough reflex.

Pharmacokinetics
Absorption: 50% absorbed from the GI tract.
Distribution: Widely distributed to tissues.
Metabolism and Excretion: Mostly metabolized by the liver via the CYP2D6 isoenzyme; 10% converted to morphine; the CYP2D6 isoenzyme exhibits genetic polymorphism (some patients [1–10% White patients, 3% Black patients, 16–28% North African/Ethiopian/Arabic patients] may be ultra-rapid metabolizers and may have ↑ morphine concentrations and an ↑ risk of adverse effects); 5–15% excreted unchanged in urine.
Half-life: 2.5–4 hr.

TIME/ACTION PROFILE (analgesia)

ROUTE	ONSET	PEAK	DURATION
PO	30–45 min	60–120 min	4 hr

Contraindications/Precautions
Contraindicated in: Hypersensitivity; Significant respiratory depression; Acute or severe bronchial asthma (in unmonitored setting or in absence of resuscitative equipment); Known or suspected GI obstruction (including paralytic ileus); Concurrent use of MAO inhibitors (or use within the past 14 days); Ultra-rapid CYP2D6 metabolizers of codeine; Lactation: Lactation; Pedi: Children <12 yr, children <18 yr following tonsillectomy and/or adenoidectomy, and children 12–18 yr who are postoperative; have obstructive sleep apnea, obesity, severe pulmonary disease, or neuromuscular disease; or are taking other medications that cause respiratory depression (↑ risk of respiratory depression and death).
Use Cautiously in: Personal or family history of substance use disorder or mental illness; Head trauma; ↑ intracranial pressure; Severe renal impairment; Severe hepatic impairment; Severe pulmonary disease; Hypothyroidism; Adrenal insufficiency; Prostatic hyperplasia; Undiagnosed abdominal pain; OB: Avoid chronic use; prolonged use of opioids during pregnancy can result in neonatal opioid withdrawal syndrome; Geri: Older adults may be more susceptible to CNS depression and constipation (dose ↓ required).

Adverse Reactions/Side Effects
CV: hypotension, bradycardia. **Derm:** flushing, sweating. **EENT:** blurred vision, diplopia, miosis. **GI:** constipation, nausea, vomiting. **GU:** urinary retention. **Neuro:** confusion, sedation, dysphoria, euphoria, floating feeling, hallucinations, headache, unusual dreams. **Resp:** RESPIRATORY DEPRESSION (INCLUDING CENTRAL SLEEP APNEA AND SLEEP-RELATED HYPOXEMIA). **Misc:** allodynia, opioid-induced hyperalgesia, physical dependence, psychological dependence, tolerance.

Interactions
Drug-Drug: MAO inhibitors ↑ risk of adverse reactions; concurrent use or use within previous 14 days contraindicated. Use with **benzodiazepines** or other **CNS depressants**, including other **opioids**, **nonbenzodiazepine sedative/hypnotics**, **anxiolytics**, **general anesthetics**, **muscle relaxants**, **antipsychotics**, and **alcohol**, may cause profound sedation, respiratory depression, coma, and death; reserve concurrent use for when alternative treatment options are inadequate. **CYP3A4 inhibitors**, including **erythromycin**, **clarithromycin**, **ketoconazole**, **itraconazole**, and **protease inhibitors**, may ↑ levels and risk of respiratory depression. **CYP3A4 inducers** may ↓ levels and effectiveness. **CYP2D6 inhibitors**, including **amiodarone** and **quinidine**, may ↓ analgesic effects. **Mixed agonist/antagonist analgesics**, including **nalbuphine** or **butorphanol**, and **partial agonist analgesics**, including **buprenorphine**, may ↓ meperidine's analgesic effects and/or precipitate opioid withdrawal in physically dependent patients. Drugs that affect serotonergic neurotransmitter systems, including **tricyclic antidepressants**, **SSRIs**, **SNRIs**, **MAO inhibitors**, **TCAs**, **tramadol**, **trazodone**, **mirtazapine**, **$5HT_3$ receptor antagonists**, **linezolid**, **methylene blue**, and **triptans**, may ↑ risk of serotonin syndrome.
Drug-Natural Products: Kava-kava, **valerian**, **skullcap**, **chamomile**, or **hops** can ↑ risk of CNS depression.

Route/Dosage
PO (Adults): *Analgesic:* 15–60 mg every 4 hr as needed (not to exceed 360 mg/day). *Antitussive:* 10–20 mg every 4–6 hr as needed (not to exceed 120 mg/day).

Renal Impairment
(Adults): *CCr 10–50 mL/min:* Administer 75% of the dose; *CCr <10 mL/min:* Administer 50% of the dose.

Availability (generic available)
Tablets: 15 mg, 30 mg, 60 mg.

NURSING IMPLICATIONS

Assessment

- Assess BP, HR, and respiratory rate before and periodically during administration. If respiratory rate <10/min, assess level of sedation. Physical stimulation may be sufficient to prevent significant hypoventilation. Dose may need to be ↓ by 25–50%. Initial drowsiness will diminish with continued use. Monitor for respiratory depression, especially during initiation or following dose ↑; serious, life-threatening, or fatal respiratory depression may occur. May cause sleep-related breathing disorders (central sleep apnea, sleep-related hypoxemia).
- Assess bowel function routinely. Prevention of constipation should be instituted with ↑ intake of fluids, bulk, and laxatives to minimize constipating effects. Stimulant laxatives should be administered routinely if opioid use >2–3 days, unless contraindicated. Consider drugs for opioid-induced constipation.
- Assess risk for opioid addiction, abuse, or misuse prior to administration.
- **Pain:** Assess type, location, and intensity of pain before and 1 hr (peak) after administration. When titrating opioid doses, ↑ of 25–50% should be administered until there is either a 50% ↓ in the patient's pain rating on a numerical or visual analogue scale or the patient reports satisfactory pain relief. A repeat dose can be safely administered at the time of the peak if previous dose is ineffective and side effects are minimal.
- An equianalgesic chart (see Appendix I) should be used when changing routes or when changing from one opioid to another.
- Monitor patients for opioid-induced hyperalgesia occurs when an opioid paradoxically causes an ↑ in pain, or an ↑ in sensitivity to pain. Opioid-induced hyperalgesia differs from tolerance, which is the need for ↑ doses of opioids to maintain a defined effect. Symptoms of opioid-induced hyperalgesia include ↑ levels of pain upon opioid dosage ↑, ↓ levels of pain upon opioid dosage ↓, or pain from ordinarily nonpainful stimuli. If opioid-induced hyperalgesia suspected, consider ↓ codeine dose.
- Prolonged use may lead to physical and psychological dependence and tolerance, which should not prevent patient from receiving adequate analgesia. Most patients who receive codeine for pain do not develop psychological dependence. If progressively higher doses are required, consider conversion to a stronger opioid.
- **Cough:** Assess cough and lung sounds during antitussive use.

Lab Test Considerations

- May cause ↑ amylase and lipase concentrations.

Toxicity and Overdose

- If an opioid antagonist is required to reverse respiratory depression or coma, naloxone is the antidote. Dilute the 0.4-mg ampule of naloxone in 10 mL of 0.9% NaCl and administer 0.5 mL (0.02 mg) by IV push every 2 min. For children and patients weighing <40 kg, dilute 0.1 mg of naloxone in 10 mL of 0.9% NaCl for a concentration of 10 mcg/mL and administer 0.5 mcg/kg every 2 min. Titrate dose to avoid withdrawal, seizures, and severe pain.

Implementation

- ***High Alert:*** Accidental overdosage of opioid analgesics has resulted in fatalities. Before administering, clarify all ambiguous orders.
- Explain therapeutic value of medication before administration to enhance the analgesic effect.
- Regularly administered doses may be more effective than prn administration. Analgesic is more effective if given before pain becomes severe.
- Coadministration with nonopioid analgesics may have additive analgesic effects and permit lower doses.
- ***REMS:*** FDA strongly encourages health care providers to complete a REMS-compliant education program that includes all the elements of the FDA Education *Blueprint for Health Care Providers Involved in the Management or Support of Patients with Pain,* available at www.fda.gov/OpioidAnalgesicREMSBlueprint. Information on programs can be found at 1-800-503-0784 or www.opioidanalgesicrems.com.
- Discuss availability of naloxone for emergency treatment of opioid overdose with the patient and caregiver and assess the potential need for access to naloxone, both when initiating and renewing therapy, especially if patient has household members (including children) or other close contacts at risk for accidental exposure or overdose. Consider prescribing naloxone, based on the patient's risk factors for overdose, such as concurrent use of CNS depressants, a history of opioid use disorder, or prior opioid overdose. However, the presence of risk factors for overdose should not prevent the proper management of pain in any patient.
- When combined with nonopioid analgesics (aspirin, acetaminophen), #2 = 15 mg, #3 = 30 mg, #4 = 60 mg codeine. Codeine as an individual drug is a Schedule II substance. In combination with other drugs, tablet form is Schedule III, and elixir or cough suppressant is Schedule V (see Appendix H).
- **PO:** Oral doses may be administered with food or milk to ↓ GI irritation.
- If administered regularly for ≥1 wk, discontinue by tapering dose gradually by a small enough increment (not >10%–25% of total daily dose) to avoid withdrawal symptoms, and proceed with

dose-lowering at an interval of every 2–4 wk or longer. Monitor for withdrawal symptoms (restlessness; lacrimation; rhinorrhea; yawning; perspiration; chills; myalgia; mydriasis; irritability; anxiety; backache; joint pain; weakness; abdominal cramps; insomnia; nausea; anorexia; vomiting; diarrhea; ↑ BP, respiratory rate, or HR) during taper. If withdrawal symptoms occur, it may be necessary to pause the taper for a period of time or raise the dose of the opioid analgesic to the previous dose and then proceed with a slower taper. Monitor for changes in mood, emergence of suicidal thoughts, or use of other substances.

Patient/Family Teaching

- Instruct patient on how and when to ask for and take pain medication. Do not stop abruptly without consulting health care provider.
- ***REMS:*** Instruct patient on risk of addiction, abuse, and misuse, which could lead to death. Discuss safe use, risks, and proper storage and disposal of opioid analgesics with patients and caregivers with each Rx. The Patient Counseling Guide is available at www.fda.gov/OpioidAnalgesicREMSPCG. Advise patient not to share codeine with others and to protect from theft or misuse.
- Advise patient that codeine is a drug with known abuse potential. Protect it from theft, and never give to anyone other than the individual for whom it was prescribed. Store out of sight and reach of children, and in a location not accessible by others.
- Educate patients and caregivers on how to recognize respiratory depression and emphasize the importance of calling 911 or getting emergency medical help right away in the event of a known or suspected overdose. Inform patients and caregivers about various ways to obtain naloxone as permitted by individual state naloxone dispensing and prescribing requirements or guidelines (by prescription, directly from a pharmacist, or as part of a community-based program).
- May cause drowsiness or dizziness. Advise patient to call for assistance when ambulating or smoking. Caution ambulatory patient to avoid driving or other activities requiring alertness until response to medication is known.
- Advise patient to change positions slowly to minimize orthostatic hypotension.
- Caution patient to avoid concurrent use of alcohol or other CNS depressants with this medication.
- Encourage patient to turn, cough, and breathe deeply every 2 hr to prevent atelectasis.
- Advise patient that good oral hygiene, frequent mouth rinses, and sugarless gum or candy may decrease dry mouth.
- Rep: Advise patient to notify health care provider if pregnancy is planned or suspected or if breastfeeding. Inform patient of potential for neonatal opioid withdrawal syndrome with prolonged use during pregnancy. Monitor neonate for signs and symptoms of withdrawal symptoms (irritability, hyperactivity and abnormal sleep pattern, high-pitched cry, tremor, vomiting, diarrhea, failure to gain weight); usually occur the first days after birth. Monitor infants exposed to codeine through breast milk for excess sedation and respiratory depression.

Evaluation/Desired Outcomes

- Decrease in severity of pain without a significant alteration in level of consciousness or respiratory status.
- Suppression of cough.

HIGH ALERT

colchicine (kol-chi-seen)

Colcrys, Gloperba, Lodoco, Mitigare

Classification

Therapeutic: antigout agents

Indications

Treatment of gout flares (Colcrys and generic tablets only). Prophylaxis of gout flares (Gloperba, Mitigare, and generic capsules only). Familial Mediterranean fever (Colcrys and generic tablets only). To reduce the risk of MI, stroke, coronary revascularization, and cardiovascular death in patients with established atherosclerotic disease or with multiple risk factors for cardiovascular disease (Lodoco only).

Action

Interferes with the functions of WBCs in initiating and perpetuating the inflammatory response to monosodium urate crystals. **Therapeutic Effects:** Decreased pain and inflammation in acute attacks of gout. Reduced number of attacks of gout and familial Mediterranean fever. Reduction in risk of MI, stroke, coronary revascularization, and cardiovascular death in patients with established atherosclerotic disease or with multiple risk factors for cardiovascular disease.

Pharmacokinetics

Absorption: 45% absorbed from the GI tract; then re-enters GI tract from biliary secretions, when more absorption may occur.
Distribution: Extensively distributed to tissues.
Metabolism and Excretion: Partially metabolized by the liver by the CYP3A4 isoenzyme; also a substrate for P-glycoprotein (P-gp). Secreted in bile

back into GI tract; eliminated in the feces. 40–65% excreted in the urine as unchanged drug.
Half-life: 19–31 hr.

TIME/ACTION PROFILE (anti-inflammatory activity)

ROUTE	ONSET	PEAK	DURATION
PO	12 hr	24–72 hr	unknown

Contraindications/Precautions

Contraindicated in: Hypersensitivity; Concurrent use of P-gp inhibitors or strong CYP3A4 inhibitors in patients with renal or hepatic impairment (generic tablets or Colcrys only); Concurrent use of drugs that inhibit both P-gp and CYP3A4 in patients with renal or hepatic impairment (Gloperba or Mitigare only); Concurrent use of strong P-glycoprotein inhibitors or strong CYP3A4 inhibitors (Lodoco only); Presence of both renal and hepatic impairment (Gloperba and Mitigare only); Renal failure (CCr <15 mL/min) (Lodoco only); Severe hepatic impairment (Lodoco only); Pre-existing blood dyscrasias (Lodoco only).
Use Cautiously in: Renal impairment (↓ dose); OB: Use during pregnancy only if potential maternal benefit justifies potential fetal risk; Lactation: Use while breastfeeding only if potential maternal benefit justifies potential risk to infant; Pedi: Safety and effectiveness not established in children (for gout or cardiovascular risk reduction); Geri: ↑ risk of toxicity in older adults with renal impairment.

Adverse Reactions/Side Effects

Derm: alopecia. **GI:** diarrhea, nausea, vomiting, abdominal pain. **Hemat:** AGRANULOCYTOSIS, APLASTIC ANEMIA, leukopenia, thrombocytopenia. **MS:** myalgia, RHABDOMYOLYSIS. **Neuro:** peripheral neuritis.

Interactions

Drug-Drug: **Strong CYP3A4 inhibitors**, including **atazanavir**, **clarithromycin**, **darunavir/ritonavir**, **itraconazole**, **ketoconazole**, **lopinavir/ritonavir**, **nefazodone**, **nelfinavir**, **ritonavir**, or **tipranavir/ritonavir**, may ↑ levels and risk of toxicity; ↓ colchicine dose in patients with normal renal or hepatic function; concurrent use in patients with renal or hepatic impairment is contraindicated; concurrent use with Lodoco is contraindicated. **Strong P-gp inhibitors**, including **cyclosporine** or **ranolazine**, may ↑ levels and risk of toxicity; ↓ colchicine dose in patients with normal renal or hepatic function; concurrent use in patients with renal or hepatic impairment is contraindicated; concurrent use with Lodoco is contraindicated. **Moderate CYP3A4 inhibitors**, including **aprepitant**, **diltiazem**, **erythromycin**, **fluconazole**, **fosamprenavir**, or **verapamil**, may ↑ levels and risk of toxicity; ↓ colchicine dose in patients with normal renal or hepatic function; avoid concurrent use of Lodoco in patients with renal or hepatic impairment. Additive bone marrow depression may occur with **bone marrow depressants** or **radiation therapy**. ↑ risk of rhabdomyolysis with **HMG-CoA reductase inhibitors**, **gemfibrozil**, **fenofibrate**, **digoxin**, or **cyclosporine**. Additive adverse GI effects with **NSAIDs**. May cause reversible malabsorption of **vitamin B_{12}**.
Drug-Food: Grapefruit juice may ↑ levels and risk of toxicity; ↓ colchicine dose (for all formulations, except Lodoco); avoid concurrent use with Lodoco.

Route/Dosage

Treatment of Gout Flares (Colcrys and Generic Tablets Only)

PO (Adults): 1.2 mg initially; then 0.6 mg 1 hr later (maximum dose of 1.8 mg in 1 hr); *Concurrent use of strong CYP3A4 inhibitors in patients with normal renal and hepatic function (atazanavir, clarithromycin, darunavir/ritonavir, itraconazole, ketoconazole, lopinavir/ritonavir, nefazodone, nelfinavir, ritonavir, tipranavir/ritonavir):* 0.6 mg initially; then 0.3 mg 1 hr later (do not repeat treatment course for ≥3 days); *Concurrent use of moderate CYP3A4 inhibitors (aprepitant, diltiazem, erythromycin, fluconazole, fosamprenavir, grapefruit juice, verapamil):* 1.2 mg as single dose (do not repeat for ≥3 days); *Concurrent use of strong P-gp inhibitors (cyclosporine, ranolazine) in patients with normal renal and hepatic function:* 0.6 mg as single dose (do not repeat for ≥3 days).

Renal Impairment

PO (Adults): *CCr <30 mL/min:* 1.2 mg initially; then 0.6 mg 1 hr later; do not repeat treatment course for ≥2 wk; *Dialysis:* 0.6 mg as single dose; do not repeat treatment course for ≥2 wk.

Prevention of Gout Flares (Gloperba, Mitigare, and Generic Capsules Only)

PO (Adults): 0.6 mg once or twice daily; *Concurrent use of strong CYP3A4 inhibitors (atazanavir, clarithromycin, darunavir/ritonavir, itraconazole, ketoconazole, lopinavir/ritonavir, nefazodone, nelfinavir, ritonavir, tipranavir/ritonavir) or strong P-gp inhibitors (cyclosporine, ranolazine) in patients with normal renal and hepatic function:* If original dose was 0.6 mg twice daily, ↓ to 0.3 mg once daily; if original dose was 0.6 mg once daily, ↓ to 0.3 mg every other day; *Concurrent use of moderate CYP3A4 inhibitors (aprepitant, diltiazem, erythromycin, fluconazole, fosamprenavir, grapefruit juice, verapamil):* If original dose was 0.6 mg twice daily, ↓ to 0.3 mg twice daily or 0.6 mg once daily; if original dose was 0.6 mg once daily, ↓ to 0.3 mg once daily.

C

Renal Impairment

PO (Adults): *CCr <30 mL/min:* 0.3 mg once daily; *Dialysis:* 0.3 mg twice weekly.

Familial Mediterranean Fever (Colcrys and Generic Tablets Only)

PO (Adults and Children >12 yr): 1.2–2.4 mg/day (in 1–2 divided doses); may ↑ or ↓ dose in 0.3-mg/day increments based on safety and efficacy; *Concurrent use of strong CYP3A4 inhibitors (atazanavir, clarithromycin, darunavir/ritonavir, itraconazole, ketoconazole, lopinavir/ritonavir, nefazodone, nelfinavir, ritonavir, tipranavir/ritonavir) or strong P-gp inhibitors (cyclosporine, ranolazine) in patients with normal renal and hepatic function:* Do not exceed 0.6 mg/day (may be given as 0.3 mg twice daily); *Concurrent use of moderate CYP3A4 inhibitors (aprepitant, diltiazem, erythromycin, fluconazole, fosamprenavir, grapefruit juice, verapamil):* Do not exceed 1.2 mg/day (may be given as 0.6 mg twice daily).

PO (Children 6–12 yr): 0.9–1.8 mg/day (in 1–2 divided doses).

PO (Children 4–6 yr): 0.3–1.8 mg/day (in 1–2 divided doses).

Renal Impairment

PO (Adults): *CCr 30–50 mL/min:* Dose ↓ may be necessary; *CCr <30 mL/min or dialysis:* 0.3 mg/day.

Reduction in Risk of MI, Stroke, Coronary Revascularization, and Cardiovascular Death (Lodoco only)

PO (Adults): 0.5 mg once daily.

Availability (generic available)

Tablets (Colcrys): 0.6 mg. **Tablets (Lodoco):** 0.5 mg. **Capsules (Mitigare):** 0.6 mg. **Oral solution (cherry flavor) (Gloperba):** 0.6 mg/5 mL. ***In combination with:*** probenecid.

NURSING IMPLICATIONS

Assessment

- Monitor intake and output. Fluids should be encouraged to promote a urinary output of ≥2000 mL/day.
- **Gout:** Assess involved joints for pain, mobility, and edema throughout therapy. During initiation of therapy, monitor for drug response every 1–2 hr.
- **Familial Mediterranean fever:** Assess for signs and symptoms of familial Mediterranean fever (abdominal pain, chest pain, fever, chills, recurrent joint pain, red and swollen skin lesions) periodically during therapy.

Lab Test Considerations

- In patients receiving prolonged therapy, monitor baseline and periodic CBC with differential; report significant ↓ in values. May cause ↓ platelet count, leukopenia, aplastic anemia, and agranulocytosis.
- May ↑ AST and alkaline phosphatase.
- May cause false-positive results for urine hemoglobin.
- May interfere with results of urinary 17-hydroxycorticosteroid concentrations.

Toxicity and Overdose

- ***High Alert:*** Assess patient for toxicity (muscle pain or weakness; tingling or numbness in fingers or toes; pale or gray color to lips, tongue, or palms of hands; severe diarrhea or vomiting; unusual bleeding, bruising, sore throat, fatigue, malaise, or weakness or tiredness). If these symptoms occur, discontinue colchicine and treat symptomatically.

Implementation

- Do not confuse colchicine with Cortrosyn.
- Intermittent therapy with 3 days between courses may be used to ↓ risk of toxicity.
- **PO:** Administer without regard to meals.
- Use an accurate calibrated measuring device for solution; a teaspoon is not accurate. Oral solution is slightly hazy red liquid with a cherry odor.

Patient/Family Teaching

- Explain the purpose and side effects to patient. Instruct patient to take colchicine as directed. Review medication administration schedule. Take missed doses as soon as remembered unless almost time for next dose. Do not double doses. Advise patient to read *Patient Information* before starting and with each Rx refill in case of changes.
- Instruct patients taking prophylactic doses not to ↑ to therapeutic doses during an acute attack to prevent toxicity. An NSAID or corticosteroid should be used to treat acute attacks.
- Advise patient to avoid grapefruit and grapefruit juice during therapy; may ↑ risk of toxicity.
- Advise patient to follow recommendations of health care professional regarding weight loss, diet, and alcohol consumption.
- Instruct patient to report muscle pain or weakness; tingling or numbness in fingers or toes; pale or gray color to lips, tongue, or palms of hands; severe diarrhea or vomiting; or unusual bleeding, bruising, sore throat, fatigue, malaise, or weakness or tiredness promptly. Hold colchicine if symptoms of toxicity occur.
- Instruct patient to notify health care professional of all Rx or OTC medications, vitamins, or herbal products being taken and to notify health care professional before taking any other Rx, OTC, or herbal products.

- Surgery may precipitate an acute attack of gout. Advise patient to confer with health care professional regarding dose 3 days before surgical or dental procedures.
- Rep: Advise women of reproductive potential to notify health care professional if pregnancy is planned or suspected or if breastfeeding. Monitor breastfed infants for diarrhea. Inform men that colchicine may cause infertility that reverses when colchicine is stopped.

Evaluation/Desired Outcomes

- Decrease in pain and swelling in affected joints within 12 hr.
- Relief of symptoms within 24–48 hr.
- Prevention of acute gout attacks.
- Reduced number of attacks of familial Mediterranean fever.
- Reduction in risk of MI, stroke, coronary revascularization, and cardiovascular death in patients with established atherosclerotic disease or with multiple risk factors for cardiovascular disease.

CONTRACEPTIVES, HORMONAL

MONOPHASIC ORAL CONTRACEPTIVES

estetrol/drospirenone (**es**-te-trol/droe-**spy**-re-nown)
Nextstellis

ethinyl estradiol/desogestrel (**eth**-in-il es-tra-**dye**-ole/dess-oh-**jess**-trel)
Apri-28, Averi, Cyred EQ, Enskyce, Isibloom, Juleber, Kalliga, Reclipsen

ethinyl estradiol/drospirenone (**eth**-in-il es-tra-**dye**-ole/droe-**spy**-re-nown)
Beyaz, Jasmiel, Lo-Zumandimine, Loryna, Nikki, Safyral, Syeda, Tydemy, Vestura, Yasmin, Yaz, Zumandimine

ethinyl estradiol/ethynodiol (**eth**-in-il es-tra-**dye**-ole/e-thye-noe-**dye**-ole)
Kelnor 1/35, Kelnor 1/50, Zovia 1/35

ethinyl estradiol/levonorgestrel (**eth**-in-il es-tra-**dye**-ole/lee-voe-nor-**jess**-trel)
Afirmelle, Altavera, Aubra EQ, Aviane, Ayuna, Balcoltra, Chateal EQ, Falmina, Joyeaux, Kurvelo, Lessina, Levora-28, Lutera, Marlissa, Portia-28, Sronyx, Tyblume, Vienva

ethinyl estradiol/norethindrone (**eth**-in-il es-tra-**dye**-ole/nor-eth-**in**-drone)
Alyacen 1/35, Aurovela 1/20, Aurovela 1.5/30, Aurovela 24 Fe, Aurovela Fe 1/20, Aurovela Fe 1.5/30, Balziva, Blisovi 24 Fe, Blisovi Fe 1/20, Blisovi Fe 1.5/30, Briellyn, Charlotte 24 Fe, Cyonanz, Dasetta 1/35, Femlyv, Finzala, Fyavolv, Gemmily, Generess Fe, Hailey 1.5/30, Hailey 24 Fe, Hailey Fe 1/20, Hailey Fe 1.5/30, Jinteli, Junel 1/20, Junel 1.5/30, Junel Fe 1/20, Junel Fe 1.5/30, Junel Fe 24, Kaitlib Fe, Larin 1/20, Larin 1.5/30, Larin 24 Fe, Larin Fe 1/20, Larin Fe 1.5/30, Layolis Fe, Loestrin 1/20, Loestrin 1.5/30, Loestrin Fe 1/20, Loestrin Fe 1.5/30, Merzee, Mibelas 24 Fe, Microgestin 1/20, Microgestin 1.5/30, Microgestin 24 Fe, Microgestin Fe 1/20, Microgestin Fe 1.5/30, Minastrin 24 Fe, Necon 0.5/35, Nexesta Fe, Nortrel 0.5/35, Nortrel 1/35, Nylia 1/35, Oshih, Philith, Tarina 24 Fe, Tarina Fe 1/20 EQ, Taysofy, Taytulla, Tilia Fe, Vyfemla, Wera, Wymzya Fe, Zenchent Fe

ethinyl estradiol/norgestimate (**eth**-in-il es-tra-**dye**-ole/nor-**jes**-ti-mate)
Estarylla, Mili, Mono-Linyah, Nymyo, Previfem, Sprintec-28, VyLibra

ethinyl estradiol/norgestrel (**eth**-in-il es-tra-**dye**-ole/nor-**jess**-trel)
Cryselle-28, Elinest, Low-Ogestrel

BIPHASIC ORAL CONTRACEPTIVES

ethinyl estradiol/desogestrel (**eth**-in-il es-tra-**dye**-ole/dess-oh-**jess**-trel)
Azurette, Bekyree, Kariva, Mircette, Pimtrea, Simliya, Viorele, Volnea

ethinyl estradiol/norethindrone (**eth**-in-il es-tra-**dye**-ole/nor-eth-**in**-drone)
Lo Loestrin Fe

TRIPHASIC ORAL CONTRACEPTIVES

ethinyl estradiol/desogestrel (**eth**-in-il es-tra-**dye**-ole/dess-oh-**jess**-trel)
Velivet

ethinyl estradiol/levonorgestrel (**eth**-in-il ess-tra-**dye**-ole/lee-voe-nor-**jess**-trel)
Enpresse-28, Levonest, Trivora-28

ethinyl estradiol/norethindrone (**eth**-in-il es-tra-**dye**-ole/nor-eth-**in**-drone)
Alyacen 7/7/7, Aranelle, Dasetta 7/7/7, Leena, Nortrel 7/7/7, Nylia 7/7/7, Tri-Legest Fe

ethinyl estradiol/norgestimate (**eth**-in-il es-tra-**dye**-ole/nor-**jess**-ti-mate)
Tri-Estarylla, Tri-Linyah, Tri-Lo-Estarylla, Tri-Lo-Marzia, Tri-Lo-Mili, Tri-Lo-Sprintec, Tri-Mili, Tri-Nymyo, Tri-Sprintec, Tri-VyLibra, Tri-VyLibra Lo

FOURPHASIC ORAL CONTRACEPTIVES

estradiol valerate/dienogest (es-tra-**dye**-ole **val**-er-ate/dye-**en**-oh-jest)
Natazia

EXTENDED-CYCLE ORAL CONTRACEPTIVE

ethinyl estradiol/levonorgestrel (**eth**-in-il ess-tra-**dye**-ole/lee-voe-nor-**jess**-trel)
Amethia, Amethyst, Ashlyna, Camrese, Camrese Lo, Daysee, Dolishale, Iclevia, Introvale, Jaimiess, Jolessa, LoJaimiess, LoSeasonique, Quartette, Rivelsa, Seasonique, Setlakin, Simpesse

PROGESTIN-ONLY ORAL CONTRACEPTIVES

norethindrone (nor-eth-**in**-drone)
Aygestin, Camila, Deblitane, Emzahh, Errin, Heather, Incassia, Jencycla, Lyleq, Nora-BE, Sharobel

drospirenone
Slynd

norgestrel
Opill

CONTRACEPTIVE IMPLANT

etonogestrel (e-toe-no-**jess**-trel)
Nexplanon

EMERGENCY CONTRACEPTIVE

levonorgestrel (**lee**-voe-nor-**jess**-trel)
Aftera, Athentia Next, Curae, EContra One-Step, Her Style, My Choice, My Way, New Day, Opcicon One-Step, Plan B One-Step, Take Action

ulipristal (**u-li-priss-tal**)
Ella

INJECTABLE CONTRACEPTIVE

medroxyprogesterone (me-**drox**-ee-proe-**jess**-te-rone)
Depo-Provera, Depo-subQ Provera 104

INTRAUTERINE CONTRACEPTIVE

levonorgestrel (**lee**-voe-nor-**jess**-trel)
Kyleena, Liletta, Mirena, Skyla

VAGINAL RING CONTRACEPTIVE

ethinyl estradiol/etonogestrel (**eth**-in-il ess-tra-**dye**-ole/e-toe-noe-**jess**-trel)
EluRyng, Enilloring, Haloette, NuvaRing

TRANSDERMAL CONTRACEPTIVE

ethinyl estradiol/levonorgestrel (**eth**-in-il ess-tra-**dye**-ole/**lee**-voe-nor-**jess**-trel)
Twirla

ethinyl estradiol/norelgestromin
(**eth**-in-il ess-tra-**dye**-ole/nor-el-**jess**-troe-min)
Xulane, Zafemy
Classification
Therapeutic: contraceptive hormones

Indications

Prevention of pregnancy. Regulation of menstrual cycle. Emergency contraception (some products). Treatment of heavy menstrual bleeding in women who choose to use intrauterine contraception as their method of contraception. Treatment of heavy menstrual bleeding in women who choose to use an oral contraceptive as their method of contraception. Treatment of premenstrual dysphoric disorder. Management of acne in women >14 yr who desire contraception, have no health problems, and have failed topical treatment. Increase folate levels in women who desire oral contraception to reduce the risk of neural tube defects in a pregnancy that occurs while taking or shortly after discontinuing the product.

Action

Monophasic Oral Contraceptives: Provide a fixed dosage of estrogen/progestin over a 21-day cycle. Ovulation is inhibited by suppression of follicle-stimulating hormone (FSH) and luteinizing hormone (LH). May alter cervical mucus and the endometrial environment, preventing penetration by sperm and implantation of the egg. **Biphasic Oral Contraceptives:** Ovulation is inhibited by suppression of FSH and LH. May alter cervical mucus and the endometrial environment, preventing penetration by sperm and implantation of the egg. In addition, smaller dose of progestin in phase 1 allows for proliferation of endometrium. Larger amount in phase 2 allows for adequate secretory development. **Triphasic Oral Contraceptives:** Ovulation is inhibited by suppression of FSH and LH. May alter cervical mucus and the endometrial environment, preventing penetration by sperm and implantation of the egg. Varying doses of estrogen/progestin may more closely mimic natural hormonal fluctuations. **Fourphasic Oral Contraceptives:** Ovulation is inhibited by suppression of FSH and LH. May alter cervical mucus and the endometrial environment, preventing penetration by sperm and implantation of the egg. Doses of estrogen decrease while doses of progestin increase over the 28-day cycle. **Extended Cycle:** Provides continuous estrogen/progestin for 84 days, then off for 7 days (low-dose estrogen-only tablet taken during these 7 days with LoSeasonique and Seasonique), resulting in 4 menstrual periods/yr. **Progressive Estrogen:** Contains constant amount of progestin with 3 progressive doses of estrogen. **Progestin-Only Contraceptives/Contraceptive Implant/Intrauterine Levonorgestrel/Medroxyprogesterone Injection:** Mechanism not clearly known. May alter cervical mucus and the endometrial environment, preventing penetration by sperm and implantation of the egg. Ovulation may also be suppressed. **Emergency Contraceptive Pills:** Inhibit ovulation/fertilization; may also alter tubal transport of sperm/egg and prevent implantation. **Vaginal Ring, Transdermal Patch:** Inhibits ovulation, decreases sperm entry into uterus, decreases likelihood of implantation. **Anti-Acne effect:** Combination of estrogen/progestin may increase sex hormone binding globulin, resulting in decreased unbound testosterone, which may be a cause of acne. **Therapeutic Effects:** Prevention of pregnancy. Decreased severity of acne. Decrease in menstrual blood loss. Decrease in premenstrual dysphoric disorder. Decrease in vasomotor symptoms or symptoms of vulvar and vaginal atrophy due to menopause. Increase in folate levels and prevention of neural tube defects.

Pharmacokinetics

Absorption: *Ethinyl estradiol:* Rapidly absorbed; *Norethindrone:* 65% absorbed; *Desogestrel and levonorgestrel:* 100% absorbed; *Dienogest:* 91% absorbed. Others are well absorbed after oral administration. Slowly absorbed from implant, SUBQ, or IM injection. Some absorption follows intrauterine implantation.
Distribution: Unknown.
Protein Binding: *Ethinyl estradiol:* 97–98%; *Drospirenone:* 97%; *Dienogest:* 90%; *Ulipristal:* >94%.
Metabolism and Excretion: *Ethinyl estradiol and norethindrone:* Undergo extensive first-pass hepatic metabolism. *Desogestrel:* Is rapidly metabolized to 3-keto-desogestrel, the active metabolite. Most agents are metabolized by the liver.
Half-life: *Ethinyl estradiol:* 6–20 hr; *Levonorgestrel:* 45 hr; *Norethindrone:* 5–14 hr; *Desogestrel (metabolite):* 38 ± 20 hr; *Drospirenone:* 30 hr; *Norgestimate (metabolite):* 12–20 hr; *Dienogest:* 11 hr; *Others:* unknown; *Ulipristal:* 32 hr.

TIME/ACTION PROFILE (prevention of pregnancy)

ROUTE	ONSET	PEAK	DURATION
PO	1 mo	1 mo	1 mo†
Implant	1 mo	1 mo	5 yr
Intrauterine system	1 mo	1 mo	5 yr
IM	1 mo	1 mo	3 mo
SUBQ	unknown	1 wk	3 mo

† Only during mo of taking contraceptive.

Contraindications/Precautions

Contraindicated in: Hypersensitivity; History of cigarette smoking and age >35 yr (↑ risk of cardiovascular or thromboembolic phenomenon);

C

History of deep vein thrombosis (DVT) or pulmonary embolism (PE); Inherited or acquired coagulopathies; Cerebrovascular disease; Coronary artery disease; Thrombogenic valvular heart disease or thrombogenic heart rhythms; Major surgery with extended periods of immobility; Diabetes and >35 yr old; diabetes with hypertension, vascular disease, or end-organ damage; or diabetes for >20 yr; Headache with focal neurological symptoms or migraine headaches with aura; Women >35 yr old with migraine headaches; Uncontrolled hypertension or hypertension with vascular disease; Breast cancer, endometrial cancer, or any other estrogen- or progestin-sensitive cancer (current or history of); Abnormal genital bleeding; Cholestatic jaundice of pregnancy or jaundice with prior contraceptive use; Hepatic adenoma or carcinoma; Hypersensitivity to and parabens (injectable only); *Drospirenone-containing products only:* Renal impairment, liver disease, or adrenal insufficiency (↑ risk of hyperkalemia); *Intrauterine levonorgestrel only:* Intrauterine anomaly, postpartum endometriosis, multiple sexual partners, pelvic inflammatory disease, liver disease, genital actinomycosis, immunosuppression, IV drug abuse, untreated genitourinary infection, or history of ectopic pregnancy; *Ethinyl estradiol/levonorgestrel and ethinyl estradiol/norelgestromin transdermal patches only:* Body mass index ≥30 kg/m^2 (↑ risk of venous thromboembolism); Concurrent use of combinations containing ombitasvir/paritaprevir/ritonavir (with or without dasabuvir); OB: Pregnancy; Lactation: Avoid use; ↑ risk of uterine rupture/perforation with intrauterine levonorgestrel.

Use Cautiously in: Presence of other cardiovascular risk factors (obesity, hyperglycemia, hypertension); History or family history of hypertriglyceridemia (↑ risk of pancreatitis); Diabetes mellitus, bleeding disorders, concurrent anticoagulant therapy or headaches; Hereditary angioedema; Chloasma; *Estetrol/drospirenone:* BMI >30 k g/m^2 (↓ effectiveness); *Ethinyl estradiol/norelgestromin transdermal patch only:* Weight >90 kg (↓ effectiveness); *Ethinyl estradiol/levonorgestrel transdermal patch only:* BMI 25–<30 kg/m^2 (↓ effectiveness); Pedi: Avoid use before menarche.

Adverse Reactions/Side Effects

CV: DVT, edema, hypertension, Raynaud phenomenon, thrombophlebitis. **Derm:** melasma, rash. **EENT:** contact lens intolerance, optic neuritis, retinal thrombosis. **Endo:** hyperglycemia. **F and E** *Drospirenone-containing products only:* hyperkalemia. **GI:** abdominal cramps, bloating, cholestatic jaundice, gallbladder disease, liver tumors, nausea, PANCREATITIS, vomiting. **GU:** *Intrauterine levonorgestrel only:*, amenorrhea, breakthrough bleeding, dysmenorrhea, spotting, uterine imbedment/uterine rupture. **MS:** *Injectable medroxyprogesterone only:* bone loss. **Neuro:** depression, headache. **Resp:** PE. **Misc:** BREAST CANCER (ESPECIALLY WITH PROLONGED USE), HYPERSENSITIVITY REACTIONS (INCLUDING ANAPHYLAXIS AND ANGIOEDEMA), weight change.

Interactions

Drug-Drug: Concurrent use of combinations containing **ombitasvir/paritaprevir/ritonavir** with combination hormonal contraceptives may ↑ risk of elevated liver enzymes; concurrent use contraindicated. Effectiveness may be ↓ by **penicillins**, **chloramphenicol**, **barbiturates**, chronic **alcohol** use, **carbamazepine**, **oxcarbazepine**, **bosentan**, **felbamate**, systemic **corticosteroids**, **phenytoin**, **topiramate**, **primidone**, **modafinil**, **rifampin**, **rifabutin**, **nelfinavir**, **ritonavir**, **darunavir/ritonavir**, **fosamprenavir/ritonavir**, **lopinavir/ritonavir**, **tipranavir/ritonavir**, **nevirapine**, **efavirenz**, **colesevelam**, or **tetracyclines**. **CYP3A4 inducers**, including **barbiturates**, **bosentan**, **carbamazepine**, **oxcarbazepine**, **phenytoin**, **topiramate**, **felbamate**, **rifampin**, may ↓ effectiveness of ulipristal; avoid concurrent use. May ↑ levels and risk of toxicity of some **benzodiazepines**, **beta blockers**, **corticosteroids**, **cyclosporine**, **tizanidine**, **theophylline**, and **voriconazole**. May ↑ risk of hepatotoxicity with **dantrolene** (estrogen only). **Atazanavir/ritonavir**, **cobicistat**, **etravirine**, **itraconazole**, **ketoconazole**, **fluconazole**, **voriconazole**, **ritonavir**, **rosuvastatin**, and **atorvastatin** may ↑ levels and risk of toxicity. **Smoking** ↑ risk of thromboembolic phenomena (estrogen only). May ↓ levels and effectiveness of **acetaminophen**, **temazepam**, **lamotrigine**, **lorazepam**, **oxazepam**, or **morphine**. Concurrent use of combinations containing **glecaprevir/pibrentasvir** with ethinyl estradiol-containing products may ↑ risk of elevated liver enzymes; avoid concurrent use. Concurrent use of drospirenone-containing products with **NSAIDs**, **potassium-sparing diuretics**, **potassium supplements**, **ACE inhibitors**, **aldosterone receptor antagonists**, or **angiotensin II receptor antagonists** may ↑ risk of hyperkalemia. Concurrent use of drospirenone-containing products with strong **CYP3A4 inhibitors**, including **ketoconazole**, **itraconazole**, **voriconazole**, **protease inhibitors**, or **clarithromycin**, may ↑ risk of hyperkalemia. Ulipristal may ↑ levels and risk of toxicity of **P-glycoprotein substrates**, including **dabigatran** and **digoxin**.

Drug-Natural Products: St. John's wort may ↓ levels and effectiveness.

Drug-Food: Grapefruit juice may ↑ levels and risk of toxicity.

Route/Dosage

Monophasic Oral Contraceptives

PO (Adults): On 21-day regimen, take 1st tablet on 1st Sunday after menses begins (take on Sunday if menses begins on Sunday) for 21 days; then skip 7 days and begin again. Regimen may also be started on 1st day of menses; continue for 21 days and then skip 7 days and begin again. Some regimens contain 7 placebo tablets so that 1 tablet is taken every day for 28 days.

Biphasic Oral Contraceptives

PO (Adults): Given in 2 phases. 1st phase is 10 days of smaller amount of progestin. 2nd phase is larger amount of progestin. Amount of estrogen remains constant for same length of time (total of 21 days); then skip 7 days and begin again. Some regimens contain 7 placebo tablets for 28-day regimen.

Triphasic Oral Contraceptives

PO (Adults): Progestin amount varies throughout 21-day cycle. Estrogen component stays the same or may vary. Some regimens contain 7 placebo tablets for 28-day regimen.

Fourphasic Oral Contraceptives

PO (Adults): Given in 4 phases. 1st phase contains higher amount of estrogen and no progestin. 2nd and 3rd phases contain lower amount of estrogen, and increasing amounts of progestin. 4th phase contains low dose of estrogen only. Also contains 2 placebo tablets to complete 28-day regimen.

Extended-Cycle Contraceptive

PO (Adults): *Daysee, LoSeasonique, Quartette,* and *Seasonique:* Start taking 1st active pill on 1st Sunday after menses begins (if 1st day is Sunday, begin then); continue for 84 days of active pill, followed by 7 days of placebo tablets (low-dose estrogen tablets for Daysee, LoSeasonique, Quartette, and Seasonique); then resume 84/7 cycle again.

Progestin-Only Oral Contraceptives

PO (Adults): Start on 1st day of menses. Taken daily and continuously.

Progressive Estrogen Oral Contraceptives

PO (Adults): Estrogen amount ↑ every 7 days throughout 21-day cycle. Progestin component stays the same. Some regimens contain 7 placebo tablets for 28-day regimen.

Emergency Contraceptive

PO (Adults and Adolescents): *Levonorgestrel:* 1 tablet within 72 hr of unprotected intercourse; *Lo/Ovral:* 4 white tablets within 72 hr of unprotected intercourse followed by 4 more white tablets 12 hr later; *Ulipristal:* 1 tablet as soon as possible within 120 hr (5 days) after unprotected intercourse or known/suspected contraceptive failure.

Injectable Contraceptive

Medroxyprogesterone (Depo-Provera)

IM (Adults): 150 mg within 1st 5 days of menses or within 5 days postpartum, if not breastfeeding. If breastfeeding, give 6 wk postpartum; repeat every 3 mo.

Medroxyprogesterone (Depo-Sub Q Provera 104)

SUBQ (Adults): 104 mg within 1st 5 days of menses or within 5 days postpartum, if not breastfeeding. If breastfeeding, give 6 wk postpartum; repeat every 12–14 wk.

Intrauterine Contraceptive

Intrauterine: (Adults): Insert one device into uterine cavity within 7 days of menses or immediately after 1st trimester abortion. Skyla should be removed or replaced after 3 yr. Kyleena should be removed or replaced after 5 yr. Mirena and Liletta should be removed or replaced after 5 yr (for treatment of heavy menstrual bleeding) or 8 yr (contraception).

Vaginal Ring Contraceptive

Vag (Adults): One ring inserted on or prior to day 5 of menstrual cycle. Ring is left in place for 3 wk and then removed for 1 wk; then a new ring is inserted.

Transdermal Patch

Transdermal (Adults): *Ethinyl estradiol/norelgestromin transdermal patch:* Patch is applied on Day 1 of menstrual cycle (or convenient day in 1st wk) and changed weekly thereafter for 3 wk. Wk 4 is patch-free. Cycle is then repeated. *Ethinyl estradiol/levonorgestrel transdermal patch:* Patch is applied during first 24 hr of menstruation and then changed weekly thereafter for 3 wk. Wk 4 is patch-free. Cycle is then repeated.

Acne

PO (Adults): Take daily for 21 days, off for 7 days.

Availability

Combination Estrogen/Progestin Oral Contraceptives (generic available)

Tablets: Usually in monthly packs with enough (21) active tablets to complete a 28-day cycle. Some contain 7 inert tablets to complete the cycle with or without supplemental iron, Beyaz and Safyral contain 0.451 mg of levomefolate calcium/tablet.

Extended-Cycle Contraceptive

Tablets: *LoSeasonique:* Active tablets containing 0.02 mg ethinyl estradiol, 0.1 mg levonorgestrel, and 7 tablets containing 0.01 mg ethinyl estradiol, *Quartette:* 42 tablets containing 0.02 mg ethinyl estradiol and 0.15 mg levonorgestrel, 21 tablets containing 0.025 mg ethinyl estradiol and 0.15 mg levonorgestrel, 21 tablets containing 0.03 mg ethinyl estradiol and 0.15 mg levonorgestrel, and 7 tablets containing 0.01 mg ethinyl estradiol, *Daysee* and *Seasonique:*

active tablets containing 0.03 mg ethinyl estradiol, 0.15 mg levonorgestrel, and 7 tablets containing 0.01 mg ethinyl estradiol.

Norgestrel
Tablets: 0.075 mg OTC.

Levonorgestrel (generic available)
Emergency contraceptive: 1.5 mg OTC. **Intrauterine system (Kyleena):** contains 19.5 mg levonorgestrel (releases 9 mcg/day). **Intrauterine system (Liletta):** contains 52 mg levonorgestrel (releases 14.7 mcg/day). **Intrauterine system (Mirena):** contains 52 mg levonorgestrel (releases 20 mcg/day). **Intrauterine system (Skyla):** contains 13.5 mg levonorgestrel (releases 14 mcg/day).

Etonogestrel
Implant: Rod contains 68 mg etonogestrel.

Ulipristal
Tablets: 30 mg.

Medroxyprogesterone (generic available)
Injectable IM: 150 mg/mL. **Injectable SUBQ:** 104 mg/0.65 mL (in prefilled syringes).

Vaginal Ring Contraceptive
Ring: delivers 0.015 mg ethinyl estradiol and 0.120 mg etonogestrel/day.

Transdermal Patch
Patch (Xulane or Onsura): Contains 0.53 mg ethinyl estradiol and 4.86 mg of norelgestromin; releases 35 mcg ethinyl estradiol/150 mcg norelgestromin per 24 hr. **Patch (Twirla):** Contains 2.3 mg ethinyl estradiol and 2.6 mg of levonorgestrel; releases 30 mcg ethinyl estradiol/120 mcg levonorgestrel per 24 hr.

NURSING IMPLICATIONS

Assessment
- Assess BP before and periodically during therapy.
- Monitor intake and output and weekly weight. Report significant discrepancies or steady weight gain.
- Monitor for signs and symptoms of venous thromboembolism, such as PE (chest pain, dyspnea, tachycardia) or DVT (calf pain or tenderness, lower extremity edema, localized warmth or erythema), or emerging cardiovascular disease, such as MI (chest pain, dyspnea, diaphoresis, dizziness, nausea) or stroke (weakness, slurred speech, confusion, dizziness). *If thromboembolic event suspected,* discontinue therapy.
- Monitor for breast tenderness, lumps, or discharge. Perform baseline mammogram before starting treatment.
- If persistent or recurring abnormal genital bleeding occur in postmenopausal women, directed or random endometrial sampling may need to be performed to rule out malignancy.
- Monitor for fluid retention; may exacerbate conditions such as HF or renal impairment.
- **Acne:** Assess skin lesions before and periodically during therapy.
- **Menopause:** Assess frequency and severity of vasomotor symptoms. Monitor individual clinical response and severity of vulvar and vaginal atrophy.
- **Emergency Contraception:** Assess history and/or physical exam and/or negative pregnancy test to exclude the possibility of pregnancy. Perform a follow-up physical or pelvic examination if there is any doubt concerning pregnancy status or concern for ectopic.
- **Amenorrhea:** Assess patient's usual menstrual history. Administration of drug usually begins 8–10 days before anticipated menstruation. Withdrawal bleeding usually occurs 48–72 hr after course of therapy. Therapy should be discontinued if menses occur during injection series.
- **Dysfunctional Bleeding:** Monitor pattern and amount of vaginal bleeding (pad count). Bleeding should end by 6th day of therapy. Discontinue therapy if menses occur during injection series.

Lab Test Considerations
- Verify negative pregnancy test before starting therapy. Monitor hepatic function periodically during therapy.
- *Estrogens only:* May ↑ serum glucose, sodium, triglyceride, HDL-C, total cholesterol, prothrombin, and factors VII, VIII, IX, and X levels. May ↓ LDL-C and antithrombin III levels. May also ↑ cortisol levels and ↓ serum folate and pyridoxine.
- May cause false interpretations of thyroid function tests.
- *Progestins only:* May ↑ LDL-C. May ↓ serum alkaline phosphatase and HDL-C.
- *Estrogens*and *progestins* may ↓ pregnanediol excretion concentrations.
- *Drospirenone-containing contraceptives:* Monitor serum potassium during 1st treatment cycle in women on long-term treatment with strong CYP3A4 inhibitors; may ↑ serum potassium concentrations.

Implementation
- Do not confuse Slynd with Syeda. Do not confuse Yasmin with Yaz.
- *Estrogen* plus *progestin* therapy should not be used for the prevention of cardiovascular disease or dementia.
- Discontinue of oral *progestins* ≥4–6 wk prior to surgical procedures associated with an ↑ risk of thromboembolism or prolonged immobilization.

- **PO:** Oral doses may be administered with or immediately after food to ↓ nausea. Chewable tablets may be swallowed whole or chewed; if chewed, follow with 8 ounces of liquid.
- For extended-cycle tablets, *Amethia, Camrese, CamreseLo, Daysee, Introvale, Jaimiess, Jolessa, Quartette, Rivelsa, Setlakin,* or *Simpesse*, take active tablets for 84 days followed by the placebo tablets for 7 days.
- For *Emergency Contraception:* Tablets are taken as soon as possible and within 72 hr after unprotected intercourse. Two doses are taken 12 hr apart. Emergency contraception products are available without a prescription to all women of reproductive potential.
- *Ulipristal:* Administer 1 tablet as soon as possible within 120 hr (5 days) after unprotected intercourse or a known or suspected contraceptive failure. May be taken without regard to food. If vomiting occurs within 3 hr of dose, may repeat. May be taken at any time during the menstrual cycle. Ulipristal may be less effective in women with a body mass index >30 kg/m^2. Health care providers who are actively trying to conceive, who are pregnant or may become pregnant, and who are breastfeeding should avoid handling ulipristal.
- **SUBQ**: Shake vigorously before use to form a uniform suspension. Inject slowly (over 5–7 sec) at a 45° angle into fatty area of anterior thigh or abdomen every 12–14 wk. If >14 wk elapse between injections, rule out pregnancy prior to administration. Do not rub area after injection.
- When switching from other hormonal contraceptives, administer within dosing period (7 days after taking last active pill, removing patch or ring, or within the dosing period for IM injection).
- **IM:** Prepare wearing double gloves and a protective gown. If possible, prepare in a biological safety cabinet or a compounding aseptic containment isolator; eye, face, and respiratory protection may be needed. Shake vial vigorously just before use to ensure uniform suspension. Administer deep IM into gluteal or deltoid muscle. If period between injections is >14 wk, determine that patient is not pregnant before administering the drug. During administration, if there is a potential that the substance could splash or if the patient may resist, use eye and face protection.
- Injectable medroxyprogesterone may lead to bone loss, especially in women <21 yr. Injectable medroxyprogesterone should be used for >2 yr only if other methods of contraception are inadequate. If used long term, women should use supplemental calcium and vitamin D and monitor bone mineral density.
- **Intrauterine system:** Health care providers are advised to become thoroughly familiar with the insertion instructions before attempting insertion. Following insertion, counsel patient on what to expect. Give patient *Follow-up Reminder Card* provided with product. Discuss expected bleeding patterns during the first mo of use. Prescribe analgesics, if indicated. Patients should be reexamined and evaluated 4–12 wk after insertion and once a year thereafter or more frequently, if clinically indicated.
- **Transdermal:** When switching from oral form, begin transdermal therapy 1 wk after the last dose or when symptoms reappear.
- Wearing double gloves, place *Climara* patch on clean, dry skin, preferably on the lower abdomen, upper quadrant of the buttock, or outer aspect of the hip; do not apply to the breasts or waistline; press firmly in place for ≥10 sec, making sure there is good contact, especially around the edges; rotate sites of application with 1 wk between applications to a particular site.

Patient/Family Teaching

- Explain the purpose and side effects of hormonal contraceptives. Instruct patient to take as directed at the same time each day. Pills should be taken in proper sequence and kept in the original container. Advise patient not to skip pills even if not having sex very often. Never share oral contraceptives; doing so can be dangerous. Keep out of children's reach. Advise patient to read *Patient Guide* before starting and with each Rx refill in case of changes.
- Emphasize the importance of routine follow-up physical exams including BP; breast, abdomen, and pelvic examinations; and Papanicolaou smears every 6–12 mo.
- *If single daily dose is missed:* Take as soon as remembered; if not until next day, take 2 tablets and continue on regular dosing schedule. *If 2 days in a row are missed:* Take 2 tablets a day for the next 2 days and continue on regular dosing schedule, using a 2nd method of birth control for the remaining cycle. *If 3 days in a row are missed:* Discontinue medication and use another form of birth control until period begins or pregnancy is ruled out; then begin a new cycle of tablets. *For 28-day dosing schedule:* If schedule is followed for 1st 21 days and one dose is missed of the last 7 tablets, it is important to take the 1st tablet of next month's cycle on the regularly scheduled day. Advise patient taking *Natazia* to follow *Patient Guide* for what to do if a pill is missed.
- Advise patient taking *Amethia, Camrese, CamreseLo, Daysee, Introvale, Jaimiess, Jolessa, Quartette, Rivelsa, Setlakin,* or *Simpesse* that withdrawal bleeding should occur during the 7 days following discontinuation of the active tablets. If withdrawal bleeding does not occur, notify health care provider.
- For initial use of *Amethia, Camrese, CamreseLo, Daysee, Introvale, Jaimiess, Jolessa, Quartette, Rivelsa, Setlakin,* or *Simpesse*, caution patient to

use a nonhormonal method of contraception until they have taken the 1st 7 days of active tablets. Each 91-day cycle should start on the same day of the week. If started later than the proper day or ≥2 days are missed, a 2nd nonhormonal method of contraception should be used until they have taken the pink tablet for 7 days. Transient spotting or bleeding may occur. If bleeding is persistent or prolonged, notify health care provider.

- Advise patient taking extended cycle tablets that spotting or light bleeding may occur, especially during 1st 3 mo. Continue medication; notify health care provider if bleeding lasts >70 days.
- Advise patient of the need to use another form of contraception for the 1st 3 wk when beginning to use *oral contraceptives*.
- Instruct patient to notify health care provider of all Rx or OTC medications, vitamins, or herbal products being taken and consult health care provider before taking any new medications.
- Advise patient that a 2nd method of birth control should also be used during each cycle in which any of the following are used: *Oral contraceptives:* ampicillin, corticosteroids, antiretroviral protease inhibitors, barbiturates, carbamazepine, chloramphenicol, dihydroergotamine, corticosteroids (systemic), mineral oil, oral neomycin, oxcarbazepine, penicillin VK, primidone, rifampin, sulfonamides, tetracyclines, topiramate, bosentan, or valproic acid.
- Explain dose schedule and maintenance routine. Discontinuing medication suddenly may cause withdrawal bleeding.
- If nausea becomes a problem, advise patient that eating solid food often provides relief. If nausea persists or vomiting or diarrhea occurs, use a nonhormonal method of contraception and notify health care provider.
- Advise patient to report signs and symptoms of fluid retention (swelling of ankles and feet, weight gain), thromboembolic disorders (pain, swelling, tenderness in extremities, headache, chest pain, blurred vision), depression, hepatic impairment (yellowed skin or eyes, pruritus, dark urine, light-colored stools), or abnormal vaginal bleeding. Women with a strong family history of breast cancer, fibrocystic breast disease, abnormal mammograms, or cervical dysplasia should be monitored for breast cancer at least yearly. Risk of thromboembolism is highest in 1st yr of use and ↑ when a combination hormonal contraceptive is restarted after a break in use of ≥4 wk.
- Caution patient that cigarette smoking during estrogen therapy may ↑ risk of serious side effects, especially for women over age 35.
- Caution patients to use sunscreen and protective clothing to prevent increased pigmentation.
- Caution patient that hormonal contraceptives do not protect against HIV or other sexually transmitted diseases.
- Advise patient to notify health care provider of medication regimen before treatment or surgery.
- **Emergency Contraception:** Instruct patient to take emergency contraceptive as directed. Advise patient that they should not take emergency contraceptives if they know or suspect they are pregnant; emergency contraceptives are not for use to end an existing pregnancy. Advise patient to contact health care provider if they vomit within 3 hr after taking *ulipristal*.
- Inform patient that *ulipristal* may ↓ effectiveness of hormonal contraceptives. Advise patient to use a nonhormonal contraceptive during that menstrual cycle. Advise patient to wait ≥5 days after taking *ulipristal* to resume taking hormonal contraceptives.
- Advise patient to notify health care provider and consider the possibility of pregnancy if their period is delayed by >1 wk beyond the expected date after taking *ulipristal*.
- Inform patient that emergency contraceptives are not to be used as a routine form of contraception or to be used repeatedly within the same menstrual cycle.
- Advise patient to notify health care provider that if severe lower abdominal pain occurs 3–5 wk after taking *ulipristal*, she should be evaluated for an ectopic pregnancy.
- Advise patient to avoid breastfeeding if taking *ulipristal*.
- **IM, SUBQ**: Advise patient to maintain adequate amounts of dietary calcium and vitamin D to help prevent bone loss.
- **Transdermal:** Instruct patient on application of patch. 1st patch should be applied within 24 hr of menstrual period. If applied after Day 1 of menstrual period, a nonhormonal method of contraception should be used for the next 7 days. Day of application becomes *Patch Change Day*. Patches are worn for 1 wk and changed on the same day of each wk for 3 wk. Wk 4 is patch-free. Withdrawal bleeding is expected during this time.
- Apply patch to clean, dry, intact, healthy skin on buttock, abdomen, upper outer arm, or upper torso in a place where it won't be rubbed by tight clothing. Do not place on skin that is red, irritated, or cut, and do not place on breasts. Do not apply makeup, creams, lotions, powders, or other topical products to area of patch application.
- To apply patch, open foil pouch by tearing along edge using fingers. Peel pouch apart and open flat. Grasp a corner of the patch firmly and remove

gently from foil pouch. Use fingernail to lift one corner of the patch and peel patch **and** the plastic liner off the foil liner. Do not remove clear liner as patch is removed. Peel away half of the clear liner without touching sticky surface. Apply the sticky surface and remove the rest of the liner. Press down firmly with palm of hand for 10 sec; make sure the edges stick well.

- On *Patch Change Day* remove patch and apply new one immediately. Used patch still contains some active hormones; fold in half so it sticks to itself and throw away. Apply new patches to a new spot to prevent skin irritation; may be applied in same anatomic area.
- Following patch-free week, apply a new patch on *Patch Change Day*, the day after Day 28, no matter when the menstrual cycle begins.
- If patch becomes partially or completely detached for <1 day, reapply patch or apply new patch. If patch is detached for >1 day, apply a new patch immediately and use a nonhormonal form of contraception for the next 7 days. Cycle will now start over with a new *Patch Change Day*. If patch is no longer sticky, apply a new patch; do not use tape or wraps to keep patch in place.
- If patch is not changed on *Patch Change Day* in the first week of the cycle, apply new patch immediately upon remembering and use a nonhormonal method of contraception for next 7 days. If patch change is missed for 1–2 days during Wk 2 or 3, apply new patch immediately and apply next patch on usual *Patch Change Day*. No backup contraception is needed. If patch change is missed for >2 days during Wk 2 or 3, stop the cycle and start a new 4-wk contraceptive cycle by applying new patch immediately and using a nonhormonal method of contraception for the next 7 days. If patch is not removed on *Patch Change Day* in Wk 4, remove as soon as remembered and start next cycle on usual *Patch Change Day*. No additional contraception is needed.
- Advise patient referred for MRI test to discuss patch with referring health care provider and MRI facility to determine if removal of patch is necessary prior to test and for directions for replacing patch.
- **NuvaRing:** *If a hormonal contraceptive was not used in the past month*, insert *NuvaRing* between Days 1 and 5 of the menstrual cycle (Day 1 = 1st day of menstrual period), even if bleeding has not finished. Use a nonhormonal method of birth control other than a diaphragm during the 1st 7 days of ring use. *If switching from a combination estrogen/progesterone oral contraceptive*, insert *NuvaRing* any time during 1st 7 days after last tablet and no later than the day a new pill cycle would have started. No extra birth control is needed. *If switching from a mini-pill*, start using *NuvaRing* on any day of the month; do not skip days between last pill and 1st day of *NuvaRing* use. *If switching from an implant*, start using *NuvaRing* on same day implant is removed. *If switching from an injectable contraceptive*, start using *NuvaRing* on the day when next injection is due. *If switching from a progestin-containing IUD*, start using *NuvaRing* on the same day as IUD is removed. A nonhormonal method of contraception, other than the diaphragm, should be used for the 1st 7 days of *NuvaRing* use when switching from the mini-pill, implant, injectable contraceptive, or IUD.
- *NuvaRing* comes in a reclosable foil pouch. Instruct patient to wash hands; then remove *NuvaRing* from pouch; keep pouch for ring disposal. Using a position of comfort (lying down, squatting, or standing with one leg up), hold *NuvaRing* between thumb and index finger and press opposite sides of the ring together. Gently push folded ring into vagina. Exact position is not important for function of *NuvaRing*. Most women do not feel *NuvaRing* once it is in place. If discomfort is felt, *NuvaRing* may not be inserted far enough into vagina; use finger to push further into vagina. *There is no danger of NuvaRing being pushed in too far or getting lost*. Once inserted, leave *NuvaRing* in place for 3 wk.
- Remove ring 3 wk after insertion on same day and time of insertion. Remove by hooking finger under forward rim or by holding ring between index and middle finger and pulling out. Place ring in foil pouch and dispose; do not throw in toilet. Menstrual period will usually start 2–3 days after ring is removed and may not have finished before next ring is inserted. To continue contraceptive protection, new ring must be inserted 1 wk after last one was removed, even if menstrual period has not stopped.
- If *NuvaRing* slips out of vagina and has been out <3 hr, contraceptive protection is still in place. *NuvaRing* can be rinsed in cool to tepid water and should be reinserted as soon as possible. If ring is lost, insert a new ring and continue same schedule as lost ring. If *NuvaRing* has been out of vagina for >3 hr, a nonhormonal method of contraception, other than a diaphragm, should be used for the next 7 days.
- *If NuvaRing has been left in for an extra week or less (≤4 wk)*, remove and insert a new ring after a 1-week ring-free break. If *NuvaRing* has been left in place for >4 wk, woman should check to be sure she is not pregnant. A nonhormonal method of contraception, other than a diaphragm, must be used for the next 7 days.
- Advise patient to avoid using other female barrier contraceptives (diaphragm, cervical cap, female condom) with *NuvaRing*.
- **Intrauterine system:** Advise patient to notify health care provider if pelvic pain or pain during

sex, unusual vaginal discharge or genital sores, unexplained fever, exposure to sexually transmitted infections, very severe or migraine headaches, yellowing of skin or whites of the eyes, or very severe vaginal bleeding or bleeding that lasts a long time occurs; if a menstrual period is missed; or if *Mirena*'s threads cannot be felt.

- Rep: Instruct patient to stop taking medication and notify health care provider if pregnancy is suspected.

Evaluation/Desired Outcomes

- Prevention of pregnancy.
- Regulation of the menstrual cycle.
- Decrease in menstrual blood loss.
- Decrease in acne.
- Decrease in symptoms of premenstrual dysphoric disorder.
- Decrease in vasomotor symptoms or symptoms of vulvar and vaginal atrophy due to menopause.

CORTICOSTEROIDS (INHALATION)

beclomethasone
(be-kloe-**meth**-a-sone)
✱ QVAR, QVAR Redihaler

budesonide (byoo-**dess**-oh-nide)
Pulmicort Flexhaler, ✱ Pulmicort Nebuamp, Pulmicort Respules, ✱ Pulmicort Turbuhaler

ciclesonide (inhalation)
(si-**kless**-o-nide)
Alvesco

fluticasone (floo-**ti**-ka-sone)
✱ Aermony Respiclick, Arnuity Ellipta, ~~Flovent Diskus, Flovent HFA~~

mometasone (mo-**met**-a-sone)
Asmanex HFA, Asmanex Twisthaler

Classification
Therapeutic: antiasthmatics, anti-inflammatories (steroidal)
Pharmacologic: corticosteroids (inhalation)

Indications

Maintenance treatment of asthma as prophylactic therapy. May decrease the need for or eliminate use of systemic corticosteroids in patients with asthma.

Action

Potent, locally acting anti-inflammatory and immune modifier. **Therapeutic Effects:** Decreased frequency and severity of asthma attacks. Improves asthma symptoms.

Pharmacokinetics

Absorption: *Beclomethasone:* 20%; *budesonide:* 6–13% (Flexhaler), 6% (Respules); *ciclesonide:* negligible; *fluticasone:* <7% (aerosol), 8–14% (powder); *mometasone:* <1%. Action is primarily local after inhalation.

Distribution: All cross the placenta and enter breast milk in small amounts.

Metabolism and Excretion: *Beclomethasone:* After inhalation, beclomethasone dipropionate is converted to beclomethasone monopropionate, an active metabolite that adds to its potency, primarily excreted in feces (<10% excreted in urine; *budesonide, fluticasone, mometasone:* Metabolized by the liver (primarily by CYP3A4) after absorption from lungs; *budesonide:* 60% excreted in urine, 40% in feces; *ciclesonide:* Converted by esterases to des-ciclesonide, the active drug, which is subsequently metabolized by the liver. Some further metabolites may be pharmacologically active. Mostly eliminated in feces via biliary excretion; <20% of des-ciclesonide is excreted in urine; *fluticasone:* Primarily excreted in feces (<5% excreted in urine); *bometasone:* 75% excreted in feces.

Half-life: *Beclomethasone:* 2.8 hr; *budesonide:* 2–3.6 hr; *ciclesonide:* 0.7 hr (ciclesonide); 6–7 hr (des-ciclesonide); *fluticasone:* 7.8 hr (propionate); 24 hr (furoate); *mometasone:* 5 hr.

TIME/ACTION PROFILE (improvement in symptoms)

ROUTE	ONSET	PEAK	DURATION
Inhalation	within 24 hr‡	1–4 wk†	unknown

† Improvement in pulmonary function; ↓ airway responsiveness may take longer.
‡ 2–8 days for budesonide respule.

Contraindications/Precautions

Contraindicated in: Some products contain alcohol or lactose and should be avoided in patients with known hypersensitivity or intolerance; Acute attack of asthma/status asthmaticus.

Use Cautiously in: Active untreated infections; Diabetes or glaucoma; Underlying immunosuppression (due to disease or concurrent therapy); Systemic corticosteroid therapy (should not be abruptly discontinued when inhalation therapy is started; additional corticosteroids needed in stress or trauma); Hepatic impairment (fluticasone); OB/Lactation: Safety not established; Pedi: Prolonged or high-dose therapy may lead to complications.

Adverse Reactions/Side Effects

EENT: dysphonia, hoarseness, cataracts, glaucoma, nasal congestion, pharyngitis, sinusitis. **Endo:** ↓

bone mineral density, ↓ growth (children), adrenal suppression (↑ dose, long-term therapy only).
GI: diarrhea, dry mouth, dyspepsia, esophageal candidiasis, nausea, taste disturbances. **MS:** back pain. **Neuro:** headache, agitation, depression, dizziness, fatigue, insomnia, restlessness. **Resp:** bronchospasm, cough, wheezing. **Misc:** CHURG-STRAUSS SYNDROME, HYPERSENSITIVITY REACTIONS (INCLUDING ANAPHYLAXIS, LARYNGEAL EDEMA, URTICARIA, AND BRONCHOSPASM).

Interactions

Drug-Drug: Strong **CYP3A4 inhibitors**, including **ritonavir**, **atazanavir**, **clarithromycin**, **conivaptan**, **itraconazole**, **ketoconazole**, **lopinavir**, **nefazodone**, **nelfinavir**, and **voriconazole**, may ↑ levels and risk of toxicity of budesonide, mometasone, and fluticasone; concurrent use with fluticasone not recommended.

Route/Dosage

Beclomethasone

Inhaln (Adults and Children ≥12 yr): *No prior treatment with inhaled corticosteroid:* 40–80 mcg twice daily (max dose = 320 mcg twice daily); *Prior treatment with inhaled corticosteroid:* 40–320 mcg twice daily (starting dose should be based on dose of previous inhaled corticosteroid and disease severity) (max dose = 320 mcg twice daily).
Inhaln (Children 4–11 yr): *No prior treatment with inhaled corticosteroid:* 40 mcg twice daily (max = 80 mcg twice daily); *Prior treatment with inhaled corticosteroid:* 40 mcg twice daily (max = 80 mcg twice daily).

Budesonide (Pulmicort Flexhaler)

Inhaln (Adults): 180–360 mcg twice daily (not to exceed 720 mcg twice daily).
Inhaln (Children ≥6 yr): 180–360 mcg twice daily (not to exceed 360 mcg twice daily).

Budesonide (Pulmicort Respules)

Inhaln (Children 1–8 yr): *Previously on bronchodilators alone:* 0.5 mg once daily or 0.25 mg twice daily (not to exceed 0.5 mg/day); *Previously on other inhaled corticosteroids:* 0.5 mg once daily or 0.25 mg twice daily (not to exceed 1 mg/day); *Previously on oral corticosteroids:* 1 mg once daily or 0.5 mg twice daily (not to exceed 1 mg/day).

Ciclesonide

Inhaln (Adults and Children ≥12 yr): *Previous therapy with bronchodilators alone:* 80 mcg twice daily; may ↑ to 160 mcg twice daily; *Previous therapy with inhaled corticosteroids:* 80 mcg twice daily; may ↑ to 320 mcg twice daily; *Previous therapy with oral corticosteroids:* 320 mcg twice daily.

Fluticasone (Aerosol Inhaler)

Inhaln (Adults and Children ≥12 yr): *Previously on bronchodilators alone:* 88 mcg twice daily initially; may ↑ up to 440 mcg twice daily; *Previously on other inhaled corticosteroids:* 88–220 mcg twice daily initially; may ↑ up to 440 mcg twice daily; *Previously on oral corticosteroids:* 440 mcg twice daily initially; may ↑ up to 880 mcg twice daily.
Inhaln (Children 4–11 yr): 88 mcg twice daily (not to exceed 88 mcg twice daily).

Fluticasone (Dry Powder Inhaler)

Inhaln (Adults and Children ≥12 yr): *No prior treatment with inhaled corticosteroid:* Propionate (Flovent Diskus generic): 100 mcg twice daily initially; may ↑ dose in 2 wk if not adequately responding (max dose = 1000 mcg twice daily); Furoate: 100 mcg once daily; may ↑ dose in 2 wk to 200 mcg once daily if not adequately responding (max dose = 200 mcg once daily); *Prior treatment with inhaled corticosteroid:* Furoate: 100–200 mcg once daily (max dose = 200 mcg once daily).
Inhaln (Children 5–11 yr): Furoate: 50 mcg once daily.
Inhaln (Children 4–11 yr): *No prior treatment with inhaled corticosteroid:* Propionate (Flovent Diskus generic): 50 mcg twice daily initially; may ↑ dose in 2 wk to 100 mcg twice daily if not adequately responding (max dose = 100 mcg twice daily).

Mometasone (Aerosol Inhaler)

Inhaln (Adults and Children ≥12 yr): *Previously on medium-dose inhaled corticosteroids:* Two 100-mcg inhalations twice daily; *Previously on high-dose inhaled corticosteroids or oral corticosteroids:* Two 200-mcg inhalations twice daily (not to exceed 800 mcg/day).

Mometasone (Dry Powder Inhaler)

Inhaln (Adults and Children ≥12 yr): *Previously on bronchodilators or other inhaled corticosteroids:* 220 mcg once daily in evening, up to 440 mcg/day as a single dose or 2 divided doses; *Previously on oral corticosteroids:* 440 mcg twice daily (not to exceed 880 mcg/day).
Inhaln (Children 4–11 yr): 110 mcg once daily in evening (not to exceed 110 mcg/day).

Availability

Beclomethasone

Inhalation aerosol: 40 mcg/metered inhalation in 10.6-g canister (delivers 120 metered inhalations), 🍁 50 mcg/metered inhalation in 6.5-g canister (delivers 100 metered inhalations) and 12.4-g canister (delivers 200 metered inhalations), 80 mcg/metered inhalation in 10.6-g canister (delivers 120 metered inhalations), 🍁 100 mcg/metered inhalation in 6.5-g canister (delivers 100 metered inhalations) and 12.4-g canister (delivers 200 metered inhalations).

Budesonide (generic available)

Inhalation powder (Flexhaler): 90 mcg/metered inhalation (delivers 60 metered inhalations), 180 mcg/metered inhalation (delivers 120 metered inhalations). **Inhalation powder (Turbuhaler):** ✱ 100 mcg/metered inhalation (delivers 200 metered inhalations), ✱ 200 mcg/metered inhalation (delivers 200 metered inhalations), ✱ 400 mcg/metered inhalation (delivers 200 metered inhalations). **Inhalation suspension (Respules):** 0.25 mg/2 mL in single-dose ampules (5 ampules/envelope), 0.5 mg/2 mL in single-dose ampules (5 ampules/envelope), 1 mg/2 mL in single-dose ampules (5 ampules/envelope). ***In combination with:*** albuterol (Airsupra); formoterol (Breyna, Symbicort); formoterol and glycopyrrolate (Breztri Aerosphere). See Appendix N.

Ciclesonide

Inhalation aerosol (contains HFA-134A as a propellant): 80 mcg/actuation in 6.1-g canisters of 60 actuations, 160 mcg/actuation in 6.1-g canisters of 60 actuations.

Fluticasone

Inhalation aerosol (propionate) (Flovent-HFA generic): 44 mcg/metered inhalation in 10.6-g canisters (delivers 120 metered inhalations), ✱ 50 mcg/metered inhalation in 13-g canisters (delivers 120 metered inhalations), 110 mcg/metered inhalation in 12-g canisters (delivers 120 metered inhalations), ✱ 125 mcg/metered inhalation in 7.5-g canisters (delivers 60 metered inhalations) and 13-g canisters (delivers 120 metered inhalations), 220 mcg/metered inhalation in 12-g canisters (delivers 120 metered inhalations), ✱ 250 mcg/metered inhalation in 7.5-g canisters (delivers 60 metered inhalations) and 13-g canisters (delivers 120 metered inhalations). **Powder for inhalation (propionate) (Flovent Diskus generic):** 50 mcg/blister, 100 mcg/blister, 250 mcg/blister, ✱ 500 mcg/blister. **Powder for inhalation (furoate) (Arnuity Ellipta):** 50 mcg/blister, 100 mcg/blister, 200 mcg/blister. ***In combination with:*** salmeterol (Advair Diskus, Advair HFA, Wixhela Inhub); vilanterol (Breo Ellipta); umeclidinium and vilanterol (Trelegy Ellipta). See Appendix N.

Mometasone

Inhalation aerosol (Asmanex HFA): 50 mcg/metered inhalation in 13-g canisters (120 metered inhalations), 100 mcg/metered inhalation in 13-g canisters (120 metered inhalations), 200 mcg/metered inhalation in 13-g canisters (120 metered inhalations). **Powder for inhalation (Asmanex Twisthaler):** ✱ 100 mcg/metered inhalation (30 metered inhalations), 110 mcg (delivers 100 mcg/metered inhalation; in packages of 7 and 30 inhalation units), ✱ 200 mcg/metered inhalation (60 metered inhalations), 220 mcg (delivers 200 mcg/metered inhalation; in packages of 14, 30, 60, and 120 inhalation units), ✱ 400 mcg/metered inhalation (30 and 60 metered inhalations). ***In combination with:*** formoterol (Dulera). See Appendix N.

NURSING IMPLICATIONS

Assessment

- Monitor respiratory status and lung sounds. Assess pulmonary function tests periodically during and for several months after switching from systemic to inhalation corticosteroids.
- Assess patients changing from systemic corticosteroids to inhalation corticosteroids for signs/symptoms of adrenal insufficiency (anorexia, nausea, weakness, fatigue, hypotension, hypoglycemia) during initial therapy and periods of stress. *If signs/symptoms of adrenal insufficiency occur,* notify health care provider immediately; condition may be life-threatening.
- Monitor for withdrawal symptoms (joint or muscular pain, lassitude, depression) during withdrawal from oral corticosteroids.
- Pedi: Monitor growth rate in children receiving chronic therapy; use lowest possible dose.
- May cause ↓ bone mineral density during prolonged therapy. Monitor patients with ↑ risk (prolonged immobilization, family history of osteoporosis, postmenopausal status, tobacco use, advanced age, poor nutrition, chronic use of drugs that can ↓ bone mass [anticonvulsants, oral corticosteroids]) for fractures.
- Monitor for signs/symptoms of hypersensitivity reactions (rash, pruritus, swelling of face and neck, dyspnea) periodically during therapy. Implement supportive measures (epinephrine) as indicated.

Lab Test Considerations

- Periodic adrenal function tests may be ordered to assess degree of hypothalamic-pituitary-adrenal (HPA) axis suppression in chronic therapy. Children and patients using higher than recommended doses are at highest risk for HPA suppression.
- May ↑ serum and urine glucose concentrations if significant absorption occurs.

Implementation

- Do not confuse Flovent with Flonase.
- After desired clinical effect has been obtained, attempts should be made to ↓ dose to lowest amount required to control symptoms. Gradually ↓ dose every 2–4 wk as long as desired effect is maintained. If symptoms return, dose may briefly return to starting dose.
- **Inhaln:** Allow >1 min between inhalations.

Patient/Family Teaching

- Explain purpose and side effects of medication to patient. Advise patient to read *Patient Information* before starting therapy. Advise to take as directed. Take missed doses as soon as remembered unless almost time for next dose. Advise patient not to discontinue medication without consulting health care provider; gradual ↓ is required.
- Advise patient to notify health care provider of all Rx or OTC medications, vitamins, or herbal products being taken and to consult with health care provider before taking other medications.
- Advise patients using inhalation corticosteroids and bronchodilator to use bronchodilator 1st and to allow 5 min to elapse before administering the corticosteroid, unless otherwise directed by health care provider.
- Advise patient that inhalation corticosteroids should not be used to treat an acute asthma attack but should be continued even if other inhalation agents are used.
- Patients using inhalation corticosteroids to control asthma may require systemic corticosteroids for acute attacks. Advise patient to use regular peak flow monitoring to determine respiratory status.
- Advise patient to avoid smoking, known allergens, and other respiratory irritants.
- Advise patient to notify health care provider if sore throat or sore mouth occurs.
- Advise patient to stop using medication and notify health care provider immediately if signs and symptoms of hypersensitivity reactions occur.
- Advise patient whose systemic corticosteroids have been recently ↓ or withdrawn to carry a warning card indicating the need for supplemental systemic corticosteroids in the event of stress or severe asthma attack unresponsive to bronchodilators.
- Advise patient to have regular eye exams. May ↑ risk for eye problems (glaucoma, cataracts, blurred vision).
- **Metered-Dose Inhaler:** Advise patient in proper use of metered-dose inhaler. Most inhalers require priming before 1st use. Shake inhaler well. Exhale completely, and then close lips firmly around mouthpiece. While breathing in deeply and slowly, press down on canister. Hold breath for as long as possible to ensure deep instillation of medication. Remove inhaler from mouth and breathe out gently. Allow 1–2 min between inhalations. Rinse mouth with water or mouthwash after each use to minimize fungal infections, dry mouth, and hoarseness. Clean mouthpiece weekly with clean, dry tissue or cloth. Do not place in water (see Appendix C).
- **Pulmicort Flexhaler:** Advise patient to follow instructions supplied. Before 1st-time use, prime unit by turning cover and lifting off; hold upright with mouthpiece up and twist brown grip fully to right and then fully to left until it clicks. To administer dose, hold upright and twist brown grip fully to right and then fully to left until it clicks. Turn head away from inhaler and exhale (do not blow into inhaler). Do not shake inhaler. Place mouthpiece between lips and inhale deeply and forcefully. Remove inhaler from mouth and exhale (do not exhale into mouthpiece). Repeat procedure if 2nd dose required. Replace cover; rinse mouth with water (do not swallow).
- **Pulmicort Respules:** Administer with a jet nebulizer connected to adequate air flow, equipped with a mouthpiece or face mask. Adjust face mask to avoid exposing eyes to nebulized medication. Wash face after use of face mask. Ultrasonic nebulizers are not adequate for administration and not recommended. Store respules upright, away from heat, and protected from light. Do not refrigerate or freeze. Respules are stable for 2 wk at room temperature after opening aluminum foil envelope. Open respules must be used promptly. Unused respules should be returned to aluminum foil envelope.
- **Arnuity Ellipta:** Do not use with a spacer. Exhale completely and then close lips firmly around mouthpiece. While breathing in deeply and slowly, press down on canister. Hold breath for as long as possible to ensure deep instillation of medication. Remove inhaler from mouth and breathe out gently. Allow 1–2 min between inhalations. After inhalation, rinse mouth with water and spit out (see Appendix C). Never wash the mouthpiece or any part of the Diskus inhaler. Discard Diskus inhaler device (Flovent Diskus) 6 wk (50-mcg strength) or 2 mo (100-mcg and 250-mcg strengths) or blister tray (Arnuity Ellipta) 6 wk after removal from protective foil overwrap pouch or after all blisters have been used (whichever comes 1st).
- **Asmanex Twisthaler:** Advise patient to remove cap while device is in upright position. To administer dose, exhale fully; then place mouthpiece between lips and inhale deeply and forcefully. Remove device from mouth and hold breath for 10 sec before exhaling (do not exhale into mouthpiece). Wipe the mouthpiece dry, if necessary, and replace the cap on the device. Rinse mouth with water. Advise patient to discard twisthaler 45 days from opening or when dose counter reads "00," whichever comes 1st.
- Rep: Advise women of reproductive potential to notify health care provider if pregnancy is planned or suspected or if breastfeeding.

Evaluation/Desired Outcomes

- Decreased frequency and severity of asthma attacks.
- Improves asthma symptoms.

CORTICOSTEROIDS (NASAL)

beclomethasone (be-kloe-**meth**-a-sone)
~~Beconase AQ~~, QNASL, 🍁 ~~Rivanase AQ~~

budesonide (byoo-**dess**-oh-nide)
Rhinocort Allergy, 🍁 Rhinocort Aqua

ciclesonide (sye-**kles**-oh-nide)
Omnaris, ~~Zetonna~~

fluticasone (floo-**ti**-ka-sone)
🍁 Avamys, Flonase Allergy Relief, Flonase Sensimist Allergy Relief, Xhance

mometasone (moe-**met**-a-sone)
~~Nasonex~~

triamcinolone (trye-am-**sin**-oh-lone)
Nasacort Allergy 24 HR, 🍁 Nasacort AQ

Classification
Therapeutic: anti-inflammatories (steroidal)
Pharmacologic: corticosteroids (nasal)

Indications

Seasonal or perennial allergic rhinitis. Nonallergic rhinitis (fluticasone). Chronic rhinosinusitis with nasal polyps.

Action

Potent, locally acting anti-inflammatory and immune modifier. **Therapeutic Effects:** ↓ in symptoms of allergic or nonallergic rhinitis. ↓ in symptoms of nasal polyps.

Pharmacokinetics

Absorption: *Beclomethasone:* 27–44% absorbed; *budesonide:* 34% absorbed; *ciclesonide, fluticasone, mometasone:* Negligible absorption. Action of all agents is primarily local following nasal use.
Distribution: Unknown.
Metabolism and Excretion: Following absorption from nasal mucosa, corticosteroids are rapidly and extensively metabolized by the liver.
Half-life: *Beclomethasone:* 2.7 hr; *budesonide:* 2–3 hr; *ciclesonide:* unknown; *fluticasone:* 7.8 hr; *mometasone:* 5.8 hr; *triamcinolone:* 3–5.4 hr.

TIME/ACTION PROFILE (improvement in symptoms)

ROUTE	ONSET	PEAK	DURATION
Beclomethasone	1–3 days	up to 2 wk	unknown
Budesonide	1–2 days	2 wk	unknown
Ciclesonide	1–2 days	2–5 wk	unknown
Flunisolide	few days	up to 3 wk	unknown
Fluticasone	few days	unknown	unknown
Mometasone	within 2 days	1–2 wk	unknown
Triamcinolone	few days	3–4 days	unknown

Contraindications/Precautions

Contraindicated in: Some products contain alcohol, propylene, or polyethylene glycol and should be avoided in patients with known hypersensitivity or intolerance.
Use Cautiously in: Active untreated infections; Diabetes or glaucoma; Underlying immunosuppression (due to disease or concurrent therapy); Systemic corticosteroid therapy (should not be abruptly discontinued when intranasal therapy is started); History of ↑ intraocular pressure, glaucoma, or cataracts; Recent nasal trauma, septal ulcers, or surgery (wound healing may be impaired by nasal corticosteroids); OB: Safety not established in pregnancy; Lactation: Safety not established in breastfeeding; Pedi: Safety and effectiveness not established in children <12 yr (beclomethasone]), <6 yr (budesonide, ciclesonide), <4 yr (fluticasone [Flonase Allergy Relief]), or <2 yr (fluticasone [Flonase Sensimist], mometasone, triamcinolone).

Adverse Reactions/Side Effects

Derm: rash (fluticasone), urticaria (fluticasone). **EENT:** ↑ intraocular pressure, blurred vision, cataracts, epistaxis, glaucoma, nasal burning, nasal congestion, nasal irritation, nasal perforation, nasal ulceration, pharyngitis, rhinorrhea, sneezing, tearing eyes. **Endo:** adrenal suppression (high-dose, long-term therapy only), growth suppression (children). **GI:** dry mouth, esophageal candidiasis, nausea, vomiting. **Neuro:** dizziness, headache. **Resp:** bronchospasm, cough. **Misc:** HYPERSENSITIVITY REACTIONS (INCLUDING ANAPHYLAXIS AND ANGIOEDEMA).

Interactions

Drug-Drug: Strong CYP3A4 inhibitors, including **atazanavir**, **clarithromycin**, **cobicistat**, **itraconazole**, **ketoconazole**, **nefazodone**, **nelfinavir**, and **ritonavir**, may ↑ levels and risk of toxicity of budesonide, ciclesonide, fluticasone, and mometasone.

Route/Dosage

Beclomethasone

Intranasal (Adults and Children ≥12 yr): 2 sprays in each nostril once daily.

🍁 = Canadian drug name. ⚕ = Genetic implication. V = Vesicant. Boxed warning.
~~Strikethrough~~ = Discontinued. *CAPITALS = life-threatening. Underline = most frequent.

Intranasal (Children 4–11 yr): 1 spray in each nostril once daily.

Budesonide

Intranasal (Adults and Children ≥12 yr): 1 spray in each nostril once daily (not to exceed 4 sprays in each nostril once daily). For OTC use, administer 2 sprays in each nostril once daily; once symptoms improve, ↓ to 1 spray in each nostril once daily.
Intranasal (Children 6–11 yr): 1 spray in each nostril once daily (not to exceed 2 sprays in each nostril once daily).

Ciclesonide

Intranasal (Adults and Children ≥12 yr): 2 sprays in each nostril once daily (not to exceed 2 sprays in each nostril/day);
Intranasal (Adults and Children ≥6 yr): 2 sprays in each nostril once daily (not to exceed 2 sprays in each nostril/day).

Flunisolide

Intranasal (Adults and Children >14 yr): 2 sprays in each nostril twice daily; may ↑ to 2 sprays in each nostril 3 times daily if greater effect needed after 4–7 days (not to exceed 8 sprays in each nostril/day).
Intranasal (Children 6–14 yr): 1 spray in each nostril 3 times daily or 2 sprays in each nostril twice daily (not to exceed 4 sprays in each nostril/day).

Fluticasone

Intranasal (Adults): *Fluticasone Rx:* 2 sprays in each nostril once daily or 1 spray in each nostril twice daily (not to exceed 2 sprays in each nostril/day); after several days, attempt to ↓ dose to 1 spray in each nostril once daily. *Xhance:* 1 spray in each nostril twice daily; may adjust to 2 sprays in each nostril twice daily.
Intranasal (Adults and Children ≥12 yr): *Flonase Sensimist Allergy Relief (OTC) and Flonase Allergy Relief (OTC):* 2 sprays in each nostril once daily; after 1 wk, may adjust to 1–2 sprays in each nostril once daily; discuss with health care provider if need to continue >6 mo.
Intranasal (Children 4–11 yr): *Flonase Allergy Relief (OTC):* 1 spray in each nostril once daily; discuss with health care provider if need to continue >2 mo.
Intranasal (Children ≥4 yr): *Fluticasone Rx:* 1 spray in each nostril once daily; may ↑ to 2 sprays in each nostril once daily if no response; once symptoms controlled, attempt to ↓ dose to 1 spray in each nostril once daily.
Intranasal (Children 2–11 yr): *Flonase Sensimist Allergy Relief (OTC):* 1 spray in each nostril once daily; discuss with health care provider if need to continue >2 mo.

Mometasone

Intranasal (Adults and Children >12 yr): *Treatment of seasonal and perennial allergic rhinitis:* 2 sprays in each nostril once daily (not to exceed 2 sprays in each nostril once daily).
Intranasal (Adults): *Nasal polyps:* 2 sprays in each nostril twice daily (not to exceed 2 sprays in each nostril twice daily).
Intranasal (Children 2–11 yr): *Treatment of seasonal and perennial allergic rhinitis:* 1 spray in each nostril once daily.

Triamcinolone

Intranasal (Adults and Children ≥12 yr): 2 sprays in each nostril once daily; not to be used in children for >2 mo.
Intranasal (Children 6–11 yr): 1 spray in each nostril once daily (not to exceed 2 sprays in each nostril/day); not to be used for >2 mo.
Intranasal (Children 2–5 yr): 1 spray in each nostril once daily not to be used for >2 mo.

Availability

Beclomethasone

Nasal spray: 40 mcg/metered spray in 4.9-g bottles (delivers 60 metered sprays), 80 mcg/metered spray in 8.7-g bottles (delivers 120 metered sprays).

Budesonide (generic available)

Nasal spray (Rhinocort Allergy): 32 mcg/metered spray in 5-mL bottle (delivers 60 metered sprays)OTC, and 8.43-mL bottle (delivers 120 metered sprays)OTC. **Nasal spray (Rhinocort Aqua):** ✱ 64 mcg/metered spray (delivers 120 metered sprays).

Ciclesonide

Nasal suspension: 50 mcg/metered spray in 12.5-g bottle (delivers 120 metered sprays).

Flunisolide (generic available)

Nasal solution: 25 mcg/actuation in 25-mL bottle (delivers 200 metered sprays).

Fluticasone (generic available)

Nasal spray: 50 mcg/metered spray in 16-g bottle (delivers 120 metered sprays). **Nasal spray (Flonase Allergy Relief):** 50 mcg/metered spray in 9.9-mL bottle (delivers 60 metered sprays)OTC. **Nasal spray (Flonase Sensimist Allergy Relief):** 27.5 mcg/spray in 9.9-mL bottle (delivers 60 metered sprays)OTC. **Nasal spray (Avamys):** ✱ 27.5 mcg/spray in 4.5-g bottle (delivers 30 metered sprays) and 10-g bottle (delivers 120 metered sprays). **Nasal spray (Xhance):** 93 mcg/spray in 16-mL bottle (delivers 120 metered sprays).
In combination with: azelastine (Dymista); see Appendix N.

Mometasone (generic available)
Nasal spray (scent-free): 50 mcg/metered spray in 17-g bottle (delivers 120 metered sprays). ***In combination with:*** olopatadine (Ryaltris). See Appendix N.

Triamcinolone (generic available)
Nasal spray: 55 mcg/metered spray in 6.7-mL bottle (delivers 30 metered sprays)[OTC], 10.8-mL bottle (delivers 60 metered sprays)[OTC], and 16.9-mL bottle (delivers 120 metered sprays)[OTC].

NURSING IMPLICATIONS

Assessment

- Assess degree of nasal stuffiness, amount and color of nasal discharge, and frequency of sneezing.
- Assess for hypersensitivity reactions (anaphylaxis); if occur, implement supportive measures (epinephrine) as indicated.
- Assess for signs of adverse effects on nasal mucosa (nasal discomfort, epistaxis, nasal ulceration, *Candida albicans* infection, nasal septal perforation, impaired wound healing) periodically during therapy. Avoid use in patients with recent nasal ulcers, nasal surgery, or nasal trauma.
- Patients on long-term therapy should have periodic otolaryngologic examinations to monitor nasal mucosa and passages for infection or ulceration.
- Pedi: Monitor growth rate in children receiving chronic therapy; use lowest possible dose.

Lab Test Considerations

- Periodic adrenal function tests may be ordered to assess degree of hypothalamic-pituitary-adrenal (HPA) axis suppression in chronic therapy. Children and patients using higher than recommended doses are at highest risk for HPA suppression.

Implementation

- Do not confuse Flonase with Flovent.
- After desired clinical effect is obtained, ↓ dose to lowest effective amount. Gradually ↓ dose every 2–4 wk as long as desired effect is maintained. If symptoms return, dose may briefly return to starting dose.
- **Intranasal:** Patients also using a nasal decongestant should be given decongestant 5–15 min before corticosteroid nasal spray. If patient is unable to breathe freely through nasal passages, instruct patient to blow nose gently in advance of medication administration.

Patient/Family Teaching

- Explain purpose and side effects of medication to patient. Advise patient to read *Patient Information* before starting therapy. Advise to take as directed. Take missed doses as soon as remembered unless almost time for next dose.
- Advise patient to notify health care provider of all Rx or OTC medications, vitamins, or herbal products being taken and to consult with health care provider before taking other medications.
- Advise patient not to exceed maximal daily dose of nasal spray.
- Educate patient on correct technique for administering nasal spray (see Appendix C). Most nasal sprays include directions with pictures. Instruct patient to read patient information sheet prior to use. Most nasal sprays require priming before 1st use or use after 7 days. Shake well before use. Warn patient that temporary nasal stinging may occur.
- Advise patient to gently blow nose to clear nostrils prior to administering dose.
- Advise patient to stop medication and notify health care provider immediately if signs/symptoms of anaphylaxis (rash, hives, difficulty breathing, swollen lips or throat) or if changes in vision occur.
- Advise patient to notify health care provider if symptoms do not improve within 1 mo, if symptoms worsen, or if sneezing or nasal irritation occurs.
- Rep: Advise women of reproductive potential to notify health care provider if pregnancy is planned or suspected or if breastfeeding.

Evaluation/Desired Outcomes

- ↓ in symptoms of allergic or nonallergic rhinitis.
- ↓ in symptoms of nasal polyps.

CORTICOSTEROIDS (SYSTEMIC)

short-acting corticosteroids

hydrocortisone (hye-droe-**kor**-ti-sone)
Alkindi Sprinkle, Cortef, Cortenema, Solu-CORTEF

intermediate-acting corticosteroids

methylPREDNISolone (meth-ill-pred-**niss**-oh-lone)
Depo-Medrol, Medrol, Solu-MEDROL

prednisoLONE (pred-**niss**-oh-lone)
~~Orapred~~, Millipred, Orapred ODT, Pediapred

predniSONE (**pred**-ni-sone)
~~Rayos~~, ✤Winipred

triamcinolone (trye-am-**sin**-oh-lone)

Hexatrione, Kenalog, ✱ Trispan, Zilretta

long-acting corticosteroids

betamethasone (bay-ta-**meth**-a-sone)

~~Betaject~~, Celestone Soluspan, ~~Celestone~~

budesonide (byoo-**dess**-oh-nide)

✱ Cortiment, ✱ Entocort, ✱ Jorveza, ~~Entocort EC~~, Ortikos, Tarpeyo, Uceris

dexAMETHasone (dex-a-**meth**-a-sone)

~~Decadron~~, Hemady

Classification

Therapeutic: antiasthmatics, corticosteroids

Pharmacologic: corticosteroids (systemic)

Indications

Hydrocortisone: Adrenocortical insufficiency. **Betamethasone, dexamethasone, hydrocortisone, prednisolone, prednisone, methylprednisolone, triamcinolone:** Used systemically and locally in a wide variety of chronic diseases, including: Inflammatory, Allergic, Hematologic, Neoplastic, Autoimmune disorders. **Methylprednisolone, prednisone:** With other immunosuppressants in the prevention of organ rejection in transplantation surgery. Asthma. **Dexamethasone:** Cerebral edema, Diagnostic agent in adrenal disorders, Multiple myeloma (in combination with other anti-myeloma agents). **Budesonide (3-mg Delayed-Release Capsules and Ortikos):** Mild to moderate Crohn disease involving ileum and/or ascending colon. **Budesonide (3-mg Delayed-Release Capsules and Ortikos):** Maintenance of clinical remission for up to 3 mo of mild to moderate Crohn disease involving ileum and/or ascending colon. **Budesonide (Uceris):** Induction of remission of active, mild to moderate ulcerative colitis. **Budesonide (Tarpeyo):** Reduction of proteinuria in patients with primary immunoglobulin A nephropathy who are at risk of rapid disease progression (i.e., a urine protein-to-creatinine ratio [UPCR] ≥ 1.5 g/g). **Unlabeled Use:** Short-term administration to high-risk mothers before delivery to prevent respiratory distress syndrome in the newborn (betamethasone, dexamethasone). Adjunctive therapy of hypercalcemia (prednisone, prednisolone, methylprednisolone). Acute spinal cord injury (methylprednisolone). Adjunctive management of nausea and vomiting from chemotherapy (dexamethasone, prednisone, prednisolone, methylprednisolone). Croup (dexamethasone). Airway edema prior to extubation (dexamethasone). Facilitation of ventilator weaning in neonates with bronchopulmonary dysplasia (dexamethasone).

Action

In pharmacologic doses, all agents suppress inflammation and the normal immune response. All agents have numerous intense metabolic effects (see Adverse Reactions/Side Effects). Suppress adrenal function at chronic doses of *betamethasone:* 0.6 mg/day; *hydrocortisone:* 20 mg/day; *dexamethasone:* 0.75 mg/day; *methylprednisolone, triamcinolone:* 4 mg/day; *prednisone/prednisolone:* 5 mg/day. **Hydrocortisone:** Replace endogenous cortisol in deficiency states. **Hydrocortisone:** Have potent mineralocorticoid (sodium-retaining) activity. **Prednisolone, prednisone:** Have minimal mineralocorticoid activity. **Betamethasone, dexamethasone, methylprednisolone, triamcinolone:** Have negligible mineralocorticoid activity. **Budesonide:** Local anti-inflammatory activity in the lumen of the GI tract in Crohn disease and ulcerative colitis; modulates activity of B cells in ileum to decrease production of galactose-deficient IgA1 antibodies, which cause IgA nephropathy. **Therapeutic Effects:** Suppression of inflammation and modification of the normal immune response. Replacement therapy in adrenal insufficiency. **Budesonide:** Improvement in symptoms/sequelae of Crohn disease, induction of remission of ulcerative colitis, and reduction in UPCR.

Pharmacokinetics

Absorption: Well absorbed after oral administration (except budesonide). Sodium phosphate and sodium succinate salts are rapidly absorbed after IM administration. Acetate and acetonide salts are slowly but completely absorbed after IM administration. Absorption from local sites (intra-articular, intralesional) is slow but complete. Bioavailability of budesonide is 9–21%.

Distribution: All are widely distributed.

Metabolism and Excretion: All are metabolized mostly by the liver to inactive metabolites. *Prednisone* is converted by the liver to prednisolone, which is then metabolized by the liver.

Half-life: *Betamethasone:* 3–5 hr (plasma), 36–54 hr (tissue). *budesonide:* 2.0–3.6 hr (3-mg delayed-release capsules, Ortikos, Uceris); 5–6.8 hr (Tarpeyo). *dexamethasone:* 3–4.5 hr (plasma), 36–54 hr (tissue). *hydrocortisone:* 1.5–2 hr (plasma), 8–12 hr (tissue). *methylprednisolone:* >3.5 hr (plasma), 18–36 hr (tissue). *prednisolone:* 2.1–3.5 hr (plasma), 18–36 hr (tissue). *prednisone:* 3.4–3.8 hr (plasma), 18–36 hr (tissue). *triamcinolone:* 2–5 hr (plasma), 18–36 hr (tissue).

TIME/ACTION PROFILE (anti-inflammatory activity)

ROUTE	ONSET	PEAK	DURATION
Betamethasone IM (acetate/sodium phosphate)	1–3 hr	unknown	1 wk
Budesonide PO	unknown	unknown	unknown
Dexamethasone PO	unknown	1–3 hr	2.75 days
Dexamethasone IM, IV (sodium phosphate)	rapid	unknown	2.75 days
Hydrocortisone PO	unknown	1–2 hr	1.25–1.5 days
Hydrocortisone IM (sodium succinate)	rapid	1 hr	variable
Hydrocortisone IV (sodium succinate)	rapid	unknown	unknown
Methylprednisolone PO	unknown	1–2 hr	1.25–1.5 days
Methylprednisolone IM (acetate)	6–48 hr	4–8 days	1–4 wk
Methylprednisolone IM, IV (sodium succinate)	rapid	unknown	unknown
Prednisolone PO	unknown	1–2 hr	1.25–1.5 days
Prednisone PO	unknown	1–2 hr	1.25–1.5 days
Triamcinolone IM (acetonide)	24–48 hr	unknown	1–6 wk
Triamcinolone Intralesional (hexacetonide)	slow	unknown	4 days–4 wk

Contraindications/Precautions

Contraindicated in: Active untreated infections (may be used in patients being treated for some forms of meningitis); Lactation: Avoid chronic use; Known alcohol, bisulfite, cow's milk, or tartrazine hypersensitivity or intolerance (some products contain these and should be avoided in susceptible patients); Administration of live-virus vaccines.

Use Cautiously in: Chronic treatment (will lead to adrenal suppression; use lowest possible dose for shortest period of time); Hypothyroidism; Immunosuppression; Cirrhosis; Stress (surgery, infections); supplemental doses may be needed; Potential infections may mask signs (fever, inflammation); Traumatic brain injury (high doses may be associated with ↑ mortality); OB: Safety not established in pregnancy; Pedi: Chronic use in children will result in ↓ growth; use lowest possible dose for shortest period of time; Pedi: Neonates (avoid use of benzyl alcohol containing injectable preparations; use preservative-free formulations).

Adverse Reactions/Side Effects

Adverse reactions/side effects are much more common with high-dose/long-term therapy.

CV: hypertension. **Derm:** ↓ wound healing, acne, ecchymoses, fragility, hirsutism, petechiae. **EENT:** ↑ intraocular pressure, cataracts. **Endo:** adrenal suppression, cushingoid appearance (moon face, buffalo hump), hyperglycemia, PHEOCHROMOCYTOMA. **F and E:** fluid retention (long-term high doses), hypokalemia, hypokalemic alkalosis. **GI:** anorexia, nausea, PEPTIC ULCERATION, vomiting. **Hemat:** leukocytosis, THROMBOEMBOLISM, thrombophlebitis. **Metab:** weight gain. **MS:** muscle wasting, osteoporosis, avascular necrosis of joints, muscle pain. **Neuro:** depression, euphoria, ↑ intracranial pressure (children only), headache, personality changes, psychoses, restlessness. **Misc:** ↑ susceptibility to infection.

Interactions

Drug-Drug: ↑ risk of hypokalemia with **thiazide** and **loop diuretics**, or **amphotericin B**. Hypokalemia may ↑ risk of **digoxin** toxicity. May ↑ requirement for **insulin** or **oral hypoglycemic agents**. **Phenytoin**, **phenobarbital**, and **rifampin** may ↓ levels and effectiveness. **Hormonal contraceptives** may ↓ levels and effectiveness. ↑ risk of adverse GI effects with **NSAIDs** (including aspirin). At chronic doses that suppress adrenal function, may ↓ antibody response to and ↑ risk of adverse reactions from **live-virus vaccines**. May ↑ levels and risk of toxicity of **cyclosporine** and **tacrolimus**. May ↑ risk of tendon rupture from **fluoroquinolones**. **Antacids** ↓ absorption of prednisone and dexamethasone. **CYP3A4 inhibitors**, including **clarithromycin**, **cobicistat**, **itraconazole**, **ketoconazole**, or **ritonavir**, may ↑ levels and risk of toxicity. May ↓ levels and effectiveness of **isoniazid**. May antagonize the effects of **anticholinergic agents** in myasthenia gravis.

Drug-Food: **Grapefruit juice** ↑ levels and risk of toxicity of budesonide; avoid concurrent use.

Route/Dosage

Betamethasone

IM (Adults): 0.5–9 mg as betamethasone sodium phosphate/acetate suspension. *Prevention of respiratory distress syndrome in newborn:* 12 mg once daily for 2–3 days before delivery (unlabeled).

IM (Children): *Adrenocortical insufficiency:* 17.5 mcg/kg/day (500 mcg/m²/day) in 3 divided doses every 3rd day or 5.8–8.75 mcg/kg (166–250 mcg/m²)/day as a single dose.

Budesonide

PO (Adults): *Active Crohn disease:* 9 mg once daily in the morning for up to 8 wk; may repeat 8-wk course for recurring episodes. *Maintenance of remission of Crohn disease:* 6 mg once daily for up to 3 mo; once symptoms are controlled, taper to complete cessation; *Induction of remission of ulcerative colitis:* 9 mg once daily for up to 8 wk; once symptoms are controlled, taper to complete cessation; *Reduction in proteinuria associated with primary immunoglobulin A nephropathy:* 16 mg once daily in the morning for 9 mo, then 8 mg once daily in the morning for 2 wk.

PO (Children 8–17 yr and >25 kg): *Active Crohn disease:* 9 mg once daily in the morning for up to 8 wk, then 6 mg once daily in the morning for 2 wk.

Hepatic Impairment

(Adults): *Moderate hepatic impairment:* 3 mg once daily in the morning.

Dexamethasone

PO, IM, IV (Adults): *Anti-inflammatory:* 0.75–9 mg/day divided every 6–12 hr. *Airway edema or extubation:* 0.5–2 mg/kg/day divided every 6 hr; begin 24 hr prior to extubation and continue for 24 hr postextubation. *Cerebral edema:* 10 mg IV initially, then 4 mg IM or IV every 6 hr until maximal response achieved; then switch to PO regimen and taper over 5–7 days.

PO, IM, IV (Children): *Airway edema or extubation:* 0.5–2 mg/kg/day divided every 6 hr; begin 24 hr prior to extubation and continue for 24 hr postextubation. *Anti-inflammatory:* 0.08–0.3 mg/kg/day or 2.5–10 mg/m²/day divided every 6–12 hr. *Physiologic replacement:* 0.03–0.15 mg/kg/day or 0.6–0.75 mg/m²/day divided every 6–12 hr.

PO (Adults): *Suppression test:* 1 mg at 11 pm or 0.5 mg every 6 hr for 48 hr. *Multiple myeloma:* 20–40 mg once daily on specific days (based on protocol being used).

IV (Children): *Chemotherapy-induced emesis:* 5–20 mg given 15–30 min before treatment; *Cerebral edema:* Loading dose of 1–2 mg/kg followed by 1–1.5 mg/kg/day divided every 4–6 hr for 5 days (not to exceed 16 mg/day); then taper over 1–6 wk; *Bacterial meningitis:* 0.6 mg/kg/day divided every 6 hr for 4 days (start at time of 1st antibiotic dose).

IV, PO (Adults): *Chemotherapy-induced emesis:* 10–20 mg given 15–30 min before each treatment or 10 mg every 12 hr on each treatment day; *Delayed nausea/vomiting:* 4–10 mg PO 1–2 times/day for 2–4 days *or* 8 mg PO every 12 hr for 2 days, then 4 mg PO every 12 hr for 2 days *or* 20 mg PO 1 hr before chemotherapy, then 10 mg PO every 12 hr after chemotherapy, then 8 mg PO every 12 hr for 2 days, then 4 mg PO every 12 hr for 2 days.

IS (Adults): 0.4–6 mg/day.

Hydrocortisone

PO (Adults): 20–240 mg/day in 1–4 divided doses.

PO (Children): *Adrenocortical insufficiency/replacement therapy:* 8–10 mg/m²/day in 2–3 divided doses; *Anti-inflammatory or immunosuppressive:* 2.5–10 mg/kg/day or 75–300 mg/m²/day in 3–4 divided doses.

IM, IV (Adults): 100–500 mg every 2–6 hr (range 100–8000 mg/day).

IM, IV (Children): *Adrenocortical insufficiency:* 0.186–0.28 mg/kg/day (10–12 mg/m²/day) in 3 divided doses. *Other uses:* 0.666–4 mg/kg (20–120 mg/m²) every 12–24 hr.

Rect (Adults): *Retention enema:* 100 mg nightly for 21 days or until remission occurs.

Methylprednisolone

PO (Adults): *Multiple sclerosis:* 160 mg/day for 7 days, then 64 mg every other day for 1 mo. *Other uses:* 2–60 mg/day as a single dose or in 2–4 divided doses. *Asthma exacerbations:* 120–180 mg/day in divided doses 3–4 times/day for 48 hr, then 60–80 mg/day in 2 divided doses.

PO (Children): *Anti-inflammatory/Immunosuppressive:* 0.5–1.7 mg/kg/day (5–25 mg/m²/day) in divided doses every 6–12 hr. *Asthma exacerbations:* 1 mg/kg every 6 hr for 48 hr, then 1–2 mg/kg/day (maximum: 60 mg/day) divided twice daily.

IM, IV (Adults): *Most uses: methylprednisolone sodium succinate:* 40–250 mg every 4–6 hr. *High-dose "pulse" therapy (methylprednisolone sodium succinate):* 30 mg/kg IV every 4–6 hr for up to 72 hr. *Status asthmaticus (methylprednisolone sodium succinate):* 2 mg/kg IV, then 0.5–1 mg/kg IV every 6 hr for up to 5 days. *Multiple sclerosis (methylprednisolone sodium succinate):* 160 mg/day for 7 days, then 64 mg every other day for 1 mo. *Adjunctive therapy of Pneumocystis jiroveci pneumonia in patients with AIDS (methylprednisolone sodium succinate):* 30 mg twice daily for 5 days, then 30 mg once daily for 5 days, then 15 mg once daily for 10 days. *Acute spinal cord injury (methylprednisolone sodium succinate):* 30 mg/kg IV over 15 min initially, followed in 45 min with a continuous infusion of 5.4 mg/kg/hr for 23 hr (unlabeled).

IM, IV (Children): *Anti-inflammatory/Immunosuppressive:* 0.5–1.7 mg/kg/day (5–25 mg/m²/day) in divided doses every 6–12 hr. *Acute spinal cord injury (methylprednisolone sodium succinate):* 30 mg/kg IV over 15 min initially, followed in 45 min with a continuous infusion of 5.4 mg/kg/hr for 23 hr (unlabeled). *Status asthmaticus:* 2 mg/kg IV, then 0.5–1 mg/kg IV every 6 hr. *Lupus nephritis:* 30 mg/kg IV every other day for 6 doses.

IM (Adults): *Methylprednisolone acetate:* 40–120 mg daily, weekly, or every 2 wk.

Prednisolone

PO (Adults): *Most uses:* 5–60 mg/day as a single dose or in divided doses. *Multiple sclerosis:* 200 mg/day for 7 days, then 80 mg every other day for 1 mo. *Asthma exacerbations:* 120–180 mg/day in divided doses 3–4 times/day for 48 hr, then 60–80 mg/day in 2 divided doses.

PO (Children): *Anti-inflammatory/Immunosuppressive:* 0.1–2 mg/kg/day in 1–4 divided doses; *Nephrotic syndrome:* 2 mg/kg/day (60 mg/m²/day) in 1–3 divided doses daily (maximum dose: 80 mg/day) until urine is protein-free for 4–6 wk, followed by 2 mg/kg/dose (40 mg/m²/dose) every other day in the morning; gradually taper off over 4–6 wk; *Asthma exacerbations:* 1 mg/kg every 6 hr for 48 hr, then 1–2 mg/kg/day (maximum: 60 mg/day) divided twice daily.

Prednisone

PO (Adults): *Most uses:* 5–60 mg/day as a single dose or in divided doses (delayed-release tablets should be administered once daily). *Multiple sclerosis:* 200 mg/day for 1 wk; then 80 mg every other day for 1 mo. *Adjunctive therapy of Pneumocystis jiroveci pneumonia in patients with AIDS:* 40 mg twice daily for 5 days; then 40 mg once daily for 5 days; then 20 mg once daily for 10 days.

PO (Children): *Nephrotic syndrome:* 2 mg/kg/day initially given in 1–3 divided doses (maximum 80 mg/day; delayed-release tablets should be administered once daily) until urine is protein-free for 4–6 wk. Maintenance dose of 2 mg/kg/day every other day in the morning; gradually taper off after 4–6 wk. *Asthma exacerbation:* 1 mg/kg every 6 hr for 48 hr; then 1–2 mg/kg/day (maximum 60 mg/day) in divided doses twice daily.

Triamcinolone

IM (Adults): *Triamcinolone acetonide:* 40–80 mg every 4 wk.

Intra-articular: (Adults): *Triamcinolone hexacetonide:* 2–20 mg every 3–4 wk (dose depends on size of joint to be injected, amount of inflammation, and amount of fluid present); *Triamcinolone acetonide:* 32 mg as a single dose into the knee joint.

IM (Children): *Triamcinolone acetonide:* 40 mg every 4 wk or 30–200 mcg/kg (1–6.25 mg/m²) every 1–7 days.

Availability

Betamethasone (generic available)

Suspension for injection (sodium phosphate and acetate): 6 mg (total)/mL.

Budesonide (generic available)

Delayed-release capsules: 3 mg. **Delayed-release capsules (Tarpeyo):** 4 mg. **Extended-release capsules (Ortikos):** 6 mg, 9 mg. **Extended-release tablets (Uceris):** 9 mg. **Orally disintegrating tablets (Jorveza):** 🍁 1 mg.

Dexamethasone (generic available)

Tablets: 0.5 mg, 0.75 mg, 1 mg, 1.5 mg, 2 mg, 4 mg, 6 mg, 20 mg. **Elixir (raspberry flavor):** 0.5 mg/5 mL. **Oral solution (cherry flavor):** 0.5 mg/5 mL, 1 mg/mL. **Solution for injection (sodium phosphate):** 4 mg/mL, 10 mg/mL.

Hydrocortisone (generic available)

Tablets: 5 mg, 10 mg, 20 mg. **Oral granules (Alkindi Sprinkle):** 0.5 mg, 1 mg, 2 mg, 5 mg. **Enema:** 100 mg/60 mL. **Lyophilized powder for injection (sodium succinate):** 100 mg/vial, 250 mg/vial, 500 mg/vial, 1 g.

Methylprednisolone (generic available)

Tablets: 2 mg, 4 mg, 8 mg, 16 mg, 32 mg. **Powder for injection (sodium succinate):** 40 mg/vial, 125 mg/vial, 500 mg/vial, 1 g/vial, 2 g/vial. **Suspension for injection (acetate):** 20 mg/mL, 40 mg/mL, 80 mg/mL.

Prednisolone (generic available)

Tablets: 5 mg. **Orally disintegrating tablets (grape flavor):** 10 mg, 15 mg, 30 mg. **Oral solution:** 5 mg/5 mL, 10 mg/5 mL, 15 mg/5 mL, 20 mg/5 mL, 25 mg/5 mL.

Prednisone (generic available)

Tablets: 1 mg, 2.5 mg, 5 mg, 10 mg, 20 mg, 50 mg. **Delayed-release tablets:** 1 mg, 2 mg, 5 mg. **Oral solution:** 5 mg/5 mL, 5 mg/mL.

Triamcinolone (generic available)

Extended-release suspension for intra-articular injection (acetonide) (requires reconstitution) (Zilretta): 32 mg/vial. **Suspension for intra-articular injection (hexacetonide):** 20 mg/mL. **Suspension for intramuscular injection (acetonide):** 10 mg/mL, 40 mg/mL, 80 mg/mL.

NURSING IMPLICATIONS

Assessment

- Assess for signs/symptoms of adrenal insufficiency (hypotension, weight loss, weakness, nausea, vomiting, anorexia, lethargy, confusion, restlessness) before and periodically during therapy. When switching other oral hydrocortisone formulations to *Alkindi Sprinkle*, use the same total daily hydrocortisone dose. Closely monitor patient after switching to *Alkindi Sprinkle* for signs/symptoms of adrenocortical insufficiency. If signs/symptoms of adrenal insufficiency occur after switching, ↑ total daily dose of *Alkindi Sprinkle*.

- Monitor intake, output, and daily weights. Observe for peripheral edema, steady weight gain, rales/crackles, or dyspnea. Notify health care provider if these occur.
- Pedi: Children should have periodic evaluations of growth; may slow growth.
- **Cerebral Edema:** Assess for changes in level of consciousness and headache during therapy.
- **Budesonide:** Assess signs of Crohn disease and ulcerative colitis (diarrhea, crampy abdominal pain, fever, bleeding from rectum) during therapy. Monitor frequency and consistency of bowel movements periodically during therapy.
- **Rect:** Assess symptoms of ulcerative colitis (diarrhea, bleeding, weight loss, anorexia, fever, leukocytosis) periodically during therapy.

Lab Test Considerations

- Verify negative pregnancy test before starting therapy with *Hemady*. Monitor serum electrolytes, CBC, and glucose. May cause hyperglycemia, especially in patients with diabetes. May ↓ WBCs. May ↓ potassium and calcium and ↑ sodium.
- Guaiac-test stools. Promptly report presence of guaiac-positive stools.
- May ↑ cholesterol. May ↓ uptake of thyroid ^{123}I or ^{131}I.
- May suppress reactions to allergy skin tests.
- Periodic adrenal function tests may be ordered to assess degree of hypothalamic-pituitary-adrenal axis suppression in systemic and chronic topical therapy.
- **Dexamethasone Suppression Test:** To diagnose Cushing syndrome: Obtain baseline cortisol level; administer dexamethasone at 11 PM and obtain cortisol levels at 8 AM the next day. Normal response is a ↓ cortisol level. Alternative method: Obtain baseline 24-hr urine for 17-hydroxycorticosteroid concentrations; then begin 48-hr administration of dexamethasone. Second 24-hr urine for 17-hydroxycorticosteroid is obtained after 24 hr of dexamethasone.

Implementation

- Do not confuse prednisone with prednisolone. Do not confuse dexamethasone with dexmedetomidine. Do not confuse methylprednisolone with medroxyprogesterone or methyltestosterone. Do not confuse Solu-Cortef with Solu-Medrol. Do not confuse Depo-Medrol with Solu-Medrol.
- If dose is ordered daily or every other day, administer in the morning to coincide with the body's normal secretion of cortisol.
- Periods of stress, such as surgery, may require supplemental systemic corticosteroids.
- Patients with mild to moderate Crohn disease may be switched from oral prednisolone without adrenal insufficiency by gradually ↓ prednisolone doses and adding budesonide.
- **PO:** Administer with meals to minimize GI irritation.
- ***DNC:*** Swallow *Ortikos* (budesonide) tablets whole; do not crush or chew. Other tablets may be crushed and administered with food or fluids for patients with difficulty swallowing. ***DNC:*** Capsules and extended-release tablets should be swallowed whole; do not open, crush, break, or chew.
- *Entocort EC* (budesonide) capsules can be opened and contents sprinkled onto 1 tablespoon (15 mL) of applesauce for patients unable to swallow capsule. Applesauce must not be hot and must be soft enough to swallow without chewing. Mix granules with applesauce and consume entire contents within 30 min of mixing. Do not chew or crush the granules. Do not save the applesauce and granules for future use. Follow with 8 ounces of cool water to ensure complete swallowing of granules.
- *Alkindi Sprinkle* (hydrocortisone) are granules in capsules. Do not swallow capsules; do not crush or chew granules. Do not use with nasogastric or gastric tubes; may cause blockage of tube. To open capsule, hold capsule so that printed strength is at the top and tap to ensure all granules are in the lower half of the capsule. Squeeze bottom of capsule gently and twist off top of capsule. Granules may be poured directly onto patient's tongue, poured onto a spoon and placed in patient's mouth, or sprinkled onto a spoonful of cold or room temperature soft food (yogurt or fruit puree). Swallow granules within 5 min to avoid bitter taste, as the outer taste-masking cover can dissolve. Tap capsule to ensure all granules are removed. Avoid wetting capsule on the tongue or soft food; may result in granules remaining in capsule. Immediately follow administration with fluids (water, milk, breast milk, formula) to ensure all granules are swallowed. Do not add granules to liquid; may result in ↓ of dose administered and may result in a bitter taste.
- Use calibrated measuring device to ensure accurate dose of liquid forms.
- For orally disintegrating tablets, remove tablet from blister just prior to dosing. Peel blister pack open, and place tablet on tongue; may be swallowed whole or allowed to dissolve in mouth, with or without water. Tablets are friable; do not cut, split, or break.
- Avoid consumption of grapefruit juice during therapy with budesonide or methylprednisolone.
- **IM, SUBQ**: Shake suspension well before drawing up. IM doses should not be administered when rapid effect is desirable. Do not dilute with other solution or admix. Do not administer suspensions IV.

Dexamethasone

IV Administration

- **IV Push: Dilution:** May be given undiluted. **Rate:** Administer over 1–4 min if dose is <10 mg.

- **Intermittent Infusion: Dilution:** High-dose therapy should be added to D5W or 0.9% NaCl solution. Solution is clear and colorless to light yellow; use diluted solution within 24 hr. **Concentration:** 10 mg/mL. **Rate:** Infuse over 15–30 min.
- **Y-Site Compatibility:** acetaminophen, acyclovir, allopurinol, amikacin, aminocaproic acid, aminophylline, amphotericin B liposomal, anidulafungin, argatroban, arsenic trioxide, ascorbic acid, atracurium, atropine, azithromycin, aztreonam, benztropine, bivalirudin, bleomycin, bumetanide, buprenorphine, butorphanol, cangrelor, carboplatin, carmustine, cefazolin, cefepime, cefiderocol, cefotaxime, cefotetan, cefoxitin, ceftaroline, ceftazidime, ceftobiprole, ceftolozane/tazobactam, ceftriaxone, chlorothiazide, cisatracurium, cisplatin, cladribine, clindamycin, cyanocobalamin, cyclophosphamide, cyclosporine, cytarabine, dacarbazine, dactinomycin, daptomycin, dexmedetomidine, digoxin, diltiazem, dimenhydrinate, docetaxel, dopamine, doxorubicin hydrochloride, doxorubicin liposomal, edetate calcium disodium, enalaprilat, ephedrine, epinephrine, epoetin alfa, eptifibatide, ertapenem, etoposide, etoposide phosphate, famotidine, fentanyl, filgrastim, fluconazole, fludarabine, fluorouracil, folic acid, fosaprepitant, foscarnet, fosphenytoin, furosemide, ganciclovir, gemcitabine, glycopyrrolate, granisetron, heparin, hydrocortisone, hydromorphone, ifosfamide, imipenem/cilastatin, imipenem/cilastatin/relebactam, indomethacin, insulin, regular, irinotecan, isoproterenol, ketorolac, leucovorin, levofloxacin, lidocaine, linezolid, lorazepam, mannitol, melphalan, meropenem, meropenem/vaborbactam, mesna, methadone, methohexital, methylprednisolone, metoclopramide, metoprolol, metronidazole, milrinone, mitomycin, morphine, moxifloxacin, multivitamins, nafcillin, nalbuphine, naloxone, nitroglycerin, nitroprusside, norepinephrine, octreotide, ondansetron, oxaliplatin, oxytocin, paclitaxel, palonosetron, pamidronate, pemetrexed, penicillin G, pentobarbital, phenobarbital, phenylephrine, phytonadione, piperacillin/tazobactam, plazomicin, potassium acetate, potassium chloride, procainamide, prochlorperazine, propofol, propranolol, pyridoxine, remifentanil, rituximab, sargramostim, sodium acetate, sodium bicarbonate, succinylcholine, sufentanil, tacrolimus, tedizolid, telavancin, theophylline, thiamine, thiotepa, tigecycline, tirofiban, trastuzumab, vancomycin, vasopressin, vecuronium, verapamil, vinblastine, vincristine, vinorelbine, voriconazole, zidovudine, zoledronic acid.
- **Y-Site Incompatibility:** alemtuzumab, amiodarone, amphotericin deoxycholate, blinatumomab, caspofungin, cefuroxime, ciprofloxacin, dacarbazine, dantrolene, daunorubicin, diazepam, diphenhydramine, dobutamine, doxycycline, epirubicin, esmolol, gemtuzumab ozogamicin, haloperidol, idarubicin, labetalol, magnesium sulfate, midazolam, minocycline, mitoxantrone, mycophenolate, nicardipine, pantoprazole, papaverine, pentamidine, phenytoin, prochlorperazine, protamine, tobramycin, topotecan, trimethoprim/sulfamethoxazole.

C

Hydrocortisone Sodium Succinate

IV Administration

- **IV Push: Reconstitution:** Reconstitute with provided solution (Act-O-Vials) or 2 mL of bacteriostatic water or saline for injection. **Concentration:** 50 mg/mL. **Rate:** Administer each 100 mg over >30 sec. Doses ≥500 mg should be pushed over ≥10 min.
- **Intermittent/Continuous Infusion: Dilution:** May be added to 50–1000 mL of D5W, 0.9% NaCl, or D5/0.9% NaCl. Diluted solutions should be used within 24 hr. **Concentration:** 1–5 mg/mL. Concentrations of up to 60 mg/mL have been used in fluid restricted adults. **Rate:** Infuse over 20–30 min or at prescribed rate.
- **Y-Site Compatibility:** acetaminophen, acyclovir, alemtuzumab, allopurinol, amikacin, aminophylline, amphotericin B liposomal, anidulafungin, argatroban, ascorbic acid, atracurium, atropine, azithromycin, aztreonam, benztropine, bivalirudin, bleomycin, bumetanide, buprenorphine, butorphanol, cangrelor, carboplatin, carmustine, caspofungin, cefazolin, cefepime, cefiderocol, cefotaxime, cefotetan, cefoxitin, ceftaroline, ceftazidime, ceftobiprole, ceftolozane/tazobactam, ceftriaxone, cefuroxime, chloramphenicol, chlorothiazide, chlorpromazine, cisatracurium, cisplatin, cladribine, clindamycin, cyanocobalamin, cyclophosphamide, cyclosporine, cytarabine, dactinomycin, daptomycin, daunorubicin, defibrotide, dexamethasone, dexmedetomidine, dexrazoxane, digoxin, docetaxel, dopamine, doxorubicin hydrochloride, doxorubicin liposomal, droperidol, edetate calcium disodium, enalaprilat, ephedrine, epinephrine, epirubicin, epoetin alfa, eptifibatide, ertapenem, erythromycin, estrogens, conjugated, etoposide, famotidine, fentanyl, filgrastim, fluconazole, fludarabine, fluorouracil, folic acid, foscarnet, fosphenytoin, furosemide, gemcitabine, glycopyrrolate, granisetron, heparin, hydromorphone, ifosfamide, imipenem/cilastatin, imipenem/cilastatin/relebactam, indomethacin, insulin, regular, irinotecan, isoproterenol, ketamine, ketorolac, leucovorin, levofloxacin, lidocaine,

linezolid, lorazepam, mannitol, melphalan, meropenem/vaborbactam, mesna, methadone, methohexital, methotrexate, methylergonovine, metoclopramide, metoprolol, metronidazole, milrinone, mitoxantrone, morphine, moxifloxacin, multivitamins, nafcillin, naloxone, neostigmine, nitroglycerin, nitroprusside, norepinephrine, octreotide, ondansetron, oxacillin, oxaliplatin, oxytocin, paclitaxel, palonosetron, pamidronate, pantoprazole, pemetrexed, penicillin G, pentobarbital, phenobarbital, phentolamine, phenylephrine, phytonadione, piperacillin/tazobactam, plazomicin, potassium acetate, potassium chloride, procainamide, prochlorperazine, propofol, propranolol, pyridostigmine, remifentanil, rituximab, scopolamine, sodium acetate, sodium bicarbonate, succinylcholine, sufentanil, tacrolimus, tedizolid, telavancin, theophylline, thiotepa, tigecycline, tirofiban, topotecan, trastuzumab, vasopressin, vecuronium, verapamil, vinblastine, vincristine, vinorelbine, voriconazole, zoledronic acid.

- **Y-Site Incompatibility:** amphotericin B deoxycholate, ampicillin/sulbactam, azathioprine, ciprofloxacin, dantrolene, diazepam, diazoxide, dobutamine, doxycycline, ganciclovir, gemtuzumab ozogamicin, haloperidol, idarubicin, labetalol, midazolam, mycophenolate, nalbuphine, pentamidine, phenytoin, protamine, pyridoxine, rocuronium, sargramostim, thiamine, trimethoprim/sulfamethoxazole.

Methylprednisolone Sodium Succinate

IV Administration

- **IV Push: Reconstitution:** Reconstitute with provided solution (Act-O-Vials, Univials) or 2 mL of bacteriostatic water (with benzyl alcohol) for injection. Use preservative-free diluent for use in neonates. Acetate injection is not for IV use. **Concentration:** 125 mg/mL. **Rate:** Low dose (<1.8 mg/kg or <125 mg/dose): May be administered IV push over 1 to several min.
- **Intermittent/Continuous Infusion: Dilution:** May be diluted further in D5W, 0.9% NaCl, or D5/0.9% NaCl. Solution may form a haze upon dilution. **Concentration:** 2.5 mg/mL. **Rate:** Moderate dose (2 mg/kg or 250 mg/dose): Infuse over 15–30 min. High dose (15 mg/kg or 500 mg/dose): Infuse over 30 min. Doses >15 mg/kg or 1 g: Infuse over 1 hr.
- **Y-Site Compatibility:** acetaminophen, acyclovir, alprostadil, amikacin, aminophylline, amphotericin B liposomal, anidulafungin, argatroban, arsenic trioxide, ascorbic acid, atracurium, atropine, azithromycin, aztreonam, benztropine, bivalirudin, bleomycin, bumetanide, buprenorphine, butorphanol, cangrelor, carboplatin, carmustine, cefazolin, cefepime, cefotetan, ceftaroline, ceftazidime, ceftobiprole, ceftolozane/tazobactam, ceftriaxone, cefuroxime, chloramphenicol, chlorpromazine, cisplatin, cladribine, clindamycin, cyanocobalamin, cyclophosphamide, cyclosporine, cytarabine, dactinomycin, daptomycin, dexamethasone, dexmedetomidine, digoxin, dobutamine, dopamine, doxorubicin liposomal, enalaprilat, ephedrine, epinephrine, epoetin alfa, eptifibatide, ertapenem, erythromycin, etoposide, fentanyl, fluconazole, fludarabine, fluorouracil, folic acid, fosaprepitant, furosemide, gentamicin, glycopyrrolate, granisetron, hydromorphone, ifosfamide, imipenem/cilastatin, imipenem/cilastatin/relebactam, insulin, regular, isoproterenol, ketorolac, labetalol, levofloxacin, linezolid, lorazepam, mannitol, melphalan, meropenem/vaborbactam, mesna, methadone, methotrexate, metoclopramide, metoprolol, metronidazole, milrinone, mitomycin, morphine, moxifloxacin, multivitamins, nafcillin, naloxone, nitroglycerin, nitroprusside, norepinephrine, octreotide, oxaliplatin, oxytocin, pamidronate, pemetrexed, penicillin G, pentobarbital, phenobarbital, phenylephrine, piperacillin/tazobactam, potassium acetate, procainamide, prochlorperazine, propranolol, remifentanil, rituximab, sodium acetate, sodium bicarbonate, succinylcholine, sufentanil, tacrolimus, tedizolid, theophylline, thiotepa, tirofiban, tobramycin, topotecan, trastuzumab, vasopressin, verapamil, vincristine, voriconazole, zoledronic acid.
- **Y-Site Incompatibility:** alemtuzumab, allopurinol, amphotericin B deoxycholate, ampicillin/sulbactam, blinatumomab, calcium chloride, calcium gluconate, caspofungin, cefotaxime, cefoxitin, ciprofloxacin, dacarbazine, dantrolene, daunorubicin, dexrazoxane, diazepam, diazoxide, diphenhydramine, docetaxel, doxycycline, epirubicin, etoposide phosphate, filgrastim, foscarnet, ganciclovir, gemcitabine, gemtuzumab ozogamicin, haloperidol, hydralazine, idarubicin, irinotecan, isavuconazonium, leucovorin, magnesium sulfate, mitoxantrone, mycophenolate, nalbuphine, paclitaxel, palonosetron, pantoprazole, papaverine, pentamidine, phenytoin, promethazine, propofol, protamine, pyridoxine, rocuronium, sargramostim, thiamine, trimethoprim/sulfamethoxazole, vancomycin, vecuronium, vinorelbine.

Patient/Family Teaching

- Explain purpose and side effects of medication to patient. Advise patient to read *Patient Information* before starting therapy.
- Advise patient to notify health care provider of all Rx or OTC medications, vitamins, or herbal products being taken and to consult with health care provider before taking other medications.
- Advise patient to take medication as directed. Take missed doses as soon as remembered unless almost time for next dose. Do not double doses. If

full dose is not administered due to regurgitating or vomiting of granules, instruct patients and/or caregivers to contact their health care provider. A repeat dose may be required to avoid adrenal insufficiency. Stopping the medication suddenly may result in adrenal insufficiency (anorexia, nausea, weakness, fatigue, dyspnea, hypotension, hypoglycemia). If these signs appear, notify health care provider immediately. This can be life-threatening.

- Advise patient to avoid consumption of grapefruit juice during therapy with *budesonide* or *methylprednisolone*.
- Corticosteroids cause immunosuppression and may mask symptoms of infection. Advise patient to avoid people with known contagious illnesses and to report possible infections immediately.
- *Pediapred* solution may be refrigerated.
- Advise patient to avoid vaccinations without first consulting health care provider.
- Advise patient to inform health care provider promptly if severe abdominal pain or tarry stools occur. Patient should also report unusual swelling, weight gain, tiredness, bone pain, bruising, nonhealing sores, visual disturbances, or behavior changes.
- Advise patient to notify health care provider if signs and symptoms of hypercorticism (acne; thicker or more hair on body and face; bruise easily; fatty pad or hump between shoulders [buffalo hump], rounding of face [moon face], pink or purple stretch marks on skin of abdomen, thighs, breasts, and arms; ankle swelling), adrenal suppression (tiredness, weakness, nausea and vomiting, low blood pressure), worsening of allergies (eczema, rhinitis), and infection (fever, chills, pain, feeling tired, aches, nausea, and vomiting). May worsen existing tuberculosis, fungal, bacterial, viral, or parasitic infections or ocular herpes simplex.
- Advise patient to notify health care provider immediately if exposed to chickenpox or measles.
- Advise patient to notify health care provider of medication regimen before treatment or surgery.
- Discuss possible effects on body image. Explore coping mechanisms.
- Advise patient to inform health care provider if symptoms of underlying disease return or worsen.
- Advise patient to carry identification describing disease process and medication regimen in the event of emergency in which patient cannot relate medical history.
- **Long-Term Therapy:** Encourage patient to eat a diet high in protein, calcium, and potassium and low in sodium and carbohydrates (see Appendix J). Alcohol should be avoided during therapy; may ↑ risk of GI irritation.
- If rectal dose used 21 days, ↓ to every other night for 2–3 wk to ↓ gradually.
- Rep: Advise women of reproductive potential to notify health care provider if pregnancy is planned or suspected or if breastfeeding. *Hemady* may cause fetal harm. Advise women taking *Hemady* to use effective contraception during and for ≥1 mo after last dose. Monitor infants born to mothers who have received substantial doses of corticosteroids during pregnancy for signs of hypoglycemia and hypoadrenalism. Advise women to avoid breastfeeding during and for 2 wk after last dose. May impair male fertility.

Evaluation/Desired Outcomes

- Suppression of inflammation and modification of the normal immune response.
- Replacement therapy in adrenal insufficiency.
- **Budesonide:** Improvement in symptoms/sequelae of Crohn disease, induction of remission of ulcerative colitis, and reduction in UPCR.

CORTICOSTEROIDS (TOPICAL)

alclometasone (al-kloe-**met**-a-sone)
~~Aclovate~~

amcinonide (am-**sin**-oh-nide)

betamethasone (bay-ta-**meth**-a-sone)
✱Betaderm, ✱Beteflam, ✱Celestoderm V, ✱Celestoderm V/2, Diprolene, ~~Diprolene AF~~, ✱Diprosone, Sernivo

clobetasol (kloe-**bay**-ta-sol)
Clobex, Clodan, ✱Dermovate, Impoyz, Olux-E, ~~Temovate~~, ~~Temovate E~~, Tovet

clocortolone (kloe-**kore**-toe-lone)
Cloderm

desonide (**des**-oh-nide)
~~Desonate~~, DesOwen, Tridesilon, Verdeso

desoximetasone (dess-ox-i-**met**-a-sone)
Topicort

diflorasone (dye-**flor**-a-sone)
Apexicon E

fluocinolone (floo-oh-**sin**-oh-lone)
Derma-Smoothe/FS, Synalar

fluocinonide
(floo-oh-**sin**-oh-nide)
🍁 Lidemol, 🍁 Lyderm, 🍁 Tiamol, Vanos

flurandrenolide
(flure-an-**dren**-oh-lide)
Cordran, ~~Cordran SP~~

fluticasone (floo-**ti**-ka-sone)
~~Cutivate~~

halcinonide (hal-**sin**-oh-nide)
Halog

halobetasol (hal-oh-**bay**-ta-sol)
Bryhali, Lexette, Ultravate

hydrocortisone
(hye-droe-**kor**-ti-sone)
Ala-Cort, Ala-Scalp, Anusol HC, 🍁 Barriere-HC, Cortaid, Cortifoam, 🍁 Cortoderm, 🍁 Hyderm, 🍁 Hydroval, Locoid, 🍁 Sarna HC, Texacort

mometasone (moe-**met**-a-sone)
🍁 Elocom, ~~Elocon~~

triamcinolone
(trye-am-**sin**-oh-lone)
🍁 Aristocort C, 🍁 Aristocort R, Kenalog, 🍁 Triaderm, Triderm, Tritocin

Classification
Therapeutic: anti-inflammatories (steroidal)
Pharmacologic: corticosteroids (topical)

Indications
Moderate to severe plaque psoriasis. Inflammation and pruritus associated with corticosteroid-responsive dermatoses.

Action
Suppress normal immune response and inflammation. **Therapeutic Effects:** Suppression of dermatologic inflammation and immune processes. Clearing of plaques

Pharmacokinetics
Absorption: Minimal. Prolonged use on large surface areas, application of large amounts, or use of occlusive dressings may ↑ systemic absorption.
Distribution: Remain primarily at site of action.
Metabolism and Excretion: Usually metabolized in skin; some have been modified to resist local metabolism and have a prolonged local effect.
Half-life: *Betamethasone:* 3–5 hr (plasma), 36–54 hr (tissue); *dexamethasone:* 3–4.5 hr (plasma), 36–54 hr (tissue); *hydrocortisone:* 1.5–2 hr (plasma), 8–12 hr (tissue); *triamcinolone:* 2–>5 hr (plasma), 18–36 hr (tissue).

TIME/ACTION PROFILE (response depends on condition being treated)

ROUTE	ONSET	PEAK	DURATION
Topical	min–hr	hr–days	hr–days

Contraindications/Precautions
Contraindicated in: Hypersensitivity or known intolerance to corticosteroids or components of vehicles (ointment or cream base, preservative, alcohol); Untreated bacterial or viral infections.
Use Cautiously in: Hepatic impairment; Diabetes mellitus, cataracts, glaucoma, or tuberculosis (use of large amounts of high-potency agents may worsen condition); Patients with pre-existing skin atrophy; OB: Lactation: Chronic use at high dosages may result in adrenal suppression in mother and growth suppression in children; Pedi: Children may be more susceptible to adrenal and growth suppression. Clobetasol not recommended for children <18 yr (cream, lotion, shampoo, spray) or <12 yr (foam, gel, ointment, solution); desoximetasone not recommended for children <10 yr (cream, ointment, gel) or <18 yr (spray); halobetasol not recommended for children <12 yr.

Adverse Reactions/Side Effects
Derm: allergic contact dermatitis, atrophy, burning, dryness, edema, folliculitis, hypersensitivity reactions, hypertrichosis, hypopigmentation, irritation, maceration, miliaria, perioral dermatitis, secondary infection, striae. **EENT:** cataracts, glaucoma. **Endo:** adrenal suppression (↑ dose, long-term therapy).

Interactions
Drug-Drug: None significant.

Route/Dosage
Topical: (Adults and Children): 1–4 times daily (depends on product, preparation, and condition being treated).
Rect (Adults): hydrocortisone: *Aerosol foam:* 90 mg 1–2 times/day for 2–3 wk; then adjusted.

Availability
Alclometasone (generic available)
Cream: 0.05%. **Ointment:** 0.05%.

Amcinonide (generic available)
Cream: 0.1%. **Lotion:** 0.1%. **Ointment:** 0.1%.

Betamethasone (generic available)
Aerosol foam: 0.12%. **Cream:** 0.05%, 0.1%. **Gel:** 0.05%. **Lotion:** 0.05%, 0.1%. **Ointment:** 0.05%, 0.1%. **Spray:** 0.05%. ***In combination with:*** calcipotriene (Enstilar, Taclonex, Wynzora), clotrimazole (Lotrisone); see Appendix N.

Clobetasol (generic available)
Cream: 0.025%, 0.05%. **Foam:** 0.05%. **Gel:** 0.05%. **Lotion:** 0.05%. **Ointment:** 0.05%. **Scalp solution:** 0.05%. **Shampoo:** 0.05%. **Spray:** 0.05%.

C

Clocortolone (generic available)

Cream: 0.1%.

Desonide (generic available)

Cream: 0.05%. **Foam:** 0.05%. **Gel:** 0.05%. **Lotion:** 0.05%. **Ointment:** 0.05%.

Desoximetasone (generic available)

Cream: 0.05%, 0.25%. **Gel:** 0.05%. **Ointment:** 0.05%, 0.25%. **Spray:** 0.25%.

Diflorasone (generic available)

Cream: 0.05%. **Ointment:** 0.05%.

Fluocinolone (generic available)

Cream: 0.01%, 0.025%. **Oil:** 0.01%. **Ointment:** 0.025%. **Solution:** 0.01%. ***In combination with:*** hydroquinone and tretinoin (Tri-Luma); neomycin (Neo-Synalar). See Appendix N.

Fluocinonide (generic available)

Cream: 0.05%, 0.1%. **Gel:** 0.05%. **Ointment:** 0.05%. **Solution:** 0.05%.

Flurandrenolide (generic available)

Lotion: 0.05%. **Ointment:** 0.05%. **Tape:** 4 mcg/cm^2.

Fluticasone (generic available)

Cream: 0.05%. **Lotion:** 0.05%. **Ointment:** 0.005%.

Halcinonide (generic available)

Cream: 0.1%. **Ointment:** 0.1%. **Solution:** 0.1%.

Halobetasol (generic available)

Cream: 0.05%. **Foam:** 0.05%. **Lotion:** 0.01%, 0.05%. **Ointment:** 0.05%. ***In combination with:*** tazarotene (Duobrii). See Appendix N.

Hydrocortisone (generic available)

Cream: 0.1%, 0.2%, 0.5%$^{Rx, OTC}$, 1%$^{Rx, OTC}$, 2.5%. **Gel:** 2%$^{Rx, OTC}$. **Lotion:** 0.1%, 1%$^{Rx, OTC}$, 2%. **Ointment:** 0.1%, 0.2%, 0.5%$^{Rx, OTC}$, 1%$^{Rx, OTC}$, 2.5%. **Rectal cream:** 1%, 2.5%. **Solution:** 0.1%, 1%, 2.5%. ***In combination with:*** acetic acid, antifungals, anti-infectives, antihistamines, urea, and benzoyl peroxide in various otic and topical preparations. See Appendix N.

Mometasone (generic available)

Cream: 0.1%. **Ointment:** 0.1%. **Lotion:** 🍁 0.1%. **Solution:** 0.1%.

Triamcinolone (generic available)

Cream: 0.025%, 0.1%, 0.5%. **Lotion:** 0.025%, 0.1%. **Ointment:** 0.025%, 0.05%, 0.1%, 0.5%. **Spray:** 0.147 mg/g. ***In combination with:*** acetic acid, antifungals, anti-infectives, antihistamines, urea, and benzoyl peroxide in various otic and topical preparations. See Appendix N.

NURSING IMPLICATIONS

Assessment

- Assess affected skin before and daily during therapy. Note degree of inflammation, pruritus, and/or plaques. Notify health care provider if symptoms of infection (↑ pain, erythema, purulent exudate) develop.

Lab Test Considerations

- Adrenal function tests may be ordered to assess degree of hypothalamic-pituitary-adrenal (HPA) axis suppression in long-term topical therapy. Children and patients with dose applied to a large area, using an occlusive dressing, or using high-potency products are at highest risk for HPA suppression.
- May ↑ serum and urine glucose concentrations if significant absorption occurs.

Implementation

- Choice of vehicle depends on site and type of lesion. Ointments are more occlusive and preferred for dry, scaly lesions. Creams should be used on oozing or intertriginous areas, where the occlusive action of ointments might cause folliculitis or maceration. Creams may be preferred for esthetic reasons even though they may dry skin more than ointments. Gels, aerosols, lotions, and solutions are useful in hairy areas.
- **Topical:** Apply *ointments, creams,* or *gels* sparingly as a thin film to clean, slightly moist skin. Wear gloves. Apply occlusive dressing only if specified by health care provider.
- Apply *lotion, solution,* or *gel* to hair by parting hair and applying a small amount to affected area. Rub in gently. Protect area from washing, clothing, or rubbing until medication has dried. Hair may be washed as usual but not right after applying medication.
- Use *aerosols* by shaking well and spraying on affected area, holding container 3–6 inches away. Spray for about 2 sec to cover an area the size of a hand. Do not inhale. If spraying near face, cover eyes.
- Shake *Sernivo spray* before using. Spray affected area and rub in gently. Discontinue if control not achieved or after 4 wk of use.

Patient/Family Teaching

- Explain purpose and side effects of medication to patient. Advise patient to read *Patient Information* before starting therapy.
- Advise patient to notify health care provider of all Rx or OTC medications, vitamins, or herbal products being taken and to consult with health care provider before taking other medications.
- Advise patient on correct technique of medication administration. Emphasize importance of avoiding the eyes. Apply missed doses as soon as remembered unless almost time for the next dose.
- Advise patient to use only as directed. Avoid using cosmetics, bandages, dressings, or other skin products over the treated area unless directed by health care provider.

- Advise patient to consult health care provider before using medicine for condition other than indicated.
- Advise patient to inform health care provider if symptoms of underlying disease return or worsen or if symptoms of infection develop.
- **Fluticasone:** Advise patient to avoid excessive natural or artificial exposure (tanning booth, sun lamp) to areas where lotion is applied.
- Pedi: Advise parents/caregivers of pediatric patients not to apply tight-fitting diapers or plastic pants on a child treated in the diaper area; these garments work as an occlusive dressing and may cause more of the drug to be absorbed.
- Rep: Advise women of reproductive potential to notify health care provider if pregnancy is planned or suspected or if breastfeeding. Advise women of reproductive potential that medication should not be used extensively, in large amounts, or for protracted periods if they are pregnant or planning to become pregnant.

Evaluation/Desired Outcomes

- Suppression of dermatologic inflammation and immune processes.
- Clearing of plaques.

cyanocobalamin

(sye-an-oh-koe-**bal**-a-min)

~~Nascobal~~

Classification

Therapeutic: antianemics, vitamins

Pharmacologic: water soluble vitamins

Indications

Vitamin B_{12} deficiency (parenteral products or nasal spray should be used when deficiency is due to malabsorption). Pernicious anemia (parenteral products should be used for initial therapy; nasal or oral products are not indicated until patients have achieved hematologic remission following parenteral therapy and have no signs of CNS involvement). Part of the Schilling test (vitamin B_{12} absorption test) (diagnostic).

Action

Necessary coenzyme for metabolic processes, including fat and carbohydrate metabolism and protein synthesis. Required for cell reproduction and hematopoiesis. **Therapeutic Effects:** Corrects manifestations of pernicious anemia (megaloblastic indices, GI lesions, neurologic damage). Corrects vitamin B_{12} deficiency. Schilling test confirms impaired vitamin B_{12} absorption.

Pharmacokinetics

Absorption: Oral absorption in GI tract requires intrinsic factor and calcium; well absorbed after IM, SUBQ, and nasal administration.

Distribution: Stored in the liver and bone marrow.

Metabolism and Excretion: Primarily excreted unchanged in urine.

Half-life: 6 days (400 days in liver).

TIME/ACTION PROFILE (reticulocytosis)

ROUTE	ONSET	PEAK	DURATION
IM	unknown	3–10 days	unknown
SUBQ	unknown	3–10 days	unknown
Nasal	unknown	3–10 days	unknown

Contraindications/Precautions

Contraindicated in: Hypersensitivity; Pedi: Avoid using preparations containing benzyl alcohol in premature infants (associated with fatal gasping syndrome).

Use Cautiously in: Hereditary optic nerve atrophy (accelerates nerve damage); Renal impairment (when using aluminum-containing products); Uremia, folic acid deficiency, concurrent infection, iron deficiency (response to vitamin B_{12} will be impaired).

Adverse Reactions/Side Effects

CV: HF. **Derm:** itching, swelling of the body. **F and E** hypokalemia. **GI:** diarrhea. **Hemat:** thrombocytosis. **Local:** pain at IM site. **Neuro:** headache. **Resp:** pulmonary edema. **Misc:** HYPERSENSITIVITY REACTIONS (INCLUDING ANAPHYLAXIS).

Interactions

Drug-Drug: Chloramphenicol and **antineoplastics** may ↓ hematologic response. **Colchicine**, **aminosalicylic acid**, or excessive intake of **alcohol** or **vitamin C** may ↓ absorption/effectiveness.

Route/Dosage

Oral products are usually not recommended due to poor absorption and should be used only if patient refuses the intramuscular, deep SUBQ, or intranasal route of administration.

Vitamin B_{12} Deficiency

PO (Adults and Children): Amount depends on deficiency (up to 1000 mcg/day have been used).

IM, SUBQ (Adults): 30 mcg/day for 5–10 days; then 100–200 mcg/mo.

IM, SUBQ (Children): 0.2 mcg/kg for 2 days; then 1000 mcg/day for 2–7 days; then 100 mcg/wk for 1 mo.

Intranasal (Adults): 500 mcg (one spray) in one nostril once weekly.

Pernicious Anemia

IM, SUBQ (Adults): 100 mcg/day for 6–7 days; if improvement, give same dose every other day for 7 doses; then every 3–4 days for 2–3 wk; once hematologic values return to normal (remission), can give maintenance dose of 100 mcg/mo (doses up to 1000 mcg have been used for maintenance) (could alternatively use oral or intranasal formulations below for maintenance at specified doses).

PO (Adults): *For hematologic remission only:* 1000–2000 mcg/day.
Intranasal (Adults): *For hematologic remission only:* 500 mcg (one spray) in one nostril once weekly.
IM, SUBQ (Children): 30–50 mcg/day for 2 or more wk (to a total dose of 1000–5000 mcg); then give maintenance dose of 100 mcg/mo (doses up to 1000 mcg have been used for maintenance).

Schilling Test

IM, SUBQ (Adults): Flushing dose is 1000 mcg.

Availability (generic available)

Tablets: 100 mcg[OTC]250 mcg[OTC], 500 mcg[OTC], 1000 mcg[OTC]. **Extended-release tablets:** 1000 mcg[OTC]. **Sublingual tablets:** 2500 mcg [OTC]. **Lozenges:** 50 mcg[OTC], 100 mcg[OTC], 250 mcg[OTC], 500 mcg[OTC]. **Nasal spray:** 500 mcg/0.1 mL actuation (8 sprays/bottle). **Solution for injection:** 1000 mcg/mL.

NURSING IMPLICATIONS

Assessment

- Assess patient for signs of vitamin B_{12} deficiency (pallor; neuropathy; psychosis; red, inflamed tongue) and folate deficiency (fatigue, mouth sores, confusion, neuropathy) before and periodically during therapy.
- Polycythemia vera can be masked by vitamin B_{12} deficiency; assess for headaches, fatigue, dizziness, blurred vision, night sweats, and pruritus.
- Monitor for signs and symptoms of hypersensitivity reactions (rash, urticaria, pruritus, flushing, dizziness, vomiting, abdominal pain) and angioedema (swelling of throat, lips, tongue, or face; dyspnea; wheezing; hoarseness). Discontinue cyanocobalamin immediately and provide supportive care. In patients with suspected cobalamin hypersensitivity, consider administering an intradermal test dose of parenteral vitamin B_{12} prior to use.

Lab Test Considerations

- Obtain hematocrit; reticulocyte count; and vitamin B_{12}, folate, and iron levels prior to therapy, 1 mo after the start of therapy, and then every 3–6 mo.
- Evaluate serum potassium level in patients receiving vitamin B_{12} for pernicious anemia for hypokalemia during the first 48 hr of treatment. Serum potassium levels and platelet counts should be monitored routinely during the course of therapy.
- *Nasal Spray:* Obtain serum B_{12} levels and CBC 1 mo after treatment initiation and then every 3–6 mo. Assess serum B_{12} level 1 mo after each dose adjustment.

Implementation

- Usually administered in combination with other vitamins; solitary vitamin B_{12} deficiencies are rare.
- Administration of vitamin B_{12} by the oral route is useful only for nutritional deficiencies. Patients with small-bowel disease, malabsorption syndrome, or gastric or ileal resections require parenteral administration.
- **IM, SUBQ**: Vials should be protected from light.
- If SUBQ route used, deep SUBQ administration is preferred.
- **PO:** Administer with meals to ↑ absorption.
- May be mixed with fruit juices. Administer immediately after mixing; ascorbic acid alters stability.
- Do not give extended-release tablets within 2 hr of other medications.
- **Intranasal** Dose should not be administered within 1 hr of hot foods or liquids (these substances may result in the formation of nasal secretions, which may ↓ effectiveness of nasal spray).
- Nasal spray unit must be primed with three strokes on first use. Unit must be primed with one stroke before each remaining dose. Advise patient to clear nose; then place tip approximately 1 in into nostril and press pump once, firmly and quickly. After dose, remove unit from nose and massage dosed nostril gently for a few seconds. Vial delivers 8 doses. Unit should be stored at room temperature and protected from light.

Patient/Family Teaching

- Teach patient reason for vitamin B_{12} therapy and side effects. Explain that they should take oral forms with food for best absorption and avoid alcohol during therapy. Advise patient to read *Medication Guide* before starting and periodically during therapy in case of changes.
- Encourage patient to comply with diet recommendations of health care professional. Explain that the best source of vitamins is a well-balanced diet. Foods high in vitamin B_{12} include meats, seafood, egg yolk, and fermented cheeses.
- Patients self-medicating with vitamin supplements should be cautioned not to exceed RDA. Effectiveness of megadoses for treatment of various medical conditions is unproven and may cause side effects.
- Inform patients with pernicious anemia of the lifelong need for vitamin B_{12} replacement.
- Emphasize the importance of follow-up exams to evaluate progress.
- Advise patient to notify health care professional of all Rx or OTC medications, vitamins, or herbal products being taken and to consult with health care professional before taking other medications. Counsel patient to avoid alcohol while taking this drug.
- Rep: Advise patient to notify health care professional if pregnancy is planned or suspected or if breastfeeding.

Evaluation/Desired Outcomes

- Resolution of the symptoms of vitamin B_{12} deficiency.
- Increase in reticulocyte count.
- Improvement in manifestations of pernicious anemia.
- Schilling test confirms impaired vitamin B_{12} absorption.

BEERS

cyclobenzaprine

(sye-kloe-**ben**-za-preen)

Amrix, Fexmid, ~~Flexeril~~

Classification

Therapeutic: skeletal muscle relaxants (centrally acting)

Indications

Acute painful musculoskeletal conditions associated with muscle spasm. **Unlabeled Use:** Fibromyalgia.

Action

Reduces tonic somatic muscle activity at the level of the brain stem. Structurally similar to tricyclic antidepressants. **Therapeutic Effects:** Reduction in muscle spasm and hyperactivity without loss of function.

Pharmacokinetics

Absorption: Well absorbed from the GI tract.
Distribution: Unknown.
Protein Binding: 93%.
Metabolism and Excretion: Mostly metabolized by the liver.
Half-life: 1–3 days.

TIME/ACTION PROFILE (skeletal muscle relaxation)

ROUTE	ONSET	PEAK†	DURATION
PO	within 1 hr	3–8 hr	12–24 hr
Extended release	unknown	unknown	24 hr

† Full effects may not occur for 1–2 wk.

Contraindications/Precautions

Contraindicated in: Hypersensitivity; Concurrent use of or use within 14 days of MAO inhibitor therapy; Immediate period after MI; Severe or symptomatic cardiovascular disease; Cardiac conduction disturbances; Hyperthyroidism.
Use Cautiously in: Cardiovascular disease; OB: Use during pregnancy only if potential maternal benefit justifies potential fetal risk; Lactation: Use while breastfeeding only if potential maternal benefit justifies potential risk to infant; Pedi: Children <15 yr (safety and effectiveness not established); Geri: Appears on Beers list. ↑ risk of anticholinergic adverse reactions, sedation, and fractures in older adults. Avoid use in older adults.

Adverse Reactions/Side Effects

CV: arrhythmias. **EENT:** dry mouth, blurred vision. **GI:** constipation, dyspepsia, nausea, unpleasant taste. **GU:** urinary retention. **Neuro:** dizziness, drowsiness, confusion, fatigue, headache, nervousness.

Interactions

Drug-Drug: Avoid use within 14 days of **MAO inhibitors** (hyperpyretic crisis, seizures, and death may occur). Additive CNS depression with other **CNS depressants**, including **alcohol**, **antihistamines**, **opioid analgesics**, and **sedative/hypnotics**. Additive anticholinergic effects with **drugs possessing anticholinergic properties**, including **antihistamines**, **antidepressants**, **atropine**, **disopyramide**, **haloperidol**, and **phenothiazines**. Drugs that affect serotonergic neurotransmitter systems, including **tricyclic antidepressants**, **SSRIs**, **SNRIs**, **fentanyl**, **buspirone**, **tramadol**, and **triptans**, may ↑ risk of serotonin syndrome.
Drug-Natural Products: Kava-kava, valerian, chamomile, or **hops** can ↑ CNS depression.

Route/Dosage

PO (Adults and Children ≥15 yr): *Acute painful musculoskeletal conditions:* Immediate release: 10 mg 3 times daily (range 20–40 mg/day in 2–4 divided doses; not to exceed 60 mg/day); Extended release: 15–30 mg once daily. *Fibromyalgia:* 5–40 mg at bedtime (unlabeled).

Availability (generic available)

Immediate-release tablets: 5 mg, 7.5 mg, 10 mg. **Extended-release capsules (Amrix):** 15 mg, 30 mg.

NURSING IMPLICATIONS

Assessment

- Assess for pain, muscle stiffness, and range of motion before and periodically during therapy.
- Geri: Assess older adults for anticholinergic effects (sedation and weakness).
- Assess for serotonin syndrome (mental changes [agitation, hallucinations, coma], autonomic instability [tachycardia, labile BP, hyperthermia], neuromuscular aberrations [hyperreflexia, incoordination], GI symptoms [nausea, vomiting, diarrhea]), especially in patients taking other serotonergic drugs (SSRIs, SNRIs, triptans). *If symptoms occur,* discontinue cyclobenzaprine and any other serotonergic drugs immediately.

Implementation

- **PO:** Administer doses at same time each day. May be administered with meals to minimize gastric irritation.
- ***DNC:*** Swallow extended-release capsules whole; do not crush or chew. Capsules may be opened and contents sprinkled onto applesauce; swallow immediately without chewing. Rinse mouth to make sure contents have been swallowed.

Patient/Family Teaching

- Explain purpose and side effects of medication. Advise patient to read *Patient Information* before starting therapy.
- Instruct patient to take missed doses within 1 hr of scheduled time; otherwise, return to normal dose schedule. Do not double doses. Do not stop abruptly.
- Medication may cause drowsiness, dizziness, and blurred vision. Caution patient to avoid driving or other activities requiring alertness until response to drug is known.
- Advise patient to avoid concurrent use of alcohol or other CNS depressants.
- If constipation occurs, advise patient to ↑ fluid and fiber intake; notify health care professional if constipation persists.
- Instruct patient to notify health care professional of all Rx or OTC medications, vitamins, or herbal products being taken and to consult health care professional before taking any other Rx, OTC, or herbal products.
- Advise patient to notify health care professional if symptoms of urinary retention (distended abdomen, feeling of fullness, overflow incontinence, voiding small amounts) occur.
- Instruct patient to notify health care professional immediately if signs and symptoms of serotonin syndrome, irregular or abnormal heartbeat, fast heartbeat, or allergic reaction (difficulty breathing, hives, swelling of face or tongue, itching) occur.
- Inform patient that good oral hygiene, frequent mouth rinses, and sugarless gum or candy may help relieve dry mouth.
- Rep: Advise women of reproductive potential to notify health care professional if pregnancy is planned or suspected or if breastfeeding.

Evaluation/Desired Outcomes

- Relief of muscular spasm in acute skeletal muscle conditions. Maximum effects may not be evident for 1–2 wk. Use is usually limited to 2–3 wk; however, has been effective for ≥12 wk in the management of fibromyalgia.

HIGH ALERT

cycloPHOSphamide

(sye-kloe-**fos**-fa-mide)

~~Cytoxan~~, ✱ Procytox

Classification

Therapeutic: antineoplastics, immunosuppressants,

Pharmacologic: alkylating agents

C

Indications

Alone or with other modalities in the management of: Hodgkin disease, malignant lymphomas, multiple myeloma, leukemias, mycosis fungoides, neuroblastoma, ovarian carcinoma, breast carcinoma, and a variety of other tumors. Minimal change nephrotic syndrome in children. **Unlabeled Use:** Severe active rheumatoid arthritis or granulomatosis with polyangiitis.

Action

Interferes with DNA replication and RNA transcription, ultimately disrupting protein synthesis (cell-cycle phase-nonspecific). **Therapeutic Effects:** Death of rapidly replicating cells, particularly malignant ones. Also has immunosuppressant action in smaller doses.

Pharmacokinetics

Absorption: Inactive parent drug is well absorbed from the GI tract. IV administration results in complete bioavailability.

Distribution: Widely distributed. Limited penetration of the blood-brain barrier.

Metabolism and Excretion: Converted to active drug by the liver; 30% eliminated unchanged by the kidneys.

Half-life: 4–6.5 hr.

TIME/ACTION PROFILE (effects on blood counts)

ROUTE	ONSET	PEAK	DURATION
PO, IV	7 days	7–15 days	21 days

Contraindications/Precautions

Contraindicated in: Hypersensitivity; OB: Pregnancy; Lactation: Lactation.

Use Cautiously in: Active infections; Bone marrow depression; Other chronic debilitating illnesses; Rep: Women of reproductive potential.

Adverse Reactions/Side Effects

CV: hypotension, MYOCARDIAL FIBROSIS. **Derm:** alopecia. **Endo:** gonadal suppression, syndrome of inappropriate antidiuretic hormone (SIADH). **GI:** anorexia, nausea, vomiting. **GU:** hematuria, ↓ fertility, HEMORRHAGIC CYSTITIS. **Hemat:** thrombocytopenia, anemia, LEUKOPENIA. **Metab:** hyperuricemia. **Resp:** PULMONARY FIBROSIS. **Misc:** SECONDARY MALIGNANCY.

Interactions

Drug-Drug: Phenobarbital or **rifampin** may ↑ toxicity of cyclophosphamide. Concurrent **allopurinol** or **thiazide diuretics** may exaggerate bone marrow depression. May prolong neuromuscular blockade from **succinylcholine**. Cardiotoxicity may be additive with other **cardiotoxic agents** (e.g.

✱ = Canadian drug name. ⧖ = Genetic implication. V = Vesicant. Boxed warning.
~~Strikethrough~~ = Discontinued. *CAPITALS = life-threatening. Underline = most frequent.

cytarabine, **daunorubicin**, **doxorubicin**). May ↓ **digoxin** levels and effectiveness. Additive bone marrow depression with other **antineoplastics** or **radiation therapy**. May potentiate the effects of **warfarin**. May ↓ antibody response to **live-virus vaccines** and ↑ risk of adverse reactions. Prolongs the effects of **cocaine**.

Route/Dosage

PO (Adults): *Induction and maintenance:* 1–5 mg/kg/day.

PO (Children): *Induction:* 2–8 mg/kg/day (60–250 mg/m^2/day) in divided doses for 6 days or longer. *Maintenance:* 2–5 mg/kg (50–150 mg/m^2/day) twice weekly.

IV (Adults): 40–50 mg/kg in divided doses over 2–5 days *or* 10–15 mg/kg every 7–10 days *or* 3–5 mg/kg twice weekly *or* 1.5–3 mg/kg/day. Other regimens may use larger doses.

IV (Children): *Induction:* 2–8 mg/kg/day (60–250 mg/m^2/day) in divided doses for 6 days or longer. Total dose for 7 days may be given as a single weekly dose. *Maintenance:* 10–15 mg/kg every 7–10 days or 30 mg/kg every 3–4 wk.

Availability (generic available)

Capsules: 25 mg, 50 mg. **Tablets:** 25 mg, 50 mg. **Lyophilized powder for injection:** 🍁 200 mg/vial, 500 mg/vial, 1 g/vial, 2 g/vial. **Solution for injection:** 100 mg/mL, 200 mg/mL, 500 mg/mL.

NURSING IMPLICATIONS

Assessment

- Monitor vital signs frequently during administration. Report significant changes.
- Monitor urinary output frequently during therapy. To ↓ the risk of hemorrhagic cystitis and to promote excretion of uric acid, fluid intake should be ≥3000 mL/day for adults and ≥1000–2000 mL/day for children. May be administered with mesna. Alkalinization of the urine may be used to help prevent uric acid nephropathy.
- Monitor for bone marrow depression. Assess for bleeding (bleeding gums; bruising; petechiae; guaiac stools, urine, and emesis) and avoid IM injections and taking rectal temperatures if platelet count is low. Apply pressure to venipuncture sites for 10 min. Assess for signs of infection during neutropenia. Anemia may occur. Monitor for ↑ fatigue, dyspnea, and orthostatic hypotension.
- Assess nausea, vomiting, and appetite. Weigh weekly. Antiemetics may be given 30 min before administration of medication to minimize GI effects. Anorexia and weight loss can be minimized by feeding frequent light meals.
- Assess cardiac and respiratory status for dyspnea, rales/crackles, cough, weight gain, or edema. Pulmonary toxicity may occur after prolonged therapy. Cardiotoxicity may occur early in therapy and is characterized by symptoms of HF.

Lab Test Considerations

- Monitor CBC with differential before and periodically during therapy. The nadir of leukopenia occurs in 7–12 days (recovery in 17–21 days). Leukocytes should be maintained at 2500–4000/mm^3. May also cause thrombocytopenia (nadir 10–15 days) and rarely causes anemia.
- Monitor BUN, serum creatinine, and uric acid before and frequently during therapy to detect nephrotoxicity.
- Monitor ALT, AST, LDH, and serum bilirubin before and frequently during therapy to detect hepatotoxicity.
- Urinalysis should be evaluated before initiating therapy and frequently during therapy to detect hematuria or change in specific gravity indicative of SIADH.
- May suppress positive reactions to skin tests for *Candida*, mumps, *Trichophyton*, and tuberculin purified-protein derivative. May also produce false-positive results in Papanicolaou smears.

Implementation

- ***High Alert:*** Fatalities have occurred with chemotherapeutic agents. Before administering, clarify all ambiguous orders; double-check single, daily, and course-of-therapy dose limits; have second practitioner independently double-check original order, calculations, and infusion pump settings.
- Do not confuse cyclophosphamide with cyclosporine or cycloserine.
- Administer antiemetics before dosing with cyclophosphamide.
- **PO:** Administer in the morning. ***DNC:*** Swallow tablets whole; do not crush, break, or chew.

IV Administration

- Provide adequate fluids (PO or IV) during or immediately after IV administration to force diuresis and ↓ risk of urinary tract toxicity.
- **IV:** Wear gloves, gown, and mask while handling medication. If powder or solution comes in contact with skin or mucosa, wash thoroughly with soap and water. Discard equipment in specially designated containers.
- Cyclophosphamide is an irritant. If extravasation occurs, immediately stop infusion. Leave needle/cannula in place temporarily but do not flush the line. Gently aspirate extravasated solution; then remove needle/cannula. Elevate patient's extremity.
- **IV Push: Reconstitution:** Reconstitute each vial of lyophilized powder for injection with 25 mL (500 mg vial), 50 mL (1000 mg vial), or 100 mL (2000 mg vial) of 0.9% NaCl. Do not reconstitute with sterile water for injection; results in a hypotonic solution not suitable for IV push. Solution is clear, colorless to slight yellow; do not administer

solutions that are cloudy, discolored, or contain particulate matter. Reconstituted solution can be stored at room temperature for up to 24 hr or in the refrigerator for up to 6 days. **Concentration:** 20 mg/mL. **Rate:** Inject very slowly.

- **Intermittent Infusion: Reconstitution:** Reconstitute each vial of lyophilized powder for injection with 25 mL (500 mg vial), 50 mL (1000 mg vial), or 100 mL (2000 mg vial) of 0.9% NaCl. Reconstituted solution can be stored at room temperature for up to 24 hr or in the refrigerator for up to 6 days. **Concentration:** 20 mg/mL. **Dilution:** Withdraw prescribed dose from vial and dilute with D5/0.9% NaCl, 0.45% NaCl, or D5W. Swirl gently to dissolve. Solutions diluted with 0.45% NaCl may be stored at room temperature for 24 hr or if refrigerated for 6 days. Solutions diluted with D5W or D5/0.9% NaCl are stable up to 24 hr at room temperature or 36 hr if refrigerated. **Concentration:** 2 mg/mL. **Rate:** Infuse very slowly; based on protocol.
- **Y-Site Compatibility:** acyclovir, alemtuzumab, allopurinol, amikacin, aminocaproic acid, aminophylline, amiodarone, amphotericin B liposomal, ampicillin/sulbactam, anidulafungin, argatroban, arsenic trioxide, atracurium, atropine, azithromycin, aztreonam, bivalirudin, bleomycin, bumetanide, buprenorphine, butorphanol, calcium chloride, calcium gluconate, carboplatin, carmustine, caspofungin, cefazolin, cefepime, cefotaxime, cefotetan, cefoxitin, ceftazidime, ceftriaxone, cefuroxime, chloramphenicol, chlorpromazine, chlorothiazide, ciprofloxacin, cisatracurium, cisplatin, cladribine, clindamycin, cyclosporine, cytarabine, dacarbazine, dactinomycin, daptomycin, daunorubicin, dexamethasone, dexmedetomidine, dexrazoxane, digoxin, diltiazem, diphenhydramine, dobutamine, docetaxel, dopamine, doxorubicin hydrochloride, doxorubicin liposomal, doxycycline, droperidol, enalaprilat, ephedrine, epinephrine, epirubicin, ertapenem, erythromycin, esmolol, etoposide, etoposide phosphate, famotidine, fentanyl, filgrastim, fluconazole, fludarabine, fluorouracil, foscarnet, fosphenytoin, furosemide, ganciclovir, gemcitabine, gentamicin, granisetron, haloperidol, heparin, hetastarch, hydralazine, hydrocortisone, hydromorphone, idarubicin, imipenem/cilastatin, insulin, regular, irinotecan, isoproterenol, ketorolac, labetalol, leucovorin, levofloxacin, lidocaine, linezolid, lorazepam, magnesium sulfate, mannitol, melphalan, meperidine, meropenem, mesna, methadone, methotrexate, methylprednisolone, metoclopramide, metoprolol, metronidazole, midazolam, milrinone, minocycline, mitomycin, mitoxantrone, morphine, moxifloxacin, nafcillin, nalbuphine, naloxone, nicardipine, nitroglycerin, nitroprusside, norepinephrine, octreotide, ondansetron, oxacillin, oxaliplatin, oxytocin, paclitaxel, palonosetron, pamidronate, pantoprazole, pemetrexed, penicillin G, pentamidine, pentobarbital, phenobarbital, phentolamine, phenylephrine, piperacillin/tazobactam, potassium acetate, potassium chloride, potassium phosphates, procainamide, prochlorperazine, promethazine, propofol, propranolol, remifentanil, rituximab, rocuronium, sargramostim, sodium acetate, sodium bicarbonate, sodium phosphates, succinylcholine, sufentanil, tacrolimus, theophylline, thiotepa, tigecycline, tirofiban, tobramycin, topotecan, trastuzumab, trimethoprim/sulfamethoxazole, vancomycin, vasopressin, vecuronium, verapamil, vinblastine, vincristine, vinorelbine, voriconazole, zidovudine, zoledronic acid.
- **Y-Site Incompatibility:** amphotericin B deoxycholate, diazepam, gemtuzumab ozogamicin, phenytoin.

Patient/Family Teaching

- Instruct patient to take dose in early morning. Emphasize need for adequate fluid intake for 72 hr after therapy. Patient should void frequently to ↓ bladder irritation from metabolites excreted by the kidneys. Report hematuria immediately. If a dose is missed, contact health care provider. Advise caregivers to use gloves when handling capsules. If capsule opens, wash hands thoroughly.
- Instruct patient to notify health care provider promptly if fever; sore throat; signs of infection; lower back or side pain; difficult or painful urination; sores in the mouth or on the lips; yellow discoloration of skin or eyes; bleeding gums; bruising; petechiae; blood in urine, stool, or emesis; unusual swelling of ankles or legs; joint pain; shortness of breath; cough; palpitations; weight gain >5 lb in 24 hr; dizziness; loss of consciousness; or confusion occurs. Caution patient to avoid crowds and persons with known infections. Instruct patient to use soft toothbrush and electric razor and to avoid falls. Patient should also be cautioned not to drink alcoholic beverages or to take products containing aspirin or NSAIDs; may precipitate GI hemorrhage.
- Discuss with patient the possibility of hair loss. Explore methods of coping. May also cause darkening of skin and fingernails.
- Instruct patient not to receive any vaccinations without advice of health care provider.
- Rep: May cause fetal harm. Advise women of reproductive potential to use highly effective contraceptive measures for up to 1 yr after last dose and to avoid breastfeeding during and for 1–6 wk after last dose. Advise men with female partners of reproductive potential to wear condoms during

and for ≥4 mo after last dose of therapy. Advise patient or notify health care provider if pregnancy is planned or suspected. Patients treated for rheumatic and musculoskeletal diseases should consider discontinuing cyclophosphamide 3–6 mo prior to conception to allow for disease monitoring and potential change to another immunosuppressant. Discontinue cyclophosphamide 12 wk before attempting conception in patients with rheumatic and musculoskeletal diseases who are planning to father a child. Inform patient that this medication may cause sterility and menstrual irregularities or cessation of menses.

Evaluation/Desired Outcomes

- Decrease in size or spread of malignant tumors.
- Improvement of hematologic status in patients with leukemia. Maintenance therapy is instituted if leukocyte count remains between 2500 and 4000/mm^3 and if patient does not demonstrate serious side effects.
- Management of minimal change nephrotic syndrome in children.

cycloSPORINE
(**sye**-kloe-spor-een)

Gengraf, Neoral, SandIMMUNE

Classification

Therapeutic: immunosuppressants, antirheumatics (DMARD)

Pharmacologic: polypeptides (cyclic)

See Appendix B for ophthalmic use

Indications

PO, IV: Prevention and treatment of rejection in renal, cardiac, and hepatic transplantation (with corticosteroids). **PO:** Severe active rheumatoid arthritis (Gengraf and Neoral only). Severe recalcitrant psoriasis in nonimmunocompromised patients (Gengraf and Neoral only). **Unlabeled Use:** Recalcitrant ulcerative colitis. Steroid-resistant nephrotic syndrome. Severe steroid-resistant autoimmune disease. Prevention and treatment of graft-versus-host disease in bone marrow transplant patients.

Action

Inhibits normal immune responses (cellular and humoral) by inhibiting interleukin-2, a factor necessary for initiation of T-cell activity. **Therapeutic Effects:** Prevention of rejection reactions. Slowed progression of rheumatoid arthritis or psoriasis.

Pharmacokinetics

Absorption: Erratically absorbed (range 10–60%) after oral administration, with significant first-pass metabolism by the liver. Microemulsion (Gengraf or Neoral) has better bioavailability than Sandimmune. IV administration results in complete bioavailability.

Distribution: Widely distributed, mainly into extracellular fluid and blood cells.

Protein Binding: 90–98%.

Metabolism and Excretion: Extensively metabolized by the liver by the CYP3A4 isoenzyme (first pass); excreted in bile, small amounts excreted unchanged in urine.

Half-life: *Children:* 7 hr; *Adults:* 19 hr.

TIME/ACTION PROFILE (plasma concentrations)

ROUTE	ONSET	PEAK	DURATION
PO	unknown†	2–6 hr	unknown
IV	unknown	end of infusion	unknown

† Onset of action in rheumatoid arthritis is 4–8 wk and may last 4 wk after discontinuation; for psoriasis, onset is 2–6 wk and lasts 6 wk following discontinuation.

Contraindications/Precautions

Contraindicated in: Hypersensitivity to cyclosporine or polyoxyethylated castor oil (vehicle for IV form); Disulfiram therapy or known alcohol intolerance (IV and oral liquid dose forms contain alcohol); Patients with psoriasis receiving immunosuppressants or radiation; Renal impairment (in rheumatoid arthritis or psoriasis); Uncontrolled hypertension; Lactation: Lactation.

Use Cautiously in: Renal impairment (frequent dose changes may be necessary); Severe hepatic impairment (↓ dose); Active infection; OB: An acceptable immunosuppressant when used following a kidney, heart, or liver transplant; not a preferred agent for other indications; Pedi: Larger or more frequent doses may be required in children.

Adverse Reactions/Side Effects

CV: hypertension. **Derm:** hirsutism, acne, psoriasis. **F and E** hyperkalemia, hypomagnesemia. **GI:** diarrhea, nausea, vomiting, abdominal discomfort, anorexia, HEPATOTOXICITY, PANCREATITIS. **GU:** nephrotoxicity. **Hemat:** anemia, leukopenia, thrombocytopenia. **Metab:** hyperlipidemia, hyperuricemia. **MS:** lower extremity pain. **Neuro:** tremor, confusion, flushing, headache, hyperesthesia, paresthesia, POSTERIOR REVERSIBLE ENCEPHALOPATHY SYNDROME (PRES), PROGRESSIVE MULTIFOCAL LEUKOENCEPHALOPATHY (PML), psychiatric problems, SEIZURES. **Misc:** gingival hyperplasia, hypersensitivity reactions, infection (including activation of latent viral infections such as BK virus-associated nephropathy), MALIGNANCY.

Interactions

Drug-Drug: **Azithromycin, clarithomycin, allopurinol, amiodarone, bromocriptine, colchicine, danazol, digoxin, diltiazem, erythromycin, fluconazole, fluoroquinolones, imatinib, itraconazole, ketoconazole, voriconazole, metoclopramide, methylprednisolone,**

nefazodone, **nicardipine**, **protease inhibitors**, **verapamil**, or **hormonal contraceptives** may ↑ levels and risk of toxicity. ↑ immunosuppression with other **immunosuppressants** (cyclophosphamide, azathioprine, corticosteroids). **Carbamazepine**, **nafcillin**, **octreotide**, **orlistat**, **oxcarbazepine**, **phenobarbital**, **phenytoin**, **rifampin**, **rifabutin**, or **terbinafine** may ↓ levels and effectiveness. **Bosentan** may significantly ↓ levels and effectiveness; avoid concurrent use. ↑ risk of hyperkalemia with **potassium-sparing diuretics**, **potassium supplements**, or **ACE inhibitors**. May ↑ levels and risk of toxicity of **aliskiren**, **bosentan**, **colchicine**, **digoxin**, **etoposide**, **HMG-CoA reductase inhibitors**, **methotrexate**, **nifedipine**, **repaglinide**, and **sirolimus**. May ↑ levels and risk of toxicity of **ambrisentan**; do not titrate dose of ambrisentan up to maximum daily dose. May ↑ levels of and risk of bleeding with **dabigatran**; avoid concurrent use. May ↓ antibody response to **live-virus vaccines** and ↑ risk of adverse reactions; avoid concurrent use. Concurrent use with **tacrolimus** should be avoided. ↑ risk of renal impairment with **ciprofloxacin**, **aminoglycosides**, **vancomycin**, **trimethoprim/sulfamethoxazole**, **melphalan**, **amphotericin B**, **ketoconazole**, **colchicine**, **NSAIDs**, **cimetidine**, or **fibric acid derivatives**.

Drug-Natural Products: Echinacea and **melatonin** may interfere with immunosuppression. **St. John's wort** may ↓ levels and effectiveness.

Drug-Food: Grapefruit or grapefruit juice may ↑ levels and risk of toxicity; avoid concurrent use. **Food** ↓ absorption of microemulsion products (Neoral).

Route/Dosage

- Sandimmune cannot be used interchangeably with Gengraf or Neoral because they are not bioequivalent.

Prevention of Transplant Rejection (Sandimmune)

PO (Adults and Children): 14–18 mg/kg/dose 4–12 hr before transplant; then 5–15 mg/kg/day divided every 12–24 hr postoperatively; taper by 5% weekly to maintenance dose of 3–10 mg/kg/day.
IV (Adults and Children): 5–6 mg/kg/dose 4–12 hr before transplant; then 2–10 mg/kg/day in divided doses every 8–24 hr; change to PO as soon as possible.

Prevention of Transplant Rejection (Gengraf or Neoral)

PO (Adults and Children): 4–12 mg/kg/day divided every 12 hr (dose varies depending on organ transplanted).

Rheumatoid Arthritis (Gengraf or Neoral)

PO (Adults and Children): 2.5 mg/kg/day given in 2 divided doses; may ↑ by 0.5–0.75 mg/kg/day after 8 and 12 wk, up to 4 mg/kg/day. ↓ dose by 25–50% if adverse reactions occur.

Severe Psoriasis (Gengraf or Neoral)

PO (Adults): 2.5 mg/kg/day given in 2 divided doses, for at least 4 wk; then may ↑ by 0.5 mg/kg/day every 2 wk, up to 4 mg/kg/day. ↓ dose by 25–50% if adverse reactions occur.

Autoimmune Diseases (Neoral only)

PO (Adults and Children): 1–3 mg/kg/day.

Availability (generic available)

Microemulsion soft gelatin capsules (Gengraf, Neoral): 25 mg, 50 mg, 100 mg. **Microemulsion oral solution (Neoral):** 100 mg/mL. **Soft gelatin capsules (Sandimmune):** 25 mg, 100 mg. **Solution for injection (Sandimmune):** 50 mg/mL.

NURSING IMPLICATIONS

Assessment

- Monitor intake and output, daily weight, and BP during therapy. Report significant changes.
- Assess for any new signs or symptoms that may be suggestive of PML, an opportunistic infection of the brain caused by the JC virus that may be fatal; withhold dose and notify health care provider promptly. PML symptoms may begin gradually (hemiparesis, apathy, confusion, cognitive deficiencies, ataxia) and may include deteriorating renal function and renal graft loss.
- Monitor for signs and symptoms of PRES (impaired consciousness; convulsions; visual disturbances, including blindness; loss of motor function; movement disorders and psychiatric disturbances; papilledema; visual impairment). Usually reversible with discontinuation of cyclosporine. Occurs more often in patients with liver transplant than kidney transplant.
- **Prevention of Transplant Rejection:** Assess for symptoms of organ rejection during therapy.
- **IV:** Monitor for signs and symptoms of hypersensitivity (wheezing, dyspnea, flushing of face or neck) continuously during at least the 1st 30 min of each treatment and frequently thereafter. Oxygen, epinephrine, and equipment for treatment of anaphylaxis should be available with each IV dose.
- **Arthritis:** Assess pain and limitation of movement before and during administration.
- Perform a baseline physical exam including BP on two occasions before starting therapy. Monitor BP every 2 wk during initial 3 mo and then monthly if stable. If hypertension occurs, ↓ dose.
- **Psoriasis:** Assess skin lesions prior to and during therapy.

Lab Test Considerations

- Monitor BUN, serum creatinine, CBC, magnesium, potassium, uric acid, and lipids at baseline, every 2 wk during initial therapy, and then monthly if stable. Nephrotoxicity may occur.
- May cause hepatotoxicity; monitor for ↑ AST, ALT, alkaline phosphatase, amylase, and bilirubin.
- May ↑ serum potassium, lipid, and uric acid levels and ↓ serum magnesium levels.

Toxicity and Overdose

- Evaluate serum cyclosporine levels periodically during therapy. Dose may be adjusted daily in response to levels during initiation of therapy. Guidelines for desired serum levels will vary among institutions.

Implementation

- Do not confuse cyclosporine with cyclophosphamide or cycloserine. Do not confuse Sandimmune with Sandostatin.
- Only health care providers experienced in immunosuppressive therapy and management of organ transplant patients should prescribe cyclosporine.
- Administer initial dose 4–12 hr before transplantation.
- Given with adrenal corticosteroids; avoid other immunosuppressive agents. Protect transplant patients from staff and visitors who may carry infection. Maintain protective isolation as indicated.
- **PO:** Draw up oral solution in the syringe provided; do not rinse syringe either before or after use. Introduction of water into the product by any means will cause variation in dose. Mix oral solution with milk, chocolate milk, apple juice, or orange juice, preferably at room temperature. Stir well and drink at once. Use a glass container and rinse with more diluent to ensure that total dose is taken. Administer oral doses with meals.

IV Administration

- Due to risk of anaphylaxis, IV dose should be reserved for patients who are unable to take the soft gelatin capsules or oral solution.
- **Intermittent Infusion: Dilution:** Dilute each 1 mL (50 mg) of IV concentrate immediately before use with 20–100 mL of D5W or 0.9% NaCl for injection. Solution is stable for 24 hr in D5W. In 0.9% NaCl, it is stable for 6 hr in a polyvinylchloride container and 12 hr in a glass container at room temperature. **Concentration:** 2.5 mg/mL. **Rate:** Infuse slowly over 2–6 hr via infusion pump.
- **Continuous Infusion:** May be administered over 24 hr.
- **Y-Site Compatibility:** alemtuzumab, amikacin, aminocaproic acid, aminophylline, amiodarone, anidulafungin, argatroban, arsenic trioxide, ascorbic acid, atropine, azathioprine, azithromycin, aztreonam, benztropine, bivalirudin, bleomycin, bumetanide, buprenorphine, butorphanol, calcium chloride, calcium gluconate, carboplatin, carmustine, caspofungin, cefazolin, cefotaxime, cefotetan, cefoxitin, ceftaroline, ceftazidime, ceftriaxone, cefuroxime, chloramphenicol, chlorpromazine, cisplatin, clindamycin, cyclophosphamide, cytarabine, dacarbazine, dactinomycin, daptomycin, daunorubicin, defibrotide, dexamethasone, dexmedetomidine, dexrazoxane, digoxin, diltiazem, dimenhydrinate, diphenhydramine, dobutamine, docetaxel, dopamine, doxorubicin hydrochloride, doxorubicin liposomal, doxycycline, enalaprilat, ephedrine, epinephrine, epirubicin, epoetin alfa, eptifibatide, ertapenem, erythromycin, esmolol, etoposide, etoposide phosphate, famotidine, fentanyl, fluconazole, fludarabine, fluorouracil, folic acid, foscarnet, fosphenytoin, furosemide, ganciclovir, gemcitabine, gentamicin, glycopyrrolate, granisetron, heparin, hetastarch, hydrocortisone, hydromorphone, ifosfamide, imipenem/cilastatin, indomethacin, irinotecan, isoproterenol, ketorolac, labetalol, leucovorin, levofloxacin, lidocaine, linezolid, lorazepam, mannitol, meperidine, meropenem, methadone, methotrexate, methylprednisolone, metoclopramide, metoprolol, metronidazole, micafungin, midazolam, milrinone, minocycline, mitomycin, mitoxantrone, morphine, moxifloxacin, multivitamins, nafcillin, nicardipine, nitroglycerin, nitroprusside, norepinephrine, octreotide, ondansetron, oxacillin, oxaliplatin, oxytocin, paclitaxel, palonosetron, pamidronate, papaverine, pemetrexed, penicillin G, pentamidine, phentolamine, phenylephrine, phytonadione, piperacillin/tazobactam, potassium acetate, potassium chloride, procainamide, prochlorperazine, promethazine, propofol, propranolol, protamine, pyridoxine, sargramostim, sodium acetate, sodium bicarbonate, succinylcholine, sufentanil, tacrolimus, theophylline, thiamine, thiotepa, tigecycline, tirofiban, tobramycin, topotecan, vancomycin, vasopressin, vecuronium, verapamil, vinblastine, vincristine, vinorelbine, zoledronic acid.
- **Y-Site Incompatibility:** amphotericin B liposomal, ceftolozane/tazobactam, cyanocobalamin, dantrolene, diazepam, diazoxide, gemtuzumab ozogamicin, idarubicin, isavuconazonium, nalbuphine, pentobarbital, phenobarbital, phenytoin, rituximab, tedizolid, trastuzumab, trimethoprim/sulfamethoxazole, voriconazole.

Patient/Family Teaching

- Explain purpose and side effects of medication to patient. Advise patient to read *Patient Information* before starting therapy. Instruct patient to take at the same time each day with meals, as directed. Take missed doses as soon as remembered within 12 hr. Do not skip doses or double up on missed doses, and do not discontinue medication without

advice of health care provider. Emphasize the importance of follow-up exams and lab tests.
- Advise patient to notify health care provider of all Rx or OTC medications, vitamins, or herbal products being taken and to consult health care provider before taking other medications.
- Reinforce the need for lifelong therapy to prevent transplant rejection. Review symptoms of rejection for transplanted organ, and stress need to notify health care provider immediately if they occur.
- Instruct patient and/or caregiver to notify health care provider if diarrhea develops; ↓ absorption of cyclosporine and can result in rejection.
- Instruct patient to avoid grapefruit and grapefruit juice to prevent interaction with cyclosporine.
- Advise patient of common side effects (nephrotoxicity, ↑ BP, hand tremors, ↑ facial and body hair, gingival hyperplasia). Advise patient that if hair growth is excessive, depilatories or waxing can be used.
- Teach patient the correct method for monitoring BP. Instruct patient to notify health care provider of significant changes in BP or if hematuria, ↑ urinary frequency, cloudy urine, ↓ urine output, fever, sore throat, tiredness, or unusual bruising occur.
- Instruct patient on proper oral hygiene. Meticulous oral hygiene and dental examinations for teeth cleaning and plaque control every 3 mo will help ↓ gingival inflammation and hyperplasia.
- Rep: Advise patient to notify health care provider if pregnancy is planned or suspected and to avoid breastfeeding.

Evaluation/Desired Outcomes
- Prevention of rejection reactions.
- Slow progression of rheumatoid arthritis or psoriasis.

HIGH ALERT

cytarabine (sye-**tare**-a-been)

~~Cytosar-U~~

Classification

Therapeutic: antineoplastics

Pharmacologic: antimetabolites

Indications
IV: Treatment of leukemias and non-Hodgkin lymphomas (in combination with other agents). **IT:** Prophylaxis and treatment of meningeal leukemia.

Action
Inhibits DNA synthesis by inhibiting DNA polymerase (cell-cycle S-phase-specific). **Therapeutic Effects:** Death of rapidly replicating cells, particularly malignant ones.

Pharmacokinetics
Absorption: Absorption occurs from SUBQ sites, but blood levels are lower than with IV administration; IT administration results in negligible systemic exposure.
Distribution: Widely distributed; IV- and SUBQ-administered cytarabine crosses the blood-brain barrier but not in significant quantities.
Metabolism and Excretion: Metabolized mostly by the liver; <10% excreted unchanged by the kidneys. Metabolism to inactive drug in the CSF is negligible because the enzyme that metabolizes it is present in very low concentrations in the CSF.
Half-life: *IV, SUBQ:* 1–3 hr; *IT:* 100–236 hr.

TIME/ACTION PROFILE (IV, SUBQ: Effects on WBCs; IT: Concentrations in CSF)

ROUTE	ONSET	PEAK	DURATION
SUBQ, IV (1st phase)	24 hr	7–9 days	12 days
SUBQ, IV (2nd phase)	15–24 days	15–24 days	25–34 days
IT	rapid	5 hr	14–28 days

Contraindications/Precautions
Contraindicated in: Hypersensitivity; Active meningeal infection (IT only); OB: Pregnancy; Lactation: Lactation.
Use Cautiously in: Active infection; ↓ bone marrow reserve; Renal impairment; Hepatic impairment; Rep: Women of reproductive potential.

Adverse Reactions/Side Effects
CV: edema. **Derm:** alopecia, rash. **EENT:** corneal toxicity (high dose), hemorrhagic conjunctivitis (high dose), visual disturbances (including blindness). **GI:** <u>nausea</u>, <u>vomiting</u>, abdominal pain, diarrhea, GI ulceration (high dose), HEPATOTOXICITY, stomatitis. **GU:** sterility, urinary incontinence. **Hemat: (less with IT use):** <u>anemia</u>, <u>leukopenia</u>, <u>thrombocytopenia</u>. **Metab:** hyperuricemia. **Neuro:** **IT:** abnormal gait, CHEMICAL ARACHNOIDITIS, CNS dysfunction (high dose), confusion, drowsiness, headache. **Resp:** PULMONARY EDEMA (HIGH DOSE). **Misc:** cytarabine syndrome, fever.

Interactions
Drug-Drug: ↑ risk of bone marrow depression with other **antineoplastics** or **radiation therapy**. ↑ risk of cardiomyopathy when used in high-dose regimens with **cyclophosphamide**. May ↓ antibody response to **live-virus vaccines** and ↑ risk of adverse reactions. May ↓ absorption and effectiveness of **digoxin**. May ↓ the effectiveness of **gentamicin** when used to treat *Klebsiella pneumoniae* infections. Recent treatment with **asparaginase** may ↑ risk of pancreatitis. ↑ risk of neurotoxicity with concurrently administered **IT antineoplastics** (IT only).

Route/Dosage

Dose regimens vary widely

IV (Adults): *Induction dose:* 200 mg/m²/day for 5 days every 2 wk as a single agent *or* 2–6 mg/kg/day (100–200 mg/m²/day) as a single daily dose *or* in 2–3 divided doses for 5–10 days or until remission occurs as part of combination chemotherapy. *Maintenance:* 70–200 mg/m²/day for 2–5 days monthly. *Refractory leukemias/lymphomas:* 3 g/m² every 12 hr for up to 12 doses.

SUBQ (Adults): *Maintenance:* 1–1.5 mg/kg every 1–4 wk.

IT (Adults): Usual dose = 30 mg/m² every 4 days; range = 5–75 mg/m² once daily for 4 days or every 4 days until CNS findings normalize, followed by one additional treatment.

Availability (generic available)

Solution for injection: 20 mg/mL, 100 mg/mL. ***In combination with:*** daunorubicin (Vyxeos). See Appendix N.

NURSING IMPLICATIONS

Assessment

- Monitor for signs of bone marrow depression (↑ bleeding and bruising; petechiae; blood in stool, urine, or emesis). Avoid IM injections and rectal temperatures if platelet count is low. Apply pressure to venipuncture sites for 10 min. Assess for signs of neutropenia and anemia (infection, fatigue, dyspnea, orthostatic hypotension).
- Monitor intake and output and daily weights. Report significant changes.
- Monitor for symptoms of gout (joint pain, edema). Encourage patient to drink ≥2 L of fluid each day.
- Assess nutritional status. Nausea and vomiting may occur within 1 hr of initiation, especially if rapidly administered. Premedicate with antiemetic and periodically throughout therapy.
- Monitor for cytarabine syndrome (fever, myalgia, bone pain, chest pain, maculopapular rash, conjunctivitis, malaise); occurs 6–12 hr after administration. Use corticosteroids for treatment or prevention. If symptoms improve, continue cytarabine and corticosteroids.
- Assess for respiratory distress and pulmonary edema. Occurs with high doses rarely.
- Monitor for signs of anaphylaxis (rash, dyspnea, swelling). Keep epinephrine, corticosteroids, and resuscitation equipment nearby.
- **IT** Assess CSF flow prior to IT therapy. Chemical arachnoiditis (nausea, vomiting, headache, fever, back pain, CSF pleocytosis, neck rigidity, neck pain) is expected with IT therapy. Incidence and severity of symptoms may be ↓ with coadministration of dexamethasone 4 mg PO or IV twice daily for 5 days beginning on day of injection.
- Monitor patients receiving IT therapy continuously for neurotoxicity (myelopathy, personality changes, dysarthria, ataxia, confusion, somnolence, coma). *If symptoms occur,* ↓ subsequent doses; discontinue cytarabine if neurotoxicity persists.
- Monitor injection site for signs and symptoms of thrombophlebitis.

Lab Test Considerations

- Monitor CBC with differential before and frequently during therapy. WBC count ↓ 24 hr after dose; 1st nadir occurs in 7–9 days, and 2nd deeper nadir occurs in 15–24 days. Platelets ↓ 5 days after dose, with a nadir at 12–15 days. WBC and platelet counts usually ↑ 10 days after the nadirs. *If WBC count <1000/mm³ or platelet count <50,000/mm³,* consider stopping therapy. Bone marrow aspirations are recommended every 2 wk until remission occurs.
- Monitor renal (BUN, serum creatinine) and hepatic (AST, ALT, bilirubin, alkaline phosphatase, LDH) function before and routinely during therapy.
- May ↑ uric acid levels. Allopurinol may ↓ levels. Alkalinization of urine may ↑ excretion of uric acid.

Implementation

- ***High Alert:*** Fatalities have occurred with chemotherapeutic agents. Before administering, clarify all ambiguous orders; double-check single, daily, and course-of-therapy dose limits; have second practitioner independently double-check original order, calculations, and infusion pump settings.
- ***High Alert:*** Do not confuse high-dose and regular therapy. Fatalities have occurred with high-dose therapy.
- ***High Alert:*** Administer under supervision of a physician experienced in use of cancer chemotherapeutic agents.
- For induction therapy, patients should be treated in a facility with laboratory and supportive resources sufficient to monitor drug tolerance and protect and maintain a patient compromised by drug toxicity.
- The health care provider must judge possible benefit to the patient against known toxic effects of this drug in considering the advisability of therapy with cytarabine.
- Solution should be prepared in a biologic cabinet. Wear gloves, gown, and mask while handling. Discard IV equipment in specially designated containers.

IV Administration

- **IV Push: Dilution:** Administer undiluted. **Concentration:** 100 mg/mL. **Rate:** Administer each 100 mg over 1–3 min
- **Intermittent Infusion: Dilution:** May be further diluted in 250–1000 mL of 0.9% NaCl, D5W,

D10W, D5/0.9% NaCl, Ringer's solution, LR, or D5/LR.. **Rate:** Infuse over 15–30 min.

- **Continuous Infusion:** Rate and concentration for IV infusion are ordered individually.
- **Y-Site Compatibility:** acyclovir, alemtuzumab, amikacin, aminocaproic acid, aminophylline, amphotericin B liposomal, ampicillin, ampicillin/sulbactam, anidulafungin, argatroban, arsenic trioxide, atracurium, azithromycin, aztreonam, bivalirudin, bleomycin, bumetanide, buprenorphine, butorphanol, calcium chloride, calcium gluconate, carboplatin, carmustine, cefazolin, cefepime, cefotaxime, cefotetan, cefoxitin, ceftazidime, ceftriaxone, cefuroxime, chlorpromazine, ciprofloxacin, cisatracurium, cisplatin, cladribine, clindamycin, cyclophosphamide, cyclosporine, dacarbazine, daunorubicin, dexamethasone, dexmedetomidine, dexrazoxane, digoxin, diltiazem, diphenhydramine, dobutamine, docetaxel, dopamine, doxorubicin hydrochloride, doxorubicin liposomal, doxycycline, droperidol, enalaprilat, ephedrine, epinephrine, ertapenem, erythromycin, esmolol, etoposide, etoposide phosphate, famotidine, fentanyl, filgrastim, fluconazole, fludarabine, foscarnet, fosphenytoin, furosemide, gemcitabine, gemtuzumab ozogamicin, gentamicin, granisetron, haloperidol, heparin, hydrocortisone, hydromorphone, hydroxyzine, idarubicin, ifosfamide, imipenem/cilastatin, insulin, regular, irinotecan, isoproterenol, ketorolac, labetalol, leucovorin, levofloxacin, lidocaine, linezolid, lorazepam, magnesium sulfate, mannitol, melphalan, meperidine, meropenem, mesna, methadone, methohexital, methotrexate, methylprednisolone, metoclopramide, metoprolol, metronidazole, midazolam, milrinone, minocycline, mitoxantrone, morphine, moxifloxacin, nalbuphine, naloxone, nicardipine, nitroglycerin, nitroprusside, norepinephrine, octreotide, ondansetron, oxaliplatin, paclitaxel, palonosetron, pamidronate, pantoprazole, pemetrexed, pentamidine, pentobarbital, phenobarbital, phenylephrine, piperacillin/tazobactam, potassium acetate, potassium chloride, potassium phosphates, procainamide, prochlorperazine, promethazine, propofol, propranolol, remifentanil, rituximab, rocuronium, sargramostim, sodium acetate, sodium bicarbonate, sodium phosphates, succinylcholine, sufentanil, tacrolimus, theophylline, thiotepa, tigecycline, tirofiban, tobramycin, trastuzumab, trimethoprim/sulfamethoxazole, vancomycin, vasopressin, vecuronium, verapamil, vincristine, vinorelbine, voriconazole, zidovudine, zoledronic acid.
- **Y-Site Incompatibility:** allopurinol, amiodarone, amphotericin B deoxycholate, daptomycin, diazepam, ganciclovir, phenytoin.
- **IT: Reconstitution:** Reconstitute with preservative-free 0.9% NaCl or autologous spinal fluid. Use immediately to prevent bacterial contamination.
- **Rate:** Inject slowly over 1–5 min.
- Following injection patient should lie flat for 1 hr. Monitor for immediate toxic reactions.

Patient/Family Teaching

- Explain purpose and side effects of medication. Advise patient to read *Patient Information* before starting therapy.
- Advise patient to notify health care provider of all Rx or OTC medications, vitamins, or herbal products being taken and to consult health care provider before taking other medications.
- Caution patient to avoid crowds and persons with known infections. Report symptoms of infection (fever, chills, cough, hoarseness, sore throat, lower back or side pain, painful or difficult urination) immediately to health care provider.
- Instruct patient to report unusual bleeding and to use soft toothbrush and electric razor, avoid falls, and avoid drinking alcohol or taking medication containing aspirin or NSAIDs.
- Instruct patient to drink ≥2 L of fluid daily.
- Emphasize the need for periodic lab tests to monitor for side effects.
- Instruct patient to inspect oral mucosa for redness and ulceration. If mouth sores occur, use sponge brush and rinse mouth with water after eating and drinking.
- Instruct patient not to receive vaccinations without advice of health care provider.
- Rep: May cause fetal harm. Advise patient to use contraception during and for ≥4 mo after therapy is complete. Advise women of reproductive potential to notify health care provider if pregnancy is planned or suspected and to avoid breastfeeding during therapy.
- **IT:** Advise patient to expect headache, nausea, vomiting and fever. Instruct patient to notify health care provider if early signs of neurotoxicity occur.

Evaluation/Desired Outcomes

- Improvement of hematopoietic values in leukemias.
- ↓ in size and spread of non-Hodgkin lymphoma tumors. Therapy is continued every 2 wk until complete remission or platelets or leukocytes fall below acceptable levels.
- Treatment of lymphomatous meningitis.

BEERS HIGH ALERT

dabigatran (da-bi-**gat**-ran)

Pradaxa

Classification

Therapeutic: anticoagulants

Pharmacologic: thrombin inhibitors

Indications

Reduction in the risk of stroke/systemic embolization associated with nonvalvular atrial fibrillation (AF). Treatment of venous thromboembolic events (VTE) (including deep vein thrombosis [DVT] or pulmonary embolism [PE]) in patients who have been treated with a parenteral anticoagulant for ≥5 days. Reduction in the risk of recurrence of VTE in patients who have been previously treated. Prevention of DVT and PE following hip replacement surgery.

Action

Acts as a direct inhibitor of thrombin. **Therapeutic Effects:** Reduced risk of thrombotic sequelae (stroke and systemic embolism) in nonvalvular AF. Reduced risk of recurrent PE and DVT. Resolution of DVT and PE.

Pharmacokinetics

Absorption: 3–7% absorbed following oral administration. Bioavailability of oral pellets higher than that of capsules in adults.

Distribution: Unknown.

Metabolism and Excretion: Of the amount absorbed, mostly excreted by kidneys (80%); 86% of ingested dose is eliminated in feces due to poor bioavailability.

Half-life: 12–17 hr.

TIME/ACTION PROFILE (effects on coagulation)

ROUTE	ONSET	PEAK	DURATION
PO	within hr	unknown	2 days†

† Following discontinuation, 3–5 days in renal impairment.

Contraindications/Precautions

Contraindicated in: Hypersensitivity; Active pathologic bleeding; Prosthetic heart valves (mechanical or bioprosthetic); Triple-positive antiphospholipid syndrome (↑ risk of thrombosis); OB: Pregnancy; Lactation: Lactation.

Use Cautiously in: Neuroaxial spinal anesthesia or spinal puncture, especially if concurrent with an indwelling epidural catheter, drugs affecting hemostasis, history of traumatic/repeated spinal puncture, or spinal deformity (↑ risk of spinal hematoma); Concurrent medications/pre-existing conditions that ↑ bleeding risk (other anticoagulants, antiplatelet agents, fibrinolytics, heparins, chronic NSAID use, labor and delivery); Renal impairment; Surgical procedures (discontinue 1–2 days prior if CCr ≥50 mL/min or 3–4 days prior if CCr <50 mL/min); Rep: Women of reproductive potential; Pedi: Safety and effectiveness in children <3 mo (treatment and reduction in risk of VTE) and <18 yr (all other indications) not established; Geri: Appears on Beers list. ↑ risk of bleeding in older adults. Use caution in selecting dabigatran over apixaban for long-term treatment of nonvalvular AF or VTE.

Adverse Reactions/Side Effects

GI: abdominal pain, diarrhea, dyspepsia, gastritis, esophageal ulceration, nausea. **Hemat:** BLEEDING, thrombocytopenia. **Misc:** HYPERSENSITIVITY REACTIONS (INCLUDING ANAPHYLAXIS AND ANGIOEDEMA).

Interactions

Drug-Drug: Concurrent use of other **anticoagulants, antiplatelet agents, fibrinolytics, heparins, prasugrel,** or **clopidogrel** or chronic use of **NSAIDs** ↑ risk of bleeding. **P-glycoprotein (P-gp) inducers,** including **rifampin,** may ↓ levels and effectiveness; avoid concurrent use. **P-gp inhibitors,** including **dronedarone, ketoconazole (systemic), verapamil, quinidine,** and **ticagrelor,** may ↑ levels and risk of bleeding; avoid concurrent use in patients with CCr 15–30 mL/min.

Route/Dosage

Do not interchange capsules and oral pellets on a milligram-to-milligram basis, and do not combine these dose forms to achieve the total dose.

Reduction in Risk of Stroke/Systemic Embolism in Nonvalvular Atrial Fibrillation

PO (Adults): *Capsules:* 150 mg twice daily.

Renal Impairment

PO (Adults): *CCr 30–50 mL/min and taking dronedarone or systemic ketoconazole:* Capsules: 75 mg twice daily; *CCr <30 mL/min and taking P-gp inhibitor:* Avoid concurrent use; *CCr 15–30 mL/min:* Capsules: 75 mg twice daily; *CCr <15 mL/min or on dialysis:* Not recommended.

Treatment of and Reduction in Risk of Recurrence of Deep Vein Thrombosis or Pulmonary Embolism

Capsules

PO (Adults): 150 mg twice daily.

PO (Children 8–<18 yr and ≥81 kg actual body weight): 260 mg (one 150-mg capsule + one 110-mg capsule *or* one 110-mg capsule + two 75-mg capsules) twice daily.

PO (Children 8–<18 yr and 61–<81 kg actual body weight): 220 mg (two 110-mg capsules) twice daily.

PO (Children 8–<18 yr and 41–<61 kg actual body weight): 185 mg (one 110-mg capsule + one 75-mg capsule) twice daily.

PO (Children 8–<18 yr and 26–<41 kg actual body weight): 150 mg (one 150-mg capsule *or* two 75-mg capsules) twice daily.
PO (Children 8–<18 yr and 16–<26 kg actual body weight): 110 mg (one 110-mg capsule) twice daily.
PO (Children 8–<18 yr and 11–<16 kg actual body weight): 75 mg (one 75-mg capsule) twice daily.

Oral Pellets

PO (Children 2–<12 yr and ≥41 kg actual body weight): 260 mg (one 110-mg pkt + one 150-mg pkt) twice daily.
PO (Children 2–<12 yr and 21–<41 kg actual body weight): 220 mg (two 110-mg pkts) twice daily.
PO (Children 2–<12 yr and 16–<21 kg actual body weight): 170 mg (one 20-mg pkt + one 150-mg pkt) twice daily.
PO (Children 2–<12 yr and 13–<16 kg actual body weight): 140 mg (one 30-mg pkt + one 110-mg pkt) twice daily.
PO (Children 2–<12 yr and 11–<13 kg actual body weight): 110 mg (one 110-mg pkt) twice daily.
PO (Children 2–<12 yr and 9–<11 kg actual body weight): 90 mg (one 40-mg pkt + one 50-mg pkt) twice daily.
PO (Children 2–<12 yr and 7–<9 kg actual body weight): 70 mg (one 30-mg pkt + one 40-mg pkt) twice daily.
PO (Children 18 mo–<2 yr and 21–<26 kg actual body weight): 180 mg (one 30-mg pkt + one 150-mg pkt) twice daily.
PO (Children 12 mo–<2 yr and 16–<21 kg actual body weight): 140 mg (one 30-mg pkt + one 110-mg pkt) twice daily.
PO (Children 11 mo–<2 yr and 13–<16 kg actual body weight): 140 mg (one 30-mg pkt + one 110-mg pkt) twice daily.
PO (Children 10 mo–<11 mo and 13–<16 kg actual body weight): 100 mg (two 50-mg pkts) twice daily.
PO (Children 18 mo–<2 yr and 11–<13 kg actual body weight): 110 mg (one 110-mg pkt) twice daily.
PO (Children 8 mo–<18 mo and 11–<13 kg actual body weight): 100 mg (two 50-mg pkts) twice daily.
PO (Children 11 mo–<2 yr and 9–<11 kg actual body weight): 90 mg (one 40-mg pkt + one 50-mg pkt) twice daily.
PO (Children 6–<11 mo and 9–<11 kg actual body weight): 80 mg (two 40-mg pkts) twice daily.
PO (Children 5–<6 mo and 9–<11 kg actual body weight): 60 mg (two 30-mg pkts) twice daily.
PO (Children 9 mo–<2 yr and 7–<9 kg actual body weight): 70 mg (one 30-mg pkt + one 40-mg pkt) twice daily.
PO (Children 4–<9 mo and 7–<9 kg actual body weight): 60 mg (two 30-mg pkts) twice daily.
PO (Children 3–<4 mo and 7–<9 kg actual body weight): 50 mg (one 50-mg pkt) twice daily.
PO (Children 5 mo–<2 yr and 5–<7 kg actual body weight): 50 mg (one 50-mg pkt) twice daily.
PO (Children 3–<5 mo and 5–<7 kg actual body weight): 40 mg (one 40-mg pkt) twice daily.
PO (Children 3–<10 mo and 4–<5 kg actual body weight): 40 mg (one 40-mg pkt) twice daily.
PO (Children 3–<6 mo and 3–<4 kg actual body weight): 30 mg (one 30-mg pkt) twice daily.

Renal Impairment

PO (Adults): *CCr <50 mL/min and taking P-gp inhibitor:* Avoid concurrent use; *CCr <30 mL/min or on dialysis:* Not recommended.

Renal Impairment

(Children 8–<18 yr and ≥11 kg): *eGFR <50 mL/min/1.73 m²:* Not recommended.

Prevention of Deep Vein Thrombosis and Pulmonary Embolism Following Hip Replacement Surgery

PO (Adults): *Capsules:* 110 mg taken 1–4 hr after surgery and once hemostasis achieved; then 220 mg once daily for 28–35 days; if unable to start on day of surgery, once hemostasis achieved, start with 220 mg once daily.

Renal Impairment

PO (Adults): *CCr <50 mL/min and taking P-gp inhibitor:* Avoid concurrent use; *CCr ≤30 mL/min or on dialysis:* Not recommended.

Availability (generic available)

Capsules: 75 mg, 110 mg, 150 mg. **Oral pellets:** 20 mg/pkt, 30 mg/pkt, 40 mg/pkt, 50 mg/pkt, 110 mg/pkt, 150 mg/pkt.

NURSING IMPLICATIONS

Assessment

- Assess for symptoms of stroke or peripheral vascular disease periodically during therapy.
- Assess for symptoms of bleeding and blood loss; may be fatal.

Lab Test Considerations

- Use aPTT or ecarin clotting time (ECT), not INR, to assess anticoagulant activity, if needed.
- Monitor renal function prior to and periodically during therapy. Patients with renal impairment may require dose ↓ or discontinuation.

Toxicity and Overdose

- Should dabigatran need to be reversed, the reversal agent is idarucizumab; has not been tested in pediatric patients.

Implementation

- Do not confuse dabigatran with vigabatrin. Do not confuse Pradaxa with Plavix.

- Do not exchange capsule for oral pellets. Doses are not equal.
- *Converting from warfarin to dabigatran:* Discontinue warfarin and start dabigatran when INR <2.0.
- *Converting from dabigatran to warfarin:* Adjust starting time based on CCr. For *CCr >50 mL/min*, start warfarin 3 days before discontinuing dabigatran. For *CCr 31–50 mL/min*, start warfarin 2 days before discontinuing dabigatran. For *CCr 15–30 mL/min*, start warfarin 1 day before discontinuing dabigatran. For *CCr <15 mL/min*, no recommendations can be made. INR will better reflect warfarin's effect after dabigatran has been stopped for >2 days.
- *Converting from parenteral anticoagulants to dabigatran:* Start dabigatran up to 2 hr before next dose of parenteral drug is due or at time of discontinuation of parenteral therapy.
- *Converting from dabigatran to parenteral anticoagulants:* Wait 12 hr (if CCr ≥30 mL/min) or 24 hr (if CCr <30 mL/min) after last dose of dabigatran before initiating parenteral anticoagulant therapy.
- *For surgery:* Discontinue dabigatran 1–2 days (if CCr ≥50 mL/min) or 3–5 days (if CCr <50 mL/min) before invasive or surgical procedures; consider longer times for major surgery, spinal puncture, or placement of a spinal or epidural catheter. If surgery cannot be delayed, bleeding risk ↑. Assess bleeding risk with ECT or aPTT if ECT is not available.
- **PO:** Administer twice daily, at the same time each day, about 12 hr apart with a full glass of water without regard to food. Give with food to ↓ GI distress. ***DNC:*** Swallow capsule whole; do not open, crush, or chew; may result in ↑ exposure.
- Administer pellets immediately after mixing or within 30 min after mixing. If not administered within 30 min of mixing, discard dose, and prepare a new dose. Mix pellets with 2 teaspoons of soft food (mashed carrots, applesauce, mashed banana) at room temperature, or spoon pellets directly into mouth and swallow with apple juice or added to 1–2 ounces of apple juice for drinking. Do not administer pellets via syringes or feeding tubes or with milk, milk products, or soft foods containing milk products.
- If dabigatran is discontinued, consider starting another anticoagulant; discontinuation of dabigatran ↑ risk of thromboembolic events.

Patient/Family Teaching

- Explain purpose and side effects of medication to patient. Advise patient to read *Patient Information* before starting therapy. Instruct patient to take as directed. Take missed doses as soon as remembered within 6 hr. If <6 hr until next dose, skip dose and take next dose when scheduled; do not double doses. Do not discontinue without consulting health care provider; may ↑ risk of stroke, DVT, or PE. If temporarily discontinued, restart as soon as possible. Store dabigatran at room temperature. After opening bottle, use within 4 mo; discard unused dabigatran after 4 mo.
- Instruct patient to notify health care provider of all Rx or OTC medications, vitamins, or herbal products being taken and consult health care provider before taking any new medications, especially aspirin or NSAIDs.
- Inform patient having had neuraxial anesthesia or spinal puncture to watch for signs and symptoms of spinal or epidural hematoma (numbness or weakness of legs, bowel or bladder dysfunction). Notify health care provider immediately if symptoms occur.
- Inform patient that they may bleed more easily or longer than usual. Advise patient to notify health care provider immediately if signs of bleeding (unusual bruising, pink or brown urine, red or black tarry stools, coughing up blood, vomiting blood, pain or swelling in a joint, headache, dizziness, weakness, recurring nosebleeds, unusual bleeding from gums, heavier-than-normal menstrual bleeding, dyspepsia, abdominal pain, epigastric pain) occur.
- Advise patient to notify health care provider of medication regimen prior to treatment or surgery.
- Rep: May cause fetal harm. Advise women of reproductive potential to notify health care provider if pregnancy is planned or suspected and to avoid breastfeeding during therapy. May ↑ risk of bleeding in the fetus and neonate. Monitor neonates for bleeding. May ↑ risk of uterine bleeding; advise patient to notify health care provider if significant uterine bleeding occurs.

Evaluation/Desired Outcomes

- Reduction in the risk of stroke and systemic embolism associated with nonvalvular AF.
- Reduced risk of recurrent PE and DVT.
- Resolution of DVT and PE.

HIGH ALERT

dabrafenib (da-**braf**-e-nib)

Tafinlar

Classification

Therapeutic: antineoplastics

Pharmacologic: kinase inhibitors

Indications

Metastatic or unresectable melanoma in patients with the BRAF V600E mutation (as monotherapy). Metastatic or unresectable melanoma in patients with the BRAF V600E or V600K mutation (in combination with trametinib). Adjuvant treatment of melanoma in patients with the BRAF V600E or V600K mutation and lymph node involvement following complete resection (in combination with trametinib). Metastatic non-small cell lung cancer

(NSCLC) in patients with the BRAF V600E mutation (in combination with trametinib). Locally advanced or metastatic anaplastic thyroid cancer in patients with the BRAF V600E mutation and no satisfactory locoregional treatment options (in combination with trametinib). Unresectable or metastatic solid tumors with the BRAF V600E mutation in patients who have progressed following prior treatment and have no satisfactory alternative treatment options (in combination with trametinib). Low-grade glioma with a BRAF V600E mutation in patients who require systemic therapy (in combination with trametinib).

Action

Inhibits kinase, an enzyme that promotes cell proliferation. **Therapeutic Effects:** Decreased spread/progression of melanoma, NSCLC, anaplastic thyroid cancer, low-grade gliomas, and other solid tumors.

Pharmacokinetics

Absorption: Well absorbed (95%) following oral administration.
Distribution: Unknown.
Protein Binding: 99.7%.
Metabolism and Excretion: Mostly metabolized by the CYP2C8 and CYP3A4 isoenzymes; two metabolites (hydroxy-dabrafenib and desmethyl-1-dabrafenib) have antineoplastic activity. Excreted as metabolites in feces (72%) and urine (23%).
Half-life: *Dabrafenib:* 8 hr; *hydroxy-dabrafenib:* 10 hr, *desmethyl-1-dabrafenib:* 21–22 hr.

TIME/ACTION PROFILE (progression-free survival)

ROUTE	ONSET	PEAK	DURATION
PO	within 1 mo	1–2 mo	8 mo

Contraindications/Precautions

Contraindicated in: BRAF wild-type solid tumors (may ↑ proliferation); OB: Pregnancy; Lactation: Lactation.
Use Cautiously in: History of glucose-6-phosphate dehydrogenase (G6PD) deficiency (may cause hemolytic anemia); Diabetes; Moderate or severe hepatic impairment; Moderate or severe renal impairment; Rep: Women of reproductive potential and men with female partners of reproductive potential; Pedi: Safety and effectiveness not established in children <18 yr (as monotherapy) or <1 yr (in combination with trametinib for unresectable or metastatic solid tumors or low-grade gliomas with BRAF V600E mutation).

Adverse Reactions/Side Effects

CV: HF. **Derm:** alopecia, hyperkeratosis, palmar-plantar erythrodysesthesia, papilloma, cutaneous squamous cell carcinoma, DRUG REACTION WITH EOSINOPHILIA AND SYSTEMIC SYMPTOMS (DRESS), photosensitivity, STEVENS-JOHNSON SYNDROME. **EENT:** iritis, retinal detachment, uveitis. **Endo:** hyperglycemia. **F and E:** hypophosphatemia, hyponatremia. **GI:** constipation, PANCREATITIS. **Hemat:** BLEEDING, hemophagocytic lymphohistiocytosis. **MS:** arthralgia, back pain, myalgia. **Neuro:** headache, fatigue, peripheral neuropathy. **Resp:** cough, nasopharyngitis. **Misc:** fever (including serious febrile reactions), chills, MALIGNANCY.

D

Interactions

Drug-Drug: Strong CYP3A4 inhibitors or **strong CYP2C8 inhibitors**, including **ketoconazole**, **nefazodone**, **clarithromycin**, and **gemfibrozil**, may ↑ levels and ↑ risk of toxicity; avoid concurrent use. **Strong CYP3A4 inducers** or **strong CYP2C8 inducers**, including **carbamazepine**, **phenobarbital**, **phenytoin**, and **rifampin**, may ↓ levels and effectiveness. **Drugs that ↑ gastric pH**, including **antacids**, **H_2-receptor antagonists**, and **proton pump inhibitors**, may ↓ levels and effectiveness. May ↓ effectiveness of other **CYP3A4 substrates** and **CYP2C9 substrates**, including **midazolam**, **warfarin**, **dexamethasone**, and **hormonal contraceptives**.
Drug-Natural Products: St. John's wort ↓ levels and effectiveness; avoid concurrent use.

Route/Dosage

Treatment of Unresectable/Metastatic Melanoma, Metastatic Non-Small Cell Lung Cancer, or Locally Advanced/Metastatic Anaplastic Thyroid Cancer

Capsules

PO (Adults): 150 mg twice daily; continue until disease progression or unacceptable toxicity.

Tablets for Oral Suspension

PO (Adults ≥51 kg): 150 mg twice daily; continue until disease progression or unacceptable toxicity.
PO (Adults 46–50 kg): 130 mg twice daily; continue until disease progression or unacceptable toxicity.
PO (Adults 42–45 kg): 110 mg twice daily; continue until disease progression or unacceptable toxicity.
PO (Adults 38–41 kg): 100 mg twice daily; continue until disease progression or unacceptable toxicity.
PO (Adults 34–37 kg): 90 mg twice daily; continue until disease progression or unacceptable toxicity.
PO (Adults 30–33 kg): 80 mg twice daily; continue until disease progression or unacceptable toxicity.
PO (Adults 26–29 kg): 70 mg twice daily; continue until disease progression or unacceptable toxicity.
PO (Adults 22–25 kg): 60 mg twice daily; continue until disease progression or unacceptable toxicity.
PO (Adults 18–21 kg): 50 mg twice daily; continue until disease progression or unacceptable toxicity.
PO (Adults 14–17 kg): 40 mg twice daily; continue until disease progression or unacceptable toxicity.

PO (Adults 10–13 kg): 30 mg twice daily; continue until disease progression or unacceptable toxicity.
PO (Adults 8–9 kg): 20 mg twice daily; continue until disease progression or unacceptable toxicity.

Adjuvant Treatment of Unresectable/Metastatic Melanoma

Capsules

PO (Adults): 150 mg twice daily; continue until disease recurrence or unacceptable toxicity for up to 1 yr.

Tablets for Oral Suspension

PO (Adults ≥51 kg): 150 mg twice daily continue until disease progression or unacceptable toxicity for up to 1 yr.
PO (Adults 46–50 kg): 130 mg twice daily; continue until disease progression or unacceptable toxicity for up to 1 yr.
PO (Adults 42–45 kg): 110 mg twice daily; continue until disease progression or unacceptable toxicity for up to 1 yr.
PO (Adults 38–41 kg): 100 mg twice daily; continue until disease progression or unacceptable toxicity for up to 1 yr.
PO (Adults 34–37 kg): 90 mg twice daily; continue until disease progression or unacceptable toxicity for up to 1 yr.
PO (Adults 30–33 kg): 80 mg twice daily; continue until disease progression or unacceptable toxicity for up to 1 yr.
PO (Adults 26–29 kg): 70 mg twice daily; continue until disease progression or unacceptable toxicity for up to 1 yr.
PO (Adults 22–25 kg): 60 mg twice daily; continue until disease progression or unacceptable toxicity for up to 1 yr.
PO (Adults 18–21 kg): 50 mg twice daily; continue until disease progression or unacceptable toxicity for up to 1 yr.
PO (Adults 14–17 kg): 40 mg twice daily; continue until disease progression or unacceptable toxicity for up to 1 yr.
PO (Adults 10–13 kg): 30 mg twice daily; continue until disease progression or unacceptable toxicity for up to 1 yr.
PO (Adults 8–9 kg): 20 mg twice daily; continue until disease progression or unacceptable toxicity for up to 1 yr.

Treatment of Unresectable/Metastatic Solid Tumors

Capsules

PO (Adults): 150 mg twice daily; continue until disease progression or unacceptable toxicity.
PO (Children ≥1 yr and ≥51 kg): 150 mg twice daily; continue until disease progression or unacceptable toxicity.
PO (Children ≥1 yr and 38–50 kg): 100 mg twice daily; continue until disease progression or unacceptable toxicity.
PO (Children ≥1 yr and 26–37 kg): 75 mg twice daily; continue until disease progression or unacceptable toxicity.

Tablets for Oral Suspension

PO (Adults and Children ≥1 yr and ≥51 kg): 150 mg twice daily; continue until disease progression or unacceptable toxicity.
PO (Adults and Children ≥1 yr and 46–50 kg): 130 mg twice daily; continue until disease progression or unacceptable toxicity.
PO (Adults and Children ≥1 yr and 42–45 kg): 110 mg twice daily; continue until disease progression or unacceptable toxicity.
PO (Adults and Children ≥1 yr and 38–41 kg): 100 mg twice daily; continue until disease progression or unacceptable toxicity.
PO (Adults and Children ≥1 yr and 34–37 kg): 90 mg twice daily; continue until disease progression or unacceptable toxicity.
PO (Adults and Children ≥1 yr and 30–33 kg): 80 mg twice daily; continue until disease progression or unacceptable toxicity.
PO (Adults and Children ≥1 yr and 26–29 kg): 70 mg twice daily; continue until disease progression or unacceptable toxicity.
PO (Adults and Children ≥1 yr and 22–25 kg): 60 mg twice daily; continue until disease progression or unacceptable toxicity.
PO (Adults and Children ≥1 yr and 18–21 kg): 50 mg twice daily; continue until disease progression or unacceptable toxicity.
PO (Adults and Children ≥1 yr and 14–17 kg): 40 mg twice daily; continue until disease progression or unacceptable toxicity.
PO (Adults and Children ≥1 yr and 10–13 kg): 30 mg twice daily; continue until disease progression or unacceptable toxicity.
PO (Adults and Children ≥1 yr and 8–9 kg): 20 mg twice daily; continue until disease progression or unacceptable toxicity.

Treatment of Low-Grade Glioma

Capsules

PO (Children ≥1 yr and ≥51 kg): 150 mg twice daily; continue until disease progression or unacceptable toxicity.
PO (Children ≥1 yr and 38–50 kg): 100 mg twice daily; continue until disease progression or unacceptable toxicity.
PO (Children ≥1 yr and 26–37 kg): 75 mg twice daily; continue until disease progression or unacceptable toxicity.

Tablets for Oral Suspension

PO (Children ≥1 yr and ≥51 kg): 150 mg twice daily; continue until disease progression or unacceptable toxicity.

PO (Children ≥1 yr and 46–50 kg): 130 mg twice daily; continue until disease progression or unacceptable toxicity.
PO (Children ≥1 yr and 42–45 kg): 110 mg twice daily; continue until disease progression or unacceptable toxicity.
PO (Children ≥1 yr and 38–41 kg): 100 mg twice daily; continue until disease progression or unacceptable toxicity.
PO (Children ≥1 yr and 34–37 kg): 90 mg twice daily; continue until disease progression or unacceptable toxicity.
PO (Children ≥1 yr and 30–33 kg): 80 mg twice daily; continue until disease progression or unacceptable toxicity.
PO (Children ≥1 yr and 26–29 kg): 70 mg twice daily; continue until disease progression or unacceptable toxicity.
PO (Children ≥1 yr and 22–25 kg): 60 mg twice daily; continue until disease progression or unacceptable toxicity.
PO (Children ≥1 yr and 18–21 kg): 50 mg twice daily; continue until disease progression or unacceptable toxicity.
PO (Children ≥1 yr and 14–17 kg): 40 mg twice daily; continue until disease progression or unacceptable toxicity.
PO (Children ≥1 yr and 10–13 kg): 30 mg twice daily; continue until disease progression or unacceptable toxicity.
PO (Children ≥1 yr and 8–9 kg): 20 mg twice daily; continue until disease progression or unacceptable toxicity.

Availability

Capsules: 50 mg, 75 mg. **Tablets for oral suspension:** 10 mg.

NURSING IMPLICATIONS

Assessment

- Perform skin examination at baseline, every 2 mo during therapy, and for 6 mo after completion of therapy. *If intolerable Grade 2–4 skin toxicity occurs,* hold dabrafenib for up to 3 wk. If improved, resume at ↓ dose. If not improved, permanently discontinue dabrafenib.
- Monitor temperature. *If temperature >100.3°F,* hold dabrafenib or dabrafenib and trametinib. Evaluate for signs and symptoms of infection and renal impairment during and following pyrexia. Restart dabrafenib and trametinib when pyrexia resolved for ≥24 hr, either at the same or ↓ dose. Administer antipyretics as secondary prophylaxis when resuming therapy. Administer prednisone 10 mg once daily for ≥5 days for 2nd or subsequent episode of pyrexia if fever does not resolve within 3 days of onset or for pyrexia associated with complications (dehydration, hypotension, renal failure, severe chills/rigors) and with no evidence of active infection.
- Monitor for signs and symptoms of ocular toxicity (blurred or ↓ vision, seeing colored dots or halos, swelling, redness, photophobia, eye pain). May require steroid and mydriatic ophthalmic drops. *If iritis occurs,* administer ocular therapy; do not modify dose. *If severe uveitis or mild to moderate uveitis that does not respond to ocular therapy occurs,* hold and treat as indicated for up to 6 wk. If improved to Grade ≤1, resume at same or ↓ dose. *If Grade ≥2 uveitis persists for >6 wk,* permanently discontinue dabrafenib.
- Monitor left ventricular ejection fraction (LVEF) by ECG or MUGA scan before starting therapy with dabrafenib and trametinib, 1 mo after initiation, and then every 2–3 mo during therapy. *If symptomatic HF occurs with absolute ↓ in LVEF >20% from baseline that is below lower limit of normal (LLN),* hold dabrafenib until improved to LLN and absolute ↓ to ≤10% of baseline; then resume at same dose.
- Assess for bleeding (headache, dizziness, weakness, hemoptysis, hematemesis, red or black tarry stool) during therapy. *If Grade 3 hemorrhagic event occurs,* hold dabrafenib and trametinib for up to 3 wk; if improved, resume at ↓ dose. *If Grade 4 hemorrhagic event occurs,* permanently discontinue dabrafenib and trametinib.

Lab Test Considerations

- Verify negative pregnancy test prior to initiation.
- Confirm presence of BRAF V600E mutation in tumor specimens prior to therapy with dabrafenib, and confirm BRAF V600E or V600K mutation in tumor specimens prior to therapy with dabrafenib and trametinib. Information on FDA-approved tests for the detection of BRAF V600E mutations in ATC, melanoma, and NSCLC is available at https://www.fda.gov/CompanionDiagnostics.
- May cause hyperglycemia, requiring ↑ dose of or initiation of insulin or oral hypoglycemic. Monitor serum glucose in patients with pre-existing diabetes or hyperglycemia.
- May cause hypophosphatemia, ↑ alkaline phosphatase, and hyponatremia.
- Monitor for hemolytic anemia in patients with G6PD deficiency.

Implementation

- **Dose reduction recommendations: Adults:** *If taking 75 mg twice daily,* 1st dose reduction, 50 mg twice daily. Permanently discontinue if unable to tolerate 50 mg twice daily. *If taking 100 mg twice daily,* 1st dose reduction, 75 mg twice daily; 2nd dose reduction, 50 mg twice daily. Permanently discontinue if unable to tolerate 50 mg twice daily. *If taking 150 mg twice daily,* 1st dose reduction, 100 mg twice daily; 2nd dose reduction, 75 mg twice daily; 3rd dose reduction, 50 mg twice daily. Permanently discontinue if unable to tolerate 50 mg twice daily. **Pediatric Patients:** *If 8–9 kg, taking 20 mg twice daily,* 1st dose reduction, 10 mg twice daily. *If 10–13 kg, taking 30 mg twice daily,* 1st dose reduction, 20 mg twice daily; 2nd dose reduction, 10 mg twice daily. *If 14–17 kg, taking 40 mg twice daily,* 1st dose reduction, 30 mg twice daily; 2nd dose reduction, 20 mg twice daily; 3rd dose reduction, 10 mg twice daily. *If 18–21 kg, taking 50 mg twice daily,* 1st dose reduction, 30 mg twice daily; 2nd dose reduction, 20 mg twice daily; 3rd dose reduction, 10 mg twice daily. *If 22–25 kg, taking 60 mg twice daily,* 1st dose reduction, 40 mg twice daily; 2nd dose reduction, 30 mg twice daily; 3rd dose reduction, 20 mg twice daily. *If 26–29 kg, taking 70 mg twice daily,* 1st dose reduction, 50 mg twice daily; 2nd dose reduction, 40 mg twice daily; 3rd dose reduction, 20 mg twice daily. *If 30–33 kg, taking 80 mg twice daily,* 1st dose reduction, 50 mg twice daily; 2nd dose reduction, 40 mg twice daily; 3rd dose reduction, 30 mg twice daily. *If 34–37 kg, taking 90 mg twice daily,* 1st dose reduction, 60 mg twice daily; 2nd dose reduction, 50 mg twice daily; 3rd dose reduction, 30 mg twice daily. *If 38–41 kg, taking 100 mg twice daily,* 1st dose reduction, 70 mg twice daily; 2nd dose reduction, 50 mg twice daily; 3rd dose reduction, 30 mg twice daily. *If 42–45 kg, taking 110 mg twice daily,* 1st dose reduction, 70 mg twice daily; 2nd dose reduction, 60 mg twice daily; 3rd dose reduction, 40 mg twice daily. *If 46–50 kg, taking 130 mg twice daily,* 1st dose reduction, 90 mg twice daily; 2nd dose reduction, 70 mg twice daily; 3rd dose reduction, 40 mg twice daily. *If ≥51 kg, taking 150 mg twice daily,* 1st dose reduction, 100 mg twice daily; 2nd dose reduction, 80 mg twice daily; 3rd dose reduction, 50 mg twice daily.

- **PO:** Administer capsules about 12 hr apart at the same time each day. Administer on empty stomach ≥1 hr before or 2 hr after food. ***DNC:*** Swallow capsules whole; do not open, crush, break, or chew.
- When administered with trametinib, administer once-daily dose of trametinib at same time each day with either morning or evening dose of dabrafenib.
- For tablets for oral suspension, only use dosing cups provided. Administer on an empty stomach ≥1 hr before or 2 hr after food. ***DNC:*** Do not swallow tablets for oral suspension whole; do not open, crush, break, or chew. Breast milk or infant formula may be given on demand if infant is unable to tolerate fasting conditions. Add cool drinking water to markings on cup. For 1–4 tablets, use 5 mL water; for 5–15 tablets, use 10 mL water. Put tablets in cup with water and gently stir until tablets break apart; may take 3 min. Suspension is cloudy white and may contain small pieces. Administer suspension within 30 min of preparing; if >30 min, dispose of suspension. To access medicine residue in cup, add 5 mL of drinking water, stir, and drink the water and residual mixture. If 1–4 tablets were used, rinse and drink once; if 5–15 tablets used, repeat rinse procedure twice.
- For tablets for oral suspension for use with oral syringe or feeding tube, use directions for oral suspension above. If dose is 1–3 tablets, use ≥10 French. If dose is 4–15 tablets, use ≥12 French. Flush feeding tube before administering; then draw up all suspension from dosing cup with syringe and administer according to manufacturer's instructions. If using an oral syringe, place the tip pointing toward the inside of the cheek. Slowly push the plunger until full dose administered. Add 5 mL water to dosing cup and stir to loosen medicine residue. Draw up mixture and administer via feeding tube or orally. Repeat procedure 3 times.

Patient/Family Teaching

- Explain purpose and side effects of medication. Advise patient to read *Patient Information* before starting therapy.
- Take missed dose as soon as remembered unless within 6 hr of next dose; then omit and take regularly scheduled dose. If vomiting occurs after administration, do not take additional dose.
- Inform patient that dabrafenib ↑ risk of developing new cutaneous malignancies and to notify health care provider immediately if new lesions (wart, skin sore, or reddish bump that bleeds or does not heal) or changes in size or color of existing moles or lesions occur.
- Caution patient to use sunscreen and protective clothing to prevent photosensitivity reactions.
- Advise patient to notify health care provider of all Rx or OTC medications, vitamins, or herbal products being taken and to consult with health care provider before taking other medications, especially St. John's wort.
- Advise patient to notify health care provider if fever; ↑ thirst, appetite, or urination; fruity breath; visual changes; eye pain or swelling; ↑ bleeding; skin blisters, sores, or peeling; high fever; flu-like symptoms; enlarged lymph nodes; or HF occur.
- Rep: Advise women of reproductive potential and men (including those who have had vasectomies) with female partners of reproductive potential to use a highly effective nonhormonal contraception during and for ≥2 wk after last dose. Dabrafenib may ↓ effectiveness of hormonal contraceptives. Advise patient to notify health care provider if pregnancy is suspected and to avoid breastfeeding during and for 2 wk after

last dose. Advise patients to seek counseling on fertility and family planning before beginning therapy; may permanently impair fertility in both sexes.

Evaluation/Desired Outcomes

- Decrease in progression of malignant melanoma, NSCLC, anaplastic thyroid cancer, low-grade gliomas, and other solid tumors.

HIGH ALERT

dacarbazine (da-kar-ba-zeen)

Classification

Therapeutic: antineoplastics

Pharmacologic: alkylating agents

Indications

Metastatic malignant melanoma. Hodgkin disease as second-line therapy (in combination with other agents).

Action

Disrupts DNA and RNA synthesis (cell-cycle phase-nonspecific). **Therapeutic Effects:** Death of rapidly growing tissue cells, especially malignant ones.

Pharmacokinetics

Absorption: IV administration results in complete bioavailability.

Distribution: Widely distributed to tissues; probably concentrates in liver; some CNS penetration.

Metabolism and Excretion: 50% metabolized by the liver; 50% excreted unchanged by the kidneys.

Half-life: 5 hr (↑ in renal and hepatic impairment).

TIME/ACTION PROFILE (effects on blood counts)

ROUTE	ONSET	PEAK	DURATION
IV (WBCs)	16–20 days	21–25 days	3–5 days
IV (platelets)	unknown	16 days	3–5 days

Contraindications/Precautions

Contraindicated in: Hypersensitivity; OB: Pregnancy; Lactation: Lactation.

Use Cautiously in: Active infection; Bone marrow depression; Renal impairment; Hepatic impairment; Pedi: Safety and effectiveness not established in children.

Adverse Reactions/Side Effects

Derm: alopecia, facial flushing, photosensitivity, rash. **Endo:** gonadal suppression. **GI:** anorexia, nausea, vomiting, diarrhea, HEPATIC NECROSIS, hepatic vein thrombosis. **Hemat:** anemia, leukopenia, thrombocytopenia. **Local:** pain at IV site, phlebitis at IV site, tissue necrosis. **MS:** myalgia. **Neuro:** facial paresthesia, malaise. **Misc:** ANAPHYLAXIS, fever, flu-like syndrome.

Interactions

Drug-Drug: Additive bone marrow depression with other **antineoplastics**. **Carbamazepine**, **phenobarbital**, and **rifampin** may ↓ levels and effectiveness. **Amiodarone**, **ciprofloxacin**, **fluvoxamine**, **ketoconazole**, **ofloxacin**, **isoniazid**, or **miconazole** may ↑ levels and risk of toxicity. May ↓ antibody response to **live-virus vaccines** and ↑ risk of adverse reactions.

Route/Dosage

Malignant Melanoma

IV (Adults): 2–4.5 mg/kg/day for 10 days administered every 4 wk *or* 250 mg/m²/day for 5 days administered every 3 wk.

Hodgkin Disease

IV (Adults): 150 mg/m²/day for 5 days (in combination with other agents) administered every 4 wk *or* 375 mg/m² (in combination with other agents) administered every 15 days.

Availability (generic available)

Powder for injection: 100 mg/vial, 200 mg/vial.

NURSING IMPLICATIONS

Assessment

- Monitor vital signs prior to and frequently during therapy.
- Monitor for bone marrow suppression. Assess for bleeding (bleeding gums; bruising; petechiae; guaiac stools, urine, and emesis), and avoid IM injections and rectal temperatures if platelet count is low. Apply pressure to venipuncture sites for 10 min. Assess for signs of infection during neutropenia. Anemia may occur. Monitor for ↑ fatigue, dyspnea, and orthostatic hypotension.
- Monitor intake and output, appetite, and nutritional intake. Assess for nausea and vomiting, which may be severe and last 1–12 hr. Administering an antiemetic prior to and periodically during therapy, restricting oral intake for 4–6 hr before administration, and adjusting diet as tolerated may help maintain fluid and electrolyte balance and nutritional status. Nausea usually ↓ on subsequent doses.

Lab Test Considerations

- Monitor CBC with differential prior to and periodically throughout therapy. The nadir of thrombocytopenia occurs in 16 days. The nadir of leukopenia occurs in 3–4 wk. Recovery begins in 5 days. Withhold dose and notify physician if platelet count <100,000/mm³ or WBC count <4000/mm³.
- Monitor for ↑ AST, ALT, BUN, and serum creatinine. May cause hepatic necrosis.

Implementation

- ***High Alert:*** Fatalities have occurred with chemotherapeutic agents. Before administering, clarify all ambiguous orders; double-check single, daily, and course-of-therapy dose limits; have second practitioner independently double-check original order, calculations, and infusion pump settings.
- ***High Alert:*** Administer under supervision of a physician experienced in use of cancer chemotherapeutic agents.

IV Administration

- Wear gloves, gown, and mask while handling medication. Discard equipment in designated containers. Dacarbazine is an irritant. If extravasation occurs, immediately stop infusion. Leave needle/cannula in place temporarily but do not flush the line. Gently aspirate extravasated solution; then remove needle/cannula. Elevate patient's extremity and apply dry cold compresses for 20 min 4 times day for 1–2 days.
- **Intermittent Infusion: Reconstitution:** Reconstitute each 100 mg and 200 mg vial with 9.9 mL and 19.7 mL, respectively, of sterile water for injection. Solution is colorless or clear yellow. Do not use solution that has turned pink. Solution is stable for 8 hr at room temperature and for 72 hr if refrigerated. **Concentration:** 10 mg/mL. **Dilution:** Further dilute reconstituted solution with 250 mL of D5W or 0.9% NaCl. Stable for 24 hr if refrigerated or 8 hr at room temperature. **Rate:** Administer over 15–60 min.
- **Y-Site Compatibility:** alemtuzumab, aminocaproic acid, aminophylline, amiodarone, anidulafungin, argatroban, atracurium, azithromycin, aztreonam, bivalirudin, bleomycin, bumetanide, buprenorphine, busulfan, butorphanol, calcium chloride, calcium gluconate, carboplatin, carmustine, caspofungin, cefotetan, cefoxitin, ceftazidime, cefuroxime, chlorpromazine, cisatracurium, cisplatin, clindamycin, cyclophosphamide, cyclosporine, cytarabine, dactinomycin, daptomycin, daunorubicin, dexmedetomidine, dexrazoxane, digoxin, diltiazem, diphenhydramine, docetaxel, doxorubicin hydrochloride, doxorubicin liposomal, doxycycline, droperidol, enalaprilat, ephedrine, epirubicin, ertapenem, erythromycin, esmolol, etoposide, etoposide phosphate, famotidine, fentanyl, filgrastim, fluconazole, fludarabine, fluorouracil, foscarnet, fosphenytoin, gemcitabine, gemtuzumab ozogamicin, glycopyrrolate, granisetron, haloperidol, hydralazine, hydromorphone, idarubicin, ifosfamide, insulin, regular, irinotecan, isoproterenol, labetalol, leucovorin, levofloxacin, lidocaine, linezolid, lorazepam, magnesium sulfate, mannitol, melphalan, meperidine, methadone, metoclopramide, metoprolol, metronidazole, midazolam, milrinone, mitoxantrone, morphine, moxifloxacin, nalbuphine, naloxone, nicardipine, nitroglycerin, nitroprusside, octreotide, ondansetron, oxaliplatin, paclitaxel, palonosetron, pamidronate, pentamidine, pentobarbital, phenobarbital, phentolamine, phenylephrine, potassium acetate, potassium chloride, potassium phosphates, procainamide, prochlorperazine, promethazine, propranolol, remifentanil, rocuronium, sargramostim, sodium acetate, sodium bicarbonate, sodium phosphates, succinylcholine, sufentanil, tacrolimus, theophylline, thiotepa, tigecycline, tirofiban, topotecan, vancomycin, vasopressin, vecuronium, verapamil, vinblastine, vincristine, vinorelbine, voriconazole, zidovudine, zoledronic acid.
- **Y-Site Incompatibility:** acyclovir, allopurinol, amikacin, amphotericin B deoxycholate, amphotericin B liposomal, ampicillin, ampicillin/sulbactam, cefazolin, ceftriaxone, cefepime, cefotaxime, chloramphenicol, dantrolene, dexamethasone, diazepam, dobutamine, dopamine, epinephrine, ganciclovir, gentamicin, imipenem/cilastatin, ketorolac, meropenem, mesna, methohexital, methotrexate, methylprednisolone, minocycline, mitomycin, nafcillin, norepinephrine, pantoprazole, pemetrexed, phenytoin, piperacillin/tazobactam, tobramycin, trimethoprim/sulfamethoxazole.

Patient/Family Teaching

- Explain purpose and side effects of medication to patient. Advise patient to read *Patient Information* before starting therapy.
- Advise patient to notify health care provider of all Rx or OTC medications, vitamins, or herbal products being taken and to consult health care provider before taking other medications.
- Instruct patient to notify health care provider if fever; chills; sore throat; signs of infection; bleeding gums; bruising; petechiae; abdominal pain; yellowing of eyes; or blood in urine, stool, or emesis occur. Caution patient to avoid crowds and persons with known infections. Instruct patient to use soft toothbrush and electric razor. Patients should be cautioned not to drink alcoholic beverages or take products containing aspirin or NSAIDs; may increase GI irritation.
- May cause photosensitivity. Instruct patient to avoid sunlight or wear protective clothing and use sunscreen for 2 days after therapy.
- Instruct patient to inform health care provider if flu-like syndrome occurs. Symptoms include fever, myalgia, and general malaise. May occur after several courses of therapy. Usually occurs 1 wk after administration. May persist for 1–3 wk. Acetaminophen may be used for relief of symptoms.
- Discuss with patient the possibility of hair loss. Explore coping strategies.

- Instruct patient not to receive any vaccinations without advice of health care provider.
- Rep: May cause fetal harm. Advise women of reproductive potential to notify health care provider if pregnancy is planned or suspected and to avoid breastfeeding during therapy. Advise patient of the need for a nonhormonal method of contraception.

Evaluation/Desired Outcomes

- Death of rapidly growing tissue cells, especially malignant ones.

dalbavancin (dal-ba-**van**-sin)

Dalvance, ✱ Xydalba

Classification

Therapeutic: anti-infectives

Pharmacologic: lipoglycopeptides

Indications

Acute bacterial skin/skin structure infections due to susceptible bacteria.

Action

Binds to bacterial cell wall resulting in cell death. **Therapeutic Effects:** Bactericidal action against susceptible bacteria with resolution of infection. **Spectrum:** Active against *Staphylococcus aureus* (including methicillin-susceptible and methicillin-resistant strains), *Streptococcus agalactiae*, *Streptococcus dysgalactiae*, *Streptococcus anginosus* (including *S. anginosus*, *S. intermedius*, and *S. constellatus*), *Streptococcus pyogenes*, and *Enterococcus faecalis* (only isolates susceptible to vancomycin).

Pharmacokinetics

Absorption: IV administration results in complete bioavailability.

Distribution: Penetrates tissues and fluids.

Metabolism and Excretion: 33% eliminated unchanged in urine; 12% eliminated as inactive metabolite; 20% excreted in feces.

Half-life: 346 hr.

TIME/ACTION PROFILE (plasma concentrations)

ROUTE	ONSET	PEAK	DURATION
IV	unknown	end of infusion	1 wk

Contraindications/Precautions

Contraindicated in: Hypersensitivity.

Use Cautiously in: Renal impairment (dose adjustment required for adults with CCr <30 mL/min and not receiving hemodialysis); Moderate to severe hepatic impairment; OB: Safety not established in pregnancy; Lactation: Safety not established in breastfeeding; Geri: Consider age-related ↓ in renal function in older adults.

Adverse Reactions/Side Effects

Derm: pruritus, rash. **GI:** ↑ liver enzymes, CLOSTRIDIOIDES DIFFICILE-ASSOCIATED DIARRHEA (CDAD), nausea. **Neuro:** headache. **Misc:** HYPERSENSITIVITY REACTIONS (INCLUDING ANAPHYLAXIS), infusion reactions (including infusion-related reaction resembling vancomycin flushing syndrome).

Interactions

Drug-Drug: None reported.

Route/Dosage

IV (Adults): 1500 mg as a single dose *or* 1000 mg followed 1 wk later by 500 mg.

IV (Children 6–<18 yr): *CCr >30 mL/min/1.73 m^2:* 18 mg/kg (max dose = 1500 mg) as a single dose.

IV (Children Birth–<6 yr): *CCr ≥30 mL/min/1.73 m^2:* 22.5 mg/kg (max dose = 1500 mg) as a single dose.

Renal Impairment

IV (Adults): *CCr <30 mL/min (with no hemodialysis):* 1125 mg as a single dose *or* 750 mg followed 1 wk later by 375 mg.

Availability

Lyophilized powder for injection: 500 mg/vial.

NURSING IMPLICATIONS

Assessment

- Assess for infection (vital signs; appearance of wound, sputum, urine, and stool; WBC) at beginning of and during therapy.
- Obtain specimens for culture and sensitivity prior to therapy. First dose may be given before receiving results.
- Monitor bowel function. Diarrhea, abdominal cramping, fever, and bloody stools should be reported to health care professional promptly as a sign of CDAD. May begin up to 2 mo following cessation of therapy.
- Monitor for infusion reactions (infusion-related reaction resembling vancomycin flushing syndrome: flushing of upper body, urticaria, pruritus, rash, back pain). May resolve with stopping or slowing infusion.

Lab Test Considerations

- Monitor hepatic function. May ↑ ALT, AST, and bilirubin.

Implementation

IV Administration

- **Intermittent Infusion: Reconstitution:** Reconstitute each vial with 25 mL of sterile water or D5W. Alternate gentle swirling and inverting to avoid foaming until completely dissolved. Do not shake.

Reconstituted vial contains a clear colorless to yellow solution. Do not administer solutions that are discolored or contain particulate matter. **Dilution:** Transfer reconstituted solution into D5W. Discard unused solution. May be refrigerated or kept at room temperature; do not freeze. Infuse within 48 hr of reconstitution. Do not administer solutions containing particulate matter. **Concentration:** 1–5 mg/mL. **Rate:** Infuse over 30 min. Flush line before and after infusion with D5W; saline solutions may cause precipitation.

- **Y-Site Incompatibility:** Do not administer other drugs through same IV line.

Patient/Family Teaching

- Explain purpose and side effects of medication to patient. Advise patient to read *Patient Information* before starting therapy.
- Advise patient to notify health care professional of all Rx or OTC medications, vitamins, or herbal products being taken and to consult with health care professional before taking other medications.
- Instruct patient to notify health care professional if signs and symptoms of hypersensitivity reactions (rash, hives, dyspnea, facial swelling) occur.
- Instruct patient to notify health care professional immediately if diarrhea, abdominal cramping, fever, or bloody stools occur and not to treat with antidiarrheals without consulting health care professionals.
- Instruct the patient to notify health care professional if symptoms do not improve.
- Rep: Advise women of reproductive potential to notify health care professional if pregnancy is planned or suspected or if breastfeeding.

Evaluation/Desired Outcomes

- Bactericidal action against susceptible bacteria with resolution of infection.

dalfampridine

(dal-**fam**-pri-deen)

Ampyra, ✱ Fampyra

Classification

Therapeutic: anti-multiple sclerosis agents

Pharmacologic: potassium channel blockers

Indications

To improve walking speed in patients with multiple sclerosis.

Action

Acts as a potassium channel blocker, which may increase conduction of action potentials.

Therapeutic Effects: Increased walking speed in patients with multiple sclerosis.

Pharmacokinetics

Absorption: Rapidly and completely absorbed.

Distribution: Unknown.

Metabolism and Excretion: 96% eliminated in urine; 0.5% in feces.

Half-life: 5.2–6.5 hr.

TIME/ACTION PROFILE (improvement in walking speed)

ROUTE	ONSET	PEAK	DURATION
PO	unknown	3–4 hr	24 hr

Contraindications/Precautions

Contraindicated in: Hypersensitivity; History of seizures; Moderate to severe renal impairment (CCr ≤50 mL/min) (↑ risk of seizures).

Use Cautiously in: Mild renal impairment (CCr 51–80 mL/min) (↑ risk of seizures); OB: Safety not established in pregnancy; Lactation: Safety not established in breastfeeding; Pedi: Safety and effectiveness not established in children; Geri: Consider age-related ↓ in renal function in older adults.

Adverse Reactions/Side Effects

EENT: nasopharyngitis, pharyngolaryngeal pain. **GI:** constipation, dyspepsia, nausea. **GU:** urinary tract infection. **MS:** back pain. **Neuro:** dizziness, headache, insomnia, multiple sclerosis relapse, paresthesia, SEIZURES, vertigo, weakness. **Misc:** ANAPHYLAXIS.

Interactions

Drug-Drug: Cimetidine may ↑ levels and ↑ risk of seizures.

Route/Dosage

PO (Adults): 10 mg twice daily.

Availability (generic available)

Extended-release tablets: 10 mg.

NURSING IMPLICATIONS

Assessment

- Assess walking speed in patients with multiple sclerosis before starting and periodically during therapy.
- Monitor for seizures during therapy; risk ↑ with ↑ dose. May occur without seizure history and within days to wks of initiation. *If seizure occurs, discontinue therapy.*
- Monitor for signs and symptoms of anaphylaxis (dyspnea, wheezing, urticaria, angioedema, hoarseness) during therapy; discontinuation and supportive care may be required.

Lab Test Considerations

- Monitor CCr before starting and at least yearly during therapy; renal impairment may require dose ↓ or discontinuation.

Implementation

- Administer tablets twice daily approximately 12 hr apart without regard to food. ***DNC:*** Swallow tablets whole; do not break, crush, chew, or dissolve.

Patient/Family Teaching

- Explain the purpose and side effects of dalfampridine to patient. Instruct patient to take as directed, with approximately 12 hr between tablets. If a dose is missed, omit and take next scheduled dose on time; do not double doses or take >two tablets within 24 hr. May ↑ risk of seizures. Advise patient to read *Medication Guide* before beginning therapy and with each Rx refill in case of changes.
- May cause vertigo, dizziness, and seizures. Caution patient to avoid driving and other activities requiring alertness until response to the drug is known.
- Instruct patient to notify health care professional or call 911 immediately to seek medical care if swelling of face, eyes, lips, or tongue or if difficulty swallowing or breathing occur. Do not restart medication without further evaluation.
- If a seizure occurs, advise patient to notify health care professional immediately, to discontinue dalfampridine, and to not restart medication.
- Advise patient to notify health care professional of all Rx or OTC medications, vitamins, or herbal products being taken and to consult with health care professional before taking other medications.
- Rep: Advise women of reproductive potential to notify health care professional if pregnancy is planned or suspected or if breastfeeding.

Evaluation/Desired Outcomes

- Improved walking and increased walking speed in patients with multiple sclerosis.

dalteparin, See HEPARINS (LOW MOLECULAR WEIGHT).

BEERS

dapagliflozin (dap-a-gli-**floe**-zin)

Farxiga, 🍁 Forxiga

Classification

Therapeutic: antidiabetics

Pharmacologic: sodium-glucose co-transporter 2 (SGLT2) inhibitors

Indications

Type 2 diabetes mellitus (as adjunct to diet and exercise). To reduce the risk of hospitalization for HF in patients with type 2 diabetes mellitus and established cardiovascular disease or multiple cardiovascular risk factors. To reduce the risk of cardiovascular death, hospitalization for HF, and urgent visits for HF in patients with HF. To reduce the risk of sustained eGFR decline, end-stage kidney disease, cardiovascular death, and hospitalization for HF in patients with chronic kidney disease at risk of progression.

Action

Inhibits proximal renal tubular sodium-glucose cotransporter 2 (SGLT2), which determines reabsorption of glucose from the tubular lumen. Inhibits reabsorption of glucose, lowers renal threshold for glucose, and increases excretion of glucose in urine. **Therapeutic Effects:** Improved glycemic control. Reduction in risk of HF hospitalizations in patients with type 2 diabetes mellitus. Reduction in risk of cardiovascular death, HF hospitalizations, and urgent visits for HF in patients with HF. Reduction in risk of sustained eGFR decline, end-stage kidney disease, cardiovascular death, and HF hospitalizations in patients with chronic kidney disease at risk of progression.

Pharmacokinetics

Absorption: 78% absorbed following oral administration.

Distribution: Unknown.

Metabolism and Excretion: Extensively metabolized by UGT1A9 to inactive metabolites, which are primarily excreted in urine. 15% excreted in feces as unchanged drug.

Half-life: 12.9 hr.

TIME/ACTION PROFILE (↓ in A1c)

ROUTE	ONSET	PEAK	DURATION
PO	within 4 wk	12 wk	unknown

Contraindications/Precautions

Contraindicated in: Hypersensitivity; Moderate renal impairment (eGFR <45 mL/min/1.73 m^2) (use not recommended to improve glycemic control in patients with type 2 diabetes mellitus); Dialysis; Type 1 diabetes; Diabetic ketoacidosis; Active bladder cancer; OB: Not recommended for use during 2nd and 3rd trimesters of pregnancy (may cause adverse renal effects in infant); Lactation: Lactation.

Use Cautiously in: History of pancreatitis, pancreatic surgery, reduced caloric intake due to illness or surgery, or alcohol abuse (↑ risk of ketoacidosis); Renal impairment (eGFR <60 mL/min/1.73 m^2), age >65 yr, or concurrent use of loop diuretics (↑ risk of hypovolemia and hypotension); History of bladder cancer; Polycystic kidney disease or recent history of immunosuppressive therapy for kidney disease (use not recommended for treatment of chronic kidney disease); OB: Use during 1st trimester of pregnancy only if potential maternal benefit justifies potential fetal risk (other agents recommended in pregnancy); Pedi: Safety and effectiveness not established in children <10 yr (type 2 diabetes) or <18 yr (all other indications); Geri: Appears on Beers list. Older adults may have ↑ risk of urogenital infections (especially women in the 1st mo of treatment) and euglycemic diabetic ketoacidosis. Use with caution in older adults.

Adverse Reactions/Side Effects

Endo: hypoglycemia (↑ with other medications).
F and E: hyperphosphatemia, hypovolemia, KETOACIDOSIS.
GU: ↑ urination, acute kidney injury, genital mycotic infections, NECROTIZING FASCIITIS OF PERINEUM (FOURNIER GANGRENE), renal impairment, urinary tract infection (including pyelonephritis), UROSEPSIS. **Misc:** HYPERSENSITIVITY REACTIONS (INCLUDING ANAPHYLAXIS OR ANGIOEDEMA).

Interactions

Drug-Drug: ↑ risk of hypoglycemia with **insulin** or **insulin secretagogues**; dose adjustments may be required. **Loop diuretics** may ↑ risk of hypovolemia and associated complications. May ↓ levels and effectiveness of **lithium**.

Route/Dosage

Type 2 Diabetes Mellitus (for Glycemic Control)

PO (Adults and Children ≥10 yr): 5 mg once daily; may ↑ to 10 mg once daily, if needed.

Renal Impairment

PO (Adults and Children ≥10 yr): *eGFR <45 mL/min/1.73 m^2:* Use not recommended.

Type 2 Diabetes (for Reduction in Risk of HF Hospitalizations), HF, or Chronic Kidney Disease

PO (Adults): 10 mg once daily.

Renal Impairment

PO (Adults): *eGFR <25 mL/min/1.73 m^2:* Initiation of therapy not recommended; however, patients currently taking dapagliflozin may continue with 10 mg once daily.

Availability (generic available)

Tablets: 5 mg, 10 mg. ***In combination with:*** metformin XR (Xigduo XR); saxagliptin (generic only). See Appendix N.

NURSING IMPLICATIONS

Assessment

- Observe for signs and symptoms of hypoglycemia (sweating, hunger, weakness, dizziness, tremor, tachycardia, anxiety), especially in patients taking insulin or other hypoglycemic agents.
- Assess volume status and correct before starting therapy. Monitor BP at initiation and periodically, as hypotension may occur. Patients with renal impairment (eGFR <60 mL/min/1.73 m^2), older adults, or patients on loop diuretics may be at ↑ risk for volume depletion or hypotension.
- Monitor for signs and symptoms of urinary tract infection (burning during urination, frequent urination, urgency, pain in pelvis, blood in urine, fever, back pain, nausea, vomiting) during therapy. *If urinary tract infection occurs,* treat promptly.
- Monitor for signs and symptoms of necrotizing fasciitis of the perineum (Fournier gangrene: tenderness, redness, or swelling of the genitals or perineum; fever, malaise, perineal skin discoloration or gangrenous appearance; drainage; sores; blisters; foul odor). *If necrotizing fasciitis of the perineum suspected,* permanently discontinue dapagliflozin; start treatment immediately with broad-spectrum antibiotics, and if necessary, perform surgical debridement.

Lab Test Considerations

- Verify negative pregnancy test prior to initiation. Monitor serum glucose and A1c periodically during therapy to evaluate effectiveness of treatment. Evaluate renal function prior to and periodically during therapy; May ↑ serum creatinine.
- May ↑ hematocrit and phosphorous. Monitor for ketoacidosis, especially during prolonged fasting for illness or surgery. Hold therapy for ≥3 days prior to surgery, if possible. Can resume therapy once patient stable and has resumed oral intake.
- Will cause urine to test positive for glucose; consider testing for urine ketones.

Toxicity and Overdose

- Overdose is manifested by symptoms of hypoglycemia. Mild hypoglycemia may be treated with administration of oral glucose. Treat severe hypoglycemia with IV push 50% dextrose in water followed by continuous IV infusion of 10% dextrose in water at a rate sufficient to keep serum glucose at approximately 100 mg/dL.

Implementation

- Do not confuse Farxiga with Fetzima.
- Patients stabilized on a diabetic regimen who are exposed to stress, fever, trauma, infection, or surgery may require administration of insulin.
- **PO:** Administer once daily in the morning without regard to food.

Patient/Family Teaching

- Explain purpose and side effects of dapagliflozin. Instruct patient to take medication at same time each day. Take missed doses as soon as remembered unless almost time for next dose; do not double doses. Advise patient to read *Medication Guide* before starting and with each Rx refill in case of changes.
- Explain to patient that this medication controls hyperglycemia but does not cure diabetes. Therapy is long term. Emphasize the importance of routine follow-up exams.
- Inform patient that dapagliflozin may cause dehydration and hypotension. Maintain adequate

hydration and notify health care provider if dizziness, fainting, weakness, or orthostatic hypotension occurs. Notify health care provider if fluid loss from nausea, vomiting, and diarrhea occurs.

- Advise patient to notify health care provider if signs and symptoms of urinary tract infections or genital mycotic infections (women: vaginal odor, white or yellowish vaginal discharge, vaginal itching; men: rash or redness of glans or foreskin of penis, foul-smelling discharge from penis, pain in skin around penis) occur. Instruct patient on treatment options and when to notify health care provider.
- Review signs of hypoglycemia and hyperglycemia with patient. If hypoglycemia occurs, advise patient to drink a glass of orange juice or ingest 2–3 teaspoons of sugar, honey, or corn syrup dissolved in water or an appropriate number of glucose tablets and notify health care provider.
- Encourage patient to follow prescribed diet, medication, and exercise regimen to prevent hypoglycemic or hyperglycemic episodes.
- Instruct patient in proper testing of serum glucose and ketones, especially during periods of stress or illness. Inform patient that dapagliflozin will cause a positive test result when testing for urine glucose. Notify health care provider if significant changes occur.
- Advise patient to notify health care provider immediately if new pain or tenderness, sores or ulcers, or infections involving the leg or foot occur and to immediately seek care if pain or tenderness, redness, or swelling of the genitals or area from the genitals back to the rectum, along with a temperature >100.4°F or malaise, occur.
- Advise patient to notify health care provider of all Rx or OTC medications, vitamins, or herbal products being taken and to consult with health care provider before taking other medications.
- Advise patient to inform health care provider of dapagliflozin use prior to treatment or surgery.
- Advise patients and family to call 911 and immediately seek treatment for signs and symptoms of hypersensitivity reactions, such as difficulty breathing; chest tightness; hives; rash; feeling light-headed; itching; or swelling of the face, lips, tongue, or throat.
- Advise patient to carry a form of sugar (glucose tablets or gel, sugar packets, candy) and identification describing disease process and medication regimen at all times.
- Rep: May cause fetal harm. Insulin is the recommended method of controlling blood sugar during pregnancy. Advise patient to notify health care provider if pregnancy is planned or suspected and to avoid breastfeeding during therapy. Advise women that dapagliflozin use is not recommended during the 2nd and 3rd trimesters of pregnancy.

Evaluation/Desired Outcomes

- Control of blood glucose levels without the appearance of hypoglycemic or hyperglycemic episodes.
- Reduction in risk of HF hospitalizations.
- Reduction in risk of sustained eGFR decline, end-stage kidney disease, cardiovascular death, and HF hospitalizations in patients with chronic kidney disease at risk of progression.

D

DAPTOmycin (dap-to-**mye**-sin)

~~Cubicin, Cubicin RF~~

Classification

Therapeutic: anti-infectives

Pharmacologic: cyclic lipopeptide antibacterial agents

Indications

Complicated skin and skin structure infections caused by gram-positive bacteria. *Staphylococcus aureus* bacteremia, including right-sided infective endocarditis caused by methicillin-susceptible and methicillin-resistant strains (in adults). *Staphylococcus aureus* bacteremia (in pediatric patients).

Action

Causes rapid depolarization of membrane potential following binding to bacterial membrane; this results in inhibition of protein, DNA, and RNA synthesis. **Therapeutic Effects:** Death of bacteria with resolution of infection. **Spectrum:** Active against *Staphylococcus aureus* (including methicillin-resistant strains), *Streptococcus pyogenes*, *Streptococcus agalactiae*, some *Streptococcus dysgalactiae*, and *Enterococcus faecalis* (vancomycin-susceptible strains).

Pharmacokinetics

Absorption: IV administration results in complete bioavailability.
Distribution: Unknown.
Protein Binding: 92%.
Metabolism and Excretion: Metabolism not known; mostly excreted by kidneys.
Half-life: 8.1 hr.

TIME/ACTION PROFILE

ROUTE	ONSET	PEAK	DURATION
IV	rapid	end of infusion	24 hr

Contraindications/Precautions

Contraindicated in: Hypersensitivity.
Use Cautiously in: Severe renal impairment (↓ dose); Moderate to severe renal impairment (may have ↓ clinical response); OB: Safety not established in pregnancy; Lactation: Safety not established in breastfeeding; Pedi: Children <1 yr (↑ risk of muscular, neuromuscular, and

CNS effects; avoid use); Geri: Older adults may have ↓ clinical response with ↑ risk of adverse reactions.

Adverse Reactions/Side Effects

CV: hypertension, hypotension. **Derm:** DRUG RASH WITH EOSINOPHILIA AND SYSTEMIC SYMPTOMS (DRESS), pruritus, rash. **GI:** ↑ liver enzymes, CLOSTRIDIOIDES DIFFICILE-ASSOCIATED DIARRHEA (CDAD), constipation, diarrhea, nausea, vomiting. **GU:** renal impairment. **Hemat:** anemia. **Local:** injection site reactions. **MS:** ↑ CK. **Neuro:** dizziness. **Resp:** dyspnea, EOSINOPHILIC PNEUMONIA. **Misc:** ANGIOEDEMA, fever.

Interactions

Drug-Drug: Tobramycin may ↑ levels and risk of toxicity. **HMG-CoA reductase inhibitors** may ↑ risk of myopathy; consider discontinuing statin before starting daptomycin; if used with statin, closely monitor CK levels.

Route/Dosage

Complicated Skin/Skin Structure Infections

IV (Adults): 4 mg/kg every 24 hr for 7–14 days.
IV (Children 12–17 yr): 5 mg/kg every 24 hr for up to 14 days.
IV (Children 7–11 yr): 7 mg/kg every 24 hr for up to 14 days.
IV (Children 2–6 yr): 9 mg/kg every 24 hr for up to 14 days.
IV (Children 1–<2 yr): 10 mg/kg every 24 hr for up to 14 days.

Renal Impairment

IV (Adults): *CCr <30 mL/min:* 4 mg/kg every 48 hr for 7–14 days; *Hemodialysis and CAPD:* 4 mg/kg every 48 hr for 7–14 days, with dose administered after hemodialysis on hemodialysis days.

Staphylococcus aureus Bacteremia/Right-Sided Infective Endocarditis

IV (Adults): 6 mg/kg every 24 hr for 2–6 wk.

Renal Impairment

IV (Adults): *CCr <30 mL/min:* 6 mg/kg every 48 hr for 2–6 wk; *Hemodialysis and CAPD:* 6 mg/kg every 48 hr for 2–6 wk, with dose administered after hemodialysis on hemodialysis days.

Staphylococcus aureus Bacteremia

IV (Children 12–17 yr): 7 mg/kg every 24 hr for up to 42 days.
IV (Children 7–11 yr): 9 mg/kg every 24 hr for up to 42 days.
IV (Children 1–6 yr): 12 mg/kg every 24 hr for up to 42 days.

Availability (generic available)

Lyophilized powder for injection: 350 mg/vial, 500 mg/vial. **Premixed infusion:** 350 mg/50 mL 0.9% NaCl, 500 mg/50 mL 0.9% NaCl, 700 mg/100 mL 0.9% NaCl, 1000 mg/100 mL 0.9% NaCl.

NURSING IMPLICATIONS

Assessment

- Assess for infection (vital signs; appearance of wound, sputum, urine, and stool; WBC) at beginning of and during therapy.
- Monitor bowel function. Diarrhea, abdominal cramping, fever, and bloody stools should be reported to health care professional promptly as a sign of CDAD. May begin up to several wk following cessation of therapy.
- Monitor for signs and symptoms of eosinophilic pneumonia (new onset or worsening fever, dyspnea, difficulty breathing, new infiltrates on chest imaging studies). Discontinue daptomycin if symptoms occur.
- Monitor for signs and symptoms of DRESS (fever, rash, lymphadenopathy, facial swelling), associated with involvement of other organ systems (hepatitis, nephritis, hematologic abnormalities, myocarditis, myositis) during therapy. May resemble an acute viral infection. Eosinophilia is often present. Discontinue therapy if signs occur.
- Monitor for development of muscle pain or weakness, particularly of distal extremities. Discontinue daptomycin in patients with unexplained signs and symptoms of myopathy in conjunction with CK >1000 units/L, or in patients without reported symptoms who have marked elevations in CK >2000 units/L. Consider temporarily suspending agents associated with rhabdomyolysis (HMG-CoA reductase inhibitors) in patients receiving daptomycin.
- Monitor for signs and symptoms of peripheral neuropathy during use.

Lab Test Considerations

- Monitor CK weekly, more frequently in patients with unexplained ↑. Discontinue daptomycin if CK >1000 units/L and signs and symptoms of myopathy occur. In patients with renal impairment, monitor both renal function and CK more frequently.
- May cause false ↑ PT and INR.
- Monitor renal function before and periodically during therapy. If new or worsening renal impairment occurs, evaluate renal function. If tubulointerstitial nephritis is suspected, discontinue daptomycin and begin treatment.

Implementation

- Do not confuse daptomycin with dactinomycin.

IV Administration

- **IV Push: Reconstitution:** Reconstitute 500-mg vial with 10 mL of 0.9% NaCl inserted toward wall of vial. Rotate vial gently to wet powder. Allow to stand for 10 min undisturbed. Swirl vial gently to completely reconstitute solution. Reconstituted vials are stable for 12 hr at room temperature or 48 hr if refrigerated. **Concentration:** 50 mg/mL. **Rate:** Administer over 2 min (for adults only).

- **Intermittent Infusion:** *Adults and children ≥7 yr:* **Dilution:** Dilute contents of reconstituted vial in 50 mL of 0.9% NaCl. Solution is stable for 12 hr at room temperature or 48 hr if refrigerated. Do not administer solutions that are cloudy or contain a precipitate. **Rate:** Infuse over 30 min.
- **Intermittent Infusion:** *Children 1–6 yr:* **Dilution:** Dilute contents of reconstituted vial in 25 mL of 0.9% NaCl. **Rate:** Infuse over 60 min.
- **Y-Site Compatibility:** amikacin, aminocaproic acid, aminophylline, amiodarone, amphotericin B liposomal, ampicillin, ampicillin/sulbactam, argatroban, arsenic trioxide, atracurium, azithromycin, aztreonam, bivalirudin, bleomycin, bumetanide, buprenorphine, busulfan, butorphanol, calcium chloride, calcium gluconate, cangrelor, carboplatin, carmustine, caspofungin, cefazolin, cefepime, cefotaxime, cefotetan, cefoxitin, ceftazidime, ceftazidime/avibactam, ceftolozane/tazobactam, ceftriaxone, cefuroxime, chloramphenicol, chlorpromazine, ciprofloxacin, cisatracurium, cisplatin, clindamycin, cyclophosphamide, cyclosporine, dacarbazine, dactinomycin, daunorubicin, dexamethasone, dexmedetomidine, dexrazoxane, digoxin, diltiazem, diphenhydramine, dobutamine, docetaxel, dopamine, doxorubicin hydrochloride, doxorubicin liposomal, doxycycline, droperidol, enalaprilat, ephedrine, epinephrine, epirubicin, eptifibatide, ertapenem, erythromycin, esmolol, etoposide, etoposide phosphate, famotidine, fentanyl, fluconazole, fludarabine, fluorouracil, foscarnet, fosphenytoin, furosemide, ganciclovir, gentamicin, glycopyrrolate, granisetron, haloperidol, heparin, hydralazine, hydrocortisone, hydromorphone, idarubicin, ifosfamide, insulin, regular, irinotecan, isavuconazonium, isoproterenol, ketorolac, labetalol, letermovir, leucovorin calcium, levofloxacin, lidocaine, linezolid, lorazepam, magnesium sulfate, mannitol, melphalan, meperidine, meropenem, mesna, methadone, methylprednisolone, metoclopramide, metoprolol, midazolam, milrinone, mitoxantrone, morphine, moxifloxacin, mycophenolate, nafcillin, nalbuphine, naloxone, nicardipine, nitroprusside, norepinephrine, octreotide, ondansetron, oxaliplatin, oxytocin, paclitaxel, palonosetron, pamidronate, pemetrexed, pentamidine, phenobarbital, phentolamine, phenylephrine, piperacillin/tazobactam, posaconazole, potassium acetate, potassium chloride, potassium phosphate, procainamide, prochlorperazine, promethazine, propranolol, rifampin, rocuronium, sodium acetate, sodium bicarbonate, sodium phosphate, succinylcholine, sufentanil, tacrolimus, tedizolid, theophylline, thiotepa, tigecycline, tirofiban, tobramycin, topotecan, trimethoprim/sulfamethoxazole, vasopressin, vecuronium, verapamil, vinblastine, vincristine, vinorelbine, voriconazole, zidovudine, zoledronic acid.
- **Y-Site Incompatibility:** acyclovir, alemtuzumab, allopurinol, blinatumomab, cytarabine, D5W, dantrolene, gemcitabine, gemtuzumab ozogamicin, imipenem/cilastatin, meropenem/vaborbactam, methotrexate, metronidazole, minocycline, mitomycin, nitroglycerin, pantoprazole, pentobarbital, phenytoin, plazomicin, remifentanil, sufentanil, sulbactam/durlobactam, vancomycin.

D

Patient/Family Teaching

- Explain the purpose and side effects of daptomycin. Advise patient to read *Medication Guide* before starting and periodically during therapy in case of changes.
- Instruct patient to notify health care professional if fever and diarrhea develop, especially if stool contains blood, pus, or mucus. Advise patient not to treat diarrhea without consulting health care professional.
- May cause dizziness. Caution patient to avoid driving or other activities requiring alertness until response to medication is known.
- Advise patient to notify health care professional immediately if weakness, numbness, or tingling in forearms and lower legs or signs and symptoms of eosinophilic pneumonia or DRESS occur.
- Advise patient to notify health care professional of all Rx or OTC medications, vitamins, or herbal products being taken and to consult with health care professional before taking other medications. Instruct patient to avoid using HMG-CoA reductase inhibitors (cholesterol-lowering agents such as atorvastatin, fluvastatin, lovastatin, pitavastatin, simvastatin) unless approved by health care professional, as concurrent use with daptomycin may ↑ risk of myopathy.
- Rep: Advise women of reproductive potential to notify health care professional if pregnancy is planned or suspected or if breastfeeding. Monitor breastfed infants exposed to daptomycin for GI disturbances.

Evaluation/Desired Outcomes

- Resolution of the signs and symptoms of infection. Length of time for complete resolution depends on the organism and site of infection.

HIGH ALERT

daratumumab

(dar-a-**toom**-ue-mab)

Darzalex

Classification

Therapeutic: antineoplastics

Pharmacologic: monoclonal antibodies

Indications

Multiple myeloma in patients whose disease has relapsed or is refractory despite receiving ≥1 prior therapy (in combination with lenalidomide and dexamethasone). Multiple myeloma in patients who have received ≥1 prior therapy (in combination with bortezomib and dexamethasone). Multiple myeloma in patients whose disease has relapsed or is refractory despite receiving 1–3 previous drug therapies (in combination daratumumab and dexamethasone). Multiple myeloma in patients who received ≥2 lines of therapy including lenalidomide and a proteasome inhibitor (in combination with pomalidomide and dexamethasone). Multiple myeloma in patients who have received ≥3 prior lines of therapy including a proteasome inhibitor and an immunomodulatory agent or who are double-refractory to a proteasome inhibitor and an immunomodulatory agent. Newly diagnosed multiple myeloma in patients who are ineligible for autologous stem cell transplant (in combination with bortezomib, melphalan, and prednisone). Newly diagnosed multiple myeloma in patients who are ineligible for autologous stem cell transplant (in combination with lenalidomide and dexamethasone). Newly diagnosed multiple myeloma in patients who are eligible for autologous stem cell transplant (in combination with bortezomib, thalidomide, and dexamethasone).

Action

Binds to CD38 on tumor cells causing apoptosis, thereby inhibiting growth of CD38-expressing tumor cells. **Therapeutic Effects:** Improved survival and decreased progression of multiple myeloma.

Pharmacokinetics

Absorption: IV administration results in complete bioavailability.

Distribution: Monoclonal antibodies cross the placenta.

Metabolism and Excretion: Unknown.

Half-life: 18 days (as monotherapy); 23 days (when used as combination therapy).

TIME/ACTION PROFILE (plasma concentrations)

ROUTE	ONSET	PEAK	DURATION
IV	unknown	end of infusion	unknown

Contraindications/Precautions

Contraindicated in: Severe hypersensitivity; OB: Pregnancy; Lactation: Lactation.

Use Cautiously in: Chronic obstructive pulmonary disease; Rep: Women of reproductive potential; Pedi: Safety and effectiveness not established in children.

Adverse Reactions/Side Effects

CV: hypertension, peripheral edema. **EENT:** nasal congestion. **GI:** diarrhea, nausea, vomiting. **Hemat:** anemia, lymphopenia, neutropenia, thrombocytopenia. **Metab:** ↓ appetite. **MS:** arthralgia, muscle spasms, pain. **Neuro:** headache, peripheral neuropathy. **Resp:** cough, dyspnea. **Misc:** fatigue, fever, INFUSION REACTIONS (INCLUDING ANAPHYLAXIS).

Interactions

Drug-Drug: None reported.

Route/Dosage

During Week 1 ONLY, the 16 mg/kg dose may administered in one dose or may be split into two doses (8 mg/kg) administered over 2 days (Days 1 and 2).

Combination Therapy with Bortezomib, Melphalan, and Prednisone

IV (Adults): 16 mg/kg every wk starting at Week 1 through Week 6 (total of 6 doses), then 16 mg/kg every 3 wk starting at Week 7 until Week 54 (total of 16 doses), then 16 mg/kg every 4 wk starting at Week 55 and onward; continue until disease progression or unacceptable toxicity.

Monotherapy and Combination Therapy with Lenalidomide or Pomalidomide and Dexamethasone

IV (Adults): 16 mg/kg every wk starting at Week 1 through Week 8 (total of 8 doses), then 16 mg/kg every 2 wk starting at Week 9 until Week 24 (total of 8 doses), then 16 mg/kg every 4 wk starting at Week 25 and onward; continue until disease progression or unacceptable toxicity.

Combination Therapy with Bortezomib and Dexamethasone

IV (Adults): 16 mg/kg every wk starting at Week 1 through Week 9 (total of 9 doses), then 16 mg/kg every 3 wk starting at Week 10 until Week 24 (total of 5 doses), then 16 mg/kg every 4 wk starting at Week 25 and onward; continue until disease progression or unacceptable toxicity.

Combination Therapy with Bortezomib, Thalidomide, and Dexamethasone

IV (Adults): *Induction treatment:* 16 mg/kg every wk starting at Week 1 through Week 8 (total of 8 doses), then 16 mg/kg every 2 wk starting at Week 9 until Week 16 (total of 4 doses), then stop for high-dose chemotherapy and autologous stem cell transplant; *Consolidation treatment (following autologous stem cell treatment):* 16 mg/kg every 2 wk starting at Week 1 through Week 8 (total of 4 doses).

Combination Therapy with Carfilzomib and Dexamethasone

IV (Adults): 8 mg/kg once daily for 2 days (Days 1 and 2 of Week 1), then 16 mg/kg every wk starting at Week 2 through Week 8 (total of 7 doses), then 16 mg/kg every 2 wk starting at Week 9 until Week 24 (total of 8 doses), then 16 mg/kg every 4 wk starting at Week 25 and onward; continue until disease progression or unacceptable toxicity.

Availability

Solution for injection: 20 mg/mL. ***In combination with:*** hyaluronidase (Darzalex Faspro). See Appendix N.

NURSING IMPLICATIONS

Assessment

- Frequently monitor for signs and symptoms of infusion reactions (bronchospasm, hypoxia, dyspnea, hypertension, cough, wheezing, larynx and throat tightness, laryngeal edema, pulmonary edema, nasal congestion, allergic rhinitis, hypotension, headache, rash, urticaria, pruritus, nausea, vomiting, chills) during therapy; occur frequently, usually during or within 4 hr of infusion. Premedicate with antihistamines, antipyretics, and corticosteroids and medicate postinfusion to prevent delayed infusion reactions.
- Monitor for ocular adverse reactions (acute myopia and narrowing of the anterior chamber angle due to ciliochoroidal effusions with potential for increased intraocular pressure, glaucoma). If ocular symptoms occur, interrupt infusion and seek immediate ophthalmologic evaluation prior to restarting therapy.

Lab Test Considerations

- Verify negative pregnancy test before starting therapy.
- Type and screen before starting therapy. Therapy results in a positive indirect antiglobulin test (Coombs' test), which interferes with antibody screening and cross matching for blood transfusions; may persist for up to 6 mo.
- Monitor CBC periodically during therapy. May cause anemia, thrombocytopenia, neutropenia, and lymphopenia. Monitor patient with neutropenia for signs and symptoms of infection. Consider holding daratumumab until neutrophil recovery or recovery of platelets.

Implementation

- Administer by a health care professional with immediate access to emergency equipment and medical support.
- **Monotherapy:** *Preinfusion:* Administer methylprednisolone 100 mg or equivalent intermediate-acting or long-acting corticosteroid plus PO antipyretics (acetaminophen 650–1000 mg) plus PO or IV antihistamine (diphenhydramine 25–50 mg or equivalent) 1–3 hr prior to each infusion. Following second infusion, methylprednisolone dose may be ↓ to 60 mg IV. *Postinfusion:* Following infusion, administer methylprednisolone 20 mg PO or equivalent on 1st and 2nd day after all infusions to ↓ risk of infusion reactions.
- **Combination Therapy:** *Preinfusion:* Administer dexamethasone 20 mg (or equivalent) PO or IV plus PO antipyretics (acetaminophen 650–1000 mg) plus PO or IV antihistamine (diphenhydramine 25–50 mg or equivalent) 1–3 hr prior to each infusion. When dexamethasone is the background regimen-specific corticosteroid, the dexamethasone dose that is part of the background regimen will serve as premedication on days of infusion. Do not administer background regimen-specific corticosteroids (e.g., prednisone) on infusion days when patients have received dexamethasone (or equivalent) as a premedication. *Postinfusion:* Consider administering PO methylprednisolone at a dose ≤20 mg (or an equivalent dose of an intermediate- or long-acting corticosteroid) starting the day after administration of daratumumab infusion. If a background regimen-specific corticosteroid (e.g., dexamethasone, prednisone) is administered the day after the infusion, additional corticosteroids may not be needed.
- For patients with a history of COPD, consider postinfusion short- and long-acting bronchodilators, and inhaled corticosteroids. After first 4 infusions, if no major infusion reactions occurred, may be discontinued.
- Initiate antiviral prophylaxis to prevent herpes zoster reactivation within 1 wk of starting therapy and continue for 3 mo following therapy with daratumumab. May also result in hepatitis B virus (HBV) reactivation.
- If a planned dose is missed, administer as soon as possible and adjust dosing to maintain same treatment interval.

IV Administration

- **Intermittent Infusion: Dilution:** Calculate volume of dose of daratumumab solution required based on patient body weight. Remove volume from polyvinyl chloride (PVC), polypropylene (PP), polyethylene (PE), or polyolefin bag of 0.9% NaCl equal to required volume. Withdraw required amount of daratumumab solution and add to 0.9% NaCl. *For Single Dose Infusion:* Dilute first infusion in 1000 mL, second and third infusions in 500 mL of 0.9% NaCl. *For Split Dose Infusion:* Dilute all infusions in 500 mL of 0.9% NaCl. Discard unused portion. Invert gently to mix; do not shake. Stable for up to 24 hr if refrigerated and protected from light; do not freeze. Allow to come to room temperature before administration. Solution is colorless to pale yellow and may develop very small, translucent to white proteinaceous particles; do not administer solution if discolored or contains opaque particulate matter.

- **Rate:** *Infuse first and second infusion* at an initial rate of 50 mL/hr through an infusion set fitted with a flow regulator and in-line, sterile, nonpyrogenic, low protein-binding polyethersulfone filter (pore size 0.22 or 0.2 micrometer). Administration sets must be either polyurethane, polybutadiene, PVC, PP, or PE. If no infusion reactions ≥Grade 1 during first 3 hr of first infusion, ↑ rate by 50 mL/hr for a maximum rate of 200 mL/hr. *Infuse subsequent infusions* at an initial rate of 100 mL/hr. If no infusion reactions ≥Grade 1 during first 3 hr of first infusion, ↑ rate by 50 mL/hr for a maximum rate of 200 mL/hr. Complete infusion within 15 hr.
- *Grade 1–2 (mild to moderate) infusion reactions:* Once reaction symptoms resolve, resume infusion at ≤ half the rate at which reaction occurred. If no further reactions experienced, resume at increments and intervals as appropriate.
- *Grade 3 (severe) infusion reactions:* If intensity of reaction ↓ to ≤Grade 2, consider restarting infusion at ≤ half rate at which reaction occurred. If no further reactions experienced, resume infusion rate escalation at appropriate increments and intervals. Repeat procedure if Grade 3 reaction recurs. If third ≥Grade 3 reaction occurs, permanently discontinue daratumumab.
- *Grade 4 (life-threatening) infusion reactions:* Permanently discontinue therapy.
- **Y-Site Incompatibility:** Do not administer in same IV line with other agents.

Patient/Family Teaching

- Instruct patient to read the *Patient Information* sheet prior to therapy.
- Advise patient to notify health care professional immediately if signs and symptoms of infusion reactions (itchy, runny, or blocked nose; chills; nausea; throat irritation; cough; headache; shortness of breath; difficulty breathing), bleeding, bruising, or fever occur.
- Advise patient to inform blood transfusion centers/personnel they are taking daratumumab in the event of a planned transfusion.
- Instruct patient to notify health care professional of all Rx or OTC medications, vitamins, or herbal products being taken and consult health care professional before taking any new medications.
- Rep: May cause fetal harm. Advise females of reproductive potential to use effective contraception during and for 3 mo after completion of therapy and to avoid breastfeeding during therapy. Immunoglobulin G1 monoclonal antibodies are transferred across the placenta. May cause fetal myeloid or lymphoid-cell depletion and decreased bone density. Defer administering live vaccines to neonates and infants exposed to daratumumab in utero until a hematology evaluation is completed.

Evaluation/Desired Outcomes

- Improved survival and decreased progression of multiple myeloma.

darbepoetin (dar-be-**poh**-e-tin)

Aranesp

Classification

Therapeutic: antianemics

Pharmacologic: erythropoiesis stimulating agents **(ESA)**

Indications

Anemia associated with chronic kidney disease (CKD). Chemotherapy-induced anemia in patients with nonmyeloid malignancies when there is ≥2 additional mo of planned chemotherapy.

Action

Stimulates erythropoiesis (production of RBCs). **Therapeutic Effects:** Maintains and may elevate RBC counts, decreasing the need for transfusions.

Pharmacokinetics

Absorption: 30–50% following SUBQ administration; IV administration results in complete bioavailability.

Distribution: Confined to the intravascular space.

Metabolism and Excretion: Unknown.

Half-life: *SUBQ:* 49 hr; *IV:* 21 hr.

TIME/ACTION PROFILE (↑ in RBCs)

ROUTE	ONSET	PEAK	DURATION
IV, SUBQ	2–6 wk	unknown	unknown

Contraindications/Precautions

Contraindicated in: Hypersensitivity; Uncontrolled hypertension; Patients with cancer receiving hormonal agents, biologic products, or radiotherapy, unless also receiving concurrent myelosuppressive chemotherapy; Patients receiving chemotherapy when anticipated outcome is cure; Patients with cancer receiving myelosuppressive chemotherapy in whom the anemia can be managed by transfusion; Patients who require immediate correction of anemia when RBC transfusions can be used instead.

Use Cautiously in: Cardiovascular disease or stroke; Underlying hematologic diseases, including hemolytic anemia, sickle-cell anemia, thalassemia, and porphyria (safety not established); OB: Use during pregnancy only if potential maternal benefit justifies potential fetal risk; Lactation: Safety not established in breastfeeding.

Adverse Reactions/Side Effects

CV: hypertension, hypotension, chest pain, DEEP VEIN THROMBOSIS (ESPECIALLY WITH HGB >11 G/DL), edema, HF, MI. **Derm:** ERYTHEMA MULTIFORME, pruritus, STEVENS-JOHNSON SYNDROME (SJS), TOXIC EPIDERMAL NECROLYSIS (TEN). **GI:** abdominal pain, diarrhea, nausea, vomiting, constipation. **Hemat:** pure red cell aplasia. **MS:** myalgia, arthralgia, back pain, limb pain. **Neuro:** dizziness, fatigue, headache, SEIZURES, STROKE, weakness. **Resp:** cough, dyspnea, bronchitis, PULMONARY EMBOLISM (ESPECIALLY WITH HGB >11 G/DL). **Misc:** fever, ↑ MORTALITY AND ↑ TUMOR GROWTH (ESPECIALLY WITH HGB >11 G/DL), HYPERSENSITIVITY REACTIONS (INCLUDING ANAPHYLAXIS AND ANGIOEDEMA), sepsis.

Interactions

Drug-Drug: None reported.

Route/Dosage

Anemia Due to Chronic Kidney Disease

(Do not initiate if Hgb ≥10 g/dL; should only consider initiating therapy in patients not on dialysis if rate of hemoglobin ↓ indicates likelihood of requiring a RBC transfusion and a goal is to ↓ the risk of alloimmunization and/or RBC transfusion risks.)

IV: SUBQ (Adults): *Starting treatment with darbepoetin (no previous epoetin):* 0.45 mcg/kg once weekly or 0.75 mcg/kg every 2 wk (for patients on dialysis); 0.45 mcg/kg every 4 wk (for patients not on dialysis); use lowest dose sufficient to ↓ the need for RBC transfusions (do not exceed Hgb of 10 g/dL [patients not on dialysis] or 11 g/dL [patients on dialysis]); if Hgb ↑ by >1 g/dL in 2 wk, ↓ dose by 25%; if Hgb ↑ by <1 g/dL after 4 wk of therapy (with adequate iron stores), ↑ dose by 25%; do not ↑ dose more frequently than every 4 wk. *Conversion from epoetin to darbepoetin:* weekly epoetin dose <2500 units = 6.25 mcg/wk darbepoetin; weekly epoetin dose 2500–4999 units = 12.5 mcg/wk darbepoetin; weekly epoetin dose 5000–10,999 units = 25 mcg/wk darbepoetin; weekly epoetin dose 11,000–17,999 units = 40 mcg/wk darbepoetin; weekly epoetin dose 18,000–33,999 units = 60 mcg/wk darbepoetin; weekly epoetin dose 34,000–89,999 units = 100 mcg/wk darbepoetin; weekly epoetin dose >90,000 units = 200 mcg/wk darbepoetin.

IV: SUBQ (Children): *Starting treatment with darbepoetin (no previous epoetin):* 0.45 mcg/kg once weekly (may also start with 0.75 mcg/kg every 2 wk in patients not on dialysis); use lowest dose sufficient to ↓ the need for RBC transfusions (do not exceed Hgb of 12 g/dL; if Hgb ↑ by >1.0 g/dL in 2 wk, ↓ dose by 25%; if Hgb ↑ by <1 g/dL after 4 wk of therapy (with adequate iron stores), ↑ dose by 25%; do not ↑ dose more frequently than every 4 wk.

Anemia Due to Chemotherapy

Use only for chemotherapy-related anemia, and discontinue when chemotherapy course is completed; do not initiate if Hgb ≥10 g/dL.

SUBQ (Adults): 2.25 mcg/kg weekly or 500 mcg every 3 wk; target Hgb should not exceed 12 g/dL. If Hgb ↑ by >1 g/dL in 2 wk or reaches a level needed to avoid RBC transfusions, ↓ dose by 40%; if Hgb ↑ by <1 g/dL after 6 wk of therapy, ↑ dose to 4.5 mcg/kg weekly.

Availability

Solution for injection (single-dose vials): 25 mcg/mL, 40 mcg/mL, 60 mcg/mL, 100 mcg/mL, 200 mcg/mL. **Solution for injection (prefilled syringes):** 10 mcg/0.4 mL, 25 mcg/0.42 mL, 40 mcg/0.4 mL, 60 mcg/0.3 mL, 100 mcg/0.5 mL, 150 mcg/0.3 mL, 200 mcg/0.4 mL, 300 mcg/0.6 mL, 500 mcg/1 mL.

NURSING IMPLICATIONS

Assessment

- Monitor BP before and during therapy. *If BP becomes difficult to control,* ↓ or hold darbepoetin. Treat with antihypertensives as indicated.
- Monitor for improving symptoms of anemia.
- Monitor dialysis shunts (thrill and bruit) and status of artificial kidney during hemodialysis. May need to ↑ heparin dose to prevent clotting. Monitor patients with underlying vascular disease for impaired circulation.
- Monitor for allergic reactions (rash, urticaria). *If anaphylaxis (dyspnea, laryngeal swelling) occurs,* permanently discontinue darbepoetin.
- Assess patient for skin rash frequently during therapy. *If rash or signs of SJS or TEN occur,* discontinue darbepoetin at first sign. Treat symptomatically.

Lab Test Considerations

- May ↑ WBC and platelets. May ↓ bleeding time.
- Monitor serum ferritin, transferrin, and iron levels prior to and during therapy to assess need for concurrent iron therapy. *If transferrin saturation <20% or serum ferritin <100 mcg/mL,* begin iron supplementation.
- **Anemia due to Chemotherapy:** Monitor Hgb before and weekly during initial therapy, for 4 wk after a change in dose, and regularly after target range has been reached and maintenance dose is determined. Monitor CBC with differential and platelets before and periodically during therapy. *If Hgb ↑ by >1 g/dL in any 2-wk period or Hgb reaches a level needed to avoid RBC transfusion,* ↓ dose by 40%. *If Hgb exceeds level needed to avoid RBC transfusion,* hold dose until Hgb approaches level where RBC transfusion required and reinitiate at a dose 40% below the previous dose. *If Hgb ↑ by <1 g/dL and remains <10 g/dL after 6 wk of therapy,* ↑

dose to 4.5 mcg/kg/wk (if on weekly therapy) or do not adjust dose (if on every 3-wk schedule). *If no Hgb response or RBC transfusions are still required after 8 wk of therapy,* discontinue darbepoetin. Hgb >11 g/dL ↑ likelihood of life-threatening cardiovascular complications, cardiac arrest, seizures, stroke, hypertension, HF, vascular thrombosis/ischemia, MI, and fluid overload.

- **Anemia of CKD:** Monitor Hgb at least weekly until stable and then at least monthly. Do not ↑ dose more frequently than once every 4 wk. Dose ↓ can be made more frequently. Avoid frequent dose adjustments. *If Hgb ↑ by >1 g/dL in 2-wk period,* ↓ dose by ≥25%. *If Hgb ↑ by <1 g/dL over 4 wk (and iron stores adequate),* ↑ dose by 25%. *If no response after 12 wk of escalation,* further dose ↑ is unlikely to improve response and may ↑ risks. Use lowest dose to maintain Hgb level sufficient to ↓ need for RBC transfusion.
- **Adults with Anemia of CKD on Dialysis:** Start therapy when Hgb >10 g/dL. If Hgb ≥11 g/dL, ↓ or hold dose.
- **Adults with Anemia of CKD Not on Dialysis:** Start therapy only when Hgb <10 g/dL AND rate of Hgb ↓ indicates likelihood of requiring a RBC transfusion AND ↓ risk of alloimmunization and/or other RBC transfusion-related risks is a goal. If Hgb level >10 g/dL, ↓ or hold dose, and use lowest darbepoetin dose sufficient to ↓ need for RBC transfusion.
- **Children with Anemia of CKD:** Start therapy only when Hgb <10 g/dL. If Hgb level >12 g/dL, ↓ or hold dose.
- Monitor renal function and electrolytes closely; patient. ↑ BUN, serum creatinine, uric acid, phosphorus, and potassium may occur.

Implementation

- Transfusions may be required for severe symptomatic anemia. Supplemental iron should be initiated with darbepoetin and continued during therapy. Correct deficiencies of folic acid or vitamin B_{12} prior to therapy.
- Institute seizure precautions for patients with a >1 g/dL ↑ in Hgb in a 2-wk period or exhibit any change in neurologic status.
- *For conversion from epoetin to darbepoetin,* if epoetin was administered 2–3 times/wk, administer darbepoetin once/wk. If epoetin was administered once/wk, administer darbepoetin once every 2 wk. Route of administration should remain consistent.
- Dose adjustments should not be more frequent than once/mo.
- Do not shake vial. Do not administer if solution is discolored or contains particulates.
- **SUBQ**: This route is often used for patients not requiring dialysis.

IV Administration

- **IV Push:** Administer undiluted. **Rate:** May be administered as direct injection or bolus over 1–3 min into IV tubing or via venous line at end of dialysis session.
- **Y-Site Incompatibility:** Do not administer other drugs through same IV line.

Patient/Family Teaching

- Explain purpose and side effects of medication. Advise patient to read *Patient Information* before starting therapy.
- Instruct patient on the appropriate steps for measuring accurate dose, administration technique, and disposal of equipment, if self-administration is appropriate.
- Advise patient to notify health care professional if new-onset seizure, premonitory symptoms, or change in seizure frequency occur. Discuss ways of preventing self-injury in patients with seizures. Driving and activities requiring continuous alertness should be avoided.
- Advise patient to stop darbepoetin and notify health care professional immediately if severe skin reactions (skin rash with itching, blisters, skin sores, peeling, areas of skin coming off) or signs and symptoms of serious allergic reactions (rash, itching, shortness of breath, wheezing, dizziness and fainting due to ↓ in BP, swelling around mouth or eyes, fast pulse, sweating) occur.
- Inform patient that use of darbepoetin may result in shortened overall survival and/or ↓ time to tumor progression. May also cause MI or stroke. Advise patient to notify health care professional immediately of chest pain; shortness of breath; pain in legs, with or without swelling; a cool or pale extremity; confusion; trouble speaking or understanding others; numbness or weakness of face or extremity; visual changes; ↓ coordination; dizziness; fainting; or if hemodialysis vascular access stops working.
- Advise patient to notify health care professional of darbepoetin therapy prior to surgery.
- Advise patient to notify health care professional of all Rx or OTC medications, vitamins, or herbal products being taken and to consult health care professional before taking other medications.
- **Rep:** Advise women of reproductive potential to notify health care professional if pregnancy is planned or suspected or if breastfeeding.
- **Anemia of CKD:** Stress importance of compliance with dietary restrictions, medications, and dialysis. Darbepoetin will result in ↑ sense of well-being but does not cure underlying disease.

Evaluation/Desired Outcomes

- Increase in Hgb not to exceed 11 g/dL with improvement in symptoms of anemia in patients with CKD or chemotherapy-induced anemia.

daridorexant (dar-i-doe-rex-ant)

Quviviq

Classification

Therapeutic: sedative/hypnotics

Pharmacologic: orexin receptor antagonists

Schedule IV

Indications

Insomnia associated with difficulty in sleep onset and/or maintenance.

Action

Antagonizes the effects of orexins A and B, naturally occurring neuropeptides that promote wakefulness, by binding to their receptors. **Therapeutic Effects:** Improved sleep.

Pharmacokinetics

Absorption: 62% absorbed following oral administration; a high-fat meal will delay absorption and sleep onset.

Distribution: Well distributed to tissues.

Protein Binding: 99.7%.

Metabolism and Excretion: Primarily metabolized in the liver via the CYP3A4 isoenzyme. Primarily excreted as metabolites in the feces (57%), with some excretion in the urine (28%).

Half-life: 8 hr.

TIME/ACTION PROFILE (sleep)

ROUTE	ONSET	PEAK	DURATION
PO	30 min	unknown	6 hr†

† Excess sedation may persist for several days after discontinuation.

Contraindications/Precautions

Contraindicated in: Hypersensitivity; Narcolepsy; Severe hepatic impairment.

Use Cautiously in: History of substance abuse or drug dependence; Depression; Underlying pulmonary disease; Moderate hepatic impairment (↓ dose); OB: Safety not established in pregnancy; Lactation: Use while breastfeeding only if potential maternal benefit justifies potential risk to infant; Pedi: Safety and effectiveness not established in children; Geri: ↑ risk of falls in older adults.

Adverse Reactions/Side Effects

GI: nausea, vomiting. **Neuro:** drowsiness, cataplexy, complex sleep behaviors (including sleep driving, sleep walking, or engaging in other activities while sleeping), dizziness, hallucinations (during sleep), headache, sleep paralysis, SUICIDAL IDEATION, worsening of depression. **Misc:** hypersensitivity reactions (including angioedema).

Interactions

Drug-Drug: Strong CYP3A4 inhibitors, including **itraconazole**, ↑ levels and risk of toxicity; concurrent use not recommended. **Moderate CYP3A4 inhibitors**, including **diltiazem**, may ↑ levels and risk of toxicity; ↓ daridorexant dose. **Strong CYP3A4 inducers**, including **rifampin**, and **moderate CYP3A4 inducers**, including **efavirenz**, ↓ levels and effectiveness; concurrent use not recommended. Risk of CNS depression, next-day impairment, sleep-driving, and other complex behaviors while not fully awake ↑ with other **CNS depressants**, including **alcohol**, some **antihistamines**, **opioids**, other **sedative/hypnotics** (including **benzodiazepines**), and **tricyclic antidepressants**; concurrent alcohol use should be avoided; for patients receiving other CNS depressants, dose adjustments of daridexorant and/or CNS depressants may be necessary.

Route/Dosage

PO (Adults): 25–50 mg within 30 min of going to bed; dose may not be repeated on a single night and should be taken when ≥7 hr of sleep time is anticipated before planned awakening. *Concurrent use of moderate CYP3A4 inhibitors:* 25 mg within 30 min of going to bed; dose may not be repeated on a single night and should be taken when ≥7 hr of sleep time is anticipated before planned awakening.

Hepatic Impairment

PO (Adults): *Moderate hepatic impairment:* 25 mg within 30 min of going to bed; dose may not be repeated on a single night and should be taken when ≥7 hr of sleep time is anticipated before planned awakening.

Availability

Tablets: 25 mg, 50 mg.

NURSING IMPLICATIONS

Assessment

- Assess sleep patterns prior to and during administration. Continued insomnia after 7–10 days of therapy may indicate primary psychiatric or mental illness.
- Assess mental status and potential for abuse prior to administration. Prolonged use of >7–10 days may lead to physical and psychological dependence. Limit amount of drug available to the patient.
- Monitor for signs and symptoms of hypersensitivity reactions (angioedema, rash, urticaria) during therapy. If severe reaction occurs, treat symptomatically and discontinue daridorexant.

Implementation

- **PO:** Administer within 30 min of going to bed with ≥7 hr remaining prior to planned awakening. Time to sleep onset may be delayed if taken with or soon after a meal.

Patient/Family Teaching

- Instruct patient to take daridorexant within 30 min of going to bed, as directed. Do not take daridorexant if alcohol was consumed that evening. Do not increase dose or discontinue without notifying health care professional. CNS-depressant effects may persist in some patients for up to several days after discontinuing. Advise patient to read *Medication Guide* before starting therapy and with each Rx refill in case of changes.

- May cause daytime and next-day drowsiness. Caution patient to avoid driving or other activities requiring alertness until response to medication is known.
- Caution patient that daridorexant may cause complex sleep behaviors (sleep walking, sleep driving, making and eating food, talking on the phone, having sex) while unaware. Patient may not remember anything done during the night; increased risk with alcohol or other CNS depressants. Discontinue daridorexant immediately and notify health care professional if complex sleep behaviors occur.
- Inform patients and their families that daridorexant may cause sleep paralysis, an inability to move or speak for several min during sleep-wake transitions and hypnagogic/hypnopompic hallucinations, including vivid and disturbing perceptions.
- Advise patient that daridorexant is a drug with known abuse potential. Protect it from theft, and never give to anyone other than the individual for whom it was prescribed. Store out of sight and reach of children, and in a location not accessible by others.
- Instruct patient to notify health care professional of all Rx or OTC medications, vitamins, or herbal products being taken and to consult health care professional before taking any other Rx, OTC, or herbal products.
- Caution patient to avoid concurrent use of alcohol or other CNS depressants, including opioids.
- Advise patient to notify health care professional if signs and symptoms of allergic reaction (swelling of tongue or throat, trouble breathing, nausea and vomiting) occur.
- Rep: Advise females of reproductive potential to notify health care professional if pregnancy is planned or suspected or if breastfeeding. Infants exposed to daridorexant through breast milk should be monitored for excessive sedation. Inform females there is a pregnancy exposure registry that monitors pregnancy outcomes in females exposed to daridorexant during pregnancy. Pregnant women exposed to daridorexant and health care professionals are encouraged to call Idorsia Pharmaceuticals Ltd at 1-833-400-9611.

Evaluation/Desired Outcomes

- Improved sleep.

darifenacin (dar-i-fen-a-sin)

Enablex

Classification

Therapeutic: urinary tract antispasmodics

Pharmacologic: anticholinergics

Indications

Overactive bladder with symptoms (urge incontinence, urgency, frequency).

Action

Acts as a muscarinic (cholinergic) receptor antagonist; antagonizes bladder smooth muscle contraction. **Therapeutic Effects:** Decreased symptoms of overactive bladder.

Pharmacokinetics

Absorption: 15–19% absorbed.

Distribution: Unknown.

Protein Binding: 98%.

Metabolism and Excretion: Extensively metabolized in the liver by the CYP2D6 isoenzyme, with some metabolism by the CYP3A4 isoenzyme; the CYP2D6 isoenzyme exhibits genetic polymorphism (~7% of population may be poor metabolizers and may have significantly ↑ darifenacin concentrations and an ↑ risk of adverse effects). 60% excreted by the kidneys as metabolites, 40% in feces as metabolites.

Half-life: 13–19 hr.

TIME/ACTION PROFILE

ROUTE	ONSET	PEAK	DURATION
PO	unknown	7 hr	24 hr

Contraindications/Precautions

Contraindicated in: Hypersensitivity; Urinary retention; Gastric retention; Uncontrolled angle-closure glaucoma; Severe hepatic impairment.

Use Cautiously in: Moderate hepatic impairment (↓ dose); Bladder outflow obstruction; GI obstructive disorders, ↓ GI motility, severe constipation, or ulcerative colitis; Myasthenia gravis; Angle-closure glaucoma; OB: Safety not established in pregnancy; Lactation: Safety not established in breastfeeding; Pedi: Safety and effectiveness not established in children.

Adverse Reactions/Side Effects

EENT: blurred vision. **GI:** constipation, dry mouth, dyspepsia, nausea. **Metab:** heat intolerance. **Neuro:** confusion, dizziness, drowsiness, hallucinations, headache. **Misc:** ANGIOEDEMA.

Interactions

Drug-Drug: Strong CYP3A4 inhibitors, including **ketoconazole, itraconazole, ritonavir, nelfinavir, clarithromycin**, and **nefazodone** may ↑ levels and risk of toxicity; do not exceed dose of 7.5 mg/day. Concurrent use of **moderate CYP3A4 inhibitors**, especially those with narrow therapeutic indices, including **flecainide, thioridazine**, and **tricyclic antidepressants**, should be undertaken with caution.

Route/Dosage
PO (Adults): 7.5 mg once daily, may ↑ after 2 wk to 15 mg once daily.

Hepatic Impairment
PO (Adults): *Moderate hepatic impairment:* Not to exceed 7.5 mg once daily.

Availability (generic available)
Extended-release tablets: 7.5 mg, 15 mg.

NURSING IMPLICATIONS
Assessment
- Monitor voiding pattern and assess symptoms of overactive bladder (urinary urgency, incontinence, frequency) before and periodically during therapy.
- Monitor for anticholinergic effects (constipation, urinary retention, blurred vision), including CNS effects (headache, confusion, hallucinations, somnolence), especially with therapy initiation or dose ↑. *If CNS effects occur,* consider dose ↓ or discontinue darifenacin.

Implementation
- **PO:** Administer once daily with water, without regard to food. ***DNC:*** Swallow extended-release tablets whole; do not break, crush, or chew.

Patient/Family Teaching
- Instruct patient to take darifenacin as directed. If dose is missed, omit and take next day; do not take two doses in same day. Advise patient to read *Patient Information* before starting therapy and with each Rx refill in case of changes.
- May cause dizziness, drowsiness, confusion, and blurred vision. Caution patient to avoid driving and other activities that require alertness until response to medication is known.
- Inform patient that darifenacin may cause heat stroke in hot environments. Notify health care professional for ↓ sweating, dizziness, fatigue, nausea, fever.
- Advise patient to immediately notify emergency health care professional for symptoms of angioedema (swelling of face, lips, tongue, or throat).
- Instruct patient to notify health care professional of all Rx or OTC medications, vitamins, or herbal products being taken and consult health care professional before taking any new medications.
- Rep: Advise women of reproductive potential to notify health care professional if pregnancy is planned or suspected or if breastfeeding.

Evaluation/Desired Outcomes
- Decreased symptoms of overactive bladder.

HIGH ALERT

darolutamide
(dar-oh-loo-ta-mide)

Nubeqa

Classification

Therapeutic: antineoplastics

Pharmacologic: androgen receptor inhibitors

D

Indications
Nonmetastatic castration resistant prostate cancer. Metastatic hormone-sensitive prostate cancer (as monotherapy or in combination with docetaxel).

Action
Acts as an androgen receptor inhibitor, preventing the binding of androgen; decreases proliferation and induces cell death of prostate cancer cells. **Therapeutic Effects:** Decreased growth and spread of prostate cancer.

Pharmacokinetics
Absorption: 30% absorbed following oral administration; absorption ↑ with food.
Distribution: Extensively distributed to tissues.
Protein Binding: *Darolutamide:* 92%; *Keto-darolutamide:* 99.8%.
Metabolism and Excretion: Primarily metabolized in the liver by the CYP3A4 isoenzyme as well as by UGT1A1 and UGT1A9 to an active metabolite (keto-darolutamide). Primarily excreted in urine (63%, 7% as unchanged drug) and 32% excreted in feces (30% as unchanged drug).
Half-life: 20 hr.

TIME/ACTION PROFILE (plasma concentrations)

ROUTE	ONSET	PEAK	DURATION
PO	unknown	4 hr	unknown

Contraindications/Precautions
Contraindicated in: End-stage renal disease; Severe hepatic impairment.
Use Cautiously in: Severe renal impairment (↓ dose); Moderate hepatic impairment (↓ dose); Rep: Men with female partners of reproductive potential; Pedi: Safety and effectiveness not established in children.

Adverse Reactions/Side Effects
CV: HF, ISCHEMIC HEART DISEASE. **Derm:** rash. **GI:** ↑ liver enzymes, hyperbilirubinemia. **Hemat:** NEUTROPENIA. **Neuro:** fatigue, SEIZURES.

Interactions

Drug-Drug: Combined P-glycoprotein and strong or moderate CYP3A4 inducers, including **rifampin**, may ↓ levels and effectiveness; avoid concurrent use. **Combined P-glycoprotein and strong CYP3A4 inhibitors**, including **itraconazole**, may ↑ levels and risk of toxicity; avoid concurrent use. May ↑ levels and risk of toxicity of **breast cancer resistance protein substrates**, including **rosuvastatin**; avoid concurrent use.

Route/Dosage

Patients should also be taking a gonadotropin-releasing hormone (GnRH) analog or should have undergone a bilateral orchiectomy.

PO (Adults): 600 mg twice daily; continue until disease progression or unacceptable toxicity.

Renal Impairment

PO (Adults): *CCr 15–29 mL/min:* 300 mg twice daily; continue until disease progression or unacceptable toxicity.

Hepatic Impairment

PO (Adults): *Moderate hepatic impairment:* 300 mg twice daily; continue until disease progression or unacceptable toxicity.

Availability

Tablets: 300 mg.

NURSING IMPLICATIONS

Assessment

- Monitor for fatigue, pain in extremities, and rash during therapy.
- Monitor for signs and symptoms of ischemic heart disease. Optimally manage hypertension, diabetes, and dyslipidemia. *If Grade 3–4 ischemic heart disease occurs,* permanently discontinue darolutamide.

Lab Test Considerations

- May cause neutropenia, ↑ AST, and ↑ bilirubin.

Implementation

- Patients with bilateral orchiectomy should take a GnRH analog concurrently.
- When darolutamide is used concurrently with docetaxel for metastatic castration-sensitive prostate cancer, administer the 1st of 6 cycles of docetaxel within 6 wk after the initiation of darolutamide.
- **PO:** Administer twice daily with food. ***DNC:*** Swallow tablets whole; do not crush, break, or chew.

Patient/Family Teaching

- Explain purpose and side effects of medication. Advise patient to read *Patient Information* before starting therapy.
- Instruct patient to take missed dose as soon as remembered, but do not double doses.
- Advise patient that therapy may ↑ risk of seizures. Avoid activities where a sudden loss of consciousness could cause serious harm to self or others. Notify health care provider immediately if seizure symptoms occur.
- Advise patient to immediately notify health care provider of chest pain or difficulty breathing.
- Advise patient to notify health care provider of all Rx or OTC medications, vitamins, or herbal products being taken and to consult with health care provider before taking other medications.
- Rep: May cause fetal harm. Advise men with female partners of reproductive potential to use effective contraception for 1 wk after last dose. Inform patient that darolutamide may impair fertility.

Evaluation/Desired Outcomes

- Decreased growth and spread of prostate cancer.

darunavir (da-**ru**-na-veer)

Prezista

Classification

Therapeutic: antiretrovirals

Pharmacologic: protease inhibitors

Indications

HIV infection (in combination with ritonavir and other antiretrovirals).

Action

Inhibits HIV-1 protease, selectively inhibiting the cleavage of HIV-encoded specific polyproteins in infected cells. This prevents the formation of mature virus particles.

Therapeutic Effects: Increased CD4 cell counts and decreased viral load with subsequent slowed progression of HIV infection and its sequelae.

Pharmacokinetics

Absorption: *Without ritonavir:* 37% absorbed following oral administration; *with ritonavir:* 82%. Food ↑ absorption by 30%.

Distribution: Unknown.

Protein Binding: 95%.

Metabolism and Excretion: Extensively metabolized by the CYP3A isoenzymes. 41% eliminated unchanged in feces, 8% in urine.

Half-life: 15 hr.

TIME/ACTION PROFILE

ROUTE	ONSET	PEAK	DURATION
PO	unknown	2.5–4 hr	12 hr

Contraindications/Precautions

Contraindicated in: Concurrent use of alfuzosin, dronedarone, colchicine (in renal/hepatic impairment), elbasvir/grazoprevir, ergot derivatives, ivabradine, lomitapide, lovastatin, lurasidone, midazolam (PO), naloxegol, pimozide, ranolazine, rifampin, sildenafil

(Revatio), simvastatin, triazolam, or St. John's wort; Lactation: Avoid breastfeeding in mothers with HIV.
Use Cautiously in: Hepatic impairment; Sulfa allergy; OB: Considered a preferred protease inhibitor (when combined with ritonavir) for pregnant females living with HIV who are antiretroviral-naive (as initial therapy), who have had antiretroviral therapy in the past but are restarting, or who require a new antiretroviral regimen (due to poor tolerance or poor virologic response of current regimen); Pedi: Children <3 yr (safety and effectiveness not established); Geri: Consider age-related impairment in hepatic function, concurrent chronic disease states, and drug therapy in older adults.

Adverse Reactions/Side Effects

Based on concurrent use with ritonavir

Derm: ACUTE GENERALIZED EXANTHEMATOUS PUSTULOSIS, rash, DRUG RASH WITH EOSINOPHILIA AND SYSTEMIC SYMPTOMS (DRESS), STEVENS-JOHNSON SYNDROME, TOXIC EPIDERMAL NECROLYSIS. **Endo:** Graves' disease, hyperglycemia. **GI:** autoimmune hepatitis, constipation, diarrhea, HEPATOTOXICITY, nausea, vomiting. **Metab:** body fat redistribution. **MS:** polymyositis. **Neuro:** Guillan-Barré syndrome. **Misc:** immune reconstitution syndrome.

Interactions

Drug-Drug: May ↑ levels and risk of toxicity from **alfuzosin**, **dronedarone**, **elbasvir/grazoprevir**, **ergot derivatives (dihydroergotamine**, **ergotamine**, **methylergonovine)**, **ivabradine**, **lomitapide**, **lovastatin**, **lurasidone**, **midazolam (oral)**, **pimozide**, **ranolazine**, **sildenafil (Revatio)**, **simvastatin**, and **triazolam**; concurrent use contraindicated. May ↑ **naloxegol** levels, which can precipitate opioid withdrawal symptoms; concurrent use contraindicated. May ↑ **colchicine** levels and cause serious/life-threatening reactions; ↓ dose of colchicine; concurrent use contraindicated in patients with renal or hepatic impairment. **Rifampin** ↑ metabolism and may ↓ antiretroviral effectiveness; concurrent use is contraindicated. ↑ levels and risk of myopathy from **atorvastatin**, **rosuvastatin**, or **pravastatin**; use lowest dose of these agents; do not exceed atorvastatin dose of 20 mg/day. Concurrent use with **efavirenz** results in ↓ darunavir levels and ↑ efavirenz levels; use combination cautiously. **Lopinavir/ritonavir** may ↓ levels; concurrent use not recommended. May ↑ **maraviroc** levels; ↓ maraviroc dose to 150 mg twice daily. May ↑ levels of **lidocaine**, **quinidine**, **disopyramide**, **mexiletine**, **propafenone**, **flecainide**, and **amiodarone**; use cautiously and with available blood level monitoring. ↑ **digoxin** levels; blood level monitoring recommended. May ↑ **carbamazepine** levels; blood level monitoring recommended. May ↓ **phenytoin** or **phenobarbital** levels; blood level monitoring recommended. May ↑ **clonazepam** levels. May ↓ levels of **warfarin**; monitor INR. May ↑ levels of **trazodone**, **amitriptyline**, **desipramine**, **imipramine**, and **nortriptyline**; use cautiously and ↓ dose if necessary. May ↑ levels of **clarithromycin**; ↓ dose of clarithromycin if CCr ≤60 mL/min. May ↑ levels of **ketoconazole**, **isavuconazonium**, and **itraconazole**; do not exceed itraconazole or ketoconazole dose >200 mg/day. **Ketoconazole**, **isavuconazole**, **itraconazole**, and **posaconazole** may ↑ levels. May ↓ levels of **voriconazole**; concurrent use not recommended. Concurrent use with **rifabutin** ↑ rifabutin levels and ↑ darunavir levels (may be due to ritonavir); ↓ rifabutin dose to 150 mg every other day. **Rifapentin** may ↓ levels; concurrent use not recommended. May ↑ levels of **beta blockers**; may need to ↓ dose. May ↑ levels of **amlodipine**, **diltiazem**, **felodipine**, **nifedipine**, **nicardipine**, or **verapamil**; monitor clinical response carefully. **Dexamethasone** may ↓ levels/effects; consider use of alternative corticosteroid, such as beclomethasone or prednisolone. May ↑ levels of **corticosteroids** (all routes of administration) primarily metabolized by the CYP3A isoenzyme (e.g., **betamethasone**, **budesonide**, **ciclesonide**, **fluticasone**, **methylprednisolone**, **mometasone**, or **triamcinolone**), which may ↑ the risk of Cushing's disease and adrenal suppression; consider alternative corticosteroid such as beclomethasone, prednisone, or prednisolone. May ↑ levels of **cyclosporine**, **tacrolimus**, or **sirolimus**; blood level monitoring recommended. May ↑ levels of **everolimus**; concurrent use not recommended. May ↑ levels of **irinotecan**; discontinue darunavir/ritonavir ≥1 wk before starting irinotecan therapy. May ↓ levels of **methadone**; may need to ↑ dose. May ↑ **risperidone** and **thioridazine** levels; may need to ↓ dose. May ↑ levels of **sildenafil**, **vardenafil**, **tadalafil**, or **avanafil**; single dose should not exceed the following (sildenafil 25 mg in 48 hr; vardenafil 2.5 mg in 72 hr; tadalafil 10 mg in 72 hr); concurrent use with avanafil not recommended. May ↓ levels of **sertraline** and **paroxetine**; adjust dose by clinical response. May ↓ levels and contraceptive efficacy of some combined **hormonal contraceptives** and **progestin-only contraceptives** (alternative methods of nonhormonal contraception recommended). May ↑ risk of hyperkalemia when used with **drospirenone**. May ↑ levels of **salmeterol**; concurrent use not recommended. May ↑ **bosentan** levels; initiate bosentan at 62.5 mg once daily or every other day once patient receiving darunavir for ≥10 days; if patient already receiving bosentan, discontinue bosentan ≥36 hr before initiation of darunavir and then restart bosentan ≥10 days later at 62.5 mg once daily or every other day. May ↑ **tadalafil (Adcirca)** levels; initiate tadalafil

(Adcirca) at 20 mg once daily once patient receiving darunavir for ≥1 wk; if patient already receiving tadalafil (Adcirca), discontinue tadalafil (Adcirca) ≥24 hr before initiation of darunavir and then restart tadalafil (Adcirca) ≥7 days later at 20 mg once daily. May ↑ **lumefantrine** levels and risk of QT interval prolongation. May ↑ **quetiapine** levels; consider alternative antipsychotic therapy; if not possible, ↓ quetiapine dose to ⅙ of current dose. May ↑ levels of and risk of bleeding with **apixaban**, **dabigatran**, **edoxaban**, and **rivaroxaban**; concurrent use with rivaroxaban not recommended. May ↑ **dasatinib** and **nilotinib** levels; may need to ↓ dose or ↑ dosing interval of dasatinib and nilotinib. May ↑ **vinblastine** and **vincristine** levels; may need to temporarily hold darunavir-ritonavir or initiate another antiretroviral regimen. May ↑ levels of **buspirone**, **diazepam**, **estazolam**, **midazolam (IV)**, and **zolpidem**; ↓ dose of sedative. May ↓ **omeprazole** levels; consider ↑ omeprazole dose (not to exceed 40 mg/day). May ↑ levels of **glecaprevir/pibrentasvir**; concurrent use not recommended. May ↑ **ticagrelor** levels and risk of bleeding; concurrent use not recommended. May ↓ antiplatelet effects of **clopidogrel**; concurrent use not recommended. May ↑ **fesoterodine** and **solifenacin** levels; should not exceed fesoterodine dose of 4 mg once daily or solifenacin dose of 5 mg once daily. May ↑ levels/risk of respiratory depression with opioids including **buprenorphine**, **buprenorphine/naloxone**, **fentanyl**, and **tramadol**; carefully monitor **opioid** effects when cobicistat with darunavir is initiated; dose adjustment of opioid may be necessary.
Drug-Natural Products: **St. John's wort** ↑ metabolism and may ↓ antiretroviral effectiveness; concurrent use contraindicated.

Route/Dosage

Genotypic testing of the baseline virus is recommended prior to initiating treatment in therapy-experienced patients. This testing is performed to screen for darunavir resistance associated substitutions, which may be helpful in determining whether the patient's HIV will be susceptible to darunavir.

PO (Adults): *Therapy-naive:* 800 mg once daily with ritonavir 100 mg once daily; *Therapy-experienced (with no darunavir resistance associated substitution):* 800 mg once daily with ritonavir 100 mg once daily; *Therapy-experienced (with ≥1 darunavir resistance associated substitution or if genotypic testing not performed):* 600 mg twice daily with ritonavir 100 mg twice daily; *Pregnancy:* 600 mg twice daily with ritonavir 100 mg twice daily; if patient taking 800 mg once daily with ritonavir 100 mg once daily before pregnancy, may continue with this regimen if they are virologically suppressed (HIV-1 RNA <50 copies/mL), and if switch to twice daily regimen may compromise tolerability or compliance.

PO (Oral suspension or tablets): (Children 3–17 yr and ≥40 kg): *Therapy-naive:* 800 mg once daily with ritonavir 100 mg once daily; *Therapy-experienced (with no darunavir resistance associated substitution):* 800 mg once daily with ritonavir 100 mg once daily; *Therapy-experienced (with ≥1 darunavir resistance associated substitution or if genotypic testing not performed):* 600 mg twice daily with ritonavir 100 mg twice daily.

PO (Oral suspension or tablets): (Children 3–17 yr and 30–39.9 kg): *Therapy-naive:* 675 mg once daily with ritonavir 100 mg once daily; *Therapy-experienced (with no darunavir resistance associated substitution):* 675 mg once daily with ritonavir 100 mg once daily; *Therapy-experienced (with ≥1 darunavir resistance associated substitution or if genotypic testing not performed):* 450 mg twice daily with ritonavir 60 mg twice daily.

PO (Oral suspension or tablets): (Children 3–17 yr and 15–29.9 kg): *Therapy-naive:* 600 mg once daily with ritonavir 100 mg once daily; *Therapy-experienced (with no darunavir resistance associated substitution):* 600 mg once daily with ritonavir 100 mg once daily; *Therapy-experienced (with ≥1 darunavir resistance associated substitution or if genotypic testing not performed):* 375 mg twice daily with ritonavir 48 mg twice daily.

PO (Oral suspension only): (Children 3–17 yr and 14–14.9 kg): *Therapy-naive:* 490 mg once daily with ritonavir 96 mg once daily; *Therapy-experienced (with no darunavir resistance associated substitution):* 490 mg once daily with ritonavir 96 mg once daily; *Therapy-experienced (with ≥1 darunavir resistance associated substitution or if genotypic testing not performed):* 280 mg twice daily with ritonavir 48 mg twice daily.

PO (Oral suspension only): (Children 3–17 yr and 13–13.9 kg): *Therapy-naive:* 455 mg once daily with ritonavir 80 mg once daily; *Therapy-experienced (with no darunavir resistance associated substitution):* 455 mg once daily with ritonavir 80 mg once daily; *Therapy-experienced (with ≥1 darunavir resistance associated substitution or if genotypic testing not performed):* 260 mg twice daily with ritonavir 40 mg twice daily.

PO (Oral suspension only): (Children 3–17 yr and 12–12.9 kg): *Therapy-naive:* 420 mg once daily with ritonavir 80 mg once daily; *Therapy-experienced (with no darunavir resistance associated substitution):* 420 mg once daily with ritonavir 80 mg once daily; *Therapy-experienced (with ≥1 darunavir resistance associated substitution or if genotypic testing not performed):* 240 mg twice daily with ritonavir 40 mg twice daily.

PO (Oral suspension only): (Children 3–17 yr and 11–11.9 kg): *Therapy-naive:* 385 mg once daily with ritonavir 64 mg once daily; *Therapy-experienced (with no darunavir resistance associated substitution):* 385 mg once daily with ritonavir 64 mg once daily; *Therapy-experienced (with ≥1 darunavir resistance associated substitution or if genotypic testing not

performed): 220 mg twice daily with ritonavir 32 mg twice daily.
PO (Oral suspension only): (Children 3–17 yr and 10–10.9 kg): *Therapy-naive:* 350 mg once daily with ritonavir 64 mg once daily; *Therapy-experienced (with no darunavir resistance associated substitution):* 350 mg once daily with ritonavir 64 mg once daily; *Therapy-experienced (with ≥1 darunavir resistance associated substitution or if genotypic testing not performed):* 200 mg twice daily with ritonavir 32 mg twice daily.

Availability (generic available)

Oral suspension: 100 mg/mL. **Tablets:** 75 mg, 150 mg, 600 mg, 800 mg. ***In combination with:*** cobicistat (Prezcobix); cobicistat, emtricitabine, tenofovir alafenamide (Symtuza). See Appendix N.

NURSING IMPLICATIONS

Assessment

- Assess patient for change in severity of HIV symptoms and for symptoms of opportunistic infections during therapy.
- Assess for allergy to sulfonamides.
- Monitor patient for development of rash; usually maculopapular and self-limited. May cause Stevens-Johnson syndrome or toxic epidermal necrolysis. Discontinue therapy if severe or if accompanied with fever, general malaise, fatigue, muscle or joint aches, blisters, oral lesions, conjunctivitis, hepatitis, and/or eosinophilia.
- Monitor for signs and symptoms of DRESS (fever, rash, lymphadenopathy, and/or facial swelling) associated with involvement of other organ systems (hepatitis, nephritis, hematologic abnormalities, myocarditis, myositis) during therapy. May resemble an acute viral infection. Eosinophilia is often present. Discontinue therapy if signs occur.

Lab Test Considerations

- Obtain HIV genotypic testing for antiretroviral treatment experienced patients prior to starting therapy.
- Monitor viral load and CD4 counts regularly during therapy.
- May cause ↑ serum AST, ALT, GGT, total bilirubin, alkaline phosphatase, pancreatic amylase, pancreatic lipase, triglycerides, total cholesterol, and uric acid concentrations. Monitor hepatic function prior to and periodically during therapy. Hepatotoxicity may require interruption or discontinuation of therapy.

Implementation

- **PO:** Must be administered with a meal or light snack along with ritonavir 100 mg to be effective. The type of food is not important.
- Administer oral suspension 8 mL dose as two 4-mL doses using syringe provided along with ritonavir and food.

Patient/Family Teaching

- Emphasize the importance of taking darunavir with ritonavir exactly as directed, at evenly spaced times throughout day. Do not take more than prescribed amount and do not stop taking without consulting health care professional. If a dose of darunavir or ritonavir is missed by more than 6 hr, wait and take next dose at regularly scheduled time. If missed by less than 6 hr, take darunavir and ritonavir immediately and then take next dose at regularly scheduled time. If a dose is skipped, do not double doses. Advise patient to read the *Patient Information* sheet before starting therapy and with each Rx renewal in case changes have been made.
- Instruct patient that darunavir should not be shared with others.
- Instruct patient to notify health care professional of all Rx or OTC medications, vitamins, or herbal products being taken and consult health care professional before taking any new medications, especially St. John's wort.
- Inform patient that darunavir does not cure AIDS or prevent associated or opportunistic infections. Darunavir may reduce the risk of transmission of HIV to others through sexual contact or blood contamination. Caution patient to use a condom during sexual contact and to avoid sharing needles or donating blood to prevent spreading HIV to others. Advise patient that the long-term effects of darunavir are unknown at this time.
- Inform patient that darunavir may cause hyperglycemia, hepatotoxicity, and severe skin reactions. Advise patient to notify health care professional promptly if signs of hyperglycemia (increased thirst or hunger; unexplained weight loss; increased urination; fatigue; or dry, itchy skin), hepatotoxicity (unexplained fatigue, anorexia, nausea, jaundice, abdominal pain, or dark urine), DRESS, or rash occur.
- Advise patient to notify health care professional if signs and symptoms of immune reconstitution syndrome (signs and symptoms of an infection) occur.
- Inform patient that redistribution and accumulation of body fat may occur, causing central obesity, dorsocervical fat enlargement (buffalo hump), peripheral wasting, breast enlargement, and cushingoid appearance. The cause and long-term effects are not known.
- Rep: Instruct females of reproductive potential using hormonal contraceptives to use an alternative nonhormonal method of contraception. Advise patient to notify health care professional if pregnancy is planned or suspected and to avoid breastfeeding. If pregnant patient is exposed to darunavir, register patient in *Antiretroviral Pregnancy Registry* by calling 1-800-258-4263 to monitor pregnancy outcomes.

- Emphasize the importance of regular follow-up exams and blood counts to determine progress and monitor for side effects.

Evaluation/Desired Outcomes

- Delayed progression of HIV and decreased opportunistic infections in patients with HIV.
- Decrease in viral load and improvement in CD4 cell counts.

darunavir/cobicistat/emtricitabine/tenofovir alafenamide (da-**roo**-na-veer/koe-**bik**-i-stat/em-tri-**si**-ti-been/te-**noe**-fo-veer al-a-**fen**-a-mide)

Symtuza

Classification

Therapeutic: antiretrovirals, pharmacoenhancers

Pharmacologic: protease inhibitors, enzyme inhibitors, nucleoside reverse transcriptase inhibitors

Indications

HIV-1 infection in patients who have no prior antiretroviral treatment history or who are virologically suppressed (HIV-1 RNA <50 copies/mL) on a stable antiretroviral regimen for ≥6 mo and have no known substitutions associated with resistance to darunavir or tenofovir.

Action

Darunavir: Inhibits HIV-1 protease, selectively inhibiting the cleavage of HIV-encoded specific polyproteins in infected cells. This prevents the formation of mature virus particles. *Cobicistat:* Strongly inhibits CYP3A enzymes, enhancing systemic exposure to darunavir. *Emtricitabine:* Phosphorylated intracellularly, where it inhibits HIV reverse transcriptase, resulting in viral DNA chain termination. *Tenofovir alafenamide:* Phosphorylated intracellularly, where it inhibits HIV reverse transcriptase, resulting in disruption of DNA synthesis.
Therapeutic Effects: Increased CD4 cell counts and decreased viral load with subsequent slowed progression of HIV infection and its sequelae.

Pharmacokinetics

Darunavir

Absorption: Food enhances oral absorption.
Distribution: Unknown.
Protein Binding: 95%.
Metabolism and Excretion: Extensively metabolized by the liver via the CYP3A isoenzyme; 41% excreted unchanged in feces, 8% in urine.
Half-life: 9.4 hr.

Cobicistat

Absorption: Absorption follows oral administration.
Distribution: Unknown.
Protein Binding: 97–98%.
Metabolism and Excretion: Metabolized by the liver primarily by the CYP3A isoenzyme and to a lesser extent by the CYP2D6 isoenzyme; 86.2% excreted in feces, 8.2% in urine.
Half-life: 3.2 hr.

Emtricitabine

Absorption: 93% absorbed following oral administration.
Distribution: Unknown.
Metabolism and Excretion: Not significantly metabolized; 86% excreted in urine, 14% in feces.
Half-life: 7.5 hr.

Tenofovir Alafenamide

Absorption: Tenofovir alafenamide is a prodrug, which is hydrolyzed into tenofovir, the active component; absorption enhanced by high-fat meals.
Distribution: Unknown.
Metabolism and Excretion: Tenofovir is phosphorylated to tenofovir diphosphate (active metabolite); 32% excreted in feces, <1% in urine.
Half-life: 0.5 hr.

TIME/ACTION PROFILE (plasma concentrations)

ROUTE	ONSET	PEAK	DURATION
Darunavir (PO)	unknown	3 hr	24 hr
Cobicistat (PO)	unknown	3 hr	24 hr
Emtricitabine (PO)	rapid	1.5 hr	24 hr
Tenofovir (PO)	unknown	0.5 hr	24 hr

Contraindications/Precautions

Contraindicated in: Concurrent use of alfuzosin, carbamazepine, dronedarone, colchicine (in renal/hepatic impairment), elbasvir/grazoprevir, ergot derivatives, ivabradine, lomitapide, lovastatin, lurasidone, midazolam (PO), naloxegol, phenobarbital, phenytoin, pimozide, ranolazine, rifampin, sildenafil (Revatio), simvastatin, triazolam, or St. John's wort; Severe renal impairment; Severe hepatic impairment; OB: Pregnancy (significantly lower concentrations of darunavir and cobicistat during 2nd and 3rd trimesters); Lactation: Breastfeeding not recommended in women with HIV.
Use Cautiously in: Chronic hepatitis B virus (HBV) infection (may exacerbate following discontinuation); Sulfonamide allergy; Hemophilia (↑ risk of bleeding); Pedi: Children <40 kg (safety and effectiveness not established); Geri: Consider age-related impairment in hepatic function and concurrent chronic disease states and drug therapy in older adults.

Adverse Reactions/Side Effects

Derm: <u>rash</u>, ACUTE GENERALIZED EXANTHEMATOUS PUSTULOSIS, DRUG REACTION WITH EOSINOPHILIA AND SYSTEMIC SYMPTOMS (DRESS), STEVENS-JOHNSON SYNDROME (SJS), TOXIC EPIDERMAL NECROLYSIS (TEN). **Endo:** Graves'

disease, hyperglycemia. **GI:** abdominal pain, ACUTE EXACERBATION OF HBV, autoimmune hepatitis, diarrhea, flatulence, HEPATOTOXICITY, LACTIC ACIDOSIS/HEPATOMEGALY WITH STEATOSIS, nausea. **GU:** acute renal failure, Fanconi syndrome, proximal renal tubulopathy. **Metab:** body fat redistribution, hyperlipidemia. **MS:** polymyositis. **Neuro:** Guillain-Barré syndrome, fatigue, headache. **Misc:** immune reconstitution syndrome.

Interactions

Drug-Drug: ↑ levels and risk of toxicity from **alfuzosin**, **dronedarone**, **elbasvir/grazoprevir**, **ergot derivatives (dihydroergotamine, ergotamine, methylergonovine)**, **ivabradine**, **lomitapide**, **lovastatin**, **lurasidone**, **midazolam (oral)**, **pimozide**, **ranolazine**, **sildenafil (Revatio)**, **simvastatin**, and **triazolam**; concurrent use contraindicated. May ↑ **naloxegol** levels, which can precipitate opioid withdrawal symptoms; concurrent use contraindicated. **Strong CYP3A4 inducers**, including **carbamazepine**, **phenobarbital**, **phenytoin**, and **rifampin**, may ↓ levels and effectiveness of cobicistat, darunavir, and tenofovir; concurrent use contraindicated. May ↑ levels and risk of toxicity of **colchicine**; concurrent use in patients with renal/hepatic impairment contraindicated; for others ↓ dose (*for gout flare:* 0.6 mg followed by 0.3 mg 1 hr later; may repeat no sooner than 3 days; *for prophylaxis of gout flare:* if dose was originally 0.6 mg twice daily, ↓ to 0.3 mg once daily; if original regimen was 0.6 mg once daily, ↓ to 0.3 mg every other day; *for treatment of familial Mediterranean fever:* not to exceed 0.6 mg once daily or 0.3 mg twice daily). **Clarithromycin** and **erythromycin** may ↑ levels and risk of toxicity of darunavir and cobicistat; consider alternative anti-infectives. May ↑ levels and risk of toxicity of **dasatinib**, **nilotinib**, **vinblastine**, and **vincristine**; careful monitoring for toxicity and dose adjustments recommended. May ↑ bleeding risk with **apixaban** and **rivaroxaban**; may need to adjust apixaban dose; avoid concurrent use with rivaroxaban. Effect on **warfarin** is not known; monitor INR. **Oxcarbazepine** and **eslicarbazepine** may ↓ levels and effectiveness of cobicistat and tenofovir; consider alternative anticonvulsant or antiretroviral therapy. May ↑ levels and risk of toxicity of **clonazepam**; careful anticonvulsant monitoring recommended. May ↑ levels and risk of toxicity of **tricyclic antidepressants** and **trazodone**; careful dosing of antidepressants recommended (effect on **SSRIs** is unknown). May ↑ levels and risk of toxicity of **ketoconazole**, **isavuconazonium**, and **itraconazole**; effect on **voriconazole** unknown; concurrent use with voriconazole not recommended. Effects are unknown with **artemether/lumefantrine**; monitor for ↓ antimalarial activity or QT interval prolongation. May ↑ levels and risk of toxicity of **rifabutin**; ↓ rifabutin dose to 150 mg every other day. **Rifapentine** may ↓ levels and effectiveness of darunavir and tenofovir; concurrent use not recommended. May ↑ levels and risk of toxicity of **neuroleptics metabolized by CYP3A or CYP2D6**, including **perphenazine**, **risperidone**, and **thioridazine**; ↓ dose of neuroleptic may be necessary. May ↑ levels and risk of toxicity of **quetiapine**; if taking quetiapine when initiating therapy, consider alternative antiretroviral therapy or ↓ quetiapine dose to 1/6 of the original dose and monitor for adverse effects. May ↑ levels and risk of toxicity of **beta blockers metabolized by CYP2D6**, including **metoprolol**, **carvedilol**, and **timolol**; clinical monitoring recommended. May ↑ levels and risk of toxicity of **calcium channel blockers metabolized by CYP3A**, including **amlodipine**, **diltiazem**, **felodipine**, **nifedipine**, or **verapamil**; careful monitoring recommended. May ↑ levels and risk of toxicity of **antiarrhythmics**, including **amiodarone**, **disopyramide**, **flecainide**, **mexiletine**, **propafenone**, and **quinidine**; careful monitoring and titration is recommended. May ↑ levels and risk of toxicity of **digoxin**; closely monitor digoxin levels and adjust dose as needed. **Dexamethasone** may ↓ levels and effectiveness of cobicistat and darunavir; consider use of alternative corticosteroid, such as prednisone or prednisolone. May ↑ levels of **corticosteroids** (all routes of administration) primarily metabolized by the CYP3A isoenzyme (e.g., **betamethasone**, **budesonide**, **ciclesonide**, **fluticasone**, **methylprednisolone**, **mometasone**, or **triamcinolone**), which may ↑ the risk of Cushing disease and adrenal suppression; consider alternative corticosteroid, such as beclomethasone, prednisone, or prednisolone. **Bosentan** may ↑ levels and risk of toxicity of bosentan and ↓ levels and effectiveness of darunavir and cobicistat; dose alteration is required (*initiating bosentan in patients already receiving darunavir/cobicistat/emtricitabine/tenofovir alafenamide for ≥10 days:* bosentan 62.5 mg daily or every other day, depending on tolerance; *initiating darunavir/cobicistat/emtricitabine/tenofovir alafenamide in patient already receiving bosentan:* discontinue bosentan for 10 days; resume bosentan at 62.5 mg daily or every other day, depending on tolerance). May ↑ levels and risk of toxicity of **glecaprevir/pibrentasvir**; concurrent use not recommended.

D

Nephrotoxic agents, including **NSAIDs**, ↑ risk of nephrotoxicity; avoid concurrent use. May ↓ levels and contraceptive efficacy of some combined **hormonal contraceptives**; additional or alternative methods of nonhormonal contraception recommended. May ↑ risk of hyperkalemia when used with **drospirenone**. May ↑ levels and risk of toxicity of **immunosuppressants metabolized by CYP3A**, including **cyclosporine**, **everolimus**, **sirolimus**, and **tacrolimus**; therapeutic monitoring recommended. May ↑ levels and risk of toxicity of **irinotecan**; discontinue darunavir/cobicistat/emtricitabine/tenofovir alafenamide ≥1 wk before starting irinotecan therapy. May ↑ levels and risk of toxicity of **salmeterol** ; concurrent use not recommended. May ↑ levels and risk of myopathy from **atorvastatin**, **fluvastatin**, **pitavastatin**, **pravastatin**, or **rosuvastatin**; use lowest dose of these agents; do not exceed atorvastatin or rosuvastatin dose of 20 mg/day. May ↑ levels and risk of respiratory depression with opioids, including **buprenorphine**, **buprenorphine/naloxone**, **fentanyl**, **oxycodone**, and **tramadol**; carefully monitor for **opioid** effects; dose adjustment of opioid may be necessary. May ↑ levels and risk of toxicity of **PDE-5 inhibitors**, including **avanafil**, **sildenafil**, **tadalafil**, and **vardenafil**; **avanafil** use is not recommended; *sildenafil:* use for pulmonary hypertension is contraindicated; when used for erectile dysfunction, single dose should not exceed 25 mg/48 hr; *tadalafil:* for pulmonary hypertension, initiating tadalafil in patients receiving darunavir/cobicistat/emtricitabine/tenofovir alafenamide for ≥7 days: 20 mg once daily initially; may be titrated to 40 mg once daily; initiating darunavir/cobicistat/emtricitabine/tenofovir alafenamide in patients receiving tadalafil: discontinue tadalafil 24 hr prior to initiating therapy; after 7 days reinstitute tadalafil at 20 mg once daily; may be ↑ to 40 mg once daily; for erectile dysfunction, single dose should not exceed 10 mg/72 hr; *vardenafil:* for erectile dysfunction, single dose should not exceed 2.5 mg/72 hr. May ↑ levels and risk of bleeding with **ticagrelor**; concurrent use not recommended. May ↓ antiplatelet effects of **clopidogrel**; concurrent use not recommended. May ↑ levels and risk of excess sedation/respiratory depression from some **sedative/hypnotics metabolized by CYP3A**, including **buspirone**, **diazepam**, and **parenteral midazolam**; concurrent with **other sedative/hypnotics metabolized by CYP3A** should be undertaken with caution; dose ↓ may be necessary. May ↑ levels and risk of toxicity of **fesoterodine** and **solifenacin**; should not exceed fesoterodine dose of 4 mg once daily or solifenacin dose of 5 mg once daily.

Drug-Natural Products: **St. John's wort** may ↓ levels and effectiveness of cobicistat, darunavir, and tenofovir levels; concurrent use contraindicated.

Route/Dosage

PO (Adults and Children ≥40 kg): One tablet (darunavir 800 mg/cobicistat 150 mg/emtricitabine 200 mg/tenofovir alafenamide 10 mg) once daily.

Availability

Tablets: darunavir 800 mg/cobicistat 150 mg/emtricitabine 200 mg/tenofovir alafenamide 10 mg.

NURSING IMPLICATIONS

Assessment

- Assess patient for change in severity of HIV symptoms and for symptoms of opportunistic infections during therapy.
- Assess for allergy to sulfonamides.
- Monitor for development of rash. May cause SJS or TEN. Discontinue therapy if severe or if accompanied with fever, general malaise, fatigue, muscle or joint aches, blisters, oral lesions, conjunctivitis, hepatitis, or eosinophilia.

Lab Test Considerations

- Monitor viral load and CD4 count before and routinely during therapy to determine response.
- Assess for HBV. *Symtuza* is not approved for administration in patients with HIV and HBV. If therapy is discontinued, may cause severe exacerbation of HBV. Monitor liver function in coinfected patients for several months after stopping therapy.
- Monitor liver function tests prior to, during, and following therapy.
- Lactic acidosis may occur with hepatotoxicity causing hepatic steatosis; may be fatal, especially in women. Discontinue therapy if symptoms occur.
- May ↑ LDL-C, total cholesterol, and triglycerides.
- Monitor serum creatinine, CCr, urine glucose, and urine protein before and periodically during therapy and when clinically indicated. In patients with chronic kidney disease, assess serum creatinine, CCr, serum phosphorus, urine glucose, and urine protein before and periodically during therapy. May cause hypophosphatemia in patients with renal impairment.
- May cause hyperglycemia and glycosuria.

Implementation

- **PO:** Administer once daily with food. For patients who are unable to swallow the whole tablet, may be split into two pieces using a tablet cutter; consume entire dose immediately after splitting.

Patient/Family Teaching

- Explain purpose and side effects of medication to patient. Advise to read *Patient Information* before starting therapy and with each Rx refill in case of changes. Instruct patient to take as directed, even if feeling better. Do not take more than prescribed amount, and do not stop taking without consulting health care provider. Discontinuing therapy may lead to severe exacerbations. Take missed doses as soon as remembered unless almost time for next dose; do not double doses. Caution patient not to share or trade tablets with others.

- Instruct patient to notify health care provider of all Rx or OTC medications, vitamins, or herbal products being taken and consult health care provider before taking any new medications, especially St. John's wort.
- Inform patient of importance of HBV testing before starting antiretroviral therapy.
- Inform patient that *Symtuza* does not cure HIV and may ↓ risk of transmission of HIV to others through sexual contact or blood contamination. Caution patient to use a condom and avoid sharing needles or donating blood to prevent spreading HIV to others.
- Advise patient to notify health care provider immediately if symptoms of lactic acidosis (nausea; vomiting; unusual or unexpected stomach discomfort; unusual muscle pain; difficulty breathing; feeling cold, especially in arms and legs; dizziness, fast or irregular heartbeat; weakness or tiredness), liver problems (yellow skin or whites of eyes, dark urine, light-colored stools, loss of appetite, nausea, stomach pain), or signs of immune reconstitution syndrome (signs and symptoms of an infection or inflammation) occur.
- Inform patient that redistribution and accumulation of body fat may occur, causing central obesity, dorsocervical fat enlargement (buffalo hump), peripheral wasting, breast enlargement, and cushingoid appearance. The cause and long-term effects are not known.
- Emphasize the importance of regular follow-up exams and blood counts to determine progress.
- Rep: Advise women of reproductive potential to notify health care provider if pregnancy is planned or suspected. Encourage pregnant women to enroll in the Antiretroviral Pregnancy Registry by calling 1-800-258-4263 to monitor pregnancy outcomes. Advise patient that pregnancy is not recommended during treatment and to avoid breastfeeding during therapy.

Evaluation/Desired Outcomes

- Increased CD4 cell counts and a decrease in viral load with subsequent slowed progression of HIV infection and its sequelae.

HIGH ALERT

V DAUNOrubicin hydrochloride

(daw-noe-**roo**-bi-sin **hye**-dro-**klor**-ide)

✱ Cerubidine

Classification

Therapeutic: antineoplastics

Pharmacologic: anthracyclines

Indications

Remission induction of various leukemias.

Action

Forms a complex with DNA, which subsequently inhibits DNA and RNA synthesis (cell-cycle phase-nonspecific). **Therapeutic Effects:** Death of rapidly replicating cells, particularly malignant ones.

Pharmacokinetics

Absorption: IV administration results in complete bioavailability.

Distribution: Widely distributed to tissues.

Metabolism and Excretion: Extensively metabolized by the liver. Converted partially to a compound that also has antineoplastic activity (daunorubicinol); 40% eliminated by biliary excretion.

Half-life: *Daunorubicin:* 18.5 hr. *Daunorubicinol:* 26.7 hr.

TIME/ACTION PROFILE (effects on blood counts)

ROUTE	ONSET	PEAK	DURATION
IV	7–10 days	10–14 days	21 days

Contraindications/Precautions

Contraindicated in: Hypersensitivity to daunorubicin or any other components in the formulation; Symptomatic HF or arrhythmias; OB: Pregnancy; Lactation: Lactation.

Use Cautiously in: Active infections or decreased bone marrow reserve; Previous radiation therapy (may reactivate skin lesions); Renal impairment (↓ dose); Hepatic impairment (↓ dose); Previous anthracycline therapy or underlying cardiovascular disease (↑ risk of cardiotoxicity); Rep: Women of reproductive potential; Geri: ↓ dose recommended for patients ≥60 yr.

Adverse Reactions/Side Effects

CV: arrhythmias, CARDIOTOXICITY. **Derm:** alopecia. **EENT:** rhinitis, abnormal vision, sinusitis. **GI:** nausea, vomiting, esophagitis, hepatoxicity, stomatitis. **GU:** red urine, gonadal suppression. **Hemat:** anemia, leukopenia, thrombocytopenia. **Local:** phlebitis at IV site. **Metab:** hyperuricemia. **Misc:** chills, fever.

Interactions

Drug-Drug: Additive myelosuppression with other **antineoplastics**. May ↓ antibody response to **live-virus vaccines** and ↑ risk of adverse reactions. **Cyclophosphamide** and **trastuzumab** may ↑ risk of cardiotoxicity; avoid use of daunorubicin for up to 7 mo after discontinuing trastuzumab. May ↑ risk of hepatotoxicity with other **hepatotoxic agents**.

Route/Dosage

In adults, cumulative dose should not exceed 550 mg/m² (450 mg/m² if previous chest radiation).

IV (Adults <60 yr): 45 mg/m²/day for 3 days in 1st course, then for 2 days of 2nd course (as part of combination regimen).
IV (Adults ≥60 yr): 30 mg/m²/day for 3 days in 1st course, then for 2 days of 2nd course (as part of combination regimen).
IV (Children >2 yr): 25 mg/m² once weekly (as part of combination regimen). In children <2 yr or BSA <0.5 m², dose should be determined on a mg/kg basis.

Renal Impairment
IV (Adults): *CCr 30–50 mL/min:* Administer 75% of normal dose; *CCr <30 mL/min or hemodialysis:* Administer 50% of normal dose.

Hepatic Impairment
IV (Adults): *Serum bilirubin 1.2–3 mg/dL:* Administer 75% of normal dose; *Serum bilirubin >3 mg/dL:* Administer 50% of normal dose.

Availability (generic available)
Solution for injection: 5 mg/mL.

NURSING IMPLICATIONS
Assessment
- Monitor vital signs before and frequently during therapy.
- Monitor for bone marrow suppression. Assess for bleeding (bleeding gums; bruising; petechiae; guaiac stools, urine, and emesis) and avoid IM injections and taking rectal temperatures if platelet count is low. Apply pressure to venipuncture sites for 10 min. Assess for signs of infection during neutropenia. Anemia may occur. Monitor for ↑ fatigue, dyspnea, and orthostatic hypotension.
- Monitor intake and output, appetite, and nutritional intake. Assess for nausea and vomiting, which, although mild, may persist for 24–48 hr. Administrating an antiemetic before and periodically during therapy and adjusting diet as tolerated may help maintain fluid and electrolyte balance and nutritional status. Encourage fluid intake of 2000–3000 mL/day. Allopurinol and alkalinization of the urine may be used to help prevent urate stone formation.
- Assess for evidence of cardiotoxicity, which manifests as HF (peripheral edema, dyspnea, rales/crackles, weight gain, JVD) and usually occurs 1–6 mo after initiation of therapy. Obtain chest x-ray, echocardiography, ECGs, and radionuclide angiography determination of left ventricular ejection fraction (LVEF) before each course of therapy and periodically during therapy. A 30% ↓ in QRS voltage and ↓ in LVEF are early signs of cardiotoxicity. Patients who receive total cumulative doses >550/mm², who have a history of cardiac disease, or who have received mediastinal radiation are at ↑ risk of developing cardiotoxicity. Cardiotoxicity may develop if cumulative dose >400–550 mg/m² in adults, 300 mg/m² in children >2 yr, or 10 mg/kg in children <2 yr. May be irreversible and fatal, but usually responds to early treatment.

Lab Test Considerations
- Monitor uric acid levels periodically during therapy.
- Monitor CBC and differential before and frequently during therapy. The leukocyte count nadir occurs 10–14 days after administration. Recovery usually occurs within 21 days after administration of daunorubicin.
- Monitor AST, ALT, LDH, and serum bilirubin prior to each course of therapy. May transiently ↑ serum alkaline phosphatase, bilirubin, and AST concentrations.
- Monitor renal function before each course of therapy.

Implementation
- ***High Alert:*** Fatalities have occurred with chemotherapeutic agents. Before administering, clarify all ambiguous orders; double-check single, daily, and course-of-therapy dose limits; have second practitioner independently double-check original order, calculations, and infusion pump settings.
- Do not confuse daunorubicin hydrochloride with doxorubicin or idarubicin. To prevent confusion, orders should include generic and brand name.
- ***High Alert:*** Administer under supervision of a physician experienced in use of cancer chemotherapeutic agents.
- Provide antiemetics before each infusion.

IV Administration
- **V** Daunorubicin is a vesicant. If extravasation occurs, immediately stop infusion. Leave needle/cannula in place temporarily but do not flush the line. Gently aspirate extravasated solution; then remove needle/cannula. Elevate patient's extremity and apply dry cold compresses for 20 min 4 times day for 1–2 days. Initiate antidote (dexrazoxane or topical dimethyl sulfoxide) based on time frame of noting extravasation. *If extravasation is noted ≤6 hr of daunorubicin infusion,* administer dexrazoxane 1000 mg/m² over 1–2 hr on Days 1 and 2 (max dose = 2000 mg/day), followed by 500 mg/m² over 1–2 hr on Day 3 (max dose = 1000 mg/day). Hold cold compresses 15 min before initiating and after completing dexrazoxane infusion. Concurrent treatment with topical dimethyl sulfoxide should not be used with dexrazoxane because it may ↓ dexrazoxane's effectiveness. *If extravasation is noted >6 hr after completion of daunorubicin infusion,* apply dimethyl sulfoxide by saturating a gauze pad and painting on an area twice the size of the extravasation. Allow site to air-dry and repeat application every 8 hr for 7 days. Do not cover the area with dressing.

- Wear gloves, gown, and mask while handling IV medication. Discard IV equipment in specially designated containers.
- **IV Push: Dilution:** Dilute appropriate volume of drug solution in 10–15 mL of 0.9% NaCl. Administer IV push through Y-site into free-flowing infusion of 0.9% NaCl or D5W.
- **Rate:** Administer over 2–3 min. Rapid administration rate may cause facial flushing or erythema along the vein.
- **Intermittent Infusion: Dilution:** Appropriate volume of drug solution may also be diluted in 50–100 mL of 0.9% NaCl. **Rate:** Infuse 50 mL over 10–15 min or 100 mL over 30–45 min.
- **Y-Site Compatibility:** alemtuzumab, amikacin, amiodarone, anidulafungin, argatroban, arsenic trioxide, atracurium, bivalirudin, bleomycin, bumetanide, buprenorphine, butorphanol, calcium chloride, calcium gluconate, carboplatin, carmustine, caspofungin, chlorpromazine, ciprofloxacin, cisatracurium, cisplatin, cyclophosphamide, cyclosporine, cytarabine, dacarbazine, dactinomycin, daptomycin, dexmedetomidine, dexrazoxane, digoxin, diltiazem, diphenhydramine, dobutamine, docetaxel, dopamine, doxycycline, droperidol, enalaprilat, ephedrine, epinephrine, erythromycin, esmolol, etoposide, etoposide phosphate, famotidine, fentanyl, filgrastim, fluconazole, gemcitabine, gemtuzumab ozogamicin, gentamicin, glycopyrrolate, granisetron, haloperidol, hydralazine, hydrocortisone, hydromorphone, idarubicin, imipenem/cilastatin, insulin regular, irinotecan, isoproterenol, labetalol, leucovorin, lidocaine, linezolid, lorazepam, magnesium sulfate, mannitol, melphalan, meperidine, meropenem, methadone, methotrexate, metoclopramide, metoprolol, metronidazole, midazolam, milrinone, minocycline, mitomycin, morphine, moxifloxacin, nalbuphine, naloxone, nitroglycerin, norepinephrine, octreotide, ondansetron, oxaliplatin, paclitaxel, palonosetron, pentamidine, phentolamine, phenylephrine, potassium acetate, potassium chloride, potassium phosphates, procainamide, prochlorperazine, promethazine, propranolol, remifentanil, rituximab, sodium acetate, sodium bicarbonate, sodium phosphates, succinylcholine, sufentanil, tacrolimus, theophylline, thiotepa, tigecycline, tobramycin, topotecan, trastuzumab, vancomycin, vecuronium, verapamil, vinblastine, vincristine, vinorelbine, voriconazole, zidovudine, zoledronic acid.
- **Y-Site Incompatibility:** acyclovir, allopurinol, aminophylline, amphotericin B deoxycholate, amphotericin B liposomal, ampicillin, ampicillin/sulbactam, aztreonam, cefazolin, cefepime, cefotaxime, cefotetan, cefoxitin, ceftazidime, ceftriaxone, cefuroxime, chloramphenicol, clindamycin, dantrolene, dexamethasone, diazepam, ertapenem, fludarabine, foscarnet, fosphenytoin, furosemide, ganciclovir, heparin, indomethacin, ketorolac, levofloxacin, methohexital, methylprednisolone, mitoxantrone, nafcillin, nitroprusside, pantoprazole, pemetrexed, pentobarbital, phenobarbital, phenytoin, piperacillin/tazobactam, trimethoprim/sulfamethoxazole.

D

Patient/Family Teaching

- Explain purpose and side effects of medication to patient. Advise patient to read *Patient Information* before starting therapy.
- Advise patient to notify health care provider of all Rx or OTC medications, vitamins, or herbal products being taken and to consult health care provider before taking other medications, especially products containing aspirin or NSAIDs.
- Instruct patient to notify health care provider if fever; chills; sore throat; signs of infection; bleeding gums; bruising; petechiae; or blood in urine, stool, or emesis occurs. Caution patient to avoid crowds and persons with known infections. Instruct patient to use soft toothbrush and electric razor. Patient should be cautioned not to drink alcoholic beverages.
- Instruct patient to inspect oral mucosa for erythema and ulceration. If ulceration occurs, advise patient to use sponge brush and rinse mouth with water after eating and drinking. Stomatitis pain may require management with opioid analgesics. Period of highest risk is 3–7 days after administration of dose.
- Instruct patient to notify health care provider immediately if irregular heartbeat, shortness of breath, or swelling of lower extremities occurs.
- Discuss possibility of hair loss with patient. Explore methods of coping. Regrowth of hair usually begins within 5 wk after discontinuing therapy.
- Inform patient that medication may turn urine reddish color for 1–2 days after administration.
- Instruct patient not to receive any vaccinations without advice of health care provider.
- Emphasize the need for periodic lab tests to monitor for side effects.
- Rep: May cause fetal harm. Advise women of reproductive potential and men with female partners of reproductive potential to use effective contraception during therapy and for >4 mo after last dose. Advise women to avoid breastfeeding during therapy. May impair fertility.

Evaluation/Desired Outcomes

- Death of rapidly replicating cells, particularly malignant ones.

deferoxamine (de-fer-**ox**-a-meen)

Desferal

Classification

Therapeutic: antidotes

Pharmacologic: heavy metal antagonists

Indications

Acute toxic iron ingestion. Secondary iron overload syndromes associated with multiple transfusion therapy.

Action

Chelates unbound iron, forming a water-soluble complex (ferrioxamine) in plasma that is easily excreted by the kidneys. **Therapeutic Effects:** Removal of excess iron. Also chelates aluminum.

Pharmacokinetics

Absorption: Poorly absorbed after oral administration. Well absorbed after IM administration and SUBQ administration. IV administration results in complete bioavailability.

Distribution: Appears to be widely distributed.

Metabolism and Excretion: Metabolized by tissues and plasma enzymes. Unchanged drug and chelated form excreted by the kidneys; 33% of iron removed is eliminated in the feces via biliary excretion.

Half-life: 1 hr.

TIME/ACTION PROFILE (effects on hematologic parameters)

ROUTE	ONSET	PEAK	DURATION
IV	rapid	unknown	unknown
IM	unknown	unknown	unknown
SUBQ	unknown	unknown	unknown

Contraindications/Precautions

Contraindicated in: Severe renal impairment; Anuria; Lactation: Lactation.

Use Cautiously in: OB: Safety not established in pregnancy. Treatment should not be withheld in pregnant women with acute iron toxicity; Pedi: Children <3 yr (safety and effectiveness not established).

Adverse Reactions/Side Effects

CV: hypotension, tachycardia. **Derm:** erythema, flushing, urticaria. **EENT:** blurred vision, cataracts, ototoxicity. **GI:** abdominal pain, diarrhea. **GU:** red urine. **Local:** induration at injection site, pain at injection site. **MS:** leg cramps. **Misc:** fever, HYPERSENSITIVITY REACTIONS (INCLUDING ANAPHYLAXIS), shock (after rapid IV administration).

Interactions

Drug-Drug: Ascorbic acid may ↑ effectiveness of deferoxamine but may also risk of ↑ cardiac iron toxicity.

Route/Dosage

Acute Iron Ingestion

IM, IV (Adults and Children ≥3 yr): 1 g initially; then 500 mg every 4 hr for 2 doses. Additional doses of 500 mg every 4–12 hr may be needed (not to exceed 6 g/24 hr).

Chronic Iron Overload

IM, IV (Adults and Children ≥3 yr): 500 mg–1 g daily IM; additional doses of 2 g should be given IV for each unit of blood transfused (not to exceed 1 g/day in absence of transfusions; 6 g/day if patient receives transfusions).

SUBQ (Adults and Children ≥3 yr): 1–2 g/day (20–40 mg/kg/day).

Availability (generic available)

Powder for injection: 500 mg/vial, 2 g/vial.

NURSING IMPLICATIONS

Assessment

- In acute poisoning, assess time, amount, and type of iron preparation ingested.
- Monitor for signs of iron toxicity: early acute (abdominal pain, bloody diarrhea, emesis) and late acute (↓ level of consciousness, shock, metabolic acidosis).
- Monitor vital signs closely, especially during IV administration, for hypersensitivity reactions. Report hypotension, erythema, urticaria, or signs of allergic reaction. Keep epinephrine, an antihistamine, and resuscitation equipment close by in the event of an anaphylactic reaction.
- May cause oculotoxicity or ototoxicity. Report ↓ visual acuity or hearing loss. Audiovisual exams should be performed every 3 mo in patients with chronic iron overload.
- Monitor intake and output and urine color. Inform health care professional if patient is anuric. Chelated iron is excreted primarily by the kidneys; urine may turn red.

Lab Test Considerations

- Monitor serum iron, total iron binding capacity (TIBC), and ferritin levels, as well as urinary iron excretion before and periodically during therapy.
- Monitor liver function to assess damage from iron poisoning.

Implementation

- IM route is preferred in acute iron intoxication unless patient is in shock.
- **IM** Administer deep IM and massage well. Rotate sites. IM administration may cause transient severe pain.
- **Reconstitution:** Reconstitute 500-mg vial with 2 mL and 2-g vial with 8 mL of sterile water for injection. Reconstituted solution is yellow and stable for 1 wk after reconstitution if protected

from light. Discard unused portion. **Concentration:** 213 mg/mL.

- Used in conjunction with induction of emesis or gastric aspiration and lavage with sodium bicarbonate and supportive measures for shock and metabolic acidosis in acute poisoning.
- **SUBQ: Reconstitution:** Reconstitute 500-mg vial with 5 mL and 2-g vial with 20 mL of sterile water for injection. **Concentration:** 95 mg/mL. SUBQ route used to treat chronically elevated iron therapy is administered into abdominal SUBQ tissue via infusion pump for 8–24 hr per treatment.

IV Administration

- **IV: Reconstitution:** Reconstitute 500-mg vial with 5 mL and 2-g vial with 20 mL of sterile water for injection. Reconstituted solution is clear and colorless to slightly yellow. Administer <3 hr of reconstitution or 24 hr if prepared under laminar flow hood. Discard unused portion. **Concentration:** 95 mg/mL. **Dilution:** Further dilute reconstituted solution in D5W, 0.9% NaCl, 0.45% NaCl, or LR. **Concentration:** 3–3.5 mg/mL.
- **Rate:** Maximum infusion rate is 15 mg/kg/hr for first 1000 mg. May be followed by 500 mg infused over 4 hr at a slower rate, not to exceed 125 mg/hr. Rapid infusion rate may cause hypotension, erythema, urticaria, wheezing, convulsions, tachycardia, or shock.
- May be administered at the same time as blood transfusion in persons with chronically ↑ serum iron levels. Use separate site for administration.

Patient/Family Teaching

- Explain purpose and side effects of medication to patient. Advise to read *Patient Information* before starting therapy.
- Advise patient to notify health care professional of all Rx or OTC medications, vitamins, or herbal products being taken and to consult health care professional before taking other medications.
- Reassure patient that red coloration of urine is expected and reflects excretion of excess iron.
- May cause dizziness or impairment of vision or hearing. Caution patient to avoid driving or other activities requiring alertness until response from medication is known.
- Advise patient not to take vitamin C preparations without consulting health care professional. May ↑ tissue toxicity.
- Encourage patients requiring chronic therapy to keep follow-up appointments for lab tests. Eye and hearing exams may be monitored every 3 mo.
- Rep: Advise women of reproductive potential to notify health care professional if pregnancy is planned or suspected. Breastfeeding should be avoided during therapy and for 1 wk after the last dose.

Evaluation/Desired Outcomes

- Removal of excess iron. Also chelates aluminum.

delafloxacin, See FLUOROQUINOLONES.

D

REMS

denosumab (de-no-su-mab)

Jubbonti, Osenvelt, Ospomyv, Prolia, Stoboclo, Wyost, Xbryk, Xgeva

Classification

Therapeutic: bone resorption inhibitors

Pharmacologic: monoclonal antibodies

Indications

Jubbonti, Ospomyv, Prolia, or Stoboclo: Treatment of osteoporosis in postmenopausal women who are at high risk for fracture or those who have failed/are intolerant of conventional osteoporosis therapy. To increase bone mass in men with osteoporosis who are at high risk for fracture or those who have failed/are intolerant of conventional osteoporosis therapy. Treatment of glucocorticoid-induced osteoporosis in men and women at high risk for fracture who are initiating or continuing systemic glucocorticoids at a daily dosage of ≥7.5 mg of prednisone and are expected to remain on glucocorticoids for ≥6 mo. To increase bone mass in men receiving androgen deprivation therapy for nonmetastatic prostate cancer who are at high risk for fracture. To increase bone mass in women receiving adjuvant aromatase inhibitor therapy for breast cancer who are at high risk for fracture. **Osenvelt, Xbryk, Xgeva, or Wyost:** Prevention of skeletal-related events in patients with multiple myeloma and in patients with bone metastases from solid tumors. Giant cell tumor of bone that is unresectable or where surgical resection is likely to result in severe morbidity. Hypercalcemia of malignancy that is refractory to bisphosphonate therapy.

Action

A monoclonal antibody that binds specifically to the human receptor activator of nuclear factor kappa-B-ligand (RANKL), which is required for formation, function, and survival of osteoclasts. Binding inhibits osteoclast formation, function, and survival. **Therapeutic Effects:** ↓ bone resorption with ↓ occurrence of fractures (vertebral, nonvertebral, hip) or other skeletal-related events (e.g., radiation therapy to bone, surgery to bone, spinal cord compression). ↑ bone mass.

Pharmacokinetics

Absorption: Well absorbed following SUBQ administration.
Distribution: Unknown.
Metabolism and Excretion: Unknown.
Half-life: 25.4 days.

TIME/ACTION PROFILE (effects on bone resorption)

ROUTE	ONSET	PEAK	DURATION
SUBQ	1 mo	unknown†	12 mo‡

† Maximum ↓ in serum calcium occurs at 10 days.
‡ Following discontinuation.

Contraindications/Precautions

Contraindicated in: Hypersensitivity; Hypocalcemia (correct before administration); OB: Pregnancy; Lactation: Lactation.
Use Cautiously in: Hypoparathyroidism, previous thyroid/parathyroid surgery, malabsorption syndromes, history of small intestinal excision, concurrent use of calcium-lowering medications, or severe renal impairment/hemodialysis (↑ risk of hypocalcemia; patients with severe renal impairment, including those on dialysis or with mineral bone disorder, at ↑ risk of severe hypocalcemia); Invasive dental procedures; cancer; receiving chemotherapy, corticosteroids, or angiogenesis inhibitors; poor oral hygiene; diabetes; gingival infections; periodontal disease; dental disease; anemia; coagulopathy; infection; or poorly fitting dentures (↑ risk of jaw osteonecrosis); History of osteoporosis or prior fractures (↑ risk of multiple vertebral fractures upon drug discontinuation); Concurrent use of immunosuppressants or diseases resulting in immunosuppression (↑ risk of infection); Rep: Women of reproductive potential; Pedi: Safety and effectiveness not established in children; Geri: Older adults may be more sensitive to drug effects.

Adverse Reactions/Side Effects

Derm: dermatitis, eczema, rash. **F and E** HYPOCALCEMIA, hypophosphatemia, hypercalcemia. **GI:** diarrhea, nausea, PANCREATITIS. **GU:** cystitis. **Metab:** hypercholesterolemia. **MS:** back pain, musculoskeletal pain, atypical femoral fracture, osteonecrosis of the jaw, suppression of bone turnover. **Neuro:** headache. **Resp:** dyspnea, cough. **Misc:** HYPERSENSITIVITY REACTIONS (INCLUDING ANAPHYLAXIS), infection.

Interactions

Drug-Drug: Immunosuppressants may ↑ risk of infection. **Calcimimetic drugs** may ↑ risk of hypocalcemia.

Route/Dosage

Jubbonti, Ospomyv, Prolia, or Stoboclo

SUBQ (Adults): 60 mg every 6 mo.

Osenvelt, Xbryk, Xgeva, or Wyost

SUBQ (Adults): *Multiple myeloma or bone metastasis from solid tumors:* 120 mg every 4 wk; *Giant cell tumor of bone:* 120 mg every 4 wk, with additional doses of 120 mg given on Days 8 and 15 of first month of therapy; *Hypercalcemia of malignancy:* 120 mg every 4 wk, with additional doses of 120 mg given on Days 8 and 15 of first month of therapy.

Availability (generic available)

Solution for injection (Jubbonti, Ospomyv, Prolia, or Stoboclo) (prefilled syringe): 60 mg/mL.
Solution for injection (Osenvelt, Xbryk, Xgeva, or Wyost): 120 mg/1.7 mL.

NURSING IMPLICATIONS

Assessment

- Assess via bone density study for low bone mass before and periodically during therapy.
- Perform a routine oral exam before initiation of therapy. Dental exam with appropriate preventative dentistry should be considered before therapy. Patients with history of tooth extraction, poor oral hygiene, gingival infections, diabetes, or use of a dental appliance or those taking immunosuppressive therapy, angiogenesis inhibitors, or systemic corticosteroids are at greater risk for osteonecrosis of the jaw.
- Assess for signs and symptoms of pancreatitis (severe abdominal pain, fever, nausea/vomiting, jaundice).
- Monitor for signs and symptoms of hypersensitivity reactions (hypotension, dyspnea, upper airway edema, lip swelling, rash, pruritus, urticaria). Treat symptomatically and discontinue medication if symptoms occur.

Lab Test Considerations

- Verify negative pregnancy status before starting therapy.
- Assess calcium, phosphorous, and magnesium levels before and periodically during therapy, especially during 1st wk of therapy. Correct hypocalcemia and vitamin D deficiency before starting therapy. May cause mild, transient ↑ of calcium and phosphate. Supplement with calcium, magnesium, and vitamin D as needed.
- In patients with advanced chronic kidney disease (eGFR <30 mL/min/1.73 m^2), assess for presence of metabolic bone disorder by evaluating intact parathyroid hormone, serum calcium, and vitamin D levels before starting therapy.
- May cause hypercalcemia within the year following discontinuation. Monitor for signs and symptoms of hypercalcemia, assess serum calcium periodically, reevaluate the patient's calcium and vitamin D supplementation requirements, and manage as clinically necessary.
- May cause anemia.
- May cause hypercholesterolemia.

Implementation

- Use of Prolia in patients with advanced chronic kidney disease should be supervised by a health care provider with expertise in the diagnosis and management of chronic kidney disease-metabolic bone disorder.
- ***REMS:*** The FDA-approved REMS consists of a communication plan and a timetable for REMS assessments that must be submitted to the FDA. More information is available at https://www.proliahcp.com/risk-evaluation-mitigation-strategy or by calling Amgen at 1-800-772-6436.
- **SUBQ**: Should be administered by a health care provider. Remove from refrigerator and bring to room temperature (15–30 min) before administration; do not warm in any other way. Do not shake. Administer using a 27-gauge needle in the upper arm, upper thigh, or abdomen. Solution is clear and colorless to pale yellow and may contain trace amounts of translucent to white proteinaceous particles. Do not use if solution is discolored, cloudy, or contains many particles. Manually activate the green safety guard *after* the injection is given, not before.
- Patients should receive calcium 1000 mg and vitamin D 400 units daily.

Patient/Family Teaching

- Explain purpose and side effects of medication to patient. Do not stop receiving drug without consulting health care provider. If an appointment is missed, contact health care provider as soon as possible to reschedule. Advise patient to read *Patient Information* before starting therapy.
- Advise patient to notify health care provider of all Rx or OTC medications, vitamins, or herbal products being taken and to consult health care provider before taking other medications.
- Advise patient once treatment is stopped, there may be an ↑ risk of having broken bones in the spine, especially in patients who have had a fracture or who have had osteoporosis. Advise patients not to interrupt therapy without advice from a health care provider. If denosumab is discontinued, consider another bone resorption inhibitor.
- Advise patient to eat a balanced diet and consult health care provider about the need for supplemental calcium and vitamin D (see Appendix J).
- Advise patient to notify health care provider immediately if signs of hypersensitivity, hypocalcemia (spasms, twitches, or cramps in muscles; numbness or tingling in fingers, toes, or around mouth), infection (fever; chills; skin that is red, swollen, hot, or tender to touch; severe abdominal pain; frequent or urgent need to urinate or burning during urination), skin reactions (redness, itching, rash, dry or leathery feeling, blisters that ooze or become crusty, peeling), or osteonecrosis of the jaw (pain; numbness; swelling of or drainage from the jaw, mouth, or teeth) occur.
- Encourage patient to participate in regular exercise and to modify behaviors that ↑ the risk of osteoporosis (stop smoking, reduce alcohol consumption).
- Advise patient to perform oral hygiene of teeth and gums (brush and floss regularly) and to inform health care provider of therapy before dental surgery.
- Rep: Advise women of reproductive potential to use highly effective contraception during and for >5 mo after therapy is completed. Advise patient to notify health care provider if pregnancy is planned or suspected or if breastfeeding.

Evaluation/Desired Outcomes

- ↓ bone resorption with ↓ occurrence of fractures (vertebral, nonvertebral, hip) or other skeletal-related events (e.g., radiation therapy to bone, surgery to bone, spinal cord compression).
- ↑ bone mass.

D

BEERS

desipramine (dess-**ip**-ra-meen)

Norpramin

Classification

Therapeutic: antidepressants

Pharmacologic: tricyclic antidepressants

Indications

Depression. **Unlabeled Use:** Chronic pain syndromes. Anxiety. Insomnia.

Action

Potentiates the effect of serotonin and norepinephrine in the CNS. Has significant anticholinergic properties. **Therapeutic Effects:** Antidepressant action (may develop only over several wk).

Pharmacokinetics

Absorption: Well absorbed from the GI tract.
Distribution: Widely distributed.
Protein Binding: 90–92%.
Metabolism and Excretion: Mostly metabolized by the liver by the CYP2D6 isoenzyme; one metabolite is pharmacologically active (2-hydroxydesipramine); the CYP2D6 enzyme system exhibits genetic polymorphism; ~7% of population may be poor metabolizers and may have significantly ↑ desipramine concentrations and an ↑ risk of adverse effects. Small amounts enter breast milk.
Half-life: 12–27 hr.

TIME/ACTION PROFILE (antidepressant effect)

ROUTE	ONSET	PEAK	DURATION
PO	2–3 wk	2–6 wk	days–wk

Contraindications/Precautions

Contraindicated in: Angle-closure glaucoma; Recent MI, HF, or known history of QTc interval prolongation.

Use Cautiously in: Pre-existing cardiovascular disease; Family history of sudden death, cardiac arrhythmias, or conduction disturbances; Prostatic hyperplasia (↑ susceptibility to urinary retention); History of seizures (threshold may be ↓; seizures may precede the development of cardiac arrhythmias or death); May ↑ risk of suicide attempt/ideation, especially during early treatment or dose adjustment; risk may be greater in children or adolescents; Hypovolemia or dehydration (↑ risk of syndrome of inappropriate antidiuretic hormone secretion [SIADH]); OB: Use during pregnancy only if potential maternal benefit outweighs potential fetal risk; Lactation: Use while breastfeeding only if potential maternal benefit outweighs risk to infant; Pedi: Children <12 yr (safety not established); Geri: Appears on Beers list. ↑ risk of adverse reactions in older adults, including falls secondary to sedative and anticholinergic effects, orthostatic hypotension, and SIADH. Avoid use in older adults.

Adverse Reactions/Side Effects

CV: hypotension, ARRHYTHMIAS, ECG changes. **Derm:** photosensitivity. **EENT:** blurred vision, dry eyes. **Endo:** changes in blood glucose, gynecomastia.
F and E hyponatremia, SIADH. **GI:** constipation, dry mouth, hepatitis, paralytic ileus. **GU:** ↓ libido, urinary retention. **Hemat:** blood dyscrasias. **Metab:** ↑ appetite, weight gain. **Neuro:** drowsiness, fatigue, SUICIDAL THOUGHTS/BEHAVIORS.

Interactions

Drug-Drug: CYP2D6 inhibitors, including **cimetidine**, **quinidine**, **amiodarone**, and **ritonavir**, may ↑ levels and risk of toxicity. May cause hypotension, tachycardia, and potentially fatal reactions when used with **MAO inhibitors**; avoid concurrent use; discontinue 2 wk before starting desipramine. **SSRIs** may result in ↑ toxicity; avoid concurrent use. Fluoxetine should be stopped 5 wk before starting desipramine. **Clonidine** may ↑ risk of hypertensive crisis; avoid concurrent use. **Phenytoin** may ↓ levels and effectiveness; ↑ doses of desipramine may be required. **Levodopa** may ↑ risk of extrapyramidal reactions and hypertension. **Rifampin**, **carbamazepine**, **barbiturates**, and **cigarette smoking** may ↓ levels and effectiveness. Concurrent use with **moxifloxacin** may ↑ risk of adverse cardiovascular reactions. ↑ CNS depression with other **CNS depressants**, including **alcohol**, **antihistamines**, **clonidine**, **opioid analgesics**, and **sedative/hypnotics**. **Adrenergic** and **anticholinergic** side effects may be ↑ with other **agents having these properties**. **Hormonal contraceptives** may ↑ levels and risk of toxicity. **Diuretics** may ↑ risk of SIADH.
Drug-Natural Products: Kava-kava, **valerian**, or **chamomile** can ↑ CNS depression. ↑ anticholinergic effects with **jimson weed** and **scopolia**.

Route/Dosage

PO (Adults): 100–200 mg/day as a single dose or in divided doses (up to 300 mg/day).
PO (Geriatric Patients): 25–50 mg/day in divided doses (up to 150 mg/day).
PO (Children >12 yr): 25–50 mg/day in divided doses; may ↑ as needed up to 100 mg/day.
PO (Children 6–12 yr): 10–30 mg/day (1–5 mg/kg/day) in divided doses.

Availability (generic available)

Tablets: 10 mg, 25 mg, 50 mg, 75 mg, 100 mg, 150 mg.

NURSING IMPLICATIONS

Assessment

- Monitor for weight gain. Obtain weight and body mass index initially; at 3, 6, and 12 mo; and then yearly in all patients and if receiving combination therapy.
- Monitor BP and HR at baseline, with significant dose ↑, and every 3–6 mo once stabilized. Notify health care provider of ↓ in BP (by 10–20 mm Hg) or sudden ↑ in HR. Monitor ECG prior to and periodically during therapy in patients taking high doses or with a history of cardiovascular disease.
- Assess for signs and symptoms of serotonin syndrome (confusion, delirium, agitation, coma, dilated pupils, tachycardia, hyperthermia, shivering, hyperreflexia, muscle rigidity, hypertension, vomiting, diarrhea, seizures). ↑ risk of serotonin syndrome with concurrent use of other serotonergic drugs (SSRIs, SNRIs, triptans); monitoring recommended; discontinuation may be required.
- Assess for signs and symptoms of SIADH (hyponatremia, headache, muscle cramps or weakness, tremors).
- **Depression:** Monitor mental status (orientation, mood behavior) frequently. Assess for suicidal tendencies, especially during early therapy. Restrict amount of drug available to patient. Risk may be ↑ in children, adolescents, and adults ≤24 yr. After starting therapy, children, adolescents, and young adults should be seen by health care provider at least weekly for 4 wk, every 3 wk for next 4 wk, and on advice of health care provider thereafter.
- **Pain:** Assess intensity, quality, and location of pain periodically during therapy.

Lab Test Considerations

- Assess CBC with differential, liver function, and serum glucose periodically. May ↑ serum bilirubin and alkaline phosphatase. May cause bone marrow depression. Serum glucose may be ↑ or ↓.

- Assess sodium level at baseline and after 3–4 wk in high-risk patients (>65 yr, previous history of antidepressant-induced hyponatremia, ↓ body weight, concurrent use of thiazides or other hyponatremia-inducing agents).
- Serum levels may be monitored in patients who fail to respond to usual therapeutic dose; therapeutic reference range is 100–300 ng/mL when used as an antidepressant.
- Assess fasting blood glucose and cholesterol levels for overweight/obese individuals.

Implementation

- Do not confuse despiramine with disopyramide.
- Begin dose ↑ at bedtime due to sedation. Dose titration is a slow process; may take wk to mo. May give entire dose at bedtime.
- When discontinuing, taper to avoid withdrawal effects. ↓ dose by 50% for 3 days; then ↓ again by 50% for 3 days; then discontinue. May require 2–4 wk to discontinue.
- **PO:** Administer medication with or immediately after a meal to minimize gastric upset. Tablet may be crushed and given with food or fluids.

Patient/Family Teaching

- Explain the purpose and side effects of desipramine. Instruct patient to take as directed. Take missed doses as soon as possible unless almost time for next dose; if regimen is a single dose at bedtime, do not take in the morning because of side effects. Advise patient that drug effects may not be noticed for ≥2 wk. Abrupt discontinuation may cause nausea; vomiting; diarrhea; headache; trouble sleeping, with vivid dreams; and irritability; ↓ dose gradually. Instruct patient to read the *Medication Guide* prior to starting and with each Rx refill in case of changes.
- Therapy for depression is usually prolonged. Emphasize the importance of follow-up exams to monitor effectiveness and side effects and to improve coping skills.
- May cause drowsiness and blurred vision. Caution patient to avoid driving and other activities requiring alertness until response to drug is known.
- Orthostatic hypotension, SIADH, sedation, and confusion are common during early therapy, especially in older adults. Protect patient from falls and advise patient to make position changes slowly. Institute fall precautions. Advise patient to make position changes slowly.
- Advise patient to avoid alcohol or other CNS depressant drugs, including opioids, during and for 3–7 days after therapy has been discontinued.
- Advise patient, family, and caregivers to look for suicidality, especially during early therapy or dose changes. Notify health care provider immediately if thoughts about suicide or dying, attempts to commit suicide, new or worse depression or anxiety, agitation or restlessness, panic attacks, insomnia, new or worse irritability, aggressiveness, acting on dangerous impulses, mania, or other changes in mood or behavior occur.
- Instruct patient to notify health care provider if urinary retention, dry mouth, or constipation persists. Sugarless candy or gum may diminish dry mouth, and an ↑ in fluids or bulk may prevent constipation. If symptoms persist, dose ↓ or discontinuation may be necessary. Consult health care provider if dry mouth persists for >2 wk.
- Caution patient to use sunscreen and protective clothing to prevent photosensitivity reactions.
- Inform patient of need to monitor dietary intake. ↑ in appetite may lead to undesired weight gain. Refer as appropriate for nutrition/weight management and medical management.
- Alert patient that medication may turn urine blue-green in color.
- Advise patient to notify health care provider of medication regimen prior to treatment or surgery.
- Rep: Advise women of reproductive potential to notify health care provider if pregnancy is planned or suspected or if breastfeeding. Enroll pregnant patients in National Pregnancy Registry for Antidepressants by calling 1-844-405-6185 or visiting https://womensmentalhealth.org/clinical-and-researchprograms/pregnancyregistry/antidepressants to monitor outcomes in women exposed to antidepressants.

Evaluation/Desired Outcomes

- Increased sense of well-being.
- Renewed interest in surroundings.
- Increased appetite. Improved energy level.
- Improved sleep.
- Decrease in chronic pain symptoms.
- Full therapeutic effects may be seen 2–6 wk after initiating therapy.

BEERS

desmopressin

(des-moe-**press**-in)

✱ Bipazen, DDAVP, ✱ DDAVP Melt, Nocdurna, ✱ Octostim

Classification

Therapeutic: hormones

Pharmacologic: antidiuretic hormones

Indications

PO, SL SUBQ IV: Intranasal Central diabetes insipidus caused by a deficiency of vasopressin.

IV: Bleeding in certain types of hemophilia and von Willebrand disease. **Intranasal sublingual** Nocturia due to nocturnal polyuria in patients who awaken ≥2 times per night to void (Nocdurna only). **PO, SL** Primary nocturnal enuresis.

Action

An analogue of naturally occurring vasopressin (antidiuretic hormone). Primary action is enhanced reabsorption of water in the kidneys. **Therapeutic Effects:** Prevention of nocturnal enuresis. Reduction in number of episodes of nocturia. Maintenance of appropriate body water content in diabetes insipidus. Control of bleeding in certain types of hemophilia or von Willebrand disease.

Pharmacokinetics

Absorption: <1% absorbed following oral or SL administration; 3–4% absorbed following intranasal administration.

Distribution: Distribution not fully known.

Metabolism and Excretion: Primarily excreted in urine.

Half-life: *PO:* 1.5–2.5 hr; *SL:* 2.8 hr; *IV:* 75 min (↑ in renal impairment); *Intranasal:* 1.8–3.5 hr.

TIME/ACTION PROFILE (PO, intranasal = antidiuretic effect; IV = effect on factor VIII activity)

ROUTE	ONSET	PEAK	DURATION
PO	1 hr	4–7 hr	unknown
SL	unknown	unknown	unknown
Intranasal	1 hr	1–5 hr	8–20 hr
IV	within min	15–30 min	3 hr†

† 4–24 hr in mild hemophilia A.

Contraindications/Precautions

Contraindicated in: Hypersensitivity; Hypersensitivity to chlorobutanol; Patients with severe type I, type IIB, or platelet-type (pseudo) von Willebrand disease; hemophilia A with factor VIII levels <5%; or hemophilia B; Renal impairment (CCr <50 mL/min); Current or a history of hyponatremia; Excessive fluid intake, concurrent use of loop diuretics or systemic/inhaled glucocorticoids, or conditions that can lead to electrolyte or fluid imbalances (↑ risk of hyponatremia); Polydipsia; Known or suspected syndrome of inappropriate antidiuretic hormone secretion; HF (New York Heart Association class II–IV); Uncontrolled hypertension; OB: Nocdurna not recommended for treatment of nocturia in pregnancy.

Use Cautiously in: Angina pectoris; Hypertension; Patients at risk for hyponatremia; Patients at risk for ↑ intracranial hypertension; Urinary retention (Nocdurna only); Women (↑ risk of hyponatremia; require ↓ dose); Patients who require use of other intranasal medications; Pedi: Safety and effectiveness not established in children (Nocdurna only); Geri: Appears on Beers list. ↑ risk of hyponatremia in older adults. Avoid use for treatment of nocturia or nocturnal polyuria in older adults.

Adverse Reactions/Side Effects

CV: edema, hypertension, hypotension, tachycardia (large IV doses only). **Derm:** flushing. **EENT: intranasal:** epistaxis, nasal congestion, nasal discomfort, rhinitis, sneezing. **F and E:** HYPONATREMIA. **GI:** dry mouth, mild abdominal cramps, nausea. **GU:** vulval pain. **Local:** phlebitis at IV site. **MS:** back pain. **Neuro:** dizziness, drowsiness, headache, listlessness, SEIZURES. **Resp:** dyspnea.

Interactions

Drug-Drug: **Loop diuretics, systemic glucocorticoids,** or **inhaled glucocorticoids** ↑ risk of severe hyponatremia; concurrent use contraindicated. **Carbamazepine, chlorpromazine, lamotrigine, NSAIDs, opioids, SSRIs, sulfonylureas, TCAs,** or **thiazide diuretics** may ↑ risk of fluid retention and hyponatremia. **Demeclocycline, lithium,** or **norepinephrine** may diminish the antidiuretic response to desmopressin. Large doses may enhance the effects of **vasopressors.**

Route/Dosage

Primary Nocturnal Enuresis

PO (Adults and Children ≥6 yr): 0.2 mg at bedtime; may be titrated up to 0.6 mg at bedtime to achieve desired response.

sublingual (Adults and Children): 120 mcg 1 hr before bedtime; may be titrated up to 360 mcg at bedtime to achieve desired response.

Diabetes Insipidus

PO (Adults and Children): 0.05 mg twice daily; adjusted as needed (usual range: 0.1–1.2 mg/day for adults or 0.1–0.8 mg/day for children in 2–3 divided doses).

Sublingual (Adults and Children): 60 mcg 3 times daily; adjusted as needed (usual range: 120–720 mcg/day in 2–3 divided doses).

Intranasal (Adults and Children ≥12 yr): *DDAVP:* 5–40 mcg (0.0.05–0.4 mL) in 1–3 divided doses.

Intranasal (Children 3 mo–12 yr): *DDAVP:* 5–30 mcg (0.05–0.3 mL) in 1–2 divided doses.

SUBQ IV (Adults and Children ≥12 yr): 2–4 mcg/day in 2 divided doses.

SUBQ IV (Children <12 yr): 0.1–1 mcg/day in 1–2 divided doses.

Hemophilia A/von Willebrand Disease

IV (Adults and Children >3 mo): 0.3 mcg/kg, repeated as needed.

Nocturia

Sublingual: (Adults): *Women:* 27.7 mcg 1 hr before bedtime; *Men:* 55.3 mcg 1 hr before bedtime.

Availability (generic available)

Tablets: 0.1 mg, 0.2 mg. **Sublingual tablet (Nocdurna):** 27.7 mcg, 55.3 mcg ✱ 60 mcg ✱ 120 mcg. **Nasal spray:** 10 mcg/spray in 5-mL bottle (contains 50 sprays). **Solution for injection:** 4 mcg/mL ✱ 15 mcg/mL.

NURSING IMPLICATIONS

Assessment

- Restrict free water intake and monitor for hyponatremia.
- Assess nasal mucosa for atrophy or acute or chronic rhinitis; dose interruption may be necessary. If nasal mucosal scarring and edema occur (may lead to erratic and unreliable absorption), discontinue and use IV until nasal problems resolve.
- **Nocturnal Enuresis:** Monitor frequency of enuresis during therapy. Use cautiously in patients at risk for water intoxication with hyponatremia.
- **Nocturia:** Assess for possible causes of nocturia (adults who awaken ≥two times per night to void), including excessive fluid intake before bedtime, and address other treatable causes of nocturia.
- **Diabetes Insipidus:** Assess for symptoms of dehydration (excessive thirst, dry skin and mucous membranes, tachycardia, poor skin turgor). Weigh daily and assess for edema. Closely monitor volume status in patients with New York Heart Association Class I HF.
- **Hemophilia:** Assess for signs of bleeding.
- Monitor BP and HR during IV infusion.
- Monitor intake and output and adjust fluid intake (especially in children and older adults) to avoid overhydration.

Lab Test Considerations

- Do not start or resume intranasal or SL desmopressin unless serum sodium concentration is normal. Measure serum sodium within 7 days and approximately 1 mo after initiating therapy and periodically during treatment. More frequent monitoring in patients ≥65 yr and in patients at ↑ risk of hyponatremia. *If hyponatremia occurs,* may need to temporarily or permanently discontinue desmopressin.
- Monitor renal function in older adults.
- *Diabetes insipidus:* Monitor urine osmolality and, in some cases, plasma osmolality during therapy.
- *Nocdurna:* Obtain a 24-hr urine collection to confirm diagnosis of nocturnal polyuria before starting therapy.
- *Hemophilia:* Monitor levels of factor VIII coagulant activity, factor VIII antigen, factor VIII ristocetin cofactor (von Willebrand factor), and activated partial thromboplastin time (aPTT). *Hemophilia A:* Determine factor VIII coagulant activity before giving desmopressin for hemostasis. *von Willebrand Disease:* Response to therapy may be assessed by blood sample 45–60 min after the completion of infusion; also monitor skin bleeding time. Do not use in patients with type IIB von Willebrand disease; may induce platelet aggregation.

Toxicity and Overdose

- Signs and symptoms of water intoxication include confusion, drowsiness, headache, weight gain, difficulty urinating, seizures, and coma.
- Treatment of overdose includes ↓ dose and, if symptoms are severe, administration of furosemide.

Implementation

- Do not confuse desmopressin with vasopressin.
- IV desmopressin has 10 times the antidiuretic effect of intranasal desmopressin.
- **PO:** Begin oral doses 12 hr after last intranasal dose. Monitor response closely.
- **Sublingual:** Administer 1 hr before bedtime. Place tablet under tongue until dissolved completely. Limit fluid intake for ≥1 hr before until 8 hr after administration. Use without fluid restriction may lead to fluid retention and hyponatremia.
- **Intranasal:** If intranasal dose is used preoperatively, administer 2 hr before procedure. Prime nasal spray pump prior to use by pressing down four times; will remain primed for up to 1 wk. Discard after 50 sprays because <10 mcg will be delivered thereafter. Doses <0.1 mL (10 mcg) should be administered with the rhinal tube delivery system. Store upright.
- Do not use intranasal form for nocturnal enuresis.
- **Diabetes Insipidus:** Parenteral dose for antidiuretic effect is administered IV push or SUBQ.
- **Hemophilia:** Parenteral dose for control of bleeding is administered via IV infusion. If used preoperatively, administer 30 min prior to procedure.

IV Administration

- **IV Push:** *(for diabetes insipidus)* **Dilution:** Administer undiluted. **Concentration:** 4 mcg/mL.
- **Rate:** Administer over 1 min.
- **Intermittent Infusion:** *(for hemophilia and von Willebrand disease)* **Dilution:** Dilute each dose in 50 mL of 0.9% NaCl for adults and children >10 kg and in 10 mL in children <10 kg. Inspect solution; do not administer solutions that are cloudy, discolored, or contain particulate matter. **Concentration:** Maximum = 0.5 mcg/mL.
- **Rate:** Infuse slowly over 15–30 min.
- **Y-Site Compatibility:** naloxone.

Patient/Family Teaching

- Explain purpose and side effects of desmopressin to patient. Teach patient or caregiver of child proper technique for administration based on product prescribed. Counsel patient that fluid restriction is necessary, and give details based on indication and product prescribed. Instruct patient to take missed doses as soon as remembered but not if it is almost time for the next dose. Do not double doses. Advise patient to read *Patient Information* before starting and with each Rx refill in case of changes.

- **Nocturia:** Instruct patient to place tablet under tongue 1 hr before bedtime and empty bladder immediately before bedtime. Advise patient to limit fluid intake before bedtime and to avoid caffeine and alcohol before bedtime.
- **Diabetes Insipidus:** If nasal spray is used, prime pump prior to first use by pressing down four times. Caution patient that nasal spray should not be used beyond the labeled number of sprays; subsequent sprays may not deliver accurate dose. Do not attempt to transfer remaining solution to another bottle.
- Advise patient to report symptoms of hyponatremia (headache, feeling restless, drowsiness, muscle cramps, nausea or vomiting, fatigue, dizziness, change in mental condition [hallucinations, confusion, ↓ awareness or alertness]), water intoxication, or fluid retention.
- Advise patient that rhinitis or upper respiratory infection may ↓ effectiveness of intranasal therapy. If ↑ urine output occurs, patient should contact health care provider for dose adjustment.
- Instruct patient to notify health care provider if fever, infection, or diarrhea occurs. May need to hold medication.
- Advise patient to notify health care provider if bleeding is not controlled or if headache, dyspnea, heartburn, nausea, abdominal cramps, vulval pain, or severe nasal congestion or irritation occurs.
- Patients with diabetes insipidus should carry identification at all times describing disease process and medication regimen.
- Instruct patient to notify health care provider of all Rx or OTC medications, vitamins, or herbal products being taken and to consult with health care provider before taking other medications. Caution patient to avoid concurrent use of alcohol with this medication.
- Rep: Advise women of reproductive potential to notify health care provider if pregnancy is planned or suspected or if breastfeeding.

Evaluation/Desired Outcomes

- Decreased frequency of nocturnal enuresis.
- Decrease in urine volume.
- Relief of polydipsia.
- Increased urine osmolality.
- Control of bleeding in hemophilia and von Willebrand disease.
- Reduced frequency of episodes of nocturia.

desonide, See CORTICOSTEROIDS (TOPICAL).

desoximetasone, See CORTICOSTEROIDS (TOPICAL).

BEERS

desvenlafaxine

(**des**-ven-la-**fax**-een)

~~Khedezla~~, Pristiq

Classification

Therapeutic: antidepressants

Pharmacologic: selective serotonin norepinephrine reuptake inhibitors

Indications

Major depressive disorder.

Action

Inhibits serotonin and norepinephrine reuptake in the CNS. **Therapeutic Effects:** Decrease in depressive symptomatology, with fewer relapses/recurrences.

Pharmacokinetics

Absorption: 80% absorbed following oral administration.

Distribution: Widely distributed to tissues.

Metabolism and Excretion: 55% metabolized by the liver; 45% excreted unchanged in urine.

Half-life: 10 hr.

TIME/ACTION PROFILE (plasma concentrations)

ROUTE	ONSET	PEAK	DURATION
PO	unknown	7.5 hr	24 hr

Contraindications/Precautions

Contraindicated in: Hypersensitivity to venlafaxine or desvenlafaxine; Concurrent use of MAO inhibitors or MAO-like drugs (linezolid or methylene blue); Should not be used concurrently with venlafaxine.

Use Cautiously in: Untreated cerebrovascular or cardiovascular disease, including untreated hypertension (control BP before initiating therapy); May ↑ risk of suicide attempt/ideation, especially during early treatment or dose adjustment; this risk appears to be greater in adolescents or children; Bipolar disorder (may activate mania/hypomania); Moderate or severe renal impairment; History of seizures or neurologic impairment; Moderate or severe hepatic impairment; Angle-closure glaucoma; OB: Safety not established in pregnancy; Lactation: Use while breastfeeding only if potential maternal benefit justifies potential risk to infant; Pedi: Safety and effectiveness not established in children; Geri: Appears on Beers list. May worsen or cause syndrome of inappropriate antidiuretic hormone (SIADH) secretion and/or hyponatremia in older adults. Use with caution in older adults and closely monitor sodium concentrations when starting therapy or ↑ dose.

Adverse Reactions/Side Effects

CV: hypertension. **Derm:** sweating, ERYTHEMA MULTIFORME, STEVENS-JOHNSON SYNDROME (SJS), TOXIC EPIDERMAL NECROLYSIS. **EENT:** ↑ intraocular pressure, mydriasis. **Endo:** SIADH. **F and E:** hyponatremia. **GI:** constipation, nausea, PANCREATITIS. **GU:** ↓ libido, delayed/absent orgasm, ejaculatory delay/failure, erectile dysfunction. **Hemat:** BLEEDING. **Metab:** ↓ appetite, hyperlipidemia. **Neuro:** anxiety, dizziness, drowsiness, insomnia, headache, NEUROLEPTIC MALIGNANT SYNDROME, SEIZURES, SUICIDAL THOUGHTS/BEHAVIORS, teeth grinding, vertigo. **Resp:** eosinophilic pneumonia, interstitial lung disease. **Misc:** discontinuation syndrome, SEROTONIN SYNDROME.

Interactions

Drug-Drug: MAO inhibitors may result in serious, potentially fatal reactions; wait ≥2 wk after stopping MAO inhibitor before initiating desvenlafaxine; wait ≥1 wk after stopping desvenlafaxine before starting an MAO inhibitor. **MAO-inhibitor-like drugs**, such as **linezolid** or **methylene blue**, may ↑ risk of serotonin syndrome; concurrent use contraindicated; do not start therapy in patients receiving **linezolid** or **methylene blue**; if **linezolid** or **methylene blue** need to be started in a patient receiving desvenlafaxine, immediately discontinue desvenlafaxine and monitor for signs/symptoms of serotonin syndrome for 2 wk or until 24 hr after last dose of linezolid or methylene blue, whichever comes first (may resume desvenlafaxine therapy 24 hr after last dose of linezolid or methylene blue). ↑ risk of bleeding with **NSAIDs**, **aspirin**, **clopidogrel**, **prasugrel**, **ticagrelor**, **dabigatran**, **apixaban**, **edoxaban**, **rivaroxaban**, or **warfarin**. Use cautiously with other **CNS-active drugs**, including **alcohol** or **sedative/hypnotics**; effects of combination are unknown. Drugs that affect serotonergic neurotransmitter systems, including **tricyclic antidepressants**, **SNRIs**, **fentanyl**, **lithium**, **buspirone**, **tramadol**, **meperidine**, **methadone**, **amphetamines**, and **triptans**, may ↑ risk of serotonin syndrome. **Ketoconazole** may ↑ levels and risk of toxicity. May ↑ levels and risk of toxicity of **CYP2D6 substrates**, including **desipramine**, **atomoxetine**, **dextromethorphan**, **metoprolol**, **nebivolol**, **perphenazine**, and **tolterodine**; if using desvenlafaxine at dose of 400 mg/day, ↓ dose of CYP2D6 substrate by 50%.

Route/Dosage

PO (Adults): 50 mg once daily (range = 50–400 mg/day).

Renal Impairment

PO (Adults): *CCr 30–50 mL/min:* 50 mg once daily; *CCr <30 mL/min:* 50 mg every other day or 25 mg once daily.

Hepatic Impairment

PO (Adults): *Moderate to severe hepatic impairment:* 50 mg once daily (not to exceed 100 mg/day).

Availability (generic available)

Extended-release tablets: 25 mg, 50 mg, 100 mg.

NURSING IMPLICATIONS

Assessment

- Assess mental status and mood changes, especially during initial few mo of therapy and during dose changes. Inform health care provider if patient demonstrates significant ↑ in signs of depression (depressed mood, loss of interest in usual activities, significant change in weight and/or appetite, insomnia or hypersomnia, psychomotor agitation or retardation, ↑ fatigue, feelings of guilt or worthlessness, slowed thinking or impaired concentration, suicide attempt or suicidal ideation).
- Assess for suicidal tendencies, especially during early therapy and dose changes. Restrict amount of drug available to patient. Risk may be ↑ in children, adolescents, and adults ≤24 yr. After starting therapy, young adults should be seen by health care provider at least weekly for 4 wk, every 3 wk for the next 4 wk, and on advice of health care provider thereafter.
- Monitor BP before and periodically during therapy. Sustained hypertension may be dose related; ↓ dose or discontinue therapy if this occurs.
- Monitor appetite and nutritional intake; weigh weekly. Report continued weight loss. Adjust diet as tolerated to support nutritional status.
- Assess for signs and symptoms of serotonin syndrome (confusion, delirium, agitation, coma, dilated pupils, tachycardia, hyperthermia, shivering, hyperreflexia, muscle rigidity, hypertension, vomiting, diarrhea, seizures). ↑ risk of serotonin syndrome with concurrent use of other serotonergic drugs (SSRIs, SNRIs, triptans); monitoring recommended; discontinuation may be required.
- Assess patient for skin rash frequently during therapy. Discontinue at first sign of rash; may be life-threatening. Erythema multiforme, SJS, or TEN may develop. Treat symptomatically; may recur once treatment is stopped.
- Assess sexual function before starting therapy. Assess for changes in sexual function during treatment, including timing of onset; patient may not report.

Lab Test Considerations

- May ↑ fasting serum total cholesterol, LDL-C, and triglycerides. May cause transient proteinuria, not usually associated with ↑ BUN or serum creatinine.

- May cause hyponatremia. Monitor sodium levels at baseline and after 3–4 wk in high-risk patients (>65 yr, previous history of antidepressant-induced hyponatremia, ↓ body weight, concurrent use of thiazides or other hyponatremia-inducing agents).
- May cause false-positive immunoassay screening tests for phencyclidine and amphetamine.

Implementation

- **PO:** Administer at the same time each day, with or without food. ***DNC:*** Swallow tablets whole; do not crush, break, chew, or dissolve.

Patient/Family Teaching

- Explain the purpose and side effects of desvenlafaxine. Instruct to take medication exactly as directed at the same time each day. Take missed doses as soon as possible unless almost time for next dose. Do not double doses or discontinue abruptly; gradually ↓ dose before discontinuation to prevent dizziness, nausea, headache, irritability, insomnia, diarrhea, anxiety, fatigue, abnormal dreams, and hyperhidrosis; discontinuation may take several mo. Advise patient to read *Patient Information* before starting and with each Rx refill in case of changes.
- Emphasize the importance of follow-up exams to monitor progress.
- Advise patient, family, and caregivers to look for suicidality, especially during early therapy or dose changes. Notify health care provider immediately if thoughts about suicide or dying, attempts to commit suicide, new or worse depression or anxiety, agitation or restlessness, panic attacks, insomnia, new or worse irritability, aggressiveness, acting on dangerous impulses, mania, or other changes in mood or behavior occur.
- May cause drowsiness or dizziness. Caution patient to avoid driving or other activities requiring alertness until response to the drug is known.
- Counsel patient to report symptoms of serotonin syndrome (agitation, confusion, diaphoresis, hallucinations, hyper-reflexia).
- Caution patient to avoid taking alcohol or other CNS-depressant drugs, including opioids, during therapy and of ↑ risk of bleeding with concurrent use of NSAIDs, aspirin, or other drugs that affect coagulation. Instruct patient to notify health care provider of all Rx or OTC medications, vitamins, or herbal products being taken, especially St. John's wort, and to consult health care provider before taking other Rx, OTC, or herbal products.
- Instruct patient to notify health care provider if signs of allergy (rash, hives, swelling, difficulty breathing) occur.
- Inform patient that desvenlafaxine may cause symptoms of sexual dysfunction. In men, ejaculatory delay or failure, ↓ libido, and erectile dysfunction may occur. In women, may result in ↓ libido and delayed or absent orgasm. Advise patient to notify health care provider if symptoms occur.
- Inform patient that remains of tablet may pass into stool, but medication has already been absorbed.
- Rep: Advise women of reproductive potential to notify health care provider if pregnancy is planned or suspected or if breastfeeding. Exposure to desvenlafaxine in mid- to late pregnancy may ↑ risk for pre-eclampsia and exposure near delivery and may ↑ risk of postpartum hemorrhage. Fetal exposure late in pregnancy may lead to ↑ risk for neonatal complications requiring prolonged hospitalization, respiratory support, and tube feeding. Monitor neonates exposed to desvenlafaxine in the 3rd trimester for drug discontinuation syndrome. Inform patient of pregnancy exposure registry to monitor pregnancy outcomes in women exposed to antidepressants during pregnancy. Register patients by calling the National Pregnancy Registry for Antidepressants at 1-866-961-2388.

Evaluation/Desired Outcomes

- Increased sense of well-being.
- Renewed interest in surroundings. Need for therapy should be periodically reassessed. Therapy is usually continued for several mo.

deucravacitinib
(doo-krav-a-**sye**-ti-nib)

Sotyktu

Classification

Therapeutic: antipsoriatics

Pharmacologic: kinase inhibitors

Indications

Moderate to severe plaque psoriasis in patients who are candidates for systemic therapy or phototherapy.

Action

Acts as a inhibitor of tyrosine kinase 2. Its exact mechanism for effect in plaque psoriasis is unknown. **Therapeutic Effects:** Decreased formation and spread of plaques.

Pharmacokinetics

Absorption: Well absorbed (99%) following oral administration.

Distribution: Extensively distributed to tissues.

Protein Binding: 82–90%.

Metabolism and Excretion: Primarily metabolized by the liver via the CYP1A2 isoenzyme to form an active metabolite (BMT-153261). Also metabolized by CYP2B6, CYP2D6, carboxylesterase 2, and UGT1A9. 26% and 13% excreted in feces and urine, respectively, as unchanged drug.

Half-life: 10 hr.

TIME/ACTION PROFILE (plasma concentrations)

ROUTE	ONSET	PEAK	DURATION
PO	unknown	2–3 hr	24 hr

Contraindications/Precautions

Contraindicated in: Hypersensitivity; Active or serious infection (including tuberculosis [TB] and hepatitis B/C); Severe hepatic impairment.
Use Cautiously in: Chronic or recurrent infection, exposure to tuberculosis, history of opportunistic infection, underlying conditions that predispose to infection; Malignancy (other than successfully treated nonmelanoma skin cancer); OB: Safety not established in pregnancy; Lactation: Use while breastfeeding only if potential maternal benefit justifies potential risk to infant; Pedi: Safety and effectiveness not established in children.

Adverse Reactions/Side Effects

Derm: acne. **GI:** ↑ liver enzymes, mouth ulcers. **Metab:** hypertriglyceridemia. **MS:** ↑ CK, RHABDOMYOLYSIS. **Misc:** INFECTION, HYPERSENSITIVITY REACTIONS (INCLUDING ANGIOEDEMA), MALIGNANCY (INCLUDING LYMPHOMA).

Interactions

Drug-Drug: Avoid concurrent use with **live vaccines**.

Route/Dosage

PO (Adults): 6 mg once daily.

Availability

Tablets: 6 mg.

NURSING IMPLICATIONS

Assessment

- Assess skin lesions and concurrent symptoms (absence of itch, pain, burning, stinging, and skin tightness) before and periodically during therapy.
- Monitor for signs and symptoms of hypersensitivity (angioedema). *If symptoms occur,* discontinue therapy.
- Assess for signs and symptoms of infection, especially pneumonia and COVID-19, during and after treatment. *If serious infection occurs,* discontinue therapy until infection resolved. *If viral reactivation of herpes zoster or hepatitis B/C occurs,* consult specialist.

Lab Test Considerations

- May cause rhabdomyolysis and asymptomatic CK ↑. *If markedly ↑ CK occurs or myopathy suspected,* discontinue deucravacitinib.
- Periodically evaluate serum triglycerides during therapy. May ↑ triglycerides.
- Consider viral hepatitis screening and monitoring for reactivation at baseline and during therapy.
- Assess liver enzymes at baseline and periodically during therapy in patients with known or suspected liver disease. *If drug-induced ↑ in liver enzymes occurs,* interrupt therapy until a diagnosis of liver injury is excluded.

Implementation

- Evaluate for acute and latent TB before starting therapy. *For latent TB,* initiate treatment before starting deucravacitinib. *For active TB,* do not administer deucravacitinib.
- Update age-appropriate immunizations before starting therapy, including herpes zoster vaccination. Avoid use of live vaccines during therapy.
- **PO:** Administer tablet once daily without regard to food. ***DNC:*** Swallow tablets whole; do not break, crush, or chew.

Patient/Family Teaching

- Explain purpose and side effects of medication. Advise patient to read *Patient Information* before starting therapy.
- Instruct patients to promptly report unexplained muscle pain, tenderness or weakness, particularly if accompanied by malaise or fever.
- Advise patient to notify health care professional and stop deucravacitinib immediately for serious hypersensitivity reactions (difficulty breathing; swelling of face, mouth, or neck).
- Advise patient to avoid live vaccines during therapy.
- Advise patient to notify health care professional of all Rx or OTC medications, vitamins, or herbal products being taken and to consult with health care professional before taking other medications.
- Inform patient that medication may ↑ risk of malignancy, including lymphomas.
- Caution patient to avoid crowds and persons with known infections. Notify health care professional immediately if symptoms of infection occur.
- Rep: Advise women of reproductive potential to notify health care professional if pregnancy is planned or suspected or if breastfeeding. If pregnancy occurs, report pregnancies to the Bristol-Myers Squibb Company's Adverse Event reporting line: 1-800-721-5072.

Evaluation/Desired Outcomes

- Absence or decrease in psoriatic symptoms.

D

deuruxolitinib

(due-**rux**-oh-**li**-ti-nib)

Leqselvi

Classification

Therapeutic: none assigned

Pharmacologic: kinase inhibitors

Indications
Severe alopecia areata.

Action
Inhibits Janus kinase, which is involved in the signaling of hematopoiesis and immune processes. **Therapeutic Effects:** Improved scalp hair coverage.

Pharmacokinetics
Absorption: 90% absorbed following oral administration.
Distribution: Well distributed to tissues.
Metabolism and Excretion: Primarily metabolized in the liver via the CYP2C9 and CYP3A4 isoenzymes and to a lesser extent by the CYP1A2 isoenzyme. The CYP2C9 isoenzyme exhibits genetic polymorphism; poor metabolizers (PMs) may have significantly ↑ deuruxolitinib concentrations and an ↑ risk of adverse effects.
Half-life: 4 hr.

TIME/ACTION PROFILE (plasma concentrations)

ROUTE	ONSET	PEAK	DURATION
PO	unknown	1.5 hr	12 hr

Contraindications/Precautions
Contraindicated in: CYP2C9 PMs; Concurrent use of strong or moderate CYP2C9 inhibitors; Active, serious infection; ↑ risk of thrombosis; History of MI or stroke; Hgb <8 g/dL; ANC <1000 cells/mm^3; Lymphocytes <500 cells/mm^3; Severe renal impairment or end-stage renal disease; Severe hepatic impairment; OB: Pregnancy; Lactation: Lactation.
Use Cautiously in: Chronic or recurrent infection; Exposed to tuberculosis (TB); History of serious or opportunistic infection; Resided or traveled in areas of endemic TB or endemic mycoses; Predisposition to infection; >50 yr old and with ≥1 cardiovascular risk factor (may have ↑ risk of mortality, cardiovascular death, nonfatal MI, or nonfatal stroke); Current or past history of smoking (↑ risk of malignancy, cardiovascular death, MI, or stroke); Known malignancy; History of diverticulitis (↑ risk of GI perforation); Rep: Women of reproductive potential; Pedi: Safety and effectiveness not established in children.

Adverse Reactions/Side Effects
CV: ARTERIAL THROMBOSIS, CARDIOVASCULAR DEATH, DEEP VEIN THROMBOSIS (DVT), MI. **Derm:** acne. **EENT:** nasopharyngitis. **GI:** GI PERFORATION. **Hemat:** anemia, lymphopenia, neutropenia, thrombocytosis. **Metab:** hyperlipidemia, hypertriglyceridemia, weight gain. **MS:** ↑ CK. **Neuro:** headache, fatigue, STROKE. **Resp:** PULMONARY EMBOLISM (PE). **Misc:** DEATH, INFECTION (INCLUDING REACTIVATION TB AND OTHER OPPORTUNISTIC INFECTIONS DUE TO BACTERIAL, FUNGAL, VIRAL, AND MYCOBACTERIAL PATHOGENS), MALIGNANCY.

Interactions
Drug-Drug: Strong CYP2C9 inhibitors or **moderate CYP2C9 inhibitors**, including **fluconazole**, may ↑ levels and risk of toxicity; concurrent use contraindicated. **Strong CYP3A4 inducers**, including **rifampin**, may ↓ levels and effectiveness; avoid concurrent use. **Strong CYP2C9 inducers** or **moderate CYP2C9 inducers**, including **rifampin**, may ↓ levels and effectiveness; avoid concurrent use. ↑ risk of immunosuppression when used concurrently with other potent **immunosuppressants**, including **azathioprine**, **cyclosporine**, **tacrolimus**, **antineoplastics**, or **radiation therapy**.

Route/Dosage
PO (Adults): 8 mg twice daily.

Availability
Tablets: 8 mg.

NURSING IMPLICATIONS
Assessment
- Assess for signs and symptoms of infection, including opportunistic infections and TB, prior to and periodically during therapy. *If sepsis or serious infection occurs,* interrupt therapy and provide appropriate diagnostic testing, antimicrobial therapy, and close monitoring. Most common are pneumonia, cellulitis, herpes zoster, urinary tract infection, diverticulitis, and appendicitis. Infections may be fatal, especially in patients taking immunosuppressive therapy.
- Assess for signs and symptoms of systemic fungal infections (fever, malaise, weight loss, sweats, cough, dyspnea, pulmonary infiltrates, serious systemic illness with or without concurrent shock). Ascertain if patient lives in or has traveled to areas of endemic mycoses. Consider empiric antifungal treatment for patients at risk of histoplasmosis and other invasive fungal infections until pathogen identified. Consult with infectious diseases specialist. Consider stopping deuruxolitinib until the infection has been diagnosed and adequately treated.
- Monitor for thrombosis, including PE, DVT, and arterial thrombi. *If symptoms of thrombosis occur,* permanently discontinue deuruxolitinib.

Lab Test Considerations
- Determine CYP2C9 genotype variant prior to initiation. An FDA-approved test is not currently available.
- Complete tuberculin skin test prior to initiation of therapy. Treatment of latent TB should be started before therapy with deuruxolitinib.

Screen for viral hepatitis according to guidelines. Monitor CBC with differential periodically during therapy. *If lymphocytes <500 cells/mm^3, ANC <1000 cells/mm^3, or Hgb <8 g/dL,* hold therapy until ≥500 cells/mm³, ≥1000 cells/mm³, or ≥8 g/dL respectively; then resume deuruxolitinib. Asses lipid panel at baseline and periodically during therapy. May ↑ CK.

Implementation

- Update all age-appropriate vaccines, including herpes zoster, according to guidelines before initiation of therapy.
- **PO:** Administer tablet without regard to food.

Patient/Family Teaching

- Explain purpose and side effects of medication. Advise patient to read *Patient Information* before starting therapy.
- Advise patient if dose is missed to omit and resume at next scheduled dose.
- Inform patient of ↑ risk of malignancy, including skin cancer, and that periodic skin exams are recommended.
- Advise patient to notify health care provider immediately if signs of infection (fever; sweating; chills; muscle aches; cough; shortness of breath; blood in phlegm; weight loss; warm, red, or painful skin or sores; diarrhea or stomach pain; burning on urination or urinating more often than normal; feeling very tired) occur.
- Inform patient of ↑ risk of MI, stroke, DVT, PE, and cardiovascular death, especially in current or past smokers, and to notify health care provider if symptoms (chest pain, shortness of breath, nausea, palpitations, fainting, trouble speaking/understanding, unilateral numbness/weakness, visual changes, headache, discoordination; pain/swelling/cramping/pallor of extremity) occur.
- Inform patient ≥50 yr of age with ≥1 cardiovascular risk factor that risk of death from all causes is ↑ with deuruxolitinib use. They should discontinue therapy if they experience heart attack or stroke.
- Inform patient that risk of malignancy and lymphoproliferative disorders is ↑ with deuruxolitinib use and periodic cancer screens, including skin assessments, are recommended.
- Advise patient to notify health care provider promptly for symptoms of GI perforation (stomach pain, fever, chills, nausea, vomiting).
- Advise patient not to receive live vaccines during therapy.
- Advise patient to notify health care provider of all Rx or OTC medications, vitamins, or herbal products being taken and to consult health care provider before taking other medications.
- Rep: May cause fetal harm. Advise women of reproductive potential to notify health care provider if pregnancy is planned or suspected. Avoid breastfeeding during therapy and for 1 day after last dose. Encourage patient to report pregnancy exposure to Sun Pharmaceutical Industries Inc. at 1-800-818-4555.

Evaluation/Desired Outcomes

- Improved scalp hair coverage.

D

deutetrabenazine

(due-tet-ra-**ben**-a-zeen)

Austedo, Austedo XR

Classification

Therapeutic: antichoreas

Pharmacologic: reversible monoamine depleters

Indications

Chorea due to Huntington Disease. Tardive dyskinesia.

Action

Its major metabolites act as reversible inhibitors of the vesicle monoamine transporter type 2 (VMAT-2), resulting in decreased reuptake of monoamines (including serotonin, norepinephrine, and dopamine) into vesicles in presynaptic neurons and depletion of monoamine stores. **Therapeutic Effects:** Decreased chorea due to Huntington Disease. Reduced severity of tardive dyskinesia.

Pharmacokinetics

Absorption: ≥80% absorbed following oral administration.

Distribution: Extensively distributed to tissues.

Metabolism and Excretion: Metabolized in liver to two active metabolites (α-dihydrotetrabenazine (α-HTBZ) and β-HTBZ), which are subsequently metabolized primarily via CYP2D6 (and to lesser extent by CYP1A2 and CYP3A4/5) to several minor metabolites (the CYP2D6 enzyme system exhibits genetic polymorphism; 7% of population may be poor metabolizers and may have significantly ↑ concentrations and an ↑ risk of adverse effects). Primarily excreted in the urine as metabolites.

Half-life: 9–10 hr.

TIME/ACTION PROFILE (plasma concentrations)

ROUTE	ONSET	PEAK	DURATION
PO	unknown	3–4 hr	12 hr
PO-XR	unknown	3 hr	24 hr

Contraindications/Precautions

Contraindicated in: Hepatic impairment; Concurrent use of MAO inhibitors, tetrabenazine, or valbenazine; Patients who are suicidal or have untreated or inadequately treated depression; Congenital long QT syndrome or cardiac arrhythmias.

Use Cautiously in: History of/propensity for depression, psychiatric illness, or suicidality; Poor CYP2D6 metabolizers; initial dose ↓ required; Bradycardia, hypokalemia, hypomagnesemia, or concurrent use of QT-interval prolonging drugs; History of breast cancer; OB: Use during pregnancy only when potential maternal benefit justifies potential fetal risk; Lactation: Use while breastfeeding only when potential maternal benefit justifies potential risk to infant; Pedi: Safety and effectiveness not established in children.

Adverse Reactions/Side Effects

CV: QTc interval prolongation. **Endo:** hyperprolactinemia. **GI:** constipation, diarrhea, dry mouth. **GU:** urinary tract infection. **MS:** bradykinesia. **Neuro:** akathisia, sedation/somnolence, agitation, anxiety, depression, dizziness, fatigue, gait disturbances, insomnia, NEUROLEPTIC MALIGNANT SYNDROME, parkinsonism, restlessness, SUICIDAL THOUGHTS/BEHAVIOR, tremor.

Interactions

Drug-Drug: MAO inhibitors ↑ risk of serious adverse reactions and are contraindicated; wait ≥14 days after discontinuing to initiate deutetrabenazine. Concurrent use of **tetrabenazine** or **valbenazine** is contraindicated. **Strong CYP2D6 inhibitors**, including **bupropion**, **fluoxetine**, **paroxetine**, and **quinidine**, may ↑ levels and risk of toxicity; ↓ dose of deutetrabenazine. **QTc interval prolonging drugs** may ↑ risk of QTc interval prolongation. **Dopamine antagonists** or **antipsychotics** may ↑ risk of neuroleptic malignant syndrome and extrapyramidal disorders. **Alcohol** or other **CNS depressants** may ↑ risk of CNS depression.

Route/Dosage

When switching between immediate-release and extended-release formulations, use same total daily dose.

Huntington Disease

PO (Adults): *Immediate-release tablets:* 6 mg twice daily; may ↑ dose by 6 mg/day at weekly intervals (max dose = 48 mg/day) based on tolerability to ↓ chorea. *Extended-release tablets:* 12 mg once daily; may ↑ dose by 6 mg/day at weekly intervals (max dose = 48 mg/day) based on tolerability to ↓ chorea. *Concurrent use of strong CYP2D6 inhibitors or poor CYP2D6 metabolizers:* Do not exceed dose of 36 mg/day.

Tardive Dyskinesia

PO (Adults): *Immediate-release tablets:* 6 mg twice daily; may ↑ dose by 6 mg/day at weekly intervals (max dose = 48 mg/day) based on tolerability to ↓ tardive dyskinesia. *Extended-release tablets:* 12 mg once daily; may ↑ dose by 6 mg/day at weekly intervals (max dose = 48 mg/day) based on tolerability to ↓ tardive dyskinesia. *Concurrent use of strong CYP2D6 inhibitors or poor CYP2D6 metabolizers:* Do not exceed dose of 36 mg/day.

Availability (generic available)

Immediate-release tablets (Austedo): 6 mg, 9 mg, 12 mg. **Extended-release tablets (Austedo XR):** 6 mg, 12 mg, 18 mg, 24 mg, 30 mg, 36 mg, 42 mg, 48 mg.

NURSING IMPLICATIONS

Assessment

- Assess signs of Huntington disease (changes in mood, cognition, chorea, rigidity, and functional capacity) periodically during therapy. Re-evaluate need for deutetrabenazine periodically by assessing beneficial effect and side effects; determination may require dose ↓ or discontinuation. Underlying chorea may improve over time, ↓ need for deutetrabenazine.
- Monitor closely for new or worsening depression or suicidality. If depression or suicidality occurs, ↓ dose and may initiate or ↑ dose of antidepressants.
- Monitor for signs of neuroleptic malignant syndrome (fever, muscle rigidity, altered mental status, irregular HR or BP, tachycardia, diaphoresis, cardiac arrhythmia) periodically during therapy. If symptoms occur, discontinue deutetrabenazine and manage symptomatically. If reintroduction of deutetrabenazine is considered, monitor carefully; recurrences of neuroleptic malignant syndrome have occurred.
- Monitor for onset of akathisia (restlessness or desire to keep moving) and parkinsonism (difficulty speaking or swallowing, loss of balance control, pill rolling of hands, mask-like face, shuffling gait, rigidity, tremors). Notify health care provider if these symptoms occur; ↓ dose or discontinue therapy.

Lab Test Considerations

- Monitor electrolytes and ECG because of risk of QT interval prolongation.

Implementation

- **PO:** Administer with food. ***DNC:*** Swallow tablet whole; do not crush, break, or chew.
- Administer extended-release tablet without regard to food.
- If switching from *Austedo to Austedo XR*, switch to the same total daily dose.
- **To switch from tetrabenazine to deutetrabenazine, stop tetrabenazine and administer deutetrabenazine the following day.**
- **Switching from tetrabenazine to deutetrabenazine immediate-release tablets:** *If taking 12.5 mg of tetrabenazine,* give deutetrabenazine 6 mg once daily. *If taking 25 mg tetrabenazine,* give deutetrabenazine 6 mg twice daily. *If taking 37.5 mg tetrabenazine,* give deutetrabenazine 9 mg twice daily. *If taking 50 mg tetrabenazine,* give deutetrabenazine 12 mg twice daily. *If taking 62.5 mg tetrabenazine,* give deutetrabenazine 15 mg twice daily. *If taking 75 mg tetrabenazine,* give deutetrabenazine

18 mg twice daily. *If taking 87.5 mg tetrabenazine,* give deutetrabenazine 21 mg twice daily. *If taking 100 mg tetrabenazine,* give deutetrabenazine 24 mg twice daily.

- **Switching from tetrabenazine to deutetrabenazine extended-release tablets:** *If taking 12.5 mg of tetrabenazine,* give deutetrabenazine 6 mg once daily. *If taking 25 mg tetrabenazine,* give deutetrabenazine 12 mg once daily. *If taking 37.5 mg tetrabenazine,* give deutetrabenazine 18 mg once daily. *If taking 50 mg tetrabenazine,* give deutetrabenazine 24 mg once daily. *If taking 62.5 mg tetrabenazine,* give deutetrabenazine 30 mg once daily. *If taking 75 mg tetrabenazine,* give deutetrabenazine 36 mg once daily. *If taking 87.5 mg tetrabenazine,* give deutetrabenazine 42 mg once daily. *If taking 100 mg tetrabenazine,* give deutetrabenazine 48 mg once daily.
- Dose adjustments can be made weekly.
- Deutetrabenazine may be stopped without taper. If therapy interrupted >1 wk, retitrate when resuming therapy. If <1 wk since discontinuation, may restart at previous dose.

Patient/Family Teaching

- Explain purpose and side effects of medication. Advise patient to read *Patient Information* before starting therapy. Instruct patient to take as directed.
- Advise patient to notify health care provider of all Rx or OTC medications, vitamins, or herbal products being taken and to consult health care provider before taking other medications.
- Advise patient and caregiver to monitor for changes, especially sudden changes in mood, behaviors, thoughts, or feelings. If new or worse feelings of sadness; crying spells; lack of interest in friends or activities; sleeping a lot more or less; feelings of unimportance, guilt, hopelessness, or helplessness; irritability or aggression; more or less hunger; difficulty paying attention; or thoughts of self-harm or suicide occur, notify health care provider promptly.
- Advise patient to notify health care provider if signs and symptoms of neuroleptic malignant syndrome, akathisia, or irregular heartbeat occur.
- Advise patient to avoid driving and other activities requiring alertness until response to medication is known.
- Inform patient of potential side effects and instruct patient to notify health care provider if side effects occur.
- Advise patient to avoid alcohol or sedating drugs; may ↑ drowsiness.
- Inform patients not to be concerned if they occasionally notice something that looks like a tablet shell in their stool when taking *Austedo XR*.
- Rep: Advise women of reproductive potential to notify health care provider if pregnancy is planned or suspected or if breastfeeding.

Evaluation/Desired Outcomes

- Decreased chorea due to Huntington disease.
- Reduced severity of tardive dyskinesia.

D

dexAMETHasone, See CORTICOSTEROIDS (SYSTEMIC).

BEERS

dexlansoprazole

(dex-lan-**soe**-pra-zole)

Dexilant

Classification

Therapeutic: antiulcer agents

Pharmacologic: proton pump inhibitors

Indications

Erosive esophagitis. Maintenance of healed erosive esophagitis and relief of heartburn. Treatment of heartburn from nonerosive gastroesophageal reflux disease (GERD).

Action

Binds to an enzyme in the presence of acidic gastric pH, preventing the final transport of hydrogen ions into the gastric lumen. **Therapeutic Effects:** Diminished accumulation of acid in the gastric lumen, with lessened acid reflux.

Pharmacokinetics

Absorption: Well absorbed following oral administration.

Distribution: Unknown.

Protein Binding: 96–99%.

Metabolism and Excretion: Extensively metabolized by the liver, primarily by the CYP2C19 and CYP3A4 isoenzymes; the CYP2C19 isoenzyme exhibits genetic polymorphism (15–20% of Asian patients and 3–5% of White and Black patients may be poor metabolizers and may have significantly ↑ dexlansoprazole concentrations and an ↑ risk of adverse effects); no active metabolites. No renal elimination.

Half-life: 1–2 hr.

TIME/ACTION PROFILE (plasma concentrations)

ROUTE	ONSET	PEAK*	DURATION
PO	unknown	1–2 hr (1st); 4–5 hr (2nd)	24 hr

* Reflects effects of delayed release capsule.

Contraindications/Precautions

Contraindicated in: Hypersensitivity to dexlansoprazole or related drugs (benzimidazoles); Severe hepatic impairment; Concurrent use of rilpivirine.
Use Cautiously in: Moderate hepatic impairment; Patients using high doses for >1 yr (↑ risk of hip, wrist, or spine fractures and fundic gland polyps); Patients using therapy for >3 yr (↑ risk of vitamin B_{12} deficiency); Pre-existing risk of hypocalcemia; OB: Safety not established in pregnancy; Lactation: Safety not established in breastfeeding; Pedi: Children <12 yr (safety and effectiveness not established); ↑ risk of heart valve thickening in children <2 yr; Geri: Appears on Beers list. ↑ risk of *Clostridioides difficile* infection, pneumonia, GI malignancies, bone loss, and fractures in older adults. Avoid scheduled use for >8 wk in older adults unless for high-risk patients (e.g., oral corticosteroid or chronic NSAID use) or patients with erosive esophagitis, Barrett esophagitis, pathological hypersecretory condition, or demonstrated need for maintenance therapy (e.g., failure of H_2 antagonist).

Adverse Reactions/Side Effects

Derm: ACUTE GENERALIZED EXANTHEMATOUS PUSTULOSIS, cutaneous lupus erythematosus, DRUG REACTION WITH EOSINOPHILIA AND SYSTEMIC SYMPTOMS (DRESS), STEVENS-JOHNSON SYNDROME (SJS), TOXIC EPIDERMAL NECROLYSIS (TEN). **F and E** hypocalcemia (especially if treatment duration ≥3 mo), hypokalemia (especially if treatment duration ≥3 mo), hypomagnesemia (especially if treatment duration ≥3 mo). **GI:** abdominal pain, diarrhea, CLOSTRIDIOIDES DIFFICILE-ASSOCIATED DIARRHEA (CDAD), flatulence, fundic gland polyps, nausea, vomiting. **GU:** acute tubulointerstitial nephritis. **Hemat:** vitamin B_{12} deficiency. **MS:** bone fracture. **Misc:** HYPERSENSITIVITY REACTIONS (INCLUDING ANAPHYLAXIS, ANGIOEDEMA, OR ACUTE TUBULOINTERSTITIAL NEPHRITIS), systemic lupus erythematosus.

Interactions

Drug-Drug: May ↓ absorption of drugs requiring acid pH, including **ketoconazole**, **itraconazole**, **atazanavir**, **nelfinavir**, **rilpivirine**, **ampicillin esters**, **iron salts**, **erlotinib**, and **mycophenolate mofetil**; concurrent use with rilpivirine contraindicated; avoid concurrent use with atazanavir and nelfinavir. May ↑ levels of **digoxin**, **methotrexate**, and **tacrolimus**. May ↑ effect of **warfarin**. Hypomagnesemia and hypokalemia ↑ risk of **digoxin** toxicity.

Route/Dosage

PO (Adults and Children ≥12 yr): *Healing of erosive esophagitis:* 60 mg once daily for up to 8 wk; *Maintenance of healed erosive esophagitis:* 30 mg once daily for up to 6 mo (adults) and up to 16 wk (12–17 yr); *GERD:* 30 mg once daily for 4 wk.

Hepatic Impairment

PO (Adults): *Moderate hepatic impairment:* Not to exceed 30 mg/day.

Availability (generic available)

Delayed-release capsules: 30 mg, 60 mg.

NURSING IMPLICATIONS

Assessment

- Monitor for positive response after therapy is complete. *If response is suboptimal or early symptomatic relapse occurs,* consider diagnostic testing for gastric malignancy, including endoscopy.
- Monitor for diarrhea, abdominal pain, fever, and bloody stools, especially in hospitalized patients. *If diarrhea occurs and does not improve,* evaluate for CDAD.
- Monitor for acute tubulointerstitial nephritis (↓ renal function, malaise, nausea, anorexia, fever, rash, arthralgias) periodically during therapy. *If signs or symptoms occur,* discontinue dexlansoprazole and evaluate.
- Monitor for severe cutaneous adverse reactions (SJS, TEN, DRESS). Discontinue dexlansoprazole at first sign of severe skin reactions and consider further evaluation.
- Assess for new signs and symptoms or exacerbation of cutaneous and systemic lupus erythematosus. *If signs or exacerbation occur,* discontinue dexlansoprazole and refer to specialist for evaluation.

Lab Test Considerations

- May cause abnormal liver function tests, including ↑ AST or ALT and ↑ or ↓ serum bilirubin.
- May ↓ vitamin B_{12}.
- May ↑ BUN and serum creatinine.
- May ↑ blood glucose.
- May ↑ serum potassium and ↓ serum magnesium. Consider monitoring magnesium and calcium levels prior to starting and periodically during therapy in patients with a pre-existing risk of hypocalcemia (hypoparathyroidism). Supplement with magnesium and/or calcium as needed. If hypocalcemia is refractory to treatment, consider discontinuing therapy.
- May ↓ platelets.
- Monitor INR and prothrombin time in patients taking warfarin.

Implementation

- Do not confuse Dexilant with duloxetine.
- **PO:** May be administered without regard to food. ***DNC:*** Swallow capsules whole or may be opened and sprinkled on 1 tablespoon of applesauce and swallowed immediately, without crushing or chewing, for patients with difficulty swallowing.
- Capsules may be opened and granules emptied into 20 mL water. Withdraw entire mixture into syringe; swirl gently to mix. Administer mixture into mouth or nasogastric tube immediately; do not save for later.

Rinse syringe with 10 mL of water twice to ensure all medication administered.
- Use for shortest time possible to ↓ risk of osteoporosis-related fractures, cutaneous or systemic lupus erythematosus, vitamin B_{12} deficiency, and fundic gland polyps.

Patient/Family Teaching

- Explain purpose and side effects of medication. Advise patient to read *Patient Information* before starting therapy.
- Instruct patient to take missed dose as soon as remembered but not if just before next scheduled dose; do not double doses.
- Advise patient to avoid alcohol, products containing aspirin or NSAIDs, and foods that may cause GI irritation.
- Advise patient to report onset of black, tarry stools; diarrhea; or abdominal pain to health care professional promptly, especially if accompanied by fever or bloody stools. Do not treat with antidiarrheals without consulting health care professional.
- Advise patient to notify health care professional if signs and symptoms of hypomagnesemia (seizure, dizziness, abnormal or fast heartbeat, jitteriness, jerking movements or shaking, muscle weakness, spasms of hands and feet, muscle aches, voice box spasm) occur.
- Instruct patient to notify health care professional of all Rx or OTC medications, vitamins, or herbal products being taken and to consult with health care professional before taking other medications.
- Rep: Advise women of reproductive potential to notify health care professional if pregnancy is planned or suspected or if breastfeeding.

Evaluation/Desired Outcomes

- Decrease in abdominal pain, heartburn, gastric irritation, and bleeding in patients with GERD; may require up to 4 wk of therapy.
- Healing in patients with erosive esophagitis; may require up to 8 wk of therapy for healing and 6 mo of therapy for maintenance.

HIGH ALERT

dexmedeTOMIDine

(dex-me-de-**to**-mi-deen)

Igalmi, Precedex

Classification

Therapeutic: sedative/hypnotics

Pharmacologic: alpha adrenergic agonists

Indications

IV: Sedation of initially intubated and mechanically ventilated patients during treatment in an intensive care setting; should not be used for >24 hr. **IV:** Sedation of nonintubated patients before and/or during surgical and other procedures. **Buccal, SL:** Acute treatment of agitation associated with schizophrenia or bipolar I or II disorder.

Action

Acts as a relatively selective alpha-2 adrenergic agonist with sedative properties. **Therapeutic Effects:** Sedation. Decreased agitation.

Pharmacokinetics

Absorption: IV administration results in complete bioavailability. 72% absorbed following SL administration; 82% absorbed following buccal administration.

Distribution: Widely distributed to extravascular tissues.

Protein Binding: 94%.

Metabolism and Excretion: Mostly metabolized by the liver; some metabolism by P450 enzyme system. Metabolites are mostly excreted in urine.

Half-life: *IV:* 2 hr; *SL/buccal:* 2.8 hr.

TIME/ACTION PROFILE (sedation)

ROUTE	ONSET	PEAK	DURATION
IV	rapid	unknown	unknown
SL/buccal	20–30 min	60–90 min	2 hr

Contraindications/Precautions

Contraindicated in: Hypersensitivity; Hypotension; Advanced heart block; Severe left ventricular dysfunction; History of syncope; QT interval prolongation, arrhythmias, symptomatic bradycardia, hypokalemia, hypomagnesemia, or concurrent use of QT interval prolonging medications.

Use Cautiously in: Hepatic impairment (lower doses may be required); Hypovolemia, diabetes, or chronic hypertension (↑ risk of hypotension and bradycardia); OB: Safety not established in pregnancy; Lactation: Use while breastfeeding only if potential maternal benefit justifies potential risk to infant; Pedi: Children <1 mo (safety and effectiveness not established); Geri: ↑ risk of bradycardia and hypotension in older adults (consider dose ↓).

Adverse Reactions/Side Effects

CV: hypotension, BRADYCARDIA, QT interval prolongation, SINUS ARREST, transient hypertension. **GI:** dry mouth, nausea, oral numbness, vomiting. **Hemat:** anemia. **Neuro:** somnolence, dizziness. **Resp:** hypoxia. **Misc:** fever, hyperthermia.

Interactions

Drug-Drug: Sedation is enhanced by **anesthetics**, other **sedative/hypnotics**, and **opioid analgesics**. **QT interval prolonging medications** may ↑ risk of

QT interval prolongation and torsades de pointes; avoid concurrent use.
Drug-Natural Products: Kava-kava, valerian, skullcap, chamomile, or **hops** can ↑ CNS depression.

Route/Dosage

ICU Sedation

IV (Adults): *Loading infusion:* 1 mcg/kg over 10 min, followed by *maintenance infusion* of 0.2–0.7 mcg/kg/hr for maximum of 24 hr; rate is adjusted to achieve desired level of sedation.

Procedural Sedation

IV (Adults): *Loading infusion:* 1 mcg/kg (0.5 mcg/kg for ophthalmic surgery or patients >65 yr) over 10 min, followed by *maintenance infusion* of 0.6 mcg/kg/hr; rate is adjusted to achieve desired level of sedation (usual range 0.2–1 mcg/kg/hr) (maintenance infusion of 0.7 mcg/kg/hr recommended for fiberoptic intubation until endotracheal tube secured).
IV (Children ≥2 yr): *Loading infusion:* 2 mcg/kg over 10 min, followed by *maintenance infusion* of 1.5 mcg/kg/hr; rate is adjusted to achieve desired level of sedation (usual range 0.5–1.5 mcg/kg/hr).
IV (Children 1 mo–<2 yr): *Loading infusion:* 1.5 mcg/kg over 10 min, followed by *maintenance infusion* of 1.5 mcg/kg/hr; rate is adjusted to achieve desired level of sedation (usual range 0.5–1.5 mcg/kg/hr).

Acute Treatment of Agitation Associated with Schizophrenia or Bipolar I or II Disorder.

Buccal, SL (Adults <65 yr): *Mild or moderate agitation:* 120 mcg initially; if agitation continues, up to two additional doses of 60 mcg may be administered ≥2 hr apart (max total dose = 240 mcg/day). *Severe agitation:* 180 mcg initially; if agitation continues, up to two additional doses of 90 mcg may be administered ≥2 hr apart (max total dose = 360 mcg/day).
Buccal, SL (Geriatric Patients ≥65 yr): *Mild, moderate, or severe agitation:* 120 mcg initially; if agitation continues, up to two additional doses of 60 mcg may be administered ≥2 hr apart (max total dose = 240 mcg/day).

Hepatic Impairment

Buccal: sublingual (Adults): *Mild or moderate hepatic impairment:* Mild or moderate agitation: 90 mcg initially; if agitation continues, up to two additional doses of 60 mcg may be administered ≥2 hr apart (max total dose = 210 mcg/day). Severe agitation: 120 mcg initially; if agitation continues, up to two additional doses of 60 mcg may be administered ≥2 hr apart (max total dose = 240 mcg/day). *Severe hepatic impairment:* Mild or moderate agitation: 60 mcg initially; if agitation continues, up to two additional doses of 60 mcg may be administered ≥2 hr apart (max total dose = 180 mcg/day). *Severe agitation:* 120 mcg initially; if agitation continues, up to two additional doses of 60 mcg may be administered ≥2 hr apart (max total dose = 240 mcg/day).

Availability (generic available)

Sublingual/buccal film (Igalmi): 120 mcg, 180 mcg. **Premixed infusion (in 0.9% NaCl):** 80 mcg/20 mL, 200 mcg/50 mL, 400 mcg/100 mL, 1000 mcg/250 mL. **Solution for injection:** 🍁 4 mcg/mL, 100 mcg/mL.

NURSING IMPLICATIONS

Assessment

- Assess level of sedation during therapy. Adjust dose as clinically indicated.
- Monitor ECG and BP continuously during therapy. *If hypotension, bradycardia, or sinus arrest occur,* provide clinically indicated intervention (↓ or stop dexmedetomidine, ↑ IV fluid rate, elevate lower extremities, administer vasopressor agent, administer anticholinergic).
- Monitor for hypotension, orthostatic hypotension, and bradycardia. Ensure patient is adequately hydrated and keep in sitting or lying position until stable. If unable to sit or lie down, take precautions to prevent falls.
- Monitor for signs and symptoms of withdrawal (nausea, vomiting, agitation); may lead to tachycardia and hypertension. Usually occur within 24–48 hr of discontinuing dexmedetomidine. Treat symptomatically.

Toxicity and Overdose:

- Atropine or glycopyrrolate IV may be used to modify the vagal tone in dexmedetomidine-induced bradycardia.

Implementation

- Do not confuse dexmedetomidine with dexamethasone.
- Dexmedetomidine should be administered only in intensive care settings with continuous monitoring.
- A loading dose may not be required when converting patient from another sedative.
- **Buccal: sublingual** Monitor vital signs and alertness after administration to prevent falls and syncope. Open pouch and instruct patient to remove film with clean dry hands. *For SL dose,* instruct patient to place under tongue; film will stick in place. Advise patient not to eat or drink for 15 min after dose. *For buccal dose,* instruct patient to place behind lower lip; film will stick in place. Advise patient not to eat or drink for 1 hr after dose. Instruct patient to close their mouth; allow film to dissolve. Do not chew or swallow film.

IV Administration

- **Continuous Infusion: Dilution:** To prepare infusion, withdraw 2 mL of dexmedetomidine and add to 48 mL of 0.9% NaCl for a total of 50 mL. Shake gently. **Concentration:** 4 mcg/mL. Solution should be clear; do not administer if discolored or contains particulates. Ampules and vials are for single use only.

- **Rate:** Administer *loading infusion* over 10 min, followed by *maintenance infusion* of 0.2–0.7 mcg/kg/hr for ICU sedation and 0.2–1.0 mcg/kg/hr for procedural sedation. Adjust dose to achieve desired level of sedation. Administer via infusion pump to ensure accurate rate.
- **Y-Site Compatibility:** acetaminophen, acyclovir, alemtuzumab, allopurinol, amikacin, aminocaproic acid, aminophylline, amiodarone, amphotericin B liposomal, ampicillin, ampicillin/sulbactam, anidulafungin, argatroban, arsenic trioxide, atracurium, atropine, azithromycin, aztreonam, bivalirudin, bleomycin, buprenorphine, busulfan, butorphanol, caffeine citrate, calcium chloride, calcium gluconate, carboplatin, carmustine, caspofungin, cefazolin, cefepime, cefotaxime, cefotetan, cefoxitin, ceftazidime, ceftazidime/avibactam, ceftolozane/tazobactam, ceftriaxone, cefuroxime, chlorpromazine, ciprofloxacin, cisatracurium, cisplatin, clindamycin, cyclophosphamide, cyclosporine, cytarabine, D5W, dacarbazine, dactinomycin, daptomycin, daunorubicin, dexamethasone, dexrazoxane, digoxin, diltiazem, diphenhydramine, dobutamine, docetaxel, dopamine, doxorubicin hydrochloride, doxorubicin liposome, doxycycline, droperidol, enalaprilat, ephedrine, epinephrine, eravacycline, ertapenem, erythromycin, esmolol, etomidate, etoposide, etoposide phosphate, famotidine, fentanyl, fluconazole, fludarabine, fluorouracil, foscarnet, fosphenytoin, furosemide, ganciclovir, gemcitabine, gentamicin, glycopyrrolate, granisetron, haloperidol, heparin, hetastarch, hydrocortisone, hydromorphone, hydroxyzine, idarubicin, ifosfamide, imipenem/cilastatin, imipenem/cilastatin/relebactam, insulin, regular, isavuconazonium, isoproterenol, ketorolac, labetalol, LR, leucovorin calcium, levetiracetam, levofloxacin, lidocaine, linezolid, lorazepam, magnesium sulfate, mannitol, meperidine, meropenem, meropenem/vaborbactam, mesna, methadone, methohexital, methotrexate, methylprednisolone, metoclopramide, metoprolol, metronidazole, midazolam, milrinone, mitomycin, mitoxantrone, morphine, moxifloxacin, mycophenolate, nalbuphine, naloxone, nicardipine, nitroglycerin, nitroprusside, norepinephrine, 0.9% NaCl, octreotide, ondansetron, oritavancin, oxaliplatin, oxytocin, paclitaxel, palonosetron, pamidronate, pemetrexed, pentamidine, pentobarbital, phenobarbital, phenylephrine, piperacillin/tazobactam, plazomicin, potassium acetate, potassium chloride, potassium phosphates, procainamide, prochlorperazine, promethazine, propofol, propranolol, remifentanil, remimazolam, sildenafil, sodium acetate, sodium bicarbonate, sodium phosphate, succinylcholine, sufentanil, sulbactam/durlobactam, tacrolimus, tedizolid, theophylline, thiotepa, tigecycline, tirofiban, tobramycin, topotecan, trimethoprim/sulfamethoxazole, vancomycin, vasopressin, vecuronium, verapamil, vinblastine, vincristine, vinorelbine, voriconazole, zidovudine, zoledronic acid.
- **Y-Site Incompatibility:** amphotericin B, diazepam, gemtuzumab ozogamicin, irinotecan, ketamine, pantoprazole, phenytoin.

D

Patient/Family Teaching

- Explain purpose and side effects of medication and that dexmedetomidine administration will be supervised by a health care professional. Advise patient to read *Patient Information* before starting therapy.
- May cause drowsiness. Caution patient to avoid driving and other activities requiring alertness until response to drug is known.
- **Rep:** Advise women of reproductive potential to notify health care professional if pregnancy is suspected or if breastfeeding. Advise patient to monitor breastfed infants for irritability.

Evaluation/Desired Outcomes

- Sedation for up to 24 hr.
- Decreased agitation.

dexmethylphenidate

(dex-meth-ill-**fen**-i-date)

Focalin, Focalin XR

Classification

Therapeutic: central nervous system stimulants

Schedule II

Indications

Attention-deficit hyperactivity disorder (ADHD).

Action

Produces CNS and respiratory stimulation with weak sympathomimetic activity. **Therapeutic Effects:** Increased attention span in ADHD.

Pharmacokinetics

Absorption: Readily absorbed following oral administration.

Distribution: Unknown.

Metabolism and Excretion: Mostly metabolized by the liver; inactive metabolites are renally excreted.

Half-life: 2.2 hr.

TIME/ACTION PROFILE (improvement in symptoms)

ROUTE	ONSET	PEAK	DURATION
PO	7 days	1 mo	unknown

Contraindications/Precautions

Contraindicated in: Hypersensitivity; Hyperexcitable states (marked anxiety, agitation, or tension); Hyperthyroidism; Psychotic personalities or suicidal or homicidal tendencies; Glaucoma; Concurrent use or use within 14 days of MAO inhibitors or MAO-like drugs (linezolid or methylene blue); Psychoses (may exacerbate symptoms).

Use Cautiously in: Cardiovascular disease (sudden death has occurred in children with structural cardiac abnormalities or other serious heart problems); Hyperthyroidism; Hypertension; Diabetes mellitus; History of substance abuse; Continual use (may produce psychological dependence or physical addiction); Seizure disorders (may ↓ seizure threshold); Open-angle glaucoma or elevated intraocular pressure; Tics or family history/diagnosis of Tourette syndrome (may worsen condition); OB: Use during pregnancy only if potential maternal benefit outweighs potential fetal risk; Lactation: Use while breastfeeding only if potential maternal benefit outweighs potential risk to infant; Pedi: Children <6 yr (safety not established).

Adverse Reactions/Side Effects

CV: peripheral vasculopathy, SUDDEN DEATH, tachycardia. **EENT:** ↑ intraocular pressure, angle closure glaucoma, visual disturbances. **GI:** abdominal pain, anorexia, nausea. **GU:** libido changes, priapism. **Metab:** growth suppression, weight loss (may occur with prolonged use). **MS:** RHABDOMYOLYSIS. **Neuro:** behavioral disturbances, hallucinations, insomnia, mania, nervousness, thought disorder, tics, Tourette syndrome, twitching. **Misc:** fever, HYPERSENSITIVITY REACTIONS (INCLUDING ANAPHYLAXIS AND ANGIOEDEMA), physical dependence, psychological dependence.

Interactions

Drug-Drug: Concurrent use with **MAO inhibitors** or **MAO-inhibitor-like drugs**, such as **linezolid** or **methylene blue**, may result in serious, potentially fatal reactions; wait at least 14 days following discontinuation of MAO inhibitor before initiation of amphetamine mixtures. Drugs that affect serotonergic neurotransmitter systems, including **MAO inhibitors**, **tricyclic antidepressants**, **SSRIs**, **SNRIs**, **fentanyl**, **buspirone**, **tramadol**, **lithium**, and **triptans**, may ↑ risk of serotonin syndrome. May ↓ effects of **antihypertensives**. May ↑ effects of **vasopressors**. May ↑ effects of **warfarin**, **phenobarbital**, **phenytoin**, and some **antidepressants**; dosage adjustments may be necessary. **Risperidone** may ↑ risk of extrapyramidal symptoms.

Route/Dosage

Tablets

PO (Adults and Children ≥6 yr): *Patients not previously taking methylphenidate:* 2.5 mg twice daily; may be ↑ weekly as needed up to 10 mg twice daily; *Patients currently taking methylphenidate:* Starting dose is ½ of the methylphenidate dose, up to 10 mg twice daily.

Extended-Release Capsules

PO (Adults): *Patients not previously taking methylphenidate:* 10 mg once daily; may be ↑ by 10 mg up to 40 mg/day; *Patients currently taking methylphenidate:* Starting dose is ½ of the methylphenidate dose, up to 40 mg/day given as a single daily dose; *Patients currently taking dexmethylphenidate:* Give same daily dose as a single dose.

PO (Children ≥6 yr): *Patients not previously taking methylphenidate:* 5 mg once daily; may be ↑ by 5 mg weekly up to 30 mg/day; *Patients currently taking methylphenidate:* Starting dose is ½ of the methylphenidate dose, up to 30 mg/day, given as a single daily dose; *Patients currently taking dexmethylphenidate:* Give same daily dose as a single dose.

Availability (generic available)

Extended-release capsules: 5 mg, 10 mg, 15 mg, 20 mg, 25 mg, 30 mg, 35 mg, 40 mg. **Immediate-release tablets:** 2.5 mg, 5 mg, 10 mg. ***In combination with:*** serdexmethylphenidate (Azstarys). See Appendix N.

NURSING IMPLICATIONS

Assessment

- Assess child's attention span, impulse control, and interactions with others. Therapy may be interrupted at intervals to determine whether symptoms are sufficient to continue therapy.
- Monitor BP, HR, and respiratory rate before administering and periodically during therapy. Obtain a history (including assessment of family history of sudden death or ventricular arrhythmia), physical exam to assess for cardiac disease, and further evaluation (ECG and echocardiogram), if indicated. If exertional chest pain, unexplained syncope, or other cardiac symptoms occur, evaluate promptly.
- Monitor weight biweekly and inform health care provider of significant loss. Pedi: Monitor height periodically in children; report growth inhibition. Growth suppression may occur in children with long-term use.
- Monitor closely for behavior changes.
- Assess for risk of abuse, misuse, or addiction prior to starting therapy and during therapy. Has high dependence and abuse or misuse potential. Misuse and abuse of CNS stimulants can result in overdose and death; this risk is ↑ with higher doses or unapproved methods of administration, such as snorting or injection. Tolerance to medication occurs rapidly; do not ↑ dose.

- Assess patient's fingers periodically for signs of peripheral vasculopathy (digital ulceration, soft tissue breakdown).
- Monitor for signs of anaphylaxis (wheezing, shortness of breath, rash) during therapy.

Lab Test Considerations

- Monitor CBC, differential, and platelet count periodically in patients receiving prolonged therapy.

Implementation

- Do not confuse dexmethylphenidate with methadone.
- **PO:** Administer twice daily at least 4 hr apart without regard to meals.
- Administer XR tablets once daily in the morning. Swallow capsules whole. For patients with difficulty swallowing, capsules can be opened and sprinkled on a spoonful of applesauce. Consume immediately; do not store for future use.

Patient/Family Teaching

- Instruct patient to take medication as directed. If more than prescribed amount is taken, notify health care provider immediately. If a dose is missed, take the remaining doses for that day at regularly spaced intervals; do not double doses. Take the last dose before 6 pm to minimize the risk of insomnia. Instruct patient not to alter dose without consulting health care provider. Abrupt cessation with high doses may cause extreme fatigue and mental depression. Advise patient and parents to read the *Medication Guide* prior to starting therapy and with each Rx refill.
- Advise patient that dexmethylphenidate is a drug with known potential for abuse, misuse, and/or addiction. Store in safe place, protect it from theft, and never give to anyone other than the individual for whom it was prescribed.
- Inform patients starting therapy of risk of peripheral vasculopathy. Instruct patients to notify health care provider of any new numbness; pain; skin color change from pale to blue to red; or coolness or sensitivity to temperature in fingers or toes and to call if unexplained wounds appear on fingers or toes. May require rheumatology consultation.
- Advise patient to check weight 2–3 times weekly and report weight loss to health care provider.
- Instruct patient to notify health care provider of all Rx or OTC medications, vitamins, or herbal products being taken and to consult health care provider before taking other Rx, OTC, or herbal products.
- May rarely cause dizziness or drowsiness. Caution patient to avoid driving or activities requiring alertness until response to medication is known.
- Advise patient to notify health care provider if nervousness, restlessness, insomnia, dizziness, anorexia, or dry mouth becomes severe. Pedi: If reduced appetite and weight loss are a problem, advise parents to provide high-calorie meals when drug levels are low (at breakfast and or bedtime).
- Advise patient and/or caregivers to notify health care provider of behavioral changes.
- Inform patient that health care provider may order periodic holidays from the drug to assess progress and to decrease dependence.
- Rep: May cause fetal harm. Advise women of reproductive potential to notify health care provider if pregnancy is planned or suspected and to avoid breastfeeding during therapy. May ↑ risk or premature birth and low birth weight. Monitor infants born to mothers taking amphetamines for symptoms of withdrawal (feeding difficulties, irritability, agitation, excessive drowsiness). Encourage patients exposed to amphetamines during pregnancy to join the registry. Health care providers may call the National Pregnancy Registry for Psychiatric Medications at 1-866-961-2388 or online at https://womensmentalhealth.org/clinical-and-research-programs/pregnancyregistry/othermedications/ to register patients.
- Emphasize the importance of routine follow-up exams to monitor progress.
- **Home Care Issues:** Advise parents to notify school nurse of medication regimen.

Evaluation/Desired Outcomes

- Improved attention span and decreased impulsiveness and hyperactivity in ADHD. If improvement is not seen within 1 mo, discontinue dexmethylphenidate. Effectiveness has not been tested beyond 6 wk. Re-evaluate usefulness for prolonged therapy.

dexrazoxane (dex-ra-**zox**-ane)

~~Totect~~, Zinecard

Classification

Therapeutic: cardioprotective agents

Indications

Reducing incidence and severity of cardiomyopathy from doxorubicin in women with metastatic breast cancer who have already received a cumulative dose of doxorubicin >300 mg/m^2 and who will continue to receive doxorubicin therapy to maintain tumor control. Treatment of extravasation resulting from IV anthracycline chemotherapy.

Action

Acts as an intracellular chelating agent. **Therapeutic Effects:** Diminishes the cardiotoxic effects of doxorubicin. Decreased damage from extravasation of anthracyclines.

Pharmacokinetics

Absorption: IV administration results in complete bioavailability.
Distribution: Well distributed to tissues.
Metabolism and Excretion: Some metabolism occurs; 42% eliminated in urine.
Half-life: 2.1–2.5 hr.

TIME/ACTION PROFILE (cardioprotective effect)

ROUTE	ONSET	PEAK	DURATION
IV	rapid	unknown	unknown

Contraindications/Precautions

Contraindicated in: Any other type of chemotherapy except other anthracyclines (doxorubicin-like agents); Hepatic impairment (for treatment of extravasation only); OB: Pregnancy; Lactation: Lactation.
Use Cautiously in: Renal impairment (CCr <40 mL/min) (↓ dose); Rep: Women of reproductive potential and men with female partners of reproductive potential; Pedi: Safety and effectiveness not established in children.

Adverse Reactions/Side Effects

GU: ↓ fertility (men). **Hemat:** leukopenia, NEUTROPENIA, thrombocytopenia. **Local:** pain at injection site. **Misc:** HYPERSENSITIVITY REACTIONS (INCLUDING ANAPHYLAXIS AND ANGIOEDEMA), MALIGNANCY.

Interactions

Drug-Drug: Myelosuppression may be ↑ by **antineoplastics** or **radiation therapy**. Antitumor effects of concurrent combination chemotherapy with **fluorouracil** and **cyclophosphamide** may be ↓ by dexrazoxane.

Route/Dosage

Cardioprotective

IV (Adults): 10 mg of dexrazoxane/1 mg doxorubicin.

Renal Impairment

IV (Adults): *CCr <40 mL/min:* ↓ dose by 50%.

Extravasation Treatment

IV (Adults): 1000 mg/m² (maximum 2000 mg) given on Days 1 and 2, followed by a dose of 500 mg/m² (maximum 1000 mg) on Day 3.

Renal Impairment

IV (Adults): *CCr <40 mL/min:* ↓ dose by 50%.

Availability (generic available)

Lyophilized powder for injection: 250 mg/vial, 500 mg/vial.

NURSING IMPLICATIONS

Assessment

- **Cardioprotective:** Assess extent of cardiomyopathy (cardiomegaly on x-ray, basilar rales, S_3 gallop, dyspnea, decline in left ventricular ejection fraction) before and periodically during therapy.
- **Extravasation protection:** Assess site of extravasation for pain, burning, swelling, and redness. Assess site during and after therapy until resolution. Dexrazoxane is not effective against the effects of vesicants other than anthracyclines.
- Assess for hypersensitivity reactions (rash, pruritus, flushing, shortness of breath). *If anaphylaxis occurs,* implement support measures (epinephrine), and treat symptoms accordingly.

Lab Test Considerations

- Verify negative pregnancy test before starting therapy.
- Monitor CBC with differential before each course of therapy and frequently during therapy. Thrombocytopenia, leukopenia, and neutropenia from chemotherapy may be more severe at nadir with dexrazoxane therapy.
- Monitor liver function tests periodically during therapy. May ↑ liver enzymes.

Implementation

IV Administration

- Wear gloves, gown, and mask while handling IV medication. Discard IV equipment in specially designated containers.
- **Extravasation Protection:** Administer as soon as possible within 6 hr of extravasation in a large-caliber vein in an extremity/area other than the one affected by the extravasation. Remove cooling procedures, such as ice packs, >15 min before administration to allow sufficient blood flow to area of extravasation. Start treatment on Day 2 and Day 3 at same hr (+/–3 hr) as on first day.
- **Intermittent Infusion: Reconstitution:** Reconstitute each vial with 50 mL of sterile water for injection. Reconstituted solution is slightly yellow. Do not administer solutions that are discolored or contain particulate matter. **Concentration:** 10 mg/mL. **Dilution:** Withdraw dose volume within 30 min of reconstitution and inject into 1000 mL bag of LR. Solution is stable for 4 hr at room temperature or 12 hr if refrigerated. **Rate:** Infuse over 1–2 hr.
- **Cardioprotective:** Doxorubicin should be administered within 30 min following dexrazoxane administration.
- **Intermittent Infusion: Reconstitution:** Reconstitute with 25 mL or 50 mL of sterile water for injection for 250-mg or 500-mg vial, respectively. Reconstituted solution is slightly yellow. Do not administer solutions that are discolored or contain particulate matter. **Concentration:** 10 mg/mL. **Dilution:** Dilute reconstituted solution further in LR. Solution is stable for 1 hr at

room temperature or 4 hr if refrigerated. **Concentration:** 1.3–3 mg/mL. **Rate:** Infuse over 15 min.

- **Y-Site Compatibility:** alemtuzumab, amikacin, amiodarone, ampicillin, ampicillin/sulbactam, anidulafungin, argatroban, arsenic trioxide, atracurium, azithromycin, aztreonam, bivalirudin, bleomycin, bumetanide, buprenorphine, busulfan, butorphanol, calcium chloride, calcium gluconate, carboplatin, carmustine, caspofungin, cefazolin, cefotaxime, cefotetan, cefoxitin, ceftazidime, ceftriaxone, cefuroxime, chloramphenicol, chlorpromazine, ciprofloxacin, cisatracurium, cisplatin, clindamycin, cyclophosphamide, cyclosporine, cytarabine, dacarbazine, dactinomycin, daptomycin, daunorubicin, dexmedetomidine, digoxin, diltiazem, diphenhydramine, docetaxel, dopamine, doxorubicin hydrochloride, doxorubicin liposomal, doxycycline, droperidol, enalaprilat, ephedrine, epinephrine, epirubicin, eptifibatide, ertapenem, erythromycin, esmolol, etoposide, etoposide phosphate, famotidine, fentanyl, fluconazole, fludarabine, fluorouracil, foscarnet, fosphenytoin, gemcitabine, gentamicin, glycopyrrolate, granisetron, haloperidol, heparin, hetastarch, hydralazine, hydrocortisone, hydromorphone, idarubicin, ifosfamide, imipenem/cilastatin, insulin, regular, irinotecan, isoproterenol, ketorolac, labetalol, leucovorin calcium, levofloxacin, lidocaine, linezolid, lorazepam, magnesium sulfate, mannitol, melphalan, meperidine, meropenem, mesna, metoclopramide, metoprolol, midazolam, milrinone, mitoxantrone, morphine, moxifloxacin, mycophenolate, nalbuphine, naloxone, nicardipine, nitroglycerin, nitroprusside, norepinephrine, octreotide, ondansetron, oxaliplatin, paclitaxel, palonosetron, pamidronate, pemetrexed, pentamidine, phenobarbital, phentolamine, phenylephrine, piperacillin/tazobactam, polmyxin B, potassium acetate, potassium chloride, potassium phosphates, procainamide, prochlorperazine, promethazine, propranolol, remifentanil, rituximab, rocuronium, sodium acetate, sodium bicarbonate, succinylcholine, sufentanil, tacrolimus, theophylline, thiotepa, tigecycline, tirofiban, tobramycin, topotecan, vancomycin, vasopressin, vecuronium, verapamil, vinblastine, vincristine, vinorelbine, voriconazole, zoledronic acid
- **Y-Site Incompatibility:** acyclovir, allopurinol, aminophylline, amphotericin B liposomal, cefepime, dantrolene, diazepam, dobutamine, furosemide, ganciclovir, gemtuzumab ozogamicin, methotrexate, methylprednisolone, mitomycin, nafcillin, pantoprazole, pentobarbital, phenytoin, sodium phosphate, trimethoprim/sulfamethoxazole, zidovudine

Patient/Family Teaching

- Explain purpose and side effects of medication. Advise patient to read *Patient Information* before starting therapy.
- Advise patient to notify health care professional of all Rx or OTC medications, vitamins, or herbal products being taken and to consult health care professional before taking other medications.
- Advise patient about neutropenia precautions; educate to avoid crowded places and people with flu-like symptoms and to use personal hygiene practices such as hand hygiene and oral care.
- Advise patient to notify health care professional if hypersensitivity reactions occur and to seek immediate medical attention if necessary.
- Advise patient to notify health care professional of unexplained weight loss, persistent fatigue, lumps, or abnormal bleeding.
- Emphasize the need for continued monitoring of cardiac function.
- Rep: May cause fetal harm. Advise women of reproductive potential to use highly effective contraception during therapy and for 6 mo after last dose of dexrazoxane and to avoid breastfeeding during therapy and for 2 wk after last dose. Advise men with female partners of reproductive potential to use highly effective contraception during and for 3 mo after last dose. Advise patient to notify health care professional immediately if pregnancy is suspected. May impair fertility in men.

Evaluation/Desired Outcomes

- Diminishes the cardiotoxic effects of doxorubicin.
- Decreased damage from extravasation of anthracyclines.

dextromethorphan

(dex-troe-meth-**or**-fan)

✱ Balminil DM, ✱ Benylin DM, ✱ Bronchophan Forte DM, ✱ Buckley's DM, ✱ Cough Syrup DM, Creo-Terpin, Creomulsion Adult Formula, Creomulsion for Children, Delsym, ✱ Delsym DM, ✱ DM Children's Cough Syrup, ✱ DM Cough Syrup, ✱ Dry Cough Syrup, Father John's, Hold DM, ✱ Koffex DM, ✱ Neocitran Thin Strips Cough, Pediacare Children's Long-Acting Cough, Robafin Cough, Robitussin Children's Cough Long-Acting, Robitussin Cough Long-Acting, Robitussin CoughGels Long-Acting, Robitussin Lingering Cold Long-Acting CoughGels, Scot-Tussin Diabetes, ✱ Sedatuss

DM, ✱ Sucrets Cough Control, ✱ Sucrets DM, ✱ Triaminic DM, ✱ Triaminic Long-Acting Cough, Triaminic Thin Strips Children's Long-Acting Cough, Triaminic Children's Cough Long-Acting, Vicks 44 Cough Relief, ✱ Vicks Custom Care Dry Cough, Vicks DayQuil Cough, Vicks Nature Fusion Cough

Classification

Therapeutic: allergy, cold, and cough remedies antitussives

Indications

Symptomatic relief of coughs caused by minor viral upper respiratory tract infections or inhaled irritants.

Action

Suppresses the cough reflex by a direct effect on the cough center in the medulla. Related to opioids structurally but has no analgesic properties. **Therapeutic Effects:** Relief of irritating nonproductive cough.

Pharmacokinetics

Absorption: Rapidly absorbed from the GI tract. Extended-release product is slowly absorbed.
Distribution: Unknown.
Metabolism and Excretion: Metabolized to dextrorphan, an active metabolite. Dextromethorphan and dextrorphan are renally excreted.
Half-life: Unknown.

TIME/ACTION PROFILE (cough suppression)

ROUTE	ONSET	PEAK	DURATION
PO	15–30 min	unknown	3–6 hr†
PO-ER	unknown	unknown	9–12 hr

† Up to 8 hr for gelcaps.

Contraindications/Precautions

Contraindicated in: Hypersensitivity; Should not be used for chronic productive coughs; Some products contain alcohol and should be avoided in patients with known intolerance.
Use Cautiously in: Cough that lasts >1 wk or is accompanied by fever, rash, or headache: health care professional should be consulted; History of drug abuse or drug-seeking behavior (capsules have been abused, resulting in deaths); Diabetes (some products contain sucrose); Lactation: Lactation; Pedi: Children <4 yr (OTC cough and cold products containing this medication should be avoided).

Adverse Reactions/Side Effects

GI: nausea. **Neuro:** *high dose:* dizziness, sedation.

Interactions

Drug-Drug: Use with **MAO inhibitors** or **SSRIs** may result in serotonin syndrome (nausea, confusion, changes in BP); concurrent use should be avoided. ↑ CNS depression with **antihistamines**, **alcohol**, **antidepressants**, **sedative/hypnotics**, or **opioids**. **Amiodarone**, **fluoxetine**, or **quinidine** may ↑ levels and risk of toxicity.

Route/Dosage

PO (Adults and Children >12 yr): 10–20 mg every 4 hr *or* 30 mg every 6–8 hr *or* 60 mg of extended-release preparation every 12 hr (not to exceed 120 mg/day).
PO (Children 6–12 yr): 5–10 mg every 4 hr *or* 15 mg every 6–8 hr *or* 30 mg of extended-release preparation every 12 hr (not to exceed 60 mg/day).
PO (Children 4–6 yr): 2.5–5 mg every 4 hr *or* 7.5 mg every 6–8 hr *or* 15 mg of extended-release preparation every 12 hr (not to exceed 30 mg/day).

Availability (generic available)

Gelcaps: 30 mg^{OTC}. **Lozenges (cherry):** 2.5 mg^{OTC}, 5 mg^{OTC}. **Liquid (cherry, grape):** 3.5 mg/5 mL^{OTC}, 5 mg/5 mL, 7.5 mg/5 mL^{OTC}, 15 mg/5 mL^{OTC}, 30 mg/5 mL^{OTC}. **Syrup (cherry, cherry bubblegum):** 7.5 mg/5 mL^{OTC}, 15 mg/15 mL^{OTC}, 10 mg/5 mL^{OTC}. **Extended-release suspension (orange):** 30 mg/5 mL^{OTC}. **Drops (Grape):** 7.5 mg/0.8 mL^{OTC}, 7.5 mg/1 mL^{OTC}. **Orally disintegrating strips (cherry, grape):** 7.5 mg^{OTC}, 15 mg^{OTC}. ***In combination with:*** antihistamines, decongestants, and expectorants in cough and cold preparations^{OTC}; bupropion (Auvelity); quinidine sulfate (Nuedexta). See Appendix N.

NURSING IMPLICATIONS

Assessment

- Assess frequency and nature of cough, lung sounds, and amount and type of sputum produced. Unless contraindicated, maintain fluid intake of 1500–2000 mL to ↓ viscosity of bronchial secretions.

Implementation

- **PO:** Administer with or without food. Take with food if an upset stomach occurs. Do not give fluids immediately after administering to prevent dilution of vehicle. Shake oral suspension well before administration. Only use dosing cup provided to measure liquid doses.

Patient/Family Teaching

- Explain purpose and side effects of medication. Advise patient to read *Patient Information* before starting therapy.
- Advise patient to notify health care professional of all Rx or OTC medications, vitamins, or herbal products being taken and to consult health care professional before taking other medications.

- Instruct patient to cough effectively. Sit upright and take several deep breaths before attempting to cough.
- Advise patient to minimize cough by avoiding irritants, such as cigarette smoke, fumes, and dust. Humidification of environmental air, frequent sips of water, and sugarless hard candy may also ↓ the frequency of dry, irritating cough.
- Caution patient to avoid taking more than the recommended dose or taking alcohol or other CNS depressants concurrently with this medication; fatalities have occurred. Caution parents to avoid OTC cough and cold products while breastfeeding or giving them to children <4 yr.
- May occasionally cause dizziness. Caution patient to avoid driving or other activities requiring alertness until response to the medication is known.
- Advise patient that any cough lasting >1 wk or accompanied by fever, chest pain, persistent headache, or skin rash warrants medical attention.
- Rep: Advise women of reproductive potential to notify health care professional if pregnancy is planned or suspected or if breastfeeding.

Evaluation/Desired Outcomes

- Relief of irritating nonproductive cough.

BEERS

V diazePAM (dye-az-e-pam)

Diastat, Libervant, Valium, Valtoco

Classification

Therapeutic: antianxiety agents, anticonvulsants, sedative/hypnotics, skeletal muscle relaxants (centrally acting)

Pharmacologic: benzodiazepines

Schedule IV

Indications

Anxiety disorders. Preoperative sedation. Conscious sedation (provides light anesthesia and anterograde amnesia). Status epilepticus/uncontrolled seizures. Acute treatment of intermittent, stereotypic episodes of frequent seizure activity that are distinct from a patient's usual seizure pattern (not status epilepticus) (nasal spray or buccal film). Skeletal muscle spasms. Alcohol withdrawal.

Action

Depresses the CNS, probably by potentiating GABA, an inhibitory neurotransmitter. Produces skeletal muscle relaxation by inhibiting spinal polysynaptic afferent pathways. Has anticonvulsant properties due to enhanced presynaptic inhibition. **Therapeutic Effects:** Relief of anxiety. Sedation. Amnesia. Skeletal muscle relaxation. Decreased seizure activity.

Pharmacokinetics

Absorption: Rapidly absorbed from the GI tract. Absorption from IM sites may be slow and unpredictable. Well absorbed from rectal mucosa (90%) and nasal mucosa (97%). IV administration results in complete bioavailability.

Distribution: Widely distributed. Crosses the blood-brain barrier.

Metabolism and Excretion: Primarily metabolized in the liver via the CYP2C19 and CYP3A4 isoenzymes; the CYP2C19 isoenzyme exhibits genetic polymorphism; 5–20% of Asian patients and 3–5% of White and Black patients may be poor metabolizers and may have significantly ↑ diazepam concentrations and an ↑ risk of adverse effects. Some products of metabolism are active as CNS depressants.

Half-life: *Neonates:* 50–95 hr; *Infants (1 mo–2 yr):* 40–50 hr; *Children 2–12 yr:* 15–21 hr; *Children 12–16 yr:* 18–20 hr; *Adults:* 20–50 hr (up to 100 hr for metabolites).

TIME/ACTION PROFILE (sedation)

ROUTE	ONSET	PEAK	DURATION
PO	30–60 min	1–2 hr	up to 24 hr
IM	within 20 min	0.5–1.5 hr	unknown
IV	1–5 min	15–30 min	15–60 min†
Rectal	2–10 min	1–2 hr	4–12 hr

† In status epilepticus, anticonvulsant duration is 15–20 min.

Contraindications/Precautions

Contraindicated in: Hypersensitivity; Cross-sensitivity with other benzodiazepines may occur; Comatose patients; Myasthenia gravis; Severe pulmonary impairment; Sleep apnea; Severe hepatic impairment; Pre-existing CNS depression; Uncontrolled severe pain; Angle-closure glaucoma; Some products contain alcohol, propylene glycol, or tartrazine and should be avoided in patients with known hypersensitivity or intolerance; Lactation: Lactation; Pedi: Children <6 mo (for oral; safety not established).

Use Cautiously in: History of suicide attempt or drug dependence; Debilitated patients (↓ dose); Hypoalbuminemia; Severe renal impairment; OB: Use late in pregnancy can result in sedation (respiratory depression, lethargy, hypotonia) and/or withdrawal symptoms (hyperreflexia, irritability, restlessness, tremors, inconsolable crying, feeding difficulties) in neonates; Pedi: Metabolites can accumulate in neonates. Injection contains benzyl alcohol, which can cause potentially fatal gasping syndrome in neonates; Geri: Appears on Beers list. ↑ risk of cognitive impairment, delirium, falls, fractures, and motor vehicle accidents. If possible, avoid use in older adults.

Adverse Reactions/Side Effects

CV: hypotension (IV). **Derm:** rash. **EENT:** ↑ intraocular pressure, blurred vision, epistaxis (nasal spray), nasal congestion (nasal spray), nasal discomfort (nasal spray). **GI:** constipation, diarrhea (may be caused by propylene glycol content in oral solution), nausea, vomiting. **Local:** pain (IM), phlebitis (IV). **Metab:** weight gain. **Neuro:** dizziness, drowsiness, lethargy, ataxia, depression, dysgeusia (nasal spray), hangover, headache, paradoxical excitation, slurred speech. **Resp:** RESPIRATORY DEPRESSION. **Misc:** physical dependence, psychological dependence, tolerance.

Interactions

Drug-Drug: Use with **opioids** or other **CNS depressants**, including other **benzodiazepines**, **nonbenzodiazepine sedative/hypnotics**, **anxiolytics**, **general anesthetics**, **muscle relaxants**, **antipsychotics**, and **alcohol**, may cause profound sedation, respiratory depression, coma, and death; reserve concurrent use for when alternative treatment options are inadequate. **Cimetidine**, **hormonal contraceptives**, **disulfiram**, **fluoxetine**, **isoniazid**, **ketoconazole**, **metoprolol**, **propranolol**, or **valproic acid** may ↑ levels and risk of toxicity. May ↓ the effectiveness of **levodopa**. **Rifampin** or **barbiturates** may ↓ levels and effectiveness. Sedative effects may be ↓ by **theophylline**. Concurrent use of **ritonavir** is not recommended.
Drug-Natural Products: Kava-kava, **valerian**, or **chamomile** can ↑ risk of CNS depression.

Route/Dosage

Anxiety

PO (Adults): 2–10 mg 2–4 times daily.
IM, IV (Adults): 2–10 mg; may repeat in 3–4 hr as needed.
PO (Children >6 mo): 1–2.5 mg 3–4 times daily.
IM, IV (Children >1 mo): 0.04–0.3 mg/kg/dose every 2–4 hr to a maximum of 0.6 mg/kg within an 8-hr period if necessary.

Pre-Endoscopy

IV (Adults): 2.5–20 mg.
IM (Adults): 5–10 mg 30 min pre-endoscopy.

Pediatric Conscious Sedation for Procedures

PO (Children >6 mo): 0.2–0.3 mg/kg (not to exceed 10 mg/dose) 45–60 min prior to procedure.

Status Epilepticus/Acute Seizure Activity

Buccal (Children 2–5 yr and 26–30 kg): 15 mg as a single dose. May administer another dose, if needed, ≥4 hr after initial dose (max = 2 doses/seizure episode).
Buccal (Children 2–5 yr and 21–25 kg): 12.5 mg as a single dose. May administer another dose, if needed, ≥4 hr after initial dose (max = 2 doses/seizure episode).
Buccal (Children 2–5 yr and 16–20 kg): 10 mg as a single dose. May administer another dose, if needed, ≥4 hr after initial dose (max = 2 doses/seizure episode).
Buccal (Children 2–5 yr and 11–15 kg): 7.5 mg as a single dose. May administer another dose, if needed, ≥4 hr after initial dose (max = 2 doses/seizure episode).
Buccal (Children 2–5 yr and 6–10 kg): 5 mg as a single dose. May administer another dose, if needed, ≥4 hr after initial dose (max = 2 doses/seizure episode).
IV (Adults): 5–10 mg; may repeat every 10–15 min to a total of 30 mg; may repeat regimen again in 2–4 hr (IM route may be used if IV route unavailable); larger doses may be required.
IM, IV (Children ≥5 yr): 0.05–0.3 mg/kg/dose given over 3–5 min every 15–30 min to a total dose of 10 mg; repeat every 2–4 hr.
IM, IV (Children 1 mo–5 yr): 0.05–0.3 mg/kg/dose given over 3–5 min every 15–30 min to maximum dose of 5 mg; repeat in 2–4 hr if needed.
IV (Neonates): 0.1–0.3 mg/kg/dose given over 3–5 min every 15–30 min to maximum dose of 2 mg.
Intranasal (Adults and Children ≥12 yr and ≥76 kg): 0.2 mg/kg as a single dose (total dose = 20 mg; administered using two 10-mg spray devices, with one spray [10 mg] from each device administered into each nostril). May administer another dose, if needed, ≥4 hr after initial dose (max = 2 doses/seizure episode).
Intranasal (Adults and Children ≥12 yr and 51–75 kg): 0.2 mg/kg as a single dose (total dose = 15 mg; administered using two 7.5-mg spray devices, with one spray [7.5 mg] from each device administered into each nostril). May administer another dose, if needed, ≥4 hr after initial dose (max = 2 doses/seizure episode).
Intranasal (Adults and Children ≥12 yr and 28–50 kg): 0.2 mg/kg as a single dose (total dose = 10 mg; administered using one 10-mg spray device, with one spray [10 mg] from device administered into one nostril). May administer another dose, if needed, ≥4 hr after initial dose (max = 2 doses/seizure episode).
Intranasal (Adults and Children ≥12 yr and 14–27 kg): 0.2 mg/kg as a single dose (total dose = 5 mg; administered using one 5-mg spray device, with one spray [5 mg] from device administered into one nostril). May administer another dose, if needed, ≥4 hr after initial dose (max = 2 doses/seizure episode).
Intranasal (Children 6–11 yr and 56–74 kg): 0.3 mg/kg as a single dose (total dose = 20 mg; administered using two 10-mg spray devices, with one spray [10 mg] from each device administered into each nostril). May administer another dose, if needed, ≥4 hr after initial dose (max = 2 doses/seizure episode).
Intranasal (Children 6–11 yr and 38–55 kg): 0.3 mg/kg as a single dose (total dose = 15 mg; administered using two 7.5-mg spray devices, with one spray [7.5 mg] from each device administered into each nostril). May administer another dose, if needed, ≥4 hr after initial dose (max = 2 doses/seizure episode).

Intranasal (Children 6–11 yr and 19–37 kg): 0.3 mg/kg as a single dose (total dose = 10 mg; administered using one 10-mg spray device, with one spray [10 mg] from device administered into one nostril). May administer another dose, if needed, ≥4 hr after initial dose (max = 2 doses/seizure episode).
Intranasal (Children 6–11 yr and 10–18 kg): 0.3 mg/kg as a single dose (total dose = 5 mg; administered using one 5-mg spray device, with one spray [5 mg] from device administered into one nostril). May administer another dose, if needed, ≥4 hr after initial dose (max = 2 doses/seizure episode).
Intranasal (Children 2–5 yr and 23–33 kg): 0.5 mg/kg as a single dose (total dose = 15 mg; administered using two 7.5-mg spray devices, with one spray [7.5 mg] from each device administered into each nostril). May administer another dose, if needed, ≥4 hr after initial dose (max = 2 doses/seizure episode).
Intranasal (Children 2–5 yr and 12–22 kg): 0.5 mg/kg as a single dose (total dose = 10 mg; administered using one 10-mg spray device, with one spray [10 mg] from device administered into one nostril). May administer another dose, if needed, ≥4 hr after initial dose (max = 2 doses/seizure episode).
Intranasal (Children 2–5 yr and 6–11 kg): 0.5 mg/kg as a single dose (total dose = 5 mg; administered using one 5-mg spray device, with one spray [5 mg] from device administered into one nostril). May administer another dose, if needed, ≥4 hr after initial dose (max = 2 doses/seizure episode).
Rect (Adults and Children >12 yr): 0.2 mg/kg; may repeat 4–12 hr later.
Rect (Children 6–11 yr): 0.3 mg/kg; may repeat 4–12 hr later.
Rect (Children 2–5 yr): 0.5 mg/kg; may repeat 4–12 hr later.

Febrile Seizure Prophylaxis

PO (Children >1 mo): 1 mg/kg/day divided every 8 hr at 1st sign of fever and continue for 24 hr after fever is gone.

Skeletal Muscle Relaxation

PO (Adults): 2–10 mg 3–4 times daily.
PO (Geriatric Patients or Debilitated Patients): 2–2.5 mg 1–2 times daily initially.
PO (Children >6 mo): 1–2.5 mg 3–4 times daily.
IM, IV (Adults): 5–10 mg; may repeat in 2–4 hr (larger doses may be required for tetanus).
IM, IV: (Geriatric Patients or Debilitated Patients): 2–5 mg; may repeat in 2–4 hr (larger doses may be required for tetanus).
IM, IV (Children ≥5 yr): *Tetanus:* 5–10 mg every 3–4 hr.
IM, IV (Children >1 mo): *Tetanus:* 1–2 mg every 3–4 hr.

Alcohol Withdrawal

PO (Adults): 10 mg 3–4 times in first 24 hr; ↓ to 5 mg 3–4 times daily.
IM IV (Adults): 10 mg initially; then 5–10 mg in 3–4 hr as needed; larger or more frequent doses have been used.

D

Availability (generic available)

Tablets: 2 mg, 5 mg, 10 mg. **Oral solution:** 1 mg/mL, 5 mg/mL (Intensol). **Buccal film (Libervant):** 5 mg, 7.5 mg, 10 mg, 12.5 mg, 15 mg. **Rectal gel delivery system:** 2.5 mg, 10 mg, 20 mg. **Nasal spray (Valtoco):** 5 mg/device, 7.5 mg/device, 10 mg/device. **Solution for injection:** 5 mg/mL (contains 10% alcohol and 40% propylene glycol).

NURSING IMPLICATIONS

Assessment

- Monitor BP, HR, respiratory rate, and level of sedation (ataxia, dizziness, slurred speech) before and periodically during therapy and frequently during IV therapy.
- Assess IV site frequently during administration; may cause phlebitis.
- Assess risk for addiction, abuse, or misuse prior to administration. Prolonged high-dose therapy may lead to psychological or physical dependence. Restrict amount of drug available to patient. Observe depressed patients closely for suicidal tendencies.
- Pedi: Monitor neonates exposed to diazepam during pregnancy or labor for signs of sedation and withdrawal; manage as indicated.
- Geri: Assess risk of falls and institute fall prevention strategies.
- **Anxiety:** Assess orientation, mood, behavior, and degree of anxiety.
- **Seizures:** Observe and record intensity, duration, and location of seizure activity. The initial dose offers seizure control for 15–20 min after administration. Institute seizure precautions.
- **Muscle Spasms:** Assess muscle spasm, associated pain, and limitation of movement prior to and during therapy.
- **Alcohol Withdrawal:** Assess for tremor, agitation, delirium, and hallucinations.

Lab Test Considerations

- Evaluate hepatic and renal function and CBC periodically during prolonged therapy. May ↑ AST, ALT, and alkaline phosphatase.

Toxicity and Overdose

- Flumazenil is an adjunct in the management of toxicity or overdose. Flumazenil may induce seizures in patients with a history of seizure disorder or who are on tricyclic antidepressants.

Implementation

- ***High Alert:*** Do not confuse diazepam with diltiazem.
- Patient should be kept on bedrest and observed for ≥3 hr following parenteral administration.
- If opioid analgesics are used concurrently with parenteral diazepam, ↓ opioid dose by 1/3 and titrate to effect.
- Use lowest effective dose. Taper by 2 mg every 3 days to ↓ withdrawal symptoms. Some patients may require longer taper periods.
- **PO:** Tablets may be crushed and taken with food or water.
- **Buccal: *Libervant*:** Open pouch by tearing along perforation. Remove film from foil pouch. Place film flat against inside of cheek; do not place against teeth or rub into cheek. Mouth can be open or closed while medication dissolves. If film is accidentally swallowed or chewed, do not administer a replacement dose. Do not administer with liquids.
- **Intranasal:** Device delivers entire contents upon activation. Do not prime or use device for more than one dose. A 2nd dose may be administered >4 hr after initial dose; use a new blister pack. Do not use >2 doses to treat a single episode and no more than one episode every 5 days and no more than 5 episodes per month.
- **IM:** IM injections are painful and erratically absorbed. If IM route is used, inject deeply into deltoid muscle for maximum absorption.

IV Administration

- **V** IV diazepam is a vesicant. Administer into a large vein. If extravasation occurs, immediately stop infusion. Leave needle/cannula in place temporarily but do not flush the line. Gently aspirate extravasated solution; then remove needle/cannula. Elevate patient's extremity and apply dry cold or warm compresses.
- **IV:** Resuscitation equipment should be available when diazepam is administered IV.
- **IV Push: Dilution:** Do not dilute or mix with any other drug. If IV push is not feasible, administer into tubing as close to insertion site as possible. Continuous infusion is not recommended due to precipitation in IV fluids and absorption into infusion bags and tubing. **Concentration:** 5 mg/mL. **Rate:** Administer slowly at 5 mg/min in adults and 1–2 mg/min in infants and children. Rapid injection may cause apnea, hypotension, bradycardia, or cardiac arrest.
- **Y-Site Compatibility:** docetaxel, methadone, piperacillin/tazobactam.
- **Y-Site Incompatibility:** acetaminophen, acyclovir, alemtuzumab, amikacin, aminocaproic acid, aminophylline, amiodarone, amphotericin B deoxycholate, amphotericin B liposomal, ampicillin, ampicillin/sulbactam, anidulafungin, argatroban, arsenic trioxide, ascorbic acid, atracurium, atropine, azathioprine, azithromycin, aztreonam, benztropine, bivalirudin, bleomycin, bumetanide, buprenorphine, butorphanol, calcium chloride, calcium gluconate, cangrelor, carboplatin, carmustine, caspofungin, cefazolin, cefepime, cefotaxime, cefotetan, cefoxitin, ceftaroline, ceftazidime, ceftobiprole, ceftriaxone, cefuroxime, chloramphenicol, chlorpromazine, cisplatin, clindamycin, cyanocobalamin, cyclophosphamide, cyclosporine, cytarabine, dacarbazine, dactinomycin, dantrolene, daunorubicin, dexamethasone, dexmedetomidine, dexrazoxane, diazoxide, digoxin, diltiazem, dimenhydrinate, diphenhydramine, dopamine, doxorubicin hydrochloride, doxorubicin liposomal, doxycycline, enalaprilat, ephedrine, epinephrine, epirubicin, epoetin alfa, eptifibatide, ertapenem, erythromycin, esmolol, etoposide, etoposide phosphate, famotidine, fluconazole, fludarabine, fluorouracil, folic acid, foscarnet, fosphenytoin, furosemide, ganciclovir, gemcitabine, gemtuzumab ozogamicin, gentamicin, glycopyrrolate, granisetron, haloperidol, heparin, hetastarch, hydralazine, hydrocortisone, idarubicin, ifosfamide, imipenem/cilastatin, indomethacin, insulin, regular, irinotecan, isoproterenol, ketorolac, labetalol, leucovorin, levofloxacin, lidocaine, linezolid, magnesium sulfate, mannitol, meperidine, meropenem, mesna, methotrexate, methylprednisolone, metoclopramide, metoprolol, metronidazole, midazolam, milrinone, minocycline, mitomycin, mitoxantrone, multivitamins, mycophenolate, nalbuphine, naloxone, nicardipine, nitroglycerin, nitroprusside, norepinephrine, octreotide, oxacillin, oxaliplatin, oxytocin, paclitaxel, palonosetron, pamidronate, pantoprazole, papaverine, pemetrexed, penicillin G, pentamidine, pentobarbital, phenobarbital, phentolamine, phenylephrine, phenytoin, phytonadione, potassium acetate, potassium chloride, procainamide, prochlorperazine, promethazine, propofol, propranolol, protamine, pyridoxine, rocuronium, sodium acetate, sodium bicarbonate, succinylcholine, tacrolimus, theophylline, thiamine, thiotepa, tigecycline, tirofiban, tobramycin, topotecan, trimethoprim/sulfamethoxazole, vancomycin, vasopressin, vecuronium, verapamil, vinblastine, vincristine, vinorelbine, voriconazole, zoledronic acid.
- **Rect:** Upon receipt of syringe, confirm correct prescribed dose is visible in display window, and the green "ready" band is visible prior to rectal administration.

Patient/Family Teaching

- Explain purpose and side effects of medication. Advise patient to read *Patient Information* before starting therapy.

- Instruct patient and caregiver on appropriate steps for administration technique, disposal of equipment, and monitoring of patient for buccal, intranasal, and rectal preparations, if appropriate. Instruct patient not to ↑ dose if less effective after a few weeks without checking with health care provider.
- Caution patient not to stop taking diazepam without consulting health care provider. Abrupt withdrawal may cause sweating, vomiting, muscle cramps, tremors, and seizures; may be life-threatening.
- Advise patient that diazepam is a drug with known abuse potential. Protect it from theft, and never give to anyone other than the individual for whom it was prescribed. Store out of sight and reach of children and in a location not accessible by others.
- Advise patient to avoid driving or other activities requiring alertness until response to medication is known. Geri: Advise older adults of ↑ risk for CNS effects and potential for falls.
- Advise patient to avoid the use of alcohol or other CNS depressants, including opioids, concurrently with diazepam; may cause respiratory depression and overdose.
- Advise patient to notify health care provider of all Rx or OTC medications, vitamins, or herbal products being taken and to consult health care provider before taking other medications.
- Rep: May cause fetal harm. Advise women of reproductive potential to notify health care provider if pregnancy is planned or suspected or if breastfeeding. Use in late pregnancy can result in sedation (respiratory depression, lethargy, hypotonia) and/or withdrawal symptoms (hyperreflexia, irritability, restlessness, tremors, inconsolable crying, feeding difficulties) in the neonate. Monitor neonates exposed to diazepam during pregnancy or labor for signs of sedation or withdrawal. Monitor infants exposed to diazepam through breast milk for sedation, poor feeding, and poor weight gain. Encourage pregnant patient to enroll in the North American Antiepileptic Drug Pregnancy Registry to monitor outcomes of diazepam exposure: 1-888-233-2334; https://www.aedpregnancyregistry.org.
- Emphasize the importance of follow-up examinations to determine effectiveness of therapy.
- **Seizures:** Patients on anticonvulsant therapy should carry identification describing disease process and medication regimen at all times.

Evaluation/Desired Outcomes

- Decrease in anxiety level. Full therapeutic antianxiety effects occur after 1–2 wk of therapy.
- Decreased recall of surgical or diagnostic procedures.
- Control of seizures.
- Decreased muscle spasm.
- Decreased tremulousness and more rational ideation when used for alcohol withdrawal.

BEERS

D

DICLOFENAC (dye-**kloe**-fen-ak)

diclofenac potassium (oral)
Cambia, ~~Cataflam~~, Lofena, Zipsor

diclofenac sodium (oral)
✱ Voltaren, ✱ Voltaren SR, ~~Voltaren-XR~~

diclofenac sodium (topical gel)
~~Solaraze~~, Aspercreme Arthritis Pain, Voltaren Arthritis Pain

diclofenac sodium (topical solution)
Pennsaid

diclofenac epolamine (topical patch)
Flector, Licart

Classification
Therapeutic: antirheumatics, nonopioid analgesics
Pharmacologic: nonsteroidal anti-inflammatory drugs (NSAIDs)

See Appendix B for ophthalmic use

Indications

PO: Management of inflammatory disorders, including: Rheumatoid arthritis, Osteoarthritis, Ankylosing spondylitis. Primary dysmenorrhea. Relief of mild to moderate pain. Acute treatment of migraines (powder for oral solution). **Topical:** Management of: Actinic keratosis (3% gel), Osteoarthritis (1% gel or solution). Acute pain due to minor strains, sprains, and contusions (patch).

Action

Inhibits prostaglandin synthesis. **Therapeutic Effects:** Suppression of pain and inflammation. Relief of acute migraine attacks. **Topical (3% gel):** Clearance of actinic keratosis lesions.

Pharmacokinetics

Absorption: Undergoes first-pass metabolism by liver, which results in 50% bioavailability. Oral diclofenac sodium is a delayed-release dose form. Diclofenac potassium is an immediate-release dose form. 6–10% of topical gel is systemically absorbed.
Distribution: Crosses the placenta.
Protein Binding: >99%.
Metabolism and Excretion: Primarily metabolized by the liver via the CYP2C9 isoenzyme to several metabolites; 65% excreted in urine, 35% in bile.
Half-life: 2 hr.

TIME/ACTION PROFILE

ROUTE	ONSET	PEAK	DURATION
PO (inflammation)	few days–1 wk	≥2 wk	unknown
PO (pain)	30 min	unknown	up to 8 hr
Top (gel and patch)	unknown	10–20 hr	unknown
Top (solution)	unknown	unknown	unknown

Contraindications/Precautions

Contraindicated in: Hypersensitivity to diclofenac or other components of formulation; Cross-sensitivity may occur with other NSAIDs, including aspirin; Active GI bleeding/ulcer disease; Coronary artery bypass graft surgery; Recent MI; HF; Exudative dermatitis, eczema, infectious lesions, burns, or wounds; OB: Avoid use after 30 wk gestation.

Use Cautiously in: Severe renal impairment; Severe hepatic impairment; History of porphyria; Cardiovascular disease or risk factors for cardiovascular disease (may ↑ risk of serious cardiovascular thrombotic events, MI, and stroke, especially with prolonged use or use of higher doses); History of long duration of NSAID use, smoking, alcohol use, advanced liver disease, coagulopathy, or poor general health (↑ risk of GI bleeding); History of peptic ulcer disease and/or GI bleeding; Bleeding tendency or concurrent anticoagulant therapy; OB: Use at or after 20 wk gestation may cause fetal or neonatal renal impairment; if treatment is necessary between 20 wk and 30 wk gestation, limit use to the lowest effective dose and shortest duration possible; Pedi: Safety and effectiveness only established for patch in children ≥6 yr and diclofenac potassium (Zipsor) in children ≥12 yr; Geri: Appears on Beers list. ↑ risk GI bleeding or peptic ulcer disease in older adults. Avoid chronic use unless other alternatives are not effective and the patient can take a gastroprotective agent; avoid short-term use in combination with oral or parenteral corticosteroids, anticoagulants, or antiplatelet agents unless other alternatives are not effective and the patient can take a gastroprotective agent.

Adverse Reactions/Side Effects

CV: edema, HF, hypertension, MI. **Derm:** pruritus, rash, DRUG REACTION WITH EOSINOPHILIA AND SYSTEMIC SYMPTOMS (DRESS), eczema, EXFOLIATIVE DERMATITIS, GENERALIZED BULLOUS FIXED DRUG ERUPTION, photosensitivity, STEVENS-JOHNSON SYNDROME (SJS), TOXIC EPIDERMAL NECROLYSIS (TEN). **EENT:** tinnitus. **F and E** hyperkalemia. **GI:** abdominal pain, constipation, diarrhea, dyspepsia, flatulence, GI BLEEDING, GI PERFORATION, GI ULCERATION, heartburn, HEPATOTOXICITY, nausea, vomiting. **GU:** acute renal failure, hematuria. **Hemat:** anemia, prolonged bleeding time. **Local:** **Topical only:** contact dermatitis, dry skin, exfoliation. **Neuro:** dizziness, headache, STROKE. **Misc:** HYPERSENSITIVITY REACTIONS (INCLUDING ANAPHYLAXIS AND SERIOUS SKIN REACTIONS).

Interactions

Primarily noted for oral administration

Drug-Drug: May ↓ effectiveness of **diuretics** or **antihypertensives**. May ↑ levels and risk of toxicity from **cyclosporine**, **lithium**, or **methotrexate**. ↑ risk of GI bleeding with **anticoagulants**, **aspirin**, **clopidogrel**, **ticagrelor**, **prasugrel**, **corticosteroids**, **fibrinolytics**, **SNRIs**, or **SSRIs**. **CYP2C9 inhibitors**, including **voriconazole**, may ↑ levels and risk of toxicity. **CYP2C9 inducers**, including **rifampin**, may ↓ levels and effectiveness. Concurrent use of oral **NSAIDs** during topical diclofenac therapy should be minimized.
Drug-Natural Products: ↑ bleeding risk with **arnica**, **chamomile**, **clove**, **dong quai**, **feverfew**, **garlic**, **ginger**, **ginkgo**, *Panax ginseng*, and others.

Route/Dosage

Different formulations of oral diclofenac (diclofenac sodium enteric-coated tablets, diclofenac sodium extended-release tablets, and diclofenac potassium immediate-release tablets) are not bioequivalent and should not be substituted on a mg-to-mg basis.

Diclofenac Potassium

PO (Adults): *Analgesic/antidysmenorrheal (immediate-release tablets):* 100 mg initially; then 50 mg 3 times daily as needed; *Mild to moderate acute pain (Zipsor):* 25 mg 4 times daily; *Rheumatoid arthritis (immediate-release tablets):* 50 mg 3–4 times daily; *Osteoarthritis (immediate-release tablets):* 50 mg 2–3 times daily; *Osteoarthritis (Cambia):* one packet (50 mg) given as a single dose.
PO (Children ≥12 yr): *Mild to moderate acute pain (Zipsor):* 25 mg 4 times daily.

Diclofenac Sodium

PO (Adults): *Rheumatoid arthritis (delayed-release [enteric-coated] tablets):* 50 mg 3–4 times daily *or* 75 mg twice daily (usual maintenance dose 25 mg 3 times daily). *Rheumatoid arthritis (extended-release tablets):* 100 mg once daily; if unsatisfactory response, dose may be ↑ to 100 mg twice daily. *Osteoarthritis (delayed-release [enteric-coated] tablets):* 50 mg 2–3 times daily *or* 75 mg twice daily. *Osteoarthritis (extended-release tablets):* 100 mg once daily. *Ankylosing spondylitis (delayed-release [enteric-coated] tablets):* 25 mg 4 times daily, with an additional 25 mg given at bedtime, if necessary.
Topical (Adults): *3% topical gel:* Apply to lesions twice daily for 60–90 days; *Voltaren gel:* Lower extremities (knees, ankles, feet): Apply 4 g to affected area 4 times daily (maximum of 16 g per joint/day); Upper extremities (elbows, wrists, hands): Apply 2 g to affected area 4 times daily (maximum of 8 g per joint/day). Maximum total body dose should not exceed 32 g/day; *Topical solution:* Apply 40 drops to affected knee(s) 4 times daily.

Diclofenac Epolamine

Topical: (Adults and Children ≥6 yr): *Flector:* Apply 1 patch to most painful area twice daily. *Licart:* Apply 1 patch to most painful area once daily.

Availability (generic available)

Diclofenac potassium immediate-release tablets: 25 mg, 50 mg. **Diclofenac potassium liquid-filled capsules (Zipsor):** 25 mg. **Diclofenac potassium powder for oral solution (Cambia):** 50 mg/packet. **Diclofenac sodium delayed-release (enteric-coated) tablets:** 25 mg, 50 mg, 75 mg. **Diclofenac sodium extended-release tablets:** ✱ 75 mg, and 100 mg. **Diclofenac sodium topical gel:** 1%OTC, 3%. **Diclofenac sodium topical solution:** 1.5%, 2%. **Diclofenac epolamine topical patch:** 1.3%. ***In combination with:*** misoprostol (Arthrotec). See Appendix N.

NURSING IMPLICATIONS

Assessment

- Patients who have asthma, aspirin-induced allergy, and nasal polyps are at ↑ risk for developing hypersensitivity reactions.
- Monitor BP closely during initiation of treatment and periodically during therapy in patients with hypertension.
- Assess patient for skin rash and blisters/erosions frequently during therapy. Discontinue at first sign of these symptoms; may be life-threatening. Exfoliative dermatitis, generalized bullous fixed drug eruption, SJS, and TEN may develop. Treat symptomatically; may recur once treatment is stopped.
- Monitor for signs and symptoms of DRESS (fever, rash, lymphadenopathy, facial swelling) periodically during therapy. Discontinue therapy if symptoms occur.
- **Pain:** Assess pain and limitation of movement; note type, location, and intensity before and 30–60 min after administration.
- **Migraine:** Assess pain location, character, intensity, and duration and associated symptoms (photophobia, phonophobia, nausea, vomiting) during migraine attack.
- **Arthritis:** Assess arthritic pain (note type, location, intensity) and limitation of movement before and periodically during therapy.
- **Actinic Keratosis:** Assess lesions before and periodically during therapy.

Lab Test Considerations

- Diclofenac has minimal effect on bleeding time and platelet aggregation.
- May ↓ in hemoglobin and hematocrit.
- Monitor CBC and liver function tests within 4–8 wk of initiating and periodically during therapy. May ↑ serum alkaline phosphatase, LDH, AST, and ALT levels.
- Monitor BUN and serum creatinine periodically during therapy. May ↑ BUN and serum creatinine.

Implementation

- Various brands and dose forms are not interchangeable.
- Administration at higher than recommended doses does not provide ↑ effectiveness but may cause ↑ risk of side effects. Use lowest effective dose for shortest period of time.
- **PO:** Take with food or milk to minimize gastric irritation.
- May take first 1–2 doses on an empty stomach for more rapid onset. ***DNC:*** Do not crush or chew enteric-coated or extended-release tablets.
- **Dysmenorrhea:** Administer as soon as possible after the onset of menses. Prophylactic treatment has not been shown to be effective.
- **Migraine:** Empty contents of one packet into a cup containing 1–2 ounces or 30–60 mL of water; mix well and drink immediately. Do not use liquids other than water. Take on empty stomach; food may ↓ effectiveness. Use only for acute migraine pain; not indicated for prophylaxis.
- **Topical: Gel:** Apply to intact skin; do not use on open wounds. An adequate amount of gel should be applied to cover the entire lesion.
- **Topical: Solution:** Dispense 10 drops at a time either directly onto knee or first into the hand and then onto knee. Spread solution evenly around front, back, and sides of the knee. Repeat until 40 drops have been applied and knee is completely covered with solution.
- **Topical:** Apply patch to the most painful area once (*Licart*) or twice (*Flector*) a day. Do not apply to nonintact or damaged skin resulting from any etiology (exudative dermatitis, eczema, infected lesion, burns, wounds). Avoid contact with eyes; wash hands after applying, handling, or removing patch.

Patient/Family Teaching

- Explain purpose and side effects of medication to patient. Advise patient to read *Patient Information* before starting therapy. Instruct patient to take as directed and not take more than recommended.
- Instruct patient to notify health care provider of all Rx or OTC medications, vitamins, or herbal products being taken and to consult with health care provider before taking other medications, especially other NSAIDs, aspirin, and acetaminophen.
- Caution patient to avoid concurrent use of alcohol.
- *Migraine:* Advise patient that overuse (use >10 days/mo) may lead to exacerbation of headache (migraine-like daily headaches, or as a marked ↑ in frequency of migraine attacks). May require gradual withdrawal of diclofenac and treatment of symptoms (transient worsening of headache).

- Instruct patient to notify health care provider of medication regimen before treatment or surgery.
- Inform patient of ↑ risk of MI and stroke. Use lowest effective dose for shortest time. Advise patient to notify health care provider immediately if signs and symptoms (shortness of breath or trouble breathing, chest pain, weakness in one part or side of body, slurred speech, swelling of the face or throat) occur.
- Advise patient to notify health care provider promptly if signs or symptoms of GI toxicity (abdominal pain, black stools) occur.
- Advise patient to notify health care provider promptly if signs or symptoms of skin (exfoliative dermatitis, SJS, TEN) or hypersensitivity (anaphylaxis) reactions. May occur without warning symptoms.
- Advise patient to notify health care provider promptly if unexplained weight gain, swelling of arms and legs or hands and feet, nausea, fatigue, lethargy, rash, pruritus, yellowing of skin or eyes, itching, stomach pain, vomiting blood, bloody or tarry stools, or flu-like symptoms occur.
- Rep: May cause fetal harm. Advise women of reproductive potential to notify health care provider if pregnancy is planned or suspected or if breastfeeding. Advise patients to avoid diclofenac in the 3rd trimester of pregnancy (after 29 wk); may cause premature closure of the fetal ductus arteriosus. Use of diclofenac after 20 wk of gestation may cause fetal renal impairment leading to oligohydramnios. May cause reversible infertility in women attempting to conceive; may consider discontinuing diclofenac.
- **PO:** Instruct patient to take diclofenac with a full glass of water and to remain in an upright position for 15–30 min after administration. Take missed doses as soon as possible within 1–2 hr if taking once or twice a day or unless almost time for next dose if taking more than twice a day. Do not double doses.
- May cause drowsiness or dizziness. Caution patient to avoid driving or other activities requiring alertness until response to medication is known.
- Caution patient to wear sunscreen and protective clothing to prevent photosensitivity reactions.
- **Topical:** ***Pennsaid:*** Instruct patient to avoid touching treated knee and allowing another person to touch knee until completely dry. Cover knee with clothing until completely dry. Avoid covering lesion with occlusive dressing or tight clothing, and avoid applying sunscreen, insect repellent, lotion, moisturizer, or cosmetics to the affected area. Do not use heating pads, sunlamps, and tanning beds. Protect treated knee from sunlight; wear protective clothes when in sunlight. Avoid showers or baths for >30 min after application.
- *Voltaren:* Measure dose using the dosing card supplied in the drug product carton. Dosing card is clear polypropylene; use for each application. Apply gel within the rectangular area of the dosing card up to the 2-g or 4-g line (2 g for each elbow, wrist, or hand, and 4 g for each knee, ankle, or foot). Apply gel using dosing card. Use hands to gently rub gel into skin. After using dosing card, hold with fingertips, rinse, and dry. If treatment site is the hands, patient should wait >1 hr to wash hands.
- *3% gel:* Advise patient that it may take 60–90 days for complete healing of the lesion to occur.
- Instruct patient on correct application procedure for patch. Apply patch to most painful area. Change patch every 24 hr (*Licart*) or 12 hr (*Flector*). Remove patch if irritation occurs. Fold used patches so adhesive sticks to itself and discard where children and pets cannot get them. Encourage patient to read the *NSAID Patient Information* that accompanies the prescription.
- Do not wear patch during bathing or showering. Bathing should take place between scheduled patch removal and application.
- Instruct patients if patch begins to peel off to tape the edges. Patient may overlay the topical system with a mesh netting sleeve to secure topical systems applied to ankles, knees, or elbows. Mesh netting sleeve (Curad® Hold Tite™, Surgilast® Tubular Elastic Dressing) must allow air to pass through and not be occlusive.
- Advise patient referred for MRI test to discuss patch with referring health care provider and MRI facility to determine if removal of patch is necessary prior to test and for directions for replacing patch.

Evaluation/Desired Outcomes

- Suppression of pain and inflammation.
- Relief of acute migraine attacks.
- **Topical (3% gel):** Clearance of actinic keratosis lesions.

dicloxacillin, See PENICILLINS, PENICILLINASE RESISTANT.

BEERS

dicyclomine

(dye-**sye**-kloe-meen)

~~Bentyl~~

Classification

Therapeutic: antispasmodics

Pharmacologic: anticholinergics

Indications

Irritable bowel syndrome in patients who do not respond to usual interventions (sedation/change in diet).

Action

May have a direct and local effect on GI smooth muscle, reducing motility and tone. **Therapeutic Effects:** Decreased GI motility.

Pharmacokinetics
Absorption: Well absorbed after oral and IM administration.
Distribution: Unknown.
Metabolism and Excretion: 80% eliminated in urine, 10% in feces.
Half-life: 9–10 hr.

TIME/ACTION PROFILE (antispasmodic effect)

ROUTE	ONSET	PEAK	DURATION
PO, IM	unknown	unknown	unknown

Contraindications/Precautions
Contraindicated in: Hypersensitivity; Obstruction of the GI or genitourinary tract; Reflux esophagitis; Severe ulcerative colitis (↑ risk of paralytic ileus); Unstable cardiovascular status; Glaucoma; Myasthenia gravis; Lactation: Lactation; Pedi: Infants <6 mo.
Use Cautiously in: High environmental temperatures (risk of heat prostration); Renal impairment; Hepatic impairment; Autonomic neuropathy; Cardiovascular disease; Prostatic hyperplasia; OB: Safety not established in pregnancy; Geri: Appears on Beers list. ↑ risk of adverse reactions in older adults due to anticholinergic effects. Avoid use in older adults.

Adverse Reactions/Side Effects
CV: palpitations, tachycardia. **Derm:** ↓ sweating. **EENT:** ↑ intraocular pressure, blurred vision. **Endo:** ↓ lactation. **GI:** constipation, heartburn, ↓ salivation, dry mouth, nausea, PARALYTIC ILEUS, vomiting. **GU:** erectile dysfunction, urinary hesitancy, urinary retention. **Local:** pain/redness at IM site. **Neuro:** confusion, delirium, drowsiness, light-headedness (IM only), psychosis. **Misc:** HYPERSENSITIVITY REACTIONS (INCLUDING ANAPHYLAXIS).

Interactions
Drug-Drug: Additive anticholinergic effects with other **anticholinergics**, including **antihistamines**, **quinidine**, and **disopyramide**. May alter the absorption of **other orally administered drugs** by slowing motility of the GI tract. **Antacids** or **adsorbent antidiarrheals** ↓ the absorption of anticholinergics. May ↑ GI mucosal lesions in patients taking oral **potassium chloride** tablets.

Route/Dosage
PO (Adults): 10–20 mg 3–4 times daily (up to 160 mg/day).
PO (Children ≥2 yr): 10 mg 3–4 times daily, adjusted as tolerated.
PO (Children 6 mo–2 yr): 5–10 mg 3–4 times daily, adjusted as tolerated.
IM (Adults): 20 mg every 4–6 hr, adjusted as tolerated.

Availability (generic available)
Tablets: 🍁 10 mg, 20 mg. **Capsules:** 10 mg. **Oral solution (cherry flavor):** 10 mg/5 mL. **Solution for injection:** 10 mg/mL.

D

NURSING IMPLICATIONS
Assessment
- Assess for symptoms of irritable bowel syndrome (abdominal cramping, alternating constipation and diarrhea, mucus in stools) before and periodically during therapy.
- Assess patient routinely for abdominal distention and auscultate for bowel sounds. If constipation becomes a problem, ↑ fluids and adding bulk to the diet may help alleviate the constipating effects of the drug. Notify health care provider for further diagnostics to rule out a paralytic ileus if symptoms occur.
- Monitor intake and output; may cause urinary retention.
- Monitor for peripheral and central nervous system side effects (dry mouth with difficulty in swallowing and talking; thirst; ↓ bronchial secretions; mydriasis with loss of accommodation [cycloplegia] and photophobia; flushing and dry skin; transient bradycardia followed by tachycardia, with palpitations and arrhythmias; difficulty in micturition; ↓ in tone and motility of GI tract, leading to constipation). Symptoms are caused by inhibitory effect on muscarinic receptors within the autonomic nervous system. Effects are dose-related and usually reversible when therapy is discontinued.
- Assess for hypersensitivity reactions (rash, pruritus, flushing, shortness of breath, anaphylaxis); implement support measures (epinephrine) if indicated, and treat symptoms as needed.

Lab Test Considerations
- Antagonizes effects of pentagastrin and histamine during the gastric acid secretion test. Avoid administration for 24 hr preceding the test.

Toxicity and Overdose
- Severe anticholinergic symptoms may be reversed with neostigmine.

Implementation
- **PO:** Administer dicyclomine without regard to food.
- **IM:** Monitor patient after administration; may cause light-headedness and irritation at injection site. Do not administer IV; may cause thrombosis and thrombophlebitis.

Patient/Family Teaching
- Explain purpose and side effects of medication. Advise patient to read *Patient Information* before starting therapy. Instruct patient to take exactly as

directed and not to take more than the prescribed amount. Take missed doses as soon as remembered if not just before next dose.

- Instruct patient to notify health care professional of all Rx or OTC medications, vitamins, or herbal products being taken and to consult health care professional before taking other Rx, OTC, or herbal products.
- Medication may cause drowsiness and blurred vision. Caution patient to avoid driving or other activities requiring alertness until response to the medication is known.
- Caution patient to avoid extremes of temperature. This medication ↓ the ability to sweat and may ↑ the risk of heat stroke. Advise patient to stay in temperature-controlled rooms. Fever and extremes of heat may cause confusional state, disorientation, amnesia, hallucinations, dysarthria, ataxia, coma, euphoria, fatigue, insomnia, agitation and mannerisms, inappropriate affect, psychosis, and delirium. Usually resolves 12–24 hr after discontinuation of dicyclomine.
- Inform patient that frequent oral rinses, sugarless gum or candy, and good oral hygiene may help relieve dry mouth. Consult health care professional regarding use of saliva substitute if dry mouth persists for >2 wk.
- Advise patient receiving dicyclomine to make position changes slowly to minimize the effects of drug-induced orthostatic hypotension.
- Advise patient to notify health care professional immediately if eye pain or ↑ sensitivity to light occurs. Emphasize the importance of routine eye exams throughout therapy.
- Rep: Advise women of reproductive potential to notify health care professional if pregnancy is planned or suspected and to avoid breastfeeding.

Evaluation/Desired Outcomes

- Decreased GI motility.

diflorasone, See CORTICOSTEROIDS (TOPICAL).

BEERS HIGH ALERT

digoxin (di-jox-in)

Lanoxin

Classification

Therapeutic: antiarrhythmics, inotropics

Pharmacologic: digitalis glycosides

Indications

HF. Atrial fibrillation and atrial flutter (slows ventricular rate). Paroxysmal atrial tachycardia.

Action

Increases the force of myocardial contraction. Prolongs refractory period of the AV node. Decreases conduction through the SA and AV nodes. **Therapeutic Effects:** Increased cardiac output (positive inotropic effect) and slowing of the heart rate (negative chronotropic effect).

Pharmacokinetics

Absorption: 60–80% absorbed after oral administration of tablets; 70–85% absorbed after administration of elixir; 80% absorbed from IM sites (IM route not recommended due to pain/irritation). IV administration results in complete bioavailability.

Distribution: Widely distributed to tissues.

Metabolism and Excretion: Excreted almost entirely unchanged by the kidneys.

Half-life: 36–48 hr (↑ in renal impairment).

TIME/ACTION PROFILE (antiarrhythmic or inotropic effects, provided that a loading dose has been given)

ROUTE	ONSET	PEAK	DURATION
PO	30–120 min	2–8 hr	2–4 days†
IM	30 min	4–6 hr	2–4 days†
IV	5–30 min	1–4 hr	2–4 days†

† Duration listed is that for normal renal function; in impaired renal function, duration will be longer.

Contraindications/Precautions

Contraindicated in: Hypersensitivity; Uncontrolled ventricular arrhythmias; Heart block (in absence of pacemaker); Idiopathic hypertrophic subaortic stenosis; Constrictive pericarditis; Known alcohol intolerance (elixir only).

Use Cautiously in: Hypokalemia (↑ risk of digoxin toxicity); Hypercalcemia (↑ risk of toxicity, especially with mild hypokalemia); Hypomagnesemia (↑ risk of digoxin toxicity); Diuretic use (may cause electrolyte abnormalities including hypokalemia and hypomagnesemia); Hypothyroidism; MI; Renal impairment (↓ dose); Obesity (base dose on ideal body weight); OB: Monitor neonates for signs/symptoms of digoxin toxicity; monitor levels in mother during pregnancy, as levels may fluctuate during pregnancy and postpartum periods; may lead to ↑ risk of arrhythmias during labor and delivery; Lactation: Use with caution while breastfeeding; Geri: Appears on Beers list. Avoid use as first-line therapy for rate control in atrial fibrillation or for HF in older adults; if used, avoid using dose >0.125 mg/day.

Adverse Reactions/Side Effects

CV: bradycardia, ARRHYTHMIAS, ECG changes, heart block. **EENT:** blurred vision, yellow or green vision. **GI:** anorexia, nausea, vomiting, diarrhea. **Hemat:** thrombocytopenia. **Neuro:** fatigue, headache, weakness.

Interactions

Drug-Drug: Thiazide and **loop diuretics**, **piperacillin/tazobactam**, **amphotericin B**, **corticosteroids**, and excessive use of **laxatives** may cause hypokalemia, which may ↑ risk of toxicity. **Quinidine** and **ritonavir** may ↑ levels and lead to toxicity; ↓ digoxin dose by 30–50%. **Amiodarone** and **dronedarone** may ↑ levels and lead to toxicity; ↓ digoxin dose by 50%. **Cyclosporine**, **itraconazole**, **mirabegron**, **propafenone**, **quinine**, **spironolactone**, and **verapamil** may ↑ levels and lead to toxicity; serum level monitoring/dose ↓ may be required. Levels may be ↓ by some **antineoplastics** (**bleomycin**, **carmustine**, **cyclophosphamide**, **cytarabine**, **doxorubicin**, **methotrexate**, **procarbazine**, **vincristine**), **activated charcoal**, **cholestyramine**, **colestipol**, **metoclopramide**, **penicillamine**, **rifampin**, or **sulfasalazine**. In a small percentage (10%) of patients, gut bacteria metabolize digoxin to inactive compounds; **macrolide anti-infectives** (**erythromycin**, **azithromycin**, **clarithromycin**) and **tetracyclines**, by killing these bacteria, will cause ↑ levels and toxicity; dose may need to be ↓ for up to 9 wk. Additive bradycardia may occur with **beta blockers**, **diltiazem**, **verapamil**, **clonidine**, **ivabradine**, and other **antiarrhythmics** (**quinidine**, **disopyramide**). Concurrent use of **sympathomimetics** may ↑ risk of arrhythmias. **Thyroid hormones** may ↓ therapeutic effects.
Drug-Natural Products: Licorice and stimulant natural products (**aloe**) may ↑ risk of potassium depletion. **St. John's wort** may ↓ levels and effect.
Drug-Food: Concurrent ingestion of a **high-fiber meal** may ↓ absorption. Administer digoxin 1 hr before or 2 hr after such a meal.

Route/Dosage

For rapid effect, a larger initial loading dose should be given in several divided doses over 12–24 hr. Maintenance doses are determined for digoxin by renal function. All dosing must be evaluated by individual response. In general, doses required for atrial arrhythmias are higher than those for inotropic effect.

IV, IM (Adults): *Loading dose:* 0.5–1 mg given as 50% of the dose initially and ¼ of the initial dose in each of 2 subsequent doses at 6–12 hr intervals.

IV, IM (Children >10 yr): *Loading dose:* 8–12 mcg/kg given as 50% of the dose initially and ¼ of the initial dose in each of 2 subsequent doses at 6–12 hr intervals.

IV, IM (Children 5–10 yr): *Loading dose:* 15–30 mcg/kg given as 50% of the dose initially and ¼ of the initial dose in each of 2 subsequent doses at 6–12 hr intervals.

IV, IM (Children 2–5 yr): *Loading dose:* 25–35 mcg/kg given as 50% of the dose initially and ¼ of the initial dose in each of 2 subsequent doses at 6–12 hr intervals.

IV, IM (Children 1–24 mo): *Loading dose:* 30–50 mcg/kg given as 50% of the dose initially and ¼ of the initial dose in each of 2 subsequent doses at 6–12 hr intervals.

IV, IM (Infants: full term): *Loading dose:* 20–30 mcg/kg given as 50% of the dose initially and ¼ of the initial dose in each of 2 subsequent doses at 6–12 hr intervals.

IV, IM (Infants: premature): *Loading dose:* 15–25 mcg/kg given as 50% of the dose initially and ¼ of the initial dose in each of 2 subsequent doses at 6–12 hr intervals.

PO (Adults): *Loading dose:* 0.75–1.5 mg given as 50% of the dose initially and ¼ of the initial dose in each of 2 subsequent doses at 6–12 hr intervals. *Maintenance dose:* 0.125–0.5 mg/day depending on patient's lean body weight, renal function, and serum level.

PO (Geriatric Patients): Initial daily dose should not exceed 0.125 mg.

PO (Children >10 yr): *Loading dose:* 10–15 mcg/kg given as 50% of the dose initially and ¼ of the initial dose in each of 2 subsequent doses at 6–12 hr intervals. *Maintenance dose:* 2.5–5 mcg/kg given daily as a single dose.

PO (Children 5–10 yr): *Loading dose:* 20–35 mcg/kg given as 50% of the dose initially and ¼ of the initial dose in each of 2 subsequent doses at 6–12 hr intervals. *Maintenance dose:* 5–10 mcg/kg given daily in 2 divided doses.

PO (Children 2–5 yr): *Loading dose:* 30–40 mcg/kg given as 50% of the dose initially and ¼ of the initial dose in each of 2 subsequent doses at 6–12 hr intervals. *Maintenance dose:* 7.5–10 mcg/kg given daily in 2 divided doses.

PO (Children 1–24 mo): *Loading dose:* 35–60 mcg/kg given as 50% of the dose initially and of the initial dose in each of 2 subsequent doses at 6–12 hr intervals. *Maintenance dose:* 10–15 mcg/kg given daily in 2 divided doses.

PO (Infants: full term): *Loading dose:* 25–35 mcg/kg given as 50% of the dose initially and of the initial dose in each of 2 subsequent doses at 6–12 hr intervals. *Maintenance dose:* 6–10 mcg/kg given daily in 2 divided doses.

PO (Infants: premature): *Loading dose:* 20–30 mcg/kg given as 50% of the dose initially and of the initial dose in each of 2 subsequent doses at 6–12 hr intervals. *Maintenance dose:* 5–7.5 mcg/kg given daily in 2 divided doses.

Availability (generic available)

Tablets: 0.0625 mg, 0.125 mg, 0.25 mg. **Oral solution (lime flavor):** 50 mcg/mL. **Solution for injection:** 0.25 mg/mL. **Solution for injection (pediatric):** 0.1 mg/mL.

NURSING IMPLICATIONS

Assessment

- Monitor HR for 1 full min before administering. Hold dose and notify health care provider if HR is <60 bpm in an adult, <70 bpm in a child, or <90 bpm in

an infant. Notify health care provider promptly of any significant changes in rate, rhythm, or quality of pulse.
- Pedi: HR varies in children depending on age; ask health care provider to specify at what HR digoxin should be withheld.
- Monitor BP periodically in patients receiving IV digoxin.
- Monitor ECG during IV administration and 6 hr after each dose. Notify health care provider if bradycardia or new arrhythmias occur.
- Observe IV site for redness or infiltration; extravasation can lead to tissue irritation and sloughing.
- Monitor intake and output and daily weights. Assess for peripheral edema, and auscultate lungs for rales/crackles during therapy.
- Before administering initial loading dose, determine whether patient has taken any digoxin in the preceding 2–3 wk.

Lab Test Considerations
- Evaluate serum electrolyte levels (especially potassium, magnesium, and calcium) and renal and hepatic function periodically during therapy. Notify health care provider before giving dose if patient is hypokalemic. Hypokalemia, hypomagnesemia, or hypercalcemia may make the patient more susceptible to digoxin toxicity. Pedi: Neonates may have falsely elevated serum digoxin concentrations due to a naturally occurring substance chemically similar to digoxin.

Toxicity and Overdose
- Therapeutic serum digoxin concentrations range from 0.5–2 ng/mL. Serum levels may be drawn 6–8 hr after a dose is administered; usually drawn immediately before the next dose. Geri: Older adults are at ↑ risk for toxic effects of digoxin (on Beers list) due to age-related ↓ renal clearance; may exist even when serum creatinine is normal. Digoxin requirements in older adult may change and a formerly therapeutic dose can become toxic.
- Observe for signs and symptoms of toxicity. *In adults and older children,* 1st symptoms of toxicity usually include abdominal pain, anorexia, nausea, vomiting, visual disturbances, bradycardia, and other arrhythmias. *In infants and small children,* 1st signs of toxicity are usually cardiac arrhythmias. If these appear, withhold drug and notify health care provider immediately.
- If signs of toxicity occur and are not severe, discontinuation of digoxin may be all that is required.
- Correct electrolyte abnormalities, thyroid dysfunction, and concurrent medications. Administer potassium to maintain serum potassium between 4.0 and 5.5 mEq/L. Monitor ECG for evidence of potassium toxicity (peaked T waves).
- Treatment of life-threatening arrhythmias may include administration of digoxin immune fab *(Digibind)*, which binds to the digitalis glycoside molecule in the blood and is excreted by the kidneys.

Implementation
- Do not confuse Lanoxin with levothyroxine or naloxone.
- ***High Alert:*** Digoxin has a narrow therapeutic range. Medication errors associated with digoxin include miscalculation of pediatric doses and insufficient monitoring of digoxin levels.
- For rapid digitalization, initial dose is higher than maintenance dose; 50% of total digitalizing dose is given initially. Administer remainder of dose in 25% increments at 4–8 hr intervals.
- When changing from parenteral to oral dose forms, dose adjustments may be necessary because of pharmacokinetic variations in percentage of digoxin absorbed: 100 mcg (0.1 mg) digoxin injection = 125 mcg (0.125 mg) tablet or 125 mcg (0.125 mg) of elixir.
- **PO:** Administer oral preparations consistently with regard to meals. Tablets can be crushed and administered with food or fluids if patient has difficulty swallowing. Use calibrated measuring device for elixir; calibrated dropper is not accurate for doses of <0.2 mL or 10 mcg.
- **IM:** Administer deep into gluteal muscle and massage well to reduce painful local reactions. Do not administer >2 mL of digoxin in each IM site. IM administration is not generally recommended.

IV Administration
- IV digoxin is a vesicant. If extravasation occurs, immediately stop infusion. Leave needle/cannula in place temporarily but do not flush the line. Gently aspirate extravasated solution; then remove needle/cannula. Elevate patient's extremity and apply dry warm or cold compresses. Initiate hyaluronidase antidote for refractory cases in addition to supportive management. For hyaluronidase, inject a total of 1 mL (15 units/mL) intradermally or SUBQ as five separate 0.2-mL injections (using a tuberculin syringe) around the site of extravasation; if IV catheter remains in place, administer IV through the infiltrated catheter; may repeat in 30–60 min if no resolution.
- **IV Push: Dilution:** May be administered undiluted. May also dilute 1 mL of digoxin in 4 mL of sterile water for injection, D5W, or 0.9% NaCl. Less diluent will cause precipitation. Use diluted solution immediately. **Rate:** Administer over ≥5 min.
- **Y-Site Compatibility:** acyclovir, alemtuzumab, amikacin, aminocaproic acid, aminophylline, anidulafungin, argatroban, arsenic trioxide, ascorbic acid, atracurium, atropine, azathioprine, azithromycin, aztreonam, benztropine, bivalirudin, bleomycin, bumetanide, buprenorphine, butorphanol, calcium chloride, calcium gluconate, cangrelor, carboplatin, carmustine, cefazolin, cefiderocol, cefotaxime, cefotetan, cefoxitin, ceftaroline, ceftazidime, ceftobiprole, ceftolozane/tazobactam, ceftriaxone, cefuroxime,

chloramphenicol, chlorothiazide, chlorpromazine, ciprofloxacin, cisatracurium, cisplatin, clindamycin, cyanocobalamin, cyclophosphamide, cyclosporine, cytarabine, dacarbazine, dactinomycin, daptomycin, daunorubicin, dexamethasone, dexmedetomidine, dexrazoxane, diltiazem, dimenhydrinate, diphenhydramine, dobutamine, docetaxel, dopamine, doxorubicin liposomal, doxycycline, enalaprilat, ephedrine, epinephrine, epirubicin, epoetin alfa, eptifibatide, ertapenem, erythromycin, esmolol, etoposide, etoposide phosphate, famotidine, fentanyl, fludarabine, fluorouracil, folic acid, fosphenytoin, furosemide, ganciclovir, gemcitabine, gentamicin, glycopyrrolate, granisetron, heparin, hetastarch, hydrocortisone, hydromorphone, ifosfamide, imipenem/cilastatin, imipenem/cilastatin/relebactam, indomethacin, irinotecan, isavuconazonium, isoproterenol, ketamine, ketorolac, labetalol, LR, leucovorin, levofloxacin, lidocaine, linezolid, lorazepam, magnesium sulfate, mannitol, meperidine, meropenem, meropenem/vaborbactam, mesna, methadone, methohexital, methotrexate, methylprednisolone, metoclopramide, metoprolol, metronidazole, midazolam, milrinone, mitomycin, morphine, moxifloxacin, multivitamins, mycophenolate, nafcillin, nalbuphine, naloxone, nicardipine, nitroglycerin, nitroprusside, norepinephrine, octreotide, ondansetron, oxacillin, oxaliplatin, oxytocin, palonosetron, pamidronate, pantoprazole, papaverine, pemetrexed, penicillin G, pentobarbital, phenobarbital, phentolamine, phenylephrine, phytonadione, piperacillin/tazobactam, plazomicin, potassium acetate, potassium chloride, procainamide, prochlorperazine, promethazine, propranolol, protamine, pyridoxine, remifentanil, rituximab, rocuronium, sodium acetate, sodium bicarbonate, streptomycin, succinylcholine, sufentanil, sulbactam/durlobactam, tacrolimus, tedizolid, theophylline, thiamine, thiotepa, tigecycline, tirofiban, tobramycin, trastuzumab, vancomycin, vasopressin, vecuronium, verapamil, vinblastine, vincristine, vinorelbine, voriconazole, zoledronic acid.

- **Y-Site Incompatibility:** amiodarone, amphotericin B deoxycholate, amphotericin B liposomal, caspofungin, dantrolene, diazepam, doxorubicin hydrochloride, foscarnet, gemtuzumab ozogamicin, idarubicin, minocycline, mitoxantrone, paclitaxel, pentamidine, phenytoin, propofol, telavancin, topotecan, trimethoprim/sulfamethoxazole.

Patient/Family Teaching

- Instruct patient to take medication as directed, at same time each day. Teach parents or caregivers of infants and children how to accurately measure medication. Take missed doses within 12 hr of scheduled dose or omit. Do not double doses. Consult health care provider if doses for >2 days are missed. Do not discontinue medication without consulting health care provider.
- Teach patient to take HR and to contact health care provider before taking medication if HR is <60 bpm or >100 bpm.
- Pedi: Teach parents or caregivers that changes in HR, especially bradycardia, are among the 1st signs of digoxin toxicity in infants and children. Instruct parents or caregivers in apical HR assessment and ask them to notify health care provider if HR is outside of range set by health care provider before administering the next scheduled dose.
- Review signs and symptoms of digoxin toxicity with patient and family. Advise patient to notify health care provider immediately if these or symptoms of HF occur. Inform patient that these symptoms may be mistaken for those of colds or flu.
- Instruct patient to keep digoxin tablets in their original container and not to mix in pill boxes with other medications; may look similar to and may be mistaken for other medications.
- Advise patient that sharing of this medication can be dangerous.
- Instruct patient to notify health care provider of all Rx or OTC medications, vitamins, or herbal products being taken and to consult health care provider before taking other Rx, OTC, or herbal products, especially St. John's wort. Advise patient to avoid taking antacids or antidiarrheals within 2 hr of digoxin.
- Advise patient to notify health care provider of this medication regimen before treatment.
- Patients taking digoxin should carry identification describing disease process and medication regimen at all times.
- Geri: Review fall prevention strategies with older adults and their families.
- Rep: Advise women of reproductive potential to notify health care provider if pregnancy is planned or suspected; may ↑ risk for low birth weight or preterm birth. Digoxin is recommended as a first-line agent for chronic treatment of highly symptomatic supraventricular tachycardia in pregnancy. Monitor for maternal arrhythmias during labor and delivery. Monitor maternal serum digoxin concentrations; may require dose adjustments during pregnancy and postpartum; may lead to ↑ risk of arrhythmias during labor and delivery. Monitor neonates for signs and symptoms of digoxin toxicity (vomiting, cardiac arrhythmias). Monitor neonates for signs/symptoms of digoxin toxicity.
- Emphasize the importance of routine follow-up exams to determine effectiveness and to monitor for toxicity.

Evaluation/Desired Outcomes
- Decrease in severity of HF.
- Increase in cardiac output.
- Decrease in ventricular response in atrial fibrillation or atrial flutter.
- Termination of paroxysmal atrial tachycardia.

diltiazem,
See CALCIUM CHANNEL BLOCKERS.

dimethyl fumarate
(dye-**meth**-il **fue**-ma-rate)
Tecfidera
Classification
Therapeutic: anti-multiple sclerosis agents

Indications
Relapsing forms of multiple sclerosis (MS), including clinically isolated syndrome, relapsing-remitting disease, and active secondary progressive disease.

Action
Activates nuclear factor-like 2 pathway involved in cellular response to oxidative stress. **Therapeutic Effects:** Decreased incidence/severity of relapse with decreased progression of lesions and disability.

Pharmacokinetics
Absorption: Rapidly converted to active metabolite monomethyl fumarate (MMF) by enzymes in GI tract, blood, and tissue.
Distribution: Unknown.
Metabolism and Excretion: MMF is metabolized by the tricarboxylic acid cycle. 60% eliminated via exhalation of CO_2. Minor amounts eliminated by renal (16%) and fecal (1%) routes; trace amounts in urine.
Half-life: *MMF:* 1 hr

TIME/ACTION PROFILE (effects on disability)

ROUTE	ONSET	PEAK	DURATION
PO	24 wk	60 wk	Unknown

Contraindications/Precautions
Contraindicated in: Hypersensitivity.
Use Cautiously in: Serious infections (treatment may be withheld); Persistent lymphopenia (>6 mo) (↑ risk of progressive multifocal leukoencephalopathy [PML]); OB: Other agents preferred when disease-modifying therapy needed; Lactation: Safety not established in breastfeeding; Pedi: Safety and effectiveness not established in children.

Adverse Reactions/Side Effects
Derm: flushing, erythema, pruritus, rash. **GI:** abdominal pain, diarrhea, nausea, dyspepsia, GI HEMORRHAGE, GI OBSTRUCTION, GI PERFORATION, GI ULCERATION, HEPATOTOXICITY, ↑ liver enzymes, vomiting. **Hemat:** lymphopenia. **Neuro:** PML. **Misc:** HYPERSENSITIVITY REACTIONS (INCLUDING ANAPHYLAXIS AND ANGIOEDEMA), INFECTION (BACTERIAL, VIRAL [ESPECIALLY HERPES ZOSTER], AND FUNGAL).

Interactions
Drug-Drug: None reported.

Route/Dosage
PO (Adults): 120 mg twice daily for one wk, then 240 mg twice daily.

Availability (generic available)
Extended-release capsules: 120 mg, 240 mg.

NURSING IMPLICATIONS
Assessment
- Monitor for signs and symptoms of infections (fever, sore throat, herpes zoster, fungal and bacterial infections). Consider withholding medication until serious infections are resolved.
- Monitor for signs and symptoms of PML (progressive weakness on one side of body or clumsiness of limbs, disturbance of vision, changes in thinking, memory, and orientation causing confusion and personality changes). Symptoms are diverse, progress over days to wks. Withhold medication and obtain diagnostic evaluation.
- Monitor for signs and symptoms of hypersensitivity reactions (difficulty breathing, urticaria, swelling of throat and tongue) during therapy.
- Monitor for new or worsening severe GI signs and symptoms (vomiting, abdominal pain, GI bleeding). Discontinue therapy if severe GI signs or symptoms develop.

Lab Test Considerations
- Monitor CBC with lymphocyte count before initiating therapy, after 6 mo, and every 6–12 mo thereafter. If lymphocyte count is $<0.5 \times 10^9$/L for >6 mo, may interrupt therapy. Consider withholding therapy for patients with serious infections.
- Assess AST, ALT, alkaline phosphatase, and total bilirubin levels prior to starting therapy and as clinically indicated. May cause ↑ AST and ALT. Discontinue therapy if clinically significant liver injury is suspected.
- May cause transient ↑ mean eosinophil count during first 2 mo of therapy.

Implementation
- **PO:** Administer 120 mg twice daily for 7 days then increase to maintenance dose of 240 mg twice daily without regard to food. For patients with difficulty tolerating maintenance dose, may temporarily decrease to 120 mg twice daily; resume maintenance dose within 4 wk. ***DNC:*** Swallow capsules whole; do not open, crush, chew, or sprinkle on food. Discard any unused capsules 90 days after opening.

D

Patient/Family Teaching

- Instruct patient to take dimethyl fumarate as directed. Advise patient to read *Patient Information* before starting therapy and with each Rx refill in case of changes.
- Caution patient not to share medication with others, even if they have the same symptoms; may be dangerous.
- May cause flushing (warmth, redness, itching, and/or burning sensation). Usually begins after starting and resolves over time. Administration of dimethyl fumarate with food or administration of nonenteric coated aspirin (up to a dose of 325 mg) 30 min prior to dimethyl fumarate dosing may decrease incidence or severity of flushing.
- Advise patient to notify health care professional if signs or symptoms of infections or liver injury (fatigue, anorexia, right upper abdominal discomfort, dark urine, jaundice) occur.
- Advise patient to notify health care professional promptly if signs and symptoms of PML (new or worsening weakness; trouble using their arms or legs; changes to thinking, eyesight, strength, or balance), GI events (rectal bleeding, bloody diarrhea, vomiting blood, severe abdominal pain, severe vomiting, severe diarrhea), or hypersensitivity reactions (difficulty breathing, urticaria, swelling of throat and tongue) occur.
- Advise patient to notify health care professional of all Rx or OTC medications, vitamins, or herbal products being taken and to consult with health care professional before taking other medications.
- Rep: Advise female patients to notify health care professional if pregnancy is planned or suspected or if breastfeeding.

Evaluation/Desired Outcomes

- Decreased incidence/severity of relapse of MS.

dinoprostone

(dye-noe-**prost**-one)

Cervidil, Prepidil

Classification

Therapeutic: cervical ripening agent

Pharmacologic: oxytocics, prostaglandins

Indications

Used to "ripen" the cervix in pregnancy at or near term when induction of labor is indicated.

Action

Produces contractions similar to those occurring during labor at term by stimulating the myometrium (oxytocic effect). Initiates softening, effacement, and dilation of the cervix ("ripening"). Also stimulates GI smooth muscle. **Therapeutic Effects:** Initiation of labor.

Pharmacokinetics

Absorption: Rapidly absorbed.
Distribution: Unknown. Action is mostly local.
Metabolism and Excretion: Metabolized by enzymes in lung, kidneys, spleen, and liver tissue.
Half-life: 2.5–5 min.

TIME/ACTION PROFILE

ROUTE	ONSET	PEAK	DURATION
Cervical ripening (gel)	rapid	30–45 min	unknown
Cervical ripening (insert)	rapid	unknown	12 hr

Contraindications/Precautions

Contraindicated in: Hypersensitivity to prostaglandins or additives in the gel or suppository; Should be avoided in situations in which prolonged uterine contractions should be avoided, including: Previous cesarean section or uterine surgery; Cephalopelvic disproportion; Traumatic delivery or difficult labor; Multiparity (≥6 term pregnancies); Hyperactive or hypertonic uterus; Fetal distress (if delivery is not imminent); Unexplained vaginal bleeding; Placenta previa; Vasa previa; Active herpes genitalis; Obstetric emergency requiring surgical intervention; Situations in which vaginal delivery is contraindicated; Presence of acute pelvic inflammatory disease or ruptured membranes; Concurrent oxytocic therapy (wait for 30 min after removing insert before using oxytocin).
Use Cautiously in: Uterine scarring; Asthma; Hypotension; Cardiac disease; Adrenal disorders; Anemia; Jaundice; Diabetes mellitus; Seizure disorders; Glaucoma; Renal impairment; Hepatic impairment; Pulmonary disease; Multiparity (up to five previous term pregnancies); Women >30 yr, those with complications during pregnancy, and those with a gestational age >40 wk (↑ risk of disseminated intravascular coagulation).

Adverse Reactions/Side Effects

GU: uterine contractile abnormalities, warm feeling in vagina. **MS:** back pain. **Misc:** AMNIOTIC FLUID EMBOLISM, fever.

Interactions

Drug-Drug: Augments the effects of other **oxytocics**.

Route/Dosage

vag (Adults, Cervical): *Endocervical gel:* 0.5 mg; if response is unfavorable, may repeat in 6 hr (not to exceed 1.5 mg/24 hr). *Vaginal insert:* One 10-mg insert.

Availability

Endocervical gel (Prepidil): 0.5 mg dinoprostone in 3 g of gel vehicle in a prefilled syringe with catheters. **Vaginal insert (Cervidil):** 10 mg.

NURSING IMPLICATIONS

Assessment

- Monitor uterine activity, fetal status, and cervical dilation and effacement continuously throughout therapy. Assess for hypertonus, sustained uterine contractility, and fetal distress throughout treatment and after removal for ≥15 min. Insert should be removed at the onset of active labor. Discontinue use if uterine tachysystole or uterine hypersystole/hypertonicity with or without fetal HR changes occurs.
- Monitor for signs and symptoms of amniotic fluid embolism syndrome (rare but fatal) (dyspnea, tachypnea, rales, rhonchi, chills, hypotension, mental status changes, abnormal bleeding, fetal distress) during treatment; notify health care provider immediately and provide supportive care.
- Women ≥30 yr who had complications during pregnancy and with a gestational age >40 wk have an ↑ risk of postpartum disseminated intravascular coagulation; Monitor for evolving fibrinolysis during the immediate postpartum period.

Implementation

- Dinoprostone is a potent oxytocic agent and should be used with strict adherence to recommended dosages and only by medically trained personnel in a hospital setting that can provide immediate intensive care and acute surgical facilities.
- **Vaginal Insert:** Place vaginal insert transversely in the posterior vaginal fornix immediately after removing from foil package. Warming of insert and sterile conditions are not required. Use vaginal insert only with a retrieval system. Use minimal amount of water-soluble lubricant during insertion; avoid excess because it may hamper release of dinoprostone from insert. Patient should remain supine for 2 hr after insertion; then may ambulate. Store vaginal inserts in freezer.
- Vaginal insert delivers dinoprostone 0.3 mg/hr over 12 hr. Remove insert at the onset of active labor, before amniotomy, or after 12 hr.
- Oxytocin should not be used during or <30 min after removal of insert.
- **Endocervical Gel:** Determine degree of effacement before insertion of the endocervical catheter. Do not administer above the level of the internal os. Use a 20-mm endocervical catheter if no effacement is present and a 10-mm catheter if the cervix is 50% effaced.
- Use caution to prevent contact of dinoprostone gel with skin. Wash hands thoroughly with soap and water after administration.
- Bring gel to room temperature just before administration. Do not force warming with external sources (e.g., water bath, microwave). Remove peel-off seal from end of syringe; then remove the protective end cap and insert end cap into plunger stopper assembly in barrel of syringe. Aseptically remove catheter from package. Firmly attach catheter hub to syringe tip; click is evidence of attachment. Fill catheter with sterile gel by pushing plunger to expel air from catheter before administration to patient. Gel is stable for 24 mo if refrigerated.
- Patient should be in dorsal position with cervix visualized using a speculum. Introduce gel with catheter into cervical canal using sterile technique. Administer gel by gentle expulsion from syringe and then remove catheter. Do not attempt to administer small amount of gel remaining in syringe. Use syringe for only one patient; discard syringe, catheter, and unused package contents after using.
- Patient should remain supine for 15–30 min after administration to minimize leakage from cervical canal.
- Oxytocin may be administered 6–12 hr after desired response from dinoprostone gel. If no cervical/uterine response to initial dose of dinoprostone is obtained, repeat dose may be administered in 6 hr.

Patient/Family Teaching

- Explain purpose and side effects of medication and vaginal exams. Advise patient to read *Medication Guide* before starting and periodically during therapy in case of changes.
- **Cervical Ripening:** Inform patient they may experience a warm feeling in their vagina during administration.
- Advise patient to notify health care professional if contractions become prolonged.
- Advise patient to notify health care professional of all Rx or OTC medications, vitamins, or herbal products being taken and to consult with health care professional before taking other medications.

Evaluation/Desired Outcomes

- Cervical ripening and induction of labor.

BEERS

diphenhydrAMINE

(dye-fen-**hye**-dra-meen)

✱ Aller-Aide, ✱ Allerdryl, ✱ Allergy Formula, AllerMax, ✱ Allernix, Banophen, Benadryl Dye-Free Allergy, Benadryl Allergy, Benadryl, ✱ Benylin, ✱ Calmex, Compoz, Compoz Nighttime Sleep Aid, ✱ Dimetane Allergy, Diphen AF, Diphen Cough, ✱ Diphenhist, ✱ Dormex, ✱ Dormiphen, Genahist, 40 Winks, Hyrexin-50, ✱ Insomnal, Maximum Strength Nytol, Maximum Strength Sleepinal, Midol PM, Miles Nervine, ✱ Nadryl, Nighttime Sleep Aid, Nytol, Scot-Tussin Allergy DM, Siladril, Silphen, Sleep-Eze 3, Sleepwell 2-night, Sominex, Snooze Fast, Sominex, Tusstat, Twilite, Unisom Nighttime Sleep-Aid

Classification

Therapeutic: allergy, cold, and cough remedies, antihistamines, antitussives

Indications

Relief of allergic symptoms caused by histamine release, including: Anaphylaxis, Seasonal and perennial allergic rhinitis, Allergic dermatoses. Parkinson disease and dystonic reactions from medications. Mild nighttime sedation. Prevention of motion sickness. Antitussive (syrup only).

Action

Antagonizes the effects of histamine at H_1-receptor sites; does not bind to or inactivate histamine. Significant CNS depressant and anticholinergic properties. **Therapeutic Effects:** Decreased symptoms of histamine excess (sneezing, rhinorrhea, nasal and ocular pruritus, ocular tearing and redness, urticaria). Relief of acute dystonic reactions. Prevention of motion sickness. Suppression of cough.

Pharmacokinetics

Absorption: Well absorbed after oral or IM administration, but 40–60% of an oral dose reaches systemic circulation due to first-pass metabolism.

Distribution: Widely distributed to tissues.

Metabolism and Excretion: 95% metabolized by the liver.

Half-life: 2.4–7 hr.

TIME/ACTION PROFILE (antihistaminic effects)

ROUTE	ONSET	PEAK	DURATION
PO	15–60 min	2–4 hr	4–8 hr
IM	20–30 min	2–4 hr	4–8 hr
IV	rapid	unknown	4–8 hr

D

Contraindications/Precautions

Contraindicated in: Hypersensitivity; Acute attacks of asthma; Known alcohol intolerance (some liquid products); Lactation: Lactation.

Use Cautiously in: Severe hepatic impairment; Angle-closure glaucoma; Seizure disorders; Prostatic hyperplasia; Peptic ulcer; Hyperthyroidism; OB: Safety not established in pregnancy; Geri: Appears on Beers list. ↑ risk of anticholinergic adverse reactions in older adults, including falls, delirium, and dementia. Avoid use of oral formulations in older adults.

Adverse Reactions/Side Effects

CV: hypotension, palpitations. **Derm:** photosensitivity. **EENT:** blurred vision, tinnitus. **GI:** <u>anorexia</u>, <u>dry mouth</u>, constipation, nausea. **GU:** dysuria, urinary frequency, urinary retention. **Local:** pain at IM site. **Neuro:** <u>drowsiness</u>, dizziness, headache, paradoxical excitation (↑ in children). **Resp:** chest tightness, thickened bronchial secretions, wheezing.

Interactions

Drug-Drug: ↑ risk of CNS depression with other **antihistamines**, **alcohol**, **opioid analgesics**, and **sedative/hypnotics**. ↑ risk of anticholinergic effects with **tricyclic antidepressants**, **quinidine**, or **disopyramide**. **MAO inhibitors** intensify and prolong the anticholinergic effects of antihistamines.

Drug-Natural Products: Kava-kava, **valerian**, or **chamomile** can ↑ CNS depression.

Route/Dosage

PO (Adults and Children >12 yr): *Antihistaminic/antiemetic/antivertiginic:* 25–50 mg every 4–6 hr (not to exceed 300 mg/day). *Antitussive:* 25 mg every 4 hr as needed (not to exceed 150 mg/day). *Antidyskinetic:* 25–50 mg every 4 hr (not to exceed 400 mg/day). *Sedative/hypnotic:* 50 mg 20–30 min before bedtime.

PO (Children 6–12 yr): *Antihistaminic/antiemetic/antivertiginic:* 12.5–25 mg every 4–6 hr (not to exceed 150 mg/day). *Antidyskinetic:* 1–1.5 mg/kg every 6–8 hr as needed (not to exceed 300 mg/day). *Antitussive:* 12.5 mg every 4 hr (not to exceed 75 mg/day). *Sedative/hypnotic:* 1 mg/kg/dose 20–30 min before bedtime (not to exceed 50 mg).

PO (Children 2–6 yr): *Antihistaminic/antiemetic/antivertiginic:* 6.25–12.5 mg every 4–6 hr (not to exceed 37.5 mg/day). *Antidyskinetic:* 1–1.5 mg/kg every

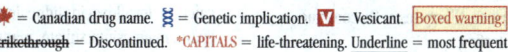

4–6 hr as needed (not to exceed 300 mg/day). *Antitussive:* 6.25 mg every 4 hr (not to exceed 37.5 mg/24 hr). *Sedative/hypnotic:* 1 mg/kg/dose 20–30 min before bedtime (not to exceed 50 mg).
IM, IV (Adults): 25–50 mg every 4 hr as needed (may need up to 100-mg dose; not to exceed 400 mg/day).
IM, IV (Children): 1.25 mg/kg (37.5 mg/m^2) 4 times daily (not to exceed 300 mg/day).
Topical (Adults and Children ≥2 yr): Apply to affected area up to 3–4 times daily.

Availability (generic available)

Capsules: 25 mg[Rx, OTC], 50 mg[Rx, OTC]. **Tablets:** 🍁 12.5 mg[Rx, OTC], 25 mg[Rx, OTC], 50 mg[Rx, OTC]. **Chewable tablets (grape flavor):** 25 mg[Rx, OTC]. **Orally disintegrating strips (cherry and grape flavor):** 12.5 mg[Rx, OTC], 25 mg[OTC]. **Orally disintegrating tablets:** 12.5 mg[OTC], 25 mg[OTC], 50 mg[Rx, OTC]. **Elixir (cherry and other flavors):** 12.5 mg/5 mL[Rx, OTC].
Syrup(cherry and raspberry flavor): 🍁 6.25 mg/5 mL[Rx, OTC], 12.5 mg/5 mL[Rx, OTC]. **Cream:** 1%[Rx, OTC], 2%[Rx, OTC]. **Topical gel:** 2%[OTC]. **Topical spray:** 2%[OTC]. **Topical stick:** 2%[OTC]. **Solution for injection:** 50 mg/mL. ***In combination with:*** analgesics, decongestants, and expectorants, in OTC pain, sleep, cough, and cold preparations. See Appendix N.

NURSING IMPLICATIONS

Assessment

- Diphenhydramine has multiple uses. Determine why the medication was ordered and assess symptoms that apply to the individual patient.
- Geri: Appears in the *Beers list.* May cause sedation and confusion due to ↑ risk of sensitivity to anticholinergic effects. Monitor carefully; assess for confusion, delirium, other anticholinergic side effects, and fall risk. Institute measures to prevent falls.
- **Prevention and Treatment of Anaphylaxis:** Assess for urticaria and patency of airway.
- **Allergic Rhinitis:** Assess degree of nasal stuffiness, rhinorrhea, and sneezing.
- **Parkinsonism and Extrapyramidal Reactions:** Assess movement disorder before and after administration.
- **Insomnia:** Assess sleep patterns.
- **Motion Sickness:** Assess nausea, vomiting, bowel sounds, and abdominal pain.
- **Cough Suppressant:** Assess frequency and nature of cough, lung sounds, and amount and type of sputum produced. Unless contraindicated, maintain fluid intake of 1500–2000 mL daily to ↓ viscosity of bronchial secretions.
- **Pruritus:** Assess degree of itching, skin rash, and inflammation.

Lab Test Considerations

- May ↓ skin response to allergy tests. Discontinue 4 days before skin testing.

Implementation

- Do not confuse Benadryl with benazepril. Do not confuse diphenhydramine with dimenhydrinate.
- When used for insomnia, administer 20–30 min before bedtime and schedule activities to minimize interruption of sleep.
- When used for prophylaxis of motion sickness, administer ≥30 min and preferably 1–2 hr before exposure to conditions that may precipitate motion sickness.
- **PO:** Administer with meals or milk to ↓ GI irritation. Capsule may be emptied and contents taken with water or food.
- Orally disintegrating tablets and strips should be left in the package until use. Remove from the blister pouch. Do not push tablet through the blister; peel open the blister pack with dry hands and place tablet on tongue. Tablet will dissolve rapidly and be swallowed with saliva. No liquid is needed to take the orally disintegrating tablet.
- **IM:** Administer 50 mg/mL into well-developed muscle. Avoid SUBQ injections.

IV Administration

- **IV Push:** Dilution: May be further diluted in 0.9% NaCl, 0.45% NaCl, D5W, D10W, dextrose/saline combinations, Ringer's solution, LR, or dextrose/Ringer's combinations. Concentration: 25 mg/mL. Rate: Infuse at a rate not to exceed 25 mg/min. For pediatric patients, may further dilute as an intermittent infusion over 10–15 min.
- **Y-Site Compatibility:** acetaminophen, aldesleukin, alemtuzumab, amikacin, aminocaproic acid, amiodarone, amphotericin B liposomal, anidulafungin, argatroban, ascorbic acid, atracurium, atropine, azithromycin, benztropine, bivalirudin, bleomycin, bumetanide, buprenorphine, butorphanol, calcium chloride, calcium gluconate, carboplatin, carmustine, caspofungin, ceftaroline, ceftolozane/tazobactam, chlorpromazine, ciprofloxacin, cisatracurium, cisplatin, cladribine, clindamycin, cyanocobalamin, cyclophosphamide, cyclosporine, cytarabine, dacarbazine, dactinomycin, daptomycin, daunorubicin, dexmedetomidine, dexrazoxane, digoxin, diltiazem, dobutamine, docetaxel, dopamine, doxorubicin hydrochloride, doxorubicin liposomal, doxycycline, enalaprilat, ephedrine, epinephrine, epirubicin, epoetin alfa, eptifibatide, ertapenem, erythromycin, esmolol, etoposide, etoposide phosphate, famotidine, fentanyl, filgrastim, fluconazole, fludarabine, folic acid, fosphenytoin, gemcitabine, gemtuzumab ozogamicin, gentamicin, glycopyrrolate, granisetron, hetastarch, hydromorphone, hydroxyzine, idarubicin, ifosfamide, imipenem/cilastatin, irinotecan, isoproterenol, ketamine, labetalol, LR, leucovorin calcium, levofloxacin, lidocaine, linezolid, lorazepam, magnesium sulfate, mannitol, melphalan,

meperidine, meropenem, mesna, methadone, methotrexate, metoclopramide, metoprolol, metronidazole, midazolam, mitomycin, mitoxantrone, morphine, moxifloxacin, multiple vitamins, mycophenolate, nalbuphine, naloxone, nicardipine, nitroglycerin, norepinephrine, octreotide, ondansetron, oxaliplatin, oxytocin, paclitaxel, palonosetron, pamidronate, papaverine, pemetrexed, penicillin G, pentamidine, phentolamine, phenylephrine, phytonadione, piperacillin/tazobactam, plazomicin, potassium acetate, potassium chloride, procainamide, prochlorperazine, promethazine, propofol, propranolol, protamine, pyridoxine, remifentanil, rituximab, rocuronium, sargramostim, sodium acetate, succinylcholine, sufentanil, sulbactam/durlobactam, tacrolimus, theophylline, thiamine, thiotepa, tigecycline, tirofiban, tobramycin, topotecan, trastuzumab, vancomycin, vasopressin, vecuronium, verapamil, vinblastine, vincristine, vinorelbine, voriconazole, zoledronic acid.

- **Y-Site Incompatibility:** allopurinol, aminophylline, amphotericin B deoxycholate, ampicillin, azathioprine, cefazolin, cefepime, cefotaxime, cefotetan, cefoxitin, ceftazidime, ceftriaxone, cefuroxime, chloramphenicol, dantrolene, dexamethasone, diazepam, fluorouracil, foscarnet, furosemide, ganciclovir, heparin, indomethacin, insulin, regular, ketorolac, meropenem/vaborbactam, methylprednisolone, milrinone, nitroprusside, oxacillin, pantoprazole, pentobarbital, phenobarbital, phenytoin, sodium bicarbonate, tedizolid, trimethoprim/sulfamethoxazole.
- **Topical:** Apply a thin coat and rub gently until absorbed. Only for topical use; avoid ingestion.

Patient/Family Teaching

- Explain the purpose and side effects of diphenhydramine. Instruct patient to take medication as directed; do not exceed recommended amount. Caution patient not to use oral OTC diphenhydramine products with any other product containing diphenhydramine, including products used topically. Patient should not use topical form on eyes or eyelid and avoid applying occlusive dressings. Advise patient to read *Medication Guide* before starting and periodically during therapy.
- May cause drowsiness. Caution patient to avoid driving or other activities requiring alertness until response to drug is known.
- Advise patients taking diphenhydramine in OTC preparations to notify health care professional if symptoms worsen or persist for >7 days.
- May cause dry mouth. Inform patient that frequent oral rinses, good oral hygiene, and sugarless gum or candy may minimize this effect. Notify health care professional if dry mouth persists for >2 wk.
- Teach sleep hygiene techniques (dark room, quiet, bedtime ritual, limit daytime napping, avoidance of nicotine and caffeine) to patients taking diphenhydramine to aid sleep.
- Advise patient to notify health care professional of all Rx or OTC medications, vitamins, or herbal products being taken and to consult with health care professional before taking other medications. Caution patient to avoid use of alcohol and other CNS depressants, including opioids, concurrently with this medication.
- Pedi: Can cause excitation in children. Caution parents or caregivers about proper dose calculation; overdose, especially in infants and children, can cause hallucinations, seizures, or death. Caution parents to avoid OTC cough and cold products while breastfeeding or to children <4 yr.
- Geri: Instruct older adults to avoid OTC products that contain diphenhydramine due to ↑ risk of sensitivity to anticholinergic effects and potential for adverse reactions related to these effects.
- Rep: Advise women of reproductive potential to notify health care professional if pregnancy is planned or suspected and to avoid breastfeeding during therapy.

Evaluation/Desired Outcomes

- Prevention of, or decreased urticaria in, anaphylaxis or other allergic reactions.
- Decreased dyskinesia in parkinsonism and extrapyramidal reactions.
- Sedation when used as a sedative/hypnotic.
- Prevention of or decrease in nausea and vomiting caused by motion sickness.
- Decrease in frequency and intensity of cough without eliminating cough reflex.

DIURETICS (LOOP)

bumetanide (byoo-**met**-a-nide)
Bumex, ✱ Burinex

furosemide (fur-**oh**-se-mide)
Furoscix, Lasix, ✱ Lasix Special

torsemide (**tore**-se-mide)
~~Demadex~~, Soaanz

Classification
Therapeutic: diuretics
Pharmacologic: loop diuretics

Indications

Edema due to: HF, Hepatic or renal disease. Hypertension. Edema due to chronic HF (SUBQ furosemide only). **Unlabeled Use: Furosemide:** Hypercalcemia of malignancy.

Action

Inhibit the reabsorption of sodium and chloride from the loop of Henle and distal renal tubule. Increase renal excretion of water, sodium, chloride, magnesium, hydrogen, and calcium. May have renal and peripheral vasodilatory effects. Effectiveness persists in impaired renal function. **Therapeutic Effects:** Diuresis and subsequent mobilization of excess fluid (edema, pleural effusions). Decreased BP.

Pharmacokinetics

Absorption: *Bumetanide:* well absorbed after oral or IM administration. *Furosemide:* 60–75% absorbed following oral administration; also absorbed from IM sites; IV administration results in complete availability; 99.6% absorbed after SUBQ administration. *Torsemide:* 80% absorbed following oral administration.
Distribution: *Bumetanide and Torsemide:* well distributed to tissues.
Protein Binding: All are >91%.
Metabolism and Excretion: *Bumetanide:* Partially metabolized by the liver; 50% eliminated unchanged by the kidneys; 20% excreted in feces. *Furosemide:* Some metabolism by liver (30–40%), some nonhepatic metabolism, and some renal excretion as unchanged drug. *Torsemide:* Primarily metabolized by CYP2C9, with minor metabolism via CYP2C8 and CYP2C18. 80% metabolized by liver; 20% excreted in urine.
Half-life: *Bumetanide:* 60–90 min (6–15 hr in neonates); *Furosemide:* 30–120 min (↑ in renal impairment and neonates, markedly ↑ in hepatic impairment); *Torsemide:* 210 min.

TIME/ACTION PROFILE (diuretic effect)

ROUTE	ONSET	PEAK	DURATION
Bumetanide–PO	30–60 min	1–2 hr	3–6 hr
Bumetanide–IM	40 min	1–2 hr	4–6 hr
Bumetanide–IV	within min	15–45 min	3–6 hr
Furosemide–PO	30–60 min	1–2 hr	6–8 hr
Furosemide–IM	10–30 min	unknown	4–8 hr
Furosemide–IV	5 min	30 min	2 hr
Furosemide–SUBQ	unknown	unknown	8 hr
Torsemide–PO	within 60 min	60–120 min	6–8 hr

Contraindications/Precautions

Contraindicated in: Hypersensitivity; Cross-sensitivity with thiazides and sulfonamides may occur; Hepatic coma; Anuria; Hepatic cirrhosis (SUBQ only); Some liquid furosemide products may contain alcohol and should be avoided in patients with known intolerance.

Use Cautiously in: Severe hepatic impairment (may precipitate hepatic coma; concurrent use with potassium-sparing diuretics may be necessary); Electrolyte depletion; Diabetes; Hypoproteinemia or severe renal impairment (↑ risk of ototoxicity); OB/ Lactation/ Pedi: Safety and effectiveness of torsemide not established in children; bumetanide is a potent displacer of bilirubin and should be used cautiously in critically ill or jaundiced neonates due to risk of kernicterus; Geri: Older adults may have ↑ risk of side effects, especially hypotension and electrolyte imbalance.

Adverse Reactions/Side Effects

CV: hypotension. **Derm:** ERYTHEMA MULTIFORME (EM), photosensitivity, pruritus, rash, STEVENS-JOHNSON SYNDROME, TOXIC EPIDERMAL NECROLYSIS, urticaria. **EENT:** hearing loss, tinnitus. **Endo:** hyperglycemia. **F and E:** dehydration, hypochloremia, hypokalemia, hypomagnesemia, hyponatremia, hypovolemia, metabolic alkalosis. **GI:** ↑ liver enzymes (furosemide), constipation, diarrhea, dry mouth, dyspepsia, nausea, vomiting. **GU:** acute renal failure, renal impairment, excessive urination. **Hemat:** blood dyscrasias (furosemide). **Metab:** hypercholesterolemia, hypertriglyceridemia, hyperuricemia. **MS:** arthralgia (torsemide), muscle cramps, myalgia (torsemide). **Neuro:** dizziness, encephalopathy (bumetanide and furosemide), headache, insomnia (torsemide), nervousness (torsemide).

Interactions

Drug-Drug: ↑ risk of hypotension with **antihypertensives**, **nitrates**, or acute ingestion of **alcohol**. ↑ risk of hypokalemia with other **diuretics**, **piperacillin/tazobactam**, **amphotericin B**, **stimulant laxatives**, and **corticosteroids**. Hypokalemia may ↑ risk of **digoxin** toxicity. May ↑ levels and risk of toxicity of **lithium**. ↑ risk of ototoxicity with **aminoglycosides** or **cisplatin**. ↑ risk of nephrotoxicity with other **nephrotoxic drugs**, including **aminoglycosides**, **cisplatin**, **NSAIDs**, **ACE inhibitors**, **angiotensin II receptor blockers**, and **radiocontrast agents**. May ↑ levels and risk of toxicity of **methotrexate**. **Cyclosporine** may ↑ risk of gouty arthritis. May ↑ risk of bleeding with **warfarin**, **thrombolytic agents**, or **anticoagulants**. **CYP2C9 inhibitors**, including **amiodarone**, **fluconazole**, **miconazole**, and **oxandrolone**, may ↑ levels and risk of toxicity of torsemide. **CYP2C9 inducers**, including **rifampin**, may ↓ levels and effectiveness of torsemide. Torsemide may ↑ levels and risk of toxicity of **CYP2C9 substrates**, including **celecoxib**, **phenytoin**, or **warfarin**.

Route/Dosage

Bumetanide

PO (Adults): 0.5–2 mg/day as a single dose. Up to 2 additional doses may be given during the day every 4–5 hr (up to 10 mg/day). Alternate-day or every-2–3-day regimens may also be used.

IM, IV (Adults): 0.5–1 mg; may be repeated every 2–3 hr as needed (up to 10 mg/day).

Furosemide

PO (Adults): *Edema:* 20–80 mg/day as a single dose initially; may repeat in 6–8 hr; may ↑ dose by 20–40 mg every 6–8 hr until desired response. Maintenance doses may be given once or twice daily or intermittently for 2–4 days/wk (doses up to 2.5 g/day have been used in patients with HF or renal disease). *Hypertension:* 40 mg twice daily initially (when added to regimen, ↓ dose of other antihypertensives by 50%); adjust further dosing based on response; *Hypercalcemia:* 120 mg/day in 1–3 doses.
PO (Children): 2 mg/kg as a single dose; may ↑ by 1–2 mg/kg every 6–8 hr (1–2 mg/kg/day initially, up to 5–6 mg/kg/day). Longer dosage intervals are recommended in neonates.
IM, IV (Adults): *Edema:* 20–40 mg; may repeat in 2 hr and ↑ by 20 mg every 2 hr until response is obtained; maintenance dose may be given once or twice daily; *Acute pulmonary edema:* 40 mg; after 1 hr may give additional 80 mg (in HF and renal failure, daily doses of up to 2.5 g have been used); *Hypercalcemia:* 80–120 mg; may repeat every 1–4 hr; titrate by response.
IM, IV (Children): 1 mg/kg; may ↑ by 1 mg/kg every 2 hr (not to exceed 6 mg/kg).
SUBQ (Adults): 30 mg over the 1st hr, then 12.5 mg per hr over the next 4 hr with the single-use on-body infusor. Replace with oral diuretic therapy as soon as possible.

Torsemide

PO (Adults): *HF:* Generic or Sooanz: 20 mg once daily; may double dose until desired effect obtained (max = 200 mg/day). *Chronic renal failure:* Generic or Soaanz: 20 mg once daily; may double dose until desired effect obtained (max = 200 mg/day). *Hepatic cirrhosis:* Generic only: 5–10 mg once daily (with aldosterone antagonist or potassium-sparing diuretic); may double dose until desired effect obtained (max = 40 mg/day). *Hypertension:* 5 mg once daily; may ↑ to 10 mg once daily after 4–6 wk (if still not effective, add another agent).

Availability

Bumetanide

Tablets: 0.5 mg, 1 mg, 2 mg, 🍁 5 mg. **Solution for injection:** 0.25 mg/mL.

Furosemide

Tablets: 20 mg, 40 mg, 80 mg, 🍁 500 mg. **Oral solution (10 mg/mL: orange flavor, 8 mg/mL: pineapple-peach flavor):** 8 mg/mL, 10 mg/mL. **Solution for intravenous/intramuscular injection:** 10 mg/mL. **Solution for SUBQ injection (Furoscix) (prefilled cartridges):** 80 mg/10 mL.

Torsemide

Tablets: 5 mg, 10 mg, 20 mg, 40 mg, 60 mg, 100 mg.

NURSING IMPLICATIONS

Assessment

- Assess fluid status during therapy. Monitor daily weight, intake and output ratios, amount and location of edema, lung sounds, skin turgor, and mucous membranes. Notify health care provider if thirst, dry mouth, lethargy, weakness, hypotension, or oliguria occurs.
- Monitor BP and HR before starting and throughout therapy.
- Assess for rash frequently with signs and symptoms of SJS, TEN, or EM during therapy (fever, general malaise, fatigue, muscle or joint aches, blisters, oral lesions, conjunctivitis, hepatitis, eosinophilia). Discontinue immediately and provide supportive care; may be life-threatening. May recur once treatment is stopped.
- Assess patients receiving digoxin for anorexia, nausea, vomiting, muscle cramps, paresthesia, and confusion; ↑ risk of digoxin toxicity because of the potassium-depleting effect of the diuretic. Potassium supplements or potassium-sparing diuretics may be used concurrently to prevent hypokalemia.
- Assess for tinnitus and hearing loss. Audiometry is recommended for patients receiving prolonged high-dose IV therapy. Hearing loss is most common following rapid or high-dose IV administration in patients with renal impairment or those taking other ototoxic drugs.
- Geri: Diuretic use is associated with ↑ risk for falls in older adults. Assess risk and implement fall prevention strategies.
- Assess for allergy to sulfonamides.

Lab Test Considerations

- Monitor electrolytes before and regularly during therapy. May ↓ sodium, potassium, calcium, and magnesium concentrations.
- Monitor renal and hepatic function, serum glucose, and uric acid levels before and periodically during therapy. May ↑ BUN, serum glucose, creatinine, and uric acid.

Implementation

- Do not confuse Lasix with Wakix.
- If given in excessive amounts, furosemide can lead to significant diuresis with water and electrolyte depletion. Careful medical supervision is required, and dose regimen must be adjusted to the individual patient's needs.
- Administer *loop diuretics* in the morning to prevent disruption of sleep cycle. If administering twice daily, give last dose no later than 5 pm.

- IV is preferred over IM for parenteral administration.
- **PO:** Administer orally with food or milk to minimize GI irritation. *Torsemide* may be administered without regard to meals. *Furosemide* tablets may be crushed if patient has difficulty swallowing.
- **SUBQ**: The single-use on-body *infusor* with prefilled cartridge is preprogrammed to deliver 30 mg over 1st hr followed by 12.5 mg/hr for the subsequent 4 hr. Inspect fluid in prefilled cartridge; solution is clear to slightly yellow; do not administer if discolored or cloudy. Load prefilled cartridge and close. Peel adhesive liner on the *infusor* and apply to clean, dry skin of the abdomen between top of beltline and bottom of rib cage (>2½ inches from beltline or bottom of rib cage) that is not tender, bruised, red or indurated. Start injection by firmly pressing and releasing the start button. Do not remove until the injection is complete (signaled by the solid green status light, beeping sound, and white plunger rod filling the cartridge window). Rotate the site of each SUBQ administration. Patient must limit activity during administration. The *infusor* cannot be immersed fluids (water, sweat, blood, etc.) to prevent malfunction. Keep *infusor* >12 inches away from electronic devices or wireless accessories (TV remote, Bluetooth devices). *Infusor* must be removed prior to MRI. SUBQ route is not for chronic use; replace with oral diuretics as soon as practical.

IV Administration

Bumetanide

- **IV Push:** Administer undiluted. **Rate:** Administer slowly over 1–2 min. **Concentration:** 0.25 mg/mL.
- **Intermittent Infusion: Dilution:** Dilute in D5W, 0.9% NaCl, or LR. Protect from light. Infusion stable for 24 hr. **Concentration:** ≤0.25 mg/mL. **Rate:** Infuse over 5 min. May be administered over 12 hr for patients with renal impairment.
- **Y-Site Compatibility:** acyclovir, allopurinol, alprostadil, amikacin, aminocaproic acid, aminophylline, amphotericin B liposomal, anidulafungin, argatroban, arsenic trioxide, ascorbic acid, atracurium, atropine, azithromycin, aztreonam, benztropine, bivalirudin, bleomycin, buprenorphine, butorphanol, calcium gluconate, cangrelor, carboplatin, carmustine, caspofungin, cefazolin, cefepime, cefiderocol, cefotaxime, cefotetan, cefoxitin, ceftaroline, ceftazidime, ceftobiprole, ceftolozane/tazobactam, ceftriaxone, cefuroxime, chloramphenicol, cisatracurium, cisplatin, cladribine, clindamycin, cyanocobalamin, cyclophosphamide, cyclosporine, cytarabine, dacarbazine, dactinomycin, daptomycin, daunorubicin, dexamethasone, dexrazoxane, digoxin, diltiazem, diphenhydramine, dobutamine, docetaxel, dopamine, doxorubicin hydrochloride, doxorubicin liposomal, doxycycline, enalaprilat, ephedrine, epirubicin, epoetin alfa, eptifibatide, eravacycline, ertapenem, erythromycin, esmolol, etoposide, etoposide phosphate, famotidine, fentanyl, filgrastim, fluconazole, fludarabine, fluorouracil, folic acid, foscarnet, fosphenytoin, furosemide, gemcitabine, gentamicin, glycopyrrolate, granisetron, hydrocortisone, idarubicin, ifosfamide, imipenem/cilastatin, imipenem/cilastatin/relebactam, insulin, regular, irinotecan, isoproterenol, ketorolac, labetalol, leucovorin, levofloxacin, lidocaine, linezolid, lorazepam, magnesium sulfate, mannitol, melphalan, meperidine, meropenem/vaborbactam, mesna, methadone, methotrexate, methylprednisolone, metoclopramide, metoprolol, metronidazole, micafungin, milrinone, mitomycin, mitoxantrone, morphine, moxifloxacin, multivitamins, mycophenolate, nafcillin, nalbuphine, naloxone, nicardipine, nitroglycerin, nitroprusside, norepinephrine, octreotide, omadacycline, ondansetron, oxacillin, oxaliplatin, oxytocin, paclitaxel, palonosetron, pamidronate, pantoprazole, pemetrexed, penicillin G, pentobarbital, phenobarbital, phentolamine, phenylephrine, phytonadione, piperacillin/tazobactam, plazomicin, potassium acetate, potassium chloride, procainamide, prochlorperazine, promethazine, propofol, propranolol, protamine, pyridoxine, remifentanil, rifampin, rituximab, sodium acetate, sodium bicarbonate, succinylcholine, sufentanil, sulbactam/durlobactam, tacrolimus, tedizolid, theophylline, thiamine, thiotepa, tigecycline, tirofiban, tobramycin, trastuzumab, vancomycin, vasopressin, vecuronium, verapamil, vinblastine, vincristine, vinorelbine, voriconazole, zoledronic acid.
- **Y-Site Incompatibility:** alemtuzumab, amphotericin B deoxycholate, azathioprine, chlorpromazine, dantrolene, diazepam, diazoxide, ganciclovir, gemtuzumab ozogamicin, haloperidol, oritavancin, papaverine, pentamidine, phenytoin, sildenafil, topotecan, trimethoprim/sulfamethoxazole.

Furosemide

- When using furosemide for hypercalcemia, replace extracellular volume and NaCl to maintain fluid volume and increase calcium excretion effectively.
- **IV Push: Dilution:** Administer undiluted. **Concentration:** 10 mg/mL. **Rate:** Administer slowly at 20 mg/min. Pedi: Administer at a maximum rate of 0.5–1 mg/kg/min (for doses <120 mg) with infusion not exceeding 10 min.
- **Intermittent Infusion: Dilution:** Dilute larger doses in D5W, D10W, D20W, D5/0.9% NaCl, D5/LR,

0.9% NaCl, 3% NaCl, 1/6 M sodium lactate, or LR. Infusion stable for 24 hr at room temperature. Do not refrigerate. Protect from light. **Concentration:** 1 mg/mL. **Rate:** Administer at a rate not to exceed 4 mg/min (for doses >120 mg) in adults to prevent ototoxicity. Pedi: Not to exceed 1 mg/kg/min with infusion not exceeding 10 min. Use an infusion pump to ensure accurate dose.

- **Y-Site Compatibility:** acyclovir, allopurinol, alprostadil, amikacin, aminocaproic acid, aminophylline, amphotericin B liposomal, anidulafungin, argatroban, arsenic trioxide, ascorbic acid, atropine, azathioprine, aztreonam, bivalirudin, bleomycin, bumetanide, calcium chloride, calcium gluconate, cangrelor, carboplatin, carmustine, cefazolin, cefepime, cefiderocol, cefotaxime, cefotetan, cefoxitin, ceftaroline, ceftazidime, ceftazidime/avibactam, ceftobiprole, ceftolozane/tazobactam, ceftriaxone, cefuroxime, chloramphenicol, chlorothiazide, cisplatin, cladribine, clindamycin, cyanocobalamin, cyclophosphamide, cyclosporine, cytarabine, dactinomycin, daptomycin, dexamethasone, dexmedetomidine, digoxin, docetaxel, doxorubicin liposomal, edetate calcium disodium, enalaprilat, ephedrine, epinephrine, epoetin alfa, ertapenem, esomeprazole, etoposide, etoposide phosphate, fentanyl, fludarabine, fluorouracil, folic acid, foscarnet, fosphenytoin, ganciclovir, granisetron, heparin, hydrocortisone, ibuprofen lysine, ifosfamide, imipenem/cilastatin, imipenem/cilastatin/relebactam, indomethacin, insulin aspart, recombinant, ketorolac, letermovir, leucovorin, lidocaine, linezolid, lorazepam, mannitol, melphalan, meropenem, meropenem/vaborbactam, mesna, methohexital, methotrexate, methylprednisolone, metoprolol, metronidazole, micafungin, mitomycin, multivitamins, nafcillin, naloxone, nitroprusside, octreotide, oxacillin, oxaliplatin, oxytocin, paclitaxel, palonosetron, pamidronate, pemetrexed, penicillin G, pentobarbital, phenobarbital, phytonadione, piperacillin/tazobactam, plazomicin, potassium acetate, potassium chloride, procainamide, propofol, propranolol, remdesivir, sargramostim, sodium acetate, sodium bicarbonate, succinylcholine, sufentanil, sulbactam/durlobactam, tedizolid, theophylline, thiotepa, tigecycline, tirofiban, tobramycin, topotecan, voriconazole, zoledronic acid.
- **Y-Site Incompatibility:** acetaminophen, alemtuzumab, atracurium, benztropine, blinatumomab, butorphanol, caffeine citrate, caspofungin, ciprofloxacin, dantrolene, daunorubicin, dexrazoxane, diazepam, diazoxide, diltiazem, dimenhydrinate, diphenhydramine, doxycycline, droperidol, epirubicin, eptifibatide, eravacycline, filgrastim, gemcitabine, gemtuzumab ozogamicin, glycopyrrolate, haloperidol, idarubicin, irinotecan, isavuconazonium, ketamine, levofloxacin, milrinone, mitoxantrone, moxifloxacin, mycophenolate, nalbuphine, nicardipine, ondansetronoritavancin papaverine, pentamidine, phenytoin, posaconazole, potassium phosphates, prochlorperazine, protamine, pyridoxine, remimazolam, rituximab, rocuronium, sildenafil, telavancin, thiamine, trastuzumab, trimethoprim/sulfamethoxazole, vancomycin, vecuronium, verapamil, vinblastine, vinorelbine.

Patient/Family Teaching

- Explain purpose and side effects of loop diuretics. Instruct to take as directed. Take missed doses as soon as possible; do not double doses. Advise patient to read *Patient Information* before starting and with each Rx refill in case of changes.
- Emphasize the importance of routine follow-up examinations. Periodic lab tests will be needed.
- **Hypertension:** Advise patients on antihypertensive regimen to continue taking medication, even if feeling better. *Furosemide* and *torsemide* control but do not cure hypertension.
- Reinforce the need to continue additional therapies for hypertension (weight loss, exercise, restricted sodium intake, stress reduction, regular exercise, moderation of alcohol consumption, cessation of smoking).
- Caution patient to make position changes slowly to minimize orthostatic hypotension. Caution patient that the use of alcohol, exercise during hot weather, or standing for long periods during therapy may enhance orthostatic hypotension.
- Instruct patient to consult health care provider regarding a diet high in potassium (see Appendix J).
- Advise patient to contact health care provider of gain >3 lb in one day.
- Instruct patient to notify health care provider of all Rx or OTC medications, vitamins, or herbal products being taken and to consult health care provider before taking any OTC medications concurrently with this therapy.
- Instruct patient to notify health care provider of medication regimen prior to treatment or surgery.
- Caution patient to use sunscreen and protective clothing to prevent photosensitivity reactions.
- Advise patient to contact health care provider immediately if rash, muscle weakness, cramps, nausea, dizziness, numbness, or tingling of extremities occurs.
- Advise patient taking *furosemide* tablets not to change brands when refilling prescription; bioavailability among brands is variable.

- Advise patients with diabetes to monitor blood sugar closely, because loop diuretics may cause ↑ blood sugar levels.
- Geri: Caution older patients or their caregivers about ↑ risk for falls. Suggest strategies for fall prevention.
- Rep: Advise women of reproductive potential to notify health care provider if pregnancy is planned or suspected or if breastfeeding. Loop diuretics are not recommended for use during pregnancy, except when necessary for treating pulmonary edema in HF. Monitor fetal growth during pregnancy; ↑ risk for higher birth weights.

Evaluation/Desired Outcomes

- Diuresis and subsequent mobilization of excess fluid (edema, pleural effusions).
- Decrease in edema.
- Decrease in abdominal girth. Increase in urinary output.
- Decrease in BP.
- Decrease in serum calcium when used to manage hypercalcemia.

DIURETICS (THIAZIDE)

chlorothiazide
(klor-oh-**thye**-a-zide)
Diuril

chlorthalidone (thiazide-like)
(klor-**thal**-i-doan)
Hemiclor, Thalitone

hydroCHLOROthiazide
(hye-droe-klor-oh-**thye**-a-zide)
Inzirqo, ~~Microzide~~

Classification
Therapeutic: antihypertensives diuretics
Pharmacologic: thiazide diuretics

Indications

- Hypertension. Treatment of edema associated with: HF, Renal impairment, Cirrhosis, Glucocorticoid therapy, Estrogen therapy.

Action

Increases excretion of sodium and water by inhibiting sodium reabsorption in the distal tubule. Promotes excretion of chloride, potassium, magnesium, and bicarbonate. May produce arteriolar dilation. **Therapeutic Effects:** Lowering of BP in hypertensive patients and diuresis with mobilization of edema.

Pharmacokinetics

Absorption: All are rapidly absorbed after oral administration.
Distribution: Well distributed to tissues.
Metabolism and Excretion: All are excreted mainly unchanged by the kidneys.
Half-life: *Chlorothiazide:* 1–2 hr; *chlorthalidone:* 35–50 hr; *hydrochlorothiazide:* 6–15 hr.

TIME/ACTION PROFILE (diuretic effect)

ROUTE	ONSET	PEAK	DURATION
Chlorothiazide PO	2 hr	4 hr	6–12 hr
Chlorothiazide IV	15 min	30 min	2 hr
Chlorthalidone	2 hr	2 hr	48–72 hr
Hydrochlorothiazide†	2 hr	3–6 hr	6–12 hr

† Onset of antihypertensive effect is 3–4 days and does not become maximal for 7–14 days of dosing.

Contraindications/Precautions

Contraindicated in: Hypersensitivity (cross-sensitivity with other thiazides or sulfonamides may exist); Some products contain tartrazine and should be avoided in patients with known intolerance; Anuria; Lactation: Lactation.
Use Cautiously in: Renal impairment; Hepatic impairment; OB: Pregnancy (jaundice or thrombocytopenia may be seen in the newborn).

Adverse Reactions/Side Effects

CV: hypotension. **Derm:** photosensitivity, rash, SKIN CANCER (NONMELANOMA), STEVENS-JOHNSON SYNDROME (SJS). **EENT:** acute angle-closure glaucoma (hydrochlorothiazide), acute myopia (hydrochlorothiazide). **Endo:** hyperglycemia. **F and E** hypokalemia, dehydration, hypercalcemia, hypochloremic alkalosis, hypomagnesemia, hyponatremia, hypophosphatemia, hypovolemia. **GI:** anorexia, cramping, hepatitis, nausea, pancreatitis, vomiting. **Hemat:** thrombocytopenia. **Metab:** hypercholesterolemia, hyperuricemia. **MS:** muscle cramps. **Neuro:** dizziness, drowsiness, lethargy, weakness.

Interactions

Drug-Drug: Additive hypotension with other **antihypertensives**, acute ingestion of **alcohol**, or **nitrates**. Additive hypokalemia with **corticosteroids**, **amphotericin B**, or **piperacillin/tazobactam**. May ↑ levels and risk of toxicity of **lithium**. **Cholestyramine** or **colestipol** may ↓ absorption. Hypokalemia ↑ risk of **digoxin** toxicity. **NSAIDs** may ↓ effectiveness.

Route/Dosage

When used as a diuretic in adults, generally given daily, but may be given every other day or 2–3 days/wk.

Chlorothiazide

PO (Adults): 125 mg–2 g/day in 1–2 divided doses.
PO (Children >6 mo): 20 mg/kg/day in 1–2 divided doses (maximum dose = 1 g/day).
PO (Neonates ≤6 mo): 10–20 mg/kg every 12 hr (maximum dose = 375 mg/day).
IV (Adults): 500 mg–1 g/day in 1–2 divided doses.

IV (Children >6 mo): 4 mg/kg/day in 1–2 divided doses (maximum dose = 20 mg/kg/day) (unlabeled use).
IV (Neonates ≤6 mo): 1–4 mg/kg every 12 hr (maximum dose = 20 mg/kg/day) (unlabeled use).

Chlorthalidone

PO (Adults): 12.5–100 mg once daily (daily doses above 25 mg are associated with greater likelihood of electrolyte abnormalities).

Hydrochlorothiazide

PO (Adults): 12.5–100 mg/day in 1–2 divided doses (up to 200 mg/day); not to exceed 50 mg/day for hypertension; daily doses above 25 mg are associated with greater likelihood of electrolyte abnormalities.
PO (Children >6 mo): 1–3 mg/kg/day in 2 divided doses (not to exceed 37.5 mg/day).
PO (Children <6 mo): 1–3 mg/kg/day in 2 divided doses.

Availability

Chlorothiazide

Oral suspension: 250 mg/5 mL. **Powder for injection:** 500 mg/vial.

Chlorthalidone

Tablets: 12.5 mg, 15 mg, 25 mg, 50 mg. ***In combination with:*** atenolol (Tenoretic); azilsartan (Edarbyclor). See Appendix N. Hydrochlorothiazide **Tablets:** 12.5 mg, 25 mg, 50 mg, 🍁 100 mg. **Capsules:** 12.5 mg. **Oral suspension (caramel-mint flavor):** 10 mg/mL. ***In combination with:*** numerous antihypertensive agents. See Appendix N.

NURSING IMPLICATIONS

Assessment

- Monitor BP, intake, output, and daily weight and assess feet, legs, and sacral area for edema daily.
- Assess for anorexia, nausea, vomiting, muscle cramps, paresthesia, and confusion, especially if taking digoxin. Notify health care provider if these signs of electrolyte imbalance occur. Patients taking digoxin are at risk of digoxin toxicity because of the potassium-depleting effect of the diuretic.
- If hypokalemia occurs, consideration may be given to potassium supplements or ↓ dose of diuretic.
- Assess for allergy to sulfonamides.
- Assess for skin rash frequently during therapy. Discontinue diuretic at 1st sign of rash; may be life-threatening. SJS may develop. Treat symptomatically; may recur once treatment is stopped.
Hypertension: Monitor BP before and periodically during therapy.

Lab Test Considerations

- Monitor electrolytes (especially potassium), blood glucose, BUN, serum creatinine, and uric acid before and periodically during therapy. May ↑ serum and urine glucose in patients with diabetes.
- May ↑ serum bilirubin, calcium, creatinine, and uric acid, and ↓ serum magnesium, potassium, sodium, and urinary calcium.
- May ↑ cholesterol, low-density lipoprotein, and triglyceride.

Implementation

- Do not confuse hydrochlorothiazide with hydroxyzine, hydralazine, or hydroxychloroquine.
- Administer in the morning to prevent disruption of sleep cycle.
- Intermittent dose schedule may be used for continued control of edema.
- **PO:** May give with food or milk to minimize GI irritation. Tablets may be crushed and mixed with fluid to facilitate swallowing.

IV Administration

- **Intermittent Infusion: Reconstitution:** Reconstitute chlorothiazide with 18 mL of sterile water for injection. Shake to dissolve. Solution is stable for 24 hr at room temperature. **Dilution:** May be given undiluted or may be diluted further with D5W or 0.9% NaCl. **Concentration:** Up to 28 mg/mL. **Rate:** If administered undiluted, may give by IV push over 3–5 min. If diluted, may infuse over 30 min.
- **Y-Site Compatibility:** alprostadil, aminophylline, atropine, calcium chloride, calcium gluconate, chloramphenicol, cyclophosphamide, dexamethasone, digoxin, edetate calcium disodium, epinephrine, erythromycin, furosemide, gentamicin, heparin, hydrocortisone, isoproterenol, lidocaine, methohexital, norepinephrine, oxytocin, penicillin G, phenobarbital, phentolamine, potassium chloride, procainamide, propranolol, succinylcholine.
- **Y-Site Incompatibility:** chlorpromazine, hydralazine, multivitamins, prochlorperazine, promethazine.

Patient/Family Teaching

- Explain purpose and side effects of medication to patient. Advise patient to read *Patient Information* before starting therapy. Advise patient to take medication at the same time each day. Take missed dose as soon as remembered but not just before next dose is due. Do not double doses.
- Advise patient to notify health care provider of all Rx or OTC medications, vitamins, or herbal products being taken and to consult health care provider before taking other medications, especially cold preparations.

- Advise patient to monitor weight biweekly and notify health care provider of significant changes.
- Caution patient to change positions slowly to minimize orthostatic hypotension. This may be potentiated by alcohol.
- Advise patient to use sunscreen and protective clothing to prevent photosensitivity reactions. Advise patient of importance of regular skin cancer screenings.
- Instruct patient to discuss dietary potassium requirements with health care provider (see Appendix J).
- Instruct patient to notify health care provider of medication regimen before treatment or surgery.
- Advise patient to report rash, muscle weakness, cramps, nausea, vomiting, diarrhea, or dizziness to health care provider.
- **Hypertension:** Advise patient to continue taking the medication even if feeling better. Medication controls but does not cure hypertension.
- Encourage patient to comply with additional interventions for hypertension (weight reduction, low-sodium diet, regular exercise, smoking cessation, moderation of alcohol consumption, stress management).
- Instruct patient and family/caregivers in correct technique for monitoring weekly BP.
- Rep: Advise women of reproductive potential to notify health care provider if pregnancy is planned or suspected or if breastfeeding.

Evaluation/Desired Outcomes

- Lowering of BP in hypertensive patients and diuresis with mobilization of edema.

divalproex sodium, **See VALPROATES.**

HIGH ALERT

DOBUTamine

(doe-**byoo**-ta-meen)

~~Dobutrex~~

Classification

Therapeutic: inotropics

Pharmacologic: adrenergics

Indications

Short-term management of HF caused by depressed contractility from organic heart disease or surgical procedures.

Action

Stimulates $beta_1$ (myocardial)-adrenergic receptors to improve cardiac contractility. **Therapeutic Effects:** Increased cardiac output.

Pharmacokinetics

Absorption: IV administration results in complete bioavailability.

Distribution: Unknown.

Metabolism and Excretion: Metabolized by the liver and other tissues.

Half-life: 2 min.

TIME/ACTION PROFILE (inotropic effects)

ROUTE	ONSET	PEAK	DURATION
IV	1–2 min	10 min	brief (min)

Contraindications/Precautions

Contraindicated in: Hypersensitivity to dobutamine or bisulfites; Idiopathic hypertrophic subaortic stenosis.

Use Cautiously in: Hypertension (↑ risk of exaggerated pressor response); MI; Atrial fibrillation; History of ventricular atopic activity (may be exacerbated); Hypovolemia (correct before administration); OB: Safety not established in pregnancy; Lactation: Safety not established in breastfeeding.

Adverse Reactions/Side Effects

CV: hypertension, premature ventricular contractions, tachycardia, angina, arrhythmias, hypotension, palpitations. **GI:** nausea, vomiting. **Local:** phlebitis. **Neuro:** headache. **Resp:** dyspnea. **Misc:** hypersensitivity reactions, nonanginal chest pain.

Interactions

Drug-Drug: Beta blockers may negate the effect of dobutamine. ↑ risk of arrhythmias or hypertension with some **anesthetics (cyclopropane, halothane), MAO inhibitors, oxytocics,** or **tricyclic antidepressants.**

Route/Dosage

IV (Adults and Children): 2.5–15 mcg/kg/min; titrate to response (max dose = 40 mcg/kg/min).

IV (Neonates): 2–15 mcg/kg/min.

Availability (generic available)

Solution for injection (requires dilution): 12.5 mg/mL. **Premixed infusion:** 250 mg/250 mL, 500 mg/250 mL, 1000 mg/250 mL.

NURSING IMPLICATIONS

Assessment

- Monitor BP, HR, ECG, pulmonary capillary wedge pressure (PCWP), cardiac output, central venous pressure (CVP), and urinary output continuously during the administration. Report significant changes in vital signs or arrhythmias. Consult physician for parameters for HR, BP, or ECG changes for adjusting dose or discontinuing medication.
- Palpate peripheral pulses and assess appearance of extremities routinely during dobutamine administration. Notify health care provider if quality of pulse deteriorates or if extremities become cold or mottled.

Lab Test Considerations

- Monitor potassium during therapy; may cause hypokalemia. Monitor electrolytes, BUN, and serum creatinine weekly during prolonged therapy.

Implementation

- ***High Alert:*** IV vasoactive medications are potentially dangerous. Have second practitioner independently check original order, dose calculations, and infusion pump settings. Do not confuse dobutamine with dopamine. If available as floor stock, store in separate areas.
- Correct hypovolemia with volume expanders before initiating dobutamine therapy.

IV Administration

- V Dobutamine is a vesicant. Administer into a large vein. If extravasation occurs, immediately stop infusion. Leave needle/cannula in place temporarily but do not flush the line. Gently aspirate extravasated solution; then remove needle/cannula. Elevate patient's extremity and apply dry warm compresses. Initiate phentolamine antidote for refractory cases in addition to supportive management. For phentolamine, dilute 5–10 mg in 10 mL of 0.9% NaCl and administer SUBQ into extravasation site as soon as possible after extravasation; if IV catheter remains in place, administer initial dose IV through the infiltrated catheter. May repeat in 60 min if patient remains symptomatic. Nitroglycerin 2% topical ointment (1-inch strip applied to site of ischemia to cover affected area; may repeat every 8 hr as necessary) or terbutaline (dilute 1 mg in 10 mL of 0.9% NaCl and administer SUBQ into extravasation site; may repeat in 15 min if necessary) may be used as alternatives to phentolamine.
- **Continuous Infusion: Dilution:** Vials must be diluted before use. Dilute 250–1000 mg in 250–500 mL of D5W, 0.9% NaCl, 0.45% NaCl, D5/0.45% NaCl, D5/0.9% NaCl, LR, or D5/LR. Admixed infusions stable for 24 hr at room temperature and 48 hr if refrigerated. Premixed infusions are already diluted and ready to use. A pink color may occur due to oxidation of the drug; there is no significant loss of potency over 24 hr. **Concentration:** 0.25–5 mg/mL. **Rate:** Based on patient's weight (see Route/Dosage section). Administer via infusion pump to ensure precise amount delivered. Titrate to patient response (HR, presence of ectopic activity, BP, urine output, CVP, PCWP, cardiac index). Dose should be titrated so HR does not increase by >10% of baseline.
- **Y-Site Compatibility:** alemtuzumab, alprostadil, amikacin, aminocaproic acid, anidulafungin, argatroban, arsenic trioxide, ascorbic acid, atracurium, atropine, azithromycin, aztreonam, benztropine, bleomycin, buprenorphine, butorphanol, calcium chloride, calcium gluconate, cangrelor, carboplatin, caspofungin, ceftolozane/tazobactam, chlorpromazine, ciprofloxacin, cisatracurium, cisplatin, cladribine, clevidipine, clindamycin, cyanocoblamin, cyclophosphamide, cyclosporine, cytarabine, dactinomycin, daptomycin, daunorubicin, dexmedetomidine, digoxin, diltiazem, dimenhydrinate, diphenhydramine, docetaxel, dopamine, doxorubicin hydrochloride, doxorubicin liposomal, doxycycline, enalaprilat, ephedrine, epinephrine, epirubicin, epoetin alfa, eptifibatide, eravacycline, erythromycin, esmolol, etoposide phosphate, famotidine, fentanyl, fluconazole, fludarabine, gemcitabine, gentamicin, glycopyrrolate, granisetron, hetastarch, hydromorphone, hydroxyzine, idarubicin, ifosfamide, insulin aspart, irinotecan, isavuconazonium, isoproterenol, ketamine, labetalol, leucovorin, levofloxacin, lidocaine, linezolid, lorazepam, magnesium sulfate, mannitol, meperidine, mesna, methylprednisolone, metoclopramide, metoprolol, metronidazole, milrinone, mitoxantrone, morphine, moxifloxacin, multivitamins, mycophenolate, nafcillin, nalbuphine, naloxone, nicardipine, nitroglycerin, norepinephrine, octreotide, ondansetron, oritavancin, oxaliplatin, oxytocin, paclitaxel, palonosetron, pamidronate, papaverine, pentamidine, phentolamine, phenylephrine, plazomicin, posaconazole, potassium acetate, potassium chloride, procainamide, prochlorperazine, promethazine, propranolol, protamine, pyridoxine, remifentanil, rituximab, rocuronium, sodium acetate, succinylcholine, sufentanil, sulbactam/durlobactam, tacrolimus, televancin, theophylline, thiamine, thiotepa, tigecycline, tirofiban, tobramycin, topotecan, trastuzumab, vancomycin, vasopressin, vecuronium, verapamil, vinblastine, vincristine, vinorelbine, voriconazole, zidovudine, zoledronic acid.
- **Y-Site Incompatibility:** acyclovir, alteplase, aminophylline, amphotericin B deoxycholate, amphotericin B liposomal, ampicillin, ampicillin/sulbactam, azathioprine, bivalirudin, carmustine, cefazolin, cefotaxime, cefotetan, cefoxitin, ceftriaxone, cefuroxime, chloramphenicol, dacarbazine, dantrolene, dexamethasone, dexrazoxane, diazoxide, ertapenem, fluorouracil, folic acid, foscarnet, fosphenytoin, ganciclovir, gemtuzumab ozogamicin, hydrocortisone, hydroxocobalamin, ketorolac, meropenem, meropenem/vaborbactam, methotrexate, micafungin, mitomycin, oxacillin, pantoprazole, pemetrexed, penicillin G, pentobarbital, phenobarbital, phenytoin, piperacillin/tazobactam, sodium bicarbonate, tedizolid, trimethoprim/sulfamethoxazole.

Patient/Family Teaching

- Explain the purpose and side effects of dobutamine and the need for frequent monitoring.
- Advise patient to inform nurse immediately if chest pain; dyspnea; or numbness, tingling, or burning of extremities occurs.
- Instruct patient to notify nurse immediately of pain or discomfort at the site of IV administration.
- Advise patient to notify health care provider of all Rx or OTC medications, vitamins, or herbal products being taken and to consult with health care provider before taking other medications.
- **Home Care Issues:** Instruct caregiver on proper care of IV equipment.
- Instruct caregiver to report signs of worsening HF (shortness of breath, orthopnea, ↓ exercise tolerance), abdominal pain, and nausea or vomiting to health care provider promptly.
- Rep: Advise women of reproductive potential to notify health care provider if pregnancy is planned or suspected or if breastfeeding.

Evaluation/Desired Outcomes

- Increase in cardiac output.
- Improved hemodynamic parameters. Increased urine output.

HIGH ALERT

DOCEtaxel (doe-se-**tax**-el)

Docivyx, ~~Taxotere~~

Classification

Therapeutic: antineoplastics

Pharmacologic: taxoids

Indications

Locally advanced or metastatic breast cancer after failure of prior chemotherapy. Adjuvant treatment of operable node-positive breast cancer (in combination with doxorubicin and cyclophosphamide). Locally advanced or metastatic non-small cell lung cancer (NSCLC) after failure of prior platinum-based regimen. Unresectable, locally advanced, or metastatic NSCLC in patients who have not previously received chemotherapy for this condition (in combination with cisplatin). Metastatic castration-resistant prostate cancer (in combination with prednisone). Locally advanced squamous cell carcinoma of the head and neck (in combination with cisplatin and fluorouracil). Advanced gastric adenocarcinoma (including adenocarcinoma of the gastroesophageal junction) in patients who have not received prior chemotherapy for advanced disease (in combination with cisplatin and fluorouracil).

Action

Interferes with normal cellular microtubule function required for interphase and mitosis. **Therapeutic Effects:** Death of rapidly replicating cells, particularly malignant ones.

Pharmacokinetics

Absorption: IV administration results in complete bioavailability.

Distribution: Widely distributed to tissues.

Metabolism and Excretion: Extensively metabolized by the liver via the CYP3A isoenzyme; metabolites undergo fecal elimination.

Half-life: 116 hr.

TIME/ACTION PROFILE (effect on blood counts)

ROUTE	ONSET	PEAK	DURATION
IV	rapid	5–9 days	7 days

Contraindications/Precautions

Contraindicated in: Hypersensitivity to docetaxel, paclitaxel, or medications formulated with polysorbate 80; Neutrophil count <1500/mm^3; Hepatic impairment (serum bilirubin > upper limit of normal [ULN], ALT and/or AST >1.5 times ULN, with alkaline phosphatase >2.5 times ULN) (↑ risk of serious adverse reactions); Known alcohol intolerance; OB: Pregnancy; Lactation: Lactation.

Use Cautiously in: Rep: Women of reproductive potential and men with female partners of reproductive potential; Pedi: Safety and effectiveness not established in children.

Adverse Reactions/Side Effects

CV: peripheral edema, CARDIAC TAMPONADE, PERICARDIAL EFFUSION. **Derm:** alopecia, edema, rash, ACUTE GENERALIZED EXANTHEMATOUS PUSTULOSIS (AGEP), dermatitis, desquamation, erythema, nail disorders, STEVENS-JOHNSON SYNDROME (SJS), TOXIC EPIDERMAL NECROLYSIS (TEN). **EENT:** cystoid macular edema. **GI:** diarrhea, nausea, stomatitis, vomiting, ASCITES, ENTEROCOLITIS, NEUTROPENIC COLITIS. **GU:** ↓ fertility (men), amenorrhea. **Hemat:** anemia, leukopenia, thrombocytopenia. **Local:** injection site reactions. **MS:** myalgia, arthralgia. **Neuro:** fatigue, weakness, alcohol intoxication, neurosensory deficits, peripheral neuropathy. **Resp:** ACUTE RESPIRATORY DISTRESS SYNDROME, bronchospasm, dyspnea, INTERSTITIAL LUNG DISEASE, PULMONARY EDEMA, PULMONARY FIBROSIS. **Misc:** HYPERSENSITIVITY REACTIONS (INCLUDING ANAPHYLAXIS), MALIGNANCY (INCLUDING LEUKEMIAS, MYELODYSPLASTIC SYNDROME, NON-HODGKIN LYMPHOMA, AND RENAL CANCER), tumor lysis syndrome.

Interactions

Drug-Drug: ↑ bone marrow depression may occur with other **antineoplastics** or **radiation therapy**. Strong inhibitors of CYP3A4, including **atazanavir**, **clarithromycin**, **itraconazole**, **ketoconazole**,

nefazodone, **nelfinavir**, **ritonavir**, or **voriconazole**, may ↑ levels and risk of toxicity; avoid concurrent use. If concurrent use unavoidable, ↓ docetaxel dose by 50%.

Route/Dosage

Locally Advanced or Metastatic Breast Cancer

IV (Adults): 60–100 mg/m^2 every 3 wk.

Adjuvant Treatment of Operable Node-Positive Breast Cancer

IV (Adults): 75 mg/m^2 every 3 wk for 6 cycles.

Non-Small Cell Lung Cancer, Metastatic Castration-Resistant Prostate Cancer, or Advanced Gastric Adenocarcinoma

IV (Adults): 75 mg/m^2 every 3 wk.

Locally Advanced Squamous Cell Carcinoma of the Head and Neck

IV (Adults): 75 mg/m^2 every 3 wk for 3–4 cycles.

Availability (generic available)

Solution for injection (concentrate): 10 mg/mL (dose of 100 mg/m^2 contains 0.15 g/m^2 of ethanol), 20 mg/mL (dose of 100 mg/m^2 contains 1.975 g/m^2 of ethanol).

NURSING IMPLICATIONS

Assessment

- Monitor vital signs before and after administration.
- Monitor for signs and symptoms of hypersensitivity reactions (bronchospasm, hypotension, erythema) continuously during infusion; most common after 1st and 2nd doses of docetaxel. Treat mild to moderate reactions symptomatically and slow or stop infusion until reaction subsides. Discontinue therapy if severe reactions occur. Do not readminister docetaxel to patients with previous severe reactions. Severe edema may also occur. Weigh patients before each treatment. Fluid accumulation may result in edema, ascites, and pleural or pericardial effusions. Pretreatment with corticosteroids is recommended to minimize edema and hypersensitivity reactions. PO furosemide may be used to treat edema. For hormone-refractory metastatic prostate cancer (given with prednisone), premedicate with dexamethasone.
- Monitor for bone marrow depression. Assess for bleeding (bleeding gums; bruising; petechiae; guaiac stools, urine, and emesis) and avoid IM injections and taking rectal temperatures if platelet count is low. Apply pressure to venipuncture sites for 10 min. Assess for signs of infection during neutropenia. Anemia may occur. Monitor for ↑ fatigue, dyspnea, and orthostatic hypotension.
- Assess for rash. May occur on feet or hands but may also occur on arms, face, or thorax, usually with pruritus. Rash usually occurs within 1 wk after infusion and resolves before next infusion. May cause SJS, TEN, and AGEP; permanently discontinue docetaxel if severe cutaneous reactions occur.
- Assess for development of neurosensory deficit (paresthesia, dysesthesia, pain, burning). May also cause weakness. Pyridoxine may be used to minimize symptoms. Severe symptoms may require dose ↓ or discontinuation.
- Assess for arthralgia and myalgia, which are usually relieved by nonopioid analgesics but may be severe enough to require treatment with opioid analgesics.
- Assess for diarrhea and stomatitis, especially in patients receiving docetaxel with cisplatin and fluorouracil. *If Grade 3 diarrhea occurs,* 1st episode: ↓ fluorouracil dose by 20%; 2nd episode: ↓ docetaxel dose by 20%. *If Grade 4 diarrhea occurs,* 1st episode: ↓ docetaxel and fluorouracil doses by 20%; 2nd episode: Discontinue treatment. *If Grade 3 stomatitis/mucositis occurs,* 1st episode: ↓ fluorouracil dose by 20%; 2nd episode: Stop fluorouracil only, at all subsequent cycles; 3rd episode: ↓ docetaxel dose by 20%. *If Grade 4 stomatitis/mucositis occurs,* 1st episode: Stop fluorouracil only, at all subsequent cycles; 2nd episode: ↓ docetaxel dose by 20%.
- Monitor for tumor lysis syndrome due to rapid ↓ in tumor volume (acute renal failure, hyperkalemia, hypocalcemia, hyperuricemia, or hypophosphatemia). Risks are higher in patients with greater tumor burden and rapidly proliferating tumors; may be fatal. Correct electrolyte abnormalities, monitor renal function and fluid balance, and administer supportive care, including dialysis, as indicated.
- Monitor for signs and symptoms of fluid retention (edema, weight gain); usually begins with peripheral edema in lower extremities. May be treated with sodium restriction and diuretics.
- Monitor patients for second primary malignancies.

Lab Test Considerations

- Verify negative pregnancy test before starting therapy.

Monitor CBC and differential before each treatment. Frequently causes neutropenia (<2000 neutrophils/mm^3); may require dose adjustment. *If neutrophil count <1500/mm^3,* hold dose. Neutropenia is reversible and not cumulative. The nadir is 8 days, with a duration of 7 days. May also cause thrombocytopenia and anemia.

- Monitor liver function studies (AST, ALT, alkaline phosphatase, bilirubin) before each cycle. *If AST/ALT >2.5–≤5 times ULN and alkaline phosphatase ≤2.5 times ULN, or AST/ALT >1.5–≤5 times ULN, and alkaline phosphatase >2.5–≤5 times ULN,* ↓ dose by 20%. *If AST/ALT >5 times ULN and/or alkaline phosphatase >5 times ULN,* discontinue therapy.

Implementation

- ***High Alert:*** Fatalities have occurred with chemotherapeutic agents. Before administering, clarify all ambiguous orders; double-check single, daily, and course-of-therapy dose limits; have second practitioner independently double-check original order, calculations, and infusion pump settings.
- Do not confuse docetaxel with paclitaxel.
- Premedicate with dexamethasone 8 mg twice daily for 3 days starting 1 day before docetaxel infusion to ↓ incidence and severity of fluid retention and hypersensitivity reactions. Premedicate patients with hormone-refractory metastatic prostate cancer with PO dexamethasone 8 mg, at 12 hr, 3 hr, and 1 hr before docetaxel infusion.

IV Administration

- **V** Docetaxel is a vesicant. If extravasation occurs, immediately stop infusion. Leave needle/cannula in place temporarily but do not flush the line. Gently aspirate extravasated solution; then remove needle/cannula. Elevate patient's extremity and apply dry cold compresses for 20 min 4 times day for 1–2 days. Solution should be prepared in a biologic cabinet. Wear gloves, gown, and mask while handling medication. If powder or solution comes in contact with skin or mucosa, wash thoroughly with soap and water. Discard equipment in specially designated containers.
- **Intermittent Infusion:** *One-vial formulation:* Do not dilute one-vial formulation. Solution is ready to add to infusion solution. *For injection concentrate:* Before dilution, allow vials to stand at room temperature for 5 min. Solution is pale yellow to brownish yellow. Use a 21-gauge needle to withdraw docetaxel from vial; larger bore needles may result in stopper coring and rubber particles. **Dilution:** Withdraw required amount and inject into 250-mL bag of 0.9% NaCl or D5W. If a dose >200 mg is required, use a larger volume diluent so that concentration of 0.74 mg/mL is not exceeded. Rotate gently to mix. Do not administer solutions that are cloudy or contain a precipitate. Diluted solution must be infused within 6 hr. **Concentration:** 0.3 mg/mL to 0.74 mg/mL. Solution is supersaturated and may crystallize over time. If crystals appear, solution must be discarded. **Rate:** Administer over 1 hr.
- **Y-Site Compatibility:** acyclovir, allopurinol, amikacin, aminocaproic acid, aminophylline, amiodarone, ampicillin, ampicillin/sulbactam, anidulafungin, argatroban, atracurium, azithromycin, aztreonam, bivalirudin, bleomycin, bumetanide, buprenorphine, busulfan, butorphanol, calcium chloride, calcium gluconate, carboplatin, carmustine, caspofungin, cefazolin, cefepime, cefotaxime, cefotetan, cefoxitin, ceftazidime, ceftriaxone, cefuroxime, chloramphenicol, chlorpromazine, ciprofloxacin, cisatracurium, cisplatin, clindamycin, cyclophosphamide, cyclosporine, cytarabine, dacarbazine, dactinomycin, daptomycin, daunorubicin, dexamethasone, dexmedetomidine, dexrazoxane, diazepam, digoxin, diltiazem, diphenhydramine, dobutamine, dopamine, doxorubicin hydrochloride, doxycycline, droperidol, enalaprilat, ephedrine, epinephrine, epirubicin, ertapenem, erythromycin, esmolol, etoposide, etoposide phosphate, famotidine, fentanyl, fluconazole, fludarabine, fluorouracil, foscarnet, fosphenytoin, furosemide, ganciclovir, gemcitabine, gentamicin, glycopyrrolate, granisetron, haloperidol, heparin, hetastarch, hydralazine, hydrocortisone, hydromorphone, ifosfamide, imipenem/cilastatin, insulin, regular, irinotecan, isoproterenol, ketorolac, labetalol, leucovorin, levofloxacin, lidocaine, linezolid, lorazepam, magnesium sulfate, mannitol, meperidine, meropenem, mesna, methadone, methotrexate, metoclopramide, metoprolol, metronidazole, midazolam, milrinone, minocycline, mitoxantrone, morphine, moxifloxacin, nafcillin, naloxone, nicardipine, nitroglycerin, nitroprusside, norepinephrine, octreotide, ondansetron, oxaliplatin, palonosetron, pamidronate, pantoprazole, pemetrexed, pentamidine, pentobarbital, phenobarbital, phentolamine, phenylephrine, piperacillin/tazobactam, potassium acetate, potassium chloride, potassium phosphates, procainamide, prochlorperazine, promethazine, propranolol, remifentanil, rituximab, rocuronium, sodium acetate, sodium bicarbonate, sodium phosphates, succinylcholine, sufentanil, tacrolimus, theophylline, thiotepa, tigecycline, tirofiban, tobramycin, topotecan, trastuzumab, trimethoprim/sulfamethoxazole, vancomycin, vasopressin, vecuronium, verapamil, vinblastine, vincristine, vinorelbine, voriconazole, zidovudine, zoledronic acid.
- **Y-Site Incompatibility:** amphotericin B deoxycholate, amphotericin B liposomal, dantrolene, doxorubicin liposomal, idarubicin, methylprednisolone, mitomycin, nalbuphine, phenytoin.

Patient/Family Teaching

- Explain purpose of docetaxel to patient.
- Instruct patient to report symptoms of hypersensitivity reactions (trouble breathing; sudden swelling of face, lips, tongue, or throat; trouble swallowing; hives; rash; redness all over body) to health care provider immediately.
- Advise patient to notify health care provider if fever >101°F; chills; sore throat; signs of infection; bleeding gums; bruising; petechiae; or blood in urine, stool, or emesis occur. Caution patient to avoid crowds and persons with known infections. Instruct patient to use soft toothbrush and electric razor.

- Patient should be cautioned to avoid alcohol and products containing aspirin or NSAIDs.
- Fatigue is a frequent side effect of docetaxel. Advise patient that frequent rest periods and pacing of activities may minimize fatigue.
- Instruct patient to notify health care provider if signs of fluid retention (peripheral edema in the lower extremities, weight gain, dyspnea), colitis (abdominal pain or tenderness, diarrhea, with or without fever), yellow skin, weakness, paresthesia, gait disturbances, swelling of the feet, or joint or muscle aches occur.
- Alcohol content of docetaxel may impair CNS. Caution patient to avoid driving or other activities requiring alertness until response to medication is known.
- Instruct patient to inspect oral mucosa for redness and ulceration. If mouth sores occur, advise patient to use sponge brush and rinse mouth with water after eating and drinking.
- Instruct patient to notify health care provider of all Rx or OTC medications, vitamins, or herbal products being taken and consult health care provider before taking any new medications.
- Advise patient to notify health care provider if changes in vision occur. Obtain a prompt and comprehensive ophthalmologic examination. May require discontinuation of docetaxel and use of a nontaxane cancer therapy.
- Discuss with patient the possibility of hair loss. Complete hair loss usually begins after 1 or 2 treatments and is reversible after discontinuation of therapy. Explore coping strategies.
- Instruct patient not to receive any vaccinations without advice of health care provider.
- Rep: May cause fetal harm. Advise women of reproductive potential to use effective contraception during and for 2 mo after last dose of therapy and to avoid breastfeeding during and for 1 wk after last dose. Advise men with female partners of reproductive potential to use effective contraception during and for 4 mo after last dose of therapy. May impair fertility in male patients.
- Emphasize the need for periodic lab tests to monitor for side effects.

Evaluation/Desired Outcomes

- Decrease in size or spread of malignancy in women with advanced breast cancer.
- Decrease in size or spread of malignancy in locally advanced or metastatic non-small cell lung cancer, squamous cell carcinoma of the head and neck, and gastric adenocarcinoma.
- Decreased size or spread of advanced metastatic hormone-refractory prostate cancer.

DOCUSATE (dok-yoo-sate)
docusate calcium
docusate sodium

Colace, DOK, Dulcolax Stool Softener, Enemeez Mini, ✱ Selax, Silace, ✱ Soflax

Classification
Therapeutic: laxatives
Pharmacologic: stool softeners

Indications

PO: Prevention of constipation (in patients who should avoid straining, such as after MI or rectal surgery). **Rect:** Used as enema to soften fecal impaction.

Action

Promotes incorporation of water into stool, resulting in softer fecal mass. May also promote electrolyte and water secretion into the colon. **Therapeutic Effects:** Softening and passage of stool.

Pharmacokinetics

Absorption: Small amounts may be absorbed from the small intestine after oral administration. Absorption from the rectum is not known.
Distribution: Unknown.
Metabolism and Excretion: Amounts absorbed after oral administration are eliminated in bile.
Half-life: Unknown.

TIME/ACTION PROFILE (softening of stool)

ROUTE	ONSET	PEAK	DURATION
PO	12–72 hr	unknown	unknown
Rectal	2–15 min	unknown	unknown

Contraindications/Precautions

Contraindicated in: Hypersensitivity; Abdominal pain, nausea, or vomiting, especially when associated with fever or other signs of an acute abdomen.
Use Cautiously in: Excessive or prolonged use may lead to dependence; Should not be used if prompt results are desired.

Adverse Reactions/Side Effects

Derm: rash. **EENT:** throat irritation. **GI:** diarrhea, mild cramps.

Interactions

Drug-Drug: None significant.

Route/Dosage

Docusate Calcium

PO (Adults): 240 mg once daily.

Docusate Sodium

PO (Adults and Children >12 yr): 50–400 mg in 1–4 divided doses.
PO (Children 6–12 yr): 40–150 mg in 1–4 divided doses.
PO (Children 3–6 yr): 20–60 mg in 1–4 divided doses.
PO (Children <3 yr): 10–40 mg in 1–4 divided doses.
PO (Infants): 5 mg/kg/day in 1–4 divided doses.
Rect (Adults): 50–100 mg or 1 unit containing 283 mg docusate sodium, soft soap, and glycerin.

Availability (generic available)

Docusate Calcium

Capsules: 240 mg[OTC].

Docusate Sodium

Tablets: 100 mg[OTC]. **Capsules:** 100 mg[OTC], 250 mg[OTC]. **Syrup:** 60 mg/15 mL[OTC]. **Liquid:** 50 mg/5 mL[OTC], 100 mg/10 mL[OTC]. **Enema:** 283 mg/5 mL[OTC]. ***In combination with:*** stimulant laxatives[OTC]. See Appendix N.

NURSING IMPLICATIONS

Assessment

- Assess for abdominal distention, presence of bowel sounds, and usual pattern (frequency) of bowel function.
- Assess color, consistency, and amount of stool produced.
- Monitor for signs and symptoms of rectal bleeding (bright red blood mixed with stool, tarry stool) or ileus (↑ abdominal distention, constipation, ↓ or absent bowel sounds) after use; discontinuation may be necessary.

Implementation

- Do not confuse Colace with Cozaar. Do not confuse Dulcolax (docusate sodium) with Dulcolax (bisacodyl).
- This medication does not stimulate intestinal peristalsis; stimulant laxative may be required for constipation.
- **PO:** Administer with a full glass of water or juice. May be administered on an empty stomach for more rapid results.
- Oral solution may be diluted in milk, infant formula, or fruit juice to ↓ bitter taste.
- Do not administer within 2 hr of other laxatives, especially mineral oil. May cause ↑ absorption.
- **Rect:** Administer as a retention or flushing enema.

Patient/Family Teaching

- Explain the purpose and side effects of docusate. Instruct them to take medication as directed. Advise patient that results may take as long as 3–5 days. Patient should report if no bowel movement occurs after use. Do not share medication with others, even if they have similar symptoms; may be harmful. Advise patient to read *Patient Information* before starting and with each Rx refill in case of changes.
- Tell patient not to take docusate or any other laxative if experiencing acute abdominal pain, nausea, vomiting, fever, or a sudden change of bowel habits of over 2 wk.
- Advise patients that laxatives should be used only for short-term therapy. Long-term therapy may cause electrolyte imbalance and dependence.
- Encourage patients to use other forms of bowel regulation, such as ↑ bulk in the diet, fluid intake (6–8 full glasses/day), and mobility. Normal bowel habits are variable and may vary from 3 times/day to 3 times/wk.
- Instruct patients with cardiac disease to avoid straining during bowel movements (Valsalva maneuver).
- Advise patient not to take docusate within 2 hr of other laxatives.
- Advise patient to notify health care provider of all Rx or OTC medications, vitamins, or herbal products being taken and to consult with health care provider before taking other medications.
- Rep: Advise women of reproductive potential to notify health care provider if pregnancy is planned or suspected or if breastfeeding. Docusate is excreted in breast milk and may cause ↑ bowel activity in nursing infants.

Evaluation/Desired Outcomes

- A soft, formed bowel movement, usually within 24–48 hr. Therapy may take 3–5 days for results. Rectal dose forms produce results within 2–15 min.

dolutegravir

(doe-loo-**teg**-ra-vir)
Tivicay, Tivicay PD

Classification
Therapeutic: antiretrovirals
Pharmacologic: integrase strand transfer inhibitors (INSTI)

Indications

HIV-1 infection (in combination with other antiretrovirals). HIV-1 infection in patients to replace the current antiretroviral regimen in those who are virologically suppressed (HIV-1 RNA <50 copies/mL) on a stable antiretroviral regimen for ≥6 mo with no history of treatment failure or known substitutions associated with resistance to either dolutegravir or rilpivirine (in combination with rilpivirine).

Action

Inhibits HIV-1 integrase, which is required for viral replication. **Therapeutic Effects:** Evidence of decreased viral replication and reduced viral load with slowed progression of HIV and its sequelae.

Pharmacokinetics

Absorption: Bioavailability is unknown.
Distribution: Enters CSF.
Protein Binding: >98.9%.
Metabolism and Excretion: Metabolized primarily by the UGT1A1 enzyme system with some metabolism by the CYP3A4 isoenzyme. 53% excreted unchanged in feces. Metabolites are renally excreted; minimal renal elimination of unchanged drug. 🧬 Poor UGT1A1 metabolizers have ↑ dolutegravir concentrations and an ↑ risk of adverse effects.
Half-life: 14 hr

TIME/ACTION PROFILE (plasma concentrations)

ROUTE	ONSET	PEAK	DURATION
PO	unknown	2–3 hr	12–24 hr†

† Depends on concurrent use of metabolic inducers.

Contraindications/Precautions

Contraindicated in: Concurrent use of dofetilide; Severe hepatic impairment.
Use Cautiously in: Underlying hepatic disease, including hepatitis B or C (↑ risk of hepatotoxicity); End-stage renal disease requiring dialysis; Lactation: Safety not established in breastfeeding; breastfeeding should be supported in people with HIV who are taking antiretroviral therapy, as prescribed, and are maintaining an undetectable amount of virus in the body; Pedi: Children <4 wk, <3 kg, or INSTI-experienced with resistance documented to other INSTIs (safety and effectiveness not established); Geri: Consider age-related ↓ in cardiac, renal, and hepatic function; chronic disease states; and concurrent medications in older adults.

Adverse Reactions/Side Effects

Derm: pruritus. **GI:** HEPATOTOXICITY (↑ WITH HEPATITIS B OR C). **GU:** renal impairment. **MS:** myositis. **Neuro:** headache, insomnia, fatigue. **Misc:** hypersensitivity reactions (including rash, constitutional symptoms, and liver injury), immune reconstitution syndrome.

Interactions

Drug-Drug: May ↑ levels and risk of toxicity of **dofetilide**; concurrent use contraindicated. **Etravirine** may ↓ levels and effectiveness; should not be used concurrently without atazanavir/ritonavir, darunavir/ritonavir, or lopinavir/ritonavir. **Efavirenz, fosamprenavir/ritonavir, tipranavir/ritonavir, carbamazepine,** and **rifampin** may ↓ levels and effectiveness; ↑ dose of dolutegravir. **Nevirapine** may ↓ levels and effectiveness; avoid concurrent use. May ↑ levels and risk of toxicity of **metformin**. **Oxcarbazepine, phenobarbital,** and **phenytoin** may ↓ levels and effectiveness; avoid concurrent use. Cation-containing **antacids** or **laxatives,** as well as **buffered medications** or **sucralfate,** may ↓ absorption and effectiveness; dolutegravir should be taken 2 hr before or 6 hr after these medications. **Calcium supplements** (oral) or **iron supplements** (oral) may ↓ absorption and effectiveness; under fasting conditions, dolutegravir should be taken 2 hr before or 6 hr after these medications; when taken with food, dolutegravir and calcium or iron supplements may be taken at the same time. May ↑ **dalfampridine** levels and risk of seizures.
Drug-Natural Products: St. John's wort may ↓ levels and effectiveness; avoid concurrent use.

Route/Dosage

Tablets (Tivicay) and tablets for oral suspension (Tivicay PD) are not interchangeable.

PO (Adults): *Treatment-naive or treatment-experienced INSTI-naive patients or virologically suppressed (HIV RNA <50 copies/mL) patients switching to dolutegravir plus rilpivirine:* 50 mg once daily; *Treatment-naive or treatment-experienced INSTI-naive patients currently receiving efavirenz, fosamprenavir/ritonavir, tipranavir/ritonavir, carbamazepine, or rifampin:* 50 mg twice daily; *INSTI-experienced with certain INSTI-associated resistance substitutions or clinically suspected INSTI resistance (consider other combinations that do not include metabolic inducers):* 50 mg twice daily.
PO (Children ≥20 kg): *Treatment-naive or treatment-experienced INSTI-naive patients:* Tivicay PD: 30 mg once daily; Tivicay tablets: 50 mg once daily; *Treatment-naive or treatment-experienced INSTI-naive patients currently receiving efavirenz, fosamprenavir/ritonavir, tipranavir/ritonavir, carbamazepine, or rifampin:* Tivicay PD: 25 mg twice daily; Tivicay tablets: 50 mg twice daily.
PO (Children 14–<20 kg): *Treatment-naive or treatment-experienced INSTI-naive patients:* Tivicay PD (preferred): 25 mg once daily; Tivicay tablets: 40 mg once daily; *Treatment-naive or treatment-experienced INSTI-naive patients currently receiving efavirenz, fosamprenavir/ritonavir, tipranvir/ritonavir, carbamazepine, or rifampin:* Tivicay PD (preferred): 25 mg twice daily; Tivicay tablets: 40 mg twice daily.
PO (Children 10–<14 kg): *Treatment-naive or treatment-experienced INSTI-naive patients:* Tivicay PD: 20 mg once daily; *Treatment-naive or treatment-experienced INSTI-naive patients currently receiving efavirenz, fosamprenavir/ritonavir, tipranavir/ritonavir, carbamazepine, or rifampin:* Tivicay PD: 20 mg twice daily.
PO (Children ≥4 wk and 6–<10 kg): *Treatment-naive or treatment-experienced INSTI-naive*

D

patients: Tivicay PD: 15 mg once daily; *Treatment-naive or treatment-experienced INSTI-naive patients currently receiving efavirenz, fosamprenavir/ritonavir, tipranavir/ritonavir, carbamazepine, or rifampin:* Tivicay PD: 15 mg twice daily.
PO (Children ≥4 wk and 3–<6 kg): *Treatment-naive or treatment-experienced INSTI-naive patients:* Tivicay PD: 5 mg once daily; *Treatment-naive or treatment-experienced INSTI-naive patients currently receiving efavirenz, fosamprenavir/ritonavir, tipranavir/ritonavir, carbamazepine, or rifampin:* Tivicay PD: 5 mg twice daily.

Availability (generic available)
Tablets (Tivicay): 🍁 10 mg, 🍁 25 mg, 50 mg. **Tablets for oral suspension (Tivicay PD):** 5 mg. ***In combination with:*** abacavir and lamivudine (Triumeq, Triumeq PD); lamivudine (Dovato); rilpivirine (Juluca). See Appendix N.

NURSING IMPLICATIONS
Assessment
- Assess patient for change in severity of HIV symptoms and for symptoms of opportunistic infections during therapy.
- Monitor for signs and symptoms of hypersensitivity reactions (rash, fever, malaise, fatigue, muscle or joint aches, blisters or peeling of skin, oral blisters or lesions, conjunctivitis, facial edema, hepatitis, eosinophilia, angioedema, difficulty breathing). Discontinue therapy and do not restart.

Lab Test Considerations
- Monitor viral load and CD4 counts regularly during therapy.
- May cause ↓ ANC, hemoglobin, total neutrophils, and platelet counts.
- Monitor liver function periodically during therapy. May cause ↑ serum glucose, lipase, AST, ALT, total bilirubin, CK concentrations.

Implementation
- **PO:** May be administered without regard to food.
- Tablets for oral suspension are preferred for patients weighing <20 kg. ***DNC:*** Administer by swallowing tablets for oral suspension whole; do not crush, break, cut, or chew. Tablets for oral suspension may also be dispersed in 5 mL (for 1 or 3 tablets for oral suspension) or 10 mL (for 4–6 tablets for oral suspension) of drinking water. Disperse in cup provided; swirl suspension so no lumps remain. After dispersion, administer within 30 min of mixing.
- Administer 2 hr before or 6 hr after calcium and iron supplements.

Patient/Family Teaching
- Emphasize the importance of taking dolutegravir as directed. Do not take more than prescribed amount, and do not stop taking without consulting health care professional. Take missed doses as soon as remembered unless within 4 hr of next dose; then skip dose. Do not double doses. Advise patient to read *Patient Information* before starting therapy and with each Rx renewal in case of changes.
- Instruct patient that dolutegravir should not be shared with others.
- Instruct patient to notify health care professional of all Rx or OTC medications, vitamins, or herbal products being taken and consult health care professional before taking any new medications, especially St. John's wort.
- Inform patient that dolutegravir does not cure HIV or prevent associated or opportunistic infections. Dolutegravir may reduce the risk of transmission of HIV to others through sexual contact or blood contamination. Caution patient to use a condom during sexual contact and to avoid sharing needles or donating blood to prevent spreading HIV to others. Advise patient that the long-term effects of dolutegravir are unknown at this time.
- Advise patient to notify health care professional if signs and symptoms of hypersensitivity occur.
- Advise patient to notify health care professional if signs and symptoms of immune reconstitution syndrome (signs and symptoms of an infection) occur.
- Rep: Advise females of reproductive potential to notify health care professional if pregnancy is planned or suspected or if breastfeeding is planned. Enroll pregnant patients in the Antiretroviral Pregnancy Registry by calling 1-800-258-4263.
- Emphasize the importance of regular follow-up exams and blood counts to determine progress and monitor for side effects.

Evaluation/Desired Outcomes
- Delayed progression of HIV and decreased opportunistic infections in patients with HIV.
- Decrease in viral load and improvement in CD4 cell counts.

dolutegravir/lamivudine
(doe-loo-**teg**-ra-vir/la-**mi**-vyoo-deen)

Dovato

Classification
Therapeutic: antiretrovirals
Pharmacologic: integrase strand transfer inhibitors (INSTI) nucleoside reverse transcriptase inhibitors

Indications
HIV-1 infection in patients with no antiretroviral treatment history and with no known substitutions associated with resistance to dolutegravir or lamivudine. HIV-1 infection as a replacement for the current antiretroviral regimen in patients

who are virologically suppressed (HIV-1 RNA <50 copies/mL), taking a stable antiretroviral regimen, have no history of treatment failure, and have no known substitutions associated with resistance to dolutegravir or lamivudine.

Action

Dolutegravir: Inhibits HIV-1 integrase, which is required for viral replication. *Lamivudine:* After intracellular conversion to its active form (lamivudine-5-triphosphate), inhibits viral DNA synthesis by inhibiting the enzyme reverse transcriptase. **Therapeutic Effects:** Evidence of decreased viral replication and reduced viral load with slowed progression of HIV and its sequelae.

Pharmacokinetics

Dolutegravir

Absorption: Bioavailability unknown.
Distribution: Unknown.
Protein Binding: >98.9%.
Metabolism and Excretion: Metabolized primarily by the UGT1A1 enzyme system with some metabolism by the CYP3A4 isoenzyme. Poor UGT1A1 metabolizers have ↑ dolutegravir concentrations and an ↑ risk of adverse effects. 64% excreted in feces (53% as unchanged drug); 31% excreted in urine (<1% as unchanged drug).
Half-life: 14 hr.

Lamivudine

Absorption: Well absorbed after oral administration.
Distribution: Unknown.
Metabolism and Excretion: Mostly excreted unchanged in urine (70% as unchanged drug).
Half-life: 13–19 hr.

TIME/ACTION PROFILE (plasma concentrations)

ROUTE	ONSET	PEAK	DURATION
Dolutegravir (PO)	unknown	2.5 hr	24 hr
Lamivudine (PO)	unknown	1 hr	24 hr

Contraindications/Precautions

Contraindicated in: Prior hypersensitivity reaction to dolutegravir; Concurrent use of dofetilide; Severe renal impairment; Severe hepatic impairment.
Use Cautiously in: Coinfected with hepatitis B virus (HBV) (severe acute exacerbations of HBV may recur after discontinuation of lamivudine); Underlying hepatic disease, including HBV or hepatitis C (↑ risk of hepatotoxicity); Women and obesity (↑ risk of lactic acidosis and severe hepatomegaly with steatosis); OB: The Health and Human Services perinatal HIV guidelines do not recommend use of this fixed-dose 2-drug combination as a complete regimen in pregnant patients with HIV who are antiretroviral-naive, who have had antiretroviral therapy (ART) in the past but are restarting, or who require a new ART regimen (due to poor tolerance or poor virologic response of current regimen). Use may continue in pregnant patients who are virologically suppressed and are already using this 2-drug regimen; Lactation: Safety not established in breastfeeding; breastfeeding should be supported in people with HIV who are taking antiretroviral therapy as prescribed and are maintaining an undetectable amount of virus in the body; Pedi: Children <12 yr (safety and effectiveness not established); Geri: Consider age-related ↓ in cardiac, renal and hepatic function, chronic disease states, and concurrent medications in older adults.

Adverse Reactions/Side Effects

Endo: hyperglycemia. **F and E** hypophosphatemia, LACTIC ACIDOSIS. **GI:** ↑ lipase, ↑ liver enzymes, diarrhea, HEPATOMEGALY WITH STEATOSIS, HEPATOTOXICITY (↑ WITH HBV OR HEPATITIS C), nausea. **Metab:** hyperlipidemia. **MS:** ↑ CK. **Neuro:** dizziness, fatigue, headache, insomnia. **Misc:** hypersensitivity reactions (including rash, constitutional symptoms, and liver injury), immune reconstitution syndrome.

Interactions

Drug-Drug: May ↑ levels and risk of toxicity of **dofetilide**; concurrent use contraindicated. May ↑ levels and risk of toxicity of **metformin**. **Carbamazepine** and **rifampin** may ↓ levels and effectiveness of dolutegravir; additional 50-mg dose of dolutegravir should be given 12 hr after dose of dolutegravir/lamivudine. **Oxcarbazepine**, **phenobarbital**, and **phenytoin** may ↓ levels and effectiveness of dolutegravir; avoid concurrent use. Absorption and effectiveness may be ↓ by cation-containing **antacids** or **laxatives**, as well as **buffered medications** or **sucralfate**; dolutegravir should be taken 2 hr before or 6 hr after these medications. Absorption and effectiveness may be ↓ by **calcium supplements** (oral) or **iron supplements** (oral); under fasting conditions, dolutegravir should be taken 2 hr before or 6 hr after these medications; when taken with food, dolutegravir and calcium or iron supplements may be taken at the same time. May ↑ **dalfampridine** levels and risk of seizures. **Sorbitol** may ↓ levels and effectiveness of lamivudine; avoid concurrent use. May ↑ **dalfampridine** levels and risk of seizures.
Drug-Natural Products: St. John's wort may ↓ levels and effectiveness of dolutegravir; avoid concurrent use.

Route/Dosage

PO (Adults and Children ≥12 yr and ≥25 kg): One tablet (dolutegravir 50 mg/lamivudine 300 mg) once daily.

Availability

Tablets: dolutegravir 50 mg/lamivudine 300 mg.

NURSING IMPLICATIONS

Assessment

- Assess for change in severity of HIV symptoms and for symptoms of opportunistic infections during therapy.
- Monitor for signs and symptoms of hypersensitivity reactions (rash, fever, malaise, fatigue, muscle or joint aches, blisters or peeling of skin, oral blisters or lesions, conjunctivitis, facial edema, hepatitis, eosinophilia, angioedema, difficulty breathing). Discontinue therapy and do not restart.

Lab Test Considerations

- Monitor viral load and CD4 counts regularly during therapy. Assess for HBV. *Dovato* is not approved for administration in patients with HIV and HBV. If therapy is discontinued, may cause severe exacerbation of HBV. Monitor liver function in coinfected patients for several months after stopping therapy.
- Monitor liver function periodically. May cause ↑ levels of AST, ALT, and alkaline phosphatase, which usually resolve after interruption of therapy. Patients with concurrent hepatitis B or C should be followed for at least several months after stopping therapy. Lactic acidosis may occur with hepatic toxicity, causing hepatic steatosis; may be fatal, especially in women.
- May cause ↑ LDL cholesterol, total cholesterol, and triglyceride concentrations.

Implementation

- **PO:** Administer once daily without regard to food.
- Iron and calcium supplements may be taken with dolutegravir/lamivudine and food. If taken separately, administer dolutegravir/lamivudine ≥2 hr before or ≥6 hr after iron and calcium supplements.

Patient/Family Teaching

- Instruct patient on the importance of taking medication as directed, even if feeling better. Take missed dose as soon as remembered; do not double doses. Do not take more than prescribed amount and do not stop taking without consulting health care provider. Advise patient to read *Patient Information* prior to starting therapy and with each Rx refill in case of changes. Caution patient not to share or trade *Dovato* with others.
- Advise patient that discontinuing therapy may lead to severe exacerbations of HBV.
- Inform patient of importance of HBV testing before starting antiretroviral therapy.
- Inform patient that *Dovato* does not cure HIV and may ↓ the risk of transmission of HIV to others through sexual contact or blood contamination. Caution patient to use a condom and avoid sharing needles or donating blood to prevent spreading HIV to others.
- Advise patient to notify health care provider immediately if symptoms of hypersensitivity reactions, lactic acidosis (nausea; vomiting; unusual or unexpected stomach discomfort; unusual muscle pain; difficulty breathing; feeling cold, especially in arms and legs; dizziness; fast or irregular heartbeat; weakness or tiredness), liver problems (yellow skin or whites of eyes, dark urine, light-colored stools, loss of appetite, nausea, stomach pain), or signs of immune reconstitution syndrome (signs and symptoms of an infection or inflammation) occur.
- Instruct patient to notify health care provider of all Rx or OTC medications, vitamins, or herbal products being taken and consult health care provider before taking any new medications, especially St. John's wort.
- Rep: Advise women of reproductive potential to notify health care provider if pregnancy is planned or suspected or if breastfeeding is planned. Enroll pregnant patients in the Antiretroviral Pregnancy Registry by calling 1-800-258-4263.
- Emphasize the importance of regular follow-up exams and blood counts to determine progress and monitor for side effects.

Evaluation/Desired Outcomes

- Slowed progression of HIV infection and decreased occurrence of sequelae.

donanemab (doe-**nan**-e-mab)

Kisunla

Classification

Therapeutic: anti-alzheimers agents

Pharmacologic: monoclonal antibodies, anti-amyloid monoclonal antibodies

Indications

Alzheimer disease (with mild cognitive impairment or mild dementia).

Action

Acts as a monoclonal antibody directed against aggregated insoluble forms of amyloid beta. **Therapeutic Effects:** Reduction in clinical decline. Reduction in amyloid beta plaques in the brain.

Pharmacokinetics

Absorption: IV administration results in complete bioavailability.

Distribution: Not widely distributed to extravascular tissues.

Metabolism and Excretion: Degraded into small peptides and amino acids via catabolic pathways.

Half-life: 12.1 days.

TIME/ACTION PROFILE (plasma concentrations)

ROUTE	ONSET	PEAK	DURATION
IV	rapid	end of infusion	4 wk

Contraindications/Precautions

Contraindicated in: Hypersensitivity.

Use Cautiously in: Apolipoprotein E ∊4 (Apo E ∊4) homozygotes (15% of patients with Alzheimer disease) (↑ risk of amyloid-related imaging abnormalities); OB: Safety not established in pregnancy; Lactation: Safety not established in breastfeeding; Pedi: Safety and effectiveness not established in children.

Adverse Reactions/Side Effects

Neuro: AMYLOID-RELATED IMAGING ABNORMALITIES (ARIA) (INCLUDING EDEMA AND HEMOSIDERIN DEPOSITION), headache, INTRACRANIAL HEMORRHAGE. **Misc:** HYPERSENSITIVITY REACTIONS (INCLUDING ANAPHYLAXIS AND ANGIOEDEMA), infusion-related reactions.

Interactions

Drug-Drug: Anticoagulant drugs and **thrombolytics** may ↑ risk of intracerebral hemorrhage.

Route/Dosage

IV (Adults): 700 mg every 4 wk for three doses; then 1400 mg every 4 wk.

Availability

Solution for injection: 17.5 mg/mL.

NURSING IMPLICATIONS

Assessment

- Monitor during and for ≥30 min after infusion for signs and symptoms of hypersensitivity reaction, including anaphylaxis and angioedema. *If symptoms occur,* promptly stop infusion and treat as clinically indicated.
- Monitor during and for ≥30 min after therapy for infusion-related reaction (chills, erythema, nausea/vomiting, dyspnea, diaphoresis, hypertension, headache, chest pain, hypotension). *If infusion reaction occurs,* ↓ infusion rate or stop infusion and treat as clinically indicated. Consider pretreatment with antihistamine, acetaminophen, or corticosteroid prior to subsequent dose.
- Monitor for intracerebral hemorrhage. *If hemorrhage >1 cm in diameter occurs,* hold until MRI findings stabilize and symptoms; if present, resolve. Resume dosing per clinical judgment.
- Monitor for signs and symptoms of ARIA with edema (ARIA-E) or with hemosiderin deposition (ARIA-H). ARIA usually occur early in therapy and are asymptomatic or may include headache, confusion, visual changes, dizziness, nausea, and gait changes. ARIA-E can cause focal neurologic deficits that can mimic ischemic stroke.
- *If mild, asymptomatic ARIA-E occur,* continue scheduled dosing. *If moderate or severe asymptomatic ARIA-E occur,* hold until MRI indicates resolution; resume dosing per clinical judgment. *If mild ARIA-E occur without symptoms disruptive to daily activities,* resume dosing per clinical judgment. *If moderate or severe ARIA-E occur with or without symptoms disruptive to daily activities,* hold until MRI findings and symptoms resolve; resume dosing per clinical judgment and consider follow-up MRI in 2–4 mo.
- *If mild asymptomatic ARIA-H occur,* continue scheduled dosing. *If moderate asymptomatic or mild to moderate symptomatic ARIA-H occur,* hold until MRI findings stabilize and symptoms resolve; resume dosing per clinical judgment. *If severe asymptomatic or symptomatic ARIA-H occur,* hold until MRI findings stabilize and symptoms resolve; continue or permanently discontinue donanemab per clinical judgment. Consider a follow-up MRI in 2–4 mo for all moderate to severe findings.
- Monitor PET imaging for ↓ in amyloid plaques. *For amyloid levels less than predefined thresholds,* consider holding therapy.

Lab Test Considerations

- Obtain Apo E ∊4 status prior to initiating therapy to inform risk of developing ARIA.

Implementation

- Confirm presence of amyloid beta pathology prior to initiating therapy.
- Obtain brain MRI at baseline and prior to 2nd, 3rd, 4th, and 7th infusions.
- If infusion is missed, resume every 4 wk at same dose as soon as possible.

IV Administration

- **Intermittent Infusion: Dilution:** Bring to room temperature. Solution is clear to opalescent, colorless to slightly yellow or brown. Do not use if discolored or contains particulates. **For 700 mg dose:** Inject 40 mL of donanemab (2 vials) into 30–135 mL of 0.9% NaCl for a total volume of 70–175 mL. **For 1400 mg dose:** Inject 80 mL of donanemab (4 vials) into 60–270 mL of 0.9% NaCl for a total volume of 140–350 mL. Gently invert to mix completely. Do not shake. If not used immediately, store at room temperature for ≤12 hr or refrigerate for ≤72 hr. Storage times include duration of infusion. **Concentration:** 4–10 mg/mL. **Rate:** Infuse over 30 min.
- **Y-Site Incompatibility:** Do not administer other drugs through same IV line.

Patient/Family Teaching

- Explain purpose and side effects of medication. Advise patient to read *Patient Information* before starting therapy.

- Inform patient of ↑ risk for ARIA if they are Apo E ∈4 homozygote, and encourage testing for Apo E ∈4 status prior to therapy initiation. Prior to testing, discuss risk of ARIA across genotypes and implications of genetic testing results.
- Inform patient that symptoms of ARIA can mimic ischemic stroke and to notify a health care provider immediately of stroke symptoms (sudden weakness or numbness, difficulty speaking or understanding, visual changes, severe headache, dizziness) occur.
- Advise patient to carry information that they are being treated with donanemab.
- Encourage patient to enroll in registry to help further the understanding of Alzheimer disease and the impact of therapy. Call 1-800-545-5979.
- Advise patient to immediately notify health care provider if signs of hypersensitivity (difficulty breathing, swelling of face) or infusion reaction occurs.
- Advise patient to notify health care provider of all Rx or OTC medications, vitamins, or herbal products being taken and to consult health care provider before taking other medications.
- Rep: Advise women of reproductive potential to notify health care provider if pregnancy is planned or suspected or if breastfeeding.

Evaluation/Desired Outcomes

- Reduction in clinical decline.
- Reduction in amyloid beta plaques in the brain.

donepezil (doe-**nep**-i-zil)

Adlarity, Aricept, ~~Aricept ODT~~

Classification

Therapeutic: anti-alzheimer's agents
Pharmacologic: cholinergics (cholinesterase inhibitors)

Indications

Mild, moderate, or severe dementia/neurocognitive disorder associated with Alzheimer disease.

Action

Inhibits acetylcholinesterase, thus improving cholinergic function by making more acetylcholine available. **Therapeutic Effects:** May temporarily lessen some of the dementia associated with Alzheimer disease. Enhances cognition. Does not cure the disease.

Pharmacokinetics

Absorption: Well absorbed after oral administration. Bioavailability of transdermal formulation comparable to that of oral tablets.
Distribution: Widely distributed to extravascular tissues.
Protein Binding: 96%.
Metabolism and Excretion: Partially metabolized by the liver (CYP2D6 and CYP3A4 isoenyzmes) and partially excreted by kidneys (17% unchanged). Two metabolites are pharmacologically active. The CYP2D6 enzyme system exhibits genetic polymorphism (~7% of population may be poor metabolizers and may have significantly ↑ donepezil concentrations and an ↑ risk of adverse effects).
Half-life: *Oral:* 70 hr. *Transdermal:* 91 hr.

TIME/ACTION PROFILE (improvement in symptoms)

ROUTE	ONSET	PEAK	DURATION
PO	unknown	several wk	6 wk†
Transdermal	unknown	several wk	6 wk†

† Return to baseline after discontinuation.

Contraindications/Precautions

Contraindicated in: Hypersensitivity to donepezil or piperidine derivatives; History of allergic contact dermatitis with transdermal donepezil.
Use Cautiously in: Underlying cardiac disease, especially sick sinus syndrome or supraventricular conduction defects; History of ulcer disease or currently taking NSAIDs; History of seizures; History of asthma or obstructive pulmonary disease; OB: Safety not established in pregnancy; Lactation: Use while breastfeeding only if potential maternal benefit justifies potential risk to infant; Pedi: Safety and effectiveness not established in children.

Adverse Reactions/Side Effects

CV: atrial fibrillation, hypertension, hypotension, vasodilation. **Derm:** allergic contact dermatitis (transdermal), ecchymoses. **Endo:** hot flashes. **GI:** diarrhea, nausea, anorexia, vomiting. **GU:** frequent urination. **Metab:** weight loss. **MS:** arthritis, muscle cramps. **Neuro:** headache, abnormal dreams, depression, dizziness, drowsiness, fatigue, insomnia, syncope.

Interactions

Drug-Drug: Exaggerates muscle relaxation from **succinylcholine**. Interferes with the action of **anticholinergics**. ↑ risk of cholinergic effects with **bethanechol**. May ↑ risk of GI bleeding from **NSAIDs**. **Quinidine** and **ketoconazole** may ↑ levels and risk of toxicity. **Rifampin**, **carbamazepine**, **dexamethasone**, **phenobarbital**, and **phenytoin** may ↓ levels and effectiveness.
Drug-Natural Products: **Jimson weed** and **scopolia** may antagonize cholinergic effects.

Route/Dosage

Mild to Moderate Alzheimer Disease

PO (Adults): 5 mg once daily; may ↑ to 10 mg once daily after 4–6 wk (dose should not exceed 5 mg/day in frail older women).
Transdermal (Adults): Apply one 5 mg/day transdermal system once weekly; may ↑ to one 10 mg/day

transdermal system once weekly after 4–6 wk. *Switching from oral to transdermal donepezil:* If patient taking 5 mg/day of oral donepezil, switch to one 5 mg/day transdermal system applied once weekly; if receiving 5 mg/day of oral donepezil for ≥4–6 wk, can switch to one 10 mg/day transdermal system applied once weekly. If patient taking 10 mg/day of oral donepezil, switch to one 10 mg/day transdermal system applied once weekly.

Severe Alzheimer Disease

PO (Adults): 5 mg once daily; may ↑ to 10 mg once daily after 4–6 wk; after 3 mo, may then ↑ to 23 mg once daily.
Transdermal (Adults): Apply one 5 mg/day transdermal system once weekly; may ↑ to one 10 mg/day transdermal system once weekly after 4–6 wk. *Switching from oral to transdermal donepezil:* If patient taking 5 mg/day of oral donepezil, switch to one 5 mg/day transdermal system applied once weekly; if receiving 5 mg/day of oral donepezil for ≥4–6 wk, can switch to one 10 mg/day transdermal system applied once weekly. If patient taking 10 mg/day of oral donepezil, switch to one 10 mg/day transdermal system applied once weekly.

Availability (generic available)

Tablets: 5 mg, 10 mg, 23 mg. **Orally disintegrating tablets:** 5 mg, 10 mg. **Transdermal patch (Adlarity):** 5 mg/day, 10 mg/day. ***In combination with:*** memantine (Namzaric). See Appendix N.

NURSING IMPLICATIONS

Assessment

- Assess cognitive function (memory, attention, reasoning, language, ability to perform simple tasks) periodically during therapy.
- Monitor HR periodically during therapy. May cause bradycardia or heart block.
- Monitor for nausea and vomiting, especially during therapy initiation and dose ↑.

Implementation

- Do not confuse Aricept with Aciphex or Azilect.
- **PO:** Administer in the evening just before going to bed. May be taken without regard to food.
- ***Orally disintegrating tablets*** should be allowed to dissolve on tongue; follow with water.
- Swallow *23-mg tablet* whole. ***DNC:*** Do not split, crush, or chew; may ↑ rate of absorption.
- **Transdermal:** Take patch from refrigerator and allow to reach room temperature; do not use external heat source to warm. Do not apply a cold transdermal patch. Apply to back; avoid the spine or a site that may be rubbed by tight clothing. May use upper buttocks or upper outer thigh. Do not use same location for application site for ≥2 wk. Do not apply after cream, lotion, or powder has recently been applied. Do not apply to red, irritated, or open skin. Do not shave site. Press down firmly for 30 sec to ensure good contact with skin at edges of patch. May be worn while bathing or in hot weather. Avoid long exposure to external heat sources. If patch falls off or a dose is missed, apply a new patch immediately and then replace 7 days later to start a new 1-wk cycle.

Patient/Family Teaching

- Explain purpose and side effects of medication. Advise patient to read *Patient Information* before starting therapy. Missed doses should be skipped and regular schedule returned to the next day. Do not take more than prescribed; higher doses do not ↑ effectiveness but may ↑ side effects.
- Inform patient/family that it may take weeks before improvement in baseline behavior is observed.
- Caution patient and caregiver that donepezil may cause dizziness and to avoid driving and other activities requiring alertness until response to medication is known.
- Advise patient and caregiver to notify health care professional if significant weight loss, inability to urinate, bronchospasm, or seizures occur.
- Advise patient and caregiver to notify health care professional if nausea, vomiting, diarrhea, or blood in stool occur or if noted symptoms ↑ in severity.
- Instruct patient to notify health care professional of all Rx or OTC medications, vitamins, or herbal products being taken and to consult health care professional before taking other Rx, OTC, or herbal products.
- Advise patient and caregiver to notify health care professional of medication regimen before treatment or surgery.
- Rep: Advise women of reproductive potential to notify health care professional if pregnancy is planned or suspected or if breastfeeding.
- Emphasize the importance of follow-up exams to monitor progress.
- **Transdermal:** Instruct patients or caregivers to fold the patch in half after use and discard it in the trash, out of the reach and sight of children and pets. Inform patients or caregivers that drug still remains in the patch after 7-day usage and that patches should not be flushed down the toilet.

Evaluation/Desired Outcomes

- Improvement in cognitive function (memory, attention, reasoning, language, ability to perform simple tasks).

HIGH ALERT

V DOPamine (dope-a-meen)

Classification

Therapeutic: inotropics, vasopressors

Pharmacologic: adrenergics

Indications

Adjunct to standard measures to improve: BP, Cardiac output, Urine output in treatment of shock unresponsive to fluid replacement. Increase renal perfusion (low doses).

Action

Small doses (0.5–3 mcg/kg/min) stimulate dopaminergic receptors, producing renal vasodilation. Larger doses (2–10 mcg/kg/min) stimulate dopaminergic and beta$_1$-adrenergic receptors, producing cardiac stimulation and renal vasodilation. Doses >10 mcg/kg/min stimulate alpha-adrenergic receptors and cause vasoconstriction. **Therapeutic Effects:** Increased cardiac output, increased BP, and improved renal blood flow.

Pharmacokinetics

Absorption: IV administration results in complete bioavailability.

Distribution: Widely distributed to tissues but does not cross the blood-brain barrier.

Metabolism and Excretion: Metabolized in liver, kidneys, and plasma.

Half-life: 2 min.

TIME/ACTION PROFILE (hemodynamic effects)

ROUTE	ONSET	PEAK	DURATION
IV	1–2 min	up to 10 min	<10 min

Contraindications/Precautions

Contraindicated in: Tachyarrhythmias; Pheochromocytoma; Hypersensitivity to bisulfites (some products).

Use Cautiously in: Hypovolemia; MI; Occlusive vascular diseases; OB: Safety not established in pregnancy; Lactation: Safety not established in breastfeeding; Geri: Older adults may be more susceptible to adverse effects.

Adverse Reactions/Side Effects

CV: arrhythmias, hypotension, angina, palpitations, vasoconstriction. **EENT:** mydriasis (high dose). **GI:** nausea, vomiting. **Local:** irritation at IV site. **Neuro:** headache. **Resp:** dyspnea.

Interactions

Drug-Drug: Use with **MAO inhibitors, ergot alkaloids (ergotamine)**, or some **antidepressants** results in severe hypertension. Use with IV **phenytoin** may cause hypotension and bradycardia. Use with **general anesthetics** may result in arrhythmias. **Beta blockers** may antagonize cardiac effects.

Route/Dosage

IV (Adults): *Dopaminergic (renal vasodilation) effects:* 1–5 mcg/kg/min continuous infusion. *Beta-adrenergic (cardiac stimulation) effects:* 5–10 mcg/kg/min continuous infusion. *Alpha-adrenergic (increased peripheral vascular resistance) effects:* >10 mcg/kg/min continuous infusion; infusion rate may be ↑ as needed.

IV (Children and Infants): 1–20 mcg/kg/min continuous infusion, depending on desired response (1–5 mcg/kg/min has been used to improve renal blood flow).

IV (Neonates): 1–20 mcg/kg/min continuous infusion.

Availability (generic available)

Solution for injection: 40 mg/mL. **Premixed infusion:** 200 mg/250 mL, 400 mg/250 mL, 400 mg/500 mL, 800 mg/250 mL, 800 mg/500 mL.

NURSING IMPLICATIONS

Assessment

- Monitor BP, HR, ECG, pulmonary capillary wedge pressure (PCWP), cardiac output, central venous pressure (CVP), and urinary output continuously during administration. *If hypotension occurs,* ↑ rate of infusion. *If hypotension continues,* consider using other vasopressors (e.g., norepinephrine). *If hypotension occurs with abrupt cessation of infusion,* restart infusion and gradually ↓ infusion rate while administering IV fluids. *If arrhythmia occurs,* treat according to guidelines.
- Monitor urine output frequently throughout administration. Report decreases in urine output promptly.
- Palpate peripheral pulses and assess skin appearance of extremities routinely during infusion, especially at infusion site.
- Monitor for hypersensitivity reaction (anaphylaxis, reactive airway episodes). *If signs of hypersensitivity occur,* treat as clinically indicated.

Implementation

- ***High Alert:*** IV vasoactive medications are potentially dangerous. Have second practitioner independently check original order, dose calculations, and infusion pump settings.
- Do not confuse dopamine with dobutamine. Store in separate areas.
- Correct hypovolemia with volume expanders before initiating therapy.

IV Administration

- V Dopamine is a vesicant. Central line administration is preferred; extravasation may cause severe ischemic necrosis. If central line is not available, may administer for <72 hr through a peripheral IV catheter placed in a large vein at a proximal site (e.g., in or proximal to antecubital fossa). If extravasation occurs, immediately stop infusion. Leave needle/cannula in place temporarily but do not flush the line. Gently aspirate extravasated solution; then remove needle/cannula. Elevate patient's extremity and apply dry warm compresses. Initiate phentolamine antidote for refractory cases in addition to supportive management. For phentolamine, dilute 5–10 mg in 10 mL of 0.9% NaCl and administer SUBQ into extravasation site as soon as possible after extravasation; if IV catheter remains in place, administer initial dose IV through the infiltrated catheter. May repeat in 60 min if patient remains symptomatic. Nitroglycerin 2% topical ointment (1-inch strip applied to site of ischemia to cover affected area; may repeat every 8 hr as necessary) or terbutaline may be used as alternatives to phentolamine. For terbutaline, for large areas of extravasation, dilute 1 mg in 10 mL of 0.9% NaCl and administer SUBQ into extravasation site; may repeat in 15 min if necessary; for small areas of extravasation, dilute 1 mg in 1 mL of 0.9% NaCl and administer 0.5 mg (0.5 mL) SUBQ into extravasation site; may repeat in 15 min if necessary.

- **Continuous Infusion: Dilution:** Vials must be diluted before use. Dilute 200–800 mg in 250–500 mL of 0.9% NaCl, D5W, D5/LR, D5/0.45% NaCl, D5/0.9% NaCl, or LR. Admixture is stable for 24 hr. Discard solution if cloudy, discolored, or contains precipitate. Premixed infusions are already diluted and ready to use. **Concentration:** 0.8–3.2 mg/mL. **Rate:** Based on patient's weight (see Route/Dosage section). Infusion must be administered via infusion pump to ensure precision. Titrate to response (BP, HR, urine output, peripheral perfusion, presence of ectopic activity, PCWP, CVP, cardiac index). ↓ infusion rate gradually when discontinuing to prevent marked ↓ in BP.
- **Y-Site Compatibility:** alemtuzumab, alprostadil, amikacin, aminocaproic acid, aminophylline, amiodarone, anidulafungin, argatroban, arsenic trioxide, ascorbic acid, atracurium, atropine, azithromycin, aztreonam, benztropine, bivalirudin, bleomycin, bumetanide, buprenorphine, butorphanol, caffeine citrate, calcium chloride, calcium gluconate, cangrelor, carboplatin, carmustine, caspofungin, cefotaxime, cefotetan, cefoxitin, ceftaroline, ceftazidime, ceftazidime/avibactam, ceftolozane/tazobactam, ceftriaxone, cefuroxime, chlorpromazine, ciprofloxacin, cisatracurium, cisplatin, cladribine, clindamycin, cyanocobalamin, cyclophosphamide, cyclosporine, cytarabine, dactinomycin, daptomycin, daunorubicin, dexamethasone, dexmedetomidine, dexrazoxane, digoxin, diltiazem, diphenhydramine, dobutamine, docetaxel, doxorubicin hydrochloride, doxorubicin liposomal, doxycycline, droperidol, enalaprilat, ephedrine, epinephrine, epirubicin, epoetin alpha, eptifibatide, eravacycline, ertapenem, erythromycin, esmolol, etoposide, etoposide phosphate, famotidine, fentanyl, fluconazole, fludarabine, fluorouracil, folic acid, foscarnet, gemcitabine, gemtuzumab ozogamicin, gentamicin, glycopyrrolate, granisetron, heparin, hetastarch, hydrocortisone, hydromorphone, hydroxyzine, idarubicin, ifosfamide, imipenem/cilastatin, imipenem/cilastatin/relebactam, insulin aspart, irinotecan, isavuconazonium, isoproterenol, ketamine, ketorolac, labetalol, LR, leucovorin, levofloxacin, lidocaine, linezolid, lorazepam, magnesium sulfate, mannitol, meperidine, meropenem/vaborbactam, mesna, methadone, methylprednisolone, metoclopramide, metoprolol, metronidazole, micafungin, midazolam, milrinone, mitoxantrone, morphine, moxifloxacin, mycophenolate, nafcillin, nalbuphine, naloxone, nicardipine, nitroglycerin, nitroprusside, norepinephrine, octreotide, ondansetron, oritavancin, oxacillin, oxaliplatin, oxytocin, paclitaxel, palonosetron, pamidronate, papaverine, pemetrexed, penicillin G, pentamidine, pentobarbital, phenobarbital, phentolamine, phenylephrine, phytonadione, piperacillin/tazobactam, plazomicin, potassium acetate, potassium chloride, procainamide, prochlorperazine, promethazine, propranolol, protamine, pyridoxine, remifentanil, rituximab, rocuronium, sargramostim, sildenafil, sodium acetate, succinylcholine, sufentanil, sulbactam/durlobactam, tacrolimus, tedizolid, telavancin, theophylline, thiamine, thiotepa, tigecycline, tirofiban, tobramycin, topotecan, trastuzumab, valproic acid, vancomycin, vasopressin, vecuronium, verapamil, vinblastine, vincristine, vinorelbine, voriconazole, warfarin, zidovudine, zoledronic acid.
- **Y-Site Incompatibility:** acyclovir, alteplase, amphotericin B deoxycholate, amphotericin B liposomal, azathioprine, cefazolin, dacarbazine, dantrolene, diazepam, diazoxide, esomeprazole, ganciclovir, ibuprofen lysine, indomethacin, methotrexate, mitomycin, phenytoin, sodium bicarbonate, trimethoprim/sulfamethoxazole.

Patient/Family Teaching

- Explain purpose of dopamine to patient and the need for frequent monitoring.
- Advise patient to inform health care provider immediately if chest pain; dyspnea; or numbness, tingling, or burning of extremities occurs.

- Instruct patient to inform health care provider immediately of pain or discomfort at the site of administration.
- Advise patient to notify health care provider of all Rx or OTC medications, vitamins, or herbal products currently being taken.
- Rep: Advise women of reproductive potential to notify health care provider if pregnancy is planned or suspected or if breastfeeding.

Evaluation/Desired Outcomes

- Increase in BP.
- Increase in peripheral circulation.
- Increase in urine output.

doravirine/lamivudine/tenofovir disoproxil fumarate

(**dor**-a-**vir**-een/la-**mi**-vyoo-deen/te-**noe**-fo-veer dye-soe-**prox**-il **fue**-ma-rate)

Delstrigo

Classification

Therapeutic: antiretrovirals

Pharmacologic: non-nucleoside reverse transcriptase inhibitors, nucleoside reverse transcriptase inhibitors

Indications

HIV-1 infection in patients with no prior antiretroviral treatment history. To replace the current antiretroviral regimen in patients with HIV-1 infection who are virologically suppressed (HIV-1 RNA <50 copies/mL), receiving a stable antiretroviral regimen with no history of treatment failure, and have no known substitutions associated with resistance to doravirine, lamivudine, or tenofovir disoproxil fumarate.

Action

Doravirine: Binds to the enzyme reverse transcriptase, which results in disrupted viral DNA synthesis. *Lamivudine:* After intracellular conversion to its active form (lamivudine-5-triphosphate), inhibits viral DNA synthesis by inhibiting the enzyme HIV reverse transcriptase. *Tenofovir disoproxil fumarate:* Phosphorylated intracellularly, where it inhibits HIV reverse transcriptase, resulting in disruption of DNA synthesis. **Therapeutic Effects:** Evidence of decreased viral replication and reduced viral load with slowed progression of HIV and its sequelae.

Pharmacokinetics

Doravirine

Absorption: 64% absorbed following oral administration.

Distribution: Extensively distributed to tissues.

Metabolism and Excretion: Primarily metabolized in the liver by CYP3A enzymes. Primarily excreted in feces (as metabolites); 6% unchanged in urine.

Half-life: 15 hr.

Lamivudine

Absorption: 86% absorbed after oral administration.

Distribution: Extensively distributed to tissues.

Metabolism and Excretion: 71% excreted unchanged in urine by glomerular filtration and active tubular secretion.

Half-life: 5–7 hr.

Tenofovir Disoproxil Fumarate

Absorption: 25% absorbed after oral administration.

Distribution: Extensively distributed to tissues.

Metabolism and Excretion: 70–80% excreted unchanged in urine by glomerular filtration and active tubular secretion.

Half-life: 17 hr.

TIME/ACTION PROFILE (plasma concentrations)

ROUTE	ONSET	PEAK	DURATION
Doravirine (PO)	unknown	2 hr	24 hr
Lamivudine (PO)	unknown	unknown	24 hr
Tenofovir (PO)	unknown	1 hr	24 hr

Contraindications/Precautions

Contraindicated in: Previous hypersensitivity reaction to lamivudine; Concurrent use of carbamazepine, enzalutamide, mitotane, oxcarbazepine, phenobarbital, phenytoin, rifampin, rifapentine, and St. John's wort; CCr <50 mL/min; Lactation: Breastfeeding not recommended in women with HIV.

Use Cautiously in: Coinfected with hepatitis B virus (HBV) (severe acute exacerbations of HBV may recur after discontinuation of lamivudine or tenofovir disoproxil fumarate); Severe hepatic impairment; OB: Safety of doravirine not established in pregnancy; Pedi: Children <35 kg (safety and effectiveness not established); Geri: Consider age-related ↓ in organ function and body mass, concurrent disease states and medications in older adults.

Adverse Reactions/Side Effects

Derm: rash, STEVENS-JOHNSON SYNDROME (SJS), TOXIC EPIDERMAL NECROLYSIS (TEN). **Endo:** Graves' disease. **GI:** ↑ lipase, ↑ liver enzymes, autoimmune hepatitis, diarrhea, HEPATOTOXICITY (↑ WITH HBV OR HEPATITIS C), hyperbilirubinemia, nausea. **GU:** ↑ serum creatinine, ACUTE RENAL FAILURE/FANCONI SYNDROME. **MS:** ↓ bone mineral density, ↑ CK, arthralgia, muscle weakness, myalgia, osteomalacia, polymyositis. **Neuro:** abnormal dreams, dizziness, Guillan-Barré syndrome, insomnia, sedation. **Misc:** immune reconstitution syndrome.

Interactions

Drug-Drug: **Strong CYP3A inducers**, including **carbamazepine**, **enzalutamide**, **mitotane**, **oxcarbazepine**, **phenobarbital**, **phenytoin**, **rifampin**, and **rifapentine**, may significantly ↓ levels and effectiveness of doravirine; concurrent use contraindicated; should discontinue these medications for ≥4 wk before initiating doravirine/lamivudine/tenofovir disoproxil fumarate therapy. **Rifabutin** may ↓ levels and effectiveness of doravirine; take one doravirine 100-mg tablet 12 hr after doravirine/lamivudine/tenofovir disoproxil fumarate dose. Nephrotoxic drugs, including **acyclovir**, **aminoglycosides**, **cidofovir**, **ganciclovir**, **NSAIDs**, **valacyclovir**, or **valganciclovir**, may ↑ risk of nephrotoxicity; avoid recent or concurrent use. **Ledipasvir/sofosbuvir** and **sofosbuvir/velpatasvir** may ↑ tenofovir levels and risk of toxicity; closely monitor. Medications containing **sorbitol** may ↓ lamivudine levels and effectiveness; avoid concurrent use.

Drug-Natural Products: **St. John's wort** may significantly ↓ levels and effectiveness of doravirine; concurrent use contraindicated; should discontinue this medication for ≥4 wk before initiating doravirine therapy.

Route/Dosage

PO (Adults and Children ≥35 kg): One tablet (doravirine 100 mg/lamivudine 300 mg/tenofovir disoproxil fumarate 300 mg) once daily.

Availability

Tablets: doravirine 100 mg/lamivudine 300 mg/tenofovir disoproxil fumarate 300 mg.

NURSING IMPLICATIONS

Assessment

- Assess for change in severity of HIV symptoms and for symptoms of opportunistic infections during therapy.
- Assess bone mineral density in patients with HIV who have a history of pathologic bone fracture or other risk factors for osteoporosis or bone loss. Consider supplementation with calcium and vitamin D.
- Monitor for severe skin reactions including signs of SJS and TEN. *If a painful rash with mucosal involvement or a progress rash occurs,* discontinue therapy immediately and monitor closely.

Lab Test Considerations

- Monitor viral load and CD4 cell count regularly during therapy.
- Assess for HBV. Not approved for administration in patients with HIV and HBV. If therapy is discontinued, may cause severe exacerbation of hepatitis B. Monitor liver function in coinfected patients for several months after stopping therapy.
- Monitor liver function periodically. May ↑ levels of AST, ALT, and alkaline phosphatase, which usually resolve after interruption of therapy. Patients with concurrent hepatitis B or C should be followed for at least several months after stopping therapy. Lactic acidosis may occur with hepatic toxicity, causing hepatic steatosis; may be fatal, especially in women.
- May ↑ LDL cholesterol, total cholesterol, and triglyceride concentrations.
- Assess serum creatinine, CCr, urine glucose, and urine protein before starting and periodically during therapy. Assess serum phosphorous in patients with chronic kidney disease, especially if taking nephrotoxic agents including NSAIDs.

Implementation

- Do not confuse lamivudine with lamotrigine. Do not confuse tenofovir disoproxil fumarate with tenofovir alafenamide.
- Administer once daily without regard to meals.

Patient/Family Teaching

- Explain purpose and side effects of medication. Advise patient to read *Patient Information* before starting therapy. Instruct patient on the importance of taking medication as directed, even if feeling better. Take missed doses as soon as remembered unless almost time for next dose; do not double doses. Caution patient not to share or trade medication with others.
- Advise patient that discontinuing therapy may lead to severe exacerbations of HBV.
- Inform patient of importance of HBV testing before starting antiretroviral therapy.
- Emphasize the importance of regular follow-up exams and blood counts to determine progress and monitor for side effects.
- Inform patient that medication does not cure HIV and may ↓ risk of transmission of HIV to others. Caution patient to use condoms and avoid sharing needles or donating blood.
- Advise patient to notify health care provider if bone pain that does not go away or worsens, pain in extremities, broken bones, or muscle pain or weakness occurs.
- Advise patient to notify health care provider if signs and symptoms of immune reconstitution syndrome (inflammation from prior infection, symptoms of infection) occur.
- Instruct patient to notify health care provider of all Rx or OTC medications, vitamins, or herbal products being taken and consult health care provider before taking any new medications, especially St. John's wort.

- Rep: Advise women of reproductive potential to notify health care provider if pregnancy is planned or suspected and to avoid breastfeeding during therapy. Encourage pregnant patients to enroll in the Antiretroviral Pregnancy Registry: 1-800-258-4263.

Evaluation/Desired Outcomes
- Delayed progression of HIV infection and decreased opportunistic infections in patients with HIV.
- Decrease in viral load and increase in CD4 cell counts.

BEERS

doxazosin (dox-**ay**-zoe-sin)
Cardura, Cardura XL

Classification
Therapeutic: antihypertensives
Pharmacologic: peripherally acting antiadrenergics

Indications
Hypertension (as monotherapy or in combination with other antihypertensive agents) (immediate release only). Symptomatic benign prostatic hyperplasia (BPH).

Action
Dilates both arteries and veins by blocking postsynaptic $alpha_1$-adrenergic receptors. **Therapeutic Effects:** Lowering of BP. Increased urine flow and decreased symptoms of BPH.

Pharmacokinetics
Absorption: Well absorbed following oral administration.
Distribution: Unknown.
Protein Binding: 98–99%.
Metabolism and Excretion: Extensively metabolized by the liver.
Half-life: 22 hr.

TIME/ACTION PROFILE

ROUTE	ONSET	PEAK	DURATION
PO†	1–2 hr	2–6 hr	24 hr
PO-XL‡	5 wk	unknown	unknown

† Antihypertensive effect.
‡ Improved urinary flow and BPH symptoms.

Contraindications/Precautions
Contraindicated in: Hypersensitivity.
Use Cautiously in: Hepatic impairment; GI narrowing (XL only); Patients undergoing cataract surgery (↑ risk of intraoperative floppy iris syndrome); OB: Not a preferred antihypertensive during pregnancy ; Pedi: Safety and effectiveness not established in children; Geri: Appears on Beers list. ↑ risk of orthostatic hypotension in older adults. Avoid use for treatment of hypertension in older adults.

Adverse Reactions/Side Effects
CV: first-dose orthostatic hypotension, arrhythmias, chest pain, edema, palpitations. **Derm:** flushing, rash, urticaria. **EENT:** blurred vision, conjunctivitis, epistaxis, intraoperative floppy iris syndrome. **GI:** abdominal discomfort, constipation, diarrhea, dry mouth, flatulence, nausea, vomiting. **GU:** ↓ libido, priapism, sexual dysfunction. **MS:** arthralgia, myalgia. **Neuro:** dizziness, headache, depression, drowsiness, fatigue, nervousness, weakness. **Resp:** dyspnea.

Interactions
Drug-Drug: ↑ risk of hypotension with **sildenafil**, **tadalafil**, **vardenafil**, other **antihypertensives**, **nitrates**, or acute ingestion of **alcohol**. **NSAIDs**, **sympathomimetics**, or **estrogens** may ↓ effects of antihypertensive therapy.

Route/Dosage
Hypertension
PO (Adults): 1 mg once daily; may be gradually ↑ at 2-wk intervals to 2–16 mg/day; incidence of postural hypotension greatly ↑ at doses >4 mg/day.

Benign Prostatic Hyperplasia
PO (Adults): *Immediate release:* 1 mg once daily; may be ↑ every 1–2 wk up to 8 mg/day; *Extended release:* 4 mg once daily (with breakfast); may be ↑ in 3–4 wk to 8 mg/day.

Availability (generic available)
Tablets: 1 mg, 2 mg, 4 mg, 8 mg. **Extended-release tablets:** 4 mg, 8 mg.

NURSING IMPLICATIONS
Assessment
- Monitor BP and HR 2–6 hr after 1st dose, with each ↑ in dose, and periodically during therapy. Report significant changes.
- Assess for 1st dose orthostatic hypotension and syncope. Incidence may be dose related. Observe patient closely during this period and take precautions to prevent injury.
- Monitor intake and output and daily weight, and assess for edema daily, especially at beginning of therapy. Report weight gain or edema.
- **BPH:** Assess patient for symptoms of prostatic hyperplasia (urinary hesitancy, feeling of incomplete bladder emptying, interruption of urinary stream, impairment of size and force of urinary stream, terminal urinary dribbling, straining to start flow, dysuria, urgency) before and periodically during therapy.

Implementation
- **PO:** Administer daily dose at bedtime.
- *DNC:* XL tablets should be swallowed whole; do not break, crush, or chew.
- **Hypertension:** May be administered concurrently with a diuretic or other antihypertensive.

Patient/Family Teaching

- Explain purpose and side effects of medication. Advise patient to read *Patient Information* before starting therapy. Emphasize the importance of continuing to take this medication, even if feeling well. Instruct to take at the same time each day. Take missed doses as soon as remembered unless almost time for next dose. Do not double doses.
- Instruct patient to notify health care professional of all Rx or OTC medications, vitamins, or herbal products being taken and to avoid concurrent use of alcohol or OTC medications and herbal products without consulting health care professional, especially cough, cold, or allergy remedies.
- May cause drowsiness or dizziness. Advise patient to avoid driving or other activities requiring alertness until response to medication is known.
- Caution patient to change positions slowly to ↓ orthostatic hypotension. May cause syncopal episodes, especially within 1st 24 hr of therapy, with dose ↑, and with resumption of therapy after interruption.
- Advise patient to notify other physicians of drug therapy.
- Advise male patient to notify health care professional if priapism or erection lasts >4 hr; may lead to permanent impotence if not treated.
- Emphasize the importance of follow-up visits to determine effectiveness of therapy.
- **Hypertension:** Instruct patient and caregiver on proper technique for BP monitoring. Advise them to check BP weekly and report significant changes.
- Encourage patient to comply with additional interventions for hypertension (weight reduction, low-sodium diet, smoking cessation, moderation of alcohol consumption, regular exercise, stress management).
- Rep: Advise women of reproductive potential to notify health care professional if pregnancy is planned or suspected or if breastfeeding.

Evaluation/Desired Outcomes

- Lowering of BP.
- Increased urine flow and decreased symptoms of BPH.

doxercalciferol, See VITAMIN D COMPOUNDS.

HIGH ALERT

V DOXOrubicin hydrochloride

(dox-oh-**roo**-bi-sin)

Adriamycin, ✱ Caelyx

Classification

Therapeutic: antineoplastics

Pharmacologic: anthracyclines

Indications

Breast cancer. Acute lymphoblastic leukemia. Acute myeloblastic leukemia. Hodgkin lymphoma. Non-Hodgkin lymphoma. Metastatic Wilms tumor. Metastatic neuroblastoma. Metastatic soft tissue sarcoma. Metastatic bone sarcoma. Metastatic ovarian carcinoma.

Action

Inhibits DNA and RNA synthesis by forming a complex with DNA; action is cell-cycle S-phase specific. Also has immunosuppressive properties. **Therapeutic Effects:** Death of rapidly replicating cells, particularly malignant ones.

Pharmacokinetics

Absorption: IV administration results in complete bioavailability.

Distribution: Widely distributed to tissues; does not cross the blood-brain barrier.

Metabolism and Excretion: Primarily metabolized by the liver via the CYP2D6 and CYP3A4 isoenzymes to an active metabolite. Excreted predominantly in the bile, 50% as unchanged drug. <5% eliminated unchanged in the urine.

Half-life: 16.7 hr.

TIME/ACTION PROFILE (effect on blood counts)

ROUTE	ONSET	PEAK	DURATION
IV	10 days	14 days	21–24 days

Contraindications/Precautions

Contraindicated in: Hypersensitivity; OB: Pregnancy; Lactation: Lactation.

Use Cautiously in: History of cardiac disease or high cumulative doses of anthracyclines; Depressed bone marrow reserve; Hepatic impairment (↓ dose if serum bilirubin >1.2 mg/dL); Rep: Women of reproductive potential and men with female partners of reproductive potential; Pedi/Geri: Children, older adults, mediastinal radiation, or concurrent cyclophosphamide (↑ risk of cardiotoxicity).

Adverse Reactions/Side Effects

CV: CARDIOMYOPATHY, ECG changes. **Derm:** alopecia, photosensitivity. **Endo:** prepubertal growth failure with temporary gonadal impairment (children only). **GI:** diarrhea, esophagitis, nausea, stomatitis, vomiting. **GU:** red urine, sterility. **Hemat:** ANEMIA, LEUKOPENIA, THROMBOCYTOPENIA. **Local:** phlebitis, tissue necrosis. **Metab:** hyperuricemia. **Resp:** recall pneumonitis. **Misc:** hypersensitivity reactions, SECOND MALIGNANCY.

Interactions

Drug-Drug: CYP2D6 inhibitors, CYP3A4 inhibitors, and **P-glycoprotein inhibitors** may ↑ levels and risk of toxicity; avoid concurrent use. **CYP2D6 inducers**, **CYP3A4 inducers**, and **P-glycoprotein inducers** may ↓ levels and effectiveness; avoid concurrent use. ↑ risk of bone marrow depression with other **antineoplastics** or **radiation therapy**. Pediatric patients who have received concurrent doxorubicin and **dactinomycin** have an ↑ risk of recall pneumonitis at variable times following local radiation therapy. May ↑ skin reactions at previous **radiation therapy** sites. If **paclitaxel** is administered first, clearance of doxorubicin is ↓ and the incidence and severity of neutropenia and stomatitis are ↑ (problem is diminished if doxorubicin is administered 1st). Hematologic toxicity is ↑ and prolonged by concurrent use of **cyclosporine**; risk of coma and seizures is also ↑. Incidence and severity of neutropenia and thrombocytopenia are ↑ by concurrent **progesterone**. May ↑ levels and risk of toxicity of **phenytoin**. May ↑ risk of hemorrhagic cystitis from **cyclophosphamide**. May ↑ risk of hepatotoxicity from **mercaptopurine**. Cardiac toxicity may be ↑ by **radiation therapy** or **cyclophosphamide**. ↑ risk of cardiac toxicity with **trastuzumab**; avoid use of doxorubicin for up to 7 mo after discontinuing trastuzumab. If **dexrazoxane** is administered at initiation of doxorubicin-containing regimens, may ↑ risk of therapeutic failure and tumor progression. May ↓ antibody response to **live-virus vaccines** and ↑ risk of adverse reactions.

Route/Dosage

IV (Adults): 60–75 mg/m² daily, repeat every 21 days; or 25–30 mg/m² daily for 2–3 days, repeat every 3–4 wk or 20 mg/m²/wk. Total cumulative dose should not exceed 550 mg/m² without monitoring of cardiac function or 400 mg/m² in patients with previous chest radiation or other cardiotoxic chemotherapy.
IV (Children): 30 mg/m²/day for 3 days every 4 wk.

Hepatic Impairment

IV (Adults): *Serum bilirubin 1.2–3 mg/dL:* ↓ dose by 50%; *Serum bilirubin 3.1–5 mg/dL:* ↓ dose by 75%.

Availability (generic available)

Powder for injection: 10 mg/vial, 50 mg/vial. 🍁 150 mg/vial. **Solution for injection:** 2 mg/mL.

NURSING IMPLICATIONS

Assessment

- Monitor BP, HR, respiratory rate, and temperature frequently during administration.
- Monitor for bone marrow depression. Assess for bleeding (bleeding gums; bruising; petechiae; guaiac stools, urine, and emesis) and avoid IM injections and taking rectal temperatures if platelet count is low. Apply pressure to venipuncture sites for 10 min. Assess for signs of infection during neutropenia. Anemia may occur. Monitor for ↑ fatigue, dyspnea, and orthostatic hypotension.
- Monitor intake and output. Encourage fluid intake of 2000–3000 mL/day. Allopurinol and alkalinization of the urine may be used to ↓ serum uric acid levels and to help prevent urate stone formation.
- Severe and protracted nausea and vomiting may occur as early as 1 hr after therapy and may last 24 hr. Administer parenteral antiemetics 30–45 min before therapy and routinely around the clock for the next 24 hr as indicated. Monitor amount of emesis and notify health care provider if emesis exceeds guidelines to prevent dehydration.
- Monitor for development of signs of cardiac toxicity, which may be either acute and transient (ST segment depression, flattened T wave, sinus tachycardia, extrasystoles) or late onset (usually occurs 1–6 mo after initiation of therapy) and characterized by intractable HF (peripheral edema, dyspnea, rales/crackles, weight gain). Chest x-ray, echocardiography, ECG, and radionuclide angiography may be ordered before and periodically during therapy. Cardiotoxicity is more prevalent in children <2 yr and older adults and when cumulative dose >300 mg/m². Dexrazoxane may be used to prevent cardiotoxicity in patients receiving cumulative doses of >300 mg/m².
- Assess oral mucosa frequently for development of stomatitis. ↑ dosing interval and/or ↓ dose is recommended if lesions are painful or interfere with nutrition.

Lab Test Considerations

- Verify negative pregnancy test before starting therapy.
- Monitor CBC with differential before and periodically during therapy. WBC nadir occurs 10–14 days after administration, and recovery usually occurs by the 21st day. Thrombocytopenia and anemia may also occur. ↑ dosing interval and/or ↓ dose is recommended if ANC is <1000 cells/mm³ and/or platelet count is <50,000 cells/mm³.
- Monitor renal (BUN and serum creatinine) and hepatic (AST, ALT, LDH, and serum bilirubin) function before and periodically during therapy. Dose ↓ is required for bilirubin >1.2 mg/dL or serum creatinine >3 mg/dL.
- May ↑ serum and urine uric acid concentrations.

Implementation

- ***High Alert:*** Fatalities have occurred with incorrect administration of chemotherapeutic agents. Before administering, clarify all ambiguous orders; double-check single, daily, and course-of-therapy dose limits; have 2nd practitioner independently double-check original order, calculations, and infusion pump settings.
- ***High Alert:*** Do not confuse doxorubicin hydrochloride with doxorubicin liposomal, daunorubicin hydrochloride, or idarubicin. Clarify orders that do not include both generic and brand names.

- ***High Alert:*** Administer under supervision of a physician experienced in use of cancer chemotherapeutic agents.
- Monitor cumulative dose of doxorubicin and other anthracyclines received; risk for cardiomyopathy ↑ as the cumulative dose ↑ (>250 mg/m² in pediatric patients <18 yr and 550 mg/m² in patients >18 yr).
- Wear gloves, gown, and mask while handling medication. Discard IV equipment in specially designated containers.
- Aluminum needles may be used to administer doxorubicin but should not be used during storage, because prolonged contact results in discoloration of solution and formation of a dark precipitate. Solution is red.

IV Administration

- V Doxorubicin hydrochloride is a vesicant. If extravasation occurs, immediately stop infusion. Leave needle/cannula in place temporarily but do not flush the line. Gently aspirate extravasated solution; then remove needle/cannula. Elevate patient's extremity and apply dry cold compresses for 20 min 4 times day for 1–2 days. Initiate antidote (dexrazoxane or topical dimethyl sulfoxide) based on time frame of noting extravasation. *If extravasation is noted ≤6 hr of doxorubicin hydrochloride infusion,* administer dexrazoxane 1000 mg/m² over 1–2 hr on Days 1 and 2 (max dose = 2000 mg/day), followed by 500 mg/m² over 1–2 hr on Day 3 (max dose = 1000 mg/day). Hold cold compresses 15 min before initiating and after completing dexrazoxane infusion. Concurrent treatment with topical dimethyl sulfoxide should not be used with dexrazoxane because it may ↓ dexrazoxane's effectiveness. *If extravasation is noted >6 hr after completion of doxorubicin hydrochloride infusion,* apply dimethyl sulfoxide by saturating a gauze pad and painting on an area twice the size of the extravasation. Allow site to air-dry and repeat application every 8 hr for 7 days. Do not cover the area with dressing.
- **IV Push: Reconstitution:** Reconstitute each 10 mg vial with 5 mL of 0.9% NaCl (nonbacteriostatic) for injection. Shake to dissolve completely. Do not add to IV solution. Reconstituted medication is stable for 24 hr at room temperature and 48 hr if refrigerated. Protect from sunlight. **Concentration:** 2 mg/mL. **Rate:** Administer each dose over 3–10 min through Y-site of a free-flowing infusion of 0.9% NaCl or D5W. Facial flushing and erythema along involved vein frequently occur when administration is too rapid.
- **Intermittent Infusion:** May be further diluted in 50–1000 mL of D5W or 0.9% NaCl. **Rate:** Infuse over 30–60 min.
- **Y-Site Compatibility:** alemtuzumab, amikacin, anidulafungin, argatroban, arsenic trioxide, aztreonam, bivalirudin, bleomycin, bumetanide, buprenorphine, butorphanol, calcium chloride, calcium gluconate, carboplatin, carmustine, caspofungin, chlorpromazine, ciprofloxacin, cisplatin, cladribine, clindamycin, cyclophosphamide, cyclosporine, cytarabine, dacarbazine, dactinomycin, daptomycin, dexamethasone, dexmedetomidine, dexrazoxane, diltiazem, diphenhydramine, dobutamine, docetaxel, dopamine, doxycycline, droperidol, enalaprilat, ephedrine, epinephrine, erythromycin, esmolol, etoposide, etoposide phosphate, famotidine, fentanyl, filgrastim, fluconazole, fludarabine, gemcitabine, gentamicin, granisetron, haloperidol, hetastarch, hydrocortisone, hydromorphone, ifosfamide, imipenem/cilastatin, irinotecan, isoproterenol, ketorolac, labetalol, leucovorin, lidocaine, linezolid, lorazepam, mannitol, melphalan, meperidine, mesna, methadone, methotrexate, metoclopramide, metoprolol, metronidazole, midazolam, milrinone, mitomycin, morphine, moxifloxacin, nalbuphine, naloxone, nicardipine, nitroglycerin, nitroprusside, 0.9% NaCl, octreotide, ondansetron, oxaliplatin, paclitaxel, palonosetron, pamidronate, phenylephrine, potassium acetate, potassium chloride, procainamide, prochlorperazine, promethazine, propranolol, sargramostim, sodium acetate, sufentanil, tacrolimus, theophylline, thiotepa, tigecycline, tirofiban, tobramycin, topotecan, trastuzumab, vancomycin, vasopressin, vecuronium, verapamil, vinblastine, vincristine, vinorelbine, zidovudine, zoledronic acid.
- **Y-Site Incompatibility:** acyclovir, allopurinol, aminophylline, amiodarone, amphotericin B deoxycholate, amphotericin B liposomal, ampicillin, ampicillin/sulbactam, azithromycin, cefazolin, cefepime, cefotaxime, cefotetan, cefoxitin, ceftazidime, ceftriaxone, cefuroxime, diazepam, digoxin, ertapenem, foscarnet, fosphenytoin, ganciclovir, gemtuzumab ozogamicin, magnesium sulfate, meropenem, methohexital, minocycline, pantoprazole, pemetrexed, pentamidine, pentobarbital, phenobarbital, phenytoin, piperacillin/tazobactam, potassium phosphates, propofol, rituximab, sodium phosphates, trimethoprim/sulfamethoxazole, voriconazole.

Patient/Family Teaching

- Explain purpose and side effects of medication. Advise patient to read *Patient Information* before starting therapy.
- Instruct patient to notify health care provider of all Rx or OTC medications, vitamins, or herbal products being taken and to consult health care provider before taking other Rx, OTC, or herbal products.

D

- Instruct patient to notify health care provider promptly if fever; sore throat; signs of infection; bleeding gums; bruising; petechiae; blood in stools, urine, or emesis; ↑ fatigue; dyspnea; or orthostatic hypotension occurs. Caution patient to avoid crowds and persons with known infections. Instruct patient to use soft toothbrush and electric razor and to avoid falls. Caution patient not to drink alcoholic beverages or take medication containing aspirin or NSAIDs, because these may precipitate gastric bleeding.
- Instruct patient to report pain at injection site immediately.
- Instruct patient to inspect oral mucosa for erythema and ulceration. If ulceration occurs, advise patient to use sponge brush, rinse mouth with water after eating and drinking, and confer with health care provider if mouth pain interferes with eating. Pain may require treatment with opioid analgesics. The risk of developing stomatitis is greatest 5–10 days after a dose; usual duration is 3–7 days.
- Instruct patient to notify health care provider immediately if irregular heartbeat, shortness of breath, swelling of lower extremities, or skin irritation (swelling, pain, or redness of feet or hands) occurs.
- Discuss the possibility of hair loss with patient. Explore methods of coping. Regrowth usually occurs 2–3 mo after discontinuation of therapy.
- Instruct patient not to receive any vaccinations without advice of health care provider.
- Inform patient that medication may cause urine to appear red for 1–2 days.
- Instruct patient to notify health care provider if skin irritation occurs at site of previous radiation therapy.
- Advise family and/or caregivers to take precautions (i.e., latex gloves) in handling body fluids for >5 days post-treatment.
- Inform patient that doxorubicin may ↑ risk of developing secondary cancers.
- Emphasize the need for periodic lab tests to monitor for side effects.
- Rep: May cause fetal harm. Advise women of reproductive potential to use effective contraception during therapy and for 6 mo after last dose and to avoid breastfeeding during therapy and for 10 days–6 wk after last dose. Advise men with female partners of reproductive potential to use effective contraception during therapy and for 3–6 mo after last dose of doxorubicin. A pregnancy registry is available for all cancers diagnosed during pregnancy at Cooper Health (877-635-4499). Inform patient before initiating therapy that this medication may cause irreversible gonadal suppression, irreversible amenorrhea, or early menopause.

Evaluation/Desired Outcomes

- Death of rapidly replicating cells, particularly malignant ones.

V doxycycline (dox-i-sye-kleen)

Acticlate, ✦ Apprilon, Doryx, Doryx MPC, Doxy, ✦ Doxycin, ✦ Doxytab, Oracea, ✦ Periostat, Targadox, ~~Vibramycin~~

Classification

Therapeutic: anti-infectives

Pharmacologic: tetracyclines

Indications

Treatment of various infections caused by unusual organisms, including: *Mycoplasma, Chlamydia, Rickettsia, Borellia burgdorferi*. Treatment of inhalational anthrax (postexposure) and cutaneous anthrax. Treatment of gonorrhea and syphilis in penicillin-allergic patients. Prevention of exacerbations of chronic bronchitis. Treatment of acne. Treatment of inflammatory lesions associated with rosacea (Oracea only). Malaria prophylaxis.

Action

Inhibits bacterial protein synthesis at the level of the 30S bacterial ribosome. Low-dose products used in the management of periodontitis inhibit collagenase. **Therapeutic Effects:** Bacteriostatic action against susceptible bacteria. **Spectrum:** Includes activity against some gram-positive pathogens: *Bacillus anthracis* (anthrax), *Clostridium perfringens, Clostridium tetani, Listeria monocytogenes, Nocardia, Propionibacterium acnes, Actinomyces israelii*. Active against some gram-negative pathogens: *Haemophilus influenzae, Legionella pneumophila, Yersinia enterocolitica, Yersinia pestis, Neisseria gonorrhoeae, Neisseria meningitidis*. Also active against several other pathogens, including: *Mycoplasma, Treponema pallidum, Chlamydia, Rickettsia, Borrelia burgdorferi*.

Pharmacokinetics

Absorption: Well absorbed from the GI tract.
Distribution: Widely distributed, some CSF and good bone penetration.
Metabolism and Excretion: 20–40% excreted unchanged in urine; some inactivation in intestine and some enterohepatic circulation with excretion in bile and feces.
Half-life: 14–17 hr (↑ in severe renal impairment).

TIME/ACTION PROFILE (plasma concentrations)

ROUTE	ONSET	PEAK	DURATION
PO	1–2 hr	1.5–4 hr	12 hr
IV	rapid	end of infusion	12 hr

Contraindications/Precautions

Contraindicated in: Hypersensitivity; Some products contain alcohol or bisulfites and should be avoided in patients with known hypersensitivity or intolerance;

OB: ↑ risk of bone growth inhibition and permanent staining of teeth in infant if used during 2nd or 3rd trimesters; may be used to treat anthrax in pregnant women due to the seriousness of the disease; Lactation: Lactation.

Use Cautiously in: Rep: Women of reproductive potential (↑ risk of intracranial hypertension if overweight or have a previous history of intracranial hypertension); Pedi: Children <8 yr (may cause permanent staining of teeth) (may be used to treat anthrax or Rocky Mountain spotted fever in children <8 yr due to the seriousness of these diseases).

Adverse Reactions/Side Effects

Derm: photosensitivity, DRUG RASH WITH EOSINOPHILIA AND SYSTEMIC SYMPTOMS (DRESS), ERYTHEMA MULTIFORME, EXFOLIATIVE DERMATITIS, rash, STEVENS-JOHNSON SYNDROME (SJS), TOXIC EPIDERMAL NECROLYSIS (TEN). **GI:** diarrhea, nausea, vomiting, CLOSTRIDIOIDES DIFFICILE-ASSOCIATED DIARRHEA (CDAD), dysphagia, esophagitis, glossitis, HEPATOTOXICITY, PANCREATITIS. **Hemat:** blood dyscrasias. **Local:** phlebitis. **Neuro:** headache, intracranial hypertension. **Misc:** hypersensitivity reactions, superinfection.

Interactions

Drug-Drug: May ↑ effect of **warfarin**. May ↓ effectiveness of **estrogen-containing oral contraceptives**. **Antacids**, **calcium**, **iron**, and **magnesium** form insoluble compounds (chelates) and ↓ absorption and effectiveness of tetracyclines; this effect is minimal with doxycycline. **Cholestyramine**, **colestipol**, and **bismuth subsalicylate** may ↓ absorption and effectiveness. **Barbiturates**, **carbamazepine**, or **phenytoin** may ↓ effectiveness. **Isotretinoin** may ↑ risk of intracranial hypertension; avoid concurrent use.

Drug-Food: Calcium in foods or **dairy products** may ↓ absorption by forming insoluble compounds (chelates); this effect is minimal with doxycycline.

Route/Dosage

More Common Infections

PO (Adults and Children >8 yr and >45 kg): *Most infections:* 100 mg every 12 hr on the 1st day, then 100–200 mg once daily or 50–100 mg every 12 hr. *Gonorrhea:* 100 mg every 12 hr for 7 days or 200 mg once daily for 7 days (delayed-release tablets) or 300 mg followed 1 hr later by another 300-mg dose. *Uncomplicated urethral, endocervical, or rectal infection caused by Chlamydia trachomatis:* 100 mg every 12 hr for 7 days. *Syphilis (early):* 100 mg every 12 hr for 14 days. *Syphilis (>1 yr duration):* 100 mg every 12 hr for 4 wk. *Malaria prophylaxis:* 100 mg once daily (2 mg/kg once daily for children >8 yr). *Lyme disease:* 100 mg twice daily; *Periodontitis:* 20 mg twice daily; *Rosacea:* 40 mg once daily in morning.

PO (Children >8 yr and <45 kg): *Less severe infections:* 2.2 mg/kg every 12 hr on the 1st day, then 2.2–4.4 mg/kg once daily or 1.1–2.2 mg/kg every 12 hr.

PO (Children >45 kg): *Severe or life-threatening infections (Rocky Mountain spotted fever):* 100 mg every 12 hr.

PO (Children <45 kg): *Severe or life-threatening infections (Rocky Mountain spotted fever):* 2.2 mg/kg every 12 hr.

Inhalational Anthrax (Postexposure)

PO, IV (Adults and Children >45 kg): 100 mg IV every 12 hr; change to 100 mg PO every 12 hr when clinically appropriate for a total of 60 days; one or two other anti-infectives may be added initially, depending on clinical situation.

PO, IV (Children ≤45 kg): 2.2 mg/kg IV every 12 hr; change to 2.2 mg/kg PO every 12 hr when clinically appropriate for a total of 60 days; one or two other anti-infectives may be added initially, depending on clinical situation.

Cutaneous Anthrax

PO (Adults): 100 mg every 12 hr for 60 days; some patients may require IV therapy initially depending on clinical situation.

PO (Children >8 yr and >45 kg): 100 mg every 12 hr; some patients may require IV therapy initially depending on clinical situation.

PO (Children >8 yr and ≤45 kg): 2.2 mg/kg every 12 hr; some patients may require IV therapy initially depending on clinical situation.

PO (Children ≤8 yr): 2.2 mg/kg every 12 hr; some patients may require IV therapy initially depending on clinical situation.

Availability (generic available)

Immediate-release tablets: 20 mg, 50 mg, 75 mg, 100 mg, 150 mg. **Immediate-release capsules:** 50 mg, 75 mg, 100 mg, 150 mg. **Delayed-release tablets:** 50 mg, 60 mg, 75 mg, 100 mg, 150 mg, 200 mg. **Delayed-release capsules (Oracea):** 40 mg. **Oral suspension (raspberry flavor):** 25 mg/5 mL. **Oral syrup (raspberry-apple flavor):** 50 mg/5 mL. **Powder for injection:** 100 mg/vial.

NURSING IMPLICATIONS

Assessment

- **Infection:** Assess for infection (vital signs; appearance of wound, sputum, urine, and stool; WBC) at beginning of and during therapy.
- Obtain specimens for culture and sensitivity before starting therapy. First dose may be given before receiving results.

D

- Monitor bowel function. Diarrhea, abdominal cramping, fever, and bloody stools should be reported to health care provider promptly as a sign of CDAD. May begin up to several weeks following cessation of therapy.
- Assess for rash periodically during therapy. May cause SJS or TEN. Discontinue therapy if severe or if accompanied with fever, general malaise, fatigue, muscle or joint aches, blisters, oral lesions, conjunctivitis, hepatitis, or eosinophilia.
- **IV:** Assess IV site frequently; may cause thrombophlebitis.

Lab Test Considerations

- Monitor renal and hepatic function and CBC periodically during long-term therapy.
- May ↑ AST, ALT, serum alkaline phosphatase, bilirubin, and amylase.
- May cause false ↑ in urinary catecholamine levels.

Implementation

- Do not confuse Oracea with Orencia.
- May cause yellow-brown discoloration and softening of teeth and bones if administered prenatally or during early childhood. Not recommended for children <8 yr of age or during pregnancy or lactation, unless used for the treatment of anthrax.
- *Oracea* is only indicated for rosacea, not for infections.
- **PO:** Administer around the clock, ≥1 hr before or 2 hr after meals. May be taken with food or milk if GI irritation occurs. Administer with 8 ounces (240 mL) of liquid and ≥1 hr before going to bed to avoid esophageal ulceration. Use calibrated measuring device for liquid preparations. Shake liquid preparations well. Do not administer within 1–3 hr of other medications.
- Capsules may also be administered by carefully opening and sprinkling capsule contents on a spoonful of applesauce. The applesauce should be swallowed immediately without chewing and followed with an 8-ounce glass of cool water to ensure complete swallowing of the capsule contents. The applesauce should not be hot, and it should be soft enough to be swallowed without chewing. If mixture cannot be taken immediately, discard; do not store for later use.
- ***DNC:*** Do not open, break, crush, or chew extended-release capsules and tablets.
- *To prepare doses for infants and children exposed to anthrax (used only in a Declared Public Health Emergency):* Place one 100-mg tablet in a small bowl and crush to a fine powder with a metal spoon, leaving no large pieces. Add 4 level teaspoons of low-fat milk, low-fat chocolate milk, regular chocolate milk, chocolate pudding, or an apple juice and sugar mixture made by combining 4 teaspoons of sugar and 4 teaspoons of apple juice. Mix food or drink and doxycycline powder until powder dissolves. Mixture is stable in a covered container for 24 hr if refrigerated (if made with milk or pudding) or at room temperature (if made with juice). Number of teaspoons to administer/dose is based on child's weight (0–12.5 lbs: ½ teaspoon; 12.5–25 lbs: 1 teaspoon; 25–37.5 lbs: 1½ teaspoons; 37.5–50 lbs: 2 teaspoons; 50–62.5 lbs: 2½ teaspoons; 62.5–75 lbs: 3 teaspoons; 75–87.5 lbs: 3½ teaspoons; 87.5–100 lbs: 4 teaspoons).
- Avoid administration of calcium, antacids, magnesium-containing medications, sodium bicarbonate, or iron supplements within 1–3 hr of oral doxycycline.

IV Administration

- **V** IV doxycycline is a vesicant. If extravasation occurs, immediately stop infusion. Leave needle/cannula in place temporarily but do not flush the line. Gently aspirate extravasated solution; then remove needle/cannula. Elevate patient's extremity and apply dry warm compresses. Initiate hyaluronidase antidote for refractory cases in addition to supportive management. For hyaluronidase, inject a total of 1 mL (15 units/mL) intradermally or SUBQ as five separate 0.2-mL injections (using a tuberculin syringe) around the site of extravasation; if IV catheter remains in place, administer IV through the infiltrated catheter; may repeat in 30–60 min if no resolution.
- **Intermittent Infusion: Reconstitution:** Reconstitute each 100 mg with 10 mL of sterile water or 0.9% NaCl for injection. **Dilution:** Dilute reconstituted solution further in 100–1000 mL of 0.9% NaCl, D5W, D5/LR, Ringer's, or lactated Ringer's solution. Solution is stable for 12 hr at room temperature and 72 hr if refrigerated. If diluted with D5/LR or lactated Ringer's solution, administer within 6 hr. Protect solution from direct sunlight. **Concentration:** Concentrations <1 mcg/mL or >1 mg/mL are not recommended. **Rate:** Administer over a minimum of 1–4 hr. Avoid rapid administration. Avoid extravasation.
- **Y-Site Compatibility:** acyclovir, alemtuzumab, amikacin, aminophylline, amiodarone, anidulafungin, argatroban, arsenic trioxide, ascorbic acid, atracurium, atropine, azithromycin, aztreonam, benztropine, bivalirudin, bleomycin, bumetanide, buprenorphine, butorphanol, calcium chloride, calcium gluconate, cangrelor, carboplatin, carmustine, caspofungin, cefotaxime, ceftolozane/tazobactam, ceftriaxone, chlorpromazine, cisatracurium, cisplatin, clindamycin, cyanocobalamin, cyclophosphamide, cyclosporine, cytarabine, dacarbazine, dactinomycin, daptomycin, daunorubicin, dexmedetomidine, dexrazoxane, digoxin, diltiazem, diphenhydramine, dobutamine, docetaxel, dopamine, doxorubicin hydrochloride, edetate disodium, enalaprilat, ephedrine, epinephrine, epirubicin, epoetin alfa, eptifibatide, ertapenem, esmolol, etoposide,

etoposide phosphate, famotidine, fentanyl, filgrastim, fluconazole, fludarabine, fosphenytoin, gemcitabine, gentamicin, glycopyrrolate, granisetron, hydromorphone, idarubicin, ifosfamide, imipenem/cilastatin, imipenem/cilastatin/relebactam, insulin, regular, irinotecan, isavuconazonium, isoproterenol, labetalol, leucovorin, levofloxacin, lidocaine, linezolid, lorazepam, magnesium sulfate, mannitol, melphalan, meperidine, meropenem/vaborbactam, mesna, methadone, metoclopramide, metoprolol, metronidazole, midazolam, milrinone, minocycline, mitoxantrone, morphine, multivitamins, mycophenolate, nalbuphine, naloxone, nicardipine, nitroglycerin, nitroprusside, norepinephrine, octreotide, ondansetron, oxaliplatin, oxytocin, paclitaxel, pamidronate, pantoprazole, papaverine, pentamidine, phentolamine, phenylephrine, phytonadione, plazomicin, potassium chloride, procainamide, prochlorperazine, promethazine, propofol, propranolol, protamine, pyridoxine, remifentanil, rituximab, rocuronium, sargramostim, sodium acetate, succinylcholine, sufentanil, sulbactam/durlobactam, tacrolimus, telavancin, theophylline, thiamine, thiotepa, tirofiban, tobramycin, topotecan, trastuzumab, vancomycin, vasopressin, vecuronium, verapamil, vinblastine, vincristine, vinorelbine, voriconazole, zoledronic acid.

- **Y-Site Incompatibility:** allopurinol, aminocaproic acid, amphotericin B deoxycholate, amphotericin B liposomal, ampicillin, ampicillin/sulbactam, azathioprine, cefazolin, cefiderocol, cefotetan, cefoxitin, ceftazidime, cefuroxime, chloramphenicol, dantrolene, dexamethasone, diazepam, diazoxide, erythromycin, fluorouracil, folic acid, furosemide, ganciclovir, gemtuzumab ozogamicin, heparin, hydrocortisone, indomethacin, ketorolac, methotrexate, methylprednisolone, mitomycin, nafcillin, oxacillin, palonosetron, pemetrexed, penicillin G, pentobarbital, phenobarbital, phenytoin, piperacillin/tazobactam, potassium acetate, sodium bicarbonate, trimethoprim/sulfamethoxazole, tedizolid.

Patient/Family Teaching

- Explain purpose and side effects of medication to patient. Advise patient to read *Patient Information* before starting therapy. Instruct patient to take medication around the clock and to finish the drug completely as directed, even if feeling better. Take missed doses as soon as possible unless it is almost time for next dose; do not double doses. Advise patient that sharing of this medication may be dangerous.
- Advise patient to notify health care provider of all Rx or OTC medications, vitamins, or herbal products being taken and to consult with health care provider before taking other medications.
- Advise patient to avoid taking antacids, calcium, magnesium-containing medications, sodium bicarbonate, and iron supplements within 1–3 hr of oral doxycycline.
- Instruct patient to notify health care provider immediately if rash, diarrhea, abdominal cramping, fever, or bloody stools occur and not to treat with antidiarrheals without consulting health care providers.
- Advise patient to use sunscreen and protective clothing to prevent photosensitivity reactions.
- Advise patient to report the signs of superinfection (black, furry overgrowth on the tongue; vaginal itching or discharge; loose or foul-smelling stools) or intracranial hypertension (headache, blurred vision, diplopia, vision loss). Women who are overweight, are of childbearing age, or have a history of intracranial hypertension are at greater risk for developing doxycycline-associated intracranial hypertension. Skin rash, pruritus, and urticaria should also be reported.
- Instruct patient to notify health care provider of medication regimen before treatment or surgery.
- Caution patient to discard outdated or decomposed doxycycline; they may be toxic.
- Rep: Advise women of reproductive potential to use a nonhormonal method of contraception while taking doxycycline and until next menstrual period. Advise patient to notify health care provider promptly if pregnancy is planned or suspected or if breastfeeding. May be used for short term. Consider developmental and health benefits of breastfeeding with the mother's clinical need for doxycycline and any potential adverse effects on the breastfed child from doxycyline or from the underlying maternal condition.
- Instruct patient to notify health care provider if symptoms do not improve within a few days for systemic preparations.
- **Malaria Prophylaxis:** Advise patient to avoid being bitten by mosquitoes by using protective measures, especially from dusk to dawn (staying in well-screened areas, using mosquito nets, covering the body with clothing, using an effective insect repellent). Doxycycline prophylaxis should begin 1–2 days before travel to the malarious area and continued daily while in the malarious area; after leaving the malarious area, it should be continued for 4 more weeks to avoid development of malaria. Do not exceed 4 mo.

Evaluation/Desired Outcomes

- Bacteriostatic action against susceptible bacteria.

D

doxylamine/pyridoxine

(dox-**il**-a-meen peer-ih-**dox**-een)

Bonjesta, Diclegis, ✤ Diclectin

Classification

Therapeutic: antiemetics

Pharmacologic: antihistamines, vitamin B6 analogues

Indications

Treatment of nausea and vomiting during pregnancy that has not responded to conservative management.

Action

Combination of an antihistamine and a vitamin B_6 analog. Mechanism not known. **Therapeutic Effects:** Decreased nausea and vomiting associated with pregnancy.

Pharmacokinetics

Absorption: Well absorbed following oral administration. Food delays/↓ absorption.

Distribution: Unknown.

Metabolism and Excretion: Doxylamine is mostly metabolized by the liver; inactive metabolites are renally excreted. Pyridoxine is a prodrug, converted to its active metabolite by the liver.

Half-life: *Doxylamine:* 12.5 hr; *pyridoxine:* 0.4–0.5 hr

TIME/ACTION PROFILE (antiemetic effect)

ROUTE	ONSET	PEAK	DURATION
PO	unknown	unknown	8–24 hr

Contraindications/Precautions

Contraindicated in: Hypersensitivity to doxylamine or pyridoxine; Concurrent use of MAO inhibitors; Lactation: Lactation.

Use Cautiously in: ↑ intraocular pressure or narrow-angle glaucoma; Stenosing peptic ulcer or pyloroduodenal obstruction; Urinary bladder-neck obstruction; Pedi: Safety and effectiveness not established in children.

Adverse Reactions/Side Effects

Neuro: drowsiness.

Interactions

Drug-Drug: MAO inhibitors ↑ intensity/duration of adverse CNS (anticholinergic) reactions; concurrent use contraindicated. ↑ risk of CNS depression with other **CNS depressants**, including **alcohol**, other **antihistamines**, **opioid analgesics**, and **sedative/hypnotics**.

Route/Dosage

Delayed-Release Tablets

PO (Adults): *Day 1:* Two tablets (doxylamine 10 mg/pyridoxine 10 mg) at bedtime; if symptoms are controlled, continue this regimen; *Days 2 and 3, if symptoms persist into afternoon on day 2:* Two tablets at bedtime on Day 2 and then one tablet in the morning and two tablets in the evening on Day 3; if symptoms are controlled, continue this regimen; *Day 4, if symptoms persist:* One tablet in the morning, one tablet midafternoon, and two tablets at bedtime (not to exceed four tablets/day).

Extended-Release Tablets

PO (Adults): *Day 1:* One tablet (doxylamine 20 mg/pyridoxine 20 mg) at bedtime; if symptoms are controlled, continue this regimen; *Day 2, if symptoms persist on day 2:* One tablet in the morning and one tablet at bedtime on Day 2; if symptoms are controlled, continue this regimen (not to exceed two tablets/day).

Availability (generic available)

Delayed-release tablets (Diclegis): doxylamine 10 mg/pyridoxine 10 mg. **Extended-release tablets (Bonjesta):** doxylamine 20 mg/pyridoxine 20 mg.

NURSING IMPLICATIONS

Assessment

- Assess for frequency and amount of emesis daily during therapy. Reassess need for medication as pregnancy progresses.
- Monitor hydration status to prevent dehydration.

Lab Test Considerations

- May cause false-positive urine screening tests for methadone, opioids, and PCP.

Implementation

- **PO:** Administer on an empty stomach with a full glass of water; food delays onset of medication. ***DNC:*** Swallow tablets whole; do not crush, break, or chew.

Patient/Family Teaching

- Explain purpose and side effects of medication. Advise patient to read *Patient Information* before starting therapy. Instruct to take as directed. Do not take more than prescribed amount.
- Instruct patient to notify health care professional of all Rx or OTC medications, vitamins, or herbal products being taken and consult health care professional before taking any new medications.
- May cause drowsiness. Caution patient to avoid driving and other activities requiring alertness until response to medication is known.
- Advise patient to avoid alcohol and CNS depressants, including sedatives, tranquilizers, antihistamines, opioids, and some cough and cold medications with doxylamine pyridoxine.
- Advise women that a result of a false-positive urine drug screening for methadone, opioids, and PCP may occur.
- Rep: Advise women to avoid breastfeeding during therapy.

Evaluation/Desired Outcomes

- Decreased nausea and vomiting associated with pregnancy.

drospirenone, See CONTRACEPTIVES, HORMONAL.

dulaglutide (doo-la-gloo-tide)

Trulicity

Classification

Therapeutic: antidiabetics

Pharmacologic: glucagon-like peptide-1 (GLP-1) receptor agonists

Indications

Type 2 diabetes (as adjunct to diet and exercise). To reduce the risk of major cardiovascular events in patients with type 2 diabetes who have established cardiovascular disease or multiple risk factors for cardiovascular disease.

Action

Acts as an acylated human glucagon-like peptide-1 (GLP-1, an incretin) receptor agonist; increases intracellular cyclic AMP (cAMP), leading to insulin release when glucose is elevated, which then subsides as blood glucose decreases toward euglycemia. Also decreases glucagon secretion and delays gastric emptying. **Therapeutic Effects:** Improved glycemic control. Reduction in risk of cardiovascular death, nonfatal MI, or nonfatal stroke.

Pharmacokinetics

Absorption: *0.75 mg dose:* 65% absorbed following SUBQ administration; *1.5 mg dose:* 47% absorbed following SUBQ administration.

Distribution: Unknown.

Metabolism and Excretion: Degraded by protein catabolic processes.

Half-life: 5 days.

TIME/ACTION PROFILE (↓ in A1c)

ROUTE	ONSET	PEAK	DURATION
SUBQ	within 4 wk	13 wk	unknown

Contraindications/Precautions

Contraindicated in: Hypersensitivity; Personal or family history of medullary thyroid carcinoma; Multiple endocrine neoplasia syndrome type 2; History of pancreatitis; Type 1 diabetes; Diabetic ketoacidosis; Severe GI disease (including severe gastroparesis).

Use Cautiously in: History of angioedema or anaphylaxis to another GLP-1 receptor agonist; Hepatic/renal impairment; Diabetic retinopathy (may ↑ risk of complications); Undergoing elective surgery or procedure requiring general anesthesia or deep sedation; OB: Use during pregnancy only if potential maternal benefit justifies potential fetal risk; Lactation: Use while breastfeeding only if potential maternal benefit justifies potential risk to infant; Pedi: Children <10 yr (safety and effectiveness not established).

Adverse Reactions/Side Effects

Derm: pruritus, rash. **Endo:** THYROID C-CELL TUMORS. **GI:** abdominal pain, nausea, vomiting, cholecystitis, cholelithiasis, constipation, diarrhea, dyspepsia, PANCREATITIS. **GU:** acute renal failure. **Local:** injection site reactions. **Metab:** ↓ appetite. **Neuro:** fatigue. **Resp:** aspiration. **Misc:** HYPERSENSITIVITY REACTIONS (INCLUDING ANAPHYLAXIS AND ANGIOEDEMA).

Interactions

Drug-Drug: Concurrent use with **insulin** or **agents that increase insulin secretion**, including **sulfonylureas**, may ↑ the risk of serious hypoglycemia; use cautiously and consider dose ↓ of insulin or agents increasing insulin secretion. May alter absorption of concurrently administered **oral medications** due to delayed gastric emptying.

Route/Dosage

Type 2 Diabetes

SUBQ (Adults): 0.75 mg once weekly; after ≥4 wk, may ↑ to 1.5 mg once weekly to obtain glycemic control; if additional glycemic control still needed, may then ↑ to 3 mg once weekly after ≥4 wk; if additional glycemic control still needed, may then ↑ to 4.5 mg once weekly after ≥4 wk.

SUBQ (Children ≥10 yr): 0.75 mg once weekly; after ≥4 wk, may ↑ to 1.5 mg once weekly to obtain glycemic control.

Risk Reduction of Major Cardiovascular Events

SUBQ (Adults): 0.75 mg once weekly; after ≥4 wk, may ↑ to 1.5 mg once weekly to obtain glycemic control; if additional glycemic control still needed, may then ↑ to 3 mg once weekly after ≥4 wk; if additional glycemic control still needed, may then ↑ to 4.5 mg once weekly after ≥4 wk.

Availability

Solution for injection (prefilled pens): 0.75 mg/0.5 mL, 1.5 mg/0.5 mL, 3 mg/0.5 mL, 4.5 mg/0.5 mL.

NURSING IMPLICATIONS

Assessment

- Observe patient taking concurrent insulin for signs and symptoms of hypoglycemia (sweating, hunger, weakness, dizziness, tremor, tachycardia, anxiety, headache, blurred vision, slurred speech, irritability).
- If thyroid nodules or ↑ serum calcitonin are noted, refer patient to endocrinology.

- Monitor for pancreatitis (persistent severe abdominal pain that may radiate to back, with or without vomiting). *If pancreatitis suspected,* discontinue dulaglutide; if confirmed, do not restart.

Lab Test Considerations
- Monitor A1c periodically during therapy to evaluate effectiveness.
- May ↑ lipase and amylase.

Implementation
- Do not confuse Trulicity with Tanzeum, Toujeo, Tradjenta, or Tresiba.
- Patients stabilized on a diabetic regimen who are exposed to stress, fever, trauma, infection, or surgery may require administration of insulin.
- **SUBQ**: Administer once weekly at any time of day, without regard to food. Day of wk may be changed as long as ≥72 hr before next dose. Inject into abdomen, thigh, or upper arm. Solution is clear and colorless; do not administer if discolored or contains particulates.

Patient/Family Teaching
- Instruct patient on manufacturer's instructions for use of pen and to take dulaglutide as directed. Pen should never be shared between patients, even if needle is changed. Store pen in refrigerator; do not freeze. After initial use, pen may be stored at room temperature up to 14 days. Advise patient to read the *Medication Guide* before starting dulaglutide and with each Rx refill in case of changes.
- Take missed dose as soon as remembered; if ≤72 hr until next scheduled dose, omit and take next dose as scheduled.
- Inform patient that nausea is the most common side effect but usually ↓ over time.
- Advise patient to never mix insulin and dulaglutide together. Both injections may be given in the same body area but not right next to each other.
- Explain to patient that this medication controls hyperglycemia but does not cure diabetes. Therapy is long term.
- Review signs of hypoglycemia and hyperglycemia. If hypoglycemia occurs, advise patient to take a glass of orange juice or 2–3 teaspoons of sugar, honey, or corn syrup dissolved in water and notify health care professional.
- Encourage patient to follow prescribed diet, medication, and exercise regimen to prevent hypoglycemia or hyperglycemia.
- Instruct patient in proper testing of serum glucose and ketones. These tests should be closely monitored during periods of stress or illness, and health care professional should be notified if significant changes occur.
- Advise patient to notify health care professional if changes in vision occur during therapy.
- Advise patient to notify health care professional of all Rx or OTC medications, vitamins, or herbal products being taken and consult health care professional before taking any new medications.
- Advise patient to notify health care professional immediately if signs of pancreatitis (nausea, vomiting, abdominal pain) or hypersensitivity (swelling of face, lips, tongue or throat; problems breathing or swallowing; severe rash or itching; fainting or feeling dizzy; very rapid heartbeat) occur.
- Inform patient of risk of benign and malignant thyroid C-cell tumors. Advise patient to notify health care professional if symptoms of thyroid tumors (lump in neck, hoarseness, trouble swallowing, shortness of breath) or allergic reaction (swelling of face, lips, tongue, or throat; fainting or feeling dizzy; very rapid heartbeat; problems breathing or swallowing; severe rash or itching) occur.
- Advise patient to inform health care professional of medication regimen before procedures or surgery due to ↑ risk of aspiration with general or deep sedation.
- Advise patient to carry a form of sugar (sugar packets, candy) and identification describing disease process and medication regimen at all times.
- Rep: Insulin is the preferred method of controlling blood glucose during pregnancy. Advise women of reproductive potential to notify health care professional if pregnancy is planned or suspected or if breastfeeding.
- Emphasize importance of routine follow-up exams.

Evaluation/Desired Outcomes
- Improved glycemic control.
- Reduction in risk of cardiovascular death, nonfatal MI, or nonfatal stroke.

BEERS

DULoxetine (do-**lox**-e-teen)

~~Cymbalta~~

Classification

Therapeutic: antidepressants

Pharmacologic: selective serotonin/norepinephrine reuptake inhibitors

Indications
Major depressive disorder. Diabetic peripheral neuropathic pain. Generalized anxiety disorder. Chronic musculoskeletal pain (including chronic lower back pain and chronic pain from osteoarthritis). Fibromyalgia.

Action
Inhibits serotonin and norepinephrine reuptake in the CNS. Both antidepressant and pain inhibition are centrally mediated. **Therapeutic Effects:** Decreased depressive

symptomatology. Decreased neuropathic pain. Decreased symptoms of anxiety. Decreased pain.

Pharmacokinetics

Absorption: Well absorbed following oral administration.

Distribution: Unknown.

Protein Binding: >90%.

Metabolism and Excretion: Primarily metabolized in the liver via the CYP2D6 and CYP1A2 isoenzymes; the CYP2D6 isoenzyme exhibits genetic polymorphism; ~7% of population may be poor metabolizers and may have significantly ↑ duloxetine concentrations and an ↑ risk of adverse effects.

Half-life: 12 hr.

TIME/ACTION PROFILE (plasma concentrations)

ROUTE	ONSET	PEAK	DURATION
PO	unknown	6 hr	12 hr

Contraindications/Precautions

Contraindicated in: Hypersensitivity; Concurrent use of MAO inhibitors or MAO-like drugs (linezolid or methylene blue); Severe renal impairment; Hepatic impairment or substantial alcohol use (↑ risk of hepatitis).

Use Cautiously in: May ↑ risk of suicide attempt/ideation, especially during early treatment or dose adjustment; this risk appears to be greater in adolescents or children; History of mania (may activate mania/hypomania); History of seizure disorder; Diabetes (may worsen glycemic control); Angle-closure glaucoma; OB: Use during 3rd trimester may result in neonatal serotonin syndrome, requiring prolonged hospitalization and respiratory and nutritional support; may ↑ risk of postpartum hemorrhage in mother when used in the month before delivery; Lactation: Use while breastfeeding only if potential maternal benefit justifies potential risk to infant; Pedi: Safety and effectiveness not established in children <7 yr (generalized anxiety disorder) or <13 yr (fibromyalgia); Geri: Appears on Beers list. May worsen or cause syndrome of inappropriate antidiuretic hormone (SIADH) secretion and/or hyponatremia in older adults. Use with caution in older adults and closely monitor sodium concentrations when starting therapy or ↑ dose.

Adverse Reactions/Side Effects

CV: hypertension, orthostatic hypotension. **Derm:** ↑ sweating, ERYTHEMA MULTIFORME, pruritus, rash, STEVENS-JOHNSON SYNDROME (SJS). **EENT:** ↑ intraocular pressure, blurred vision. **Endo:** SIADH. **F and E** hyponatremia. **GI:** constipation, dry mouth, nausea, ↑ liver enzymes, diarrhea, gastritis, HEPATOTOXICITY, PANCREATITIS, vomiting. **GU:** dysuria, ↓ libido, delayed/absent orgasm, ejaculatory delay/failure, erectile dysfunction, urinary retention. **Hemat:** BLEEDING. **Metab:** ↓ appetite. **Neuro:** drowsiness, fatigue, insomnia, activation of mania, dizziness, fainting, falls, NEUROLEPTIC MALIGNANT SYNDROME, nightmares, SEIZURES, SUICIDAL THOUGHTS/BEHAVIORS, tremor. **Misc:** SEROTONIN SYNDROME.

Interactions

Drug-Drug: Concurrent use with **MAO inhibitors** may result in serious potentially fatal reactions; do not use within 14 days of discontinuing MAO inhibitor; wait at least 5 days after stopping duloxetine to start MAO inhibitor. Concurrent use with **MAO-inhibitor-like drugs**, such as **linezolid** or **methylene blue**, may ↑ risk of serotonin syndrome; concurrent use contraindicated; do not start therapy in patients receiving **linezolid** or **methylene blue**; if **linezolid** or **methylene blue** need to be started in a patient receiving duloxetine, immediately discontinue duloxetine and monitor for signs/symptoms of serotonin syndrome for 5 days or until 24 hr after last dose of linezolid or methylene blue, whichever comes first (may resume duloxetine therapy 24 hr after last dose of linezolid or methylene blue). ↑ risk of hepatotoxicity with alcohol use disorder/**alcohol** abuse. Drugs that affect serotonergic neurotransmitter systems, including **tricyclic antidepressants**, **SNRIs**, **fentanyl**, **lithium**, **buspirone**, **tramadol**, **meperidine**, **methadone**, **amphetamines**, and **triptans**, may ↑ risk of serotonin syndrome. **Strong CYP1A2 inhibitors**, including **cimetidine**, **ciprofloxacin**, and **fluvoxamine**, may ↑ levels and risk of toxicity; avoid concurrent use. **CYP2D6 inhibitors**, including **paroxetine**, **fluoxetine**, and **quinidine**, may ↑ levels and risk of toxicity. May ↑ levels and risk of toxicity of **CYP2D6 substrates**, including **TCAs**, **phenothiazines**, and **class Ic antiarrhythmics** (**propafenone** and **flecainide**); concurrent use should be undertaken with caution. ↑ risk of serious arrhythmias with **thioridazine**; avoid concurrent use. ↑ risk of bleeding with **NSAIDs**, **aspirin**, **clopidogrel**, **prasugrel**, **ticagrelor**, **dabigatran**, **apixaban**, **edoxaban**, **rivaroxaban**, or **warfarin**.

Drug-Natural Products: St. John's wort may ↑ risk of serotonin syndrome.

Route/Dosage

Major Depressive Disorder

PO (Adults): 40–60 mg/day (as 20 mg or 30 mg twice daily or as 60 mg once daily) as initial therapy; then 60 mg once daily as maintenance therapy.

Generalized Anxiety Disorder

PO (Adults ≥65 yr): 30 mg once daily for 2 wk; may then consider ↑ to 60 mg once daily; then may ↑ by 30 mg once daily to maintenance dose of 60–120 mg once daily.

PO (Adults <65 yr): 30–60 mg once daily as initial therapy (if initiated on 30 mg once daily, should titrate to

60 mg once daily after 1 wk); may then ↑ by 30 mg once daily to maintenance dose of 60–120 mg once daily.
PO (Children ≥7 yr): 30 mg once daily for 2 wk; may then consider ↑ to 60 mg once daily; recommended maintenance dose = 30–60 mg once daily (not to exceed 120 mg once daily).

Diabetic Peripheral Neuropathic Pain
PO (Adults): 60 mg once daily.

Fibromyalgia
PO (Adults): 30 mg once daily for 1 wk; then ↑ to 60 mg once daily.
PO (Children ≥13 yr): 30 mg once daily; may ↑ to 60 mg once daily based on response and tolerability.

Chronic Musculoskeletal Pain
PO (Adults): 30 mg once daily for 1 wk; then ↑ to 60 mg once daily.

Availability (generic available)
Delayed-release capsules: 20 mg, 30 mg, 40 mg, 60 mg.

NURSING IMPLICATIONS
Assessment
- Monitor BP before and periodically during therapy. Sustained hypertension may be dose related; ↓ dose or discontinue therapy if this occurs.
- Monitor appetite and nutritional intake. Weigh weekly. Report continued weight loss. Adjust diet as tolerated to support nutritional status.
- Assess sexual function before starting duloxetine. Assess for changes in sexual function during treatment, including timing of onset; patient may not report.
- Assess mental status and mood changes. Inform health care provider if patient demonstrates significant ↑ in anxiety, nervousness, or insomnia.
- Assess for suicidal tendencies, especially during early therapy. Restrict amount of drug available to patient. Risk may be ↑ in children, adolescents, and adults ≤24 yr. After starting therapy, children, adolescents, and young adults should be seen by health care provider at least weekly for 4 wk, every 3 wk for next 4 wk, and on advice of health care provider thereafter.
- Assess for serotonin syndrome (mental changes [agitation, hallucinations, coma], autonomic instability [tachycardia, labile BP, hyperthermia], neuromuscular aberrations [hyperreflexia, incoordination], or GI symptoms [nausea, vomiting, diarrhea]), especially in patients taking other serotonergic drugs (SSRIs, SNRIs, triptans).
- Assess for rash periodically during therapy. May cause SJS. Discontinue therapy if severe or if accompanied with fever, general malaise, fatigue, muscle or joint aches, blisters, oral lesions, conjunctivitis, hepatitis, or eosinophilia.
- **Depression or Anxiety:** Assess mental status (orientation, mood, behavior). Inform health care provider if patient demonstrates significant ↑ in anxiety, nervousness, or insomnia.
- **Pain or Fibromyalgia:** Assess intensity, quality, and location of pain periodically during therapy. May require several wk for effects to be seen.

Lab Test Considerations
- May cause ↑ ALT, AST, bilirubin, CK, and alkaline phosphatase.
- May cause hyponatremia.
- Monitor blood sugar and A1c. May cause slight ↑ in blood glucose.

Implementation
- Do not confuse duloxetine with fluoxetine, paroxetine, or Dexilant. Do not confuse Cymbalta with Symbyax.
- **PO:** May be administered without regard to meals. ***DNC:*** Swallow capsules whole; do not crush, chew, or open and sprinkle contents on food or liquids.

Patient/Family Teaching
- Explain purpose and side effects of medication to patient. Advise patient to read *Patient Information* before starting therapy. Instruct patient to take as directed at the same time each day. Take missed doses as soon as possible unless time for next dose. Do not stop abruptly; may cause dizziness, headache, nausea, diarrhea, paresthesia, irritability, vomiting, insomnia, anxiety, hyperhidrosis, and fatigue; must be ↓ gradually. Advise patients they may notice improvement within 1–4 wk, but should be advised to continue therapy as directed. Therapy is usually continued for several months.
- Instruct patient to notify health care provider of all Rx or OTC medications, vitamins, or herbal products being taken and to consult with health care provider before taking other medications, especially NSAIDs or aspirin.
- Advise patient, family, and caregivers to look for suicidality, especially during early therapy or dose changes. Notify health care provider immediately if thoughts about suicide or dying, attempts to commit suicide, new or worse depression or anxiety, agitation or restlessness, panic attacks, insomnia, new or worse irritability, aggressiveness, acting on dangerous impulses, mania, or other changes in mood or behavior occur.
- May cause drowsiness. Caution patient to avoid driving or other activities requiring alertness until response to medication is known.
- Geri: Advise patient to make position changes slowly to minimize orthostatic hypotension and falls, especially in older adults and those taking antihypertensive medications.
- Instruct patient to notify health care provider if signs of serotonin syndrome (mental status changes: agitation, hallucinations, coma),

autonomic instability (tachycardia, labile BP, hyperthermia), neuromuscular aberrations (hyperreflexia, incoordination), gastrointestinal symptoms (nausea, vomiting, diarrhea), liver damage (pruritus, dark urine, jaundice, right upper quadrant tenderness, unexplained flu-like symptoms), bleeding (ecchymoses, hematomas, epistaxis, petechiae, hemorrhage), or rash occur.
- Advise patient to avoid taking alcohol during therapy.
- Inform patient that duloxetine may cause symptoms of sexual dysfunction. In men, ejaculatory delay or failure, ↓ libido, and erectile dysfunction may occur. In women, may result in ↓ libido and delayed or absent orgasm. Advise patient to notify health care provider if symptoms occur.
- Rep: May cause fetal harm. Advise women of reproductive potential to notify health care provider if pregnancy is planned or suspected or if breastfeeding. Use late in 3rd trimester may result in neonatal serotonin syndrome requiring prolonged hospitalization, respiratory support, and tube feeding; may occur immediately upon delivery. Symptoms include respiratory distress, cyanosis, apnea, seizures, temperature instability, feeding difficulty, vomiting, hypoglycemia, hypotonia, hypertonia, hyperreflexia, tremor, jitteriness, irritability, and constant crying. Use of duloxetine in last month of pregnancy may ↑ risk of postpartum hemorrhage. There is a pregnancy exposure registry that monitors pregnancy outcomes in women exposed to antidepressants during pregnancy. Encourage health care providers to register patients by contacting the National Pregnancy Registry for Antidepressants at 1-866-961-2388 or online at https://womensmentalhealth.org/research/pregnancyregistry/. Monitor infants exposed to duloxetine via breastfeeding for sedation, poor feeding, and poor weight gain.

Evaluation/Desired Outcomes
- Decreased depressive symptomatology.
- Decreased neuropathic pain.
- Decrease pain.
- Decrease anxiety.

dupilumab (doo-**pil**-ue-mab)

Dupixent

Classification

Therapeutic: anti-inflammatories, antiasthmatics

Pharmacologic: interleukin antagonists

Indications
Moderate to severe atopic dermatitis not controlled by other prescription therapies or when these therapies cannot be used (with or without topical corticosteroids). Add-on maintenance treatment of moderate to severe asthma that is of an eosinophilic phenotype or that is dependent on oral corticosteroids. Add-on maintenance treatment of inadequately controlled chronic rhinosinusitis with nasal polyps. Eosinophilic esophagitis. Prurigo nodularis. Patients with inadequately controlled chronic obstructive pulmonary disease (COPD) and an eosinophilic phenotype (as add-on maintenance treatment). Chronic spontaneous urticaria in patients who remain symptomatic despite H_1 antihistamine treatment. Bullous pemphigoid.

Action
Monoclonal antibody that inhibits interleukin-4 (IL-4) and IL-13, which inhibits cytokine-induced inflammatory responses. Mechanism in asthma not fully established. **Therapeutic Effects:** Decreased severity of atopic dermatitis. Decreased incidence of asthma and COPD exacerbations. Reduction in nasal polyps and nasal congestion. Achievement of remission and reduction in dysphagia in eosinophilic esophagitis. Reduction in itching associated with prurigo nodularis and chronic spontaneous urticaria. Achievement of remission in bullous pemphigoid.

Pharmacokinetics
Absorption: 61–64% absorbed following SUBQ administration.
Distribution: Minimally distributed to tissues.
Metabolism and Excretion: Degraded by proteolytic enzymes located throughout the body.
Half-life: Unknown.

TIME/ACTION PROFILE (plasma concentrations)

ROUTE	ONSET	PEAK	DURATION
SUBQ	unknown	1 wk	unknown

Contraindications/Precautions
Contraindicated in: Hypersensitivity; Acute bronchospasm or status asthmaticus.
Use Cautiously in: Pre-existing helminth infections; OB: Use during pregnancy only if potential maternal benefit justifies potential fetal risk; Lactation: Use while breastfeeding only if potential maternal benefit justifies potential risk to infant; Pedi: Safety and effectiveness not established in children <6 mo (atopic dermatitis), <1 yr (eosinophilic esophagitis), <6 yr (asthma), <12 yr (chronic rhinosinusitis with nasal polyps, chronic spontaneous urticaria), or <18 yr (COPD, prurigo nodularis, bullous pemphigoid).

Adverse Reactions/Side Effects

CV: eosinophilic granulomatosis with polyangiitis, vasculitis. **Derm:** psoriasis. **EENT:** conjunctivitis, keratitis. **Hemat:** eosinophilia. **Local:** injection site reactions. **MS:** arthralgia, psoriatic arthritis. **Resp:** eosinophilic pneumonia. **Misc:** HYPERSENSITIVITY REACTIONS (INCLUDING ANAPHYLAXIS AND ANGIOEDEMA).

Interactions

Drug-Drug: Avoid use of **live vaccines**.

Route/Dosage

Atopic Dermatitis

SUBQ (Adults and Children ≥6 yr and ≥60 kg): 600 mg (given as two 300-mg injections) initially, then 300 mg in 2 wk, then 300 mg every 2 wk.
SUBQ (Children ≥6 yr and 30–<60 kg): 400 mg (given as two 200-mg injections) initially, then 200 mg in 2 wk, then 200 mg every 2 wk.
SUBQ (Children ≥6 yr and 15–<30 kg): 600 mg (given as two 300-mg injections) initially, then 300 mg in 4 wk, then 300 mg every 4 wk.
SUBQ (Children 6 mo–5 yr and 15–<30 kg): 300 mg every 4 wk.
SUBQ (Children 6 mo–5 yr and 5–<15 kg): 200 mg every 4 wk.

Asthma

SUBQ (Adults): 400 mg (given as two 200-mg injections) initially, then 200 mg in 2 wk, then 200 mg every 2 wk *or* 600 mg (given as two 300-mg injections) initially, then 300 mg in 2 wk, then 300 mg every 2 wk. *Patients with oral corticosteroid-dependent asthma, concurrent moderate to severe atopic dermatitis, or concurrent chronic rhinosinusitis with nasal polyps:* 600 mg (given as two 300-mg injections) initially, then 300 mg in 2 wk, then 300 mg every 2 wk.
SUBQ (Children ≥12 yr): 400 mg (given as two 200-mg injections) initially, then 200 mg in 2 wk, then 200 mg every 2 wk *or* 600 mg (given as two 300-mg injections) initially, then 300 mg in 2 wk, then 300 mg every 2 wk. *Patients with oral corticosteroid-dependent asthma or concurrent moderate to severe atopic dermatitis:* 600 mg (given as two 300-mg injections) initially, then 300 mg in 2 wk, then 300 mg every 2 wk.
SUBQ (Children 6–11 yr and ≥30 kg): 200 mg every 2 wk. *Patients with concurrent moderate to severe atopic dermatitis:* 400 mg (given as two 200-mg injections) initially, then 200 mg in 2 wk, then 200 mg every 2 wk.
SUBQ (Children 6–11 yr and 15–<30 kg): 300 mg every 4 wk. *Patients with concurrent moderate to severe atopic dermatitis:* 600 mg (given as two 300-mg injections) initially, then 300 mg in 4 wk, then 300 mg every 4 wk.

Chronic Rhinosinusitis with Nasal Polyps

SUBQ (Adults and Children ≥12 yr): 300 mg every 2 wk.

Eosinophilic Esophagitis

SUBQ (Adults and Children ≥1 yr and ≥40 kg): 300 mg once weekly.
SUBQ (Adults and Children ≥1 yr and 30–<40 kg): 300 mg every 2 wk.
SUBQ (Adults and Children ≥1 yr and 15–<30 kg): 200 mg every 2 wk.

Prurigo Nodularis or Bullous Pemphigoid

SUBQ (Adults): 600 mg (given as two 300-mg injections) initially, then 300 mg in 2 wk, then 300 mg every 2 wk.

Chronic Obstructive Pulmonary Disease

SUBQ (Adults): 300 mg every 2 wk.

Chronic Spontaneous Urticaria

SUBQ (Adults and Children 12–17 yr and ≥60 kg): 600 mg (given as two 300-mg injections) initially, then 300 mg in 2 wk, then 300 mg every 2 wk.
SUBQ (Children 12–17 yr and 30–<60 kg): 400 mg (given as two 200-mg injections) initially, then 200 mg in 2 wk, then 200 mg every 2 wk.

Availability

Solution for injection (prefilled syringes or pens): 200 mg/1.14 mL, 300 mg/2 mL.

NURSING IMPLICATIONS

Assessment

- Monitor for signs and symptoms of hypersensitivity reactions (anaphylaxis, acute generalized exanthematous pustulosis, angioedema, rash, urticaria, erythema nodosum, serum sickness, and erythema multiforme) during therapy. *If any reaction occurs,* treat symptomatically and discontinue therapy.
- Monitor for signs and symptoms of conjunctivitis and keratitis (eye redness or irritation) periodically during therapy.
- Monitor for signs and symptoms of rhinosinusitis periodically during therapy.
- Assess for new-onset of psoriasis. If symptoms persist or worsen, consider dermatologic evaluation and/or discontinue therapy.
- Assess for new-onset of arthralgia and psoriatic arthritis. If symptoms persist or worsen, consider rheumatological evaluation and/or discontinue therapy.
- **Atopic Dermatitis and Bullous Pemphigoid:** Monitor skin lesions before starting and periodically during therapy.
- **Asthma/COPD:** Assess lung sounds, BP, and HR before administration and during peak of medication. Note amount, color, and character of sputum produced.

Lab Test Considerations

- May ↑ eosinophil count. Monitor before and during treatment. May ↓ IgE. Monitor in patients with severe allergic asthma.

Implementation

- Complete all age-appropriate vaccinations as recommended by current immunization guidelines before starting therapy.
- Prefilled pen is for adults and children ≥2 yr; prefilled syringe is for adults and children ≥6 mo.
- Before injection, remove dupilumab from the refrigerator and allow to reach room temperature (45 min for 300 mg/2 mL prefilled syringe or prefilled pen, 30 min for 200 mg/1.14 mL prefilled syringe or prefilled pen) without removing the needle cap. After removal from the refrigerator, must be used within 14 days or discarded.
- **Bullous pemphigoid:** Use dupilumab in combination with a tapering course of oral corticosteroids. Once disease control has occurred, gradually taper corticosteroids, after which dupilumab can be continued as monotherapy. If relapse occurs, consider reinitiation of corticosteroid therapy.
- **SUBQ**: Dose must be divided into two injections for 400 mg and 600 mg doses. Administer at different sites. Thigh and abdomen may be used if patient administers dose. May also use upper arm if administered by caregiver. Rotate site with each injection; do not inject in skin that is tender, damaged, bruised, or scarred. Solution is clear to slightly opalescent, colorless to pale yellow; do not administer solutions that are cloudy, discolored, or contain particulate matter.

Patient/Family Teaching

- Explain purpose and side effects of medication to patient. Advise patient to read *Patient Information* before starting therapy. Instruct patient and caregiver in correct injection technique and disposal of equipment. If a weekly dose is missed, administer dose as soon as possible, and start a new weekly schedule from the date of the last administered dose. If every-other-wk dose is missed, administer within 7 days from the missed dose; then resume original schedule. If missed dose is not administered within 7 days, administer dose, starting a new schedule based on this date. If every-4-wk dose is missed, administer injection within 7 days from missed dose and resume original schedule. If missed dose is not administered within 7 days, administer dose and start a new schedule based on this date.
- Instruct patient to notify health care provider of all Rx or OTC medications, vitamins, or herbal products being taken and to consult health care provider before taking other Rx, OTC, or herbal products.
- Advise patient to discontinue dupilumab and seek immediate medical attention if any hypersensitivity reactions occur.
- Advise patient not to discontinue systemic or inhaled corticosteroids unless directed. The ↓ in corticosteroid dose may cause systemic withdrawal symptoms and/or unmask conditions.
- Inform patient that dupilumab is not used for acute asthma symptoms or acute COPD exacerbations. Instruct patient to notify health care provider if asthma/COPD symptoms remain uncontrolled or worsen after starting therapy.
- Advise patient to notify health care provider if new onset or worsening eye symptoms occur.
- Advise patient to avoid live vaccines during therapy.
- Advise patient to have helminth infections treated before starting therapy. If patient becomes infected while receiving treatment with dupilumab and does not respond to antihelminth treatment, discontinue treatment with dupilumab until infection resolves.
- Rep: Advise women of reproductive potential to notify health care provider if pregnancy is planned or suspected or if breastfeeding. Inform patient of pregnancy exposure registry that monitors outcomes in women exposed to dupilumab. Health care providers and patients may call 1-877-311-8972 or go to https://mothertobaby.org/ongoing-study/dupixent/ to enroll or to obtain information about the registry.

Evaluation/Desired Outcomes

- Decreased severity of atopic dermatitis.
- Decreased incidence of asthma and COPD exacerbations.
- Reduction in nasal polyps and nasal congestion.
- Achievement of remission and reduction in dysphagia in eosinophilic esophagitis.
- Reduction in itching associated with prurigo nodularis and chronic spontaneous urticaria.
- Achievement of remission in bullous pemphigoid.

HIGH ALERT

durvalumab

(dur-**val**-ue-mab)

Imfinzi

Classification

Therapeutic: antineoplastics

Pharmacologic: monoclonal antibodies, programmed death ligand 1 (PD-L1) inhibitors

Indications

Unresectable stage III non-small cell lung cancer (NSCLC) in patients whose disease has not progressed with concurrent platinum-containing chemotherapy and radiation. Metastatic NSCLC in patients with no sensitizing epidermal growth factor receptor (EGFR) mutations or anaplastic lymphoma kinase (ALK) genomic tumor aberrations (in combination with tremelimumab and platinum-based chemotherapy). Resectable (tumors ≥4 cm and/or node positive) NSCLC with no known EGFR mutations or ALK rearrangements (in combination with platinum-containing chemotherapy as neoadjuvant treatment, followed by monotherapy as adjuvant treatment after surgery). First-line treatment of extensive-stage small cell lung cancer (in combination with etoposide and either carboplatin or cisplatin). Limited-stage small cell lung cancer in patients whose disease has not progressed following concurrent platinum-based chemotherapy and radiation therapy. Locally advanced or metastatic biliary tract cancer (in combination with gemcitabine and cisplatin). Unresectable hepatocellular carcinoma (in combination with tremelimumab). Primary advanced or recurrent endometrial cancer that is mismatch repair deficient (dMMR) (in combination with carboplatin and paclitaxel followed by monotherapy). Muscle invasive bladder cancer (in combination with gemcitabine and cisplatin as neoadjuvant treatment, followed by single agent durvalumab as adjuvant treatment following radical cystectomy).

Action

Binds to programmed death ligand 1 (PD-L1) to prevent its interaction with the programmed cell death-1 (PD-1) and CD80 (B7.1) receptors, which activates the antitumor immune response. **Therapeutic Effects:** Decreased spread of NSCLC with improved overall survival and progression-free survival. Improved overall survival in small cell lung cancer, biliary tract cancer, hepatocellular carcinoma, and bladder cancer. Improved progression-free survival in endometrial cancer.

Pharmacokinetics

Absorption: IV administration results in complete bioavailability.
Distribution: Minimally distributed to tissues.
Metabolism and Excretion: Unknown.
Half-life: 18 days.

TIME/ACTION PROFILE (plasma concentrations)

ROUTE	ONSET	PEAK	DURATION
IV	unknown	unknown	unknown

Contraindications/Precautions

Contraindicated in: OB: Pregnancy; Lactation: Lactation.

Use Cautiously in: Allogeneic hematopoietic stem cell transplantation recipients (↑ risk of transplant-related complications); Solid organ transplant recipients (↑ risk of rejection); Prior thoracic radiation (↑ risk of pneumonitis); Rep: Women of reproductive potential; Pedi: Safety and effectiveness not established in children.

Adverse Reactions/Side Effects

CV: peripheral edema, MYOCARDITIS, pericarditis, vasculitis. **Derm:** pruritus, rash, DRUG REACTION WITH EOSINOPHILIA AND SYSTEMIC SYMPTOMS (DRESS), STEVENS-JOHNSON SYNDROME (SJS), TOXIC EPIDERMAL NECROLYSIS (TEN). **EENT:** keratitis, uveitis. **Endo:** hyperglycemia, immune-mediated hypothyroidism, immune-mediated adrenal insufficiency, immune-mediated hyperthyroidism, immune-mediated hypophysitis, immune-mediated type 1 diabetes mellitus. **F and E** hyperkalemia, hypocalcemia, hyponatremia, hypercalcemia, hypermagnesemia, hypokalemia. **GI:** ↓ appetite, abdominal pain, constipation, nausea, gastritis, hypoalbuminemia, immune-mediated colitis, IMMUNE-MEDIATED HEPATITIS, pancreatitis. **GU:** immune-mediated nephritis. **Hemat:** lymphopenia, anemia, hemolytic anemia, NEUTROPENIA. **MS:** pain, myositis, RHABDOMYOLYSIS. **Neuro:** fatigue, autoimmune neuropathy, ENCEPHALITIS, Guillain-Barré syndrome, MENINGITIS, myasthenic syndrome, myelitis. **Resp:** cough, dyspnea, IMMUNE-MEDIATED PNEUMONITIS. **Misc:** fever, INFECTION, INFUSION-RELATED REACTIONS.

Interactions

Drug-Drug: None reported.

Route/Dosage

Unresectable Stage III Non-Small Cell Lung Cancer

IV (Adults ≥30 kg): 10 mg/kg every 2 wk *or* 1500 mg every 4 wk; continue until disease progression, unacceptable toxicity, or a maximum of 12 mo.
IV (Adults <30 kg): 10 mg/kg every 2 wk; continue until disease progression, unacceptable toxicity, or a maximum of 12 mo.

Metastatic Non-Small Cell Lung Cancer

IV (Adults ≥30 kg): *Nonsquamous:* Cycles 1–4: 1500 mg on Day 1 every 3 wk (administered prior to platinum-based chemotherapy and following tremelimumab); Cycle 5 (3 wk after previous durvalumab dose): 1500 mg on Day 1 (administered prior to pemetrexed [if being used for maintenance]); Cycle 6 (4 wk after previous durvalumab dose): 1500 mg on Day 1 (administered prior to pemetrexed [if being used for maintenance] and following tremelimumab); Cycle 7 (4 wk after previous durvalumab dose) and beyond: 1500 mg on Day 1 every 4 wk (administered prior to pemetrexed [if being used for maintenance]); continue until disease progression or unacceptable toxicity. *Squamous:* Cycles 1–4: 1500 mg on Day 1 every 3 wk (administered prior to platinum-based chemotherapy and following tremelimumab); Cycle 5 (3 wk after previous durvalumab dose): 1500 mg on Day 1 (as monotherapy); Cycle 6 (4 wk after previous durvalumab dose): 1500 mg on Day 1 (administered following tremelimumab); Cycle 7 (4 wk after previous durvalumab dose) and beyond: 1500 mg on Day 1 every 4 wk (as monotherapy); continue until disease progression or unacceptable toxicity.

IV (Adults <30 kg): *Nonsquamous:* Cycles 1–4: 20 mg/kg on Day 1 every 3 wk (administered prior to platinum-based chemotherapy and following tremelimumab); Cycle 5 (3 wk after previous durvalumab dose): 20 mg/kg on Day 1 (administered prior to pemetrexed [if being used for maintenance]); Cycle 6 (4 wk after previous durvalumab dose): 20 mg/kg on Day 1 (administered prior to pemetrexed [if being used for maintenance] and following tremelimumab); Cycle 7 (4 wk after previous durvalumab dose) and beyond: 20 mg/kg on Day 1 every 4 wk (administered prior to pemetrexed [if being used for maintenance]); continue until disease progression or unacceptable toxicity. *Squamous:* Cycles 1–4: 20 mg/kg on Day 1 every 3 wk (administered prior to platinum-based chemotherapy and following tremelimumab); Cycle 5 (3 wk after previous durvalumab dose): 20 mg/kg on Day 1 (as monotherapy); Cycle 6 (4 wk after previous durvalumab dose): 20 mg/kg on Day 1 (administered following tremelimumab); Cycle 7 (4 wk after previous durvalumab dose) and beyond: 20 mg/kg on Day 1 every 4 wk (as monotherapy); continue until disease progression or unacceptable toxicity.

Neoadjuvant and Adjuvant Treatment of Resectable Non-Small Cell Lung Cancer

IV (Adults ≥30 kg): *Neoadjuvant therapy:* 1500 mg every 3 wk (administered prior to platinum-containing chemotherapy); continue for up to 4 cycles prior to surgery. *Adjuvant therapy:* 1500 mg every 4 wk (as monotherapy); continue for up to 12 cycles after surgery.

IV (Adults <30 kg): *Neoadjuvant therapy:* 20 mg/kg every 3 wk (administered prior to platinum-containing chemotherapy); continue for up to 4 cycles prior to surgery. *Adjuvant therapy:* 20 mg/kg every 4 wk (as monotherapy); continue for up to 12 cycles after surgery.

Extensive-Stage Small Cell Lung Cancer

IV (Adults ≥30 kg): 1500 mg every 3 wk for 4 cycles (administered prior to etoposide and either carboplatin or cisplatin on the same day); then 1500 mg every 4 wk (as monotherapy); continue until disease progression or unacceptable toxicity.

IV (Adults <30 kg): 20 mg/kg every 3 wk for 4 cycles (administered prior to etoposide and either carboplatin or cisplatin on the same day); then 20 mg/kg every 4 wk (as monotherapy); continue until disease progression or unacceptable toxicity.

Limited-Stage Small Cell Lung Cancer

IV (Adults ≥30 kg): 1500 mg every 4 wk; continue until disease progression, unacceptable toxicity, or a maximum of 24 mo.

IV (Adults <30 kg): 20 mg/kg every 4 wk; continue until disease progression, unacceptable toxicity, or a maximum of 24 mo.

Biliary Tract Cancer

IV (Adults ≥30 kg): 1500 mg every 3 wk for up to 8 cycles (administered prior to gemcitabine and cisplatin on the same day); then 1500 mg every 4 wk (as monotherapy); continue until disease progression or unacceptable toxicity.

IV (Adults <30 kg): 20 mg/kg every 3 wk for up to 8 cycles (administered prior to gemcitabine and cisplatin on the same day); then 20 mg/kg every 4 wk (as monotherapy); continue until disease progression or unacceptable toxicity.

Hepatocellular Carcinoma

IV (Adults ≥30 kg): 1500 mg administered following a single dose of tremelimumab on Day 1 of Cycle 1; then 1500 mg every 4 wk (as monotherapy); continue until disease progression or unacceptable toxicity.

IV (Adults <30 kg): 20 mg/kg administered following a single dose of tremelimumab on Day 1 of Cycle 1; then 20 mg/kg every 4 wk (as monotherapy); continue until disease progression or unacceptable toxicity.

dMMR Endometrial Cancer

IV (Adults ≥30 kg): 1120 mg every 3 wk for 6 cycles (administered prior to carboplatin and paclitaxel on the same day); then 1500 mg every 4 wk as monotherapy; continue until disease progression or unacceptable toxicity.

IV (Adults <30 kg): 15 mg/kg every 3 wk for 6 cycles (administered prior to carboplatin and paclitaxel on the same day); then 20 mg/kg every 4 wk as monotherapy; continue until disease progression or unacceptable toxicity.

Muscle Invasive Bladder Cancer

IV (Adults ≥30 kg): *Neoadjuvant therapy:* 1500 mg every 3 wk (administered prior to gemcitabine and cisplatin); continue for 4 cycles prior to surgery. *Adjuvant therapy:* 1500 mg every 4 wk

D

(as monotherapy); continue for up to 8 cycles after surgery.

IV (Adults <30 kg): *Neoadjuvant therapy:* 20 mg/kg every 3 wk (administered prior to gemcitabine and cisplatin); continue for 4 cycles prior to surgery. *Adjuvant therapy:* 20 mg/kg every 4 wk (as monotherapy); continue for up to 8 cycles after surgery.

Availability

Solution for injection: 50 mg/mL.

NURSING IMPLICATIONS

Assessment

- Monitor for signs and symptoms of pneumonitis (new or worsening cough, chest pain, dyspnea). *If Grade 2 pneumonitis occurs,* hold durvalumab and administer prednisone 1–2 mg/kg/day (or equivalent); resume durvalumab when pneumonitis is Grade ≤1 after corticosteroid taper over ≥1 mo. *If no partial or complete resolution occurs 12 wk after corticosteroid initiation, inability to ↓ dose to ≤10 mg prednisone equivalent per day within 12 wk of corticosteroid initiation when part of tremelimumab containing regimen, or for Grade 3 or 4 pneumonitis,* permanently discontinue durvalumab.
- Assess for signs and symptoms of colitis (diarrhea, severe abdominal pain, bloody or tarry stools) and intestinal perforation. *If Grade 2 or 3 colitis occurs,* hold durvalumab and administer prednisone 1–2 mg/kg/day (or equivalent); resume durvalumab when colitis is Grade ≤1 after corticosteroid taper over ≥1 mo. *For Grade 3 when part of tremelimumab containing regimen, Grade 4 colitis, or any Grade perforation,* permanently discontinue durvalumab.
- Monitor for signs and symptoms of adrenal insufficiency, diabetes, hyperthyroidism, hypothyroidism, and hypophysitis periodically. *If Grade 3–4 symptoms occur,* hold durvalumab and treat as clinically indicated until stable or permanently discontinue durvalumab depending on severity.
- Assess for rash periodically during therapy. Topical emollients and/or topical corticosteroids may be adequate to treat mild to moderate nonexfoliative rashes. *If SJS, TEN, or DRESS suspected,* hold durvalumab and initiate prednisone 1–2 mg/kg/day (or equivalent) followed by taper, until Grade ≤1 and ≤10 mg/day of prednisone (or equivalent) within 12 wk of corticosteroid initiation when part of tremelimumab containing regimen. *If SJS, TEN, or DRESS confirmed,* permanently discontinue durvalumab.
- Monitor for signs and symptoms of infection (fever, cough, frequent urination, pain with urination, flu-like symptoms) prior to and periodically during therapy. *If Grade 3 or 4 infection occurs,* hold durvalumab until clinically stable.
- Monitor for signs and symptoms of infusion-related reactions (fever, chills, flushing, itching or rash, dizziness, dyspnea, wheezing, back pain, neck pain, feeling faint, facial swelling). *For Grade 1 or 2 infusion-related reactions when part of tremelimumab containing regimen,* hold or slow rate of infusion. *For Grade 3 or 4 infusion-related reactions when part of tremelimumab containing regimen,* stop infusion and permanently discontinue durvalumab.
- Monitor for other immune-mediated reactions (aseptic meningitis, hemolytic anemia, immune thrombocytopenic purpura, myositis, uveitis, keratitis). *For Grade 2 immune-mediated reactions,* exclude other causes and initiate corticosteroids as indicated. *For Grade 3 or 4 immune-mediated reactions,* administer prednisone 1–4 mg/kg/day (or equivalent), followed by taper. Hold or permanently discontinue durvalumab for severe reaction.
- Monitor for signs and symptoms of myocarditis (chest pain, irregular heartbeats, shortness of breath, swelling of ankles). *If Grade 2, 3, or 4 myocarditis occurs when part of tremelimumab containing regimen,* permanently discontinue durvalumab.
- Monitor for signs and symptoms of neurological toxicities (meningitis, encephalitis, myelitis, myasthenic syndrome/myasthenia gravis including exacerbation, Guillain-Barré syndrome, nerve paresis, neuropathy). *If Grade 2 neurological toxicities occur when part of tremelimumab containing regimen,* hold durvalumab and begin prednisone 1–2 mg/kg/day (or equivalent) until Grade ≤1; then initiate corticosteroid taper over ≥1 mo. *If Grade 3 or 4 neurological toxicities occur,* permanently discontinue durvalumab.

Lab Test Considerations

- Verify negative pregnancy test before starting therapy.
- Select patients for treatment of endometrial cancer based on presence of dMMR in tumor specimen. FDA-approved tests for dMMR status is available at https://www.fda.gov/companiondiagnostics.
- Monitor for signs and symptoms of hepatitis. **In patients with no hepatic tumor involvement:** *For ALT or AST >3 but ≤8 times upper limit of normal (ULN) or total bilirubin >1.5 but ≤3 times ULN when part of tremelimumab containing regimen,* hold durvalumab until Grade ≤1 and administer prednisone ≤10 mg/day (or equivalent). *For ALT or AST >8 times ULN or total bilirubin >3 times ULN,* permanently discontinue durvalumab. **In patients with hepatic tumor involvement:** *If AST or ALT >1 but <3 times ULN at baseline and ↑ to >5 but <10 times ULN OR AST or ALT >3 but*

<5 times ULN at baseline and ↑ to >8 but <10 times ULN when part of tremelimumab containing regimen, hold dose and administer prednisone 1–2 mg/kg/day (or equivalent) until Grade ≤1; then initiate corticosteroid taper over ≥1 mo. *If AST or ALT ↑ to >10 times ULN or total bilirubin ↑ to >3 times ULN,* permanently discontinue durvalumab.

- Monitor thyroid function prior to and periodically during therapy.
- Monitor blood glucose periodically during therapy. May cause hypoglycemia.
- Monitor renal function prior to and during therapy. Initiate prednisone 1–2 mg/kg/day (or equivalent) for Grade 2–4 nephritis, followed by taper. *If Grade 2 or 3 ↑ serum creatinine occurs when part of tremelimumab containing regimen,* hold durvalumab until Grade ≤1 and ≤10 mg/day of prednisone (or equivalent) needed. *If Grade 4 ↑ serum creatinine occurs,* permanently discontinue durvalumab.
- May cause hypocalcemia, hyponatremia, and hyperkalemia.

Implementation

- Weigh patient before each infusion.

IV Administration

- **Intermittent Infusion: Dilution:** Dilute with 0.9% NaCl or D5W. Invert gently to mix; do not shake. Solution is clear to opalescent, colorless to slightly yellow. Do not administer solutions that are cloudy, discolored, or contain particulates. **Concentration:** 1–15 mg/mL. Administer immediately after preparation. May be stored for up to 28 hr in refrigerator or up to 8 hr at room temperature. Do not freeze. **Rate:** Administer over 60 min through a sterile, low-protein-binding 0.2- or 0.22-micron in-line filter.
- **Y-Site Incompatibility:** Do not administer other drugs through same IV line.

Patient/Family Teaching

- Explain purpose and side effects of medication. Advise patient to read *Patient Information* before starting therapy.
- Advise patient to notify health care provider immediately if signs and symptoms of pneumonitis, hepatitis (jaundice, severe nausea or vomiting, pain on right side of abdomen, lethargy, easy bruising or bleeding, dark urine, light-colored stools), colitis, adrenal insufficiency (prolonged or unusual headache, feeling cold, extreme tiredness, constipation, weight gain or loss, deepening voice, dizziness or fainting, ↑ urination, ↑ hunger or thirst, nausea or vomiting, hair loss, abdominal pain, changes in mood or behavior, ↓ sex drive, irritability, forgetfulness), nephritis (↓ urine output, hematuria, ankle edema, loss of appetite, rash, itching, skin blistering), or infusion-related reactions occur.
- Advise patient to inform health care provider if neck stiffness, fatigue, excessive bleeding or bruising, confusion, muscle weakness or pain, fever, vision changes, chest pain, shortness of breath, irregular heartbeat, eye pain or redness, or mood or behavior changes occur.
- Advise patient to notify health care provider of all Rx or OTC medications, vitamins, or herbal products being taken and to consult with health care provider before taking other medications.
- Rep: May cause fetal harm. Advise women of reproductive potential to use effective contraception and avoid breastfeeding during therapy and for ≥3 mo after last dose. Advise women of reproductive potential to notify health care provider if pregnancy is planned or suspected or if breastfeeding.

Evaluation/Desired Outcomes

- Improved overall survival in NSCLC, small cell lung cancer, biliary tract cancer, hepatocellular carcinoma, and bladder cancer.
- Improved progression-free survival in endometrial cancer.

dutasteride (doo-tas-te-ride)

Avodart

Classification

Therapeutic: benign prostatic hyperplasia (BPH) agents

Pharmacologic: androgen inhibitors

Indications

Management of the symptoms of benign prostatic hyperplasia (BPH) in men with an enlarged prostate gland (as monotherapy or in combination with tamsulosin).

Action

Inhibits the enzyme 5-alpha-reductase, which is responsible for converting testosterone to its potent metabolite 5-alpha-dihydrotestosterone in the prostate gland and other tissues. 5-alpha-dihydrotestosterone is partly responsible for prostatic hyperplasia. **Therapeutic Effects:** Reduced prostate size with associated decrease in urinary symptoms.

Pharmacokinetics

Absorption: Well absorbed (60%) following oral administration; also absorbed through skin.

Distribution: 11.5% of serum concentration partitions into semen.

Protein Binding: 99% bound to albumin; 96.6% bound to alpha-1 glycoprotein.
Metabolism and Excretion: Mostly metabolized by the liver via the CYP3A4 isoenzyme; metabolites are excreted in feces.
Half-life: 5 wk.

TIME/ACTION PROFILE (↓ in dihydrotestosterone levels†)

ROUTE	ONSET	PEAK	DURATION
PO	unknown	1–2 wk	unknown

† Symptoms may only improve over 3–12 mo.

Contraindications/Precautions

Contraindicated in: Hypersensitivity; Cross-sensitivity with other 5-alpha-reductase inhibitors may occur.
Use Cautiously in: Hepatic impairment.

Adverse Reactions/Side Effects

Derm: rash, urticaria. **Endo:** gynecomastia. **GU:** ↓ libido, ejaculation disorders, erectile dysfunction, PROSTATE CANCER (HIGH-GRADE), testicular pain, testicular swelling. **Neuro:** depression. **Misc:** HYPERSENSITIVITY REACTIONS (INCLUDING ANGIOEDEMA).

Interactions

Drug-Drug: CYP3A4 inhibitors, including **ritonavir**, **ketoconazole**, **verapamil**, **diltiazem**, **cimetidine**, and **ciprofloxacin**, may ↑ levels and risk of toxicity.

Route/Dosage

PO (Adults): 0.5 mg once daily.

Availability (generic available)

Soft gelatin capsules: 0.5 mg. ***In combination with:*** tamsulosin (Jalyn); see Appendix N.

NURSING IMPLICATIONS

Assessment

- Assess patient for symptoms of BPH (urinary hesitancy, feeling of incomplete bladder emptying, interruption of urinary stream, impairment of size and force of urinary stream, terminal urinary dribbling, straining to start flow, dysuria, urgency) before and periodically during therapy.
- Digital rectal examinations should be performed before and periodically during therapy for BPH.

Lab Test Considerations

- Serum prostate-specific antigen (PSA) concentrations, used to screen for prostate cancer, ↓ by about 20% within the 1st mo of therapy and stabilize at about 50% of the pretreatment level within 6 mo. New baseline PSA concentrations should be established at 3 and 6 mo of therapy and evaluated periodically during therapy. Any ↑ in PSA during dutasteride therapy may be a sign of prostate cancer and should be evaluated, even those within normal limits. Isolated PSA values from men taking dutasteride for 3 mo or more should be doubled for comparison in untreated men.

Implementation

- Capsules should only be handled and administered with gloved hands.
- **PO:** Administer once daily with or without meals. ***DNC:*** Do not break, crush, or chew capsule.

Patient/Family Teaching

- Explain the purpose and side effects. Instruct patient to take dutasteride at the same time each day as directed, even if symptoms improve or are unchanged. Take missed doses as soon as remembered later in the day or omit dose. Do not make up by taking double doses the next day. Swallow capsule whole; do not chew or open capsule, to avoid mouth and throat irritation. Advise patient to read *Patient Information* before starting and with each Rx refill in case of changes.
- Caution patient that sharing of dutasteride may be dangerous.
- Inform patient that the volume of ejaculate may be ↓ during therapy but that this will not interfere with normal sexual function.
- Advise patient to avoid donating blood for ≥6 mo after last dose of dutasteride to prevent a pregnant woman from receiving dutasteride through a blood transfusion.
- Inform patient of potential ↑ risk in high-grade prostate cancer.
- Emphasize the importance of periodic follow-up exams to determine whether a clinical response has occurred.
- Rep: Caution patient that dutasteride poses a potential risk to a male fetus. Women who are pregnant or may become pregnant should avoid exposure to semen of a partner taking dutasteride and should not handle dutasteride because of the potential for absorption. If a pregnant woman comes into contact with dutasteride, wash the area immediately with soap and water.

Evaluation/Desired Outcomes

- Decrease in urinary symptoms of BPH.

econazole, See ANTIFUNGALS (TOPICAL).

REMS

eculizumab (e-ku-liz-ue-mab)

Bkemv, Epysqli, Soliris

Classification

Therapeutic: hemostatic agents

Pharmacologic: complement inhibitors

Indications

Bkemv, Epysqli, and Soliris: Treatment of the following conditions: Paroxysmal nocturnal hemoglobinuria; Atypical hemolytic uremic syndrome. **Soliris and Epysqli:** Generalized myasthenia gravis in patients who are antiacetylcholine receptor antibody positive. **Soliris:** Neuromyelitis optica spectrum disorder in patients who are anti-aquaporin-4 antibody positive.

Action

Eculizumab is a monoclonal antibody that binds to complement protein C5. This binding inhibits complement activation, a necessary step in the initiation of hemolysis due to paroxysmal nocturnal hemoglobinuria and the development of thrombotic microangiopathy in atypical hemolytic uremic syndrome. Its mechanism of effect in generalized myasthenia gravis and neuromyelitis optica spectrum disorder is unknown. **Therapeutic Effects:** Decreased hemolysis associated with paroxysmal nocturnal hemoglobinuria. Reduced complement-mediated thrombotic microangiopathy in atypical hemolytic uremic syndrome. Improved ability to perform activities of daily living in generalized myasthenia gravis. Decreased relapse rates in neuromyelitis optica spectrum disorder.

Pharmacokinetics

Absorption: IV administration results in complete bioavailability.

Distribution: Distributed to tissues.

Metabolism and Excretion: Unknown.

Half-life: 272 hr.

TIME/ACTION PROFILE

ROUTE	ONSET	PEAK	DURATION
IV	rapid	end of infusion	1–2 wk

Contraindications/Precautions

Contraindicated in: Unresolved serious *Neisseria meninigitidis* infection; Patients not vaccinated against *Neisseria meninigitidis* (unless risk of delaying treatment outweighs risks of developing a meningococcal infection) (vaccinate ≥2 wk prior to 1st dose).

Use Cautiously in: Systemic infection; OB: Use during pregnancy only if potential maternal benefit justifies potential fetal risk; Lactation: Safety not established in breastfeeding; Pedi: Safety and effectiveness not established for treatment of paroxysmal nocturnal hemoglobinuria or generalized myasthenia gravis in children.

Adverse Reactions/Side Effects

CV: hypertension, tachycardia, peripheral edema. **EENT:** nasopharyngitis, sinusitis, vertigo. **GI:** diarrhea, nausea, vomiting, constipation. **Hemat:** anemia, leukopenia. **MS:** back pain, extremity pain, myalgia. **Neuro:** headache, insomnia, fatigue. **Resp:** cough. **Misc:** fever, *Haemophilus influenzae* infection, herpes simplex infection, influenza-like illness, MENINGOCOCCAL INFECTIONS, *Neisseria gonorrhoeae* infection, *Streptococcus pneumoniae* infection.

Interactions

Drug-Drug: Plasma exchange, plasmapheresis, or **fresh frozen plasma** may ↓ levels and effectiveness; administer supplemental dose of eculizumab. **Neonatal Fc receptor blockers** may ↓ levels and effectiveness.

Route/Dosage

Paroxysmal Nocturnal Hemoglobinuria

IV (Adults): *Bkemv, Epysqli, or Soliris:* 600 mg once weekly during Weeks 1–4 (total of 4 doses); then 900 mg one wk later during Week 5; then 900 mg every 2 wk.

Atypical Hemolytic Uremic Syndrome

IV (Adults): *Bkemv, Epysqli, or Soliris:* 900 mg once weekly during Weeks 1–4 (total of 4 doses); then 1200 mg one wk later during Week 5; then 1200 mg every 2 wk; *Supplemental dose if patient receiving plasmapheresis or plasma exchange:* Bkemv, Epysqli, or Soliris: 600 mg per each plasmapheresis or plasma exchange session; *Supplemental dose if patient receiving fresh frozen plasma infusion:* Bkemv, Epysqli, or Soliris: 300 mg per infusion of fresh frozen plasma.

IV (Children<18 yr and ≥40 kg): *Bkemv, Epysqli, or Soliris:* 900 mg once weekly during Weeks 1–4 (for a total of 4 doses); then 1200 mg one wk later during Week 5; then 1200 mg every 2 wk; *Supplemental dose if patient receiving plasmapheresis or plasma exchange:* Bkemv, Epysqli, or Soliris: 600 mg per each plasmapheresis or plasma exchange session; *Supplemental dose if patient receiving fresh frozen plasma infusion:* Bkemv, Epysqli, or Soliris: 300 mg per infusion of fresh frozen plasma.

IV (Children<18 yr and 30–<40 kg): *Bkemv, Epysqli, or Soliris:* 600 mg once weekly during Weeks 1 and 2 (total of 2 doses); then 900 mg one wk later during Week 3; then 900 mg every 2 wk; *Supplemental dose if patient receiving plasmapheresis or plasma*

exchange: Bkemv, Epysqli, or Soliris: 600 mg per each plasmapheresis or plasma exchange session; *Supplemental dose if patient receiving fresh frozen plasma infusion:* Bkemv, Epysqli, or Soliris: 300 mg per infusion of fresh frozen plasma.
IV (Children<18 yr and 20–<30 kg): *Bkemv, Epysqli, or Soliris:* 600 mg once weekly during Weeks 1 and 2 (total of 2 doses); then 600 mg one wk later during Week 3; then 600 mg every 2 wk; *Supplemental dose if patient receiving plasmapheresis or plasma exchange:* Bkemv, Epysqli, or Soliris: 600 mg per each plasmapheresis or plasma exchange session; *Supplemental dose if patient receiving fresh frozen plasma infusion:* Bkemv, Epysqli, or Soliris: 300 mg per infusion of fresh frozen plasma.
IV (Children<18 yr and 10–<20 kg): *Bkemv, Epysqli, or Soliris:* 600 mg initially during Week 1; then 300 mg one wk later during Week 2; then 300 mg every 2 wk; *Supplemental dose if patient receiving plasmapheresis or plasma exchange:* Bkemv, Epysqli, or Soliris: 300 mg per each plasmapheresis or plasma exchange session; *Supplemental dose if patient receiving fresh frozen plasma infusion:* Bkemv, Epysqli, or Soliris: 300 mg per infusion of fresh frozen plasma.
IV (Children<18 yr and 5–<10 kg): *Bkemv, Epysqli, or Soliris:* 300 mg initially during Week 1; then 300 mg one wk later during Week 2; then 300 mg every 3 wk; *Supplemental dose if patient receiving plasmapheresis or plasma exchange:* Bkemv, Epysqli, or Soliris: 300 mg per each plasmapheresis or plasma exchange session; *Supplemental dose if patient receiving fresh frozen plasma infusion:* Bkemv, Epysqli, or Soliris: 300 mg per infusion of fresh frozen plasma.

Generalized Myasthenia Gravis

IV (Adults): *Epysqli or Soliris:* 900 mg once weekly during Weeks 1–4 (total of 4 doses); then 1200 mg one wk later during Week 5; then 1200 mg every 2 wk; *Supplemental dose if patient receiving plasmapheresis or plasma exchange:* Epysqli or Soliris: 600 mg per each plasmapheresis or plasma exchange session; *Supplemental dose if patient receiving fresh frozen plasma infusion:* Epysqli or Soliris: 300 mg per infusion of fresh frozen plasma.

Neuromyelitis Optica Spectrum Disorder

IV (Adults): *Soliris: Soliris:* 900 mg once weekly during Weeks 1–4 (total of 4 doses); then 1200 mg one wk later during Week 5; then 1200 mg every 2 wk.

Availability

Solution for injection: 10 mg/mL.

NURSING IMPLICATIONS

Assessment

- Monitor for hypersensitivity reactions, including anaphylaxis and infusion-related reactions, during infusion and for ≥1 hr following. *If reactions occur,* infusion may be slowed or stopped, if infusion completed within 2 hr.
- Monitor for early signs and symptoms of meningococcal infections. Evaluate immediately if infection is suspected. Consider discontinuation of therapy during treatment of serious meningococcal infections.
- Patients who discontinue eculizumab are at ↑ risk for serious hemolysis (serum LDH levels > pretreatment level with either >25% absolute ↓ in paroxysmal nocturnal hemoglobinuria clone size [in the absence of dilution due to transfer] in ≤1 wk, hemoglobin <5 g/dL, or ↓ in hemoglobin of >4 g/dL in ≤1 wk), angina, change in mental status, 50% ↑ in serum creatinine level, or thrombosis. Monitor patients who discontinue therapy for ≥8 wk to detect serious hemolysis or other reactions. *If serious reactions occur,* consider blood transfusion (packed RBCs) or exchange transfusion if the paroxysmal nocturnal hemoglobinuria RBCs are >50% of total RBCs by flow cytometry, anticoagulation, corticosteroids, or reinstitution of eculizumab.

Lab Test Considerations

- Serum LDH levels ↑ during hemolysis and may assist in monitoring effects of eculizumab, including response to discontinuation of therapy. Monitor patients after discontinuing for ≥8 wk to detect hemolysis.

Implementation

- ***REMS:*** Only available through enrollment in restricted programs. *Bkemv* REMS: 1-866-718-6927 or www.bkemvrems.com. *Epysqli* REMS: 1-866-318-8144 or www.epysqlirems.com Ultomiris *and Soliris* REMS: 1-888-SOLIRIS 1-888-765-4747 or www.ultsolrems.com.
- Vaccinate patient with meningococcal vaccine ≥2 wk prior to 1st dose; revaccinate according to current medical guidelines. If eculizumab must be started immediately and patient is not up to date with vaccine, provide antibacterial drug prophylaxis and administer meningococcal vaccine as soon as possible. Children should also be vaccinated for *Streptococcus pneumoniae* and *Haemophilus influenza* type b prior to treatment with eculizumab.

IV Administration

- **Intermittent Infusion:** Withdraw required amount of eculizumab from vial into sterile syringe and transfer to an infusion bag. **Dilution:** Dilute with equal amount of drug volume to 0.9% NaCl, 0.45% NaCl, D5W, or LR. Final admixture is 60 mL for 300-mg dose, 120 mL for 600-mg dose, 180 mL for 900-mg dose, or 240 mL for 1200-mg dose. Gently invert bag to ensure thorough mixing; discard unused portion in vial. Prior to administration, allow admixture to adjust to room temperature. Solution is clear to opalescent and colorless to slightly yellow; do not use solutions that are discolored or contain particulates. Solution is stable for 24 hr at room temperature or if refrigerated. **Concentration:** 5 mg/mL. **Rate:** Administer over 35 min (not to exceed 2 hr) for adults and 1–4 hr for children.

- **Y-Site Incompatibility:** Do not administer other drugs through same IV line.

Patient/Family Teaching

- Explain the risks and benefits of eculizumab to patient. Instruct patient to read the *Medication Guide* before starting therapy and with each dose in case of changes.
- Instruct patient to obtain required meningococcal vaccination ≥2 wk prior to therapy and revaccinate according to guidelines. Caution patient to report symptoms of meningococcal infection (moderate to severe headache with nausea or vomiting, headache, fever, or stiff neck or back; fever ≥103°F; rash; confusion; severe muscle aches with flu-like symptoms; eyes sensitive to light). Inform patient or caregiver that vaccination does not eliminate risk of serious meningococcal infections, despite development of antibodies.
- Inform patients that eculizumab may ↑ risk of other infections. Encourage patient and caregiver to notify health care professional of signs and symptoms of infection and maintain current vaccinations.
- Advise patient to notify health care professional of all Rx or OTC medications, vitamins, or herbal products being taken and to consult with health care professional before taking other medications.
- Inform patient to carry the *Patient Safety Card* at all times during and for 3 mo following therapy due to ↑ risk of meningococcal infection.
- Advise patient with paroxysmal nocturnal hemoglobinuria of potential for serious hemolysis when eculizumab is discontinued and of need for monitoring by health care professional for ≥8 wk following discontinuation. Caution patient to notify health care professional immediately if a large ↓ in RBC count causing anemia, confusion, chest pain, kidney problems, and blood clots occurs.
- Advise patient with atypical hemolytic uremic syndrome of potential for serious thrombotic microangiopathy when eculizumab is discontinued and of need for monitoring by health care professional for ≥12 wk following discontinuation. Caution patient to notify health care professional immediately if changes in mental status, seizures, angina, dyspnea, or thrombosis occur.
- Rep: Advise women of reproductive potential to notify health care professional if pregnancy is planned or suspected or if breastfeeding.

Evaluation/Desired Outcomes

- Reduced hemolysis resulting in improvements in anemia (↑ hemoglobin stabilization, ↓ need for RBC transfusions), ↓ fatigue, and improved health-related quality of life.
- Inhibition of complement-mediated thrombotic microangiopathy in patients with atypical hemolytic uremic syndrome.
- Improved ability to perform activities of daily living in generalized myasthenia gravis.
- Decreased relapse rates in neuromyelitis optica spectrum disorder.

E

HIGH ALERT

edoxaban (e-dox-a-ban)

Lixiana, Savaysa

Classification

Therapeutic: anticoagulants

Pharmacologic: factor Xa inhibitors

Indications

Reduction of stroke/systemic embolization risk associated with nonvalvular atrial fibrillation (AF). Treatment of deep vein thrombosis (DVT) and pulmonary embolism (PE) following 5–10 days of initial therapy with a parenteral anticoagulant.

Action

Selective inhibitor of factor Xa. Does not inhibit platelet aggregation directly, but does inhibit thrombin-induced platelet aggregation. Decreases thrombin generation and thrombus development. **Therapeutic Effects:** Decreased thrombotic events associated with AF, including stroke and systemic embolization. Resolution of DVT and PE.

Pharmacokinetics

Absorption: 62% absorbed following oral administration.

Distribution: Widely distributed to tissues.

Metabolism and Excretion: Minimal metabolism; one metabolite is pharmacologically active. Excreted mostly unchanged in urine.

Half-life: 10–14 hr.

TIME/ACTION PROFILE (anticoagulant effect)

ROUTE	ONSET	PEAK	DURATION
PO	unknown	1–2 hr	24 hr

Contraindications/Precautions

Contraindicated in: Active bleeding; CCr >95 mL/min (↓ effectiveness); Concurrent use of other anticoagulants or rifampin; Presence of mechanical heart valves or severe mitral stenosis; Moderate to severe hepatic impairment; Triple-positive antiphospholipid syndrome (↑ risk of thrombosis); Lactation: Lactation.

Use Cautiously in: Elective/planned invasive/surgical procedures (discontinue at least 24 hr prior to ↓ risk of bleeding); Premature discontinuation (↑ risk of ischemic events); Neuroaxial spinal anesthesia or spinal puncture, especially if concurrent with an indwelling epidural catheter; drugs affecting hemostasis; history of traumatic/repeated spinal puncture; or spinal deformity (↑ risk of spinal hematoma); Renal impairment (↓ dose for CCr 15–50 mL/min); Deteriorating or improving renal function (may require dose change); Body weight ≤60 kg (requires lower dose); Rep: Women of reproductive potential; OB: Use during pregnancy only if potential maternal benefit justifies potential fetal risk; Pedi: Safety and effectiveness not established in children.

Adverse Reactions/Side Effects

GI: ↑ liver enzymes. **Hemat:** anemia, BLEEDING.

Interactions

Drug-Drug: **Rifampin** may ↓ levels and effectiveness; concurrent use contraindicated. ↑ risk of bleeding with other **anticoagulants, aspirin, clopidogrel, ticagrelor, prasugrel, fibrinolytics, NSAIDs, SNRIs**, or **SSRIs. P-glycoprotein (P-gp) inhibitors**, including **azithromycin, clarithromycin, erythromycin, itraconazole** (oral), **ketoconazole** (oral), **quinidine**, or **verapamil**, may ↑ levels and risk of bleeding; lower dose required.

Route/Dosage

Treatment of Nonvalvular Atrial Fibrillation

PO (Adults): 60 mg once daily.

Renal Impairment

PO (Adults): *CCr 15–50 mL/min:* 30 mg once daily.

Treatment of Deep Vein Thrombosis/Pulmonary Embolism

PO (Adults >60 kg): 60 mg once daily. *Concurrent use of P-gp inhibitors (verapamil, quinidine, azithromycin, clarithromycin, erythromycin, itraconazole [PO], or ketoconazole [PO]):* 30 mg once daily.
PO (Adults ≤60 kg): 30 mg once daily.

Renal Impairment

PO (Adults): *CCr 15–50 mL/min:* 30 mg once daily.

Availability

Tablets: 15 mg, 30 mg, 60 mg.

NURSING IMPLICATIONS

Assessment

- Monitor for bleeding. Discontinue edoxaban if active bleeding occurs. Anticoagulant effects of edoxaban persist for about 24 hr after last dose. Anticoagulant effects cannot be reliably monitored with standard laboratory tests. No reversal agent is available; protamine sulfate, vitamin K, and tranexamic acid do not reverse anticoagulant activity. May consider prothrombin complex concentrate (PCC) or other procoagulant reversal agents such as activated prothrombin complex concentrate or recombinant factor VIIa. If PCC is used, monitoring anticoagulation effect of edoxaban using clotting test (PT, INR, or aPTT) or anti-FXa activity is not useful. Hemodialysis does not significantly contribute to edoxaban clearance.
- Calculate a HAS-BLED score (hypertension, abnormal renal and liver function, stroke, bleeding, labile INRs, elderly, and drugs or alcohol) in high-risk patients at every follow-up to assess the risk of major bleeding during therapy.
- Monitor frequently for signs and symptoms of neurological impairment (numbness or weakness of legs, bowel or bladder dysfunction, back pain, tingling, muscle weakness); if noted, urgent treatment is required. Intrathecal or epidural catheters should not be removed earlier than 12 hr after last dose of edoxaban. Next dose of edoxaban should not be given <2 hr after removal of catheter.

Lab Test Considerations

- Assess renal function before starting therapy and periodically during treatment; frequency of monitoring depends on individual patient factors, including baseline renal function, concurrent drug therapy, comorbidities, and age. Monitor at least every 6 mo, every 3–6 mo in patients with renal impairment (CCr < 60 mL/min), or during an acute illness that may worsen renal function. Assess CCr using Cockcroft-Gault equation CCr = (140 − age) × (weight in kg) × (0.85 if female)/(72 × serum creatinine in mg/dL). Assess liver function at baseline and then yearly in healthy patients (every 3–6 mo in patients at risk of hepatic impairment or at-risk older adult patients [≥75 yr]). Assess CBC during initiation and at regular intervals (at least yearly) to assess trends in hemoglobin/hematocrit; assess more frequently if needed, especially in patients with active bleeding symptoms.

Implementation

- Discontinue edoxaban ≥24 hr prior to invasive or surgical procedures; may ↑ risk of bleeding. Edoxaban may be restarted as soon as adequate hemostasis is established; time to onset of pharmacodynamic effect is 1–2 hr.
- **PO:** Tablets may be crushed and mixed with 2–3 ounces of water and immediately administered by mouth or through a gastric tube. May also be mixed with applesauce and administered immediately.
- *If transitioning from warfarin or other vitamin K antagonists to edoxaban,* discontinue warfarin and start edoxaban when INR ≤2.5. *If transitioning from oral anticoagulants other than warfarin or other vitamin K antagonists to edoxaban,* discontinue current oral anticoagulant and start edoxaban at time of next scheduled dose of other oral anticoagulant. *If transitioning from low molecular weight heparin*

(LMWH) to edoxaban, discontinue LMWH and start edoxaban at time of next scheduled administration of LMWH. *If transitioning from unfractionated heparin to edoxaban,* discontinue infusion and start edoxaban 4 hr later.

- *If transitioning from edoxaban to warfarin:* **Oral Option:** For patients taking 60 mg of edoxaban, ↓ dose to 30 mg and begin warfarin concurrently. For patients taking 30 mg of edoxaban, ↓ dose to 15 mg and begin warfarin concurrently. Measure INR at least weekly and just prior to daily dose of edoxaban to minimize influence of edoxaban on INR measurements. Once stable INR ≥2.0 achieved, discontinue edoxaban and continue warfarin. **Parenteral Option:** Discontinue edoxaban and administer a parenteral anticoagulant and warfarin at time of next scheduled edoxaban dose. Once stable INR ≥2.0 achieved, discontinue parenteral anticoagulant and continue warfarin. *If transitioning from edoxaban to non-vitamin-K dependent oral anticoagulant,* discontinue edoxaban and start other oral anticoagulant at time of next dose of edoxaban. *If transitioning from edoxaban to parenteral anticoagulant,* discontinue edoxaban and start parenteral anticoagulant at time of next dose of edoxaban.
- If edoxaban is discontinued, consider starting another anticoagulant; discontinuation of edoxaban ↑ risk of thromboembolic events.

Patient/Family Teaching

- Explain purpose and side effects of medication to patient. Instruct patient to take as directed. Take missed doses as soon as remembered on same day. Return to regular schedule next day. Do not double doses in one day. Do not discontinue without consulting health care provider; may ↑ risk of stroke, DVT, or PE. If temporarily discontinued, restart as soon as possible. Advise patient to read *Medication Guide* before starting therapy and with each Rx refill in case of changes.
- Caution patient that they may bleed more easily, longer, or bruise more easily during therapy. Advise patient to notify health care provider immediately if bleeding or a fall, especially with head injury, occurs.
- Advise patient to notify health care provider of all Rx or OTC medications, vitamins, or herbal products being taken and to consult with health care provider before taking other medications, especially aspirin or NSAIDs.
- Inform patient having had neuraxial anesthesia or spinal puncture to watch for signs and symptoms of spinal or epidural hematoma (numbness or weakness of legs, bowel or bladder dysfunction). Notify health care provider immediately if symptoms occur.
- Advise patient to notify health care provider of therapy before surgery, medical, or dental procedures are scheduled.
- Rep: Advise women of reproductive potential to notify health care provider if pregnancy is planned or suspected and to avoid breastfeeding during therapy. May ↑ risk of uterine bleeding in women of reproductive potential and those with abnormal uterine bleeding. Monitor neonates for bleeding.

Evaluation/Desired Outcomes

- Decreased thrombotic events (stroke and systemic embolization) associated with nonvalvular AF.
- Treatment of deep vein thrombosis DVT and pulmonary embolism PE.

efinaconazole, See ANTIFUNGALS (TOPICAL).

elagolix (el-a-goe-lix)

Orilissa

Classification

Therapeutic: analgesics

Pharmacologic: GnRH antagonist

Indications

Moderate to severe pain associated with endometriosis.

Action

Competitively binds to and inhibits gonadotropin-releasing hormone receptors in the pituitary gland, causing a decrease in the release of estradiol and progesterone by the ovaries. **Therapeutic Effects:** Reduction in dysmenorrhea and nonmenstrual pelvic pain.

Pharmacokinetics

Absorption: Rapidly absorbed.

Distribution: Unknown.

Metabolism and Excretion: Primarily metabolized in the liver via the CYP3A isoenzyme with some metabolism by the CYP2D6 and CYP2C8 isoenzymes as well as UGT. 90% of dose excreted in feces; <3% in urine.

Half-life: 4–6 hr.

TIME/ACTION PROFILE (plasma concentrations)

ROUTE	ONSET	PEAK	DURATION
PO	unknown	1 hr	24 hr

Contraindications/Precautions

Contraindicated in: Hypersensitivity; Osteoporosis (may ↑ risk of bone loss); Severe hepatic impairment; Concurrent use of strong organic anion transporting polypeptide (OATP) 1B1 inhibitors; OB: Pregnancy.

Use Cautiously in: History of low-trauma fracture or other risk factors for osteoporosis; History of suicidal thoughts/behaviors or depression; Moderate hepatic impairment (use lower dose); Lactation: Use while breastfeeding only if potential maternal benefit justifies potential risk to infant; Rep: Women of reproductive potential; Pedi: Safety and effectiveness not established in children.

Adverse Reactions/Side Effects

Derm: rash. **Endo:** hot flush, night sweats. **GI:** nausea, ↑ liver enzymes, abdominal pain, constipation, diarrhea. **GU:** ↓ libido, menstrual irregularities. **Metab:** dyslipidemia, weight gain. **MS:** ↓ bone density, arthralgia. **Neuro:** headache, anxiety, depression, dizziness, insomnia, mood swings, SUICIDAL THOUGHTS/BEHAVIOR. **Misc:** HYPERSENSITIVITY REACTIONS (INCLUDING ANAPHYLAXIS AND ANGIOEDEMA).

Interactions

Drug-Drug: **Strong OATP1B1 inhibitors**, including **cyclosporine** and **gemfibrozil**, may significantly ↑ levels and risk of toxicity; concurrent use contraindicated. **Estrogen-containing oral contraceptives** may ↓ effectiveness; impact of **progestin-containing oral contraceptives** on effectiveness unknown; recommended to use nonhormonal contraceptives. May ↑ estrogen exposure when used with **estrogen-containing contraceptives**, which may ↑ risk of thromboembolic events. May ↓ levels and effectiveness of **levonorgestrel-containing oral contraceptives**. May ↓ levels and effectiveness of **CYP3A substrates**, including **midazolam**. May ↑ levels and risk of toxicity of **CYP2C19 substrates**, including **omeprazole**; consider ↓ omeprazole dose when using higher doses (>40 mg/day). May ↑ levels and risk of toxicity of **P-glycoprotein substrates**, including **digoxin**; closely monitor digoxin levels. **Strong CYP3A inhibitors** may ↑ levels and risk of toxicity; limit concurrent use with elagolix 200 mg twice daily to ≤1 mo; limit concurrent use with elagolix 150 mg once daily to ≤6 mo. **CYP3A inducers**, including **rifampin**, may ↓ levels and effectiveness; concurrent use with elagolix 200 mg twice daily not recommended; limit concurrent use with elagolix 150 mg once daily to ≤6 mo. May ↓ levels and effectiveness of **rosuvastatin**; consider ↑ rosuvastatin dose.

Route/Dosage

PO (Adults): *No dyspareunia:* 150 mg once daily for max duration of 24 mo.; *Coexisting dyspareunia:* 200 mg twice daily for max duration of 6 mo.

Hepatic Impairment

PO (Adults): *Moderate hepatic impairment:* 150 mg once daily for max duration of 6 mo.

Availability

Tablets: 150 mg, 200 mg. ***In combination with:*** estradiol/norethindrone (Oriahnn). See Appendix N.

NURSING IMPLICATIONS

Assessment

- Evaluate baseline pain levels and symptomatic response to therapy.
- Assess bone mineral density in patients with a history of a low-trauma fracture or other risk factors for osteoporosis or bone loss. Vitamin D and calcium supplements may be considered. Use lowest effective dose for limited duration to minimize bone loss, which may not be completely reversible after therapy discontinuation.
- Monitor for signs and symptoms of hepatotoxicity (fatigue, nausea, upper abdominal pain, jaundice, scleral icterus, dark urine, clay-colored stools).
- Assess for depression and mood changes during therapy. Refer patients with new or worsening depression, anxiety or other mood changes, or suicidal ideation and behavior to a mental health professional. Consider benefits and risks of continuing elagolix.

Lab Test Considerations

- Verify negative pregnancy test before starting therapy.
- Monitor liver function tests periodically during therapy. May ↑ AST and ALT. Use lowest effective dose and assess risks versus benefit of continuing therapy if ↑ transaminase occurs.
- May ↑ lipid levels during first 2 mo of therapy; then usually remains stable.

Implementation

- **PO:** Administer at the same time each day without regard to food.

Patient/Family Teaching

- Explain the purpose and side effects of elagolix. Instruct patient to take as directed at approximately the same time each day. Take missed doses as soon as remembered if same day as missed dose; then return to regular dosing schedule; do not double doses. Advise patient to read *Medication Guide* before starting and with each Rx refill in case of changes.
- Inform patient that elagolix may change menstrual periods (irregular bleeding or spotting, ↓ in menstrual bleeding, no bleeding at all) and make pregnancy difficult to detect. Watch for other signs of pregnancy (breast tenderness, weight gain, nausea).
- May cause depression or suicide. Instruct patients and caregivers to monitor for emergence of suicidal thoughts and behaviors. Notify health care professional immediately if suicidal thoughts; new or worsening depression; anxiety; changes in behavior or mood; thoughts of suicide, dying, or hurting self; or acting on dangerous impulses occur. Instruct patient to carry wallet card and to call the National Suicide Prevention Lifeline at 1-800-273-8255 or visit www.988lifeline.org if they experience suicidal thoughts.
- Advise patient and family to notify health care professional if signs and symptoms of liver problems

(yellowing of skin or whites of eyes, dark amber-colored urine, feeling tired, nausea and vomiting, generalized swelling, right upper abdomen pain, bruising easily) occur.

- Instruct patient to maintain adequate intake of calcium and vitamin D during therapy due to the risk of bone loss.
- Advise patient to notify health care professional of all Rx or OTC medications, vitamins, or herbal products being taken and to consult with health care professional before taking other medications, especially birth control pills.
- Rep: May result in pregnancy loss if used in early pregnancy. Advise women of reproductive potential to use effective nonhormonal contraception during therapy and for 28 days after last dose. Hormonal contraceptives may ↓ effectiveness of elagolix and may ↑ risk of thromboembolic and vascular disorders. Advise patient to notify health care professional if pregnancy is planned or suspected or if breastfeeding. Encourage patient to enroll in pregnancy registry to monitor outcomes while taking elagolix by calling 1-833-782-7241 or by visiting bloompregnancyregistry.com. Discontinue elagolix if pregnancy occurs.

Evaluation/Desired Outcomes

- Reduction in dysmenorrhea and nonmenstrual pelvic pain.

elagolix/estradiol/norethindrone

(**el**-a-**goe**-lix/es-tra-**dye**-ole/nor-eth-**in**-drone)

Oriahnn

Classification

Therapeutic: hemostatic agents, hormones

Pharmacologic: GnRH antagonist, estrogens, progestins

Indications

Heavy menstrual bleeding associated with uterine fibroids in premenopausal women.

Action

Elagolix: Competitively binds to and inhibits gonadotropin-releasing hormone receptors in the pituitary gland, causing a decrease in the release of estradiol and progesterone by the ovaries, reducing bleeding associated with uterine fibroids. *Estradiol:* Binds to estrogen receptors and reduces the increase in bone resorption and potential bone loss associated with elagolix. *Norethindrone:* Protects uterus from potential adverse endometrial effects caused by unopposed estrogen use. **Therapeutic Effects:** Reduced menstrual blood loss.

Pharmacokinetics

Elagolix

Absorption: Rapidly absorbed following oral administration.

Distribution: Unknown.

Metabolism and Excretion: Primarily metabolized in the liver via the CYP3A isoenzyme with some metabolism by the CYP2D6 and CYP2C8 isoenzymes as well as UGT. 90% of dose excreted in feces; <3% in urine.

Half-life: 4–6 hr.

Estradiol

Absorption: Well absorbed following oral administration.

Distribution: Widely distributed.

Protein Binding: 98%.

Metabolism and Excretion: Metabolized by the liver via the CYP3A isoenzyme; also undergoes sulfation and glucuronidation. Enterohepatic recirculation occurs; more absorption may occur from the GI tract.

Half-life: 8–20 hr.

Norethindrone

Absorption: Rapidly absorbed following oral administration.

Distribution: Unknown.

Protein Binding: 97%.

Metabolism and Excretion: Metabolized by the liver via the CYP3A isoenzyme.

Half-life: 5–13 hr.

TIME/ACTION PROFILE (plasma concentrations)

ROUTE	ONSET	PEAK	DURATION
PO	rapid	1–2 hr	unknown

Contraindications/Precautions

Contraindicated in: Hypersensitivity to elagolix, estradiol, or norethindrone; History of cigarette smoking and age >35 yr (↑ risk of cardiovascular or thromboembolic phenomenon); Thromboembolic disease (e.g., deep vein thrombosis [DVT], pulmonary embolism [PE], MI, stroke); Uncontrolled hypertension; Cerebrovascular disease, coronary artery disease, or peripheral vascular disease; Valvular heart disease or thrombogenic heart rhythms; Protein C, protein S, or antithrombin deficiency or other thrombophilic disorder; Headache with focal neurological symptoms or migraine headaches with aura in women >35 yr; Major surgery with extended periods of immobility; Osteoporosis (may ↑ risk of bone loss); Breast cancer or other hormone-sensitive malignancy; ↑ risk for hormone sensitive malignancy; Hepatic impairment; Undiagnosed abnormal uterine bleeding;

Concurrent use of strong organic anion transporting polypeptide (OATP) 1B1 inhibitors; OB: Pregnancy.
Use Cautiously in: Aspirin hypersensitivity (contains tartrazine, which may cause allergic reaction); History of low-trauma fracture or other risk factors for osteoporosis; History of suicidal thoughts/behaviors or depression; Controlled hypertension; Diabetes; Hypertriglyceridemia (↑ risk of pancreatitis); Lactation: Use while breastfeeding only if potential maternal benefit justifies potential risk to infant; Rep: Women of reproductive potential; Pedi: Safety and effectiveness not established in children.

Adverse Reactions/Side Effects

CV: ↑ BP, alopecia, DVT, MI. **Endo:** hot flush, hyperglycemia. **GI:** ↑ liver enzymes, cholelithiasis, vomiting. **GU:** ↓ libido, metrorrhagia. **Metab:** hyperlipidemia, weight gain. **MS:** ↓ bone density, arthralgia. **Neuro:** depression, headache, mood swings, STROKE, SUICIDAL THOUGHTS/BEHAVIOR. **Resp:** PE. **Misc:** fatigue, MALIGNANCY (BREAST, ENDOMETRIAL, OVARIAN).

Interactions

Drug-Drug: **Strong OATP1B1 inhibitors**, including **rifampin**, may significantly ↑ elagolix levels and risk of toxicity; concurrent use contraindicated. **Corticosteroids**, **anticonvulsants**, and **proton pump inhibitors** may ↑ risk for bone loss. Elagolix may ↓ levels and effectiveness of **CYP3A substrates**, including **midazolam**; consider ↑ midazolam dose. Elagolix may ↑ levels and risk of toxicity of **CYP2C19 substrates**, including **omeprazole**; consider ↓ omeprazole dose when using higher doses (>40 mg/day). Elagolix may ↑ levels and risk of toxicity of **P-glycoprotein substrates**, including **digoxin**; closely monitor digoxin levels. May ↓ **rosuvastatin** levels and effectiveness; consider ↑ rosuvastatin dose. **Strong CYP3A inhibitors** may ↑ elagolix, estradiol, and norethindrone levels and risk of toxicity; concurrent use not recommended. **Strong CYP3A inducers** may ↓ elagolix, estradiol, and norethindrone levels and effectiveness.

Route/Dosage

PO (Adults): One morning capsule (elagolix 300 mg/estradiol 1 mg/norethindrone 0.5 mg) every morning and one evening capsule (elagolix 300 mg) every evening. Continue for no longer than 24 mo.

Availability

Capsules: elagolix 300 mg/estradiol 1 mg/norethindrone 0.5 mg (morning capsule); elagolix 300 mg (evening capsule).

NURSING IMPLICATIONS

Assessment

- Monitor amount of menstrual bleeding during therapy.
- Monitor for signs and symptoms of thromboembolic disorders and vascular events (pain, swelling, or tenderness in extremities; headache; chest pain; blurred vision; sudden, unexplained partial or complete loss of vision; proptosis; diplopia; papilledema retinal vascular lesions) during therapy. *If symptoms occur,* discontinue therapy and evaluate for retinal vein thrombosis if visual changes occur.
- Assess bone mineral density by dual-energy x-ray absorptiometry (DXA) at baseline and periodically during therapy. *If risk associated with bone loss exceeds benefit of therapy,* consider discontinuing therapy and recommending calcium and vitamin D supplementation.
- Assess for new or worsening depression, anxiety, or other mood changes periodically during therapy. *If symptoms occur,* refer to mental health professional and reevaluate benefits and risks of therapy.
- Monitor BP prior to and periodically during therapy. Hold therapy for significant ↑ in BP.

Lab Test Considerations

- Verify negative pregnancy test within 7 days from onset of menses.
- May ↑ AST and ALT.
- May ↑ blood glucose levels. Monitor blood glucose more frequently in patient with prediabetes and diabetes.
- Monitor lipid levels periodically during therapy. May ↑ total cholesterol, LDL-C, HDL-C, and triglycerides.

Implementation

- **PO:** Administer morning and evening doses at same times each day without regard to food.

Patient/Family Teaching

- Explain purpose and side effects of medication. Advise patient to read *Patient Information* before starting therapy.
- Instruct patient to take missed doses within 4 hr of original time; then take next scheduled dose. If missed dose is >4 hr of original time, omit and take next scheduled dose.
- Advise patient to stop taking medication and notify health care provider immediately if signs and symptoms of cardiovascular conditions (leg pain or swelling that will not go away; sudden shortness of breath; double vision; bulging of the eyes; sudden blindness, partial or complete; pain or pressure in chest, arm, or jaw; sudden, severe headache unlike usual headaches; weakness or numbness in an arm or leg; trouble speaking) occur.
- Inform patient of risk of bone loss. Advise patient to take supplementary calcium and vitamin D and to avoid taking iron supplements at same time.
- Instruct patient to pay attention to changes in mood, behaviors, thoughts, or feelings. Advise patients to notify health care provider immediately if signs and symptoms of suicidal ideation and behavior changes (thoughts about suicide or dying, suicide attempts, new or worse depression, new or worse anxiety) occur.
- Advise patient to notify health care provider if signs and symptoms of liver injury (jaundice, dark amber-colored urine, feeling tired, nausea and

vomiting, generalized swelling, right upper stomach area pain, bruising easily) occur.

- Advise patient that alopecia and hair thinning in no specific pattern may occur and may not completely resolve after discontinuing therapy. Advise patient to consult health care provider with concerns about changes to hair.
- Caution patient that cigarette smoking during estrogen therapy may ↑ risk of serious side effects, especially for women over age 35.
- Instruct patient to notify health care provider of all Rx or OTC medications, vitamins, or herbal products being taken and to avoid concurrent use of Rx, OTC, and herbal products without consulting health care provider.
- Dispose unused medication via a take-back option if available. Otherwise, follow FDA instructions for disposing medication in the household trash: www.fda.gov/drugdisposal. Do NOT flush down the toilet.
- Rep: Inform patient that therapy may ↓ menstrual bleeding or result in no bleeding, making it hard to detect pregnancy; watch for other signs of pregnancy (breast tenderness, weight gain, nausea). May result in pregnancy loss if used in early pregnancy. Advise women of reproductive potential to use effective nonhormonal contraception during therapy and for 1 wk after last dose. Hormonal contraceptives may ↓ effectiveness of elagolix and ↑ risk of thromboembolic and vascular events. Advise patient to notify health care provider if pregnancy is planned or suspected or if breastfeeding. Encourage patients who become pregnant during therapy to enroll in pregnancy exposure registry: 1-833-782-7241; https://www.bloompregnancyregistry.com.

Evaluation/Desired Outcomes

- Reduced menstrual blood loss.

elexacaftor/tezacaftor/ivacaftor

(e-lex-a-**kaf**-tor/tez-a-**kaf**-tor/**eye**-va-**kaf**-tor)

Trikafta

Classification

Therapeutic: cystic fibrosis therapy adjuncts

Pharmacologic: transmembrane conductance regulator potentiators

Indications

Cystic fibrosis (CF) in patients who have ≥1 F508del mutation in the cystic fibrosis transmembrane conductance regulator (CFTR) gene or a mutation in the CFTR gene that is responsive based on clinical and/or in vitro data.

Action

Elexacaftor and tezacaftor: Facilitate the cellular processing and trafficking of F508del-CFTR to increase the amount of mature CFTR protein delivered to the cell surface. *Ivacaftor:* Acts as a potentiator of the CFTR protein (a chloride channel on the surface of endothelial cells), facilitating chloride transport by increasing the channel-open probability (gating). **Therapeutic Effects:** Improved lung function.

Pharmacokinetics

Elexacaftor

Absorption: Well absorbed (88%) following oral administration; absorption is enhanced 2-fold by moderate-fat-containing foods.
Distribution: Well distributed to tissues.
Protein Binding: >99%.
Metabolism and Excretion: Primarily metabolized in liver via the CYP3A4 and CYP3A5 isoenzymes; one metabolite (M23) is pharmacologically active; 87% excreted in feces (primarily as metabolite); <1% excreted in urine.
Half-life: 30 hr.

Tezacaftor

Absorption: Some absorption following oral administration.
Distribution: Widely distributed to tissues.
Protein Binding: >99%.
Metabolism and Excretion: Primarily metabolized in liver via the CYP3A4 and CYP3A5 isoenzymes; one metabolite (M1) is pharmacologically active; 72% excreted in feces as unchanged drug or metabolite; 14% excreted in urine (primarily as metabolite).
Half-life: 15 hr.

Ivacaftor

Absorption: Some absorption following oral administration; absorption is enhanced 3-fold by fat-containing foods.
Distribution: Widely distributed to tissues.
Protein Binding: >99%.
Metabolism and Excretion: Primarily metabolized in liver via the CYP3A4 and CYP3A5 isoenzymes; one metabolite (M1) is pharmacologically active; 87.8% eliminated in feces; negligible urinary elimination.
Half-life: 14 hr.

TIME/ACTION PROFILE (plasma concentrations)

ROUTE	ONSET	PEAK	DURATION
Elexacaftor (PO)	unknown	6 hr	24 hr
Tezacaftor (PO)	unknown	4 hr	12 hr
Ivacaftor (PO)	unknown	6 hr	12 hr

Contraindications/Precautions

Contraindicated in: Severe hepatic impairment.
Use Cautiously in: Moderate hepatic impairment (not recommended; if necessary, use only if benefit outweighs risk; dose ↓ recommended); Severe renal impairment or end-stage renal disease; OB: Safety not established in pregnancy; Lactation: Safety not established in breastfeeding; Pedi: Children <6 yr (safety and effectiveness not established).

Adverse Reactions/Side Effects

Derm: rash. **EENT:** nasal congestion, cataracts, rhinitis, rhinorrhea, sinusitis. **GI:** ↑ liver enzymes, abdominal pain, diarrhea, HEPATOTOXICITY, hyperbilirubinemia. **MS:** ↑ CK. **Neuro:** headache. **Resp:** upper respiratory tract infection. **Misc:** HYPERSENSITIVITY REACTIONS (INCLUDING ANAPHYLAXIS), influenza.

Interactions

Drug-Drug: Strong CYP3A inducers, including **carbamazepine**, **phenobarbital**, **phenytoin**, **rifabutin**, and **rifampin**, may ↓ elexacaftor, tezacaftor, and ivacaftor levels and effectiveness; avoid concurrent use. **Strong CYP3A inhibitors**, including **clarithromycin**, **itraconazole**, **ketoconazole**, **posaconazole**, and **voriconazole**, and **moderate CYP3A inhibitors**, including **erythromycin** and **fluconazole**, may ↑ elexacaftor, tezacaftor, and ivacaftor levels and risk of toxicity; dose adjustment recommended. May ↑ levels and risk of bleeding with **warfarin**; monitor INR closely. May ↑ levels and risk of hypoglycemia with **glimepiride** or **glipizide**. May ↑ levels of **P-glycoprotein substrates**, including **cyclosporine**, **digoxin**, **everolimus**, **sirolimus**, and **tacrolimus**. May ↑ levels of **glyburide**, **nateglinide**, **repaglinide**, and **statins**. **Hormonal contraceptives** may ↑ risk of rash.
Drug-Natural Products: St. John's wort may ↓ elexacaftor, tezacaftor, and ivacaftor levels and effectiveness; avoid concurrent use.
Drug-Food: Grapefruit juice may ↑ elexacaftor, tezacaftor, and ivacaftor levels; avoid concurrent use.

Route/Dosage

PO (Adults and Children ≥12 yr): Two elexacaftor 100-mg/tezacaftor 50-mg/ivacaftor 75-mg tablets in am and one ivacaftor 150-mg tablet in pm (approximately 12 hr apart) with fat-containing food. *Concurrent use of strong CYP3A inhibitor:* Two elexacaftor 100-mg/tezacaftor 50-mg/ivacaftor 75-mg tablets given twice weekly (3–4 days apart) in am. Do not give pm ivacaftor dose on any of the days. *Concurrent use of moderate CYP3A inhibitor:* Two elexacaftor 100-mg/tezacaftor 50-mg/ivacaftor 75-mg tablets in am on Day 1; then one ivacaftor 150-mg tablet in am on Day 2; continue this regimen on alternate days in am. Do not give pm ivacaftor dose on any of the days.
PO (Children 6–11 yr and ≥30 kg): Two elexacaftor 100-mg/tezacaftor 50-mg/ivacaftor 75-mg tablets in am and one ivacaftor 150-mg tablet in pm (approximately 12 hr apart) with fat-containing food. *Concurrent use of strong CYP3A inhibitor:* Two elexacaftor 100-mg/tezacaftor 50-mg/ivacaftor 75-mg tablets given twice weekly (3–4 days apart) in am. Do not give pm ivacaftor dose on any of the days. *Concurrent use of moderate CYP3A inhibitor:* Two elexacaftor 100-mg/tezacaftor 50-mg/ivacaftor 75-mg tablets in am on Day 1; then one ivacaftor 150-mg tablet in am on Day 2; continue this regimen on alternate days in am. Do not give pm ivacaftor dose on any of the days.
PO (Children 6–11 yr and <30 kg): Two elexacaftor 50-mg/tezacaftor 25-mg/ivacaftor 37.5-mg tablets in am and one ivacaftor 75-mg tablet in pm (approximately 12 hr apart) with fat-containing food. *Concurrent use of strong CYP3A inhibitor:* Two elexacaftor 50-mg/tezacaftor 25-mg/ivacaftor 37.5-mg tablets given twice weekly (3–4 days apart) in am. Do not give pm ivacaftor dose on any of the days. *Concurrent use of moderate CYP3A inhibitor:* Two elexacaftor 50-mg/tezacaftor 25-mg/ivacaftor 37.5-mg tablets in am on Day 1; then one ivacaftor 75-mg tablet in am on Day 2; continue this regimen on alternate days in am. Do not give pm ivacaftor dose on any of the days.
PO (Children 2–5 yr and ≥14 kg): One packet (containing elexacaftor 100 mg/tezacaftor 50 mg/ivacaftor 75 mg oral granules) in am and one packet (containing ivacaftor 75-mg oral granules) in pm (approximately 12 hr apart) with fat-containing food. *Concurrent use of strong CYP3A inhibitor:* One packet (containing elexacaftor 100 mg/tezacaftor 50 mg/ivacaftor 75 mg oral granules) twice weekly (given 3–4 days apart). Do not give pm ivacaftor dose on any of the days. *Concurrent use of moderate CYP3A inhibitor:* One packet (containing elexacaftor 100 mg/tezacaftor 50 mg/ivacaftor 75 mg oral granules) in am on Day 1; then one packet (containing ivacaftor 75-mg oral granules) in am on Day 2; continue this regimen on alternate days in am. Do not give pm ivacaftor dose on any of the days.
PO (Children 2–5 yr and <14 kg): One packet (containing elexacaftor 80 mg/tezacaftor 40 mg/ivacaftor 60 mg oral granules) in am and one packet (containing ivacaftor 59.5-mg oral granules) in pm (approximately 12 hr apart) with fat-containing food. *Concurrent use of strong CYP3A inhibitor:* One packet (containing elexacaftor 80 mg/tezacaftor 40 mg/ivacaftor 60 mg oral granules) twice weekly (given 3–4 days apart). Do not give pm ivacaftor dose on any of the days. *Concurrent use of moderate CYP3A inhibitor:* One packet (containing elexacaftor 80 mg/tezacaftor 40 mg/ivacaftor 60 mg oral granules) in am on Day 1; then one packet (containing ivacaftor 59.5-mg oral granules) in am on Day 2; continue this regimen on alternate days in am. Do not give pm ivacaftor dose on any of the days.

Hepatic Impairment

(Adults and Children ≥12 yr): *Moderate hepatic impairment:* Two elexacaftor 100-mg/tezacaftor 50-mg/ivacaftor 75-mg tablets in am on Day 1; then one elexacaftor 100-mg/tezacaftor 50-mg/ivacaftor 75-mg tablet in am on Day 2. Continue this regimen on alternate days in am. Do not give ivacaftor 150-mg tablet in pm on any day.

Hepatic Impairment

(Adults and Children 6–11 yr and ≥30 kg): *Moderate hepatic impairment:* Two elexacaftor 100-mg/tezacaftor 50-mg/ivacaftor 75-mg tablets in am on Day 1; then one elexacaftor 100-mg/tezacaftor 50-mg/ivacaftor 75-mg tablet in am on Day 2. Continue this regimen on alternate days in am. Do not give ivacaftor 150-mg tablet in pm on any day.

Hepatic Impairment

(Adults and Children 6–11 yr and <30 kg): *Moderate hepatic impairment:* Two elexacaftor 50-mg/tezacaftor 25-mg/ivacaftor 37.5-mg tablets in am on Day 1; then one elexacaftor 50-mg/tezacaftor 25-mg/ivacaftor 37.5-mg tablet in am on Day 2. Continue this regimen on alternate days in am. Do not give ivacaftor 75-mg tablet in pm on any day.

Hepatic Impairment

(Adults and Children 2–5 yr and ≥14 kg): *Moderate hepatic impairment:* One packet (containing elexacaftor 100 mg/tezacaftor 50 mg/ivacaftor 75 mg oral granules) in am on Days 1–3. No dose on Day 4. One packet (containing elexacaftor 100 mg/tezacaftor 50 mg/ivacaftor 75 mg oral granules) in am on Days 5 and 6. No dose on Day 7. Continue this weekly dosing schedule in am. Do not give pm ivacaftor dose on any day of weekly dosing schedule.

Hepatic Impairment

(Adults and Children 2–5 yr and <14 kg): *Moderate hepatic impairment:* One packet (containing elexacaftor 80 mg/tezacaftor 40 mg/ivacaftor 60 mg oral granules) in am on Days 1–3. No dose on Day 4. One packet (containing elexacaftor 80 mg/tezacaftor 40 mg/ivacaftor 60 mg oral granules) in am on Days 5 and 6. No dose on Day 7. Continue this weekly dosing schedule in am. Do not give pm ivacaftor dose on any day of weekly dosing schedule.

Availability

Tablets: elexacaftor 50 mg/tezacaftor 25 mg/ivacaftor 37.5 mg (combo) + ivacaftor 75 mg (separate tablets), elexacaftor 100 mg/tezacaftor 50 mg/ivacaftor 75 mg (combo) + ivacaftor 150 mg (separate tablets). **Oral granules:** elexacaftor 80 mg/tezacaftor 40 mg/ivacaftor 60 mg (combo) + ivacaftor 59.5 mg (separate oral granules), elexacaftor 100 mg/tezacaftor 50 mg/ivacaftor 75 mg (combo) + ivacaftor 75 mg (separate oral granules).

NURSING IMPLICATIONS

Assessment

- Monitor lung function (FEV, lung sounds) before and periodically during therapy.
- Assess eyes for cataracts/opacities prior to and periodically during therapy.
- Monitor for signs and symptoms of hypersensitivity reactions (rash, urticaria, pruritus, flushing, dizziness, vomiting, abdominal pain) and angioedema (swelling of throat, lips, tongue, or face; dyspnea; wheezing; hoarseness). Discontinue immediately and provide supportive care.
- Monitor for signs and symptoms of hepatic impairment (fatigue, nausea, upper abdominal pain, jaundice, scleral icterus, dark urine, clay-colored stools).

Lab Test Considerations

- Determine patient's genotype prior to starting therapy. If genotype is unknown, use an FDA-cleared CF mutation test to detect the presence of a CFTR mutation, followed by verification with bidirectional sequencing when recommended by the mutation test instructions for use.
- Prior to initiation, obtain liver function (ALT, AST, alkaline phosphatase, and bilirubin) for all patients; then monitor every 3 mo during the 1st yr and annually thereafter. May cause ↑ serum transaminases and bilirubin. More frequent monitoring may be warranted in patients with a history of hepatobiliary disease or ↑ liver function tests. ALT or AST >5 times upper limit of normal (ULN) or ALT or AST >3 times ULN with bilirubin >2 times ULN and/or clinical symptoms suggestive of liver injury; hold therapy. Once AST or ALT have returned to normal, consider benefits and risks before resuming therapy.

Implementation

- **PO:** Administer tablets twice daily, 12 hr apart, with fat-containing food (meals or snacks that contain fat are those prepared with butter or oils or those containing eggs, cheeses, nuts, whole milk, or meats). ***DNC:*** Swallow tablets whole; do not crush, break, or chew.
- Administer oral granules immediately before or after ingestion of fat-containing food. Mix entire contents of each packet of oral granules with one teaspoon (5 mL) of age-appropriate soft food or liquid (pureed fruits or vegetables, yogurt, applesauce, water, milk, juice) that is at or below room temperature. Once mixed, consume product completely within 1 hr.

Patient/Family Teaching

- Explain the purpose and side effects of elexacaftor/tezacaftor/ivacaftor. Instruct patient to tablet take as directed with a fat-containing meal to ↑ absorption. Examples of fat-containing foods include whole milk, eggs, avocado, butter, peanut butter, or cheese pizza. Instruct patient or caregiver to mix entire contents of the granule packet with one teaspoon of soft food (pureed fruits or vegetables, yogurt, pudding, applesauce) or liquid (whole milk, breast milk, infant formula, juice) that is at or below room temperature and consume within 1 hr. Take missed doses within 6 hr of missed dose. If >6 hr since missed morning dose, take missed dose as soon as possible and omit the evening dose. Take next scheduled morning dose at usual time. If missed evening dose, omit the missed dose. Take next scheduled morning dose at usual time. Do not take morning and evening doses at same time. Advise patient or caregiver to read *Patient Information* before starting therapy and with each Rx refill in case of changes.
- Emphasize importance of regular follow-up, blood tests to monitor liver function, and eye examinations.
- Advise patient to avoid eating grapefruit or drinking grapefruit juice during therapy.
- May cause dizziness. Advise patient to avoid driving and other activities requiring alertness until response to medication is known.
- Advise patient to notify health care provider immediately if symptoms of liver problems (pain or discomfort in right abdominal area, yellowing of skin or whites of eyes, loss of appetite, nausea, vomiting, dark amber-colored urine) occur.
- Instruct patient to notify health care provider of all Rx or OTC medications, vitamins, or herbal products being taken and to consult with health care provider before taking other medications, especially St. John's wort.
- Rep: Advise women of reproductive potential to notify health care provider if pregnancy is planned or suspected or if breastfeeding.

Evaluation/Desired Outcomes

- Improved lung function.

eltrombopag (el-trom-bo-pag)

Alvaiz, Promacta, Revolade

Classification

Therapeutic: antithrombocytopenics

Pharmacologic: thrombopoietin receptor agonists

Indications

Promacta or Alvaiz: Treatment of the following: Persistent or chronic immune thrombocytopenia in patients who have had an inadequate response to corticosteroids, immunoglobulins, or splenectomy (should only be used in patients with an ↑ risk of bleeding); Thrombocytopenia in patients with chronic hepatitis C to allow the initiation and maintenance of interferon-based therapy; Severe aplastic anemia in patients who have had an inadequate response to immunosuppressive therapy. **Promacta:** First-line treatment of severe aplastic anemia (in combination with standard immunosuppressive therapy).

Action

Increases platelet production by initiating proliferation and differentiation of megakaryocytes from bone marrow progenitor cells. **Therapeutic Effects:** Increased blood counts.

Pharmacokinetics

Absorption: 52% absorbed following oral administration.

Distribution: Unknown.

Protein Binding: >99%.

Metabolism and Excretion: Extensively metabolized; 59% eliminated in feces, 20% as unchanged drug; 31% excreted in urine as metabolites.

Half-life: 21–35 hr.

TIME/ACTION PROFILE (effect on platelet count)

ROUTE	ONSET	PEAK	DURATION
PO	1 wk	2 wk	1 wk

Contraindications/Precautions

Contraindicated in: Lactation: Lactation.

Use Cautiously in: Myelodysplastic syndromes (may ↑ risk of hematologic malignancy); Patients of East/Southeast Asian ancestry (may require lower doses); Hepatic impairment (↓ initial dose); OB: Use during pregnancy only if potential maternal benefit justifies potential fetal risk; Pedi: Safety and effectiveness not established in children <6 yr (Alvaiz) or <1 yr (Promacta); Geri: Older adults may be more sensitive to drug effects; ↑ dose cautiously and consider age-related ↓ in renal and hepatic function, concurrent disease states and drug therapy.

Adverse Reactions/Side Effects

CV: DEEP VEIN THROMBOSIS (DVT), MI. **EENT:** development/worsening of cataracts. **GI:** HEPATOTOXICITY. **Neuro:** STROKE. **Resp:** PULMONARY EMBOLISM (PE).

Interactions

Drug-Drug: ↓ availability and absorption of **iron, calcium, aluminum, magnesium, selenium,** and **zinc** by chelation; give eltrombopag ≥2 hr before or 4 hr after medications containing these and other polyvalent cations. **Ribavirin and interferon** may ↑ risk of hepatic decompensation.

Drug-Food: ↓ availability and absorption of **iron, calcium, aluminum, magnesium, selenium,** and

zinc by chelation; do not administer within 4 hr of foods containing these and other polyvalent cations.

Route/Dosage

Promacta and Alvaiz should NOT be substituted for each other.

Persistent or Chronic Immune Thrombocytopenia

PO (Adults and Children ≥6 yr): *Promacta:* 50 mg once daily; may ↑ to achieve platelet count ≥50 × 10^9/L (not to exceed 75 mg/day); *Alvaiz:* 36 mg once daily; may ↑ to achieve platelet count ≥50 × 10^9/L (not to exceed 54 mg/day). *Patients of East/Southeast Asian ancestry: Promacta:* 25 mg once daily initially; may ↑ to achieve platelet count ≥50 × 10^9/L (not to exceed 75 mg/day); *Alvaiz:* 18 mg once daily initially; may ↑ to achieve platelet count ≥50 × 10^9/L (not to exceed 54 mg/day).

PO (Children 1–5 yr): *Promacta:* 25 mg once daily; may ↑ to achieve platelet count ≥50 × 10^9/L (not to exceed 75 mg/day).

Hepatic Impairment

(Adults): *Mild, moderate, or severe hepatic impairment:* Promacta: 25 mg once daily initially; may ↑ to achieve platelet count ≥50 × 10^9/L (not to exceed 75 mg/day); Alvaiz: 18 mg once daily initially; may ↑ to achieve platelet count ≥50 × 10^9/L (not to exceed 54 mg/day). *Patients of East/Southeast Asian ancestry with mild, moderate, or severe hepatic impairment: Promacta:* 12.5 mg once daily initially; may ↑ to achieve platelet count ≥50 × 10^9/L (not to exceed 75 mg/day); *Alvaiz:* 9 mg once daily initially; may ↑ to achieve platelet count ≥50 × 10^9/L (not to exceed 54 mg/day).

Chronic Hepatitis C-Associated Thrombocytopenia

PO (Adults): *Promacta:* 25 mg once daily; may ↑ by 25 mg every 2 wk to achieve the target platelet count required to initiate antiviral therapy; during antiviral therapy, adjust dose to avoid dose ↓ of peginterferon (not to exceed 100 mg/day); *Alvaiz:* 18 mg once daily; may ↑ by 18 mg every 2 wk to achieve the target platelet count required to initiate antiviral therapy; during antiviral therapy, adjust dose to avoid dose ↓ of peginterferon (not to exceed 72 mg/day).

First-Line Treatment of Severe Aplastic Anemia

PO (Adults and Children ≥12 yr): *Promacta:* 150 mg once daily for 6 mo. *Patients of East/Southeast Asian ancestry: Promacta:* 75 mg once daily for 6 mo.

PO (Children 6–11 yr): *Promacta:* 75 mg once daily for 6 mo. *Patients of East/Southeast Asian ancestry: Promacta:* 37.5 mg once daily for 6 mo.

PO (Children 2–5 yr): *Promacta:* 2.5 mg/kg once daily for 6 mo. *Patients of East/Southeast Asian ancestry: Promacta:* 1.25 mg/kg once daily for 6 mo.

Hepatic Impairment

PO (Adults and Children ≥12 yr): *Mild, moderate, or severe hepatic impairment: Promacta:* 75 mg once daily for 6 mo.

Hepatic Impairment

PO (Adults and Children 6–11 yr): *Mild, moderate, or severe hepatic impairment: Promacta:* 37.5 mg once daily for 6 mo.

Hepatic Impairment

PO (Adults and Children 2–5 yr): *Mild, moderate, or severe hepatic impairment: Promacta:* 1.25 mg/kg once daily for 6 mo.

Refractory Severe Aplastic Anemia

PO (Adults): *Promacta:* 50 mg once daily; may ↑ by 50 mg every 2 wk to achieve platelet count ≥50 × 10^9/L (not to exceed 150 mg/day); *Alvaiz:* 36 mg once daily; may ↑ by 36 mg every 2 wk to achieve platelet count ≥50 × 10^9/L (not to exceed 108 mg/day). *Patients of East/Southeast Asian ancestry: Promacta:* 25 mg once daily; may ↑ by 50 mg every 2 wk to achieve platelet count ≥50 × 10^9/L (not to exceed 150 mg/day); *Alvaiz:* 18 mg once daily; may ↑ by 36 mg every 2 wk to achieve platelet count ≥50 × 10^9/L (not to exceed 108 mg/day).

Hepatic Impairment

(Adults): *Mild, moderate, or severe hepatic impairment: Promacta:* 25 mg once daily; may by 50 mg every 2 wk to achieve platelet count ≥50 × 109/L (not to exceed 150 mg/day); *Alvaiz:* 18 mg once daily; may ↑ by 36 mg every 2 wk to achieve platelet count ≥50 × 109/L (not to exceed 108 mg/day).

Availability (generic available)

Powder for oral suspension (Promacta): 12.5 mg/pkt, 25 mg/pkt. **Tablets (Promacta):** 12.5 mg, 25 mg, 50 mg, 75 mg. **Tablets (Alvaiz):** 9 mg, 18 mg, 36 mg, 54 mg.

NURSING IMPLICATIONS

Assessment

- Monitor for unusual bleeding and bruising, thromboembolic events (DVT, PE, stroke, MI) and signs of hepatotoxicity during therapy. *If thromboembolism occurs,* discontinue eltrombopag and continue horse antithymocyte globulin (h-ATG) and cyclosporine.
- Monitor for signs and symptoms of cataracts. Perform baseline ocular examination prior to administration and periodically during therapy.

Lab Test Considerations

- May cause laboratory discoloration and interference with accurate results. Many tests may be impacted including bilirubin, serum creatinine, total protein, albumin, and others. Communicate to the lab that the patient is taking eltrombopag and consider retesting using other methods to determine validity of results.
- **For Chronic Immune Thrombocytopenia (*Promacta*):** Monitor CBC with differential weekly until platelets stable at ≥50 × 10^9/L. Modify dose based on platelet count. *If platelets <50 × 10^9/L following ≥2 wk of therapy*, ↑ daily dose by 25 mg (max = 75 mg/day). For dose of 12.5 mg once daily, ↑ to 25 mg once daily before ↑ daily dose by 25 mg. *If platelets 200 × 10^9/L–400 × 10^9/L*, ↓ daily dose by 25 mg. For dose of 25 mg once daily, ↓ to 12.5 once daily. Wait 2 wk to assess effects of dose adjustment. *If platelets >400 × 10^9/L*, stop *Promacta* and ↑ monitoring of platelets to twice weekly. Once platelets <150 × 10^9/L, reinitiate therapy by ↓ dose by 25 mg/day. For dose of 25 mg once daily, reinitiate at 12.5 mg once daily. *If platelets >400 × 10^9/L after 2 wk of therapy at lowest dose*, permanently discontinue *Promacta*. Discontinue *Promacta* if platelets do not ↑ to a level sufficient to avoid clinically important bleeding after 4 wk of therapy at max dose of 75 mg/day.
- **For Chronic Immune Thrombocytopenia (*Alvaiz*):** Monitor CBC with differential weekly until platelets stable at ≥50 × 10^9/L. Modify dose based on platelet count. *If platelets <50 × 10^9/L following ≥2 wk of therapy*, ↑ daily dose by 18 mg (max = 54 mg/day). For dose of 9 mg once daily, ↑ to 18 mg once daily before ↑ daily dose by 18 mg. *If platelets 200 × 10^9/L–400 × 10^9/L*, ↓ daily dose by 18 mg. For dose of 18 mg once daily, ↓ to 9 mg once daily. Wait 2 wk to assess effects of dose adjustment. *If platelets >400 × 10^9/L*, stop *Alvaiz* and ↑ monitoring of platelets to twice weekly. Once platelets <150 × 10^9/L, reinitiate therapy by ↓ dose by 18 mg/day. For dose of 18 mg once daily, reinitiate at 9 mg once daily. *If platelets >400 × 10^9/L after 2 wk of therapy at lowest dose*, permanently discontinue *Alvaiz*. Discontinue *Alvaiz* if platelets do not ↑ to a level sufficient to avoid clinically important bleeding after 4 wk of therapy at max dose of 54 mg/day.
- **Chronic Hepatitis C-Associated Thrombocytopenia (*Promacta*):** Monitor platelet counts every week prior to starting antiviral therapy. Goal is to achieve and maintain platelet count necessary to initiate and maintain antiviral therapy with pegylated interferon and ribavirin. Modify dose based on platelet count. Adjust dose in 25-mg increments every 2 wk as necessary for target platelet count required to initiate antiviral therapy. During antiviral therapy, adjust dose to avoid dose ↓ of peginterferon. Monitor CBC with differential weekly during antiviral therapy until stable platelet count achieved. Monitor platelet counts monthly thereafter. *If platelets <50 × 10^9/L following ≥2 wk of therapy*, ↑ daily dose by 25 mg (max = 100 mg/day). *If platelets 200 × 10^9/L–400 × 10^9/L*, ↓ daily dose by 25 mg. Wait 2 wk to assess effects of dose adjustment. *If platelets >400 × 10^9/L*, stop *Promacta*; ↑ monitoring of platelets to twice weekly. Once platelets <150 × 10^9/L, reinitiate therapy by ↓ dose by 25 mg/day. For dose of 25 mg once daily, reinitiate at 12.5 mg once daily. *If platelets >400 × 10^9/L after 2 wk of therapy at lowest dose*, permanently discontinue *Promacta*. Discontinue *Promacta* when antiviral therapy is discontinued.
- **Chronic Hepatitis C-Associated Thrombocytopenia (*Alvaiz*):** Monitor platelet counts every week prior to starting antiviral therapy. Goal is to achieve and maintain platelet count necessary to initiate and maintain antiviral therapy with pegylated interferon and ribavirin. Modify dose based on platelet count. Adjust dose in 18-mg increments every 2 wk as necessary for target platelet count required to initiate antiviral therapy. During antiviral therapy, adjust dose to avoid dose ↓ of peginterferon. Monitor CBC with differentials weekly during antiviral therapy until stable platelet count achieved. Monitor platelet counts monthly thereafter. *If platelets <50 × 10^9/L following ≥2 wk of therapy*, ↑ daily dose by 18 mg (max = 72 mg/day). *If platelets 200 × 10^9/L–400 × 10^9/L*, ↓ daily dose by 18 mg. Wait 2 wk to assess effects of dose adjustment. *If platelets >400 × 10^9/L*, stop *Alvaiz*; ↑ monitoring of platelets to twice weekly. Once platelets <150 × 10^9/L, reinitiate therapy by ↓ dose by 18 mg/day. For dose of 18 mg once daily, reinitiate at 9 mg once daily. *If platelets >400 × 10^9/L after 2 wk of therapy at lowest dose*, permanently discontinue *Alvaiz*. Discontinue *Alvaiz* when antiviral therapy is discontinued.
- **Aplastic Anemia (*Promacta*):** Goal is platelet count >50 × 10^9/L. Modify dose based on platelet count. *If platelets <50 × 10^9/L following ≥2 wk of therapy*, ↑ daily dose by 50 mg. For dose of 25 mg once daily, ↑ to 50 mg once daily before ↑ daily dose by 50 mg (max = 150 mg/day). *If platelets 200 × 10^9/L–400 × 10^9/L*, ↓ daily dose by 50 mg. Wait 2 wk to assess effects of dose adjustment. *If platelets >400 × 10^9/L*, stop *Promacta* for 1 wk. Once platelets <150 × 10^9/L, reinitiate therapy by ↓ dose by 50 mg/day. *If platelets >400 × 10^9/L after 2 wk of therapy at lowest dose*, permanently discontinue *Promacta*. If no hematologic response after 16 wk of therapy, discontinue *Promacta*.
- **Aplastic Anemia (*Alvaiz*):** Goal is platelet count >50 × 10^9/L. Modify dose based on platelet count. *If platelets <50 × 10^9/L following ≥2 wk of therapy*, ↑ daily dose by 36 mg. For dose of 18 mg once daily, ↑ to 36 mg once daily before ↑ daily dose by 50 mg (max = 150 mg/day). *If platelets 200 × 10^9/L–400 × 10^9/L*, ↓ daily dose by 50 mg. Wait 2 wk to assess

effects of dose adjustment. *If platelets >400 × 10⁹/L,* stop *Alvaiz* for 1 wk. Once platelets <150 × 10⁹/L, reinitiate therapy by ↓ dose by 50 mg/day. *If platelets >400 × 10⁹/L after 2 wk of therapy at lowest dose,* permanently discontinue *Alvaiz*. If no hematologic response after 16 wk of therapy, discontinue *Alvaiz*.

- When switching between *Promacta* oral suspension and tablet, assess platelet count weekly for 2 wk; then follow standard monthly monitoring.
- Monitor AST, ALT, and serum bilirubin before starting therapy, every 2 wk during dose adjustment, and monthly following stable dose. *If bilirubin ↑,* perform fractionation. *If transaminases abnormal,* repeat test in 3–5 days. *If abnormalities confirmed,* monitor serum transaminases weekly until resolved, stabilized, or returned to baseline. Discontinue eltrombopag if ALT levels ≥3 times upper limit of normal (ULN) in patients with normal liver function or ≥3 times baseline or >5 times ULN and progressively ↑, or persistent for ≥4 wk, or accompanied by ↑ direct bilirubin or symptoms of liver injury or hepatic decompensation.
- **First-line treatment of aplastic anemia (*Promacta*):** Measure ALT, AST, and bilirubin before starting therapy, every other day while hospitalized for h-ATG therapy, and then every 2 wk during therapy. Do not start *Promacta* if AST or ALT ≥6 times ULN. Once AST or ALT <5 times ULN, restart *Promacta* at same dose. *If AST or ALT >6 times ULN after restarting therapy,* discontinue therapy and monitor ALT or AST at least every 3–4 days. Once ALT or AST <5 times ULN, restart *Promacta* at dose ↓ from previous dose by 25 mg/day. *If AST or ALT >6 times ULN with ↓ dose,* ↓ daily dose by 25 mg until AST or ALT <5 times ULN. *In pediatric patient <12 yr,* ↓ daily dose by ≥15% to nearest dose that can be administered.

Implementation

- **PO:** Administer on an empty stomach or with food low in calcium (≤50 mg). *DNC:* Swallow tablets whole; do not crush, break, chew, or mix with food/liquids.
- Prepare oral suspension of *Promacta* with water only, using 40-mL reconstitution vessel and threaded closure with syringe-port capability provided; do not use hot water to prepare the suspension. Powder for suspension is reddish-brown to yellow. Administer suspension immediately after preparation with single-use oral syringe provided. Discard any suspension not administered within 30 min after preparation.
- Allow ≥4 hr between *Promacta* or *Alvaiz* and other medications (antacids), calcium-rich foods (containing >50 mg calcium [dairy products, calcium-fortified juices, certain fruits and vegetables]), and supplements containing polyvalent cations (iron, calcium, aluminum, magnesium, zinc, selenium).

Patient/Family Teaching

- Explain purpose and side effects of medication. Advise patient to read *Patient Information* before starting therapy.
- Instruct patient to avoid taking eltrombopag within 4 hr of food, mineral supplements, and antacids containing iron, calcium, aluminum, magnesium, zinc, and selenium.
- Advise patients to avoid activities and medications that may ↑ risk of bleeding.
- Advise patient of need for baseline ocular exam before starting therapy and monitoring for signs and symptoms of cataracts during therapy.
- Advise patient to notify health care provider of all Rx or OTC medications, vitamins, or herbal products being taken and to consult health care provider before taking other medications.
- Instruct patient to notify health care provider if symptoms of liver problems (yellowing of skin or whites of eyes, unusual darkening of urine, tiredness, pain or swelling in right upper abdomen, confusion) occur.
- Rep: May cause fetal harm. Advise women of reproductive potential to use effective contraception during and for ≥7 days after last dose, to notify health care provider promptly if pregnancy is planned or suspected, and to avoid breastfeeding.
- Emphasize the importance of routine lab tests to determine effectiveness and monitor for side effects.

Evaluation/Desired Outcomes

- Increased platelet counts and ↓ risk of bleeding. Platelet counts usually ↑ within 1–2 wk of starting and ↓ within 1–2 wk of discontinuing therapy.
- Increased blood counts. For patients with aplastic anemia, if no hematologic response after 16 wk of therapy, discontinue therapy.

elvitegravir/cobicistat/emtricitabine/tenofovir alafenamide

(el-vi-**teg**-ra-vir/koe-**bik**-i-stat/em-trye-**sye**-ta-been/ten-**of**-oh-vir al-a-**fen**-a-mide)

Genvoya

Classification

Therapeutic: antiretrovirals

Pharmacologic: integrase strand transfer inhibitors (INSTI), enzyme inhibitors, nucleoside reverse transcriptase inhibitors

Indications

HIV infection in treatment-naive adults. HIV infection in patients with HIV-1 RNA <50 copies/mL (to replace their current antiretroviral regimen) who are on a stable antiretroviral regimen for ≥6 mo, have no history of treatment failure, and have no known substitutions associated with resistance to the individual medications in the combination product.

Action

Elvitegravir: An integrase strand transfer inhibitor that inhibits an enzyme necessary for viral replication. *Cobicistat:* A pharmacokinetic enhancer (inhibits the CYP3A and CYP2D6 isoenzymes) that increases systemic exposure to elvitegravir. *Emtricitabine:* Phosphorylated intracellularly, where it inhibits HIV reverse transcriptase, resulting in viral DNA chain termination. *Tenofovir alafenamide:* Phosphorylated intracellularly, where it inhibits HIV reverse transcriptase resulting in disruption of DNA synthesis. When compared to tenofovir disoproxil fumarate, tenofovir alafenamide is associated with fewer episodes of renal impairment and reductions in bone mineral density. **Therapeutic Effects:** Slowed progression of HIV infection and decreased occurrence of sequelae.

Pharmacokinetics

Elvitegravir
Absorption: Absorption follows oral administration.
Distribution: Unknown.
Protein Binding: 98–99%.
Metabolism and Excretion: Metabolized by the liver via the CYP3A isoenzyme; 94.5% eliminated in feces; 6.7% in urine.
Half-life: 12.9 hr.

Cobicistat
Absorption: Absorption follows oral administration.
Distribution: Unknown.
Protein Binding: 97–98%.
Metabolism and Excretion: Metabolized by the liver via the CYP3A isoenzyme and to a lesser extent by the CYP2D6 isoenzyme; 86.2% eliminated in feces; 8.2% in urine.
Half-life: 3.5 hr.

Emtricitabine
Absorption: 93% absorbed following oral administration.
Distribution: Unknown.
Metabolism and Excretion: Some metabolism; 86% eliminated in urine; 14% in feces.
Half-life: 10 hr.

Tenofovir Alafenamide
Absorption: Tenofovir alafenamide is a prodrug that is hydrolyzed into tenofovir, the active component; absorption enhanced by high-fat meals.
Distribution: Unknown.
Metabolism and Excretion: Tenofovir is phosphorylated to tenofovir diphosphate (active metabolite); 32% excreted in feces; <1% in urine.
Half-life: 0.51 hr.

TIME/ACTION PROFILE (plasma concentrations)

ROUTE	ONSET	PEAK	DURATION
Elvitegravir PO	unknown	4 hr	24 hr
Cobicistat PO	unknown	3 hr	24 hr
Emtricitabine PO	rapid	1–2 hr	24 hr
Tenofovir alafenamide PO	unknown	0.5 hr	24 hr

Contraindications/Precautions

Contraindicated in: Severe hepatic impairment; Concurrent use of alfuzosin, carbamazepine, ergot derivatives, lomitapide, lovastatin, lurasidone, phenobarbital, phenytoin, pimozide, rifampin, sildenafil (Revatio), simvastatin, triazolam, or St. John's wort; Severe renal impairment or end-stage renal disease not receiving hemodialysis; Severe hepatic impairment; OB: Not recommended in pregnancy (significantly lower concentrations of elvitegravir and cobicistat); Lactation: Breastfeeding not recommended in women with HIV.
Use Cautiously in: Women or obese patients (may be at ↑ risk for lactic acidosis/hepatic steatosis); Chronic hepatitis B virus (HBV) infection (may exacerbate following discontinuation); Concurrent use of nephrotoxic drugs (↑ risk of renal impairment); Pedi: Children <25 kg (safety and effectiveness not established); Geri: Older adults may be more sensitive to drug effects; consider age-related ↓ in renal, hepatic, and cardiovascular function, as well as concurrent disease states and medications.

Adverse Reactions/Side Effects

Endo: Graves disease. **F and E** hypophosphatemia. **GI:** nausea, autoimmune hepatitis, diarrhea, LACTIC ACIDOSIS/HEPATOMEGALY WITH STEATOSIS. **GU:** proteinuria, ACUTE RENAL FAILURE/FANCONI SYNDROME. **Metab:** hyperlipidemia. **MS:** polymyositis. **Neuro:** Guillain-Barré syndrome, headache. **Misc:** fatigue, immune reconstitution syndrome.

Interactions

Drug-Drug: May significantly ↑ levels and risk of toxicity of **alfuzosin**, **dihydroergotamine**, **ergotamine**, **lomitapide**, **lovastatin**, **lurasidone**, **methylergonovine**, **pimozide**, **sildenafil** (when used for pulmonary hypertension), **simvastatin**, and **triazolam**; concurrent use contraindicated. **Carbamazepine**, **phenobarbital**, **phenytoin**, or **rifampin** may significantly ↓ levels and effectiveness of cobicistat and elvitegravir and ↑ risk of resistance; concurrent use contraindicated. Nephrotoxic agents, including **NSAIDs** and **aminoglycosides**, may ↑ risk of nephrotoxicity; avoid concurrent use.

Acyclovir, **cidofovir**, **ganciclovir**, **valacyclovir**, and **valganciclovir** may ↑ levels and risk of toxicity of emtricitabine and tenofovir alafenamide. May ↑ levels and risk of toxicity of **amiodarone**, **digoxin**, **disopyramide**, **flecainide**, **lidocaine**, **mexiletine**, **propafenone** and **quinidine**; careful monitoring recommended. May alter effects of **warfarin**; careful monitoring of INR recommended. Concurrent use with **clarithromycin** may ↑ levels and risk of toxicity of clarithromycin and/or cobicistat; for patients with CCr 50–60 mL/min, ↓ dose of clarithromycin by 50%. May ↑ levels and risk of toxicity of **ethosuximide**. **Oxcarbazepine** may ↓ levels and effectiveness of cobicistat, elvitegravir, and tenofovir alafenamide; consider using alternative anticonvulsant. May ↑ levels and risk of toxicity of **SSRIs** (except sertraline), **tricyclic antidepressants**, and **trazodone**. Concurrent use with **itraconazole**, **ketoconazole**, or **voriconazole** may ↑ levels and risk of toxicity of itraconazole, ketoconazole, voriconazole, elvitegravir, and cobicistat (max dose of ketoconazole or itraconazole = 300 mg/day; assess risk vs. benefit before using voriconazole). May ↑ levels and risk of toxicity of **colchicine**; concurrent use contraindicated in renal or hepatic impairment; *dosing adjustment for gout flares:* 0.6 mg; then 0.3 mg 1 hr later; do not repeat for ≥3 days; *dosing adjustment for gout flare prophylaxis:* 0.3 mg once daily if original regimen was 0.6 mg twice daily; 0.3 mg every other day if original regimen was 0.6 mg once daily; *dosing adjustment for treatment of familial Mediterranean fever:* not to exceed 0.6 mg daily; may be given as 0.3 mg twice daily. **Rifabutin** or **rifapentine** may ↓ levels and effectiveness of cobicistat, elvitegravir, and tenofovir alafenamide and may foster resistance; concurrent use not recommended. May ↑ levels and risk of toxicity of **beta blockers**; ↓ beta blocker dose, if necessary. May ↑ levels and risk of toxicity of **calcium channel blockers**. **Corticosteroids** that are CYP3A inducers, including **betamethasone**, **budesonide**, **ciclesonide**, **dexamethasone**, **fluticasone**, **methylprednisolone**, **mometasone**, **prednisone**, and **triamcinolone**, may ↓ levels and effectiveness and ↑ risk of resistance to elvitegravir; consider use of other corticosteroids, such as beclomethasone or prednisolone. **Corticosteroids** that are CYP3A substrates, including **betamethasone**, **budesonide**, **ciclesonide**, **dexamethasone**, **fluticasone**, **methylprednisolone**, **mometasone**, **prednisone**, and **triamcinolone**, may ↑ risk of Cushing disease and adrenal suppression; consider use of other corticosteroids, such as beclomethasone or prednisolone. May ↑ levels and risk of toxicity of **bosentan**; initiate bosentan at 62.5 mg once daily or every other day if already receiving elvitegravir/cobicistat/emtricitabine/tenofovir alafenamide for ≥10 days; if already receiving bosentan, discontinue bosentan ≥36 hr prior to starting elvitegravir/cobicistat/emtricitabine/tenofovir alafenamide; after 10 days, bosentan may be restarted at 62.5 mg once daily or every other day. May ↑ levels and risk of toxicity of **atorvastatin**; initiate atorvastatin at lowest dose titrate cautiously; do not exceed dose of 20 mg/day. May ↑ levels and risk of toxicity of **norgestimate** and ↓ levels and effectiveness of **ethinyl estradiol**; due to unpredictable effects, nonhormonal contraceptive methods should be considered. ↑ risk of hyperkalemia with contraceptives containing **drospirenone**; closely monitor serum potassium concentrations. May ↑ levels and risk of toxicity of **immunosuppressants**, including **cyclosporine**, **sirolimus**, and **tacrolimus**. **Cyclosporine** may ↑ levels and risk of toxicity of cobicistat and elvitegravir. May ↑ levels and risk of toxicity of **buprenorphine** and ↓ levels and effectiveness of **naloxone**. May ↑ levels and risk of toxicity of **fentanyl**, and **tramadol**; consider ↓ tramadol dose. May ↑ levels of and risk of adverse cardiovascular effects with **salmeterol**; concurrent use not recommended. ↑ levels and risk of toxicity of **neuroleptics**, including **perphenazine**, **risperidone**, and **thioridazine**; may need to ↓ dose of neuroleptic. May ↑ levels and risk of toxicity of **quetiapine**; if taking quetiapine when initiating therapy, consider alternative antiretroviral therapy or ↓ quetiapine dose to ⅙ of the original dose and monitor for adverse effects. May ↑ levels and risk of toxicity of **PDE5 inhibitors**, including **sildenafil**, **tadalafil**, and **vardenafil**; *dosing adjustment for pulmonary hypertension:* sildenafil is contraindicated; in patients who have received elvitegravir/cobicistat/emtricitabine/tenofovir alafenamide for ≥7 days, start tadalafil at 20 mg once daily and carefully titrate if tolerating to 40 mg once daily; in patients already receiving tadalafil, discontinue tadalafil for ≥24 hr before initiating elvitegravir/cobicistat/emtricitabine/tenofovir alafenamide; after ≥1 wk, resume tadalafil at 20 mg once daily and titrate if tolerating to 40 mg once daily; *dosing adjustment for erectile dysfunction:* sildenafil dose should not exceed 25 mg in 48 hr, vardenafil dose should not exceed 2.5 mg in 72 hr, and tadalafil dose should not exceed 10 mg in 72 hr. May ↑ levels and risk of toxicity of **sedative/hypnotics**, including **midazolam** (parenteral), **diazepam**, **buspirone**, and **zolpidem**; consider dose ↓ of parenteral midazolam; clinical monitoring and dose ↓, if necessary, is recommended for other sedative/hypnotics. May ↑ bleeding risk with **rivaroxaban**; avoid concurrent use. May ↑ bleeding risk with **apixaban**; if taking apixaban 5–10 mg twice daily, ↓ apixaban dose by 50%; if taking apixaban 2.5 mg twice daily, avoid concurrent use. May ↑ bleeding risk with **dabigatran**; may need to avoid concurrent use if patient has moderate or severe renal impairment (depends on dabigatran indication). May ↑ bleeding risk with **edoxaban**; ↓ edoxaban dose by 50% when used for treatment of venous thromboembolism in patients with moderate or severe renal impairment. May ↑ bleeding risk with **ticagrelor**; concurrent use not recommended. May ↓ antiplatelet effects of **clopidogrel** and ↑ risk of thromboembolic events; concurrent use not recommended. Medications containing polyvalent cations, including **calcium**, **magnesium**, **aluminum**, **iron**, or **zinc**, may ↓ levels and effectiveness of elvitegravir; separate administration by ≥2 hr.

Drug-Natural Products: St. John's wort may significantly ↓ levels and effectiveness of cobicistat and elvitegravir and ↑ risk of resistance; concurrent use contraindicated.

Route/Dosage

PO (Adults and Children ≥25 kg): One tablet once daily.

Renal Impairment

PO (Adults): *CCr <15 mL/min AND receiving chronic hemodialysis:* One tablet once daily (give after dialysis on dialysis days).

Availability

Tablets: elvitegravir 150 mg/cobicistat 150 mg/ emtricitabine 200 mg/tenofovir alafenamide 10 mg.

NURSING IMPLICATIONS

Assessment

- Assess patient for change in severity of HIV symptoms and for symptoms of opportunistic infections during therapy.
- Monitor for an inflammatory response to residual opportunistic infections during the initial phase of therapy. *If signs and symptoms of immune reconstitution syndrome occur,* evaluate and treat as clinically indicated.

Lab Test Considerations

- Monitor viral load and CD4 count before and routinely during therapy to determine response.
- Assess for HBV. *Genvoya* is not approved for administration in patients with HIV and HBV. If therapy is discontinued, may cause severe exacerbation of HBV. Monitor liver function in coinfected patients for several months after stopping therapy.
- Monitor liver function tests prior to, during, and following therapy.
- Lactic acidosis may occur with hepatic toxicity causing hepatic steatosis; may be fatal. Discontinue therapy if symptoms occur.
- May ↑ LDL-C, total cholesterol, and triglycerides.
- Calculate serum creatinine, CCr, urine glucose, and urine protein prior to and periodically during therapy and as clinically indicated. In patients with chronic kidney disease, additionally assess serum phosphorus. *For serum creatinine >0.4 mg/dL from baseline,* monitor renal status closely. *For clinically significant ↓ in renal function or evidence of Fanconi syndrome,* discontinue *Genvoya.*
- May cause hyperglycemia and glycosuria.

Implementation

- Do not confuse elvitegravir, cobicistat, emtricitabine, and tenofovir alafenamide with elvitegravir, cobicistat, emtricitabine, and tenofovir disoproxil fumarate.
- **PO:** Administer once daily with food.

Patient/Family Teaching

- Instruct patient not to take more than prescribed amount and not to stop taking without consulting health care provider. Take missed doses as soon as remembered unless almost time for next dose; do not double dose. Advise patient to read *Patient Information* prior to starting therapy. Caution patient not to share or trade *Genvoya* with others.
- Do not stop taking without consulting health care provider. Discontinuing therapy may lead to severe exacerbations. Inform patient of importance of HBV testing before starting antiretroviral therapy.
- Advise patient to take antacids containing aluminum, magnesium hydroxide, or calcium carbonate ≥2 hr before or after *Genvoya.*
- Instruct patient to notify health care provider of all Rx or OTC medications, vitamins, or herbal products being taken and consult health care provider before taking any new medications, especially St. John's wort.
- Advise patient to notify health care provider immediately if symptoms of lactic acidosis (nausea; vomiting; unusual stomach discomfort; muscle pain; difficulty breathing; feeling cold, especially in extremities; dizziness; fast or irregular heartbeat; weakness or tiredness), liver problems (yellow skin or whites of eyes, dark urine, light-colored stools, loss of appetite, nausea, stomach pain), or signs of immune reconstitution syndrome occur.
- Inform patient that *Genvoya* does not cure AIDS and may ↓ risk of transmission of HIV to others. Caution patient to use a condom and avoid sharing needles or donating blood to prevent spreading HIV to others.
- Rep: Advise women of reproductive potential to notify health care provider if pregnancy is planned or suspected. Monitor viral load closely during pregnancy. Encourage patients who become pregnant during therapy to join the Antiretroviral Pregnancy Registry. Enroll patient by calling 1-800-258-4263. Advise patient to avoid breastfeeding during therapy.
- Emphasize the importance of regular follow-up exams and blood counts to determine progress and monitor for side effects.

Evaluation/Desired Outcomes

- Delayed progression of AIDS and decreased opportunistic infections in patients with HIV.
- Decreased viral load and increased CD4 cell counts.

emicizumab (em-i-siz-ue-mab)

Hemlibra

Classification

Therapeutic: hemostatic agents

Pharmacologic: monoclonal antibodies

Indications

Routine prophylaxis to prevent or reduce the frequency of bleeding in patients with hemophilia A (congenital factor VIII deficiency) (with or without factor VIII inhibitors).

Action

Bridges activated factor IX and factor X to restore the function of missing activated factor VIII that is needed for effective hemostasis. **Therapeutic Effects:** Prevention or reduction in frequency of bleeding.

Pharmacokinetics

Absorption: 80–93% absorbed following SUBQ administration.

Distribution: Minimally distributed to tissues.

Metabolism and Excretion: Unknown.

Half-life: 27 days.

TIME/ACTION PROFILE (plasma concentrations)

ROUTE	ONSET	PEAK	DURATION
SUBQ	unknown	unknown	unknown

Contraindications/Precautions

Contraindicated in: None known.

Use Cautiously in: Severe renal impairment; Severe hepatic impairment; OB: Use during pregnancy only if potential maternal benefit outweighs potential fetal risk; Lactation: Safety not established in breastfeeding; Rep: Women of reproductive potential.

Adverse Reactions/Side Effects

GI: diarrhea. **Hemat:** THROMBOEMBOLISM, THROMBOTIC MICROANGIOPATHY. **Local:** injection site reactions. **MS:** arthralgia. **Neuro:** headache. **Misc:** antibody development, fever.

Interactions

Drug-Drug: ↑ risk of thrombotic microangiopathy and thromboembolism when used with **activated prothrombin complex concentrate** for up to 6 mo after last dose of emicizumab.

Route/Dosage

SUBQ (Adults and Children): 3 mg/kg once weekly for 4 wk, followed by maintenance dose of 1.5 mg/kg once weekly *or* 3 mg/kg every 2 wk *or* 6 mg/kg every 4 wk.

Availability

Solution for injection: 30 mg/mL, 60 mg/0.4 mL, 105 mg/0.7 mL, 150 mg/mL.

NURSING IMPLICATIONS

Assessment

- Monitor for signs and symptoms of thrombotic angiopathy (thrombocytopenia, microangiopathic hemolytic anemia, acute kidney injury). *If signs or symptoms occur,* discontinue therapy immediately; may resolve within 1 wk.
- Monitor for signs and symptoms of thromboembolism (swelling, erythema or pain in extremities, dizziness, headache, dyspnea, numbness in face, chest pain or tightness, eye pain or swelling, tachycardia, vision changes, hemoptysis) during therapy. *If signs or symptoms occur,* discontinue therapy immediately; may resolve within 1 mo.
- Monitor for signs of loss of efficacy (↑ breakthrough bleeding). *If neutralizing anti-emicizumab antibodies suspected,* assess cause and consider changing therapy.

Lab Test Considerations

- Monitor plasma factor VIII inhibition activity to determine dosing for factor replacement or anticoagulation. Do not use activated clotting time, activated partial thromboplastin time (aPTT), or all assays based on aPTT, such as one-stage factor VIII activity, to monitor activity due to the effects of emicizumab. Assess patient for signs of bleeding.

Implementation

- May continue factor VIII products for prophylaxis during 1st wk of therapy. Discontinue prophylactic use of bypassing agents the day before starting therapy.
- **SUBQ:** Do not combine vials of different concentrations in a single injection. Solution is colorless to slight yellow; do not administer if discolored or contains particulates. Refrigerate and protect from light; do not freeze or shake. May store at room temperature for ≤7 days. Administer ≤1-mL dose with a 1-mL syringe and doses >1 mL with a 2-mL or 3-mL syringe of transparent polypropylene or polycarbonate with Luer-Lock tip, graduation 0.01 mL, sterile, for injection only, single-use, latex-free, and nonpyrogenic. Use an 18 gauge, 1–1½ inch, single bevel or semiblunted tip needle for transfer and a 25–27 gauge, ⅜–½ inch needle for injection. Administer into upper outer arm, thigh, or any quadrant of abdomen; rotate sites with

each dose. Avoid moles, scars, or areas where the skin is tender, bruised, red, hard, or not intact.

Patient/Family Teaching

- Explain purpose and side effects of medication. Advise patient to read *Patient Information* before starting therapy.
- Instruct patient and caregiver in the correct technique for preparation, injection, and how to dispose of materials. Take missed doses as soon as possible; do not take two doses on the same day.
- Advise patient to notify health care provider immediately if signs and symptoms of thrombotic microangiopathy (confusion, abdomen or back pain, weakness, nausea, vomiting, swelling of extremities, yellowing of skin and eyes, ↓ urination) or thromboembolism occur.
- Advise patient to notify health care provider of therapy before blood tests or procedures.
- Advise patient to notify health care provider of all Rx or OTC medications, vitamins, or herbal products being taken and to consult with health care provider before taking other medications.
- Rep: Advise women of reproductive potential to use contraception during therapy and notify health care provider if pregnancy is planned or suspected or if breastfeeding.

Evaluation/Desired Outcomes

- Prevention or reduction in frequency of bleeding.

BEERS

empagliflozin

(em-pa-gli-**floe**-zin)

Jardiance

Classification

Therapeutic: antidiabetics

Pharmacologic: sodium-glucose co-transporter 2 (SGLT2) inhibitors

Indications

Type 2 diabetes (as adjunct to diet and exercise). To reduce risk of cardiovascular death in patients with type 2 diabetes and established cardiovascular disease. To reduce the risk of cardiovascular death and hospitalization for HF in patients with HF. To reduce the risk of sustained decline in eGFR, end-stage kidney disease, cardiovascular death, and hospitalization in adults with chronic kidney disease at risk of progression.

Action

Inhibits proximal renal tubular sodium-glucose cotransporter 2 (SGLT2), which determines reabsorption of glucose from the tubular lumen. Inhibits reabsorption of glucose, lowers renal threshold for glucose, and increases excretion of glucose in urine. **Therapeutic Effects:** Improved glycemic control. Reduced death due to cardiovascular causes in patients with type 2 diabetes and cardiovascular disease. Reduced death due to cardiovascular causes and hospitalizations due to HF in patients with HF. Reduced risk of sustained decline in eGFR, end-stage kidney disease, cardiovascular death, and hospitalization in adults with chronic kidney disease at risk of progression.

Pharmacokinetics

Absorption: Well absorbed following oral administration.

Distribution: Enters red blood cells; remainder of distribution unknown.

Metabolism and Excretion: Minimally metabolized; excreted in feces (41.2% mostly as unchanged drug) and urine (54.4% half as unchanged drug, half as metabolites).

Half-life: 12.4 hr.

TIME/ACTION PROFILE (↓ in A1c)

ROUTE	ONSET	PEAK	DURATION
PO	within 6 wk	12 wk	unknown

Contraindications/Precautions

Contraindicated in: Hypersensitivity; Severe renal impairment (eGFR <30 mL/min/1.73 m² [patients with type 2 diabetes] or eGFR <20 mL/min/1.73 m² [patients with heart failure]) or receiving dialysis; Type 1 diabetes; Diabetic ketoacidosis; Lactation: Lactation.

Use Cautiously in: eGFR <60 mL/min/1.73 m² or concurrent use of loop diuretics (↑ risk of volume depletion or hypotension); History of pancreatitis, pancreatic surgery, reduced caloric intake due to illness or surgery, surgical procedures, or alcohol abuse (↑ risk of ketoacidosis); Peripheral arterial disease, diabetic foot infection, or osteomyelitis (↑ risk of lower limb amputation); OB: Use during pregnancy only if potential maternal benefit justifies potential fetal risk; Pedi: Children <10 yr (safety and effectiveness not established); Geri: Appears on Beers list. Older adults may have ↑ risk of urogenital infections (especially women in the 1st mo of treatment) and euglycemic diabetic ketoacidosis. Use with caution in older adults.

Adverse Reactions/Side Effects

CV: hypotension, volume depletion. **Endo:** hypoglycemia (↑ with other medications). **F and E:** hyperphosphatemia, KETOACIDOSIS. **GU:** ↑ urination, acute kidney injury, genital mycotic infections, NECROTIZING FASCIITIS OF PERINEUM (FOURNIER'S GANGRENE), renal impairment, urinary tract infection (including pyelonephritis), UROSEPSIS. **Metab:** hyperlipidemia. **MS:** lower limb amputation. **Misc:** HYPERSENSITIVITY REACTIONS (INCLUDING ANGIOEDEMA).

Interactions

Drug-Drug: ↑ risk of hypotension with **antihypertensives or diuretics.** ↑ risk of hypoglycemia with other

antidiabetics (dose adjustments may be required). ↑ risk of acute kidney injury with **diuretics**, **ACE inhibitors**, **angiotensin II receptor blockers**, or **NSAIDs**. May ↓ **lithium** levels and effectiveness.

Route/Dosage

Type 2 Diabetes

PO (Adults and Children ≥10 yr): 10 mg once daily in the morning;, may ↑ to 25 mg once daily for additional glycemic control.

Type 2 Diabetes in Patients with Established Cardiovascular Disease, Heart Failure, and Chronic Kidney Disease

PO (Adults): 10 mg once daily in the morning.

Availability (generic available)

Tablets: 10 mg, 25 mg. ***In combination with:*** linagliptin (Glyxambi); linagliptin and metformin XR (Trijardy XR); metformin (Synjardy); metformin XR (Synjardy XR). See Appendix N.

NURSING IMPLICATIONS

Assessment

- Observe patient for signs and symptoms of hypoglycemic reactions (sweating, hunger, weakness, dizziness, confusion, headache, tremor, tachycardia, irritability, drowsiness).
- Monitor for signs and symptoms of volume depletion (dizziness, feeling faint, weakness, orthostatic hypotension) after initiating therapy, especially in elderly patients and patients with renal impairment, low systolic BP, or on diuretics.
- Monitor for signs and symptoms of urinary tract infection during therapy. Treat promptly.
- Monitor for infection (pain or burning on urination, frequency), new pain, tenderness, erythema, swelling, sores, ulcers involving genital or perianal area, with fever or malaise, or ulcers involving lower limbs; assess for necrotizing fasciitis. If suspected, start treatment immediately with broad-spectrum antibiotics and, if necessary, surgical debridement. Discontinue empagliflozin if these occur.
- Assess for ketoacidosis in patients presenting with signs and symptoms of dehydration and metabolic acidosis (nausea, vomiting, abdominal pain, malaise, shortness of breath), regardless of blood glucose level. Discontinue empagliflozin and treat promptly (insulin, fluid and caloric replacement) if suspected. Consider risk factors for ketoacidosis (pancreatic insulin deficiency, caloric restriction, alcohol abuse) before starting empagliflozin.

Lab Test Considerations

- Monitor A1c prior to and periodically during therapy.
- May ↑ serum creatinine and ↓ eGFR. Monitor renal function prior to starting and periodically during therapy. Do not begin therapy if eGFR <30 mL/min/1.73 m^2. Discontinue therapy if eGFR is persistently <30 mL/min/1.73 m^2.
- May cause ↑ serum phosphate levels. Monitor electrolytes periodically during therapy.
- May cause ↑ LDL-cholesterol. Monitor serum lipid levels periodically during therapy.
- May cause ↑ hematocrit.
- Monitor for ketoacidosis, especially during prolonged fasting for illness or surgery. May require temporary discontinuation of therapy.

Implementation

- Patients stabilized on a diabetic regimen who are exposed to stress, fever, trauma, infection, or surgery may require administration of insulin. Discontinue empagliflozin for at least 3 days before surgery; therapy can be resumed once patient is clinically stable following surgery and has resumed oral intake.
- Correct volume depletion before starting therapy with empagliflozin.
- **PO:** Administer once daily in the morning with or without food.

Patient/Family Teaching

- Instruct patient to take empagliflozin as directed. Take missed doses as soon as remembered, unless it is almost time for next dose; do not double doses. Advise patient to read the *Medication Guide* before starting and with each Rx refill in case of changes.
- Explain to patient that empagliflozin helps control hyperglycemia but does not cure diabetes. Therapy is usually long term.
- Instruct patient not to share this medication with others, even if they have the same symptoms; it may harm them.
- Encourage patient to follow prescribed diet, medication, and exercise regimen to prevent hyperglycemic or hypoglycemic episodes.
- Review signs of hypoglycemia and hyperglycemia with patient. If hypoglycemia occurs, advise patient to take a glass of orange juice or 2–3 teaspoons of sugar, honey, or corn syrup dissolved in water, and notify health care professional.
- Instruct patient in proper testing of serum glucose and ketones, especially during periods of stress or illness. Inform patient that empagliflozin will cause a positive test result when testing for urine glucose. Notify health care professional if significant changes occur.
- Advise patient to inform health care professional of therapy before surgery. Empagliflozin should be discontinued for at least 3 days before surgery. Monitor for ketoacidosis during and after surgery. Advise patient to discontinue empagliflozin and to

notify health care professional immediately if signs and symptoms of ketoacidosis occur.

- Advise patient to notify health care professional immediately if new pain or tenderness, sores or ulcers, or infections involving the leg or foot occur and to immediately seek care if pain or tenderness, redness, or swelling of the genitals or area from the genitals back to the rectum, along with a fever above 100.4°F or malaise, occur.
- Advise patient to notify health care professional if signs and symptoms of hypotension occur and to maintain adequate hydration as dehydration may increase risk of hypotension.
- Inform patient that empagliflozin may cause mycotic (yeast) infections. Women may have signs and symptoms of a vaginal yeast infection (vaginal odor, white or yellow vaginal discharge [may be lumpy or look like cottage cheese], vaginal itching). Men may have signs and symptoms of a yeast infection of the penis (redness, itching, or swelling of penis; rash on penis; foul-smelling discharge from penis; pain in skin around penis). Advise patient to notify health care professional if yeast infection occurs.
- Advise patient to notify health care professional if signs and symptoms of urinary tract infection (burning feeling when passing urine, cloudy urine, pain in pelvis or back) occur.
- Advise patient to notify health care professional of all Rx or OTC medications, vitamins, or herbal products being taken and to consult with health care professional before taking other medications, especially other oral hypoglycemic medications.
- Advise patient to notify health care professional promptly if signs and symptoms of hypersensitivity reactions (rash; raised red patches on skin; swelling of face, lips, tongue, throat; difficulty breathing or swallowing) occur.
- Rep: Insulin is the recommended method of controlling blood sugar during pregnancy. Advise females of reproductive potential to notify health care professional if pregnancy is planned or suspected and to avoid breastfeeding during therapy.
- Emphasize importance of routine follow up with routine lab tests for blood glucose and renal function.

Evaluation/Desired Outcomes

- Improved A1c and glycemic control in adults and children >10 yr with type 2 diabetes.
- Reduced risk of cardiovascular death in patients with type 2 diabetes and established cardiovascular disease.
- Reduced death due to cardiovascular causes and hospitalizations due to HF in patients with HF.
- Reduced risk of sustained decline in eGFR, end-stage kidney disease, cardiovascular death, and hospitalization in adults with chronic kidney disease at risk of progression.

emtricitabine/rilpivirine/tenofovir alafenamide

(em-tri-**sye**-ti-been/**ril**-pi-vir-een/te-**noe**-fo-veer al-a-**fen**-a-mide)

Odefsey

Classification

Therapeutic: antiretrovirals

Pharmacologic: nucleoside reverse transcriptase inhibitors, non-nucleoside reverse transcriptase inhibitors

Indications

HIV infection in treatment-naive patients with HIV-1 RNA <100,000 copies/mL at the start of therapy (for use as a complete regimen). HIV infection in patients on a stable antiretroviral regimen with HIV-1 RNA <50 copies/mL for ≥6 mo and have no history of treatment failure or no known substitutions associated with resistance to the individual components of the medication (to replace their current antiretroviral regimen).

Action

Emtricitabine: Phosphorylated intracellularly, where it inhibits HIV reverse transcriptase, resulting in viral DNA chain termination. *Rilpivirine:* Inhibits HIV-replication by noncompetitively inhibiting HIV reverse transcriptase. *Tenofovir:* Phosphorylated intracellularly, where it inhibits HIV reverse transcriptase, resulting in disruption of DNA synthesis. **Therapeutic Effects:** Slowed progression of HIV infection and decreased occurrence of sequelae.

Pharmacokinetics

Emtricitabine

Absorption: 93% absorbed following oral administration.

Distribution: Unknown.

Metabolism and Excretion: Some metabolism, 86% renally excreted; 14% fecal excretion.

Half-life: 10 hr.

Rilpivirine

Absorption: Well absorbed following oral administration.

Distribution: Unknown.

Protein Binding: 99.7%.

Metabolism and Excretion: Primarily metabolized by the liver via the CYP3A isoenzyme; 25% excreted in feces unchanged; <1% excreted unchanged in urine.

Half-life: 50 hr.

Tenofovir Alafenamide

Absorption: Tenofovir alafenamide is a prodrug, which is hydrolyzed into tenofovir, the active component; absorption enhanced by high-fat meals.

Distribution: Unknown.

Metabolism and Excretion: Tenofovir is phosphorylated to tenofovir diphosphate (active metabolite); 32% excreted in feces; <1% in urine.
Half-life: 0.51 hr.

TIME/ACTION PROFILE (plasma concentrations)

ROUTE	ONSET	PEAK	DURATION
Emtricitabine PO	rapid	1–2 hr	24 hr
Rilpivirine PO	unknown	4–5 hr	24 hr
Tenofovir PO	unknown	1 hr	24 hr

Contraindications/Precautions

Contraindicated in: Concurrent use of carbamazepine, oxcarbazepine, phenobarbital, phenytoin, rifampin, rifapentine, proton pump inhibitors, dexamethasone (>1 dose), or St. John's wort; Severe renal impairment or end-stage renal disease not receiving hemodialysis; Lactation: Breastfeeding is not recommended in patients with HIV.
Use Cautiously in: Chronic hepatitis B virus (HBV) infection (may exacerbate following discontinuation); History of suicidal ideation or depression; HIV-1 RNA >100,000 copies/mL (↑ risk of virologic failure); Renal impairment or receiving nephrotoxic medications (↑ risk of renal impairment); Severe hepatic impairment; OB: Monitor viral load closely when used during pregnancy; Pedi: Children <25 kg (safety and effectiveness not established).

Adverse Reactions/Side Effects

CV: QT interval prolongation. **Derm:** DRUG REACTION WITH EOSINOPHILIA AND SYSTEMIC SYMPTOMS (DRESS). **Endo:** Graves disease. **GI:** ACUTE EXACERBATION OF HBV, autoimmune hepatitis, HEPATOTOXICITY, LACTIC ACIDOSIS/HEPATOMEGALY WITH STEATOSIS. **GU:** ACUTE RENAL FAILURE/FANCONI SYNDROME. **Metab:** hyperlipidemia. **MS:** polymyositis. **Neuro:** depression, Guillain-Barré syndrome, headache, sleep disturbances, SUICIDAL ATTEMPTS/THOUGHTS. **Misc:** immune reconstitution syndrome.

Interactions

Drug-Drug: Strong CYP3A4 inducers, including **carbamazepine**, **oxcarbazepine**, **phenobarbital**, **phenytoin**, **dexamethasone** (more than a single dose), **rifampin**, and **rifapentine**, may ↓ levels and effectiveness of rilpivirine; concurrent use contraindicated. **Proton pump inhibitors**, including **esomeprazole**, **lansoprazole**, **omeprazole**, **pantoprazole**, and **rabeprazole**, ↑ gastric pH and may ↓ levels and effectiveness of rilpivirine; concurrent use contraindicated. **QT interval prolonging medications** may ↑ risk of torsades de pointes. Medications that compete for active tubular secretion, including **acyclovir**, **cidofovir**, **ganciclovir**, **valacyclovir**, **valganciclovir**, or **aminoglycosides**, may ↑ levels and risk of toxicity of emtricitabine and tenofovir; avoid concurrent use. **Antacids** including **aluminum hydroxide**, **magnesium hydroxide**, and **calcium carbonate** ↑ gastric pH and may ↓ levels and effectiveness of rilpivirine; administer antacid ≥2 hr before or ≥4 hr after. **H_2-antagonists**, including **cimetidine**, **famotidine**, and **nizatidine**, ↑ gastric pH and may ↓ levels and effectiveness of rilpivirine; administer ≥12 hr before or ≥4 hr after rilpivirine. Nephrotoxic agents, including **NSAIDs**, may ↑ risk of nephrotoxicity; avoid concurrent use. **Rifabutin** may ↓ levels and effectiveness of rilpivirine and tenofovir; concurrent use not recommended. **Fluconazole**, **itraconazole**, **ketoconazole**, **posaconazole**, and **voriconazole** may ↑ levels and risk of toxicity of rilpivirine and tenofovir. May ↓ levels and effectiveness of **ketoconazole**. May alter requirements for **methadone** maintenance. **Clarithromycin** or **erythromycin** may ↑ levels and risk of toxicity of rilpivirine; consider azithromycin as an alternative. **Ledipasvir/sofosbuvir**, **sofosbuvir/velpatasvir**, and **sofosbuvir/velpatasvir/voxilaprevir** may ↑ levels and risk of toxicity of tenofovir.
Drug-Natural Products: St. John's wort may ↓ levels and effectiveness of rilpivirine; concurrent use contraindicated.

Route/Dosage

PO (Adults and Children ≥25 kg): One tablet once daily.

Renal Impairment

PO (Adults and Children ≥25 kg): *End-stage renal disease (CCr <15 mL/min) AND receiving hemodialysis:* One tablet once daily (to be given after hemodialysis).

Availability

Tablets: emtricitabine 200 mg/rilpivirine 25 mg/tenofovir alafenamide 25 mg.

NURSING IMPLICATIONS

Assessment

- Assess for change in severity of HIV symptoms and for symptoms of opportunistic infections during therapy.
- Monitor for signs and symptoms of DRESS (fever, rash, blisters, mucosal lesions, conjunctivitis), lymphadenopathy, or facial swelling associated with involvement of other organs (hepatitis, nephritis, blood dyscrasias, myocarditis, myositis) during therapy. *If symptoms occur,* discontinue *Odefsey*.
- Assess mental status (orientation, mood, behavior) before and periodically during therapy. Monitor closely for notable changes in behavior that could indicate the emergence or worsening of suicidal thoughts or behavior or depression.

Lab Test Considerations

- Monitor viral load and CD4 cell count regularly during therapy.
- Assess for HBV. *Odefsey* is not approved for use in patients with HIV and HBV. If therapy is discontinued in HBV-positive patient, may cause severe exacerbation of HBV. Monitor liver function in coinfected patients for several months after stopping therapy.
- Monitor liver function tests prior to, during, and following therapy.
- May ↑ total cholesterol, LDL-C, and triglycerides. May cause lactic acidosis and severe hepatomegaly with steatosis. These events are more likely to occur if patient is female, obese, or receiving nucleoside analogue medications for extended periods. *If clinical or laboratory signs of lactic acidosis occur,* discontinue therapy.
- Assess serum creatinine, CCr, urine glucose, and urine protein before starting and periodically during therapy. Monitor serum phosphorous in patients with chronic kidney disease.

Implementation

- **PO:** Administer once daily with food.

Patient/Family Teaching

- Explain purpose and side effects of medication. Advise patient to read *Patient Information* before starting therapy.
- Caution patient that missing doses may result in development of resistance.
- Do not stop taking without consulting health care provider. Discontinuing therapy may lead to severe exacerbation. Inform patient of importance of HBV testing before starting antiretroviral therapy.
- Instruct patient that *Odefsey* should not be shared with others.
- Inform patient that *Odefsey* does not cure HIV but may ↓ risk of transmission. Caution patient to use a condom and avoid sharing needles or donating blood to prevent spreading HIV.
- Advise patient to notify health care provider immediately if symptoms of lactic acidosis (nausea, vomiting, unusual or unexpected stomach discomfort, weakness), hypersensitivity (swelling of face, eyes, lips, mouth, tongue, or throat; difficulty breathing), liver disease (yellow skin or conjunctiva, dark urine, light-colored stool, loss of appetite, nausea, abdominal pain), or DRESS occur.
- Inform patient of risk of suicidal thoughts and behavior and advise that behavioral changes, worsening signs of depression, mood changes, or suicidal thoughts or behavior should be reported to health care provider immediately.
- Immune reconstitution syndrome may trigger opportunistic infections or autoimmune disorders. Notify health care provider if symptoms (infection or inflammation) occur.
- Advise patient to notify health care provider of all Rx or OTC medications, vitamins, or herbal products being taken and to consult with health care provider before taking other medications, especially St. John's wort.
- Rep: Advise women of reproductive potential to notify health care provider if pregnancy is planned or suspected and to avoid breastfeeding during therapy. Monitor viral load closely during pregnancy. Encourage women who become pregnant during therapy to join the Antiviral Pregnancy Registry that monitors outcomes. Enroll patient by calling 1-800-258-4263.

Evaluation/Desired Outcomes

- Delayed progression of HIV and ↓ opportunistic infections.
- Decrease in viral load and ↑ in CD4 cell counts.

enalapril/enalaprilat, See ANGIOTENSIN-CONVERTING ENZYME (ACE) INHIBITORS.

HIGH ALERT

encorafenib

(en-koe-**raf**-e-nib)

Braftovi

Classification

Therapeutic: antineoplastics

Pharmacologic: kinase inhibitors

Indications

Metastatic or unresectable melanoma in patients with a BRAF V600E or V600K mutation (in combination with binimetinib). Metastatic colorectal cancer in patients with a BRAF V600E mutation (in combination with cetuximab and mFOLFOX6). Metastatic colorectal cancer in patients with a BRAF V600E mutation (in combination with cetuximab). Metastatic non-small cell lung cancer (NSCLC) in patients with a BRAF V600E mutation (in combination with binimetinib).

Action

Kinase inhibitor that targets BRAF V600E, a mutated enzyme that promotes tumor cell proliferation. **Therapeutic Effects:** Improvement in progression-free survival and overall survival in patients with melanoma and colorectal cancer. Decreased progression of NSCLC.

Pharmacokinetics

Absorption: Well absorbed (86%) following oral administration.

Distribution: Extensively distributed to tissues.

Metabolism and Excretion: Primarily metabolized by the liver via the CYP3A4 and CYP2C19 isoenzymes. Primarily excreted as metabolites in feces (42%) and urine (45%).

Half-life: 3.5 hr

TIME/ACTION PROFILE (plasma concentrations)

ROUTE	ONSET	PEAK	DURATION
PO	unknown	2 hr	24 hr

Contraindications/Precautions

Contraindicated in: Wild-type BRAF melanoma (may ↑ proliferation); Long QT syndrome, bradyarrhythmias, severe or decompensated HF, hypokalemia, or hypomagnesemia (↑ risk of QT interval prolongation); Concurrent use of QT-interval prolonging medications; Baseline QTc interval >500 msec; OB: Pregnancy; Lactation: Lactation.

Use Cautiously in: Left ventricular ejection fraction (LVEF) <50%; Moderate or severe hepatic impairment; Severe renal impairment; Rep: Women of reproductive potential; Pedi: Safety and effectiveness not established in children.

Adverse Reactions/Side Effects

CV: CARDIOMYOPATHY, QT interval prolongation. **Derm:** alopecia, dry skin, hyperkeratosis, pruritus, rash, BASAL CELL CARCINOMA, CUTANEOUS SQUAMOUS CELL CARCINOMA, nodule formation, photosensitivity. **EENT:** uveitis. **Endo:** hyperglycemia. **F and E** hypermagnesemia, hyponatremia. **GI:** ↑ liver enzymes, abdominal pain, constipation, nausea, vomiting, GI HEMORRHAGE, PANCREATITIS. **GU:** ↑ serum creatinine, ↓ fertility (men). **Hemat:** anemia, BLEEDING, leukopenia, lymphopenia, neutropenia. **MS:** arthralgia, myalgia. **Neuro:** dizziness, fatigue, headache, peripheral neuropathy, facial paralysis, INTRACRANIAL HEMORRHAGE. **Misc:** fever, HYPERSENSITIVITY REACTIONS, MALIGNANCY.

Interactions

Drug-Drug: **QT interval prolonging drugs** may ↑ the risk of QT interval prolongation and torsades de pointes; avoid concurrent use. **Strong or moderate CYP3A4 inhibitors**, including **diltiazem** and **posaconazole**, may ↑ levels and risk of toxicity; avoid concurrent use. If concurrent use unavoidable, ↓ encorafenib dose. **Strong CYP3A4 inducers** may ↓ levels and effectiveness; avoid concurrent use. May ↓ effectiveness of **hormonal contraceptives**; avoid concurrent use. May ↑ levels and risk of toxicity of **OATP1B1 substrates**, **OATP1B3 substrates**, or **BCRP substrates**.

Drug-Natural Products: St. John's wort may ↓ levels and effectiveness; avoid concurrent use.

Drug-Food: Grapefruit juice may ↑ levels and risk of toxicity; avoid concurrent use.

Route/Dosage

BRAF V600E or V600K Mutation-Positive Unresectable or Metastatic Melanoma and BRAF V600E Mutation-Positive Metastatic NSCLC

PO (Adults): 450 mg once daily until disease progression or unacceptable toxicity. *Concurrent use of moderate CYP3A4 inhibitor:* 225 mg once daily (if planned dose 450 mg once daily); 150 mg once daily (if planned dose 300 mg once daily); 75 mg once daily (if planned dose 225 mg once daily). *Concurrent use of strong CYP3A4 inhibitor:* 150 mg once daily (if planned dose 450 mg once daily); 75 mg once daily (if planned dose 300 mg once daily or 225 mg once daily).

BRAF V600E Mutation-Positive Metastatic Colorectal Cancer

PO (Adults): 300 mg once daily until disease progression or unacceptable toxicity. *Concurrent use of moderate CYP3A4 inhibitor:* 150 mg once daily (if planned dose 300 mg once daily); 75 mg once daily (if planned dose 225 mg once daily or 150 mg once daily). *Concurrent use of strong CYP3A4 inhibitor:* 75 mg once daily (if planned dose 300 mg once daily, 225 mg once daily, or 150 mg once daily).

Availability

Capsules: 75 mg.

NURSING IMPLICATIONS

Assessment

- Assess for signs and symptoms of HF (dyspnea, cough, paroxysmal nocturnal dyspnea, peripheral edema, S_3 gallop, rales) before and frequently during therapy. Assess LVEF by echocardiogram or MUGA scan before starting therapy, 1 mo after starting therapy, and then every 2–3 mo throughout treatment. If symptomatic HF or absolute ↓ in LVEF of >20% from baseline that is also below the lower limit of normal develops, ↓ dose by one level. If LVEF improves to at least institutional lower limit of normal and absolute ↓ is ≤10% compared to baseline, continue encorafenib at the reduced dose. If no improvement in LVEF after dose ↓, hold encorafenib until LVEF improves to at least institutional lower limit of normal and absolute ↓ is ≤10% compared to baseline, and then resume at the ↓ dose or ↓ dose an additional dose level.
- Assess skin for lesions before starting, every 2 mo during and for up to 6 mo following discontinuation of therapy. Manage suspicious skin lesions with excision and dermatopathologic evaluation. *For Grade 2 reactions,* if no improvement in 2 wk, hold encorafenib until Grade ≤1; then resume at same dose. *For Grade 3 reactions,* hold encorafenib until Grade ≤1.

E

Resume at same dose if 1st occurrence or ↓ dose if recurrent. *For Grade 4 reactions,* permanently discontinue encorafenib.

- Monitor for noncutaneous RAS mutation-positive malignancies. Permanently discontinue encorafenib if these malignancies occur.
- Monitor for signs and symptoms of hemorrhage (bleeding GI, rectal, anal, hemorrhoidal) periodically during therapy. *If Grade 2 or 1st occurrence of Grade 3 hemorrhagic event,* hold encorafenib for up to 4 wk. If improves to Grade ≤1, resume at ↓ dose. If no improvement, permanently discontinue encorafenib. *If 1st occurrence of Grade 4 hemorrhagic event,* permanently discontinue encorafenib or hold for up to 4 wk. If improves to Grade ≤1, resume at ↓ dose. If no improvement, permanently discontinue encorafenib. *If recurrent Grade 3 hemorrhagic event,* consider permanently discontinuing encorafenib. *If recurrent Grade 4 hemorrhagic event,* permanently discontinue encorafenib.
- Monitor ECG in patients who already have or are at risk of QTc interval prolongation, including patients with known long QT syndrome, clinically significant bradyarrhythmias, severe or uncontrolled HF, and those taking other medications leading to QT interval prolongation. *If QTcF interval >500 msec and ≤60 msec ↑ from baseline,* hold encorafenib until QTcF interval ≤500 msec. Resume at ↓ dose. If occurs more than once, permanently discontinue encorafenib. *If QTcF interval >500 msec and >60 msec ↑ from baseline,* permanently discontinue encorafenib.
- Assess for signs and symptoms of uveitis (visual changes, eye pain) during therapy. Perform ophthalmologic exam regularly and for new or worsening visual disturbances; follow new or persistent ophthalmologic findings. *If Grade 1 or 2 does not respond to ocular therapy or for Grade 3 uveitis,* hold encorafenib for up to 6 wk. If improved, resume at same or ↓ dose. If not improved, permanently discontinue encorafenib. *If Grade 4 uveitis occurs,* permanently discontinue encorafenib.

Lab Test Considerations

- Verify a negative pregnancy test before starting therapy.
- Confirm presence of a BRAF V600E or V600K mutation in tumor specimens before starting therapy for melanoma and of BRAF V600E mutation before starting therapy for colorectal cancer or NSCLC. Information on FDA-approved tests for the detection of BRAF V600E and V600K mutations is available at http://www.fda.gov/CompanionDiagnostics.
- Monitor serum electrolytes periodically during therapy. Correct hypokalemia and hypomagnesemia before and during therapy. May also cause hyponatremia and hyperglycemia.
- May cause anemia, leukopenia, lymphopenia, and neutropenia.
- Monitor liver function periodically during therapy. May ↑ GGT, AST, ALT, and alkaline phosphatase. *If Grade 2 AST or ALT ↑ occurs,* continue dose. If no improvement within 4 wk, hold encorafenib until Grade ≤1; then resume at same dose. If no improvement, permanently discontinue encorafenib. *If Grade 3 AST or ALT ↑ occurs,* consider permanently discontinuing encorafenib. *If Grade 4 AST or ALT ↑ occurs,* permanently discontinue encorafenib.

Implementation

- **Melanoma and NSCLC Dose Reduction Recommendations:** If binimetinib is held, ↓ encorafenib dose to max of 300 mg once daily until binimetinib is resumed. *1st dose reduction:* 300 mg (four 75-mg capsules) once daily. *2nd dose reduction:* 225 mg (three 75-mg capsules) once daily. *Subsequent modification:* Permanently discontinue if unable to tolerate encorafenib 225 mg (three 75-mg capsules) once daily.
- **Colorectal Cancer Dose Reduction Recommendations:** If cetuximab is discontinued, discontinue encorafenib. *1st dose reduction:* 225 mg (three 75-mg capsules) once daily. *2nd dose reduction:* 150 mg (two 75-mg capsules) once daily. *Subsequent modification:* Permanently discontinue if unable to tolerate encorafenib 150 mg (two 75-mg capsules) once daily.
- **PO:** Administer once daily without regard to food. Store in original bottle, tightly capped, at room temperature; do not remove desiccant; protect from moisture.

Patient/Family Teaching

- Explain purpose and side effects of medication to patient. Advise patient to read *Patient Information* before starting therapy. Instruct patient to take as directed. Take missed dose within 12 hr of missed dose; do not take dose within 12 hr of next dose. If vomiting occurs, skip dose; continue with next scheduled dose.
- Advise patient to notify health care professional of all Rx or OTC medications, vitamins, or herbal products being taken and to consult with health care professional before taking other medications, especially St. John's wort.
- Inform patient to avoid grapefruit and grapefruit juice during therapy.
- Instruct patient to notify health care professional promptly if new onset or worsening shortness of breath; cough; swelling of the ankles, legs, or face; palpitations; or weight gain of >5 pounds in 24 hr occur.
- Inform patient of the ↑ risk of developing new cutaneous malignancies. Notify health care professional immediately if new lesions (wart, skin sore or reddish bump that bleeds or does not heal) or changes in size or color of existing moles or lesions occur.

- Advise patient to notify health care professional immediately if signs and symptoms of bleeding (headaches, dizziness, weakness, coughing up blood or blood clots, vomiting blood or vomit looks like coffee grounds, red or black tarry stools), liver dysfunction (yellow skin or whites of eyes, feeling tired, dark or brown urine, nausea or vomiting, loss of appetite, pain on right side of stomach), changes in heart rhythm (feeling faint, light-headed, or dizzy; heart beating irregularly or fast), or eye problems (blurred vision, loss of vision, other vision changes, seeing colored dots, seeing halos or blurred outline around objects, eye pain, swelling, redness) occur.
- Inform patient that regular assessments of skin and assessments for signs and symptoms of other malignancies must be done every 2 mo during and for up to 6 mo after therapy. Advise patient to notify health care professional immediately if any changes in skin occur.
- Rep: May cause fetal harm, and may ↓ effectiveness of hormonal contraceptives. Advise women to use a highly effective nonhormonal form of contraception during and for 2 wk after last dose. Advise patient to notify health care professional if pregnancy is suspected and to avoid breastfeeding during therapy and for >2 wk after last dose. May impair fertility in men.

Evaluation/Desired Outcomes

- Improvement in progression-free survival and overall survival in patients with melanoma and colorectal cancer.
- Decreased progression of NSCLC.

HIGH ALERT

enfortumab vedotin

(en-**fort**-ue-mab ve-**doe**-tin)

Padcev

Classification

Therapeutic: antineoplastics

Pharmacologic: drug-antibody conjugates

Indications

Locally advanced or metastatic urothelial cancer in patients who are not eligible for cisplatin-containing chemotherapy (in combination with pembrolizumab). Locally advanced or metastatic urothelial cancer in patients who have previously received a programmed death receptor-1 (PD-1) or programmed death-ligand 1 (PD-L1) inhibitor and a platinum-containing chemotherapy. Locally advanced or metastatic urothelial cancer in patients who are not eligible for cisplatin-containing chemotherapy and have previously received ≥1 line of therapy.

Action

Acts as an antibody-drug conjugate (ADC) composed of a humanized IgG1 monoclonal antibody directed against Nectin-4 (an adhesion protein located on cell surface), a cleavable linker, and monomethyl auristatin E (MMAE) (an agent that disrupts microtubles and subsequently causes apoptosis). **Therapeutic Effects:** Reduced progression of locally advanced or metastatic urothelial cancer.

E

Pharmacokinetics

Absorption: IV administration results in complete bioavailability.

Distribution: Minimally distributed to extravascular tissues.

Metabolism and Excretion: Monoclonal antibody component is degraded into smaller peptides via catabolism. MMAE is primarily metabolized in the liver via the CYP3A4 isoenzyme. 17% of MMAE excreted in feces; 6% excreted in urine, primarily as unchanged drug.

Half-life: *ADC:* 3.4 days; *MMAE:* 2.4 days.

TIME/ACTION PROFILE (plasma concentrations)

ROUTE	ONSET	PEAK	DURATION
IV	unknown	ADC: end of infusion; MMAE: 2 days	unknown

Contraindications/Precautions

Contraindicated in: Moderate or severe hepatic impairment; OB: Pregnancy; Lactation: Lactation.

Use Cautiously in: Patients with or at risk for diabetes mellitus (↑ risk of hyperglycemia); Rep: Women of reproductive potential and men with female partners of reproductive potential; Pedi: Safety and effectiveness not established in children.

Adverse Reactions/Side Effects

Derm: alopecia, dry skin, palmar-plantar erythrodysesthesia, pruritus, rash, cellulitis, STEVENS-JOHNSON SYNDROME (SJS), TOXIC EPIDERMAL NECROLYSIS (TEN). **EENT:** blurred vision, dry eye, keratitis. **Endo:** HYPERGLYCEMIA, DIABETIC KETOACIDOSIS. **F and E:** hypokalemia, hypophosphatemia, hyponatremia. **GI:** ↓ appetite, ↑ lipase, diarrhea, nausea, vomiting. **GU:** ↑ serum creatinine, ↓ fertility (men), acute kidney injury, urinary tract infection. **Hemat:** anemia, leukopenia, lymphocytopenia, neutropenia. **Local:** extravasation. **Metab:** hyperuricemia. **Neuro:** dysgeusia, fatigue, peripheral neuropathy. **Resp:** PNEUMONITIS/INTERSTITIAL LUNG DISEASE, dyspnea. **Misc:** herpes zoster infection.

Interactions

Drug-Drug: Strong CYP3A4 inhibitors, including **ketoconazole**, may ↑ levels and risk of toxicity of MMAE; monitor closely.

Route/Dosage

IV (Adults ≥100 kg): 125 mg on Days 1, 8, and 15 of a 28-day cycle; continue until disease progression or unacceptable toxicity.

IV (Adults <100 kg): 1.25 mg/kg on Days 1, 8, and 15 of a 28-day cycle; continue until disease progression or unacceptable toxicity.

Availability

Lyophilized powder for injection: 20 mg/vial, 30 mg/vial.

NURSING IMPLICATIONS

Assessment

- Monitor for symptoms of new or worsening peripheral neuropathy (burning, numbness, or tingling in hands or feet; muscle weakness) during therapy. *If Grade 2 neuropathy occurs,* hold medication until Grade ≤1; then resume therapy at same dose (if 1st occurrence). For a recurrence, withhold until Grade ≤1; then resume therapy by ↓ one dose level. *If Grade 3 neuropathy occurs,* permanently discontinue enfortumab vedotin.
- Monitor for signs and symptoms of skin reactions (maculopapular rash, pruritus) during therapy. Consider topical corticosteroids and antihistamines as clinically indicated. *For persistent or recurrent Grade 2 skin reactions,* consider holding dose until Grade ≤1; then resume treatment at the same dose level or ↓ dose by one dose level. *If Grade 3 skin reactions occur,* hold dose until Grade ≤1; then resume treatment at same dose level or ↓ dose by one dose level. *If SJS or TEN is suspected,* immediately hold dose; consult a specialist to confirm diagnosis. If not SJS/TEN, see Grade 2–4 skin reactions. *If confirmed SJS or TEN and Grade 4 or recurrent Grade 3 skin reactions occur,* permanently discontinue enfortumab vedotin.
- Monitor for ocular disorders. Consider artificial tears for prophylaxis of dry eyes and ophthalmologic evaluation if ocular symptoms occur or do not resolve. May use ophthalmic topical steroids, if indicated, after an ophthalmic exam. Consider interrupting therapy or ↓ dose for symptomatic ocular disorders.

Lab Test Considerations

- Verify negative pregnancy test before starting therapy.
- Monitor blood glucose closely in patients with or at risk for hyperglycemia or diabetes mellitus. *If blood glucose >250 mg/dL,* hold medication until blood glucose <250 mg/dL; then resume therapy at same dose.
- May ↓ hemoglobin, lymphocytes, neutrophils, and leukocytes.

Implementation

IV Administration

- ***High Alert:*** Fatalities have occurred with chemotherapeutic agents. Before administering, clarify all ambiguous orders; double-check single, daily, and course-of-therapy dose limits; have second practitioner independently double-check original order, calculations, and infusion pump settings.
- Wear gloves, gown, and mask while handling medication. If powder or solution comes in contact with skin or mucosa, wash thoroughly with soap and water. Discard equipment in specially designated containers.
- **Dose Reduction Schedule:** *1st dose reduction:* 1 mg/kg (up to 100 mg). *2nd dose reduction:* 0.75 mg/kg (up to 75 mg). *3rd dose reduction:* 0.5 mg/kg (up to 50 mg).
- Enfortumab vedotin is an irritant. If extravasation occurs, immediately stop infusion. Leave needle/cannula in place temporarily but do not flush the line. Gently aspirate extravasated solution; then remove needle/cannula. Elevate patient's extremity.
- **Intermittent Infusion: Reconstitution:** Reconstitute 20 mg vial with 2.3 mL and 30 mg vial with 3.3 mL of sterile water for injection. Direct stream to walls of vial, not to powder. Swirl vial to dissolve contents. Allow vial to settle for ≥1 min until bubbles are gone. Do not shake or expose to direct sunlight. Solution is clear to slightly opalescent, colorless to light yellow; do not administer solutions that are cloudy, discolored, or contain particulate matter. **Dilution:** Withdraw required volume of reconstituted solution and transfer to bag containing D5W, 0.9% NaCl, or LR. Mix diluted solution by gently inverting; do not shake or expose to direct sunlight. Solution is stable for up to 8 hr if refrigerated; do not freeze. **Concentration:** 0.3–4 mg/mL.
- **Rate:** Infuse over 30 min.
- **Y-Site Incompatibility:** Do not administer other drugs through same IV line.

Patient/Family Teaching

- Explain purpose and side effects of medication. Advise patient to read *Patient Information* before starting therapy.
- Instruct patient to notify health care provider of all Rx or OTC medications, vitamins, or herbal products being taken and consult health care provider before taking any new medications.
- Advise patient to notify health care provider if signs and symptoms of hyperglycemia (frequent urination, ↑ thirst, blurred vision, confusion, drowsiness, loss of

appetite, fruity breath smell, nausea, vomiting, stomach pain), difficulty controlling blood sugar, peripheral neuropathy, ocular disorders (visual changes), skin reactions, or infusion site reactions occur.

- Discuss with patient the possibility of hair loss. Explore methods of coping.
- Rep: May cause fetal harm. Advise women of reproductive potential to use effective contraception during and for 2 mo after last dose and men with female partners of reproductive potential to use effective contraception for 4 mo after last dose. Advise patient to avoid breastfeeding during and for >3 wk after last dose. Advise patient to notify health care provider immediately if pregnancy is suspected. May reversibly impair female fertility and may impair male fertility.

Evaluation/Desired Outcomes

- Reduced progression of locally advanced or metastatic urothelial cancer.

enoxaparin, See HEPARINS (LOW MOLECULAR WEIGHT).

entacapone (en-tak-a-pone)

Comtan

Classification

Therapeutic: antiparkinson agents

Pharmacologic: catechol-*O*-methyltransferase (COMT) inhibitors

Indications

Parkinson disease when signs and symptoms of end-of-dose wearing-off (so-called fluctuating patients) occur (in combination with levodopa/carbidopa).

Action

Acts as a selective and reversible inhibitor of the enzyme catechol *O*-methyltransferase (COMT). Inhibition of COMT prevents the breakdown of levodopa, increasing availability to the CNS. **Therapeutic Effects:** Prolongs duration of response to levodopa with end-of-dose motor fluctuations. Decreased signs and symptoms of Parkinson disease.

Pharmacokinetics

Absorption: 35% absorbed following oral administration; absorption is rapid.

Distribution: Widely distributed to tissues.

Protein Binding: 98%.

Metabolism and Excretion: Minimal amounts excreted unchanged; highly metabolized followed by biliary excretion.

Half-life: *Initial phase:* 0.4–0.7 hr; *second phase:* 2.4 hr.

TIME/ACTION PROFILE (inhibition of COMT)

ROUTE	ONSET	PEAK	DURATION
PO	unknown	unknown	up to 8 hr

Contraindications/Precautions

Contraindicated in: Hypersensitivity; Psychotic disorder.

Use Cautiously in: Hepatic impairment; OB: Safety not established in pregnancy; Lactation: Safety not established in breastfeeding; Pedi: Safety and effectiveness not established in children.

Adverse Reactions/Side Effects

CV: hypotension. **Derm:** MELANOMA. **GI:** abdominal pain, colitis, diarrhea, nausea (during initiation), retroperitoneal fibrosis. **GU:** brownish-orange discoloration of urine. **MS:** dyskinesia, RHABDOMYOLYSIS. **Neuro:** aggressive behavior, agitation, confusion, delirium, disorientation, dizziness, hallucinations, NEUROLEPTIC MALIGNANT SYNDROME, paranoid ideation, syncope, urges (gambling, sexual). **Resp:** pleural effusion, pleural thickening, pulmonary infiltrates.

Interactions

Drug-Drug: Concurrent use with selective **MAO inhibitors** is not recommended; both agents inhibit the metabolic pathways of catecholamines. Drugs that are metabolized by COMT, including **isoproterenol**, **epinephrine**, **norepinephrine**, **dopamine**, and **dobutamine**, may ↑ risk of tachycardia, ↑ BP, and arrhythmias. **Probenecid**, **cholestyramine**, **erythromycin**, **rifampin**, **ampicillin**, and **chloramphenicol** may interfere with biliary elimination of entacapone; use concurrently with caution.

Route/Dosage

PO (Adults): 200 mg with each dose of levodopa/carbidopa up to a maximum of 8 times daily.

Availability (generic available)

Tablets: 200 mg. ***In combination with:*** levodopa/carbidopa (Stalevo); see Appendix N.

NURSING IMPLICATIONS

Assessment

- Assess parkinsonian and extrapyramidal symptoms (restlessness or desire to keep moving, rigidity, tremors, pill rolling, mask-like face, shuffling gait, muscle spasms, twisting motions, difficulty speaking or swallowing, loss of balance control) prior to and during therapy. Dyskinesia may ↑ with therapy.
- Monitor for development of diarrhea. Usually occurs within 4–12 wk of start of therapy, but may occur as early as the 1st wk and as late as months after initiation of therapy.

- Monitor for signs and symptoms of neuroleptic malignant syndrome (↑ temperature, muscular rigidity, altered consciousness, ↑ CK). Symptoms have been associated with rapid dose ↓ or withdrawal of other dopaminergic drugs. Withdrawal should be gradual.

Implementation

- **PO:** Always administer entacapone with levodopa/carbidopa. Entacapone has no antiparkinsonism effects of its own.

Patient/Family Teaching

- Explain purpose and side effects of medication. Advise patient to read *Patient Information* before starting therapy. Instruct to take as directed. Take missed doses as soon as possible, up to 2 hr before the next dose. Taper gradually when discontinuing or a withdrawal reaction may occur.
- Advise patient to notify health care professional of all Rx or OTC medications, vitamins, or herbal products being taken and to consult health care professional before taking other medications.
- May cause dizziness or hallucinations. Advise patient to avoid driving or other activities that require alertness until response to the drug is known.
- Inform patient that nausea may occur, especially at initiation of therapy, and diarrhea. Advise patient with diarrhea to drink fluids to maintain adequate hydration and monitor for weight loss. If diarrhea is prolonged, may resolve with discontinuation. Therapy may cause change in urine color to brownish orange.
- Caution patient to change positions slowly to minimize orthostatic hypotension.
- Advise patient to notify health care professional if suspicious or unusual skin changes; agitation; aggression; delirium; hallucinations; or new or ↑ gambling, sexual, or other intense urges occur.
- Emphasize the importance of routine follow-up exams.
- Rep: Advise women of reproductive potential to notify health care professional if pregnancy is planned or suspected or if breastfeeding.

Evaluation/Desired Outcomes

- Prolongs duration of response to levodopa with end-of-dose motor fluctuations.
- Decreased signs and symptoms of Parkinson disease.

entecavir (en-**tek**-aveer)

Baraclude

Classification

Therapeutic: antivirals

Pharmacologic: nucleoside analogues

Indications

Chronic hepatitis B virus (HBV) infection with evidence of active viral replication and either persistent elevations in AST or ALT or histologically active disease.

Action

Phosphorylated intracellularly to active form, which acts as an analogue of guanosine, interfering with viral DNA synthesis. **Therapeutic Effects:** Decreased hepatic damage due to chronic HBV infection.

Pharmacokinetics

Absorption: Well absorbed following oral administration.

Distribution: Extensive tissue distribution.

Metabolism and Excretion: 62–73% excreted unchanged by kidneys.

Half-life: *Plasma:* 128–149 hr; *intracellular:* 15 hr.

TIME/ACTION PROFILE (plasma concentrations)

ROUTE	ONSET	PEAK	DURATION
PO	rapid	0.5–1 hr	24 hr

Contraindications/Precautions

Contraindicated in: Hypersensitivity.

Use Cautiously in: Renal impairment (↓ dose if CCr <50 mL/min; Liver transplant recipients (careful monitoring of renal function recommended); Patients coinfected with HIV (unless receiving highly active antiretroviral therapy; at ↑ risk for resistance); OB: Other agents preferred for treatment of HBV during pregnancy; Lactation: Use during breastfeeding only if benefit to patient outweighs potential risk to infant; Pedi: Children <2 yr (safety and effectiveness not established); Geri: ↑ risk of toxicity in older adults due to age-related ↓ in renal function.

Adverse Reactions/Side Effects

Derm: alopecia, rash. **F and E** LACTIC ACIDOSIS. **GI:** HEPATOMEGALY (WITH STEATOSIS), dyspepsia, nausea. **Neuro:** dizziness, fatigue, headache.

Interactions

Drug-Drug: Concurrent use of drugs that may impair renal function may ↑ levels and risk of toxicity.

Route/Dosage

PO (Adults): *Compensated liver disease:* 0.5 mg once daily; *Decompensated liver disease or history of lamivudine resistance:* 1 mg once daily.

PO (Children ≥2 yr and >30 kg): 0.5 mg once daily (1 mg once daily if history of lamivudine resistance).

PO (Children ≥2 yr and >26–30 kg): 0.45 mg once daily (0.9 mg once daily if history of lamivudine resistance).

PO (Children ≥2 yr and >23–26 kg): 0.4 mg once daily (0.8 mg once daily if history of lamivudine resistance).

PO (Children ≥2 yr and >20–23 kg): 0.35 mg once daily (0.7 mg once daily if history of lamivudine resistance).
PO (Children ≥2 yr and >17–20 kg): 0.3 mg once daily (0.6 mg once daily if history of lamivudine resistance).
PO (Children ≥2 yr and >14–17 kg): 0.25 mg once daily (0.5 mg once daily if history of lamivudine resistance).
PO (Children ≥2 yr and >11–14 kg): 0.2 mg once daily (0.4 mg once daily if history of lamivudine resistance).
PO (Children ≥2 yr and 10–11 kg): 0.15 mg once daily (0.3 mg once daily if history of lamivudine resistance).

Renal Impairment
PO (Adults): *CCr 30–<50 mL/min:* 0.25 mg once daily or 0.5 mg every 48 hr (0.5 mg once daily or 1 mg every 48 hr if lamivudine-resistant or decompensated liver disease). *CCr 10–<30 mL/min:* 0.15 mg once daily or 0.5 mg every 72 hr (0.3 mg once daily or 1 mg every 72 hr if lamivudine-resistant or decompensated liver disease). *CCr <10 mL/min, hemodialysis, or CAPD:* 0.05 mg once daily or 0.5 mg every 7 days (0.1 mg once daily or 1 mg every 7 days if lamivudine-resistant or decompensated liver disease).

Availability (generic available)
Oral solution (orange flavor): 0.05 mg/mL. **Tablets:** 0.5 mg, 1 mg.

NURSING IMPLICATIONS
Assessment
- Monitor signs of HBV (jaundice, fatigue, anorexia, pruritus) during and for several months following discontinuation of therapy. Exacerbations may occur when therapy is discontinued.
- Monitor patient for signs of lactic acidosis and severe hepatomegaly with steatosis (↑ serum lactate levels, ↑ liver enzymes, liver enlargement on palpation). Suspend therapy if clinical or laboratory signs occur.

Lab Test Considerations
- Monitor liver function tests closely during and for several months following discontinuation of therapy. May ↑ serum AST, ALT, bilirubin, amylase, lipase, creatinine, and glucose. May ↓ albumin.

Implementation
- **PO:** Administer on an empty stomach >2 hr before or after a meal. Use oral solution for dose <0.5 mg and children up to 30 kg. Children >30 kg can use oral solution or tablet. Oral solution is ready to use; do not dilute or mix with water or any other liquid. Hold dosing spoon in a vertical position and fill gradually to mark corresponding to prescribed dose; rinse dosing spoon with water after each daily dose. Store in outer carton at room temperature. After opening, solution can be used until expiration date on bottle.

Patient/Family Teaching
- Explain purpose and side effects of medication. Advise patient to read *Patient Information* before starting therapy. Instruct patient to take as directed. Take missed doses as soon as possible unless almost time for next dose. Do not double doses. Emphasize the importance of compliance with full course of therapy and not taking more than the prescribed amount. Caution patient not to share medication with others.
- Do not stop taking without consulting health care provider. Discontinuing therapy may lead to severe exacerbations.
- Instruct patient to notify health care provider of all Rx or OTC medications, vitamins, or herbal products being taken and to consult with health care provider before taking other medications.
- Inform patient that entecavir does not cure HBV but may ↓ the amount of HBV in the body, ↓ the ability of HBV to multiply and infect new liver cells, and improve the condition of the liver. Entecavir does not ↓ the risk of transmission of HBV to others through sexual contact or blood contamination. Caution patient to use a condom during sexual contact and avoid sharing needles or donating blood to prevent spreading HBV to others.
- Advise patient to notify health care provider promptly if signs of lactic acidosis (weakness or tiredness; unusual muscle pain; trouble breathing; stomach pain with nausea and vomiting; feeling cold, especially in arms or legs; dizziness; fast or irregular heartbeat) or hepatotoxicity (jaundice, dark urine, light-colored bowel movements, anorexia, nausea, lower stomach pain) occur.
- May cause dizziness. Caution patient to avoid driving or other activities requiring alertness until response to medication is known.
- Discuss the possibility of hair loss with patient. Explore methods of coping.
- Emphasize the importance of regular follow-up exams and blood tests to determine progress and monitor for side effects.
- Rep: Advise women of reproductive potential to notify health care provider if pregnancy is planned or suspected and to avoid breastfeeding during therapy. Encourage pregnant women to enroll in the Antiretroviral Pregnancy Registry by calling 1-800-258-4263.

Evaluation/Desired Outcomes
- Decreased hepatic damage due to chronic HBV infection.

HIGH ALERT

enzalutamide
(en-za-**loo**-ta-mide)

Xtandi

Classification

Therapeutic: antineoplastics

Pharmacologic: androgen receptor inhibitors

Indications
Castration-resistant prostate cancer. Metastatic, castration-sensitive prostate cancer. Nonmetastatic castration-sensitive prostate cancer with biochemical recurrence at high risk for metastasis.

Action
Acts as an androgen receptor inhibitor, preventing the binding of androgen; also inhibits androgen nuclear translocation and DNA interaction. Decreases proliferation and induces cell death of prostate cancer cells. **Therapeutic Effects:** Decreased growth and spread of prostate cancer.

Pharmacokinetics
Absorption: Well absorbed following oral administration.

Distribution: Widely distributed to tissues.

Protein Binding: *Enzalutamide:* 97–98%; *N-desmethylenzalutamide:* 95%.

Metabolism and Excretion: Extensively metabolized by the liver via the CYP2C8 and CYP3A4 isoenzymes; one metabolite (N-desmethylenzalutamide) has antineoplastic activity. Metabolites are primarily renally excreted, only minimal amounts as unchanged drug.

Half-life: *Enzalutamide:* 5.8 days; *N-desmethylenzalutamide:* 7.8–8.6 days.

TIME/ACTION PROFILE (improved survival)

ROUTE	ONSET	PEAK	DURATION
PO	3 mo	unknown	unknown

Contraindications/Precautions
Contraindicated in: None.

Use Cautiously in: History of seizures, underlying brain pathology, cerebrovascular accident, transient ischemic attack (within 12 mo), brain metastases, or brain arteriovenous malformation (↑ risk of seizures); Dysphagia; Rep: Men with female partners of reproductive potential; Geri: Older adults may be more sensitive to drug effects.

Adverse Reactions/Side Effects
CV: peripheral edema, hypertension, ISCHEMIC HEART DISEASE. **Derm:** dry skin, pruritus. **EENT:** epistaxis. **Endo:** hot flush. **GI:** diarrhea. **GU:** hematuria, urinary frequency. **MS:** arthralgia, fracture, musculoskeletal pain, muscular stiffness, muscular weakness. **Neuro:** headache, weakness, anxiety, dizziness, hallucinations, hypoesthesia, insomnia, paresthesia, POSTERIOR REVERSIBLE ENCEPHALOPATHY SYNDROME (PRES), SEIZURES, SPINAL CORD COMPRESSION/CAUDA EQUINA SYNDROME. **Misc:** falls, HYPERSENSITIVITY REACTIONS (INCLUDING ANGIOEDEMA).

Interactions
Drug-Drug: Strong CYP2C8 inhibitors, including **gemfibrozil**, may ↑ levels and risk of toxicity; avoid concurrent use (if concurrent administration necessary, ↓ enzalutamide dose). **Strong CYP3A4 inducers**, including **carbamazepine**, **phenobarbital**, **phenytoin**, **rifabutin**, **rifampin**, and **rifapentine**, may ↓ levels and effectiveness; avoid concurrent use. If concurrent use necessary, ↑ enzalutamide dose. May ↓ levels and effectiveness of **CYP3A4, CYP2C9, and CYP2C19 substrates** that have narrow therapeutic indexes, including **cyclosporine**, **fentanyl**, **phenytoin**, **sirolimus**, **tacrolimus**, and **warfarin**; avoid concurrent use. **Drugs that ↓ seizure threshold** may ↑ risk of seizures.

Drug-Natural Products: St. John's wort may ↓ levels and effectiveness; avoid concurrent use. If concurrent use necessary, ↑ enzalutamide dose.

Route/Dosage
Patients with castration-resistant prostate cancer or metastatic castration-sensitive prostate cancer should also receive gonadotropin-releasing hormone (GnRH) analog concurrently or should have had bilateral orchiectomy. Patients with nonmetastatic castration-sensitive prostate cancer with biochemical recurrence at high risk for metastasis may receive enzalutamide with or without a GnRH analog.

PO (Adults): 160 mg once daily. *Concurrent use of strong CYP2C8 inhibitors:* 80 mg once daily; *Concurrent use of strong CYP3A4 inducers:* 240 mg once daily.

Availability (generic available)
Capsules: 40 mg. **Film-coated tablets:** 40 mg, 80 mg.

NURSING IMPLICATIONS
Assessment
- Monitor for seizures. Implement seizure precautions. If a seizure occurs during therapy, permanently discontinue enzalutamide therapy.
- Monitor all patients for signs and symptoms of PRES (visual disturbance, seizure, headaches, altered mentation); discontinue enzalutamide and report immediately. Diagnosis is made with MRI.
- Monitor for signs and symptoms of hypersensitivity reactions (rash, urticaria, pruritus, flushing, dizziness, vomiting, abdominal pain) and angioedema (swelling of throat, lips, tongue, or face; dyspnea; wheezing; hoarseness). Discontinue enzalutamide immediately and provide supportive care.

- Monitor for signs and symptoms of ischemic heart disease (chest pain, fainting, dyspnea). *If Grade 3 or 4 ischemic heart disease symptoms occur,* permanently discontinue enzalutamide.
- Assess risk of falls and fractures periodically during therapy. May consider bone-targeted agents.

Lab Test Considerations

- May cause hematuria.

Implementation

- ***High Alert:*** During administration, wear double chemotherapy gloves and protective gown when handling uncoated, cut, or crushed tablets. Eye/face protection is need if there is risk of patient vomiting or spitting up. Single chemotherapy gloves are appropriate if handling and administering intact tablets from a unit-dose package. Health care providers who are actively trying to conceive, who are pregnant or may become pregnant, and who are breastfeeding should avoid handling enzalutamide.
- **PO:** Administer (two 80-mg tablets or four 40-mg tablets or four 40-mg capsules) once daily without regard to food. ***DNC:*** Swallow capsules and tablets whole; do not open, dissolve, or chew capsules, and do not cut, crush, or chew tablets. Discontinue if patient cannot swallow due to capsule or tablet size; severe dysphagia or choking could be life-threatening.
- Treatment can be suspended if prostate-specific antigen (PSA) is undetectable (<0.2 ng/mL) after 36 wk of therapy. Reinitiate enzalutamide when PSA has ↑ to ≥2.0 ng/mL for patients who had prior radical prostatectomy or ≥5.0 ng/mL for patients who had prior primary radiation therapy.
- *If Grade ≥3 toxicity or intolerable side effects occur,* hold dose for 1 wk or until symptoms improve to Grade <2; then resume at same or reduced dose (120 mg or 80 mg).

Patient/Family Teaching

- Explain the purpose and side effects of enzalutamide. Instruct patient to take as directed at the same time each day. Take missed doses as soon as remembered within the same day. If a whole day is missed, omit dose and take next day's scheduled dose; do not double doses. Advise patient not to interrupt, modify dose, or stop taking enzalutamide without consulting health care professional. Warn patient to report difficulty swallowing capsules or tablets. Advise patient to read *Patient Information* before starting therapy and with each Rx refill in case of changes.
- May cause seizures, dizziness, mental impairment, paresthesia, hypoesthesia, falls, and hallucinations. Caution patient to avoid driving and other activities requiring alertness until response to medication is known. Notify health care professional immediately if loss of consciousness, seizure, chest pain, signs and symptoms of PRES, or hypersensitivity reactions occur.
- Inform patient of common side effects associated with enzalutamide: asthenia/fatigue, back pain, diarrhea, arthralgia, hot flush, peripheral edema, musculoskeletal pain, headache, upper and lower respiratory infection, muscular weakness, dizziness, insomnia, spinal cord compression, cauda equina syndrome, hematuria, paresthesia, anxiety, and hypertension. Notify health care professional if falls or problems thinking clearly occur or if side effects are bothersome.
- Instruct patient to notify health care professional of all Rx or OTC medications, vitamins, or herbal products being taken and to consult health care professional before taking other Rx, OTC, or herbal products, especially St. John's wort.
- Rep: May cause fetal harm and loss of pregnancy. Instruct women of reproductive potential to avoid handling enzalutamide tablets. Advise men with female partners of reproductive potential to use a condom and effective contraception during and for 3 mo after last dose. May impair fertility in men.

Evaluation/Desired Outcomes

- Decreased growth and spread of prostate cancer.

HIGH ALERT

V EPINEPHrine (ep-i-**nef**-rin)

Adrenaclick, Adrenalin, ✱ Allerject, ✱ Anapen, ✱ Anapen Junior, ~~AsthmaNefrin~~, Auvi-Q, ✱ Emerade, EpiPen, Neffy, Primatene Mist, ✱ S-2 (racepinephrine), Symjepi, ~~Twin-Jeet~~

Classification

Therapeutic: antiasthmatics, bronchodilators, vasopressors

Pharmacologic: adrenergics

See Appendix B for ophthalmic use

Indications

Intranasal, SUBQ, IM, IV: Severe allergic reactions. **IV:** Hypotension associated with septic shock. **Inhaln:** Upper airway obstruction and croup (racemic epinephrine). Temporary relief of mild symptoms of intermittent asthma (over-the-counter). **Local/Spinal:** Adjunct in the localization/prolongation of anesthesia. **Unlabeled Use: IV, intracardiac, intratracheal, intraosseous (part of advanced cardiac life support [ACLS], and pediatric advanced life support [PALS] guidelines):** Cardiac arrest. **SUBQ, IM:** Reversible airway disease due to asthma or COPD.

Action

Results in the accumulation of cyclic adenosine monophosphate (cAMP) at beta-adrenergic receptors. Affects both $beta_1$ (cardiac)-adrenergic receptors and $beta_2$ (pulmonary)-adrenergic receptor sites. Produces bronchodilation. Also has alpha-adrenergic agonist properties, which result in vasoconstriction. Inhibits the release of mediators of immediate hypersensitivity reactions from mast cells. **Therapeutic Effects:** Bronchodilation. Maintenance of HR and BP. Localization/prolongation of local/spinal anesthetic.

Pharmacokinetics

Absorption: IV administration results in complete bioavailability; well absorbed following SUBQ and intranasal administration; some absorption may occur following repeated inhalation of large doses.
Distribution: Does not cross the blood-brain barrier.
Metabolism and Excretion: Action is rapidly terminated by metabolism and uptake by nerve endings.
Half-life: Unknown.

TIME/ACTION PROFILE (bronchodilation)

ROUTE	ONSET	PEAK	DURATION
Inhaln	1 min	unknown	1–3 hr
SUBQ	5–10 min	20 min	<1–4 hr
IM	6–12 min	unknown	<1–4 hr
IV	rapid	20 min	20–30 min
Intranasal	5–10 min	20–30 min	1 hr

Contraindications/Precautions

Contraindicated in: Hypersensitivity to adrenergic amines; Some products may contain bisulfites and should be avoided in patients with known hypersensitivity or intolerance.
Use Cautiously in: Cardiac disease (angina, tachycardia, MI); Hypertension; Hyperthyroidism; Parkinson disease; Pheochromocytoma; Diabetes; Cerebral arteriosclerosis; Glaucoma (except for ophthalmic use); Excessive use may lead to tolerance and paradoxical bronchospasm (inhaler); Structural or anatomic nasal conditions (intranasal only); OB: Use during pregnancy only if potential maternal benefit justifies potential fetal risk; use for anaphylaxis should not be delayed in pregnancy; Lactation: High IV doses of epinephrine might ↓ milk production or letdown. Low-dose epidural, topical, inhaled, intranasal, or ophthalmic epinephrine are unlikely to interfere with breastfeeding; Pedi: Safety and effectiveness not established in children <12 yr (over-the-counter product only) or <15 kg (intranasal only); Geri: Older adults more susceptible to adverse reactions; may require ↓ dose.

Adverse Reactions/Side Effects

CV: angina, arrhythmias, hypertension, tachycardia. **Derm:** skin and soft tissue infections (including necrotizing fasciitis and myonecrosis). **EENT:** intranasal paresthesia (nasal spray), nasal discomfort (nasal spray), throat irritation (nasal spray), nasal congestion (nasal spray), nasal pruritus (nasal spray), rhinorrhea (nasal spray), sneezing (nasal spray). **Endo:** hyperglycemia. **GI:** abdominal pain (nasal spray), nausea, vomiting. **GU:** renal impairment. **Neuro:** dizziness (nasal spray), headache, nervousness, restlessness, tremor, insomnia. **Resp:** PARADOXICAL BRONCHOSPASM (WITH EXCESSIVE USE OF INHALERS), pulmonary edema.

Interactions

Drug-Drug: Adrenergic agents will cause additive adrenergic side effects. Use with **MAO inhibitors** may lead to hypertensive crisis. **Beta blockers** may negate therapeutic effect. **Tricyclic antidepressants** enhance pressor response to epinephrine. Use of intranasal product may ↑ absorption of other **intranasal products** and ↑ risk of toxicity.
Drug-Natural Products: Use with caffeine-containing herbs (**cola nut, guarana, mate, tea, coffee**) ↑ stimulant effect.

Route/Dosage

SUBQ, IM (Adults and Children ≥30 kg): *Severe anaphylaxis:* 0.3–0.5 mg (not to exceed 0.5 mg/dose); may repeat every 10–15 min as needed.
SUBQ (Children <30 kg): *Severe anaphylaxis:* 0.01 mg/kg (not to exceed 0.3 mg/dose); may repeat every 10–15 min as needed; *Auvi-Q or Symjepi (15–30 kg):* 0.15 mg; may repeat if anaphylactic symptoms persist; *Auvi-Q (7.5–15 kg):* 0.1 mg; may repeat if anaphylactic symptoms persist.
IV (Adults): *Severe anaphylaxis:* 0.1–0.25 mg every 5–15 min; may be followed by 1–4 mcg/min continuous infusion; *Cardiopulmonary resuscitation (ACLS guidelines):* 1 mg every 3–5 min; *Bradycardia (ACLS guidelines):* 2–10 mcg/min continuous infusion; *Hypotension associated with septic shock:* 0.05–2 mcg/kg/min continuous infusion; titrate every 10–15 min by 0.05–0.2 mcg/kg/min to achieve desired mean arterial pressure.
IV (Children): *Severe anaphylaxis:* 0.1 mg (less in younger children); may be followed by 0.1 mcg/kg/min continuous infusion (may ↑ up to 1.5 mcg/kg/min); *Symptomatic bradycardia/pulseless arrest (PALS guidelines):* 0.01 mg/kg; may repeat every 3–5 min; higher doses (up to 0.1–0.2 mg/kg) may be considered; may also be given by the intraosseous route. May also be given by the endotracheal route in doses of 0.1–0.2 mg/kg diluted to a volume of 3–5 mL with normal saline followed by several positive pressure ventilations.
Inhaln (Adults): *Inhalation solution:* 1 inhalation of 1% solution; may repeat after 1–2 min; additional doses may be given every 3 hr; *Racepinephrine:* Via hand nebulizer, 2–3 inhalations of 2.25% solution; may repeat in 5 min with 2–3 more inhalations, up to 4–6 times daily.

Inhaln: (Adults and Children ≥12 yr): *Over-the-counter inhaler:* 1–2 inhalations every 4 hr as needed (max = 8 inhalations/day).
Inhaln: (Children >1 mo): 0.25–0.5 mL of 2.25% racemic epinephrine solution diluted in 3 mL normal saline.
Intranasal (Adults and Children ≥4 yr and ≥30 kg): One spray (2 mg) administered into one nostril; if no clinical improvement in 5 min, may administer another spray (2 mg) in same nostril.
Intranasal (Adults and Children ≥4 yr and 15–<30 kg): One spray (1 mg) administered into one nostril; if no clinical improvement in 5 min, may administer another spray (1 mg) in same nostril.
IV, Intratracheal **(Neonates):** 0.01–0.03 mg/kg every 3–5 min as needed.
Intracardiac (Adults): 0.3–0.5 mg.
Endotracheal: (Adults): *Cardiopulmonary resuscitation (ACLS guidelines):* 2–2.5 mg.
Topical (Adults and Children ≥6 yr): *Nasal decongestant:* Apply 1% solution as drops, spray, or with a swab.
Intraspinal: (Adults and Children): 0.2–0.4 mL of 1:1000 solution.
With Local Anesthetics: (Adults and Children): Use 1:200,000 solution with local anesthetic.

Availability (generic available)

Inhalation aerosol: 0.125 mg/inhalation (160 metered inhalations)OTC. **Inhalation solution (racepinephrine):** 🍁 2.25%. **Nasal spray:** 1 mg/0.1 mL, 2 mg/0.1 mL. **Premixed infusion:** 2 mg/250 mL 0.9% NaCl, 4 mg/250 mL 0.9% NaCl, 5 mg/250 mL 0.9% NaCl, 8 mg/250 mL 0.9% NaCl, 10 mg/250 mL 0.9% NaCl. **Solution for injection:** 1 mg/mL (1:1000). **Solution for injection (autoinjectors) (Adrenaclick, Auvi-Q, EpiPen):** 0.1 mg/0.1 mL (1:1000), 0.15 mg/0.15 mL (1:1000), 0.15 mg/0.3 mL (1:2000), 0.3 mg/0.3 mL (1:1000). **Solution for injection (prefilled syringes):** 0.1 mg/mL (1:10,000), 0.15 mg/0.3 mL (1:2000), 0.3 mg/0.3 mL (1:1000).

NURSING IMPLICATIONS

Assessment

- **Bronchodilator:** Assess lung sounds, respiratory pattern, HR, and BP before administration and during peak. Note amount, color, and character of sputum produced.
- Monitor pulmonary function tests before and periodically during therapy.
- Observe for paradoxical bronchospasm (wheezing). *If condition occurs,* hold epinephrine and provide appropriate intervention.
- Assess for drug tolerance, especially if >3 inhalations in 24 hr needed. *If minimal or no relief is in 6–12 hr,* further treatment with aerosol alone is not recommended.
- Assess for hypersensitivity reaction (rash; urticaria; swelling of face, lips, or eyelids). *If condition occurs,* hold epinephrine.
- **Vasopressor:** Monitor BP, HR, ECG, respiratory rate, and urine output continuously during IV administration. *If chest pain, arrhythmia, HR >110 bpm, or hypertension occur,* consider dose adjustment or discontinue epinephrine depending on severity of symptoms.
- **Shock:** Assess volume status. Correct hypovolemia prior to administering epinephrine IV.
- **Nasal Decongestant:** Assess for nasal and sinus congestion prior to and periodically during therapy.

Lab Test Considerations

- May cause transient ↓ in potassium with nebulization or at higher than recommended doses.
- May ↑ blood glucose and lactic acid.

Toxicity and Overdose

- Symptoms of overdose include persistent agitation, chest pain or discomfort, ↓ BP, dizziness, hyperglycemia, hypokalemia, seizures, tachyarrhythmia, persistent trembling, and vomiting.
- Treatment includes discontinuing adrenergic bronchodilator and other beta-adrenergic agonists and symptomatic, supportive therapy. Cardioselective beta blockers are used cautiously because they may induce bronchospasm.

Implementation

- Do not confuse epinephrine with ephedrine.
- ***High Alert:*** Patient harm or fatalities have occurred from medication errors with epinephrine. Epinephrine is available in various concentrations, strengths, and percentages and used for different purposes. Packaging labels may be confused or products incorrectly diluted. Dilutions should be prepared by a pharmacist. IV doses should be expressed in milligrams, not ampules, concentration, or volume. Prior to administration, have second practitioner independently check original order, dose calculations, concentration, route of administration, and infusion pump settings.
- Medication should be administered promptly at the onset of bronchospasm.
- Use a tuberculin syringe with a 26-gauge ½-in. needle for SUBQ injection to ensure that correct amount of medication is administered.
- Tolerance may develop with prolonged or excessive use. Effectiveness may be restored by discontinuing for a few days and then readministering.
- Do not use solutions that are pinkish or brownish or that contain precipitates.
- For anaphylactic shock, volume replacement should be administered concurrently with epinephrine.

Antihistamines and corticosteroids may be used in conjunction with epinephrine.

- **Intranasal:** Administer one spray into either nostril. If no clinical improvement or symptoms worsen, administer 2nd dose to same nostril 5 min after first dose.
- **Inhaln:** Place 10 drops of 1% base solution in the reservoir of the nebulizer.
- The 2.25% inhalation solution of racepinephrine must be diluted for use in the combination nebulizer/respirator.
- Allow 1–2 min to elapse between inhalations of epinephrine inhalation solution to make certain the 2nd inhalation is necessary.
- When epinephrine is used concurrently with corticosteroid or ipratropium inhalations, administer bronchodilator 1st and other medications 5 min apart to prevent toxicity from inhaled fluorocarbon propellants.
- **IM, SUBQ**: Administer into anterolateral thigh, through clothing if necessary, for anaphylaxis. Hold leg firmly to limit movement during injection to prevent lacerations, bent needles, and broken/embedded needles. Avoid injecting into gluteal muscle; may not be effective for anaphylaxis and may cause infection. Rotate injection sites to prevent tissue irritation or necrosis. Massage injection sites well after administration to enhance absorption and ↓ local vasoconstriction.

IV Administration

- **V** IV epinephrine is a vesicant. Central line administration is preferred; extravasation may cause severe ischemic necrosis. If central line is not available, may administer for <72 hr through a peripheral IV catheter placed in a large vein at a proximal site (e.g., in or proximal to antecubital fossa). If extravasation occurs, immediately stop infusion. Leave needle/cannula in place temporarily but do not flush the line. Gently aspirate extravasated solution; then remove needle/cannula. Elevate patient's extremity and apply dry warm compresses. Initiate phentolamine antidote for refractory cases in addition to supportive management. For phentolamine, dilute 5–10 mg in 10 mL of 0.9% NaCl and administer SUBQ into extravasation site as soon as possible after extravasation; if IV catheter remains in place, administer initial dose IV through the infiltrated catheter. May repeat in 60 min if patient remains symptomatic. Nitroglycerin 2% topical ointment (1-inch strip applied to site of ischemia to cover affected area; may repeat every 8 hr as necessary) or terbutaline may be used as alternatives to phentolamine. For terbutaline, for large areas of extravasation, dilute 1 mg in 10 mL of 0.9% NaCl and administer SUBQ into extravasation site; may repeat in 15 min if necessary; for small areas of extravasation, dilute 1 mg in 1 mL of 0.9% NaCl and administer 0.5 mg (0.5 mL) SUBQ into extravasation site; may repeat in 15 min if necessary.
- **IV Push: Dilution:** 1:10,000 solution can be administered undiluted. Dilute 1 mg (1 mL) of a 1:1000 solution in 9 mL of 0.9% NaCl to prepare a 1:10,000 solution. **Concentration:** 0.1 mg/mL (1:10,000). **Rate:** Administer each 1 mg (10 mL) of a 1:10,000 solution over ≥1 min; more rapid administration may be used during cardiac resuscitation. Follow each dose with 20 mL IV saline flush.
- **Continuous Infusion: Dilution:** Dilute 1 mg (1 mL) of a 1:1000 solution in 250 mL of D5W or 0.9% NaCl. Protect from light. Infusion stable for 24 hr. **Concentration:** 4 mcg/mL. **Rate:** See Route/Dosage section. Titrate to response.
- **Y-Site Compatibility:** alprostadil, amikacin, aminocaproic acid, amiodarone, amphotericin B liposomal, angiotensin II, anidulafungin, argatroban, arsenic trioxide, ascorbic acid, asparaginase, atracurium, atropine, azithromycin, aztreonam, benztropine, bivalirudin, bleomycin, buprenorphine, butorphanol, caffeine citrate, calcium chloride, calcium gluconate, cangrelor, carboplatin, caspofungin, cefazolin, cefiderocol, cefotaxime, cefotetan, cefoxitin, ceftazidime, ceftolozane/tazobactam, ceftriaxone, cefuroxime, chloramphenicol, chlorothiazide, chlorpromazine, cisatracurium, cisplatin, clindamycin, cyanocobalamin, cyclophosphamide, cyclosporine, cytarabine, dactinomycin, daptomycin, daunorubicin, dexamethasone, dexmedetomidine, dexrazoxane, digoxin, diltiazem, diphenhydramine, dobutamine, docetaxel, dopamine, doxorubicin hydrochloride, doxorubicin liposomal, doxycycline, edetate calcium disodium, enalaprilat, ephedrine, epirubicin, epoetin alfa, eptifibatide, eravacycline, ertapenem, erythromycin, esmolol, etoposide, etoposide phosphate, famotidine, fentanyl, fluconazole, fludarabine, folic acid, foscarnet, fosphenytoin, furosemide, gemcitabine, gentamicin, glycopyrrolate, granisetron, heparin, hydrocortisone, hydromorphone, ibuprofen lysine, idarubicin, ifosfamide, imipenem/cilastatin, imipenem/cilastatin/relebactam, irinotecan, isavuconazonium, isoproterenol, ketamine, ketorolac, labetalol, leucovorin, levofloxacin, lidocaine, linezolid, lorazepam, magnesium sulfate, mannitol, meperidine, meropenem, meropenem/vaborbactam, mesna, methadone, methotrexate, methylprednisolone, metoclopramide, metoprolol, metronidazole, midazolam, milrinone, minocycline, mitomycin, mitoxantrone, morphine, moxifloxacin, multivitamins, mycophenolate, nafcillin, nalbuphine, naloxone, nicardipine, nitroglycerin, nitroprusside, norepinephrine, octreotide, ondansetron, oritavancin, oxacillin, oxaliplatin, oxytocin, paclitaxel, palonosetron, pamidronate, papaverine, pemetrexed, penicillin G, pentamidine, phentolamine, phenylephrine, phytonadione, piperacillin/tazobactam, plazomicin, potassium acetate, potassium chloride, procainamide, prochlorperazine, promethazine, propranolol, protamine, pyridoxine, remifentanil, remimazolam,

rocuronium, sildenafil, sodium acetate, succinylcholine, sulbactam/durlobactam, tacrolimus, tedizolid, theophylline, thiamine, thiotepa, tigecycline, tirofiban, tobramycin, topotecan, vancomycin, vasopressin, vecuronium, verapamil, vinblastine, vincristine, vinorelbine, voriconazole, zoledronic acid.

- **Y-Site Incompatibility:** acyclovir, alemtuzumab, amphotericin B deoxycholate, azathioprine, carmustine, clevidipine, dacarbazine, dantrolene, diazepam, diazoxide, fluorouracil, ganciclovir, gemtuzumab ozogamicin, indomethacin, micafungin, pentobarbital, phenobarbital, phenytoin, sodium bicarbonate, sulfamethoxazole/trimethoprim.
- **Endotracheal:** Epinephrine can be injected directly into the bronchial tree via the endotracheal tube if the patient has been intubated. Perform 5 rapid insufflations; forcefully administer 10 mL containing 2–2.5 mg epinephrine (1 mg/mL) directly into tube; follow with 5 quick insufflations.

Patient/Family Teaching

- Explain purpose and side effects of medication. Advise patient to read *Patient Information* before starting therapy.
- Instruct patient to take medication exactly as directed. If on a scheduled dosing regimen, take a missed dose as soon as possible; space remaining doses at regular intervals. Do not double doses.
- Instruct patient to seek emergency care immediately if shortness of breath is not relieved, worsens, or is accompanied by diaphoresis, dizziness, palpitations, or chest pain.
- Advise patient to notify health care provider of all Rx or OTC medications, vitamins, or herbal products being taken and to consult health care provider before taking other medications or alcohol. Caution patient also to avoid smoking and other respiratory irritants.
- Rep: Advise women of reproductive potential to notify health care provider if pregnancy is planned or suspected or if breastfeeding.
- **Inhaln:** Review correct administration technique (aerosolization, IPPB) with patient.
- Do not spray inhaler near eyes.
- Advise patient to use bronchodilator 1st if using other inhalation medications, and allow 5 min to elapse before administering other inhalant medications, unless otherwise directed.
- Advise patient to rinse mouth with water after each inhalation dose to minimize dry mouth.
- Advise patient to maintain adequate fluid intake (2000–3000 mL/day) to help liquefy tenacious secretions.
- **Autoinjector or intranasal:** Advise patient using epinephrine for anaphylaxis to always carry device with them. Instruct in appropriate administration and disposal. *For use of autoinjector,* instruct patient to remove gray safety cap, placing black tip on thigh at right angle to leg. Press hard into thigh until autoinjector functions, hold in place for 10 sec, remove, and discard properly. Massage injected area for 10 sec. *For use of intranasal preparation,* instruct patient to administer single dose in either nostril. If 2nd dose is needed, use same nostril 5 min after initial dose. Do not sniff during or after use. Pedi: Teach caregivers signs and symptoms of anaphylaxis, correct administration techniques, and to get the child to a hospital as soon as possible. Instruct caregivers to teach child how to manage their allergy, how to self-administer, and what to do in an emergency. For children too young to administer epinephrine and who will be separated from caregiver, tell caregivers to always discuss allergy and use of medication with responsible adult.

Evaluation/Desired Outcomes

- Prevention or relief of bronchospasm.
- Increase in ease of breathing.
- Prevention of bronchospasm or reduced frequency of acute asthma attacks in patients with chronic asthma.
- Prevention of exercise-induced asthma.
- Reversal of signs and symptoms of anaphylaxis.
- ↑ in cardiac rate and output, when used in cardiac resuscitation.
- ↑ BP, when used as a vasopressor.
- Localization of local anesthetic.
- ↓ sinus and nasal congestion.

eplerenone (e-ple-re-none)

Inspra

Classification

Therapeutic: antihypertensives

Pharmacologic: aldosterone antagonists

Indications

Hypertension (as monotherapy or in combination with other antihypertensive agents). Symptomatic HF with reduced ejection fraction (≤40%) after an acute MI.

Action

Blocks the effects of aldosterone by attaching to mineralocorticoid receptors. **Therapeutic Effects:** Lowering of BP. Improved survival in patients with evidence of HF post-MI.

Pharmacokinetics

Absorption: Well absorbed following oral administration.

Distribution: Unknown.

Metabolism and Excretion: Primarily metabolized by the liver via the CYP3A isoenzyme; <5% excreted unchanged by the kidneys.
Half-life: 4–6 hr.

TIME/ACTION PROFILE (antihypertensive effect)

ROUTE	ONSET	PEAK	DURATION
PO	unknown	4 wk	unknown

Contraindications/Precautions

Contraindicated in: Serum potassium >5.5 mEq/L; Type 2 diabetes with microalbuminuria (for patients with hypertension; ↑ risk of hyperkalemia); Serum creatinine >2 mg/dL in men or >1.8 mg/dL in women (for patients with hypertension); CCr ≤30 mL/min (for all patients); CCr <50 mL/min (for patients with hypertension); Concurrent use of potassium supplements or potassium-sparing diuretics (for patients with hypertension); Concurrent use of strong inhibitors of the CYP3A4 enzyme system; Lactation: Lactation.
Use Cautiously in: Moderate hepatic impairment; OB: Use during pregnancy only if potential maternal benefit justifies potential fetal risk; Pedi: Safety and effectiveness not established in children; Geri: ↑ risk of hyperkalemia in older adults due to age-related ↓ in renal function.

Adverse Reactions/Side Effects

Endo: gynecomastia. **F and E:** HYPERKALEMIA. **GI:** ↑ liver enzymes, abdominal pain, diarrhea. **GU:** abnormal vaginal bleeding, albuminuria. **Metab:** hypercholesterolemia, hypertriglyceridemia. **Neuro:** dizziness, fatigue. **Misc:** flu-like symptoms.

Interactions

Drug-Drug: Strong CYP3A inhibitors, including **ketoconazole**, **itraconazole**, **nefazodone**, **clarithromycin**, **ritonavir**, or **nelfinavir**, may ↑ levels and risk of toxicity; concurrent use contraindicated. Moderate CYP3A inhibitors, including **erythromycin**, **fluconazole**, or **verapamil**, may ↑ levels and risk of toxicity; ↓ eplerenone dose. **NSAIDs** may ↓ antihypertensive effects. **ACE inhibitors** or **angiotensin II receptor blockers** may ↑ risk of hyperkalemia.

Route/Dosage

Hypertension

PO (Adults): 50 mg once daily initially; may ↑ to 50 mg twice daily; *Concurrent use of moderate CYP3A4 inhibitors (erythromycin, verapamil, or fluconazole):* 25 mg once daily initially; may ↑ to 25 mg twice daily.

Heart Failure with Reduced Ejection Fraction Post–Myocardial Infarction

PO (Adults): 25 mg daily once initially; ↑ in 4 wk to 50 mg once daily; *Concurrent use of moderate CYP3A4 inhibitors (erythromycin, verapamil, or fluconazole):* Do not exceed 25 mg once daily.

Availability (generic available)

Tablets: 25 mg, 50 mg.

NURSING IMPLICATIONS

Assessment

- Monitor BP periodically during therapy.

Lab Test Considerations

- May cause hyperkalemia. Monitor serum potassium before starting therapy, within the 1st wk, at 1 mo following start of therapy or dose adjustment, and periodically thereafter. Monitor serum potassium and serum creatinine in 3–7 days in patients who start taking a moderate CYP3A4 inhibitor.
- May ↓ serum sodium and ↑ serum triglyceride, cholesterol, ALT, GGT, creatinine, and uric acid levels.

Implementation

- Do not confuse Inspra with Spiriva.
- **PO:** Administer once daily with or without food.

Patient/Family Teaching

- Explain purpose and side effects of medication. Advise patient to read *Patient Information* before starting therapy. Instruct patient to take medication as directed at the same time each day, even if feeling well.
- Advise patient to notify health care professional of all Rx or OTC medications, vitamins, or herbal products being taken and to consult health care professional before taking other medications. Inform patient not to use potassium supplements, salt substitutes containing potassium, or other Rx, OTC, or herbal products without consulting health care professional.
- Encourage patient to comply with additional interventions for hypertension (weight ↓, smoking cessation, moderation of alcohol consumption, regular exercise, stress management). Medication controls but does not cure hypertension.
- Instruct patient and caregiver on correct technique for monitoring BP. Advise them to monitor BP at least weekly, and notify health care professional of significant changes.
- May cause dizziness. Caution patient to avoid driving or other activities requiring alertness until response to medication is known.
- Advise patient to notify health care professional if dizziness, diarrhea, vomiting, rapid or irregular heartbeat, lower extremity edema, or difficulty breathing occur.
- Advise patient to inform health care professional of treatment regimen before treatment or surgery.
- Emphasize the importance of follow-up exams to check serum potassium.
- Rep: Advise women of reproductive potential to notify health care professional if pregnancy is planned or suspected and to avoid breastfeeding during therapy. May impair male fertility.

Evaluation/Desired Outcomes

- Lowering of BP.
- Improved survival in patients with evidence of HF post-MI.

epoetin alfa (e-poe-e-tin)

Epogen, ✱ Eprex, Procrit, Retacrit

Classification

Therapeutic: antianemics

Pharmacologic: hormones, erythropoiesis stimulating agents (ESA)

Indications

Anemia associated with chronic kidney disease. Anemia secondary to zidovudine therapy in patients infected with HIV. Anemia from chemotherapy in patients with nonmyeloid malignancies when there is ≥2 additional mo of planned chemotherapy. Reduction of need for allogeneic RBC transfusions in patients undergoing elective, noncardiac, nonvascular surgery.

Action

Stimulates erythropoiesis (production of RBCs).
Therapeutic Effects: Maintains and may elevate RBCs, decreasing the need for transfusions.

Pharmacokinetics

Absorption: Well absorbed after SUBQ administration.
Distribution: Concentrated in kidneys, liver, and bone marrow.
Metabolism and Excretion: Unknown.
Half-life: *Children and Adults:* 4–13 hr; *Neonates:* 11–17 hr.

TIME/ACTION PROFILE (↑ in RBCs)

ROUTE	ONSET†	PEAK	DURATION
IV, SUBQ	7–10 days	within 2 mo	2 wk‡

† Increase in reticulocytes.
‡ After discontinuation.

Contraindications/Precautions

Contraindicated in: Hypersensitivity to albumin or mammalian cell–derived products; Uncontrolled hypertension; Erythropoietin levels >200 mUnits/mL; Patients with cancer receiving hormonal agents, biologic products, or radiotherapy, unless also receiving concurrent myelosuppressive chemotherapy; Patients receiving chemotherapy when anticipated outcome is cure; Patients with cancer receiving myelosuppressive chemotherapy in whom the anemia can be managed by transfusion; Patients who require immediate correction of anemia when RBC transfusions can be used instead; Patients scheduled for surgery who are willing to donate autologous blood; Patients undergoing cardiac or vascular surgery; OB: Lactation: Multidose vials should not be used in pregnancy or during breastfeeding, as they contain benzyl alcohol and may cause fatal gasping syndrome in fetus in utero and breastfed infants; Pedi: Neutropenia in newborns; multidose vials should not be used in neonates and infants, as they contain benzyl alcohol, which can cause potentially fatal gasping syndrome.
Use Cautiously in: History of seizures or stroke; Cardiovascular disease; History of porphyria; Lactation: Use while breastfeeding only if potential maternal benefit justifies potential risk to infant.

E

Adverse Reactions/Side Effects

CV: <u>hypertension</u>, DEEP VEIN THROMBOSIS (DVT) (ESPECIALLY WITH HGB >11 G/DL), HF, MI. **Derm:** ERYTHEMA MULTIFORME, STEVENS-JOHNSON SYNDROME (SJS), TOXIC EPIDERMAL NECROLYSIS (TEN), transient rash. **Endo:** restored fertility, resumption of menses. **Neuro:** headache, SEIZURES, STROKE. **Resp:** PULMONARY EMBOLISM (PE) (ESPECIALLY WITH HGB >11 G/DL). **Misc:** ↑ MORTALITY AND ↑ TUMOR GROWTH (ESPECIALLY WITH HGB >12 G/DL).

Interactions

Drug-Drug: May ↑ requirement for **heparin** anticoagulation during hemodialysis.

Route/Dosage

Anemia of Chronic Kidney Disease

(Do not initiate if Hgb ≥10 g/dL)
SUBQ, IV (Adults): 50–100 units/kg 3 times weekly initially; use lowest dose sufficient to ↓ the need for RBC transfusions (do not exceed Hgb of 11 g/dL [patients on dialysis] or 10 g/dL [patients not on dialysis]); if Hgb ↑ by >1.0 g/dL in 2 wk, ↓ dose by 25%; if Hgb ↑ by <1.0 g/dL after 4 wk of therapy (with adequate iron stores), ↑ dose by 25%; do not ↑ dose more frequently than every 4 wk.
SUBQ IV (Children 1 mo–16 yr): 50 units/kg 3 times weekly initially; use lowest dose sufficient to ↓ the need for RBC transfusions (do not exceed Hgb of 12 g/dL); if Hgb ↑ by >1.0 g/dL in 2 wk, ↓ dose by 25%; if Hgb ↑ by <1.0 g/dL after 4 wk of therapy (with adequate iron stores), ↑ dose by 25%; do not ↑ dose more frequently than every 4 wk.

Anemia Secondary to Zidovudine Therapy

SUBQ, IV (Adults): 100 units/kg 3 times weekly for 8 wk; if inadequate response, may ↑ by 50–100 units/kg every 4–8 wk (max: 300 units/kg 3 times weekly).
SUBQ, IV (Children 8 mo–17 yr): 50–400 units/kg 2–3 times weekly.

Anemia from Chemotherapy

(Use only for chemotherapy-related anemia and discontinue when chemotherapy course is completed; do not initiate if Hgb ≥10 g/dL.)

SUBQ (Adults): 150 units/kg 3 times weekly or 40,000 units weekly; adjust dose to maintain lowest Hgb level sufficient to avoid RBC transfusions (do not exceed Hgb of 12 g/dL); if Hgb ↑ by >1.0 g/dL in 2 wk or reaches a level needed to avoid RBC transfusions, ↓ dose by 25%; if Hgb ↑ by <1.0 g/dL (and remains <10 g/dL) after initial 4 wk of therapy (with adequate iron stores), ↑ dose to 300 units/kg 3 times weekly or 60,000 units weekly.

IV (Children 5–18 yr): 600 units/kg weekly; adjust dose to maintain lowest hemoglobin level sufficient to avoid RBC transfusions (do not exceed Hgb of 12 g/dL); if Hgb ↑ by >1.0 g/dL in 2 wk or reaches a level needed to avoid RBC transfusions, ↓ dose by 25%; if Hgb ↑ by <1.0 g/dL (and remains <10 g/dL) after initial 4 wk of therapy (with adequate iron stores), ↑ dose to 900 units/kg (maximum = 60,000 units) weekly.

Surgery

SUBQ (Adults): 300 units/kg/day for 10 days before surgery, day of surgery, and 4 days after *or* 600 units/kg 21, 14, and 7 days before surgery and on day of surgery.

Availability

Solution for injection: 2000 units/mL, 3000 units/mL, 4000 units/mL, 10,000 units/mL, 20,000 units/mL, 40,000 units/mL. **Solution for injection (prefilled syringes):** 🍁 1000 units/0.5 mL, 🍁 2000 units/0.5 mL, 🍁 3000 units/0.3 mL, 🍁 4000 units/0.4 mL, 🍁 5000 units/0.5 mL, 🍁 6000 units/0.6 mL, 🍁 8000 units/0.8 mL, 🍁 10,000 units/1 mL, 🍁 20,000 units/0.5 mL, 🍁 30,000 units/0.75 mL, 🍁 40,000 units/1 mL.

NURSING IMPLICATIONS

Assessment

- Monitor BP before and during therapy. Inform health care professional if severe hypertension is present or if BP begins to ↑. Additional antihypertensive therapy may be required during initiation of therapy.
- Monitor for symptoms of anemia (fatigue, dyspnea, pallor).
- Monitor dialysis shunts (thrill and bruit) and status of artificial kidney during hemodialysis. Heparin dose may need to be increased to prevent clotting. Monitor patients with underlying vascular disease for impaired circulation.
- Monitor patients for signs and symptoms of severe cutaneous adverse reactions, including SJS (fever, general malaise, fatigue, muscle or joint aches, blisters, oral lesions, conjunctivitis) and TEN (prodrome of fever, flu-like symptoms, mucosal lesions, progressive skin rash, lymphadenopathy). If a severe cutaneous adverse reaction is suspected, discontinue therapy and provide supportive care.
- Monitor for signs and symptoms of venous thromboembolism such as PE (chest pain, dyspnea, tachycardia), DVT (calf pain or tenderness, lower extremity edema, localized warmth or erythema), or stroke (headache, facial numbness, unilateral weakness, aphasia, eye pain or swelling, vision changes). Discontinue therapy if suspected.

Lab Test Considerations

- May cause ↑ WBCs and platelets. May ↓ bleeding times.
- Monitor serum ferritin, transferrin, and iron levels to assess need for concurrent iron therapy. Administer supplemental iron therapy when serum ferritin <100 mcg/L or when serum transferrin saturation <20%.
- Monitor Hgb weekly until the Hgb level is stable and sufficient to minimize the need for RBC transfusion after starting therapy and after each dose adjustment.
- **Anemia of Chronic Kidney Disease:** Monitor Hgb at least weekly until stable and then at least monthly. Do not ↑ dose more frequently than once every 4 wk. A ↓ in dose can be made more frequently. Avoid frequent dose adjustments. *If Hgb ↑ >12 g/dL in a 2-wk period,* ↓ dose by 25% or more. *If Hgb ↑ by <1 g/dL over 4 wk (and iron stores are adequate),* ↑ dose by 25%. If no response after 12 wk of escalation, further dose ↑ is unlikely to improve response and may ↑ risks. Use lowest dose that will maintain Hgb level sufficient to reduce need for RBC transfusions.
- **Adults with Anemia of Chronic Kidney Disease on Dialysis:** Start epoetin when Hgb >10 g/dL. If Hgb ≥11 g/dL, ↓ or hold dose.
- **Adults with Anemia of Chronic Kidney Disease Not on Dialysis:** Start epoetin only when Hgb <10 g/dL AND rate of Hgb decline indicates likelihood of requiring a RBC transfusion AND ↓ risk of alloimmunization and/or other RBC transfusion-related risks is a goal. If Hgb level >10 g/dL, ↓ or hold dose, and use lowest epoetin dose sufficient to ↓ need for RBC transfusions.
- **Children with Anemia of Chronic Kidney Disease:** Start epoetin only when Hgb <10 g/dL. If Hgb level >12 g/dL, ↓ or hold dose.
- Monitor renal function and electrolytes closely; resulting ↑ sense of well-being may lead to ↓ compliance with other therapies for renal failure. ↑ in BUN, serum creatinine, uric acid, phosphorus, and potassium may occur.
- **Anemia Secondary to Zidovudine Therapy:** Before initiating therapy, determine serum erythropoietin level before transfusion. Patients receiving zidovudine with endogenous serum erythropoietin levels >500 mUnits/mL may not respond to therapy. *If Hgb does not ↑ after 8 wk of therapy,* ↑ dose by 50–100 units/kg at 4–8 wk intervals until Hgb reaches level needed to avoid RBC transfusions or 300 units/kg.

If Hgb ≥12 g/dL, hold dose until Hgb ↓ to <11 g/dL; then ↓ dose by 25%. *If ↑ in Hgb is not achieved at a dose of 300 Units/kg for 8 wk,* discontinue therapy.

- **Anemia from Chemotherapy:** Start epoetin only if Hgb ≥10 g/dL and there is an additional 2 mo of planned chemotherapy. Patients with lower baseline serum erythropoietin levels may respond more rapidly; not recommended if levels >200 mUnits/mL. *If Hgb ↑ by >1 g/dL in any 2-wk period or Hgb reaches level needed to avoid RBC transfusion,* ↓ dose by 25%. *If Hgb ↑ by <1 g/dL after 4 wk in absence of RBC transfusion and remains <10 g/dL,* ↑ dose to 300 units/kg three times per wk in adults or 60,000 units weekly (adults) or 900 units/kg (max: 60,000 units) in children. *If no response in Hgb levels or if RBC transfusions are still required after 8 wk of therapy,* discontinue epoetin.
- **Surgery:** Implement prophylaxis of venous thromboembolism during therapy.

Implementation

IV Administration

- Transfusions are still required for severe symptomatic anemia. Supplemental iron should be initiated with epoetin alfa and continued throughout therapy.
- Institute seizure precautions in patients who experience greater than a 4-point ↑ in hematocrit in a 2-wk period or exhibit any change in neurologic status. Risk of seizures is greatest during the 1st 90 days of therapy.
- Do not shake vial; inactivation of medication may occur. Solution is clear and colorless; do not administer solutions that are discolored, cloudy, or contain a precipitate. Discard vial immediately after withdrawing dose from single-use 1-mL vial. Refrigerate multidose vials; stable for 21 days after initial entry.
- **SUBQ:** This route is often used for patients not requiring dialysis.
- May be admixed in syringe immediately before administration with 0.9% NaCl with benzyl alcohol 0.9% in a 1:1 ratio to prevent injection site discomfort.
- **IV Push: Dilution:** Administer undiluted or dilute with an equal amount of 0.9% NaCl. **Concentration:** 1000–40,000 units/mL. **Rate:** May be administered as direct injection or bolus over 1–3 min into IV tubing or via venous line at end of dialysis session.
- **Y-Site Compatibility:** amikacin, aminophylline, ascorbic acid, atracurium, atropine, azathioprine, aztreonam, benztropine, bumetanide, buprenorphine, butorphanol, calcium chloride, calcium gluconate, cefazolin, cefotaxime, cefotetan, cefoxitin, ceftazidime, ceftriaxone, cefuroxime, chloramphenicol, clindamycin, cyanocobalamin, cyclosporine, dexamethasone, digoxin, diphenhydramine, dobutamine, dopamine, doxycycline, enalaprilat, ephedrine, epinephrine, erythromycin, esmolol, famotidine, fentanyl, fluconazole, folic acid, furosemide, ganciclovir, gentamicin, glycopyrrolate, heparin, hydrocortisone, imipenem/cilastatin, indomethacin, insulin, regular, isoproterenol, ketorolac, labetalol, LR, lidocaine, magnesium sulfate, mannitol, meperidine, methylprednisolone, metoclopramide, metoprolol, morphine, multivitamins, nafcillin, nalbuphine, naloxone, nitroglycerin, nitroprusside, norepinephrine, ondansetron, oxacillin, oxytocin, penicillin G, pentobarbital, phenobarbital, phentolamine, phenylephrine, phytonadione, potassium chloride, procainamide, promethazine, propranolol, protamine, pyridoxine, sodium bicarbonate, succinylcholine, sufentanil, theophylline, tobramycin, vasopressin, verapamil.
- **Y-Site Incompatibility:** amphotericin B deoxycholate, chlorpromazine, dantrolene, diazepam, haloperidol, midazolam, minocycline, pentamidine, phenytoin, prochlorperazine, trimethoprim/sulfamethoxazole, vancomycin.

Patient/Family Teaching

- Explain the purpose and side effects of epoetin alfa. Do not stop receiving drug without consulting health care professional. If an appointment is missed, contact health care professional as soon as possible to reschedule. Advise patient to read *Medication Guide* before starting and periodically during therapy in case of changes. Patient must sign the patient–health care provider acknowledgment form before each course of therapy.
- Explain rationale for concurrent iron therapy (↑ RBC production requires iron).
- Advise patient to notify health care professional immediately if signs and symptoms of blood clots (chest pain; trouble breathing or shortness of breath; pain in the legs, with or without swelling; a cool or pale arm or leg; sudden confusion; trouble speaking or trouble understanding others' speech; sudden numbness or weakness in the face, arm, or leg, especially on one side of the body; sudden trouble seeing; sudden trouble walking; dizziness; loss of balance or coordination; loss of consciousness or fainting; hemodialysis vascular access stops working), allergic reactions (rash, itching, shortness of breath, wheezing, dizziness and fainting, swelling around mouth or eyes, fast pulse, sweating), skin reactions (blisters, skin sores, peeling, or areas of skin coming off) occur.
- Inform patient that use of epoetin alfa may result in shortened overall survival and/or ↓ time to tumor progression.
- Advise patient to notify health care professional of all Rx or OTC medications, vitamins, or herbal products being taken and to consult with health care professional before taking other medications. Advise patient

E

to inform health care professional of medication prior to treatment or surgery.

- **Anemia of Chronic Kidney Disease:** Stress importance of compliance with dietary restrictions, medications, and dialysis. Foods high in iron and low in potassium include liver, pork, veal, beef, mustard and turnip greens, peas, eggs, broccoli, kale, blackberries, strawberries, apple juice, watermelon, oatmeal, and enriched bread. Epoetin alfa will result in ↑ sense of well-being, but it does not cure underlying disease.
- **Home Care Issues:** Home dialysis patients determined to be able to safely and effectively administer epoetin alfa should be taught proper dosage, administration technique, and disposal of equipment. *Information for Home Dialysis Patients* should be provided to patient along with medication.
- Rep: Discuss possible return of menses and fertility with health care professional. Advise women of reproductive potential to notify health care professional if pregnancy is planned or suspected or if breastfeeding.

Evaluation/Desired Outcomes

- Increase in hematocrit to 30–36% with improvement in symptoms of anemia in patients with chronic renal failure.
- Increase in hematocrit in anemia secondary to zidovudine therapy.
- Increase in hematocrit in patients with anemia resulting from chemotherapy.
- Reduction of need for RBC transfusions after surgery.

HIGH ALERT

eptifibatide (ep-ti-**fib**-a-tide)

~~Integrilin~~

Classification

Therapeutic: antiplatelet agents

Pharmacologic: glycoprotein IIb/IIIa inhibitors

Indications

Acute coronary syndrome (unstable angina/non-ST-elevation MI), including patients who will be managed medically and those who will undergo percutaneous coronary intervention (PCI). Patients undergoing PCI, including intracoronary stenting.

Action

Decreases platelet aggregation by reversibly antagonizing the binding of fibrinogen to the glycoprotein IIb/IIIa binding site on platelet surfaces. **Therapeutic Effects:** Reduction in risk of death or new MI in patients with acute coronary syndrome. Reduction in risk of death, new MI, or need for urgent intervention in patients undergoing PCI.

Pharmacokinetics

Absorption: IV administration results in complete bioavailability.

Distribution: Unknown.

Metabolism and Excretion: 50% excreted by the kidneys.

Half-life: 2.5 hr.

TIME/ACTION PROFILE (effects on platelet function)

ROUTE	ONSET	PEAK	DURATION
IV	immediate	following bolus	brief†

† Inhibition is reversible following cessation of infusion.

Contraindications/Precautions

Contraindicated in: Hypersensitivity; Active internal bleeding or history of bleeding within previous 30 days; Severe uncontrolled hypertension (systolic BP >200 mm Hg and/or diastolic BP >110 mm Hg); Major surgical procedure within 6 wk; History of hemorrhagic stroke or other stroke within 30 days; Concurrent use of other glycoprotein IIb/IIIa receptor antagonists; Platelet count <100,000/mm^3; Severe renal impairment (serum creatinine ≥4 mg/dL) or dependency on renal dialysis.

Use Cautiously in: Renal impairment (↓ infusion rate if CCr <50 mL/min); OB: Safety not established in pregnancy; Lactation: Safety not established in breastfeeding; Pedi: Safety and effectiveness not established in children; Geri: ↑ risk of bleeding in older adults.

Adverse Reactions/Side Effects

Noted for patients receiving heparin and aspirin in addition to eptifibatide.

CV: hypotension. **Hemat:** BLEEDING (INCLUDING GI AND INTRACRANIAL BLEEDING, HEMATURIA, AND HEMATOMAS), thrombocytopenia.

Interactions

Drug-Drug: ↑ risk of bleeding with other drugs that affect hemostasis (**heparins, warfarin, NSAIDs, thrombolytic agents, dipyridamole, clopidogrel,** some **cephalosporins, valproates**).

Drug-Natural Products: ↑ bleeding risk with **arnica, chamomile, clove, dong quai, feverfew, garlic, ginger, ginkgo,** and ***Panax ginseng***.

Route/Dosage

Acute Coronary Syndrome

IV (Adults): 180 mcg/kg (max = 22.6 mg) as a bolus dose, followed by 2 mcg/kg/min (max = 15 mg/hr) infusion until hospital discharge or initiation of coronary artery bypass graft surgery (up to 72 hr). If a patient is to undergo PCI, the infusion should be continued until hospital discharge or for up to 18–24 hr after the PCI, whichever comes first, allowing for up to 96 hr of therapy.

Renal Impairment

IV (Adults): *CCr <50 mL/min:* 180 mcg/kg (max = 22.6 mg) as a bolus dose, followed by 1 mcg/kg/min (max = 7.4 mg/hr) infusion until hospital discharge or initiation of coronary artery bypass graft surgery (up to 72 hr). If a patient is to undergo PCI, the infusion should be continued until hospital discharge or for up to 18–24 hr after the PCI, whichever comes first, allowing for up to 96 hr of therapy.

Percutaneous Coronary Intervention

IV (Adults): 180 mcg/kg (max = 22.6 mg) as a bolus dose immediately before PCI, followed by 2 mcg/kg/min (max = 15 mg/hr) infusion; a 2nd bolus of 180 mcg/kg (max = 22.6 mg) is given 10 min after 1st bolus. Infusion should be continued until hospital discharge or for up to 18–24 hr, whichever comes first (minimum of 12 hr).

Renal Impairment

(Adults): *CCr <50 mL/min:* 180 mcg/kg (max = 22.6 mg) bolus followed by 1 mcg/kg/min (max = 7.4 mg/hr) infusion; a 2nd bolus of 180 mcg/kg (max = 22.6 mg) is given 10 min after 1st bolus.

Availability (generic available)

Solution for injection: 20 mg/10 mL, 75 mg/100 mL, 200 mg/100 mL.

NURSING IMPLICATIONS

Assessment

- Assess for bleeding. Most common sites are arterial access site for cardiac catheterization or GI or genitourinary tract. Minimize arterial and venous punctures; IM injections; and use of urinary catheters, nasotracheal intubation, and nasogastric tubes. Avoid noncompressible sites for IV access. If bleeding cannot be controlled with pressure, discontinue eptifibatide and heparin immediately.

Lab Test Considerations

- Prior to eptifibatide therapy, assess hemoglobin or hematocrit, platelet count, serum creatinine, and PT/aPTT. Activated clotting time (ACT) should also be measured in patients undergoing PCI. Maintain the aPTT between 50 and 70 sec unless PCI is to be performed. Maintain ACT between 200 and 300 sec during PCI.
- Arterial sheath should not be removed unless aPTT <45 sec or ACT < 150 sec.
- If platelet count decreases to <100,000/mm^3 and is confirmed, discontinue eptifibatide and heparin and monitor and treat condition.

Implementation

- ***High Alert:*** Accidental overdose of antiplatelet medications has resulted in patient harm or death from internal hemorrhage or intracranial bleeding. Have second practitioner independently check original order, dose calculations, and infusion pump settings.
- Most patients receive heparin and aspirin concurrently with eptifibatide.
- After PCI, femoral artery sheath may be removed during eptifibatide treatment only after heparin has been discontinued and its effects mostly reversed.
- Do not administer solutions that are discolored or contain particulate matter. Discard unused portion.

IV Administration

- **IV Push:** ***High Alert:*** **Dilution:** Withdraw appropriate loading dose from bolus vial (20 mg/10-mL vial) into a syringe. Administer undiluted. **Concentration:** 2 mg/mL. **Rate:** Administer over 1–2 min.
- **Continuous Infusion: Dilution:** Administer undiluted directly from the 100-mL vial via an infusion pump. **Concentration:** 0.75 mg/mL or 2 mg/mL (depends on vial used). **Rate:** Based on patient's weight (see Route/Dosage section).
- **Y-Site Compatibility:** alemtuzumab, alteplase, amikacin, aminophylline, amphotericin B liposomal, ampicillin, ampicillin/sulbactam, anidulafungin, argatroban, arsenic trioxide, atracurium, atropine, azithromycin, aztreonam, bivalirudin, bumetanide, buprenorphine, butorphanol, calcium chloride, calcium gluconate, cangrelor, cefazolin, cefepime, cefotaxime, cefotetan, cefoxitin, ceftazidime, ceftolozane/tazobactam, ceftriaxone, cefuroxime, ciprofloxacin, cisatracurium, clindamycin, cyclosporine, daptomycin, dexamethasone, dexrazoxane, D5/0.9% NaCl, digoxin, diltiazem, diphenhydramine, dobutamine, dopamine, doxorubicin liposomal, doxycycline, droperidol, enalaprilat, ephedrine, epinephrine, ertapenem, erythromycin, esmolol, famotidine, fentanyl, fluconazole, foscarnet, fosphenytoin, ganciclovir, gentamicin, granisetron, haloperidol, heparin, hydrocortisone, hydromorphone, imipenem/cilastatin, isavuconazonium, isoproterenol, ketorolac, labetalol, leucovorin calcium, levofloxacin, lidocaine, linezolid, lorazepam, magnesium sulfate, mannitol, meperidine, meropenem, meropenem/vaborbactam, methylprednisolone, metoclopramide, metoprolol, metronidazole, micafungin, midazolam, milrinone, morphine, nalbuphine, naloxone, nicardipine, nitroglycerin, nitroprusside, octreotide, ondansetron, oxytocin, palonosetron, pemetrexed, pentobarbital, phenobarbital, phenylephrine, piperacillin/tazobactam, plazomicin, potassium acetate, potassium chloride, potassium phosphates, procainamide, prochlorperazine, promethazine, propranolol, remifentanil, rocuronium, sodium bicarbonate, sodium phosphates, succinylcholine, sufentanil, sulfamethoxazole/trimethoprim, tedizolid, theophylline, tigecycline,

tirofiban, tobramycin, vancomycin, vecuronium, verapamil, zidovudine, zoledronic acid.

- **Y-Site Incompatibility:** acyclovir, amphotericin B deoxycholate, chlorpromazine, diazepam, furosemide, gemtuzumab ozogamicin, methohexital, mycophenolate, pentamidine, phenytoin.

Patient/Family Teaching

- Inform patient of the purpose and side effects of eptifibatide. Inform patient bedrest may be required during infusion and for several hr postinfusion.
- Instruct patient to notify health care professional immediately if any bleeding is noted.
- Advise patient to notify health care professional of all Rx or OTC medications, vitamins, or herbal products being taken and to consult with health care professional before taking other medications.
- Rep: Advise women of reproductive potential to notify health care professional if pregnancy is planned or suspected or if breastfeeding.

Evaluation/Desired Outcomes

- Reduction in risk of death or new MI in patients with acute coronary syndrome.
- Reduction in risk of death, new MI, or need for urgent intervention in patients undergoing PCI.

erenumab (e-ren-ue-mab)

Aimovig

Classification

Therapeutic: vascular headache suppressants

Pharmacologic: calcitonin gene related peptide receptor antagonists monoclonal antibodies

Indications

Migraine prevention.

Action

Monoclonal antibody that binds to the calcitonin gene-related peptide (CGRP) receptor, which reduces the neuroinflammatory and vasodilatory effects of CGRP. **Therapeutic Effects:** Reduction in frequency of migraines.

Pharmacokinetics

Absorption: 82% absorbed following SUBQ administration.

Distribution: Some tissue distribution.

Metabolism and Excretion: *Low concentrations:* Eliminated through saturable binding to CGRP receptor; *High concentrations:* Eliminated through nonspecific, nonsaturable proteolytic pathway.

Half-life: 28 days.

TIME/ACTION PROFILE (plasma concentrations)

ROUTE	ONSET	PEAK	DURATION
SUBQ	unknown	6 days	1 mo

Contraindications/Precautions

Contraindicated in: Hypersensitivity.

Use Cautiously in: Hypertension; Raynaud phenomenon; OB: Safety not established in pregnancy; Lactation: Safety not established in breastfeeding; Pedi: Safety and effectiveness not established in children; Geri: Choose dose carefully in older adults, considering concurrent disease states, drug therapy, and age-related ↓ in hepatic and renal function.

Adverse Reactions/Side Effects

CV: hypertension, Raynaud phenomenon. **GI:** constipation. **Local:** injection site reactions. **MS:** muscle spasm. **Misc:** HYPERSENSITIVITY REACTIONS (INCLUDING ANAPHYLAXIS AND ANGIOEDEMA).

Interactions

Drug-Drug: Medications that ↓ GI motility may ↑ risk of more severe constipation.

Route/Dosage

SUBQ (Adults): 70 mg once monthly; may ↑ dose, if needed, to 140 mg once monthly.

Availability

Solution for injection (prefilled syringes and autoinjectors): 70 mg/mL, 140 mg/mL.

NURSING IMPLICATIONS

Assessment

- Assess frequency and intensity of migraines. Evaluate efficacy after a minimum of 3 consecutive months of treatment and continue as long as needed. May consider trial off of treatment on case-by-case basis after 12–18 mo.
- Assess for latex allergy. Needle shield within white or orange cap of prefilled autoinjector and gray needle cap of prefilled syringe contain dry natural rubber (a derivative of latex); may cause allergic reactions in individuals sensitive to latex.
- Monitor for new-onset hypertension or worsening of pre-existing hypertension. May require discontinuation.
- Monitor for signs and symptoms of hypersensitivity reactions (rash, urticaria, pruritus, flushing, dizziness, vomiting, abdominal pain) and angioedema (swelling of throat, lips, tongue, or face; dyspnea; wheezing; hoarseness); usually occur within hours of injection but can occur >1 wk after injection. If reaction is severe, discontinue erenumab and treat as needed.
- Monitor for signs and symptoms of severe constipation, especially if on concurrent medications that ↓ GI mobility; manage as needed.
- Monitor for Raynaud phenomenon and recurrence or worsening of pre-existing Raynaud phenomenon. May require discontinuation.

Implementation

- **SUBQ:** Prior to use, allow vial to sit at room temperature for ≥30 min; protect from direct sunlight. Do not use other methods to warm solution (hot water or microwave). Do not shake. Solution is clear to opalescent, colorless to light yellow; do not administer solutions that are discolored, cloudy, or contain particulates. Store in refrigerator in original carton to protect from light; do not freeze. May be stored up to 7 days at room temperature.

- Inject entire contents into abdomen, thigh, or upper arm. Do not inject into areas where the skin is tender, bruised, red, or hard.

Patient/Family Teaching

- Explain the purpose and side effects of erenumab. Instruct patient to take as directed. Administer missed doses as soon as possible and schedule next dose 1 mo from last dose administered. Educate patient and/or caregiver on correct technique for injection and disposal of equipment. Advise patient to read *Patient Information* before starting therapy and with each Rx refill in case of changes.
- Instruct patient to notify health care provider immediately or call 911 if signs and symptoms of hypersensitivity reaction (swelling of face, mouth, tongue, or throat; trouble breathing; rash) occur.
- Advise patient to notify health care provider if severe constipation occurs; may cause serious complications.
- Advise patient to notify health care provider of all Rx or OTC medications, vitamins, or herbal products being taken and to consult with health care provider before taking other medications.
- Rep: Advise women of reproductive potential to notify health care provider if pregnancy is planned or suspected or if breastfeeding. Inform patient of pregnancy registry that monitors outcomes in women exposed to erenumab. Encourage patients to enroll by calling 1-833-244-4083 or visiting www.genesispregnancyregistry.com.

Evaluation/Desired Outcomes

- Decrease in frequency and intensity of migraines.

ergocalciferol, See VITAMIN D COMPOUNDS.

HIGH ALERT

erlotinib (er-lo-ti-nib)

Tarceva

Classification

Therapeutic: antineoplastics

Pharmacologic: enzyme inhibitors

Indications

Treatment of metastatic non-small cell lung cancer (NSCLC) that has epidermal growth factor exon 19 deletions or exon 21 substitution mutations in patients who are receiving first-line, maintenance, or second- or greater line treatment after progression following ≥1 previous chemotherapy regimen. First-line therapy for locally advanced, surgically unresectable, or metastatic pancreatic cancer (in combination with gemcitabine).

Action

Inhibits the enzyme tyrosine kinase, which is associated with human epidermal growth factor receptor (EGFR); blocks growth stimulation signals in cancer cells. **Therapeutic Effects:** Decreased spread of lung or pancreatic cancer with increased survival.

Pharmacokinetics

Absorption: 60% absorbed; bioavailability ↑ to 100% with food.

Distribution: Unknown.

Protein Binding: 93%.

Metabolism and Excretion: Mostly metabolized by the liver, primarily by the CYP3A4 isoenzyme. 83% excreted in feces (<1% as unchanged drug); 8% excreted in urine (<1% as unchanged drug).

Half-life: 36 hr.

TIME/ACTION PROFILE (plasma concentrations)

ROUTE	ONSET	PEAK	DURATION
PO	unknown	4 hr	24 hr

Contraindications/Precautions

Contraindicated in: OB: Pregnancy; Lactation: Lactation.

Use Cautiously in: Hepatic impairment; Previous chemotherapy/radiation, pre-existing lung disease, metastatic lung disease (may ↑ risk of interstitial lung disease); Rep: Women of reproductive potential; Pedi: Safety and effectiveness not established in children.

Adverse Reactions/Side Effects

CV: MYOCARDIAL INFARCTION/ISCHEMIA (PATIENTS WITH PANCREATIC CANCER). **Derm:** rash, BULLOUS AND EXFOLIATIVE SKIN DISORDERS, dry skin, pruritus. **EENT:** ↓ tear production, abnormal eyelash growth, conjunctivitis, corneal perforation, corneal ulceration, keratitis. **GI:** diarrhea, HEPATOTOXICITY, ↑ liver enzymes, abdominal pain, anorexia, GI PERFORATION, nausea, stomatitis, vomiting. **GU:** RENAL FAILURE. **Hemat:** microangiopathic hemolytic anemia with thrombocytopenia (pancreatic cancer patients). **Neuro:** CEREBROVASCULAR ACCIDENT (PANCREATIC CANCER PATIENTS), fatigue. **Resp:** dyspnea, cough, INTERSTITIAL LUNG DISEASE (ILD).

Interactions

Drug-Drug: Strong CYP3A4 inhibitors, including **atazanavir**, **clarithromycin**, **itraconazole**, **ketoconazole**, **nefazodone**, **nelfinavir**, **ritonavir**, or **voriconazole**, may ↑ levels and risk of toxicity; consider alternative therapy or ↓ erlotinib dose. **Strong CYP3A4 inducers**, including **rifampin**, **rifabutin**, **rifapentine**, **phenytoin**, **carbamazepine**, or **phenobarbital**, may ↓ levels and effectiveness; consider alternative therapy or ↑ erlotinib dose. **CYP1A2 inhibitors**, including **ciprofloxacin**, may ↑ levels and risk of toxicity; consider ↓ erlotinib dose if used with CYP3A4 inhibitor. **Smoking** may ↓ levels and effectiveness; avoid smoking during therapy or consider ↑ erlotinib dose if smoking continues. **Moderate CYP1A2 inducers**, including **teriflunomide**, **rifampin**, or **phenytoin**, may ↓ levels and effectiveness; avoid concurrent use or ↑ erlotinib dose. May ↓ **midazolam** levels. May ↑ risk of bleeding with **warfarin**. **Proton pump inhibitors**, **H_2 blockers**, and **antacids** may ↓ levels and effectiveness; avoid concurrent use with **proton pump inhibitors**; take 10 hr after **H_2 antagonist** and ≥2 hr before next dose of **H_2 antagonist**; separate from **antacid** by several hr.
Drug-Natural Products: St. John's wort may ↓ levels and effectiveness; consider alternative therapy or ↑ erlotinib dose.
Drug-Food: Grapefruit juice or **grapefruit** may ↑ levels and risk of toxicity; consider ↓ erlotinib dose.

Route/Dosage

Non-Small Cell Lung Cancer

PO (Adults): 150 mg once daily; *Concurrent use of strong CYP3A4 inhibitor or concurrent use of CYP3A4 and CYP1A2 inhibitor (e.g., ciprofloxacin):* Consider ↓ dose in 50-mg increments (avoid concurrent use if possible); *Concurrent use of strong CYP3A4 inducer:* Consider ↑ dose by 50 mg every 2 wk (max dose = 450 mg/day) (avoid concurrent use if possible); *Concurrent cigarette smoking or concurrent use of moderate CYP1A2 inducer:* ↑ dose by 50 mg every 2 wk (max dose = 300 mg/day); immediately ↓ dose to recommended initial dose for indication upon smoking cessation.

Pancreatic Cancer

PO (Adults): 100 mg once daily. *Concurrent use of strong CYP3A4 inhibitor or concurrent use of CYP3A4 and CYP1A2 inhibitor (e.g., ciprofloxacin):* Consider ↓ dose in 50-mg increments (avoid concurrent use if possible); *Concurrent use of strong CYP3A4 inducer:* Consider ↑ dose by 50 mg every 2 wk (max dose = 450 mg/day) (avoid concurrent use if possible); *Concurrent cigarette smoking or concurrent use of moderate CYP1A2 inducer:* ↑ dose by 50 mg every 2 wk (max dose = 300 mg/day); immediately ↓ dose to recommended initial dose for indication upon smoking cessation.

Availability (generic available)

Tablets: 25 mg, 100 mg, 150 mg.

NURSING IMPLICATIONS

Assessment

- Assess respiratory status before and periodically during therapy. *If dyspnea, cough, or fever occur,* hold and evaluate until resolved to Grade ≤1; resume therapy with ↓ dose by 50 mg. *If ILD confirmed,* discontinue erlotinib.
- Assess for GI pain and diarrhea. *If diarrhea unresponsive to loperamide or dehydration occurs,* hold erlotinib. *If GI perforation occurs,* discontinue erlotinib.
- Assess skin during therapy. *If severe rash unresponsive to medical management occurs,* hold until resolved to Grade ≤1; resume therapy with ↓ dose by 50 mg. *If bullous and exfoliative skin disorders occur,* discontinue erlotinib.
- Assess for ocular changes periodically during therapy. *If Grade 3 or 4 keratitis (or Grade 2 keratitis lasting >2 wk), or acute or worsening eye pain or disorders occurs,* hold erlotinib until resolved to Grade ≤1; resume therapy with ↓ dose by 50 mg. *If corneal perforation or ulcers occur,* discontinue erlotinib.

Lab Test Considerations

- Test patients for EGFR exon 19 deletions or exon 21 (L858R) substitution mutations in plasma or tumor specimens prior to starting therapy; presence is required for therapy. Information on FDA-approved tests is available at: http://www.fda.gov/CompanionDiagnostics.
- Monitor AST, ALT, bilirubin, and alkaline phosphatase periodically during therapy. If tripling of transaminase levels in *patients with pre-existing hepatic impairment* or total bilirubin ≥3 times upper limit of normal (ULN) and/or transaminases ≥5 times ULN in *patients without pre-existing hepatic impairment,* consider dose ↓ by 50 mg.
- Monitor renal function and serum electrolytes periodically during therapy. *If Grade 3 or 4 renal toxicity occurs,* hold erlotinib and evaluate until resolved to Grade ≤1; resume therapy with ↓ dose by 50 mg or discontinue erlotinib.
- Monitor INR regularly in patients taking warfarin.

Implementation

- Do not confuse Tarceva with Tresiba.
- **PO:** Administer at ≥1 hr before or 2 hr after food.

Patient/Family Teaching

- Explain purpose and side effects of medication. Advise patient to read *Patient Information* before starting therapy.
- Advise patient to notify health care professional if severe or persistent diarrhea, nausea, anorexia, vomiting, rash, unexplained dyspnea or cough, eye irritation, or signs and symptoms of a cerebrovascular accident (sudden weakness, paralysis or numbness of face or extremities, confusion, trouble speaking or

understanding, visual changes, problems breathing, dizziness, loss of balance or coordination, unexplained falls, loss of consciousness, sudden and severe headache) occur.

- Instruct patient to avoid proton pump inhibitors. If antacids are necessary, separate antacids and erlotinib by several hr. If therapy with H_2 antagonists is required, take erlotinib 10 hr after H_2 antagonist and ≥2 hr before next H_2 antagonist dose.
- Advise patient to notify health care professional of all Rx or OTC medications, vitamins, or herbal products being taken and consult health care professional before taking any new medications.
- Advise patient to wear sunscreen and protective clothing to ↓ skin reactions.
- Instruct patient to discontinue smoking during therapy.
- Rep: May cause fetal harm. Caution women of reproductive potential to use highly effective contraceptive during therapy and for ≥1 mo after last dose and to avoid breastfeeding during and for ≥2 wk following last dose. Advise women to notify health care professional if pregnancy is planned or suspected.

Evaluation/Desired Outcomes

- Decrease in spread of non-small cell lung or pancreatic cancer with increased survival.

ertapenem (er-ta-pen-em)

~~INVanz~~

Classification

Therapeutic: anti-infectives

Pharmacologic: carbapenems

Indications

Complicated intra-abdominal infections. Complicated skin and skin structure infections (including diabetic foot infections with osteomyelitis). Community-acquired pneumonia. Complicated urinary tract infections (including pyelonephritis). Acute pelvic infections (including postpartum endomyometritis, septic abortion, and post-surgical gynecologic infections). Prophylaxis of surgical site infection following elective colorectal surgery.

Action

Binds to bacterial cell wall, resulting in cell death. Ertapenem resists the actions of many enzymes that degrade most other penicillins and penicillin-like anti-infectives. **Therapeutic Effects:** Bactericidal action against susceptible bacteria. **Spectrum:** Active against the following aerobic gram-positive organisms: *Staphylococcus aureus* (methicillin-susceptible strains only), *Staphylococcus epidermidis*, *Streptococcus agalactiae*, *S. pneumoniae* (penicillin-susceptible strains only), and *S. pyogenes*. Also active against the following gram-negative aerobic organisms: *Escherichia coli*, *Haemophilus influenzae* (beta-lactamase negative strains), *Klebsiella pneumonia*, *Moraxella catarrhalis*, and *Providencia rettgeri*. Additional anaerobic spectrum includes *Bacteroides fragilis*, *B. distasonis*, *B. ovatus*, *B. thetaiotamicron*, *B. uniformis*, *B. vulgatis*, *Clostridioides clostrioforme*, *Eubacterium lentum*, *Peptostreptococcus*, *Porphyromonas asaccharolytica*, and *Prevotella bivia*.

E

Pharmacokinetics

Absorption: 90% absorbed following IM administration. IV administration results in complete bioavailability.

Distribution: Minimally distributed to tissues.

Metabolism and Excretion: Mostly excreted by the kidneys.

Half-life: 1.8 hr (↑ in renal impairment).

TIME/ACTION PROFILE (plasma concentrations)

ROUTE	ONSET	PEAK	DURATION
IM	rapid	2 hr	24 hr
IV	rapid	end of infusion	24 hr

Contraindications/Precautions

Contraindicated in: Hypersensitivity; Cross-sensitivity may occur with penicillins, cephalosporins, and other carbapenems; Hypersensitivity to lidocaine (may be used as a diluent for IM administration).

Use Cautiously in: History of multiple hypersensitivity reactions; Seizure disorders; Renal impairment; OB: Safety not established in pregnancy; Lactation: Use during breastfeeding only if potential maternal benefit to patient justifies potential risk to infant; Pedi: Safety and effectiveness not established in children; Geri: ↑ sensitivity due to age-related ↓ in renal function in older adults.

Adverse Reactions/Side Effects

Derm: ACUTE GENERALIZED EXANTHEMATOUS PUSTULOSIS. **GI:** CLOSTRIDIOIDES DIFFICILE-ASSOCIATED DIARRHEA (CDAD), diarrhea, nausea, vomiting. **GU:** vaginitis. **Local:** pain at IM site, phlebitis at IV site. **Neuro:** headache, SEIZURES. **Misc:** HYPERSENSITIVITY REACTIONS (INCLUDING ANAPHYLAXIS).

Interactions

Drug-Drug: Probenecid ↓ excretion and ↑ levels. May ↓ **valproate** levels and ↑ risk of seizures.

Route/Dosage

IV, IM (Adults and Children ≥13 yr): 1 g once daily for up to 14 days (IV) or 7 days (IM).

IV, IM (Children 3 mo–12 yr): 15 mg/kg twice daily (not to exceed 1 g/day) for up to 14 days (IV) or 7 days (IM).

Renal Impairment

IM, IV (Adults): *CCr ≤30 mL/min/1.73 m²:* 500 mg once daily.

Availability (generic available)

Powder for injection: 1 g/vial.

NURSING IMPLICATIONS

Assessment

- Assess for infection (vital signs; appearance of wound, sputum, urine, and stool; WBC) at baseline and during therapy.
- Obtain a history before initiating therapy to determine previous use of and reactions to penicillins, cephalosporins, or carbapenems.
- Monitor for signs and symptoms of hypersensitivity reaction, including anaphylaxis. *If a serious reaction occurs,* immediately discontinue ertapenem and provide treatment as clinically indicated. Keep epinephrine, an antihistamine, and resuscitative equipment close by during therapy.
- Monitor for signs and symptoms of seizure during therapy. *If focal tremors, myoclonus, or seizures occur,* evaluate and place on anticonvulsant as indicated. Consider ↓ dose or discontinuing ertapenem.
- Monitor for diarrhea, abdominal cramping, fever, and bloody stools during therapy and for 2 mo after last dose. *If CDAD suspected or confirmed,* treat as clinically indicated and consider discontinuation of antibiotic therapy not directed against CDAD.

Lab Test Considerations

- Obtain specimens for culture and sensitivity before initiating therapy. First dose may be given before receiving results.
- Monitor renal and hepatic function during prolonged therapy. May ↑ AST, ALT, and serum alkaline phosphatase.
- May ↑ platelets and eosinophils.

Implementation

- **IM:** Reconstitute 1-g vial with 3.2 mL of 1% lidocaine without epinephrine. Shake well. Immediately withdraw contents and inject deep into large muscle. Use reconstituted solution within 1 hr.

IV Administration

- **Intermittent Infusion: Reconstitution:** Reconstitute 1-g vial with 10 mL of sterile water for injection or 0.9% NaCl using 21-gauge or smaller diameter needle and shake well. **Dilution:** *For adults and pediatric patients ≥13 yr:* further dilute in 50 mL of 0.9% NaCl. *For pediatric patients 3 mo–12 yr,* immediately withdraw volume equal to 15 mg/kg (not to exceed 1 g/day) and dilute in 0.9% NaCl to a final concentration ≤20 mg/mL. Administer within 6 hr of reconstitution. **Rate:** Infuse over 30 min.
- **Y-Site Compatibility:** acyclovir, amikacin, aminocaproic acid, aminophylline, amphotericin B liposomal, argatroban, arsenic trioxide, atracurium, azithromycin, aztreonam, bivalirudin, bleomycin, bumetanide, buprenorphine, busulfan, butorphanol, calcium chloride, calcium gluconate, cangrelor, carboplatin, carmustine, ceftazidime/avibactam, ceftolozane/tazobactam, cisatracurium, cisplatin, cyclophosphamide, cyclosporine, cytarabine, dacarbazine, dactinomycin, daptomycin, dexamethasone, dexmedetomidine, dexrazoxane, digoxin, diltiazem, diphenhydramine, docetaxel, dopamine, doxorubicin liposomal, doxycycline, enalaprilat, ephedrine, epinephrine, eptifibatide, erythromycin, esmolol, etoposide, etoposide phosphate, famotidine, fluconazole, fludarabine, fluorouracil, foscarnet, fosphenytoin, furosemide, ganciclovir, gemcitabine, gemtuzumab ozogamicin, gentamicin, glycopyrrolate, granisetron, haloperidol, heparin, hetastarch, hydrocortisone, hydromorphone, ifosfamide, insulin, regular, irinotecan, isoproterenol, ketorolac, labetalol, leucovorin, levofloxacin, lidocaine, linezolid, lorazepam, magnesium sulfate, mannitol, melphalan, meperidine, meropenem, meropenem/vaborbactam, mesna, methadone, methotrexate, methylprednisolone, metoclopramide, metronidazole, milrinone, mitomycin, morphine, moxifloxacin, nalbuphine, naloxone, nitroglycerin, nitroprusside, norepinephrine, octreotide, oxaliplatin, oxytocin, paclitaxel, pamidronate, pantoprazole, pemetrexed, pentobarbital, phenobarbital, phentolamine, phenylephrine, plazomicin, potassium acetate, potassium chloride, potassium phosphate, procainamide, propranolol, remifentanil, rocuronium, sodium acetate, sodium bicarbonate, sodium phosphate, succinylcholine, sufentanil, sulbactam/durlobactam, tacrolimus, telavancin, theophylline, thiotepa, tigecycline, tirofiban, tobramycin, trimethoprim/sulfamethoxazole, vancomycin, vasopressin, vecuronium, vinblastine, vincristine, vinorelbine, voriconazole, zidovudine, zoledronic acid.
- **Y-Site Incompatibility:** alemtuzumab, allopurinol, amiodarone, anidulafungin, caspofungin, chlorpromazine, dantrolene, daunorubicin, diazepam, dobutamine, doxorubicin hydrochloride, droperidol, epirubicin, hydralazine, hydroxyzine, idarubicin, isavuconazonium, midazolam, minocycline, mitoxantrone, nicardipine, ondansetron, pentamidine, phenytoin, prochlorperazine, promethazine, topotecan, verapamil.

Patient/Family Teaching

- Explain purpose and side effects of medication. Advise patient to read *Patient Information* before starting therapy.
- Advise patient to report signs of superinfection (black, furry overgrowth on tongue; vaginal itching or discharge; loose or foul-smelling stools) and allergy.

- Caution patient to notify health care professional if fever and diarrhea occur, especially if stool contains blood, pus, or mucus. Advise patient not to treat diarrhea without consulting health care professional.
- Instruct patient to notify health care professional of all Rx or OTC medications, vitamins, or herbal products being taken and to consult health care professional before taking any new medications.
- Rep: Advise women of reproductive potential to notify health care professional if pregnancy is planned or suspected or if breastfeeding.

Evaluation/Desired Outcomes

- Resolution of the signs and symptoms of infection. Length of time for complete resolution depends on the organism and site of infection.

ERYTHROMYCIN

(eh-rith-roe-**mye**-sin)

erythromycin base

~~E-Mycin~~, ✦ Eryc, Ery-Tab, ~~PCE~~

erythromycin ethylsuccinate

E.E.S, EryPed

erythromycin lactobionate

Erythrocin

erythromycin (topical)

~~Erygel~~

Classification

Therapeutic: anti-infectives

Pharmacologic: macrolides

See Appendix B for ophthalmic use

Indications

IV, PO: Infections caused by susceptible organisms, including: Upper and lower respiratory tract infections, Otitis media (with sulfonamides), Skin and skin structure infections, Pertussis, Diphtheria, Erythrasma, Intestinal amebiasis, Pelvic inflammatory disease, Nongonococcal urethritis, Syphilis, Legionnaires' disease, Rheumatic fever. Useful when penicillin is the most appropriate drug but cannot be used because of hypersensitivity, including: Streptococcal infections, Syphilis or gonorrhea. **Topical:** Acne.

Action

Suppresses protein synthesis at the level of the 50S bacterial ribosome. **Therapeutic Effects:** Bacteriostatic action against susceptible bacteria. **Spectrum:** Active against many gram-positive cocci, including: streptococci, Staphylococci. Gram-positive bacilli, including: *Clostridioides*, *Corynebacterium*. Several gram-negative pathogens, notably: *Neisseria*, *Legionella pneumophila*. *Mycoplasma* and *Chlamydia* are also usually susceptible.

Pharmacokinetics

Absorption: Variable absorption from the duodenum after oral administration (dependent on salt form). Absorption of enteric-coated products is delayed. Minimal absorption may follow topical or ophthalmic use.

Distribution: Widely distributed. Minimal CNS penetration.

Protein Binding: 70–80%.

Metabolism and Excretion: Partially metabolized by the liver, excreted mainly unchanged in the bile; small amounts excreted unchanged in the urine.

Half-life: Neonates: 2.1 hr; Adults: 1.4–2 hr.

TIME/ACTION PROFILE (plasma concentrations)

ROUTE	ONSET	PEAK	DURATION
PO	1 hr	1–4 hr	6–12 hr
IV	rapid	end of infusion	6–12 hr

Contraindications/Precautions

Contraindicated in: Hypersensitivity; Concurrent use of dihydroergotamine, ergotamine, lovastatin, pimozide, or simvastatin; Long QT syndrome; Hypokalemia; Hypomagnesemia; HR <50 bpm; Known alcohol intolerance (most topicals); Tartrazine sensitivity (some products contain tartrazine: FDC yellow dye #5); Pedi: Products containing benzyl alcohol should be avoided in neonates.

Use Cautiously in: Renal impairment; Hepatic impairment; Myasthenia gravis (may worsen symptoms); OB: May be used in pregnancy to treat chlamydial infections or syphilis; Geri: ↑ risk of ototoxicity if parenteral dose >4 g/day and ↑ risk of QTc interval prolongation in older adults.

Adverse Reactions/Side Effects

CV: QT interval prolongation, TORSADES DE POINTES, VENTRICULAR ARRHYTHMIAS. **Derm:** rash. **EENT:** ototoxicity. **GI:** nausea, vomiting, abdominal pain, CLOSTRIDIOIDES DIFFICILE-ASSOCIATED DIARRHEA (CDAD), cramping, diarrhea, hepatitis, infantile hypertrophic pyloric stenosis, pancreatitis (rare). **GU:** interstitial nephritis. **Local:** phlebitis. **Misc:** HYPERSENSITIVITY REACTIONS (INCLUDING ANAPHYLAXIS).

Interactions

Drug-Drug: **Pimozide** may ↑ levels and risk for serious arrhythmias; concurrent use contraindicated; similar effects may occur with **diltiazem**, **verapamil**, **ketoconazole**, **itraconazole**, **nefazodone**, and **protease inhibitors**; concurrent use with pimozide contraindicated. May ↑ levels and risk for ergot toxicity of **ergotamine** and **dihydroergotamine**; concurrent use contraindicated. **Lovastatin** or **simvastatin** may ↑ risk of rhabdomyolysis; concurrent use contraindicated. **Amiodarone**, **dofetilide**, or **sotalol** may ↑ risk of torsades de pointes; avoid concurrent use. May ↑ **verapamil** levels and risk for hypotension, bradycardia, and lactic acidosis. May ↑ levels and risk of toxicity of **sildenafil**, **tadalafil**, and **vardenafil**; use lower doses. **Rifabutin** or **rifampin** may ↓ levels and effectiveness. May ↑ levels and risk of toxicity of **alprazolam**, **bromocriptine**, **carbamazepine**, **cyclosporine**, **cilostazol**, **diazepam**, **disopyramide**, **ergot alkaloids**, **felodipine**, **methylprednisolone**, **midazolam**, **quinidine**, **rifabutin**, **tacrolimus**, **triazolam**, or **vinblastine**. May ↑ levels and risk of toxicity of **digoxin**. **Theophylline** may ↓ levels and effectiveness. May ↑ levels and risk of toxicity of **colchicine**; use lower starting and maximum dose of colchicine. May ↑ levels and risk of toxicity of **theophylline**; ↓ theophylline dose. May ↑ levels of and risk of bleeding with **warfarin**.

Route/Dosage

250 mg of erythromycin base = 400 mg of erythromycin ethylsuccinate.

Most Infections

PO (Adults): *Base:* 250 mg every 6 hr, *or* 333 mg every 8 hr, *or* 500 mg every 12 hr. *Ethylsuccinate:* 400 mg every 6 hr *or* 800 mg every 12 hr.
PO (Children >1 mo): *Base and ethylsuccinate:* 30–50 mg/kg/day divided every 6–8 hr (max = 2 g/day as base or 3.2 g/day as ethylsuccinate).
PO (Neonates): *Ethylsuccinate:* 20–50 mg/kg/day divided every 6–12 hr.
IV (Adults): 250–500 mg (up to 1 g) every 6 hr.
IV (Children >1 mo): 15–50 mg/kg/day divided every 6 hr (max = 4 g/day).

Acne

Topical (Adults and Children >12 yr): 2% gel, solution, or pledgets twice daily.

Availability (generic available)

Erythromycin Base

Delayed-release capsules: 🍁 250 mg, 🍁 333 mg. **Delayed-release tablets:** 250 mg, 333 mg, 500 mg.

Erythromycin Ethylsuccinate

Oral suspension (fruit, cherry, orange, or banana flavor): 200 mg/5 mL, 400 mg/5 mL. **Tablets:** 400 mg.

Erythromycin Lactobionate

Powder for injection (requires reconstitution and dilution): 500 mg/vial, 🍁 1 g.

Erythromycin Topical Preparations

Gel: 2%. **Pledgets:** 2%. **Solution:** 2%. ***In combination with:*** benzoyl peroxide (Benzamycin). See Appendix N.

NURSING IMPLICATIONS

Assessment

- Assess for resolving infection (vital signs; appearance of wound, sputum, urine, and stool; WBC) during therapy.
- Monitor bowel function. Diarrhea, abdominal cramping, fever, and bloody stools should be reported to health care provider promptly as a sign of CDAD. May begin up to several weeks following cessation of therapy.

Lab Test Considerations

- Obtain specimens for culture and sensitivity before initiating therapy. 1st dose may be given before receiving results.
- Monitor liver function tests periodically in patients receiving high-dose, long-term therapy. May ↑ bilirubin, AST, ALT, and alkaline phosphatase.
- Assess CBC to monitor for therapeutic response.
- May cause false ↑ of urinary catecholamines.

Implementation

- **PO:** Administer around the clock. *Erythromycin film-coated tablets (base)* are absorbed better on an empty stomach, >1 hr before or 2 hr after meals; may be taken with food if GI irritation occurs. *Enteric-coated erythromycin (base)* may be taken without regard to meals. *Erythromycin ethylsuccinate* is best absorbed when taken with meals. Take each dose with a full glass of water.
- Use calibrated measuring device for liquid preparations. Shake well before using.
- ***DNC:*** Do not crush or chew delayed-release capsules or tablets; swallow whole. *Erythromycin base delayed-release capsules* may be opened and sprinkled on applesauce, jelly, or ice cream immediately before ingestion. Entire contents of the capsule should be taken.

IV Administration

- **Intermittent Infusion: Reconstitution:** Add 10 mL of sterile water for injection without preservatives to 250-mg or 500-mg vials and 20 mL to 1-g vial. Reconstituted solution can be stored in refrigerator for 2 wk or at room temperature for 24 hr. **Concentration:** 50 mg/mL. **Dilution:** Further dilute reconstituted solution in 0.9% NaCl, LR, or Normosol-R. **Concentration:** 1–5 mg/mL. **Rate:** Administer slowly over 20–60 min to avoid phlebitis. Assess for pain along vein; slow rate if pain occurs; apply ice and notify health care provider if unable to relieve pain.
- **Continuous Infusion: Dilution:** 0.9% NaCl, D5W, or LR. **Concentration:** 1 g/L. **Rate:** Administer over 4 hr.
- **Y-Site Compatibility:** acyclovir, alemtuzumab, amikacin, aminocaproic acid, aminophylline, amiodarone, anidulafungin, argatroban, arsenic trioxide, atracurium, atropine, azathioprine, benztropine, bivalirudin,

bleomycin, bumetanide, buprenorphine, butorphanol, calcium chloride, calcium gluconate, cangrelor, carboplatin, carmustine, caspofungin, cefotaxime, ceftriaxone, cefuroxime, chlorothiazide, chlorpromazine, cisplatin, cyanocobalamin, cyclophosphamide, cyclosporine, cytarabine, dacarbazine, dactinomycin, daptomycin, daunorubicin, dexmedetomidine, dexrazoxane, digoxin, diltiazem, diphenhydramine, dobutamine, docetaxel, dopamine, doxapram, doxorubicin hydrochloride, doxorubicin liposomal, edetate calcium disodium, enalaprilat, ephedrine, epinephrine, epirubicin, epoetin alfa, eptifibatide, ertapenem, esmolol, etoposide, etoposide phosphate, famotidine, fentanyl, fluconazole, fludarabine, fluorouracil, folic acid, foscarnet, fosphenytoin, gemcitabine, gentamicin, glycopyrrolate, granisetron, hydrocortisone, hydromorphone, idarubicin, ifosfamide, imipenem/cilastatin, insulin, regular, irinotecan, isoproterenol, labetalol, leucovorin, levofloxacin, lidocaine, lorazepam, mannitol, meperidine, meropenem, mesna, methadone, methohexital, methotrexate, methylprednisolone, metoclopramide, metoprolol, metronidazole, midazolam, milrinone, mitomycin, mitoxantrone, morphine, multivitamins, mycophenolate, nafcillin, nalbuphine, naloxone, nicardipine, nitroglycerin, norepinephrine, octreotide, ondansetron, oxacillin, oxaliplatin, oxytocin, paclitaxel, palonosetron, pamidronate, papaverine, pentamidine, phentolamine, phenylephrine, phytonadione, piperacillin/tazobactam, potassium acetate, potassium chloride, procainamide, prochlorperazine, promethazine, propranolol, protamine, pyridoxine, sodium acetate, sodium bicarbonate, succinylcholine, sufentanil, tacrolimus, theophylline, thiamine, thiotepa, tigecycline, tirofiban, tobramycin, topotecan, vancomycin, vasopressin, vecuronium, verapamil, vinblastine, vincristine, vinorelbine, voriconazole, zidovudine, zoledronic acid.

- **Y-Site Incompatibility:** amphotericin B deoxycholate, amphotericin B liposomal, ascorbic acid, aztreonam, cefazolin, cefepime, cefotetan, cefoxitin, dantrolene, diazepam, diazoxide, doxycycline, ganciclovir, gemtuzumab ozogamicin, indomethacin, ketorolac, nitroprusside, pemetrexed, pentobarbital, phenytoin, trimethoprim/sulfamethoxazole.
- **Topical:** Cleanse area before application. Wear gloves during application.

Patient/Family Teaching

- Explain purpose and side effects of erythromycin. Instruct patient to take medication around the clock and to finish the drug completely as directed, even if feeling better. Take missed doses as soon as remembered, with remaining doses evenly spaced throughout day. Advise patient to read *Patient Information* before starting therapy.
- Pedi: Teach parents or caregivers to calculate and measure doses accurately. Reinforce importance of using measuring device supplied by pharmacy or with product, not household items.
- Instruct the patient to notify health care provider if symptoms do not improve.
- Advise patient to report the signs of superinfection (furry overgrowth on the tongue, vaginal itching or discharge, loose or foul-smelling stools) and allergy.
- Instruct patient to notify health care provider immediately if diarrhea, abdominal cramping, fever, or bloody stools occur and not to treat with antidiarrheals without consulting health care provider.
- Advise patient to notify health care provider of all Rx or OTC medications, vitamins, or herbal products being taken and to consult health care provider before taking other medications.
- May cause nausea, vomiting, diarrhea, or stomach cramps; notify health care provider if these effects persist or if severe abdominal pain, yellow discoloration of the skin or eyes, darkened urine, pale stools, or unusual tiredness develops. May cause infantile hypertrophic pyloric stenosis in infants; notify health care provider if vomiting and irritability occur.
- Rep: Advise women of reproductive potential to notify health care provider if pregnancy is planned or suspected or if breastfeeding.

Evaluation/Desired Outcomes

- Bacteriostatic action against susceptible bacteria.
- Resolution of the signs and symptoms of infection. Length of time for complete resolution depends on the organism and site of infection.
- Treatment of acne (topical).

BEERS

escitalopram

(ess-sit-**al**-o-pram)

Cipralex, Lexapro

Classification

Therapeutic: antidepressants

Pharmacologic: selective serotonin reuptake inhibitors (SSRIs)

Indications

Major depressive disorder. Generalized anxiety disorder. **Unlabeled Use:** Panic disorder. Obsessive-compulsive disorder. Post-traumatic stress disorder. Social anxiety disorder (social phobia). Premenstrual dysphoric disorder.

Action

Selectively inhibits the reuptake of serotonin in the CNS.
Therapeutic Effects: Antidepressant action.

Pharmacokinetics

Absorption: 80% absorbed following oral administration.
Distribution: Widely distributed to tissues.
Metabolism and Excretion: Mostly metabolized by the liver, primarily by the CYP3A4 and CYP2C19 isoenzymes; 7% excreted unchanged by kidneys.
Half-life: 27–32 hr (↑ in older adults and hepatic impairment).

TIME/ACTION PROFILE (antidepressant effect)

ROUTE	ONSET	PEAK	DURATION
PO	within 1–4 wk	unknown	unknown

Contraindications/Precautions

Contraindicated in: Hypersensitivity; Concurrent use of pimozide; Concurrent use of MAO inhibitors or MAO-like drugs (linezolid or methylene blue); Concurrent use of citalopram; Angle-closure glaucoma.
Use Cautiously in: Personal or family history of bipolar disorder, mania, or hypomania (may activate mania/hypomania); History of seizures; May ↑ risk of suicide attempt/ideation especially during early treatment or dose adjustment; this risk appears to be greater in adolescents or children; Hepatic impairment; Severe renal impairment; OB: Use during pregnancy only if potential maternal benefit justifies potential fetal risk; Lactation: Use while breastfeeding only if potential maternal benefit justifies potential risk to infant; Pedi: May ↑ risk of suicide attempt/ideation especially during early treatment or dose adjustment; safety not established in children <12 yr (major depressive disorder) or <7 yr (generalized anxiety disorder); Geri: Appears on Beers list. May worsen or cause syndrome of inappropriate antidiuretic hormone (SIADH) secretion and/or hyponatremia in older adults. Use with caution in older adults and closely monitor sodium concentrations when starting therapy or ↑ dose.

Adverse Reactions/Side Effects

Derm: sweating. **Endo:** SIADH. **F and E** hyponatremia. **GI:** <u>diarrhea</u>, <u>nausea</u>, abdominal pain, constipation, dry mouth, indigestion. **GU:** ↓ libido, delayed/absent orgasm, ejaculatory delay/failure, erectile dysfunction. **Hemat:** BLEEDING. **Metab:** ↑ appetite. **Neuro:** <u>insomnia</u>, dizziness, drowsiness, fatigue, NEUROLEPTIC MALIGNANT SYNDROME, SUICIDAL THOUGHTS/BEHAVIORS. **Misc:** SEROTONIN SYNDROME.

Interactions

Drug-Drug: May cause serious, potentially fatal reactions when used with **MAO inhibitors**; allow ≥14 days between escitalopram and **MAO inhibitors**. Concurrent use with **MAO-inhibitor-like drugs**, such as **linezolid** or **methylene blue**, may ↑ risk of serotonin syndrome; concurrent use contraindicated; do not start therapy in patients receiving **linezolid** or **methylene blue**; if **linezolid** or **methylene blue** need to be started in a patient receiving escitalopram, immediately discontinue escitalopram and monitor for signs/symptoms of serotonin syndrome for 2 wk or until 24 hr after last dose of linezolid or methylene blue, whichever comes first (may resume escitalopram therapy 24 hr after last dose of linezolid or methylene blue). Concurrent use with **pimozide** may result in prolongation of the QT interval and is contraindicated. Use cautiously with other **centrally acting drugs**, including **alcohol**, **antihistamines**, **opioid analgesics**, and **sedative/hypnotics**; concurrent use with **alcohol** is not recommended. Drugs that affect serotonergic neurotransmitter systems, including **tricyclic antidepressants**, **SNRIs**, **fentanyl**, **lithium**, **buspirone**, **tramadol**, **meperidine**, **methadone**, **amphetamines**, and **triptans**, may ↑ risk of serotonin syndrome. **Cimetidine** may ↑ levels and risk of toxicity. Serotonergic effects may be ↑ by **lithium**; concurrent use should be carefully monitored. **Carbamazepine** may ↓ levels and effectiveness. May ↑ levels and risk of toxicity of **metoprolol**. ↑ risk of bleeding with **NSAIDs**, **aspirin**, **clopidogrel**, **prasugrel**, **ticagrelor**, **dabigatran**, **apixaban**, **edoxaban**, **rivaroxaban**, or **warfarin**.
Drug-Natural Products: ↑ risk of serotonin syndrome with **St. John's wort** and **SAMe**.

Route/Dosage

Major Depressive Disorder

PO (Adults): 10 mg once daily; may ↑ to 20 mg once daily after 1 wk.
PO (Geriatric Patients): 10 mg once daily.
PO (Children ≥12 yr): 10 mg once daily; may ↑ to 20 mg once daily after 3 wk.

Hepatic Impairment

PO (Adults): 10 mg once daily.

Generalized Anxiety Disorder

PO (Adults): 10 mg once daily; may ↑ to 20 mg once daily after 1 wk.
PO (Geriatric Patients): 10 mg once daily.
PO (Children ≥7 yr): 10 mg once daily; may ↑ to 20 mg once daily after 2 wk.

Hepatic Impairment

PO (Adults): 10 mg once daily.

Availability (generic available)

Tablets: 5 mg, 10 mg, 20 mg. **Orally disintegrating tablets:** ✱ 10 mg, ✱ 20 mg. **Oral solution (peppermint flavor):** 1 mg/mL.

NURSING IMPLICATIONS

Assessment

- Screen patient for a personal or family history of bipolar disorder, mania, or hypomania before starting therapy; may precipitate a mixed/manic episode.
- Monitor mood changes and level of anxiety during therapy.
- Assess for suicidal tendencies, especially during early therapy. Restrict amount of drug available to patient. Risk may be ↑ in children, adolescents, and adults ≤24 yr. After starting therapy, children, adolescents, and young adults should be seen by health care provider face-to-face at least weekly for 4 wk, then every other wk for next 4 wk, then at 12 wk, and then on advice of health care provider thereafter.
- Assess sexual function before starting escitalopram. Assess for changes in sexual function during treatment, including timing of onset; patient may not report.
- Assess for serotonin syndrome (mental changes [agitation, hallucinations, coma], autonomic instability [tachycardia, labile BP, hyperthermia], neuromuscular aberrations [hyperreflexia, incoordination], or GI symptoms [nausea, vomiting, diarrhea]), especially in patients taking other serotonergic drugs (SSRIs, SNRIs, triptans).

Implementation

- Do not confuse escitalopram with citalopram.
- Do not administer escitalopram and citalopram concurrently. When discontinuing therapy, taper to avoid potential withdrawal reactions (↓ dose by 50% for 3 days; then again by 50% for 3 days; then discontinue).
- **PO:** Administer as a single dose in the morning or evening without regard to meals.

Patient/Family Teaching

- Instruct patient to take escitalopram as directed. Take missed doses on the same day as soon as remembered and consult health care provider. Resume regular dosing schedule next day. Do not double doses. Do not stop abruptly; should be discontinued gradually. Instruct patient to read *Medication Guide* before starting and with each Rx refill in case of changes.
- May cause dizziness. Caution patient to avoid driving or other activities requiring alertness until response to medication is known.
- Advise patient, family, and caregivers to look for suicidality, especially during early therapy or dose changes. Notify health care provider immediately if thoughts about suicide or dying, attempts to commit suicide, new or worse depression or anxiety, agitation or restlessness, panic attacks, insomnia, new or worse irritability, aggressiveness, acting on dangerous impulses, mania, or other changes in mood or behavior.
- Advise patient and caregivers to immediately notify health care provider if symptoms of serotonin syndrome occur.
- Instruct patient to notify health care provider of all Rx or OTC medications, vitamins, or herbal products being taken and to consult health care provider before taking any other Rx, OTC, or herbal products, especially St. John's wort, alcohol, or other CNS depressants.
- Inform patient that escitalopram may cause symptoms of sexual dysfunction. In men, ejaculatory delay or failure, ↓ libido, and erectile dysfunction may occur. In women, may result in ↓ libido and delayed or absent orgasm. Advise patient to notify health care provider if symptoms occur.
- Rep: Advise women of reproductive potential to notify health care provider if pregnancy is planned or suspected or if breastfeeding. Use late in 3rd trimester may result in neonatal serotonin syndrome requiring prolonged hospitalization, respiratory support, and tube feeding; may occur immediately upon delivery. Symptoms include respiratory distress, cyanosis, apnea, seizures, temperature instability, feeding difficulty, vomiting, hypoglycemia, hypotonia, hypertonia, hyperreflexia, tremor, jitteriness, irritability, and constant crying. Use of escitalopram in last months of pregnancy may ↑ risk of postpartum hemorrhage. Encourage pregnant patients to enroll in pregnancy exposure registry that monitors outcomes of women exposed to antidepressants during pregnancy by contacting National Pregnancy Registry for Antidepressants at 1-866-961-2388 or visiting online at https://womensmentalhealth.org/research/pregnancyregistry/antidepressants/. Monitor infants exposed to escitalopram via breastfeeding for sedation, poor feeding, and poor weight gain.
- Emphasize importance of follow-up exams to monitor progress.

Evaluation/Desired Outcomes

- Increased sense of well-being.
- Renewed interest in surroundings. May require 1–4 wk of therapy to obtain antidepressant effects. Full antidepressant effects occur in 4–6 wk.
- Decrease in anxiety.

REMS

esketamine (es-**ket**-a-meen)

Spravato

Classification

Therapeutic: antidepressants

Pharmacologic: N-methyl-D-aspartate antagonist

Schedule III

Indications

Treatment-resistant depression (as monotherapy or in combination with an oral antidepressant). Depressive symptoms in patients with major depressive disorder with acute suicidal ideation or behavior (in combination with an oral antidepressant).

Action

Acts as a noncompetitive N-methyl-D-aspartate receptor antagonist; the exact mechanism by which it exerts its antidepressant effect is unknown. **Therapeutic Effects:** Decreased severity of depressive symptoms and prolonged time to relapse.

Pharmacokinetics

Absorption: 48% absorbed following nasal administration.
Distribution: Extensively distributed to tissues.
Metabolism and Excretion: Primarily metabolized to noresketamine (active metabolite) in liver by CYP2B6 and CYP3A4 isoenzymes and to lesser extent by CYP2C9 and CYP2C19 isoenzymes. Primarily excreted in urine (≥78%; <1% as unchanged drug); ≤2% excreted in feces.
Half-life: 7–12 hr.

TIME/ACTION PROFILE (plasma concentrations)

ROUTE	ONSET	PEAK	DURATION
Intranasal	unknown	20–40 min	unknown

Contraindications/Precautions

Contraindicated in: Hypersensitivity to esketamine or ketamine; Aneurysmal vascular disease (including thoracic and abdominal aorta, intracranial and peripheral arterial vessels) or arteriovenous malformation; History of intracerebral hemorrhage; Severe hepatic impairment; OB: Pregnancy; Lactation: Lactation.
Use Cautiously in: May ↑ risk of suicide attempt/ideation especially during early treatment or dose adjustment; this risk appears to be greater in adolescents or children; History of hypertensive encephalopathy; Psychosis; Substance use disorder; Moderate hepatic impairment; Rep: Women of reproductive potential; Pedi: Safety and effectiveness not established in children.

Adverse Reactions/Side Effects

CV: ↑ BP, tachycardia. **Derm:** ↑ sweating. **EENT:** nasal irritation, throat irritation. **GI:** nausea, vomiting, constipation, diarrhea, dry mouth. **GU:** urinary tract infection. **Neuro:** anxiety, depersonalization, derealization, dissociative changes, dizziness, dysgeusia, fatigue, headache, hypoesthesia, sedation, vertigo, cognitive impairment, insomnia, loss of consciousness, slurred/slow speech, SUICIDAL THOUGHTS/BEHAVIORS, tremor. **Resp:** RESPIRATORY DEPRESSION. **Misc:** physical dependence, psychological dependence, tolerance.

Interactions

Drug-Drug: Concurrent use with **psychostimulants**, including **amphetamines**, **methylphenidate**, **modafanil**, or **armodafanil**, as well as **MAO inhibitors**, may ↑ BP. Use with **opioids** or other **CNS depressants**, including **benzodiazepines**, **nonbenzodiazepine sedative/hypnotics**, **anxiolytics**, **general anesthetics**, **muscle relaxants**, **antipsychotics**, and **alcohol**, may cause profound sedation.

Route/Dosage

Treatment-Resistant Depression

Intranasal (Adults): *Induction phase (Wk 1–4):* 56 mg (2 sprays in each nostril) or 84 mg (3 sprays in each nostril) twice weekly. *Maintenance phase (Wk 5–8):* 56 mg (2 sprays in each nostril) or 84 mg (3 sprays in each nostril) once weekly. *Maintenance phase (Wk 9 and beyond):* 56 mg (2 sprays in each nostril) or 84 mg (3 sprays in each nostril) once weekly or every other wk (use least frequent dosing to maintain remission/response).

Depressive Symptoms in Patients with Major Depressive Disorder with Acute Suicidal Ideation or Behavior

Intranasal (Adults): 84 mg (3 sprays in each nostril) twice weekly for 4 wk; may ↓ dosage to 56 mg (2 sprays in each nostril) twice weekly based on tolerability. Reevaluate patient for continued need for treatment after 4 wk.

Availability

Nasal spray: 28 mg/device (14 mg/spray).

NURSING IMPLICATIONS

Assessment

- Monitor patient for sedation and respiratory depression for ≥2 hr after each dose.
- Monitor BP before and 40 min after each dose and then periodically for ≥2 hr after administration. *If BP elevated before administration,* may hold dose. *If BP elevated following dose,* continue monitoring.
- Assess for history of psychosis and dissociative or perceptual changes (distortion of time, space, and illusions), derealization, and depersonalization at baseline and for ≥2 hr after each dose.
- Monitor for worsening or emergence of suicidal thoughts and behaviors, especially during initial few months of therapy and with dose changes.
- Monitor for urinary tract and bladder symptoms during therapy. *If symptoms of ulcerative or interstitial cystitis occur,* consult specialist as clinically indicated.
- Assess for risk of abuse or misuse prior to administration, and monitor for these behaviors as well

as drug-seeking behaviors and dependence during treatment.

Implementation

- Do not confuse Spravato with Steglatro.
- *REMS:* Due to risks of serious adverse outcomes from sedation, dissociation, abuse, and misuse, esketamine is available only through a restricted program under *Spravato REMS.* Health care settings and pharmacies must be certified, and patients must be enrolled in REMS program. Esketamine is only administered in health care settings under direct observation of health care provider, and patients must be monitored for ≥2 hr after administration.
- Advise patient to avoid food for ≥2 hr and liquids for 30 min prior to administration.
- If nasal corticosteroid or nasal decongestant is administered on a dosing day, administer ≥1 hr before esketamine administration.
- Esketamine may be given as monotherapy or in conjunction with an oral antidepressant.
- **Intranasal:** Use 2 devices (for a 56-mg dose) or 3 devices (for an 84-mg dose), with a 5-min rest between use of each device. Do not prime device. Advise patient to gently blow nose before 1st dose. Check that indicator shows two or three green dots. Instruct patient to recline head back 45°, insert device into nostril until nose rest is between nostrils, close opposite nostril, and sniff gently after administering dose. After administration, confirm no green dots. Instruct patient to recline and rest for 5 min between doses and to not blow their nose. Repeat for each dose. Discard according to institution guidelines for Schedule III drugs. Observe patient for ≥2 hr after dose until stable for discharge.

Patient/Family Teaching

- *REMS:* Explain purpose of esketamine, administration procedure, and *Spravato REMS* program to patient. Advise patient to read *Medication Guide* before starting therapy. If a treatment session is missed and no worsening of depressive symptoms occurs, continue current dosing schedule. If depressive symptoms worsen, may return to previous dosing schedule.
- Advise patient that esketamine is a controlled substance and can lead to dependence and has abuse potential.
- Caution patient to avoid driving or activities requiring alertness until next day after a restful sleep.
- Advise patient, family, and caregivers to look for changes in behavior and suicidality, especially during early therapy or dose changes. Notify health care provider immediately of thoughts about suicide or dying, suicide attempts, new or worse depression or anxiety, agitation or restlessness, panic attacks, insomnia, new or worse irritability, aggressiveness, acting on dangerous impulses, mania, or other changes in mood or behavior.
- Instruct patient to notify health care provider of all Rx or OTC medications, vitamins, or herbal products being taken and to avoid concurrent use of Rx, OTC, and herbal products without consulting health care provider.
- Rep: May cause fetal harm. Advise women of reproductive potential to use effective contraception during therapy and to avoid breastfeeding. Notify health care provider promptly if pregnancy is planned or suspected. Inform patients who become pregnant during therapy of pregnancy registry that monitors pregnancy outcomes. Enroll patients by contacting the National Pregnancy Registry for Antidepressants at 1-866-961-2388 or online at https://womensmentalhealth.org/clinical-and-researchprograms/pregnancyregistry/antidepressants/.

Evaluation/Desired Outcomes

- Decreased severity of depressive symptoms and prolonged time to relapse.

HIGH ALERT

V esmolol (es-moe-lol)

Brevibloc

Classification

Therapeutic: antiarrhythmics (class II)

Pharmacologic: beta blockers

Indications

Sinus tachycardia. Supraventricular arrhythmias.

Action

Blocks stimulation of $beta_1$ (myocardial)-adrenergic receptors. Does not usually affect $beta_2$ (pulmonary, vascular, or uterine)-receptor sites. **Therapeutic Effects:** Decreased heart rate. Decreased AV conduction.

Pharmacokinetics

Absorption: IV administration results in complete bioavailability.

Distribution: Rapidly and widely distributed.

Metabolism and Excretion: Metabolized by enzymes in RBCs and liver.

Half-life: 9 min.

TIME/ACTION PROFILE (antiarrhythmic effect)

ROUTE	ONSET	PEAK	DURATION
IV	within min	unknown	1–20 min

Contraindications/Precautions

Contraindicated in: Uncompensated HF; Pulmonary edema; Cardiogenic shock; Bradycardia or heart block; Known alcohol intolerance; Lactation: Lactation.

Use Cautiously in: Thyrotoxicosis (may mask symptoms); Diabetes mellitus (may mask symptoms of hypoglycemia); Patients with a history of severe allergic reactions (intensity of reactions may be ↑); OB: Use during pregnancy only if potential maternal benefit justifies potential fetal risk; may cause fetal bradycardia, ↓ uterine blood flow, and fetal hypoxia if used during the last trimester; Pedi: Safety and effectiveness not established in children; Geri: Older adults may have ↑ sensitivity to the effects of beta blockers.

Adverse Reactions/Side Effects

CV: hypotension, peripheral ischemia. **Derm:** sweating. **Endo:** hypoglycemia. **F and E** hyperkalemia. **GI:** nausea, vomiting. **Local:** injection site reactions. **Neuro:** fatigue, agitation, confusion, dizziness, drowsiness, weakness.

Interactions

Drug-Drug: General anesthesia, IV **phenytoin**, and **verapamil** may cause additive myocardial depression. Additive bradycardia may occur with **digoxin**. Additive hypotension may occur with other **antihypertensives**, acute ingestion of **alcohol**, or **nitrates**. Concurrent use with **amphetamine**, **cocaine**, **ephedrine**, **epinephrine**, **norepinephrine**, **phenylephrine**, or **pseudoephedrine** may result in unopposed alpha-adrenergic stimulation (excessive hypertension, bradycardia). Concurrent **thyroid hormone** administration may ↓ effectiveness. May alter the effectiveness of **insulins** or **oral hypoglycemic agents** (dose adjustments may be necessary). May ↓ effectiveness of **theophylline**. May ↓ beneficial beta cardiovascular effects of **dopamine** or **dobutamine**. Use cautiously within 14 days of **MAO inhibitor** therapy (may result in hypertension).

Route/Dosage

IV (Adults): *Antiarrhythmic:* 500-mcg/kg loading dose over 1 min initially, followed by 50-mcg/kg/min infusion for 4 min; if no response within 5 min, give 2nd loading dose of 500 mcg/kg over 1 min; then ↑ infusion to 100 mcg/kg/min for 4 min. If no response, repeat loading dose of 500 mcg/kg over 1 min and ↑ infusion rate by 50-mcg/kg/min increments (not to exceed 200 mcg/kg/min for 48 hr). As therapeutic end point is achieved, eliminate loading doses and decrease dose increments to 25 mg/kg/min. *Intraoperative antihypertensive/antiarrhythmic:* 250–500-mcg/kg loading dose over 1 min initially, followed by 50-mcg/kg/min infusion for 4 min; if no response within 5 min, give 2nd loading dose of 250–500 mcg/kg over 1 min; then ↑ infusion to 100 mcg/kg/min for 4 min. If no response, repeat loading dose of 250–500 mcg/kg over 1 min and ↑ infusion rate by 50-mcg/kg/min increments (not to exceed 200 mcg/kg/min for 48 hr).

IV (Children): *Antiarrhythmic:* 50 mcg/kg/min; may be ↑ every 10 min up to 300 mcg/kg/min.

Availability (generic available)

Solution for injection (for use as loading dose): 10 mg/mL. **Premixed infusion:** 2000 mg/100 mL, 2500 mg/250 mL.

NURSING IMPLICATIONS

Assessment

- Monitor BP, ECG, and HR frequently during dose adjustment period and regularly during therapy. The risk of hypotension is greatest within the 1st 30 min of starting infusion. Hold therapy for severe bradycardia or 2nd/3rd-degree heart block.
- Monitor for bronchospasm in patients with asthma or COPD.
- Monitor intake, output, and daily weights. Assess routinely for signs and symptoms of HF (dyspnea, rales/crackles, weight gain, peripheral edema, jugular venous distention). Hold therapy if cardiogenic shock or decompensated HF develops.
- Assess infusion site frequently during therapy. Concentrations >10 mg/mL may cause injection site reaction (redness, swelling, skin discoloration, and burning at the injection site). Do not use small veins or butterfly needles for administration. If venous irritation occurs, stop the infusion and resume at another site.
- Monitor for signs/symptoms of hypoglycemia (sweating, nausea, tachycardia). Tachycardia may be prevented by esmolol. If hypoglycemia occurs, seek emergency treatment.
- Assess electrolytes regularly during therapy; may cause life-threatening hyperkalemia (↑ risk if renal impairment).

Toxicity and Overdose

- Monitor patients for signs/symptoms of overdose (bradycardia, severe hypotension, severe dizziness or fainting, severe drowsiness, dyspnea, bluish fingernails or palms, seizures).
- IV glucagon and symptomatic care are used in the treatment of esmolol overdose. Because of the short action of esmolol, discontinuation of therapy may relieve acute toxicity.

Implementation

- ***High Alert:*** IV vasoactive medications are inherently dangerous. Esmolol is available in different concentrations; fatalities have occurred when loading dose vial is confused with concentrated solution for injection, which contains 2500 mg in 10 mL (250 mg/mL) and must be diluted. Before administering, have 2nd practitioner independently check original order, dose calculations, and infusion pump settings.
- ***High Alert:*** Do not confuse Brevibloc with Brevital. If both are available as floor stock, store in separate areas.

IV Administration

- V Esmolol is a vesicant. Infuse into a large vein. If extravasation occurs, immediately stop infusion. Leave needle/cannula in place temporarily but do not flush the line. Gently aspirate extravasated solution; then remove needle/cannula. Elevate patient's extremity and apply dry warm compresses. Initiate hyaluronidase antidote for refractory cases in addition to supportive management. For hyaluronidase, inject a total of 1 mL (15 units/mL) intradermally or SUBQ as five separate 0.2-mL injections (using a tuberculin syringe) around the site of extravasation; if IV catheter remains in place, administer IV through the infiltrated catheter; may repeat in 30–60 min if no resolution.
- **IV Push: Dilution:** The 10-mg/mL vial should be used for the loading dose. These vials are already diluted. No further dilution is needed. **Rate:** Administer 1 mg/kg over 30 sec or 500 mcg/kg over 1 min.
- **Continuous Infusion: Dilution:** Premixed infusions are already diluted and ready to use. Solution is clear, colorless to light yellow; do not administer solutions that are discolored or contain particulate matter. Do not remove overwrap until ready to use. Use within 24 hr once opened. **Concentration:** Premixed 10 mg/mL and 20 mg/mL. **Rate:** Based on patient's weight (see Route/Dosage section). Titration of dose is based on desired HR or undesired ↓ in BP. Infusion should not be abruptly discontinued; the infusion rate should be tapered.
- **Y-Site Compatibility:** acetaminophen, albumin, human, alemtuzumab, amikacin, aminophylline, amiodarone, amphotericin B liposomal, anidulafungin, argatroban, ascorbic acid, atracurium, atropine, azithromycin, aztreonam, benztropine, bivalirudin, bleomycin, bumetanide, buprenorphine, butorphanol, calcium chloride, calcium gluconate, cangrelor, carboplatin, carmustine, caspofungin, cefazolin, cefepime, cefotaxime, cefoxitin, ceftazidime, ceftolozane/tazobactam, ceftriaxone, cefuroxime, chlorpromazine, cisatracurium, cisplatin, clindamycin, cyanocobalamin, cyclophosphamide, cyclosporine, cytarabine, dacarbazine, dactinomycin, daptomycin, daunorubicin, dexmedetomidine, dexrazoxane, digoxin, diltiazem, diphenhydramine, dobutamine, docetaxel, dopamine, doxorubicin hydrochloride, doxorubicin liposomal, doxycycline, enalaprilat, ephedrine, epinephrine, epoetin alfa, eptifibatide, eravacycline, ertapenem, erythromycin, etoposide, etoposide phosphate, famotidine, fentanyl, fluconazole, fludarabine, fluorouracil, folic acid, foscarnet, fosphenytoin, gemcitabine, gentamicin, glycopyrrolate, granisetron, heparin, hydromorphone, idarubicin, ifosfamide, imipenem/cilastatin, insulin, regular, irinotecan, isavuconazonium, isoproterenol, labetalol, leucovorin, levofloxacin, levothyroxine, lidocaine, linezolid, lorazepam, magnesium sulfate, mannitol, meperidine, meropenem, meropenem/vaborbactam, mesna, methadone, methotrexate, metoclopramide, metoprolol, metronidazole, micafungin, midazolam, mitoxantrone, morphine, moxifloxacin, multivitamins, mycophenolate, nalbuphine, naloxone, nicardipine, nitroglycerin, nitroprusside, norepinephrine, octreotide, ondansetron, oxaliplatin, oxytocin, paclitaxel, palonosetron, papaverine, pemetrexed, penicillin G, pentamidine, phentolamine, phenylephrine, phytonadione, piperacillin/tazobactam, plazomicin, potassium acetate, potassium chloride, potassium phosphates, procainamide, prochlorperazine, promethazine, propofol, propranolol, protamine, pyridoxine, remifentanil, rocuronium, sodium acetate, sodium bicarbonate, succinylcholine, sufentanil, tacrolimus, theophylline, thiamine, thiotepa, tigecycline, tirofiban, tobramycin, topotecan, vancomycin, vasopressin, vecuronium, verapamil, vinblastine, vincristine, voriconazole, zoledronic acid.
- **Y-Site Incompatibility:** acyclovir, amphotericin B deoxycholate, azathioprine, cefotetan, dantrolene, dexamethasone, diazepam, furosemide, ganciclovir, gemtuzumab ozogamicin, ibuprofen, indomethacin, ketorolac, milrinone, mitomycin, oxacillin, pantoprazole, pentobarbital, phenobarbital, tedizolid, warfarin.

Patient/Family Teaching

- Explain purpose and side effects of esmolol to patient.
- May cause drowsiness. Caution patients receiving esmolol to call for assistance during ambulation or transfer.
- Advise patients to change positions slowly to minimize orthostatic hypotension.
- Patients with diabetes should closely monitor blood glucose, especially if weakness, malaise, irritability, or fatigue occurs. Medication does not block dizziness or sweating as signs of hypoglycemia.
- Advise patient to call right away for chest pain, trouble breathing, nausea, unusual sweating, light-headedness, feeling faint, itchiness, numbness in hands or feet, or warmth/redness in upper body (face, neck, arms, chest).
- Rep: May cause fetal harm. Advise women of reproductive potential to notify health care provider if pregnant. Avoid breastfeeding during therapy. May cause fetal bradycardia.

Evaluation/Desired Outcomes

- Control of arrhythmias without appearance of detrimental side effects.

BEERS

esomeprazole

(es-oh-**mep**-ra-zole)

NexIUM, NexIUM 24hr

Classification

Therapeutic: antiulcer agents

Pharmacologic: proton-pump inhibitors

Indications

PO, IV: GERD/erosive esophagitis (IV therapy should only be used if PO therapy is not possible/appropriate). **IV:** Reduction in risk of rebleeding following therapeutic endoscopy for acute bleeding gastric or duodenal ulcers. **PO:** Hypersecretory conditions, including Zollinger-Ellison syndrome. **PO:** Eradication of *Helicobacter pylori* in duodenal ulcer disease or history of duodenal ulcer disease (in combination with amoxicillin and clarithromycin). **PO:** Reduction in risk of gastric ulcer during continuous NSAID therapy. **OTC:** Heartburn occurring at least twice/wk.

Action

Binds to an enzyme on gastric parietal cells in the presence of acidic gastric pH, preventing the final transport of hydrogen ions into the gastric lumen. **Therapeutic Effects:** Diminished accumulation of acid in the gastric lumen with lessened gastroesophageal reflux. Healing of duodenal ulcers. Decreased incidence of gastric ulcer during continuous NSAID therapy.

Pharmacokinetics

Absorption: 90% absorbed following oral administration; food ↓ absorption.

Distribution: Unknown.

Protein Binding: 97%.

Metabolism and Excretion: Primarily metabolized by the liver via the CYP2C19 isoenzyme, with some metabolism by the CYP3A4 isoenzyme; (the CYP2C19 enzyme system exhibits genetic polymorphism; 15–20% of Asian patients and 3–5% of White and Black patients may be poor metabolizers and may have significantly ↑ esomeprazole concentrations and an ↑ risk of adverse effects); <1% excreted unchanged in urine.

Half-life: *Children 1–11 yr:* 0.42–0.88 hr; *Adults:* 1.0–1.5 hr.

TIME/ACTION PROFILE (plasma concentrations*)

ROUTE	ONSET	PEAK	DURATION
PO	rapid	1.6 hr	24 hr
IV	rapid	end of infusion	24 hr

* Resolution of symptoms takes 5–8 days.

Contraindications/Precautions

Contraindicated in: Hypersensitivity to esomeprazole or related drugs (benzimidazoles); Hypersensitivity; Concurrent use of rilpivirine.

Use Cautiously in: Severe hepatic impairment; Patients using high doses for >1 yr (↑ risk of hip, wrist, or spine fractures and fundic gland polyps); Patients using therapy for >3 yr (↑ risk of vitamin B_{12} deficiency); Pre-existing risk of hypocalcemia; OB: Safety not established in pregnancy; Lactation: Safety not established in breastfeeding; Geri: Appears on Beers list. ↑ risk of *Clostridioides difficile* infection, pneumonia, GI malignancies, bone loss, and fractures in older adults. Avoid scheduled use for >8 wk in older adults unless for high-risk patients (e.g., oral corticosteroid or chronic NSAID use) or patients with erosive esophagitis, Barrett esophagitis, pathological hypersecretory condition, or demonstrated need for maintenance therapy (e.g., failure of H_2 antagonist).

Adverse Reactions/Side Effects

Derm: ACUTE GENERALIZED EXANTHEMATOUS PUSTULOSIS, cutaneous lupus erythematosus, DRUG REACTION WITH EOSINOPHILIA AND SYSTEMIC SYMPTOMS (DRESS), STEVENS-JOHNSON SYNDROME, TOXIC EPIDERMAL NECROLYSIS. **F and E** hypocalcemia (especially if treatment duration ≥3 mo), hypokalemia (especially if treatment duration ≥3 mo), hypomagnesemia (especially if treatment duration ≥3 mo). **GI:** abdominal pain, CLOSTRIDIOIDES DIFFICILE-ASSOCIATED DIARRHEA (CDAD), constipation, diarrhea, dry mouth, flatulence, fundic gland polyps, nausea. **GU:** acute tubulointerstitial nephritis. **Hemat:** vitamin B_{12} deficiency. **MS:** bone fracture. **Neuro:** headache. **Misc:** HYPERSENSITIVITY REACTIONS (INCLUDING ANAPHYLAXIS, ANGIOEDEMA, OR TUBULOINTERSTITIAL NEPHRITIS), systemic lupus erythematosus.

Interactions

Drug-Drug: May significantly ↓ levels and effectiveness of **rilpivirine**; concurrent use contraindicated. May ↓ levels and effectiveness of **atazanavir** and **nelfinavir**; avoid concurrent use. May ↓ absorption and effectiveness of drugs requiring acidic pH, including **ketoconazole**, **itraconazole**, **ampicillin esters**, **iron salts**, **erlotinib**, and **mycophenolate mofetil**. May ↑ levels and risk of toxicity of **digoxin** and **methotrexate**. May ↑ risk of bleeding with **warfarin**; monitor INR and PT. **Voriconazole** may ↑ levels and risk of toxicity. May ↓ the antiplatelet effects of **clopidogrel**; avoid concurrent use. May ↑ levels and risk of toxicity of **cilostazol**; consider ↓ dose of cilostazol from 100 mg twice daily to 50 mg twice daily. **Rifampin** may ↓ levels and effectiveness; avoid concurrent use. Hypomagnesemia and hypokalemia ↑ risk of **digoxin** toxicity. May ↑ levels and risk of toxicity of **tacrolimus** and **methotrexate**.

Drug-Natural Products: St. John's wort may ↓ levels and effectiveness; avoid concurrent use.

Route/Dosage

Gastroesophageal Reflux Disease

PO (Adults): *Healing of erosive esophagitis:* 20 mg or 40 mg once daily for 4–8 wk; *Maintenance of healing of erosive esophagitis:* 20 mg once daily; *Symptomatic GERD:* 20 mg once daily for 4 wk (additional 4 wk may be considered for nonresponders); *Heartburn:* 20 mg once daily for 2 wk.

PO (Children 12–17 yr): *Short-term treatment of GERD:* 20–40 mg once daily for up to 8 wk.

PO (Children 1–11 yr): *Short-term treatment of GERD:* 10 mg once daily for up to 8 wk; *Healing of erosive esophagitis:* <20 kg: 10 mg once daily for 8 wk; ≥20 kg: 10–20 mg once daily for 8 wk.

PO (Infants and Children 1 mo–<1 yr): *>7.5–12 kg:* 10 mg once daily for up to 6 wk; *>5–7.5 kg:* 5 mg once daily for up to 6 wk; *3–5 kg:* 2.5 mg once daily for up to 6 wk.

IV (Adults): 20 or 40 mg once daily.

IV (Children 1–17 yr): *<55 kg:* 10 mg once daily; *≥55 kg:* 20 mg once daily.

IV (Children 1 mo–<1 yr): 0.5 mg/kg once daily.

Hepatic Impairment

PO IV (Adults): *Severe hepatic impairment:* Dose should not exceed 20 mg/day.

Reduction of Risk of Rebleeding of Gastric or Duodenal Ulcers After Therapeutic Endoscopy

IV (Adults): 80 mg over 30 min; then 8 mg/hr continuous infusion for 71.5 hr.

Hepatic Impairment

IV (Adults): *Mild to moderate hepatic impairment:* Do not exceed continuous infusion rate of 6 mg/hr; *Severe hepatic impairment:* Do not exceed continuous infusion rate of 4 mg/hr.

H. pylori Eradication to Reduce the Risk of Duodenal Ulcer Recurrence (Triple Therapy)

PO (Adults): 40 mg once daily for 10 days with amoxicillin 1000 mg twice daily for 10 days and clarithromycin 500 mg twice daily for 10 days.

Hepatic Impairment

PO (Adults): *Severe hepatic impairment:* Dose should not exceed 20 mg/day.

Reduction in Risk of Gastric Ulcer During Continuous NSAID Therapy

PO (Adults): 20 or 40 mg once daily for up to 6 mo.

Hepatic Impairment

PO (Adults): *Severe hepatic impairment:* Dose should not exceed 20 mg/day.

Pathological Hypersecretory Conditions, Including Zollinger-Ellison Syndrome

PO (Adults): 40 mg twice daily.

Hepatic Impairment

PO, (Adults): *Severe hepatic impairment:* Dose should not exceed 20 mg/day.

E

Availability (generic available)

Delayed-release tablets: 20 mg[OTC]. **Delayed-release capsules:** 20 mg[Rx, OTC], 40 mg. **Delayed-release oral suspension packets:** 2.5 mg/pkt, 5 mg/pkt, 10 mg/pkt, 20 mg/pkt, 40 mg/pkt. **Powder for injection:** 40 mg/vial. ***In combination with:*** naproxen (generic only).

NURSING IMPLICATIONS

Assessment

- Assess routinely for epigastric or abdominal pain and frank or occult blood in the stool, emesis, or gastric aspirate.
- Monitor bowel function. Diarrhea, abdominal cramping, fever, and bloody stools should be reported to health care professional promptly as a sign of CDAD.

Lab Test Considerations

- May ↑ serum creatinine, uric acid, total bilirubin, alkaline phosphatase, AST, and ALT. May alter hemoglobin, WBC, platelets, serum sodium, potassium, and thyroxine levels.
- Monitor serum magnesium and calcium before and periodically during therapy. May ↓ magnesium and calcium.
- May cause false positive results in diagnostic investigations for neuroendocrine tumors due to ↑ serum chromogranin A (CgA) levels secondary to drug-induced ↓ gastric acidity. Temporarily stop esomeprazole >14 days before assessing CgA levels and consider repeating test if initial CgA levels are high.

Implementation

- ***High Alert:*** Do not confuse Nexium with Nexavar.
- Antacids may be used while taking esomeprazole.
- **PO:** Administer >1 hr before meals. ***DNC:*** Swallow tablets and capsules whole. Do not chew or crush.
- *Delayed-release capsules:* For patients with difficulty swallowing, place 15 mL of applesauce in an empty bowl. Open capsule and empty the pellets inside onto applesauce. Mix pellets with applesauce and swallow immediately. Applesauce should not be hot and should be soft enough to swallow without chewing. Do not store applesauce mixture for future use. Tap water, orange juice, apple juice, and yogurt have also been used. Do not crush or chew pellets.

- *For delayed-release capsules for NG tube,* hold enteral nutrition 30–60 min before administering, if applicable. Delayed-release capsules can be opened and intact granules emptied into a 60-mL syringe and mixed with 50 mL of water. Replace plunger and shake syringe vigorously for 15 sec. Hold syringe with tip up and check for granules in tip. Attach syringe to NG tube and administer solution. After administering, flush syringe with additional water. Do not administer if granules have dissolved or disintegrated. Administer immediately after mixing.
- *For delayed-release oral suspension*, mix contents of packet with 15 mL of water; leave 2–3 min to thicken, and then stir and drink within 30 min.
- *For delayed-release oral suspension for NG or gastric tube,* add 15 mL of water to a syringe and then add contents of packet. Shake syringe; leave 2–3 min to thicken. Shake syringe and inject through NG or gastric tube within 30 min.

IV Administration

- **IV Push: Reconstitution:** Reconstitute each vial with 5 mL of 0.9% NaCl. Do not administer solutions that are discolored or contain a precipitate. Stable at room temperature for up to 12 hr. Do not administer with other medication or solutions. Flush line with 0.9% NaCl before and after administration. **Rate:** Administer over ≥3 min.
- **Intermittent Infusion: Dilution:** Dilute reconstituted solution to a volume of 45 mL with *D5W, 0.9% NaCl, or LR for adults* or *with 0.9% NaCl for pediatric patients.* **Concentration:** 0.8 mg/mL (40-mg vial) or 0.4 mg/mL (20-mg vial). Solutions diluted with 0.9% NaCl or LR are stable for 12 hr; those diluted with D5W are stable for 6 hr at room temperature. **Rate:** Administer over 10–30 min.
- **Continuous Infusion: Reconstitution:** *For 80-mg loading dose,* reconstitute two 40-mg vials with 5 mL of 0.9% NaCl. *For 80-mg continuous infusion,* reconstitute two 40-mg vials with 5 mL of 0.9% NaCl. **Dilution:** Further dilute 80-mg loading dose or dose for continuous infusion in 100 mL 0.9% NaCl. **Concentration:** 0.8 mg/mL. **Rate:** Administer *loading dose* over 30 min. Follow loading dose with infusion at a rate of 8 mg/hr for 71.5 hr.
- **Y-Site Compatibility:** ceftaroline, ceftolozane/tazobactam, cisatracurium, D5W, epinephrine, fentanyl, flumazenil, furosemide, hydrocortisone, imipenem/cilastatin/relebactam, insulin, regular, LR, meropenem/vaborbactam, methadone, metoprolol, nitroglycerin, somatostatin, sulbactam/durlobactam, tedizolid.
- **Y-Site Incompatibility:** dobutamine, dopamine, esmolol, isavuconazonium, labetalol, midazolam, plazomicin, tacrolimus, telavancin, tigecycline.

Patient/Family Teaching

- Explain purpose and side effects of medication. Advise patient to read *Patient Information* before starting therapy. Instruct to take medication as directed. Take missed doses as soon as remembered but not if almost time for next dose. Do not double doses.
- Instruct patient to notify health care professional of all Rx or OTC medications, vitamins, or herbal products being taken and consult health care professional before taking any new medications, especially St. John's wort.
- Advise patient to avoid alcohol, products containing aspirin or NSAIDs, and foods that may cause an ↑ in GI irritation.
- Advise patient to report onset of black, tarry stools; diarrhea; abdominal pain; or persistent headache to health care professional promptly.
- Advise patient to notify health care professional if signs of hypomagnesemia (seizures, dizziness, abnormal or fast heartbeat, jitteriness, jerking movements or shaking, muscle weakness, spasms of the hands and feet, cramps or muscle aches, spasm of the voice box) occur.
- Caution patient to notify health care professional if fever and diarrhea occur, especially if stool contains blood, pus, or mucus. Advise patient not to treat diarrhea without consulting health care professional.
- Rep: Advise women of reproductive potential to notify health care professional if pregnancy is planned or suspected or if breastfeeding.

Evaluation/Desired Outcomes

- Diminished accumulation of acid in the gastric lumen with lessened gastroesophageal reflux.
- Healing of duodenal ulcers.
- Decreased incidence of gastric ulcer during continuous NSAID therapy.

estetrol/drospirenone, See CONTRACEPTIVES, HORMONAL.

estradiol valerate/dienogest, See CONTRACEPTIVES, HORMONAL.

ESTRADIOL (es-tra-**dye**-ole)

estradiol cypionate
Depo-Estradiol
estradiol tablets
Estrace
estradiol transdermal gel
Divigel, Elestrin, EstroGel

estradiol transdermal spray
EvaMist
estradiol transdermal system
~~Alora~~, Climara, Dotti, ~~Estraderm~~, ✱ Estradot, Lyllana, Menostar, Minivelle, ✱ Oesclim, Vivelle-Dot
estradiol vaginal cream
Estrace
estradiol vaginal insert
Imvexxy
estradiol vaginal ring
Estring, Femring
estradiol vaginal tablet
Vagifem, Yuvafem
estradiol valerate
Delestrogen

Classification
Therapeutic: hormones
Pharmacologic: estrogens

Indications

PO, IM, TRANSDERMAL: Replacement of estrogen to diminish moderate to severe vasomotor symptoms of menopause and of various estrogen deficiency states, including: Female hypogonadism, Ovariectomy, Primary ovarian failure. Treatment and prevention of postmenopausal osteoporosis (not vaginal dose forms). **PO:** Inoperable metastatic postmenopausal breast or prostate carcinoma. **Vag:** Management of: Atrophic vaginitis due to menopause, Moderate to severe dyspareunia due to menopause.

Action

Estrogens promote growth and development of female sex organs and the maintenance of secondary sex characteristics in women. Metabolic effects include reduced blood cholesterol, protein synthesis, and sodium and water retention. **Therapeutic Effects:** Restoration of hormonal balance in various deficiency states, including menopause. Treatment of hormone-sensitive tumors.

Pharmacokinetics

Absorption: Well absorbed after oral administration. Readily absorbed through skin and mucous membranes.
Distribution: Widely distributed to tissues.
Metabolism and Excretion: Mostly metabolized by the liver and other tissues. Enterohepatic recirculation occurs, and more absorption may occur from the GI tract.
Half-life: Gel: 36 hr.

TIME/ACTION PROFILE (estrogenic effects)

ROUTE	ONSET	PEAK	DURATION
PO	unknown	unknown	unknown
IM	unknown	unknown	unknown
Transdermal	unknown	unknown	3–4 days (Estraderm), 7 days (Climara)
Topical	unknown	unknown	unknown
Vaginal insert	unknown	unknown	3–4 days
Vaginal ring	unknown	unknown	90 days

Contraindications/Precautions

Contraindicated in: History of anaphylaxis or angioedema to estradiol; Hepatic impairment; Thromboembolic disease (e.g., deep vein thrombosis, pulmonary embolism, MI, stroke); Protein C, protein S, or antithrombin deficiency or other thrombophilic disorder; History of breast cancer; History of estrogen-dependent cancer; Undiagnosed vaginal bleeding; OB: Pregnancy.
Use Cautiously in: Long-term use (more than 4–5 yr); may ↑ risk of MI, stroke, invasive breast cancer, pulmonary emboli (PE), deep vein thrombosis (DVT), and dementia in postmenopausal women; Underlying cardiovascular disease; Severe renal impairment; History of porphyria; History of hereditary angioedema; Lactation: Use while breastfeeding only if potential maternal benefit justifies potential risk to infant.

Adverse Reactions/Side Effects

CV: edema, hypertension, DVT, MI. **Derm:** oily skin, acne, pigmentation, urticaria. **EENT:** intolerance to contact lenses, worsening of myopia or astigmatism. **Endo:** gynecomastia (men), hyperglycemia. **F and E** hypercalcemia, sodium and water retention. **GI:** nausea, weight changes, anorexia, jaundice, vomiting. **GU: women:** amenorrhea, dysmenorrhea, breakthrough bleeding, cervical erosions, loss of libido, vaginal candidiasis; **men:** erectile dysfunction, testicular atrophy. **Metab:** ↑ appetite. **MS:** leg cramps. **Neuro:** headache, dementia, dizziness, lethargy, STROKE. **Resp:** PE. **Misc:** breast tenderness, MALIGNANCY (BREAST, ENDOMETRIAL, OVARIAN).

Interactions

Drug-Drug: May alter requirement for **warfarin**, **oral hypoglycemic agents**, or **insulins**. **Barbiturates** or **rifampin** may ↓ effectiveness. **Smoking** ↑ risk of adverse CV reactions.

Route/Dosage

Estrogens should be used in the lowest doses for the shortest period of time consistent with desired therapeutic outcome. Concurrent use of progestin is recommended during cyclical therapy to ↓ the risk of endometrial carcinoma in patients with an intact uterus.

Symptoms of Menopause, Atrophic Vaginitis, Moderate to Severe Dyspareunia, Female Hypogonadism, Ovarian Failure/Osteoporosis

PO (Adults): 0.45–2 mg once daily or in a cycle.
IM (Adults): 1–5 mg monthly (estradiol cypionate) *or* 10–20 mg (estradiol valerate) monthly.
Topical Gel: (Adults): Apply contents of one packet *(Divigel)* or one actuation from pump *(EstroGel, Elestrin)* once daily.
Topical Spray *EvaMist*: (Adults): 1 spray once daily; may be ↑ to 2–3 sprays once daily.
Transdermal (Adults): *Climara:* 25 mcg/24-hr transdermal patch applied weekly. *Vivelle-Dot:* 25–50 mcg/24-hr transdermal patch applied twice weekly. *Menostar:* 14 mcg/24-hr transdermal patch applied every 7 days. Progestin may be administered for 10–14 days of each mo. *Dotti, Lyllana, or Minivelle:* 37.5 mcg/24-hr transdermal patch applied twice weekly (for treatment of vasomotor symptoms); 25 mcg/24-hr transdermal patch applied twice weekly (for prevention of postmenopausal osteoporosis).
Vag (Adults): *Cream:* 2–4 g (0.2–0.4 mg estradiol) once daily for 1–2 wk; then ↓ to 1–2 g/day for 1–2 wk; then maintenance dose of 1 g 1–3 times weekly for 3 wk; then off for 1 wk; then repeat cycle once vaginal mucosa has been restored; *Vaginal ring (Estring):* 2-mg (releases 7.5 mcg estradiol/24 hr) every 3 mo; *Vaginal ring (Femring):* 12.4 mg (releases 50 mcg estradiol/24 hr) every 3 mo or 24.8 mg (releases 100 mcg estradiol/24 hr) every 3 mo (*Femring* requires concurrent progesterone); *Vaginal insert (Vagifem, Yuvafem, or Imvexxy):* 1 insert once daily for 2 wk; then 1 insert twice weekly.

Postmenopausal Breast Cancer

PO (Adults): 10 mg 3 times daily.

Prostate Cancer

PO (Adults): 1–2 mg 3 times daily.
IM (Adults): 30 mg every 1–2 wk (estradiol valerate).

Availability (generic available)

Estradiol

Tablets: 0.5 mg, 1 mg, 2 mg. ***In combination with:*** dienogest (Natazia); drospirenone (Angeliq); elagolix/norethindrone (Oriahnn); norethindrone (Activella, Amabelz, Mimvey); norgestimate (Prefest); progesterone (Bijuva); relugolix/norethindrone (Myfembree). See Appendix N.

Estradiol Cypionate

Injection (in oil): 5 mg/mL.

Estradiol Transdermal Preparations

Gel packet (Divigel): 0.25 mg/pkt, 0.5 mg/pkt, 0.75 mg/pkt, 1 mg/pkt, 1.25 mg/pkt. **Gel pump (Elestrin):** 0.52 mg/actuation. **Gel pump (Estrogel):** 0.75 mg/actuation. **Transdermal patch:** 14 mcg/24-hr release rate, 25 mcg/24-hr release rate, 37.5 mcg/24-hr release rate, 50 mcg/24-hr release rate, 60 mcg/24-hr release rate, 75 mcg/24-hr release rate, 100 mcg/24-hr release rate. **Spray:** 1.53 mg/spray. ***In combination with:*** levonorgestrel (Climara Pro); norethindrone (Combipatch). See Appendix N.

Estradiol Vaginal Preparations

Vaginal cream: 0.01%. **Vaginal tablet (Vagifem or Yuvafem):** 10 mcg. **Vaginal insert (Imvexxy):** 4 mcg, 10 mcg. **Vaginal ring (Estring):** 2 mg (releases 7.5 mcg/day over 90 days). **Vaginal ring (Femring):** 12.4 mg (releases 50 mcg/day over 90 days), 24.8 mg (releases 100 mcg/day over 90 days).

Estradiol Valerate

Injection (in oil): 10 mg/mL, 20 mg/mL, 40 mg/mL.

NURSING IMPLICATIONS

Assessment

- Assess BP before and periodically during therapy.
- Monitor intake and output and weekly weight. Report significant discrepancies or steady weight gain.
- Monitor for signs and symptoms of venous thromboembolism, such as PE (chest pain, dyspnea, tachycardia) or DVT (calf pain or tenderness, lower extremity edema, localized warmth or erythema), or emerging cardiovascular disease, such as MI (chest pain, dyspnea, diaphoresis, dizziness, nausea) or stroke (weakness, slurred speech, confusion, dizziness); discontinue therapy in all patients if PE, DVT, stroke, or MI are suspected.
- If persistent or recurring abnormal genital bleeding occurs in postmenopausal women, directed or random endometrial sampling may need to be performed to rule out malignancy.
- **Menopause:** Assess frequency and severity of vasomotor symptoms. Monitor individual clinical response and severity of vulvar and vaginal atrophy.

Lab Test Considerations

- May ↑ HDL-C and triglycerides and ↓ LDL-C and total cholesterol concentrations.
- May ↑ serum glucose, sodium, cortisol, prolactin, prothrombin, and factor VII, VIII, IX, and X levels. May ↓ serum folate, pyridoxine, antithrombin III, and urine pregnanediol concentrations.
- Monitor hepatic function before and periodically during therapy.
- May cause false interpretations of thyroid function tests, false ↑ in norepinephrine platelet-induced aggregability, and false ↓ in metyrapone tests.
- May cause hypercalcemia in patients with metastatic bone lesions.

Implementation

- Topical and vaginal products may be administered by the patient or health care provider.
- Health care providers should use double gloves and a protective gown to prepare and administer oral,

vaginal, transdermal patches, topical gels, and injections. If possible, prepare in a biological safety cabinet or a compounding aseptic containment isolator; eye, face, and respiratory protection may be needed. Prepare and administer in a closed-system drug transfer device. During administration, if there is a potential that the substance could splash or if the patient may resist, use eye and face protection.

- **PO:** Administer with or immediately after food to reduce nausea.
- **Vag:** Measure prescribed dose using manufacturer supplied applicator; dose is marked on the applicator. Gently insert into the vagina as far as it can comfortably go without force and press plunger. Wash applicator with mild soap and warm water after each use.
- **Transdermal:** When switching from PO form, begin transdermal therapy 1 wk after the last dose or when symptoms reappear.
- Wearing double gloves, place *Climara* patch on clean, dry skin, preferably on the lower abdomen, upper quadrant of the buttock, or outer aspect of the hip; do not apply to the breasts or waistline; press firmly in place for ≥10 sec, making sure there is good contact, especially around the edges; rotate sites of application with 1 wk between applications to a particular site.
- **Topical:** Wearing double gloves, apply *Divigel* individual-use once-daily packets of quick-drying gel to an area measuring 5 inches × 7 inches (size of two palm prints) on the thigh. Do not wash area for ≥1 hr after gel has dried.
- Wearing double gloves, start with one pump daily and apply *Elestrin* to skin of upper arm to shoulder in a thin layer.
- Before first use of *Estrogel*, remove large canister cover and fully depress pump five times wearing double gloves. Discard unused gel by rinsing down the sink or placing it in the household trash. After priming, pump is ready to use. Apply a thin layer over the entire arm on the inside and outside from wrist to shoulder.
- Handle spray pumps and administer with double gloved hands, eye, face, and respiratory protection. Spray *EvaMist* on inside of forearm at the same time each day. Do not massage or rub the spray into the skin. Allow to dry for 2 min before dressing and ≥1 hr before washing. Never spray *EvaMist* around breast or vagina. Do not use >56 doses, even if fluid remains in pump.
- **IM:** Prepare wearing double gloves and a protective gown. If possible, prepare in a biological safety cabinet or a compounding aseptic containment isolator; eye, face, and respiratory protection may be needed. Injection has oil base. Roll syringe to ensure even dispersion. Administer deep IM. Avoid IV administration. During administration, if there is a potential that the substance could splash or if the patient may resist, use eye and face protection.

Patient/Family Teaching

- Explain the purpose and side effects of estradiol to patient. Instruct patient on correct method of administration. Instruct patient to take medication as directed. Take missed doses as soon as remembered as long as it is not just before next dose. If taking a bath or shower or using a sauna, apply dose afterward. Dry skin completely before application. Apply dose at the same time each day. If a dose of *EvaMist* is missed, apply if >12 hr before next dose; if <12 hr, omit dose and return to regular schedule. Do not double doses. Advise patient to read *Patient Information* before starting and with each Rx refill in case of changes.
- Explain dose schedule and maintenance routine. Discontinuing medication suddenly may cause withdrawal bleeding.
- If nausea becomes a problem, advise patient that eating solid food often provides relief.
- Advise patient to report signs and symptoms of fluid retention (swelling of ankles and feet, weight gain), mental depression, or hepatic impairment (yellowed skin or eyes, pruritus, dark urine, light-colored stools) to health care provider.
- Advise patient to report signs and symptoms of thromboembolic disorders (pain, swelling, tenderness in extremities, headache, chest pain, blurred vision).
- Inform postmenopausal women that long-term use may ↑ risk of MI, stroke, invasive breast cancer, PE, DVT, and dementia.
- Emphasize the importance of routine follow-up physical exams, including BP check; breast, abdomen, and pelvic examinations; Papanicolaou smears every 6–12 mo; and mammogram every 12 mo or as directed. Health care provider will evaluate possibility of discontinuing medication every 3–6 mo. If on continuous (not cyclical) therapy or without concurrent progestins, endometrial biopsy may be recommended, if uterus is intact.
- Advise patient to notify health care provider of medication regimen before treatment or surgery.
- Caution patient that cigarette smoking during estrogen therapy may cause ↑ risk of serious side effects, especially for women >35 yr.
- Caution patient to use sunscreen and protective clothing to prevent ↑ pigmentation.
- Advise patient treated for osteoporosis that exercise has been found to arrest and reverse bone loss. Patient should discuss any exercise limitations with health care provider before beginning program.
- Inform patient that estrogens should not be used to ↓ risk of cardiovascular disease or dementia. Estrogens may ↑ risk of cardiovascular disease (MI, stroke), dementia, and breast cancer.

- Rep: Instruct women of reproductive potential to stop taking medication and notify health care provider if pregnancy is planned or suspected or if breastfeeding.
- **Vag:** Instruct patient in the correct use of applicator. Patient should remain recumbent for ≥30 min after administration. May use sanitary napkin to protect clothing, but do not use tampon. If a dose is missed, do not use the missed dose, but return to regular dosing schedule.
- Instruct patient to use applicator provided with vaginal tablet. Insert as high up in the vagina as comfortable, without using force.
- **Vaginal Ring:** Instruct patient to press ring into an oval and insert into the upper third of the vaginal vault. Exact position is not critical. Once ring is inserted, patient should not feel anything. If discomfort is felt, ring is probably not in far enough; gently push farther into vagina. Leave in place continuously for 90 days. Ring does not interfere with sexual intercourse. If straining at defecation makes ring move to lower vagina, push up with finger. If expelled totally, rinse ring with lukewarm water and reinsert. To remove, hook a finger through the ring and pull it out.
- **Transdermal:** Instruct patient to wash and dry hands first. Apply disc to intact skin on hairless portion of abdomen; do not apply to breasts or waistline. Apply patch to lower abdomen or buttocks. Press disc/patch for 10 sec to ensure contact with skin (especially around edges). Avoid areas where clothing may rub disc loose. Change site with each administration to prevent skin irritation. Remove carefully and slowly, fold in half, and throw it away. If any adhesive remains on the skin, allow the area to dry for 15 min; then gently rub with an oil-based cream or lotion to remove residue. Do not reuse site for 1 wk; disc may be reapplied if it falls off.
- Advise patient referred for MRI test to discuss patch with referring health care provider and MRI facility to determine if removal of patch is necessary prior to test and for directions for replacing patch.
- ***Evamist:*** Caution patient to make sure children are not exposed to *Evamist* and do not come into contact with any skin area where the drug was applied. Women who cannot avoid contact with children should wear a garment with long sleeves to cover the application site.

Evaluation/Desired Outcomes

- Resolution of menopausal vasomotor symptoms.
- Decreased vaginal and vulvar itching, inflammation, or dryness associated with menopause.
- Normalization of estrogen levels in patients with ovariectomy or hypogonadism.
- Control of the spread of advanced metastatic breast or prostate cancer.
- Prevention of osteoporosis.

BEERS

estrogens, conjugated

(ess-troe-jenz con-joo-gae-ted)

C.E.S, Premarin

Classification

Therapeutic: hormones

Pharmacologic: estrogens

Indications

PO: Moderate to severe vasomotor symptoms of menopause. Vulvar and vaginal atrophy associated with menopause. Estrogen deficiency states, including: Female hypogonadism, Ovariectomy, Primary ovarian failure. Prevention of postmenopausal osteoporosis. Advanced inoperable metastatic breast and prostatic carcinoma. **IM IV:** Uterine bleeding resulting from hormonal imbalance. **Vag:** Atrophic vaginitis. Moderate to severe dyspareunia due to menopause. Concurrent use of progestin is recommended during cyclical therapy to ↓ the risk of endometrial carcinoma in patients with an intact uterus.

Action

Estrogens promote the growth and development of female sex organs and the maintenance of secondary sex characteristics in women. **Therapeutic Effects:** Restoration of hormonal balance in various deficiency states and treatment of hormone-sensitive tumors.

Pharmacokinetics

Absorption: Well absorbed after oral administration. Readily absorbed through skin and mucous membranes. IV administration results in complete bioavailability.

Distribution: Widely distributed to tissues.

Metabolism and Excretion: Mostly metabolized by liver via the CYP3A4 isoenzyme. Enterohepatic recirculation occurs, with more absorption from GI tract.

Half-life: Unknown.

TIME/ACTION PROFILE (estrogenic effects†)

ROUTE	ONSET	PEAK	DURATION
PO	rapid	unknown	24 hr
IM	delayed	unknown	6–12 hr
IV	rapid	unknown	6–12 hr

† Tumor response may take several wk.

Contraindications/Precautions

Contraindicated in: History of anaphylaxis or angioedema to estrogen; Hepatic impairment; Thromboembolic disease (e.g., deep vein thrombosis [DVT], pulmonary embolism [PE], MI, stroke); Undiagnosed vaginal bleeding; History of breast cancer; History of estrogen-dependent cancer; Protein C, protein S, or antithrombin deficiency or other thrombophilic disorder; OB: Pregnancy; Lactation: Lactation.

Use Cautiously in: Long-term use (more than 4–5 yr); may ↑ risk of MI, stroke, invasive breast cancer, PE, DVT, and dementia in postmenopausal women; Underlying cardiovascular disease; Hypertriglyceridemia; History of hereditary angioedema; Geri: Appears on Beers list. ↑ risk of breast and endometrial cancer, heart disease, thromboembolic events, and dementia in older adults. Avoid use of systemic estrogens in older adults. Vaginal cream is acceptable to use for treatment of dyspareunia, recurrent lower urinary tract infections, and other vaginal symptoms in older adults.

Adverse Reactions/Side Effects

(Systemic use)

CV: edema, hypertension, DVT, MI. **Derm:** acne, oily skin, pigmentation, urticaria. **Endo:** gynecomastia (men), hyperglycemia. **F and E** hypercalcemia. **GI:** nausea, anorexia, jaundice, vomiting. **GU: women:** amenorrhea, breakthrough bleeding, breast tenderness, dysmenorrhea, cervical erosion, loss of libido, vaginal candidiasis**men:** erectile dysfunction, testicular atrophy. **Metab:** weight changes, ↑ appetite. **MS:** leg cramps. **Neuro:** headache, dementia, depression, dizziness, insomnia, lethargy, STROKE. **Resp:** PE. **Misc:** ANAPHYLAXIS, ANGIOEDEMA, MALIGNANCY (BREAST, ENDOMETRIAL, OVARIAN).

Interactions

Drug-Drug: May alter requirement for **warfarin**, **oral hypoglycemic agents**, or **insulins**. **Barbiturates**, **carbamazepine**, or **rifampin** may ↓ levels and effectiveness. **Smoking** ↑ risk of adverse CV reactions. **Erythromycin**, **clarithromycin**, **itraconazole**, **ketoconazole**, and **ritonavir** may ↑ levels and risk of toxicity.

Drug-Food: **Grapefruit juice** may ↑ levels and risk of toxicity.

Route/Dosage

Estrogens should be used in the lowest doses for the shortest period of time consistent with desired therapeutic outcome. Concurrent use of progestin is recommended during cyclical therapy to ↓ the risk of endometrial carcinoma in patients with an intact uterus.

Ovariectomy, Primary Ovarian Failure

PO (Adults): 1.25 mg once daily administered cyclically (3 wk on, 1 wk off).

Osteoporosis/Menopausal Symptoms

PO (Adults): 0.3–1.25 mg once daily or in a cycle.

Female Hypogonadism

PO (Adults): 0.3–0.625 mg once daily administered cyclically (3 wk on, 1 wk off).

Inoperable Breast Carcinoma: Men and Postmenopausal Women

PO (Adults): 10 mg 3 times daily.

Inoperable Prostate Carcinoma

PO (Adults): 1.25–2.5 mg 3 times daily.

Uterine Bleeding

IM IV (Adults): 25 mg as single dose; may repeat in 6–12 hr if necessary.

Atrophic Vaginitis

PO (Adults): 0.3–1.25 mg once daily.

vaginal **(Adults):** 0.5–2 g cream (0.3125 mg–1.25 g conjugated estrogens) once daily for 3 wk, off for 1 wk, then repeat.

Moderate to Severe Dyspareunia

Vaginal (Adults): 0.5 g cream (0.3125 mg conjugated estrogens) twice weekly continuously or daily for 3 wk, off for 1 wk, then repeat.

Availability

Tablets: 0.3 mg, 0.45 mg, 0.625 mg, 0.9 mg, 1.25 mg. **Powder for injection:** 25 mg/vial. **Vaginal cream:** 0.625 mg/g. ***In combination with:*** bazedoxifene (Duavee); medroxyprogesterone (Prempro and Premphase [compliance package]). See Appendix N.

NURSING IMPLICATIONS

Assessment

- Assess BP before and periodically during therapy.
- Monitor for signs and symptoms of venous thromboembolism, such as PE (chest pain, dyspnea, tachycardia) or DVT (calf pain or tenderness, lower extremity edema, localized warmth or erythema), or emerging cardiovascular disease, such as MI (chest pain, dyspnea, diaphoresis, dizziness, nausea) or stroke (weakness, slurred speech, confusion, dizziness); discontinue therapy in all patients if PE, DVT, stroke, or MI is suspected.
- If persistent or recurring abnormal genital bleeding occurs in postmenopausal women, directed or random endometrial sampling may need to be performed to rule out malignancy.
- Monitor for breast tenderness, lumps, or discharge. Perform baseline mammogram before starting treatment.
- Assess for signs of anaphylactic reactions and angioedema (hives; pruritus; swollen lips, tongue, or face) within minutes to hours after administration. Implement emergency medical management as needed.
- Monitor intake and output and weekly weight. Report significant discrepancies or steady weight gain.
- **Menopause:** Assess frequency and severity of vasomotor symptoms.

Lab Test Considerations

- May ↑ HDL and triglycerides and ↓ LDL and total cholesterol concentrations.
- May ↑ serum glucose, sodium, cortisol, prolactin, prothrombin, and factor VII, VIII, IX, and X levels. May ↓ serum folate, pyridoxine, antithrombin III, and urine pregnanediol concentrations.
- Monitor hepatic function before and periodically during therapy.
- May cause false interpretations of thyroid function tests.
- May cause hypercalcemia in patients with metastatic bone lesions.

Implementation

- Estrogens should be used in the lowest doses for the shortest period of time consistent with desired therapeutic outcome.
- **PO:** Administer with or immediately after food to ↓ nausea.
- **Vag:** Manufacturer provides applicator with cream. Dose is marked on the applicator. Wash applicator with mild soap and warm water after each use.
- **IM:** To reconstitute, withdraw ≥5 mL of air from dry container and then slowly introduce the sterile diluent (bacteriostatic water for injection) against the container side. Gently agitate container to dissolve; do not shake vigorously. Solution is stable for 60 days if refrigerated. Do not use solution if precipitate is present or if darkened.
- IV is preferred parenteral route because of rapid response.

IV Administration

- **IV Push: Reconstitution:** Reconstitute as for IM. Inject into distal port tubing of free-flowing IV of 0.9% NaCl, D5W, or lactated Ringer's solution. **Concentration:** 5 mg/mL. **Rate:** Administer slowly (no faster than 5 mg/min) to prevent flushing.
- **Y-Site Compatibility:** heparin, hydrocortisone, potassium chloride.
- **Y-Site Incompatibility:** pantoprazole.

Patient/Family Teaching

- Explain purpose and side effects of medication. Advise patient to read *Patient Information* before starting therapy. Instruct patient to take oral medication as directed. Take missed doses as soon as remembered, but not just before next dose. Do not double doses.
- **Vag:** Instruct patient in the correct use of applicator. Patient should remain recumbent for >30 min after administration. May use sanitary napkin to protect clothing, but do not use tampon. If a dose is missed, do not use the missed dose, but return to regular dosing schedule.
- Advise patient to notify health care provider of all Rx or OTC medications, vitamins, or herbal products being taken and to consult health care provider before taking other medications. Advise patient to avoid drinking grapefruit juice during therapy.
- Explain dose schedule and maintenance routine. Discontinuing medication suddenly may cause withdrawal bleeding. Bleeding is anticipated during the wk when conjugated estrogens are withheld.
- If nausea becomes a problem, advise patient that eating solid food often provides relief.
- Inform postmenopausal women that long-term use may ↑ risk of MI, stroke, invasive breast cancer, PE, DVT, and dementia.
- Advise patient to report signs and symptoms of fluid retention (swelling of ankles and feet, weight gain), depression, hepatic dysfunction (yellowed skin or eyes, pruritus, dark urine, light-colored stools), or abnormal vaginal bleeding to health care provider.
- Advise patient to report signs and symptoms of thromboembolic disorders (pain, swelling, tenderness in extremities, headache, chest pain, blurred vision).
- Caution patient that cigarette smoking during estrogen therapy may ↑ risk of serious side effects, especially for women over age 35.
- Inform patient that *Premarin* tablet may appear in stool; this is not harmful.
- Caution patient to use sunscreen and protective clothing to prevent ↑ pigmentation.
- Advise patient to notify health care provider of medication regimen before treatment or surgery.
- Advise patient treated for osteoporosis that exercise has been found to arrest and reverse bone loss. The patient should discuss any exercise limitations with health care provider before beginning program.
- Emphasize the importance of routine follow-up physical exams, including BP check; breast, abdomen, and pelvic examinations; Papanicolaou smears every 6–12 mo; and mammogram every 12 mo or as directed. Health care provider will evaluate possibility of discontinuing medication every 3–6 mo. If on continuous (not cyclical) therapy or without concurrent progestins, endometrial biopsy may be recommended, if uterus is intact.
- Rep: May cause fetal harm. Advise women of reproductive potential patient to stop taking medication and notify health care provider if pregnancy is planned or suspected and to avoid breastfeeding during therapy.

Evaluation/Desired Outcomes

- Restoration of hormonal balance in various deficiency states and treatment of hormone-sensitive tumors.

BEERS

eszopiclone (es-zop-i-klone)

Lunesta

Classification

Therapeutic: sedative/hypnotics

Pharmacologic: cyclopyrrolones

Schedule IV

Indications
Insomnia.

Action
Interacts with GABA-receptor complexes; not a benzodiazepine. **Therapeutic Effects:** Improved sleep with decreased latency and increased maintenance of sleep.

Pharmacokinetics
Absorption: Rapidly absorbed after oral administration.
Distribution: Unknown.
Metabolism and Excretion: Extensively metabolized by the liver by the CYP3A4 and CYP2E1 isoenzymes; metabolites are renally excreted; <10% excreted unchanged in urine.
Half-life: 6 hr.

TIME/ACTION PROFILE (plasma concentrations)

ROUTE	ONSET	PEAK	DURATION
PO	rapid	1 hr	6 hr

Contraindications/Precautions
Contraindicated in: Hypersensitivity; History of experiencing complex sleep behaviors with zolpidem.
Use Cautiously in: Conditions that may alter metabolic or hemodynamic function; Severe hepatic impairment (↓ dose); OB: Safety not established in pregnancy; Lactation: Occasional use while breastfeeding an older infant should pose little risk; Pedi: Safety and effectiveness not established in children; Geri: Appears on Beers list. ↑ risk of cognitive impairment, delirium, falls, fractures, and motor vehicle accidents in older adults. Avoid use in older adults.

Adverse Reactions/Side Effects
CV: chest pain, peripheral edema. **Derm:** rash.
GI: dry mouth, unpleasant taste. **Neuro:** abnormal thinking, behavior changes, COMPLEX SLEEP BEHAVIORS (INCLUDING SLEEP DRIVING, SLEEPWALKING, OR ENGAGING IN OTHER ACTIVITIES WHILE SLEEPING), depression, hallucinations, headache, next-day impairment.

Interactions
Drug-Drug: ↑ risk of CNS depression and next-day impairment with other **CNS depressants**, including **antihistamines**, **antidepressants**, **opioids**, **sedative/hypnotics**, and **antipsychotics**. **CYP3A4 inhibitors**, including **ketoconazole**, **itraconazole**, **clarithromycin**, **nefazodone**, **ritonavir**, and **nelfinavir**, may ↑ levels and risk of CNS depression. **CYP3A4 inducers**, including **rifampin**, may ↓ levels and effectiveness.

Route/Dosage
PO (Adults): 1 mg immediately before bedtime; may ↑ to 2–3 mg if needed; *Concurrent use of CYP3A4 inhibitors:* 1 mg immediately before bedtime; may ↑ to 2 mg if needed.
PO (Geriatric Patients): 1 mg immediately before bedtime; may ↑ to 2 mg if needed.

Hepatic Impairment
PO (Adults): *Severe hepatic impairment:* 1 mg immediately before bedtime; may ↑ to 2 mg if needed.

Availability (generic available)
Tablets: 1 mg, 2 mg, 3 mg.

NURSING IMPLICATIONS
Assessment
- Assess sleep patterns before and during administration. Continued insomnia after 7–10 days of therapy may indicate primary psychiatric or mental illness.
- Assess mental status and potential for abuse before administration. Prolonged use of >7–10 days may lead to physical and psychological dependence. Limit amount of drug available to the patient.

Implementation
- Do not confuse Lunesta with Neulasta.
- **PO:** Onset is rapid. Administer immediately before going to bed or after patient has gone to bed and has experienced difficulty falling asleep, only on nights when patient is able to get >8 hr of sleep before being active again.
- ***DNC:*** Swallow tablet whole; do not break, crush, or chew.
- Eszopiclone is more effective if not taken with or before a high-fat, heavy meal.

Patient/Family Teaching
- Explain purpose and side effects of medication. Advise patient to read *Patient Information* before starting therapy.
- Instruct patient to take eszopiclone immediately before going to bed, as directed. May result in short-term memory impairment, hallucinations, impaired coordination, and dizziness. Do not take eszopiclone if alcohol consumed that evening. Do not ↑ dose or discontinue without notifying health care provider. Dose may need to be ↓ gradually to minimize withdrawal symptoms. Rebound insomnia and/or anxiety may occur upon discontinuation and usually resolves within 1–2 nights.
- Instruct patient to notify health care provider of all Rx or OTC medications, vitamins, or herbal products being taken and to consult health care provider before taking any other Rx, OTC, or herbal products.
- May cause daytime and next-day drowsiness. Caution patient to avoid driving or other activities requiring alertness until response to medication is known.

- Caution patient that eszopiclone may cause complex sleep behaviors (sleepwalking, sleep driving, making and eating food, talking on the phone, having sex) while unaware. Patient may not remember anything done during the night; ↑ risk with alcohol or other CNS depressants. Discontinue eszopiclone immediately and notify health care provider if complex sleep behaviors occur.
- Caution patient to avoid concurrent use of alcohol or other CNS depressants, including opioids.
- Advise patient to notify health care provider if signs and symptoms of allergic reaction (swelling of tongue or throat, trouble breathing, nausea, vomiting) occur.
- Rep: Advise women of reproductive potential to notify health care provider if pregnancy is planned or suspected or if breastfeeding.

Evaluation/Desired Outcomes

- Improved sleep with decreased latency and increased maintenance of sleep.

etanercept (e-tan-er-sept)

Brenzys, Enbrel, Erelzi, Rymti

Classification

Therapeutic: antirheumatics (DMARDs)
Pharmacologic: anti-TNF agents

Indications

Moderately to severely active rheumatoid arthritis (as monotherapy or in combination with methotrexate). Moderate to severely active polyarticular juvenile idiopathic arthritis. Active ankylosing spondylitis. Psoriatic arthritis (as monotherapy or in combination with methotrexate). Active juvenile psoriatic arthritis. Moderate to severe chronic plaque psoriasis in patients who are candidates for systemic therapy or phototherapy.

Action

Binds to tumor necrosis factor (TNF), making it inactive. TNF is a mediator of inflammatory response. **Therapeutic Effects:** Decreased pain and swelling with decreased rate of joint destruction in patients with rheumatoid arthritis, psoriatic arthritis, juvenile psoriatic arthritis, juvenile idiopathic arthritis, and ankylosing spondylitis. Reduced severity of plaques.

Pharmacokinetics

Absorption: 60% absorbed after SUBQ administration.
Distribution: Unknown.
Metabolism and Excretion: Unknown.
Half-life: 115 hr (range 98–300 hr).

TIME/ACTION PROFILE (symptom reduction)

ROUTE	ONSET	PEAK	DURATION
SUBQ	2–4 wk	unknown	unknown

Contraindications/Precautions

Contraindicated in: Hypersensitivity; Active infection (including localized); Untreated infections; Granulomatosis with polyangiitis (receiving immunosuppressive agents); Concurrent cyclophosphamide or anakinra.
Use Cautiously in: History of chronic or recurrent infection or underlying illness/treatment predisposing to infection (including advanced or poorly controlled diabetes); History of exposure to tuberculosis; History of opportunistic infection; History of hepatitis B virus (HBV); Patients residing or who have resided where tuberculosis, histoplasmosis, coccidioidomycoses, or blastomycosis is endemic; Pre-existing or recent demyelinating disorders (multiple sclerosis, myelitis, optic neuritis); Latex allergy (needle cover of diluent syringe contains latex); OB: Use during pregnancy only if potential maternal benefit justifies potential fetal risk; Lactation: Use while breastfeeding only if potential maternal benefit justifies potential risk to infant; Pedi: Children with significant exposure to varicella virus (temporarily discontinue etanercept; consider varicella zoster immune globulin); ↑ risk of lymphoma (including hepatosplenic T-cell lymphoma [HSTCL]), leukemia, and other malignancies; Pedi: Safety and effectiveness not established in children <2 yr (juvenile idiopathic arthritis) or <4 yr (plaque psoriasis); Geri: Older adults may have ↑ risk of infection.

Adverse Reactions/Side Effects

Derm: psoriasis, rash. **EENT:** rhinitis, pharyngitis. **GI:** abdominal pain, dyspepsia. **Hemat:** pancytopenia. **Local:** injection site reactions. **Neuro:** headache, dizziness, weakness. **Resp:** upper respiratory tract infection, cough, respiratory disorder. **Misc:** HYPERSENSITIVITY REACTIONS (INCLUDING ANAPHYLAXIS), INFECTION (INCLUDING REACTIVATION TUBERCULOSIS AND OTHER OPPORTUNISTIC INFECTIONS DUE TO BACTERIAL, INVASIVE FUNGAL, VIRAL, MYCOBACTERIAL, AND PARASITIC PATHOGENS), MALIGNANCY (INCLUDING LYMPHOMA, HSTCL, LEUKEMIA, AND SKIN CANCER), SARCOIDOSIS.

Interactions

Drug-Drug: Concurrent use with **anakinra** ↑ risk of serious infections (not recommended). Concurrent use of **cyclophosphamide** may ↑ risk of malignancies. Concurrent use with **azathioprine** and/or **methotrexate** may ↑ risk of HSTCL. May ↓ antibody response to **live-virus vaccine** and ↑ risk of adverse reactions (do not administer concurrently).

Route/Dosage

Rheumatoid Arthritis, Psoriatic Arthritis, and Ankylosing Spondylitis

SUBQ (Adults): 50 mg once weekly.

Plaque Psoriasis

SUBQ (Adults): 50 mg twice weekly for 3 mo, then 50 mg once weekly; may also be given as 25–50 mg once weekly as an initial dose.

SUBQ (Children ≥4 yr and ≥63 kg): 50 mg once weekly.
SUBQ (Children ≥4 yr and <63 kg): *Enbrel:* 0.8 mg/kg once weekly.

Juvenile Idiopathic Arthritis and Juvenile Psoriatic Arthritis

SUBQ (Children ≥2 yr and ≥63 kg): 50 mg once weekly.
SUBQ (Children ≥2 yr and <63 kg): 0.8 mg/kg once weekly.

Availability

Powder for injection: 25 mg/vial. **Solution for injection:** 25 mg/0.5 mL (prefilled syringe and single-dose vial), 50 mg/mL (prefilled syringe and autoinjector).

NURSING IMPLICATIONS

Assessment

- Assess range of motion, degree of swelling, and pain in affected joints before and periodically during therapy.
- Assess for injection site reaction (erythema, pain, itching, swelling). Reactions are usually mild to moderate and last 3–5 days after injection.
- Closely monitor patients who develop a new infection while taking etanercept. Discontinue therapy in patients who develop a serious infection or sepsis. Do not start etanercept in patients with active infections.
- Assess for signs and symptoms of systemic fungal infections (fever, malaise, weight loss, sweats, cough, dyspnea, pulmonary infiltrates, serious systemic illness with or without shock). Ascertain whether patient lives in or has traveled to areas of endemic mycoses. Consult with an infectious diseases specialist to evaluate patients at risk of invasive fungal infections for empiric treatment until the pathogens are identified. Consider stopping etanercept until infection has been diagnosed and adequately treated.
- Assess for signs and symptoms of active HBV infection in patients at risk or previously infected (fever, fatigue, abdominal pain, nausea, vomiting, dark urine, clay-colored stools, jaundice).

Lab Test Considerations

- Monitor CBC with differential periodically during therapy. May cause leukopenia, neutropenia, thrombocytopenia, and pancytopenia. Discontinue etanercept if symptoms of blood dyscrasias (persistent fever) occur.
- Monitor hepatic function periodically during therapy.
- Obtain HBV panel in patients at risk or previously infected with HBV throughout therapy and for several mo after discontinuation.

Implementation

- Do not confuse Enbrel with Levbid.
- Administer a tuberculin skin test prior to therapy; patients with active latent TB should be treated for TB before starting therapy.
- **SUBQ**: Prepare injection with single-dose prefilled syringe, single-dose vial, or multidose vial for reconstitution.
- Allow solution in prefilled syringe to reach room temperature (15–30 min); do not remove needle cap during this time.
- *For single-dose vial,* allow solution to reach room temperature for at least 30 min before injecting. Solution may contain small white particles of protein; do not use if discolored, cloudy, or contains other particulate matter. Discard unused solution. Individual single-dose prefilled syringes, SureClick autoinjectors, single-dose vials, or Enbrel Mini cartridges can also be stored at room temperature for up to 30 days.
- *For multidose vial,* reconstitute with 1 mL of the bacteriostatic sterile water supplied by manufacturer for a concentration of 25 mg/mL. If the vial is used for multiple doses, use a 25-gauge needle for reconstituting and withdrawing solution, and apply "Mixing Date" sticker with date of reconstitution entered. Inject diluent slowly into vial to avoid foaming. Some foaming will occur. Swirl gently for dissolution; do not shake or vigorously agitate to prevent excess foaming. Solution should be clear and colorless; do not administer solution that is discolored or contains particulate matter. Dissolution usually takes <10 min. Withdraw solution into syringe. Some foam may remain in vial. Amount in syringe should approximate 1 mL. Do not filter reconstituted solution during preparation or administration. Attach a 27-gauge needle to inject. Administer as soon as possible after reconstitution; stable up to 6 hr if refrigerated. Solution from single-dose vials and prefilled syringes are stable if refrigerated and used within 14 days.
- May be injected into abdomen, thigh, or upper arm. Rotate sites. Do not administer within 1 inch of an old site or into area that is tender, red, hard, or bruised.

Patient/Family Teaching

- Explain purpose and side effects of medication to patient. Advise patient to read *Patient Information* before starting therapy and with each Rx refill in case of changes.
- Advise patient to notify health care professional of all Rx or OTC medications, vitamins, or herbal products being taken and to consult health care professional before taking other medications.
- Instruct patient on self-administration technique, storage, and disposal of equipment. First injection should be administered under the supervision of health care professional. Provide patient with a puncture-proof container for used equipment.

- Explain need for continued medical follow-up to assess effectiveness and possible side effects of medication. Periodic lab tests will be needed.
- Advise patient not to receive live vaccines during therapy. Parents should be advised that children should complete immunizations to date before starting etanercept. Patients with significant exposure to varicella virus (chickenpox) should temporarily discontinue therapy, and varicella immune globulin should be considered.
- Advise patient that methotrexate, analgesics, NSAIDs, corticosteroids, and salicylates may be continued during therapy.
- Instruct patient to notify health care professional if upper respiratory or other infections occur. Therapy may need to be discontinued if serious infection occurs.
- Advise patient of risk of malignancies such as HSTCL. Instruct patient to report signs and symptoms (splenomegaly, hepatomegaly, abdominal pain, persistent fever, night sweats, weight loss) to health care professional promptly.
- Advise patient with history of HBV infection that reactivation can occur; report signs and symptoms of fever, fatigue, abdominal pain, nausea, vomiting, dark urine, clay-colored stools, or jaundice
- Rep: Instruct females of reproductive potential to notify health care professional if pregnancy is planned or suspected or if breastfeeding during therapy. Advise patients who become pregnant during therapy to notify health care professional. May limit administration of live vaccines to infant. May continue breastfeeding if potential maternal benefit justifies potential risk to infant.

Evaluation/Desired Outcomes

- Reduction in symptoms of rheumatoid arthritis. Symptoms may return within 1 mo of discontinuation of therapy.
- Reduced severity of plaques in chronic plaque psoriasis.

ethambutol (e-tham-byoo-tole)

Etibi, ~~Myambutol~~

Classification

Therapeutic: antituberculars

Indications

Active tuberculosis or other mycobacterial diseases (in combination with ≥1 other drug).

Action

Inhibits the growth of mycobacteria. **Therapeutic Effects:** Tuberculostatic effect against susceptible organisms.

Pharmacokinetics

Absorption: 80% absorbed following oral administration.

Distribution: Widely distributed to tissues; crosses blood-brain barrier in small amounts.

Metabolism and Excretion: 50% metabolized by the liver; 50% eliminated unchanged by the kidneys.

Half-life: 3.3 hr (↑ in renal or hepatic impairment).

TIME/ACTION PROFILE (plasma concentrations)

ROUTE	ONSET	PEAK	DURATION
PO	rapid	2–4 hr	24 hr

Contraindications/Precautions

Contraindicated in: Hypersensitivity; Optic neuritis.

Use Cautiously in: Renal impairment (↓ dose); Severe hepatic impairment (↓ dose); OB: Although safety not established, ethambutol has been used with isoniazid in pregnant women without fetal adverse effects; Lactation: Use while breastfeeding only if potential maternal benefit justifies potential risk to infant.

Adverse Reactions/Side Effects

EENT: <u>optic neuritis</u>. **GI:** abdominal pain, anorexia, HEPATITIS, nausea, vomiting. **Metab:** hyperuricemia. **MS:** joint pain. **Neuro:** confusion, dizziness, hallucinations, headache, malaise, peripheral neuritis. **Resp:** pulmonary infiltrates. **Misc:** anaphylactoid reactions, fever.

Interactions

Drug-Drug: Neurotoxicity may be ↑ with other **neurotoxic agents**. **Aluminum hydroxide** may ↓ absorption (space doses 4 hr apart).

Route/Dosage

PO (Adults and Children >13 yr): 15–25 mg/kg/day (max = 2.5 g/day) *or* 50 mg/kg (up to 2.5 g) twice weekly *or* 25–30 mg/kg (up to 2.5 g) 3 times weekly.

PO (Children 1 mo–13 yr): *HIV negative:* 15–20 mg/kg/day once daily (max = 1 g/day) or 50 mg/kg/dose twice weekly (max = 2.5 g/dose); *HIV-exposed/-infected:* 15–25 mg/kg/day once daily (max = 2.5 g/day); *MAC, secondary prophylaxis, or treatment in HIV-exposed/-infected:* 15–25 mg/kg/day once daily (max = 2.5 g/day) with clarithromycin (or azithromycin) with or without rifabutin; *Nontuberculous mycobacterial infection:* 15–25 mg/kg/day once daily (max = 2.5 g/day).

Availability (generic available)

Tablets: 100 mg, 400 mg.

NURSING IMPLICATIONS

Assessment

- Mycobacterial studies and susceptibility tests should be performed before and periodically during therapy to detect possible resistance. Perform chest x-ray after 2–3 mo and at end of treatment in patients with negative initial cultures.

- Assess lung sounds and character and amount of sputum periodically during therapy.
- Assessments of visual function should be made frequently during therapy. Advise patient to report blurring of vision, constriction of visual fields, or changes in color perception immediately. Visual impairment, if not identified early, may lead to permanent sight impairment.
- Monitor for signs and symptoms of hepatotoxicity (fatigue, nausea, upper abdominal pain, jaundice, scleral icterus, dark urine, clay-colored stools).

Lab Test Considerations

- Monitor renal and hepatic function, CBC, and uric acid levels at baseline and routinely. Frequently ↑ uric acid, which may precipitate an attack of gout.
- Obtain acid-fast bacilli smear and culture from sputum monthly until two consecutive specimens are negative.

Implementation

- Ethambutol is given as a single daily dose and should be taken at the same time each day. Some regimens require dosing 2–3 times/wk. Usually administered concurrently with other antitubercular medications to prevent development of bacterial resistance.
- Do not administer within 4 hr of aluminum hydroxide-containing antacids to prevent ↓ absorption.
- **PO:** Administer with food or milk to minimize GI irritation.
- **PO:** Tablets may be crushed and mixed with apple juice or applesauce.

Patient/Family Teaching

- Explain the purpose and side effects of ethambutol. Instruct patient to take as directed without regard to food, but food or milk may prevent GI upset. Take missed doses as soon as possible unless almost time for next dose; do not double up on missed doses. A full course of therapy may take mo to yr. Do not discontinue without consulting health care professional, even though symptoms may disappear. Advise patient to read *Patient Information* before starting and with each Rx refill in case of changes.
- Instruct patient to notify health care professional if no improvement is seen in 2–3 wk. Health care professional should also be notified if unexpected weight gain or ↓ urine output occurs.
- Explain need for continued medical follow-up to assess effectiveness and possible side effects of medication. Periodic lab tests will be needed. Emphasize the importance of routine ophthalmic examinations, especially if signs of optic neuritis occur.
- Advise patient to notify health care professional of all Rx or OTC medications, vitamins, or herbal products being taken and to consult with health care professional before taking other medications. Advise patient to avoid aluminum hydroxide-containing antacids within 4 hr of taking ethambutol; may ↓ absorption.
- Rep: Advise women of reproductive potential to notify health care professional if pregnancy is planned or suspected or if breastfeeding.

Evaluation/Desired Outcomes

- Resolution of clinical symptoms of tuberculosis.
- Decrease in acid-fast bacteria in sputum samples.
- Improvement seen in chest x-rays. Therapy for tuberculosis is usually continued for at least 1–2 yr.

ethinyl estradiol/desogestrel, See CONTRACEPTIVES, HORMONAL.

ethinyl estradiol/drospirenone, See CONTRACEPTIVES, HORMONAL.

ethinyl estradiol/ethynodiol, See CONTRACEPTIVES, HORMONAL.

ethinyl estradiol/etonogestrel, See CONTRACEPTIVES, HORMONAL.

ethinyl estradiol/levonorgestrel, See CONTRACEPTIVES, HORMONAL.

ethinyl estradiol/norelgestromin, See CONTRACEPTIVES, HORMONAL.

ethinyl estradiol/norethindrone, See CONTRACEPTIVES, HORMONAL.

ethinyl estradiol/norgestimate, See CONTRACEPTIVES, HORMONAL.

ethinyl estradiol/norgestrel, See CONTRACEPTIVES, HORMONAL.

etonogestrel, See CONTRACEPTIVES, HORMONAL.

HIGH ALERT

everolimus (e-ver-**oh**-li-mus)

Afinitor, Afinitor Disperz, Zortress

Classification

Therapeutic: antineoplastics immunosuppressants,

Pharmacologic: kinase inhibitors

Indications

Afinitor: Advanced renal cell carcinoma that has failed treatment with sunitinib or sorafenib. Subependymal giant cell astrocytoma associated with tuberous sclerosis complex in patients who are not candidates for curative surgical resection. Tuberous sclerosis complex–associated partial-onset seizures (adjunctive treatment). Progressive neuroendocrine tumors of pancreatic origin in patients with unresectable, locally advanced, or metastatic disease. Progressive, well-differentiated, nonfunctional neuroendocrine tumors of GI or lung origin in patients with unresectable, locally advanced, or metastatic disease. Renal angiomyolipoma with tuberous sclerosis complex in patients not requiring immediate surgery. Treatment of postmenopausal women with advanced hormone receptor-positive, HER2-negative breast cancer after failure of treatment with letrozole or anastrozole (in combination with exemestane). **Zortress:** Prevention of organ rejection in patients who have received a kidney transplant and are at low to moderate immunologic risk. Prevention of organ rejection in patients who have received a liver transplant.

Action

Acts as a kinase inhibitor, decreasing cell proliferation. Inhibits activation and proliferation of T and B lymphocytes. **Therapeutic Effects:** Decreased spread of renal cell carcinoma and breast cancer. Improvement in progression-free survival in patients with progressive neuroendocrine tumors. Decreased volume of subependymal giant cell astrocytoma and angiomyolipoma lesions. Prevention of kidney and liver transplant rejection. Reduction in seizure frequency.

Pharmacokinetics

Absorption: Well absorbed following oral administration.

Distribution: 20% confined to plasma.

Metabolism and Excretion: Mostly metabolized by liver via the CYP3A4 isoenzyme; metabolites are mostly excreted in feces (80%) and urine (5%).

Half-life: 30 hr.

TIME/ACTION PROFILE (plasma concentrations)

ROUTE	ONSET	PEAK	DURATION
PO	unknown	1–2 hr	24 hr

Contraindications/Precautions

Contraindicated in: Hypersensitivity to everolimus or other rapamycins; Severe hepatic impairment; use only if benefit exceeds risk for renal cell carcinoma, progressive neuroendocrine tumors, breast cancer, and renal angiomyolipoma with tuberous sclerosis complex; Heart transplantation (Zortress) (↑ risk of mortality); Functional carcinoid tumors; OB: Pregnancy; Lactation: Lactation.

Use Cautiously in: Mild or moderate hepatic impairment (dose ↓ required); Exposure to sunlight/UV light (may ↑ risk of malignant skin changes); Patients undergoing radiation treatment before, during, or after therapy (↑ risk of radiation sensitization and radiation recall); Rep: Women of reproductive potential and men with female partners of reproductive potential; Pedi: Safety not established in children for indications other than SEGA and TSC-associated partial-onset seizures; Geri: Older adults may be more sensitive to drug effects; consider age-related ↓ in hepatic function, concurrent disease states, and drug therapy.

Adverse Reactions/Side Effects

CV: peripheral edema. **Derm:** delayed wound healing, dry skin, pruritus, rash. **Endo:** hyperglycemia. **GI:** anorexia, constipation, diarrhea, mouth ulcers, mucositis, nausea, stomatitis, vomiting, HEPATIC ARTERY THROMBOSIS. **GU:** ↓ fertility, acute renal failure, amenorrhea, KIDNEY ARTERIAL/VENOUS THROMBOSIS (ZORTRESS), menstrual irregularities, proteinuria. **Hemat:** anemia, leukopenia, thrombocytopenia, HEMOLYTIC UREMIC SYNDROME, THROMBOTIC MICROANGIOPATHY, THROMBOTIC THROMBOCYTOPENIC PURPURA. **Metab:** hyperlipidemia, hypertriglyceridemia. **MS:** extremity pain. **Neuro:** fatigue, weakness, dysgeusia, headache. **Resp:** cough, dyspnea, pulmonary embolism, INTERSTITIAL LUNG DISEASE, PULMONARY HYPERTENSION. **Misc:** fever, HYPERSENSITIVITY REACTIONS (INCLUDING ANAPHYLAXIS AND ANGIOEDEMA), INFECTION (INCLUDING ACTIVATION OF LATENT VIRAL INFECTIONS SUCH AS BK VIRUS-ASSOCIATED NEPHROPATHY), LYMPHOMA/SKIN CANCER (ZORTRESS).

Interactions

Drug-Drug: P-glycoprotein (P-gp) inhibitors and **strong CYP3A4 inhibitors**, including **atazanavir**, **clarithromycin**, **itraconazole**, **ketoconazole**, **nefazodone**, **nelfinavir**, **ritonavir**, and **voriconazole**, may ↑ levels and risk of toxicity;

avoid concurrent use. **P-gp inhibitors** and **moderate CYP3A4 inhibitors**, including **aprepitant**, **diltiazem**, **erythromycin**, **fluconazole**, **fosamprenavir**, and **verapamil**, may ↑ levels and risk of toxicity; ↓ dose of everolimus (Afinitor). **P-gp inducers** and **strong CYP3A4 inducers**, including **carbamazepine**, **dexamethasone**, **phenobarbital**, **phenytoin**, **rifabutin**, and **rifampin**, may ↓ levels and effectiveness; avoid concurrent use, if possible. If concurrent use unavoidable, ↑ dose of everolimus may be required. ↑ risk of nephrotoxicity with **aminoglycosides**, **amphotericin B**, **cisplatin**, or **cyclosporine**. **ACE inhibitors** may ↑ risk of angioedema. May ↓ antibody formation and ↑ risk of adverse reactions from **live-virus vaccines**; avoid use of live-virus vaccines during treatment. **Cannabidiol** may ↑ levels and risk of toxicity; consider ↓ everolimus dose.

Drug-Natural Products: St. John's wort may ↓ levels and effectiveness; avoid concurrent use.

Drug-Food: Grapefruit juice may ↑ levels and risk of toxicity; avoid concurrent use.

Route/Dosage

Advanced Renal Cell Carcinoma, Advanced Progressive Neuroendocrine Tumors, Advanced Neuroendocrine Tumors, Advanced Hormone Receptor-Positive, HER2-Negative Breast Cancer, and Renal Angiomyolipoma with Tuberous Sclerosis Complex (Afinitor)

PO (Adults): 10 mg once daily until disease progression or unacceptable toxicity; *Concurrent use of P-gp inhibitor and moderate CYP3A4 inhibitor:* 2.5 mg once daily until disease progression or unacceptable toxicity; *Concurrent use of P-gp inducer and strong CYP3A4 inducer:* ↑ dose in 5 mg increments up to 20 mg once daily; continue until disease progression or unacceptable toxicity.

Hepatic Impairment

PO (Adults): *Mild hepatic impairment:* 7.5 mg once daily until disease progression or unacceptable toxicity; may ↓ to 5 mg once daily if not well tolerated; *Moderate hepatic impairment:* 5 mg once daily until disease progression or unacceptable toxicity; may ↓ to 2.5 mg once daily if not well tolerated; *Severe hepatic impairment:* 2.5 mg once daily until disease progression or unacceptable toxicity.

Subependymal Giant Cell Astrocytoma with Tuberous Sclerosis Complex (Afinitor)

PO (Adults and Children ≥1 yr): 4.5 mg/m² once daily. Titrate as needed at 2-wk intervals to achieve recommended whole blood trough concentration. Continue until disease progression or unacceptable toxicity; *Concurrent use of P-gp inhibitor and moderate CYP3A4 inhibitor:* 2.25 mg/m² once daily. Titrate as needed at 2-wk intervals to achieve recommended whole blood trough concentration. Continue until disease progression or unacceptable toxicity; *Concurrent use of P-gp inducer and strong CYP3A4 inducer:* 9 mg/m² once daily. Titrate as needed at 2-wk intervals to achieve recommended whole blood trough concentration. Continue until disease progression or unacceptable toxicity.

Hepatic Impairment

PO (Adults and Children ≥1 yr): *Severe hepatic impairment:* 2.5 mg/m² once daily. Titrate as needed at 2-wk intervals to achieve recommended whole blood trough concentration. Continue until disease progression or unacceptable toxicity.

Tuberous Sclerosis Complex-Associated Partial-Onset Seizures (Afinitor)

PO (Adults and Children ≥2 yr): 5 mg/m² once daily. Titrate as needed at 2-wk intervals to achieve recommended whole blood trough concentration. Continue until disease progression or unacceptable toxicity; *Concurrent use of P-gp inhibitor and moderate CYP3A4 inhibitor:* 2.5 mg/m² once daily. Titrate as needed at 2-wk intervals to achieve recommended whole blood trough concentration. Continue until disease progression or unacceptable toxicity; *Concurrent use of P-gp inducer and strong CYP3A4 inducer:* 10 mg/m² once daily. Titrate as needed, at 2-wk intervals to achieve recommended whole blood trough concentration. Continue until disease progression or unacceptable toxicity.

Hepatic Impairment

PO (Adults and Children ≥2 yr): *Severe hepatic impairment:* 2.5 mg/m² once daily. Titrate as needed at 2-wk intervals to achieve recommended whole blood trough concentration. Continue until disease progression or unacceptable toxicity.

Kidney Transplantation (Zortress)

PO (Adults): 0.75 mg twice daily (with reduced-dose cyclosporine); titrate to achieve recommended whole blood trough concentration.

Hepatic Impairment

PO (Adults): *Mild hepatic impairment:* ↓ daily dose by 33%; *Moderate or severe hepatic impairment:* ↓ daily dose by 50%.

Liver Transplantation (Zortress)

PO (Adults): 1 mg twice daily (with reduced-dose tacrolimus) (start ≥30 days post-transplant);

E

titrate to achieve recommended whole blood trough concentration.

Hepatic Impairment

PO (Adults): *Mild hepatic impairment:* ↓ daily dose by 33%; *Moderate or severe hepatic impairment:* ↓ daily dose by 50%.

Availability (generic available)

Tablets (Afinitor): 2.5 mg, 5 mg, 7.5 mg, 10 mg. **Tablets for oral suspension (Afinitor Disperz):** 2 mg, 3 mg, 5 mg. **Tablets (Zortress):** 0.25 mg, 0.5 mg, 0.75 mg, 1 mg.

NURSING IMPLICATIONS

Assessment

- Assess for symptoms of noninfectious pneumonitis (hypoxia, pleural effusion, cough, dyspnea) during therapy. If symptoms are mild, therapy may continue. *If Grade 2 pneumonitis occurs,* hold therapy until Grade ≤1; reinitiate everolimus at 50% of previous dose. Permanently discontinue if does not resolve or improve to Grade 1 within 4 wk. *If Grade 3 pneumonitis occurs,* hold therapy until Grade ≤1; resume at 50% of previous dose. Change to every other day if dose is lower than lowest available strength. Permanently discontinue everolimus if Grade 3 pneumonitis recurs. *If Grade 4 pneumonitis occurs,* permanently discontinue everolimus.
- Assess for mouth ulcers, stomatitis, or oral mucositis; usually occurs within first 8 wk of therapy. Begin dexamethasone alcohol-free oral solution as a swish-and-spit mouthwash when starting therapy to reduce incidence and severity of stomatitis. Topical treatments may be used; avoid peroxide-containing mouthwashes and antifungals unless fungal infection has been diagnosed. *If Grade 2 stomatitis occurs,* hold therapy until Grade ≤1; resume at previous dose. If Grade 2 recurs, withhold until Grade ≤1; resume at 50% of previous dose. Change to every other day if dose is lower than lowest available strength. *If Grade 3 stomatitis occurs,* hold therapy until Grade ≤1; hold until Grade 0–1; resume at 50% of previous dose. Change to every other day if dose is lower than lowest available strength. *If Grade 4 stomatitis occurs,* permanently discontinue everolimus.
- Assess for signs and symptoms of systemic fungal infections (fever, malaise, weight loss, sweats, cough, dyspnea, pulmonary infiltrates, serious systemic illness with or without concurrent shock). Withhold therapy until infection has been diagnosed and adequately treated.
- Monitor for signs and symptoms of hypersensitivity reactions (anaphylaxis, dyspnea, flushing, chest pain, angioedema) during therapy. *If severe hypersensitivity reaction occurs,* permanently discontinue everolimus.

Lab Test Considerations

- Verify negative pregnancy test before starting therapy. Monitor renal function before and periodically during therapy. May ↑ BUN, serum creatinine, and proteinuria.
- Monitor fasting serum glucose and lipid profile prior to and periodically during therapy. May ↑ cholesterol, triglycerides, and glucose. Attempt to achieve optimal glucose and lipid control prior to therapy. *If Grade 3 metabolic events (hyperglycemia, dyslipidemia) occur,* hold until improvement to Grade ≤2. Resume at 50% of previous dose. Change to every other day if dose is lower than lowest available strength.
- Monitor CBC before and every 6 mo for 1st yr of therapy and annually thereafter; may ↓ hemoglobin, lymphocytes, neutrophils, and platelets. *If Grade 2 thrombocytopenia occurs,* hold dose until Grade ≤1; resume at same dose. *If Grade 3 or 4 thrombocytopenia occurs,* hold until improvement to Grade ≤2. Resume at 50% of previous dose. Change to every other day if dose is lower than lowest available strength. *If Grade 3 neutropenia occurs,* hold dose until Grade ≤1; resume at same dose. *If Grade 4 neutropenia occurs,* hold until improvement to Grade ≤2. Resume at 50% of previous dose. Change to every other day if dose is lower than lowest available strength. *If Grade 3 febrile neutropenia occurs,* hold until improvement to Grade ≤2 and no fever. Resume at 50% of previous dose. Change to every other day if dose is lower than lowest available strength. *If Grade 4 febrile neutropenia occurs,* permanently discontinue everolimus.
- May ↑ AST, ALT, phosphate, and bilirubin.
- **Afinitor:** Monitor *Afinitor* trough levels 2 wk after initiation of therapy, a change in dose, a change in coadministration of CYP3A4 and/or P-gp inducers or inhibitors, change in hepatic function, or change in dose form between everolimus tablets and *Disperz*. Once at a stable dose, monitor trough concentrations every 3–6 mo in patients with changing body surface area or every 6–12 mo in patients with stable body surface area for duration of treatment. Therapeutic blood concentrations are 5–15 ng/mL (*Afinitor*). If trough concentration <5 ng/mL, ↑ daily dose by 2.5 mg in patients taking tablets and 2 mg for *Disperz*. If trough concentration >15 ng/mL, ↓ daily dose by 2.5 mg in patients taking tablets and 2 mg for *Disperz*. If dose ↓ is required with lowest dose, administer every other day. Do not combine dose forms to achieve dose.
- **Zortress:** Therapeutic blood concentrations are 3–8 ng/mL via the LCMSMS assay. Base dose adjustments of *Zortress* on trough concentrations obtained 4 or 5 days after a previous dosing change. Adjust dose if trough concentration <3

ng/mL by doubling dose using available tablet strengths (0.25 mg, 0.5 mg, or 0.75 mg). If trough concentration >8 ng/mL on two consecutive measures, ↓ dose of *Zortress* by 0.25 mg twice daily.

- **Zortress (Kidney Transplantation):** Both cyclosporine doses and the target range for whole blood trough concentrations should be ↓ when given in a regimen with *Zortress* in order to minimize the risk of nephrotoxicity. The recommended cyclosporine therapeutic ranges when administered with *Zortress* are 100–200 ng/mL through Month 1 post-transplant, 75–150 ng/mL at Months 2 and 3 post-transplant, 50–100 ng/mL at Month 4 post-transplant, and 25–50 ng/mL from Month 6 through Month 12 post-transplant. Cyclosporine, USP Modified is to be administered as oral capsules twice daily unless cyclosporine oral solution or IV administration of cyclosporine cannot be avoided. Cyclosporine, USP Modified should be initiated as soon as possible and no later than 48 hr after reperfusion of the graft and dose adjusted to target concentrations from Day 5 onward. If impairment of renal function is progressive, the treatment regimen should be adjusted. In renal transplant patients, the cyclosporine dose should be based on cyclosporine whole blood trough concentrations. Prior to dose ↓ of cyclosporine, steady-state everolimus whole blood trough concentration should be ≥3 ng/mL. Everolimus concentrations may ↓ if cyclosporine exposure is ↓.
- **Zortress (Liver Transplantation):** Both tacrolimus doses and the target range for whole blood trough concentrations should be ↓ when administered with *Zortress* in order to minimize the potential risk of nephrotoxicity. The recommended tacrolimus therapeutic range when administered with *Zortress* are whole blood trough concentrations of 3–5 ng/mL by 3 wk after the first dose of *Zortress* (approximately Month 2) and through Month 12 post-transplant. Tacrolimus is to be administered as oral capsules twice daily unless IV administration of tacrolimus cannot be avoided. In liver transplant patients, the tacrolimus dose should be based on tacrolimus whole blood trough concentrations. Prior to dose ↓ of tacrolimus, steady-state everolimus whole blood trough concentration should be ≥3 ng/mL. Tacrolimus does not affect everolimus trough concentrations; everolimus concentrations do not ↓ if the tacrolimus exposure is ↓.

Implementation

- May impair wound healing. Hold everolimus for ≥1 wk before and ≥2 wk after elective surgery to ensure adequate wound healing.
- **Zortress:** Antimicrobial prophylaxis for *Pneumocystis jiroveci* pneumonia and prophylaxis for cytomegalovirus is recommended in transplant recipients.
- **PO:** Administer at the same time each day consistently with or without food, followed by a whole glass of water. ***DNC:*** Swallow tablets whole; do not break, crush, or chew.
- Do not combine the two dose forms (*Afinitor Tablets* and *Afinitor Disperz*) to achieve the desired total dose. Use one dose form or the other.
- Administer *Disperz*, dispersible tablet, as a suspension only. Wear gloves to avoid possible contact with everolimus when preparing suspensions for another person. Place dose in 10 mL syringe; do not exceed 10 mg/syringe. If higher dose required, use additional syringe. Do not break or crush tablets. Draw 5 mL water and 4 mL of air into syringe. Place filled syringe into container (tip up) for 3 min until tablets are in suspension. Invert syringe five times immediately prior to administration. Administer immediately after preparation; discard suspension if not administered within 60 min after preparation. After administration, draw 5 mL of water and 4 mL of air into same syringe, and swirl contents to suspend remaining particles. Administer entire contents of syringe. Can also be dispersed using same technique and 25 mL water in small glass.

Patient/Family Teaching

- Instruct patient to take everolimus at the same time each day as directed. Take missed doses as soon as remembered up to 6 hr after time of normal dose. If >6 hr after normal dose, omit dose for that day and take next dose next day; do not take two doses to make up missed dose. Do not eat grapefruit or drink grapefruit juice during therapy. Advise patient to read *Patient Information* prior to beginning therapy and with each Rx refill in case of new information.
- Advise patient to report worsening respiratory symptoms or signs of infection (new or worsening cough, shortness of breath, chest pain, difficulty breathing or wheezing, fever, chills, skin rash, joint pain and inflammation, tiredness, loss of appetite, nausea, pale stool or dark urine, yellowing of the skin, pain in upper right side) or severe allergic reaction (rash; itching; hives; flushing; trouble breathing or swallowing; chest pain; dizziness; trouble breathing; swelling of tongue, mouth, or throat) to health care provider promptly.
- Inform patient that mouth sores may occur. Consult health care provider for treatment if pain, discomfort, or open sores in mouth occur. May require special mouthwash or gel.

- Instruct patient to avoid use of live vaccines and close contact with those who have received live vaccines.
- Instruct patient to notify health care provider of all Rx or OTC medications, vitamins, or herbal products being taken and to consult with health care provider before taking other medications, especially St. John's wort.
- Notify health care provider of everolimus therapy before treatment or surgery. May require temporarily stopping everolimus.
- Rep: May cause fetal harm. Advise women of reproductive potential to use effective contraception during and for up to 8 wk after last dose, male patients with female partners of reproductive potential to use effective contraception during and for up to 4 wk after last dose, and to notify health care provider if pregnancy is planned or suspected. Advise female patients to avoid breastfeeding during and for 2 wk after last dose. May impair fertility in female and male patients.
- Emphasize the importance of routine blood tests to determine effectiveness and side effects.

Evaluation/Desired Outcomes

- Decreased spread of tumor. Continue treatment as long as clinical benefit is observed or until unacceptable toxicity occurs.
- Prevention of kidney or liver transplant rejection.
- Reduced seizure frequency.

evolocumab (e-vo-**lo**-kyoo-mab)

Repatha

Classification

Therapeutic: lipid-lowering agents

Pharmacologic: proprotein convertase subtilisin kexin type 9 (PCSK9) inhibitors monoclonal antibodies

Indications

Primary hyperlipidemia (including heterozygous familial hypercholesterolemia [HeFH]) in adults (as an adjunct to diet as monotherapy or in combination with other low-density lipoprotein cholesterol [LDL-C]-lowering therapies). Homozygous familial hypercholesterolemia (in combination with other LDL-C lowering therapies). HeFH in pediatric patients ≥10 yr (as an adjunct to diet in combination with other LDL-C-lowering therapies). To reduce the risk of cardiovascular death, MI, stroke, unstable angina requiring hospitalization, and coronary revascularization in patients with cardiovascular disease.

Action

A human monoclonal immunoglobulin produced in genetically engineered Chinese hamster ovary cells that binds to PCSK9, inhibiting its binding to the low-density lipoprotein receptor (LDLR), resulting in ↑ number of LDLRs available to clear LDL-C from blood. **Therapeutic Effects:** Reduction in LDL-C. Reduction in the risk of MI, stroke, and coronary revascularization.

Pharmacokinetics

Absorption: Well absorbed (72%) following SUBQ administration.

Distribution: Minimally distributed to tissues.

Metabolism and Excretion: Eliminated by binding to PCSK9 and by proteolytic degradation.

Half-life: 11–17 days.

TIME/ACTION PROFILE (effect on circulating unbound PCSK9)

ROUTE	ONSET	PEAK	DURATION
SUBQ	rapid	4 hr	2–4 wk

Contraindications/Precautions

Contraindicated in: Hypersensitivity.

Use Cautiously in: Hypersensitivity to latex (use preparation that does not contain dry natural rubber); Severe renal impairment; Severe hepatic impairment; OB: Safety not established in pregnancy; Lactation: Safety not established in breastfeeding; Pedi: Children <10 yr (safety and effectiveness not established); Geri: Older adults may be more sensitive to drug effects.

Adverse Reactions/Side Effects

Local: injection site reactions. **MS:** back pain. **Misc:** HYPERSENSITIVITY REACTIONS (INCLUDING ANGIOEDEMA).

Interactions

Drug-Drug: None reported.

Route/Dosage

Established Cardiovascular Disease or Primary Hyperlipidemia

SUBQ (Adults): 140 mg every 2 wk *or* 420 mg once monthly.

Heterozygous Familial Hypercholesterolemia

SUBQ (Children ≥10 yr): 140 mg every 2 wk *or* 420 mg once monthly.

Homozygous Familial Hypercholesterolemia

SUBQ (Adults and Children ≥10 yr): 420 mg once monthly; if inadequate response after 12 wk, may ↑ to 420 mg every 2 wk. *Patients on lipid apheresis:* 420 mg every 2 wk (administered after apheresis session completed).

Availability

Solution for injection (some needle covers contains latex derivative) (prefilled syringes and autoinjectors): 140 mg/mL.

NURSING IMPLICATIONS

Assessment

- Obtain a diet history, especially with regard to saturated fat consumption.
- Monitor for signs and symptoms of hypersensitivity reactions (rash, urticaria, dyspnea) during therapy. *If symptoms occur,* discontinue therapy.

Lab Test Considerations

- Assess LDL-C levels within 4–8 wk of initiating; response to therapy depends on degree of LDLR function. For patients on a monthly regimen, measure LDL-C just prior to next scheduled dose.

Implementation

- Some needle cover of glass single-dose prefilled syringe and single-dose prefilled autoinjector contain latex; avoid with latex allergies.
- **SUBQ**: To administer the 140-mg or 420-mg dose, give one injection (140-mg dose) or give three injections (420-mg dose) using three separate pens/syringes in three separate sites, consecutively within 30 min. When switching dose regimens, administer 1st dose of new regimen on next scheduled date of prior regimen. If stored in refrigerator, allow solution to warm to room temperature for ≥30 min before injecting. May also be stored at room temperature for 30 days. Solution is clear to opalescent and colorless to pale yellow; do not administer solutions that are cloudy or contain particulates. Do not shake. Stretch or pinch skin. Inject into thigh, abdomen, or upper arm at a 90° angle. Injection may take 15 sec. Window turns from clear to yellow when the injection is done. Rotate sites with each injection. Do not inject into areas that are tender, bruised, red, or indurated. Do not reuse prefilled pen or syringe. Do not administer other injectable drugs at same site.

Patient/Family Teaching

- Explain the purpose and side effects of evolocumab. Instruct patient to take as directed. Advise patient to read the *Medication Guide* before starting and with each refill in case of changes.
- Instruct patient in correct technique for self-injection and care and disposal of equipment. Administer missed doses within 7 days; then resume original schedule. If not administered within 7 days, wait until next dose on original schedule.
- Advise patient that this medication should be used in conjunction with diet restrictions (fat, cholesterol, carbohydrates, alcohol), exercise, and cessation of smoking.
- Instruct patient to notify health care professional of all Rx or OTC medications, vitamins, or herbal products being taken and to consult health care professional before taking any other Rx, OTC, or herbal products.
- Advise patient to notify health care professional of medication regimen prior to treatment or surgery.
- Rep: Advise women of reproductive potential to notify health care professional if pregnancy is planned or suspected or if breastfeeding. Inform patients of pregnancy safety study that monitors pregnancy outcomes in women exposed to evolocumab during pregnancy. Enroll patient by contacting Amgen at 1-800-77-AMGEN (1-800-772-6436).

Evaluation/Desired Outcomes

- Decreased LDL-C levels.
- Reduction in the risk of cardiovascular death, MI, stroke, unstable angina requiring hospitalization and coronary revascularization.

HIGH ALERT

exemestane (ex-e-**mes**-tane)

Aromasin

Classification

Therapeutic: antineoplastics

Pharmacologic: aromatase inhibitors

Indications

Adjuvant treatment of breast cancer in postmenopausal women who have estrogen-receptor positive early disease and who have already received 2–3 yr of tamoxifen and are then switched to exemestane to complete a total of 5 yr of adjuvant therapy. Advanced postmenopausal breast cancer that has progressed despite tamoxifen therapy.

Action

Inhibits aromatase, an enzyme responsible for the conversion of androgen to estrogen. In postmenopausal women, the primary source of estrogen is androgen. Decreases circulating estrogen. **Therapeutic Effects:** Decreased spread of estrogen-sensitive breast cancer.

Pharmacokinetics

Absorption: 42% absorbed following oral administration.

Distribution: Extensively distributed to tissues.

Metabolism and Excretion: Primarily metabolized by the liver via the CYP3A4 isoenzyme; metabolites are excreted in urine (40%) and feces (40%); <1% excreted unchanged in urine.

Half-life: 24 hr.

TIME/ACTION PROFILE (suppression of circulating estrogen)

ROUTE	ONSET	PEAK	DURATION
PO	unknown	2–3 days	4–5 days

Contraindications/Precautions

Contraindicated in: Hypersensitivity; Premenopausal status; OB: Pregnancy; Lactation: Lactation.
Use Cautiously in: Rep: Women of reproductive potential.

Adverse Reactions/Side Effects

CV: hypertension, DEEP VEIN THROMBOSIS. **Derm:** ↑ sweating, alopecia, hot flush, dermatitis. **EENT:** visual disturbances. **GI:** diarrhea, nausea. **GU:** endometrial hyperplasia, uterine polyps. **MS:** arthralgia, carpal tunnel syndrome, muscle cramps, osteoporosis, pain. **Neuro:** fatigue, depression, insomnia, neuropathy, paresthesia. **Resp:** PULMONARY EMBOLISM (PE).

Interactions

Drug-Drug: Strong CYP3A4 inducers, including **rifampin** or **phenytoin**, may ↓ levels and effectiveness. **Estrogens** can interfere with action.

Route/Dosage

PO (Adults): 25 mg once daily; *Concurrent use of strong CYP3A4 inducers:* 50 mg once daily.

Availability (generic available)

Tablets: 25 mg.

NURSING IMPLICATIONS

Assessment

- Assess for pain and other side effects periodically during therapy.
- Assess for ↑ risk of osteoporosis and fractures (↓ dietary calcium intake, tobacco use, body weight <57 kg, early menopause ≤45 yr, women >65 yr, T-score <−2.5, vertebral compression fracture, osteopenia on x-ray). Monitor for bone mineral density loss and treat as appropriate.
- Monitor for signs and symptoms of venous thromboembolism such as PE (chest pain, dyspnea, tachycardia), DVT (calf pain or tenderness, lower extremity edema, localized warmth or erythema), or stroke (headache, facial numbness, unilateral weakness, aphasia, eye pain or swelling, vision changes). Discontinue therapy if suspected.

Lab Test Considerations

- Verify negative pregnancy test within 7 days of starting exemestane. Assess bone mineral density panel (serum albumin, calcium, phosphate, alkaline phosphatase) at baseline in patients with or at risk for osteoporosis. Perform dual energy x-ray absorptiometry scan at baseline and every 1–2 yr to monitor for osteoporosis and fractures.
- May ↑ GGT, AST, ALT, bilirubin, and serum creatinine levels.
- Assess 25-hydroxy vitamin D levels prior to starting therapy. Supplement vitamin D deficiency with vitamin D due to high prevalence of vitamin D deficiency in women with early breast cancer.

Implementation

- Handle intact tablets or capsules with single gloves.
- **PO:** Give tablet after a meal.

Patient/Family Teaching

- Explain the purpose and side effects of exemestane. Instruct patient to take as directed at the same time each day. Take missed doses as soon as remembered unless it is almost time for next dose. Do not double doses. Advise patient to read the *Patient Information* leaflet before starting and with each Rx refill in case of changes.
- Explain need for follow-up blood tests to check liver and kidney function.
- Advise patient not to take other estrogen-containing agents because they may interfere with action of exemestane.
- Inform patient that lower level of estrogen may lead to ↓ bone mineral density over time and ↑ risk of osteoporosis and fracture. Women with or at risk for osteoporosis should have their bone mineral density formally assessed by bone densitometry every 1–2 yr.
- Advise patient to notify health care professional immediately if chest pain or signs of HF or stroke occur.
- Advise patient to notify health care professional of all Rx or OTC medications, vitamins, or herbal products being taken and to consult with health care professional before taking other medications.
- Rep: May cause fetal harm. Advise women of reproductive potential to use effective contraception and avoid breastfeeding during therapy and for ≥1 mo after last dose. May impair fertility.

Evaluation/Desired Outcomes

- Slowing of disease progression in women with breast cancer.

ezetimibe (e-zet-i-mibe)

✱ Ezetrol, Zetia

Classification
Therapeutic: lipid-lowering agents
Pharmacologic: cholesterol absorption inhibitors

Indications

Primary hyperlipidemia, including heterozygous familial hypercholesterolemia (as monotherapy [in adults only] or in combination with a statin). Mixed hyperlipidemia (in combination with fenofibrate). Homozygous familial hypercholesterolemia (in combination with a statin and other LDL-C-lowering therapies). Familial sitosterolemia.

Action

Inhibits absorption of cholesterol in the small intestine. **Therapeutic Effects:** Reduction of LDL-C concentrations. Reduction of sitosterol and campesterol concentrations.

Pharmacokinetics

Absorption: Following absorption, rapidly converted to ezetimibe-glucuronide, which is active. Bioavailability is variable.

Distribution: Unknown.

Metabolism and Excretion: Undergoes enterohepatic recycling, mostly eliminated in feces; minimal renal excretion.

Half-life: 22 hr.

TIME/ACTION PROFILE

ROUTE	ONSET	PEAK	DURATION
PO	unknown	unknown	unknown

Contraindications/Precautions

Contraindicated in: Hypersensitivity; When a statin, fenofibrate, or other LDL-C-lowering therapy is contraindicated (when used in combination with statin, fenofibrate, or other LDL-C-lowering therapy); Moderate or severe hepatic impairment.

Use Cautiously in: OB: Safety not established in pregnancy; Lactation: Safety not established in breastfeeding; Pedi: Children <10 yr (safety and effectiveness not established).

Adverse Reactions/Side Effects

Derm: rash. **GI:** ↑ liver enzymes, cholecystitis, cholelithiasis, nausea, pancreatitis. **MS:** myopathy, RHABDOMYOLYSIS. **Misc:** ANGIOEDEMA.

Interactions

Drug-Drug: Cholestyramine or other **bile acid sequestrants** may ↓ effectiveness. **Fibrates** may ↑ levels and risk of cholelithiasis. **Cyclosporine** may ↑ levels and risk of toxicity. **HMG CoA-reductase inhibitors** may ↑ risk of rhabdomyolysis.

Route/Dosage

PO: (Adults): 10 mg once daily.

Renal Impairment

PO: (Adults): *CCr <60 mL/min and concurrent use with simvastatin:* Not to exceed simvastatin dose of 20 mg/day.

Availability (generic available)

Tablets: 10 mg. ***In combination with:*** bempedoic acid (Nexlizet); simvastatin (Vytorin); see Appendix N.

NURSING IMPLICATIONS

Assessment

- Obtain a diet history, especially with regard to fat consumption.
- Monitor for signs and symptoms of rhabdomyolysis (malaise, myalgia, muscle cramps/weakness, dark or tea-colored urine). *If myopathy suspected,* discontinue ezetimibe.

Lab Test Considerations

- Evaluate lipid panel before initiating, after 2–4 wk of therapy, and periodically thereafter.
- May ↑ liver transaminases when administered with HMG-CoA reductase inhibitors. Monitor liver enzymes prior to initiation and during therapy according to recommendations of HMG-CoA reductase inhibitor. Elevations are usually asymptomatic and return to baseline with continued therapy. Consider discontinuation of ezetimibe if ↑ ALT or AST ≥3 times upper limit of normal persists.

Implementation

- Do not confuse Zetia with Zestril.
- **PO:** Administer without regard to meals. May be taken at the same time as HMG-CoA reductase inhibitors or fenofibrate. Administer ≥2 hr before or ≥4 hr after bile acid sequestrants.

Patient/Family Teaching

- Explain the purpose and side effects of ezetimibe. Instruct patient to take as directed, at the same time each day. Take missed doses as soon as remembered, but do not take more than one dose per day. Medication helps control but does not cure elevated serum cholesterol levels. Advise patient to read *Patient Information* before starting therapy and with each Rx refill in case of change.
- Emphasize the importance of follow-up exams to determine effectiveness and to monitor for side effects.
- Advise patient that this medication should be used in conjunction with diet restrictions (fat, cholesterol, carbohydrates, alcohol), exercise, and cessation of smoking. Ezetimibe does not assist with weight loss.
- Instruct patient to notify health care professional if unexplained muscle pain, tenderness, or weakness occur. Risk may ↑ when used with HMG-CoA reductase inhibitors.
- Instruct patient to notify health care professional of all Rx or OTC medications, vitamins, or herbal products being taken and to consult health care professional before taking any other Rx, OTC, or herbal products.
- Advise patient to notify health care professional of medication regimen prior to treatment or surgery.
- Rep: Advise women of reproductive potential to notify health care professional promptly if pregnancy is planned or suspected or if breastfeeding. If regimen includes HMG-CoA reductase inhibitors, they are contraindicated in pregnancy.

Evaluation/Desired Outcomes

- Decrease in serum LDL-C and total cholesterol levels.

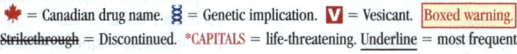

famciclovir (fam-**sye**-kloe-veer)

~~Famvir~~

Classification

Therapeutic: antivirals

Indications

Acute herpes zoster infections (shingles). Treatment/suppression of recurrent herpes genitalis in immunocompetent patients. Treatment of recurrent herpes labialis (cold sores) in immunocompetent patients. Treatment of recurrent mucocutaneous herpes simplex virus (HSV) infection in patients with HIV.

Action

Inhibits viral DNA synthesis in herpes-infected cells only. **Therapeutic Effects:** Decreased duration of herpes zoster infection with decreased duration of viral shedding. Decreased time to healing for cold sores. Decreased lesion formation and improved healing in recurrent HSV infection.

Pharmacokinetics

Absorption: Following absorption, famciclovir is rapidly converted in the intestinal wall to penciclovir, the active compound.

Distribution: Unknown.

Metabolism and Excretion: Penciclovir is mostly excreted by the kidneys.

Half-life: *Penciclovir:* 2.1–3 hr (↑ in renal impairment).

TIME/ACTION PROFILE (penciclovir plasma concentrations)

ROUTE	ONSET	PEAK	DURATION
PO	rapid	0.9 hr	8–12 hr

Contraindications/Precautions

Contraindicated in: Hypersensitivity.

Use Cautiously in: Renal impairment (↑ dose interval/↓ dose if CCr <40–60 mL/min); OB: Use during pregnancy only if potential maternal benefit justifies potential fetal risk; Lactation: Use during breastfeeding only if potential maternal benefit justifies potential risk to infant; Pedi: Safety and effectiveness not established in children; Geri: Consider age-related ↓ in renal function in older adults.

Adverse Reactions/Side Effects

CV: palpitations. **Derm:** hypersensitivity vasculitis. **GI:** diarrhea, nausea, vomiting. **GU:** ↓ fertility (men). **Neuro:** headache, dizziness, fatigue, SEIZURES. **Misc:** ANAPHYLAXIS.

Interactions

Drug-Drug: Probenecid ↑ levels of penciclovir.

Route/Dosage

Herpes Zoster

PO (Adults): 500 mg every 8 hr for 7 days.

Renal Impairment

PO (Adults): *CCr 40–59 mL/min:* 500 mg every 12 hr; *CCr 20–39 mL/min:* 500 mg every 24 hr; *CCr <20 mL/min:* 250 mg every 24 hr; *Hemodialysis:* 250 mg after each dialysis.

Recurrent Genital Herpes Simplex Infections

PO (Adults): 1000 mg twice daily for one day.

Renal Impairment

PO (Adults): *CCr 40–59 mL/min:* 500 mg twice daily for 1 day; *CCr 20–39 mL/min:* 500 mg as a single dose; *CCr <20 mL/min:* 250 mg as a single dose; *Hemodialysis:* 250 mg as a single dose after dialysis.

Suppression of Recurrent Herpes Simplex Infections

PO (Adults): 250 mg every 12 hr for up to 1 yr.

Renal Impairment

PO (Adults): *CCr 20–39 mL/min:* 125 mg every 12 hr for 5 days; *CCr <20 mL/min:* 125 mg every 24 hr for 5 days; *Hemodialysis:* 125 mg after each dialysis.

Recurrent Herpes Labialis Infections (Cold Sores)

PO (Adults): 1500 mg as a single dose.

Renal Impairment

PO (Adults): *CCr 40–59 mL/min:* 750 mg as a single dose; *CCr 20–39 mL/min:* 500 mg as a single dose; *CCr <20 mL/min:* 250 mg as a single dose; *Hemodialysis:* 250 mg as a single dose after dialysis.

Herpes Simplex in Patients with HIV

PO (Adults): 500 mg every 12 hr for 7 days.

Renal Impairment

PO (Adults): *CCr 20–39 mL/min:* 500 mg every 24 hr for 7 days; *CCr <20 mL/min:* 250 mg every 24 hr for 7 days; *Hemodialysis:* 250 mg after each dialysis.

Availability (generic available)

Tablets: 125 mg, 250 mg, 500 mg.

NURSING IMPLICATIONS

Assessment

- Assess lesions prior to and during therapy to evaluate efficacy.
- Assess patient for postherpetic neuralgia periodically during and following therapy.

Lab Test Considerations

- Assess renal function as indicated, especially in underlying renal impairment.

Implementation

- Famciclovir therapy should be started as soon as herpes zoster is diagnosed, at least within 72 hr, preferably within 48 hr.
- **PO:** Administer without regard to food.

Patient/Family Teaching

- Explain purpose and side effects of medication. Advise patient to read *Patient Information* before starting therapy.
- Advise patient to notify health care professional of all Rx or OTC medications, vitamins, or herbal products being taken and to consult health care professional before taking other medications.
- Instruct patient to take famciclovir as directed for the full course of therapy. Take missed doses as soon as remembered, if not just before next dose.
- Inform patient that famciclovir does not prevent the spread of infection to others. Until all lesions have crusted, precautions should be taken around others who have not had chickenpox or varicella vaccine or in people who are immunosuppressed.
- May cause nausea, headache, or dizziness. Caution patient to avoid driving and other activities requiring alertness until response to medication is known.
- Advise patient to notify health care professional immediately if seizures or signs and symptoms of anaphylaxis (rash, facial swelling, difficulty breathing) occur.
- Instruct patients with genital herpes to have yearly Papanicolaou (Pap) smears due to ↑ risk of cervical cancer.
- Rep: Advise women of reproductive potential to notify health care professional if pregnancy is planned or suspected or if breastfeeding. Advise patient to use condoms during sexual contact and to avoid sexual contact while lesions are present.

Evaluation/Desired Outcomes

- Decrease in time to full crusting, loss of vesicles, loss of ulcers, and loss of crusts in patients with acute herpes zoster (shingles).
- Crusting over and healing of lesions in herpes labialis, genital herpes, and in recurrent mucocutaneous HSV infection in patients with HIV.
- Prevention of recurrence of herpes genitalis.
- Decreased time to healing for cold sores.

famotidine (fa-moe-ti-deen)

~~Pepcid~~, Pepcid AC

Classification

Therapeutic: antiulcer agents

Pharmacologic: histamine H_2 antagonists

Indications

Short-term treatment of active duodenal ulcers and benign gastric ulcers. Maintenance therapy for duodenal ulcers after healing of active ulcer(s). Gastroesophageal reflux disease (GERD). Heartburn, acid indigestion, and sour stomach (OTC use). Gastric hypersecretory states (Zollinger-Ellison syndrome). Prevention and treatment of stress-induced upper GI bleeding in critically ill patients. **Unlabeled Use:** GI symptoms associated with the use of NSAIDs. Prevention of stress ulceration or aspiration pneumonitis. Management of urticaria.

Action

Inhibits the action of histamine at the H_2-receptor site located primarily in gastric parietal cells, resulting in inhibition of gastric acid secretion. **Therapeutic Effects:** Healing and prevention of ulcers. Decreased symptoms of GERD. Decreased secretion of gastric acid.

Pharmacokinetics

Absorption: 40–45% absorbed following oral administration.

Distribution: Enters cerebrospinal fluid.

Metabolism and Excretion: Up to 70% excreted unchanged by the kidneys; 30–35% metabolized by the liver.

Half-life: *Infants:* 4.5–15 hr; *Children:* 3.3–5.7 hr; *Adults:* 2.5–3.5 hr.

TIME/ACTION PROFILE

ROUTE	ONSET	PEAK	DURATION
PO	within 60 min	1–4 hr	6–12 hr
IV	within 60 min	0.5–3 hr	8–15 hr

Contraindications/Precautions

Contraindicated in: Hypersensitivity; Phenylketonuria (chewable tablets only).

Use Cautiously in: Renal impairment (more susceptible to adverse CNS reactions; ↑ dosage interval recommended if CCr <10 mL/min); OB: Use during pregnancy only if potential maternal benefit outweighs potential fetal risk; Lactation: Use while breastfeeding only if potential maternal benefit outweighs potential risk to infant; Pedi: Injection contains benzyl alcohol, which has been associated with gasping syndrome in neonates; Geri: Older adults are more susceptible to adverse CNS reactions; dose ↓ recommended.

Adverse Reactions/Side Effects

CV: ARRHYTHMIAS. **Endo:** gynecomastia. **GI:** constipation, diarrhea, nausea. **GU:** ↓ sperm count, erectile dysfunction. **Hemat:** AGRANULOCYTOSIS, APLASTIC ANEMIA, anemia, neutropenia, thrombocytopenia. **Neuro:** confusion, dizziness, drowsiness, hallucinations, headache.

Interactions

Drug-Drug: May ↓ absorption and effectiveness of **ketoconazole**, **itraconazole**, **atazanavir**, and **gefitinib**.

Route/Dosage

PO (Adults): *Short-term treatment of active ulcers:* 40 mg/day at bedtime or 20 mg twice daily for up to 8 wk. *Duodenal ulcer prophylaxis:* 20 mg once daily at bedtime. *GERD:* 20 mg twice daily for up

to 6 wk; up to 40 mg twice daily for up to 12 wk for esophagitis with erosions, ulcerations, and continuing symptoms. *Gastric hypersecretory conditions:* 20 mg every 6 hr initially, up to 160 mg every 6 hr. *OTC use:* 10 mg for relief of symptoms; for prevention: 10 mg 60 min before eating or take 10 mg as chewable tablet 15 min before heartburn-inducing foods or beverages (not to exceed 20 mg/24 hr for up to 2 wk).
PO, IV (Children 1–12 yr): *Peptic ulcer:* 0.5 mg/kg/day as a single bedtime dose or in divided doses twice daily (maximum: 40 mg daily); *GERD:* 1 mg/kg/day in divided doses twice daily (maximum: 80 mg daily).
PO (Infants >3 mo–1 yr): *GERD:* 0.5 mg/kg/dose twice daily.
PO (Infants and neonates <3 mo): *GERD:* 0.5 mg/kg/dose once daily.
IV (Adults): 20 mg every 12 hr.

Renal Impairment
PO (Adults): *CCr 10–50 mL/min:* Administer normal dose every 24 hr or 50% dose at normal dosing interval; *CCr <10 mL/min:* 20 mg at bedtime; interval may need to be ↑ to every 36–48 hr.

Availability (generic available)
Tablets: 10 mg^{OTC}, 20 mg$^{\text{Rx, OTC}}$, 40 mg. **Oral suspension (cherry-banana-mint flavor):** 40 mg/5 mL. **Premixed infusion:** 20 mg/50 mL 0.9% NaCl. **Solution for injection:** 10 mg/mL. ***In combination with:*** calcium carbonate/magnesium hydroxide (Pepcid Complete). See Appendix N.

NURSING IMPLICATIONS
Assessment
- Assess for epigastric or abdominal pain and frank or occult blood in stool, emesis, or gastric aspirate.
- Geri: Monitor routinely for CNS reactions (confusion, delirium, hallucination, agitation, seizure, lethargy).

Lab Test Considerations
- Monitor CBC with differential periodically during therapy.
- Antagonizes effects of pentagastrin and histamine during gastric acid secretion testing. Avoid administration for 24 hr preceding the test.
- May cause false-negative results in skin tests using allergenic extracts. Discontinue 24 hr prior to the test.
- May ↑ AST, ALT, and serum creatinine.
- May cause false-positive results for urine protein; test with sulfosalicylic acid.

Implementation
- **PO:** Administer with meals or immediately afterward and at bedtime to prolong effect.
- Administer once daily doses at bedtime to prolong effect.
- Shake oral suspension prior to administration. Discard unused suspension after 30 days.

IV Administration
- **IV Push: Dilution:** Mix 20 mg famotidine with 0.9% NaCl for a total volume of 5 or 10 mL. **Concentration:** Not >4 mg/mL. **Rate:** Administer over ≥2 min. Rapid administration may cause hypotension.
- **Intermittent Infusion: Dilution:** Dilute each 20 mg in 100 mL of 0.9% NaCl, D5W, D10W, or LR. **Concentration:** 0.2 mg/mL. Diluted solution is stable for 48 hr at room temperature. Do not use solution that is discolored or contains particulates. **Rate:** Administer over 15–30 min.
- **Y-Site Compatibility:** acyclovir, alemtuzumab, allopurinol, amikacin, aminocaproic acid, aminophylline, amiodarone, amphotericin B liposomal, anakinra, anidulafungin, argatroban, arsenic trioxide, ascorbic acid, atracurium, atropine, aztreonam, benztropine, bleomycin, bumetanide, buprenorphine, butorphanol, calcium chloride, calcium gluconate, cangrelor, carboplatin, carmustine, caspofungin, cefotaxime, ceftaroline, ceftazidime, ceftolozane/tazobactam, cefuroxime, chlorpromazine, cisatracurium, cisplatin, cladribine, clindamycin, cyanocobalamin, cyclophosphamide, cyclosporine, cytarabine, dacarbazine, dactinomycin, daptomycin, daunorubicin, dexamethasone, dexmedetomidine, dexrazoxane, dextran 40, digoxin, diltiazem, diphenhydramine, dobutamine, docetaxel, dopamine, doxorubicin hydrochloride, doxorubicin liposomal, doxycycline, droperidol, enalaprilat, ephedrine, epinephrine, epirubicin, epoetin alfa, eptifibatide, ertapenem, erythromycin, esmolol, etoposide, etoposide phosphate, fentanyl, filgrastim, fluconazole, fludarabine, fluorouracil, folic acid, foscarnet, fosphenytoin, gemcitabine, gentamicin, glycopyrrolate, granisetron, heparin, hetastarch, hydrocortisone, hydromorphone, hydroxyzine, idarubicin, ifosfamide, imipenem/cilastatin, irinotecan, isavuconazonium, isoproterenol, ketorolac, labetalol, letermovir, leucovorin, levofloxacin, lidocaine, linezolid, lorazepam, magnesium sulfate, mannitol, melphalan, meperidine, meropenem/vaborbactam, mesna, methadone, methotrexate, methylprednisolone, metoclopramide, metoprolol, metronidazole, midazolam, milrinone, mitoxantrone morphine, moxifloxacin, mycophenolate, nafcillin, nalbuphine, naloxone, nicardipine, nitroglycerin, nitroprusside, norepinephrine, octreotide, ondansetron, oritavancin, oxacillin, oxaliplatin, oxytocin, paclitaxel, palonosetron, pamidronate, papaverine, pemetrexed, penicillin G, pentamidine, pentobarbital, phenobarbital, phentolamine, phenylephrine, phytonadione, plazomicin, posaconazole, potassium acetate, potassium chloride, potassium phosphate, procainamide, prochlorperazine, promethazine, propofol, propranolol, protamine, pyridoxine, remifentanil, rituximab, sargramostim, sodium

acetate, sodium bicarbonate, succinylcholine, sufentanil, sulbactam/durlobactam, tacrolimus, tedizolid, telavancin, theophylline, thiamine, thiotepa, tigecycline, tirofiban, tobramycin, topotecan, trastuzumab, vancomycin, vasopressin, vecuronium, verapamil, vinblastine, vincristine, vinorelbine, voriconazole, zoledronic acid.

- **Y-Site Incompatibility:** amphotericin B deoxycholate, azathioprine, cefepime, dantrolene, diazepam, diazoxide, ganciclovir, gemtuzumab ozogamicin, indomethacin, minocycline, mitomycin, pantoprazole, piperacillin/tazobactam, trimethoprim/sulfamethoxazole.

Patient/Family Teaching

- Explain purpose and side effects of medication. Advise patient to read *Patient Information* before starting therapy and take missed doses as soon as remembered but do not double doses.
- Advise patient to notify health care professional of all Rx or OTC medications, vitamins, or herbal products being taken and to consult health care professional before taking other medications.
- Advise patient taking OTC preparation not to take the maximum dose continuously for >2 wk without consulting health care professional. Notify health care professional if difficulty swallowing occurs or abdominal pain persists.
- Inform patient that smoking interferes with the action of histamine antagonists. Encourage patient to quit smoking or not to smoke after last dose of the day.
- May cause drowsiness or dizziness. Caution patient to avoid driving or other activities requiring alertness until response to the drug is known.
- Advise patient to avoid alcohol, products containing aspirin or NSAIDs, and foods that may cause ↑ GI irritation.
- Inform patient that ↑ fluid and fiber intake and exercise may minimize constipation.
- Advise patient to report onset of black, tarry stools; fever; sore throat; diarrhea; dizziness; rash; confusion; or hallucinations to health care professional promptly.
- Rep: Advise women of reproductive potential to notify health care professional if pregnancy is planned or suspected or if breastfeeding.

Evaluation/Desired Outcomes

- Decrease in abdominal pain, heartburn, acid indigestion, and sour stomach.
- Prevention of gastric irritation and bleeding. Healing of duodenal ulcers can be seen by endoscopy. Therapy is continued for ≥6 wk in treatment of ulcers but not usually >8 wk.
- Decreased symptoms of GERD.

HIGH ALERT

fam-trastuzumab deruxtecan

(fam tras-**tu**-zoo-mab de-**rux**-te-can)

Enhertu

Classification

Therapeutic: antineoplastics

Pharmacologic: monoclonal antibodies, enzyme inhibitors

Indications

Unresectable or metastatic human epidermal growth factor receptor 2 (HER2)-positive (IHC 3+ or ISH+) breast cancer in patients who have previously received an anti-HER2-based regimens either in the metastatic setting or in the neoadjuvant or adjuvant setting and have developed disease recurrence during or within 6 mo of completing therapy. Unresectable or metastatic hormone receptor-positive HER2-low (IHC 1+ or IHC 2+/ISH-) or HER2-ultralow (IHC 0 with membrane staining) breast cancer that has progressed on ≥1 endocrine therapies in the metastatic setting. Unresectable or metastatic HER2-low (IHC 1+ or IHC 2+/ISH-) breast cancer in patients who have previously received chemotherapy in the metastatic setting or developed disease recurrence during or within 6 mo of completing adjuvant chemotherapy. Locally advanced or metastatic HER2-positive (IHC 3+ or 2+/ISH+) gastric or gastroesophageal junction adenocarcinoma in patients who have previously received a trastuzumab-based regimen. Unresectable or metastatic non-small cell lung cancer (NSCLC) in patients whose tumors have activating HER2 (ERBB2) mutations and who have received a prior systemic therapy. Unresectable or metastatic HER2-positive (IHC 3+) solid tumors in patients who have received prior systemic treatment and have no satisfactory alternative treatment options.

Action

Acts as a HER2-directed antibody-drug conjugate composed of a humanized IgG1 monoclonal antibody (which has the same amino acid sequence as trastuzumab [and targets HER2]), a cleavable linker, and a topoisomerase I inhibitor (DXd) (the cytotoxic component that causes DNA damage and apoptosis). **Therapeutic Effects:** Regression of breast cancer and metastases. Improved survival in gastric or gastroesophageal junction adenocarcinoma. Decreased spread of NSCLC.

F

Pharmacokinetics

Absorption: IV administration results in complete bioavailability.
Distribution: Minimally distributed to extravascular tissues.
Protein Binding: 97%.
Metabolism and Excretion: Monoclonal antibody component is degraded into smaller peptides via catabolism. DXd primarily metabolized by the liver via CYP3A4 isoenzyme. Excretion pathway unknown.
Half-life: *Fam-trastuzumab deruxtecan:* 5.7 days; *DXd:* 5.8 days.

TIME/ACTION PROFILE (plasma concentrations)

ROUTE	ONSET	PEAK	DURATION
IV	unknown	unknown	unknown

Contraindications/Precautions

Contraindicated in: OB: Pregnancy; Lactation: Lactation.
Use Cautiously in: Severe renal impairment; Severe hepatic impairment (total bilirubin >3–10 times upper limit of normal [ULN] or AST > ULN); Rep: Women of reproductive potential and men with female partners of reproductive potential; Pedi: Safety and effectiveness not established in children; Geri: Older adults may have ↑ risk of adverse reactions.
Exercise Extreme Caution in: Pre-existing cardiac dysfunction.

Adverse Reactions/Side Effects

CV: ↓ left ventricular ejection fraction (LVEF), HF. **Derm:** alopecia, rash. **EENT:** dry eye, epistaxis. **F and E:** hypokalemia. **GI:** ↓ appetite, ↑ liver enzymes, abdominal pain, constipation, diarrhea, dyspepsia, nausea, stomatitis, vomiting. **GU:** ↓ fertility (men). **Hemat:** anemia, leukopenia, NEUTROPENIA, thrombocytopenia. **Neuro:** dizziness, fatigue, headache. **Resp:** cough, dyspnea, INTERSTITIAL LUNG DISEASE (ILD)/PNEUMONITIS, upper respiratory tract infection.

Interactions

Drug-Drug: None reported.

Route/Dosage

Do NOT substitute fam-trastuzumab deruxtecan with trastuzumab or ado-trastuzumab emtansine.

Metastatic Breast Cancer, Unresectable/Metastatic Non-Small Cell Lung Cancer, or Unresectable/Metastatic Solid Tumors

IV (Adults): 5.4 mg/kg every 3 wk; continue until disease progression or unacceptable toxicity.

Locally Advanced or Metastatic Gastric or Gastroesophageal Junction Adenocarcinoma

IV (Adults): 6.4 mg/kg every 3 wk; continue until disease progression or unacceptable toxicity.

Availability

Lyophilized powder for injection: 100 mg/vial.

NURSING IMPLICATIONS

Assessment

- Assess for signs and symptoms of ILD/pneumonitis (cough, dyspnea, fever) periodically during therapy. *If asymptomatic,* hold until resolved to Grade 0; if resolved in <28 days, maintain dose. If resolved in >28 days, ↓ dose one level. Consider corticosteroid therapy as soon as ILD/pneumonitis is suspected. *If symptomatic ILD/pneumonitis occurs,* permanently discontinue fam-trastuzumab deruxtecan and start corticosteroid therapy.
- Assess for signs and symptoms of left ventricular dysfunction before starting and at regular intervals during therapy as clinically indicated. *If LVEF >45% and absolute ↓ from baseline is 10–20%,* continue therapy. *If LVEF is 40–45% and absolute ↓ from baseline is <10%,* continue therapy and repeat LVEF assessment in 3 wk. *If LVEF is 40–45% and absolute ↓ from baseline is 10–20%,* hold therapy and repeat LVEF assessment in 3 wk. If LVEF has not recovered to within 10% from baseline, permanently discontinue fam-trastuzumab deruxtecan. If LVEF recovers to within 10% from baseline, resume therapy at same dose. *If LVEF <40% or absolute ↓ from baseline >20%,* hold therapy and repeat LVEF assessment in 3 wk. If LVEF <40% or absolute ↓ from baseline >20% is confirmed, permanently discontinue fam-trastuzumab deruxtecan. *If symptomatic HF occurs,* permanently discontinue fam-trastuzumab deruxtecan.

Lab Test Considerations

- Verify negative pregnancy test before starting therapy.
- Select patients for treatment of: **(1) Locally advanced or metastatic HER2-positive gastric cancer** based on HER2 protein overexpression or HER2 gene amplification (IHC 3+ or IHC 2+/ISH+). Reassess HER2 status if it is feasible to obtain a new tumor specimen after prior trastuzumab-based therapy and before initiating treatment with fam-trastuzumab deruxtecan. **(2) Unresectable or metastatic HER2-low or HER2-ultralow breast cancer** based on HER2 expression (IHC 0, IHC 1+ or IHC 2+/ISH-). **(3) Unresectable or metastatic HER2-mutant NSCLC** based on the presence of activating HER2 (ERBB2) mutations in tumor or plasma specimens. If no mutation is detected in a plasma specimen, test tumor tissue. **(4) Unresectable or metastatic HER2-positive solid tumor** based on HER2-positive (IHC 3+) specimens. An FDA-approved test for detection of HER2-positive (IHC 3+) solid tumors for treatment with fam-trastuzumab deruxtecan is not currently available.

Information on FDA-approved tests available at http://www.fda.gov/CompanionDiagnostics.

- Monitor CBC before starting therapy, before each dose, and as clinically indicated. *If Grade 3 neutropenia (ANC<1.0–0.5 × 10⁹/L) occurs,* hold therapy until resolved to Grade ≤2; then resume at same dose. *If Grade 4 neutropenia (ANC < 0.5 × 10⁹/L) occurs,* hold therapy until resolved to Grade ≤2; then ↓ dose by one level. *If febrile neutropenia (ANC <1.0 × 10⁹/L and temperature >38.3°C or a sustained temperature of ≥38°C for >1 hr),* hold therapy until resolved; then ↓ dose by one level. *If Grade 3 thrombocytopenia (platelets <50–25 × 10⁹/L) occurs,* hold therapy until resolved to Grade ≤1; then resume at same dose. *If Grade 4 thrombocytopenia (platelets <25 × 10⁹/L) occurs,* hold therapy until resolved to Grade ≤1; then ↓ dose by one level.

Implementation

- Do not substitute fam-trastuzumab deruxtecan for or with trastuzumab or ado-trastuzumab.
- Fam-trastuzumab deruxtecan is highly emetogenic and may cause delayed nausea and/or vomiting. Administer prophylactic antiemetics per local institutional guidelines for prevention of chemotherapy-induced nausea and vomiting.
- **Dose reduction schedule:** *Breast cancer, NSCLC, or solid tumors:* 1st dose reduction: 4.4 mg/kg. 2nd dose reduction: 3.2 mg/kg. If further dose ↓ needed, discontinue fam-trastuzumab deruxtecan. Do not re-escalate dose after dose ↓ is made. *Gastric cancer:* 1st dose reduction: 5.4 mg/kg. 2nd dose reduction: 4.4 mg/kg. If further dose ↓ needed, discontinue fam-trastuzumab deruxtecan. Do not re-escalate dose after dose ↓ is made.

IV Administration

- **Intermittent Infusion: Reconstitution:** Reconstitute each 100 mg vial with 5 mL of sterile water for injection. **Concentration:** 20 mg/mL. Swirl gently to dissolve; do not shake. Solution is clear and colorless to light yellow; do not use if cloudy, discolored, or contains particulates. **Dilution:** Further dilute reconstituted solution in 100 mL of D5W; do not dilute with 0.9% NaCl. Gently invert to mix; do not shake. Cover infusion bag to protect from light. Diluted solution is stable for 4 hr at room temperature and up to a maximum of 24 hr from reconstitution through infusion if refrigerated; do not freeze. Allow refrigerated solution to reach room temperature before infusion. **Rate:** Infuse 1st infusion over 90 min via an infusion set of polyolefin or polybutadiene and a 0.20- or 0.22-micron in-line polyethersulfone or polysulfone filter. If tolerated, subsequent infusions can be infused over 30 min. Slow rate or interrupt infusion if patient develops infusion-related symptoms. If reaction is severe, discontinue therapy. Do not administer IV push or bolus.
- **Y-Site Incompatibility:** Do not administer other drugs through same IV line.

Patient/Family Teaching

- Explain purpose of therapy to patient. Advise patient to read *Medication Guide* before starting therapy.
- Advise patient to notify health care provider immediately if signs and symptoms of lung problems (cough, trouble breathing, shortness of breath, fever) occur.
- Advise patient to notify health care provider immediately if signs and symptoms of infection (fever, chills) or heart problems (new or worsening shortness of breath, coughing, feeling tired, swelling of ankles or legs, irregular heartbeat, sudden weight gain, dizziness or light-headedness, loss of consciousness) occur.
- Instruct patient to notify health care provider of all Rx or OTC medications, vitamins, or herbal products being taken and to consult with health care provider before taking other medications.
- Rep: May cause fetal harm. Advise women of reproductive potential to use effective contraception and avoid breastfeeding during therapy and for ≥7 mo after last dose. Advise men with female partners of reproductive potential to use effective contraception during and for ≥4 mo after last dose. May impair male fertility.

Evaluation/Desired Outcomes

- Regression of breast cancer and metastases.
- Improved survival in gastric or gastroesophageal junction adenocarcinoma.
- Decreased spread of NSCLC.

febuxostat (fe-**bux**-o-stat)

Uloric

Classification

Therapeutic: antigout agents

Pharmacologic: xanthine oxidase inhibitors

Indications

Chronic management of hyperuricemia in patients with gout who have an inadequate response to a maximally titrated dose of allopurinol, who are intolerant to allopurinol, or in whom allopurinol is not an appropriate treatment option.

Action

Decreases production of uric acid by inhibiting xanthine oxidase. **Therapeutic Effects:** Lowering of serum uric acid levels with resultant decrease in gouty attacks.

Pharmacokinetics

Absorption: 49% absorbed following oral administration.
Distribution: Widely distributed to tissues.
Protein Binding: 99.2%.
Metabolism and Excretion: Extensively metabolized by the liver; minimal renal excretion of unchanged drug; 45% eliminated in feces as unchanged drug; remainder is eliminated in urine and feces as inactive metabolites.
Half-life: 5–8 hr.

TIME/ACTION PROFILE (plasma concentrations)

ROUTE	ONSET	PEAK	DURATION
PO	rapid	1–1.5 hr*	24 hr

* Maximum lowering of uric acid may take 2 wk.

Contraindications/Precautions

Contraindicated in: Concurrent use of azathioprine or mercaptopurine.
Use Cautiously in: Cardiovascular disease (↑ risk of cardiovascular death compared to allopurinol) (consider using low-dose aspirin when using febuxostat in these patients); Previous skin reaction with allopurinol; Severe renal impairment; Severe hepatic impairment; OB: Use during pregnancy only when potential maternal benefit justifies potential fetal risk; Lactation: Safety not established in breastfeeding; Pedi: Safety and effectiveness not established in children.

Adverse Reactions/Side Effects

Derm: DRUG REACTION WITH EOSINOPHILIA AND SYSTEMIC SYMPTOMS (DRESS), rash, STEVENS-JOHNSON SYNDROME, TOXIC EPIDERMAL NECROLYSIS. **GI:** ↑ liver enzymes, nausea. **MS:** arthralgia, gout flare.

Interactions

Drug-Drug: Significantly ↑ levels of and risk of serious toxicity from **azathioprine** and **mercaptopurine**; concurrent use contraindicated. May ↑ levels and risk of toxicity of **theophylline**; use cautiously together.

Route/Dosage

Should only be used in patients who have an inadequate response to a maximally titrated dose of allopurinol, who are intolerant to allopurinol, or for whom treatment with allopurinol is not advisable.
PO (Adults): 40 mg once daily initially; if serum uric acid does not ↓ to <6 mg/dL, ↑ to 80 mg once daily.

Renal Impairment

PO (Adults): *CCr <30 mL/min:* Maximum dose = 40 mg/day.

Availability (generic available)

Tablets: 40 mg, 80 mg.

NURSING IMPLICATIONS

Assessment

- Assess for gout flares (joint pain, swelling), especially during early therapy. Use prophylactic NSAID or colchicine therapy for up to 6 mo. *If a gout flare occurs,* continue febuxostat therapy and treat flare concurrently.
- Monitor for signs and symptoms of MI and stroke.
- Assess patient for skin reactions throughout therapy. Reactions may be severe and life-threatening. *If severe reaction suspected,* discontinue febuxostat.

Lab Test Considerations

- Monitor serum uric acid levels prior to therapy, 2 wk after initiating, and periodically thereafter. *If serum uric acid levels ≥6 mg/dL after 2 wk of daily 40 mg therapy,* ↑ dose to 80 mg daily.
- Monitor liver function at 2 and 4 mo of therapy and periodically thereafter. May cause ↑ AST, ALT, CK, LDH, and alkaline phosphatase.
- May cause prolonged aPTT and PT and ↓ hematocrit, hemoglobin, RBC, platelet count, lymphocyte count, and neutrophil counts. May cause ↑ or ↓ WBC.
- May ↓ serum bicarbonate and ↑ serum sodium, glucose, potassium, and TSH.
- May ↑ serum cholesterol, triglycerides, amylase, and low-density lipoprotein cholesterol.
- May cause ↑ BUN and serum creatinine and proteinuria.

Implementation

- **PO:** May be taken with or without food and with antacids.

Patient/Family Teaching

- Explain purpose and side effects of medication. Advise patient to read *Patient Information* before starting therapy.
- Advise patient if a gout flare occurs to continue febuxostat and notify a health care provider.
- Advise patient to notify health care provider if rash, chest pain, shortness of breath, dizziness, rapid or irregular heartbeat, or stroke symptoms (weakness, blurred vision, headache, confusion, slurred speech) occur or if side effects are persistent or bothersome.
- Instruct patient to notify health care provider of all Rx or OTC medications, vitamins, or herbal products being taken and to consult health care provider before taking any other Rx, OTC, or herbal products.

- Rep: Advise women of reproductive potential to notify health care provider if pregnancy is planned or suspected or if breastfeeding.
- Emphasize the importance of follow-up lab tests to monitor therapy.

Evaluation/Desired Outcomes

- Reduction in serum uric acid levels and resultant gout attacks.

felodipine, See CALCIUM CHANNEL BLOCKERS.

fenofibrate (fen-o-fi-brate)

Antara, ~~Fenoglide,~~ ✽ Lipidil EZ, ✽ Lipidil Supra, Lipofen, ~~Tricor,~~ ~~Triglide,~~ Trilipix

Classification

Therapeutic: lipid-lowering agents

Pharmacologic: fibric acid derivatives

Indications

Severe hypertriglyceridemia (triglycerides ≥500 mg/dL) (as adjunct to diet). Primary hyperlipidemia to lower LDL-C when use of recommended LDL-C-lowering therapy is not possible.

Action

Fenofibric acid primarily inhibits triglyceride synthesis. **Therapeutic Effects:** Lowering of triglycerides and LDL-C.

Pharmacokinetics

Absorption: Well absorbed (60%) after oral administration; absorption ↑ by food.

Distribution: Unknown.

Protein Binding: 99%.

Metabolism and Excretion: Rapidly converted to fenofibric acid, which is the active metabolite; fenofibric acid is metabolized by the liver. Fenofibric acid and its metabolites are primarily excreted in urine (60%).

Half-life: 20 hr.

TIME/ACTION PROFILE (lowering of triglycerides)

ROUTE	ONSET	PEAK	DURATION
PO	unknown	2 wk	unknown

Contraindications/Precautions

Contraindicated in: Hypersensitivity; Hepatic impairment (including primary biliary cirrhosis); Pre-existing gallbladder disease; Severe renal impairment; Lactation: Lactation.

Use Cautiously in: OB: Safety not established in pregnancy; Pedi: Safety and effectiveness not established in children; Geri: Age-related ↓ in renal function may make older patients more susceptible to adverse reactions.

Adverse Reactions/Side Effects

CV: arrhythmias, DEEP VEIN THROMBOSIS. **Derm:** rash, DRUG REACTION WITH EOSINOPHILIA AND SYSTEMIC SYMPTOMS (DRESS), STEVENS-JOHNSON SYNDROME, TOXIC EPIDERMAL NECROLYSIS, urticaria. **GI:** ↑ liver enzymes, cholelithiasis, HEPATOTOXICITY, pancreatitis. **Metab:** ↓ HDL-C. **MS:** RHABDOMYOLYSIS. **Neuro:** fatigue, headache. **Resp:** INTERSTITIAL LUNG DISEASE, PULMONARY EMBOLISM. **Misc:** HYPERSENSITIVITY REACTIONS (INCLUDING ANAPHYLAXIS AND ANGIOEDEMA).

Interactions

Drug-Drug: ↑ risk of bleeding with **warfarin**. Absorption ↓ by **bile acid sequestrants**; give fenofibrate ≥1 hr before or 4–6 hr after. ↑ risk of nephrotoxicity with **cyclosporine**. **Colchicine** may ↑ risk of rhabdomyolysis.

Route/Dosage

Hypertriglyceridemia

PO (Adults): *Antara:* 43–130 mg once daily. *Generic tablets:* 40–160 mg once daily. *Lipofen:* 50–150 mg once daily. *Trilipix:* 45–135 mg once daily.

Renal Impairment

PO (Adults): *CCr 30–<60 mL/min: Antara:* 43 mg once daily initially; may titrate, if needed, up to 130 mg once daily. *Lipofen:* 50 mg once daily initially; may titrate, if needed, up to 150 mg once daily. *Generic tablets:* 40–48 mg once daily initially; may titrate, if needed, up to 120–145 mg once daily. *Trilipix:* 45 mg once daily; may titrate, if needed, up to 135 mg once daily.

Primary Hyperlipidemia

PO (Adults): *Generic tablets:* 120–145 mg once daily. *Lipofen:* 150 mg once daily. *Trilipix:* 135 mg once daily.

Renal Impairment

PO (Adults): *CCr 30–<60 mL/min: Generic tablets:* 40–48 mg once daily; may titrate, if needed, up to 120–145 mg once daily. *Lipofen:* 50 mg once daily initially; may titrate, if needed, up to 150 mg once daily. *Trilipix:* 45 mg once daily; may titrate, if needed, up to 135 mg once daily.

Availability (generic available)

Capsules (generic): 43 mg, 50 mg, 67 mg, 130 mg, 134 mg, 150 mg, 200 mg. **Capsules (Lipofen):** 50 mg, 150 mg. **Micronized capsules (Antara):** 30 mg, 90 mg. **Delayed-release**

capsules (Trilipix): 45 mg, 135 mg. **Tablets (generic):** 40 mg, 48 mg, 54 mg, 120 mg, 145 mg, 160 mg.

NURSING IMPLICATIONS

Assessment

- Before starting therapy with fenofibrate, obtain a diet history. Assess for hyperlipidemia-contributing diseases (hypothyroidism, diabetes mellitus) and medications (estrogen therapy, thiazide diuretics, beta blockers). Intervene as indicated.
- Assess for cholelithiasis. *If symptoms occur,* complete gallbladder studies; discontinue therapy if gallstones found.
- Assess for skin reactions throughout therapy. Reactions may be severe and life-threatening. *If severe reaction or moderate rash with systemic symptoms occurs,* discontinue fenofibrate.

Lab Test Considerations

- Assess serum lipids, including triglycerides, before and periodically during therapy.
- Monitor AST, ALT, and total bilirubin at baseline and periodically during therapy. *If signs of liver injury occur or if elevated enzyme levels persist (ALT or AST >3 times upper limit of normal, or if accompanied by ↑ bilirubin),* discontinue fenofibrate. Do not restart fenofibrate if there is no alternative explanation for hepatotoxicity.
- Assess renal function before and periodically during therapy.
- Monitor for rhabdomyolysis. *If markedly ↑ CK occurs or myopathy suspected,* permanently discontinue fenofibrate.
- May cause mild to moderate ↓ in hemoglobin, hematocrit, and WBC count. Monitor for hematologic changes periodically during 1st 12 mo of therapy. Levels usually stabilize during long-term therapy.
- Monitor PT/INR levels frequently until levels stabilize in patients taking warfarin concurrently.

Implementation

- Encourage a triglyceride-lowering diet before and throughout therapy.
- Dose may be ↑ after repeated serum triglyceride levels every 4–8 wk. Discontinue if response is not adequate after 2 mo of therapy.
- Brands are not interchangeable.
- **PO:** Administer *Lipofen* with food. *Antara* and *Trilipix* may be administered any time of day and without regard to food. ***DNC:*** Swallow capsules and tablets whole; do not open, break, dissolve, or chew.

Patient/Family Teaching

- Explain purpose and side effects of medication to patient. Advise patient to read *Patient Information* before starting therapy.
- Instruct patient to omit missed dose and resume with next scheduled dose; do not double dose.
- Advise patient to follow diet restrictions (fat, cholesterol, carbohydrates, alcohol) and exercise regimen and to stop smoking.
- Instruct patient to notify health care provider if signs and symptoms of liver injury (jaundice, abdominal pain, nausea, malaise, dark urine, abnormal stool, pruritus) or unexplained muscle pain, tenderness, or weakness occurs, especially if accompanied by fever or malaise.
- Instruct patient to notify health care provider of all Rx or OTC medications, vitamins, or herbal products being taken and to consult health care provider before taking other Rx, OTC, or herbal products, especially bile acid sequestrants to avoid impeding absorption.
- Rep: Advise women of reproductive potential to notify health care provider promptly if pregnancy is planned or suspected and to avoid breastfeeding during therapy and for ≥5 days after last dose.
- Emphasize the importance of follow-up exams to determine effectiveness or need for change in dosing and to monitor for side effects.

Evaluation/Desired Outcomes

- ↓ serum triglycerides and cholesterol to normal levels.

HIGH ALERT

fentaNYL (parenteral)

(**fen**-ta-nil)

~~Sublimaze~~

Classification

Therapeutic: opioid analgesics

Pharmacologic: opioid agonists

Schedule II

Indications

Analgesic supplement to general anesthesia, usually with other agents (ultra-short-acting barbiturates, neuromuscular blocking agents, and inhalation anesthetics) to produce balanced anesthesia. Induction/maintenance of anesthesia (in combination with oxygen or oxygen/nitrous oxide and a neuromuscular blocking agent). Neuroleptanalgesia/neuroleptanesthesia (with or without nitrous oxide). Supplement to regional/local anesthesia. Preoperative and postoperative analgesia. **Unlabeled Use:** Continuous IV infusion as part of patient-controlled analgesia.

Action

Binds to opiate receptors in the CNS, altering the response to and perception of pain. Produces CNS depression. **Therapeutic Effects:** Supplement in anesthesia. Decreased pain.

Pharmacokinetics

Absorption: Well absorbed after IM administration. IV administration results in complete bioavailability.

Distribution: Extensively distributed to CNS and tissues.

Metabolism and Excretion: Primarily metabolized by the liver via the CYP3A4 isoenzyme; 10–25% excreted unchanged by the kidneys.

Half-life: *Children:* Bolus dose: 2.4 hr; long-term continuous infusion: 11–36 hr; *Adults:* 2–4 hr (↑ after cardiopulmonary bypass and in geriatric patients).

TIME/ACTION PROFILE (analgesia*)

ROUTE	ONSET	PEAK	DURATION
IM	7–15 min	20–30 min	1–2 hr
IV	1–2 min	3–5 min	0.5–1 hr

* Respiratory depression may last longer than analgesia.

Contraindications/Precautions

Contraindicated in: Hypersensitivity; cross-sensitivity among agents may occur; Known intolerance; Concurrent use of MAO inhibitors.

Use Cautiously in: Personal or family history of substance use disorder or mental illness; Diabetes; Severe renal impairment; Severe hepatic impairment; Severe pulmonary disease; CNS tumors; ↑ intracranial pressure; Head trauma; Adrenal insufficiency; Undiagnosed abdominal pain; Hypothyroidism; Cardiac disease (arrhythmias); OB: Use during pregnancy only if potential maternal benefit justifies potential fetal risk. Chronic maternal treatment with opioids during pregnancy may result in neonatal opioid withdrawal syndrome; Lactation: Use while breastfeeding only if potential maternal benefit justifies potential risk to infant (may cause infant sedation and/or respiratory depression); Geri: Older adults may be more sensitive to effects and may have an ↑ risk of adverse reactions; titrate dosage carefully.

Adverse Reactions/Side Effects

CV: arrhythmias, bradycardia, hypotension. **Derm:** facial itching. **EENT:** blurred/double vision. **Endo:** adrenal insufficiency. **GI:** biliary spasm, nausea, vomiting. **MS:** skeletal and thoracic muscle rigidity (with rapid IV infusion). **Neuro:** confusion, paradoxical excitation/delirium, postoperative drowsiness. **Resp:** allergic bronchospasm, APNEA, LARYNGOSPASM, RESPIRATORY DEPRESSION (INCLUDING CENTRAL SLEEP APNEA AND SLEEP-RELATED HYPOXEMIA). **Misc:** allodynia, opioid-induced hyperalgesia, physical dependence, psychological dependence.

Interactions

Drug-Drug: Concurrent use or within previous 14 days of **MAO inhibitors** may produce unpredictable, potentially fatal reactions and is contraindicated. **CYP3A4 inhibitors**, including **ritonavir**, **ketoconazole**, **itraconazole**, **clarithromycin**, **nelfinavir**, **nefazodone**, **diltiazem**, **aprepitant**, **fluconazole**, **fosamprenavir**, **verapamil**, and **erythromycin**, may ↑ levels and risk of CNS and respiratory depression. **CYP3A4 inducers**, including **barbiturates**, **carbamazepine**, **efavirenz**, **corticosteroids**, **modafinil**, **nevirapine**, **oxcarbazepine**, **phenobarbital**, **phenytoin**, **rifabutin**, or **rifampin**, may ↓ levels and analgesia; if inducers are discontinued or dosage ↓, patients should be monitored for signs of opioid toxicity, and necessary dose adjustments should be made. Use with **benzodiazepines** or other **CNS depressants**, including other **opioids**, **nonbenzodiazepine sedative/hypnotics**, **anxiolytics**, **general anesthetics**, **muscle relaxants**, **antipsychotics**, and **alcohol**, may cause profound sedation, respiratory depression, coma, and death; reserve concurrent use for when alternative treatment options are inadequate. ↑ risk of hypotension with **benzodiazepines**. **Nalbuphine** or **buprenorphine** may ↓ analgesia. Drugs that affect serotonergic neurotransmitter systems, including **tricyclic antidepressants**, **SSRIs**, **SNRIs**, **MAO inhibitors**, **TCAs**, **tramadol**, **trazodone**, **mirtazapine**, **5-HT$_3$ receptor antagonists**, **linezolid**, **methylene blue**, and **triptans**, ↑ risk of serotonin syndrome.

Drug-Food: Grapefruit juice may ↑ levels and the risk of respiratory and CNS depression.

Route/Dosage

Preoperative Use

IM, IV (Adults and Children >12 yr): 50–100 mcg 30–60 min before surgery.

Adjunct to General Anesthesia

IM, IV (Adults and Children >12 yr): *Low dose: minor surgery:* 2 mcg/kg. *Moderate dose: major surgery:* 2–20 mcg/kg. *High dose: major surgery:* 20–50 mcg/kg.

Adjunct to Regional Anesthesia

IM, IV (Adults and Children >12 yr): 50–100 mcg.

Postoperative Use (Recovery Room)

IM, IV (Adults and Children >12 yr): 50–100 mcg; may repeat in 1–2 hr.

General Anesthesia

IV (Adults and Children >12 yr): 50–100 mcg/kg (up to 150 mcg/kg).

IV (Children 1–12 yr): 2–3 mcg/kg.

Sedation/Analgesia

IV (Adults and Children >12 yr): 0.5–1 mcg/kg/dose; may repeat after 30–60 min.

IV (Children 1–12 yr): *Bolus:* 1–2 mcg/kg/dose; may repeat at 30–60 min intervals. *Continuous infusion:* 1–5 mcg/kg/hr following bolus dose.

IV (Neonates): *Bolus:* 0.5–3 mcg/kg/dose. *Continuous infusion:* 0.5–2 mcg/kg/hr following bolus dose. *Continuous infusion during ECMO:* 5–10 mcg/kg bolus followed by 1–5 mcg/kg/hr; may require up to 20 mcg/kg/hr after 5 days of therapy.

Availability (generic available)

Solution for injection: 50 mcg/mL.

NURSING IMPLICATIONS

Assessment

- Assess type, location, and intensity of pain prior to and 30 min following IM and 5 min (peak) following IV administration. When titrating opioid doses, increases of 25–50% should be administered until there is either a 50% ↓ in the patient's pain rating on a numerical or visual analogue scale or the patient reports satisfactory pain relief.
- Assess BP, HR, and respiratory rate before and periodically during administration. If respiratory rate <10/min, assess level of sedation. Dose may need to be ↓ by 25–50%. Respiratory depression does not ↑ in severity, only in duration, with ↑ dose. Monitor for respiratory depression, especially during initiation or following dose ↑; serious, life-threatening, or fatal respiratory depression may occur. The respiratory depressant effects of fentanyl may last longer than the analgesic effects. May cause sleep-related breathing disorders (central sleep apnea, sleep-related hypoxemia).
- Geri: Opioids have been associated with ↑ risk of falls in older adults. Assess risk and implement fall prevention strategies.
- Assess type, location, and intensity of pain before and 30 min after IM administration or 3–5 min after IV administration when fentanyl is used to treat pain.
- Assess for opioid-induced hyperalgesia, which can appear as ↑ levels of pain upon increasing the dose of the opioid, ↓ levels of pain upon decreasing the dose of the opioid, or pain from ordinarily nonpainful stimuli (allodynia). This condition is different from tolerance. If a patient is suspected to be experiencing opioid-induced hyperalgesia, consider ↓ the dose of the current opioid or switching to a different opioid analgesic.
- Assess risk for opioid addiction, abuse, or misuse prior to administration.

Lab Test Considerations

- May cause ↑ serum amylase and lipase concentrations.

Toxicity and Overdose

- Symptoms of toxicity include respiratory depression, hypotension, arrhythmias, bradycardia, and asystole. Atropine may be used to treat bradycardia. If respiratory depression persists after surgery, prolonged mechanical ventilation may be required. If an opioid antagonist is required to reverse respiratory depression or coma, naloxone is the antidote. Dilute the 0.4-mg ampule of naloxone in 10 mL of 0.9% NaCl and administer 0.5 mL (0.02 mg) by IV push every 2 min. Pedi: For children and patients weighing <40 kg, dilute 0.1 mg of naloxone in 10 mL of 0.9% NaCl for a concentration of 10 mcg/mL and administer 0.5 mcg/kg every 2 min. Titrate dose to avoid withdrawal, seizures, and severe pain. Administration of naloxone in these circumstances, especially in cardiac patients, has resulted in hypertension and tachycardia, occasionally causing left ventricular failure and pulmonary edema.

Implementation

- ***High Alert:*** Accidental overdosage of opioid analgesics has resulted in fatalities. Before administering, clarify all ambiguous orders; have second practitioner independently check original order, dose calculations, route of administration, and infusion pump programming.
- Do not confuse fentanyl with sufentanil.
- Benzodiazepines may be administered before or after administration of fentanyl to reduce the induction dose requirements, ↓ the time to loss of consciousness, and produce amnesia. This combination may also ↑ the risk of hypotension and respiratory depression.
- Explain therapeutic value of medication prior to administration to enhance the analgesic effect.
- Regularly administered doses may be more effective than prn administration. Analgesic is more effective if given before pain becomes severe.
- Coadministration with nonopioid analgesics may have additive analgesic effects and permit lower opioid doses.
- Medication should be discontinued gradually after long-term use to prevent withdrawal symptoms.
- May cause muscle rigidity, particularly involving muscles of respiration; effects are related to the dose and speed of injection. Effects can be reduced by (1) administration of up to ¼ of the full paralyzing dose of a nondepolarizing neuromuscular blocking agent just prior to administration of fentanyl; (2) administration of a full paralyzing dose of a neuromuscular blocking agent following loss of eyelash reflex when fentanyl is used in anesthetic doses titrated by slow intravenous infusion; or (3) simultaneous administration of fentanyl and a full paralyzing dose of a neuromuscular blocking agent when fentanyl is used in rapidly administered anesthetic doses.

IV Administration

- **IV Push: Dilution:** Administer undiluted. **Concentration:** 50 mcg/mL. **Rate:** Inject slowly over 1–3 min. Administer doses >5 mcg/kg over 5–10 min. Slow IV administration may ↓ the incidence and severity of muscle rigidity, bradycardia, or hypotension. Neuromuscular blocking agents may be administered concurrently to ↓ chest wall muscle rigidity.

- **Intermittent Infusion: Dilution:** May be diluted in D5W or 0.9% NaCl. **Concentration:** Up to 50 mcg/mL. **Rate:** See IV Push.
- **Y-Site Compatibility:** acyclovir, alemtuzumab, alprostadil, amikacin, aminocaproic acid, aminophylline, amphotericin B liposomal, anidulafungin, argatroban, arsenic trioxide, ascorbic acid, atracurium, atropine, azathioprine, aztreonam, benztropine, bivalirudin, bleomycin, bumetanide, buprenorphine, butorphanol, calcium chloride, calcium gluconate, cangrelor, carboplatin, carmustine, caspofungin, cefazolin, cefiderocol, cefotaxime, cefotetan, cefoxitin, ceftaroline, ceftazidime, ceftobiprole, ceftolozane/tazobactam, ceftriaxone, cefuroxime, chloramphenicol, chlorpromazine, cisatracurium, cisplatin, clindamycin, cyanocobalamin, cyclophosphamide, cyclosporine, cytarabine, dacarbazine, dactinomycin, daptomycin, daunorubicin, dexamethasone, dexmedetomidine, dexrazoxane, digoxin, diltiazem, diphenhydramine, dobutamine, docetaxel, dopamine, doxorubicin hydrochloride, doxorubicin liposomal, doxycycline, enalaprilat, ephedrine, epinephrine, epirubicin, epoetin alfa, eptifibatide, eravacycline, erythromycin, esmolol, etomidate, etoposide, etoposide phosphate, famotidine, fluconazole, fludarabine, fluorouracil, folic acid, foscarnet, fosphenytoin, furosemide, ganciclovir, gemcitabine, gentamicin, glycopyrrolate, granisetron, heparin, hetastarch, hydrocortisone, hydromorphone, idarubicin, ifosfamide, imipenem/cilastatin, imipenem/cilastatin/relebactam, indomethacin, insulin, regular, irinotecan, isavuconazonium, isoproterenol, ketorolac, labetalol, letermovir, leucovorin, levofloxacin, lidocaine, linezolid, lorazepam, magnesium sulfate, mannitol, meperidine, meropenem, meropenem/vaborbactam, mesna, methotrexate, methylprednisolone, metoclopramide, metoprolol, metronidazole, midazolam, milrinone, minocycline, mitomycin, mitoxantrone, morphine, multivitamins, mycophenolate, nafcillin, nalbuphine, naloxone, nicardipine, nitroglycerin, nitroprusside, norepinephrine, octreotide, ondansetron, oritavancin, oxacillin, oxaliplatin, oxytocin, paclitaxel, palonosetron, pamidronate, papaverine, pemetrexed, penicillin G, pentamidine, pentobarbital, phenobarbital, phentolamine, phenylephrine, phytonadione, piperacillin/tazobactam, plazomicin, potassium acetate, potassium chloride, procainamide, prochlorperazine, promethazine, propofol, propranolol, protamine, pyridoxine, remdesivir, remifentanil, remimazolam, rituximab, rocuronium, sargramostim, scopolamine, sodium acetate, sodium bicarbonate, succinylcholine, sufentanil, sulbactam/durlobactam, tacrolimus, tedizolid, theophylline, thiamine, thiotepa, tigecycline, tirofiban, tobramycin, topotecan, trastuzumab, vancomycin, vasopressin, vecuronium, verapamil, vinblastine, vincristine, vinorelbine, voriconazole, zoledronic acid.
- **Y-Site Incompatibility:** dantrolene, diazoxide, gemtuzumab ozogamicin, phenytoin, trimethoprim/sulfamethoxazole.

F

Patient/Family Teaching

- Discuss the use of anesthetic agents and the sensations to expect with the patient before surgery.
- Instruct patient on how and when to ask for pain medication. Explain pain assessment scale to patient.
- Advise patient to notify health care provider if pain control is not adequate or if side effects occur.
- Caution patient to change positions slowly to minimize orthostatic hypotension. Geri: Older adults may be at a greater risk for orthostatic hypotension and consequently falls. Teach patient to take precautions until drug effects have completely resolved.
- Medication causes dizziness and drowsiness. Advise patient to call for assistance during ambulation and transfer and to avoid driving or other activities requiring alertness for 24 hr after administration during outpatient surgery.
- Instruct patient to notify health care provider of all Rx or OTC medications, vitamins, or herbal products being taken and consult health care provider before taking any new medications.
- Encourage patient to turn, cough, and breathe deeply every 2 hr to prevent atelectasis.
- Instruct patient to avoid alcohol or other CNS depressants for 24 hr after administration for outpatient surgery.
- Rep: Advise women of reproductive potential to notify health care provider if pregnancy is planned or suspected or if breastfeeding. Inform patient of potential for neonatal opioid withdrawal syndrome with prolonged use during pregnancy. Monitor neonate for signs and symptoms of withdrawal symptoms (irritability, hyperactivity and abnormal sleep pattern, high-pitched cry, tremor, vomiting, diarrhea, failure to gain weight); usually occur the first days after birth. Monitor infants exposed to fentanyl through breast milk for excess sedation and respiratory depression.

Evaluation/Desired Outcomes

- General quiescence.
- Reduced motor activity.
- Pronounced analgesia.

REMS HIGH ALERT

fentaNYL (transdermal)

(**fen**-ta-nil)

~~Duragesic~~

Classification

Therapeutic: opioid analgesics

Pharmacologic: opioid agonists

Schedule II

Indications

Moderate to severe chronic pain in opioid-tolerant patients requiring use of daily, around-the-clock long-term opioid treatment and for which alternative treatment options are inadequate (extended release). Transdermal fentanyl is not recommended for the control of postoperative, mild, or intermittent pain, and it should not be used for short-term pain relief.

Action

Binds to opiate receptors in the CNS, altering the response to and perception of pain. **Therapeutic Effects:** Decrease in severity of chronic pain.

Pharmacokinetics

Absorption: Well absorbed (92% of dose) through skin surface under transdermal patch, creating a depot in the upper skin layers. Release from transdermal system into systemic circulation ↑ gradually to a constant rate, providing continuous delivery for 72 hr.

Distribution: Widely distributed to tissues.

Metabolism and Excretion: Mostly metabolized by the liver via the CYP3A4 isoenzyme; 10–25% excreted unchanged by the kidneys.

Half-life: 17 hr after removal of a single application patch; ↑ to 21 hr after removal of multiple patches (because of continued release from deposition of drug in skin layers).

TIME/ACTION PROFILE (analgesia)

ROUTE	ONSET	PEAK	DURATION
Transdermal	6 hr†	12–24 hr	72 hr‡

† Achievement of plasma concentrations associated with analgesia. Maximal response and dose titration may take up to 6 days.

‡ While patch is worn.

Contraindications/Precautions

Contraindicated in: Hypersensitivity to fentanyl or adhesives; Patients who are not opioid tolerant; Acute, mild, intermittent, or postoperative pain; Significant respiratory depression; Acute or severe bronchial asthma; Paralytic ileus; Severe hepatic or renal impairment; Alcohol intolerance (small amounts of alcohol released into skin); OB: Not recommended during labor and delivery; Lactation: Lactation.

Use Cautiously in: Personal or family history of substance use disorder or mental illness; Diabetes; Patients with severe pulmonary disease; Mild or moderate hepatic or renal impairment; CNS tumors; ↑ intracranial pressure; Head trauma; Adrenal insufficiency; Undiagnosed abdominal pain; Hypothyroidism; Cardiac disease (particularly bradyarrhythmias); Fever or situations that ↑ body temperature (↑ release of fentanyl from delivery system); Cachectic or debilitated patients (dose ↓ suggested because of altered drug disposition); OB: Avoid chronic use; prolonged use of opioids during pregnancy can result in neonatal opioid withdrawal syndrome; Pedi: Children <2 yr (safety not established); pediatric patients initiating therapy at 25 mcg/hr should be opioid tolerant and receiving at least 60 mg oral morphine equivalents per day; Geri: ↑ risk of respiratory depression in older adults (dose ↓ suggested).

Adverse Reactions/Side Effects

CV: bradycardia, hypotension. **Derm:** sweating, erythema. **Endo:** adrenal insufficiency. **GI:** anorexia, constipation, dry mouth, nausea, vomiting. **Local:** application site reactions. **MS:** skeletal and thoracic muscle rigidity. **Neuro:** confusion, sedation, weakness, dizziness, restlessness. **Resp:** APNEA, bronchoconstriction, laryngospasm, RESPIRATORY DEPRESSION (INCLUDING CENTRAL SLEEP APNEA AND SLEEP-RELATED HYPOXEMIA). **Misc:** allodynia, opioid-induced hyperalgesia, physical dependence, psychological dependence.

Interactions

Drug-Drug: Avoid use in patients who have received **MAO inhibitors** within the previous 14 days (may produce unpredictable, potentially fatal reactions). Concurrent use of **CYP3A4 inhibitors**, including **ritonavir**, **ketoconazole**, **itraconazole**, **clarithromycin**, **nelfinavir**, **nefazodone**, **amiodarone**, **diltiazem**, **aprepitant**, **fluconazole**, **fosamprenavir**, **verapamil**, and **erythromycin**, may result in ↑ levels and ↑ risk of CNS and respiratory depression. **CYP3A4 inducers**, including **barbiturates**, **carbamazepine**, **efavirenz**, **corticosteroids**, **modafinil**, **nevirapine**, **oxcarbazepine**, **phenobarbital**, **phenytoin**, **rifabutin**, or **rifampin**, may ↓ levels and analgesia; if inducers are discontinued or dosage ↓, patients should be monitored for signs of opioid toxicity and necessary dose adjustments should be made. Use with **benzodiazepines** or other **CNS depressants**, including other **opioids**, **nonbenzodiazepine sedative/hypnotics**, **anxiolytics**, **general anesthetics**, **muscle relaxants**, **antipsychotics**, and **alcohol**, may cause profound sedation, respiratory depression, coma, and death; reserve concurrent use for when alternative treatment options are inadequate. **Mixed agonist/antagonist analgesics**, including **nalbuphine** or **butorphanol**, and **partial agonist analgesics**, including **buprenorphine**, may ↓ fentanyl's analgesic effects and/or precipitate opioid withdrawal in physically dependent patients. Drugs that affect serotonergic neurotransmitter systems, including **tricyclic antidepressants, SSRIs, SNRIs, MAO inhibitors, TCAs, tramadol, trazodone, mirtazapine, 5-HT$_3$ receptor antagonists, linezolid, methylene blue**, and **triptans**, ↑ risk of serotonin syndrome.

Drug-Natural Products: Concurrent use of **kava-kava, valerian,** or **chamomile** can ↑ CNS depression.

Drug-Food: Grapefruit juice may ↑ levels and the risk of respiratory and CNS depression. Careful monitoring and dose adjustment is recommended.

Route/Dosage

Transdermal (Adults): 25 mcg/hr is the initial dose; patients who have not been receiving opioids should receive not more than 25 mcg/hr. To calculate the dose of transdermal fentanyl required in patients who are already receiving opioid analgesics, assess the 24-hr requirement of currently used opioid. Using the equianalgesic table in Appendix I, convert this to an equivalent amount of morphine/24 hr. Conversion to fentanyl transdermal may be accomplished by using the fentanyl conversion table (Appendix I). During dose titration, additional short-acting opioids should be available for breakthrough pain. Morphine 10 mg IM or 60 mg PO every 4 hr (60 mg/24 hr IM or 360 mg/24 hr PO) is considered to be approximately equivalent to transdermal fentanyl 100 mcg/hr. Transdermal patch lasts 72 hr in most patients. Some patients require a new patch every 48 hr.

Transdermal (Adults >60 yr, Debilitated, or Cachectic Patients): Initial dose should be 25 mcg/hr unless previous opioid use was >135 mg morphine PO/day (or other opioid equivalent).

Hepatic Impairment

Transdermal (Adults): *Mild to moderate hepatic impairment:* 12 mcg/hr is the initial dose.

Renal Impairment

Transdermal (Adults): *Mild to moderate renal impairment:* 12 mcg/hr is the initial dose.

Availability (generic available)

Transdermal systems: 12.5 mcg/hr, 25 mcg/hr, 37.5 mcg/hr, 50 mcg/hr, 62.5 mcg/hr, 75 mcg/hr, 87.5 mcg/hr, 100 mcg/hr.

NURSING IMPLICATIONS

Assessment

- Assess type, location, and intensity of pain before and 24 hr after application and periodically during therapy. Monitor pain frequently during initiation of therapy and dose changes to assess need for supplementary analgesics for breakthrough pain.
- Assess BP, HR, and respiratory rate before and periodically during administration. If respiratory rate <10/min, assess level of sedation. Dose may need to be ↓ by 25–50%. Respiratory depression does not ↑ in severity, only in duration, with ↑ dose. Monitor for respiratory depression, especially during initiation or following dose ↑; serious, life-threatening, or fatal respiratory depression may occur. May cause sleep-related breathing disorders (central sleep apnea, sleep-related hypoxemia).
- Prolonged use may lead to physical and psychological dependence and tolerance. This should not prevent patient from receiving adequate analgesia. Most patients who receive opioid analgesics for pain rarely develop psychological dependence.
- Assess for opioid-induced hyperalgesia, which can appear as ↑ levels of pain upon increasing the dose of the opioid, ↓ levels of pain upon decreasing the dose of the opioid, or pain from ordinarily nonpainful stimuli (allodynia). This condition is different from tolerance. If a patient is suspected to be experiencing opioid-induced hyperalgesia, consider ↓ the dose of the current opioid or switching to a different opioid analgesic.
- Progressively higher doses may be required to relieve pain with long-term therapy. It may take up to 6 days after ↑ doses to reach equilibrium, so patients should wear higher dose through two applications before ↑ dose again. ↑ doses and prolonged use may ↑ risk of overdose. Prolonged use of opioids should be reserved for patients whose pain remains severe enough to require them and alternative treatment options continue to be inadequate. Many acute pain conditions treated in the outpatient setting require no more than a few days of an opioid pain medicine.
- Assess bowel function routinely. Prevent constipation with increased intake of fluids and bulk, and laxatives to minimize constipating effects. Administer stimulant laxatives routinely if opioid use exceeds 2–3 days, unless contraindicated. Consider drugs for opioid-induced constipation.
- Assess risk for opioid addiction, abuse, or misuse prior to administration. Misuse or abuse of *transdermal fentanyl* by chewing, swallowing, snorting, or injecting fentanyl extracted from transdermal system will result in the uncontrolled delivery of fentanyl and risk of overdose and death.

Lab Test Considerations

- May ↑ plasma amylase and lipase levels.

Toxicity and Overdose

- If an opioid antagonist is required to reverse respiratory depression or coma, naloxone is the antidote. Dilute the 0.4-mg ampule of naloxone in 10 mL of 0.9% NaCl and administer 0.5 mL

F

(0.02 mg) by IV push every 2 min. For patients weighing <40 kg, dilute 0.1 mg of naloxone in 10 mL of 0.9% NaCl for a concentration of 10 mcg/mL and administer 0.5 mcg/kg every 2 min. Titrate dose to avoid withdrawal, seizures, and severe pain. Monitor patient closely; dose may need to be repeated or may need to be administered as an infusion because of long duration of action despite removal of patch.

Implementation

- Do not confuse fentanyl with sufentanil.
- ***High Alert:*** Accidental overdose of opioid analgesics has resulted in fatalities. Before administering, confirm patient is opioid tolerant and clarify ambiguous orders.
- 12-mcg patch delivers 12.5 mcg/hr of fentanyl. Use supplemental doses of short-acting opioid analgesics to manage pain until relief is obtained with the transdermal system. Patients may continue to require supplemental opioids for breakthrough pain. If >100 mcg/hr is required, use multiple transdermal systems.
- Titrate dose based on patient's report of pain until adequate analgesia (50% ↓ in patient's pain rating on numerical or visual analogue scale or patient reports satisfactory relief) is attained. Determine dose by calculating the previous 24-hr analgesic requirement and converting to the equianalgesic morphine dose using Appendix I. The conversion ratio from morphine to transdermal fentanyl is conservative; 50% of patients may require a dose ↑ after initial application. ↑ after 3 days based on required daily doses of supplemental analgesics. Base increases on ratio of 45 mg/24 hr of oral morphine to 12.5 mcg/hr ↑ in transdermal fentanyl dose.
- Coadministration with nonopioid analgesics may have additive analgesic effects and permit lower opioid doses.
- To convert to another opioid analgesic, remove transdermal fentanyl system and begin treatment with half the equianalgesic dose of the new analgesic in 12–18 hr.
- Discontinue medication gradually after long-term use to prevent withdrawal symptoms. May be necessary to provide patient with a lower dose strength for a successful taper. Monitor frequently to manage pain and withdrawal symptoms (restlessness; lacrimation; rhinorrhea; yawning; perspiration; chills; myalgia; mydriasis; irritability; anxiety; backache; joint pain; weakness; abdominal cramps; insomnia; nausea; anorexia; vomiting; diarrhea; or ↑ BP, respiratory rate, or heart rate). If withdrawal symptoms occur, pause the taper for a period of time or ↑ the dose of opioid analgesic to the previous dose, and then proceed with a slower taper. Also, monitor patients for changes in mood, emergence of suicidal thoughts, or use of other substances. A multimodal approach to pain management may optimize the treatment of chronic pain and assist with the successful tapering of the opioid analgesic.
- ***REMS:*** FDA strongly encourages health care providers to complete a REMS-compliant education program that includes all the elements of the FDA Education *Blueprint for Health Care Providers Involved in the Management or Support of Patients with Pain,* available at www.fda.gov/OpioidAnalgesicREMSBlueprint. Information on programs can be found at 1-800-503-0784 or www.opioidanalgesicrems.com.
- Discuss availability of naloxone for emergency treatment of opioid overdose with the patient and caregiver and assess the potential need for access to naloxone, both when initiating and renewing therapy, especially if patient has household members (including children) or other close contacts at risk for accidental exposure or overdose. Consider prescribing naloxone, based on the patient's risk factors for overdose, such as concurrent use of CNS depressants, a history of opioid use disorder, or prior opioid overdose. However, the presence of risk factors for overdose should not prevent the proper management of pain in any patient.
- **Transdermal:** Apply system to flat, nonirritated, and nonirradiated site such as chest, back, flank, or upper arm. If skin preparation is necessary, use clear water and clip (do not shave) hair. Allow skin to dry completely before application. Apply immediately after removing from package. Do not alter the system (cut) in any way before application. Remove liner from adhesive layer and press firmly in place with palm of hand for 30 sec, especially around the edges, to make sure contact is complete. Remove used system and fold so that adhesive edges are together. Follow the institutional disposal policy following removal of the patch. Apply new system to a different site.

Patient/Family Teaching

- ***REMS:*** Instruct patient in how and when to ask for and take pain medication. Do not ↑ doses without discussing with health care provider; may lead to overdose. Discuss safe use, risks, and proper storage and disposal of opioid analgesics with patients and caregivers with each Rx. The Patient Counseling Guide is available at www.fda.gov/OpioidAnalgesicREMSPCG. Advise patient to read *Medication Guide* before starting therapy and with each Rx refill in case of changes.
- Instruct patient in correct method for application and disposal of transdermal system. Fatalities have occurred from children having access to improperly discarded patches. May be worn while bathing, showering, or swimming.
- Advise patient to avoid grapefruit juice during therapy.

- Advise patient that fentanyl is a drug with known abuse potential. Protect it from theft, and never give to anyone other than the individual for whom it was prescribed. Store out of sight and reach of children and in a location not accessible by others.
- Educate patients and caregivers on how to recognize respiratory depression and emphasize the importance of calling 911 or getting emergency medical help right away in the event of a known or suspected overdose. Inform patients and caregivers about various ways to obtain naloxone as permitted by individual state naloxone dispensing and prescribing requirements or guidelines (by prescription, directly from a pharmacist, or as part of a community-based program).
- May cause drowsiness or dizziness. Caution patient to call for assistance when ambulating or smoking and to avoid driving or other activities requiring alertness until response to medication is known.
- Advise patient to change positions slowly to minimize dizziness.
- Caution patient to avoid concurrent use of alcohol or other CNS depressants with this medication.
- Caution patient that fever, electric blankets, heating pads, saunas, hot tubs, and heated water beds ↑ the release of fentanyl from the patch and can result in fatal overdose.
- Advise patient that good oral hygiene, frequent mouth rinses, and sugarless gum or candy may ↓ dry mouth.
- Advise patient to notify health care provider of all Rx or OTC medications, vitamins, or herbal products being taken and to consult with health care provider before taking other medications.
- Advise patient referred for MRI test to discuss patch with referring health care provider and MRI facility to determine if removal of patch is necessary prior to test and for directions for replacing patch.
- Rep: Advise women of reproductive potential to notify health care provider if pregnancy is planned or suspected and to avoid breastfeeding during therapy. Inform patient of potential for neonatal opioid withdrawal syndrome with prolonged use during pregnancy. Monitor neonate for signs and symptoms of withdrawal symptoms (irritability, hyperactivity and abnormal sleep pattern, high-pitched cry, tremor, vomiting, diarrhea, failure to gain weight); usually occur the first days after birth. Monitor infants exposed to fentanyl through breast milk for excess sedation and respiratory depression. Chronic use may ↓ fertility in women and men.

Evaluation/Desired Outcomes

- Decrease in severity of pain without a significant alteration in level of consciousness, respiratory status, or BP.

ferrous sulfate (30% elemental iron)

(fer-us sul-fate)

Classification

Therapeutic: antianemics

Pharmacologic: iron supplements

Indications

PO: Treatment and prevention of iron deficiency anemia.

Action

An essential mineral found in hemoglobin, myoglobin, and many enzymes. Enters the bloodstream and is transported to the organs of the reticuloendothelial system (liver, spleen, bone marrow) where it becomes part of iron stores. **Therapeutic Effects:** Resolution or prevention of iron deficiency anemia.

Pharmacokinetics

Absorption: Approximately 5–10% of dietary iron is absorbed (up to 30% in deficiency states). Therapeutically administered PO iron is up to 60% absorbed via active and passive transport processes.

Distribution: Remains in the body for many months.

Protein Binding: ≥90%.

Metabolism and Excretion: Mostly recycled; small daily losses occurring via desquamation, sweat, urine, and bile.

Half-life: Unknown.

TIME/ACTION PROFILE (effects on erythropoiesis)

ROUTE	ONSET	PEAK	DURATION
PO	4 days	7–10 days	2–4 mo

Contraindications/Precautions

Contraindicated in: Hypersensitivity to iron products; Anemia not due to iron deficiency; Hemochromatosis; Hemosiderosis.

Use Cautiously in: Peptic ulcer disease; Ulcerative colitis or regional enteritis (condition may be aggravated); Alcoholism; Severe renal impairment. Severe hepatic impairment.

Adverse Reactions/Side Effects

GI: constipation, dark stools, epigastric pain, nausea, GI bleeding, vomiting. **Neuro:** dizziness, headache, syncope. **Misc:** temporary staining of teeth (liquid preparations).

Interactions

Drug-Drug: May ↓ absorption and effects of **tetracyclines**, **fluoroquinolones**, **bisphosphonates**, **levodopa**, **levothyroxine**, **mycophenolate mofetil**, and **penicillamine**; avoid simultaneous administration. Concurrent administration of **proton pump inhibitors**, **H_2 antagonists**, and **cholestyramine** may ↓ absorption of iron. Doses of **ascorbic acid** ≥200 mg may ↑ absorption of iron by up to 30%. **Chloramphenicol** and **vitamin E** may ↓ hematologic response to iron therapy.
Drug-Food: Iron absorption is ↓ 33–50% by concurrent administration of food.

Route/Dosage

Oral iron dosages are expressed as mg of elemental iron. Multiple salt forms exist; see approximate equivalent doses below or consider % elemental iron of each salt for dose conversions.
Approximate Equivalent Doses (mg of iron salt): ***Ferrous fumarate:*** **197;** ***Ferrous gluconate:*** **560;** ***Ferrous sulfate:*** **324;** ***Ferrous sulfate, exsiccated:*** **217.**
PO (Adults): *Deficiency:* 2–3 mg/kg/day in 2–4 divided doses or 60–100 mg elemental iron twice daily. *Prophylaxis:* 60–100 mg elemental iron daily.
PO (Infants and Children): *Severe deficiency:* 4–6 mg/kg/day in 3 divided doses. *Mild to moderate deficiency:* 3 mg/kg/day in 1–2 divided doses. *Prophylaxis:* 1–2 mg/kg/day in 1–2 divided dose (maximum: 15 mg/day).
PO (Neonates, premature): 2–4 mg/kg/day in 1–2 divided doses, maximum of 15 mg/day.

Availability (generic available)

Tablets: 325 mg^{OTC}. **Delayed-release tablets:** 142 mg^{OTC}, 160 mg^{OTC}, 325 mg^{OTC}. **Solution:** 75 mg/mL^{OTC}, 300 mg/5 mL^{OTC}. **Elixir:** 220 mg/5 mL^{OTC}.

NURSING IMPLICATIONS

Assessment

- Assess nutritional status and dietary history to determine possible cause of anemia and need for patient teaching.
- Assess bowel function for constipation or diarrhea. Notify health care professional and use appropriate nursing measures should these occur.

Lab Test Considerations

- Monitor hemoglobin, hematocrit, and reticulocyte values prior to and every 3 wk during the 1st 2 mo of therapy and periodically thereafter. Serum ferritin and iron levels may also be monitored to assess effectiveness of therapy. Occult blood in stools may be obscured by black coloration of iron in stool. Guaiac test results may occasionally be false-positive. Benzidine test results are not affected by iron preparations.

Toxicity and Overdose

- Early symptoms of overdose include stomach pain, fever, nausea, vomiting (may contain blood), and diarrhea. Late symptoms include bluish lips, fingernails, and palms; drowsiness; weakness; tachycardia; seizures; metabolic acidosis; hepatic injury; and cardiovascular collapse. Patient may appear to recover prior to the onset of late symptoms. Therefore, hospitalization continues for 24 hr after patient becomes asymptomatic to monitor for delayed onset of shock or GI bleeding. Late complications of overdose include intestinal obstruction, pyloric stenosis, and gastric scarring.
- If patient is comatose or seizing, gastric lavage with sodium bicarbonate is performed. Deferoxamine is the antidote. Additional supportive treatments to maintain fluid and electrolyte balance and correction of metabolic acidosis are also indicated.

Implementation

- Discontinue oral iron preparations before parenteral administration.
- **PO:** Administer 1 hr before or 2 hr after meals. If GI irritation occurs, administer with meals. Take tablets with 8 ounces of water or juice. ***DNC:*** Do not crush or chew enteric-coated tablets.
- Liquid preparations may stain teeth. Dilute in water or fruit juice (240 mL for adults and 120 mL for children) and administer with a straw or place drops at back of throat.
- Avoid using antacids, coffee, tea, dairy products, eggs, or whole-grain breads with or within 1 hr after administration of ferrous sulfate. Iron absorption is ↓ by 33% if iron is given with meals.

Patient/Family Teaching

- Explain purpose and side effects of medication. Advise patient to read *Patient Information* before starting therapy. Instruct patient to take as directed. Take missed doses as soon as remembered within 12 hr; otherwise, return to regular dosing schedule. Do not double doses.
- Advise patient to notify health care professional of all Rx or OTC medications, vitamins, or herbal products being taken and to consult health care professional before taking other medications.
- Advise patient that stools may become dark green or black.
- Instruct patient to follow a diet high in iron (see Appendix J).
- Pedi: Discuss with caregivers the risk of a child overdosing on iron. Medication should be stored in the

original childproof container and kept out of reach of children. Do not refer to vitamins as candy. In the event of a suspected overdose, caregivers should contact poison control center (1-800-222-1222) or seek emergency medical treatment immediately.

- Rep: Advise women of reproductive potential to notify health care professional if pregnancy is planned or suspected or if breastfeeding.

Evaluation/Desired Outcomes

- Resolution or prevention of iron deficiency anemia.

fesoterodine

(fes-oh-**ter**-o-deen)

Toviaz

Classification

Therapeutic: urinary tract antispasmodics

Pharmacologic: anticholinergics

Indications

Overactive bladder with symptoms of urinary frequency, urgency, and urge incontinence. Neurogenic detrusor overactivity.

Action

Acts as a competitive muscarinic receptor antagonist resulting in inhibition of cholinergically mediated bladder contraction. **Therapeutic Effects:** Decreased urinary frequency, urgency, and urge incontinence in overactive bladder. Increase in maximum cystometric bladder capacity in neurogenic detrusor overactivity.

Pharmacokinetics

Absorption: Rapidly absorbed following oral administration but is rapidly converted to its active metabolite (bioavailability of metabolite 52%).

Distribution: Unknown.

Metabolism and Excretion: Primarily metabolized in the liver via the CYP2D6 and CYP3A4 isoenzymes; the CYP2D6 enzyme system exhibits genetic polymorphism; ~7% of population may be poor metabolizers and may have significantly ↑ fesoterodine concentrations and an ↑ risk of adverse effects. 16% of active metabolite is excreted in urine; most of the remainder of inactive metabolites are renally excreted. 7% excreted in feces.

Half-life: 7 hr.

TIME/ACTION PROFILE (plasma concentrations of active metabolite)

ROUTE	ONSET	PEAK	DURATION
O	rapid	5 hr	24 hr

Contraindications/Precautions

Contraindicated in: Hypersensitivity; Urinary retention; Significant bladder outlet obstruction (↑ risk of retention); Gastric retention; ↓ GI motility including severe constipation; Severe hepatic impairment; Uncontrolled narrow-angle glaucoma; Pedi: eGFR <15 mL/min/1.73 m² or requiring dialysis (children ≥6 yr and >35 kg); Pedi: eGFR <30 mL/min/1.73 m² or requiring dialysis (children ≥6 yr and 25–35 kg).

Use Cautiously in: CCr <30 mL/min (dose adjustment required in adults); Treated narrow-angle glaucoma (use only if benefits outweigh risks); Myasthenia gravis; OB: Safety not established in pregnancy; Lactation: Safety not established in breastfeeding; Pedi: Safety and effectiveness not established in children <18 yr (overactive bladder) or <6 yr or <25 kg (neurogenic detrusor overactivity); Geri: ↑ risk of anticholinergic side effects in patients >75 yr.

Adverse Reactions/Side Effects

CV: tachycardia (dose related). **GI:** <u>dry mouth</u>, constipation, nausea, upper abdominal pain. **GU:** dysuria, urinary retention. **MS:** back pain. **Neuro:** dizziness, drowsiness, headache. **Misc:** HYPERSENSITIVITY REACTIONS (INCLUDING ANGIOEDEMA).

Interactions

Drug-Drug: Strong CYP3A4 inhibitors, including **ketoconazole**, **itraconazole**, and **clarithromycin**, may ↑ levels and risk of toxicity; daily dose should not exceed 4 mg in adults and children ≥6 yr and >35 kg; avoid concurrent use in children ≥6 yr and 25–35 kg. Additive anticholinergic effects with other **anticholinergic drugs**, including **antihistamines**, **phenothiazines**, **quinidine**, **disopyramide**, and **tricyclic antidepressants**.

Route/Dosage

Overactive Bladder

PO (Adults): 4 mg once daily initially; may ↑ to 8 mg/daily, if needed based on response and tolerability; *Concurrent use of strong CYP3A4 inhibitors:* Do not exceed 4 mg/day.

Renal Impairment

PO (Adults): *CCr <30 mL/min:* Do not exceed 4 mg/day.

Neurogenic Detrusor Overactivity

PO (Children ≥6 yr and >35 kg): 4 mg once daily; then ↑ to 8 mg once daily after 1 wk; *Concurrent use of strong CYP3A4 inhibitors:* Do not exceed 4 mg/day.

PO (Children ≥6 yr and 25–35 kg): 4 mg once daily; ↑ to 8 mg once daily, if needed; *Concurrent use of strong CYP3A4 inhibitors:* Use not recommended.

Renal Impairment

PO (Children ≥6 yr and >35 kg): *eGFR 15–29 mL/min/1.73 m²:* Do not exceed 4 mg/day; *eGFR <15 mL/min/1.73 m² or requiring dialysis:* Use not recommended

Renal Impairment

PO (Children ≥6 yr and 25–35 kg): *eGFR 30–89 mL/min/1.73 m2:* Do not exceed 4 mg/day; *eGFR <30 mL/min/1.73 m² or requiring dialysis:* Use not recommended

Availability (generic available)

Extended-release tablets: 4 mg, 8 mg.

NURSING IMPLICATIONS

Assessment

- Assess for urinary urgency, frequency, and urge incontinence periodically during therapy.
- Monitor for signs and symptoms of angioedema (swelling of face, lips, tongue, or larynx). May occur with 1st or subsequent doses. *If angioedema occurs,* discontinue therapy and provide supportive therapy. Have epinephrine, corticosteroids, and resuscitation equipment available.

Lab Test Considerations

- May ↑ ALT and GGT.

Implementation

- **PO:** Administer with liquid without regard to food.
- ***DNC:*** Swallow extended-release tablets whole; do not break, crush, or chew.

Patient/Family Teaching

- Explain purpose and side effects of medication to patient. Advise patient to read *Patient Information* before starting therapy. Instruct to take as directed. If a dose is missed, omit and begin taking again the next day; do not take two doses on the same day.
- Instruct patient to notify health care professional of all Rx or OTC medications, vitamins, or herbal products being taken and to consult with health care professional before taking other medications.
- May cause drowsiness, dizziness, and blurred vision. Caution patient to avoid driving or other activities requiring alertness until response to medication is known.
- Advise patient to avoid alcohol; may ↑ drowsiness.
- Advise patient to use caution in hot environments; may cause ↓ sweating and severe heat illness.
- Advise patient to stop medication and notify health care professional immediately if signs and symptoms of angioedema occur or seek emergent medical care.
- Rep: Advise women of reproductive potential to notify health care professional if pregnancy is planned or suspected or if breastfeeding.

Evaluation/Desired Outcomes

- Decreased urinary frequency, urgency, and urge incontinence.
- Increase in maximum cystometric bladder capacity in neurogenic detrusor overactivity.

fexofenadine

(fex-oh-**fen**-a-deen)

~~Allegra~~, Allegra Allergy, Children's Allegra Allergy, ~~Children's Allegra Hives, Mucinex Allergy~~

Classification

Therapeutic: allergy, cold, and cough remedies

Pharmacologic: antihistamines

Indications

Relief of symptoms of seasonal allergic rhinitis. Chronic idiopathic urticaria.

Action

Antagonizes the effects of histamine at peripheral histamine-1 (H_1) receptors, including pruritus and urticaria. Also has a drying effect on the nasal mucosa. **Therapeutic Effects:** Decreased sneezing, rhinorrhea, itchy eyes, nose, and throat associated with seasonal allergies. Decreased urticaria.

Pharmacokinetics

Absorption: Rapidly absorbed after oral administration.

Distribution: Unknown.

Metabolism and Excretion: 80% excreted in urine; 11% excreted in feces.

Half-life: 14.4 hr (↑ in renal impairment).

TIME/ACTION PROFILE (antihistaminic effect)

ROUTE	ONSET	PEAK	DURATION
PO	within 1 hr	2–3 hr	12–24 hr

Contraindications/Precautions

Contraindicated in: Hypersensitivity.

Use Cautiously in: Renal impairment (↑ dosing interval recommended); OB: Use only if potential maternal benefit justifies potential fetal risk; Lactation Safety not established in breastfeeding.

Adverse Reactions/Side Effects

GI: dyspepsia. **GU:** dysmenorrhea. **Neuro:** drowsiness, fatigue.

Interactions

Drug-Drug: Magnesium and aluminum-containing antacids may ↓ absorption and effectiveness.

Drug-Food: Apple, orange, and **grapefruit juice** may ↓ absorption and effectiveness.

Route/Dosage

PO (Adults and Children ≥12 yr): 60 mg twice daily *or* 180 mg once daily.

PO (Children 2–11 yr): 30 mg twice daily.

PO (Children 6 mo–2 yr): 15 mg twice daily.

Renal Impairment

PO (Adults): 60 mg once daily.

PO (Children 6–11 yr): 30 mg once daily.

Availability (generic available)

Tablets: 60 mg^{OTC}, 🍁 120 mg^{OTC}, 180 mg^{OTC}. **Orally disintegrating tablets:** 30 mg^{OTC}. **Suspension (berry flavor):** 30 mg/5 mL^{OTC}. ***In combination with:*** pseudoephedrine (Allegra-D). See Appendix N.

NURSING IMPLICATIONS

Assessment

- Assess allergy symptoms (rhinitis, conjunctivitis, hives) before and periodically during therapy.
- Assess lung sounds and character of bronchial secretions. Maintain fluid intake of 1500–2000 mL/day to ↓ viscosity of secretions.

Lab Test Considerations

- Will cause false-negative reactions on allergy skin tests; discontinue 3 days before testing.

Implementation

- Do not confuse Allegra with Viagra. Do not confuse Allegra (fexofenadine) with Allegra Anti-Itch Cream (diphenhydramine/allantoin).
- **PO:** Administer with food or milk to ↓ GI irritation. Administer capsules and tablets with water or milk, not juice. Shake solution bottle well before use.

Patient/Family Teaching

- Explain purpose and side effects of medication. Advise patient to read *Patient Information* before starting therapy. Instruct patient to take medication as directed. Take missed doses as soon as remembered unless almost time for next dose. Do not take more than recommended.
- Advise patient to notify health care professional of all Rx or OTC medications, vitamins, or herbal products being taken and to consult health care professional before taking other medications.
- Instruct patient or caregivers to avoid taking fexofenadine with fruit juices (apple, orange, grapefruit) or antacids containing aluminum or magnesium; may ↓ effectiveness.
- Inform patient that fexofenadine may cause drowsiness, although it is less likely to occur than with other antihistamines. Avoid driving or other activities requiring alertness until response to drug is known.
- Rep: Advise women of reproductive potential to notify health care professional if pregnancy is planned or suspected or if breastfeeding.

Evaluation/Desired Outcomes

- Decreased sneezing, rhinorrhea, itchy eyes, nose, and throat associated with seasonal allergies.
- Decreased urticaria.

fezolinetant (fez-oh-lin-e-tant)

Veozah

Classification

Therapeutic: menopausal agents

Pharmacologic: neurokinin 3 receptor antagonists

Indications

Moderate to severe vasomotor symptoms due to menopause.

Action

Acts as a neurokinin 3 receptor antagonist that blocks neurokinin B binding on the kisspeptin/neurokinin B/dynorphin neuron to regulate neuronal activity in the thermoregulatory center. **Therapeutic Effects:** Reduction in frequency and severity of vasomotor symptoms due to menopause.

Pharmacokinetics

Absorption: Extent of absorption unknown.

Distribution: Extensively distributed to tissues.

Metabolism and Excretion: Primarily metabolized by the liver via the CYP1A2 isoenzyme, with some metabolism by the CYP2C9 and CYP2C19 isoenzymes. Primarily excreted in the urine (77%; 1% as unchanged drug), with 15% excreted in the feces (<1% as unchanged drug).

Half-life: 9.6 hr.

TIME/ACTION PROFILE (plasma concentrations)

ROUTE	ONSET	PEAK	DURATION
PO	unknown	1–4 hr	24 hr

Contraindications/Precautions

Contraindicated in: Cirrhosis; Severe renal impairment or end-stage renal disease; AST, ALT, or total bilirubin ≥2 times upper limit of normal (ULN); Concurrent use with CYP1A2 inhibitors.

Use Cautiously in: None.

Adverse Reactions/Side Effects

Derm: hot flush. **GI:** ↑ liver enzymes, abdominal pain, diarrhea, HEPATOTOXICITY. **MS:** back pain. **Neuro:** insomnia.

Interactions

Drug-Drug: **CYP1A2 inhibitors**, including **fluvoxamine**, **mexiletine**, and **cimetidine**, may ↑ levels and risk of toxicity; concurrent use contraindicated.

Route/Dosage

PO (Adults): 45 mg once daily.

Availability

Tablets: 45 mg.

NURSING IMPLICATIONS

Assessment

- Assess vasomotor symptoms (feelings of warmth in the face, neck, and chest) or sudden intense feelings of heat and sweating (hot flashes or hot flushes) before starting and periodically during therapy.
- Assess for signs and symptoms of hepatotoxicity (new onset fatigue, nausea, vomiting, pruritus, jaundice, pale feces, dark urine, right upper quadrant pain).

Lab Test Considerations

- Monitor ALT, AST, alkaline phosphatase, and bilirubin (total and direct) before starting therapy and then monthly for the 1st 3 mo, 6 mo, and 9 mo after starting therapy. *If AST/ALT >3 times upper limit of normal (ULN),* monitor hepatic function frequently until resolution. *If AST/ALT >5 times ULN, OR AST/ALT >3 times ULN and total bilirubin > 2 times ULN.* permanently discontinue fezolinetant.

Implementation

- **PO:** Administer once daily with or without food, at the same time each day. ***DNC:*** Swallow tablets whole. Do not break, crush, or chew.

Patient/Family Teaching

- Explain purpose and side effects of medication to patient. Advise patient to read *Patient Information* before starting therapy. Instruct patient to take as directed. Take missed doses as soon as remembered, unless there is <12 hr before next dose is due. Return to regular schedule next day.
- Instruct patient to notify health care provider of all Rx or OTC medications, vitamins, or herbal products being taken and to consult with health care provider before taking other medications.
- Advise patient to discontinue fezolinetant immediately and seek medical attention if signs or symptoms of liver abnormalities (new onset fatigue, ↓ appetite, nausea, vomiting, pruritus, jaundice, pale feces, dark urine, abdominal pain) occur.

Evaluation/Desired Outcomes

- Reduction in frequency and severity of vasomotor symptoms due to menopause.

fidaxomicin (fi-dax-oh-**mye**-sin)

Dificid

Classification

Therapeutic: anti-infectives

Pharmacologic: macrolides

Indications

Diarrhea associated with *Clostridioides difficile*.

Action

Bactericidal action mostly against clostridia; inhibits RNA synthesis. Acts locally in the GI tract to eliminate *Clostridioides difficile*. **Therapeutic Effects:** Elimination of diarrhea caused by *Clostridioides difficile*.

Pharmacokinetics

Absorption: Minimal systemic absorption.

Distribution: Stays primarily in the GI tract.

Metabolism and Excretion: Mostly transformed via hydrolysis in the GI tract to OP-1118, its active metabolite. Eliminated mostly (>92%) in feces: <1% excreted in urine.

Half-life: *Fidaxomicin:* 11.7 hr; *OP-1118:* 11.2 hr.

TIME/ACTION PROFILE

ROUTE	ONSET	PEAK	DURATION
PO	unknown	unknown	unknown

Contraindications/Precautions

Contraindicated in: Hypersensitivity to fidaxomicin or macrolides (cross-sensitivity may occur).

Use Cautiously in: OB: Use during pregnancy only if potential maternal benefit justifies potential fetal risk; Lactation: Use while breastfeeding only if potential maternal benefit justifies potential risk to infant; Pedi: Children <6 mo (safety and effectiveness not established).

Adverse Reactions/Side Effects

GI: nausea, abdominal pain, GI HEMORRHAGE. **Hemat:** anemia, neutropenia. **Misc:** HYPERSENSITIVITY REACTIONS (INCLUDING ANGIOEDEMA).

Interactions

Drug-Drug: None reported.

Route/Dosage

PO (Adults): 200 mg twice daily for 10 days.

PO (Children ≥6 mo and ≥12.5 kg): *Tablets:* 200 mg twice daily for 10 days (if unable to swallow tablets, use granules for oral suspension).

PO (Children ≥6 mo and 9–<12.5 kg): *Granules for oral suspension:* 160 mg twice daily for 10 days.

PO (Children ≥6 mo and 7–<9 kg): *Granules for oral suspension:* 120 mg twice daily for 10 days.

PO (Children ≥6 mo and 4–<7 kg): *Granules for oral suspension:* 80 mg twice daily for 10 days.

Availability (generic available)

Granules for oral suspension(berry flavor): 40 mg/mL. **Tablets:** 200 mg.

NURSING IMPLICATIONS

Assessment

- Monitor bowel function for diarrhea, abdominal cramping, fever, and bloody stools. May begin up to several wk following cessation of antibiotic therapy.
- Monitor for signs and symptoms of hypersensitivity reactions (dyspnea, pruritus, rash, angioedema of mouth, throat, and face) periodically during therapy. Risk ↑ with a macrolide allergy.

Lab Test Considerations

- May cause ↑ serum alkaline phosphatase, and hepatic enzymes.
- May cause ↓ serum bicarbonate, ↓ platelet count, anemia, and neutropenia.
- May cause hyperglycemia and metabolic acidosis.

Implementation

- **PO:** Administer twice daily, about 12 hr apart, without regard to food.
- For oral suspension, shake the glass bottle to ensure the granules move around freely and no caking has occurred. Measure 130 mL of purified water, add to glass bottle, and cap tightly. Hold bottle in a horizontal position and shake bottle vigorously in that position for ≥2 min. Verify that suspension is homogeneous; shake again. Once suspension is homogeneous, shake an additional 30 sec. Let bottle stand for 1 min. Verify that suspension is still homogeneous. If not, repeat previous steps. Once reconstituted, oral suspension is white to yellowish white. Write discard date (current date plus 12 days) on the bottle. Stable in refrigerator for up to 12 days; discard after 12 days. Remove bottle from refrigerator 15 min before administration. Shake vigorously until suspension is homogenous. Administer orally with or without food using an oral dosing syringe to ensure accurate dose.

Patient/Family Teaching

- Instruct patient to take fidaxomicin twice daily, 12 hr apart, as directed for the full course of therapy, even if feeling better. Skipping doses or not completing full course of therapy may ↓ effectiveness of therapy and ↑ risk that bacteria will develop resistance and not be treatable in the future.
- Advise patient to notify health care professional of all Rx or OTC medications, vitamins, or herbal products being taken and to consult with health care professional before taking other medications.
- Rep: Advise females of reproductive potential to notify health care professional if pregnancy is planned or suspected or if breastfeeding.

Evaluation/Desired Outcomes

- Decrease in diarrhea caused by *Clostridioides difficile*.

F

filgrastim (fil-gra-stim)

Granix, ✱ Grastofil, Neupogen, Nivestym, Nypozi, Releuko, Zarxio

Classification

Therapeutic: colony-stimulating factors

Indications

Granix, Neupogen, Nivestym, Nypozi, Releuko, Zarxio: Prevention of febrile neutropenia and associated infection in patients who have received bone marrow–depressing antineoplastics for the treatment of nonmyeloid malignancies. **Neupogen, Nivestym, Nypozi, Releuko, Zarxio:** Management of the following: Reduction of time for neutrophil recovery and duration of fever in patients undergoing induction and consolidation chemotherapy for acute myelogenous leukemia. Reduction of time to neutrophil recovery and sequelae of neutropenia in patients with nonmyeloid malignancies undergoing myeloablative chemotherapy followed by bone marrow transplantation. Severe neutropenia in symptomatic patients with congenital neutropenia cyclic neutropenia or idiopathic neutropenia. Mobilization of hematopoietic progenitor cells into peripheral blood for collection by leukapheresis. **Neupogen, Nypozi, Releuko, Zarxio:** Survival improvement in patients acutely exposed to myelosuppressive doses of radiation.

Action

Binds to and stimulates immature neutrophils to divide and differentiate. Also activates mature neutrophils. **Therapeutic Effects:** Decreased incidence of infection in patients who are neutropenic from chemotherapy or other causes. Improved harvest of progenitor cells for bone marrow transplantation. Improved survival in patients exposed to myelosuppressive doses of radiation.

Pharmacokinetics

Absorption: Well absorbed after SUBQ administration.

Distribution: Unknown.

Metabolism and Excretion: Unknown.

Half-life: *Adults:* 3.5 hr; *Neonates:* 4.4 hr.

TIME/ACTION PROFILE

ROUTE	ONSET	PEAK	DURATION
IV, SUBQ	unknown	unknown	4 days†

† Return of neutrophil count to baseline.

Contraindications/Precautions

Contraindicated in: Hypersensitivity to filgrastim or *Escherichia coli*–derived proteins.

Use Cautiously in: Congenital neutropenia (↑ risk of myelodysplastic syndrome or acute myeloid leukemia); Patients with breast or lung cancer receiving chemotherapy and/or radiotherapy (↑ risk of myelodysplastic syndrome or acute myeloid leukemia); Sickle cell disease (↑ risk of sickle cell crisis); Malignancy with myeloid characteristics; Pre-existing cardiac disease; OB: Use during pregnancy only if potential maternal benefit justifies potential fetal risk; Lactation: Use while breastfeeding only if potential maternal benefit justifies potential risk to infant.

Adverse Reactions/Side Effects

CV: aortitis, vasculitis. **GI:** SPLENIC RUPTURE, splenomegaly. **GU:** glomerulonephritis. **Hemat:** ACUTE MYELOID LEUKEMIA, excessive leukocytosis, MYELODYSPLASTIC SYNDROME, sickle cell crises, thrombocytopenia. **Local:** pain at injection site. **MS:** medullary bone pain. **Resp:** ACUTE RESPIRATORY DISTRESS SYNDROME, hemoptysis, pulmonary infiltrates. **Misc:** HYPERSENSITIVITY REACTIONS (INCLUDING ANAPHYLAXIS).

Interactions

Drug-Drug: Simultaneous use with **antineoplastics** may have adverse effects on rapidly proliferating neutrophils; avoid use for 24 hr before and 24 hr after chemotherapy. **Lithium** may potentiate the release of neutrophils; concurrent use should be undertaken cautiously.

Route/Dosage

Receiving Myelosuppressive Chemotherapy

IV: SUBQ (Adults and Children): *Granix, Neupogen, Nivestym, Nypozi, Releuko, Zarxio:* 5 mcg/kg/day as a single SUBQ injection, by short IV infusion, or via continuous IV infusion for up to 2 wk or until ANC reaches 10,000/mm³. Initiate ≥24 hr after chemotherapy. May ↑ by 5 mcg/kg during each cycle of chemotherapy, depending on blood counts.

Receiving Induction and/or Consolidation Chemotherapy for Acute Myelogenous Leukemia

IV, SUBQ (Adults and Children): *Neupogen, Nivestym, Nypozi, Releuko, Zarxio:* 5 mcg/kg/day as a single SUBQ injection, by short IV infusion, or via continuous IV infusion for up to 2 wk or until ANC reaches 10,000/mm³. Initiate ≥24 hr after chemotherapy. May ↑ by 5 mcg/kg during each cycle of chemotherapy, depending on blood counts.

After Bone Marrow Transplantation

IV (Adults): *Neupogen, Nivestym, Nypozi, Releuko, Zarxio:* 10 mcg/kg/day as a continuous IV infusion for up to 24 hr; initiate ≥24 hr after chemotherapy and ≥24 hr after bone marrow transplantation. Subsequent dose is adjusted according to blood counts.

Peripheral Blood Progenitor Cell Collection and Therapy

SUBQ (Adults): *Neupogen, Nivestym, Nypozi, Releuko, Zarxio:* 10 mcg/kg/day for ≥4 days before 1st leukapheresis and continued until last leukapheresis. Discontinue if WBC >100,000 cells/mm³.

Severe Neutropenia

SUBQ (Adults): *Neupogen, Nivestym, Nypozi, Releuko, Zarxio:* Congenital neutropenia: 6 mcg/kg twice daily. Idiopathic/cyclical neutropenia: 5 mcg/kg daily (↓ if ANC remains >10,000/mm³).

After Myelosuppressive Radiation

SUBQ (Adults): *Neupogen, Nypozi, Releuko, Zarxio:* 10 mcg/kg once daily; initiate as soon as possible after exposure to radiation doses >2 gray (Gy); continue until ANC remains >1000/mm³ for three consecutive blood counts (performed every 3 days) or is >10,000/mm³ after a radiation-induced nadir.

Availability

Solution for injection (prefilled syringes): 300 mcg/0.5 mL, 480 mcg/0.8 mL. **Solution for injection (vials):** 300 mcg/1 mL, 480 mcg/1.6 mL.

NURSING IMPLICATIONS

Assessment

- Monitor HR, BP, and respiratory status before and periodically during therapy.
- Assess bone pain during therapy. May pretreat with loratadine 10 mg PO to prevent bone pain. *If mild to moderate pain occurs,* consider treating with nonopioid or opioid analgesics, especially in patients receiving high-dose IV therapy.
- Monitor for signs and symptoms of severe allergic reaction, including anaphylaxis, especially on initial exposure. *If severe allergic reaction occurs,* permanently discontinue filgrastim and provide symptomatic medical treatment. Symptoms may recur days after discontinuation of antiallergy treatment.
- Assess for signs and symptoms of acute respiratory distress syndrome (fever, lung infiltrates, respiratory distress). *If symptoms of acute respiratory distress syndrome occur,* hold until symptoms resolve or discontinue therapy.
- Monitor for signs and symptoms of splenic enlargement or rupture (left upper abdominal or shoulder pain).
- Monitor for transient positive bone-imaging changes.

- Monitor for signs and symptoms of myelodysplastic syndrome and acute myeloid leukemia (tiredness, fever, easy bruising or bleeding) in patient with severe chronic neutropenia, breast, or lung cancer.

Lab Test Considerations

- Obtain CBC with differential, including examination for presence of blast cells, after chemotherapy and before initiating filgrastim and then twice weekly during therapy. Do not discontinue therapy until ANC >10,000/mm³. *For chronic severe neutropenia,* monitor CBC with differential twice weekly during initial 4 wk of therapy and for 2 wk after any dose adjustment. *For myelosuppressive doses of radiation,* obtain baseline CBC and then every 3rd day until ANC >1000/mm³ for three serial CBCs or ANC >10,000/mm³ after radiation-induced nadir.
- *After bone marrow transplant,* the daily dose is titrated by the neutrophil response. When the ANC >1000/mm³ for 3 consecutive days, ↓ dose to 5 mcg/kg/day. If the ANC remains >1000/mm³ for ≥3 consecutive days, discontinue filgrastim. If the ANC ↓ to <1000/mm³, resume filgrastim at 5 mcg/kg/day.
- May cause ↓ platelets and transient ↑ in uric acid, LDH, and alkaline phosphatase.

Implementation

- Administer no earlier than 24 hr after cytotoxic chemotherapy, ≥24 hr after bone marrow infusion, and not during the 24 hr before administration of chemotherapy.
- **SUBQ**: May be administered in upper outer arm, abdomen, thigh, or upper outer buttock. If dose is >1 mL in volume, may be divided into two injection sites. Do not use prefilled syringe for dose <0.3 mL.
- Cap of needle contains latex; avoid administration by persons with latex allergy.
- Refrigerate; do not freeze. Do not shake. Warm to room temperature for ≥30 min–24 hr before injection. Solution is clear and colorless to yellowish. Do not administer if discolored or contains particulates. If not used immediately, may be stored at room temperature for ≤8 days. Discard any unused portion.
- May also be administered as a continuous SUBQ infusion over 24 hr after bone marrow transplantation.

IV Administration

- **Continuous Infusion:** Refrigerate; do not freeze. Do not shake. Warm to room temperature for ≥30 min–8 days before dilution. **Dilution:** Dilute in D5W; do not dilute with 0.9% NaCl (will precipitate). **Concentration:** >5 mcg/mL. Protect from adsorption to plastics by adding human albumin to final concentration of 2 mg/mL; then filgrastim is compatible with glass, polyvinylchloride, polyolefin, and polypropylene. Diluted solution from *prefilled syringe* may be stored at room temperature ≤24 hr and *vial* ≤4 hr, including infusion time, or *vial* may be refrigerated ≤24 hr. **Rate:** *After chemotherapy,* dose is administered via infusion over 15–60 min.
- *After chemotherapy,* dose may also be administered as a continuous infusion.
- *After bone marrow transplant,* administer dose as an infusion over 4–24 hr.
- **Y-Site Compatibility:** acyclovir, allopurinol, amikacin, aminophylline, ampicillin, ampicillin/sulbactam, aztreonam, bleomycin, bumetanide, buprenorphine, butorphanol, calcium gluconate, carboplatin, carmustine, cefazolin, cefotetan, ceftazidime, ceftolozane/tazobactam, chlorpromazine, cisplatin, cyclophosphamide, cytarabine, dacarbazine, daunorubicin, dexamethasone, diphenhydramine, doxorubicin hydrochloride, doxycycline, droperidol, enalaprilat, famotidine, floxuridine, fluconazole, fludarabine, ganciclovir, granisetron, haloperidol, hydrocortisone, hydromorphone, idarubicin, ifosfamide, leucovorin, levofloxacin, lorazepam, melphalan, meperidine, mesna, methotrexate, metoclopramide, minocycline, mitoxantrone, morphine, nalbuphine, ondansetron, posaconazole, potassium chloride, promethazine, rituximab, sodium acetate, sodium bicarbonate, tobramycin, trastuzumab, trimethoprim/sulfamethoxazole, vancomycin, vinblastine, vincristine, vinorelbine, zidovudine.
- **Y-Site Incompatibility:** aminocaproic acid, amphotericin B deoxycholate, cefepime, cefotaxime, cefoxitin, ceftaroline, ceftobiprole, ceftriaxone, cefuroxime, clindamycin, dactinomycin, etoposide, fluorouracil, furosemide, heparin, isavuconazonium, letermovir, mannitol, methylprednisolone, metronidazole, mitomycin, prochlorperazine, thiotepa.

Patient/Family Teaching

- Explain purpose and side effects of medication. Advise patient to read *Patient Information* before starting therapy.
- Instruct patient on correct technique for injection, care, and disposal of equipment. Advise patient to notify health care provider regarding when to give a missed dose.
- Instruct patient to notify health care provider immediately if signs and symptoms of spleen enlargement or rupture, allergic reaction, acute respiratory distress syndrome, glomerulonephritis (swelling of face or ankles, dark-colored urine or blood in urine, ↓ urine production), myelodysplastic syndrome, acute myeloid leukemia, or vasculitis (skin redness, purple spots on skin) occur. Discuss risk of sickle cell crisis with patients with sickle cell disease before administering.

- Advise patient to notify health care provider of all Rx or OTC medications, vitamins, or herbal products being taken and to consult with health care provider before taking other medications.
- Rep: Advise women of reproductive potential to notify health care provider if pregnancy is planned or suspected or if breastfeeding.
- **Home Care Issues:** Instruct patient on correct technique and proper disposal for home administration. Caution patient not to reuse needle, vial, or syringe. Provide patient with a puncture-proof container for needle and syringe disposal.

Evaluation/Desired Outcomes

- Decreased incidence of infection in patients who receive bone marrow–depressing antineoplastics.
- Reduction of duration and sequelae of neutropenia after bone marrow transplantation.
- Reduction of the incidence and duration of sequelae of neutropenia in patients with severe chronic neutropenia.
- Improved harvest of progenitor cells for bone marrow transplantation.
- Improved survival in patients exposed to myelosuppressive doses of radiation.

finasteride (fi-nas-ter-ide)

Propecia, Proscar

Classification
Therapeutic: benign prostatic hyperplasia (BPH) agents, hair regrowth stimulants
Pharmacologic: androgen inhibitors

Indications

Benign prostatic hyperplasia (BPH); can be used with doxazosin. Androgenetic alopecia (male pattern baldness) in men only.

Action

Inhibits the enzyme 5-alpha-reductase, which is responsible for converting testosterone to its potent metabolite 5-alpha-dihydrotestosterone in prostate, liver, and skin; 5-alpha-dihydrotestosterone is partially responsible for prostatic hyperplasia and hair loss. **Therapeutic Effects:** Reduced prostate size with associated decrease in urinary symptoms. Decreases hair loss; promotes hair regrowth.

Pharmacokinetics

Absorption: 63% absorbed following oral administration.
Distribution: Enters prostatic tissue and crosses the blood-brain barrier. Remainder of distribution not known.
Protein Binding: 90%.
Metabolism and Excretion: Mostly metabolized; 39% excreted in urine as metabolites; 57% excreted in feces.
Half-life: 6 hr (range 6–15 hr; slightly ↑ in patients >70 yr).

TIME/ACTION PROFILE (↓ in dihydrotestosterone levels†)

ROUTE	ONSET	PEAK	DURATION
PO	rapid	8 hr	2 wk

† Clinical effects as noted by urinary tract symptoms and hair regrowth may not be evident for several months and remain for 4 mo after discontinuation.

Contraindications/Precautions

Contraindicated in: Hypersensitivity.
Use Cautiously in: Hepatic impairment; Obstructive uropathy.

Adverse Reactions/Side Effects

Endo: gynecomastia. **GU:** ↓ libido, ↓ volume of ejaculate, erectile dysfunction, infertility, PROSTATE CANCER (HIGH-GRADE). **Misc:** ANGIOEDEMA, BREAST CANCER.

Interactions

Drug-Drug: None reported.

Route/Dosage

Benign Prostatic Hypertrophy

PO (Adults): *Proscar:* 5 mg once daily.

Androgenetic Alopecia

PO (Adults): *Propecia:* 1 mg once daily.

Availability (generic available)

Tablets (Proscar): 5 mg. **Tablets (Propecia):** 1 mg. ***In combination with:*** tadalafil (Entadfi). See Appendix N.

NURSING IMPLICATIONS

Assessment

- Assess for symptoms of prostatic hyperplasia (urinary hesitancy, feeling of incomplete bladder emptying, interruption of urinary stream, impairment of size and force of urinary stream, terminal urinary dribbling, straining to start flow, dysuria, urgency) before and periodically during therapy.
- Digital rectal examinations should be performed before and periodically during therapy for BPH.

Lab Test Considerations

- Establish a new baseline serum prostate-specific antigen (PSA) concentration ≥6 mo after initiating treatment and periodically during therapy. Finasteride may cause a ↓ in serum PSA levels. Any confirmed ↑ from lowest PSA value while on *Propecia* may be a sign of prostate cancer and should be evaluated, even if PSA levels are within the normal range for men not taking a 5 -reductase inhibitor.

Implementation

- Do not confuse Proscar with Prograf or Provera.

- When cutting, crushing, or handling tablets, wear double chemotherapy gloves, protective gown, and hair and shoe covers. Prepare in a ventilated engineering control, if possible, and consider crushing tablets in a pill pouch. Use respiratory (N95) protection and eye and face protection, if not prepared in a ventilated engineering control. During administration, wear double chemotherapy gloves and protective gown when handling uncoated, cut, or crushed tablets. Eye/face protection is need if there is risk of patient vomiting or spitting up. Single chemotherapy gloves are appropriate if handling and administering intact tablets from a unit-dose package. Those who are actively trying to conceive, who are pregnant or may become pregnant, and who are breastfeeding should avoid handling finasteride.
- **PO:** Administer once daily with or without meals.

Patient/Family Teaching

- Explain the purpose and side effects of finasteride. Instruct patient to take as directed, even if symptoms improve or are unchanged. ≥6–12 mo of therapy may be necessary to determine whether or not an individual will respond to finasteride. If a dose is missed, omit and take next tablet at usual time. Advise patient to read the *Patient Information* prior to starting therapy and with each Rx refill in case of changes.
- Emphasize the importance of periodic follow-up exams to determine whether a clinical response has occurred.
- Inform patient that the volume of ejaculate may be ↓ and erectile dysfunction and ↓ libido may occur during therapy and after therapy is completed.
- Advise patient to notify health care professional promptly if changes in breasts (lumps, pain, nipple discharge) occur.
- Inform patient that there is an ↑ risk of high-grade prostate cancer in men taking this drug.
- Advise patient to notify health care professional of all Rx or OTC medications, vitamins, or herbal products being taken and to consult with health care professional before taking other medications.
- Rep: May cause fetal harm. Caution patient that finasteride poses a potential risk to a male fetus. Women who are pregnant or may become pregnant should avoid exposure to semen of a partner taking finasteride and should not handle crushed finasteride due to potential absorption.

Evaluation/Desired Outcomes

- Decrease in urinary symptoms of benign prostatic hyperplasia.
- Hair regrowth in androgenetic alopecia. Evidence of hair growth usually requires ≥3 mo. Continued use is recommended to sustain benefit. Withdrawal leads to reversal of effect within 12 mo.

finerenone (fin-er-e-none)

Kerendia

Classification

Therapeutic: none assigned

Pharmacologic: mineralocorticoid receptor antagonists (non-steroidal)

Indications

Chronic kidney disease (CKD) associated with type 2 diabetes.

Action

Acts as a nonsteroidal, selective antagonist of the mineralocorticoid receptor, which results in reduction in sodium reabsorption and a reduction in fibrosis and inflammation in the heart, blood vessels, and kidneys. **Therapeutic Effects:** Reduction in the risk of a sustained eGFR decline, end-stage kidney disease, cardiovascular death, nonfatal MI, and hospitalization for HF in CKD associated with type 2 diabetes.

Pharmacokinetics

Absorption: 44% absorbed following oral administration.

Distribution: Widely distributed to tissues.

Protein Binding: 92%.

Metabolism and Excretion: Primarily metabolized in the liver via the CYP3A4 isoenzyme and to a lesser extent by the CYP2C8 isoenzyme to inactive metabolites. Primarily excreted in the urine (80%) as metabolites, with 20% being excreted in feces.

Half-life: 2–3 hr.

TIME/ACTION PROFILE (plasma concentrations)

ROUTE	ONSET	PEAK	DURATION
PO	rapid	30 min–1.25 hr	unknown

Contraindications/Precautions

Contraindicated in: Concurrent use of strong CYP3A4 inhibitors; Adrenal insufficiency; Hyperkalemia (serum potassium >5 mEq/L); eGFR <25 mL/min/m²; Severe hepatic impairment; Lactation: Lactation.

Use Cautiously in: Renal impairment (↑ risk of hyperkalemia) (adjust dose); Moderate hepatic impairment; OB: Safety not established in pregnancy; Pedi: Safety and effectiveness not established in children.

Adverse Reactions/Side Effects

CV: hypotension. **F and E:** <u>hyperkalemia</u>, hyponatremia.

Interactions

Drug-Drug: **Strong CYP3A4 inhibitors** may significantly ↑ levels and risk of hyperkalemia; concurrent use contraindicated. **Moderate CYP3A4 inhibitors**, including **erythromycin**, or **weak CYP3A4 inhibitors**, including **amiodarone**, may ↑ levels and risk of hyperkalemia; closely monitor serum potassium levels after initiation of or after dosage adjustment of either the CYP3A4 inhibitor or finerenone. **Strong CYP3A4 inducers**, including **rifampin**, or **moderate CYP3A4 inducers**, including **efavirenz**, may ↓ levels and effectiveness; avoid concurrent use. Use with **ACE inhibitors**, **NSAIDs**, **potassium supplements**, **angiotensin II receptor antagonists**, **potassium-sparing diuretics**, **angiotensin converting enzyme inhibitors**, or **cyclosporine** ↑ risk of hyperkalemia.
Drug-Food: **Grapefruit juice** or **grapefruit** may ↑ levels and risk of hyperkalemia; avoid concurrent use.

Route/Dosage

PO (Adults): 20 mg once daily.

Renal Impairment

PO (Adults): *eGFR 25–<60 mL/min/m2:* 10 mg once daily; after 4 wk, may ↑ to 20 mg once daily if serum potassium ≤ 4.8 mEq/L.

Availability

Tablets: 10 mg, 20 mg.

NURSING IMPLICATIONS

Assessment

- Monitor for signs and symptoms of hyperkalemia (fatigue, muscle weakness, paresthesia, confusion, dyspnea, cardiac arrhythmias) during therapy. If symptoms occur, confirm with serum potassium.

Lab Test Considerations

- Measure serum potassium levels and eGFR before starting therapy. Do not start therapy if serum potassium >5.0 mEq/L. Measure serum potassium 4 wk after starting therapy and adjust dose. If serum potassium ≤4.8 mEq/L, ↑ dose to 20 mg/day if at 10 mg/day or maintain 20 mg/day dose. If serum potassium >4.8–5.5 mEq/L, maintain current 10 mg/day or 20 mg/day dose. If serum potassium >5.5 mEq/L, hold finerenone dose; if at 10 mg/day dose, consider restarting at 10 mg/day once serum potassium ≤5.0 mEq/L; if at 20 mg/day dose, restart at 10 mg/day when serum potassium ≤5.0 mEq/L. Monitor serum potassium 4 wk after a dose adjustment and throughout treatment, and adjust the dose as needed.

Implementation

- **PO:** For patients unable to swallow tablets whole, tablets may be crushed and mixed with water or soft foods (applesauce) immediately before use.

Patient/Family Teaching

- Explain the purpose and side effects of finerenone. Instruct patient to take as directed. Take missed dose as soon as remembered, but only on same day. Do not double doses. Advise patient to read *Patient Information* before starting and with each Rx refill in case of changes.
- Emphasize the importance of regular lab tests to monitor potassium levels.
- Advise patient to notify health care professional of all Rx or OTC medications, vitamins, or herbal products being taken and to consult with health care professional before taking other medications. Advise patients to consult with health care professional before using potassium supplements or salt substitutes containing potassium. Caution patient to avoid grapefruit and grapefruit juice during therapy; may increase the plasma concentration of finerenone.
- Rep: Advise women of reproductive potential to notify health care professional if pregnancy is planned or suspected and to avoid breastfeeding during therapy and for 1 day after last dose.

Evaluation/Desired Outcomes

- Reduction of the risk of sustained eGFR decline, end-stage kidney disease, cardiovascular death, nonfatal MI, and hospitalization for HF in patients with CKD associated with type 2 diabetes.

fingolimod (fin-go-li-mod)

Gilenya, Tascenso ODT

Classification

Therapeutic: anti-multiple sclerosis agents
Pharmacologic: receptor modulators

Indications

Relapsing forms of multiple sclerosis (MS), including clinically isolated syndrome, relapsing-remitting disease, and active secondary progressive disease.

Action

Converted by sphingosine kinase to the active metabolite fingolimod-phosphate, which binds to sphingosine 1-phosphate receptors, resulting in ↓ migration of lymphocytes into peripheral blood. This may ↓ lymphocyte migration into the CNS. **Therapeutic Effects:** ↓ frequency of relapses/delayed accumulation of disability.

Pharmacokinetics

Absorption: 93% absorbed following oral administration.
Distribution: Extensively distributed to body tissues; 86% of parent drug distributes into red blood cells; active metabolite uptake 17%.
Protein Binding: >99.7%.

Metabolism and Excretion: Converted to its active metabolite, then metabolized mostly by the CYP4F2 isoenzyme, with further degradation by other enzyme systems. Most inactive metabolites excreted in urine (81%); <2.5% excreted as fingolimod and fingolimod-phosphate in feces.
Half-life: 6–9 days.

TIME/ACTION PROFILE

ROUTE	ONSET	PEAK	DURATION
PO	unknown	1–2 mo*	2 mo†

* Time to steady state plasma concentrations, peak plasma concentrations after a single dose at 12–16 hr.
† Time for complete elimination.

Contraindications/Precautions

Contraindicated in: Hypersensitivity; MI, unstable angina, stroke, transient ischemic attack, or class III or IV HF within previous 6 mo; 2nd- or 3rd-degree heart block or sick sinus syndrome (in the absence of a pacemaker); QT interval ≥500 msec; Cardiac arrhythmias requiring use of class Ia or III antiarrhythmics; Active acute/chronic untreated infections; OB: Pregnancy.
Use Cautiously in: History of ischemic heart disease, MI, HF, cerebrovascular disease, uncontrolled hypertension, AV or SA heart block, symptomatic bradycardia, recurrent syncope, cardiac arrest, or severe untreated sleep apnea (↑ risk of bradycardia/heart block); QT interval prolongation before or during observation period (>450 msec in adult and pediatric males, >470 msec in adult females, >460 msec in pediatric females), hypokalemia, hypomagnesemia, congenital long QT syndrome, or concurrent use of QT interval prolonging medications (↑ risk of QT interval prolongation); Severe hepatic impairment; Diabetes mellitus/history of uveitis (↑ risk of macular edema); Negative history for chickenpox or vaccination against varicella zoster virus (VZV) vaccination; Lactation: Use while breastfeeding only if potential maternal benefit justifies potential risk to infant; Rep: Women of reproductive potential; Pedi: Children <10 yr (safety and effectiveness not established); Geri: Risk of adverse reactions may be ↑ in older adults; consider age-related ↓ in cardiac/renal/hepatic function, chronic illnesses, and concurrent drug therapy.

Adverse Reactions/Side Effects

CV: ASYSTOLE, BRADYCARDIA, HEART BLOCK, QT interval prolongation, hypertension, syncope. **Derm:** BASAL/SQUAMOUS CELL CARCINOMA, MELANOMA. **EENT:** blurred vision, eye pain, macular edema. **GI:** ↑ liver enzymes, diarrhea, HEPATOTOXICITY. **Hemat:** leukopenia, lymphopenia. **MS:** back pain. **Neuro:** headache, POSTERIOR REVERSIBLE ENCEPHALOPATHY SYNDROME (PRES), PROGRESSIVE MULTIFOCAL LEUKOENCEPHALOPATHY (PML), tumefactive MS. **Resp:** cough, ↓ pulmonary function. **Misc:** HYPERSENSITIVITY REACTIONS (INCLUDING ANGIOEDEMA), IMMUNE RECONSTITUTION INFLAMMATORY SYNDROME (IRIS), INFECTION (INCLUDING BACTERIAL, VIRAL AND FUNGAL), LYMPHOMA.

Interactions

Drug-Drug: **Class Ia or class III antiarrhythmics** may ↑ risk of serious arrhythmias; concurrent use contraindicated. Concurrent use of **beta blockers, diltiazem, verapamil, ivabradine, clonidine,** or **digoxin** may ↑ risk of bradycardia; careful monitoring recommended. Concurrent use of **QT-interval prolonging medications** may ↑ risk of QT interval prolongation and torsades de pointes. Concurrent use of **ketoconazole** may ↑ levels and risk of toxicity. ↑ risk of immunosuppression with **antineoplastics, immunosuppressants,** or **immune-modulating therapies**. **Live-attenuated vaccines** ↑ risk of infection.

Route/Dosage

PO (Adults and Children ≥10 yr and >40 kg): 0.5 mg once daily.
PO (Children ≥10 yr and ≤40 kg): 0.25 mg once daily.

Availability (generic available)

Capsules: 0.25 mg, 0.5 mg. **Orally disintegrating tablets:** 0.25 mg, 0.5 mg.

NURSING IMPLICATIONS

Assessment

- Perform *first-dose monitoring* when starting therapy, when restarting therapy after drug was discontinued for ≥ 14 days, when therapy is interrupted ≥1 day in first 2 wk or >7 days during wk 3 and 4, and in pediatric patients when increasing dose.
- *First-dose monitoring:* Monitor pulse and BP hourly for ≥6 hr following first dose and periodically during therapy. Obtain ECG prior to first dose and at end of observation period. *If the patient develops* a HR <45 bpm in adults, <55 bpm in children ≥12 yr, <60 bpm in children 10–11 yr; lowest postdose HR is at the end of the 6-hr observation period; or routine postdose ECG shows new ≥ 2nd-degree AV block, monitor until abnormality resolves. *If bradycardia is symptomatic,* monitor with continuous ECG until resolved. *If pharmacological intervention is required,* repeat first-dose monitoring for second dose. *If the patient has preexisting heart or cerebrovascular conditions, prolonged QTc interval prior to or during therapy, or uses drugs that may prolong QT interval or slow HR/AV conduction,* monitor with continuous ECG overnight in an appropriate medical facility.

- Monitor for signs of infection during and for 2 mo after discontinuation of therapy. Consider suspending therapy if serious infection develops.
- *If clinical signs of PML (progressive unilateral body weakness; changes in vision, memory, orientation, personality) or MRI changes occur,* immediately withhold therapy and perform appropriate diagnostics. *If PML is confirmed*, permanently discontinue fingolimod and monitor for IRIS (rapid neurologic clinical decline, characteristic MRI changes). The time to onset of IRIS in patients with PML was generally within a few mo after receptor modulator discontinuation. *If IRIS occurs,* initiate appropriate medical treatment.
- Perform baseline ophthalmologic exam of the fundus, including the macula, at start of therapy, then at 3–4 mo, periodically during therapy, and if any visual changes occur. *If macular edema occurs,* consider discontinuing fingolimod based on benefits and risks for the individual patient.
- Monitor for signs and symptoms of liver injury. *If ALT >3 × upper limit of normal (ULN) with total bilirubin >2 × ULN,* withhold fingolimod and discontinue if alternative etiology for liver injury cannot be established.
- Monitor for symptoms of PRES (sudden onset headache, altered metal status, visual changes and seizures). *If symptoms occur,* discontinue fingolimod.
- Evaluate pulmonary function with spirometry and diffusion lung capacity for carbon monoxide when indicated clinically.
- Perform baseline skin exam and periodically thereafter. Evaluate suspicious skin lesions promptly.
- Monitor patients for ↑ in disability 12–24 wk following discontinuation.
- Review current and past medications. If patient is currently taking or has taken antineoplastic, immunosuppressive, or immune-modulating therapies, consider possible unintended additive immunosuppressive effects before initiating treatment.

Lab Test Considerations

- Verify negative pregnancy test before starting therapy.
- Obtain baseline AST, ALT, and total bilirubin periodically during and for 2 mo after therapy discontinued. *If ALT >3 × ULN with total bilirubin >2 × ULN,* withhold fingolimod and discontinue if alternative etiology for liver injury cannot be established.
- Obtain baseline CBC within 6 mo of initiating therapy. May cause lymphocytopenia for up to 2 mo following discontinuation.
- Assess for VZV antibodies before starting therapy.

Implementation

- Before initiating therapy (≥ 1 mo), administer VZV vaccine to patients who are antibody negative and complete all immunizations, including human papilloma virus, according to current guidelines for pediatric patients. Cancer screening, including Papanicolaou (Pap) test, is recommended before starting therapy.
- **PO:** Administer once daily without regard to food.
- **Orally disintegrating tablet (ODT):** Open blister pack with dry hands. Peel back foil over one blister and gently remove ODT; do not push through foil. Place ODT on tongue, allowing it to dissolve before swallowing. May be taken with or without water. Take immediately after opening blister pack. Do not store ODT outside blister pack for future use.

Patient/Family Teaching

- Instruct patient to take fingolimod as directed. Do not discontinue therapy without consulting health care professional; may cause severe ↑ in disability. If a dose is missed, contact health care professional before taking next dose; may need to be observed by a health care professional for >6 hr after taking next dose. Advise patient to read *Medication Guide* prior to starting therapy and with each Rx refill in case of changes.
- Advise patient to notify health care professional if they develop signs and symptoms of liver dysfunction, infection, PML, new onset of dyspnea, PRES (sudden headache, confusion, seizures, loss of vision, weakness), hypersensitivity reactions (rash or itchy hives; swelling of lips, tongue, or face), skin lesions, nodules (shiny pearly nodules), patches or open sores that do not heal within wks, or changes in vision.
- Instruct patient not to receive live-attenuated vaccines during and for 2 mo after treatment due to risk of life-threatening infection. Advise patients who have not had a health care professional–confirmed history of chickenpox or a full course vaccination to be tested for antibodies to VZV before starting therapy.
- Advise patient to notify health care professional of all Rx or OTC medications, vitamins, or herbal products being taken and to consult with health care professional before taking other medications.
- Caution patient to avoid exposure to sunlight and ultraviolet light, wear protective clothing, and use sunscreen with a high protection factor to minimize risk of cutaneous malignancies.
- Rep: May cause fetal harm. Advise females of reproductive potential to use contraception during and for ≥2 mo after discontinuation of therapy and to notify health care professional immediately if pregnancy is planned or suspected or if breastfeeding. Inform pregnant patients of registry that monitors outcomes in women exposed to fingolimod during pregnancy. To enroll patient in the pregnancy registry, call 1-877-598-7237 or visit www.gilenyapregnancyregistry.com.

Evaluation/Desired Outcomes

- Delayed disability progression and decreased frequency of relapses.

flibanserin (flib-an-ser-in)

Addyi

Classification

Therapeutic: sexual dysfunction agents

Indications

Premenopausal women with hypoactive sexual desire disorder unrelated to concurrent medical/psychiatric diagnoses, relationship issues, or substance abuse (does not enhance sexual performance).

Action

May be explained by agonist activity at 5-HT_{1A} receptors and antagonist activity at 5-HT_{2A} receptors; also has moderate antagonist activity at 5-HT_{2B}, 5-HT_{2C}, and dopamine D_4 receptors. **Therapeutic Effects:** Improved sexual desire with decreased distress and interpersonal dysfunction.

Pharmacokinetics

Absorption: Moderately absorbed (33%) following oral administration.

Distribution: Unknown.

Protein Binding: 98%.

Metabolism and Excretion: Primarily metabolized in the liver, via the CYP3A4 isoenzyme, and to a lesser extent by the CYP2C19 isoenzyme; the CYP2C19 isoenzyme exhibits genetic polymorphism; poor metabolizers may have significantly ↑ flibanserin concentrations and an ↑ risk of adverse effects. 44% excreted in urine, 51% in feces almost entirely as metabolites, which do not appear to be pharmacologically active.

Half-life: 11 hr.

TIME/ACTION PROFILE (plasma concentrations)

ROUTE	ONSET	PEAK	DURATION
PO	within 1 hr	1 hr	24 hr

Contraindications/Precautions

Contraindicated in: Hypersensitivity; Concurrent use of strong/moderate CYP3A4 inhibitors; Hepatic impairment; Lactation: Lactation.

Use Cautiously in: Alcohol ingestion within 2 hr of flibanserin dose (excess risk of hypotension/ syncope); CYP2C19 poor metabolizers (↑ risk of adverse reactions including hypotension, syncope, and drowsiness); OB: Safety not established in pregnancy.

Adverse Reactions/Side Effects

CV: HYPOTENSION/SYNCOPE. **Derm:** rash. **GI:** nausea, constipation, dry mouth. **Neuro:** dizziness, drowsiness, anxiety, fatigue, insomnia, vertigo. **Misc:** HYPERSENSITIVITY REACTIONS (INCLUDING ANAPHYLAXIS AND ANGIOEDEMA).

Interactions

Drug-Drug: **Strong CYP3A4 inhibitors** or **moderate CYP3A4 inhibitors**, including **atazanavir**, **ciprofloxacin**, **clarithromycin**, **conivaptan**, **diltiazem**, **erythromycin**, **fluconazole**, **fosamprenavir**, **itraconazole**, **ketoconazole**, **nelfinavir**, **posaconazole**, **ritonavir**, and **verapamil**, significantly ↑ levels and risk of toxicity; concurrent use contraindicated. Wait 2 wk after discontinuing inhibitor before initiating flibanserin. If initiating inhibitor, wait 2 days after last dose of flibanserin. Concurrent use with **alcohol** ↑ risk of hypotension/syncope and excess sedation; wait ≥2 hr after consuming 1–2 standard alcoholic drinks before taking dose at bedtime; skip bedtime dose if consumed ≥3 standard alcoholic drinks. **Oral hormonal contraceptives** and **weak CYP3A4 inhibitors**, including **cimetidine**, and **fluoxetine**, may ↑ levels and risk of toxicity; avoid concurrent use with multiple weak CYP3A4 inhibitors. **Strong CYP2C19 inhibitors**, including **proton pump inhibitors**, **SSRIs**, **benzodiazepines**, and **antifungals**, may ↑ levels and risk of toxicity; undertake concurrent use with caution. **CYP3A4 inducers**, including **carbamazepine**, **phenobarbital**, **phenytoin**, **rifabutin**, **rifampin**, and **rifapentine**, may ↓ levels and effectiveness; concurrent use not recommended. May ↑ levels and risk of toxicity of **digoxin** and **sirolimus**; careful monitoring recommended. May ↑ risk of CNS depression with other **CNS depressants**, including **alcohol**, **antihistamines**, **opioids**, **sedative/hypnotics**, some **anti-anxiety agents**, **antidepressants**, and **antipsychotics**.

Gingko may ↑ levels and risk of toxicity; avoid use with other weak CYP3A4 inhibitors. **St. John's wort** may ↓ levels and effectiveness; concurrent use not recommended. **Drug-Food:** **Grapefruit juice** may ↑ levels and risk of toxicity; concurrent ingestion contraindicated.

Route/Dosage

PO (Adults): 100 mg once daily at bedtime.

Availability

Tablets: 100 mg.

NURSING IMPLICATIONS

Assessment

- Assess sexual desire and related distress and interpersonal dysfunction before and periodically during therapy; discontinue treatment after 8 wk if no improvement
- Monitor for hypotension and syncope. Have patient lie supine if dizziness occurs.
- Assess likelihood of patient following alcohol restrictions, taking into account the patient's current and past drinking behavior and other pertinent

social and medical history. Counsel patients who are prescribed flibanserin about the importance of following guidelines for alcohol use; interaction with alcohol ↑ risk of hypotension and syncope.

Implementation

- Administer once daily at bedtime; administration during waking hours ↑ risks of hypotension, syncope, accidental injury, and CNS depression.

Patient/Family Teaching

- Explain the purpose and side effects of fliabanserin. Instruct patient to take flibanserin only at bedtime as directed. If dose is missed, omit and take next dose at bedtime on next day. Advise patient to read *Medication Guide* before starting therapy and with each Rx refill in case of changes.
- Advise patient to avoid grapefruit juice during therapy.
- Caution patient to follow alcohol guidelines during therapy. Wait ≥2 hr after drinking one or two standard alcoholic drinks (one 12-oz regular beer; 5 oz of wine; 1.5 oz or a shot of brandy, gin, rum, tequila, vodka, or whiskey) before taking flibanserin at bedtime. If you drink ≥3 standard alcoholic drinks in the evening, skip your flibanserin dose at bedtime. After you have taken your flibanserin at bedtime, do not drink alcohol until the following day. Alcohol ↑ hypotensive effects. May cause dizziness and fainting.
- Advise patient if dizziness occurs, immediately lie supine and promptly seek medical help if symptoms do not resolve.
- May cause drowsiness. Caution patient to avoid driving and other activities requiring alertness until 6 hr after each dose or until response to medication is known.
- Advise patient to stop taking flibanserin and notify health care provider immediately if signs and symptoms of hypersensitivity reaction (swelling of the face, lips, and mouth; pruritus; urticaria) occur.
- Instruct patient to notify health care provider of all Rx or OTC medications, vitamins, or herbal products being taken and consult health care provider before taking any new medications, especially St. John's wort.
- Rep: Advise women of reproductive potential to notify health care provider if pregnancy is planned or suspected or if breastfeeding.

Evaluation/Desired Outcomes

- Increase in sexual desire in premenopausal women.

fluconazole (floo-**kon**-a-zole)

Diflucan

Classification

Therapeutic: antifungals (systemic)

Pharmacologic: azoles

Indications

PO, IV: Fungal infections caused by susceptible organisms, including: Oropharyngeal or esophageal candidiasis, Serious systemic candidal infections, Urinary tract infections, Peritonitis, Cyptococcal meningitis. Prevention of candidiasis in patients who have undergone bone marrow transplantation. **PO:** Single-dose oral treatment of vaginal candidiasis. **Unlabeled Use:** Prevention of recurrent vaginal yeast infections.

Action

Inhibits synthesis of fungal sterols, a necessary component of the cell membrane. **Therapeutic Effects:** Fungistatic action against susceptible organisms. May be fungicidal in higher concentrations. **Spectrum:** *Cryptococcus neoformans. Candida* spp.

Pharmacokinetics

Absorption: Well absorbed after oral administration.
Distribution: Widely distributed; good penetration into CSF, saliva, sputum, vaginal fluid, skin, eye, and peritoneum.
Metabolism and Excretion: >80% excreted unchanged by the kidneys; <10% metabolized by the liver.
Half-life: *Premature neonates:* 46–74 hr; *Children:* 19–25 hr (PO) and 15–17 hr (IV); *Adults:* 30 hr (↑ in renal impairment).

TIME/ACTION PROFILE (plasma concentrations)

ROUTE	ONSET	PEAK	DURATION
PO	unknown	2–4 hr	24 hr
IV	rapid	end of infusion	24 hr

Contraindications/Precautions

Contraindicated in: Hypersensitivity to fluconazole or other azole antifungals; Concurrent use with pimozide, erythromycin, or quinidine; OB: Pregnancy; may consider using for severe or life-threatening fungal infection if anticipated maternal benefit justifies potential fetal risk.
Use Cautiously in: Renal impairment (dose ↓ required if CCr <50 mL/min); Underlying liver disease; Structural heart disease, electrolyte abnormalities, or concurrent use of other QT interval-prolonging medications; Geri: ↑ risk of adverse reactions in older adults; consider age-related ↓ in renal function in determining dose.

Adverse Reactions/Side Effects

CV: QT interval prolongation, TORSADES DE POINTES. **Derm:** STEVENS-JOHNSON SYNDROME (SJS), TOXIC EPIDERMAL NECROLYSIS (TEN). **Endo:** adrenal insufficiency, hypertriglyceridemia, hypokalemia. **GI:** abdominal discomfort, diarrhea, HEPATOTOXICITY, nausea, vomiting. **Neuro:** dizziness, headache, seizures. **Misc:** HYPERSENSITIVITY REACTIONS (INCLUDING ANAPHYLAXIS).

Interactions

Drug-Drug: May ↑ levels of **pimozide**, **erythromycin**, and **quinidine**, which can prolong the QT interval and ↑ the risk of torsades de pointes; concurrent use contraindicated. May ↑ levels of **amiodarone** (especially with high-dose fluconazole [800 mg]), which can cause QT interval prolongation. May ↑ levels of and the risk of bleeding with **warfarin**. **Rifampin**, **rifabutin**, and **isoniazid** may ↓ levels and effectiveness. ↑ hypoglycemic effects of **glyburide** or **glipizide**. ↑ levels and risk of toxicity from **cyclosporine**, **carbamazepine**, **celecoxib**, **rifabutin**, **tacrolimus**, **sirolimus**, **theophylline**, **zidovudine**, and **phenytoin**. ↑ levels and risk of toxicity of **benzodiazepines**, **amlodipine**, **felodipine**, **isradipine**, **nifedipine**, **nisoldipine**, **verapamil**, **atorvastatin**, **fluvastatin**, **lovastatin**, **simvastatin**, **methadone**, **prednisone**, **tricyclic antidepressants**, and **losartan**. ↑ levels and risk of toxicity of **tofacitinib**; ↓ tofacitinib dose to 5 mg once daily. May ↑ levels and risk of toxicity of **ivacaftor**; ↓ ivacaftor dose. May ↑ levels and risk of toxicity of **lurasidone**; ↓ lurasidone dose. May antagonize effects of **amphotericin B**. May ↑ levels and risk of toxicity of **abrocitinib**, **lemborexant**, and **voriconazole**; avoid concurrent use. May ↑ levels and risk of toxicity of **olaparib**; concurrent use not recommended. May ↑ levels and risk of toxicity of **ibrutinib**; ↓ ibrutinib dose. May ↑ levels and risk of toxicity of **tolvaptan**; ↓ tolvaptan dose. May ↑ levels and risk of toxicity of **ivacaftor**; ↓ ivacaftor dose. May ↑ levels and risk of toxicity of **lurasidone**; ↓ lurasidone dose.

Route/Dosage

Oropharyngeal Candidiasis

PO, IV (Adults): 200 mg initially, then 100 mg daily for at least 2 wk.

PO, IV (Children ≥6 mo): 6 mg/kg initially, then 3 mg/kg once daily for ≥2 wk.

Renal Impairment

PO, IV (Adults and Children ≥6 mo): *CCr ≤50 mL/min (no hemodialysis):* Give 50% of the usual dose; *Hemodialysis:* Give 100% of the usual dose after each dialysis session; give reduced dose based on CCr on nondialysis days.

Esophageal Candidiasis

PO, IV (Adults): 200 mg initially, then 100 mg once daily for at least 3 wk (up to 400 mg/day).

PO, IV (Children ≥6 mo): 6 mg/kg initially, then 3 mg/kg once daily/day for ≥3 wk.

Renal Impairment

PO, IV (Adults and Children ≥6 mo): *CCr ≤50 mL/min (no hemodialysis):* Give 50% of the usual dose; *Hemodialysis:* Give 100% of the usual dose after each dialysis session; give reduced dose based on CCr on nondialysis days.

Vaginal Candidiasis

PO (Adults): 150-mg single dose; prevention of recurrence (unlabeled): 150 mg daily for 3 days then weekly for 6 mo.

Systemic Candidiasis

PO, IV (Adults): 400 mg/day initially, then 200–800 mg/day for 28 days.

PO, IV (Children ≥3 mo): 25 mg/kg initially (max = 800 mg), then 12 mg/kg once daily (max = 400 mg/day) for ≥3 wk.

PO, IV (Neonates and Children Birth to 3 mo postnatal age and ≥30 wk gestational age): 25 mg/kg initially, then 12 mg/kg once daily for ≥3 wk.

PO, IV (Neonates and Children Birth to 3 mo postnatal age and <30 wk gestational age): 25 mg/kg initially, then 9 mg/kg once daily for ≥3 wk.

Renal Impairment

PO, IV (Adults and Children): *CCr ≤50 mL/min (no hemodialysis):* Give 50% of the usual dose; *Hemodialysis:* Give 100% of the usual dose after each dialysis session; give reduced dose based on CCr on nondialysis days.

Cryptococcal Meningitis

PO, IV (Adults): *Treatment:* 400 mg once daily until favorable clinical response, then 200–800 mg once daily for at least 10–12 wk after clearing of CSF; change to oral therapy as soon as possible. *Suppressive therapy:* 200 mg once daily.

PO, IV (Children): 12 mg/kg initially, then 6–12 mg/kg once daily for ≥10–12 wk after clearing of CSF; change to oral therapy as soon as possible. *Suppressive therapy:* 6 mg/kg/day.

Renal Impairment

PO, IV (Adults and Children): *CCr ≤50 mL/min (no hemodialysis):* Give 50% of the usual dose; *Hemodialysis:* Give 100% of the usual dose after each dialysis session; give reduced dose based on CCr on nondialysis days.

Prevention of Candidiasis After Bone Marrow Transplant

PO, IV (Adults): 400 mg once daily; begin several days before procedure if severe neutropenia is expected, and continue for 7 days after ANC >1000 /mm^3.

PO, IV (Children >14 days): 10–12 mg/kg/day, not to exceed 600 mg/day.

Renal Impairment

PO, IV (Adults): *CCr ≤50 mL/min (no hemodialysis):* Give 50% of the usual dose; *Hemodialysis:* Give 100% of the usual dose after each dialysis session; give reduced dose based on CCr on nondialysis days.

F

Availability (generic available)

Tablets: 50 mg, 100 mg, 150 mg, 200 mg. **Powder for oral suspension (orange flavor):** 10 mg/mL, 40 mg/mL. **Premixed infusion:** 100 mg/50 mL 0.9% NaCl, 200 mg/100 mL 0.9% NaCl, 400 mg/200 mL 0.9% NaCl.

NURSING IMPLICATIONS

Assessment

- Assess infected area and monitor CSF cultures before and periodically during therapy.
- Obtain specimens for culture before instituting therapy. Therapy may be started before results are obtained.
- Assess patient for rash (mild to moderate rash usually occurs in the 2nd wk of therapy and resolves within 1–2 wk of continued therapy). If rash is severe (extensive erythematous or maculopapular rash with moist desquamation or angioedema), accompanied by systemic symptoms (serum sickness-like reaction, SJS, TEN), or occurs during treatment for a superficial fungal infection, therapy must be discontinued immediately.

Lab Test Considerations

- Monitor BUN and serum creatinine before and periodically during therapy.
- Monitor liver function tests before and periodically during therapy. May cause ↑ AST, ALT, serum alkaline phosphate, and bilirubin concentrations.

Implementation

- Do not confuse Diflucan with Diprivan.
- **PO:** Administer at the same time each day. Shake oral suspension well before administration.

IV Administration

- **Intermittent Infusion: Dilution:** Premixed infusions are prediluted and ready to use. Do not unwrap until ready to use. Some opacity of the plastic is normal and does not affect the solution quality or safety; opacity will diminish gradually. Do not administer solution that is cloudy or has a precipitate. Check for leaks by squeezing inner bag. If leaks are found, discard container as unsterile. **Concentration:** 2 mg/mL. **Rate:** Infuse over 1–2 hr. Do not exceed a rate of 200 mg/hr. Pedi: For children receiving doses >6 mg/kg/day, give over 2 hr.
- **Y-Site Compatibility:** acyclovir, aldesleukin, alemtuzumab, allopurinol, amikacin, aminocaproic acid, aminophylline, amiodarone, anidulafungin, argatroban, arsenic trioxide, ascorbic acid, atracurium, atropine, azathioprine, azithromycin, aztreonam, benztropine, bivalirudin, bleomycin, bumetanide, buprenorphine, butorphanol, calcium chloride, cangrelor, carboplatin, carmustine, caspofungin, cefazolin, cefepime, cefiderocol, cefotetan, cefoxitin, ceftaroline, ceftobiprole, chlorpromazine, cisatracurium, cisplatin, cyanocobalamin, cyclophosphamide, cyclosporine, cytarabine, dacarbazine, dactinomycin, daptomycin, daunorubicin, defibrotide, dexamethasone, dexmedetomidine, dexrazoxane, diltiazem, diphenhydramine, dobutamine, docetaxel, dopamine, doxorubicin hydrochloride, doxorubicin liposomal, doxycycline, droperidol, enalaprilat, ephedrine, epinephrine, epirubicin, epoetin alfa, eptifibatide, eravacycline, ertapenem, erythromycin, esmolol, etoposide, etoposide phosphate, famotidine, fentanyl, filgrastim, fludarabine, fluorouracil, folic acid, foscarnet, fosphenytoin, ganciclovir, gemcitabine, gentamicin, glycopyrrolate, granisetron, heparin, hetastarch, hydrocortisone, hydromorphone, idarubicin, ifosfamide, imipenem/cilastatin/relebactam, immune globulin, indomethacin, insulin, regular, irinotecan, isoproterenol, ketorolac, labetalol, LR, letermovir, leucovorin calcium, levofloxacin, lidocaine, linezolid, lorazepam, magnesium sulfate, mannitol, melphalan, meperidine, meropenem, mesna, methadone, methotrexate, methylprednisolone, metoclopramide, metoprolol, metronidazole, midazolam, milrinone, mitomycin, mitoxantrone, morphine, multivitamins, mycophenolate, nafcillin, nalbuphine, naloxone, nicardipine, nitroglycerin, nitroprusside, norepinephrine, octreotide, ondansetron, oritavancin, oxacillin, oxaliplatin, oxytocin, paclitaxel, palonosetron, pamidronate, papaverine, pemetrexed, penicillin G, pentobarbital, phenobarbital, phentolamine, phenylephrine, phytonadione, piperacillin/tazobactam, plazomicin, potassium acetate, potassium chloride, procainamide, prochlorperazine, promethazine, propofol, propranolol, protamine, pyridoxine, remifentanil, rituximab, rocuronium, sargramostim, sodium acetate, sodium bicarbonate, succinylcholine, sufentanil, sulbactam/durlobactam, tacrolimus, telavancin, theophylline, thiotepa, tigecycline, tirofiban, tobramycin, topotecan, trastuzumab, vancomycin, vasopressin, vecuronium, verapamil, vinblastine, vincristine, vinorelbine, voriconazole, zidovudine, zoledronic acid.
- **Y-Site Incompatibility:** amphotericin B deoxycholate, ampicillin, dantrolene, diazepam, diazoxide, gemtuzumab ozogamicin, pantoprazole, trimethoprim/sulfamethoxazole.

Patient/Family Teaching

- Instruct patient to take medication as directed, at the same time each day, even if feeling better. Take missed doses as soon as remembered, but not if almost time for next dose. Do not double doses.
- May cause dizziness or seizures. Caution patient to avoid driving and other activities requiring alertness until response to fluconazole is known.
- Instruct patient to notify health care professional if skin rash, abdominal pain, fever, or diarrhea becomes pronounced; if signs and symptoms of liver dysfunction (unusual fatigue, anorexia, nausea, vomiting, jaundice, dark urine, or pale stools) occur; if unusual bruising or bleeding occur; or if no improvement is seen within a few days of therapy.

- Rep: May cause fetal harm. Advise females of reproductive potential to use effective contraception during and for 1 wk after last dose. Advise patient to notify health care professional if pregnancy is planned or suspected or if breastfeeding.

Evaluation/Desired Outcomes

- Resolution of clinical and laboratory indications of fungal infections. Full course of therapy may require wk or mo of treatment after resolution of symptoms.
- Prevention of candidiasis in patients who have undergone bone marrow transplantation.
- Decrease in skin irritation and vaginal discomfort in patients with vaginal candidiasis. Diagnosis should be reconfirmed with smears or cultures before a second course of therapy to rule out other pathogens associated with vulvovaginitis. Recurrent vaginal infections may be a sign of systemic illness.

fludrocortisone

(floo-droe-**kor**-ti-sone)

✦ Florinef

Classification

Therapeutic: hormones

Pharmacologic: corticosteroids (mineralocorticoid)

Indications

Sodium loss and hypotension associated with adrenocortical insufficiency (in combination with hydrocortisone or cortisone). Sodium loss due to congenital adrenogenital syndrome (congenital adrenal hyperplasia). **Unlabeled Use:** Idiopathic orthostatic hypotension (with increased sodium intake). Type IV renal tubular acidosis.

Action

Causes sodium reabsorption, hydrogen and potassium excretion, and water retention by its effects on the distal renal tubule. **Therapeutic Effects:** Maintenance of sodium balance and BP in patients with adrenocortical insufficiency.

Pharmacokinetics

Absorption: Well absorbed following oral administration.

Distribution: Widely distributed to tissues.

Metabolism and Excretion: Mostly metabolized by the liver.

Half-life: 3.5 hr.

TIME/ACTION PROFILE (mineralocorticoid activity)

ROUTE	ONSET	PEAK	DURATION
PO	unknown	unknown	1–2 days

Contraindications/Precautions

Contraindicated in: Hypersensitivity.

Use Cautiously in: HF; Addison's disease (patients may have exaggerated response); OB: Safety not established in pregnancy; Lactation: Safety not established in breastfeeding; Pedi: Safety and effectiveness not established in children.

Adverse Reactions/Side Effects

CV: arrhythmias, edema, HF, hypertension. **Endo:** adrenal suppression. **F and E:** hypokalemia, hypokalemic alkalosis. **GI:** anorexia, nausea. **Metab:** weight gain. **MS:** arthralgia, muscular weakness, tendon contractures. **Neuro:** ascending paralysis, dizziness, headache. **Misc:** hypersensitivity reactions.

Interactions

Drug-Drug: Use with **thiazide diuretics, loop diuretics**, or **amphotericin B** may ↑ risk of hypokalemia. Hypokalemia may ↑ risk of **digoxin** toxicity. May produce prolonged neuromuscular blockade following the use of **nondepolarizing neuromuscular blocking agents. Phenobarbital** or **rifampin** may ↓ levels and effectiveness.

Drug-Food: Large amounts of **salt** or **sodium-containing foods** may cause excessive sodium retention and potassium loss.

Route/Dosage

PO (Adults): *Adrenocortical insufficiency:* 0.1 mg/day (range 0.1 mg 3 times weekly: 0.2 mg daily). Doses as small as 0.05 mg daily may be required by some patients. Use with 10–30 mg hydrocortisone daily. *Adrenogenital syndrome:* 0.1–0.2 mg/day. *Idiopathic hypotension:* 0.05–0.2 mg/day (unlabeled).

PO (Children): 0.05–0.1 mg/day.

Availability (generic available)

Tablets: 0.1 mg.

NURSING IMPLICATIONS

Assessment

- Monitor BP periodically during therapy. Report significant changes. Hypotension may indicate insufficient dose.
- Monitor for fluid retention (peripheral edema, rales/crackles, dyspnea, daily weight gain, jugular venous distention). Notify health care provider should these occur.
- Monitor patients with Addison's disease closely and stop treatment if a significant ↑ in weight or BP, edema, or cardiac enlargement occurs. Patients with Addison's disease are more sensitive to the action of fludrocortisone and may have an exaggerated response.

Lab Test Considerations

- Monitor serum electrolytes periodically during therapy. Fludrocortisone causes ↓ serum potassium.

Implementation

- **PO:** Administer without regard to food; take with food if GI upset occurs. Tablets are scored and may be broken if dose adjustment is necessary. May require higher doses when subject to stress.

Patient/Family Teaching

- Explain the purpose and side effects of fludrocortisone. Instruct patient to take medication as directed. Take missed doses as soon as remembered but not just before next dose is due. Explain that lifelong therapy may be necessary. Patient should keep an adequate supply available at all times. Discontinue gradually if needed. Advise patient to read *Patient Information* before starting and with each Rx refill in case of changes.
- Advise patient to follow dietary modification prescribed by health care professional. Instruct patient to follow a diet high in potassium (see Appendix J). Amount of sodium allowed in diet varies with pathophysiology.
- Instruct patient to inform health care professional if weight gain or edema, muscle weakness, cramps, nausea, anorexia, or dizziness occurs.
- Stopping the medication suddenly may result in adrenal insufficiency (anorexia, nausea, weakness, fatigue, dyspnea, hypotension, hypoglycemia). If these signs appear, notify health care professional immediately, as this condition can be life-threatening. Medical ID describing disease process and medication regimen should be worn in case of emergencies.
- Caution patient to avoid vaccinations without first consulting health care professional.
- Advise patient to notify health care professional of all Rx or OTC medications, vitamins, or herbal products being taken and to consult with health care professional before taking other medications.
- Rep: Advise women of reproductive potential to notify health care professional if pregnancy is planned or suspected or if breastfeeding. Monitor newborns of patients taking fludrocortisone during pregnancy for hypoadrenalism.

Evaluation/Desired Outcomes

- Normalization of fluid and electrolyte balance without the development of hypokalemia or hypertension.

flumazenil (flu-maz-e-nil)

~~Romazicon~~

Classification
Therapeutic: antidotes

Indications

Complete/partial reversal of effects of benzodiazepines used as general anesthetics or during diagnostic or therapeutic procedures. Intentional or accidental overdose of benzodiazepines.

Action

Flumazenil is a benzodiazepine derivative that antagonizes the CNS depressant effects of benzodiazepine compounds. It has no effect on CNS depression from other causes, including opioids, alcohol, barbiturates, or general anesthetics. **Therapeutic Effects:** Reversal of benzodiazepine effects.

Pharmacokinetics

Absorption: IV administration results in complete bioavailability.

Distribution: Unknown.

Metabolism and Excretion: Primarily metabolized in the liver. Primarily excreted in feces and urine (<1% as unchanged drug).

Half-life: *Children:* 20–75 min; *Adults:* 41–79 min.

TIME/ACTION PROFILE (reversal of benzodiazepine effects)

ROUTE	ONSET	PEAK	DURATION
IV	1–2 min	6–10 min	1–2 hr†

† Depends on dose/concentration of benzodiazepine and dose of flumazenil.

Contraindications/Precautions

Contraindicated in: Hypersensitivity to flumazenil or benzodiazepines; Patients receiving benzodiazepines for life-threatening medical problems, including status epilepticus or ↑ intracranial pressure; Serious cyclic antidepressant overdosage.

Use Cautiously in: Mixed CNS depressant overdose (effects of other agents may emerge when benzodiazepine effect is removed); History of seizures (seizures are more likely to occur in patients who are experiencing sedative/hypnotic withdrawal, who have recently received repeated doses of benzodiazepines, or who have a previous history of seizure activity); Head injury (may ↑ intracranial pressure and risk of seizures); Severe hepatic impairment; OB: Safety not established in pregnancy; Lactation: Safety not established in breastfeeding; Pedi: Children <1 yr (safety and effectiveness not established).

Adverse Reactions/Side Effects

CV: arrhythmias, chest pain, hypertension. **Derm:** flushing, sweating. **EENT:** abnormal hearing, abnormal vision, blurred vision. **GI:** nausea, vomiting, hiccups. **Local:** pain/injection-site reactions, phlebitis. **Neuro:** dizziness, agitation, confusion, drowsiness, emotional lability, fatigue, headache, paresthesia, SEIZURES, sleep disorders. **Misc:** rigors, shivering.

Interactions

Drug-Drug: None reported.

Route/Dosage

Reversal of Conscious Sedation or General Anesthesia

IV (Adults): 0.2 mg initially. Additional doses may be given at 1-min intervals until desired results are obtained, up to a total dose of 1 mg. If resedation occurs, regimen may be repeated at 20-min intervals, not to exceed 3 mg/hr.
IV (Children): 0.01 mg/kg (up to 0.2 mg); if the desired level of consciousness is not obtained after waiting an additional 45 sec, further injections of 0.01 mg/kg (up to 0.2 mg) can be administered and repeated at 1-min intervals when necessary (up to a max of 4 additional times) to a max total dose of 0.05 mg/kg or 1 mg, whichever is lower. The dose should be individualized based on the patient's response.

Suspected Benzodiazepine Overdose

IV (Adults): 0.2 mg initially. Additional 0.3 mg may be given 30 sec later. Further doses of 0.5 mg may be given at 1-min intervals, if necessary, to a total dose of 3 mg. Usual dose required is 1–3 mg. If resedation occurs, additional doses of 0.5 mg/min for 2 min may be given at 20-min intervals (given no more than 1 mg at a time, not to exceed 3 mg per hr).
IV (Children): *Unlabeled:* 0.01 mg/kg (maximum dose 0.2 mg) with repeat doses every min up to a cumulative dose of 1 mg. As an alternative to repeat doses, continuous infusions of 0.005–0.01 mg/kg/hr have been used.

Availability (generic available)

Solution for injection: 0.1 mg/mL.

NURSING IMPLICATIONS

Assessment

- Assess level of consciousness and respiratory status before and during therapy. Observe patient for ≥2 hr after administration for the appearance of resedation. Hypoventilation may occur.
- **Overdose:** Attempt to determine time of ingestion and amount and type of benzodiazepine taken. Knowledge of agent ingested allows an estimate of duration of CNS depression.
- Monitor for seizure activity associated with benzodiazepine withdrawal. Institute seizure precautions as indicated. Seizures are more likely to occur in patients who are experiencing sedative/hypnotic withdrawal, those who have recently received repeated doses of benzodiazepines, or those who have a previous history of seizure activity. Seizures may be treated with benzodiazepines, barbiturates, or phenytoin. Larger than normal doses of benzodiazepines may be required.

Implementation

- Do not confuse flumazenil with influenza virus vaccine.
- Ensure that patient has a patent airway before administration of flumazenil.
- Observe IV site frequently for redness or irritation. Administer through a free-flowing IV infusion into a large vein to minimize pain at the injection site.
- Optimal emergence should be undertaken slowly to decrease undesirable effects including confusion, agitation, emotional lability, and perceptual distortion.
- **Suspected Benzodiazepine Overdose:** If no effects are seen after administration of flumazenil, consider other causes of decreased level of consciousness (alcohol, barbiturates, opioid analgesics).

IV Administration

- **IV Push: Dilution:** May be administered undiluted or diluted in syringe with D5W, 0.9% NaCl, or LR. Diluted solution should be discarded after 24 hr. **Concentration:** Up to 0.1 mg/mL. **Rate:** Administer 0.1 mg over 15–30 sec into free-flowing IV in a large vein. Do not exceed 0.2 mg/min in children or 0.5 mg/min in adults.
- **Y-Site Compatibility:** esomeprazole, remimazolam.

Patient/Family Teaching

- Explain the purpose and side effects. Flumazenil does not consistently reverse the amnestic effects of benzodiazepines. Provide patient and family with written instructions for postprocedure care.
- Inform family that patient may appear alert at the time of discharge but the sedative effects of the benzodiazepine may recur. Instruct patient to avoid driving or other activities requiring alertness for ≥24 hr after discharge.
- Instruct patient not to take any alcohol or nonprescription drugs for at least 18–24 hr after discharge.
- Resumption of usual activities should occur only when no residual effects of the benzodiazepine remain.
- Advise patient to notify health care provider if dizziness, headache, upset stomach, vomiting, blurred eyesight, dry mouth, sweating a lot, feeling nervous and excitable, shakiness, or trouble sleeping occur.
- Rep: Advise women of reproductive potential to notify health care provider if pregnancy is planned or suspected or if breastfeeding.

Evaluation/Desired Outcomes

- Improved level of consciousness.
- Decrease in respiratory depression caused by benzodiazepines.

fluocinolone, See CORTICOSTEROIDS (TOPICAL).

fluocinonide, See CORTICOSTEROIDS (TOPICAL).

FLUOROQUINOLONES
(floor-oh-**kwin**-oh-lones)

ciprofloxacin† (sip-roe-**flox**-a-sin)
Cipro, ~~Cipro XR~~

delafloxacin (del-a-**floks**-a-sin)
Baxdela

levofloxacin (le-voe-**flox**-a-sin)
~~Levaquin~~

moxifloxacin† (mox-i-**flox**-a-sin)
~~Avelox~~

ofloxacin† (oh-**flox**-a-sin)
~~Floxin~~

Classification
Therapeutic: anti-infectives
Pharmacologic: fluoroquinolones

† See Appendix B for ophthalmic use

Indications
PO, IV: Treatment of the following bacterial infections: Urinary tract infections (UTIs), including cystitis and prostatitis (ciprofloxacin, levofloxacin, ofloxacin) (should be used for acute uncomplicated cystitis only when there are no other alternative treatment options); Gonorrhea (may not be considered first-line agents due to increasing resistance); Gynecologic infections (ciprofloxacin, ofloxacin); Respiratory tract infections, including acute sinusitis, acute exacerbations of chronic bronchitis, and pneumonia (should be used for acute sinusitis or acute bacterial exacerbations of chronic bronchitis only when there are no other alternative treatment options); Skin and skin structure infections (delafloxacin, levofloxacin, moxifloxacin, ciprofloxacin, ofloxacin); Bone and joint infections (ciprofloxacin); Infectious diarrhea (ciprofloxacin); Intra-abdominal infections (ciprofloxacin, moxifloxacin). Febrile neutropenia (ciprofloxacin). Postexposure treatment of inhalational anthrax (ciprofloxacin, levofloxacin). Treatment and prophylaxis of plague (ciprofloxacin, levofloxacin, moxifloxacin).

Action
Inhibit bacterial DNA synthesis by inhibiting DNA gyrase. **Therapeutic Effects:** Death of susceptible bacteria. **Spectrum:** Broad activity includes many gram-positive pathogens: Staphylococci including methicillin-resistant *Staphylococcus aureus*, *Staphylococcus epidermidis*, *Staphylococcus saprophyticus*, *Streptococcus pneumoniae*, *Streptococcus pyogenes*, and *Bacillus anthracis*. Gram-negative spectrum notable for activity against: *Escherichia coli*, *Klebsiella*, *Enterobacter*, *Salmonella*, *Shigella*, *Proteus*, *Providencia*, *Morganella morganii*, *Pseudomonas aeruginosa*, *Serratia*, *Haemophilus*, *Acinetobacter*, *Neisseria gonorrhoeae*, *Moraxella catarrhalis*, *Campylobacter*, and *Yersinia pestis*. Additional spectrum includes: *Chlamydia pneumoniae*, *Legionella pneumoniae*, and *Mycoplasma pneumoniae*.

Pharmacokinetics
Absorption: Well absorbed after oral administration (*ciprofloxacin:* 70%; *delafloxacin:* 59%; *moxifloxacin:* 90%; *levofloxacin:* 99%; *ofloxacin:* 98%).
Distribution: Widely distributed. High tissue and urinary levels are achieved. *Ciprofloxacin* and *ofloxacin* enter breast milk.
Metabolism and Excretion: *Ciprofloxacin:* 15% metabolized by the liver, 40–50% excreted unchanged by the kidneys; *delafloxacin:* primarily undergoes glucuronidation; 50–65% excreted unchanged by the kidneys; 28–48% excreted unchanged in feces; *levofloxacin:* 87% excreted unchanged in urine, small amounts metabolized; *moxifloxacin:* mostly metabolized by the liver, 20% excreted unchanged in urine, 25% excreted unchanged in feces; *ofloxacin:* 70–80% excreted unchanged by the kidneys.
Half-life: *Ciprofloxacin:* 4 hr; *delafloxacin:* 3.7 hr (IV); 4.2–8.5 hr (PO); *levofloxacin:* 8 hr; *moxifloxacin:* 12 hr; *ofloxacin:* 5–7 hr (all are ↑ in renal impairment).

TIME/ACTION PROFILE (blood levels)

ROUTE	ONSET	PEAK	DURATION
Ciprofloxacin: PO	rapid	1–2 hr	12 hr
Ciprofloxacin: IV	rapid	end of infusion	12 hr
Delafloxacin: PO	rapid	1 hr	12 hr
Delafloxacin: IV	rapid	end of infusion	12 hr
Levofloxacin: PO	rapid	1–2 hr	24 hr
Levofloxacin: IV	rapid	end of infusion	24 hr
Moxifloxacin: PO	within 1 hr	1–3 hr	24 hr
Moxifloxacin: IV	rapid	end of infusion	24 hr
Ofloxacin: PO	rapid	1–2 hr	12 hr
Ofloxacin: IV	rapid	end of infusion	12 hr

Contraindications/Precautions
Contraindicated in: Hypersensitivity. Cross-sensitivity among agents within class may occur; History of myasthenia gravis (may worsen symptoms including muscle weakness and breathing problems); History of tendon disorders, including tendinitis or tendon rupture; History of peripheral neuropathy; Patients with or at ↑ risk for aortic aneurysm (use only if no alternatives); **Moxifloxacin:** Concurrent use of Class

IA antiarrhythmics (disopyramide, quinidine, procainamide) or Class III antiarrhythmics (amiodarone, sotalol) (↑ risk of QTc interval prolongation and torsades de pointes); Known QT interval prolongation or concurrent use of agents causing prolongation; **Ciprofloxacin:** Concurrent use with tizanidine; **Delafloxacin:** End-stage renal disease (eGFR <15 mL/min); OB: Do not use unless potential benefit outweighs potential fetal risk (delafloxacin, moxifloxacin, ofloxacin); Lactation: Avoid breastfeeding during treatment and for 2 days after final dose (for ciprofloxacin and levofloxacin, applies for all indications other than postexposure prophylaxis of inhalational anthrax); Pedi: Use only for treatment of anthrax, plague, and complicated UTIs in children 1–17 yr due to possible arthropathy.

Use Cautiously in: Known or suspected CNS disorder; Depression; Renal impairment (dose ↓ if CCr ≤50 mL/min for ciprofloxacin, levofloxacin, ofloxacin); Cirrhosis (levofloxacin, moxifloxacin); Concurrent use of corticosteroids, strenuous exercise, or rheumatoid arthritis (↑ risk of tendinitis/tendon rupture); Kidney, heart, or lung transplant patients (↑ risk of tendinitis/tendon rupture); Diabetes; **Moxifloxacin:** Concurrent use of erythromycin, antipsychotics, and tricyclic antidepressants (↑ risk of QTc prolongation and torsades de pointes); **Moxifloxacin:** Bradycardia; **Moxifloxacin:** Acute myocardial ischemia; **Delafloxacin:** Severe renal impairment (dose ↓ if eGFR 15–29 mL/min) (IV diluent may accumulate and ↑ serum creatinine) (↑ risk of tendon rupture in renal failure); OB: Use during pregnancy only if potential maternal benefit outweighs potential fetal risk (ciprofloxacin and levofloxacin only); Lactation: Can be used while breastfeeding for postexposure prophylaxis of anthrax if potential maternal benefit justifies potential risk to infant (ciprofloxacin and levofloxacin only); Geri: ↑ risk of adverse reactions in older adults.

Adverse Reactions/Side Effects

CV: AORTIC ANEURYSM/DISSECTION, myocardial ischemia, QT interval prolongation (levofloxacin, moxifloxacin), TORSADES DE POINTES, vasodilation. **Derm:** ACUTE GENERALIZED EXANTHEMATOUS PUSTULOSIS, photosensitivity, rash, STEVENS-JOHNSON SYNDROME (SJS). **Endo:** hyperglycemia, hypoglycemia. **GI:** diarrhea, nausea, ↑ liver enzymes (ciprofloxacin, moxifloxacin), abdominal pain, CLOSTRIDIOIDES DIFFICILE-ASSOCIATED DIARRHEA (CDAD), HEPATOTOXICITY (CIPROFLOXACIN), vomiting. **GU:** vaginitis. **Local:** phlebitis. **MS:** arthralgia, myalgia, tendinitis, tendon rupture. **Neuro:** dizziness, headache, insomnia, ↑ INTRACRANIAL PRESSURE (INCLUDING PSEUDOTUMOR CEREBRI), acute psychoses, agitation, anxiety, attention disturbances, confusion, depression, drowsiness, hallucinations, light-headedness, memory impairment, nightmares, paranoia, peripheral neuropathy, SEIZURES, SUICIDAL THOUGHTS/BEHAVIORS, toxic psychosis, tremor. **Misc:** HYPERSENSITIVITY REACTIONS (INCLUDING ANAPHYLAXIS).

Interactions

Drug-Drug: Ciprofloxacin may ↑ **tizanidine** levels and risk of hypotension and sedation; concurrent use contraindicated. **QT interval-prolonging medications** may ↑ risk of QT interval prolongation and torsades de pointes; avoid concurrent use. Ciprofloxacin may ↑ **theophylline** levels and risk of CNS toxicity; avoid concurrent use; if concurrent use cannot be avoided, closely monitor serum theophylline levels. Ciprofloxacin may ↑ levels and risk of toxicity of **CYP1A2 substrates**, including **ropinirole**, **clozapine**, **olanzapine**, and **zolpidem**; avoid concurrent use with zolpidem. **Antacids**, **iron salts**, **bismuth subsalicylate**, **sucralfate**, **sevelemer**, **lanthanum**, and **zinc salts** may ↓ absorption of fluoroquinolones; separate administration of medications. May ↑ levels of and risk of bleeding from **warfarin**. Ciprofloxacin may alter levels and the effects of **phenytoin**. **Probenecid** may ↑ levels and risk of toxicity. May ↑ risk of nephrotoxicity from **cyclosporine**. Concurrent use of ciprofloxacin with **NSAIDs** may ↑ risk of seizures. **Corticosteroids** may ↑ risk of tendon rupture. May ↑ risk of hypoglycemia when used with **antidiabetic agents**.

Drug-Natural Products: **Fennel** ↓ the absorption of ciprofloxacin.

Drug-Food: Absorption is impaired by **concurrent tube feeding** (because of metal cations). Absorption is ↓ if taken with **dairy products** or calcium-fortified juices.

Route/Dosage

Ciprofloxacin

PO (Adults): *Most infections:* 500–750 mg every 12 hr. *Complicated UTIs:* 500 mg every 12 hr for 7–14 days. *Uncomplicated UTIs:* 250 mg every 12 hr for 3 days. *Gonorrhea:* 250-mg single dose. *Inhalational anthrax (postexposure) or cutaneous anthrax:* 500 mg every 12 hr for 60 days; *Plague:* 500–750 mg every 12 hr for 14 days.

PO (Children 1–17 yr): *Complicated UTIs:* 10–15 mg/kg every 12 hr (max = 750 mg/dose) for 10–21 days. *Inhalational anthrax (postexposure) or cutaneous anthrax:* 10–15 mg/kg every 12 hr (max = 500 mg/dose) for 60 days; *Plague:* 15 mg/kg every 8–12 hr (max = 500 mg/dose) for 14 days.

IV (Adults): *Most infections:* 400 mg every 12 hr. *Complicated UTIs:* 400 mg every 12 hr for 7–14 days. *Uncomplicated UTIs:* 200 mg every 12 hr for

7–14 days. *Inhalational anthrax (postexposure):* 400 mg every 12 hr for 60 days; *Plague:* 400 mg every 8–12 hr for 14 days.
IV (Children 1–17 yr): *Inhalational anthrax (postexposure):* 10 mg/kg every 12 hr (not to exceed 400 mg/dose) for 60 days; *Complicated UTIs:* 6–10 mg/kg every 8 hr (max = 400 mg/dose) for 10–21 days; *Plague:* 10 mg/kg every 8–12 hr (max = 400 mg/dose) for 10–21 days.

Renal Impairment

PO (Adults): *CCr 30–50 mL/min:* 250–500 mg every 12 hr; *CCr 5–29 mL/min:* 250–500 mg every 18 hr.
IV (Adults): *CCr 5–29 mL/min:* 200–400 mg every 18–24 hr.

Delafloxacin

IV (Adults): 300 mg every 12 hr for 5–14 days (for acute bacterial skin and skin structure infections) or 5–10 days (for community-acquired pneumonia [CAP]) *or* 300 mg every 12 hr followed by switching to oral regimen (at dose stated below) for a total of 5–14 days (for acute bacterial skin and skin structure infections) or 5–10 days (for CAP).
PO (Adults): 450 mg every 12 hr for 5–14 days (for acute bacterial skin and skin structure infections) or 5–10 days (for CAP).

Renal Impairment

IV (Adults): *eGFR 15–29 mL/min:* 200 mg every 12 hr for 5–14 days (for acute bacterial skin and skin structure infections) or 5–10 days (for CAP) *or* 200 mg every 12 hr followed by switching to oral regimen (450 mg every 12 hr) for a total of 5–14 days (for acute bacterial skin and skin structure infections) or 5–10 days (for CAP); *eGFR <15 mL/min:* Not recommended.

Levofloxacin

PO, IV (Adults): *Most infections:* 250–750 mg every 24 hr; *Inhalational anthrax (postexposure):* 500 mg once daily for 60 days.
PO, IV (Children >50 kg): *Inhalational anthrax (postexposure):* 500 mg once daily for 60 days; *Plague:* 500 mg once daily for 10–14 days.
PO, IV (Children <50 kg and ≥6 mo): *Inhalational anthrax (postexposure):* 8 mg/kg (max: 250 mg/dose) every 12 hr for 60 days. *Plague:* 8 mg/kg (max: 250 mg/dose) every 12 hr for 10–14 days; *Other infections:* 10 mg/kg/dose every 24 hr (max: 500 mg/dose).

Renal Impairment

PO, IV (Adults): *Normal renal function dosing of 750 mg/day: CCr 20–49 mL/min:* 750 mg every 48 hr; *CCr 10–19 mL/min:* 750 mg initially, then 500 mg every 48 hr; *Normal renal function dosing of 500 mg/day: CCr 20–49 mL/min:* 500 mg initially then 250 mg every 24 hr; *CCr 10–19 mL/min:* 500 mg initially then 250 mg every 48 hr. *Normal renal function dosing of 250 mg/day: CCr 10–19 mL/min:* 250 mg every 48 hr.

Moxifloxacin

PO, IV (Adults): *Bacterial sinusitis:* 400 mg once daily for 10 days; *CAP:* 400 mg once daily for 7–14 days. *Acute bacterial exacerbation of chronic bronchitis:* 400 mg once daily for 5 days. *Complicated intra-abdominal infection:* 400 mg once daily for 5–14 days. *Skin/skin structure infections:* 400 mg/day for 7–21 days. *Treatment/prevention of plague:* 400 mg once daily for 10–14 days.

Ofloxacin

PO (Adults): *Most infections:* 400 mg every 12 hr. *Prostatitis:* 300 mg every 12 hr for 6 wk. *Uncomplicated UTIs:* 200 mg every 12 hr for 3–7 days. *Complicated UTIs:* 200 mg every 12 hr for 10 days. *Gonorrhea:* 400-mg single dose.

Renal Impairment

PO, IV (Adults): *CCr 20–50 mL/min:* 100% of the usual dose every 24 hr; *CCr <20 mL/min:* 50% of the usual dose every 24 hr.

Availability

Ciprofloxacin (generic available)

Immediate-release tablets: 100 mg, 250 mg, 500 mg, 750 mg. **Oral suspension (strawberry flavor):** 250 mg/5 mL, 500 mg/5 mL. **Premixed infusion:** 200 mg/100 mL D5W, 400 mg/200 mL D5W. **Solution for injection:** 10 mg/mL. ***In combination with:*** fluocinolone (Otovel); hydrocortisone (Cipro HC) (see Appendix N).

Delafloxacin

Tablets: 450 mg. **Lyophilized powder for injection:** 300 mg/vial.

Levofloxacin (generic available)

Tablets: 250 mg, 500 mg, 750 mg. **Oral solution:** 25 mg/mL. **Solution for injection:** 25 mg/mL. **Premixed infusion:** 250 mg/50 mL D5W, 500 mg/100 mL D5W, 750 mg/150 mL D5W.

Moxifloxacin (generic available)

Tablets: 400 mg. **Premixed infusion:** 400 mg/250 mL 0.8% NaCl.

Ofloxacin (generic available)

Tablets: 200 mg, 300 mg, 400 mg.

NURSING IMPLICATIONS

Assessment

- Assess for resolving infection (vital signs; appearance of wound, sputum, urine, and stool; WBC) during therapy.
- Monitor for signs/symptoms of tuberculosis (TB) (cough, bloody sputum, fever) during *moxifloxacin* and *levofloxacin* therapy. *Negative initial TB*

cultures: Obtain AFB smear every month until 2 consecutive negative tests; obtain chest x-ray at 2–3 mo and end of treatment. *Positive initial cultures:* Obtain AFB smear every 2 wk until 2 consecutive negative tests.

- Assess cardiac history and ECG at baseline; avoid use in patients with long QT syndrome or cardiac arrhythmias associated with prolonged QT interval.
- Monitor bowel function. Diarrhea, abdominal cramping, fever, and bloody stools should be reported to health care provider promptly as a sign of CDAD. May begin up to several weeks following cessation of therapy.
- Monitor for signs/symptoms of hypersensitivity reactions (rash, urticaria, pruritus, flushing, dizziness, vomiting, abdominal pain) and angioedema (swelling of throat, lips, tongue, or face; dyspnea; wheezing; hoarseness). Discontinue drug immediately and provide supportive care.
- Assess for rash periodically during therapy. May cause SJS. Discontinue therapy if severe or if accompanied with fever, general malaise, fatigue, muscle or joint aches, blisters, oral lesions, conjunctivitis, hepatitis, or eosinophilia.
- Assess for signs/symptoms of peripheral neuropathy (pain, burning, tingling, numbness, and/or weakness or other alterations of sensation, including light touch, pain, temperature, position sense, and vibratory sensation) periodically during therapy. Symptoms may be irreversible; discontinue fluoroquinolone if symptoms occur.
- Assess for suicidal tendencies, depression, or changes in behavior periodically during therapy.

Lab Test Considerations

- Obtain specimens for culture and sensitivity before initiating therapy. 1st dose may be given before receiving results. Monitor CBC to assess therapeutic response. May ↑ AST, ALT, LDH, bilirubin, and alkaline phosphatase. Discontinue fluoroquinolone immediately if hepatitis occurs. May ↑ or ↓ serum glucose, especially in patients with diabetes. Monitor renal function. Monitor prothrombin time closely in patients receiving fluoroquinolones and warfarin; may enhance the anticoagulant effects of warfarin.

Implementation

- Do not confuse levofloxacin with levetiracetam.
- Assure adequate hydration prior to fluoroquinolone therapy to avoid crystalluria.
- **PO:** Administer *ofloxacin* on an empty stomach 1 hr before or 2 hr after meals, with a full glass of water. *Moxifloxacin, ciprofloxacin, delafloxacin* and *levofloxacin* may be administered without regard to food and with a full glass of water, at the same time each day. Should be taken ≥2 hr (4 hr for *moxifloxacin* and *ofloxacin*) before or 2 hr (6 hr for *ciprofloxacin* and *delafloxacin,* 8 hr for *moxifloxacin*) after antacids or other products containing calcium, iron, zinc, magnesium, or aluminum.
- If gastric irritation occurs, *ciprofloxacin* may be administered with meals. Food slows and may slightly ↓ absorption. Regular tablets can be crushed for patients unable to swallow.
- Use a calibrated measuring device to ensure accurate dosing of *ciprofloxacin* suspension and *levofloxacin* solution; shake well before measuring dose.
- *Ciprofloxacin* oral suspension and *levofloxacin* solution should not be administered through a feeding tube or with enteral feedings; may ↓ absorption and *ciprofloxacin* suspension can clog tube. If enteral route is unavoidable for *ciprofloxacin,* slurry can alternatively be prepared by crushing regular *ciprofloxacin* tablets and mixing with ≥20 mL water; allow to dissolve over 2 min. Stop enteral feed, flush tube with 15–30 mL of water 1 hr before, and resume 2 hr after administration. For *levofloxacin* solution, stop enteral feed, flush tube with 15–30 mL of water 2 hr before, and resume 4 hr after administration.

Ciprofloxacin

IV Administration

- **Intermittent Infusion: Dilution:** Dilute with D5W, 0.9% NaCl, or LR. Stable for 24 hr at room temperature or 72 hr if refrigerated. **Concentration:** 1–2 mg/mL. **Rate:** Administer over 60 min into a large vein to minimize venous irritation.
- **Y-Site Compatibility:** alemtuzumab, amiodarone, anidulafungin, argatroban, arsenic trioxide, aztreonam, bivalirudin, bleomycin, caffeine citrate, calcium gluconate, carboplatin, carmustine, caspofungin, ceftaroline, ceftazidime, ceftolozane/tazobactam, cisatracurium, cisplatin, cyclophosphamide, cytarabine, dactinomycin, daptomycin, daunorubicin, defibrotide, dexmedetomidine, dexrazoxane, digoxin, diltiazem, dimenhydrinate, diphenhydramine, dobutamine, docetaxel, dopamine, doxorubicin hydrochloride, doxorubicin liposomal, epirubicin, eptifibatide, eravacycline, ertapenem, etoposide, etoposide phosphate, fludarabine, fosphenytoin, gemcitabine, gentamicin, granisetron, hydromorphone, idarubicin, ifosfamide, irinotecan, isavuconazonium, labetalol, leucovorin, lidocaine, linezolid, lorazepam, meperidine, mesna, methadone, methotrexate, metoclopramide, metoprolol, metronidazole, midazolam, milrinone, mitomycin, mitoxantrone, mycophenolate, naloxone, nicardipine, octreotide, ondansetron, oritavancin, oxaliplatin, oxytocin, paclitaxel, palonosetron,

pamidronate, plazomicin, posaconazole, potassium acetate, potassium chloride, promethazine, remifentanil, rifampin, rocuronium, sildenafil, tacrolimus, tedizolid, telavancin, thiotepa, tigecycline, tirofiban, tobramycin, topotecan, trastuzumab, vancomycin, vasopressin, vecuronium, verapamil, vinblastine, vincristine, vinorelbine, voriconazole, zoledronic acid.

- **Y-Site Incompatibility:** acyclovir, aminocaproic acid, aminophylline, amphotericin B liposomal, ampicillin/sulbactam, blinatumomab, cangrelor, cefepime, dexamethasone, esmolol, fluorouracil, foscarnet, furosemide, gemtuzumab ozogamicin, heparin, letermovir, meropenem, meropenem/vaborbactam, methylprednisolone, pantoprazole, pemetrexed, phenytoin, piperacillin/tazobactam, potassium phosphates, propofol, rituximab, sodium phosphates, sulbactam/durlobactam.

Delafloxacin

IV Administration

- **Intermittent Infusion:** Reconstitute each vial with 10.5 mL of D5W or 0.9% NaCl. Shake vigorously to completely dissolve. **Concentration:** 25 mg/mL. Solution is clear yellow to amber; do not administer solutions that are discolored or contain particulate matter. Reconstituted solution is stable if refrigerated or at room temperature for 24 hr. **Dilution:** Dilute to volume of 250 mL with 0.9% NaCl or D5W. **Concentration:** 1.2 mg/mL. Diluted solution is stable if refrigerated or at room temperature for 24 hr. **Rate:** Infuse over 60 min.
- **Y-Site Incompatibility:** Do not administer other drugs through same IV line.

Levofloxacin

IV Administration

- **Intermittent Infusion:** **Dilution:** Dilute with 0.9% NaCl, D5W, or dextrose/saline combinations. Also available in premixed bottles and flexible containers with D5W, which need no further dilution. **Concentration:** 5 mg/mL. Discard unused solution. Diluted solution is stable for 72 hr at room temperature and 14 days if refrigerated. Store at room temperature and protect from light. Do not freeze. Discard any unused solution. **Rate:** Infuse 250-mg or 500-mg doses over 60 min and 750-mg dose over 90 min. Avoid rapid bolus injection to prevent hypotension.
- **Y-Site Compatibility:** alemtuzumab, amikacin, aminocaproic acid, aminophylline, ampicillin, ampicillin/sulbactam, anidulafungin, argatroban, arsenic trioxide, atracurium, aztreonam, bivalirudin, bleomycin, bumetanide, buprenorphine, busulfan, butorphanol, caffeine citrate, calcium gluconate, cangrelor, carboplatin, carmustine, caspofungin, cefepime, cefiderocol, cefotetan, ceftaroline, ceftazidime, ceftolozane/tazobactam, ceftriaxone, cefuroxime, chlorpromazine, cisatracurium, cisplatin, clindamycin, cyclophosphamide, cyclosporine, cytarabine, dacarbazine, dactinomycin, daptomycin, dexamethasone, dexmedetomidine, dexrazoxane, digoxin, diltiazem, diphenhydramine, dobutamine, docetaxel, dopamine, doxorubicin liposomal, doxycycline, droperidol, enalaprilat, ephedrine, epinephrine, epirubicin, eptifibatide, eravacycline, ertapenem, erythromycin, esmolol, etoposide, etoposide phosphate, famotidine, fentanyl, filgrastim, floxuridine, fluconazole, fludarabine, foscarnet, fosphenytoin, gemcitabine, gemtuzumab ozogamicin, gentamicin, granisetron, haloperidol, hydrocortisone, hydromorphone, idarubicin, ifosfamide, imipenem/cilastatin, imipenem/cilastatin/relebactam, irinotecan, isavuconazonium, isoproterenol, labetalol, leucovorin, lidocaine, linezolid, mannitol, meperidine, meropenem/vaborbactam, mesna, methadone, methylprednisolone, metoclopramide, metoprolol, metronidazole, midazolam, milrinone, mitomycin, mitoxantrone, mycophenolate, nalbuphine, naloxone, nicardipine, norepinephrine, octreotide, ondansetron, oxacillin, oxaliplatin, oxytocin, paclitaxel, palonosetron, pamidronate, pemetrexed, penicillin G sodium, pentamidine, phenylephrine, posaconazole, potassium acetate, potassium chloride, promethazine, propranolol, remifentanil, rocuronium, sargramostim, sodium acetate, sodium bicarbonate, succinylcholine, sufentanil, tacrolimus, tedizolid, theophylline, thiotepa, tigecycline, tirofiban, tobramycin, topotecan, trimethoprim/sulfamethoxazole, vancomycin, vasopressin, vecuronium, verapamil, vinblastine, vincristine, vinorelbine, voriconazole, zidovudine, zoledronic acid.
- **Y-Site Incompatibility:** acyclovir, alprostadil, amphotericin deoxycholate, amphotericin B liposomal, cefoxitin, daunorubicin, diazepam, fluorouracil, furosemide, ganciclovir, heparin, indomethacin, ketorolac, letermovir, methotrexate, micafungin, nitroglycerin, nitroprusside, pantoprazole, pentobarbital, phenytoin, piperacillin/tazobactam, plazomicin, prochlorperazine, propofol, rituximab, sulbactam/durlobactam, telavancin, trastuzumab.

Moxifloxacin

IV Administration

- **Intermittent Infusion:** **Dilution:** Premixed bags are diluted in sodium chloride 0.8% and should not be further diluted. Use transfer set whose piercing pin does not require excessive force; insert with a gentle twisting motion until pin is firmly seated. **Concentration:** 1.6 mg/mL. **Rate:** Administer over 60 min. Avoid rapid or bolus infusion.
- **Y-Site Compatibility:** alemtuzumab, aminocaproic acid, amiodarone, anidulafungin, argatroban, arsenic trioxide, atracurium, bivalirudin, bleomycin,

bumetanide, busulfan, calcium acetate, calcium chloride, calcium gluconate, cangrelor, carboplatin, carmustine, caspofungin, ceftaroline, chlorpromazine, cisatracurium, cisplatin, cyclophosphamide, cyclosporine, cytarabine, dacarbazine, dactinomycin, daptomycin, daunorubicin, dexamethasone, dexmedetomidine, dexrazoxane, digoxin, diltiazem, diphenhydramine, dobutamine, docetaxel, dopamine, doxorubicin hydrochloride, doxorubicin liposomal, droperidol, enalaprilat, epinephrine, epirubicin, ertapenem, esmolol, etoposide, etoposide phosphate, famotidine, fludarabine, gemcitabine, gemtuzumab ozogamicin, glycopyrrolate, granisetron, haloperidol, heparin, hydralazine, hydrocortisone, idarubicin, ifosfamide, insulin, regular, irinotecan, isoproterenol, ketorolac, labetalol, leucovorin, lidocaine, magnesium sulfate, mannitol, melphalan, mesna, methadone, methotrexate, methylprednisolone, metoclopramide, metoprolol, milrinone, mitomycin, mitoxantrone, mycophenolate, naloxone, nicardipine, nitroglycerin, norepinephrine, octreotide, ondansetron, oxaliplatin, oxytocin, paclitaxel, palonosetron, pamidronate, pemetrexed, phentolamine, phenylephrine, potassium acetate, potassium chloride, potassium phosphates, procainamide, prochlorperazine, promethazine, propranolol, rocuronium, sodium acetate, sodium bicarbonate, sodium phosphates, succinylcholine, tacrolimus, theophylline, thiotepa, tigecycline, tirofiban, topotecan, vasopressin, vecuronium, verapamil, vinblastine, vincristine, vinorelbine, zoledronic acid.

- **Y-Site Incompatibility:** allopurinol, aminophylline, ceftobiprole, dantrolene, fluorouracil, fosphenytoin, furosemide, nitroprusside, pantoprazole, phenytoin, vancomycin, voriconazole.

Patient/Family Teaching

- Explain the purpose and side effects of fluoroquinolones. Instruct to take medication as directed at evenly spaced times and to finish drug completely, even if feeling better. Take missed doses as soon as possible, unless almost time (within 6 hr for ciprofloxacin; 8 hr for moxifloxacin) for next dose. Do not double doses. Advise that sharing of this medication may be dangerous. Advise patient to read *Patient Information* before starting therapy.
- Instruct the patient to notify health care provider if symptoms do not improve.
- Advise patients to notify health care provider immediately if they are taking theophylline.
- Encourage patient to maintain a fluid intake of ≥1500–2000 mL/day to prevent crystalluria.
- Advise that antacids or medications containing iron or zinc will ↓ absorption. *Ciprofloxacin, levofloxacin,* and *ofloxacin* should be taken ≥2 hr before (4 hr for *moxifloxacin*) or 2 hr after (6 hr for *ciprofloxacin,* and *delafloxacin*, 8 hr for *moxifloxacin*) these products.
- May cause dizziness and drowsiness. Caution patient to avoid driving or other activities requiring alertness until response to medication is known.
- Advise patient to notify health care provider of any personal or family history of QTc prolongation or proarrhythmic conditions such as recent hypokalemia, significant bradycardia, or recent myocardial ischemia or if fainting spells or palpitations occur.
- Advise patient to report signs/symptoms of superinfection (furry overgrowth on the tongue, vaginal itching or discharge, loose or foul-smelling stools).
- Instruct patient to notify health care provider immediately if diarrhea, abdominal cramping, fever, or bloody stools occur and not to treat with antidiarrheals without consulting health care provider.
- Advise patient to immediately report signs and symptoms of hepatotoxicity (fatigue, nausea, upper abdominal pain, yellowing of skin or eyes, dark urine, light-colored stools).
- Advise patients and family to call 911 and seek urgent treatment for signs and symptoms of hypersensitivity reactions (difficulty breathing; chest tightness; hives; rash; feeling light-headed; itching; swelling of the face, lips, tongue, or throat).
- Caution patient to use sunscreen and protective clothing to prevent phototoxicity reactions during and for 5 days after therapy. Notify health care provider if a sunburn-like reaction or skin eruption occurs.
- Instruct patients being treated for gonorrhea that partners also must be treated.
- Advise patient to notify health care provider of all Rx or OTC medications, vitamins, or herbal products being taken and to consult with health care provider before taking other medications.
- Instruct patient to notify health care provider immediately if serious CNS effects (seizures, agitation, insomnia, anxiety, nightmares, paranoia, dizziness, confusion, tremors, hallucinations, depression, suicidal ideations/thoughts); peripheral neuropathy (pain, burning, tingling, numbness, weakness, other alterations in sensation); or tendon (shoulder, hand, Achilles, other) pain, swelling, or inflammation occur.
- Inform patient that fluoroquinolones may cause worsening of myasthenia gravis symptoms (muscle weakness, breathing problems). Advise patient to notify health care provider immediately if symptoms occur.
- Rep: Advise patient to notify health care provider if pregnancy is planned or suspected. Advise women of reproductive potential to use effective contraception during delafloxacin, moxifloxacin,

F

and ofloxacin therapy and to avoid breastfeeding during therapy with delafloxacin, moxifloxacin, ofloxacin and during and for 2 days after last dose of ciprofloxacin or levofloxacin.

Evaluation/Desired Outcomes

- Resolution of the signs and symptoms of infection. Time for complete resolution depends on organism and site of infection.
- Death of susceptible bacteria.
- Postexposure treatment of inhalational anthrax or cutaneous anthrax (ciprofloxacin and levofloxacin).
- Prevention and treatment of plague (ciprofloxacin, levofloxacin, and moxifloxacin).
- Febrile neutropenia prophylaxis (ciprofloxacin).

HIGH ALERT

fluorouracil

(flure-oh-**yoor**-a-sill)

Carac, Efudex, Tolak

Classification

Therapeutic: antineoplastics

Pharmacologic: antimetabolites

Indications

IV: Used alone and in combination with other modalities (surgery, radiation therapy, other antineoplastics) in the treatment of: Colorectal adenocarcinoma, Breast adenocarcinoma, Gastric adenocarcinoma, Pancreatic adenocarcinoma. **Topical:** Multiple actinic (solar) keratoses and superficial basal cell carcinomas.

Action

Inhibits DNA and RNA synthesis by preventing thymidine production (cell-cycle S-phase-specific). **Therapeutic Effects:** Death of rapidly replicating cells, particularly malignant ones.

Pharmacokinetics

Absorption: Minimal absorption (5–10%) after topical application.
Distribution: Widely distributed; concentrates and persists in tumors.
Metabolism and Excretion: Metabolized by dihydropyrimidine dehydrogenase to a less toxic compound; inactive metabolites are excreted primarily in urine.
Half-life: 20 hr.

TIME/ACTION PROFILE (IV = effects on blood counts, Top = dermatologic effects)

ROUTE	ONSET	PEAK	DURATION
IV	1–9 days	9–21 days (nadir)	30 days
Top	2–3 days	2–6 wk	1–2 mo

Contraindications/Precautions

Contraindicated in: Hypersensitivity; Dihydropyrimidine dehydrogenase deficiency (↑ risk of toxicity); OB: Pregnancy; Lactation: Lactation.
Use Cautiously in: Infection; Depressed bone marrow reserve; Other chronic debilitating illnesses; Obese patients, patients with edema or ascites (dose should be based on ideal body weight); Pedi: Safety and effectiveness not established in children.

Adverse Reactions/Side Effects

More likely to occur with systemic use than with topical use

CV: CARDIOTOXICITY. **Derm:** alopecia, maculopapular rash, local inflammatory reactions (topical only), melanosis of nails, nail loss, palmar-plantar erythrodysesthesia, phototoxicity. **Endo:** sterility. **GI:** diarrhea, nausea, stomatitis, vomiting. **Hemat:** anemia, leukopenia, thrombocytopenia. **Local:** thrombophlebitis. **Neuro:** acute cerebellar dysfunction. **Misc:** fever.

Interactions

Drug-Drug: Combination chemotherapy with **irinotecan** may produce unacceptable toxicity (dehydration, neutropenia, sepsis). Additive bone marrow depression with other **bone marrow depressants**, including other **antineoplastics** and **radiation therapy**. May ↓ antibody response to **live-virus vaccines** and ↑ risk of adverse reactions.

Route/Dosage

Advanced Colorectal Cancer

IV (Adults): *In combination with leucovorin alone or leucovorin + oxaliplatin or irinotecan:* 400 mg/m² as IV bolus on Day 1, then 2400–3000 mg/m² continuous infusion every 2 wk; *In combination with leucovorin:* 500 mg/m² as IV bolus 1 hr after leucovorin on Days 1, 8, 15, 22, 29, and 36 every 8 wk.

Breast Cancer

IV (Adults): *In combination with cyclophosphamide + epirubicin or cyclophosphamide + methotrexate:* 500 mg/m² or 600 mg/m² on Days 1 and 28 every 28 days for 6 cycles.

Gastric Adenocarcinoma

IV (Adults): *As part of platinum-containing regimen:* 200–1000 mg/m² as IV infusion (frequency of administration and number of cycles depends on specific regimen used).

Pancreatic Adenocarcinoma

IV (Adults): *In combination with leucovorin or as part of multidrug regimen:* 400 mg/m² as IV bolus on Day 1, then 2400 mg/m² continuous infusion every 2 wk.

Actinic (Solar) Keratoses

Topical (Adults): *Carac:* Apply 0.5% cream to lesions once daily for up to 4 wk; *Efudex:* Apply 2% or 5% solution or cream to lesions twice daily for 2–4 wk.

Superficial Basal Cell Carcinomas

Topical (Adults): *Efudex:* Apply 5% solution or cream to lesions twice daily for 3–6 wk (up to 12 wk).

Availability (generic available)

Solution for injection: 50 mg/mL. **Topical cream:** 0.5%, 4%, 5%. **Topical solution:** 2%, 5%.

NURSING IMPLICATIONS

Assessment

- Monitor vital signs before and frequently during therapy.
- Assess mucous membranes, number and consistency of stools, and frequency of vomiting. Assess for signs of infection (fever, chills, sore throat, cough, hoarseness, pain in lower back or side, difficult or painful urination). Assess for bleeding (bleeding gums; bruising; petechiae; and guaiac test stools, urine, and emesis). Avoid IM injections and taking rectal temperatures. Apply pressure to venipuncture sites for 10 min. Notify health care provider if Grade 3 or 4 toxicity (stomatitis or esophagopharyngitis, uncontrollable vomiting, diarrhea, GI bleeding, myocardial ischemia, leukocyte count <3500/mm^3, platelet count <100,000/mm^3, or hemorrhage from any site) occurs; hold fluorouracil until resolution to Grade ≤1. May be reinitiated at a lower dose when side effects have subsided.
- Assess skin for palmar-plantar erythrodysesthesia (tingling of hands and feet followed by pain, erythema, swelling, desquamation) throughout therapy. Occurs more frequently with continuous infusion. Usually occurs after 8–9 wk of therapy, but may occur earlier. Hold fluorouracil for Grades 2 or 3 and resume at lower dose when resolved or Grade 1.
- Monitor intake and output, appetite, and nutritional intake. GI effects usually occur on 4th day of therapy. Adjusting diet as tolerated and administering antidiarrheal agents may help maintain fluid and electrolyte balance and nutritional status. May cause severe diarrhea. Withhold therapy if Grade 3 or 4 diarrhea occurs and until resolved or decreased to Grade 1; then resume at reduced dose.
- Monitor for cerebellar dysfunction (ataxia, confusion, disorientation, visual disturbances). This may persist after discontinuation of therapy.
- Monitor for angina, myocardial infarction/ischemia, arrhythmia, and HF in patients with no history of coronary artery disease or cardiac dysfunction. Discontinue therapy if symptoms occur.
- Monitor for signs and symptoms of hyperammonemic encephalopathy (altered mental status, confusion, disorientation, coma, ataxia) with ↑ serum ammonia level within 72 hr of start of infusion. Discontinue fluorouracil and initiate ammonia-lowering therapy.
- Assess for mucositis, stomatitis, and esophagopharyngitis during therapy. May lead to mucosal sloughing or ulceration. Occurs more frequently with IV bolus doses. If Grade 3 or 4 mucositis occurs, withhold dose and resume at reduced dose when resolved or reduced to Grade 1.
- **Topical:** Inspect involved skin before and throughout therapy.

Lab Test Considerations

- May cause ↓ in plasma albumin.
- 🧬 Consider testing for genetic variants of the *DPYD* gene prior to initiating fluorouracil to reduce the risk of serious adverse reactions. Patients with certain variants in this gene may have dihydropyrimidine dehydrogenase deficiency, which can result in serious adverse reactions including mucositis, <u>diarrhea</u>, neutropenia, and neurotoxicity.
- Monitor hepatic (AST, ALT, LDH, and serum bilirubin), renal, and hematologic (hematocrit, hemoglobin, leukocyte, platelet count) functions before each treatment and periodically during therapy.
- Monitor CBC daily during IV therapy. Report WBC of <3500/mm^3 or platelets <100,000/mm^3 immediately; they are criteria for discontinuation. Nadir of leukopenia usually occurs in 9–14 days, with recovery by day 30. May also cause thrombocytopenia. Hold doses if Grade 4 myelosuppression occurs. Resume at ↓ dose when resolved or improved to Grade 1.
- May cause ↑ in urine excretion of 5-hydroxyindoleacetic acid.

Implementation

- ***High Alert:*** Fatalities have occurred with incorrect administration of chemotherapeutic agents. Before administering, clarify all ambiguous orders; double-check single, daily, and course-of-therapy dose limits; have second practitioner independently double-check original order, calculations, and infusion pump settings.
- When administering fluorouracil via IV push, 30 min of cryotherapy is recommended to prevent oral mucositis.

IV Administration

- Fluorouracil is an irritant. If extravasation occurs, immediately stop infusion. Leave needle/cannula in place temporarily but do not flush the line. Gently aspirate extravasated solution; then remove needle/cannula. Elevate patient's extremity and apply dry cold compresses for 20 min 4 times day for 1–2 days.
- **IV Push: Dilution:** May be administered undiluted. **Concentration:** 50 mg/mL. **Rate:** Rapid IV push administration (over 1–2 min) is most effective, but there is a more rapid onset of toxicity.

- **Intermittent Infusion: Dilution:** May be diluted with D5W or 0.9% NaCl.
- Use plastic IV tubing and IV bags to maintain greater stability of medication. Solution is stable for 24 hr at room temperature; do not refrigerate. Solution is colorless to faint yellow. Discard highly discolored or cloudy solution. If crystals form, dissolve by warming solution to 140°F, shaking vigorously, and cooling to body temperature. **Concentration:** Up to 50 mg/mL. **Rate:** Onset of toxicity is greatly delayed by administering an infusion over 2–8 hr.
- **Y-Site Compatibility:** acyclovir, allopurinol, amikacin, aminophylline, amphotericin B liposomal, ampicillin, ampicillin/sulbactam, anidulafungin, argatroban, atracurium, azithromycin, aztreonam, bivalirudin, bleomycin, bumetanide, butorphanol, calcium gluconate, carboplatin, carmustine, cefazolin, cefepime, cefotaxime, cefotetan, cefoxitin, ceftazidime, ceftriaxone, cefuroxime, cisatracurium, cisplatin, clindamycin, cyclophosphamide, cyclosporine, dacarbazine, daptomycin, dexamethasone, dexmedetomidine, dexrazoxane, digoxin, docetaxel, dopamine, doxorubicin liposomal, enalaprilat, ephedrine, ertapenem, erythromycin, esmolol, etoposide phosphate, famotidine, fentanyl, fluconazole, fludarabine, foscarnet, fosphenytoin, furosemide, ganciclovir, gemcitabine, gentamicin, granisetron, heparin, hetastarch, hydrocortisone, hydromorphone, ifosfamide, imipenem/cilastatin, isoproterenol, ketorolac, labetalol, leucovorin, lidocaine, linezolid, magnesium sulfate, mannitol, melphalan, meperidine, meropenem, mesna, methohexital, methotrexate, methylprednisolone, metoprolol, metronidazole, milrinone, mitomycin, mitoxantrone, morphine, nalbuphine, naloxone, nitroglycerin, nitroprusside, octreotide, paclitaxel, palonosetron, pamidronate, pantoprazole, pemetrexed, pentobarbital, phenobarbital, phenylephrine, piperacillin/tazobactam, potassium acetate, potassium chloride, potassium phosphates, procainamide, propofol, propranolol, remifentanil, rituximab, sargramostim, sodium acetate, sodium bicarbonate, sodium phosphates, succinylcholine, sufentanil, tenoposide, theophylline, thiotepa, tigecycline, tirofiban, tobramycin, trastuzumab, trimethoprim/sulfamethoxazole, vasopressin, vecuronium, vinblastine, vincristine, voriconazole, zidovudine, zoledronic acid.
- **Y-Site Incompatibility:** aldesleukin, amiodarone, amphotericin B deoxycholate, buprenorphine, calcium chloride, caspofungin, chlorpromazine, ciprofloxacin, diazepam, diltiazem, diphenhydramine, dobutamine, doxycycline, droperidol, epinephrine, epirubicin, filgrastim, haloperidol, idarubicin, irinotecan, levofloxacin, lorazepam, methadone, midazolam, minocycline, moxifloxacin, nicardipine, pentamidine, phenytoin, prochlorperazine, promethazine, topotecan, vancomycin, verapamil, vinorelbine.
- **Topical:** Consult health care provider before administering topical preparations to determine which skin preparation regimen should be followed. Avoid tight occlusive dressings because of irritation to surrounding healthy tissue. A loose gauze dressing for cosmetic purposes is usually preferred. Wear gloves when applying medication. Do not use metallic applicator.

Patient/Family Teaching

- Explain purpose of fluorouracil to patient.
- Instruct patient to notify health care provider if fever; chills; sore throat; signs of infection; yellowing of skin or eyes; abdominal pain; joint or flank pain; swelling of feet or legs; bleeding gums; bruising; petechiae; or blood in urine, stool, or emesis occurs. Caution patient to avoid crowds and persons with known infections. Instruct patient to use soft toothbrush and electric razor. Patients should be cautioned not to drink alcoholic beverages or take products containing aspirin or NSAIDs.
- Advise patient to rinse mouth with clear water after eating and drinking and to avoid flossing to minimize stomatitis. Viscous lidocaine may be used if mouth pain interferes with eating. Stomatitis pain may require treatment with opioid analgesics.
- Discuss with patient the possibility of hair loss. Explore methods of coping.
- Caution patient to use sunscreen and protective clothing to prevent phototoxicity reactions.
- Instruct patient not to receive any vaccinations without advice of health care provider.
- Instruct patient to notify health care provider of all Rx or OTC medications, vitamins, or herbal products being taken and consult health care provider before taking any new medications. ↑ dietary intake of thiamine may be recommended.
- Rep: May cause fetal harm. Advise women of reproductive potential and men with female partners of reproductive potential to use effective contraception during therapy and for at least 3 mo following completion of therapy and to avoid breastfeeding during therapy. Inform patients that fertility may be impaired during therapy.
- Emphasize the importance of routine follow-up lab tests to monitor progress and to check for side effects.
- **Topical:** Instruct patient in correct application of solution or cream. Emphasize importance of avoiding the eyes; caution should also be used when applying medication near mouth and nose. If patient uses clean finger to self-administer, emphasize importance of washing hands thoroughly after application. Explain that erythema, scaling, and blistering with pruritus and burning sensation are expected. Advise

patient to avoid sunlight or ultraviolet light (tanning booths) as much as possible; may increase side effects. Therapy is discontinued when erosion, ulceration, and necrosis occur in 2–6 wk (10–12 wk for basal cell carcinomas). Skin heals 4–8 wk later.

- Fluorouracil may be fatal if ingested by pets. Do not allow pets to be in contact with the container or the skin where fluorouracil topical has been applied. Store out of reach of pets. Safely discard or clean any cloth or applicator that may retain fluorouracil and avoid leaving any residues on your hands, clothing, carpeting, or furniture.

Evaluation/Desired Outcomes

- Tumor regression.
- Removal of solar keratoses or superficial basal cell skin cancers.

BEERS

FLUoxetine (floo-**ox**-uh-teen)

PROzac, ~~Sarafem~~

Classification

Therapeutic: antidepressants

Pharmacologic: selective serotonin reuptake inhibitors (SSRIs)

Indications

Major depressive disorder. Obsessive compulsive disorder (OCD). Bulimia nervosa. Panic disorder. Acute treatment of depressive episodes associated with bipolar I disorder (when used with olanzapine). Treatment-resistant depression (when used with olanzapine). Premenstrual dysphoric disorder (PMDD). **Unlabeled Use:** Anorexia nervosa, Diabetic neuropathy, Fibromyalgia, Obesity, Raynaud phenomenon, Social anxiety disorder (social phobia), Post-traumatic stress disorder.

Action

Selectively inhibits the reuptake of serotonin in the CNS. **Therapeutic Effects:** Antidepressant action. Decreased behaviors associated with: panic disorder, bulimia. Decreased mood alterations associated with PMDD.

Pharmacokinetics

Absorption: Well absorbed after oral administration.
Distribution: Crosses the blood-brain barrier.
Protein Binding: 94.5%.
Metabolism and Excretion: Converted by the liver to norfluoxetine (primarily by the CYP2D6 isoenzyme), another antidepressant compound; the CYP2D6 enzyme system exhibits genetic polymorphism (~7% of population may be poor metabolizers and may have significantly ↑ fluoxetine concentrations and an ↑ risk of adverse effects). Fluoxetine and norfluoxetine are mostly metabolized by the liver; 12% excreted by kidneys as unchanged fluoxetine, 7% as unchanged norfluoxetine.
Half-life: 1–3 days (norfluoxetine 5–7 days).

TIME/ACTION PROFILE (antidepressant effect)

ROUTE	ONSET	PEAK	DURATION
PO	1–4 wk	unknown	2 wk

F

Contraindications/Precautions

Contraindicated in: Hypersensitivity; Concurrent use of MAO inhibitors or MAO-like drugs (linezolid or methylene blue); Concurrent use of pimozide; Concurrent use of thioridazine (fluoxetine should be discontinued ≥5 wk before thioridazine therapy is initiated).
Use Cautiously in: History of seizures; Debilitated patients (↑ risk of seizures); Diabetes mellitus; Patients with concurrent chronic illness or multiple drug therapy (dose adjustments may be necessary); Hepatic impairment (↓ doses/↑ dosing interval may be necessary); May ↑ risk of suicide attempt/ideation especially during early treatment or dose adjustment; this risk appears to be greater in adolescents or children; Congenital long QT syndrome, history of QT interval prolongation, family history of long QT syndrome or sudden cardiac death, concurrent use of QT interval prolonging drugs, hypokalemia, hypomagnesemia, recent MI, uncompensated HF, or bradycardia; Angle-closure glaucoma; OB: Use during pregnancy only if potential maternal benefit justifies potential fetal risk. Use during 1st trimester may ↑ risk of cardiovascular malformations in infant. Use during 3rd trimester may result in neonatal serotonin syndrome requiring prolonged hospitalization and respiratory and nutritional support. Use may also be associated with persistent pulmonary hypertension in newborn. May cause sedation in infant; Lactation: Use while breastfeeding only if potential maternal benefit justifies potential risk to infant; Pedi: May ↑ risk of suicide attempt/ideation especially during early treatment or dose adjustment; children <7 yr (safety and effectiveness not established); Geri: Appears on Beers list. May worsen or cause syndrome of inappropriate antidiuretic hormone (SIADH) secretion and/or hyponatremia in older adults. Use with caution in older adults and closely monitor sodium concentrations when starting therapy or ↑ dose.

Adverse Reactions/Side Effects

CV: chest pain, palpitations, QT interval prolongation, TORSADES DE POINTES. **Derm:** ↑ sweating, pruritus, erythema nodosum, flushing, rash. **EENT:** mydriasis, stuffy nose, visual disturbances. **Endo:** SIADH, dysmenorrhea, hot flush. **F and E:** hyponatremia. **GI:** diarrhea, abdominal pain, abnormal taste, anorexia, constipation, dry mouth, dyspepsia, nausea, vomiting, weight loss. **GU:** ↓ libido, delayed/absent orgasm, ejaculatory delay/failure, erectile dysfunction, urinary frequency. **Hemat:** BLEEDING. **MS:** arthralgia, back pain, myalgia. **Neuro:** anxiety, drowsiness, headache, insomnia, nervousness, tremor, abnormal dreams, dizziness, fatigue, hypomania, mania, NEUROLEPTIC MALIGNANT SYNDROME, SEIZURES, SUICIDAL THOUGHTS/BEHAVIORS, weakness. **Resp:** cough. **Misc:** fever, flu-like syndrome, hypersensitivity reactions, SEROTONIN SYNDROME.

Interactions

Drug-Drug: Discontinue use of **MAO inhibitors** for 14 days before fluoxetine therapy; combined therapy may result in confusion, agitation, seizures, hypertension, and hyperpyrexia (serotonin syndrome). Fluoxetine should be discontinued for ≥5 wk before MAO inhibitor therapy is initiated. **MAO-inhibitor-like drugs**, such as **linezolid** or **methylene blue** may ↑ risk of serotonin syndrome; concurrent use contraindicated. Do not start therapy in patients receiving **linezolid** or **methylene blue**; if **linezolid** or **methylene blue** need to be started in a patient receiving fluoxetine, immediately discontinue fluoxetine and monitor for signs/symptoms of serotonin syndrome for 2 wk or until 24 hr after last dose of linezolid or methylene blue, whichever comes first; may resume fluoxetine therapy 24 hr after last dose of linezolid or methylene blue. **Pimozide** may ↑ risk of QT interval prolongation; concurrent use contraindicated. May ↑ levels of **thioridazine** and risk of QT interval prolongation; concurrent use contraindicated. Fluoxetine should be discontinued for ≥5 wk before thioridazine is initiated. **QT interval prolonging drugs** may ↑ the risk of QT interval prolongation with arrhythmias; avoid concurrent use. **Ritonavir** and **efavirenz** may ↑ the risk of developing the serotonin syndrome. For concurrent use with **ritonavir**, ↓ fluoxetine dose by 70%; if initiating fluoxetine, start with 10 mg/day dose. May ↑ levels and risk of toxicity of **alprazolam**; ↓ alprazolam dose by 50%. Drugs that affect serotonergic neurotransmitter systems, including **tricyclic antidepressants**, **SNRIs**, **fentanyl**, **lithium**, **buspirone**, **tramadol**, **meperidine**, **methadone**, **amphetamines**, and **triptans**, ↑ risk of serotonin syndrome. ↑ CNS depression with **alcohol**, **antihistamines**, other **antidepressants**, **opioid analgesics**, or **sedative/hypnotics**. ↑ risk of side effects and adverse reactions with other **antidepressants**, **risperidone**, or **phenothiazines**. May ↑ levels and risk of toxicity of **carbamazepine**, **clozapine**, **digoxin**, **haloperidol**, **phenytoin**, **lithium**, or **warfarin**. May ↓ the effects of **buspirone**. **Cyproheptadine** may ↓ or reverse effects of fluoxetine. May ↑ sensitivity to **adrenergics** and ↑ the risk of serotonin syndrome. ↑ risk of bleeding with **NSAIDs**, **aspirin**, **clopidogrel**, **prasugrel**, **ticagrelor**, **dabigatran**, **apixaban**, **edoxaban**, **rivaroxaban**, or **warfarin**.
Drug-Natural Products: ↑ risk of serotonin syndrome with **St. John's wort** and **SAMe**.

Route/Dosage

Depression

PO (Adults): 20 mg once daily in the morning. After several wk, may ↑ by 20 mg/day at weekly intervals. Doses >20 mg/day should be given in 2 divided doses, in the morning and at noon (not to exceed 80 mg/day). Patients who have been stabilized on the 20 mg/day dose may be switched over to delayed-release capsules at dose of 90 mg once weekly, initiated 7 days after the last 20-mg dose.
PO (Geriatric Patients): 10 mg once daily in the morning initially; may be ↑ (not to exceed 60 mg/day).
PO (Children 7–17 yr): *Adolescents and higher weight children:* 10 mg once daily; may ↑ after 2 wk to 20 mg once daily; additional dosage ↑ may be made after several more wk (range: 20–60 mg/day); *Lower-weight children:* 10 mg once daily initially; may ↑ after several more wk (range: 20–30 mg/day).

Obsessive Compulsive Disorder

PO (Adults): 20 mg once daily in the morning. After several wk, may ↑ by 20 mg/day at weekly intervals. Doses >20 mg/day should be given in 2 divided doses, in the morning and at noon (not to exceed 80 mg/day). Patients who have been stabilized on the 20 mg/day dose may be switched over to delayed-release capsules at dose of 90 mg once weekly, initiated 7 days after the last 20-mg dose.
PO (Children 7–17 yr): *Adolescents and higher weight children:* 10 mg once daily; may ↑ after 2 wk to 20 mg once daily; additional dosage ↑ may be made after several more wk (range: 20–60 mg/day); *Lower-weight children:* 10 mg once daily initially; may ↑ after several more wk (range: 20–30 mg/day).

Panic Disorder

PO (Adults): 10 mg once daily initially; may ↑ after 1 wk to 20 mg once daily (may ↑ as needed/tolerated up to 60 mg/day).

Bulimia Nervosa

PO (Adults): 60 mg once daily.

Premenstrual Dysphoric Disorder

PO (Adults): 20 mg once daily (not to exceed 80 mg/day) *or* 20 mg once daily starting 14 days prior to expected onset on menses, continued through 1st full day of menstruation, repeated with each cycle.

Depressive Disorders Associated with Bipolar I Disorder

PO (Adults): 20 mg once daily with olanzapine 5 mg/day (both given in evening); may ↑ fluoxetine dose up to 50 mg/day and olanzapine dose up to 12.5 mg/day.

PO (Children 10–17 yr): 20 mg once daily with olanzapine 2.5 mg/day (both given in evening); may ↑ fluoxetine dose up to 50 mg once daily and olanzapine dose up to 12 mg/day.

Treatment-Resistant Depression

PO (Adults): 20 mg once daily with olanzapine 5 mg/day (both given in evening); may ↑ fluoxetine dose up to 50 mg once daily and olanzapine dose up to 20 mg/day.

Availability (generic available)

Tablets: 10 mg, 20 mg, 60 mg. **Capsules:** 10 mg, 20 mg, 40 mg, 🍁 60 mg. **Delayed-release capsules:** 90 mg. **Oral solution(mint flavor):** 20 mg/5 mL. ***In combination with:*** olanzapine (generic).

NURSING IMPLICATIONS

Assessment

- Monitor mood changes to determine effectiveness.
- Assess for suicidal tendencies, especially during early therapy. Restrict amount of drug available to patient. Risk may be ↑ in children, adolescents, and adults ≤24 yr. After starting therapy, children, adolescents, and young adults should be seen by health care provider face-to-face at least weekly for 4 wk, then every other wk for next 4 wk, then at 12 wk, and then on advice of health care provider thereafter.
- Monitor appetite and nutritional intake. Weigh weekly and adjust diet as tolerated to support nutritional status.
- Assess for hypersensitivity reaction (urticaria, fever, arthralgia, edema, carpal tunnel syndrome, rash, hives, lymphadenopathy, respiratory distress). *If rash or other symptoms occur,* discontinue fluoxetine and treat as indicated.
- Assess baseline sexual function and for changes in sexual function during therapy.
- Monitor for neuroleptic malignant syndrome (fever, respiratory distress, tachycardia, seizures, diaphoresis, arrhythmias, hypertension or hypotension, pallor, tiredness, severe muscle stiffness, loss of bladder control). *If signs or symptoms occur,* discontinue fluoxetine and treat as indicated.
- Assess for serotonin syndrome (mental changes [agitation, hallucinations, coma], autonomic instability [tachycardia, labile BP, hyperthermia], neuromuscular aberrations [hyperreflexia, incoordination], and/or GI symptoms [nausea, vomiting, diarrhea]), especially in patients taking other serotonergic drugs (SSRIs, SNRIs, triptans). *If signs and symptoms occur,* discontinue fluoxetine and any concurrent serotonergic drugs; treat as indicated.
- **OCD:** Assess for frequency of obsessive-compulsive behaviors. Note degree to which these thoughts and behaviors interfere with daily functioning.
- **Bulimia Nervosa:** Assess frequency of binge eating and vomiting during therapy.

Lab Test Considerations

- Monitor CBC and differential periodically during therapy and clotting times as clinically indicated. May ↑ risk of bleeding.
- Proteinuria and ↑ AST may occur during hypersensitivity reaction.
- May ↑alkaline phosphatase, ALT, BUN, and CK; may cause hyperuricemia, hypocalcemia, hypoglycemia, hyperglycemia, and hyponatremia.
- May cause hypoglycemia in patient with diabetes.

Implementation

- Do not confuse fluoxetine with duloxetine or paroxetine. Do not confuse Prozac with Prilosec, Prograf, or Provera.
- **PO:** Administer as a single dose in the morning. Some patients may require ↑ amounts, with a 2nd dose at noon.
- May be administered with food to minimize GI irritation. ***DNC:*** Do not open, dissolve, chew, or crush delayed-release capsules.
- Delayed release capsules may be started after last dose of *PROzac* 20 mg. May ↑ dose after several wk if no clinically significant improvement.

Patient/Family Teaching

- Explain purpose and side effects of medication. Advise patient to read *Patient Information* before starting therapy.
- Instruct patient to take missed dose as soon as remembered unless almost time for next dose; then omit and return to regular schedule. Do not double doses or discontinue without consulting health care provider; discontinuation may cause anxiety, insomnia, or nervousness.
- May cause drowsiness, dizziness, impaired judgment, and blurred vision. Caution patient to avoid driving and other activities requiring alertness until response is known.
- Advise patient, family, and caregivers to watch for suicidality, especially during early therapy or dose changes. Notify health care provider immediately if thoughts about suicide or dying, attempts to commit suicide, new or worse depression or anxiety, agitation or restlessness, panic attacks, insomnia, new or worse irritability, aggressiveness, acting on dangerous impulses, mania, or other changes in mood or behavior occur.
- Advise patient and caregivers to immediately notify health care provider if symptoms of serotonin syndrome occur.

- Instruct patient to notify health care provider of all Rx or OTC medications, vitamins, or herbal products being taken and consult health care provider before taking any new medications. Advise patient to avoid taking other CNS depressants, including opioids, or alcohol. Advise patient that concurrent use of aspirin, NSAIDs, or anticoagulants may ↑ bleeding risk.
- Caution patient to change positions slowly to minimize dizziness.
- Inform patient that frequent mouth rinses, good oral hygiene, and sugarless gum or candy may minimize dry mouth. If dry mouth persists for >2 wk, consult health care provider regarding use of saliva substitute.
- Caution patient to wear protective clothing and use sunscreen to prevent photosensitivity reactions.
- Advise patient to notify health care provider if symptoms of hypersensitivity reaction occur or if headache, nausea, anorexia, anxiety, or insomnia persist.
- Inform patient that fluoxetine may cause symptoms of sexual dysfunction. Advise patient to notify health care provider if ejaculatory delay or failure, ↓ libido, erectile dysfunction, or delayed/absent orgasm occur.
- Rep: May cause fetal harm. Advise women of reproductive potential to notify health care provider if pregnancy is planned or suspected or if breastfeeding. Use during 1st trimester may ↑ risk of cardiovascular malformations in infant. Monitor infants exposed to fluoxetine during 3rd trimester for respiratory distress, cyanosis, apnea, seizures, temperature instability, feeding difficulty, vomiting, hypoglycemia, hypotonia, hypertonia, hyperreflexia, tremors, jitteriness, irritability, and constant crying. May ↑ risk of postpartum hemorrhage. Monitor infants exposed to fluoxetine via breast milk for agitation, irritability, poor feeding, and poor weight gain. Inform patient of pregnancy exposure registry. Register patient in the National Pregnancy Registry for Antidepressants at 1-844-405-6185 or https://womensmentalhealth.org/clinical-and-researchprograms/pregnancyregistry/antidepressants/.
- Emphasize the importance of follow-up exams to monitor progress.

Evaluation/Desired Outcomes

- Increased sense of well-being.
- Renewed interest in surroundings. May require 1–4 wk of therapy to obtain antidepressant effects.
- Decrease in obsessive-compulsive behaviors.
- Decrease in binge eating and vomiting in patients with bulimia nervosa.
- Decreased incidence frequency of panic attacks.
- Decreased mood alterations associated with PMDD.

flurandrenolide, See CORTICOSTEROIDS (TOPICAL).

fluticasone, See CORTICOSTEROIDS (INHALATION).

fluticasone, See CORTICOSTEROIDS (NASAL).

fluticasone, See CORTICOSTEROIDS (TOPICAL).

fluticasone/umeclidinium/vilanterol

(floo-**tik**-a-sone/ue-mek-li-**din**-ee-um/vye-**lan**-ter-ol)

Trelegy Ellipta

Classification

Therapeutic: bronchodilators

Pharmacologic: corticosteroids, anticholinergics, adrenergics

Indications

Maintenance treatment of COPD. Maintenance treatment of asthma.

Action

Fluticasone: decreases airway inflammation; *umeclidinium:* acts as an anticholinergic by inhibiting M3 muscarinic receptors in bronchial smooth muscle resulting in bronchodilation; *vilanterol:* $beta_2$-adrenergic agonist that stimulates adenyl cyclase, resulting in accumulation of cyclic adenosine monophosphate and subsequent bronchodilation. **Therapeutic Effects:** Improved airflow and ↓ exacerbations in COPD and asthma.

Pharmacokinetics

Fluticasone

Absorption: 15.2% systemically absorbed from lungs following inhalation; minimal absorption from swallowing.

Distribution: Unknown.

Protein Binding: >99%.

Metabolism and Excretion: Primarily metabolized by the CYP3A4 isoenzyme to inactive metabolites; parent drug and metabolites excreted primarily in feces, 1–2% excreted in urine.

Half-life: 24 hr

Umeclidinium

Absorption: Mostly absorbed from lungs; minimal oral absorption.

Distribution: Unknown.

Metabolism and Excretion: Primarily metabolized by the CYP2D6 isoenzyme to inactive metabolites;

parent drug and metabolites excreted in feces (58%) and urine (22%).
Half-life: 11 hr.

Vilanterol
Absorption: Mostly absorbed from lungs; minimal oral absorption.
Distribution: Unknown.
Protein Binding: 94%.
Metabolism and Excretion: Primarily metabolized by the CYP3A4 isoenzyme to inactive metabolites; parent drug and metabolites excreted in urine (70%) and feces (30%).
Half-life: 11 hr.

TIME/ACTION PROFILE (bronchodilation)

ROUTE	ONSET	PEAK	DURATION
Inhalation	1 hr	2–12 hr	24 hr

Contraindications/Precautions

Contraindicated in: Hypersensitivity to any components or severe hypersensitivity to milk proteins; Acute attack of COPD or asthma or status asthmaticus (onset of action is delayed).
Use Cautiously in: Active untreated infections; Cardiovascular disease; Prolonged immobilization, family history of osteoporosis, postmenopausal status, tobacco use, advanced age, poor nutrition, or chronic use of anticonvulsants or oral corticosteroids (↑ risk of ↓ bone mineral density); Narrow-angle glaucoma (may cause acute angle closure); Cataracts; Urinary retention, prostatic hyperplasia, or bladder-neck obstruction; History of seizures, thyrotoxicosis, diabetes mellitus, or ketacidosis; Renal impairment; Hepatic impairment; OB: Safety not established in pregnancy; Lactation: Use while breastfeeding only if potential maternal benefit outweighs potential risk to infant; Pedi: Safety and effectiveness not established in children; Geri: Older adults may be more sensitive to drug effects.
Exercise Extreme Caution in: Concurrent use of MAO inhibitors, tricyclic antidepressants, or QTc interval prolonging drugs.

Adverse Reactions/Side Effects

CV: ARRHYTHMIAS, hypertension, QTc interval prolongation, tachycardia. **EENT:** cataracts, dysphonia, glaucoma, oral candidiasis. **Endo:** adrenal suppression, hyperglycemia. **F and E:** hypokalemia. **GI:** constipation, diarrhea. **GU:** urinary retention. **MS:** ↓ bone mineral density, arthralgia, back pain. **Neuro:** dysgeusia, headache. **Resp:** ↑ risk of pneumonia, paradoxical bronchospasm. **Misc:** HYPERSENSITIVITY REACTIONS (INCLUDING ANAPHYLAXIS AND ANGIOEDEMA).

Interactions

Drug-Drug: **CYP3A4 inhibitors**, including **clarithromycin**, **conivaptan**, **itraconazole**, **ketoconazole**, **lopinavir**, **nefazodone**, **nelfinavir**, **ritonavir**, or **voriconazole**, may ↑ fluticasone and vilanterol levels and risk of corticosteroid effects or adverse cardiovascular reactions; concurrent use should be undertaken with caution. **MAO inhibitors**, **tricyclic antidepressants**, or **QTc interval prolonging drugs** may ↑ risk of cardiovascular reactions from vilanterol; exercise extreme caution when considering concurrent use or use within 2 wk of discontinuing above drugs. **Beta blockers** may ↓ effectiveness of vilanterol and ↑ risk of severe bronchospasm; consider use of cardioselective beta blocker. ↑ risk of hypokalemia with **loop diuretics** or **thiazide diuretics**. ↑ risk of anticholinergic adverse reactions with other **anticholinergics**; avoid concurrent use.

F

Route/Dosage

COPD

Inhaln (Adults): One inhalation (fluticasone 100 mcg/umeclidinium 62.5 mcg/vilanterol 25 mcg) once daily.

Asthma

Inhaln (Adults): One inhalation (either fluticasone 100 mcg/umeclidinium 62.5 mcg/vilanterol 25 mcg or fluticasone 200 mcg/umeclidinium 62.5 mcg/vilanterol 25 mcg) once daily. If inadequate response to fluticasone 100 mcg/umeclidinium 62.5 mcg/vilanterol 25 mcg once daily, may ↑ to one inhalation (fluticasone 200 mcg/umeclidinium 62.5 mcg/vilanterol 25 mcg) once daily.

Availability

Powder for inhalation (contains lactose): fluticasone 100 mcg/umeclidinium 62.5 mcg/vilanterol 25 mcg in a two-strip blister per dose, fluticasone 200 mcg/umeclidinium 62.5 mcg/vilanterol 25 mcg in a two-strip blister per dose.

NURSING IMPLICATIONS

Assessment

- Monitor respiratory status, including lung sounds. Assess pulmonary function tests periodically during and for several months after a transfer from systemic to inhalation corticosteroids.
- Assess for severe milk allergy prior to therapy; contains lactose.
- Monitor for signs and symptoms of hypersensitivity reaction (rash, pruritus, swelling of face and neck, dyspnea) periodically during therapy.
- Monitor ECG, BP, and HR periodically during therapy. May cause ↑ HR, ↑ BP, prolonged QTc interval, ST segment depression, supraventricular tachycardia, and extrasystoles.
- Observe for paradoxical bronchospasm (wheezing, dyspnea, chest tightness) and hypersensitivity

reaction (rash; urticaria; swelling of face, lips, or eyelids). *If bronchospasm or hypersensitivity reaction occurs,* hold therapy and support as clinically indicated.

- Assess patients changing from systemic to inhalation corticosteroids for signs of adrenal insufficiency (anorexia, nausea, weakness, fatigue, hypotension, hypoglycemia) during initial therapy and periods of stress. *If signs of adrenal insufficiency appear,* notify health care provider immediately; condition may be life-threatening.
- Monitor for withdrawal symptoms (joint or muscular pain, lassitude, depression) during withdrawal from systemic corticosteroids.
- Monitor bone mineral density in patients on prolonged therapy and/or with ↑ risk (prolonged immobilization, family history of osteoporosis, postmenopausal status, tobacco use, advanced age, poor nutrition, chronic use of drugs that can reduce bone mass [anticonvulsants, oral corticosteroids]) for fractures.

Lab Test Considerations

- May cause hypokalemia and hyperglycemia.

Implementation

- **Inhaln:** Administer once daily at the same time each day. Do not open cover of inhaler until ready to use. Discard inhaler 6 wk after opening; inhaler is not reusable.
- See Appendix C for administration of inhalation medications.

Patient/Family Teaching

- Explain purpose and side effects of medication. Advise patient to read *Patient Information* before starting therapy and to follow instructions in Medication Guide for use of inhaler.
- Advise patient to take medication as directed. If a dose is missed, take as soon as remembered unless almost time for next dose. Advise patient not to discontinue medication without consulting a health care provider; gradual ↓ is required.
- Advise patient to rinse mouth with water without swallowing after administration to ↓ risk of oropharyngeal candidiasis.
- Caution patient not to use medication to treat acute symptoms. A rapid-acting inhaled beta-adrenergic bronchodilator should be used for relief of acute asthma attacks. Notify health care provider immediately if symptoms worsen or more inhalations than usual are needed from rescue inhaler.
- Advise patient to stop using medication and notify health care provider immediately if signs and symptoms of hypersensitivity reaction occur.
- Instruct patient not to use additional long-acting beta$_2$ agonists.
- Caution patient to avoid smoking, known allergens, and other respiratory irritants.
- Advise patient to notify health care provider if signs and symptoms of pneumonia (fever, chills, shortness of breath, increased cough, increased sputum production or change in mucus color), urinary retention (difficulty passing urine, painful urination), or sore throat or mouth occur.
- Instruct patient to notify health care provider immediately if exposed to chickenpox or measles. Inform patients of potential worsening of existing tuberculosis; fungal, bacterial, viral, or parasitic infections; or ocular herpes simplex.
- Advise patient to notify health care provider of all Rx or OTC medications, vitamins, or herbal products being taken and consult health care provider before taking other Rx, OTC, or herbal products.
- Advise patient to have regular eye examinations. Instruct patient to notify health care provider immediately if signs and symptoms of glaucoma (eye pain or discomfort, blurred vision, visual halos or colored images in association with red eyes from conjunctival congestion corneal edema) occur.
- Rep: Advise women of reproductive potential to notify health care provider if pregnancy is planned or suspected or if breastfeeding.

Evaluation/Desired Outcomes

- Improved airflow and ↓ exacerbations in COPD and asthma.

fluticasone/vilanterol

(floo-**tik**-a-sone vye-**lan**-ter-ol)

Breo Ellipta

Classification

Therapeutic: bronchodilators

Pharmacologic: corticosteroids, adrenergics

Indications

Maintenance treatment of COPD. Maintenance treatment of asthma.

Action

Fluticasone: decreases airway inflammation. *Vilanterol:* relaxes bronchial smooth muscle. **Therapeutic Effects:** Improved airflow and ↓ exacerbations in COPD. Reduction in asthma exacerbations.

Pharmacokinetics

Fluticasone

Absorption: 15.2% systemically absorbed from lungs following inhalation; minimal absorption from swallowing (swallowed drug undergoes extensive first-pass hepatic metabolism).

Distribution: Unknown.

Protein Binding: 99.6%.

Metabolism and Excretion: Primarily metabolized by the liver via the CYP3A4 isoenzyme to inactive metabolites; primarily excreted in feces.

Half-life: 24 hr.

Vilanterol

Absorption: 27.3% systemically absorbed from lungs following inhalation; minimal absorption from swallowing (swallowed drug undergoes extensive first-pass hepatic metabolism).

Distribution: Unknown.

Protein Binding: 93.9%.

Metabolism and Excretion: Primarily metabolized by the CYP3A4 isoenzyme to inactive metabolites. Primarily excreted in urine (70%), with 30% excreted in feces.

Half-life: 21.3 hr.

TIME/ACTION PROFILE (bronchodilation)

ROUTE	ONSET	PEAK	DURATION
Fluticasone/vilanterol (inhaln)	within 1 hr	1–2 hr	24 hr

Contraindications/Precautions

Contraindicated in: Hypersensitivity to any components or severe hypersensitivity to milk proteins; Acute attack of asthma or COPD (onset of action is delayed); Patients not receiving a long-term asthma-control medication (e.g., inhaled corticosteroid); Patients whose asthma is currently controlled on low- or medium-dose inhaled corticosteroid therapy.

Use Cautiously in: Moderate to severe hepatic impairment (↑ fluticasone levels may lead to systemic corticosteroid effects); Cardiovascular history; Glaucoma or cataracts; History of seizures, thyrotoxicosis, diabetes mellitus, or ketacidosis; OB: Safety not established in pregnancy; Lactation: Use while breastfeeding only if potential maternal benefit outweighs potential risk to infant; Pedi: Safety and effectiveness not established in children <18 yr (COPD) or <5 yr (asthma); Geri: Older adults may be more sensitive to effects.

Exercise Extreme Caution in: Concurrent use of MAO inhibitors or tricyclic antidepressants.

Adverse Reactions/Side Effects

EENT: cataracts, glaucoma, nasopharyngitis, oral candidiasis. **Endo:** adrenal suppression, ↓ growth (in children), hyperglycemia. **F and E:** hypokalemia. **MS:** ↓ bone mineral density. **Neuro:** headache. **Resp:** ↑ risk of pneumonia, paradoxical bronchospasm, upper respiratory tract infection. **Misc:** HYPERSENSITIVITY REACTIONS (INCLUDING ANAPHYLAXIS, ANGIOEDEMA, AND URTICARIA).

Interactions

Drug-Drug: ↑ risk of corticosteroid effects or adverse cardiovascular reactions with **CYP3A4 inhibitors**, including **clarithromycin**, **conivaptan**, **itraconazole**, **ketoconazole**, **lopinavir**, **nefazodone**, **nelfinavir**, **ritonavir**, or **voriconazole**; concurrent use should be undertaken with extreme caution. **Beta blockers** may ↓ effectiveness of vilanterol and ↑ risk of severe bronchospasm. ↑ risk of hypokalemia with **non-potassium-sparing diuretics**.

Route/Dosage

COPD

Inhaln (Adults): One inhalation (fluticasone 100 mcg/vilanterol 25 mcg) once daily.

Asthma

Inhaln (Adults): One inhalation of either fluticasone 100 mcg/vilanterol 25 mcg or fluticasone 200 mcg/vilanterol 25 mcg once daily (base decision on severity of asthma); not to exceed dosage of one inhalation of fluticasone 200 mcg/vilanterol 25 mcg once daily.

Inhaln (Children 12–17 yr): One inhalation (fluticasone 100 mcg/vilanterol 25 mcg) once daily.

Inhaln (Children 5–11 yr): One inhalation (fluticasone 50 mcg/vilanterol 25 mcg) once daily.

Availability

Powder for inhalation (contains lactose): fluticasone 50 mcg/vilanterol 25 mcg/inhalation in a two-strip blister per dose, fluticasone 100 mcg/vilanterol 25 mcg/inhalation in a two-strip blister per dose, fluticasone 200 mcg/vilanterol 25 mcg/inhalation in a two-strip blister per dose.

NURSING IMPLICATIONS

Assessment

- Monitor respiratory status, including lung sounds. Assess pulmonary function tests periodically during and for several months after a transfer from systemic to inhalation corticosteroids.
- Assess for severe milk allergy prior to initiation; contains lactose.
- Monitor for signs and symptoms of hypersensitivity reactions (rash, pruritus, swelling of face and neck, dyspnea) periodically during therapy.
- Monitor ECG, BP, and HR periodically during therapy. May cause ↑ HR, ↑ BP, prolonged QTc interval, ST segment depression, supraventricular tachycardia, and extrasystoles.
- Observe for paradoxical bronchospasm (wheezing, dyspnea, chest tightness) and hypersensitivity reaction (rash; urticaria; swelling of face, lips, or eyelids). *If bronchospasm or hypersensitivity reaction occurs,* hold therapy and support as clinically indicated.
- Assess patients changing from systemic to inhalation corticosteroids for signs of adrenal insufficiency (anorexia, nausea, weakness,

fatigue, hypotension, hypoglycemia) during initial therapy and periods of stress. *If signs of adrenal insufficiency appear,* notify health care provider immediately; condition may be life-threatening.

- Monitor for withdrawal symptoms (joint or muscular pain, lassitude, depression) during withdrawal from systemic corticosteroids.
- Monitor bone mineral density in patients on prolonged therapy and/or with ↑ risk (prolonged immobilization, family history of osteoporosis, postmenopausal status, tobacco use, advanced age, poor nutrition, chronic use of drugs that can reduce bone mass [anticonvulsants, oral corticosteroids]) for fractures.

Lab Test Considerations

- May cause hypokalemia and hyperglycemia.

Implementation

- **Inhaln:** Administer once daily at the same time each day. Do not open cover of inhaler until ready to use. Discard inhaler 6 wk after opening; inhaler is not reusable.
- See Appendix C for administration of inhalation medications.

Patient/Family Teaching

- Explain purpose and side effects of medication. Advise patient to read *Patient Information* before starting therapy and to follow instructions in Medication Guide for use of inhaler.
- Advise patient to take medication as directed. If a dose is missed, take as soon as remembered unless almost time for next dose. Advise patient not to discontinue medication without consulting a health care provider; gradual ↓ is required.
- Advise patient to rinse mouth with water without swallowing after administration to ↓ risk of oropharyngeal candidiasis.
- Caution patient not to use medication to treat acute symptoms. A rapid-acting inhaled beta-adrenergic bronchodilator should be used for relief of acute asthma attacks. Notify health care provider immediately if symptoms worsen or more inhalations than usual are needed from rescue inhaler.
- Advise patient to stop using medication and notify health care provider immediately if signs and symptoms of hypersensitivity reaction occur.
- Instruct patient not to use additional long-acting beta$_2$ agonists.
- Caution patient to avoid smoking, known allergens, and other respiratory irritants.
- Advise patient to notify health care provider if signs and symptoms of pneumonia or sore throat or mouth occur.
- Instruct patient to notify health care provider immediately if exposed to chickenpox or measles. Inform patients of potential worsening of existing tuberculosis; fungal, bacterial, viral, or parasitic infections; or ocular herpes simplex.
- Advise patient to notify health care provider of all Rx or OTC medications, vitamins, or herbal products being taken and to consult health care provider before taking other Rx, OTC, or herbal products.
- Advise patient to have regular eye examinations. Instruct patient to notify health care provider immediately if signs and symptoms of glaucoma (eye pain or discomfort, blurred vision, visual halos or colored images in association with red eyes from conjunctival congestion corneal edema) occur.
- Rep: Advise women of reproductive potential to notify health care provider if pregnancy is planned or suspected or if breastfeeding.
- Pedi: Advise caretakers to have a health care provider monitor growth regularly during therapy and to titrate to lowest effective dose.

Evaluation/Desired Outcomes

- Improved airflow and ↓ exacerbations in COPD.
- Reduction in asthma exacerbations.

fluvastatin, See HMG-CoA REDUCTASE INHIBITORS (statins)

BEERS

fluvoxaMINE

(floo-**voks**-a-meen)

Luvox, ~~Luvox CR~~

Classification

Therapeutic: antidepressants, antiobsessive agents

Pharmacologic: selective serotonin reuptake inhibitors (SSRIs)

Indications

Obsessive-compulsive disorder. **Unlabeled Use:** Depression. Generalized anxiety disorder. Social anxiety disorder. Post-traumatic stress disorder.

Action

Inhibits the reuptake of serotonin in the CNS. **Therapeutic Effects:** Decrease in obsessive-compulsive behaviors.

Pharmacokinetics

Absorption: 53% absorbed after oral administration.
Distribution: Enters the CNS. Remainder of distribution not known.
Metabolism and Excretion: Mostly metabolized by the liver via the CYP2D6 isoenzyme; the CYP2D6 isoenzyme exhibits genetic polymorphism; ~7% of population may be poor metabolizers and may have

significantly ↑ fluvoxamine concentrations and an ↑ risk of adverse effects.
Half-life: 13.6–15.6 hr.

TIME/ACTION PROFILE (improvement on obsessive-compulsive behaviors)

ROUTE	ONSET	PEAK	DURATION
PO	within 2–3 wk	several mo	unknown

Contraindications/Precautions

Contraindicated in: Hypersensitivity to fluvoxamine or other SSRIs; Concurrent use of MAO inhibitors (or within 14 days of discontinuing fluvoxamine), MAO-inhibitor-like drugs (linezolid or methylene blue), alosetron, pimozide, thioridazine, or tizanidine.
Use Cautiously in: Hepatic impairment; May ↑ risk of suicide attempt/ideation especially during early treatment or dose adjustment; this risk appears to be greater in adolescents or children; Angle-closure glaucoma; OB: Neonates exposed to SSRI in 3rd trimester may develop drug discontinuation syndrome, including respiratory distress, feeding difficulty, and irritability; Lactation: Use while breastfeeding only if potential maternal benefit justifies potential risk to infant; Pedi: May ↑ risk of suicide attempt/ideation especially during early treatment or dose adjustment; safety and effectiveness not established in children <18 yr (controlled release) and <8 yr (immediate release); Geri: Appears on Beers list. May worsen or cause syndrome of inappropriate antidiuretic hormone (SIADH) secretion and/or hyponatremia in older adults. Use with caution in older adults and closely monitor sodium concentrations when starting therapy or ↑ dose.

Adverse Reactions/Side Effects

CV: edema, hypertension, palpitations, postural hypotension, tachycardia. **Derm:** ↑ sweating. **EENT:** sinusitis. **Endo:** SIADH. **F and E:** hyponatremia. **GI:** constipation, diarrhea, dry mouth, dyspepsia, nausea, ↑ liver enzymes, anorexia, dysphagia, flatulence, vomiting, weight loss. **GU:** ↓ libido, delayed/absent orgasm, ejaculatory delay/failure, erectile dysfunction. **Hemat:** BLEEDING. **Metab:** weight gain. **MS:** hypertonia, myoclonus/twitching. **Neuro:** dizziness, drowsiness, headache, insomnia, nervousness, weakness, agitation, anxiety, apathy, depression, emotional lability, hypokinesia/hyperkinesia, manic reactions, NEUROLEPTIC MALIGNANT SYNDROME, psychotic reactions, sedation, SUICIDAL THOUGHTS/BEHAVIORS, syncope, tremor. **Resp:** cough, dyspnea. **Misc:** chills, flu-like symptoms, hypersensitivity reactions, SEROTONIN SYNDROME, tooth disorder/caries, yawning.

Interactions

Drug-Drug: Concurrent use with **MAO inhibitors** may result in serious potentially fatal reactions; MAO inhibitors should be stopped at least 14 days before fluvoxamine therapy; fluvoxamine should be stopped at least 14 days before MAO inhibitor therapy. Concurrent use with **MAO-inhibitor-like drugs**, such as **linezolid** or **methylene blue**, may ↑ risk of serotonin syndrome; concurrent use contraindicated; do not start therapy in patients receiving **linezolid** or **methylene blue**; if **linezolid** or **methylene blue** need to be started in a patient receiving fluvoxamine, immediately discontinue fluvoxamine and monitor for signs/symptoms of serotonin syndrome for 2 wk or until 24 hr after last dose of linezolid or methylene blue, whichever comes first (may resume fluvoxamine therapy 24 hr after last dose of linezolid or methylene blue). May ↑ **thioridazine** and **pimozide** levels and risk of QT interval prolongation and torsades de pointes; concurrent use contraindicated. May ↑ levels and risk of toxicity of **tizanidine** and **alosetron**; concurrent use contraindicated. **Smoking** may ↓ levels and effectiveness. **Tricyclic antidepressants** may ↑ levels and risk of toxicity. Drugs that affect serotonergic neurotransmitter systems, including **tricyclic antidepressants**, **SNRIs**, **fentanyl**, **lithium**, **buspirone**, **tramadol**, **meperidine**, **methadone**, **amphetamines**, and **triptans**, may ↑ risk of serotonin syndrome. May ↑ levels and risk of toxicity of some **beta blockers** (**propranolol**), some **benzodiazepines** (avoid concurrent **diazepam**), **carbamazepine**, **methadone**, **lithium**, **theophylline** (↓ dose to 33% of usual dose), **ramelteon** (avoid concurrent use), **warfarin**, and **L-tryptophan**. May ↑ risk of bleeding with **NSAIDs**, **aspirin**, **clopidogrel**, **prasugrel**, **ticagrelor**, **dabigatran**, **apixaban**, **edoxaban**, **rivaroxaban**, or **warfarin**. May ↑ levels and risk of toxicity of **clozapine**; dose adjustments may be necessary.
Drug-Natural Products: St. John's wort may ↑ risk of of serotonin syndrome.

Route/Dosage

PO (Adults): *Immediate release:* 50 mg once daily at bedtime; ↑ by 50 mg every 4–7 days until desired effect is achieved. If daily dose >100 mg, give in 2 equally divided doses or give a larger dose at bedtime (not to exceed 300 mg/day); *Controlled release:* 100 mg once daily at bedtime; ↑ by 50 mg every 7 days until desired effect is achieved, not to exceed 300 mg/day.
PO (Children 8–17 yr): *Immediate release:* 25 mg once daily at bedtime; may ↑ by 25 mg/day every 4–7 days (not to exceed 200 mg/day; daily doses >50 mg should be given in divided doses with a larger dose at bedtime).

Hepatic Impairment

PO (Adults): *Immediate release:* 25 mg once daily at bedtime initially; slower titration and longer dosing intervals should be used.

F

Availability (generic available)

Tablets: 25 mg, 50 mg, 100 mg. **Controlled-release capsules:** 100 mg, 150 mg.

NURSING IMPLICATIONS

Assessment

- Monitor mood changes. Assess frequency of obsessive-compulsive behaviors. Note degree to which these thoughts and behaviors interfere with daily functioning. Inform health care provider if patient demonstrates significant ↑ in anxiety, nervousness, or insomnia.
- Assess for suicidal tendencies, especially during early therapy. Restrict amount of drug available to patient. Risk may be ↑ in children, adolescents, and adults ≤24 yr. After starting therapy, children, adolescents, and young adults should be seen by health care provider at least weekly for 4 wk, every 3 wk for next 4 wk, and on advice of health care provider thereafter.
- Monitor appetite and nutritional intake. Weigh weekly. Report significant changes in weight. Adjust diet as tolerated to support nutritional status.
- Assess for bleeding (hemoptysis; coffee grounds vomit; hematuria; black, red, or tarry stools; bleeding from the gums; abnormal vaginal bleeding; bruises without a cause).
- Assess sexual function before starting fluvoxamine. Assess for changes in sexual function during treatment, including timing of onset; patient may not report.
- Assess for serotonin syndrome (mental changes [agitation, hallucinations, coma], autonomic instability [tachycardia, labile BP, hyperthermia], neuromuscular aberrations [hyperreflexia, incoordination], GI symptoms [nausea, vomiting, diarrhea]), especially in patients taking other serotonergic drugs (SSRIs, SNRIs, triptans).

Lab Test Considerations

- Monitor liver and renal function tests.

Toxicity and Overdose

- Common symptoms of toxicity include drowsiness, vomiting, diarrhea, and dizziness. Coma, tachycardia, bradycardia, hypotension, ECG abnormalities, liver function abnormalities, and convulsions may also occur. Treatment is symptomatic and supportive.

Implementation

- Do not confuse fluvoxamine with fluphenazine or flavoxate.
- Taper to avoid withdrawal effects. ↓ dose by 50% for 3 days; then ↓ by 50% for 3 days; then discontinue.
- **PO:** Initial therapy is administered as a single bedtime dose. May be ↑ every 4–7 days as tolerated.
- Administer without regard to meals. ***DNC:*** Swallow capsules whole. Do not open, break, crush, or chew controlled-release capsules.

Patient/Family Teaching

- Explain purpose and side effects of medication to patient. Advise patient to read *Patient Information* before starting therapy. Instruct patient to take as directed. Do not skip or double up on missed doses. Improvement in symptoms may be noticed in 2–3 wk, but medication should be continued as directed.
- Instruct patient to notify health care provider of all Rx or OTC medications, vitamins, or herbal products being taken and consult health care provider before taking any new medications, especially St. John's wort. Advise patient to avoid taking other CNS depressants, including opioids, or alcohol.
- May cause drowsiness and dizziness. Caution patient to avoid driving and other activities requiring alertness until response to medication is known.
- Advise patient, family, and caregivers to look for suicidality, especially during early therapy or dose changes. Notify health care provider immediately if thoughts about suicide or dying, attempts to commit suicide, new or worse depression or anxiety, agitation or restlessness, panic attacks, insomnia, new or worse irritability, aggressiveness, acting on dangerous impulses, mania, or other changes in mood or behavior occur or if symptoms of serotonin syndrome occur.
- Advise patient to report any signs of uncontrolled bleeding.
- Advise patient to notify health care provider if rash or hives occur or if headache, nausea, anorexia, anxiety, or insomnia persists.
- Advise patient to avoid use of caffeine (chocolate, tea, cola).
- Inform patient that fluvoxamine may cause symptoms of sexual dysfunction. In men, ejaculatory delay or failure, ↓ libido, and erectile dysfunction may occur. In women, may result in ↓ libido and delayed or absent orgasm. Advise patient to notify health care provider if symptoms occur.
- Rep: May cause fetal harm. Advise women of reproductive potential to notify health care provider if pregnancy is planned or suspected or if breastfeeding. Monitor infants exposed to fluvoxamine during 3rd trimester for respiratory distress, cyanosis, apnea, seizures, temperature instability, feeding difficulty, vomiting, hypoglycemia, hypotonia, hypertonia, hyperreflexia, tremors, jitteriness, irritability, and constant crying. May ↑ risk of postpartum hemorrhage. Monitor infants exposed to fluvoxamine via breast milk for agitation, irritability, poor feeding, and poor weight gain. Inform patient of pregnancy exposure registry that monitors pregnancy outcomes in women exposed to antidepressants during pregnancy. Register patient by calling the National Pregnancy Registry for Antidepressants at 1-866-961-2388 or visiting online at https://womensmentalhealth.org/clinical-and-researchprograms/pregnancyregistry/antidepressants/.

Evaluation/Desired Outcomes
- Decrease in obsessive-compulsive behaviors.

folic acid (foe-lik a-sid)

Classification

Therapeutic: antianemics, vitamins

Pharmacologic: water soluble vitamins

Indications
Prevention and treatment of megaloblastic and macrocytic anemias. Given during pregnancy to promote normal fetal development.

Action
Required for protein synthesis and red blood cell function. Stimulates the production of red blood cells, white blood cells, and platelets. Necessary for normal fetal development. **Therapeutic Effects:** Restoration and maintenance of normal hematopoiesis.

Pharmacokinetics
Absorption: Well absorbed from the GI tract and IM and SUBQ sites.
Distribution: Half of all stores are in the liver. Enters breast milk. Crosses the placenta.
Metabolism and Excretion: Converted by the liver to its active metabolite, dihydrofolate reductase. Excess amounts are excreted unchanged by the kidneys.
Half-life: Unknown.

TIME/ACTION PROFILE (↑ in reticulocyte count)

ROUTE	ONSET	PEAK	DURATION
PO, IM, SUBQ, IV	30–60 min	1 hr	unknown

Contraindications/Precautions
Contraindicated in: Uncorrected pernicious, aplastic, or normocytic anemias (neurologic damage will progress despite correction of hematologic abnormalities); Pedi: Preparations containing benzyl alcohol should not be used in newborns.
Use Cautiously in: Undiagnosed anemias.

Adverse Reactions/Side Effects
Derm: rash. **Neuro:** confusion, difficulty sleeping, irritability, malaise. **Misc:** fever.

Interactions
Drug-Drug: Pyrimethamine, methotrexate, trimethoprim, and **triamterene** prevent the activation of folic acid (leucovorin should be used instead to treat overdoses of these drugs). **Sulfonamides** (including **sulfasalazine**), **antacids**, and **cholestyramine** may ↓ absorption. Folic acid requirements are ↑ by **estrogens, phenytoin, phenobarbital, primidone, carbamazepine**, or **corticosteroids**. May ↓ levels and effectiveness of **phenytoin**.

Route/Dosage
Therapeutic Dose (Folic acid deficiency)
PO, IM, IV: SUBQ (Adults and Children >11 yr): 1 mg/day initially, then 0.5 mg/day maintenance dose.
PO, IM, IV: SUBQ (Children >1 yr): 1 mg/day initially, then 0.1–0.4 mg/day maintenance dose.
PO, IM, IV: SUBQ (Infants): 15 mcg/kg/dose daily or 50 mcg/day.

Recommended Daily Allowance
PO (Adults and Children >15 yr): 0.2 mg/day.
PO (Adults): *Women of reproductive potential:* 0.4–0.8 mg/day.
PO (Children 11–14 yr): 0.15 mg/day.
PO (Children 7–10 yr): 0.1 mg/day.
PO (Children 4–6 yr): 0.075 mg/day.
PO (Infants 6 mo–3 yr): 0.05 mg/day.

Availability (generic available)
Solution for injection: 5 mg/mL. **Tablets:** 0.4 mg, 0.8 mg, 1 mg, 🍁5 mg, 🍁25 mg. ***In combination with:*** other vitamins and minerals as multiple vitamins[Rx, OTC].

NURSING IMPLICATIONS
Assessment
- Assess for signs of megaloblastic anemia (fatigue, weakness, dyspnea) before and periodically throughout therapy.

Lab Test Considerations
- Monitor folic acid, hemoglobin, hematocrit, and reticulocyte count before and periodically during therapy.
- May ↓ serum concentrations of other B complex vitamins when given in high continuous doses.

Implementation
- Because of infrequency of solitary vitamin deficiencies, combinations are commonly administered (see Appendix N).
- May be given SUBQ, deep IM, or IV when PO route is not feasible.
- **PO:** Antacids should be given >2 hr after folic acid; folic acid should be given 2 hr before or 4–6 hr after cholestyramine. A 50-mcg/mL oral solution may be extemporaneously prepared by pharmacy for use in neonates and infants.
- **IV:** Solution ranges from yellow to orange-yellow in color.

IV Administration
- **IV Push: Dilution:** Dilute with dextrose or 0.9% NaCl. **Concentration:** 0.1 mg/mL. **Rate:** 5 mg/min.

- **Continuous Infusion: Dilution:** May be added to hyperalimentation solution.
- **Y-Site Compatibility:** aminophylline, ascorbic acid, atracurium, atropine, azathioprine, aztreonam, benztropine, bumetanide, calcium gluconate, cefazolin, cefotaxime, cefotetan, cefoxitin, ceftazidime, ceftriaxone, cefuroxime, chloramphenicol, cimetidine, clindamycin, cyanocobalamin, cyclosporine, dexamethasone, digoxin, diphenhydramine, dopamine, enalaprilat, ephedrine, epinephrine, epoetin alfa, erythromycin, esmolol, famotidine, fentanyl, fluconazole, furosemide, ganciclovir, glycopyrrolate, heparin, hydrocortisone, imipenem/cilastatin, indomethacin, insulin regular, ketorolac, labetalol, letermovir, lidocaine, magnesium sulfate, mannitol, meperidine, methylprednisolone, metoclopramide, metoprolol, midazolam, multivitamins, naloxone, nitroglycerin, nitroprusside, ondansetron, oxacillin, penicillin G, pentobarbital, phenobarbital, phentolamine, phenylephrine, phytonadione, potassium chloride, procainamide, propranolol, sodium bicarbonate, succinylcholine, sufentanil, theophylline, vancomycin, vasopressin.
- **Y-Site Incompatibility:** amikacin, calcium chloride, chlorpromazine, dantrolene, diazepam, diazoxide, dobutamine, doxycycline, gentamicin, haloperidol, hydralazine, minocycline, morphine, nafcillin, nalbuphine, norepinephrine, pentamidine, phenytoin, prochlorperazine, promethazine, protamine, pyridoxine, tacrolimus, thiamine, tobramycin, trimethoprim/sulfamethoxazole, verapamil.

Patient/Family Teaching

- Explain purpose and side effects of medication to patient. Advise patient to read *Patient Information* before starting therapy.
- Advise patient to notify health care provider of all Rx or OTC medications, vitamins, or herbal products being taken and to consult health care provider before taking other medications.
- Encourage patient to comply with diet recommendations of health care provider. Explain that the best source of vitamins is a well-balanced diet with foods from the four basic food groups. A diet low in vitamin B and folate will be used to diagnose folic acid deficiency without concealing pernicious anemia.
- Foods high in folic acid include vegetables, fruits, and organ meats; heat destroys folic acid in foods.
- Patients self-medicating with vitamin supplements should be cautioned not to exceed RDA. The effectiveness of megadoses for treatment of various medical conditions is unproven and may cause side effects.
- Explain that folic acid may make urine more intensely yellow.
- Instruct patient to notify health care provider if rash occurs, which may indicate hypersensitivity.
- Rep: Folic acid in early pregnancy is necessary to prevent neural tube defects. Advise women of reproductive potential to notify health care provider if pregnancy is planned or suspected or if breastfeeding.

Evaluation/Desired Outcomes

- Restoration and maintenance of normal hematopoiesis.

HIGH ALERT

fondaparinux

(fon-da-**par**-i-nux)

Arixtra

Classification

Therapeutic: anticoagulants

Pharmacologic: active factor X inhibitors

Indications

Prevention and treatment of deep vein thrombosis (DVT) and pulmonary embolism (PE). **Unlabeled Use:** Systemic anticoagulation for other diagnoses.

Action

Binds selectively to antithrombin III (AT III). This binding potentiates the neutralization (inactivation) of active factor X (Xa). **Therapeutic Effects:** Interruption of the coagulation cascade resulting in inhibition of thrombus formation. Prevention of thrombus formation decreases the risk of pulmonary emboli.

Pharmacokinetics

Absorption: 100% absorbed following SUBQ administration.

Distribution: Distributes mainly throughout the intravascular space.

Metabolism and Excretion: Eliminated mainly unchanged in urine.

Half-life: 17–21 hr.

TIME/ACTION PROFILE (anticoagulant effect)

ROUTE	ONSET	PEAK	DURATION
SUBQ	rapid	3 hr	24 hr

Contraindications/Precautions

Contraindicated in: Hypersensitivity; Severe renal impairment (↑ risk of bleeding); Body weight <50 kg (for prophylaxis) (markedly ↑ risk of bleeding); Active major bleeding; Bacterial endocarditis; Thrombocytopenia due to fondaparinux antibodies.

Use Cautiously in: Mild to moderate renal impairment; Untreated hypertension; Recent history of ulcer disease; Body weight <50 kg (for treatment of DVT or PE) (may ↑ risk of bleeding); Malignancy; History of heparin-induced thrombocytopenia; OB: Use during pregnancy should be limited to those who have severe allergic reactions to heparin, including eparin-induced thrombocytopenia; Lactation: Safety not established in breastfeeding; Pedi: Children <1 yr (safety and effectiveness not established); Geri: ↑ risk of bleeding in older adults.

Exercise Extreme Caution in: History of congenital or acquired bleeding disorder; Severe uncontrolled hypertension; Hemorrhagic stroke; Recent CNS or ophthalmologic surgery; Active GI bleeding/ulceration; Retinopathy (hypertensive or diabetic); Neuroaxial spinal anesthesia or spinal puncture, especially if concurrent with an indwelling epidural catheter; drugs affecting hemostasis; history of traumatic/repeated spinal puncture; or spinal deformity (↑ risk of spinal hematoma).

Adverse Reactions/Side Effects

CV: edema, hypotension. **Derm:** bullous eruption, hematoma, purpura, rash. **F and E:** hypokalemia. **GI:** ↑ liver enzymes, constipation, diarrhea, dyspepsia, nausea, vomiting. **GU:** urinary retention. **Hemat:** BLEEDING, thrombocytopenia. **Neuro:** confusion, dizziness, headache, insomnia. **Misc:** fever, HYPERSENSITIVITY REACTIONS (INCLUDING ANGIOEDEMA).

Interactions

Drug-Drug: Warfarin or **drugs that affect platelet function**, including **aspirin**, **NSAIDs**, **dipyridamole**, some **cephalosporins**, **valproates**, **clopidogrel**, **prasugrel**, **ticagrelor**, **eptifibatide**, **tirofiban**, and **dextran** may ↑ risk of bleeding.

Drug-Natural Products: ↑ risk of bleeding with **arnica**, **chamomile**, **clove**, **dong quai**, **feverfew**, **garlic**, **ginger**, **gingko**, ***Panax ginseng***, and others.

Route/Dosage

Treatment of Deep Vein Thrombosis/ Pulmonary Embolism

SUBQ (Adults >100 kg): 10 mg once daily for ≥5 days until therapeutic anticoagulation with warfarin is achieved (INR >2 for 2 consecutive days); warfarin may be started within 72 hr of fondaparinux.

SUBQ (Adults 50–100 kg): 7.5 mg once daily for ≥5 days until therapeutic anticoagulation with warfarin is achieved (INR >2 for 2 consecutive days).

SUBQ (Adults <50 kg): 5 mg once daily for ≥5 days until therapeutic anticoagulation with warfarin is achieved (INR >2 for 2 consecutive days); warfarin may be started within 72 hr of fondaparinux (has been used for up to 26 days).

SUBQ (Children ≥1 yr and >60 kg): 7.5 mg once daily.

SUBQ (Children ≥1 yr and >40–60 kg): 5 mg once daily. Adjust dose based on fondaparinux-based anti-Xa assay with a therapeutic goal range of 0.5–1 mg/L (not to exceed 7.5 mg/day).

SUBQ (Children ≥1 yr and >20–40 kg): 2.5 mg once daily. Adjust dose based on fondaparinux-based anti-Xa assay with a therapeutic goal range of 0.5–1 mg/L (not to exceed 7.5 mg/day).

SUBQ (Children ≥1 yr and 10–20 kg): 0.1 mg/kg (rounded to the nearest 0.1 mg) once daily. Adjust dose based on fondaparinux-based anti-Xa assay with a therapeutic goal range of 0.5–1 mg/L (not to exceed 7.5 mg/day).

Prevention of Deep Vein Thrombosis/ Pulmonary Embolism

SUBQ (Adults): 2.5 mg once daily, starting 6–8 hr after surgery, continuing for 5–9 days (up to 11 days) following abdominal surgery or knee/hip replacement or continuing for 24 days following hip fracture surgery (up to 32 days).

Availability (generic available)

Solution for injection (prefilled syringes): 2.5 mg/0.5 mL, 5 mg/0.4 mL, 7.5 mg/0.6 mL, 10 mg/0.8 mL.

NURSING IMPLICATIONS

Assessment

- Assess for signs of bleeding and hemorrhage (bleeding gums; nosebleed; ↑ bruising; black, tarry, guaiac positive stools; hematuria; ↓ hematocrit; sudden ↓ in BP). *If unexpected changes in coagulation parameters or major bleeding occurs,* discontinue fondaparinux.
- Assess for therapy effectiveness by monitoring for signs and symptoms of additional or ↑ thrombi.
- Monitor neurological status frequently, especially in patients with indwelling epidural catheters or concurrent use of other drugs affecting hemostasis. Risk is ↑ by traumatic or repeated epidural or spinal puncture. May require urgent treatment.

Lab Test Considerations

- Monitor platelets closely. *If platelets <100,000/ mm³,* discontinue fondaparinux.
- PT, aPTT, and international standards of heparin or low-molecular-weight heparins are not sensitive measures of the activity of fondaparinux.
- Monitor CBC and stool occult blood routinely during therapy.
- Assess renal function periodically during therapy. Anticoagulant effects may last >4 days after therapy discontinued in patients with renal impairment.
- May ↑ AST and ALT.
- May ↑ aPTT temporally associated with bleeding with or without concurrent administration of other anticoagulants and thrombocytopenia with thrombosis similar to heparin-induced thrombocytopenia. Anti-factor Xa activity can be measured by anti-Xa assay, as clinically indicated.

Implementation

- *High Alert:* Do not confuse Arixtra with Arista AH (absorbable hemostatic agent).
- Fondaparinux cannot be used interchangeably with heparin, low-molecular-weight heparins, or heparinoids.
- Initial dose should be administered 6–8 hr after surgery. Administration <6 hr after surgery carries ↑ risk of hemorrhage.
- Do not expel air bubble from prefilled syringe before injection to prevent loss of drug.
- **SUBQ**: Administer using single-dose prefilled syringe or pharmacist-prepared syringe if alternate dose is required. Inject SUBQ into fatty tissue, alternating sites between right and left anterolateral or posterolateral abdomen. Insert entire length of needle at 45° or 90° angle into a skin fold held between thumb and forefinger. Do not aspirate or massage. Rotate sites frequently. Do not administer IM. Solution is clear; do not use if cloudy or contains particulates. Do not mix with other injections.

Patient/Family Teaching

- Explain purpose and side effects of medication. Advise patient to read *Patient Information* before starting therapy. Instruct patient on appropriate steps for administration technique and disposal of equipment, if self-administration is appropriate.
- Advise patient to report any symptoms of easy bleeding or bruising, dizziness, itching, rash, fever, swelling, or difficulty breathing to health care provider immediately.
- Inform patient having had neuraxial anesthesia or spinal puncture to watch for signs and symptoms of spinal or epidural hematoma (numbness or weakness of legs, bowel or bladder dysfunction). Notify health care provider immediately if symptoms occur.
- Instruct patient not to take aspirin or NSAIDs without consulting health care provider during therapy and to notify health care provider of all Rx or OTC medications, vitamins, or herbal products being taken and before taking other medications.
- Inform patient that packaging contains latex and to notify health care provider of latex allergy prior to therapy initiation.
- Rep: Advise women of reproductive potential to notify health care provider if pregnancy is planned or suspected or if breastfeeding.

Evaluation/Desired Outcomes

- Prevention and treatment of DVT and PE.

foscarnet (foss-**kar**-net)

Foscavir, ✱ Vocarvi

Classification

Therapeutic: antivirals

Indications

Cytomegalovirus (CMV) retinitis in patients with HIV (alone or in combination with ganciclovir). Acyclovir-resistant mucocutaneous herpes simplex virus (HSV) infections in immunocompromised patients.

Action

Prevents viral replication by inhibiting viral DNA polymerase and reverse transcriptase. **Therapeutic Effects:** Virustatic action against susceptible viruses, including CMV.

Pharmacokinetics

Absorption: IV administration results in complete bioavailability.

Distribution: Variable penetration into CSF. May concentrate in and be slowly released from bone.

Metabolism and Excretion: 80–90% excreted unchanged in urine.

Half-life: 3 hr (normal renal function); longer half life of 90 hr may reflect release of drug from bone.

TIME/ACTION PROFILE

ROUTE	ONSET	PEAK	DURATION
IV	rapid	end of infusion	8–24 hr

Contraindications/Precautions

Contraindicated in: Hypersensitivity; HF (due to sodium content); Patients on sodium-restricted diets; Hemodialysis; Lactation: Lactation.

Use Cautiously in: Renal impairment (dose ↓ required if CCr ≤1.4 mL/min/kg); Seizure disorders; QT interval prolongation or cardiovascular disease; Hypokalemia or hypomagnesemia (must be corrected prior to therapy); OB: Safety not established in pregnancy; Pedi: Safety and effectiveness not established in children.

Adverse Reactions/Side Effects

CV: chest pain, edema, palpitations, QT interval prolongation, TORSADES DE POINTES. **Derm:** ↑ sweating, pruritus, rash, skin ulceration. **EENT:** conjunctivitis, eye pain, vision abnormalities. **F and E:** hypocalcemia, hypokalemia, hypomagnesemia, hyperphosphatemia, hypophosphatemia. **GI:** diarrhea, nausea, vomiting, abdominal pain, abnormal taste sensation, anorexia, constipation, dyspepsia. **GU:** RENAL FAILURE, albuminuria, dysuria, nocturia, polyuria, urinary retention. **Hemat:** anemia, leukopenia, neutropenia. **Local:** pain/inflammation at injection site. **MS:** arthralgia, myalgia, back pain, involuntary muscle contraction. **Neuro:** headache, anxiety, ataxia, confusion, depression, dizziness, fatigue, hypoesthesia, neuropathy, paresthesia, SEIZURES, tremor, weakness. **Resp:** cough, dyspnea. **Misc:** fever, chills, flu-like syndrome, HYPERSENSITIVITY REACTIONS (INCLUDING ANAPHYLAXIS, URTICARIA, AND ANGIOEDEMA), MALIGNANCY.

nteractions

)rug-Drug: QT interval prolonging medications, ıcluding **quinidine, procainamide, amiodarone,** **otalol, chlorpromazine, thioridazine, moxifloxa-** **in, pentamidine,** and **methadone,** may ↑ risk of QT ıterval prolongation; avoid concurrent use. Parenteral **entamidine** may result in severe, life-threatening ıypocalcemia. Risk of nephrotoxicity may be ↑ by **neph-** **otoxic agents,** including **amphotericin B, amino-** **lycosides, cyclosporine, acyclovir, methotrexate,** **acrolimus,** and **pentamidine (IV).**

₹oute/Dosage

;ytomegalovirus Retinitis

V (Adults): 60 mg/kg every 8 hr or 90 mg/kg every 12 hr for 2–3 wk as induction therapy; then 0–120 mg/kg once daily as maintenance therapy.

₹enal Impairment

V (Adults): *CCr >1–1.4 mL/min/kg:* 45 mg/kg every 8 hr or 70 mg/kg every 12 hr for 2–3 wk as ıduction therapy; then 70–90 mg/kg once daily as naintenance therapy; *CCr >0.8–1 mL/min/kg:* 50 mg/ g every 12 hr for 2–3 wk as induction therapy; then 0–65 mg/kg once daily as maintenance therapy; *CCr >0.6–0.8 mL/min/kg:* 40 mg/kg every 12 hr or 80 mg/ g once daily for 2–3 wk as induction therapy; then 0–105 mg/kg every 48 hr as maintenance therapy; *Cr >0.5–0.6 mL/min/kg:* 60 mg/kg once daily for –3 wk as induction therapy; then 60–80 mg/kg every 8 hr as maintenance therapy; *CCr >0.4–0.5 mL/ nin/kg:* 50 mg/kg once daily for 2–3 wk as induction herapy; then 50–65 mg/kg every 48 hr as maintenance herapy; *CCr <0.4 mL/min/kg:* Not recommended.

Ierpes Simplex Virus

V (Adults): 40 mg/kg every 8–12 hr for 2–3 wk or ıntil healing occurs.

₹enal Impairment

V (Adults): *CCr >1–1.4 mL/min/kg:* 30 mg/kg every 8–12 hr for 2–3 wk or until healing occurs; *CCr >0.8–1 mL/min/kg:* 20–35 mg/kg every 8–12 hr for –3 wk or until healing occurs; *CCr >0.6–0.8 mL/ nin/kg:* 25 mg/kg every 12 hr or 35 mg/kg once daily or 2–3 wk or until healing occurs; *CCr >0.5– .6 mL/min/kg:* 25–40 mg/kg once daily for 2–3 wk r until healing occurs; *CCr >0.4–0.5 mL/min/kg:* 0–35 mg/kg once daily for 2–3 wk or until healing ccurs; *CCr <0.4 mL/min/kg:* Not recommended.

Availability (generic available)

olution for injection: 24 mg/mL.

JURSING IMPLICATIONS

Assessment

Monitor ECG periodically during therapy for QT interval prolongation and arrhythmias.

- **CMV Retinitis:** Diagnosis of CMV retinitis should be determined by ophthalmoscopy before treatment with foscarnet. Ophthalmologic examinations should be performed at the conclusion of induction and every 4 wk during maintenance therapy.
- Culture for CMV (urine, blood, throat) may be taken before administration, but a negative CMV culture does not rule out CMV retinitis.
- **HSV Infections:** Assess lesions before and daily during therapy.
- Monitor for seizure activity. Implement seizure precautions if necessary.
- Assess for hypersensitivity reactions (anaphylaxis, urticaria, angioedema). Implement supportive medical treatment (epinephrine) as indicated.

Lab Test Considerations

- Monitor serum creatinine before and 2–3 times weekly during induction therapy and at least once every 1–2 wk during maintenance therapy. Monitor 24-hr CCr before and periodically throughout therapy. If CCr drops below 0.4 mL/min/kg, discontinue foscarnet.
- Monitor serum calcium, magnesium, potassium, and phosphorus before and 2–3 times weekly during induction therapy and at least weekly during maintenance therapy. May cause hypocalcemia, hypomagnesemia, hypokalemia, and hypophosphatemia.
- May cause anemia, granulocytopenia, leukopenia, and thrombocytopenia. May cause ↑ AST and ALT levels and abnormal A-G ratios.

Implementation

- Adequately hydrate patient with 750–1000 mL of 0.9% NaCl or D5W before 1st infusion to establish diuresis; then administer 750–1000 mL with 120 mg/kg of foscarnet or 500 mL with 40–60 mg/kg of foscarnet with each dose to prevent renal toxicity.

IV Administration

- **Intermittent Infusion: Dilution:** May be administered via central line undiluted. If administered via peripheral line, *must* be diluted with D5W or 0.9% NaCl to prevent vein irritation. Do not administer solution that is discolored or contains particulate matter. Do not refrigerate or freeze; stable for 24 hr at room temperature. Use diluted solution within 24 hr. **Concentration:** Undiluted: 24 mg/mL; Diluted: 12 mg/mL.
- Dose is based on patient weight; excess solution may be discarded from bottle before administration to prevent overdosage.
- Patients who experience progression of CMV retinitis during maintenance therapy may be retreated with induction therapy followed by maintenance therapy. **Rate:** Administer at a rate not to exceed 1 mg/kg/min.

- Infuse solution via infusion pump to ensure accurate infusion rate.
- **Y-Site Compatibility:** aldesleukin, alemtuzumab, amikacin, aminocaproic acid, aminophylline, amphotericin B liposomal, ampicillin, ampicillin/sulbactam, anidulafungin, argatroban, arsenic trioxide, atracurium, azithromycin, aztreonam, bivalirudin, bleomycin, bumetanide, buprenorphine, busulfan, butorphanol, carboplatin, carmustine, cefazolin, cefepime, cefotaxime, cefotetan, cefoxitin, ceftazidime, ceftriaxone, cefuroxime, chloramphenicol, cisatracurium, cisplatin, clindamycin, cyclophosphamide, cyclosporine, cytarabine, dacarbazine, dactinomycin, daptomycin, defibrotide, dexamethasone, dexmedetomidine, dexrazoxane, diltiazem, docetaxel, dopamine, doxorubicin liposomal, enalaprilat, ephedrine, epinephrine, eptifibatide, ertapenem, erythromycin, esmolol, etoposide, etoposide phosphate, famotidine, fentanyl, fluconazole, flucytosine, fludarabine, fluorouracil, fosphenytoin, furosemide, gemcitabine, gemtuzumab ozogamicin, gentamicin, glycopyrrolate, granisetron, heparin, hetastarch, hydrocortisone, hydromorphone, ifosfamide, imipenem/cilastatin, insulin, regular, irinotecan, isoproterenol, ketorolac, levofloxacin, lidocaine, linezolid, magnesium sulfate, mannitol, melphalan, meperidine, meropenem, mesna, methadone, methotrexate, metoclopramide, metoprolol, metronidazole, milrinone, mitomycin, morphine, nafcillin, nalbuphine, naloxone, nitroglycerin, nitroprusside, octreotide, oxacillin, oxaliplatin, oxytocin, paclitaxel, palonosetron, pamidronate, pantoprazole, pemetrexed, penicillin G potassium, pentobarbital, phenobarbital, phentolamine, phenylephrine, piperacillin/tazobactam, potassium acetate, potassium chloride, potassium phosphates, procainamide, propranolol, remifentanil, rocuronium, sodium acetate, sodium bicarbonate, sodium phosphates, succinylcholine, sufentanil, tacrolimus, theophylline, thiotepa, tigecycline, tirofiban, tobramycin, vecuronium, vinblastine, vincristine, voriconazole, zidovudine, zoledronic acid.
- **Y-Site Incompatibility:** acyclovir, allopurinol, amiodarone, amphotericin B deoxycholate, calcium chloride, calcium gluconate, caspofungin, chlorpromazine, ciprofloxacin, dantrolene, daunorubicin, diazepam, digoxin, diphenhydramine, dobutamine, doxorubicin hydrochloride, droperidol, epirubicin, ganciclovir, haloperidol, hydralazine, idarubicin, labetalol, leucovorin, methylprednisolone, midazolam, minocycline, mitoxantrone, mycophenolate, nicardipine, norepinephrine, ondansetron, pentamidine, prochlorperazine, promethazine, topotecan, verapamil, vinorelbine.

Patient/Family Teaching

- Explain purpose and side effects of medication to patient. Advise patient to read *Patient Information* before starting therapy. Inform patient that foscarnet is not a cure for CMV retinitis. Progression of retinitis may continue in immunocompromised patients during and after therapy. Advise patients to have regular ophthalmologic exams.
- Advise patient to notify health care provider of all Rx or OTC medications, vitamins, or herbal products being taken and to consult health care provider before taking other medications.
- May cause dizziness and seizures. Caution patient to avoid driving or other activities requiring alertness until response to medication is known.
- Advise patient to notify health care provider immediately if perioral tingling or numbness in the extremities or paresthesia occurs during or after infusion. If these signs of electrolyte imbalance occur during administration, infusion should be stopped and lab samples for serum electrolyte concentrations obtained immediately.
- Rep: Advise women of reproductive potential to notify health care provider if pregnancy is planned or suspected and to avoid breastfeeding.

Evaluation/Desired Outcomes

- Virustatic action against susceptible viruses, including CMV.

fosinopril, See ANGIOTENSIN-CONVERTING ENZYME (ACE) INHIBITORS.

fosphenytoin

(foss-**fen**-i-toyn)

Cerebyx

Classification

Therapeutic: anticonvulsants

Indications

Short-term (<5 day) parenteral management of generalized, tonic-clonic status epilepticus when use of phenytoin is not feasible. Treatment and prevention of seizures during neurosurgery when use of phenytoin is not feasible. Short-term substitution for oral phenytoin in patients ≥2 yr old.

Action

Limits seizure propagation by altering ion transport. May also decrease synaptic transmission. Fosphenytoin is rapidly converted to phenytoin, which is responsible for its pharmacologic effects. **Therapeutic Effects:** Diminished seizure activity.

Pharmacokinetics

Absorption: Rapidly converted to phenytoin after IV administration and completely absorbed after IM administration.
Distribution: Distributes into CSF and other body tissues and fluids. Preferentially distributes into fatty tissue.
Protein Binding: *Fosphenytoin:* 95–99%; *phenytoin:* 90–95%.
Metabolism and Excretion: Mostly metabolized by the liver via the CYP2C9 isoenzyme and to a lesser extent by the CYP2C19 isoenzyme; the CYP2C9 isoenzyme exhibits genetic polymorphism (intermediate or poor metabolizers may have significantly ↑ fosphenytoin concentrations and an ↑ risk of adverse reactions); minimal amounts excreted in the urine.
Half-life: *Fosphenytoin:* 15 min; *phenytoin:* 22 hr (range 7–42 hr).

TIME/ACTION PROFILE (anticonvulsant effect)

ROUTE	ONSET	PEAK	DURATION
IM	unknown	30 min	up to 24 hr
IV	15–45 min	15–60 min	up to 24 hr

Contraindications/Precautions

Contraindicated in: Hypersensitivity; Sinus bradycardia, sinoatrial block, 2nd- or 3rd-degree AV heart block or Adams-Stokes syndrome; Prior acute hepatotoxicity due to fosphenytoin or phenytoin.
Use Cautiously in: Renal impairment; Hepatic impairment (↓ dose); CYP2C9 intermediate or poor metabolizers (↑ risk of phenytoin toxicity); OB: ↑ risk of congenital anomalies; ↑ risk of hemorrhage in newborn if used at term; Lactation: Use while breastfeeding only if potential maternal benefit justifies potential risk to infant.
Exercise Extreme Caution in: Patients positive for HLA-B* 1502 allele or carriers of CYP2C9* 3 variant (unless benefits clearly outweigh the risks) (↑ risk of serious skin reactions).

Adverse Reactions/Side Effects

CV: hypotension (with rapid IV administration), tachycardia. **Derm:** pruritus, ACUTE GENERALIZED EXANTHEMATOUS PUSTULOSIS, DRUG REACTION WITH EOSINOPHILIA AND SYSTEMIC SYMPTOMS (DRESS), purple glove syndrome, rash, STEVENS-JOHNSON SYNDROME, TOXIC EPIDERMAL NECROLYSIS. **EENT:** amblyopia, deafness, diplopia, tinnitus. **GI:** dry mouth, nausea, taste perversion, tongue disorder, vomiting. **Hemat:** lymphadenopathy, megaloblastic anemia, pure red cell aplasia. **MS:** back pain. **Neuro:** ataxia, dizziness, drowsiness, nystagmus, agitation, brain edema, dysarthria, extrapyramidal syndrome, headache, hypoesthesia, incoordination, paresthesia, stupor, tremor, vertigo. **Misc:** ANGIOEDEMA, pelvic pain.

Interactions

Drug-Drug: Disulfiram, acute ingestion of **alcohol**, **amiodarone**, **capecitabine**, **chloramphenicol**, **chlordiazepoxide**, **cimetidine**, **diazepam**, **estrogens**, **ethosuximide**, **felbamate**, **fluconazole**, **fluorouracil**, **fluoxetine**, **fluvastatin**, **fluvoxamine**, **halothane**, **isoniazid**, **itraconazole**, **ketoconazole**, **methylphenidate**, **miconazole**, **omeprazole**, **oxcarbazepine**, **phenothiazines**, **salicylates**, **sertraline**, **sulfonamides**, **topiramate**, **trazodone**, **voriconazole**, and **warfarin** may ↑ phenytoin levels. **Barbiturates**, **bleomycin**, **carbamazepine**, **carboplatin**, **cisplatin**, **diazoxide**, **doxorubicin**, **folic acid**, **fosamprenavir**, **methotrexate**, **nelfinavir**, **rifampin**, **ritonavir**, **theophylline**, **vigabatrin**, and chronic ingestion of **alcohol** may ↓ phenytoin levels. Phenytoin may ↓ levels and effectiveness of **albendazole**, **amiodarone**, **atorvastatin**, **benzodiazepines**, **carbamazepine**, **chloramphenicol**, **clozapine**, **corticosteroids**, **cyclosporine**, **digoxin**, **disopyramide**, **doxycycline**, **efavirenz**, **estrogens**, **felbamate**, **fluconazole**, **fluvastatin**, **folic acid**, **furosemide**, **irinotecan**, **itraconazole**, **ketoconazole**, **lamotrigine**, **lopinavir/ritonavir**, **methadone**, **mexiletine**, **nelfinavir**, **nifedipine**, **nimodipine**, **nisoldipine**, **oral contraceptives**, **oxcarbazepine**, **paclitaxel**, **paroxetine**, **posaconazole**, **propafenone**, **quetiapine**, **quinidine**, **rifampin**, **ritonavir**, **sertraline**, **simvastatin**, **tacrolimus**, **theophylline**, **topiramate**, **tricyclic antidepressants**, **verapamil**, **vitamin D**, **voriconazole**, **warfarin**, and **zonisamide**.
Drug-Natural Products: St. John's wort may ↓ levels and effectiveness.

Route/Dosage

Note: Doses of fosphenytoin should be expressed as phenytoin sodium equivalents [PE].

Status Epilepticus

IV (Adults and Children): 15–20 mg PE/kg.

Nonemergent and Maintenance Dosing

IV, IM (Adults and Children >16 yr): *Loading dose:* 10–20 mg PE/kg. *Maintenance dose:* 4–6 mg PE/kg/day (start 12 hr after loading dose; administer in 2–3 divided doses).
IV (Children Birth to 16 yr): *Loading dose:* 10–15 mg PE/kg. *Maintenance dose:* 2–4 mg PE/kg given 12 hr after loading dose; then 4–8 mg PE/kg/day (in 2 divided doses).

Availability (generic available)

Solution for injection: 50 mg PE/mL, 🍁75 mg PE/mL.

NURSING IMPLICATIONS

Assessment

- Assess location, duration, frequency, and characteristics of seizure activity. EEG may be monitored periodically during therapy.
- Monitor BP, ECG, and respiratory function continuously during administration of fosphenytoin and during period when peak serum phenytoin levels occur (10–20 min after administration).
- Monitor patients for development of severe cutaneous adverse reactions such as exfoliative, purpuric, bullous rashes; lupus erythematosus; DRESS; SJS; and TEN. Advise patients of signs and symptoms of these reactions (prodrome of fever, flu-like symptoms, mucosal lesions, progressive skin rash, lymphadenopathy). If a severe cutaneous adverse reaction is suspected, interrupt therapy until etiology of reaction is determined. Drug may be resumed if rash determined not drug-related. If rash reappears, avoid further use of fosphenytoin. Stevens-Johnson syndrome and toxic epidermal necrolysis are significantly more common in patients with a particular HLA allele, HLA-B* 1502 (occurs almost exclusively in patients with Asian ancestry, including Han Chinese, Filipinos, Malaysians, South Asian Indians, and Thais) and/or CYP2C9* 3 carriers. Avoid using fosphenytoin as an alternative to carbamazepine for patients who test positive for these genetic variations.
- Assess mental status (orientation, mood, behavior) before and periodically during therapy. Monitor closely for notable changes in behavior that could indicate the emergence or worsening of suicidal thoughts or behavior or depression.
- Monitor injection site for edema, discoloration, and pain distal to the site of injection (described as "purple glove syndrome") frequently during therapy. May or may not be associated with extravasation. The syndrome may not develop for several days after injection of fosphenytoin.

Lab Test Considerations

- Fosphenytoin contains 0.0037 mmol phosphate per mg PE. Monitor serum phosphate concentrations in patients with renal insufficiency; may cause ↑ phosphate concentrations.
- May cause ↑ serum alkaline phosphatase, GGT, and glucose levels.
- Fosphenytoin therapy may be monitored using phenytoin levels. Optimal total plasma phenytoin concentrations are typically 10–20 mcg/mL (unbound plasma phenytoin concentrations of 1–2 mcg/mL).

Toxicity and Overdose

- Serum phenytoin levels should not be monitored until complete conversion from fosphenytoin to phenytoin has occurred (2 hr after IV or 4 hr after IM administration).
- Initial signs and symptoms of phenytoin toxicity include nystagmus, ataxia, confusion, nausea, slurred speech, and dizziness.

Implementation

- Do not confuse Cerebyx with Celebrex or Celexa.
- Do not confuse concentration of fosphenytoin with total amount of drug in vial.
- When substituting *fosphenytoin* for oral *phenytoin* therapy, the same total daily dose may be given as a single dose. Unlike parenteral phenytoin, fosphenytoin may be given safely by the IM route.
- The anticonvulsant effect of fosphenytoin is not immediate. Additional measures (including parenteral benzodiazepines) are usually required in the immediate management of status epilepticus. Loading dose of *fosphenytoin* should be followed with the institution of maintenance anticonvulsant therapy.

IV Administration

- **IV Push: Dilution:** D5W or 0.9% NaCl. **Concentration:** 1.5–25 mg PE/mL. May be refrigerated for up to 48 hr. **Rate:** Administer at a rate of <150 mg PE/min in adults and <0.4 mg/kg/min in children 2–17 yr to minimize risk of hypotension and arrhythmias.
- **Y-Site Compatibility:** acyclovir, alemtuzumab, allopurinol, amikacin, aminocaproic acid, aminophylline, amphotericin B liposomal, ampicillin, ampicillin/sulbactam, anidulafungin, argatroban, arsenic trioxide, azithromycin, aztreonam, bivalirudin, bleomycin, bumetanide, buprenorphine, busulfan, butorphanol, carboplatin, carmustine, cefazolin, cefepime, cefotaxime, cefotetan, cefoxitin, ceftazidime, ceftolozane/tazobactam, ceftriaxone, cefuroxime, ciprofloxacin, cisatracurium, cisplatin, clindamycin, cyclophosphamide, cyclosporine, cytarabine, dacarbazine, dactinomycin, daptomycin, dexamethasone, dexmedetomidine, dexrazoxane, digoxin, diltiazem, diphenhydramine, docetaxel, doxorubicin liposomal, doxycycline, enalaprilat, ephedrine, epinephrine, eptifibatide, ertapenem, erythromycin, esmolol, etoposide, etoposide phosphate, famotidine, fentanyl, fluconazole, fludarabine, fluorouracil, foscarnet, furosemide, ganciclovir, gemcitabine, gemtuzumab ozogamicin, gentamicin, glycopyrrolate, granisetron, heparin, hetastarch, hydrocortisone, hydromorphone, ifosfamide, imipenem/cilastatin, insulin, regular, isoproterenol, ketotolac, labetalol, leucovorin, levetiracetam, levofloxacin, lidocaine, linezolid, lorazepam, magnesium sulfate, mannitol, melphalan, meperidine, meropenem, meropenem/vaborbactam, mesna, methadone, methotrexate,

methylprednisolone, metoclopramide, metoprolol, metronidazole, milrinone, mitomycin, morphine, nafcillin, nalbuphine, naloxone, nitroglycerin, nitroprusside, norepinephrine, octreotide, ondansetron, oxaliplatin, oxytocin, paclitaxel, palonosetron, pamidronate, pantoprazole, pemetrexed, pentobarbital, phenobarbital, phentolamine, phenylephrine, piperacillin/tazobactam, plazomicin, potassium acetate, potassium chloride, potassium phosphate, procainamide, propranolol, remifentanil, rocuronium, sodium acetate, sodium bicarbonate, sodium phosphate, succinylcholine, sufentanil, sulbactam/durlobactam, tacrolimus, tedizolid, theophylline, thiotepa, tigecycline, tirofiban, tobramycin, trimethoprim/sulfamethoxazole, vancomycin, vasopressin, vecuronium, vinblastine, vincristine, vinorelbine, voriconazole, zidovudine, zoledronic acid.

- **Y-Site Incompatibility:** amiodarone, amphotericin B deoxycholate, calcium chloride, calcium gluconate, caspofungin, chlorpromazine, dantrolene, daunorubicin hydrochloride, diazepam, dobutamine, doxorubicin hydrochloride, droperidol, epirubicin, haloperidol, hydralazine, hydroxyzine, idarubicin, irinotecan, isavuconazonium, midazolam, mitoxantrone, moxifloxacin, mycophenolate, nicardipine, pentamidine, phenytoin, polymyxin B, prochlorperazine, topotecan, verapamil.

Patient/Family Teaching

- Explain purpose and side effects of fosphenytoin to patient. Advise patient against sudden discontinuation of drug, as this may ↑ seizure frequency. Advise patient to read *Medication Guide* before starting and periodically during therapy in case of changes.
- Emphasize the importance of routine exams to monitor progress. Patient should have routine physical exams, especially monitoring skin and lymph nodes, and EEG testing.
- Instruct patient to notify health care provider if any rash (particularly with fever, flu-like symptoms, or swollen lymph nodes) develops during the 1–2 wk of therapy.
- Advise patient and family to notify health care provider if thoughts about suicide or dying, attempts to commit suicide, new or worse depression, behavioral changes, new or worse anxiety, feeling very agitated or restless, panic attacks, trouble sleeping, new or worse irritability, acting aggressive, being angry or violent, acting on dangerous impulses, an extreme ↑ in activity and talking, or other unusual changes in behavior or mood occur.
- Medical ID describing disease process and medication regimen should be worn at all times in case of emergencies.
- May cause drowsiness or dizziness. Caution patient to avoid driving or other activities requiring alertness until response to medication is known. Do not resume driving until physician gives clearance based on control of seizure disorder.
- Advise patient to notify health care provider of all Rx or OTC medications, vitamins, or herbal products being taken and to consult with health care provider before taking other medications, especially St. John's wort. Avoid drinking alcohol during treatment.
- Rep: May cause fetal harm. Advise women of reproductive potential to use an additional nonhormonal method of contraception during therapy and until next menstrual period. Instruct patient to notify health care provider if pregnancy is planned or suspected or if breastfeeding. To prevent a potentially life-threatening bleeding disorder related to ↓ levels of vitamin K–dependent clotting factors in newborns exposed to phenytoin in utero, administer vitamin K to the mother before delivery and to the neonate after birth. Encourage patients who become pregnant to enroll in the North American Antiepileptic Drug Pregnancy Registry by calling 1-888-233-2334 or on the web at www.aedpregnancyregistry.org. Enrollment must be done by patients themselves.

Evaluation/Desired Outcomes

- Decrease or cessation of seizures without excessive sedation.

fremanezumab

(free-ma-**nez**-ue-mab)

Ajovy

Classification

Therapeutic: vascular headache suppressants

Pharmacologic: monoclonal antibodies, calcitonin gene-related peptide receptor antagonists

Indications

Migraine prevention.

Action

Monoclonal antibody that binds to the calcitonin gene-related peptide (CGRP) receptor, which reduces the neuroinflammatory and vasodilatory effects of CGRP. **Therapeutic Effects:** Reduction in frequency of migraines.

F

Pharmacokinetics

Absorption: Unknown.
Distribution: Minimal distribution to tissues.
Metabolism and Excretion: Degraded by enzymatic proteolysis into small peptides and amino acids.
Half-life: 31 days.

TIME/ACTION PROFILE (plasma concentrations)

ROUTE	ONSET	PEAK	DURATION
SUBQ	unknown	5–7 days	1 mo

Contraindications/Precautions

Contraindicated in: Hypersensitivity.
Use Cautiously in: OB: Safety not established in pregnancy; Lactation: Safety not established in breastfeeding; Pedi: Safety and effectiveness not established in children.

Adverse Reactions/Side Effects

Local: injection site reactions. **Misc:** HYPERSENSITIVITY REACTIONS (INCLUDING ANAPHYLAXIS AND ANGIOEDEMA).

Interactions

Drug-Drug: None reported.

Route/Dosage

SUBQ (Adults): 225 mg once monthly *or* 675 mg every 3 mo.

Availability

Solution for injection (prefilled syringes and autoinjectors): 225 mg/1.5 mL.

NURSING IMPLICATIONS

Assessment

- Assess frequency and intensity of migraines.
- Monitor for signs and symptoms of hypersensitivity reactions (rash, urticaria, pruritus, flushing, dizziness, vomiting, abdominal pain) and angioedema (swelling of throat, lips, tongue, or face; dyspnea; wheezing; hoarseness). May occur up to 1 mo after administration. *If reaction is severe,* discontinue fremanezumab and treat as needed.

Implementation

- **SUBQ**: Prior to use, allow vial to sit at room temperature for ≥30 min; protect from direct sunlight. Do no use other methods to warm solution (hot water or microwave). Do not shake. Solution is clear to opalescent, colorless to light yellow; do not administer solutions that are discolored, cloudy, or contain particulate matter. Store in refrigerator in original carton to protect from light; do not freeze. May be stored up to 7 days at room temperature; discard if at room temperature >7 days.
- Inject entire contents into abdomen, thigh, or upper arm. Do not inject into areas where the skin is tender, bruised, red, or hard.

Patient/Family Teaching

- Explain the purpose and side effects. Instruct patient to take as directed. Administer missed doses as soon as possible and schedule next dose from date last dose administered. Educate patient and/or caregiver on correct technique for injection and disposal of equipment. Advise patient to read *Patient Information* before starting therapy and with each Rx refill in case of changes.
- Instruct patient to notify health care provider or call 911 immediately to seek medical care if signs and symptoms of hypersensitivity reaction (itching, rash, hives, swelling of face, mouth, tongue or throat, trouble breathing) occur.
- Advise patient to notify health care provider of all Rx or OTC medications, vitamins, or herbal products being taken and to consult with health care provider before taking other medications.
- Rep: Advise women of reproductive potential to notify health care provider if pregnancy is planned or suspected or if breastfeeding. Women with migraines may be at ↑ risk of preeclampsia and gestational hypertension during pregnancy. Inform patient of pregnancy exposure registry that monitors outcomes in women exposed to fremanezumab. Enrollment can be done by health care provider or patient by calling 1-833-927-2605 or visiting www.tevamigrainepregnancyregistry.com.

Evaluation/Desired Outcomes

- Decrease in frequency of migraines.

furosemide, See DIURETICS (LOOP).

gabapentin (ga-ba-**pen**-tin)

Gabarone, Gralise, Horizant, Neurontin

Classification

Therapeutic: analgesics, anticonvulsants, mood stabilizers

Pharmacologic: gamma aminobutyric acid (GABA) analogues

Schedule V (only schedule V in some states)

Indications

Partial seizures (adjunct treatment) (immediate release only). Postherpetic neuralgia. Restless legs syndrome (Horizant only). **Unlabeled Use:** Neuropathic pain. Prevention of migraine headache.

Action

Mechanism of action is not known. May affect transport of amino acids across and stabilize neuronal membranes. **Therapeutic Effects:** Decreased incidence of seizures. Decreased postherpetic pain. Decreased leg restlessness.

Pharmacokinetics

Absorption: Well absorbed after oral administration by active transport. At larger doses, transport becomes saturated and absorption ↓ (bioavailability ranges from 60% for a 300-mg dose to 35% for a 1600-mg dose).

Distribution: Well distributed to tissues; crosses blood-brain barrier.

Metabolism and Excretion: Eliminated mostly by renal excretion of unchanged drug.

Half-life: *Adults:* 5–7 hr (normal renal function); up to 132 hr in anuria; *Children:* 4.7 hr.

TIME/ACTION PROFILE (plasma concentrations)

ROUTE	ONSET	PEAK	DURATION
PO-IR	rapid	2–4 hr	8 hr
PO-SR	unknown	5–8 hr	24 hr

Contraindications/Precautions

Contraindicated in: Hypersensitivity.

Use Cautiously in: All patients (may ↑ risk of suicidal thoughts/behaviors); Renal impairment (↓ dose and/or ↑ dosing interval if CCr ≤60 mL/min); Respiratory impairment (↑ risk of respiratory depression); OB: Safety not established in pregnancy; Lactation: Use while breastfeeding only if potential maternal benefit justifies potential risk to infant; Pedi: Safety and effectiveness not established in children <18 yr (sustained/extended release) or <3 yr (immediate release); Geri: Older adults may be more susceptible to toxicity due to age-related ↓ in renal function.

Adverse Reactions/Side Effects

Derm: bullous pemphigoid, STEVENS-JOHNSON SYNDROME. **EENT:** abnormal vision, nystagmus. **GI:** anorexia, flatulence, gingivitis. **Metab:** weight gain. **MS:** ↑ CK, arthralgia, RHABDOMYOLYSIS. **Neuro:** ataxia, confusion, depression, dizziness, drowsiness, altered reflexes, anxiety, concentration difficulties (children), emotional lability (children), hostility, hyperkinesia (children), malaise, paresthesia, sedation, SUICIDAL THOUGHTS, vertigo, weakness. **Misc:** HYPERSENSITIVITY REACTIONS (INCLUDING ANAPHYLAXIS OR ANGIOEDEMA).

Interactions

Drug-Drug: Antacids may ↓ absorption. ↑ risk of CNS and respiratory depression with other **CNS depressants**, including **alcohol**, **antihistamines**, **opioids**, and **sedative/hypnotics**. May ↓ levels and effectiveness of **hydrocodone**.

Drug-Natural Products: Kava-kava, **valerian**, or **chamomile** can ↑ risk of CNS depression.

Route/Dosage

The sustained-/extended-release formulations should not be interchanged with the immediate-release products.

Partial Seizures

PO (Adults and Children >12 yr): 300 mg 3 times daily initially. Titration may be continued until desired effect achieved (range is 900–1800 mg/day in 3 divided doses; dosage interval should not exceed 12 hr). Doses up to 2400–3600 mg/day have been well tolerated.

PO (Children ≥5–12 yr): 10–15 mg/kg/day in 3 divided doses initially titrated upward over 3 days to 25–35 mg/kg/day in 3 divided doses; dosage interval should not exceed 12 hr (doses up to 50 mg/kg/day have been used).

PO (Children 3–4 yr): 10–15 mg/kg/day in 3 divided doses initially titrated upward over 3 days to 40 mg/kg/day in 3 divided doses; dosage interval should not exceed 12 hr (doses up to 50 mg/kg/day have been used).

Renal Impairment

PO (Adults and Children >12 yr): *CCr 30–59 mL/min:* 200–700 mg twice daily; *CCr 15–29 mL/min:* 200–700 mg once daily; *CCr 15 mL/min:* 100–300 mg once daily; *CCr <15 mL/min:* ↓ daily dose in proportion to CCr.

Postherpetic Neuralgia

PO (Adults): *Immediate release:* 300 mg once daily on Day 1, then 300 mg twice daily on Day 2, then 300 mg 3 times daily on Day 3; may titrate as needed up to 600 mg 3 times/day; *Sustained release (Gralise):* 300 mg once daily on Day 1, then 600 mg once daily on Day 2, then 900 mg once daily on Days 3–6, then 1200 mg once daily on Days 7–10, then 1500 mg once daily on Days 11–14, then 1800 mg once daily thereafter; *Extended release (Horizant):* 600 mg once daily in the morning on Days 1–3, then 600 mg twice daily thereafter.

Renal Impairment

PO (Adults): *CCr 30–59 mL/min:* 200–700 mg twice daily (immediate release); 600–1800 mg once daily (sustained release [Gralise]); 300 mg once daily in the morning on Days 1–3, then 300 mg twice daily thereafter (may ↑ to 600 mg twice daily, as needed) (extended release [Horizant]); *CCr 15–29 mL/min:* 200–700 mg once daily (immediate release); sustained release (Gralise) not recommended; 300 mg in the morning on Days 1 and 3, then 300 mg once daily in the morning thereafter (may ↑ to 300 mg twice daily, as needed) (extended release [Horizant]); *CCr 15 mL/min:* 100–300 mg once daily (immediate release); sustained release (Gralise) not recommended; *CCr <15 mL/min:* ↓ daily dose in proportion to CCr (immediate release); sustained release (Gralise) not recommended; 300 mg every other day in the morning (may ↑ to 300 mg once daily in the morning, as needed) (extended release [Horizant]); *CCr <15 mL/min (on hemodialysis):* 300 mg after each dialysis session (may ↑ to 600 mg after each dialysis session, as needed) (extended release [Horizant]).

Restless Legs Syndrome

PO (Adults): *Extended release (Horizant):* 600 mg once daily at 5 pm.

Renal Impairment

(Adults): *CCr 30–59 mL/min:* 300 mg once daily at 5 pm; may ↑ to 600 mg once daily at 5 pm as needed; *CCr 15–29 mL/min:* 300 mg once daily at 5 pm; *CCr <15 mL/min:* 300 mg every other day; *CCr <15 mL/min (on hemodialysis):* Not recommended.

Neuropathic Pain (unlabeled use)

PO (Adults): 100 mg 3 times daily initially. Titrate weekly by 300 mg/day up to 900–2400 mg/day (maximum: 3600 mg/day).

PO (Children): 5 mg/kg/dose at bedtime initially; then ↑ to 5 mg/kg twice daily on Day 2 and 5 mg/kg 3 times daily on Day 3. Titrate to effect up to 8–35 mg/kg/day in 3 divided doses.

Availability (generic available)

Immediate-release capsules: 100 mg, 300 mg, 400 mg. **Immediate-release tablets:** 100 mg, 400 mg, 600 mg, 800 mg. **Extended-release tablets (Horizant):** 300 mg, 600 mg. **Sustained-release tablets (Gralise):** 300 mg, 450 mg, 600 mg, 750 mg, 900 mg. **Oral solution (cool strawberry anise flavor):** 250 mg/5 mL.

NURSING IMPLICATIONS

Assessment

- Monitor closely for notable changes in behavior that could indicate the emergence or worsening of suicidal thoughts or behavior or depression.
- If administered with CNS depressants, including opioids, monitor for respiratory depression and sedation. Consider starting gabapentin at a low dose.
- Monitor for signs and symptoms of rhabdomyolysis (malaise, myalgia, muscle cramps or weakness, dark or tea-colored urine).
- **Seizures:** Assess location, duration, and characteristics of seizure activity. Institute seizure precautions as indicated.
- **Postherpetic Neuralgia and Neuropathic Pain:** Assess location, characteristics, and intensity of pain periodically during therapy.
- **Migraine Prophylaxis:** Monitor frequency and intensity of pain on pain scale.
- **Restless Leg Syndrome:** Assess frequency and intensity of restless leg syndrome prior to and periodically during therapy.

Lab Test Considerations

- May cause false-positive readings when testing for urinary protein with *Ames N-Multistix SG* dipstick test; use sulfosalicylic acid precipitation procedure.
- May cause leukopenia.

Implementation

- Do not confuse gabapentin with gemfibrozil. Do not confuse Neurontin with Motrin.
- Doses of *Gralise* and *Horizant* are not interchangeable with other dose forms of gabapentin.
- **PO:** May be administered without regard to meals.
- 600-mg and 800-mg tablets are scored and can be broken to administer a half-tablet. If half-tablet is used, administer other half at the next dose. Discard half-tablets not used within 28 days.
- Immediate-release capsules may be opened and mixed with 4 ounces of applesauce, 120 mL of orange juice, or 4 ounces of fat-free chocolate pudding.
- Administer *Gralise* with evening meal. ***DNC:*** Swallow tablet whole; do not crush, break, or chew.
- Administer *Horizant for Restless Leg Syndrome* with evening meal at 5 pm. *Horizant for Postherpetic Neuralgia* is administered twice daily. ***DNC:*** Swallow tablet whole; do not crush, break, or chew.
- Discontinue gabapentin gradually over ≥1 wk. If dose is 600 mg/day, may discontinue without tapering. If >600 mg/day, titrate daily to 600 mg for 1 wk; then discontinue. If patient is taking

600 mg twice daily, taper to once daily before discontinuing. Abrupt discontinuation may cause ↑ in seizure frequency.

Patient/Family Teaching

- Explain the purpose and side effects. Instruct patient to take medication exactly as directed. Patients on 3-times-daily dosing should not exceed 12 hr between doses. Take missed doses as soon as possible; if <2 hr until next dose, take dose immediately and take next dose 1–2 hr later; then resume regular dosing schedule. Do not double dose. Do not discontinue abruptly; may cause ↑ in frequency of seizures. Advise patient to read *Patient Information* before starting and with each Rx refill in case of changes.
- Advise patient not to take gabapentin within 2 hr of an antacid.
- Gabapentin may cause dizziness and drowsiness. Caution patient to avoid driving or activities requiring alertness until response to medication is known. Patients with seizure should not resume driving until health care provider gives clearance based on control of seizure disorder.
- Instruct patient to notify health care provider of all Rx or OTC medications, vitamins, or herbal products being taken and consult health care provider before taking any new medications.
- Caution patients about risk of respiratory depression when taken with CNS depressants, including opioids and alcohol, or in patients with underlying respiratory impairment. Teach patients how to recognize respiratory depression and advise them to seek medical attention immediately if it occurs.
- Advise patient and family to notify health care provider if thoughts about suicide or dying, attempts to commit suicide, new or worse depression, new or worse anxiety, feeling very agitated or restless, panic attacks, trouble sleeping, new or worse irritability, acting aggressive, being angry or violent, acting on dangerous impulses, an extreme ↑ in activity and talking, or other unusual changes in behavior or mood occur.
- Instruct patient to notify health care provider of medication regimen before treatment or surgery.
- Medical ID describing disease process and medication regimen should be worn at all times in case of emergencies.
- Rep: Advise women of reproductive potential to notify health care provider if pregnancy is planned or suspected or if breastfeeding. Encourage patients who become pregnant to enroll in the North American Antiepileptic Drug Pregnancy Registry by calling 1-888-233-2334 or on the web at www.aedpregnancyregistry.org.

Evaluation/Desired Outcomes

- Decreased frequency of or cessation of seizures.
- Decreased postherpetic neuralgia pain.
- Decreased intensity of neuropathic pain.
- Decreased frequency of migraine headaches.
- Decreased effects of restless leg syndrome.

G

galantamine
(ga-**lant**-a-meen)

~~Razadyne, Razadyne ER~~

Classification
Therapeutic: anti-Alzheimer's agents
Pharmacologic: cholinergics (cholinesterase inhibitors)

Indications

Mild to moderate dementia/neurocognitive disorder of the Alzheimer type.

Action

Enhances cholinergic function by reversible inhibition of cholinesterase. **Therapeutic Effects:** Decreased dementia/cognitive decline (temporary) associated with Alzheimer disease. Cognitive enhancer.

Pharmacokinetics

Absorption: Well absorbed (90%) following oral administration.
Distribution: Unknown.
Metabolism and Excretion: Primarily metabolized by the liver via the CYP2D6 and CYP3A4 isoenzymes; the CYP2D6 enzyme system exhibits genetic polymorphism; ~7% of population may be poor metabolizers and may have significantly ↑ galantamine concentrations and an ↑ risk of adverse effects. 20% excreted unchanged in urine.
Half-life: 7 hr.

TIME/ACTION PROFILE (anticholinesterase activity)

ROUTE	ONSET	PEAK	DURATION
PO	unknown	1 hr	12 hr
PO-ER	unknown	1 hr	24 hr

Contraindications/Precautions

Contraindicated in: Hypersensitivity; Severe renal impairment; Severe hepatic impairment.
Use Cautiously in: Supraventricular cardiac conduction defects or concurrent use of drugs that may slow heart rate (↑ risk of bradycardia); History of ulcer disease/GI bleeding/concurrent NSAID use;

Severe asthma or obstructive pulmonary disease; Mild to moderate renal impairment; Mild to moderate hepatic impairment (cautious dose titration recommended); OB: Safety not established in pregnancy; Lactation: Use while breastfeeding only if potential maternal benefit justifies potential risk to infant; Pedi: Safety and effectiveness not established in children.

Adverse Reactions/Side Effects

CV: bradycardia, chest pain. **Derm:** ACUTE GENERALIZED EXANTHEMATOUS PUSTULOSIS, STEVENS-JOHNSON SYNDROME. **GI:** nausea, vomiting, anorexia, diarrhea, dyspepsia, flatulence. **GU:** bladder outflow obstruction, incontinence. **Metab:** weight loss. **Neuro:** dizziness, extrapyramidal symptoms, fatigue, headache, syncope, tremor.

Interactions

Drug-Drug: ↑ neuromuscular blockade from **succinylcholine-type neuromuscular blocking agents.** May ↑ effects of other **cholinesterase inhibitors** or other **cholinergic agonists**, including **bethanechol**. May ↓ effectiveness of **anticholinergic medications**. **Ketoconazole**, **paroxetine**, **amitriptyline**, **fluvoxamine**, or **quinidine** may ↑ levels and risk of toxicity.

Route/Dosage

PO (Adults): *Immediate-release tablets:* 4 mg twice daily initially; may ↑ dose in increments of 4 mg at 4 wk intervals, up to 12 mg twice daily. Doses up to 16 mg twice daily have been used (range 16–32 mg/day); *Extended-release capsules:* 8 mg once daily in the morning; may ↑ to 16 mg once daily in the morning after 4 wk, then up to 24 mg once daily in the morning after 4 wk.

Renal Impairment

PO (Adults): *Moderate renal impairment:* Not to exceed 16 mg/day.

Hepatic Impairment

PO (Adults): *Moderate hepatic impairment:* Not to exceed 16 mg/day.

Availability (generic available)

Immediate-release tablets: 4 mg, 8 mg, 12 mg. **Extended-release capsules:** 8 mg, 16 mg, 24 mg. **Oral solution:** 4 mg/mL.

NURSING IMPLICATIONS

Assessment

- Assess cognitive function at baseline and periodically during therapy.
- Assess for seizure activity at baseline and throughout therapy.
- Monitor HR periodically during therapy for bradycardia and heart block.
- Monitor respiratory function (reactive airway or obstructive disease) during therapy.

Implementation

- Patient should be maintained on a stable dose for ≥4 wk prior to ↑ dose.
- For dose interruption ≥3 days, restart at lowest dose and titrate up to current dose.
- **PO:** Administer without regard to food. Administration with food, an antiemetic, and adequate fluid intake may ↓ nausea and vomiting. Do not take with alcohol. ***DNC:*** Swallow whole; do not split, open, crush, or chew.
- *For oral solution,* use measuring device that comes with drug. Mix dose with 3–4 ounces (100 mL) liquid. Stir well and drink right away. Do not store for future use.

Patient/Family Teaching

- Explain purpose and side effects of medication. Advise patient and caregiver to read *Patient Information* before starting therapy.
- Emphasize the importance of taking galantamine daily. Instruct patient and caregiver to review *Oral Solution Instruction Sheet* as indicated. Omit missed dose and return to regular schedule; do not double doses. If doses missed for >3 days, restart at lowest dose. Do not discontinue abruptly.
- Caution patient and caregiver that galantamine may cause dizziness. Monitor and assist with ambulation and caution patient to avoid driving and other activities requiring alertness until response to medication is known.
- Instruct patient to maintain adequate fluid intake during therapy.
- Advise patient and caregiver to stop taking galantamine and notify health care provider immediately if rash occurs.
- Advise patient and caregiver to monitor weight during therapy and notify health care provider if nausea, vomiting, or diarrhea persists >7 days or if weight loss or signs of GI bleeding occur.
- Advise patient to notify health care provider of all Rx or OTC medications, vitamins, or herbal products being taken and to consult health care provider before taking other medications.
- Inform patient and caregiver that effects of anesthesia may be blocked while using galantamine; notify health care provider prior to surgery.
- Inform patient and caregiver that improvements in cognitive functioning may take weeks to months.
- Rep: Advise women of reproductive potential to notify health care provider if pregnancy is planned or suspected or if breastfeeding.
- Emphasize the importance of follow-up exams to monitor progress.

Evaluation/Desired Outcomes

- Improvement in cognitive function in patients with Alzheimer disease.

galcanezumab
(gal-ka-nez-ue-mab)

Emgality

Classification

Therapeutic: vascular headache suppressants

Pharmacologic: monoclonal antibodies, calcitonin gene related peptide receptor antagonists

Indications
Migraine prevention. Treatment of episodic cluster headaches.

Action
Monoclonal antibody that binds to the calcitonin gene-related peptide (CGRP) receptor, which reduces the neuroinflammatory and vasodilatory effects of CGRP. **Therapeutic Effects:** Reduction in frequency of migraines and cluster headaches.

Pharmacokinetics
Absorption: Unknown.
Distribution: Some tissue distribution.
Metabolism and Excretion: Degraded into small peptides and amino acids via catabolic pathways.
Half-life: 27 days.

TIME/ACTION PROFILE (plasma concentrations)

ROUTE	ONSET	PEAK	DURATION
SUBQ	unknown	5 days	1 mo

Contraindications/Precautions
Contraindicated in: Hypersensitivity.
Use Cautiously in: OB: Safety not established in pregnancy; Lactation: Use while breastfeeding only if potential maternal benefit justifies potential risk to infant; Pedi: Safety and effectiveness not established in children.

Adverse Reactions/Side Effects
Local: injection site reactions. **Misc:** HYPERSENSITIVITY REACTIONS (INCLUDING ANAPHYLAXIS AND ANGIOEDEMA).

Interactions
Drug-Drug: None reported.

Route/Dosage
Migraine Prevention
SUBQ (Adults): 240 mg once initially as loading dose, then 120 mg once monthly.

Episodic Cluster Headache
SUBQ (Adults): 300 mg once at the onset of the cluster period, then 300 mg once monthly until the end of the cluster period.

Availability
Solution for injection (prefilled pens and prefilled syringes): 100 mg/mL, 120 mg/mL.

NURSING IMPLICATIONS
Assessment
- Assess frequency and intensity of migraines and cluster headaches at baseline and during therapy.
- Monitor for signs and symptoms of hypersensitivity reaction including anaphylaxis (rash, urticaria, dyspnea, angioedema) during therapy. *If severe reaction occurs,* discontinue galcanezumab and treat as indicated.

Implementation
- **SUBQ**: Bring prefilled pen or syringe to room temperature for ≥30 min; protect from direct sunlight. Do not shake. Solution is clear to opalescent, colorless to light yellow; do not administer if discolored, cloudy, or contains particulates. Do not freeze. May be stored in original carton to protect from light for ≤7 days at room temperature; do not re-refrigerate.
- Inject entire contents SUBQ into abdomen, thigh, or upper arm. Do not inject into areas where skin is tender, bruised, red, or hard.
- Loading doses require multiple SUBQ injections to attain appropriate dose.

Patient/Family Teaching
- Explain purpose and side effects of medication. Advise patient to read *Patient Information* before starting therapy.
- Instruct patient on correct technique for preparation, SUBQ injection and disposal of equipment.
- Instruct patient to notify health care provider immediately if signs and symptoms of hypersensitivity reaction (itching; rash; hives; swelling of face, mouth, tongue, or throat; trouble breathing) occur.
- Advise patient to notify health care provider of all Rx or OTC medications, vitamins, or herbal products being taken and to consult with health care provider before taking other medications.
- Rep: Advise women of reproductive potential to notify health care provider if pregnancy is planned or suspected or if breastfeeding. Inform patient of pregnancy exposure registry. Health care providers or the pregnant patient may enroll by calling 1-833-464-4724 or visiting www.migrainepregnancyregistry.com.

Evaluation/Desired Outcomes
- Reduction in frequency of migraines and cluster headaches.

G

ganciclovir (gan-sye-kloe-vir)

Cytovene

Classification
Therapeutic: antivirals

Indications
Treatment of cytomegalovirus (CMV) retinitis in immunocompromised patients, including patients with HIV (may be used in combination with foscarnet). Prevention of CMV infection in transplant patients at risk. Congenital CMV infection in neonates.

Action
CMV converts ganciclovir to its active form (ganciclovir phosphate) inside the host cell, where it inhibits viral DNA polymerase. **Therapeutic Effects:** Antiviral effect directed preferentially against CMV-infected cells.

Pharmacokinetics
Absorption: IV administration results in complete bioavailability.
Distribution: Widely distributed; enters CSF.
Protein Binding: 1–2%.
Metabolism and Excretion: 90% excreted unchanged by the kidneys.
Half-life: *Adults:* 2.9 hr; *Children 9 mo–12 yr:* 2.4 ±0.7 hr; *Neonates:* 2.4 hr (↑ in renal impairment).

TIME/ACTION PROFILE (antiviral levels)

ROUTE	ONSET	PEAK	DURATION
IV	rapid	end of infusion	12–24 hr

Contraindications/Precautions
Contraindicated in: Hypersensitivity to ganciclovir or acyclovir; Bone marrow depression or immunosuppression or thrombocytopenia (do not administer if absolute neutrophil count [ANC] <500/mm^3, hemoglobin <8 g/dL, or platelet count <25,000/mm^3); OB: Ganciclovir is not the preferred systemic therapy during pregnancy; Lactation: Lactation.
Use Cautiously in: Renal impairment (dose ↓ required if CCr <80 mL/min); Rep: Women of reproductive potential and men with female partners of reproductive potential; Geri: Dose ↓ recommended in older adults.

Adverse Reactions/Side Effects
CV: arrhythmias, edema, hypertension, hypotension. **Derm:** alopecia, photosensitivity, pruritus, rash, urticaria. **Endo:** hypoglycemia. **GI:** ↑ liver enzymes, abdominal pain, GI BLEEDING, nausea, vomiting. **GU:** ↓ fertility, gonadal suppression, hematuria, renal impairment. **Hemat:** NEUTROPENIA, THROMBOCYTOPENIA, ANEMIA, eosinophilia. **Local:** pain/phlebitis at IV site. **Neuro:** abnormal dreams, ataxia, confusion, dizziness, drowsiness, headache, malaise, nervousness, SEIZURES, tremor. **Resp:** dyspnea. **Misc:** fever.

Interactions
Drug-Drug: Toxicity may be ↑ by **probenecid**. ↑ risk of seizures with **imipenem/cilastatin**; concurrent use not recommended. Concurrent use of **cyclosporine** or **amphotericin B** ↑ risk of nephrotoxicity. ↑ risk of nephrotoxicity and hematological toxicity with **mycophenolate mofetil**. Concurrent use with **dapsone**, **doxorubicin**, **flucytosine**, **hydroxyurea**, **pentamidine**, **tacrolimus**, **trimethoprim/sulfamethoxazole**, **vinblastine**, **vincristine**, or **zidovudine** ↑ risk of nephrotoxicity and myelosuppression.

Route/Dosage
IV (Adults and Children >3 mo): *Induction:* 5 mg/kg every 12 hr for 14–21 days. *Maintenance regimen:* 5 mg/kg/day or 6 mg/kg for 5 days of each wk. If progression occurs, ↑ to every 12 hr regimen. *Prevention:* 5 mg/kg every 12 hr for 7–14 days; then 5 mg/kg/day or 6 mg/kg for 5 days of each wk.
IV (Neonates): *Congenital CMV infection:* 12 mg/kg/day divided every 12 hr for 6 wk.

Renal Impairment
IV (Adults and Children): *Induction:* CCr 50–69 mL/min: 2.5 mg/kg/dose every 12 hr; CCr 25–49 mL/min: 2.5 mg/kg/dose every 24 hr; CCr 10–24 mL/min: 1.25 mg/kg/dose every 24 hr; CCr <10 mL/min: 1.25 mg/kg 3 times/wk after hemodialysis. *Maintenance:* CCr 50–69 mL/min: 2.5 mg/kg/dose every 24 hr; CCr 25–49 mL/min: 1.25 mg/kg/dose every 24 hr; CCr 10–24 mL/min: 0.625 mg/kg/dose every 24 hr; CCr <10 mL/min: 0.625 mg/kg 3 times/wk after hemodialysis.

Availability (generic available)
Lyophilized powder for injection: 500 mg/vial. **Solution for injection:** 50 mg/mL. **Premixed infusion:** 500 mg/250 mL.

NURSING IMPLICATIONS

Assessment
- Diagnosis of CMV retinitis should be determined by ophthalmoscopy before treatment with ganciclovir. Visual acuity and measurement of intraocular pressure can be done when appropriate. Follow-up ophthalmoscopy should be conducted at the end of induction (or reinduction) therapy and on a monthly basis thereafter; monthly fundus photographs can help identify early relapse. For patients who achieve immune recovery, the frequency of ophthalmic examinations may be ↓ to every 3 mo.
- Culture for CMV (urine, blood, throat) may be taken before administration, but a negative CMV culture does not rule out CMV retinitis. If symptoms

do not respond after several weeks, resistance to ganciclovir may have occurred.

- Assess for signs of infection (fever, chills, cough, hoarseness, lower back or side pain, sore throat, difficult or painful urination). Notify health care provider if these symptoms occur.
- Assess for bleeding (bleeding gums; bruising; petechiae; guaiac stools, urine, and emesis). Avoid IM injections and taking rectal temperatures. Apply pressure to venipuncture sites for 10 min.

Lab Test Considerations

- Verify negative pregnancy test prior to starting therapy.
- Monitor CBC with differential at least every 2 days during twice daily therapy and weekly thereafter. Granulocytopenia usually occurs during the first 2 wk of treatment but may occur anytime during therapy. Recovery begins within 3–7 days of discontinuation of therapy.
- Monitor renal function (BUN and serum creatinine) twice weekly during induction therapy and then at least once weekly throughout therapy.
- Monitor liver function tests (AST, ALT, serum bilirubin, alkaline phosphatase) periodically during therapy. May ↑ levels.
- Monitor serum electrolytes twice weekly during induction therapy and then at least once weekly throughout therapy.
- May ↓ blood glucose.

Implementation

- Do not administer SUBQ or IM; severe tissue irritation may result.
- **IV:** Observe infusion site for phlebitis. Rotate infusion site to prevent phlebitis.
- Maintain adequate hydration throughout therapy.

IV Administration

- Because ganciclovir is considered to be carcinogenic, it should be handled and disposed of based on guidelines issued for antineoplastic drugs. Use double gloves and a protective gown to prepare and administer. If possible, prepare in a biologic safety cabinet or a compounding aseptic containment isolator; eye, face, and respiratory protection may be needed. Prepare and administer in a closed-system drug transfer device. During administration, if there is a potential that the substance could splash or if the patient may resist, use eye and face protection. Discard IV equipment in specially designated containers.
- **Intermittent Infusion: Reconstitution:** Reconstitute each vial with 10 mL of sterile water for injection. Do not reconstitute with bacteriostatic water with parabens; precipitation will occur. Shake well to dissolve completely. Discard vial if particulate matter or discoloration occurs. Reconstituted solution is stable for 12 hr at room temperature; do not refrigerate. **Concentration:** 50 mg/mL
- **Dilution:** Dilute reconstituted solution or solution for injection in 100 mL of D5W, 0.9% NaCl, LR. Once diluted for infusion, solution should be used within 24 hr. Refrigerate but do not freeze. **Concentration:** 10 mg/mL. **Rate:** Administer slowly, via infusion pump, over 1 hr using an in-line filter. Rapid administration may ↑ risk of toxicity.
- **Y-Site Compatibility:** alemtuzumab, allopurinol, anidulafungin, argatroban, arsenic trioxide, atropine, azithromycin, bivalirudin, bleomycin, calcium chloride, calcium gluconate, carboplatin, carmustine, caspofungin, cisplatin, cyanocobalamin, cyclophosphamide, cyclosporine, dactinomycin, daptomycin, defibrotide, dexamethasone, dexmedetomidine, digoxin, docetaxel, doxorubicin liposomal, enalaprilat, epoetin alfa, eptifibatide, ertapenem, etoposide, etoposide phosphate, fentanyl, filgrastim, fluconazole, fluorouracil, folic acid, fosphenytoin, furosemide, glycopyrrolate, granisetron, heparin, hetastarch, hydromorphone, ifosfamide, indomethacin, insulin, regular, labetalol, LR, letermovir, leucovorin, linezolid, lorazepam, mannitol, melphalan, methotrexate, metoprolol, milrinone, mitoxantrone, nafcillin, naloxone, nitroglycerin, nitroprusside, octreotide, oxytocin, paclitaxel, pamidronate, pantoprazole, pemetrexed, pentobarbital, phenobarbital, phytonadione, potassium chloride, propranolol, protamine, remifentanil, rituximab, rocuronium, sodium acetate, sufentanil, thiotepa, tigecycline, tirofiban, trastuzumab, vasopressin, vinblastine, vincristine, voriconazole, zoledronic acid.
- **Y-Site Incompatibility:** aldesleukin, amikacin, aminocaproic acid, aminophylline, amiodarone, amphotericin B deoxycholate, ampicillin, ampicillin/sulbactam, ascorbic acid, atracurium, azathioprine, aztreonam, benztropine, bumetanide, butorphanol, cefazolin, cefepime, cefotaxime, cefotetan, cefoxitin, ceftazidime, ceftriaxone, cefuroxime, chloramphenicol, chlorpromazine, clindamycin, cytarabine, dacarbazine, dantrolene, daunorubicin, dexrazoxane, diazepam, diazoxide, diltiazem, diphenhydramine, dobutamine, dopamine, doxorubicin hydrochloride, doxycycline, ephedrine, epinephrine, epirubicin, erythromycin, esmolol, famotidine, fludarabine, foscarnet, gemcitabine,

G

gemtuzumab ozogamicin, gentamicin, haloperidol, hydralazine, hydrocortisone, idarubicin, imipenem/cilastatin, irinotecan, isoproterenol, ketorolac, levofloxacin, lidocaine, magnesium sulfate, meperidine, mesna, methadone, methylprednisolone, metoclopramide, metronidazole, midazolam, minocycline, mitomycin, morphine, multivitamins, mycophenolate, nalbuphine, nicardipine, norepinephrine, ondansetron, oxacillin, palonosetron, papaverine, penicillin G, pentamidine, phentolamine, phenylephrine, phenytoin, piperacillin/tazobactam, posaconazole, potassium acetate, procainamide, prochlorperazine, promethazine, pyridoxine, sargramostim, sodium bicarbonate, succinylcholine, tacrolimus, theophylline, thiamine, tobramycin, topotecan, trimethoprim/sulfamethoxazole, vancomycin, vecuronium, verapamil, vinorelbine.

Patient/Family Teaching

- Explain the purpose and side effects of ganciclovir. Do not stop receiving drug without consulting health care provider. If an appointment is missed, contact health care provider as soon as possible to reschedule. Advise patient to read *Medication Guide* before starting and periodically during therapy in case of changes.
- Inform patient that ganciclovir is not a cure for CMV retinitis. Progression of retinitis may continue in immunocompromised patients during and after therapy. Advise patients to have regular ophthalmic exams at least every 6 wk. Duration of therapy for CMV prevention is based on the duration and degree of immunosuppression.
- Emphasize the importance of frequent follow-up exams to monitor blood counts.
- Advise patient to notify health care provider if fever; chills; sore throat; other signs of infection; bleeding gums; bruising; petechiae; or blood in urine, stool, or emesis occurs. Caution patient to avoid crowds and persons with known infections. Instruct patient to use soft toothbrush and electric razor. Patient should be cautioned not to drink alcoholic beverages or take products containing aspirin or NSAIDs.
- Caution patient to use sunscreen and protective clothing to prevent photosensitivity reactions.
- Advise patient to notify health care provider of all Rx or OTC medications, vitamins, or herbal products being taken and to consult with health care provider before taking other medications.
- Rep: May cause fetal harm. Advise women of reproductive potential to use a nonhormonal method of contraception during therapy and for ≥30 days after last dose and to avoid breastfeeding during therapy. Advise men to use condoms during and for ≥90 days after therapy. May ↓ fertility.

Evaluation/Desired Outcomes

- Treatment of the symptoms of CMV retinitis in immunocompromised patients.
- Prevention of CMV retinitis in transplant patients at risk.

HIGH ALERT

gemcitabine (jem-site-a-been)

Avgemsi, ~~Gemzar~~

Classification

Therapeutic: antineoplastics

Pharmacologic: antimetabolites, nucleoside analogues

Indications

Pancreatic cancer (locally advanced or metastatic). Inoperable locally advanced/metastatic non-small cell lung cancer (with cisplatin). Metastatic breast cancer after failure of prior anthracycline-containing adjuvant chemotherapy (unless anthracycline therapy contraindicated) (with paclitaxel). Advanced ovarian cancer that has relapsed 6 mo after completion of platinum-based therapy (with carboplatin).

Action

Interferes with DNA synthesis (cell-cycle phase-specific). **Therapeutic Effects:** Death of rapidly replicating cells, particularly malignant ones.

Pharmacokinetics

Absorption: IV administration results in complete bioavailability.

Distribution: Unknown.

Metabolism and Excretion: Converted in cells to active diphosphate and triphosphate metabolites; these are excreted primarily by the kidneys.

Half-life: 32–94 min.

TIME/ACTION PROFILE (effect on blood counts)

ROUTE	ONSET	PEAK	DURATION
IV	unknown	unknown	unknown

Contraindications/Precautions

Contraindicated in: Hypersensitivity; OB: Pregnancy (may cause fetal harm); Lactation: Lactation.

Use Cautiously in: History of cardiovascular disease; Renal impairment; Hepatic impairment; Rep: Women of reproductive potential and men with female partners of reproductive potential; Pedi: Safety and effectiveness not established in children.

Adverse Reactions/Side Effects

CV: edema, ARRHYTHMIAS, CAPILLARY LEAK SYNDROME, CEREBROVASCULAR ACCIDENT, hypertension, MI. **Derm:** alopecia, ACUTE GENERALIZED EXANTHEMATOUS PUSTULOSIS, DRUG REACTION WITH EOSINOPHILIA AND SYSTEMIC

SYMPTOMS (DRESS), rash, STEVENS-JOHNSON SYNDROME (SJS), TOXIC EPIDERMAL NECROLYSIS (TEN). **GI:** ↑ liver enzymes, diarrhea, nausea, stomatitis, vomiting, HEPATOTOXICITY. **GU:** hematuria, proteinuria, ↓ fertility (men), HEMOLYTIC UREMIC SYNDROME, renal failure, thrombotic microangiopathy. **Hemat:** anemia, leukopenia, thrombocytopenia, thrombotic microangiopathy. **Local:** injection site reactions. **Neuro:** paresthesias, POSTERIOR REVERSIBLE ENCEPHALOPATHY SYNDROME (PRES). **Resp:** dyspnea, ADULT RESPIRATORY DISTRESS SYNDROME, bronchospasm, pulmonary edema, PULMONARY FIBROSIS. **Misc:** flu-like symptoms, anaphylactoid reactions, fever.

Interactions

Drug-Drug: ↑ bone marrow depression with other **antineoplastics** or **radiation therapy**. May ↓ antibody response to **live-virus vaccines** and ↑ risk of adverse reactions.

Route/Dosage

Pancreatic Cancer

IV (Adults): 1000 mg/m² once weekly for 7 wk, followed by a week of rest, and then 1000 mg/m² on Days 1, 8, and 15 of each 28-day cycle.

Non-Small Cell Lung Cancer

IV (Adults): 1000 mg/m² on Days 1, 8, and 15 of each 28-day cycle (cisplatin is also given on day 1) *or* 1250 mg/m² on Days 1 and 8 of each 21-day cycle (cisplatin is also given on Day 1).

Breast Cancer

IV (Adults): 1250 mg/m² on Days 1 and 8 of each 21-day cycle (paclitaxel is also given on Day 1).

Ovarian Cancer

IV (Adults): 1000 mg/m² on Days 1 and 8 of each 21-day cycle (carboplatin is also given on Day 1).

Availability (generic available)

Powder for injection: 200 mg/vial, 1 g/vial, 2 g/vial. **Solution for injection:** 200 mg/5.26 mL, 1 g/26.3 mL, 2 g/52.6 mL, 100 mg/mL.

NURSING IMPLICATIONS

Assessment

- Monitor vital signs before and frequently during therapy.
- Monitor for bone marrow depression. Assess for bleeding (bleeding gums; bruising; petechiae; guaiac stools, urine, and emesis) and avoid IM injections and taking rectal temperatures if platelet count is low. Apply pressure to venipuncture sites for 10 min. Assess for signs of infection during neutropenia. Anemia may occur. Monitor for ↑ fatigue, dyspnea, and orthostatic hypotension.
- Monitor intake and output, appetite, and nutritional intake. Mild to moderate nausea and vomiting occur frequently. Antiemetics may be used prophylactically.
- Assess for signs/symptoms of capillary leak syndrome (severe hypotension, hypoalbuminemia, hemoconcentration). *If capillary leak syndrome symptoms occur,* discontinue gemcitabine.
- Monitor respiratory status during therapy. *If unexplained dyspnea or other evidence of severe pulmonary toxicity occurs,* discontinue gemcitabine. May occur up to 2 wk after last dose.
- Monitor for signs/symptoms of PRES (headache, seizure, lethargy, hypertension, confusion, blindness, other visual and neurologic disturbances) during therapy. Confirm diagnosis of PRES with MRI. *If PRES occurs,* discontinue gemcitabine.
- Monitor for signs/symptoms of exanthematous pustulosis (itching; burning; fever; nonfollicular pustular rash on a red base in the armpits, groin, behind the knees, on the inner elbows, or on the face that spreads to other areas), which can occur within 1–2 days of taking the medication but can take up to 2 wk. *If exanthematous pustulosis occurs,* discontinue gemcitabine.
- Monitor for signs/symptoms of severe cutaneous adverse reactions (prodrome of fever, flu-like symptoms, mucosal lesions, progressive skin rash, lymphadenopathy), including DRESS, SJS, and TEN. *If severe cutaneous adverse reaction suspected,* hold gemcitabine until etiology is determined. *If severe cutaneous adverse reaction confirmed,* permanently discontinue gemcitabine.

Lab Test Considerations

- Verify negative pregnancy test before starting therapy. Monitor CBC with differential before each dose. ***For single-agent use:*** *If ANC >1000 cells/mm³ and platelets >100,000 cells/mm³,* administer full dose. *If ANC 500–999 cells/mm³ or platelets 50,000–99,000 cells/mm³,* administer 75% of dose. *If ANC <500 cells/mm³ or platelets <50,000 cells/mm³,* hold gemcitabine. ***For gemcitabine with paclitaxel (breast cancer):*** *If ANC >1200 cells/mm³ and platelets >75,000 cells/mm³,* administer full dose. *If ANC 1000–1199 cells/mm³ or platelets 50,000–75,000 cells/mm³,* administer 75% of dose. *If ANC 700–999 cells/mm³ or platelets ≥50,000 cells/mm³,* administer 50% of dose. *If ANC <700 cells/mm³ or platelets <50,000 cells/mm³,* hold gemcitabine. ***For gemcitabine with carboplatin (ovarian cancer):*** *If ANC >1500 cells/mm³ and platelets >100,000 cells/mm³,* administer full dose. *If ANC 1000–1499 cells/mm³ or platelets 75,000–99,000*

G

cells/mm^3, administer 75% of dose. *If ANC <1000 cells/mm*^{3} *or platelets <75,000 cells/mm*^{3}, hold gemcitabine.

- Monitor serum creatinine, potassium, calcium, and magnesium in patients taking cisplatin with gemcitabine.
- Monitor hepatic and renal function before and periodically during therapy. May transiently ↑ in AST, ALT, alkaline phosphatase, and bilirubin concentrations. *If severe hepatic toxicity or hemolytic-uremic syndrome occurs,* discontinue gemcitabine.
- May cause ↑ BUN and serum creatinine, proteinuria, and hematuria.

Implementation

- ***High Alert:*** Fatalities have occurred with incorrect administration of chemotherapeutic agents. Before administering, clarify all ambiguous orders; double-check single, daily, and course-of-therapy dose limits; have 2nd practitioner independently double-check original order, calculations, and infusion pump settings.

IV Administration

- Use double gloves and a protective gown to prepare and administer. Prepare in a biological safety cabinet or a compounding aseptic containment isolator; eye, face, and respiratory protection should be worn while handling IV medication. Prepare compounds in a closed-system drug transfer device. Administer certain dosage forms via a closed-system drug transfer device. During administration, if there is a potential that the substance could splash or if the patient may resist, use eye and face protection. Discard IV equipment in specially designated containers.
- Gemcitabine is an irritant. If extravasation occurs, immediately stop infusion. Leave needle/cannula in place temporarily but do not flush the line. Gently aspirate extravasated solution; then remove needle/cannula. Elevate patient's extremity.
- **Intermittent Infusion: Reconstitution:** Add 5 mL of 0.9% NaCl without preservatives to 200-mg vial, 25 mL of 0.9% NaCl to the 1-g vial, or 50 mL of 0.9% NaCl to the 2-g vial. **Concentration:** 38 mg/mL. Incomplete dissolution may result in concentrations >40 mg/mL. **Dilution:** May be further diluted with 0.9% NaCl. Solution is colorless to light straw color. Do not administer solutions that are discolored or contain particulate matter. Solution is stable for 24 hr at room temperature. Discard unused portions. Do not refrigerate; crystallization may occur. **Rate:** Administer dose over 30 min. If two bags required, infuse total of both bags over 30 min. Infusions >60 min have a greater incidence of toxicity.
- **Y-Site Compatibility:** alemtuzumab, allopurinol, amikacin, aminocaproic acid, aminophylline, amiodarone, ampicillin, ampicillin/sulbactam, anidulafungin, argatroban, atracurium, azithromycin, aztreonam, bivalirudin, bleomycin, bumetanide, buprenorphine, butorphanol, calcium acetate, calcium chloride, calcium gluconate, carboplatin, carmustine, caspofungin, cefazolin, cefotetan, cefoxitin, ceftazidime, ceftriaxone, cefuroxime, chlorpromazine, ciprofloxacin, cisatracurium, cisplatin, clindamycin, cyclophosphamide, cyclosporine, cytarabine, dacarbazine, dactinomycin, dexamethasone, dexmedetomidine, dexrazoxane, digoxin, diltiazem, diphenhydramine, dobutamine, docetaxel, dopamine, doxorubicin hydrochloride, doxycycline, droperidol, enalaprilat, ephedrine, epinephrine, epirubicin, ertapenem, erythromycin, esmolol, etoposide, etoposide phosphate, famotidine, fentanyl, fluconazole, fludarabine, fluorouracil, foscarnet, fosphenytoin, gemtuzumab ozogamicin, gentamicin, glycopyrrolate, granisetron, haloperidol, heparin, hydralazine, hydrocortisone, hydromorphone, idarubicin, ifosfamide, insulin, regular, isoproterenol, labetalol, leucovorin, levofloxacin, lidocaine, linezolid, lorazepam, magnesium sulfate, mannitol, meperidine, meropenem, mesna, methadone, metoclopramide, metoprolol, metronidazole, midazolam, milrinone, mitoxantrone, morphine, moxifloxacin, nalbuphine, naloxone, nicardipine, nitroglycerin, nitroprusside, norepinephrine, octreotide, ondansetron, oxaliplatin, paclitaxel, paclitaxel protein-bound, palonosetron, pamidronate, pentamidine, pentobarbital, phenobarbital, phentolamine, potassium acetate, potassium chloride, potassium phosphates, procainamide, promethazine, propranolol, remifentanil, rituximab, rocuronium, sodium acetate, sodium bicarbonate, sodium phosphates, succinylcholine, sufentanil, tacrolimus, theophylline, thiotepa, tigecycline, tirofiban, tobramycin, topotecan, trastuzumab, trimethoprim/sulfamethoxazole, vancomycin, vasopressin, vecuronium, verapamil, vinblastine, vincristine, vinorelbine, voriconazole, zidovudine, zoledronic acid.
- **Y-Site Incompatibility:** acyclovir, amphotericin B liposomal, cefepime, cefotaxime, chloramphenicol, dantrolene, daptomycin, diazepam, doxorubicin liposomal, furosemide, ganciclovir, imipenem-cilastatin, irinotecan, ketorolac, methotrexate, methylprednisolone, mitomycin, nafcillin, pantoprazole, pemetrexed, phenytoin, piperacillin/tazobactam, prochlorperazine.

Patient/Family Teaching

- Explain purpose and side effects of gemcitabine to patient. Do not stop receiving drug without consulting health care provider. If an appointment is missed, contact health care provider as soon as possible to reschedule. Advise patient to read *Medication Guide* before starting and periodically during therapy in case of changes.

- Emphasize the need for periodic lab tests to monitor for side effects.
- Instruct patient to notify health care provider if fever; chills; sore throat; signs of infection; bleeding gums; bruising; petechiae; or blood in urine, stool, or emesis occurs. Caution patient to avoid crowds and persons with known infections. Instruct patient to use soft toothbrush and electric razor. Patient should be cautioned not to drink alcoholic beverages or take products containing aspirin or NSAIDs.
- Instruct patient to inspect oral mucosa for erythema and ulceration. If ulceration occurs, advise patient to use sponge brush and rinse mouth with water after eating and drinking. Stomatitis pain may require management with opioid analgesics.
- Instruct patient to notify health care provider if flu-like symptoms (fever, anorexia, headache, cough, chills, myalgia), swelling of feet or legs, signs and symptoms of pulmonary toxicity (shortness of breath, wheezing, cough), hemolytic-uremic syndrome (changes in color or volume of urine output, ↑ bruising or bleeding), or hepatotoxicity (jaundice, pain/tenderness in right upper abdominal quadrant) occur.
- Instruct patient to notify health care provider if any rash (particularly with fever, flu-like symptoms, swollen lymph nodes) develops within 1–2 wk of starting therapy.
- Discuss with patient the possibility of hair loss. Explore methods of coping.
- Instruct patient not to receive any vaccinations without advice of health care provider.
- Rep: May cause fetal harm. Advise women of reproductive potential to use effective contraception during therapy and for 6 mo after final dose and to avoid breastfeeding during therapy and for ≥1 wk after last dose. Advise men with female partners of reproductive potential to use effective contraception during therapy and for 3 mo after last dose. May cause male infertility.

Evaluation/Desired Outcomes

- Palliative, symptomatic improvement in patients with pancreatic cancer.
- Decrease in size and spread of malignancy in lung, ovarian, and breast cancer.

gentamicin, See AMINOGLYCOSIDES.

gepotidacin (jep-oh-ti-day-sin)

Blujepa

Classification

Therapeutic: anti-infectives

Pharmacologic: triazaacenaphthylenes

Indications

Uncomplicated urinary tract infections in female patients.

Action

Acts as a triazaacenaphthylene antibacterial that inhibits type II topoisomerases including bacterial topoisomerase II (DNA gyrase) and topoisomerase IV, which then inhibits DNA replication. Also acts as a reversible acetylcholinesterase inhibitor. **Therapeutic Effects:** Death of susceptible bacteria with resolution of infection. **Spectrum:** Active against *Escherichia coli*, *Klebsiella pneumoniae*, *Citrobacter freundii*, *Staphylococcus saprophyticus*, and *Enterococcus faecalis*.

Pharmacokinetics

Absorption: IV administration results in complete bioavailability.

Distribution: Widely distributed to tissues.

Metabolism and Excretion: Primarily metabolized by the liver via the CYP3A isoenzyme. 52% excreted in feces (30% as unchanged drug); 31% excreted in urine (20% as unchanged drug).

Half-life: 9 hr.

TIME/ACTION PROFILE (plasma concentrations)

ROUTE	ONSET	PEAK	DURATION
IV	rapid	end of infusion	unknown

Contraindications/Precautions

Contraindicated in: Severe hypersensitivity; QT interval prolongation or pre-existing cardiac disease; Severe renal impairment or end-stage renal disease; Severe hepatic impairment.

Use Cautiously in: OB: Safety not established in pregnancy; Lactation: Safety not established in breastfeeding; Pedi: Children <12 yr and <40 kg (safety and effectiveness not established; Geri: Consider age-related impairment of renal function in older adults.

Adverse Reactions/Side Effects

CV: QT interval prolongation. **GI:** <u>diarrhea</u>, abdominal pain, CLOSTRIDIOIDES DIFFICILE-ASSOCIATED DIARRHEA (CDAD), flatulence, nausea, vomiting. **GU:** vulvovaginal candidiasis. **Neuro:** dizziness, headache. **Misc:** HYPERSENSITIVITY REACTIONS (INCLUDING ANAPHLYAXIS).

Interactions

Drug-Drug: Antiarrhythmics and **QT interval prolonging medications** may ↑ risk of QT interval prolongation; avoid concurrent use. **Strong CYP3A4 inhibitors**, including **itraconazole** or **ketoconazole**, may ↑ levels and risk of QT interval prolongation; avoid concurrent use. **Strong CYP3A4 inducers**, including **rifampin**, may ↓ levels and effectiveness; avoid concurrent use. May ↑ levels and risk of toxicity of **CYP3A4 substrates**, including **cyclosporine**, **midazolam**, or **quinidine**; avoid concurrent use. May ↑ levels and risk of toxicity of **digoxin**; closely monitor digoxin levels. May exaggerate the neuromuscular effects of **succinylcholine**. May ↑ risk of cholinergic adverse effects of other **acetylcholinesterase inhibitors**, including **donepezil**. May antagonize the effects of **anticholinergic drugs**, including **benztropine** or **oxybutynin** and **non-depolarizing neuromuscular blockers**.

Route/Dosage

PO (Adults and Children ≥12 yr and ≥40 kg): 1,500 mg twice daily for 5 days.

Availability

Film-coated tablets: 750 mg.

NURSING IMPLICATIONS

Assessment

- Assess for signs/symptoms of resolving infection (worsening urinary tract infection include fever, dysuria, polyuria, hematuria, flank pain, suprapubic pain or pressure) during therapy.
- Assess cardiac history baseline; avoid use in patients with long QT syndrome or cardiac arrhythmias associated with prolonged QT interval. If administration cannot be avoided in these patients, correct serum electrolyte abnormalities and collect an ECG prior to administration, during treatment, and as clinically indicated.
- Observe for signs and symptoms of anaphylaxis (rash, pruritus, laryngeal edema, wheezing). Have epinephrine, antihistamine, and resuscitative equipment close by. *If hypersensitivity reaction occurs,* immediately discontinue gepotidacin and treat as clinically indicated.
- Monitor for signs/symptoms of excess acetylcholinesterase inhibition including dysarthria, presyncope, muscle spasms, diarrhea, nausea, vomiting, abdominal pain, hypersalivation, and hyperhidrosis, especially if administered with drugs with additive cholinergic effects.
- Monitor for signs/symptoms of CDAD including watery diarrhea with mucus, fever, abdominal pain or cramping, anorexia, nausea, and in severe cases, dehydration, and blood or pus in the stool. May occur >2 mo after therapy. Report promptly to health care provider.

Lab Test Considerations

- Obtain specimen for culture and sensitivity before initiating therapy. First dose may be given before receiving results.
- Monitor serum electrolytes including potassium, calcium, and magnesium in patients with QT interval prolongation.

Implementation

- **PO:** Administer after a meal to ↓ GI intolerance.

Patient/Family Teaching

- Explain purpose and side effects of gepotidacin. Instruct patient to take medication as directed after a meal. If a dose is missed, take it as soon as possible; do not double the dose to make up for the missed dose. Keep out of children's reach. Do not share medication with others, even if they have similar symptoms; may be harmful. Advise patient to read *Patient Information* before starting therapy.
- Warn patient to report symptoms of arrhythmias and QT interval prolongation (fast heart beat, skipped beats, palpitations, dizziness, lightheaded, trouble breathing, faintness).
- Advise the patient to report signs and symptoms of excessive cholinergic symptoms such as dizziness, trouble breathing, sweating a lot, feeling very weak, stomach cramps, nausea, vomiting, diarrhea, or drooling.
- Advise patients and family to call 911 and seek urgent treatment for signs and symptoms of hypersensitivity reactions such as difficulty breathing, chest tightness, hives, rash, feeling lightheaded, itching, swelling of the face, lips, tongue or throat.
- Instruct patient to notify health care professional immediately if diarrhea, abdominal cramping, fever, or bloody stools occur and not to treat with antidiarrheals without consulting health care professionals.
- Advise patient to notify health care professional of all Rx or OTC medications, vitamins, or herbal products being taken and to consult health care professional before taking other medications.
- Rep: Advise women of reproductive potential to notify health care professional if pregnancy is planned or suspected or if breastfeeding. Encourage pregnant patient to enroll in registry that monitors outcomes in women exposed to gepotidacin during pregnancy by calling 1-888-825-5249.

Evaluation/Desired Outcomes

- Death of susceptible bacteria with resolution of infection.
- Resolution of uncomplicated urinary tract infections in female patients.

glecaprevir/pibrentasvir (glek-a-pre-vir/pi-brent-as-vir)

Maviret, Mavyret

Classification

Therapeutic: antivirals

Pharmacologic: NS5A inhibitors protease inhibitors

Indications

Acute or chronic hepatitis C virus (HCV) genotypes 1, 2, 3, 4, 5, or 6 infection without cirrhosis or with compensated cirrhosis. Chronic HCV genotype 1 infection in patients who have previously received treatment with a regimen containing an HCV NS5A inhibitor or an NS3/4A protease inhibitor, but not both.

Action

Glecaprevir: Inhibits the HCV NS3/4A protease, resulting in inhibition of viral replication; *Pibrentasvir:* Inhibits the HCV NS5A protein, resulting in inhibition of viral replication. **Therapeutic Effects:** Decreased levels of HCV with sustained virologic response and lessened sequelae of chronic HCV infection.

Pharmacokinetics

Glecaprevir

Absorption: Well absorbed following oral administration; absorption ↑ by high-fat meal.
Distribution: Unknown.
Protein Binding: 97.5%.
Metabolism and Excretion: Partially metabolized by the liver via the CYP3A4 isoenzyme; 92% excreted in feces; <1% eliminated in urine.
Half-life: 6 hr.

Pibrentasvir

Absorption: Well absorbed following oral administration.
Distribution: Unknown.
Protein Binding: >99.9%.
Metabolism and Excretion: Not metabolized; 97% excreted in feces.
Half-life: 13 hr.

TIME/ACTION PROFILE (plasma concentrations)

ROUTE	ONSET	PEAK	DURATION
glecaprevir (PO)	unknown	5 hr	24 hr
pibrentasvir (PO)	unknown	5 hr	24 hr

Contraindications/Precautions

Contraindicated in: Moderate or severe hepatic impairment or any prior history of hepatic decompensation (↑ risk of hepatic decompensation/failure); Concurrent use of atazanavir or rifampin.
Use Cautiously in: Receiving immunosuppressant or chemotherapy medications (↑ risk of hepatitis B virus [HBV] reactivation); OB: Safety not established in pregnancy; Lactation: Safety not established in breastfeeding; Pedi: Children <3 yr (safety and effectiveness not established).

Adverse Reactions/Side Effects

Derm: pruritus. **GI:** diarrhea, HBV REACTIVATION, hyperbilirubinemia, nausea. **Neuro:** fatigue, headache.

Interactions

Drug-Drug: **Atazanavir** may ↑ levels and risk of liver enzyme elevation; concurrent use contraindicated. **Rifampin** may ↓ levels and effectiveness; concurrent use contraindicated. **Strong CYP3A inducers**, including **carbamazepine** or **efavirenz**, may ↓ levels and effectiveness; concurrent use not recommended. **Darunavir**, **lopinavir**, or **ritonavir** may ↑ levels and risk of toxicity; concurrent use not recommended. May ↑ levels and risk of myopathy of **atorvastatin**, **fluvastatin**, **lovastatin**, **pitavastatin**, **pravastatin**, **rosuvastatin**, and **simvastatin**; concurrent use with atorvastatin, lovastatin, and simvastatin not recommended; ↓ dose of pravastatin by 50%; do not exceed rosuvastatin dose of 10 mg/day; use lowest possible dose of fluvastatin or pitavastatin. May ↑ levels and risk of bleeding of **dabigatran**; avoid concurrent use. May ↑ levels and risk of toxicity of **digoxin**; ↓ digoxin dose by 50% when initiating glecaprevir/pibrentasvir therapy. **Ethinyl estradiol-containing oral contraceptives** may ↑ risk of liver enzyme elevation; concurrent use with products containing >20 mcg of ethinyl estradiol not recommended. **Cyclosporine** may ↑ levels and risk of toxicity; concurrent use not recommended if patients require cyclosporine dose >100 mg/day. May cause fluctuations in INR when used with **warfarin**; closely monitor INR. ↑ risk of hypoglycemia with use of certain **antidiabetic agents**.
Drug-Natural Products: St. John's wort may ↓ levels and effectiveness; concurrent use not recommended.

Route/Dosage

PO (Adults and Children ≥12 yr or ≥45 kg): *Genotype 1, 2, 3, 4, 5, or 6: Treatment-naive with no cirrhosis or with compensated cirrhosis:* Three 100-mg/40-mg tablets once daily for 8 wk *or* six 50-mg/20-mg pellet packets once daily for 8 wk; *Genotype 1: Treatment-experienced with NS5A inhibitor (with no cirrhosis or with compensated cirrhosis):* Three 100-mg/40-mg tablets once daily for

16 wk *or* six 50-mg/20-mg pellet packets once daily for 16 wk; *Genotype 1: Treatment-experienced with NS3/4A protease inhibitor (with no cirrhosis or with compensated cirrhosis):* Three 100-mg/40-mg tablets once daily for 12 wk *or* six 50-mg/20-mg pellet packets once daily for 12 wk; *Genotype 1, 2, 4, 5, or 6: Treatment-experienced with regimens containing interferon, pegylated interferon, ribavirin, and/or sofosbuvir (no cirrhosis):* Three 100-mg/40-mg tablets once daily for 8 wk *or* six 50-mg/20-mg pellet packets once daily for 8 wk; *Genotype 1, 2, 4, 5, or 6: Treatment-experienced with regimens containing interferon, pegylated interferon, ribavirin, and/or sofosbuvir (with compensated cirrhosis):* Three 100-mg/40-mg tablets once daily for 12 wk *or* six 50-mg/20-mg pellet packets once daily for 12 wk; *Genotype 3: Treatment-experienced with regimens containing interferon, pegylated interferon, ribavirin, and/or sofosbuvir (with no cirrhosis or with compensated cirrhosis):* Three 100-mg/40-mg tablets once daily for 16 wk *or* six 50-mg/20-mg pellet packets once daily for 16 wk; *Liver or kidney transplant recipients:* Three 100-mg/40-mg tablets once daily for 12 wk (16 wk for those with genotype 1 who are treatment experienced with NS5A inhibitor without prior treatment with an NS3/4A protease inhibitor; 16 wk for those with genotype 3 who are treatment experienced with regimens containing interferon, pegylated interferon, ribavirin, and/or sofosbuvir) *or* six 50-mg/20-mg pellet packets once daily for 12 wk (16 wk for those with genotype 1 who are treatment experienced with NS5A inhibitor without prior treatment with an NS3/4A protease inhibitor; 16 wk for those with genotype 3 who are treatment experienced with regimens containing interferon, pegylated interferon, ribavirin, and/or sofosbuvir).

PO (Children 3–<12 yr and 30–<45 kg): *Genotype 1, 2, 3, 4, 5, or 6: Treatment-naive with no cirrhosis or with compensated cirrhosis:* Five 50-mg/20-mg pellet packets once daily for 8 wk; *Genotype 1: Treatment-experienced with NS5A inhibitor (with no cirrhosis or with compensated cirrhosis):* Five 50-mg/20-mg pellet packets once daily for 16 wk; *Genotype 1: Treatment-experienced with NS3/4A protease inhibitor (with no cirrhosis or with compensated cirrhosis):* Five 50-mg/20-mg pellet packets once daily for 12 wk; *Genotype 1, 2, 4, 5, or 6: Treatment-experienced with regimens containing interferon, pegylated interferon, ribavirin, and/or sofosbuvir (no cirrhosis):* Five 50-mg/20-mg pellet packets once daily for 8 wk; *Genotype 1, 2, 4, 5, or 6: Treatment-experienced with regimens containing interferon, pegylated interferon, ribavirin, and/or sofosbuvir (with compensated cirrhosis):* Five 50-mg/20-mg pellet packets once daily for 12 wk; *Genotype 3: Treatment-experienced with regimens containing interferon, pegylated interferon, ribavirin, and/or sofosbuvir (with no cirrhosis or with compensated cirrhosis):* Five 50-mg/20-mg pellet packets once daily for 16 wk; *Liver or kidney transplant recipients:* Five 50-mg/20-mg pellet packets once daily for 12 wk (16 wk for those with genotype 1 who are treatment experienced with NS5A inhibitor without prior treatment with an NS3/4A protease inhibitor; 16 wk for those with genotype 3 who are treatment experienced with regimens containing interferon, pegylated interferon, ribavirin, and/or sofosbuvir).

PO (Children 3–<12 yr and 20–<30 kg): *Genotype 1, 2, 3, 4, 5, or 6: Treatment-naive with no cirrhosis or with compensated cirrhosis:* Four 50-mg/20-mg pellet packets once daily for 8 wk; *Genotype 1: Treatment-experienced with NS5A inhibitor (with no cirrhosis or with compensated cirrhosis):* Four 50-mg/20-mg pellet packets once daily for 16 wk; *Genotype 1: Treatment-experienced with NS3/4A protease inhibitor (with no cirrhosis or with compensated cirrhosis):* Four 50-mg/20-mg pellet packets once daily for 12 wk; *Genotype 1, 2, 4, 5, or 6: Treatment-experienced with regimens containing interferon, pegylated interferon, ribavirin, and/or sofosbuvir (no cirrhosis):* Four 50-mg/20-mg pellet packets once daily for 8 wk; *Genotype 1, 2, 4, 5, or 6: Treatment-experienced with regimens containing interferon, pegylated interferon, ribavirin, and/or sofosbuvir (with compensated cirrhosis):* Four 50-mg/20-mg pellet packets once daily for 12 wk; *Genotype 3: Treatment-experienced with regimens containing interferon, pegylated interferon, ribavirin, and/or sofosbuvir (with no cirrhosis or with compensated cirrhosis):* Four 50-mg/20-mg pellet packets once daily for 16 wk; *Liver or kidney transplant recipients:* Four 50-mg/20-mg pellet packets once daily for 12 wk (16 wk for those with genotype 1 who are treatment experienced with NS5A inhibitor without prior treatment with an NS3/4A protease inhibitor; 16 wk for those with genotype 3 who are treatment experienced with regimens containing interferon, pegylated interferon, ribavirin, and/or sofosbuvir).

PO (Children 3–<12 yr and <20 kg): *Genotype 1, 2, 3, 4, 5, or 6: Treatment-naive with no cirrhosis or with compensated cirrhosis:* Three 50-mg/20-mg pellet packets once daily for 8 wk; *Genotype 1: Treatment-experienced with NS5A inhibitor (with no cirrhosis or with compensated cirrhosis):* Three 50-mg/20-mg pellet packets once daily for 16 wk; *Genotype 1: Treatment-experienced with NS3/4A protease inhibitor (with no cirrhosis or with compensated cirrhosis):* Three 50-mg/20-mg pellet packets once daily for 12 wk; *Genotype 1, 2, 4, 5, or 6: Treatment-experienced with regimens containing interferon, pegylated interferon, ribavirin, and/*

or sofosbuvir (no cirrhosis): Three 50-mg/20-mg pellet packets once daily for 8 wk; *Genotype 1, 2, 4, 5, or 6: Treatment-experienced with regimens containing interferon, pegylated interferon, ribavirin, and/or sofosbuvir (with compensated cirrhosis):* Three 50-mg/20-mg pellet packets once daily for 12 wk; *Genotype 3: Treatment-experienced with regimens containing interferon, pegylated interferon, ribavirin, and/or sofosbuvir (with no cirrhosis or with compensated cirrhosis):* Three 50-mg/20-mg pellet packets once daily for 16 wk; *Liver or kidney transplant recipients:* Three 50-mg/20-mg pellet packets once daily for 12 wk (16 wk for those with genotype 1 who are treatment experienced with NS5A inhibitor without prior treatment with an NS3/4A protease inhibitor; 16 wk for those with genotype 3 who are treatment experienced with regimens containing interferon, pegylated interferon, ribavirin, and/or sofosbuvir).

Availability

Tablets: glecaprevir 100 mg/pibrentasvir 40 mg. **Oral pellets:** glecaprevir 50 mg/pibrentasvir 20 mg per pkt.

NURSING IMPLICATIONS

Assessment

- Monitor for signs and symptoms of HBV reactivation or hepatitis (jaundice, dark urine, light-colored stools, fatigue, weakness, loss of appetite, nausea, vomiting, stomach pain) during therapy.

Lab Test Considerations

- Assess for current or prior HBV infection before starting HCV therapy; may cause HBV reactivation. Assess hepatitis B surface antigen (HBsAg) and hepatitis core antibody (anti-HBc), and for clinical and laboratory signs of hepatitis flare (↑ AST, ALT, bilirubin, liver failure) or HBV reactivation (rapid ↑ in serum HBV DNA level) during HCV treatment and post-treatment follow-up.
- 🧬 Test patient with HCV genotype 1a infection for presence of virus with NS5A resistance-associated polymorphisms prior to starting therapy to determine dose regimen and duration.

Implementation

- **PO:** Administer once daily with food.
- **Oral Pellets:** Take oral pellets together with food once daily. Oral pellets may also be sprinkled on a small amount of soft food with low water content that will stick to a spoon and should be swallowed without chewing (peanut butter, chocolate hazelnut spread, cream cheese, thick jam, Greek yogurt). Entire mixture of food and oral pellets should be swallowed within 15 min of preparation. ***DNC:*** Do not crush or chew oral pellets. Liquids or foods that would drip or slide off the spoon are not recommended, as the drug may dissolve quickly and become less effective.

Patient/Family Teaching

- Explain purpose and side effects of medication. Advise patient to read *Patient Information* before starting therapy.
- Instruct patient to take missed dose if <18 hr from scheduled time. If >18 hr from usual time of scheduled dose, omit dose and take next dose at usual time. Do not stop medication without consulting health care provider.
- Advise patient to notify health care provider of any history of HBV. May cause reactivation.
- Advise patient to notify health care provider of all Rx or OTC medications, vitamins, or herbal products being taken and to consult health care provider before taking other medications, especially St. John's wort.
- Rep: Advise women of reproductive potential to notify health care provider if pregnancy is planned or suspected or if breastfeeding.

Evaluation/Desired Outcomes

- Decreased levels of HCV with sustained virologic response and lessened sequelae of chronic HCV infection.

glimepiride, See SULFONYLUREAS.

glipiZIDE, See SULFONYLUREAS.

glucagon (gloo-ka-gon)

Baqsimi, ~~GlucaGen~~, Gvoke

Classification

Therapeutic: hormones

Pharmacologic: pancreatics

Indications

Acute management of severe hypoglycemia. Facilitation of radiographic examination of the GI tract. **Unlabeled Use:** Beta blocker overdose. Calcium channel blocker overdose.

Action

Stimulates hepatic production of glucose from glycogen stores (glycogenolysis). Relaxes the musculature of the GI tract (stomach, duodenum, small

bowel, colon), temporarily inhibiting movement. Has positive inotropic and chronotropic effects.
Therapeutic Effects: Increase in blood glucose. Relaxation of GI musculature, facilitating radiographic examination.

Pharmacokinetics

Absorption: Well absorbed following IM, intranasal, and SUBQ administration; IV administration results in complete bioavailability.
Distribution: Extensively distributed to tissues.
Metabolism and Excretion: Extensively metabolized by the liver, plasma, and kidneys.
Half-life: 8–18 min.

TIME/ACTION PROFILE

ROUTE	ONSET	PEAK	DURATION
IM (hyperglycemic action)	within 10 min	30 min	12–27 min
IV (hyperglycemic action)	1 min	5 min	9–17 min
SUBQ (hyperglycemic action)	within 10 min	30–45 min	60–90 min
Intranasal (hyperglycemic action)	within 15 min	unknown	unknown
IV (effect on GI musculature)	45 sec (for 0.25–2-mg dose)	unknown	9–17 min (0.25–0.5-mg dose); 22–25 min (2-mg dose)
IM (effect on GI musculature)	8–10 min (1-mg dose); 4–7 min (2-mg dose)	unknown	9–27 min (1-mg dose); 21–32 min (2-mg dose)

Contraindications/Precautions

Contraindicated in: Hypersensitivity; Pheochromocytoma; Insulinoma.
Use Cautiously in: Prolonged fasting, starvation, adrenal insufficiency, or chronic hypoglycemia (low levels of releasable glucose); OB: Use during pregnancy only if potential maternal benefit justifies potential fetal risk; Lactation: Safety not established in breastfeeding; Pedi: Children <1 yr (safety and effectiveness of nasal powder not established).

Adverse Reactions/Side Effects

CV: hypotension. **Derm:** necrolytic migratory erythema. **EENT:** epistaxis, eye redness, itchy eyes, itchy throat, nasal congestion, nasal discomfort, nasal itching, rhinorrhea, sneezing, watery eyes. **GI:** nausea, vomiting. **Neuro:** headache. **Resp:** cough. **Misc:** HYPERSENSITIVITY REACTIONS (INCLUDING ANAPHYLAXIS).

Interactions

Drug-Drug: Large doses may ↑ the effect of **warfarin**. Negates the response to **insulin** or **oral hypoglycemic agents. Phenytoin** inhibits the stimulant effect of glucagon on insulin release. Hyperglycemic effect is intensified and prolonged by **epinephrine**. Patients on **beta blocker** therapy may have a greater ↑ in HR and BP.

Route/Dosage

Hypoglycemia

IV, IM, SUBQ (Adults and Children >25 kg): 1 mg; may repeat in 15 min if necessary.
SUBQ (Adults and Children ≥12 yr): *Gvoke:* 1 mg; may repeat in 15 min if necessary.
IV, IM, SUBQ (Children <25 kg): 0.5 mg or 0.02–0.03 mg/kg; may repeat in 15 min if necessary.
IV, IM, SUBQ (Children >6 yr and unknown weight): 1 mg; may repeat in 15 min if necessary.
IV, IM, SUBQ (Children <6 yr and unknown weight): 0.5 mg or 0.02–0.03 mg/kg; may repeat in 15 min if necessary.
SUBQ (Children 2–12 yr and ≥45 kg): *Gvoke:* 1 mg; may repeat in 15 min if necessary.
SUBQ (Children 2–12 yr and <45 kg): *Gvoke:* 0.5 mg; may repeat in 15 min if necessary.
Intranasal (Adults and Children ≥1 yr): 3 mg (one actuation) in one nostril; may repeat in 15 min if necessary.

Radiographic Examination of the GI Tract

IV, IM, (Adults): 0.25–2 mg, depending on location and duration of examination (0.5 mg IV or 2 mg IM for relaxation of stomach; for examination of the colon, 2 mg IM 10 min before procedure).

Beta Blocker or Calcium Channel Blocker Overdose

IV (Adults): *Beta blocker overdose:* 50–150 mcg (0.05–0.15 mg)/kg, followed by 1–5 mg/hr infusion. *Calcium channel blocker overdose:* 2 mg; additional doses determined by response.

Availability (generic available)

Nasal powder: 3 mg/device. **Lyophilized powder for injection:** 1 mg/vial. **Solution for SUBQ injection (Gvoke) (prefilled syringes and prefilled autoinjectors):** 0.5 mg/0.1 mL, 1 mg/0.2 mL.

NURSING IMPLICATIONS

Assessment

- Assess for signs of hypoglycemia (sweating, hunger, weakness, headache, dizziness, tremor, irritability, tachycardia, anxiety) before and periodically during therapy.
- Assess for hypersensitivity reactions (anaphylaxis, rash, hives, itching, wheezing, trouble breathing) and implement supportive measures (epinephrine) as indicated.

- Assess neurologic status during therapy. Institute safety precautions to protect patient from injury caused by seizures, falling, or aspiration. For insulin shock therapy, 0.5–1 mg is administered after 1 hr of coma; patient usually awakens in 10–25 min. If no response occurs, repeat the dose. Feed patient supplemental carbohydrates orally to replenish liver glycogen and prevent secondary hypoglycemia as soon as possible after awakening, especially in pediatric patients.
- Assess nutritional status. Patients who lack liver glycogen stores (starvation, chronic hypoglycemia, adrenal insufficiency) will require glucose instead of glucagon.
- Assess for nausea and vomiting after administration of dose. Protect patients with depressed level of consciousness from aspiration by positioning on side; ensure that a suction unit is available. Notify health care provider if vomiting occurs; patient will require parenteral glucose to prevent recurrent hypoglycemia.

Lab Test Considerations

- Monitor serum glucose levels throughout episode, during treatment, and for 3–4 hr after patient regains consciousness. Use of bedside fingerstick blood glucose determination methods is recommended for rapid results. Follow-up lab results may be ordered to validate fingerstick values, but do not delay treatment while awaiting lab results, as this could result in neurologic injury or death.
- Large doses of glucagon may ↓ potassium.

Implementation

- Administer supplemental carbohydrates IV or PO to ↑ serum glucose levels.
- **SUBQ**: *Gvoke* solution is clear and colorless to pale yellow; do not administer if solution is discolored or contains particulate matter. Inject in lower abdomen, outer thigh, or outer upper arm.
- **Intranasal** Administer by inserting tip into one nostril and pressing device plunger all the way in until green line is no longer showing. Dose does not need to be inhaled. Call for emergency assistance immediately after administering dose. When patient responds to treatment, give oral carbohydrates.

IV Administration

- **IV Push: Reconstitution:** Reconstitute each vial with 1 mL of an appropriate diluent. For doses ≤2 mg, use diluent provided by manufacturer. For doses >2 mg, use sterile water for injection instead of diluent supplied by manufacturer to minimize risk of thrombophlebitis, CNS toxicity, and myocardial depression from phenol preservative in diluent supplied by manufacturer. Reconstituted vials should be used immediately. **Concentration:** ≤1 mg/mL. **Rate:** Administer at a rate ≤1 mg/min. May be administered through IV line containing D5W.
- **Continuous Infusion: Reconstitution:** Reconstitute vials as per directions above (use sterile water for injection). **Dilution:** Further dilute 10 mg of glucagon in 100 mL of D5W. **Concentration:** 0.1 mg/mL.
- **Rate:** See Route/Dosage section.
- **Y-Site Compatibility:** naloxone.

Patient/Family Teaching

- Explain purpose and side effects of medication to patient. Advise patient to read *Patient Information* before starting therapy.
- Instruct patient to notify health care provider of all Rx or OTC medications, vitamins, or herbal products being taken and to consult health care provider before taking other Rx, OTC, or herbal products.
- Educate patient and family/caregivers on signs and symptoms of hypoglycemia. Instruct patient to take oral glucose as soon as symptoms of hypoglycemia occur; glucagon is reserved for episodes when patient is unable to swallow because of ↓ level of consciousness.
- **Home Care Issues:** Instruct family/caregivers on correct technique to prepare, draw up, and administer injection. Health care provider must be contacted immediately after each dose for orders regarding further therapy or adjustment of insulin dose or diet.
- Advise patient, family, and caregivers of hypersensitivity reactions and to seek immediate medical attention if any occur.
- Instruct family/caregivers to position patient on side until fully alert. Explain that glucagon may cause nausea and vomiting. Aspiration may occur if patient vomits while lying on back.
- Instruct patient to check expiration date monthly and to replace outdated medication immediately.
- Review hypoglycemic medication regimen, diet, and exercise programs.
- Patients with diabetes mellitus should carry a source of sugar (such as a packet of sugar or candy) and identification describing disease process and treatment regimen at all times.
- Rep: Advise women of reproductive potential to notify health care provider if pregnancy is planned or suspected or if breastfeeding.

Evaluation/Desired Outcomes

- Increase in blood glucose.
- Relaxation of GI musculature, facilitating radiographic examination.

glyBURIDE, See SULFONYLUREAS.

glycopyrrolate (systemic)

(glye-koe-**pye**-roe-late)

Cuvposa, Glycate, Glyrx-PF, Robinul

Classification

Therapeutic: antispasmodics

Pharmacologic: anticholinergics

Indications

Inhibits salivation and excessive respiratory secretions when given preoperatively. Reverses some of the secretory and vagal actions of cholinesterase inhibitors used to treat nondepolarizing neuromuscular blockade (cholinergic adjunct). Adjunctive management of peptic ulcer disease. **Oral solution:** Reduce chronic severe drooling in children with neurologic conditions associated with drooling.

Action

Inhibits the action of acetylcholine at postganglionic sites located in smooth muscle, secretory glands, and the CNS (antimuscarinic activity). Low doses decrease sweating, salivation, and respiratory secretions. Larger doses decrease GI and GU tract motility. **Therapeutic Effects:** Decreased GI and respiratory secretions.

Pharmacokinetics

Absorption: Incompletely absorbed (<10%) after oral administration. Well absorbed after IM administration. IV administration results in complete bioavailability.

Distribution: Distribution not fully known. Does not significantly cross the blood-brain barrier or eye.

Metabolism and Excretion: Eliminated primarily unchanged in the urine and bile.

Half-life: 1.7 hr (0.6–4.6 hr).

TIME/ACTION PROFILE (anticholinergic effects)

ROUTE	ONSET	PEAK	DURATION
PO	1 hr	unknown	8–12 hr
IM	15–30 min	30–45 min	2–7 hr*
IV	1–10 min	unknown	2–7 hr*

* Antisecretory effect lasts up to 7 hr; vagal blockade lasts 2–3 hr.

Contraindications/Precautions

Contraindicated in: Hypersensitivity; Angle-closure glaucoma; Acute hemorrhage; Tachycardia secondary to cardiac insufficiency or thyrotoxicosis; Severe ulcerative colitis; Toxic megacolon; Myasthenia gravis; Obstructive uropathy; Paralytic ileus; Concurrent use of oral potassium chloride dose forms (oral solution only).

Use Cautiously in: Patients who may have intra-abdominal infections; Prostatic hyperplasia; Chronic renal, hepatic, pulmonary, or cardiac disease; Hyperthyroidism; Down syndrome and children with spastic paralysis or brain damage (may be hypersensitive to antimuscarinic effects); OB: Safety not established in pregnancy; Lactation: Use while breastfeeding only if potential maternal benefit justifies potential risk to infant; Pedi: ↑ sensitivity to anticholinergic effects and adverse reactions; Geri: ↑ sensitivity to anticholinergic effects and adverse reactions.

Adverse Reactions/Side Effects

CV: tachycardia, orthostatic hypotension, palpitations. **Derm:** flushing. **EENT:** nasal congestion, blurred vision, cycloplegia, dry eyes, mydriasis. **GI:** dry mouth, vomiting, constipation. **GU:** urinary hesitancy, urinary retention. **Neuro:** headache, confusion, drowsiness..

Interactions

Drug-Drug: May ↑ GI mucosal lesions in patients taking oral **potassium chloride** tablets; concurrent use with oral glycopyrrolate solution contraindicated. Additive anticholinergic effects with other **anticholinergics**, including **antihistamines, phenothiazines, meperidine, amantadine, tricyclic antidepressants, quinidine**, and **disopyramide**. May alter the absorption of other **orally administered drugs** by slowing motility of the GI tract. May ↑ GI transit time of oral **digoxin** and ↑ digoxin levels. **Antacids** or **adsorbent antidiarrheal agents** ↓ absorption of anticholinergics. May ↑ GI mucosal lesions in patients taking oral **potassium chloride** tablets. May ↑ **atenolol** and **metformin** levels. May ↓ levels and effectiveness of **haloperidol** and **levodopa**. May ↓ absorption of **ketoconazole**; administer 2 hr after ketoconazole.

Route/Dosage

Control of Secretions During Surgery

IM (Adults): 4.4 mcg/kg 30–60 min before surgery (not to exceed 0.1 mg).

IM (Children >2 yr): 4.4 mcg/kg 30–60 min before surgery.

IM (Children <2 yr): 4.4–8.8 mcg/kg 30–60 min before surgery.

Control of Secretions (chronic)

IM, IV (Children): 4–10 mcg/kg/dose every 3–4 hr.

PO (Children): 40–100 mcg/kg/dose 3–4 times/day.

Cholinergic Adjunct

IV (Adults and Children): 200 mcg for each 1 mg of neostigmine or 5 mg of pyridostigmine given at the same time.

Peptic Ulcer

PO (Adults): 1–2 mg 2–3 times daily. An additional 2 mg may be given at bedtime; may be ↓ to 1 mg twice daily (not to exceed 8 mg/day).
IM, IV (Adults): 100–200 mcg every 4 hr up to 4 times daily.

Chronic Severe Drooling

PO (Children 3–16 yr): *Oral solution:* 0.02 mg/kg 3 times daily; may ↑ by 0.02 mg/kg 3 times daily every 5–7 days (not to exceed 0.1 mg/kg 3 times daily or 1.5–3 mg/dose).

Availability (generic available)

Tablets: 1 mg, 1.5 mg, 2 mg. **Oral solution (cherry flavor):** 1 mg/5 mL. **Solution for injection:** 200 mcg (0.2 mg)/mL. ***In combination with:*** neostigmine (Prevduo). See Appendix N.

NURSING IMPLICATIONS

Assessment

- Assess HR, BP, and respiratory rate before and periodically during parenteral therapy.
- Monitor intake and output in older adults or surgical patients; glycopyrrolate may cause urinary retention. Instruct patient to void before parenteral administration.
- Assess routinely for abdominal distention and auscultate for bowel sounds. If constipation occurs, ↑ fluids and add high-fiber foods into diet to help alleviate it.
- Periodic intraocular pressure determinations should be made for patients receiving long-term therapy.
- Pedi: Monitor amount and frequency of drooling periodically during therapy.
- Assess for hyperexcitability, a paradoxical response that may occur in children.

Lab Test Considerations

- Antagonizes effects of pentagastrin and histamine during the gastric acid secretion test. Avoid administration for 24 hr preceding the test.
- May ↓ uric acid levels in patients with gout or hyperuricemia.

Toxicity and Overdose

- If overdose occurs, neostigmine is the antidote.

Implementation

- Do not administer cloudy or discolored solution.
- **PO:** Administer 30–60 min before meals to maximize absorption. Do not administer within 1 hr of antacids or antidiarrheal medications.
- For drooling: Administer >1 hr before or 2 hr after meals.
- Oral dose is 10 times the parenteral dose.
- **IM:** Dilution: Undiluted. Concentration: 200 mcg/mL.

IV Administration

- **IV Push:** Dilution: Undiluted or diluted with D5W, D10W, 0.9% NaCl, D5W/0.9% NaCl, or D5W/0.45% NaCl. Concentration: 200 mcg/mL. Rate: Administer at a maximum rate of 20 mcg over 1–2 min.
- **Y-Site Compatibility:** acyclovir, alemtuzumab, amikacin, aminophylline, amiodarone, anidulafungin, argatroban, arsenic trioxide, ascorbic acid, atracurium, atropine, azathioprine, aztreonam, benztropine, bivalirudin, bleomycin, bumetanide, buprenorphine, butorphanol, calcium chloride, calcium gluconate, carmustine, caspofungin, cefazolin, cefotaxime, cefotetan, cefoxitin, ceftazidime, ceftriaxone, cefuroxime, chloramphenicol, chlorpromazine, cisplatin, clindamycin, cyanocobalamin, cyclosporine, dacarbazine, dactinomycin, daptomycin, daunorubicin, dexamethasone, dexmedetomidine, dexrazoxane, digoxin, diltiazem, diphenhydramine, dobutamine, docetaxel, dopamine, doxorubicin liposomal, doxycycline, enalaprilat, ephedrine, epinephrine, epoetin alfa, ertapenem, erythromycin, esmolol, etoposide, etoposide phosphate, famotidine, fentanyl, fluconazole, fludarabine, folic acid, foscarnet, fosphenytoin, ganciclovir, gemcitabine, gemtuzumab ozogamicin, gentamicin, granisetron, heparin, hydrocortisone, hydromorphone, idarubicin, imipenem/cilastatin, isoproterenol, ketorolac, labetalol, leucovorin, lidocaine, linezolid, lorazepam, magnesium sulfate, mannitol, meperidine, mesna, methadone, methylprednisolone, metoclopramide, metoprolol, metronidazole, midazolam, milrinone, minocycline, mitoxantrone, morphine, moxifloxcin, multivitamins, mycophenolate, nafcillin, nalbuphine, naloxone, nitroglycerin, nitroprusside, norepinephrine, octreotide, ondansetron, oxacillin, oxaliplatin, oxytocin, paclitaxel, palonosetron, pamidronate, papaverine, pemetrexed, penicillin G, pentamidine, pentobarbital, phenobarbital, phentolamine, phenylephrine, phytonadione, potassium acetate, potassium chloride, procainamide, prochlorperazine, promethazine, propofol, propranolol, protamine, pyridoxine, rocuronium, sodium bicarbonate, succinylcholine, sufentanil, tacrolimus, theophylline, thiamine, thiotepa, tigecycline, tirofiban, tobramycin, topotecan, vancomycin, vasopressin, vecuronium, verapamil, vinblastine, vinorelbine, voriconazole, zoledronic acid.
- **Y-Site Incompatibility:** amphotericin B deoxycholate, dantrolene, diazepam, diazoxide, furosemide, indomethacin, insulin, regular, irinotecan, mitomycin, pantoprazole, phenytoin, piperacillin/tazobactam, trimethoprim/sulfamethoxazole.

G

Patient/Family Teaching

- Explain purpose and side effects of medication to patient. Advise patient to read *Patient Information* before starting therapy. Instruct patient to take as directed and not to take more than the prescribed amount. Take missed doses as soon as remembered if not just before next dose.
- Advise patient to notify health care provider of all Rx or OTC medications, vitamins, or herbal products being taken and to consult health care provider before taking other medications.
- Medication may cause drowsiness and blurred vision. Caution patient to avoid driving or other activities requiring alertness until response to the medication is known.
- Inform patient that frequent oral rinses, sugarless gum or candy, and good oral hygiene may help relieve dry mouth. Consult health care provider regarding use of saliva substitute if dry mouth persists for >2 wk.
- Advise patient to change positions slowly to minimize the effects of drug-induced orthostatic hypotension.
- Caution caregivers and patient to avoid extremes of temperature. This medication ↓ the ability to sweat and may ↑ the risk of heat stroke.
- Advise patient to notify health care provider immediately if eye pain or ↑ sensitivity to light occurs. Emphasize the importance of routine eye exams throughout therapy.
- Rep: Advise women of reproductive potential to notify health care provider if pregnancy is planned or suspected or if breastfeeding.
- Geri: Advise older adults about ↑ susceptibility to side effects and to call health care provider immediately if they occur.
- Pedi: Instruct caregivers to use a calibrated measuring device with solution for accurate dosing.
- Advise caregivers to stop glycopyrrolate and notify health care provider if constipation, signs of urinary retention (inability to urinate, dry diapers or undergarments, irritability, crying), rash, hives, or an allergic reaction occurs.

Evaluation/Desired Outcomes

- Decreased GI and respiratory secretions.

golimumab (go-li-mu-mab)

Simponi, Simponi Aria,
✱ Simponi IV

Classification
Therapeutic: antirheumatics
Pharmacologic: DMARDs monoclonal antibodies anti-TNF agents

Indications

Simponi and Simponi Aria: Treatment of the following conditions: Moderately to severely active rheumatoid arthritis (in combination with methotrexate), Active psoriatic arthritis, Active ankylosing spondylitis. **Simponi:** Moderately to severely active ulcerative colitis in patients who have demonstrated corticosteroid dependence or have responded inadequately to immunosuppressants such as aminosalicylates, corticosteroids, azathioprine, or 6-mercaptopurine. **Simponi Aria:** Active polyarticular juvenile idiopathic arthritis.

Action

Inhibits binding of TNF-α to receptors, inhibiting activity and resulting in anti-inflammatory and antiproliferative activity. **Therapeutic Effects:** Decreased pain and swelling with decreased joint destruction in patients with rheumatoid arthritis, psoriatic arthritis, ankylosing spondylitis, and polyarticular juvenile idiopathic arthritis. Induction and maintenance of clinical remission of ulcerative colitis.

Pharmacokinetics

Absorption: Well absorbed following SUBQ administration. IV administration results in complete bioavailability.
Distribution: Distributed primarily in the circulatory system with limited extravascular distribution.
Metabolism and Excretion: Unknown.
Half-life: 2 wk.

TIME/ACTION PROFILE (improvement)

ROUTE	ONSET	PEAK	DURATION
SUBQ	within 3 mo	2–7 days†	unknown
IV	within 3 mo	unknown	unknown

† Blood levels.

Contraindications/Precautions

Contraindicated in: Active infection (including localized).
Use Cautiously in: History of chronic or recurrent infection or underlying illness/treatment predisposing to infection; History of exposure to tuberculosis (TB); History of opportunistic infection; Patients residing or who have resided where TB, histoplasmosis, coccidioidomycoses, or blastomycosis is endemic; History of HF (may worsen); Pre-existing CNS demyelinating disorders (including multiple sclerosis or Guillain-Barré syndrome); History of cytopenias (may worsen); History of psoriasis (may worsen); Hepatitis B virus (HBV) carriers (risk of reactivation); OB: Use during pregnancy only if potential maternal benefit justifies potential fetal risk; Lactation: Use while breastfeeding only if potential maternal benefit justifies potential risk to infant; Pedi: Safety and effectiveness not established in children <18 yr (rheumatoid arthritis, ankylosing spondylitis, or ulcerative colitis) or <2 yr (psoriatic

arthritis or polyarticular juvenile idiopathic arthritis); ↑ risk of lymphoma (including HSTCL), leukemia, and other malignancies in children; Geri: ↑ risk of infection in older adults.

Adverse Reactions/Side Effects

CV: HF, hypertension. **Derm:** psoriasis. **EENT:** nasopharyngitis, optic neuritis. **GI:** ↑ liver enzymes. **Hemat:** agranulocytosis, aplastic anemia, leukopenia, neutropenia, pancytopenia, thrombocytopenia. **Local:** injection site reactions. **Neuro:** CNS DEMYELINATING DISORDERS, Guillain-Barré syndrome, multiple sclerosis, paresthesia. **Resp:** upper respiratory tract infection. **Misc:** fever, HYPERSENSITIVITY REACTIONS (INCLUDING ANAPHYLAXIS), INFECTION (INCLUDING REACTIVATION TB AND OTHER OPPORTUNISTIC INFECTIONS DUE TO BACTERIAL, INVASIVE FUNGAL, VIRAL, MYCOBACTERIAL, AND PARASITIC PATHOGENS), lupus-like syndrome, MALIGNANCY (INCLUDING LYMPHOMA, HSTCL, LEUKEMIA, AND SKIN CANCER).

Interactions

Drug-Drug: Abatacept, anakinra, corticosteroids, or **methotrexate** ↑ risk of serious infections; concurrent use with anakinra or abatacept not recommended. **Live-virus vaccines** or therapeutic infectious agents may ↑ risk of infection; avoid concurrent use. **Azathioprine** or **6-mercaptopurine** may ↑ risk of HSTCL. May normalize previously suppressed levels of CYP450 enzymes; following initiation or discontinuation of golimumab, effects of substrates of this system may be altered and should be monitored, including **warfarin**, **theophylline**, and **cyclosporine**.

Route/Dosage

Rheumatoid Arthritis and Ankylosing Spondylitis

SUBQ (Adults): 50 mg once monthly.
IV (Adults): 2 mg/kg initially and 4 wk later, then 2 mg/kg every 8 wk.

Psoriatic Arthritis

SUBQ (Adults): 50 mg once monthly.
IV (Adults): 2 mg/kg initially and 4 wk later, then 2 mg/kg every 8 wk.
IV (Children ≥2 yr): 80 mg/m^2 initially and 4 wk later, then 80 mg/m^2 every 8 wk.

Ulcerative Colitis

SUBQ (Adults): 200 mg initially, then 100 mg 2 wk later, then 100 mg every 4 wk.

Polyarticular Juvenile Idiopathic Arthritis

IV (Children ≥2 yr): 80 mg/m^2 initially and 4 wk later, then 80 mg/m^2 every 8 wk.

Availability

Solution for SUBQ injection (prefilled syringes and autoinjectors): 50 mg/0.5 mL, 100 mg/mL. **Solution for intravenous injection (Simponi Aria):** 12.5 mg/mL.

NURSING IMPLICATIONS

Assessment

- Assess for signs and symptoms of infection (fever, dyspnea, flu-like symptoms, frequent or painful urination, redness or swelling at the site of a wound) before, during, and after therapy. Discontinue therapy if serious or opportunistic infection or sepsis occurs. If new infection develops during therapy, assess patient and institute antimicrobial therapy. Patients who tested negative for latent TB before therapy may develop TB during therapy. Initiate treatment for latent TB before starting therapy.
- Test for HBV before therapy and monitor carriers of HBV for signs of reactivation during and for several months after therapy. If reactivation occurs, discontinue golimumab and institute antiviral therapy.
- Monitor patients with HF for new or worsening symptoms. Discontinue therapy if symptoms occur.
- Assess for exacerbations and new onset psoriasis. Discontinue therapy if these occur.
- Assess patient for latex allergy. Needle cover of syringe contains latex and should not be handled by persons sensitive to latex.
- Assess for signs and symptoms of systemic fungal infections (fever, malaise, weight loss, sweats, cough, dyspnea, pulmonary infiltrates, serious systemic illness with or without concurrent shock). Ascertain if patient lives in or has traveled to areas of endemic mycoses. Consider empiric antifungal treatment for patients at risk of histoplasmosis and other invasive fungal infections until the pathogens are identified. Consult with an infectious diseases specialist. Consider stopping golimumab until the infection has been diagnosed and adequately treated.
- Observe for signs and symptoms of anaphylaxis (rash, pruritus, laryngeal edema, wheezing). Implement supportive medical treatment (epinephrine, resuscitation equipment) if needed.
- **Rheumatoid Arthritis:** Assess pain and range of motion before and periodically during therapy.
- **Ulcerative Colitis:** Assess for signs and symptoms before, during, and after therapy.

Lab Test Considerations

- Monitor liver function tests periodically during therapy. May ↑ AST and ALT.

- Monitor CBC with differential periodically during therapy. May cause leukopenia, neutropenia, thrombocytopenia, and pancytopenia. Discontinue golimumab if symptoms of blood dyscrasias (persistent fever) occur.
- Monitor for HBV blood tests before starting, during, and for several months after therapy is completed.

Implementation

- Administer a tuberculin skin test before administration of golimumab. Assess if treatment for latent TB is needed; an induration of >5 mm is a positive tuberculin skin test, even for patients previously vaccinated with Bacille Calmette-Guerin. Consider antituberculosis therapy before therapy in patients with a history of latent or active tuberculosis if an adequate course of treatment cannot be confirmed and for patients with risk factors for TB infection.
- Update immunizations before starting therapy following current immunization guidelines for patients receiving immunosuppressive agents.
- Initial injection should be supervised by health care provider.
- Refrigerate solution; do not freeze. Allow prefilled syringe or autoinjector to sit at room temperature for 30 min before injection; do not warm in any other way. Do not shake. Solution is clear to slightly opalescent and colorless to light yellow. Do not administer solutions that are discolored, cloudy, or contain particulate matter. Discard unused solution.
- **SUBQ**: Remove the needle cover or autoinjector cap just before injection; both caps contain latex. Inject into front of middle thigh or lower part of abdomen 2 inches from navel. Do not inject in areas where skin is tender, bruised, red, scaly, or hard; avoid scars or stretch marks. Press a cotton ball or gauze over injection site for 10 sec; do not rub.
- *Autoinjector:* Press open end of autoinjector against skin at 90° angle. Press button with fingers or thumb; button will stay pressed and does not need to be held. Injection will begin following a loud click. Keep holding the autoinjector against skin until a 2nd loud click is heard (usually 3–6 sec, but may take up to 15 sec). Lift autoinjector from skin following 2nd click. Yellow indicator in viewing window indicates autoinjector worked correctly. If yellow does not appear in viewing window, call 1-800-526-7736 for help.
- *Prefilled syringe:* Hold body of syringe between thumb and index finger. Do not pull back on plunger at any time. Pinch skin. Inject all medication by pushing plunger until plunger head is between needle guard wings. Take needle out of skin and let go of skin. Slowly take thumb off plunger to allow empty syringe to move up until entire needle is covered by needle guard.

IV Administration

- **Intermittent Infusion:** Calculate dose and number of vials needed for dose. Solution in vial is colorless to light yellow; may contain a few fine translucent particles of protein. Do not use if opaque particles, discoloration, or other particles present.
- **Dilution:** Withdraw volume of dose from 100 mL bag of 0.9% NaCl or 0.45% NaCl and discard. Add golimumab dose to infusion bag; mix gently. Solution is stable for 4 hr at room temperature. **Concentration:** 12.5 mg/mL. **Rate:** Infuse through an in-line, sterile, nonpyrogenic, low-protein-binding filter with ≤0.22-micrometer pore size over 30 min.
- **Y-Site Incompatibility:** Do not administer other drugs through same IV line.

Patient/Family Teaching

- Explain purpose and side effects of medication to patient. Advise patient to read *Patient Information* before starting therapy.
- Advise patient to notify health care provider of all Rx or OTC medications, vitamins, or herbal products being taken and to consult health care provider before taking other medications.
- Instruct patient on correct technique for administration, and disposal of equipment into a puncture-resistant container. Inject missed doses as soon as remembered; then return to regular schedule.
- Inform patient of ↑ risk of infections, malignancies, and cardiac and CNS disorders during therapy.
- Caution patient to notify health care provider promptly if any signs of infection, including TB, invasive fungal infections (fever, malaise, weight loss, sweats, cough, dyspnea, pulmonary infiltrates, serious systemic illness with or without concurrent shock), reactivation of HBV (muscle aches, clay-colored bowel movements, feeling very tired, fever, dark urine, chills, skin or eyes look yellow, stomach discomfort, little or no appetite, skin rash, vomiting), hypersensitivity reactions, or nervous system problems (vision changes, weakness in arms or legs, numbness or tingling in any part of the body) develop.
- Advise patient to examine skin periodically during therapy and notify health care provider of any changes in appearance of skin or growths on skin.
- Inform patient to avoid receiving live vaccinations; other vaccinations may be given.
- Inform patient of ↑ risk of cancer. Advise patient of need for screening for dysplasia (colonoscopy, skin cancer examinations, biopsy) periodically during therapy.

- Rep: Advise women of reproductive potential to notify health care provider if pregnancy is planned or suspected or if breastfeeding. Advise women to notify health care provider if they recently had a baby while taking golimumab. Infants have an ↑ chance of getting an infection for up to 6 mo after birth; avoid administration of live vaccines to infants for 6 mo after mother's last dose.

Evaluation/Desired Outcomes

- Decreased pain and swelling with decreased joint destruction in patients with rheumatoid arthritis, psoriatic arthritis, ankylosing spondylitis, and polyarticular juvenile idiopathic arthritis.
- Induction and maintenance of clinical remission of ulcerative colitis.

HIGH ALERT

goserelin (goe-se-rel-lin)

Zoladex, Zoladex LA

Classification

Therapeutic: antineoplastics hormones

Pharmacologic: gonadotropin-releasing hormones

Indications

Palliative treatment of advanced prostate cancer. Locally confined stage T2b–T4 (stage B2–C) prostate cancer (in combination with flutamide). Palliative treatment of advanced breast cancer in perimenopausal and postmenopausal women. Endometriosis. Produces thinning of the endometrium before endometrial ablation for dysfunctional uterine bleeding.

Action

Acts as a synthetic form of luteinizing hormone-releasing hormone (LHRH, GnRH). Inhibits the production of gonadotropins by the pituitary gland. Initially, levels of luteinizing hormone (LH), follicle-stimulating hormone (FSH), and testosterone increase. Continued administration leads to decreased production of testosterone and estradiol. **Therapeutic Effects:** Decreased spread of cancer of the prostate or breast. Regression of endometriosis with decreased pain. Thinning of the endometrium.

Pharmacokinetics

Absorption: Well absorbed from SUBQ implant. Absorption is slower in first 8 days and then faster and continuous for remainder of 28-day dosing cycle.
Distribution: Unknown.
Metabolism and Excretion: Some metabolism by the liver (<10%), some excretion by kidneys (>90%, only 20% as unchanged drug).
Half-life: 4.2 hr.

TIME/ACTION PROFILE (↓ in serum testosterone concentrations)

ROUTE	ONSET	PEAK	DURATION
SUBQ	unknown	2–4 wk	length of therapy

Contraindications/Precautions

Contraindicated in: Hypersensitivity; Undiagnosed vaginal bleeding; OB: Pregnancy; Lactation: Lactation.
Use Cautiously in: Congenital long QT syndrome, HF, hypokalemia, or hypomagnesemia; Concurrent use of other drugs known to prolong the QTc interval; Low body mass index (↑ risk of bleeding complications); Concurrent use of anticoagulant therapy (↑ risk of bleeding complications); Pedi: Safety and effectiveness not established in children.

Adverse Reactions/Side Effects

CV: vasodilation, chest pain, hypertension, MI, palpitations, peripheral edema, QT interval prolongation. **Derm:** hot flushing, sweating, acne, rash. **Endo:** ↓ libido, erectile dysfunction, breast swelling, breast tenderness, infertility, ovarian cysts, ovarian hyperstimulation syndrome (with gonadotropins). **GI:** anorexia, constipation, diarrhea, nausea, ulcer, vomiting. **GU:** renal insufficiency, urinary obstruction. **Hemat:** anemia. **Local:** injection site/vascular injury. **Metab:** ↑ weight, gout, hyperglycemia, hyperlipidemia. **MS:** ↑ bone pain, ↓ bone density, arthralgia. **Neuro:** headache, anxiety, depression (women), dizziness, fatigue, insomnia, mood swings, SEIZURES, STROKE, SUICIDAL IDEATION/BEHAVIOR (WOMEN), weakness. **Resp:** dyspnea. **Misc:** chills, fever.

Interactions

Drug-Drug: None reported.

Route/Dosage

SUBQ (Adults): 3.6 mg every 4 wk or 10.8 mg every 12 wk. *Endometrial thinning:* 1 or 2 depots given 4 wk apart; if 1 depot used, surgery is performed at 4 wk; if 2 depots used, surgery is performed 2–4 wk after 2nd depot.

Availability

Implant: 3.6 mg, 10.8 mg.

NURSING IMPLICATIONS

Assessment

- Monitor for signs and symptoms of injection site injury/abdominal hemorrhage (abdominal pain, abdominal distension, dyspnea, dizziness, hypotension, any altered levels of consciousness) following administration.
- Assess for signs and symptoms of MI or stroke (chest pain, palpations, shortness of breath, facial droop, weakness, altered mental status).

- Monitor mental status (orientation, mood behavior, depression) frequently. Assess for suicidal thoughts, behaviors or tendencies.
- Observe for characteristics of seizure activity. Implement seizure precautions if needed.
- **Cancer:** Monitor patients with vertebral metastases for ↑ back pain and ↓ sensory/motor function.
- Monitor intake and output and assess for bladder distention in patients with urinary tract obstruction during initiation of therapy.
- **Endometriosis:** Assess for signs and symptoms of endometriosis before and periodically during therapy. Amenorrhea usually occurs within 8 wk of initial administration and menses usually resume 8 wk after completion.

Lab Test Considerations

- Initially ↑ and then ↓ LH and FSH. This leads to castration levels of testosterone in men 2–4 wk after initial ↑ in concentrations.
- Monitor serum acid phosphatase and prostate-specific antigen concentrations periodically during therapy. May cause transient ↑ in serum acid phosphatase concentrations, which usually return to baseline by the 4th wk of therapy and may ↓ to below baseline or return to baseline if ↑ before therapy.
- May cause hypercalcemia in patients with breast or prostate cancer with bony metastases.
- May ↑ serum HDL, LDL, and triglycerides.
- May cause hyperglycemia. Monitor blood glucose and A1c periodically during therapy.

Implementation

- **SUBQ**: Implant is inserted in upper SUBQ tissue of anterior abdominal wall below the navel line every 28 days. Local anesthesia may be used before injection.
- If the implant needs to be removed for any reason, it can be located by ultrasound.

Patient/Family Teaching

- Explain purpose and side effects of medication to patient. Advise patient to read *Patient Information* before starting therapy. Emphasize importance of adhering to the schedule of monthly or every-3-mo administration.
- Advise patient to notify health care provider of all Rx or OTC medications, vitamins, or herbal products being taken and to consult health care provider before taking other medications.
- Advise patient that bone pain may ↑ at initiation of therapy. This will resolve with time. Patient should discuss use of analgesics to control pain with health care provider.
- Advise female patients to notify health care provider if regular menstruation persists.
- Inform patients with diabetes of potential for hyperglycemia. Encourage close monitoring of serum glucose.
- Advise patient that medication may cause hot flashes. Notify health care provider if these become bothersome. Hormone replacement therapy may be added to ↓ vasomotor symptoms and vaginal dryness without compromising beneficial effect.
- Advise patient and caregivers to monitor for suicidal thoughts or behaviors or depression and to notify health care provider immediately if these occur.
- Instruct patient to notify health care provider promptly if difficulty urinating, symptoms of MI or stroke (chest pain, difficulty breathing, weakness, loss of consciousness), or seizures occur.
- Rep: May cause fetal harm. Advise women of reproductive potential to notify health care provider if pregnancy is planned or suspected and to avoid breastfeeding. Effective nonhormonal contraception should be used during and for 12 wk after treatment ends.

Evaluation/Desired Outcomes

- Decreased spread of cancer of the prostate or breast.
- Regression of endometriosis with decreased pain.
- Thinning of the endometrium.

granisetron (gra-ni-se-tron)

~~Kytril~~, Sancuso, Sustol

Classification

Therapeutic: antiemetics

Pharmacologic: 5-HT_3 agonists

Indications

PO: Prevention of nausea and vomiting due to emetogenic chemotherapy or radiation therapy. **IV:** Prevention of nausea and vomiting due to emetogenic chemotherapy. **IV:** Prevention and treatment of postoperative nausea and vomiting. **SUBQ**: Prevention of acute and delayed nausea and vomiting due to moderately emetogenic chemotherapy or anthracycline/cyclophosphamide combination chemotherapy (in combination with dexamethasone). **Transdermal:** Prevention of nausea and vomiting due to moderately/highly emetogenic chemotherapy.

Action

Blocks the effects of serotonin at receptor sites (selective antagonist) located in vagal nerve terminals and in the chemoreceptor trigger zone in the CNS. **Therapeutic Effects:** Decreased incidence and severity of nausea and vomiting following emetogenic chemotherapy, radiation therapy, or surgery.

Pharmacokinetics

Absorption: 50% absorbed following oral administration; transdermal enters systemic circulation via passive diffusion through intact skin. IV administration results in complete bioavailability.
Distribution: Distributes into erythrocytes; remainder of distribution is unknown.
Metabolism and Excretion: Mostly metabolized by the liver; 12% excreted unchanged in urine.
Half-life: *Patients with cancer:* 10–12 hr (range 0.9–31.1 hr); *healthy volunteers:* 3–4 hr (range 0.9–15.2 hr); *older adults:* 7.7 hr (range 2.6–17.7 hr); *SUBQ:* 24 hr.

TIME/ACTION PROFILE (plasma concentrations)

ROUTE	ONSET	PEAK	DURATION
PO	rapid	60 min	24 hr
IV	1–3 min	30 min	up to 24 hr
TD	unknown	48 hr	unknown
SUBQ	unknown	12 hr	7 days

Contraindications/Precautions

Contraindicated in: Hypersensitivity; Some products contain benzyl alcohol; avoid use in neonates; Severe renal impairment (SUBQ).
Use Cautiously in: History of arrhythmias or conduction disorders; Recent abdominal surgery (SUBQ); Moderate renal impairment (↓ frequency of administration); Lactation: Safety not established in breastfeeding; Pedi: Safety and effectiveness not established in children <18 yr (oral, SUBQ, or transdermal) or <2 yr (IV).

Adverse Reactions/Side Effects

CV: hypertension, QT interval prolongation. **Derm:** **Topical:** application site reactions, photosensitivity. **GI:** constipation, ↑ liver enzymes, abdominal pain, diarrhea, dyspepsia. **Local:** injection site reactions (SUBQ). **Neuro:** headache, agitation, anxiety, CNS stimulation, dizziness, drowsiness, dysgeusia, headache, insomnia, weakness. **Misc:** fever, HYPERSENSITIVITY REACTIONS (INCLUDING ANAPHYLAXIS).

Interactions

Drug-Drug: ↑ risk of extrapyramidal reactions with other **agents causing extrapyramidal reactions**. ↑ risk of QT interval prolongation with other **agents causing QT interval prolongation**. Drugs that affect serotonergic neurotransmitter systems, including **SSRIs**, **SNRIs**, **tricyclic antidepressants**, **MAO inhibitors**, **fentanyl**, **lithium**, **buspirone**, **tramadol**, **methylene blue**, and **triptans**, may ↑ risk of serotonin syndrome

Route/Dosage

Prevention of Nausea and Vomiting Due to Emetogenic Chemotherapy

PO (Adults): 1 mg twice daily; 1st dose given ≥60 min prior to chemotherapy and 2nd dose 12 hr later only on days when chemotherapy is administered; may also be given as 2 mg once daily ≥60 min prior to chemotherapy.
IV (Adults and Children 2–16 yr): 10 mcg/kg given within 30 min prior to chemotherapy or 20–40 mcg/kg/day divided once or twice daily (maximum: 3 mg/dose or 9 mg/day).
Transdermal (Adults): One patch applied up to 48 hr prior to chemotherapy; leave in place for ≥24 hr following chemotherapy; may be left in place for a total of 7 days.

Prevention of Nausea and Vomiting Associated with Radiation Therapy

PO (Adults): 2 mg taken once daily within 1 hr of radiation therapy.

Prevention and Treatment of Postoperative Nausea and Vomiting

IV (Adults): *Prevention:* 1 mg prior to induction of anesthesia or just prior to reversal of anesthesia; *Treatment:* 1 mg as a single dose.
IV (Children ≥4 yr): 20–40 mcg/kg as a single dose (maximum: 1 mg).

Prevention of Acute and Delayed Nausea and Vomiting Due to Emetogenic Chemotherapy

SUBQ (Adults): 10 mg given ≥30 min prior to chemotherapy (with dexamethasone) on Day 1 of chemotherapy; do not administer more frequently than every 7 days.

Renal Impairment

SUBQ (Adults): *CCr 30–59 mL/min:* Do not administer more frequently than every 14 days.

Availability (generic available)

Tablets: 1 mg. **Solution for intravenous injection:** 1 mg/mL. **Solution for SUBQ injection (prefilled syringes) (Sustol):** 10 mg/0.4 mL. **Transdermal patch:** 3.1 mg/24 hr.

NURSING IMPLICATIONS

Assessment

- Assess for nausea, vomiting, abdominal distention, and constipation prior to and following administration. Monitor for signs and symptoms of ileus (abdominal distention, ↓ or absent bowel sounds).
- Assess for extrapyramidal symptoms (involuntary movements, facial grimacing, rigidity, shuffling walk, trembling of hands) during therapy. This occurs

rarely and is usually associated with concurrent use of other drugs known to cause this effect.

- Assess cardiac history and monitor ECG in patients with HF, bradycardia, underlying heart disease, or renal impairment and in older adults.
- Assess for signs and symptoms of serotonin syndrome (confusion, delirium, agitation, coma, dilated pupils, tachycardia, hyperthermia, shivering, hyperreflexia, muscle rigidity, hypertension, vomiting, diarrhea, seizures). *If symptoms of serotonin syndrome occur,* discontinue granisetron and treat symptomatically.
- Monitor for signs and symptoms of hypersensitivity reactions (rash, urticaria, pruritus, flushing, dizziness, vomiting, abdominal pain) and angioedema (swelling of throat, lips, tongue, or face; dyspnea; wheezing; hoarseness). Discontinue immediately and provide supportive care.
- **Transdermal:** Monitor application site. If allergic, erythematous, macular, or papular rash or pruritus occurs, remove patch.

Lab Test Considerations

- May ↑ AST and ALT.

Implementation

- Correct hypokalemia and hypomagnesemia before administering.
- For chemotherapy or radiation, granisetron is administered only on the day(s) chemotherapy or radiation is given. Continued treatment when not on chemotherapy or radiation therapy has not been found to be useful.
- **PO:** Administer 1st dose up to 1 hr before chemotherapy or radiation therapy and 2nd dose 12 hr after 1st dose.
- **SUBQ**: Use kit and components provided by manufacturer. Injection should be administered by health care provider. Remove kit from refrigerator and allow to warm to room temperature for 60 min. Activate one syringe warming pouch, and wrap syringe in warming pouch for 5–6 min to warm to body temperature. Do not inject solutions that contain particulate matter. Inject in back of upper arm or in skin of abdomen ≥1 inch away from umbilicus. Avoid injecting in areas where skin is burned, hardened, inflamed, or swollen. Topical anesthesia may be used at injection site prior to injection. Solution is viscous and requires a slow, sustained injection over 20–30 sec. Pressing the plunger harder will NOT expel medication faster.

IV Administration

- **IV Push: Dilution:** May be administered undiluted or diluted in 20–50 mL of 0.9% NaCl or D5W. Solution should be prepared at time of administration but is stable for 24 hr at room temperature. **Concentration:** Up to 1 mg/mL. **Rate:** Administer undiluted granisetron over 30 sec or as a diluted solution over 5 min.
- **Y-Site Compatibility:** acetaminophen, alemtuzumab, allopurinol, amikacin, aminocaproic acid, aminophylline, amiodarone, amphotericin B liposomal, ampicillin, ampicillin/sulbactam, anidulafungin, argatroban, arsenic trioxide, atracurium, azithromycin, aztreonam, bivalirudin, bleomycin, bumetanide, buprenorphine, busulfan, butorphanol, calcium acetate, calcium chloride, calcium gluconate, carboplatin, carmustine, caspofungin, cefazolin, cefepime, cefotaxime, cefotetan, cefoxitin, ceftaroline, ceftazidime, ceftobiprole, ceftriaxone, cefuroxime, chloramphenicol, chlorpromazine, ciprofloxacin, cisatracurium, cisplatin, cladribine, clindamycin, cyclophosphamide, cyclosporine, cytarabine, dacarbazine, dactinomycin, daptomycin, daunorubicin, dexamethasone, dexmedetomidine, dexrazoxane, digoxin, diltiazem, diphenhydramine, dobutamine, docetaxel, dopamine, doxorubicin hydrochloride, doxorubicin liposomal, doxycycline, droperidol, enalaprilat, ephedrine, epinephrine, epirubicin, eptifibatide, ertapenem, erythromycin, esmolol, etoposide, etoposide phosphate, famotidine, fentanyl, filgrastim, floxuridine, fluconazole, fludarabine, fluorouracil, fosaprepitant, foscarnet, fosphenytoin, furosemide, ganciclovir, gemcitabine, gentamicin, glycopyrrolate, haloperidol, heparin, hydralazine, hydrocortisone, hydromorphone, idarubicin, ifosfamide, imipenem/cilastatin, insulin, regular, irinotecan, isoproterenol, ketorolac, labetalol, leucovorin, levofloxacin, lidocaine, linezolid, lorazepam, magnesium sulfate, mannitol, melphalan, meperidine, meropenem, mesna, methadone, methotrexate, methylprednisolone, metoclopramide, metoprolol, metronidazole, midazolam, milrinone, mitomycin, mitoxantrone, morphine, moxifloxacin, mycophenolate, nafcillin, nalbuphine, naloxone, nicardipine, nitroglycerin, nitroprusside, norepinephrine, octreotide, oxaliplatin, oxytocin, paclitaxel, pamidronate, pantoprazole, pemetrexed, pentamidine, pentobarbital, phenobarbital, phentolamine, phenylephrine, piperacillin/tazobactam, potassium acetate, potassium chloride, potassium phosphates, procainamide, prochlorperazine, promethazine, propofol, propranolol, remifentanil, rituximab, rocuronium, sargramostim, sodium acetate, sodium bicarbonate, sodium phosphates, succinylcholine, sufentanil, tacrolimus, theophylline, thiotepa, tigecycline, tirofiban, tobramycin, topotecan, trastuzumab, trimethoprim/sulfamethoxazole, vancomycin, vasopressin, vecuronium, verapamil, vinblastine, vincristine, vinorelbine, voriconazole, zidovudine, zoledronic acid.

- **Y-Site Incompatibility:** amphotericin B deoxycholate, dantrolene, diazepam, gemtuzumab ozogamicin, phenytoin.
- **Transdermal:** Apply system to clear, dry, intact healthy skin on upper outer arm 24–48 hr before chemotherapy. Do not use creams, lotions, or oils that may keep patch from sticking. Do not apply to skin that is red, irritated, or damaged. Apply immediately after removing from package. Do not cut patch into pieces. Remove liner from adhesive layer and press firmly in place with palm of hand for 30 sec, especially around the edges, to make sure contact is complete. Patch should be worn throughout chemotherapy. If patch does not stick, bandages or medical adhesive tape may be applied on edges of patch; do not cover patch with tape or bandages or wrap completely around arm. Patient may shower and wash normally while wearing patch; avoid swimming, strenuous exercise, sauna, or whirlpool during patch use. Remove patch gently ≥24 hr after completion of chemotherapy; may be worn for up to 7 days. Fold so that adhesive edges are together. Throw away in garbage, out of reach of children and pets. Do not reuse patch. Use soap and water to remove remaining adhesive; do not use alcohol or acetone.

Patient/Family Teaching

- Explain the purpose and side effects of granisetron. Instruct patient to take as directed. Advise patient to read *Patient Information* before starting and with each Rx refill in case of changes.
- Advise patient to notify health care provider immediately if involuntary movement of eyes, face, or limbs occurs.
- May cause dizziness and drowsiness. Caution patient to avoid driving and other activities requiring alertness until response to medication is known.
- Warn patient to report symptoms of arrhythmias and QT prolongation (fast heartbeat, skipped beats, palpitations, dizziness, light-headedness, trouble breathing, faintness).
- Instruct patient to report symptoms of abdominal pain, bloating, constipation, nausea, vomiting.
- Counsel patient to report symptoms of serotonin syndrome (confusion, sweating, fast heart rate, fever, vomiting, hallucinations, muscle spasms, tremors, twitching).
- Advise patient to notify health care provider of all Rx or OTC medications, vitamins, or herbal products being taken and to consult with health care provider before taking other medications.
- **Transdermal:** Instruct patient on correct application, removal, and disposal of patch. Inform patient that additional granisetron should not be taken during patch application unless directed by health care provider. Advise patient to avoid using a heating pad near or over patch and to cover patch application site with clothing to avoid exposure to sunlight, sunlamp, or tanning beds during and for 10 days following removal of patch. Instruct patient to notify health care provider if pain or swelling in the abdomen occurs or if redness at patch removal site remains for >3 days. Advise patient referred for MRI test to discuss patch with referring health care provider and MRI facility to determine if removal of patch is necessary prior to test and for directions for replacing patch.
- Rep: Advise women of reproductive potential to notify health care provider if pregnancy is planned or suspected or if breastfeeding.

Evaluation/Desired Outcomes

- Prevention of nausea and vomiting associated with emetogenic cancer chemotherapy or radiation therapy.
- Prevention and treatment of postoperative nausea and vomiting.

guaiFENesin (gwye-**fen**-e-sin)

Alfen Jr, Altarussin, ✱ Balminil Expectorant, ✱ Benylin Chest Congestion Extra Strength, Breonesin, ✱ Bronchophan Expectorant, ✱ Chest Congestion, ✱ Cough Syrup Expectorant, Diabetic Tussin, ✱ Expectorant Syrup, Ganidin NR, Guiatuss, Hytuss, Hytuss-2X, ✱ Jack & Jill Expectorant, Mucinex, Naldecon Senior EX, Organidin NR, Robitussin, Scot-tussin Expectorant, Siltussin SA, Siltussin DAS, ✱ Vicks Chest Congestion Relief, ✱ Vicks Dayquil Mucus Control

Classification

Therapeutic: allergy, cold, and cough remedies, expectorant

Indications

Cough associated with viral upper respiratory tract infections.

Action

Reduces viscosity of tenacious secretions by increasing respiratory tract fluid. **Therapeutic Effects:** Mobilization and subsequent expectoration of mucus.

Pharmacokinetics

Absorption: Well absorbed after oral administration.
Distribution: Unknown.
Metabolism and Excretion: Renally excreted as metabolites.
Half-life: Unknown.

TIME/ACTION PROFILE (expectorant action)

ROUTE	ONSET	PEAK	DURATION
PO	30 min	unknown	4–6 hr
PO-ER	unknown	unknown	12 hr

Contraindications/Precautions

Contraindicated in: Hypersensitivity; Some products contain alcohol; avoid in patients with known intolerance; Some products contain aspartame and should be avoided in patients with phenylketonuria.
Use Cautiously in: Cough lasting >1 wk or accompanied by fever, rash, or headache; Patients receiving disulfiram (liquid products may contain alcohol); Diabetes (some products may contain sugar); OB: Although safety has not been established, guaifenesin has been used without adverse effects; Lactation: Safety not established in breastfeeding; Pedi: OTC cough and cold products containing this medication should be avoided in children <4 yr.

Adverse Reactions/Side Effects

Derm: rash, urticaria. **GI:** diarrhea, nausea, stomach pain, vomiting. **Neuro:** dizziness, headache.

Interactions

Drug-Drug: None reported.

Route/Dosage

PO (Adults): *Immediate release:* 200–400 mg every 4 hr; *Extended release:* 600–1200 mg every 12 hr; not to exceed 2400 mg/day.
PO (Children 6–12 yr): *Immediate release:* 100–200 mg every 4 hr. *Extended release:* 600 mg every 12 hr; not to exceed 1200 mg/day.
PO (Children 4–6 yr): *Immediate release:* 50–100 mg every 4 hr (not to exceed 600 mg/day).

Availability (generic available)

Immediate-release capsules: 200 mg[OTC]. **Immediate-release tablets:** 100 mg[OTC], 200 mg[Rx, OTC], 1200 mg. **Extended-release tablets (Mucinex):** 600 mg, 1200 mg. **Oral solution:** 100 mg/5 mL[Rx, OTC], 200 mg/5 mL[OTC]. **Syrup:** 100 mg/5 mL[OTC]. ***In combination with:*** analgesics/antipyretics, antihistamines, decongestants, and cough suppressants. See Appendix N.

NURSING IMPLICATIONS

Assessment

- Assess lung sounds, frequency and type of cough, and character of bronchial secretions periodically during therapy. Maintain fluid intake of 1500–2000 mL/day to ↓ viscosity of secretions.

Implementation

- ***High Alert:*** Do not confuse guaifenesin with guanfacine.
- **PO:** Administer each dose of guaifenesin followed by a full glass of water to ↓ viscosity of secretions.
- ***DNC:*** Extended-release tablets should be swallowed whole; do not open, break, crush, or chew.

Patient/Family Teaching

- Instruct patient to cough effectively. Patient should sit upright and take several deep breaths before attempting to cough.
- Caution parents to avoid OTC cough and cold products in children <4 yr.
- Advise patient that guaifenesin is a drug with known abuse potential. Protect it from theft, and never give to anyone other than the individual for whom it was recommended. Store out of sight and reach of children, and in a location not accessible by others.
- Inform patient that drug may occasionally cause dizziness. Avoid driving or other activities requiring alertness until response to drug is known.
- Advise patient to limit talking, stop smoking, maintain moisture in environmental air, and take some sugarless gum or hard candy to help alleviate the discomfort caused by a chronic nonproductive cough.
- Instruct patient to contact health care professional if cough persists longer than 1 wk or is accompanied by fever, rash, or persistent headache or sore throat.
- Rep: Advise females of reproductive potential to notify health care professional if pregnancy is planned or suspected, or if breastfeeding.

Evaluation/Desired Outcomes

- Easier mobilization and expectoration of mucus from cough associated with upper respiratory infection.

BEERS

guanFACINE (gwahn-fa-seen)

Intuniv, Intuniv XR, ~~Tenex~~

Classification
Therapeutic: antihypertensives, agents for attention deficit hyperactivity disorder (ADHD)
Pharmacologic: alpha adrenergic agonists

Indications
Hypertension (in combination with thiazide-type diuretics) (immediate-release). Attention-deficit hyperactivity disorder (ADHD) (as monotherapy or as adjunctive therapy to stimulants) (extended-release).

Action
Stimulates CNS $alpha_2$-adrenergic receptors, producing a decrease in sympathetic outflow to heart, kidneys, and blood vessels. Result is decreased BP and peripheral resistance, a slight decrease in heart rate, and no change in cardiac output. Mechanism of action in ADHD is unknown. **Therapeutic Effects:** Lowering of BP in hypertension. Increased attention span in ADHD.

Pharmacokinetics
Absorption: Immediate-release is well absorbed (80%); extended-release has lower rate and extent of absorption (↑ absorption with high-fat meals).
Distribution: Appears to be widely distributed.
Metabolism and Excretion: 50% metabolized by the liver, 50% excreted unchanged by the kidneys.
Half-life: 17 hr.

TIME/ACTION PROFILE (antihypertensive effect)

ROUTE	ONSET	PEAK	DURATION
PO (single dose)	unknown	8–12 hr	24 hr
PO (multiple doses)	within 1 wk	1–3 mo	unknown

Contraindications/Precautions
Contraindicated in: Hypersensitivity.
Use Cautiously in: Severe coronary artery disease or recent MI; Cerebrovascular disease; Severe renal impairment; Severe hepatic impairment; History of hypotension, heart block, bradycardia, or cardiovascular disease; OB: Other agents preferred for treatment of hypertension or ADHD in pregnancy; Lactation: Use while breastfeeding only if potential maternal benefit justifies potential risk to infant; Pedi: Children <6 yr (safety and effectiveness not established); Geri: Appears on Beers list. ↑ risk of CNS effects, orthostatic hypotension, and bradycardia in older adults. Avoid use for treatment of hypertension in older adults.

Adverse Reactions/Side Effects
CV: bradycardia, chest pain, hypotension, palpitations, rebound hypertension, syncope. **EENT:** tinnitus. **GI:** constipation, dry mouth, abdominal pain, nausea. **GU:** erectile dysfunction. **Neuro:** drowsiness, headache, weakness, depression, dizziness, fatigue, insomnia, irritability. **Resp:** dyspnea.

Interactions
Drug-Drug: ↑ hypotension with other **antihypertensives**, **nitrates**, and acute ingestion of **alcohol**. ↑ CNS depression may occur with other **CNS depressants**, including **alcohol**, **antihistamines**, **opioid analgesics**, **tricyclic antidepressants**, and **sedative/hypnotics**. **NSAIDs** may ↓ effectiveness. **Adrenergics** may ↓ effectiveness. ↑ risk of hypotension and bradycardia with strong and moderate **CYP3A4 inhibitors**, including **ketoconazole** and **fluconazole** (↓ in dose of guanfacine may be needed). Strong and moderate **CYP3A4 inducers**, including **rifampin**, **efavirenz**, and **carbamazepine** may ↓ effects (an ↑ in dose of guanfacine may be needed). May ↑ levels of **valproic acid**.

Route/Dosage
Immediate-release and extended-release tablets should not be interchanged.

Hypertension
PO (Adults): *Immediate-release:* 1 mg once daily given at bedtime, may be ↑ if necessary at 3–4 wk intervals up to 2 mg/day; may also be given in 2 divided doses.

ADHD
PO (Adults and Children ≥6 yr): *Extended-release:* 1 mg once daily in morning or evening; may be ↑ by 1 mg/day at weekly intervals to achieve dose of 1–4 mg/day (6–12 yr) or 1–7 mg-day (13–17 yr) when used as monotherapy or 1–4 mg/day when used as adjunctive therapy. *Concurrent strong or moderate CYP3A4 inhibitor:* ↓ initial and maintenance dose by 50%; *Concurrent strong or moderate CYP3A4 inducer:* Consider ↑ initial and maintenance dose up to double the recommended level (maintenance dose can be ↑ over period of 1–2 wk).

Availability (generic available)
Immediate-release tablets: 1 mg, 2 mg. **Extended-release tablets (Intuniv):** 1 mg, 2 mg, 3 mg, 4 mg.

NURSING IMPLICATIONS
Assessment
- **Hypertension:** Monitor BP (lying and standing) and pulse frequently during initial dose adjustment and periodically during therapy. Report significant changes.
- Monitor frequency of prescription refills to determine adherence.
- **ADHD:** Assess attention span, impulse control, and interactions with others.
- Monitor BP and heart rate prior to starting therapy, following dose increases, and periodically during

therapy. May cause hypotension, orthostatic hypotension, and bradycardia.

Lab Test Considerations

- May cause temporary, clinically insignificant ↑ in plasma growth hormone levels.
- May cause ↓ in urinary catecholamines and vanillylmandelic acid levels.

Implementation

- Do not confuse guanfacine with guaifenesin. Do not confuse Intuniv with Invega.
- Do not substitute extended-release tablets for immediate-release tablets on a mg-mg basis. Doses are not the same.
- **PO:** *For hypertension:* Administer daily dose at bedtime to minimize daytime sedation.
- *For ADHD:* Administer once daily in the morning or evening. ***DNC:*** Swallow extended-release tablets whole; do not crush, break, or chew. Do not administer with high fat meals, due to increased exposure.

Patient/Family Teaching

- Instruct patient/caregiver to take guanfacine as directed. Advise patient and parents to read the *Medication Guide* prior to starting therapy and with each Rx refill in case of changes. Instruct patients/caregivers not to discontinue guanfacine without consulting health care provider. Monitor blood pressure and pulse when reducing dose or discontinuing the drug. Taper the daily dose in decrements of no >1 mg every 3 to 7 days to minimize risk of rebound hypertension. If two or more doses are missed, may need to decrease dose and titrate to usual dose.
- Advise patient to notify health care professional of all Rx or OTC medications, vitamins, or herbal products being taken and to consult with health care professional before taking other medications, especially cough, cold, or allergy remedies.
- Caution patient to avoid alcohol and other CNS depressants, including opioids, while taking guanfacine.
- Advise patient to notify health care professional if dry mouth or constipation persists. Frequent mouth rinses, good oral hygiene, and sugarless gum or candy may minimize dry mouth. Increase in fluid and fiber intake and exercise may decrease constipation.
- Instruct patient to notify health care professional of medication regimen prior to treatment or surgery.
- Advise patient to notify health care professional if dizziness, prolonged drowsiness, fatigue, weakness, depression, headache, sexual dysfunction, mental depression, or sleep pattern disturbance occurs. Discontinuation may be required if drug-related mental depression occurs.
- Rep: May cause fetal harm. Advise females of reproductive potential to notify health care professional if pregnancy is planned or suspected, or if breastfeeding. Monitor breastfed infants exposed to guanfacine through breast milk for sedation, lethargy, and poor feeding. Inform patient about pregnancy exposure registry that monitors pregnancy outcomes in women exposed to ADHD medications during pregnancy. Health care providers are encouraged to register patients by calling the National Pregnancy Registry for ADHD Medications at 1-866-961-2388.
- Emphasize the importance of follow-up exams to evaluate effectiveness of medication.
- **Hypertension:** Emphasize the importance of continuing to take medication as directed, even if feeling well. Medication controls but does not cure hypertension. Instruct patient to take medication at the same time each day. Take missed doses as soon as remembered; do not double doses. If 2 or more doses are missed, consult health care professional. Do not discontinue abruptly; may cause sympathetic overstimulation (nervousness, anxiety, rebound hypertension, chest pain, tachycardia, increased salivation, nausea, trembling, stomach cramps, sweating, difficulty sleeping). These effects may occur 2–7 days after discontinuation, although rebound hypertension is rare and more likely to occur with high doses.
- Advise patient to make sure enough medication is available for weekends, holidays, and vacations. A written prescription may be kept in wallet in case of emergency.
- Encourage patient to comply with additional interventions for hypertension (weight reduction, low-sodium diet, smoking cessation, moderation of alcohol consumption, regular exercise, and stress management).
- Instruct patient and family on proper technique for BP monitoring. Advise them to check BP at least weekly and to report significant changes.
- May cause drowsiness or dizziness. Advise patient to avoid driving or other activities requiring alertness until response to the medication is known.
- **ADHD:** Instruct patient to take medication as directed at the same time each day. Take missed doses as soon as possible, but should not take more than the total daily amount in any 24-hr period. Do not stop taking abruptly; discontinue gradually at no more than 1 mg every 3–7 days. Monitor heart rate and BP during discontinuation. Advise patient and parents to read the *Medication Guide* prior to starting therapy and with each Rx refill.
- Inform patient that sharing this medication may be dangerous.
- Pedi: Advise parents to notify school nurse of medication regimen.

Evaluation/Desired Outcomes

- Decrease in BP without excessive side effects.
- Improved attention span and social interactions in ADHD. Re-evaluate use if used for >9 wk.

guselkumab (gue-sel-koo-mab)

Tremfya

Classification

Therapeutic: antipsoriatics

Pharmacologic: interleukin antagonists, monoclonal antibodies

Indications

Moderate to severe plaque psoriasis in patients who are candidates for phototherapy or systemic therapy. Active psoriatic arthritis (as monotherapy or in combination with a conventional disease-modifying antirheumatic drug). Moderately to severely active ulcerative colitis. Moderately to severely active Crohn disease.

Action

Binds to the p19 protein subunit of the interleukin (IL)-23 cytokine to prevent its interaction with the IL-23 receptor. This cytokine is normally involved in inflammatory and immune responses. Binding to ILs antagonizes their effects, inhibiting the release of proinflammatory cytokines and chemokines. **Therapeutic Effects:** Decrease in area and severity of psoriatic lesions. Decreased pain and swelling with decreased rate of joint destruction in psoriatic arthritis. Induction of clinical remission of ulcerative colitis and Crohn disease.

Pharmacokinetics

Absorption: 49% absorbed following SUBQ administration.

Distribution: Well distributed to tissues.

Metabolism and Excretion: Broken down by catabolic processes into peptides and amino acids.

Half-life: 15–18 days

TIME/ACTION PROFILE (plasma concentrations)

ROUTE	ONSET	PEAK	DURATION
SUBQ	unknown	5.5 days	8 wk

Contraindications/Precautions

Contraindicated in: Hypersensitivity; Active, untreated infection.

Use Cautiously in: History of tuberculosis (TB) (possibility of reactivation); OB: Safety not established in pregnancy; Lactation: Use while breastfeeding only if potential maternal benefit justifies potential risk to infant; Pedi: Safety and effectiveness not established in children.

Exercise Extreme Caution in: Chronic infection or history of recurrent infection.

Adverse Reactions/Side Effects

GI: ↑ liver enzymes, diarrhea, HEPATOTOXICITY. **Local:** injection site reactions. **MS:** arthralgia. **Neuro:** headache. **Misc:** <u>infection</u>, HYPERSENSITIVITY REACTIONS (INCLUDING ANAPHYLAXIS).

Interactions

Drug-Drug: May ↓ antibody response to and ↑ risk of adverse reactions from **live vaccines**; avoid use during therapy. May affect the activity of CYP450 drug-metabolizing enzymes; appropriate monitoring and dose adjustment should be carried out when treatment is started in patients receiving concurrent treatment with **CYP450 substrate**, especially those with a narrow therapeutic index, including **warfarin** and **cyclosporine**.

Route/Dosage

Plaque Psoriasis and Psoriatic Arthritis

SUBQ (Adults): 100 mg initially and 4 wk later; then 100 mg every 8 wk.

Ulcerative Colitis

IV, SUBQ (Adults): *Induction:* 200 mg IV infusion initially; then 200 mg IV infusion 4 wk later (Wk 4); then 200 mg IV infusion 4 wk later (Wk 8); then continue with maintenance dosing. *Maintenance:* 100 mg SUBQ 8 wk after last induction IV dose (Wk 16); then 100 mg SUBQ every 8 wk OR 200 mg SUBQ 4 wk after last induction IV dose (Wk 12); then 200 mg SUBQ every 4 wk.

Crohn Disease

IV, SUBQ (Adults): *Induction:* 200 mg IV infusion initially; then 200 mg IV infusion 4 wk later (Wk 4); then 200 mg IV infusion 4 wk later (Wk 8) OR 400 mg SUBQ initially; then 400 mg SUBQ 4 wk later (Wk 4); then 400 mg SUBQ 4 wk later (Wk 8); then continue with maintenance dosing. *Maintenance:* 100 mg SUBQ 8 wk after last induction IV dose (Wk 16); then 100 mg SUBQ every 8 wk OR 200 mg SUBQ 4 wk after last induction IV dose (Wk 12); then 200 mg SUBQ every 4 wk.

Availability

Solution for SUBQ injection (prefilled syringes, prefilled pens, and patient-controlled injectors): 100 mg/mL. **Solution for IV injection:** 10 mg/mL.

NURSING IMPLICATIONS

Assessment

- **Plaque Psoriasis and Psoriatic Arthritis:** Assess affected area(s) prior to and periodically during therapy and evaluate for therapeutic

G

response based on reduced surface area affected and improved physical function.

- **Ulcerative Colitis and Crohn disease:** Assess for therapeutic response to treatment based on ↓ in signs and symptoms, clinical remission, mucosal healing, and ↓ corticosteroid use.
- Assess patient for latent TB with a tuberculin skin test prior to initiation of therapy. Treatment of latent TB should be started before therapy with guselkumab.
- Assess for signs of infection (fever, dyspnea, flu-like symptoms, frequent or painful urination, redness or swelling at the site of a wound), including TB, prior to injection. Monitor new infections closely; most common are upper respiratory tract infections, bronchitis, and urinary tract infections.
- Monitor for signs and symptoms of hepatotoxicity (fatigue, nausea, upper abdominal pain, jaundice, scleral icterus, dark urine, clay-colored stools). Discontinuation may be required.
- Monitor for signs and symptoms of hypersensitivity reactions (rash, urticaria, pruritus, flushing, dizziness, vomiting, abdominal pain) and angioedema (swelling of throat, lips, tongue, or face; dyspnea; wheezing; hoarseness). Discontinue guselkumab immediately and provide supportive care.

Lab Test Considerations

- Monitor liver enzymes and bilirubin prior to starting therapy and then as clinically indicated for 16 wk during therapy and periodically thereafter in patients with ulcerative colitis and Crohn disease. May ↑ liver enzymes.

Implementation

- Update immunizations to current prior to initiating therapy. Patients may receive concurrent vaccinations, except for live vaccines.
- **SUBQ:** Allow syringe and solution to reach room temperature for 30 min before injecting. Solution is clear and colorless to light yellow and may contain small translucent particles; do not administer solutions that are cloudy, discolored, or contain large particles. Store solution in refrigerator in original carton to protect from light; do not shake or freeze. Inject full amount (1 mL) of One-Press injector in front of thigh, abdomen, or upper arm. Avoid areas that are tender, bruised, red, hard, thick, scaly, or affected by psoriasis.

IV Administration

- **Intermittent Infusion: *Induction for ulcerative colitis and Crohn disease:* Dilution:** Guselkumab is a clear and colorless to light yellow solution that may contain small translucent particles. Withdraw and then discard 20 mL of 0.9% NaCl from a 250-mL infusion bag, which is equal to the volume of guselkumab to be added. Withdraw 20 mL of guselkumab from the vial and add it to the 250-mL IV infusion bag of 0.9% NaCl. Gently mix the diluted solution. Discard the vial with any remaining solution. Do not administer solutions that are discolored or contain particulate matter. Diluted solution is stable for 10 hr at room temperature. Do not freeze. **Concentration:** 0.8 mg/mL. **Rate:** Administer diluted solution over ≥1 hr using only an infusion set with an in-line, sterile, nonpyrogenic, low-protein-binding filter (pore size 0.2 micrometer). Infusion should be completed within 10 hr after the dilution in the infusion bag.
- **Y-Site Incompatibility:** Do not administer other drugs through same IV line.

Patient/Family Teaching

- Explain the purpose and side effects of guselkumab to patient. Do not stop receiving drug without consulting health care provider. If an appointment is missed, contact health care provider as soon as possible to reschedule. Instruct patient on correct technique for self-injection, care, and disposal of equipment. If a dose is missed, administer the dose as soon as possible. Thereafter, resume dosing at the regular scheduled time. Review *Medication Guide* with patient before starting therapy and with each injection.
- Advise patient to notify health care provider if signs and symptoms of infection (fever, chills, sore throat, painful urination) occur.
- Instruct patient to avoid receiving live vaccines during therapy.
- Advise patient to immediately report signs and symptoms of hepatotoxicity (fatigue, nausea, upper abdominal pain, yellowing of skin or eyes, dark urine, light-colored stools).
- Advise patient to notify health care provider immediately if signs and symptoms of hypersensitivity reaction (feel faint; swelling of face, eyelids, lips, mouth, tongue, or throat; trouble breathing; throat tightness; chest tightness; skin rash; hives) occur.
- Instruct patient to notify health care provider of all Rx or OTC medications, vitamins, or herbal products being taken and consult health care provider before taking any new medications.
- Instruct patient to notify health care provider of medication regimen prior to treatment or surgery.
- Rep: Advise women of reproductive potential to notify health care provider if pregnancy is planned or suspected or if breastfeeding. Inform patient of pregnancy registry that monitors outcomes in women exposed to guselkumab during pregnancy. Encourage patients to enroll by calling 1-877-311-8972 or visiting https://www.mothertobaby.org/ongoing-study/tremfya-guselkumab.

Evaluation/Desired Outcomes

- Decrease in extent and severity of psoriatic lesions.
- Decreased pain and swelling with decreased rate of joint destruction in psoriatic arthritis.
- Induction of clinical remission of ulcerative colitis.
- Induction of clinical remission of Crohn disease.

halcinonide, See CORTICOSTEROIDS (TOPICAL).

halobetasol, See CORTICOSTEROIDS (TOPICAL).

BEERS

haloperidol (ha-loe-per-i-dole)

~~Haldol, Haldol Decanoate~~

Classification
Therapeutic: antipsychotics
Pharmacologic: butyrophenones

Indications

Acute and chronic psychotic disorders including: schizophrenia, manic states, drug-induced psychoses. Patients with schizophrenia who require long-term parenteral (IM) antipsychotic therapy. Agitation or aggressive behavior. Tourette syndrome. Severe behavioral problems in children that may be accompanied by: unprovoked, combative, explosive hyperexcitability; hyperactivity accompanied by conduct disorders (short-term use when other modalities have failed). **Unlabeled Use:** Nausea and vomiting from surgery or chemotherapy.

Action

Alters the effects of dopamine in the CNS. Also has anticholinergic and alpha-adrenergic blocking activity. **Therapeutic Effects:** Diminished signs and symptoms of psychoses. Improved behavior in children with Tourette syndrome or other behavioral problems.

Pharmacokinetics

Absorption: Well absorbed following PO/IM administration. Decanoate salt is slowly absorbed and has a long duration of action.
Distribution: Concentrates in liver.
Protein Binding: 92%.
Metabolism and Excretion: Mostly metabolized by the liver.
Half-life: 21–24 hr.

TIME/ACTION PROFILE (antipsychotic activity)

ROUTE	ONSET	PEAK	DURATION
PO	2 hr	2–6 hr	8–12 hr
IM	20–30 min	30–45 min	4–8 hr†
IM (decanoate)	3–9 days	unknown	1 mo

† Effect may persist for several days.

Contraindications/Precautions

Contraindicated in: Hypersensitivity; Angle-closure glaucoma; Bone marrow depression; CNS depression; Parkinsonism; Severe hepatic or cardiovascular disease (↑ risk of QT interval prolongation); Some products contain tartrazine, sesame oil, or benzyl alcohol and should be avoided in patients with known intolerance or hypersensitivity; Lactation: Lactation.
Use Cautiously in: Debilitated patients (↓ dose); Cardiac disease (↑ risk of QT interval prolongation with high doses); Diabetes; Respiratory disease; Prostatic hyperplasia; CNS tumors; Intestinal obstruction; Seizures; Patients at risk for falls; History of breast cancer; OB: Neonates at ↑ risk for extrapyramidal symptoms and withdrawal after delivery when exposed during the 3rd trimester; use during pregnancy only if potential maternal benefit justifies potential fetal risk; Geri: Appears on Beers list. ↑ risk of stroke, cognitive decline, and mortality in older adults with dementia. Avoid use in older adults, except for schizophrenia, bipolar disorder, or for short-term use as an antiemetic.

Adverse Reactions/Side Effects

CV: hypotension, QT interval prolongation, tachycardia, TORSADES DE POINTES, ventricular arrhythmias. **Derm:** diaphoresis, photosensitivity, rash. **EENT:** blurred vision, dry eyes. **Endo:** amenorrhea, galactorrhea, gynecomastia, hyperprolactinemia. **GI:** constipation, dry mouth, anorexia, hepatitis, ileus. **GU:** impotence, urinary retention. **Hemat:** AGRANULOCYTOSIS, anemia, leukopenia, neutropenia. **Metab:** weight gain. **Neuro:** extrapyramidal reactions, confusion, drowsiness, restlessness, SEIZURES, tardive dyskinesia. **Resp:** respiratory depression. **Misc:** hypersensitivity reactions, NEUROLEPTIC MALIGNANT SYNDROME.

Interactions

Drug-Drug: Concurrent use with **QT interval prolonging drugs** may ↑ risk of QT interval prolongation. ↑ hypotension with **antihypertensives**, **nitrates**, or acute ingestion of **alcohol**. ↑ anticholinergic effects with **drugs having anticholinergic properties**, including **antihistamines**, **antidepressants**, **atropine**, **phenothiazines**, **quinidine**, and **disopyramide**. ↑ CNS depression with other **CNS depressants**, including **alcohol**, **antihistamines**, **opioid analgesics**, and **sedative/hypnotics**. Concurrent use with **epinephrine** may result in severe hypotension and tachycardia. May ↓ therapeutic effects of **levodopa**. Acute encephalopathic syndrome may occur when used with **lithium**.
Drug-Natural Products: **Kava-kava**, **valerian**, or **chamomile** can ↑ CNS depression.

Route/Dosage

Haloperidol

PO (Adults): 0.5–5 mg 2–3 times daily. Patients with severe symptoms may require up to 100 mg/day.
PO (Geriatric Patients): 0.5–2 mg twice daily initially; may be gradually ↑ as needed.
PO (Children 3–12 yr or 15–40 kg): 0.25–0.5 mg/day given in 2–3 divided doses; ↑ by 0.25–0.5 mg every 5–7 days; max dose: 0.15 mg/kg/day (up to 0.75 mg/kg/day for Tourette syndrome or 0.15 mg/kg/day for psychoses).
IM (Adults): *Haloperidol lactate:* 2–5 mg every 1–8 hr (not to exceed 100 mg/day).
IM (Children 6–12 yr): *Haloperidol lactate:* 1–3 mg/dose every 4–8 hr to a maximum of 0.15 mg/kg/day.
IV (Adults): *Haloperidol lactate:* 0.5–5 mg, may be repeated every 30 min (unlabeled).

Haloperidol Decanoate

IM (Adults): 10–15 times the previous daily PO dose but not to exceed 100 mg initially, given monthly (not to exceed 300 mg/mo).

Availability (generic available)

Tablets: 0.5 mg, 1 mg, 2 mg, 5 mg, 10 mg, 20 mg. **Oral concentrate:** 2 mg/mL. **Solution for intramuscular injection (decanoate):** 50 mg/mL, 100 mg/mL. **Solution for intravenous injection (lactate):** 5 mg/mL.

NURSING IMPLICATIONS

Assessment

- Assess mental status (orientation, mood, behavior) prior to and periodically during therapy.
- Assess positive (hallucination, delusions) and negative (social isolation) symptoms of schizophrenia.
- Assess weight and BMI initially and during therapy. Refer as appropriate for nutritional/weight and medical management.
- Monitor BP (sitting, standing, lying) and HR prior to and frequently during the period of dose adjustment.
- Observe patient carefully when administering oral medication to ensure that medication is actually taken and not hoarded.
- Assess cardiac history and ECG at baseline; may cause QT interval prolongation. Use of IV haloperidol requires continuous ECG monitoring via telemetry.
- Monitor intake and output and daily weight. Assess patient for signs and symptoms of dehydration (↓ thirst, lethargy, hemoconcentration), especially in older adults.
- Assess fluid intake and bowel function. ↑ bulk and fluids in the diet help minimize constipating effects.
- Monitor patient for onset of akathisia (restlessness or desire to keep moving), which may appear within 6 hr of 1st dose and may be difficult to distinguish from psychotic agitation. Benztropine may be used to differentiate agitation from akathisia. Observe closely for extrapyramidal side effects (*parkinsonian:* difficulty speaking or swallowing, loss of balance control, pill rolling of hands, masklike face, shuffling gait, rigidity, tremors; and *dystonic:* muscle spasms, twisting motions, twitching, inability to move eyes, weakness of arms or legs). Trihexyphenidyl or benzotropine may be used to control these symptoms. Benzodiazepines may alleviate akathisia.
- Monitor for tardive dyskinesia (uncontrolled rhythmic movement of mouth, face, and extremities; lip smacking or puckering; puffing of cheeks; uncontrolled chewing; rapid or worm-like movements of tongue, excessive eye blinking). Report immediately; may be irreversible.
- Monitor for symptoms related to hyperprolactinemia (menstrual abnormalities, galactorrhea, sexual dysfunction).
- Monitor for development of neuroleptic malignant syndrome (fever, respiratory distress, tachycardia, seizures, diaphoresis, hypertension or hypotension, pallor, tiredness, severe muscle stiffness, loss of bladder control). Report symptoms and immediately discontinue; manage as medically indicated.
- Assess for falls risk. Drowsiness, orthostatic hypotension, and motor and sensory instability ↑ risk. Institute falls prevention if indicated.

Lab Test Considerations

- Monitor CBC with differential and liver function tests periodically during therapy. If ANC ≤1000/mm^3, discontinue therapy until WBC count recovers.
- Monitor serum prolactin prior to and periodically during therapy. May cause ↑ serum prolactin levels.

Implementation

- Avoid skin contact with oral solution; may cause contact dermatitis.
- **PO:** Administer with food or full glass of water or milk to minimize GI irritation.
- Use calibrated measuring device for accurate dose. Do not dilute concentrate with coffee or tea; may cause precipitation. May be given undiluted or mixed with water or juice.
- **IM:** Inject slowly, using 2-in, 21-gauge needle into well-developed muscle via Z-track technique. Do not exceed 3 mL per injection site. Slight yellow color does not indicate altered potency. Keep patient recumbent for ≥30 min following injection to minimize hypotensive effects.

IV Administration

- **IV:** Haloperidol decanoate should not be administered IV.
- **IV Push: Dilution:** May be administered undiluted for rapid control of acute psychosis or delirium. **Concentration:** 5 mg/mL. **Rate:** Administer at a rate of 5 mg/min.
- **Intermittent Infusion: Dilution:** May be diluted in 30–50 mL of D5W. **Rate:** Infuse over 30 min.
- **Continuous Infusion: Dilution:** May be diluted in D5W or 0.9% normal saline. **Concentration:** 3 mg/mL in D5W or 0.75 mg/mL in 0.9% normal saline.
- **Rate:** Infuse at 3–25 mg/hr initially; titrate upward by 5 mg/hr to a max of 40 mg/hr.
- **Y-Site Compatibility:** acetaminophen, alemtuzumab, aminocaproic acid, amphotericin B liposomal, anidulafungin, argatroban, arsenic trioxide, azithromycin, bleomycin, cangrelor, carboplatin, carmustine, caspofungin, ceftaroline, cisatracurium, cisplatin, cladribine, clonidine, cyclophosphamide, cytarabine, dacarbazine, dactinomycin, daptomycin, daunorubicin, dexmedetomidine, dexrazoxane, diltiazem, docetaxel, doxorubicin hydrochloride, doxorubicin liposomal, epirubicin, eptifibatide, ertapenem, etoposide, etoposide phosphate, filgrastim, fludarabine, gemcitabine, granisetron, hydromorphone, idarubicin, ifosfamide, irinotecan, ketamine, leucovorin, levofloxacin, linezolid, lorazepam, melphalan, mesna, methadone, metronidazole, milrinone, mitoxantrone, morphine, moxifloxacin, mycophenolate, nicardipine, octreotide, oritavancin, oxaliplatin, paclitaxel, palonosetron, pamidronate, pemetrexed, potassium acetate, propofol, remifentanil, rituximab, rocuronium, sodium acetate, tacrolimus, thiotepa, tigecycline, tirofiban, topotecan, trastuzumab, vecuronium, vinblastine, vincristine, vinorelbine, voriconazole, zoledronic acid.
- **Y-Site Incompatibility:** acyclovir, allopurinol, aminophylline, amphotericin B deoxycholate, ampicillin, ampicillin/sulbactam, azathioprine, bumetanide, calcium chloride, cefazolin, cefepime, cefotaxime, cefotetan, cefoxitin, ceftazidime, ceftobiprole, ceftriaxone, cefuroxime, chloramphenicol, clindamycin, dantrolene, dexamethasone, diazepam, diazoxide, epoetin alfa, fluorouracil, folic acid, foscarnet, fosphenytoin, furosemide, ganciclovir, gemtuzumab ozogamicin, heparin, hydralazine, hydrocortisone, imipenem/cilastatin, imipenem/cilastatin/relebactam, indomethacin, ketorolac, magnesium sulfate, methylprednisolone, minocycline, mitomycin, nafcillin, oxacillin, pantoprazole, penicillin G, pentobarbital, phenobarbital, phenytoin, piperacillin/tazobactam, potassium chloride, sargramostim, sodium bicarbonate, trimethoprim/sulfamethoxazole.

Patient/Family Teaching

- Explain the purpose and side effects. Advise patient to take medication as directed. Take missed doses as soon as remembered, with remaining doses evenly spaced throughout the day. May require several weeks to obtain desired effects. Do not ↑ dose or discontinue medication without consulting health care provider. Abrupt withdrawal may cause dizziness; nausea; vomiting; GI upset; trembling; or uncontrolled movements of mouth, tongue, or jaw. Advise patient to read *Patient Information* before starting and with each Rx refill in case of changes.
- Emphasize the importance of routine follow-up exams to monitor response to medication and detect side effects.
- Inform patient of possibility of extrapyramidal symptoms, tardive dyskinesia, and neuroleptic malignant syndrome. Caution patient to report symptoms immediately.
- Advise patient to change positions slowly to minimize orthostatic hypotension. Protect from falls.
- May cause drowsiness. Caution patient to avoid driving or other activities requiring alertness until response to medication is known.
- Instruct patient to notify health care provider of all Rx or OTC medications, vitamins, or herbal products being taken and to consult with health care provider before taking other medications.
- Caution patient to avoid taking alcohol or other CNS depressants, including opioids, concurrently with this medication.
- Advise patient to use sunscreen and protective clothing when exposed to the sun to prevent photosensitivity reactions. Extremes of temperature should also be avoided; drug impairs body temperature regulation.
- Instruct patient to use frequent mouth rinses, good oral hygiene, and sugarless gum or candy to minimize dry mouth.
- Advise patient to notify health care provider of medication regimen prior to treatment or surgery.
- Instruct patient to notify health care provider promptly if weakness, tremors, visual disturbances, dark-colored urine or clay-colored stools, sore throat, fever, menstrual abnormalities, galactorrhea, or sexual dysfunction occur.
- Rep: Advise women of reproductive potential to notify health care provider if pregnancy is planned or suspected and to avoid breastfeeding during therapy. Monitor neonates exposed to haloperidol during the 3rd trimester of pregnancy

H

for extrapyramidal and/or withdrawal symptoms following delivery. There have been reports of agitation, hypertonia, hypotonia, tremor, somnolence, respiratory distress, and feeding disorder in these neonates. Inform patient of the National Pregnancy Registry for Psychiatric Medications, which monitors the safety of psychiatric medications taken by women during pregnancy. Encourage patient to contact the registry at https://womensmentalhealth.org/clinical-and-research-programs/pregnancyregistry or by phone at 1-866-961-2388. Monitor breastfed infants for excessive drowsiness, lethargy, and developmental delays.

Evaluation/Desired Outcomes

- Decrease in hallucinations, insomnia, agitation, hostility, and delusions.
- Decreased tics and vocalization in Tourette syndrome.
- Improved behavior in children with severe behavioral problems. If no therapeutic effects are seen in 2–4 wk, dosage may be increased.

HIGH ALERT

heparin (hep-a-rin)

Classification
Therapeutic: anticoagulants
Pharmacologic: antithrombotics

Indications

Prophylaxis and treatment of various thromboembolic disorders, including: Deep vein thrombosis (DVT), Pulmonary embolism (PE), Atrial fibrillation with embolization, Acute and chronic consumptive coagulopathies, Peripheral arterial thromboembolism. Used in very low doses (10–100 units) to maintain patency of IV catheters (heparin flush).

Action

Potentiates the inhibitory effect of antithrombin on factor Xa and thrombin. In low doses, prevents the conversion of prothrombin to thrombin by its effects on factor Xa. Higher doses neutralize thrombin, preventing the conversion of fibrinogen to fibrin. **Therapeutic Effects:** Prevention of thrombus formation. Prevention of extension of existing thrombi (full dose).

Pharmacokinetics

Absorption: Erratically absorbed following SUBQ or IM administration. IV administration results in complete bioavailability.
Distribution: Widely distributed to tissues.
Metabolism and Excretion: Probably removed by the reticuloendothelial system (lymph nodes, spleen).
Half-life: 1–2 hr (↑ with ↑ dose); affected by obesity, renal and hepatic function, malignancy, presence of PE, and infections.

TIME/ACTION PROFILE (anticoagulant effect)

ROUTE	ONSET	PEAK	DURATION
SUBQ	20–60 min	2 hr	8–12 hr
IV	immediate	5–10 min	2–6 hr

Contraindications/Precautions

Contraindicated in: Hypersensitivity; Uncontrolled bleeding; History of heparin-induced thrombocytopenia (HIT); Severe thrombocytopenia; Pedi: Avoid use of products containing benzyl alcohol in premature infants.
Use Cautiously in: Severe renal impairment; Severe hepatic impairment; Retinopathy (hypertensive or diabetic); Ulcer disease; Spinal cord or brain injury; History of congenital or acquired bleeding disorder; Malignancy; Diabetes mellitus, chronic renal failure, metabolic acidosis, increased serum potassium, or concurrent use of potassium-sparing drugs (↑ risk of hyperkalemia); Allergy to pork products; OB: Use during pregnancy only if potential maternal benefit justifies potential fetal risk; avoid use of products containing benzyl alcohol; Lactation: Use while breastfeeding only if potential maternal benefit justifies potential risk to infant; avoid use of products containing benzyl alcohol; Geri: Women >60 yr have ↑ risk of bleeding.
Exercise Extreme Caution in: Severe uncontrolled hypertension; Bacterial endocarditis, bleeding disorders; GI bleeding/ulceration/pathology; Hemorrhagic stroke; History of thrombocytopenia related to heparin; Recent CNS or ophthalmologic surgery; Active GI bleeding/ulceration.

Adverse Reactions/Side Effects

Derm: alopecia (long-term use), rash, urticaria. **F and E** hyperkalemia. **GI:** ↑ liver enzymes. **Hemat:** anemia, BLEEDING, HIT (WITH OR WITHOUT THROMBOSIS). **Local:** pain at injection site. **MS:** osteoporosis (long-term use). **Misc:** fever, hypersensitivity reactions.

Interactions

Heparin is frequently used concurrently or sequentially with other agents affecting coagulation. The risk of potentially serious interactions is greatest with full anticoagulation.
Drug-Drug: Aspirin, NSAIDs, clopidogrel, dipyridamole, some **penicillins, eptifibatide, tirofiban,** and **dextran** may ↑ risk of bleeding. **Quinidine, cefotetan,** and **valproic acid** may ↑ risk of bleeding. **Thrombolytics** may ↑ risk of bleeding. **Digoxin, tetracyclines, nicotine,** and **antihistamines** may ↓ effects.
Drug-Natural Products: ↑ risk of bleeding with **arnica, anise, chamomile, clove, dong quai, feverfew, garlic, ginger,** and **Panax ginseng.**

Route/Dosage

Therapeutic Anticoagulation

IV (Adults): *Intermittent bolus:* 10,000 units initially, followed by 5000–10,000 units every 4–6 hr. *Continuous infusion:* 5000 units (35–70 units/kg) initially, followed by 1000 units/hr or 15–18 units/kg/hr; adjust to maintain therapeutic aPTT.

IV (Children >1 yr): *Intermittent bolus:* 50–100 units/kg initially, followed by 50–100 units/kg every 4 hr. *Continuous infusion:* 75 units/kg initially, followed by 20 units/kg/hr; adjust to maintain therapeutic aPTT.

IV (Children <1 yr): *Continuous infusion:*75 units/kg initially, followed by 28 units/kg/hr; adjust to maintain therapeutic aPTT.

SUBQ (Adults): 5000 units IV, followed by initial SUBQ dose of 10,000–20,000 units; then 8000–10,000 units every 8 hr or 15,000–20,000 units every 12 hr.

Prophylaxis of Thromboembolism

SUBQ (Adults): 5000 units every 8–12 hr (may be started 2 hr prior to surgery).

Cardiovascular Surgery

IV (Adults): At least 150 units/kg (300 units/kg if procedure <60 min; 400 units/kg if >60 min).

IA (Neonates, Infants, and Children): 100–150 units/kg via an artery prior to cardiac catheterization.

Line Flushing

IV (Adults and Children): 10–100 units/mL (10 units/mL for infants <10 kg; 100 units/mL for all others) solution to fill heparin lock set to needle hub; replace after each use.

Total Parenteral Nutrition

IV (Adults and Children): 0.5–1 units/mL (final solution concentration) to maintain line patency.

Arterial Line Patency

IA (Neonates): 0.5–2 units/mL.

Availability (generic available)

Premixed infusion: 1000 units/500 mL of 0.9% NaCl or D5W; 2000 units/1000 mL of 0.9% NaCl or D5W; 12,500 units/250 mL of 0.45% NaCl or D5W; 25,000 units/250 mL of 0.45% NaCl or D5W; 25,000 units/500 mL of 0.45% NaCl or D5W. **Solution for injection:** 10 units/mL, 100 units/mL, 1000 units/mL, 5000 units/mL, 7500 units/mL, 10,000 units/mL, 20,000 units/mL, 40,000 units/mL.

NURSING IMPLICATIONS

Assessment

- Assess for signs of bleeding and hemorrhage (bleeding gums; nosebleed; unusual bruising; black, tarry stools; hematuria; ↓ hematocrit or ↓ BP; guaiac-positive stools).
- Monitor for signs of HIT and HITT (DVT; PE; cerebral vein thrombosis; limb ischemia, gangrene, and necrosis; stroke; MI; other arterial or venous thrombi). *If arterial or venous thrombosis suspected,* evaluate with platelet count and treat as clinically indicated.
- Monitor for signs and symptoms of ↑ heparin resistance, especially in patients with fever, thrombosis, thrombophlebitis, infection, MI, cancer, and antithrombin III deficiency or who are postsurgical. *If resistance is suspected,* closely monitor coagulation tests and consider adjustment of heparin dose based on anti-factor Xa levels.
- Assess for evidence of effective therapy. Symptoms depend on area of original thrombus involvement.
- Monitor for hypersensitivity reaction. *If chills, fever, or urticaria occur,* discontinue therapy, evaluate, and treat as clinically indicated.
- Assess injection sites for hematomas, ecchymosis, and erythema.

Lab Test Considerations

- Monitor aPTT and hematocrit prior to and periodically during therapy. For *intermittent IV* therapy, draw aPTT 30 min before each dose during initial therapy and then periodically. For *continuous* therapy, monitor aPTT levels every 4 hr. aPTT is typically not monitored when therapy is administered SUBQ.
- Obtain platelet counts before and periodically during heparin therapy. Thrombocytopenia may occur 2 days to several weeks after initiation and discontinuation. A ↓ in platelet count >50% from baseline is considered indicative of HIT. *For platelets <100,000/mm³ or recurrent thrombosis,* promptly discontinue heparin, evaluate for HIT or HITT, and administer another anticoagulant as needed.
- Monitor potassium before initiating therapy in patients at high risk for hyperkalemia and periodically in patients treated for >5 days.
- May ↑ AST and ALT.

Toxicity and Overdose

- Protamine sulfate is the antidote. Due to short half-life, overdose can often be treated by withdrawing heparin.

Implementation

- ***High Alert:*** Fatal hemorrhages have occurred in pediatric patients when heparin sodium injection vials were confused with heparin flush vials. Carefully examine all heparin vials to confirm the correct vial choice. Have second practitioner independently check original order, dose calculation, and infusion pump settings. Unintended concurrent use of two heparin products (unfractionated heparin and low-molecular-weight heparins) has resulted in serious harm or death. Review patients' recent (emergency department, operating room) and current medication records before administering any heparin product.

- ***High Alert:*** Do not confuse heparin with Hespan. Do not confuse vials of heparin with vials of insulin.
- Inform all personnel caring for patient of anticoagulant therapy. Venipunctures and injection sites require application of pressure to prevent bleeding or hematoma formation. Avoid IM injections of other medications.
- In patients requiring long-term anticoagulation, warfarin therapy should be instituted 4–5 days prior to discontinuing heparin therapy.
- **SUBQ**: Administer deep into SUBQ tissue. Alternate injection sites between arm and left and right abdominal wall above the iliac crest. Inject entire length of needle at a 45° or 90° angle into a skin fold held between thumb and forefinger; hold skin fold throughout injection. Do not aspirate or massage. Rotate sites frequently. Do not inject solution containing particulates.

IV Administration

- **IV Push: Dilution:** Administer loading dose undiluted. **Concentration:** Varies depending upon vial used. **Rate:** Administer over ≥1 min. Loading dose is given before continuous infusion.
- **Continuous Infusion: Dilution:** Dilute 25,000 units of heparin in 250–500 mL of 0.9% NaCl or D5W. Premixed infusions are already diluted and ready to use. Admixed solutions stable for 24 hr at room temperature or refrigerated. Premixed infusion stable for 30 days once overwrap removed. **Concentration:** 50–100 units/mL. **Rate:** See Route/Dosage section. Adjust to maintain therapeutic aPTT. Use an infusion pump to ensure accuracy.
- **Flush:** To prevent clot formation in intermittent infusion (heparin lock) sets, inject dilute heparin solution of 10–100 units/0.5–1 mL after each medication injection or every 8–12 hr. To prevent incompatibility of heparin with medication, flush lock set with sterile water or 0.9% NaCl for injection before and after medication is administered.
- **Y-Site Compatibility:** acetaminophen, acetylcysteine, acyclovir, alemtuzumab, allopurinol, alprostadil, aminocaproic acid, aminophylline, amphotericin B liposomal, anidulafungin, argatroban, arsenic trioxide, ascorbic acid, atropine, azathioprine, azithromycin, aztreonam, benztropine, bivalirudin, bleomycin, buprenorphine, butorphanol, caffeine citrate, cangrelor, carboplatin, carmustine, cefazolin, cefiderocol, cefotaxime, cefotetan, cefoxitin, ceftaroline, ceftazidime, ceftazidime/avibactam, ceftobiprole, ceftolozane/tazobactam, ceftriaxone, cefuroxime, chlorothiazide, cisplatin, cladribine, clevidipine, clindamycin, cyanocobalamin, cyclophosphamide, cyclosporine, cytarabine, dactinomycin, daptomycin, defibrotide, dexamethasone, dexmedetomidine, dexrazoxane, digoxin, docetaxel, dopamine, doxorubicin liposomal, edetate calcium disodium, enalaprilat, ephedrine, epinephrine, epoetin alfa, eptifibatide, eravacycline, ergonovine, ertapenem, esmolol, etoposide, etoposide phosphate, famotidine, fentanyl, fluconazole, fludarabine, fluorouracil, folic acid, foscarnet, fosphenytoin, ganciclovir, gemcitabine, gemtuzumab ozogamicin, glycopyrrolate, granisetron, hydrocortisone, hydromorphone, ibuprofen lysine, ifosfamide, imipenem/cilastatin, imipenem/cilastatin/relebactam, indomethacin, irinotecan, isoproterenol, ketorolac, leucovorin, lidocaine, linezolid, lorazepam, magnesium sulfate, mannitol, melphalan, meropenem, meropenem/vaborbactam, mesna, methadone, methohexital, methotrexate, metoclopramide, metoprolol, metronidazole, micafungin, midazolam, milrinone, mitomycin, minocycline, mitomycin, morphine, moxifloxacin, multivitamins, nafcillin, nalbuphine, naloxone, neostigmine, nitroglycerin, nitroprusside, norepinephrine, octreotide, omadacycline, ondansetron, oxacillin, oxaliplatin, oxytocin, paclitaxel, palonosetron, pamidronate, pemetrexed, penicillin G, pentobarbital, phenobarbital, phentolamine, phenylephrine, phytonadione, piperacillin/tazobactam, potassium acetate, potassium chloride, procainamide, prochlorperazine, propofol, propranolol, pyridostigmine, pyridoxine, remdesevir, remifentanil, rituximab, rocuronium, sargramostim, sodium acetate, sodium bicarbonate, succinylcholine, sufentanil, sulbactam/durlobactam, tacrolimus, tedizolid, theophylline, thiamine, thiotepa, tigecycline, tirofiban, topotecan, tranexamic acid, trastuzumab, vasopressin, vecuronium, verapamil, vinblastine, vincristine, voriconazole, zidovudine, zoledronic acid.
- **Y-Site Incompatibility:** alteplase, amiodarone, blinatumomab, caspofungin, ciprofloxacin, dantrolene, daunorubicin, diazepam, diazoxide, doxycycline, epirubicin, filgrastim, haloperidol, idarubicin, isavuconazonium, ketamine, levofloxacin, mitoxantrone, mycophenolate, oritavancin, palifermin, papaverine, pentamidine, phenytoin, plazomicin, protamine.

Patient/Family Teaching

- Explain purpose and side effects of medication. Advise patient to read *Patient Information* before starting therapy.

- Advise patient to report any symptoms of unusual bleeding or bruising to health care provider immediately.
- Instruct patient not to take medications containing aspirin or NSAIDs while on heparin.
- Caution patient to avoid IM injections and activities leading to injury and to use a soft toothbrush and electric razor during therapy.
- Advise patient to inform health care provider of heparin regimen prior to treatment or surgery.
- Advise patient to notify health care provider of all Rx or OTC medications, vitamins, or herbal products being taken and to consult health care provider before taking other medications.
- Rep: Advise women of reproductive potential to notify health care provider if pregnancy is planned or suspected or if breastfeeding.

Evaluation/Desired Outcomes

- Prolonged aPTT of 1.5–2.5 times the control without signs of hemorrhage.
- Prevention of DVT and PE.
- Patency of IV catheters.

HIGH ALERT

HEPARINS (LOW MOLECULAR WEIGHT)

dalteparin (dal-**te**-pa-rin)
Fragmin

enoxaparin (e-nox-a-**pa**-rin)
✱ Elonox, Enoxiluv Kit, ✱ Inclunox, Lovenox, ✱ Noromby, ✱ Redesca

Classification
Therapeutic: anticoagulants
Pharmacologic: antithrombotics

Indications

Enoxaparin and dalteparin: Prevention of venous thromboembolism (VTE) (deep vein thrombosis [DVT] and/or pulmonary embolism [PE]) in surgical or medical patients. **Dalteparin only:** Extended treatment of symptomatic DVT and/or PE in patients with cancer. **Enoxaparin only:** Treatment of DVT with or without PE (in combination with warfarin). **Enoxaparin and dalteparin:** Prevention of ischemic complications (with aspirin) from unstable angina and non–ST-segment-elevation MI. **Enoxaparin only:** Treatment of acute ST-segment-elevation MI (with thrombolytics or percutaneous coronary intervention).

Action

Potentiate the inhibitory effect of antithrombin on factor Xa and thrombin. **Therapeutic Effects:** Prevention of thrombus formation.

Pharmacokinetics

Absorption: Well absorbed after SUBQ administration (87% for dalteparin, 92% for enoxaparin).
Distribution: Minimally distributed to tissues.
Metabolism and Excretion: *Dalteparin:* Unknown; *enoxaparin:* Primarily eliminated renally.
Half-life: *Dalteparin:* 2.1–2.3 hr; *enoxaparin:* 3–6 hr (all are ↑ in renal insufficiency).

TIME/ACTION PROFILE (anticoagulant effect)

ROUTE	ONSET	PEAK	DURATION
Dalteparin SUBQ	rapid	4 hr	up to 24 hr
Enoxaparin SUBQ	unknown	3–5 hr	12 hr

Contraindications/Precautions

Contraindicated in: Hypersensitivity to specific agents, unfractionated heparin, or pork products; cross-sensitivity may occur; Some products contain sulfites or benzyl alcohol and should be avoided in patients with known hypersensitivity or intolerance; Active major bleeding; *Enoxaparin:* History of immune-mediated heparin-induced thrombocytopenia (HIT) within the past 100 days or in the presence of circulating antibodies; *Dalteparin:* History of HIT; *Dalteparin:* Regional anesthesia during treatment for unstable angina/non–ST-segment elevation MI.
Use Cautiously in: Severe renal impairment (adjust dose of enoxaparin if CCr <30 mL/min); Severe hepatic impairment; Women <45 kg or men <57 kg; Retinopathy (hypertensive or diabetic); Untreated hypertension; *Enoxaparin:* History of HIT >100 days ago and no circulating antibodies present; Recent history of ulcer disease; History of congenital or acquired bleeding disorder; OB: Safety not established in pregnancy; should not be used in pregnant patients with prosthetic heart valves or inherited/acquired thrombophilias without careful monitoring; if enoxaparin used during pregnancy, use preservative-free formulation; Lactation: Use while breastfeeding only if potential maternal benefit justifies potential risk to infant; Pedi: Safety and effectiveness not established in children; enoxaparin multidose vial contains benzyl alcohol, which can cause potentially fatal gasping syndrome in neonates; Geri: Older adults may have ↑ risk of bleeding due to age-related ↓ in renal function; Geri: *Dalteparin:* ↑ mortality in patients >70 yr with renal impairment.
Exercise Extreme Caution in: Neuroaxial spinal anesthesia or spinal puncture, especially if concurrent with an indwelling epidural catheter, drugs affecting hemostasis, history of traumatic/repeated spinal puncture, or spinal deformity (↑ risk of spinal hematoma); Severe uncontrolled hypertension; Bacterial endocarditis; Bleeding disorders.

Adverse Reactions/Side Effects

CV: edema. **Derm:** alopecia, ecchymoses, pruritus, rash, urticaria. **GI:** ↑ liver enzymes, constipation, nausea, vomiting. **GU:** urinary retention. **Hemat:** anemia, BLEEDING, eosinophilia, thrombocytopenia. **Local:** erythema at injection site, hematoma, irritation, pain at injection site. **MS:** osteoporosis. **Neuro:** dizziness, headache, insomnia. **Misc:** fever.

Interactions

Drug-Drug: Warfarin, **aspirin**, **thrombolytic agents**, **NSAIDs**, **dipyridamole**, some **penicillins**, **clopidogrel**, **eptifibatide**, **tirofiban**, and **dextran** may ↑ risk of bleeding.
Drug-Natural Products: ↑ bleeding risk with **arnica**, **chamomile**, **clove**, **feverfew**, **garlic**, **ginger**, **ginkgo**, **Panax ginseng**, and others.

Route/Dosage

Dalteparin

SUBQ (Adults): *Prophylaxis of DVT following abdominal surgery:* 2500 units 1–2 hr before surgery, then once daily for 5–10 days; *Prophylaxis of VTE in high-risk patients undergoing abdominal surgery:* 5000 units evening before surgery, then once daily for 5–10 days *OR* in patients with malignancy, 2500 units 1–2 hr before surgery, another 2500 units 12 hr later, then 5000 units once daily for 5–10 days; *Prophylaxis of VTE in patients undergoing hip replacement surgery:* 2500 units within 2 hr before surgery, then 2500 units 4–8 hr after surgery, then 5000 units once daily (start ≥6 hr after postsurgical dose) for 5–10 days *OR* 5000 units evening before surgery (10–14 hr before surgery), then 5000 units 4–8 hr after surgery, then 5000 units once daily for 5–10 days *or* 2500 units 4–8 hr after surgery, then 5000 units once daily (start ≥6 hr after postsurgical dose); *Prophylaxis of VTE in medical patients with severely restricted mobility during acute illness:* 5000 units once daily for 12–14 days. *Unstable angina/non–ST-segment-elevation MI:* 120 units/kg (not to exceed 10,000 units) every 12 hr for 5–8 days with concurrent aspirin; *Extended treatment of symptomatic VTE in cancer patients:* 200 units/kg (not to exceed 18,000 units) once daily for first 30 days, followed by 150 units/kg (not to exceed 18,000 units) once daily for Months 2–6.

Renal Impairment

SUBQ (Adults): *Cancer patients receiving extended treatment of symptomatic VTE with CCr <30 mL/min:* Monitor anti-Xa levels (target 0.5–1.5 IU/mL).

Enoxaparin

SUBQ (Adults): *VTE prophylaxis in patients undergoing knee replacement surgery:* 30 mg every 12 hr starting 12–24 hr postop for 7–10 days; *VTE prophylaxis in patients undergoing hip replacement surgery:* 30 mg every 12 hr starting 12–24 hr postop *OR* 40 mg once daily starting 12 hr before surgery (either dose may be continued for 7–14 days; continued prophylaxis with 40 mg once daily may be continued for up to 3 wk); *VTE prophylaxis following abdominal surgery:* 40 mg once daily starting 2 hr before surgery and then continued for 7–12 days or until ambulatory (up to 14 days); *VTE prophylaxis in medical patients with acute illness:* 40 mg once daily for 6–14 days; *Treatment of DVT/PE (outpatient):* 1 mg/kg every 12 hr. Warfarin should be started within 72 hr; enoxaparin may be continued for a minimum of 5 days and until therapeutic anticoagulation with warfarin is achieved (INR >2 for 2 consecutive days); *Treatment of DVT/PE (inpatient):* 1 mg/kg every 12 hr *or* 1.5 mg/kg once daily. Warfarin should be started within 72 hr; enoxaparin may be continued for a minimum of 5 days and until therapeutic anticoagulation with warfarin is achieved (INR >2 for two consecutive days); *Unstable angina/non–ST-segment-elevation MI:* 1 mg/kg every 12 hr for 2–8 days (with aspirin).
IV, SUBQ (Adults <75 yr): *Acute ST-segment-elevation MI:* Administer single IV bolus of 30 mg plus 1 mg/kg SUBQ dose (maximum of 100 mg for first 2 doses only), followed by 1 mg/kg SUBQ every 12 hr. The usual duration of treatment is 2–8 days. In patients undergoing percutaneous coronary intervention, if last SUBQ dose was <8 hr before balloon inflation, no additional dosing needed; if last SUBQ dose was ≥8 hr before balloon inflation, administer single IV bolus of 0.3 mg/kg.
SUBQ (Adults ≥75 yr): *Acute ST-segment-elevation MI:* 0.75 mg/kg every 12 hr (no IV bolus needed) (maximum of 75 mg for first 2 doses only no initial bolus). The usual duration of treatment is 2–8 days.

Renal Impairment

SUBQ (Adults CCr <30 mL/min): *VTE prophylaxis for abdominal or knee/hip replacement surgery:* 30 mg once daily. *Treatment of DVT/PE:* 1 mg/kg once daily. *Unstable angina/non–ST-segment-elevation MI:* 1 mg/kg once daily. *Acute ST-segment-elevation MI (patients <75 yr):* Single IV bolus of 30 mg plus 1 mg/kg SUBQ dose, followed by 1 mg/kg SUBQ once daily. *Acute ST-segment-elevation MI (patients ≥75 yr):* 1 mg/kg once daily (no initial bolus).

Availability

Dalteparin

Solution for injection (prefilled syringes): 2500 units/0.2 mL, 🍁 3500 units/0.28 mL, 5000 units/0.2 mL, 7500 units/0.3 mL, 🍁 10,000 units/0.4 mL, 10,000 units/1 mL, 12,500 units/0.5 mL

15,000 units/0.6 mL, ✱ 16,500 units/0.66 mL, 18,000 units/0.72 mL. **Solution for injection (multidose vials):** 25,00 units/mL, ✱ 10,000 units/mL, 25,000 units/mL.

Enoxaparin (generic available)

Solution for injection (prefilled syringes): 30 mg/0.3 mL, 40 mg/0.4 mL, 60 mg/0.6 mL, 80 mg/0.8 mL, 100 mg/1 mL, 120 mg/0.8 mL, 150 mg/mL. **Solution for injection (multidose vials):** 100 mg/mL.

NURSING IMPLICATIONS

Assessment

- Assess for signs/symptoms of bleeding and hemorrhage (bleeding gums; nosebleed; unusual bruising; black, tarry stools; hematuria; ↓ hematocrit or BP; guaiac-positive stools; bleeding from surgical site). Notify health care provider if these occur.
- Assess for evidence of additional or ↑ thrombosis. Symptoms depend on area of involvement. Monitor neurological status frequently for signs of neurological impairment. May require urgent treatment.
- Monitor for hypersensitivity reactions (chills, fever, urticaria). Report signs to health care provider.
- Monitor patients with epidural catheters frequently for signs/symptoms of neurologic impairment. Delay placement or removal of catheter for ≥12 hr after administration of lower doses (30 mg once or twice daily or 40 mg once daily) and ≥24 hr after administration of higher doses (0.75 mg/kg twice daily, 1 mg/kg twice daily, or 1.5 mg/kg once daily) of enoxaparin. Do not give 2nd enoxaparin dose in twice-daily regimen to patients receiving 0.75 mg/kg twice-daily dose or 1 mg/kg twice-daily dose to allow a longer delay before catheter placement or removal; then delay next dose for ≥4 hr. *For patients with CCr <30 mL/min,* double timing of removal of catheter, ≥24 hr for lower dose (30 mg once daily) and ≥48 hr for higher dose (1 mg/kg/day). Monitor for signs and symptoms of neurological impairment (midline back pain, sensory and motor deficits [numbness or weakness in lower limbs], bowel or bladder dysfunction) frequently if epidural or spinal anesthesia or lumbar puncture is done during therapy.
- **SUBQ**: Observe injection sites for hematomas, ecchymosis, or inflammation.

Lab Test Considerations

- Monitor CBC and stools for occult blood periodically during therapy. *If thrombocytopenia occurs (platelets <100,000 cells/mm³),* discontinue therapy. *If hematocrit ↓ unexpectedly,* assess patient for potential bleeding sites. For *dalteparin* use for extended treatment of symptomatic VTE in cancer patients, if platelets ↓ to 50,000–100,000 cells/mm³, ↓ dose to 2500 units once daily until recovery to ≥100,000 cells/mm³; if platelets <50,000 cells/mm³, discontinue until count returns to ≥50,000 cells/mm³.
- Special monitoring of aPTT is not necessary.
- Monitoring of antifactor Xa levels may be considered in patients who are obese or have renal impairment (for *enoxaparin,* obtain 4 hr after injection). Pregnant women with mechanical prosthetic heart valve should have antifactor Xa peak and trough monitored frequently due to ↑ risk of thrombosis; obtain 4–6 hr after *enoxaparin* injection.
- Monitoring of antifactor Xa levels may be necessary to titrate *enoxaparin* doses in pediatric patients (therapeutic range 0.5–1 unit/mL) and periodically in pediatrics patients on *dalteparin*; obtain 4 hr after injection.
- May ↑ AST and ALT.
- May cause hyperkalemia.

Toxicity and Overdose

- For *enoxaparin* overdose, protamine sulfate 1 mg for each mg of *enoxaparin* should be administered by slow IV injection. For *dalteparin* overdose, protamine sulfate 1 mg for each 100 antifactor Xa units of *dalteparin* should be administered by slow IV injection. If the aPTT measured 2–4 hr after protamine administration remains prolonged, a 2nd infusion of protamine 0.5 mg/100 antifactor Xa units of *dalteparin* may be administered.

Implementation

- ***High Alert:*** Unintended concurrent use of two heparin products (unfractionated heparin and low molecular weight heparins) has resulted in serious harm and death. Review patient's recent and current medication administration records before administering any heparin or low-molecular-weight heparin product.
- Cannot be used interchangeably (unit for unit) with unfractionated heparin or other low molecular weight heparins.
- Multiple-dose vials contain benzyl alcohol, which can cause fatal gasping syndrome in neonates and low-birth-weight infants.
- Assess for latex allergy in all persons handling prefilled syringe; dalteparin prefilled syringe needle shield may contain latex.
- **SUBQ**: Administer deep SUBQ while patient is sitting or lying down. To avoid loss of drug, do not expel the air bubble. For *dalteparin,* inject into the abdominal wall inferior, lateral to the umbilicus,

the upper outer side of the thigh, or the upper outer quadrant of the buttock. Rotate injection sites daily. For *enoxaparin*, inject between the left and right anterolateral and left and right posterolateral abdominal wall. Insert entire length of needle at a 45° or 90° angle while lifting and holding skin between thumb and forefinger. Do not aspirate or massage. Do not administer IM because of danger of hematoma formation. Do not administer solutions that are discolored or contain particulate matter. May be stored at room temperature.

- If excessive bruising occurs, ice cube massage of site before injection may lessen bruising.
- Use a tuberculin syringe when using multidose vials to ensure correct dose.
- To minimize risk of bleeding with enoxaparin after vascular instrumentation for unstable angina, recommended intervals between doses should be followed closely. Leave vascular access sheath in place for 6–8 hr after enoxaparin dose. Give next enoxaparin dose ≥6–8 hr after sheath removal. Observe site for bleeding or hematoma formation.

Enoxaparin

IV Administration

- **IV Push:** (for treatment of STEMI only) Use multiple-dose vial. Inject via IV line. Flush with 0.9% NaCl or D5W prior to and following administration to avoid mixture with other drugs and clear the port of the drug. May be administered with 0.9% NaCl or D5W. When administered with a thrombolytic, administer enoxaparin between 15 min before and 30 min after start of fibrinolytic therapy. **Rate:** Inject as a bolus.
- **Y-Site Incompatibility:** Do not administer other drugs through same IV line.

Patient/Family Teaching

- Explain purpose and side effects of low molecular weight heparins. Instruct patient in correct technique for self-injection and care and disposal of equipment. Advise patient to read *Patient Information* before starting therapy.
- Advise patient to report any symptoms of unusual bleeding or bruising, dizziness, itching, rash, fever, swelling, or difficulty breathing to health care provider immediately.
- Instruct patient to notify health care provider of all Rx or OTC medications, vitamins, or herbal products being taken and to consult health care provider before taking any other Rx, OTC, or herbal products. Instruct not take aspirin or NSAIDs without consulting health care provider.
- Inform patient having had neuraxial anesthesia or spinal puncture to watch for signs and symptoms of spinal or epidural hematoma (numbness or weakness of legs, bowel or bladder dysfunction). Notify health care provider immediately if symptoms occur.
- Advise patient to notify health care provider of medication regimen prior to treatment or surgery.
- Rep: Advise women of reproductive potential to notify health care provider if pregnancy is planned or suspected or if breastfeeding. Monitor for evidence of bleeding or excessive anticoagulation. Consider use of a shorter acting anticoagulant (e.g., heparin) as delivery approaches. Women with mechanical prosthetic heart valves may be at ↑ risk for thromboembolism during pregnancy and, when pregnant, have an ↑ rate of fetal loss from stillbirth, spontaneous abortion, and premature delivery. Frequently monitor peak and trough anti-factor Xa levels; adjustment of dose may be needed. Use caution when administering low molecular weight heparins preserved with benzyl alcohol to pregnant women; benzyl alcohol may cross the placenta. Large amounts of benzyl alcohol (99–404 mg/kg/day) ↑ risk of gasping syndrome (CNS depression, metabolic acidosis, gasping respirations) in premature infants. If anticoagulation with low molecular weight heparins is needed during pregnancy, use preservative-free formulations where possible.

Evaluation/Desired Outcomes

- Prevention of DVT and PE (enoxaparin and dalteparin).
- Resolution of DVT and PE (enoxaparin only).
- Prevention of ischemic complications (with aspirin) in patients with unstable angina or non–ST-segment-elevation MI (enoxaparin and dalteparin).
- Treatment of acute ST-segment-elevation MI (enoxaparin only).
- Treatment of symptomatic VTE in pediatric patients (dalteparin only).
- Decreased incidence of death or recurrent MI (dalteparin only).
- Extended treatment of symptomatic VTE, DVT, and/or PE in patients with cancer (dalteparin only).

HMG-CoA REDUCTASE INHIBITORS (statins)

atorvastatin (a-**tore**-va-stat-in)
Atorvaliq, Lipitor

fluvastatin (**floo**-va-sta-tin)
~~Lescol~~, Lescol XL

lovastatin (**loe**-va-sta-tin)
~~Mevacor~~

pitavastatin (pi-**tava**-sta-tin)
Livalo, Zypitamag
pravastatin (**pra**-va-sta-tin)
~~Pravachol~~
rosuvastatin (roe-**soo**-va-sta-tin)
Crestor, Ezallor Sprinkle
simvastatin (**sim**-va-sta-tin)
FloLipid, Zocor

Classification
Therapeutic: lipid-lowering agents
Pharmacologic: HMG-CoA reductase inhibitors

Indications

Adjunctive management of primary hypercholesterolemia and mixed dyslipidemias. **Atorvastatin:** Primary prevention of cardiovascular disease (↓ risk of MI or stroke) in patients with multiple risk factors for coronary heart disease (CHD) or type 2 diabetes mellitus (also ↓ risk of angina or revascularization procedures in patients with multiple risk factors for CHD). **Atorvastatin and pravastatin:** Secondary prevention of cardiovascular disease (↓ risk of MI, stroke, revascularization procedures, angina, and hospitalizations for HF) in patients with clinically evident CHD. **Fluvastatin:** Secondary prevention of coronary revascularization procedures in patients with clinically evident CHD. **Fluvastatin and lovastatin:** Slow progression of coronary atherosclerosis in patients with CHD. **Lovastatin:** Primary prevention of CHD (↓ risk of MI, unstable angina, and coronary revascularization) in patients without symptomatic cardiovascular disease with ↑ total and low-density lipoprotein cholesterol (LDL-C) and ↓ high-density lipoprotein cholesterol (HDL-C). **Pravastatin:** Primary prevention of CHD (↓ risk of MI, coronary revascularization, and cardiovascular mortality) in patients without clinically evident CHD. **Simvastatin:** Secondary prevention of cardiovascular events (↓ risk of MI, coronary revascularization, stroke, and cardiovascular mortality) in patients with clinically evident CHD or those at high-risk for CHD (history of diabetes, peripheral arterial disease, or stroke). **Rosuvastatin:** Slow progression of coronary atherosclerosis. **Rosuvastatin:** To reduce the risk of major adverse cardiovascular events (cardiovascular death, nonfatal MI, nonfatal stroke, or an arterial revascularization procedure) in patients without established coronary heart disease who are at increased risk of cardiovascular disease based on age, high-sensitivity C-reactive protein ≥2 mg/L, and at least one additional cardiovascular risk factor. **Rosuvastatin:** Adjunctive therapy to diet and exercise for the reduction of LDL-C in children 8–17 yr with heterozygous familial hypercholesterolemia if after diet therapy fails the following still exist: LDL-C remains >190 mg/dL or remains >160 mg/dL (with family history of premature cardiovascular disease or ≥2 risk factors for cardiovascular disease).

Action

Inhibit an enzyme, 3-hydroxy-3-methylglutaryl-coenzyme A (HMG-CoA) reductase, which is responsible for catalyzing an early step in the synthesis of cholesterol. **Therapeutic Effects:** Lower total and LDL-C and triglycerides. Slightly increase HDL-C. Slow the progression of coronary atherosclerosis with resultant decrease in CHD-related events.

Pharmacokinetics

Absorption: *Atorvastatin:* Rapidly absorbed but undergoes extensive GI and hepatic metabolism, resulting in 14% bioavailability; *Fluvastatin:* 98% absorbed after oral administration, but undergoes extensive first-pass metabolism resulting in 24% bioavailability; *Lovastatin, Pravastatin:* Poorly and variably absorbed after oral administration; *Pitavastatin:* well absorbed (51%) after oral administration; *Rosuvastatin:* 20% absorbed following oral administration; *Simvastatin:* 85% absorbed but rapidly metabolized.
Distribution: *Atorvastatin:* probably enters breast milk. *Fluvastatin:* enters breast milk. *Lovastatin:* crosses the blood-brain barrier and placenta. *Pravastatin:* small amounts enter breast milk. *Pitavastatin, Rosuvastatin, and Simvastatin:* unknown.
Protein Binding: *Atorvastatin, Fluvastatin, Pitavastatin, and Simvastatin:* >98%.
Metabolism and Excretion: All agents are extensively metabolized by the liver; amount excreted unchanged in urine: *Atorvastatin:* <2%, *Lovastatin:* 10%, *Fluvastatin:* 5%, *Pitavastatin:* 15%, *Pravastatin:* 20%, and *Simvastatin:* 13%.
Half-life: *Atorvastatin:* 14 hr; *Fluvastatin:* 1.2 hr; *Lovastatin:* 3 hr; *Pitavastatin:* 12 hr; *Pravastatin:* 1.3–2.7 hr; *Rosuvastatin:* 19 hr; *Simvastatin:* unknown.

TIME/ACTION PROFILE (cholesterol-lowering effect)

ROUTE	ONSET	PEAK	DURATION*
Atorvastatin	unknown	unknown	20–30 hr
Fluvastatin	1–2 wk	4–6 wk	unknown
Lovastatin	2 wk	4–6 wk	6 wk
Pitavastatin	within 4 wk	4 wk	unknown
Pravastatin	several days	2–4 wk	unknown
Rosuvastatin	unknown	2–4 wk	unknown
Simvastatin	several days	2–4 wk	unknown

* After discontinuation.

H

Contraindications/Precautions

Contraindicated in: Hypersensitivity; Active liver failure or decompensated cirrhosis; *Simvastatin and lovastatin:* Concurrent use of strong CYP3A4 inhibitors (↑ risk of myopathy/rhabdomyolysis); *Pitavastatin:* Concurrent use of cyclosporine; *Pitavastatin:* severe renal impairment; *Simvastatin:* Concurrent use of cyclosporine, gemfibrozil, or danazol (↑ risk of myopathy/rhabdomyolysis); *Simvastatin:* Chinese patients receiving ≥1 g/day of niacin (↑ risk of myopathy); Lactation: Lactation.

Use Cautiously in: History of liver disease; Alcoholism; *Rosuvastatin:* Patients with Asian ancestry (may have ↑ blood levels and ↑ risk of rhabdomyolysis); *Pitavastatin:* Hypothyroidism (higher risk of myopathy/rhabdomyolysis); Renal impairment; OB: Use statin therapy during pregnancy only if potential maternal benefit justifies potential fetal risk (if needed, consider using a more water-soluble agent [pravastatin or rosuvastatin] that is less likely to cross the placenta); Rep: Women of reproductive potential; Pedi: Safety and effectiveness not established in children <18 yr (fluvastatin, pitavastatin), <10 yr (atorvastatin, lovastatin, simvastatin), or <8 yr (pravastatin, rosuvastatin); Geri: *Atorvastatin and pitavastatin:* ↑ risk of myopathy in older adults.

Adverse Reactions/Side Effects

CV: chest pain, peripheral edema. **Derm:** rash, pruritus. **EENT:** rhinitis, blurred vision (lovastatin). **Endo:** hyperglycemia. **GI:** abdominal cramps, constipation, diarrhea, flatus, heartburn, ↑ liver enzymes, altered taste, drug-induced hepatitis, dyspepsia, nausea, pancreatitis. **GU:** erectile dysfunction. **MS:** arthralgia, arthritis, immune-mediated necrotizing myopathy (IMNM), myalgia, myopathy (↑ with simvastatin 80 mg/day dose), RHABDOMYOLYSIS. **Neuro:** amnesia, confusion, dizziness, headache, insomnia, memory loss, weakness. **Resp:** bronchitis. **Misc:** HYPERSENSITIVITY REACTIONS (INCLUDING ANGIOEDEMA AND URTICARIA).

Interactions

Atorvastatin, lovastatin, simvastatin, and rosuvastatin are metabolized by the CYP3A4 metabolic pathway. Fluvastatin is metabolized by CYP2C9. Pravastatin is not metabolized by the CYP P450 system.

Drug-Drug: Risk of myopathy with lovastatin is ↑ by **strong CYP3A4 inhibitors**, including **ketoconazole**, **itraconazole**, **posaconazole**, **voriconazole protease inhibitors**, **clarithromycin**, **erythromycin**, **nefazodone**, and **cobicistat-containing products**; concurrent use contraindicated. Risk of myopathy with simvastatin is ↑ by **cyclosporine**, **gemfibrozil**, **danazol**, **erythromycin**, **clarithromycin**, **protease inhibitors**, **nefazodone**, **ketoconazole**, **itraconazole**, **voriconazole**, **posaconazole**, and **cobicistat-containing products**; concurrent use contraindicated. Risk of myopathy with pitavastatin is ↑ by **cyclosporine**; concurrent use contraindicated. Bioavailability and effectiveness may be ↓ by **cholestyramine** and **colestipol**. Risk of myopathy with atorvastatin is ↑ by **clarithromycin**, **colchicine**, **cyclosporine**, **darunavir/ritonavir**, **elbasvir/grazoprevir**, **erythromycin**, **fosamprenavir**, **fosamprenavir/ritonavir gemfibrozil**, **glecaprevir/pibrentasvir**, **itraconazole**, **ledipasvir/sofosbuvir**, **letermovir**, **lopinavir/ritonavir**, **nelfinavir**, **niacin** (>1 g/day), or **tipranavir/ritonavir**; avoid concurrent use with **cyclosporine**, **gemfibrozil**, **glecaprevir/pibrentasvir**, or **tipranavir/ritonavir**; use lowest dose with **lopinavir/ritonavir**; use ↓ doses with clarithromycin, darunavir/ritonavir, elbasvir/grazoprevir, fosamprenavir, fosamprenavir/ritonavir, itraconazole, letermovir, or nelfinavir. Risk of myopathy with fluvastatin is ↑ by **gemfibrozil**, **erythromycin**, **colchicine**, **cyclosporine**, **azole antifungal agents**, or large doses of **niacin**; avoid concurrent use with gemfibrozil; use ↓ doses with cyclosporine and fluconazole. Risk of myopathy with lovastatin is ↑ by **amiodarone cyclosporine**, **gemfibrozil**, **diltiazem**, **verapamil**, **danazol**, and large doses of **niacin**; avoid concurrent use with gemfibrozil or cyclosporine; use ↓ doses with danazol, amiodarone, diltiazem, or verapamil. Risk of myopathy with pitavastatin is ↑ by **erythromycin**, **rifampin**, **colchicine**, **fibrates**, or large doses of **niacin**; avoid concurrent use with gemfibrozil; use ↓ doses with erythromycin, rifampin, and niacin. Risk of myopathy with pravastatin is ↑ by **cyclosporine**, **fibrates**, **colchicine**, **erythromycin**, **clarithromycin**, **azithromycin**, or large doses of **niacin**; avoid concurrent use with gemfibrozil; consider lower dose with niacin. Risk of myopathy with rosuvastatin is ↑ by **atazanavir/ritonavir**, **capmatinib**, **colchicine**, **cyclosporine**, **darolutamide**, **dasabuvir/ombitasvir/paritaprevir/ritonavir**, **elbasvir/grazoprevir**, **enasidenib**, **febuxostat**, **fibrates**, **fostamatinib**, **glecaprevir/pibrentasvir**, **lopinavir/ritonavir**, **niacin** (large doses), **regorafenib**, **sofosbuvir/velpatasvir**, **tafamidis**, **teriflunomide**, and **ticagrelor**; avoid concurrent use with gemfibrozil; use ↓ doses with atazanavir/ritonavir, capmatinib, cyclosporine, darolutamide, dasabuvir/ombitasvir/paritaprevir/ritonavir, elbasvir/grazoprevir, enasidenib, fostamatinib, glecaprevir/pibrentasvir, lopinavir/ritonavir, regorafenib, sofosbuvir/velpatasvir, tafamidis, and teriflunomide. Risk of myopathy with simvastatin is ↑ by **amiodarone**, **amlodipine**, **daptomycin**, **diltiazem**, **dronedarone**, **verapamil**, **ranolazine**, **lomitapide**, or **niacin**; avoid concurrent use with niacin at doses of ≥1 g/day in Chinese patients; temporarily suspend

simvastatin therapy during treatment with daptomycin; use ↓ doses with amiodarone, amlodipine, diltiazem, dronedarone, lomitapide, ranolazine, or verapamil. Atorvastatin, fluvastatin, and simvastatin may slightly ↑ **digoxin** levels. Atorvastatin and rosuvastatin may ↑ levels and risk of toxicity of **hormonal contraceptives**. Atorvastatin, fluvastatin, lovastatin, rosuvastatin, and simvastatin may ↑ risk of bleeding with **warfarin**. **Alcohol**, **cimetidine**, and **omeprazole** may ↑ levels and risk of toxicity of fluvastatin. **Rifampin** may ↓ levels and effectiveness of fluvastatin. **Antacids** may ↓ absorption of rosuvastatin; administer 2 hr after rosuvastatin. Fluvastatin ↑ levels of and risk of hypoglycemia with **glyburide**.
Drug-Natural Products: St. John's wort may ↓ levels and effectiveness of lovastatin and simvastatin.
Drug-Food: Large quantities of **grapefruit juice** may ↑ levels and risk of rhabdomyolysis with atorvastatin, lovastatin, and simvastatin; concurrent use contraindicated. **Food** ↑ levels of lovastatin.

Route/Dosage

Atorvastatin

PO (Adults): 10–20 mg once daily initially; may start with 40 mg/day if LDL-C needs to be ↓ by >45%; may ↑ every 2–4 wk up to 80 mg/day; *Concurrent use of nelfinavir:* Dose should not exceed 40 mg/day; *Concurrent use of clarithromycin, itraconazole, letermovir, darunavir/ritonavir, fosamprenavir, fosamprenavir/ritonavir, or elbasvir/grazoprevir:* Dose should not exceed 20 mg/day.
PO (Children ≥10 yr): 10 mg/day initially; may ↑ every 4 wk up to 20 mg/day; *Concurrent use of nelfinavir:* Dose should not exceed 40 mg/day; *Concurrent use of clarithromycin, itraconazole, darunavir/ritonavir, fosamprenavir, fosamprenavir/ritonavir therapy, or elbasvir/grazoprevir:* Dose should not exceed 20 mg/day.

Fluvastatin

PO (Adults): 20–40 mg (immediate release) once daily at bedtime. May ↑ to 40 mg twice daily (immediate release) or 80 mg once daily (extended release); *Concurrent use of fluconazole or cyclosporine:* Dose should not exceed 20 mg twice daily.

Lovastatin

PO (Adults): 20 mg once daily with evening meal. May ↑ at 4-wk intervals to a maximum of 80 mg/day; *Concurrent use of danazol, verapamil, or diltiazem:* Initiate at 10 mg once daily; do not exceed 20 mg/day; *Concurrent use of amiodarone:* Dose should not exceed 40 mg/day.
PO (Children ≥10 yr): *Familial heterozygous hypercholesterolemia:* 10–40 mg/day adjusted at 4-wk intervals.

Renal Impairment

PO (Adults): *CCr <30 mL/min:* Dose should not exceed 20 mg/day unless carefully titrated.

Pitavastatin

PO (Adults): 2 mg once daily initially; may ↑ up to 4 mg once daily depending on response. *Concurrent erythromycin therapy:* Dose should not exceed 1 mg/day; *Concurrent use of rifampin:* Dose should not exceed 2 mg/day.

Renal Impairment

PO (Adults): *CCr 30–<60 mL/min:* 1 mg once daily initially; may ↑ up to 2 mg daily.

Pravastatin

PO (Adults): 40 mg once daily at bedtime; may ↑ after 4 wk, if needed to 80 mg once daily at bedtime; *Concurrent use of cyclosporine:* Initiate therapy with 10 mg once daily at bedtime; may ↑ after 4 wk, if needed, to 20 mg once daily at bedtime (max dose = 20 mg/day); *Concurrent use of clarithromycin:* Dose should not exceed 40 mg/day.
PO (Children 14–18 yr): 40 mg once daily (max dose = 40 mg/day).
PO (Children 8–13 yr): 20 mg once daily (max dose = 20 mg/day).

Renal Impairment

PO (Adults): *CCr <30 mL/min:* Initiate therapy with 10 mg once daily at bedtime; may titrate at 4-wk intervals as needed (max dose = 80 mg/day).

Rosuvastatin

PO (Adults): 10 mg once daily initially (range 5–20 mg initially) (20 mg initial dose may be considered for patients with LDL-C >190 mg/dL or homozygous familial hypercholesterolemia); dose may be adjusted at 2–4 wk intervals, some patients may require up to 40 mg/day, however this dose is associated with ↑ risk of rhabdomyolysis; 🧬 *Patients with Asian ancestry:* Initial dose should be 5 mg; *Concurrent use of cyclosporine or darolutamide:* Dose should not exceed 5 mg/day. *Concurrent use of capmatinib, enasidenib, regorafenib, or teriflunomide:* Dose should not exceed 10 mg/day. *Concurrent use of gemfibrozil:* Avoid concurrent use. If concurrent use necessary, initiate at 5 mg once daily; dose should not exceed 10 mg/day. *Concurrent use of atazanavir/ritonavir, dasabuvir/ombitasvir/paritaprevir/ritonavir, elbasvir/grazoprevir, glecaprevir/pibrentasvir, lopinavir/ritonavir, or sofosbuvir/velpatasvir:* Initial dose should be 5 mg once daily; dose should not exceed 10 mg/day. *Concurrent use of tafamidis:* Avoid concurrent use. If concurrent use necessary, initiate at 5 mg once daily; dose should not exceed 20 mg/day.

PO (Children 10–17 yr): *Heterozygous familial hypercholesterolemia:* 5–20 mg once daily; *Patients with Asian ancestry:* Initial dose should be 5 mg; *Concurrent use of cyclosporine:* Dose should not exceed 5 mg/day; *Concurrent use of atazanavir/ritonavir, glecaprevir/pibrentasvir, lopinavir/ritonavir, or sofosbuvir/velpatasvir:* Dose should not exceed 10 mg/day.
PO (Children 8–<10 yr): *Heterozygous familial hypercholesterolemia:* 5–10 mg once daily; *Patients with Asian ancestry:* Initial dose should be 5 mg; *Concurrent use of cyclosporine:* Dose should not exceed 5 mg/day; *Concurrent use of atazanavir/ritonavir, lopinavir/ritonavir, or sofosbuvir/velpatasvir:* Dose should not exceed 10 mg/day.
PO (Children 7–17 yr): *Homozygous familial hypercholesterolemia:* 20 mg once daily. *Patients with Asian ancestry:* Initial dose should be 5 mg; *Concurrent use of cyclosporine:* Dose should not exceed 5 mg/day; *Concurrent use of atazanavir/ritonavir, lopinavir/ritonavir, or sofosbuvir/velpatasvir:* Dose should not exceed 10 mg/day.

Renal Impairment

PO (Adults): *CCr <30 mL/min:* 5 mg once daily initially; dose may be ↑ but should not exceed 10 mg/day.

Simvastatin

The 80-mg dose should be restricted to patients who have been taking this dose for ≥12 mo without evidence of muscle toxicity.
PO (Adults): 20–40 mg once daily in the evening; if LDL-C goal cannot be achieved with 40 mg/day dose, add another lipid-lowering therapy (do not ↑ simvastatin dose to 80 mg/day). *Concurrent use of verapamil, diltiazem, or dronedarone:* Dose should not exceed 10 mg/day. *Concurrent use of amiodarone, amlodipine, or ranolazine:* Dose should not exceed 20 mg/day; *Concurrent use of lomitapide:* ↓ dose by 50% (dose should not exceed 20 mg/day or 40 mg/day for patients who previously received 80 mg/day chronically [for ≥12 mo] without evidence of myopathy).
PO (Children 10–17 yr): 10 mg once daily in the evening initially; may ↑ at 4-wk intervals up to 40 mg/day. *Concurrent use of verapamil or diltiazem:* Dose should not exceed 10 mg/day. *Concurrent use of amiodarone, amlodipine, or ranolazine:* Dose should not exceed 20 mg/day.

Renal Impairment

PO (Adults): *CCr 15–29 mL/min:* 5 mg once daily in the evening initially, titrate carefully.

Availability

Atorvastatin (generic available)

Tablets: 10 mg, 20 mg, 40 mg, 80 mg. **Oral suspension (orange flavor):** 20 mg/5 mL. ***In combination with:*** amlodipine (Caduet). See Appendix N.

Fluvastatin (generic available)

Immediate-release capsules: 20 mg, 40 mg. **Extended-release tablets:** 80 mg.

Lovastatin (generic available)

Immediate-release tablets: 10 mg, 20 mg, 40 mg.

Pitavastatin (generic available)

Tablets: 1 mg, 2 mg, 4 mg.

Pravastatin (generic available)

Tablets: 10 mg, 20 mg, 40 mg, 80 mg.

Rosuvastatin (generic available)

Tablets (Crestor): 5 mg, 10 mg, 20 mg, 40 mg. **Sprinkle capsules (Ezallor):** 5 mg, 10 mg, 20 mg, 40 mg. ***In combination with:*** ezetimibe (Roszet). See Appendix N.

Simvastatin (generic available)

Tablets (Zocor): 5 mg, 10 mg, 20 mg, 40 mg, 80 mg. **Oral suspension (FloLipid):** 20 mg/5 mL, 40 mg/5 mL. ***In combination with:*** ezetimibe (Vytorin). See Appendix N.

NURSING IMPLICATIONS

Assessment

- Obtain a dietary history, especially with regard to fat consumption.
- Monitor for signs/symptoms of myopathy or rhabdomyolysis (malaise, myalgia, muscle cramps or weakness, dark or tea-colored urine). Predisposing factors for myopathy include ≥65 yr, female patients, uncontrolled hypothyroidism, and renal impairment. Asian patients may be at ↑ risk for myopathy.
- Pedi: In pediatric patients, monitor growth, development (with Tanner staging), and sexual maturation during therapy.

Lab Test Considerations

- Monitor lipid panel (total cholesterol, HDL-C, LDL-C, triglycerides) at baseline, after 2–4 wk of therapy, 2–4 wk after dose adjustments, and periodically.
- Monitor liver function tests, including AST and ALT, before initiating therapy and if signs of liver injury (fatigue, anorexia, right upper abdominal discomfort, dark urine, jaundice) occur. May also ↑ alkaline phosphatase and bilirubin levels.
- If patient develops muscle tenderness during therapy, monitor CK levels. If CK levels are >10 times the upper limit of normal or myopathy occurs, therapy should be discontinued. Monitor for signs and symptoms of IMNM (proximal muscle weakness, ↑ serum CK), persisting despite discontinuation of statin therapy. Perform muscle biopsy to diagnose; shows necrotizing myopathy without

significant inflammation. Treat with immunosuppressive agents.
- May ↑ A1c.

Implementation

- Do not confuse Lipitor with lisinopril or Zyrtec. Do not confuse Zocor with Cozaar or Zyrtec. Do not confuse atorvastatin with atomoxetine. Do not confuse pravastatin with pitavastatin. Do not confuse HMG-CoA reductase inhibitors ("statins") with nystatin.
- **PO:** Administer *lovastatin* with food. Administration on an empty stomach ↓ absorption by approximately 30%. Initial once-daily dose is administered with the evening meal.
- Administer extended-release tablets at bedtime. ***DNC:*** Extended-release tablets should be swallowed whole; do not break, crush, chew, or open capsules.
- Administer *fluvastatin, pravastatin,* and *simvastatin* once daily in the evening without regard to food. Do not administer two 40-mg *fluvastatin* tablets at one time (should be 2 divided doses/day). *Atorvastatin, pitavastatin,* and *rosuvastatin* can be administered any time of day without regard to food.
- Use a calibrated measuring device to ensure accurate dosing of *atorvastatin* and *simvastatin* oral suspensions. Shake well before using. Administer once daily at any time of day, only on an empty stomach (1 hr before or 2 hr after a meal). Use the 40-mg/5-mL strength for doses of ≥40 mg *simvastatin* oral suspension.
- Administer *Ezallor Sprinkle* (rosuvastatin) as a single dose at any time of day without regard to food. ***DNC:*** Swallow capsules whole; do not crush or chew. For patients who cannot swallow capsules, they may be opened, emptied, and swallowed along with a small amount (1 teaspoon) of soft food, such as applesauce or pudding, without chewing within 60 min.
- *Ezallor Sprinkle* (rosuvastatin) may be administered via 16-French nasogastric tube. Open the capsule and empty the intact granules into a 60-mL catheter tipped syringe and add 40 mL of water. Replace the plunger and shake the syringe vigorously for 15 seconds; the granules may start dissolving. Deliver the contents of the syringe immediately through the nasogastric tube; then flush with 20 mL of additional water. Use with any other liquids not recommended.
- Avoid grapefruit and grapefruit juice during therapy; may ↑ risk of toxicity.
- If *fluvastatin* or *pravastatin* is administered in conjunction with bile acid sequestrants (cholestyramine, colestipol), administer ≥4 hr after bile acid sequestrant.
- If *rosuvastatin* is administered concurrently with magnesium or aluminum-containing antacids, administer antacid ≥2 hr after *rosuvastatin*.

Patient/Family Teaching

- Explain the purpose and side effects of statins. Instruct to take as directed and not to skip doses or double up on missed doses. Take missed doses as soon as remembered but not if <12 hr before next dose. Advise patient to avoid drinking more than 1 quart of grapefruit juice/day during therapy. Medication helps control but does not cure ↑ serum cholesterol levels. Advise patient to read *Patient Information* before starting and with each Rx refill in case of changes.
- Emphasize the importance of follow-up exams to determine effectiveness and to monitor for side effects.
- Advise patient that this medication should be used in conjunction with diet restrictions (fat, cholesterol, carbohydrates, alcohol), exercise, and cessation of smoking.
- Instruct patient to notify health care provider if unexplained muscle pain, tenderness, or weakness, especially if accompanied by fever or malaise, or signs and symptoms of liver injury (fatigue, anorexia, right upper abdominal discomfort, dark urine, jaundice) occur.
- Advise patient to notify health care provider of all Rx or OTC medications, vitamins, or herbal products being taken and to consult with health care provider before taking other medications, especially St. John's wort.
- Inform patient that statins may ↑ A1c. Advise patient to maintain lifestyle measures (regular exercise, maintaining healthy body weight, making healthy food choices).
- Advise patient to wear sunscreen and protective clothing to prevent photosensitivity reactions (rare).
- Advise patient to notify health care provider of medication regimen before treatment or surgery.
- Rep: Advise patient to notify health care provider promptly if pregnancy is planned or suspected. Use statin therapy during pregnancy only if potential maternal benefit justifies potential fetal risk (if needed, consider using a more water-soluble agent [pravastatin or rosuvastatin] that is less likely to cross the placenta). Advise patients to avoid breastfeeding during therapy.

Evaluation/Desired Outcomes

- Decrease in LDL-C and total cholesterol levels.
- Increase in HDL-C levels.

H

- Decrease in triglyceride levels.
- Slowing of the progression of CHD.
- Prevention of cardiovascular disease.

hydrALAZINE
(hye-**dral**-a-zeen)

Apresoline

Classification

Therapeutic: antihypertensives

Pharmacologic: vasodilators

Indications
Moderate to severe hypertension. **Unlabeled Use:** New York Heart Associated Class III or IV HF with reduced ejection fraction (in combination with isosorbide dinitrate).

Action
Direct-acting peripheral arteriolar vasodilator. **Therapeutic Effects:** Lowering of BP in hypertensive patients and decreased afterload in patients with HF.

Pharmacokinetics
Absorption: Rapidly absorbed following oral administration; well absorbed from IM sites. IV administration results in complete bioavailability.
Distribution: Widely distributed.
Metabolism and Excretion: Mostly metabolized by the GI mucosa and liver by N-acetyltransferase (rate of acetylation is genetically determined [slow acetylators have ↑ hydralazine levels and ↑ risk of toxicity; fast acetylators have ↓ hydralazine levels and ↓ response]).
Half-life: 2–8 hr.

TIME/ACTION PROFILE (antihypertensive effect)

ROUTE	ONSET	PEAK	DURATION
PO	45 min	2 hr	2–4 hr
IM	10–30 min	1 hr	3–8 hr
IV	5–20 min	15–30 min	2–6 hr

Contraindications/Precautions
Contraindicated in: Hypersensitivity; Some products contain tartrazine and should be avoided in patients with known intolerance.
Use Cautiously in: Cardiovascular or cerebrovascular disease; Severe renal impairment (dose modification may be necessary); Severe hepatic impairment (dose modification may be necessary).

Adverse Reactions/Side Effects
CV: tachycardia, angina, arrhythmia, edema, orthostatic hypotension. **Derm:** rash. **GI:** diarrhea, nausea, vomiting. **MS:** arthralgias, arthritis. **Neuro:** dizziness, drowsiness, headache, peripheral neuropathy. **Misc:** drug-induced lupus syndrome.

Interactions
Drug-Drug: ↑ hypotension with acute ingestion of **alcohol**, other **antihypertensives**, or **nitrates**. **MAO inhibitors** may exaggerate hypotension. May ↓ pressor response to **epinephrine**. **NSAIDs** may ↓ antihypertensive response. **Beta blockers** ↓ tachycardia from hydralazine (therapy may be combined for this reason). **Metoprolol** and **propranolol** may ↑ levels and risk of toxicity. May ↑ levels and risk of toxicity of **metoprolol** and **propranolol**.

Route/Dosage
PO (Adults): *Hypertension:* 10 mg 4 times daily initially. After 2–4 days, may ↑ to 25 mg 4 times daily for the rest of the 1st wk; may then ↑ to 50 mg 4 times daily (up to 300 mg/day). Once maintenance dose is established, twice-daily dosing may be used. *HF:* 25–37.5 mg 4 times daily; may be ↑ up to 300 mg/day in 3–4 divided doses.
PO (Children >1 mo): 0.75–1 mg/kg/day in 2–4 divided doses (max = 25 mg/dose) initially; may ↑ gradually to 5 mg/kg/day in infants and 7.5 mg/kg/day in children (max = 200 mg/day) in 2–4 divided doses.
IM, IV (Adults): *Hypertension:* 5–40 mg repeated as needed. *Eclampsia:* 5 mg every 15–20 min; if no response after a total of 20 mg, consider an alternative agent.
IM, IV (Children >1 mo): 0.1–0.2 mg/kg/dose every 4–6 hr (max = 20 mg/dose) as needed, up to 1.7–3.5 mg/kg/day in 4–6 divided doses.

Availability (generic available)
Tablets: 10 mg, 25 mg, 50 mg, 100 mg. **Injection:** 20 mg/mL. ***In combination with:*** isosorbide dinitrate (BiDil). See Appendix N.

NURSING IMPLICATIONS
Assessment
- Monitor BP and HR frequently during initial dose adjustment and periodically during therapy (20 min after each dose). BP may start to fall within a few min after injection, with maximal effect in 10–80 min. Monitor the patient for ≥30–60 min prior to discharge from an ambulatory setting; monitoring time may vary based on the individual patient's response and any setting specific clinical guidelines. Observe for potential side effects, such as hypotension or reflex tachycardia.
- About 50–65% of White, Black, South Indian, and Mexican people are slow acetylators at risk for ↑ levels and toxicity, while 80–90% of Inuit, Japanese, and Chinese people are rapid acetylators at risk for ↓ levels and treatment failure.

Lab Test Considerations

- Monitor CBC, electrolytes, and ANA titer prior to and periodically during prolonged therapy.
- May cause a positive direct Coombs test result.

Implementation

- Do not confuse hydralazine with hydroxyzine, hydromorphone, or hydrochlorothiazide.
- IM or IV route should be used only when drug cannot be given orally.
- May be administered concurrently with diuretics or beta blockers to permit lower doses and minimize side effects.
- **PO:** Administer with meals consistently to enhance absorption.
- Pharmacist may prepare oral solution from hydralazine injection for patients with difficulty swallowing.

IV Administration

- **IV Push: Dilution:** Administer undiluted. Use solution as quickly as possible after drawing through needle into syringe. **Concentration:** 20 mg/mL. **Rate:** Administer over ≥1 min. Pedi: Administer at a rate of 0.2 mg/kg/min in children. Monitor BP and HR in all patients frequently after injection.
- **Y-Site Compatibility:** alemtuzumab, amiodarone, anidulafungin, argatroban, arsenic trioxide, bivalirudin, bleomycin, carmustine, cyclophosphamide, dacarbazine, dactinomycin, daptomycin, daunorubicin hydrochloride, dexrazoxane, diltiazem, docetaxel, etoposide, etoposide phosphate, fludarabine, gemcitabine, granisetron, hetastarch, hydromorphone, idarubicin, irinotecan, LR, leucovorin calcium, linezolid, mesna, methadone, metronidazole, milrinone, mitomycin, mitoxantrone, moxifloxacin, mycophenolate, octreotide, oxaliplatin, paclitaxel, palonosetron, pamidronate, prochlorperazine, 0.9% NaCl, 0.45% NaCl, tacrolimus, thiotepa, tirofiban, topotecan, vecuronium, vinblastine, vincristine, vinorelbine, voriconazole, zoledronic acid.
- **Y-Site Incompatibility:** acyclovir, ampicillin/sulbactam, ascorbic acid, azathioprine, aztreonam, cefazolin, cefotaxime, cefotetan, cefoxitin, ceftazidime, ceftriaxone, cefuroxime, D5W, dantrolene, diazepam, doxorubicin liposomal, ertapenem, folic acid, foscarnet, fosphenytoin, ganciclovir, gemtuzumab ozogamicin, haloperidol, indomethacin, lorazepam, meropenem, methylprednisolone, minocycline, multivitamins, nafcillin, nitroprusside, oxacillin, pantoprazole, pemetrexed, pentobarbital, phenytoin, piperacillin/tazobactam, potassium acetate, sodium acetate, tigecycline, trimethoprim/sulfamethoxazole.

Patient/Family Teaching

- Explain the purpose and side effects of hydralazine to patient. Emphasize the importance of continuing to take this medication, even if feeling well. Instruct patient to take medication at the same time each day; last dose of the day should be taken at bedtime. Take missed doses as soon as remembered; do not double doses. If >2 doses in a row are missed, consult health care professional. Must be discontinued gradually to avoid sudden ↑ in BP. Hydralazine controls but does not cure hypertension. Advise patient to read *Patient Information* before starting and periodically during therapy in case of changes.
- Emphasize the importance of follow-up exams to evaluate effectiveness of medication.
- Encourage patient to comply with additional interventions for hypertension (weight ↓, low-sodium diet, smoking cessation, moderation of alcohol intake, regular exercise, stress management). Instruct patient and family on proper technique for BP monitoring. Advise them to check BP at least weekly and report significant changes.
- Patients should weigh themselves twice weekly and assess feet and ankles for fluid retention.
- May occasionally cause drowsiness. Advise patient to avoid driving or other activities requiring alertness until response to medication is known.
- Caution patient to avoid sudden changes in position to minimize orthostatic hypotension.
- Advise patient to notify health care professional of all Rx or OTC medications, vitamins, or herbal products being taken and to consult with health care professional before taking other medications, especially cough, cold, or allergy remedies.
- Instruct patient to notify health care professional of medication prior to treatment or surgery.
- Advise patient to notify health care professional immediately if general tiredness; fever; muscle or joint aching; chest pain; skin rash; sore throat; or numbness, tingling, pain, or weakness of hands and feet occurs. Vitamin B_6 (pyridoxine) may be used to treat peripheral neuritis.
- Rep: Advise women of reproductive potential to notify health care professional if pregnancy is planned or suspected or if breastfeeding.

Evaluation/Desired Outcomes

- Decrease in BP without appearance of side effects.
- Decreased afterload in patients with HF.

H

hydralazine/isosorbide dinitrate

(hye-**dral**-a-zeen eye-so-**sor**-bide di-**ni**-trate)

BiDil

Classification

Therapeutic: vasodilators

Pharmacologic: vasodilators, nitrates

Indications

HF with reduced ejection fraction in Black patients.

Action

BiDil is a fixed-dose combination of **isosorbide dinitrate**, a vasodilator with effects on both arteries and veins, and **hydralazine**, a predominantly arterial vasodilator. **Therapeutic Effects:** Improved survival, increased time to hospitalization, and decreased symptoms of HF in Black patients.

Pharmacokinetics

Hydralazine

Absorption: 10–26% absorbed following oral administration; absorption can be saturated, leading to large ↑ in absorption with higher doses.

Distribution: Widely distributed to tissues.

Metabolism and Excretion: Mostly metabolized by GI mucosa and liver.

Half-life: 4 hr.

Isosorbide Dinitrate

Absorption: Variable absorption (10–90%) following oral administration, reflecting first-pass hepatic metabolism.

Distribution: Accumulates in muscle and venous wall.

Metabolism and Excretion: Undergoes extensive first-pass metabolism in the liver, mostly metabolized by the liver; some metabolites are vasodilators.

Half-life: 2 hr.

TIME/ACTION PROFILE (effect on BP)

ROUTE	ONSET	PEAK	DURATION
hydralazine (PO)	45 min	2 hr	2–4 hr
isosorbide (PO)	15–40 min	unknown	4 hr

Contraindications/Precautions

Contraindicated in: Hypersensitivity to either component; Concurrent use of PDE-5 inhibitor (avanafil, sildenafil, tadalafil, vardenafil) or riociguat.

Use Cautiously in: Severe renal impairment (dose modification may be necessary); Severe hepatic impairment (dose modification may be necessary); Head trauma or cerebral hemorrhage; OB: Safety not established in pregnancy; Lactation: Use while breastfeeding only if potential maternal benefit justifies potential risk to infant; Pedi: Safety and effectiveness not established in children; Geri: Start with lower doses in older adults.

Adverse Reactions/Side Effects

Hydralazine

CV: tachycardia, angina, arrhythmias, edema, orthostatic hypotension. **Derm:** rash. **GI:** diarrhea, nausea, vomiting. **MS:** arthralgias, arthritis. **Neuro:** dizziness, headache, drowsiness, peripheral neuritis, weakness. **Misc:** drug-induced lupus syndrome.

Isosorbide Dinitrate

CV: hypotension, tachycardia, paradoxical bradycardia, syncope. **GI:** abdominal pain, nausea, vomiting. **Misc:** flushing, tolerance.

Interactions

Drug-Drug: Avanafil, sildenafil, tadalafil, vardenafil, or riociguat may ↑ risk of severe hypotension; concurrent use contraindicated. ↑ risk of hypotension with other **antihypertensives**, acute ingestion of **alcohol**, and **phenothiazines**. **MAO inhibitors** may exaggerate hypotension. May ↓ the pressor response to **epinephrine**. **Beta blockers** ↓ tachycardia from hydralazine (therapy may be combined for this reason). **Metoprolol** and **propranolol** may ↑ hydralazine levels and risk of toxicity. Hydralazine may ↑ levels and risk of toxicity of **metoprolol** and **propranolol**.

Route/Dosage

PO (Adults): 1 tablet 3 times daily; may ↑ to 2 tablets 3 times daily.

Availability

Tablets: hydralazine 37.5 mg/isosorbide dinitrate 20 mg.

NURSING IMPLICATIONS

Assessment

- Monitor BP and HR routinely during period of dose adjustment. Symptomatic hypotension may occur even with small doses. Use caution with patients who are volume or sodium depleted or hypotensive.
- Assess for signs and symptoms of peripheral neuritis (paresthesia, numbness, tingling) periodically during therapy. Adding pyridoxine may cause symptoms to ↓.

Lab Test Considerations

- If symptoms of systemic lupus erythematosus (SLE) occur, obtain a CBC and ANA titer. If positive for SLE, carefully weigh risks/benefits of continued therapy.

Implementation

- Dose may be titrated rapidly over 3–5 days, but may need to ↓ if side effects occur. May ↓ to one-half tablet 3 times daily if intolerable side effects occur. Titrate up as soon as side effects subside.

Patient/Family Teaching

- Explain the purpose and side effects of hydralazine/isosorbide dinitrate. Instruct patient to take as directed on a regular schedule. Advise patient to read *Patient Information* before starting and with each Rx refill in case of changes.

- Caution patient to make position changes slowly to minimize orthostatic hypotension.
- May cause dizziness. Caution patient to avoid driving or other activities requiring alertness until response to medication is known.
- Advise patient to notify health care provider of all Rx or OTC medications, vitamins, or herbal products being taken and to consult with health care provider before taking other medications. Advise patient to avoid concurrent use of alcohol or medications for erectile dysfunction with this medication.
- Caution patient that inadequate fluid intake or excessive fluid loss from perspiration, diarrhea, or vomiting may lead to a ↓ in BP, dizziness, or syncope. If syncope occurs, discontinue medication and notify health care provider promptly.
- Inform patient that headache is a common side effect that should ↓ with continuing therapy. Aspirin or acetaminophen may be ordered to treat headache. Notify health care provider if headache is persistent or severe. Do not alter dose to avoid headache.
- Advise patient to notify health care provider if symptoms of SLE occur (arthralgia, fever, chest pain, prolonged malaise, other unexplained symptoms).
- Rep: Advise women of reproductive potential to notify health care provider if pregnancy is planned or suspected or if breastfeeding.

Evaluation/Desired Outcomes

- Improved survival, increased time to hospitalization, and decreased symptoms of HF in Black patients.

hydroCHLOROthiazide, See DIURETICS (THIAZIDE).

REMS HIGH ALERT

HYDROcodone

(hye-droe-**koe**-done)
Hysingla ER, ~~Zohydro ER~~

HYDROcodone/Acetaminophen
~~Anexsia, Norco, Vicodin~~

HYDROcodone/Ibuprofen
~~Reprexain~~

Classification
Therapeutic: allergy, cold, and cough remedies (antitussive), opioid analgesics
Pharmacologic: opioid agonists/nonopioid analgesic combinations

Schedule II

For information on the acetaminophen and ibuprofen components of these formulations, see the acetaminophen and ibuprofen monographs.

Indications

Extended-release product: Pain that is severe enough to warrant daily, around-the-clock, long-term opioid treatment for which alternative treatment options are inadequate. **Combination products:** Moderate to severe pain. Antitussive (usually in combination products with decongestants).

Action

Bind to opiate receptors in the CNS. Alter the perception of and response to painful stimuli while producing generalized CNS depression.
Suppress the cough reflex via a direct central action.
Therapeutic Effects: Decrease in severity of moderate pain. Suppression of the cough reflex.

Pharmacokinetics

Absorption: Well absorbed following oral administration.
Distribution: Unknown.
Metabolism and Excretion: Mostly metabolized by the liver; eliminated in the urine (50–60% as metabolites, 10% as unchanged drug).
Half-life: 2.2 hr; *Extended release:* 8 hr.

TIME/ACTION PROFILE (analgesic effect)

ROUTE	ONSET	PEAK	DURATION
PO	10–30 min	30–60 min	4–6 hr
PO-ER	unknown	unknown	unknown

Contraindications/Precautions

Noted for hydrocodone only; see acetaminophen/ibuprofen monographs for specific information on individual components.

Contraindicated in: Hypersensitivity to hydrocodone (cross-sensitivity may exist to other opioids); Significant respiratory depression; Paralytic ileus; Acute or severe bronchial asthma or hypercarbia; Congenital long QT syndrome (Hysingla only); Products containing alcohol, aspartame, saccharin, sugar, or tartrazine (FDC yellow dye #5) should be avoided in patients who have hypersensitivity or intolerance to these compounds; Lactation: Lactation.
Use Cautiously in: Personal or family history of substance use disorder or mental illness; Head trauma; ↑ intracranial pressure; Severe renal, hepatic, or pulmonary disease; Difficulty swallowing;

Undiagnosed abdominal pain; Prostatic hyperplasia; OB: Use during pregnancy only if potential maternal benefit justifies potential fetal risk. Chronic maternal treatment with opioids during pregnancy may result in neonatal opioid withdrawal syndrome. Geri: Older adults are more prone to CNS depression and constipation (initial dose ↓ required).

Adverse Reactions/Side Effects

Noted for hydrocodone only; see acetaminophen/ibuprofen monographs for specific information on individual components.

CV: hypotension, bradycardia, QT interval prolongation (Hysingla only). **Derm:** sweating. **EENT:** blurred vision, diplopia, miosis. **Endo:** adrenal insufficiency. **GI:** constipation, dyspepsia, nausea, choking, dysphagia, esophageal obstruction, vomiting. **GU:** urinary retention. **Neuro:** confusion, dizziness, sedation, euphoria, hallucinations, headache, unusual dreams. **Resp:** RESPIRATORY DEPRESSION (INCLUDING CENTRAL SLEEP APNEA AND SLEEP-RELATED HYPOXEMIA). **Misc:** allodynia, opioid-induced hyperalgesia, physical dependence, psychological dependence, tolerance.

Interactions

Drug-Drug: Use with extreme caution in patients receiving **MAO inhibitors**; may produce severe, unpredictable reactions; do not use within 14 days of each other. **CYP3A4 inhibitors**, including **ritonavir**, **ketoconazole**, **itraconazole**, **fluconazole**, **clarithromycin**, **erythromycin**, **nefazodone**, **diltiazem**, **verapamil**, **nelfinavir**, and **fosamprenavir**, may ↑ levels and risk of opioid toxicity; careful monitoring during initiation, dose changes, or discontinuation of the inhibitor is recommended. **CYP3A4 inducers**, including **barbiturates**, **carbamazepine**, **efavirenz**, **corticosteroids**, **modafinil**, **nevirapine**, **oxcarbazepine**, **phenobarbital**, **phenytoin**, **rifabutin**, or **rifampin**, may ↓ levels and analgesia; if inducers are discontinued or dosage ↓, patients should be monitored for signs of opioid toxicity and necessary dose adjustments should be made. Use with **benzodiazepines** or other **CNS depressants**, including other **opioids**, **nonbenzodiazepine sedative/hypnotics**, **anxiolytics**, **general anesthetics**, **muscle relaxants**, **antipsychotics**, and **alcohol**, may cause profound sedation, respiratory depression, coma, and death; reserve concurrent use for when alternative treatment options are inadequate. **Mixed agonist/antagonist analgesics**, including **nalbuphine** or **butorphanol**, and **partial agonist analgesics**, including **buprenorphine**, may ↓ analgesic effects and/or precipitate opioid withdrawal in physically dependent patients. **Anticholinergic drugs** may ↑ risk of urinary retention and constipation. Drugs that affect serotonergic neurotransmitter systems, including **tricyclic antidepressants**, **SSRIs**, **SNRIs**, **MAO inhibitors**, **TCAs**, **tramadol**, **trazodone**, **mirtazapine**, **5-HT$_3$ receptor antagonists**, **linezolid**, **methylene blue**, and **triptans**, may ↑ risk of serotonin syndrome.
Drug-Natural Products: **Kava-kava**, **valerian**, **skullcap**, **chamomile**, or **hops** can ↑ risk of CNS depression.

Route/Dosage

PO (Adults): *Analgesic (in combo products):* 2.5–10 mg every 3–6 hr as needed; if using combination products, acetaminophen dose should not exceed 4 g/day and should not exceed 5 tablets/day of ibuprofen-containing products; *Antitussive:* 5 mg every 4–6 hr as needed; *Extended-release capsules:* 10 mg every 12 hr; may ↑ as needed in increments of 10 mg every 12 hr every 3–7 days; *Extended-release tablets:* 20 mg once daily; may ↑ as needed in increments of 10–20 mg/day every 3–5 days.

Renal Impairment

PO (Adults): *CCr <45 mL/min:* Extended-release tablets: ↓ initial dose by 50%.

Hepatic Impairment

PO (Adults): *Extended-release tablets:* ↓ initial dose by 50%.

Availability

Hydrocodone (generic available)

Extended-release capsules: 10 mg, 15 mg, 20 mg, 30 mg, 40 mg, 50 mg. **Extended-release tablets (Hysingla ER) (abuse deterrent):** 20 mg, 30 mg, 40 mg, 60 mg, 80 mg, 100 mg, 120 mg. ***In combination with:*** chlorpheniramine.

Hydrocodone/Acetaminophen (generic available)

Tablets: 5 mg hydrocodone/325 mg acetaminophen, 7.5 mg hydrocodone/325 mg acetaminophen, 10 mg hydrocodone/325 mg acetaminophen. **Elixir/oral solution:** 7.5 mg hydrocodone plus 325 mg acetaminophen/15 mL, 10 mg hydrocodone plus 325 mg acetaminophen/15 mL.

Hydrocodone/Ibuprofen (generic available)

Tablets: 5 mg hydrocodone/200 mg ibuprofen, 7.5 mg hydrocodone/200 mg ibuprofen, 10 mg hydrocodone/200 mg ibuprofen.

NURSING IMPLICATIONS

Assessment

- Assess BP, HR, and respiratory rate before and periodically during administration. If respiratory rate <10/min, assess level of sedation. Dose may need to be ↓ by 25–50%. Respiratory depression does not ↑ in severity, only in duration, with ↑ dose. Monitor for respiratory depression, especially during initiation or following dose ↑; serious, life-threatening, or fatal respiratory depression may occur. May cause sleep-related breathing disorders (central sleep apnea, sleep-related hypoxemia).

- **Pain:** Assess type, location, and intensity of pain prior to and 1 hr (peak) following administration. When titrating opioid doses, ↑ of 25–50% should be administered until there is either a 50% ↓ in the patient's pain rating on a numerical or visual analogue scale or the patient reports satisfactory pain relief. A repeat dose can be safely administered at the time of the peak if previous dose is ineffective and side effects are minimal.
- Patients taking extended-release hydrocodone may require additional short-acting or rapid-onset opioid doses for breakthrough pain. Doses of short-acting opioids should be equivalent to 10–20% of 24 hr total and given every 2 hr as needed.
- Assess for opioid-induced hyperalgesia, which can appear as ↑ levels of pain upon increasing the dose of the opioid, ↓ levels of pain upon decreasing the dose of the opioid, or pain from ordinarily nonpainful stimuli (allodynia). This condition is different from tolerance. If a patient is suspected to be experiencing opioid-induced hyperalgesia, consider ↓ the dose of the current opioid or switching to a different opioid analgesic.
- An equianalgesic chart (see Appendix I) should be used when changing routes or when changing from one opioid to another.
- Prolonged use may lead to physical and psychological dependence and tolerance. This should not prevent patient from receiving adequate analgesia. Patients who receive opioids for pain rarely develop psychological dependence. If progressively higher doses are required, consider conversion to a stronger opioid. Prolonged use of opioids should be reserved for patients whose pain remains severe enough to require them and alternative treatment options continue to be inadequate. Many acute pain conditions treated in the outpatient setting require no more than a few days of an opioid pain medicine.
- Assess risk for opioid addiction, abuse, or misuse prior to administration. Abuse or misuse of extended-release preparations by crushing, chewing, snorting, or injecting dissolved product will result in uncontrolled delivery of hydrocodone and can result in overdose and death. Hysingla ER is an abuse deterrent formulation that is difficult to crush and, if crushed, results in a gel.
- **Cough:** Assess cough and lung sounds during antitussive use.

Lab Test Considerations

- May cause ↑ plasma amylase and lipase concentrations.

Toxicity and Overdose

- If an opioid antagonist is required to reverse respiratory depression or coma, naloxone is the antidote. Dilute the 0.4-mg ampule of naloxone in 10 mL of 0.9% NaCl and administer 0.5 mL (0.02 mg) by IV push every 2 min. For children and patients weighing <40 kg, dilute 0.1 mg of naloxone in 10 mL of 0.9% NaCl for a concentration of 10 mcg/mL and administer 0.5 mcg/kg every 2 min. Titrate dose to avoid withdrawal, seizures, and severe pain.

Implementation

- ***High Alert:*** Do not confuse hydrocodone with oxycodone.
- ***High Alert:*** Ensure accuracy when prescribing, dispensing, and administering hydrocodone bitartrate and acetaminophen oral solution. Dosing errors due to confusion between mg and mL can result in accidental overdose and death.
- Explain therapeutic value of medication prior to administration to enhance the analgesic effect.
- Regularly administered doses may be more effective than prn administration. Analgesic is more effective if given before pain becomes severe.
- Combination with nonopioid analgesics may have additive analgesic effects and permit lower doses. Maximum doses of nonopioid agents limit the titration of hydrocodone doses.
- Medication should be discontinued gradually after long-term use to prevent withdrawal symptoms. For patients on long-acting agents who are physically opioid-dependent, initiate the taper by a smalql enough increment (e.g., no greater than 10–25% of total daily dose) to avoid withdrawal symptoms, and proceed with dose-lowering at an interval of every 2–4 wk. May be necessary to provide patient with a lower dose strength for a successful taper. Monitor frequently to manage pain and withdrawal symptoms (restlessness; lacrimation; rhinorrhea; yawning; perspiration; chills; myalgia; mydriasis; irritability; anxiety; backache; joint pain; weakness; abdominal cramps; insomnia; nausea; anorexia; vomiting; diarrhea; or increased blood pressure, respiratory rate, or heart rate). If withdrawal symptoms occur, pause the taper for a period of time or ↑ the dose of opioid analgesic to the previous dose, and then proceed with a slower taper. Also, monitor patients for changes in mood, emergence of suicidal thoughts, or use of other substances. A multimodal approach to pain management may optimize the treatment of chronic pain and assist with the successful tapering of the opioid analgesic.
- ***REMS:*** FDA strongly encourages health care providers to complete a REMS-compliant education

program that includes all the elements of the FDA Education *Blueprint for Health Care Providers Involved in the Management or Support of Patients with Pain,* available at www.fda.gov/OpioidAnalgesicREMSBlueprint. Information on programs can be found at 1-800-503-0784 or www.opioidanalgesicrems.com.

- Discuss availability of naloxone for emergency treatment of opioid overdose with the patient and caregiver and assess the potential need for access to naloxone, both when initiating and renewing therapy, especially if patient has household members (including children) or other close contacts at risk for accidental exposure or overdose. Consider prescribing naloxone, based on the patient's risk factors for overdose, such as concurrent use of CNS depressants, a history of opioid use disorder, or prior opioid overdose. However, the presence of risk factors for overdose should not prevent the proper management of pain in any patient.
- **PO:** May be administered with food or milk to minimize GI irritation.
- *DNC:* Swallow extended-release capsules whole; do not open, crush, dissolve, or chew.

Patient/Family Teaching

- *REMS:* Advise patient to take medication as directed and not to take more than the recommended amount. Severe and permanent liver damage may result from prolonged use or high doses of acetaminophen. Renal damage may occur with prolonged use of acetaminophen or ibuprofen. Doses of nonopioid agents should not exceed the maximum recommended daily dose. Do not stop taking without discussing with health care provider; may cause withdrawal symptoms if discontinued abruptly after prolonged use. Do not ↑ doses without discussing with health care provider; may lead to overdose. Discuss safe use, risks, and proper storage and disposal of opioid analgesics with patients and caregivers with each Rx. The Patient Counseling Guide is available at www.fda.gov/OpioidAnalgesicREMSPCG.
- Instruct patient on how and when to ask for and take pain medication.
- Advise patient that hydrocodone is a drug with known abuse potential. Protect it from theft, and never give to anyone other than the individual for whom it was prescribed. Store out of sight and reach of children, and in a location not accessible by others.
- Educate patients and caregivers on how to recognize respiratory depression and emphasize the importance of calling 911 or getting emergency medical help right away in the event of a known or suspected overdose. Inform patients and caregivers about various ways to obtain naloxone as permitted by individual state naloxone dispensing and prescribing requirements or guidelines (by prescription, directly from a pharmacist, or as part of a community-based program).
- May cause drowsiness or dizziness. Advise patient to call for assistance when ambulating or smoking. Caution patient to avoid driving or other activities requiring alertness until response to the medication is known.
- Advise patient to notify health care provider if pain control is not adequate or if severe or persistent side effects occur.
- Advise patient to change positions slowly to minimize orthostatic hypotension.
- Caution patient to avoid concurrent use of alcohol or other CNS depressants with this medication; may lead to overdose.
- Instruct patient to notify health care provider of all Rx or OTC medications, vitamins, or herbal products being taken and consult health care provider before taking any new medications.
- Emphasize the importance of aggressive prevention of constipation with the use of hydrocodone.
- Encourage patient to turn, cough, and breathe deeply every 2 hr to prevent atelectasis.
- Advise patient that good oral hygiene, frequent mouth rinses, and sugarless gum or candy may decrease dry mouth.
- Rep: Advise women of reproductive potential to notify health care provider if pregnancy is planned or suspected or if breastfeeding. Inform patient of potential for neonatal opioid withdrawal syndrome with prolonged use during pregnancy. Monitor neonate for signs and symptoms of withdrawal symptoms (irritability, hyperactivity and abnormal sleep pattern, high-pitched cry, tremor, vomiting, diarrhea, failure to gain weight); usually occur the first days after birth. Monitor infants exposed to hydrocodone through breast milk for excess sedation and respiratory depression. Chronic use may ↓ fertility in women and men.

Evaluation/Desired Outcomes

- Decrease in severity of pain without a significant alteration in level of consciousness or respiratory status.
- Suppression of nonproductive cough.

hydrocortisone, See CORTICOSTEROIDS (SYSTEMIC).

hydrocortisone, See CORTICOSTEROIDS (TOPICAL).

REMS HIGH ALERT

HYDROmorphone

(hye-droe-**mor**-fone)

Dilaudid, ~~Dilaudid-HP, Exalgo,~~

✱ Hydromorph Contin

Classification

Therapeutic: opioid analgesics

Pharmacologic: opioid agonists

Schedule II

Indications

Moderate to severe pain (alone and in combination with nonopioid analgesics). Moderate to severe chronic pain in opioid-tolerant patients requiring use of daily, around-the-clock long-term opioid treatment and for which alternative treatment options are inadequate (extended release).

Action

Binds to opiate receptors in the CNS. Alters the perception of and response to painful stimuli while producing generalized CNS depression. Suppresses the cough reflex via a direct central action. **Therapeutic Effects:** Decrease in moderate to severe pain.

Pharmacokinetics

Absorption: Well absorbed following oral, rectal, SUBQ, and IM administration. Extended-release product results in an initial release of drug, followed by a 2nd sustained phase of absorption.

Distribution: Widely distributed to tissues.

Metabolism and Excretion: Mostly metabolized by the liver.

Half-life: *Oral (immediate release) or injection:* 2–4 hr; *Oral (extended release):* 8–15 hr.

TIME/ACTION PROFILE (analgesic effect)

ROUTE	ONSET	PEAK	DURATION
PO-IR	30 min	30–90 min	4–5 hr
PO-ER	unknown	unknown	unknown
SUBQ	15 min	30–90 min	4–5 hr
IM	15 min	30–60 min	4–5 hr
IV	10–15 min	15–30 min	2–3 hr
Rect	15–30 min	30–90 min	4–5 hr

Contraindications/Precautions

Contraindicated in: Hypersensitivity; Some products contain bisulfites and should be avoided in patients with known hypersensitivity; Severe respiratory depression (in absence of resuscitative equipment) (extended release only); Acute or severe bronchial asthma (extended release only); Paralytic ileus (extended release only); Acute, mild, intermittent, or postoperative pain (extended release only); Prior GI surgery or narrowing of GI tract (extended release only); Opioid-intolerant patients (extended release only); Severe hepatic impairment (extended release only).

Use Cautiously in: Personal or family history of substance use disorder or mental illness; Head trauma; ↑ intracranial pressure; Severe pulmonary disease; Moderate or severe renal impairment (extended release only) (dose ↓ recommended); Moderate hepatic impairment (extended release only) (dose ↓ recommended); Hypothyroidism; Seizure disorder; Adrenal insufficiency; Undiagnosed abdominal pain; Prostatic hypertrophy; Biliary tract disease (including pancreatitis); OB: Use during pregnancy only if potential maternal benefit justifies potential fetal risk. Chronic maternal treatment with opioids during pregnancy may result in neonatal opioid withdrawal syndrome; Lactation: Use while breastfeeding only if potential maternal benefit justifies potential risk to infant; Geri: Older adults may have ↑ risk of respiratory depression; dose ↓ suggested.

Adverse Reactions/Side Effects

CV: hypotension, bradycardia. **Derm:** flushing, sweating. **EENT:** blurred vision, diplopia, miosis. **Endo:** adrenal insufficiency. **GI:** constipation, dry mouth, nausea, vomiting. **GU:** urinary retention. **Neuro:** confusion, sedation, dizziness, dysphoria, euphoria, floating feeling, hallucinations, headache, unusual dreams. **Resp:** RESPIRATORY DEPRESSION (INCLUDING CENTRAL SLEEP APNEA AND SLEEP-RELATED HYPOXEMIA). **Misc:** allodynia, opioid-induced hyperalgesia, physical dependence, psychological dependence, tolerance.

Interactions

Drug-Drug: Exercise extreme caution with **MAO inhibitors**; may produce severe, unpredictable reactions; reduce initial dose of hydromorphone to 25% of usual dose; discontinue MAO inhibitors 2 wk prior to hydromorphone. Use with **benzodiazepines** or other **CNS depressants**, including other **opioids**, **nonbenzodiazepine sedative/hypnotics**, **anxiolytics**, **general anesthetics**, **muscle relaxants**, **antipsychotics**, and **alcohol**, may cause profound sedation, respiratory depression, coma, and death; reserve concurrent use for when alternative treatment options are inadequate. **Mixed agonist/antagonist analgesics**, including **nalbuphine** or **butorphanol**, and **partial agonist analgesics**, including **buprenorphine**, may ↓ hydromorphone's analgesic effects and/or precipitate opioid withdrawal in physically dependent patients. Drugs that affect serotonergic neurotransmitter systems, including **tricyclic antidepressants**, **SSRIs**, **SNRIs**, **MAO inhibitors**, **TCAs**, **tramadol**, **trazodone**, **mirtazapine**, **5-HT$_3$**

receptor antagonists, **linezolid**, **methylene blue**, and **triptans**, ↑ risk of serotonin syndrome.
Drug-Natural Products: Concurrent use of **kava-kava**, **valerian**, **chamomile**, or **hops** can ↑ CNS depression.

Route/Dosage

Doses depend on level of pain and tolerance. Larger doses may be required during chronic therapy.
PO (Adults ≥50 kg): *Immediate release:* 4–8 mg every 3–4 hr initially (some patients may respond to doses as small as 2 mg initially); *or* once 24-hr opioid requirement is determined, convert to *extended release* by administering total daily oral dose once daily.
PO (Adults and Children <50 kg): 0.06 mg/kg every 3–4 hr initially; younger children may require smaller initial doses of 0.03 mg/kg. Maximum dose 5 mg.
IV, IM, SUBQ (Adults ≥50 kg): 1.5 mg every 3–4 hr as needed initially; may be ↑.
IV, IM, SUBQ (Adults and Children <50 kg): 0.015 mg/kg every 3–4 hr as needed initially; may be ↑.
IV (Adults): *Continuous infusion (unlabeled):* 0.2–3 mg/hr depending on previous opioid use. An initial bolus of twice the hourly rate in mg may be given with subsequent breakthrough boluses of 50–100% of the hourly rate in mg.
Rect (Adults): 3 mg every 6–8 hr initially as needed.

Hepatic Impairment

PO (Adults): *Moderate hepatic impairment (extended release):* ↓ initial dose by 75%.

Renal Impairment

PO (Adults): *Moderate renal impairment (extended release):* ↓ initial dose by 50%; *Severe renal impairment (extended release):* ↓ initial dose by 75%.

Availability (generic available)

Immediate-release tablets: 2 mg, 4 mg, 8 mg. **Extended-release capsules:** 🍁 3 mg 🍁 4.5 mg 🍁 6 mg 🍁 9 mg 🍁 12 mg 🍁 18 mg 🍁 24 mg 🍁 30 mg. **Extended-release tablets (abuse deterrent):** 8 mg, 12 mg, 16 mg, 32 mg. **Oral solution:** 1 mg/mL. **Solution for injection:** 0.2 mg/mL, 1 mg/mL, 2 mg/mL, 4 mg/mL, 10 mg/mL. **Rectal suppositories:** 3 mg.

NURSING IMPLICATIONS

Assessment

- Assess type, location, and intensity of pain prior to and 1 hr following IM or PO and 5 min (peak) following IV administration. When titrating opioid doses, ↑ of 25–50% should be administered until there is either a 50% ↓ in the patient's pain rating on a numerical or visual analogue scale or the patient reports satisfactory pain relief. When titrating doses of short-acting hydromorphone, a repeat dose can be safely administered at the time of the peak if previous dose is ineffective and side effects are minimal.
- Assess BP, HR, and respiratory rate before and periodically during administration. If respiratory rate <10/min, assess level of sedation. Dose may need to be ↓ by 25–50%. Respiratory depression does not ↑ in severity, only in duration, with ↑ dose. Monitor for respiratory depression, especially during initiation or following dose ↑; serious, life-threatening, or fatal respiratory depression may occur. May cause sleep-related breathing disorders (central sleep apnea, sleep-related hypoxemia).
- Patients on a continuous infusion should have additional bolus doses provided every 15–30 min as needed for breakthrough pain. The bolus dose is usually set to the amount of drug infused each hr by continuous infusion.
- Patients taking extended-release hydromorphone may require additional short-acting or rapid-onset opioid doses for breakthrough pain. Doses of short-acting opioids should be equivalent to 10–20% of 24 hr total and given every 2 hr as needed.
- An equianalgesic chart (see Appendix I) should be used when changing routes or when changing from one opioid to another.
- Geri/Pedi: Assess geriatric and pediatric patients frequently; they are more sensitive to the effects of opioid analgesics and may experience side effects and respiratory complications more frequently.
- Assess for opioid-induced hyperalgesia, which can appear as ↑ levels of pain upon increasing the dose of the opioid, ↓ levels of pain upon decreasing the dose of the opioid, or pain from ordinarily nonpainful stimuli (allodynia). This condition is different from tolerance. If a patient is suspected to be experiencing opioid-induced hyperalgesia, consider ↓ the dose of the current opioid or switching to a different opioid analgesic.
- Prolonged use may lead to physical and psychological dependence and tolerance. This should not prevent patient from receiving adequate analgesia. Patients who receive hydromorphone for pain rarely develop psychological dependence. Progressively higher doses may be required to relieve pain with long-term therapy; may ↑ risk of overdose. Prolonged use of opioids should be reserved for patients whose pain remains severe enough to require them and alternative treatment options continue to be inadequate. Many acute pain conditions treated in the outpatient setting require no more than a few days of an opioid pain medicine.

- Assess bowel function routinely. Institute prevention of constipation with increased intake of fluids and bulk, and laxatives to minimize constipating effects. Administer stimulant laxatives routinely if opioid use exceeds 2–3 days, unless contraindicated. Consider drugs for opioid-induced constipation.
- Assess risk for opioid addiction, abuse, or misuse prior to administration. Abuse or misuse of extended-release preparations by crushing, chewing, snorting, or injecting dissolved product will result in uncontrolled delivery of morphine and can result in overdose and death.

Lab Test Considerations

- May ↑ plasma amylase and lipase levels.

Toxicity and Overdose

- If an opioid antagonist is required to reverse respiratory depression or coma, naloxone (Narcan) is the antidote. Dilute the 0.4-mg ampule of naloxone in 10 mL of 0.9% NaCl and administer 0.5 mL (0.02 mg) by IV push every 2 min. For children and patients weighing <40 kg, dilute 0.1 mg of naloxone in 10 mL of 0.9% NaCl for a concentration of 10 mcg/mL and administer 0.5 mcg every 2 min. Titrate dose to avoid withdrawal, seizures, and severe pain.

Implementation

- ***High Alert:*** Accidental overdose of opioid analgesics has resulted in fatalities. Before administering, check infusion pump settings. Pedi: Medication errors with opioid analgesics are common in pediatric patients; calculate doses carefully. Use appropriate measuring devices.
- ***High Alert:*** Do not confuse hydromorphone with buprenorphine, hydralazine, hydroxyzine, morphine, or oxymorphone; fatalities have occurred. Do not confuse high-potency dose forms with regular-dose forms.
- Explain therapeutic value of medication prior to administration to enhance the analgesic effect.
- Regularly administered doses may be more effective than prn administration. Analgesic is more effective if given before pain becomes severe.
- Coadministration with nonopioid analgesics may have additive analgesic effects and permit lower opioid doses.
- When converting from immediate-release to extended-release hydromorphone, administer total daily oral hydromorphone dose once daily; dose of extended-release product can be titrated every 3–4 days (see Appendix I). To convert from another opioid to extended-release hydromorphone, convert to total daily dose of hydromorphone and then administer 50% of this dose as extended-release hydromorphone once daily; can then titrate dose every 3–4 days. When converting from transdermal fentanyl, initiate extended-release hydromorphone 18 hr after removing transdermal fentanyl patch; for each 25 mcg/hr fentanyl transdermal dose, the equianalgesic dose of extended-release hydromorphone is 12 mg once daily (should initiate at 50% of this calculated total daily dose given once daily).
- Medication should be discontinued gradually after long-term use to prevent withdrawal symptoms. For patients on long-acting agents who are physically opioid-dependent, initiate the taper by a small enough increment (not >10%–25% of total daily dose) to avoid withdrawal symptoms, and proceed with dose-lowering at an interval of every 2–4 wk. May be necessary to provide patient with a lower dose strength for a successful taper. Monitor frequently to manage pain and withdrawal symptoms (restlessness; lacrimation; rhinorrhea; yawning; perspiration; chills; myalgia; mydriasis; irritability; anxiety; backache; joint pain; weakness; abdominal cramps; insomnia; nausea; anorexia; vomiting; diarrhea; or increased blood pressure, respiratory rate, or heart rate). If withdrawal symptoms occur, pause taper for a period of time or raise the dose of opioid analgesic to the previous dose, and then proceed with a slower taper. Monitor patients for changes in mood, emergence of suicidal thoughts, or use of other substances. A multimodal approach to pain management may optimize the treatment of chronic pain and assist with the successful tapering of the opioid analgesic.
- ***REMS:*** FDA strongly encourages health care providers to complete a REMS-compliant education program that includes all the elements of the FDA Education *Blueprint for Health Care Providers Involved in the Management or Support of Patients with Pain,* available at www.fda.gov/OpioidAnalgesicREMSBlueprint. Information on programs can be found at 1-800-503-0784 or www.opioidanalgesicrems.com.
- Discuss availability of naloxone for emergency treatment of opioid overdose with the patient and caregiver and assess the potential need for access to naloxone, both when initiating and renewing therapy, especially if patient has household members (including children) or other close contacts at risk for accidental exposure or overdose. Consider prescribing naloxone based on the patient's risk factors for overdose, such as concurrent use of CNS depressants, a history of opioid use disorder, or prior opioid overdose. However, the presence

of risk factors for overdose should not prevent the proper management of pain in any patient.

- **PO:** May be administered with food or milk to minimize GI irritation.
- ***DNC:*** Swallow extended-release tablets whole; do not break, crush, dissolve, or chew.

IV Administration

- **IV Push:** Administer undiluted. Inspect solution for particulate matter. Slight yellow color does not alter potency. Store at room temperature. **Rate:** Administer slowly over 2–3 min. ***High Alert:*** Rapid administration may lead to increased respiratory depression, hypotension, and circulatory collapse.
- For other clinical situations (sedation in mechanically ventilated patient), a continuous infusion may also be administered.
- **Y-Site Compatibility:** acetaminophen, acyclovir, alemtuzumab, allopurinol, amikacin, aminocaproic acid, aminophylline, amiodarone, amphotericin B deoxycholate, amphotericin B liposomal, ampicillin/sulbactam, anidulafungin, argatroban, arsenic trioxide, atracurium, atropine, azithromycin, aztreonam, bivalirudin, bleomycin, busulfan, calcium chloride, calcium gluconate, cangrelor, carboplatin, carmustine, caspofungin, cefepime, cefiderocol, cefotaxime, cefotetan, cefoxitin, ceftaroline, ceftazidime, ceftolozane/tazobactam, ceftriaxone, cefuroxime, chloramphenicol, chlorpromazine, ciprofloxacin, cisatracurium, cisplatin, cladribine, clindamycin, cyclophosphamide, cyclosporine, cytarabine, dacarbazine, dactinomycin, daptomycin, daunorubicin, dexamethasone, dexmedetomidine, dexrazoxane, digoxin, diltiazem, diphenhydramine, dobutamine, docetaxel, dopamine, doxorubicin hydrochloride, doxorubicin liposomal, doxycycline, droperidol, enalaprilat, ephedrine, epinephrine, epirubicin, eptifibatide, eravacycline, ertapenem, erythromycin, esmolol, etoposide, etoposide phosphate, famotidine, fentanyl, filgrastim, fluconazole, fludarabine, fluorouracil, foscarnet, fosphenytoin, ganciclovir, gemcitabine, gemtuzumab ozogamicin, gentamicin, glycopyrrolate, granisetron, haloperidol, heparin, hetastarch, hydralazine, hydrocortisone, idarubicin, ifosfamide, imipenem/cilastatin, insulin, regular, irinotecan, isavuconazonium, isoproterenol, ketorolac, labetalol, leucovorin, levofloxacin, lidocaine, linezolid, lorazepam, magnesium sulfate, mannitol, melphalan, meropenem, meropenem/vaborbactam, mesna, methohexital, methotrexate, methylprednisolone, metoclopramide, metoprolol, metronidazole, micafungin, midazolam, milrinone, mitomycin, mitoxantrone, morphine, mycophenolate, nafcillin, naloxone, nicardipine, nitroglycerin, nitroprusside, norepinephrine, octreotide, ondansetron, oxacillin, oxaliplatin, oxytocin, paclitaxel, palonosetron, pamidronate, pemetrexed, penicillin G potassium, pentamidine, pentobarbital, phenylephrine, piperacillin/tazobactam, plazomicin, posaconazole, potassium acetate, potassium chloride, potassium phosphates, procainamide, prochlorperazine, promethazine, propofol, propranolol, remdesivir, remifentanil, rituximab, sodium acetate, sodium phosphates, succinylcholine, sulbactam/durlobactam, tacrolimus, tedizolid, theophylline, thiotepa, tigecycline, tirofiban, tobramycin, topotecan, trastuzumab, trimethoprim/sulfamethoxazole, vancomycin, vasopressin, vecuronium, verapamil, vinblastine, vincristine, vinorelbine, zidovudine, zoledronic acid.
- **Y-Site Incompatibility:** clevidipine, dantrolene, dimenhydrinate, minocycline, phenytoin, sargramostim.

Patient/Family Teaching

- ***REMS:*** Instruct patient on how and when to ask for pain medication. Do not stop taking without discussing with health care provider; may cause withdrawal symptoms if discontinued abruptly after prolonged use. Do not ↑ doses without discussing with health care provider; may lead to overdose. Discuss safe use, risks, and proper storage and disposal of opioid analgesics with patients and caregivers with each Rx. The Patient Counseling Guide is available at www.fda.gov/OpioidAnalgesicREMSPCG.
- Advise patient that hydromorphone is a drug with known abuse potential. Protect it from theft, and never give to anyone other than the individual for whom it was prescribed. Store out of sight and reach of children, and in a location not accessible by others.
- Educate patients and caregivers on how to recognize respiratory depression and emphasize the importance of calling 911 or getting emergency medical help right away in the event of a known or suspected overdose. Inform patients and caregivers about ways to obtain naloxone as permitted by individual state naloxone dispensing and prescribing requirements or guidelines (by prescription, directly from a pharmacist, or as part of a community-based program).
- May cause drowsiness or dizziness. Advise patient to call for assistance when ambulating or smoking. Caution patient to avoid driving or other activities requiring alertness until response to medication is known.
- Advise patient to notify health care provider if pain control is not adequate or if side effects occur.
- Advise patient to change positions slowly to minimize orthostatic hypotension.
- Instruct patient to avoid concurrent use of alcohol or other CNS depressants.

- Instruct patient to notify health care provider of all Rx or OTC medications, vitamins, or herbal products being taken and consult health care provider before taking any new medications.
- Encourage patient to turn, cough, and breathe deeply every 2 hr to prevent atelectasis.
- Rep: Advise patient to notify health care provider if pregnancy is planned or suspected or if breast-feeding. Inform patient of potential for neonatal opioid withdrawal syndrome with prolonged use during pregnancy. Monitor neonate for signs and symptoms of withdrawal symptoms (irritability, hyperactivity and abnormal sleep pattern, high-pitched cry, tremor, vomiting, diarrhea, failure to gain weight); usually occur the first days after birth. Monitor infants exposed to hydromorphone through breast milk for excess sedation and respiratory depression. Chronic use may ↓ fertility in women and men.
- **Home Care Issues:** ***High Alert:*** Explain to patient and family how and when to administer hydromorphone; discuss safe storage of medication and proper care of infusion equipment. Pedi: Teach parents or caregivers how to accurately measure liquid medication and to use only measuring device dispensed with medication.
- Emphasize the importance of aggressive prevention of constipation with the use of hydromorphone.

Evaluation/Desired Outcomes

- Decrease in severity of pain without a significant alteration in level of consciousness or respiratory status.

hydroxychloroquine

(hye-drox-ee-**klor**-oh-kwin)

Plaquenil, Sovuna

Classification

Therapeutic: antimalarials, antirheumatics (DMARDs)

Indications

Treatment of uncomplicated malaria in geographic areas where chloroquine resistance is not reported. Prophylaxis of malaria in geographic areas where chloroquine resistance is not reported. Acute and chronic rheumatoid arthritis. Chronic discoid lupus erythematosus and systemic lupus erythematosus.

Action

Inhibits protein synthesis in susceptible organisms by inhibiting DNA and RNA polymerase. **Therapeutic Effects:** Death of plasmodia responsible for causing malaria. Also has anti-inflammatory properties. **Spectrum:** Active against chloroquine-sensitive strains of: *Plasmodium falciparum*, *Plasmodium malariae*, *Plasmodium ovale*, and *Plasmodium vivax*.

Pharmacokinetics

Absorption: Highly variable (31–100%) following oral administration.

Distribution: Widely distributed; high concentrations in RBCs.

Metabolism and Excretion: Partially metabolized by the liver to active metabolites; partially excreted unchanged by the kidneys.

Half-life: 40 days.

TIME/ACTION PROFILE (plasma concentrations)

ROUTE	ONSET	PEAK	DURATION
PO	rapid†	1–2 hr	days–wk

† Onset of antirheumatic action may take 6 wk.

Contraindications/Precautions

Contraindicated in: Hypersensitivity to hydroxychloroquine or chloroquine; Previous visual damage from hydroxychloroquine or chloroquine.

Use Cautiously in: Concurrent use of hepatotoxic drugs; Hepatic impairment or alcoholism; Use of high doses (>5 mg/kg/day), duration of use >5 yr, renal impairment, concurrent use of tamoxifen, or macular disease (↑ risk of retinopathy); Glucose-6-phosphate dehydrogenase deficiency; Psoriasis; Porphyria; Bone marrow depression; Obesity (determine dose by ideal body weight); Pedi: Safety and effectiveness for treatment of rheumatoid arthritis, chronic discoid lupus erythematosus, or systemic lupus erythematosus not established in children; Geri: ↓ renal function may ↑ risk of adverse reactions in older adults.

Adverse Reactions/Side Effects

CV: heart block, HF, QT interval prolongation, TORSADES DE POINTES. **Derm:** acute generalized exanthematous pustulosis, alopecia, DRUG REACTION WITH EOSINOPHILIA AND SYSTEMIC SYMPTOMS (DRESS), ERYTHEMA MULTIFORME, hair color changes, hyperpigmentation, photosensitivity, pruritus, rash, STEVENS-JOHNSON SYNDROME (SJS), TOXIC EPIDERMAL NECROLYSIS, urticaria. **EENT:** corneal deposits, nystagmus, retinopathy, tinnitus, vertigo, visual disturbances. **Endo:** hypoglycemia. **GI:** ↑ liver enzymes, abdominal pain, anorexia, diarrhea, HEPATOTOXICITY, nausea, vomiting. **GU:** proteinuria. **Hemat:** AGRANULOCYTOSIS, APLASTIC ANEMIA, leukopenia, thrombocytopenia. **Metab:** weight loss. **Neuro:** aggressiveness, anxiety, ataxia, dizziness, dyskinesia, dystonia, fatigue, headache, irritability, neuromyopathy, nightmares, peripheral neuritis, personality changes, psychoses, SEIZURES, SUICIDAL THOUGHTS/BEHAVIORS, tremor. **Resp:** bronchospasm, PULMONARY HYPERTENSION. **Misc:** ANGIOEDEMA.

Interactions

Drug-Drug: QT interval-prolonging drugs may ↑ risk of torsades de pointes. May ↑ risk of hypoglycemia when used with **antidiabetic agents**. **Mefloquine** may ↑ risk of seizures. **Antacids** may bind to and ↓ the absorption of hydroxychloroquine; separate administration by ≥4 hr. **Cimetidine** may ↑ levels and risk of toxicity; avoid concurrent use. May ↑ levels and risk of toxicity of **digoxin** or **cyclosporine**. May ↑ risk of adverse effects with **methotrexate**. Effectiveness may be ↓ by **rifampin**; avoid concurrent use. May ↓ levels and effectiveness of **ampicillin** and **praziquantel**.

Route/Dosage

Malaria

PO (Adults): *Prophylaxis:* 400 mg once weekly; start 2 wk prior to entering malarious area; continue for 4 wk after leaving area. *Treatment:* 800 mg initially, then 400 mg at 6 hr, 24 hr, and 48 hr after initial dose.

PO (Children ≥31 kg): *Prophylaxis:* 6.5 mg/kg (not to exceed 400 mg) once weekly; start 2 wk prior to entering malarious area; continue for 4 wk after leaving area. *Treatment:* 13 mg/kg (not to exceed 800 mg) initially, then 6.5 mg/kg (not to exceed 400 mg) at 6 hr, 24 hr, and 48 hr after initial dose.

Rheumatoid Arthritis

PO (Adults): 400–600 mg per day in 1–2 divided doses; once adequate response obtained, may ↓ dose to maintenance dose of 200–400 mg per day in 1–2 divided doses.

Lupus Erythematosus

PO (Adults): 200–400 mg per day in 1–2 divided doses.

Availability (generic available)

Tablets: 100 mg, 200 mg, 300 mg, 400 mg.

NURSING IMPLICATIONS

Assessment

- Assess deep tendon reflexes periodically to determine muscle weakness. Therapy may be discontinued should this occur.
- Obtain baseline ocular exam within first yr of therapy. Patients on prolonged high-dose therapy should have eye exams prior to and every 3–6 mo during therapy to detect retinal damage. Monitor patients without risk factors every 5 yr. Retinal changes may progress even after therapy is completed.
- Monitor ECG for cardiomyopathy and QT prolongation periodically during therapy.
- Monitor for signs and symptoms of DRESS (fever, rash, lymphadenopathy, and/or facial swelling), associated with involvement of other organ systems (hepatitis, nephritis, hematologic abnormalities, myocarditis, myositis) during therapy. May resemble an acute viral infection. Eosinophilia is often present. Discontinue therapy if signs occur.
- Assess for rash periodically during therapy. May cause SJS. Discontinue therapy if severe or if accompanied with fever, general malaise, fatigue, muscle or joint aches, blisters, oral lesions, conjunctivitis, hepatitis and/or eosinophilia.
- Assess for suicidal tendencies, depression, or changes in behavior periodically during therapy.
- **Malaria or Lupus Erythematosus:** Assess patient for improvement in signs and symptoms of condition daily throughout course of therapy.
- **Rheumatoid Arthritis:** Assess patient monthly for pain, swelling, and range of motion.

Lab Test Considerations

- Monitor CBC and platelet count periodically during therapy. May cause ↓ RBC, WBC, and platelet counts. If severe ↓ occur that are not related to the disease process, discontinue hydroxychloroquine.
- Monitor liver function tests periodically during therapy.
- May cause hypoglycemia.

Implementation

- Do not confuse hydroxychloroquine with hydrochlorothiazide or hydroxyurea.
- **PO:** Administer with milk or meals to minimize GI distress.
- Tablets may be crushed and placed inside empty capsules for patients with difficulty swallowing. Contents of capsules may also be mixed with a teaspoonful of jam, jelly, or Jell-O prior to administration.
- **Malaria Prophylaxis:** Hydroxychloroquine therapy should be started 2 wk prior to potential exposure and continued for 4–6 wk after leaving the malarious area.

Patient/Family Teaching

- Instruct patient to take medication as directed and continue full course of therapy even if feeling better. Take missed doses as soon as remembered unless it is almost time for next dose. Do not double doses.
- Advise patients to avoid use of alcohol while taking hydroxychloroquine.
- Caution patient to keep hydroxychloroquine out of reach of children; fatalities have occurred with ingestion of three or four tablets.
- Explain need for periodic ophthalmic exams for patients on prolonged high-dose therapy. Advise patient that the risk of ocular damage may be

decreased by the use of dark glasses in bright light. Protective clothing and sunscreen should also be used to reduce risk of dermatoses.

- Advise patient to notify health care professional promptly if sore throat, fever, unusual bleeding or bruising, blurred vision, visual changes, ringing in the ears, difficulty hearing, or muscle weakness occurs.
- Rep: Advise females of reproductive potential to notify health care professional if pregnancy is planned or suspected or if breastfeeding. Inform patient of pregnancy exposure registry that monitors pregnancy outcomes in women exposed to hydroxychloroquine during pregnancy. Encourage patients to register by calling 1-877-311-8972.
- **Malaria Prophylaxis:** Review methods of minimizing exposure to mosquitoes with patients receiving hydroxychloroquine prophylactically (use repellent, wear long-sleeved shirt and long trousers, use screen or netting).
- Advise patient to notify health care professional if fever develops while traveling or within 2 mo of leaving an endemic area.
- **Rheumatoid Arthritis:** Instruct patient to contact health care professional if no improvement is noticed within a few days. Treatment for rheumatoid arthritis may require up to 6 mo for full benefit.

Evaluation/Desired Outcomes

- Prevention or resolution of malaria.
- Improvement in signs and symptoms of rheumatoid arthritis.
- Improvement in symptoms of lupus erythematosus.

BEERS

hydrOXYzine (hye-**drox**-i-zeen)

✱ Atarax, Vistaril

Classification

Therapeutic: antianxiety agents, sedative/hypnotics

Pharmacologic: antihistamines

Indications

Anxiety. Preoperative sedation. Nausea and vomiting. Pruritus. Urticaria.

Action

Acts as a CNS depressant at the subcortical level of the CNS. Has anticholinergic, antihistaminic, and antiemetic properties. Blocks histamine-1 receptors. **Therapeutic Effects:** Sedation. Relief of anxiety. Decreased nausea and vomiting. Decreased allergic symptoms associated with release of histamine, including pruritus and urticaria.

Pharmacokinetics

Absorption: Well absorbed following oral and IM administration.

Distribution: Unknown.

Metabolism and Excretion: Completely metabolized by the liver; eliminated in the feces via biliary excretion.

Half-life: 3 hr.

TIME/ACTION PROFILE (sedative, antiemetic, antipruritic effects)

ROUTE	ONSET	PEAK	DURATION
PO	15–30 min	2–4 hr	4–6 hr
IM	15–30 min	2–4 hr	4–6 hr

H

Contraindications/Precautions

Contraindicated in: Hypersensitivity; QT interval prolongation; OB: Pregnancy; Lactation: Lactation.

Use Cautiously in: Severe hepatic impairment; Congenital long QT syndrome, family history of long QT syndrome, recent MI, HF, hypokalemia, hypomagnesemia, bradycardia, or concurrent use of antiarrhythmics; Pedi: Injection contains benzyl alcohol, which can cause potentially fatal gasping syndrome in neonates; Geri: Appears on Beers list. ↑ risk of anticholinergic adverse reactions in older adults, including falls, delirium, and dementia. Avoid use in older adults.

Adverse Reactions/Side Effects

CV: QT interval prolongation, TORSADES DE POINTES. **Derm:** acute generalized exanthematous pustulosis, flushing, rash. **GI:** dry mouth, bitter taste, constipation, nausea. **GU:** urinary retention **Local:** pain (at IM site), abscesses at IM sites. **Neuro:** drowsiness, agitation, ataxia, dizziness, headache, weakness. **Resp:** wheezing.

Interactions

Drug-Drug: Additive CNS depression with other **CNS depressants**, including **alcohol**, **antidepressants**, **antihistamines**, **opioid analgesics**, and **sedative/hypnotics**. Concurrent use of **QT interval prolonging medications** may ↑ risk of QT interval prolongation and torsades de pointes. Additive anticholinergic effects with other **drugs possessing anticholinergic properties**, including **antihistamines**, **antidepressants**, **atropine**, **haloperidol**, **phenothiazines**, **quinidine**, and **disopyramide**. Can antagonize the vasopressor effects of **epinephrine**.

Drug-Natural Products: Kava-kava, **valerian**, or **chamomile** can ↑ CNS depression. ↑ anticholinergic effects with **angel's trumpet**, **jimson weed**, and **scopolia**.

Route/Dosage

PO: (Adults): *Antianxiety:* 25–100 mg 4 times/day, not to exceed 600 mg/day. *Preoperative sedation:* 50–100 mg single dose. *Antipruritic:* 25 mg 3–4 times daily.
PO (Children): 2 mg/kg/day divided every 6–8 hr.
IM (Adults): *Preoperative sedation:* 25–100 mg single dose. *Antiemetic, adjunct to opioid analgesics:* 25–100 mg every 4–6 hr as needed.
IM (Children): 0.5–1 mg/kg every 4–6 hr as needed.

Availability (generic available)

Tablets: 10 mg, 25 mg, 50 mg. **Capsules:** 🍁 10 mg, 25 mg, 50 mg, 100 mg. **Syrup:** 10 mg/5 mL. **Solution for injection:** 25 mg/mL, 50 mg/mL.

NURSING IMPLICATIONS

Assessment

- Assess sedation levels and monitor for oversedation or confusion; provide safety precautions as indicated (side rails up, bed in low position, call light within reach, bed alarms, supervision of ambulation and transfer). Geri: Older adults are more sensitive to CNS and anticholinergic effects (delirium, acute confusion, dizziness, dry mouth, blurred vision, urinary retention, constipation, tachycardia). Monitor for drowsiness, agitation, oversedation, and other systemic side effects. Assess falls risk and implement prevention strategies.
- **Anxiety:** Assess mental status (orientation, mood, and behavior).
- **Nausea and Vomiting:** Assess degree of nausea and frequency and amount of emesis.
- **Pruritus:** Assess degree of itching and character of involved skin.

Lab Test Considerations

- May cause false-negative skin test results using allergen extracts. Discontinue hydroxyzine at least 72 hr before test.

Implementation

- Do not confuse hydroxyzine with hydralazine, hydrochlorothiazide, hydromorphone, or hydroxyurea.
- **PO:** Tablets may be crushed and capsules opened and administered with food or fluids for patients having difficulty swallowing.
- **IM:** Administer *only* IM deep into well-developed muscle; preferably the upper outer quadrant of the buttock in adults or the midlateral thigh in adults and children. Aspirate to avoid inadvertent injection into blood vessels. Injection is extremely painful. Do not use deltoid site. Significant tissue damage, necrosis, and sloughing may result from SUBQ or intra-arterial injections. Hemolysis may result from IV injections. Rotate injection sites frequently.

Patient/Family Teaching

- Explain the purpose and side effects of hydroxyzine. Instruct patient to take as directed. Take missed doses as soon as remembered unless it is almost time for next dose; do not double doses. Do not share medication with others, even if they have similar symptoms; may be harmful. Advise patient to read *Patient Information* before starting and with each Rx refill in case of changes.
- May cause drowsiness or dizziness. Caution patient to avoid driving and other activities requiring alertness until response to medication is known. Geri: Warn patients or caregivers that older adults are at ↑ risk for CNS effects and falls.
- Advise patient to notify health care provider of all Rx or OTC medications, vitamins, or herbal products being taken and to consult with health care provider before taking other medications. Advise patient to avoid concurrent use of alcohol or other CNS depressants with this medication.
- Inform patient that frequent mouth rinses, good oral hygiene, and sugarless gum or candy may help ↓ dry mouth. If dry mouth persists for >2 wk, consult dentist about saliva substitute.
- Rep: Advise women of reproductive potential to avoid use during early pregnancy or use effective contraception and to avoid breastfeeding during therapy. Instruct to notify health care provider if pregnancy is planned or suspected or if breastfeeding.

Evaluation/Desired Outcomes

- Decrease in anxiety.
- Relief of nausea and vomiting.
- Decreased allergic symptoms associated with release of histamine, including pruritus and urticaria.
- Sedation when used as a sedative/hypnotic.

ibandronate (i-ban-dro-nate)

~~Boniva~~

Classification

Therapeutic: bone resorption inhibitors
Pharmacologic: bisphosphonates

Indications

Treatment/prevention of postmenopausal osteoporosis.

Action

Inhibits resorption of bone by inhibiting osteoclast activity. **Therapeutic Effects:** Reversal/prevention of progression of osteoporosis with decreased fractures.

Pharmacokinetics

Absorption: 0.6% absorbed following oral administration (significantly ↓ by food).
Distribution: Rapidly binds to bone.
Protein Binding: 90.9–99.5%.
Metabolism and Excretion: 50–60% excreted in urine; unabsorbed drug is eliminated in feces.
Half-life: *PO:* 10–60 hr; *IV:* 4.6–25.5 hr.

TIME/ACTION PROFILE

ROUTE	ONSET	PEAK	DURATION
PO	unknown	0.5–2 hr	up to 1 mo
IV	unknown	3 hr	up to 3 mo

Contraindications/Precautions

Contraindicated in: Hypersensitivity; Abnormalities of the esophagus that delay esophageal emptying (e.g., strictures, achalasia); Uncorrected hypocalcemia; Inability to stand/sit upright for ≥60 min; Severe renal impairment; OB: Pregnancy.
Use Cautiously in: History of upper GI disorders; Invasive dental procedures, cancer, receiving chemotherapy, corticosteroids, or angiogenesis inhibitors, poor oral hygiene, periodontal disease, dental disease, anemia, coagulopathy, infection, or poorly fitting dentures (may ↑ risk of jaw osteonecrosis); Lactation: Safety not established in breastfeeding; Pedi: Safety and effectiveness not established in children; Geri: Consider age-related ↓ in body mass, renal and hepatic function, concurrent disease states, and drug therapy in older adults.

Adverse Reactions/Side Effects

Derm: ERYTHEMA MULTIFORME, STEVENS-JOHNSON SYNDROME. **GI:** diarrhea, dyspepsia, dysphagia, ESOPHAGEAL CANCER, esophageal/gastric ulcer, esophagitis. **Local:** injection site reactions. **MS:** musculoskeletal pain, pain in arms/legs, femur fractures, osteonecrosis (primarily of jaw). **Resp:** asthma exacerbation. **Misc:** ANAPHYLAXIS.

Interactions

Drug-Drug: Calcium-, aluminum-, magnesium-, and **iron-**containing products, including **antacids**, ↓ absorption; give ibandronate 60 min before these medications. **NSAIDs**, including **aspirin**, may ↑ risk of gastric irritation.
Drug-Food: Food may ↓ absorption.

Route/Dosage

PO (Adults): 150 mg once monthly.
IV (Adults): 3 mg every 3 mo.

Availability (generic available)

Tablets: 150 mg. **Injection (prefilled syringes):** 1 mg/mL.

NURSING IMPLICATIONS

Assessment

- **Osteoporosis:** Monitor bone mass before and periodically during therapy and re-evaluate need for ibandronate. *If low risk for fracture,* consider discontinuation after 3–5 yr of therapy.
- **IV:** Monitor for signs and symptoms of anaphylaxis (swelling of face, lips, mouth, or tongue; dyspnea; wheezing; rash; syncope; tachycardia; diaphoresis) during therapy. *If symptoms occur,* immediately discontinue ibandronate and begin supportive treatment.
- Perform routine oral exam prior to initiation and periodically during therapy. *If osteonecrosis of the jaw occurs,* consult oral surgeon and consider discontinuing ibandronate.

Lab Test Considerations

- Assess serum calcium before and periodically during therapy. Treat hypocalcemia and vitamin D deficiency before initiating ibandronate therapy.
- Obtain serum creatinine prior to each IV injection and as clinically indicated.
- May ↓ alkaline phosphatase.
- May cause hypercholesterolemia.

Implementation

- **PO:** Administer ≥60 min before the 1st food, drink, or other medications of the day with 6–8 ounces of plain water. Take while standing or sitting upright; avoid lying down for ≥60 min after swallowing tablet. ***DNC:*** Tablet should be swallowed whole; do not break, crush, or chew.

IV Administration

- **IV:** Administer using prefilled syringe. Do not administer if solution is discolored or contains particulates.

- **Rate:** Administer as a 15–30 sec bolus.
- **Y-Site Incompatibility:** Do not administer with calcium-containing solutions or other IV drugs.

Patient/Family Teaching

- Explain purpose and side effects of medication. Advise patient to read *Patient Information* before starting therapy.
- Instruct patient to take tablet on the same day each month. If dose missed >7 days before next scheduled dose, take the morning after remembered; if ≤7 days before next scheduled dose, omit missed dose. In both cases return to scheduled dosing.
- Advise patient that IV doses should not be administered sooner than every 3 mo. If a dose is missed, have health care provider administer as soon as possible; next injection should be scheduled 3 mo from last injection.
- Advise patient to notify health care provider of all Rx or OTC medications, vitamins, or herbal products being taken and to consult health care provider before taking other medications.
- Advise patient to eat a balanced diet and consult health care provider for supplemental calcium and vitamin D need.
- Encourage patient to participate in regular exercise and to modify behaviors (smoking, alcohol consumption) that ↑ risk of osteoporosis.
- Inform patient that severe musculoskeletal pain may occur within days, months, or years after starting ibandronate. Symptoms may or may not resolve completely after discontinuation. Notify health care provider if severe pain occurs.
- Advise patient to have routine dental exams and notify health care provider if rash or other signs and symptoms of osteonecrosis of the jaw (pain, numbness, swelling of, or drainage from the jaw, mouth, or teeth) occur.
- Instruct patient to notify health care provider if chest pain, new or worsening heartburn, or trouble or pain when swallowing occurs.
- Advise patient to inform health care provider of ibandronate therapy prior to dental surgery.
- **Rep:** Advise women of reproductive potential to notify health care provider if pregnancy is planned or suspected or if breastfeeding.

Evaluation/Desired Outcomes

- Prevention of or ↓ in the progression of osteoporosis in postmenopausal women. Discontinuation after 3–5 yr should be considered for women with low risk for fractures.

BEERS

ibuprofen (eye-byoo-**proe**-fen)

Advil, Advil Infants, Advil Junior Strength, Advil Migraine, Children's Advil, ✱ Children's Europrofen, Children's Motrin, ✱ Motrin, Motrin IB, Motrin Infants Drops, Motrin Junior Strength, PediaCare IB Ibuprofen

ibuprofen (injection)

Caldolor, NeoProfen (ibuprofen lysine)

Classification

Therapeutic: antipyretics antirheumatics nonopioid analgesics

Pharmacologic: nonsteroidal anti-inflammatory drugs (NSAIDs)

Indications

PO, IV: Treatment of: Mild to moderate pain, Fever. **PO:** Treatment of: Inflammatory disorders, including rheumatoid arthritis (including juvenile) and osteoarthritis, Dysmenorrhea. **IV:** Moderate to severe pain with opioid analgesics. Closure of a clinically significant patent ductus arteriosus (PDA) in neonates weighing 500–1500 g and ≤32 wk gestational age (ibuprofen lysine only).

Action

Inhibits prostaglandin synthesis. **Therapeutic Effects:** Decreased pain and inflammation. Reduction of fever. Closure of PDA.

Pharmacokinetics

Absorption: Oral formulation is well absorbed (80%) from the GI tract; IV administration results in complete bioavailability.

Distribution: Well distributed to tissues.

Protein Binding: 99%.

Metabolism and Excretion: Mostly metabolized by the liver; small amounts (1%) excreted unchanged by the kidneys.

Half-life: *Neonates:* 26–43 hr; *Children:* 1–2 hr; *Adults:* 2–4 hr.

TIME/ACTION PROFILE

ROUTE	ONSET	PEAK	DURATION
PO (antipyretic)	0.5–2.5 hr	2–4 hr	6–8 hr
PO (analgesic)	30 min	1–2 hr	4–6 hr
PO (anti-inflammatory)	≤7 days	1–2 wk	unknown
IV (analgesic)	unknown	unknown	6 hr
IV (antipyretic)	within 2 hr	10–12 hr†	4–6 hr

† With repeated dosing.

Contraindications/Precautions

Contraindicated in: Hypersensitivity (cross-sensitivity may exist with other NSAIDs, including aspirin); Active GI bleeding or ulcer disease; Chewable tablets contain aspartame and should not be used in patients with phenylketonuria; Coronary artery bypass graft surgery; Recent MI; HF; OB: Avoid use after 30 wk gestation; Pedi: Ibuprofen lysine: Preterm neonates with untreated infection, congenital heart disease where patency of PDA is necessary for pulmonary or systemic blood flow, bleeding, thrombocytopenia, coagulation defects, necrotizing enterocolitis, or significant renal dysfunction.

Use Cautiously in: Cardiovascular disease or risk factors for cardiovascular disease (may ↑ risk of serious cardiovascular thrombotic events, MI, and stroke, especially with prolonged use or use of higher doses); Renal or hepatic disease, dehydration, or patients on nephrotoxic drugs (may ↑ risk of renal toxicity); Aspirin triad patients (asthma, nasal polyps, and aspirin intolerance); can cause fatal anaphylactoid reactions; History of long duration of NSAID use, smoking, alcohol use, advanced liver disease, coagulopathy, or poor general health (↑ risk of GI bleeding); History of peptic ulcer disease and/or GI bleeding; Bleeding tendency or concurrent anticoagulant therapy; OB: Use at or after 20 wk gestation may cause fetal or neonatal renal impairment; if treatment is necessary between 20 wk and 30 wk gestation, limit use to the lowest effective dose and shortest duration possible; Lactation: Use while breastfeeding only if potential maternal benefit justifies potential risk to infant; Pedi: Safety and effectiveness not established for children <6 mo (oral) or <3 mo (IV Caldolor); hyperbilirubinemia in neonates (may displace bilirubin from albumin-binding sites); safety and effectiveness of ibuprofen lysine only established in premature infants; Geri: Appears on Beers list. ↑ risk GI bleeding or peptic ulcer disease in older adults. Avoid chronic use unless other alternatives are not effective and the patient can take a gastroprotective agent; avoid short-term use in combination with oral or parenteral corticosteroids, anticoagulants, or antiplatelet agents unless other alternatives are not effective and the patient can take a gastroprotective agent.

Exercise Extreme Caution in: History of GI bleeding or GI ulcer disease.

Adverse Reactions/Side Effects

CV: arrhythmias, edema, HF, hypertension, MI. **Derm:** ACUTE GENERALIZED EXANTHEMATOUS PUSTULOSIS (AGEP), DRUG REACTION WITH EOSINOPHILIA AND SYSTEMIC SYMPTOMS (DRESS), EXFOLIATIVE DERMATITIS, GENERALIZED BULLOUS FIXED DRUG ERUPTION, rash, STEVENS-JOHNSON SYNDROME (SJS), TOXIC EPIDERMAL NECROLYSIS (TEN). **EENT:** amblyopia, blurred vision, tinnitus. **F and E:** hyperkalemia. **GI:** constipation, dyspepsia, nausea, vomiting, abdominal discomfort, GI BLEEDING, GI PERFORATION, GI ULCERATION, HEPATITIS, necrotizing enterocolitis (ibuprofen lysine). **GU:** cystitis, hematuria, renal failure. **Hemat:** anemia, blood dyscrasias, prolonged bleeding time. **Local:** injection site reaction. **Neuro:** headache, dizziness, drowsiness, intraventricular hemorrhage (ibuprofen lysine), psychic disturbances, STROKE. **Misc:** HYPERSENSITIVITY REACTIONS (INCLUDING ANAPHYLAXIS AND SERIOUS SKIN REACTIONS).

Interactions

Drug-Drug: May limit the cardioprotective (antiplatelet) effects of low-dose **aspirin**. **Aspirin** may ↓ effectiveness of ibuprofen. Additive adverse GI side effects with **aspirin**, **oral potassium**, other **NSAIDs**, **corticosteroids**, or **alcohol**. Chronic use with **acetaminophen** may ↑ risk of adverse renal reactions. May ↓ effectiveness of **diuretics**, **ACE inhibitors**, or other **antihypertensives**. May ↑ hypoglycemic effects of **insulin** or **oral hypoglycemic agents**. May ↑ levels and risk of toxicity of **lithium**. ↑ risk of toxicity from **methotrexate**. **Probenecid** may ↑ risk of toxicity. ↑ risk of GI bleeding with **anticoagulants**, **aspirin**, **clopidogrel**, **ticagrelor**, **prasugrel**, **corticosteroids**, **fibrinolytics**, **SNRIs**, or **SSRIs**. ↑ risk of adverse hematologic reactions with **antineoplastics** or **radiation therapy**. ↑ risk of nephrotoxicity with **cyclosporine**. May ↑ levels and the risk of toxicity of **amikacin**.

Drug-Natural Products: ↑ bleeding risk with **arnica**, **chamomile**, **feverfew**, **garlic**, **ginger**, **ginkgo**, **Panax ginseng**, and others.

Route/Dosage

Analgesia/Anti-inflammatory/Antipyretic

PO (Adults): *Anti-inflammatory:* 400–800 mg 3–4 times daily (not to exceed 3200 mg/day). *Analgesic/antidysmenorrheal/antipyretic:* 200–400 mg every 4–6 hr (not to exceed 1200 mg/day).

PO (Children 6 mo–12 yr): *Anti-inflammatory:* 30–50 mg/kg/day in 3–4 divided doses (maximum dose: 2.4 g/day). *Antipyretic:* 5 mg/kg for temperature <102.5°F or 10 mg/kg for higher temperatures (not to exceed 40 mg/kg/day); may be repeated every 4–6 hr.

PO (Infants and Children): *Analgesic:* 4–10 mg/kg/dose every 6–8 hr.

IV (Adults): *Analgesic (Caldolor):* 400–800 mg every 6 hr as needed (not to exceed 3200 mg/day); *Antipyretic (Caldolor):* 400 mg initially, then 400 mg every 4–6 hr or 100–200 mg every 4 hr as needed (not to exceed 3200 mg/day).

IV (Children 12–17 yr): *Analgesic and antipyretic (Caldolor):* 400 mg every 4–6 hr as needed (not to exceed 2400 mg/day).

IV (Children 6 mo–12 yr): *Analgesic and antipyretic (Caldolor):* 10 mg/kg (not to exceed 400 mg) every 4–6 hr as needed (not to exceed 40 mg/kg/day or 2400 mg/day, whichever is less).
IV (Children 3–<6 mo): *Analgesic and antipyretic (Caldolor):* 10 mg/kg (not to exceed 100 mg) as a single dose.

Pediatric OTC Dosing

PO (Children 11 yr/72–95 lb): 300 mg every 6–8 hr.
PO (Children 9–10 yr/60–71 lb): 250 mg every 6–8 hr.
PO (Children 6–8 yr/48–59 lb): 200 mg every 6–8 hr.
PO (Children 4–5 yr/36–47 lb): 150 mg every 6–8 hr.
PO (Children 2–3 yr/24–35 lb): 100 mg every 6–8 hr.
PO (Children 12–23 mo/18–23 lb): 75 mg every 6–8 hr.
PO (Infants 6–11 mo/12–17 lb): 50 mg every 6–8 hr.

Patent Ductus Arteriosus Closure

IV (Neonates Gestational age ≤32 wk, 500–1500 g): *Neoprofen:* 10 mg/kg followed by two doses of 5 mg/kg at 24 and 48 hr after initial dose.

Availability (generic available)

Tablets: 200 mg^OTC, 400 mg, 600 mg, 800 mg. **Capsules (liquigels):** 200 mg^OTC. **Chewable tablets (fruit, grape, orange, and citrus flavor):** 100 mg^OTC. **Oral solution (berry flavor):** 50 mg/1.25 mL^OTC. **Oral suspension (fruit, berry, grape flavor):** 100 mg/5 mL^OTC. **Solution for injection:** 10 mg/mL (NeoProfen), 100 mg/mL (Caldolor). **Premixed infusion (Caldolor):** 800 mg/200 mL. ***In combination with:*** decongestants^OTC, hydrocodone.

NURSING IMPLICATIONS

Assessment

- Monitor for hypersensitivity reactions, including anaphylaxis. Patients who have asthma, aspirin-induced allergy, and nasal polyps are at ↑ risk.
- Assess for signs and symptoms of GI bleeding (tarry stools, dizziness, hypotension), renal impairment (↑ BUN and serum creatinine, ↓ urine output), and hepatic impairment (↑ liver enzymes, jaundice) periodically during therapy. Geri: Older adults have higher risk for poor outcomes or death from GI bleeding. Age-related renal impairment ↑ risk of hepatic and renal toxicity.
- Assess patient for rash (SJS, TEN, generalized bullous fixed drug eruption) frequently during therapy. *At first sign of rash,* discontinue ibuprofen and treat as indicated; may recur once therapy is stopped.
- Monitor for signs and symptoms of DRESS (fever, rash, lymphadenopathy, facial swelling, eosinophilia) periodically during therapy. *If symptoms occur,* discontinue ibuprofen.
- **Pain:** Assess pain (note type, location, and intensity) prior to and 1–2 hr following administration.
- **Arthritis:** Assess pain and range of motion prior to and 1–2 hr following administration.
- **Fever:** Monitor temperature; note signs associated with fever (diaphoresis, tachycardia, malaise).
- **PDA Closure:** Monitor preterm neonates for signs of bleeding, infection, and ↓ urine output. Monitor IV site for signs of extravasation. If PDA closes or size significantly ↓, 2nd and 3rd doses are unnecessary.

Lab Test Considerations

- Monitor BUN, serum creatinine, CBC, and liver function tests periodically during prolonged therapy.
- May ↑ potassium, BUN, serum creatinine, alkaline phosphatase, LDH, AST, and ALT. May ↓ blood glucose, hemoglobin, hematocrit, leukocytes, platelets, and CCr.
- May cause prolonged bleeding time.
- **PDA Closure:** If urinary output <0.6 mL/kg/hr at time of 2nd or 3rd dose, hold dose until renal function has returned to normal.

Implementation

- Do not confuse Motrin with Neurontin.
- Administration of higher than recommended doses does not provide ↑ pain relief but may ↑ incidence of side effects.
- Ensure appropriate hydration before initiation and during therapy to prevent renal toxicity.
- Use lowest effective dose for shortest period of time, especially in older adults, to minimize risk of cardiovascular thrombotic events.
- Coadministration with opioid analgesics may have additive analgesic effects, permitting lower opioid doses.
- **PO:** For rapid initial effect, administer 30 min before or 2 hr after food. May be administered with food, milk, or antacids to ↓ GI irritation. Tablets may be crushed and mixed with fluids or food; 800-mg tablet can be dissolved in water.
- **Dysmenorrhea:** Administer as soon as possible after the onset of menses.

IV Administration

- **Intermittent Infusion:** *Ibuprofen injection:* **Dilution:** Dilute 800-mg dose in ≥200 mL and 100-mg, 200-mg, and 400-mg doses in ≥100 mL of 0.9% NaCl, D5W, or LR. **Concentration:** ≤4 mg/mL. *Ibuprofen lysine:* **Dilution:** Dilute in appropriate volume of D5W or 0.9% NaCl. Administer within 30 min of dilution. Do not administer solutions that are discolored or contain particulates.

Stable for up to 24 hr at room temperature. Discard remaining solution. Rate: Infuse *Ibuprofen injection* over ≥30 min for adults and ≥10 min for children for *Caldolor* or over 15 min for *NeoProfen*. Infuse *Ibuprofen lysine* over 15 min.

Ibuprofen

- **Y-Site Compatibility:** hydrocortisone, metoprolol.
- **Y-Site Incompatibility:** caffeine citrate, esmolol, labetalol, sildenafil.

Ibuprofen Lysine

- **Y-Site Compatibility:** ceftazidime, epinephrine, furosemide, heparin, insulin regular, phenobarbital, potassium chloride, sodium bicarbonate.
- **Y-Site Incompatibility:** amikacin, caffeine citrate, dobutamine, dopamine, isoproterenol, midazolam, vancomycin, vecuronium.

Patient/Family Teaching

- Explain purpose and side effects of medication. Advise patient to read *Patient Information* before starting therapy.
- Advise patients to take ibuprofen with a full glass of water and to remain upright for 15–30 min after administration.
- Pedi: Teach caregivers to calculate and measure doses accurately and to use measuring device supplied with product.
- May cause drowsiness or dizziness. Advise patient to avoid driving or other activities requiring alertness until response to medication is known.
- Caution patient to avoid the concurrent use of alcohol, aspirin (including low-dose aspirin), acetaminophen, and other OTC or herbal products without consulting health care provider.
- Advise patient to notify health care provider of all Rx or OTC medications, vitamins, or herbal products being taken and to consult health care provider before taking other medications or undergoing surgery.
- Instruct patient not to take OTC ibuprofen preparations >10 days for pain or >3 days for fever and to consult health care provider if symptoms persist or worsen. Many OTC products contain ibuprofen; avoid duplication.
- Caution patient that use of ibuprofen with ≥3 glasses of alcohol per day may ↑ the risk of GI bleeding.
- Inform patient of ↑ risk of MI and stroke. Use lowest effective dose for shortest time. Advise patient to notify health care provider immediately if signs and symptoms (shortness of breath or trouble breathing, chest pain, weakness in one part or side of body, slurred speech, swelling of the face or throat) occur.
- Advise patient to notify health care provider promptly if signs or symptoms of GI toxicity (abdominal pain, black stools) occur.
- Pedi: Advise parents or caregivers not to administer ibuprofen to children who may be dehydrated (can occur with vomiting, diarrhea, or poor fluid intake); dehydration ↑ risk of renal impairment.
- Rep: May cause fetal harm. Advise women of reproductive potential to notify health care provider if pregnancy is planned or suspected and to avoid ibuprofen starting at 20 wk gestation due to risk of oligohydramnios and 30 wk gestation because of risk of premature closing of the fetal ductus arteriosus. If NSAIDs are necessary between 20 and 30 wk gestation, limit use to the lowest effective dose and shortest duration possible. Consider ultrasound monitoring of amniotic fluid for NSAID therapy >48 hr. Discontinue ibuprofen if oligohydramnios occurs and follow up with infant. Use during labor or delivery may delay birth and ↑ risk of stillbirth. Advise patient to notify health care provider if breastfeeding. May cause temporary infertility in women.

Evaluation/Desired Outcomes

- Decrease in severity of pain.
- Improved joint mobility. Partial arthritic relief is usually seen within 7 days, but maximum effectiveness may require 1–2 wk of continuous therapy. Patients who do not respond to one NSAID may respond to another.
- Reduction in fever.
- Closure of PDA.

idaruCIZUmab

(eye-da-roo-**siz**-ue-mab)

Praxbind

Classification

Therapeutic: antidotes

Pharmacologic: monoclonal antibodies

Indications

To counteract the anticoagulant effect of dabigatran for emergency surgery/urgent procedures or life-threatening uncontrolled bleeding.

Action

Human monoclonal antibody fragment that selectively binds to dabigatran and its metabolites, preventing its binding to thrombin and negating its anticoagulant effects. Does not reverse any other anticoagulants. **Therapeutic Effects:** Reversal of the anticoagulant effect of dabigatran.

Pharmacokinetics

Absorption: IV administration results in complete bioavailability.
Distribution: Minimally distributed to tissues.
Metabolism and Excretion: Biodegraded to smaller molecules. 60% excreted in urine, remainder via protein catabolism primarily in the kidneys.
Half-life: 10.3 hr.

TIME/ACTION PROFILE (plasma concentrations)

ROUTE	ONSET	PEAK	DURATION
IV	immediate	unknown	24 hr

Contraindications/Precautions

Contraindicated in: None reported.
Use Cautiously in: OB: Safety not established in pregnancy; Lactation: Safety not established in breastfeeding; Pedi: Safety and effectiveness not established in children; Geri: Older adults may be more sensitive to drug effects.
Exercise Extreme Caution in: Hereditary fructose intolerance (risk of serious adverse reactions due to sorbitol excipient); History of serious hypersensitivity (including anaphylactoid reactions) to idarucizumab.

Adverse Reactions/Side Effects

CV: DEEP VEIN THROMBOSIS (DVT). **F and E:** hypokalemia. **GI:** constipation. **Neuro:** delirium. **Resp:** PULMONARY EMBOLISM (PE). **Misc:** fever, HYPERSENSITIVITY REACTIONS (INCLUDING ANAPHYLAXIS).

Interactions

Drug-Drug: None reported.

Route/Dosage

IV (Adults): 5 g as single dose.

Availability

Solution for injection (contains sorbitol): 2.5 g/50 mL.

NURSING IMPLICATIONS

Assessment

- Monitor for thromboembolism (DVT, PE). Resume anticoagulant therapy as soon as medically appropriate to ↓ thromboembolic risk. Dabigatran can be reinstituted 24 hr after idarucizumab infusion.
- Monitor for signs and symptoms of hypersensitivity (rash, urticaria, fever, pruritus, dyspnea, orofacial swelling). *If symptoms occur,* discontinue idarucizumab and treat symptomatically. Contains sorbitol; reactions in patients with hereditary fructose intolerance have included hypoglycemia, hypophosphatemia, metabolic acidosis, ↑ uric acid, and acute liver failure.

Lab Test Considerations

- Monitor coagulation parameters (aPTT, ecarin clotting time [ECT]) 12–24 hr after infusion. *If ↑ coagulation parameters occur with bleeding recurrence or an additional emergency procedure,* consider administration of an additional 5-g dose of idarucizumab.
- May cause hypokalemia.

Implementation

- Do not confuse idarucizumab with idarubicin.

IV Administration

- **Intermittent Infusion:** Solution is clear to opalescent, colorless to slightly yellow; do not administer if discolored or contains precipitates. May store vials at room temperature ≤6 hr. Administer within 1 hr after solution is removed from vials. Flush IV line with 0.9% NaCl prior to and following infusion. Administer as 2 consecutive infusions or inject both vials consecutively via syringe as bolus. Infusion of each vial should take no longer than 5–10 min with the 2nd vial of 2.5 g administered no later than 15 min after the end of the 1st 2.5-g vial.
- **Y-Site Incompatibility:** Do not administer other drugs through same IV line.

Patient/Family Teaching

- Explain purpose and side effects of idarucizumab to patient.
- Instruct patient to notify health care provider immediately if bleeding or signs and symptoms of hypersensitivity occur.
- Inform patient that reversal of dabigatran therapy exposes them to the thromboembolic risk of their underlying disease, and resumption of anticoagulant therapy should be considered as soon as possible once they are stable.
- Rep: Advise women of reproductive potential to notify health care provider if pregnancy is planned or suspected or if breastfeeding.

Evaluation/Desired Outcomes

- Reversal of the anticoagulant effect of dabigatran.

HIGH ALERT

ifosfamide (eye-foss-fam-ide)

Ifex

Classification
Therapeutic: antineoplastics
Pharmacologic: alkylating agents

Indications

Germ cell testicular carcinoma (with other chemotherapy agents and with mesna, which prevents ifosfamide-induced hemorrhagic cystitis).

Action

Following conversion to active compounds, interferes with DNA replication and RNA transcription, ultimately disrupting protein synthesis (cell-cycle phase-nonspecific). **Therapeutic Effects:** Death of rapidly replicating cells, particularly malignant ones.

Pharmacokinetics

Absorption: IV administration results in complete bioavailability.
Distribution: Minimally distributed to tissues.
Metabolism and Excretion: Metabolized by the liver to active antineoplastic compounds.
Half-life: 15 hr.

TIME/ACTION PROFILE (effects on blood counts)

ROUTE	ONSET	PEAK	DURATION
IV	unknown	7–14 days	21 days

Contraindications/Precautions

Contraindicated in: Hypersensitivity; Active infections; WBC count <2000/mm³; Platelet count <50,000/mm³; OB: Pregnancy; Lactation: Lactation.
Use Cautiously in: Renal impairment (↑ risk of nephrotoxicity); High ifosfamide dose, hypoalbuminemia, renal impairment, poor performance status, or bulky abdominal-pelvic disease (↑ risk of encephalopathy); Bladder radiation (↑ risk of hemorrhagic cystitis); Rep: Women of reproductive potential; Pedi: Safety and effectiveness not established in children; Geri: Drug may accumulate in older adults due to age-related renal impairment.

Adverse Reactions/Side Effects

CV: cardiotoxicity. **Derm:** alopecia, impaired wound healing. **EENT:** blurred vision. **GI:** nausea, vomiting, anorexia, constipation, diarrhea, hepatotoxicity. **GU:** HEMORRHAGIC CYSTITIS, dysuria, RENAL FAILURE, sterility, urinary incontinence. **Hemat:** ANEMIA, LEUKOPENIA, THROMBOCYTOPENIA. **Local:** phlebitis. **Neuro:** confusion, sedation, dizziness, ENCEPHALOPATHY, extrapyramidal symptoms, hallucinations, psychosis, SEIZURES. **Misc:** HYPERSENSITIVITY REACTIONS (INCLUDING ANAPHYLAXIS).

Interactions

Drug-Drug: CYP3A4 inhibitors, including **ketoconazole**, **fluconazole**, **itraconazole**, **sorafenib**, and **aprepitant**, may ↓ its effectiveness. **CYP3A4 inducers**, including **carbamazepine**, **phenytoin**, **phenobarbital**, and **rifampin**, may ↑ the formation of a toxic metabolite and may ↑ risk of toxicity. ↑ risk of myelosuppression with other **antineoplastics** or **radiation therapy**. Toxicity may be ↑ by **allopurinol** or **phenobarbital**. **Nephrotoxic drugs** (including **cisplatin**), **CNS depressants**, or **alcohol** may ↑ risk of encephalopathy. **Busulfan** may ↑ risk of hemorrhagic cystitis. May ↓ antibody response to and ↑ risk of adverse reactions from **live-virus vaccines**.
Drug-Food: Grapefruit juice may ↑ levels; avoid concurrent use.

Route/Dosage

IV (Adults): 1.2 g/m²/day for 5 days; coadminister with mesna. May repeat cycle every 3 wk.

Availability (generic available)

Powder for injection: 1 g/vial, 3 g/vial. **Solution for injection:** 50 mg/mL.

NURSING IMPLICATIONS

Assessment

- Monitor BP, HR, respiratory rate, and temperature frequently during administration.
- Monitor urinary output frequently during therapy.
- Monitor for signs and symptoms of encephalopathy (confusion, somnolence, hallucinations, blurred vision, psychotic behavior, extrapyramidal symptoms, incontinence, seizures) during and for hours to days after administration. *If CNS signs/symptoms occur,* treat as clinically indicated and consider methylene blue until complete resolution. Dose interruption or permanent discontinuation may be required based on individual safety and tolerability.
- Assess nausea, vomiting, and appetite. Weigh weekly. Premedication with an antiemetic may be used to minimize GI effects. Adjust diet as tolerated.
- Monitor for myelosuppression. Assess for bleeding (bleeding gums; bruising; petechiae; guaiac stools, urine, or emesis) and avoid IM injections and rectal temperatures. Apply pressure to venipuncture sites for 10 min. Assess for signs of infection during neutropenia. Anemia may occur. Monitor for fatigue, dyspnea, and orthostatic hypotension.

Lab Test Considerations

- Monitor CBC with differential prior to and periodically during therapy. Leukocyte nadir usually occurs in 2nd wk after administration. *For WBC <2000/µL, platelets <50,000/µL, active infection, or signs of severe immunosuppression,* delayed administration may be required. Nadir of leukopenia and thrombocytopenia occurs within 7–14 days and usually recovers within 21 days of therapy.
- Monitor AST, ALT, serum alkaline phosphatase, bilirubin, and LDH prior to and periodically during therapy. May ↑ liver enzymes and bilirubin.
- Monitor serum and urine phosphorus and potassium, sediment for the presence of erythrocytes, and serum creatinine prior to initiation and as indicated during therapy. Obtain urinalysis prior to

each dose. *If microscopic hematuria (>10 RBCs per high-power field) present,* hold therapy until complete resolution; may resume with vigorous oral or parenteral hydration. Avoid administration with active urinary tract infection.

Implementation

- Prior to initiating therapy, correct urinary tract obstructions.
- Administer with extensive hydration of ≥2 L of oral or IV fluid per day to ↓ incidence or severity of bladder toxicity.
- Administer with mesna to ↓ incidence or severity of hemorrhagic cystitis.
- Prepare solution in a biologic cabinet. Wear gloves, gown, and mask while handling IV medication. Discard IV equipment in specially designated containers.

IV Administration

- Ifosfamide is an irritant. If extravasation occurs, immediately stop infusion. Leave needle/cannula in place temporarily but do not flush the line. Gently aspirate extravasated solution; then remove needle/cannula. Elevate patient's extremity and apply dry cold compresses for 20 min 4 times day for 1–2 days.
- **IV: Dilution:** Dilute 1-g vial with 20 mL and 3-g vial with 60 mL sterile water or bacteriostatic water for injection; shake to dissolve completely. Do not infuse solution if cloudy, discolored or contains particulates. **Concentration:** 50 mg/mL.
- **Intermittent Infusion: Dilution:** Dilute 1-g vial with 20 mL and 3-g vial with 60 mL sterile water or bacteriostatic water for injection (resulting concentration = 50 mg/mL) ; shake to dissolve completely. Do not infuse solution if cloudy, discolored, or contains particulates. May be further diluted in D5W, 0.9% NaCl, LR, or sterile water for injection. **Concentration:** 0.6–20 mg/mL. Refrigerate reconstituted and further diluted solutions and use within 24 hr. **Rate:** Administer over ≥30 min.
- **Y-Site Compatibility:** acyclovir, alemtuzumab, allopurinol, amikacin, aminocaproic acid, aminophylline, amiodarone, amphotericin B deoxycholate, amphotericin B liposomal, ampicillin, ampicillin/sulbactam, anidulafungin, argatroban, arsenic trioxide, atracurium, azithromycin, aztreonam, bivalirudin, bleomycin, bumetanide, buprenorphine, butorphanol, calcium chloride, calcium gluconate, carboplatin, caspofungin, cefazolin, cefotaxime, cefotetan, cefoxitin, ceftazidime, ceftriaxone, cefuroxime, chlorpromazine, ciprofloxacin, cisatracurium, cisplatin, clindamycin, cyclosporine, cytarabine, dacarbazine, dactinomycin, daptomycin, dexamethasone, dexmedetomidine, dexrazoxane, digoxin, diltiazem, diphenhydramine, dobutamine, docetaxel, dopamine, doxorubicin hydrochloride, doxorubicin liposomal, doxycycline, droperidol, enalaprilat, ephedrine, epinephrine, epirubicin, ertapenem, erythromycin, esmolol, etoposide, etoposide phosphate, famotidine, fentanyl, filgrastim, fluconazole, fludarabine, fluorouracil, foscarnet, fosphenytoin, furosemide, ganciclovir, gemcitabine, gemtuzumab ozogamicin, gentamicin, granisetron, haloperidol, heparin, hydrocortisone, hydromorphone, idarubicin, imipenem/cilastatin, insulin regular, isoproterenol, ketorolac, labetalol, leucovorin, levofloxacin, lidocaine, linezolid, lorazepam, magnesium sulfate, mannitol, melphalan, meperidine, meropenem, mesna, methadone, methohexital, methylprednisolone, metoclopramide, metoprolol, metronidazole, midazolam, milrinone, minocycline, mitomycin, mitoxantrone, morphine, moxifloxacin, nalbuphine, naloxone, nicardipine, nitroglycerin, nitroprusside, norepinephrine, octreotide, ondansetron, oxaliplatin, paclitaxel, palonosetron, pamidronate, pemetrexed, pentamidine, pentobarbital, phenobarbital, phenylephrine, piperacillin/tazobactam, potassium acetate, potassium chloride, procainamide, prochlorperazine, promethazine, propofol, propranolol, remifentanil, rituximab, rocuronium, sargramostim, sodium acetate, sodium bicarbonate, sodium phosphates, succinylcholine, sufentanil, tacrolimus, theophylline, thiotepa, tigecycline, tirofiban, tobramycin, topotecan, trastuzumab, trimethoprim/sulfamethoxazole, vancomycin, vasopressin, vecuronium, verapamil, vinblastine, vincristine, vinorelbine, voriconazole, zidovudine, zoledronic acid.
- **Y-Site Incompatibility:** cefepime, diazepam, methotrexate, pantoprazole, phenytoin, potassium phosphates.

Patient/Family Teaching

- Explain purpose and side effects of medication. Advise patient to read *Patient Information* before starting therapy.
- Emphasize need for adequate fluid intake throughout therapy and to void frequently to ↓ bladder irritation. Notify health care provider immediately if blood in the urine occurs.
- Advise patient to avoid grapefruit and grapefruit juice during therapy.
- Instruct patient to notify health care provider promptly if fever; chills; cough; hoarseness; sore throat; signs of infection; lower back or side pain; painful or difficult urination; bleeding gums; bruising; petechiae; blood in urine, stool, or emesis; or confusion occurs.
- Caution patient to avoid crowds and persons with known infections. Instruct patient to use soft toothbrush and electric razor and to avoid falls. Patient should also be cautioned not to drink alcoholic beverages or take products containing aspirin or NSAIDs, as these may cause GI hemorrhage.

- Advise patient to notify health care provider immediately if confusion, sedation, hallucination, blurred vision, psychotic behavior, extrapyramidal symptoms, urinary incontinence, or seizure occur.
- Discuss with patient the possibility of hair loss. Explore methods of coping.
- Instruct patient to notify health care provider of all Rx or OTC medications, vitamins, or herbal products being taken and to consult with health care provider before taking other medications.
- Instruct patient not to receive any vaccinations without advice of health care provider; ifosfamide may ↓ antibody response to and ↑ risk of adverse reactions from live-virus vaccines.
- Rep: May cause fetal harm. Advise women of reproductive potential to notify health care provider if pregnancy is planned or suspected. Instruct women of reproductive potential and men with female partners of reproductive potential to use contraception during and for ≥6 mo after therapy and to avoid breastfeeding during and for 1 wk after last dose. Caution patient about potential for amenorrhea, premature menopause, and sterility.

Evaluation/Desired Outcomes

- Decrease in size or spread of malignant germ cell testicular carcinoma.

BEERS

iloperidone

(eye-loe-**per**-i-done)

Fanapt

Classification

Therapeutic: antipsychotics

Pharmacologic: benzisoxazoles

Indications

Schizophrenia. Acute treatment of manic or mixed episodes associated with bipolar I disorder.

Action

May act by antagonizing dopamine and serotonin in the CNS. **Therapeutic Effects:** Decreased symptoms of schizophrenia or bipolar mania.

Pharmacokinetics

Absorption: Well absorbed (96%) following oral administration.

Distribution: Unknown.

Metabolism and Excretion: Extensively metabolized by the liver, primarily by the CYP3A4 and CYP2D6 isoenzymes. The CYP2D6 enzyme system exhibits genetic polymorphism (7–10% of White patients and 3–8% of Black patients are considered poor metabolizers [PM]). Two major metabolites (P88 and P95) may be partially responsible for pharmacologic activity. 58% excreted in urine as metabolites in extensive metabolizers (EM) and 45% in PM; 20% eliminated in feces in EM and 22.1% in PM.

Half-life: *EMs:* iloperidone: 18 hr, P88: 26 hr, P95: 23 hr; *PMs:* iloperidone: 33 hr, P88: 37 hr, P95: 31 hr.

TIME/ACTION PROFILE (antipsychotic effect)

ROUTE	ONSET	PEAK	DURATION
PO	2–4 wk	2–4 hr†	unknown

† Blood level.

Contraindications/Precautions

Contraindicated in: Hypersensitivity; Bradycardia, recent MI, or uncompensated HF (↑ risk of serious arrhythmias); Congenital long QT syndrome, QTc interval >500 msec, or history of cardiac arrhythmias; Electrolyte abnormalities, especially hypomagnesemia or hypokalemia (correct prior to therapy); Severe hepatic impairment; Lactation: Lactation.

Use Cautiously in: Known cardiovascular disease including HF, history of MI/ischemia, conduction abnormalities, cerebrovascular disease, or other conditions known to predispose to hypotension, including dehydration, hypovolemia, and concurrent antihypertensive therapy (↑ risk of orthostatic hypotension); Known ↓ WBC or history of drug-induced leukopenia/neutropenia; Circumstances that may result in ↑ body temperature, including strenuous exercise, exposure to extreme heat, concurrent anticholinergic activity, or dehydration (may impair thermoregulation); At risk for aspiration or falls; History of breast cancer; Moderate hepatic impairment; Undergoing cataract or glaucoma surgery (↑ risk of intraoperative floppy iris syndrome); OB: Neonates at ↑ risk for extrapyramidal symptoms and withdrawal after delivery when exposed during the 3rd trimester; use only if potential maternal benefit justifies potential fetal risk; Pedi: Safety and effectiveness not established in children; Geri: Appears on Beers list. ↑ risk of stroke, cognitive decline, and mortality in older adults with dementia. Avoid use in older adults, except for schizophrenia.

Adverse Reactions/Side Effects

CV: orthostatic hypotension, tachycardia, palpitations, QT interval prolongation. **EENT:** nasal congestion, intraoperative floppy iris syndrome. **Endo:** hyperglycemia, hyperprolactinemia. **GI:** dry mouth, nausea, abdominal discomfort, diarrhea. **GU:** priapism, urinary incontinence. **Metab:** weight gain, dyslipidemia, weight loss. **MS:** ↓ bone density, musculoskeletal stiffness. **Neuro:** dizziness, drowsiness, fatigue, agitation, cognitive impairment, delusions, extrapyramidal disorders, NEUROLEPTIC MALIGNANT SYNDROME, restlessness, tardive dyskinesia. **Misc:** HYPERSENSITIVITY REACTIONS (INCLUDING ANAPHYLAXIS AND ANGIOEDEMA).

Interactions

Drug-Drug: QT interval prolonging medications, including **quinidine**, **procainamide**, **amiodarone**, **sotalol**, **chlorpromazine**, **thioridazine**, **moxifloxacin**, **pentamidine**, and **methadone**, may ↑ risk of QT interval prolongation; avoid concurrent use. **Strong CYP2D6 inhibitors**, including **fluoxetine** and **paroxetine**, may ↑ levels and the risk of toxicity; ↓ iloperidone dose. **Strong CYP3A4 inhibitors**, including **ketoconazole** and **clarithromycin**, may ↑ levels and the risk of toxicity; ↓ iloperidone dose. **Antihypertensives**, including **diuretics**, may ↑ risk of orthostatic hypotension. **Anticholinergics** may ↑ risk of impaired thermoregulation.

Route/Dosage

Schizophrenia

PO (Adults): 1 mg twice daily on Day 1, then 2 mg twice daily on Day 2; then ↑ by 2 mg/day every day until a target dose of 12–24 mg/day given in two divided doses is reached; retitration is required if iloperidone is discontinued >3 days. *Concurrent use of strong CYP2D6 and/or CYP3A4 inhibitors:* ↓ dose by 50%; if inhibitor is withdrawn, ↑ iloperidone dose to previous amount. *CYP2D6 PMs:* 1 mg twice daily on Day 1, then 2 mg twice daily on Day 2; then ↑ by 2 mg/day every day until a target dose of 6–12 mg/day given in two divided doses is reached.

Acute Manic or Mixed Episodes Associated with Bipolar I Disorder

PO (Adults): 1 mg twice daily on Day 1, then 3 mg twice daily on Day 2; then ↑ by 3 mg/day every day until a target dose of 12 mg twice daily is reached; retitration is required if iloperidone is discontinued >3 days. *Concurrent use of strong CYP2D6 and/or CYP3A4 inhibitors:* ↓ dose by 50%; if inhibitor is withdrawn ↑ dose to previous amount. *CYP2D6 PMs:* 1 mg twice daily on Day 1, then 3 mg twice daily on Day 2; then ↑ by 3 mg/day every day until a target dose of 6 mg twice daily is reached.

Availability (generic available)

Tablets: 1 mg, 2 mg, 4 mg, 6 mg, 8 mg, 10 mg, 12 mg.

NURSING IMPLICATIONS

Assessment

- Monitor mental status (delusions, hallucinations, behavior) before and periodically during therapy. Monitor closely for notable changes in behavior that could indicate the emergence or worsening of suicidal thoughts or behavior or depression, especially during early therapy. Restrict amount of drug available to patient.
- Assess weight and BMI initially and throughout therapy. Refer as appropriate for nutritional/weight and medical management.
- Obtain ECG at baseline. Monitor BP (sitting, standing, lying down) and HR before and periodically during therapy. May cause QT interval prolongation, tachycardia, hypertension, and orthostatic hypotension.
- Monitor for signs and symptoms of hyperglycemia (polydipsia, polyuria, polyphagia, nausea, weakness) during treatment.
- Monitor for extrapyramidal side effects (*akathisia:* restlessness; *dystonia:* muscle spasms and twisting motions; or *pseudoparkinsonism:* masklike face, rigidity, tremors, drooling, shuffling gait, dysphagia). Report these symptoms; ↓ dose or discontinuation of medication may be necessary.
- Monitor for tardive dyskinesia (involuntary rhythmic movement of mouth, face, and extremities). Report immediately and discontinue therapy; may be irreversible.
- Monitor for development of neuroleptic malignant syndrome (fever, muscle rigidity, delirium, respiratory distress, tachycardia, seizures, diaphoresis, hypertension or hypotension, cardiac arrhythmia, pallor, tiredness). *If these symptoms occur, discontinue iloperidone immediately.*
- Monitor for symptoms related to hyperprolactinemia (menstrual abnormalities, galactorrhea, sexual dysfunction, changes in libido, erectile or ejaculatory dysfunction).
- Assess for falls risk. Drowsiness, orthostatic hypotension, and motor and sensory instability ↑ risk. Institute prevention if indicated.

Lab Test Considerations

- Monitor fasting blood glucose at baseline, at Wk 12, and annually in all patients; monitor more frequently for patients with risk factors for diabetes mellitus; patients with diabetes should be closely monitored for worsening glucose control.
- Monitor cholesterol levels at baseline, at Wk 12, and every 5 yr thereafter.
- Monitor potassium and magnesium in patients at risk for electrolyte disturbances.
- Monitor serum prolactin prior to and periodically during therapy. May ↑ prolactin.
- Monitor CBC frequently during initial months of therapy in patients with pre-existing or history of low WBC. May cause leukopenia, neutropenia, or agranulocytosis. *If any of these occur,* discontinue therapy.

Implementation

- Do not confuse Fanapt with Xanax.
- **PO:** Administer twice daily without regard to food. Observe patient when administering medication to ensure that medication is actually swallowed and not hoarded or cheeked.

Patient/Family Teaching

- Explain purpose and side effects of iloperidone to patient. Instruct patient to take medication exactly as directed. Do not share medication with others, even if they have similar symptoms; may be harmful. Keep out of children's reach. If doses are missed for >3 days, restart at initiation dose. Advise patient that appearance of tablets in stool is normal and not of concern. Advise patient to read *Patient Information* before starting and with each Rx refill in case of changes.

- Emphasize the importance of routine follow-up exams and lab tests to monitor side effects and continued participation in psychotherapy to improve coping skills.
- Inform patient of the possibility of extrapyramidal symptoms, neuroleptic malignant syndrome, and tardive dyskinesia. Instruct patient to report these symptoms immediately to health care provider.
- Advise patient to change positions slowly to minimize orthostatic hypotension. Protect from falls.
- Inform patient of potential for weight gain and hyperglycemia and the need for monitoring weight and blood glucose periodically during therapy.
- May cause drowsiness. Caution patient to avoid driving or other activities requiring alertness until response to medication is known.
- Extremes in temperature should also be avoided; this drug impairs body temperature regulation.
- Instruct patient to notify health care provider promptly if sore throat, fever, unusual bleeding or bruising, rash, tremors, palpitations, fainting, menstrual abnormalities, galactorrhea, or sexual dysfunction occur.
- Advise patient and family to notify health care provider if thoughts about suicide or dying, attempts to commit suicide, new or worse depression, new or worse anxiety, feeling very agitated or restless, panic attacks, trouble sleeping, new or worse irritability, acting aggressive, being angry or violent, acting on dangerous impulses, an extreme ↑ in activity and talking, or other unusual changes in behavior or mood occur.
- Advise patient to notify health care provider of all Rx or OTC medications, vitamins, or herbal products being taken and to consult with health care provider before taking other medications. Caution patient to avoid concurrent use of alcohol and other CNS depressants.
- Advise patient to notify health care provider of medication regimen before treatment or surgery (especially cataract surgery).
- Rep: Advise women of reproductive potential to notify health care provider if pregnancy is planned or suspected and to avoid breastfeeding during therapy. Monitor neonates exposed to iloperidone during the 3rd trimester of pregnancy for extrapyramidal and/or withdrawal symptoms following delivery. There have been reports of agitation, hypertonia, hypotonia, tremor, somnolence, respiratory distress, and feeding disorder in these neonates. Monitor breastfed infants for excessive drowsiness, lethargy, and developmental delays. Encourage women who become pregnant while taking iloperidone to enroll in the National Pregnancy Registry for Atypical Antipsychotics at 1-866-961-2388 or visit https://womensmentalhealth.org/clinical-and-research-programs/pregnancyregistry/.

Evaluation/Desired Outcomes

- Decrease in excited, paranoid, or withdrawn behavior.

I

HIGH ALERT

imatinib (i-mat-i-nib)

Gleevec, Imkeldi

Classification

Therapeutic: antineoplastics

Pharmacologic: enzyme inhibitors

Indications

Newly diagnosed Philadelphia positive (Ph+) chronic myeloid leukemia (CML) in chronic phase. CML in blast crisis, accelerated phase, or in chronic phase after failure of interferon-alpha treatment. Kit (CD117)-positive metastatic/unresectable malignant GI stromal tumors. Adjuvant treatment following resection of Kit (CD117)-positive GI stromal tumors. Relapsed or refractory Ph+ acute lymphoblastic leukemia (ALL). Newly diagnosed Ph+ ALL (in combination with chemotherapy). Myelodysplastic/myeloproliferative disease associated with platelet-derived growth factor receptor gene rearrangements. Aggressive systemic mastocytosis without the D816V c-Kit mutation or with c-Kit mutational status unknown. Hypereosinophilic syndrome and/or chronic eosinophilic leukemia in patients who have the FIP1L1-PDGFRα fusion kinase and for patients with hypereosinophilic syndrome and/or chronic eosinophilic leukemia who are FIP1L1-PDGFRα fusion kinase negative or unknown. Unresectable, recurrent, or metastatic dermatofibrosarcoma protuberans.

Action

Inhibits kinases, which may be produced by malignant cell lines. **Therapeutic Effects:** Inhibits production of malignant cell lines with decreased proliferation of leukemic cells in CML, hypereosinophilic syndrome, and/or chronic eosinophilic leukemia, and ALL and malignant cells in GI stromal tumor, myelodysplastic/myeloproliferative disease, aggressive systemic mastocytosis, and dermatofibrosarcoma protuberans.

Pharmacokinetics

Absorption: Well absorbed (98%) following oral administration.
Distribution: Unknown.
Protein Binding: 95%.
Metabolism and Excretion: Primarily metabolized by the liver via the CYP3A4 isoenzyme to N-demethyl imatinib, which is as active as imatinib. Excreted mostly in feces as metabolites. 5% excreted unchanged in urine.
Half-life: *Imatinib:* 18 hr; *N-desmethyl imatinib:* 40 hr.

TIME/ACTION PROFILE (plasma concentrations of imatinib)

ROUTE	ONSET	PEAK	DURATION
PO	unknown	2–4 hr	24 hr

Contraindications/Precautions

Contraindicated in: Hypersensitivity; OB: Pregnancy; Lactation: Lactation.
Use Cautiously in: Hepatic impairment (dose ↓ recommended if bilirubin >3 times upper limit of normal [ULN] or AST/ALT >5 times ULN); Cardiac disease (severe HF and left ventricular dysfunction may occur); Renal impairment, diabetes, hypertension, or HF (↑ risk of nephrotoxicity); Rep: Women of reproductive potential; Pedi: Children <1 yr (safety and effectiveness not established); Geri: ↑ risk of edema in older adults.

Adverse Reactions/Side Effects

CV: edema, HF. **Derm:** petechiae, pruritus, rash, DRUG RASH WITH EOSINOPHILIA AND SYSTEMIC SYMPTOMS (DRESS). **EENT:** epistaxis, nasopharyngitis, blurred vision. **Endo:** ↓ growth (in children), hypothyroidism. **GI:** abdominal pain, anorexia, constipation, diarrhea, dyspepsia, nausea, vomiting, HEPATOTOXICITY. **GU:** nephrotoxicity. **Hemat:** BLEEDING, NEUTROPENIA, THROMBOCYTOPENIA. **Metab:** weight gain. **MS:** arthralgia, muscle cramps, myalgia, pain. **Neuro:** fatigue, headache, weakness, dizziness, somnolence. **Resp:** cough, dyspnea, pneumonia. **Misc:** fever, night sweats, TUMOR LYSIS SYNDROME.

Interactions

Drug-Drug: Strong CYP3A4 inhibitors, including **ketoconazole, itraconazole, clarithromycin, atazanavir, nefazodone, nelfinavir, ritonavir,** or **voriconazole**, may ↑ levels and risk of toxicity. **Strong CYP3A4 inducers**, including **dexamethasone, phenytoin, carbamazepine, rifampin, rifabutin**, and **phenobarbital**, may ↓ levels and effectiveness; if used concurrently, ↑ imatinib dose by 50%. May ↑ levels and risk of toxicity of **benzodiazepines, simvastatin**, and **calcium channel blockers**.
Drug-Food: Grapefruit juice may ↑ levels and risk of toxicity; avoid concurrent use.

Route/Dosage

Chronic Myeloid Leukemia

PO (Adults): *Chronic phase:* 400 mg once daily; may ↑ to 600 mg once daily; *Accelerated phase or blast crisis:* 600 mg once daily; may ↑ to 800 mg/day given as 400 mg twice daily based on response and circumstances.
PO (Children): *Newly diagnosed Ph+ CML:* 340 mg/m^2 once daily (not to exceed 600 mg).

Hepatic Impairment

PO (Adults): *Severe hepatic impairment:* ↓ dose by 25%.

Renal Impairment

PO (Adults): *CCr 40–59 mL/min:* Do not exceed dose of 600 mg/day; *CCr 20–39 mL/min:* ↓ initial dose by 50%; ↑ as tolerated.

Gastrointestinal Stromal Tumors

PO (Adults): *Metastatic or unresectable:* 400 mg once daily; may ↑ to 400 mg twice daily if well tolerated and response insufficient; *Adjuvant treatment after resection:* 400 mg once daily.

Hepatic Impairment

PO (Adults): *Severe hepatic impairment:* ↓ dose by 25%.

Renal Impairment

PO (Adults): *CCr 40–59 mL/min:* Do not exceed dose of 600 mg/day; *CCr 20–39 mL/min:* ↓ initial dose by 50%; ↑ as tolerated.

Ph+ Acute Lymphoblastic Leukemia

PO (Adults): 600 mg once daily.
PO (Children): 340 mg/m^2 once daily (not to exceed 600 mg).

Hepatic Impairment

PO (Adults): *Severe hepatic impairment:* ↓ dose by 25%.

Renal Impairment

PO (Adults): *CCr 40–59 mL/min:* Do not exceed dose of 600 mg/day; *CCr 20–39 mL/min:* ↓ initial dose by 50%; ↑ as tolerated.

Myelodysplastic/Myeloproliferative Diseases

PO (Adults): 400 mg once daily.

Hepatic Impairment

PO (Adults): *Severe hepatic impairment:* ↓ dose by 25%.

Renal Impairment

PO (Adults): *CCr 40–59 mL/min:* Do not exceed dose of 600 mg/day; *CCr 20–39 mL/min:* ↓ initial dose by 50%; ↑ as tolerated.

Aggressive Systemic Mastocytosis

PO (Adults): 400 mg once daily. *Patients with eosinophilia:* 100 mg once daily; ↑ to 400 mg once daily if well tolerated and response insufficient.

Hepatic Impairment

PO (Adults): *Severe hepatic impairment:* ↓ dose by 25%.

Renal Impairment

PO (Adults): *CCr 40–59 mL/min:* Do not exceed dose of 600 mg/day; *CCr 20–39 mL/min:* ↓ initial dose by 50%; ↑ as tolerated.

Hypereosinophilic Syndrome and/or Chronic Eosinophilic Leukemia

PO (Adults): *For patients who are FIP1L1-PDGFRα fusion kinase negative or unknown:* 400 mg once daily. *For patients with FIP1L1-PDGFRa fusion kinase:* 100 mg once daily; ↑ to 400 mg once daily if well tolerated and response insufficient.

Hepatic Impairment

PO (Adults): *Severe hepatic impairment:* ↓ dose by 25%.

Renal Impairment

PO (Adults): *CCr 40–59 mL/min:* Do not exceed dose of 600 mg/day; *CCr 20–39 mL/min:* ↓ initial dose by 50%; ↑ as tolerated.

Dermatofibrosarcoma Protuberans

PO (Adults): 400 mg twice daily.

Hepatic Impairment

PO (Adults): *Severe hepatic impairment:* ↓ dose by 25%.

Renal Impairment

PO (Adults): *CCr 40–59 mL/min:* Do not exceed dose of 600 mg/day; *CCr 20–39 mL/min:* ↓ initial dose by 50%; ↑ as tolerated.

Availability (generic available)

Tablets: 100 mg, 400 mg. **Oral solution (strawberry flavor):** 80 mg/mL.

NURSING IMPLICATIONS

Assessment

- Monitor for fluid retention. Weigh regularly, and assess for signs of pleural effusion, pericardial effusion, pulmonary edema, or ascites (dyspnea, periorbital edema, swelling in feet and ankles, weight gain). Evaluate unexpected weight gain. General fluid retention is usually dose related, more common in accelerated phase or blast crisis, and more common in older adults. Treatment usually involves diuretics, supportive therapy, and interruption of imatinib.
- Monitor vital signs; may cause fever.
- Monitor for tumor lysis syndrome (malignant disease progression, ↑ WBC counts, hyperuricemia, hyperkalemia, hyperphosphatemia, hypocalcemia, dehydration). Prevent by maintaining adequate hydration and correcting uric acid levels before starting imatinib.
- Monitor for signs and symptoms of DRESS (fever, rash, lymphadenopathy, facial swelling), associated with involvement of other organ systems (hepatitis, nephritis, hematologic abnormalities, myocarditis, myositis) during therapy. May resemble an acute viral infection. Eosinophilia is often present. *If signs/symptoms of DRESS occur,* discontinue therapy.
- Pedi: Monitor for ↓ growth rate in children and adolescents.

Lab Test Considerations

- Verify negative pregnancy status in women with reproductive potential before starting therapy.
- Monitor liver enzymes before and monthly during treatment or when clinically indicated. May ↑ AST/ALT and bilirubin, which usually lasts 1 wk. *If bilirubin >3 times ULN or AST/ALT >5 times ULN,* hold dose until bilirubin <1.5 times ULN and AST/ALT <2.5 times ULN. Resume at ↓ dose (patients on 400 mg/day should receive 300 mg/day and patients receiving 600 mg/day should receive 400 mg/day).
- May cause hypokalemia.
- Monitor CBC weekly for the 1st mo, biweekly for the 2nd mo, and periodically during therapy. May cause neutropenia and thrombocytopenia, usually lasting 2–3 wk or 3–4 wk, respectively, and anemia.
- **Aggressive Systemic Mastocytosis with Eosinophilia or Hypereosinophilic Syndrome and/or Chronic Eosinophilic Leukemia with FIP1L1-PDGFRα Fusion Kinase:** *If ANC <1 × 10^9/L and/or platelets <50 × 10^9/L,* stop imatinib until ANC ≥1.5 × 10^9/L and platelets ≥75 × 10^9/L. Resume at previous dose.
- **Chronic Phase CML, Myelodysplastic/Myeloproliferative Disease, Aggressive Systemic Mastocytosis, Hypereosinophilic Syndrome, and/or Chronic Eosinophilic Leukemia (FIP1L1-PDGFRα fusion kinase negative or unknown), and Gastrointestinal Stromal Tumor:** *If ANC <1 × 10^9/L and/or platelets <50 × 10^9/L,* stop imatinib until ANC ≥1.5 × 10^9/L and platelets ≥75 × 10^9/L. Resume at 400 mg once daily. If recurrence, stop imatinib until resolved; then ↓ dose to 300 mg once daily.
- **Ph+ CML Accelerated Phase and Blast Crisis or Ph+ ALL:** *If ANC <0.5 × 10^9/L and/or platelets <10 × 10^9/L,* determine if cytopenia is related to leukemia (with marrow aspirate or biopsy). If cytopenia is unrelated to leukemia, ↓ dose to 400 mg once daily. If cytopenia persists for 2 wk, ↓ dose to 300 mg once daily. If cytopenia persists for 4 wk and is still unrelated to leukemia, stop

imatinib until ANC ≥1 × 10^9/L and platelets ≥20 × 10^9/L; then resume at 300 mg once daily.

- **Dermatofibrosarcoma Protuberans:** *If ANC <1 × 10^9/L and/or platelets <50 × 10^9/L,* stop imatinib until ANC ≥1.5 × 10^9/L and platelets ≥75 × 10^9/L. Resume at 600 mg once daily. If recurrence, stop until resolved, and then ↓ dose to 400 mg once daily.
- **Newly Diagnosed Chronic Phase CML:** *If ANC <1 × 10^9/L and/or platelets <50 × 10^9/L,* stop imatinib until ANC ≥1.5 × 10^9/L and platelets ≥75 × 10^9/L. Resume at previous dose. If recurrence, stop until resolved; then ↓ dose to 260 mg/m^2 once daily.

Implementation

- ***High Alert:*** Fatalities have occurred with incorrect administration of chemotherapeutic agents. Before administering, clarify all ambiguous orders; double-check single, daily, and course-of-therapy dose limits; have second practitioner independently double-check original order and dose calculations. Therapy should be initiated by physician experienced in the treatment of patients with chronic myeloid leukemia.
- Patients requiring anticoagulation should receive low molecular weight or standard heparin, not warfarin.
- Treatment should be continued as long as patient continues to benefit.
- **PO:** Administer with food and 8 ounces of water to minimize GI irritation.
- If difficulty swallowing, tablets may be dispersed in 50 mL (100 mg) or 100 mL (400 mg) of water or apple juice and stirred with a spoon. Administer immediately after suspension.
- Administer doses >800 mg/day as 400 mg twice daily to ↓ exposure to iron.
- Pedi: Doses may be given once daily or divided into two doses, one in morning and one in evening.

Patient/Family Teaching

- Explain purpose and side effects of medication to patient. Advise patient to read *Patient Information* before starting therapy. Instruct to take as directed. If a dose is missed, take next dose at regular scheduled time. Do not double doses. Provide instructions for measuring correct dose and to use appropriate press-in bottle adapter and oral dispensing syringe if indicated.
- Advise patient to notify health care provider of all Rx or OTC medications, vitamins, or herbal products being taken and to consult health care provider before taking other medications.
- Advise patient to avoid grapefruit and grapefruit juice during therapy.
- May cause drowsiness or dizziness. Caution patient to avoid driving or other activities requiring alertness until response to medication is known.
- Inform patient of possibility of edema and fluid retention. Advise patient to notify health care provider if unexpected rapid weight gain occurs.
- Advise patient to notify health care provider if signs and symptoms of liver failure (jaundice, anorexia, bleeding or bruising) or DRESS occur.
- Pedi: Advise patient/caregiver that the long-term effects of prolonged treatment with imatinib on growth in children are unknown. Advise that children will be closely monitored during treatment.
- Rep: Advise women of reproductive potential to use effective contraception during and for >14 days after last dose, to notify health care provider if pregnancy is planned or suspected, and to avoid breastfeeding for >1 mo after last dose.

Evaluation/Desired Outcomes

- Inhibits production of malignant cell lines with decreased proliferation of leukemic cells in CML, hypereosinophilic syndrome, and/or chronic eosinophilic leukemia and ALL and malignant cells in GI stromal tumor, myelodysplastic/myeloproliferative disease, aggressive systemic mastocytosis, and dermatofibrosarcoma protuberans.

imipenem/cilastatin

(i-me-**pen**-em/sye-la-**stat**-in)

Primaxin

Classification

Therapeutic: anti-infectives

Pharmacologic: carbapenems

Indications

Treatment of: Lower respiratory tract infections, Urinary tract infections, Abdominal infections, Gynecologic infections, Skin and skin structure infections, Bone and joint infections, Bacteremia, Endocarditis, Polymicrobic infections.

Action

Imipenem inhibits bacterial cell wall synthesis. Combination with cilastatin prevents renal inactivation of imipenem, resulting in high urinary concentrations. Imipenem resists the actions of many enzymes that degrade most other penicillins and penicillin-like anti-infectives. **Therapeutic Effects:** Bactericidal action against susceptible bacteria. **Spectrum:** Spectrum is broad. Active against most gram-positive aerobic cocci: *Streptococcus pneumoniae*, Group A beta-hemolytic streptococci, *Enterococcus*, *Staphylococcus aureus*. Active against many gram-negative bacillary organisms: *Escherichia coli*, *Klebsiella*, *Acinetobacter*, *Proteus*, *Serratia*, *Pseudomonas aeruginosa*. Also displays activity against: *Salmonella*, *Shigella*, *Neisseria gonorrhoeae*, Numerous anaerobes.

Pharmacokinetics

Absorption: IV administration results in complete bioavailability.

Distribution: Widely distributed to tissues.

Metabolism and Excretion: 70% excreted unchanged by the kidneys.

Half-life: 1 hr (↑ in renal impairment).

TIME/ACTION PROFILE (plasma concentrations)

ROUTE	ONSET	PEAK	DURATION
IV	rapid	end of infusion	6–8 hr

Contraindications/Precautions

Contraindicated in: Hypersensitivity; Cross-sensitivity may occur with penicillins and cephalosporins.

Use Cautiously in: Previous history of multiple hypersensitivity reactions; Seizure disorders; Renal impairment (↓ dose if CCr ≤90 mL/min); OB: Safety not established in pregnancy; Lactation: Use during breastfeeding only if potential maternal benefit justifies potential risk to infant; Pedi: Children with CNS infections (↑ risk of seizures) or children <30 kg with renal impairment (safety and effectiveness not established); Geri: Older adults may be at ↑ risk for adverse reactions due to age-related ↓ in renal function.

Adverse Reactions/Side Effects

CV: hypotension. **Derm:** rash, pruritus, sweating, urticaria. **GI:** diarrhea, nausea, vomiting, CLOSTRIDIOIDES DIFFICILE-ASSOCIATED DIARRHEA (CDAD). **Hemat:** eosinophilia. **Local:** phlebitis at IV site. **Neuro:** dizziness, SEIZURES, somnolence. **Misc:** fever, HYPERSENSITIVITY REACTIONS (INCLUDING ANAPHYLAXIS), superinfection.

Interactions

Drug-Drug: Do not admix with **aminoglycosides**; inactivation may occur. **Probenecid** ↓ renal excretion and ↑ levels. ↑ risk of seizures with **ganciclovir** or **cyclosporine**; avoid concurrent use with ganciclovir. May ↓ **valproate** levels and ↑ risk of seizures.

Route/Dosage

IV (Adults): *If infection is suspected or proven to be due to a susceptible bacterial species:* 500 mg every 6 hr *or* 1 g every 8 hr; *If infection is suspected or proven to be due to bacterial species with intermediate susceptibility:* 1 g every 6 hr.

IV (Children ≥3 mo): 15–25 mg/kg every 6 hr; higher doses have been used in older children with cystic fibrosis.

IV (Children 4 wk–3 mo): 25 mg/kg every 6 hr.

IV (Children 1–4 wk): 25 mg/kg every 8 hr.

IV (Children <1 wk): 25 mg/kg every 12 hr.

Renal Impairment

IV (Adults): If infection is suspected or proven to be due to a susceptible bacterial species: *CCr 60–89 mL/min:* 400 mg every 6 hr *or* 500 mg every 6 hr; *CCr 30–59 mL/min:* 300 mg every 6 hr *or* 500 mg every 8 hr; *CCr 15–29 mL/min:* 200 mg every 6 hr *or* 500 mg every 12 hr; *CCr <15 mL/min receiving hemodialysis:* 200 mg every 6 hr *or* 500 mg every 12 hr; **If infection is suspected or proven to be due to bacterial species with intermediate susceptibility:** *CCr 60–89 mL/min:* 750 mg every 8 hr; *CCr 30–59 mL/min:* 500 mg every 6 hr; *CCr 15–29 mL/min:* 500 mg every 12 hr; *CCr <15 mL/min receiving hemodialysis:* 500 mg every 12 hr.

I

Availability (generic available)

Powder for injection: 250 mg imipenem/250 mg cilastatin, 500 mg imipenem/500 mg cilastatin.

NURSING IMPLICATIONS

Assessment

- Monitor infection (vital signs; appearance of wound, sputum, urine, and stool; WBC) at baseline and throughout therapy.
- Obtain a history before initiating therapy to determine previous use of and reactions to penicillins or cephalosporins. Persons with a negative history of sensitivity may still have an allergic response.
- Observe for signs and symptoms of anaphylaxis (rash, pruritus, laryngeal edema, wheezing). Have epinephrine, antihistamine, and resuscitative equipment close by. *If hypersensitivity reaction occurs,* immediately discontinue imipenem/cilastatin and treat as clinically indicated.
- Monitor for CNS changes. *If focal tremors, myoclonus, or seizures occur,* evaluate, place on anticonvulsant other than valproic acid, and consider dose ↓ or discontinuing imipenem/cilastatin.
- Monitor for diarrhea, abdominal cramping, fever, and bloody stools during and for several weeks after therapy. *If CDAD is suspected or confirmed,* discontinue imipenem/cilastatin and treat as clinically indicated.

Lab Test Considerations

- Obtain specimen for culture and sensitivity before initiating therapy. First dose may be given before receiving results.
- May transiently ↑ BUN, AST, ALT, LDH, alkaline phosphatase, bilirubin, and serum creatinine.
- May ↓ hemoglobin and hematocrit.
- May cause positive direct Coombs test.

Implementation

IV Administration

- **Intermittent Infusion:** Reconstitute each 250- or 500-mg vial with 10 mL of D5W, D5/0.9% NaCl,

0.9% NaCl, or D5/0.45% NaCl and shake well. **Dilution:** Further dilute in 100 mL of D5W or 0.9% NaCl. Solution may range from clear to yellow in color. Infusion is stable for 4 hr at room temperature and 24 hr refrigerated. **Concentration:** 2.5–5 mg/mL. **Rate:** Infuse doses ≤500 mg over 20–30 min. Infuse doses ≥750 mg over 40–60 min. Pedi: Infuse doses ≤500 mg over 15–30 min. Infuse doses >500 mg over 40–60 min.

- If rapid infusion causes nausea and vomiting, slow infusion.
- **Y-Site Compatibility:** acyclovir, amikacin, aminocaproic acid, anidulafungin, argatroban, arsenic trioxide, ascorbic acid, atracurium, atropine, benztropine, bivalirudin, bleomycin, bumetanide, buprenorphine, butorphanol, carboplatin, carmustine, caspofungin, cefazolin, cefepime, cefotaxime, cefotetan, cefoxitin, ceftazidime, ceftazidime/avibactam, ceftolozane/tazobactam, cefuroxime, chloramphenicol, cisatracurium, cisplatin, clindamycin, cyanocobalamin, cyclophosphamide, cyclosporine, cytarabine, dactinomycin, daunorubicin, defibrotide, dexamethasone, dexmedetomidine, dexrazoxane, digoxin, diltiazem, diphenhydramine, docetaxel, dopamine, doxorubicin hydrochloride, doxorubicin liposomal, doxycycline, enalaprilat, ephedrine, epinephrine, epirubicin, epoetin alfa, eptifibatide, eravacycline, erythromycin, esmolol, etoposide, famotidine, fentanyl, fludarabine, fluorouracil, folic acid, foscarnet, fosphenytoin, furosemide, gemtuzumab ozogamicin, gentamicin, glycopyrrolate, granisetron, heparin, hydrocortisone, hydromorphone, idarubicin, ifosfamide, indomethacin, insulin regular, irinotecan, isavuconazonium, isoproterenol, ketorolac, labetalol, leucovorin, levofloxacin, lidocaine, linezolid, magnesium sulfate, melphalan, meropenem, meropenem/vaborbactam, mesna, methadone, methotrexate, methylprednisolone, metoclopramide, metoprolol, metronidazole, mitomycin, mitoxantrone, morphine, multivitamins, nafcillin, naloxone, nitroglycerin, norepinephrine, octreotide, ondansetron, oxacillin, oxaliplatin, oxytocin, paclitaxel, pamidronate, pantoprazole, pemetrexed, penicillin G, pentobarbital, phentolamine, phenylephrine, phytonadione, plazomicin, potassium acetate, potassium chloride, propofol, propranolol, protamine, remifentanil, rituximab, rocuronium, sodium acetate, succinylcholine, sufentanil, sulbactam/durlobactam, tacrolimus, tedizolid, theophylline, thiotepa, tigecycline, tirofiban, tobramycin, trastuzumab, vasopressin, verapamil, vinblastine, vincristine, vinorelbine, voriconazole, zidovudine, zoledronic acid.
- **Y-Site Incompatibility:** alemtuzumab, allopurinol, amiodarone, amphotericin B liposomal, azathioprine, blinatumomab, ceftriaxone, chlorpromazine, dacarbazine, dantrolene, daptomycin, diazepam, diazoxide, etoposide phosphate, ganciclovir, gemcitabine, haloperidol, lorazepam, mannitol, milrinone, minocycline, mycophenolate, nalbuphine, nicardipine, palonosetron, phenytoin, prochlorperazine, pyridoxine, sargramostim, sodium bicarbonate, thiamine, topotecan, trimethoprim/sulfamethoxazole, vecuronium.

Patient/Family Teaching

- Explain purpose and side effects of medication. Advise patient to read *Patient Information* before starting therapy.
- Advise patient to notify health care provider for signs of superinfection (black, furry overgrowth on tongue; vaginal itching or discharge; loose or foul-smelling stools) and allergy.
- Caution patient to notify health care provider if fever and diarrhea occur, especially if stool contains blood, pus, or mucus. Advise patient not to treat diarrhea without consulting health care provider. May occur up to several weeks after discontinuation of medication.
- Advise patient to notify health care provider for history of stroke, seizure, or valproic acid use prior to initiating therapy.
- Advise patient to notify health care provider of all Rx or OTC medications, vitamins, or herbal products being taken and to consult health care provider before taking other medications.
- Rep: Advise women of reproductive potential to notify health care provider if pregnancy is planned or suspected or if breastfeeding.

Evaluation/Desired Outcomes

- Resolution of signs and symptoms of infection. Length of time for complete resolution depends on organism and site of infection.

imipenem/cilastatin/relebactam

(i-me-**pen**-em/sye-la-**stat**-in/**rel**-e-**bak**-tam)

Recarbrio

Classification

Therapeutic: anti-infectives

Pharmacologic: carbapenems, beta-lactamase inhibitors

Indications

Complicated urinary tract infections, including pyelonephritis (for patients with limited or no alternative treatment options). Complicated intra-abdominal infections (for patients with limited or no alternative treatment options). Hospital-acquired or ventilator-associated pneumonia.

Action
Imipenem inhibits bacterial cell wall synthesis. Cilastatin is a renal dehydropeptidase inhibitor that prevents renal inactivation of imipenem (does not have antibacterial properties). Relebactam inhibits beta-lactamase, which is an enzyme that can destroy beta-lactam antibiotics. **Therapeutic Effects:** Bactericidal action against susceptible bacteria. **Spectrum:** Spectrum is broad. Active against many gram-negative aerobic bacteria: *Acinetobacter calcoaceticus-baumannii complex*, *Citrobacter freundii*, *Enterobacter cloacae*, *Escherichia coli*, *Haemophilus influenzae*, *Klebsiella aerogenes*, *Klebsiella oxytoca*, *Klebsiella pneumoniae*, *Pseudomonas aeruginosa*, *Serratia marcescens*. Also active against the following gram-negative anaerobic bacteria: *Bacteroides caccae*, *Bacteroides fragilis*, *Bacteroides ovatus*, *Bacteroides stercoris*, *Bacteroides thetaiotaomicron*, *Bacteroides uniformis*, *Bacteroides vulgatus*, *Fusobacterium nucleatum*.

Pharmacokinetics
Absorption: IV administration results in complete bioavailability.
Distribution: Widely distributed to tissues.
Metabolism and Excretion: Minimally metabolized. Primarily excreted unchanged by the kidneys (imipenem 63%, cilastatin 77%, relebactam >90%).
Half-life: 1–1.2 hr.

TIME/ACTION PROFILE (plasma concentrations)

ROUTE	ONSET	PEAK	DURATION
IV	unknown	end of infusion	6 hr

Contraindications/Precautions
Contraindicated in: Hypersensitivity (cross-sensitivity may occur with penicillins and cephalosporins).
Use Cautiously in: Seizure disorders; Renal impairment (↓ dose if CCr <90 mL/min); OB: Use during pregnancy only if potential maternal benefit justifies potential fetal risk; Lactation: Use while breastfeeding only if potential maternal benefit justifies potential risk to infant; Pedi: Safety and effectiveness not established in children; Geri: Older adults may be at ↑ risk for adverse reactions due to age-related renal impairment.

Adverse Reactions/Side Effects
CV: hypertension. **GI:** ↑ lipase, ↑ liver enzymes, CLOSTRIDIOIDES DIFFICILE-ASSOCIATED DIARRHEA (CDAD), diarrhea, nausea, vomiting. **Hemat:** anemia. **Local:** phlebitis. **Neuro:** headache, SEIZURES. **Misc:** fever, HYPERSENSITIVITY REACTIONS (INCLUDING ANAPHYLAXIS).

Interactions
Drug-Drug: May ↓ **valproate** levels and ↑ risk of seizures. ↑ risk of seizures with **ganciclovir**; avoid concurrent use.

Route/Dosage
IV (Adults): 1.25 g every 6 hr.

Renal Impairment
IV (Adults): *CCr 60–89 mL/min:* 1 g every 6 hr; *CCr 30–59 mL/min:* 750 mg every 6 hr; *CCr 15–29 mL/min:* 500 mg every 6 hr; *CCr <15 mL/min on hemodialysis:* 500 mg every 6 hr (on dialysis days, administer doses after hemodialysis).

Availability
Powder for injection: imipenem 500 mg/cilastatin 500 mg/250 mg relebactam.

NURSING IMPLICATIONS
Assessment
- Monitor infection (vital signs; appearance of wound, sputum, urine, and stool; WBC) at baseline and during therapy.
- Obtain a history before initiating therapy to determine previous use of and reactions to penicillins or cephalosporins. Persons with a negative history of sensitivity may still have an allergic response.
- Observe patient for signs and symptoms of anaphylaxis (rash, pruritus, laryngeal edema, wheezing). Have epinephrine, antihistamine, and resuscitative equipment close by. *If hypersensitivity reaction occurs,* immediately discontinue therapy and treat as clinically indicated.
- Monitor for CNS changes. *If focal tremors, myoclonus, or seizures occur,* evaluate, place on anticonvulsant other than valproic acid, and consider dose ↓ or discontinuing therapy.
- Monitor for diarrhea, abdominal cramping, fever, and bloody stools during and for several weeks after therapy. *If CDAD is suspected or confirmed,* discontinue imipenem/cilastatin/relebactam, and treat as clinically indicated.

Lab Test Considerations
- Obtain specimen for culture and sensitivity before initiating therapy. 1st dose may be given before receiving results.
- May transiently ↑ BUN, AST, ALT, LDH, alkaline phosphatase, bilirubin, and serum creatinine.
- May ↓ hemoglobin and hematocrit.
- May cause positive direct Coombs test.

Implementation
IV Administration
- **Intermittent Infusion: Reconstitution:** Reconstitute with 0.9% NaCl, D5W, D5/0.9% NaCl, D5/0.45% NaCl, or D5/0.225% NaCl. **Dilution:** *Step 1:* For diluent available in 100-mL prefilled infusion bag, proceed to step 2. For diluent not available in 100-mL prefilled infusion bag, withdraw 100 mL of diluent and transfer to an empty

infusion bag. *Step 2:* Withdraw 20 mL (as two 10-mL aliquots) of diluent from infusion bag and reconstitute vial with one 10-mL aliquot diluent. *Step 3:* Shake vial well and transfer suspension into remaining 80 mL diluent in infusion bag. *Step 4:* Add second 10-mL aliquot of diluent to vial and shake well to ensure complete transfer of vial contents; repeat transfer of resulting suspension to infusion bag before administering. Agitate bag until clear. Solution is colorless to yellow; do not use if discolored or contains particulates. Stable for 2 hr at room temperature or 24 hr refrigerated; do not freeze. **Rate:** Infuse over 30 min.

- **Y-Site Compatibility:** acyclovir, albumin, human, amikacin, ampicillin/sulbactam, anidulafungin, azithromycin, aztreonam, bumetanide, calcium chloride, calcium gluconate, caspofungin, ceftolozane/tazobactam, cisatracurium, clindamycin, dexamethasone, dexmedetomidine, digoxin, diltiazem, diphenhydramine, dobutamine, dopamine, doxycycline, enalaprilat, epinephrine, eptifibatide, esmolol, esomeprazole, famotidine, fentanyl, fluconazole, fosphenytoin, furosemide, gentamicin, heparin, hydrocortisone, insulin aspart, insulin glulisine, insulin lispro, insulin regular, isavuconazonium, ketorolac, labetalol, levofloxacin, lidocaine, linezolid, magnesium sulfate, mesna, methylprednisolone, metoclopramide, metoprolol, metronidazole, micafungin, midazolam, milrinone, morphine, naloxone, nitroglycerin, norepinephrine, ondansetron, pantoprazole, phenylephrine, potassium phosphates, rocuronium, sulbactam/durlobactam, tedizolid, tigecycline, tobramycin, vancomycin, vasopressin, voriconazole.
- **Y-Site Incompatibility:** amphotericin B deoxycholate, haloperidol, phenytoin, posaconazole.

Patient/Family Teaching

- Explain purpose and side effects of medication. Advise patient to read *Patient Information* before starting therapy.
- Advise patient to notify health care provider for signs of superinfection (black, furry overgrowth on tongue; vaginal itching or discharge; loose or foul-smelling stools) and allergy.
- Instruct patient to notify health care provider of all Rx or OTC medications, vitamins, or herbal products being taken and consult health care provider before taking any new medications, especially valproate.
- Caution patient to notify health care provider if fever and diarrhea occur, especially if stool contains blood, pus, or mucus. Advise patient not to treat diarrhea without consulting health care provider. May occur up to several weeks after discontinuation of medication.
- Advise patient to notify health care provider for history of stroke, seizure, or valproic acid use prior to initiating therapy.
- Rep: Advise women of reproductive potential to notify health care provider if pregnancy is planned or suspected or if breastfeeding.

Evaluation/Desired Outcomes

- Resolution of signs and symptoms of infection. Length of time for complete resolution depends on organism and site of infection.

BEERS

imipramine (im-ip-ra-meen)

~~Tofranil~~

Classification

Therapeutic: antidepressants

Pharmacologic: tricyclic antidepressants

Indications

Major depressive disorder. Enuresis in children. **Unlabeled Use:** Adjunct in the management of chronic pain, incontinence (in adults), vascular headache prophylaxis, cluster headache, or insomnia.

Action

Potentiates the effect of serotonin and norepinephrine. Has significant anticholinergic properties. **Therapeutic Effects:** Antidepressant action that develops slowly over several weeks. Diminished incidence of enuresis.

Pharmacokinetics

Absorption: Well absorbed from the GI tract.
Distribution: Widely distributed to tissues.
Protein Binding: 89–95%.
Metabolism and Excretion: Mostly metabolized by the liver (CYP2D6 isoenzyme) to desipramine; the CYP2D6 enzyme system exhibits genetic polymorphism; ~7% of population may be poor metabolizers and may have significantly ↑ imipramine concentrations and an ↑ risk of adverse effects.
Half-life: 8–16 hr.

TIME/ACTION PROFILE (antidepressant effect)

ROUTE	ONSET	PEAK	DURATION
PO	hours	2–6 wk	weeks

Contraindications/Precautions

Contraindicated in: Hypersensitivity; Angle-closure glaucoma; Hypersensitivity to tartrazine or sulfites (in some preparations); Recent MI, known history of QT interval prolongation, HF; Concurrent use of MAO inhibitors or MAO-like drugs (linezolid or methylene blue); Lactation: Lactation.
Use Cautiously in: Pre-existing cardiovascular disease; Seizures or history of seizure disorder; Hypovolemia or dehydration (↑ risk of syndrome of inappropriate antidiuretic hormone secretion

[SIADH]); May ↑ risk of suicide attempt/ideation, especially during early treatment or dose adjustment; risk may be greater in children or adolescents; OB: Use during pregnancy only if potential maternal benefit justifies potential fetal risk; Pedi: Children <6 yr (safety and effectiveness not established); Geri: Appears on Beers list. ↑ risk of adverse reactions in older adults, including falls secondary to sedative and anticholinergic effects, orthostatic hypotension, and SIADH. Avoid use in older adults.

Adverse Reactions/Side Effects

CV: hypotension, ARRHYTHMIAS, ECG changes. **Derm:** photosensitivity. **EENT:** blurred vision, dry eyes. **Endo:** gynecomastia, SIADH. **F and E:** hyponatremia. **GI:** constipation, dry mouth, nausea, paralytic ileus. **GU:** ↓ libido, urinary retention. **Hemat:** blood dyscrasias. **Metab:** weight gain. **Neuro:** drowsiness, fatigue, agitation, confusion, hallucinations, insomnia, SUICIDAL THOUGHTS/BEHAVIORS.

Interactions

Drug-Drug: Concurrent use with **MAO inhibitors** may result in serious, potentially fatal reactions; MAO inhibitors should be stopped ≥14 days before imipramine therapy; imipramine should be stopped ≥14 days before MAO inhibitor therapy. Concurrent use with **MAO-inhibitor-like drugs**, such as **linezolid** or **methylene blue**, may ↑ risk of serotonin syndrome; concurrent use contraindicated; do not start therapy in patients receiving **linezolid** or **methylene blue**; if **linezolid** or **methylene blue** need to be started in a patient receiving imipramine, immediately discontinue imipramine and monitor for signs/symptoms of serotonin syndrome for 2 wk or until 24 hr after last dose of linezolid or methylene blue, whichever comes first (may resume imipramine therapy 24 hr after last dose of linezolid or methylene blue). Concurrent use with **SSRIs** may result in ↑ toxicity and should be avoided; **fluoxetine** should be stopped 5 wk before starting imipramine. Hypertensive crisis may occur with **clonidine**. **CYP2D6 inhibitors**, including **cimetidine**, **quinidine**, **amiodarone**, and **ritonavir**, may ↑ levels and risk of toxicity. Concurrent use with **levodopa** may result in delayed/↓ absorption of levodopa or hypertension. **Rifampin** and **phenobarbital** may ↓ levels and effectiveness. ↑ risk of CNS depression with other CNS **depressants**, including **alcohol**, **antihistamines**, **clonidine**, **opioids**, and **sedative/hypnotics**. **Adrenergic** and **anticholinergic** side effects may be ↑ with other **agents having these properties**. **Phenothiazines** or **hormonal contraceptives** may ↑ levels and risk of toxicity. **Cigarette smoking (nicotine)** may ↓ levels and effectiveness. Drugs that affect serotonergic neurotransmitter systems, including **SSRIs**, **SNRIs**, **fentanyl**, **buspirone**, **tramadol**, and **triptans**, may ↑ risk of serotonin syndrome.
Drug-Natural Products: St. John's wort may ↑ risk of serotonin syndrome. **Kava-kava**, **valerian**, or **chamomile** may ↑ risk of CNS depression. ↑ anticholinergic effects with **jimson weed** and **scopolia**.

Route/Dosage

Major Depressive Disorder

PO (Adults): 25–50 mg 3–4 times daily (not to exceed 300 mg/day); total daily dose may be given at bedtime.
PO (Geriatric Patients): 25 mg at bedtime initially, up to 100 mg/day in divided doses.
PO (Children >12 yr): 25–50 mg/day in divided doses (not to exceed 100 mg/day).
PO (Children 6–12 yr): 10–30 mg/day in 2 divided doses.

Enuresis

PO (Children ≥6 yr): 25 mg once daily 1 hr before bedtime; ↑ if necessary by 25 mg at weekly intervals to 50 mg in children <12 yr, up to 75 mg in children >12 yr.

Availability (generic available)

Tablets: 10 mg, 25 mg, 50 mg, ✱ 75 mg. **Capsules:** 75 mg, 100 mg, 125 mg, 150 mg.

NURSING IMPLICATIONS

Assessment

- Monitor BP and HR before and during initial therapy.
- Monitor weight and BMI initially and periodically throughout therapy.
- Assess for sexual dysfunction (↓ libido; erectile dysfunction).
- Assess for suicidal tendencies, especially during early therapy. Restrict amount of drug available to patient. Risk may be ↑ in children, adolescents, and adults ≤24 yr. After starting therapy, children, adolescents, and young adults should be seen by health care provider face-to-face at least weekly for 4 wk, every 3 wk for next 4 wk, and on advice of health care provider thereafter.
- Pedi, Geri: Monitor baseline and periodic ECG in older adults or patients with heart disease and before ↑ dose with children treated for enuresis. May cause prolonged PR and QT intervals and may flatten T waves.
- **Depression:** Assess mental status (orientation, mood, behavior) frequently. Confusion, agitation, and hallucinations may occur during initiation of therapy and may require dose ↓.
- **Enuresis:** Assess frequency of bed-wetting during therapy. Ask patient or caretaker to maintain diary.

- **Pain:** Assess location, duration, and severity of pain periodically during therapy. Use pain scale to monitor effectiveness of therapy.

Lab Test Considerations

- Assess WBC and differential blood counts and renal and hepatic functions before and periodically during prolonged or high-dose therapy.
- Serum levels may be monitored in patients who fail to respond to usual therapeutic dose. Therapeutic plasma concentration range for depression is 150–300 ng/mL.
- May cause alterations in blood glucose levels and hyponatremia.

Toxicity and Overdose

- Symptoms of acute overdose include disturbed concentration, confusion, restlessness, agitation, seizures, drowsiness, mydriasis, arrhythmias, fever, hallucinations, vomiting, and dyspnea.
- Treatment of overdose includes gastric lavage, activated charcoal, and a stimulant cathartic. Maintain respiratory and cardiac function (monitor ECG for >5 days) and temperature. Treatment may also include antiarrhythmics and anticonvulsants.

Implementation

- Dose ↑ should be made at bedtime because of sedation. Dose titration is a slow process; may take weeks to months to see therapeutic effect. May be given as a single dose at bedtime to minimize sedation during the day.
- When discontinuing therapy, taper to avoid withdrawal effects. Gradually taper dose over 2–4 wk to prevent withdrawal effects.
- **PO:** Administer with or immediately following a meal to minimize gastric irritation.
- For enuresis, administer dose 1 hr before bedtime; for early night bed-wetters, drug has been shown to be more effective if given earlier and in divided amounts (25 mg in midafternoon and repeated at bedtime).

Patient/Family Teaching

- Explain purpose and side effects of medication to patient. Advise patient to read *Patient Information* before starting therapy. Instruct patient to take as directed. Take missed doses as soon as possible unless almost time for next dose; if regimen is a single dose at bedtime, do not take in the morning because of side effects. Advise patient that drug effects may not be noticed for ≥2 wk. Abrupt discontinuation may cause nausea, vomiting, diarrhea, headache, trouble sleeping with vivid dreams, and irritability.
- Advise patient to notify health care provider of all Rx or OTC medications, vitamins, or herbal products being taken and to consult health care provider before taking other medications.
- May cause drowsiness and blurred vision. Caution patient to avoid driving and other activities requiring alertness until response to drug is known.
- Instruct patient to notify health care provider if visual changes occur. Inform patient that periodic glaucoma testing may be needed during long-term therapy.
- Caution patient to change positions slowly to minimize orthostatic hypotension.
- Advise patient, family, and caregivers to look for suicidality, especially during early therapy or dose changes. Notify health care provider immediately if thoughts about suicide or dying, attempts to commit suicide, new or worse depression or anxiety, agitation or restlessness, panic attacks, insomnia, new or worse irritability, aggressiveness, acting on dangerous impulses, mania, or other changes in mood or behavior occur.
- Advise patient, family, and caregivers to notify health care provider immediately if symptoms of serotonin syndrome occur.
- Advise patient to avoid alcohol or other CNS depressant drugs during therapy and for ≥3–7 days after therapy has been discontinued.
- Instruct patient to notify health care provider if urinary retention, dry mouth, or constipation persists. Sugarless candy or gum may diminish dry mouth and an increase in fluid intake or bulk may prevent constipation. If symptoms persist, dose ↓ or discontinuation may be necessary. Consult health care provider if dry mouth persists for >2 wk.
- Caution patient to use sunscreen and protective clothing to prevent photosensitivity reactions.
- Alert patient that urine may turn blue-green in color.
- Inform patient of need to monitor dietary intake, as possible ↑ in appetite may lead to undesired weight gain. Inform patient that ↑ amounts of riboflavin in the diet may be required; consult health care provider.
- Advise patient to notify health care provider of medication regimen before treatment or surgery.
- Therapy for depression is usually prolonged. Emphasize the importance of follow-up exams to evaluate progress and improve coping skills.
- Rep: Advise women of reproductive potential to notify health care provider if pregnancy is planned or suspected and to avoid breastfeeding.
- Pedi: Inform caregivers that the side effects most likely to occur include nervousness, insomnia, unusual tiredness, and mild nausea and vomiting. Notify health care provider if these symptoms become pronounced.
- Advise patients to keep medication out of reach of children to prevent inadvertent overdose.

Evaluation/Desired Outcomes

- Antidepressant action that develops slowly over several weeks.
- Diminished incidence of enuresis.

HIGH ALERT

inavolisib (in-a-voe-lis-ib)

Itovebi

Classification

Therapeutic: antineoplastics

Pharmacologic: kinase inhibitors

Indications

Endocrine-resistant, PIK3CA-mutated, hormone receptor-positive, human epidermal growth factor receptor 2-negative, locally advanced or metastatic breast cancer (in combination with palbociclib and fulvestrant).

Action

Acts as an inhibitor of phosphatidylinositol 3-kinase (PI3K). Mutations in the gene encoding the catalytic α-subunit of PI3K (PI3KCA) lead to activation of PI3Kα and Akt-signaling, cellular transformation, and tumor generation. Inavolisib inhibits phosphorylation of PI3K downstream targets (including Akt) and demonstrated activity in cell lines harboring a PIK3CA mutation. Activating mutations in PIK3CA may induce overgrowths and malformations in PIK3CA-related overgrowth spectrum. **Therapeutic Effects:** Decreased progression of breast cancer.

Pharmacokinetics

Absorption: 76% absorbed following oral administration.

Distribution: Well distributed to tissues.

Metabolism and Excretion: Primarily metabolized via hydrolysis; minimally metabolized by the CYP3A4 isoenzyme. 49% excreted in urine (40% as unchanged drug); 48% excreted in feces (11% as unchanged drug).

Half-life: 15 hr.

TIME/ACTION PROFILE (plasma concentrations)

ROUTE	ONSET	PEAK	DURATION
PO	unknown	3 hr	24 hr

Contraindications/Precautions

Contraindicated in: OB: Pregnancy; Lactation: Lactation.

Use Cautiously in: Diabetes mellitus; Moderate renal impairment (↓ dose); Rep: Women of reproductive potential and men with female partners of reproductive potential; Pedi: Safety and effectiveness not established in children; Geri: Older adults may be more sensitive to drug effects.

Adverse Reactions/Side Effects

Derm: alopecia, dry skin, rash. **Endo:** hyperglycemia. **F and E:** hypocalcemia, hypokalemia, hypomagnesemia, hyponatremia. **GI:** ↑ lipase, ↑ liver enzymes, diarrhea, nausea, stomatitis, vomiting. **GU:** ↑ serum creatinine, ↓ fertility. **Hemat:** anemia, lymphopenia, neutropenia, thrombocytopenia. **Metab:** ↓ appetite, weight loss. **Neuro:** fatigue, headache. **Misc:** infection.

Interactions

Drug-Drug: None reported.

Route/Dosage

PO (Adults): 9 mg once daily; continue until disease progression or unacceptable toxicity.

Renal Impairment

PO (Adults): 6 mg once daily; continue until disease progression or unacceptable toxicity.

Availability

Tablets: 3 mg, 9 mg.

I

NURSING IMPLICATIONS

Assessment

- Monitor patients for diarrhea. Correct any significant fluid and/or electrolyte abnormalities in patients with significant diarrhea. Early management of diarrhea with antidiarrheal agents should be considered. *If Grade 1 diarrhea occurs,* no adjustment required. *If Grade 2 diarrhea occurs,* hold until recovery to Grade ≤1; then resume at same dose level. *If recurrent Grade 2 diarrhea occurs,* hold until recovery to Grade ≤1; then resume at one lower dose level. *If Grade 3 diarrhea occurs,* hold until recovery to Grade ≤1; then resume at one lower dose level. *If Grade 4 diarrhea occurs,* permanently discontinue inavolisib.
- Monitor patients for signs and symptoms of stomatitis. Treat mild to moderate mucositis with bland oral rinses with 0.9% saline, sodium bicarbonate, and water. Treat moderate to severe mucositis with topical anesthetics (2% viscous lidocaine), systemic opioids, or steroids. Patients with mucositis and moderate xerostomia may receive sugarless candy/mints or pilocarpine/cevimeline to stimulate salivary gland function. Patients who are receiving myelosuppressive therapy may receive prophylactic antiviral and antifungal agents to prevent infections. Topical oral antimicrobial mouthwashes, rinses, pastilles, or lozenges may be used to ↓ the risk of infection. *If Grade 1 stomatitis occurs,* no adjustment required. *If Grade 2 stomatitis occurs,* hold until recovery to Grade ≤1. *If recurrent Grade 2 stomatitis occurs,* hold until recovery to Grade ≤1; then resume at one lower dose level. *If Grade 3 stomatitis occurs,* hold until recovery to Grade ≤1; then resume at one lower dose level. *If Grade 4 stomatitis occurs,* permanently discontinue inavolisib.

Lab Test Considerations

- Verify a negative pregnancy test before starting therapy.

- May cause severe hyperglycemia. Monitor fasting plasma or blood glucose every 3 days for the 1st wk, then once every wk for the next 3 wk, then once every 2 wk for the next 8 wk, then once every 4 wk thereafter, and as clinically indicated. *If glucose ≤160 mg/dL,* no adjustment required. *If glucose >160–250 mg/dL,* hold inavolisib and initiate or intensify antihyperglycemic medications; if glucose ↓ to ≤160 mg/dL within 7 days, resume at the same dose level; if glucose ↓ to ≤160 mg/dL in ≥8 days, resume at one lower dose level. *If glucose >250–500 mg/dL,* hold inavolisib and initiate or intensify antihyperglycemic medications; if glucose ↓ to ≤160 mg/dL within 7 days, resume at same dose level; if glucose ↓ to ≤160 mg/dL in ≥8 days, resume at one lower dose level ; if glucose >250–500 mg/dL recurs within 30 days, hold until glucose ↓ to ≤160 mg/dL and resume at one lower dose level. *If glucose >500 mg/dL,* hold inavolisib and initiate or intensify antihyperglycemic medications; if glucose ↓ to ≤ 160 mg/dL, resume at one lower dose level; if glucose >500 mg/dL recurs within 30 days, permanently discontinue inavolisib.
- Monitor A1c every 3 mo and as clinically indicated.
- Assess renal function (BUN and serum creatinine) at baseline.

Implementation

- **PO:** Administer without regard to food at the same time each day. ***DNC:*** Do not chew, crush, or split tablets prior to swallowing.
- **Dose Reduction for Adverse Reactions:** *1st dose reduction:* 6 mg once daily; *2nd dose reduction:* 3 mg once daily.

Patient/Family Teaching

- Explain purpose and side effects of inavolisib. Advise patient to take as directed. Swallow tablets whole, with or without food, at the same time each day; do not chew, crush, or split tablets prior to swallowing. If ≤9 hr from when dose is missed, take the missed dose as soon as possible; if >9 hr since missed dose, skip the dose and take the next dose at the scheduled time. If a dose is vomited, do not take an additional dose on that day and resume the usual dosing schedule the next day. Advise patient to read *Patient Information* before starting therapy.
- Teach patient to report symptoms of hyperglycemia (↑ thirst, frequent urination, headache, blurred vision, fatigue).
- Advise patient to report symptoms of stomatitis (painful mouth ulcers, sores, or blisters; bad breath; discomfort with eating and drinking). Sugar-free hard candies or mints can be used to prevent dry mouth. Teach patient about maintaining good oral hygiene and hydration.
- Instruct patient to report severe diarrhea; advise patient to drink plenty of fluid to prevent dehydration.
- Advise patient to notify health care professional of all Rx or OTC medications, vitamins, or herbal products being taken and to consult health care professional before taking other medications.
- Rep: May cause fetal harm. Advise women of reproductive potential to notify health care professional if pregnancy is planned or suspected and to avoid breastfeeding during therapy. Advise women of reproductive potential to use effective nonhormonal contraception during treatment and for 1 wk after last dose. Advise men with female partners of reproductive potential to use effective contraception during treatment and for 1 wk after last dose.

Evaluation/Desired Outcomes

- Decreased progression of breast cancer.

BEERS

indomethacin
(in-doe-**meth**-a-sin)

Indocin, ~~Tivorbex~~

Classification

Therapeutic: antirheumatics ductus arteriosus patency adjuncts (IV only), nonopioid analgesics
Pharmacologic: nonsteroidal anti-inflammatory drugs (NSAIDs)

Indications

PO: Inflammatory disorders, including: Rheumatoid arthritis, Gouty arthritis, Osteoarthritis, Ankylosing spondylitis. Mild to moderate acute pain. **IV:** Alternative to surgery in the management of patent ductus arteriosus (PDA) in premature neonates.

Action

Inhibits prostaglandin synthesis. In the treatment of PDA, decreased prostaglandin production allows the ductus to close. **Therapeutic Effects: PO:** Suppression of pain and inflammation. **IV:** Closure of PDA.

Pharmacokinetics

Absorption: Well absorbed after oral administration in adults; incomplete oral absorption in neonates.
Distribution: Crosses the blood-brain barrier.
Protein Binding: 99%.
Metabolism and Excretion: Mostly metabolized by the liver.
Half-life: *Neonates <2 wk:* 20 hr; *Neonates >2 wk:* 11 hr; *Adults:* 2.6–11 hr.

TIME/ACTION PROFILE

ROUTE	ONSET	PEAK	DURATION
PO (analgesic)	30 min	0.5–2 hr	4–6 hr
PO-ER (analgesic)	30 min	unknown	4–6 hr
PO (anti-inflammatory)	up to 7 days	1–2 wk	4–6 hr
PO-ER (anti-inflammatory)	up to 7 days	1–2 wk	4–6 hr
IV (closure of PDA)	up to 48 hr	unknown	unknown

Contraindications/Precautions

Contraindicated in: Hypersensitivity; Known alcohol intolerance (suspension); Cross-sensitivity may exist with other NSAIDs, including aspirin; Active GI bleeding; Ulcer disease; Proctitis or recent history of rectal bleeding; Intraventricular hemorrhage; Thrombocytopenia; Coronary artery bypass graft surgery; Recent MI; HF; OB: Avoid use after 30 wk gestation (may cause premature closure of fetal ductus arteriosus); Pedi: ↑ risk of necrotizing enterocolitis and bowel perforation in premature infants with PDA.

Use Cautiously in: Severe renal impairment; Severe hepatic impairment; Cardiovascular disease or risk factors for cardiovascular disease (may ↑ risk of serious cardiovascular thrombotic events, MI, and stroke, especially with prolonged use or use of higher doses); History of long duration of NSAID use, smoking, alcohol use, advanced liver disease, coagulopathy, or poor general health (↑ risk of GI bleeding); History of peptic ulcer disease and/or GI bleeding; Bleeding tendency or concurrent anticoagulant therapy; Seizure disorders; Hypertension; OB: Use at or after 20 wk gestation may cause fetal renal impairment leading to oligohydramnios and, possibly neonatal renal impairment; if treatment is necessary between 20 wk and 30 wk gestation, limit use to the lowest effective dose and shortest duration possible; Geri: Appears on Beers list. ↑ risk GI bleeding or peptic ulcer disease in older adults. Avoid chronic use unless other alternatives are not effective and the patient can take a gastroprotective agent; avoid short-term use in combination with oral or parenteral corticosteroids, anticoagulants, or antiplatelet agents unless other alternatives are not effective and the patient can take a gastroprotective agent.

Adverse Reactions/Side Effects

CV: edema, HF, hypertension, MI. **Derm:** EXFOLIATIVE DERMATITIS, GENERALIZED BULLOUS FIXED DRUG ERUPTION, rash, STEVENS-JOHNSON SYNDROME (SJS), TOXIC EPIDERMAL NECROLYSIS (TEN). **EENT:** blurred vision, tinnitus. **Endo: IV:** hypoglycemia. **F and E:** hyperkalemia **IV:** hyponatremia. **GI:** constipation, dyspepsia, nausea, vomiting, discomfort **PO:** GI BLEEDING, GI PERFORATION, GI ULCERATION, HEPATOTOXICITY, necrotizing enterocolitis, PANCREATITIS. **GU:** cystitis, hematuria, renal failure. **Hemat:** blood dyscrasias, prolonged bleeding time, thrombocytopenia. **Local:** phlebitis at IV site. **Neuro:** dizziness, drowsiness, headache, psychic disturbances, STROKE. **Misc:** HYPERSENSITIVITY REACTIONS (INCLUDING ANAPHYLAXIS AND SERIOUS SKIN REACTIONS).

Interactions

Drug-Drug: Concurrent use with **aspirin** may ↓ effectiveness. ↑ risk of GI bleeding with **anticoagulants, aspirin, clopidogrel, ticagrelor, prasugrel, corticosteroids, fibrinolytics, SNRIs,** or **SSRIs.** Chronic use of **acetaminophen** ↑ risk of adverse renal reactions. May ↓ effectiveness of **diuretics** or **antihypertensives**. May ↑ hypoglycemia from **insulins** or **oral hypoglycemic agents**. May ↑ risk of toxicity from **lithium** or **zidovudine** (avoid concurrent use with zidovudine). ↑ risk of toxicity from **methotrexate**. **Probenecid** ↑ risk of toxicity from indomethacin. ↑ risk of adverse hematologic reactions with **antineoplastics** or **radiation therapy**. ↑ risk of nephrotoxicity with **cyclosporine**. Concurrent use with **potassium-sparing diuretics** may result in hyperkalemia. May ↑ levels of **digoxin, methotrexate, lithium,** and **aminoglycosides** when used IV in neonates.

Drug-Natural Products: ↑ bleeding risk with **anise, arnica, chamomile, clove, dong quai, feverfew, garlic, ginger, ginkgo,** and **Panax ginseng**.

Route/Dosage

Anti-inflammatory

PO (Adults): *Arthritis (immediate release):* 25–50 mg 2–4 times daily (max dose = 200 mg/day). A single bedtime dose of 100 mg may alternatively be used; *Arthritis (extended release):* 75 mg once or twice daily (max dose = 150 mg/day). *Gout:* 100 mg initially, followed by 50 mg 3 times daily for relief of pain; then ↓ further.

PO (Children >2 yr): 1–2 mg/kg/day in 2–4 divided doses (not to exceed 4 mg/kg/day or 150–200 mg/day).

PDA Closure

IV (Neonates): *Treatment:* 0.2 mg/kg initially, then 2 subsequent doses at 12–24 hr intervals of 0.1 mg/kg if age <48 hr at time of initial dose; 0.2 mg/kg if 2–7 days at initial dose; 0.25 mg/kg if age >7 days at initial dose. *Prophylaxis:* 0.1–0.2 mg/kg initially, then 0.1 mg/kg every 12–24 hr for 2 doses.

Availability (generic available)

Capsules: 25 mg, 50 mg. **Extended-release capsules:** 75 mg. **Oral suspension (fruit mint, pineapple, coconut, mint flavors):** 25 mg/5 mL. **Powder for injection:** 1 mg/vial. **Rectal suppository:** 50 mg, ✱ 100 mg.

NURSING IMPLICATIONS

Assessment

- Monitor for rhinitis, asthma, and urticaria. Patients who have asthma, aspirin-induced allergy, and nasal polyps are at ↑ risk for developing hypersensitivity reactions.
- Assess for SJS, TEN, and generalized bullous fixed drug eruption. Discontinue indomethacin at 1st sign of rash and treat as indicated.
- Monitor BP during initiation and periodically thereafter.
- **Arthritis:** Assess limitation of movement and pain; note type, location, and intensity before and 1–2 hr after administration.

I

- **PDA:** Monitor respiratory status, HR, BP, echocardiogram, and heart sounds routinely throughout therapy.
- Monitor intake and output. Fluid restriction is usually instituted throughout therapy.
- **Acute pain:** Assess type, location, and intensity of pain prior to and 2 hr (peak) following administration.

Lab Test Considerations

- Evaluate BUN, serum creatinine, CBC, potassium, and liver function tests periodically in patients receiving prolonged therapy.
- May alter blood glucose values.
- May ↓ hemoglobin, hematocrit, leukocytes, platelets, and CCr. Bleeding time may be prolonged for several days after last dose.
- May cause ↑ in urine glucose and protein concentrations.

Implementation

- If prolonged therapy is used, dose should be ↓ to the lowest level that controls symptoms to minimize risk of cardiovascular thrombotic events.
- **PO:** Administer after meals, with food, or with antacids to ↓ GI irritation. ***DNC:*** Do not break, crush, or chew sustained-release capsules.
- Shake suspension before administration. Do not mix with antacid or any other liquid.

IV Administration

- **IV Push: Reconstitution:** Reconstitute with 1–2 mL of preservative-free 0.9% NaCl or sterile water. Reconstitute immediately before use and discard any unused solution. Do not dilute further or admix. **Concentration:** 0.5–1 mg/mL. **Rate:** Administer over 20–30 min. Do not administer via umbilical catheter into vessels near the superior mesenteric artery, as these can cause vasoconstriction and compromise blood flow to the intestines. Do not administer intra-arterially.
- **Y-Site Compatibility:** aminophylline, ascorbic acid, atropine, bumetanide, caffeine citrate, cefazolin, cefotaxime, cefoxitin, ceftazidime, ceftriaxone, cefuroxime, chloramphenicol, cisplatin, clindamycin, cyanocobalamin, cyclosporine, dexamethasone, digoxin, enalaprilat, ephedrine, epoetin alfa, fentanyl, fluconazole, folic acid, furosemide, ganciclovir, heparin, hydrocortisone, imipenem/cilastatin, insulin regular, ketorolac, lidocaine, mannitol, metoclopramide, metoprolol, multivitamins, nafcillin, nitroglycerin, nitroprusside, penicillin G, pentobarbital, phenobarbital, phytonadione, potassium chloride, procainamide, sodium bicarbonate, theophylline.
- **Y-Site Incompatibility:** amikacin, atracurium, aztreonam, benztropine, buprenorphine, butorphanol, calcium chloride, calcium gluconate, cefotetan, chlorpromazine, dactinomycin, dantrolene, daunorubicin, diazepam, diazoxide, diphenhydramine, dobutamine, dopamine, doxycycline, epinephrine, erythromycin, esmolol, etoposide, famotidine, gentamicin, glycopyrrolate, haloperidol, hydralazine, isoproterenol, labetalol, levofloxacin, magnesium sulfate, meperidine, midazolam, minocycline, morphine, nalbuphine, norepinephrine, ondansetron, oxytocin, paclitaxel, pantoprazole, papaverine, pentamidine, phenylephrine, phenytoin, prochlorperazine, promethazine, propranolol, protamine, pyridoxine, succinylcholine, sufentanil, thiamine, tobramycin, trimethoprim/sulfamethoxazole, vancomycin, vasopressin, verapamil.

Patient/Family Teaching

- Explain purpose and side effects of medication. Advise patient to read *Patient Information* before starting therapy.
- Advise patient to take this medication with a full glass of water and to remain in an upright position for 15–30 min after administration.
- May cause drowsiness or dizziness. Advise patient to avoid driving or other activities requiring alertness until response to medication is known.
- Advise patient to notify health care provider of all Rx or OTC medications, vitamins, or herbal products being taken and to consult health care provider before taking other medications. Avoid concurrent use of alcohol, aspirin and other NSAIDs.
- Caution patient to wear sunscreen and protective clothing to prevent photosensitivity reactions.
- Advise patient to inform health care provider of medication regimen before treatment or surgery.
- Inform patient of ↑ risk of MI and stroke. Use lowest effective dose for shortest time. Advise patient to notify health care provider immediately if signs and symptoms (shortness of breath or trouble breathing, chest pain, weakness in one part or side of body, slurred speech, swelling of the face or throat) occur.
- Advise patient to notify health care provider promptly if signs or symptoms of GI toxicity (abdominal pain, black stools) occur.
- Instruct patient to notify health care provider immediately if signs and symptoms of hepatotoxicity (nausea, fatigue, lethargy, diarrhea, pruritus, jaundice, right upper quadrant tenderness, flu-like symptoms), rash, itching, chills, fever, muscle aches, visual disturbances, weight gain, edema, or persistent headache occurs.
- Rep: May cause fetal harm. Advise women of reproductive potential to notify health care provider if pregnancy is planned or suspected or if breastfeeding. Advise women to avoid indomethacin in the 3rd trimester of pregnancy (after 29 wk); may cause premature closure of the fetal ductus arteriosus. Use of indomethacin after 20 wk may cause fetal renal dysfunction

leading to oligohydramnios. May cause temporary infertility in women.

Evaluation/Desired Outcomes

- Decrease in severity of mild to moderate pain.
- Improved joint mobility. Partial arthritic relief is usually seen within 2 wk, but maximum effectiveness may require up to 1 mo of continuous therapy. Patients who do not respond to one NSAID may respond to another.
- Successful PDA closure.

inFLIXimab (in-flix-i-mab)

Avsola, Inflectra, Ixifi, Remicade, Renflexis, Remsima, Zymfentra

Classification

Therapeutic: antirheumatics (DMARDs), gastrointestinal anti-inflammatories

Pharmacologic: monoclonal antibodies

Indications

IV, SUBQ: Treatment of the following conditions: Moderately to severely active rheumatoid arthritis (in combination with methotrexate); Moderately to severely active Crohn's disease in patients with an inadequate response to conventional therapy. **IV:** Treatment of the following conditions: Active psoriatic arthritis; Active ankylosing spondylitis; Moderately to severely active ulcerative colitis in patients with an inadequate response to conventional therapy; Chronic severe plaque psoriasis in patients who are candidates for systemic therapy and when other systemic therapies are less appropriate.

Action

Neutralizes and prevents the activity of tumor necrosis factor-alpha (TNF-alpha), resulting in anti-inflammatory and antiproliferative activity. **Therapeutic Effects:** Decreased signs and symptoms, decreased rate of joint destruction, and improved physical function in rheumatoid arthritis and psoriatic arthritis. Decreased signs and symptoms and induction and maintenance of clinical remission in Crohn's disease. Reduction in number of fistulas and maintenance of closure of fistulae in Crohn's disease. Decreased signs and symptoms in ankylosing spondylitis. Decreased signs and symptoms, maintenance of clinical remission and mucosal healing, and eliminating corticosteroid use in ulcerative colitis. Decreased induration, scaling, and erythema of psoriatic lesions.

Pharmacokinetics

Absorption: IV administration results in complete bioavailability; 23% absorbed following SUBQ administration.

Distribution: Predominantly distributed within the vascular compartment.

Metabolism and Excretion: Unknown.

Half-life: *IV:* 9.5 days; *SUBQ:* 13.8 days.

TIME/ACTION PROFILE (symptoms of Crohn's disease)

ROUTE	ONSET	PEAK	DURATION
IV	1–2 wk	unknown	12–48 wk†

† After infusion.

Contraindications/Precautions

Contraindicated in: Hypersensitivity to infliximab, murine (mouse) proteins, or other components in the formulation; Moderate to severe HF (doses >5 mg/kg); Concurrent anakinra or abatacept.

Use Cautiously in: History of chronic or recurrent infection or underlying illness/treatment predisposing to infection; Patients being retreated after 2 yr without treatment (↑ risk of adverse reactions); History of tuberculosis or exposure (latent tuberculosis should be treated prior to infliximab therapy); History of opportunistic infection; Moderate to severe HF (doses ≤5 mg/kg); Patients residing or who have resided where tuberculosis, histoplasmosis, coccidioidomycoses, or blastomycosis is endemic; Chronic obstructive pulmonary disease (↑ risk of malignancy); History of hepatitis B; OB: Use only if potential maternal benefit justifies potential fetal risk; infants exposed in utero may be at ↑ risk for infection or agranulocytosis; Lactation: Use while breastfeeding only if potential maternal benefit justifies potential risk to infant; Pedi: Children <6 yr (safety not established); ↑ risk of lymphoma (including hepatosplenic T-cell lymphoma [HSTCL] in patients with Crohn's disease or ulcerative colitis), leukemia, and other malignancies; Geri: ↑ risk of adverse reactions, including serious infections, in older adults.

Adverse Reactions/Side Effects

CV: ARRHYTHMIAS, chest pain, edema, HF, hypertension, hypotension, MYOCARDIAL ISCHEMIA/INFARCTION, pericardial effusion, tachycardia, vasculitis. **Derm:** acne, alopecia, dry skin, ecchymosis, eczema, erythema, flushing, hematoma, hot flushing, pruritus, psoriasis, rash, sweating, urticaria. **EENT:** conjunctivitis, vision loss. **GI:** abdominal pain, nausea, vomiting, constipation, diarrhea, dyspepsia, flatulence, hepatitis B virus reactivation, hepatotoxicity, intestinal obstruction, oral pain, tooth pain, ulcerative stomatitis. **GU:** dysuria, urinary frequency, urinary tract infection. **Hemat:** neutropenia. **Local:** injection site reaction. **MS:** arthralgia, arthritis, back pain, involuntary muscle contractions, myalgia. **Neuro:** fatigue, headache, anxiety, depression, dizziness, insomnia, paresthesia, STROKE. **Resp:** upper respiratory tract infection, bronchitis, cough, dyspnea, laryngitis, pharyngitis, respiratory tract allergic reaction, rhinitis, sinusitis. **Misc:** fever, infusion reactions, chills, flu-like syndrome, HYPERSENSITIVITY REACTIONS (INCLUDING ANAPHYLAXIS), INFECTION (INCLUDING REACTIVATION TUBERCULOSIS AND OTHER OPPORTUNISTIC INFECTIONS DUE TO BACTERIAL, INVASIVE FUNGAL, VIRAL, MYCOBACTERIAL, AND PARASITIC PATHOGENS), lupus-like syndrome, MALIGNANCY (INCLUDING LYMPHOMA, HSTCL, LEUKEMIA, SKIN CANCER, AND CERVICAL CANCER), pain, SARCOIDOSIS.

Interactions

Drug-Drug: Concurrent use with **anakinra** or **abatacept** ↑ risk of serious infections (not recommended). Concurrent use with **azathioprine** or **methotrexate** may ↑ risk of HSTCL. Use of **live-virus vaccines** or therapeutic infectious agents may ↑ risk of infection; avoid concurrent use; wait for ≥6 mo before administering any live vaccines to infants exposed in utero.

Route/Dosage

Rheumatoid Arthritis

IV (Adults): 3 mg/kg initially; then repeat at 2 and 6 wk after initial infusion; then repeat every 8 wk; dose may be adjusted in partial responders up to 10 mg/kg or treatment as often as every 4 wk (to be used with methotrexate).
SUBQ (Adults): 120 mg every 2 wk starting at wk 10 after receiving induction treatment with IV therapy. If patient responding to maintenance IV therapy, can also be switched to SUBQ therapy by administering the first SUBQ dose in place of the next scheduled IV dose and then giving the SUBQ dose every 2 wk thereafter.

Crohn's Disease

IV (Adults): 5 mg/kg initially; then repeat at 2 and 6 wk after initial infusion; then maintenance dose of 5 mg/kg every 8 wk; dose may be adjusted up to 10 mg/kg in patients who initially respond and then lose their response.
SUBQ (Adults): 120 mg every 2 wk starting at wk 10 after receiving induction treatment with IV therapy. If patient responding to maintenance IV therapy, can also be switched to SUBQ therapy by administering the first SUBQ dose in place of the next scheduled IV dose and then giving the SUBQ dose every 2 wk thereafter.
IV (Children): 5 mg/kg initially; then repeat at 2 and 6 wk after initial infusion; then maintenance dose of 5 mg/kg every 8 wk.

Ankylosing Spondylitis

IV (Adults): 5 mg/kg initially; then repeat at 2 and 6 wk after initial infusion; then maintenance dose of 5 mg/kg every 6 wk.

Psoriatic Arthritis

IV (Adults): 5 mg/kg initially; then repeat at 2 and 6 wk after initial infusion; then maintenance dose of 5 mg/kg every 8 wk (to be used with or without methotrexate).

Ulcerative Colitis

IV (Adults and Children ≥6 yr): 5 mg/kg initially; then repeat at 2 and 6 wk after initial infusion; then maintenance dose of 5 mg/kg every 8 wk.

Plaque Psoriasis

IV (Adults): 5 mg/kg initially; then repeat at 2 and 6 wk after initial infusion; then maintenance dose of 5 mg/kg every 8 wk.

Availability (generic available)

Lyophilized powder for IV injection: 100 mg/vial. **Solution for SUBQ injection (Zymfentra) (prefilled pens and syringes):** 120 mg/mL.

NURSING IMPLICATIONS

Assessment

- Assess for infusion-related reactions (fever, chills, urticaria, pruritus) during and for 2 hr after infusion. Symptoms usually resolve when infusion is discontinued. Reactions are more common after 1st or 2nd infusion. Frequency of reactions may be reduced with immunosuppressant agents.
- Monitor patients who develop a new infection while taking infliximab closely. Discontinue therapy in patients who develop a serious infection or sepsis. Do not initiate therapy in patients with active infections.
- Assess for signs and symptoms of systemic infections (fever, malaise, weight loss, sweats, cough, dyspnea, pulmonary infiltrates, serious systemic illness with or without concomitant shock). Ascertain if patient lives in or has traveled to areas of endemic mycoses. Consider empiric antifungal treatment for patients at risk of histoplasmosis and other invasive fungal infections until the pathogens are identified. Consult with an infectious diseases specialist. Consider stopping infliximab until the infection has been diagnosed and adequately treated.
- Assess for latent tuberculosis with a tuberculin skin test prior to initiation of and during therapy. Treatment of latent tuberculosis should be initiated prior to therapy with infliximab.
- Monitor patient for hypersensitivity reactions (urticaria, dyspnea, hypotension) during infusion. Discontinue infliximab if severe reaction occurs. Have medications (antihistamines, acetaminophen, corticosteroids, epinephrine) and equipment readily available in the event of a severe reaction.
- **Rheumatoid Arthritis:** Assess pain and range of motion prior to and periodically during therapy.
- **Crohn's Disease and Ulcerative Colitis:** Assess for signs and symptoms before, during, and after therapy.
- **Psoriasis:** Assess lesions periodically during therapy.

Lab Test Considerations

- May cause ↑ in positive ANA. Frequency may be decreased with baseline immunosuppressant therapy.
- Monitor liver function tests periodically during therapy. May cause mild to moderate AST and ALT ↑ without progressing to liver dysfunction. If patient develops jaundice or liver enzyme elevations ≥5 times the upper limits of normal, discontinue infliximab.
- Monitor CBC with differential periodically during therapy. May cause leukopenia, neutropenia, thrombocytopenia, and pancytopenia. Discontinue infliximab if symptoms of blood dyscrasias (persistent fever) occur.

Implementation

- Do not confuse infliximab with rituximab.
- Ensure vaccinations are brought up to date in adult and pediatric patients before starting therapy.
- **SUBQ:** All patients must complete an IV induction regimen with an infliximab product before starting SUBQ therapy with *Zymfentra*. Allow prefilled pen or syringe to sit at room temperature for 30 min prior to injection; do not use other methods of warming. Solution is clear to opalescent and colorless to pale brown. Do not inject solutions that are discolored or contain particulate matter. Administer injection into abdomen, thigh, or upper arm. Rotate injection sites with each injection. Avoid areas of tenderness, bruising, redness, or hardness. Refrigerate prefilled pens and syringes prior to use; do not freeze or shake. Avoid exposure to heat. May be stored at room temperature if protected from sunlight for up to 14 days. Once the prefilled pen or syringe has reached room temperature, do not put back into refrigerator.

IV Administration

- **Intermittent Infusion:** Calculate the total number of vials needed. **Reconstitution:** Reconstitute each vial with 10 mL of sterile water for injection using a syringe with a 21-gauge needle or smaller. Direct stream to sides of vial. Do not use if vacuum is not present in vial. Gently swirl solution by rotating vial to dilute; do not shake. May foam on reconstitution; allow to stand for 5 min. Solution is colorless to light yellow and opalescent; a few translucent particles may develop because infliximab is a protein. Do not use if opaque particles, discoloration, or other particles occur. **Dilution:** Withdraw volume of total infliximab dose from infusion container containing 250 mL with 0.9% NaCl. Slowly add total dose of infliximab. Do not dilute with other solutions. **Concentration:** 0.4 to 4 mg/mL. Mix gently. Infusion should begin within 3 hr (4 hr for *Renflexis*) of preparation. Solution is incompatible with polyvinyl chloride equipment. Prepare in glass infusion bottle or polypropylene or polyolefin bags. Do not reuse or store any portion of infusion solution. Unopened vials are stable for 6 mo at room temperature; once removed from refrigerator, cannot be returned to the refrigerator. Diluted solution is stable for 4 hr at room temperature, 34 days if refrigerated, and 6 hr at room temperature when removed from refrigerator.
- **Rate:** Administer over at least 2 hr through polyethylene-lined administration set with an in-line, sterile, nonpyrogenic, low-protein-building filter with ≤1.2-micron pore size.
- **Y-Site Incompatibility:** Do not administer concurrently in the same line with any other agents.

Patient/Family Teaching

- Explain purpose of infliximab to patient.
- Instruct patient in correct technique for SUBQ injection, care, and disposal of equipment. If a SUBQ dose is missed, instruct patient to administer as soon as possible; then take next dose according to regular schedule.
- Advise patient that adverse reactions (myalgia, rash, fever, polyarthralgia, pruritus) may occur 3–12 days after delayed (>2 yr) retreatment with infliximab. Symptoms usually decrease or resolve within 1–3 days. Instruct patient to notify health care professional if symptoms occur.
- May cause dizziness. Caution patient to avoid driving or other activities requiring alertness until response to medication is known.
- Advise patient to notify health care professional promptly if symptoms of fungal infection occur.
- Instruct patient to notify health care professional of all Rx or OTC medications, vitamins, or herbal products being taken and consult health care professional before taking any new medications.
- Advise patient of risk of malignancies such as hepatosplenic T-cell lymphoma. Instruct patient to report signs and symptoms (splenomegaly, hepatomegaly, abdominal pain, persistent fever, night sweats, weight loss) to health care professional promptly.
- Advise patient to examine skin periodically during therapy and notify health care professional of any changes in appearance of skin or growths on skin.
- Instruct patient not to receive live vaccines during therapy.
- Advise females to continue regular PAP smears for cervical cancer screening.
- **Rep:** Advise females of reproductive potential to notify health care professional if pregnancy is planned or suspected or if breastfeeding. Infants exposed to infliximab in utero should wait at least 6 mo before receiving any live vaccine; may be at increased risk of infection.

Evaluation/Desired Outcomes

- Decreased pain and swelling with decreased rate of joint destruction and improved physical function

in patients with ankylosing spondylitis, psoriatic, or rheumatoid arthritis.
- Decrease in the signs and symptoms of Crohn's disease and a decrease in the number of draining enterocutaneous fistulas. Decreased symptoms, maintaining remission, and mucosal healing with decreased corticosteroid use in ulcerative colitis.
- Decrease in induration, scaling, and erythema of psoriatic lesions.

HIGH ALERT

INSULIN (mixtures) (in-su-lin)

insulin aspart protamine suspension/insulin aspart injection mixtures, rDNA origin

NovoLOG Mix 70/30, NovoLOG Mix 70/30 FlexPen

insulin lispro protamine suspension/insulin lispro injection mixtures, rDNA origin

HumaLOG Mix 75/25, HumaLOG Mix 50/50

NPH/regular insulin mixtures

HumuLIN 70/30, NovoLIN 70/30

Classification

Therapeutic: antidiabetics, hormones

Pharmacologic: pancreatics

See Appendix K for more information concerning insulins.

Indications

Type 1 or type 2 diabetes mellitus.

Action

Lower blood glucose by: stimulating glucose uptake in skeletal muscle and fat, inhibiting hepatic glucose production. Other actions: inhibition of lipolysis and proteolysis, enhanced protein synthesis. **Therapeutic Effects:** Control of hyperglycemia in diabetic patients.

Pharmacokinetics

Absorption: Well absorbed from SUBQ administration sites.

Distribution: Widely distributed to tissues.

Metabolism and Excretion: Metabolized by liver, spleen, kidney, and muscle.

Half-life: 5–6 min (prolonged in patients with diabetes; biologic half-life is 1–1.5 hr).

TIME/ACTION PROFILE (hypoglycemic effect)

ROUTE	ONSET	PEAK	DURATION
Insulin aspart protamine suspension/insulin aspart injection mixture SUBQ	15 min	1–4 hr	18–24 hr
Insulin lispro protamine suspension/ insulin lispro injection mixture SUBQ	15–30 min	2.8 hr	24 hr
NPH/regular insulin mixture SUBQ	30 min	2–12 hr	24 hr

Contraindications/Precautions

Contraindicated in: Hypoglycemia; Allergy or hypersensitivity to a particular type of insulin, preservatives, or other additives.

Use Cautiously in: Stress and infection (may temporarily ↑ insulin requirements); Renal impairment (may ↓ insulin requirements); Hepatic impairment (may ↓ insulin requirements); OB: Pregnancy may temporarily ↑ insulin requirements; Lactation: Use while breastfeeding only if potential maternal benefit justifies potential risk to infant; Pedi: Safety of Humalog not established.

Adverse Reactions/Side Effects

Endo: HYPOGLYCEMIA. **F and E:** hypokalemia. **Local:** cutaneous amyloidosis, erythema, lipodystrophy, pruritus, swelling. **Misc:** HYPERSENSITIVITY REACTIONS (INCLUDING ANAPHYLAXIS).

Interactions

Drug-Drug: Beta blockers and **clonidine** may mask some of the signs and symptoms of hypoglycemia. **Corticosteroids, thyroid supplements, estrogens, isoniazid, niacin, phenothiazines,** and **rifampin** may ↑ insulin requirements. **Alcohol, ACE inhibitors, MAO inhibitors, octreotide, oral hypoglycemic agents,** and **salicylates** may ↓ insulin requirements. **Pioglitazone** may ↑ risk of fluid retention and worsening HF.

Drug-Natural Products: Glucosamine may worsen blood glucose control. **Fenugreek, chromium,** and **coenzyme Q-10** may produce additive hypoglycemic effects.

Route/Dosage

SUBQ (Adults and Children): 0.5–1 unit/kg/day. *Adolescents during rapid growth:* 0.8–1.2 units/kg/day.

Availability

Insulin aspart protamine suspension/insulin aspart injection mixture: 70% insulin aspart protamine suspension and 30% insulin aspart injection: NovoLog Mix 70/30 100 units/mL (vials and prefilled pens). **Insulin lispro protamine suspension/insulin lispro injection mixture:** 75% insulin lispro protamine suspension and 25% insulin lispro injection: Humalog Mix 75/25 100 units/mL (vials and prefilled pens), 50% insulin lispro protamine suspension and 50% insulin lispro injection: Humalog Mix 50/50 100 units/mL (vials and prefilled pens). **NPH insulin/regular insulin suspension mixture:** 70 units NPH/30 units regular insulin/mL: Novolin 70/30, Humulin 70/30 (100 units/mL total) (vials and prefilled pens).

NURSING IMPLICATIONS

Assessment

- Assess for signs/symptoms of hypoglycemia (anxiety; restlessness; mood changes; tingling in hands, feet, lips, or tongue; chills; cold sweats; confusion; cool, pale skin; difficulty concentrating; drowsiness; nightmares or trouble sleeping; excessive hunger; headache; irritability; nausea; nervousness; tachycardia; tremor; weakness; unsteady gait) and hyperglycemia (confusion; drowsiness; flushed, dry skin; fruit-like breath odor; rapid, deep breathing; polyuria; loss of appetite; nausea; vomiting; tiredness; unusual thirst) periodically during therapy.
- Monitor body weight periodically. Changes in weight, meal patterns, and physical activity levels may necessitate changes in insulin dose.
- Assess for signs/symptoms of allergic reactions (rash, shortness of breath, wheezing, rapid HR, sweating, low BP) during therapy.

Lab Test Considerations

- Monitor blood glucose every 6 hr during therapy, more frequently in ketoacidosis and times of stress. Monitor A1c twice yearly or every 3 mo when not meeting glycemic goals or at change in therapy.
- Monitor serum potassium in patients at risk for hypokalemia (those using potassium-lowering agents, those receiving IV insulin) periodically during therapy.

Toxicity and Overdose

- Overdose is manifested by symptoms of hypoglycemia. Mild hypoglycemia may be treated by ingestion of oral glucose. Severe hypoglycemia is a life-threatening emergency; treatment consists of IV dextrose or glucagon. Octreotide may help stabilize blood glucose concentrations after prolonged hypoglycemia. Early signs of hypoglycemia may be less pronounced by long duration of diabetes, diabetic nerve disease, and use of beta blockers; may result in loss of consciousness prior to patient's awareness of hypoglycemia.

Implementation

- ***High Alert:*** Insulin-related medication errors have resulted in patient harm and death. Clarify ambiguous orders; do not accept orders using the abbreviation "u" for units (can be misread as a zero or the numeral 4; has resulted in tenfold overdoses).
- Insulins are available in different types and strengths. Check type, dose, and expiration date with another licensed nurse. Do not interchange insulins without consulting health care provider.
- Do not confuse Humulin 70/30 with Humalog Mix 75/25. Do not confuse Novolin 70/30 with Novolog Mix 70/30. Do not confuse Novolog Mix 70/30 Flexpen with Novolog Flexpen.
- Use *only* insulin syringes to draw up dose. The unit markings on the insulin syringe must match the insulin's units/mL.
- Insulin should be stored in a cool place but does not need to be refrigerated. Follow manufacturer's instructions regarding storage of insulin and insulin pens before and after use. Do not use if cloudy, discolored, or unusually viscous.
- NPH insulins should not be used in the management of ketoacidosis.
- **SUBQ:** Rotate injection sites to prevent lipodystrophy and cutaneous amyloidosis. Repeated insulin injections into areas of localized cutaneous amyloidosis may cause hyperglycemia; a sudden change to an unaffected injection site may cause hypoglycemia.
- Administer into abdominal wall, thigh, or upper arm SUBQ.

Patient/Family Teaching

- Explain the purpose and side effects of insulin mixtures. Instruct patient on proper technique for administration. Include type of insulin, equipment (syringe, cartridge pens, alcohol swabs), storage, and place to discard syringes. Discuss the importance of not changing brands of insulin or syringes, selection and rotation of injection sites, and compliance with therapeutic regimen. Keep out of children's reach. Advise patient to read *Patient Information* before starting and with each Rx refill in case of changes.
- Emphasize the importance of regular follow-up to assess effectiveness, especially during 1st few weeks of therapy. Periodic lab tests will be needed.
- Caution patient not to share pen device with another person, even if needle is changed and clean needles are used; may be harmful and ↑ risk of transmitting of bloodborne pathogens.
- Explain to patient that this medication controls hyperglycemia but does not cure diabetes. Therapy is long term.
- Instruct patient in proper testing of serum glucose and ketones. These tests should be closely monitored during periods of stress or illness and health care provider notified of significant changes.
- Emphasize the importance of compliance with nutritional guidelines and regular exercise as directed by health care provider.
- Instruct patient to notify health care provider of all Rx or OTC medications, vitamins, or herbal products being taken and to consult health care provider before taking other Rx, OTC, herbal products, or alcohol.
- Advise patient to notify health care provider of medication regimen prior to treatment or surgery.

- Advise patient to notify health care provider if nausea, vomiting, or fever develops; if unable to eat regular diet; or if blood glucose levels are not controlled.
- Instruct patient on signs and symptoms of hypoglycemia and hyperglycemia and what to do if they occur.
- Patients with diabetes mellitus should carry a source of sugar (candy, glucose gel) and identification describing their disease and treatment regimen at all times.
- Rep: Advise women to notify health care provider if pregnancy is planned or suspected or if breastfeeding.

Evaluation/Desired Outcomes

- Control of blood glucose levels in diabetic patients without the appearance of hypoglycemic or hyperglycemic episodes.

HIGH ALERT

insulin NPH (isophane insulin suspension)

HumuLIN N, HumuLIN N KwikPen, NovoLIN N, NovoLIN N FlexPen

Classification

Therapeutic: antidiabetics, hormones

Pharmacologic: pancreatics

See Appendix K for more information concerning insulins.

Indications

Control of hyperglycemia in patients with diabetes mellitus.

Action

Lowers blood glucose by stimulating glucose uptake in skeletal muscle and fat, inhibiting hepatic glucose production. Other actions of insulin: inhibition of lipolysis and proteolysis, enhanced protein synthesis. **Therapeutic Effects:** Control of hyperglycemia in diabetic patients.

Pharmacokinetics

Absorption: Rapidly absorbed from SUBQ administration sites. Presence of protamine delays peak effect and prolongs action.
Distribution: Identical to endogenous insulin.
Metabolism and Excretion: Metabolized by liver, spleen, kidney, and muscle.
Half-life: Unknown.

TIME/ACTION PROFILE (hypoglycemic effect)

ROUTE	ONSET	PEAK	DURATION
NPH SUBQ	2–4 hr	4–10 hr	10–16 hr
70% NPH/30% regular insulin mixture	30 min	2–12 hr	24 hr

Contraindications/Precautions

Contraindicated in: Hypoglycemia; Allergy or hypersensitivity to a particular type of insulin, preservatives, or other additives.
Use Cautiously in: Stress or infection (may temporarily ↑ insulin requirements); Renal impairment (may ↓ insulin requirements); Hepatic impairment (may ↓ insulin requirements); OB: Pregnancy may temporarily ↑ insulin requirements; Lactation: Use while breastfeeding only if potential maternal benefit justifies potential risk to infant.

Adverse Reactions/Side Effects

Endo: HYPOGLYCEMIA. **F and E:** hypokalemia. **Local:** cutaneous amyloidosis, erythema, lipodystrophy, pruritus, swelling. **Misc:** HYPERSENSITIVITY REACTIONS (INCLUDING ANAPHYLAXIS).

Interactions

Drug-Drug: Beta blockers and **clonidine** may mask some of the signs and symptoms of hypoglycemia. **Corticosteroids**, **thyroid supplements**, **estrogens**, **isoniazid**, **niacin**, **phenothiazines**, and **rifampin** may ↑ insulin requirements. **Alcohol**, **ACE inhibitors**, **MAO inhibitors**, **octreotide**, **oral hypoglycemic agents**, and **salicylates** may ↓ insulin requirements. **Pioglitazone** may ↑ risk of fluid retention and worsening HF.
Drug-Natural Products: Glucosamine may worsen blood glucose control. **Fenugreek**, **chromium**, and **coenzyme Q-10** may produce additive hypoglycemic effects.

Route/Dosage

SUBQ (Adults and Children): 0.5–1 unit total insulin/kg/day. *Adolescents during rapid growth:* 0.8–1.2 units total insulin/kg/day.

Availability

Solution for injection (vials and prefilled pens): 100 units/mL.

NURSING IMPLICATIONS

Assessment

- Assess for signs/symptoms of hypoglycemia (anxiety; restlessness; tingling in hands, feet, lips, or tongue; chills; cold sweats; confusion; cool, pale skin; difficulty in concentration; drowsiness; nightmares or trouble sleeping; excessive hunger; headache; irritability; nausea; nervousness; tachycardia; tremor; weakness; unsteady gait) and hyperglycemia (confusion, drowsiness; flushed, dry skin; fruit-like breath odor; rapid, deep breathing; polyuria; loss of appetite; unusual thirst) during therapy.
- Monitor for hypersensitivity reactions (anaphylaxis, rash, hives, itching, wheezing, tightness in the chest or throat, trouble breathing or swallowing). Implement supportive measures (epinephrine) if needed.

- Monitor body weight periodically. Changes in weight may necessitate changes in insulin dose.

Lab Test Considerations
- Monitor blood glucose every 6 hr during therapy and more frequently during changes to insulin regimen, ketoacidosis, and times of stress. A1c may be monitored every 3–6 mo to determine effectiveness.
- Monitor serum potassium in patients at risk for hypokalemia (those using potassium-lowering agents, those receiving IV insulin) periodically during therapy.

Toxicity and Overdose
- Overdose is manifested by symptoms of hypoglycemia. Mild hypoglycemia may be treated by ingestion of oral glucose. Severe hypoglycemia is a life-threatening emergency; treatment consists of IV glucose, glucagon, or epinephrine.

Implementation
- ***High Alert:*** Medication errors involving insulins have resulted in serious patient harm and death. Clarify all ambiguous orders and do not accept orders using the abbreviation "u" for units, which can be misread as a zero or the numeral 4 and has resulted in tenfold overdoses. Insulins are available in different types and strengths. Check type, dose, and expiration date with another licensed nurse. Do not interchange insulins without consulting another health care provider.
- Do not confuse Humulin with Humalog or Novolin. Do not confuse Novolin N with Novolog.
- Use *only* insulin syringes to draw up dose. The unit markings on the insulin syringe must match the insulin's units/mL. Special syringes for doses <50 units are available. Before withdrawing dose, rotate vial between palms to ensure uniform solution; do not shake.
- When mixing insulins, draw regular insulin or insulin lispro into syringe first to avoid contamination of regular insulin vial.
- Follow manufacturer's instructions regarding storage of insulin and insulin pens before and after use.
- When transferring from once-daily NPH human insulin to ***insulin glargine***, the dose usually remains unchanged. When transferring from twice-daily NPH human insulin to insulin glargine, the initial dose of insulin glargine is usually ↓ by 20%.
- NPH insulin should not be used in the management of ketoacidosis.
- **SUBQ:** Administer NPH insulin within 30–60 min before a meal. Inject SUBQ in abdomen, thigh, upper arm, or buttocks. Rotate injection sites to ↓ risk of lipodystrophy or localized cutaneous amyloidosis. Repeated insulin injections into areas of lipodystrophy or localized cutaneous amyloidosis may result in hyperglycemia. A sudden change in the injection site (to an unaffected area) may result in hypoglycemia.

Patient/Family Teaching
- Explain purpose and side effects of medication. Advise patient to read *Patient Information* before starting therapy.
- Advise patient to notify health care professional of all Rx or OTC medications, vitamins, or herbal products being taken and to consult health care professional before taking other medications.
- Instruct patient on proper technique for administration. Include type of insulin, equipment (syringe, cartridge pens, alcohol swabs), storage, and place to discard syringes. Discuss the importance of not changing brands of insulin or syringes, selection and rotation of injection sites, and compliance with therapeutic regimen. Caution patient that insulin pens should not be shared with others, even if clean needles are used.
- Demonstrate technique for mixing insulins by drawing up regular insulin or insulin lispro first and rolling intermediate-acting insulin vial between palms to mix rather than shaking (may cause inaccurate dose).
- Explain to patient that this medication controls hyperglycemia but does not cure diabetes. Therapy is long term.
- Instruct patient in proper testing of serum glucose and ketones. These tests should be closely monitored during periods of stress or illness and health care professional notified of significant changes.
- Emphasize the importance of compliance with nutritional guidelines and regular exercise as directed by health care professional.
- Advise patient to notify health care professional of medication regimen prior to treatment or surgery.
- Advise patient to notify health care professional if nausea, vomiting, or fever develops; if unable to eat regular diet; or if blood glucose levels are not controlled.
- Instruct patient on signs and symptoms of hypoglycemia, hyperglycemia, and hypersensitivity reactions and what to do if they occur.
- Patients with diabetes mellitus should carry a source of sugar (candy, glucose gel) and identification describing their disease and treatment regimen at all times.
- Rep: Advise women of reproductive potential to notify health care professional if pregnancy is planned or suspected or if breastfeeding.

Evaluation/Desired Outcomes
- Control of hyperglycemia in diabetic patients.

BEERS HIGH ALERT

insulin regular (in-su-lin)

Entuzity Kwikpen, HumuLIN R, HumuLIN R U-500 (Concentrated), HumuLIN R U-500 KwikPen (Concentrated), Myxredlin, NovoLIN R, NovoLIN R FlexPen

Classification

Therapeutic: antidiabetics, hormones

Pharmacologic: pancreatics

See Appendix K for more information concerning insulins.

Indications

Type 1 or type 2 diabetes mellitus. **Concentrated regular insulin U-500:** Only for use in patients with insulin requirements >200 units/day. **Unlabeled Use:** Hyperkalemia.

Action

Lowers blood glucose by: stimulating glucose uptake in skeletal muscle and fat, inhibiting hepatic glucose production. Other actions of insulin: inhibition of lipolysis and proteolysis, enhanced protein synthesis. **Therapeutic Effects:** Control of hyperglycemia in patients with diabetes.

Pharmacokinetics

Absorption: Rapidly absorbed from SUBQ administration sites. U-100 regular insulin is absorbed slightly more quickly than U-500. IV administration results in complete bioavailability.

Distribution: Identical to endogenous insulin.

Metabolism and Excretion: Metabolized by liver, spleen, kidney, and muscle.

Half-life: 30–60 min.

TIME/ACTION PROFILE (hypoglycemic effect)

ROUTE	ONSET	PEAK	DURATION
IV	10–30 min	15–30 min	30–60 min
SUBQ	30–60 min	2–4 hr	5–7 hr

Contraindications/Precautions

Contraindicated in: Hypoglycemia; Allergy or hypersensitivity to a particular type of insulin, preservatives, or other additives.

Use Cautiously in: Stress or infection (may temporarily ↑ insulin requirements); Renal impairment (may ↓ insulin requirements); Hepatic impairment (may ↓ insulin requirements); OB: Pregnancy may temporarily ↑ insulin requirements; Geri: Appears on Beers list. ↑ risk of hypoglycemia in older adults. Avoid use of regimens containing only short- or rapid-acting insulin without concurrent use of basal or long-acting insulin.

Adverse Reactions/Side Effects

Endo: HYPOGLYCEMIA. **F and E:** hypokalemia. **Local:** cutaneous amyloidosis, erythema, lipodystrophy, pruritus, swelling. **Misc:** HYPERSENSITIVITY REACTIONS (INCLUDING ANAPHYLAXIS).

Interactions

Drug-Drug: Beta blockers and **clonidine** may mask some of the signs and symptoms of hypoglycemia. **Corticosteroids, thyroid supplements, estrogens, isoniazid, niacin, phenothiazines,** and **rifampin** may ↑ insulin requirements. **Alcohol, ACE inhibitors, MAO inhibitors, octreotide, oral hypoglycemic agents,** and **salicylates** may ↓ insulin requirements. Concurrent use with **pioglitazone** may ↑ risk of fluid retention and worsening HF.

Drug-Natural Products: Glucosamine may worsen blood glucose control. **Fenugreek, chromium,** and **coenzyme Q-10** may produce additive hypoglycemic effects.

Route/Dosage

Ketoacidosis: Regular (100 units/mL) Insulin Only

IV (Adults): 0.1 unit/kg/hr as a continuous infusion.

IV (Children): Loading dose of 0.1 unit/kg, then maintenance continuous infusion 0.05–0.2 unit/kg/hr; titrate to optimal rate of ↓ of serum glucose of 80–100 mg/dL/hr.

Maintenance Therapy

SUBQ (Adults and Children): 0.5–1 unit/kg/day in divided doses. *Adolescents during rapid growth:* 0.8–1.2 unit/kg/day in divided doses.

Treatment of Hyperkalemia

SUBQ, IV (Adults and Children): Dextrose 0.5–1 g/kg combined with insulin 1 unit for every 4–5 g dextrose given.

Availability

Premixed infusion: 100 units/100 mL 0.9% NaCl. **Solution for injection (vials and prefilled pens):** 100 units/mL[OTC]. **Solution for injection (concentrated) (vials and prefilled pens):** 500 units/mL. ***In combination with:*** NPH insulins (Humulin 70/30, Novolin 70/30).

NURSING IMPLICATIONS

Assessment

- Assess for symptoms of hypoglycemia (anxiety; restlessness; tingling in hands, feet, lips, or tongue; chills; cold sweats; confusion; cool, pale skin; difficulty in concentration; drowsiness; nightmares or trouble sleeping; excessive hunger; headache; irritability; nausea; nervousness; tachycardia; tremor; weakness; unsteady gait) and hyperglycemia (confusion; drowsiness; flushed, dry skin; fruit-like breath odor; rapid, deep breathing; polyuria; loss of appetite; unusual thirst) during therapy.

- Monitor body weight periodically. Changes in weight may necessitate changes in insulin dose.
- Monitor for hypersensitivity reactions (anaphylaxis, hives). Implement supportive medical treatment (epinephrine) if necessary.

Lab Test Considerations

- Monitor blood glucose every 6 hr during therapy and more frequently in ketoacidosis and times of stress. A1c may be monitored every 3–6 mo to determine effectiveness.
- Monitor potassium in patients at risk for hypokalemia (those using potassium-lowering agents, those receiving IV insulin) periodically during therapy.

Toxicity and Overdose

- Overdose is manifested by symptoms of hypoglycemia. Mild hypoglycemia may be treated by ingestion of oral glucose. Severe hypoglycemia is a life-threatening emergency; treatment consists of IV glucose, glucagon, or epinephrine.

Implementation

- ***High Alert:*** Medication errors involving insulins have resulted in serious patient harm and death. Clarify all ambiguous orders and do not accept orders using the abbreviation "u" for units, which can be misread as a zero or the numeral 4; errors have resulted in tenfold overdoses. Insulins are available in different types and strengths. Check type, dose, and expiration date with another licensed nurse. Do not intechange insulins without consulting health care provider. Do not confuse regular concentrated (U-500) insulin with regular insulin. To prevent errors between regular U-100 insulin and concentrated U-500 insulin, concentrated U-500 insulin is marked with a band of diagonal brown strips and "U-500" is highlighted in red on the label; a conversion chart should always be available.
- Do not confuse Humulin with Humalog or Novolin. Do not confuse Novolin with Novolog.
- Use *only* insulin syringes to draw up dose. The unit markings on the insulin syringe must match the insulin's units/mL. Special syringes for doses <50 units and U-500 insulin are available. Prior to withdrawing dose, rotate vial between palms to ensure uniform solution; do not shake.
- When mixing insulins, draw regular insulin into syringe first to avoid contamination of regular insulin vial.
- Insulin should be stored in a cool place but does not need to be refrigerated. Once opened, store at room temperature. Follow manufacturer's instructions regarding storage of insulin and insulin pens before and after use.
- **SUBQ:** Administer regular insulin within 30 min before a meal into the thigh, upper arm, abdomen, or buttocks. Rotate sites with each injection to prevent lipodystrophy and cutaneous amyloidosis. Repeated insulin injections into areas of localized cutaneous amyloidosis may cause hyperglycemia; a sudden change to an unaffected injection site may cause hypoglycemia.

IV Administration

- **IV:** Do not use if cloudy, discolored, or unusually viscous. ***High Alert:*** Do not administer regular (concentrated) insulin U-500 IV.
- **IV Push: Dilution:** May be administered IV undiluted directly into vein or through Y-site. **Rate:** Administer up to 50 units over 1 min.
- **Continuous Infusion: Dilution:** May be diluted in 0.9% NaCl using polyvinyl chloride infusion bags. **Concentration:** 0.1 unit/mL to 1 unit/mL in infusion systems with the infusion fluids. **Rate:** Place on an IV pump for accurate administration.
- Rate of administration should be ↓ when serum glucose level reaches 250 mg/dL.
- **Y-Site Compatibility:** acetaminophen, acyclovir, aminophylline, anidulafungin, argatroban, arsenic trioxide, ascorbic acid, atropine, azathioprine, aztreonam, benztropine, bivalirudin, bleomycin, bumetanide, buprenorphine, calcium chloride, calcium gluconate, carboplatin, carmustine, caspofungin, cefazolin, cefepime, cefiderocol, ceftaroline, ceftazidime, ceftolozane/tazobactam, ceftriaxone, cefuroxime, chloramphenicol, cisatracurium, clevidipine, clindamycin, cyanocobalamin, cyclophosphamide, cytarabine, dacarbazine, dactinomycin, daptomycin, daunorubicin, dexamethasone, dexmedetomidine, dexrazoxane, docetaxel, doxorubicin liposomal, doxycycline, enalapril, ephedrine, epirubicin, epoetin alfa, eravacycline, ertapenem, erythromycin, esmolol, esomeprazole, etoposide, etoposide phosphate, fentanyl, fluconazole, fludarabine, folic acid, foscarnet, fosphenytoin, ganciclovir, gemcitabine, granisetron, hydrocortisone, hydromorphone, ibuprofen lysine, idarubicin, ifosfamide, imipenem/cilastatin, indomethacin, irinotecan, isavuconazonium, ketorolac, letermovir, leucovorin, lidocaine, linezolid, lorazepam, magnesium sulfate, mannitol, meperidine, meropenem, meropenem/vaborbactam, mesna, methadone, methotrexate, methylprednisolone, metoclopramide, metoprolol, metronidazole, milrinone, mitoxantrone, moxifloxacin, mycophenolate, nalbuphine, naloxone, nitroglycerin, nitroprusside, octreotide, oritavancin, oxacillin, oxaliplatin, paclitaxel, palonosetron, pamidronate, papaverine, pemetrexed, penicillin G, pentobarbital, phenobarbital, phytonadione, plazomicin, potassium acetate, potassium chloride, procainamide, promethazine, propofol, pyridoxine, remifentanil, sodium bicarbonate, sufentanil, sulbactam/durlobactam, tacrolimus, tedizolid, terbutaline, theophylline, thiamine, thiotepa, tigecycline,

tirofiban, topotecan, vancomycin, vecuronium, verapamil, vinblastine, vincristine, vinorelbine, voriconazole, zoledronic acid.

- **Y-Site Incompatibility:** alemtuzumab, butorphanol, cefoxitin, ceftobiprole, chlorpromazine, cisplatin, dantrolene, diazepam, diphenhydramine, gemtuzumab ozogamicin, glycopyrrolate, isoproterenol, ketamine, labetalol, micafungin, minocycline, mitomycin, pentamidine, phentolamine, phenylephrine, phenytoin, piperacillin/tazobactam, prochlorperazine, propranolol, protamine, remimazolam, rocuronium, trimethoprim/sulfamethoxazole.
- **Additive Compatibility:** May be added to total parenteral nutrition solutions.

Patient/Family Teaching

- Explain purpose and side effects of medication to patient. Advise patient to read *Patient Information* before starting therapy. Instruct patient on proper technique for administration. Include type of insulin, equipment (syringe, cartridge pens, alcohol swabs), storage, and place to discard syringes. Discuss the importance of not changing brands of insulin or syringes, selection and rotation of injection sites, and compliance with therapeutic regimen. Opened, unused insulin vials should be discarded 1 mo after opening.
- Advise patient to notify health care provider of all Rx or OTC medications, vitamins, or herbal products being taken and to consult health care provider before taking other medications.
- Demonstrate technique for mixing insulins by drawing up regular insulin 1st and rolling intermediate-acting insulin vial between palms to mix rather than shaking (may cause inaccurate dose).
- Caution patient not to share pen device with another person, even if needle is changed; may risk transmission of bloodborne pathogens.
- Explain to patient that this medication controls hyperglycemia but does not cure diabetes. Therapy is long term.
- Instruct patient in proper testing of serum glucose and ketones. These tests should be closely monitored during periods of stress or illness and health care provider notified of significant changes.
- Emphasize the importance of compliance with nutritional guidelines and regular exercise as directed by health care provider.
- Advise patient to notify health care provider of medication regimen prior to treatment or surgery.
- Advise patient to notify health care provider if nausea, vomiting, or fever develops; if unable to eat regular diet; or if blood glucose levels are not controlled.
- Instruct patient on signs and symptoms of hypoglycemia and hyperglycemia and what to do if they occur.
- Patients with diabetes mellitus should carry a source of sugar (candy, glucose gel) and identification describing their disease and treatment regimen at all times.
- Rep: Advise women of reproductive potential to notify health care provider if pregnancy is planned or suspected or if breastfeeding.

Evaluation/Desired Outcomes

- Control of hyperglycemia in patients with diabetes.

HIGH ALERT

INSULINS (long-acting)

(**in**-su-lin)

insulin degludec

Tresiba, Tresiba FlexTouch

insulin glargine

Basaglar KwikPen, Basaglar Tempo Pen, Lantus, ~~Lantus SoloStar~~, Rezvoglar KwikPen, Semglee, Toujeo Max SoloStar, Toujeo SoloStar

Classification

Therapeutic: antidiabetics, hormones

Pharmacologic: pancreatics

See Appendix K for more information concerning insulins.

Indications

Control of hyperglycemia in patients with type 1 or type 2 diabetes mellitus.

Action

Lower blood glucose by stimulating glucose uptake in skeletal muscle and fat, inhibiting hepatic glucose production. Other actions: inhibition of lipolysis and proteolysis, enhanced protein synthesis. **Therapeutic Effects:** Control of hyperglycemia in patients with diabetes.

Pharmacokinetics

Absorption: Physiochemical characteristics of long-acting insulins result in delayed and prolonged absorption.

Distribution: Widely distributed.

Metabolism and Excretion: Metabolized by liver, spleen, kidney, and muscle.

Half-life: 5–6 min (prolonged in patients with diabetes); biologic half-life is 1–1.5 hr; *insulin degludec* 25 hr.

TIME/ACTION PROFILE (hypoglycemic effect)

ROUTE	ONSET	PEAK	DURATION
Insulin degludec	within 2 hr	12 hr	up to 42 hr*
Insulin glargine	3–4 hr	none†	24 hr

* Following discontinuation after chronic use.
† Small amounts of insulin glargine are slowly released resulting in a relatively constant effect over time.
‡ Duration is dose dependent; duration ↑ as dose ↑.

Contraindications/Precautions

Contraindicated in: Hypoglycemia; Allergy or hypersensitivity to a particular type of insulin, preservatives, or other additives.

Use Cautiously in: Stress and infection (may temporarily ↑ insulin requirements); Renal/hepatic impairment (may ↓ insulin requirements); Patients with visual impairment who may rely on audible clicks to dial their dose (Toujeo and Tresiba); OB: Pregnancy may temporarily ↑ insulin requirements; Pedi: Children <18 yr (Toujeo), <6 yr (Basaglar, Rezvoglar, or Semglee), or <1 yr (degludec) (safety not established).

Adverse Reactions/Side Effects

Endo: HYPOGLYCEMIA. **F and E:** hypokalemia. **Local:** cutaneous amyloidosis, erythema, lipodystrophy, pruritus, swelling. **Misc:** HYPERSENSITIVITY REACTIONS (INCLUDING ANAPHYLAXIS).

Interactions

Drug-Drug: Beta blockers and **clonidine** may mask some of the signs and symptoms of hypoglycemia. **Corticosteroids, thyroid supplements, estrogens, isoniazid, niacin, phenothiazines,** and **rifampin** may ↑ insulin requirements. **Alcohol, ACE inhibitors, MAO inhibitors, octreotide, oral hypoglycemic agents,** and **salicylates** may ↓ insulin requirements. **Pioglitazone** may ↑ risk of fluid retention and worsening HF.

Drug-Natural Products: Glucosamine may worsen blood glucose control. **Fenugreek, chromium,** and **coenzyme Q-10** may produce additive hypoglycemic effects.

Route/Dosage

Toujeo has a lower glucose-lowering effect than Basaglar, Rezvoglar, or Semglee on a unit-to-unit basis.

Insulin Degludec

SUBQ (Adults): *Type 1 diabetes (insulin naive):* ⅓–½ of the total daily insulin dose given once daily; then adjust on the basis of patient's needs (remainder of insulin dose should be given as a short-acting insulin and divided between each daily meal) (usual starting total daily insulin dose = 0.2–0.4 units/kg); *Type 2 diabetes (insulin naive):* 10 units once daily; then adjust on the basis of patient's needs; *Type 1 or 2 diabetes (and already on insulin):* Give the same dose as the total daily dose of the long-acting or intermediate-acting insulin once daily; then adjust on the basis of patient's needs.

SUBQ (Children ≥1 yr): *Type 1 or 2 diabetes (and already on insulin):* Give 80% of the total daily dose of the long-acting or intermediate-acting insulin once daily; then adjust on the basis of patient's needs.

Insulin Glargine (Basaglar, Rezvoglar, or Semglee)

SUBQ (Adults and Children ≥6 yr): *Type 1 diabetes (insulin naive):* ⅓ of the total daily insulin dose given once daily; then adjust on the basis of patient's needs (remainder of insulin dose should be given as a short-acting insulin) (usual starting total daily insulin dose = 0.2–0.4 units/kg); *Type 2 diabetes (insulin naive):* 0.2 units/kg or up to 10 units once daily; then adjust on the basis of patient's needs; *Type 1 or 2 diabetes (and converting from Toujeo):* Give 80% of Toujeo dose as Basaglar or Semglee once daily; then adjust on the basis of patient's needs; *Type 1 or 2 diabetes (and converting from once daily NPH):* Give the same dose once daily; then adjust on the basis of patient's needs; *Type 1 or 2 diabetes (and converting from twice daily NPH):* Give 80% of the total daily NPH dose once daily; then adjust on the basis of patient's needs.

Insulin Glargine (Toujeo)

SUBQ (Adults): *Type 1 diabetes (insulin naive):* ⅓–½ of the total daily insulin dose given once daily; then adjust on the basis of patient's needs (range = 1–80 units/day) (remainder of insulin dose should be given as a short-acting insulin) (usual starting total daily insulin dose = 0.2–0.4 units/kg); *Type 2 diabetes (insulin naive):* 0.2 units/kg once daily; then adjust on the basis of patient's needs; *Type 1 or 2 diabetes (and converting from intermediate or long-acting insulin):* Use same total daily dose and give once daily; then adjust on the basis of patient's needs; *Type 1 or 2 diabetes (and converting from NPH insulin):* Use 80% of the total daily NPH and give once daily; then adjust on the basis of patient's needs.

Availability

Insulin Degludec

Solution for injection: 100 units/mL (prefilled pens and vials), 200 units/mL (prefilled pens). ***In combination with:*** liraglutide (Xultophy). See Appendix N.

Insulin Glargine

Solution for injection (Basaglar, Rezvoglar): 100 units/mL (prefilled pens). **Solution for injection (Semglee):** 100 units/mL (prefilled pens and vials). **Solution for injection (Toujeo):** 300 units/mL (prefilled pens). ***In combination with:*** lixisenatide (Soliqua). See Appendix N.

NURSING IMPLICATIONS

Assessment

- Assess for signs/symptoms of hypoglycemia (anxiety; restlessness; mood changes; tingling in hands, feet, lips, or tongue; chills; cold sweats; confusion; cool, pale skin; difficulty concentrating; drowsiness; nightmares or trouble sleeping; excessive hunger; headache; irritability; nausea; nervousness; tachycardia; tremor; weakness; unsteady gait) and hyperglycemia (confusion; drowsiness; flushed, dry skin; fruit-like breath odor; rapid, deep breathing; polyuria; loss of appetite; nausea; vomiting; tiredness; unusual thirst) periodically during therapy.

- Monitor body weight periodically. Changes in weight may necessitate changes in insulin dose.
- Assess for signs/symptoms of allergic reactions (rash, shortness of breath, wheezing, rapid HR, sweating, low BP) during therapy.

Lab Test Considerations

- Monitor blood glucose every 6 hr during therapy, more frequently in ketoacidosis and times of stress.
- Monitor A1c twice yearly or every 3 mo when not meeting glycemic goals or change in therapy.
- Monitor serum potassium in patients at risk for hypokalemia (those using potassium-lowering agents, those receiving IV insulin) periodically during therapy.

Toxicity and Overdose

- Overdose is manifested by symptoms of hypoglycemia. Mild hypoglycemia may be treated by ingestion of oral glucose. Severe hypoglycemia is a life-threatening emergency; treatment consists of IV dextrose or glucagon. Octreotide may help stabilize blood glucose concentrations after prolonged hypoglycemia. Early signs of hypoglycemia may be less pronounced due to long duration of diabetes, diabetic nerve disease, and use of beta blockers; may result in loss of consciousness prior to patient's awareness of hypoglycemia.

Implementation

- ***High Alert:*** Insulin-related medication errors have resulted in patient harm and death. Clarify ambiguous orders; do not accept orders using the abbreviation "u" for units (can be misread as a zero or the numeral 4; has resulted in tenfold overdoses).
- Insulins are available in different types and strengths. Check type, dose, and expiration date with another licensed nurse. Do not interchange insulins without consulting health care provider.
- Do not confuse Toujeo with Tradjenta, Tresiba, or Trulicity. Do not confuse Tresiba with Tarceva, Toujeo, Tradjenta, or Trulicity.
- Use *only* insulin syringes to draw up dose. The unit markings on the insulin syringe must match the insulin's units/mL. Special syringes for doses <50 units are available. Before withdrawing dose, rotate vial between palms to ensure uniform solution; do not shake.
- Pedi: Use 100 units/mL vial for children requiring <5 units of insulin degludec each day.
- ***High Alert:*** Do not mix *insulin glargine* with any other insulin or solution or use syringes containing any other medicinal product or residue. If giving with a short-acting insulin, use separate syringes and different injection sites. Solution should be clear and colorless with no particulate matter.
- Do not use if cloudy, discolored, or unusually viscous. Store unopened vials and cartridges of *insulin glargine* in the refrigerator; do not freeze. If unable to refrigerate, the 10-mL vial of *insulin glargine* can be kept in a cool place unrefrigerated for up to 28 days. Once the cartridge is placed in a pen, do not refrigerate. *Insulin degludec* pens may be stored in the refrigerator or kept at room temperature for up to 56 days. Do not store in-use cartridges and prefilled syringes in refrigerator or with needle in place. Keep away from direct heat and sunlight.
- When transferring from once-daily NPH human insulin to *insulin glargine*, the dose usually remains unchanged. When transferring from twice-daily NPH human insulin to insulin glargine, the initial dose of insulin glargine is usually ↓ by 20%.
- **SUBQ:** Inject in abdominal area, thigh, buttocks, or upper arms, and rotate injection sites with each injection to reduce the risk of lipodystrophy and localized cutaneous amyloidosis. Repeated insulin injections into areas of localized cutaneous amyloidosis may cause hyperglycemia; a sudden change to an unaffected injection site may cause hypoglycemia.
- Administer *insulin glargine* and *insulin degludec* once daily at the same time each day.
- Do not administer *insulin degludec* or *insulin glargine* IV or in insulin pumps.

Patient/Family Teaching

- Explain purpose and side effects of medication to patient. Advise patient to read *Patient Information* before starting therapy. Advise patient on proper technique for administration. Include type of insulin, equipment (syringe, cartridge pens, alcohol swabs), storage, and place to discard syringes. Discuss the importance of not changing brands of insulin or syringes, selection and rotation of injection sites, and compliance with therapeutic regimen.
- Advise patient to notify health care provider of all Rx or OTC medications, vitamins, or herbal products being taken and to consult with health care provider before taking other medications.
- Advise patient not to share pen device with another person, even if needle is changed; may risk transmission of bloodborne pathogens.
- Advise to patient that this medication controls hyperglycemia but does not cure diabetes. Therapy is long term.
- Advise patient in proper testing of serum glucose and ketones. These tests should be closely monitored during periods of stress or illness and health care provider notified of significant changes.
- Emphasize the importance of compliance with nutritional guidelines and regular exercise as directed by health care provider.
- Advise patient to notify health care provider of medication regimen prior to treatment or surgery.

- Advise patient to notify health care provider if nausea, vomiting, or fever develops; if unable to eat regular diet; or if blood glucose levels are not controlled.
- Advise patient on signs and symptoms of hypoglycemia and hyperglycemia and what to do if they occur.
- Patients with diabetes mellitus should carry a source of sugar (candy, glucose gel) and identification describing their disease and treatment regimen at all times.
- Emphasize the importance of regular follow-up, especially during 1st few weeks of therapy.
- Rep: Advise women of reproductive potential to notify health care provider if pregnancy is planned or suspected or if breastfeeding.

Evaluation/Desired Outcomes

- Control of hyperglycemia in patients with diabetes.

HIGH ALERT

INSULINS (rapid-acting)

(in-su-lin)

insulin aspart

Fiasp, Fiasp FlexTouch, Fiasp PenFill, Fiasp PumpCart, ✦ Kirsty, Merilog, Merilog SoloStar, NovoLOG, NovoLOG FlexPen, NovoLOG PenFill, ✦ NovoRapid, ✦ Trurapi, ✦ Trurapi Solostar

insulin glulisine

Apidra, Apidra SoloStar

insulin lispro

Admelog, Admelog SoloStar, HumaLOG, HumaLOG Junior KwikPen, HumaLOG KwikPen, HumaLOG Tempo Pen, Lyumjev, Lyumjev KwikPen, Lyumjev Tempo Pen

Classification

Therapeutic: antidiabetics, hormones
Pharmacologic: pancreatics

See Appendix K for more information concerning insulins.

Indications

Type 1 or type 2 diabetes mellitus.

Action

Lower blood glucose by stimulating glucose uptake in skeletal muscle and fat, inhibiting hepatic glucose production. Other actions: inhibition of lipolysis and proteolysis, enhanced protein synthesis. These are rapid-acting insulins with a more rapid onset and shorter duration than regular insulin; should be used with an intermediate- or long-acting insulin. **Therapeutic Effects:** Control of hyperglycemia in diabetic patients.

Pharmacokinetics

Absorption: Very rapidly absorbed from SUBQ administration sites.
Distribution: Widely distributed to tissues.
Metabolism and Excretion: Metabolized by liver, spleen, kidney, and muscle.
Half-life: *Insulin aspart:* 1–1.5 hr; *Insulin glulisine:* 42 min; *Insulin lispro:* 1 hr.

TIME/ACTION PROFILE (hypoglycemic effect)

ROUTE	ONSET	PEAK	DURATION
Insulin aspart	within 15 min	1–2 hr	3–4 hr
Insulin glulisine	within 15 min	1–2 hr	3–4 hr
Insulin lispro	within 15 min	1–2 hr	3–4 hr

Contraindications/Precautions

Contraindicated in: Hypoglycemia; Allergy or hypersensitivity to a particular type of insulin, preservatives, or other additives.
Use Cautiously in: Stress and infection (may temporarily ↑ insulin requirements); Renal impairment (may ↓ insulin requirements); Hepatic impairment (may ↓ insulin requirements); OB: Pregnancy may temporarily ↑ insulin requirements; Pedi: Safety not established in children <1 yr (Lyumjev), <3 yr (Admelog and Humalog), <4 yr (insulin glulisine), or <6 yr (for insulin aspart).

Adverse Reactions/Side Effects

Endo: HYPOGLYCEMIA. **F and E:** hypokalemia. **Local:** cutaneous amyloidosis, erythema, lipodystrophy, pruritus, swelling. **Misc:** HYPERSENSITIVITY REACTIONS (INCLUDING ANAPHYLAXIS).

Interactions

Drug-Drug: Beta blockers and **clonidine** may mask some of the signs and symptoms of hypoglycemia. **Corticosteroids, thyroid supplements, estrogens, isoniazid, niacin, phenothiazines,** and **rifampin** may ↑ insulin requirements. **Alcohol, ACE inhibitors, MAO inhibitors, octreotide, oral hypoglycemic agents,** and **salicylates** may ↓ insulin requirements. **Pioglitazone** may ↑ risk of fluid retention and worsening HF.
Drug-Natural Products: Glucosamine may worsen blood glucose control. **Fenugreek, chromium,** and **coenzyme Q-10** may produce additive hypoglycemic effects.

Route/Dosage

Dose depends on blood glucose, response, and many other factors. Only insulin aspart and insulin glulisine can be administered IV. Lyumjev has faster onset of action and greater blood glucose-lowering effect than Admelog or Humalog on a unit-to-unit basis.

SUBQ (Adults and Children): Total insulin dose determined by needs of patient; generally 0.5–1 unit/kg/day; 50–70% of this dose may be given as meal-related boluses of rapid-acting insulin, and the remainder as an intermediate or long-acting insulin. *SUBQ infusion pump:* ~50% of total dose can be given as meal-related boluses and ~50% of total dose can be given as basal infusion.

Availability

Insulin Aspart

Solution for injection: 100 units/mL (vials, prefilled cartridges, and prefilled pens).

Insulin Glulisine

Solution for injection: 100 units/mL (vials and prefilled pens).

Insulin Lispro

Solution for injection (Admelog): 100 units/mL (vials, prefilled cartridges, and prefilled pens). **Solution for injection (Humalog, Lyumjev):** 100 units/mL (vials, prefilled cartridges, and prefilled pens), 200 units/mL (prefilled pens).

NURSING IMPLICATIONS

Assessment

- Assess for signs/symptoms of hypoglycemia (anxiety; restlessness; mood changes; tingling in hands, feet, lips, or tongue; chills; cold sweats; confusion; cool, pale skin; difficulty in concentration; drowsiness; nightmares or trouble sleeping; excessive hunger; headache; irritability; nausea; nervousness; tachycardia; tremor; weakness; unsteady gait) and hyperglycemia (confusion; drowsiness; flushed, dry skin; fruit-like breath odor; rapid, deep breathing; polyuria; loss of appetite; nausea; vomiting; tiredness; unusual thirst) periodically during therapy.
- Monitor body weight periodically. Changes in weight, meal patterns, and physical activity levels may necessitate changes in insulin dose.
- Assess patient for signs of allergic reactions (rash, shortness of breath, wheezing, rapid HR, sweating, low BP) during therapy.

Lab Test Considerations

- Monitor blood glucose every 6 hr during therapy, more frequently in ketoacidosis and times of stress.
- Monitor serum A1c twice yearly or every 3 mo when not meeting glycemic goals or change in therapy.
- Monitor serum potassium in patients at risk for hypokalemia (those using potassium-lowering agents, those receiving IV insulin) periodically during therapy.

Toxicity and Overdose

- Overdose is manifested by symptoms of hypoglycemia. Mild hypoglycemia may be treated by ingestion of oral glucose. Severe hypoglycemia is a life-threatening emergency; treatment consists of IV dextrose or glucagon. Octreotide may help stabilize blood glucose concentrations after prolonged hypoglycemia. Early signs of hypoglycemia may be less pronounced due to long duration of diabetes, diabetic nerve disease, and use of beta blockers; may result in loss of consciousness prior to patient's awareness of hypoglycemia.

Implementation

- ***High Alert:*** Insulin-related medication errors have resulted in patient harm and death. Clarify ambiguous orders; do not accept orders using the abbreviation "u" for units (can be misread as a zero or the numeral 4; has resulted in tenfold overdoses).
- Insulins are available in different types and strengths. Check type, dose, and expiration date with another licensed nurse. Do not interchange insulins without consulting health care provider.
- Do not confuse Humalog with Humulin or Novolog. Do not confuse Novolog with Novolin. Do not confuse Apidra with Spiriva.
- Use *only* insulin syringes to draw up dose. The unit markings on the insulin syringe must match the insulin's units/mL. Special syringes for doses <50 units are available. Do not draw up dose into a syringe from the Kwik Pens; syringe markings do not match up and could lead to a medication error. Use *only* U-100 insulin syringes to draw up ***insulin lispro*** dose. Prior to withdrawing dose, rotate vial between palms to ensure uniform solution; do not shake.
- ***Insulin aspart, insulin glulisine,*** and ***insulin lispro*** may be mixed with NPH insulin. When mixing insulins, draw insulin aspart, insulin glulisine, or insulin lispro into syringe first to avoid contamination of rapid-acting insulin vial. Mixed insulins should never be used in a pump or for IV infusion.
- Store vials in refrigerator. Vials may also be kept at room temperature for up to 28 days. Do not use if cloudy, discolored, or unusually viscous. Store cartridges and pens at room temperature and use within 28 days. Never use the *PenFill* cartridge after the expiration date on the *PenFill* cartridge or on the box.
- Because of their short duration, ***insulin lispro, insulin glulisine,*** and ***insulin aspart*** must be used with a longer-acting insulin or insulin infusion pump. In patients with type 2 diabetes, ***insulin lispro*** may be used without a longer-acting insulin when used in combination with an oral sulfonylurea agent.

- Humalog U-200 and Lyumjev U-200 should not be mixed with other insulins, administered IV, or used in insulin pumps.
- **SUBQ:** Administer into abdominal wall, thigh, or upper arm SUBQ. Rotate injection sites to prevent lipodystrophy and cutaneous amyloidosis. Repeated insulin injections into areas of localized cutaneous amyloidosis may cause hyperglycemia; a sudden change to an unaffected injection site may cause hypoglycemia.
- Administer *insulin aspart* within 5–10 min before a meal. Administer *Fiasp* at the start of a meal or within 20 min after starting a meal.
- When used as meal-time insulin, administer *insulin glulisine* 15 min before or within 20 min after starting a meal.
- Administer *insulin lispro: Admelog* and *Humalog* within 15 min before or immediately after a meal. Administer *Lyumjev* at the start of a meal or within 20 min after starting a meal.
- May also be administered SUBQ via external insulin pump. Do not mix with other insulins or solution when used with a pump. Change the solution in the reservoir at least every 6 days (Lyumjev at least every 9 days), change the infusion set, and the infusion set insertion site at least every 3 days. Do not mix with other insulins or with a diluent when used in the pump.

IV Administration

Insulin Aspart

- **IV:** May be administered IV in selected situations under appropriate medical supervision. **Dilution:** Dilute with 0.9% NaCl or D5W in infusion systems using polypropylene infusion bags; stable for 24 hr at room temperature. **Concentration:** 0.05–1 unit/mL.
- **Y-Site Compatibility:** imipenem/cilastatin/relebactam.
- **Y-Site Incompatibility:** posaconazole.

IV Administration

Insulin Glulisine

- **IV:** May be administered IV in selected situations under appropriate medical supervision. **Dilution:** Dilute with 0.9% NaCl, using polyvinyl chloride (PVC) Viaflex infusion bags and PVC tubing (Clearlink System Continu-Flo solution set) with a dedicated infusion line. **Concentration:** 0.05–1 unit/mL.
- **Y-Site Compatibility:** imipenem/cilastatin/relebactam.

IV Administration

Insulin Lispro

- **IV:** Insulin lispro (100 units/mL) can be administered IV under medical supervision ONLY with close monitoring of blood glucose and potassium levels to avoid hypoglycemia and hypokalemia. **Concentration:** 0.1–1 unit/mL. **Dilution:** 0.9% NaCl. Solution can be stored for 48 hr in refrigerator and then used at room temperature for another 48 hr.
- **Y-Site Compatibility:** ceftaroline, imipenem/cilastatin/relebactam.

Patient/Family Teaching

- Explain the purpose and side effects of rapid-acting insulins. Instruct patient on proper technique for administration. Tell patient to administer <15 min before or <20 min after starting a meal, depending on product. Include type of insulin, equipment (syringe, cartridge pens, external pump, alcohol swabs), storage, and place to discard syringes. Discuss the importance of not changing brands of insulin or syringes, selection and rotation of injection sites, and compliance with therapeutic regimen. Keep out of children's reach. Advise patient to read *Patient Information* before starting and with each Rx refill in case of changes.
- Instruct patient using an external insulin pump to change the insulin in the reservoir at least every 7 days or according to the pump user manual. Patient should not use mixed or diluted insulin in a pump. An alternate source of insulin should be available in case of pump failure.
- Emphasize the importance of regular follow-up to assess effectiveness, especially during first few weeks of therapy. Periodic lab tests will be needed.
- Demonstrate technique for mixing insulins by drawing up insulin aspart, insulin glulisine, or insulin lispro first. Roll intermediate-acting insulin vial between palms to mix rather than shaking (may cause inaccurate dose).
- Caution patient not to share pen device with another person, even if needle is changed and clean needles are used; may be harmful and ↑ risk of transmitting bloodborne pathogens.
- Instruct patient in prompt identification and correction of the cause of hyperglycemia or ketosis. Pump or infusion set malfunctions can lead to a rapid onset of hyperglycemia and ketoacidosis. Interim therapy with SUBQ injection may be required. Patients using continuous SUBQ insulin infusion pump therapy must be trained to administer insulin by injection and have alternate insulin therapy available in case of pump failure.
- Explain to patient that this medication controls hyperglycemia but does not cure diabetes. Therapy is long term.
- Instruct patient in proper testing of serum glucose and ketones. These tests should be closely

monitored during periods of stress or illness and health care provider notified of significant changes.

- Emphasize the importance of compliance with nutritional guidelines and regular exercise as directed by health care provider.
- Advise patient to notify health care provider of all Rx or OTC medications, vitamins, or herbal products being taken and to consult with health care provider before taking other medications or alcohol.
- Advise patient to notify health care provider of medication regimen prior to treatment or surgery.
- Advise patient to notify health care provider if nausea, vomiting, or fever develops; if unable to eat regular diet; or if blood glucose levels are not controlled.
- Instruct patient on signs and symptoms of hypoglycemia and hyperglycemia and what to do if they occur.
- Patients with diabetes mellitus should carry a source of sugar (candy, glucose gel) and identification describing their disease and treatment regimen at all times.
- Rep: Advise women to notify health care provider if pregnancy is planned or suspected or if breastfeeding.

Evaluation/Desired Outcomes

- Control of blood glucose levels without the appearance of hypoglycemic or hyperglycemic episodes.

HIGH ALERT

ipilimumab (i-pil-li-moo-mab)

Yervoy

Classification

Therapeutic: antineoplastics

Pharmacologic: monoclonal antibodies, cytotoxic T-lymphocyte antigen 4 inhibitors

Indications

Unresectable/metastatic melanoma (as monotherapy or in combination with nivolumab). Adjuvant treatment of cutaneous melanoma with pathologic involvement of regional lymph nodes >1 mm in patients who have undergone complete resection, including total lymphadenectomy. Previously untreated advanced renal cell carcinoma in patients who are at intermediate or poor risk (in combination with nivolumab). Microsatellite instability-high (MSI-H) or mismatch repair deficient (dMMR) metastatic colorectal cancer that has progressed following treatment with a fluoropyrimidine, oxaliplatin, and irinotecan. Hepatocellular carcinoma in patients who have been previously treated with sorafenib (in combination with nivolumab). First-line treatment of metastatic non-small cell lung cancer (NSCLC) in patients whose tumors express PD-L1 (≥1%) and have no epidermal growth factor receptor (EGFR) or anaplastic lymphoma kinase (ALK) genomic tumor aberrations (in combination with nivolumab). First-line treatment of metastatic or recurrent NSCLC in patients whose tumors have no EGFR or ALK genomic tumor aberrations (in combination with nivolumab and two cycles of platinum-based chemotherapy). First-line treatment of unresectable malignant pleural mesothelioma (in combination with nivolumab). First-line treatment of unresectable advanced or metastatic esophageal squamous cell carcinoma in patients whose tumors express PD-L1 (≥1) (in combination with nivolumab).

Action

Binds to cytotoxic T-lymphocyte-associated antigen 4 (CTLA-4) and prevents it from binding to CD80/CD86 ligands. CTLA-4 is a negative regulator of T-cell activation; binding results in augmented T-cell activation and proliferation as well as enhanced T-cell responsiveness. **Therapeutic Effects:** ↓ spread or recurrence of melanoma and improved survival. Improved survival with renal cell carcinoma, NSCLC, malignant pleural mesothelioma, and esophageal squamous cell carcinoma. ↓ progression of MSI-H or dMMR metastatic colorectal cancer. ↓ progression of hepatocellular carcinoma.

Pharmacokinetics

Absorption: IV administration results in complete bioavailability.

Distribution: Unknown.

Metabolism and Excretion: Unknown.

Half-life: 14.7 days.

TIME/ACTION PROFILE

ROUTE	ONSET	PEAK	DURATION
IV	unknown	unknown	unknown

Contraindications/Precautions

Contraindicated in: Lactation: Lactation.

Use Cautiously in: Patients undergoing allogeneic hematopoietic stem cell transplantation (↑ risk of graft-versus-host disease; OB: Use only if potential maternal benefit justifies potential risk to the fetus; Rep: Women of reproductive potential; Pedi: Children <12 yr (safety and effectiveness not established).

Adverse Reactions/Side Effects

CV: MYOCARDITIS, pericarditis, vasculitis. **Derm:** pruritus, rash, DRUG REACTION WITH EOSINOPHILIA AND SYSTEMIC SYMPTOMS (DRESS), STEVENS-JOHNSON SYNDROME (SJS), TOXIC EPIDERMAL NECROLYSIS (TEN). **EENT:** hearing loss, immune-mediated iritis, immune-mediated uveitis. **Endo:** immune-mediated hypothyroidism, IMMUNE-MEDIATED ADRENAL INSUFFICIENCY, immune-mediated hyperthyroidism, immune-mediated hypoparathyroidism, immune-mediated hypophysitis, immune-mediated type 1 diabetes. **GI:** diarrhea, IMMUNE-MEDIATED COLITIS, immune-mediated gastritis, IMMUNE-MEDIATED HEPATITIS, immune-mediated pancreatitis. **GU:** immune-mediated nephritis. **Hemat:** immune-mediated hemolytic anemia. **MS:** immune-mediated myositis, IMMUNE-MEDIATED RHABDOMYOLYSIS. **Neuro:** fatigue, autoimmune neuropathy, Guillain-Barré syndrome, IMMUNE-MEDIATED ENCEPHALITIS, IMMUNE-MEDIATED MENINGITIS, immune-mediated myasthenic syndrome, immune-mediated myelitis. **Resp:** IMMUNE-MEDIATED PNEUMONITIS. **Misc:** INFUSION REACTIONS.

Interactions

Drug-Drug: Concurrent use with **vemurafenib** may ↑ risk of hepatic impairment.

Route/Dosage

Unresectable/Metastatic Melanoma

IV (Adults and Children ≥12 yr): *As monotherapy:* 3 mg/kg every 3 wk for up to 4 doses. *In combination with nivolumab:* 3 mg/kg every 3 wk for up to 4 doses or unacceptable toxicity (administer after nivolumab on same day); after completing 4 doses of the combination, give nivolumab alone until disease progression or unacceptable toxicity.

Adjuvant Treatment of Melanoma

IV (Adults and Children ≥12 yr): 3 mg/kg every 3 wk for up to 4 doses, then 3 mg/kg every 12 wk for up to 4 additional doses.

Advanced Renal Cell Carcinoma

IV (Adults): 1 mg/kg every 3 wk for up to 4 doses (administer after nivolumab on same day); after completing 4 doses of the combination, give nivolumab alone until disease progression or unacceptable toxicity.

Colorectal Cancer

IV (Adults): 1 mg/kg every 3 wk for 4 doses (administer after nivolumab on same day); after completing 4 doses of the combination, give nivolumab alone until disease progression or unacceptable toxicity.

Hepatocellular Carcinoma

IV (Adults): 3 mg/kg every 3 wk for 4 doses (administer after nivolumab on same day); after completing 4 doses of the combination, give nivolumab alone until disease progression or unacceptable toxicity.

Metastatic or Recurrent Non-Small Cell Lung Cancer

IV (Adults): 1 mg/kg every 6 wk until disease progression, unacceptable toxicity, or for up to 2 yr (if no disease progression) (administer after nivolumab, but before platinum-based chemotherapy [if being given] on same day).

Malignant Pleural Mesothelioma

IV (Adults): 1 mg/kg every 6 wk until disease progression, unacceptable toxicity, or for up to 2 yr (if no disease progression) (administer after nivolumab on same day).

Esophageal Squamous Cell Carcinoma

IV (Adults): 1 mg/kg every 6 wk until disease progression, unacceptable toxicity, or for up to 2 yr (administer after nivolumab on same day).

Availability

Solution for injection: 5 mg/mL.

NURSING IMPLICATIONS

Assessment

- Monitor for signs and symptoms of colitis (diarrhea, abdominal pain, mucus or blood in stool, with or without fever) and bowel perforation (peritoneal signs, ileus). Rule out infection and consider endoscopic evaluation. *If Grade 2 colitis occurs,* hold therapy and administer corticosteroids (initial dose of 1–2 mg/kg/day prednisone or equivalent, followed by a corticosteroid taper). Resume therapy if Grade ≤1 after corticosteroid taper. Permanently discontinue ipilimumab if no complete or partial resolution within 12 wk of last dose or inability to reduce prednisone to ≤10 mg per day (or equivalent) within 12 wk of initiating steroids. *If Grade 3 or 4 colitis occurs,* permanently discontinue ipilimumab.
- Assess for skin reactions, including SJS, TEN, and DRESS (prodrome of fever, malaise, mucosal lesions, progressive skin rash, blisters, lymphadenopathy, conjunctivitis, myalgias, hepatitis, eosinophilia), during therapy. Treat mild to moderate nonexfoliative rashes with topical emollients and/or topical corticosteroids. *If SJS, TEN, or DRESS is suspected,* hold ipilimumab. *If SJS, TEN, or DRESS is confirmed,* permanently discontinue ipilimumab.
- Monitor for signs and symptoms of pneumonitis (new or worsening cough, chest pain, shortness of breath) during therapy. Evaluate with x-ray. Administer corticosteroids (initial dose of 1–2 mg/kg/day prednisone or equivalent, followed by a corticosteroid taper). *For Grade 2 pneumonitis,* hold ipilimumab and resume if complete or partial resolution (Grade ≤1) after corticosteroid taper. *For Grade 3 or 4 or recurrent Grade 2 pneumonitis,* permanently discontinue ipilimumab.
- Monitor for signs and symptoms of neurologic toxicity (headache, neck stiffness, change in consciousness, weakness) periodically during therapy. *If Grade 2 symptoms occur,* hold ipilimumab. *If Grade 3 or 4 symptoms occur,* permanently discontinue ipilimumab.
- Monitor for signs and symptoms of hypophysitis (headache, photophobia, visual field defects) during therapy. May cause hypopituitarism. Begin

hormone replacement therapy. Hold or permanently discontinue ipilimumab based on severity.

- Assess eyes for signs and symptoms of uveitis, iritis, or episcleritis. Administer corticosteroid eye drops if these occur. Consider Vogt-Koyanagi-Harada-like syndrome if uveitis occurs with other immune-mediated adverse reactions. May require treatment with systemic steroids to ↓ the risk of permanent vision loss. *If Grade 2–4 ophthalmologic symptoms occur that do not improve to Grade 1 within 2 wk while receiving topical therapy or that requires systemic treatment,* permanently discontinue ipilimumab.
- Monitor for signs and symptoms of infusion-related reactions (fever, chills, flushing, hypotension, dyspnea, wheezing, back pain, abdominal pain, urticaria) during infusion. *If Grade 1 or 2 infusion-related reactions occur,* interrupt or slow rate of infusion. *If Grade 3 or 4 infusion-related reactions occur,* stop infusion and permanently discontinue ipilimumab.
- Monitor for signs and symptoms of cardiovascular events during therapy. Assess left ventricular ejection fraction at baseline and periodically during therapy. Manage cardiovascular risk factors (hypertension, diabetes, dyslipidemia). *If Grade 2–4 cardiovascular events occur,* permanently discontinue ipilimumab.
- Monitor for signs and symptoms of graft-versus-host disease (fatigue, rash, pruritus, nausea, vomiting, diarrhea, jaundice, scleral icterus, xerostomia, arthralgias).

Lab Test Considerations

- Patient selection with metastatic NSCLC or unresectable advanced or metastatic esophageal squamous cell carcinoma for treatment with ipilimumab in combination with nivolumab is based on PD-L1 expression. Information on FDA-approved tests for the determination of PD-L1 expression is available at https://www.fda.gov/CompanionDiagnostics.
- Verify negative pregnancy status before starting therapy.
- May cause hepatitis; monitor liver function tests prior to therapy and before each dose during therapy. *If levels ↑,* administer corticosteroids (initial dose of 1–2 mg/kg/day prednisone or equivalent, followed by a corticosteroid taper). **For hepatitis with no tumor involvement of the liver or hepatitis with tumor involvement of liver/nonhepatocellular carcinoma:** *If AST or ALT ↑ >3–<5 times upper limit of normal (ULN) or total bilirubin ↑ >1.5–<3 times ULN,* hold ipilimumab and resume with complete or partial resolution (Grade 0–1) after corticosteroid taper. *If AST or ALT >5 times ULN or total bilirubin >3 times ULN,* permanently discontinue ipilimumab. **For hepatitis with tumor involvement of the liver/hepatocellular carcinoma:** *If baseline AST or ALT >1–<3 times ULN and ↑ to >5–<10 times ULN or if baseline AST or ALT >3–<5 times ULN and ↑ to >8 to <10 times ULN,* hold ipilimumab and resume with complete or partial resolution (Grade 0–1) after corticosteroid taper. *If AST or ALT >10 times ULN or if total bilirubin >3 times ULN,* permanently discontinue ipilimumab.
- Monitor for signs and symptoms of adrenal insufficiency, including but not limited to hypothyroidism, hyperthyroidism, adrenal insufficiency, and hyperglycemia during and after treatment. Administer corticosteroids as appropriate, followed by a corticosteroid taper. *If Grade 3 or 4 endocrinopathies occur,* hold ipilimumab until clinically stable or permanently discontinue ipilimumab based on severity.
- May cause nephritis; monitor for ↑ serum creatinine before and periodically during therapy. Administer corticosteroids (initial dose of 1–2 mg/kg/day prednisone or equivalent, followed by a corticosteroid taper). *If Grade 2 or 3 ↑ serum creatinine occurs,* hold ipilimumab and resume with complete or partial resolution (Grade 0–1) of nephritis and renal impairment after corticosteroid taper. *If Grade 4 ↑ serum creatinine occurs,* permanently discontinue ipilimumab.

Implementation

- For unresectable/metastatic melanoma, doses may be delayed in the event of toxicity, but must be administered within 16 wk from 1st dose. For adjuvant treatment of melanoma, doses can be omitted, but not delayed in the event of toxicity.

IV Administration

- Allow vial to stand at room temperature for 5 min prior to preparation of infusion. Withdraw amount of ipilimumab required and transfer to IV bag. **Dilution:** Dilute with 0.9% NaCl or D5W. **Concentration:** 1–2 mg/mL. Mix slowly by gentle inversion; do not shake. Solution is clear, pale yellow, and may contain translucent to white amorphous particles; do not administer if cloudy, discolored, or contains particulate matter. Store for up to 24 hr at room temperature or refrigerated; do not freeze; protect from light. Discard partially used vials.
- **Rate:** Infuse through a sterile, nonpyrogenic, low-protein-binding in-line filter. Flush the IV line with 0.9% NaCl or D5W after each dose. *Unresectable or metastatic melanoma:* Infuse over 30 min; *Adjuvant treatment of melanoma:* Infuse over 90 min; *Renal cell carcinoma, hepatocellular carcinoma, NSCLC, malignant pleural mesothelioma, esophageal squamous cell carcinoma, or colorectal cancer:* Infuse over 30 min immediately following nivolumab infusion.
- **Y-Site Incompatibility:** Do not administer other drugs through same IV line.

Patient/Family Teaching

- Explain purpose and potential adverse effects of ipilimumab to patient. Do not stop receiving drug without consulting health care provider. If an appointment is missed, contact health care provider as soon as possible to reschedule. Advise patient to read *Medication Guide* before starting and periodically during therapy in case of changes.
- Inform patient of the risk of immune-mediated reactions due to T-cell activation and proliferation. Advise patients these reactions may be severe and fatal. Advise patient to notify health care provider if signs and symptoms of colitis (diarrhea; black, tarry, sticky, bloody, or mucus in stools; severe abdominal pain or tenderness), hepatitis (yellowing of skin or the whites of eyes, severe nausea or vomiting, pain on right side of abdomen), skin reactions (rash; itching; skin blistering or peeling; painful sores in mouth, nose, throat, or genital area), endocrinopathies (persistent or unusual headache, eye sensitivity to light, eye problems, rapid heartbeat, ↑ sweating, extreme tiredness, weight gain or weight loss, feeling hungrier or thirstier than usual, urinating more often than usual, hair loss, feeling cold, constipation, deepening of voice, dizziness or fainting, changes in mood or behavior, ↓ sex drive, irritability, forgetfulness), pneumonitis (new or worsening cough, shortness of breath, chest pain), nephritis (↓ in amount of urine, blood in urine, swelling of ankles, loss of appetite), or eye problems (blurry vision, double vision, other vision problems, eye pain or redness) occur.
- Instruct patient to notify health care provider of all Rx or OTC medications, vitamins, or herbal products being taken and to consult health care provider before taking other Rx, OTC, herbal products.
- Rep: May cause fetal harm. Advise women of reproductive potential to use effective contraception and avoid breastfeeding during therapy and for 3 mo following last dose. Encourage women who become pregnant during therapy to contact Bristol Myers Squibb by calling 1-844-593-7869.

Evaluation/Desired Outcomes

- ↓ spread or recurrence of melanoma and improved survival.
- Improved survival with renal cell carcinoma, NSCLC, malignant pleural mesothelioma, and esophageal squamous cell carcinoma.
- ↓ progression of MSI-H or dMMR metastatic colorectal cancer.
- ↓ progression of hepatocellular carcinoma.

ipratropium (i-pra-**troe**-pee-um)

Atrovent HFA

Classification

Therapeutic: allergy, cold, and cough remedies, bronchodilators

Pharmacologic: anticholinergics

Indications

Inhaln: Maintenance therapy of reversible airway obstruction due to COPD, including chronic bronchitis and emphysema. **Intranasal:** Rhinorrhea associated with allergic and nonallergic perennial rhinitis (0.03% solution) or the common cold (0.06% solution). **Unlabeled Use: Inhaln:** Adjunctive management of bronchospasm caused by asthma.

Action

Inhaln: Inhibits cholinergic receptors in bronchial smooth muscle, resulting in decreased concentrations of cyclic guanosine monophosphate (cGMP). Decreased levels of cGMP produce local bronchodilation. **Intranasal:** Local application inhibits secretions from glands lining the nasal mucosa. **Therapeutic Effects: Inhaln:** Bronchodilation without systemic anticholinergic effects. **Intranasal:** Decreased rhinorrhea.

Pharmacokinetics

Absorption: Minimal systemic absorption (2% for inhalation solution; 20% for inhalation aerosol; <20% following nasal use).

Distribution: 15% of dose reaches lower airways after inhalation.

Metabolism and Excretion: Small amounts absorbed are metabolized by the liver.

Half-life: 2 hr.

TIME/ACTION PROFILE (bronchodilation)

ROUTE	ONSET	PEAK	DURATION
Inhalation	1–3 min	1–2 hr	4–6 hr
Intranasal	15 min	unknown	6–12 hr

Contraindications/Precautions

Contraindicated in: Hypersensitivity to ipratropium, atropine, belladonna alkaloids, or bromide; Acute bronchospasm.

Use Cautiously in: Bladder-neck obstruction, prostatic hyperplasia, glaucoma, or urinary retention; Lactation: Safety not established in breastfeeding; Geri: Older adults may be more sensitive to effects.

Adverse Reactions/Side Effects

CV: hypotension, palpitations. **Derm:** rash. **EENT:** blurred vision, sore throat**nasal only:** epistaxis, nasal dryness/irritation. **GI:** GI irritation, nausea. **Neuro:**

dizziness, headache, nervousness. **Resp:** bronchospasm, cough. **Misc:** HYPERSENSITIVITY REACTIONS (INCLUDING ANAPHYLAXIS).

Interactions

Drug-Drug: ↑ anticholinergic effects with other **drugs having anticholinergic properties**, including **antihistamines, phenothiazines**, and **disopyramide**.

Route/Dosage

Inhaln (Adults and Children >12 yr): *Metered-dose inhaler (nonacute):* 2 inhalations 4 times daily (not to exceed 12 inhalations/24 hr or more frequently than every 4 hr). *Metered-dose inhaler (acute exacerbations):* 4–8 puffs using a spacer device as needed. *Nebulization (nonacute):* 500 mcg 3–4 times daily. *Nebulization (acute exacerbations):* 500 mcg every 30 min for 3 doses, then every 2–4 hr as needed.
Inhaln (Adults and Children 5–12 yr): *Metered-dose inhaler (nonacute):* 1–2 inhalations every 6 hr as needed (not to exceed 12 inhalations/24 hr). *Metered-dose inhaler (acute exacerbations):* 4–8 puffs as needed. *Nebulization (nonacute):* 250–500 mcg 4 times daily given every 6 hr. *Nebulization (acute exacerbations):* 250 mcg every 20 min for 3 doses, then every 2–4 hr as needed.
Inhaln (Infants): *Nebulization:* 125–250 mcg 3 times a day.
Inhaln (Neonates): *Nebulization:* 25 mcg/kg/dose 3 times a day.
Intranasal (Adults and Children >6 yr): *0.03% solution:* 2 sprays in each nostril 2–3 times daily (21 mcg/spray).
Inhaln (Adults and Children >5 yr): *0.06% solution:* 2 sprays in each nostril 3–4 times daily (42 mcg/spray).

Availability (generic available)

Aerosol inhaler (HFA) (chlorofluorocarbon-free): 17 mcg/inhalation in 12.9-g canister (200 inhalations). **Inhalation solution:** 🍁 0.0125%, 0.02%, 🍁 0.025%. **Nasal spray:** 0.03% solution: 21 mcg/spray in 30-mL bottle (345 sprays/bottle), 0.06% solution: 42 mcg/spray in 15-mL bottle (165 sprays). ***In combination with:*** albuterol (Combivent Respimat). See Appendix N.

NURSING IMPLICATIONS

Assessment

- Assess for allergy to atropine and belladonna alkaloids; patients with these allergies may also be sensitive to ipratropium.
- **Inhaln:** Assess respiratory status (rate, breath sounds, degree of dyspnea) before administration and at peak of medication. Consult health care provider about alternative medication if severe bronchospasm is present; onset of action is too slow for patients in acute distress. *If hypersensitivity reactions or paradoxical bronchospasm (wheezing) occurs,* withhold medication and implement supportive measures (epinephrine).
- **Nasal Spray:** Assess patient for rhinorrhea.

Implementation

- **Inhaln:** See Appendix C for administration of inhalation medications.
- When ipratropium is administered concurrently with other inhalation medications, administer adrenergic bronchodilators first, followed by ipratropium, and then corticosteroids. Wait 5 min between medications.
- Solution for *nebulization* can be diluted with preservative-free 0.9% NaCl. Diluted solution should be used within 24 hr at room temperature or 48 hr if refrigerated. Solution can be mixed with preservative-free albuterol or cromolyn if used within 1 hr of mixing.

Patient/Family Teaching

- Explain purpose and side effects of medication to patient. Advise patient to read *Patient Information* before starting therapy. Instruct patient in proper use of inhaler, nebulizer, or nasal spray and to take medication as directed. Take missed doses as soon as remembered unless almost time for the next dose; space remaining doses evenly during day. Do not double doses.
- Advise patient to notify health care provider of all Rx or OTC medications, vitamins, or herbal products being taken and to consult health care provider before taking other medications.
- Advise patient that rinsing mouth after using inhaler, proper oral hygiene, and sugarless gum or candy may minimize dry mouth. Health care provider should be notified if stomatitis occurs or if dry mouth persists for >2 wk.
- **Inhalation:** Caution patient not to exceed 12 doses within 24 hr. Patient should notify health care provider if symptoms do not improve within 30 min after administration of medication or if condition worsens.
- Explain need for pulmonary function tests before and periodically during therapy to determine effectiveness of medication.
- Caution patient to avoid spraying medication in eyes; may cause blurring of vision or irritation.
- Advise patient to inform health care provider if cough, nervousness, headache, dizziness, nausea, or GI distress occurs.
- **Nasal Spray:** Instruct patient in proper use of nasal spray. Clear nasal passages gently before administration. Do not inhale during administration, so medication remains in nasal passages.

Prime pump initially with 7 actuations. If used regularly, no further priming is needed. If not used in 24 hr, prime with 2 actuations. If not used for >7 days, prime with 7 actuations.

- Advise patient to contact health care provider if symptoms do not improve within 1–2 wk or if condition worsens.
- Advise patient if hypersensitivity reactions occur (anaphylaxis) to seek immediate medical assistance.
- Rep: Advise women of reproductive potential to notify health care provider if pregnancy is planned or suspected or if breastfeeding.

Evaluation/Desired Outcomes

- Bronchodilation without systemic anticholinergic effects.
- Decreased rhinorrhea.

irbesartan, See ANGIOTENSIN II RECEPTOR ANTAGONISTS.

HIGH ALERT

irinotecan

(eye-ri-noe-**tee**-kan)

Camptosar

Classification

Therapeutic: antineoplastics

Pharmacologic: enzyme inhibitors

Indications

First-line therapy of metastatic colorectal cancer (in combination with 5-fluorouracil and leucovorin). Metastatic colorectal cancer that has recurred or progressed following initial fluorouracil-based therapy.

Action

Interferes with DNA synthesis by inhibiting the enzyme topoisomerase. **Therapeutic Effects:** Death of rapidly replicating cells, particularly malignant ones.

Pharmacokinetics

Absorption: IV administration results in complete bioavailability.

Distribution: Unknown.

Protein Binding: *Irinotecan:* 30–68%; *SN-38 (active metabolite):* 95%.

Metabolism and Excretion: Converted by the liver to SN-38, its active metabolite, which is metabolized by the liver by UDP-glucuronosyl 111 transferase 1A1 (UGT1A1) and CYP3A4. Small amounts excreted by kidneys.

Half-life: 6 hr.

TIME/ACTION PROFILE (hematologic effects)

ROUTE	ONSET	PEAK	DURATION
IV	unknown	21–29 days	27–34 days

Contraindications/Precautions

Contraindicated in: Hypersensitivity; Hereditary fructose intolerance (contains sorbitol); OB: Pregnancy; Lactation: Lactation.

Use Cautiously in: Previous pelvic or abdominal irradiation or age ≥65 yr (↑ risk of myelosuppression); Presence of infection, underlying bone marrow depression, or concurrent chronic illness; History of prior pelvic/abdominal irradiation and serum bilirubin >1–2 mg/dL (initial dose ↓ recommended); Hepatic impairment; Previous severe myelosuppression or diarrhea (reinstitute at lower dose following resolution); Homozygous for UGT1A1*28 [*28/*28] or UGT1A1*6 [*6/*6] alleles or compound heterozygous for UGT1A1*28 or UGT1A1*6 [*6/*28] alleles (poor UGT1A1 metabolizers) or heterozygous for either the UGT1A1*28 or UGT1A1*6 alleles (*1/*28, *1/*6) (intermediate UGT1A1 metabolizers) (↑ risk of severe or life-threatening neutropenia); Rep: Women of reproductive potential and men with female partners of reproductive potential; Pedi: Safety and effectiveness not established in children; Geri: ↑ sensitivity to adverse effects (myelosuppression) in older adults; initiate at lower dose.

Adverse Reactions/Side Effects

CV: edema, vasodilation. **Derm:** alopecia, rash, sweating. **EENT:** rhinitis. **F and E:** dehydration. **GI:** abdominal pain/cramping, anorexia, constipation, DIARRHEA, dyspepsia, flatulence, nausea, stomatitis, vomiting, weight loss, ↑ liver enzymes, abdominal enlargement, colonic ulceration. **GU:** ↓ fertility, menstrual abnormalities. **Hemat:** ANEMIA, NEUTROPENIA, THROMBOCYTOPENIA. **Local:** injection site reactions. **MS:** back pain. **Neuro:** dizziness, headache, insomnia, weakness. **Resp:** coughing, dyspnea, INTERSTITIAL LUNG DISEASE (ILD). **Misc:** chills, fever, INFECTION.

Interactions

Drug-Drug: ↑ bone marrow depression may occur with other **antineoplastics** or **radiation therapy**. Strong **CYP3A4 inhibitors**, including **ketoconazole, clarithromycin, itraconazole, lopinavir, nefazodone, nelfinavir, ritonavir**, and **voriconazole**, and strong **UGT1A1 inhibitors**, including **atazanavir** and **gemfibrozil**, may ↑ levels and risk of toxicity of irinotecan and its active metabolite; discontinue ≥1 wk before initiating irinotecan. **Phenobarbital, phenytoin, carbamazepine, rifampin**, or **rifabutin** may ↓ levels of irinotecan

and its active metabolite; consider using an alternative anticonvulsant at least 2 wk before initiating irinotecan. **Laxatives** should be avoided; diarrhea may be ↑. **Diuretics** ↑ risk of dehydration; may discontinue during therapy. **Dexamethasone** may ↑ risk of hyperglycemia and lymphocytopenia. **Prochlorperazine** given on the same day as irinotecan may risk of akathisia. May ↓ antibody response to and ↑ risk of adverse reactions from **live-virus vaccines**.
Drug-Natural Products: St. John's wort ↓ levels of irinotecan and the active metabolite; discontinue ≥2 wk before initiating irinotecan.

Route/Dosage

Other regimens are used; careful modification required for all levels of toxicity/tolerance.

Single Agent

IV (Adults): *Weekly dosage schedule:* 125 mg/m² once weekly for 4 wk, followed by a 2-wk rest period. Cycle may be repeated using doses that depend on patient tolerance and degree of toxicity encountered. *Once-every-3-wk schedule:* 350 mg/m² once every 3 wk. Cycle may be repeated using doses that depend on patient tolerance and degree of toxicity encountered.
IV (Geriatric Patients >70 yr): *Weekly dosage schedule:* 125 mg/m² once weekly for 4 wk, followed by a 2-wk rest period. Cycle may be repeated using doses that depend on patient tolerance and degree of toxicity encountered. *Once-every-3-wk schedule:* 300 mg/m² once every 3 wk. Cycle may be repeated using doses that depend on patient tolerance and degree of toxicity encountered.
IV (Adults Homozygous for UGT1A1*28 [*28/*28] or UGT1A1*6 [*6/*6] Alleles or Compound Heterozygous for UGT1A1*28 or UGT1A1*6 [*6/*28] Alleles): *Weekly dosage schedule:* 100 mg/m² once weekly for 4 wk, followed by a 2-wk rest period. Cycle may be repeated using doses that depend on patient tolerance and degree of toxicity encountered. *Once-every-3-wk schedule:* 300 mg/m² once every 3 wk. Cycle may be repeated using doses that depend on patient tolerance and degree of toxicity encountered.

Hepatic Impairment

IV (Adults): *Bilirubin 1–2 mg/dL and history of prior pelvic/abdominal irradiation: Weekly dosage schedule:* Initiate therapy at lower dose (100 mg/m²); once weekly for 4 wk, followed by a 2-wk rest period. Cycle may be repeated with dose adjusted as tolerated. *Once-every-3-wk schedule:* 300 mg/m² once every 3 wk. Cycle may be repeated with dose adjusted as tolerated.

As Part of Combination Therapy with Leucovorin and 5-Fluorouracil

IV (Adults): *Regimen 1 (Bolus regimen):* 125 mg/m² once weekly for 4 wk, followed by a 2-wk rest period. Cycle may be repeated using doses that depend on patient tolerance and degree of toxicity encountered; *Regimen 2 (Infusional regimen):* 180 mg/m² every 2 wk for 3 doses, followed by a 3-wk rest period. Cycle may be repeated using doses that depend on patient tolerance and degree of toxicity encountered.
IV (Adults Homozygous for UGT1A1*28 [*28/*28] or UGT1A1*6 [*6/*6] Alleles or Compound Heterozygous for UGT1A1*28 or UGT1A1*6 [*6/*28] Alleles): *Regimen 1 (Bolus regimen):* 100 mg/m² once weekly for 4 wk, followed by a 2-wk rest period. Cycle may be repeated using doses that depend on patient tolerance and degree of toxicity encountered; *Regimen 2 (Infusional regimen):* 150 mg/m² every 2 wk for 3 doses, followed by a 3-wk rest period. Cycle may be repeated using doses that depend on patient tolerance and degree of toxicity encountered.

Availability (generic available)

Solution for injection: 20 mg/mL.

NURSING IMPLICATIONS

Assessment

- Monitor vital signs frequently during administration.
- Monitor for bone marrow suppression. Assess for bleeding (bleeding gums; bruising; petechiae; guaiac stools, urine, and emesis). Avoid IM injections and taking rectal temperatures if platelet count is low. Apply pressure to venipuncture sites for 10 min. Assess for signs of infection during neutropenia. Anemia may occur. Monitor for ↑ fatigue, dyspnea, and orthostatic hypotension.
- Monitor closely for the development of diarrhea. Two types may occur. The early type occurs within 24 hr of administration and may be preceded by cramps and sweating. Atropine 0.25–1 mg IV or SUBQ may be given to ↓ symptoms. Potentially life-threatening diarrhea may occur >24 hr after a dose; may be accompanied by severe dehydration and electrolyte imbalance. Loperamide 4 mg initially, followed by 2 mg every 2 hr until diarrhea ceases for >12 hr (or 4 mg every 4 hr if given during sleeping hours) should be administered promptly to treat late-occurring diarrhea. Do not administer loperamide at these doses for >48 hr. Careful fluid and electrolyte replacement should be instituted to prevent complications. *If diarrhea of 2–3 stools/day pretreatment occurs,* maintain dose. *If 4–6 stools/day more than pretreatment occurs during a cycle,* ↓ by 25 mg/m². *If 4–6 stools/day more than pretreatment occurs at the beginning of a weekly cycle or at the beginning of a once-every-3-wk cycle,* maintain dose. *If 7–9 stools/day more than pretreatment occurs during a cycle,* hold dose until resolved to Grade ≤2; then ↓ by 25 mg/m². *If 7–9 stools/day more*

than pretreatment occurs at the beginning of a weekly cycle, ↓ by 25 mg/m². *If 7–9 stools/day more than pretreatment occurs at the beginning of a once-every-3-wk cycle,* ↓ by 50 mg/m². *If ≥10 stools/day more than pretreatment occurs during a cycle,* hold dose until resolved to Grade ≤2; then ↓ by 50 mg/m². *If ≥10 stools/day more than pretreatment occurs at the beginning of a weekly cycle or at the beginning of a once-every-3-wk cycle,* ↓ by 50 mg/m². *If ileus, fever, or severe neutropenia occurs,* initiate antibiotic therapy.

- *If signs of pulmonary toxicity (dyspnea, cough, fever) occur,* interrupt therapy. *If ILD is confirmed,* permanently discontinue irinotecan.
- Assess for cholinergic symptoms (rhinitis, ↑ salivation, miosis, lacrimation, diaphoresis, flushing, abdominal cramping) during therapy. Atropine 0.25–1 mg SUBQ or IV may be used to prevent or treat symptoms.

Lab Test Considerations

- Consider laboratory test to determine the UGT1A1 status. Testing can detect the UGT1A1 *6 and *28, genotypes.
- Verify negative pregnancy test before starting therapy.
- Monitor CBC with differential and platelet count before each dose. *If neutropenia with ANC 1500–1999/mm³ occurs,* maintain dose. *If ANC 1000–1499/mm³ occurs during a cycle,* ↓ dose by 25 mg/m². *If ANC 1000–1499/mm³ occurs at beginning of cycle,* maintain dose. *If ANC 500–999/mm³ occurs during a cycle,* hold dose until resolved to Grade ≤2; then ↓ by 25 mg/m². *If ANC 500–999/mm³ occurs at the beginning of a weekly cycle,* ↓ dose by 25 mg/m². *If ANC 500–999/mm³ occurs at the beginning of a once-every-3-wk cycle,* ↓ dose by 50 mg/m². *If ANC <500/mm³ occurs during a cycle,* hold dose until resolved to Grade ≤2; then ↓ by 50 mg/m². *If ANC 500–999/mm³ occurs at the beginning of a weekly cycle or at the beginning of a once-every-3-wk cycle,* ↓ dose by 50 mg/m². *If neutropenic fever occurs during a cycle,* hold dose until resolved; then ↓ by 50 mg/m² when resolved. *If neutropenic fever occurs at the beginning of a weekly cycle or at the beginning of a once-every-3-wk cycle,* ↓ by 50 mg/m². Administration of a colony-stimulating factor may be considered if clinically significant ↓ in WBC (<2000/mm³), neutrophil count (<1000/mm³), hemoglobin (<9 g/dL), or platelet count (<100,000 cells/mm³) occur.
- May ↑ serum alkaline phosphatase and AST.

Implementation

IV Administration

- Wear gloves, gown, and mask while handling IV medication. Discard IV equipment in specially designated containers.
- Nausea and vomiting are common. Pretreatment with dexamethasone 10 mg along with agents such as ondansetron or granisetron should be started on the same day as irinotecan >30 min before administration. Prochlorperazine may be used on subsequent days but may ↑ risk of akathisia if given on the same day as irinotecan.
- Irinotecan is an irritant. If extravasation occurs, immediately stop infusion. Leave needle/cannula in place temporarily but do not flush the line. Gently aspirate extravasated solution; then remove needle/cannula. Elevate patient's extremity and apply dry cold compresses for 20 min 4 times day for 1–2 days.
- **Intermittent Infusion: Dilution:** Dilute with 500 mL of D5W or 0.9% NaCl. **Concentration:** 0.12–2.8 mg/mL. Solution is pale yellow. Do not administer solutions that are cloudy, discolored, or contain particulate matter. Solution is stable for 24 hr if refrigerated. **Rate:** Infuse over 90 min.
- **Y-Site Compatibility:** alemtuzumab, amikacin, aminocaproic acid, aminophylline, amiodarone, ampicillin, ampicillin/sulbactam, anidulafungin, argatroban, atracurium, azithromycin, aztreonam, bivalirudin, bleomycin, bumetanide, buprenorphine, butorphanol, calcium chloride, calcium gluconate, carboplatin, caspofungin, cefazolin, cefotetan, cefoxitin, ceftazidime, cefuroxime, ciprofloxacin, cisatracurium, cisplatin, clindamycin, cyclophosphamide, cyclosporine, cytarabine, dacarbazine, daptomycin, daunorubicin, dexamethasone, dexrazoxane, digoxin, diltiazem, diphenhydramine, dobutamine, docetaxel, dopamine, doxorubicin hydrochloride, doxorubicin liposomal, doxycycline, enalaprilat, ephedrine, epinephrine, ertapenem, erythromycin, esmolol, etoposide, etoposide phosphate, famotidine, fentanyl, fluconazole, foscarnet, gemtuzumab ozogamicin, gentamicin, granisetron, haloperidol, heparin, hetastarch, hydralazine, hydrocortisone, hydromorphone, idarubicin, imipenem/cilastatin, insulin regular, isoproterenol, ketorolac, labetalol, leucovorin, levofloxacin, levoleucovorin, lidocaine, linezolid, lorazepam, magnesium sulfate, mannitol, meperidine, meropenem, mesna, methadone, metoclopramide, metoprolol, metronidazole, midazolam, milrinone, mitoxantrone, morphine, moxifloxacin, nalbuphine, naloxone, nicardipine, nitroglycerin, norepinephrine, octreotide,

ondansetron, oxaliplatin, paclitaxel, palonosetron, pantoprazole, pentamidine, pentobarbital, phenobarbital, phentolamine, phenylephrine, potassium acetate, potassium chloride, potassium phosphates, procainamide, prochlorperazine, promethazine, propranolol, remifentanil, rituximab, rocuronium, sodium acetate, sodium bicarbonate, sodium phosphates, succinylcholine, sufentanil, tacrolimus, theophylline, thiotepa, tigecycline, tirofiban, tobramycin, trimethoprim/sulfamethoxazole, vancomycin, vasopressin, vecuronium, verapamil, vinblastine, vinorelbine, voriconazole, zidovudine, zoledronic acid.

- **Y-Site Incompatibility:** acyclovir, allopurinol, amphotericin B liposomal, cefepime, cefotaxime, ceftriaxone, chloramphenicol, chlorpromazine, dantrolene, dexmedetomidine, diazepam, droperidol, fluorouracil, fosphenytoin, furosemide, ganciclovir, gemcitabine, glycopyrrolate, methohexital, methylprednisolone, mitomycin, nafcillin, nitroprusside, pemetrexed, phenytoin, piperacillin/tazobactam, trastuzumab.

Patient/Family Teaching

- Explain purpose and side effects of medication to patient. Advise patient to read *Patient Information* before starting therapy.
- Advise patient to notify health care provider of all Rx or OTC medications, vitamins, or herbal products being taken and to consult health care provider before taking other medications.
- Instruct patient to report occurrence of diarrhea to health care provider immediately if diarrhea occurs for 1st time during treatment; black or bloody stools; symptoms of dehydration such as light-headedness, dizziness, or faintness; inability to take fluids by mouth due to nausea or vomiting; or inability to get diarrhea under control within 24 hr. Diarrhea may be accompanied by severe dehydration and electrolyte imbalance. It may be life-threatening; treat promptly. Loperamide may be used for treatment up to 48 hr.
- Instruct patient to monitor their temperature and to notify health care provider promptly if fever; chills; sore throat; signs of infection; bleeding gums; bruising; petechiae; or blood in urine, stool, or emesis occurs. Caution patient to avoid crowds and persons with known infections. Instruct patient to monitor temperature frequently and use soft toothbrush and electric razor. Caution patient not to drink alcoholic beverages or take products containing aspirin or other NSAIDs.
- Instruct patient to notify nurse of pain at injection site immediately.
- Instruct patient to notify health care provider if vomiting, fainting, or dizziness occurs.
- Discuss with patient possibility of hair loss. Explore methods of coping.
- Instruct patient not to receive any vaccinations without consulting health care provider.
- Rep: May cause fetal harm. Advise women of reproductive potential to notify health care provider if pregnancy is planned or suspected, to use highly effective contraception during and for 6 mo after last dose of therapy, and to avoid breastfeeding during therapy and for 7 days after final dose. Advise men with female partners of reproductive potential to use condoms during and for 3 mo after last dose. May impair female and male infertility.

Evaluation/Desired Outcomes

- Death of rapidly replicating cells, particularly malignant ones.

iron sucrose (eye-ern su-krose)

Venofer

Classification

Therapeutic: antianemics

Pharmacologic: iron supplements

Indications

Iron deficiency anemia in chronic kidney disease.

Action

Enters the bloodstream and is transported to the organs of the reticuloendothelial system (liver, spleen, bone marrow), where it becomes separated from the sucrose complex and becomes part of iron stores. **Therapeutic Effects:** Resolution of iron deficiency anemia associated with chronic kidney disease.

Pharmacokinetics

Absorption: Following IV administration, the uptake of iron by the reticuloendothelial system is constant at about 40–60 mg/hr. Following IM doses, 60% is absorbed after 3 days and 90% after 1–3 wk; the balance is absorbed slowly over months.

Distribution: Taken up by the reticuloendothelial system.

Metabolism and Excretion: Most sucrose is eliminated in urine. Most of the iron remains stored and used on demand. Small amounts eliminated in urine.

Half-life: 6 hr.

TIME/ACTION PROFILE (effects on erythropoiesis)

ROUTE	ONSET	PEAK	DURATION
IV	days	1–2 wk	Weeks to months

Contraindications/Precautions

Contraindicated in: Anemia not due to iron deficiency; Hemochromatosis, hemosiderosis, or other evidence of iron overload; Hypersensitivity to iron sucrose.

Use Cautiously in: Any evidence of tissue iron overload; OB: Severe hypersensitivity reactions may occur that can lead to bradycardia in fetus, especially during 2nd and 3rd trimesters; safety not established during 1st trimester; Lactation: Use during breastfeeding only if potential maternal benefit justifies potential risk to infant; Pedi: Children <2 yr (safety and effectiveness not established).

Adverse Reactions/Side Effects

CV: chest pain, HF, hypertension, hypotension. **Derm:** pruritus. **F and E:** hypervolemia. **GI:** diarrhea, nausea, vomiting, ↑ liver enzymes, abdominal pain. **Local:** injection site reactions. **MS:** leg cramps, musculoskeletal pain. **Neuro:** headache, dizziness, dysgeusia, weakness. **Resp:** cough, dyspnea. **Misc:** fever, HYPERSENSITIVITY REACTIONS (INCLUDING ANAPHYLAXIS), sepsis.

Interactions

Drug-Drug: Chloramphenicol and **vitamin E** may ↓ hematologic response to iron therapy.

Route/Dosage

IV (Adults): *Hemodialysis dependent patients:* 100 mg during each dialysis session for 10 doses (total of 1000 mg); may repeat if iron deficiency recurs; *Non-dialysis-dependent patients:* 200 mg on 5 different days within a 14-day period to a total of 1000 mg; may also be given as infusion of 500 mg on day 1 and day 14; may repeat if iron deficiency recurs; *Peritoneal dialysis patients:* Administered in a total cumulative dose of 1000 mg in 3 divided doses, 14 days apart within a 28-day period with first 2 doses of 300 mg and third dose of 400 mg; may repeat if iron deficiency recurs.

IV (Children ≥2 yr): *Hemodialysis dependent patients (for iron maintenance therapy):* 0.5 mg/kg (max = 100 mg/dose) every 2 wk for 12 wk; may repeat if necessary; *Non-dialysis-dependent patients or peritoneal dialysis patients who are receiving erythropoietin for iron maintenance therapy:* 0.5 mg/kg (max = 100 mg/dose) every 4 wk for 12 wk; may repeat if necessary.

Availability

Solution for injection: 20 mg/mL.

NURSING IMPLICATIONS

Assessment

- Assess for hypersensitivity reactions and anaphylaxis (rash, dyspnea, loss of consciousness, hypotension, collapse, convulsions) for ≥30 min after injection. Resuscitation medication and equipment should be readily available.
- Monitor for hypotension and other symptoms related to rapid infusion (headache, vomiting, nausea, dizziness, arthralgia, paresthesia, abdominal pain, edema, cardiovascular shock). *If symptoms occur,* ↓ infusion rate and administer IV fluids, corticosteroids, and/or antihistamines.

Lab Test Considerations

- Monitor hemoglobin, hematocrit, serum ferritin, and transferrin saturation before and periodically during therapy. Transferrin saturation values ↑ rapidly after administration; therefore, serum iron values may be reliably obtained 48 hr after administration. *If iron overload occurs,* hold therapy.
- May ↑ AST and ALT.

Implementation

- Do not confuse Venofer with Vfend or Vimpat.
- Do not administer iron sucrose concurrently with oral iron; will ↓ oral iron absorption.
- Solution is brown. Do not administer if discolored or contains particulates. Stable for 7 days at room temperature or refrigerated in syringe.
- Pedi: Exercise caution when calculating and administering dose; overdose can be fatal.

IV Administration

Hemodialysis-Dependent Patient

- **IV Push:** Administer undiluted. **Rate:** Administer 100 mg over 2–5 min into dialysis line within the 1st hr of dialysis session, not to exceed one vial per injection. Discard any unused portion.
- **Intermittent Infusion: Dilution:** Dilute 100 mg iron sucrose in ≤100 mL of 0.9% NaCl. **Rate:** Infuse over ≥15 min.

Non-Dialysis-Dependent Patients

- **IV Push:** Administer undiluted. **Rate:** Administer 200 mg over 2–5 min.
- **Intermittent Infusion:** Dilute 200 mg in 100 mL of 0.9% NaCl or 500 mg in 250 mL of 0.9% NaCl. **Rate:** Infuse 200 mg over 15 min. Infuse 500 mg over 3.5–4 hr on days 1 and 14.

Peritoneal Dialysis Patients

- **Intermittent Infusion: Dilution:** Dilute each dose in ≤250 mL of 0.9% NaCl. **Rate:** Infuse 300 mg over 1.5 hr or 400 mg over 2.5 hr.

Pediatric Patients

- **IV Push:** Administer undiluted. **Rate:** Administer 0.5 mg/kg, not to exceed 100 mg, over 5 min.
- **Intermittent Infusion:** Dilute in 0.9% NaCl. **Concentration:** 1–2 mg/mL. **Rate:** Infuse over 5–60 min.
- **Y-Site Incompatibility:** cefiderocol, dopamine, tacrolimus.

Patient/Family Teaching

- Explain purpose and side effects of medication. Advise patient to read *Patient Information* before starting therapy.

- Instruct patient to report symptoms of hypersensitivity reaction to health care provider immediately.
- Rep: Advise women of reproductive potential to notify health care provider if pregnancy is planned or suspected or if breastfeeding. Maternal hypersensitivity reactions following use of parenteral iron may result in fetal bradycardia, especially during the 2nd and 3rd trimesters. Monitor breastfed infants for GI toxicity (constipation, diarrhea).

Evaluation/Desired Outcomes

- Improvement in anemia of chronic kidney disease.

isavuconazonium

(eye-sa-vue-kon-a-**zoe**-nee-um)

Cresemba

Classification

Therapeutic: antifungals

Pharmacologic: azoles

Indications

Invasive aspergillosis. Mucormycosis.

Action

A prodrug that is converted (rapidly hydrolyzed) to isavuconazole. Inhibits the synthesis of ergosterol, a key component of fungal cell walls. **Therapeutic Effects:** Resolution of invasive fungal infections. **Spectrum:** Active against *Aspergillus flavus*, *Aspergillus fumigatus*, *Aspergillus niger*, and Mucormycetes species, including *Rhizopus oryzae*.

Pharmacokinetics

Absorption: Prodrug is rapidly converted to isavuconazole, the active component. 98% absorbed following oral administration. IV administration results in complete bioavailability.

Distribution: Extensively distributed.

Protein Binding: >99%

Metabolism and Excretion: Extensively metabolized by liver by the CYP3A4 and CYP3A5 isoenzymes; inactive metabolites are mostly renally eliminated. <1% excreted unchanged in urine.

Half-life: 130 hr

TIME/ACTION PROFILE (plasma concentrations)

ROUTE	ONSET	PEAK	DURATION
PO	unknown	2 hr	unknown
IV	unknown	end of infusion	unknown

Contraindications/Precautions

Contraindicated in: Hypersensitivity; Strong CYP3A4 inhibitors; Familial short QT syndrome; Strong CYP3A4 inducers; OB: Pregnancy; Lactation: Lactation.

Use Cautiously in: Severe hepatic impairment (use only if benefits outweigh risks; monitor carefully for adverse reactions); Rep: Women of reproductive potential; Pedi: Safety and effectiveness not established in children <1 yr (IV) or <6 yr and <16 kg (PO).

Adverse Reactions/Side Effects

CV: peripheral edema, chest pain, hypotension. **Derm:** pruritus, rash, STEVENS-JOHNSON SYNDROME (SJS). **F and E:** hypokalemia, hypomagnesemia. **GI:** ↑ liver enzymes, constipation, diarrhea, nausea, vomiting, ↓ appetite, dyspepsia. **GU:** renal failure. **Local:** injection site reactions. **MS:** back pain. **Neuro:** fatigue, headache, insomnia, anxiety, delirium. **Resp:** cough, dyspnea, respiratory failure. **Misc:** HYPERSENSITIVITY REACTIONS (INCLUDING ANAPHYLAXIS), infusion-related reactions.

Interactions

Drug-Drug: Strong CYP3A4 inhibitors, including **ketoconazole** or high-dose **ritonavir**, ↑ levels and risk of toxicity; concurrent use contraindicated. **Strong CYP3A4 inducers**, including long-acting **barbiturates**, **carbamazepine**, or **rifampin**, may ↓ levels and effectiveness; concurrent use contraindicated. **Lopinavir/ritonavir** significantly ↑ levels and risk of toxicity; concurrent use should be undertaken with caution. Isavuconazonium ↓ levels and effectiveness of **lopinavir/ritonavir**. Isavuconazonium ↑ levels and risk of toxicity of **atorvastatin**, **cyclosporine**, **digoxin**, **midazolam**, **mycophenolate**, **sirolimus**, and **tacrolimus**; undertake concurrent use with caution, monitoring drug effects and making adjustments if necessary. ↓ levels and effectiveness of **bupropion**; bupropion dose may need to be ↑ but should not exceed maximum recommended dose.

Drug-Natural Products: St. John's wort ↓ levels and effectiveness; concurrent use contraindicated.

Route/Dosage

PO, IV (Adults≥18 yr): *Loading dose:* 372 mg isavuconazonium (PO as either two 186 mg capsules or five 74.5 mg capsules; equivalent to 200 mg isavuconazole) every 8 hr for six doses; *Maintenance dose:* 372 mg isavuconazonium (PO as either two 186 mg capsules or five 74.5 mg capsules; equivalent to 200 mg isavuconazole) once daily starting 12–24 hr after last loading dose.

IV (Children 3–<18 yr and ≥37 kg): *Loading dose:* 372 mg isavuconazonium (equivalent to 200 mg isavuconazole) every 8 hr for six doses; *Maintenance dose:* 372 mg isavuconazonium (equivalent to 200 mg isavuconazole) once daily starting 12–24 hr after last loading dose.

IV (Children 3–<18 yr and <37 kg): *Loading dose:* 10 mg/kg isavuconazonium every 8 hr for six doses; *Maintenance dose:* 10 mg/kg

isavuconazonium once daily starting 12–24 hr after last loading dose.
IV (Children 1–<3 yr and <18 kg): *Loading dose:* 15 mg/kg isavuconazonium every 8 hr for six doses; *Maintenance dose:* 15 mg/kg isavuconazonium once daily starting 12–24 hr after last loading dose.
PO (Children 6–<18 yr and ≥32 kg): *Loading dose:* 372 mg isavuconazonium (five 74.5 mg capsules; equivalent to 200 mg isavuconazole) every 8 hr for six doses; *Maintenance dose:* 372 mg isavuconazonium (five 74.5 mg capsules; equivalent to 200 mg isavuconazole) once daily starting 12–24 hr after last loading dose.
PO (Children 6–<18 yr and 25–<32 kg): *Loading dose:* 298 mg isavuconazonium (four 74.5 mg capsules; equivalent to 160 mg isavuconazole) every 8 hr for six doses; *Maintenance dose:* 298 mg isavuconazonium (four 74.5 mg capsules; equivalent to 160 mg isavuconazole) once daily starting 12–24 hr after last loading dose.
PO (Children 6–<18 yr and 18–<25 kg): *Loading dose:* 223.5 mg isavuconazonium (three 74.5 mg capsules; equivalent to 120 mg isavuconazole) every 8 hr for six doses; *Maintenance dose:* 223.5 mg isavuconazonium (three 74.5 mg capsules; equivalent to 120 mg isavuconazole) once daily starting 12–24 hr after last loading dose.
PO (Children 6–<18 yr and 16–<18 kg): *Loading dose:* 149 mg isavuconazonium (two 74.5 mg capsules; equivalent to 80 mg isavuconazole) every 8 hr for six doses; *Maintenance dose:* 149 mg isavuconazonium (two 74.5 mg capsules; equivalent to 80 mg isavuconazole) once daily starting 12–24 hr after last loading dose.

Availability

Capsules: 74.5 mg isavuconazonium (equivalent to 40 mg isavuconazole), 186 mg isavuconazonium (equivalent to 100 mg isavuconazole). **Lyophilized powder for injection:** 372 mg isavuconazonium (equivalent to 200 mg isavuconazole)/vial.

NURSING IMPLICATIONS

Assessment

- Monitor signs and symptoms of infection (fever, cough) periodically during therapy.
- Obtain specimens for culture and sensitivity prior to therapy. First dose may be given before receiving results.
- Monitor for signs and symptoms of infusion-related reactions (hypotension, dyspnea, chills, dizziness, paresthesia, hypoesthesia) periodically during therapy. Discontinue infusion if symptoms occur.
- Monitor skin for hypersensitivity reactions during therapy such as SJS.

Lab Test Considerations

- Verify negative pregnancy test before starting therapy.
- Monitor LFTs, BUN, serum creatinine, and electrolytes at baseline and periodically during therapy. If severe hepatic impairment occurs, discontinue therapy.

Implementation

- Oral and IV formulations are bioequivalent; may be used interchangeably. Loading dose is not needed when switching.
- **PO:** Administer without regard to food. ***DNC:*** Swallow capsule whole; do not open, dissolve, crush, or chew.
- To administer via NG tube, reconstitute one vial isavuconazonium for injection (equivalent to 200 mg isavuconazonium) with 5 mL of water for injection. Withdraw the entire contents (5 mL) of vial using a syringe and needle. Discard the needle and cap the syringe. To administer, remove cap from syringe containing the reconstituted solution and connect the syringe to NG tube to deliver dose. After administering, administer three 5 mL rinses to NG tube with water. Administer reconstituted solution via NG tube within 1 hr of reconstitution. Do not administer capsules via NG tube.

IV Administration

- **Reconstitution:** Reconstitute by adding 5 mL sterile water to vial. Shake gently to dissolve powder completely. Solution should be clear and colorless; do not administer solutions that are discolored or contain particulate matter. Solution is stable for 1 hr at room temperature.
- **Intermittent Infusion: Dilution:** Remove 5 mL of reconstituted solution from vial and add to 250 mL 0.9% NaCl or D5W. **Concentration:** ≤1.5 mg isavuconazonium/mL. Diluted solution may show visible translucent to white particulates; removed with in-line filter. Roll bag to mix gently; avoid shaking. Solution is stable if infused at room temperature within 6 hr; may refrigerate for up to 24 hr; do not freeze. Flush line with 0.9% NaCl or D5W prior to and following infusion.
- **Rate:** Infuse over at least 1 hr to minimize infusion-related reactions. Infuse through a 0.2–1.2 micron in-line filter. Do not administer as a bolus injection.
- **Y-Site Compatibility:** amikacin, amiodarone, anidulafungin, aztreonam, calcium chloride, calcium gluconate, caspofungin, ceftolozane/tazobactam, ciprofloxacin, cisatracurium, daptomycin, dexamethasone, dexmedetomidine, digoxin, diltiazem, diphenhydramine, dobutamine,

I

dopamine, doxycycline, epinephrine, eptifibatide, esmolol, famotidine, fentanyl, gentamicin, hydrocortisone, hydromorphone, imipenem/cilastatin, insulin regular, labetalol, levofloxacin, lidocaine, linezolid, lorazepam, magnesium sulfate, mannitol, meperidine, mesna, metoclopramide, midazolam, milrinone, morphine, mycophenolate, naloxone, nicardipine, nitroglycerin, nitroprusside, norepinephrine, octreotide, ondansetron, pantoprazole, phenylephrine, plazomicin, potassium chloride, rocuronium, sulbactam/durlobactam, tacrolimus, tigecycline, tobramycin, vancomycin, vasopressin, vecuronium.

- **Y-Site Incompatibility:** albumin, human, amphotericin B deoxycholate, amphotericin B liposome, ampicillin/sulbactam, cefazolin, cefepime, ceftaroline, ceftazidime, ceftriaxone, cefuroxime, cyclosporine, ertapenem, esomeprazole, filgrastim, fosphenytoin, furosemide, heparin, meropenem, meropenem/vaborbactam, methylprednisolone, micafungin, phenytoin, potassium phosphate, propofol, sodium bicarbonate, sodium phosphates, tedizolid.

Patient/Family Teaching

- Explain purpose and side effects of isavuconazonium to patient. Instruct patient to take isavuconazonium as directed. Do not stop taking isavuconazonium without consulting heath care professional. If missed dose, take as soon as remembered or resume regular dose if almost time; do not take extra dose. Advise patient to read *Patient Information* before starting and with each Rx refill in case of changes.
- Advise patient to notify health care professional promptly of signs and symptoms of liver disease (itchy skin, nausea, vomiting, yellowing of eyes, dark urine, feeling very tired, stomach pain), infusion-related reactions (flu-like symptoms, dizziness, numb/tingling skin), or hypersensitivity reactions (blistering, peeling, red skin rash) occur.
- Instruct patient to notify health care professional of all Rx or OTC medications, vitamins, or herbal products being taken and consult health care professional before taking any new medications.
- Rep: May cause fetal harm. Advise females of reproductive potential to use effective contraception during therapy and for 28 days after final dose and to avoid breastfeeding during therapy. Advise patient to notify health care professional if pregnancy is planned or suspected.
- Emphasize the importance of lab tests to monitor for side effects during therapy.

Evaluation/Desired Outcomes

- Resolution of signs and symptoms of invasive aspergillosis.
- Resolution of signs and symptoms of mucormycosis.

☒ isoniazid (eye-soe-**nye**-a-zid)

Classification
Therapeutic: antituberculars

Indications
First-line therapy of active tuberculosis (TB) (in combination with other agents). Prevention of TB in patients exposed to active disease (as monotherapy).

Action
Inhibits mycobacterial cell wall synthesis and interferes with metabolism. **Therapeutic Effects:** Bacteriostatic or bactericidal action against susceptible mycobacteria.

Pharmacokinetics
Absorption: Well absorbed following PO/IM administration.
Distribution: Widely distributed; readily crosses the blood-brain barrier.
Metabolism and Excretion: 50% metabolized by the liver by N-acetyltransferase ☒ (rate of acetylation is genetically determined [slow acetylators have ↑ isoniazid levels and ↑ risk of toxicity; fast acetylators have ↓ isoniazid levels and ↑ risk for treatment failure]); 50% excreted unchanged by the kidneys.
Half-life: 1–4 hr in patients with normal renal and hepatic function; ☒ 0.5–1.6 hr in fast acetylators; 2–5 hr in slow acetylators.

TIME/ACTION PROFILE (plasma concentrations)

ROUTE	ONSET	PEAK	DURATION
PO	rapid	1–2 hr	up to 24 hr
IM	rapid	1–2 hr	up to 24 hr

Contraindications/Precautions
Contraindicated in: Hypersensitivity; Acute liver disease; History of hepatitis from previous use.
Use Cautiously in: History of liver damage, chronic alcohol ingestion, or use of illicit injectable drugs; Black and Hispanic women, women in the postpartum period, or patients >50 yr (↑ risk of drug-induced hepatitis); Severe renal impairment (dose ↓ may be necessary); Malnourished patients, patients with diabetes, or chronic alcoholics (↑ risk of neuropathy).

Adverse Reactions/Side Effects
Derm: ACUTE GENERALIZED EXANTHEMATOUS PUSTULOSIS, DRUG REACTION WITH EOSINOPHILIA AND SYSTEMIC SYMPTOMS (DRESS), rash, STEVENS-JOHNSON SYNDROME, TOXIC EPIDERMAL NECROLYSIS. **EENT:** visual disturbances. **Endo:** gynecomastia. **GI:** HEPATOTOXICITY, nausea, vomiting. **Hemat:** blood dyscrasias. **Neuro:** peripheral neuropathy, cerebellar syndrome, psychosis, seizures. **Misc:** fever.

Interactions

Drug-Drug: Additive CNS toxicity with other **antituberculars**. **BCG vaccine** may not be effective during isoniazid therapy. Isoniazid may ↑ levels and risk of toxicity of **phenytoin**. **Aluminum-containing antacids** may ↓ absorption. Psychotic reactions and coordination difficulties may result with **disulfiram**. Concurrent administration of **pyridoxine** may prevent neuropathy.

↑ risk of hepatotoxicity with other **hepatotoxic agents**, including **alcohol**, **acetaminophen**, and **rifampin**. Isoniazid may ↓ levels and effectiveness of **ketoconazole**. May ↑ **carbamazepine** levels and risk of hepatotoxicity. May ↓ effectiveness of **clopidogrel**; avoid concurrent use.

Drug-Food: Severe reactions may occur with ingestion of foods containing high concentrations of **tyramine** (see Appendix J).

Route/Dosage

PO, IM (Adults): 5 mg/kg/day (max dose = 300 mg once daily) *or* 15 mg/kg (max dose = 900 mg) 2–3 times weekly.

PO, IM (Children <40 kg): *Latent TB infection:* 10–20 mg/kg/day (max dose = 300 mg once daily) *or* 20–40 mg/kg (max dose = 900 mg) 2 times weekly; *Active TB infection:* 10–15 mg/kg/day (max dose = 300 mg once daily) *or* 20–40 mg/kg (max dose = 900 mg) 2 times weekly.

Availability (generic available)

Tablets: 100 mg, 300 mg. **Oral solution (orange, raspberry flavor):** 50 mg/5 mL. **Solution for injection:** 100 mg/mL.

NURSING IMPLICATIONS
Assessment

- Monitor for signs and symptoms of hypersensitivity reaction (fever, rash) including severe skin eruptions (morbilliform, maculopapular, purpuric, exfoliative).
- Monitor for signs and symptoms of DRESS (fever, rash, lymphadenopathy, angioedema, hepatitis, nephritis, hematologic abnormalities, myocarditis, myositis) during therapy. *If symptoms occur,* discontinue isoniazid.
- Assess for neurotoxicity (peripheral neuropathy, seizures, encephalopathy, optic neuritis, memory loss, psychosis) during therapy.

Lab Test Considerations

- ☒ Mycobacterial studies and susceptibility tests should be performed prior to and periodically during therapy to detect possible resistance. About 50–65% of White, Black, South Indian, and Mexican patients are slow acetylators at risk for toxicity,

while 80–90% of Inuit, Japanese, and Chinese patients are rapid acetylators at risk for ↓ levels and treatment failure.

- ☒ Monitor hepatic function prior to therapy, monthly throughout, and as indicated. *If AST, ALT, or serum bilirubin >3–5 times upper limit of normal or if signs/symptoms of hepatotoxicity occur,* hold and consider alternate drug. If isoniazid must be used, resume only after symptoms and lab values have returned to baseline. Restart in small, gradually ↑ doses and discontinue immediately if liver toxicity recurs. Black, Hispanic, pregnant, and postpartal women and patients ≥35 yr are at highest risk. Isoniazid-associated hepatotoxicity usually occurs during 1st 3 mo of treatment.
- May cause agranulocytosis, anemia, thrombocytopenia, and eosinophilia.
- May ↓ vitamin B$_6$ and vitamin B$_3$.
- May cause hyperglycemia and metabolic acidosis.

Toxicity and Overdose

- If isoniazid overdose occurs, treat with pyridoxine and other supportive measures as indicated.

Implementation

- **PO:** Administer on an empty stomach.
- **IM** Medication may cause discomfort at injection site. Massage site after administration and rotate injection sites.
- Solution may form crystals at low temperatures; crystals will redissolve upon warming to room temperature.

Patient/Family Teaching

- Explain purpose and side effects of medication. Advise patient to read *Patient Information* before starting therapy.
- Advise patient to take missed doses as soon as possible unless almost time for next dose; do not double doses. Emphasize the importance of continuing therapy even after symptoms have subsided. Therapy may be continued for 6 mo–2 yr.
- Advise patient to notify health care provider of all Rx or OTC medications, vitamins, or herbal products being taken and to consult health care provider before taking other medications.
- Advise patient to notify health care provider immediately if signs and symptoms of hepatotoxicity (yellow eyes and skin, nausea, vomiting, abdominal tenderness, anorexia, dark urine, rash, fatigue, weakness, or fever >3 days) occur.
- Advise patient to notify health care provider immediately if signs and symptoms of peripheral neuritis (numbness, tingling, paresthesia) or visual changes (pain, blurred vision, ↓ acuity) occur. Pyridoxine may be used concurrently to prevent neuropathy.

☀ = Canadian drug name. ☒ = Genetic implication. **V** = Vesicant. Boxed warning. ~~Strikethrough~~ = Discontinued. *CAPITALS = life-threatening. Underline = most frequent.

- Caution patient to avoid the use of alcohol during therapy, as this may ↑ risk of hepatotoxicity. Avoid ingestion of Swiss or Cheshire cheeses, fish (tuna, skipjack, sardines), and tyramine-containing foods (see Appendix J).
- Rep: Caution pregnant patient that isoniazid may ↑ risk of peripheral neurotoxicity and pyridoxine supplementation is recommended. Advise patient to notify health care provider and discontinue breastfeeding if jaundice occurs in the breastfed infant. Pyridoxine supplementation is recommended for breastfed infants.
- Emphasize the importance of regular follow-up including laboratory tests, and physical and ophthalmic exams.

Evaluation/Desired Outcomes

- Resolution of signs and symptoms of TB.
- Negative sputum culture.
- Prevention of activation of TB in persons known to have been exposed.

ISOSORBIDE

isosorbide dinitrate
(eye-soe-**sor**-bide dye-**nye**-trate)
~~Dilatrate-SR~~, Isordil

isosorbide mononitrate
(eye-soe-**sor**-bide mo-noe-**nye**-trate) ✦
~~Imdur~~, ✦ Imdur, ~~Ismo~~

Classification
Therapeutic: antianginals
Pharmacologic: nitrates

Indications

Prophylactic management of angina pectoris. **Unlabeled Use:** Chronic HF (unlabeled).

Action

Produce vasodilation (venous greater than arterial). Decrease left ventricular end-diastolic pressure and left ventricular end-diastolic volume (preload). Net effect is reduced myocardial oxygen consumption. Increase coronary blood flow by dilating coronary arteries and improving collateral flow to ischemic regions. **Therapeutic Effects:** Prevention of anginal attacks.

Pharmacokinetics

Absorption: Isosorbide dinitrate undergoes extensive first-pass metabolism by the liver, resulting in 25% bioavailability; isosorbide mononitrate has 100% bioavailability (does not undergo first-pass metabolism).
Distribution: Unknown.
Metabolism and Excretion: Isosorbide dinitrate is metabolized by the liver to 2 active metabolites (5-mononitrate and 2-mononitrate). Isosorbide mononitrate is primarily metabolized by the liver to inactive metabolites; primarily excreted in urine as metabolites.
Half-life: *Isosorbide dinitrate:* 1 hr; *isosorbide mononitrate:* 5 hr.

TIME/ACTION PROFILE (cardiovascular effects)

ROUTE	ONSET	PEAK	DURATION
ISDN-PO	45–60 min	unknown	4 hr
ISMN-ER	unknown	unknown	12 hr

Contraindications/Precautions

Contraindicated in: Hypersensitivity; Concurrent use of PDE-5 inhibitor or riociguat.
Use Cautiously in: Volume-depleted patients; Right ventricular infarction; Hypertrophic cardiomyopathy; OB: Safety not established in pregnancy; Lactation: Safety not established in breastfeeding; Pedi: Safety and effectiveness not established in children; Geri: Initial dose ↓ required in older adults due to ↑ potential for hypotension.

Adverse Reactions/Side Effects

CV: hypotension, tachycardia, paradoxic bradycardia, syncope. **Derm:** flushing. **GI:** nausea, vomiting. **Neuro:** dizziness, headache. **Misc:** tolerance.

Interactions

Drug-Drug: **Avanafil**, **sildenafil**, **tadalafil**, or **vardenafil** may result in severe hypotension (do not use within 24 hr of isosorbide dinitrate or mononitrate); concurrent use contraindicated. **Riociguat** may result in severe hypotension; concurrent use contraindicated. Additive hypotension with **antihypertensives**, acute ingestion of **alcohol**, **beta blockers**, **calcium channel blockers**, and **phenothiazines**.

Route/Dosage

Isosorbide Dinitrate

PO (Adults): *Prophylaxis of angina pectoris:* 5–20 mg 2–3 times daily; usual maintenance dose is 10–40 mg every 6 hr.

Isosorbide Mononitrate

PO (Adults): 30–60 mg once daily; may ↑ to 120 mg once daily (maximum dose = 240 mg/day).

Availability

Isosorbide Dinitrate (generic available)

Tablets: 5 mg, 10 mg, 20 mg, 30 mg, 40 mg. ***In combination with:*** hydralazine (BiDil). See Appendix N.

Isosorbide Mononitrate (generic available)

Extended-release tablets: 30 mg, 60 mg, 120 mg.

NURSING IMPLICATIONS

Assessment

- Assess location, duration, intensity, and precipitating factors of anginal pain.
- Monitor BP and HR routinely during period of dose adjustment.

Lab Test Considerations

- Excessive doses may ↑ methemoglobin concentrations.

Implementation

Isosorbide Dinitrate

- **PO:** Do not administer around the clock to prevent tolerance to nitrate effect; allow nitrate-free interval for ≥14 hr. Twice-daily dosing may be administered at 8 AM and 2 PM and 3 times daily dosing may be given at 8 AM, 1 PM, and 6 PM.

Isosorbide Mononitrate

- **PO:** Do not administer around the clock. Administer extended-release tablet once daily in the morning upon rising with 4 ounces of fluid. ***DNC:*** Swallow extended-release tablets whole; do not break, crush, or chew. Extended-release tablets that are scored may be split.

Patient/Family Teaching

- Explain purpose and side effects of medication to patient. Advise patient to read *Patient Information* before starting therapy. Advise patient to take as directed, even if feeling better. Take missed doses as soon as remembered; doses of isosorbide dinitrate should be taken > 2 hr apart. Do not double doses. Do not discontinue abruptly.
- Advise patient to notify health care provider of all Rx or OTC medications, vitamins, or herbal products being taken and to consult with health care provider before taking other medications.
- Advise patient to take last dose of day (when taking 2–4 doses/day) no later than 7 pm to prevent the development of tolerance.
- Advise patient to make position changes slowly to minimize orthostatic hypotension.
- May cause dizziness. Advise patient to avoid driving or other activities requiring alertness until response to medication is known.
- Advise patient to avoid alcohol while taking this medication.
- Advise patient that headache is a common side effect that should ↓ with continuing therapy. Aspirin or acetaminophen may be ordered to treat headache. Notify health care provider if headache is persistent or severe. Do not alter dose to avoid headache.
- Advise patient to notify health care provider if dry mouth or blurred vision occurs.
- Rep: Advise women of reproductive potential to notify health care provider if pregnancy is planned or suspected or if breastfeeding.

Evaluation/Desired Outcomes

- Prevention of anginal attacks.

REMS

ISOtretinoin

(eye-soe-**tret**-i-noyn)

Absorica, Absorica LD, Accutane, Amnesteem, Claravis, ✱ Clarus, ✱ Epuris, ~~Myorisan~~, Zenatane

Classification

Therapeutic: antiacne agents

Pharmacologic: retinoids

Indications

Severe recalcitrant nodular acne in patients with multiple inflammatory nodules having a diameter of ≥5 mm and that are unresponsive to more conventional therapy, including systemic antibiotics.

Action

A metabolite of vitamin A (retinol) reduces sebaceous gland size and differentiation. **Therapeutic Effects:** Diminution and resolution of severe acne. May also prevent abnormal keratinization.

Pharmacokinetics

Absorption: Rapidly absorbed following (23–25%) oral administration (bioavailability of Absorica LD higher than that of Absorica); absorption ↑ when taken with a high-fat meal.

Distribution: Widely distributed to tissues.

Protein Binding: 99.9%.

Metabolism and Excretion: Metabolized by the liver and excreted in the urine and feces.

Half-life: 10–20 hr.

TIME/ACTION PROFILE (diminution of acne)

ROUTE	ONSET	PEAK	DURATION
PO	unknown	up to 8 wk	unknown

Contraindications/Precautions

Contraindicated in: Hypersensitivity to retinoids, glycerin, soybean oil, or parabens; Patients planning to donate blood; OB: Pregnancy; Lactation: Lactation.

Use Cautiously in: Pre-existing hypertriglyceridemia; Diabetes mellitus; History of alcohol abuse, psychosis, depression, or suicide attempt; Obese patients; Inflammatory bowel disease; Rep: Women of reproductive potential; Pedi: Children <12 yr (safety and effectiveness not established).

Adverse Reactions/Side Effects

CV: edema. **Derm:** pruritus, palmar desquamation, photosensitivity, skin infections, STEVENS-JOHNSON SYNDROME (SJS), thinning of hair, TOXIC EPIDERMAL NECROLYSIS (TEN). **EENT:** conjunctivitis, epistaxis, ↓ night vision, blurred vision, contact lens intolerance, corneal opacities, dry eyes. **Endo:** hyperglycemia. **F and E:** ↑ thirst. **GI:** cheilitis, dry mouth, nausea, vomiting, abdominal pain, anorexia, hepatitis, pancreatitis. **Hemat:** anemia. **Metab:** ↓ HDL-C, hypercholesterolemia, hypertriglyceridemia, ↑ appetite, hyperuricemia. **MS:** arthralgia, back pain, muscle/bone pain (↑ in adolescents), hyperostosis. **Neuro:** behavior changes, depression, PSEUDOTUMOR CEREBRI, psychosis, SUICIDAL THOUGHTS/BEHAVIORS.

Interactions

Drug-Drug: Additive toxicity with **vitamin A** and **drugs having anticholinergic properties**. ↑ risk of pseudotumor cerebri with **tetracycline** or **minocycline**. **Alcohol** ↑ risk of hypertriglyceridemia. Drying effects ↑ by concurrent use of **benzoyl peroxide, sulfur, tretinoin**, and **other topical agents**.
Drug-Food: Excessive ingestion of **foods high in vitamin A** may result in additive toxicity.

Route/Dosage

Absorica and Absorica LD are not interchangeable.
PO (Adults and Children ≥12 yr): 0.5–1 mg/kg/day (may use up to 2 mg/kg/day for very severe disease) in 2 divided doses for 15–20 wk. Once discontinued, if relapse occurs, therapy may be reinstituted after an 8-wk rest period. *Absorica LD:* 0.4–0.8 mg/kg/day (may use up to 1.6 mg/kg/day for very severe disease) in 2 divided doses for 15–20 wk. Once discontinued, if relapse occurs, therapy may be reinstituted after an 8-wk rest period.

Availability (generic available)

Capsules: 10 mg, 20 mg, 25 mg, 30 mg, 35 mg, 40 mg. **Capsules (Absorica LD):** 8 mg, 16 mg, 24 mg, 32 mg.

NURSING IMPLICATIONS

Assessment

- Assess skin prior to and periodically during therapy. Transient worsening of acne may occur at initiation. Note number and severity of cysts, degree of skin dryness, erythema, and itching.
- Assess for allergy to parabens; capsules contain parabens as a preservative.
- Monitor for behavioral changes (depression, psychosis, aggression, suicidal ideation). *If behavioral changes occur,* immediately discontinue isotretinoin and treat as indicated.
- Monitor for signs and symptoms of intracranial hypertension. *If signs of pseudotumor cerebri with papilledema occur,* immediately discontinue isotretinoin and refer to neurologist.
- Assess for rash periodically during therapy. May cause SJS or TEN. *If severe rash or rash associated with generalized symptoms occurs,* discontinue isotretinoin.

Lab Test Considerations

- Verify two negative sequential serum or urine pregnancy tests with a sensitivity ≥25 mIU/mL before receiving initial Rx and monthly before each new Rx.
- Monitor liver enzymes (AST, ALT, LDH) before starting therapy, after 1 mo of therapy, and periodically thereafter. *If hepatitis suspected,* discontinue isotretinoin.
- Monitor fasting serum cholesterol, HDL-C, and triglycerides before initiating therapy, at 1–2 wk intervals until lipid response is established, and periodically thereafter.
- Obtain baseline and periodic CBC, urinalysis, and metabolic panel. May ↑ blood glucose, CK, platelets, sedimentation rate, and uric acid. May ↓ RBC and WBC. May cause proteinuria, RBCs and WBCs in urine.

Implementation

- Do not confuse isotretinoin with tretinoin.
- ***REMS:*** Health care providers who prescribe and pharmacies who dispense isotretinoin must enroll in iPLEDGE REMS (www.ipledgeprogram.com, 1-866-495-0654), and patients must meet all requirements.
- **PO:** Administer without regard to food. Administer with a full glass of liquid to ↓ risk of esophageal irritation. ***DNC:*** Do not crush or open capsules.

Patient/Family Teaching

- ***REMS:*** Explain purpose and side effects of medication as well as *iPLEDGE REMS* and its requirements. The patient must read *Patient Information* and sign consent form prior to initiation of therapy.
- Advise patient to omit dose if missed and then resume as scheduled; do not double doses.
- Explain to patient that a temporary worsening of acne may occur at beginning of therapy.
- Advise patient and family to notify health care provider if rash, visual or hearing changes, headache, nausea or vomiting, or mood changes (suicidal ideation or attempt, depression, anxiety, agitation, restlessness, insomnia) occur.

- May cause sudden ↓ in night vision. Caution patient to avoid driving at night until response is known.
- Advise patient to consult with health care provider before using other acne preparations while taking isotretinoin.
- Advise patient to notify health care provider of all Rx or OTC medications, vitamins, or herbal products being taken and to consult with health care provider before taking other medications, especially St. John's wort.
- Instruct patient not to take vitamin A supplements and to avoid excessive ingestion of foods high in vitamin A (liver, fish liver oils, egg yolks, yellow-orange fruits and vegetables, dark green leafy vegetables, whole milk, vitamin A–fortified skim milk, butter, margarine) to avoid vitamin A toxicity.
- Advise patient to avoid alcoholic beverages during therapy, as this may further ↑ triglycerides.
- Inform patient that dry skin and chapped lips will occur. Lubricant to lips may help cheilitis.
- Instruct patient that oral rinses, good oral hygiene, and sugarless gum or candy may help minimize dry mouth and to notify health care provider if dry mouth persists >2 wk.
- Discuss possibility of excessively dry eyes with patients who wear contact lenses. Patient should contact health care provider about eye lubricant and may need to switch to glasses during and for up to 2 wk following therapy.
- Caution patient to use sunscreen and protective clothing to prevent photosensitivity reactions. Consult health care provider about sunscreen, as some sunscreens may worsen acne.
- Inform patients with diabetes that difficulty controlling blood glucose may occur.
- Instruct patient to report burning of eyes, abdominal pain, and diarrhea, to health care provider.
- Advise patient not to donate blood during and for ≥1 mo after therapy to prevent a pregnant patient from receiving the blood.
- Rep: May cause fetal harm. Instruct women of reproductive potential to use 2 forms of contraception 1 mo before, during, and for ≥1 mo after discontinuation of therapy. Advise that patient must have 2 negative pregnancy tests before initiating therapy. 1st test is when decision is made to prescribe isotretinoin; 2nd test is after 2 forms of contraception are used for 1 mo and during 1st 5 days of menstrual period immediately preceding beginning of therapy. For patients with amenorrhea, 2nd test should be done 11 days after last act of unprotected sexual intercourse. Pregnancy test must be repeated every month prior to receiving prescription. Patient should discontinue medication and inform health care provider immediately if pregnancy is suspected during or 1 mo after therapy. If pregnancy occurs, report immediately to the FDA via MedWatch (1-800-FDA-1088) and also to the iPLEDGE pregnancy registry (1-866-495-0654 or www.ipledgeprogram.com). Recommended consent form prepared by manufacturer stresses fetal risk. Parents of minors should also read and sign form. Yellow self-adhesive qualification stickers completed by prescriber must accompany prescription. Advise patient to avoid breastfeeding during and for ≥8 days after last dose.
- Inform patient of need for medical follow-up. Periodic lab tests may be required.

Evaluation/Desired Outcomes

- Decrease in the number and severity of cysts in severe acne. Therapy may take 4–5 mo before full effects are seen. Therapy is discontinued when the number of cysts is ↓ by 70% or after 5 mo. Improvement may occur after discontinuation of therapy; therefore, a delay of ≥8 wk is recommended before a second course of therapy is considered.

isradipine, See CALCIUM CHANNEL BLOCKERS.

ivabradine (eye-vab-ra-deen)

Corlanor, ✱ Lancora

Classification

Therapeutic: heart failure agents

Pharmacologic: hyperpolarization-activated cyclic nucleotide-gated channel blockers

Indications

To decrease the need for hospitalization due to worsening HF in patients with stable but symptomatic chronic HF (ejection fraction <35%, sinus rhythm ≥70 bpm, receiving highest tolerated doses of beta blockers or are unable to tolerate beta blockers). Stable symptomatic HF due to dilated cardiomyopathy in pediatric patients ≥6 mo old who are in sinus rhythm with an elevated heart rate.

Action

Inhibits the cardiac pacemaker I_f-current by acting as a hyperpolarization-activated cyclic nucleoside-gated channel blocker, resulting in ↓ spontaneous pacemaker activity of sinus node. Decreases heart rate without affecting contractility or ventricular repolarization. **Therapeutic Effects:** Lowering of heart rate with reduced need for hospitalization in patients with HF.

Pharmacokinetics

Absorption: 40% absorbed following oral administration (undergoes first-pass metabolism); food delays absorption and ↑ levels.
Distribution: Unknown.
Metabolism and Excretion: Extensively metabolized, primarily by the CYP3A4 enzyme system. The major metabolite is pharmacologically active and has the same potency as ivabradine. Metabolites excreted equally in urine and feces; 4% excreted unchanged in urine.
Half-life: 6 hr.

TIME/ACTION PROFILE (plasma concentrations)

ROUTE	ONSET	PEAK	DURATION
PO	unknown	1 hr	12 hr

Contraindications/Precautions

Contraindicated in: Acute decompensated HF; Clinically significant hypotension; Sick sinus syndrome, sinoatrial block, or 2nd- or 3rd-degree heart block (unless a functioning demand pacemaker is in place, ↑ risk of bradycardia); Clinically significant bradycardia; Severe hepatic impairment; Pacemaker dependence; Concurrent use of strong CYP3A4 inhibitors; OB: Pregnancy; Lactation: Lactation.
Use Cautiously in: Rep: Women of reproductive potential; Pedi: Children <6 mo (safety and effectiveness not established).

Adverse Reactions/Side Effects

CV: atrial fibrillation, bradycardia, heart block, hypertension, QT interval prolongation, sinus arrest, TORSADE DE POINTES. **EENT:** phosphenes (luminous phenomena).

Interactions

Drug-Drug: Strong CYP3A4 inhibitors, including **azole antifungals**, **macolides**, **protease inhibitors**, and **nefazodone**, may ↑ levels; concurrent use contraindicated. **Moderate CYP3A4 inhibitors**, including **diltiazem** and **verapamil**, may ↑ levels and risk of bradycardia; avoid concurrent use. **CYP3A4 inducers**, including **barbiturates**, **phenytoin**, and **rifampin**, may ↓ levels and effectiveness; avoid concurrent use. ↑ risk of bradycardia with **negative chronotropes**, including **amiodarone**, **beta blockers**, **digoxin**, and **clonidine**; monitor heart rate. **QT-interval prolonging drugs** may ↑ risk of QT interval prolongation and torsade de pointes.
Drug-Natural Products: St. John's wort may ↓ levels and effectiveness; avoid concurrent use.
Drug-Food: Grapefruit juice may ↑ levels and risk of toxicity; avoid concurrent use.

Route/Dosage

PO (Adults): 5 mg twice daily for 2 wk; dose may then be adjusted based on HR; not to exceed 7.5 mg twice daily; *Patients with conduction defects or bradycardia:* 2.5 mg twice daily initially.
PO (Children ≥6 mo and ≥40 kg): *Tablets:* 2.5 mg twice daily; adjust dose at 2-wk intervals by 2.5 mg twice daily to achieve HR ↓ of ≥20%; not to exceed 7.5 mg twice daily.
PO (Children ≥6 mo and <40 kg): *Oral solution:* 0.05 mg/kg twice daily; adjust dose at 2-wk intervals by 0.05 mg/kg twice daily to achieve a HR ↓ of ≥20%; not to exceed 0.2 mg/kg twice daily (6 mo–<1 yr) or 0.3 mg/kg twice daily (≥1 yr) up to max of 7.5 mg twice daily.

Availability (generic available)

Tablets: 5 mg, 7.5 mg. **Oral solution:** 1 mg/mL.

NURSING IMPLICATIONS

Assessment

- Assess HR before, after 2 wk, and periodically during therapy. Adjust dose for a resting HR of 50–60 bpm. *If HR >60 bpm,* ↑ dose by 2.5 mg twice daily, up to 7.5 mg twice daily. *If HR 50–60 bpm,* maintain dose. *If HR <50 bpm or signs and symptoms of bradycardia (dizziness, fatigue, hypotension) occur,* ↓ dose by 2.5 mg twice daily; if current dose is 2.5 mg given twice daily, discontinue ivabradine.
- Monitor ECG periodically during therapy. May cause atrial fibrillation and torsade de pointes. *If atrial fibrillation occurs,* discontinue ivabradine.

Implementation

- **PO:** Administer twice daily with meals.
- For oral solution, empty entire contents of ampule(s) into a medication cup. With a calibrated oral syringe, measure prescribed dose and administer orally. Discard unused oral solution; do not store or reuse. Solution is colorless.

Patient/Family Teaching

- Explain purpose and side effects of medication to patient. Advise patient to read *Patient Information* before starting therapy. Instruct patient to take as directed. If dose is missed or patient spits out drug, omit dose; do not double doses.
- Advise patient to notify health care provider of all Rx or OTC medications, vitamins, or herbal products being taken and to consult health care provider before taking other medications, especially St. John's wort.
- Advise patient to avoid taking grapefruit juice during therapy; may ↑ risk of side effects.
- Advise patient to notify health care provider if signs and symptoms of irregular or rapid heartbeat (heart pounding or racing, chest pressure, worsened shortness of breath, near fainting or fainting)

or slower than normal HR (dizziness, fatigue, lack of energy) occur. In young children, signs and symptoms of slow HR include poor feeding, difficulty breathing, and turning blue.

- Inform patient that ivabradine may cause phosphenes or luminous phenomena, a transiently enhanced brightness in a limited area of the visual field, halos, image decomposition, colored bright lights, or multiple images. Phosphenes are usually triggered by sudden variations in light intensity. Usually begin within 1st 2 mo of therapy; may occur repeatedly of mild to moderate intensity and resolve after therapy is discontinued.
- Rep: May cause fetal harm. Advise women of reproductive potential to use effective contraception during therapy and to avoid breastfeeding during therapy. Advise patient to notify health care provider immediately if pregnancy is suspected.

Evaluation/Desired Outcomes

- Lowering of heart rate with reduced need for hospitalization in patients with HF.

ixekizumab (ix-ee-**kiz**-ue-mab)

Taltz

Classification

Therapeutic: antipsoriatics

Pharmacologic: interleukin antagonists

Indications

Moderate to severe plaque psoriasis in patients who are candidates for systemic therapy or phototherapy. Active psoriatic arthritis (as monotherapy or in combination with a nonbiologic DMARD). Active ankylosing spondylitis. Active nonradiographic axial spondyloarthritis in patients with objective signs of inflammation.

Action

A monoclonal antibody that acts as an antagonist of interleukin (IL)-17A by selectively binding to it and preventing its interaction with the IL-17 receptor. Antagonism prevents the production of inflammatory cytokines and chemokines. **Therapeutic Effects:** Decreased plaque formation and spread in plaque psoriasis. Decreased pain and swelling with decreased joint destruction in psoriatic arthritis. Decreased disease activity in ankylosing spondylitis and nonradiographic axial spondyloarthritis.

Pharmacokinetics

Absorption: Well absorbed (60–81%) following SUBQ administration.

Distribution: Minimally distributed to tissues.

Metabolism and Excretion: Catabolized into small peptides and amino acids.

Half-life: 13 days.

TIME/ACTION PROFILE (plasma concentrations)

ROUTE	ONSET	PEAK	DURATION
SUBQ	unknown	4 days	unknown

Contraindications/Precautions

Contraindicated in: Hypersensitivity; Active tuberculosis.

Use Cautiously in: Inflammatory bowel disease (may lead to exacerbations); OB: Safety not established in pregnancy; Lactation: Use while breastfeeding only if potential maternal benefit justifies potential risk to infant; Pedi: Children <6 yr (safety and effectiveness not established).

Adverse Reactions/Side Effects

Derm: eczematous eruptions. **GI:** inflammatory bowel disease, nausea. **Hemat:** neutropenia, thrombocytopenia. **Local:** injection site reactions. **Misc:** INFECTION (INCLUDING REACTIVATION TUBERCULOSIS [TB]), HYPERSENSITIVITY REACTIONS (INCLUDING ANAPHYLAXIS, ANGIOEDEMA, AND URTICARIA).

Interactions

Drug-Drug: May ↓ antibody response to **live-virus vaccine** and ↑ risk of adverse reactions; do not administer concurrently.

Route/Dosage

Plaque Psoriasis

SUBQ (Adults): 160 mg (as two 80-mg injections) at Wk 0; then 80 mg at Wk 2, 4, 6, 8, 10, and 12; then 80 mg every 4 wk.

SUBQ (Children ≥6 yr and >50 kg): 160 mg (as two 80-mg injections) at Wk 0; then 80 mg every 4 wk.

SUBQ (Children ≥6 yr and 25–50 kg): 80 mg at Wk 0; then 40 mg every 4 wk.

SUBQ (Children ≥6 yr and <25 kg): 40 mg at Wk 0; then 20 mg every 4 wk.

Psoriatic Arthritis and Ankylosing Spondylitis

SUBQ (Adults): 160 mg (as two 80-mg injections) initially; then 80 mg every 4 wk.

Nonradiographic Axial Spondyloarthritis

SUBQ (Adults): 80 mg every 4 wk.

Availability

Solution for injection (prefilled autoinjectors): 80 mg/mL. **Solution for injection (prefilled syringes):** 20 mg/0.25 mL, 40 mg/0.5 mL, 80 mg/mL.

NURSING IMPLICATIONS

Assessment

- Assess for TB infection before starting therapy; do not administer to patient with active TB infection. Initiate treatment of latent TB before administering ixekizumab. In patient with previous history of TB in whom an adequate course cannot be confirmed, consider anti-TB therapy before starting ixekizumab.
- Monitor for signs and symptoms of infection (fever; sweats; chills; muscle aches; cough; dyspnea; blood in mucus; weight loss; warm, red, or painful skin or sores; diarrhea or stomach pain; burning or frequency of urination) before and periodically during therapy.
- Monitor for signs and symptoms of hypersensitivity (urticaria; feeling faint; swelling of face, eyelids, lips, mouth, tongue, or throat; dyspnea; throat tightness; chest tightness; rash) during therapy. If hypersensitivity reaction occurs, discontinue ixekizumab immediately and begin supportive therapy.
- Monitor for signs and symptoms of severe eczematous eruptions (dry, cracked, crusty, scaly, thickened, or blistered skin; red rash or red patches; pruritus). Discontinuation and/or hospitalization may be necessary.
- Monitor for onset or exacerbation of inflammatory bowel disease (abdominal pain, diarrhea with or without blood, weight loss) during therapy.

Lab Test Considerations

- May cause neutropenia and thrombocytopenia.

Implementation

- Complete all age-appropriate vaccinations as recommended by current immunization guidelines before starting therapy.
- Adult patients may self-inject, or caregivers may administer 80-mg injections; doses of 20 mg or 40 mg must be administered by a health care professional.
- **SUBQ**: Allow to reach room temperature (30 min) before injection; do not microwave, run under hot water, or leave in sunlight to warm. Solution is clear and colorless to slightly yellow; do not administer solutions that are cloudy, discolored, or contain a precipitate. Place *autoinjector* flat against skin at injection site before injecting. Avoid areas where skin is bruised, tender, erythematous, indurated, or affected by psoriasis. Rotate injection sites. Store in refrigerator in original box to protect from light; may be stored at room temperature for up to 5 days. Do not return to refrigerator once stored at room temperature. For *prefilled syringe*, pinch skin and inject into upper arm, thigh, or abdomen at a 45° angle; let go of skin pinch before injecting. Rotate injection sites. To prepare 20-mg or 40-mg doses, expel contents of 80-mg prefilled syringe into sterile vial and withdraw the prescribed dose using a 0.5 mL or 1 mL disposable syringe; do not shake or swirl the vial. Do not add other medications. Remove the needle from the syringe and replace it with a 27-gauge needle for administration. Prepared 20-mg or 40-mg doses may be stored at room temperature for up to 4 hr.
- Pedi: For children ≤50 kg, after withdrawing dose from vial, change to a 27-gauge needle for administration.

Patient/Family Teaching

- Explain the purpose and side effects of ixekizumab to patient. Instruct patient and caregiver in proper technique for self-injection and care and disposal of equipment. Administer missed doses as soon as possible and resume regular dosing schedule. Advise patient to read *Medication Guide and Instructions for Use* prior to starting therapy and with each Rx refill in case of changes.
- Advise patient to notify health care professional if signs and symptoms of allergic reaction, infection, or inflammatory bowel disease occur.
- Advise patient to avoid use of live vaccines during therapy.
- Instruct patient to notify health care professional of all Rx or OTC medications, vitamins, or herbal products being taken and consult health care professional before taking any new medications. May be used with conventional disease-modifying antirheumatic drugs, corticosteroids, NSAIDs, and/or analgesics.
- Rep: Advise female patients of reproductive potential to notify health care professional if pregnancy is planned or suspected, or if breastfeeding. There is a pregnancy exposure registry that monitors pregnancy outcomes in women exposed to ixekizumab during pregnancy. Pregnant women exposed to ixekizumab are encouraged to enroll in the pregnancy exposure registry that monitors pregnancy outcomes in women exposed to ixekizumab, by calling the *Taltz* Pregnancy Registry at 1-800-284-1695 or contacting the registry at https://www.taltz.com.

Evaluation/Desired Outcomes

- Decreased plaque formation and spread in patients with plaque psoriasis.
- Decreased pain and swelling with decreased joint destruction in psoriatic arthritis.
- Decreased disease activity in ankylosing spondylitis and nonradiographic axial spondyloarthritis.

HIGH ALERT

ketamine (ket-a-meen)

Ketalar

Classification

Therapeutic: general anesthetics

Indications

Induction and maintenance of general anesthesia. **Unlabeled Use:** Provides sedation, analgesia, and anxiolytic effects.

Action

Blocks afferent impulses of pain perception. Suppresses spinal cord activity. Affects CNS transmitter systems. **Therapeutic Effects:** Anesthesia with profound analgesia, minimal respiratory depression, and minimal skeletal muscle relaxation.

Pharmacokinetics

Absorption: Rapidly absorbed after IM administration. IV administration results in complete bioavailability.

Distribution: Rapidly distributed. Enters the CNS.

Metabolism and Excretion: Mostly metabolized by the liver. Some conversion to another active compound.

Half-life: 2.5 hr.

TIME/ACTION PROFILE (anesthesia)

ROUTE	ONSET	PEAK	DURATION
IV	30 sec	unknown	5–10 min
IM	3–4 min	unknown	12–25 min

Contraindications/Precautions

Contraindicated in: Hypersensitivity; Psychiatric disturbances; Uncontrolled hypertension; ↑ intracranial pressure; OB: May affect child's brain development when used during 3rd trimester; Lactation: Lactation.

Use Cautiously in: Cardiovascular disease; Procedures involving larynx, pharynx, or bronchial tree (muscle relaxants required); Gastroesophageal reflux; History of alcohol abuse; Cerebral trauma; Intracerebral mass or hemorrhage; Hyperthyroidism; History of psychiatric problems; ↑ intraocular pressure; Severe eye trauma; Hepatic impairment; Pedi: Children <3 yr (may affect brain development).

Adverse Reactions/Side Effects

CV: hypertension, tachycardia, arrhythmias, bradycardia, hypotension. **Derm:** erythema, rash. **EENT:** ↑ intraocular pressure, diplopia, nystagmus. **GI:** excessive salivation, hepatotoxicity, nausea, vomiting. **GU:** cystitis. **Local:** pain at injection site. **MS:** ↑ skeletal muscle tone. **Neuro:** emergence reactions, ↑ intracranial pressure. **Resp:** laryngospasm, respiratory depression and apnea (rapid IV administration of large doses).

Interactions

Drug-Drug: Barbiturates, hydroxyzine or **opioid analgesics** may result in prolonged recovery time. **Halothane** may result in ↓ BP, cardiac output, and HR. **Nondepolarizing neuromuscular blocking agents** may result in prolonged respiratory depression. **Levothyroxine** may ↑ risk of tachycardia and hypertension. **Diazepam** may ↓ incidence of emergence reaction. **Atropine** may ↑ incidence of unpleasant dreams. **Aminophylline** or **theophylline** may ↑ risk of seizures; consider using alternative to ketamine. **Vasopressin** or **sympathomimetics** may ↑ ketamine's sympathomimetic effects.

K

Route/Dosage

General Anesthesia

IV (Adults): *Induction:* 1–2 mg/kg (range 1–4.5 mg/kg) produces 5–10 min of surgical anesthesia or 1–2 mg/kg as a single injection or infused at 0.5 mg/min. May be used with concurrent diazepam. *Maintenance:* Increments of ½ to the full induction dose may be repeated as needed. If given with concurrent diazepam, an infusion of 0.1–0.5 mg/min may be used, augmented by 2–5 mg doses of diazepam.

IV (Children): 0.5–2 mg/kg, use smaller doses (0.5–1 mg/kg) for minor procedures.

IM (Adults): 3–8 mg/kg (10 mg/kg produces 12–25 min of surgical anesthesia).

IM (Children): 3–7 mg/kg.

PO (Children): 6–10 mg/kg for 1 dose (mix in cola or other beverage) 30 min prior to procedure.

Sedation/Analgesia (Unlabeled)

IV (Adults): 0.2–0.75 mg/kg over 2–3 min initially, followed by 0.005–0.02 mg/kg/min as an infusion.

IV (Children): 0.005–0.02 mg/kg/min as an infusion.

IM (Adults): 2–4 mg/kg initially, then 0.005–0.02 mg/kg/min as an IV infusion.

Availability (generic available)

Solution for injection: 10 mg/mL, 50 mg/mL, 100 mg/mL.

NURSING IMPLICATIONS

Assessment

- Assess level of consciousness frequently throughout therapy. Ketamine produces a dissociative state. The patient does not appear to be asleep and experiences a feeling of dissociation from the environment.

- Monitor for development of emergence delirium, which may result in confusion or agitation during the recovery period.
- Monitor BP, ECG, and respiratory status frequently during therapy. May cause hypertension and tachycardia. May ↑ cerebrospinal fluid pressure and intraocular pressure.

Lab Test Considerations

- Monitor baseline liver function tests (alkaline phosphatase, gamma glutamyl transferase) in patients receiving recurrent doses of ketamine.

Toxicity and Overdose

- Respiratory depression or apnea may be treated with mechanical ventilation.

Implementation

- Do not confuse Ketalar with ketorolac. Do not confuse ketamine with ketorolac.
- May be administered concurrently with a drying agent (atropine, scopolamine); ketamine ↑ salivary and tracheobronchial mucous gland secretions. Atropine may ↑ the incidence of unpleasant dreams.
- Patients may experience a state of confusion (emergence delirium) during recovery from ketamine. Administering a benzodiazepine and minimizing verbal, tactile, and visual stimulation may prevent emergence delirium. Severe emergence delirium may be treated with short- or ultra-short-acting barbiturates.
- **PO:** Administer on an empty stomach to prevent vomiting and aspiration. Use 100 mg/mL IV solution and mix appropriate dose in 0.2–0.3 mL/kg of cola or other beverage.

IV Administration

- **IV Push: Dilution:** Dilute 100 mg/mL with equal parts of sterile water for injection, 0.9% NaCl, or D5W. **Concentration:** Max = 50 mg/mL for slow IV push. **Rate:** Administer over 60 sec unless a rapid-sequence induction technique is indicated. More rapid administration may cause respiratory depression, apnea, and hypertension. Do not exceed 0.5 mg/kg/min.
- **Continuous Infusion: Dilution:** Dilute 10 mL of 50 mg/mL or 5 mL of 100 mg/mL with 500 mL of 0.9% NaCl or D5W and mix well. **Concentration:** 1–2 mg/mL. **Rate:** Administer at 0.5 mg/kg/min for induction. Maintenance infusion may be administered at a 1–2 mg/min or 0.1–0.5 mg/min given concurrently with diazepam. Titrate dose according to individual patient requirements. Tonic-clonic movements during anesthesia do not indicate the need for more ketamine.
- **Y-Site Compatibility:** acetaminophen, albumin, alprostadil, amikacin, amiodarone, arsenic trioxide, atropine, caffeine citrate, calcium gluconate, cefazolin, cefepime, cefotaxime, ceftazidime, cefuroxime, chlorpromazine, clindamycin, clonidine, digoxin, dimenhydrinate, diphenhydramine, dobutamine, dopamine, epinephrine, gentamicin, haloperidol, hydrocortisone, magnesium sulfate, meperidine, metoclopramide, metronidazole, midazolam, milrinone, morphine, multivitamins, naloxone, oxytocin, penicillin G, piperacillin/tazobactam, potassium chloride, promethazine, propofol, sufentanil, tobramycin.
- **Y-Site Incompatibility:** acyclovir, ampicillin, cisatracurium, dexmedetomidine, furosemide, heparin, insulin, regular, meropenem, phenytoin, potassium phosphates, rocuronium, sodium bicarbonate, trimethoprim/sulfamethoxazole.

Patient/Family Teaching

- Explain purpose and side effects of ketamine to patient.
- Psychomotor impairment may last for 24 hr after anesthesia. Advise patient to avoid driving or other activities requiring alertness until response to medication is known.
- Advise patient to avoid alcohol or other CNS depressants for 24 hr after anesthesia.
- Rep: Advise women of reproductive potential to notify health care provider if pregnancy is planned or suspected. Ketamine is not recommended for use during pregnancy or delivery.

Evaluation/Desired Outcomes

- Anesthesia with profound analgesia, minimal respiratory depression, and minimal skeletal muscle relaxation.

ketoconazole, See ANTIFUNGALS (TOPICAL).

BEERS

ketorolac (kee-toe-role-ak)

Sprix, ~~Toradol~~, ✱ Toradol

Classification

Therapeutic: nonopioid analgesics

Pharmacologic: nonsteroidal anti-inflammatory drugs (NSAIDs)

See Appendix B for ophthalmic use.

Indications

Short-term management of pain.

Action

Inhibits prostaglandin synthesis, producing peripherally mediated analgesia. Also has antipyretic and anti-inflammatory properties. **Therapeutic Effects:** Decreased pain.

Pharmacokinetics

Absorption: Rapidly and completely absorbed following all routes of administration.
Distribution: Well distributed to tissues.
Protein Binding: 99%.
Metabolism and Excretion: Primarily metabolized by the liver. Primarily excreted by the kidneys (92%); 6% excreted in feces.
Half-life: 4.5 hr (range 3.8–6.3 hr; ↑ in older adults and patients with renal impairment).

TIME/ACTION PROFILE (analgesic effects)

ROUTE	ONSET	PEAK	DURATION
PO	unknown	2–3 hr	4–6 hr or longer
IM, IV	10 min	1–2 hr	6 hr or longer
IN	unknown	unknown	6–8 hr or longer

Contraindications/Precautions

Contraindicated in: Hypersensitivity; Cross-sensitivity with other NSAIDs may exist; Preoperative use; Active or history of peptic ulcer disease or GI bleeding; Known alcohol intolerance (injection only); Coronary artery bypass graft surgery; Recent MI; HF; Cerebrovascular bleeding; Advanced renal impairment or at risk for renal failure due to volume depletion; Concurrent use of pentoxifylline or probenecid; OB: Avoid use of after 30 wk gestation; may inhibit labor and ↑ maternal bleeding at delivery.
Use Cautiously in: Cardiovascular disease or risk factors for cardiovascular disease (may ↑ risk of serious cardiovascular thrombotic events, MI, and stroke, especially with prolonged use or use of higher doses); History of long duration of NSAID use, smoking, alcohol use, advanced liver disease, coagulopathy, or poor general health (↑ risk of GI bleeding); History of peptic ulcer disease and/or GI bleeding; Bleeding tendency or concurrent anticoagulant therapy; Mild to moderate renal impairment (↓ dose may be required); Hepatic impairment; OB: Use at or after 20 wk gestation may cause fetal or neonatal renal impairment; if treatment is necessary between 20 wk and 30 wk gestation, limit use to the lowest effective dose and shortest duration possible; Lactation: Use while breastfeeding only if potential maternal benefit justifies potential risk to infant; Pedi: Safety and effectiveness not established in neonates; Geri: Appears on Beers list. ↑ risk of GI bleeding or peptic ulcer disease in older adults. Avoid chronic use unless other alternatives are not effective and the patient can take a gastroprotective agent; avoid short-term use in combination with oral or parenteral corticosteroids, anticoagulants, or antiplatelet agents unless other alternatives are not effective and the patient can take a gastroprotective agent.

Adverse Reactions/Side Effects

CV: edema, HF, MI. **Derm:** ↑ sweating, DRUG REACTION WITH EOSINOPHILIA AND SYSTEMIC SYMPTOMS (DRESS), EXFOLIATIVE DERMATITIS, GENERALIZED BULLOUS FIXED DRUG ERUPTION, pruritus, purpura, rash, STEVENS-JOHNSON SYNDROME (SJS), TOXIC EPIDERMAL NECROLYSIS (TEN), urticaria. **EENT:** ↑ lacrimation (nasal spray), nasal discomfort (nasal spray), throat irritation (nasal spray). **F and E** hyperkalemia. **GI:** ↑ liver enzymes, abdominal pain, abnormal taste, diarrhea, dry mouth, dyspepsia, GI BLEEDING, GI PERFORATION, GI ULCERATION, nausea. **GU:** oliguria, renal toxicity, urinary frequency. **Hemat:** prolonged bleeding time. **Local:** injection site pain. **Neuro:** drowsiness, abnormal thinking, dizziness, euphoria, headache, paresthesia, STROKE. **Resp:** asthma, dyspnea. **Misc:** HYPERSENSITIVITY REACTIONS (INCLUDING ANAPHYLAXIS AND SERIOUS SKIN REACTIONS).

K

Interactions

Drug-Drug: **Probenecid** ↑ levels and risk of toxicity; concurrent use contraindicated. ↑ risk of bleeding with **pentoxifylline**; concurrent use contraindicated. **Aspirin** may ↓ effectiveness. ↑ risk of GI bleeding with **anticoagulants**, **aspirin**, **clopidogrel**, **ticagrelor**, **prasugrel**, **corticosteroids**, **fibrinolytics**, **SNRIs**, or **SSRIs**. May ↓ effectiveness of **diuretics** or **antihypertensives**. May ↑ levels and risk of toxicity of **lithium**. May ↑ levels and risk of toxicity of **methotrexate**. ↑ risk of adverse hematologic reactions with **antineoplastics** or **radiation therapy**. May ↑ risk of nephrotoxicity from **cyclosporine**.
Drug-Natural Products: ↑ bleeding risk with **arnica**, **chamomile**, **clove**, **dong quai**, **feverfew**, **garlic**, **ginger**, **ginkgo**, or **Panax ginseng**.

Route/Dosage

Oral therapy is indicated only as a continuation of parenteral therapy. Total duration of therapy by all routes should not exceed 5 days.
PO (Adults <65 yr): 20 mg initially, followed by 10 mg every 4–6 hr (not to exceed 40 mg/day).
PO (Adults ≥65 yr, <50 kg, or with renal impairment): 10 mg every 4–6 hr (not to exceed 40 mg/day).
PO (Children 2–16 yr, <50 kg): 1 mg/kg as a single dose. No data available for multiple doses.
IM (Adults <65 yr): *Single dose:* 60 mg. *Multiple dosing:* 30 mg every 6 hr (not to exceed 120 mg/day).
IM (Adults ≥65 yr, <50 kg, or with renal impairment): *Single dose:* 30 mg. *Multiple dosing:* 15 mg every 6 hr (not to exceed 60 mg/day).
IM (Children 2–16 yr, <50 kg): *Single dose:* 0.4–1 mg/kg (maximum: 30 mg/dose). *Multiple dosing:* 0.5 mg/kg every 6 hr.

IV (Adults <65 yr): *Single dose:* 30 mg. *Multiple dosing:* 30 mg every 6 hr (not to exceed 120 mg/day).
IV (Adults ≥65 yr, <50 kg, or with renal impairment): *Single dose:* 15 mg. *Multiple dosing:* 15 mg every 6 hr (not to exceed 60 mg/day).
IV (Children 2–16 yr, <50 kg): *Single dose:* 0.4–1 mg/kg (maximum: 15 mg/dose). *Multiple dosing:* 0.5 mg/kg every 6 hr.
Intranasal (Adults <65 yr): One spray in each nostril every 6–8 hr (not to exceed 4 sprays in each nostril/day).
Intranasal (Adults ≥65 yr, <50 kg, or with renal impairment): One spray in only one nostril every 6–8 hr (not to exceed 4 sprays in one nostril/day).

Availability (generic available)

Tablets: 10 mg. **Nasal spray (Sprix):** 15.75 mg/spray in 1.7-g bottle (delivers 8 sprays). **Solution for injection:** 15 mg/mL, 30 mg/mL.

NURSING IMPLICATIONS

Assessment

- Assess pain (type, location, intensity) prior to and 1–2 hr following administration.
- Assess for hypersensitivity reaction (rhinitis, asthma, urticaria), including anaphylaxis. Patients who have asthma, aspirin-induced allergy, and nasal polyps are at ↑ risk for hypersensitivity. *If symptoms occur,* immediately discontinue therapy and initiate symptomatic treatment.
- Assess for serious skin reactions (exfoliative dermatitis, SJS, TEN, generalized bullous fixed drug eruption) periodically during therapy. *If severe rash occurs or is accompanied by fever, malaise, fatigue, myalgia, arthralgia, blisters, oral lesions, conjunctivitis, hepatitis or eosinophilia,* discontinue therapy.
- Monitor BP and edema during initiation and periodically during therapy.
- Monitor for signs and symptoms of DRESS (fever, rash, lymphadenopathy, facial swelling) periodically during therapy. *If symptoms occur,* discontinue therapy.

Lab Test Considerations

- Assess AST, ALT, CBC, and chemistry panel periodically during prolonged therapy.
- May cause prolonged bleeding time that may persist for 24–48 hr following discontinuation of therapy.
- May ↑ BUN, serum creatinine, and potassium.

Implementation

- Do not confuse ketorolac with Ketalar, ketamine, or methadone.
- Administration in higher-than-recommended doses does not provide ↑ effectiveness but may cause ↑ side effects. Duration of ketorolac therapy by all routes combined should not exceed 5 days.
- Use lowest effective dose for shortest period of time to minimize risk of cardiovascular thrombotic events.
- Coadministration with opioid analgesics may have additive analgesic effects and may permit lower opioid doses.
- Correct volume status in dehydrated or hypovolemic patients prior to initiating.
- **PO:** Use oral route *only* as a continuation of parenteral therapy.
- **IM:** Solution is clear, colorless, and slightly yellow; do not use if cloudy, discolored, or contains particulates. Protect single-dose vial from light until use. Inject slowly and deeply into large muscle.

IV Administration

- **IV Push:** Administer undiluted. **Concentration:** 15–30 mg/mL. **Rate:** Administer over ≥15 sec.
- **Y-Site Compatibility:** amikacin, aminocaproic acid, aminophylline, amphotericin B liposomal, anidulafungin, argatroban, ascorbic acid, atracurium, atropine, aztreonam, benztropine, bivalirudin, bleomycin, bumetanide, buprenorphine, butorphanol, carboplatin, carmustine, cefazolin, cefotaxime, cefotetan, cefoxitin, ceftazidime, ceftriaxone, cefuroxime, chloramphenicol, cisplatin, clindamycin, cyanocobalamin, cyclophosphamide, cyclosporine, cytarabine, dactinomycin, daptomycin, dexamethasone, dexmedetomidine, dexrazoxane, digoxin, docetaxel, dopamine, doxorubicin hydrochloride, doxorubicin liposomal, enalaprilat, ephedrine, epinephrine, epoetin alfa, eptifibatide, ertapenem, etoposide, etoposide phosphate, famotidine, fentanyl, fluconazole, fludarabine, fluorouracil, folic acid, foscarnet, fosphenytoin, furosemide, gentamicin, glycopyrrolate, granisetron, heparin, hydrocortisone, hydromorphone, ifosfamide, imipenem/cilastatin, imipenem/cilastatin/relebactam, indomethacin, insulin regular, irinotecan, isoproterenol, leucovorin, lidocaine, linezolid, lorazepam, magnesium sulfate, mannitol, meperidine, mesna, methadone, methotrexate, methylprednisolone, metoclopramide, metoprolol, metronidazole, milrinone, mitomycin, mitoxantrone, morphine, moxifloxacin, nafcillin, naloxone, nitroglycerin, nitroprusside, norepinephrine, octreotide, ondansetron, oxacillin, oxaliplatin, oxytocin, paclitaxel, palonosetron, pamidronate, pemetrexed, penicillin G, phenobarbital, phenylephrine, phytonadione, piperacillin/tazobactam, potassium acetate, potassium chloride, procainamide, propranolol, remifentanil, sodium acetate, sodium bicarbonate, succinylcholine, sufentanil, tacrolimus, theophylline, thiotepa, tigecycline, tirofiban, tobramycin, vasopressin,

verapamil, vinblastine, vincristine, voriconazole, zoledronic acid.

- **Y-Site Incompatibility:** acyclovir, alemtuzumab, amiodarone, amphotericin B deoxycholate, azathioprine, calcium chloride, caspofungin, chlorpromazine, dacarbazine, dantrolene, daunorubicin, diazepam, diazoxide, diltiazem, diphenhydramine, dobutamine, doxycycline, epirubicin, erythromycin, esmolol, ganciclovir, gemcitabine, gemtuzumab ozogamicin, haloperidol, idarubicin, labetalol, levofloxacin, midazolam, minocycline, mycophenolate, nalbuphine, nicardipine, pantoprazole, papaverine, pentamidine, phentolamine, phenytoin, prochlorperazine, promethazine, protamine, pyridoxine, rocuronium, topotecan, trimethoprim/sulfamethoxazole, vancomycin, vecuronium, vinorelbine.
- **Intranasal:** Activate pump before 1st use by holding bottle arm's length away with index finger and middle finger resting on top of finger flange and thumb supporting base. Press down evenly and release pump 5 times to activate. Prior to each use, blow nose gently. Sit up straight or stand. Tilt head slightly forward. Insert tip of container into nostril. Point container away from center of nose. Push down to spray. Discard bottle no more than 24 hr after taking 1st dose, even if some liquid remains.

Patient/Family Teaching

- Explain purpose and side effects of medication. Advise patient to read *Patient Information* before starting therapy.
- Instruct patient to take missed doses as soon as remembered if not almost time for next dose. Do not double doses. Do not take more than prescribed or for >5 days. Advise patient to notify health care provider of all Rx or OTC medications, vitamins, or herbal products being taken and to consult health care provider before taking other medications, especially the concurrent use of alcohol, aspirin, NSAIDs, or acetaminophen.
- May cause drowsiness or dizziness. Advise patient to avoid driving or other activities requiring alertness until response to the medication is known.
- Advise patient to inform health care provider of medication regimen prior to treatment or surgery.
- Inform patient of ↑ risk of MI and stroke. Use lowest effective dose for shortest time. Advise patient to notify health care provider immediately if signs and symptoms (shortness of breath or trouble breathing, chest pain, weakness in one part or side of body, slurred speech, swelling of the face or throat) occur.
- Advise patient to notify health care provider promptly if signs or symptoms of GI toxicity (abdominal pain, black stools) occur.
- Inform patient to discontinue ketorolac and notify health care provider if signs and symptoms of hepatotoxicity (nausea, fatigue, lethargy, diarrhea, pruritus, jaundice, abdominal pain, flu-like symptoms) occur.
- Advise patient to consult health care provider if rash, visual disturbances, tinnitus, weight gain, edema, persistent headache, chills, fever, or muscle aches occurs.
- Rep: May cause fetal harm. Advise women of reproductive potential to notify health care provider if pregnancy is planned or suspected or if breastfeeding. Advise pregnant patients to avoid ketorolac in the 3rd trimester of pregnancy (after 29 wk); may cause premature closure of fetal ductus arteriosus. Use of ketorolac after 20 wk may cause fetal renal impairment leading to oligohydramnios. Avoid use of ketorolac in labor and delivery; may adversely affect fetal circulation and inhibit uterine contractions. The risk of uterine hemorrhage may be ↑. May cause reversible infertility in women attempting to conceive.

Evaluation/Desired Outcomes

- Decrease in severity of pain. Patients who do not respond to one NSAID may respond to another.

K

labetalol, See BETA BLOCKERS (nonselective).

lacosamide (la-kose-a-mide)

Motpoly XR, Vimpat

Classification

Therapeutic: anticonvulsants

Schedule V

Indications

Partial-onset seizures (as either monotherapy or adjunctive therapy). Primary generalized tonic-clonic seizures (as adjunctive therapy).

Action

Mechanism is not known, but may involve enhancement of slow inactivation of sodium channels with resultant membrane stabilization **Therapeutic Effects:** Decreased incidence and severity of partial-onset seizures generalized tonic-clonic seizures.

Pharmacokinetics

Absorption: 100% absorbed following oral administration; IV administration results in complete bioavailability.

Distribution: Unknown.

Protein Binding: <15%.

Metabolism and Excretion: Partially metabolized by the liver; 40% excreted in urine as unchanged drug; 30% as a metabolite.

Half-life: 13 hr.

TIME/ACTION PROFILE (plasma concentrations)

ROUTE	ONSET	PEAK	DURATION
PO-IR	unknown	1–4 hr	12 hr
PO-XR	unknown	7 hr	24 hr
IV	unknown	end of infusion	12 hr

Contraindications/Precautions

Contraindicated in: Hypersensitivity; Severe hepatic impairment.

Use Cautiously in: CCr <30 mL/min (use lower daily dose); All patients (may ↑ risk of suicidal thoughts/behaviors); Mild to moderate hepatic impairment; Severe renal impairment; Known cardiac conduction problems (heart block or sick sinus syndrome without a pacemaker), severe cardiac disease (MI or HF), Brugada syndrome, or taking medications that affect cardiac conduction; Diabetic neuropathy or cardiac disease (↑ risk for atrial fibrillation/flutter); OB: Use during pregnancy only if potential maternal benefit justifies potential fetal risk; Lactation: Use while breastfeeding only if potential maternal benefit justifies potential risk to infant; Pedi: Children <1 mo (safety and effectiveness not established); Geri: Titrate dose carefully in older adults.

Adverse Reactions/Side Effects

CV: atrial fibrillation/flutter, bradycardia, heart block, syncope, VENTRICULAR ARRHYTHMIAS. **Derm:** DRUG REACTION WITH EOSINOPHILIA AND SYSTEMIC SYMPTOMS (DRESS), rash, STEVENS-JOHNSON SYNDROME (SJS), TOXIC EPIDERMAL NECROLYSIS. **EENT:** diplopia. **GI:** nausea, vomiting. **Hemat:** AGRANULOCYTOSIS. **Neuro:** dizziness, headache, ataxia, hallucinations, SUICIDAL THOUGHTS, syncope, vertigo. **Misc:** physical dependence, psychological dependence.

Interactions

Drug-Drug: Use cautiously with other drugs that affect cardiac conduction, including **sodium channel blockers, beta blockers, diltiazem, verapamil, potassium channel blockers**, and **PR-interval prolonging medications**.

Route/Dosage

Partial-Onset Seizures

PO, IV (Adults): *Monotherapy (immediate-release PO or IV):* 100 mg twice daily; may ↑ weekly by 100 mg/day in 2 divided doses up to a maintenance dose of 150–200 mg twice daily; may also initiate therapy with 200-mg single loading dose followed 12 hr later by 100 mg twice daily for 1 wk; may then ↑ weekly by 100 mg/day in 2 divided doses up to a maintenance dose of 150–200 mg twice daily. *Monotherapy (extended-release PO):* 200 mg once daily; may ↑ weekly by 100 mg once daily up to a maintenance dose of 300–400 mg once daily; *Adjunctive therapy (immediate-release PO or IV):* 50 mg twice daily; may ↑ weekly by 100 mg/day in 2 divided doses up to a maintenance dose of 100–200 mg twice daily; may also initiate therapy with 200-mg single loading dose followed 12 hr later by 100 mg twice daily for 1 wk; may then ↑ weekly by 100 mg/day in 2 divided doses up to a maintenance dose of 100–200 mg twice daily. *Adjunctive therapy (extended-release PO):* 100 mg once daily; may ↑ weekly by 100 mg once daily up to a maintenance dose of 200–400 mg once daily.

PO, IV (Children ≥1 mo and ≥50 kg): *Monotherapy (immediate-release PO or IV):* 50 mg twice daily; may ↑ weekly by 100 mg/day in 2 divided doses up to a maintenance dose of 150–200 mg twice daily; may also initiate therapy with 200-mg single loading dose followed 12 hr later by 100 mg twice daily for 1 wk; may then ↑ weekly by 100 mg/day in 2 divided doses up to a maintenance dose of 150–200 mg twice daily. *Monotherapy (extended-release PO):* 100 mg once daily; may ↑ weekly by 100 mg once daily up to a maintenance dose of 300–400 mg once daily. *Adjunctive therapy (immediate-release PO or IV):* 50 mg twice daily; may ↑ weekly by 100 mg/day in 2 divided doses up to

a maintenance dose of 100–200 mg twice daily; may also initiate therapy with 200-mg single loading dose followed 12 hr later by 100 mg twice daily for 1 wk; may then ↑ weekly by 100 mg/day in 2 divided doses up to a maintenance dose of 100–200 mg twice daily. *Adjunctive therapy (extended-release PO):* 100 mg once daily; may ↑ weekly by 100 mg once daily up to a maintenance dose of 200–400 mg once daily.
PO, IV (Children ≥1 mo and 30–<50 kg): *Monotherapy or adjunctive therapy (immediate-release PO or IV):* 1 mg/kg twice daily; may ↑ weekly by 2 mg/kg/day in 2 divided doses up to a maintenance dose of 2–4 mg/kg twice daily; may also initiate therapy with 4 mg/kg single loading dose followed 12 hr later by 2 mg/kg twice daily for 1 wk; may then ↑ weekly by 2 mg/kg/day in 2 divided doses up to a maintenance dose of 2–4 mg/kg twice daily.
PO, IV (Children ≥1 mo and 6–<30 kg): *Monotherapy or adjunctive therapy (immediate-release PO or IV):* 1 mg/kg twice daily; may ↑ weekly by 2 mg/kg/day in 2 divided doses up to a maintenance dose of 3–6 mg/kg twice daily; may also initiate therapy with 4.5 mg/kg single loading dose followed 12 hr later by 3 mg/kg twice daily for 1 wk; may then ↑ weekly by 2 mg/kg/day in 2 divided doses up to a maintenance dose of 3–6 mg/kg twice daily.
PO (Children ≥1 mo and <6 kg): *Monotherapy or adjunctive therapy (immediate-release PO or IV):* 1 mg/kg twice daily; may ↑ weekly by 2 mg/kg/day in 2 divided doses up to a maintenance dose of 3.75–7.5 mg/kg twice daily; may also initiate therapy with 3.75 mg/kg twice daily for 1 wk; may then ↑ weekly by 2 mg/kg/day in 2 divided doses up to a maintenance dose of 3.75–7.5 mg/kg twice daily.
IV (Children ≥1 mo and <6 kg): *Monotherapy or adjunctive therapy (immediate-release PO or IV):* 0.66 mg/kg 3 times daily; may ↑ weekly by 2 mg/kg/day in 3 divided doses up to a maintenance dose of 2.5–5 mg/kg 3 times daily; may also initiate therapy with 2.5 mg/kg 3 times daily for 1 wk; may then ↑ weekly by 2 mg/kg/day in 3 divided doses up to a maintenance dose of 2.5–5 mg/kg 3 times daily.

Renal Impairment

PO, IV (Adults and Children ≥1 mo): *CCr ≤30 mL:* Monotherapy or adjunctive therapy (immediate-release PO or IV): ↓ maximum dose by 25%. Monotherapy or adjunctive therapy (extended-release PO): Not to exceed maximum dose of 300 mg once daily.

Hepatic Impairment

PO, IV (Adults and Children ≥1 mo): *Mild or moderate hepatic impairment:* Monotherapy or adjunctive therapy (immediate-release PO or IV): ↓ maximum dose by 25%. Monotherapy or adjunctive therapy (extended-release PO): Not to exceed dose of 300 mg once daily.

Primary Generalized Tonic-Clonic Seizures

PO, IV (Adults): *Adjunctive therapy (immediate-release PO or IV):* 50 mg twice daily; may ↑ weekly by 100 mg/day in 2 divided doses up to a maintenance dose of 100–200 mg twice daily; may also initiate therapy with 200-mg single loading dose followed 12 hr later by 100 mg twice daily; may ↑ weekly by 100 mg/day in 2 divided doses up to a maintenance dose of 100–200 mg twice daily. *Adjunctive therapy (extended-release PO):* 100 mg once daily; may ↑ weekly by 100 mg once daily up to a maintenance dose of 200–400 mg once daily.
PO, IV (Children ≥4 yr and ≥50 kg): *Adjunctive therapy (immediate-release PO or IV):* 50 mg twice daily; may ↑ weekly by 100 mg/day in 2 divided doses up to a maintenance dose of 100–200 mg twice daily; may also initiate therapy with 200-mg single loading dose followed 12 hr later by 100 mg twice daily; may ↑ weekly by 100 mg/day in 2 divided doses up to a maintenance dose of 100–200 mg twice daily. *Adjunctive therapy (extended-release PO):* 100 mg once daily; may ↑ weekly by 100 mg once daily up to a maintenance dose of 200–400 mg once daily.
PO, IV (Children ≥4 yr and 30–<50 kg): *Adjunctive therapy (immediate-release PO or IV):* 1 mg/kg twice daily; may ↑ weekly by 2 mg/kg/day in 2 divided doses up to a maintenance dose of 2–4 mg/kg twice daily; may also initiate therapy with 4 mg/kg single loading dose followed 12 hr later by 2 mg/kg twice daily; may ↑ weekly by 2 mg/kg/day in 2 divided doses up to a maintenance dose of 2–4 mg/kg twice daily.
PO, IV (Children ≥4 yr and 11–<30 kg): *Adjunctive therapy (immediate-release PO or IV):* 1 mg/kg twice daily; may ↑ weekly by 2 mg/kg/day in 2 divided doses up to a maintenance dose of 3–6 mg/kg twice daily; may also initiate therapy with 4.5 mg/kg single loading dose followed 12 hr later by 3 mg/kg twice daily; may ↑ weekly by 2 mg/kg/day in 2 divided doses up to a maintenance dose of 3–6 mg/kg twice daily.

Renal Impairment

PO, IV (Adults and Children ≥4 yr): *CCr ≤30 mL/min:* Adjunctive therapy (immediate-release PO or IV): ↓ maximum dose by 25%. Adjunctive therapy (extended-release PO): Not to exceed dose of 300 mg once daily.

Hepatic Impairment

PO, IV (Adults and Children ≥4 yr): *Mild or moderate hepatic impairment:* Adjunctive therapy (immediate-release PO or IV): ↓ maximum dose by 25%. Adjunctive therapy (extended-release PO): Not to exceed dose of 300 mg once daily.

L

Availability (generic available)

Immediate-release tablets: 50 mg, 100 mg, 150 mg, 200 mg. **Extended-release capsules:** 100 mg, 150 mg, 200 mg. **Oral solution:** 10 mg/mL. **Solution for injection:** 10 mg/mL.

NURSING IMPLICATIONS

Assessment

- Assess location, duration, and characteristics of seizure activity. Institute seizure precautions.
- Monitor for changes in behavior that could indicate the emergence or worsening of suicidal thoughts or behavior or depression.
- Assess patient for skin rash frequently during therapy. Discontinue at first sign of rash; may be life-threatening. SJS may develop. Treat symptomatically; may recur once treatment is stopped.
- Monitor for signs and symptoms of DRESS (fever, rash, lymphadenopathy, facial swelling), associated with involvement of other organ systems (hepatitis, nephritis, hematologic abnormalities, myocarditis, myositis), during therapy. May resemble an acute viral infection. Eosinophilia is often present. Discontinue therapy if signs occur.
- **IV:** Assess ECG prior to therapy in patients with pre-existing cardiac disease before starting and after titration to steady-state maintenance. Closely monitor patients with cardiac conduction problems or on medications that affect conduction. IV lacosamide may cause bradycardia or AV block.

Lab Test Considerations

- May cause ↑ ALT, which may return to normal without treatment.
- Monitor CBC and platelets periodically during therapy.

Implementation

- Do not confuse Vimpat with Venofer or Vfend.
- **IV:** IV administration is indicated for short-term replacement (up to 5 days) when PO is not feasible. When switching from PO to IV, initial total daily dose should be equivalent to total daily dose and frequency of PO therapy. At end of IV period, may switch to PO at equivalent daily dose and frequency.
- When switching from another antiepileptic drug to lacosamide, administer 150–200 mg twice daily for at least 3 days before beginning withdrawal of other antiepileptic drug. Gradually ↓ other antiepileptic drug over 6 wk.
- When administering loading dose, closely monitor for CNS and cardiovascular adverse reactions.
- When discontinuing lacosamide, gradually ↓ dose over 1 wk.
- **PO:** May be administered with or without food. ***DNC:*** Swallow tablets whole with liquid; do not crush, break, or chew.
- Use a calibrated measuring device for accurate dosing of oral solution; household measures are not accurate. Discard any unused solution 6 mo after opening bottle.
- Oral solution may also be given via nasogastric tube or gastrostomy tube.

IV Administration

- **Intermittent Infusion: Dilution:** May be administered undiluted or diluted with 0.9% NaCl, D5W, or LR. **Concentration:** 10 mg/mL. Solution is clear and colorless; do not administer if cloudy, discolored, or contains precipitates. Solution is stable for 4 hr at room temperature. Discard unused portion. **Rate:** Infuse over 15–60 min, preferably 30–60 min. Do not infuse over less than 30 min in children.

Patient/Family Teaching

- Explain purpose and side effects of medication to patient. Advise patient to read *Patient Information* before starting therapy.
- Advise patient to notify health care professional of all Rx or OTC medications, vitamins, or herbal products being taken and to consult health care professional before taking other medications.
- Instruct patient to take lacosamide around the clock, as directed. Medication should be gradually discontinued over >1 wk to prevent seizures.
- May cause dizziness, ataxia, and syncope. Caution patient to avoid driving or other activities requiring alertness until response to medication is known. Tell patient not to resume driving until health care professional gives clearance based on control of seizure disorder. If syncope occurs, advise patient to lie down with legs raised until recovered and notify health care professional.
- Inform patients and families of risk of suicidal thoughts and behavior. Advise that behavior or mood changes; worsening or emergent symptoms of depression, suicidal or self-harm thoughts or behavior; or rash should be reported to health care professional immediately.
- Instruct patient to notify health care professional if signs of multiorgan hypersensitivity reactions (fever, rash, fatigue, jaundice, dark urine) occur.
- Rep: Advise females of reproductive potential to notify health care professional if pregnancy is planned or suspected or if breastfeeding. Monitor infants exposed to lacosamide through breast milk for excess sedation. Encourage pregnant patients to enroll in the North American Antiepileptic Drug registry by calling 1-888-233-2334; call must be made by patient. Information on registry can be found at http://www.aedpregnancyregistry.org/.

Evaluation/Desired Outcomes

- Decreased seizure activity.

lactic acid/citric acid/potassium bitartrate

(lak-tik as-id/sit-rik as-id/poe-tas-ee-um bye-tar-trate)

Phexx

Classification

Therapeutic: contraceptive nonhormonals

Indications

Rep: Prevention of pregnancy in women of reproductive potential as an on-demand form of contraception.

Action

Lowers the pH in the vagina, which subsequently reduces sperm motility. **Therapeutic Effects:** Prevention of pregnancy.

Pharmacokinetics

Absorption: Systemic absorption not expected following vaginal administration.
Distribution: Systemic absorption not expected following vaginal administration.
Metabolism and Excretion: Unknown.
Half-life: Unknown.

TIME/ACTION PROFILE

ROUTE	ONSET	PEAK	DURATION
Vag	unknown	unknown	unknown

Contraindications/Precautions

Contraindicated in: Hypersensitivity; OB: Pregnancy; Rep: History of recurrent urinary tract infection or urinary tract abnormalities.
Use Cautiously in: Lactation: Safety not established in breastfeeding.

Adverse Reactions/Side Effects

GU: vulvovaginal burning, vulvovaginal pruritus, bacterial vaginosis, cystitis, dysuria, genital discomfort, pyelonephritis, urinary tract infection, vagina discharge, vulvovaginal candidiasis, vulvovaginal pain. **Misc:** hypersensitivity reactions.

Interactions

Drug-Drug: Avoid use with **vaginal rings**.

Route/Dosage

Vag (Adults and Children [women of reproductive potential]): One prefilled applicator (5 g) immediately before or up to 1 hr before **each** act of vaginal intercourse. If ≥1 act of vaginal intercourse occurs within 1 hr, must insert another prefilled applicator.

Availability

Vaginal gel: lactic acid 90 mg/citric acid 50 mg/potassium bitartrate 20 mg in each 5-g prefilled applicator.

NURSING IMPLICATIONS

Assessment

- Assess patient for history of recurrent urinary tract infections or urinary tract abnormalities. May cause cystitis and pyelonephritis.

Implementation

- **Vag:** Administer one prefilled applicator vaginally immediately before or up to 1 hr before each act of vaginal intercourse. If >1 act of vaginal intercourse occurs within 1 hr, apply an additional dose.

Patient/Family Teaching

- Explain the purpose and side effects. Instruct patient in correct timing and technique for vaginal administration **before** vaginal sex. May be used during any part of menstrual cycle and as soon as it is safe to resume vaginal intercourse after childbirth, abortion, or miscarriage. Advise patient to read *Patient Information* before starting and with each Rx refill in case of changes.
- Advise patient that *Phexx* is not effective at preventing pregnancy when used **after** vaginal sex.
- Inform patient that *Phexx* may be used with hormonal contraceptives; latex, polyurethane, and polyisoprene condoms; and vaginal diaphragms. Avoid use with vaginal rings. May also be used concurrently with other products for vaginal infections (miconazole, metronidazole, tioconazole).
- Advise patient to notify health care provider if severe or prolonged genital irritation or symptoms of urinary tract infection (burning feeling when passing urine, cloudy urine, pain in the pelvis, back pain) occur. May also cause burning, itching, and pain in male partner.
- Inform patient that *Phexx* does not protect against HIV or other sexually transmitted infections.
- Advise patient to notify health care provider of all Rx or OTC medications, vitamins, or herbal products being taken and to consult with health care provider before taking other medications.
- Rep: Advise women of reproductive potential to notify health care provider if pregnancy is planned or suspected or if breastfeeding. There is no use for *Phexx* in pregnancy; discontinue use.

Evaluation/Desired Outcomes

- Prevention of pregnancy.

L

lactulose (lak-tyoo-lose)

Constulose, Enulose, Generlac, Kristalose

Classification
Therapeutic: laxatives
Pharmacologic: osmotics

Indications

Chronic constipation. Adjunct in the management of portal-systemic (hepatic) encephalopathy.

Action

Increases water content and softens the stool. Lowers the pH of the colon, which inhibits the diffusion of ammonia from the colon into the blood, thereby reducing blood ammonia levels. **Therapeutic Effects:** Relief of constipation. Decreased blood ammonia levels with improved mental status in portal-systemic encephalopathy.

Pharmacokinetics

Absorption: Less than 3% absorbed after oral administration.
Distribution: Unknown.
Metabolism and Excretion: Absorbed lactulose is excreted unchanged in the urine. Unabsorbed lactulose is metabolized by colonic bacteria to lactic, acetic, and formic acids.
Half-life: Unknown.

TIME/ACTION PROFILE (relief of constipation)

ROUTE	ONSET	PEAK	DURATION
PO	24–48 hr	unknown	unknown

Contraindications/Precautions

Contraindicated in: Patients on low-galactose diets.
Use Cautiously in: Diabetes mellitus; Excessive or prolonged use (may lead to dependence); Lactation: Safety not established in breastfeeding.

Adverse Reactions/Side Effects

Endo: hyperglycemia (patients with diabetes). **GI:** belching, cramps, distention, flatulence, diarrhea.

Interactions

Drug-Drug: Should not be used with other **laxatives** in the treatment of hepatic encephalopathy (leads to inability to determine optimal dose of lactulose). **Anti-infectives** may ↓ effectiveness in treatment of hepatic encephalopathy.

Route/Dosage

Constipation

PO (Adults): 15–30 mL/day up to 60 mL/day as liquid or 10–20 g as powder for oral solution (up to 40 g/day has been used).
PO (Children): 7.5 mL once daily after breakfast (unlabeled).

Portal-Systemic Encephalopathy

PO (Adults): 30–45 mL 3–4 times/day; may be given every 1–2 hr initially to induce laxation.
PO (Infants): 2.5–10 mL/day in 3–4 divided doses (unlabeled).
PO (Children): 40–90 mL/day in 3–4 divided doses (unlabeled).
Rect (Adults): 300 mL diluted and administered as a retention enema every 4–6 hr.

Availability (generic available)

Oral solution: 10 g/15 mL. **Single-use packets (Kristalose):** 10 g (equal to 15 mL liquid lactulose), 20 g (equal to 30 mL liquid lactulose).

NURSING IMPLICATIONS

Assessment

- Assess patient for abdominal distention, presence of bowel sounds, and normal pattern of bowel function.
- Assess color, consistency, and amount of stool produced. **Portal-Systemic Encephalopathy:** Assess mental status (orientation, level of consciousness) before and periodically throughout course of therapy.

Lab Test Considerations

- Should ↓ blood ammonia concentrations by 25–50%.
- May ↑ blood glucose levels in patients with diabetes.
- Monitor serum electrolytes periodically when used chronically. May cause diarrhea with resulting hypokalemia and hypernatremia.

Implementation

- When used in hepatic encephalopathy, adjust dose until patient averages 2–3 soft bowel movements per day. During initial therapy, 30–45 mL may be given hourly to induce rapid laxation.
- Darkening of solution does not alter potency.
- **PO:** Mix with fruit juice, water, milk, or carbonated citrus beverage to improve flavor. Administer with a full glass (240 mL) of water or juice. May be administered on an empty stomach for more rapid results.
- Dissolve single dose packets (*Kristalose*) in 4 ounces of water. Solution should be colorless to slightly pale yellow.
- **Rect:** To administer enema, use rectal balloon catheter. Mix 300 mL of lactulose with 700 mL of water or 0.9% NaCl. Enema should be retained for 30–60 min. If inadvertently evacuated, may repeat administration.

Patient/Family Teaching

- Explain purpose and side effects of lactulose to patient. Instruct patient to take lactulose as directed. May mix drug with fruit juice, water, or milk. If patient is using drug to relieve constipation, inform patient that drug effects may not be seen for 24–48 hr. Advise patient to read *Patient Information* before starting and with each Rx refill in case of changes.

- Encourage patients to use other forms of bowel regulation, such as ↑ bulk in the diet, fluid intake, and mobility. Normal bowel habits are individualized and may vary from 3 times/day to 3 times/wk.
- Caution patients that this medication may cause belching, flatulence, or abdominal cramping. Health care provider should be notified if this becomes bothersome or if diarrhea occurs.
- Advise patient to notify health care provider of all Rx or OTC medications, vitamins, or herbal products being taken and to consult with health care provider before taking other medications. Use with other laxatives is not recommended.
- Rep: Advise women of reproductive potential to notify health care provider if pregnancy is planned or suspected or if breastfeeding.

Evaluation/Desired Outcomes

- Passage of a soft, formed bowel movement, usually within 24–48 hr.
- Clearing of confusion, apathy, and irritation and improved mental status in portal-systemic encephalopathy. Improvement may occur within 2 hr after enema and 24–48 hr after oral administration.

lamiVUDine (la-mi-vyoo-deen)

Epivir, ~~Epivir-HBV~~

Classification

Therapeutic: antiretrovirals antivirals

Pharmacologic: nucleoside reverse transcriptase inhibitors

Indications

HIV infection (in combination with other antiretrovirals). Chronic hepatitis B virus (HBV) infection. **Unlabeled Use:** HIV-postexposure prophylaxis (in combination with other antiretrovirals).

Action

After intracellular conversion to its active form (lamivudine-5-triphosphate), inhibits viral DNA synthesis by inhibiting the enzyme reverse transcriptase. **Therapeutic Effects:** Slows the progression of HIV infection and decreases the occurrence of its sequelae. Increases CD4 cell counts and decreases viral load. Protection from liver damage caused by chronic HBV infection; decreases viral load.

Pharmacokinetics

Absorption: Well absorbed after oral administration (86% in adults, 66% in infants and children).

Distribution: Distributes into the extravascular space. Some penetration into CSF; remainder of distribution unknown.

Metabolism and Excretion: Mostly excreted unchanged in urine; <5% metabolized by the liver.

Half-life: 5–7 hr.

TIME/ACTION PROFILE (plasma concentrations)

ROUTE	ONSET	PEAK	DURATION
PO	unknown	0.9 hr†	12 hr

† On an empty stomach; peak levels occur at 3.2 hr if lamivudine is taken with food. Food does not affect total amount of drug absorbed.

Contraindications/Precautions

Contraindicated in: Hypersensitivity; Concurrent use of antiretroviral combination products containing lamivudine or emtricitabine.

Use Cautiously in: Renal impairment (↑ dosing interval/↓ dose if CCr <50 mL/min); Women and obesity (↑ risk of lactic acidosis and severe hepatomegaly with steatosis); Chronic hepatitis B virus (HBV) infection (may exacerbate following discontinuation); OB: Considered a preferred nucleoside reverse transcriptase inhibitor (NRTI) for pregnant patients with HIV infection who are antiretroviral-naive, who have had antiretroviral therapy in the past but are restarting, or who require a new antiretroviral regimen; use has also been studied in pregnant women with HBV; Lactation: Breastfeeding should be supported in people with HIV who are taking antiretroviral therapy, as prescribed, and are maintaining an undetectable amount of virus in the body; Pedi: Safety and effectiveness not established in children <3 mo (HIV) or <2 yr (HBV); Geri: ↓ dose may be necessary in older adults due to age-related ↓ in renal function.

Exercise Extreme Caution in: Pedi: Pediatric patients with a history of or significant risk factors for pancreatitis (use only if no alternative).

Adverse Reactions/Side Effects

Derm: alopecia, erythema multiforme, rash, urticaria. **Endo:** hyperglycemia. **F and E:** lactic acidosis. **GI:** anorexia, diarrhea, nausea, vomiting, ↑ liver enzymes, abdominal discomfort, dyspepsia, HEPATOMEGALY WITH STEATOSIS, PANCREATITIS (↑ IN PEDIATRIC PATIENTS). **Hemat:** anemia, neutropenia, pure red cell aplasia. **MS:** musculoskeletal pain, arthralgia, muscle weakness, myalgia, rhabdomyolysis. **Neuro:** fatigue, headache, insomnia, malaise, neuropathy, depression, dizziness, SEIZURES. **Resp:** cough. **Misc:** HYPERSENSITIVITY REACTIONS (INCLUDING ANAPHYLAXIS), immune reconstitution syndrome.

Interactions

Drug-Drug: Trimethoprim/sulfamethoxazole may ↑ levels and risk of toxicity; dose alteration may be necessary in renal impairment. ↑ risk of pancreatitis with concurrent use of other **drugs causing pancreatitis.** ↑ risk of neuropathy with concurrent use of other **drugs causing neuropathy**. Combination therapy with **tenofovir** and **abacavir** may lead to virologic nonresponse and should not be used. **Sorbitol** may ↓ levels and effectiveness; avoid concurrent use.

Route/Dosage

HIV-1 Infection

PO (Adults): 150 mg twice daily or 300 mg once daily.
PO (Children ≥3 mo): *Oral solution:* 5 mg/kg twice daily or 10 mg/kg once daily (max dose = 300 mg/day); *Tablets:* 14–19 kg: 75 mg twice daily or 150 mg once daily; 20–24 kg: 75 mg in AM, 150 mg in PM (or 225 mg once daily); ≥25 kg: 150 mg twice daily or 300 mg once daily.

Renal Impairment

(Adults and Children ≥25 kg): *CCr 30–49 mL/min:* 150 mg once daily; *CCr 15–29 mL/min:* 150 mg initially; then 100 mg once daily; *CCr 5–14 mL/min:* 150 mg initially; then 50 mg once daily; *CCr <5 mL/min:* 50 mg initially; then 25 mg once daily.

Chronic Hepatitis B

PO (Adults): 100 mg once daily.
PO (Children 2–17 yr): 3 mg/kg once daily (up to 100 mg/day).

Renal Impairment

PO (Adults): *CCr 30–49 mL/min:* 100 mg first dose; then 50 mg once daily; *CCr 15–29 mL/min:* 100 mg first dose; then 25 mg once daily; *CCr 5–14 mL/min:* 35 mg first dose; then 15 mg once daily; *CCr <5 mL/min:* 35 mg first dose; then 10 mg once daily.

Availability (generic available)

Tablets: 100 mg, 150 mg, 300 mg. **Oral solution(strawberry-banana flavor):** 10 mg/mL.
In combination with: abacavir; abacavir and dolutegravir (Triumeq, Triumeq PD); abacavir and zidovudine; doravirine and tenofovir disoproxil fumarate (Delstrigo); efavirenz and tenofovir disoproxil fumarate (Symfi, Symfi Lo); dolutegravir (Dovato); tenofovir disoproxil fumarate (Cimduo); zidovudine. See Appendix N.

NURSING IMPLICATIONS

Assessment

- Assess patient, especially pediatric patients, for signs of pancreatitis (nausea, vomiting, abdominal pain) periodically during therapy. May require discontinuation of therapy.
- **HIV:** Assess for change in severity of symptoms of HIV infection and for symptoms of opportunistic infection during therapy.
- Monitor for signs and symptoms of peripheral neuropathy (tingling, burning, numbness, or pain in hands or feet); may be difficult to differentiate from peripheral neuropathy of severe HIV disease. May require discontinuation of therapy. **Chronic Hepatitis B Infection:** Monitor for signs of hepatitis (jaundice, fatigue, anorexia, pruritus) during therapy.

Lab Test Considerations

- Monitor viral load and CD4 levels before and periodically during therapy.
- Monitor serum amylase, lipase, and triglycerides periodically during therapy. ↑ levels may indicate pancreatitis and require discontinuation.
- Monitor liver function. May ↑ AST, ALT, CK, bilirubin, and alkaline phosphatase. If therapy is discontinued, may cause severe exacerbation of HBV. Monitor liver function in coinfected patients for several months after stopping therapy.
- Lactic acidosis may occur with hepatotoxicity causing hepatic steatosis; may be fatal, especially in women.
- May rarely cause neutropenia and anemia.

Implementation

- Do not confuse lamivudine with lamotrigine.
- **PO:** May be administered without regard to food.
- Epivir scored tablet is preferred for HIV-1-infected pediatric patients weighing ≥14 kg and able to swallow pills; solution is associated with higher resistance rates. Before prescribing, assess for ability to swallow tablets. For patients unable to safely and reliably swallow tablets, oral solution may be used.
- The dosage of lamivudine for HIV is higher than that used for HBV. If a decision is made to administer lamivudine to patients coinfected with HIV and HBV, the higher dose of lamivudine should be used as part of an appropriate combination regimen.

Patient/Family Teaching

- Instruct patient to take lamivudine as directed. Emphasize the importance of compliance with full course of therapy and not taking more than the prescribed amount. Take missed doses as soon as possible unless almost time for next dose. Do not double doses. Caution patient not to share medication with others. Advise patient to read *Patient Information* before starting and with each Rx refill in case of changes.
- Do not stop taking without consulting health care provider. Discontinuing therapy may lead to severe exacerbations. Inform patient of importance of HBV testing before starting antiretroviral therapy.
- Inform patient that lamivudine does not cure HIV or prevent associated or opportunistic infections. Lamivudine may ↓ risk of transmission of HIV to others through sexual contact or blood contamination. Caution patient to use a condom during sexual contact and avoid sharing needles or donating blood to prevent spreading HIV to others. Advise patient that the long-term effects of lamivudine are unknown at this time.

- Instruct patient to notify health care provider promptly if signs of peripheral neuropathy, pancreatitis, lactic acidosis (feel very weak or tired; feel cold, especially in arms and legs; unusual muscle pain; feel dizzy or light-headed; trouble breathing; fast or irregular heartbeat; stomach pain with nausea and vomiting), liver problems (yellowing of skin or white part of eyes; loss of appetite; nausea; dark or tea-colored urine; pain, aching, or tenderness on right side of abdomen; light-colored stools), or immune reconstitution syndrome (signs and symptoms of an infection, *Mycobacterium avium* infection, cytomegalovirus, *Pneumocystis jirovecii* pneumonia, tuberculosis) occur.
- Inform patient that redistribution and accumulation of body fat may occur, causing central obesity, dorsocervical fat enlargement (buffalo hump), peripheral wasting, breast enlargement, and cushingoid appearance. The cause and long-term effects are not known.
- Instruct patient to notify health care provider of all Rx or OTC medications, vitamins, or herbal products being taken and to consult health care provider before taking other Rx, OTC, or herbal products.
- Rep: Advise women of reproductive potential using hormonal contraceptives to use an alternative nonhormonal method of contraception. Advise patient to notify health care provider if pregnancy is planned or suspected. If pregnant patient is exposed to lamivudine, register patient in *Antiretroviral Pregnancy Registry* by calling 1-800-258-4263.
- Emphasize the importance of regular follow-up exams and blood tests to determine progress and monitor for side effects.

Evaluation/Desired Outcomes

- Slowing of the progression of HIV infection and its sequelae.
- Decrease in viral load and improvement in CD4 levels in patients with advanced HIV infection.
- Protection from liver damage caused by chronic hepatitis B infection; decrease in viral load.

lamoTRIgine (la-moe-tri-jeen)

LaMICtal, LaMICtal ODT, LaMICtal XR, Subvenite

Classification

Therapeutic: anticonvulsants

Indications

Adjunct treatment of partial seizures in adults and children with epilepsy (immediate-release, extended-release, chewable, and orally disintegrating tablets). Lennox-Gastaut syndrome (immediate-release, chewable, and orally disintegrating tablets only). Adjunct treatment of primary generalized tonic-clonic seizures in adults and children (immediate-release, extended-release, chewable, and orally disintegrating tablets). Conversion to monotherapy in adults with partial seizures receiving carbamazepine, phenytoin, phenobarbital, primidone, or valproate as the single antiepileptic drug (immediate-release, extended-release, chewable, and orally disintegrating tablets only). Maintenance treatment of bipolar disorder (immediate-release, chewable, and orally disintegrating tablets only).

Action

Stabilizes neuronal membranes by inhibiting sodium transport. **Therapeutic Effects:** Decreased incidence of seizures. Delayed time to recurrence of mood episodes in bipolar disorder.

Pharmacokinetics

Absorption: 98% absorbed following oral administration.

Distribution: Highly bound to melanin-containing tissues (eyes, pigmented skin).

Metabolism and Excretion: Mostly metabolized by the liver via glucuronidation to inactive metabolites; 10% excreted unchanged by the kidneys.

Half-life: *Children taking enzyme-inducing anticonvulsants:* 7–10 hr; *Children taking enzyme inducers and valproic acid:* 15–27 hr; *Children taking valproic acid:* 44–94 hr; *Adults:* 25.4 hr (during chronic therapy of lamotrigine alone).

TIME/ACTION PROFILE (plasma concentrations)

ROUTE	ONSET	PEAK	DURATION
PO	unknown	1.4–4.8 hr; 4–10 hr (XR)	unknown

Contraindications/Precautions

Contraindicated in: Hypersensitivity; Acute manic or mixed episodes; Second- or third-degree heart block, ventricular arrhythmias, ischemic heart disease, HF, valvular heart disease, congenital heart disease, or Brugada syndrome.

Use Cautiously in: All patients (may ↑ risk of suicidal thoughts/behaviors); Renal impairment (lower maintenance doses may be required); Hepatic impairment (lower maintenance doses may be required); Prior history of rash to lamotrigine; OB: Exposure during 1st trimester may ↑ risk of cleft lip/palate; Lactation: Use while breastfeeding only if potential maternal benefit justifies potential risk to infant; Pedi: Safety and effectiveness not established in children <13 yr

L

(extended-release tablets) and <2 yr (immediate-release, chewable, and orally disintegrating tablets).

Adverse Reactions/Side Effects

CV: arrhythmias, bradycardia, CARDIAC ARREST, heart block, QRS interval prolongation. **Derm:** photosensitivity, rash (higher incidence in children, patients taking valproic acid, high initial doses, or rapid dose ↑), DRUG REACTION WITH EOSINOPHILIA AND SYSTEMIC SYMPTOMS (DRESS), STEVENS-JOHNSON SYNDROME (SJS), TOXIC EPIDERMAL NECROLYSIS (TEN). **EENT:** blurred vision, double vision, rhinitis. **GI:** nausea, vomiting, HEPATIC FAILURE. **GU:** vaginitis. **Hemat:** HEMOPHAGOCYTIC LYMPHOHISTIOCYTOSIS. **MS:** arthralgia. **Neuro:** ataxia, dizziness, headache, ASEPTIC MENINGITIS, behavior changes, depression, drowsiness, insomnia, SUICIDAL THOUGHTS, tremor.

Interactions

Drug-Drug: May ↑ levels of an active metabolite of **carbamazepine**. Concurrent use with drugs that induce glucuronidation, including **phenobarbital, phenytoin, primidone, carbamazepine, estrogen-containing oral contraceptives, rifampin, lopinavir/ritonavir**, or **atazanavir/ritonavir** may ↓ levels and effectiveness; lamotrigine dose adjustments may be necessary when starting and stopping oral contraceptive or atazanavir/ritonavir therapy. Concurrent use with drugs that inhibit glucuronidation, including **valproic acid**, may ↑ levels and incidence of rash; may also ↓ valproic acid levels (↓ lamotrigine dose by ≥50%). **Amiodarone, disopyramide, dronedarone, flecainide, lidocaine, mexiletine, procainamide, propafenone**, or **quinidine** may ↑ risk of proarrhythmia; avoid concurrent use.

Route/Dosage

Epilepsy

In Combination with Other Antiepileptic Agents

PO (Adults and Children >12 yr; Immediate-Release, Chewable, or Orally Disintegrating Tablets): *Patients taking anticonvulsant drugs other than carbamazepine, phenobarbital, phenytoin, primidone, or valproate:* 25 mg once daily for 1st 2 wk, then 50 mg once daily for next 2 wk; then ↑ by 50 mg/day every 1–2 wk to maintenance dose of 225–375 mg/day (in 2 divided doses); *Patients taking carbamazepine, phenobarbital, phenytoin, or primidone (and not valproate):* 50 mg once daily for 1st 2 wk, then 50 mg twice daily for next 2 wk; then ↑ by 100 mg/day every 1–2 wk to maintenance dose of 300–500 mg/day (in 2 divided doses); *Patients taking regimen containing valproate:* 25 mg every other day for 1st 2 wk, then 25 mg once daily for next 2 wk; then ↑ by 25–50 mg/day every 1–2 wk to maintenance dose of 100–400 mg/day (in 1–2 divided doses) (maintenance dose of 100–200 mg/day if receiving valproate alone).

PO (Adults and Children ≥13 yr; Extended-Release Tablets): *Patients taking anticonvulsant drugs other than carbamazepine, phenobarbital, phenytoin, primidone, or valproate:* 25 mg once daily for 1st 2 wk, then 50 mg once daily for next 2 wk, then 100 mg once daily for 1 wk, then 150 mg once daily for 1 wk, then 200 mg once daily for 1 wk; then ↑ by 100 mg/day every wk to maintenance dose of 300–400 mg once daily; *Patients taking carbamazepine, phenobarbital, phenytoin, or primidone (and not valproate):* 50 mg once daily for 1st 2 wk, then 100 mg once daily for next 2 wk, then 200 mg once daily for 1 wk, then 300 mg once daily for 1 wk, then 400 mg once daily for 1 wk; then ↑ by 100 mg/day every wk to maintenance dose of 400–600 mg once daily; *Patients taking regimen containing valproate:* 25 mg every other day for 1st 2 wk, then 25 mg once daily for next 2 wk, then 50 mg once daily for 1 wk, then 100 mg once daily for 1 wk, then 150 mg once daily for 1 wk, then maintenance dose of 200–250 mg once daily.

PO (Children 2–12 yr; Immediate-Release, Chewable, or Orally Disintegrating Tablets): *Patients taking anticonvulsant drugs other than carbamazepine, phenobarbital, phenytoin, primidone, or valproate:* 0.3 mg/kg/day in 1–2 divided doses (rounded down to nearest whole tablet) for 1st 2 wk, then 0.6 mg/kg/day in 2 divided doses (rounded down to nearest whole tablet) for next 2 wk; then ↑ by 0.6 mg/kg/day (rounded down to nearest whole tablet) every 1–2 wk to maintenance dose of 4.5–7.5 mg/kg/day (not to exceed 300 mg/day in 2 divided doses); *Patients taking carbamazepine, phenobarbital, phenytoin, or primidone (and not valproate):* 0.6 mg/kg/day in 2 divided doses (rounded down to nearest whole tablet) for 1st 2 wk, then 1.2 mg/kg/day in 2 divided doses (rounded down to nearest whole tablet) for next 2 wk; then ↑ by 1.2 mg/kg/day (rounded down to nearest whole tablet) every 1–2 wk to maintenance dose of 5–15 mg/kg/day (not to exceed 400 mg/day in 2 divided doses). *Patients taking regimen containing valproate:* 0.15 mg/kg/day in 1–2 divided doses (rounded down to nearest whole tablet) for 1st 2 wk, then 0.3 mg/kg in 1–2 divided doses (rounded down to nearest whole tablet) for next 2 wk; then ↑ by 0.3 mg/kg/day (rounded down to nearest whole tablet) every 1–2 wk to maintenance dose of 1–5 mg/kg/day (not to exceed 200 mg/day in 1–2 divided doses) (maintenance dose of 1–3 mg/kg/day if receiving valproate alone).

Conversion to Monotherapy

PO (Adults and Children ≥16 yr; Immediate-Release, Chewable, or Orally Disintegrating Tablets): *Patients taking carbamazepine, phenobarbital, phenytoin, or primidone (and not valproate):* After achieving a dose of 500 mg/day (as per dosing guidelines above), ↓ dose of other antiepileptic by 20% weekly over 4 wk; *Patients taking regimen containing* *alproate:* After achieving a dose of 200 mg/day (as er dosing guidelines above), ↓ valproate dose by 00 mg/day on a weekly basis until a dose of 500 mg/ ay is achieved. Maintain the valproate dose of 500 mg/ ay and the lamotrigine dose of 500 mg/day for 1 wk. hen ↑ lamotrigine dose to 300 mg/day and ↓ valproate ose to 250 mg/day, and maintain these doses for 1 wk. hen discontinue valproate and ↑ lamotrigine dose by 00 mg/day every wk until maintenance dose of 500 mg/ ay is achieved.

O (Adults and Children ≥13 yr; Extended- elease Tablets): *Patients taking carbamazepine, henobarbital, phenytoin, or primidone (and not alproate):* After achieving a dose of 500 mg/day (as per osing guidelines above), ↓ dose of other antiepileptic y 20% weekly over 4 wk. 2 wk later, ↓ dose of lamo- igine by 100 mg/day every wk to achieve maintenance ose of 250–300 mg/day; *Patients taking regimen ontaining valproate:* After achieving a dose of 150 mg/ ay (as per dosing guidelines above), ↓ valproate dose y 500 mg/day on a weekly basis until a dose of 500 mg/ ay is achieved. Maintain the valproate dose of 500 mg/ ay and the lamotrigine dose of 150 mg/day for 1 wk. hen ↑ lamotrigine dose to 200 mg/day and ↓ valproate ose to 250 mg/day, and maintain these doses for 1 wk. hen discontinue valproate and ↑ lamotrigine dose 250–300 mg/day; *Patients taking anticonvulsant rugs other than carbamazepine, phenobarbital, phe- ytoin, primidone, or valproate:* After achieving a dose f 250–300 mg/day (as per dosing guidelines above), ↓ ose of other antiepileptic by 20% weekly over 4 wk.

ipolar Disorder

scalation Regimen

O (Adults Immediate-Release, Chewable, or rally Disintegrating Tablets): *Patients not taking arbamazepine, phenobarbital, phenytoin, primi- one, rifampin, or valproate:* 25 mg once daily for 1st wk, then 50 mg once daily for next 2 wk, then 100 mg nce daily for 1 wk, then 200 mg once daily; *Patients aking valproate:* 25 mg every other day for first 2 wk, en 25 mg once daily for next 2 wk, then 50 mg once aily for 1 wk, then 100 mg once daily; *Patients taking arbamazepine, phenobarbital, phenytoin, primi- one, or rifampin (and not valproate):* 50 mg once aily for 1st 2 wk, then 100 mg/day (in divided doses) r next 2 wk, then 200 mg/day (in divided doses) for ne wk, then 300 mg/day (in divided doses) for 1 wk, en up to 400 mg/day (in divided doses).

osage Adjustment Following iscontinuation of Other Psychotropics

O (Adults Immediate-Release, Chewable, or rally Disintegrating Tablets): *Following discon- nuation of valproate (if current dose 100 mg/day):* ↑ to 150 mg/day for 1 wk, then 200 mg/day; *Following discontinuation of carbamazepine, phenobarbital, phenytoin, primidone, or rifampin (if current dose 400 mg/day):* 400 mg/day for 1 wk, then 300 mg/day for 1 wk, then 200 mg/day; *Following discontinuation of other psychotropics:* maintain previous dose.

Availability (generic available)

Immediate-release tablets: 25 mg, 100 mg, 150 mg, 200 mg. **Extended-release tablets:** 25 mg, 50 mg, 100 mg, 200 mg, 250 mg, 300 mg. **Orally disintegrating tablets:** 25 mg, 50 mg, 100 mg, 200 mg. **Tablets for oral suspension (berry flavor):** 5 mg, 25 mg.

NURSING IMPLICATIONS

Assessment

- Monitor closely for changes in behavior that could indicate the emergence or worsening of suicidal thoughts or behavior or depression.
- Monitor for severe cutaneous adverse reactions, including SJS and TEN. Frequently assess for progressive rash or symptoms such as fever, malaise, lymphadenopathy, joint/muscle pain, blisters, oral lesions, and conjunctivitis. Discontinue lamotrigine at the 1st sign of rash, as SJS/TEN may be life-threatening. Risk is highest within the first 2–8 wk. Risk factors include valproate coadministration, exceeding initial dose, or rapid titration. While benign rashes occur, severity is unpredictable; discontinue lamotrigine unless rash is clearly unrelated. Pedi: Serious rashes, including fatal cases, are more common in pediatric patients.
- Monitor for signs and symptoms of multiorgan hypersensitivity reactions: DRESS (rash, fever, lymphadenopathy). May be associated with other organ involvement (hepatitis, hepatic failure, blood dyscrasias, acute multiorgan failure). If cause cannot be determined, discontinue lamotrigine immediately.
- **Seizures:** Assess location, duration, and characteristics of seizure activity. Institute seizure precautions as indicated.
- **Bipolar disorders:** Assess mood, ideation, and behaviors frequently. Initiate suicide precautions if indicated.

Lab Test Considerations

- Lamotrigine plasma concentrations may be monitored periodically during therapy, especially in patients concurrently taking other anticonvulsants. Therapeutic plasma concentration range include: *Seizures:* 2.5–15 mcg/mL; *Treatment-resistant depression:* 3.25–15 mcg/mL.
- May cause false-positive results for phencyclidine in some rapid urine drug screens. Use a more specific analytical method to confirm results.

Implementation

- Do not confuse lamotrigine with labetalol, lamivudine, levetiracetam, or levothyroxine. Do not confuse Lamictal with labetalol.
- When converting from immediate-release to XR form, initial dose of XR should match the total daily dose of immediate-release lamotrigine; monitor closely and adjust as needed.
- **PO:** May be administered without regard to meals. *DNC:* Swallow XR tablets whole; do not break, crush, or chew.
- Lamotrigine should be discontinued gradually over ≥2 wk, unless safety concerns require a more rapid withdrawal. Abrupt discontinuation may cause increase in seizure frequency.
- **chewable:** May be swallowed whole, chewed, or dispersed in 5 mL of water or fruit juice. If dispersed, wait 1 min and swirl; then administer immediately. If chewed, follow with water or fruit juice to aid in swallowing. Only use whole tablets; do not attempt to administer partial quantities of dispersible tablets.
- **Orally Disintegrating Tablets:** Place on the tongue and move around the mouth. Tablet will rapidly disintegrate; can be swallowed with or without water, and can be taken with or without food.

Patient/Family Teaching

- Explain the purpose and side effects of lamotrigine. Instruct patient to take as directed. Take missed doses as soon as possible unless almost time for next dose. Do not double doses. Do not discontinue abruptly; may cause increase in frequency of seizures. Instruct patient to read the *Medication Guide* before starting and with each Rx refill, changes may occur.
- Advise patient to notify health care provider immediately if skin rash, fever, or swollen lymph glands occur or if frequency of seizures increases.
- May cause dizziness, drowsiness, and blurred vision. Caution patient to avoid driving or activities requiring alertness until response to medication is known. Do not resume driving until physician gives clearance based on control of seizure disorder.
- Caution patient to wear sunscreen and protective clothing to prevent photosensitivity reactions.
- Advise patient and family to notify health care provider if thoughts about suicide or dying, attempts to commit suicide, new or worse depression, new or worse anxiety, feeling very agitated or restless, panic attacks, trouble sleeping, new or worse irritability, acting aggressive, being angry or violent, acting on dangerous impulses, an extreme ↑ in activity and talking, or other unusual changes in behavior or mood occur or if symptoms of aseptic meningitis (headache, fever, nausea, vomiting, nuchal rigidity, rash, photophobia, myalgia, chills, altered consciousness, somnolence) or cardiac symptoms (fast, slow, or pounding heartbeat; heart skipping beats; shortness of breath; chest pain; feeling light-headed) occur.
- Advise patient to notify health care provider of all Rx or OTC medications, vitamins, or herbal products being taken and to consult with health care provider before taking other medications.
- Instruct patient to notify health care provider of medication regimen prior to treatment or surgery.
- Medical ID describing disease process and medication regimen should be worn at all times in case of emergencies.
- Advise patient to notify health care provider immediately if signs and symptoms of hemophagocytic lymphohistiocytosis (fever, hepatosplenomegaly, rash, lymphadenopathy, neurologic symptoms, cytopenias, ↑ serum ferritin, hypertriglyceridemia liver function, coagulation abnormalities) occur. Symptoms usually occur between 8 and 24 days. May be fatal.
- Rep: Advise women of reproductive potential to use a nonhormonal form of contraception while taking lamotrigine, avoid breastfeeding, and notify health care provider if pregnancy is planned or suspected. Encourage patients who become pregnant to enroll in the North American Antiepileptic Drug Pregnancy Registry. Must be done by patients themselves by calling 1-888-233-2334 or visiting http://www.aedpregnancyregistry.org. Enrollment in the registry must be done prior to any prenatal diagnostic tests and before fetal outcome is known.
- Rep: *Seizure Disorder Pregnancy Monitoring and Dosage Adjustments:* Optimally establish a therapeutic baseline prior to pregnancy. Due to the possibility of ↑ lamotrigine clearance during pregnancy, monitor plasma concentrations approximately every 4 wk. If plasma concentration falls below an established therapeutic baseline, ↑ dose by 20– 25% and recheck plasma concentration after 4–5 wk. *After Pregnancy:* Measure plasma concentration within the 1st wk after birth If there is no ↑ in plasma concentration, recheck after 1–2 wk. If plasma concentration is higher than therapeutic baseline, ↓ dose by 20–25%, and recheck plasma concentration every 1–2 wk until stable at therapeutic baseline. In patients who had ≥3–4 dose ↑ during pregnancy, ↓ dose by 20–25% on the 1st days after birth. Thereafter, if the plasma concentration is higher than the established therapeutic baseline, ↓ dose by 20–25%, and recheck plasma concentration every 1–2 wk until stable at baseline.

Evaluation/Desired Outcomes

- Decrease in the frequency of or cessation of seizures
- Delay in time to occurrence of mood episodes (depression, mania, hypomania, mixed episodes) in patients with bipolar I disorder.

lanadelumab
(lan-a-del-ue-mab)
Takhzyro

Classification
Therapeutic: antiangioedema agents
Pharmacologic: kallikrein inhibitors, monoclonal antibodies

ndications
revention of hereditary angioedema attacks.

ction
cts as a selective, reversible inhibitor of kallikrein, ereby inhibiting its action in initiating bradykinin roduction, part of the cascade of events in hereditary ngioedema. **Therapeutic Effects:** Reduction in umber of hereditary angioedema attacks.

harmacokinetics
bsorption: Well absorbed following SUBQ admintration.
istribution: Well distributed to tissues.
etabolism and Excretion: Unknown.
alf-life: 14–15 days.

IME/ACTION PROFILE (plasma oncentrations)

OUTE	ONSET	PEAK	DURATION
JBQ	unknown	4–5 days	unknown

ontraindications/Precautions
ontraindicated in: OB: Pregnancy.
se Cautiously in: Lactation: Use while breasteding only if potential maternal benefit justifies otential risk to infant; Pedi: Children <2 yr (safety nd effectiveness not established).

dverse Reactions/Side Effects
erm: rash. **GI:** diarrhea, ↑ liver enzymes. **Local:** jection site reactions. **Neuro:** headache, dizziness. **esp:** upper respiratory infection. **MS:** myalgia. **isc:** HYPERSENSITIVITY REACTIONS (INCLUDING ANAPHYXIS).

teractions
rug-Drug: None reported.

oute/Dosage
UBQ (Adults and Children ≥12 yr): 300 mg every wk. If patient has been free of attacks for >6 mo, can ljust regimen to 300 mg every 4 wk.
UBQ (Children 6–<12 yr): 150 mg every 2 wk. If tient has been free of attacks for >6 mo, can adjust gimen to 150 mg every 4 wk.
SUBQ (Children 2–<6 yr): 150 mg every 4 wk.

Availability
Solution for injection (prefilled syringes): 150 mg/mL.

NURSING IMPLICATIONS

Assessment
- Assess for signs (facial, laryngeal, or abdominal swelling; dyspnea; pain; nausea; vomiting; cramps; diarrhea) and frequency of hereditary angioedema attacks.
- Monitor for signs and symptoms of hypersensitivity reactions (rash, urticaria, pruritus, flushing, dizziness, vomiting, abdominal pain) and angioedema (swelling of throat, lips, tongue, or face; dyspnea; wheezing; hoarseness) during or after injection. Discontinue immediately and provide supportive care.

Implementation
- **SUBQ:** Remove prefilled syringe from refrigerator 15 min before injecting to allow to warm to room temperature. Do not shake prefilled syringe. Inject dose slowly into abdomen, thigh, or upper arm over 10–60 sec. Discard unused portion of prefilled syringe.

Patient/Family Teaching
- Explain the purpose and side effects of lanadelumab to patient. Do not stop receiving drug without consulting health care professional. May be administered by patient or caregiver to adults and children ≥12 yr; should be administered by health care professional or caregiver in children 2–<12 yr. Instruct patient or caregiver in correct technique for injection, storage, and place to discard syringes and needles. Advise patient to read *Patient Information* before starting and with each Rx refill in case of changes.
- Advise patient to notify health care professional immediately if signs and symptoms of hypersensitivity reaction occur (rash, hives, itchiness, flushing, dizziness, vomiting, abdominal pain). If angioedema occurs (swelling of throat, lips, tongue, or face; trouble breathing; wheezing; hoarseness), notify health care professional and call 911 immediately.
- May cause dizziness. Caution patient to avoid driving or other activities requiring alertness until response to medication is known.
- Rep: Advise patient to notify health care professional if pregnancy is planned or suspected or if breastfeeding.

Evaluation/Desired Outcomes
- Decrease in frequency, intensity, and duration of symptoms of hereditary angioedema attacks.

L

BEERS

lansoprazole (lan-soe-pra-zole)

Prevacid, ~~Prevacid 24 Hr~~, Prevacid SoluTab

Classification

Therapeutic: antiulcer agents

Pharmacologic: proton-pump inhibitors

Indications

Erosive esophagitis. Duodenal ulcers (with or without anti-infectives for *Helicobacter pylori*). Active benign gastric ulcer. Short-term treatment of symptomatic GERD. Healing and risk reduction of NSAID-associated gastric ulcer. Pathologic hypersecretory conditions, including Zollinger-Ellison syndrome. **OTC:** Heartburn occurring at least twice per week.

Action

Binds to an enzyme in the presence of acidic gastric pH, preventing the final transport of hydrogen ions into the gastric lumen. **Therapeutic Effects:** Diminished accumulation of acid in the gastric lumen, with lessened acid reflux. Healing of duodenal ulcers and esophagitis.

Pharmacokinetics

Absorption: 80% absorbed after oral administration.
Distribution: Unknown.
Protein Binding: 97%.
Metabolism and Excretion: Extensively metabolized by the liver to inactive compounds. Converted intracellularly to at least two other antisecretory compounds.
Half-life: *Children:* 1.2–1.5 hr; *Adults:* 1.3–1.7 hr (↑ in older adults and patients with hepatic impairment).

TIME/ACTION PROFILE (acid suppression)

ROUTE	ONSET	PEAK	DURATION
PO	rapid	1.7 hr	>24 hr

Contraindications/Precautions

Contraindicated in: Hypersensitivity to lansoprazole or related drugs (benzimidazoles); Concurrent use of rilpivirine-containing products.
Use Cautiously in: Phenylketonuria (solutabs contain aspartame); Severe hepatic impairment (do not exceed 30 mg/day); Patients using high doses for >1 yr (↑ risk of hip, wrist, or spine fractures and fundic gland polyps); Patients using therapy for >3 yr (↑ risk of vitamin B_{12} deficiency); Pre-existing risk of hypocalcemia; Lactation: Safety not established in breastfeeding; Pedi: Children <1 yr (↑ risk of heart valve thickening); Geri: Appears on Beers list. ↑ risk of *Clostridioides difficile* infection, pneumonia, GI malignancies, bone loss, and fractures in older adults. Avoid scheduled use for >8 wk in older adults unless for high-risk patients (e.g., oral corticosteroid or chronic NSAID use) or patients with erosive esophagitis, Barrett esophagitis, pathological hypersecretory condition, or demonstrated need for maintenance therapy (e.g., failure of H_2 antagonist).

Adverse Reactions/Side Effects

Derm: ACUTE GENERALIZED EXANTHEMATOUS PUSTULOSIS, cutaneous lupus erythematosus, DRUG REACTION WITH EOSINOPHILIA AND SYSTEMIC SYMPTOMS (DRESS), rash, STEVENS-JOHNSON SYNDROME (SJS), TOXIC EPIDERMAL NECROLYSIS (TEN). **F and E:** hypocalcemia (especially if treatment duration ≥3 mo), hypokalemia (especially if treatment duration ≥3 mo), hypomagnesemia (especially if treatment duration ≥3 mo). **GI:** diarrhea, abdominal pain, CLOSTRIDIOIDES DIFFICILE-ASSOCIATED DIARRHEA (CDAD), fundic gland polyps, nausea. **GU:** acute tubulointerstitial nephritis. **Hemat:** vitamin B_{12} deficiency. **MS:** bone fracture. **Neuro:** dizziness, headache. **Misc:** HYPERSENSITIVITY REACTIONS (INCLUDING ANAPHYLAXIS, ANGIOEDEMA, OR ACUTE TUBULOINTERSTITIAL NEPHRITIS), systemic lupus erythematosus.

Interactions

Drug-Drug: May ↓ **rilpivirine** levels and ↑ risk of resistance; concurrent use contraindicated. **Sucralfate** ↓ absorption of lansoprazole; take 30 min before sucralfate. May ↓ absorption of drugs requiring acid pH including **ketoconazole**, **itraconazole**, **atazanavir**, **nelfinavir**, **ampicillin esters**, **iron salts**, **erlotinib**, and **mycophenolate mofetil**; avoid concurrent use with **atazanavir** and **nelfinavir**.
May ↑ levels and risk of toxicity of **digoxin**, **tacrolimus**, and **methotrexate**. May ↑ risk of bleeding with **warfarin**; monitor INR/PT. Hypomagnesemia and hypokalemia ↑ risk of **digoxin** toxicity.

Route/Dosage

Erosive Esophagitis

PO (Adults): *Short-term treatment:* 30 mg once daily for up to 8 wk (8 additional wk may be necessary); *Maintenance of healing:* 15 mg once daily.
PO (Children 12–17 yr): 30 mg once daily for up to 8 wk.
PO (Children 1–11 yr and >30 kg): 30 mg once daily for up to 12 wk.
PO (Children 1–11 yr and ≤30 kg): 15 mg once daily for up to 12 wk.

Duodenal Ulcer

PO (Adults): *Short-term treatment:* 15 mg once daily for 4 wk; *H. pylori eradication to ↓ risk of duodenal ulcer recurrence:* 30 mg twice daily with clarithromycin 500 mg twice daily and amoxicillin 1000 mg twice daily for 10–14 days (triple therapy) or 30 mg 3 times daily with 1000 mg amoxicillin 3 times daily for 14 days (dual therapy); *Maintenance of healed duodenal ulcers:* 15 mg once daily.

Gastric Ulcer
PO (Adults): *Short-term treatment of gastric ulcers/healing of NSAID-associated gastric ulcer:* 30 mg once daily for up to 8 wk; *Risk ↓ of NSAID-associated gastric ulcer:* 15 mg once daily for up to 12 wk.

GERD
PO (Adults): *Short-term treatment:* 15 mg once daily for up to 8 wk.
PO (Children 12–17 yr): 15 mg once daily for up to 8 wk.
PO (Children 1–11 yr and >30 kg): 30 mg once daily for up to 12 wk.
PO (Children 1–11 yr and ≤30 kg): 15 mg once daily for up to 12 wk.

Pathologic Hypersecretory Conditions
PO (Adults): 60 mg once daily initially, up to 90 mg twice daily (daily dose >120 mg should be given in divided doses).

Heartburn (OTC Use)
PO (Adults): *OTC:* 15 mg once daily for up to 14 days (14 day course may be repeated every 4 mo).

Availability (generic available)
Delayed-release capsules: 15 mg[Rx, OTC], 30 mg. **Delayed-release orally disintegrated tablets (SoluTabs):** 15 mg[Rx, OTC], 30 mg. ***In combination with:*** amoxicillin and clarithromycin as part of a compliance package (Prevpac). See Appendix N.

NURSING IMPLICATIONS
Assessment
- Monitor for positive response after therapy is complete. *If response is suboptimal or early symptomatic relapse occurs,* consider diagnostic testing for gastric malignancy, including endoscopy.
- Monitor for diarrhea, abdominal pain, fever, and bloody stools, especially in hospitalized patients. *If diarrhea occurs and does not improve,* evaluate for CDAD.
- Monitor for acute tubulointerstitial nephritis (↓ renal function, malaise, nausea, anorexia, fever, rash, arthralgias) periodically during therapy. *If signs or symptoms occur,* discontinue lansoprazole and evaluate.
- Monitor for severe cutaneous adverse reactions (SJS, TEN, DRESS). Discontinue lansoprazole at 1st sign of severe skin reactions and consider further evaluation.
- Assess for new signs and symptoms or exacerbation of cutaneous and systemic lupus erythematosus. *If signs or exacerbation occur,* discontinue lansoprazole and refer to specialist for evaluation.

Lab Test Considerations
- May ↑ AST, ALT, alkaline phosphatase, LDH, and bilirubin.
- May ↑ serum creatinine and ↓ potassium and magnesium levels.
- May alter RBCs, WBCs, and platelets.
- May ↑ gastrin levels, abnormal A/G ratio, hyperlipidemia, and ↑ or ↓ cholesterol.
- Monitor INR and prothrombin time in patients taking warfarin.
- May cause vitamin B_{12} deficiency with long-term use (>3 yr).
- May ↑ serum chromogranin levels, which may interfere with diagnosis of neuroendocrine tumors.

Implementation
- **PO:** *Delayed-release capsules:* Administer before meals. ***DNC:*** Swallow whole; do not crush or chew capsule contents. Capsules may be opened and intact granules may be sprinkled on 1 tablespoon of soft food, including applesauce, and swallowed immediately. Capsules may be opened and intact granules may be mixed in a small volume of either apple juice, orange juice, or tomato juice (60 mL/2 ounces); administer immediately.
- For patients with a nasogastric (NG) tube, capsules may be opened and intact granules may be mixed in 40 mL of apple juice and injected through the NG tube into stomach. Flush NG tube with additional apple juice to clear tube.
- *Orally disintegrating tablets* may be placed on tongue, allowed to disintegrate, and swallowed with or without water. Do not cut or break tablet. For administration via oral syringe or NG tube, *Prevacid SoluTab* can be administered by placing a 15-mg tablet in oral syringe and drawing up 4 mL of water or a 30-mg tablet in oral syringe and drawing up 10 mL of water. Shake gently to allow for a quick dispersal. After tablet has dispersed, administer the contents within 15 min. Refill syringe with 2 mL (5 mL for the 30-mg tablet) of water, shake gently, and administer any remaining contents; then flush NG tube.
- Antacids may be used concurrently.
- Use for shortest time possible to ↓ risk of osteoporosis-related fractures, cutaneous or systemic lupus erythematosus, vitamin B_{12} deficiency, and fundic gland polyps.

Patient/Family Teaching
- Explain purpose and side effects of medication. Advise patient to read *Patient Information* before starting therapy.
- Instruct patient to take missed dose as soon as remembered but not if just before next scheduled dose; do not double doses.
- May occasionally cause dizziness. Caution patient to avoid driving and other activities that require alertness until response to medication is known.

L

- Advise patient to avoid alcohol, products containing aspirin or NSAIDs, and foods that may cause an ↑ in GI irritation.
- Advise patient to report onset of black, tarry stools; diarrhea; or abdominal pain to health care provider promptly. Instruct patient to notify health care provider immediately if rash, diarrhea, abdominal cramping, fever, or bloody stools occur and not to treat with antidiarrheals without consulting health care provider.
- Instruct patient to notify health care provider of all Rx or OTC medications, vitamins, or herbal products being taken and consult health care provider before taking any new medications.
- Advise patient to notify health care provider if signs and symptoms of hypomagnesemia (seizure, dizziness, abnormal or fast heartbeat, jitteriness, jerking movements or shaking, muscle weakness, spasms of hands and feet, muscle aches, voice box spasm) occur.
- Rep: Advise women of reproductive potential to notify health care provider if pregnancy is planned or suspected or if breastfeeding.

Evaluation/Desired Outcomes

- Decrease in abdominal pain or prevention of gastric irritation and bleeding. Healing of duodenal ulcers can be seen on x-ray examination or endoscopy. Therapy for pathologic hypersecretory conditions may be long term.
- Healing in patients with erosive esophagitis.

lanthanum (lan-than-um)

Fosrenol

Classification

Therapeutic: hypophosphatemics

Pharmacologic: phosphate binders

Indications

Hyperphosphatemia in end-stage kidney disease.

Action

Dissociates in the upper GI tract, forming lanthanate ions, which form an insoluble complex with phosphate. **Therapeutic Effects:** Decreased serum phosphate levels.

Pharmacokinetics

Absorption: Negligible absorption.

Distribution: Stays within the GI tract.

Metabolism and Excretion: Eliminated almost entirely in feces.

Half-life: 53 hr (in plasma).

TIME/ACTION PROFILE (effect on phosphate levels)

ROUTE	ONSET	PEAK	DURATION
PO	unknown	2–3 wk	unknown

Contraindications/Precautions

Contraindicated in: Hypersensitivity; Bowel obstruction; Ileus; Fecal impaction; OB: Pregnancy; Lactation: Lactation; Pedi: Use in children not recommended (potential negative effect on developing bone).

Use Cautiously in: Patients with risk factors for GI obstruction or perforation, including history of GI surgery, colon cancer, GI ulceration, diverticular disease, peritonitis, constipation, ileus, diabetic gastroparesis, or taking medications that cause constipation.

Adverse Reactions/Side Effects

F and E: hypocalcemia. **GI:** <u>nausea</u>, <u>vomiting</u>, diarrhea, fecal impaction, GI obstruction, GI perforation, ileus.

Interactions

Drug-Drug: May ↓ absorption of **fluoroquinolones**, **tetracyclines**, and **levothyroxine**; administer ≥1 hr before or 3 hr after lanthanum.

Route/Dosage

PO (Adults): 1500 mg/day in divided doses; may be titrated upward every 2–3 wk in increments of 750 mg/day up to 4500 mg/day (usual range 1500–3000 mg/day).

Availability (generic available)

Chewable tablets: 🍁 250 mg, 500 mg, 750 mg, 1000 mg. **Oral powder:** 750 mg/pkt, 1000 mg/pkt.

NURSING IMPLICATIONS

Assessment

- Assess for GI adverse reactions (GI obstruction, ileus, subileus, GI perforation, fecal impaction). May require discontinuation of therapy in patients without another explanation for severe GI symptoms.
- Assess for nausea and vomiting during therapy.

Lab Test Considerations

- Monitor serum phosphate levels prior to and periodically during therapy.

Implementation

- Do not confuse lanthanum carbonate with lithium carbonate.
- Divide total daily dose and administer with meals.
- May bind with other orally administered drugs; consider separating the administration of other oral medications.
- **PO:** Administer with or immediately after meals. Tablets should be crushed or chewed completely before swallowing; intact tablets should not be swallowed.
- Sprinkle powder on small quantity of applesauce or other similar food; consume immediately. Consider powder formulation for patients with poor dentition or who have difficulty chewing tablets.

Patient/Family Teaching

- Educate patient on reason for lanthanum and side effects. Instruct patient to take lanthanum as directed. Do not swallow intact tablets. Do not premix future powder doses, open packet in advance, or attempt to mix with liquids. Discuss need to separate the administration of other oral medications with health care provider. Advise patient to read *Patient Information* before starting therapy and with each Rx refill in case of changes.
- Advise patient to take antacids or thyroid medicine (levothyroxine) 2 hr before or after lanthanum carbonate and antibiotics 1 hr before or 4 hr after lanthanum carbonate.
- Advise patient to notify health care professional of all Rx or OTC medications, vitamins, or herbal products being taken and to consult with health care professional before taking other medications.
- Advise patient to notify health care professional of medication regimen before an abdominal x-ray or if they have a history of GI disease.
- Rep: May cause fetal harm. Advise women of reproductive potential to notify health care professional if pregnancy is planned or suspected and to avoid breastfeeding during therapy.

Evaluation/Desired Outcomes

- Decrease in serum phosphate to below 6 mg/dL in patients with end-stage renal disease.

HIGH ALERT

☒ lapatinib (la-pat-i-nib)
Tykerb

Classification
Therapeutic: antineoplastics
Pharmacologic: enzyme inhibitors kinase inhibitors

Indications

☒ Advanced or metastatic breast cancer with tumor overexpression of the human epidermal receptor type 2 (HER2) and past therapy with an anthracycline, a taxane, and trastuzumab (in combination with capecitabine). ☒ Hormone-receptor positive metastatic breast cancer that overexpresses HER2 in postmenopausal women for whom hormonal therapy is indicated (in combination with letrozole).

Action

☒ Acts as an inhibitor of intracellular tyrosine kinase, affecting epidermal growth factor (EGFR, ErbB1) and HER2 (ErbB2). Inhibits the growth of ErbB-driven tumors. Effect is additive with capecitabine. **Therapeutic Effects:** Decreased/slowed spread of metastatic breast cancer.

Pharmacokinetics

Absorption: Incompletely and variably absorbed following oral administration; levels ↑ by food.
Distribution: Unknown.
Protein Binding: >99%.
Metabolism and Excretion: Extensively metabolized by the liver via the CYP3A4 and CYP3A5 isoenzymes; <2% excreted by kidneys.
Half-life: 24 hr.

TIME/ACTION PROFILE (plasma concentrations)

ROUTE	ONSET	PEAK	DURATION
PO	unknown	4 hr	24 hr

Contraindications/Precautions

Contraindicated in: Hypersensitivity; ↓ left ventricular ejection fraction (LVEF) (Grade ≥2); OB: Pregnancy; Lactation: Lactation.
Use Cautiously in: Severe hepatic impairment (dose ↓ recommended); Known QTc interval prolongation or coexisting risk factors for QTc interval prolongation including hypokalemia, hypomagnesemia, concurrent antiarrhythmics, or medications that are known to prolong the QTc interval; Rep: Women of reproductive potential and men with female partners of reproductive potential; Pedi: Safety and effectiveness not established in children; Geri: Older adults may be more sensitive to effects.

Adverse Reactions/Side Effects

CV: ↓ LVEF, QT interval prolongation. **Derm:** palmar-plantar erythrodysesthesia, rash, dry skin, ERYTHEMA MULTIFORM (EM), nail disorders, STEVENS-JOHNSON SYNDROME (SJS), TOXIC EPIDERMAL NECROLYSIS (TEN). **GI:** nausea, vomiting, ↑ liver enzymes, DIARRHEA, dyspepsia, HEPATOTOXICITY, stomatitis. **Hemat:** neutropenia. **MS:** pain. **Neuro:** fatigue, insomnia. **Resp:** dyspnea, INTERSTITIAL LUNG DISEASE (ILD).

Interactions

Drug-Drug: May ↑ effects of **midazolam, paclitaxel**, and **digoxin**. **Strong CYP3A4 inhibitors**, including **ketoconazole, itraconazole, clarithromycin, atazanavir, nefazodone, nelfinavir, ritonavir**, and **voriconazole**, may ↑ levels and risk of toxicity; avoid concurrent use; if concurrent use unavoidable, ↓ lapatinib dose. **Strong CYP3A4 inducers**, including **dexamethasone, phenytoin, carbamazepine, rifampin, rifabutin, rifapentin**, and **phenobarbital**, may ↓ levels and effectiveness; avoid concurrent use; if concurrent use unavoidable, ↑ lapatinib dose.
Drug-Natural Products: St. John's wort may ↓ levels and effectiveness; avoid concurrent use; if concurrent use unavoidable, ↑ lapatinib dose.

☀ = Canadian drug name. ☒ = Genetic implication. **V** = Vesicant. Boxed warning.
~~Strikethrough~~ = Discontinued. *CAPITALS = life-threatening. Underline = most frequent.

L

Drug-Food: Grapefruit juice may ↑ levels and risk of toxicity; avoid concurrent use.

Route/Dosage

HER2-Positive Metastatic Breast Cancer (Past Therapy with an Anthracycline, a Taxane and Trastuzumab)

PO (Adults): 1250 mg once daily on Days 1–21 of 21-day cycle; continue until disease progression or unacceptable toxicity; *Concurrent use of strong CYP3A4 inhibitors:* 500 mg once daily on Days 1–21 of 21-day cycle; continue until disease progression or unacceptable toxicity; *Concurrent use of strong CYP3A4 inducers:* Gradually titrate dose from 1250 mg once daily up to 4500 mg once daily as tolerated; administer dose on Days 1–21 of 21-day cycle and continue until disease progression or unacceptable toxicity.

Hepatic Impairment

PO (Adults): *Severe hepatic impairment:* 750 mg once daily on Days 1–21 of 21-day cycle; continue until disease progression or unacceptable toxicity.

Hormone Receptor-Positive, HER2-Positive Metastatic Breast Cancer (Hormone Therapy Indicated)

PO (Adults): 1500 mg once daily on Days 1–21 of 21-day cycle; continue until disease progression or unacceptable toxicity; *Concurrent use of strong CYP3A4 inhibitors:* 500 mg once daily on Days 1–21 of 21-day cycle; continue until disease progression or unacceptable toxicity; *Concurrent use of strong CYP3A4 inducers:* Gradually titrate dose from 1500 mg once daily up to 5500 mg once daily as tolerated; administer dose on Days 1–21 of 21-day cycle and continue until disease progression or unacceptable toxicity.

Hepatic Impairment

PO (Adults): *Severe hepatic impairment:* 1000 mg once daily on Days 1–21 of 21-day cycle; continue until disease progression or unacceptable toxicity.

Availability (generic available)

Tablets: 250 mg.

NURSING IMPLICATIONS

Assessment

- Evaluate LVEF before and periodically during therapy. *If LVEF ↓ to Grade ≥2,* discontinue therapy. If asymptomatic and LVEF returns to normal after 2 wk, resume therapy at ↓ dose of 1000 mg/day (with capecitabine) or 1250 mg/day (with letrozole).
- Monitor for diarrhea; usually occurs within first 6 days of therapy and lasts 4–5 days. *If Grade 3 or Grades 1–2 diarrhea with complicating factors occurs,* hold therapy until Grade ≤1; may resume at ↓ dose from 1500 mg/day to 1250 mg/day or from 1250 mg/day to 1000 mg/day. *If Grade 4 diarrhea occurs,* permanently discontinue lapatinib.
- Monitor ECG during therapy to assess QTc interval in patients who have or may develop QTc interval prolongation (hypokalemia, hypomagnesemia, congenital long QT syndrome, antiarrhythmics, cumulative high-dose anthracyclines).
- Monitor respiratory status. *If Grade ≥3 ILD or pneumonitis occurs,* discontinue lapatinib.
- Monitor for signs and symptoms of skin reactions (progressive rash, blisters, mucosal lesions). *If EM, SJS, or TEN suspected,* discontinue lapatinib.

Lab Test Considerations

- Verify negative pregnancy test before starting therapy. Monitor liver enzymes before starting therapy, every 4–6 wk during therapy, and then as clinically indicated. If severe hepatic toxicity occurs during therapy, permanently discontinue lapatinib. Hepatotoxicity may occur days to several months after initiation of treatment.
- Monitor serum potassium and magnesium before starting and periodically during therapy.

Implementation

- Correct hypokalemia and hypomagnesemia before starting therapy.
- **PO:** Administer ≥1 hr before or 1 hr after a meal. Do not divide daily dose.

Patient/Family Teaching

- Explain purpose and side effects of medication. Advise patient to read *Patient Information* before starting therapy. If a dose is missed, take as soon as remembered that day. If a day is missed, omit; do not double doses.
- Advise patient to avoid drinking grapefruit juice or eating grapefruit during therapy.
- Advise patient to notify health care provider if symptoms of ↓ LVEF (shortness of breath, palpitations, fatigue) or rash occur.
- Advise patient to notify health care provider of all Rx or OTC medications, vitamins, or herbal products being taken and to consult health care provider before taking other medications, especially St. John's wort.
- Advise patient that lapatinib may cause diarrhea, which may become severe. Instruct patient in how to prevent and manage diarrhea and to notify health care provider if severe.
- Rep: May cause fetal harm. Advise women of reproductive potential and men with female partners of reproductive potential to use effective contraception during therapy and for 1 wk after last dose and to avoid breastfeeding for 1 wk after last dose. Advise patient to notify health care provider if pregnancy is planned or suspected.

Evaluation/Desired Outcomes

- Decreased/slowed spread of metastatic breast cancer.

HIGH ALERT

lazertinib (laz-er-ti-nib)

Lazcluze

Classification

Therapeutic: antineoplastics

Pharmacologic: kinase inhibitors

Indications

First-line treatment of locally advanced or metastatic non-small cell lung cancer (NSCLC) with epidermal growth factor receptor (EGFR) exon 19 deletions or exon 21 L858R substitution mutations (in combination with amivantamab).

Action

Acts as a kinase inhibitor of EGFR that inhibits EGFR exon 19 deletions and exon 21 L858R substitution mutations, contributing to antitumor activity. **Therapeutic Effects:** Improved progression-free survival of NSCLC.

Pharmacokinetics

Absorption: Unknown.

Distribution: Extensively distributed to tissues.

Protein Binding: 99%.

Metabolism and Excretion: Primarily metabolized by glutathione conjugation as well as by the CYP3A4 isoenzyme. 86% excreted in feces (<5% as unchanged drug) and 4% excreted in urine.

Half-life: 3.7 days.

TIME/ACTION PROFILE (plasma concentrations)

ROUTE	ONSET	PEAK	DURATION
PO	unknown	2–4 hr	24 hr

Contraindications/Precautions

Contraindicated in: OB: Pregnancy; Lactation: Lactation.

Use Cautiously in: Severe renal impairment or end-stage renal disease; Severe hepatic impairment; Rep: Women of reproductive potential and men with female partners of reproductive potential; Pedi: Safety and effectiveness not established in children.

Adverse Reactions/Side Effects

CV: DEEP VEIN THROMBOSIS (DVT), edema. **Derm:** dry skin, nail toxicity, pruritus, rash, dermatitis acneiform. **EENT:** conjunctivitis, keratitis. **F and E:** hypermagnesemia, hypocalcemia, hypokalemia, hypomagnesemia, hyponatremia. **GI:** ↓ appetite, ↑ liver enzymes, abdominal pain, constipation, diarrhea, hemorrhoids, hypoalbuminemia, nausea, stomatitis, vomiting. **GU:** ↑ serum creatinine, ↓ fertility. **Hemat:** anemia, hemorrhage, leukopenia, neutropenia, thrombocytopenia. **MS:** pain. **Neuro:** dizziness, fatigue, headache, insomnia, paresthesia. **Resp:** cough, dyspnea, PULMONARY EMBOLISM (PE), INTERSTITIAL LUNG DISEASE (ILD)/PNEUMONITIS. **Misc:** fever.

Interactions

Drug-Drug: Strong CYP3A4 inducers, including **rifampin**, and **moderate CYP3A4 inducers**, including **efavirenz**, may ↓ levels and effectiveness; avoid concurrent use. May ↑ levels and risk of toxicity of **CYP3A4 substrates**, including **midazolam**. May ↑ levels and risk of toxicity of **breast cancer resistance protein substrates**, including **rosuvastatin**.

Route/Dosage

PO (Adults): 240 mg once daily; continue until disease progression or unacceptable toxicity.

Availability

Tablets: 80 mg, 240 mg.

NURSING IMPLICATIONS

Assessment

- Assess for signs/symptoms of venous thromboembolism such as PE (chest pain, dyspnea, tachycardia) or DVT (calf pain or tenderness, lower extremity edema, localized warmth or erythema). *If Grade 2 or 3 thromboembolic event occurs,* hold lazertinib and amivantamab; administer anticoagulant treatment as clinically indicated, then resume lazertinib and amivantamab at same dose. *If Grade 4 or recurrent Grade 2 or 3 thromboembolic events occurs despite therapeutic level anticoagulation,* hold lazertinib and permanently discontinue amivantamab; administer anticoagulant treatment as clinically indicated, then treatment can continue with lazertinib at same dose.
- Monitor for signs/symptoms of ILD or pneumonitis such as dyspnea, cough, hypoxia, fever. CT scan or chest x-ray can confirm. *If ILD or pneumonitis suspected,* hold lazertinib. *If ILD or pneumonitis confirmed,* permanently discontinue lazertinib.
- Monitor for dermatologic reactions including dermatitis, pruritus, dry skin, and acneiform during therapy; may occur ≥ 2 mo after therapy is complete. Treat as indicated with topical corticosteroids and topical and/or oral antibiotics. *If Grade 2 dermatologic reaction occurs,* if no improvement after 2 wk, ↓ amivantamab dose and continue lazertinib at same dose; reassess every 2 wk. If no improvement, ↓ lazertinib dose until reaction is Grade ≤1. *If Grade 3 dermatologic reaction occurs,* administer oral corticosteroids and hold lazertinib and amivantamab

L

until recovery to Grade ≤2. Resume lazertinib at same or ↓ dose, resume amivantamab at ↓ dose. Permanently discontinue lazertinib and amivantamab if no improvement within 2 wk. *If Grade 4 dermatologic reaction occurs,* permanently discontinue amivantamab and hold lazertinib until recovery to Grade ≤2. Resume lazertinib at ↓ dose.

- Monitor for ocular toxicity such as keratitis or conjunctivitis during therapy. Promptly refer patients presenting with new or worsening eye symptoms to an ophthalmologist. *If ocular toxicity confirmed,* ↓ lazertinib dose, or permanently discontinue amivantamab and continue lazertinib based on severity.

Lab Test Considerations

- Verify negative pregnancy status before starting therapy.
- Screen for the presence of EGFR exon 19 deletions and exon 21 L858R substitution mutations in tumor specimens with an FDA-approved companion diagnostic test.

Implementation

- Administer anticoagulant prophylaxis to prevent venous thromboembolic events for the 1st 4 mo of treatment when initiating lazertinib in combination with amivantamab. Vitamin K antagonist not recommended.
- **PO:** Administer lazertinib with or without food any time prior to amivantamab when given on the same day. ***DNC:*** Swallow tablets whole; do not crush, split, or chew.
- **Dose Reductions for Adverse Reactions:** *1st Dose ↓:* 160 mg once daily; *2nd Dose ↓:* 80 mg once daily; *3rd Dose ↓:* Discontinue lazertinib.

Patient/Family Teaching

- Explain purpose and side effects of lazertinib. Advise patient to take as directed. If dose missed <12 hr of scheduled time, instruct patient to take the missed dose. If >12 hr since the dose was to be given, instruct the patient to take the next dose at its scheduled time. If vomiting occurs any time after taking dose, instruct patient to take the next dose at its next regularly scheduled time. Advise patient to read *Patient Information* before starting therapy and with each Rx refill in case of changes.
- Emphasize need for continued medical follow-up to assess effectiveness and possible side effects of medication. Periodic lab tests and eye exams may be needed.
- Advise patient to notify health care professional and promptly seek treatment for signs/symptoms of DVT or PE such as chest pain, trouble breathing, fast heart beat, calf pain or tenderness, lower leg swelling.
- Instruct patient to notify health care professional promptly of any new rash, nail changes, or eye symptoms.
- Inform patient to immediately report signs/symptoms of ILD or pneumonitis such as cough, trouble breathing, or fever.
- Advise patient to apply alcohol free emollient cream to dry skin.
- Encourage patients to limit sun exposure during and for 2 mo after treatment, to wear protective clothing, and use broad-spectrum UVA/UVB sunscreen to ↓ risk of dermatologic adverse reactions.
- Advise patient to notify health care professional of all Rx or OTC medications, vitamins, or herbal products being taken and to consult health care professional before taking other medications.
- Rep: May cause fetal harm. Advise women of reproductive potential to notify health care professional if pregnancy is planned or suspected or if breastfeeding. Advise women of reproductive potential to use effective contraception and not to breastfeed during treatment and for 3 wk after final dose. Advise men with female partners of reproductive potential to use effective contraception during treatment and for 3 wk after final dose.

Evaluation/Desired Outcomes

- Improved progression-free survival of NSCLC.

lecanemab (lek-an-e-mab)

Leqembi

Classification

Therapeutic: anti alzheimers agents
Pharmacologic: monoclonal antibodies, anti amyloid monoclonal antibodies

Indications

Alzheimer disease (with mild cognitive impairment or mild dementia).

Action

Acts as a monoclonal antibody directed against aggregated soluble and insoluble forms of amyloid beta. **Therapeutic Effects:** Reduction in clinical decline. Reduction in amyloid beta plaques in the brain.

Pharmacokinetics

Absorption: IV administration results in complete bioavailability.
Distribution: Not widely distributed to extravascular tissues.
Metabolism and Excretion: Degraded into small peptides and amino acids via catabolic pathways.
Half-life: 5–7 days.

TIME/ACTION PROFILE (plasma concentrations)

ROUTE	ONSET	PEAK	DURATION
IV	rapid	unknown	2 wk

Contraindications/Precautions

Contraindicated in: Hypersensitivity.
Use Cautiously in: Apolipoprotein E ∊4 homozygotes (15% of patients with Alzheimer disease) (↑ risk of amyloid-related imaging abnormalities); OB: Safety not established in pregnancy; Lactation: Safety not established in breastfeeding; Pedi: Safety and effectiveness not established in children.

Adverse Reactions/Side Effects

CV: atrial fibrillation. **GI:** diarrhea. **Hemat:** lymphopenia. **Neuro:** AMYLOID-RELATED IMAGING ABNORMALITIES (ARIA) (INCLUDING EDEMA AND HEMOSIDERIN DEPOSITION), headache, INTRACRANIAL HEMORRHAGE, SEIZURES. **Resp:** cough. **Misc:** HYPERSENSITIVITY REACTIONS (INCLUDING ANAPHYLAXIS AND ANGIOEDEMA), infusion-related reactions.

Interactions

Drug-Drug: Anticoagulant drugs and **thrombolytics** may ↑ risk of intracerebral hemorrhage.

Route/Dosage

IV (Adults): 10 mg/kg every 2 wk. After 18 mo, may continue with 10 mg/kg every 2 wk or transition to maintenance regimen of 10 mg/kg every 4 wk.

Availability

Solution for injection: 100 mg/mL.

NURSING IMPLICATIONS

Assessment

- Baseline brain MRI and periodic monitoring with MRI are recommended. Enhanced clinical vigilance for ARIA is recommended during the 1st 14 wk of therapy.
- May cause amyloid related imaging abnormalities edema (ARIA-E) and hemosiderin deposition (ARIA-H). **For patients with ARIA-E severity on MRI:** *If asymptomatic and mild severity,* continue dosing. *If asymptomatic and moderate or severe severity,* suspend dosing. *If symptoms are mild (discomfort noticed, but no disruption of normal daily activity) with mild severity,* may continue dosing based on clinical judgment. *If symptoms are mild with moderate or severe severity,* suspend dosing. *If symptoms are moderate (discomfort sufficient to reduce or affect normal daily activity) or severe (incapacitating, with inability to work or to perform normal daily activity),* suspend dosing. Suspend until MRI demonstrates radiographic resolution and symptoms, if present, resolve; consider a follow-up MRI to assess for resolution 2–4 mo after initial identification. Use clinical judgment when considering resumption of dosing.
- **For patients with ARIA-H severity on MRI:** *If asymptomatic and mild severity,* continue dosing. *If asymptomatic and moderate or severe severity,* suspend dosing. *If symptomatic,* suspend dosing. *For mild or moderate severity,* suspend until MRI demonstrates radiographic stabilization and symptoms resolve; use clinical judgment regarding resumption of dosing; consider a follow-up MRI to assess for stabilization 2–4 mo after initial identification. *For severe ARIA-H severity on MRI,* suspend until MRI demonstrates radiographic stabilization and symptoms resolve; use clinical judgment in considering whether to continue or permanently discontinue therapy.
- If patient develops an intracerebral hemorrhage >1 cm in diameter during therapy, suspend dosing until MRI demonstrates radiographic stabilization and symptoms resolve. Use clinical judgment in considering whether to continue or permanently discontinue therapy.
- Monitor for signs or symptoms of infusion-related reactions (fever and flu-like symptoms [chills, generalized aches, feeling shaky, joint pain], nausea, vomiting, hypotension, hypertension, oxygen desaturation) during therapy. The infusion rate may be ↓, or the infusion may be discontinued, and appropriate therapy administered. Consider premedication at subsequent dosing with antihistamines, NSAIDs, or corticosteroids.
- Monitor for hypersensitivity reactions (angioedema, bronchospasm, anaphylaxis). *If hypersensitivity reaction occurs,* discontinue infusion and initiate appropriate therapy (epinephrine) as indicated.

Lab Test Considerations

- Confirm the presence of amyloid beta pathology before starting therapy.

Implementation

- Obtain a recent (within 1 yr) brain magnetic resonance imaging (MRI) before starting therapy. Obtain an MRI before the 5th, 7th, and 14th infusions.

IV Administration

- **Intermittent Infusion: Dilution:** Dilute an appropriate volume of solution from vial in 250 mL of 0.9% NaCl. Solution is clear to opalescent and colorless to pale yellow; do not administer solution that is discolored, cloudy, or contains particulate matter. Gently invert to mix; do not shake. Solution is stable for 4 hr at room temperature or if refrigerated; do not freeze. Allow solution to warm to room temperature before infusing. **Concentration:** 100 mg/mL. **Rate:** Infuse over 1 hr through a terminal low-protein-binding 0.2-micron in-line filter. Flush infusion line to ensure all medication is administered.

L

- **Y-Site Incompatibility:** Do not administer other drugs through same IV line.

Patient/Family Teaching

- Explain purpose and side effects of medication. Advise patient to read *Patient Information* before starting therapy. If an infusion is missed, schedule next infusion as soon as possible.
- Advise patient to notify health care provider of all Rx or OTC medications, vitamins, or herbal products being taken and to consult health care provider before taking other medications.
- Inform patient of ↑ risk for ARIA if they are ApoE 4 homozygote, and encourage testing for ApoE 4 status prior to therapy initiation. Prior to testing, discuss risk of ARIA across genotypes and implications of genetic testing results.
- Inform patient that symptoms of ARIA can mimic ischemic stroke and to notify a health care provider immediately of stroke symptoms (sudden weakness or numbness, difficulty speaking or understanding, visual changes, severe headache, dizziness) occur.
- Advise patient to seek immediate medical attention if they experience any symptoms of serious or severe hypersensitivity reactions.
- Advise patients that the Alzheimer's Network for Treatment and Diagnostics (ALZ-NET) is a voluntary provider-enrolled patient registry that collects information on treatments for Alzheimer disease, including *Leqembi*. Encourage patients to participate in the ALZ-NET registry.
- Rep: Advise women of reproductive potential to notify health care provider if pregnancy is planned or suspected or if breastfeeding.

Evaluation/Desired Outcomes

- Reduction in clinical decline.
- Reduction in amyloid beta plaques in the brain.

leflunomide (le-flu-noe-mide)

Arava

Classification

Therapeutic: antirheumatics (DMARDs)
Pharmacologic: immune response modifiers pyrimidine synthesis inhibitors

Indications

Rheumatoid arthritis.

Action

Inhibits an enzyme required for pyrimidine synthesis; has antiproliferative and anti-inflammatory effects.
Therapeutic Effects: Decreased pain and inflammation, slowed structural progression, and improved physical function.

Pharmacokinetics

Absorption: 80% absorbed following oral administration.
Distribution: Well distributed to tissues.
Protein Binding: 99%.
Metabolism and Excretion: Extensively metabolized in the liver to teriflunomide, which is responsible for pharmacologic activity; metabolites excreted in urine (43%) and feces (48%). Also undergoes biliary recycling.
Half-life: 14–18 days.

TIME/ACTION PROFILE (antirheumatic effect)

ROUTE	ONSET	PEAK	DURATION
PO	1 mo	3–6 mo	wk–mos†

† Due to persistence of active metabolite.

Contraindications/Precautions

Contraindicated in: Hypersensitivity to leflunomide or teriflunomide; Compromised immune function, including bone marrow dysplasia or severe uncontrolled infection; Concurrent vaccination with live vaccines; Severe hepatic impairment, pre-existing acute or chronic liver disease, or ALT >2 times upper limit of normal (ULN); OB: Pregnancy; Lactation: Lactation.
Use Cautiously in: Renal impairment; History of interstitial lung disease (ILD); Patients >60 yr, with diabetes, or taking neurotoxic medications (↑ risk of peripheral neuropathy); Rep: Women of reproductive potential; Pedi: Safety and effectiveness not established in children.
Exercise Extreme Caution in: Concurrent use of other hepatotoxic agents (↑ risk of hepatotoxicity).

Adverse Reactions/Side Effects

CV: chest pain, hypertension. **Derm:** alopecia, rash, DRUG REACTION WITH EOSINOPHILIA AND SYSTEMIC SYMPTOMS (DRESS), dry skin, eczema, pruritus, skin ulcers, STEVENS-JOHNSON SYNDROME (SJS), TOXIC EPIDERMAL NECROLYSIS (TEN). **EENT:** pharyngitis, rhinitis, sinusitis. **F and E:** hypokalemia. **GI:** diarrhea, nausea, ↑ liver enzymes, abdominal pain, anorexia, dyspepsia, gastroenteritis, HEPATOTOXICITY, mouth ulcers, vomiting. **GU:** urinary tract infection. **Metab:** weight loss. **MS:** arthralgia, back pain, joint disorder, leg cramps, synovitis, tenosynovitis. **Neuro:** headache, dizziness, paresthesia, peripheral neuropathy, weakness. **Resp:** bronchitis, cough, ILD, pneumonia. **Misc:** INFECTION (INCLUDING SEPSIS AND TUBERCULOSIS [TB] REACTIVATION).

Interactions

Drug-Drug: Cholestyramine and **activated charcoal** cause a rapid and significant ↓ in levels of the active metabolite. **Methotrexate** and other **hepatotoxic drugs** ↑ risk of hepatotoxicity. **Rifampin** ↑ levels of the active metabolite. May ↑ risk of bleeding with **warfarin**. May ↓ response to and ↑ risk of adverse reactions from **live vaccines**; avoid live vaccinations and consider long half-life of leflunomide's active metabolite before administering once leflunomide discontinued.

Route/Dosage

PO (Adults): *Loading dose:* 100 mg once daily for 3 days; then initiate maintenance dose; *Maintenance dose:* 20 mg once daily (if intolerance occurs, may ↓ to 10 mg once daily).

Availability (generic available)

Tablets: 10 mg, 20 mg.

NURSING IMPLICATIONS

Assessment

- Obtain baseline BP. Monitor throughout therapy.
- Assess for skin ulcers. If ulcers do not resolve, consider discontinuing therapy and use accelerated drug elimination procedure (see Implementation).
- Assess range of motion and degree of swelling and pain in affected joints before and periodically during therapy.
- Monitor for signs and symptoms of ILD (new onset or worsening cough or dyspnea, associated with fever). May require discontinuation of therapy; consider drug elimination procedure if needed.
- Assess for rash periodically during therapy. May cause SJS or TEN. Discontinue therapy if severe or if accompanied with fever, general malaise, fatigue, muscle or joint aches, blisters, oral lesions, conjunctivitis, hepatitis, or eosinophilia.
- Monitor for signs and symptoms of DRESS (fever, rash, lymphadenopathy, facial swelling), associated with involvement of other organ systems (hepatitis, nephritis, hematologic abnormalities, myocarditis, myositis) during therapy. May resemble an acute viral infection. Eosinophilia is often present. Discontinue therapy if signs occur.

Lab Test Considerations

- Verify negative pregnancy test before starting therapy. Monitor liver function throughout therapy. Assess ALT at baseline, then monthly during initial 6 mo of therapy, then every 6–8 wk. If given concurrently with methotrexate, monitor ALT, AST, and serum albumin monthly. May ↑ ALT and AST, which are usually reversible with ↓ in dose or discontinuation, but may be fatal. *If ALT is 2–3 times ULN,* ↓ dose to 10 mg once daily. Monitor closely after dose ↓; plasma concentrations may not ↓ for several weeks due to long half-life. *If ALT ↑ of 2–3 times ULN persists despite dose reduction or if ALT >3 times ULN occurs,* discontinue leflunomide and begin accelerated drug elimination procedure (see Implementation).
- Monitor CBC monthly for 6 mo following initiation of therapy and every 6–8 wk thereafter. If used with methotrexate or other immunosuppressive therapy, continue monitoring monthly. If bone marrow depression occurs, discontinue leflunomide and begin accelerated drug elimination procedure (see Implementation).
- May rarely ↑ alkaline phosphatase and bilirubin.

Implementation

- Administer a tuberculin skin test prior to administration of leflunomide. Patients with active latent TB should be treated for TB prior to therapy.
- **Accelerated Drug Elimination Procedure:** Recommended to achieve nondetectable plasma teriflunomide concentrations <0.02 mg/L after stopping treatment with leflunomide. Administer cholestyramine 8 g 3 times daily orally for 11 days (days do not need to be consecutive unless rapid lowering of levels is desired). Alternatively, can administer activated charcoal powder 50 g (made into a suspension) orally every 12 hr for 11 days. Verify plasma teriflunomide concentrations <0.02 mg/L by two separate tests ≥14 days apart. If plasma teriflunomide concentrations >0.02 mg/L, consider additional cholestyramine treatment. Plasma teriflunomide concentrations may take up to 2 yr to reach nondetectable levels without drug elimination procedure.

Patient/Family Teaching

- Explain purpose and side effects of medication to patient. Advise patient to read *Patient Information* before starting therapy.
- Advise patient to notify health care provider of all Rx or OTC medications, vitamins, or herbal products being taken and to consult health care provider before taking other medications. Aspirin, NSAIDs, or low-dose corticosteroids may be continued during therapy, but other agents for treatment of rheumatoid arthritis may require discontinuation.
- Advise patient if a dose is missed to take as soon as remembered. Do not take two doses at the same time.
- May cause dizziness. Caution patient to avoid driving or other activities requiring alertness until response to medication is known.
- Discuss the possibility of hair loss with patient. Explore methods of coping.
- Advise patient to notify health care provider if rash, mucous membrane lesions, unusual tiredness, abdominal pain, jaundice, or symptoms of ILD occur.

L

- Instruct patient to avoid vaccinations with live vaccines during and following therapy without consulting health care provider.
- Emphasize the importance of routine lab tests to monitor for side effects.
- Rep: May cause fetal harm. Advise women of reproductive potential to use effective contraception. If pregnancy is planned or suspected or if breastfeeding, notify health care provider immediately; an accelerated elimination procedure (see Implementation) must be used to ↓ levels more rapidly. Advise patient to avoid breastfeeding during therapy.

Evaluation/Desired Outcomes

- Decrease in signs and symptoms of rheumatoid arthritis and slowing of structural damage as evidenced by x-ray erosions and joint narrowings.
- Improved physical function.

lenacapavir
(len-uh-**kap**-uh-veer)
Sunlenca, Yeztugo

Classification
Therapeutic: antiretrovirals
Pharmacologic: capsid inhibitors

Indications
Sunlenca: HIV-1 infection in heavily treatment-experienced patients with multidrug-resistant HIV-1 infection who are failing their current antiretroviral regimen due to resistance, intolerance, or safety issues (in combination with other antiretrovirals). **Yeztugo:** Pre-exposure prophylaxis (PrEP) to reduce the risk of sexually acquired HIV-1 infection in at-risk individuals.

Action
Inhibits HIV-1 capsid function, which interferes with multiple early- to late-stage processes of the viral life cycle, including nuclear transport, virus assembly and release, and capsid assembly. **Therapeutic Effects:** Increase in CD4 cell counts and reduction in viral load with subsequent slowed progression of HIV and its sequelae. Reduction in risk of sexually acquired HIV infection in at-risk individuals.

Pharmacokinetics
Absorption: 6–10% absorbed following oral administration; 91% absorbed following SUBQ administration.
Distribution: Extensively distributed to tissues.
Protein Binding: >98.5%.
Metabolism and Excretion: Primarily metabolized by the liver with some metabolism by the CYP3A isoenzyme and UGT1A1. Primarily excreted in feces (33% as unchanged drug), with <1% excreted in urine.
Half-life: *Oral:* 10–12 days; *SUBQ:* 8–12 wk.

TIME/ACTION PROFILE (plasma concentrations)

ROUTE	ONSET	PEAK	DURATION
PO	unknown	4 hr	unknown
SUBQ	unknown	77–84 days	unknown

Contraindications/Precautions
Contraindicated in: Concurrent use of strong CYP3A inducers (Sunlenca only); Unknown or positive HIV status (Yeztugo only); End-stage renal disease; Severe hepatic impairment; Lactation: Breastfeeding not recommended for patients with HIV (Sunlenca only).
Use Cautiously in: OB: Safety not established in pregnancy; not a recommended antiretroviral agent in pregnancy (Sunlenca only); Lactation: Use while breastfeeding only if potential maternal benefit justifies potential risk to infant (Yeztugo only); Pedi: Safety and effectiveness not established in children <18 yr (Sunlenca) or <35 kg (Yeztugo).

Adverse Reactions/Side Effects
Endo: hyperglycemia. **GI:** ↑ liver enzymes, diarrhea, nausea, vomiting. **GU:** ↑ serum creatinine, glycosuria, proteinuria. **Local:** injection site reactions. **Neuro:** dizziness, headache. **Misc:** immune reconstitution syndrome.

Interactions
Because of long half-life of SUBQ lenacapavir, levels and risk of toxicity of CYP3A substrates initiated within 9 mo of last SUBQ dose may remain elevated.
Drug-Drug: **Strong CYP3A inducers**, including **carbamazepine**, **phenytoin**, or **rifampin**, significantly ↓ levels and effectiveness; concurrent use with Sunlenca contraindicated; administer supplemental Yeztugo doses. **Moderate CYP3A inducers**, including **efavirenz**, **nevirapine**, **oxcarbazepine**, **phenobarbital**, **rifabutin**, **rifapentine**, and **tipranavir/ritonavir**, may ↓ levels and effectiveness; concurrent use with Sunlenca not recommended; administer supplemental Yeztugo doses. **Combined p-glycoprotein, UGT1A1, and strong CYP3A inhibitors**, including **atazanavir**, **cobicistat**, **darunavir**, **ergot derivatives**, **ritonavir**, and **voriconazole**, may ↑ levels and risk of toxicity; concurrent use not recommended. May ↑ levels and risk of toxicity of **digoxin**; monitor levels closely. May ↑ levels and risk of bleeding of **dabigatran**, **edoxaban**, and **rivaroxaban**. May ↑ levels and risk of toxicity of **buprenorphine**, **dexamethasone**, **fentanyl**, **hydrocortisone**, **lovastatin**, **methadone**, **oxycodone**, **simvastatin**, **tramadol**, and **triazolam**. May ↑ levels and risk of toxicity of **naloxegol**; avoid concurrent use, if possible. If concurrent use is unavoidable, ↓ naloxegol dose. May ↑ levels and risk of toxicity of **sildenafil**,

tadalafil, and **vardenafil**; concurrent use with tadalafil for pulmonary arterial hypertension not recommended. **Drug-Natural Products: St. John's wort** significantly ↓ levels and effectiveness; concurrent use contraindicated.

Route/Dosage

Sunlenca

Treatment can be initiated with *either* the 2-day or 15-day initiation regimen.

2-Day Initiation Regimen

PO SUBQ (Adults): *Day 1:* 600 mg orally as single dose **AND** 927 mg SUBQ as single dose. *Day 2:* 600 mg orally as single dose. *Maintenance dosing:* Starting 6 mo following date of last injection, administer 927 mg SUBQ every 6 mo (26 wk ± 2 wk).

15-Day Initiation Regimen

PO SUBQ (Adults): *Day 1:* 600 mg orally as single dose. *Day 2:* 600 mg orally as single dose. *Day 8:* 300 mg orally as single dose. *Day 15:* 927 mg SUBQ as single dose. *Maintenance dosing:* Starting 6 mo following date of last injection, administer 927 mg SUBQ every 6 mo (26 wk ± 2 wk).

Yeztugo

PO SUBQ (Adults and Children ≥35 kg): *Initiation (Day 1):* 927 mg SUBQ as single dose AND 600 mg orally as single dose; *Initiation (Day 2):* 600 mg orally as single dose; *Continuation:* Starting 6 mo following date of last injection, administer 927 mg SUBQ every 6 mo (26 wk ± 2 wk). *Concurrent use of strong CYP3A inducer:* Continue to administer 927 mg SUBQ every 6 mo as previously scheduled PLUS administer the following supplemental doses: **On day strong CYP3A inducer initiated (should be ≥2 days after Yeztugo 1st initiated):** Step 1: Administer 927 mg SUBQ as single dose AND 600 mg orally as single dose; **On day after strong CYP3A inducer initiated:** Step 2: Administer 600 mg orally as single dose; **If strong CYP3A inducer coadministered for >6 mo:** Every 6 mo from initiation of strong CYP3A inducer, continue to administer supplemental doses as outlined above in Steps 1 and 2. **Concurrent use of moderate CYP3A inducer:** Continue to administer 927 mg SUBQ every 6 mo as previously scheduled PLUS administer the following supplemental doses; **On day moderate CYP3A inducer initiated:** Administer 463.5 mg SUBQ as single dose; **If moderate CYP3A inducer coadministered for >6 mo:** Every 6 mo from initiation of moderate CYP3A inducer, continue to administer a supplemental dose.

Availability

Tablets: 300 mg. **Solution for SUBQ injection:** 463.5 mg/1.5 mL.

NURSING IMPLICATIONS

Assessment

- Assess for change in severity of HIV symptoms during therapy.
- Assess for immune reconstitution syndrome. Monitor for signs and symptoms of fever, localized inflammation, confusion, and respiratory issues and for symptoms of opportunistic infections during therapy.
- Assess SUBQ injection sites for reactions (erythema, pain, induration, nodules).

Lab Test Considerations

- Obtain baseline HIV RNA levels.
- Monitor viral load and CD4 count.
- Obtain baseline ALT, AST, and bilirubin. May cause hepatotoxicity.
- Monitor serum creatinine during routine assessment.
- Monitor for metabolic abnormalities such as lipid or glucose changes.
- *Yeztugo:* Perform HIV-1 screening before starting, before each subsequent injection, and as clinically appropriate. Do not initiate therapy unless negative infection status is confirmed.

Implementation

- **PO:** Administer with or without food.
- **SUBQ**: Use aseptic technique. Visually inspect the solution in the vials and prepared syringe for particulate matter and discoloration before administration. Solution is a yellow color. Do not use if the solution is discolored or contains particulate matter.
- Withdraw 1.5 mL from each vial using provided syringes and withdrawal needles or vial access devices; two 1.5-mL injections are required for each dose. Prepared syringes should be administered as soon as possible. Discard any solution remaining in vial.
- Administer each injection at separate sites apart in the abdomen (≥2 in from the navel). Do not administer intradermally due to risk of serious injection site reactions.
- *Planned missed injections:* If a patient plans to miss a scheduled 6-mo injection visit by >2 wk during the maintenance period, lenacapavir 300 mg orally once every 7 days may be taken for up to 6 mo until injections resume. Resume maintenance injection dosage within 7 days after the last PO dose.
- *Unplanned missed Sunlenca injections:* If >28 wk since the last injection during the maintenance period, if lenacapavir oral tablets have not been taken, and if clinically appropriate to continue treatment, restart starting dosage regimen from Day 1, using either 2-day or 15-day initiation. *Unplanned missed Yeztugo injection:* If >28 wk since the last injection and tablets have not been taken, restart initiation from Day 1, if clinically appropriate.

L

- *Discontinuation of therapy:* Residual concentrations of lenacapavir long-acting injection may remain in the systemic circulation of patients for ≥12 mo; consider this if therapy is discontinued. To minimize the potential risk of resistance development, an alternative fully suppressive antiretroviral regimen should be initiated when possible, no later than 28 wk after final injection.
- **Yeztugo:** *Missed PO Initiation Dose:* If Day 2 PO initiation dose (600 mg) is missed, take it as soon as possible. Do not take Day 1 and Day 2 PO initiation doses on the same day.

Patient/Family Teaching

- Explain purpose and side effects of medication. Advise patient to read *Patient Information* before starting therapy. Advise patient to contact health care provider if dose is missed or plan to miss a scheduled injection visit and that oral therapy may be used for up to 6 mo to replace missed injections.
- Advise patient to notify health care provider of all Rx or OTC medications, vitamins, or herbal products being taken and to consult health care provider before taking other medications, especially St. John's wort. If therapy is discontinued, advise patient that lenacapavir may remain in the body and affect certain other drugs for up to 9 mo after receiving the last injection.
- Advise patient to inform their health care provider immediately of any symptoms of infection; signs and symptoms of inflammation from previous infections may occur soon after anti-HIV treatment is started.
- Advise patient that injection site reactions (swelling, pain, erythema, nodule, induration, pruritus, extravasation, mass) may occur. Nodules and indurations at the injection site may take longer to resolve than other reactions and may be persistent.
- Advise patient about the importance of continued medication adherence and scheduled visits to maintain viral suppression and to ↓ risk of loss of virologic response and development of resistance. Advise patient to contact health care provider immediately if they stop taking therapy or any other drug in their antiretroviral regimen.
- Advise patient taking *Yeztugo* about the potential risk of developing resistance to lenacapavir if HIV-1 is acquired either before or when receiving or following discontinuation of therapy. Advise that testing will be done before each injection and additionally as clinically appropriate to confirm HIV-1 negative status. If HIV-1 is acquired while receiving Yeztugo, discontinue therapy, and treatment should be changed to a full HIV-1 regimen.
- Advise patient taking *Yeztugo* on adhering to the required initiation and continuation dosing schedule, safe sex practices (condoms), and other measures to reduce the risk of sexually transmitted infections.
- Rep: Advise women of reproductive potential to notify health care provider if pregnancy is planned or suspected and to avoid breastfeeding during therapy. Enroll all patients exposed to antiretroviral medications as early in pregnancy as possible in the Antiretroviral Pregnancy Registry (1-800-258-4263).

Evaluation/Desired Outcomes

- Increase in CD4 cell counts and reduction in viral load with subsequent slowed progression of HIV and its sequelae.
- Reduction in risk of sexually acquired HIV infection in at-risk individuals.

REMS HIGH ALERT

lenalidomide

(le-na-**lid**-o-mide)

Revlimid

Classification

Therapeutic: antineoplastics

Pharmacologic: immunomodulatory agents

Indications

Transfusion-dependent anemia due to specific myelodysplastic syndromes associated with deletion 5q cytogenetic abnormality. Multiple myeloma (in combination with dexamethasone). Maintenance therapy in patients with multiple myeloma after autologous hematopoietic stem cell transplantation. Mantle cell lymphoma patients whose disease has relapsed or progressed after 2 prior therapies, including bortezomib. Previously treated follicular lymphoma (in combination with rituximab). Previously treated marginal zone lymphoma (in combination with rituximab).

Action

Lenalidomide is a structural analog of thalidomide. Inhibits secretion of pro-inflammatory cytokines and increases secretion of anti-inflammatory cytokines. **Therapeutic Effects:** Decreased anemia in certain myelodysplastic syndromes with a decreased requirement for transfusions. Slowed progression of multiple myeloma and mantle cell lymphoma. Improved progression-free survival in follicular lymphoma and marginal zone lymphoma.

Pharmacokinetics

Absorption: Well absorbed following oral administration. Levels are higher in patients with multiple myeloma.

Distribution: Unknown.

Metabolism and Excretion: 66% excreted unchanged in urine, some renal excretion involves active secretion.

Half-life: 3 hr.

TIME/ACTION PROFILE (↓ need for transfusions)

ROUTE	ONSET	PEAK	DURATION
PO	within 3 mo	unknown	unknown

Contraindications/Precautions

Contraindicated in: Hypersensitivity; Chronic lymphocytic leukemia (↑ risk of mortality); Concurrent use of pembrolizumab in patients with multiple myeloma (↑ risk of mortality); OB: Pregnancy; Lactation: Lactation.

Use Cautiously in: Renal impairment (may ↑ risk of adverse reactions; dose ↓ recommended if CCr <60 mL/min); Patients with mantle cell lymphoma with high tumor burden, high mantle cell lymphoma International Prognostic Index at diagnosis, and high white blood cell count at baseline (↑ risk of early mortality); Rep: Women of reproductive potential and men with female partners of reproductive potential; Pedi: Safety and effectiveness not established in children; Geri: Consider age-related ↓ in renal function in older adults.

Adverse Reactions/Side Effects

CV: edema, chest pain, DEEP VEIN THROMBOSIS (DVT), MI, palpitations. **Derm:** pruritus, rash, DRUG REACTION WITH EOSINOPHILIA AND SYSTEMIC SYMPTOMS (DRESS), dry skin, STEVENS-JOHNSON SYNDROME (SJS), sweating, TOXIC EPIDERMAL NECROLYSIS (TEN). **Endo:** hyperthyroidism, hypothyroidism. **F and E:** hypokalemia, hypomagnesemia. **GI:** abdominal pain, constipation, diarrhea, nausea, vomiting, abnormal taste, anorexia, dry mouth, HEPATOTOXICITY. **Hemat:** NEUTROPENIA, THROMBOCYTOPENIA. **MS:** arthralgia, myalgia. **Neuro:** dizziness, fatigue, headache, depression, insomnia, STROKE. **Resp:** cough, pharyngitis, PULMONARY EMBOLISM (PE). **Misc:** fever, TUMOR FLARE REACTION, chills, HYPERSENSITIVITY REACTIONS (INCLUDING ANAPHYLAXIS AND ANGIOEDEMA), MALIGNANCY, tumor lysis syndrome.

Interactions

Drug-Drug: Risk of neutropenia and thrombocytopenia may ↑ with **antineoplastics, immunosuppressants,** and **radiation therapy.** May ↑ levels and risk of toxicity of **digoxin. Erythropoeitin, darbepoeitin,** and **estrogens** may ↑ risk of thromboembolic events.

Route/Dosage

Myelodysplastic Syndromes

PO (Adults): 10 mg once daily.

Renal Impairment

PO (Adults): *CCr 30–60 mL/min:* 5 mg once daily; *CCr <30 mL/min (not on dialysis):* 2.5 mg once daily; *CCr <30 mL/min (requiring dialysis):* 2.5 mg once daily (give after dialysis on dialysis days).

Multiple Myeloma

PO (Adults): 25 mg once daily on Days 1–21 of repeated 28-day cycles (with dexamethasone); if patients not eligible for auto-hematopoietic stem-cell transplantation (HSCT), continue treatment until disease progression or unacceptable toxicity; for patients eligible for auto-HSCT, hematopoietic stem cell mobilization should take place within 4 cycles.

Renal Impairment

PO (Adults): *CCr 30–60 mL/min:* 10 mg once daily; if patient tolerates initial dose, may ↑ to 15 mg once daily after 2 cycles; *CCr <30 mL/min (not on dialysis):* 15 mg every 48 hr; *CCr <30 mL/min (requiring dialysis):* 5 mg once daily (give after dialysis on dialysis days).

Maintenance Therapy for Multiple Myeloma Following Autologous Hematopoietic Stem Cell Transplantation

PO (Adults): After adequate hematologic recovery (ANC ≥1000/mcL and/or platelet counts ≥75,000/mcL), initiate therapy with 10 mg once daily continuously on Days 1–28 of repeated 28-day cycles; after 3 cycles, dose may be ↑ to 15 mg once daily, if tolerated; continue treatment until disease progression or unacceptable toxicity.

Renal Impairment

PO (Adults): *CCr 30–60 mL/min:* 5 mg once daily; *CCr <30 mL/min (not on dialysis):* 2.5 mg once daily; *CCr <30 mL/min (requiring dialysis):* 2.5 mg once daily (give after dialysis on dialysis days).

Mantle Cell Lymphoma

PO (Adults): 25 mg once daily on Days 1–21 of repeated 28-day cycles; continue treatment until disease relapse or unacceptable toxicity develops.

Renal Impairment

PO (Adults): *CCr 30–60 mL/min:* 10 mg once daily; *CCr <30 mL/min (not on dialysis):* 15 mg every 48 hr; *CCr <30 mL/min (requiring dialysis):* 5 mg once daily (give after dialysis on dialysis days).

Follicular Lymphoma or Marginal Zone Lymphoma

PO (Adults): 20 mg once daily on Days 1–21 of repeated 28-day cycles for up to 12 cycles.

Renal Impairment

PO (Adults): *CCr 30–60 mL/min:* 10 mg once daily; if patient tolerates initial dose, may ↑ to 15 mg once daily after 2 cycles; *CCr <30 mL/min (not on dialysis):* 5 mg once daily; *CCr <30 mL/min (requiring dialysis):* 5 mg once daily (give after dialysis on dialysis days).

Availability (generic available)

Capsules: 2.5 mg, 5 mg, 10 mg, 15 mg, 20 mg, 25 mg.

NURSING IMPLICATIONS

Assessment

- Assess for signs of DVT and PE (dyspnea, chest pain, arm or leg swelling) periodically during therapy; risk is greater when lenalidomide is administered with dexamethasone. Venous thromboembolism prophylaxis is recommended in patients receiving lenalidomide; prophylaxis regimen should be based on assessment of the patient's underlying risks.
- Assess for SJS, DRESS, and TEN. *If Grade 2–3 rash occurs,* consider holding or discontinuing therapy. *If SJS, DRESS, or TEN is suspected or Grade 4 rash occurs,* permanently discontinue lenalidomide.
- Monitor for signs and symptoms of tumor flare reaction (tender lymph node swelling, low-grade fever, pain rash); may mimic mantle cell lymphoma progression. *If Grade 1–2 tumor flare reaction occurs,* may continue lenalidomide without interruption or modification, at health care provider's discretion. May also be treated with corticosteroids, NSAIDs, and/or opioid analgesics. *If Grade 3–4 tumor flare reaction occurs,* hold lenalidomide until reaction resolves to Grade ≤1.

Lab Test Considerations

- Verify negative pregnancy status before starting therapy. In women of reproductive potential, obtain two negative pregnancy tests before starting lenalidomide. Pregnancy tests with a sensitivity of ≥50 mIU/mL must be done 10–14 days and 24 hr before starting therapy; then verify negative pregnancy test weekly during 1st 4 wk of use, every 4 wk if menstrual cycle is regular, and every 2 wk if cycle is irregular.
- *Patients taking lenalidomide for multiple myeloma with dexamethasone or as maintenance therapy:* Monitor CBC every 7 days for 1st 2 cycles, on days 1 and 15 of Cycle 3, and every 28 days thereafter. *Patients taking lenalidomide for myelodysplastic syndrome:* Monitor CBC with differential weekly for 1st 8 wk of therapy and at least monthly thereafter. *Patients taking lenalidomide for mantle cell lymphoma:* Monitor CBC weekly for 1st 28 days, every 2 wk during Cycles 2–4, and monthly thereafter. May require dose interruption and/or ↓ and support with blood or growth factors.
- May cause neutropenia with an average onset of 42 days and recovery time of 17 days. **Multiple myeloma:** *For ANC <1000/mcL,* hold and follow CBC weekly until ANC ≥1000/mcL and neutropenia is the only toxicity; resume at initial dose. If concurrent toxicity present, resume at next lower dose. *For each subsequent occurrence of ANC <1000/mcL,* hold until ANC ≥1000/mcL; then resume at next lower dose. Do not administer doses below 2.5 mg once daily. **Myelodysplastic syndromes:** *For neutropenia that develops ≤4 wk of starting at a dose of 10 mg once daily with baseline ANC ≥1000/mcL and ↓ to <750/mcL,* hold until ANC ≥1000/mcL; then resume at 5 mg once daily. *If baseline ANC <1000/mcL and ↓ to <500/mcL,* hold until ANC ≥500/mcL; then resume at 5 mg once daily. *For neutropenia that develops after 4 wk of therapy at a dose of 10 mg once daily and ANC <500/mcL for ≥7 days or <500/mcL with fever ≥38.5°C,* hold until ANC ≥500/mcL; then resume at 5 mg once daily. *For neutropenia that develops at dose of 5 mg once daily and ANC <500/mcL for ≥7 days or <500/mcL with fever ≥38.5°C,* hold until ANC ≥500/mcL; then resume at 2.5 mg once daily. **Mantle cell lymphoma:** *For ANC <1000/mcL for ≥7 days or <1000/mcL with fever ≥38.5°C or <500/mcL,* hold and follow CBC weekly until ANC ≥1000/mcL; then ↓ dose by 5 mg/day. Do not administer doses <5 mg once daily. **Marginal zone lymphoma or follicular lymphoma:** *For ANC <1000/mcL for ≥7 days or <1000/mcL with fever ≥38.5° C or <500/mcL,* hold and follow CBC weekly until ANC ≥1000/mcL. If starting dose was 20 mg daily, ↓ dose by 5 mg/day. Do not administer doses <5 mg/day If starting dose was 10 mg daily, ↓ dose by 5 mg/day. Do not administer doses <2.5 mg/day.
- May cause thrombocytopenia with an onset of 28 days (range 8–290 days) and a recovery in 22 days (range 5–224 days). **Multiple myeloma:** *If platelets <30,000/mcL,* hold and follow CBC weekly. When platelets ≥30,000/mcL, restart lenalidomide at next lower dose. For each subsequent drop in platelets to <30,000/mcL, interrupt therapy. When platelets ≥30,000/mcL, resume at next lower dose. Do not administer doses below 2.5 mg once daily. **Myelodysplastic syndrome:** *If thrombocytopenia develops within 4 wk of starting a dose of 10 mg once daily with a platelet baseline of ≥100,000/mcL and ↓to <50,000/mcL,* hold and resume at 5 mg once daily when platelets >50,000/mcL. *If platelet baseline <100,000/mcL and ↓ to 50% of baseline,* hold therapy. If platelet baseline ≥60,000/mcL and returns to ≥50,000/mcL or if platelet baseline <60,000/mcL and returns to ≥30,000/mcL, resume at 5 mg once daily. *If thrombocytopenia develops after 4 wk of treatment at 10 mg once daily and platelets <30,000/mcL or <50,000/mcL with platelet transfusions,* hold therapy. When platelets return

to ≥30,000/mcL without hemostatic failure, resume therapy at 2.5 mg once daily. **Mantle cell lymphoma:** *If platelets fall to <50,000/mcL,* hold and follow CBC weekly. If platelets return to ≥50,000/mcL, ↓ dose by 5 mg/day. Do not administer doses <5 mg/day. **Follicular lymphoma or marginal cell lymphoma:** *If platelets <50,000/mcL,* hold and follow CBC weekly. When platelets return to ≥50,000/mcL, if starting dose was 20 mg daily, ↓ dose by 5 mg/day; do not administer doses <5 mg/day. If starting dose was 10 mg daily, ↓ dose by 5 mg/day; do not administer doses <2.5 mg/day.

- Monitor liver enzymes periodically during therapy. Stop therapy if enzymes are ↑; may resume when return to normal or ↓ dose.
- May cause anemia and leukopenia.
- May cause hypokalemia and hypomagnesemia.
- Monitor thyroid function before starting and periodically during therapy.

Implementation

- ***REMS:*** Patients must sign a patient-physician agreement form and must meet the following conditions before receiving therapy: they must understand the risks and be able to carry out instructions, must be capable of complying with patient registration and patient survey in the *Lenalidomide REMS program*, must comply with contraceptive measures, have received both oral and written warnings of the risks of contraception failure and the need for two reliable forms of contraception (women) or the risks of exposing a fetus to the drug and the need to use a latex condom during sexual intercourse with a woman of reproductive potential, and acknowledge understanding of these warnings in writing. If patient is 12–18 yr, their parent or legal guardian is to read the educational materials and agree to try to ensure compliance with conditions. Lenalidomide can only be prescribed by health care providers and dispensed by a pharmacy registered in the *Lenalidomide REMS program*.
- Patients with multiple myeloma who are eligible for autologous stem cell transplantation should have stem cell mobilization performed within 4 cycles of therapy.
- **PO:** Administer without regard to food at the same time each day with water. ***DNC:*** Swallow capsules whole; do not open, break, or chew.

Patient/Family Teaching

- Explain purpose and side effects of medication. Advise patient to read *Patient Information* before starting therapy.
- Instruct patient to take missed doses as soon as remembered within 12 hr. If >12 hr, omit and return to next scheduled dose; do not administer 2 doses within 12 hr.
- ***REMS:*** Instruct patient to comply with all aspects of the *Lenalidomide REMS program*. Inform patient that they are required to participate in a telephone survey and patient registry while taking lenalidomide. Details available at www.lenalidomiderems.com.
- Advise patient to notify health care provider if signs/symptoms of thromboembolism (shortness of breath, chest pain, arm or leg swelling), infection (fever, dyspnea) or bleeding occur.
- Advise patient to notify health care provider if rash, signs and symptoms of liver failure (yellow skin or eyes, dark or brown urine, upper right abdominal pain, fatigue, unusual bleeding or bruising), or hypersensitivity (swelling of lips, mouth, tongue, or throat; trouble breathing or swallowing; hives; very fast heartbeat; feeling dizzy or faint) occur.
- May cause dizziness. Caution patient to avoid driving and other activities requiring alertness until response to medication is known.
- Inform patient that lenalidomide may ↑ risk of death in patients with mantle cell lymphoma and may ↑ risk of new cancers.
- Instruct patient to notify health care provider of all Rx or OTC medications, vitamins, or herbal products being taken and consult health care provider before taking any new medications.
- Advise patient that they cannot donate blood during and for 1 mo following therapy and male patients cannot donate sperm while taking lenalidomide.
- Rep: May cause fetal harm. Inform women of reproductive potential that they must use one highly effective method (IUD, hormonal contraceptive, tubal ligation, vasectomy) and one additional method (latex or synthetic condom, diaphragm, cervical cap) AT THE SAME TIME for ≥4 wk before, during therapy and interruptions of therapy, and for 4 wk following discontinuation of therapy, even with a history of infertility unless due to hysterectomy or patient has been postmenopausal naturally for 24 consecutive mo. Advise patient to avoid breastfeeding during therapy. Men with female partners of reproductive potential must always use a latex or synthetic condom during therapy and for up to 4 wk following last dose, even with a successful vasectomy. Men taking lenalidomide must not donate sperm during and for 4 wk after last dose. Lenalidomide must be discontinued if pregnancy is suspected or confirmed. Suspected fetal exposure must be reported to FDA via MedWatch

at 1-800-FDA-1088 and to Celgene Corporation at 1-888-423-5436. Inform women who are pregnant to enroll in the Pregnancy Exposure Registry that monitors outcomes by contacting 1-888-423-5436 or visiting www.lenalidomiderems.com.

Evaluation/Desired Outcomes

- Decreased anemia in myelodysplastic syndromes with a decreased requirement for transfusions.
- Slowing of multiple myeloma progression.
- Slowing progression of mantle cell lymphoma.
- Improved progression-free survival in follicular lymphoma and marginal zone lymphoma.

HIGH ALERT

lenvatinib (len-**va**-ti-nib)

Lenvima

Classification

Therapeutic: antineoplastics

Pharmacologic: kinase inhibitors

Indications

Locally recurrent or metastatic/progressive, radioactive-iodine-refractory differentiated thyroid cancer. Advanced renal cell carcinoma following one previous antiangiogenic therapy (in combination with everolimus). First-line treatment of advanced renal cell carcinoma (in combination with pembrolizumab). Unresectable hepatocellular carcinoma. Advanced endometrial carcinoma that is mismatch repair proficient (pMMR) or not microsatellite instability-high (MSI-H) in patients who have disease progression following prior systemic therapy in any setting and are not candidates for curative surgery or radiation (in combination with pembrolizumab).

Action

Acts as a receptor tyrosine kinase inhibitor; inhibits kinase activities of various vascular endothelial growth factor receptors, resulting in decreased pathogenic angiogenesis and tumor growth and spread. **Therapeutic Effects:** Decreased progression and improved survival of differentiated thyroid cancer, endometrial cancer, renal cell carcinoma, and hepatocellular carcinoma.

Pharmacokinetics

Absorption: Well absorbed following oral administration.
Distribution: Unknown.
Protein Binding: 98–99%.
Metabolism and Excretion: Metabolized primarily by the CYP3A isoenzyme and aldehyde oxidase; 64% eliminated in feces; 25% in urine.
Half-life: 28 hr

TIME/ACTION PROFILE (improvement in progression-free survival)

ROUTE	ONSET	PEAK	DURATION
PO	within 2 mo	8 mo	throughout treatment

Contraindications/Precautions

Contraindicated in: OB: Pregnancy; Lactation: Lactation.
Use Cautiously in: Hypertension (control BP before initiating treatment; may need to withhold/discontinue for life-threatening elevation); History of HF (may need to withhold/discontinue for worsening HF); History of congenital long QTc syndrome, HF, bradyarrhythmias, and concurrent use of drugs that prolong QTc, including Class Ia and III antiarrhythmics (↑ risk of further QTc prolongation and serious arrhythmias; may require interruption/discontinuation of lenvatinib); Severe hepatic or renal impairment (↓ dose); Dehydration/volume depletion (↑ risk of renal impairment; may need to withhold/discontinue for worsening renal function); Hypocalcemia (replace calcium; if persistent may require dose adjustment/interruption); History of reversible posterior leukoencephalopathy syndrome (may require dose adjustment/interruption); Invasive dental procedures, concurrent use of bisphosphonates or denosumab, or dental disease (may ↑ risk of osteonecrosis of the jaw [ONJ]); Rep: Women and men of reproductive potential; Pedi: Safety and effectiveness not established in children.

Adverse Reactions/Side Effects

CV: hypertension, HF, hypotension, MI, QT interval prolongation. **Derm:** alopecia, palmar-plantar erythrodysesthesia syndrome, rash, hyperkeratosis, impaired wound healing. **EENT:** dysphonia, epistaxis. **Endo:** hyperglycemia, hypoglycemia, hypothyroidism. **F and E:** hypercalcemia, hyperkalemia, hypermagnesemia, hypocalcemia, hypokalemia, hypomagnesemia, hyponatremia, hypophosphatemia, dehydration. **GI:** ↓ appetite, ↑ amylase, ↑ lipase, ↑ liver enzymes, abdominal pain, diarrhea, dry mouth, nausea, stomatitis, vomiting, weight loss, GI PERFORATION/FISTULA FORMATION, HEPATOTOXICITY. **GU:** ↑ serum creatinine, proteinuria, ↓ fertility, NEPHROTIC SYNDROME. **Hemat:** anemia, BLEEDING, leukopenia, lymphopenia, neutropenia, thrombocytopenia. **Metab:** hypercholesterolemia, hypertriglyceridemia, hypoalbuminemia. **MS:** ↑ CK, arthralgia/myalgia, osteonecrosis (primarily of jaw). **Neuro:** dysgeusia, fatigue, headache, insomnia, CAROTID ARTERY HEMORRHAGE, REVERSIBLE POSTERIOR LEUKOENCEPHALOPATHY SYNDROME (RPLS), STROKE. **Resp:** cough.

Interactions

Drug-Drug: QT interval prolonging drugs, including **Class Ia and III antiarrhythmics,** may ↑

risk of further QTc prolongation and serious arrhythmias (may require interruption/discontinuation of lenvatinib). **Alendronate**, **denosumab**, **ibandronate**, **pamidronate**, **risedronate**, or **zoledronic acid** may ↑ risk of ONJ.

Route/Dosage

Differentiated Thyroid Cancer

PO (Adults): 24 mg once daily until disease progression or unacceptable toxicity.

Renal Impairment

PO (Adults): *CCr <30 mL/min:* 14 mg once daily until disease progression or unacceptable toxicity.

Hepatic Impairment

PO (Adults): *Severe hepatic impairment:* 14 mg once daily until disease progression or unacceptable toxicity.

Renal Cell Carcinoma

PO (Adults): *First-line treatment of advanced renal cell carcinoma:* 20 mg once daily (in combination with pembrolizumab) until disease progression, unacceptable toxicity, or up to 2 yr. After 2 yr of combination therapy, continue 20 mg once daily (as monotherapy) until disease progression or unacceptable toxicity. *Previously treated renal cell carcinoma:* 18 mg once daily until disease progression or unacceptable toxicity.

Renal Impairment

PO (Adults): *CCr <30 mL/min:* First-line treatment of advanced renal cell carcinoma: 10 mg once daily (in combination with pembrolizumab) until disease progression, unacceptable toxicity, or up to 2 yr. After 2 yr of combination therapy, continue 10 mg once daily (as monotherapy) until disease progression or unacceptable toxicity. Previously treated renal cell carcinoma: 10 mg once daily until disease progression or unacceptable toxicity.

Hepatic Impairment

PO (Adults): *Severe hepatic impairment:* 10 mg once daily until disease progression or unacceptable toxicity.

Hepatocellular Carcinoma

PO (Adults ≥60 kg): 12 mg once daily until disease progression or unacceptable toxicity.

PO (Adults <60 kg): 8 mg once daily until disease progression or unacceptable toxicity.

Endometrial Carcinoma

PO (Adults): 20 mg once daily until disease progression or unacceptable toxicity.

Renal Impairment

PO (Adults): *CCr <30 mL/min:* 10 mg once daily until disease progression or unacceptable toxicity.

Hepatic Impairment

PO (Adults): *Severe hepatic impairment:* 10 mg once daily until disease progression or unacceptable toxicity.

Availability

Capsules: 4 mg, 10 mg.

NURSING IMPLICATIONS

Assessment

- Assess BP before starting therapy and after 1 wk, then every 2 wk for 1st 2 mo, and then at least monthly thereafter during therapy. Control preexisting hypertension before starting therapy. *If Grade 3 hypertension persists despite antihypertensive therapy,* hold lenvatinib until BP is controlled or Grade ≤2; then resume therapy at ↓ dose. *If life-threatening hypertension occurs,* discontinue lenvatinib.
- Monitor for clinical signs and symptoms of cardiac dysfunction (shortness of breath, swollen ankles) during therapy. *If Grade 3 cardiac dysfunction occurs,* hold lenvatinib until improved to Grade ≤1; then resume at ↓ dose or discontinue depending on severity and persistence of cardiac dysfunction.
- Monitor for signs and symptoms of arterial thromboembolic events (chest pain, acute neurologic symptoms of MI or stroke) during therapy. *If arterial thromboembolic events occurs,* discontinue lenvatinib.
- Assess for signs and symptoms of GI perforation or fistula formation (severe abdominal pain) during therapy. *If GI perforation/fistula occurs,* discontinue lenvatinib.
- Monitor ECG for patients with congenital long QT syndrome, HF, bradyarrhythmias, or those taking QT interval prolonging medications. *If QT interval >500 msec or ↑ by 60 msec from baseline,* hold lenvatinib until QT interval ≤480 msec; then resume at ↓ dose.
- Monitor for signs and symptoms of RPLS (severe headache, seizures, weakness, confusion, blindness or change in vision) during therapy. *If signs/symptoms of RPLS occur,* confirm diagnosis with MRI. *If RPLS confirmed,* hold lenvatinib until fully resolved; then resume at ↓ dose or discontinue depending on severity and persistence of neurologic symptoms.
- Monitor for bleeding (severe and persistent nosebleeds, vomiting blood, red or black stools, coughing up blood or blood clots, heavy or new onset vaginal bleeding) during therapy. *If Grade 3 hemorrhage occurs,* hold lenvatinib until Grade ≤1; then resume at ↓ dose or discontinue depending on severity and persistence of hemorrhage. *If Grade 4 hemorrhage occurs,* discontinue lenvatinib.
- Obtain an oral exam prior to and periodically during therapy. Hold lenvatinib for ≥1 wk before scheduled dental surgery or invasive dental procedures, if possible. Discontinuation of bisphosphonate therapy may ↓ risk of ONJ. Hold lenvatinib if ONJ develops and restart after adequate resolution.

L

Lab Test Considerations

- Verify negative pregnancy test before starting therapy.
- For pMMR/not MSI-H advanced endometrial carcinoma, select patients for therapy with lenvatinib in combination with pembrolizumab based on MSI or MMR status in tumor specimens. Information on FDA-approved tests for patient selection is available at http://www.fda.gov/CompanionDiagnostics.
- Monitor ALT and AST before starting therapy, every 2 wk for 1st 2 mo, and at least monthly thereafter during therapy. May cause hypoalbuminemia, ↑ alkaline phosphatase, and hyperbilirubinemia. Permanently discontinue for hepatic failure. *If Grade 3–4 hepatotoxicity occurs,* hold lenvatinib until ALT/AST ↓ Grade ≤1; then resume at ↓ dose.
- Monitor for proteinuria prior to and periodically during therapy. If urine dipstick proteinuria ≥2+ is detected, obtain 24 hr urine protein. *If ≥2 g proteinuria/24 hr occurs,* hold lenvatinib until proteinuria <2 g/24 hr; then resume at ↓ dose. *If nephrotic syndrome occurs,* discontinue lenvatinib.
- Monitor BUN and serum creatinine before starting and periodically during therapy. *If Grade 3 or 4 renal failure/impairment occurs,* hold lenvatinib until resolved to Grade ≤1; then resume at ↓ dose or discontinue depending on severity and persistence of renal impairment.
- Monitor and correct electrolyte abnormalities. Monitor calcium at least monthly and replace calcium as needed during therapy. Interrupt and adjust lenvatinib dose based on severity, presence of ECG changes, and persistence of hypocalcemia. May cause hypokalemia, hypomagnesemia, hypoglycemia, hypercalcemia, and hyperkalemia.
- Monitor TSH monthly and adjust thyroid replacement medication as needed in patients with ↓ thyroid levels.
- May ↑ lipase and amylase and may cause hypercholesterolemia.
- May cause anemia, neutropenia, leukopenia, and thrombocytopenia.

Implementation

- **Recommended Dose Modifications: Differentiated thyroid cancer:** *1st dose reduction:* 20 once daily; *2nd dose reduction:* 14 mg once daily; *3rd dose reduction:* 10 mg once daily. **Renal cell carcinoma and endometrial carcinoma:** *1st dose reduction:* 14 mg once daily; *2nd dose reduction:* 10 mg once daily; *3rd dose reduction:* 8 mg once daily. **Hepatocellular carcinoma (weight ≥60 kg):** *1st dose reduction:* 8 mg once daily; *2nd dose reduction:* 4 mg once daily; *3rd dose reduction:* 4 mg every other day. **Hepatocellular carcinoma (weight <60 kg):** *1st dose reduction:* 4 mg once daily; *2nd dose reduction:* 4 mg every other day; *3rd dose reduction:* Discontinue lenvatinib.
- Hold therapy for ≥1 wk before elective surgery and for ≥2 wk after major surgery, until adequate wound healing occurs.
- During administration and when preparing tablets, wear double chemotherapy gloves, protective gown, and hair and shoe covers. Respiratory (N95) protection and eye/face protection is needed if there is risk of patient vomiting or spitting up. Single chemotherapy gloves are appropriate if handling and administering intact tablets from a unit-dose package. Health care providers who are actively trying to conceive, who are pregnant or may become pregnant, and who are breastfeeding should avoid handling lenvatinib.
- **PO:** Administer two 10-mg capsules and one 4-mg capsule to make 24 mg at the same time each day without regard to food. ***DNC:*** Swallow capsules whole; do not open, crush, or chew. For patients with difficulty swallowing, measure 1 tablespoon (about 15 mL) of water or apple juice and put capsule in liquid without breaking or crushing. Leave capsule in liquid for ≥10 min. Stir for ≥3 min; then drink mixture. After drinking, add same amount (1 tablespoon) of water or apple juice to glass. Swirl contents and swallow additional liquid. *For administration via feeding tube:* Place required number of capsules, up to a maximum of 5, in a small container (20 mL capacity) or syringe (20 mL). Do not break or crush capsules. Add 3 mL of liquid to container or syringe. Wait 10 min for the capsule shell (outer surface) to disintegrate; then stir or shake mixture for 3 min until capsules are fully disintegrated and administer the entire contents. Add an additional 2 mL of liquid to container or syringe using a 2nd syringe or dropper, swirl or shake, and administer. Repeat this step at least once and until there is no visible residue to ensure all of the medication is taken. Suspension is stable for 24 hr if covered and refrigerated; discard suspension after 24 hr.

Patient/Family Teaching

- Explain the purpose a side effects of lenvatinib. Instruct patient to take as directed at the same time each day. Take missed dose within 12 hr or omit and take next dose at usual time; do not double doses. Keep out of children's reach. Advise patient to read *Patient Information* before starting therapy and with each Rx refill in case of changes.
- Explain need for continued medical follow-up to assess effectiveness and possible side effects of medication. Emphasize importance of lab tests to monitor for adverse reactions.
- Advise patient to immediately report signs and symptoms of hepatotoxicity (fatigue, nausea, upper abdominal pain, yellowing of skin or eyes, dark urine, light-colored stools).
- Advise patient to notify health care provider promptly if signs and symptoms of high BP, heart problems,

blood clots (severe chest pain or pressure; pain in arms, back, or jaw; shortness of breath; numbness or weakness on one side of body; trouble talking; sudden severe headache; sudden vision changes), severe stomach pain, RPLS, or bleeding occur.

- Instruct patient to notify health care provider of therapy before any elective surgery or dental procedure. Lenvatinib must be stopped ≥1 wk before and for ≥2 wk after major surgery until wound healing occurs.
- Advise patient to practice good mouth care during therapy and to notify health care provider if signs and symptoms of ONJ (jaw pain, toothache, sores on gums) occur.
- Advise patient to notify health care provider of all Rx or OTC medications, vitamins, or herbal products being taken and to consult with health care provider before taking other medications.
- Rep: May cause fetal harm. Advise women of reproductive potential to use effective contraception during and for ≥30 days following last dose of therapy and to notify health care provider if pregnancy is suspected. Advise patient to avoid breastfeeding during and for ≥1 wk after last dose. May impair fertility in men and women.

Evaluation/Desired Outcomes

- Decreased progression and improved survival of differentiated thyroid cancer, endometrial cancer, renal cell carcinoma, and hepatocellular carcinoma.

HIGH ALERT

☒ letrozole (let-roe-zole)
Femara
Classification
Therapeutic: antineoplastics
Pharmacologic: aromatase inhibitors

Indications

☒ First-line or second-line treatment of postmenopausal women with hormone receptor positive or hormone receptor unknown advanced breast cancer. ☒ Adjuvant treatment of postmenopausal women with hormone receptor positive early breast cancer. Extended adjuvant treatment of postmenopausal early breast cancer already treated with 5 yr of tamoxifen.

Action

Inhibits the enzyme aromatase, which is partially responsible for conversion of precursors to estrogen. **Therapeutic Effects:** Lowers levels of circulating estrogen, which may halt progression of estrogen-sensitive breast cancer. Decreased risk of recurrence/metastatic disease.

Pharmacokinetics

Absorption: Rapidly and completely absorbed.
Distribution: Well distributed to tissues.
Metabolism and Excretion: Mostly metabolized by the liver. Primarily excreted in the urine (90%), with 6% being excreted as unchanged drug.
Half-life: 2 days.

TIME/ACTION PROFILE (effect on lowering of serum estradiol concentrations)

ROUTE	ONSET	PEAK	DURATION
PO	unknown	2–3 days	unknown

Contraindications/Precautions

Contraindicated in: Hypersensitivity; Premenopausal women; OB: Pregnancy; Lactation: Lactation.
Use Cautiously in: Severe hepatic impairment; Rep: Women of reproductive potential; Pedi: Safety and effectiveness not established in children.

Adverse Reactions/Side Effects

CV: chest pain, DEEP VEIN THROMBOSIS (DVT), edema, hypertension. **Derm:** ↑ sweating, alopecia, hot flush, pruritus, rash. **F and E:** hypercalcemia. **GI:** nausea, abdominal pain, anorexia, constipation, diarrhea, dyspepsia, vomiting. **GU:** ↓ fertility. **Metab:** hypercholesterolemia, weight gain. **MS:** musculoskeletal pain, ↓ bone density, arthralgia, fracture. **Neuro:** anxiety, depression, dizziness, drowsiness, fatigue, headache, STROKE/TRANSIENT ISCHEMIC ATTACK (TIA), vertigo, weakness. **Resp:** cough, dyspnea, pleural effusion, PULMONARY EMBOLISM (PE).

Interactions

Drug-Drug: None reported.

Route/Dosage

PO (Adults): 2.5 mg once daily.

Hepatic Impairment
PO (Adults): *Severe hepatic impairment:* 2.5 mg every other day.

Availability (generic available)

Tablets: 2.5 mg.

NURSING IMPLICATIONS
Assessment

- Assess for musculoskeletal pain and risk for fractures periodically during therapy.
- Monitor bone mineral density periodically during therapy.
- Assess for altered mental status, confusion, chest pain, swelling and redness in legs, shortness of breath, or hypertension. Symptoms may indicate stroke/TIA, PE, or DVT.

✚ = Canadian drug name. ☒ = Genetic implication. **V** = Vesicant. Boxed warning.

Lab Test Considerations
- Verify negative pregnancy test before starting therapy. May ↑ AST, ALT, alkaline phosphatase, bilirubin, GGT, and cholesterol.

Implementation
- **PO:** May be taken without regard to food.

Patient/Family Teaching
- Explain purpose and side effects of medication to patient. Advise patient to read *Patient Information* before starting therapy. Instruct to take medication as directed.
- Advise patient to notify health care provider of all Rx or OTC medications, vitamins, or herbal products being taken and to consult health care provider before taking other medications.
- May cause dizziness and fatigue. Caution patient to avoid driving and other activities requiring awareness until response to medication is known.
- Advise patient to notify health care provider of signs and symptoms of stroke/TIA, PE, or DVT and to seek immediate medical attention if needed.
- Encourage patient to consume calcium and vitamin D supplements to improve bone health.
- Rep: May cause fetal harm. Advise women of reproductive potential to use effective contraception and to avoid breastfeeding during therapy and for >3 wk after last dose. May impair fertility in men and women. Caution women who are perimenopausal or who recently became menopausal to use adequate contraception during therapy.

Evaluation/Desired Outcomes
- Lowers levels of circulating estrogen, which may halt progression of estrogen-sensitive breast cancer.
- Decreased risk of recurrence/metastatic disease.

leucovorin (loo-koe-**vor**-in)

Classification

Therapeutic: antidotes (for methotrexate) vitamins

Pharmacologic: folic acid analogues

Indications
Minimizes hematologic effects of high-dose methotrexate therapy (leucovorin rescue). Advanced colorectal carcinoma (with 5-fluorouracil). Management of overdoses/prevention of toxicity from folic acid antagonists (pyrimethamine, trimethoprim). Folic acid deficiency (megaloblastic anemia) unresponsive to oral replacement.

Action
The reduced form of folic acid that serves as a cofactor in the synthesis of DNA and RNA. **Therapeutic Effects:** Reversal of toxic effects of folic acid antagonists. Reversal of folic acid deficiency.

Pharmacokinetics
Absorption: 38% absorbed following oral administration. ↓ bioavailability with larger doses. Oral absorption is saturated at doses >25 mg. Well absorbed following IM administration. IV administration results in complete bioavailability.
Distribution: Widely distributed to tissues. Concentrates in the CNS and liver.
Metabolism and Excretion: Extensively converted to tetrahydrofolic derivatives, including 5-methyltetrahydrofolate, a major storage form.
Half-life: 3.5 hr.

TIME/ACTION PROFILE (serum folate concentrations)

ROUTE	ONSET	PEAK	DURATION
PO	20–30 min	unknown	3–6 hr
IM	10–20 min	unknown	3–6 hr
IV	<5 min	unknown	3–6 hr

Contraindications/Precautions
Contraindicated in: Hypersensitivity; Pedi: Preparations containing benzyl alcohol should not be used in neonates.
Use Cautiously in: Undiagnosed anemia (may mask the progression of pernicious anemia); Ascites; Renal failure; Dehydration; Pleural effusions; Urine pH <7; OB: Safety not established in pregnancy; Lactation: Safety not established in breastfeeding.

Adverse Reactions/Side Effects
Hemat: thrombocytosis. **Misc:** allergic reactions (rash, urticaria, wheezing).

Interactions
Drug-Drug: May ↓ anticonvulsant effect of **barbiturates**, **phenytoin**, or **primidone**. May ↓ effectiveness of **trimethoprim/sulfamethoxazole** when used to treat *Pneumocystis jirovecii* pneumonia in patients with HIV. May ↑ effects and toxicity of **fluorouracil**; therapy may be combined for this purpose.

Route/Dosage
High-Dose Methotrexate: Leucovorin Rescue
Must start within 24 hr of methotrexate.
PO IM IV (Adults and Children): *Normal methotrexate elimination:* 10 mg/m² every 6 hr (1st dose IV/IM; then change to PO) until methotrexate concentration $<5 \times 10^{-8}$ M (0.05 micromolar). Larger doses/longer duration may be required in patients with aciduria, ascites, dehydration, renal impairment, GI obstruction, or pleural/peritoneal effusions. Dose of leucovorin

should be determined based on the plasma methotrexate concentrations.

Advanced Colorectal Cancer

IV (Adults): 200 mg/m², followed by 5-fluorouracil 370 mg/m², or leucovorin 20 mg/m², followed by 5-fluorouracil 425 mg/m². Regimen is given daily for 5 days every 4–5 wk.

Prevention of Hematologic Toxicity from Pyrimethamine

PO IV (Adults and Children): 5–15 mg/day.

Inadvertent Overdose of Folic Acid Antagonists

IM IV (Adults and Children): *Methotrexate, large doses:* 75 mg IV followed by 12 mg IM every 6 hr for 4 doses; *Methotrexate, average doses:* 6–12 mg IM every 6 hr for 4 doses; *Other folic acid antagonists:* Amount equal in mg to folic acid antagonist.

Megaloblastic Anemia

PO IM IV (Adults and Children): Up to 1 mg/day (up to 6 mg/day for dihydrofolate reductase deficiency).

Availability (generic available)

Tablets: 5 mg, 10 mg, 15 mg, 25 mg. **Powder for injection:** 50 mg/vial, 100 mg/vial, 200 mg/vial, 350 mg/vial, 500 mg/vial. **Solution for injection (preservative-free):** 10 mg/mL.

NURSING IMPLICATIONS

Assessment

- Assess for nausea and vomiting secondary to methotrexate therapy or folic acid antagonist (pyrimethamine and trimethoprim) overdose. Parenteral route may be necessary to ensure that patient receives dose.
- Monitor for development of allergic reactions (rash, urticaria, wheezing). Notify health care provider if these occur and implement supportive measures as needed. **Megaloblastic Anemia:** Assess degree of weakness and fatigue.

Lab Test Considerations

- **Leucovorin rescue:** Monitor serum methotrexate concentrations to determine dose and effectiveness of therapy. Leucovorin concentration should be equal to or greater than methotrexate concentrations. Rescue continues until serum methotrexate concentration <5 × 10 M.
- Monitor CCr and serum creatinine before and every 24 hr during therapy to detect methotrexate toxicity. An ↑ of >50% over the pretreatment concentration at 24 hr is associated with severe renal toxicity.
- Monitor urine pH every 6 hr during therapy; pH should be maintained at >7 to ↓ nephrotoxic effects of high-dose methotrexate. Sodium bicarbonate or acetazolamide may be ordered to alkalinize urine.
- *Megaloblastic anemia:* Monitor folic acid, hemoglobin, hematocrit, and reticulocyte count before and periodically during therapy.

Implementation

- Do not confuse leucovorin with levoleucovorin. Do not confuse leucovorin with Leukeran.
- Make sure leucovorin is available before administering high-dose methotrexate. Administration must be initiated within 24 hr of methotrexate therapy.
- Administer as soon as possible after toxic dose of folic acid antagonist (pyrimethamine and trimethoprim). Effectiveness of therapy begins to ↓ 1 hr after overdose.
- **PO:** Parenteral therapy should be used in patients with GI toxicity, with nausea and vomiting, or with doses >25 mg.
- **IM** IM route is preferred for treatment of megaloblastic anemia. Ampules of leucovorin injection for IM use do not require reconstitution.

L

IV Administration

- **IV Push: Reconstitution:** Reconstitute with bacteriostatic water or sterile water. Do not use product containing benzyl alcohol. Use immediately if reconstituted with sterile water for injection. Stable for 7 days when reconstituted with bacteriostatic water. **Concentration:** Reconstitute 50-mg, 100-mg, and 200-mg vials to a concentration of 10 mg/mL; reconstitute 350-mg vial to a concentration of 20 mg/mL. Do not administer with methotrexate; start leucovorin 24 hr after start of methotrexate. **Rate:** Administer by slow injection over ≥3 min (not to exceed 160 mg/min).
- **Intermittent Infusion: Dilution:** May be diluted in 100–500 mL of D5W, D10W, 0.9% NaCl, Ringer's, or LR. Stable for 24 hr.
- **Y-Site Compatibility:** acyclovir, alemtuzumab, allopurinol, amikacin, aminocaproic acid, aminophylline, ampicillin, ampicillin/sulbactam, anidulafungin, argatroban, arsenic trioxide, atracurium, azithromycin, aztreonam, bivalirudin, bleomycin, bumetanide, buprenorphine, busulfan, butorphanol, calcium chloride, calcium gluconate, carmustine, caspofungin, cefazolin, cefepime, cefotaxime, cefotetan, cefoxitin, ceftazidime, cefuroxime, chloramphenicol, ciprofloxacin, cisatracurium, cisplatin, cladribine, clindamycin, cyclophosphamide, cyclosporine, cytarabine, dacarbazine, dactinomycin, daptomycin, daunorubicin, dexamethasone, dexmedetomidine, dexrazoxane, digoxin, diltiazem, diphenhydramine, dobutamine, docetaxel, dopamine, doxorubicin hydrochloride, doxorubicin liposomal, doxycycline, enalaprilat, ephedrine, epinephrine, eptifibatide, ertapenem, erythromycin, esmolol, etoposide, etoposide phosphate, famotidine, fentanyl, filgrastim,

fluconazole, fludarabine, fluorouracil, fosphenytoin, furosemide, ganciclovir, gemcitabine, gentamicin, glycopyrrolate, granisetron, haloperidol, heparin, hydralazine, hydrocortisone, hydromorphone, idarubicin, ifosfamide, imipenem/cilastatin, insulin regular, irinotecan, isoproterenol, ketorolac, labetalol, levofloxacin, lidocaine, linezolid, lorazepam, magnesium sulfate, mannitol, melphalan, meperidine, meropenem, mesna, methadone, methotrexate, metoclopramide, metoprolol, metronidazole, midazolam, milrinone, minocycline, mitomycin, mitoxantrone, morphine, moxifloxacin, mycophenolate, nafcillin, nalbuphine, nicardipine, nitroglycerin, nitroprusside, norepinephrine, octreotide, ondansetron, oxaliplatin, oxytocin, paclitaxel, palonosetron, pemetrexed, pentobarbital, phenobarbital, phentolamine, phenylephrine, piperacillin/tazobactam, potassium acetate, potassium chloride, procainamide, prochlorperazine, promethazine, propranolol, remifentanil, rituximab, rocuronium, sodium acetate, sodium phosphates, succinylcholine, sufentanil, tacrolimus, theophylline, thiotepa, tigecycline, tirofiban, tobramycin, topotecan, trastuzumab, trimethoprim/sulfamethoxazole, vasopressin, vecuronium, verapamil, vinblastine, vincristine, vinorelbine, voriconazole, zidovudine.

- **Y-Site Incompatibility:** amiodarone, amphotericin B deoxycholate, amphotericin B liposomal, carboplatin, ceftriaxone, chlorpromazine, dantrolene, diazepam, droperidol, epirubicin, foscarnet, gemtuzumab ozogamicin, methylprednisolone, naloxone, pamidronate, pantoprazole, pentamidine, phenytoin, potassium phosphates, sodium bicarbonate, vancomycin.

Patient/Family Teaching

- Explain purpose and side effects of medication to patient. Advise patient to read *Patient Information* before starting therapy. Emphasize need to take exactly as ordered. Advise patient to contact health care provider if a dose is missed.
- Advise patient to notify health care provider of all Rx or OTC medications, vitamins, or herbal products being taken and to consult health care provider before taking other medications.
- **Leucovorin Rescue:** Instruct patient to drink >3 liters of fluid each day during leucovorin rescue.
- **Folic Acid Deficiency:** Encourage patient to eat a diet high in folic acid (meat proteins, bran, dried beans, green leafy vegetables).
- Rep: Advise women of reproductive potential to notify health care provider if pregnancy is planned or suspected or if breastfeeding.

Evaluation/Desired Outcomes

- Reversal of toxic effects of folic acid antagonists.
- Reversal of folic acid deficiency.

HIGH ALERT

leuprolide (loo-proe-lide)

Camcevi, Eligard, Fensolvi, ~~Lupron~~, Lupron Depot, Lupron Depot-Ped, ✦ Zeulide Depot

Classification

Therapeutic: antineoplastics

Pharmacologic: hormones, gonadotropin-releasing hormones

Indications

Advanced prostate cancer. Central precocious puberty. Endometriosis (as monotherapy or in combination with norethindrone). Uterine fibroids (in combination with iron).

Action

Acts as an agonist of gonadotropin releasing hormone (GnRH) receptors. Initially causes a transient increase in testosterone; however, with continuous administration, testosterone levels are decreased. Reduces gonadotropins, testosterone, and estradiol. **Therapeutic Effects:** Decreased testosterone levels and resultant decrease in spread of prostate cancer. Reduction of pain/lesions in endometriosis. Decreased growth of fibroids. Delayed puberty.

Pharmacokinetics

Absorption: Rapidly and almost completely absorbed following SUBQ administration. More slowly absorbed following IM administration of depot form.

Distribution: Unknown.

Metabolism and Excretion: Unknown.

Half-life: 3 hr.

TIME/ACTION PROFILE (effect on hormone concentration)

ROUTE	ONSET†	PEAK‡	DURATION§
SUBQ	within 1st wk	2–4 wk	4–12 wk
IM	within 1st wk	2–4 wk	4–12 wk
IM-depot	within 1st wk	2–4 wk	4–12 wk

† Initial transient ↑ in testosterone and estradiol concentrations.

‡ Maximum decline in testosterone and estradiol concentrations.

§ Restoration of normal pituitary-gonadal function; in amenorrheic patients, normal menses usually returns 60–90 days after treatment is discontinued.

Contraindications/Precautions

Contraindicated in: Hypersensitivity to GnRH agonists; OB: Pregnancy; Lactation: Lactation.

Use Cautiously in: Hypersensitivity to benzyl alcohol (results in induration and erythema at SUBQ site); Congenital long QT syndrome, HF, electrolyte abnormalities, or concurrent use of other drugs known to prolong the QT interval; Seizures, cerebrovascular disorders, CNS tumor, or concurrent use of bupropion or SSRIs; Rep: Women of reproductive potential; Pedi: Children <1 yr (safety and effectiveness not established).

Adverse Reactions/Side Effects

CV: angina, arrhythmias, DEEP VEIN THROMBOSIS (DVT), edema, MI. **Depot:** QT interval prolongation. **Derm: Depot:** hair growth, rash, ACUTE GENERALIZED EXANTHEMATOUS PUSTULOSIS (AGEP), DRUG REACTION WITH EOSINOPHILIA AND SYSTEMIC SYMPTOMS (DRESS), ERYTHEMA MULTIFORME, STEVENS-JOHNSON SYNDROME (SJS), TOXIC EPIDERMAL NECROLYSIS (TEN). **SUBQ:** dry skin, hair loss, pigmentation, skin cancer, skin lesions. **EENT:** blurred vision. **Depot:** epistaxis, throat nodules. **SUBQ:** hearing disorder. **Endo:** hot flushes, breast swelling, breast tenderness, hyperglycemia. **F and E:** hypercalcemia. **GI:** anorexia, diarrhea, dysphagia, nausea, vomiting. **Depot:** gingivitis, HEPATOTOXICITY, nonalcoholic fatty liver disease. **SUBQ:** GI BLEEDING, hepatic impairment, peptic ulcer, rectal polyps. **GU:** ↓ fertility (men), ↓ libido, ↓ testicular size, dysuria, incontinence, testicular pain. **Depot:** cervix disorder. **SUBQ:** bladder spasm, penile swelling, prostate pain, urinary obstruction. **Local:** burning, itching, swelling at injection site. **Metab: Depot:** hyperlipidemia, hyperuricemia. **MS:** fibromyalgia, ↑ bone pain (transient; prostate cancer only). **Depot:** ↓ bone density. **SUBQ:** ankylosing spondylitis, joint pain, pelvic fibrosis, temporal bone pain. **Neuro: SUBQ:** aggression, anger, anxiety, dizziness, dysgeusia, headache, impatience, intracranial hypertension (children), irritability, lethargy, memory disorder, mood swings, peripheral neuropathy, SEIZURES, STROKE, syncope. **Depot:** depression, drowsiness, intracranial hypertension (children), personality disorder. **Resp:** hemoptysis, PULMONARY EMBOLISM (PE). **SUBQ:** cough, pleural rub, pulmonary fibrosis, pulmonary infiltrate. **Misc:** chills, fever, tumor flare. **Depot:** body odor.

Interactions

Drug-Drug: ↑ antineoplastic effects with **antiandrogens (megestrol, flutamide)**. **Bupropion** or **SSRIs** may ↑ risk of seizures. **QT interval prolonging drugs** may ↑ risk of QT interval prolongation.

Route/Dosage

Advanced Prostate Cancer

SUBQ (Adults): *Leuprolide acetate:* 1 mg/day; *Eligard:* 7.5 mg once monthly, 22.5 mg every 3 mo, 30 mg every 4 mo, or 45 mg every 6 mo. *Camcevi:* 42 mg every 6 mo.
IM (Adults): *Lupron Depot:* 7.5 mg once monthly *or* 22.5 mg every 3 mo *or* 30 mg every 4 mo *or* 45 mg every 6 mo.

Endometriosis

IM (Adults): *Lupron Depot:* 3.75 mg once monthly for up to 6 mo *or* 11.25 mg every 3 mo for up to 2 doses; if symptoms recur after initial course of therapy, may administer a 2nd course of therapy.

Uterine Fibroids

IM (Adults): *Lupron Depot:* 3.75 mg once monthly for up to 3 mo *or* 11.25 mg single injection.

Central Precocious Puberty

SUBQ (Children ≥2 yr): *Leuprolide acetate:* 50 mcg/kg/day; may ↑ by 10 mcg/kg/day as required. *Fensolvi:* 45 mg every 6 mo.
IM (Children ≥1 yr and >37.5 kg): *Lupron Depot-Ped (monthly formulation):* 15 mg every 4 wk; may ↑ by 3.75 mg every 4 wk as required.
IM (Children ≥1 yr and 26–37.5 kg): *Lupron Depot-Ped (monthly formulation):* 11.25 mg every 4 wk; may ↑ by 3.75 mg every 4 wk as required.
IM (Children ≥1 yr and ≤25 kg): *Lupron Depot-Ped (monthly formulation):* 7.5 mg every 4 wk; may ↑ by 3.75 mg every 4 wk as required.
IM (Children ≥1 yr): *Lupron Depot-Ped (3-month formulation):* 11.25 or 30 mg every 3 mo.
IM (Children ≥1 yr): *Lupron Depot-Ped (6-month formulation):* 45 mg every 6 mo.

Availability (generic available)

Emulsion for injection (Camcevi) (prefilled syringe): 42 mg. **Lyophilized microspheres for depot injection (Lupron Depot):** 3.75 mg, 7.5 mg, 11.25 mg, 22.5 mg, 30 mg, 45 mg. **Lyophilized microspheres for depot injection (Lupron Depot-Ped):** 7.5 mg, 11.25 mg, 15 mg, 30 mg, 45 mg. **Lyophilized powder for injection (Fensolvi):** 45 mg/vial. **Polymeric matrix injectable formulation for injection (Eligard):** 7.5 mg, 22.5 mg, 30 mg, 45 mg. **Solution for injection (leuprolide acetate):** 1 mg/0.2 mL.

NURSING IMPLICATIONS

Assessment

- Monitor ECG periodically in patients at risk for QT interval prolongation. Assess for palpitations, change in heartbeat, dizziness, shortness of breath, and fainting. Assess for signs of thromboembolic events (DVT, PE, MI, stroke).
- Assess skin for AGEP (small red-white or red elevations with pus). Assess for DRESS (rash with fever, lymphadenopathy, hepatitis, hematologic abnormalities). Assess for TEN (red, painful raw skin near eyes, mouth/throat, and gentials/urethra/anus). Assess for SJS (flu-like symptoms, rash with blisters). Assess for erythema multiforme (target or bull's-eye lesions, red

circular patches with concentric rings on hands, feet, face, and mucous membranes).
- Monitor for seizure activity. Implement seizure precautions if indicated.
- **Prostate Cancer:** Assess for an ↑ in bone pain, especially during the 1st few weeks of therapy. Monitor patients with vertebral metastases for ↑ back pain and ↓ sensory/motor function.
- Monitor intake and output; assess for bladder distention in patients with urinary tract obstruction during initiation of therapy. **Fibroids:** Assess for severity of symptoms (bloating, pelvic pain, pressure, excessive vaginal bleeding) periodically during therapy.
- **Endometriosis:** Assess for endometrial pain prior to and periodically during therapy.
- **Central Precocious Puberty:** Before therapy, confirm diagnosis of central precocious puberty by onset of secondary sex characteristics in girls <8 yr or boys <9 yr. A complete physical and endocrinologic examination, including height, weight, and hand and wrist x-ray; total sex steroid level (estradiol or testosterone); adrenal steroid level; beta human chorionic gonadotropin level; GnRH stimulation test; and computerized tomography of the head must be performed. These parameters are monitored after 1–2 mo and every 3–6 mo during therapy.
- Assess for signs of precocious puberty (menses, breast development, testicular growth) periodically during therapy. Dose is ↑ until no progression of the disease is noted either clinically or by lab test parameters and then usually maintained throughout therapy. Discontinuation of therapy should be considered before age 11 in girls and age 12 in boys.

Lab Test Considerations
- Verify negative pregnancy test before starting therapy.
- Initially ↑ and then ↓ luteinizing hormone and follicle-stimulating hormone. This leads to castration levels of testosterone in boys 2–4 wk after initial ↑ in concentrations.
- Monitor testosterone, prostatic acid phosphate, and prostate-specific antigen levels to evaluate response to therapy. Transient ↑ in levels may occur during the 1st mo of therapy for prostate cancer.
- Monitor electrolytes before starting and periodically during therapy. May cause ↑ BUN, calcium, uric acid, hypoproteinemia, LDH, alkaline phosphatase, AST, hyperglycemia, hyperlipidemia, hyperphosphatemia, WBC, PT, or aPTT. May ↓ platelets and potassium.
- Monitor blood sugar and A1c periodically during therapy.

Implementation
- Do not confuse Lupron Depot with Lupron Depot-Ped.
- Norethindrone acetate 5 mg daily may be used to prevent bone density loss from leuprolide.
- Correct electrolyte abnormalities before starting therapy.
- **SUBQ** *Camcevi:* Must be administered by a health care provider. Allow prefilled syringe to stand at room temperature for 30 min before injection. Wear gloves during preparation and administration. Inject into upper or midabdominal area with sufficient soft or loose SUBQ tissue that has not recently been used. Clean the injection site with an alcohol swab. Do NOT inject in areas with brawny or fibrous SUBQ tissue or locations that can be rubbed or compressed (with a belt or clothing waistband). Avoid applying heat directly to the site of injection. Pinch skin and inject at 90° angle; release skin and inject full contents of syringe.
- *Eligard SUBQ formulation:* Bring to room temperature before mixing. **Reconstitution:** Assemble the *Eligard* kit and reconstitute solution using syringes provided, as directed by manufacturer. Wearing gloves, mix in syringes as directed by manufacturer; do not shake. Solution must reach room temperature before administration and must be administered within 30 min of mixing or discarded. Solution is light tan to tan in color. Inject into abdomen, upper buttocks, or anywhere that has adequate amounts of SUBQ tissue without excessive pigment, nodules, lesions, or hair. Vary site with each injection. Store in refrigerator; may also be stored at room temperature in original packing for up to 8 wk before mixing.
- *Fensolvi:* Must be administered by a health care provider. Allow to reach room temperature before reconstitution. **Reconstitution:** Follow manufacturer's instructions for assembling syringes and mixing. **Concentration:** 45 mg/0.375 mL. Administer within 30 min or discard. Inject into abdomen or upper buttocks. Avoid areas that have excessive pigment, nodules, lesions, or hair. Pinch skin and inject at 90° angle. Release skin and inject slowly. Rotate injection sites.
- **IM:** Use syringe supplied by manufacturer. Rotate sites.
- Leuprolide depot is *only* for IM injection.
- *Lupron Depot formulation* and *Lupron Depot-Ped* must be administered by a health care provider. **Reconstitution:** To prepare for injection, screw white plunger into end stopper until stopper begins to turn. Hold syringe upright; release diluent by slowly pushing, over 6–8 sec, until the first stopper is at the blue line in the middle of the barrel. Keep syringe upright. Mix microspheres by shaking syringe until power forms a unified suspension. Tap syringe if caking or clumping occurs. Do not combine syringes or partial syringes to arrive at a dose of *Lupron Depot-Ped*. Suspension will appear milky. Do not use if powder does not go into suspension. Keep syringe upright; remove cap and expel air. Inject at 90° angle in gluteal area, anterior thigh, or deltoid; aspirate and discard if blood in

syringe. Suspension settles very quickly; mix and administer immediately. Administer within 2 hr or discard. Rotate injection sites.

Patient/Family Teaching

- Explain purpose and side effects of medication. Advise patient to read *Patient Information* before starting therapy.
- Advise patient to notify health care provider of all Rx or OTC medications, vitamins, or herbal products being taken and to consult health care provider before taking other medications.
- Advise patient that medication may cause hot flushes. Notify health care provider if these become bothersome.
- Leuprolide depot usually causes a temporary discontinuation of menstruation. Advise patient to notify health care provider if menstruation persists or if intermittent bleeding occurs.
- Inform patient of the possibility of the development or worsening of depression and occurrence of memory disorders.
- Advise patient of the risk of MI, stroke, and other thromboembolic events. Advise to immediately report signs and symptoms associated with these events to their health care provider for evaluation or seek immediate medical attention.
- Inform patient of the risk of seizures. Advise to immediately contact their health care provider if they experience any seizure activity.
- Rep: May cause fetal harm. Advise women of reproductive potential to use effective contraception during therapy. Advise patient to notify health care provider if pregnancy is planned or suspected or if breastfeeding. Advise patient that leuprolide may impair fertility.
- **Prostate Cancer:** Instruct patient and family on SUBQ injection technique. Review patient insert provided with leuprolide patient administration kit.
- Instruct patient to take medication exactly as directed. Take missed doses as soon as remembered unless not remembered until next day.
- Inform patient that bone pain may ↑ at initiation of therapy, but will resolve with time. Advise patient to discuss use of analgesics to control pain with health care provider.
- Instruct patient to notify health care provider promptly if difficulty urinating, weakness, or numbness occurs.
- **Endometriosis:** Advise patient to use a form of contraception other than oral contraceptives during therapy. Inform patient that amenorrhea is expected but does not guarantee contraception. Advise patient that breastfeeding should be avoided during therapy.
- **Central Precocious Puberty:** Instruct patient and caregivers on the proper technique for SUBQ injection. Emphasize the importance of administering the medication at the same time each day. Rotate injection sites periodically.
- Inform patient and caregivers that if injections are not given daily, pubertal process may be reactivated.
- Advise patient and caregivers that during the 1st 2 mo of therapy, patient may experience a light menstrual flow or spotting. Health care provider should be notified if this continues beyond 2nd mo.
- Instruct patient and caregivers to notify health care provider immediately if irritation at the injection site or unusual signs or symptoms occur.

Evaluation/Desired Outcomes

- Decreased testosterone levels and resultant decrease in spread of prostate cancer.
- Reduction of pain/lesions in endometriosis.
- Decreased growth of fibroids.
- Delayed puberty.

levalbuterol

(lev-al-**byoo**-ter-ole)

Xopenex HFA

Classification

Therapeutic: bronchodilators

Pharmacologic: adrenergics

Indications

Bronchospasm due to reversible airway disease (short-term control agent).

Action

R-enantiomer of racemic albuterol. Binds to beta-2 adrenergic receptors in airway smooth muscle, leading to activation of adenylcyclase and increased levels of cyclic-3′, 5′-adenosine monophosphate (cAMP). Increases in cAMP activate kinases, which inhibit the phosphorylation of myosin and decrease intracellular calcium. Decreased intracellular calcium relaxes bronchial smooth muscle. **Therapeutic Effects:** Relaxation of airway smooth muscle with subsequent bronchodilation. Relatively selective for beta-2 (pulmonary) receptors.

Pharmacokinetics

Absorption: Some absorption occurs following inhalation.

Distribution: Unknown.

Metabolism and Excretion: Metabolized in the liver to an inactive sulfate; 3–6% excreted unchanged in the urine.

Half-life: 3.3–4 hr.

TIME/ACTION PROFILE (bronchodilation)

ROUTE	ONSET	PEAK	DURATION
Inhaln	10–17 min	90 min	5–6 hr

Contraindications/Precautions

Contraindicated in: Hypersensitivity to levalbuterol or albuterol.

Use Cautiously in: Cardiovascular disorders (including coronary insufficiency, hypertension, and arrhythmias); History of seizures; Hypokalemia; Hyperthyroidism; Diabetes mellitus; Unusual sensitivity to adrenergic amines; OB: Safety not established in pregnancy; Lactation: Use while breastfeeding only if potential maternal benefit justifies potential risk to infant; Pedi: Safety and effectiveness not established in children <6 yr (nebulized solution) or <4 yr (metered-dose inhaler).

Exercise Extreme Caution in: Concurrent use or use within 2 wk of **tricyclic antidepressants** or **MAO inhibitors** may ↑ risk of adverse cardiovascular reactions.

Adverse Reactions/Side Effects

CV: tachycardia. **EENT:** turbinate edema. **Endo:** hyperglycemia. **F and E:** hypokalemia. **GI:** dyspepsia, vomiting. **Neuro:** anxiety, dizziness, headache, nervousness, tremor. **Resp:** cough, PARADOXICAL BRONCHOSPASM (EXCESSIVE USE OF INHALERS).

Interactions

Drug-Drug: Concurrent use or use within 2 wk of **tricyclic antidepressants** or **MAO inhibitors** may ↑ risk of adverse cardiovascular reactions (use with extreme caution). **Beta blockers** block the beneficial pulmonary effects of adrenergic bronchodilators; choose cardioselective beta blockers if necessary and with caution. May ↑ risk of hypokalemia from **thiazide diuretics** and **loop diuretics**. May ↓ **digoxin** levels. May ↑ risk of arrhythmias with **hydrocarbon inhalation anesthetics** or **cocaine**.

Drug-Natural Products: Use with caffeine-containing herbs **(guarana, tea, coffee)** ↑ stimulant effect.

Route/Dosage

Inhaln: (Adults and Children ≥4 yr): 2 inhalations every 4–6 hr; some patients may respond to 1 inhalation every 4 hr.

Inhaln: (Adults and Children >12 yr): 0.63 mg via nebulization 3 times daily (every 6–8 hr); may be ↑ to 1.25 mg 3 times daily (every 6–8 hr).

Inhaln: (Children 6–11 yr): 0.31 mg via nebulization 3 times daily (not to exceed 0.63 mg 3 times daily).

Availability (generic available)

Inhalation aerosol: 45 mcg/actuation in 15-g canisters (200 metered actuations). **Inhalation solution:** 0.31 mg/3 mL, 0.63 mg/3 mL, 1.25 mg/3 mL, 1.25 mg/0.5 mL.

NURSING IMPLICATIONS

Assessment

- Assess lung sounds, pulse, and BP before administration and during peak of medication. Note amount, color, and character of sputum produced. Closely monitor patients on higher dose for adverse effects.
- Monitor cardiac status (chest pain) and for ECG changes (flattening T wave, prolongation of QTc interval, and ST segment depression). Should be used with caution in patients with ischemic heart disease, arrhythmias, and hypertension.
- Monitor pulmonary function tests before initiating therapy and periodically during course to determine effectiveness of medication.
- Observe for paradoxical bronchospasm (wheezing, dyspnea, tightness in chest). If condition occurs, withhold medication and notify health care provider immediately.

Lab Test Considerations

- May cause ↑ serum glucose and ↓ serum potassium.

Implementation

- **Inhaln:** Allow at least 1 min between inhalations of aerosol medication.
- For *metered-dose inhaler*, shake well before using. Prime inhaler before using for the 1st time or if not used for >3 days; release 4 sprays into the air away from face. Use actuator that is supplied with the product. Clean actuator with warm water and let air-dry completely at least once a wk.
- For *nebulization*, concentrated solution should be diluted with 2.5 mL of NS prior to use, or per prescriber's order. Once the foil pouch is opened, vials must be used within 2 wk; open vials may be stored for 1 wk and should be protected from light. Discard vial if solution is not clear or colorless.

Patient/Family Teaching

- Instruct patient in the proper use and side effects of inhalation aerosol nebulizer (see Appendix C) and to take levalbuterol as directed. Caution patient not to exceed recommended dose; may cause adverse effects, paradoxical bronchospasm, or loss of effectiveness of medication.
- Advise patient to read *Patient Information* before starting therapy.
- Instruct patient to notify health care professional of all Rx or OTC medications, vitamins, or herbal products being taken and to consult health care

professional before taking any OTC medications or alcoholic beverages concurrently with this therapy. Caution patient also to avoid smoking and other respiratory irritants.

- Instruct patient to contact health care professional immediately if shortness of breath is not relieved by medication or is accompanied by diaphoresis, dizziness, palpitations, or chest pain.
- Advise patients to use levalbuterol first if using other inhalation medications, and allow 5 min to elapse before administering other inhalant medications unless otherwise directed.
- Advise patient to rinse mouth with water after each inhalation dose to minimize dry mouth.
- Instruct patient to seek medical attention immediately if symptoms become worse, treatment is less effective for symptomatic relief, or the use of the product is more frequent than usual.
- Rep: Advise females of reproductive potential to notify health care professional if pregnancy is planned or suspected or if breastfeeding. Encourage women who become pregnant while taking levalbuterol to enroll in the Asthma & Pregnancy Study to monitor pregnancy outcomes in women exposed to asthma medications by calling 1-877-311-8972 or visiting www.mothertobaby.org/ongoing-study/asthma.
- Pedi: Children should use under adult supervision, as instructed by patient's physician.

Evaluation/Desired Outcomes

- Prevention or relief of bronchospasm.

levETIRAcetam

(le-ve-teer-**a**-se-tam)

Keppra, Keppra XR, Roweepra, Spritam

Classification

Therapeutic: anticonvulsants

Pharmacologic: pyrrolidines

Indications

Partial onset seizures (as monotherapy or adjunctive therapy). Primary generalized tonic-clonic seizures (adjunct) (immediate release and injection only). Myoclonic seizures in patients with juvenile myoclonic epilepsy (adjunct) (immediate release and injection only). **Unlabeled Use:** Status epilepticus.

Action

Appears to inhibit burst firing without affecting normal neuronal excitability and may selectively prevent hypersynchronization of epileptiform burst firing and propagation of seizure activity. **Therapeutic Effects:** Decreased incidence and severity of seizures.

Pharmacokinetics

Absorption: Rapidly and completely absorbed following oral administration. IV administration results in complete bioavailability.

Distribution: Well distributed to tissues.

Metabolism and Excretion: 66% excreted unchanged by the kidneys; some metabolism by the liver (metabolites inactive).

Half-life: 7.1 hr (↑ in renal impairment).

TIME/ACTION PROFILE (plasma concentrations)

ROUTE	ONSET	PEAK	DURATION
PO	rapid	1–1.5 hr†‡	12 hr
IV	rapid	end of infusion	unknown

† 1 hr in the faszting state, 1.5 hr when taken with food.
‡ 4 hr with extended release.

Contraindications/Precautions

Contraindicated in: Hypersensitivity.

Use Cautiously in: All patients (may ↑ risk of suicidal thoughts/behaviors); Renal impairment (↓ dose if CCr ≤80 mL/min); OB: Use during pregnancy only if potential maternal benefit justifies potential fetal risk; blood levels may be ↓ during pregnancy (especially during 3rd trimester); Lactation: Safety not established in breastfeeding; Pedi: Safety and effectiveness not established in children <1 mo (immediate-release tablets, tablets for oral suspension, oral solution, and injection), <12 yr (extended-release tablets); Geri: Older adults may have ↓ renal elimination (dose ↓ may be necessary).

Adverse Reactions/Side Effects

CV: hypertension. **Derm:** DRUG REACTION WITH EOSINOPHILIA AND SYSTEMIC SYMPTOMS (DRESS), STEVENS-JOHNSON SYNDROME (SJS), TOXIC EPIDERMAL NECROLYSIS. **Hemat:** AGRANULOCYTOSIS, anemia, eosinophilia, neutropenia, thrombocytopenia. **Neuro:** aggression, agitation, anger, anxiety, apathy, depersonalization, depression, dizziness, drowsiness, fatigue, hostility, irritability, personality disorder, psychosis, weakness, coordination difficulties (adults only), hyperkinesia, SUICIDAL THOUGHTS. **Misc:** HYPERSENSITIVITY REACTIONS (INCLUDING ANAPHYLAXIS AND ANGIOEDEMA).

Interactions

Drug-Drug: None reported.

Route/Dosage

Only the oral solution should be used in patients ≤20 kg.

Partial Onset Seizures

PO IV (Adults and Children ≥16 yr): 500 mg twice daily initially; may ↑ by 1000 mg/day at 2-wk intervals up to 3000 mg/day in 2 divided doses.
PO (Adults and Children 4–15 yr): *Oral solution:* 10 mg/kg twice daily; ↑ by 20 mg/kg/day at 2-wk intervals to recommended dose of 30 mg/kg twice daily (not to exceed 1500 mg twice daily). *Immediate-release tablets or tablets for oral suspension (for patients >40 kg):* 500 mg twice daily; may ↑ by 1000 mg/day at 2-wk intervals up to 3000 mg/day in 2 divided doses. *Immediate-release tablets or tablets for oral suspension (for patients 20–40 kg):* 250 mg twice daily; may ↑ by 500 mg/day at 2-wk intervals up to 1500 mg/day in 2 divided doses.
PO (Adults and Children ≥12 yr and ≥50 kg): *Extended release:* 1000 mg once daily; may ↑ by 1000 mg/day at 2-wk intervals up to 3000 mg once daily.
IV (Children 4–15 yr): 10 mg/kg twice daily; ↑ by 20 mg/kg/day at 2-wk intervals to recommended dose of 30 mg/kg twice daily (not to exceed 1500 mg twice daily).
PO IV (Children 6 mo–3 yr): 10 mg/kg twice daily; ↑ by 20 mg/kg/day at 2-wk intervals to recommended dose of 25 mg/kg twice daily.
PO, IV (Children 1–5 mo): 7 mg/kg twice daily; ↑ by 14 mg/kg/day at 2-wk intervals to recommended dose of 21 mg/kg twice daily.

Renal Impairment

PO IV (Adults): *CCr 50–80 mL/min:* 500–1000 mg twice daily (1000–2000 mg once daily for extended release); *CCr 30–50 mL/min:* 250–750 mg twice daily (500–1500 mg once daily for extended release); *CCr <30 mL/min:* 250–500 mg twice daily (500–1000 mg once daily for extended release); *Dialysis (immediate release and injection):* 500–1000 mg once daily with a 250–500-mg supplemental dose after dialysis.

Primary Generalized Tonic-Clonic Seizures

PO IV (Adults and Children ≥16 yr): 500 mg twice daily initially; ↑ by 1000 mg/day at 2-wk intervals to recommended dose of 3000 mg/day.
PO (Adults and Children ≥6 yr and >40 kg): *Tablets for oral suspension:* 500 mg twice daily; may ↑ by 1000 mg/day at 2-wk intervals up to 3000 mg/day in 2 divided doses.
PO IV (Children 6–15 yr): 10 mg/kg twice daily; ↑ by 20 mg/kg/day at 2-wk intervals to recommended dose of 30 mg/kg twice daily.
PO (Children ≥6 yr and 20–40 kg): *Tablets for oral suspension:* 250 mg twice daily; may ↑ by 500 mg/day at 2-wk intervals up to 1500 mg/day in 2 divided doses.

Renal Impairment

PO IV (Adults): *CCr 50–80 mL/min (immediate release and injection):* 500–1000 mg twice daily; *CCr 30–50 mL/min (immediate release and injection):* 250–750 mg twice daily; *CCr <30 mL/min (immediate release and injection):* 250–500 mg twice daily; *Dialysis (immediate release and injection):* 500–1000 mg once daily with a 250–500-mg supplemental dose after dialysis.

Myoclonic Seizures

PO IV (Adults and Children ≥12 yr): 500 mg twice daily initially; ↑ by 1000 mg/day at 2-wk intervals to recommended dose of 3000 mg/day (in 2 divided doses).

Renal Impairment

PO IV (Adults): *CCr 50–80 mL/min (immediate release and injection):* 500–1000 mg twice daily; *CCr 30–50 mL/min (immediate release and injection):* 250–750 mg twice daily; *CCr <30 mL/min (immediate release and injection):* 250–500 mg twice daily; *Dialysis (immediate release and injection):* 500–1000 mg once daily with a 250–500-mg supplemental dose after dialysis.

Status Epilepticus

IV (Infants and Children <16 yr): 50 mg/kg as a loading dose followed by maintenance dose of 30–55 mg/kg/day IV/PO in 2 divided doses.
IV (Neonates): 20–30 mg/kg as a loading dose followed by neonatal seizure dosing.

Availability (generic available)

Immediate-release tablets: 250 mg, 500 mg, 750 mg, 1000 mg. **Extended-release tablets:** 500 mg, 750 mg. **Oral solution (grape flavored):** 100 mg/mL. **Tablets for oral suspension (Spritam)(spearmint flavored):** 250 mg, 500 mg, 750 mg, 1000 mg. **Premixed infusion:** 250 mg/50 mL 0.82% NaCl, 500 mg/100 mL 0.82% NaCl, 1000 mg/100 mL 0.75% NaCl, 1500 mg/100 mL 0.54% NaCl. **Solution for injection (requires dilution):** 100 mg/mL.

NURSING IMPLICATIONS

Assessment

- Assess type, location, duration, and characteristics of seizure activity.
- Assess patient for CNS adverse effects during therapy, such as somnolence, fatigue (asthenia), coordination difficulties (ataxia, abnormal gait, incoordination), and behavioral abnormalities (agitation, hostility, anxiety, apathy, emotional lability, depersonalization, depression), which usually occur during the 1st 4 wk of therapy.
- Monitor mood and behavior changes. Assess for suicidality, especially during early therapy. Restrict amount of drug available to patient.
- Assess for rash or signs/symptoms of SJS periodically during therapy (fever, general malaise, fatigue, muscle or joint aches, blisters,

oral lesions, conjunctivitis). *If severe rash occurs,* discontinue levetiracetam and provide supportive care.

- Monitor for signs/symptoms of DRESS (fever, rash, lymphadenopathy, facial swelling) or organ system injury such as hepatitis, nephritis, hematologic abnormalities, myocarditis, or myositis during therapy. Usually occurs 2–8 wk after starting therapy. May resemble an acute viral infection. Eosinophilia is often present. *If signs/symptoms of DRESS occur,* discontinue levetiracetam.
- Monitor for signs/symptoms of anaphylaxis (dyspnea, wheezing, facial swelling). *If anaphylaxis occurs,* discontinue levetiracetam.
- Pedi: Monitor patients 1 mo–<4 yr of age for ↑ in diastolic BP.

Lab Test Considerations

- May cause ↓ RBC and WBC and abnormal liver function tests.

Implementation

- Do not confuse Keppra with Kaletra. Do not confuse levetiracetam with lamotrigine, levocarnitine, or levofloxacin.
- IV doses should be used temporarily when oral route is not feasible. To convert IV to PO, equivalent dose and frequency may be used.
- **PO:** May be administered without regard to meals.
- ***DNC:*** Administer tablets whole; do not administer partial tablets. Do not break, crush, or chew XR tablets.
- *Tablets for oral suspension (Spritam)* can be administered by placing tablet on tongue with a dry hand; follow with a sip of liquid and swallow only after tablet disintegrates; do not swallow tablet intact. Do not administer partial tablets. *Spritam* disintegrates in about 11 sec in the mouth when taken with a sip of liquid. May also add whole tablet to a small volume of liquid in a cup (one tablespoon or enough to cover tablets). Allow the tablet to disperse before consuming the entire contents immediately. After administration of suspension, resuspend any residue by adding an additional small volume of liquid and swallowing the full amount. Do not administer partial quantities of dispersed tablets. Peel foil to access tablet; do not push through foil. May also administer *Spritam* down nasogastric or gastrostomy tube by placing the number of whole tablets needed for the prescribed dose in a small dosing cup. Add 10 mL of room temperature water to the cup, and then swirl the cup until the tablets disperse in the liquid. Draw up the mixture into a 10-mL oral catheter-tip syringe, and then administer immediately via the nasogastric or gastrostomy tube. After administration, add another 10 mL of room temperature water to the dosing cup that contained the dispersion, and swirl the cup to resuspend any tablet residue. Draw up the mixture into the same oral syringe and immediately push through the feeding tube to flush it.
- Pedi: Patients <20 kg should receive oral solution. Administer with calibrated measuring device for accurate dose.
- Discontinue gradually to minimize the risk of increase in seizure frequency.

IV Administration

- **Intermittent Infusion: Dilution:** Dilute dose in 100 mL of 0.9% NaCl, D5W, or LR. **Concentration:** <15 mg/mL. Do not administer solutions that are cloudy or contain particulate matter.
- Stable for 4 hr once diluted. Discard unused portions. **Rate:** Infuse over 15 min.
- **Y-Site Compatibility:** caffeine citrate, cefazolin, cefotaxime, cisatracurium, dexmedetomidine, fosphenytoin, norepinephrine, propofol, sildenafil, vancomycin, vasopressin.
- **Y-Site Incompatibility:** heparin, posaconazole.

Patient/Family Teaching

- Explain purpose and side effects of levetiracetam to patient.
- Instruct patient to take medication as directed. Pedi: Explain to parents the importance of using calibrated measuring device for accurate dosing. Take missed doses as soon as possible unless almost time for next dose. Do not double doses. Do not discontinue abruptly; may cause ↑ in frequency of seizures. Advise patient and parents to read the *Medication Guide* prior to starting therapy and with each Rx refill in case of changes.
- May cause dizziness and somnolence. Caution patient to avoid driving or activities requiring alertness until response to medication is known. Do not resume driving until physician gives clearance based on control of seizure disorder.
- Emphasize importance of regular follow-ups and that medical ID describing disease process and medication regimen should be worn at all times in case of emergencies.
- Advise patient and family to notify health care provider if thoughts about suicide or dying, suicide attempts, new or worse depression, new or worse anxiety, feeling very agitated or restless, panic attacks, trouble sleeping, new or worse irritability, acting aggressive, being angry or violent, acting on

L

dangerous impulses, an extreme ↑ in activity and talking, or other unusual changes in behavior or mood occur.

- Teach the patient to immediately report signs and symptoms of SJS (rash, fever, fatigue, muscle and joint pain, blisters, oral lesions, conjunctivitis) or DRESS (fever, rash, swollen face or lymph nodes, abdominal pain, jaundice, nausea, dark urine, chest pain, shortness of breath, flu-like symptoms).
- Advise patient to notify health care provider of all Rx or OTC medications, vitamins, or herbal products being taken and to consult with health care provider before taking other medications.
- Instruct patient to notify health care provider of medication regimen prior to treatment or surgery.
- Rep: Advise women of reproductive potential to notify health care provider if pregnancy is planned or suspected or if breastfeeding. Encourage pregnant patients to enroll in the North American Antiepileptic Drug Pregnancy Registry by calling 1-888-233-2334 or visiting www.aedpregnancyregistry.org. Levetiracetam levels may ↓ during pregnancy, especially in the 3rd trimester. Dose adjustments may be necessary to maintain clinical response.

Evaluation/Desired Outcomes

- Decrease in the frequency of or cessation of seizures.

levocetirizine

(lee-vo-se-**teer**-i-zeen)

~~Xyzal~~, Xyzal Allergy 24HR

Classification

Therapeutic: allergy cold cough remedies

Pharmacologic: antihistamines

Indications

Seasonal/perennial allergic rhinitis. Chronic idiopathic urticaria.

Action

Antagonizes the effects of histamine at H_1 receptor sites; does not bind to or inactivate histamine.

Therapeutic Effects: Decreased symptoms of histamine excess (rhinitis, itching).

Pharmacokinetics

Absorption: Well absorbed following oral administration.

Distribution: Unknown.

Metabolism and Excretion: Excreted mostly unchanged by the kidneys (85%).

Half-life: 8 hr.

ROUTE	ONSET	PEAK	DURATION
PO	rapid	0.9 hr	24 hr

Contraindications/Precautions

Contraindicated in: Hypersensitivity to levocetirizine or cetirizine; Severe renal impairment (CCr <10 mL/min).

Use Cautiously in: OB: Other 2nd-generation antihistamines preferred in pregnancy; Lactation: Other 2nd-generation antihistamines preferred in breastfeeding; Pedi: Children <6 mo (safety and effectiveness not established); Geri: Consider age-related ↓ in renal function and concurrent disease states in older adults.

Adverse Reactions/Side Effects

Derm: acute generalized exanthematous pustulosis. **GI:** dry mouth. **GU:** urinary retention. **Neuro:** drowsiness, fatigue, weakness.

Interactions

Drug-Drug: May ↑ levels and risk of toxicity of **ritonavir**. ↑ CNS depression may occur with **alcohol**, **opioid analgesics**, or **sedative hypnotics**.

Route/Dosage

PO (Adults and Children ≥12 yr): 5 mg once daily in the evening; some patients may respond to 2.5 mg once daily.

PO (Children 6–11 yr): 2.5 mg once daily in the evening.

PO (Children 6 mo–5 yr): 1.25 mg (oral solution) once daily in the evening.

Renal Impairment

(Adults and Children ≥12 yr): *CCr 50–80 mL/min:* 2.5 mg once daily; *CCr 30–50 mL/min:* 2.5 mg every other day; *CCr 10–30 mL/min:* 2.5 mg twice weekly (every 3–4 days).

Availability (generic available)

Tablets: 5 mg [OTC]. **Oral solution (tutti-frutti, grape, and bubble gum flavors):** 2.5 mg/5 mL[OTC].

NURSING IMPLICATIONS

Assessment

- Assess allergy symptoms (rhinitis, conjunctivitis, hives) before and periodically during therapy.
- Assess lung sounds and character of bronchial secretions. Maintain fluid intake of 1500–2000 mL/day to ↓ viscosity of secretions.

Lab Test Considerations

- May cause false-negative result in allergy skin testing.
- May cause transient ↑ in serum bilirubin and transaminases.

Implementation

- **PO:** Administer once daily in the evening without regard to food. Oral solution is clear and colorless; administer undiluted.

Patient/Family Teaching

- Explain purpose and side effects of medication to patient. Advise patient to read *Patient Information* before starting therapy. Instruct to take medication as directed. Do not ↑ doses; may cause ↑ drowsiness.
- Advise patient to notify health care provider of all Rx or OTC medications, vitamins, or herbal products being taken and to consult health care provider before taking other medications.
- May cause drowsiness. Caution patient to avoid driving or other activities requiring alertness until response to medication is known.
- Advise patient to avoid taking alcohol or other CNS depressants concurrently with this drug.
- Advise patient that good oral hygiene, frequent rinsing of mouth with water, and sugarless gum or candy may minimize dry mouth. Patient should notify dentist if dry mouth persists >2 wk.
- Rep: Advise women of reproductive potential to notify health care provider if pregnancy is planned or suspected or if breastfeeding.

Evaluation/Desired Outcomes

- Decreased symptoms of histamine excess (rhinitis, itching).

levofloxacin, See FLUOROQUINOLONES.

levonorgestrel, See CONTRACEPTIVES, HORMONAL.

levothyroxine

(lee-voe-thye-**rox**-een)

🍁 Eltroxin, Ermeza, Levo-T, Levoxyl, Synthroid, Thyquidity, Tirosint, Tirosint-SOL, Unithroid

Classification

Therapeutic: hormones

Pharmacologic: thyroid preparations

Indications

Thyroid supplementation in hypothyroidism. Treatment or suppression of euthyroid goiters. Adjunctive treatment for thyrotropin-dependent thyroid cancer. Should NOT be used for the treatment of obesity or for weight loss.

Action

Synthetic form of thyroxine (T_4). Replacement of or supplementation to endogenous thyroid hormones. Principal effect is increasing metabolic rate of body tissues: Promote gluconeogenesis, Increase utilization and mobilization of glycogen stores, Stimulate protein synthesis, Promote cell growth and differentiation, Aid in the development of the brain and CNS. **Therapeutic Effects:** Replacement in hypothyroidism to restore normal hormonal balance. Suppression of thyroid cancer.

Pharmacokinetics

Absorption: Levothyroxine is variably (40–80%) absorbed from the GI tract.

Distribution: Distributed into most body tissues.

Protein Binding: >99%.

Metabolism and Excretion: Metabolized by the liver and other tissues to active T3. Thyroid hormone undergoes enterohepatic recirculation and is excreted in the feces via the bile.

Half-life: 6–7 days.

ROUTE	ONSET	PEAK	DURATION
PO	unknown	1–3 wk	1–3 wk
IV	6–8 hr	24 hr	unknown

Contraindications/Precautions

Contraindicated in: Hypersensitivity; Recent MI; Hyperthyroidism.

Use Cautiously in: Cardiovascular disease (initiate therapy with lower doses); Severe renal impairment; Uncorrected adrenocortical disorders; Pedi: Monitor neonates and infants for cardiac overload, arrhythmias, and aspiration during 1st 2 wk of therapy; Geri: Older adults are extremely sensitive to thyroid hormones; initial dose should be ↓.

Adverse Reactions/Side Effects

Usually only seen when excessive doses cause iatrogenic hyperthyroidism.

CV: angina, arrhythmias, tachycardia. **Derm:** sweating. **Endo:** heat intolerance, hyperthyroidism, menstrual irregularities. **GI:** abdominal cramps, diarrhea, vomiting. **Metab:** weight loss. **MS:** accelerated bone maturation in children. **Neuro:** headache, insomnia, irritability.

Interactions

Drug-Drug: Cholestyramine, colesevelam, colestipol, and **sodium polystyrene sulfonate** may bind to and ↓ absorption of orally administered levothyroxine; administer levothyroxine ≥4 hr prior to these medications or monitor TSH levels. **Phosphate binders**, including **calcium carbonate, ferrous sulfate, lanthanum carbonate**, and **sevelemer**, may bind to and ↓ absorption of orally administered levothyroxine; administer levothyroxine ≥4 hr apart from these medications. Absorption may be ↓ by **orlistat**, **proton pump inhibitors**, **sucralfate**, **antacids**, and **simethicone**. **Phenobarbital** and **rifampin** may ↓ levels and effectiveness; may need to ↑ levothyroxine dosage. May ↑ the risk of bleeding with **warfarin**. May ↑ requirement for **insulin** or **oral hypoglycemic agents** in patients with diabetes. May ↓ effects of **digoxin**; may need to ↑ digoxin dosage. Concurrent use with **ketamine** may lead to significant hypertension and tachycardia. ↑ cardiovascular effects with **adrenergics (sympathomimetics)**. **Biotin** may interfere with thyroid function test assays; discontinue biotin or biotin-containing supplements for ≥2 days before assessing TSH and/or T4 levels.

Drug-Food: Foods or supplements containing calcium, iron, magnesium, or zinc may bind levothyroxine and prevent complete absorption. Absorption may be delayed when used with **grapefruit juice**.

Route/Dosage

PO (Adults): *Hypothyroidism:* 1.6 mcg/kg once daily; may ↑ by 12.5–25 mcg/day every 4–6 wk until patient clinically euthyroid based on signs/symptoms and TSH levels.

PO (Geriatric Patients and Patients with Cardiac Disease): 12.5–25 mcg once daily; may ↑ by 12.5–25 mcg/day every 6–8 wk until patient clinically euthyroid based on signs/symptoms and TSH levels.

PO (Children >12 yr): 2–3 mcg/kg/day (≥150 mcg/day).

PO (Children 6–12 yr): 4–5 mcg/kg/day (100–125 mcg/day).

PO (Children 1–5 yr): 5–6 mcg/kg/day (75–100 mcg/day).

PO (Children 6–12 mo): 6–8 mcg/kg/day (50–75 mcg/day).

PO (Infants 3–6 mo): 8–10 mcg/kg/day (25–50 mcg/day).

PO (Infants 0–3 mo or Infants at Risk for Cardiac Failure): 10–15 mcg/kg/day or 25 mcg/day; may ↑ after 4–6 wk to 50 mcg.

IM IV (Adults): *Hypothyroidism:* 50–100 mcg/day as a single dose. *Myxedema coma/stupor:* 300–500 mcg IV; additional 100–300 mcg may be given on 2nd day, followed by daily administration of smaller doses.

IM IV (Children): *Hypothyroidism:* 50–80% of the oral dose.

Availability (generic available)

Tablets: 25 mcg, 50 mcg, 75 mcg, 88 mcg, 100 mcg, 112 mcg, 125 mcg, 137 mcg, 150 mcg, 175 mcg, 200 mcg, 300 mcg. **Capsules (Tirosint):** 13 mcg, 25 mcg, 50 mcg, 75 mcg, 88 mcg, 100 mcg, 112 mcg, 125 mcg, 137 mcg, 150 mcg, 175 mcg, 200 mcg. **Oral solution:** 13 mcg/mL, 20 mcg/mL, 25 mcg/mL, 50 mcg/mL, 75 mcg/mL, 88 mcg/mL, 100 mcg/mL, 112 mcg/mL, 125 mcg/mL, 137 mcg/mL, 150 mcg/mL, 175 mcg/mL, 200 mcg/mL. **Powder for injection:** 100 mcg/vial, 200 mcg/vial, 500 mcg/vial. **Solution for injection:** 20 mcg/mL, 40 mcg/mL, 100 mcg/mL.

NURSING IMPLICATIONS

Assessment

- Assess BP and HR prior to and periodically during therapy. Assess for tachyarrhythmias and chest pain.
- **Children:** Monitor height, weight, and psychomotor development.

Lab Test Considerations

- Monitor thyroid function studies prior to and during therapy. For adults, monitor serum TSH levels in adults 6–8 wk after change in dose or changing from one brand to another. When on a stable dose, evaluate TSH every 6–12 mo and with clinical changes. For pediatric patients, monitor TSH and total or free T4 2 and 4 wk after start of therapy, 2 wk after any change in dose, and then every 3–12 mo after dose stabilization until growth is completed.
- Monitor blood and urine glucose in patients with diabetes. Insulin or oral hypoglycemic dose may need to be ↑.

Toxicity and Overdose

- Overdose is manifested as hyperthyroidism (tachycardia, chest pain, nervousness, insomnia, diaphoresis, tremors, weight loss). Usual treatment is to withhold dose for 2–6 days and then resume at a lower dose. Acute overdose is treated by induction of emesis or gastric lavage, followed by activated charcoal. Sympathetic overstimulation may be controlled by antiadrenergic drugs (beta blockers), such as propranolol. Oxygen and supportive measures to control symptoms are also used.

Implementation

- ***High Alert:*** Do not confuse levothyroxine with lamotrigine, Lanoxin, or liothyronine.
- Levothyroxine should NOT be used for the treatment of obesity or for weight loss. Doses within the range of daily hormonal requirements are ineffective for weight reduction in patients who are euthyroid. Larger doses may produce serious or even life-threatening manifestations of toxicity.
- **PO:** Administer with a full glass of water, on an empty stomach, 30–60 min before breakfast, to prevent insomnia.
- Initial dose is low, especially in patients with cardiac disease and older adults. Dose is ↑ gradually based on thyroid function tests.

- For patients with difficulty swallowing, tablets can be crushed and placed in 5–10 mL of water and administered immediately via dropper or spoon; do not store suspension.

IV Administration

- **IV Push: Reconstitution:** Reconstitute the 200-mcg and 500-mcg vials with 2 or 5 mL, respectively, of 0.9% NaCl without preservatives (diluent usually provided). **Concentration:** 100 mcg/mL. Shake well to dissolve completely. Administer solution immediately after preparation; discard unused portion. **Rate:** Administer at a rate of 100 mcg over 1 min. Do not add to IV infusions; may be administered through Y-tubing.
- **Y-Site Compatibility:** esmolol, hydrocortisone, labetalol, metoprolol.
- **Y-Site Incompatibility:** tacrolimus.

Patient/Family Teaching

- Explain purpose and side effects of levothyroxine to patient.
- Instruct patient to take medication as directed at the same time each day. Take missed doses as soon as remembered unless almost time for next dose. If more than 2–3 doses are missed, notify health care provider. Do not discontinue without consulting health care provider.
- Explain to patient that medication does not cure hypothyroidism; it provides a thyroid hormone supplement. Therapy is lifelong.
- Advise patient to notify health care provider if headache, nervousness, diarrhea, excessive sweating, heat intolerance, chest pain, ↑ HR, palpitations, weight loss >2 lb/wk, or any unusual symptoms occur.
- Caution patient to avoid taking other medications concurrently with thyroid preparations unless instructed by health care provider. Advise patient to take 4 hr apart from antacids, iron, and calcium supplements. Advise patient to stop biotin-containing supplements ≥ 2 days before assessing TSH or T4 levels.
- Instruct patient to inform health care providers of thyroid therapy.
- Rep: Advise women of reproductive potential to notify health care provider if pregnancy is planned or suspected or if breastfeeding. Pregnancy may ↑ thyroid requirements. Monitor serum TSH levels and adjust levothyroxine dose accordingly during pregnancy. Since postpartum TSH levels are similar to preconception values, levothyroxine dose should return to prepregnancy dose immediately after delivery.
- Emphasize importance of follow-up exams to monitor effectiveness of therapy. Thyroid function tests are performed at least yearly.
- Pedi: Discuss with parents the need for routine follow-up studies to ensure correct development. Inform patient that partial hair loss may be experienced by children on thyroid therapy. This is usually temporary.

Evaluation/Desired Outcomes

- Resolution of symptoms of hypothyroidism and normalization of hormone levels.

HIGH ALERT

LIDOCAINE

lidocaine (parenteral)
(lye-doe-kane)
Xylocaine, ✱ Xylocard

lidocaine (local anesthetic)
Xylocaine

lidocaine (mucosal)
✱ Jampocaine Viscous, Xylocaine Viscous

lidocaine (topical)
✱ Betacaine, ✱ Cathejell, Glydo, ✱ Lidodan, Lidoderm, L-M-X 4, L-M-X 5, ✱ Lyracaine, ✱ Maxilene, ✱ Stallion, ✱ Topicaine, Xylocaine, ZTLido

Classification
Therapeutic: anesthetics topical local, antiarrhythmics (class IB)

Indications

IV: Ventricular arrhythmias. **Local:** Infiltration/mucosal/topical anesthetic. **Topical:** Pain due to postherpetic neuralgia.

Action

IV: Suppresses automaticity and spontaneous depolarization of the ventricles during diastole by altering the flux of sodium ions across cell membranes with little or no effect on heart rate. **Local:** Produces local anesthesia by inhibiting transport of ions across neuronal membranes, thereby preventing initiation and conduction of normal nerve impulses. **Therapeutic Effects:** Control of ventricular arrhythmias. Local anesthesia.

Pharmacokinetics

Absorption: IV administration results in complete bioavailability; some absorption follows local use.
Distribution: Widely distributed to tissues. Concentrates in adipose tissue. Crosses the blood-brain barrier.

Metabolism and Excretion: Mostly metabolized by the liver; <10% excreted in urine as unchanged drug.
Half-life: Biphasic: initial phase, 7–30 min; terminal phase, 90–120 min; ↑ in HF and hepatic impairment.

TIME/ACTION PROFILE (IV = antiarrhythmic effects; local = anesthetic effects)

ROUTE	ONSET	PEAK	DURATION
IV	immediate	immediate	10–20 min (up to several hr after continuous infusion)
Local	rapid	unknown	1–3 hr

Contraindications/Precautions

Contraindicated in: Hypersensitivity; cross-sensitivity may occur; 3rd-degree heart block; Wolff-Parkinson-White syndrome; Pedi: Children <3 yr (↑ risk of seizures, cardiac arrest, and death with viscous lidocaine); viscous lidocaine should not be used for teething pain; should only be used for other indications when safer alternatives are not available or have failed.
Use Cautiously in: Glucose-6-phosphate dehydrogenase deficiency, history of methemoglobinemia, cardiac or pulmonary disease, or concurrent exposure to oxidizing agents (or metabolites of these agents) (↑ risk of methemoglobinemia); Liver disease, HF, patients <50 kg, and older adults (↓ bolus and/or maintenance dose); Respiratory depression; Shock; 1st- or 2nd-degree heart block; OB: Use during pregnancy only if the potential maternal benefit justifies potential fetal risk; Lactation: Use while breastfeeding only if potential maternal benefit justifies potential risk to infant; Pedi: Infants <6 mo (↑ risk of methemoglobinemia); safety of topical patch not established in children.

Adverse Reactions/Side Effects

CV: arrhythmias, bradycardia, CARDIAC ARREST, heart block, hypotension. **EENT: mucosal use:** ↓ or absent gag reflex. **GI:** nausea, vomiting. **Hemat:** methemoglobinemia. **Local:** stinging, burning, contact dermatitis, erythema. **MS:** chondrolysis. **Neuro:** confusion, drowsiness, agitation, blurred vision, dizziness, paresthesia, SEIZURES, slurred speech, tremor. **Resp:** bronchospasm. **Misc:** HYPERSENSITIVITY REACTIONS (INCLUDING ANAPHYLAXIS).

Interactions

Drug-Drug: Acetaminophen, **benzocaine**, **bupivacaine**, **chloroquine**, **cyclophosphamide**, **dapsone**, **flutamide**, **hydroxyurea**, **ifosfamide**, **metoclopramide**, **nitrofurantoin**, **nitroglycerin**, **nitroprusside**, **nitrous oxide**, **phenobarbital**, **phenytoin**, **prilocaine**, **primaquine**, **procaine**, **quinine**, **rasburicase**, **ropivacaine**, **sulfonamides**, **tetracaine**, and **valproate** may ↑ risk of methemoglobinemia; monitor closely. ↑ cardiac depression and toxicity with **phenytoin**, **amiodarone**, **quinidine**, **procainamide**, or **propranolol**. **Cimetidine**, **azole antifungals**, **clarithromycin**, **erythromycin**, **fluoxetine**, **fluvoxamine**, **nefazodone**, **paroxetine**, **protease inhibitors**, **propofol**, **ritonavir**, **verapamil**, and **propranolol** may ↑ levels and risk of toxicity. Lidocaine may ↑ levels and risk of toxicity of **calcium channel blockers**, certain **benzodiazepines**, **cyclosporine**, **fluoxetine**, **lovastatin**, **simvastatin**, **mirtazapine**, **paroxetine**, **ritonavir**, **tacrolimus**, **theophylline**, **tricyclic antidepressants**, and **venlafaxine**. **Carbamazepine**, **phenobarbital**, **phenytoin**, and **rifampin** may ↓ levels and effectiveness.

Route/Dosage

Ventricular Tachycardia (with a Pulse) or Pulseless Ventricular Tachycardia/ Ventricular Fibrillation

IV (Adults): 1–1.5 mg/kg bolus; may repeat doses of 0.5–0.75 mg/kg every 5–10 min up to a total dose of 3 mg/kg; may then start continuous infusion of 1–4 mg/min.
Endotracheal: (Adults): Give 2–2.5 times the IV loading dose down the endotracheal tube, followed by a 10-mL saline flush.
IV (Children): 1 mg/kg bolus (not to exceed 100 mg), followed by 20–50 mcg/kg/min continuous infusion (range 20–50 mcg/kg/min); may administer 2nd bolus of 0.5–1 mg/kg if delay between bolus and continuous infusion.
Endotracheal: (Children): Give 2–3 mg/kg down the endotracheal tube followed by a 5-mL saline flush.

Local

Infiltration: (Adults and Children): Infiltrate affected area as needed (↑ amount and frequency of use ↑ likelihood of systemic absorption and adverse reactions).
Topical: (Adults): *Cream/ointment/gel/solution/ jelly:* Apply to affected area 2–3 times daily. *Patch:* Up to 3 patches may be applied once for up to 12 hr in any 24-hr period; consider smaller areas of application in older adults.
Mucosal: (Adults): *For anesthetizing oral surfaces:* 20 mg as 2 sprays/quadrant (not to exceed 30 mg/quadrant) may be used. 15 mL of the viscous solution may be used every 3 hr for oral or pharyngeal pain. *For anesthetizing the female urethra:* 3–5 mL of the jelly or 20 mg as 2% solution may be used. *For anesthetizing the male urethra:* 5–10 mL of the jelly or 5–15 mL of 2% solution may be used before catheterization or 30 mL of jelly before cystoscopy or similar procedures. Topical solutions may be used to anesthetize mucous membranes of the larynx, trachea, or esophagus.

Mucosal: (Children ≥3 yr): Do not exceed 4.5 mg/kg/dose (or 300 mg/dose) of viscous solution; swish in the mouth and spit out no more frequently than every 3 hr (maximum: 4 doses per 12-hr period).
Mucosal: (Children <3 yr): ≤1.2 mL applied to area with a cotton-tipped applicator no more frequently than every 3 hr (maximum: 4 doses per 12-hr period); use only if the underlying condition requires treatment with product volume of ≤1.2 mL.

Availability (generic available)

Solution for injection: 5 mg/mL (0.5%), 10 mg/mL (1%), 15 mg/mL (1.5%), 20 mg/mL (2%). **Premixed infusion:** 1000 mg/250 mL D5W (0.4%), 2000 mg/500 mL D5W (0.4%), 2000 mg/250 mL D5W (0.8%). **Injection for local infiltration/nerve block:** 0.5%, 1%, 2%, 4%. **Topical cream:** 4%OTC, 5%. **Topical gel:** 2%OTC, 3%, 4%, 5%OTC. **Topical jelly:** 2%. **Topical liquid:** 2.5%. **Topical ointment:** 4%, 5%. **Topical patch:** 1.8%, 3.5%, 4%, 5%. **Topical solution:** 2%, 4%. **Topical spray:** 2%, 4%. **Viscous solution:** 2%. ***In combination with:*** diclofenac (Diclona); epinephrine (Xylocaine with Epinephrine); prilocaine (Oraquix).

NURSING IMPLICATIONS

Assessment

- **Antiarrhythmic:** Monitor ECG continuously and BP and respiratory status frequently during administration.
- **Anesthetic:** Assess degree of numbness of affected part. Local or regional anesthesia is indicative of efficacy.
- **Topical:** Monitor for pain intensity in affected area periodically during therapy.
- Monitor for seizure activity or CNS toxicity (restlessness, anxiety, tinnitus, dizziness, blurred vision, tremors, depression, drowsiness), which may occur with repeated dosing. Institute seizure precautions.
- Monitor for signs/symptoms of malignant hyperthermia (*early signs:* tachycardia, tachypnea, muscle rigidity; *late signs:* hyperpyrexia, diaphoresis, altered mental status, rhabdomyolysis, dark urine, cardiac arrhythmia). *If malignant hyperthermia occurs,* discontinue lidocaine and treat patient with cooling measures, IV fluids, and dantrolene.
- Monitor for signs/symptoms of methemoglobinemia (cyanosis, fatigue, weakness, headache, dyspnea, dark brown or chocolate-colored blood), which may occur immediately or may be delayed a few hr after exposure. *If methemoglobinemia occurs,* discontinue lidocaine and any other oxidizing agents. Initiate oxygen therapy. Treat with methylene blue. A medical toxicologist should be consulted.

Lab Test Considerations

- Serum electrolyte levels should be monitored periodically during prolonged therapy.

Toxicity and Overdose

- Monitor serum lidocaine levels periodically during prolonged or high-dose IV therapy. Therapeutic serum lidocaine levels range from 1.5–5 mcg/mL.
- Signs/symptoms of toxicity include confusion, excitation, blurred or double vision, nausea, vomiting, ringing in ears, tremors, twitching, seizures, difficulty breathing, severe dizziness or fainting, and unusually slow heart rate.
- *If symptoms of overdose occur,* stop infusion and monitor patient closely. Consider IV lipid therapy early for patients with ventricular arrhythmias or hypotension.

Implementation

- ***High Alert:*** Lidocaine is readily absorbed through mucous membranes. Inadvertent overdose of lidocaine jelly and spray has resulted in patient harm or death from neurologic and/or cardiac toxicity. Do not exceed recommended doses.
- **Throat Spray:** Patient should be positioned upright to avoid aspiration. Ensure that gag reflex is intact before allowing patient to drink or eat.

IV Administration

- **IV Push:** Only 1% and 2% solutions are used for IV push injection. **Dilution:** Administer undiluted. **Rate:** Administer loading dose over 2–3 min. Follow by IV continuous infusion.
- **Continuous Infusion:** **Dilution:** Lidocaine vials need to be further diluted. Dilute 2 g of lidocaine in 250 mL or 500 mL of D5W or 0.9% NaCl. Admixed infusion stable for 24 hr at room temperature. Premixed infusions are already diluted and ready to use. **Concentration:** 4–8 mg/mL.
- **Rate:** See Route/Dosage section. Administer via infusion pump for accurate dose.
- **Y-Site Compatibility:** acetaminophen, alemtuzumab, alteplase, amikacin, aminocaproic acid, aminophylline, amiodarone, amphotericin B liposomal, anidulafungin, argatroban, arsenic trioxide, ascorbic acid, atracurium, atropine, azithromycin, aztreonam, benztropine, bivalirudin, bleomycin, bumetanide, buprenorphine, butorphanol, calcium chloride, calcium gluconate, cangrelor, carboplatin, carmustine, caspofungin, cefazolin, cefiderocol, cefotaxime, cefotetan, cefoxitin, ceftaroline, ceftazidime, ceftolozane/tazobactam, ceftriaxone, cefuroxime, chloramphenicol, chlorpromazine, chlorothiazide, ciprofloxacin, cisatracurium, cisplatin, clindamycin, cyanocobalamin, cyclophosphamide, cyclosporine, cytarabine, dacarbazine, dactinomycin, daptomycin,

daunorubicin, dexamethasone, dexmedetomidine, dexrazoxane, digoxin, diltiazem, diphenhydramine, dobutamine, docetaxel, dopamine, doxorubicin hydrochloride, doxorubicin liposomal, doxycycline, edetate calcium disodium, enalaprilat, ephedrine, epinephrine, epirubicin, epoetin alfa, eptifibatide, ertapenem, erythromycin, esmolol, etomidate, etoposide, etoposide phosphate, famotidine, fentanyl, fluconazole, fludarabine, fluorouracil, folic acid, foscarnet, fosphenytoin, furosemide, ganciclovir, gemcitabine, gentamicin, glycopyrrolate, granisetron, heparin, hydrocortisone, hydromorphone, idarubicin, ifosfamide, imipenem/cilastatin, imipenem/cilastatin/relebactam, indomethacin, insulin regular, irinotecan, isavuconazonium, isoproterenol, ketorolac, labetalol, leucovorin, levofloxacin, linezolid, lorazepam, magnesium sulfate, mannitol, meperidine, meropenem/vaborbactam, mesna, methadone, methotrexate, methylprednisolone, metoclopramide, metronidazole, micafungin, midazolam, minocycline, mitomycin, mitoxantrone, morphine, moxifloxacin, multivitamins, mycophenolate, nafcillin, nalbuphine, naloxone, nicardipine, nitroglycerin, nitroprusside, norepinephrine, octreotide, ondansetron, oxacillin, oxaliplatin, oxytocin, paclitaxel, palonosetron, pamidronate, papaverine, pemetrexed, penicillin G, pentamidine, phentolamine, phenylephrine, phytonadione, piperacillin/tazobactam, plazomicin, potassium acetate, potassium chloride, procainamide, prochlorperazine, promethazine, propranolol, protamine, pyridoxine, remifentanil, rocuronium, sodium acetate, sodium bicarbonate, succinylcholine, sufentanil, sulbactam/durlobactam, tacrolimus, tedizolid, theophylline, thiamine, thiotepa, tigecycline, tirofiban, tobramycin, topotecan, vancomycin, vasopressin, vecuronium, verapamil, vinblastine, vincristine, vinorelbine, voriconazole, zoledronic acid.

- **Y-Site Incompatibility:** acyclovir, amphotericin B deoxycholate, azathioprine, caspofungin, dantrolene, diazepam, ganciclovir, gemtuzumab ozogamicin, milrinone, pantoprazole, pentobarbital, phenobarbital, phenytoin, trimethoprim/sulfamethoxazole. **Infiltration:** Lidocaine with epinephrine may be used to minimize systemic absorption and prolong local anesthesia.
- **Topical:** When used concurrently with other products containing local anesthetic agents, consider amount absorbed from all formulations.
- *Lidoderm* and *ZTLido* are not interchangeable.

Patient/Family Teaching

- Explain purpose and side effects of lidocaine. Instruct them to use medication as directed. Explain to parents the importance of using calibrated measuring device for accurate dosing. Keep out of children's reach. Advise patient to read *Patient Information* before starting and with each Rx refill in case of changes.
- May cause drowsiness and dizziness. Advise patient to call for assistance during ambulation and transfer.
- Advise patient to notify health care provider of all Rx or OTC medications, vitamins, or herbal products being taken and to consult with health care provider before taking other medications.
- **Topical:** Apply *Lidoderm Patch* to intact skin to cover the most painful area. Patch may be cut to smaller sizes with scissors before removing release liner. Clothing may be worn over patch. Avoid contact with water (bathing, swimming, showering); may not stick if it gets wet. If irritation or burning sensation occurs during application, remove patch until irritation subsides. Wash hands after application; avoid contact with eyes. Dispose of used patch to avoid access by children or pets.
- Apply *ZTLido* to intact skin to cover the most painful area. Apply immediately after removing from envelope. System may be cut to smaller sizes with scissors before removing release liner. Clothing may be worn over patch. May be used during moderate exercise (e.g., biking for 30 min). May be exposed to water (showering for 10 min or immersion for 15 min). Dry by gently patting the skin, not by rubbing skin or topical system. If edges have lifted, press firmly on edges. If system detaches, may be reapplied as originally directed. If system will not stick, dispose by folding adhesive sides together and discard where children or pets cannot get to them. Apply a new system for total duration of 12 hr of used and new system together. If irritation or a burning sensation occurs during application, remove and reapply when irritation subsides.
- Caution women to consult health care provider before using a topical anesthetic for a mammogram or other procedures. If recommended, use lowest drug concentration, and apply sparingly. Do not apply to broken or irritated skin, do not wrap skin, and do not apply heat to area (heating pad/electric blanket) to decrease chance that drug may be absorbed into the body. May result in seizures, cardiac arrhythmias, respiratory failure, coma, and death.
- Advise patient referred for MRI test to discuss patch with referring health care provider and MRI facility to determine if removal of patch is necessary prior to test and for directions for replacing patch.
- **Mucosal:** Caution parent to administer as directed, not to use more or more often than directed, and to use measuring device for accurate dose in children <3 yr if safer alternatives are ineffective. Lidocaine hydrochloride 2% viscous solution should not be used for teething pain or in children <3 yr. Advise parent that if signs and symptoms of toxicity (lethargy, shallow breathing, seizure activity) occur to seek emergency attention and not to administer more lidocaine.
- Caution parents that oral lidocaine causes numbness and may impair swallowing; do not administer

food and/or chewing gum for at least 60 min after administration.

- Rep: Advise women of reproductive potential to notify health care provider if pregnancy is planned or suspected or if breastfeeding. Consider total drug doses of all lidocaine-containing formulations used concurrently during pregnancy. If maternal hypotension or fetal bradycardia develop, place patient in left lateral decubitus position; continuous fetal monitoring is recommended.

Evaluation/Desired Outcomes
- Decrease in ventricular arrhythmias.
- Local anesthesia.

linaCLOtide (lin-a-**kloe**-tide)
✱ Constella, Linzess

Classification
Therapeutic: anti-irritable bowel syndrome agents
Pharmacologic: guanylate cyclase-C agonists

Indications
Irritable bowel syndrome with constipation (IBS-C). Chronic idiopathic constipation (CIC). Functional constipation.

Action
Locally increases levels of cyclic guanosine monophosphate (cGMP); accelerates transit time, increases intestinal fluid, and decreases pain sensation. **Therapeutic Effects:** Increased frequency of bowel movements with decreased pain associated with IBS-C, CIC, or functional constipation.

Pharmacokinetics
Absorption: Minimally absorbed, action is primarily local.
Distribution: Stays within the GI tract with minimal distribution.
Metabolism and Excretion: Converted to its principal active metabolite within the GI tract; subsequently locally degraded to smaller peptides and amino acids; 3–5% found in stool, mostly as the active metabolite.
Half-life: Unknown.

TIME/ACTION PROFILE (improvement in GI symptoms)

ROUTE	ONSET	PEAK	DURATION
PO	unknown	6–9 wk	1 wk†

† Following discontinuation.

Contraindications/Precautions
Contraindicated in: Known/suspected mechanical GI obstruction; Pedi: Children <2 yr (↑ risk of severe dehydration).
Use Cautiously in: OB: Use during pregnancy only if potential maternal benefit justifies potential fetal risk; Pedi: Children ≥2 yr (safety and effectiveness not established).

Adverse Reactions/Side Effects
GI: diarrhea, abdominal distention, abdominal pain, flatulence, gastrointestinal reflux, vomiting. **Neuro:** fatigue.

Interactions
Drug-Drug: None reported.

Route/Dosage
Irritable Bowel Syndrome with Constipation
PO (Adults): 290 mcg once daily.

Chronic Idiopathic Constipation
PO (Adults): 145 mcg once daily; 72 mcg once daily may be used based on patient presentation or tolerability.

Functional Constipation
PO (Children ≥6 yr): 72 mcg once daily.

Availability (generic available)
Capsules: 72 mcg, 145 mcg, 290 mcg.

NURSING IMPLICATIONS
Assessment
- Assess patient for symptoms of IBS (abdominal pain or discomfort, bloating, constipation). If severe diarrhea occurs, hold therapy and rehydrate patient. May require IV fluids.

Implementation
- Do not confuse linaclotide with linagliptin.
- **PO:** Administer once daily on an empty stomach, 30 min before eating first meal of the day. ***DNC:*** Swallow capsules whole; do not open, break, dissolve, or chew.
- For patients with difficulty swallowing, open capsule and sprinkle entire capsule contents in one teaspoon applesauce or 30 mL water. For applesauce, consume immediately; do not chew beads or store for later. For water, swirl water and beads gently for at ≥20 sec. Swallow entire mixture immediately. Add another 30 mL of water to any beads remaining in cup, swirl for 20 sec, and swallow immediately. Do not store mixture for later use. Water method may also be used for NG or G-tube administration.

Patient/Family Teaching

- Explain the purpose and side effects of linaclotide. Instruct patient to take as directed. Keep capsules in original bottle with desiccant packet to help keep medication dry; keep bottle tightly closed. If a dose is missed, omit and take next dose at regular time; do not double doses. Advise patient to read *Patient Information* before starting and with each Rx refill in case of changes.
- Inform patient that diarrhea often begins within first 2 wk of therapy. Stop taking and notify health care provider if severe diarrhea occurs. Contact health care provider and go to nearest hospital emergency room immediately if bright-red bloody stools or black stools that look like tar occur.
- Advise patient to notify health care provider of all Rx or OTC medications, vitamins, or herbal products being taken and to consult with health care provider before taking other medications.
- OB: Advise women of reproductive potential to notify health care provider if pregnancy is planned or suspected.

Evaluation/Desired Outcomes

- Increased frequency of bowel movements with decreased pain associated with IBS-C or CIC.
- Increased frequency of bowel movements in pediatric patients 6–17 yr of age with functional constipation.

linaGLIPtin (lin-a-**glip**-tin)

Tradjenta, Trajenta

Classification

Therapeutic: antidiabetics

Pharmacologic: dipeptidyl peptidase-4 (DDP-4) inhibitors, enzyme inhibitors

Indications

Type 2 diabetes mellitus (as adjunct to diet and exercise).

Action

Inhibits the enzyme dipeptidyl peptidase-4 (DPP-4), which slows the inactivation of incretin hormones, resulting in increased levels of active incretin hormones. These hormones are released by the intestine throughout the day and are involved in regulation of glucose. Increased/prolonged incretin levels increase insulin release and decrease glucagon levels. **Therapeutic Effects:** Improved control of blood glucose and A1c.

Pharmacokinetics

Absorption: 30% absorbed following oral administration.

Distribution: Extensively distributed to tissues.

Metabolism and Excretion: Minimally metabolized; primarily excreted in feces (80%) and urine (5%) as unchanged drug.

Half-life: >100 hr (due to saturable binding to DPP-4).

TIME/ACTION PROFILE

ROUTE	ONSET	PEAK	DURATION
PO	unknown	1.5 hr†	24 hr

† Blood level.

Contraindications/Precautions

Contraindicated in: Hypersensitivity (cross-sensitivity may exist with sitagliptin, alogliptin, or saxagliptin); Type 1 diabetes mellitus; Diabetic ketoacidosis.

Use Cautiously in: History of pancreatitis; History of HF or renal impairment (↑ risk of HF); OB: Use during pregnancy only if potential maternal benefit justifies potential fetal risk; Lactation: Use while breastfeeding only if potential maternal benefit justifies potential risk to infant; Pedi: Safety and effectiveness not established in children; Geri: Older adults may have ↑ risk of hypoglycemia.

Adverse Reactions/Side Effects

CV: HF. **Derm:** bullous pemphigoid, localized exfoliation, urticaria. **Endo:** hypoglycemia. **GI:** ↑ lipase, PANCREATITIS. **Metab:** hypertriglyceridemia. **MS:** arthralgia, RHABDOMYOLYSIS. **Resp:** bronchial hyperreactivity. **Misc:** HYPERSENSITIVITY REACTIONS (INCLUDING ANAPHYLAXIS, ANGIOEDEMA, AND EXFOLIATIVE SKIN CONDITIONS).

Interactions

Drug-Drug: ↑ risk of hypoglycemia with **sulfonylureas** or **insulin**; dose ↓ of sulfonylurea or insulin may be necessary. Concurrent use of **P-glycoprotein inducers** or **CYP3A4 inducers**, including **rifampin**, may ↓ levels and effectiveness; avoid concurrent use.

Route/Dosage

PO (Adults): 5 mg once daily.

Availability (generic available)

Tablets: 5 mg. ***In combination with:*** empagliflozin (Glyxambi); empagliflozin and metformin XR (Trijardy XR); metformin (Jentadueto); metformin XR (Jentadueto XR). See Appendix N.

NURSING IMPLICATIONS

Assessment

- Assess for signs and symptoms of hypoglycemic reactions (abdominal pain, sweating, hunger, weakness, dizziness, headache, tremor, tachycardia, anxiety), especially with use of insulin or an insulin secretagogue; dose adjustment may be required.
- Assess for signs of HF (dyspnea, peripheral edema, rales/crackles, jugular venous distension) during therapy. Notify provider; may need to discontinue therapy.

- Monitor for signs of pancreatitis (nausea; vomiting; anorexia; persistent severe abdominal pain, sometimes radiating to the back) during therapy. If pancreatitis occurs, discontinue linagliptin and monitor serum and urine amylase, amylase/CCr ratio, electrolytes, serum calcium, glucose, and lipase.
- Monitor for arthralgia. Severe joint pain usually disappears with discontinuation of linagliptin; however, may reoccur with another DPP-4 inhibitor.

Lab Test Considerations

- Monitor A1c twice yearly, every 3 mo when not meeting glycemic goals, or with change in therapy.
- May cause ↑ uric acid levels.

Implementation

- Do not confuse linagliptin with linaclotide. Do not confuse Tradjenta with Toujeo, Tresiba, or Trulicity.
- Patients stabilized on a diabetic regimen who are exposed to stress, fever, trauma, infection, or surgery may require administration of insulin.
- **PO:** May be administered without regard to food.

Patient/Family Teaching

- Explain the purpose and side effects of linagliptin. Instruct patient to take as directed. Take missed doses as soon as remembered, unless it is almost time for next dose; do not double doses. Advise patient to read the *Medication Guide* before starting and with each Rx refill in case of changes.
- Explain to patient that linagliptin helps control hyperglycemia but does not cure diabetes. Therapy is usually long term. Emphasize the importance of routine follow-up exams.
- Instruct patient not to share this medication with others, even if they have the same symptoms; it may harm them.
- Encourage patient to follow prescribed diet, medication, and exercise regimen to prevent hyperglycemic or hypoglycemic episodes.
- Review signs of hypoglycemia and hyperglycemia with patient. If hypoglycemia occurs, advise patient to take a glass of orange juice or 2–3 teaspoons of sugar, honey, or corn syrup dissolved in water, and notify health care provider.
- Instruct patient in proper testing of blood glucose and urine ketones. These tests should be monitored closely during periods of stress or illness and health care provider notified if significant changes occur.
- Warn patient to report symptoms and seek treatment for HF (trouble breathing, leg swelling, lung congestion, rapid weight gain).
- Advise patient to notify health care provider promptly if signs and symptoms of pancreatitis or if rash; hives; blisters; or swelling of face, lips, or throat occur.
- Advise patient to report severe and persistent joint pain; onset can occur 1 day to years after initiation and may require discontinuation of therapy.
- Advise patient to notify health care provider of all Rx or OTC medications, vitamins, or herbal products being taken and to consult with health care provider before taking other medications, especially other oral hypoglycemic medications.
- Rep: Insulin is the recommended method of controlling blood sugar during pregnancy. Advise women of reproductive potential to notify health care provider if pregnancy is planned or suspected or if breastfeeding.

Evaluation/Desired Outcomes

- Improved A1c, fasting plasma glucose, and 2-hr postprandial glucose levels.

L

linezolid (li-nez-o-lid)

Zyvox, ✱ Zyvoxam

Classification

Therapeutic: anti-infectives

Pharmacologic: oxazolidinones

Indications

Nosocomial pneumonia. Community-acquired pneumonia. Complicated skin and skin structure infections. Uncomplicated skin and skin structure infections. Infections caused by vancomycin-resistant *Enterococcus faecium*.

Action

Inhibits bacterial protein synthesis at the level of the 23S ribosome of the 50S subunit. **Therapeutic Effects:** Bactericidal action against streptococci; bacteriostatic action against enterococci and staphylococci. **Spectrum:** Active against gram-positive pathogens, including: *Staphylococcus aureus* (methicillin-susceptible and methicillin-resistant), *Streptococcus agalactiae*, *Streptococcus pneumoniae*, *Streptococcus pyogenes*, *Enterococcus faecium*.

Pharmacokinetics

Absorption: Rapidly and extensively (100%) absorbed following oral administration. IV administration results in complete bioavailability.

Distribution: Readily distributes to well-perfused tissues.

Metabolism and Excretion: 65% metabolized, mostly by the liver; 30% excreted unchanged by the kidneys.

Half-life: 6.4 hr.

TIME/ACTION PROFILE

ROUTE	ONSET	PEAK	DURATION
PO	rapid	1–2 hr	12 hr
IV	rapid	end of infusion	12 hr

Contraindications/Precautions

Contraindicated in: Hypersensitivity; Phenylketonuria (suspension contains phenylalanine); Uncontrolled hypertension, pheochromocytoma, thyrotoxicosis, or concurrent use of sympathomimetic agents, vasopressors, or dopaminergic agents (↑ risk of hypertensive response); Concurrent or recent (<2 wk) use of MAO inhibitors (↑ risk of hypertensive response); Carcinoid syndrome or concurrent use of SSRIs, SNRIs, TCAs, triptans, opioids, bupropion, or buspirone (↑ risk of serotonin syndrome).
Use Cautiously in: Thrombocytopenia, concurrent use of antiplatelet agents, bleeding diathesis, severe renal impairment, or moderate/severe hepatic impairment (platelet counts should be monitored more frequently); Diabetes (↑ risk of hypoglycemia); OB: Use during pregnancy only if potential maternal benefit justifies potential fetal risk; Lactation: Use while breastfeeding only if potential maternal benefit justifies potential risk to infant.

Adverse Reactions/Side Effects

CV: headache, insomnia. **Derm:** TOXIC EPIDERMAL NECROLYSIS. **EENT:** teeth discoloration, tongue discoloration. **Endo:** hypoglycemia, syndrome of inappropriate diuretic hormone (SIADH) secretion. **F and E:** hyponatremia, lactic acidosis. **GI:** ↑ liver enzymes, CLOSTRIDIOIDES DIFFICILE-ASSOCIATED DIARRHEA (CDAD), diarrhea, nausea, vomiting. **Hemat:** anemia, leukopenia, thrombocytopenia. **MS:** RHABDOMYOLYSIS. **Neuro:** dysgeusia, optic neuropathy, peripheral neuropathy. **Misc:** SEROTONIN SYNDROME.

Interactions

Drug-Drug: ↑ risk of hypertensive crisis with **MAO inhibitors**, **sympathomimetics** (e.g., **pseudoephedrine**), **vasopressors** (e.g., **epinephrine**, **norepinephrine**), and **dopaminergic agents** (e.g., **dopamine**, **dobutamine**); concurrent or recent use should be avoided. ↑ risk of serotonin syndrome with **SSRIs**, **SNRIs**, **TCAs**, **triptans**, **opioids**, **bupropion**, or **buspirone**; avoid concurrent use. **Rifampin**, **carbamazepine**, **phenytoin**, and **phenobarbital** may ↓ levels and effectiveness. **Oral hypoglycemics** or **insulin** may ↑ risk of hypoglycemia.
Drug-Food: Because of MAO inhibitory properties, consumption of large amounts of foods or beverages containing tyramine should be avoided (↑ risk of pressor response; see Appendix J).

Route/Dosage

Vancomycin-Resistant *Enterococcus faecium* Infections

PO, IV (Adults): 600 mg every 12 hr for 14–28 days.
PO, IV (Children ≤11 yr): In the first wk of life, preterm neonates may initially receive 10 mg/kg every 12 hr.

Pneumonia or Complicated Skin/Skin Structure Infections

PO, IV (Adults): 600 mg every 12 hr for 10–14 days.
PO, IV (Children ≤11 yr): 10 mg/kg every 8 hr for 10–14 days (in the first wk of life, preterm neonates may initially receive 10 mg/kg every 12 hr).

Uncomplicated Skin/Skin Structure Infections

PO, (Adults): 400 mg every 12 hr for 10–14 days.
PO, IV (Children 5–11 yr): 10 mg/kg every 12 hr for 10–14 days.
PO, IV (Children <5 yr): 10 mg/kg every 8 hr for 10–14 days (in the first wk of life, preterm neonates may initially receive 10 mg/kg every 12 hr).

Availability (generic available)

Tablets: 600 mg. **Oral suspension: (orange flavored):** 100 mg/5 mL (each 5 mL contains phenylalanine 20 mg). **Premixed infusion:** 200 mg/100 mL, 600 mg/300 mL.

NURSING IMPLICATIONS

Assessment

- Assess for infection (vital signs; appearance of wound, sputum, urine, and stool) at beginning of and during therapy.
- Monitor for signs of lactic acidosis. *If repeated nausea and vomiting, unexplained acidosis or low bicarbonate level occurs,* initiate immediate evaluation.
- Monitor visual function in patients receiving linezolid for ≥3 mo or who report visual symptoms (changes in acuity or color vision, blurred vision, visual field defect) regardless of length of therapy. *If optic neuropathy occurs,* reconsider therapy.
- Monitor bowel function for signs and symptoms of CDAD (diarrhea, abdominal cramping, fever, bloody stool). May begin up to several weeks following cessation of therapy. *If CDAD suspected or confirmed,* ongoing antibacterial drug use not directed against *C. difficile* may need to be discontinued. Fluid and electrolyte management, protein supplementation, and surgical evaluation should be instituted as clinically indicated.
- Monitor patient taking serotonergic drugs for signs of serotonin syndrome (hyperthermia, rigidity, myoclonus, autonomic instability, mental status changes, extreme agitation progressing to delirium and coma) for 2 wk (5 wk if fluoxetine was taken) or until 24 hr after the last dose of linezolid, whichever comes first.
- Monitor for rhabdomyolysis. *If rhabdomyolysis occurs,* discontinue linezolid and initiate appropriate treatment.

Lab Test Considerations

- Obtain specimens for culture and sensitivity prior to initiating therapy. 1st dose may be given before obtaining specimens. May cause myelosuppression. Monitor CBC weekly, especially in patients at risk for ↑ bleeding, with pre-existing bone marrow suppression, with severe renal impairment or moderate/severe hepatic impairment, receiving concurrent medications that may cause myelosuppression, or requiring >2 wk of therapy. *If bone marrow suppression occurs or worsens,* consider discontinuing therapy.
- May ↑ AST, ALT, LDH, alkaline phosphatase, and BUN.
- May cause hypoglycemia, requiring ↓ in dose of antidiabetic agent or discontinuation of linezolid.
- Monitor serum sodium levels regularly in older adults, patients taking diuretics, and other patients at risk of hyponatremia and/or SIADH. *If signs and symptoms of hyponatremia and/or SIADH (confusion, somnolence, generalized weakness, respiratory failure, death) occur,* discontinue linezolid, and institute supportive measures.

Implementation

- ***High Alert:*** Do not confuse Zyvox with Zovirax.
- Dose adjustment is not necessary when switching from IV to oral dose.
- **PO:** Administer without regard to food.
- Before using oral solution, gently invert 3–5 times to mix; do not shake. Store at room temperature; use within 21 days of constitution.

IV Administration

- **Intermittent Infusion: Dilution:** Premixed infusions are already diluted and ready to use. Solution is yellowish in color, which may intensify over time without affecting its potency. **Concentration:** 2 mg/mL. Do not use in series connections. **Rate:** Infuse over 30–120 min. Flush line before and after infusion.
- **Y-Site Compatibility:** acetaminophen, acyclovir, alemtuzumab, allopurinol, amikacin, aminocaproic acid, aminophylline, amiodarone, amphotericin B liposomal, ampicillin, ampicillin/sulbactam, anidulafungin, argatroban, arsenic trioxide, azithromycin, aztreonam, bivalirudin, bleomycin, bumetanide, buprenorphine, busulfan, butorphanol, caffeine citrate, calcium chloride, calcium gluconate, cangrelor, carboplatin, carmustine, caspofungin, cefazolin, cefepime, cefiderocol, cefotaxime, cefotetan, cefoxitin, ceftazidime, ceftazidime/avibactam, ceftolozane/tazobactam, ceftriaxone, cefuroxime, chloramphenicol, ciprofloxacin, cisatracurium, cisplatin, clindamycin, cyclophosphamide, cyclosporine, cytarabine, dacarbazine, dactinomycin, daptomycin, daunorubicin, dexamethasone, dexmedetomidine, dexrazoxane, digoxin, diltiazem, diphenhydramine, dobutamine, docetaxel, dopamine, doxorubicin hydrochloride, doxorubicin liposomal, doxycycline, droperidol, enalaprilat, ephedrine, epinephrine, epirubicin, eptifibatide, eravacycline, ertapenem, esmolol, etoposide, etoposide phosphate, famotidine, fentanyl, fluconazole, fludarabine, fluorouracil, foscarnet, fosphenytoin, furosemide, ganciclovir, gemcitabine, gemtuzumab ozogamicin, gentamicin, glycopyrrolate, granisetron, haloperidol, heparin, hydralazine, hydrocortisone, hydromorphone, idarubicin, ifosfamide, imipenem/cilastatin, imipenem/cilastatin/relebactam, insulin regular, irinotecan, isavuconazonium, isoproterenol, ketorolac, labetalol, leucovorin, levofloxacin, lidocaine, lorazepam, magnesium sulfate, mannitol, melphalan, meperidine, meropenem, meropenem/vaborbactam, mesna, methadone, methotrexate, methylprednisolone, metoclopramide, metoprolol, metronidazole, midazolam, milrinone, minocycline, mitomycin, mitoxantrone, morphine, mycophenolate, nafcillin, nalbuphine, naloxone, nicardipine, nitroglycerin, nitroprusside, norepinephrine, octreotide, ondansetron, oxaliplatin, oxytocin, paclitaxel, palonosetron, pamidronate, pemetrexed, pentobarbital, phenobarbital, phenylephrine, piperacillin/tazobactam, plazomicin, potassium acetate, potassium chloride, potassium phosphates, procainamide, prochlorperazine, promethazine, propranolol, remifentanil, rocuronium, sodium acetate, sodium bicarbonate, sodium phosphates, succinylcholine, sufentanil, sulbactam/durlobactam, tacrolimus, theophylline, thiotepa, tigecycline, tirofiban, tobramycin, topotecan, trimethoprim/sulfamethoxazole, vancomycin, vasopressin, vecuronium, verapamil, vinblastine, vincristine, vinorelbine, voriconazole, zidovudine, zoledronic acid.
- **Y-Site Incompatibility:** chlorpromazine, dantrolene, diazepam, erythromycin, pantoprazole, pentamidine, phenytoin.

Patient/Family Teaching

- Explain purpose and side effects of medication. Advise patient to read *Patient Information* before starting therapy.
- Instruct patient taking oral linezolid to take as directed for full course of therapy, even if feeling better. Take missed dose as soon as remembered unless almost time for next dose; do not double dose.
- Instruct patient to avoid large quantities of foods or beverages containing tyramine (see Appendix J). May cause hypertensive response.
- Instruct patient to notify health care provider if they have a history of hypertension, seizures, or diabetes.

- Advise patient to notify health care provider of all Rx or OTC medications, vitamins, or herbal products being taken and to consult with health care provider before taking other medications, especially cold remedies, decongestants, or antidepressants.
- Instruct patient to notify health care provider if changes in vision occur or if diarrhea, abdominal cramping, fever, or bloody stools occur and not to treat with antidiarrheals without consulting health care provider.
- Advise patient to notify health care provider if signs of rhabdomyolysis (muscle pain or weakness, dark urine) occur.
- Advise patient to notify health care provider promptly if signs and symptoms of SIADH (confusion, somnolence, generalized weakness, respiratory failure) occur. May be fatal.
- Rep: Advise women of reproductive potential to notify health care provider if pregnancy is planned or suspected or if breastfeeding. Advise lactating women to monitor breastfed infant for diarrhea and vomiting. May reversibly impair fertility in men.
- Advise patient to notify health care provider if no improvement is seen in a few days.

Evaluation/Desired Outcomes

- Resolution of signs and symptoms of infection. Length of time for complete resolution depends on organism and site of infection.

liraglutide (lir-a-gloo-tide)

Saxenda, Victoza

Classification

Therapeutic: antidiabetics

Pharmacologic: glucagon-like peptide-1 (GLP-1) receptor agonists

Indications

Victoza: Type 2 diabetes mellitus (as adjunct to diet and exercise). To reduce the risk of major adverse cardiovascular events (cardiovascular death, nonfatal MI, nonfatal stroke) in patients with type 2 diabetes mellitus and established cardiovascular disease. **Saxenda:** Chronic weight management in adults who are obese (body mass index [BMI] $\geq$30 kg/m^2) or are overweight (BMI $\geq$27 kg/m^2) with $\geq$1 weight-related comorbid condition (e.g., hypertension, dyslipidemia, type 2 diabetes) (as adjunct to reduced-calorie diet and increased physical activity). **Saxenda:** Chronic weight management in children $\geq$12 yr old with a body weight >60 kg and an initial BMI corresponding to $\geq$30 kg/m^2 for adults (obese) by international cutoffs (Cole Criteria) (as adjunct to reduced-calorie diet and increased physical activity).

Action

Acts as an acylated human glucagon-like peptide-1 (GLP-1, an incretin) receptor agonist; increases intracellular cyclic AMP leading to insulin release when glucose is elevated, which then subsides as blood glucose decreases toward euglycemia. Also decreases glucagon secretion and delays gastric emptying. Also helps to suppress appetite, leading to decreased caloric intake.
Therapeutic Effects: Improved glycemic control. Reduction in body weight. Reduction in cardiovascular death, nonfatal MI, or nonfatal stroke.

Pharmacokinetics

Absorption: 55% absorbed following SUBQ injection.
Distribution: Unknown.
Protein Binding: >98%.
Metabolism and Excretion: Endogenously metabolized.
Half-life: 13 hr.

ROUTE	ONSET	PEAK	DURATION
SUBQ	within 4 wk† within 2 wk‡	8 wk† 40 wk‡	unknown†‡

† ↓ in A1c.
‡ ↓ in body weight.

Contraindications/Precautions

Contraindicated in: Hypersensitivity; Personal or family history of medullary thyroid carcinoma; Multiple endocrine neoplasia syndrome type 2; Type 1 diabetes (Victoza only); Diabetic ketoacidosis (Victoza only); Concurrent use with other weight-loss products (Saxenda only); History of suicidal attempts or suicidal thoughts (Saxenda only); Undergoing elective surgery or procedure requiring general anesthesia or deep sedation; Severe GI disease (including severe gastroparesis); OB: Weight loss not recommended during pregnancy (Saxenda only); Lactation: Lactation; Pedi: Children $\geq$12 yr with type 2 diabetes (safety and effectiveness not established) (Saxenda only).
Use Cautiously in: History of pancreatitis; History of angioedema or anaphylaxis to another GLP-1 receptor agonist; Hepatic impairment; Renal impairment; OB: Use during pregnancy only if potential maternal benefit justifies potential fetal risk (Victoza only); Pedi: Safety and effectiveness not established in children <12 yr (Saxenda) and children <10 yr (Victoza); ↑ risk of hypoglycemia with use of either Saxenda or Victoza in children.

Adverse Reactions/Side Effects

CV: tachycardia. **Derm:** cutaneous amyloidosis, pruritus, rash. **Endo:** hypoglycemia, THYROID C-CELL TUMORS. **GI:** diarrhea, nausea, vomiting, cholecystitis, cholelithiasis, constipation, PANCREATITIS. **GU:** acute renal failure. **Local:** injection site reactions. **Neuro:** headache, SUICIDAL BEHAVIOR/IDEATION (SAXENDA ONLY).

Resp: aspiration. **Misc:** HYPERSENSITIVITY REACTIONS (INCLUDING ANAPHYLAXIS AND ANGIOEDEMA).

Interactions

Drug-Drug: Insulin secretagogues, including **sulfonylureas** and **insulin**, may ↑ risk of serious hypoglycemia; use cautiously and consider ↓ dose of agent ↑ insulin secretion. May alter absorption of concurrently administered **oral medications** due to delayed gastric emptying.

Route/Dosage

Victoza

Type 2 Diabetes Mellitus

SUBQ (Adults): 0.6 mg once daily for 1 wk, then 1.2 mg once daily for 1 wk; may then ↑ dose, if needed, up to 1.8 mg once daily.
SUBQ (Children ≥10 yr): 0.6 mg once daily for 1 wk; may then ↑, if needed, to 1.2 mg once daily; after 1 wk, if additional glycemic control needed, may then ↑ to 1.8 mg once daily.

Reduction in Risk of Major Adverse Cardiovascular Events

SUBQ (Adults): 0.6 mg once daily for 1 wk, then 1.2 mg once daily for 1 wk; may then ↑, if needed, up to 1.8 mg once daily.

Saxenda

SUBQ (Adults): 0.6 mg once daily for 1 wk (Wk 1), then 1.2 mg once daily for 1 wk (Wk 2), then 1.8 mg once daily for 1 wk (Wk 3), then 2.4 mg once daily for 1 wk (Wk 4), then 3 mg once daily. Discontinue if patient cannot tolerate dose of 3 mg once daily.
SUBQ (Children ≥12 yr): 0.6 mg once daily for 1 wk (Wk 1), then 1.2 mg once daily for 1 wk (Wk 2), then 1.8 mg once daily for 1 wk (Wk 3), then 2.4 mg once daily for 1 wk (Wk 4), then 3 mg once daily. If patient cannot tolerate dose of 3 mg once daily, ↓ to 2.4 mg once daily; discontinue if patient cannot subsequently tolerate dose of 2.4 mg once daily.

Availability (generic available)

Solution for injection (Saxenda) (prefilled pens): 18 mg/3 mL (delivers doses of 0.6 mg, 1.2 mg, 1.8 mg, 2.4 mg, or 3 mg). **Solution for injection (Victoza) (prefilled pens):** 18 mg/3 mL (delivers doses of 0.6 mg, 1.2 mg, or 1.8 mg). ***In combination with:*** insulin degludec (Xultophy). See Appendix N

NURSING IMPLICATIONS

Assessment

- Assess for thyroid C-cell tumors (mass in neck, dysphagia, dyspnea, persistent hoarseness). Monitor for elevated serum calcitonin. If noted, refer to an endocrinologist.
- Monitor for pancreatitis during therapy (persistent severe abdominal pain, sometimes radiating to the back, with or without vomiting). *If pancreatitis is suspected,* discontinue liraglutide; if confirmed, do not restart liraglutide.
- Monitor for hypersensitivity reactions (swelling of face, lips, tongue, or throat; fainting or feeling dizzy; very rapid heartbeat; problems breathing or swallowing; severe rash or itching). *If hypersensitivity reaction occurs,* discontinue liraglutide, treat per standard of care, and monitor until symptoms resolve.
- **Victoza:** Observe patient taking concurrent insulin for signs and symptoms of hypoglycemic reactions (sweating, hunger, weakness, dizziness, tremor, tachycardia, anxiety).
- **Saxenda:** Monitor for weight loss and adjust concurrent medications (antihypertensives, antidiabetics, lipid-lowering agents) as needed. Assess for suicidal thoughts or behaviors (depression, anxiety, agitation, irritability).

Lab Test Considerations

- Monitor A1c periodically during therapy to evaluate effectiveness.
- Monitor renal function and triglycerides.

Implementation

- Patients stabilized on a diabetic regimen who are exposed to stress, fever, trauma, infection, or surgery may require administration of insulin.
- **SUBQ**: Administer once daily at any time of the day, without regard to food. Inject at a 90° angle into abdomen, thigh, or upper arm. Apply light pressure but do not rub injection site. Solution should be clear and colorless; do not administer solutions that are discolored or contain particulate matter. Rotate injection sites within the same region to ↓ risk of cutaneous amyloidosis. Use a new needle for each injection. Store in refrigerator before 1st dose; after 1st dose, may be stored for 30 days at room temperature or in refrigerator.

Patient/Family Teaching

- Explain purpose and side effects of medication to patient. Advise patient to read *Patient Information* before starting therapy. Explain this medication controls hyperglycemia but does not cure diabetes. Therapy is long term. Emphasize the importance of routine follow-up exams. Advise patient if a dose is missed to omit and take next dose as scheduled; do not double doses. If missed >3 days, reinitiate with 0.6 mg dose; titrate at direction of health care provider.
- Advise patient to notify health care provider of all Rx or OTC medications, vitamins, or herbal products

L

being taken and to consult with health care provider before taking other medications.

- Educate on use of the pen injector. Pen should never be shared between patients, even if needle is changed.
- Inform patient that nausea is the most common side effect but usually ↓ over time.
- Advise patient to never mix another insulin and liraglutide together. Give as two separate injections. Both injections may be given in the same body area but should not be given right next to each other.
- Review signs of hypoglycemia and hyperglycemia with patient. If hypoglycemia occurs, advise patient to take a glass of orange juice or 2–3 teaspoons of sugar, honey, or corn syrup dissolved in water and notify health care provider. Advise patient to carry a form of sugar (sugar packets, candy) and identification describing disease process and medication regimen at all times.
- Encourage patient to follow prescribed diet, medication, and exercise regimen to prevent hypoglycemic or hyperglycemic episodes.
- Instruct patient in proper testing of serum glucose and ketones. These tests should be closely monitored during periods of stress or illness, and health care provider should be notified if significant changes occur.
- Advise patient to discontinue liraglutide and seek medical advice immediately if signs/symptoms of thyroid tumors (mass in neck, difficulty swallowing or breathing, persistent hoarseness) occur.
- Advise patient to discontinue liraglutide and seek medical advice immediately if signs and symptoms of pancreatitis or hypersensitivity reactions (anaphylaxis) occur.
- Advise patient to inform health care provider of medication regimen before treatment or surgery.
- Advise patients taking *Saxenda* about suicidal behavior or thoughts. Discontinue if occur, and seek medical advice.
- Advise adult patients to discontinue *Saxenda* if they have not lost ≥4% of body weight by 16 wk of treatment. Instruct caregivers of pediatric patients >12 yr to discontinue *Saxenda* if they have not achieved a BMI ↓ of ≥1% from baseline after 12 wk on the maintenance dose.
- Rep: Insulin is the preferred method of controlling blood glucose during pregnancy. Counsel women of reproductive potential to notify health care provider if pregnancy is planned or suspected or if breastfeeding. *Saxenda* is contraindicated in pregnancy, as weight loss during pregnancy may cause fetal harm.

Evaluation/Desired Outcomes

- Improved glycemic control.
- Reduction in body weight.
- Reduction in cardiovascular death, nonfatal MI, or nonfatal stroke.

lisdexamfetamine

(lis-dex-am-**fet**-a-meen)

Arynta, Vyvanse

Classification

Therapeutic: central nervous system stimulants

Pharmacologic: sympathomimetics

Schedule II

Indications

Attention-deficit hyperactivity disorder (ADHD). Moderate to severe binge eating disorder.

Action

Blocks reuptake and increases release of norepinephrine and dopamine resulting in increased levels in extraneuronal space. **Therapeutic Effects:** Improved attention span in ADHD. Reduction in number of binge eating days per wk.

Pharmacokinetics

Absorption: Rapidly absorbed and converted to dextroamphetamine, the active drug.

Distribution: Unknown.

Metabolism and Excretion: 42% excreted in urine as amphetamine.

Half-life: <1 hr.

ROUTE	ONSET	PEAK	DURATION
PO	rapid	1 hr	24 hr

Contraindications/Precautions

Contraindicated in: Hypersensitivity to lisdexamfetamine or other sympathomimetic amines; Advanced arteriosclerosis; Serious structural cardiac abnormalities, cardiomyopathy, serious cardiac arrhythmia, coronary artery disease, or other serious cardiac disease (may ↑ risk of sudden death); Moderate to severe hypertension; Glaucoma; Agitation; Concurrent use or use within 14 days of MAO inhibitors or MAO-like drugs (linezolid or methylene blue); Lactation: Lactation.

Use Cautiously in: History of pre-existing psychosis, bipolar disorder, aggression, or seizures (may exacerbate condition); Tics or family history/diagnosis of Tourette syndrome (may worsen condition); History of substance abuse; Continual use (may result in psychological or physical dependence); Severe renal impairment (↓ maximum daily dose); OB: Use during pregnancy only if potential maternal benefit outweighs potential fetal risk; Pedi: Children <6 yr (safety and effectiveness not established); growth suppression may occur in children with long-term use.

Adverse Reactions/Side Effects

CV: hypertension, tachycardia, Raynaud phenomenon, SUDDEN DEATH. **Derm:** alopecia, rash. **EENT:** blurred vision, poor accommodation. **GI:** ↓ appetite, abdominal pain, dry mouth, intestinal ischemia, nausea, vomiting, weight loss (especially with prolonged use). **GU:** ↓ libido, priapism. **Metab:** growth suppression (especially with prolonged use). **MS:** RHABDOMYOLYSIS. **Neuro:** behavioral disturbances, dizziness, hallucinations, insomnia, irritability, mania, paresthesia, psychomotor hyperactivity, thought disorder, tics, Tourette syndrome. **Misc:** physical dependence, psychological dependence, SEROTONIN SYNDROME.

Interactions

Drug-Drug: Concurrent use with **MAO inhibitors** or **MAO-inhibitor-like drugs**, such as **linezolid** or **methylene blue**, may result in serious, potentially fatal reactions; wait ≥14 days following discontinuation of MAO inhibitor before initiation of amphetamine mixtures. Drugs that affect serotonergic neurotransmitter systems, including **MAO inhibitors**, **tricyclic antidepressants**, **SSRIs**, **SNRIs**, **fentanyl**, **buspirone**, **tramadol**, **lithium**, and **triptans**, may ↑ risk of serotonin syndrome. **Sympathomimetic amines** may result in additive effects and ↑ risk of adverse reactions. **Urinary acidifying agents**, including **sodium acid phosphate**, ↑ excretion and ↓ levels and may result in ↓ effectiveness. May ↓ effectiveness of **adrenergic blockers**. ↑ risk of adverse cardiovascular reactions with **tricyclic antidepressants**. May ↓ sedating effects of **antihistamines**. May ↓ effectiveness of **antihypertensives**. Effects may be ↓ by **haloperidol**, **lithium**, or **chlorpromazine**. May ↓ absorption of **phenobarbital** or **phenytoin**.

Route/Dosage

Attention-Deficit Hyperactivity Disorder

PO (Adults and Children ≥6 yr): 30 mg once daily; may ↑ by 10–20 mg/day at weekly intervals, up to 70 mg/day.

Renal Impairment

PO (Adults and Children ≥6 yr): *CCr 15–29 mL/min:* Do not exceed 50 mg/day; *CCr <15 mL/min:* Do not exceed 30 mg/day.

Binge Eating Disorder

PO (Adults): 30 mg once daily; may ↑ by 20 mg/day at weekly intervals, up to target dose of 50–70 mg/day.

Availability (generic available)

Capsules: 10 mg, 20 mg, 30 mg, 40 mg, 50 mg, 60 mg, 70 mg. **Chewable tablets:** 10 mg, 20 mg, 30 mg, 40 mg, 50 mg, 60 mg. **Oral solution (Arynta):** 10 mg/mL.

NURSING IMPLICATIONS

Assessment

- Monitor BP, HR, and respiratory rate before administering and periodically during therapy. Obtain a history (including assessment of family history of sudden death or ventricular arrhythmia), physical exam to assess for cardiac disease, and further evaluation (ECG and echocardiogram), if indicated. If exertional chest pain, unexplained syncope, or other cardiac symptoms occur, evaluate and treat promptly.
- Assess for risk of abuse, misuse, or addiction prior to starting therapy and during therapy. Has high dependence and abuse or misuse potential. Misuse and abuse of CNS stimulants can result in overdose and death; this risk is ↑ with higher doses or unapproved methods of administration, such as snorting or injection. Tolerance to medication occurs rapidly; do not ↑ dose.
- Screen patients with bipolar disorder for risk of manic episode (comorbid or history of depressive symptoms or a family history of suicide, bipolar disorder, or depression) prior to starting therapy.
- Pedi: Monitor growth, both height and weight, in children on long-term therapy. May need to interrupt therapy in patients who are not growing or gaining height or weight as expected.
- Monitor closely for behavior change.
- Assess for signs/symptoms of serotonin syndrome (mental changes [agitation, hallucinations, coma], autonomic instability [tachycardia, labile BP, hyperthermia], neuromuscular aberrations [hyperreflexia, incoordination], or GI symptoms [nausea, vomiting, diarrhea]), especially in patients taking other serotonergic drugs (SSRIs, SNRIs, triptans).
- **ADHD:** Assess child's attention span, impulse control, and interactions with others. Therapy may be interrupted at intervals to determine whether symptoms are sufficient to continue therapy.
- **Binge Eating Disorder:** Monitor frequency and amount of binge eating.

Lab Test Considerations

- May cause ↑ plasma corticosteroid levels interfering with urinary steroid determinations.

Implementation

- **PO:** Administer in the morning without regard to meals. Avoid afternoon doses due to potential for insomnia. Capsules may be swallowed whole or opened and the entire contents dissolved in yogurt, water, or orange juice. If solution method is used, consume immediately; do not store for future use. Do not divide capsules or take less than one capsule per day. Chewable tablets must be chewed thoroughly. Tablets and chewable tablets can be substituted on a unit per unit/mg per mg basis.
- For oral solution, use oral dosing syringe and adapter provided with the bottle. Ensure that the bottle adapter is firmly inserted into the bottle before 1st

L

use and keep the adapter in place for as long as bottle is used. Discard any remaining solution 30 days after initially opening the bottle.

Patient/Family Teaching

- Instruct patient to take medication as directed. Advise patient and caregivers to read *Patient Information* before therapy and with each renewal of Rx refill. If more than prescribed amount is taken, notify health care provider immediately. Instruct patient not to alter dose without consulting health care provider. Emphasize the importance of routine follow-up exams to monitor progress.
- Advise patient to notify health care provider of all Rx or OTC medications, vitamins, or herbal products being taken and to consult health care provider before taking other medications.
- Advise caregivers to notify school nurse of medication regimen.
- Advise patient that lisdexamfetamine is a drug with known potential for abuse, misuse, or addiction. Store in safe place, protect it from theft, and never give to anyone other than the individual for whom it was prescribed.
- Advise patient to store in a safe place, preferably locked, and not to share this medication with anyone.
- Advise patient to check weight 2–3 times weekly and report weight loss to health care provider. Pedi: If ↓ appetite and weight loss are a problem, advise parents to provide high-calorie meals when drug levels are low (at breakfast and or bedtime).
- Inform patients starting therapy of risk of peripheral vasculopathy. Instruct patients to notify health care provider of any new numbness; pain; skin color change, from pale to blue to red; or coolness or sensitivity to temperature in fingers or toes, and call if unexplained wounds appear on fingers or toes. May require rheumatology consultation.
- Advise caregivers to notify health care provider immediately if child has signs of heart problems (chest pain, shortness of breath, fainting) or if new or worsening mental symptoms or problems, especially seeing or hearing things that are not real or believing things that are not real or are suspicious, occur.
- May cause dizziness or blurred vision. Caution patient to avoid driving or activities requiring alertness until response to medication is known.
- Advise patient to notify health care provider if nervousness, restlessness, insomnia, dizziness, anorexia, or dry mouth becomes severe.
- Inform patient that health care provider may order periodic holidays from the drug to assess progress and to ↓ dependence.
- Rep: May cause fetal harm. Advise women of reproductive potential to notify health care provider if pregnancy is planned or suspected and to avoid breastfeeding. May cause premature delivery. Monitor infants born to mothers taking lisdexamfetamine for symptoms of withdrawal (feeding difficulties, irritability, agitation, excessive drowsiness). Inform pregnant patient of registry that monitors outcomes in women exposed to ADHD medications during pregnancy. Register patient by calling the National Pregnancy Registry for Psychostimulants at 1-866-961-2388 or visiting https://womensmentalhealth.org/clinical-and-researchprograms/pregnancyregistry/adhdmedications/.

Evaluation/Desired Outcomes

- Improved attention span, decreased impulsiveness and hyperactivity in ADHD.
- Reduction in number of binge eating days per wk.

lisinopril, See ANGIOTENSIN-CONVERTING ENZYME (ACE) INHIBITORS.

lithium (lith-ee-um)

✱ Carbolith, ✱ Lithane, ✱ Lithmax, Lithobid

Classification

Therapeutic: mood stabilizers

Indications

Acute manic and mixed episodes associated with bipolar I disorder. Maintenance treatment of bipolar I disorder.

Action

Alters cation transport in nerve and muscle. May also influence reuptake of neurotransmitters. **Therapeutic Effects:** Prevents/decreases incidence of acute manic episodes.

Pharmacokinetics

Absorption: Completely absorbed after oral administration.

Distribution: Widely distributed into many tissues and fluids; CSF levels are 50% of plasma levels.

Metabolism and Excretion: Excreted almost entirely unchanged by the kidneys.

Half-life: 20–27 hr.

TIME/ACTION PROFILE (antimanic effects)

ROUTE	ONSET	PEAK	DURATION
PO, PO-ER	5–7 days	10–21 days	days

Contraindications/Precautions

Contraindicated in: Hypersensitivity; Brugada syndrome; Some products contain alcohol or tartrazine and should be avoided in patients with known hypersensitivity or intolerance; OB: Pregnancy Lactation: Lactation.

Use Cautiously in: Significant cardiovascular disease, renal impairment, dehydration, fever, or hyponatremia (↑ risk of lithium toxicity); Diabetes mellitus; Pedi: Children <7 yr (safety and effectiveness not established); Geri: Initial dosage ↓ recommended in older adults.

Adverse Reactions/Side Effects

CV: ECG changes, arrhythmias, edema, hypotension, unmasking of Brugada syndrome. **Derm:** acneiform eruption, folliculitis, alopecia, diminished sensation, DRUG REACTION WITH EOSINOPHILIA AND SYSTEMIC SYMPTOMS (DRESS), pruritus. **EENT:** blurred vision, tinnitus. **Endo:** hypothyroidism, goiter, hyperglycemia, hyperparathyroidism, hyperthyroidism. **F and E:** hypercalcemia, hyponatremia. **GI:** abdominal pain, anorexia, bloating, diarrhea, nausea, dry mouth. **GU:** polyuria, glycosuria, nephrogenic diabetes insipidus, renal impairment. **Hemat:** leukocytosis. **Metab:** weight gain. **MS:** muscle weakness, rigidity. **Neuro:** fatigue, headache, memory impairment, tremor, aphasia, ataxia, confusion, dizziness, drowsiness, dysarthria, dysgeusia, hyperirritability, PSEUDOTUMOR CEREBRI, psychomotor retardation, restlessness, sedation, SEIZURES, stupor. **Misc:** SEROTONIN SYNDROME.

Interactions

Drug-Drug: May prolong the action of **neuromuscular blocking agents**. ↑ risk of neurologic toxicity with **calcium channel blockers**, **phenytoin**, or **carbamazepine**. **Diuretics**, **NSAIDs**, **ACE inhibitors**, **angiotensin II receptor blockers**, and **metronidazole** may ↑ levels and risk of toxicity. Hypothyroid effects may be additive with **potassium iodide** or **antithyroid agents**. **Aminophylline**, **acetazolamide**, **theophylline**, and **sodium bicarbonate** may ↑ renal elimination and ↓ effectiveness. **Psyllium** may ↓ levels. Drugs that affect serotonergic neurotransmitter systems, including **tricyclic antidepressants**, **SSRIs**, **SNRIs**, **fentanyl**, **buspirone**, **tramadol**, **amphetamines**, and **triptans**, may ↑ risk of serotonin syndrome. **Antipsychotics** may ↑ risk of developing an encephalopathic syndrome (e.g. weakness, lethargy, fever, tremulousness and confusion, extrapyramidal symptoms, leukocytosis, ↑ BUN, ↑ fasting blood glucose); monitor closely. **SGLT2 inhibitors** may ↓ levels and effectiveness.
Drug-Natural Products: Caffeine-containing herbs (**cola nut**, **guarana**, **mate**, **tea**, **coffee**) may ↓ levels and effectiveness. ↑ risk of serotonergic side effects, including serotonin syndrome, with **St. John's wort**.
Drug-Food: Large changes in **sodium** intake may ↑ renal excretion and ↓ levels and effectiveness of lithium.

Route/Dosage

Precise dosing is based on serum lithium levels. 300 mg lithium carbonate contains 8–12 mEq lithium.
PO (Adults and Children ≥7 yr and >30 kg): *Tablets/capsules/liquid:* 300 mg 3 times daily initially; ↑ by 300 mg/day every 3 days; usual dose for treatment of acute manic and mixed episodes = 600 mg 2–3 times daily; usual maintenance dose = 300–600 mg 2–3 times daily.
PO (Adults and Children >12 yr): *Extended-release tablets:* 450–900 mg twice daily *or* 300–600 mg 3 times daily initially; usual maintenance dose is 450 mg twice daily *or* 300 mg 3 times daily.
PO (Children ≥7 yr and 20–30 kg): *Tablets/capsules/liquid:* 300 mg twice daily initially; ↑ by 300 mg/wk; usual dose for treatment of acute manic and mixed episodes = 600–1500 mg/day in divided doses; usual maintenance dose = 600–1200 mg/day in divided doses.

L

Availability (generic available)

Immediate-release tablets: 300 mg. **Immediate-release capsules:** 150 mg, 300 mg, 600 mg. **Extended-release tablets:** 300 mg, 450 mg. **Oral solution:** 300 mg (8 mEq lithium)/5 mL.

NURSING IMPLICATIONS

Assessment

- Assess and monitor mental status (orientation, mood, behavior, affect). Assess for suicidal tendencies and initiate suicide precautions if indicated. Inform health care provider if patient demonstrates significant changes in mood or behavior.
- Monitor intake and output. Report significant changes in totals. Unless contraindicated, fluid intake of ≥2000–3000 mL/day should be maintained. Weight should also be monitored at least every 3 mo.
- Assess for signs and symptoms of serotonin syndrome (confusion, delirium, agitation, coma, dilated pupils, tachycardia, hyperthermia, shivering, hyperreflexia, muscle rigidity, hypertension, vomiting, diarrhea, seizures). ↑ risk of serotonin syndrome with concurrent use of other serotonergic drugs (SSRIs, SNRIs, triptans); monitoring recommended; discontinuation may be required.

Lab Test Considerations

- Evaluate renal and thyroid function, WBC with differential, electrolytes, and glucose periodically during therapy.

Toxicity and Overdose

- Lithium toxicity is closely related to serum lithium concentrations and can occur at doses close to therapeutic concentrations. Monitor serum lithium concentrations twice weekly during initiation of therapy and every 2 mo during chronic therapy. Draw blood samples in the morning, immediately before next dose. Therapeutic levels range from 0.5–1.5 mEq/L for acute mania and 0.6–1.2 mEq/L for long-term control. Serum concentrations should not exceed 2.0 mEq/L.

- Assess patient for signs and symptoms of lithium toxicity (vomiting, diarrhea, slurred speech, light-headedness, ↓ coordination, drowsiness, muscle weakness, tremor, twitching). If these occur, report before administering next dose.

Implementation

- Do not confuse lithium carbonate with lanthanum carbonate.
- **PO:** Administer with food or milk to ↓ GI irritation. ***DNC:*** Extended-release preparations should be swallowed whole; do not break, crush, or chew.

Patient/Family Teaching

- Explain the purpose and side effects of lithium. Instruct patient to take medication as directed, even if feeling well. Take missed doses as soon as remembered unless within 2 hr of next dose (6 hr if extended release). Advise patient to read *Patient Information* before starting and with each Rx refill in case of changes.
- Emphasize the importance of periodic lab tests to monitor for lithium toxicity.
- Lithium may cause dizziness or drowsiness. Caution patient to avoid driving or other activities requiring alertness until response to medication is known.
- Low sodium levels may predispose patient to toxicity. Advise patient to drink 2000–3000 mL fluid each day and follow a diet with consistent and moderate sodium intake. Excessive amounts of coffee, tea, and cola should be avoided because of diuretic effect. Avoid activities that cause excess sodium loss (heavy exertion, exercise in hot weather, saunas). Notify health care provider of fever, vomiting, and diarrhea, which also cause sodium loss.
- Advise patient that weight gain may occur. Review principles of a low-calorie diet.
- Advise patient to notify health care provider of all Rx or OTC medications, vitamins, or herbal products being taken and to consult with health care provider before taking other medications, especially NSAIDs and St. John's wort.
- Review side effects and symptoms of toxicity with patient. Instruct patient to stop medication and report signs of toxicity to health care provider promptly.
- Advise patient to notify health care provider if fainting, light-headedness, palpitations, or difficulty breathing occur, as these may be symptoms of Brugada syndrome.
- Rep: May cause fetal harm. Advise women of reproductive potential to use contraception during therapy, consult health care provider if pregnancy is planned or suspected, and avoid breastfeeding. Monitor breastfed infants for signs and symptoms of lithium toxicity (hypertonia, hypothermia, cyanosis, ECG changes).

Evaluation/Desired Outcomes

- Resolution of the symptoms of mania (hyperactivity, pressured speech, poor judgment, need for little sleep).
- Decreased incidence of mood swings in bipolar disorders.
- Improved affect in unipolar disorders. Improvement in condition may require 1–3 wk.
- Decreased incidence of acute manic episodes.

lofexidine (loe-**fex**-i-deen)

Lucemyra

Classification

Therapeutic: none assigned

Pharmacologic: adrenergics (centrally acting)

Indications

Mitigation of opioid withdrawal symptoms to facilitate abrupt opioid discontinuation in adults.

Action

Stimulates $alpha_2$-adrenergic receptors in the CNS, which results in decreased sympathetic outflow. **Therapeutic Effects:** Reduction in severity of opioid withdrawal symptoms.

Pharmacokinetics

Absorption: 72% absorbed following oral administration.

Distribution: Extensively distributed to tissues, including CNS.

Metabolism and Excretion: Primarily metabolized by the liver via the CYP2D6 isoenzyme and to a lesser extent by the CYP1A2 and CYP2C19 isoenzymes to inactive metabolites; primarily excreted in urine (15–20% as unchanged drug); the CYP2D6 isoenzyme exhibits genetic polymorphism; 7% of population may be poor metabolizers and may have significantly ↑ lofexidine concentrations and an ↑ risk of adverse effects.

Half-life: 17–22 hr.

TIME/ACTION PROFILE (plasma concentrations)

ROUTE	ONSET	PEAK	DURATION
PO	unknown	3–5 hr	unknown

Contraindications/Precautions

Contraindicated in: Congenital long QT syndrome.

Use Cautiously in: Severe cardiac or cerebrovascular disease, recent MI, chronic kidney disease, or severe bradycardia (↑ risk of hypotension, bradycardia, and/or syncope); HF, bradyarrhythmias, hepatic impairment, renal impairment, hypokalemia, hypomagnesemia, or concurrent use of QT-interval prolonging medications (↑ risk of QT interval prolongation); CYP2D6 poor metabolizers; OB: Safety not established in pregnancy; Lactation: Safety not established in breastfeeding; Pedi: Safety and effectiveness not established in children; Geri: ↑ risk of orthostatic hypotension and adverse CNS effects in older adults (↓ dose recommended).

Adverse Reactions/Side Effects

CV: bradycardia, hypotension, palpitations, QT interval prolongation, syncope, TORSADES DE POINTES. **EENT:** tinnitus. **GI:** dry mouth. **Neuro:** dizziness, drowsiness, insomnia.

Interactions

Drug-Drug: Additive hypotension with other **antihypertensives** and **nitrates**; avoid concurrent use. Additive bradycardia with **beta blockers**, **diltiazem**, **verapamil**, **digoxin**, **clonidine**, or **ivabradine**; avoid concurrent use. Additive sedation with **CNS depressants**, including **alcohol**, **antihistamines**, **opioid analgesics**, and **sedative/hypnotics**. Concurrent use with **QT interval-prolonging medications**, including **methadone**, may ↑ risk of QT interval prolongation and torsades de pointes. May ↓ **naltrexone (PO)** levels and effectiveness; separate administration by >2 hr. **CYP2D6 inhibitors**, including **paroxetine**, may ↑ levels and risk of toxicity.

Route/Dosage

PO (Adults): 0.54 mg 4 times daily (with 5–6 hr between each dose) during the period of peak withdrawal symptoms (usually the first 5–7 days after the last opioid dose); may adjust dose based on symptoms (max dose = 2.88 mg/day or 0.72 mg/dose); may be continued for up to 14 days. Must taper therapy on discontinuation (gradually ↓ dose over 2–4-day period).

Hepatic Impairment

PO (Adults): *Moderate hepatic impairment:* 0.36 mg 4 times daily (with 5–6 hr between each dose) during the period of peak withdrawal symptoms (usually the first 5–7 days after the last opioid dose); *Severe hepatic impairment:* 0.18 mg 4 times daily (with 5–6 hr between each dose) during the period of peak withdrawal symptoms (usually the first 5–7 days after the last opioid dose).

Renal Impairment

PO (Adults): *CCr 30–<90 mL/min:* 0.36 mg 4 times daily (with 5–6 hr between each dose) during the period of peak withdrawal symptoms (usually the first 5–7 days after the last opioid dose); *CCr <30 mL/min:* 0.18 mg 4 times daily (with 5–6 hr between each dose) during the period of peak withdrawal symptoms (usually the first 5–7 days after the last opioid dose).

Availability (generic available)

Tablets: 0.18 mg.

NURSING IMPLICATIONS

Assessment

- Assess vital signs and symptoms of bradycardia and orthostatic hypotension (low BP, slow HR, dizziness, light-headedness, feeling faint at rest or when standing up) before dose and as needed during therapy. May need to ↓ dose or hold/discontinue therapy if hypotension, bradycardia, or syncope occur.
- Monitor ECG when starting therapy and in patients with HF, bradyarrhythmias, hepatic impairment, renal impairment, or those taking medications (methadone) that lead to QT interval prolongation.

Lab Test Considerations

- Monitor electrolytes before starting and during therapy. Correct electrolyte abnormalities (hypokalemia, hypomagnesemia) before starting therapy.

Implementation

- ↑ risk of fatal overdose with resumed opioid use; treatment for opioid use disorder should only be performed in conjunction with a comprehensive management program.
- Abrupt discontinuation can cause a marked ↑ in BP; gradually ↓ dose. Lower doses may be appropriate as opioid withdrawal symptoms wane.
- **PO:** Administer three tablets four times daily without regard to food, with 5–6 hr between doses.

Patient/Family Teaching

- Explain the purpose and side effects of lofexidine to patient. Instruct patient to take lofexidine as directed and not to stop without consulting health care professional. Take missed doses as soon as remembered unless almost time for next dose. Abrupt discontinuation can cause diarrhea, insomnia, anxiety, chills, hyperhidrosis, and extremity pain. ↓ dose gradually. Advise patient to read *Patient Information* before starting and with each Rx refill in case of changes.

L

- Caution patients that after a period of not using opioids, they may be more sensitive to the effects of opioids and at greater risk of overdosing.
- May cause dizziness and sedation. Caution patient to avoid driving and activities requiring alertness until response to medication is known.
- Caution patient to avoid sudden changes in position to ↓ orthostatic hypotension. Use of alcohol, standing for long periods, exercising, dehydration, and hot weather may ↑ orthostatic hypotension.
- Instruct patient to notify health care professional of all Rx or OTC medications, vitamins, or herbal products being taken and to consult health care professional before taking any other Rx, OTC, or herbal products, especially benzodiazepines, barbiturates, tranquilizers, or sleeping pills.
- Caution patient to avoid concurrent use of alcohol or other CNS depressants with lofexidine.
- Rep: Advise women of reproductive potential to notify health care professional if pregnancy is planned or suspected or if breastfeeding.

Evaluation/Desired Outcomes

- Reduction in severity of opioid withdrawal symptoms.

loperamide (loe-**per**-a-mide)

Imodium A-D

Classification

Therapeutic: antidiarrheals

Indications

Adjunctive therapy of acute diarrhea. Chronic diarrhea associated with inflammatory bowel disease. Decreases the volume of ileostomy drainage.

Action

Inhibits peristalsis and prolongs transit time by a direct effect on nerves in the intestinal muscle wall. Reduces fecal volume and increases fecal viscosity and bulk while diminishing loss of fluid and electrolytes. **Therapeutic Effects:** Relief of diarrhea.

Pharmacokinetics

Absorption: Not well absorbed following oral administration.
Distribution: Does not cross the blood-brain barrier.
Protein Binding: 97%.
Metabolism and Excretion: Metabolized partially by the liver, undergoes enterohepatic recirculation; 30% eliminated in the feces. Minimal excretion in the urine.
Half-life: 10.8 hr.

TIME/ACTION PROFILE (relief of diarrhea)

ROUTE	ONSET	PEAK	DURATION
PO	1 hr	2.5–5 hr	10 hr

Contraindications/Precautions

Contraindicated in: Hypersensitivity; Patients in whom constipation must be avoided; Abdominal pain of unknown cause, especially if associated with fever; Alcohol intolerance (liquid only); Pedi: Children <2 yr (↑ risk of respiratory depression and arrhythmias).
Use Cautiously in: Hepatic impairment; OB: Safety not established in pregnancy; Geri: Older adults may have ↑ sensitivity to effects.

Adverse Reactions/Side Effects

CV: CARDIAC ARREST, QT interval prolongation, syncope, TORSADE DE POINTES. **GI:** constipation, abdominal pain/distention/discomfort, dry mouth, nausea, vomiting. **Neuro:** drowsiness, dizziness. **Misc:** HYPERSENSITIVITY REACTIONS (INCLUDING ANAPHYLAXIS).

Interactions

Drug-Drug: ↑ risk of CNS depression with other **CNS depressants**, including **alcohol, antihistamines, opioid analgesics**, and **sedative/hypnotics**. ↑ anticholinergic properties with other **drugs having anticholinergic properties**, including **antidepressants** and **antihistamines**. **Cimetidine, clarithromycin, erythromycin, gemfibrozil, itraconazole, ketoconazole, quinidine, quinine**, or **ritonavir** may ↑ levels and risk of cardiac arrhythmias.
Drug-Natural Products: Kava-kava, valerian, skullcap, chamomile, or **hops** can ↑ risk of CNS depression.

Route/Dosage

Acute Diarrhea

PO (Adults and Children ≥ 12 yr): 4 mg initially, then 2 mg after each loose stool. Maintenance dose usually 4–8 mg/day in divided doses (not to exceed 8 mg/day for OTC use or 16 mg/day for Rx use).
PO (Children 9–11 yr or 30–47 kg): 2 mg initially, then 1 mg after each loose stool (not to exceed 6 mg/24 hr; OTC use should not exceed 2 days).
PO (Children 6–8 yr or 24–30 kg): 1 mg initially, then 1 mg after each loose stool (not to exceed 4 mg/24 hr; OTC use should not exceed 2 days).
PO (Children 2–5 yr or 13–20 kg): 1 mg initially, then 0.1 mg/kg after each loose stool (not to exceed 3 mg/24 hr; OTC use should not exceed 2 days).

Chronic Diarrhea

PO (Adults): 4 mg initially, then 2 mg after each loose stool. Maintenance dose usually 4–8 mg/day in divided doses (not to exceed 16 mg/day for Rx use).
PO (Children): 0.08–0.24 mg/kg/day divided 2–3 times/day (not to exceed 2 mg/dose).

Reduction of Ileostomy Output

PO (Adults): 2 mg 2–3 times daily (tablets or capsules only); may ↑ dose in 2 mg/day increments if output remains elevated (not to exceed 16 mg/day for Rx use).

Availability (generic available)

Tablets: 2 mg[OTC]. **Capsules:** 2 mg. **Oral liquid (mint):** 1 mg/7.5 mL[OTC]. ***In combination with:*** simethicone (Imodium Multi-Symptom Relief), see Appendix N).

NURSING IMPLICATIONS

Assessment

- Assess frequency and consistency of stools and bowel sounds prior to and during therapy.
- Assess fluid and electrolyte balance and skin turgor for hydration status periodically during therapy as indicated.

Implementation

- Avoid doses higher than recommended due to ↑ risk of cardiac arrhythmias.
- **PO:** Administer with clear fluids to help prevent dehydration, which may accompany diarrhea.

Patient/Family Teaching

- Explain purpose and side effects of medication. Advise patient to read *Patient Information* before starting therapy. Do not take missed doses, and do not double doses. In acute diarrhea, medication may be ordered after each unformed stool. Advise patient not to exceed the maximum number of doses.
- May cause drowsiness. Advise patient to avoid driving or other activities requiring alertness until response to drug is known.
- Advise patient that frequent mouth rinses, good oral hygiene, and sugarless gum or candy may relieve dry mouth.
- Caution patient to avoid using alcohol and other CNS depressants concurrently with this medication.
- Instruct patient to notify health care provider if diarrhea persists or if fever, abdominal pain, or distention occurs.
- Advise patient to notify health care provider of all Rx or OTC medications, vitamins, or herbal products being taken and to consult health care provider before taking other medications.
- Rep: Advise women of reproductive potential to notify health care provider if pregnancy is planned or suspected or if breastfeeding.

Evaluation/Desired Outcomes

- Decrease in diarrhea.
- In acute diarrhea, treatment should be discontinued if no improvement is seen in 48 hr.
- In chronic diarrhea, if no improvement has occurred after ≥10 days of treatment with maximum dose, loperamide is unlikely to be effective.

loratadine (lor-a-ta-deen)

Alavert, Claritin, Claritin Allergy Childrens, Claritin Childrens, Claritin Reditabs, Loradamed

Classification

Therapeutic: allergy, cold, and cough remedies

Pharmacologic: antihistamines

Indications

Seasonal allergies. Chronic idiopathic urticaria. Hives.

Action

Blocks peripheral effects of histamine released during allergic reactions. **Therapeutic Effects:** Decreased symptoms of allergic reactions (nasal stuffiness; red, swollen eyes, itching).

Pharmacokinetics

Absorption: Rapidly absorbed after oral administration (80%).

Distribution: Unknown.

Protein Binding: *Loratadine:* 97%; *descarboethoxyloratadine:* 73–77%.

Metabolism and Excretion: Rapidly and extensively metabolized during first pass through the liver. Much is converted to descarboethoxyloratadine, an active metabolite.

Half-life: *Loratadine:* 8.4 hr; *descarboethoxyloratadine:* 28 hr.

TIME/ACTION PROFILE (antihistaminic effects)

ROUTE	ONSET	PEAK	DURATION
PO	1–3 hr	8–12 hr	>24 hr

Contraindications/Precautions

Contraindicated in: Hypersensitivity.

Use Cautiously in: Severe renal impairment (↓ dose); Hepatic impairment (↓ dose); Pedi: Children <2 yr (safety and effectiveness not established). Syrup contains sodium benzoate; avoid use in neonates; Geri: ↑ risk of adverse reactions in older adults.

Adverse Reactions/Side Effects

Derm: photosensitivity, rash. **EENT:** blurred vision. **GI:** dry mouth, GI upset. **Metab:** weight gain. **Neuro:** confusion, drowsiness (rare), paradoxical excitation.

Interactions

Drug-Drug: **MAO inhibitors** may intensify and prolong effects of antihistamines. ↑ risk of CNS depression may occur with other **CNS depressants**, including

alcohol, antidepressants, opioid analgesics, and **sedative/hypnotics.**
Drug-Natural Products: Kava-kava, valerian, or **chamomile** may ↑ risk of CNS depression.

Route/Dosage

PO (Adults and Children ≥6 yr): 10 mg once daily.
PO (Children ≥2–5 yr): 5 mg once daily.

Renal Impairment

PO (Adults): *CCr <30 mL/min:* 10 mg every other day.

Hepatic Impairment

PO (Adults): 10 mg every other day.

Availability (generic available)

Tablets: 10 mg[OTC]. **Capsules:** 10 mg[OTC]. **Chewable tablets (cool mint flavor, grape flavor, bubblegum flavor):** 5 mg[OTC]. **Orally disintegrating tablets (mint):** 10 mg[OTC]. **Oral solution (grape flavor, fruit flavor):** 5 mg/5 mL[OTC]. ***In combination with:*** pseudoephedrine (Claritin-D)[OTC]. See Appendix N.

NURSING IMPLICATIONS

Assessment

- Assess allergy symptoms (rhinitis, conjunctivitis, hives) before and periodically during therapy.
- Assess lung sounds and character of bronchial secretions. Maintain fluid intake of 1500–2000 mL/day to ↓ viscosity of secretions.

Lab Test Considerations

- May cause false-negative result on allergy skin testing.

Implementation

- **PO:** Administer once daily.
- *For rapidly disintegrating tablets (Alavert, Claritin Reditabs),* place on tongue. Tablet disintegrates rapidly. May be taken with or without water.

Patient/Family Teaching

- Explain purpose and side effects of medication. Advise patient to read *Patient Information* before starting therapy.
- May cause dizziness or drowsiness. Caution patient to avoid driving or other activities requiring alertness until response to medication is known.
- Caution patient to use sunscreen and protective clothing to prevent photosensitivity reactions.
- Advise patient to avoid taking alcohol or other CNS depressants concurrently with this drug.
- Advise patient that good oral hygiene, frequent rinsing of mouth with water, and sugarless gum or candy may minimize dry mouth and to notify dentist if dry mouth persists >2 wk.
- Instruct patient to contact health care provider immediately if dizziness, fainting, or fast or irregular heartbeat occurs or if symptoms persist.
- Advise patient to notify health care provider of all Rx or OTC medications, vitamins, or herbal products being taken and to consult health care provider before taking other medications.
- Rep: Advise women of reproductive potential to notify health care provider if pregnancy is planned or suspected or if breastfeeding.

Evaluation/Desired Outcomes

- Decrease in allergic symptoms.
- Management of chronic idiopathic urticaria.
- Management of hives.

BEERS HIGH ALERT

V LORazepam (lor-az-e-pam)

Ativan, Loreev XR

Classification

Therapeutic: analgesic adjuncts, antianxiety agents, sedative//hypnotics
Pharmacologic: benzodiazepines

Schedule IV

Indications

PO: Anxiety disorder. **IM, IV:** Status epilepticus, Preanesthetic to produce sedation, decrease preoperative anxiety, and induce amnesia.

Action

Depresses the CNS, probably by potentiating GABA, an inhibitory neurotransmitter. **Therapeutic Effects:** Sedation. Decreased anxiety. Decreased seizures.

Pharmacokinetics

Absorption: Well absorbed following oral administration. Rapidly and completely absorbed following IM administration. Sublingual absorption is more rapid than oral and is similar to IM. IV administration results in complete bioavailability.
Distribution: Widely distributed. Crosses the blood-brain barrier.
Metabolism and Excretion: Highly metabolized by the liver.
Half-life: *Full-term neonates:* 18–73 hr; *Older children:* 6–17 hr; *Adults:* 10–16 hr.

TIME/ACTION PROFILE (sedation)

ROUTE	ONSET	PEAK	DURATION
PO	15–60 min	1–6 hr	8–12 hr
PO-XR	unknown	unknown	unknown
IM	30–60 min	1–2 hr†	8–12 hr
IV	15–30 min	15–20 min	8–12 hr

† Amnestic response.

Contraindications/Precautions

Contraindicated in: Hypersensitivity; Cross-sensitivity with other benzodiazepines may exist; Comatose patients or those with pre-existing CNS depression;

Uncontrolled severe pain; Angle-closure glaucoma; Severe hypotension; Sleep apnea.

Use Cautiously in: Severe hepatic impairment; Severe renal impairment; Severe lung disease; Myasthenia gravis; Depression; Psychosis; History of suicide attempt or drug abuse/substance use disorder; COPD; Sleep apnea; OB: Use late in pregnancy can result in sedation (respiratory depression, lethargy, hypotonia) and/or withdrawal symptoms (hyperreflexia, irritability, restlessness, tremors, inconsolable crying, feeding difficulties) in neonates; Lactation: Use while breastfeeding only if potential maternal benefit outweighs potential risk to infant; Pedi: Safety and effectiveness not established in children <18 yr (IV) or <12 yr (PO); in ↑ doses, benzyl alcohol in injection may cause potentially fatal gasping syndrome in neonates; IV use may affect brain development in children <3 yr; Geri: Appears on Beers list. ↑ risk of cognitive impairment, delirium, falls, fractures, and motor vehicle accidents in older adults. If possible, avoid use in older adults.

Adverse Reactions/Side Effects

CV: bradycardia, hypotension**rapid IV use only:** APNEA, CARDIAC ARREST. **Derm:** rash. **EENT:** blurred vision. **GI:** constipation, diarrhea, nausea, vomiting. **Neuro:** dizziness, drowsiness, lethargy, ataxia, confusion, forgetfulness, hangover, headache, mental depression, rhythmic myoclonic jerking (in preterm infants), paradoxical excitation, slurred speech. **Resp:** RESPIRATORY DEPRESSION. **Misc:** physical dependence, psychological dependence, tolerance.

Interactions

Drug-Drug: Use with **opioids** or other **CNS depressants, including other benzodiazepines, nonbenzodiazepine sedative/hypnotics, anxiolytics, general anesthetics, muscle relaxants, antipsychotics**, and **alcohol**, may cause profound sedation, respiratory depression, coma, and death; reserve concurrent use for when alternative treatment options are inadequate. May ↓ the efficacy of **levodopa**. **Smoking** may ↓ levels and effectiveness. **Valproate** and **probenecid** may ↑ levels and risk of toxicity; ↓ dose by 50%. **Oral contraceptives** may ↓ levels and effectiveness.

Drug-Natural Products: kava-kava, valerian, or **chamomile** may ↑ risk of CNS depression.

Route/Dosage

Status Epilepticus

IV IM (Adults): 4 mg; may be repeated after 10–15 min.

Preanesthetic

IM (Adults): 0.05 mg/kg (not to exceed 4 mg) ≥2 hr before surgery.

IV (Adults): 0.044 mg/kg (not to exceed 2 mg) 15–20 min before surgery.

Anxiety

PO (Adults): *Immediate-release tablets:* 1–3 mg 2–3 times daily (up to 10 mg/day). *Extended-release capsules:* Give total daily dose of lorazepam immediate-release tablets (at the previous three times daily dose) and administer once daily in the morning. If dose ↑ needed, switch to lorazepam immediate-release tablets to ↑ the dose; once stable response achieved, may switch back to equivalent daily dose of lorazepam extended-release capsules.

PO (Geriatric Patients or Debilitated Patients): 0.5–2 mg/day in divided doses initially.

Availability (generic available)

Immediate-release tablets: 0.5 mg, 1 mg, 2 mg. **Extended-release capsules (Loreev XR):** 1 mg, 1.5 mg, 2 mg, 3 mg. **Concentrated oral solution:** 2 mg/mL. **Solution for injection:** 2 mg/mL, 4 mg/mL.

L

NURSING IMPLICATIONS

Assessment

- Assess continued need for therapy regularly.
- Assess risk for addiction, abuse, or misuse before administration and periodically during therapy.
- Monitor respiratory function during therapy. *If signs and symptoms of respiratory depression or apnea occur,* consider discontinuing lorazepam.
- Prolonged high-dose therapy may lead to psychological or physical dependence. Restrict the amount of drug available to patient. Assess regularly for continued need for treatment.
- Geri: Assess older adults carefully for CNS reactions and fall risk.
- **Anxiety:** Monitor degree and manifestations of anxiety and mental status (orientation, mood, behavior) prior to and periodically during therapy.
- **Status Epilepticus:** Assess location, duration, characteristics, and frequency of seizures. Institute seizure precautions.

Lab Test Considerations

- Patients on high-dose therapy should receive routine evaluation of renal, hepatic, and hematologic function. May cause leukopenia. May ↑ lactate dehydrogenase.

Toxicity and Overdose

- If overdose occurs, flumazenil is the antidote. Do not use with patients with seizure disorder. May induce seizures.

Implementation

- Do not confuse lorazepam with alprazolam, clonazepam, or Lovaza.

- Gradually taper to discontinue or ↓ dose to ↓ risk of withdrawal reactions, seizures, and status epilepticus. If a patient develops withdrawal reactions, consider pausing taper or ↑ dose to previous tapered dose level. Subsequently ↓ dose more slowly. Some patients may require longer tapering period (weeks to >12 mo).
- Following parenteral administration, keep patient supine for ≥8 hr and observe closely.
- **PO:** Tablet may also be given sublingually (unlabeled) for more rapid onset.
- Administer XR capsules with or without food. ***DNC:*** Do not crush or chew. Swallow whole or open and sprinkle the entire contents of capsule over a tablespoon of applesauce; then drink water after consuming the applesauce (without chewing). Consume entire contents of capsule within 2 hr of opening capsule.
- Take concentrated liquid solution with water, soda, pudding, or applesauce. Use calibrated dropper provided to ensure accurate dose.
- **IM,** Administer IM doses deep into muscle mass ≥2 hr before surgery for optimum effect.

IV Administration

- **V** IV lorazepam is a vesicant. If extravasation occurs, immediately stop infusion. Leave needle/cannula in place temporarily but do not flush the line. Gently aspirate extravasated solution; then remove needle/cannula. Elevate patient's extremity and apply dry cold compresses.
- **IV Push:** **Dilution:** Dilute immediately before use with an equal amount of sterile water for injection, D5W, or 0.9% NaCl for injection. Pedi: To ↓ the amount of benzyl alcohol delivered to neonates, dilute the 4 mg/mL injection with preservative-free sterile water for injection to make a 0.4 mg/mL dilution for IV use. Do not use if solution is discolored or contains particulates. **Rate:** Administer at a rate not to exceed 2 mg/min or 0.05 mg/kg over 2–5 min. Rapid IV administration may result in apnea, hypotension, bradycardia, or cardiac arrest.
- **Y-Site Compatibility:** acetaminophen, acyclovir, albumin, alemtuzumab, allopurinol, amikacin, aminocaproic acid, aminophylline, amiodarone, amphotericin B deoxycholate, anakinra, anidulafungin, argatroban, arsenic trioxide, atracurium, azithromycin, bleomycin, bumetanide, buprenorphine, busulfan, butorphanol, calcium chloride, calcium gluconate, cangrelor, carboplatin, carmustine, cefazolin, cefepime, cefotaxime, cefotetan, cefoxitin, ceftaroline, ceftazidime, ceftobiprole, ceftolozane/tazobactam, ceftriaxone, cefuroxime, chloramphenicol, chlorpromazine, ciprofloxacin, cisatracurium, cisplatin, cladribine, clindamycin, cyclophosphamide, cyclosporine, cytarabine, dacarbazine, dactinomycin, daptomycin, daunorubicin, dexamethasone, dexmedetomidine, dexrazoxane, digoxin, diltiazem, dimenhydrinate, diphenhydramine, dobutamine, docetaxel, dopamine, doxorubicin hydrochloride, doxorubicin liposomal, doxycycline, droperidol, enalaprilat, ephedrine, epinephrine, epirubicin, eptifibatide, ertapenem, erythromycin, esmolol, etomidate, etoposide phosphate, famotidine, fentanyl, filgrastim, fluconazole, fludarabine, fosphenytoin, furosemide, ganciclovir, gemcitabine, gentamicin, glycopyrrolate, granisetron, haloperidol, heparin, hydrocortisone, hydromorphone, ifosfamide, insulin regular, irinotecan, isavuconazonium, isoproterenol, ketorolac, labetalol, leucovorin, lidocaine, linezolid, magnesium sulfate, mannitol, melphalan, meropenem, meropenem/vaborbactam, mesna, methadone, methotrexate, methylprednisolone, metoclopramide, metoprolol, metronidazole, micafungin, midazolam, milrinone, mitoxantrone, morphine, mycophenolate, nafcillin, nalbuphine, nitroglycerin, nitroprusside, norepinephrine, octreotide, oritavancin, oxaliplatin, oxytocin, paclitaxel, palonosetron, pamidronate, pemetrexed, pentamidine, pentobarbital, phenobarbital, phentolamine, phenylephrine, piperacillin/tazobactam, plazomicin, posaconazole, potassium acetate, potassium chloride, procainamide, prochlorperazine, promethazine, propofol, propranolol, remifentanil, rituximab, sodium acetate, sodium bicarbonate, sodium phosphates, succinylcholine, sulbactam/durlobactam, tacrolimus, tedizolid, theophylline, thiotepa, tigecycline, tirofiban, tobramycin, topotecan, trastuzumab, trimethoprim/sulfamethoxazole, vancomycin, vasopressin, vecuronium, verapamil, vinblastine, vincristine, vinorelbine, voriconazole, zidovudine, zoledronic acid.
- **Y-Site Incompatibility:** aldesleukin, amphotericin B liposomal, ampicillin, ampicillin/sulbactam, aztreonam, dantrolene, fluorouracil, gemtuzumab ozogamicin, hydralazine, idarubicin, imipenem/cilastatin, letermovir, meperidine, mitomycin, omeprazole, ondansetron, pantoprazole, phenytoin, potassium phosphates, rocuronium, sargramostim, sufentanil.

Patient/Family Teaching

- Explain purpose and side effects of medication. Advise patient to read *Patient Information* before starting therapy.
- Instruct patient to take medication exactly as directed and not to skip or double up on missed doses. If medication is less effective after a few weeks, notify health care provider; do not ↑ dose.
- Caution patient not to stop taking lorazepam without consulting health care provider. Abrupt withdrawal may cause sweating, vomiting, muscle cramps, tremors, and seizures; may be life-threatening.

- Caution patient to notify health care provider immediately if unusual movements, seizures, sudden and severe mental or nervous system changes, depression, hallucinations, an extreme ↑ in activity or talking, or suicidal ideas or actions occur.
- Advise patient that lorazepam is a drug with known abuse potential. Protect it from theft, and never give to anyone other than the individual for whom it was prescribed. Store out of sight and reach of children and in a location not accessible by others.
- Advise patient that lorazepam is usually prescribed for short-term use and does not cure underlying problem.
- May cause drowsiness or dizziness. Advise patient to avoid driving or other activities requiring alertness until response to medication is known.
- Advise patient to avoid the use of alcohol or other CNS depressants, including opioids, concurrently with lorazepam; may cause respiratory depression and overdose. Instruct patient to consult health care provider before taking Rx, OTC, or herbal products concurrently with this medication.
- Rep: May cause fetal harm. Advise women of reproductive potential to notify health care provider immediately if pregnancy is planned or suspected or if breastfeeding. Monitor infants exposed to lorazepam during pregnancy or labor for several weeks or more prior to delivery for signs and symptoms of withdrawal (hypoactivity, hypotonia, hypothermia, respiratory depression, apnea, feeding problems, impaired metabolic response to cold stress). Notify health care provider immediately if sedation, poor feeding, or poor weight gain occurs in infants exposed to lorazepam during breastfeeding. Notify patient about the National Pregnancy Registry for Psychiatric Medications, which monitors outcomes in women exposed to psychiatric medications, including lorazepam, during pregnancy. Health care providers are encouraged to register patients by calling 1-866-961-2388 or visiting https://womensmentalhealth.org/pregnancyregistry/.
- Emphasize the importance of follow-up exams to determine effectiveness of therapy.

Evaluation/Desired Outcomes

- Increase in sense of well-being.
- Decrease in subjective feelings of anxiety without excessive sedation.
- Reduction of preoperative anxiety.
- Postoperative amnesia.
- Improvement in sleep patterns.

losartan, See ANGIOTENSIN II RECEPTOR ANTAGONISTS.

lovastatin, See HMG-CoA REDUCTASE INHIBITORS (statins).

luliconazole, See ANTIFUNGALS (TOPICAL).

⧖ lumacaftor/ivacaftor

(loo-ma-kaf-tor/eye-va-kaf-tor)

Orkambi

Classification

Therapeutic: cystic fibrosis therapy adjuncts

Pharmacologic: transmembrane conductance regulator potentiators

Indications

⧖ Cystic fibrosis (CF) in patients who are homozygous for the *F508del* mutation in the *CFTR* gene.

Action

Ivacaftor: Acts as a potentiator of the CFTR protein (a chloride channel on the surface of endothelial cells), facilitating chloride transport by increasing the channel-open probability (gating). *Lumacaftor:* Improves the conformational stability of *F508del-CFTR,* which results in increased processing and trafficking of mature protein to the cell surface. **Therapeutic Effects:** Improved lung function with increased weight; decreased exacerbations and CF symptoms.

Pharmacokinetics

Lumacaftor

Absorption: Some absorption follows oral administration; absorption is enhanced 2-fold by fat-containing foods.

Distribution: Widely distributed.

Protein Binding: >99%.

Metabolism and Excretion: Minimally metabolized via oxidation and glucuronidation; 51% excreted unchanged in feces; <1% excreted unchanged in urine.

Half-life: 26 hr.

Ivacaftor

Absorption: Some absorption follows oral administration; absorption is enhanced 3-fold by fat-containing foods.

Distribution: Unknown.
Protein Binding: >99%.
Metabolism and Excretion: Extensively metabolized by the liver, mostly by the CYP3A isoenzyme; one metabolite (M1) is pharmacologically active; 87.8% eliminated in feces; negligible urinary elimination.
Half-life: 9 hr.

TIME/ACTION PROFILE (plasma concentrations)

ROUTE	ONSET	PEAK	DURATION
Lumacaftor (PO)	within 1 wk	4 hr	12 hr
Ivacaftor (PO)	within 1 wk	4 hr	12 hr

Contraindications/Precautions

Contraindicated in: None.
Use Cautiously in: Severe renal impairment or end stage renal disease; Moderate or severe hepatic impairment (↓ dose); Advanced lung disease (↑ risk of respiratory events); OB: Use in pregnancy only if clearly needed; Lactation: Use while breastfeeding only if potential maternal benefit outweighs potential risk to infant; Pedi: Children <1 yr (safety and effectiveness not established).

Adverse Reactions/Side Effects

CV: ↑ BP. **Derm:** rash. **EENT:** cataracts, rhinorrhea. **GI:** diarrhea, nausea, ↑ liver enzymes, flatulence, hyperbilirubinemia. **GU:** amenorrhea, dysmenorrhea, menorrhagia. **MS:** ↑ CK. **Neuro:** fatigue. **Resp:** dyspnea, chest discomfort. **Misc:** HYPERSENSITIVITY REACTIONS (INCLUDING ANAPHYLAXIS AND ANGIOEDEMA).

Interactions

Drug-Drug: Strong CYP3A inducers, including **rifampin**, **rifabutin**, **phenobarbital**, **carbamazepine** and **phenytoin**, may ↓ levels and effectiveness of ivacaftor; avoid concurrent use. Lumacaftor may ↓ levels and effectiveness of **CYP3A substrates**, including **hormonal contraceptive agents**; avoid concurrent use with sensitive CYP3A substrates or those with a narrow therapeutic index, including **cyclosporine**, **everolimus**, **midazolam**, **sirolimus**, **tacrolimus**, or **triazolam**. **Strong CYP3A inhibitors**, including **ketoconazole**, **itraconazole**, **posaconazole**, **voriconazole**, and **clarithromycin**, may ↑ levels and risk of toxicity of ivacaftor; no dose adjustment required when initiating CYP3A inhibitor in patients currently receiving ivacaftor/lumacaftor; ↓ initial ivacaftor/lumacaftor dose for 1 wk when starting therapy in patient currently receiving strong CYP3A4 inhibitor and then proceed with recommended dose. Ivacaftor may ↑ levels and risk of toxicity of **CYP2C9 substrates**. May ↑ or ↓ **digoxin** or **warfarin** levels. May ↓ levels and effectiveness of **citalopram**, **clarithromycin**, **corticosteroids**, **erythromycin**, **escitalopram**, **ibuprofen**, **itraconazole**, **ketoconazole**, **montelukast**, **posaconazole**, **proton pump inhibitors**, **repaglinide**, **sertraline**, **sulfonylureas**, and **voriconazole**.
Drug-Natural Products: St. John's wort may ↓ levels and effectiveness of ivacaftor; avoid concurrent use.

Route/Dosage

PO (Adults and Children ≥12 yr): Two lumacaftor 200 mg/ivacaftor 125 mg tablets every 12 hr; *Initiation of therapy in patients receiving strong CYP3A inhibitor:* One lumacaftor 200 mg/ivacaftor 125 mg tablet once daily for 1 wk; then ↑ to two lumacaftor 200 mg/ivacaftor 125 mg tablets every 12 hr.
PO (Children 6–11 yr): Two lumacaftor 100 mg/ivacaftor 125 mg tablets every 12 hr; *Initiation of therapy in patients receiving strong CYP3A inhibitor:* One lumacaftor 100 mg/ivacaftor 125 mg tablet once daily for 1 wk; then ↑ to two lumacaftor 200 mg/ivacaftor 125 mg tablets every 12 hr.
PO (Children 2–5 yr and ≥14 kg): One lumacaftor 150 mg/ivacaftor 188 mg granule packet every 12 hr; *Initiation of therapy in patients receiving strong CYP3A inhibitor:* One lumacaftor 150 mg/ivacaftor 188 mg granule packet every other day for 1 wk; then ↑ to one lumacaftor 150 mg/ivacaftor 188 mg granule packet every 12 hr.
PO (Children 2–5 yr and <14 kg): One lumacaftor 100 mg/ivacaftor 125 mg granule packet every 12 hr; *Initiation of therapy in patients receiving strong CYP3A inhibitor:* One lumacaftor 100 mg/ivacaftor 125 mg granule packet every other day for 1 wk; then ↑ to one lumacaftor 100 mg/ivacaftor 125 mg granule packet every 12 hr.
PO (Children 1–<2 yr and ≥14 kg): One lumacaftor 150 mg/ivacaftor 188 mg granule packet every 12 hr; *Initiation of therapy in patients receiving strong CYP3A inhibitor:* One lumacaftor 150 mg/ivacaftor 188 mg granule packet every other day for 1 wk; then ↑ to one lumacaftor 150 mg/ivacaftor 188 mg granule packet every 12 hr.
PO (Children 1–<2 yr and 9–<14 kg): One lumacaftor 100 mg/ivacaftor 125 mg granule packet every 12 hr; *Initiation of therapy in patients receiving strong CYP3A inhibitor:* One lumacaftor 100 mg/ivacaftor 125 mg granule packet every other day for 1 wk; then ↑ to one lumacaftor 100 mg/ivacaftor 125 mg granule packet every 12 hr.
PO (Children 1–<2 yr and 7–<9 kg): One lumacaftor 75 mg/ivacaftor 94 mg granule packet every 12 hr; *Initiation of therapy in patients receiving strong CYP3A inhibitor:* One lumacaftor 75 mg/ivacaftor 94 mg granule packet every other day for 1 wk;

then ↑ to one lumacaftor 75 mg/ivacaftor 94 mg granule packet every 12 hr.

Hepatic Impairment

(Adults and Children ≥12 yr): *Moderate hepatic impairment:* Two lumacaftor 200 mg/ivacaftor 125 mg tablets in AM and one lumacaftor 200 mg/ivacaftor 125 mg tablet in PM; *Severe hepatic impairment:* One lumacaftor 200 mg/ivacaftor 125 mg tablet in AM and one lumacaftor 200 mg/ivacaftor 125 mg tablet in PM.

Hepatic Impairment

(Children 6–11 yr): *Moderate hepatic impairment:* Two lumacaftor 100 mg/ivacaftor 125 mg tablets in AM and one lumacaftor 100 mg/ivacaftor 125 mg tablet in PM; *Severe hepatic impairment:* One lumacaftor 100 mg/ivacaftor 125 mg tablet in AM and one lumacaftor 100 mg/ivacaftor 125 mg tablet in PM.

Hepatic Impairment

(Children 2–5 yr and ≥14 kg): *Moderate hepatic impairment:* One lumacaftor 150 mg/ivacaftor 188 mg granule packet in AM and one lumacaftor 150 mg/ivacaftor 188 mg granule packet every other PM; *Severe hepatic impairment:* One lumacaftor 150 mg/ivacaftor 188 mg granule packet in AM.

Hepatic Impairment

(Children 2–5 yr and <14 kg): *Moderate hepatic impairment:* One lumacaftor 100 mg/ivacaftor 125 mg granule packet in AM and one lumacaftor 100 mg/ivacaftor 125 mg granule packet every other PM; *Severe hepatic impairment:* One lumacaftor 100 mg/ivacaftor 125 mg granule packet in AM.

Hepatic Impairment

(Children 1–<2 yr and ≥14 kg): *Moderate hepatic impairment:* One lumacaftor 150 mg/ivacaftor 188 mg granule packet in AM and one lumacaftor 150 mg/ivacaftor 188 mg granule packet every other PM; *Severe hepatic impairment:* One lumacaftor 150 mg/ivacaftor 188 mg granule packet in AM.

Hepatic Impairment

(Children 1–<2 yr and 9–<14 kg): *Moderate hepatic impairment:* One lumacaftor 100 mg/ivacaftor 125 mg granule packet in AM and one lumacaftor 100 mg/ivacaftor 125 mg granule packet every other PM; *Severe hepatic impairment:* One lumacaftor 100 mg/ivacaftor 125 mg granule packet in AM.

Hepatic Impairment

(Children 1–<2 yr and 7–<9 kg): *Moderate hepatic impairment:* One lumacaftor 75 mg/ivacaftor 94 mg granule packet in AM and one lumacaftor 75 mg/ivacaftor 94 mg granule packet every other PM; *Severe hepatic impairment:* One lumacaftor 75 mg/ivacaftor 94 mg granule packet in AM.

Availability

Oral granules: lumacaftor 75 mg/ivacaftor 94 mg/pkt, lumacaftor 100 mg/ivacaftor 125 mg/pkt, lumacaftor 150 mg/ivacaftor 188 mg/pkt. **Tablets:** lumacaftor 100 mg/ivacaftor 125 mg, lumacaftor 200 mg/ivacaftor 125 mg.

NURSING IMPLICATIONS

Assessment

- Assess respiratory status (chest discomfort, dyspnea, abnormal respiration) before and periodically during therapy.
- Monitor BP periodically during therapy; may cause hypertension.
- Pedi: Obtain baseline and periodic ophthalmological exams on pediatric patients starting therapy; may cause cataracts.
- Monitor for hypersensitivity reactions (angioedema, anaphylaxis). *If signs or symptoms of serious hypersensitivity reactions (hives, rash, swelling of lips or face, dyspnea) occur,* discontinue lumacaftor/ivacaftor and institute appropriate therapy.

Lab Test Considerations

- Determine patient's genotype before starting therapy. If genotype is unknown, use an FDA-cleared CF mutation test to detect presence of the F508del mutation on both alleles of the CFTR gene.
- Monitor ALT, AST, and bilirubin before starting therapy, every 3 mo during 1st yr of therapy, and annually thereafter. Monitor patients with a history of ALT, AST, or bilirubin ↑ more frequently. If ↑ ALT, AST, or bilirubin occur, monitor closely until resolved. *If ALT or AST >5 times upper limit of normal (ULN),* hold lumacaftor/ivacaftor. *If ALT or AST >3 times ULN with bilirubin >2 times ULN,* hold lumacaftor/ivacaftor. Consider benefits and risks of resuming dosing once liver enzyme ↑ resolves.

Implementation

- **PO:** Administer 2 tablets every 12 hr with fat-containing food (eggs, avocados, nuts, butter, peanut butter, cheese pizza, whole-milk dairy products [whole milk, cheese, yogurt], etc.).
- To administer granules, mix entire content of single-use packet with 1 teaspoon (5 mL) of age-appropriate soft food or liquid (pureed fruits, flavored yogurt or pudding, milk, juice). Food should be at room temperature or below. Mixture is stable for 1 hr.

Patient/Family Teaching

- Explain purpose and side effects of medication to patient. Instruct patient to take medication as directed. Take missed doses within 6 hr with fat-containing food. If >6 hr after usual dosing time,

omit dose and resume normal schedule for following dose; do not double doses. Advise patient to read *Patient Information* prior to starting and with each Rx refill in case of changes.
- Advise patient to notify health care provider of all Rx or OTC medications, vitamins, or herbal products being taken and to consult with health care provider before taking other medications, especially St. John's wort.
- May cause dizziness. Avoid driving and other activities requiring alertness until response to medication is known.
- Advise patient to notify health care provider if signs and symptoms of liver problems (pain or discomfort in upper right abdomen, yellowing of skin or white of eyes, loss of appetite, nausea or vomiting, dark amber-colored urine, confusion) or respiratory problems (shortness of breath, chest tightness) occur.
- Rep: Advise women of reproductive potential to use a nonhormonal contraceptive during therapy and to notify health care provider if pregnancy is planned or suspected or if breastfeeding. Lumacaftor/ivacaftor may ↓ effectiveness of hormonal contraceptives exposure and ↓ effectiveness; do not rely upon hormonal contraceptives as effective method of contraception.

Evaluation/Desired Outcomes
- Improved lung function with increased weight and decreased exacerbations and CF symptoms.

BEERS

lurasidone (loo-ras-i-done)
Latuda

Classification
Therapeutic: antipsychotics
Pharmacologic: benzoisothiazole

Indications
Schizophrenia. Depressive episodes associated with bipolar I disorder (as monotherapy or in combination with lithium or valproate).

Action
Effect may be mediated via effects on central dopamine type 2 (D_2) and serotonin Type 2 ($5HT_{2A}$) receptor antagonism. **Therapeutic Effects:** Reduction in schizophrenic behavior. Reduction in depressive episodes in bipolar I disorder.

Pharmacokinetics
Absorption: 9–19% absorbed following oral administration.
Distribution: Unknown.
Protein Binding: >99%.
Metabolism and Excretion: Primarily metabolized by the liver via the CYP3A4 isoenzyme. Two metabolites are pharmacologically active; 80% eliminated in feces, 8% in urine primarily as metabolites.
Half-life: 18 hr.

TIME/ACTION PROFILE (plasma concentrations)

ROUTE	ONSET	PEAK	DURATION
PO	unknown	1–3 hr	24 hr

Contraindications/Precautions
Contraindicated in: Hypersensitivity; Concurrent use of strong CYP3A4 inhibitors or inducers.
Use Cautiously in: Moderate or severe renal impairment (dose adjustment recommended); Moderate or severe hepatic impairment (dose adjustment recommended); May ↑ risk of suicide attempt/ideation especially during early treatment or dose adjustment; this risk appears to be greater in adolescents or children; Diabetes mellitus; Overheating/dehydration (may ↑ risk of serious adverse reactions); Patients at risk for falls; History of leukopenia or previous drug-induced leukopenia/neutropenia; History of breast cancer; OB: Use in pregnancy only if potential maternal benefit justifies potential fetal risk; Lactation: Use while breastfeeding only if potential maternal benefit justifies potential risk to infant; Pedi: Children <10 yr (safety and effectiveness not established); Geri: Appears on Beers list. ↑ risk of stroke, cognitive decline, and mortality in older adults with dementia. Avoid use in older adults, except for schizophrenia or bipolar disorder.

Adverse Reactions/Side Effects
CV: bradycardia, orthostatic hypotension, syncope, tachycardia. **Derm:** pruritus, rash. **EENT:** blurred vision. **Endo:** hyperglycemia, hyperprolactinemia. **GI:** nausea, esophageal dysmotility. **Hemat:** AGRANULOCYTOSIS, anemia, leukopenia. **Metab:** dyslipidemia, weight gain. **Neuro:** akathisia, drowsiness, parkinsonism, agitation, anxiety, cognitive/motor impairment, dizziness, dystonia, NEUROLEPTIC MALIGNANT SYNDROME (NMS), SEIZURES, SUICIDAL THOUGHTS/BEHAVIORS, tardive dyskinesia.

Interactions
Drug-Drug: Strong CYP3A4 inhibitors, including **ketoconazole**, **clarithromycin**, **ritonavir**, and **voriconazole**, significantly ↑ levels and risk of toxicity; concurrent use contraindicated. **Strong CYP3A4 inducers**, including **rifampin**, **phenytoin**, and **carbamazepine**, significantly ↓ levels and effectiveness; concurrent use contraindicated. **Moderate CYP3A4 inhibitors**, including **diltiazem**, **atazanavir**, **erythromycin**, **fluconazole**, and **verapamil**, ↑ levels and risk of toxicity; if used concurrently, lurasidone dose should not exceed 40 mg/day. ↑ sedation may

occur with other **CNS depressants**, including **alcohol**, **sedative/hypnotics**, **opioids**, and some **antidepressants** and **antihistamines**.

Drug-Natural Products: **St. John's wort** significantly ↓ levels and effectiveness; concurrent use contraindicated.

Drug-Food: **Grapefruit juice** significantly ↑ levels and risk of toxicity; concurrent use contraindicated.

Route/Dosage

Schizophrenia

PO: (Adults): 40 mg once daily (not to exceed 160 mg once daily); *Addition of moderate CYP3A4 inhibitor to existing lurasidone therapy:* ↓ lurasidone dose by 50%; *Addition of lurasidone to existing moderate CYP3A4 inhibitor therapy:* 20 mg once daily (not to exceed 80 mg once daily).

PO (Children 13–17 yr): 40 mg once daily (not to exceed 80 mg once daily); *Addition of moderate CYP3A4 inhibitor to existing lurasidone therapy:* ↓ lurasidone dose by 50%; *Addition of lurasidone to existing moderate CYP3A4 inhibitor therapy:* 20 mg once daily (not to exceed 80 mg once daily).

Renal Impairment

PO (Adults and Children 13–17 yr): *CCr <50 mL/min:* 20 mg once daily (not to exceed 80 mg once daily).

Hepatic Impairment

(Adults and Children 13–17 yr): *Moderate hepatic impairment:* 20 mg once daily (not to exceed 80 mg once daily); *Severe hepatic impairment:* 20 mg once daily (not to exceed 40 mg once daily).

Depressive Episodes Associated with Bipolar I Disorder

PO: (Adults): 20 mg once daily (not to exceed 120 mg once daily); *Addition of moderate CYP3A4 inhibitor to existing lurasidone therapy:* ↓ lurasidone dose by 50%; *Addition of lurasidone to existing moderate CYP3A4 inhibitor therapy:* 20 mg once daily (not to exceed 80 mg once daily).

PO (Children 10–17 yr): 20 mg once daily (not to exceed 80 mg once daily); *Addition of moderate CYP3A4 inhibitor to existing lurasidone therapy:* ↓ lurasidone dose by 50%; *Addition of lurasidone to existing moderate CYP3A4 inhibitor therapy:* 20 mg once daily (not to exceed 80 mg once daily).

Renal Impairment

PO (Adults and Children 10–17 yr): *CCr <50 mL/min:* 20 mg once daily (not to exceed 80 mg once daily).

Hepatic Impairment

PO (Adults and Children 10–17 yr): *Moderate hepatic impairment:* 20 mg once daily (not to exceed 80 mg once daily); *Severe hepatic impairment:* 20 mg once daily (not to exceed 40 mg once daily).

Availability (generic available)

Tablets: 20 mg, 40 mg, 60 mg, 80 mg, 120 mg.

NURSING IMPLICATIONS

Assessment

- Monitor mental status (orientation, mood, behavior) before and periodically during therapy.
- Assess weight and BMI initially; then at 4, 8, and 12 wk; and then every 4 mo during therapy. Refer as appropriate for nutritional/weight and medical management.
- Assess for suicidal tendencies, especially during early therapy. Restrict amount of drug available to patient. Risk may be ↑ in children, adolescents, and adults ≤24 yr. After starting therapy, children, adolescents, and young adults should be seen by health care provider face-to-face at least weekly for 4 wk, then every other wk for next 4 wk, then at 12 wk, and then on advice of health care provider thereafter.
- Monitor BP (sitting, standing, lying down) and HR before and frequently during initial dose titration; repeat in 12 wk and then annually. May cause tachycardia and orthostatic hypotension. If hypotension occurs, dose may need to be ↓.
- Observe patient when administering medication to ensure medication is swallowed and not hoarded or cheeked.
- Monitor for onset of extrapyramidal side effects (*akathisia:* restlessness; *dystonia:* muscle spasms and twisting motions; or *pseudoparkinsonism:* masklike face, rigidity, tremors, drooling, shuffling gait, dysphagia). Report these symptoms; ↓ of dose or discontinuation may be necessary. Trihexyphenidyl or benztropine may be used to control symptoms.
- Monitor for tardive dyskinesia (involuntary rhythmic movement of mouth, face, and extremities) every 6 mo. Report immediately; may be irreversible.
- Monitor for symptoms related to hyperprolactinemia (menstrual abnormalities, galactorrhea, sexual dysfunction).
- Monitor for signs and symptoms of NMS (hyperpyrexia, muscle rigidity, seizures, altered mental status, evidence of autonomic instability [irregular HR or BP, tachycardia, diaphoresis, cardiac arrhythmia]). *If signs/symptoms of NMS occur,* discontinue lurasidone and notify health care provider immediately.

L

- Monitor for symptoms of hyperglycemia (polydipsia, polyuria, polyphagia, weakness) periodically during therapy.
- Assess for falls risk. Drowsiness, orthostatic hypotension, and motor and sensory instability ↑ risk. Institute prevention if indicated.

Lab Test Considerations

- May ↑ serum prolactin levels.
- May ↑ CK.
- Obtain fasting blood glucose and cholesterol initially and periodically during therapy.
- Monitor CBC frequently during initial months of therapy in patients with pre-existing or history of low WBC. May cause leukopenia, neutropenia, or agranulocytosis. Discontinue therapy if this occurs.

Implementation

- ***High Alert:*** Do not confuse Latuda with Lantus.
- **PO:** Administer once daily with food that is ≥350 calories.

Patient/Family Teaching

- Explain the purpose and side effects of lurasidone. Instruct patient to take as directed. Emphasize the caloric food needs for taking medication. Caution patient to consult health care provider before discontinuing. Advise patient to read *Medication Guide* before starting and with each Rx refill in case of changes.
- Emphasize the importance of follow-up exams to monitor progress. Laboratory tests may be needed to detect side effects.
- Inform patient of the possibility of extrapyramidal symptoms. Instruct patient to report these symptoms immediately to health care provider.
- Advise patient to change positions slowly to minimize orthostatic hypotension. Protect from falls.
- May cause drowsiness and cognitive and motor impairment. Caution patient to avoid driving or other activities requiring alertness until response to medication is known.
- Advise patient, family, and caregivers to watch for suicidality, especially during early therapy or dose changes. Notify health care provider immediately if thoughts about suicide or dying, attempts to commit suicide, new or worse depression or anxiety, agitation or restlessness, panic attacks, insomnia, new or worse irritability, aggressiveness, acting on dangerous impulses, mania, or other changes in mood or behavior occur.
- Advise patient and family to notify health care provider if new or worse depression, new or worse anxiety, feeling very agitated or restless, panic attacks, trouble sleeping, new or worse irritability, acting aggressive, being angry or violent, acting on dangerous impulses, an extreme ↑ in activity and talking, or other unusual changes in behavior or mood occur.
- Advise patient to avoid extremes in temperature; this drug impairs body temperature regulation.
- Advise patient to tell health care provider what medications they are taking and to avoid taking new Rx, OTC, vitamins, or herbal products without consulting health care provider, especially alcohol and other CNS depressants. Instruct patient to avoid grapefruit and grapefruit juice.
- Advise patient to notify health care provider of medication regimen before treatment or surgery.
- Instruct patient to notify health care provider promptly if sore throat, fever, unusual bleeding or bruising, rash, or tremors occur.
- Rep: Advise women of reproductive potential to notify health care provider if pregnancy is planned or suspected or if breastfeeding. Monitor neonates exposed to lurasidone during the 3rd trimester of pregnancy for extrapyramidal and/or withdrawal symptoms following delivery. There have been reports of agitation, hypertonia, hypotonia, tremor, somnolence, respiratory distress, and feeding disorder in these neonates. Monitor breastfed infants for excessive drowsiness, lethargy, and developmental delays. Encourage women who become pregnant while taking lurasidone to enroll in the National Pregnancy Registry for Atypical Antipsychotics at 1-866-961-2388 or visit http://womensmentalhealth.org/clinical-and-research-programs/pregnancyregistry/.

Evaluation/Desired Outcomes

- Reduction in symptoms of schizophrenia (delusions, hallucinations, social withdrawal, flat, blunted affects).
- Reduction in depressive episodes in bipolar I disorder.

macitentan (ma-si-ten-tan)

Opsumit

Classification

Therapeutic: vasodilators

Pharmacologic: endothelin receptor antagonists

Indications

Pulmonary arterial hypertension (PAH) (WHO Group I) to delay disease progression.

Action

Acts as an endothelin receptor antagonist. Endothelin mediates vasoconstriction, fibrosis, proliferation, hypertrophy, and inflammation. Antagonizing endothelin effects delays vascular hypertrophy and organ damage. **Therapeutic Effects:** Delayed sequelae of progression of PAH (death, need for initiation of parenteral prostanoids, increased frequency of hospitalization, diminished exercise tolerance, or need for other interventions)

Pharmacokinetics

Absorption: Extent of absorption unknown.
Distribution: Unknown.
Protein Binding: *Macitentan:* >99%; *active metabolite:* >99%
Metabolism and Excretion: Extensively metabolized, primarily by the CYP3A4 isoenzyme with conversion to a pharmacologically active metabolite that contributes 40% of activity. 50% excreted in urine as metabolites; 24% in feces.
Half-life: *Macitentan:* 16 hr; *active metabolite:* 48 hr

TIME/ACTION PROFILE (improvement in primary endpoints†)

ROUTE	ONSET	PEAK	DURATION
PO	within 6 mo	12–18 mo	unknown

† Worsening of PAH, death, or need for other interventions.

Contraindications/Precautions

Contraindicated in: Hypersensitivity; OB: Pregnancy; Lactation: Lactation.
Use Cautiously in: Pulmonary veno-occlusive disease (↑ risk of pulmonary edema); Rep: Women of reproductive potential; Pedi: Safety and effectiveness not established in children.

Adverse Reactions/Side Effects

Derm: pruritus, rash. **GI:** hepatotoxicity. **GU:** ↓ fertility (men). **Hemat:** anemia. **Neuro:** headache. **Resp:** pulmonary edema. **Misc:** HYPERSENSITIVITY REACTIONS (INCLUDING ANGIOEDEMA).

Interactions

Drug-Drug: Strong CYP3A4 inducers, including **rifampin**, may ↓ levels and effectiveness; avoid concurrent use. **Strong CYP3A4 inhibitors**, including **ketoconazole**, may ↑ levels and risk of toxicity; avoid concurrent use. **Moderate dual CYP3A4 and CYP2C9 inhibitors**, including **fluconazole**, as well as concurrent use with a **moderate CYP3A4 inhibitor** and a **moderate CYP2C9 inhibitor**, may ↑ levels and risk of toxicity; avoid concurrent use.

Route/Dosage

PO (Adults): 10 mg once daily.

Availability (generic available)

Tablets: 10 mg. ***In combination with:*** tadalafil (Opsynvi); see Appendix N

NURSING IMPLICATIONS

Assessment

- Monitor hemodynamic parameters and exercise tolerance prior to and periodically during therapy.
- Assess for signs and symptoms of pulmonary edema (shortness of breath, crackles, wheezing), peripheral edema, and fluid retention (weight gain; swelling of feet, ankles, or hands). If confirmed, discontinue therapy.
- Assess for hepatotoxicity (nausea, vomiting, right upper quadrant pain, fatigue, anorexia, jaundice, dark urine, fever, itching).
- Monitor for signs and symptoms of hypersensitivity reactions (angioedema, pruritus, rash). May need to discontinue therapy.

Lab Test Considerations

- Verify negative pregnancy test prior to beginning, monthly during therapy, and 1 mo following treatment.
- Monitor hepatic function periodically during therapy. May cause ↑ AST, ALT, and bilirubin. If clinically relevant ↑ of AST or ALT occur or if ↑ are accompanied by ↑ bilirubin >2 times the upper limit of normal or by clinical symptoms of hepatotoxicity, discontinue therapy. May reinitiate therapy when hepatic enzyme levels normalize in patients who have not experienced clinical symptoms of hepatotoxicity.
- Monitor CBC before starting and periodically during therapy. May ↓ hemoglobin. Avoid therapy in patients with severe anemia.

Implementation

- **PO:** Administer once daily at the same time each day. ***DNC:*** Swallow tablets whole; do not break, crush, or chew.

Patient/Family Teaching

- Explain purpose and side effects of medication to patient. Advise patient to read *Patient Information*

M

before starting therapy and with each Rx refill in case of changes. Instruct patient to take as directed. Take missed doses as soon as remembered unless almost time for next dose; do not double doses.

- Advise patient to notify health care provider of all Rx or OTC medications, vitamins, or herbal products being taken and to consult with health care provider before taking other medications.
- Advise patients to notify health care provider if signs or symptoms of hypersensitivity reactions, hepatotoxicity, pulmonary edema, or fluid retention occur.
- Rep: May cause fetal harm. Instruct women of reproductive potential to use effective contraception (intrauterine device, contraceptive implants, tubal sterilization) or a combination of methods (hormone method with a barrier method or two barrier methods) during and for ≥1 mo following discontinuation of therapy. If a partner's vasectomy is method of contraception, a hormone or barrier method must be used along with this method. Counsel patient on emergency contraception. May impair fertility in men. Advise women of reproductive potential to notify health care provider immediately if pregnancy is suspected and avoid breastfeeding during therapy. Macitentan should be discontinued as soon as possible when pregnancy is detected.

Evaluation/Desired Outcomes

- Delayed sequelae of PAH progression.

MAGNESIUM SALTS (ORAL)

magnesium chloride (12% Mg; 9.8 mEq Mg/g)
(mag-**nee**-zhum **klor**-ide)
Slo-Mag

magnesium citrate (16.2% Mg; 4.4 mEq Mg/g)
(mag-**nee**-zhum **si**-trate)
Citroma

magnesium gluconate (5.4% Mg; 4.4 mEq/g)
(mag-**nee**-zhum **gloo**-con-ate)

magnesium hydroxide (41.7% Mg; 34.3 mEq Mg/g)
(mag-**nee**-zhum hye-**drox**-ide)
Milk of Magnesia

magnesium oxide (60.3% Mg; 49.6 mEq Mg/g)
(mag-**nee**-zhum **ox**-ide)
Mag-Oxide

Classification
Therapeutic: mineral and electrolyte replacements/supplements, laxatives
Pharmacologic: salines

Indications

Treatment/prevention of hypomagnesemia. As a: Laxative, Bowel evacuant in preparation for surgical/radiographic procedures. Milk of magnesia has also been used as an antacid.

Action

Essential for the activity of many enzymes. Play an important role in neurotransmission and muscular excitability. Are osmotically active in GI tract, drawing water into the lumen and causing peristalsis. **Therapeutic Effects:** Replacement in deficiency states. Evacuation of the colon.

Pharmacokinetics

Absorption: Up to 30% may be absorbed orally.
Distribution: Widely distributed to tissues.
Metabolism and Excretion: Excreted primarily by the kidneys.
Half-life: Unknown.

TIME/ACTION PROFILE (laxative effect)

ROUTE	ONSET	PEAK	DURATION
PO	3–6 hr	unknown	unknown

Contraindications/Precautions

Contraindicated in: Hypermagnesemia; Hypocalcemia; Anuria; Heart block; OB: Unless used for preterm labor, use during active labor or within 2 hr of delivery may ↑ potential for magnesium toxicity in newborn.
Use Cautiously in: Renal impairment.

Adverse Reactions/Side Effects

Derm: flushing, sweating. **GI:** diarrhea.

Interactions

Drug-Drug: Potentiates **neuromuscular blocking agents**. May ↓ absorption of **fluoroquinolones**, **nitrofurantoin**, **tetracyclines**, and **penicillamine**.

Route/Dosage

Prevention of Deficiency (in mg of Magnesium)

PO (Adults and Children >10 yr): *Adolescent and adult men:* 270–400 mg/day; *Adolescent and adult women:* 280–300 mg/day; *Pregnant women:* 320 mg/day; *Breastfeeding women:* 340–355 mg/day.
PO (Children 7–10 yr): 170 mg/day.
PO (Children 4–6 yr): 120 mg/day.
PO (Children ≤3 yr): 40–80 mg/day.

Treatment of Deficiency (in mg of Magnesium)

PO (Adults): 200–400 mg/day in 3–4 divided doses.
PO (Children 6–11 yr): 3–6 mg/kg/day in 3–4 divided doses.

Laxative

PO (Adults): *Magnesium citrate:* 240 mL as a single dose; *Magnesium hydroxide:* 30–60 mL (as a single dose or in divided doses) or 10–20 mL as concentrate.

PO (Children 6–12 yr): *Magnesium citrate:* 100 mL as a single dose; *Magnesium hydroxide:* 15–30 mL as a single dose or in divided doses.
PO (Children 2–5 yr): *Magnesium hydroxide:* 5–15 mL as a single dose or in divided doses.

Availability

Magnesium Chloride (generic available)
Sustained-release tablets: 535 mg (64 mg magnesium)OTC.

Magnesium Citrate (generic available)
Oral solution: 240-, 296-, and 300-mL bottles (77 mEq magnesium/100 mL)OTC.

Magnesium Gluconate (generic available)
Tablets: 500 mgOTC.

Magnesium Hydroxide (generic available)
Liquid: 400 mg/5 mL (164 mg magnesium/5 mL)OTC. **Concentrated liquid:** 800 mg/5 mL (328 mg magnesium/5 mL)OTC. **Chewable tablets:** 400 mg (173 mg magnesium)OTC.

Magnesium Oxide (generic available)
Tablets: 400 mg (241.3 mg magnesium)OTC.

NURSING IMPLICATIONS

Assessment
- **Laxative:** Assess for abdominal distention, presence of bowel sounds, and usual pattern of bowel function.
- Assess color, consistency, and amount of stool produced.
- **Antacid:** Assess for heartburn and indigestion as well as location, duration, character, and precipitating factors of gastric pain.

Implementation
- **PO:** To prevent tablets entering small intestine in undissolved form, chew thoroughly before swallowing. Follow administration with ½ glass of water.
- *Magnesium citrate:* Refrigerate solutions to ensure they retain potency and palatability. May be served over ice. Magnesium citrate in an open container will lose carbonation upon standing; this will not affect potency but may reduce palatability.
- *Magnesium hydroxide:* Shake solution well before administration.
- **Antacid:** Administer 1–3 hr after meals and at bedtime.
- Powder and liquid forms are considered more effective than tablets.
- **Laxative:** Administer on empty stomach for more rapid results. Follow all oral laxative doses with a full glass of liquid to prevent dehydration and for faster effect. Do not administer at bedtime or late in the day.

Patient/Family Teaching
- Explain purpose and side effects of medication. Advise patient to read *Patient Information* before starting therapy.
- Advise patient not to take this medication within 2 hr of taking other medications, especially fluoroquinolones, nitrofurantoin, and tetracyclines.
- **Antacids:** Caution patient to consult health care provider before taking antacids for >2 wk if problem is recurring, if relief is not obtained, or if symptoms of gastric bleeding (black, tarry stools; coffee-ground emesis) occur.
- **Laxatives:** Advise patient that laxatives should be used only for short-term therapy. Long-term therapy may cause electrolyte imbalance and dependence.
- Encourage patient to use other forms of bowel regulation, such as ↑ dietary fiber, fluid intake, and mobility.
- Advise patient to notify health care provider if unrelieved constipation, rectal bleeding, or symptoms of electrolyte imbalance (muscle cramps or pain, weakness, dizziness) occur.
- Rep: Advise patient to notify health care provider if pregnancy is planned or suspected or if breastfeeding.

Evaluation/Desired Outcomes
- Relief of gastric pain and irritation.
- Passage of a soft, formed bowel movement, usually within 3–6 hr.
- Prevention and treatment of magnesium deficiency.

M

HIGH ALERT

V magnesium sulfate (parenteral)
(mag-**nee**-zhum **sul**-fate)

Classification
Therapeutic: mineral and electrolyte replacements/supplements
Pharmacologic: minerals/electrolytes

Indications
Treatment/prevention of hypomagnesemia. Prevention and treatment of seizures associated with severe eclampsia or pre-eclampsia. **Unlabeled Use:** Treatment of torsades de pointes. Adjunctive treatment for bronchodilation in moderate to severe acute asthma.

Action
Essential for the activity of many enzymes. Plays an important role in neurotransmission and muscular excitability. **Therapeutic Effects:** Replacement in deficiency states. Resolution of eclampsia.

Pharmacokinetics
Absorption: IV administration results in complete bioavailability; well absorbed from IM sites.
Distribution: Widely distributed to tissues

Metabolism and Excretion: Excreted primarily by the kidneys.
Half-life: Unknown.

TIME/ACTION PROFILE (anticonvulsant effect)

ROUTE	ONSET	PEAK	DURATION
IM	60 min	unknown	3–4 hr
IV	immediate	unknown	30 min

Contraindications/Precautions

Contraindicated in: Hypermagnesemia; Hypocalcemia; Anuria; Heart block.
Use Cautiously in: Renal impairment; OB: Avoid using for more than 5–7 days for preterm labor (may ↑ risk of hypocalcemia and bone changes in newborn); avoid continuous use during active labor or within 2 hr of delivery due to potential for magnesium toxicity in newborn; Geri: Older adults may require ↓ dosage due to age-related ↓ in renal function.

Adverse Reactions/Side Effects

CV: arrhythmias, bradycardia, hypotension. **Derm:** flushing, sweating. **GI:** diarrhea. **Metab:** hypothermia. **MS:** muscle weakness. **Neuro:** drowsiness. **Resp:** ↓ respiratory rate.

Interactions

Drug-Drug: May potentiate **calcium channel blockers** and **neuromuscular blocking agents**.

Route/Dosage

Treatment of Deficiency

IM, IV (Adults): *Severe deficiency:* 8–12 g/day in divided doses; *Mild deficiency:* 1 g every 6 hr for 4 doses or 250 mg/kg over 4 hr.
IM, IV (Children >1 mo): 25–50 mg/kg/dose every 4–6 hr for 3–4 doses (max single dose = 2 g).
IV (Neonates): 25–50 mg/kg/dose every 8–12 hr for 2–3 doses.

Seizures Associated With Eclampsia/Pre-Eclampsia

IV (Adults): 4–6 g loading dose over 15–30 min at onset of labor or induction/cesarean delivery, followed by 1–2 g/hr continuous infusion for ≥24 hr after delivery (max infusion rate = 3 g/hr). If seizure occurs while receiving magnesium, an additional bolus of 2–4 g may be administered over ≥5 min. Max dose = 40 g/24 hr.
IM (Adults): 10 g loading dose administered as 5 g in each buttock at onset of labor or induction/cesarean delivery, followed by 5 g every 4 hr for ≥24 hr after delivery.

Torsades de Pointes

IV (Adults): 1–2 g over 15 min. If no response or torsade de pointes recurs, may repeat dose up to a total of 4 g in 1 hr; may follow with a continuous IV infusion of 0.5–1 g/hr.
IV (Infants and Children): 25–50 mg/kg/dose (max dose = 2 g).

Bronchodilation

IV (Adults): 2 g single dose.
IV (Children): 25 mg/kg/dose (max dose = 2 g).

Parenteral Nutrition

IV (Adults): 4–24 mEq/day.
IV (Children): 0.25–0.5 mEq/kg/day.

Availability (generic available)

Solution for injection (8.1 mEq Mg/g): 500 mg/mL (50%). **Premixed infusion:** 1 g/100 mL, 2 g/50 mL, 4 g/50 mL, 4 g/100 mL, 20 g/500 mL, 40 g/1000 mL.

NURSING IMPLICATIONS

Assessment

- **Hypomagnesemia/Anticonvulsant:** Monitor BP, HR, respirations, and ECG frequently during administration. Respirations should be >16/min before each dose.
- Monitor neurologic status before and throughout therapy. Institute seizure precautions. Patellar reflex (knee jerk) should be tested before each dose. If response is absent, no additional doses should be administered until positive response is obtained.
- Pedi: Monitor newborn for hypotension, hyporeflexia, and respiratory depression if mother has received magnesium sulfate.

Lab Test Considerations

- Monitor serum magnesium levels and renal function periodically.

Implementation

- ***High Alert:*** Accidental overdose of IV magnesium has resulted in serious patient harm and death. Have second practitioner independently double-check original order, dose calculations, and infusion pump settings. Do not confuse milligram (mg), gram (g), or milliequivalent (mEq) doses.
- **IM:** IM route should only be used when unable to establish venous access. Administer deep IM. Administer subsequent injections in alternate sides. Dilute to a concentration of 200 mg/mL before injection.

IV Administration

- **V** Magnesium sulfate is a vesicant. If extravasation occurs, immediately stop infusion. Leave needle/cannula in place temporarily but do not flush the line. Gently aspirate extravasated solution; then remove needle/cannula. Elevate patient's extremity and apply dry cold compresses.
- **IV Push: Dilution:** 50% solution must be diluted in 0.9% NaCl or D5W to a concentration of ≤20% prior to administration. **Concentration:** ≤20%. **Rate:** Administer over several min at a rate not to exceed 150 mg/min. In patients not in cardiac arrest, rapid administration may cause hypotension and asystole.

- **Intermittent Infusion: Dilution:** 50% solution must be diluted in 0.9% NaCl or D5W to a concentration of ≤20% prior to administration. **Concentration:** ≤20%. **Rate:** *For ventricular tachycardia/torsade:* Infuse over 10–20 min; rapid infusion may cause hypotension. *For severe asthma exacerbation:* Infuse over 15–60 min.
- **Continuous Infusion: Dilution:** Dilute in D5W, 0.9% NaCl, or LR. **Concentration:** 0.5 mEq/mL (60 mg/mL) (may use max concentration of 1.6 mEq/mL) (200 mg/mL) in fluid-restricted patients. **Rate:** Infuse over 2–4 hr. Do not exceed a rate of 1 mEq/kg/hr (125 mg/kg/hr). When rapid infusions are needed (severe asthma or torsade de pointes), may infuse over 10–20 min.
- **Y-Site Compatibility:** acetaminophen, acyclovir, aldesleukin, alemtuzumab, amikacin, aminocaproic acid, argatroban, arsenic trioxide, ascorbic acid, atropine, azithromycin, aztreonam, benztropine, bivalirudin, bleomycin, bumetanide, buprenorphine, butorphanol, calcium gluconate, cangrelor, carboplatin, carmustine, caspofungin, cefiderocol, cefotaxime, cefotetan, cefoxitin, ceftazidime, ceftazidime/avibactam, chloramphenicol, chlorpromazine, cisatracurium, cisplatin, clindamycin, cyanocobalamin, cyclophosphamide, cytarabine, dacarbazine, dactinomycin, daptomycin, daunorubicin, dexmedetomidine, dexrazoxane, digoxin, diltiazem, diphenhydramine, dobutamine, docetaxel, dopamine, doxorubicin liposomal, doxycycline, enalaprilat, ephedrine, epinephrine, epoetin alfa, eptifibatide, eravacycline, ertapenem, esmolol, etoposide, etoposide phosphate, famotidine, fentanyl, fluconazole, fludarabine, fluorouracil, folic acid, foscarnet, fosphenytoin, gemcitabine, gemtuzumab ozogamicin, gentamicin, glycopyrrolate, granisetron, heparin, hydromorphone, idarubicin, ifosfamide, imipenem/cilastatin, imipenem/cilastatin/relebactam, insulin regular, irinotecan, isavuconazonium, isoproterenol, ketamine, ketorolac, labetalol, leucovorin, lidocaine, linezolid, lorazepam, mannitol, meropenem/vaborbactam, mesna, methotrexate, metoclopramide, metoprolol, metronidazole, micafungin, midazolam, milrinone, mitomycin, mitoxantrone, morphine, moxifloxacin, multivitamins, mycophenolate, nafcillin, nalbuphine, nicardipine, nitroglycerin, nitroprusside, norepinephrine, octreotide, omadacycline, ondansetron, oxaliplatin, oxytocin, paclitaxel, palonosetron, pamidronate, papaverine, pemetrexed, penicillin G, pentobarbital, phenobarbital, phentolamine, phenylephrine, piperacillin/tazobactam, plazomicin, potassium acetate, potassium chloride, procainamide, prochlorperazine, promethazine, propranolol, protamine, pyridoxine, remifentanil, rituximab, rocuronium, sargramostim, sodium acetate, sodium bicarbonate, succinylcholine, sufentanil, sulbactam/durlobactam, tacrolimus, telavancin, theophylline, thiamine, thiotepa, tigecycline, tirofiban, tobramycin, topotecan, trastuzumab, vancomycin, vasopressin, vecuronium, verapamil, vinblastine, vincristine, vinorelbine, voriconazole, zoledronic acid.
- **Y-Site Incompatibility:** aminophylline, amphotericin B liposomal, anidulafungin, azathioprine, calcium chloride, cefepime, ceftobiprole, ceftriaxone, cefuroxime, ciprofloxacin, dantrolene, dexamethasone, diazepam, diazoxide, doxorubicin hydrochloride, epirubicin, ganciclovir, haloperidol, indomethacin, methylprednisolone, pentamidine, phenytoin, phytonadione, tedizolid

Patient/Family Teaching

- Explain purpose of medication to patient and caregivers.
- Rep: Monitor vital signs, oxygen saturation, respiration, deep tendon reflexes, level of consciousness, fetal HR, maternal uterine activity, and renal function when used during pregnancy. Monitor magnesium concentrations every 4 hr in patients with renal impairment (every 2 hr if serum magnesium is elevated). Breast milk concentrations are ↑ for only 24 hr after end of therapy.

Evaluation/Desired Outcomes

- Replacement in deficiency states.
- Resolution of eclampsia.

BEERS

meclizine (mek-li-zeen)

Antivert, Bonine

Classification

Therapeutic: antiemetics, antihistamines

Indications

Motion sickness. Vertigo associated with diseases of the vestibular system.

Action

Has central anticholinergic, CNS depressant, and antihistaminic properties. Decreases excitability of the middle ear labyrinth and depresses conduction in middle ear vestibular-cerebellar pathways. **Therapeutic Effects:** Decreased motion sickness. Decreased vertigo from vestibular pathology.

Pharmacokinetics

Absorption: Absorbed after oral administration.
Distribution: Unknown.

M

Metabolism and Excretion: Primarily metabolized by liver via the CYP2D6 isoenzyme; the CYP2D6 isoenzyme exhibits genetic polymorphism (~ 7% of population may be poor metabolizers and may have significantly ↑ meclizine concentrations and an ↑ risk of adverse effects).
Half-life: 6 hr.

TIME/ACTION PROFILE (antihistaminic effects)

ROUTE	ONSET	PEAK	DURATION
PO	1 hr	unknown	8–24 hr

Contraindications/Precautions

Contraindicated in: Hypersensitivity.
Use Cautiously in: Prostatic hyperplasia; Angle-closure glaucoma; Lactation: Use while breastfeeding only if potential maternal benefit justifies potential risk to infant; Pedi: Children <12 yr (safety and effectiveness not established); Geri: Appears on Beers list. ↑ risk of anticholinergic adverse reactions in older adults, including falls, delirium, and dementia. Avoid use in older adults.

Adverse Reactions/Side Effects

EENT: blurred vision. **GI:** dry mouth. **Neuro:** drowsiness, fatigue.

Interactions

Drug-Drug: Additive CNS depression with other **CNS depressants**, including **alcohol**, other **antihistamines**, **opioid analgesics**, and **sedative/hypnotics**. Additive anticholinergic effects with other **drugs possessing anticholinergic properties**, including some **antihistamines**, **antidepressants**, **atropine**, **haloperidol**, **phenothiazines**, **quinidine**, and **disopyramide**. **CYP2D6 inhibitors** may ↑ levels and risk of toxicity.

Route/Dosage

Motion Sickness

PO (Adults and Children ≥12 yr): 25–50 mg 1 hr before exposure; may repeat in 24 hr.

Vertigo

PO (Adults and Children ≥12 yr): 25–100 mg/day in divided doses.

Availability (generic available)

Tablets: 12.5 mg, 25 mg[Rx, OTC], 50 mg. **Chewable tablets (raspberry flavor):** 25 mg[OTC].

NURSING IMPLICATIONS

Assessment

- Assess patient for level of sedation after administration.
- **Motion Sickness:** Assess for nausea and vomiting before and 60 min after administration.
- **Vertigo:** Assess degree of vertigo periodically in patients receiving meclizine for labyrinthitis.

Lab Test Considerations

- May cause false-negative results in skin tests using allergen extracts. Discontinue meclizine 72 hr before testing.

Implementation

- **PO:** Administer oral doses with food, water, or milk to minimize GI irritation. ***DNC:*** Swallow tablets whole; do not crush, break, or chew.
- Chewable tablets must be chewed or crushed completely before swallowing. Do not swallow chewable tablets whole.

Patient/Family Teaching

- Explain purpose and side effects of medication to patient. Advise patient to read *Patient Information* before starting therapy. Instruct patient to take as directed. If a dose is missed, take as soon as possible unless almost time for next dose. Do not double doses.
- Advise patient to notify health care provider of all Rx or OTC medications, vitamins, or herbal products being taken and to consult health care provider before taking other medications.
- May cause drowsiness. Caution patient to avoid driving or other activities requiring alertness until response to the medication is known.
- Advise patient that frequent mouth rinses, good oral hygiene, and sugarless gum or candy may ↓ dryness of mouth.
- Caution patient to avoid concurrent use of alcohol and other CNS depressants, including opioids, with this medication.
- Rep: Advise women of reproductive potential to notify health care provider if pregnancy is planned or suspected or if breastfeeding.
- **Motion Sickness:** When used as prophylaxis for motion sickness, advise patient to take medication >1 hr before exposure to conditions that may cause motion sickness.

Evaluation/Desired Outcomes

- Decreased motion sickness.
- Decreased vertigo from vestibular pathology.

medroxyPROGESTERone

(me-**drox**-ee-proe-**jess**-te-rone)
Depo-Provera, Depo-SubQ Provera 104, Provera

Classification
Therapeutic: antineoplastics, contraceptive hormones
Pharmacologic: hormones, progestins

Indications
Prevention of pregnancy. To decrease endometrial hyperplasia in postmenopausal women receiving concurrent estrogen (0.625 mg/day conjugated estrogens). Treatment of secondary amenorrhea and abnormal uterine bleeding caused by hormonal imbalance. **IM:** Treatment of advanced unresponsive endometrial or renal carcinoma. Prevention of pregnancy. Management of endometriosis-associated pain (Depo-Sub Q Provera 104 only).

Action
A synthetic form of progesterone; actions include secretory changes in the endometrium, increases in basal body temperature, histologic changes in vaginal epithelium, relaxation of uterine smooth muscle, mammary alveolar tissue growth, pituitary inhibition, and withdrawal bleeding in the presence of estrogen. **Therapeutic Effects:** Decreased endometrial hyperplasia in postmenopausal women receiving concurrent estrogen (combination with estrogen decreases vasomotor symptoms and prevents osteoporosis). Restoration of hormonal balance with control of uterine bleeding. Management of endometrial or renal cancer. Prevention of pregnancy.

Pharmacokinetics
Absorption: 0.6–10% absorbed after oral administration.
Distribution: Unknown.
Metabolism and Excretion: Metabolized by the liver. Primarily excreted in the urine as metabolites.
Half-life: *1st phase:* 52 min; *2nd phase:* 230 min; *biological:* 14.5 hr.

TIME/ACTION PROFILE (IM = antineoplastic effects)

ROUTE	ONSET	PEAK	DURATION
PO	unknown	unknown	unknown
IM	wk–mos	mo	unknown†
SC	unknown	1 wk	3 mo

† Contraceptive effect lasts 3 mo.

Contraindications/Precautions
Contraindicated in: Hypersensitivity; Hypersensitivity to parabens (IM suspension only); Missed abortion; Thromboembolic disease (e.g., deep vein thrombosis [DVT], pulmonary embolism [PE], MI, stroke); Cerebrovascular disease; Severe hepatic impairment; History of breast cancer; Protein C, protein S, or antithrombin deficiency or other thrombophilic disorder; Porphyria; OB: Pregnancy; Lactation: Lactation.

Use Cautiously in: Long-term use (>4–5 yr); may ↑ risk of MI, stroke, invasive breast cancer, DVT, PE, and dementia in postmenopausal women; Renal impairment; Hepatic impairment; Cardiovascular disease; Seizure disorders; Depression.

Adverse Reactions/Side Effects
CV: DVT, edema, MI, thrombophlebitis. **Derm:** chloasma, melasma, rash. **EENT:** retinal thrombosis. **Endo:** breast tenderness, galactorrhea, hyperglycemia. **GI:** drug-induced hepatitis, gingival bleeding. **GU:** amenorrhea, breakthrough bleeding, cervical erosions, changes in menstrual flow, dysmenorrhea. **Local:** injection site reactions. **Metab:** weight gain, weight loss. **MS:** bone loss. **Neuro:** dementia, depression, STROKE. **Resp:** PE. **Misc:** HYPERSENSITIVITY REACTIONS (INCLUDING ANAPHYLAXIS OR ANGIOEDEMA), MALIGNANCY (BREAST, ENDOMETRIAL, OVARIAN).

Interactions
Drug-Drug: Strong CYP3A4 inhibitors, including **ketoconazole**, **itraconazole**, **clarithromycin**, **atazanavir**, **nefazodone**, **nelfinavir**, **ritonavir**, and **voriconazole**, may ↑ levels and risk of toxicity; avoid concurrent use. **Strong CYP3A4 inducers**, including **phenytoin**, **phenobarbital**, **carbamazepine**, **rifampin**, **rifabutin**, **rifapentin**, and **phenobarbital**, may ↓ levels and effectiveness; avoid concurrent use. May ↓ effectiveness of **bromocriptine** when used concurrently for galactorrhea/amenorrhea.
Drug-Natural Products: St. John's wort may ↓ levels and effectiveness; avoid concurrent use

M

Route/Dosage
Postmenopausal Women Receiving Concurrent Estrogen
PO (Adults): 2.5–5 mg daily concurrently with 0.625 mg conjugated estrogens (monophasic regimen) *or* 5 mg daily on Days 15–28 of the cycle with 0.625 mg conjugated estrogens taken daily throughout cycle (biphasic regimen).

Secondary Amenorrhea
PO (Adults): 5–10 mg/day for 5–10 days; start at any time in cycle.

Dysfunctional Uterine Bleeding/Induction of Menses
PO (Adults): 5–10 mg/day for 5–10 days, starting on Day 16 or Day 21 of menstrual cycle.

Renal or Endometrial Carcinoma
IM (Adults): 400–1000 mg; may be repeated weekly; if improvement occurs, attempt to ↓ dose to 400 mg monthly.

Endometriosis-Associated Pain

SUBQ (Adults): 104 mg every 12–14 wk (3 mo), beginning on Day 5 of normal menses (not recommended for more than 2 yr).

Prevention of Pregnancy

IM (Adults): 150 mg within 1st 5 days of menses or within 5 days postpartum, if not breastfeeding. If breastfeeding, give 6 wk postpartum; repeat every 3 mo.
SUBQ (Adults): 104 mg within 1st 5 days of menses or within 5 days postpartum, if not breastfeeding. If breastfeeding, give 6 wk postpartum; repeat every 12–14 wk.

Availability (generic available)

Tablets: 2.5 mg, 5 mg, 10 mg, 🍁 100 mg. **Suspension for intramuscular injection:** 🍁 50 mg/mL, 150 mg/mL. **Suspension for SUBQ injection (Depo-SubQ Provera 104):** 104 mg/0.65 mL. ***In combination with***: conjugated estrogens as Prempro (single combination tablet of 0.626 mg conjugated estrogens plus 2.5 or 5 mg medroxyprogesterone) or Premphase (0.625 mg conjugated estrogens tablet for 14 days followed by combination tablet of 0.625 mg conjugated estrogens plus 5 mg medroxyprogesterone for days 15–28) in convenience packages. See Appendix N.

NURSING IMPLICATIONS

Assessment

- Monitor for signs and symptoms of venous thromboembolism, such as PE (chest pain, dyspnea, tachycardia) or DVT (calf pain or tenderness, lower extremity edema, localized warmth or erythema), or emerging cardiovascular disease, such as MI (chest pain, dyspnea, diaphoresis, dizziness, nausea) or stroke (weakness, slurred speech, confusion, dizziness); discontinue therapy in all patients if PE, DVT, stroke, or MI are suspected.
- Monitor BP periodically during therapy.
- Monitor intake and output and weekly weight. Report significant discrepancies or steady weight gain.
- Monitor for breast tenderness, lumps, or discharge. Perform baseline mammogram before starting treatment.

Lab Test Considerations

- Monitor hepatic function before and periodically during therapy.May ↑ alkaline phosphatase. May ↓ pregnanediol excretion concentrations.
- May ↑ serum LDL or ↓ HDL.
- May alter thyroid hormone assays.
- May ↓ glucose tolerance; monitor patients with diabetes closely.

Implementation

- Do not confuse Depo-Provera with Depo-SubQ Provera 104. Do not confuse Provera with Proscar or Prozac. Do not confuse medroxyprogesterone with methylprednisolone, or methyltestosterone.
- Estrogen plus progestin therapy should not be used for the prevention of cardiovascular disease or dementia.
- *Contraception:* To ensure patient is not pregnant at time of 1st injection, administer ONLY during 1st 5 days of a normal menstrual period; ONLY within 1st 5 days postpartum if not breastfeeding; and if exclusively breastfeeding, ONLY at the 6th postpartum wk. If interval between injections >13 wk, use pregnancy test to ensure patient is not pregnant before administration. Only the 150 mg/mL vial or prefilled syringe should be used for contraception.
- When switching from other hormonal contraceptives, administer within dosing period (7 days after taking last active pill, removing patch or ring, or within dosing period for IM injection).
- Injectable medroxyprogesterone may lead to bone loss, especially in women <21 yr; should be used for <2 yr only if other methods of contraception are inadequate. If used long term, women should use supplemental calcium and vitamin D and monitor bone mineral density.
- IM and SUBQ injections are to be administered by a health care provider.
- **SUBQ**: Shake vigorously before use to form a uniform suspension. Inject slowly (over 5–7 sec) at a 45° angle into fatty area of anterior thigh or abdomen every 12–14 wk. If more than 14 wk elapse between injections, rule out pregnancy prior to administration. **Do not rub area after injection.**
- **IM**: Shake vial or prefilled syringe vigorously before preparing IM dose. Administer deep IM into gluteal or deltoid muscle. Rotate sites with each injection. If period between injections >14 wk, determine that patient is not pregnant before administering the drug.
- In patients with cancer, IM dose may initially be required weekly. Once stabilized, IM dose may be required only monthly.
- Dose for contraception lasts 3 mo and should not be used >2 yr.

Patient/Family Teaching

- Explain purpose and side effects of medication to patient. Advise patient to read *Patient Information* before starting therapy and with each Rx refill or injection. Take missed doses as soon as remembered; do not double doses.
- Advise patient to notify health care provider of all Rx or OTC medications, vitamins, or herbal products being taken and to consult health care provider before taking other medications.
- Inform postmenopausal women that long-term use may ↑ risk of MI, stroke, invasive breast cancer, PE, DVT, and dementia.
- Explain the importance of adhering to every 3-mo schedule to patients using medroxyprogesterone for contraception.

- Advise patients receiving medroxyprogesterone for menstrual dysfunction to anticipate withdrawal bleeding 3–7 days after discontinuing medication.
- Advise patient to report signs and symptoms of thromboembolic disorders (pain, swelling, tenderness in extremities, headache, chest pain, blurred vision).
- Advise patient to keep a 1-mo supply of medroxyprogesterone available at all times.
- Instruct patient in correct method of monthly breast self-examination. ↑ breast tenderness may occur.
- Advise patient that gingival bleeding may occur. Instruct patient to use good oral hygiene and to receive regular dental care and examinations.
- Inform patient that medroxyprogesterone does not protect against HIV infection and other sexually transmitted infections.
- Medroxyprogesterone may cause melasma (brown patches of discoloration) on face when patient is exposed to sunlight. Advise patient to avoid sun exposure and to wear sunscreen or protective clothing when outdoors.
- Emphasize the importance of routine follow-up physical exams, including BP check; breast, abdomen, and pelvic examinations; Papanicolaou smears every 6–12 mo; and mammogram every 12 mo or as directed. Health care provider will evaluate possibility of discontinuing medication every 3–6 mo. If on continuous (not cyclical) therapy or without concurrent estrogens, endometrial biopsy may be recommended, if uterus is intact.
- Rep: Advise women of reproductive potential to notify health care provider if menstrual period is missed or if pregnancy is suspected or if breastfeeding. Patient should not attempt conception for 3 mo after discontinuing medication in order to ↓ risk to fetus. Once discontinued, may delay conception for ≥10 mo.
- **IM, SUBQ**: Advise patient to maintain adequate amounts of dietary calcium and vitamin D to help prevent bone loss.

Evaluation/Desired Outcomes

- Regular menstrual periods.
- Decrease in endometrial hyperplasia in postmenopausal women receiving concurrent estrogen.
- Management of the spread of endometrial or renal cancer.
- Prevention of pregnancy.

BEERS HIGH ALERT

megestrol (me-jess-trole)

~~Megace~~

Classification

Therapeutic: antineoplastics, hormones

Pharmacologic: progestins

Indications

Palliative treatment of endometrial and breast carcinoma, either alone or with surgery or radiation (tablets only). Anorexia, weight loss, and cachexia associated with AIDS (oral suspension only).

Action

Antineoplastic effect may result from inhibition of pituitary function. **Therapeutic Effects:** Regression of tumor. Increased appetite and weight gain in patients with AIDS.

Pharmacokinetics

Absorption: Well absorbed from the GI tract.
Distribution: Unknown.
Protein Binding: ≥90%.
Metabolism and Excretion: Completely metabolized by the liver.
Half-life: 38 hr (range 13–104 hr).

TIME/ACTION PROFILE (antineoplastic activity)

ROUTE	ONSET	PEAK	DURATION
PO	week–months	2 mo	unknown

Contraindications/Precautions

Contraindicated in: Hypersensitivity; Undiagnosed vaginal bleeding; Severe hepatic impairment; Suspension contains alcohol and should be avoided in patients with known intolerance; OB: Pregnancy; Lactation: Lactation.
Use Cautiously in: Diabetes; Mental depression; Renal impairment; History of thromboembolism; Cardiovascular disease; Seizures; Rep: Women of reproductive potential; Pedi: Safety and effectiveness not established in children; Geri: Appears on Beers list. ↑ risk of thrombotic events and possibly death in older adults. Avoid use in older adults.

Adverse Reactions/Side Effects

CV: DEEP VEIN THROMBOSIS (DVT), edema. **Derm:** alopecia. **Endo:** <u>asymptomatic adrenal suppression (chronic therapy)</u>. **GI:** GI irritation. **GU:** vaginal bleeding. **MS:** carpal tunnel syndrome. **Resp:** PULMONARY EMBOLISM (PE).

Interactions

Drug-Drug: May ↑ INR and risk of bleeding when used with **warfarin**.

Route/Dosage

Breast Carcinoma

PO (Adults): 160 mg/day as a single dose or divided doses.

Endometrial Carcinoma

PO (Adults): 40–320 mg/day in divided dose.

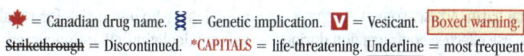

Anorexia Associated With AIDS

PO (Adults): *40 mg/mL suspension:* 800 mg once daily; may ↓ to 400 mg/day after 1 mo (range 400–800 mg/day); *125 mg/mL suspension:* 625 mg once daily.

Availability (generic available)

Oral suspension(lemon-lime flavor): 40 mg/mL, 125 mg/mL. **Tablets:** 20 mg, 40 mg, 🍁 160 mg.

NURSING IMPLICATIONS

Assessment

- Monitor for signs and symptoms of venous thromboembolism such as PE (chest pain, dyspnea, tachycardia) or DVT (calf pain or tenderness, lower extremity edema, localized warmth or erythema). Report if suspected.
- **Anorexia:** Monitor weight, appetite, and nutritional intake in patients with AIDS.

Lab Test Considerations

- Verify negative pregnancy test before starting therapy.

Implementation

- When cutting, crushing, or handling tablets, wear double chemotherapy gloves, protective gown, and hair and shoe covers. Prepare in a ventilated engineering control, if possible, and consider crushing tablets in a pill pouch. Use respiratory (N95) protection and eye and face protection, if not prepared in a ventilated engineering control. During administration, wear double chemotherapy gloves and protective gown when handling uncoated, cut, or crushed tablets. Eye/face protection is needed if there is risk of patient vomiting or spitting up. Single chemotherapy gloves are appropriate if handling and administering intact tablets from a unit-dose package.
- Because of high dose, suspension is most convenient form for patients with AIDS.
- **PO:** May be administered with meals if GI irritation becomes a problem.
- Shake suspension well before administering. Suspension is compatible to mix with water, apple juice, orange juice, or Sustacal H.C. for immediate consumption.

Patient/Family Teaching

- Explain the purpose and side effects of megestrol. Instruct patient to take as directed; do not skip or double up on missed doses. Missed doses may be taken as long as not right before next dose. Gradually decrease dose prior to discontinuation. Advise patient to read *Patient Information* before starting and with each Rx refill in case of changes.
- Advise patient to report to health care provider any unusual vaginal bleeding or signs of DVT or PE.
- Discuss with patient the possibility of hair loss. Explore methods of coping.
- Rep: May cause fetal harm. Advise women of reproductive potential to use effective contraception during and for ≥4 mo after therapy is completed. Advise patient to notify health care provider immediately if pregnancy is planned or suspected and to avoid breastfeeding during therapy.

Evaluation/Desired Outcomes

- Slowing or arresting the spread of endometrial or breast malignancy. Therapeutic effects usually occur within 2 mo of initiating therapy.
- Increased appetite and weight gain in patients with AIDS.

BEERS

meloxicam (me-**lox**-i-kam)

~~Mobic~~, Xifyrm

Classification

Therapeutic: nonopioid analgesics

Pharmacologic: nonsteroidal anti-inflammatory drugs (NSAIDs)

Indications

PO: Relief of signs and symptoms of osteoarthritis and rheumatoid arthritis (including juvenile rheumatoid arthritis). **IV:** Moderate to severe pain (as monotherapy or in combination with non-NSAID analgesics).

Action

Inhibits prostaglandin synthesis, probably by inhibiting the enzyme cyclooxygenase. **Therapeutic Effects:** Decreased pain and inflammation.

Pharmacokinetics

Absorption: Well absorbed following oral administration. IV administration results in complete bioavailability.
Distribution: Not widely distributed to tissues.
Protein Binding: 99.4%.
Metabolism and Excretion: Mostly metabolized to inactive metabolites by the liver via the CYP2C9 isoenzyme (and to a lesser extent by the CYP3A4 isoenzyme); the CYP2C9 isoenzyme exhibits genetic polymorphism (intermediate or poor metabolizers may have significantly ↑ meloxicam concentrations and an ↑ risk of adverse reactions). Metabolites are excreted in urine and feces.
Half-life: 20.1 hr.

TIME/ACTION PROFILE (plasma concentrations)

ROUTE	ONSET	PEAK	DURATION
PO	unknown	5–6 hr	24 hr
IV	rapid	end of injection	24 hr

Contraindications/Precautions

Contraindicated in: Hypersensitivity; Cross-sensitivity may occur with other NSAIDs, including aspirin; Severe renal impairment (CCr ≤15 mL/min) (oral); Moderate to severe renal impairment in patients who are at risk for renal failure due to volume depletion (IV); Concurrent use of aspirin

(↑ risk of adverse reactions); Coronary artery bypass graft surgery; Recent MI; HF OB: Avoid use after 30 wk gestation.

Use Cautiously in: Cardiovascular disease or risk factors for cardiovascular disease (may ↑ risk of serious cardiovascular thrombotic events, myocardial infarction, and stroke, especially with prolonged use or use of higher doses); History of long duration of NSAID use, smoking, alcohol use, advanced liver disease, coagulopathy, or poor general health (↑ risk of GI bleeding); History of peptic ulcer disease and/or GI bleeding; Bleeding tendency or concurrent anticoagulant therapy; Dehydration (correct deficits before initiating therapy); Renal impairment, hepatic impairment, or concurrent ACE inhibitor or diuretic therapy (↑ risk of renal impairment); Hypertension; OB: Use at or after 20 wk gestation may cause fetal or neonatal renal impairment; if treatment is necessary between 20 wk and 30 wk gestation, limit use to the lowest effective dose and shortest duration possible; Lactation: Safety not established in breastfeeding; Pedi: Children <2 yr or <60 kg (safety and effectiveness of tablets not established); safety and effectiveness of capsules and injection not established in children; Geri: Appears on Beers list. ↑ risk GI bleeding or peptic ulcer disease in older adults. Avoid chronic use unless other alternatives are not effective and the patient can take a gastroprotective agent; avoid short-term use in combination with oral or parenteral corticosteroids, anticoagulants, or antiplatelet agents unless other alternatives are not effective and the patient can take a gastroprotective agent.

Adverse Reactions/Side Effects

CV: edema, HF, hypertension, MI. **Derm:** DRUG REACTION WITH EOSINOPHILIA AND SYSTEMIC SYMPTOMS (DRESS), EXFOLIATIVE DERMATITIS, GENERALIZED BULLOUS FIXED DRUG ERUPTION, pruritus, rash, STEVENS-JOHNSON SYNDROME (SJS), TOXIC EPIDERMAL NECROLYSIS (TEN). **F and E** hyperkalemia. **GI:** ↑ liver enzymes, diarrhea, dyspepsia, GI BLEEDING, GI PERFORATION, GI ULCERATION, HEPATOTOXICITY, nausea. **GU:** delayed ovulation. **Hemat:** anemia, leukopenia, thrombocytopenia. **Neuro:** STROKE. **Misc:** HYPERSENSITIVITY REACTIONS (INCLUDING ANAPHYLAXIS AND SERIOUS SKIN REACTIONS).

Interactions

Drug-Drug: May ↓ antihypertensive effects of **ACE inhibitors**. May ↓ diuretic effects of **furosemide** or **thiazide diuretics**. Concurrent use with **aspirin** ↑ meloxicam blood levels and may ↑ risk of adverse reactions. Concurrent use with **cholestyramine** ↓ blood levels. ↑ plasma **lithium** levels; close monitoring recommended when meloxicam is introduced or withdrawn. ↑ risk of GI bleeding with **anticoagulants, aspirin, clopidogrel, ticagrelor, prasugrel, corticosteroids, fibrinolytics, SNRIs,** or **SSRIs.** Concurrent use with **sodium polystyrene sulfonate** may ↑ risk of colonic necrosis; concurrent use should be avoided.

Route/Dosage

PO (Adults): *Capsules:* 5 mg once daily; may ↑ to 10 mg once daily, if needed; *Tablets:* 7.5 mg once daily; may ↑ to 15 mg once daily, if needed.

PO (Children 2–17 yr and ≥60 kg): *Tablets:* 7.5 mg once daily.

IV (Adults): 30 mg once daily.

Availability (generic available)

Tablets: 7.5 mg, 15 mg. **Capsules:** 5 mg, 10 mg. **Oral suspension (raspberry flavor):** 7.5 mg/5 mL. **Solution for injection:** 30 mg/mL. ***In combination with:*** bupivacaine (Zynrelef Kit). See Appendix N.

M

NURSING IMPLICATIONS

Assessment

- Assess pain and range of motion prior to and 2–3 hr following administration. *If analgesic effect is delayed in the 1st 24 hr,* consider administering a short-acting, non-NSAID analgesic.
- Monitor for signs and symptoms of hypersensitivity reaction, including anaphylaxis. Patients with asthma, aspirin-induced allergy, and nasal polyps are at ↑ risk.
- Assess for rash periodically during therapy. May cause SJS, TEN, or generalized bullous fixed drug eruption. *At the 1st sign of rash,* discontinue meloxicam.
- Monitor for signs and symptoms of DRESS (fever, rash, lymphadenopathy, facial swelling) periodically during therapy. *If symptoms of DRESS occur,* immediately stop meloxicam and evaluate for DRESS.
- Monitor BP during initiation and periodically during therapy. May cause fluid retention and edema leading to new onset hypertension.
- Monitor for GI bleeding, ulceration, and perforation during extended therapy. *If serious GI event is suspected,* promptly evaluate and hold therapy until a serious GI event is ruled out.

Lab Test Considerations

- Monitor serum potassium and CBC periodically in patients receiving prolonged therapy. May cause hyperkalemia, anemia, thrombocytopenia, leukopenia, and eosinophilia.
- Monitor renal function (BUN, serum creatinine) in patients on extended therapy and those with renal or hepatic impairment, dehydration, or hypovolemia. *If signs and symptoms of hepatotoxicity occur,* immediately discontinue meloxicam.
- Bleeding time may be prolonged.

Implementation

- Correct volume status in dehydrated or hypovolemic patients prior to initiation.
- Administration in higher than recommended doses does not provide ↑ effectiveness but may cause ↑ side effects. Use lowest effective dose for shortest period of time to minimize risk of cardiovascular thrombotic events.
- **PO:** Administer without regard to food. Administer with food or milk to ↓ GI irritation.
- Shake oral suspension gently before using.

IV Administration

- **IV Push:** Single-dose vial; undiluted. Solution is clear to yellow. **Concentration:** 30 mg/mL. **Rate:** Administer over 15 sec.
- **Y-Site Incompatibility:** Do not administer other drugs through same IV line.

Patient/Family Teaching

- Explain purpose and side effects of medication. Advise patient to read *Patient Information* before starting therapy.
- Advise patient to remain in an upright position for 15–30 min after administration and to take missed doses as soon as remembered but not if almost time for the next dose. Do not double doses.
- Caution patient to avoid the concurrent use of alcohol, aspirin, acetaminophen, or other OTC medications without consulting health care provider.
- Advise patient to notify health care provider of all Rx or OTC medications, vitamins, or herbal products being taken and to consult health care provider before taking other medications, especially the concurrent use of alcohol, aspirin, NSAIDs, or acetaminophen.
- Inform patient of ↑ risk of MI and stroke. Use lowest effective dose for shortest time. Advise patient to notify health care provider immediately if signs and symptoms (shortness of breath or trouble breathing, chest pain, weakness in one part or side of body, slurred speech, swelling of the face or throat) occur.
- Advise patient to notify health care provider promptly if signs or symptoms of GI toxicity (abdominal pain, black stools) occur.
- Advise patient to consult health care provider if rash, itching, visual disturbances, weight gain, edema, or signs of hepatotoxicity (nausea, fatigue, lethargy, jaundice, upper right quadrant tenderness, flu-like symptoms) occur.
- Rep: May cause fetal harm. Advise women of reproductive potential to notify health care provider if pregnancy is planned or suspected or if breastfeeding. Advise patient to avoid meloxicam in 3rd trimester of pregnancy (after 29 wk); may cause premature closure of fetal ductus arteriosus. Use of meloxicam after 20 wk may cause fetal renal impairment leading to oligohydramnios. May cause reversible infertility in men and women attempting to conceive; may consider discontinuing meloxicam.

Evaluation/Desired Outcomes

- Relief of pain.
- Improved joint mobility. Patients who do not respond to one NSAID may respond to another.

REMS HIGH ALERT

melphalan (mel-fa-lan)

~~Alkeran~~, Evomela, Hepzato, Ivra

Classification

Therapeutic: antineoplastics

Pharmacologic: alkylating agents

Indications

IV: High-dose conditioning treatment prior to hematopoietic stem cell transplantation (Evomela only). **IV:** Palliative treatment of multiple myeloma. **Intraarterial:** Uveal melanoma in patients with unresectable hepatic metastases affecting <50% of the liver and no extrahepatic disease or extrahepatic disease limited to the bone, lymph nodes, subcutaneous tissues, or lung that is amenable to resection or radiation (Hepzato only).

Action

Inhibits DNA and RNA synthesis by alkylation (cell-cycle phase-nonspecific). **Therapeutic Effects:** Death of rapidly replicating cells, particularly malignant ones. Also has immunosuppressive properties.

Pharmacokinetics

Absorption: IV and intra-arterial administration results in complete bioavailability.

Distribution: Rapidly distributed to tissues.

Metabolism and Excretion: Rapidly metabolized in the bloodstream. Small amounts (10%) excreted unchanged by the kidneys.

Half-life: *IV:* 1.5 hr; *Intra-arterial:* 1.1 hr.

TIME/ACTION PROFILE (effects on blood counts)

ROUTE	ONSET	PEAK	DURATION
IV	unknown	2–3 wk	4–5 wk
Intra-arterial	unknown	10–13 days	2–3 wk

Contraindications/Precautions

Contraindicated in: Hypersensitivity to melphalan; History of allergy to natural rubber latex or heparin (Hepzato only); Heparin-induced thrombocytopenia (Hepzato only); History of severe allergic reaction to iodinated contrast not controlled by premedication with antihistamines and steroids (Hepzato only); Active intracranial metastases or brain lesion at risk for bleeding (Hepzato only); Liver failure, portal hypertension, or known varices at risk for bleeding (Hepzato only); Surgical or medical treatment of the liver in the past 4 wk (Hepzato only); Uncorrectable coagulopathy (Hepzato only); Unable to safely undergo general anesthesia, including active cardiac conditions (e.g. unstable coronary syndromes [unstable or severe angina or MI], worsening or new-onset HF, significant arrhythmias, or severe valvular disease) (Hepzato only); Platelets ≤100,000 cells/mm³ (Hepzato only); Hgb <10 g/dL (Hepzato only); Neutrophils ≤2000 cells/mm³ (Hepzato only); OB: Pregnancy; Lactation: Lactation.

Use Cautiously in: Active infections; ↓ bone marrow reserve; Renal impairment (↓ dose ↓ for palliative treatment only if BUN ≥30 mg/dL); Abnormal hepatic vascular or biliary anatomy or gastric acid hypersecretion syndromes (↑ risk of periprocedural complications with intra-arterial administration); Rep: Women of reproductive potential and men with female partners of reproductive potential; Pedi: Safety and effectiveness not established in children; Geri: Begin at lower end of dosing range in older adults due to potential for age-related ↓ in renal, hepatic, or cardiac function.

Adverse Reactions/Side Effects

CV: hypotension (Hepzato only), peripheral edema. **Derm:** alopecia, DEEP VEIN THROMBOSIS (DVT) (HEPZATO ONLY), pruritus, rash. **Endo:** menstrual irregularities. **F and E** hypokalemia, hypophosphatemia. **GI:** ↓ appetite, ↑ liver enzymes (Hepzato only), abdominal pain, constipation, diarrhea, hyperbilirubinemia, mucositis, nausea, vomiting. **GU:** infertility. **Hemat:** ↑ aPTT, ↑ INR, ANEMIA, LEUKOPENIA, NEUTROPENIA, THROMBOCYTOPENIA, HEMORRHAGE (HEPZATO ONLY). **Metab:** hyperuricemia. **MS:** ↑ troponin I, pain. **Neuro:** dizziness, fatigue, headache, lethargy. **Resp:** cough, dyspnea, PULMONARY EMBOLISM (PE) (HEPZATO ONLY). **Misc:** fever, HYPERSENSITIVITY REACTIONS (INCLUDING ANAPHYLAXIS), SECONDARY MALIGNANCY.

Interactions

Drug-Drug: ↑ bone marrow depression with other **antineoplastics** or **radiation therapy**. May ↓ antibody response to **live-virus vaccines** and ↑ risk of adverse reactions. **Cyclosporine** may ↑ risk of renal failure. **Apixaban, aspirin, clopidogrel, dabigatran, edoxaban, NSAIDs, prasugrel, rivaroxaban, ticagrelor,** and **warfarin** may ↑ risk of bleeding during administration of intra-arterial infusion; discontinue prior to procedure. **ACE inhibitors, calcium channel blockers,** or **alpha-1 receptor blockers** may ↑ risk of hypotension during administration of intra-arterial infusion; discontinue antihypertensives ≥5 half-lives before administration of intra-arterial infusion.

Route/Dosage

Multiple Myeloma (Palliative Treatment)

IV (Adults): 16 mg/m² every 2 wk for 4 doses, then every 4 wk.

Renal Impairment

IV (Adults): *BUN ≥30 mg/dL:* ↓ dose by up to 50%.

Multiple Myeloma (Conditioning Treatment)

IV (Adults): 100 mg/m²/day on Day 3 and Day 2 prior to autologous stem cell transplantation on Day 0.

Unresectable Hepatic Metastases in Patients With Uveal Melanoma

Intraarterial (Adults): *Hepzato:* 3 mg/kg (based on ideal body weight) (max dose = 220 mg) every 6–8 wk for a total of 6 infusions.

Availability (generic available)

Powder for injection: 50 mg/vial. **Solution for injection:** 90 mg/mL.

M

NURSING IMPLICATIONS

Assessment

- Assess for signs/symptoms of infection (fever, chills, sore throat, cough, hoarseness, headache, malaise, flu-like symptoms, lower back or side pain, dysuria, hematuria, cellulitis, erythematous nonhealing wound). Notify health care provider if these symptoms occur.
- Assess for signs/symptoms of acute hypersensitivity reactions including anaphylaxis (urticaria, pruritus, edema, rash, tachycardia, bronchospasm, dyspnea, hypotension). *If serious hypersensitivity reaction occurs,* discontinue melphalan.
- Monitor for signs/symptoms of venous thromboembolism such as PE (chest pain, dyspnea, tachycardia) or DVT (calf pain or tenderness, lower extremity edema, localized warmth or erythema). Report if suspected.
- Monitor for signs/symptoms of bleeding or hemorrhage (weakness, tachycardia, dyspnea, dizziness, pallor, fatigue, tarry stools, coffee ground emesis, bruising, bleeding gums, epistaxis). Avoid IM injections and taking rectal temperatures. Apply pressure to venipuncture sites for 10 min.
- May cause nausea and vomiting. Monitor intake and output, appetite, and nutritional intake. Prophylactic antiemetics may be used. Adjust diet as tolerated.
- Monitor for signs/symptoms of gout (joint pain, edema). Encourage patient to drink ≥2 L of fluid per day. Allopurinol may be given to ↓ uric acid levels.
- Anemia may occur. Monitor for ↑ fatigue, weakness, dizziness, pallor of skin and sclera, and dyspnea.

- Assess for allergy to chlorambucil. Patients may have cross-sensitivity.
- **Evomela:** For patients receiving *Evomela* as part of a conditioning regimen, nausea, vomiting, mucositis, and diarrhea may occur in >50% of patients. Use prophylactic antiemetic medication and provide supportive care. Provide nutritional support and analgesics for patients with severe mucositis.

Lab Test Considerations
- Verify pregnancy status before starting therapy.
- Monitor CBC and differential weekly during therapy. The nadir of leukopenia occurs in 2–3 wk. Notify health care provider if leukocyte count <3000/mm^3. The nadir of thrombocytopenia occurs in 2–3 wk. Notify health care provider if platelet count <100,000/mm^3. Recovery of leukopenia and thrombocytopenia occurs in 5–6 wk.
- Monitor liver function (AST, ALT, LDH, bilirubin) and renal function (BUN, serum creatinine) before starting and periodically during therapy.
- May ↑ uric acid. Monitor periodically during therapy.
- May ↑ 5-hydroxyindoleacetic acid concentrations as a result of tumor breakdown.

Implementation
IV Administration
- Use double chemotherapy gloves and a protective gown to prepare and administer. If possible, prepare in a biological safety cabinet or a compounding aseptic containment isolator; eye, face, and respiratory protection may be needed. Prepare and administer in a closed-system drug transfer device. During administration, if there is a potential that the substance could splash or if the patient may resist, use eye and face protection. Discard IV equipment in specially designated containers.
- If solution contacts skin or mucosa, immediately wash skin or mucosa with soap and water.
- Melphalan is an irritant. Administration by slow injection into a fast-running IV solution into an injection port or via a central line is recommended; do not administer by direct injection into a peripheral vein. If extravasation occurs, immediately stop infusion. Leave needle/cannula in place temporarily but do not flush the line. Gently aspirate extravasated solution; then remove needle/cannula. Elevate patient's extremity and apply dry cold compresses for 20 min 4 times day for 1–2 days.
- **Premedication:** Administer prophylactic antiemetics. For *Hepzato* administer a proton pump inhibitor the day prior to and the morning of the procedure.
- **Intermittent Infusion: Reconstitution:** Reconstitute with 10 mL of diluent supplied. **Concentration:** 5 mg/mL. Shake vigorously until solution is clear. **Dilution:** Dilute dose immediately with 0.9% NaCl. **Concentration:** Not to exceed 0.45 mg/mL. Administer within 60 min of reconstitution. Store at room temperature and protect from light; do not refrigerate reconstituted solution. **Rate:** Administer over 15–30 min. Keep time between reconstitution/dilution and administration to a minimum; reconstituted and diluted solutions are unstable.
- **Evomela, Intermittent Infusion:** For patients receiving *Evomela* as part of a conditioning regimen, myeloablation occurs in all patients. Do not begin the conditioning regimen if a stem cell product is not available for rescue. **Reconstitution:** Reconstitute with 8.6 mL of 0.9% NaCl. **Concentration:** 5 mg/mL. Reconstituted solution is stable for 1 hr at room temperature and 24 hr if refrigerated. Solution is clear and colorless to light yellow; do not administer solutions that are discolored or contain particulate matter. **Dilution:** Dilute dose further in 0.9% NaCl. **Concentration:** 0.45 mg/mL. Diluted solution is stable for an additional 4 hr at room temperature. **Rate:** Infuse over 30 min via injection port or central venous catheter; may cause local tissue damage if extravasation occurs. Do not administer IV push into a peripheral vein. Administer *Evomela* by injecting slowly into a fast-running IV infusion via a central venous access line.
- **Ivra, Intermittent Infusion: Dilution:** Dilute dose in appropriate volume of 0.9% NaCl. Immediately mix the contents of infusion vigorously by manual rotation. **Concentration:** 0.45 mg/mL. Diluted solution is stable for 1 hr at room temperature. **Rate:** Administer *Ivra* over 15–20 min via an injection port or central venous catheter.
- **Y-Site Compatibility:** acyclovir, alemtuzumab, amikacin, aminophylline, ampicillin, anidulafungin, argatroban, arsenic trioxide, aztreonam, bivalirudin, bleomycin, bumetanide, buprenorphine, butorphanol, calcium gluconate, carboplatin, carmustine, caspofungin, cefazolin, cefepime, cefotaxime, cefotetan, ceftazidime, ceftriaxone, cefuroxime, cisplatin, clindamycin, cyclophosphamide, cytarabine, dacarbazine, dactinomycin, daptomycin, daunorubicin, dexamethasone, dexrazoxane, diltiazem, diphenhydramine, doxorubicin hydrochloride, doxycycline, droperidol, enalaprilat, ertapenem, etoposide, famotidine, filgrastim, floxuridine, fluconazole, fludarabine, fluorouracil, foscarnet, fosphenytoin, furosemide, ganciclovir, gemtuzumab ozogamicin, gentamicin, granisetron, haloperidol, heparin, hydrocortisone, hydromorphone, idarubicin, ifosfamide, imipenem/cilastatin, leucovorin, linezolid, lorazepam, mannitol, meperidine, mesna, methadone, methotrexate, methylprednisolone, metoclopramide, metronidazole, milrinone, mitomycin, mitoxantrone, morphine, moxifloxacin, nalbuphine, octreotide, ondansetron, palonosetron, pamidronate, pentostatin, piperacillin/tazobactam, potassium acetate, potassium chloride, prochlorperazine, promethazine, sodium bicarbonate, thiotepa, tigecycline, tirofiban, tobramycin,

trimethoprim/sulfamethoxazole, vancomycin, vasopressin, vecuronium, vinblastine, vincristine, vinorelbine, voriconazole, zidovudine, zoledronic acid

- **Y-Site Incompatibility:** amiodarone, chlorpromazine, pantoprazole.
- ***Hepzato:*** ***REMS:*** *Hepzato* is part of the *Hepzato Kit Hepatic Delivery System [HDS]*, which is only available through the *Hepzato Kit Hepatic Delivery System REMS.* Health care providers must complete required *Hepzato Kit REMS* training before administering *Hepzato Kit,* and health care facilities must be certified to offer the program.
- Assess for latex allergies. The double balloon catheter component of the HDS contains natural rubber latex, which may cause allergic reactions.
- If Grade 4 neutropenia of >5 days duration despite growth factor support or associated with neutropenic fever OR Grade 4 thrombocytopenia of >5 days duration or associated with a hemorrhage that required a transfusion occurs, a dose ↓ to 2 mg/kg is recommended for subsequent treatments. Discontinue *Hepzato* if patients have life-threatening or *Hepzato*-related persistent toxicity that has not resolved to Grade ≤2 by 8 wk following treatment.
- **Intraarterial:** Rapidly (in ≤5 sec) inject 10 mL of the supplied sterile diluent into the *Hepzato* 50 mg vial using a sterile needle (≥20-gauge) and syringe. Resulting solution will contain melphalan 5 mg/mL. Immediately shake vial vigorously until a clear solution is obtained. No more than 5 sec should elapse between discharge of the syringe and shaking. Immediately further dilute the required dose with the provided 0.9% NaCl, to a concentration of <0.45 mg/mL. *For Hepzato doses <110 mg:* Dilute in 250 mL of 0.9% NaCl. *For Hepzato doses 111 mg–220 mg:* Divide total dose equally into 2 and dilute each in 250 mL of 0.9% NaCl. Solution is clear; do not administer solutions that are discolored or contain particulate matter. Administer diluted *Hepzato* intra-arterially with the Hepzato kit hepatic delivery system. Complete infusion within 30 min, followed by a 30-min washout period. Reconstituted and diluted solutions of *Hepzato* are unstable. No more than 60 min should elapse from reconstitution and completion of the intra-hepatic infusion of the diluted *Hepzato* solution. Do not refrigerate *Hepzato* once reconstituted.
- Administration of *Hepzato* requires general anesthesia and extracorporeal bypass of circulation. Ensure patient is euvolemic, but do not overhydrate. Monitor for hemorrhage, hepatocellular injury, and thromboembolic events during the procedure and for at least 72 hr following the procedure. Closely monitor BP during procedure; patients may require fluid support and vasopressors.

Patient/Family Teaching

- Explain purpose of melphalan to patient. If an appointment is missed, contact health care provider as soon as possible to reschedule. Advise patient to read *Medication Guide* before starting and periodically during therapy in case of changes.
- Emphasize need for periodic lab tests to monitor for side effects.
- Advise patient to notify health care provider if fever; chills; dyspnea; persistent cough; sore throat; signs of infection; bleeding gums; bruising; petechiae; or blood in urine, stool, or emesis occurs. Caution patient to avoid crowds and persons with known infections. Instruct patient to use soft toothbrush and electric razor. Caution patient not to drink alcoholic beverages or take products containing aspirin or other NSAIDs.
- Instruct patient to notify health care provider if skin rash, vasculitis, bleeding, fever, persistent cough, nausea, vomiting, amenorrhea, weight loss, or unusual lumps/masses occur.
- Instruct patient to inspect oral mucosa for redness and ulceration. If ulceration occurs, advise patient to use sponge brush and to rinse mouth with water after eating and drinking. Consult health care provider if pain interferes with eating. Stomatitis pain may require treatment with opioid analgesics.
- Advise patient to notify health care provider immediately if signs and symptoms of allergic reactions (skin reactions, including welts, rash, itching, and redness; fast heartbeat; shortness of breath or trouble breathing; feel light-headed or dizzy; blurry vision; swelling of face, tongue, or throat) occur.
- Instruct patient not to receive any vaccinations without advice of health care provider.
- Inform patient that melphalan may cause new cancers.
- Rep: May cause fetal harm. Advise women of reproductive potential to use effective contraception during therapy and for 6 mo after last dose and to avoid breastfeeding during therapy and for 1 wk after last dose. Advise men with a female partner of reproductive potential to use effective contraception during therapy and for 3 mo after last dose. May cause female and male infertility.

Evaluation/Desired Outcomes

- Decrease in size and spread of malignant tissue.

memantine (me-man-teen)

🍁 Ebixa, ~~Namenda, Namenda XR~~

Classification

Therapeutic: anti alzheimers agents

Pharmacologic: N-methyl-D-aspartate antagonist

M

Indications
Moderate to severe dementia/neurocognitive disorder associated with Alzheimer disease.

Action
Binds to CNS N-methyl-D-aspartate (NMDA) receptor sites, preventing binding of glutamate, an excitatory neurotransmitter. **Therapeutic Effects:** Decreased symptoms of dementia/cognitive decline. Does not slow progression. Cognitive enhancement.

Pharmacokinetics
Absorption: Well absorbed after oral administration.
Distribution: Unknown.
Metabolism and Excretion: 57–82% excreted unchanged in urine by active tubular secretion moderated by pH dependent tubular reabsorption. Remainder metabolized; metabolites are not pharmacologically active.
Half-life: 60–80 hr.

TIME/ACTION PROFILE (plasma concentrations)

ROUTE	ONSET	PEAK	DURATION
PO	unknown	3–7 hr	12 hr
PO-ER	unknown	9–12 hr	24 hr

Contraindications/Precautions
Contraindicated in: Hypersensitivity.
Use Cautiously in: Severe renal impairment (↓ dose); Severe hepatic impairment; Concurrent use of other NMDA antagonists (amantadine, rimantadine, ketamine, dextromethorphan); Conditions that ↑ urine pH including severe urinary tract infections or renal tubular acidosis (lead to ↓ excretion and ↑ levels); OB: Safety not established in pregnancy; Lactation: Use while breastfeeding only if potential maternal benefit justifies potential risk to infant; Pedi: Safety and effectiveness not established in children.

Adverse Reactions/Side Effects
CV: hypertension. **Derm:** rash. **GI:** diarrhea. **GU:** urinary frequency. **Hemat:** anemia. **Metab:** weight gain. **Neuro:** dizziness, fatigue, headache, sedation.

Interactions
Drug-Drug: Medications that ↑ urine pH (e.g. **carbonic anhydrase inhibitors, sodium bicarbonate**) may ↓ excretion and ↑ levels and risk of toxicity.

Route/Dosage
PO (Adults): *Immediate release:* 5 mg once daily initially; ↑ at weekly intervals to 10 mg/day (5 mg twice daily), then 15 mg/day (5 mg once daily, 10 mg once daily as separate doses), then to target dose of 20 mg/day (10 mg twice daily); *Extended release:* 7 mg once daily, ↑ at weekly intervals by 7 mg/day to target dose of 28 mg once daily.

Renal Impairment
(Adults): *CCr 5–29 mL/min:* Immediate release (solution): Target dose is 10 mg/day (5 mg twice daily); Extended release: Target dose is 14 mg once daily.

Availability (generic available)
Immediate-release tablets: 5 mg, 10 mg. **Extended-release capsules:** 7 mg, 14 mg, 21 mg, 28 mg. **Oral solution, sugar-free, alcohol-free (peppermint):** 2 mg/mL. ***In combination with:*** donepezil (Namzaric). See Appendix N.

NURSING IMPLICATIONS
Assessment
- Assess cognitive function (memory, attention, reasoning, language, ability to perform simple tasks) at baseline and periodically during therapy.
- Assess fall risk by evaluating history of falls, mobility, balance, strength, medications, vision, cognition, and home environment.

Lab Test Considerations
- May cause anemia.

Implementation
- Do not confuse memantine with methadone.
- Dose ↑ should occur no more frequently than weekly.
- To switch from *immediate release* to *extended release*, patients taking 10 mg twice daily of *immediate release* tablets may be switched to *extended release* 28 mg once daily capsules the day following the last dose of a 10 mg *immediate release* tablet. Patients with renal impairment may use the same procedure to switch from *immediate release* 5 mg twice daily to *extended release* 14 mg once daily.
- Discontinuation of therapy may result in worsening of cognitive function. Avoid abrupt discontinuation to minimize withdrawal symptoms (altered mental status, hallucinations, delusions, insomnia, increased anxiety, agitation). To taper memantine, use a 50% dose ↓ or stepwise ↓ via available dose formulations every 4 wk to lowest dose prior to discontinuation. Consider reinitiation if clear worsening of the condition occurs after withdrawal.
- **PO:** May be administered without regard to food.
- Administer oral solution using syringe provided. Do not dilute or mix with other fluids. Slowly squirt into corner of patient's mouth.
- ***DNC:*** Swallow extended release capsules whole; do not crush, chew, or divide. Capsules may be opened, sprinkled on applesauce, and swallowed. Entire contents of each capsule should be consumed; do not divide dose.

Patient/Family Teaching
- Explain the purpose and side effects. Instruct patient and caregiver on how and when to administer memantine and how to titrate dose. Take missed doses as soon as remembered but not just before

next dose; do not double doses. If several days of doses are missed, may need to resume at a lower dose and retitrate up to previous dose; consult health care provider. Advise patient and caregiver to read *Patient Instructions* before starting and with each Rx refill in case of changes.

- Caution patient and caregiver that memantine may cause dizziness. Monitor and assist with ambulation and caution patient to avoid driving and other activities requiring alertness until response to medication is known.
- Advise patient and caregiver to notify health care provider of all Rx or OTC medications, vitamins, or herbal products being taken and to consult with health care provider before taking other medications.
- Teach patient and caregivers that improvement in cognitive functioning may take months; degenerative process is not reversed.
- Rep: May cause fetal harm. Advise women of reproductive potential to notify health care provider if pregnancy is planned or suspected or if breastfeeding.

Evaluation/Desired Outcomes

- Improvement in neurocognitive decline (memory, attention, reasoning, language, ability to perform simple tasks) in patients with Alzheimer disease.

BEERS REMS HIGH ALERT

meperidine (me-per-i-deen)

Demerol

Classification

Therapeutic: opioid analgesics

Pharmacologic: opioid agonists

Schedule II

Indications

Moderate or severe pain (as monotherapy or in combination with nonopioid agents). Anesthesia adjunct. Analgesic during labor. Preoperative sedation. **Unlabeled Use:** Rigors.

Action

Binds to opiate receptors in the CNS. Alters the perception of and response to painful stimuli while producing generalized CNS depression. **Therapeutic Effects:** Reduction in severity of pain.

Pharmacokinetics

Absorption: 50% from the GI tract; well absorbed from IM sites. Oral doses are about half as effective as parenteral doses. IV administration results in complete bioavailability.

Distribution: Widely distributed to tissues.

Metabolism and Excretion: Mostly metabolized by the liver; some converted to normeperidine, which may accumulate and cause seizures. 5% excreted unchanged by the kidneys.

Half-life: *Neonates:* 12–39 hr; *Infants 3–18 mo:* 2.3 hr; *Children 5–8 yr:* 3 hr; *Adults:* 2.5–4 hr (↑ in impaired renal or hepatic function [7–11 hr]).

TIME/ACTION PROFILE (analgesia)

ROUTE	ONSET	PEAK	DURATION
PO	15 min	60 min	2–4 hr
IM	10–15 min	30–50 min	2–4 hr
SUBQ	10–15 min	40–60 min	2–4 hr
IV	immediate	5–7 min	2–3 hr

Contraindications/Precautions

Contraindicated in: Hypersensitivity; Hypersensitivity to bisulfites (some injectable products); Recent (within 14 days) MAO inhibitor therapy; Severe respiratory impairment; OB: Labor and delivery; Lactation: Lactation.

Use Cautiously in: Personal or family history of substance use disorder or mental illness; Head trauma; ↑ intracranial pressure; Severe renal or hepatic impairment; Acute asthma attack, COPD, hypoxia, or hypercapnea; Hypothyroidism; Adrenal insufficiency; Debilitated patients (dose ↓ suggested); Undiagnosed abdominal pain or prostatic hyperplasia; Extensive burns; High-dose or prolonged therapy (>600 mg/day or >2 days; ↑ risk of CNS stimulation and seizures due to accumulation of normeperidine); Sickle cell anemia (may require ↓ initial doses); OB: Use during pregnancy only if potential maternal benefit justifies potential fetal risk. Chronic maternal treatment with opioids during pregnancy may result in neonatal opioid withdrawal syndrome; Pedi: Syrup contains benzyl alcohol, which can cause gasping syndrome in neonates. Children have ↑ risk of seizures due to accumulation of normeperidine; Geri: Appears on Beers list. ↑ risk of delirium in older adults. Avoid use in older adults.

Adverse Reactions/Side Effects

CV: hypotension, bradycardia. **Derm:** flushing, sweating. **EENT:** blurred vision, diplopia, miosis. **Endo:** adrenal insufficiency. **GI:** constipation, nausea, vomiting. **GU:** urinary retention. **Neuro:** confusion, sedation, dysphoria, euphoria, floating feeling, hallucinations, headache, SEIZURES, unusual dreams. **Resp:** RESPIRATORY DEPRESSION (INCLUDING CENTRAL SLEEP APNEA OR SLEEP-RELATED HYPOXEMIA). **Misc:** allodynia, HYPERSENSITIVITY REACTIONS (INCLUDING ANAPHYLAXIS), opioid-induced hyperalgesia, physical dependence, psychological dependence, tolerance.

M

Interactions

Drug-Drug: Do not use in patients receiving **MAO inhibitors** or **procarbazine**; may cause fatal reaction; contraindicated within 14 days of MAO inhibitor therapy. Use with **benzodiazepines** or other **CNS depressants**, including other **opioids**, **nonbenzodiazepine sedative/hypnotics**, **anxiolytics**, **general anesthetics**, **muscle relaxants**, **antipsychotics**, and **alcohol**, may cause profound sedation, respiratory depression, coma, and death; reserve concurrent use for when alternative treatment options are inadequate. **Mixed agonist/antagonist analgesics**, including **nalbuphine** or **butorphanol**, or **partial agonist analgesics**, including **buprenorphine**, may ↓ meperidine's analgesic effects and/or precipitate opioid withdrawal in physically dependent patients. **CYP3A4 inhibitors**, including **ritonavir**, **ketoconazole**, **itraconazole**, **fluconazole**, **clarithromycin**, **erythromycin**, **nefazodone**, **diltiazem**, **verapamil**, **nelfinavir**, and **fosamprenavir**, may ↑ levels and risk of opioid toxicity; careful monitoring during initiation, dose changes, or discontinuation of the inhibitor is recommended. **CYP3A4 inducers**, including **barbiturates**, **carbamazepine**, **efavirenz**, **corticosteroids**, **modafinil**, **nevirapine**, **oxcarbazepine**, **phenobarbital**, **phenytoin**, **rifabutin**, or **rifampin**, may ↓ levels and analgesia; if inducers are discontinued or dosage ↓, patients should be monitored for signs of opioid toxicity and necessary dose adjustments should be made. **Chlorpromazine** and **thioridazine** may ↑ risk of adverse reactions; avoid concurrent use. May aggravate side effects of **isoniazid**. **Acyclovir** may ↑ levels of meperidine and normeperidine. Drugs that affect serotonergic neurotransmitter systems, including **tricyclic antidepressants**, **SSRIs**, **SNRIs**, **MAO inhibitors**, **TCAs**, **tramadol**, **trazodone**, **mirtazapine**, **5-HT_3 receptor antagonists**, **linezolid**, **methylene blue**, and **triptans**, may ↑ risk of serotonin syndrome.

Drug-Natural Products: Kava-kava, **valerian**, or **chamomile** can ↓ risk of CNS depression. **St. John's wort** may ↓ levels and analgesia; concurrent use not recommended.

Route/Dosage

PO (Adults): *Analgesia:* 50–150 mg every 3–4 hr; may ↑ as needed (not to exceed 600 mg/24 hr).

IM, SUBQ (Adults): *Analgesia:* 50–150 mg every 3–4 hr; may ↑ as needed (not to exceed 600 mg/24 hr). *Analgesia during labor:* 50–100 mg when contractions become regular; may repeat every 1–3 hr. *Preoperative sedation:* 50–100 mg 30–90 min before anesthesia.

PO (Children): *Analgesia:* 1.1–1.8 mg/kg every 3–4 hr (max = 100 mg/dose).

IM, SUBQ (Children): *Analgesia:* 1.1–1.8 mg/kg every 3–4 hr (max = 100 mg/dose). *Preoperative sedation:* 1.1–2.2 mg/kg 30–90 min before anesthesia (not to exceed adult dose).

IV (Adults): 15–35 mg/hr as a continuous infusion; *PCA:* 10 mg initially; with a range of 1–5 mg/incremental dose, recommended lockout interval is 6–10 min (minimum 5 min).

IV (Children): *Continuous infusion:* 0.5–1 mg/kg loading dose followed by 0.3 mg/kg/hr; titrate to effect up to 0.5–0.7 mg/kg/hr.

Availability (generic available)

Tablets: 50 mg. **Oral solution (banana flavor):** 50 mg/5 mL. **Solution for injection:** 25 mg/mL, 50 mg/mL, 75 mg/mL, 100 mg/mL.

NURSING IMPLICATIONS

Assessment

- Assess type, location, and intensity of pain prior to and 1 hr following PO, SUBQ, and IM doses and 5 min (peak) following IV administration. When titrating opioid doses, ↑ of 25–50% should be administered until there is either a 50% ↓ in the patient's pain rating on a numerical or visual analogue scale or the patient reports satisfactory pain relief. A repeat dose can be safely administered at the time of the peak if previous dose is ineffective and side effects are minimal.
- An equianalgesic chart (see Appendix I) should be used when changing routes or when changing from one opioid to another.
- Assess BP, HR, and respiratory rate before and periodically during administration. If respiratory rate <10/min, assess level of sedation. Dose may need to be ↓ by 25–50%. Respiratory depression does not ↑ in severity, only in duration, with ↑ dose. Monitor for respiratory depression, especially during initiation or following dose ↑; serious, life-threatening, or fatal respiratory depression may occur. May cause sleep-related breathing disorders (central sleep apnea, sleep-related hypoxemia).
- Assess bowel function routinely. Institute prevention of constipation with ↑ intake of fluids and bulk and laxatives to minimize constipating effects. Administer stimulant laxatives routinely if opioid use exceeds 2–3 days, unless contraindicated. Consider drugs for opioid-induced constipation.
- Prolonged use may lead to physical and psychological dependence and tolerance, which should not prevent patient from receiving adequate analgesia. Patients who receive meperidine for pain rarely develop psychological dependence. Progressively higher doses may be required to relieve pain with long-term therapy.
- Monitor patients on chronic or high-dose therapy for CNS stimulation (restlessness, irritability, seizures) due to accumulation of normeperidine metabolite. Risk of toxicity ↑ with doses >600 mg/24 hr, chronic administration (>2 days), and renal impairment.

- Prolonged use may lead to physical and psychological dependence and tolerance. This should not prevent patient from receiving adequate analgesia. Patients who receive opioids for pain rarely develop psychological dependence. If progressively higher doses are required, consider conversion to a stronger opioid. Prolonged use of opioids should be reserved for patients whose pain remains severe enough to require them and alternative treatment options continue to be inadequate. Many acute pain conditions treated in the outpatient setting require no more than a few days of an opioid pain medicine.
- Assess risk for opioid addiction, abuse, or misuse prior to administration.
- Geri: Meperidine has been reported to cause delirium in older adults; older adults are at ↑ risk for normeperidine toxicity. Monitor frequently.
- Pedi: Assess pediatric patient frequently; neonates, infants, and children are more sensitive to the effects of opioid analgesics and may experience respiratory complications, excitability, and restlessness more frequently.
- Assess for opioid-induced hyperalgesia, which can appear as ↑ levels of pain upon increasing the dose of the opioid, ↓ levels of pain on decreasing the dose of the opioid, or pain from ordinarily nonpainful stimuli (allodynia). This condition is different from tolerance. If a patient is suspected to be experiencing opioid-induced hyperalgesia, consider ↓ the dose of the current opioid or switching to a different opioid analgesic.

Lab Test Considerations

- May ↑ amylase and lipase.

Toxicity and Overdose

- If an opioid antagonist is required to reverse respiratory depression or coma, naloxone is the antidote to improve respiratory function without reversing analgesia. Dilute the 0.4-mg ampule of naloxone in 10 mL of 0.9% NaCl and administer 0.5 mL (0.02 mg) by IV push every 2 min. For children and patients weighing <40 kg, dilute 0.1 mg of naloxone in 10 mL of 0.9% NaCl for a concentration of 10 mcg/mL and administer 0.5 mcg/kg every 2 min. Titrate dose to avoid withdrawal, seizures, and severe pain. In patients receiving meperidine chronically, naloxone may precipitate seizures by eliminating the CNS depressant effects of meperidine, allowing the convulsant activity of normeperidine to predominate. Monitor patient closely.

Implementation

- ***High Alert:*** Accidental overdose of opioid analgesics has resulted in fatalities. Before administering, clarify all ambiguous orders; have second practitioner independently check original order, dose calculations, and infusion pump settings. Pedi: Medication errors with opioid analgesics are common in the pediatric population and include misinterpretation or miscalculation of doses and use of inappropriate measuring devices.
- Explain therapeutic value of medication prior to administration to enhance the analgesic effect.
- Regularly administered doses may be more effective than as needed administration. Analgesic is more effective if given before pain becomes severe.
- Coadministration with nonopioid analgesics may have additive analgesic effects and permit lower doses.
- Oral dose is <50% as effective as parenteral dose. When changing to oral administration, dose may need to be ↑ (see Appendix I).
- Medication should be discontinued gradually after long-term use to prevent withdrawal symptoms. For patients who are physically opioid dependent, initiate the taper by a small enough increment (no greater than 25–50% of total daily dose) to avoid withdrawal symptoms, and proceed with dose-lowering at an interval of every 2–4 days. Patients who have been taking opioids for briefer periods of time may tolerate a more rapid taper. Monitor frequently to manage pain and withdrawal symptoms (restlessness; lacrimation; rhinorrhea; yawning; perspiration; chills; myalgia; mydriasis; irritability; anxiety; backache; joint pain; weakness; abdominal cramps; insomnia; nausea; anorexia; vomiting; diarrhea; or ↑ BP, respiratory rate, or HR). If withdrawal symptoms occur, pause the taper for a period of time or ↑ dose of opioid analgesic to previous dose, and then proceed with a slower taper. Also, monitor patients for changes in mood, emergence of suicidal thoughts, or use of other substances. A multimodal approach to pain management may optimize the treatment of chronic pain and assist with the successful tapering of the opioid analgesic.
- May be administered via PCA pump.
- **PO:** Doses may be administered with food or milk to minimize GI irritation. Dilute syrup in half-full glass of water.
- **IM** Patient should be lying down when administered; IM is the preferred route for repeated doses. SUBQ administration may cause tissue irritation.
- ***REMS:*** FDA strongly encourages health care providers to complete a REMS-compliant education program that includes all the elements of the FDA Education *Blueprint for Health Care Providers Involved in the Management or Support of Patients with Pain,* available at www.fda.gov/OpioidAnalgesicREMSBlueprint. Information on programs can be found at 1-800-503-0784 or www.opioidanalgesicrems.com.
- Discuss availability of naloxone for emergency treatment of opioid overdose with the patient and caregiver and assess the potential need for access to naloxone, both when initiating and renewing

M

therapy, especially if patient has household members (including children) or other close contacts at risk for accidental exposure or overdose. Consider prescribing naloxone, based on the patient's risk factors for overdose, such as concurrent use of CNS depressants, a history of opioid use disorder, or prior opioid overdose. However, the presence of risk factors for overdose should not prevent the proper management of pain in any patient.

IV Administration

- **IV Push:** Administer undiluted. **Rate:** ***High Alert:*** Administer slowly over ≥5 min. Rapid administration may lead to ↑ respiratory depression, hypotension, and circulatory collapse.
- **Intermittent Infusion: Dilution:** Dilute with D5W, D10W, dextrose/saline combinations, dextrose/Ringer's or LR injection combinations, 0.45% NaCl, 0.9% NaCl, or LR. Administer via infusion pump. **Concentration:** 1 mg/mL. **Rate:** Administer over 15–30 min
- **Y-Site Compatibility:** acetaminophen, alemtuzumab, amikacin, aminocaproic acid, aminophylline, amiodarone, anidulafungin, argatroban, arsenic trioxide, ascorbic acid, atracurium, atropine, azithromycin, aztreonam, benztropine, bivalirudin, bleomycin, bumetanide, buprenorphine, busulfan, butorphanol, calcium chloride, calcium gluconate, cangrelor, carboplatin, carmustine, caspofungin, cefazolin, cefotaxime, cefoxitin, ceftaroline, ceftazidime, ceftolozane/tazobactam, ceftriaxone, cefuroxime, chlorpromazine, ciprofloxacin, cisatracurium, cisplatin, cladribine, clindamycin, cyanocobalamin, cyclophosphamide, cyclosporine, cytarabine, dacarbazine, dactinomycin, daptomycin, daunorubicin, dexmedetomidine, dexrazoxane, digoxin, diltiazem, diphenhydramine, dobutamine, docetaxel, dopamine, doxorubicin hydrochloride, doxycycline, droperidol, enalaprilat, ephedrine, epinephrine, epirubicin, epoetin alfa, eptifibatide, ertapenem, erythromycin, esmolol, etoposide, etoposide phosphate, famotidine, fentanyl, filgrastim, fluconazole, fludarabine, fluorouracil, folic acid, foscarnet, fosphenytoin, gemcitabine, gentamicin, glycopyrrolate, granisetron, hetastarch, hydrocortisone, ifosfamide, insulin, regular, irinotecan, isavuconazonium, isoproterenol, ketamine, ketorolac, labetalol, LR, leucovorin, levofloxacin, lidocaine, linezolid, mannitol, melphalan, meropenem/vaborbactam, mesna, methotrexate, metoclopramide, metoprolol, metronidazole, midazolam, milrinone, mitomycin, mitoxantrone, morphine, multivitamins, mycophenolate, nalbuphine, naloxone, nicardipine, nitroglycerin, nitroprusside, norepinephrine, octreotide, ondansetron, oxaliplatin, oxytocin, paclitaxel, palonosetron, pamidronate, papaverine, pemetrexed, penicillin G, pentamidine, phentolamine, phenylephrine, phytonadione, piperacillin/tazobactam, plazomicin, potassium acetate, potassium chloride, procainamide, prochlorperazine, promethazine, propofol, propranolol, protamine, pyridoxine, remifentanil, rituximab, rocuronium, sargramostim, sodium acetate, succinylcholine, sufentanil, sulbactam/durlobactam, tacrolimus, tedizolid, theophylline, thiamine, thiotepa, tigecycline, tirofiban, tobramycin, topotecan, trastuzumab, vancomycin, vasopressin, vecuronium, verapamil, vinblastine, vincristine, vinorelbine, voriconazole, zidovudine, zoledronic acid.
- **Y-Site Incompatibility:** allopurinol, amphotericin B deoxycholate, amphotericin B liposomal, azathioprine, cefepime, dantrolene, diazepam, diazoxide, ganciclovir, gemtuzumab ozogamicin, idarubicin, indomethacin, lorazepam, micafungin, nafcillin, pantoprazole, pentobarbital, phenobarbital, phenytoin, sodium bicarbonate.

Patient/Family Teaching

- Explain purpose and side effects of meperidine to patient. Advise patient to not share medication with others, even if they have similar symptoms; may be harmful. Advise patient to read *Patient Information* before starting and with each Rx refill in case of changes.
- ***REMS:*** Instruct patient to take meperidine as directed. If dose is less effective after a few wk, do not ↑ dose without consulting health care provider. Discuss safe use, risks, and proper storage and disposal of opioid analgesics with patients and caregivers with each Rx. The *Patient Counseling Guide* is available at www.fda.gov/OpioidAnalgesicREMSPCG.
- Teach parents or caregivers how to accurately measure liquid medication and to use only the measuring device dispensed with the medication
- Advise patient that meperidine is a drug with known abuse potential. Protect it from theft, and never give to anyone other than the individual for whom it was prescribed. Store out of sight and reach of children and in a location not accessible by others.
- May cause drowsiness or dizziness. Advise patient to call for assistance when ambulating and to avoid driving or other activities that require alertness until response to the medication is known.
- Educate patients and caregivers on how to recognize respiratory depression and emphasize the importance of calling 911 or getting emergency medical help right away in the event of a known or suspected overdose. Inform patients and caregivers about various ways to obtain naloxone as permitted by individual state naloxone-dispensing and prescribing requirements or guidelines (Rx, direct from pharmacist, or state programs). OTC naloxone nasal spray is available at pharmacies nationwide for overdose or accidental ingestion.
- Advise patient to change positions slowly to minimize orthostatic hypotension.

- Instruct patient to avoid concurrent use of alcohol or other CNS depressants; may lead to overdose.
- Instruct patient to notify health care provider of all Rx or OTC medications, vitamins, or herbal products being taken and consult health care provider before taking any new medications.
- Advise ambulatory patients that nausea and vomiting may be ↓ by lying down.
- Encourage patient to turn, cough, and breathe deeply every 2 hr to prevent atelectasis.
- Rep: May cause fetal harm. Advise women of reproductive potential to notify health care provider if pregnancy is planned or suspected and to avoid breastfeeding. Inform patient of potential for neonatal opioid withdrawal syndrome with prolonged use during pregnancy. Monitor neonate for signs and symptoms of withdrawal symptoms (irritability, hyperactivity and abnormal sleep pattern, high-pitched cry, tremor, vomiting, diarrhea, failure to gain weight); usually occur the first days after birth. Monitor infants exposed to meperidine through breast milk for excess sedation and respiratory depression. Chronic use may ↓ fertility in women and men.

Evaluation/Desired Outcomes

- Decrease in severity of pain without a significant alteration in level of consciousness or respiratory status.
- Resolution of rigors.

mepolizumab

(me-poe-**liz**-ue-mab)

Nucala

Classification

Therapeutic: antiasthmatics

Pharmacologic: monoclonal antibodies, interleukin antagonists

Indications

Severe asthma that is of an eosinophilic phenotype (as add-on maintenance treatment). Eosinophilic granulomatosis with polyangiitis. Hypereosinophilic syndrome with a duration of ≥6 mo that has no identifiable nonhematologic secondary cause. Chronic rhinosinusitis with nasal polyps in patients with an inadequate response to nasal corticosteroids (as add-on maintenance treatment). Chronic obstructive pulmonary disease (COPD) that is of an eosinophilic phenotype and is inadequately controlled.

Action

Interleukin-5 (IL-5) antagonist that inhibits binding of IL-5 to the surface of the eosinophil, which reduces the production and survival of eosinophils.

Therapeutic Effects: Decreased incidence of asthma and COPD exacerbations and reduction in use of maintenance oral corticosteroid therapy. Prolonged duration of remission and reduction in use of maintenance oral corticosteroid therapy in eosinophilic granulomatosis with polyangiitis. Reduction in hypereosinophilic syndrome flares. Reduction in nasal polyps and nasal obstruction.

Pharmacokinetics

Absorption: 80% absorbed following SUBQ administration.

Distribution: Minimally distributed to tissues.

Metabolism and Excretion: Degraded by proteolytic enzymes located throughout the body.

Half-life: 16–22 days.

TIME/ACTION PROFILE (plasma concentrations)

ROUTE	ONSET	PEAK	DURATION
SUBQ	unknown	unknown	unknown

Contraindications/Precautions

Contraindicated in: Hypersensitivity; Acute bronchospasm or status asthmaticus.

Use Cautiously in: OB: Safety not established in pregnancy; expected to cross the placenta (potential effects likely to be greater during 2nd and 3rd trimesters); Lactation: Safety not established in breastfeeding; Pedi: Safety and effectiveness not established in children <18 yr (eosinophilic granulomatosis with polyangiitis), <12 yr (hypereosinophilic syndrome), or <6 yr (severe asthma of an eosinophilic phenotype).

Adverse Reactions/Side Effects

Derm: flushing, rash. **Local:** injection site reactions. **MS:** back pain, myalgia. **Neuro:** <u>headache</u>, fatigue. **Misc:** herpes zoster infection, HYPERSENSITIVITY REACTIONS (INCLUDING ANAPHYLAXIS AND ANGIOEDEMA).

Interactions

Drug-Drug: None reported.

Route/Dosage

Severe Asthma

SUBQ (Adults and Children ≥12 yr): 100 mg every 4 wk.

SUBQ (Children 6–11 yr): 40 mg every 4 wk.

Eosinophilic Granulomatosis with Polyangiitis

SUBQ (Adults): 300 mg every 4 wk.

Hypereosinophilic Syndrome

SUBQ (Adults and Children ≥12 yr): 300 mg every 4 wk.

Chronic Rhinosinusitis With Nasal Polyps or COPD

SUBQ (Adults): 100 mg every 4 wk.

Availability

Lyophilized powder for injection: 100 mg/vial. **Solution for injection:** 40 mg/0.4 mL (prefilled syringes), 100 mg/mL (prefilled autoinjectors and prefilled syringes).

NURSING IMPLICATIONS

Assessment

- Assess respiratory status (rate, breath sounds, degree of dyspnea, pulse) periodically during therapy.
- Monitor for signs and symptoms of hypersensitivity, including anaphylaxis (angioedema, bronchospasm, urticaria, rash), following injection. Reactions usually occur within hours but may have a delayed onset (days). *If hypersensitivity reaction occurs,* discontinue mepolizumab.
- Assess for and treat parasitic infections prior to therapy. *If infected during therapy and unresponsive to antihelminth treatment,* discontinue mepolizumab until infection resolves.

Implementation

- Only administer in a health care setting by a health care provider able to manage anaphylaxis. Do not use to treat acute bronchospasm or status asthmaticus.
- Consider administration of varicella vaccination prior to starting therapy.
- Do not abruptly stop systemic or inhaled corticosteroids when starting therapy; may taper gradually under direct supervision of health care provider.
- **Reconstitution:** Reconstitute with 1.2 mL of sterile water for injection using a 2- or 3-mL syringe and a 21-gauge needle. **Concentration:** 100 mg/mL. Direct stream into center of cake. Swirl gently for 10 sec until powder is dissolved; do not shake. Reconstitution takes ≥5 min. Solution is clear to opalescent and colorless to pale yellow or pale brown; do not administer if discolored, cloudy, or contains particles. Stable for 8 hr if refrigerated.
- **SUBQ:** Using a 21- to 27-gauge needle, administer 1 mL for a 100-mg dose or 0.4 mL for a 40-mg dose once every 4 wk into upper arm, thigh, or abdomen. Avoid areas that are tender, bruised, red, or hard. The 100-mg/mL prefilled autoinjector and prefilled syringe are for use by adults and children ≥12 yr. The 40-mg/0.4-mL prefilled syringe is for children 6–11 yr (must be administered by health care provider or caregiver).
- Bring prefilled autoinjector to room temperature ≥30 min before injection.
- 300 mg dose must be given as three separate 100-mg injections ≥2 inches apart.

Patient/Family Teaching

- Explain purpose and side effects of medication. Advise patient to read *Patient Information* before starting therapy. Administer missed doses as soon as possible; if next dose is already due, administer as planned.
- May be self-administered by adults and adolescents ≥12 using the prefilled autoinjector and prefilled syringe. Teach the appropriate administration technique and disposal of equipment, if self-administration is appropriate.
- Inform patient of risk and signs and symptoms of anaphylaxis. Instruct patient to notify health care provider immediately if signs and symptoms of hypersensitivity reactions (swelling of face, mouth, or tongue; fainting; dizziness; hives; breathing problems; rash) occur.
- Advise patient to notify health care provider if asthma remains uncontrolled or worsens after starting therapy.
- Caution patient not to ↓ corticosteroid dose unless instructed by health care provider.
- Instruct patient to notify health care provider of all Rx or OTC medications, vitamins, or herbal products being taken and consult health care provider before taking any new medications.
- Rep: Advise women of reproductive potential to notify health care provider if pregnancy is planned or suspected and to avoid breastfeeding during therapy.

Evaluation/Desired Outcomes

- Decreased incidence of asthma or COPD exacerbations and reduction in use of maintenance oral corticosteroid therapy.
- Reduction in hypereosinophilic syndrome flares.
- Reduction in nasal polyps and nasal obstruction.

meropenem (mer-oh-**pen**-nem)

~~Merrem~~

Classification

Therapeutic: anti-infectives

Pharmacologic: carbapenems

Indications

Complicated skin and skin structure infections. Complicated intra-abdominal infections. Bacterial meningitis. **Unlabeled Use:** Febrile neutropenia. Hospital-acquired pneumonia and sepsis.

Action

Inhibits bacterial cell wall synthesis. Meropenem resists the actions of many enzymes that degrade most other penicillins and penicillin-like anti-infectives. **Therapeutic Effects:** Bactericidal action against susceptible bacteria. **Spectrum:** Active against the following gram-positive organisms: *Staphylococcus aureus*, *Streptococcus agalactiae*, *Streptococcus pneumoniae*, *Streptococcus pyogenes*, viridans group streptococci, *Enterococcus faecalis*. Also active against the following gram-negative pathogens: *Escherichia coli*, *Haemophilus influenzae*, *Klebsiella pneumoniae*, *Neisseria meningitidis*, *Proteus mirabilis*, *Pseudomonas aeruginosa*. Active against the following anaerobes: *Bacteroides fragilis*, *Bacteroides thetaiotaomicron*, *Peptostreptococcus spp.*

Pharmacokinetics

Absorption: IV administration results in complete bioavailability.
Distribution: Widely distributed to tissues; enters CSF when meninges are inflamed.
Metabolism and Excretion: Primarily metabolized by the liver; 50–75% excreted unchanged by the kidneys.
Half-life: *Premature neonates:* 3 hr; *Term neonates:* 2 hr; *Infants (3 mo–2 yr)* 1.4 hr; *Children >2 yr and Adults:* 1 hr (↑ in renal impairment).

TIME/ACTION PROFILE (plasma concentrations)

ROUTE	ONSET	PEAK	DURATION
IV	rapid	end of infusion	8 hr

Contraindications/Precautions

Contraindicated in: Hypersensitivity to meropenem or imipenem; Serious hypersensitivity to other beta-lactams (penicillins or cephalosporins; cross-sensitivity may occur).
Use Cautiously in: Renal impairment (↑ risk of thrombocytopenia and seizures; ↓ dose if CCr <50 mL/min); History of seizures, brain lesions, or meningitis; OB: Safety not established in pregnancy; Lactation: Use during breastfeeding only if potential maternal benefit outweighs potential risk to infant; Pedi: Children <3 mo (safety and effectiveness not established for complicated skin/skin structure infections and meningitis).

Adverse Reactions/Side Effects

Derm: acute generalized exanthematous pustulosis, DRUG REACTION WITH EOSINOPHILIA AND SYSTEMIC SYMPTOMS (DRESS), ERYTHEMA MULTIFORME, moniliasis (children only), pruritus, rash, STEVENS-JOHNSON SYNDROME (SJS), TOXIC EPIDERMAL NECROLYSIS (TEN). **GI:** diarrhea, nausea, vomiting, CLOSTRIDIOIDES DIFFICILE-ASSOCIATED DIARRHEA (CDAD), constipation, glossitis (↑ in children), thrush (↑ in children). **Hemat:** thrombocytopenia (↑ in renal impairment). **Local:** inflammation at injection site, phlebitis. **MS:** RHABDOMYOLYSIS. **Neuro:** dizziness, headache, paresthesias, SEIZURES. **Resp:** APNEA. **Misc:** HYPERSENSITIVITY REACTIONS (INCLUDING ANAPHYLAXIS).

Interactions

Drug-Drug: Probenecid ↓ renal excretion and ↑ levels; concurrent use not recommended. May ↓ serum **valproate** levels and ↑ risk of seizures.

Route/Dosage

Complicated Skin/Skin Structure Infections

IV (Adults): 500 mg every 8 hr or 1 g every 8 hr (if caused by *Pseudomonas aeruginosa*).
IV (Children ≥3 mo–12 yr): 10 mg/kg (max dose = 500 mg) every 8 hr or 20 mg/kg (max dose = 1 g) every 8 hr (if caused by *Pseudomonas aeruginosa*).

Renal Impairment

IV (Adults): *CCr 26–50 mL/min:* 500 mg every 12 hr; *CCr 10–25 mL/min:* 250 mg every 12 hr; *CCr <10 mL/min:* 250 mg every 24 hr.

Intra-abdominal Infections

IV (Adults): 1 g every 8 hr.
IV (Children ≥3 mo–12 yr): 20 mg/kg (max dose = 1 g) every 8 hr.
IV (Children <3 mo): *<32 wk gestational age (GA) and postnatal age (PNA) <2 wk:* 20 mg/kg every 12 hr; *<32 wk GA and PNA ≥2 wk:* 20 mg/kg every 8 hr; *≥32 wk GA and PNA <2 wk:* 20 mg/kg every 8 hr; *≥32 wk GA and PNA ≥2 wk:* 30 mg/kg every 8 hr.

Renal Impairment

IV (Adults): *CCr 26–50 mL/min:* 1 g every 12 hr; *CCr 10–25 mL/min:* 500 mg every 12 hr; *CCr <10 mL/min:* 500 mg every 24 hr.

Bacterial Meningitis

IV (Children ≥3 mo): 40 mg/kg (max dose = 2 g) every 8 hr.

Availability (generic available)

Powder for injection: 500 mg/vial, 1 g/vial, 2 g/vial.
Premixed infusion: 500 mg/50 mL 0.9% NaCl, 1 g/50 mL 0.9% NaCl.

NURSING IMPLICATIONS

Assessment

- Assess for infection (vital signs; appearance of wound, sputum, urine, and stool; WBC) at beginning of and throughout therapy.
- Obtain a history before initiating therapy to determine previous use of and reactions to penicillins.
- Monitor for diarrhea, abdominal pain, fever, and bloody stools. *If CDAD suspected,* discontinue meropenem and treat as clinically indicated. May begin up to several weeks following cessation of therapy.
- Observe for signs/symptoms of anaphylaxis (rash, pruritus, laryngeal edema, wheezing). *If symptoms occur,* immediately discontinue therapy and provide appropriate medical care. Have epinephrine, an antihistamine, and resuscitative equipment close by.
- Assess for severe cutaneous adverse reactions, including SJS, TEN, and DRESS, during therapy. *If rash or other signs/symptoms suggestive of these reactions occur,* immediately discontinue meropenem, treat as indicated, and consider alternate therapy.
- Assess for history of CNS disorders, including seizures. *If focal tremors, myoclonus, or seizures occur,* place patient on anticonvulsant therapy as

needed and assess need to ↓ meropenem dose or discontinue therapy.

- Monitor for signs and symptoms of rhabdomyolysis. *If signs of symptoms of rhabdomyolysis occur,* discontinue therapy and treat as indicated.
- Assess injection site for phlebitis, pain, and swelling periodically during administration.

Lab Test Considerations

- Obtain specimens for culture and sensitivity prior to initiating therapy. 1st dose may be given before receiving results.
- May cause transient ↑ in AST, ALT, LDH, alkaline phosphatase, bilirubin, BUN, and serum creatinine, as well as hematuria.
- May cause hypokalemia.
- May ↑ or ↓ platelets WBC, and may ↓ hemoglobin and hematocrit.
- May cause shortened prothrombin time and partial thromboplastin time.
- May cause positive direct or indirect Coombs test.

Implementation

IV Administration

- **IV Push: Reconstitution:** Reconstitute 500-mg and 1-g vials with 10 mL and 20 mL, respectively, of sterile water for injection. **Concentration:** 50 mg/mL. **Rate:** Administer over 3–5 min.
- **Intermittent Infusion: Reconstitution:** Reconstitute 500-mg and 1-g vials with 10 mL and 20 mL, respectively, of sterile water for injection, 0.9% NaCl, or D5W. Vials reconstituted with sterile water for injection are stable for 3 hr at room temperature or 13 hr if refrigerated; if reconstituted with 0.9% NaCl, stable for 1 hr at room temperature or 15 hr if refrigerated; if reconstituted with D5W, use immediately. **Dilution:** Further dilute in 0.9% NaCl or D5W. Infusions further diluted in 0.9% NaCl are stable for 4 hr at room temperature or 24 hr if refrigerated. Infusions further diluted in D5W are stable for 1 hr at room temperature or 4 hr if refrigerated. **Concentration:** 1–20 mg/mL. **Rate:** Infuse over 15–30 min
- **Y-Site Compatibility:** acetaminophen, acetylcysteine, albumin, human, alemtuzumab, amikacin, aminocaproic acid, aminophylline, ampicillin, anidulafungin, argatroban, arsenic trioxide, atropine, azithromycin, aztreonam, benztropine, bivalirudin, bleomycin, caffeine citrate, calcium chloride, cangrelor, carboplatin, carmustine, caspofungin, cefazolin, cefotaxime, cefoxitin, ceftazidime, ceftazidime/avibactam, ceftolozane/tazobactam, ceftriaxone, cefuroxime, cisplatin, clindamycin, cyclophosphamide, cytarabine, dactinomycin, daptomycin, daunorubicin, dexamethasone, dexmedetomidine, dexrazoxane, digoxin, diltiazem, dimenhydrinate, diphenhydramine, docetaxel, dopamine, doxorubicin liposomal, enalaprilat, epinephrine, eptifibatide, ertapenem, erythromycin, esmolol, etoposide, etoposide phosphate, fentanyl, fluconazole, fludarabine, fluorouracil, foscarnet, fosphenytoin, furosemide, gemcitabine, gemtuzumab ozogamicin, gentamicin, granisetron, heparin, hydrocortisone, hydromorphone, ifosfamide, imipenem, insulin aspart, insulin regular, irinotecan, isoproterenol, labetalol, leucovorin, levocarnitine, lidocaine, linezolid, magnesium sulfate, mannitol, mesna, methadone, methotrexate, methylprednisolone, metoclopramide, metoprolol, metronidazole, milrinone, mitomycin, mitoxantrone, morphine, naloxone, nitroprusside, norepinephrine, octreotide, oxaliplatin, oxytocin, paclitaxel, palonosetron, pamidronate, pemetrexed, penicillin G sodium, phenobarbital, piperacillin/tazobactam, plazomicin, posaconazole, potassium acetate, potassium chloride, potassium phosphates, procainamide, propranolol, rocuronium, sodium bicarbonate, sufentanil, sulbactam/durlobactam, tacrolimus, tedizolid, telavancin, thiotepa, tigecycline, tirofiban, tobramycin, trimethoprim/sulfamethoxazole, valproate sodium, vasopressin, vecuronium, vinblastine, vincristine, vinorelbine, voriconazole, zoledronic acid
- **Y-Site Incompatibility:** amiodarone, amphotericin B deoxycholate, blinatumomab, bupivacaine, ciprofloxacin, dacarbazine, diazepam, dobutamine, doxorubicin hydrochloride, epirubicin, eravacycline, hydralazine, idarubicin, isavuconazonium, ketamine, midazolam, mycophenolate, nicardipine, nitroglycerin, oritavancin, phenytoin, sildenafil, sodium phosphates, topotecan.

Patient/Family Teaching

- Explain purpose and side effects of medication. Advise patient to read *Patient Information* before starting therapy.
- Advise patient to report signs of superinfection (black, furry overgrowth on tongue; vaginal itching or discharge; loose or foul-smelling stools) and rash or other symptoms of allergy.
- Caution patient to avoid driving or other activities requiring alertness until response to drug is known.
- Caution patient to notify health care provider if fever and diarrhea occur, especially if stool contains blood, pus, or mucus. Advise patient not to treat diarrhea without consulting health care provider. May occur up to several weeks after discontinuation of medication.
- Advise patient to notify health care provider promptly if signs and symptoms of rhabdomyolysis (muscle pain or weakness, dark urine) occur.
- Advise patient to notify health care provider of all Rx or OTC medications, vitamins, or herbal products being taken and to consult with health care provider before taking other medications.

- Rep: Advise women of reproductive potential to notify health care provider if pregnancy is planned or suspected or if breastfeeding. Monitor breastfed infants for thrush and diarrhea.

Evaluation/Desired Outcomes

- Resolution of the signs and symptoms of infection. Length of time for complete resolution depends on the organism and site of infection.

meropenem/vaborbactam

(mer-oh-**pen**-nem/va-bor-**bak**-tam)

Vabomere

Classification

Therapeutic: anti-infectives

Pharmacologic: carbapenems beta lactamase inhibitors

Indications

Complicated urinary tract infections, including pyelonephritis.

Action

Inhibits bacterial cell wall synthesis. Addition of vaborbactam protects meropenem from being degraded by certain serine beta-lactamases, such as *Klebsiella pneumoniae* carbapenemase. **Therapeutic Effects:** Bactericidal action against susceptible bacteria. **Spectrum:** Active against the following gram-negative pathogens: *Escherichia coli*, *Enterobacter cloacae*, *Klebsiella pneumoniae*.

Pharmacokinetics

Absorption: IV administration results in complete bioavailability.

Distribution: Well distributed to tissues.

Metabolism and Excretion: Meropenem undergoes hydrolysis; vaborbactam is not metabolized. Both meropenem and vaborbactam are primarily excreted by the kidneys (40–60% of meropenem and 75–95% of vaborbactam excreted unchanged in the urine).

Half-life: *Meropenem:* 1.22 hr; *Vaborbactam:* 1.68 hr.

TIME/ACTION PROFILE (plasma concentrations)

ROUTE	ONSET	PEAK	DURATION
IV	rapid	end of infusion	8 hr

Contraindications/Precautions

Contraindicated in: Hypersensitivity to any of the carbapenems (ertapenem, imipenem, meropenem); Anaphylactic reactions to other beta-lactams (cross-sensitivity may occur); OB: Pregnancy.

Use Cautiously in: Renal impairment (↑ risk of thrombocytopenia and seizures; ↓ dose if eGFR <50 mL/min/1.73 m²); History of seizures, brain lesions, or meningitis; Rep: Women of reproductive potential; Lactation: Use while breastfeeding only if potential maternal benefit justifies potential risk to infant; Pedi: Safety and effectiveness not established in children; Geri: Older adults may be at ↑ risk for adverse reactions due to age-related ↓ in renal function.

Adverse Reactions/Side Effects

GI: CLOSTRIDIOIDES DIFFICILE-ASSOCIATED DIARRHEA (CDAD), diarrhea. **Local:** infusion site reactions, phlebitis. **MS:** RHABDOMYOLYSIS. **Neuro:** delirium, headache, paresthesias, SEIZURES. **Misc:** HYPERSENSITIVITY REACTIONS (INCLUDING ANAPHYLAXIS).

Interactions

Drug-Drug: Probenecid ↓ renal excretion of meropenem and ↑ its levels; concurrent use not recommended. May ↓ **valproate** levels and ↑ risk of seizures; concurrent use not recommended. May ↓ levels and effectiveness of **hormonal contraceptives**.

Route/Dosage

IV (Adults): 4 g (meropenem 2 g/vaborbactam 2 g) every 8 hr for up to 14 days.

Renal Impairment

IV (Adults): *eGFR 30–49 mL/min/1.73 m²:* 2 g (meropenem 1 g/vaborbactam 1 g) every 8 hr for up to 14 days; *eGFR 15–29 mL/min/1.73 m²:* 2 g (meropenem 1 g/vaborbactam 1 g) every 12 hr for up to 14 days; *eGFR <15 mL/min/1.73 m²:* 1 g (meropenem 0.5 g/vaborbactam 0.5 g) every 12 hr for up to 14 days.

Availability

Powder for injection: 2 g/vial (1 g meropenem/1 g vaborbactam).

NURSING IMPLICATIONS

Assessment

- Assess for infection (vital signs; appearance of wound, sputum, urine, and stool; WBC) at beginning of and throughout therapy.
- Obtain a history before initiating therapy to determine previous use of and reactions to penicillins.
- Monitor for diarrhea, abdominal pain, fever, and bloody stools. *If CDAD suspected,* discontinue meropenem/vaborbactam and treat as clinically indicated. May begin up to several weeks following cessation of therapy.
- Observe for anaphylaxis (rash, pruritus, laryngeal edema, wheezing). *If symptoms occur,* immediately discontinue therapy and provide appropriate

M

medical care. Have epinephrine, an antihistamine, and resuscitative equipment close by.

- Assess for severe cutaneous adverse reactions, including SJS, TEN, and DRESS, during therapy. *If rash or other signs and symptoms suggestive of these reactions occur,* immediately discontinue meropenem/vaborbactam, treat as indicated, and consider alternate therapy.
- Assess for history of CNS disorders, including seizures. *If focal tremors, myoclonus, or seizures occur,* place patient on anticonvulsant therapy as needed and assess need to ↓ meropenem/vaborbactam dose or discontinue.
- Monitor for signs and symptoms of rhabdomyolysis. *If signs of symptoms occur,* discontinue therapy and treat as indicated.
- Assess injection site for phlebitis, pain, and swelling periodically during administration.

Lab Test Considerations

- Obtain specimens for culture and sensitivity prior to initiating therapy. 1st dose may be given before receiving results.
- May ↑ AST and ALT.
- May cause hypokalemia, leukopenia and azotemia.

Implementation

- **Intermittent Infusion: Reconstitution:** Reconstitute each vial with 20 mL of 0.9% NaCl. Mix gently to dissolve. **Dilution:** Dilute further in 250 mL to 1000 mL of 0.9% NaCl. **Concentration:** 2–16 mg/mL. Solution is clear to light yellow; do not infuse solution if discolored or contains particulate. Infusion must be completed within 4 hr if stored at room temperature or 22 hr if refrigerated. **Rate:** Infuse over 3 hr.
- **Y-Site Compatibility:** amikacin, ampicillin/sulbactam, azithromycin, aztreonam, bumetanide, calcium gluconate, cefazolin, cefepime, cefiderocol, ceftazidime, ceftazidime/avibactam, ceftolozane/tazobactam, ceftriaxone, cefuroxime, cisatracurium, dexamethasone, dexmedetomidine, digoxin, diltiazem, dopamine, doxycycline, epinephrine, eptifibatide, ertapenem, esmolol, esomeprazole, famotidine, fentanyl, fosphenytoin, furosemide, gentamicin, heparin, hydrocortisone, hydromorphone, imipenem/cilastatin, insulin, regular, labetalol, levofloxacin, lidocaine, linezolid, lorazepam, magnesium sulfate, mannitol, meperidine, mesna, methylprednisolone, metoclopramide, metronidazole, micafungin, milrinone, morphine, naloxone, nitroglycerin, norepinephrine, octreotide, pantoprazole, penicillin G potassium, phenylephrine, piperacillin/tazobactam, plazomicin, potassium chloride, potassium phosphates, rocuronium, sodium bicarbonate, sodium phosphates, sulbactam/durlobactam, tedizolid, tigecycline, tobramycin, vancomycin, vasopressin, vecuronium.
- **Y-Site Incompatibility:** albumin, amiodarone, anidulafungin, calcium chloride, caspofungin, ceftaroline, ciprofloxacin, daptomycin, diphenhydramine, dobutamine, eravacycline, isavuconazonium, midazolam, nicardipine, ondansetron, phenytoin.

Patient/Family Teaching

- Explain purpose and side effects of medication. Advise patient to read *Patient Information* before starting therapy.
- Advise patient to report signs of superinfection (black, furry overgrowth on the tongue; vaginal itching or discharge; loose or foul-smelling stools) and rash or other symptoms of allergy.
- Caution patient to notify health care provider if fever and diarrhea occur, especially if stool contains blood, pus, or mucus. Advise patient not to treat diarrhea without consulting health care provider. May occur up to several weeks after discontinuation of medication.
- Advise patient to notify health care provider promptly if signs and symptoms of rhabdomyolysis (muscle pain or weakness, dark urine) occur.
- Advise patient to notify health care provider of all Rx or OTC medications, vitamins, or herbal products being taken and to consult with health care provider before taking other medications.
- Rep: Advise women of reproductive potential to use nonhormonal contraceptive and notify health care provider if pregnancy is planned or suspected or if breastfeeding. Monitor breastfed infant for thrush and diarrhea.

Evaluation/Desired Outcomes

- Resolution of the signs and symptoms of infection. Length of time for complete resolution depends on the organism and site of infection.

mesalamine (me-**sal**-a-meen)

Apriso, ~~Asacol, Asacol HD~~, Canasa, ~~Delzicol~~, Lialda, ✱ Mezavant, ✱ Mezera, ✱ Octasa, Pentasa, Rowasa, ✱ Salofalk, ✱ Teva 5-ASA

Classification

Therapeutic: gastrointestinal anti-inflammatories

Indications

Delayed-Release Capsules, Lialda, and Pentasa: Treatment and maintenance of remission of mildly to moderately active ulcerative colitis. **Apriso:** Maintenance of remission of ulcerative colitis. **Canasa:** Treatment of active ulcerative proctitis. **Rowasa:** Treatment of active mild to moderate distal ulcerative colitis, proctosigmoiditis, or proctitis.

Action

Locally acting anti-inflammatory action in the colon, where activity is probably due to inhibition of prostaglandin synthesis. **Therapeutic Effects:** Reduction in the symptoms of ulcerative colitis, proctosigmoiditis, and proctitis.

Pharmacokinetics

Absorption: 28% absorbed following oral administration; 10–30% absorbed from the colon, depending on retention time, following rectal administration.
Distribution: Unknown.
Metabolism and Excretion: Some metabolism occurs, site unknown; mostly eliminated unchanged in the feces.
Half-life: *Oral:* 12 hr (range 2–15 hr); *Rectal:* 0.5–1.5 hr.

TIME/ACTION PROFILE (clinical improvement)

ROUTE	ONSET	PEAK	DURATION
PO	unknown	unknown	6–8 hr
ER	2 hr	9–12 hr	24 hr
Rectal	3–21 days	unknown	24 hr

Contraindications/Precautions

Contraindicated in: Hypersensitivity reactions to sulfonamides, salicylates, mesalamine, or sulfasalazine; Cross-sensitivity with furosemide, sulfonylureas, or carbonic anhydrase inhibitors may exist; Hypersensitivity to bisulfites (mesalamine enema only); Urinary tract or intestinal obstruction; Porphyria.
Use Cautiously in: Renal impairment; Hepatic impairment; Atopic dermatitis or atopic eczema (↑ risk of photosensitivity); Phenylketonuria (Apriso contains phenylalanine); OB: Use tablets only if potential benefits justify potential fetal risks (enteric coating contains dibutyl phthalate, which has been shown to cause congenital malformations in animals); Lactation: Use while breastfeeding only if potential maternal benefits justify potential risk to infant; Geri: Older adults may have ↑ risk of agranulocytosis, neutropenia, and pancytopenia.

Adverse Reactions/Side Effects

CV: pericarditis. **Derm:** ACUTE GENERALIZED EXANTHEMATOUS PUSTULOSIS, DRUG REACTION WITH EOSINOPHILIA AND SYSTEMATIC SYMPTOMS (DRESS), hair loss, photosensitivity, rash, STEVENS-JOHNSON SYNDROME, TOXIC EPIDERMAL NECROLYSIS. **EENT:** pharyngitis, rhinitis. **GI:** diarrhea, eructation (oral), flatulence, HEPATOTOXICITY, nausea, pancreatitis, vomiting. **GU:** interstitial nephritis, nephrolithiasis, renal impairment. **Local:** anal irritation (enema, suppository). **MS:** back pain, myalgia. **Neuro:** headache, dizziness, malaise, weakness. **Misc:** acute intolerance syndrome, fever, HYPERSENSITIVITY REACTIONS (INCLUDING ANAPHYLAXIS AND ANGIOEDEMA).

Interactions

Drug-Drug: May ↑ myelosuppressive effects of **mercaptopurine** or **azathioprine**; avoid concurrent use, if possible. **NSAIDs** may ↑ risk of nephrotoxicity.

Route/Dosage

One 800-mg tablet is NOT bioequivalent to two 400-mg delayed-release capsules.

Treatment of Ulcerative Colitis

PO (Adults): 1.6 g (two 800-mg tablets) 3 times daily for 6 wk; *Delayed-release capsules:* 800 mg (two 400-mg capsules) 3 times daily for 6 wk; *Lialda:* 2.4–4.8 g (two to four 1.2-g tablets) once daily for up to 8 wk; *Pentasa:* 1 g (four 250-mg capsules or two 500-mg capsules) 4 times daily for up to 8 wk.
Rect (Adults): *Rowasa:* 4-g enema (60 mL) at bedtime, retained for 8 hr for 3–6 wk.
PO (Children ≥12 yr and 54–90 kg): *Delayed-release capsules:* 27–44 mg/kg/day in 2 divided doses (max dose = 2.4 g/day) for 6 wk.
PO (Children ≥12 yr and 33–53 kg): *Delayed-release capsules:* 37–61 mg/kg/day in 2 divided doses (max dose = 2 g/day) for 6 wk.
PO (Children ≥12 yr and 17–32 kg): *Delayed-release capsules:* 36–71 mg/kg/day in 2 divided doses (max dose = 1.2 g/day) for 6 wk.
PO (Children >50 kg): *Lialda:* 4.8 g (four 1.2-g tablets) once daily for 8 wk, then 2.4 g (two 1.2-g tablets) once daily.
PO (Children 36–50 kg): *Lialda:* 3.6 g (three 1.2-g tablets) once daily for 8 wk, then 2.4 g (two 1.2-g tablets) once daily.
PO (Children 24–35 kg): *Lialda:* 2.4 g (two 1.2-g tablets) once daily for 8 wk, then 1.2 g once daily.

Maintenance of Remission of Ulcerative Colitis

PO (Adults): *Apriso:* 1.5 g (four 375-mg capsules) once daily in the morning; *Delayed-release capsules:* 800 mg (two 400-mg capsules) 2 times daily; *Lialda:* 2.4 g (two 1.2-g tablets) once daily; *Pentasa:* 1 g (four 250-mg capsules or two 500-mg capsules) 4 times daily.

Treatment of Ulcerative Proctosigmoiditis

Rect (Adults): *Rowasa:* 4-g enema (60 mL) at bedtime, retained for 8 hr (treatment duration = 3–6 wk).

Treatment of Ulcerative Proctitis

Rect (Adults): *Rowasa:* 4-g enema (60 mL) at bedtime, retained for 8 hr (treatment duration = 3–6 wk); *Canasa:* Insert a 1-g suppository at bedtime, retain for at least 1–3 hr (treatment duration = 3–6 wk).

M

Availability (generic available)

Delayed-release tablets: ✱ 400 mg, ✱ 500 mg, 800 mg, ✱ 1 g, 1.2 g (Lialda), ✱ 1.6 g. **Delayed-release capsules:** 400 mg. **Extended-release capsules (Apriso) (contain phenylalanine):** 375 mg. **Extended-release capsules (Pentasa):** 250 mg, 500 mg. **Rectal enema (Rowasa):** ✱ 1 g/100 mL, ✱ 2 g/60 mL, 4 g/60 mL, ✱ 4 g/100 mL. **Rectal foam:** ✱ 1 g/actuation. **Rectal suppository (Canasa):** ✱ 500 mg, 1 g.

NURSING IMPLICATIONS

Assessment

- Assess abdominal pain and frequency, quantity, and consistency of stools at the beginning of and during therapy.
- Assess for allergy to sulfonamides and salicylates. Patients allergic to sulfasalazine may take mesalamine or olsalazine without difficulty, but therapy should be discontinued if rash or fever occurs.
- Monitor intake and output. Fluid intake should be sufficient to maintain a urine output of ≥1200–1500 mL daily to prevent crystalluria and stone formation.
- Monitor for signs/symptoms of hypersensitivity reactions including rash. *If hypersensitivity or severe cutaneous reactions occur,* discontinue mesalamine and provide appropriate medical care.
- Monitor for signs/symptoms of acute intolerance syndrome (cramping, acute abdominal pain, bloody diarrhea, sometimes fever, headache, rash) during therapy; may be difficult to distinguish from an exacerbation of ulcerative colitis. *If acute intolerance syndrome occurs,* discontinue mesalamine.

Lab Test Considerations

- Monitor urinalysis, BUN, and serum creatinine before starting and periodically during therapy. Mesalamine may cause renal toxicity. Discontinue mesalamine if renal function ↓.
- May ↑ AST, ALT, alkaline phosphatase, GGT, LDH, amylase, and lipase.

Implementation

- **PO:** Administer with a full glass of water. ***DNC:*** Swallow tablets whole; do not break the outer coating, which is designed to remain intact. Take *Lialda* tablets with a meal. Take *Apriso* capsules in the morning without regard to meals. Do not coadminister with antacids; may affect dissolution of the coating of the granules in *Apriso* capsules. Intact or partially intact tablets may occasionally be found in the stool. If this occurs repeatedly, advise patient to notify health care provider. ***DNC:*** Swallow *delayed-release* capsules whole; do not break, crush, or chew. Administer without regard to meals. If needed, may open capsule and swallow inner tablets. Intact or partially intact tablets may occasionally be found in the stool. If this occurs repeatedly, advise patient to notify health care provider. Two *delayed-release* 400-mg capsules are not equal to one *Asacol HD* (mesalamine) delayed-release 800-mg tablet. *Pentasa* capsules may be swallowed whole or opened and sprinkled onto applesauce or yogurt. Consume entire contents immediately.
- **Rect** Patient should empty bowel prior to administration of rectal dose forms.
- Avoid excessive handling of *suppository*. Remove foil wrapper and insert pointed end first into rectum with gentle pressure. Do not cut or break suppository. Retain suppository for 1–3 hr or more for maximum benefit.
- Administer 60-mL retention enema once daily at bedtime. Solution should be retained for approximately 8 hr. Prior to administration of *rectal suspension*, shake bottle well and remove the protective cap. Have patient lie on left side with the lower leg extended and the upper leg flexed for support or place the patient in knee-chest position. Gently insert the applicator tip into the rectum, pointing toward the umbilicus. Squeeze the bottle steadily to discharge most of the preparation.

Patient/Family Teaching

- Instruct patient on the correct method of administration. Advise patient to take medication as directed, even if feeling better. Take missed doses as soon as remembered unless almost time for next dose. Advise patient to read *Patient Information* before starting therapy and with each Rx refill in case of changes.
- Advise patient not to change brands of mesalamine without consulting health care provider.
- Encourage patient to drink an adequate amount of fluids to minimize risk of kidney stones. Notify health care provider if severe side or back pain or blood in urine occur.
- Inform patient of possible reddish-brown urine discoloration when in contact with surfaces or water treated with hypochlorite-containing bleach.
- May cause dizziness. Caution patient to avoid driving or other activities that require alertness until response to medication is known.
- Advise patient to notify health care provider if skin rash, sore throat, fever, mouth sores, unusual bleeding or bruising, wheezing, fever, or hives occur.
- Advise patient to avoid sun exposure, wear protective clothing, and use a broad-spectrum sunscreen when outdoors to ↓ risk of photosensitivity.
- Instruct patient to notify health care provider if symptoms do not improve after 1–2 mo of therapy.
- Instruct patient to notify health care provider if symptoms worsen. If symptoms of acute intolerance (cramping, acute abdominal pain, bloody diarrhea, fever, headache, rash) occur, discontinue therapy and notify health care provider immediately.

- Inform patient that proctoscopy and sigmoidoscopy may be required periodically during treatment to determine response.
- **Rect** Instruct patient to use *rectal suspension* at bedtime and retain suspension all night for best results.
- Rep: Advise women of reproductive potential to notify health care provider if pregnancy is planned or suspected or if breastfeeding. Monitor breastfed infants for diarrhea.

Evaluation/Desired Outcomes

- Decrease in diarrhea and abdominal pain.
- Return to normal bowel pattern in patients with inflammatory bowel disease. Effects may be seen within 3–21 days. The usual course of therapy is 3–6 wk.
- Maintenance of remission in patients with inflammatory bowel disease.

mesna (mes-na)

Mesnex, ✱ Uromitexan

Classification

Therapeutic: antidotes

Pharmacologic: ifosfamide detoxifying agents

Indications

Prevention of ifosfamide-induced hemorrhagic cystitis. **Unlabeled Use:** Prevention of cyclophosphamide-induced hemorrhagic cystitis.

Action

Binds to the toxic metabolites of ifosfamide in the kidneys. **Therapeutic Effects:** Prevents hemorrhagic cystitis from ifosfamide.

Pharmacokinetics

Absorption: IV administration results in complete bioavailability; 45–79% absorbed after oral administration. Following IV with PO dosing ↑ systemic exposure.

Distribution: Minimally distributed to tissues.

Metabolism and Excretion: Rapidly converted to mesna disulfide, then back to mesna in the kidneys, where it binds to toxic metabolites of ifosfamide (18–26% excreted as free mesna in urine after IV and PO dosing).

Half-life: *Mesna:* 0.36 hr (IV); 1.2–8.3 hr (IV followed by PO); *Mesna disulfide:* 1.17 hr.

TIME/ACTION PROFILE (detoxifying action)

ROUTE	ONSET	PEAK	DURATION
PO, IV	rapid	unknown	4 hr

Contraindications/Precautions

Contraindicated in: Hypersensitivity to mesna or other thiol (rubber) compounds; Lactation: Lactation.

Use Cautiously in: OB: Safety not established in pregnancy; Pedi: Injection contains benzyl alcohol, which can cause potentially fatal gasping syndrome in neonates.

Adverse Reactions/Side Effects

Derm: flushing. **GI:** anorexia, diarrhea, nausea, unpleasant taste, vomiting. **Local:** injection site reactions. **Neuro:** dizziness, drowsiness, headache. **Misc:** flu-like symptoms.

Interactions

Drug-Drug: None reported.

Route/Dosage

IV (Adults): Give a dose of mesna equal to 20% of the ifosfamide dose at the same time as ifosfamide and 4 and 8 hr after.

PO, IV (Adults): Give a dose of IV mesna equal to 20% of the ifosfamide dose at the same time as ifosfamide; then give PO mesna equal to 40% of the ifosfamide dose 2 and 6 hr after ifosfamide (total mesna dose is 100% of ifosfamide dose).

Availability (generic available)

Solution for injection: 100 mg/mL. **Tablets:** 400 mg.

NURSING IMPLICATIONS

Assessment

- Monitor for development of hemorrhagic cystitis in patients receiving ifosfamide.

Lab Test Considerations

- Verify negative pregnancy test before initiating therapy when given with ifosfamide.
- Causes a false-positive result when testing urinary ketones.

Implementation

- Initial IV bolus is to be given at time of ifosfamide administration.
- **PO:** If 2nd and 3rd doses are given orally, administer 2 and 6 hr after IV dose.
- If PO mesna is vomited within 2 hr of administration, repeat dose or use IV mesna.

IV Administration

- **Intermittent Infusion:** 2nd IV dose is given 4 hr later; 3rd dose is given 8 hr after initial dose. This schedule must be repeated with each subsequent dose of ifosfamide. **Dilution:** Dilute 2-, 4-, and 10-mL ampules, containing a concentration of 100 mg/mL in 8 mL, 16 mL, or 50 mL, respectively, of D5W, 0.9% NaCl, D5/0.9% NaCl, D5/0.2% NaCl, D5/0.33% NaCl, or LR. **Concentration:** 20 mg/mL. Refrigerate to store. Use within 6 hr. Discard unused solution. **Rate:** Administer over 15–30 min or as a continuous infusion.
- **Syringe Compatibility:** ifosfamide

M

- **Y-Site Compatibility:** alemtuzumab, allopurinol, amikacin, aminocaproic acid, aminophylline, amiodarone, amphotericin B liposomal, ampicillin/sulbactam, anidulafungin, argatroban, arsenic trioxide, atracurium, azithromycin, aztreonam, bivalirudin, bleomycin, bumetanide, buprenorphine, busulfan, butorphanol, calcium chloride, calcium gluconate, carmustine, caspofungin, cefazolin, cefepime, cefotaxime, cefotetan, cefoxitin, ceftazidime, ceftolozane/tazobactam, ceftriaxone, cefuroxime, chlorpromazine, ciprofloxacin, cisatracurium, cladribine, clindamycin, cyclophosphamide, cytarabine, dactinomycin, daptomycin, defibrotide, dexamethasone, dexmedetomidine, dexrazoxane, digoxin, diltiazem, diphenhydramine, dobutamine, docetaxel, dopamine, doxorubicin hydrochloride, doxorubicin liposomal, doxycycline, droperidol, enalaprilat, ephedrine, epinephrine, epirubicin, ertapenem, erythromycin, esmolol, etoposide, etoposide phosphate, famotidine, fentanyl, filgrastim, fluconazole, fludarabine, fluorouracil, foscarnet, fosphenytoin, furosemide, gemcitabine, gentamicin, glycopyrrolate, granisetron, haloperidol, heparin, hydralazine, hydrocortisone, hydromorphone, idarubicin, ifosfamide, imipenem/cilastatin, insulin, regular, irinotecan, isavuconazonium, isoproterenol, ketorolac, labetalol, leucovorin, levofloxacin, lidocaine, linezolid, lorazepam, magnesium sulfate, mannitol, melphalan, meperidine, meropenem, meropenem/vaborbactam, methadone, methotrexate, methyprednisolone, metoclopramide, metoprolol, metronidazole, micafungin, midazolam, milrinone, mitomycin, mitoxantrone, morphine, moxifloxacin, mycophenolate, nafcillin, nalbuphine, naloxone, nitroglycerin, norepinephrine, octreotide, ondansetron, oxaliplatin, paclitaxel, palonosetron, pamidronate, pantoprazole, pemetrexed, pentamidine, pentobarbital, phenobarbital, phentolamine, phenylephrine, piperacillin/tazobactam, plazomicin, potassium acetate, potassium chloride, potassium phosphates, procainamide, prochlorperazine, promethazine, propranolol, remifentanil, rituximab, rocuronium, sargramostim, sodium acetate, sodium bicarbonate, sodium phosphates, succinylcholine, sufentanil, sulbactam/durlobactam, tacrolimus, tedizolid, theophylline, thiotepa, tigecycline, tirofiban, tobramycin, topotecan, trastuzumab, trimethoprim/sulfamethoxazole, vancomycin, vasopressin, vecuronium, verapamil, vinblastine, vincristine, vinorelbine, voriconazole, zidovudine, zoledronic acid.
- **Y-Site Incompatibility:** acyclovir, amphotericin B deoxycholate, dacarbazine, dantrolene, diazepam, ganciclovir, gemtuzumab ozogamicin, nicardipine, nitroprusside, phenytoin.

Patient/Family Teaching

- Inform patient that unpleasant taste may occur during administration.
- Advise patient to notify health care provider if nausea, vomiting, or diarrhea persists or is severe.
- Rep: Advise women of reproductive potential to use effective contraception during therapy and for 6 mo after last dose and to avoid breastfeeding during therapy and for 1 wk after last dose. Advise men with female partners of reproductive potential to use effective contraception during therapy and for 3 mo after last dose. Advise patient to notify health care provider immediately if pregnancy is suspected.

Evaluation/Desired Outcomes

- Prevention of hemorrhagic cystitis associated with ifosfamide therapy.

metFORMIN (met-for-min)

Glucophage, ~~Glucophage XR~~, Glumetza

Classification

Therapeutic: antidiabetics

Pharmacologic: biguanides

Indications

Type 2 diabetes mellitus.

Action

Decreases hepatic glucose production. Decreases intestinal glucose absorption. Increases sensitivity to insulin. **Therapeutic Effects:** Maintenance of blood glucose.

Pharmacokinetics

Absorption: 50–60% absorbed after oral administration.

Distribution: Extensively distributed to tissues.

Metabolism and Excretion: Eliminated almost entirely unchanged by the kidneys.

Half-life: 17.6 hr.

TIME/ACTION PROFILE (plasma concentrations)

ROUTE	ONSET	PEAK	DURATION
PO-IR	unknown	unknown	12 hr
PO-ER	unknown	4–8 hr	24 hr

Contraindications/Precautions

Contraindicated in: Hypersensitivity; Metabolic acidosis (including diabetic ketoacidosis); Severe renal impairment (CCr <30 mL/min); Iodinated contrast imaging procedure in patients with CCr 30–60 mL/min; a history of liver disease, alcoholism, or HF; or those who will be administered intra-arterial iodinated contrast; discontinue metformin and reevaluate renal function 48 hr after imaging procedure; may restart therapy if renal function stable; Hepatic impairment; Lactation: Lactation.

Use Cautiously in: Mild to moderate renal impairment (initiation of therapy not recommended if CCr 30–45 mL/min; if CCr becomes <45 mL/min during therapy, assess risk-to-benefit of continuing therapy); Chronic alcohol use/abuse; Hypoxic states (acute HF, shock, MI, sepsis) (↑ risk of lactic acidosis); Surgery (temporarily discontinue metformin when food and/or fluid intake is restricted); Pituitary deficiency or hyperthyroidism; OB: Insulin recommended during pregnancy; Pedi: Safety and effectiveness not established in children <18 yr (extended release) or <10 yr (immediate release); Geri: Older adults may be at ↑ risk of lactic acidosis.

Adverse Reactions/Side Effects

F and E LACTIC ACIDOSIS. **GI:** abdominal bloating, diarrhea, nausea, vomiting, unpleasant metallic taste. **Hemat:** ↓ vitamin B_{12} levels.

Interactions

Drug-Drug: Acute or chronic **alcohol** ingestion, **iodinated contrast media**, **topiramate**, **zonisamide**, and **acetazolamide** may ↑ risk of lactic acidosis. **Amiloride**, **digoxin**, **morphine**, **procainamide**, **quinidine**, **triamterene**, **trimethoprim**, **calcium channel blockers**, and **vancomycin** may compete for elimination pathways with metformin. Altered responses may occur. **Cimetidine** and **furosemide** may ↑ effects of metformin. **Nifedipine** ↑ absorption and effects.

Drug-Natural Products: **Glucosamine** may worsen blood glucose control. **Chromium** and **coenzyme Q-10** may produce ↑ hypoglycemic effects.

Route/Dosage

PO (Adults): *Immediate-release tablets:* 500 mg twice daily; may ↑ by 500 mg at weekly intervals up to 2000 mg/day. If doses >2000 mg/day are required, give in 3 divided doses (not to exceed 2500 mg/day) or 850 mg once daily; may ↑ by 850 mg at 2-wk intervals (in divided doses) up to 2550 mg/day in divided doses (up to 850 mg 3 times daily); *Extended-release tablets:* 500 mg once daily with evening meal; may ↑ by 500 mg at weekly intervals up to 2000 mg once daily.

PO (Children 10–17 yr): *Immediate-release tablets:* 500 mg twice daily; may be ↑ by 500 mg/day at 1-wk intervals, up to 2000 mg/day in 2 divided doses.

Availability (generic available)

Immediate-release tablets: 500 mg, 625 mg, 850 mg, 1000 mg. **Extended-release tablets (Glumetza):** 500 mg, 750 mg, 1000 mg. **Oral solution(cherry flavor):** 500 mg/5 mL. ***In combination with:*** alogliptin (Kazano); canagliflozin (Invokamet, Invokamet XR); dapagliflozin (Xigduo XR); empagliflozin (Synjardy, Synjardy XR); empagliflozin and linagliptin (Trijardy XR); ertugliflozin (Segluromet); glipizide (generic only); glyburide (generic only); linagliptin (Jentadueto, Jentadueto XR); pioglitazone (Actoplus Met); saxagliptin (generic only); and sitagliptin (Janumet, Janumet XR, Zituvimet, Zituvimet XR). See Appendix N.

NURSING IMPLICATIONS

Assessment

- When combined with oral sulfonylureas, observe for signs and symptoms of hypoglycemia (abdominal pain, sweating, hunger, weakness, dizziness, headache, tremor, tachycardia, anxiety).
- Patients whose blood sugar has been well controlled on metformin who develop illness or laboratory abnormalities should be assessed for ketoacidosis or lactic acidosis. Assess serum electrolytes, ketones, glucose, and, if indicated, blood pH, lactate, and pyruvate levels. *If acidosis occurs,* discontinue metformin immediately and provide appropriate medical treatment.

Lab Test Considerations

- Monitor serum glucose and A1c periodically during therapy to evaluate effectiveness of therapy. May cause false-positive results for urine ketones.
- Assess renal function before starting and at least annually during therapy. Monitor patients at risk for renal impairment more frequently. Discontinue metformin if renal impairment occurs.
- Monitor serum folic acid and vitamin B_{12} levels every 1–2 yr in long-term therapy. Metformin may interfere with their absorption.

Implementation

- Do not confuse metformin with metronidazole.
- Patients stabilized on a regimen for diabetes who are exposed to stress, fever, trauma, infection, or surgery may require administration of insulin. Withhold metformin and reinstitute after resolution of acute episode.
- Temporarily discontinue metformin in patients requiring surgery involving restricted intake of food and fluids. Resume metformin when oral intake has resumed and renal function is normal.
- Hold metformin before or at the time of studies requiring IV administration of iodinated contrast media and for 48 hr after study.
- **PO:** Administer metformin with meals to minimize GI effects.
- ***DNC:*** Extended-release tablets must be swallowed whole; do not crush, dissolve, or chew. Administer *Glumetza* with the evening meal.

M

Patient/Family Teaching

- Instruct patient to take metformin at the same time each day, as directed. Take missed doses as soon as possible unless almost time for next dose. Do not double doses. Instruct parent/caregiver to read the *Medication Guide* prior to use and with each Rx refill as changes may occur.
- Explain to patient that metformin helps control hyperglycemia but does not cure diabetes. Therapy is usually long term.
- Encourage patient to follow prescribed diet, medication, and exercise regimen to prevent hyperglycemic or hypoglycemic episodes.
- Review signs of hypoglycemia and hyperglycemia with patient. If hypoglycemia occurs, advise patient to take a glass of orange juice or 2–3 teaspoons of sugar, honey, or corn syrup dissolved in water, and notify health care provider.
- Instruct patient in proper testing of blood glucose and urine ketones. These tests should be monitored closely during periods of stress or illness and health care provider notified if significant changes occur.
- Explain to patient the risk of lactic acidosis and the potential need for discontinuation of metformin therapy if a severe infection, dehydration, or severe or continuing diarrhea occurs or if medical tests or surgery is required. Symptoms of lactic acidosis (chills, diarrhea, dizziness, low BP, muscle pain, abdominal pain, sleepiness, slow heartbeat or pulse, dyspnea, weakness) should be reported to health care provider immediately.
- Advise patient to notify health care provider of all Rx or OTC medications, vitamins, or herbal products being taken and to consult with health care provider before taking other medications or alcohol.
- Inform patient that metformin may cause an unpleasant or metallic taste that usually resolves spontaneously.
- Inform patients taking extended-release tablets that inactive ingredients resembling the tablet may appear in stools.
- Advise patient to inform health care provider of medication regimen before treatment or surgery.
- Advise patient to report the occurrence of diarrhea, nausea, vomiting, and stomach pain or fullness to health care provider.
- Advise patient to carry a form of sugar (sugar packets, candy) and identification describing disease process and medication regimen at all times.
- Rep: Insulin is the recommended method of controlling blood glucose during pregnancy. Advise women of reproductive potential to notify health care provider promptly if pregnancy is planned or suspected or if breastfeeding. Caution patient that metformin may result in ovulation in some anovulatory women, leading to unintended pregnancy.
- Emphasize the importance of routine follow-up exams and regular testing of blood glucose, A1c, renal function, and hematologic parameters.

Evaluation/Desired Outcomes

- Control of blood glucose levels without the appearance of hypoglycemic or hyperglycemic episodes.

REMS HIGH ALERT

methadone (meth-a-done)

~~Dolophine~~, Metadol, Metadol-D, Methadose

Classification

Therapeutic: opioid analgesics

Pharmacologic: opioid agonists

Schedule II

Indications

Moderate to severe chronic pain in opioid-tolerant patients requiring use of daily, around-the-clock long-term opioid treatment and for which alternative treatment options are inadequate (extended release). Detoxification and maintenance therapy for opioid use disorder. **Unlabeled Use:** Neonatal abstinence syndrome.

Action

Binds to opiate receptors in the CNS. Alters the perception of and response to painful stimuli while producing generalized CNS depression. **Therapeutic Effects:** Decrease in severity of pain. Suppression of withdrawal symptoms during detoxification and maintenance from heroin and other opioids.

Pharmacokinetics

Absorption: 50% absorbed following oral administration. IV administration results in complete bioavailability.

Distribution: Widely distributed to tissues.

Protein Binding: 85–90%.

Metabolism and Excretion: Mostly metabolized by the liver; some metabolites are active and may accumulate with chronic administration. Primarily excreted in the urine (<10% as unchanged drug).

Half-life: 15–25 hr (↑ with chronic use).

TIME/ACTION PROFILE (analgesic effect)

ROUTE	ONSET	PEAK	DURATION
PO	30–60 min	90–120 min	4–12 hr
IM, IV, SUBQ	10–20 min	60–120 min	8–12 hr

Contraindications/Precautions

Contraindicated in: Hypersensitivity; Significant respiratory depression; Acute or severe bronchial asthma; Paralytic ileus; Known alcohol intolerance (some oral solutions); Concurrent MAO inhibitor therapy.

Use Cautiously in: Personal or family history of substance use disorder or mental illness (for pain management); Structural heart disease, concurrent diuretic use, hypokalemia, hypomagnesemia, history of arrhythmia/syncope, or other risk factors for arrhythmias; Head trauma; Seizure disorders; ↑ intracranial pressure; Severe renal impairment; Severe hepatic impairment; Severe pulmonary disease; Hypothyroidism; Adrenal insufficiency; Undiagnosed abdominal pain; Prostatic hyperplasia or ureteral stricture; OB: Use during pregnancy only if the potential maternal benefit justifies the potential fetal risk. Prolonged use of methadone during pregnancy can result in neonatal opioid withdrawal syndrome; Lactation: Use while breastfeeding only if potential maternal benefit justifies potential risk to infant; Geri: ↑ risk of respiratory depression in older adults (dose ↓ suggested).

Adverse Reactions/Side Effects

CV: hypotension, bradycardia, QT interval prolongation, TORSADES DE POINTES. **Derm:** flushing, sweating. **EENT:** blurred vision, diplopia, miosis. **Endo:** adrenal insufficiency. **GI:** constipation, nausea, vomiting. **GU:** urinary retention. **Neuro:** confusion, sedation, dizziness, dysphoria, euphoria, floating feeling, hallucinations, headache, unusual dreams. **Resp:** RESPIRATORY DEPRESSION (INCLUDING CENTRAL SLEEP APNEA AND SLEEP-RELATED HYPOXEMIA). **Misc:** allodynia, opioid-induced hyperalgesia, physical dependence, psychological dependence, tolerance.

Interactions

Drug-Drug: Use with extreme caution in patients receiving **MAO inhibitors**; may result in severe, unpredictable reactions; ↓ initial dose of methadone to 25% of usual dose. Use with extreme caution with any drug known to potentially prolong QT interval, including **class I and III antiarrhythmics**, some **neuroleptics** and **tricyclic antidepressants**, and **calcium channel blockers**. Concurrent use with **laxatives**, **diuretics**, or **mineralocorticoids** may ↑ risk of hypomagnesemia or hypokalemia and ↑ risk of arrhythmias. Drugs that affect serotonergic neurotransmitter systems, including **tricyclic antidepressants**, **SSRIs**, **SNRIs**, **MAO inhibitors**, **TCAs**, **tramadol**, **trazodone**, **mirtazapine**, **5-HT$_3$ receptor antagonists**, **linezolid**, **methylene blue**, and **triptans**, may ↑ risk of serotonin syndrome. **CYP3A4 inhibitors**, **CYP2C9 inhibitors**, **CYP2C19 inhibitors**, or **CYP2D6 inhibitors**, including **ritonavir**, **ketoconazole**, **itraconazole**, **fluconazole**, **clarithromycin**, **erythromycin**, **nefazodone**, **diltiazem**, **verapamil**, **nelfinavir**, **fosamprenavir**, and **fluvoxamine**, ↑ levels and risk of opioid toxicity; careful monitoring during initiation, dose changes, or discontinuation of the inhibitor is recommended. **CYP3A4 inducers**, **CYP2C9 inducers**, or **CYP2C19 inducers**, including **barbiturates**, **carbamazepine**, **efavirenz**, **corticosteroids**, **modafinil**, **nevirapine**, **oxcarbazepine**, **phenobarbital**, **phenytoin**, **rifabutin**, or **rifampin**, may ↓ levels and analgesia; if inducers are discontinued or dosage ↓, patients should be monitored for signs of opioid toxicity and necessary dose adjustments should be made. Use with **benzodiazepines** or other **CNS depressants**, including other **opioids**, **nonbenzodiazepine sedative/hypnotics**, **anxiolytics**, **general anesthetics**, **muscle relaxants**, **antipsychotics**, and **alcohol**, may cause profound sedation, respiratory depression, coma, and death; reserve concurrent use for when alternative treatment options are inadequate. **Nalbuphine** may ↓ analgesia. May ↑ levels and risk of toxicity of **zidovudine** and **desipramine**. **Mixed agonist/antagonist analgesics**, including **nalbuphine** or **butorphanol**, and **partial agonist analgesics**, including **buprenorphine**, may ↓ methadone's analgesic effects and/or precipitate opioid withdrawal in physically dependent patients.

Drug-Natural Products: St. John's wort may ↓ levels and effects; concurrent use may result in withdrawal. **Kava-kava**, **valerian**, or **chamomile** can ↑ risk of CNS depression.

Route/Dosage

Moderate to Severe Pain

PO (Adults and Children ≥50 kg): *Usual starting dose for moderate to severe pain in opioid-naive patients:* 2.5 mg every 8–12 hr.

PO (Adults and Children <50 kg): 0.1 mg/kg/dose every 4 hr for 2–3 doses, then every 6–8 hr as needed; maximum: 10 mg/dose.

PO, IV (Neonates): Initial 0.05–0.2 mg/kg/dose every 12–24 hr or 0.5 mg/kg/day divided every 8 hr; taper dose by 10–20% per wk over 1–1.5 mo.

IV: IM SUBQ (Adults and Children ≥50 kg): 10 mg every 6–8 hr.

IV: IM SUBQ (Adults and Children <50 kg): 0.1 mg/kg every 6–8 hr; maximum: 10 mg/dose.

Opioid Detoxification

PO (Adults and Children ≥50 kg): 15–40 mg once daily or amount needed to prevent withdrawal. Dose may be ↓ every 1–2 days; maintenance dose is determined on an individual basis.

PO (Adults and Children <50 kg): 0.05–0.1 mg/kg/dose every 6 hr; ↑ by 0.05 mg/kg/dose until withdrawal symptoms controlled; after 1–2 days, lengthen dosing interval to every 12–24 hr; taper by ↓ dose by 0.05 mg/kg/day.

IV: IM SUBQ (Adults and Children ≥50 kg): 15–40 mg once daily or amount needed to prevent withdrawal. May ↓ dose every 1–2 days; maintenance dose is determined on an individual basis.

Availability (generic available)

Tablets: 🍁 1 mg, 5 mg, 10 mg, 🍁 25 mg. **Tablets for oral suspension:** 40 mg (available only to licensed detoxification/maintenance programs). **Oral concentrate (cherry and unflavored):** 10 mg/mL. **Oral solution (contains alcohol) (citrus):** 5 mg/5 mL, 10 mg/5 mL. **Solution for injection:** 10 mg/mL.

NURSING IMPLICATIONS

Assessment

- **Pain:** Assess type, location, and intensity of pain prior to and 1–2 hr (peak) following administration. When titrating opioid doses, ↑ of 25–50% should be administered until there is either a 50% ↓ in the patient's pain rating on a numeric or visual analogue scale or the patient reports satisfactory pain relief. Dose ↑ should be made no more frequently than every 3–5 days because of variability in half-life between patients. Cumulative effects of this medication may require periodic dose adjustments.
- Doses of methadone for patients on methadone maintenance only prevent withdrawal symptoms; *no analgesia is provided*. Additional opioid doses are required for treatment of pain. An equianalgesic chart (see Appendix I) should be used when changing routes or when changing from one opioid to another.
- Assess BP, HR, and respiratory rate before and periodically during administration. If respiratory rate <10/min, assess level of sedation. Dose may need to be ↓ by 25–50%. Initial drowsiness will ↓ with continued use. Monitor for respiratory depression, especially during initiation or following dose ↑; serious, life-threatening, or fatal respiratory depression may occur. May cause sleep-related breathing disorders (central sleep apnea, sleep-related hypoxemia).
- Assess bowel function routinely. Prevention of constipation should be instituted with ↑ intake of fluids and bulk and with laxatives to minimize constipating effects. Stimulant laxatives should be administered routinely if opioid use exceeds 2–3 days, unless contraindicated. Consider drugs for opioid-induced constipation.
- Prolonged use may lead to physical and psychological dependence and tolerance, which should not prevent patient from receiving adequate analgesia. Patients who receive methadone for pain rarely develop psychological dependence. Progressively higher doses may be required to relieve pain with long-term therapy.
- Assess for history of structural heart disease, arrhythmia, and syncope. Obtain a pretreatment ECG to measure QTc interval and follow-up ECG within 30 days and annually. Additional ECGs recommended if dose >100 mg/day or if patients have unexplained syncope or seizures. If QTc interval >450 msec but <500 msec, discuss potential risks and benefits with patients and monitor more frequently. If the QTc interval >500 msec, consider discontinuing or ↓ dose; eliminating contributing factors (drugs that promote hypokalemia) or using an alternative therapy.
- Assess risk for opioid addiction, abuse, or misuse prior to administration. Abuse or misuse by crushing, chewing, snorting, or injecting dissolved product will result in uncontrolled delivery of methadone and can result in overdose and death.
- Assess for opioid-induced hyperalgesia, which can appear as ↑ levels of pain on increasing the dose of the opioid, ↓ levels of pain on decreasing the dose of the opioid, or pain from ordinarily nonpainful stimuli (allodynia). This condition is different from tolerance. If a patient is suspected to be experiencing opioid-induced hyperalgesia, consider ↓ the dose of the current opioid or switching to a different opioid analgesic.
- **Opioid Detoxification:** Assess patient for signs of opioid withdrawal (irritability, runny nose and eyes, abdominal cramps, body aches, sweating, loss of appetite, shivering, unusually large pupils, trouble sleeping, weakness, yawning). Methadone maintenance is undertaken only by federally approved treatment centers. This does not preclude maintenance for addicts hospitalized for other conditions and who require temporary maintenance during their care.

Lab Test Considerations

- May ↑ plasma amylase and lipase levels.

Toxicity and Overdose

- If an opioid antagonist is required to reverse respiratory depression or coma, naloxone is the antidote. Dilute the 0.4-mg ampule of naloxone in 10 mL of 0.9% NaCl and administer 0.5 mL (0.02 mg) by IV push every 2 min. For children and patients weighing <40 kg, dilute 0.1 mg of naloxone in 10 mL of 0.9% NaCl for a concentration of 10 mcg/mL and administer 0.5 mcg/kg every 2 min. Titrate dose to avoid withdrawal, seizures, and severe pain.

Implementation

- ***High Alert:*** Do not confuse methadone with dexmethylphenidate, ketorolac, memantine, methylphenidate, or metolazone.
- When used for the treatment of opioid addiction in detoxification or maintenance programs, methadone is dispensed only by opioid treatment programs certified by the Substance Abuse and Mental Health Services Administration approved by the designated state authority.

- The initial dose for patients receiving detoxification treatment should be administered under medical supervision.
- Explain therapeutic value of medication prior to administration to enhance the analgesic effect.
- Regularly administered doses may be more effective than as needed administration. Analgesic is more effective if administered before pain becomes severe. For patients in chronic severe pain, the oral solution containing 5 mg/5 mL or 10 mg/5 mL is recommended on a fixed dose schedule.
- Coadministration with nonopioid analgesics may have additive analgesic effects and may permit lower doses.
- Medication should be discontinued gradually after long-term use to prevent withdrawal symptoms. For patients on long-acting agents who are physically opioid-dependent, initiate the taper by a small enough increment (less than 10% of total daily dose) to avoid withdrawal symptoms, and proceed with dose-lowering at an interval of every 2–4 wk. Patients who have been taking opioids for briefer periods of time may tolerate a more rapid taper. Monitor frequently to manage pain and withdrawal symptoms (restlessness; lacrimation; rhinorrhea; yawning; perspiration; chills; myalgia; mydriasis; irritability; anxiety; backache; joint pain; weakness; abdominal cramps; insomnia; nausea; anorexia; vomiting; diarrhea; or ↑ BP, respiratory rate, or HR). If withdrawal symptoms occur, pause the taper for a period of time or ↑ the dose of opioid analgesic to the previous dose, and then proceed with a slower taper. Also, monitor patients for changes in mood, emergence of suicidal thoughts, or use of other substances. A multimodal approach to pain management may optimize the treatment of chronic pain, as well as assist with the successful tapering of the opioid analgesic.
- **PO:** Doses may be administered with food or milk to minimize GI irritation.
- Dilute each dose of 10 mg/mL oral concentrate with ≥30 mL of water or other liquid prior to administration.
- Diskettes (dispersible tablets) are to be dissolved and used for detoxification and maintenance treatment only. Available only to licensed detoxification/maintenance programs.
- **SUBQ IM** IM is the preferred route for repeated doses. SUBQ administration may cause tissue irritation.
- ***REMS:*** FDA strongly encourages health care providers to complete a REMS-compliant education program that includes all the elements of the FDA Education *Blueprint for Health Care Providers Involved in the Management or Support of Patients with Pain*, available at www.fda.gov/OpioidAnalgesicREMS-Blueprint. Information on programs can be found at 1-800-503-0784 or www.opioidanalgesicrems.com.
- Discuss availability of naloxone for emergency treatment of opioid overdose with the patient and caregiver and assess the potential need for access to naloxone, both when initiating and renewing therapy, especially if patient has household members (including children) or other close contacts at risk for accidental exposure or overdose. Consider prescribing naloxone, based on the patient's risk factors for overdose, such as concurrent use of CNS depressants, a history of opioid use disorder, or prior opioid overdose. However, the presence of risk factors for overdose should not prevent the proper management of pain in any patient.

IV Administration

- **IV Push:** Administer undiluted. **Rate:** Inject slowly.
- **Y-Site Compatibility:** amikacin, aminocaproic acid, aminophylline, amiodarone, amphotericin B liposomal, ampicillin, ampicillin/sulbactam, anidulafungin, argatroban, arsenic trioxide, atropine, azithromycin, aztreonam, bleomycin, bumetanide, busulfan, calcium chloride, calcium gluconate, carboplatin, carmustine, caspofungin, cefazolin, cefepime, cefotaxime, cefotetan, cefoxitin, ceftazidime, ceftriaxone, cefuroxime, chloramphenicol, chlorpromazine, ciprofloxacin, cisatracurium, cisplatin, clindamycin, cyclophosphamide, cyclosporine, cytarabine, dacarbazine, dactinomycin, daptomycin, daunorubicin, dexamethasone, dexmedetomidine, dexrazoxane, diazepam, digoxin, diltiazem, diphenhydramine, dobutamine, docetaxel, dopamine, doxorubicin hydrochloride, doxorubicin liposomal, doxycycline, droperidol, enalaprilat, ephedrine, epinephrine, epirubicin, eptifibatide, ertapenem, erythromycin, esmolol, esomeprazole, etoposide, etoposide phosphate, famotidine, fluconazole, fludarabine, foscarnet, fosphenytoin, gemcitabine, gentamicin, glycopyrrolate, granisetron, haloperidol, heparin, hydralazine, hydrocortisone, idarubicin, ifosfamide, imipenem/cilastatin, insulin regular, irinotecan, isoproterenol, ketorolac, labetalol, leucovorin, levofloxacin, lidocaine, linezolid, lorazepam, magnesium sulfate, mannitol, melphalan, meropenem, mesna, methotrexate, methylprednisolone, metoclopramide, metoprolol, metronidazole, midazolam, milrinone, mitomycin, mitoxantrone, morphine, moxifloxacin, mycophenolate, nafcillin, naloxone, nicardipine, nitroglycerin, nitroprusside, norepinephrine, octreotide, ondansetron, oxaliplatin, oxytocin, paclitaxel, palonosetron, pamidronate, pantoprazole, pemetrexed, pentamidine, phenobarbital, phenylephrine, potassium acetate, potassium chloride, potassium phosphates,

M

procainamide, prochlorperazine, promethazine, propranolol, rocuronium, sodium acetate, sodium bicarbonate, sodium phosphates, succinylcholine, tacrolimus, theophylline, thiotepa, tirofiban, tobramycin, topotecan, vancomycin, vasopressin, vecuronium, verapamil, vinblastine, vincristine, vinorelbine, voriconazole, zidovudine, zoledronic acid.

- **Y-Site Incompatibility:** acyclovir, allopurinol, amphotericin B deoxycholate, dantrolene, fluorouracil, ganciclovir, methohexital, pentobarbital, phenytoin, piperacillin/tazobactam, trimethoprim/sulfamethoxazole.

Patient/Family Teaching

- Explain purpose and side effects of methadone to patient. Instruct them to take medication as directed and when to ask for pain medication. Advise patient to read *Patient Information* before starting and with each Rx refill in case of changes.
- ***REMS:*** Instruct patient to take methadone exactly as directed. If dose is less effective after a few wk, do not ↑ dose without consulting health care provider. Discuss safe use, risks, and proper storage and disposal of opioid analgesics with patients and caregivers with each Rx. The Patient Counseling Guide is available at www.fda.gov/OpioidAnalgesicREMSPCG.
- Advise patient that methadone is a drug with known abuse potential. Protect it from theft, and never give to anyone other than the individual for whom it was prescribed. Store out of sight and reach of children, and in a location not accessible by others.
- Educate patients and caregivers on how to recognize respiratory depression and emphasize the importance of calling 911 or getting emergency medical help right away in the event of a known or suspected overdose. Inform patients and caregivers about various ways to obtain naloxone as permitted by individual state naloxone dispensing and prescribing requirements or guidelines (Rx, direct from pharmacist, or state programs). OTC naloxone nasal spray is available at pharmacies nationwide for overdose or accidental ingestion.
- Medication may cause drowsiness or dizziness. Advise patient to call for assistance when ambulating and to avoid driving or other activities that require alertness until response to the medication is known.
- Inform patient of the potential for arrhythmias and emphasize the importance of regular ECGs.
- Advise patient to notify health care provider if pain control is not adequate or if side effects occur.
- Caution patient to notify health care provider if signs of overdose (difficult or shallow breathing; extreme tiredness or sleepiness; blurred vision; inability to think, talk, or walk normally; feelings of faintness, dizziness, or confusion) occur. Methadone has a prolonged action, causing ↑ risk of overdose.
- Advise patient to change positions slowly to minimize orthostatic hypotension.
- Advise patient to tell health care provider what medications they are taking and to avoid taking new Rx, OTC, vitamins, or herbal products without consulting health care provider. Caution patient to avoid concurrent use of alcohol or other CNS depressants, including other opioids, with this medication.
- Encourage patient to turn, cough, and breathe deeply every 2 hr to prevent atelectasis.
- Emphasize the importance of aggressive prevention of constipation with the use of methadone.
- Rep: Advise patient to notify health care provider if pregnancy is planned or suspected or if breastfeeding. Inform patient of potential for neonatal opioid withdrawal syndrome with prolonged use during pregnancy. Monitor neonate for signs and symptoms of withdrawal (irritability, hyperactivity and abnormal sleep pattern, high-pitched cry, tremor, vomiting, diarrhea, failure to gain weight); usually occur the first days after birth. Monitor infants exposed to methadone through breast milk for excess sedation and respiratory depression. Chronic use may ↓ fertility in women and men. During pregnancy, a woman's methadone dose may need to be ↑ or the dosing interval ↓ due to ↑ clearance.

Evaluation/Desired Outcomes

- Decrease in severity of pain without a significant alteration in level of consciousness or respiratory status.
- Prevention of withdrawal symptoms in detoxification from heroin and other opioid analgesics.

methIMAzole (meth-im-a-zole)

Tapazole

Classification

Therapeutic: antithyroid agents

Indications

Palliative treatment of hyperthyroidism. Used as an adjunct to control hyperthyroidism in preparation for thyroidectomy or radioactive iodine therapy.

Action

Inhibits the synthesis of thyroid hormones. **Therapeutic Effects:** Decreased signs and symptoms of hyperthyroidism.

Pharmacokinetics

Absorption: Rapidly absorbed following oral administration.

Distribution: Concentrated in the thyroid gland.

Metabolism and Excretion: Mostly metabolized by the liver; <10% eliminated unchanged by the kidneys.

Half-life: 3–5 hr.

TIME/ACTION PROFILE (effect on thyroid function)

ROUTE	ONSET	PEAK	DURATION
PO	1 wk	4–10 wk	1–2 wk

Contraindications/Precautions

Contraindicated in: Hypersensitivity.
Use Cautiously in: ↓ bone marrow reserve; Patients >40 yr (↑ risk of agranulocytosis); OB: Use during pregnancy only if potential maternal benefit justifies potential fetal risk. May cause congenital malformations (especially if used during 1st trimester).

Adverse Reactions/Side Effects

Derm: rash, skin discoloration, urticaria. **GI:** diarrhea, HEPATOTOXICITY, loss of taste, nausea, parotitis, vomiting. **Hemat:** AGRANULOCYTOSIS, anemia, leukopenia, thrombocytopenia. **MS:** arthralgia. **Neuro:** drowsiness, headache, vertigo. **Misc:** fever, lymphadenopathy.

Interactions

Drug-Drug: Additive bone marrow depression with **antineoplastics** or **radiation therapy**. Antithyroid effect may be ↓ by **potassium iodide** or **amiodarone**. ↑ risk of agranulocytosis with **phenothiazines**. May alter response to **warfarin** and **digoxin**.

Route/Dosage

PO (Adults): *Initial:* 15–60 mg/day in 3 divided doses. *Maintenance:* 5–15 mg once daily.
PO (Children): *Initial:* 0.4 mg/kg/day in 3 divided doses. *Maintenance:* 0.2 mg/kg/day in single dose or 2 divided doses.

Availability (generic available)

Tablets: 5 mg, 10 mg.

NURSING IMPLICATIONS

Assessment

- Monitor for symptoms of hyperthyroidism or thyrotoxicosis (tachycardia, palpitations, nervousness, insomnia, fever, diaphoresis, heat intolerance, tremors, weight loss, diarrhea).
- Assess for development of hypothyroidism (intolerance to cold, constipation, dry skin, headache, listlessness, tiredness, weakness). Dose adjustment may be required.

Lab Test Considerations

- Monitor thyroid function tests prior to therapy, monthly during initial therapy, and every 2–3 mo during therapy.
- Monitor WBC and differential periodically during therapy. Agranulocytosis may develop rapidly; usually occurs during the 1st 2 mo and is more common in patients >40 yr and those receiving >40 mg/day. *If agranulocytosis or pancytopenia occurs,* discontinue methimazole and monitor bone marrow indices.
- May ↑ AST, ALT, LDH, alkaline phosphatase, serum bilirubin, and PT. *If clinically significant hepatotoxicity, including transaminases >3 times the upper limit of normal, occurs,* discontinue methimazole.

Implementation

- Do not confuse methimazole with metolazone or methazolamide.
- **PO:** Administer at same time in relation to food every day.

Patient/Family Teaching

- Explain purpose and side effects of medication. Advise patient to read *Patient Information* before starting therapy.
- Instruct patient to take missed doses as soon as remembered; take both doses together if almost time for next dose; check with health care provider if >1 dose is missed. Consult health care provider prior to discontinuing medication.
- Instruct patient to monitor weight 2–3 times weekly and notify health care provider of significant changes.
- May cause drowsiness. Caution patient to avoid driving or other activities requiring alertness until response to medication is known.
- Advise patient to consult health care provider regarding dietary sources of iodine (iodized salt, shellfish).
- Advise patient to report sore throat, fever, chills, headache, malaise, weakness, yellowing of eyes or skin, unusual bleeding or bruising, or symptoms of hyperthyroidism or hypothyroidism promptly.
- Advise patient to notify health care provider if signs or symptoms of vasculitis (new rash, hematuria, ↓ urine output, dyspnea, hemoptysis, headache, fatigue, numbness and tingling in extremities, weakness) occur.
- Instruct patient to notify health care provider of all Rx or OTC medications, vitamins, or herbal products being taken and to consult with health care provider before taking other medications.
- Advise patient to carry identification describing medication regimen at all times.
- Advise patient to notify health care provider of medication regimen prior to treatment or surgery.
- Rep: Advise women of reproductive potential to notify health care provider if pregnancy is planned or suspected or if breastfeeding. May cause fetal harm, especially during 1st trimester. If breastfeeding, monitor infant thyroid levels weekly or biweekly.

M

- Emphasize the importance of routine exams to monitor progress and to check for side effects.

Evaluation/Desired Outcomes

- Decrease in severity of symptoms of hyperthyroidism (↓ pulse rate and weight gain).
- Return of thyroid function studies to normal.
- May be used as short-term adjunctive therapy to prepare patient for thyroidectomy or radiation therapy, or may be used in treatment of hyperthyroidism. Treatment from 6 mo to several yr may be necessary, averaging 1 yr.

BEERS

methocarbamol

(meth-oh-**kar**-ba-mole)

Robaxin, Tanlor

Classification

Therapeutic: skeletal muscle relaxants, (centrally acting)

Indications

Adjunctive treatment of muscle spasm associated with acute painful musculoskeletal conditions (with rest and physical therapy).

Action

Skeletal muscle relaxation, probably as a result of CNS depression. **Therapeutic Effects:** Skeletal muscle relaxation.

Pharmacokinetics

Absorption: Rapidly absorbed from the GI tract.
Distribution: Widely distributed to tissues.
Metabolism and Excretion: Metabolized by the liver.
Half-life: 1–2 hr.

TIME/ACTION PROFILE (skeletal muscle relaxation)

ROUTE	ONSET	PEAK	DURATION
PO	30 min	2 hr	unknown
IM	rapid	unknown	unknown
IV	immediate	end of infusion	unknown

Contraindications/Precautions

Contraindicated in: Hypersensitivity; Hypersensitivity to polyethylene glycol (parenteral form); Renal impairment (parenteral form).
Use Cautiously in: Seizure disorders (parenteral form); OB: Safety not established in pregnancy; Lactation: Safety not established in breastfeeding; Pedi: Safety and effectiveness not established in children; Geri: Appears on Beers list. ↑ risk of anticholinergic adverse reactions, sedation, and fractures in older adults. Avoid use in older adults.

Adverse Reactions/Side Effects

CV: IV: bradycardia, hypotension. **Derm:** flushing (IV), pruritus, rash, urticaria. **EENT:** blurred vision, nasal congestion. **GI:** anorexia, GI upset, nausea. **GU:** brown, black, or green urine. **Local:** pain at IM site, phlebitis (IV). **Neuro:** dizziness, drowsiness, light-headedness, SEIZURES (IV, IM). **Misc:** fever, HYPERSENSITIVITY REACTIONS (INCLUDING ANAPHYLAXIS) (IM, IV).

Interactions

Drug-Drug: Additive CNS depression with other **CNS depressants**, including **alcohol**, **antihistamines**, **opioid analgesics**, and **sedative/hypnotics**.
Drug-Natural Products: Kava-kava, valerian, chamomile, or **hops** can ↑ risk of CNS depression.

Route/Dosage

PO (Adults): 1.5 g 4 times daily initially (up to 8 g/day) for 2–3 days, then 4–4.5 g/day in 3–6 divided doses; may be followed by maintenance dosing of 750 mg every 4 hr or 1 g 4 times daily or 1.5 g 3 times daily.
IM, IV (Adults): 1–3 g/day for not more than 3 days; course may be repeated after a 48-hr rest.

Availability (generic available)

Tablets: 500 mg, 750 mg, 1000 mg. **Solution for injection:** 100 mg/mL.

NURSING IMPLICATIONS

Assessment

- Assess pain, muscle stiffness, and range of motion before and periodically throughout therapy.
- Monitor HR and BP every 15 min during parenteral administration.
- Assess for hypersensitivity reactions (skin rash, asthma, hives, wheezing, hypotension) after parenteral administration. Implement emergent medical support (epinephrine, oxygen) if needed.
- Monitor IV site. Injection is hypertonic and may cause thrombophlebitis. Avoid extravasation.
- Monitor for seizure activity. Implement seizure precautions if needed.
- Geri: Assess older adults for anticholinergic effects (sedation and weakness).

Lab Test Considerations

- Monitor renal function periodically during prolonged parenteral therapy (>3 days), because polyethylene glycol 300 vehicle is nephrotoxic.
- May falsely ↑ urinary 5-hydroxyindoleacetic acid and vanillylmandelic acid levels.

Implementation

- Provide safety measures as indicated. Supervise ambulation and transfer of patients.
- **PO:** Administer with food to minimize GI irritation. Tablets may be crushed and mixed with food or liquids to facilitate swallowing. **NG tube:** Crush tablet and suspend in water or saline.

- **IM** Do not administer SUBQ. IM injections should contain no more than 5 mL (500 mg) at a time in the gluteal region.

IV Administration
- **IV Push: Dilution:** Administer undiluted.
- **Concentration:** 100 mg/mL **Rate:** Administer at a max rate of 180 mg/m²/min but not >3 mL (300 mg)/min.
- **Intermittent Infusion: Dilution:** Dilute each dose in no more than 250 mL of 0.9% NaCl or D5W for injection. **Concentration:** 4 mg/mL for slower infusions. Do not refrigerate after dilution.
- Have patient remain recumbent during and for >10–15 min after infusion to avoid orthostatic hypotension.
- **Y-Site Incompatibility:** Do not administer other drugs through same IV line.

Patient/Family Teaching
- Explain purpose and side effects of medication to patient. Advise patient to read *Patient Information* before starting therapy. Advise to take as directed. Take missed doses within 1 hr; if not, return to regular dosing schedule. Do not double doses.
- Advise patient to notify health care provider of all Rx or OTC medications, vitamins, or herbal products being taken and to consult health care provider before taking other medications.
- Encourage patient to comply with additional therapies prescribed for muscle spasm (rest, physical therapy, heat).
- May cause dizziness, drowsiness, and blurred vision. Advise patient to avoid driving and other activities requiring alertness until response to drug is known.
- Instruct patient to change positions slowly to minimize orthostatic hypotension.
- Advise patient to avoid concurrent use of alcohol and other CNS depressants.
- Advise patient to contact health care provider immediately for new-onset seizures, premonitory symptoms, or change in seizure frequency.
- Inform patient that urine may turn black, brown, or green, especially if left standing.
- Instruct patient to notify health care provider immediately if skin rash, itching, fever, nasal congestion, or other signs of hypersensitivity reactions occur. Advise to seek immediate medical attention if needed.
- Rep: Advise women of reproductive potential to notify health care provider if pregnancy is planned or suspected or if breastfeeding.

Evaluation/Desired Outcomes
- Skeletal muscle relaxation.

HIGH ALERT

methotrexate (meth-o-**trex**-ate)
Jylamvo, ✤ Metoject, ✤ Nordimet, Otrexup, Rasuvo, ~~Rheumatrex~~, Trexall, Xatmep

Classification
Therapeutic: antineoplastics, antirheumatics (DMARDs), immunosuppressants
Pharmacologic: antimetabolites

Indications
PO, IV: Treatment of the following conditions: Acute lymphoblastic leukemia (in combination with other chemotherapy drugs), Non-Hodgkin lymphoma (in combination with other chemotherapy drugs).
IT: Treatment and prophylaxis of meningeal leukemia.
IV: Treatment of the following conditions: Osteosarcoma (in combination with other chemotherapy drugs), Breast cancer (in combination with other chemotherapy drugs), Squamous cell carcinoma of the head and neck. **IM, IV:** Gestational trophoblastic neoplasia (in combination with other chemotherapy drugs). **PO, IM SUBQ:** Treatment of the following conditions: Severe, active rheumatoid arthritis in patients with intolerance or an inadequate response to first-line therapy, Severe, active polyarticular juvenile idiopathic arthritis in patients with intolerance or an inadequate response to first-line therapy. **PO, IM, IV, SUBQ:** Severe, recalcitrant, disabling psoriasis in patients with an inadequate response to other therapies. **PO:** Mycosis fungoides (cutaneous T-cell lymphoma) (as monotherapy or in combination with other chemotherapy drugs).

Action
Interferes with folic acid metabolism. Result is inhibition of DNA synthesis and cell reproduction (cell-cycle S-phase-specific). Also has immunosuppressive activity. **Therapeutic Effects:** Death of rapidly replicating cells, particularly malignant ones, and immunosuppression.

Pharmacokinetics
Absorption: Small doses are well absorbed from the GI tract. Larger doses incompletely absorbed.
Distribution: Actively transported across cell membranes; widely distributed. Does not reach therapeutic concentrations in the CSF. Absorption in children is variable (23–95%) and dose-dependent.
Metabolism and Excretion: Excreted mostly unchanged by the kidneys.
Half-life: *Low dose:* 3–10 hr; *High dose:* 8–15 hr (↑ in renal impairment).

M

TIME/ACTION PROFILE (effects on blood counts)

ROUTE	ONSET	PEAK	DURATION
PO, IM, IV	4–7 days	7–14 days	21 days
SUBQ	unknown	unknown	unknown

Contraindications/Precautions

Contraindicated in: Hypersensitivity; Alcoholism or hepatic impairment; Immunosuppression; ↓ bone marrow reserve; OB: Pregnancy; Lactation: Lactation; Pedi: Products containing benzyl alcohol should not be used in neonates.

Use Cautiously in: Cranial radiation (↑ risk of leukoencephalopathy); Peptic ulcer disease or ulcerative colitis; Renal impairment (CCr must be ≥60 mL/min prior to therapy); Active infections; Rep: Women of reproductive potential and men with female partners of reproductive potential; Geri: Older adults may be more sensitive to toxicity and adverse events.

Adverse Reactions/Side Effects

Derm: alopecia, ERYTHEMA MULTIFORME, painful plaque erosions (during psoriasis treatment), photosensitivity, pruritus, rash, skin ulceration, soft tissue necrosis, STEVENS-JOHNSON SYNDROME (SJS), TOXIC EPIDERMAL NECROLYSIS (TEN), urticaria. **EENT:** blurred vision, transient blindness. **GI:** anorexia, DIARRHEA, nausea, STOMATITIS, VOMITING, GI PERFORATION, HEPATOTOXICITY. **GU:** NEPHROPATHY, ↓ fertility, acute renal failure, menstrual abnormalities, oligospermia. **Hemat:** ANEMIA, LEUKOPENIA, THROMBOCYTOPENIA, APLASTIC ANEMIA. **Metab:** hyperuricemia. **MS:** hemiparesis, osteonecrosis, stress fracture. **Neuro:** arachnoiditis (IT use only), confusion, dizziness, drowsiness, dysarthria, headache, leukoencephalopathy, malaise, SEIZURES. **Resp:** INTERSTITIAL PNEUMONITIS. **Misc:** chills, fever, HYPERSENSITIVITY REACTIONS (INCLUDING ANAPHYLAXIS), INFECTION, SECONDARY MALIGNANCY, tumor lysis syndrome.

Interactions

Drug-Drug: The following drugs may ↑ hematologic toxicity of methotrexate: high-dose **salicylates**, **dapsone**, **pemetrexed**, **mercaptopurine**, **NSAIDs**, **phenytoin**, **tetracyclines**, **probenecid**, **trimethoprim/sulfamethoxazole**, **penicillins**, **pyrimethamine**, **sulfonylureas**, and **warfarin**. ↑ risk of hepatotoxicity with other **hepatotoxic drugs**, including **azathioprine**, **sulfasalazine**, and **retinoids**. ↑ risk of nephrotoxicity with other **nephrotoxic drugs**. ↑ risk of bone marrow depression with other **antineoplastics** or **radiation therapy**. **Radiation therapy** ↑ risk of soft tissue necrosis and osteonecrosis. May ↓ antibody response to **live-virus vaccines** and ↑ risk of adverse reactions. ↑ risk of neurologic reactions with **acyclovir** (IT methotrexate only). **Nitrous oxide** may ↑ risk of toxicity; avoid concurrent use. **Folic acid** may ↓ antineoplastic effects; avoid concurrent use. May ↑ levels and risk of toxicity of **theophylline**.

Drug-Natural Products: Concurrent use with **echinacea** and **melatonin** may interfere with immunosuppression. **Caffeine** may ↓ efficacy of methotrexate; similar effect may occur with **guarana**.

Route/Dosage

Acute Lymphoblastic Leukemia

IV (Adults and Children): 10–5000 mg/m² followed by leucovorin rescue (for doses >500 mg/m²). Lower doses (20–30 mg/m²/wk) may be used IM.

PO (Adults and Children): 20 mg/m² once weekly.

Meningeal Leukemia

IT (Adults and Children ≥9 yr): 12–15 mg given at intervals of 2 or more days up to twice weekly (for treatment) and no more than once weekly (for prophylaxis).

IT (Children 3–<9 yr): 12 mg given at intervals of 2 or more days up to twice weekly (for treatment) and no more than once weekly (for prophylaxis).

IT (Children 2–<3 yr): 10 mg given at intervals of 2 or more days up to twice weekly (for treatment) and no more than once weekly (for prophylaxis).

IT (Children 1–<2 yr): 8 mg given at intervals of 2 or more days up to twice weekly (for treatment) and no more than once weekly (for prophylaxis).

IT (Children <1 yr): 6 mg given at intervals of 2 or more days up to twice weekly (for treatment) and no more than once weekly (for prophylaxis).

Non-Hodgkin Lymphoma

IV (Adults and Children): *In combination with other chemotherapy agents:* 1000 mg/m² *or* 3000 mg/m² over 24 hr followed by leucovorin rescue. *CNS-directed therapy:* 8000 mg/m² over 4 hr followed by leucovorin rescue (as monotherapy) *or* 3000–8000 mg/m² followed by leucovorin rescue (in combination with immunochemotherapy).

PO (Adults): 2.5 mg 2–4 times weekly.

Osteosarcoma

IV (Adults and Children): 12 g/m² (max = 20 g/dose) over 4 hr followed by leucovorin rescue, usually as part of a combination chemotherapeutic regimen (or ↑ dose until peak serum methotrexate level is 1×10^{-3} M/L but not to exceed 15 g/m²); 12 courses are given starting 4 wk after surgery and repeated at scheduled intervals.

Breast Cancer

IV (Adults): 40 mg/m² on days 1 and 8 (with other agents; many regimens are used).

Squamous Cell Carcinoma of Head and Neck

IV (Adults): 40–60 mg/m² once weekly.

Gestational Trophoblastic Neoplasia

IV, IM (Adults): *Low-risk gestational trophoblastic neoplasia:* 30–200 mg/m².

IV (Adults): *High-risk gestational trophoblastic neoplasia:* 300 mg/m² over 12 hr (with other agents).

Mycosis Fungoides

PO (Adults): *Monotherapy:* 25–75 mg once weekly; *As part of combination regimen:* 10 mg/m² twice weekly.

Rheumatoid Arthritis

PO, IM, SUBQ (Adults): 7.5 mg once weekly (not to exceed 20 mg/wk); when optimal clinical response is obtained, dose should be ↓. Otrexup may be used when dose is 10–20 mg/wk.

Polyarticular Juvenile Idiopathic Arthritis

PO, IM, SUBQ (Children): 10 mg/m² once weekly initially; may be ↑ up to 20–30 mg/m²; however, response may be better if doses >20 mg/m² are given IM or SUBQ; Otrexup may be used when dose is 10–25 mg/wk.

Psoriasis

Therapy may be preceded by a 5–10-mg test dose **PO, IM, SUBQ, IV (Adults):** 10–25 mg once weekly (not to exceed 25 mg/wk); when optimal clinical response is obtained, dose should be ↓. Otrexup may be used when dose is 10–25 mg/wk.

Availability (generic available)

Tablets: 2.5 mg, 5 mg, 7.5 mg, 10 mg, 15 mg. **Oral solution (Jylamvo) (orange flavor):** 2 mg/mL. **Oral solution (Xatmep) (orange flavor):** 2.5 mg/mL. **Solution for SUBQ injection (Otrexup):** 10 mg/0.4 mL, 12.5 mg/0.4 mL, 15 mg/0.4 mL, 17.5 mg/0.4 mL, 20 mg/0.4 mL, 22.5 mg/0.4 mL, 25 mg/0.4 mL. **Solution for SUBQ injection (Rasuvo):** 7.5 mg/0.15 mL, 10 mg/0.2 mL, 12.5 mg/0.25 mL, 15 mg/0.3 mL, 17.5 mg/0.35 mL, 20 mg/0.4 mL, 22.5 mg/0.45 mL, 25 mg/0.5 mL, 30 mg/0.6 mL. **Powder for injection:** 1 g/vial. **Solution for injection:** 25 mg/mL. **Solution for injection (preservative-free):** 25 mg/mL.

NURSING IMPLICATIONS

Assessment

- Monitor vital signs periodically during administration.
- Monitor for abdominal pain, diarrhea, or stomatitis; therapy may need to be discontinued.
- Monitor for bone marrow depression. Assess for bleeding (bleeding gums; bruising; petechiae; guaiac stools, urine, and emesis) and avoid IM injections and taking rectal temperatures if platelet count is low. Apply pressure to venipuncture sites for 10 min. Assess for signs of infection during neutropenia. Anemia may occur. Monitor for ↑ fatigue, dyspnea, and orthostatic hypotension.
- Monitor intake and output and daily weights. Observe for peripheral edema, steady weight gain, rales/crackles, or dyspnea. Notify health care provider should these occur. Drug accumulates in third spaces (e.g., pleural effusions, ascites), which results in prolonged elimination and ↑ the risk of adverse reactions. Evacuate significant third space accumulations prior to treatment.
- Monitor for signs and symptoms of infection (fever, chills, cough, headache, malaise, flu-like symptoms, dysuria, hematuria, cellulitis, erythematous nonhealing wound). Dose interruption or discontinuation and supportive therapy may be necessary based on severity.
- Monitor for symptoms of interstitial pneumonitis, which may manifest early as a dry, nonproductive cough.
- Monitor for symptoms of gout (joint pain, edema). Encourage patient to drink ≥2 L of fluid each day. Allopurinol and alkalinization of urine may be used to ↓ uric acid levels.
- Assess nutritional status. Administering an antiemetic prior to and periodically during therapy and adjusting diet as tolerated may help maintain fluid and electrolyte balance and nutritional status.
- Assess for rash periodically during therapy. May cause SJS and TEN. Discontinue therapy if severe or if accompanied with fever, general malaise, fatigue, muscle or joint aches, blisters, oral lesions, conjunctivitis, hepatitis, or eosinophilia.
- **IT:** Assess for development of nuchal rigidity, headache, fever, confusion, drowsiness, dizziness, weakness, or seizures.
- **Rheumatoid Arthritis:** Assess for pain and range of motion prior to and periodically during therapy.
- **Psoriasis:** Assess skin lesions prior to and periodically during therapy.

Lab Test Considerations

- Verify negative pregnancy test prior to starting therapy. Monitor CBC with differential prior to and at least monthly during therapy and at least daily for high-dose regimens. The nadir of leukopenia and thrombocytopenia occurs in 7–14 days. Leukocyte and platelet counts usually recover 7 days after the nadirs. Discontinue methotrexate immediately for any sudden ↓ in values.
- Monitor renal (BUN and serum creatinine) prior to and every 1–2 mo during therapy. Urine pH should be monitored prior to high-dose methotrexate therapy and every 6 hr during leucovorin rescue. Urine pH should be maintained at >7.0 from before 1st dose through therapy to prevent renal damage.
- Monitor hepatic function (AST, ALT, bilirubin, and LDH) prior to and every 1–2 mo during therapy.

- May cause ↑ serum uric acid concentrations, especially during initial treatment of leukemia and lymphoma.
- **Rheumatoid arthritis:** Monitor serum C-reactive protein levels.

Toxicity and Overdose

- Monitor serum methotrexate levels at least daily during high-dose therapy and adjust hydration and leucovorin dosing as needed. This monitoring is essential to plan correct leucovorin dose and determine duration of rescue therapy.
- With high-dose therapy (doses ≥500 mg/m^2), patient must receive leucovorin rescue within 24–48 hr to prevent fatal toxicity. May be considered for intermediate doses of 100 mg/m^2–<500 mg/m^2. Administer IV fluids starting before 1st dose and continuing through therapy to maintain adequate hydration and urine output. Administer glucarpidase in patients who have toxic plasma methotrexate concentrations (>1 micromolar) and delayed methotrexate clearance due to impaired renal function. Glucarpidase may be used for patients with impaired renal function. If glucarpidase is used, do not administer leucovorin within 2 hr before or after glucarpidase because leucovorin is a substrate for glucarpidase. In cases of massive overdose, hydration and urinary alkalinization with sodium bicarbonate are required to prevent renal tubule damage. Leucovorin and levoleucovorin are indicated to diminish the toxicity and counteract the effect of inadvertently administered overdoses of methotrexate. Monitor fluid and electrolyte status; patients must be well hydrated. Intermittent hemodialysis using a high-flux dialyzer may be used for clearance until levels <0.05 micromolar. Methotrexate should be delayed until recovery if WBC <1500 cells/mm^3, neutrophil count <200 cells/mm^3, platelet count <75,000 cells/mm^3, serum bilirubin >1.2 mg/dL, AST >450 IU/L, mucositis is present, or until evidence of healing. If persistent pleural effusion is present, should be drained dry prior to infusion. Adequate renal function is required. Serum creatinine must be normal and CCr must be >60 mL/min before initiation of therapy. Serum creatinine must be measured before each course of therapy. If ↑ by ≥50% of a prior value, CCr must be >60 mL/min, even if serum creatinine is within normal range.

Implementation

- ***High Alert:*** Fatalities have occurred with chemotherapeutic agents. Before administering, clarify all ambiguous orders; double-check single, daily, and course-of-therapy dose limits; have second practitioner independently double-check original order, calculations, and infusion pump settings. Methotrexate for nononcologic use is given at a much lower dose and frequency: often just once a wk. Do not confuse nononcologic dosing regimens with dosing regimens for cancer patients. Do not confuse methotrexate with metolazone or MTX Patch (lidocaine/menthol). Do not confuse Trexall with Paxil.
- Administer IV fluids starting before 1st dose and continuing through therapy to maintain adequate hydration and urine output.
- Use double gloves and a protective gown to prepare and administer solutions and injections. If possible, prepare in a biological safety cabinet or a compounding aseptic containment isolator; eye, face, and respiratory protection may be needed. Prepare and administer in a closed-system drug-transfer device. During administration, if there is a potential that the substance could splash or if the patient may resist, use eye and face protection. Discard equipment in specially designated containers.
- When switching the patient's dosing regimen from a methotrexate product for PO administration to a methotrexate product for IV, IM, or SUBQ administration, an alternative dosing regimen may be necessary due to potential differences in bioavailability.
- **PO:** Use only the copackaged syringe to measure *Jylamvo* and *Xatmep*; a teaspoon is not an accurate measuring device. Solution is clear yellow; do not administer solutions that are discolored, cloudy, or contain particulate matter.
- *Otrexup* and *Rasuvo* are not indicated for treatment of neoplastic diseases and not for patients requiring PO, IM, IV, intra-arterial, or IT dosing; doses <10 mg/wk; doses >25 mg/wk; high-dose regimens; or dose adjustments of less than 5 mg increments.
- **SUBQ:** *Otrexup* and *Rasuvo* are single-dose auto-injectors. Inject once weekly in abdomen or upper thigh. Avoid areas where skin is tender, bruised, red, scaly, hard, or has scars or stretch marks. Solution is clear and yellow; do not inject solutions that are discolored or contain particulate matter.

IV Administration

- **IV Push: Reconstitution:** Reconstitute each vial with 25 mL of 0.9% NaCl. Use sterile preservative-free diluents for high-dose regimens, neonates, low-birth-weight infants, and intrathecal use to prevent complications from large amounts of benzyl alcohol. Solution is clear yellow; do not use preparations that are cloudy, discolored, or contain a precipitate. Reconstitute immediately before use. Discard unused portion. **Concentration:** <25 mg/mL for IV push and intermittent/continuous infusions. **Rate:** Administer at a rate of 10 mg/min into Y-site of a free-flowing IV.
- **Intermittent/Continuous Infusion: Dilution:** Doses >100–300 mg/m^2 may also be diluted in D5W,

D5/0.9% NaCl, or 0.9% NaCl and infused as intermittent or continuous infusion. **Rate:** Administration rates of 4–20 mg/hr have been used.

- **Y-Site Compatibility:** acyclovir, alemtuzumab, allopurinol, amikacin, aminophylline, amiodarone, amphotericin B liposomal, ampicillin, ampicillin/sulbactam, anidulafungin, argatroban, atracurium, azithromycin, aztreonam, bivalirudin, bleomycin, bumetanide, buprenorphine, butorphanol, calcium chloride, calcium gluconate, carboplatin, carmustine, cefazolin, cefepime, cefotaxime, cefotetan, cefoxitin, ceftazidime, ceftriaxone, cefuroxime, ciprofloxacin, cisatracurium, cisplatin, clindamycin, cyclophosphamide, cyclosporine, cytarabine, dactinomycin, daunorubicin, dexmedetomidine, digoxin, diphenhydramine, docetaxel, doxorubicin hydrochloride, doxorubicin liposomal, enalaprilat, ephedrine, epinephrine, epirubicin, ertapenem, erythromycin, esmolol, etoposide, etoposide phosphate, famotidine, fentanyl, filgrastim, fluconazole, fludarabine, fluorouracil, foscarnet, fosphenytoin, furosemide, ganciclovir, gemtuzumab ozogamicin, granisetron, heparin, hetastarch, hydrocortisone, hydromorphone, imipenem/cilastatin, insulin regular, isoproterenol, ketorolac, letermovir, leucovorin, lidocaine, linezolid, lorazepam, magnesium sulfate, mannitol, melphalan, meperidine, meropenem, mesna, methadone, methohexital, methylprednisolone, metoclopramide, metoprolol, metronidazole, milrinone, minocycline, mitomycin, mitoxantrone, morphine, moxifloxacin, naloxone, nitroglycerin, norepinephrine, octreotide, ondansetron, oxacillin, paclitaxel, palonosetron, pamidronate, pentobarbital, phenobarbital, phenylephrine, piperacillin/tazobactam, potassium acetate, potassium chloride, potassium phosphates, procainamide, prochlorperazine, propranolol, remifentanil, rituximab, rocuronium, sargramostim, sodium acetate, sodium bicarbonate, sodium phosphates, succinylcholine, sufentanil, tacrolimus, theophylline, thiotepa, tigecycline, tirofiban, tobramycin, trastuzumab, trimethoprim/sulfamethoxazole, vasopressin, vecuronium, verapamil, vinblastine, vincristine, vinorelbine, voriconazole, zidovudine, zoledronic acid.
- **Y-Site Incompatibility:** amiodarone, amphotericin B deoxycholate, caspofungin, chlorpromazine, dacarbazine, daptomycin, dexrazoxane, diazepam, diltiazem, dobutamine, dopamine, doxycycline, gemcitabine, gentamicin, idarubicin, ifosfamide, levofloxacin, midazolam, mycophenolate, nalbuphine, nicardipine, pantoprazole, pentamidine, phenytoin, propofol.
- **IT:** Reconstitute preservative-free methotrexate with preservative-free 0.9% NaCl, Elliot's B solution, or patient's CSF to a concentration not greater than 2 mg/mL. May be administered via lumbar puncture or Ommaya reservoir. To prevent bacterial contamination, use immediately.

Patient/Family Teaching

- Explain the purpose and side effects of methotrexate to patient. Do not stop receiving drug without consulting health care provider. Instruct patient to take medication as directed. If a dose is missed, it should be omitted. Instruct patient on correct technique for SUBQ injection and care and disposal of equipment. Consult health care provider if vomiting occurs shortly after a dose is taken. Advise patients taking PO or SUBQ therapy to read *Patient Information* before starting therapy and with each Rx refill in case of changes.
- Advise patient prescribed a once-weekly regimen that dose should be administered as directed and that mistaken daily use can lead to fatal toxicity.
- Instruct patient to notify health care provider promptly if rash, fever, chills, cough, hoarseness, sore throat, signs of infection, lower back or side pain, painful or difficult urination, ↑ fatigue, dyspnea, or orthostatic hypotension occurs. Caution patient to avoid crowds and persons with known infections.
- Instruct patient to notify health care provider promptly if bleeding gums; bruising; petechiae; or blood in stools, urine, or emesis occurs. Instruct patient to use soft toothbrush and electric razor and to avoid falls. Caution patient not to drink alcoholic beverages or take medication containing aspirin or other NSAIDs; may precipitate gastric bleeding.
- Instruct patient to inspect oral mucosa for erythema and ulceration. If ulceration occurs, advise patient to use sponge brush and to rinse mouth with water after eating and drinking. Topical therapy may be used if mouth pain interferes with eating. Stomatitis pain may require treatment with opioid analgesics.
- Advise patient to notify health care provider of all Rx or OTC medications, vitamins, or herbal products being taken and to consult with health care provider before taking other medications. Instruct patient on high-dose methotrexate to avoid aspirin, NSAIDs, and proton pump inhibitors.
- Discuss the possibility of hair loss with patient. Explore methods of coping.
- Instruct patient not to receive any vaccinations without advice of health care provider.
- Caution patient to use sunscreen and protective clothing to prevent photosensitivity reactions.
- Rep: May cause fetal harm. Advise women of reproductive potential to use effective contraception during therapy and for 6 mo after last dose and avoid breastfeeding during and for 1 wk after last dose of therapy. Advise men with female partners of reproductive

M

potential to use effective contraception during and for 3 mo after therapy. Advise patient to notify health care provider if pregnancy is planned or suspected. May impair fertility in both men and women.

- Emphasize the need for periodic lab tests to monitor for side effects.

Evaluation/Desired Outcomes

- Improvement of hematopoietic values in leukemia.
- Decrease in symptoms of meningeal involvement in leukemia.
- Decrease in size and spread of non-Hodgkin lymphomas and other solid cancers.
- Resolution of skin lesions in severe psoriasis.
- Decreased joint pain and swelling.
- Improved mobility in patients with rheumatoid arthritis.
- Regression of lesions in mycosis fungoides.

methylergonovine

(meth-ill-er-goe-**noe**-veen)

Methergine

Classification

Therapeutic: oxytocics

Pharmacologic: ergot alkaloids

Indications

Prevention and treatment of postpartum or postabortion hemorrhage caused by uterine atony or subinvolution.

Action

Directly stimulates uterine and vascular smooth muscle. **Therapeutic Effects:** Uterine contraction.

Pharmacokinetics

Absorption: Well absorbed following oral or IM administration.

Distribution: Widely distributed to tissues.

Metabolism and Excretion: Probably metabolized by the liver.

Half-life: 30–120 min.

TIME/ACTION PROFILE (effects on uterine contractions)

ROUTE	ONSET	PEAK	DURATION
PO	5–15 min	unknown	3 hr
IM	2–5 min	unknown	3 hr
IV	immediate	unknown	45 min–3 hr

Contraindications/Precautions

Contraindicated in: Hypersensitivity; Concurrent use of strong CYP3A4 inhibitors; OB: Should not be used to induce labor; Lactation: Lactation.

Use Cautiously in: Hypertensive or eclamptic patients (more susceptible to hypertensive and arrhythmogenic side effects); History of or risk factors for coronary artery disease; Severe renal impairment; Severe hepatic impairment; Sepsis.

Exercise Extreme Caution in: OB: Third stage of labor.

Adverse Reactions/Side Effects

CV: arrhythmias, chest pain, heart block, HYPERTENSION, palpitations. **Derm:** ↑ sweating. **EENT:** tinnitus. **GI:** nausea, vomiting. **GU:** cramps. **Neuro:** dizziness, headache, paresthesia, STROKE. **Resp:** dyspnea.

Interactions

Drug-Drug: **Strong CYP3A4 inhibitors**, including **erythromycin**, **clarithromycin**, **ritonavir**, **nelfinavir**, **ketoconazole**, **itraconazole**, or **voriconazole**, may ↑ levels and risk of ischemia; concurrent use contraindicated. Excessive vasoconstriction may result when used with heavy cigarette smoking (**nicotine**), other **vasopressors** (such as **dopamine**), or **beta blockers**. **Moderate CYP3A4 inhibitors**, including **nefazodone**, **fluconazole**, **fluoxetine**, **fluvoxamine**, **zileuton**, or **clotrimazole**, may ↑ levels and risk of toxicity; use concurrently with caution. **CYP3A4 inducers**, including **nevirapine** and **rifampin**, may ↓ levels and effectiveness. **Anesthetics** may ↓ its oxytocic properties. May ↓ the antianginal effects of **nitrates**.

Drug-Food: **Grapefruit juice** may ↑ levels and risk of toxicity; use concurrently with caution.

Route/Dosage

PO (Adults): 0.2–0.4 mg every 6–12 hr for 2–7 days.

IM, IV (Adults): 0.2 mg every 2–4 hr for up to 5 doses.

Availability (generic available)

Tablets: 0.2 mg. **Solution for injection:** 0.2 mg/mL.

NURSING IMPLICATIONS

Assessment

- Monitor BP every 15–30 min for 1–2 hr postdose, especially after IV administration. Monitor for hypertension, bradycardia, and chest pain.
- Assess for signs of ergotism (cold, numb fingers and toes; chest pain; nausea; vomiting; headache; muscle pain; weakness).
- Assess for signs and symptoms of stroke (vision changes, facial drooping on one side, extremity weakness, slurred speech).
- Reassess fundal firmness and lochia 15–30 min after dose, and check for ongoing hemorrhage.

Lab Test Considerations

- If no response to methylergonovine, calcium levels may need to be assessed. Effectiveness of medication is ↓ with hypocalcemia.
- May ↓ serum prolactin.

Implementation

- **PO:** Administer with or without food.
- **IM:** Administer into IM site (vastus lateralis, ventrogluteal, or dorsogluteal).

IV Administration

- **IV:** IV administration is used for emergencies only. Oral and IM routes are preferred.

- **IV Push: Dilution:** Administer undiluted or diluted in 5 mL of 0.9% NaCl and administered through Y-site. Do not add to IV solutions. Do not mix in syringe with any other drug. Refrigerate; stable for storage at room temperature for 60 days; deteriorates with age. Use only solution that is clear and colorless and that contains no precipitate. **Concentration:** 0.2 mg/mL. **Rate:** Administer slowly over >1 min.
- **Y-Site Compatibility:** heparin, hydrocortisone, potassium chloride.

Patient/Family Teaching

- Explain purpose and side effects of medication to patient. Advise patient to read *Patient Information* before starting therapy. Instruct to take as directed; do not skip or double up on missed doses. If a dose is missed, omit it and return to regular dose schedule.
- Advise patient to notify health care provider of all Rx or OTC medications, vitamins, or herbal products being taken and to consult health care provider before taking other medications.
- Advise patient to monitor BP during treatment and notify health care provider if hypertension or signs and symptoms of a stroke occur. Seek immediate medical attention if needed.
- Advise patient that medication may cause menstrual-like cramps.
- Caution patient to avoid smoking because nicotine constricts blood vessels.
- Instruct patient to notify health care provider if infection develops, as this may cause ↑ sensitivity to the medication.
- Rep: Advise women of reproductive potential to notify health care provider if pregnancy is planned or suspected. Advise women not to breastfeed during therapy and for >12 hr after last dose.

Evaluation/Desired Outcomes

- Uterine contraction.

methylnaltrexone

(me-thil-nal-**trex**-one)

Relistor

Classification

Therapeutic: laxatives

Pharmacologic: opioid antagonists

Indications

SUBQ: Opioid-induced constipation (OIC) in patients with advanced illness or pain caused by active cancer who require opioid dose escalation for palliative care. **SUBQ, PO:** OIC in patients with chronic noncancer pain, including those with chronic pain related to prior cancer or its treatment who do not require frequent (e.g., weekly) opioid dose escalation.

Action

Acts peripherally as mu-opioid receptor antagonist, blocking opioid effects on the GI tract. **Therapeutic Effects:** Blocks constipating effects of opioids on the GI tract without loss of analgesia.

Pharmacokinetics

Absorption: Rapidly absorbed after SUBQ and oral administration; oral absorption delayed by high-fat meal.
Distribution: Moderate tissue distribution, does not cross the blood-brain barrier.
Metabolism and Excretion: Some metabolism; 85% excreted unchanged in urine.
Half-life: 15 hr (oral).

TIME/ACTION PROFILE (plasma concentrations)

ROUTE	ONSET	PEAK	DURATION
SUBQ	rapid	0.5 hr	24–48 hr
PO	rapid	1.5 hr	unknown

Contraindications/Precautions

Contraindicated in: Known/suspected mechanical GI obstruction; Lactation: Lactation.
Use Cautiously in: Known/suspected lesions of GI tract (↑ risk for GI perforation); Moderate or severe renal impairment (↓ dose); Moderate or severe hepatic impairment (dose ↓ may be required); OB: Use during pregnancy only if potential maternal benefit justifies potential fetal risk; Pedi: Safety and effectiveness not established in children.

Adverse Reactions/Side Effects

Derm: ↑ sweating. **GI:** abdominal pain, flatulence, nausea, diarrhea. **Neuro:** dizziness. **Misc:** opioid withdrawal.

Interactions

Drug-Drug: None reported.

Route/Dosage

Opioid-Induced Constipation in Patients With Advanced Illness

SUBQ (Adults >114 kg): 0.15 mg/kg every other day, as needed (not to exceed one dose every 24 hr).

Renal Impairment

SUBQ (Adults >114 kg): *CCr <60 mL/min:* 0.075 mg/kg every other day, as needed (not to exceed one dose every 24 hr).

Renal Impairment

SUBQ (Adults 62–114 kg): *CCr <60 mL/min:* 6 mg every other day, as needed (not to exceed one dose every 24 hr).

Renal Impairment

SUBQ (Adults 38–<62 kg): *CCr <60 mL/min:* 4 mg every other day, as needed (not to exceed one dose every 24 hr).

Renal Impairment

SUBQ (Adults <38 kg): *CCr <60 mL/min:* 0.075 mg/kg every other day, as needed (not to exceed one dose every 24 hr).

Opioid-Induced Constipation in Patients With Noncancer Pain

SUBQ (Adults): 12 mg once daily.

PO (Adults): 450 mg once daily.

Renal Impairment

SUBQ (Adults): *CCr <60 mL/min:* 6 mg once daily.

Renal Impairment

PO (Adults): *CCr <60 mL/min:* 150 mg once daily.

Hepatic Impairment

SUBQ (Adults >114 kg): *Severe hepatic impairment:* 0.075 mg/kg once daily.

Hepatic Impairment

SUBQ (Adults 62–114 kg): *Severe hepatic impairment:* 6 mg once daily.

Hepatic Impairment

SUBQ (Adults 38–<62 kg): *Severe hepatic impairment:* 4 mg once daily.

Hepatic Impairment

SUBQ (Adults <38 kg): *Severe hepatic impairment:* 0.075 mg/kg once daily.

Hepatic Impairment

PO (Adults): *Moderate or severe hepatic impairment:* 150 mg once daily.

Availability

Tablets: 150 mg. **Solution for injection (prefilled syringes):** 8 mg/0.4 mL, 12 mg/0.6 mL. **Solution for injection (single-use vials):** 12 mg/0.6 mL.

NURSING IMPLICATIONS

Assessment

- Assess bowel sounds and frequency, quantity, and consistency of stools periodically during therapy.
- Monitor pain intensity during therapy. Methylnaltrexone does not affect pain or effects of opioid analgesics on pain control.

Lab Test Considerations

- Monitor BUN, creatinine, sodium, potassium, and magnesium.
- Monitor AST ALT, alkaline phosphatase, and bilirubin.

Implementation

- Maintenance laxative must be stopped before administration of methylnaltrexone. If response is not sufficient after 3 days, laxatives may be restarted.
- **PO:** Administer with water on an empty stomach >30 min before 1st meal of the day.
- **SUBQ:** Pinch skin and administer in upper arm, abdomen, or thigh at a 45° angle using a 1-mL syringe with a 27-gauge needle inserted the full length of the needle. Do not rub the injection site. Solution is clear and colorless to pale yellow. Do not administer solutions that are discolored or contain a precipitate. Solution is stable for 24 hr at room temperature. Protect vials from light. Do not freeze. Do not use single-use vials for more than one dose.

Patient/Family Teaching

- Explain purpose and side effects of medication to patient. Advise patient to read *Patient Information* before starting therapy. Instruct patient to take as directed and teach appropriate injection technique and syringe/needle disposal. Usual schedule is one dose every other day, as needed, but no more than one dose in a 24-hr period.
- Advise patient to notify health care provider of all Rx or OTC medications, vitamins, or herbal products being taken and to consult health care provider before taking other medications.
- Advise patient that laxation may occur within 30 min of SUBQ injection; toilet facilities should be available following administration.
- Advise patient to discontinue all maintenance laxatives; can be added if inadequate response to methylnaltrexone.
- May cause dizziness. Caution patient to avoid driving and other activities requiring alertness until response to medication is known.
- Advise patient to notify health care provider and discontinue therapy if severe or persistent diarrhea occurs or if abdominal pain, nausea, or vomiting persists or worsens.
- Instruct patient to stop taking methylnaltrexone if they stop taking opioid medications.
- Rep: Advise women of reproductive potential to notify health care provider if pregnancy is planned or suspected or if breastfeeding.

Evaluation/Desired Outcomes

- Blocks constipating effects of opioids on the GI tract without loss of analgesia.

METHYLPHENIDATE

methylphenidate (oral)

(meth-ill-**fen**-i-date)

~~Adhansia XR~~, Aptensio XR, 🍁 Biphentin, Concerta, Cotempla XR-ODT, 🍁 Foquest, Jornay PM, ~~Metadate CD~~, Methylin, Quillichew ER, Quillivant XR, Relexxii, Ritalin, Ritalin LA

methylphenidate (transdermal)

Daytrana

Classification
Therapeutic: central nervous system stimulants

Schedule II

Indications

Oral, orally disintegrating tablets, and transdermal: Attention-deficit hyperactivity disorder (ADHD) (adjunct). **Oral only:** Narcolepsy.

Action

Produces CNS and respiratory stimulation with weak sympathomimetic activity. **Therapeutic Effects:** Increased attention span in ADHD. Increased motor activity, mental alertness, and diminished fatigue in narcolepsy.

Pharmacokinetics

Absorption: Slow and incomplete after oral administration; absorption of sustained or extended-release tablet (ER) is delayed and provides continuous release; well absorbed from skin. *Aptensio XR, Concerta, Relexxii, Ritalin LA:* Provides initial rapid release followed by a second continuous release (biphasic release).
Distribution: Unknown.
Metabolism and Excretion: Mostly metabolized (80%) by the liver.
Half-life: 2–4 hr.

TIME/ACTION PROFILE (CNS stimulation)

ROUTE	ONSET	PEAK	DURATION
PO	unknown	1–3 hr	4–6 hr
PO-ER	unknown	4–7 hr	3–12 hr†
Transdermal	unknown	unknown	12 hr

† Depends on formulation.

Contraindications/Precautions

Contraindicated in: Hypersensitivity; Hyperexcitable states; Hyperthyroidism; Patients with psychotic personalities or suicidal or homicidal tendencies; Serious structural cardiac abnormalities, cardiomyopathy, serious cardiac arrhythmia, coronary artery disease, or other serious cardiac disease (may ↑ risk of sudden death); Glaucoma; Concurrent use or use within 14 days of MAO inhibitors or MAO-inhibitor-like drugs (linezolid or methylene blue); Fructose intolerance, glucose-galactose malabsorption, or sucrose-isomaltase insufficiency; Surgery.
Use Cautiously in: Tics or family history/diagnosis of Tourette syndrome (may worsen condition); Hypertension; Diabetes mellitus; History of contact sensitization with transdermal product (may be at ↑ risk for systemic sensitization reactions with oral products); History or family history of vitiligo (may be at ↑ risk for loss of skin pigmentation with transdermal product); History of substance use; Continual use (may produce psychological dependence or physical addiction); Seizure disorders (may lower seizure threshold); Concerta product should be used cautiously in patients with esophageal motility disorders or severe GI narrowing (may ↑ the risk of obstruction); OB: Use during pregnancy only if potential maternal benefit outweighs potential fetal risk; may lead to premature delivery and low birth weight infants; Lactation: Use while breastfeeding only if potential maternal benefit outweighs potential risk to infant; Pedi: Growth suppression may occur in children with long-term use for children <6 yr (↑ risk of adverse reactions, particularly weight loss in children 4–<6 yr); Geri: Safety and effectiveness of many of the products have not been evaluated in older adults.

Adverse Reactions/Side Effects

CV: hypertension, palpitations, tachycardia, hypotension, peripheral vasculopathy, SUDDEN DEATH. **Derm:** contact sensitization (erythema, edema, papules, vesicles) (transdermal), erythema, loss of skin pigmentation (transdermal), rash. **EENT:** blurred vision, ↑ intraocular pressure, teeth grinding. **GI:** anorexia, constipation, cramps, diarrhea, dry mouth, metallic taste, nausea, vomiting. **GU:** priapism. **Metab:** growth suppression (especially with prolonged use), weight loss (especially with prolonged use). **MS:** RHABDOMYOLYSIS. **Neuro:** hyperactivity, insomnia, restlessness, tremor, akathisia, behavioral disturbances, dizziness, dyskinesia, hallucinations, headache, irritability, mania, thought disorder, tics, Tourette syndrome. **Misc:** fever, HYPERSENSITIVITY REACTIONS (INCLUDING ANAPHYLAXIS AND ANGIOEDEMA), physical dependence, psychological dependence, tolerance.

Interactions

Drug-Drug: Concurrent use with **MAO inhibitors** or **MAO-inhibitor-like drugs**, such as **linezolid** or **methylene blue**, may result in serious, potentially fatal reactions; wait ≥14 days following discontinuation of MAO inhibitor before initiation of amphetamine mixtures. Drugs that affect serotonergic neurotransmitter systems, including **MAO inhibitors, tricyclic antidepressants, SSRIs, SNRIs, fentanyl, buspirone, tramadol, lithium**, and **triptans**, may ↑ risk of serotonin syndrome. ↑ sympathomimetic effects with other **adrenergics**, including **vasoconstrictors, decongestants**, and **halogenated anesthetics**. May ↑ levels and risk of toxicity of **warfarin, phenytoin, phenobarbital, primidone, SSRIs**, and **tricyclic antidepressants**. **Pimozide** may mask cause of tics; avoid concurrent use.

May ↓ the effectiveness of **antihypertensives**. **Alcohol** may ↑ rate of release of drug from some methylphenidate formulations (Metadate CD, Ritalin LA). **Risperidone** may ↑ risk of extrapyramidal symptoms.

Drug-Natural Products: Use with caffeine-containing herbs (**guarana**, **tea**, **coffee**) may ↑ stimulant effect. **St. John's wort** may ↑ risk of serotonin syndrome.

Drug-Food: Excessive use of **caffeine**-containing foods or beverages (**coffee**, **cola**, **tea**) may cause ↑ CNS stimulation.

Route/Dosage

Attention-Deficit Hyperactivity Disorder

PO (Adults <65 yr): *Immediate-release tablets:* 5–20 mg 2–3 times daily. When maintenance dose is determined, may change to extended-release formulation. *Methylphenidate SR:* May be used in place of the immediate-release tablets when the 8-hr dose corresponds to the titrated 8-hr dosage of the immediate-release tablets. *Concerta and Relexxii (patients who have not taken methylphenidate previously):* 18–36 mg once daily in the morning initially; may be titrated as needed up to 72 mg/day. *Concerta and Relexxii (patients are currently taking other forms of methylphenidate):* 18 mg once daily in the morning if previous dose was 5 mg 2–3 times daily; 36 mg once daily in the morning if previous dose was 10 mg 2–3 times daily; 54 mg once daily in the morning if previous dose was 15 mg 2–3 times daily; 72 mg once daily in the morning if previous dose was 20 mg 2–3 times daily. *Aptensio XR:* 10 mg once daily; may ↑ dose in 10-mg increments at weekly intervals (maximum dose = 60 mg/day). *Quillivant XR and Quillichew ER:* 20 mg once daily; may ↑ dose in 10–20-mg increments at weekly intervals (maximum dose = 60 mg/day). *Jornay PM:* 20 mg once daily in the evening; may ↑ dose in 20-mg increments at weekly intervals (maximum dose = 100 mg/day).

PO (Children ≥6 yr [Ritalin LA for children 6–12 yr]): *Immediate-release tablets:* 0.3 mg/kg/dose or 2.5–5 mg before breakfast and lunch; may ↑ dose by 0.1 mg/kg/dose or by 5–10 mg/day at weekly intervals (not to exceed 60 mg/day or 2 mg/kg/day). When maintenance dose is determined, may change to extended-release formulation. *Methylphenidate SR:* May be used in place of the immediate-release tablets when the 8-hr dose corresponds to the titrated 8-hr dosage of the immediate-release tablets. *Ritalin LA (patients who have not taken methylphenidate previously):* 20 mg once daily; may ↑ by 10 mg/day at weekly intervals (max = 60 mg/day). *Ritalin LA (patients currently taking other forms of methylphenidate):* Can be used in place of immediate-release twice daily regimen given once daily at same total dose or in place of SR product at same dose. *Concerta (patients who have not taken methylphenidate previously):* 18 mg once daily in the morning initially; may be titrated as needed up to 54 mg/day (children 6–12 yr old) or up to 72 mg/day (children 13–17 yr old). *Concerta (patients are currently taking other forms of methylphenidate):* 18 mg once daily in the morning if previous dose was 5 mg 2–3 times daily; 36 mg once daily in the morning if previous dose was 10 mg 2–3 times daily; 54 mg once daily in the morning if previous dose was 15 mg 2–3 times daily; 72 mg once daily in the morning if previous dose was 20 mg 2–3 times daily. *Aptensio XR:* 10 mg once daily; may ↑ dose in 10-mg increments at weekly intervals (maximum dose = 60 mg/day). *Quillivant XR and Quillichew ER:* 20 mg once daily; may ↑ dose in 10–20-mg increments at weekly intervals (maximum dose = 60 mg/day). *Jornay PM:* 20 mg once daily in the evening; may ↑ dose in 20-mg increments at weekly intervals (maximum dose = 100 mg/day). *Cotempla XR-ODT:* 17.3 mg once daily in the morning; may ↑ dose in 8.6–17.3-mg increments at weekly intervals (maximum dose = 51.8 mg/day).

Transdermal (Children ≥6 yr): Apply one 10-mg patch initially (should be applied 2 hr before desired effect and removed 9 hr after application); may be titrated based on response and tolerability; may ↑ to 15-mg patch after 1 wk, then to 20-mg patch after another wk, and then to 30-mg patch after another wk.

Narcolepsy

PO (Adults): *Immediate-release tablets:* 10 mg 2–3 times/day; maximum dose = 60 mg/day.

Availability (generic available)

Immediate-release tablets (Ritalin): 5 mg, 10 mg, 20 mg. **Extended-release capsules (Aptensio XR):** 10 mg, 15 mg, 20 mg, 30 mg, 40 mg, 50 mg, 60 mg. **Extended-release capsules (Jornay PM):** 20 mg, 40 mg, 60 mg, 80 mg, 100 mg. **Extended-release capsules (Ritalin LA):** 10 mg, 20 mg, 30 mg, 40 mg. **Extended-release capsules (Foquest):** 25 mg, 35 mg, 45 mg, 55 mg, 70 mg, 85 mg. **Extended-release tablets (Concerta):** 18 mg, 27 mg, 36 mg, 54 mg. **Extended-release tablets (Relexxii):** 18 mg, 27 mg, 36 mg, 45 mg, 54 mg, 63 mg, 72 mg. **Extended-release orally disintegrating tablets (Cotempla XR-ODT):** 8.6 mg, 17.3 mg, 25.9 mg. **Chewable tablets (grape flavor):** 2.5 mg, 5 mg, 10 mg. **Extended-release chewable tablets (Quillichew ER):** 20 mg, 30 mg, 40 mg. **Oral solution (Methylin) (grape flavor):** 5 mg/5 mL, 10 mg/5 mL. **Extended-release oral suspension (Quillivant XR) (banana flavor):** 25 mg/5 mL. **Transdermal patch:** 10 mg/9 hr, 15 mg/9 hr, 20 mg/9 hr, 30 mg/9 hr.

NURSING IMPLICATIONS

Assessment

- Assess cardiac history, BP, HR, and respiratory rate prior to and periodically during therapy. Sudden death has been reported in patients with serious cardiac disease.

- Assess for risk of abuse, misuse, or addiction prior to starting therapy and during therapy. Has high dependence and abuse or misuse potential. Misuse and abuse of CNS stimulants can result in overdose and death; this risk is ↑ with higher doses or unapproved methods of administration, such as snorting or injection. Tolerance to medication occurs rapidly; do not ↑ dose.
- Assess for pre-existing psychiatric disorders, including family and personal history of bipolar disorder, mania, depression, and suicidal ideation. Monitor for behavior or mood changes during therapy.
- Assess for pre-existing and family history of tics and Tourette syndrome. Monitor for worsening motor and verbal tics during therapy and discontinue therapy when medically appropriate.
- Monitor for signs and symptoms of peripheral vasculopathy (intermittent pain, numbness, burning or color changes in digits). May require ↓ in dose or discontinuation.
- Pedi: Monitor growth (height and weight) in children. May need to interrupt therapy in patients who are not growing as expected.
- Assess for risk of acute angle-closure glaucoma. *If at risk,* obtain ophthalmic evaluation.
- **ADHD:** Assess children for attention span, impulse control, and interactions with others. Therapy may be interrupted at intervals to determine whether symptoms are sufficient to continue therapy.
- **Narcolepsy:** Observe and document frequency of episodes.
- **Transdermal:** Assess skin for signs of contact sensitization (erythema with edema, papules, or vesicles that does not improve within 48 hr or spreads beyond patch site) during therapy. May lead to systemic sensitization to other forms of methylphenidate. *If symptoms occur,* may change to oral preparation with close monitoring.
  Monitor for signs of skin depigmentation at application site and at distant sites. Discontinue transdermal patch if depigmentation occurs.

Lab Test Considerations

- Monitor CBC with differential during prolonged therapy.

Implementation

- Do not confuse methylphenidate with methadone.
- **PO:** Administer immediate and ER tablets (with the exception of *Concerta*) on an empty stomach (30–45 min before a meal); *Concerta* may be administered without regard to food, but must be taken with water, milk, or juice. ***DNC:*** ER tablets should be swallowed whole; do not break, crush, or chew. ***Quillichew ER*** chewable tablets may be broken in half. ***Aptensio XL, Metadate CD***, and ***Ritalin LA*** capsules may be opened and sprinkled on cool applesauce; entire mixture should be ingested immediately and followed by a drink of water. Do not store for future use.
- Shake ER oral suspension for 10 sec before administering. May be given with or without food.
- **Transdermal:** Apply patch to a clean, dry site on the hip; do not apply to waistline where tight clothing may rub it. Press firmly in place with palm of hand for 30 sec to secure. Alternate site daily. Apply patch 2 hr before desired effect and remove 9 hr after applied; effects last several more hr. Do not apply or reapply with dressings, tape, or other adhesives. Do not cut patches.
- If difficulty in separating patch from release liner, tearing, or other damage occurs during removal from liner, discard patch and apply a new patch. Inspect release liner to ensure no adhesive containing medication has transferred to liner; if transfer has occurred, discard patch. Avoid touching adhesive during application; wash hands immediately after application.
- If patch does not fully adhere or partially detaches, remove and replace with another patch. Exposure to water during bathing, swimming, or showering may affect patch adherence.
- Patches may be removed earlier before ↓ dose if an unacceptable loss of appetite or insomnia occurs.
- Store patches at room temperature in safe place to prevent abuse and misuse; do not refrigerate or freeze.
- To remove patch, peel off slowly. An oil-based product (petroleum jelly, olive oil, mineral oil) may be applied gently to facilitate removal. On removal, fold so that adhesive side of patch adheres to itself and flush down toilet or dispose of in an appropriate lidded container.

Patient/Family Teaching

- Instruct patient to take medication as directed. If an oral dose is missed, take the remaining doses for that day at regularly spaced intervals; do not double doses. Take the last dose before 6 pm to minimize the risk of insomnia. Instruct patient not to alter dose without consulting health care provider. Abrupt cessation of high doses may cause extreme fatigue and mental depression. Instruct parent/caregiver to read the *Medication Guide* prior to use and with each Rx refill as changes may occur.
- Advise patient to check weight 2–3 times weekly and report weight loss to health care provider.

M

- Advise patient that methylphenidate is a drug with known potential for abuse, misuse, and/or addiction. Store in safe place, protect it from theft, and never give to anyone other than the individual for whom it was prescribed.
- May cause dizziness or blurred vision. Caution patient to avoid driving or activities requiring alertness until response to medication is known.
- Inform patient that shell of *Concerta* tablet may appear in the stool. This is no cause for concern.
- Advise patient to avoid eating or drinking caffeine-containing substances concurrently with therapy.
- Advise patient to notify health care provider if nervousness, insomnia, palpitations, vomiting, skin rash, fever, painful and prolonged erections, or peripheral circulation problems occur.
- Advise patient to notify health care provider of behavior or mood changes.
- Advise patient to notify health care provider of all Rx or OTC medications, vitamins, or herbal products being taken and to consult with health care provider before taking other medications, especially St. John's wort.
- Inform patient that health care provider may order periodic holidays from the drug to assess progress and to ↓ dependence.
- Rep: Advise women of reproductive potential to notify health care provider if pregnancy is planned or suspected or if breastfeeding. May lead to premature delivery and low-birth-weight infants. Inform patients who become pregnant while taking methylphenidate of National Pregnancy Registry of ADHD Medications, which monitors pregnancy outcomes in patients exposed to ADHD medications. Enroll by calling 1-866-961-2388 or visit online at https://womens mentalhealth.org/adhd-medications/. Monitor breastfed infants exposed to methylphenidate for agitation, insomnia, anorexia, and ↓ weight gain.
- Emphasize the importance of routine follow-up exams to monitor progress.
- **Transdermal:** Encourage parent/caregiver to use the administration chart included in package to monitor application and removal time and disposal method.
- Caution patient to avoid exposing patch to direct external heat sources (hair dryers, heating pads, etc.). May ↑ rate and extent of absorption.
- Inform parent/caregiver that skin redness, itching, and small bumps on the skin are common. If swelling or blistering occurs, the patch should not be worn and health care provider notified. Caution parent/caregiver not to apply creams or ointments prior to application.
- Advise patient to discuss patch with referring health care provider prior to undergoing an MRI.
- **Home Care Issues:** Pedi: Advise parent/caregiver to notify school nurse of medication.

Evaluation/Desired Outcomes

- Improved attention span and social interactions in ADHD.
- Decreased frequency of narcoleptic symptoms.

methylPREDNISolone, See CORTICOSTEROIDS (SYSTEMIC).

BEERS

metoclopramide

(met-oh-**kloe**-pra-mide)

Gimoti, Reglan

Classification

Therapeutic: antiemetics

Indications

PO: Gastroesophageal reflux. **PO, IV, Intranasal:** Acute and recurrent diabetic gastroparesis. **IV:** Used for the following conditions: Prevention of nausea and vomiting associated with emetogenic chemotherapy, Prevention of postoperative nausea and vomiting when nasogastric suctioning is undesirable. Facilitation of small bowel intubation in radiographic procedures. **Unlabeled Use:** Hiccups

Action

Blocks dopamine receptors in chemoreceptor trigger zone of the CNS. Stimulates motility of the upper GI tract and accelerates gastric emptying. **Therapeutic Effects:** Decreased nausea and vomiting. Decreased symptoms of gastric stasis. Easier passage of nasogastric tube into small bowel.

Pharmacokinetics

Absorption: Well absorbed from the GI tract, from rectal mucosa, and from IM sites. 47% absorbed following intranasal administration. IV administration results in complete bioavailability.
Distribution: Widely distributed into body tissues and fluids. Crosses blood-brain barrier.
Metabolism and Excretion: Partially metabolized by the liver via the CYP2D6 isoenzyme; the CYP2D6 isoenzyme exhibits genetic polymorphism (~7% of population may be poor metabolizers and may have significantly ↑ metoclopramide concentrations and an ↑ risk of adverse effects). 25% eliminated unchanged in the urine.
Half-life: 2.5–6 hr.

TIME/ACTION PROFILE (effects on peristalsis)

ROUTE	ONSET	PEAK	DURATION
PO	30–60 min	unknown	1–2 hr
IM	10–15 min	unknown	1–2 hr
Intranasal	unknown	unknown	unknown
IV	1–3 min	immediate	1–2 hr

Contraindications/Precautions

Contraindicated in: Hypersensitivity; Possible GI obstruction, perforation, or hemorrhage; Seizure disorders; Hypertension; Pheochromocytoma; History of tardive dyskinesia; Parkinson disease; Moderate or severe renal or hepatic impairment (intranasal only); 🧬 CYP2D6 poor metabolizers (↑ risk for tardive dyskinesia) (intranasal only).

Use Cautiously in: History of depression; Diabetes (may alter response to insulin); Cirrhosis or HF (↑ risk of fluid retention); Renal impairment (↓ dose if CCr <50 mL/min) (oral and IV/IM only); Chronic use >12 wk (↑ risk for tardive dyskinesia); Moderate or severe hepatic impairment; 🧬 CYP2D6 poor metabolizers (↑ risk for tardive dyskinesia) (oral and IV/IM only); OB: May cause extrapyramidal symptoms or methemoglobinemia in neonate when used during pregnancy; Lactation: May lead to diarrhea, extrapyramidal symptoms, or methemoglobinemia in infant when used during breastfeeding; Pedi: Prolonged clearance in neonates can result in high serum concentrations and ↑ risk for methemoglobinemia. Side effects are more common in children, especially extrapyramidal reactions. Avoid use of tablets and intranasal because of ↑ risk of tardive dyskinesia and methemoglobinemia (in neonates); Geri: Appears on Beers list. ↑ risk of extrapyramidal effects, including tardive dyskinesia, in older adults. Avoid use in older adults, except for gastroparesis (duration for this indication should generally not exceed 12 wk). Intranasal therapy not recommended as initial therapy in older adults (can be transitioned to intranasal therapy once stabilized on oral therapy).

Adverse Reactions/Side Effects

CV: bradycardia, hypertension, hypotension, supraventricular tachycardia. **Endo:** gynecomastia, hyperprolactinemia. **GI:** constipation, diarrhea, dry mouth, nausea. **Hemat:** agranulocytosis, leukopenia, methemoglobinemia, neutropenia. **Neuro:** drowsiness, dysgeusia (intranasal), extrapyramidal reactions, restlessness, anxiety, bradykinesia, cog-wheel rigidity, depression, irritability, NEUROLEPTIC MALIGNANT SYNDROME, tardive dyskinesia, tremor.

Interactions

Drug-Drug: MAO inhibitors may cause release of catecholamines, which may ↑ BP; avoid concurrent use. Additive CNS depression with other **CNS depressants**, including **alcohol**, **antidepressants**, **antihistamines**, **opioid analgesics**, and **sedative/hypnotics**. May ↑ absorption and risk of toxicity from **cyclosporine**. May affect the GI absorption of other **orally administered drugs** as a result of effect on GI motility. May exaggerate hypotension during **general anesthesia**. ↑ risk of tardive dyskinesia, extrapyramidal reactions, or neuroleptic malignant syndrome with **antipsychotic agents**; avoid concurrent use. **Strong CYP2D6 inhibitors**, including **bupropion**, **fluoxetine**, **paroxetine**, or **quinidine**, may ↑ levels and risk of extrapyramidal reactions; avoid concurrent use with intranasal metoclopramide; ↓ PO or IV/IM metoclopramide dose. **Opioids** and **anticholinergics** may antagonize the GI effects of metoclopramide. May ↑ neuromuscular blockade from **succinylcholine**. May ↓ effectiveness of **levodopa**. May ↑ levels and risk of toxicity of **tacrolimus**.

Route/Dosage

Prevention of Chemotherapy-Induced Nausea and Vomiting

IV (Adults and Children): 1–2 mg/kg 30 min before chemotherapy. Additional doses of 1–2 mg/kg may be given every 2–4 hr; pretreatment with diphenhydramine will ↓ risk of extrapyramidal reactions to this dose.

Facilitation of Small Bowel Intubation

IV (Adults and Children >14 yr): 10 mg over 1–2 min.

IV (Children 6–14 yr): 2.5–5 mg (dose should not exceed 0.5 mg/kg) over 1–2 min.

IV (Children <6 yr): 0.1 mg/kg over 1–2 min.

Diabetic Gastroparesis

PO, IV: IM (Adults): 10 mg 30 min before meals and at bedtime for 2–8 wk (not to exceed 40 mg/day). *CYP2D6 poor metabolizers:* 5 mg 30 min before meals and at bedtime for 2–8 wk (not to exceed 20 mg/day). *Concurrent use of strong CYP2D6 inhibitor:* 5 mg 30 min before meals and at bedtime for 2–8 wk (not to exceed 20 mg/day).

Intranasal (Adults): One spray (15 mg) in one nostril 30 min before each meal and at bedtime (not to exceed 60 mg/day) for 2–8 wk (not to exceed 12 wk).

PO, IV, IM (Geriatric Patients): 5 mg 30 min before meals and at bedtime for 2–8 wk; may titrate up to 10 mg 30 min before each meal and at bedtime based on response and tolerability (not to exceed 40 mg/day).

Intranasal (Geriatric Patients): *Patients receiving alternative metoclopramide product at stable dose of 10 mg four times daily:* One spray (15 mg) in one nostril 30 min before each meal and at bedtime (not to exceed 60 mg/day) for 2–8 wk (not to exceed 12 wk).

Renal Impairment

PO (Adults): *CCr ≤60 mL/min:* 5 mg 30 min before meals and at bedtime for 2–8 wk (not to exceed 20 mg/day). *End-stage renal disease (including hemodialysis and peritoneal dialysis):* 5 mg twice daily for 2–8 wk (not to exceed 10 mg/day).

Hepatic Impairment

PO, IV, IM (Adults): *Mild hepatic impairment:* 10 mg 30 min before meals and at bedtime for 2–8 wk (not to exceed 40 mg/day). *Moderate or severe hepatic impairment:* 5 mg 30 min before meals and at bedtime for 2–8 wk (not to exceed 20 mg/day).

Gastroesophageal Reflux

PO (Adults): 10–15 mg 30 min before each meal and at bedtime (not to exceed 60 mg/day). *CYP2D6 poor metabolizers:* 5 mg 30 min before each meal and at bedtime or 10 mg 3 times daily (not to exceed 30 mg/day). *Concurrent use of strong CYP2D6 inhibitor:* 5 mg 30 min before each meal and at bedtime or 10 mg 3 times daily (not to exceed 30 mg/day).

PO (Geriatric Patients): 5 mg 30 min before each meal and at bedtime; may titrate up to 10–15 mg 30 min before each meal and at bedtime based on response and tolerability (not to exceed 60 mg/day).

Renal Impairment

PO (Adults): *CCr ≤60 mL/min:* 5 mg 30 min before each meal and at bedtime or 10 mg 3 times daily (not to exceed 30 mg/day). *End-stage renal disease (including hemodialysis and peritoneal dialysis):* 5 mg 30 min before each meal and at bedtime or 10 mg twice daily (not to exceed 20 mg/day).

Hepatic Impairment

PO (Adults): *Mild hepatic impairment:* 10–15 mg 30 min before each meal and at bedtime (not to exceed 60 mg/day). *Moderate or severe hepatic impairment:* 5 mg 30 min before each meal and at bedtime or 10 mg 3 times daily (not to exceed 30 mg/day).

Prevention of Postoperative Nausea and Vomiting

IM, IV (Adults): 10 mg at the end of surgical procedure; repeat in 6–8 hr if needed.

Hiccups

PO, IM (Adults): 10–20 mg 4 times daily PO; may be preceded by a single 10-mg dose IM.

Availability (generic available)

Tablets: 5 mg, 10 mg. **Orally disintegrating tablets:** 5 mg, 10 mg. **Oral solution (apricot-peach flavor):** 5 mg/5 mL. **Nasal spray:** 15 mg/metered spray in 9.8-mL bottle (delivers 112 metered sprays). **Solution for injection:** 5 mg/mL.

NURSING IMPLICATIONS

Assessment

- Assess for nausea, vomiting, abdominal distention, and bowel sounds before and after administration.
- Assess for extrapyramidal side effects (*parkinsonian:* difficulty speaking or swallowing, loss of balance control, pill rolling, masklike face, shuffling gait, rigidity, tremors; and *dystonic:* muscle spasms, twisting motions, twitching, inability to move eyes, weakness of arms or legs) periodically throughout course of therapy. May occur wk to mo after initiation of therapy and are reversible on discontinuation. Dystonic reactions may occur within minutes of IV infusion and stop within 24 hr of discontinuation of metoclopramide. May be treated with 50 mg of IM diphenhydramine, or diphenhydramine 1 mg/kg IV may be administered prophylactically 15 min before metoclopramide IV infusion.
- Monitor for tardive dyskinesia (uncontrolled rhythmic movement of mouth, face, and extremities; lip smacking or puckering; puffing of cheeks; uncontrolled chewing; rapid or worm-like movements of tongue). Avoid treatment with metoclopramide (all dose forms and routes of administration) for >12 wk due to ↑ risk of developing tardive dyskinesia with longer-term use. Report immediately and discontinue metoclopramide; may be irreversible.
- Monitor for neuroleptic malignant syndrome (hyperthermia, muscle rigidity, altered consciousness, irregular HR or BP, tachycardia, diaphoresis). Report immediately.
- Assess for signs of depression periodically throughout therapy.
- Monitor for symptoms related to hyperprolactinemia (menstrual abnormalities, galactorrhea, sexual dysfunction).

Lab Test Considerations

- May alter liver function tests.
- May ↑ serum prolactin and aldosterone.

Implementation

- **PO:** Administer doses 30 min before meals and at bedtime.
- Do not remove *orally disintegrating tablets* from the bottle until just prior to dosing. Remove tablet from bottle with dry hands, immediately place on tongue to disintegrate, and swallow with saliva. Tablet typically disintegrates in 1–1.5 min. Administration with liquid is not necessary.
- **IM:** For prevention of postoperative nausea and vomiting, inject IM near the end of surgery. Do not add any other solution or drug to the syringe.
- **Intranasal:** Administer one spray in one nostril. Before administering 1st dose from a bottle, prime the pump by pressing down on the finger flange and releasing 10 sprays in the air. Place the spray nozzle tip under one nostril and lean the head slightly forward so the tip of spray nozzle is aimed away from the septum and toward the back of the nose. Close the other nostril with the other index finger. Move spray pump upward so the tip of the nozzle is in the nostril. To ensure a full dose, hold the bottle upright while pressing down firmly and completely on finger flange and release while inhaling slowly through the open nostril. Remove spray pump nozzle tip from nostril and exhale slowly through the mouth. Wipe the spray nozzle with a clean tissue. If

uncertain that spray entered the nose, do not repeat dose. Take next dose at scheduled time.

IV Administration

- **IV Push:** Administer IV dose 30 min before administration of chemotherapeutic agent. **Rate:** Doses may be given slowly over 1–2 min. Rapid administration causes a transient but intense feeling of anxiety and restlessness followed by drowsiness.
- **Intermittent Infusion: Dilution:** May be diluted for IV infusion in 50 mL of D5W, 0.9% NaCl, D5/0.45% NaCl, Ringer's solution, or LR. Diluted solution is stable for 48 hr if protected from light or 24 hr under normal light. **Concentration:** May dilute to 0.2 mg/mL or give undiluted at 5 mg/mL. **Rate:** Infuse slowly (maximum rate 5 mg/min) over ≥15–30 min.
- **Y-Site Compatibility:** acetaminophen, aldesleukin, alemtuzumab, amikacin, aminocaproic acid, aminophylline, amiodarone, anidulafungin, argatroban, arsenic trioxide, ascorbic acid, atracurium, atropine, azathioprine, azithromycin, aztreonam, benztropine, bivalirudin, bleomycin, bumetanide, buprenorphine, butorphanol, calcium chloride, calcium gluconate, cangrelor, carboplatin, caspofungin, cefazolin, cefotaxime, cefotetan, cefoxitin, ceftaroline, ceftazidime, ceftolozane/tazobactam, ceftriaxone, cefuroxime, chloramphenicol, chlorpromazine, ciprofloxacin, cisatracurium, cisplatin, cladribine, clindamycin, cyanocobalamin, cyclophosphamide, cyclosporine, cytarabine, dacarbazine, dactinomycin, daptomycin, daunorubicin, dexamethasone, dexmedetomidine, dexrazoxane, digoxin, diltiazem, diphenhydramine, dobutamine, docetaxel, dopamine, doxorubicin hydrochloride, doxycycline, droperidol, enalaprilat, ephedrine, epinephrine, epirubicin, epoetin alfa, eptifibatide, ertapenem, erythromycin, esmolol, etoposide, etoposide phosphate, famotidine, fentanyl, filgrastim, fluconazole, fludarabine, folic acid, foscarnet, fosphenytoin, gemcitabine, gentamicin, glycopyrrolate, granisetron, heparin, hydrocortisone, hydromorphone, idarubicin, ifosfamide, imipenem/cilastatin, indomethacin, insulin regular, irinotecan, isavuconazonium, isoproterenol, ketamine, ketorolac, labetalol, leucovorin, levofloxacin, lidocaine, linezolid, lorazepam, magnesium sulfate, mannitol, melphalan, meperidine, meropenem, meropenem/vaborbactam, mesna, methadone, methotrexate, methylprednisolone, metoprolol, metronidazole, midazolam, milrinone, mitomycin, mitoxantrone, morphine, moxifloxacin, multivitamins, mycophenolate, nafcillin, nalbuphine, naloxone, nicardipine, nitroglycerin, nitroprusside, norepinephrine, octreotide, ondansetron, oxacillin, oxaliplatin, oxytocin, paclitaxel, palonosetron, pamidronate, papaverine, pemetrexed, penicillin G, pentamidine, pentobarbital, phenobarbital, phentolamine, phenylephrine, phytonadione, piperacillin/tazobactam, plazomicin, potassium acetate, potassium chloride, procainamide, prochlorperazine, promethazine, propranolol, protamine, pyridoxine, remifentanil, rituximab, rocuronium, sargramostim, sodium acetate, sodium bicarbonate, succinylcholine, sufentanil, tacrolimus, tedizolid, telavancin, theophylline, thiamine, thiotepa, tigecycline, tirofiban, tobramycin, topotecan, trastuzumab, vancomycin, vasopressin, vecuronium, verapamil, vinblastine, vincristine, vinorelbine, voriconazole, zidovudine, zoledronic acid.
- **Y-Site Incompatibility:** amphotericin B deoxycholate, amphotericin B liposomal, carmustine, cefepime, dantrolene, diazepam, diazoxide, doxorubicin liposomal, ganciclovir, gemtuzumab ozogamicin, phenytoin, propofol, trimethoprim/sulfamethoxazole.

M

Patient/Family Teaching

- Explain the purpose and side effects of metoclopramide. Instruct patient to take as directed. Explain how to administer intranasal doses. Take oral missed doses as soon as remembered if not almost time for next dose. If an intranasal dose is missed, omit and take the next dose at regularly scheduled time; do not double doses. Advise patient to read the *Medication Guide* before starting therapy and with each Rx refill in case of changes.
- Pedi: Unintentional overdose has been reported in infants and children with the use of metoclopramide oral solution. Teach parents how to accurately read labels and administer medication.
- May cause drowsiness. Caution patient to avoid driving or other activities requiring alertness until response to medication is known.
- Advise patient to notify health care provider of all Rx or OTC medications, vitamins, or herbal products being taken and to consult with health care provider before taking other medications. Advise patient to avoid concurrent use of alcohol and other CNS depressants while taking this medication.
- Inform patient of risk of extrapyramidal symptoms, tardive dyskinesia, and neuroleptic malignant syndrome. Advise patient to notify health care provider immediately if involuntary or repetitive movements of eyes, face, or limbs occur.
- Rep: Advise women of reproductive potential to notify health care provider if pregnancy is planned or suspected or if breastfeeding. Monitor neonates for extrapyramidal signs and methemoglobinemia.

Evaluation/Desired Outcomes

- Prevention or relief of nausea and vomiting.
- Decreased symptoms of gastric stasis.
- Facilitation of small bowel intubation.
- Decreased symptoms of esophageal reflux.
- Metoclopramide should not be used for >12 wk due to risk of tardive dyskinesia.

metOLazone (me-tole-a-zone)

Zaroxolyn

Classification

Therapeutic: antihypertensives, diuretics
Pharmacologic: thiazide-like diuretics

Indications

Mild to moderate hypertension. Edema associated with HF or nephrotic syndrome.

Action

Increases excretion of sodium and water by inhibiting sodium reabsorption in the distal tubule. Promotes excretion of chloride, potassium, magnesium, and bicarbonate. May produce arteriolar dilation. **Therapeutic Effects:** Lowering of BP in hypertensive patients. Diuresis with subsequent mobilization of edema. Effect may continue in renal impairment.

Pharmacokinetics

Absorption: Absorption is variable.
Distribution: Extensively distributed to tissues.
Protein Binding: 95%.
Metabolism and Excretion: Excreted mainly unchanged by the kidneys.
Half-life: 6–20 hr.

TIME/ACTION PROFILE (diuretic effect†)

ROUTE	ONSET	PEAK	DURATION
PO	1 hr	2 hr	12–24 hr

† Full antihypertensive effect may take days–wk.

Contraindications/Precautions

Contraindicated in: Hypersensitivity; Cross-sensitivity with other sulfonamides may exist; Anuria; Lactation: Lactation.
Use Cautiously in: Severe hepatic impairment; OB: Use during pregnancy only if potential maternal benefit justifies potential fetal risk; may ↑ risk of hypoglycemia, hypokalemia, hyponatremia, jaundice, and thrombocytopenia in fetus; Geri: Older adults may have ↑ sensitivity to drug effects.

Adverse Reactions/Side Effects

CV: chest pain, hypotension, palpitations. **Derm:** photosensitivity, rash. **Endo:** hyperglycemia. **F and E** hypokalemia, dehydration, hypercalcemia, hypochloremic alkalosis, hypomagnesemia, hyponatremia, hypophosphatemia, hypovolemia. **GI:** anorexia, bloating, cramping, drug-induced hepatitis, nausea, pancreatitis, vomiting. **Hemat:** blood dyscrasias. **Metab:** hyperuricemia. **MS:** muscle cramps. **Neuro:** drowsiness, lethargy.

Interactions

Drug-Drug: ↑ risk of hypotension with **nitrates**, acute ingestion of **alcohol**, or other **antihypertensives**. ↑ risk of hypokalemia with **corticosteroids**, **amphotericin B**, or **piperacillin/tazobactam**. May ↑ risk of **digoxin** toxicity. May ↑ levels and risk of toxicity of **lithium**. May ↓ effectiveness of **methenamine**. **Stimulant laxatives** (including **aloe**, **senna**) may ↑ risk of potassium depletion.
Drug-Food: Food may ↑ extent of absorption.

Route/Dosage

PO (Adults): *Hypertension:* 2.5–5 mg/day; *edema:* 5–20 mg/day.
PO (Children): 0.2–0.4 mg/kg/day divided every 12–24 hr.

Availability (generic available)

Tablets: 2.5 mg, 5 mg, 10 mg.

NURSING IMPLICATIONS

Assessment

- Monitor BP, intake and output, and daily weight, and assess feet, legs, and sacral area for edema daily.
- Assess patient for allergy to sulfonamides; cross-sensitivity may occur in patients allergic to sulfonamide-derived drugs such as thiazides, sulfonylureas, or sulfasalazine.
- Assess patient for signs and symptoms of fluid and electrolyte imbalances (anorexia, nausea, vomiting, muscle cramps, paresthesia, confusion). Risk is ↑ with vomiting and diarrhea. Patients taking digoxin are at risk of digoxin toxicity because of the potassium-depleting effect of the diuretic. Notify health care provider and treat as clinically indicated.
- **Hypertension:** Monitor BP every month until control is achieved and then every 3–6 mo; monitor more closely in patients with stage 2 HTN and BP ≥160/100 mm Hg.

Lab Test Considerations

- Monitor electrolytes (especially potassium), blood glucose, BUN, serum creatinine, and uric acid levels before and periodically during therapy.
- May ↑ serum and urine glucose in patients with diabetes.
- May ↑ in serum bilirubin, calcium, creatinine, and uric acid, and ↓ serum magnesium, potassium, sodium, and urinary calcium.
- May ↑ serum cholesterol, LDL-C, and triglycerides.

Implementation

- Do not confuse metolazone with methimazole, methazolamide, methadone, or methotrexate.

- Administer in the morning to prevent disruption of sleep cycle.
- Intermittent dose schedule may be used for continued control of edema.
- **PO:** May give with food or milk to minimize GI irritation.

Patient/Family Teaching

- Explain the purpose and side effects of metolazone. Instruct patient to take at the same time each day. Take missed doses as soon as remembered but not just before next dose is due. Do not double doses. Do not share medication with others, even if they have similar symptoms; may be harmful. Advise patient to read *Patient Information* before starting and with each Rx refill in case of changes.
- Explain need for continued medical follow-up to assess effectiveness and possible side effects of medication. Periodic lab tests may be needed.
- Instruct patient to monitor weight daily and notify health care provider of significant changes.
- Caution patient to change positions slowly to minimize orthostatic hypotension; may be potentiated by alcohol.
- Advise patient to report muscle weakness, cramps, nausea, vomiting, diarrhea, or dizziness to health care provider.
- Advise patient to use sunscreen and protective clothing in the sun to prevent photosensitivity reactions.
- Instruct patient to discuss dietary potassium requirements with health care provider (see Appendix J).
- Advise patient to notify health care provider of all Rx or OTC medications, vitamins, or herbal products being taken and to consult with health care provider before taking other medications.
- Instruct patient to notify health care provider of medication regimen before treatment or surgery.
- **Hypertension:** Advise patient to continue taking the medication even if feeling better. Medication controls but does not cure hypertension.
- Encourage patient to comply with additional interventions for hypertension (weight reduction, low-sodium diet, regular exercise, smoking cessation, moderation of alcohol consumption, stress management).
- Instruct patient and family in correct technique for monitoring weekly BP.
- Rep: Advise women of reproductive potential to notify health care provider if pregnancy is planned or suspected and to avoid breastfeeding during therapy. Monitor for hypoglycemia, hypokalemia, hyponatremia, jaundice, and thrombocytopenia in the fetus or newborn following maternal use.

Evaluation/Desired Outcomes

- Decrease in BP.
- Increase in urine output.
- Decrease in edema.

metoprolol, See BETA BLOCKERS (selective).

metroNIDAZOLE
(me-troe-**ni**-da-zole)

Flagyl, Likmez, MetroCream, MetroGel, MetroLotion, ✱Nidagel, Noritate, Nuvessa, Vandazole

Classification
Therapeutic: anti-infectives, antiprotozoals, antiulcer agents

Indications

PO, IV: Treatment of the following anaerobic infections: Intra-abdominal infections (may be used with a cephalosporin), Gynecologic infections, Skin and skin structure infections, Lower respiratory tract infections, Bone and joint infections, CNS infections, Septicemia, Endocarditis. **IV:** Perioperative prophylactic agent in colorectal surgery. **PO:** Treatment of the following infections: Amebic dysentery, amebic liver abscess, and trichomoniasis; Peptic ulcer disease caused by *Helicobacter pylori*. **Topical:** Acne rosacea. vaginal Bacterial vaginosis. **Unlabeled Use:** Giardiasis. Anti-infective associated *Clostridioides difficile*-associated diarrhea (CDAD).

Action

Disrupts DNA and protein synthesis in susceptible organisms. **Therapeutic Effects:** Bactericidal, trichomonacidal, or amebicidal action. **Spectrum:** Most notable for activity against anaerobic bacteria, including *Bacteroides spp., Clostridioides difficile, Gardnerella vaginalis, Mobiluncus spp. Peptostreptococcus spp.* In addition, active against *Trichomonas vaginalis, Entamoeba histolytica, Giardia lamblia, H. pylori*.

Pharmacokinetics

Absorption: 80% absorbed after oral administration. Minimal absorption after topical or vaginal application.
Distribution: Widely distributed into most tissues and fluids, including CSF.
Metabolism and Excretion: Partially metabolized by the liver (30–60%), partially excreted unchanged in the urine; 6–15% eliminated in the feces.
Half-life: Neonates: 25–75 hr; Children and adults: 6–12 hr.

TIME/ACTION PROFILE (PO, IV = plasma concentrations; topical = improvement in rosacea)

ROUTE	ONSET	PEAK	DURATION
PO	rapid	1–3 hr	8 hr
PO-ER	rapid	unknown	up to 24 hr
IV	rapid	end of infusion	6–8 hr
Topical	3 wk	9 wk	12 hr
Vaginal	unknown	6–12 hr	12 hr

Contraindications/Precautions

Contraindicated in: Hypersensitivity; Hypersensitivity to parabens (topical only); Cockayne syndrome (↑ risk of hepatotoxicity and death); OB: 1st trimester of pregnancy.

Use Cautiously in: History of blood dyscrasias; History of seizures or neurologic problems; Severe hepatic impairment (↓ dose); Patients receiving corticosteroids or predisposed to edema (injection contains 28 mEq sodium/g metronidazole); OB: Although safety has not been established, has been used to treat trichomoniasis in 2nd- and 3rd-trimester pregnancy, but not as single-dose regimen; Lactation: If needed, use single dose and interrupt nursing for 24 hr thereafter.

Adverse Reactions/Side Effects

Derm: ACUTE GENERALIZED EXANTHEMATOUS PUSTULOSIS (AGEP), DRUG REACTION WITH EOSINOPHILIA AND SYSTEMIC SYMPTOMS (DRESS), rash, STEVENS-JOHNSON SYNDROME (SJS), TOXIC EPIDERMAL NECROLYSIS (TEN), urticaria **topical only:** burning, mild dryness, skin irritation, transient redness. **EENT:** hearing impairment, optic neuropathy, tearing (topical only). **GI:** abdominal pain, anorexia, nausea, diarrhea, dry mouth, furry tongue, glossitis, unpleasant taste, vomiting. **Hemat:** leukopenia. **Local:** phlebitis at IV site. **Neuro:** dizziness, headache, aseptic meningitis (IV), encephalopathy (IV), peripheral neuropathy, psychosis, SEIZURES. **Misc:** superinfection.

Interactions

Drug-Drug: Cimetidine may ↑ levels and risk of toxicity. **Phenobarbital** and **rifampin** may ↓ levels and effectiveness. May ↑ levels and risk of toxicity of **phenytoin**, **lithium**, and **warfarin**. Disulfiram-like reaction may occur with **alcohol** ingestion. May cause acute psychosis and confusion with **disulfiram**. ↑ risk of leukopenia with **fluorouracil** or **azathioprine**. Use with **QT interval prolonging medications** may ↑ risk of QT interval prolongation.

Route/Dosage

PO (Adults): *Anaerobic infections:* 7.5 mg/kg every 6 hr (not to exceed 4 g/day). *Trichomoniasis:* 250 mg every 8 hr for 7 days *or* single 2-g dose *or* 1 g twice daily for 1 day. *Amebiasis:* 500–750 mg every 8 hr for 5–10 days. *H. pylori:* 250 mg 4 times daily *or* 500 mg twice daily for 1–2 wk (with other agents). *CDAD:* 250–500 mg 3–4 times/day for 10–14 days.

PO (Infants and Children): *Anaerobic infections:* 30 mg/kg/day divided every 6 hr, maximum dose: 4 g/day. *Trichomoniasis:* 15–30 mg/kg/day divided every 8 hr for 7–10 days. *Amebiasis:* 35–50 mg/kg/day divided every 8 hr for 5–10 days (not to exceed 750 mg/dose). *CDAD:* 30 mg/kg/day divided every 6 hr for 7–10 days. *H. pylori:* 15–20 mg/kg/day divided twice daily for 4 wk.

IV, PO (Neonates 0–4 wk, <1200 g): 7.5 mg/kg every 48 hr. *Postnatal age <7 days, 1200–2000 g:* 7.5 mg/kg/day every 24 hr. *Postnatal age <7 days, >2000 g:* 15 mg/kg/day divided every 12 hr. *Postnatal age >7 days, 1200–2000 g:* 15 mg/kg/day divided every 12 hr. *Postnatal age >7 days, >2000 g:* 30 mg/kg/day divided every 12 hr.

IV (Adults): *Anaerobic infections:* Initial dose 15 mg/kg; then 7.5 mg/kg every 6–8 hr *or* 500 mg every 6–8 hr (not to exceed 4 g/day). *Perioperative prophylaxis:* Initial dose 15 mg/kg 1 hr before surgery; then 7.5 mg/kg 6 and 12 hr later. *Amebiasis:* 500–750 mg every 8 hr for 5–10 days.

IV (Children): *Anaerobic infections:* 30 mg/kg/day divided every 6 hr; maximum dose: 4 g/day.

Topical: (Adults): *Acne rosacea:* Apply thin film to affected area bid.

Vaginal (Adults): *0.75% vaginal gel:* One applicatorful (37.5 mg) of 0.75% gel 1–2 times daily for 5 days. *Nuvessa:* One applicatorful (65 mg) of 1.3% gel as a single dose at bedtime. *Vandazole:* One applicatorful (37.5 mg) of 0.75% gel once daily for 5 days.

Vag (Children ≥12 yr): *Nuvessa:* One applicatorful (65 mg) of 1.3% gel as a single dose at bedtime.

Vag (Children Postmenarchal): *Vandazole:* One applicatorful (37.5 mg) of 0.75% gel once daily for 5 days.

Availability (generic available)

Tablets: 250 mg, 500 mg. **Capsules:** 375 mg 🍁 500 mg. **Oral suspension (Likmez) (strawberry-peppermint flavor):** 500 mg/5 mL. **Premixed infusion:** 500 mg/100 mL. **Topical cream:** 0.75%, 1%. **Topical gel:** 0.75%, 1%. **Topical lotion:** 0.75%. **Vaginal cream:** 🍁 10% (500 mg/applicatorful). **Vaginal gel:** 0.75% (37.5 mg/5 g applicatorful), 1.3% (65 mg/5 g applicatorful). ***In combination with:*** bismuth subcitrate potassium and tetracycline (Pylera). See Appendix N.

NURSING IMPLICATIONS

Assessment

- Assess for infection (vital signs; appearance of wound, sputum, urine, and stool; WBC) at beginning of and during therapy.
- Obtain specimens for culture and sensitivity before initiating therapy. First dose may be given before receiving results.
- Monitor neurologic status during and after IV infusion.

- Monitor intake, output, and daily weight, especially for patients on sodium restriction. Each 500 mg of premixed injection for dilution contains 14 mEq of sodium.
- Assess for rash periodically during therapy. May cause SJS, AGEP, and TEN. *If severe or if accompanied by fever, general malaise, fatigue, muscle or joint aches, blisters, oral lesions, conjunctivitis, hepatitis, and/or eosinophilia,* discontinue metronidazole.
- Monitor for signs and symptoms of DRESS (fever, rash, lymphadenopathy, facial swelling), associated with involvement of other organ systems (hepatitis, nephritis, hematologic abnormalities, myocarditis, myositis) during therapy. May resemble an acute viral infection. Eosinophilia is often present. Discontinue therapy if signs occur.
- **Giardiasis:** Monitor three stool samples taken several days apart, beginning 3–4 wk after treatment.

Lab Test Considerations

- May alter results of serum AST, ALT, and LDH tests.
- Monitor CBC before, during, and after prolonged or repeated courses of metronidazole.

Implementation

- Do not confuse metronidazole with metformin.
- Metronidazole has been shown to be carcinogenic in mice and rats. Reserve metronidazole for use in the treatment of trichomoniasis, amebiasis, and anaerobic bacterial infections.
- **PO:** Administer on an empty stomach, or may administer with food or milk to minimize GI irritation. Tablets may be crushed for patients with difficulty swallowing. ***DNC:*** Swallow extended-release tablets whole; do not break, crush, or chew.
- Oral suspension is stable for 60 days after opening.

IV Administration

- **Intermittent Infusion: Dilution:** Administer premixed injection (500 mg/100 mL) undiluted. Do not refrigerate. Once taken out of overwrap, premixed infusion stable for 30 days at room temperature. **Concentration:** 5 mg/mL. **Rate:** Infuse over 30–60 min.
- **Y-Site Compatibility:** acyclovir, alemtuzumab, allopurinol, amikacin, aminocaproic acid, aminophylline, amiodarone, ampicillin, ampicillin/sulbactam, anidulafungin, argatroban, arsenic trioxide, atracurium, azithromycin, bivalirudin, bleomycin, bumetanide, buprenorphine, busulfan, butorphanol, caffeine citrate, calcium chloride, calcium gluconate, cangrelor, carboplatin, carmustine, cefazolin, cefepime, cefiderocol, cefotaxime, cefotetan, cefoxitin, ceftaroline, ceftazidime, ceftozolane/tazobactam, ceftriaxone, cefuroxime, chloramphenicol, chlorpromazine, ciprofloxacin, cisatracurium, cisplatin, clindamycin, cyclophosphamide, cyclosporine, cytarabine, dacarbazine, dactinomycin, daunorubicin, defibrotide, dexamethasone, dexmedetomidine, dexrazoxane, digoxin, diltiazem, diphenhydramine, dobutamine, docetaxel, dopamine, doxorubicin hydrochloride, doxorubicin liposomal, doxycycline, droperidol, enalaprilat, ephedrine, epinephrine, epirubicin, eptifibatide, eravacycline, ertapenem, erythromycin, esmolol, etoposide, etoposide phosphate, famotidine, fentanyl, fluconazole, fludarabine, fluorouracil, foscarnet, fosphenytoin, furosemide, gemcitabine, gemtuzumab ozogamicin, gentamicin, glycopyrrolate, granisetron, haloperidol, heparin, hetastarch, hydralazine, hydrocortisone, hydromorphone, idarubicin, ifosfamide, imipenem/cilastatin, imipenem/cilastatin/relebactam, insulin regular, irinotecan, isoproterenol, ketamine, ketorolac, labetalol, LR, leucovorin, levofloxacin, lidocaine, linezolid, lorazepam, magnesium sulfate, mannitol, melphalan, meperidine, meropenem, meropenem/vaborbactam, mesna, methadone, methotrexate, methylprednisolone, metoclopramide, metoprolol, midazolam, milrinone, mitomycin, mitoxantrone, morphine, mycophenolate, nafcillin, nalbuphine, naloxone, nicardipine, nitroglycerin, nitroprusside, norepinephrine, octreotide, ondansetron, oxaliplatin, oxytocin, paclitaxel, palonosetron, pamidronate, pentamidine, pentobarbital, phenobarbital, phentolamine, phenylephrine, piperacillin/tazobactam, plazomicin, potassium acetate, potassium chloride, potassium phosphates, prochlorperazine, promethazine, propranolol, remifentanil, remimazolam, rituximab, rocuronium, sargramostim, sildenafil, sodium acetate, sodium bicarbonate, sodium phosphates, succinylcholine, sufentanil, sulbactam/durlobactam, tacrolimus, tedizolid, theophylline, thiotepa, tigecycline, tirofiban, tobramycin, topotecan, trastuzumab, trimethoprim/sulfamethoxazole, vancomycin, vasopressin, vecuronium, verapamil, vinblastine, vincristine, vinorelbine, voriconazole, zidovudine, zoledronic acid.
- **Y-Site Incompatibility:** acetaminophen, amphotericin B deoxycholate, amphotericin B liposomal, aztreonam, blinatumomab, dantrolene, daptomycin, diazepam, filgrastim, ganciclovir, minocycline, pantoprazole, pemetrexed, phenytoin, procainamide, propofol.
- **Topical:** Cleanse affected area before application. Apply and rub in a thin film twice daily, morning and evening. Avoid contact with eyes.
- **Vag** Administer once daily dosing at bedtime.

M

Patient/Family Teaching

- Instruct patient to take medication as directed, even if feeling better. Do not double up on missed doses; take as soon as remembered if not almost time for next dose.
- Advise patients treated for trichomoniasis that sexual partners may be asymptomatic sources of reinfection and should be treated concurrently. Patient should also refrain from intercourse or use a condom to prevent reinfection.
- Caution patient to avoid intake of alcoholic beverages or preparations containing alcohol during and for ≥3 days after treatment with metronidazole, including vaginal gel. May cause serious disulfiram-like reaction (flushing, nausea, vomiting, headache, abdominal cramps).
- May cause dizziness or light-headedness. Caution patient to avoid driving or other activities requiring alertness until response to medication is known.
- Instruct patient to notify health care provider promptly if rash occurs.
- Advise patient to notify health care provider if numbness, tingling, weakness or seizures occur.
- Inform patient that medication may cause an unpleasant metallic taste.
- Advise patient to notify health care provider of all Rx or OTC medications, vitamins, or herbal products being taken and to consult with health care provider before taking other medications.
- Advise patient that frequent mouth rinses, good oral hygiene, and sugarless gum or candy may minimize dry mouth. Notify health care provider if dry mouth persists for >2 wk.
- Inform patient that medication may cause urine to turn dark.
- Advise patient to consult health care provider if no improvement in a few days or if signs and symptoms of superinfection (black, furry overgrowth on tongue; vaginal itching or discharge; loose or foul-smelling stools) develop.
- Rep: Advise women of reproductive potential to inform health care provider if pregnancy is planned or suspected and to avoid breastfeeding during therapy.
- **Vag** Instruct patient in correct technique for intravaginal instillation. Advise patient to avoid intercourse during treatment with vaginal gel.
- **Topical:** Instruct patient on correct technique for application of topical gel. Cosmetics may be used after application of gel.

Evaluation/Desired Outcomes

- Resolution of the signs and symptoms of infection. Length of time for complete resolution depends on organism and site of infection.
- Significant results should be seen within 3 wk of application of topical gel. Application may be continued for 9 wk.

micafungin (my-ka-fun-gin)

Mycamine

Classification

Therapeutic: antifungals

Pharmacologic: echinocandins

Indications

Treatment of esophageal candidiasis. Treatment of candidemia/acute disseminated candidiasis/*Candida* peritonitis and abscesses (in adults and pediatric patients ≥4 mo). Treatment of candidemia/acute disseminated candidiasis/*Candida* peritonitis and abscesses without meningoencephalitis and/or ocular dissemination (in pediatric patients <4 mo). Prophylaxis of *Candida* infections during hematopoetic stem cell transplantation.

Action

Inhibits synthesis of glucan required for the formation of fungal cell wall. **Therapeutic Effects:** Death of susceptible fungi. **Spectrum:** Active against the following *Candida* spp.: *C. albicans*, *C. glabrata*, *C. krusei*, *C. parapsilosis*, *C. tropicalis*.

Pharmacokinetics

Absorption: IV administration results in complete bioavailability.

Distribution: Primarily distributed into lung, liver, and spleen; minimal distribution to CNS and eyes.

Protein Binding: >99%.

Metabolism and Excretion: Mostly metabolized in the liver; 71% fecal elimination.

Half-life: 15 hr.

TIME/ACTION PROFILE (plasma concentrations)

ROUTE	ONSET	PEAK	DURATION
IV	rapid	end of infusion	24 hr

Contraindications/Precautions

Contraindicated in: Hypersensitivity.

Use Cautiously in: Severe hepatic impairment; OB: Use during pregnancy only if potential maternal benefit justifies potential fetal risk; Lactation: Use while breastfeeding only if potential maternal benefit justifies potential risk to infant; Pedi: Children <4 mo with meningoencephalitis and/or ocular dissemination (safety and effectiveness not established).

Adverse Reactions/Side Effects

GI: worsening hepatic function/hepatitis. **GU:** renal impairment. **Hemat:** hemolysis/hemolytic anemia. **Local:** injection site reactions. **Misc:** infusion reactions, HYPERSENSITIVITY REACTIONS (INCLUDING ANAPHYLAXIS).

Interactions

Drug-Drug: ↑ levels and risk of toxicity with **sirolimus** and **nifedipine** (dose adjustments may be necessary).

Route/Dosage

Treatment of Esophageal Candidiasis

IV (Adults): 150 mg once daily for 15 days (range 10–30 days).
IV (Children ≥4 mo and >30 kg): 2.5 mg/kg once daily (max daily dose = 150 mg).
IV (Children ≥4 mo and ≤30 kg): 3 mg/kg once daily.

Treatment of Candidemia/Acute Disseminated Candidiasis/*Candida* Peritonitis and Abscesses

IV (Adults): 100 mg once daily for 15 days (range 10–47 days).
IV (Children ≥4 mo and >30 kg): 2 mg/kg once daily (max daily dose = 100 mg).
IV (Children ≥4 mo and ≤30 kg): 2 mg/kg once daily.

Treatment of Candidemia/Acute Disseminated Candidiasis/*Candida* Peritonitis and Abscesses Without Meningoencephalitis and/or Ocular Dissemination

IV (Children <4 mo): 4 mg/kg once daily.

Prophylaxis of *Candida* Infections During Hematopoetic Stem Cell Transplantation

IV (Adults): 50 mg once daily (duration range 6–51 days).
IV (Children ≥4 mo and >30 kg): 1 mg/kg once daily (max daily dose = 50 mg).
IV (Children ≥4 mo and ≤30 kg): 1 mg/kg once daily.

Availability (generic available)

Lyophilized powder for injection: 50 mg/vial, 100 mg/vial. **Premixed infusion:** 50 mg/50 mL 0.9% NaCl, 100 mg/100 mL 0.9% NaCl, 150 mg/150 mL 0.9% NaCl.

NURSING IMPLICATIONS

Assessment

- Assess symptoms of esophageal candidiasis (dysphagia, odynophagia, retrosternal pain) prior to and during therapy.
- Monitor for signs of anaphylaxis (rash, pruritus, wheezing, laryngeal edema, abdominal pain). Discontinue micafungin and notify health care professional immediately if these occur.
- Monitor for signs and symptoms of histamine-mediated reactions (rash, pruritus, facial swelling, vasodilation) during infusion. If symptoms occur, slow infusion rate.
- Assess for injection site reactions (phlebitis, thrombophlebitis) during therapy. These occur more frequently in patients receiving micafungin via peripheral IV infusion.

Lab Test Considerations

- May cause ↑ serum alkaline phosphatase, bilirubin, ALT, AST, and LDH levels. If elevations occur, monitor for worsening liver function; may require discontinuation of therapy.
- May cause ↑ BUN and serum creatinine.
- May cause leukopenia, neutropenia, thrombocytopenia, and anemia. Monitor for worsening levels; may require discontinuation of therapy.
- May cause hypokalemia, hypocalcemia, and hypomagnesemia.

Implementation

IV Administration

- **Intermittent Infusion: Reconstitution:** *For Adults:* Reconstitute each 50-mg vial with 5 mL of 0.9% NaCl or D5W to achieve concentration of 10 mg/mL. Reconstitute each 100-mg vial with 5 mL of 0.9% NaCl or D5W to achieve concentration of 20 mg/mL. Dissolve by gently swirling vial; do not shake vigorously. **Dilution:** Directions for further dilution based on indication for use. For prophylaxis of *Candida infections*, add 50 mg of micafungin to 100 mL of 0.9% NaCl or D5W. For treatment of *esophageal candidiasis*, add 150 mg of micafungin to 100 mL of 0.9% NaCl or D5W. Reconstituted vials and infusion are stable for 24 hr at room temperature. Protect diluted solution from light. **Concentration:** 0.5–1.5 mg/mL.
- *For Children:* **Dilution:** Determine dose and divide by final concentration (10 or 20 mg/mL). Add withdrawn volume to 0.9% NaCl or D5W in IV bag or syringe. **Concentration:** 0.5–4 mg/mL. Concentrations >1.5 mg/mL should be administered via central venous catheter to minimize infusion reactions. Discard unused vials.
- **Rate:** Flush line with 0.9% NaCl prior to administration. Infuse over 1 hr. More rapid infusions may result in more frequent histamine mediated reactions.
- **Y-Site Compatibility:** aminophylline, bumetanide, calcium chloride, calcium gluconate, cangrelor, carboplatin, ceftolozane/tazobactam, cyclosporine, dopamine, eptifibatide, esmolol, etoposide, furosemide, heparin, hydromorphone, imipenem/cilastatin/relebactam, letermovir, lidocaine, lorazepam, magnesium sulfate, meropenem/vaborbactam, mesna, milrinone, nitroglycerin, nitroprusside, norepinephrine, phenylephrine, posaconazole, potassium chloride, potassium phosphates, sodium phosphates, sulbactam/durlobactam, tacrolimus, tedizolid, theophylline, vasopressin.
- **Y-Site Incompatibility:** albumin, human, amiodarone, cisatracurium, diltiazem, dobutamine,

M

epinephrine, eravacycline, insulin regular, isavuconazonium, labetalol, levofloxacin, meperidine, midazolam, morphine, mycophenolate, nicardipine, octreotide, ondansetron, phenytoin, plazomicin, rocuronium, telavancin, vecuronium.

Patient/Family Teaching

- Explain purpose and side effects of medication to patient. Advise patient to read *Patient Information* before starting therapy.
- Instruct patient to notify health care professional of all Rx or OTC medications, vitamins, or herbal products being taken and to consult health care professional before taking any other Rx, OTC, or herbal products.
- Advise patient to notify health care professional immediately if signs of anaphylaxis occur. Infusion should be discontinued if symptoms occur.
- Rep: May cause fetal harm. Advise females of reproductive potential to notify health care professional if pregnancy is planned or suspected or if breastfeeding.

Evaluation/Desired Outcomes

- Resolution of signs and symptoms of esophageal candidiasis, candidemia, acute disseminated candidiasis, candidal peritonitis, and abscesses.
- Prevention of *Candida* infections during hematopoetic stem cell transplantation.

miconazole, See ANTIFUNGALS (TOPICAL).

miconazole, See ANTIFUNGALS (VAGINAL).

BEERS HIGH ALERT

midazolam (mid-ay-zoe-lam)

Nayzilam, Seizalam, ~~Versed~~

Classification

Therapeutic: antianxiety agents, anticonvulsants, sedative/hypnotics

Pharmacologic: benzodiazepines

Schedule IV

Indications

PO: Preprocedural sedation and anxiolysis in pediatric patients. **IM, IV:** Preoperative sedation/anxiolysis/amnesia: Status epilepticus. **IV:** Provides sedation/anxiolysis/amnesia during therapeutic, diagnostic, or radiographic procedures (conscious sedation). Aids in the induction of anesthesia and as part of balanced anesthesia. As a continuous infusion, provides sedation of mechanically ventilated patients during anesthesia or in a critical care setting. **Intranasal:** Acute treatment of intermittent, stereotypic episodes of frequent seizure activity (e.g., seizure clusters, acute repetitive seizures) that are distinct from a patient's usual seizure pattern in patients with epilepsy.

Action

Acts at many levels of the CNS to produce generalized CNS depression. Effects may be mediated by GABA, an inhibitory neurotransmitter. **Therapeutic Effects:** Short-term sedation. Postoperative amnesia. Termination of seizure activity.

Pharmacokinetics

Absorption: Rapidly absorbed following oral and nasal administration; undergoes substantial intestinal and first-pass hepatic metabolism. Well absorbed following IM administration; IV administration results in complete bioavailability.

Distribution: Crosses the blood-brain barrier.

Protein Binding: 97%.

Metabolism and Excretion: Almost exclusively metabolized by the liver by the CYP3A4 isoenzyme, resulting in conversion to hydroxymidazolam, an active metabolite, and 2 other inactive metabolites; metabolites are excreted in urine.

Half-life: *Preterm neonates:* 2.6–17.7 hr; *Neonates:* 4–12 hr; *Children:* 3–7 hr; *Adults:* 2–6 hr (↑ in renal impairment, HF, or cirrhosis).

TIME/ACTION PROFILE (sedation)

ROUTE	ONSET	PEAK	DURATION
IN	5 min	10 min	30–60 min
IM	15 min	30–60 min	2–6 hr
IV	1.5–5 min	rapid	2–6 hr

Contraindications/Precautions

Contraindicated in: Hypersensitivity; Cross-sensitivity with other benzodiazepines may occur; Shock; Comatose patients or those with pre-existing CNS depression; Uncontrolled severe pain; Acute angle-closure glaucoma; Pedi: Products containing benzyl alcohol should not be used in neonates.

Use Cautiously in: All patients (may ↑ risk of suicidal thoughts/behaviors); Pulmonary disease; HF; Renal impairment; Severe hepatic impairment; Open-angle glaucoma; OB: Use late in pregnancy can result in sedation (respiratory depression, lethargy, hypotonia) and/or withdrawal symptoms (hyperreflexia, irritability, restlessness, tremors, inconsolable crying, feeding difficulties) in neonates; Lactation: Use while breastfeeding only if potential maternal benefit justifies potential risk to infant; Pedi: Obese pediatric patients (calculate dose on the basis of ideal body weight); Pedi: Rapid injection in neonates has caused severe hypotension and seizures, especially when used with fentanyl;

may affect brain development in children <3 yr; safety and effectiveness of nasal spray has not been established in children <12 yr; Geri: Appears on Beers list. ↑ risk of cognitive impairment, delirium, falls, fractures, and motor vehicle accidents in older adults. If possible, avoid use in older adults.

Adverse Reactions/Side Effects

CV: arrhythmias, CARDIAC ARREST. **Derm:** rash. **EENT:** blurred vision. **GI:** hiccups, nausea, vomiting. **Local:** phlebitis at IV site, pain at IM site. **Neuro:** agitation, drowsiness, excess sedation, headache, SUICIDAL THOUGHTS. **Resp:** APNEA, bronchospasm, cough, LARYNGOSPASM, RESPIRATORY DEPRESSION. **Misc:** physical dependence, psychological dependence, tolerance.

Interactions

Drug-Drug: Use with **opioids** or other **CNS depressants**, including other **benzodiazepines**, **nonbenzodiazepine sedative/hypnotics**, **anxiolytics**, **general anesthetics**, **muscle relaxants**, **antipsychotics**, and **alcohol**, may cause profound sedation, respiratory depression, coma, and death; reserve concurrent use for when alternative treatment options are inadequate. ↑ risk of hypotension with **antihypertensives**, **opioid analgesics**, acute ingestion of **alcohol**, or **nitrates**. **Moderate CYP3A4 inhibitors** and **strong CYP3A4 inhibitors**, including **clarithromycin**, **diltiazem**, **erythromycin**, **itraconazole**, **ketoconazole**, and **verapamil**, may ↑ levels and risk of toxicity; avoid concurrent use. **Strong CYP3A4 inducers**, including **carbamazepine**, **phenobarbital**, **phenytoin**, **rifampin**, and **rifabutin**, may ↓ levels and effectiveness.
Drug-Natural Products: **Kava-kava**, **valerian**, or **chamomile** can ↑ risk of CNS depression. Long-term use of **St. John's wort** may significantly ↓ levels and effectiveness.
Drug-Food: **Grapefruit juice** may ↑ levels and risk of toxicity.

Route/Dosage

Preoperative Sedation/Anxiolysis/Amnesia

PO (Children 6 mo–16 yr): 0.25–0.5 mg/kg; may require up to 1 mg/kg (dose should not exceed 20 mg); *Patients with cardiac/respiratory compromise or concurrent CNS depressants:* 0.25 mg/kg.
IM (Adults <60 yr, otherwise healthy): 0.07–0.08 mg/kg 1 hr before surgery (usual dose 5 mg).
IM (Adults ≥60 yr, debilitated, or chronically ill): 0.02–0.03 mg/kg 1 hr before surgery (usual dose 1–3 mg).
IM (Children): 0.1–0.15 mg/kg up to 0.5 mg/kg 30–60 min prior to procedure; not to exceed 10 mg/dose.

Conscious Sedation for Short Procedures

IV (Adults and Children >12 yr and <60 yr, otherwise healthy): 1–2.5 mg initially; dosage may be ↑ further as needed. Total doses >5 mg are rarely needed (↓ dose by 50% if other CNS depressants are used). Maintenance doses of 25% of the dose required for initial sedation may be given as necessary.
IV (Children 6–12 yr): 0.025–0.05 mg/kg initially; then titrate dose carefully; may need up to 0.4 mg/kg total; maximum dose 10 mg.
IV (Children 6 mo–5 yr): 0.05 mg/kg initially; then titrate dose carefully; may need up to 0.6 mg/kg total; maximum dose 6 mg.
IV: Geri: **(Geriatric Patients ≥60 yr, debilitated, or chronically ill):** 1–1.5 mg initially; dose may be ↑ further as needed. Total doses >3.5 mg are rarely needed (↓ dose by 30% if other CNS depressants are used). Maintenance doses of 25% of the dose required for initial sedation may be given as necessary.
Intranasal (Children): 0.2–0.3 mg/kg, may repeat in 5–15 min.

M

Status Epilepticus

IM (Adults): 10 mg single dose.
IV (Children >2 mo): 0.15 mg/kg load followed by a continuous infusion of 1 mcg/kg/min. Titrate dose upward every 5 min until seizure controlled, range: 1–18 mcg/kg/min.

Seizure Clusters

Intranasal (Adults and Children ≥12 yr): One spray (5 mg) into one nostril initially; if inadequate response after 10 min, administer one spray (5 mg) into other nostril. Not to exceed 2 doses for a single seizure episode. Should not be used to treat more than one episode every 3 days and no more than 5 episodes per mo.

Induction of Anesthesia (Adjunct)

IV (Adults <55 yr, otherwise healthy): 300–350 mcg/kg initially (up to 600 mcg/kg total). May give additional dose of 25% of initial dose if needed. If patient is premedicated, initial dose should be further ↓.
IV: Geri: **(Geriatric Patients >55 yr):** 150–300 mcg/kg as initial dose. May give additional dose of 25% of initial dose if needed. If patient is premedicated, initial dose should be further ↓.
IV (Adults, debilitated): 150–250 mcg/kg initial dose. May give additional dose of 25% of initial dose if needed. If patient is premedicated, initial dose should be further ↓.

Sedation in Critical Care Settings

IV (Adults): 0.01–0.05 mg/kg (0.5–4 mg in most adults) initially if a loading dose is required; may repeat every 10–15 min until desired effect is obtained; may be followed by infusion at 0.02–0.1 mg/kg/hr (1–7 mg/hr in most adults).

IV (Children): *Intubated patients only:* 0.05–0.2 mg/kg initially as a loading dose; follow with infusion at 0.06–0.12 mg/kg/hr (1–2 mcg/kg/min); titrate to effect, range: 0.4–6 mcg/kg/min.
IV (Neonates >32 wk): *Intubated patients only:* 0.06 mg/kg/hr (1 mcg/kg/min).
IV (Neonates <32 wk): *Intubated patients only:* 0.03 mg/kg/hr (0.5 mcg/kg/min).

Availability (generic available)

Oral syrup (cherry flavor): 2 mg/mL. **Nasal spray (Nayzilam):** 5 mg/0.1 mL single-dose unit. **Premixed infusion:** 100 mg/100 mL 0.8% NaCl, 50 mg/50 mL 0.9% NaCl, 100 mg/100 mL 0.9% NaCl. **Solution for injection:** 1 mg/mL, 5 mg/mL.

NURSING IMPLICATIONS

Assessment

- Assess level of sedation and level of consciousness during and for 2–6 hr following administration.
- Monitor BP, HR, and respiratory rate continuously during administration, especially if coadministering opioid analgesics.
- Oxygen and resuscitative equipment should be immediately available during IV administration.
- Assess risk for addiction, abuse, or misuse before starting and periodically during therapy.
- Prolonged high-dose therapy may lead to psychological or physical dependence. Restrict the amount of drug available to patient. Assess regularly for continued need for treatment.

Toxicity and Overdose

- If overdose occurs, monitor BP, HR, and respiratory rate continuously. Maintain patent airway and assist ventilation as needed. If hypotension occurs, treatment includes IV fluids, repositioning, and vasopressors.
- The effects of midazolam can be reversed with flumazenil.

Implementation

- ***High Alert:*** Accidental overdose of oral midazolam syrup in children has resulted in serious harm or death. Do not accept orders prescribed by volume (5 mL or 1 teaspoon); instead, request dose be expressed in milligrams. Have second practitioner independently check original order and dose calculations. Midazolam syrup should only be administered by health care providers authorized to administer conscious sedation.
- Supervise ambulation and transfer of patients after administration. Two side rails should be raised and call bell within reach at all times.
- Gradually taper to discontinue or ↓ dose to reduce risk of withdrawal reactions, seizure frequency, and status epilepticus. If a patient develops withdrawal reactions, consider pausing taper or ↑ dose to previous tapered dose level. Subsequently ↓ dose more slowly. Some patients may require longer tapering period (weeks to >12 mo).
- **PO:** To use the *Press-in Bottle Adaptor,* remove the cap and push bottle adaptor into neck of bottle. Close bottle tightly with cap. Solution is a clear red to purplish-red cherry-flavored syrup. Then remove cap and insert tip of oral dispenser in bottle adaptor. Push the plunger completely down toward tip of oral dispenser and insert firmly into bottle adaptor. Turn entire unit (bottle and oral dispenser) upside down. Pull plunger out slowly until desired amount of medication is withdrawn into oral dispenser. Turn entire unit right side up and slowly remove oral dispenser from the bottle. Tip of dispenser may be covered with tip of cap until time of use. Close bottle with cap after each use.
- Dispense directly into mouth. Do not mix with any liquid prior to dispensing.
- **Intranasal:** Administer 1 spray into one nostril. If no response to initial dose after 10 min, may administer 1 spray into other nostril.
- **IM:** Administer IM doses deep into mid-outer thigh (vastus lateralis muscle), maximum concentration 1 mg/mL. Solution is clear, colorless to light yellow. Do not administer solutions that are discolored or contain particulate matter.

IV Administration

- Doses of sedative medications in pediatric patients must be calculated on a mg/kg basis, and initial doses and all subsequent doses should always be titrated slowly. The initial pediatric dose of midazolam for sedation/anxiolysis/amnesia is age, procedure, and route dependent
- **IV Push: Dilution:** Administer undiluted or diluted with D5W or 0.9% NaCl. **Concentration:** Undiluted: 1 mg/mL or 5 mg/mL. Diluted: 0.03–3 mg/mL. **Rate:** Administer slowly over at least 2–5 min. Titrate dose to patient response. Rapid injection, especially in neonates, has caused severe hypotension.
- **Continuous Infusion: Dilution:** Dilute with 0.9% NaCl or D5W. **Concentration:** 0.5–1 mg/mL.
- **Rate:** Based on patient's weight (see Route/Dosage section). Titrate to desired level of sedation. Assess sedation at regular intervals and adjust rate up or down by 25–50% as needed. Dose should also be ↓ by 10–25% every few hours to find minimum effective infusion rate, which prevents accumulation of midazolam and provides more rapid recovery upon termination.
- **Y-Site Compatibility:** acetaminophen, alemtuzumab, alprostadil, amikacin, amiodarone, anidulafungin, argatroban, arsenic trioxide, atracurium, atropine, aztreonam, benztropine, bivalirudin, bleomycin, buprenorphine, caffeine

citrate, calcium chloride, calcium gluconate, carboplatin, carmustine, caspofungin, cefazolin, cefiderocol, cefotaxime, cefoxitin, ceftaroline, ceftolozane/tazobactam, ceftriaxone, chlorpromazine, ciprofloxacin, cisatracurium, cisplatin, cyanocobalamin, cyclophosphamide, cyclosporine, cytarabine, dacarbazine, dactinomycin, daptomycin, daunorubicin, dexmedetomidine, dexrazoxane, digoxin, diltiazem, diphenhydramine, docetaxel, dopamine, doxorubicin hydrochloride, doxorubicin liposomal, doxycycline, enalaprilat, ephedrine, epinephrine, epirubicin, eptifibatide, eravacycline, erythromycin, esmolol, etomidate, etoposide, etoposide phosphate, famotidine, fentanyl, fluconazole, fludarabine, folic acid, gemcitabine, gentamicin, glycopyrrolate, granisetron, hetastarch, hydromorphone, idarubicin, ifosfamide, imipenem/cilastatin/relebactam, irinotecan, isavuconazonium, isoproterenol, ketamine, labetalol, LR, leucovorin, levofloxacin, lidocaine, linezolid, lorazepam, magnesium sulfate, mannitol, meperidine, mesna, methadone, metoclopramide, metoprolol, metronidazole, milrinone, minocycline, mitoxantrone, morphine, multivitamins, mycophenolate, nalbuphine, naloxone, nicardipine, nitroglycerin, nitroprusside, norepinephrine, octreotide, ondansetron, oritavancin, oxacillin, oxaliplatin, oxytocin, paclitaxel, palonosetron, pamidronate, papaverine, pemetrexed, penicillin G, pentamidine, phentolamine, phenylephrine, phytonadione, plazomicin, potassium chloride, potassium phosphates, procainamide, promethazine, propranolol, protamine, pyridoxine, remifentanil, remimazolam, rifampin, rocuronium, sildenafil, succinylcholine, sufentanil, sulbactam/durlobactam, tacrolimus, tedizolid, theophylline, thiotepa, tigecycline, tirofiban, tobramycin, topotecan, vancomycin, vasopressin, vecuronium, verapamil, vinblastine, vincristine, vinorelbine, voriconazole, zoledronic acid.

- **Y-Site Incompatibility:** acyclovir, albumin, human, aminocaproic acid, aminophylline, amphotericin B deoxycholate, amphotericin B liposomal, ampicillin, ampicillin/sulbactam, ascorbic acid, azathioprine, azithromycin, blinatumomab, cefepime, ceftazidime, cefuroxime, chloramphenicol, dantrolene, dexamethasone, diazepam, diazoxide, epoetin alfa, ertapenem, esomeprazole, fluorouracil, foscarnet, fosphenytoin, ganciclovir, gemtuzumab ozogamicin, ibuprofen lysine, indomethacin, ketorolac, letermovir, meropenem, meropenem/vaborbactam, methotrexate, micafungin, mitomycin, pentobarbital, phenobarbital, phenytoin, piperacillin/tazobactam, potassium acetate, prochlorperazine, sodium bicarbonate, trimethoprim/sulfamethoxazole.

Patient/Family Teaching

- Inform patient that this medication will ↓ mental recall of the procedure.
- Advise patient to avoid grapefruit juice during therapy.
- May cause drowsiness or dizziness. Advise patient to request assistance prior to ambulation and transfer and to avoid driving or other activities requiring alertness for 24 hr following administration.
- Caution patient not to stop taking midazolam without consulting health care provider. Abrupt withdrawal may cause sweating, vomiting, muscle cramps, tremors, and seizures; may be life-threatening.
- Instruct patient to notify health care provider of all Rx or OTC medications, vitamins, or herbal products being taken and to consult health care provider before taking any Rx, OTC, or herbal products, especially blood pressure medicine, antibiotics, and St. John's wort.
- Advise patient that midazolam is a drug with known abuse potential. Protect it from theft, and never give to anyone other than the individual for whom it was prescribed. Store out of sight and reach of children, and in a location not accessible by others.
- Advise patient to avoid the use of alcohol or other CNS depressants, including opioids, concurrently with midazolam; may cause respiratory depression and overdose. Instruct patient to consult health care provider before taking Rx, OTC, or herbal products concurrently with this medication.
- Advise patient and family to notify health care provider if thoughts about suicide or dying, attempts to commit suicide, new or worse depression, new or worse anxiety, feeling very agitated or restless, panic attacks, trouble sleeping, new or worse irritability, acting aggressive, being angry or violent, acting on dangerous impulses, an extreme increase in activity and talking, other unusual changes in behavior or mood, or skin rash occur.
- Rep: May cause fetal harm. Advise patient to notify health care provider if pregnancy is planned or suspected or if breastfeeding. Use in late pregnancy can result in sedation (respiratory depression, lethargy, hypotonia) and/or withdrawal symptoms (hyperreflexia, irritability, restlessness, tremors, inconsolable crying, feeding difficulties) in the neonate. Monitor neonates exposed to midazolam during pregnancy or labor for signs of sedation and monitor neonates exposed to midazolam during pregnancy for signs of withdrawal. Monitor infants exposed to midazolam through breast milk for sedation, poor feeding, and poor weight gain. Encourage women who take midazolam during pregnancy to enroll in the North American Antiepileptic Drug

M

Pregnancy Registry by calling 1-888-233-2334 or visiting http://www.aedpregnancyregistry.org to monitor pregnancy outcomes in women exposed to antiepileptic drugs.

- **Nayzilam:** Instruct individual administering *Nayzilam* on how to identify seizure clusters and use product appropriately. Explain purpose and side effects of medication to patient. Advise patient to read *Patient Information* before starting therapy and with each Rx refill. Discuss safe use, risks, and proper storage and disposal with patients and caregivers.

Evaluation/Desired Outcomes

- Sedation during and amnesia following surgical, diagnostic, and radiologic procedures.
- Sedation and amnesia for mechanically ventilated patients in a critical care setting.
- Termination of seizure activity.

midodrine (mye-doe-dreen)

~~ProAmatine~~

Classification

Therapeutic: vasopressors

Indications

Symptomatic management of refractory orthostatic hypotension in patients whose lives are impaired.

Action

Activation of alpha-1-adrenergic receptors in arteries and veins. **Therapeutic Effects:** Increase in vascular tone and BP.

Pharmacokinetics

Absorption: 93% absorbed following oral administration; rapidly converted to desglymidodrine, the active metabolite.
Distribution: Desglymidodrine crosses the blood-brain barrier poorly.
Metabolism and Excretion: Desglymidodrine is 80% excreted by the kidneys.
Half-life: *Midodrine:* 25 min; *desglymidodrine:* 3–4 hr.

TIME/ACTION PROFILE (blood levels of active metabolite)

ROUTE	ONSET	PEAK	DURATION
PO	rapid	1–2 hr	2–3 hr

Contraindications/Precautions

Contraindicated in: Urinary retention; Severe organic heart disease; Acute renal disease; Persistent/excessive supine hypertension; Pheochromocytoma; Thyrotoxicosis.
Use Cautiously in: History of hypertension; Renal impairment (↓ initial dose); Hepatic impairment; Diabetes mellitus, visual problems, concurrent fludrocortisone (↑ risk of visual disturbances); OB: Safety not established in pregnancy; Lactation: Safety not established in breastfeeding; Pedi: Safety and effectiveness not established in children.

Adverse Reactions/Side Effects

CV: supine hypertension, bradycardia. **Derm:** piloerection, pruritus, facial flushing, rash. **GU:** dysuria, urinary urge/retention/frequency. **Neuro:** paresthesia, anxiety, confusion, head pressure/fullness, headache, nervousness. **Misc:** chills, pain.

Interactions

Drug-Drug: ↑ risk of bradycardia with **digoxin**, **beta blockers**, and **antipsychotics**. **Phenylephrine**, **ephedrine**, **pseudoephedrine**, **thyroid hormones**, **droxidopa**, **dihydroergotamine**, **MAO inhibitors**, or **linezolid** may significantly ↑ BP; avoid concurrent use. **Alpha-adrenergic blockers**, including **prazosin**, **terazosin**, and **doxazosin**, may ↓ effectiveness. May ↑ effects of **fludrocortisone**; ↓ initial dose of fludrocortisone or ↓ salt intake prior to midodrine.

Route/Dosage

PO (Adults): 10 mg three times daily.

Renal Impairment

PO (Adults): 2.5 mg three times daily.

Availability (generic available)

Tablets: 2.5 mg, 5 mg, 10 mg.

NURSING IMPLICATIONS

Assessment

- Monitor supine and sitting BP prior to and during therapy.

Lab Test Considerations

- Monitor renal and hepatic function prior to and periodically during therapy.

Implementation

- Because midodrine can cause marked ↑ of supine BP, it should be used in patients whose lives are considerably impaired despite standard clinical care.
- **PO:** Administer three times daily at 3–4 hr intervals. Do not administer after last meal or within 4 hr of bedtime.

Patient/Family Teaching

- Instruct patient to take midodrine as directed. 1st dose should be taken on or shortly after arising, 2nd dose at midday, and 3rd dose should be taken before evening meal and ≥4 hr before bedtime. Take missed doses as soon as remembered unless almost time for next dose; do not double doses.
- Advise patient to notify health care provider of all Rx or OTC medications, vitamins, or herbal products being taken and to consult with health care provider before taking other medications.
- Rep: Advise women of reproductive potential to notify health care provider if pregnancy is planned or suspected or if breastfeeding.

Evaluation/Desired Outcomes

- Decrease in signs and symptoms of orthostatic hypotension.
- Decrease in the incidence of urinary incontinence.

REMS

miFEPRIStone

(mi-fe-**priss**-tone)

Korlym, Mifeprex

Classification

Therapeutic: abortifacients, antidiabetics

Pharmacologic: antiprogestational agents

Indications

Mifeprex: Medical termination of intrauterine pregnancy up to day 70 of pregnancy (in combination with misoprostol). **Korlym:** Hyperglycemia secondary to hypercortisolism in patients with endogenous Cushing syndrome who have type 2 diabetes or glucose intolerance and have failed or are not candidates for surgery.

Action

Antagonizes endometrial and myometrial effects of progesterone. Sensitizes the myometrium to contraction-inducing activity of prostaglandins. Antagonizes the glucocorticoid receptor. **Therapeutic Effects:** Termination of pregnancy. Improved control of blood glucose.

Pharmacokinetics

Absorption: Rapidly absorbed following oral administration (69% bioavailability); absorption ↑ with food.

Distribution: Unknown.

Protein Binding: 98%.

Metabolism and Excretion: Primarily metabolized by the liver via the CYP3A4 isoenzyme; primarily excreted in the feces.

Half-life: 18 hr.

TIME/ACTION PROFILE (termination of pregnancy)

ROUTE	ONSET	PEAK	DURATION
PO	unknown	within 2 days	unknown

Contraindications/Precautions

Contraindicated in: Hypersensitivity; Presence of an intrauterine device (IUD) (Mifeprex); Undiagnosed adnexal mass (Mifeprex); Chronic adrenal failure (Mifeprex); Concurrent long-term corticosteroid therapy; Bleeding disorders or concurrent anticoagulant therapy (Mifeprex); Inherited porphyrias (Mifeprex); Severe hepatic impairment (Korlym); Concurrent use with simvastatin, lovastatin, cyclosporine, dihydroergotamine, ergotamine, fentanyl, pimozide, quinidine, sirolimus, or tacrolimus (Korlym); Vaginal bleeding; Endometrial hyperplasia with atypia or endometrial carcinoma (Korlym); OB: Confirmed or suspected ectopic pregnancy (Mifeprex); OB: Pregnancy (Korlym).

Use Cautiously in: Chronic medical conditions such as cardiovascular, hypertensive, hepatic, renal, or respiratory disease (Mifeprex); Women >35 yr old or who smoke ≥10 cigarettes/day (Mifeprex); Bleeding disorders or concurrent anticoagulant therapy (Korlym).

Adverse Reactions/Side Effects

CV: hypertension (Korlym), peripheral edema (Korlym), QT interval prolongation (Korlym). **Derm:** rash (Korlym). **Endo:** hypothyroidism (Korlym), ↓ HDL-C (Korlym), adrenal insufficiency (Korlym). **F and E** hypokalemia (Korlym). **GI:** abdominal pain (Mifeprex), anorexia (Korlym), constipation (Korlym), diarrhea, dry mouth (Korlym), nausea, vomiting. **GU:** uterine bleeding, uterine cramping (Mifeprex), pelvic pain (Mifeprex), ruptured ectopic pregnancy (Mifeprex). **MS:** arthralgia (Korlym), myalgia (Korlym). **Neuro:** anxiety (Korlym), dizziness, fatigue (Korlym), headache, fainting (Mifeprex), weakness (Mifeprex). **Resp:** dyspnea (Korlym). **Misc:** ANGIOEDEMA, INFECTION (MIFEPREX).

Interactions

Drug-Drug: May ↑ levels and risk of toxicity of **dihydroergotamine, ergotamine, lovastatin, simvastatin, cyclosporine, fentanyl, pimozide, quinidine, sirolimus,** or **tacrolimus**; concurrent use with Korlym contraindicated. **Strong CYP3A4 inhibitors**, including **ketoconazole, itraconazole, nefazodone, ritonavir, nelfinavir, atazanavir, fosamprenavir, clarithromycin, conivaptan, lopinavir/ritonavir, posaconazole,** or **voriconazole**, may ↑ levels and risk of toxicity; adjust dose of Korlym. **Moderate CYP3A4 inhibitors**, including **aprepitant, diltiazem, fluconazole, imatinib,** or **verapamil**, may ↑ levels and risk of toxicity; use caution with concurrent use of Korlym. **Rifampin, rifabutin dexamethasone, phenytoin, phenobarbital,** and **carbamazepine** may ↓ levels and effectiveness; avoid concurrent use with Korlym.

Drug-Natural Products: St. John's wort may ↓ levels and effectiveness; avoid concurrent use with Korlym.

Drug-Food: Grapefruit juice may ↑ levels and risk of toxicity; caution with concurrent use of Korlym.

Route/Dosage

Mifeprex

PO (Adults): *Day 1:* 200 mg as a single dose, followed on *Day 2 or Day 3 (within 24–48 hr of taking*

M

Mifeprex) by misoprostol 800 mcg (given as four 200-mcg tablets) given buccally.

Korlym

PO (Adults): 300 mg once daily; may ↑ by 300 mg/day every 2–4 wk (maximum dose = 1200 mg/day or 20 mg/kg/day); *Initiation of Korlym in patients already being treated with strong CYP3A4 inhibitor:* 300 mg once daily; may titrate up to 900 mg once daily, if needed; *Initiation of strong CYP3A4 inhibitor in patients already being treated with Korlym:* Current dose of Korlym = 300 mg once daily: No change; Current dose of Korlym = 600 mg once daily: ↓ dose to 300 mg once daily (may titrate up to 600 mg once daily, if needed); Current dose of Korlym = 900 mg once daily: ↓ dose to 600 mg once daily; Current dose of Korlym = 1200 mg once daily: ↓ dose to 900 mg once daily.

Renal Impairment

PO (Adults): 300 mg once daily; may ↑ by 300 mg/day every 2–4 wk (maximum dose = 600 mg/day).

Hepatic Impairment

PO (Adults): 300 mg once daily; may ↑ by 300 mg/day every 2–4 wk (maximum dose = 600 mg/day).

Availability (generic available)

Tablets (Korlym): 300 mg. **Tablets (Mifeprex):** 200 mg.

NURSING IMPLICATIONS

Assessment

- **Mifeprex:** Determine duration of pregnancy. Pregnancy is dated from the 1st day of the last menstrual period in a presumed 28-day cycle with ovulation occurring at midcycle and can be determined by menstrual history and clinical examination; use ultrasound if duration is uncertain or if ectopic pregnancy is suspected. Assess women who became pregnant with an IUD in place for ectopic pregnancy.
- Assess for signs and symptoms of infection (fever, abdominal pain, tachycardia).
- Assess amount of bleeding and cramping during treatment. Determine if termination is complete on day 14. Prolonged heavy bleeding may be a sign of incomplete abortion or other complications.
- **Korlym:** Monitor for changes in cushingoid appearance (acne, hirsutism, striae, body weight) during therapy.
- Monitor for signs and symptoms of adrenal insufficiency (weakness, nausea, ↑ fatigue, hypotension, hypoglycemia) during therapy. *If adrenal insufficiency is suspected,* discontinue Korlym and administer glucocorticoids immediately.

Lab Test Considerations

- **Mifeprex:** May ↓ hemoglobin, hematocrit, and RBCs in women who bleed heavily.
- Changes in quantitative human chorionic gonadotropin (hCG) levels are not accurate until ≥10 days after mifepristone administration; complete termination of pregnancy must be confirmed by clinical examination.
- **Korlym:** Verify negative pregnancy test in women prior to starting therapy or before restarting therapy if stopped for >14 days.
- Correct hypokalemia prior to starting therapy. Assess serum potassium 1–2 wk after starting or ↑ dose of Korlym and periodically thereafter.
- Monitor A1c periodically during therapy.

Implementation

- Do not confuse mifepristone with misoprostol.
- ***REMS:*** Mifeprex is only available through a restricted program, mifepristone REMS program. Prescribers and pharmacies that dispense mifepristone must be certified by the program, and patients must sign an agreement form.
- **Mifeprex:** Mifepristone should be administered only by health care providers who have read and understood the prescribing information, are able to assess gestational age of an embryo and diagnose ectopic pregnancies, and are able to provide surgical intervention in cases of incomplete abortion or severe bleeding.
- Remove any IUD prior to mifepristone administration.
- Measures to prevent rhesus immunization, similar to those of surgical abortion, should be taken.
- During administration and when preparing tablets, wear double chemotherapy gloves, protective gown, and hair and shoe covers. Respiratory (N95) protection and eye/face protection is needed if there is risk of patient vomiting or spitting up. Single chemotherapy gloves are appropriate if handling and administering intact tablets from a unit-dose package. Health care providers who are actively trying to conceive, who are pregnant or may become pregnant, and who are breastfeeding should avoid handling mifepristone.
- **PO:** On *Day 1*, after the patient has read the *Medication Guide* and signed the Patient Agreement, administer one 200-mg tablet of mifepristone as a single dose. On *Day 2 or 3*, unless abortion has occurred and been confirmed by clinical examination or ultrasound, administer four 200-mcg tablets of misoprostol buccally between 24 and 48 hr after taking mifepristone. Expulsion of pregnancy usually happens within 2–24 hr of taking misoprostol. On *Days 7–14*, confirm that termination of pregnancy has occurred by clinical examination or ultrasound. If complete expulsion has not occurred, administer another dose of misoprostil 800 mcg buccally.
- **Korlym:** Administer with a meal. ***DNC:*** Swallow tablet whole; do not crush, break, or chew.
- If Korlym therapy is interrupted, reinitiate at lowest dose (300 mg).

Patient/Family Teaching

- **Mifeprex:** Explain the purpose of medication. Advise patient of the treatment and its effects. Patients must be given a copy of the *Medication Guide and Patient Agreement.* Patient must understand the necessity of completing the treatment schedule of three office visits (Day 1, Days 2–3, and Days 7–14).
- Inform patient that vaginal bleeding and uterine cramping will probably occur and that prolonged or heavy vaginal bleeding is not proof of complete expulsion. Bleeding or spotting occurs for an average of 9–16 days but may continue for >30 days. Advise patient that if the treatment fails, there is a risk of fetal malformation; medical abortion failures are managed by surgical termination.
- Caution patient to notify health care provider immediately if heavy bleeding (soak through 2 thick full-size sanitary pads per hr for 2 consecutive hr or are concerned about heavy bleeding); abdominal pain; feeling sick (weakness, nausea, vomiting, or diarrhea with or without abdominal pain or fever more than 24 hr after taking mifepristone); or fever (≥100.4°F that lasts >4 hr; may indicate life-threatening sepsis) occurs.
- Instruct patient in the steps to take in an emergency situation, including precise instructions and a telephone number to call if they have problems or concerns.
- May cause dizziness or fainting. Caution patient to avoid driving or other activities requiring alertness until response to medication is known.
- Advise patient to notify health care provider if they smoke ≥10 cigarettes/day.
- Rep: Caution patient that pregnancy can occur following termination of pregnancy and before resumption of normal menses. Contraception can be initiated as soon as pregnancy termination is confirmed or before sexual intercourse is resumed.
- **Korlym:** Explain the purpose and side effects of medication. Instruct patient to take as directed. Advise patient to read *Medication Guide* prior to starting therapy and with each refill in case of changes.
- Caution patient to avoid drinking grapefruit juice during therapy.
- Instruct patient to notify health care provider if signs and symptoms of adrenal insufficiency, abnormal vaginal bleeding, or low potassium (muscle weakness, aches, cramps, palpitations) occur.
- Advise patient to notify health care provider of all Rx or OTC medications, vitamins, or herbal products being taken and to consult with health care provider before taking other medications. Avoid St. John's wort during treatment.
- Rep: May cause fetal harm. Advise women of reproductive potential to use a nonhormonal form of contraception during and for ≥1 mo after last dose of therapy. Notify health care provider immediately if pregnancy is suspected. Advise women to avoid breastfeeding during therapy. To minimize exposure to a breastfed infant, women who discontinue or interrupt Korlym therapy may consider pumping and discarding milk during therapy and for 18–21 days (5–6 half-lives) after last dose before breastfeeding.

Evaluation/Desired Outcomes

- **Mifeprex:** Termination of an intrauterine pregnancy of less than 70 days duration.
- **Korlym:** Improved control of blood glucose.

BEERS

milnacipran (mil-na-**sip**-ran)

Savella

Classification

Therapeutic: antifibromyalgia agents

Pharmacologic: selective norepinephrine reuptake inhibitors

M

Indications

Fibromyalgia.

Action

Inhibits neuronal reuptake of norepinephrine and serotonin. **Therapeutic Effects:** Decreased pain associated with fibromyalgia.

Pharmacokinetics

Absorption: 85–90% absorbed following oral administration.

Distribution: Unknown.

Metabolism and Excretion: Mostly excreted in urine as unchanged drug (55%) and inactive metabolites.

Half-life: *D:* isomer 8–10 hr; *L:* isomer 4–6 hr.

TIME/ACTION PROFILE (↓ in pain)

ROUTE	ONSET	PEAK	DURATION
PO	1 wk	unknown	unknown

Contraindications/Precautions

Contraindicated in: Concurrent use of MAO inhibitors or MAO-like drugs (linezolid or methylene blue); End-stage renal disease; Significant history of alcohol use/abuse; Chronic liver disease; Lactation: Lactation.

Use Cautiously in: May ↑ risk of suicide attempt/ideation especially during early treatment or dose adjustment; this risk appears to be greater in adolescents or children; History of seizures; Hypertension;

Moderate to severe renal impairment (↓ dose); Severe hepatic impairment; Obstructive uropathy (↑ risk of adverse genitourinary effects); Angle-closure glaucoma; OB: Use during pregnancy only if potential maternal benefit justifies potential fetal risk; Pedi: Safety and effectiveness not established in children; Geri: Appears on Beers list. May worsen or cause syndrome of inappropriate antidiuretic hormone (SIADH) secretion and/or hyponatremia in older adults. Use with caution in older adults and closely monitor sodium concentrations when starting therapy or ↑ dose.

Adverse Reactions/Side Effects

CV: hypertension, tachycardia. **Derm:** ↑ sweating, hot flush. **Endo:** SIADH. **F and E** hyponatremia. **GI:** ↑ liver enzymes, constipation, dry mouth, nausea, PANCREATITIS, vomiting. **GU:** ↓ libido, delayed/absent orgasm, ejaculatory delay/failure, erectile dysfunction. **Hemat:** BLEEDING. **Neuro:** dizziness, headache, insomnia, NEUROLEPTIC MALIGNANT SYNDROME, SUICIDAL THOUGHTS/BEHAVIORS. **Misc:** SEROTONIN SYNDROME.

Interactions

Drug-Drug: Concurrent use with **MAO inhibitors** may result in serious, potentially fatal reactions; wait ≥14 days following discontinuation of MAO inhibitor before initiation of milnacipran. Wait ≥5 days after discontinuing milnacipran before initiation of MAO inhibitor. Concurrent use with **MAO-inhibitor-like drugs**, such as **linezolid** or **methylene blue**, may ↑ risk of serotonin syndrome; concurrent use contraindicated; do not start therapy in patients receiving **linezolid** or **methylene blue**; if **linezolid** or **methylene blue** need to be started in a patient receiving milnacipran, immediately discontinue milnacipran and monitor for signs/symptoms of serotonin syndrome for 5 days or until 24 hr after last dose of linezolid or methylene blue, whichever comes first (may resume milnacipran therapy 24 hr after last dose of linezolid or methylene blue). Drugs that affect serotonergic neurotransmitter systems, including **tricyclic antidepressants**, **SNRIs**, **fentanyl**, **lithium**, **buspirone**, **tramadol**, **meperidine**, **methadone**, **amphetamines**, and **triptans**, may ↑ risk of serotonin syndrome. ↑ risk of bleeding with **NSAIDs**, **aspirin**, **clopidogrel**, **prasugrel**, **ticagrelor**, **dabigatran**, **apixaban**, **edoxaban**, **rivaroxaban**, or **warfarin**. May ↓ antihypertensive effectiveness of **clonidine**. ↑ risk of hypertension and arrhythmias with **epinephrine** or **norepinephrine**. ↑ risk of euphoria and hypotension when switching from **clomipramine**. Concurrent use with **digoxin** may result in adverse hemodynamics, including hypotension and tachycardia; avoid concurrent use with IV digoxin.
Drug-Natural Products: St. John's wort may ↑ risk of serotonin syndrome.

Route/Dosage

PO (Adults): *Day 1:* 12.5 mg; *Day 2–3:* 12.5 mg twice daily; *Day 4–7:* 25 mg twice daily; *After Day 7:* 50 mg twice daily. Some patients may require up to 100 mg twice daily depending on response.

Renal Impairment

PO (Adults): *CCr 5–29 mL/min:* Maintenance dose is 25 mg twice daily; some patients may require up to 50 mg twice daily depending on response.

Availability (generic available)

Tablets (contain tartrazine): 12.5 mg, 25 mg, 50 mg, 100 mg.

NURSING IMPLICATIONS

Assessment

- Assess intensity, quality, and location of pain periodically during therapy. May require several weeks to be effective.
- Monitor BP and HR before and periodically during therapy. Treat pre-existing hypertension and cardiac disease prior to therapy. *If sustained hypertension occurs,* ↓ dose or discontinue therapy.
- Assess for suicidal tendencies, especially during early therapy. Restrict amount of drug available to patient. Risk may be ↑ in adults ≤24 yr. After starting therapy, young adults should be seen by health care provider face-to-face at least weekly for 4 wk, then every other wk for next 4 wk, then at 12 wk, and then on advice of health care provider thereafter.
- Monitor for development of neuroleptic malignant syndrome (fever, respiratory distress, tachycardia, convulsions, diaphoresis, hypertension, hypotension, pallor, tiredness, severe muscle stiffness, incontinence).
- Assess sexual function before starting therapy. Assess for changes in sexual function during treatment, including timing of onset; patient may not report.

Lab Test Considerations

- May ↑ ALT, AST, and bilirubin.
- May cause hyponatremia.

Implementation

- **PO:** Administer without regard to food at the same time daily; may be more tolerable if taken with food.

Patient/Family Teaching

- Explain purpose and side effects of medication. Advise patient to read *Patient Information* before starting therapy.
- Instruct patient to take missed doses as soon as possible unless time for next dose. Do not stop abruptly; must be ↓ gradually.
- Encourage patient to maintain routine follow-up visits with health care provider to determine effectiveness.

- Advise patient to immediately notify health care provider for signs of serotonin syndrome (agitation, hallucinations, tachycardia, labile BP, dizziness, diaphoresis, flushing, tremor, rigidity, myoclonus, hyperreflexia, incoordination, seizure, nausea, vomiting, diarrhea).
- Advise patient, family, and caregivers to look for suicidality, especially during early therapy or dose changes. Notify health care provider immediately if thoughts about suicide or dying, attempts to commit suicide, new or worse depression or anxiety, agitation or restlessness, panic attacks, insomnia, new or worse irritability, aggressiveness, acting on dangerous impulses, mania, or other changes in mood or behavior.
- Encourage patient and family to be alert for emergence of anxiety, agitation, panic attacks, insomnia, irritability, hostility, impulsivity, akathisia, hypomania, or mania, especially during early antidepressant therapy. Changes may be abrupt. If symptoms occur, notify health care provider immediately.
- May cause dizziness. Caution patient to avoid driving or other activities requiring alertness until response to medication is known.
- Advise patient to notify health care provider of all Rx or OTC medications, vitamins, or herbal products being taken and to consult with health care provider before taking other medications, especially St. John's wort. Avoid use of aspirin, NSAIDs, and warfarin due to ↑ risk for bleeding.
- Instruct patient to notify health care provider if signs of liver damage (pruritus, dark urine, jaundice, right upper quadrant tenderness, unexplained flu-like symptoms) or hyponatremia (headache, difficulty concentrating, memory impairment, confusion, weakness, unsteadiness, falls), or rash occur.
- Advise patient to avoid taking alcohol during therapy.
- Inform patient that milnacipran may cause symptoms of sexual dysfunction. In men, ejaculatory delay or failure, ↓ libido, and erectile dysfunction may occur. In women, may result in ↓ libido and delayed or absent orgasm. Advise patient to notify health care provider if symptoms occur.
- Rep: Instruct women of reproductive potential to notify health care provider if pregnancy is planned or suspected or if breastfeeding. May be associated with an ↑ risk of postpartum hemorrhage. Neonates exposed to milnacipran late in the 3rd trimester have developed complications requiring prolonged hospitalization, respiratory support, and tube feeding; can arise immediately upon delivery. Symptoms may include respiratory distress, cyanosis, apnea, seizures, temperature instability, feeding difficulty, vomiting, hypoglycemia, hypotonia, hypertonia, hyperreflexia, tremor, jitteriness, irritability, and constant crying. Monitor infants exposed to milnacipran for agitation, irritability, poor feeding, and poor weight gain.

Evaluation/Desired Outcomes

- Reduction in pain and soreness associated with fibromyalgia.

HIGH ALERT

milrinone (mill-ri-none)

~~Primacor~~

Classification

Therapeutic: inotropics

Indications

Short-term treatment of HF unresponsive to conventional therapy with digoxin, diuretics, and vasodilators.

Action

Increases myocardial contractility. Decreases preload and afterload by a direct dilating effect on vascular smooth muscle. **Therapeutic Effects:** Increased cardiac output (inotropic effect).

Pharmacokinetics

Absorption: IV administration results in complete bioavailability.
Distribution: Moderately distributed to tissues.
Metabolism and Excretion: 80–90% excreted unchanged by the kidneys.
Half-life: 2.3 hr (↑ in renal impairment).

TIME/ACTION PROFILE (hemodynamic effects)

ROUTE	ONSET	PEAK	DURATION
IV	5–15 min	unknown	3–6 hr

Contraindications/Precautions

Contraindicated in: Hypersensitivity; Severe aortic or pulmonic valvular heart disease; Hypertrophic subaortic stenosis (may ↑ outflow tract obstruction).
Use Cautiously in: History of arrhythmias, electrolyte abnormalities, abnormal digoxin levels, or insertion of vascular catheters (↑ risk of ventricular arrhythmias); Renal impairment (↓ infusion rate if CCr is <50 mL/min); OB: Safety not established in pregnancy; Lactation: Safety not established in breastfeeding.

Adverse Reactions/Side Effects

CV: angina pectoris, chest pain, hypotension, supraventricular arrhythmias, VENTRICULAR ARRHYTHMIAS.

M

Derm: rash. **GI:** ↑ liver enzymes. **Hemat:** thrombocytopenia. **Neuro:** headache, tremor.

Interactions

Drug-Drug: None reported.

Route/Dosage

IV (Adults): *Loading dose:* 50 mcg/kg followed by *Continuous infusion* at 0.5 mcg/kg/min (range 0.375–0.75 mcg/kg/min).

IV (Infants and Children): *Loading dose:* 50 mcg/kg over 10 min followed by *Continuous infusion* at 0.5 mcg/kg/min (range 0.25–0.75 mcg/kg/min).

Availability (generic available)

Solution for injection: 1 mg/mL. **Premixed infusion:** 20 mg/100 mL, 40 mg/200 mL.

NURSING IMPLICATIONS

Assessment

- Monitor intake, output, and daily weight. Assess patient for resolution of signs and symptoms of HF (peripheral edema, dyspnea, rales/crackles, weight gain) and improvement in hemodynamic parameters (↑ cardiac output and cardiac index, ↓ pulmonary capillary wedge pressure). Correct effects of previous aggressive diuretic therapy to allow for optimal filling pressure.
- Monitor BP and ECG continuously during infusion. Arrhythmias are common and may be life-threatening. The risk of ventricular arrhythmias is ↑ in patients with history of arrhythmias, electrolyte abnormalities, abnormal digoxin levels, or insertion of vascular catheters. *If hypotension or arrhythmias occurs,* slow or discontinue therapy depending on severity.

Lab Test Considerations

- Monitor electrolytes and renal function frequently during therapy. Correct hypokalemia prior to administration to ↓ risk of arrhythmias.
- Monitor platelet count during therapy.

Toxicity and Overdose

- ***High Alert:*** Overdose manifests as hypotension. Dose should be ↓ or discontinued until patient is stabilized. Provide circulatory support as indicated.

Implementation

- ***High Alert:*** Accidental overdose of milrinone can cause patient harm or death. Have 2nd practitioner independently check original order, dose calculations, and infusion pump settings.

IV Administration

- **IV Push: Dilution:** Loading dose may be administered undiluted. May also be diluted in 0.9% NaCl, 0.45% NaCl, or D5W for ease of administration. **Concentration:** 1 mg/mL. **Rate:** Administer loading dose over 10 min.
- **Continuous Infusion: Dilution:** Dilute 10 mg (10 mL) in 40 mL of diluent or 20 mg (20 mL) in 80 mL of diluent. Compatible diluents include 0.45% NaCl, 0.9% NaCl, and D5W. Premixed infusions are already diluted and ready to use. Admixed solutions are stable for 72 hr at room temperature. Do not use solution that is discolored or contains particulates. **Concentration:** 200 mcg/mL.
- **Rate:** Based on patient's weight (see Route/Dosage section). Titrate according to hemodynamic and clinical response.
- **Y-Site Compatibility:** acyclovir, alemtuzumab, allopurinol, amikacin, aminocaproic acid, aminophylline, amiodarone, amphotericin B liposomal, ampicillin, anidulafungin, argatroban, arsenic trioxide, atracurium, azithromycin, aztreonam, bivalirudin, bleomycin, bumetanide, buprenorphine, busulfan, butorphanol, caffeine citrate, calcium chloride, calcium chloride, calcium gluconate, cangrelor, carboplatin, carmustine, caspofungin, cefazolin, cefepime, cefiderocol, cefotaxime, cefotetan, cefoxitin, ceftaroline, ceftazidime, ceftolozane/tazobactam, ceftriaxone, cefuroxime, chlorpromazine, ciprofloxacin, cisatracurium, cisplatin, clindamycin, cyclophosphamide, cyclosporine, cytarabine, dacarbazine, dactinomycin, daptomycin, daunorubicin, dexamethasone, dexmedetomidine, dexrazoxane, digoxin, diltiazem, dobutamine, docetaxel, dopamine, doxorubicin hydrochloride, doxorubicin liposomal, doxycycline, droperidol, enalaprilat, ephedrine, epinephrine, epirubicin, eptifibatide, ertapenem, erythromycin, etoposide, etoposide phosphate, famotidine, fentanyl, fluconazole, fludarabine, fluorouracil, foscarnet, fosphenytoin, ganciclovir, gemcitabine, gentamicin, glycopyrrolate, granisetron, haloperidol, heparin, hydralazine, hydrocortisone, hydromorphone, idarubicin, ifosfamide, insulin aspart, insulin regular, irinotecan, isavuconazonium, isoproterenol, ketamine, ketorolac, labetalol, leucovorin, levofloxacin, linezolid, lorazepam, magnesium sulfate, mannitol, melphalan, meperidine, meropenem, meropenem/vaborbactam, mesna, methadone, methohexital, methotrexate, methylprednisolone, metoclopramide, metoprolol, metronidazole, micafungin, midazolam, mitoxantrone, morphine, moxifloxacin, mycophenolate, nafcillin, nalbuphine, naloxone, nicardipine, nitroglycerin, nitroprusside, norepinephrine, octreotide, oxacillin, oxaliplatin, oxytocin, paclitaxel, palonosetron, pamidronate, pemetrexed, pentamidine, pentobarbital, phenobarbital, phenylephrine, piperacillin/tazobactam, plazomicin, potassium acetate, potassium chloride, potassium phosphates, prochlorperazine, promethazine, propofol, propranolol, remifentanil, rocuronium, sildenafil, sodium acetate, sodium bicarbonate, sodium phosphates, succinylcholine, sufentanil, sulbactam/durlobactam, tacrolimus, tedizolid, telavancin, theophylline, thiotepa, tigecycline, tirofiban, tobramycin,

topotecan, vancomycin, vasopressin, vecuronium, verapamil, vinblastine, vincristine, vinorelbine, voriconazole, zidovudine, zoledronic acid.
- **Y-Site Incompatibility:** amphotericin B deoxycholate, clevidipine, dantrolene, diazepam, diphenhydramine, esmolol, furosemide, gemtuzumab ozogamicin, imipenem/cilastatin, lidocaine, mitomycin, ondansetron, pantoprazole, phenytoin, procainamide.

Patient/Family Teaching
- Explain purpose and side effects of medication. Advise patient to read *Patient Information* before starting therapy.
- Advise patient to notify health care provider immediately if bronchospasm or other signs of anaphylaxis occur.
- Rep: Advise women of reproductive potential to notify health care provider if pregnancy is planned or suspected or if breastfeeding.

Evaluation/Desired Outcomes
- Decrease in the signs and symptoms of HF.
- Improvement in hemodynamic parameters.

mirabegron (mye-ra-**beg**-ron)
Myrbetriq

Classification
Therapeutic: urinary tract antispasmodics
Pharmacologic: beta-adrenergic agonists

Indications
Overactive bladder, including urge urinary incontinence, urgency, and frequency (either as monotherapy or in combination with solifenacin). Pediatric neurogenic detrusor overactivity.

Action
Acts as a selective beta-3 adrenergic agonist. Increases bladder capacity by relaxing detrusor smooth muscle during storage phase of bladder fill-void cycle. **Therapeutic Effects:** Decreased symptoms of overactive bladder. Improved bladder capacity in neurogenic detrusor overactivity.

Pharmacokinetics
Absorption: 29–35% absorbed following oral administration.
Distribution: Widely distributed.
Metabolism and Excretion: Extensively metabolized, 6% excreted unchanged in urine (25-mg dose); remainder excreted in urine and feces as metabolites.
Half-life: *Adults:* 50 hr; *Children:* 26–31 hr.

TIME/ACTION PROFILE (effects on bladder)

ROUTE	ONSET	PEAK	DURATION
PO	unknown	3–4 hr†	24 hr

† Blood level.

Contraindications/Precautions
Contraindicated in: Hypersensitivity; Severe uncontrolled hypertension; End-stage renal disease (eGFR <15 mL/min/1.73 m^2 or requiring dialysis); Severe hepatic impairment.
Use Cautiously in: Hypertension; Bladder outlet obstruction/concurrent antimuscarinics (↑ risk of urinary retention); Concurrent use of antimuscarinics used to treat overactive bladder; OB: Safety not established in pregnancy; Lactation: Safety not established in breastfeeding; Pedi: Children <3 yr (safety and effectiveness not established).

Adverse Reactions/Side Effects
CV: ↑ BP, tachycardia. **EENT:** nasopharyngitis. **GI:** constipation, diarrhea, nausea. **GU:** urinary tract infection. **Neuro:** dizziness, headache. **Misc:** ANGIOEDEMA.

Interactions
Drug-Drug: May ↑ levels and risk of toxicity of **CYP2D6 substrates**, including **desipramine**, **flecainide**, **metoprolol**, **propafenone**, and **thioridazine**. May ↑ levels and risk of toxicity of **digoxin**; use lowest effective level of digoxin/monitor serum levels.

Route/Dosage
The extended-release tablets and extended-release oral suspension are NOT interchangeable and should NOT be combined.

Overactive Bladder
PO (Adults): 25 mg once daily; may ↑ to 50 mg once daily, if needed, after 4–8 wk.

Renal Impairment
PO (Adults): *eGFR 15–29 mL/min/m²:* 25 mg once daily (max dose = 25 mg/day).

Hepatic Impairment
PO (Adults): *Moderate hepatic impairment:* 25 mg once daily (max dose = 25 mg/day).

Neurogenic Detrusor Overactivity
PO (Children ≥3 yr and ≥35 kg): *Extended-release tablets:* 25 mg once daily; may ↑ to 50 mg once daily, if needed, after 4–8 wk. *Extended-release oral suspension (granules):* 48 mg once daily; may ↑ to 80 mg once daily, if needed after 4–8 wk.
PO (Children ≥3 yr and 22–<35 kg): *Extended-release oral suspension (granules):* 32 mg once daily; may ↑ to 64 mg once daily, if needed after 4–8 wk.
PO (Children ≥3 yr and 11–<22 kg): *Extended-release oral suspension (granules):* 24 mg once daily; may ↑ to 48 mg once daily, if needed after 4–8 wk.

Renal Impairment
PO (Children ≥3 yr and ≥35 kg): *eGFR 15–29 mL/min/m²:* Extended-release tablets: 25 mg once daily

M

(max dose = 25 mg/day); Extended-release oral suspension (granules): 48 mg once daily (max dose = 48 mg/day).

Renal Impairment

PO (Children ≥3 yr and 22–<35 kg): *eGFR 15–29 mL/min/m²:* Extended-release oral suspension (granules): 32 mg once daily (max dose = 32 mg/day).

Renal Impairment

PO (Children ≥3 yr and 11–<22 kg): *eGFR 15–29 mL/min/m²:* Extended-release oral suspension (granules): 24 mg once daily (max dose = 24 mg/day).

Hepatic Impairment

PO (Children ≥3 yr and ≥35 kg): *Moderate hepatic impairment:* Extended-release tablets: 25 mg once daily (max dose = 25 mg/day); Extended-release oral suspension (granules): 48 mg once daily (max dose = 48 mg/day).

Hepatic Impairment

PO (Children ≥3 yr and 22–<35 kg): *Moderate hepatic impairment:* Extended-release oral suspension (granules): 32 mg once daily (max dose = 32 mg/day).

Hepatic Impairment

PO (Children ≥3 yr and 11–<22 kg): *Moderate hepatic impairment:* Extended-release oral suspension (granules): 24 mg once daily (max dose = 24 mg/day).

Availability (generic available)

Extended-release tablets: 25 mg, 50 mg. **Extended-release oral suspension (granules):** 8 mg/mL.

NURSING IMPLICATIONS

Assessment

- Assess for urinary urgency, frequency, urge incontinence, and urinary retention periodically during therapy.
- Monitor BP prior to starting and periodically during therapy; may ↑ BP.
- Monitor for signs and symptoms of angioedema (swelling of face, lips, tongue, or larynx). *If airway symptoms occur,* discontinue mirabegron and treat symptomatically.

Implementation

- Tablets and granules are different products. Do not interchange, substitute, or combine.
- **PO:** Administer without regard to food.
- ***DNC:*** Swallow tablets whole with water; do not break, crush, or chew.
- Pediatric patients weighing ≥35 kg may use tablets or granules.
- Administer granules for patients weighing <35 kg. Prepare granules as an extended-release oral suspension. Tap the closed bottle to loosen granules. Add 100 mL of water to bottle, shake vigorously for 1 min, let stand for 10–30 min, and then shake again for 1 min. Repeat shaking for 1 min if granules have not dispersed. Take with food. Store at room temperature for ≤28 days after reconstitution.

Patient/Family Teaching

- Explain purpose and side effects of medication. Advise patient to read *Patient Information* before starting therapy.
- Instruct patient to take a missed dose as soon as remembered. If >12 hr since missed dose omit and take next dose at scheduled time.
- Advise patient to have BP checked periodically during therapy to monitor for hypertension.
- May cause dizziness. Caution patient to avoid driving or other activities requiring alertness until response to medication is known.
- Advise patient to notify health care provider if difficulty emptying bladder occurs.
- Advise patient to notify health care provider of all Rx or OTC medications, vitamins, or herbal products being taken and to consult with health care provider before taking other medications.
- Advise patient to immediately discontinue mirabegron and notify health care provider if difficulty breathing or upper airway swelling occurs.
- Rep: Advise women of reproductive potential to notify health care provider if pregnancy is planned or suspected or if breastfeeding.

Evaluation/Desired Outcomes

- Decreased urinary frequency, urgency, and urge incontinence.

BEERS

mirtazapine (meer-taz-a-peen)

Remeron, ✱ Remeron RD, Remeron SolTab

Classification

Therapeutic: antidepressants

Pharmacologic: tetracyclic antidepressants

Indications

Major depressive disorder. **Unlabeled Use:** Panic disorder. Generalized anxiety disorder. Post-traumatic stress disorder.

Action

Potentiates the effects of norepinephrine and serotonin. **Therapeutic Effects:** Antidepressant action, which may develop only after several wk.

Pharmacokinetics

Absorption: Well absorbed but rapidly metabolized, resulting in 50% bioavailability.

Distribution: Unknown.

Protein Binding: 85%.

Metabolism and Excretion: Extensively metabolized by the liver by the CYP1A2, CYP2D6, and CYP3A

isoenzymes; metabolites excreted in urine (75%) and feces (15%).
Half-life: 20–40 hr.

TIME/ACTION PROFILE (antidepressant effect)

ROUTE	ONSET	PEAK	DURATION
PO	1–2 wk	6 wk or more	unknown

Contraindications/Precautions

Contraindicated in: Hypersensitivity; Concurrent use of MAO inhibitors or MAO-like drugs (linezolid or methylene blue).
Use Cautiously in: History of seizures; History of suicide attempt; May ↑ risk of suicide attempt/ideation especially during early treatment or dose adjustment; this risk appears to be greater in adolescents or children; History of mania/hypomania; Renal impairment; Hepatic impairment; Angle-closure glaucoma; OB: Other antidepressants are preferred in pregnancy; Lactation: Other antidepressants are preferred when breastfeeding; Pedi: Safety and effectiveness in children not established; Geri: Appears on Beers list. May worsen or cause syndrome of inappropriate antidiuretic hormone (SIADH) secretion and/or hyponatremia in older adults. Use with caution in older adults and closely monitor sodium concentrations when starting therapy or ↑ dose.

Adverse Reactions/Side Effects

CV: edema, hypotension. **Derm:** BULLOUS DERMATITIS, DRUG REACTION WITH EOSINOPHILIA AND SYSTEMIC SYMPTOMS (DRESS), ERYTHEMA MULTIFORME, pruritus, rash, STEVENS-JOHNSON SYNDROME (SJS), TOXIC EPIDERMAL NECROLYSIS (TEN). **EENT:** sinusitis. **Endo:** SIADH. **F and E** ↑ thirst, hyponatremia. **GI:** constipation, dry mouth, ↑ liver enzymes, abdominal pain, anorexia, nausea, vomiting. **GU:** urinary frequency. **Hemat:** AGRANULOCYTOSIS. **Metab:** ↑ appetite, weight gain, hypercholesterolemia, hypertriglyceridemia. **MS:** arthralgia, back pain, myalgia. **Neuro:** drowsiness, abnormal dreams, abnormal thinking, agitation, akathisia, anxiety, apathy, confusion, dizziness, hyperkinesia, hypoesthesia, malaise, NEUROLEPTIC MALIGNANT SYNDROME (NMS), SUICIDAL THOUGHTS/BEHAVIORS, twitching, weakness. **Resp:** cough, dyspnea. **Misc:** flu-like syndrome, SEROTONIN SYNDROME.

Interactions

Drug-Drug: May cause hypertension, seizures, and death when used with **MAO inhibitors**; do not use within 14 days of MAO inhibitor therapy. Concurrent use with **MAO-inhibitor-like drugs**, such as **linezolid** or **methylene blue**, may ↑ risk of serotonin syndrome; concurrent use contraindicated; do not start therapy in patients receiving **linezolid** or **methylene blue**; if **linezolid** or **methylene blue** need to be started in a patient receiving mirtazapine, immediately discontinue mirtazapine and monitor for signs/symptoms of serotonin syndrome for 2 wk or until 24 hr after last dose of linezolid or methylene blue, whichever comes first (may resume mirtazapine therapy 24 hr after last dose of linezolid or methylene blue). Drugs that affect serotonergic neurotransmitter systems, including **tricyclic antidepressants**, **SNRIs**, **fentanyl**, **buspirone**, **tramadol**, and **triptans**, may ↑ risk of serotonin syndrome. ↑ risk of CNS depression with other **CNS depressants**, including **alcohol** and **benzodiazepines**. **Ketoconazole**, **cimetidine**, **clarithromycin**, **erythromycin**, **itraconazole**, **nefazodone**, **nelfinavir**, or **ritonavir** may ↑ levels and risk of toxicity. **Phenobarbital**, **phenytoin**, **carbamazepine**, **rifampin**, or **rifabutin** may ↓ levels and effectiveness; may need to ↑ mirtazapine dose. May ↑ risk of bleeding from **warfarin**.
Drug-Natural Products: **Kava-kava**, **valerian**, **skullcap**, **chamomile**, or **hops** can ↑ risk of CNS depression. ↑ risk of serotonin syndrome with **St. John's wort** and **SAMe**.

Route/Dosage

PO (Adults): 15 mg/day as a single bedtime dose initially; may be ↑ every 1–2 wk up to 45 mg/day.

Availability (generic available)

Tablets: 7.5 mg, 15 mg, 30 mg, 45 mg. **Orally disintegrating tablets (orange flavor):** 15 mg, 30 mg, 45 mg.

NURSING IMPLICATIONS

Assessment

- Assess mental status (orientation, mood, behavior) frequently.
- Assess for suicidal tendencies, especially during early therapy. Restrict amount of drug available to patient. Risk may be ↑ in adults ≤24 yr. After starting therapy, young adults should be seen by health care provider face-to-face at least weekly for 4 wk, then every other wk for next 4 wk, then at 12 wk, and then on advice of health care provider thereafter.
- Assess weight and BMI initially and throughout therapy. For overweight/obese individuals, obtain fasting blood glucose and cholesterol levels. Refer as appropriate for nutritional/weight management and medical management.

M

- Monitor BP and HR periodically during initial therapy. Report significant changes.
- Monitor for seizure activity in patients with a history of seizures or alcohol abuse. Institute seizure precautions.
- Assess skin periodically during therapy. Severe skin reactions, including DRESS, SJS, bullous dermatitis, erythema multiforme, and TEN, may occur. *If signs/ symptoms of severe skin reactions occur,* discontinue mirtazapine immediately.
- Assess for serotonin syndrome (mental changes [agitation, hallucinations, coma], autonomic instability [tachycardia, labile BP, hyperthermia], neuromuscular aberrations [hyperreflexia, incoordination], GI symptoms [nausea, vomiting, diarrhea]), especially in patients taking other serotonergic drugs (SSRIs, SNRIs, triptans).
- Monitor for development of NMS (fever, respiratory distress, tachycardia, seizures, diaphoresis, hypertension or hypotension, pallor, tiredness). *If signs/ symptoms of NMS occur,* discontinue mirtazapine and notify health care provider immediately.

Lab Test Considerations

- Assess CBC, liver function, and cholesterol/triglyceride levels before and periodically during therapy.

Implementation

- Do not confuse Remeron with Rozerem.
- **PO:** Administer with or without food at bedtime to minimize excessive drowsiness or dizziness.
- **Orally disintegrating tablets:** Do not attempt to push through foil backing; with dry hands, peal back backing and remove tablet. Immediately place tablet on tongue; tablet will dissolve in seconds; then swallow with saliva. Administration with liquid is not necessary.

Patient/Family Teaching

- Explain purpose and side effects of medication to patient. Advise patient to read *Patient Information* before starting therapy. Instruct patient to take as directed. Take missed doses as soon as remembered; if almost time for next dose, skip missed dose and return to regular schedule. If single bedtime dose regimen is used, do not take missed dose in morning, but consult health care provider. Do not discontinue abruptly; gradual dose ↓ may be required.
- Advise patient to notify health care provider of all Rx or OTC medications, vitamins, or herbal products being taken and to consult with health care provider before taking other medications, especially St. John's wort.
- May cause drowsiness and dizziness. Caution patient to avoid driving and other activities requiring alertness until response to drug is known.
- Advise patient, family, and caregivers to look for suicidality, especially during early therapy or dose changes. Notify health care provider immediately if thoughts about suicide or dying, attempts to commit suicide, new or worse depression or anxiety, agitation or restlessness, panic attacks, insomnia, new or worse irritability, aggressiveness, acting on dangerous impulses, mania, or other changes in mood or behavior occur.
- Encourage patient and caregivers to be alert for emergence of anxiety, agitation, panic attacks, insomnia, irritability, hostility, impulsivity, akathisia, hypomania, or mania, especially during early antidepressant therapy. Assess symptoms on a day-to-day basis, as changes may be abrupt. If these symptoms occur, notify health care provider.
- Caution patient to change positions slowly to minimize orthostatic hypotension.
- Advise patient to avoid alcohol or other CNS depressant drugs during and for ≥3–7 days after therapy has been discontinued.
- Instruct patient to notify health care provider of signs and symptoms of serotonin syndrome (mental status changes [agitation, hallucinations, coma], autonomic instability [tachycardia, labile BP, hyperthermia], neuromuscular aberrations [hyperreflexia, incoordination], gastrointestinal symptoms [nausea, vomiting, diarrhea]) or rash occur.
- Advise patient to notify health care provider if dry mouth, urinary retention, or constipation occurs. Frequent rinses, good oral hygiene, and sugarless candy or gum may diminish dry mouth. An ↑ in fluid intake, fiber, and exercise may prevent constipation.
- Inform patient of need to monitor dietary intake. ↑ in appetite may lead to undesired weight gain.
- Advise patient to notify health care provider of medication regimen before treatment or surgery.
- Rep: Advise women of reproductive potential to notify health care provider if pregnancy is planned or suspected or if breastfeeding. Inform patient of National Pregnancy Registry for Antidepressants that monitors pregnancy outcomes in women exposed to antidepressants during pregnancy. Advise pregnant women ≤45 yr of age with a history of psychiatric illness to enroll in the National Pregnancy Registry for Antidepressants by calling (1-866-961-2388) or visiting https://womensmentalhealth.org/research/pregnancyregistry/antidepressants.

Evaluation/Desired Outcomes

- Antidepressant action, which may develop only after several wk.

miSOPROStol

(mye-soe-**prost**-ole)

Cytotec

Classification

Therapeutic: antiulcer agents, cytoprotective agents, abortifacients

Pharmacologic: prostaglandins

Indications
Prevention of gastric mucosal injury from NSAIDs, including aspirin, in high-risk patients (older adults, debilitated patients, those with a history of ulcers). Termination of pregnancy (in combination with mifepristone). **Unlabeled Use:** Treatment of duodenal ulcers. Cervical ripening and labor induction.

Action
Acts as a prostaglandin analogue, decreasing gastric acid secretion (antisecretory effect) and increasing the production of protective mucus (cytoprotective effect). Causes uterine contractions. **Therapeutic Effects:** Prevention of gastric ulceration from NSAIDs. With mifepristone, terminates pregnancy of less than 49 days.

Pharmacokinetics
Absorption: Well absorbed following oral administration.
Distribution: Unknown.
Protein Binding: 85%.
Metabolism and Excretion: Metabolized in liver to its active form (misoprostol acid); 80% excreted by the kidneys.
Half-life: 20–40 min.

TIME/ACTION PROFILE (effect on gastric acid secretion)

ROUTE	ONSET	PEAK	DURATION
PO	30 min	unknown	3–6 hr

Contraindications/Precautions
Contraindicated in: Hypersensitivity to prostaglandins; OB: Should not be used to prevent NSAID-induced gastric injury in pregnancy due to potential for fetal harm or death; Lactation: Lactation.
Use Cautiously in: Rep: Women of reproductive potential; Pedi: Safety and effectiveness not established in children.
Exercise Extreme Caution in: Late trimester pregnancy, previous cesarean section or uterine surgery, advanced gestational age, or ≥5 previous pregnancies (when used for cervical ripening or to induce abortion, may cause uterine rupture).

Adverse Reactions/Side Effects
GI: abdominal pain, diarrhea, constipation, dyspepsia, flatulence, nausea, vomiting. **GU:** miscarriage, menstrual disorders. **Neuro:** headache.

Interactions
Drug-Drug: ↑ risk of diarrhea with **magnesium-containing antacids**.

Route/Dosage
Prevention of NSAID-Induced Ulcers
PO (Adults): 200 mcg four times daily with or after meals and at bedtime, *or* 400 mcg twice daily, with the last dose at bedtime. If intolerance occurs, may ↓ dose to 100 mcg 4 times daily.

Pregnancy Termination
PO (Adults): 400 mcg single dose 2 days after mifepristone if abortion has not occurred.

Cervical Ripening and Labor Induction
Intravaginally: (Adults): 25 mcg (¼ of 100-mcg tablet); may repeat every 3–6 hr, if needed.

Availability (generic available)
Tablets: 100 mcg, 200 mcg. ***In combination with:*** diclofenac (Arthrotec). See Appendix N.

NURSING IMPLICATIONS
Assessment
- Assess for epigastric or abdominal pain and frank or occult blood in the stool, emesis, or gastric aspirate.
- **Termination of pregnancy:** Monitor uterine cramping and bleeding during therapy.
- **Cervical Ripening:** Monitor fetal HR and uterine activity continuously for ≥30 min following administration and for as long as regular uterine activity persists.

Lab Test Considerations
- Verify negative serum pregnancy test in women of reproductive potential within 2 wk before starting therapy.

Implementation
- Do not confuse misoprostol with mifepristone.
- Misoprostol therapy should be started at the onset of treatment with NSAIDs. Avoid magnesium-containing antacids to minimize diarrhea. Start on the 2nd or 3rd day of a normal menstrual period in women of reproductive potential.
- **PO:** Administer medication with meals and at bedtime to ↓ severity of diarrhea.

Patient/Family Teaching
- Explain purpose and side effects of medication to patient. Advise patient to read *Patient Information* before starting therapy. Instruct patient to take medication as directed for the full course of therapy, even if feeling better. Take missed doses as soon as possible unless next dose is due within 2 hr; do not double doses.
- Advise patient to notify health care provider of all Rx or OTC medications, vitamins, or herbal products being taken and to consult health care provider before taking other medications.

M

- Advise patient not to share misoprostol with others, even if they have similar symptoms; may be dangerous.
- Inform patient that diarrhea may occur. Health care provider should be notified if diarrhea persists for >1 wk. Also advise patient to report onset of black, tarry stools or severe abdominal pain.
- Advise patient to avoid alcohol and foods that may cause an ↑ in GI irritation.
- Rep: Administration of misoprostol to women who are pregnant can cause spontaneous abortion, birth defects, premature birth, or uterine rupture. The risk of uterine rupture ↑ with advancing gestational age and with prior uterine surgery, including cesarean delivery. Women of reproductive potential must be informed of this effect through verbal and written information and must use contraception throughout therapy. Misoprostol should not be used by pregnant women to ↓ the risk of NSAID-induced ulcers. It also should not be used in women of reproductive potential to ↓ the risk of NSAID-induced ulcers unless the patient is at high risk of complications from gastric ulcers associated with use of NSAIDs or is at high risk of developing gastric ulceration. In these patients, misoprostol may be prescribed if the patient has had a negative serum pregnancy test within 2 wk prior to beginning therapy; is capable of complying with effective contraceptive measures; has received both oral and written warnings of the hazards of misoprostol, including the risk of possible contraception failure; and will begin misoprostol only on the 2nd or 3rd day of the next normal menstrual period. If pregnancy is suspected, the woman should stop taking misoprostol and immediately notify health care provider.

Evaluation/Desired Outcomes

- Prevention of gastric ulceration from NSAIDs.
- With mifepristone, terminates pregnancy of less than 49 days.

HIGH ALERT

V mitoXANTRONE
(mye-toe-**zan**-trone)

~~Novantrone~~

Classification

Therapeutic: antineoplastics, immune modifiers

Pharmacologic: antitumor antibiotics

Indications

Acute nonlymphocytic leukemia (in combination with other antineoplastics). Initial chemotherapy for patients with pain associated with advanced hormone-refractory prostate cancer. Secondary (chronic) progressive, progressive relapsing, or worsening relapsing-remitting multiple sclerosis (MS).

Action

Inhibits DNA synthesis (cell-cycle phase-nonspecific). **Therapeutic Effects:** Death of rapidly replicating cells, particularly malignant ones. Decreased pain in patients with advanced prostate cancer. Decreased disability and slowed progression of MS.

Pharmacokinetics

Absorption: IV administration results in complete bioavailability.

Distribution: Widely distributed to tissues; limited penetration of CSF.

Metabolism and Excretion: Mostly eliminated by hepatobiliary clearance; <10% excreted unchanged by the kidneys.

Half-life: 5.8 days.

TIME/ACTION PROFILE (effects on blood counts)

ROUTE	ONSET	PEAK	DURATION
IV	unknown	10 days	21 days

Contraindications/Precautions

Contraindicated in: Hypersensitivity; Baseline neutrophils <1500 cells/mm^3 (for prostate cancer and MS only); Baseline left ventricular ejection fraction (LVEF) <50% (for MS only); OB: Pregnancy; Lactation: Lactation.

Use Cautiously in: Cardiovascular disease, previous mediastinal radiation, or use of anthracyclines (↑ risk of HF); Active infection; ↓ bone marrow reserve; Impaired hepatobiliary function; Rep: Women of reproductive potential; Pedi: Safety and effectiveness not established in children; Geri: Older adults may have ↑ sensitivity to drug effects.

Adverse Reactions/Side Effects

CV: arrhythmias, ECG changes, HF. **Derm:** alopecia, rash. **EENT:** blue-green sclera, conjunctivitis. **GI:** abdominal pain, diarrhea, HEPATOTOXICITY, nausea, stomatitis, vomiting. **GU:** blue-green urine, gonadal suppression, renal failure. **Hemat:** anemia, NEUTROPENIA, thrombocytopenia, SECONDARY LEUKEMIA. **Metab:** hyperuricemia. **Neuro:** headache, SEIZURES. **Resp:** cough, dyspnea. **Misc:** fever, HYPERSENSITIVITY REACTIONS.

Interactions

Drug-Drug: ↑ bone marrow depression with other **antineoplastics** or **radiation therapy**. Risk of cardiomyopathy ↑ by previous **anthracycline antineoplastics (daunorubicin, doxorubicin, idarubicin)** or **mediastinal radiation.** May ↓ antibody response to **live-virus vaccines** and ↑ risk of adverse reactions.

Route/Dosage

Acute Nonlymphocytic Leukemia

IV (Adults): *Induction:* 12 mg/m^2/day for 3 days; if incomplete remission occurs, a 2nd induction may be given. *Consolidation:* 12 mg/m^2/day for 2 days, given 6 wk after induction with another course 4 wk later.

Advanced Prostate Cancer
IV (Adults): 12–14 mg/m² as single dose.

Multiple Sclerosis
IV (Adults): 12 mg/m² every 3 mo.

Availability (generic available)
Solution for injection: 2 mg/mL.

NURSING IMPLICATIONS
Assessment
- Monitor for hypersensitivity reactions (rash; urticaria; bronchospasm; tachycardia; hypotension; wheezing; tightness in chest or throat; swelling of mouth, face, lips, tongue, or throat). *If signs/symptoms of hypersensitivity reaction occurs,* stop infusion and implement supportive measures (epinephrine) as indicated.
- Monitor for bone marrow suppression. Assess for bleeding (bleeding gums; bruising; petechiae; guaiac stools, urine, and emesis) and avoid IM injections and taking rectal temperatures if platelet count is low. Apply pressure to venipuncture sites for 10 min. Assess for signs of infection during neutropenia. Anemia may occur. Monitor for ↑ fatigue, dyspnea, and orthostatic hypotension.
- Monitor intake and output, appetite, and nutritional intake. Assess for nausea and vomiting. Antiemetics may be administered prophylactically. Adjust diet as tolerated to help maintain fluid and electrolyte balance and nutritional status.
- Monitor chest x-ray, ECG, echocardiography or MUGA, and radionuclide angiography to determine ejection fraction before and periodically during therapy. Patients with MS with baseline LVEF <50% should not receive mitoxantrone. May cause cardiotoxicity, especially in patients who have received daunorubicin or doxorubicin. Assess for rales/crackles, dyspnea, edema, jugular vein distention, ECG changes, arrhythmias, and chest pain. Monitor LVEF with echocardiogram or MUGA if signs of HF occur, before each dose, and yearly after stopping therapy in patients with MS. Additional doses of mitoxantrone should not be administered to patients with MS who have experienced either a ↓ in LVEF to below the lower limit of normal or a clinically significant ↓ in LVEF during therapy. Potentially fatal HF may occur during or for months or years after therapy. Risk is greater in patients receiving a cumulative dose >140 mg/m². Patients with MS should not receive cumulative dose >140 mg/m².
- Monitor for symptoms of gout (↑ uric acid levels and joint pain and swelling). Encourage patient to drink ≥2 L/day of fluid. Allopurinol may be given to ↓ uric acid levels.
- **Multiple sclerosis:** Assess frequency of exacerbations of symptoms periodically during therapy.

Lab Test Considerations
- Verify negative pregnancy test before starting therapy.
- Monitor CBC with differential before and periodically during therapy. The nadir of leukopenia usually occurs within 10 days, and recovery usually occurs within 21 days.
- Monitor liver function (AST, ALT, LDH, bilirubin) and renal function (BUN, serum creatinine) before and periodically during therapy.
- May ↑ uric acid. Monitor periodically during therapy.

Implementation
- Do not confuse mitoxantrone with mitomycin or MTX Patch (lidocaine/menthol).
- Mitoxantrone should be administered under the supervision of a physician experienced in the use of cytotoxic chemotherapy agents.
- There are lifetime maximum doses for mitoxantrone. Check manufacturer's information and patient history before administering.
- Wear gloves, gown, and mask while handling medication. Discard equipment in designated containers.
- Avoid contact with skin. Use Luer-Lok tubing to prevent accidental leakage. If contact with skin occurs, immediately wash skin with soap and water.
- Clean all spills with an aqueous solution of calcium hypochlorite. Mix solution by adding 5.5 parts (per weight) of calcium hypochlorite to 13 parts water.

IV Administration
- V Mitoxantrone is a vesicant. If extravasation occurs, immediately stop infusion. Leave needle/cannula in place temporarily but do not flush the line. Gently aspirate extravasated solution; then remove needle/cannula. Elevate patient's extremity and apply dry cold compresses for 20 min 4 times day for 1–2 days. Initiate antidote (dexrazoxane or topical dimethyl sulfoxide) based on time frame of noting extravasation. *If extravasation is noted ≤6 hr of mitoxantrone infusion,* administer dexrazoxane 1000 mg/m² over 1–2 hr on Days 1 and 2 (max dose = 2000 mg/day), followed by 500 mg/m² over 1–2 hr on Day 3 (max dose = 1000 mg/day). Hold cold compresses 15 min before initiating and after completing dexrazoxane infusion. Concurrent treatment with topical dimethyl sulfoxide should not be used with dexrazoxane because it may ↓ dexrazoxane's effectiveness. *If extravasation is noted >6 hr after completion of mitoxantrone infusion,* apply dimethyl sulfoxide by saturating a gauze pad and painting on an area twice the size of the extravasation. Allow site to air-dry and repeat application every 8 hr for 7 days. Do not cover the area with dressing.

M

- **IV Push:** **Dilution:** Dilute dark blue mitoxantrone solution in 50 mL of 0.9% NaCl or D5W. Discard unused solution. **Concentration:** 1–2 mg/mL. **Rate:** Administer slowly over >3 min into the tubing of a free-flowing IV of 0.9% NaCl or D5W.
- **Intermittent Infusion:** **Dilution:** Opened vials may be stored at room temperature for 7 days or under refrigeration for up to 14 days. May be further diluted in D5W, 0.9% NaCl, or D5/0.9%. Solutions diluted in D5W or 0.9% NaCl are stable for up to 7 days at room temperature or under refrigeration; manufacturer recommends immediate use. **Concentration:** 0.02–0.5 mg/mL. **Rate:** Administer over 15–30 min.
- **Continuous Infusion:** May also be administered over 24 hr.
- **Y-Site Compatibility:** acyclovir, alemtuzumab, allopurinol, amikacin, aminocaproic acid, aminophylline, amiodarone, anidulafungin, argatroban, arsenic trioxide, atracurium, bivalirudin, bleomycin, bumetanide, buprenorphine, butorphanol, calcium chloride, calcium gluconate, carboplatin, carmustine, caspofungin, cefotetan, chloramphenicol, chlorpromazine, ciprofloxacin, cisatracurium, cisplatin, cladribine, cyclophosphamide, cyclosporine, cytarabine, dacarbazine, dactinomycin, daptomycin, dexmedetomidine, dexrazoxane, diltiazem, diphenhydramine, dobutamine, docetaxel, dopamine, doxycycline, droperidol, enalaprilat, ephedrine, epinephrine, erythromycin, esmolol, etoposide, etoposide phosphate, famotidine, fentanyl, filgrastim, fluconazole, fludarabine, fluorouracil, ganciclovir, gemcitabine, gentamicin, glycopyrrolate, granisetron, haloperidol, hydralazine, hydrocortisone, hydromorphone, ifosfamide, imipenem/cilastatin, insulin regular, irinotecan, isoproterenol, ketorolac, labetalol, leucovorin, levofloxacin, lidocaine, linezolid, lorazepam, magnesium sulfate, mannitol, melphalan, meperidine, meropenem, mesna, methadone, methohexital, methotrexate, metoclopramide, metoprolol, metronidazole, midazolam, milrinone, minocycline, morphine, moxifloxacin, nalbuphine, naloxone, nicardipine, nitroglycerin, norepinephrine, octreotide, ondansetron, oxaliplatin, palonosetron, pamidronate, pentamidine, pentobarbital, phenobarbital, phentolamine, phenylephrine, potassium acetate, potassium chloride, procainamide, prochlorperazine, promethazine, propranolol, remifentanil, rituximab, rocuronium, sargramostim, sodium acetate, sodium bicarbonate, succinylcholine, sufentanil, tacrolimus, theophylline, thiotepa, tigecycline, tirofiban, tobramycin, topotecan, trastuzumab, trimethoprim/sulfamethoxazole, vancomycin, vasopressin, vecuronium, verapamil, vinblastine, vincristine, vinorelbine, zidovudine, zoledronic acid.
- **Y-Site Incompatibility:** amphotericin B deoxycholate, amphotericin B liposomal, ampicillin, ampicillin/sulbactam, azithromycin, aztreonam, cefazolin, cefepime, cefotaxime, cefoxitin, ceftazidime, ceftriaxone, cefuroxime, clindamycin, dantrolene, daunorubicin, dexamethasone, diazepam, digoxin, doxorubicin liposomal, ertapenem, foscarnet, fosphenytoin, furosemide, gemtuzumab ozogamicin, heparin, idarubicin, methylprednisolone, nafcillin, nitroprusside, paclitaxel, pantoprazole, pemetrexed, phenytoin, piperacillin/tazobactam, potassium phosphates, propofol, sodium phosphates, voriconazole.

Patient/Family Teaching

- Explain purpose and side effects of medication to patient. Advise patient to read *Patient Information* before starting therapy.
- Advise patient to notify health care provider of all Rx or OTC medications, vitamins, or herbal products being taken and to consult health care provider before taking other medications.
- Instruct patient to notify health care provider promptly if fever; chills; cough; hoarseness; sore throat; signs of infection; lower back or side pain; painful or difficult urination; bleeding gums; bruising; petechiae; blood in stools, urine, or emesis; ↑ fatigue; dyspnea; or orthostatic hypotension occurs. Caution patient to avoid crowds and persons with known infections. Instruct patient to use soft toothbrush and electric razor and to avoid falls. Caution patient not to drink alcoholic beverages or take medication containing aspirin or NSAIDs; may precipitate gastric bleeding.
- Instruct patient to notify health care provider if abdominal pain, yellow skin, cough, diarrhea, or ↓ urine output occurs.
- Inform patient that medication may cause the urine and sclera to turn blue-green.
- Instruct patient to inspect oral mucosa for redness and ulceration. If mouth sores occur, advise patient to use sponge brush and rinse mouth with water after eating and drinking. Topical agents may be used if pain interferes with eating. Stomatitis pain may require treatment with opioid analgesics.
- Discuss with patient the possibility of hair loss. Explore coping strategies.
- Instruct patient not to receive any vaccinations without advice of health care provider.
- Rep: May cause fetal harm. Refer patient to a facility with expertise in cancer during pregnancy. Advise patient that although mitoxantrone may cause infertility, contraception during therapy is necessary because of possible fetal harm. Discontinue breastfeeding before starting mitoxantrone.

Evaluation/Desired Outcomes

- Death of rapidly replicating cells, particularly malignant ones.

- Decreased pain in patients with advanced prostate cancer.
- Decreased disability and slowed progression of MS.

modafinil (mo-daf-i-nil)

Alertec, Provigil

Classification

Therapeutic: central nervous system stimulants

Schedule IV

Indications

Excessive daytime drowsiness due to narcolepsy, obstructive sleep apnea, or shift work sleep disorder.

Action

Produces CNS stimulation. **Therapeutic Effects:** Decreased daytime drowsiness in patients with narcolepsy and obstructive sleep apnea. Decreased drowsiness during work in patients with shift work sleep disorder.

Pharmacokinetics

Absorption: Rapidly absorbed; bioavailability unknown.

Distribution: Well distributed to tissues.

Metabolism and Excretion: Highly (90%) metabolized by the liver; <10% eliminated unchanged in the urine.

Half-life: 15 hr.

TIME/ACTION PROFILE (plasma concentrations)

ROUTE	ONSET	PEAK	DURATION
PO	rapid	2–4 hr	24 hr

Contraindications/Precautions

Contraindicated in: Hypersensitivity; History of left ventricular hypertrophy or ischemic ECG changes, chest pain, arrhythmia, or other significant manifestations of mitral valve prolapse in association with CNS stimulant use; OB: Pregnancy.

Use Cautiously in: History of MI or unstable angina; Severe hepatic impairment with or without cirrhosis (↓ dose); Lactation: Use while breastfeeding only if potential maternal benefit justifies potential risk to infant; Pedi: Safety and effectiveness not established in children; Geri: Lower doses may be necessary in older adults due to ↑ sensitivity to drug effects.

Adverse Reactions/Side Effects

CV: arrhythmias, chest pain, hypertension, hypotension, syncope. **Derm:** dry skin, rash, STEVENS-JOHNSON SYNDROME (SJS). **EENT:** rhinitis, abnormal vision, amblyopia, epistaxis, pharyngitis. **Endo:** hyperglycemia. **F and E** ↑ thirst. **GI:** ↑ liver enzymes, nausea, anorexia, diarrhea, gingivitis, mouth ulcers, vomiting. **GU:** abnormal ejaculation, albuminuria, urinary retention. **Hemat:** eosinophilia. **MS:** joint disorder, neck pain. **Neuro:** headache, aggression, amnesia, anxiety, ataxia, cataplexy, confusion, delusions, depression, dizziness, dyskinesia, hallucinations, hypertonia, insomnia, mania, paresthesia, SEIZURES, SUICIDAL IDEATION, tremor. **Resp:** dyspnea. **Misc:** HYPERSENSITIVITY REACTIONS (INCLUDING ANAPHYLAXIS AND ANGIOEDEMA), infection.

Interactions

Drug-Drug: May ↑ levels and risk of toxicity of **diazepam**, **phenytoin**, **propranolol**, and **tricyclic antidepressants**; dosage adjustments may be necessary. May ↓ levels and effectiveness of **hormonal contraceptives**, **cyclosporine**, and **theophylline**; dosage adjustments or additional methods of contraception may be necessary.

Drug-Natural Products: Cola nut, **guarana**, **mate**, **tea**, or **coffee** may ↑ stimulant effect.

Route/Dosage

PO (Adults): 200 mg once daily.

Hepatic Impairment

PO (Adults): *Severe hepatic impairment:* 100 mg once daily.

Availability (generic available)

Tablets: 100 mg, 200 mg.

NURSING IMPLICATIONS

Assessment

- Observe and document frequency of narcoleptic episodes.
- Assess BP and HR at baseline, then in 1–3 mo, and then every 6–12 mo thereafter.
- Obtain complete family and patient cardiovascular history to determine potential risk factors associated with sudden cardiac death; if indicated, consult cardiologist.
- Monitor closely for changes in behavior that could indicate the emergence or worsening of suicidal thoughts or behavior or depression.
- Assess for rash or signs/symptoms of SJS periodically during therapy (fever, general malaise, fatigue, muscle or joint aches, blisters, oral lesions, conjunctivitis). Discontinue therapy at the 1st signs of rash, unless clearly not drug-related.
- Monitor for signs/symptoms of hypersensitivity reactions (rash, urticaria, pruritus, flushing, dizziness, vomiting, abdominal pain) and angioedema (swelling

M

of throat, lips, tongue, or face; dyspnea; wheezing; hoarseness). *If signs/symptom of hypersensitivity reaction occur,* discontinue modafinil immediately and provide supportive care.

Lab Test Considerations

- May ↑ liver enzymes.

Implementation

- **PO:** Administer as a single dose in the morning for patients with narcolepsy or obstructive sleep apnea. Administer 1 hr before the start of work shift for patients with shift work sleep disorder.

Patient/Family Teaching

- Explain the purpose and side effects. Instruct patient to take medication as directed. Advise patient to read the *Medication Guide* prior to starting therapy and with each Rx refill, in case of changes.
- Medication may impair judgment. Advise patient to use caution when driving or during other activities requiring alertness.
- Advise patient that modafinil is a drug with known abuse potential. Advise patient that sharing this medication with others, even those with the same symptoms, is dangerous and illegal. Protect it from theft; store out of sight and reach of children and in a location not accessible by others.
- Encourage patient and family to be alert for emergence of anxiety, agitation, panic attacks, insomnia, irritability, hostility, impulsivity, akathisia, hypomania, mania, worsening of depression, and suicidal ideation, especially during early antidepressant therapy. Assess symptoms on a day-to-day basis as changes may be abrupt. If these symptoms occur, notify health care provider.
- Advise patient to notify health care provider immediately if rash or symptoms of anaphylaxis occur.
- Advise patient to notify health care provider of all Rx or OTC medications, vitamins, or herbal products being taken and to consult with health care provider before taking other medications. If alcohol is used during therapy, intake should be limited to moderate amounts.
- Rep: Advise women of reproductive potential to use effective nonhormonal methods of contraception during and for 1 mo following discontinuation of therapy. Instruct patient to notify health care provider promptly if pregnancy is planned or suspected or if breastfeeding. Encourage women who become pregnant to enroll in the registry that collects information about the safety of modafinil during pregnancy by calling 1-866-404-4106.

Evaluation/Desired Outcomes

- Decrease in narcoleptic symptoms and an enhanced ability to stay awake.

moexipril, **See ANGIOTENSIN-CONVERTING ENZYME (ACE) INHIBITORS.**

molnupiravir

(mol-noo-**peer**-a-veer)

Lagevrio

Classification

Therapeutic: antivirals

Pharmacologic: nucleoside analogues

Indications

Mild to moderate COVID-19 infection in nonhospitalized patients with positive results of direct SARS-CoV-2 viral testing, who are at high risk for progression to severe COVID-19, including hospitalization or death, and for whom alternative COVID-19 treatment options authorized by FDA are not accessible or clinically appropriate. An Emergency Use Authorization (EUA) has been issued for this use of molnupiravir; this drug is not FDA-approved for the above indication.

Action

As a prodrug, molnupiravir is metabolized to the active cytidine nucleoside analogue, NHC, which distributes into cells, where NHC is phosphorylated to the active ribonucleoside triphosphate (NHC-TP). NHC-TP is incorporated as NHC-monophosphate into SARS-CoV-2 RNA by the viral RNA polymerase, which results in inhibition of viral RNA replication. **Therapeutic Effects:** Reduction in hospitalization or mortality.

Pharmacokinetics

Absorption: Well absorbed.

Distribution: Widely distributed to extravascular tissues.

Metabolism and Excretion: Molnupiravir is a prodrug that is metabolized intracellularly to the active metabolite, NHC-TP. 3% excreted in urine.

Half-life: 3.3 hr.

TIME/ACTION PROFILE (plasma concentrations)

ROUTE	ONSET	PEAK	DURATION
PO	unknown	1.5 hr	12 hr

Contraindications/Precautions

Contraindicated in: Pedi: Children <18 yr (may affect bone and cartilage growth); Lactation: Lactation.

Use Cautiously in: Rep: Women and men of reproductive potential; OB: Use during pregnancy only if the potential maternal benefit outweighs potential fetal risk (has caused fetal harm in animal studies).

Adverse Reactions/Side Effects

GI: diarrhea, nausea. **Neuro:** dizziness.

Interactions

Drug-Drug: None reported.

Route/Dosage

PO (Adults): 800 mg every 12 hr for 5 days. Should be started as soon as possible after diagnosis of COVID-19 and within 5 days of symptom onset.

Availability

Capsules: 200 mg.

NURSING IMPLICATIONS

Assessment

- Assess COVID-19 symptoms (fever or chills, cough, dyspnea, wheezing, fatigue, muscle or body aches, headache, new loss of taste or smell, sore throat, congestion or runny nose, nausea or vomiting, diarrhea) during therapy.

Lab Test Considerations

- Verify negative pregnancy test before starting therapy.

Implementation

- **PO:** Administer twice daily without regard to food for 5 days. ***DNC:*** Do not open, break, or crush capsules. Start as soon as possible after COVID-19 diagnosis and within 5 days of symptom onset.
- **Administration via nasogastric (NG) or orogastric (OG) tube (≥12F):** Open four capsules and transfer contents into a clean container with a lid. Add 40 mL of water to container. Put lid on container and shake to mix the capsule contents and water thoroughly for 3 min. Capsule contents may not dissolve completely; prepared mixture may have visible undissolved particulates and are acceptable for administration. Flush NG/OG tube with 5 mL of water before administration. Using a catheter tip syringe, draw up entire contents from container and administer immediately through the NG/OG tube. Do not keep mixture for future use. If any portion of capsule contents are left in container, add 10 mL of water to container, mix, and using the same syringe draw up entire contents of the container and administer through the NG/OG. Repeat as needed until no capsule contents are left in container or syringe. Flush NG/OG tube with 5 mL of water twice (10 mL total) after administration of mixture.
- If patient requires hospitalization after starting therapy, patient may complete the full 5-day course per the health care provider's discretion.

Patient/Family Teaching

- Explain the purpose and side effects of the medication to the patient. Instruct patient to take as directed for full course of therapy. If dose is missed within 10 hr of usual time, take it as soon as possible and resume normal dosing schedule. If dose is missed by >10 hr, omit dose and take next dose at the regularly scheduled time. Do not double dose to make up for a missed dose. Advise patient to read *Patient Information* before starting therapy.
- Advise patient to discontinue therapy and notify health care provider promptly at first sign of hypersensitivity reaction (skin rash; hives or other skin reactions; rapid heartbeat; difficulty swallowing or breathing; swelling of the lips, tongue, or face; tightness of the throat; hoarseness).
- Advise patient to continue isolation in accordance with public health recommendations to maximize viral clearance and minimize transmission of SARS-CoV-2.
- Rep: May cause fetal harm. Advise women of reproductive potential to use effective contraception during therapy and avoid breastfeeding during therapy and for 4 days after last dose. Advise men with female partners of reproductive potential to use effective contraception during therapy and for 3 mo after last dose. If patient decides to take molnupiravir during pregnancy, prescribing health care provider must document that the known and potential benefits and risks of using molnupiravir during pregnancy were communicated to the pregnant individual. Encourage patient to enroll in pregnancy registry that monitors outcomes by visiting https://covid-pr.pregistry.com or calling 1-800-616-3791.

Evaluation/Desired Outcomes

- Reduction in hospitalization or mortality.

M

mometasone, See CORTICOSTEROIDS (INHALATION).

mometasone, See CORTICOSTEROIDS (NASAL).

mometasone, See CORTICOSTEROIDS (TOPICAL).

montelukast (mon-te-**loo**-kast)

Singulair

Classification

Therapeutic: allergy, cold, and cough remedies, bronchodilators

Pharmacologic: leukotriene antagonists

Indications

Prevention and chronic treatment of asthma. Seasonal or perennial allergic rhinitis (should only be used in patients with inadequate response or intolerance to other therapies). Prevention of exercise-induced bronchoconstriction.

Action

Antagonizes the effects of leukotrienes, which mediate the following: Airway edema, Smooth muscle constriction, Altered cellular activity. Result is decreased inflammatory process, which is part of asthma and allergic rhinitis. **Therapeutic Effects:** Decreased frequency and severity of acute asthma attacks. Decreased severity of allergic rhinitis. Decreased attacks of exercise-induced bronchoconstriction.

Pharmacokinetics

Absorption: Rapidly absorbed (63–73%) following oral administration.
Distribution: Minimally distributed to tissues.
Protein Binding: 99%.
Metabolism and Excretion: Mostly metabolized by the liver by the CYP3A4 and CYP2C9 isoenzymes; metabolites eliminated in feces via bile; negligible renal excretion.
Half-life: 2.7–5.5 hr.

TIME/ACTION PROFILE (improved symptoms of asthma)

ROUTE	ONSET	PEAK†	DURATION
PO (swallow)	within 24 hr	3–4 hr	24 hr
PO (chew)	within 24 hr	2–2.5 hr	24 hr

† Plasma concentrations.

Contraindications/Precautions

Contraindicated in: Hypersensitivity; Acute attacks of asthma.
Use Cautiously in: Phenylketonuria (chewable tablets contain aspartame); Hepatic impairment (may need to ↓ dose); Reduction of corticosteroid therapy (may ↑ risk of eosinophilic conditions); Pedi: Children <6 yr (exercise-induced bronchoconstriction), <2 yr (seasonal allergic rhinitis), <12 mo (asthma), <6 mo (perennial allergic rhinitis) (safety and effectiveness not established).

Adverse Reactions/Side Effects

Derm: rash, STEVENS-JOHNSON SYNDROME (SJS), TOXIC EPIDERMAL NECROLYSIS (TEN). **EENT:** epistaxis, otitis (children), rhinorrhea, sinusitis (children). **GI:** ↑ liver enzymes, abdominal pain, diarrhea (children), dyspepsia, nausea (children). **Neuro:** aggression, agitation, anxiety, attention disturbance, depression, disorientation, dream abnormalities, fatigue, hallucinations, headache, insomnia, irritability, memory impairment, obsessive-compulsive symptoms, restlessness, sleep walking, stuttering, SUICIDAL THOUGHTS/BEHAVIORS, tics, tremor, weakness. **Resp:** cough. **Misc:** EOSINOPHILIC CONDITIONS (INCLUDING CHURG-STRAUSS SYNDROME), fever.

Interactions

Drug-Drug: CYP3A4 inducers and **CYP2C9 inducers**, including **phenobarbital** and **rifampin**, may ↓ levels and effectiveness.

Route/Dosage

Asthma

PO (Adults and Children ≥15 yr): 10 mg once daily.
PO (Children 6–14 yr): *Chewable tablets:* 5 mg once daily.
PO (Children 2–5 yr): *Chewable tablets or granules:* 4 mg once daily.
PO (Children 12–23 mo): *Granules:* 4 mg once daily.

Exercise-Induced Bronchoconstriction

PO (Adults and Children ≥15 yr): 10 mg ≥2 hr before exercise. Do not take within 24 hr of another dose; if taking daily doses, do not take dose for exercise-induced bronchoconstriction.
PO (Children 6–14 yr): *Chewable tablets:* 5 mg ≥2 hr before exercise. Do not take within 24 hr of another dose; if taking daily doses, do not take dose for exercise-induced bronchoconstriction.

Allergic Rhinitis

PO (Adults and Children ≥15 yr): *Seasonal or perennial:* 10 mg once daily.
PO (Children 6–14 yr): *Seasonal or perennial:* 5 mg once daily (as chewable tablet).
PO (Children 2–5 yr): *Seasonal or perennial:* 4 mg once daily (as chewable tablet or granules).
PO (Children 6–23 mo): *Perennial only:* 4 mg once daily (as granules).

Availability (generic available)

Tablets: 10 mg. **Chewable tablets (cherry flavor):** 4 mg, 5 mg. **Oral granules:** 4 mg/pkt.

NURSING IMPLICATIONS

Assessment

- Assess lung sounds and respiratory function prior to and periodically during therapy.
- Assess allergy symptoms (rhinitis, conjunctivitis, hives) before and periodically during therapy.
- Monitor closely for changes in behavior or new neuropsychiatric symptoms that could indicate the emergence or worsening of depression or suicidal thoughts. If observed, discontinue use and contact health care provider immediately.

Lab Test Considerations

- May ↑ AST and ALT.

Implementation

- Doses of inhaled corticosteroids may be gradually ↓ with supervision of health care provider; do not discontinue abruptly.
- **PO:** For asthma, administer once daily in the evening. For allergic rhinitis, may be administered at any time of day.

- Administer granules directly into mouth; mix in a spoonful of cold or room-temperature foods (use only applesauce, mashed carrots, rice, or ice cream) or dissolved in 5 mL of cold or room-temperature baby formula or breast milk. Do not open packet until ready to use. After opening packet, administer full dose within 15 min. Do not store mixture. Discard unused portion. Do not dissolve granules in fluid, but fluid may be taken following administration. Granules may be administered without regard to meals.
- *For Exercise-Induced Bronchoconstriction:* Administer one tablet ≥2 hr before exercise; do not take within 24 hr of another dose.

Patient/Family Teaching

- Explain the purpose and side effects of the medication to the patient. Instruct patient to take medication as directed daily in the evening or ≥2 hr before exercise, even if not experiencing symptoms of asthma. If dose is missed, omit and take next dose at regularly scheduled time; do not double doses. Do not discontinue therapy without consulting health care provider. Advise patient to read *Patient Information* before starting therapy and with each Rx refill in case of changes.
- Instruct patient not to discontinue or ↓ dose of other asthma medications without consulting health care provider.
- Advise patient that montelukast is not used to treat acute asthma attacks but may be continued during an acute exacerbation. Patient should carry rapid-acting therapy for bronchospasm at all times. Advise patient to notify health care provider if more than the maximum number of short-acting bronchodilator treatments prescribed for a 24-hr period are needed.
- Advise patient to notify health care provider of all Rx or OTC medications, vitamins, or herbal products being taken and to consult health care provider before taking any new medications.
- Encourage patient and family to be alert for emergence of anxiety, agitation, panic attacks, insomnia, irritability, hostility, impulsivity, akathisia, hypomania, mania, worsening of depression, and suicidal ideation, especially during early antidepressant therapy. Assess symptoms on a day-to-day basis as changes may be abrupt. If these symptoms or rash occurs, notify health care provider.
- Rep: Advise women of reproductive potential to notify health care provider if pregnancy is planned or suspected or if breastfeeding.

Evaluation/Desired Outcomes

- Prevention of and reduction in symptoms of asthma.
- Decrease in severity of allergic rhinitis.
- Prevention of exercise-induced bronchoconstriction.

REMS HIGH ALERT

morphine (mor-feen)

~~AVINza,~~ ✱ Doloral, Duramorph, ~~Embeda~~, Infumorph, ✱ Kadian, ✱ M-Eslon, Mitigo, ~~Morphabond ER,~~ ✱ Morphine LP Epidural, MS Contin, ~~Roxanol~~

Classification

Therapeutic: opioid analgesics

Pharmacologic: opioid agonists

Schedule II

Indications

Severe pain (the 20 mg/mL oral solution concentration should only be used in opioid-tolerant patients). Pain severe enough to require daily, around-the-clock long-term opioid treatment and for which alternative treatment options are inadequate (extended release). Pulmonary edema. Pain associated with MI.

Action

Binds to opiate receptors in the CNS. Alters the perception of and response to painful stimuli while producing generalized CNS depression. **Therapeutic Effects:** Decrease in severity of pain.

Pharmacokinetics

Absorption: Variably absorbed (about 30%) following oral administration. More reliably absorbed from rectal, SUBQ, and IM sites. Following epidural administration, systemic absorption and absorption into the intrathecal space via the meninges occurs.

Distribution: Widely distributed to tissues.

Metabolism and Excretion: Mostly metabolized by the liver. Active metabolites excreted renally.

Half-life: *Premature neonates:* 10–20 hr; *Neonates:* 7.6 hr; *Infants 1–3 mo:* 6.2 hr; *Children 6 mo–2.5 yr:* 2.9 hr; *Children 3–6 yr:* 1–2 hr; *Children 6–19 yr with sickle cell disease:* 1.3 hr; *Adults:* 2–4 hr.

TIME/ACTION PROFILE (analgesia)

ROUTE	ONSET	PEAK	DURATION
PO	unknown	60 min	4–5 hr
PO-ER	unknown	3–4 hr	8–24 hr
IM	10–30 min	30–60 min	4–5 hr
SUBQ	20 min	50–90 min	4–5 hr
Rect	unknown	20–60 min	3–7 hr
IV	rapid	20 min	4–5 hr
Epidural	6–30 min	1 hr	up to 24 hr
IT	rapid (min)	unknown	up to 24 hr

M

Contraindications/Precautions

Contraindicated in: Hypersensitivity; Some products contain tartrazine, bisulfites, or alcohol and should be avoided in patients with known hypersensitivity; Acute, mild, intermittent, or postoperative pain (extended/sustained release); Significant respiratory depression (extended release); Acute or severe bronchial asthma (extended release); Paralytic ileus (extended release).

Use Cautiously in: Personal or family history of substance use disorder or mental illness; Head trauma; ↑ intracranial pressure; Severe renal impairment; Severe hepatic impairment; Severe pulmonary disease; Hypothyroidism; Seizure disorder; Adrenal insufficiency; Undiagnosed abdominal pain; Prostatic hyperplasia; Patients undergoing procedures that rapidly ↓ pain (cordotomy, radiation); long-acting agents should be discontinued 24 hr before and replaced with short-acting agents; OB: Use during pregnancy only if potential maternal benefit justifies potential fetal risk. Chronic maternal treatment with opioids during pregnancy may result in neonatal opioid withdrawal syndrome; Lactation: Use while breastfeeding only if potential maternal benefit justifies potential risk to infant; Pedi: Neonates and infants <3 mo (more susceptible to respiratory depression); Pedi: Neonates (oral solution contains sodium benzoate, which can cause potentially fatal gasping syndrome); Geri: ↑ risk of respiratory depression in older adults; dose ↓ suggested.

Adverse Reactions/Side Effects

CV: hypotension, bradycardia. **Derm:** flushing, itching, sweating. **EENT:** blurred vision, diplopia, miosis. **Endo:** adrenal insufficiency. **GI:** constipation, nausea, vomiting. **GU:** urinary retention. **Neuro:** confusion, sedation, dizziness, dysphoria, euphoria, floating feeling, hallucinations, headache, unusual dreams. **Resp:** RESPIRATORY DEPRESSION (INCLUDING CENTRAL SLEEP APNEA AND SLEEP-RELATED HYPOXEMIA). **Misc:** allodynia, opioid-induced hyperalgesia, physical dependence, psychological dependence, tolerance.

Interactions

Drug-Drug: Use with **extreme caution** in patients receiving **MAO inhibitors** within 14 days prior; may result in unpredictable, severe reactions; ↓ initial dose of morphine to 25% of usual dose. Use with **benzodiazepines** or other **CNS depressants**, including other **opioids**, **nonbenzodiazepine sedative/hypnotics**, **anxiolytics**, **general anesthetics**, **muscle relaxants**, **antipsychotics**, and **alcohol**, may cause profound sedation, respiratory depression, coma, and death; reserve concurrent use for when alternative treatment options are inadequate. Drugs that affect serotonergic neurotransmitter systems, including **tricyclic antidepressants**, **SSRIs**, **SNRIs**, **MAO inhibitors**, **TCAs**, **tramadol**, **trazodone**, **mirtazapine**, **5-HT$_3$ receptor antagonists**, **linezolid**, **methylene blue**, and **triptans**, may ↑ risk of serotonin syndrome. **Mixed agonist/antagonist analgesics**, including **nalbuphine** or **butorphanol**, and **partial agonist analgesics**, including **buprenorphine**, may ↓ morphine's analgesic effects and/or precipitate opioid withdrawal in physically dependent patients. May ↑ the anticoagulant effect of **warfarin**. **Cimetidine** may ↑ levels and risk of toxicity. IV morphine may ↓ levels and antiplatelet effects of **clopidogrel**, **prasugrel**, and **ticagrelor**; consider IV antiplatelet agent as alternative in patients with acute coronary syndrome if morphine concurrently used.

Drug-Natural Products: Kava-kava, **valerian**, or **chamomile** can ↑ risk of CNS depression.

Route/Dosage

Larger doses may be required during chronic therapy

PO, Rect (Adults ≥50 kg): *Usual starting dose for moderate to severe pain in opioid-naive patients:* 30 mg every 3–4 hr initially *or* once 24-hr opioid requirement is determined, convert to extended-release morphine by administering total daily oral morphine dose every 24 hr (as ER capsules), 50% of the total daily oral morphine dose every 12 hr (as *MS Contin*), or 33% of the total daily oral morphine dose every 8 hr (as *MS Contin*). See equianalgesic chart, Appendix I. Dose of ER capsules should not exceed 1600 mg/day because of fumaric acid in formulation.

PO, Rect (Adults and Children <50 kg): *Usual starting dose for moderate to severe pain in opioid-naive patients:* 0.3 mg/kg every 3–4 hr initially.

PO (Children >1 mo): *Prompt-release tablets and solution:* 0.2–0.5 mg/kg every 4–6 hr as needed. *Controlled-release tablet:* 0.3–0.6 mg/kg every 12 hr.

IM, IV, SUBQ (Adults ≥50 kg): *Usual starting dose for moderate to severe pain in opioid-naive patients:* 4–10 mg every 3–4 hr. *MI:* 8–15 mg, for very severe pain additional smaller doses may be given every 3–4 hr.

IM, IV, SUBQ (Adults and Children <50 kg): *Usual starting dose for moderate to severe pain in opioid-naive patients:* 0.05–0.2 mg/kg every 3–4 hr; maximum: 15 mg/dose.

IM, IV, SUBQ (Neonates): 0.05 mg/kg every 4–8 hr, maximum dose: 0.1 mg/kg. Use preservative-free formulation.

IV, SUBQ (Adults): *Continuous infusion:* 0.8–10 mg/hr; may be preceded by a bolus of 15 mg (infusion rates vary greatly; up to 80 mg/hr have been used).

IV, SUBQ (Children >1 mo): *Continuous infusion, postoperative pain:* 0.01–0.04 mg/kg/hr. *Continuous infusion, sickle cell or cancer pain:* 0.02–2.6 mg/kg/hr.

IV (Neonates): *Continuous infusion:* 0.01–0.03 mg/kg/hr.
Epidural (Adults): *Intermittent injection:* 5 mg/day (initially); if relief is not obtained at 60 min, 1–2 mg increments may be made (total dose not to exceed 10 mg/day). *Continuous infusion:* 2–4 mg/24 hr; may ↑ by 1–2 mg/day (up to 30 mg/day).
Epidural (Children >1 mo): 0.03–0.05 mg/kg, maximum dose: 0.1 mg/kg or 5 mg/24 hr. Use preservative-free formulation.
IT (Adults): 0.2–1 mg. Use preservative-free formulation.

Availability (generic available)

Immediate-release tablets: 15 mg, 30 mg. **Extended-release tablets (MS Contin):** 15 mg, 30 mg, 60 mg, 100 mg, 200 mg. **Extended-release capsules:** 10 mg, 20 mg, 30 mg, 45 mg, 50 mg, 60 mg, 75 mg, 80 mg, 90 mg, 100 mg, 120 mg. **Oral solution:** 🍁 1 mg/mL, 10 mg/5 mL, 20 mg/5 mL🍁 5 mg/mL, 100 mg/5 mL. **Rectal suppositories:** 5 mg, 10 mg, 20 mg, 30 mg. **Solution for epidural, IV injection (preservative-free):** 0.5 mg/mL, 1 mg/mL. **Solution for epidural or IT use (continuous microinfusion device; preservative-free):** 10 mg/mL, 25 mg/mL. **Solution for IM, SUBQ, IV injection:** 1 mg/mL, 2 mg/mL, 4 mg/mL, 5 mg/mL, 8 mg/mL, 10 mg/mL, 25 mg/mL, 50 mg/mL. **Solution for IV injection (PCA device):** 1 mg/mL, 2 mg/mL, 3 mg/mL, 5 mg/mL.

NURSING IMPLICATIONS

Assessment

- Assess type, location, and intensity of pain prior to and 1 hr following PO, SUBQ, and IM and 20 min (peak) following IV administration. When titrating opioid doses, ↑ of 25–50% should be administered until there is either a 50% ↓ in the patient's pain rating on a numerical or visual analogue scale or the patient reports satisfactory pain relief. When titrating doses of short-acting morphine, a repeat dose can be safely administered at the time of the peak if previous dose is ineffective and side effects are minimal.
- Assess BP, HR, and respiratory rate before and periodically during administration. If respiratory rate <10/min, assess level of sedation. Dose may need to be ↓ by 25–50%. Respiratory depression does not ↑ in severity, only in duration, with ↑ dose. Monitor for respiratory depression, especially during initiation or following dose ↑; serious, life-threatening, or fatal respiratory depression may occur. May cause sleep-related breathing disorders (central sleep apnea, sleep-related hypoxemia).
- Patients on a continuous infusion should have additional bolus doses provided every 15–30 min as needed for breakthrough pain. The bolus dose is usually set to the amount of drug infused each hr by continuous infusion.
- Patients taking extended-release morphine may require additional short-acting opioid doses for breakthrough pain. Doses of short-acting opioids should be equivalent to 10–20% of 24 hr total and given every 2 hr as needed.
- An equianalgesic chart (see Appendix I) should be used when changing routes or when changing from one opioid to another.
- Geri: Assess older adults frequently, as they may be more sensitive to the effects of opioid analgesics and may experience side effects and respiratory complications more frequently.
- Pedi: Assess pediatric patients frequently; children are more sensitive to the effects of opioid analgesics and may experience respiratory complications, excitability, and restlessness more frequently.
- Prolonged use may lead to physical and psychological dependence and tolerance. This should not prevent patient from receiving adequate analgesia. Patients who receive morphine for pain rarely develop psychological dependence. Progressively higher doses may be required to relieve pain with long-term therapy; may ↑ risk of overdose. Prolonged use of opioids should be reserved for patients whose pain remains severe enough to require them and when alternative treatment options continue to be inadequate. Many acute pain conditions treated in the outpatient setting require no more than a few days of an opioid pain medicine.
- Assess bowel function routinely. Institute prevention of constipation with ↑ intake of fluids and bulk and with laxatives to minimize constipating effects. Administer stimulant laxatives routinely if opioid use exceeds 2–3 days, unless contraindicated. Consider drugs for opioid-induced constipation.
- Assess risk for opioid addiction, abuse, or misuse prior to administration. Abuse or misuse of extended-release preparations by crushing, chewing, snorting, or injecting dissolved product will result in uncontrolled delivery of morphine and can result in overdose and death.
- Assess for opioid-induced hyperalgesia, which can appear as ↑ levels of pain on increasing the dose of the opioid, ↓ levels of pain on decreasing the dose of the opioid, or pain from ordinarily nonpainful stimuli (allodynia). This condition is different from tolerance. If a patient is suspected

M

to be experiencing opioid-induced hyperalgesia, consider ↓ the dose of the current opioid or switching to a different opioid analgesic.

Lab Test Considerations

- May ↑ amylase and lipase.

Toxicity and Overdose

- If an opioid antagonist is required to reverse respiratory depression or coma, naloxone is the antidote. Dilute the 0.4-mg ampule of naloxone in 10 mL of 0.9% NaCl and administer 0.5 mL (0.02 mg) by IV push every 2 min. For children and adults weighing <40 kg, dilute 0.1 mg of naloxone in 10 mL of 0.9% NaCl for a concentration of 10 mcg/mL and administer 0.5 mcg/kg every 2 min. Titrate dose to avoid withdrawal, seizures, and severe pain.

Implementation

- ***High Alert:*** Do not confuse MS Contin with Oxycontin. Do not confuse morphine with hydromorphone. Do not confuse morphine (nonconcentrated oral liquid) with morphine (concentrated oral liquid).
- Use only preservative-free formulations for neonates and for epidural and intrathecal routes in all patients.
- Explain therapeutic value of medication prior to administration to enhance the analgesic effect.
- Regularly administered doses may be more effective than as needed administration. Analgesic is more effective if given before pain becomes severe.
- Coadministration with nonopioid analgesics may have additive analgesic effects and may permit lower doses.
- When transferring from other opioids or other forms of morphine to extended-release tablets, administer a total daily dose of oral morphine equivalent to previous daily dose (see Appendix I) and divided every 8 hr (MS Contin), every 12 hr (MS Contin), or every 24 hr.
- Morphine should be discontinued gradually to prevent withdrawal symptoms after long-term use. For patients on long-acting agents who are physically opioid-dependent, initiate the taper by a small enough increment (no greater than 10–25% of total daily dose) to avoid withdrawal symptoms, and proceed with dose-lowering at an interval of every 2–4 wk. Patients who have been taking opioids for briefer periods of time may tolerate a more rapid taper. Monitor frequently to manage pain and withdrawal symptoms (restlessness; lacrimation; rhinorrhea; yawning; perspiration; chills; myalgia; mydriasis; irritability; anxiety; backache; joint pain; weakness; abdominal cramps; insomnia; nausea; anorexia; vomiting; diarrhea; or ↑ BP, respiratory rate, or HR). If withdrawal symptoms occur, pause the taper for a period of time or ↑ the dose of opioid analgesic to the previous dose, and then proceed with a slower taper. Also, monitor patients for changes in mood, emergence of suicidal thoughts, or use of other substances. A multimodal approach to pain management may optimize the treatment of chronic pain and assist with the successful tapering of the opioid analgesic.
- **PO:** Doses may be administered with food or milk to minimize GI irritation.
- Administer oral solution with properly calibrated measuring device; may be diluted in a glass of fruit juice just prior to administration to improve taste. Verify correct dose (mg) and correct volume (mL) prior to administration. Use an oral syringe when using 20 mg/mL concentration of oral solution.
- ***DNC:*** Swallow extended-release tablets whole; do not break, crush, dissolve, or chew (could result in rapid release and absorption of a potentially toxic dose).
- Extended-release capsules may be opened and the pellets sprinkled onto applesauce immediately prior to administration. Patients should rinse mouth and swallow to assure ingestion of entire dose. ***DNC:*** Pellets should not be chewed, crushed, or dissolved. Capsules may also be opened and sprinkled on approximately 10 mL of water and flushed while swirling through a prewetted 16 French gastrostomy tube fitted with a funnel at the port end. Additional water should be used to transfer and flush any remaining pellets. Do not administer extended-release capsules via a nasogastric tube.
- **Rect:** *MS Contin* has been administered rectally.
- **IM, SUBQ:** IM is the preferred route for repeated doses. SUBQ administration may cause tissue irritation.
- Pedi: Avoid IM administration in children. Fear of pain from IM injection may lead to inadequate pain control.
- ***REMS:*** FDA strongly encourages health care providers to complete a REMS-compliant education program that includes all the elements of the FDA Education *Blueprint for Health Care Providers Involved in the Management or Support of Patients with Pain,* available at www.fda.gov/OpioidAnalgesicREMSBlueprint. Information on programs can be found at 1-800-503-0784 or www.opioidanalgesicrems.com.
- Discuss availability of naloxone for emergency treatment of opioid overdose with the patient and caregiver and assess the potential need for access to naloxone, both when initiating and renewing therapy, especially if patient has household members (including children) or other close contacts at risk for accidental exposure or

overdose. Consider prescribing naloxone, based on the patient's risk factors for overdose, such as concurrent use of CNS depressants, a history of opioid use disorder, or prior opioid overdose. However, the presence of risk factors for overdose should not prevent the proper management of pain in any patient.

IV Administration

- **IV:** Solution is colorless; do not administer discolored solution.
- **IV Push: Dilution:** Do not dilute prior to injection. **Rate:** ***High Alert:*** Administer slowly at 2.5–15 mg over 5 min. Rapid administration may lead to ↑ respiratory depression, hypotension, and circulatory collapse.
- **Continuous Infusion: Dilution:** May be added to D5W, D10W, 0.9% NaCl, 0.45% NaCl, LR, dextrose/saline solution, or dextrose/LR. **Concentration:** 0.1–1 mg/mL or greater for continuous infusion. **Rate:** Administer via infusion pump to control the rate. Dose should be titrated to ensure adequate pain relief without excessive sedation, respiratory depression, or hypotension. May be administered via patient-controlled analgesia pump.
- **Y-Site Compatibility:** acetaminophen, aldesleukin, allopurinol, amikacin, aminocaproic acid, aminophylline, amiodarone, anidulafungin, argatroban, arsenic trioxide, ascorbic acid, atropine, aztreonam, benztropine, bivalirudin, bleomycin, bumetanide, buprenorphine, butorphanol, caffeine citrate, calcium chloride, calcium gluconate, cangrelor, carboplatin, carmustine, caspofungin, cefazolin, cefotaxime, cefotetan, cefoxitin, ceftaroline, ceftazidime, ceftolozane/tazobactam, ceftriaxone, cefuroxime, chloramphenicol, chlorpromazine, cisatracurium, cladribine, clindamycin, cyanocobalamin, cyclophosphamide, cyclosporine, cytarabine, dacarbazine, dactinomycin, daptomycin, daunorubicin, dexamethasone, dexmedetomidine, dexrazoxane, digoxin, diltiazem, diphenhydramine, dobutamine, docetaxel, dopamine, doxorubicin hydrochloride, doxycycline, enalaprilat, ephedrine, epinephrine, epirubicin, epoetin alfa, eptifibatide, eravacycline, ertapenem, erythromycin, esmolol, etomidate, etoposide, etoposide phosphate, famotidine, fentanyl, filgrastim, fluconazole, fludarabine, fluorouracil, foscarnet, fosphenytoin, gemcitabine, gentamicin, glycopyrrolate, granisetron, heparin, hetastarch, hydrocortisone, hydromorphone, idarubicin, ifosfamide, imipenem/cilastatin, imipenem/cilastatin/relebactam, irinotecan, isavuconazonium, isoproterenol, ketorolac, labetalol, LR, letermovir, leucovorin, lidocaine, linezolid, lorazepam, magnesium sulfate, mannitol, melphalan, meperidine, meropenem, meropenem/vaborbactam, mesna, methotrexate, methylprednisolone, metoclopramide, metoprolol, metronidazole, midazolam, milrinone, mitoxantrone, multivitamins, mycophenolate, nafcillin, nalbuphine, naloxone, nicardipine, nitroglycerin, nitroprusside, norepinephrine, octreotide, ondansetron, oritavancin, oxacillin, oxaliplatin, oxytocin, paclitaxel, palonosetron, pamidronate, papaverine, pemetrexed, penicillin G, phenobarbital, phentolamine, phenylephrine, phytonadione, piperacillin/tazobactam, plazomicin, posaconazole, potassium acetate, potassium chloride, procainamide, prochlorperazine, promethazine, propranolol, protamine, pyridoxine, remifentanil, rituximab, rocuronium, sildenafil, sodium acetate, sodium bicarbonate, succinylcholine, sufentanil, tacrolimus, tedizolid, theophylline, thiamine, thiotepa, tigecycline, tirofiban, tobramycin, topotecan, vancomycin, vasopressin, vecuronium, verapamil, vinblastine, vincristine, vinorelbine, voriconazole, zidovudine, zoledronic acid.
- **Y-Site Incompatibility:** alemtuzumab, amphotericin B deoxycholate, amphotericin B liposomal, azathioprine, ceftobiprole, dantrolene, diazoxide, doxorubicin liposomal, folic acid, ganciclovir, gemtuzumab ozogamicin, indomethacin, micafungin, mitomycin, pentamidine, pentobarbital, phenytoin, sargramostim, trastuzumab.
- **Epidural:** Administer undiluted. Do not use an in-line filter. Do not admix or administer other medications in epidural space for 48 hr after administration. Administer within 4 hr after removing from vial. Store in refrigerator; do not freeze.

Patient/Family Teaching

- Explain purpose and side effects of morphine to patient. Instruct them to take medication as directed. Advise patient to read *Patient Information*before starting and with each Rx refill in case of changes.
- ***REMS:*** Instruct patient how and when to ask for pain medication. Do not stop taking without discussing with health care provider; may cause withdrawal symptoms if discontinued abruptly after prolonged use. Do not ↑ doses without discussing with health care provider; may lead to overdose. Discuss safe use, risks, and proper storage and disposal of opioid analgesics with patients and caregivers with each Rx. The Patient Counseling Guide is available at www.fda.gov/OpioidAnalgesicREMSPCG.

M

- Medication may cause drowsiness or dizziness. Advise patient to call for assistance when ambulating and to avoid driving or other activities that require alertness until response to the medication is known.
- Advise patient that morphine is a drug with known abuse potential. Protect it from theft, and never give to anyone other than the individual for whom it was prescribed. Store out of sight and reach of children, and in a location not accessible by others.
- Educate patients and caregivers on how to recognize respiratory depression and emphasize the importance of calling 911 or getting emergency medical help right away in the event of a known or suspected overdose. Inform patients and caregivers about various ways to obtain naloxone as permitted by individual state naloxone dispensing and prescribing requirements or guidelines (Rx, direct from pharmacist, or state programs). OTC naloxone nasal spray is available at pharmacies nationwide for overdose or accidental ingestion.
- Advise patient to notify health care provider if pain control is not adequate or if severe or persistent side effects occur.
- Advise patient to change positions slowly to minimize orthostatic hypotension.
- Instruct patient to notify health care provider of all Rx or OTC medications, vitamins, or herbal products being taken and consult health care provider before taking any new medications.
- Emphasize the importance of aggressive prevention of constipation with the use of morphine.
- Caution patient to avoid concurrent use of alcohol or other CNS depressants with this medication.
- Encourage patients who are immobilized or on prolonged bedrest to turn, cough, and breathe deeply every 2 hr to prevent atelectasis.
- Advise patient that good oral hygiene, frequent mouth rinses, and sugarless gum or candy may decrease dry mouth.
- Rep: Advise patient to notify health care provider if pregnancy is planned or suspected or if breastfeeding. Inform patient of potential for neonatal opioid withdrawal syndrome with prolonged use during pregnancy. Monitor neonate for signs and symptoms of withdrawal (irritability, hyperactivity and abnormal sleep pattern, high-pitched cry, tremor, vomiting, diarrhea, failure to gain weight); these usually occur the first days after birth. Monitor infants exposed to morphine through breast milk for excess sedation and respiratory depression. Chronic use may ↓ fertility in women and men.
- **Home Care Issues:** ***High Alert:*** Explain to patient and family how and when to administer morphine and how to care for infusion equipment properly. Pedi: Teach parents or caregivers how to accurately measure liquid medication and to use only the measuring device dispensed with the medication.

Evaluation/Desired Outcomes

- Decrease in severity of pain without a significant alteration in level of consciousness or respiratory status.
- Decrease in symptoms of pulmonary edema.

moxifloxacin, See FLUOROQUINOLONES.

mupirocin (myoo-**peer**-oh-sin)

~~Bactroban~~

Classification

Therapeutic: anti-infectives

Indications

Impetigo. Secondarily infected traumatic skin lesions (up to 10 cm in length or 100 cm^2 area).

Action

Inhibits bacterial protein synthesis. **Therapeutic Effects:** Inhibition of bacterial growth and reproduction. **Spectrum:** Greatest activity against gram-positive organisms, including: *Staphylococcus aureus*, *Streptococcus pyogenes*.

Pharmacokinetics

Absorption: Minimal systemic absorption.
Distribution: Remains in the stratum corneum after topical use for prolonged periods of time (72 hr).
Metabolism and Excretion: Metabolized in the skin; removed by desquamation.
Half-life: 17–36 min.

TIME/ACTION PROFILE (anti-infective effect)

ROUTE	ONSET	PEAK	DURATION
Topical†	unknown	3–5 days	72 hr

† Resolution of lesions.

Contraindications/Precautions

Contraindicated in: Hypersensitivity to mupirocin or polyethylene glycol.
Use Cautiously in: Renal impairment; Burn patients.

Adverse Reactions/Side Effects

Derm: burning, itching, pain, stinging.

Interactions

Drug-Drug: None reported.

Route/Dosage

Topical: (Adults and Children ≥2 mo): *Ointment:* Apply 3–5 times daily for 5–14 days.

Topical: (Adults and Children ≥3 mo): *Cream:* Apply small amount 3 times/day for 10 days.

Availability (generic available)
Cream: 2%. **Ointment:** 2%.

NURSING IMPLICATIONS
Assessment
- Assess lesions before and daily during therapy for efficacy.
- Monitor for signs and symptoms of hypersensitivity reaction, including anaphylaxis, urticaria, angioedema, generalized rash, or local irritation. *If severe hypersensitivity reaction occurs,* discontinue therapy, treat as clinically indicated, and institute alternative therapy for infection.
- Monitor for microbial overgrowth of nonsusceptible microorganisms, including fungi.

Implementation
- **Topical:** Wash affected area with soap and water and dry thoroughly. Apply a small amount of mupirocin using a cotton swab or gauze to affected area 3 times daily and rub in gently. Treated area may be covered with gauze if desired. Do not apply to mucosa or concurrently with other lotions, creams, or ointments.

Patient/Family Teaching
- Explain purpose and side effects of medication. Advise patient to read *Patient Information* before starting therapy.
- Instruct patient on correct application procedure, as well as appropriate hygienic measures to prevent spread of impetigo. If a dose is missed, apply as soon as possible unless almost time for next dose. Avoid contact with eyes.
- Advise patient to notify health care provider of all Rx, OTC or topical medications, vitamins, or herbal products being taken and to consult health care provider before taking other medications.
- Advise patient to immediately notify health care provider if swelling of lips, face, or tongue or wheezing occurs.
- Advise patient to stop mupirocin and notify health care provider if local reaction (irritation, severe itching, rash) occurs.
- Rep: Advise women of reproductive potential to notify health care provider if pregnancy is planned or suspected or if breastfeeding. To minimize oral exposure to child, a breast treated with mupirocin should be thoroughly washed prior to breastfeeding.

Evaluation/Desired Outcomes
- Healing of skin lesions. If no clinical response is seen in 3–5 days, condition should be re-evaluated.

REMS

mycophenolate mofetil
(mye-koe-**fee**-noe-late **moe**-fe-til)
CellCept, Myhibbin

mycophenolic acid
(mye-koe-**fee**-noe-lik)
Myfortic

Classification
Therapeutic: immunosuppressants

Indications
Mycophenolate mofetil: Prevention of rejection in allogeneic kidney, liver, and heart transplantation (used concurrently with cyclosporine and corticosteroids). **Mycophenolic acid:** Prevention of rejection in allogeneic renal transplantation (used concurrently with cyclosporine and corticosteroids).

Action
Inhibits the enzyme inosine monophosphate dehydrogenase, which is involved in purine synthesis. This inhibition results in suppression of T- and B-lymphocyte proliferation. **Therapeutic Effects:** Prevention of heart, kidney, or liver transplant rejection.

Pharmacokinetics
Absorption: Following oral and IV administration, mycophenolate mofetil is rapidly hydrolyzed to mycophenolic acid (MPA), the active metabolite. Absorption of enteric-coated mycophenolic acid (Myfortic) is delayed compared with mycophenolate mofetil (CellCept).
Distribution: Widely distributed to tissues.
Protein Binding: *MPA:* 97%.
Metabolism and Excretion: MPA is extensively metabolized; <1% excreted unchanged in urine. Some enterohepatic recirculation of MPA occurs.
Half-life: *MPA:* 8–18 hr.

TIME/ACTION PROFILE (MPA plasma concentrations)

ROUTE	ONSET	PEAK	DURATION
mycophenolate mofetil-PO	rapid	0.25–1.25 hr	N/A
mycophenolic acid	rapid	1.5–2.75 hr	N/A

Contraindications/Precautions
Contraindicated in: Hypersensitivity; Hypersensitivity to polysorbate 80 (for IV mycophenolate mofetil); OB: Pregnancy

M

Use Cautiously in: Active serious pathology of the GI tract (including history of ulcer disease or GI bleeding); Phenylketonuria (oral suspension contains aspartame); Severe chronic renal impairment (dose not to exceed 1 g twice daily [CellCept] if CCr <25 mL/min/1.73 m^2); careful monitoring recommended; Delayed graft function following transplantation (observe for ↑ toxicity); Lactation: Use while breastfeeding only if potential maternal benefit justifies potential risk to infant; Rep: Women of reproductive potential and men with female partners of reproductive potential; Pedi: Safety and effectiveness not established in children <3 mo (mycophenolate mofetil) or <5 yr (mycophenolic acid); Geri: ↑ risk of adverse reactions related to immunosuppression in older adults.

Adverse Reactions/Side Effects

CV: edema, hypertension, hypotension, tachycardia. **Derm:** rash. **Endo:** hyperglycemia. **F and E** hyperkalemia, hypocalcemia, hypokalemia, hypomagnesemia. **GI:** anorexia, constipation, diarrhea, nausea, vomiting, abdominal pain, GI BLEEDING. **GU:** renal impairment. **Hemat:** leukocytosis, leukopenia, thrombocytopenia, anemia, pure red cell aplasia. **Metab:** hypercholesterolemia. **Neuro:** anxiety, confusion, dizziness, headache, insomnia, paresthesia, sedation, tremor, PROGRESSIVE MULTIFOCAL LEUKOENCEPHALOPATHY (PML). **Resp:** cough, dyspnea. **Misc:** fever, INFECTION (INCLUDING ACTIVATION OF LATENT VIRAL INFECTIONS SUCH AS POLYOMAVIRUS-ASSOCIATED NEPHROPATHY OR HEPATITIS B/C), acute inflammatory syndrome, HYPERSENSITIVITY REACTIONS (INCLUDING ANAPHYLAXIS AND ANGIOEDEMA), MALIGNANCY.

Interactions

Drug-Drug: Combined use with **azathioprine** is not recommended (effects unknown). **Acyclovir** and **ganciclovir** compete with MPA for renal excretion and, in patients with renal impairment; may ↑ each other's toxicity. **Magnesium and aluminum hydroxide** antacids ↓ the absorption of MPA; avoid concurrent use. **Proton pump inhibitors**, including **dexlansoprazole**, **esomeprazole**, **lansoprazole**, **omeprazole**, **pantoprazole**, and **rabeprazole**, may ↓ levels and effectiveness. **Cholestyramine** and **colestipol** may ↓ absorption of MPA; avoid concurrent use. May ↓ effectiveness of **oral contraceptives**; additional contraceptive method should be used. May ↓ the antibody response to and ↑ risk of adverse reactions from **live-attenuated vaccines**. **Amoxicillin/clavulanic acid** or **ciprofloxacin** may ↓ MPA trough levels and effectiveness. **Cyclosporine** may ↓ levels and effectiveness; use caution when discontinuing cyclosporine (may ↑ mycophenolate levels) or when switching from cyclosporine to another immunosuppressant, such as tacrolimus or belatacept. **Telmisartan** may ↓ levels and effectiveness.

Route/Dosage

Mycophenolate Mofetil

Kidney Transplantation

PO, IV (Adults): 1 g twice daily; IV should be started ≤24 hr after transplantation and switched to PO as soon as possible (IV not recommended for ≥14 days).
PO (Children ≥3 mo): 600 mg/m^2 twice daily (not to exceed 2 g/day).

Liver Transplantation

PO, IV (Adults): 1 g twice daily IV, or 1.5 g twice daily PO. IV should be started ≤24 hr after transplantation and switched to PO as soon as possible (IV not recommended for ≥14 days).
PO (Children ≥3 mo): 600 mg/m^2 twice daily; if well tolerated, can ↑ to 900 mg/m^2 twice daily (not to exceed 3 g/day).

Heart Transplantation

PO, IV (Adults): 1.5 g twice daily; IV should be started ≤24 hr after transplantation and switched to PO as soon as possible (IV not recommended for ≥14 days).
PO (Children ≥3 mo): 600 mg/m^2 twice daily; if well tolerated, can ↑ to 900 mg/m^2 twice daily (not to exceed 3 g/day).

Renal Impairment

PO, IV (Adults): *CCr <25 mL/min:* Daily dose should not exceed 2 g.

Mycophenolic Acid

Mycophenolate mofetil and mycophenolic acid should not be used interchangeably without the advice of a health care provider.

Kidney Transplantation

PO (Adults): 720 mg twice daily.
PO (Children 5–16 yr and ≥1.19 m^2): 400–450 mg/m^2 twice daily (not to exceed 720 mg twice daily).

Availability (generic available)

Mycophenolate Mofetil

Tablets: 500 mg. **Capsules:** 250 mg. **Oral suspension (fruit flavor):** 200 mg/mL. **Powder for injection:** 500 mg/vial.

Mycophenolic Acid

Delayed-release tablets: 180 mg, 360 mg.

NURSING IMPLICATIONS

Assessment

- Assess for symptoms of organ rejection throughout therapy.
- Assess for signs/symptoms of infection, including PML (hemiparesis, apathy, confusion, cognitive deficiencies, ataxia), periodically during therapy. *If new infection or reactivated viral infection occurs,* consider dose ↓, weighing risk to functioning allograft.

- Monitor for signs/symptoms and laboratory parameters of acute inflammatory syndrome when starting treatment with mycophenolate products or when ↑ dose. Discontinue mycophenolate and consider treatment alternatives based on risks and benefits.
- Monitor for signs/symptoms of hypersensitivity reactions (rash, urticaria, pruritus, flushing, dizziness, vomiting, abdominal pain) and angioedema (swelling of throat, lips, tongue, or face; dyspnea; wheezing; hoarseness). Discontinue mycophenolate immediately and provide supportive care.

Lab Test Considerations

- Verify negative urine pregnancy test with a specificity of 25 mIU/mL immediately prior to beginning therapy and again 8–10 days later. Repeat pregnancy tests should be performed during routine follow-up visits.
- Monitor CBC with differential weekly for 1st mo, twice monthly for the 2nd and 3rd mo of therapy, and then monthly during the 1st yr. Neutropenia occurs most frequently 31–180 days post-transplant. *If ANC <1300 × 10 cells/mm³*, hold mycophenolate or ↓ dose and manage appropriately.
- Monitor hepatic and renal function and electrolytes periodically during therapy. May ↑ alkaline phosphatase, AST, ALT, LDH, BUN, and serum creatinine. May also cause hyperkalemia, hypokalemia, hypocalcemia, hypomagnesemia, hyperglycemia, and hyperlipidemia.

Implementation

- The initial dose of mycophenolate should be given within 24 hr of transplant.
- Mycophenolate mofetil (Cellcept) and mycophenolic acid (Myfortic) are not interchangeable; rate of absorption is different.
- ***REMS:*** Mycophenolate is administered under REMS requirements. Prescribers are encouraged to complete prescriber training program and patients are encouraged to complete the *Information for Patients* to mitigate the risk of embryofetal toxicity associated with the use of mycophenolate during pregnancy.
- **PO:** Administer on an empty stomach, 1 hr before or 2 hr after meals. ***DNC:*** Swallow capsules and delayed-release tablets whole; do not open, crush, or chew. **Oral suspension:** Must be reconstituted by pharmacist. Do not mix with other medication. Can be administered by nasogastric tube (minimum size, 8 French) and is stable for 60 days refrigerated. Mycophenolate may be teratogenic; wear gloves and avoid contact with skin or mucous membranes or inhalation of contents of capsules or oral suspension powder.
- Do not administer mycophenolate concurrently with antacids containing magnesium or aluminum.

IV Administration

- **IV:** IV route should only be used for patients unable to take oral medication and should be switched to oral dose form as soon as tolerated.
- **Intermittent Infusion: Reconstitution:** Reconstitute each vial with 14 mL of D5W. Shake gently to dissolve. Solution is slightly yellow. **Dilution:** Dilute contents of 2 vials (1-g dose) further with 140 mL of D5W or 3 vials (1.5-g dose) with 210 mL of D5W. Discard if solution is discolored or contains particulates. Solution is stable for 4 hr. **Concentration:** 6 mg/mL. **Rate:** Administer via slow IV infusion over ≥2 hr. Do not administer as bolus or rapid infusion (↑ risk of phlebitis and thrombosis).
- **Y-Site Compatibility:** alemtuzumab, amikacin, amiodarone, anidulafungin, argatroban, atracurium, bivalirudin, bumetanide, buprenorphine, butorphanol, calcium chloride, caspofungin, ceftolozane/tazobactam, chlorpromazine, ciprofloxacin, cisatracurium, daptomycin, dexmedetomidine, dexrazoxane, digoxin, diltiazem, diphenhydramine, dobutamine, dopamine, doxorubicin liposomal, doxycycline, droperidol, enalaprilat, ephedrine, epinephrine, erythromycin, esmolol, famotidine, fentanyl, fluconazole, gentamicin, glycopyrrolate, granisetron, haloperidol, hydralazine, hydromorphone, insulin, regular, isavuconazonium, isoproterenol, labetalol, leucovorin, levofloxacin, lidocaine, linezolid, lorazepam, magnesium sulfate, mannitol, meperidine, mesna, methadone, metoclopramide, metoprolol, metronidazole, midazolam, milrinone, morphine, moxifloxacin, nalbuphine, naloxone, nicardipine, nitroglycerin, norepinephrine, octreotide, ondansetron, oxytocin, pamidronate, pentamidine, phentolamine, phenylephrine, potassium chloride, procainamide, prochlorperazine, promethazine, propranolol, remifentanil, rocuronium, succinylcholine, sufentanil, tacrolimus, theophylline, tigecycline, tirofiban, tobramycin, vancomycin, vasopressin, vecuronium, verapamil, voriconazole, zidovudine, zoledronic acid.
- **Y-Site Incompatibility:** acyclovir, allopurinol, aminocaproic acid, aminophylline, amphotericin B deoxycholate, amphotericin B liposomal, ampicillin, ampicillin/sulbactam, azithromycin,

M

aztreonam, calcium gluconate, cangrelor, cefazolin, cefiderocol, cefotaxime, cefotetan, cefoxitin, ceftazidime, ceftriaxone, cefuroxime, chloramphenicol, clindamycin, dantrolene, defibrotide, dexamethasone, diazepam, eptifibatide, foscarnet, fosphenytoin, furosemide, ganciclovir, gemtuzumab ozogamicin, heparin, hydrocortisone, imipenem/cilastatin, ketorolac, letermovir, meropenem, methotrexate, methylprednisolone, micafungin, nafcillin, nitroprusside, pantoprazole, pentobarbital, phenobarbital, phenytoin, piperacillin/tazobactam, potassium acetate, potassium phosphates, sodium acetate, sodium bicarbonate, sodium phosphates, trimethoprim/sulfamethoxazole.

Patient/Family Teaching

- Instruct patient to take medication as directed, at the same time each day. Take missed dose as soon as remembered, but not if within 2 hr before next dose. Do not skip or double up on missed doses. Do not discontinue without consulting health care provider. Advise patient to read *Medication Guide* before starting therapy and with each Rx refill in case of changes.
- ***REMS:*** Explain REMS program to patient.
- Reinforce the need for lifelong therapy to prevent transplant rejection. Review symptoms of rejection for the transplanted organ, and stress need to notify health care provider immediately if signs of rejection or infection occur.
- Emphasize importance of routine follow-up laboratory tests.
- May cause somnolence, confusion, dizziness, tremor, or hypotension. Caution patient to avoid driving and other activities requiring alertness until response from medication is known.
- Advise patients and family to call 911 and seek urgent treatment for signs and symptoms of hypersensitivity reactions (difficulty breathing; chest tightness; hives; rash; feeling light-headed; itching; swelling of the face, lips, tongue, or throat).
- Instruct patient to notify health care provider immediately if signs and symptoms of infection (temperature ≥100.5°F; cold symptoms [runny nose, sore throat]; flu symptoms [upset stomach, stomach pain, vomiting, diarrhea]; earache or headache; pain during urination; frequent urination; white patches in mouth or throat; unexpected bruising or bleeding; cuts, scrapes, or incisions that are red, warm, and oozing pus) or PML occur. Advise patient to avoid contact with persons with contagious diseases.
- Advise patient to avoid live-attenuated virus vaccines during therapy.
- Inform patient of the ↑ risk of lymphoma and other malignancies. Advise patient to use sunscreen and wear protective clothing to ↓ risk of skin cancer.
- Advise patient to notify health care provider of all Rx or OTC medications, vitamins, or herbal products being taken and to consult with health care provider before taking other medications.
- Instruct patient to avoid donating blood during and for >6 wk after discontinuation of therapy.
- Rep: May cause fetal harm and pregnancy loss. Discuss importance of simultaneously using two reliable nonhormonal forms of contraception or abstinence prior to beginning, during, and for 6 wk following last dose and to avoid breastfeeding. Discuss acceptable forms of contraception with health care provider. Mycophenolate may ↓ effectiveness of hormonal contraceptives. Encourage pregnant patients during or within 6 wk after therapy to enroll in registry that monitors outcomes in women exposed to mycophenolate during pregnancy by calling 1-800-617-8191 or visiting www.mycophenolateREMS.com. Instruct men with female partners of reproductive potential to use effective contraception during and for ≥90 days after last dose. Advise men to avoid semen donation during and for ≥90 days after last dose.

Evaluation/Desired Outcomes

- Prevention of rejection of transplanted organs.

nadolol, See BETA BLOCKERS (nonselective).

nafarelin (na-fare-e-lin)

Synarel

Classification

Therapeutic: hormones

Pharmacologic: gonadotropin-releasing hormones

Indications

Endometriosis. Central precocious puberty (gonadotropin-dependent) in children.

Action

Acts as a synthetic analogue of gonadotropin-releasing hormone (GnRH). Initially increases pituitary production of luteinizing hormone and follicle-stimulating hormone, which cause ovarian steroid production. Chronic administration leads to decreased production of gonadotropins. Endometriotic lesions are sensitive to ovarian hormones. **Therapeutic Effects:** Reduction in lesions and associated pain in endometriosis. Arrest and regression of puberty in children with central precocious puberty.

Pharmacokinetics

Absorption: Well absorbed following intranasal administration.

Distribution: Unknown.

Metabolism and Excretion: 20–40% excreted in feces; 3% excreted unchanged by the kidneys.

Half-life: 3 hr.

TIME/ACTION PROFILE (↓ ovarian steroid production)

ROUTE	ONSET	PEAK	DURATION
Intranasal	within 4 wk	3–4 wk	3–6 mo†

† Relief of symptoms of endometriosis following discontinuation.

Contraindications/Precautions

Contraindicated in: Hypersensitivity to GnRH, its analogues, or sorbitol; OB: Pregnancy ; Lactation: Lactation.

Use Cautiously in: Rhinitis; Seizures, cerebrovascular disorders, or CNS tumor (may ↑ risk of seizures).

Adverse Reactions/Side Effects

CV: edema, MI. **Derm:** acne, hot flushing, hirsutism, seborrhea. **EENT:** nasal irritation. **Endo:** ↓ breast size, hyperglycemia. **GU:** ↓ fertility, ↓ libido, cessation of menses, vaginal dryness. **Metab:** weight gain. **MS:** ↓ bone density, myalgia. **Neuro:** headache, aggression, anger, depression, impatience, insomnia, intracranial hypertension (children), irritability, SEIZURES, STROKE, SUICIDAL ATTEMPT/IDEATION (CHILDREN). **Misc:** hypersensitivity reactions.

Interactions

Drug-Drug: Topical nasal decongestants may ↓ absorption (administer decongestant ≥2 hr after nafarelin). **Bupropion** or **SSRIs** may ↑ risk of seizures.

Route/Dosage

Endometriosis

Intranasal (Adults): One spray (200 mcg) in one nostril in the morning and one spray in the other nostril in the evening (400 mcg/day). May ↑ to one spray in each nostril in the morning and evening (800 mcg/day).

Central Precocious Puberty

Intranasal (Children): Two sprays in each nostril in the morning and in the evening (1600 mcg/day); may ↑ up to 1800 mcg/day (three sprays in alternating nostrils three times daily).

Availability

Nasal spray: 2 mg/mL (200 mcg/spray).

NURSING IMPLICATIONS

Assessment

- **Endometriosis:** Assess for endometriotic pain periodically during therapy.
- **Central Precocious Puberty:** Prior to therapy, a complete physical and endocrinologic examination, including height, weight, hand and wrist x-ray, total sex steroid level (estradiol or testosterone), adrenal steroid level, beta human chorionic gonadotropin level, GnRH stimulation test, pelvic/adrenal/testicular ultrasound, and CT of the head, must be performed. These parameters are monitored after 6–8 wk and every 3–6 mo during therapy.
- Assess patient for signs of precocious puberty (menses, breast development, testicular growth) periodically during therapy.
- Monitor for the onset of normal puberty and assess menstrual cycle, reproductive function, and final adult height.

Implementation

- **Endometriosis:** Start therapy between Days 2 and 4 of the menstrual cycle and continue for up to 6 mo.

Patient/Family Teaching

- Explain purpose and side effects of medication. Advise patient to read *Patient Information* before starting therapy.

N

- Instruct patient on correct technique for nasal spray: Tilt head back slightly; wait 30 sec between sprays. Inform patient and caregiver that if doses are not taken as directed, pubertal process may be reactivated when treating central precocious puberty.
- Advise patient to notify health care provider if rhinitis occurs and if a topical decongestant is needed; do not use decongestant until 2 hr after nafarelin dose. If possible, avoid sneezing during and immediately after dose is administered.
- Advise patient that medication may cause hot flashes. Notify health care provider if persistent or bothersome.
- Advise patient to notify health care provider of all Rx or OTC medications, vitamins, or herbal products being taken and to consult health care provider before taking other medications.
- Inform patients with endometriosis that amenorrhea is expected and to notify health care provider if regular menstruation persists or if successive doses are missed.
- Rep: May cause fetal harm. Advise women of reproductive potential to use a form of contraception other than oral contraceptives and to avoid breastfeeding during therapy.
- Advise patient and caregiver that some signs of puberty (vaginal bleeding, breast enlargement) may occur and should resolve after 1st mo of therapy. If these signs persist after 2nd mo of therapy, notify health care provider.

Evaluation/Desired Outcomes

- Reduction in lesions and associated pain in endometriosis.
- Regression of the signs of precocious puberty. Nafarelin is discontinued when the onset of normal puberty is desired.

nafcillin, See PENICILLINS, PENICILLINASE RESISTANT.

naftifine, See ANTIFUNGALS (TOPICAL).

REMS HIGH ALERT

nalbuphine (nal-byoo-feen)

Nubain

Classification

Therapeutic: opioid analgesics

Pharmacologic: opioid agonists/analgesics

Indications

Moderate to severe pain. Supplement to balanced anesthesia. Pain control during labor. Sedation before surgery.

Action

Binds to opiate receptors in the CNS. Alters the perception of and response to painful stimuli while producing generalized CNS depression. In addition, has partial antagonist properties, which may result in opioid withdrawal in physically dependent patients. **Therapeutic Effects:** Decreased pain.

Pharmacokinetics

Absorption: Well absorbed after IM and SUBQ administration. IV administration results in complete bioavailability.

Distribution: Unknown.

Metabolism and Excretion: Mostly metabolized by the liver and eliminated in the feces via biliary excretion. Minimal amounts excreted unchanged by the kidneys.

Half-life: *Children (1–8 yr):* 0.9 hr; *Adults:* 3.5–5 hr.

TIME/ACTION PROFILE (analgesia)

ROUTE	ONSET	PEAK	DURATION
IM	<15 min	60 min	3–6 hr
SUBQ	<15 min	unknown	3–6 hr
IV	2–3 min	30 min	3–6 hr

Contraindications/Precautions

Contraindicated in: Hypersensitivity to nalbuphine or bisulfites; Patients physically dependent on opioids and who have not been detoxified (may precipitate withdrawal).

Use Cautiously in: Personal or family history of substance use disorder or mental illness; Head trauma; ↑ intracranial pressure; Severe renal impairment; Severe hepatic impairment; Severe pulmonary disease; Hypothyroidism; Adrenal insufficiency; Undiagnosed abdominal pain; Prostatic hyperplasia; Patients who have recently received opioid agonists; OB: Use during pregnancy only if potential maternal benefit justifies potential fetal risk. Has been used during labor but may cause respiratory depression in the newborn; prolonged use of opioids during pregnancy can result in neonatal opioid withdrawal syndrome; Lactation: Use while breastfeeding only if potential maternal benefit justifies potential risk to infant. May cause respiratory depression and excessive sedation in infant; Pedi: Safety and effectiveness not established in children; Geri: Dose ↓ suggested in older adults.

Adverse Reactions/Side Effects

CV: hypertension, orthostatic hypotension, palpitations. **Derm:** ↑ sweating, clammy feeling. **EENT:** blurred vision, diplopia, miosis (high doses). **Endo:** adrenal insufficiency. **GI:** dry mouth, nausea, vomiting, constipation, ileus. **GU:** urinary urgency. **Neuro:** dizziness, headache, sedation, confusion, dysphoria, euphoria, floating feeling, hallucinations, unusual dreams. **Resp:** RESPIRATORY DEPRESSION (INCLUDING CENTRAL SLEEP APNEA AND SLEEP-RELATED HYPOXEMIA). **Misc:** allodynia, opioid-induced hyperalgesia, physical dependence, psychological dependence, tolerance.

Interactions

Drug-Drug: Use with extreme caution in patients receiving **MAO inhibitors**; may result in unpredictable, severe reactions; ↓ initial dose of nalbuphine to 25% of usual dose. Use with **benzodiazepines** or other **CNS depressants**, including other **opioids**, **nonbenzodiazepine sedative/hypnotics**, **anxiolytics**, **general anesthetics**, **muscle relaxants**, **antipsychotics**, and **alcohol**, may cause profound sedation, respiratory depression, coma, and death; reserve concurrent use for when alternative treatment options are inadequate. May precipitate withdrawal in patients who are physically dependent on **opioid agonists**. Avoid concurrent use with other **opioid agonists**; may ↓ analgesic effect. Drugs that affect serotonergic neurotransmitter systems, including **tricyclic antidepressants**, **SSRIs**, **SNRIs**, **MAO inhibitors**, **tramadol**, **trazodone**, **mirtazapine**, **$5HT_3$ receptor antagonists**, **linezolid**, **methylene blue**, and **triptans**, may ↑ risk of serotonin syndrome.

Drug-Natural Products: **Kava-kava**, **valerian**, **skullcap**, **chamomile**, or **hops** may ↑ risk of CNS depression.

Route/Dosage

Analgesia

IM, SUBQ, IV (Adults): Usual dose is 10 mg every 3–6 hr (max = 20 mg/dose or 160 mg/day).

IM, SUBQ, IV (Children): 0.1–0.15 mg/kg every 3–6 hr (max = 20 mg/dose or 160 mg/day).

Supplement to Balanced Anesthesia

IV (Adults): *Initial:* 0.3–3 mg/kg over 10–15 min. *Maintenance:* 0.25–0.5 mg/kg as needed.

Availability (generic available)

Solution for injection: 10 mg/mL, 20 mg/mL.

NURSING IMPLICATIONS

Assessment

- Assess type, location, and intensity of pain before and 1 hr after IM or 30 min (peak) after IV administration. When titrating opioid doses, increases of 25–50% should be administered until there is either a 50% ↓ in the patient's pain rating on a numeric or visual analogue scale or the patient reports satisfactory pain relief. A repeat dose can be safely administered at the time of the peak if previous dose is ineffective and side effects are minimal. Patients requiring doses higher than 20 mg should be converted to an opioid agonist. Nalbuphine is not recommended for prolonged use or as first-line therapy for acute or cancer pain.
- An equianalgesic chart (see Appendix I) should be used when changing routes or when changing from one opioid to another.
- Assess BP, HR, and respiratory rate before and periodically during administration. If respiratory rate is <10/min, assess level of sedation. Physical stimulation may be sufficient to prevent significant hypoventilation. Dose may need to be ↓ by 25–50%. Monitor for respiratory depression, especially during initiation or following dose ↑; serious, life-threatening, or fatal respiratory depression may occur. May cause sleep-related breathing disorders (central sleep apnea, sleep-related hypoxemia). Nalbuphine produces respiratory depression, but this does not markedly ↑ with increased doses.
- Monitor for severe hypotension, including orthostatic hypotension and syncope, in ambulatory patients, especially in patients with compromised ability to maintain BP.
- Assess bowel function routinely. Institute prevention of constipation with ↑ intake of fluids and bulk and with laxatives to minimize constipating effects. Administer stimulant laxatives routinely if opioid use exceeds 2–3 days, unless contraindicated. Consider drugs for opioid-induced constipation.
- Assess previous analgesic history. Antagonistic properties may induce withdrawal symptoms (vomiting, restlessness, abdominal cramps, ↑ BP and temperature) in patients physically dependent on opioids.
- Although this drug has a low potential for dependence, prolonged use may lead to physical and psychological dependence and tolerance. This should not prevent patient from receiving adequate analgesia. Most patients who receive nalbuphine for pain do not develop psychological dependence. If tolerance develops, changing to an opioid agonist may be required to relieve pain.
- Assess risk for opioid addiction, abuse, or misuse prior to administration.

Lab Test Considerations

- May ↑ amylase and lipase.

Toxicity and Overdose

- If an opioid antagonist is required to reverse respiratory depression or coma, naloxone is the antidote. Dilute the 0.4-mg ampule of naloxone in 10 mL of 0.9% NaCl and administer 0.5 mL (0.02 mg) by IV push every 2 min. For children and patients weighing <40 kg, dilute 0.1 mg of naloxone in 10 mL of 0.9% NaCl for a concentration of 10 mcg/mL and administer 0.5 mcg/kg every 2 min. Titrate dose to avoid withdrawal, seizures, and severe pain.

Implementation

- ***High Alert:*** Do not confuse nalbuphine with naloxone.
- Explain therapeutic value of medication before administration to enhance the analgesic effect.
- Regularly administered doses may be more effective than as needed administration. Analgesic is more effective if administered before pain becomes severe.
- Coadministration with nonopioid analgesics may have additive effects and permit lower opioid doses.
- Nalbuphine should be discontinued gradually to prevent withdrawal symptoms after long-term use. Monitor frequently to manage pain and withdrawal symptoms (restlessness; lacrimation; rhinorrhea; yawning; perspiration; chills; myalgia; mydriasis; irritability; anxiety; backache; joint pain; weakness; abdominal cramps; insomnia; nausea; anorexia; vomiting; diarrhea; ↑ BP, respiratory rate, or HR). If withdrawal symptoms occur, pause the taper for a period of time or ↑ the dose of opioid analgesic to the previous dose, and then proceed with a slower taper. Also, monitor patients for changes in mood, emergence of suicidal thoughts, or use of other substances. A multimodal approach to pain management may optimize the treatment of chronic pain and assist with the successful tapering of the opioid analgesic.
- ***REMS:*** FDA strongly encourages health care providers to complete a REMS-compliant education program that includes all the elements of the FDA Education *Blueprint for Health Care Providers Involved in the Management or Support of Patients with Pain,* available at www.fda.gov/OpioidAnalgesic REMSBlueprint. Information on programs can be found at 1-800-503-0784 or www.opioidanalgesi crems.com.
- Discuss availability of naloxone for emergency treatment of opioid overdose with the patient and caregiver and assess the potential need for access to naloxone, both when initiating and renewing therapy, especially if patient has household members (including children) or other close contacts at risk for accidental exposure or overdose. Consider prescribing naloxone, based on the patient's risk factors for overdose, such as concurrent use of CNS depressants, a history of opioid use disorder, or prior opioid overdose. However, the presence of risk factors for overdose should not prevent the proper management of pain in any patient.
- **IM:** Administer deep into well-developed muscle. Rotate sites of injections.

IV Administration

- **IV Push:** May give IV undiluted. **Concentration:** 10–20 mg/mL. **Rate:** Administer slowly, each 10 mg over 3–5 min.
- **Y-Site Compatibility:** acetaminophen, amikacin, aminocaproic acid, aminophylline, amiodarone, argatroban, arsenic trioxide, ascorbic acid, atracurium, atropine, azithromycin, aztreonam, benztropine, bivalirudin, bleomycin, bumetanide, buprenorphine, butorphanol, calcium chloride, calcium gluconate, cangrelor, carboplatin, carmustine, caspofungin, cefazolin, cefotaxime, cefotetan, cefoxitin, ceftazidime, ceftriaxone, cefuroxime, chlorpromazine, cisatracurium, cladribine, clindamycin, cyanocobalamin, cyclophosphamide, cytarabine, dacarbazine, dactinomycin, daptomycin, daunorubicin, defibrotide, dexamethasone, dexmedetomidine, dexrazoxane, digoxin, diltiazem, diphenhydramine, dobutamine, dopamine, doxorubicin hydrochloride, doxorubicin liposomal, doxycycline, enalaprilat, ephedrine, epinephrine, epirubicin, epoetin alfa, eptifibatide, ertapenem, erythromycin, esmolol, etoposide, etoposide phosphate, famotidine, fentanyl, filgrastim, fluconazole, fludarabine, fluorouracil, foscarnet, fosphenytoin, gemcitabine, gentamicin, glycopyrrolate, granisetron, heparin, hetastarch, idarubicin, ifosfamide, insulin regular, irinotecan, isoproterenol, labetalol, LR, leucovorin, levofloxacin, lidocaine, linezolid, lorazepam, magnesium sulfate, mannitol, melphalan, meperidine, mesna, metoclopramide, metoprolol, metronidazole, midazolam, milrinone, minocycline, mitoxantrone, morphine, multivitamins, mycophenolate, naloxone, nicardipine, nitroglycerin, nitroprusside, norepinephrine, octreotide, ondansetron, oxaliplatin, oxytocin, paclitaxel, palonosetron, pamidronate, papaverine, penicillin G, phentolamine, phenylephrine, phytonadione, potassium acetate, potassium chloride, procainamide, prochlorperazine, promethazine, propofol, propranolol, protamine, pyridoxine, remifentanil, rituximab, rocuronium, sodium acetate, succinylcholine, sufentanil, tacrolimus, theophylline, thiamine, thiotepa, tigecycline, tirofiban, tobramycin, topotecan, vancomycin, vasopressin, vecuronium, verapamil, vinblastine, vincristine, vinorelbine, voriconazole, zoledronic acid.
- **Y-Site Incompatibility:** alemtuzumab, allopurinol, amphotericin B deoxycholate, amphotericin B liposomal, anidulafungin, azathioprine, blinatumomab, cefepime, chloramphenicol, cyclosporine, dantrolene, diazepam, diazoxide, docetaxel, folic acid, furosemide, ganciclovir, gemtuzumab ozogamicin, hydrocortisone, imipenem/cilastatin, indomethacin, ketorolac, methotrexate, methylprednisolone, mitomycin, pantoprazole, pemetrexed, pentamidine, pentobarbital, phenobarbital, phenytoin, piperacillin/tazobactam, sargramostim, sodium bicarbonate, trastuzumab, trimethoprim/sulfamethoxazole.

Patient/Family Teaching

- Explain purpose and side effects of nalbuphine to patient. Instruct them how and when to ask for pain medication. Do not stop taking drug without consulting health care provider. If an appointment is missed, contact health care provider as soon as possible to reschedule. Advise patient to read *Medication Guide* before starting and periodically during therapy in case of changes.
- May cause drowsiness or dizziness. Advise patient to call for assistance when ambulating and to avoid driving or other activities requiring alertness until response to the medication is known.
- Instruct patient to notify health care provider of all Rx or OTC medications, vitamins, or herbal products being taken and consult health care provider before taking any new medications.
- Advise patient to notify health care provider if pain control is not adequate or if severe or persistent side effects occur.
- Emphasize the importance of aggressive prevention of constipation with the use of nalbuphine.
- Caution patient to change positions slowly to minimize orthostatic hypotension.
- Advise patient that frequent mouth rinses, good oral hygiene, and sugarless gum or candy may ↓ dry mouth.
- Encourage patient to turn, cough, and breathe deeply every 2 hr to prevent atelectasis.
- Advise patient to avoid concurrent use of alcohol or other CNS depressants with this medication.
- Rep: Advise patient to notify health care provider if pregnancy is planned or suspected or if breastfeeding. Inform patient of potential for neonatal opioid withdrawal syndrome with prolonged use during pregnancy. Monitor neonate for signs and symptoms of withdrawal (irritability, hyperactivity and abnormal sleep pattern, high-pitched cry, tremor, vomiting, diarrhea, failure to gain weight); usually occur the first days after birth. Monitor infants exposed to nalbuphine through breast milk for excess sedation and respiratory depression. Chronic use may reduce fertility in women and men.

Evaluation/Desired Outcomes

- Decrease in severity of pain without significant alteration in level of consciousness or respiratory status.

nalmefene (nal-me-feen)

Opvee

Classification

Therapeutic: antidotes

Pharmacologic: opioid antagonists

Indications

Emergency treatment of known or suspected overdose caused by natural or synthetic opioids and characterized by respiratory and/or CNS depression.

Action

Competitively blocks the effects of opioid analgesics, including CNS and respiratory depression, without producing any agonist (opioid-like) effects. **Therapeutic Effects:** Reversal of signs of opioid excess.

Pharmacokinetics

Absorption: 82% absorbed following intranasal administration.

Distribution: Rapidly and widely distributed to tissues.

Metabolism and Excretion: Primarily metabolized by the liver via glucuronide conjugation; <5% excreted unchanged in urine; 17% in feces. Undergoes enterohepatic recycling.

Half-life: 11.4 hr.

TIME/ACTION PROFILE (reversal of opioid effects)

ROUTE	ONSET	PEAK	DURATION
Intranasal	minutes	5–15 min	unknown

Contraindications/Precautions

Contraindicated in: Known hypersensitivity.

Use Cautiously in: Overdosage of buprenorphine (may not completely reverse respiratory depression; may required repeated doses); Pedi: Children <12 yr (safety and effectiveness not established).

Exercise Extreme Caution in: Patients known to be physically dependent on opioid agents or who have undergone surgery with large doses of opioid analgesics (especially those with severe cardiovascular disease or who have received cardiovascular medications) (↑ risk of withdrawal and cardiovascular complications).

Adverse Reactions/Side Effects

CV: palpitations, hypertension, hypotension, tachycardia. **Derm:** hot flush, ↑ sweating, erythema. **EENT:** nasal discomfort, tinnitus, ear discomfort, nasal congestion, oropharyngeal pain, rhinitis, throat irritation. **GI:** ↓ appetite, nausea, vomiting, abdominal pain, dry mouth. **Neuro:** allodynia, dizziness, headache, irritability, agitation, anxiety, claustrophobia, dysgeusia, fatigue, insomnia, paresthesia, recurrent CNS depression. **Resp:** dyspnea, recurrent respiratory depression. **Misc:** chills, fever, postoperative pain.

Interactions

Drug-Drug: None reported.

N

Route/Dosage

Intranasal (Adults and Children ≥12 yr): One spray (2.7 mg) in one nostril; if desired response not achieved, may repeat dose every 2–5 min.

Availability

Nasal spray (Opvee): 2.7 mg/device.

NURSING IMPLICATIONS

Assessment

- Monitor respiratory rate, HR, ECG, BP, and level of sedation frequently. Repeat doses may be necessary for reversal of opioid-related respiratory depression.
- Assess patient for intensity of pain when nalmefene is used to treat postoperative respiratory depression. Careful titration of nalmefene can reverse respiratory depression while maintaining analgesia.
- Assess for signs/symptoms of opioid withdrawal (vomiting, restlessness, anxiety, abdominal cramps, ↑ BP and temperature). Symptoms may occur within a few minutes to 2 hr. Severity depends on dose of nalmefene, opioid involved, and degree of physical dependence. Opioid-tolerant and physically dependent patients should be monitored closely after initial and subsequent doses.
- Lack of significant improvement may indicate that symptoms are caused by a disease process or other nonopioid CNS depressants not affected by nalmefene.

Lab Test Considerations

- May ↑ AST.

Implementation

- Resuscitation equipment, oxygen, vasopressors, and mechanical ventilation should be available to supplement nalmefene therapy as needed.
- Abrupt reversal of opioid analgesics in emergency or postoperative settings may cause pulmonary edema, cardiovascular instability, hypotension, hypertension, ventricular tachycardia, and ventricular fibrillation.
- Administration of higher doses or doses at shorter intervals than recommended may ↑ incidence and severity of acute withdrawal symptoms.
- If respiratory depression recurs, titrate repeat doses based on clinical effects to avoid over-reversal.
- **Intranasal:** Administer a single spray into one nostril. If patient does not respond or responds and relapses into respiratory depression, additional doses may be given every 2–5 min in alternating nostrils until emergency medical assistance arrives.

Patient/Family Teaching

- Explain to family and patient the rationale for use and to take only as directed. Advise to read *Instructions for Use* at the time of prescription.
- Instruct patient and caregivers in the correct technique for use and disposal of provided device.
- Advise caregiver to use as quickly as possible, always seek emergency medical care after 1st dose, and monitor the patient continuously.

Evaluation/Desired Outcomes

- Reversal of respiratory depression, sedation, and hypotension caused by opioid analgesics.

naloxegol (nal-**ox**-ee-gol)

Movantik

Classification

Therapeutic: laxatives

Pharmacologic: opioid antagonists

Indications

Opioid-induced constipation in patients with chronic noncancer pain, including those with chronic pain related to prior cancer or its treatment who do not require frequent (e.g., weekly) opioid dose escalation.

Action

Acts peripherally as a mu receptor antagonist, blocking opioid receptors in the GI tract. **Therapeutic Effects:** Blocks constipating effects of opioids on the GI tract without loss of analgesia.

Pharmacokinetics

Absorption: Systemic absorption follows oral administration. High-fat meals ↑ absorption.

Distribution: Does not cross the blood-brain barrier.

Metabolism and Excretion: Primarily metabolized by the liver via the CYP3A4 isoenzyme; 68% excreted in feces, 16% in urine mostly as metabolites.

Half-life: 6–11 hr.

TIME/ACTION PROFILE (spontaneous bowel movement)

ROUTE	ONSET	PEAK	DURATION
PO	within 24 hr	unknown	unknown

Contraindications/Precautions

Contraindicated in: Hypersensitivity; Known/suspected/history of GI obstruction; Severe hepatic impairment; Concurrent use of strong CYP3A4 inhibitors, strong CYP3A4 inducers, or other opioid antagonists; Severe hepatic impairment; Lactation: Lactation.

Use Cautiously in: Infiltrative GI tract malignancy, recent GI tract surgery, diverticular disease, ischemic colitis, or concurrent use of bevacizumab (↑ risk of GI perforation); Patients with disruption of the blood-brain barrier (may precipitate opioid withdrawal); OB: Use during pregnancy only if potential maternal benefit justifies potential fetal risk; Pedi: Safety and effectiveness not established in children; Geri: Levels are ↑ in older Japanese patients.

Adverse Reactions/Side Effects

Derm: ↑ sweating. **GI:** abdominal pain, diarrhea, flatulence, GI PERFORATION, nausea, vomiting. **Neuro:** headache. **Misc:** HYPERSENSITIVITY REACTIONS (INCLUDING ANGIOEDEMA), opioid withdrawal.

Interactions

Drug-Drug: Strong CYP3A4 inhibitors, including **clarithromycin** and **ketoconazole**, may significantly ↑ levels and risk of toxicity; concurrent use contraindicated. **Strong CYP3A4 inducers**, including **rifampin**, may significantly ↓ levels and effectiveness; concurrent use contraindicated. Other **opioid antagonists** may precipitate opioid withdrawal; concurrent use contraindicated. **Moderate CYP3A4 inhibitors**, including **diltiazem**, **erythromycin**, and **verapamil**, may ↑ levels and risk of toxicity; ↓ naloxegol dose. **Methadone** for pain ↑ risk of stomach pain and diarrhea. **Bevacizumab** may ↑ risk of GI perforation.
Drug-Food: Grapefruit/grapefruit juice may ↑ levels and risk of toxicity; avoid concurrent use.

Route/Dosage

PO (Adults): 25 mg once daily; if poorly tolerated, ↓ dose to 12.5 mg once daily; *Concurrent use of moderate CYP3A4 inhibitors:* 12.5 mg once daily (careful monitoring recommended).

Renal Impairment

PO (Adults): *CCr <60 mL/min:* 12.5 mg once daily initially; may cautiously ↑ to 25 mg once daily, if necessary, with careful monitoring.

Availability

Tablets: 12.5 mg, 25 mg.

NURSING IMPLICATIONS

Assessment

- Assess bowel sounds and frequency, quantity, and consistency of stools periodically during therapy.
- Monitor for signs of opioid withdrawal in patients with disruptions to the blood-brain barrier and assess for ↓ analgesic effects in patients using concurrent opioids.
- Monitor for signs and symptoms of GI perforation (severe, persistent, or worsening abdominal pain) and diarrhea periodically during therapy. *If symptoms of GI perforation occur,* discontinue naloxegol.

Implementation

- Discontinue all maintenance laxative therapy before starting naloxegol. If a suboptimal response occurs with naloxegol, laxatives may be used after 3 days.
- **PO:** Administer on an empty stomach ≥1 hr before 1st meal in morning or 2 hr after meal. Tablet may be crushed to a powder and mixed with 4 ounces of water (120 mL). Drink mixture immediately; refill glass with 120 mL water, stir, and drink contents.
- May be administered by nasogastric (NG) tube. Flush the NG tube with 1 ounce (30 mL) of water using a 60 mL syringe. Crush tablet to a powder and mix with 2 ounces (60 mL) of water. Draw up mixture using the 60 mL syringe and administer through the NG tube. Add 2 ounces (60 mL) of water to rinse container and administer to flush NG tube and any remaining medicine from NG tube into stomach.

Patient/Family Teaching

- Explain purpose and side effects of medication. Advise patient to read *Patient Information* before starting therapy.
- Caution patient to avoid grapefruit and grapefruit juice during therapy.
- Advise patient to notify health care provider immediately if stomach pain or diarrhea that does not go away occurs.
- Advise patient to notify health care provider if signs and symptoms of opioid withdrawal (sweating, chills, diarrhea, stomach pain, anxiety, irritability, yawning) occur. Patients taking methadone for pain are at ↑ risk for stomach pain and diarrhea.
- Instruct patient to stop taking naloxegol if they stop taking opioid medications.
- Instruct patient to notify health care provider of all Rx or OTC medications, vitamins, or herbal products being taken and consult health care provider before taking any new medications.
- Rep: Advise women of reproductive potential to notify health care provider if pregnancy is planned or suspected and to avoid breastfeeding during therapy. May cause opioid withdrawal in infant.

Evaluation/Desired Outcomes

- Relief of opioid-induced constipation, especially if opioid therapy has been for ≥4 wk.

N

naloxone (nal-**ox**-one)
~~Evzio~~, Kloxxado, Narcan, Rextovy, Rezenopy, Rivive, Zimhi
Classification
Therapeutic: antidotes (for opioids)
Pharmacologic: opioid antagonists

Indications

Reversal of CNS depression and respiratory depression because of suspected opioid overdose. **Unlabeled Use:** Opioid-induced pruritus (low-dose IV infusion). Management of refractory circulatory shock.

Action

Competitively blocks the effects of opioids, including CNS and respiratory depression, without producing any agonist (opioid-like) effects. **Therapeutic Effects:** Reversal of signs of opioid excess.

Pharmacokinetics

Absorption: Well absorbed after IM or SUBQ administration. IV administration results in complete bioavailability. Rapidly absorbed from nasal mucosa.
Distribution: Rapidly distributed to tissues. Crosses the placenta.
Metabolism and Excretion: Metabolized by the liver.
Half-life: *IM, IV, or SUBQ:* 30–90 min (up to 3 hr in neonates); *Intranasal:* 2 hr.

TIME/ACTION PROFILE (reversal of opioid effects)

ROUTE	ONSET	PEAK	DURATION
IV	1–2 min	unknown	45 min
IM, SUBQ	2–5 min	unknown	>45 min
Intranasal	8–13 min	unknown	unknown

Contraindications/Precautions

Contraindicated in: Hypersensitivity.
Use Cautiously in: Cardiovascular disease; Patients physically dependent on opioids (may precipitate severe withdrawal); OB: May cause acute withdrawal syndrome in mother and fetus if mother is opioid dependent; Lactation: Safety not established in breastfeeding; Pedi: May cause acute withdrawal syndrome in neonates of opioid-dependent mothers.

Adverse Reactions/Side Effects

CV: hypertension, hypotension, VENTRICULAR ARRHYTHMIA. **GI:** nausea, vomiting.

Interactions

Drug-Drug: Can precipitate withdrawal in patients physically dependent on **opioid analgesics**. Larger doses may be required to reverse the effects of **buprenorphine**, **butorphanol**, or **nalbuphine**. Antagonizes postoperative **opioid analgesics**.

Route/Dosage

Postoperative Opioid-Induced Respiratory Depression

IV (Adults): 0.02–0.2 mg every 2–3 min until response obtained; repeat every 1–2 hr if needed.
IV (Children): 0.01 mg/kg; may repeat every 2–3 min until response obtained. Additional doses may be given every 1–2 hr if needed.
IM, IV, SUBQ (Neonates): 0.01 mg/kg; may repeat every 2–3 min until response obtained. Additional doses may be given every 1–2 hr if needed.

Opioid-Induced Respiratory Depression During Chronic (>1 wk) Opioid Use

IV, IM, SUBQ (Adults >40 kg): 20–40 mcg (0.02–0.04 mg) given as small, frequent (every min) boluses or as an infusion titrated to improve respiratory function without reversing analgesia.
IV, IM, SUBQ (Adults and Children <40 kg): 0.005–0.02 mg/dose given as small, frequent (every min) boluses or as an infusion titrated to improve respiratory function without reversing analgesia.

Overdose of Opioids

IV, IM, SUBQ (Adults): *Patients not suspected of being opioid dependent:* 0.4 mg (10 mcg/kg); may repeat every 2–3 min (IV route is preferred). Some patients may require up to 2 mg. *Patients suspected to be opioid dependent:* Initial dose should be ↓ to 0.1–0.2 mg every 2–3 min. May also be given by IV infusion at rate adjusted to patient's response.
IV, IM, SUBQ (Children >5 yr or >20 kg): 2 mg/dose; may repeat every 2–3 min.
IV, IM, SUBQ (Infants up to 5 yr or 20 kg): 0.1 mg/kg; may repeat every 2–3 min.
IM, SUBQ, (Adults and Children): *Zimbi:* 5 mg, may repeat every 2–3 min.
Intranasal (Adults and Children): 1 spray (3 mg, 4 mg, 8 mg, or 10 mg) in one nostril; may repeat dose every 2–3 min (with each subsequent dose being administered in alternate nostril).

Opioid-Induced Pruritus

IV (Children): 2 mcg/kg/hr continuous infusion, may ↑ by 0.5 mcg/kg/hr every few hrs if pruritus continues.

Availability (generic available)

Nasal spray: 3 mg/0.1 mL OTC, 4 mg/0.1 mL OTC, 4 mg/0.25 mL, 8 mg/0.1 mL, 10 mg/0.11 mL. **Solution for injection:** 0.4 mg/mL, 2 mg/2 mL (prefilled syringe), 5 mg/0.5 mL (prefilled syringe). ***In combination with:*** buprenorphine (Suboxone, Zubsolv). See Appendix N.

NURSING IMPLICATIONS

Assessment

- Monitor respiratory rate, rhythm, and depth; HR, ECG, and BP; and level of consciousness frequently for 3–4 hr after the expected peak of blood concentrations. After a moderate overdose of a short half-life opioid, physical stimulation may be enough to prevent significant hypoventilation. The effects of some opioids may last longer than the effects of naloxone, and repeat doses may be necessary.
- Patients who have been receiving opioids for >1 wk are extremely sensitive to the effects of naloxone. Dilute and administer in slow increments.

- Assess patient for level of pain after administration when used to treat postoperative respiratory depression. Naloxone ↓ respiratory depression but also reverses analgesia.
- Assess patient for signs and symptoms of opioid withdrawal (restlessness; lacrimation; rhinorrhea; yawning; perspiration; chills; myalgia; mydriasis; irritability; anxiety; backache; joint pain; weakness; abdominal cramps; insomnia; nausea; anorexia; vomiting; diarrhea; or ↑ BP, respiratory rate, or HR). Symptoms may occur within a few min to 2 hr. Severity depends on dose of naloxone, the opioid involved, and degree of physical dependence.
- Lack of significant improvement indicates that symptoms are caused by a disease process or other nonopioid CNS depressants not affected by naloxone.

Toxicity and Overdose

- Naloxone is a pure antagonist with no agonist properties and minimal toxicity.

Implementation

- Do not confuse naloxone with Lanoxin or nalbuphine.
- Larger doses of naloxone may be necessary when used to antagonize the effects of buprenorphine, butorphanol, and nalbuphine.
- Resuscitation equipment, oxygen, vasopressors, and mechanical ventilation should be available to supplement naloxone therapy as needed.
- Doses should be titrated carefully in postoperative patients to avoid interference with control of postoperative pain.
- **Intranasal:** Administer a single spray into one nostril. Do not prime or test the device prior to use. If patient does not respond or responds and relapses into respiratory depression, additional doses may be given every 2–3 min in alternating nostrils until emergency medical assistance arrives. Naloxone is not a substitute for emergency medical care.
- **SUBQ, IM:** Inject into the anterolateral aspect of the thigh with the needle facing downward; inject through clothing if necessary. Push the plunger all the way down until it clicks and hold for 2 seconds after completely embedding needle. Slide the safety guard over the needle immediately after injection.
- Visually inspect the syringe though the viewing window on device; if the solution is discolored yellow or brown color, cloudy, or contains particles, replace with a new one.
- Pedi: Pinch the child's thigh muscle while administering dose.

IV Administration

- **IV Push:** Dilution: Administer undiluted for *suspected opioid overdose*. For *opioid-induced respiratory depression*, dilute with sterile water for injection. For children or adults weighing <40 kg, dilute 0.1 mg of naloxone in 10 mL of sterile water or 0.9% NaCl for injection. **Concentration:** 0.4 mg/mL, 1 mg/mL, or 10 mcg/mL (depending on preparation used). **Rate:** Administer over 30 sec for patients with a *suspected opioid overdose*. For patients who develop *opioid-induced respiratory depression*, administer dilute solution of 0.4 mg/10 mL at a rate of 0.5 mL (0.02 mg) IV push every 2 min. Titrate to avoid withdrawal and severe pain. Excessive dose in postoperative patients may cause excitement, pain, hypotension, hypertension, pulmonary edema, ventricular tachycardia and fibrillation, and seizures. For children and adults weighing <40 kg, administer 10 mcg/mL solution at a rate of 0.5 mcg/kg every 1–2 min.
- **Continuous Infusion: Dilution:** Dilute 2 mg of naloxone in 500 mL of 0.9% NaCl or D5W. Infusion is stable for 24 hr **Concentration:** 4 mcg/mL. **Rate:** Titrate dose according to patient response.
- **Y-Site Compatibility:** acetylcysteine, amikacin, aminocaproic acid, amiodarone, anidulafungin, argatroban, arsenic trioxide, ascorbic acid, atropine, azithromycin, aztreonam, benztropine, bivalirudin, bleomycin, bumetanide, buprenorphine, butorphanol, calcium chloride, calcium gluconate, carboplatin, carmustine, caspofungin, cefotaxime, cefotetan, cefoxitin, ceftazidime, ceftolozane/tazobactam, ceftriaxone, cefuroxime, chlorpromazine, ciprofloxacin, cisplatin, clindamycin, cyanocobalamin, cyclophosphamide, cytarabine, dacarbazine, dactinomycin, daptomycin, daunorubicin, defibrotide, desmopressin, dexamethasone, dexmedetomidine, dexrazoxane, digoxin, diltiazem, diphenhydramine, dobutamine, docetaxel, dopamine, doxorubicin hydrochloride, doxorubicin liposomal, doxycycline, droperidol, enalaprilat, ephedrine, epinephrine, epirubicin, epoetin alfa, eptifibatide, ertapenem, erythromycin, esmolol, etoposide, etoposide phosphate, famotidine, fentanyl, fluconazole, fludarabine, fluorouracil, folic acid, foscarnet, fosphenytoin, furosemide, ganciclovir, gemcitabine, gentamicin, glucagon, glycopyrrolate, granisetron, heparin, hetastarch, hydrocortisone, hydromorphone, idarubicin, ifosfamide, imipenem/cilastatin, indomethacin, insulin regular, irinotecan, isavuconazonium, isoproterenol, ketamine, ketorolac, labetalol, LR, levofloxacin, lidocaine, linezolid, mannitol, meperidine, meropenem, meropenem/vaborbactam, mesna, methadone, methotrexate, methylprednisolone, metoclopramide, metoprolol, metronidazole, midazolam, milrinone, mitoxantrone, morphine,

N

moxifloxacin, multivitamins, mycophenolate, nafcillin, nalbuphine, nicardipine, nitroprusside, norepinephrine, octreotide, ondansetron, oxacillin, oxaliplatin, oxytocin, paclitaxel, palonosetron, pamidronate, papaverine, pemetrexed, penicillin G, pentamidine, pentobarbital, phenobarbital, phentolamine, phenylephrine, phytonadione, piperacillin/tazobactam, plazomicin, potassium acetate, potassium chloride, potassium phosphate, procainamide, prochlorperazine, promethazine, propofol, propranolol, protamine, pyridoxine, rocuronium, sodium acetate, sodium bicarbonate, succinylcholine, sufentanil, tacrolimus, tedizolid, theophylline, thiamine, tigecycline, tirofiban, tobramycin, topotecan, vancomycin, vasopressin, vecuronium, verapamil, vinblastine, vincristine, vinorelbine, voriconazole, zoledronic acid.

- **Y-Site Incompatibility:** alemtuzumab, amphotericin B liposomal, blinatumomab, dantrolene, diazepam, gemtuzumab ozogamicin, leucovorin calcium, mitomycin, pantoprazole, phenytoin, thiotepa.

Patient/Family Teaching

- As medication becomes effective, explain purpose and effects of naloxone to patient. Advise patient to read *Medication Guide* periodically during therapy in case of changes.
- Advise patient and caregiver that symptoms of opioid withdrawal may occur in physically dependent patients, including neonates.
- Educate patients and caregivers on how to recognize respiratory depression and emphasize the importance of calling 911 or getting emergency medical help right away in the event of a known or suspected overdose. Inform patients and caregivers about various ways to obtain naloxone as permitted by individual state naloxone dispensing and prescribing requirements or guidelines (Rx, direct from pharmacist, or state programs). OTC nasal spray is available at pharmacies nationwide for overdose or accidental ingestion.
- **Intranasal:** Instruct parents and caregivers in the correct technique for use and to seek emergency medical care immediately after use. Keep the patient under continued surveillance and to administer additional doses every 2–3 min, if necessary, until emergency care arrives.
- Intranasal side effects may include hypotension, musculoskeletal pain, headache, abdominal pain, asthenia, dizziness, headache, presyncope, nasal discomfort, dryness, edema, congestion, and inflammation.
- Rep: Advise females of reproductive potential to notify health care professional if pregnancy is planned or suspected or if breastfeeding. Monitor mother and fetus for withdrawal syndrome if mother is opioid dependent.

Evaluation/Desired Outcomes

- Adequate ventilation following opioid excess.
- Alertness without significant pain or withdrawal symptoms.
- Reversal of CNS depression and respiratory depression because of suspected opioid overdose.

naltrexone (oral) (nal-**trex**-one)

ReVia

naltrexone (injection)

Vivitrol

Classification

Therapeutic: alcohol abuse therapy adjuncts

Pharmacologic: opioid antagonists

Indications

Opioid dependence. Alcohol dependence.

Action

Competitively blocks the effects of opioids, including CNS and respiratory depression, without producing any agonist (opioid-like) effects. Mechanism in managing alcohol dependence may involve the endogenous opioid system. **Therapeutic Effects:** Blocks the effects of opioids in previously dependent patients. Reduced alcohol-dependent behavior.

Pharmacokinetics

Absorption: Well absorbed orally, but undergoes extensive first-pass hepatic metabolism, resulting in 5–40% bioavailability. Well absorbed following IM administration.

Distribution: Widely distributed to tissues.

Metabolism and Excretion: Extensively metabolized by the liver. Major metabolite (6-beta-naltrexol) has opioid antagonist activity. Metabolites are excreted in urine.

Half-life: Oral: *Naltrexone:* 4 hr; *6-beta-naltrexol:* 13 hr; IM: *Naltrexone:* 5–10 days; *6-beta-naltrexol:* 5–10 days.

TIME/ACTION PROFILE (opioid blockade)

ROUTE	ONSET	PEAK	DURATION
50 mg PO	5 min–1 hr†	unknown	24 hr†
100 mg PO	5 min–1 hr†	unknown	48 hr†
150 mg PO	5 min–1 hr†	unknown	72 hr†
IM	unknown	unknown	4 wk

† Determined by blockade of effects of 25 mg heroin IV.

Contraindications/Precautions

Contraindicated in: Hypersensitivity; Concurrent use of opioid analgesics or physiologic opioid dependence; Acute opioid withdrawal; Positive urine screen for opioids; Failure of a naloxone challenge test.

Use Cautiously in: History of depression or suicidal behavior/attempt; Moderate or severe renal impairment; History of hepatic impairment; OB: Use during pregnancy only if potential maternal benefit justifies potential fetal risk; Lactation: Use while breastfeeding only if potential maternal benefit justifies potential risk to infant; Pedi: Safety and effectiveness not established in children.

Adverse Reactions/Side Effects

CV: palpitations. **Derm:** rash. **EENT:** hoarseness, runny/stuffy nose, sinus problems, sneezing. **F and E:** ↑ thirst. **GI:** abdominal cramps/pain, nausea, ↓ appetite, constipation, diarrhea, HEPATOTOXICITY, vomiting. **GU:** delayed ejaculation, erectile dysfunction. **Hemat:** eosinophilia, thrombocytopenia. **Local:** injection site reactions. **MS:** joint pain, muscle pain. **Neuro:** anxiety, fatigue, headache, insomnia, nervousness, ↑ energy, depression, dizziness, sedation, SUICIDAL THOUGHTS/BEHAVIOR. **Resp:** EOSINOPHILIC PNEUMONIA (INJECTION), cough. **Misc:** chills.

Interactions

Drug-Drug: Thioridazine may ↑ risk of CNS depression. May prevent therapeutic effects of **opioid analgesics**, **antidiarrheals**, and **antitussives**.

Route/Dosage

Opioid Dependence

PO (Adults): Following a negative naloxone challenge and 7–10 days of opioid abstinence (longer for methadone), initial dose is 25 mg. If opioid withdrawal does not occur within 1 hr, additional 25 may be given. Maintenance dose is 50 mg once daily *or* 50 mg once daily on weekdays and 100 mg on Saturday *or* 100 mg every other day *or* 150 mg every 3rd day *or* 100 mg on Monday and Wednesday and 150 mg on Friday.
IM (Adults): 380 mg every 4 wk or once monthly.

Alcohol Dependence

PO (Adults): 50 mg once daily *or* 50 mg once daily on weekdays and 100 mg on Saturday *or* 100 mg every other day *or* 150 mg every third day *or* 100 mg on Monday and Wednesday and 150 mg on Friday.
IM (Adults): 380 mg every 4 wk or once monthly.

Availability (generic available)

Tablets: 50 mg. **Suspension for injection:** 380 mg/vial.

NURSING IMPLICATIONS

Assessment

- Assess patient from last time opioids or alcohol were taken. Patient must be free from opioids for 7–10 days prior to initiation of therapy. Does not eliminate withdrawal symptoms (anxiety, sleeplessness, yawning, fever, sweating, teary eyes, runny nose, goose bumps, shakiness, hot or cold flushes, muscle aches, muscle twitches, restlessness, nausea and vomiting, diarrhea, stomach cramps). If physical dependence on opioids is possible, a *Naloxone Challenge Test* should be used. Patients transitioning from buprenorphine, buprenorphine/naloxone, or methadone are also at risk for developing withdrawal symptoms.
- Monitor mental status, mood changes, and affect. Monitor closely for changes in behavior that could indicate the emergence or worsening of suicidal thoughts or behavior or depression.
- Assess for signs of eosinophilic pneumonia (dyspnea, hypoxia, coughing, wheezing). Advise patient to seek treatment immediately if these symptoms occur.

Lab Test Considerations

- May ↑ liver enzymes; monitor periodically during therapy.
- May ↑ eosinophils and ↓ platelets.

Implementation

- Should be used in conjunction with a comprehensive alcohol or drug program. Patient should not be actively drinking at the time of naltrexone initiation.
- If emergent analgesia is required for pain management, regional analgesia, conscious sedation with a benzodiazepine, and use of nonopioid analgesics or general anesthesia are recommended. If opioid analgesics are required, the amount may be greater than usual and the respiratory depression deeper and more prolonged. A rapidly acting opioid that minimizes the duration of respiratory depression is recommended.
- **PO:** Administer as directed. A number of dose schedules have been used.
- **IM:** Must be administered by a health care provider every 4 wk or once a month. Suspend using only diluent and needle supplied. A spare administration needle is provide in case of clogging. Do not substitute other components. Allow drug to reach room temperature, approximately 45 min, before preparing. To ease mixing, firmly tap vial on a hard surface, ensuring powder moves freely. Using the ½-inch preparation needle, withdraw 3.4 mL of clear diluent and inject into microsphere vial. Mix by shaking vigorously for approximately 1 min. Suspension is milky white without clumps and moving freely up and down the wall of the vial. Immediately after suspension, withdraw 4.2 mL of suspension using same preparation needle. Remove preparation needle and replace with 1½- or 2-inch administration needle for immediate use. Prior to administration, tap syringe to release any bubbles; then gently push

N

plunger until 4 mL of suspension remains in syringe. Activate safety sheath by pressing against hard surface to cover needle. Store in refrigerator; do not freeze. May be kept at room temperature for 7 days.

- Administer as a deep IM injection into the gluteal muscle using prepackaged 1½- or 2-inch needle specifically designed for this drug. Avoid IV or SUBQ use or administration into fatty tissue.
- If a dose is missed, patient should receive dose as soon as possible.

Patient/Family Teaching

- Explain the purpose and side effects of naltrexone. Instruct patient to take as directed. Do not stop receiving naltrexone without consulting health care provider. Inform patients that there are potentially serious consequences and possibly death if they try to overcome the effects of naltrexone with higher doses of opioids. Do not share medication with others, even if they have similar symptoms; may be harmful. Keep out of childrencs reach. Advise patient to read *Patient Information* before starting and with each Rx refill in case of changes.
- May cause injection site reactions (cellulitis, induration, hematoma, abscess, sterile abscess, necrosis). Advise patient to monitor injection site and notify health care provider if pain, swelling, tenderness, induration, bruising, pruritus, or redness at the injection site occurs and does not improve or worsens within 2 wk. Promptly refer patients with worsening injection site reactions to a surgeon.
- May cause dizziness. Advise patient to avoid driving and other activities requiring alertness until effects of the medication are known.
- Encourage patient and family to be alert for emergence of anxiety, agitation, panic attacks, insomnia, irritability, hostility, impulsivity, akathisia, hypomania, mania, worsening of depression, and suicidal ideation, especially during early antidepressant therapy. Assess symptoms on a day-to-day basis as changes may be abrupt. If these symptoms occur, notify health care provider.
- Advise patient to immediately report signs and symptoms of hepatotoxicity (fatigue, nausea, upper abdominal pain, yellowing of skin or eyes, dark urine, light-colored stools); naltrexone should be discontinued.
- Advise patient and family that patient may be more sensitive to lower doses of opioids after naltrexone treatment stops, when next dose is due, and if a dose is missed. Advise patients that they will not perceive any effects of small doses of opioids and may not experience the same effects from opioid-containing analgesics, antidiarrheals, or antitussives. May lead to overdose, including serious injury, coma, or death.
- Educate patients and caregivers on how to recognize respiratory depression and emphasize the importance of calling 911 or getting emergency medical help right away in the event of a known or suspected overdose. Inform patients and caregivers about various ways to obtain naloxone as permitted by individual state naloxone dispensing and prescribing requirements or guidelines (by prescription, directly from a pharmacist, or as part of a community-based program).
- Advise patient to notify health care provider of medication regimen prior to treatment or surgery. Medical ID describing medication regimen should be carried in case of emergencies.
- Advise patient to notify health care provider of all Rx or OTC medications, vitamins, or herbal products being taken and to consult with health care provider before taking other medications.
- Rep: Advise women of reproductive potential to notify health care provider if pregnancy is planned or suspected or if breastfeeding.

Evaluation/Desired Outcomes

- The blockade of the effects of exogenously administered opioids.
- Management of alcoholism.

BEERS

naproxen (na-prox-en)

Aleve, Anaprox, Anaprox DS, EC-Naprosyn, Naprelan, Naprosyn

Classification

Therapeutic: antipyretics, antirheumatics nonopioid analgesics

Pharmacologic: nonsteroidal anti-inflammatory drugs (NSAIDs)

Indications

Mild to moderate pain. Dysmenorrhea. Fever. Inflammatory disorders, including: Rheumatoid arthritis, Osteoarthritis.

Action

Inhibits prostaglandin synthesis. **Therapeutic Effects:** Decreased pain. Reduction of fever. Suppression of inflammation.

Pharmacokinetics

Absorption: Completely absorbed from the GI tract. Sodium salt is more rapidly absorbed.

Distribution: Well distributed to tissues.

Protein Binding: >99%.

Metabolism and Excretion: Mostly metabolized by the liver.

Half-life: *Children <8 yr:* 8–17 hr; *Children 8–14 yr:* 8–10 hr; *Adults:* 10–20 hr.

TIME/ACTION PROFILE

ROUTE	ONSET	PEAK	DURATION
PO (analgesic)	1 hr	unknown	8–12 hr
PO (anti-inflammatory)	14 days	2–4 wk	unknown

Contraindications/Precautions

Contraindicated in: Hypersensitivity; Cross-sensitivity may occur with other NSAIDs, including aspirin; Active GI bleeding; Ulcer disease; Coronary artery bypass graft surgery; Recent MI; HF; OB: Avoid use after 30 wk gestation; Lactation: Lactation.

Use Cautiously in: Cardiovascular disease or risk factors for cardiovascular disease (may ↑ risk of serious cardiovascular thrombotic events, MI, and stroke, especially with prolonged use or use of higher doses); History of long duration of NSAID use, smoking, alcohol use, advanced liver disease, coagulopathy, or poor general health (↑ risk of GI bleeding); History of peptic ulcer disease and/or GI bleeding; Bleeding tendency or concurrent anticoagulant therapy; Chronic alcohol use/abuse; Severe renal impairment; Severe hepatic impairment; OB: Use at or after 20 wk gestation may cause fetal or neonatal renal impairment; if treatment is necessary between 20 wk and 30 wk gestation, limit use to the lowest effective dose and shortest duration possible; Pedi: Children <2 yr (safety and effectiveness not established); Geri: Appears on Beers list. ↑ risk GI bleeding or peptic ulcer disease in older adults. Avoid chronic use unless other alternatives are not effective and the patient can take a gastroprotective agent; avoid short-term use in combination with oral or parenteral corticosteroids, anticoagulants, or antiplatelet agents unless other alternatives are not effective and the patient can take a gastroprotective agent.

Adverse Reactions/Side Effects

CV: edema, HF, hypertension, MI, palpitations, tachycardia. **Derm:** ↑ sweating, DRUG REACTION WITH EOSINOPHILIA AND SYSTEMIC SYMPTOMS (DRESS), EXFOLIATIVE DERMATITIS, rash, GENERALIZED BULLOUS FIXED DRUG ERUPTION, photosensitivity, pseudoporphyria (↑ in children with juvenile rheumatoid arthritis), rash, STEVENS-JOHNSON SYNDROME (SJS), TOXIC EPIDERMAL NECROLYSIS (TEN). **EENT:** tinnitus, visual disturbances. **F and E:** hyperkalemia. **GI:** constipation, dyspepsia, nausea, anorexia, diarrhea, discomfort, flatulence, GI BLEEDING, GI PERFORATION, GI ULCERATION, HEPATITIS, vomiting. **GU:** cystitis, hematuria, renal failure. **Hemat:** blood dyscrasias, prolonged bleeding time. **Neuro:** dizziness, drowsiness, headache, STROKE. **Resp:** dyspnea. **Misc:** HYPERSENSITIVITY REACTIONS (INCLUDING ANAPHYLAXIS AND SERIOUS SKIN REACTIONS).

Interactions

Drug-Drug: May limit the cardioprotective (antiplatelet) effects of **aspirin**. ↑ risk of GI bleeding with **anticoagulants, aspirin, clopidogrel, ticagrelor, prasugrel, corticosteroids, fibrinolytics, SNRIs,** or **SSRIs**. **Probenecid** may ↑ levels and risk of toxicity. May ↑ risk of toxicity from **methotrexate**, **antineoplastics**, or **radiation therapy**. May ↑ levels and risk of toxicity of **lithium**. ↑ risk of nephrotoxicity with **cyclosporine**, **ACE inhibitors**, **angiotensin II antagonists**, or chronic use of **acetaminophen**. May ↓ effectiveness of **antihypertensives** or **diuretics**. May ↑ risk of hypoglycemia with **insulin** or **oral hypoglycemic agents**. **Oral potassium supplements** may ↑ GI adverse effects.

Drug-Natural Products: ↑ risk of bleeding with **anise**, **arnica**, **chamomile**, **clove**, **dong quai**, **feverfew**, **garlic**, **ginger**, **ginkgo**, **Panax ginseng**, and **licorice**.

Route/Dosage

275 mg naproxen sodium is equivalent to 250 mg naproxen.

Anti-inflammatory/Analgesic/Antidysmenorrheal

PO (Adults): *Naproxen:* 250–500 mg twice daily (up to 1.5 g/day). *Delayed-release naproxen:* 375–500 mg twice daily. *Naproxen sodium:* 275–550 mg twice daily (up to 1.65 g/day).

PO (Children >2 yr): *Analgesia:* 5–7 mg/kg/dose every 8–12 hr. *Inflammatory disease:* 10–15 mg/kg/day divided every 12 hr, maximum: 1000 mg/day.

Gout

PO (Adults): *Naproxen:* 750 mg initially, then 250 mg every 8 hr. *Naproxen sodium:* 825 mg initially, then 275 mg every 8 hr.

OTC Use (Naproxen Sodium)

PO (Adults): 200 mg every 8–12 hr or 400 mg followed by 200 mg every 12 hr (not to exceed 600 mg/24 hr).

PO (Geriatric Patients >65 yr): Not to exceed 200 mg every 12 hr.

Availability

Naproxen (generic available)

Immediate-release tablets (Naprosyn): ✱ 125 mg, 250 mg, 375 mg, 500 mg. **Delayed-release tablets (EC-Naprosyn):** 375 mg, 500 mg. **Extended-release tablets:** ✱ 750 mg. **Oral suspension (Naprosyn):** 125 mg/5 mL. ***In combination with:*** esomeprazole (Vimovo).

Naproxen Sodium (generic available)

Immediate-release tablets (Aleve, Anaprox DS): 220 mg^OTC, 275 mg, 550 mg. **Immediate-release capsules (Maxidol):** ✱ 220 mg^OTC. **Extended-release tablets (Naprelan):** 375 mg, 500 mg, 750 mg. ***In combination with:*** pseudoephedrine (Aleve-D Sinus and Cold), sumatriptan (Treximet). See Appendix N.

NURSING IMPLICATIONS

Assessment

- Patients who have asthma, aspirin-induced allergy, and nasal polyps are at ↑ risk for developing hypersensitivity reactions. Assess for rhinitis, asthma, and urticaria.
- Monitor BP during initiation and periodically during therapy. May cause fluid retention and edema leading to new onset or worsening hypertension.
- Assess for signs and symptoms of HF (dyspnea, peripheral edema, rales/crackles, jugular venous distension) during therapy.
- Monitor patients for development of severe cutaneous adverse reactions, including exfoliative dermatitis, SJS, and TEN, including signs and symptoms of prodrome of fever, malaise, mucosal lesions, progressive skin rash, blisters, lymphadenopathy, conjunctivitis, myalgias, hepatitis, or eosinophilia. *If a severe cutaneous adverse reaction is suspected,* interrupt therapy until etiology of reaction is determined. Consultation with a dermatologist is recommended. If a severe cutaneous adverse reaction is confirmed, permanently discontinue naproxen.
- Monitor for signs and symptoms of DRESS (fever, rash, lymphadenopathy, facial swelling) periodically during therapy. *If signs/symptoms of DRESS occur,* discontinue naproxen.
- Monitor for signs/symptoms of GI bleeding, ulceration, or perforation (fatigue, weakness, pallor, hematochezia, melena, coffee ground emesis, hematemesis, abdominal pain or distention) especially with prolonged therapy.
- **Pain:** Assess pain (note type, location, and intensity) prior to and 1–2 hr following administration.
- **Arthritis:** Assess pain and range of motion prior to and 1–2 hr following administration.
- **Fever:** Monitor temperature; note signs associated with fever (diaphoresis, tachycardia, malaise).

Lab Test Considerations

- Evaluate BUN, serum creatinine, CBC, and liver function tests periodically in patients receiving prolonged therapy. May ↑ serum potassium, BUN, serum creatinine, alkaline phosphatase, LDH, AST, and ALT. May ↓ blood glucose, hemoglobin, hematocrit, WBCs, and platelets.
- May ↓ C-reactive protein levels and erythrocyte sedimentation rate in patients with rheumatoid arthritis.
- Bleeding time may be prolonged up to 4 days following discontinuation of therapy.
- May alter test results for urine 5-HIAA and urine steroid determinations.

Implementation

- Administration in higher than recommended doses does not provide ↑ effectiveness but may cause ↑ risk of side effects. Use lowest effective dose for the shortest duration possible to minimize risk of cardiovascular thrombotic events.
- Coadministration with opioid analgesics may have additive analgesic effects and may permit lower opioid doses.
- Naproxen is more effective if given before pain becomes severe.
- **PO:** For rapid initial effect, administer 30 min before or 2 hr after meals. May be administered with food, milk, or antacids to ↓ GI irritation. Food slows but does not ↓ the extent of absorption. ***DNC:*** Swallow extended-release, delayed-release, and controlled-release tablets whole; do not break, crush, or chew.
- **Dysmenorrhea:** Administer as soon as possible after the onset of menses. Prophylactic treatment has not been shown to be effective.

Patient/Family Teaching

- Explain the purpose and side effects of naproxen. Instruct patient to take medication as directed. Take missed doses as soon as remembered but not if almost time for the next dose. Do not double doses. Advise patient to read *Patient Information* before starting and with each Rx refill in case of changes.
- Advise patient to take this medication with a full glass of water and to remain in an upright position for 15–30 min after administration.
- Instruct patient not to take OTC naproxen preparations for >3 days for fever and to consult health care provider if symptoms persist or worsen.
- May cause drowsiness or dizziness. Advise patient to avoid driving or other activities requiring alertness until response to the medication is known.
- Advise patient to notify health care provider of all Rx or OTC medications, vitamins, or herbal products being taken and to consult with health care provider before taking other medications.
- Inform patient of ↑ risk of MI and stroke. Use lowest effective dose for shortest time. Advise patient to notify health care provider immediately if signs and symptoms (shortness of breath or trouble breathing, chest pain, weakness in one part or side of body, slurred speech, swelling of the face or throat) occur.
- Advise patient to notify health care provider promptly if signs or symptoms of GI toxicity (abdominal pain, black stools) occur.
- Caution patient to avoid the concurrent use of alcohol, aspirin, acetaminophen, or other OTC medications without consulting health care provider. Use of naproxen with ≥3 glasses of alcohol per day may ↑ risk of GI bleeding.
- Advise patient to inform health care provider of medication regimen prior to treatment or surgery.
- Caution patient to wear sunscreen and protective clothing to prevent photosensitivity reactions

(especially in children with juvenile rheumatoid arthritis).
- Advise patient to consult health care provider if rash, itching, visual disturbances, tinnitus, weight gain, edema, persistent headache, or flu-like syndrome (chills, fever, muscle aches, pain) occurs.
- Rep: May cause fetal harm. Advise women of reproductive potential to notify health care provider if pregnancy is planned or suspected or if breastfeeding. Advise women to avoid naproxen in the 3rd trimester of pregnancy (after 29 wk); may cause premature closure of the fetal ductus arteriosus. Use of naproxen after 20 wk may cause fetal renal impairment, leading to oligohydramnios. May cause reversible infertility in women attempting to conceive; may consider discontinuing naproxen.

Evaluation/Desired Outcomes
- Relief of pain.
- Improved joint mobility. Partial arthritic relief is usually seen within 2 wk, but maximum effectiveness may require 2–4 wk of continuous therapy. Patients who do not respond to one NSAID may respond to another.
- Reduction of fever.

REMS

natalizumab
(na-ta-li-zoo-mab)

Tyruko, Tysabri

Classification

Therapeutic: anti-multiple sclerosis agents, gastrointestinal anti-inflammatories

Pharmacologic: monoclonal antibodies

Indications
Relapsing forms of multiple sclerosis (MS), including clinically isolated syndrome, relapsing-remitting disease, and active secondary progressive disease (as monotherapy). Moderately to severely active Crohn disease in patients who have been unresponsive to conventional therapies, including tumor-necrosis factor inhibitors.

Action
Binds to integrin receptors on non-neutrophil leukocytes, which may alter adhesion and migration characteristics involved in the crossing of activated inflammatory cells into the CNS. **Therapeutic Effects:** Fewer exacerbations of relapsing MS. Induction and maintenance of remission in Crohn disease.

Pharmacokinetics
Absorption: IV administration results in complete bioavailability.
Distribution: Unknown.
Metabolism and Excretion: Unknown.
Half-life: 7–15 days.

TIME/ACTION PROFILE

ROUTE	ONSET	PEAK	DURATION
IV	unknown	unknown	unknown

Contraindications/Precautions
Contraindicated in: Hypersensitivity; History of progressive multifocal leukoencephalopathy (PML).
Use Cautiously in: Anti-JC virus antibody positive (↑ risk of PML); Prior use of immunosuppressants (↑ risk of PML); OB: Neonatal thrombocytopenia and anemia may occur in newborns with in utero exposure; Lactation: Use while breastfeeding only if potential maternal benefit justifies potential risk to infant; Pedi: Safety and effectiveness not established in children.

N

Adverse Reactions/Side Effects
Derm: MELANOMA. **EENT:** acute retinal necrosis (caused by herpes simplex virus and varicella zoster virus). **GI:** cholelithiasis, HEPATOTOXICITY. **Hemat:** immune thrombocytopenic purpura, thrombocytopenia. **Neuro:** depression, ENCEPHALITIS (CAUSED BY HERPES SIMPLEX VIRUS AND VARICELLA ZOSTER VIRUS), fatigue, JC virus granule cell neuronopathy, MENINGITIS (CAUSED BY HERPES SIMPLEX VIRUS AND VARICELLA ZOSTER VIRUS), PML. **Misc:** <u>HYPERSENSITIVITY REACTIONS (INCLUDING ANAPHYLAXIS)</u>, INFECTION, infusion-related reactions.

Interactions
Drug-Drug: ↑ risk of infection with **immunosuppressants** and **tumor necrosis factor inhibitors**; avoid concurrent use.

Route/Dosage
Multiple Sclerosis
IV (Adults): 300 mg every 4 wk.

Crohn Disease
IV (Adults): 300 mg every 4 wk; if no response after 12 wk or if patient cannot be tapered off corticosteroid therapy after 6 mo, discontinue therapy.

Availability
Solution for injection: 20 mg/mL.

NURSING IMPLICATIONS
Assessment
- Observe patient during infusion and for 1 hr after infusion is completed. For patients who have received

12 infusions without evidence of a hypersensitivity reaction, observe patients postinfusion for any subsequent infusions according to clinical judgment. During the infusion and postinfusion, assess for signs of hypersensitivity reactions (urticaria, dizziness, fever, rash, rigors, pruritus, nausea, flushing, hypotension, dyspnea, chest pain, anaphylaxis). *If signs/symptoms of hypersensitivity reaction occur,* discontinue natalizumab and treat symptoms.

- Assess for new signs/symptoms suggestive of PML, an opportunistic infection of the brain caused by the JC virus, leading to death or severe disability. Monitor during therapy and for ≥6 mo following discontinuation. PML symptoms may begin gradually but usually worsen rapidly. Symptoms vary depending on which part of the brain is infected (mental function declines rapidly and progressively, causing dementia; speaking becomes increasingly difficult; partial blindness; difficulty walking; headaches; progressive weakness on one side of body; personality changes; seizures) occur. *If signs/symptoms of PML occur,* withhold natalizumab and notify health care provider promptly. Diagnosis is usually made via gadolinium-enhanced MRI and CSF analysis. Risk of PML ↑ with presence of anti-JC virus antibodies and prior use of immunosuppressants and treatment beyond 2 yr.
- Obtain an MRI of the brain before starting therapy to help in differentiating symptoms of MS with those of PML and to identify newly developed lesions in patients with Crohn disease.
- Monitor for signs/symptoms of thrombocytopenia (easy bruising, abnormal bleeding, and petechiae) during therapy. If suspected, discontinue natalizumab promptly.
- **MS:** Assess frequency of exacerbations of symptoms periodically during therapy.
- **Crohn disease:** Assess abdominal pain and frequency, quantity, and consistency of stools at beginning and during therapy.

Lab Test Considerations

- May ↑ lymphocytes, monocytes, eosinophils, basophils, and nucleated RBCs and ↓ hemoglobin; does not usually ↑ neutrophils. These changes occur during therapy but usually return to baseline within 16 wk after last dose.
- May ↑ liver enzymes and total bilirubin; these changes may occur within 6 days after the 1st dose or for the 1st time after multiple doses. *If signs/symptoms of hepatotoxicity occur,* discontinue natalizumab.
- Monitor serum anti-JC virus antibodies periodically during therapy. Patients with a negative antibody should be retested periodically during therapy due to potential for false-positive results or a new infection. Wait ≥6 mo after patient receives IVIG in order to avoid false-positive results.

Implementation

IV Administration

- **Intermittent Infusion:** Dilution: Dilute 300 mg in 100 mL of 0.9% NaCl. Invert to mix solution; do not shake. Do not mix with other diluents. Solution is colorless and clear to slightly opalescent. Do not administer solutions that are discolored or contain particulate matter. Administer immediately after dilution or refrigerate and use within 48 hr. Concentration: 2.6 mg/mL. Rate: Infuse over 1 hr.
- **Y-Site Incompatibility:** Do not administer other drugs through same IV line.

Patient/Family Teaching

- Explain purpose and side effects of medication. Advise patient to read *Patient Information* before starting therapy. Patients must visit their health care provider/prescriber 3 and 6 mo after 1st infusion and every 6 mo thereafter for follow-up exam.
- Advise patient to notify health care provider of all Rx or OTC medications, vitamins, or herbal products being taken and to consult with health care provider before taking other medications.
- ***REMS:*** Instruct patient to read the *Medication Guide* before starting the infusion. Natalizumab is available only through a special restricted distribution program called the TOUCH® Prescribing Program, MS-TOUCH for multiple sclerosis and CD-TOUCH for Crohn disease and must be administered only to patients enrolled in this program.
- Instruct patient to report symptoms of PML (progressive weakness on one side of the body or clumsiness of limbs; disturbance of vision; changes in thinking, memory, and orientation, leading to confusion and personality changes), hypersensitivity reactions, hepatotoxicity (yellowing of the skin and eyes, unusual darkening of the urine, nausea, feeling tired or weak, vomiting), thrombocytopenia (easy bruising, prolonged bleeding from cuts, petechiae, abnormally heavy menstrual periods, new bleeding from the nose or gums), or worsening of symptoms (new or sudden change in thinking, eyesight, balance, or strength or other problems) that persist over several days to health care provider immediately.
- Instruct patient to inform all health care providers about treatment with natalizumab.
- Rep: Advise women of reproductive potential to notify health care provider if pregnancy is planned or suspected or if breastfeeding. Neonatal thrombocytopenia and anemia may occur in newborns exposed to natalizumab during pregnancy. Monitor CBC in newborns exposed to natalizumab in utero.

Evaluation/Desired Outcomes

- Fewer exacerbations of relapsing MS.
- Induction and maintenance of remission in Crohn disease.

nebivolol, See BETA BLOCKERS (selective).

neomycin, See AMINOGLYCOSIDES.

netupitant/palonosetron (oral)

(ne-**too**-pi-tant/pa-lone-**o**-se-tron)

Akynzeo

fosnetupitant/palonosetron (injection)

(fos-ne-**too**-pi-tant/pa-lone-**o**-se-tron)

Akynzeo

Classification

Therapeutic: antiemetics

Pharmacologic: neurokinin antagonists, 5-HT_3 antagonists

Indications

PO: Prevention of acute and delayed nausea and vomiting associated with initial and repeat courses of cancer chemotherapy, including but not limited to highly emetogenic chemotherapy (in combination with dexamethasone). **IV:** Prevention of acute and delayed nausea and vomiting associated with initial and repeat courses of highly emetogenic chemotherapy (in combination with dexamethasone).

Action

Netupitant: Acts as a selective antagonist at substance P/neurokinin 1 (NK1) receptors in the CNS; prevents nausea and vomiting in the acute and delayed phases after chemotherapy. *Palonosetron:* Blocks the effects of serotonin at receptor sites (selective antagonist) located in vagal nerve terminals and in the chemoreceptor trigger zones in the CNS; prevents nausea and vomiting in the acute phase. **Therapeutic Effects:** Decreased incidence and severity of nausea and vomiting following emetogenic chemotherapy.

Pharmacokinetics

Netupitant

Absorption: Extent of absorption following oral administration unknown.

Distribution: Extensively distributed to tissues.

Protein Binding: >99.5%.

Metabolism and Excretion: Primarily metabolized in the liver via the CYP3A4 isoenzyme and to a lesser extent by the CYP2C9 and CYP2D6 isoenzymes to three metabolites that have antiemetic activity; <1% excreted unchanged in urine.

Half-life: 80 hr.

Fosnetupitant

Absorption: Following IV administration, fosnetupitant is rapidly converted to netupitant, the active component. IV administration results in complete bioavailability.

Distribution: Extensively distributed to tissues.

Protein Binding: 92–95%.

Metabolism and Excretion: Netupitant is primarily metabolized in the liver via the CYP3A4 isoenzyme and to a lesser extent by the CYP2C9 and CYP2D6 isoenzymes to three metabolites that have antiemetic activity; <1% excreted unchanged in urine.

Half-life: *Netupitant:* 80 hr.

Palonosetron

Absorption: 97% absorbed following oral administration. IV administration results in complete bioavailability.

Distribution: Extensively distributed to tissues.

Metabolism and Excretion: 50% metabolized by the liver (mostly by the CYP2D6 isoenzyme) and to a lesser extent by the CYP3A4 and CYP1A2 isoenzymes; 40% excreted unchanged in urine.

Half-life: 40 hr.

TIME/ACTION PROFILE (plasma concentrations)

ROUTE	ONSET	PEAK	DURATION
PO	within 1 hr	5 hr	unknown
IV	rapid	30 min	unknown

Contraindications/Precautions

Contraindicated in: Cross-sensitivity may occur with other 5-HT_3 antagonists; Severe renal impairment; Severe hepatic impairment.

Use Cautiously in: OB: Safety not established in pregnancy; Lactation: Safety not established in breastfeeding; Pedi: Safety and effectiveness not established in children; Geri: Consider age-related ↓ in renal, hepatic, and cardiac function; concurrent disease states; and drug therapies in older adults.

Adverse Reactions/Side Effects

Derm: erythema. **GI:** constipation, dyspepsia. **Neuro:** fatigue, headache, weakness. **Misc:** HYPERSENSITIVITY REACTIONS (INCLUDING ANAPHYLAXIS), SEROTONIN SYNDROME.

N

Interactions

Drug-Drug: Netupitant is a moderate inhibitor of CYP3A4 and can ↑ levels of drugs that are **CYP3A4 substrates**, including **alprazolam**, **cyclophosphamide**, **dexamethasone**, **docetaxel**, **etoposide**, **ifosfamide**, **imatinib**, **irinotecan**, **midazolam**, **erythromycin**, **paclitaxel**, **triazolam**, **vinorelbine**, **vinblastine**, and **vincristine**; avoid concomitant use for one wk; if avoiding use not feasible, ↓ dose of CYP3A4 substrate. **CYP3A4 inducers**, including **rifampin**, may ↓ netupitant levels and effectiveness; avoid concurrent use. Drugs that affect serotonergic neurotransmitter systems, including **tricyclic antidepressants**, **SNRIs**, **fentanyl**, **buspirone**, **tramadol**, **amphetamines**, and **triptans**, ↑ risk of serotonin syndrome

Route/Dosage

Netupitant/Palonosetron

PO (Adults): *Highly emetogenic chemotherapy (included cisplatin-based):* One capsule (netupitant 300 mg/palonosetron 0.5 mg) 1 hr before chemotherapy on day 1. *Anthracycline- and cyclophosphamide-based chemotherapy and other chemotherapy not considered highly emetogenic:* One capsule (netupitant 300 mg/palonosetron 0.5 mg) 1 hr before chemotherapy on day 1.

Fosnetupitant/Palonosetron

IV (Adults): *Highly emetogenic chemotherapy (included cisplatin-based):* Fosnetupitant 235 mg/palonosetron 0.25 mg administered 30 min before chemotherapy on day 1.

Availability

Capsules: netupitant 300 mg/palonosetron 0.5 mg. **Solution for injection:** fosnetupitant 235 mg/palonosetron 0.25 mg/20 mL.

NURSING IMPLICATIONS

Assessment

- Assess patient for nausea, vomiting, abdominal distention, and bowel sounds prior to and following administration.
- Assess for serotonin syndrome (agitation, hallucinations, delirium, coma, autonomic instability, tremor, muscular rigidity, myoclonus, hyperreflexia, incoordination, seizure, GI symptoms), especially in patients taking other serotonergic drugs (SSRIs, SNRIs, triptans).

Lab Test Considerations

- May cause transient ↑ in serum bilirubin, AST, and ALT levels.

Implementation

- *For highly emetogenic chemotherapy,* administer with dexamethasone PO 12 mg 30 min prior to chemotherapy on day 1 and 8 mg PO on days 2 and 4. *For chemotherapy not considered highly emetogenic,* administer dexamethasone 30 min prior to chemotherapy on day 1 (day 2 and 4 not needed).
- **PO:** Administer netupitant/palonosetron 1 hr prior to start of chemotherapy without regard to food.

IV Administration

- **Intermittent Infusion: Dilution:** Prepare an infusion vial or bag with 30 mL D5W or 0.9% NaCl. Withdraw entire volume of *to-be-diluted vial* and transfer into prepared infusion vial or bag for a total volume of 50 mL. Gently invert bag until combined. Store final diluted solution at room temperature. Dexamethasone can be given concomitantly or added to solution.
- Ready-to-use solution does not require dilution. Insert vented IV set through vial septum and use immediately once punctured. Do not add dexamethasone to the ready-to-use injection. **Rate:** Infuse over 30 min starting 30 min before chemotherapy. At end of infusion, flush line with the same carrier solution to ensure complete drug administration.
- **Y-Site Compatibility:** dexamethasone.
- **Y-Site Incompatibility:** solutions containing calcium, solutions containing magnesium, LR, Hartmann's solution.

Patient/Family Teaching

- Instruct patient to take netupitant/palonosetron as directed. Advise patient to read *Patient Information* prior to starting therapy and with each Rx refill in case of changes.
- Advise patient to notify health care professional promptly if signs and symptoms of anaphylaxis (shortness of breath; rash; hives; swelling of mouth, throat, and lips) or serotonin syndrome occur.
- Instruct patient to notify health care professional of all Rx or OTC medications, vitamins, or herbal products being taken and consult health care professional before taking any new medications.
- Rep: May cause fetal harm. Advise females of reproductive potential to notify health care professional if pregnancy is planned or suspected or if breastfeeding.

Evaluation/Desired Outcomes

- Decrease in frequency and severity of nausea and vomiting.

niCARdipine, See CALCIUM CHANNEL BLOCKERS.

NICOTINE (nik-o-teen)

nicotine chewing gum

Nicorette

nicotine lozenge

Nicorette

nicotine nasal spray
Nicotrol NS
nicotine transdermal patch
Habitrol, Nicoderm CQ
Classification
Therapeutic: smoking deterrents

Indications
Nicotine withdrawal in patients desiring to give up cigarette smoking (as adjunct therapy with behavior modification).

Action
Provides a source of nicotine during controlled withdrawal from cigarette smoking. **Therapeutic Effects:** Lessened sequelae of nicotine withdrawal (irritability, insomnia, somnolence, headache, increased appetite).

Pharmacokinetics
Absorption: *Gum, lozenge:* Slowly absorbed from buccal mucosa during chewing/sucking. *Nasal spray:* 53% absorbed from nasal mucosa. *Transdermal:* 70% of nicotine released from the system is absorbed through the skin.
Distribution: Enter breast milk.
Metabolism and Excretion: Mostly metabolized by the liver. Small amounts are metabolized by kidneys and lungs; 10–20% excreted unchanged by kidneys.
Half-life: 1–2 hr.

TIME/ACTION PROFILE (plasma concentrations)

ROUTE	ONSET	PEAK	DURATION
Gum	rapid	15–30 min	unknown
Lozenge	unknown	unknown	unknown
Nasal spray	rapid	4–15 min	unknown
Transdermal	rapid	2–4 hr	unknown

Contraindications/Precautions
Contraindicated in: Hypersensitivity; Recent history of MI (nasal spray); Arrhythmias (nasal spray); Severe or worsening angina (nasal spray); Severe cardiovascular disease; OB: Pregnancy.
Use Cautiously in: Cardiovascular disease (including hypertension); Recent history of MI (gum, lozenge, patch); Arrhythmias (gum, lozenge, patch); Severe or worsening angina (gum, lozenge, patch); Diabetes mellitus; Pheochromocytoma; Peripheral vascular diseases; Hyperthyroidism; Continued smoking; Peptic ulcer disease; Seizures; Hepatic disease; Bronchospastic lung disease (nasal spray); Allergic reaction to adhesive tape (patch); Lactation: Use while breastfeeding only if potential maternal benefit justifies potential risk to infant; Pedi: Safety and effectiveness not established in children; Geri: Begin at lower dosages in older adults.

Adverse Reactions/Side Effects
CV: tachycardia, chest pain, hypertension. **Derm: transdermal:** burning at patch site, erythema, pruritus, cutaneous hypersensitivity, rash, sweating. **EENT:** sinusitis**gum:** pharyngitis**nasal spray:** nasopharyngeal irritation, sneezing, watering eyes, change in smell, earache, epistaxis, eye irritation, hoarseness. **Endo:** dysmenorrhea. **GI:** abdominal pain, abnormal taste, constipation, diarrhea, dry mouth, dyspepsia, hiccups, nausea, vomiting**gum:** ↑ appetite, belching, ↑ salivation, oral injury, sore mouth. **MS:** arthralgia, back pain, myalgia**gum:** jaw muscle ache. **Neuro:** paresthesia, headache, insomnia, abnormal dreams, dizziness, drowsiness, impaired concentration, nervousness, seizures, weakness. **Resp: Nasal spray:** cough, dyspnea.

Interactions
Drug-Drug: Effects of **acetaminophen**, **caffeine**, **imipramine**, **insulin**, **oxazepam**, **propranolol**, other **beta blockers**, **adrenergic antagonists** (**prazosin**, **labetalol**), and **theophylline** may be ↑ upon smoking cessation; dose ↓ at cessation may be necessary. Effects of adrenergic agonists (e.g., **isoproterenol**, **phenylephrine**) may be ↓ upon smoking cessation; dose ↑ at cessation may be necessary. Concurrent treatment with **bupropion** may cause treatment-emergent hypertension.

Route/Dosage
Gum (Adults): If 1st cigarette is desired >30 min after awakening, start with 2 mg gum; if 1st cigarette is desired <30 min after awakening, start with 4 mg gum. Patients should chew one piece of gum every 1–2 hr for 6 wk, then one piece of gum every 2–4 hr for 3 wk, then one piece of gum every 4–8 hr for 3 wk; then discontinue. Should not exceed 24 pieces of gum/day.
Lozenge (Adults): If 1st cigarette is desired >30 min after awakening, start with 2 mg lozenge; if 1st cigarette is desired <30 min after awakening, start with 4 mg lozenge. Patients should use one lozenge every 1–2 hr for 6 wk, then one lozenge every 2–4 hr for 3 wk, then one lozenge every 4–8 hr for 3 wk; then discontinue. Should not exceed 20 lozenges/day or more than 5 lozenges in 6 hr.
Intranasal (Adults): One spray in each nostril 1–2 times/hr (up to 5 times/hr); may ↑ up to maximum of 40 times/day (should not exceed 3 mo of therapy).
Transdermal (Adults): *Patients smoking >10 cigarettes/day:* Begin with Step 1 (21 mg/day) for 6 wk, followed by Step 2 (14 mg/day) for 2 wk, and then Step 3 (7 mg/day) for 2 wk; then stop (total of 10 wk) (new

N

patch should be applied every 24 hr); *Patients smoking ≤10 cigarettes/day:* Begin with Step 2 (14 mg/day) for 6 wk, followed by Step 3 (7 mg/day) for 2 wk; then stop (total of 8 wk) (new patch should be applied every 24 hr).

Availability (generic available)

Chewing gum (cinnamon, mint, spearmint, white ice, and fruit chill flavors): 2 mg^OTC^, 4 mg^OTC^. **Lozenges (original, mint, cherry, cherry peppermint, and cappuccino flavors):** 2 mg^OTC^, 4 mg^OTC^. **Nasal spray:** 0.5 mg/spray in 10-mL bottles (200 sprays). **Transdermal patch:** 7 mg/day^OTC^, 14 mg/day^OTC^, 21 mg/day^OTC^.

NURSING IMPLICATIONS

Assessment

- Assess smoking history (number of cigarettes smoked daily, smoking patterns, nicotine content of preferred brand, degree to which patient inhales smoke) before therapy.
- Assess for signs/symptoms of smoking withdrawal (irritability, drowsiness, fatigue, headache, nicotine craving) periodically during nicotine replacement therapy.
- Evaluate progress in smoking cessation periodically during therapy.

Toxicity and Overdose

- Monitor for nausea, vomiting, diarrhea, ↑ salivation, abdominal pain, headache, dizziness, auditory and visual disturbances, weakness, dyspnea, hypotension, and irregular HR.

Implementation

- **Gum:** Protect gum from light; exposure to light causes gum to turn brown.
- **Lozenge:** Lozenge should be allowed to dissolve slowly in the mouth; it should not be chewed or swallowed.
- **Transdermal:** Patch can be worn for 16 or 24 hr; the patch can be removed before the patient goes to bed (especially if patient has vivid dreams or sleep disturbances) or can remain on while the patient sleeps (especially if patient craves cigarettes upon awakening).
- **Nasal Spray:** Regular use of the spray during the 1st wk of therapy may help patient adjust to irritant effects of the spray.

Patient/Family Teaching

- Explain purpose and side effects of nicotine to patient. Advise patient to read *Patient Information* before starting therapy.
- Advise patient to notify health care provider of all Rx or OTC medications, vitamins, or herbal products being taken and to consult with health care provider before taking other medications.
- Encourage patient to participate in a smoking cessation program while using this product.
- Advise patient in proper method of disposal of unit. Emphasize need to keep out of the reach of children or pets.
- Emphasize the importance of regular visits to health care provider to monitor progress of smoking cessation.
- **Gum:** Explain purpose of nicotine gum to patient. Patient should chew one piece of gum whenever a craving for nicotine occurs or according to a fixed schedule (every 1–2 hr while awake) as directed. Chew gum slowly until a tingling sensation is felt (about 15 chews). Then, patient should stop chewing and store the gum between the cheek and gums until the tingling sensation disappears (about 1 min). Process of stopping and then resuming chewing should be repeated for approximately 30 min until most of the tingle has disappeared. Rapid, vigorous chewing may result in side effects similar to those of smoking too many cigarettes (headache, dizziness, nausea, ↑ salivation, heartburn, hiccups). For best chances of quitting, chew ≥9 pieces of gum/day during 1st 6 wk.
- Inform patient that the gum has a slight tobacco/pepper-like taste. Many patients initially find it unpleasant and slightly irritating to the mouth. This usually resolves after several days of therapy.
- Advise patient to carry gum at all times during therapy.
- Advise patient to avoid eating or drinking for 15 min before and during chewing of nicotine gum; these interfere with buccal absorption of nicotine.
- The gum usually can be chewed by denture wearers. Contact dentist if the gum adheres to bridgework.
- Advise patient that if they still feel need to use gum after completion of treatment period, advise them to contact a health care provider.
- Instruct patient not to swallow gum.
- Dispose of the gum by wrapping in wrapper to prevent ingestion by children and animals. Call the poison control center, emergency department, or health care provider immediately if a child ingests the gum.
- **Transdermal:** Instruct patient in application and use of patch. Apply patch at the same time each day. Keep patch in sealed pouch until ready to apply. Apply to clean, dry skin of upper arm or torso free of oil, hair, scars, cuts, burns, or irritation. Press patch firmly in place with palm for 10 sec, making sure there is good contact, especially around the edges. Keep patch in place during showering, bathing, or swimming; replace patches that have fallen off. Wash hands with soap and water after handling patches. Do not trim or cut patch. No more than one patch should be worn at a time. Alternate application sites. Dispose of used patches by folding adhesive sides together and

replacing in protective pouch or aluminum foil; keep out of reach of children.

- Advise patient that redness, itching, and burning at application site usually subside within 1 hr. Advise patient to notify health care provider and not apply new patch if signs of allergic reaction (urticaria, generalized rash, hives) or persistent local skin reactions (severe erythema, pruritus, edema) occur.
- May cause drowsiness or dizziness. Advise patient to avoid driving or other activities requiring alertness until response to medication is known.
- Advise patient referred for MRI test to discuss patch with referring health care provider and MRI facility to determine if removal of patch is necessary before test and for directions for replacing patch.
- **Nasal Spray:** Advise patient in proper use of spray. Tilt head back slightly. Do not sniff, swallow, or inhale through nose as spray is being administered. Patients who have successfully stopped smoking should continue to use the same dose for up to 8 wk, after which the spray should be discontinued over the next 4–6 wk.
- Discontinue nasal spray by using ½ dose (one spray at a time), using the spray less frequently, skipping a dose by not using every hr, or setting a planned stop date for use of the spray.
- Treatment should be discontinued in patients who are unable to stop smoking by the 4th wk of therapy (patient is unlikely to quit on that attempt).
- Patients who fail to stop smoking should be given a therapy holiday before another attempt.
- Advise patient to replace childproof cap after using and before disposal.
- **Lozenge:** Instruct patient to place lozenge in mouth and allow it to slowly dissolve (20–30 min). Minimize swallowing; advise patient not to chew or swallow lozenge. May cause a warm tingling sensation in mouth. Advise patient to occasionally move lozenge from side to side of mouth until completely dissolved. Instruct patient not to eat or drink 15 min before or while lozenge is in mouth. For best chances of quitting, use ≥9 lozenges/day during 1st 6 wk. Do not use more than one lozenge at a time or use continuously one after the another. Lozenge should not be used after 12 wk without consulting health care provider.
- Rep: Advise women of reproductive potential to notify health care provider if pregnancy is planned or suspected or if breastfeeding. Nicotine in any form can be harmful to a pregnant woman and/or the fetus. Assist patient in determining risk/benefit of nicotine replacement therapy and harm to the fetus versus the likelihood of stopping smoking without nicotine replacement therapy. Maternal smoking and nicotine ↑ risk of sudden infant death syndrome.

Evaluation/Desired Outcomes

- Lessened sequelae of nicotine withdrawal (irritability, insomnia, somnolence, headache, and increased appetite) during smoking cessation.

NIFEdipine, See CALCIUM CHANNEL BLOCKERS.

HIGH ALERT

nilotinib (ni-**lo**-ti-nib)

Danziten, Tasigna

Classification

Therapeutic: antineoplastics

Pharmacologic: enzyme inhibitors, kinase inhibitors

N

Indications

Newly diagnosed Philadelphia chromosome positive (Ph+) chronic myelogenous leukemia (CML) in chronic phase (capsules or tablets). Chronic or accelerated phase Ph+ CML in adult patients who are resistant or intolerant to prior treatment, including imatinib (capsules or tablets). Chronic or accelerated phase Ph+ CML in pediatric patients ≥1 yr who are resistant or intolerant to prior tyrosine-kinase inhibitor treatment (capsules only).

Action

Inhibits kinases, which may be produced by malignant cell lines. **Therapeutic Effects:** Inhibits production of malignant cells lines with decreased proliferation of leukemic cells.

Pharmacokinetics

Absorption: Well absorbed following oral administration. Levels of capsules are significantly ↑ by food.
Distribution: Unknown.
Protein Binding: 98%.
Metabolism and Excretion: Mostly metabolized by the liver via the CYP3A4 isoenzyme to inactive metabolites. Primarily excreted in the feces (93%), with 69% being excreted unchanged.
Half-life: 14–17 hr.

TIME/ACTION PROFILE (plasma concentrations)

ROUTE	ONSET	PEAK	DURATION
PO	unknown	3 hr	12 hr

Contraindications/Precautions

Contraindicated in: Hypokalemia or hypomagnesemia; Long QT syndrome; Galactose intolerance, severe lactase deficiency, or glucose-galactose malabsorption (capsules contain lactose); OB: Pregnancy; Lactation: Lactation.

Use Cautiously in: Electrolyte abnormalities; correct prior to administration to ↓ risk of arrhythmias; Hepatic impairment (↓ dose if Grade 3 elevated bilirubin, transaminases, or lipase); Total gastrectomy (may need to ↑ dose or use alterative therapy); History of pancreatitis; Patients with genetically reduced UGT1A1 activity (presence of UGT1A1*28 allele) (↑ risk of hyperbilirubinemia); Rep: Women of reproductive potential; Pedi: May affect growth and development of children; safety and effectiveness not established in children <1 yr.

Adverse Reactions/Side Effects

CV: hypertension, MI, palpitations, pericardial effusion, peripheral arterial disease, QT interval prolongation, TORSADES DE POINTES. **Derm:** pruritus, rash, alopecia, flushing. **EENT:** vertigo. **F and E:** hyperkalemia, hypocalcemia, hypokalemia, hyponatremia, hypophosphatemia. **GI:** ↑ lipase, constipation, diarrhea, nausea, vomiting, abdominal discomfort, anorexia, ascites, dyspepsia, flatulence, hepatitis B virus reactivation, HEPATOTOXICITY. **Hemat:** BLEEDING, MYELOSUPRESSION. **Metab:** hyperglycemia. **MS:** ↓ growth, musculoskeletal pain. **Neuro:** fatigue, headache, dizziness, paresthesia, STROKE. **Resp:** pleural effusion, pulmonary edema. **Misc:** fever, night sweats, tumor lysis syndrome.

Interactions

Drug-Drug: **Strong CYP3A4 inhibitors**, including **ketoconazole**, **itraconazole**, **voriconazole**, **clarithromycin**, **atazanavir**, **nelfinavir**, **ritonavir**, and **nefazodone**, may ↑ levels and risk of toxicity; avoid concurrent use. If concurrent use is necessary, ↓ nilotinib dose. **Strong CYP3A4 inducers**, including **carbamazepine**, **dexamethasone**, **phenobarbital**, **phenytoin**, **rifabutin**, **rifampin**, and **rifapentine**, may ↓ levels and effectiveness; avoid concurrent use. May ↑ levels and risk of toxicity of **CYP3A4 substrates**, including **atorvastatin**, **cyclosporine**, **dihydroergotamine**, **ergotamine**, **fentanyl**, **lovastatin**, **midazolam**, **simvastatin**, **sirolimus**, and **tacrolimus**. **QT interval prolonging drugs** may ↑ risk of QT interval prolongation and torsades de pointes; avoid concurrent use. **Proton pump inhibitors**, **H_2 receptor antagonists**, and **antacids** may ↓ absorption of nilotinib; avoid concurrent use of proton pump inhibitors; doses of H_2 receptor antagonists may be administered 10 hr before or 2 hr after nilotinib; doses of antacids may be administered 2 hr before or after nilotinib.

Drug-Natural Products: **St. John's wort** may ↓ levels and effectiveness; avoid concurrent use.

Drug-Food: **Grapefruit juice** may ↑ levels and risk of toxicity; avoid concurrent use.

Route/Dosage

Capsules should NOT be substituted with tablets on a milligram per milligram basis.

Newly Diagnosed Chronic Phase Ph+ Chronic Myelogenous Leukemia

PO (Adults): *Capsules:* 300 mg twice daily; treatment discontinuation may be considered in patients who have received nilotinib for ≥3 yr and achieved a sustained molecular response; if patients lose molecular response after discontinuing therapy, restart nilotinib within 4 wk at the dose level prior to discontinuation. *Tablets:* 142 mg twice daily; treatment discontinuation may be considered in patients who have received nilotinib for ≥3 yr and achieved a sustained molecular response; if patients lose molecular response after discontinuing therapy, restart nilotinib within 4 wk at the dose level prior to discontinuation. *Concurrent use of strong CYP3A4 inhibitors (ketoconazole, itraconazole, clarithromycin, atazanavir, nefazodone, nelfinavir, ritonavir, or voriconazole):* Capsules: 200 mg once daily; Tablets: 95 mg once daily.

PO (Children ≥1 yr): *Capsules:* 230 mg/m^2 twice daily (max single dose = 400 mg) until disease progression or unacceptable toxicity; treatment discontinuation may be considered in patients who have received nilotinib for ≥3 yr and achieved a sustained molecular response; if patients lose molecular response after discontinuing therapy, restart nilotinib within 4 wk at the dose level prior to discontinuation. *Concurrent use of strong CYP3A4 inhibitors (ketoconazole, itraconazole, clarithromycin, atazanavir, nefazodone, nelfinavir, ritonavir, or voriconazole):* 200 mg once daily.

Hepatic Impairment

PO (Adults): *Mild, moderate, or severe hepatic impairment:* Capsules: 200 mg twice daily; may ↑ to 300 mg twice daily if tolerated; Tablets: 95 mg twice daily; may ↑ to 142 mg twice daily if tolerated.

Hepatic Impairment

PO (Children ≥1 yr): *Mild, moderate, or severe hepatic impairment:* Capsules: 200 mg twice daily; may ↑ to 300 mg twice daily if tolerated.

Resistant or Intolerant Chronic or Accelerated Phase Ph+ Chronic Myelogenous Leukemia

PO (Adults): *Capsules:* 400 mg twice daily; treatment discontinuation may be considered in patients who have received nilotinib for ≥3 yr and achieved a sustained molecular response; if patients lose molecular response after discontinuing therapy, restart nilotinib within 4 wk at the dose level prior to discontinuation. *Tablets:* 190 mg twice daily; treatment discontinuation may be considered in patients who have received nilotinib for

≥3 yr and achieved a sustained molecular response; if patients lose molecular response after discontinuing therapy, restart nilotinib within 4 wk at the dose level prior to discontinuation. *Concurrent use of strong CYP3A4 inhibitors (ketoconazole, itraconazole, clarithromycin, atazanavir, nefazodone, nelfinavir, ritonavir, or voriconazole):* Capsules: 300 mg once daily; Tablets: 142 mg once daily.

PO (Children ≥1 yr): *Capsules:* 230 mg/m² twice daily (max single dose = 400 mg) until disease progression or unacceptable toxicity; treatment discontinuation may be considered in patients who have received nilotinib for ≥3 yr and achieved a sustained molecular response; if patients lose molecular response after discontinuing therapy, restart nilotinib within 4 wk at the dose level prior to discontinuation. *Concurrent use of strong CYP3A4 inhibitors (ketoconazole, itraconazole, clarithromycin, atazanavir, nefazodone, nelfinavir, ritonavir, or voriconazole):* 200 mg once daily.

Hepatic Impairment

(Adults): *Mild or moderate hepatic impairment:* Capsules: 300 mg twice daily; may ↑ to 400 mg twice daily if tolerated; Tablets: 142 mg twice daily; may ↑ to 190 mg twice daily if tolerated. *Severe hepatic impairment:* Capsules: 200 mg twice daily; may ↑ to 300 mg twice daily and eventually to 400 mg twice daily if tolerated; Tablets: 95 mg twice daily; may ↑ to 142 mg twice daily and eventually 190 mg twice daily if tolerated.

Hepatic Impairment

(Children ≥1 yr): *Mild or moderate hepatic impairment:* Capsules: 300 mg twice daily; may ↑ to 400 mg twice daily if tolerated. *Severe hepatic impairment:* Capsules: 200 mg twice daily; may ↑ to 300 mg twice daily and eventually to 400 mg twice daily if tolerated.

Hepatic Impairment

PO (Adults and Children ≥1 yr): *Mild or moderate hepatic impairment:* 300 mg twice daily; may ↑ to 400 mg twice daily if tolerated. *Severe hepatic impairment:* 200 mg twice daily; may ↑ to 300 mg twice daily and eventually to 400 mg twice daily if tolerated.

Availability (generic available)

Capsules (Tasigna): 50 mg, 150 mg, 200 mg. **Tablets (Danziten):** 71 mg, 95 mg.

NURSING IMPLICATIONS

Assessment

- Monitor ECG to assess the QTc interval at baseline, 7 days after initiation of therapy, after any dose adjustment, and periodically thereafter. *If QTc interval >480 msec,* hold nilotinib and check serum potassium and magnesium. If serum potassium and magnesium below lower limit of normal, correct to normal with supplements. Review concurrent medications for effects on electrolytes. *If QTc interval returns to <450 msec and within 20 msec of baseline within 2 wk,* return to prior dose. *If QTc interval <480 msec and >450 msec after 2 wk,* ↓ dose to 400 mg once daily. Following dose ↓ to 400 mg once daily, *if QTc interval returns to >480 msec,* discontinue nilotinib.
- Monitor for myelosuppression. Assess for bleeding (bleeding gums; bruising; petechiae; blood in stools, urine, or emesis); avoid IM injections and taking rectal temperatures if platelet count is low. Assess for signs of infection during neutropenia. Anemia may occur. Monitor for fatigue, dyspnea, and orthostatic hypotension.
- Monitor for tumor lysis syndrome (high WBC counts, hyperuricemia, hyperkalemia, hyperphosphatemia, hypocalcemia, dehydration). Prevent by maintaining adequate hydration and correcting uric acid levels prior to starting nilotinib.
- Monitor for signs/symptoms of severe fluid retention (unexpected rapid weight gain or swelling) and for signs/symptoms of respiratory or cardiac compromise (shortness of breath) periodically during therapy; evaluate cause and treat patients as needed.
- Pedi: Monitor growth and development in pediatric patients receiving nilotinib.

Lab Test Considerations

- Verify negative pregnancy test before starting therapy.
- Monitor serum electrolytes prior to and periodically during therapy. May cause hypokalemia, hypomagnesemia, hypophosphatemia, hyperkalemia, hypocalcemia, hyperglycemia, and hyponatremia.
- Monitor CBC every 2 wk for 1st 2 mo and monthly thereafter or as indicated. *If ANC <1.0 × 10⁹ cells/L and/or platelets <50 × 10⁹cells/L,* hold nilotinib and monitor blood counts. Resume within 2 wk at prior dose if ANC recover to >1.0 × 10⁹cells/L and platelets >50 × 10⁹cells/L. If blood counts remain low for >2 wk, ↓ dose to 400 mg once daily. Myelosuppression is generally reversible.
- May ↑ serum lipase or amylase. *If serum lipase or amylase ↑ to Grade ≥3,* hold nilotinib and continue to monitor serum lipase and amylase levels. If serum lipase or amylase return to Grade ≤1, resume nilotinib at 400 mg once daily (230 mg/m² once daily if prior dose was 230 mg/m² twice daily). *For pediatric patients,* hold nilotinib until serum lipase or amylase return to Grade ≤1. Resume nilotinib at 230 mg/m² once daily if prior dose was 230 mg/m² twice daily; discontinue nilotinib if prior dose was 230 mg/m² once daily.
- Monitor liver function tests monthly. May ↑ serum ALT, AST, and bilirubin. *If AST, ALT, or bilirubin ↑ to Grade ≥3,* hold nilotinib and monitor bilirubin. If AST, ALT, or bilirubin return to Grade ≤1, resume

nilotinib at 400 mg once daily. *For pediatric patients,* hold nilotinib until serum bilirubin returns to Grade ≤1; then resume nilotinib at 230 mg/m² once daily if prior dose was 230 mg/m² twice daily; discontinue nilotinib if prior dose was 230 mg/m² once daily and recovery to Grade ≤1 takes >28 days.

- Monitor lipid panel and glucose before starting and periodically during first year of therapy and then yearly during chronic therapy.
- Upon discontinuation, monitor BCR-ABL transcript levels and CBC with differential monthly for 1 yr, then every 6 wk for 2nd yr, and every 12 wk thereafter.

Implementation

- Do not confuse nilotinib with neratinib or niraparib.
- Correct hypokalemia and hypomagnesemia prior to beginning therapy.
- Indications for use and dosing differ between capsule and tablet formulations; do not substitute capsules and tablets (or vice versa) on a mg-per-mg basis.
- **PO:** Administer capsules twice daily at 12-hr intervals on an empty stomach, ≥1 hr before and 2 hr after food. Administer tablets with or without food. ***DNC:*** Swallow capsules and tablets whole with water; do not cut, crush, or chew tablets.
- Patients unable to swallow capsule may open capsule and sprinkle contents of each capsule in one teaspoon of applesauce. Swallow mixture within 15 min. Do not use more than one teaspoon of applesauce and use only applesauce.
- Avoid antacids <2 hr before or after administration; avoid H_2 antagonists < 10 hr before or <2 hr after administration.

Patient/Family Teaching

- Instruct patient to take nilotinib as directed, approximately 12 hr apart. If a dose is missed, skip dose and resume taking next prescribed dose. Nilotinib is a long-term treatment; do not stop medication or change dose without consulting health care provider. Advise patient to read the *Medication Guide* before starting and with each Rx refill, in case of changes.
- Advise patient to avoid grapefruit, grapefruit juice, or products with grapefruit extract during therapy; may cause toxicity.
- May cause dizziness. Caution patient to avoid driving or other activities requiring alertness until response to medication is known.
- Advise patient to notify health care provider of all Rx or OTC medications, vitamins, or herbal products being taken and to consult with health care provider before taking other medications, especially St. John's wort, during therapy.
- Instruct patient to notify health care provider promptly if fever; chills; cough; hoarseness; sore throat; signs of infection; lower back or side pain; painful or difficult urination; bleeding gums; bruising; petechiae; blood in stools, urine, or emesis; ↑ fatigue; dyspnea; signs of fluid retention; or orthostatic hypotension occurs. Caution patient to avoid crowds and persons with known infections. Instruct patient to use a soft toothbrush and electric razor and to avoid falls. Caution patient not to drink alcoholic beverages or take medication containing aspirin or NSAIDs; may precipitate bleeding.
- Instruct patient not to receive any vaccinations without advice of health care provider.
- Discuss the possibility of hair loss with patient. Explore methods of coping. Regrowth usually occurs 2–3 mo after discontinuation of therapy.
- Rep: May cause fetal harm. Advise women of reproductive potential to use highly effective contraception during therapy and for ≥14 days following last dose and to avoid breastfeeding for ≥14 days following last dose. Advise patient to notify health care provider immediately if pregnancy is suspected.

Evaluation/Desired Outcomes

- Decrease in production of leukemic cells.

niMODipine, See CALCIUM CHANNEL BLOCKERS.

nintedanib (nin-**ted**-a-nib)

Ofev

Classification

Therapeutic: pulmonary fibrosis agents

Pharmacologic: kinase inhibitors

Indications

Idiopathic pulmonary fibrosis. Chronic fibrosing interstitial lung diseases with a progressive phenotype. Systemic sclerosis-associated interstitial lung disease.

Action

Inhibits tyrosine kinases, which may be responsible for proliferation, migration, and transformation of fibroblasts in pulmonary fibrosis. **Therapeutic Effects:** Slowed progression of pulmonary impairment.

Pharmacokinetics

Absorption: 4.7% absorbed following oral administration (substantial first-pass effect).

Distribution: Unknown.

Protein Binding: 97.8%.

Metabolism and Excretion: Undergoes extensive metabolism and subsequent fecal/biliary elimination (93.4%). Minimal amounts excreted in urine.

Half-life: 9.5 hr.

TIME/ACTION PROFILE (effects on pulmonary function)

ROUTE	ONSET	PEAK	DURATION
PO	4–6 wk	36 wk	unknown

Contraindications/Precautions

Contraindicated in: Moderate or severe hepatic impairment; OB: Pregnancy; Lactation: Lactation.
Use Cautiously in: Recent GI surgery, history of diverticular disease, or current use of corticosteroids or NSAIDs (↑ risk of GI perforation; use only if expected benefit outweighs potential risk); Known cardiovascular risk factors, including coronary artery disease; Known risk of bleeding (use only if expected benefit outweighs potential risk); Severe renal impairment or end-stage renal disease; Low body weight (<65 kg), Asian, and female patients (↑ risk of hepatotoxicity); Rep: Women of reproductive potential; Pedi: Safety and effectiveness not established in children; Geri: Older adults may have ↑ risk of adverse reactions.

Adverse Reactions/Side Effects

CV: ARTERIAL THROMBOEMBOLIC EVENTS (INCLUDING MI), hypertension. **Endo:** hypothyroidism. **GI:** ↓ appetite, ↑ liver enzymes, abdominal pain, diarrhea, hyperbilirubinemia, nausea, vomiting, GI PERFORATION, HEPATOTOXICITY, weight loss. **GU:** proteinuria. **Hemat:** BLEEDING. **Neuro:** headache.

Interactions

Drug-Drug: P-glycoprotein and CYP3A4 inhibitors, including **erythromycin** and **ketoconazole**, may ↑ levels and risk of toxicity; close monitoring recommended. **P-glycoprotein and CYP3A4 inducers**, including **carbamazepine**, **phenytoin**, and **rifampin**, may ↓ levels and effectiveness; avoid concurrent use. **Cigarette smoking** may ↓ levels and effectiveness; encourage cessation prior to treatment. **Anticoagulants** and **antiplatelet agents** may ↑ risk of bleeding.
Drug-Natural Products: St. John's wort may ↓ levels and effectiveness; avoid concurrent use.

Route/Dosage

PO (Adults): 150 mg twice daily; may ↓ to 100 mg twice daily if adverse reactions occur.

Hepatic Impairment

PO (Adults): *Mild hepatic impairment:* 100 mg twice daily.

Availability

Capsules: 100 mg, 150 mg.

NURSING IMPLICATIONS

Assessment

- Monitor for signs/symptoms of lung disease (dyspnea, ↓ forced vital capacity, diffuse pulmonary infiltrates on chest x-ray) during therapy.
- Monitor for diarrhea, nausea, and vomiting during therapy. Diarrhea usually occurs during 1st 3 mo. Treat diarrhea, nausea, and vomiting with adequate hydration and antidiarrheal (loperamide) and antiemetic medications. Consider interruption of therapy if diarrhea or nausea and vomiting continues. Therapy may be resumed at full dose or at ↓ dose and ↑ to full dose. Discontinue therapy if diarrhea, nausea, and vomiting are severe and persist despite symptomatic therapy.
- Monitor for signs/symptoms of bleeding (weakness, fatigue, tachycardia, dyspnea, pallor, petechiae, tarry stools, coffee ground emesis, epistaxis).
- Monitor for signs/symptoms of emerging cardiovascular disease such as MI (chest pain, dyspnea, diaphoresis, dizziness, nausea).

Lab Test Considerations

- Verify negative pregnancy test prior to starting therapy.
- Obtain liver function tests (AST, ALT, bilirubin) prior to starting therapy, at regular intervals for 3 mo, and periodically thereafter as clinically indicated. Risk may be ↑ in patients with a low body weight (<65 kg) and Asian and female patients. *If AST or ALT ↑ >3 times to <5 times upper limit of normal (ULN) without signs of liver damage,* hold nintedanib. Once liver enzymes have returned to baseline, may resume therapy at a ↓ dose of 100 mg twice daily and then ↑ to full dose (150 mg twice daily). *If AST or ALT ↑ >5 times ULN or >3 times ULN with signs and symptoms of liver damage,* discontinue nintedanib.

Implementation

- **PO:** Administer with food and liquid once every 12 hr. ***DNC:*** Swallow capsule whole; do not open, crush, or chew. Contents taste bitter. If contact with capsule powder occurs, wash hands immediately.

Patient/Family Teaching

- Explain the purpose and side effects of nintedanib. Instruct patient to take as directed. If a dose is missed, omit and take next dose at scheduled time; do not double doses. Advise patient to read *Patient Information* sheet prior to starting therapy and with each Rx refill in case of changes.
- Emphasize the importance of follow-up blood tests to monitor liver function.
- Advise patient that diarrhea, nausea, and vomiting are common side effects and advise to maintain hydration

and take antidiarrheal or antiemetic medication as needed. Notify health care provider if diarrhea, nausea, or vomiting is persistent or severe.

- Encourage patient to stop smoking before therapy and to avoid smoking during therapy.
- Advise patient to notify health care provider immediately if signs and symptoms of liver dysfunction (fatigue, anorexia, skin or whites of eyes turn yellow, urine turns dark or brown [tea colored], pain on right side of stomach, unusual bleeding or bruising, lethargy), arterial thrombotic events such as heart attack (chest pain or pressure; pain in arms, back, neck, or jaw; shortness of breath), or gastric perforation (pain or swelling in stomach area) occur.
- Advise patient to notify health care provider of all Rx or OTC medications, vitamins, or herbal products being taken and to consult with health care provider before taking other medications. Avoid St. John's wort during treatment.
- Rep: May cause fetal harm. Advise women of reproductive potential to use highly effective contraception during and for ≥3 mo after last dose and to avoid breastfeeding during therapy. Patients with vomiting and/or diarrhea during therapy may have ↓ efficacy of oral hormonal contraceptives; advise these patients to use an alternate form of highly effective contraception. Notify health care provider promptly if pregnancy is suspected.

Evaluation/Desired Outcomes

- Decrease in rate of decline in forced vital capacity and extension in time to first exacerbation of pulmonary fibrosis.

nirmatrelvir/ritonavir

(nur-ma**trel**-veer/ri-**toe**-na-veer)

Paxlovid

Classification

Therapeutic: antivirals

Pharmacologic: protease inhibitors

Indications

Mild to moderate COVID-19 infection in patients who are at high risk for progression to severe COVID-19, including hospitalization or death.

Action

Nirmatrelvir acts as an inhibitor of the SARS-CoV-2 main protease (Mpro), which ultimately prevents viral replication. While ritonavir is also a protease inhibitor, this drug has no activity against Mpro. Ritonavir inhibits the CYP3A4-mediated metabolism of nirmatrelvir, resulting in increased plasma concentrations of nirmatrelvir. **Therapeutic Effects:** Reduction in COVID-19 related hospitalization or death from any cause.

Pharmacokinetics

Nirmatrelvir

Absorption: Well absorbed.

Distribution: Extensively distributed to extravascular tissues.

Metabolism and Excretion: CYP3A4 substrate; minimal metabolism by this isoenzyme when coadministered with ritonavir. Excreted in feces (49.6%) and urine (35.3%).

Half-life: 6 hr.

Ritonavir

Absorption: Well absorbed.

Distribution: Extensively distributed to extravascular tissues.

Protein Binding: 98–99%.

Metabolism and Excretion: Primarily metabolized in the liver via the CYP3A isoenzyme and to a lesser extent by the CYP2D6 isoenzyme. Primarily excreted in feces (86.4%), with 11.3% excreted in urine.

Half-life: 6 hr.

TIME/ACTION PROFILE (plasma concentrations)

ROUTE	ONSET	PEAK	DURATION
PO (nirmatrelvir)	unknown	3 hr	12 hr
PO (ritonavir)	unknown	4 hr	12 hr

Contraindications/Precautions

Contraindicated in: Hypersensitivity; Concurrent use of alfuzosin, amiodarone, apalutamide, carbamazepine, clozapine, colchicine, dihydroergotamine, dronedarone, enzalutamide, ergotamine, flecainide, lovastatin, lumacaftor/ivacaftor, lurasidone, methylergonovine, midazolam (PO), phenobarbital, phenytoin, piroxicam, pimozide, propafenone, quinidine, ranolazine, rifampin, simvastatin, sildenafil (Revatio), St. John's wort, or triazolam; Severe hepatic impairment.

Use Cautiously in: Moderate or severe renal impairment (↓ dose); OB: Use during pregnancy only if potential maternal benefit justifies potential fetal risk; Lactation: Safety not established in breastfeeding; Pedi: Safety and effectiveness not established in children.

Adverse Reactions/Side Effects

CV: hypertension. **Derm:** STEVENS-JOHNSON SYNDROME, TOXIC EPIDERMAL NECROLYSIS. **GI:** ↑ liver enzymes, abdominal pain, diarrhea, nausea, vomiting. **MS:** myalgia. **Neuro:** dysgeusia, headache. **Misc:** HYPERSENSITIVITY REACTIONS (INCLUDING ANAPHYLAXIS).

Interactions

Drug-Drug: May ↑ levels and risk of toxicity of some **antiarrhythmics (amiodarone, dronedarone, flecainide, propafenone, quinidine)**, some **antipsychotics (clozapine, pimozide, lurasidone)**,

alfuzosin, **ergot derivatives (dihydroergotamine, ergotamine, methylergonovine)**, **colchicine**, **piroxicam**, **ranolazine**, **sildenafil (Revatio)**, **midazolam (oral)**, and **triazolam**; concurrent use contraindicated. **Apalutamide**, **carbamazepine**, **enzalutamide**, **lumacaftor/ivacaftor**, **phenobarbital**, **phenytoin**, and **rifampin** may ↓ levels and effectiveness and promote resistance; concurrent use contraindicated. May ↑ levels and risk of toxicity of **lovastatin** and **simvastatin**; concurrent use contraindicated; discontinue lovastatin and simvastatin ≥12 hr before starting nirmatrelvir/ritonavir. May ↑ levels and risk of toxicity of **lidocaine**; monitor lidocaine levels closely. May ↑ levels and risk of toxicity of **digoxin**; monitor digoxin levels closely. May ↑ levels and risk of toxicity of **cyclosporine**, **sirolimus**, and **tacrolimus**; avoid concurrent use with sirolimus; monitor cyclosporine and tacrolimus levels closely. May ↑ levels and risk of toxicity of **abemaciclib**, **ceritinib**, **dasatinib**, **encorafenib**, **ibrutinib**, **ivosidenib**, **neratinib**, **nilotinib**, **venetoclax**, **vinblastine**, and **vincristine**; avoid concurrent use with encorafenib ibrutinib, ivosidenib, neratinib, and venetoclax. May ↑ or ↓ **warfarin** levels; closely monitor INR. May ↑ levels of and risk of bleeding with **rivaroxaban**; avoid concurrent use. May ↓ levels and effectiveness of **bupropion**. May ↑ levels and risk of toxicity of **trazodone**; consider ↓ trazodone dose. May ↑ levels and risk of toxicity of **quetiapine**; consider ↓ quetiapine dose. May ↑ levels and risk of toxicity of **amlodipine**, **diltiazem**, **felodipine**, **nicardipine**, and **nifedipine**; consider ↓ calcium channel blocker dose. May ↓ levels and effectiveness of **voriconazole**; avoid concurrent use. May ↑ levels and risk of toxicity of **atazanavir**, **bedaquiline**, **bictegravir**, **clarithromycin**, **darunavir**, **efavirenz**, **erythromycin**, **fentanyl**, **fosamprenavir**, **isavuconazonium**, **itraconazole**, **ketoconazole**, **maraviroc**, **midazolam (parenteral) nelfinavir**, **nevirapine**, **rifabutin**, **rosuvastatin**, **tenofovir**, and **tipranavir**. **Isavuconazonium**, **itraconazole**, and **ketoconazole** may ↑ levels and risk of toxicity. May ↓ levels and effects of **raltegravir** and **zidovudine**. May ↑ levels and risk of toxicity of **bosentan**; discontinue bosentan ≥36 hr prior to starting nirmatrelvir/ritonavir. May ↑ levels and risk of toxicity of **elbasvir/grazoprevir**, **glecaprevir/pibrentasvir**, **ombitasvir/paritaprevir/ritonavir/dasabuvir**, and **sofosbuvir/velpatasvir/voxilaprevir**; avoid concurrent use with glecaprevir/pibrentasvir. May ↑ levels and risk of toxicity of **atorvastatin** and **rosuvastatin**; consider temporarily discontinuing atorvastatin and rosuvastatin during treatment. May ↓ levels and effectiveness of oral contraceptives containing **ethinyl estradiol**; use an additional nonhormonal contraceptive during treatment. May ↑ levels and risk of toxicity of **salmeterol**; concurrent use not recommended. May ↓ levels and effectiveness of **methadone**; monitor patients closely for signs/symptoms of withdrawal. May ↑ levels and risk of toxicity of **betamethasone**, **budesonide**, **ciclesonide**, **dexamethasone**, **fluticasone**, **methylprednisolone**, **mometasone**, **prednisone**, or **triamcinolone**; consider alternative corticosteroid such as beclomethasone or prednisolone.

Drug-Natural Products: **St. John's wort** may ↓ levels and effectiveness and promote resistance; concurrent use contraindicated.

Route/Dosage

PO (Adults): Two nirmatrelvir 150-mg tablets and one ritonavir 100-mg tablet twice daily for 5 days. Should be started as soon as possible after diagnosis of COVID-19 and within 5 days of symptom onset.

Renal Impairment

PO (Adults): *eGFR 30–59 mL/min:* One nirmatrelvir 150-mg tablet and one ritonavir 100-mg tablet twice daily for 5 days. Should be started as soon as possible after diagnosis of COVID-19 and within 5 days of symptom onset. *eGFR <30 mL/min (including hemodialysis):* Two nirmatrelvir 150-mg tablets and one ritonavir 100-mg tablet as a single dose on Day 1, then one nirmatrelvir 150-mg tablet and one ritonavir 100-mg tablet once daily on Days 2–5. Administer nirmatrelvir/ritonavir after hemodialysis on hemodialysis days.

Availability

Tablets: nirmatrelvir 150 mg + ritonavir 100 mg (separate tablets).

NURSING IMPLICATIONS

Assessment

- Assess signs/symptoms of COVID-19 before starting and during therapy.

Implementation

- Prior to initiating *Paxlovid*: Review all medications taken by the patient to assess potential drug-drug interactions with strong CYP3A inhibitors and determine if concurrent medications require a dose adjustment, interruption, or additional monitoring. Consider the benefit of *Paxlovid* treatment in ↓ hospitalization and death and whether the risk of potential drug-drug interactions for an individual patient can be appropriately managed.
- Not approved for use as pre-exposure or postexposure prophylaxis of COVID-19.
- Start 5-day course as soon as possible after COVID-19 diagnosis and within 5 days of symptom onset, even if symptoms are mild. If hospitalization is required after starting treatment with *Paxlovid*, the full 5-day course should be completed.

- **PO:** Administer tablets without regard to food. Dose packs contain two nirmatrelvir tablets and one ritonavir tablet. Dose for renal impairment contains one nirmatrelvir tablet and one ritonavir tablet. Nirmatrelvir must be coadministered with ritonavir. *DNC:* Swallow tablets whole; do not break, crush, or chew. Completion of the full 5-day course of therapy and continued isolation in accordance current guidelines are important to maximize viral clearance and minimize transmission of SARS-Co-2.

Patient/Family Teaching

- Instruct patient to take *Paxlovid* as directed. If a dose is missed within 8 hr of the time it is usually taken, patient should take it as soon as possible and resume the normal dosing schedule. If the dose is missed by >8 hr, omit dose and take next dose at next scheduled time. Do not double dose. Advise patient to read *Patient Information* before starting therapy.
- Advise patient to notify health care provider and immediately discontinue therapy at the first sign or symptom of hypersensitivity reaction (skin rash; hives; difficulty swallowing or breathing; swelling of the lips, tongue, or face; hoarseness; or other symptoms of an allergic reaction).
- Instruct patient to notify health care provider of all Rx or OTC medications, vitamins, or herbal products being taken and to consult with health care provider before taking other medications, especially St. John's wort.
- Rep: Advise women of reproductive potential to notify health care provider if pregnancy is planned or suspected or if breastfeeding. Ritonavir may ↓ efficacy of hormonal contraceptives. Advise patients using hormonal contraceptives to use an effective alternative method or an additional barrier method of contraception.

Evaluation/Desired Outcomes

- Reduction in COVID-19 related hospitalization or death.

nirsevimab (nir-sev-i-mab)

Beyfortus

Classification

Therapeutic: vaccines immunizing agents

Pharmacologic: immune globulins, monoclonal antibodies

Indications

- Prevention of respiratory syncytial virus (RSV) lower respiratory tract disease in the following individuals: Neonates and infants born during or entering their first RSV season; Children up to 24 mo of age who remain vulnerable to severe RSV disease through their second RSV season.

Action

Monoclonal antibody that neutralizes RSV by inhibiting conformation changes in the F protein that are necessary for fusion of the viral and cellular membranes and viral entry. **Therapeutic Effects:** Prevention of RSV infection.

Pharmacokinetics

Absorption: 84% absorbed following IM administration.

Distribution: Not widely distributed to tissues.

Metabolism and Excretion: Degraded into small peptides by catabolic pathways.

Half-life: 71 days.

TIME/ACTION PROFILE (neutralizing antibody plasma concentrations)

ROUTE	ONSET	PEAK	DURATION
IM	unknown	6 days	unknown

Contraindications/Precautions

Contraindicated in: Serious hypersensitivity reactions; Pedi: Children >24 mo (safety and effectiveness not established).

Use Cautiously in: Thrombocytopenia any coagulation disorder or receiving anticoagulation therapy.

Adverse Reactions/Side Effects

Derm: rash **Local:** injection site reaction. **Misc:** HYPERSENSITIVITY REACTIONS (INCLUDING ANAPHYLAXIS).

Interactions

Drug-Drug: None reported.

Route/Dosage

Neonates and Infants Born During or Entering Their First RSV Season

IM (Neonates and Infants <8 mo and ≥5 kg): 100 mg as single dose; *Undergoing cardiac surgery with cardiopulmonary bypass (>90 days since initial dose):* Administer additional 50 mg as single dose; *Undergoing cardiac surgery with cardiopulmonary bypass (≤90 days since initial dose):* Administer additional 100 mg as single dose.

IM (Neonates and Infants <8 mo and <5 kg): 50 mg as single dose. *Undergoing cardiac surgery with cardiopulmonary bypass (regardless of time since initial dose):* Administer additional 50 mg as single dose.

Children Who Remain at Increased Risk for Severe RSV Disease in Their Second RSV Season

IM (Infants and Children 8–19 mo): 200 mg as a single dose. *Undergoing cardiac surgery with cardiopulmonary bypass (>90 days since initial dose):* Administer additional 100 mg as single dose; *Undergoing cardiac surgery with cardiopulmonary* *bypass (≤90 days since initial dose):* Administer additional 200 mg as single dose.

Availability

Solution for injection (prefilled syringes): 50 mg/0.5 mL, 100 mg/mL.

NURSING IMPLICATIONS

Assessment

- Assess injection site for bleeding or hematomas.
- Assess for hypersensitivity reactions (anaphylaxis, cyanosis, dyspnea, hypotonia, urticaria). If these occur, administer appropriate medications (epinephrine) and provide supportive care as required.

Implementation

- Administer by a health care professional only.
- Infants ≥8 mo and children ≤19 mo (second RSV season); if only received half dose (100 mg), give remaining 100 mg dose as soon as possible, and no later than the end of the season.
- **IM:** Prefilled syringe solution should be clear to opalescent, colorless to yellow. If <1 yr old, inject into the anterolateral thigh. If >1 yr old, can use deltoid muscle if adequate muscle mass. Use different injection sites when >one injection required. Do not inject in the gluteal muscle due to risk of damage to the sciatic nerve. Use appropriately prefilled syringe/dose. Do not split a single 100-mg prefilled syringe into two 50-mg doses, or administer two 50-mg doses in place of a single 100-mg dose. Store refrigerated. If removed from the refrigerator, use within 8 hr or discard.

Patient/Family Teaching

- Explain purpose and side effects of medication to patient's caregiver. Advise to read *Patient Information* before starting therapy.
- Advise patient's caregiver to notify health care professional of all Rx or OTC medications, vitamins, or herbal products being taken and to consult health care professional before taking other medications.
- Inform patient's caregiver of signs and symptoms of potential hypersensitivity reactions and to seek immediate medical attention if any occur.
- Advise the caregiver the child will receive one dose by IM injection by a health care professional. If the child remains at ↑ risk for RSV, a second dose may be required during the second RSV season.

Evaluation/Desired Outcomes

- Prevention of RSV infection.

nisoldipine, See CALCIUM CHANNEL BLOCKERS.

BEERS

nitrofurantoin

(nye-troe-fyoor-**an**-toyn)

Furadantin, Macrobid, Macrodantin

Classification

Therapeutic: anti-infectives

Indications

Prevention and treatment of urinary tract infections caused by susceptible organisms.

Action

Interferes with bacterial enzymes. **Therapeutic Effects:** Bactericidal or bacteriostatic action against susceptible organisms. **Spectrum:** Many gram-negative and some gram-positive organisms, specifically: *Citrobacter, Corynebacterium, Enterobacter, Escherichia coli, Klebsiella, Neisseria, Salmonella, Shigella, Staphylococcus aureus, Staphylococcus epidermidis, Enterococcus.*

Pharmacokinetics

Absorption: Readily absorbed after oral administration. Absorption is slower but more complete with macrocrystals (Macrodantin).

Distribution: Minimally distributed to tissues (concentrated in urine).

Metabolism and Excretion: Partially metabolized by the liver; 30–50% excreted unchanged by the kidneys.

Half-life: 20 min (↑ in renal impairment).

TIME/ACTION PROFILE (urine levels)

ROUTE	ONSET	PEAK	DURATION
PO	unknown	30 min	6–12 hr

Contraindications/Precautions

Contraindicated in: Hypersensitivity; Hypersensitivity to parabens (suspension); Oliguria, anuria, or significant renal impairment (CCr <60 mL/min); History of cholestatic jaundice or hepatic impairment with previous use of nitrofurantoin; OB: Pregnancy near term (38–42 wk gestation) and during labor/delivery (↑ risk of hemolytic anemia); Pedi: Infants <1 mo (↑ risk of hemolytic anemia).

Use Cautiously in: Glucose-6-phosphate dehydrogenase (G6PD) deficiency (↑ risk of hemolytic anemia, especially in Blacks and Mediterranean and Near Eastern ethnic groups); Diabetes (↑ risk of neuropathy); OB: Use during pregnancy only if potential fetal risk outweighs potential material benefit; Lactation: May cause hemolysis in infants with G6PD deficiency who are breastfed; Geri: Appears on Beers list. ↑ risk of pulmonary toxicity, hepatotoxicity, and peripheral neuropathy, especially with long-term use, in older

N

adults. Avoid use in older adults if CCr <30 mL/min or for long-term suppression of urinary tract infections.

Adverse Reactions/Side Effects

CV: chest pain. **Derm:** photosensitivity. **EENT:** nystagmus. **GI:** anorexia, nausea, vomiting, abdominal pain, CLOSTRIDIOIDES DIFFICILE-ASSOCIATED DIARRHEA (CDAD), diarrhea, HEPATOTOXICITY. **GU:** rust/brown discoloration of urine. **Hemat:** blood dyscrasias, hemolytic anemia. **Neuro:** dizziness, drowsiness, headache, peripheral neuropathy. **Resp:** PNEUMONITIS, PULMONARY FIBROSIS. **Misc:** hypersensitivity reactions.

Interactions

Drug-Drug: Probenecid prevents high urinary concentrations; may ↓ effectiveness. **Antacids** may ↓ absorption. ↑ risk of neurotoxicity with **neurotoxic drugs**. ↑ risk of hepatotoxicity with **hepatotoxic drugs**. ↑ risk of pneumonitis with **drugs having pulmonary toxicity**.

Route/Dosage

PO (Adults): *Treatment of active infection:* 50–100 mg every 6 hr *or* 100 mg every 12 hr as extended-release product. *Chronic suppression:* 50–100 mg at bedtime.

PO (Children >1 mo): *Treatment of active infection:* 5–7 mg/kg/day divided every 6 hr; maximum dose: 400 mg/day. *Chronic suppression:* 1–2 mg/kg/day in 1–2 divided doses; maximum dose: 100 mg/day (unlabeled).

Availability (generic available)

Tablets: 50 mg, 100 mg. **Capsules (Macrodantin):** 25 mg, 50 mg, 100 mg. **Extended-release capsules (Macrobid):** 100 mg. **Oral suspension:** 25 mg/5 mL, 50 mg/5 mL.

NURSING IMPLICATIONS

Assessment

- Assess for signs and symptoms of urinary tract infection (frequency, urgency, pain, and burning on urination; fever; cloudy or foul-smelling urine) before and periodically during therapy.
- Obtain specimens for culture and sensitivity before and during drug administration.
- Monitor intake and output ratios. Report significant discrepancies in totals.
- Monitor bowel function. Diarrhea, abdominal cramping, fever, and bloody stools should be reported to health care professional promptly as a sign of CDAD. May begin up to several wk following cessation of therapy.
- Assess for signs and symptoms of pulmonary reactions periodically during therapy. Acute reactions (fever, chills, cough, chest pain, dyspnea, pulmonary infiltration with consolidation or pleural effusion on x-ray, eosinophilia) usually occur within first wk of treatment and resolve when therapy is discontinued. Chronic reactions (malaise, dyspnea on exertion, cough, altered pulmonary function) may indicate pneumonitis or pulmonary fibrosis and are more common in patients taking nitrofurantoin for 6 mo or longer.

Lab Test Considerations

- Monitor CBC routinely with patients on prolonged therapy.
- Monitor liver function tests periodically during therapy. May cause ↑ serum glucose, bilirubin, and alkaline phosphatase. If hepatotoxicity occurs, discontinue therapy.
- Monitor renal function periodically during therapy. May cause ↑ BUN and serum creatinine.

Implementation

- **PO:** Take with meals to improve absorption and ↓ adverse effects.
- ***DNC:*** Do not crush tablets or open capsules (Macrobid).
- **Macrodantin** may be opened and mixed with food or juice for immediate use.
- Administer liquid preparations with calibrated measuring device. Shake well before administration. Oral suspension may be mixed with water, milk, fruit juices, or infant formula. Rinse mouth with water after administration of oral suspension to avoid staining teeth.

Patient/Family Teaching

- Explain purpose and side effects of medication to patient. Advise patient to read *Patient Information* before starting therapy. Instruct patient to take medication around the clock, as directed. Take missed doses as soon as remembered and space next dose 2–4 hr apart. Do not skip or double up on missed doses. Instruct patient to consult health care professional if no improvement is seen within a few days after initiation of therapy.
- May cause dizziness or drowsiness. Caution patient to avoid driving or other activities requiring alertness until response to medication is known.
- Inform patient that medication may cause a rust-yellow to brown discoloration of urine, which is not significant.
- Advise patient to notify health care professional if fever, chills, cough, chest pain, dyspnea, skin rash, numbness or tingling of the fingers or toes, or intolerable GI upset occurs. Signs of superinfection (milky, foul-smelling urine; perineal irritation; dysuria) should also be reported.
- Instruct patient to notify health care professional if fever and diarrhea develop, especially if stool contains blood, pus, or mucus. Advise patient not to treat diarrhea without consulting health care professional.
- Rep: May cause fetal harm. Advise females of reproductive potential to notify health care professional

if pregnancy is planned or suspected and to avoid breastfeeding during therapy and for 1 mo after last dose of therapy. May cause hemolytic anemia in pregnant patients at term (38–42 wk gestation), during labor and delivery, or when the onset of labor is imminent.

Evaluation/Desired Outcomes

- Resolution of the signs and symptoms of infection. Therapy should be continued for a minimum of 7 days and for at least 3 days after the urine has become sterile.
- Decrease in the frequency of infections in chronic suppressive therapy.

NITROGLYCERIN

(nye-tro-**gli**-ser-in)

nitroglycerin extended-release capsules

Nitro-Time

nitroglycerin intravenous

~~Nitro-Bid IV~~, ✱ Nitroject, ~~Tridil~~

nitroglycerin sublingual tablets

Nitrostat

nitroglycerin transdermal ointment

Nitro-Bid

nitroglycerin transdermal patch

Nitro-Dur, ✱ Trinipatch

nitroglycerin translingual spray

Nitrolingual

Classification

Therapeutic: antianginals

Pharmacologic: nitrates

Indications

Acute (**translingual, SL, ointment**) and long-term prophylactic (**oral, transdermal**) management of angina pectoris. **PO:** Adjunct treatment of HF. **IV:** Adjunct treatment of acute MI. Production of controlled hypotension during surgical procedures. Treatment of HF.

Action

Increases coronary blood flow by dilating coronary arteries and improving collateral flow to ischemic regions. Produces vasodilation (venous greater than arterial). Decreases left ventricular end-diastolic pressure and left ventricular end-diastolic volume (preload). Reduces myocardial oxygen consumption. **Therapeutic Effects:** Relief or prevention of anginal attacks. Increased cardiac output. Reduction of BP.

Pharmacokinetics

Absorption: Well absorbed after oral, buccal, and sublingual administration. Also absorbed through skin. Orally administered nitroglycerin is rapidly metabolized, leading to ↓ bioavailability.

Distribution: Unknown.

Metabolism and Excretion: Undergoes rapid and almost complete metabolism by the liver; also metabolized by enzymes in bloodstream.

Half-life: 1–4 min.

TIME/ACTION PROFILE (cardiovascular effects)

ROUTE	ONSET	PEAK	DURATION
SL/Translingual	1–3 min	unknown	30–60 min
PO-ER	40–60 min	unknown	8–12 hr
Oint	20–60 min	unknown	4–8 hr
Patch	40–60 min	unknown	8–24 hr
IV	immediate	unknown	several min

Contraindications/Precautions

Contraindicated in: Hypersensitivity; ↑ intracranial pressure; Severe anemia; Pericardial tamponade; Constrictive pericarditis; Uncorrected hypovolemia; Alcohol intolerance (large IV doses only); Acute circulatory failure/shock; Concurrent use of PDE-5 inhibitor (avanafil, sildenafil, tadalafil, vardenafil) or riociguat.

Use Cautiously in: Head trauma or cerebral hemorrhage; Glaucoma; Hypertrophic cardiomyopathy; Severe hepatic impairment; Malabsorption or hypermotility (PO); Cardioversion (remove transdermal patch before procedure); OB: May compromise maternal/fetal circulation; Lactation: Safety not established in breastfeeding; Pedi: Safety and effectiveness not established in children.

Adverse Reactions/Side Effects

CV: hypotension, tachycardia, syncope. **Derm:** contact dermatitis (transdermal), flushing. **EENT:** blurred vision. **GI:** abdominal pain, nausea, vomiting. **Neuro:** dizziness, headache, apprehension, restlessness, weakness.. **Misc:** alcohol intoxication (large IV doses only), tolerance.

Interactions

Drug-Drug: **Avanafil, sildenafil, tadalafil,** or **vardenafil** may result in severe hypotension (do not use within 24 hr of isosorbide dinitrate or mononitrate); concurrent use contraindicated. **Riociguat** may result in severe hypotension; concurrent use contraindicated. Additive hypotension with **antihypertensives**, acute ingestion of **alcohol**, **beta blockers**, **calcium channel blockers**, **haloperidol**, or **phenothiazines**. Agents having anticholinergic properties (**tricyclic antidepressants**, **antihistamines**,

N

✱ = Canadian drug name. ⚕ = Genetic implication. V = Vesicant. Boxed warning.
~~Strikethrough~~ = Discontinued. *CAPITALS = life-threatening. Underline = most frequent.

phenothiazines) may ↓ absorption of translingual or sublingual nitroglycerin.

Route/Dosage

SL (Adults): *Tablets:* 0.3–0.6 mg; may repeat every 5 min for 2 additional doses for acute attack; may also be used prophylactically 5–10 min before activities that may precipitate an acute attack.
Translingual Spray: (Adults): 1–2 sprays; may be repeated every 5 min for 2 additional doses for acute attack; may also be used prophylactically 5–10 min before activities that may precipitate an acute attack.
PO (Adults): 2.5–9 mg every 8–12 hr.
IV (Adults): 5 mcg/min; ↑ by 5 mcg/min every 3–5 min to 20 mcg/min; if no response, ↑ by 10–20 mcg/min every 3–5 min (dosing determined by hemodynamic parameters; max: 200 mcg/min).
Transdermal (Adults): *Ointment:* 1–2 in. every 6–8 hr. *Transdermal patch:* 0.2–0.4 mg/hr initially; may titrate up to 0.4–0.8 mg/hr. Patch should be worn 12–14 hr/day and then taken off for 10–12 hr/day.

Availability (generic available)

Extended-release capsules: 2.5 mg, 6.5 mg, 9 mg. **Sublingual tablets:** 0.3 mg, 0.4 mg, 0.6 mg. **Translingual spray:** 0.4 mg/spray in 4.9-g bottle (60 doses) or 14.6-g bottle (200 doses). **Transdermal patch:** 0.1 mg/hr, 0.2 mg/hr, 0.3 mg/hr, 0.4 mg/hr, 0.6 mg/hr, 0.8 mg/hr. **Transdermal ointment:** 2%. **Solution for injection:** 5 mg/mL. **Premixed infusion:** 25 mg/250 mL D5W, 50 mg/250 mL D5W, 100 mg/250 mL D5W.

NURSING IMPLICATIONS

Assessment

- Assess location, duration, intensity, and precipitating factors of patient's anginal pain.
- Monitor BP and HR before and after administration. Patients receiving IV nitroglycerin require continuous ECG and BP monitoring. Additional hemodynamic parameters may be monitored.

Lab Test Considerations

- May cause ↑ urine catecholamine and urine vanillylmandelic acid concentrations.
- Excessive doses may cause ↑ methemoglobin concentrations.
- May cause falsely ↑ serum cholesterol levels.

Implementation

- **PO:** Administer dose 1 hr before or 2 hr after meals with a full glass of water for faster absorption. ***DNC:*** Sustained-release preparations should be swallowed whole; do not break, crush, or chew.
- **SL:** Tablet should be held under tongue until dissolved. Avoid eating, drinking, or smoking until tablet is dissolved.
- **Translingual spray:** Spray *Nitrolingual* under tongue.

IV Administration

- **IV:** Doses must be diluted and administered as an infusion. Standard infusion sets made of polyvinyl chloride plastic may absorb up to 80% of the nitroglycerin in solution. Use glass bottles only and special tubing provided by manufacturer.
- **Continuous Infusion: Dilution:** Vials must be diluted in D5W or 0.9% NaCl. Premixed infusions already diluted in D5W and are ready to be administered (no further dilution needed). Admixed solutions stable for 48 hr at room temperature or 7 days if refrigerated. Stability of premixed solutions based on manufacturer's expiration date. **Concentration:** Should not exceed 400 mcg/mL. **Rate:** See Route/Dosage section. Administer via infusion pump to ensure accurate rate. Titrate rate according to patient response.
- **Y-Site Compatibility:** acyclovir, alemtuzumab, amikacin, aminocaproic acid, aminophylline, amiodarone, amphotericin B liposome, anidulafungin, argatroban, arsenic trioxide, ascorbic acid, atracurium, atropine, azathioprine, azithromycin, aztreonam, benztropine, bivalirudin, bleomycin, bumetanide, buprenorphine, butorphanol, calcium chloride, calcium gluconate, cangrelor, carboplatin, carmustine, caspofungin, cefazolin, cefiderocol, cefotaxime, cefotetan, cefoxitin, ceftazidime, ceftolozane/tazobactam, ceftriaxone, cefuroxime, chloramphenicol, chlorpromazine, cisatracurium, cisplatin, clevidipine, clindamycin, cyanocobalamin, cyclophosphamide, cyclosporine, cytarabine, dacarbazine, dactinomycin, daunorubicin, dexamethasone, dexmedetomidine, dexrazoxane, digoxin, diltiazem, diphenhydramine, dobutamine, docetaxel, dopamine, doxorubicin hydrochloride, doxorubicin liposomal, doxycycline, enalaprilat, ephedrine, epinephrine, epirubicin, epoetin alfa, eptifibatide, ertapenem, erythromycin, esmolol, esomeprazole, etoposide, etoposide phosphate, famotidine, fentanyl, fluconazole, fludarabine, fluorouracil, folic acid, foscarnet, fosphenytoin, ganciclovir, gemcitabine, gemtuzumab ozogamicin, gentamicin, glycopyrrolate, granisetron, heparin, hetastarch, hydrocortisone, hydromorphone, idarubicin, ifosfamide, imipenem/cilastatin, imipenem/cilastatin/relebactam, indomethacin, insulin regular, irinotecan, isavuconazonium, isoproterenol, ketorolac, labetalol, LR, leucovorin, lidocaine, linezolid, lorazepam, magnesium sulfate, mannitol, meperidine, meropenem/vaborbactam, mesna, methadone,

methotrexate, methylprednisolone, metoclopramide, metronidazole, micafungin, midazolam, milrinone, minocycline, mitomycin, mitoxantrone, morphine, moxifloxacin, multivitamins, mycophenolate, nafcillin, nalbuphine, naloxone, nicardipine, nitroprusside, norepinephrine, octreotide, ondansetron, oritavancin, oxacillin, oxaliplatin, oxytocin, paclitaxel, palonosetron, pamidronate, papaverine, pemetrexed, penicillin G, pentamidine, pentobarbital, phenobarbital, phentolamine, phenylephrine, phytonadione, piperacillin/tazobactam, plazomicin, potassium acetate, potassium chloride, procainamide, prochlorperazine, promethazine, propranolol, protamine, pyridoxine, remifentanil, remimazolam, rocuronium, sodium bicarbonate, succinylcholine, sufentanil, sulbactam/durlobactam, tacrolimus, tedizolid, theophylline, thiamine, thiotepa, tigecycline, tirofiban, tobramycin, topotecan, vancomycin, vasopressin, vecuronium, verapamil, vinblastine, vincristine, vinorelbine, voriconazole, zoledronic acid.

Y-Site Incompatibility: alteplase, dantrolene, daptomycin, diazepam, diazoxide, levofloxacin, phenytoin, trimethoprim/sulfamethoxazole.

- **Topical:** Rotate sites of topical application to prevent skin irritation. Remove patch or ointment from previous site before application.
- Doses may be ↑ to the highest dose that does not cause symptomatic hypotension.
- Apply ointment by using dose-measuring application papers supplied with ointment. Squeeze ointment onto measuring scale printed on paper. Use paper to spread ointment onto nonhairy area of skin (chest, abdomen, thighs; avoid distal extremities) in a thin, even layer, covering a 2–3-in. area. Do not allow ointment to come in contact with hands. Do not massage or rub in ointment; this will ↑ absorption and interfere with sustained action. Apply occlusive dressing if ordered.
- Transdermal patches may be applied to any hairless site (avoid distal extremities or areas with cuts or calluses). Apply firm pressure over patch to ensure contact with skin, especially around edges. Apply a new dose unit if the first one becomes loose or falls off. Units are waterproof and not affected by showering or bathing. Do not cut or trim system to adjust dosage. Do not alternate between brands of transdermal products; dose may not be equivalent. Remove patches before MRI, cardioversion, or defibrillation to prevent patient burns. Patch may be worn for 12–14 hr and removed for 10–12 hr at night to prevent development of tolerance.

Patient/Family Teaching

- Instruct patient to take medication as directed, even if feeling better. Take missed doses as soon as remembered unless next dose is scheduled within 2 hr (6 hr with extended-release preparations). Do not double doses. Do not discontinue abruptly; gradual dose ↓ may be necessary to prevent rebound angina.
- Caution patient to change positions slowly to minimize orthostatic hypotension. 1st dose should be taken while in a sitting or reclining position, especially in older adults.
- Advise patient to avoid concurrent use of alcohol with this medication. Patient should also consult health care provider before taking OTC medications while taking nitroglycerin.
- Inform patient that headache is a common side effect that should decrease with continuing therapy. Aspirin or acetaminophen may be ordered to treat headache. Notify health care provider if headache is persistent or severe.
- Advise patient to notify health care provider if dry mouth or blurred vision occurs.
- Rep: Advise women of reproductive potential to notify health care provider if pregnancy is planned or suspected or if breastfeeding.
- **Acute Anginal Attacks:** Advise patient to sit down and use medication at 1st sign of attack. Relief usually occurs within 5 min. Dose may be repeated if pain is not relieved in 5–10 min. Call health care provider or go to nearest emergency room if anginal pain is not relieved by 3 tablets in 15 min.
- **SL:** Inform patient that tablets should be kept in original glass container or in specially made metal containers, with cotton removed to prevent absorption. Tablets lose potency in containers made of plastic or cardboard or when mixed with other capsules or tablets. Exposure to air, heat, and moisture also causes loss of potency. Instruct patient not to open bottle frequently, handle tablets, or keep bottle of tablets next to body (e.g., shirt pocket) or in automobile glove compartment. Advise patient that tablets should be replaced 6 mo after opening to maintain potency.
- **Lingual Spray:** Instruct patient to lift tongue and spray dose under tongue.

Evaluation/Desired Outcomes

- Decrease in frequency and severity of anginal attacks.
- Increase in activity tolerance. During long-term therapy, tolerance may be minimized by intermittent administration in 12–14 hr or 10–12 hr off intervals.
- Controlled hypotension during surgical procedures.
- Treatment of HF associated with acute MI.

N

HIGH ALERT

nitroprusside
(nye-troe-**pruss**-ide)
✱ Nipride, Nipride RTU, ~~Nitropress~~

Classification
Therapeutic: antihypertensives
Pharmacologic: vasodilators

Indications
Hypertensive crises. Controlled hypotension during anesthesia. Cardiac pump failure or cardiogenic shock (as monotherapy or in combination with dopamine).

Action
Produces peripheral vasodilation by a direct action on venous and arteriolar smooth muscle. **Therapeutic Effects:** Rapid lowering of BP. Decreased cardiac preload and afterload.

Pharmacokinetics
Absorption: IV administration results in complete bioavailability.
Distribution: Unknown.
Metabolism and Excretion: Rapidly metabolized in RBCs and tissues to cyanide and subsequently by the liver to thiocyanate.
Half-life: 2 min.

TIME/ACTION PROFILE (hypotensive effect)

ROUTE	ONSET	PEAK	DURATION
IV	immediate	rapid	1–10 min

Contraindications/Precautions
Contraindicated in: Hypersensitivity; ↓ cerebral perfusion.
Use Cautiously in: Renal impairment (↑ risk of thiocyanate accumulation); Hepatic impairment (↑ risk of cyanide accumulation); Hypothyroidism; Hyponatremia; Vitamin B deficiency; OB: Safety not established in pregnancy; Lactation: Safety not established in breastfeeding; Geri: Older adults may have ↑ sensitivity to drug effects.

Adverse Reactions/Side Effects
CV: dyspnea, HYPOTENSION, palpitations. **EENT:** blurred vision, tinnitus. **F and E:** acidosis. **GI:** abdominal pain, nausea, vomiting **Local:** phlebitis. **Neuro:** dizziness, headache, restlessness. **Misc:** CYANIDE TOXICITY, thiocyanate toxicity.

Interactions
Drug-Drug: ↑ hypotensive effect with **ganglionic blocking agents, general anesthetics,** and other **antihypertensives. Estrogens** and **sympathomimetics** may ↓ the response to nitroprusside.

Route/Dosage
IV (Adults and Children): 0.3 mcg/kg/min initially; may ↑ as needed up to 10 mcg/kg/min (usual dose is 3 mcg/kg/min; not to exceed 10 min of therapy at 10 mcg/kg/min infusion rate).

Availability (generic available)
Premixed infusion: 20 mg/100 mL 0.9% NaCl, 50 mg/100 mL 0.9% NaCl. **Solution for injection:** 25 mg/mL.

NURSING IMPLICATIONS
Assessment
- Monitor BP, HR, and ECG frequently throughout therapy; continuous monitoring is preferred. Monitor for rebound hypertension following discontinuation of nitroprusside.
- Pulmonary capillary wedge pressure may be monitored in patients with MI or HF.

Lab Test Considerations
- May ↓ bicarbonate concentrations, pCO_2, and pH.
- May cause ↑ lactate concentrations.
- May ↑ cyanide and thiocyanate concentrations.
- Monitor serum methemoglobin concentrations in patients receiving >10 mg/kg and exhibiting signs of impaired oxygen delivery despite adequate cardiac output and arterial pCO_2 (blood is chocolate brown without change on exposure to air). Treatment of methemoglobinemia is 1–2 mg/kg of methylene blue IV administered over several minutes.

Toxicity and Overdose
- If severe hypotension occurs, drug effects are quickly reversed, within 1–10 min, by ↓ rate or temporarily discontinuing infusion. May place patient in Trendelenburg position to maximize venous return.
- Signs and symptoms of thiocyanate toxicity include tinnitus, toxic psychoses, hyperreflexia, confusion, weakness, seizures, and coma. Monitor plasma thiocyanate levels daily in patients receiving prolonged infusions at a rate >3 mcg/kg/min or 1 mcg/kg/min in patients with anuria. Thiocyanate levels should not exceed 1 mmol/L.
- Cyanide toxicity may manifest as lactic acidosis, hypoxemia, tachycardia, altered consciousness, seizures, and characteristic breath odor similar to almonds. Acute treatment of cyanide toxicity includes 4–6 mg/kg of sodium nitrite (as a 3% solution) over 2–4 min. This acts as a buffer for cyanide by converting 10% of hemoglobin to methemoglobin. If administration of sodium nitrite is delayed, inhalation of crushed ampule of amyl nitrite for 15–30 sec of every minute should be started until sodium nitrite is running. Following completion of sodium nitrite infusion, administer

sodium thiosulfate 150–200 mcg/kg (available as 25% and 50% solutions). This will convert cyanide to thiocyanate, which may then be eliminated. If required, entire regimen may be repeated in 2 hr at 50% of the initial doses.

mplementation

- If infusion of 10 mcg/kg/min for 10 min does not produce adequate ↓ in BP, manufacturer recommends nitroprusside be discontinued.
- May be administered in HF concurrently with an inotropic agent (dopamine, dobutamine) when effective doses of nitroprusside restore pump function and cause excessive hypotension.

V Administration

- **Continuous Infusion: Dilution:** Dilute 50 mg of nitroprusside in 250–1000 mL of D5W. Wrap infusion in aluminum foil to protect from light; administration set tubing need not be covered. Amber plastic bags do not offer sufficient protection from light; wrap must be opaque. Freshly prepared solution has a slight brownish tint; discard if solution is dark brown, orange, blue, green, or dark red. Solution must be used within 24 hr of preparation. **Concentration:** 50–200 mcg/mL. **Rate:** Based on patient's weight (see Route/Dosage section).
- **Y-Site Compatibility:** alemtuzumab, alprostadil, amikacin, aminocaproic acid, aminophylline, amphotericin B liposomal, anidulafungin, argatroban, arsenic trioxide, atropine, azithromycin, aztreonam, benztropine, bivalirudin, bleomycin, bumetanide, buprenorphine, butorphanol, calcium chloride, calcium gluconate, cangrelor, carboplatin, carmustine, cefazolin, cefotaxime, cefotetan, cefoxitin, ceftolozane/tazobactam, ceftriaxone, cefuroxime, chloramphenicol, cisplatin, clevidipine, clindamycin, cyanocobalamin, cyclophosphamide, cyclosporine, cytarabine, dacarbazine, dactinomycin, daptomycin, dexamethasone, dexmedetomidine, dexrazoxane, digoxin, diltiazem, docetaxel, dopamine, doxorubicin hydrochloride, doxorubicin liposomal, doxycycline, enalaprilat, ephedrine, epinephrine, epirubicin, epoetin alfa, eptifibatide, ertapenem, esmolol, etoposide, etoposide phosphate, famotidine, fentanyl, fluconazole, fludarabine, fluorouracil, folic acid, foscarnet, fosphenytoin, furosemide, ganciclovir, gemcitabine, gemtuzumab ozogamicin, gentamicin, glycopyrrolate, granisetron, heparin, hydrocortisone, hydromorphone, idarubicin, ifosfamide, indomethacin, insulin regular, isavuconazonium, isoproterenol, ketorolac, labetalol, leucovorin, lidocaine, linezolid, lorazepam, magnesium sulfate, mannitol, meperidine, meropenem, methadone, methylprednisolone, metoclopramide, metoprolol, metronidazole, micafungin, midazolam, milrinone, minocycline, morphine, multivitamins, nafcillin, nalbuphine, naloxone, nicardipine, nitroglycerin, norepinephrine, octreotide, ondansetron, oxacillin, oxaliplatin, oxytocin, paclitaxel, palonosetron, pamidronate, penicillin G, pentamidine, pentobarbital, phenobarbital, phentolamine, phenylephrine, phytonadione, piperacillin/tazobactam, plazomicin, potassium acetate, potassium chloride, potassium phosphates, procainamide, propofol, propranolol, protamine, pyridoxine, rocuronium, sodium acetate, sodium bicarbonate, succinylcholine, sufentanil, tacrolimus, theophylline, thiamine, tigecycline, tirofiban, tobramycin, topotecan, vancomycin, vasopressin, vecuronium, verapamil, vinblastine, vincristine, zoledronic acid.
- **Y-Site Incompatibility:** acyclovir, ascorbic acid, azathioprine, caspofungin, ceftazidime, chlorpromazine, dantrolene, daunorubicin, diazepam, diazoxide, diphenhydramine, erythromycin, hydralazine, irinotecan, levofloxacin, mesna, mitomycin, mitoxantrone, moxifloxacin, mycophenolate, oritavancin, papaverine, pemetrexed, phenytoin, prochlorperazine, promethazine, thiotepa, trimethoprim/sulfamethoxazole, vinorelbine, voriconazole.

Patient/Family Teaching

- Explain purpose of nitroprusside to patient.
- Advise patient to notify health care provider of all Rx or OTC medications, vitamins, or herbal products being taken and to consult health care provider before taking other medications.
- Advise patient to report the onset of tinnitus, dyspnea, dizziness, headache, or blurred vision immediately.
- Rep: Advise women of reproductive potential to notify health care provider if pregnancy is planned or suspected or if breastfeeding.

Evaluation/Desired Outcomes

- Rapid lowering of BP.
- Decreased cardiac preload and afterload.

N

HIGH ALERT

nivolumab (nye-**vol**-ue-mab)

Opdivo

Classification

Therapeutic: antineoplastics

Pharmacologic: monoclonal antibodies, programmed death-1 inhibitors

Indications

Unresectable/metastatic melanoma (as monotherapy or in combination with ipilimumab). Adjuvant treatment of patients with completely resected Stage IIB, Stage IIC, Stage III, or Stage IV melanoma. Metastatic non-small cell lung cancer (NSCLC) with progression on or after platinum-based chemotherapy. Patients with epidermal growth factor receptor (EGFR) or anaplastic lymphoma kinase (ALK) genomic tumor aberrations should have disease progression on FDA-approved therapy for these aberrations prior to receiving nivolumab. First-line treatment of metastatic NSCLC in patients whose tumors express PD-L1 (≥1%) and have no EGFR or ALK genomic tumor aberrations (in combination with ipilimumab). First-line treatment of metastatic or recurrent NSCLC in patients whose tumors have no EGFR or ALK genomic tumor aberrations (in combination with ipilimumab and two cycles of platinum-based chemotherapy). Neoadjuvant treatment of resectable (tumors ≥4 cm or node positive) NSCLC (in combination with platinum-doublet chemotherapy). Neoadjuvant treatment of resectable (tumors ≥4 cm or node positive) NSCLC in patients whose tumors have no known EGFR mutations or ALK rearrangements (in combination with platinum-doublet chemotherapy as neoadjuvant treatment and then continued as a single agent as adjuvant treatment after surgery). Advanced renal cell carcinoma in patients who have previously received antiangiogenic therapy (as monotherapy). Immediate or poor risk, previously untreated advanced renal cell carcinoma (in combination with ipilimumab). First-line treatment of advanced renal cell carcinoma (in combination with cabozantinib). Classic Hodgkin lymphoma that has relapsed or progressed after either autologous hematopoietic stem cell transplantation and brentuximab or ≥3 lines of systemic therapy that includes autologous hematopoietic stem cell transplantation. Recurrent or metastatic squamous cell carcinoma of the head and neck with progression on or after platinum-based therapy. Adjuvant treatment of urothelial carcinoma in patients who are at high risk of recurrence after undergoing radical resection of urothelial carcinoma. First-line treatment of unresectable or metastatic urothelial carcinoma (in combination with cisplatin and gemcitabine). Locally advanced or metastatic urothelial carcinoma in patients who either have progression during or following platinum-based therapy or have progression within 12 mo of neoadjuvant or adjuvant treatment with platinum-based therapy. Unresectable or metastatic microsatellite instability-high (MSI-H) or mismatch repair deficient (dMMR) colorectal cancer (in combination with ipilimumab). MSI-H or dMMR colorectal cancer that has progressed following treatment with fluoropyrimidine, oxaliplatin, and irinotecan (as monotherapy). First-line treatment of unresectable or metastatic hepatocellular carcinoma (in combination with ipilimumab). Unresectable or metastatic hepatocellular carcinoma in patients who have been previously treated with sorafenib (in combination with ipilimumab). Unresectable advanced, recurrent, or metastatic esophageal squamous cell carcinoma after prior fluoropyrimidine- and platinum-based chemotherapy. First-line treatment of unresectable advanced or metastatic esophageal squamous cell carcinoma in patients whose tumors express PD-L1 (≥1) (in combination with fluoropyrimidine- and platinum-containing chemotherapy). First-line treatment of unresectable advanced or metastatic esophageal squamous cell carcinoma in patients whose tumors express PD-L1 (≥1) (in combination with ipilimumab). Adjuvant treatment of completely resected esophageal or gastroesophageal junction cancer with residual pathologic disease in patients who have received neoadjuvant chemoradiotherapy. Advanced or metastatic gastric cancer, gastroesophageal junction cancer, and esophageal adenocarcinoma in patients whose tumors express PD-L1 (≥1) (in combination with fluoropyrimidine- and platinum-containing chemotherapy). First-line treatment of unresectable malignant pleural mesothelioma (in combination with ipilimumab).

Action

Programmed death receptor-1 (PD-1) blocking antibody (an IgG4 kappa immunoglobulin) that binds to PD-1 and blocks its interaction with its ligands, PD-L1 and PD-L2, resulting in activation of the immune system and decreased tumor growth. **Therapeutic Effects:** Decreased progression of melanoma, Hodgkin lymphoma, urothelial carcinoma, colorectal cancer, and hepatocellular carcinoma. Decreased progression of and improved survival with NSCLC and advanced renal cell carcinoma. Improved survival in squamous cell carcinoma of head and neck, esophageal cancer, gastric cancer, gastroesophageal junction cancer, esophageal adenocarcinoma, and malignant pleural mesothelioma.

Pharmacokinetics

Absorption: IV administration results in complete bioavailability.
Distribution: Unknown.
Metabolism and Excretion: Unknown.
Half-life: 26.7 days.

TIME/ACTION PROFILE

ROUTE	ONSET	PEAK	DURATION
IV	unknown	unknown	unknown

Contraindications/Precautions

Contraindicated in: OB: Pregnancy; Lactation: Lactation.

Use Cautiously in: Patients undergoing allogeneic hematopoietic stem cell transplantation before or after nivolumab therapy (↑ risk of complications); Patients with multiple myeloma receiving a thalidomide analogue and dexamethasone (↑ risk of mortality); Rep: Women of reproductive potential; Pedi: Safety and effectiveness not established in children <12 yr (microsatellite instability-high or mismatch repair deficient colorectal cancer and melanoma) or children <18 yr (all other indications).

Adverse Reactions/Side Effects

CV: MYOCARDITIS, pericarditis, peripheral edema, vasculitis. **Derm:** rash, DRUG REACTION WITH EOSINOPHILIA AND SYSTEMIC SYMPTOMS (DRESS), STEVENS-JOHNSON SYNDROME (SJS), TOXIC EPIDERMAL NECROLYSIS (TEN). **EENT:** iritis, uveitis. **Endo:** hypothyroidism, ADRENAL INSUFFICIENCY, hyperthyroidism, hypoparathyroidism, hypophysitis, type 1 diabetes. **F and E:** hyperkalemia. **GI:** COLITIS, gastritis, HEPATITIS, pancreatitis. **GU:** nephritis. **Hemat:** hemolytic anemia. **MS:** myositis, RHABDOMYOLYSIS. **Neuro:** autoimmune neuropathy, ENCEPHALITIS, Guillain-Barré syndrome, MENINGITIS, myasthenic syndrome, myelitis. **Resp:** cough, PNEUMONITIS. **Misc:** INFUSION-RELATED REACTIONS.

Interactions

Drug-Drug: None reported.

Route/Dosage

Unresectable or Metastatic Melanoma

IV (Adults and Children ≥12 yr and ≥40 kg): *As monotherapy:* 240 mg every 2 wk until disease progression or unacceptable toxicity *or* 480 mg every 4 wk until disease progression or unacceptable toxicity; *In combination with ipilimumab:* 1 mg/kg every 3 wk for a max of 4 doses or until unacceptable toxicity (whichever occurs first) (administer before ipilimumab on same day); then either 240 mg as monotherapy every 2 wk until disease progression or unacceptable toxicity *or* 480 mg as monotherapy every 4 wk until disease progression or unacceptable toxicity.

IV (Children ≥12 yr and <40 kg): *As monotherapy:* 3 mg/kg every 2 wk until disease progression or unacceptable toxicity *or* 6 mg/kg every 4 wk until disease progression or unacceptable toxicity; *In combination with ipilimumab:* 1 mg/kg every 3 wk for a max of 4 doses or until unacceptable toxicity (whichever occurs first) (administer before ipilimumab on same day); then either 3 mg/kg as monotherapy every 2 wk until disease progression or unacceptable toxicity *or* 6 mg/kg as monotherapy every 4 wk until disease progression or unacceptable toxicity.

Adjuvant Treatment of Melanoma

IV (Adults and Children ≥12 yr and ≥40 kg): 240 mg every 2 wk until disease progression or unacceptable toxicity for up to 1 yr *or* 480 mg every 4 wk until disease progression or unacceptable toxicity for up to 1 yr.

IV (Children ≥12 yr and <40 kg): 3 mg/kg every 2 wk until disease progression or unacceptable toxicity for up to 1 yr *or* 6 mg/kg every 4 wk until disease progression or unacceptable toxicity for up to 1 yr.

Hepatocellular Carcinoma

IV (Adults): 1 mg/kg every 3 wk for a max of 4 doses (administer before ipilimumab on same day); then 240 mg as monotherapy every 2 wk until disease progression, unacceptable toxicity, or up to 2 yr *or* 480 mg as monotherapy every 4 wk until disease progression, unacceptable toxicity, or up to 2 yr.

First-Line Treatment of Unresectable or Metastatic Urothelial Carcinoma

IV (Adults): *In combination with cisplatin and gemcitabine:* 360 mg every 3 wk for up to 6 cycles (administer before cisplatin and gemcitabine on same day); then either 240 mg as monotherapy every 2 wk until disease progression, unacceptable toxicity, or up to 2 yr *or* 480 mg as monotherapy every 4 wk until disease progression, unacceptable toxicity, or up to 2 yr.

Adjuvant Treatment of Urothelial Carcinoma

IV (Adults): 240 mg every 2 wk until disease progression or unacceptable toxicity for up to 1 yr *or* 480 mg every 4 wk until disease progression or unacceptable toxicity for up to 1 yr.

Classical Hodgkin Lymphoma, Urothelial Carcinoma, or Squamous Cell Carcinoma of Head and Neck

IV (Adults): 240 mg every 2 wk until disease progression or unacceptable toxicity *or* 480 mg every 4 wk until disease progression or unacceptable toxicity.

Esophageal Squamous Cell Carcinoma

IV (Adults): *As monotherapy:* 240 mg every 2 wk until disease progression or unacceptable toxicity *or* 480 mg every 4 wk until disease progression or unacceptable toxicity. *In combination with fluoropyrimidine- and platinum-containing chemotherapy:* 240 mg every 2 wk until disease progression, unacceptable toxicity, or for up to 2 yr *or* 480 mg every 4 wk until disease progression, unacceptable toxicity, or up to 2 yr. *In combination with ipilimumab:* 3 mg/kg every 2 wk until disease progression, unacceptable toxicity, or up to 2 yr (administer before ipilimumab on same day) *or* 360 mg every 3 wk until disease progression,

N

unacceptable toxicity, or up to 2 yr (administer before ipilimumab on same day).

Adjuvant Treatment of Resected Esophageal or Gastroesophageal Junction Cancer

IV (Adults): 240 mg every 2 wk until disease progression or unacceptable toxicity for a total treatment duration of 1 yr *or* 480 mg every 4 wk until disease progression or unacceptable toxicity for a total treatment duration of 1 yr.

Metastatic Non-Small Cell Lung Cancer

IV (Adults): *As monotherapy:* 240 mg every 2 wk until disease progression or unacceptable toxicity *or* 480 mg every 4 wk until disease progression or unacceptable toxicity; *In combination with ipilimumab (for metastatic tumors expressing PD-L1):* 3 mg/kg every 3 wk until disease progression, unacceptable toxicity, or up to 2 yr (if no disease progression) (administer before ipilimumab on same day). *In combination with ipilimumab (for metastatic or recurrent tumors not expressing PD-L1):* 360 mg every 3 wk until disease progression, unacceptable toxicity, or up to 2 yr (if no disease progression) (when given just with platinum-based chemotherapy on same day, administer nivolumab then platinum-based chemotherapy; when given with ipilimumab and platinum-based chemotherapy on same day, administer nivolumab, then ipilimumab, then platinum-based chemotherapy).

Neoadjuvant Treatment of Resectable Non-Small Cell Lung Cancer

IV (Adults): 360 mg every 3 wk (when given with platinum-doublet chemotherapy on same day) for 3 cycles.

Neoadjuvant and Adjuvant Treatment of Resectable Non-Small Cell Lung Cancer

IV (Adults): *Neoadjuvant treatment:* 360 mg every 3 wk (when given with platinum-doublet chemotherapy on same day) for up to 4 cycles, or until disease progression or unacceptable toxicity. *Adjuvant treatment:* 480 mg as monotherapy after surgery every 4 wk for up to 13 cycles (1 yr), or until disease recurrence or unacceptable toxicity.

Advanced Renal Cell Carcinoma

IV (Adults): *As monotherapy:* 240 mg every 2 wk until disease progression or unacceptable toxicity *or* 480 mg every 4 wk until disease progression or unacceptable toxicity; *In combination with ipilimumab:* 3 mg/kg every 3 wk for 4 doses (administer before ipilimumab on same day); then 240 mg as monotherapy every 2 wk until disease progression or unacceptable toxicity *or* 480 mg as monotherapy every 4 wk until disease progression or unacceptable toxicity. *In combination with cabozantinib:* 240 mg every 2 wk until disease progression, unacceptable toxicity, or up to 2 yr *or* 480 mg every 4 wk until disease progression, unacceptable toxicity, or up to 2 yr.

Microsatellite Instability-High or Mismatch Repair Deficient Metastatic Colorectal Cancer

IV (Adults and Children ≥12 yr and ≥40 kg): *As monotherapy:* 240 mg every 2 wk until disease progression or unacceptable toxicity *or* 480 mg every 4 wk until disease progression or unacceptable toxicity; *In combination with ipilimumab:* 240 mg every 3 wk for a max of 4 doses (administer before ipilimumab on same day); then 240 mg as monotherapy every 2 wk until disease progression, unacceptable toxicity, or up to 2 yr *or* 480 mg as monotherapy every 4 wk until disease progression, unacceptable toxicity, or up to 2 yr.

IV (Children ≥12 yr and <40 kg): *As monotherapy:* 3 mg/kg every 2 wk until disease progression or unacceptable toxicity; *In combination with ipilimumab:* 3 mg/kg every 3 wk for a max of 4 doses (administer before ipilimumab on same day), then 3 mg/kg as monotherapy every 2 wk until disease progression, unacceptable toxicity, or up to 2 yr *or* 6 mg/kg as monotherapy every 4 wk until disease progression, unacceptable toxicity, or up to 2 yr.

Gastric Cancer, Gastroesophageal Junction Cancer, and Esophageal Adenocarcinoma

IV (Adults): 240 mg every 2 wk until disease progression, unacceptable toxicity, or up to 2 yr (administer before fluoropyrimidine- and platinum-containing chemotherapy on same day) *or* 360 mg every 3 wk until disease progression, unacceptable toxicity, or up to 2 yr (administer before fluoropyrimidine- and platinum-containing chemotherapy on same day).

Malignant Pleural Mesothelioma

IV (Adults): 360 mg every 3 wk until disease progression, unacceptable toxicity, or up to 2 yr (if no disease progression) (administer before ipilimumab on same day).

Availability

Solution for injection: 10 mg/mL.

NURSING IMPLICATIONS

Assessment

- Monitor for signs/symptoms of immune-mediated pneumonitis (shortness of breath, chest pain, new or worse cough) periodically during therapy. Treat with corticosteroids 1–2 mg/kg/day of prednisone equivalents for Grade ≥2 pneumonitis followed by corticosteroid taper. *If Grade 2 pneumonitis occurs,* hold nivolumab; resume therapy when recovery to Grade ≤1. *If Grade 3 or 4 pneumonitis occurs,* permanently discontinue nivolumab.
- Assess for signs/symptoms of infusion reactions (chills or shaking, itching or rash, flushing, difficulty breathing, dizziness, fever, feeling faint) periodically during therapy. *If Grade 1 or 2 infusion reactions*

occur, hold or slow infusion. *If Grade 3 or 4 infusion reactions occur,* permanently discontinue nivolumab.

- Monitor for signs/symptoms of immune-mediated colitis (diarrhea, abdominal pain, mucus or blood in stool, with or without fever). Treat with corticosteroids at doses of 1–2 mg/kg/day of prednisone equivalents followed by corticosteroid taper for severe (Grade 3) or life-threatening (Grade 4) colitis. *If Grade 2 or 3 colitis occurs,* hold nivolumab. Resume therapy if complete or partial resolution (Grade ≤1) after corticosteroid taper. Permanently discontinue nivolumab if no complete or partial resolution within 12 wk of last dose or inability to ↓ prednisone to ≤10 mg/day (or equivalent) within 12 wk of initiating steroids. *If Grade 4 colitis occurs,* permanently discontinue nivolumab. *If administered with ipilimumab,* hold nivolumab for Grade 2 colitis. *For moderate or severe (Grade 3 or 4) or recurrent colitis,* permanently discontinue nivolumab and ipilimumab.
- Monitor for signs/symptoms of hepatitis (yellowing of skin or whites of eyes, severe nausea or vomiting, right-sided abdominal pain, drowsiness, dark urine, unusual bleeding or bruising, anorexia) periodically during therapy.
- Assess for rash periodically during therapy. Topical emollients and/or topical corticosteroids may be adequate to treat mild to moderate nonexfoliative rashes. May cause SJS and TEN. *If rash, itching, blistering, or ulcers in mouth or other mucous membranes occur and SJS, TEN, or DRESS are suspected,* hold nivolumab and refer for assessment and treatment. *If severe rash, SJS, TEN, or DRESS are confirmed,* permanently discontinue nivolumab. For immune-mediated rash, administer corticosteroids at doses of 1–2 mg/kg/day of prednisone equivalents followed by corticosteroid taper for severe (Grade 3) or life-threatening (Grade 4) rash.
- Monitor for signs/symptoms of hypophysitis (headaches, photophobia, visual field defects, extreme tiredness, weight gain or loss, dizziness or fainting, mood changes, hair loss, feeling cold, constipation, deepening voice, excessive thirst and urination) periodically during therapy. *If moderate or severe hypophysitis occurs,* hold nivolumab and administer hormone replacement and corticosteroids at a dose of 1 mg/kg/day of prednisone equivalents followed by corticosteroid taper. *If life-threatening hypophysitis occurs,* permanently discontinue nivolumab.
- Monitor for signs/symptoms of adrenal insufficiency. *If severe or life-threatening adrenal insufficiency occurs,* permanently discontinue nivolumab and administer corticosteroids at a dose of 1–2 mg/kg/day prednisone equivalents followed by corticosteroid taper.
- Monitor for signs/symptoms of encephalitis (headache, fever, tiredness or weakness, confusion, memory problems, sleepiness, hallucinations, seizures, stiff neck) periodically during therapy. *If Grade 2 neurological toxicities occur,* hold nivolumab for patients with new-onset moderate to severe neurologic symptoms during diagnosis. *If Grade 3 or 4 neurological toxicities occur,* permanently discontinue nivolumab and administer corticosteroids at dose of 1–2 mg/kg/day prednisone equivalents for immune-mediated encephalitis, followed by corticosteroid taper.
- Monitor for signs/symptoms of renal impairment (↓ in amount of urine, blood in urine, swelling in ankles, anorexia) periodically during therapy.
- Monitor for signs/symptoms of myocarditis (chest pain, dyspnea) during therapy. *If Grade 2–4 myocarditis occurs,* permanently discontinue nivolumab.

Lab Test Considerations

- Verify negative pregnancy test before starting therapy.
- Patient selection for NSCLC in combination with ipilimumab is based on PD-L1 expression. Information on FDA-approved tests for the determination of PD-L1 expression in NSCLC is available at: http://www.fda.gov/CompanionDiagnostics.
- Monitor for abnormal liver function tests prior to and periodically during therapy. ***For hepatitis with no tumor involvement:*** *If AST/ALT >3–≤8 times (or ≤5 times if given with ipilimumab) upper limit of normal (ULN) or total bilirubin >1.5–≤3 times ULN,* hold nivolumab. Resume therapy if complete or partial resolution (Grade ≤1) after corticosteroid taper. Permanently discontinue nivolumab if no complete or partial resolution within 12 wk of last dose or inability to ↓ prednisone to ≤10 mg/day (or equivalent) within 12 wk of starting steroids. *If AST or ALT >8 times (or >5 times if given with ipilimumab) ULN or total bilirubin >3 times ULN,* permanently discontinue nivolumab. **For hepatitis with tumor involvement of the liver:** *If baseline AST/ALT >1–≤3 times ULN and ↑ to >5–≤10 times ULN or baseline AST/ALT is >3–≤5 times ULN and ↑ to >8–≤10 times ULN,* hold nivolumab. *If AST/ALT >10 times ULN or total bilirubin >3 times ULN,* permanently discontinue nivolumab. *If given with cabozantinib and ALT or AST >3–≤10 times ULN with concurrent total bilirubin <2 times ULN,* hold nivolumab and cabozantinib until recovery to Grade ≤1. *If given with cabozantinib and AST or ALT >10 times ULN or >3 times with concurrent bilirubin ≥2 times ULN,* permanently discontinue nivolumab and cabozantinib.
- Monitor for ↑ serum creatinine before and periodically during therapy. *If Grade 2 or 3 ↑ in*

N

serum creatinine occurs, hold nivolumab. Resume therapy if complete or partial resolution (Grade ≤1) after corticosteroid taper. Permanently discontinue nivolumab if no complete or partial resolution within 12 wk of last dose or inability to ↓ prednisone to ≤10 mg/day (or equivalent) within 12 wk of starting steroids. *If Grade 4 ↑ in serum creatinine occurs,* permanently discontinue nivolumab.

- Monitor thyroid function prior to and periodically during therapy. Treat hypothyroidism with replacement therapy. Use medical management for hyperthyroidism. Immune-mediated thyroid dysfunction does not require dose modification of nivolumab.
- Monitor for hyperglycemia. *If severe hyperglycemia occurs,* hold nivolumab until metabolic control achieved. *If life-threatening hyperglycemia occurs,* permanently discontinue nivolumab.

Implementation

IV Administration

- **Intermittent Infusion: Dilution:** 0.9% NaCl or D5W. **Concentration:** 1–10 mg/mL. The total volume of infusion must not exceed 160 mL for patients ≥40 kg (or 4 mL/kg for patients <40 kg). Mix by gentle inversion; do not shake. Solution is clear to slightly opalescent, colorless to slightly yellow; do not administer solution if discolored or contains particulate matter other than translucent to white proteinaceous particles. Solution is stable for up to 8 hr at room temperature and 7 days if refrigerated. **Rate:** Infuse over 30 min through a sterile, nonpyrogenic, low-protein-binding 0.2–1.2-micrometer in-line filter. Flush line at end of infusion.
- **Y-Site Incompatibility:** Do not administer other drugs through same IV line.

Patient/Family Teaching

- Explain purpose and side effects of medication. Advise patient to read *Patient Information* before starting therapy. Emphasize importance of keeping scheduled appointments for blood work or other laboratory tests.
- Instruct patient to notify health care provider of all Rx or OTC medications, vitamins, or herbal products being taken and to consult with health care provider before taking other medications.
- Advise patient to notify health care provider immediately if signs and symptoms of pneumonitis, colitis, hepatitis (jaundice, severe nausea or vomiting, pain on right side of abdomen, lethargy, easy bruising or bleeding), kidney problems (↓ urine output, blood in urine, swollen ankles, loss of appetite), or hormone gland problems (rapid heartbeat, weight loss, ↑ sweating, weight gain, hair loss, feeling cold, constipation, deepening of voice, muscle aches, dizziness or fainting, persistent or unusual headache) occur.
- Rep: May cause fetal harm. Advise women of reproductive potential to use highly effective contraception and avoid breastfeeding during therapy and for 5 mo after last dose. Advise patient to notify health care provider immediately if pregnancy is planned or suspected.

Evaluation/Desired Outcomes

- Decreased progression of melanoma, Hodgkin lymphoma, urothelial carcinoma, colorectal cancer, and hepatocellular carcinoma.
- Decreased progression of and improved survival with NSCLC and advanced renal cell carcinoma.
- Improved survival in squamous cell carcinoma of head and neck, esophageal cancer, gastric cancer, gastroesophageal junction cancer, esophageal adenocarcinoma, and malignant pleural mesothelioma.

HIGH ALERT

V norepinephrine

(**nor**-ep-i-nef-rin)

Levophed

Classification

Therapeutic: vasopressors

Indications

Severe acute hypotension.

Action

Stimulates alpha-adrenergic receptors located mainly in blood vessels, causing constriction of both capacitance and resistance vessels. Also has minor beta-adrenergic activity (myocardial stimulation). **Therapeutic Effects:** Increased BP. Increased cardiac output.

Pharmacokinetics

Absorption: IV administration results in complete bioavailability.

Distribution: Concentrates in sympathetic nervous tissue. Does not cross the blood-brain barrier.

Metabolism and Excretion: Taken up and metabolized rapidly by sympathetic nerve endings.

Half-life: 2.5 min.

TIME/ACTION PROFILE (effects on BP)

ROUTE	ONSET	PEAK	DURATION
IV	immediate	rapid	1–2 min

Contraindications/Precautions

Contraindicated in: Vascular, mesenteric, or peripheral thrombosis; Hypoxia; Hypercarbia; Hypotension secondary to hypovolemia (without appropriate volume replacement); Hypersensitivity to bisulfites.

Use Cautiously in: Hypertension; Hyperthyroidism; Cardiovascular disease; OB: May ↓ uterine blood flow in pregnancy; Lactation: Safety not established in breastfeeding.

Adverse Reactions/Side Effects

CV: arrhythmia, bradycardia, chest pain, hypertension. **Endo:** hyperglycemia. **F and E:** metabolic acidosis. **GU:** ↓ urine output, renal failure **Local:** phlebitis. **Neuro:** anxiety, dizziness, headache, insomnia, restlessness, tremor, weakness. **Resp:** dyspnea. **Misc:** fever.

Interactions

Drug-Drug: Cyclopropane or **halothane anesthesia**, **digoxin**, **doxapram**, or local use of **cocaine** may ↑ myocardial irritability. Use with **MAO inhibitors** or **tricyclic antidepressants** may result in severe hypertension. **Alpha-adrenergic blockers** can prevent pressor response. **Beta blockers** may exaggerate hypertension or block cardiac stimulation. **Ergot alkaloids** (**ergotamine**, **methylergonovine**, or **oxytocin**) may result in enhanced vasoconstriction and hypertension.

Route/Dosage

IV (Adults): 0.5–1 mcg/min initially, followed by maintenance infusion of 2–12 mcg/min titrated by BP response (average rate 2–4 mcg/min, up to 30 mcg/min for refractory shock have been used).
IV (Children): 0.1 mcg/kg/min initially; may be followed by infusion titrated to BP response, up to 1 mcg/kg/min.

Availability (generic available)

Premixed infusion: 4 mg/250 mL D5W or 0.9% NaCl, 8 mg/250 mL D5W or 0.9% NaCl, 16 mg/250 mL 0.9% NaCl. **Solution for injection:** 1 mg/mL.

NURSING IMPLICATIONS

Assessment

- Monitor BP every 2–3 min until stabilized and every 5 min thereafter. Systolic BP is usually maintained at 80–100 mm Hg or 30–40 mm Hg below the previously existing systolic pressure in previously hypertensive patients. Continue to monitor BP frequently for hypotension following discontinuation of norepinephrine.
- ECG should be monitored continuously. Central venous pressure, intra-arterial pressure, pulmonary artery diastolic pressure, pulmonary capillary wedge pressure, and cardiac output may also be monitored.
- Monitor urine output and notify health care provider if it ↓ to <30 mL/hr.
- Assess IV site frequently during infusion. If prolonged therapy is required or if blanching along the course of the vein occurs, change injection sites to provide relief from vasoconstriction.

Toxicity and Overdose

- If overdose occurs, discontinue norepinephrine and administer fluid and electrolyte replacement therapy. An alpha-adrenergic blocking agent may be administered IV to treat hypertension.

Implementation

- ***High Alert:*** Vasoactive medications are inherently dangerous. Have 2nd practitioner independently check original order, dose calculations, and infusion pump programming. Establish maximum dose limits. Norepinephrine overdose can result in severe peripheral vasoconstriction with resultant ischemia and necrosis of peripheral tissue. Assess peripheral circulation frequently.
- Correct volume depletion, if possible, prior to initiation.
- May deplete plasma volume and cause ischemia of vital organs, resulting in hypotension when discontinued, if used for prolonged periods. Prolonged or large doses may also ↓ cardiac output.
- Infusion should be discontinued gradually, upon adequate tissue perfusion and maintenance of BP, to prevent hypotension. Do not resume therapy unless systolic BP falls to 70–80 mm Hg.

N

IV Administration

- **V** Norepinephrine is a vesicant. Central line administration is preferred; extravasation may cause severe ischemic necrosis. If central line is not available, may administer for <72 hr through a peripheral IV catheter placed in a large vein at a proximal site (e.g., in or proximal to antecubital fossa). May also administer through a midline catheter. If extravasation occurs, immediately stop infusion. Leave needle/cannula in place temporarily but do not flush the line. Gently aspirate extravasated solution; then remove needle/cannula. Elevate patient's extremity and apply dry warm compresses. Initiate phentolamine antidote for refractory cases in addition to supportive management. For phentolamine, dilute 5–10 mg in 10 mL of 0.9% NaCl and administer SUBQ into extravasation site as soon as possible after extravasation; if IV catheter remains in place, administer initial dose IV through the infiltrated catheter. May repeat in 60 min if patient remains symptomatic. Nitroglycerin 2% topical ointment (1-inch strip applied to site of ischemia to cover affected area; may repeat every 8 hr as necessary) or terbutaline may be used as alternatives to phentolamine. For terbutaline, for large areas of extravasation, dilute 1 mg in 10 mL of 0.9% NaCl and administer SUBQ into extravasation site; may repeat in 15 min if necessary; for small areas of extravasation, dilute 1 mg in 1 mL of 0.9% NaCl and administer 0.5 mg (0.5 mL) SUBQ into extravasation site; may repeat in 15 min if necessary.

- **Continuous Infusion: Dilution:** Dilute 4 mg in 1000 mL of D5W, D5/0.9% NaCl, or 0.9% NaCl. **Concentration:** 4 mcg/mL. Solution is colorless. Do not use discolored solutions (pink, yellow, brown) or those containing a precipitate. Solution is stable for 24 hr at room temperature. Protect from light. **Rate:** Titrate infusion rate according to patient response, using slowest possible rate to correct hypotension.
- **Y-Site Compatibility:** alemtuzumab, amikacin, anidulafungin, argatroban, arsenic trioxide, ascorbic acid, atracurium, atropine, aztreonam, benztropine, bivalirudin, bleomycin, bumetanide, buprenorphine, butorphanol, calcium chloride, calcium gluconate, cangrelor, carboplatin, carmustine, caspofungin, cefazolin, cefiderocol, cefotaxime, cefotetan, cefoxitin, ceftaroline, ceftazidime, ceftazidime/avibactam, ceftobiprole, ceftolozane/tazobactam, ceftriaxone, cefuroxime, chloramphenicol, chlorpromazine, cisatracurium, cisplatin, clindamycin, cyanocobalamin, cyclophosphamide, cyclosporine, cytarabine, dactinomycin, daptomycin, daunorubicin, dexamethasone, dexmedetomidine, dexrazoxane, digoxin, diltiazem, diphenhydramine, dobutamine, docetaxel, dopamine, doxycycline, doxorubicin liposomal, enalaprilat, ephedrine, epinephrine, epirubicin, epoetin alfa, eravacycline, ertapenem, erythromycin, esmolol, etoposide, etoposide phosphate, famotidine, fentanyl, fluconazole, fludarabine, fosphenytoin, gemcitabine, gentamicin, glycopyrrolate, granisetron, heparin, hydrocortisone, hydromorphone, idarubicin, ifosfamide, imipenem/cilastatin, imipenem/cilastatin/relebactam, irinotecan, isavuconazonium, isoproterenol, ketorolac, labetalol, letermovir, leucovorin, levetiracetam, levofloxacin, lidocaine, linezolid, lorazepam, magnesium sulfate, mannitol, meperidine, meropenem, meropenem/vaborbactam, mesna, methadone, methotrexate, methylprednisolone, metoclopramide, metoprolol, metronidazole, micafungin, midazolam, milrinone, minocycline, mitoxantrone, morphine, moxifloxacin, multivitamins, mycophenolate, nafcillin, nalbuphine, naloxone, nicardipine, nitroglycerin, nitroprusside, octreotide, ondansetron, oritavancin, oxacillin, oxaliplatin, oxytocin, paclitaxel, palonosetron, pamidronate, papaverine, pemetrexed, penicillin G, pentamidine, phentolamine, phenylephrine, phytonadione, piperacillin/tazobactam, plazomicin, posaconazole, potassium acetate, potassium chloride, procainamide, prochlorperazine, promethazine, propofol, propranolol, protamine, pyridoxine, remifentanil, succinylcholine, sufentanil, tacrolimus, tedizolid, telavancin, theophylline, thiamine, thiotepa, tigecycline, tirofiban, tobramycin, topotecan, vancomycin, vasopressin, vecuronium, verapamil, vinblastine, vincristine, vinorelbine, voriconazole, zoledronic acid.
- **Y-Site Incompatibility:** aminophylline, amphotericin B deoxycholate, azathioprine, dacarbazine, dantrolene, diazepam, folic acid, foscarnet, ganciclovir, gemtuzumab ozogamicin, indomethacin, mitomycin, pentobarbital, phenobarbital, phenytoin, sodium bicarbonate, trimethoprim/sulfamethoxazole.

Patient/Family Teaching

- Explain purpose of norepinephrine to patient.
- Instruct patient to report headache, dizziness, dyspnea, chest pain, or pain at infusion site promptly.
- Rep: Advise women of reproductive potential to notify health care provider if pregnancy is planned or suspected or if breastfeeding.

Evaluation/Desired Outcomes

- Increased BP.
- Increased cardiac output.

norethindrone, See CONTRACEPTIVES, HORMONAL.

norgestrel, See CONTRACEPTIVES, HORMONAL.

BEERS

nortriptyline (nor-trip-ti-leen)

Aventyl, ~~Pamelor~~

Classification

Therapeutic: antidepressants

Pharmacologic: tricyclic antidepressants

Indications

Major depressive disorder. **Unlabeled Use:** Chronic neuropathic pain.

Action

Potentiates the effect of serotonin and norepinephrine. Has significant anticholinergic properties. **Therapeutic Effects:** Antidepressant action that develops slowly over several weeks.

Pharmacokinetics

Absorption: Well absorbed after oral administration.

Distribution: Widely distributed to tissues.

Protein Binding: 92%.

Metabolism and Excretion: Mostly metabolized by the liver by the CYP2D6 isoenzyme; the CYP2D6 enzyme system exhibits genetic polymorphism; 7% of population may be poor metabolizers and may have

significantly ↑ nortriptyline concentrations and an ↑ risk of adverse effects.
Half-life: 18–28 hr.

TIME/ACTION PROFILE (antidepressant effect)

ROUTE	ONSET	PEAK	DURATION
PO	2–3 wk	6 wk	unknown

Contraindications/Precautions

Contraindicated in: Hypersensitivity; Angle-closure glaucoma; Alcohol intolerance (solution only); Brugada syndrome; Concurrent use of MAO inhibitors or MAO-like drugs (linezolid or methylene blue); Lactation: Lactation.
Use Cautiously in: Pre-existing cardiovascular disease; History of seizures; Asthma; May ↑ risk of suicide attempt/ideation especially during early treatment or dose adjustment; risk may be greater in children or adolescents; OB: Use during pregnancy only if potential maternal benefit justifies potential fetal risk; Pedi: Safety and effectiveness not established in children; Geri: Appears on Beers list. ↑ risk of adverse reactions in older adults, including falls secondary to sedative and anticholinergic effects and orthostatic hypotension. Avoid use in older adults.

Adverse Reactions/Side Effects

CV: hypotension, ARRHYTHMIAS, ECG changes. **Derm:** photosensitivity. **EENT:** blurred vision, dry eyes. **Endo:** gynecomastia. **GI:** constipation, dry mouth, nausea, paralytic ileus, unpleasant taste. **GU:** urinary retention. **Hemat:** blood dyscrasias. **Metab:** weight gain. **Neuro:** drowsiness, fatigue, lethargy, agitation, confusion, extrapyramidal reactions, hallucinations, headache, insomnia, SUICIDAL THOUGHTS/BEHAVIORS.

Interactions

Drug-Drug: MAO inhibitors may result in serious potentially fatal reactions (MAO inhibitors should be stopped ≥14 days before nortriptyline therapy; nortriptyline should be stopped ≥14 days before MAO inhibitor therapy). **MAO-inhibitor-like drugs**, such as **linezolid** or **methylene blue**, may ↑ risk of serotonin syndrome; concurrent use contraindicated; do not start therapy in patients receiving **linezolid** or **methylene blue**; if **linezolid** or **methylene blue** need to be started in a patient receiving nortriptyline, immediately discontinue nortriptyline and monitor for signs/symptoms of serotonin syndrome for 2 wk or until 24 hr after last dose of linezolid or methylene blue, whichever comes 1st (may resume nortriptyline therapy 24 hr after last dose of linezolid or methylene blue). May prevent the therapeutic response to most **antihypertensives**. Hypertensive crisis may occur with **clonidine**. ↑ CNS depression with other **CNS depressants**, including **alcohol**, **antihistamines**, **opioids**, and **sedative/hypnotics**. Adrenergic effects may be ↑ with other **adrenergic agents**, including **vasoconstrictors** and **decongestants**. ↑ anticholinergic effects with other **anticholinergic drugs**, including **antihistamines**, **antidepressants**, **atropine**, **haloperidol**, **phenothiazines**, **quinidine**, and **disopyramide**. **Cimetidine**, **fluoxetine**, or **hormonal contraceptives** may ↑ levels and risk of toxicity. ↑ risk of agranulocytosis with **antithyroid agents**. Drugs that affect serotonergic neurotransmitter systems, including **SSRIs**, **SNRIs**, **fentanyl**, **buspirone**, **tramadol**, and **triptans**, may ↑ risk of serotonin syndrome.
Drug-Natural Products: Kava-kava, **valerian**, or **chamomile** can ↑ risk of CNS depression. **St. John's wort** may ↑ risk of serotonin syndrome. ↑ anticholinergic effects with **jimson weed** and **scopolia**.

Route/Dosage

PO (Adults): 25 mg 3–4 times daily, up to 150 mg/day.
PO (Geriatric Patients): 30–50 mg/day in divided doses or as a single dose.

Availability (generic available)

Capsules: 10 mg, 25 mg, 50 mg, 75 mg. **Oral solution:** 10 mg/5 mL.

NURSING IMPLICATIONS

Assessment

- Monitor mental status (orientation, mood, behavior).
- Assess weight and BMI initially and throughout treatment. For overweight/obese individuals, monitor fasting blood glucose and cholesterol levels.
- Monitor BP and HR before and during initial therapy. Report significant ↓ in BP or a sudden ↑ in HR.
- Monitor baseline and periodic ECGs in older adults or patients with heart disease. May cause prolonged PR and QT intervals and may flatten T waves.
- Assess for suicidal tendencies, especially during early therapy. Restrict amount of drug available to patient. Risk may be ↑ in adults ≤24 yr. After starting therapy, young adults should be seen by health care provider face-to-face at least weekly for 4 wk, then every other wk for next 4 wk, then at 12 wk, and then on advice of health care provider thereafter.
- **Pain:** Assess type, location, and severity of pain before and periodically during therapy. Use pain scale to monitor effectiveness of medication.

Lab Test Considerations

- Assess WBC with differential, liver function, and serum glucose periodically. May ↑ serum bilirubin

N

and alkaline phosphatase. May cause bone marrow depression. May ↑ or ↓ serum glucose.

- Serum levels may be monitored in patients who fail to respond to usual therapeutic dose. Therapeutic plasma concentration range is 50–150 ng/mL.

Toxicity and Overdose

- Symptoms of acute overdose include disturbed concentration, confusion, restlessness, agitation, seizures, drowsiness, mydriasis, arrhythmias, fever, hallucinations, vomiting, and dyspnea.
- Treatment of overdose includes gastric lavage, activated charcoal, and a stimulant cathartic. Maintain respiratory and cardiac function (monitor ECG for ≥5 days) and temperature. Medications may include digoxin for HF, antiarrhythmics, and anticonvulsants.

Implementation

- Taper to avoid withdrawal effects. ↓ dose 50% for 3 days, then by 50% for 3 more days, and then discontinue.
- **PO:** Administer with meals to minimize gastric irritation.
- May be given as a single dose at bedtime to minimize sedation during the day. Dose ↑ should be made at bedtime because of sedation.

Patient/Family Teaching

- Explain purpose and side effects of medication to patient. Advise patient to read *Patient Information* before starting therapy. Advise to take as directed. Take missed doses as soon as possible unless almost time for next dose; if regimen is a single dose at bedtime, do not take in the morning because of side effects. Advise patient that drug effects may not be noticed for ≥2 wk. Abrupt discontinuation may cause nausea, vomiting, diarrhea, headache, trouble sleeping with vivid dreams, and irritability.
- Advise patient to notify health care provider of all Rx or OTC medications, vitamins, or herbal products being taken and to consult with health care provider before taking other medications.
- May cause drowsiness and blurred vision. Advise patient to avoid driving and other activities requiring alertness until response to drug is known.
- Advise patient to notify health care provider if visual changes occur. Inform patient that periodic glaucoma testing may be required during long-term therapy.
- Advise patient to make position changes slowly to minimize orthostatic hypotension. This side effect is less pronounced with this medication than with other tricyclic antidepressants.
- Advise patient, family, and caregivers to look for suicidality, especially during early therapy or dose changes. Notify health care provider immediately if thoughts about suicide or dying, attempts to commit suicide, new or worse depression or anxiety, agitation or restlessness, panic attacks, insomnia, new or worse irritability, aggressiveness, acting on dangerous impulses, mania, or other changes in mood or behavior occur.
- Advise patient to avoid alcohol or other CNS depressant drugs, including opioids, during therapy and for ≥3–7 days after therapy has been discontinued.
- Advise patient to notify health care provider if urinary retention occurs or if dry mouth or constipation persists. Sugarless candy or gum may diminish dry mouth, and an ↑ in fluid intake or fiber may prevent constipation. If symptoms persist, dose ↓ or discontinuation may be necessary. Consult health care provider if dry mouth persists for >2 wk.
- Advise patient to use sunscreen and protective clothing to prevent photosensitivity reactions.
- Alert patient that urine may turn blue-green in color.
- Advise patient of need to monitor dietary intake. ↑ in appetite may lead to undesired weight gain. Refer as appropriate for nutritional, weight, or medical management.
- Advise patient to notify health care provider of medication regimen before treatment or surgery.
- Therapy for depression is usually prolonged. Emphasize the importance of follow-up exams.
- Rep: May cause fetal harm. Advise women of reproductive potential to use effective contraception during therapy and for ≥5 mo after last dose and to avoid breastfeeding during therapy. Advise patient to notify health care provider immediately if pregnancy is planned or suspected.

Evaluation/Desired Outcomes

- Antidepressant action that develops slowly over several weeks.

NPH/regular insulin mixtures, See INSULIN (mixtures).

nystatin, See ANTIFUNGALS (TOPICAL).

nystatin (oral) (nye-**stat**-in)

Mycostatin

Classification

Therapeutic: antifungals

For other nystatin dosage forms, see antifungals (topical) and antifungals (vaginal).

Indications

Oral suspension: Local treatment of oropharyngeal candidiasis. **Oral tablet:** Treatment of nonesophageal mucus membrane gastrointestinal candidiasis.

Action

Binds to fungal cell membrane, allowing leakage of cellular contents. **Therapeutic Effects:** Fungistatic or fungicidal action. **Spectrum:** Active against most pathogenic *Candida* species, including *C. albicans*.

Pharmacokinetics

Absorption: Poorly absorbed; action is primarily local.
Distribution: Unknown.
Metabolism and Excretion: Excreted unchanged in the feces after oral administration.
Half-life: Unknown.

TIME/ACTION PROFILE (antifungal effects)

ROUTE	ONSET	PEAK	DURATION
PO	24–72 hr	unknown	unknown

Contraindications/Precautions

Contraindicated in: Hypersensitivity; Some products may contain ethyl alcohol or benzyl alcohol; avoid use in patients who may be hypersensitive to or intolerant of these additives.
Use Cautiously in: Denture wearers (dentures require soaking in nystatin suspension).

Adverse Reactions/Side Effects

Derm: contact dermatitis, STEVENS-JOHNSON SYNDROME (SJS). **GI:** diarrhea, nausea, stomach pain (large doses), vomiting.

Interactions

Drug-Drug: None reported.

Route/Dosage

Oropharyngeal Candidiasis

PO (Adults and Children): 400,000–600,000 units 4 times daily as oral suspension.
PO (Infants): 200,000 units 4 times daily or 100,000 units to each side of the mouth 4 times daily.
PO (Neonates): 100,000 units 4 times daily or 50,000 units to each side of the mouth 4 times a day.

Gastrointestinal Candidiasis

PO (Adults): 500,000–1,000,000 units 3 times daily. Continue for ≥48 hr after clinical cure to prevent relapse.

Availability (generic available)

Oral suspension: 100,000 units/mL. **Oral tablets:** 500,000 units.

NURSING IMPLICATIONS

Assessment

- Inspect oral mucous membranes before and frequently during therapy for symptomatic improvement. ↑ irritation of mucous membranes may indicate need to discontinue medication.
- Assess for rash or signs and symptoms of SJS periodically during therapy (fever, general malaise, fatigue, muscle or joint aches, blisters, oral lesions, conjunctivitis). *If signs/symptoms of SJS occur,* discontinue nystatin and provide supportive care.

Implementation

- Do not confuse nystatin with HMG-CoA reductase inhibitors (statins).
- **PO:** Administer suspension by placing of dose in each side of mouth. Patient should hold suspension in mouth or swish throughout mouth for several minutes before swallowing; then gargle and swallow. Use calibrated measuring device for liquid doses. Shake well before administration. Pedi: For neonates and infants, paint suspension into recesses of the mouth. Avoid feedings for 5–10 min following administration or administer after meals.

Patient/Family Teaching

- Explain the purpose and side effects of nystatin. Instruct patient to take as directed. If a dose is missed, take as soon as remembered but not if almost time for next dose. Do not double doses. Therapy should be continued for ≥2 days after symptoms subside. Advise patient to read *Patient Information* before starting therapy.
- Pedi: Instruct parents or caregivers of infants and children on correct dose and administration. Remind them to use only the measuring device dispensed with the product.
- Advise patient to report ↑ irritation of mucous membranes or lack of therapeutic response to health care provider.
- Advise patient to notify health care provider of all Rx or OTC medications, vitamins, or herbal products being taken and to consult with health care provider before taking other medications.
- Rep: Advise women of reproductive potential to notify health care provider if pregnancy is planned or suspected or if breastfeeding.

Evaluation/Desired Outcomes

- Decrease in stomatitis.
- Treatment of intestinal candidiasis.

N

ocrelizumab (ok-re-liz-ue-mab)

Ocrevus

Classification

Therapeutic: anti-multiple sclerosis agents

Pharmacologic: monoclonal antibodies

Indications

Relapsing forms of multiple sclerosis (MS), including clinically isolated syndrome, relapsing-remitting disease, and active secondary progressive disease. Primary progressive MS.

Action

Binds to the CD20 antigen on pre-B and mature B lymphocytes, which results in antibody-dependent and complement-mediated cell lysis. **Therapeutic Effects:** Reduction in relapse rate and decreased progression toward disability.

Pharmacokinetics

Absorption: IV administration results in complete bioavailability.

Distribution: Binds specifically to CD20 binding sites on B lymphocytes.

Metabolism and Excretion: Unknown.

Half-life: 26 days.

TIME/ACTION PROFILE

ROUTE	ONSET	PEAK	DURATION
IV	unknown	unknown	unknown

Contraindications/Precautions

Contraindicated in: Active hepatitis B virus (HBV) infection (may reactivate infection during and for several mo after treatment); Active infection; History of life-threatening infusion reaction to ocrelizumab.

Use Cautiously in: Patients who are immunocompromised or receiving other immunosuppressants; OB: Safety not established in pregnancy (may cause fetal B-cell depletion); Lactation: Safety not established in breastfeeding; Rep: Women of reproductive potential; Pedi: Safety and effectiveness not established in children.

Adverse Reactions/Side Effects

CV: peripheral edema. **GI:** diarrhea, HEPATITIS B VIRUS REACTIVATION, IMMUNE-MEDIATED COLITIS. **Hemat:** neutropenia. **MS:** back pain. **Neuro:** depression, PROGRESSIVE MULTIFOCAL LEUKOENCEPHALOPATHY (PML). **Resp:** cough. **Misc:** INFECTION, INFUSION REACTIONS (INCLUDING ANAPHYLAXIS), MALIGNANCY (PRIMARILY BREAST CANCER).

Interactions

Drug-Drug: Concurrent use with **immunosuppressive therapies** may ↑ risk of immunosuppression. May ↓ antibody response to or ↑ risk of adverse reactions to **non-live vaccines** and **live vaccines**.

Route/Dosage

IV (Adults): 300 mg initially, then 300 mg in 2 wk, then 600 mg every 6 mo.

Availability

Solution for injection: 30 mg/mL.

NURSING IMPLICATIONS

Assessment

- Assess for active infection prior to each infusion. Delay infusion until infection resolves.
- Monitor for signs and symptoms of infusion reaction (pruritus, rash, urticaria, erythema, bronchospasm, throat irritation, oropharyngeal pain, dyspnea, pharyngeal or laryngeal edema, flushing, hypotension, pyrexia, fatigue, headache, dizziness, nausea, tachycardia) during and for ≥1 hr after completion of infusion. *If mild to moderate infusion reaction occurs,* ↓ infusion rate by 50% at onset of reaction and for ≥30 min. If reduced infusion rate tolerated, ↑ rate (see Rate below). Will ↑ duration of infusion, but not total dose. *If severe reaction occurs,* immediately stop infusion and administer supportive treatment. Restart infusion only after all symptoms resolved. Restart by ↓ infusion rate by 50% at time of onset of reaction. If tolerated, ↑ rate (see Rate below). Will ↑ duration of infusion, but not total dose. *If life-threatening infusion reaction occurs,* immediately stop infusion and permanently discontinue therapy. Provide supportive treatment.
- Assess for signs and symptoms of PML (progressive weakness on one side of body or clumsiness of limbs; disturbance of vision; changes in thinking, memory, and orientation leading to confusion and personality changes) periodically during therapy. Symptoms are diverse and progress over days to wks. At first sign of PML, suspend ocrelizumab and perform diagnostic evaluation. MRI findings may be apparent before clinical signs or symptoms. If PML is confirmed, discontinue ocrelizumab.
- Monitor for signs and symptoms of immune-mediated colitis (diarrhea, abdominal pain, blood in stool) during therapy. May require systemic corticosteroids and hospitalization.

Lab Test Considerations

- Determine current or prior HBV infection by measuring hepatitis B surface antigen (HBsAg) and hepatitis B core antibody (anti-HBc) before starting therapy. Do not administer to patients with active HBV infection.
- Perform testing for quantitative serum immunoglobulins before starting therapy. May require immunology consult if serum immunoglobulins are low.

Implementation

- Administer in a health care setting by an experienced health care professional with access to appropriate medical support and equipment in case of a infusion or severe reaction. Monitor during and for ≥1 hr after infusion.

- Administer all necessary immunizations ≥4 wk before starting therapy. Avoid immunizations during therapy and after discontinuation until B-cell repletion.
- Premedicate to reduce frequency and severity of infusion reactions with methylprednisolone 100 mg IV or equivalent 30 min and an antihistamine, diphenhydramine, 30–60 min before each infusion. May add an antipyretic, acetaminophen.
- **Intermittent Infusion: Dilution:** Dilute the 300-mg dose (10 mL) in 250 mL of 0.9% NaCl and the 600-mg dose (20 mL) in 500 mL of 0.9% NaCl. Do not use other diluents. Do not shake. Allow infusion bag to come to room temperature before infusion. **Concentration:** 1.2 mg/mL. Solution is clear or slightly opalescent, and colorless to pale brown; do not administer solutions that are discolored or contain particulate matter. Solution is stable for 24 hr if refrigerated or up to 8 hr (including infusion time) at room temperature.
- **Rate:** Administer using a dedicated line with a 0.2 or 0.22 micron in-line filter. *For first 2 infusions (300 mg in 250 mL),* begin at 30 mL/hr. ↑ by 30 mL/hr every 30 min to 180 mL/hr over 2.5 hr or longer. *For subsequent infusions (600 mg in 500 mL),* begin at 40 mL/hr. ↑ by 40 mL/hr every 30 min to 200 mL/hr over 3.5 hr or longer OR start at 100 mL/hr for first 15 min. ↑ to 200 mL/hr for next 15 min. ↑ to 250 mL/hr for next 30 min. ↑ to 300 mL/hr for last 60 min. Duration 2 hr or longer.

Patient/Family Teaching

- Explain purpose and side effects of medication. Advise patient to read *Patient Information* before starting therapy. Explain the importance of maintaining a schedule to patient. If infusion is missed, administer as soon as possible; do not wait for next scheduled dose. Reset schedule for 6 mo after missed dose is given. Separate doses by ≥5 mo.
- Instruct patient to notify health care professional of all Rx or OTC medications, vitamins, or herbal products being taken and to consult health care professional before taking other Rx, OTC, or herbal products.
- Inform patient that infusion reactions may occur up to 24 hr after infusion. Advise patient to notify health care professional immediately if infusion reaction symptoms occur.
- Advise patient to notify health care professional if signs and symptoms of infection (fever, chills, constant cough, cold sore, shingles, genital sores), immune-mediated colitis (new or persistent diarrhea, abdominal pain, blood in stool) or PML (problems with thinking, balance, eyesight, strength, or using arms or legs; weakness on one side of body) occur.
- Instruct patient to avoid live vaccines during therapy. Administer any live or live-attenuated vaccines ≥4 wk prior to start of therapy and administer any non-live vaccines ≥2 wk prior to start of therapy.
- Inform patient of increased risk of malignancy. Advise patient to receive regular breast cancer screening.
- Rep: May cause fetal harm. Advise females of reproductive potential to use effective contraception during and for 6 mo after last infusion and to notify health care professional if breastfeeding. Do not administer live or live-attenuated vaccines to infants born to mothers taking ocrelizumab until recovery of B-cell counts is confirmed; may administer non-live vaccines to these infants, but should consider assessing vaccine immune responses to determine whether protective immune response developed.

Evaluation/Desired Outcomes

- Reduction in relapse rate and decreased progression toward disability in patients with MS.

O

octreotide (ok-tree-oh-tide)

Mycapssa, SandoSTATIN,
✦ SandoSTATIN LAR, SandoSTATIN LAR Depot

Classification

Therapeutic: antidiarrheals, hormones

Indications

IV, IM, SUBQ: Treatment of the following: Symptoms (flushing and diarrhea) associated with metastatic carcinoid tumors; Profuse, watery diarrhea associated with vasoactive intestinal peptide tumors (VIPomas); Acromegaly in patients who have had inadequate response to or cannot be treated with surgical resection, pituitary irradiation, and bromocriptine at maximally tolerated doses. **PO:** Long-term maintenance treatment of acromegaly in patients who have responded to and tolerated treatment with octreotide or lanreotide. **Unlabeled Use:** Management of diarrhea associated with chemotherapy or graft-versus-host disease. Gastroesophageal variceal hemorrhage.

Action

Suppresses secretion of serotonin and gastroenterohepatic peptides. Increases absorption of fluid and electrolytes from the GI tract and increases transit time. Decreases levels of serotonin metabolites. Also suppresses growth hormone, insulin, and glucagon. **Therapeutic Effects:** Normalization of growth hormone (GH) and insulin-like growth factor-1

(IGF-1) levels and maintenance of these levels. Control of severe flushing and diarrhea associated with metastatic carcinoid tumors and VIPomas.

Pharmacokinetics

Absorption: IV administration results in complete bioavailability. Well absorbed following SUBQ administration and IM administration of depot form. Food ↓ rate and extent of oral absorption.

Distribution: Some distribution to extravascular tissues.

Metabolism and Excretion: Extensive hepatic metabolism; 32% excreted unchanged in urine.

Half-life: 1.5 hr.

TIME/ACTION PROFILE (control of symptoms)

ROUTE	ONSET	PEAK	DURATION
SUBQ, IV	unknown	unknown	up to 12 hr
IM (LAR depot)	unknown	2 wk	up to 4 wk
PO	unknown	unknown	unknown

Contraindications/Precautions

Contraindicated in: Hypersensitivity.

Use Cautiously in: Gallbladder disease (↑ risk of stone formation); Renal impairment (dose ↓ may be necessary); Hyperglycemia or hypoglycemia (changes in blood glucose may occur); Fat malabsorption (may be aggravated); OB: Safety not established in pregnancy; Lactation: Safety not established in breastfeeding; Rep: Premenopausal women (may ↑ fertility and ↑ risk of pregnancy); Pedi: Safety and effectiveness of depot injection and oral formulation not established in children.

Adverse Reactions/Side Effects

CV: edema, QT interval prolongation, atrioventricular block, bradycardia, hypertension, orthostatic hypotension, palpitations. **Derm:** ↑ sweating, flushing. **EENT:** sinusitis, visual disturbances. **Endo:** hyperglycemia, hypoglycemia, hypothyroidism. **GI:** abdominal pain, cholelithiasis, diarrhea, nausea, vomiting, abdominal bloating, cholecystitis, fat malabsorption, flatulence, ILEUS, PANCREATITIS, steatorrhea, stool discoloration. **GU:** urinary tract infection. **Local:** injection-site pain. **Metab:** weight loss. **MS:** arthralgia. **Neuro:** headache, dizziness, drowsiness, fatigue, weakness. **Misc:** ↓ vitamin B_{12} levels.

Interactions

Drug-Drug: May alter requirements for **insulin** or **oral hypoglycemic agents**. May ↓ levels and effectiveness of **cyclosporine** and **digoxin**; closely monitor levels and adjust dose of cyclosporine and digoxin as needed. **Beta blockers**, **digoxin**, **diltiazem**, **ivabradine**, and **verapamil** may ↑ risk of bradycardia. **Proton pump inhibitors**, **H_2 receptor antagonists**, and **antacids** may ↓ absorption and levels of orally administered octreotide; may need to ↑ dosage of oral octreotide. May ↑ levels and risk of toxicity of **lisinopril**; closely monitor BP. May ↓ levels and effectiveness of **levonorgestrel**; advise patient to use nonhormonal contraceptive or a backup method while receiving octreotide. May ↑ levels and risk of toxicity of **bromocriptine**; may need to ↓ dose of bromocriptine. May ↓ effectiveness of **lutetium Lu 177 dotatate**; discontinue long-acting octreotide ≥4 wk and short-acting octreotide ≥24 hr prior to each dose of lutetium Lu 177 dotatate.

Route/Dosage

Carcinoid Tumors

SUBQ IV (Adults): 100–600 mcg/day in 2–4 divided doses during first 2 wk of therapy (range 50–1500 mcg/day).

IM (Adults): *Sandostatin LAR:* 20 mg every 4 wk for 2 mo; dose may be further adjusted.

VIPomas

SUBQ IV (Adults): 200–300 mcg/day in 2–4 divided doses during first 2 wk of therapy (range 150–750 mcg/day).

IM (Adults): *Sandostatin LAR:* 20 mg every 2 wk for 2 mo; dose may be further adjusted.

Acromegaly

SUBQ IV (Adults): 50–100 mcg 3 times daily; titrate to achieve GH levels <5 ng/mL or IGF-1 levels <1.9 units/mL (men) or <2.2 units/mL (women) (usual effective dose = 100–200 mcg 3 times daily).

IM (Adults): *Sandostatin LAR:* 20 mg every 4 wk for 3 mo, then adjusted on the basis of GH levels.

PO (Adults): 20 mg twice daily initially; titrate based on IGF-1 levels obtained every 2 wk by 20 mg/day. If maintenance dose = 60 mg/day, administer as 40 mg in am and 20 mg in pm; if maintenance dose = 80 mg/day, administer as 40 mg twice daily (not to exceed 80 mg/day).

Renal Impairment

PO (Adults): *End-stage renal disease:* 20 mg once daily initially; titrate based on IGF-1 levels obtained every 2 wk by 20 mg/day. If maintenance dose = 40 mg/day, administer as 20 mg twice daily; if maintenance dose = 60 mg/day, administer as 40 mg in am and 20 mg in pm; if maintenance dose = 80 mg/day, administer as 40 mg twice daily (not to exceed 80 mg/day).

Diarrhea Associated With Chemotherapy (off-label)

SUBQ, IV (Adults): 100–150 mcg SUBQ every 8 hr; may ↑ to 500–1500 mcg SUBQ or IV every 8 hr for severe diarrhea.

SUBQ (Children): 1–10 mcg/kg every 8–12 hr.

Diarrhea Associated With Graft-Versus-Host Disease (off-label)

IV (Adults): 500 mcg every 8 hr; do not continue for longer than 7 days (discontinue within 24 hr of diarrhea resolution).

SUBQ (Children): 1–10 mcg/kg every 8–12 hr.

Gastroesophageal Variceal Hemorrhage (off-label)

IV (Adults): 25–100 mcg bolus (may repeat in 1st hr if hemorrhage uncontrolled), followed by continuous infusion of 25–50 mcg/hr for 2–5 days.
IV (Children): 1–2 mcg/kg bolus, followed by continuous infusion of 1–2 mcg/kg/hr; taper dose by 50% every 12 hr when no active bleeding for 24 hr; discontinue when dose is 25% of initial dose.

Availability (generic available)

Delayed release capsules (Mycapssa): 20 mg. **Solution for IV or SUBQ injection (Sandostatin):** 50 mcg/mL, 100 mcg/mL, 200 mcg/mL, 500 mcg/mL, 1000 mcg/mL. **Suspension for IM injection (depot) (Sandostatin LAR):** 10 mg/6 mL, 20 mg/6 mL, 30 mg/6 mL.

NURSING IMPLICATIONS

Assessment

- Assess frequency and consistency of stools and bowel sounds during therapy.
- Monitor for steatorrhea, abdominal bloating, and weight loss. *If new occurrence or worsening of these symptoms occurs,* evaluate for pancreatic exocrine insufficiency and provide appropriate medical management.
- Monitor BP and HR prior to and periodically during therapy.
- Assess patient's fluid status, including skin turgor, for dehydration.
- Monitor patients with diabetes for signs of hypoglycemia. May require ↓ in requirements for insulin and sulfonylureas and treatment with diazoxide.
- Assess for right upper quadrant or radiating pain, and monitor gallbladder and bile duct ultrasound prior to and periodically during prolonged therapy.

Lab Test Considerations

- Monitor GH and IGF-1 in patients with acromegaly. *If IGF-1 levels remain above the upper limit of normal with max recommended dose or is not tolerated,* consider discontinuing octreotide.
- Monitor 5-HIAA (urinary 5-hydroxyindoleacetic acid), plasma serotonin, and plasma substance P in patients with carcinoid tumors; plasma VIP in patients with VIPoma; and free T_4 and serum glucose concentrations prior to and periodically during therapy in all patients taking octreotide.
- Monitor quantitative 72-hr fecal fat and serum carotene determinations periodically for possible drug-induced aggravations of fat malabsorption.
- May cause slight ↑ in liver enzymes.
- Monitor vitamin B12 during therapy (may ↓ levels).
- Monitor glycemic control for all patients with diabetes and adjust antidiabetic treatment as needed.

Implementation

- Do not confuse Sandostatin with Sandimmune.
- If a dose is missed, administer as soon as possible; then return to regular schedule. Do not double doses.
- **PO:** Administer with water on an empty stomach, ≥1 hr before or ≥2 hr after a meal. ***DNC:*** Swallow capsules whole; do not open, crush, or chew.
- **SUBQ:** Solution is clear and colorless; do not use if cloudy, discolored, or contains particulates. Ampules should be refrigerated but may be stored at room temperature for the days they will be used. Discard unused solution.
- Administer the smallest volume needed to achieve required dose. Rotate injection sites (hip, thigh, abdomen) at least 2 inches away from last site; avoid multiple injections in same site within short periods of time.
- Administer injections between meals and at bedtime to avoid GI side effects.
- **IM:** Should be administered by a health care professional. Mix IM solution by adding diluent included in kit. Administer immediately after mixing into the gluteus maximus. Avoid using deltoid due to pain of injection.
- Patients with carcinoid tumors and VIPomas should continue to receive SUBQ dose for 2 wk following switch to IM depot form to maintain therapeutic level.

IV Administration

- **IV Push: Dilution:** May be administered undiluted. **Rate:** Administer over 3 min or rapid bolus if emergency.
- **Intermittent Infusion: Dilution:** Dilute in 50–200 mL of 0.9% NaCl or D5W. **Concentration:** 1.5–250 mcg/mL. Store ampules in refrigerator and keep in outer carton to protect from light. **Rate:** Infuse over 15–30 min.
- **Y-Site Compatibility:** acyclovir, allopurinol, amikacin, aminocaproic acid, aminophylline, amiodarone, amphotericin B liposomal, ampicillin, ampicillin/sulbactam, anidulafungin, argatroban, arsenic trioxide, atracurium, azithromycin, aztreonam, bivalirudin, bleomycin, bumetanide, buprenorphine, busulfan, butorphanol, calcium chloride, calcium gluconate, carboplatin, carmustine, caspofungin, cefazolin, cefepime, cefotaxime, cefotetan, cefoxitin, ceftazidime, ceftolozane/tazobactam, ceftriaxone, cefuroxime, chloramphenicol, chlorpromazine, ciprofloxacin, cisatracurium, cisplatin, clindamycin, cyclophosphamide, cyclosporine, cytarabine, dacarbazine, dactinomycin, dantrolene, daptomycin, daunorubicin,

O

dexamethasone, dexmedetomidine, dexrazoxane, digoxin, diltiazem, diphenhydramine, dobutamine, docetaxel, dopamine, doxorubicin hydrochloride, doxorubicin liposomal, doxycycline, droperidol, enalaprilat, ephedrine, epinephrine, epirubicin, eptifibatide, eravacycline, ertapenem, erythromycin, esmolol, etoposide, etoposide phosphate, famotidine, fentanyl, fluconazole, fludarabine, fluorouracil, foscarnet, fosphenytoin, furosemide, ganciclovir, gemcitabine, gentamicin, glycopyrrolate, granisetron, haloperidol, heparin, hydralazine, hydrocortisone, hydromorphone, hydroxyzine, idarubicin, ifosfamide, imipenem/cilastatin, insulin aspart, insulin regular, irinotecan, isavuconazonium, isoproterenol, ketorolac, labetalol, LR, leucovorin calcium, levofloxacin, lidocaine, linezolid, lorazepam, magnesium sulfate, mannitol, melphalan, meperidine, meropenem, meropenem/vaborbactam, mesna, methadone, methohexital, methotrexate, methylprednisolone, metoclopramide, metoprolol, metronidazole, midazolam, milrinone, mitomycin, mitoxantrone, morphine, moxifloxacin, mycophenolate, nafcillin, nalbuphine, naloxone, nicardipine, nitroglycerin, nitroprusside, norepinephrine, ondansetron, oxaliplatin, paclitaxel, palonosetron, pamidronate, pemetrexed, pentamidine, pentobarbital, phenobarbital, phentolamine, phenylephrine, piperacillin/tazobactam, plazomicin, potassium acetate, potassium chloride, potassium phosphate, procainamide, prochlorperazine, promethazine, propranolol, remdesivir, remifentanil, rocuronium, sodium acetate, sodium bicarbonate, sodium phosphate, succinylcholine, sufentanil, sulbactam/durlobactam, tacrolimus, thiotepa, tigecycline, tirofiban, tobramycin, topotecan, trimethoprim/sulfamethoxazole, vancomycin, vasopressin, vecuronium, verapamil, vinblastine, vincristine, vinorelbine, voriconazole, zidovudine, zoledronic acid.

- **Y-Site Incompatibility:** dantrolene, diazepam, micafungin, phenytoin, total parenteral nutrition (TPN) solutions.

Patient/Family Teaching

- Explain purpose of octreotide to patient and instruct patient using injection form in correct technique, care, and disposal of equipment. Advise all patients to read *Medication Guide* prior to using and with each Rx refill, in case of changes.
- Advise patient to notify health care professional of all Rx or OTC medications, vitamins, or herbal products being taken and to consult health care professional before taking other medications.
- May cause dizziness, drowsiness, or visual disturbances. Caution patient to avoid driving or other activities requiring alertness until response to medication is known.
- Advise patient to change positions slowly to minimize orthostatic hypotension.
- Advise patient to notify health care professional if signs and symptoms of gallstones, hyperglycemia, hypoglycemia, thyroid dysfunction, or irregular heartbeat occur.
- Advise patient to notify health care professional if they experience new or worsening symptoms of fat in their stool, stool discoloration, loose stools, abdominal bloating, or weight loss.
- Rep: Inform women of reproductive potential that therapy with octreotide may result in improved fertility. Caution patient to use nonhormonal contraception to prevent unintended pregnancy. Advise patient to notify health care professional if pregnancy is planned or suspected or if breastfeeding.

Evaluation/Desired Outcomes

- Reduction in severity of diarrhea and improvement of electrolyte imbalances in patients with carcinoid or VIP-secreting tumors.
- Relief of symptoms and suppressed tumor growth in patients with pituitary tumors associated with acromegaly.
- Growth hormone levels <5 ng/mL or IGF-1 levels within normal reference ranges for age and sex in patients treated for acromegaly.

ofatumumab

(oh-fa-**too**-moo-mab)

Kesimpta

Classification

Therapeutic: anti-multiple sclerosis agents

Pharmacologic: monoclonal antibodies

Indications

Relapsing forms of multiple sclerosis (MS), including clinically isolated syndrome, relapsing-remitting disease, and active secondary progressive disease.

Action

A monoclonal antibody that specifically binds to CD20 molecule found on the surface of B lymphocytes, resulting in B-cell lysis. **Therapeutic Effects:** Decreased incidence of relapses in MS.

Pharmacokinetics

Absorption: Extent of absorption following SUBQ administration unknown.

Distribution: Unknown.

Metabolism and Excretion: Undergoes enzymatic degradation to smaller peptides.

Half-life: 16 days.

TIME/ACTION PROFILE (plasma concentrations)

ROUTE	ONSET	PEAK	DURATION
SUBQ	unknown	unknown	unknown

Contraindications/Precautions

Contraindicated in: Hypersensitivity; Acute hepatitis B virus (HBV) infection.
Use Cautiously in: History of HBV infection (may reactivate); OB: Safety not established in pregnancy; Lactation: Safety not established in breastfeeding; Rep: Women of reproductive potential; Pedi: Safety and effectiveness not established in children.

Adverse Reactions/Side Effects

CV: peripheral edema. **Derm:** sweating. **GI:** HBV INFECTION OR REACTIVATION, INTESTINAL OBSTRUCTION.
Hemat: anemia, neutropenia, thrombocytopenia.
Local: injection site reactions. **MS:** back pain, muscle spasm. **Neuro:** headache, PROGRESSIVE MULTIFOCAL LEUKOENCEPHALOPATHY (PML), weakness. **Misc:** INFECTION, chills, fever, HYPERSENSITIVITY REACTIONS (INCLUDING ANAPHYLAXIS AND ANGIOEDEMA), tumor lysis syndrome.

Interactions

Drug-Drug: May ↓ antibody response to and ↑ risk of adverse reactions from **live-virus vaccines**; may also interfere with effectiveness of **inactivated vaccines**. **Immunosuppressants** may ↑ risk of immunosuppression.

Route/Dosage

Relapsing Multiple Sclerosis

SUBQ (Adults): 20 mg once weekly for 3 wk (Wk 0, 1, and 2), then 20 mg once monthly starting on Wk 4.

Availability

Solution for SUBQ injection (prefilled pens and syringes): 20 mg/0.4 mL.

NURSING IMPLICATIONS

Assessment

- Assess for hypersensitivity reaction or life-threatening systemic injection-related reactions (anaphylaxis, angioedema, pruritus, rash, urticaria, erythema, bronchospasm, throat irritation, oropharyngeal pain, dyspnea, pharyngeal or laryngeal edema, flushing, hypotension, dizziness, nausea, tachycardia). Discontinue permanently if these symptoms occur.
- Monitor for mild systemic injection-related reactions (fever, headache, myalgia, chills, fatigue). If reaction is not life-threatening and rechallenge is considered appropriate, administer next injection under clinical observation.
- Monitor for PML signs and symptoms (altered mental status, hemiparesis or monoparesis, limb/gait ataxia, vision disturbances). Withhold immediately at the first sign/symptom suggestive of PML, and perform a diagnostic evaluation. Discontinue treatment if PML is confirmed.
- Assess for severe opportunistic or recurrent infections (with low immunoglobulins) or prolonged hypogammaglobulinemia requiring immunoglobulin treatment. Consider discontinuing therapy.
- Screen all patients for HBV infection before starting therapy. Monitor carriers of HBV for clinical and laboratory signs during and for ≥12 mo following discontinuation of therapy. Discontinue therapy in patients who develop viral hepatitis or reactivation of viral hepatitis and institute appropriate treatment.

Lab Test Considerations

- Monitor quantitative serum immunoglobulins at baseline, throughout treatment as clinically necessary, in patients with opportunistic or recurrent infections, and after discontinuation of therapy until B-cell repletion.
- Monitor hepatitis B surface antigen (HBsAg), hepatitis B core antibody (HBcAb), and other hepatitis B markers at baseline and as clinically necessary. Screen for hepatitis and tuberculosis in high-risk populations.

Implementation

- Administer all immunizations according to immunization guidelines ≥4 wk before starting therapy for live or live-attenuated vaccines and ≥2 wk for inactivated vaccines. Vaccines are not recommended until B-cell repletion.
- **SUBQ:** Remove from refrigerator and allow to reach room temperature for 15–30 min before use. Solution is clear to slightly opalescent and colorless to slightly brownish-yellow; do not administer solutions that are cloudy, discolored, or contain particulate matter. Administer first injection under the guidance of a health care professional. Inject in the abdomen, thigh, or outer upper arm. Do not give injection into moles, scars, stretch marks, or areas where the skin is tender, bruised, red, scaly, or hard. Pens and syringes are for one-time use; discard after use.

Patient/Family Teaching

- Explain purpose and side effects of medication. Advise patient to read *Patient Information* before starting therapy. Instruct patient about correct preparation, injection technique, and equipment disposal. Administer missed doses as soon as remembered; then administer subsequent doses at recommended intervals.
- Instruct patient to notify health care professional of all Rx or OTC medications, vitamins, or herbal products being taken and to consult health care professional before taking other Rx, OTC, or herbal products.
- Advise patient to avoid live-virus vaccines during therapy.
- Inform patients about the signs and symptoms of injection-related reactions and hypersensitivity

O

reactions. Inform patients that injection-related reactions generally occur within 24 hr and mainly after the first injection but may occur with any injection. Advise patients to contact their health care provider or seek immediate medical attention if reactions occur.

- Rep: Advise females of reproductive potential to use effective contraception during and for 6 mo after last dose and to notify health care professional if breastfeeding. May cause fetal B-cell depletion. Avoid administering live vaccines to neonates and infants exposed to ofatumumab in utero until B-cell recovery occurs.

Evaluation/Desired Outcomes

- Decreased incidence of relapses in MS.

ofloxacin, See FLUOROQUINOLONES.

BEERS REMS

OLANZapine (oh-lan-za-peen)

ZyPREXA, ZyPREXA Relprevv, ZyPREXA Zydis

Classification

Therapeutic: antipsychotics, mood stabilizers

Pharmacologic: thienobenzodiazepines

Indications

PO, IM: Schizophrenia. **PO:** Management of the following: Acute therapy of manic or mixed episodes associated with bipolar I disorder (as monotherapy [adults and adolescents] or in combination with lithium or evaporate [adults only]); Maintenance therapy of bipolar I disorder; Depressive episodes associated with bipolar I disorder (in combination with fluoxetine); Treatment-resistant depression (in combination with fluoxetine). **IM:** Acute agitation due to schizophrenia or bipolar I mania. **Unlabeled Use:** Anorexia nervosa. Treatment of nausea and vomiting related to highly emetogenic chemotherapy.

Action

Antagonizes dopamine and serotonin type 2 in the CNS. Also has anticholinergic, antihistaminic, and anti–alpha$_1$-adrenergic effects. **Therapeutic Effects:** Decreased manifestations of psychoses.

Pharmacokinetics

Absorption: Well absorbed but rapidly metabolized by first-pass effect, resulting in 60% bioavailability. Conventional tablets and orally disintegrating tablets (Zydis) are bioequivalent. IM administration results in significantly higher blood levels (5 times that of oral).

Distribution: Extensively distributed.

Protein Binding: 93%.

Metabolism and Excretion: Primarily metabolized by the liver by the CYP1A2 isoenzyme; 7% excreted unchanged in urine.

Half-life: 21–54 hr.

TIME/ACTION PROFILE (antipsychotic effects)

ROUTE	ONSET	PEAK*	DURATION
PO	unknown	6 hr	unknown
IM	rapid	15–45 min	2–4 hr

* Blood levels.

Contraindications/Precautions

Contraindicated in: Hypersensitivity; Phenylketonuria (orally disintegrating tablets contain aspartame).

Use Cautiously in: Hepatic impairment; Patients at risk for aspiration or falls; Cardiovascular or cerebrovascular disease; History of seizures; History of attempted suicide; Diabetes or risk factors for diabetes (may worsen glucose control); Presence/history of constipation, urinary retention, prostatic hypertrophy, or paralytic ileus; Low WBC or ANC or history of drug-induced neutropenia/leukopenia; Angle-closure glaucoma; History of breast cancer; OB: Use during pregnancy only if potential maternal benefit justifies potential fetal risk; neonates at ↑ risk for extrapyramidal symptoms and withdrawal after delivery when exposed during the 3rd trimester; Lactation: Use while breastfeeding only if potential maternal benefit justifies potential fetal risk; Pedi: Children <13 yr (safety and effectiveness not established); adolescents at ↑ risk for weight gain and hyperlipidemia; Geri: Appears on Beers list. ↑ risk of stroke, cognitive decline, and mortality in older adults with dementia. Avoid use in older adults, except for schizophrenia, bipolar disorder, or adjunctive treatment of major depressive disorder.

Adverse Reactions/Side Effects

CV: orthostatic hypotension, bradycardia, chest pain, syncope, tachycardia. **Derm:** DRUG REACTION WITH EOSINOPHILIA AND SYSTEMIC SYMPTOMS (DRESS), photosensitivity. **EENT:** amblyopia, rhinitis, ↑ salivation, pharyngitis. **Endo:** galactorrhea, goiter, gynecomastia, hyperglycemia, hyperprolactinemia. **F and E:** ↑ thirst. **GI:** ↑ liver enzymes, constipation, dry mouth, weight loss, abdominal pain, dysphagia, nausea. **GU:** ↓ fertility (women), ↓ libido, amenorrhea, impotence, urinary incontinence. **Hemat:** AGRANULOCYTOSIS, leukopenia, neutropenia. **Metab:** weight gain, ↑ appetite, dyslipidemia. **MS:** hypertonia, joint pain. **Neuro:** agitation, delirium, dizziness, headache, restlessness, sedation, tremor, weakness, dystonia, falls, insomnia, mood changes, NEUROLEPTIC MALIGNANT SYNDROME, personality disorder, SEIZURES, speech impairment, SUICIDAL THOUGHTS, tardive dyskinesia. **Resp:** aspiration, cough, dyspnea. **Misc:** body temperature dysregulation, fever, flu-like syndrome.

Interactions

Drug-Drug: ↑ CNS depression may occur with concurrent use of **alcohol** or other **CNS depressants**; concurrent use of IM olanzapine and parenteral benzodiazepines should be avoided. ↑ anticholinergic effects with other **anticholinergic drugs**, including **antihistamines**, **quinidine**, **disopyramide**, and **antidepressants**; avoid concurrent use. Effects may be ↓ by **carbamazepine**, **omeprazole**, or **rifampin**. **Antihypertensives** and **CNS depressants** may ↑ risk of orthostatic hypotension. May antagonize the effects of **levodopa** or other **dopamine agonists**. **Fluvoxamine** may ↑ levels and risk of toxicity. **Nicotine** can ↓ levels and effectiveness.

Route/Dosage

Schizophrenia

PO (Adults): 5–10 mg/day initially; may ↑ at weekly intervals by 5 mg/day (target dose = 10 mg/day; not to exceed 20 mg/day).

PO (Adults: Debilitated or Nonsmoking Female Patients ≥65 yr): Initiate therapy at 5 mg/day.

PO (Children 13–17 yr): 2.5–5 mg/day initially; may ↑ at weekly intervals by 2.5–5 mg/day (target dose = 10 mg/day; not to exceed 20 mg/day).

IM (Adults): *Oral olanzapine dose = 10 mg/day:* 210 mg every 2 wk or 410 mg every 4 wk for the 1st 8 wk, then 150 mg every 2 wk or 300 mg every 4 wk as maintenance therapy; *Oral olanzapine dose = 15 mg/day:* 300 mg every 2 wk for the 1st 8 wk, then 210 mg every 2 wk or 405 mg every 4 wk as maintenance therapy; *Oral olanzapine dose = 20 mg/day:* 300 mg every 2 wk for the 1st 8 wk, then 300 mg every 2 wk as maintenance therapy.

IM (Adults – Debilitated or Nonsmoking Female Patients ≥65 yr): Initiate therapy at 150 mg every 4 wk.

Acute Manic or Mixed Episodes Associated With Bipolar I Disorder

PO (Adults): 10–15 mg/day initially (use 10 mg/day when used with lithium or evaporate); may ↑ every 24 hr by 5 mg/day (not to exceed 20 mg/day).

PO (Children 13–17 yr): 2.5–5 mg/day initially; may ↑ by 2.5–5 mg/day (target dose = 10 mg/day; not to exceed 20 mg/day).

Maintenance Treatment of Bipolar I Disorder

PO (Adults): Continue at the dose required to maintain symptom remission (usual dose: 5–20 mg/day).

PO (Children 13–17 yr): Continue at the lowest dose required to maintain symptom remission.

Acute Agitation Due to Schizophrenia or Bipolar I Mania

IM (Adults): 10 mg; may repeat in 2 hr and then 4 hr later.

IM (Adults >65 yr): Initiate therapy with 5 mg.

Depressive Episodes Associated With Bipolar I Disorder

PO (Adults): 5 mg/day with fluoxetine 20 mg/day (both given in evening); may ↑ fluoxetine dose up to 50 mg/day and olanzapine dose up to 12.5 mg/day.

PO (Children 10–17 yr): 20 mg/day with olanzapine 2.5 mg/day (both given in evening); may ↑ fluoxetine dose up to 50 mg/day and olanzapine dose up to 12 mg/day.

Treatment-Resistant Depression

PO (Adults): 5 mg/day with fluoxetine 20 mg/day (both given in evening); may ↑ fluoxetine dose up to 50 mg/day and olanzapine dose up to 20 mg/day.

Availability (generic available)

Tablets: 2.5 mg, 5 mg, 7.5 mg, 10 mg, 15 mg, 20 mg. **Orally disintegrating tablets (Zyprexa Zydis):** 5 mg, 10 mg, 15 mg, 20 mg. **Powder for injection:** 10 mg/vial. **Extended-release powder for suspension for injection (Zyprexa Relprevv):** 210 mg/vial, 300 mg/vial, 405 mg/vial. ***In combination with:*** fluoxetine (generic only); samidorphan (Lybalvi). See Appendix N.

O

NURSING IMPLICATIONS

Assessment

- Assess mental status (orientation, mood, behavior) before and periodically during therapy. Monitor closely for notable changes in behavior that could indicate the emergence or worsening of suicidal thoughts or behavior or depression.
- Monitor BP (sitting, standing, lying), ECG, HR, and respiratory rate before and frequently during dose adjustment.
- Assess weight and BMI initially and throughout therapy.
- Observe patient carefully when administering medication to ensure that medication is taken and not hoarded or cheeked.
- Assess fluid intake and bowel function. ↑ of fiber and fluids may help minimize constipation.
- Monitor patient for onset of akathisia (restlessness or desire to keep moving) and extrapyramidal side effects (*parkinsonian:* difficulty speaking or swallowing, loss of balance control, pill rolling of hands, masklike face, shuffling gait, rigidity, tremors; and *dystonic:* muscle spasms, twisting motions, twitching, inability to move eyes, weakness of arms or legs) every 2 mo during therapy and 8–12 wk after therapy has been discontinued. Report these symptoms if they occur, as ↓ in dose or discontinuation of medication may be necessary. Trihexyphenidyl or benztropine may be used to control symptoms.

- Monitor for tardive dyskinesia (uncontrolled rhythmic movement of mouth, face, and extremities; lip smacking or puckering; puffing of cheeks; uncontrolled chewing; rapid or worm-like movements of tongue; excessive blinking of eyes). Discontinue olanzapine and report immediately; may be irreversible.
- Monitor for development of neuroleptic malignant syndrome (fever, respiratory distress, tachycardia, seizures, diaphoresis, hypertension or hypotension, pallor, tiredness, severe muscle stiffness, loss of bladder control). Notify health care provider immediately if these symptoms occur.
- Monitor for symptoms related to hyperprolactinemia (menstrual abnormalities, galactorrhea, sexual dysfunction).
- Assess for falls risk. Drowsiness, orthostatic hypotension, and motor and sensory instability ↑ risk. Institute prevention if indicated.
- Monitor for signs and symptoms of DRESS (fever, rash, lymphadenopathy, facial swelling), associated with involvement of other organ systems (hepatitis, nephritis, hematologic abnormalities, myocarditis, myositis) during therapy. May resemble an acute viral infection. Eosinophilia is often present. Discontinue therapy if signs occur.
- *Zyprexa Relprevv*: Observe for signs and symptoms of postinjection delirium/sedation syndrome (dizziness, confusion, disorientation, slurred speech, altered gait, difficulty ambulating, weakness, agitation, extrapyramidal symptoms, hypertension, convulsion, reduced level of consciousness ranging from mild sedation to coma) for ≥3 hr after injection.

Lab Test Considerations

- Monitor liver function tests, and ocular examinations periodically during therapy. May ↑ bilirubin, AST, ALT, GGT, CK, and alkaline phosphatase.
- Monitor blood glucose before and periodically during therapy.
- Monitor serum prolactin before and periodically during therapy. May ↑ serum prolactin levels.
- Monitor CBC frequently during initial months of therapy in patients with pre-existing or history of low WBC. May cause leukopenia, neutropenia, or agranulocytosis. Discontinue therapy if this occurs.
- May cause hyperlipidemia; monitor serum lipids before and periodically during therapy.

Implementation

- Do not confuse Zyprexa with Celexa, Zyrtec, Zestril, or Zelapar. Do not confuse olanzapine with quetiapine.
- ***REMS:*** *Zyprexa Relprevv* is only prescribed through *Zyprexa Relprevv Patient Care Program*. Prescribers, pharmacies, and patients must be educated about the program and must comply with the program requirements.
- **PO:** Administer without regard to meals.
- *For orally disintegrating tablets,* peel back foil on blister; do not push tablet through foil. Using dry hands, remove from foil and place entire tablet in mouth. Tablet will disintegrate with or without liquid.
- **IM: Reconstitution:** Reconstitute with 2.1 mL of sterile water for injection. Solution should be clear and yellow; do not administer solutions that are discolored or contain particulate matter. **Concentration:** 5 mg/mL. Inject slowly, deep into muscle. Do not administer IV or SUBQ. Administer within 1 hr of reconstitution. Discard unused solution.
- **Zyprexa Relprevv**: Use gloves when preparing; solution may be irritating to skin. **Reconstitution:** Use only diluent provided by manufacturer. Reconstitute 150-mg or 210-mg dose with 1.3 mL, 300-mg dose with 1.8 mL, and 405-mg dose with 2.3 mL of diluent. Loosen powder by tapping vial; inject diluent into powder. Remove needle from vial, holding vial upright to prevent loss of solution. Engage needle safety device as explained by manufacturer. Pad a hard surface and tap vial repeatedly until no powder or dry yellow clumps are visible. Shake vial vigorously until suspension appears smooth and consistent in color and texture. Solution will be yellow and opaque. Allow foam to dissipate. Suspension is stable for 24 hr at room temperature; if not used immediately, shake to resuspend. **Concentration:** 150 mg/mL. Replace needle with 19-gauge, 1½-inch or 2-inch needle for obese patients. Slowly withdraw desired amount from vial; 150 mg = 1 mL, 210 mg = 1.4 mL, 300 mg = 2 mL, 405 mg = 2.7 mL. Administer immediately deep IM gluteal after withdrawing. Do not massage injection site. Patient must be observed for ≥3 hr after injection for postinjection delirium/sedation syndrome.

Patient/Family Teaching

- ***REMS:*** Explain purpose and side effects of medication to patient. Advise patient to read *Patient Information* before starting therapy. Advise to take as directed and not to skip doses or double up on missed doses. May need to discontinue gradually. Explain the *Zyprexa Relprevv Patient Care Program* to patient and encourage patient to enroll in the *Zyprexa Relprevv Patient Care Program* registry.
- Emphasize the importance of routine follow-up exams and continued participation in psychotherapy.
- Advise patient to notify health care provider of all Rx or OTC medications, vitamins, or herbal products being taken and to consult with health care provider before taking other medications and alcohol.
- Advise patient of possibility of extrapyramidal symptoms and tardive dyskinesia. Advise patient to report these symptoms immediately to health care provider.
- Advise patient to change positions slowly to minimize orthostatic hypotension. Protect from falls.

- Medication may cause drowsiness. Advise patient to avoid driving or other activities requiring alertness until response to the medication is known. Patients receiving *Zyprexa Relprevv* should not drive for 24 hr following injection.
- Advise patient and family/caregiver to notify health care provider if thoughts about suicide or dying, attempts to commit suicide, new or worse depression, new or worse anxiety, feeling very agitated or restless, panic attacks, trouble sleeping, new or worse irritability, acting aggressive, being angry or violent, acting on dangerous impulses, an extreme ↑ in activity and talking, or other unusual changes in behavior or mood occur.
- Advise patient to use sunscreen and protective clothing when exposed to the sun. Extremes of temperature (exercise, hot weather, hot baths or showers) should also be avoided; this drug impairs body temperature regulation.
- Advise patient to use saliva substitute, frequent mouth rinses, good oral hygiene, and sugarless gum or candy to minimize dry mouth. Consult dentist if dry mouth continues for >2 wk.
- Advise patient to notify health care provider of medication regimen before treatment or surgery.
- Advise patient to notify health care provider promptly if sore throat, fever, unusual bleeding or bruising, rash, symptoms of postinjection delirium/sedation syndrome, weakness, tremors, visual disturbances, dark-colored urine, clay-colored stools, menstrual abnormalities, galactorrhea, or sexual dysfunction occur.
- Rep: Advise women of reproductive potential to notify health care provider if pregnancy is planned or suspected and to avoid breastfeeding during therapy. Encourage women who become pregnant while taking olanzapine to enroll in the National Pregnancy Registry for Atypical Antipsychotics at 1-866-961-2388 or visit https://womensmentalhealth.org/research/pregnancyregistry/. Monitor neonates for extrapyramidal and/or withdrawal symptoms and manage symptoms appropriately. Monitor infants exposed through breastfeeding for excess sedation, irritability, poor feeding, and extrapyramidal symptoms (tremors and abnormal muscle movements).

Evaluation/Desired Outcomes

- Decreased manifestations of psychoses.

HIGH ALERT

olaparib (oh-lap-a-rib)

Lynparza

Classification

Therapeutic: antineoplastics

Pharmacologic: enzyme inhibitors

Indications

Maintenance treatment of recurrent epithelial ovarian, fallopian tube, or primary peritoneal cancer in patients who are in a complete or partial response to platinum-based chemotherapy. First-line maintenance treatment of deleterious/suspected deleterious germline or somatic *BRCA*-mutated recurrent epithelial ovarian, fallopian tube, or primary peritoneal cancer in patients who are in a complete or partial response to first-line platinum-based chemotherapy. First-line maintenance treatment of advanced epithelial ovarian, fallopian tube, or primary peritoneal cancer in patients who are in a complete or partial response to first-line platinum-based chemotherapy and whose cancer is associated with homologous recombination deficiency positive status defined by either a deleterious/suspected deleterious *BRCA* mutation and/or genomic instability (in combination with bevacizumab). Adjuvant treatment of deleterious or suspected deleterious germline *BRCA*-mutated human epidermal growth factor receptor 2 (HER2)-negative high-risk early breast cancer in patients who have been treated with neoadjuvant or adjuvant chemotherapy. Deleterious/suspected deleterious germline *BRCA*-mutated HER2-negative metastatic breast cancer in patients who have been treated with chemotherapy in the neoadjuvant, adjuvant, or metastatic setting (should have been previously treated with or considered intolerant to an endocrine therapy). First-line maintenance treatment of deleterious/suspected deleterious germline *BRCA*-mutated metastatic pancreatic adenocarcinoma in patients whose disease has not progressed on ≥16 wk of a first-line platinum-based chemotherapy regimen. Deleterious/suspected deleterious germline or somatic homologous recombination repair (HRR) gene-mutated metastatic castration-resistant prostate cancer in patients who have progressed following previous treatment with enzalutamide or abiraterone. Deleterious/suspected deleterious *BRCA*-mutated metastatic castration-resistant prostate cancer (in combination with abiraterone and prednisolone [or prednisone]).

Action

Acts as a poly (ADP-ribose) polymerase (PARP) inhibitor; disrupts DNA transcription, cell cycle regulation, and DNA repair. **Therapeutic Effects:** Improved progression-free survival in ovarian, fallopian tube, primary peritoneal, breast, pancreatic, and prostate cancer.

Pharmacokinetics

Absorption: Well absorbed following oral administration.

Distribution: Unknown.

Metabolism and Excretion: Extensively metabolized (mostly by the CYP3A isoenzyme); 15% excreted unchanged in urine, 6% in feces.

Half-life: 14.9 hr.

O

TIME/ACTION PROFILE (plasma concentrations)

ROUTE	ONSET	PEAK	DURATION
PO	unknown	1–3 hr	12 hr

Contraindications/Precautions

Contraindicated in: OB: Pregnancy; Lactation: Lactation.

Use Cautiously in: Moderate or severe hepatic impairment; Moderate or severe renal impairment (CCr <50 mL/min) (dose ↓ may be needed); Rep: Women of reproductive potential and men with female partners of reproductive potential; Pedi: Safety and effectiveness not established in children.

Adverse Reactions/Side Effects

CV: DEEP VEIN THROMBOSIS. **Derm:** dermatitis/rash. **GI:** abdominal pain, diarrhea, dyspepsia, nausea, vomiting. **Hemat:** anemia, lymphopenia, neutropenia, thrombocytopenia, MYELODYSPLASTIC SYNDROME (MDS)/ACUTE MYELOID LEUKEMIA (AML). **Metab:** ↓ appetite. **MS:** arthralgia, back pain, myalgia. **Neuro:** fatigue, headache, dysgeusia, weakness. **Resp:** cough, PNEUMONITIS, PULMONARY EMBOLISM.

Interactions

Drug-Drug: ↑ risk of prolonged myelosuppression with other **antineoplastics**. Concurrent use with **strong CYP3A4 inhibitors**, including **clarithromycin, itraconazole, ketoconazole, lopinavir/ritonavir, nefazodone, nelfinavir, posaconazole, ritonavir**, or **voriconazole**, ↑ levels and risk of toxicity; avoid concurrent use if possible but if necessary, ↓ olaparib dose. Concurrent use with **moderate CYP3A4 inhibitors**, including **aprepitant, atazanavir, ciprofloxacin, crizotinib, darunavir/ritonavir, diltiazem, erythromycin, fluconazole, fosamprenavir, imatinib**, or **verapamil**, ↑ levels and risk of toxicity; avoid concurrent use if possible but if necessary, ↓ olaparib dose. Concurrent use with **strong CYP3A inducers**, including **carbamazepine, phenytoin**, and **rifampin**, ↓ blood levels and effectiveness and should be avoided. Concurrent use with **moderate CYP3A inducers**, including **bosentan, efavirenz, etravirine, modafinil**, and **nafcillin**, ↓ blood levels and effectiveness; avoid if possible.

Drug-Natural Products: St. John's wort may ↓ blood levels and effectiveness and should be avoided.

Drug-Food: Concurrent ingestion of **grapefruit** and **Seville oranges** may ↑ blood levels and the risk of toxicity and should be avoided.

Route/Dosage

First-Line Maintenance Treatment of *BRCA*-Mutated Advanced Ovarian Cancer or Advanced Ovarian Cancer (in Combination with Bevacizumab)

PO (Adults): 300 mg twice daily until disease progression, unacceptable toxicity, or completion of 2 yr of treatment. If complete response achieved after 2 yr of treatment (i.e., no radiological evidence of disease), can stop therapy. If evidence of disease at 2 yr, may continue therapy. *Concurrent use of strong CYP3A4 inhibitor:* 100 mg twice daily until disease progression, unacceptable toxicity, or completion of 2 yr of treatment. If complete response achieved after 2 yr of treatment (i.e., no radiological evidence of disease), can stop therapy. If evidence of disease at 2 yr, may continue therapy. *Concurrent use of moderate CYP3A4 inhibitor:* 150 mg twice daily until disease progression, unacceptable toxicity, or completion of 2 yr of treatment. If complete response achieved after 2 yr of treatment (i.e., no radiological evidence of disease), can stop therapy. If evidence of disease at 2 yr, may continue therapy.

Renal Impairment

PO (Adults): *CCr 31–50 mL/min:* 200 mg twice daily until disease progression, unacceptable toxicity, or completion of 2 yr of treatment. If complete response achieved after 2 yr of treatment (i.e., no radiological evidence of disease), can stop therapy. If evidence of disease at 2 yr, may continue therapy.

Adjuvant Treatment of Germline *BRCA*-Mutated HER2-Negative High-Risk Early Breast Cancer

PO (Adults): 300 mg twice daily for 1 yr or until disease recurrence or unacceptable toxicity, whichever occurs first. *Concurrent use of strong CYP3A4 inhibitor:* 100 mg twice daily for 1 yr or until disease recurrence or unacceptable toxicity, whichever occurs first. *Concurrent use of moderate CYP3A4 inhibitor:* 150 mg twice daily for 1 yr or until disease recurrence or unacceptable toxicity, whichever occurs first.

Renal Impairment

PO (Adults): *CCr 31–50 mL/min:* 200 mg twice daily for 1 yr or until disease recurrence or unacceptable toxicity, whichever occurs first.

Recurrent Ovarian Cancer, Germline *BRCA*-Mutated HER2-Negative Metastatic Breast Cancer, Germline *BRCA*-Mutated Metastatic Pancreatic Adenocarcinoma, HRR Gene-Mutated Metastatic Castration-Resistant Prostate Cancer, *BRCA*-Mutated Metastatic Castration-Resistant Prostate Cancer

PO (Adults): 300 mg twice daily until disease progression or unacceptable toxicity. *Concurrent use of strong CYP3A4 inhibitor:* 100 mg twice daily until disease progression or unacceptable toxicity. *Concurrent use of moderate CYP3A4 inhibitor:* 150 mg twice daily until disease progression or unacceptable toxicity.

Renal Impairment

PO (Adults): *CCr 31–50 mL/min:* 200 mg twice daily until disease progression or unacceptable toxicity.

Availability
Tablets: 100 mg, 150 mg.

NURSING IMPLICATIONS
Assessment
- Monitor for signs and symptoms of pneumonitis (new or worsening respiratory symptoms, dyspnea, fever, cough, wheezing, radiological abnormality) during therapy. Interrupt therapy; if pneumonitis confirmed, discontinue therapy.
- Monitor for signs and symptoms of deep vein thrombosis and pulmonary embolism and treat as medically appropriate. May require long-term anticoagulation.

Lab Test Considerations
- Patient selection is based on the presence of deleterious or suspected deleterious HRR gene mutations, including BRCA mutations, or genomic instability based on the indication, biomarker, and sample type. Information on FDA-approved tests for the detection of genetic mutations is available at http://www.fda.gov/companiondiagnostics.
- Verify negative pregnancy test prior to starting therapy.
- Monitor CBC at baseline and monthly during therapy. Do not start olaparib until patient has recovered from hematological toxicities from previous chemotherapy (≤CTCAE Grade 1). *For prolonged hematological toxicities,* interrupt olaparib and monitor CBC weekly until recovery. If levels have not recovered to Grade ≤1 after 4 wk, refer to hematologist. Discontinue olaparib if MDS or AML is confirmed.
- May cause ↓ hemoglobin, neutrophils, platelets, and lymphocytes. May cause ↑ mean corpuscular volume and serum creatinine.

Implementation
- **PO:** Administer twice daily, about 12 hr apart, without regard to food. ***DNC:*** Swallow tablets whole; do not break, chew, or dissolve tablets.

Patient/Family Teaching
- Explain purpose and side effects of medication. Advise patient to read *Patient Information* before starting therapy. Instruct patient to take as directed. If a dose is missed, do not take another to make up; omit dose and take next scheduled dose. Emphasize importance of routine lab tests.
- Instruct patient to notify health care professional of all Rx or OTC medications, vitamins, or herbal products being taken and to consult with health care professional before taking other medications, especially St. John's wort.
- Inform patient that mild to moderate nausea and/or vomiting is common. Notify a health care professional for antiemetic options if this is problematic.
- Advise patient to avoid grapefruit, grapefruit juice, Seville oranges, and Seville orange juice during therapy.
- Advise patient to notify health care professional if signs and symptoms of pneumonitis or hematological toxicity (weakness, feeling tired, fever, weight loss, frequent infections, bruising, bleeding easily, shortness of breath, blood in urine or stool, low blood cell counts on laboratory findings, need for blood transfusions) occur. May also be MDS or AML.
- Rep: May cause fetal harm and ↑ risk for loss of pregnancy. Advise females of reproductive potential to use effective contraception during therapy and for ≥6 mo after last dose and to avoid breastfeeding for 1 mo after last dose. Advise patient to notify health care professional if pregnancy is planned or suspected. Advise males with female partners of reproductive potential to use effective contraception during and for 3 mo after last dose. Advise male patients not to donate sperm during therapy and for 3 mo following the last dose.

Evaluation/Desired Outcomes
- Improved progression-free survival in ovarian, fallopian tube, primary peritoneal, breast, pancreatic, and prostate cancer.

O

olmesartan, See ANGIOTENSIN II RECEPTOR ANTAGONISTS.

olsalazine (ole-sal-a-zeen)
Dipentum

Classification
Therapeutic: gastrointestinal anti-inflammatories

Indications
Ulcerative colitis (when patients cannot tolerate sulfasalazine).

Action
Locally acting anti-inflammatory action in the colon, where activity is probably due to inhibition of prostaglandin synthesis. **Therapeutic Effects:** Reduction in the symptoms of inflammatory bowel disease.

Pharmacokinetics
Absorption: Acts locally in colon, where 98–99% is converted to mesalamine (5-aminosalicylic acid).
Distribution: Action is primarily local and remains in the colon.
Metabolism and Excretion: 2% absorbed into systemic circulation is rapidly metabolized; mostly eliminated as mesalamine in the feces.
Half-life: 0.9 hr.

TIME/ACTION PROFILE (plasma concentrations)

ROUTE	ONSET	PEAK	DURATION
PO	unknown	1 hr; 4–8 hr	12 hr

Contraindications/Precautions

Contraindicated in: Hypersensitivity reaction to salicylates; Cross-sensitivity with furosemide, sulfonylureas, or carbonic anhydrase inhibitors may exist; Glucose-6-phosphate dehydrogenase (G6PD) deficiency; Urinary tract or intestinal obstruction; Porphyria; Lactation: Lactation.

Use Cautiously in: Severe hepatic or renal impairment; Renal impairment (↑ risk of renal tubular damage); OB: Safety not established in pregnancy; Pedi: Children <2 yr (safety and effectiveness not established); Geri: ↑ risk of blood dyscrasias (agranulocytosis, neutropenia, pancytopenia) in older adults. Consider ↓ hepatic/renal/cardiac function, concomitant illnesses, and drug therapies.

Adverse Reactions/Side Effects

Derm: ACUTE GENERALIZED EXANTHEMATOUS PUSTULOSIS (AGEP), DRUG REACTION WITH EOSINOPHILIA AND SYSTEMIC SYMPTOMS (DRESS), itching, photosensitivity, rash, STEVENS-JOHNSON SYNDROME (SJS), TOXIC EPIDERMAL NECROLYSIS (TEN). **GI:** diarrhea, abdominal pain, anorexia, exacerbation of colitis, HEPATOTOXICITY, nausea, vomiting. **GU:** interstitial nephritis, nephrolithiasis, renal impairment. **Hemat:** blood dyscrasias. **Neuro:** ataxia, confusion, depression, dizziness, drowsiness, headache, psychosis, restlessness. **Misc:** acute intolerance syndrome, hypersensitivity reactions.

Interactions

Drug-Drug: ↑ risk of bleeding after neuraxial anesthesia with **low molecular weight heparins** and **heparin**; discontinue olsalazine before initiation of therapy or monitor closely if discontinuation not possible. May ↑ levels of and risk of bleeding from **warfarin**; closely monitor INR. May ↑ myelosuppressive effects of **mercaptopurine** or **azathioprine**; avoid concurrent use, if possible. Concurrent use with **NSAIDs** may ↑ risk of nephrotoxicity. ↑ risk of developing Reye syndrome; avoid olsalazine during 6 wk after **varicella vaccine**.

Route/Dosage

PO (Adults): 500 mg twice daily.

Availability

Capsules: 250 mg.

NURSING IMPLICATIONS

Assessment

- Assess abdominal pain and frequency, quantity, and consistency of stools at the beginning of and during therapy.
- Monitor for hypersensitivity reactions; may present as internal organ involvement (myocarditis, pericarditis, nephritis, hepatitis, pneumonitis, hematologic abnormalities). Discontinue olsalazine if hypersensitivity reactions occur.
- Assess patient for allergy to sulfonamides and salicylates. Patients allergic to sulfasalazine may take mesalamine or olsalazine without difficulty, but therapy should be discontinued if rash or fever occur.
- Monitor intake and output ratios. Fluid intake should be sufficient to maintain a urine output of ≥1200–1500 mL daily to prevent crystalluria and stone formation.
- Assess for severe cutaneous adverse reactions (SJS, TEN, DRESS, and AGEP). Discontinue olsalazine at first sign of severe cutaneous reactions.

Lab Test Considerations

- Monitor urinalysis, BUN, and serum creatinine prior to and periodically during therapy. If renal function declines during therapy, discontinue olsalazine.
- May cause ↑ AST and ALT levels.
- Monitor CBC prior to and every 3–6 mo during prolonged therapy. Discontinue olsalazine if blood dyscrasias occur.

Implementation

- Maintain adequate hydration during therapy.
- **PO:** Administer with food in evenly divided doses every 12 hr.

Patient/Family Teaching

- Instruct patient to take medication as directed, even if feeling better. Take missed doses as soon as remembered unless almost time for next dose.
- Inform patient of possible reddish-brown urine discoloration when in contact with surfaces or water treated with hypochlorite-containing bleach.
- May cause dizziness. Caution patient to avoid driving or other activities that require alertness until response to medication is known.
- Advise patient to notify health care professional if skin rash, sore throat, fever, mouth sores, unusual bleeding or bruising, wheezing, fever, or hives occurs.
- Advise patient to avoid sun exposure and to wear sunscreen and protective clothing when outdoors due to ↑risk of photosensitivity reactions.
- Instruct patient to notify health care professional if symptoms do not improve after 1–2 mo of therapy.
- Instruct patient to notify health care professional if symptoms worsen or do not improve. If symptoms of acute intolerance (cramping, acute abdominal pain, bloody diarrhea, fever, headache, rash) occur, discontinue therapy and notify health care professional immediately.
- Rep: Advise females of reproductive potential to use effective contraception and to notify health care professional if pregnancy is planned or suspected and to

avoid breastfeeding during therapy. Monitor breastfed infants for diarrhea.

- Inform patient that proctoscopy and sigmoidoscopy may be required periodically during treatment to determine response.

Evaluation/Desired Outcomes

- Decrease in diarrhea and abdominal pain.
- Return to normal bowel pattern in patients with inflammatory bowel disease. Effects may be seen within 3–21 days. The usual course of therapy is 3–6 wk.
- Maintenance of remission in patients with inflammatory bowel disease.

omalizumab (o-ma-liz-ue-mab)

Omlyclo, Xolair

Classification

Therapeutic: antiasthmatics

Pharmacologic: monoclonal antibodies

Indications

Moderate to severe persistent asthma in patients who have a positive skin test or in vitro reactivity to a perennial aeroallergen and whose symptoms are not controlled by inhaled corticosteroids. Chronic spontaneous urticaria in patients who remain symptomatic despite antihistamine treatment. IgE-mediated food allergy. Add-on maintenance treatment of chronic rhinosinusitis with nasal polyps in patients who have had an inadequate response to nasal corticosteroids.

Action

Inhibits binding of IgE to receptors on mast cells and eosinophils, preventing the release of mediators of the allergic response. Also lowers amount of IgE and decreases amount of IgE receptors on basophils. **Therapeutic Effects:** Decreased incidence of exacerbations of asthma. Decreased severity of itching and quantity of hives. Reduction of type I allergic reactions, including anaphylaxis. Decreased size of nasal polyps and decreased severity of nasal congestion.

Pharmacokinetics

Absorption: 62% absorbed slowly from SUBQ sites.
Distribution: Unknown.
Metabolism and Excretion: Degraded similarly to IgG via binding degradation, reticuloendothelial system and the liver.
Half-life: 26 days.

TIME/ACTION PROFILE (effects on IgE levels)

ROUTE	ONSET	PEAK	DURATION
SUBQ	within 1 hr	unknown	up to 1 yr

Contraindications/Precautions

Contraindicated in: Hypersensitivity; Acute bronchospasm or status asthmaticus.
Use Cautiously in: History of anaphylaxis to foods, medications, or other causes (↑ risk of anaphylaxis); Pedi: Children <6 yr (safety and effectiveness not established).

Adverse Reactions/Side Effects

CV: DEEP VENOUS THROMBOSIS, MI, transient ischemic attack. **Local:** injection site reactions. **Resp:** PULMONARY EMBOLISM. **Misc:** HYPERSENSITIVITY REACTIONS (INCLUDING ANAPHYLAXIS), MALIGNANCY.

Interactions

Drug-Drug: None reported.

Route/Dosage

Asthma

SUBQ (Adults and Children ≥12 yr, Pretreatment serum IgE ≥30–100 units/mL and >90–150 kg): 300 mg every 4 wk.
SUBQ (Adults and Children ≥12 yr, Pretreatment serum IgE ≥30–100 units/mL and 30–90 kg): 150 mg every 4 wk.
SUBQ (Adults and Children ≥12 yr, Pretreatment serum IgE >100–200 units/mL and >90–150 kg): 225 mg every 2 wk.
SUBQ (Adults and Children ≥12 yr, Pretreatment serum IgE >100–200 units/mL and 30–90 kg): 300 mg every 4 wk.
SUBQ (Adults and Children ≥12 yr, Pretreatment serum IgE >200–300 units/mL and >90–150 kg): 300 mg every 2 wk.
SUBQ (Adults and Children ≥12 yr, Pretreatment serum IgE >200–300 units/mL and >60–90 kg): 225 mg every 4 wk.
SUBQ (Adults and Children ≥12 yr, Pretreatment serum IgE >200–300 units/mL and 30–60 kg): 300 mg every 4 wk.
SUBQ (Adults and Children ≥12 yr, Pretreatment serum IgE >300–400 units/mL and >70–90 kg): 300 mg every 2 wk.
SUBQ (Adults and Children ≥12 yr, Pretreatment serum IgE >300–400 units/mL and 30–70 kg): 225 mg every 2 wk.
SUBQ (Adults and Children ≥12 yr, Pretreatment serum IgE >400–500 units/mL and >70–90 kg): 375 mg every 2 wk.
SUBQ (Adults and Children ≥12 yr, Pretreatment serum IgE >400–500 units/mL and 30–70 kg): 300 mg every 2 wk.
SUBQ (Adults and Children ≥12 yr, Pretreatment serum IgE >500–600 units/mL and >60–70 kg): 375 mg every 2 wk.

O

SUBQ (Adults and Children ≥12 yr, Pretreatment serum IgE >500–600 units/mL and 30–60 kg): 300 mg every 2 wk.

SUBQ (Adults and Children ≥12 yr, Pretreatment serum IgE >600–700 units/mL and 30–60 kg): 375 mg every 2 wk.

SUBQ (Children 6–11 yr, Pretreatment serum IgE ≥30–100 units/mL and >90–150 kg): 300 mg every 4 wk.

SUBQ (Children 6–11 yr, Pretreatment serum IgE ≥30–100 units/mL and >40–90 kg): 150 mg every 4 wk.

SUBQ (Children 6–11 yr, Pretreatment serum IgE ≥30–100 units/mL and 20–40 kg): 75 mg every 4 wk.

SUBQ (Children 6–11 yr, Pretreatment serum IgE >100–200 units/mL and >125–150 kg): 300 mg every 2 wk.

SUBQ (Children 6–11 yr, Pretreatment serum IgE >100–200 units/mL and >90–125 kg): 225 mg every 2 wk.

SUBQ (Children 6–11 yr, Pretreatment serum IgE >100–200 units/mL and >40–90 kg): 300 mg every 4 wk.

SUBQ (Children 6–11 yr, Pretreatment serum IgE >100–200 units/mL and 20–40 kg): 150 mg every 4 wk.

SUBQ (Children 6–11 yr, Pretreatment serum IgE >200–300 units/mL and >125–150 kg): 375 mg every 2 wk.

SUBQ (Children 6–11 yr, Pretreatment serum IgE >200–300 units/mL and >90–125 kg): 300 mg every 2 wk.

SUBQ (Children 6–11 yr, Pretreatment serum IgE >200–300 units/mL and >60–90 kg): 225 mg every 2 wk.

SUBQ (Children 6–11 yr, Pretreatment serum IgE >200–300 units/mL and >40–60 kg): 300 mg every 4 wk.

SUBQ (Children 6–11 yr, Pretreatment serum IgE >200–300 units/mL and >30–40 kg): 225 mg every 4 wk.

SUBQ (Children 6–11 yr, Pretreatment serum IgE >200–300 units/mL and 20–30 kg): 150 mg every 4 wk.

SUBQ (Children 6–11 yr, Pretreatment serum IgE >300–400 units/mL and >70–90 kg): 300 mg every 2 wk.

SUBQ (Children 6–11 yr, Pretreatment serum IgE >300–400 units/mL and >40–70 kg): 225 mg every 2 wk.

SUBQ (Children 6–11 yr, Pretreatment serum IgE >300–400 units/mL and >30–40 kg): 300 mg every 4 wk.

SUBQ (Children 6–11 yr, Pretreatment serum IgE >300–400 units/mL and 20–30 kg): 225 mg every 4 wk.

SUBQ (Children 6–11 yr, Pretreatment serum IgE >400–500 units/mL and >70–90 kg): 375 mg every 2 wk.

SUBQ (Children 6–11 yr, Pretreatment serum IgE >400–500 units/mL and >50–70 kg): 300 mg every 2 wk.

SUBQ (Children 6–11 yr, Pretreatment serum IgE >400–500 units/mL and >30–50 kg): 225 mg every 2 wk.

SUBQ (Children 6–11 yr, Pretreatment serum IgE >400–500 units/mL and >25–30 kg): 300 mg every 4 wk.

SUBQ (Children 6–11 yr, Pretreatment serum IgE >400–500 units/mL and 20–25 kg): 225 mg every 4 wk.

SUBQ (Children 6–11 yr, Pretreatment serum IgE >500–600 units/mL and >60–70 kg): 375 mg every 2 wk.

SUBQ (Children 6–11 yr, Pretreatment serum IgE >500–600 units/mL and >40–60 kg): 300 mg every 2 wk.

SUBQ (Children 6–11 yr, Pretreatment serum IgE >500–600 units/mL and >30–40 kg): 225 mg every 2 wk.

SUBQ (Children 6–11 yr, Pretreatment serum IgE >500–600 units/mL and 20–30 kg): 300 mg every 4 wk.

SUBQ (Children 6–11 yr, Pretreatment serum IgE >600–700 units/mL and >50–60 kg): 375 mg every 2 wk.

SUBQ (Children 6–11 yr, Pretreatment serum IgE >600–700 units/mL and >40–50 kg): 300 mg every 2 wk.

SUBQ (Children 6–11 yr, Pretreatment serum IgE >600–700 units/mL and >25–40 kg): 225 mg every 2 wk.

SUBQ (Children 6–11 yr, Pretreatment serum IgE >600–700 units/mL and 20–25 kg): 300 mg every 4 wk.

SUBQ (Children 6–11 yr, Pretreatment serum IgE >700–900 units/mL and >40–50 kg): 375 mg every 2 wk.

SUBQ (Children 6–11 yr, Pretreatment serum IgE >700–900 units/mL and >30–40 kg): 300 mg every 2 wk.

SUBQ (Children 6–11 yr, Pretreatment serum IgE >700–900 units/mL and 20–30 kg): 225 mg every 2 wk.

SUBQ (Children 6–11 yr, Pretreatment serum IgE >900–1100 units/mL and >30–40 kg): 375 mg every 2 wk.

SUBQ (Children 6–11 yr, Pretreatment serum IgE >900–1100 units/mL and >25–30 kg): 300 mg every 2 wk.

SUBQ (Children 6–11 yr, Pretreatment serum IgE >900–1100 units/mL and 20–25 kg): 225 mg every 2 wk.

SUBQ (Children 6–11 yr, Pretreatment serum IgE >1100–1200 units/mL and 20–30 kg): 300 mg every 2 wk.
SUBQ (Children 6–11 yr, Pretreatment serum IgE >1200–1300 units/mL and >25–30 kg): 375 mg every 2 wk.
SUBQ (Children 6–11 yr, Pretreatment serum IgE >1200–1300 units/mL and 20–25 kg): 300 mg every 2 wk.

Chronic Idiopathic Urticaria

SUBQ (Adults and Children ≥12 yr): 150 or 300 mg every 4 wk.

IgE-Mediated Food Allergy

SUBQ (Adults and Children ≥1 yr, Pretreatment serum IgE ≥30–100 units/mL and >90–150 kg): 300 every 4 wk.
SUBQ (Adults and Children ≥1 yr, Pretreatment serum IgE ≥30–100 units/mL and >40–90 kg): 150 mg every 4 wk.
SUBQ (Adults and Children ≥1 yr, Pretreatment serum IgE ≥30–100 units/mL and ≥10–40 kg): 75 mg every 4 wk.
SUBQ (Adults and Children ≥1 yr, Pretreatment serum IgE >100–200 units/mL and >125–150 kg): 600 mg every 4 wk.
SUBQ (Adults and Children ≥1 yr, Pretreatment serum IgE >100–200 units/mL and >90–125 kg): 450 mg every 4 wk.
SUBQ (Adults and Children ≥1 yr, Pretreatment serum IgE >100–200 units/mL and >40–90 kg): 300 mg every 4 wk.
SUBQ (Adults and Children ≥1 yr, Pretreatment serum IgE >100–200 units/mL and >20–40 kg): 150 mg every 4 wk.
SUBQ (Adults and Children ≥1 yr, Pretreatment serum IgE >100–200 units/mL and ≥10–20 kg): 75 mg every 4 wk.
SUBQ (Adults and Children ≥1 yr, Pretreatment serum IgE >200–300 units/mL and >125–150 kg): 375 mg every 2 wk.
SUBQ (Adults and Children ≥1 yr, Pretreatment serum IgE >200–300 units/mL and >90–125 kg): 600 mg every 4 wk.
SUBQ (Adults and Children ≥1 yr, Pretreatment serum IgE >200–300 units/mL and >60–90 kg): 450 mg every 4 wk.
SUBQ (Adults and Children ≥1 yr, Pretreatment serum IgE >200–300 units/mL and >40–60 kg): 300 mg every 4 wk.
SUBQ (Adults and Children ≥1 yr, Pretreatment serum IgE >200–300 units/mL and >30–40 kg): 225 mg every 4 wk.
SUBQ (Adults and Children ≥1 yr, Pretreatment serum IgE >200–300 units/mL and >15–30 kg): 150 mg every 4 wk.
SUBQ (Adults and Children ≥1 yr, Pretreatment serum IgE >200–300 units/mL and ≥10–15 kg): 75 mg every 4 wk.
SUBQ (Adults and Children ≥1 yr, Pretreatment serum IgE >300–400 units/mL and >125–150 kg): 525 mg every 2 wk.
SUBQ (Adults and Children ≥1 yr, Pretreatment serum IgE >300–400 units/mL and >90–125 kg): 450 mg every 2 wk.
SUBQ (Adults and Children ≥1 yr, Pretreatment serum IgE >300–400 units/mL and >70–90 kg): 600 mg every 4 wk.
SUBQ (Adults and Children ≥1 yr, Pretreatment serum IgE >300–400 units/mL and >40–70 kg): 450 mg every 4 wk.
SUBQ (Adults and Children ≥1 yr, Pretreatment serum IgE >300–400 units/mL and >30–40 kg): 300 mg every 4 wk.
SUBQ (Adults and Children ≥1 yr, Pretreatment serum IgE >300–400 units/mL and >20–30 kg): 225 mg every 4 wk.
SUBQ (Adults and Children ≥1 yr, Pretreatment serum IgE >300–400 units/mL and ≥10–20 kg): 150 mg every 4 wk.
SUBQ (Adults and Children ≥1 yr, Pretreatment serum IgE >400–500 units/mL and >125–150 kg): 600 mg every 2 wk.
SUBQ (Adults and Children ≥1 yr, Pretreatment serum IgE >400–500 units/mL and >90–125 kg): 525 mg every 2 wk.
SUBQ (Adults and Children ≥1 yr, Pretreatment serum IgE >400–500 units/mL and >70–90 kg): 375 mg every 2 wk.
SUBQ (Adults and Children ≥1 yr, Pretreatment serum IgE >400–500 units/mL and >50–70 kg): 600 mg every 4 wk.
SUBQ (Adults and Children ≥1 yr, Pretreatment serum IgE >400–500 units/mL and >30–50 kg): 450 mg every 4 wk.
SUBQ (Adults and Children ≥1 yr, Pretreatment serum IgE >400–500 units/mL and >25–30 kg): 300 mg every 4 wk.
SUBQ (Adults and Children ≥1 yr, Pretreatment serum IgE >400–500 units/mL and >15–25 kg): 225 mg every 4 wk.
SUBQ (Adults and Children ≥1 yr, Pretreatment serum IgE >400–500 units/mL and ≥10–15 kg): 150 mg every 4 wk.
SUBQ (Adults and Children ≥1 yr, Pretreatment serum IgE >500–600 units/mL and >90–125 kg): 600 mg every 2 wk.

O

SUBQ (Adults and Children ≥1 yr, Pretreatment serum IgE >500–600 units/mL and >70–90 kg): 450 mg every 2 wk.
SUBQ (Adults and Children ≥1 yr, Pretreatment serum IgE >500–600 units/mL and >60–70 kg): 375 mg every 2 wk.
SUBQ (Adults and Children ≥1 yr, Pretreatment serum IgE >500–600 units/mL and >40–60 kg): 600 mg every 4 wk.
SUBQ (Adults and Children ≥1 yr, Pretreatment serum IgE >500–600 units/mL and >30–40 kg): 450 mg every 4 wk.
SUBQ (Adults and Children ≥1 yr, Pretreatment serum IgE >500–600 units/mL and >20–30 kg): 300 mg every 4 wk.
SUBQ (Adults and Children ≥1 yr, Pretreatment serum IgE >500–600 units/mL and >15–20 kg): 225 mg every 4 wk.
SUBQ (Adults and Children ≥1 yr, Pretreatment serum IgE >500–600 units/mL and ≥10–15 kg): 150 mg every 4 wk.
SUBQ (Adults and Children ≥1 yr, Pretreatment serum IgE >600–700 units/mL and >80–90 kg): 525 mg every 2 wk.
SUBQ (Adults and Children ≥1 yr, Pretreatment serum IgE >600–700 units/mL and >60–80 kg): 450 mg every 2 wk.
SUBQ (Adults and Children ≥1 yr, Pretreatment serum IgE >600–700 units/mL and >50–60 kg): 375 mg every 2 wk.
SUBQ (Adults and Children ≥1 yr, Pretreatment serum IgE >600–700 units/mL and >40–50 kg): 600 mg every 4 wk.
SUBQ (Adults and Children ≥1 yr, Pretreatment serum IgE >600–700 units/mL and >30–40 kg): 450 mg every 4 wk.
SUBQ (Adults and Children ≥1 yr, Pretreatment serum IgE >600–700 units/mL and >25–30 kg): 225 mg every 2 wk.
SUBQ (Adults and Children ≥1 yr, Pretreatment serum IgE >600–700 units/mL and >20–25 kg): 300 mg every 4 wk.
SUBQ (Adults and Children ≥1 yr, Pretreatment serum IgE >600–700 units/mL and >15–20 kg): 225 mg every 4 wk.
SUBQ (Adults and Children ≥1 yr, Pretreatment serum IgE >600–700 units/mL and ≥10–15 kg): 150 mg every 2 wk.
SUBQ (Adults and Children ≥1 yr, Pretreatment serum IgE >700–800 units/mL and >80–90 kg): 600 mg every 2 wk.
SUBQ (Adults and Children ≥1 yr, Pretreatment serum IgE >700–800 units/mL and >70–80 kg): 525 mg every 2 wk.
SUBQ (Adults and Children ≥1 yr, Pretreatment serum IgE >700–800 units/mL and >50–70 kg): 450 mg every 2 wk.
SUBQ (Adults and Children ≥1 yr, Pretreatment serum IgE >700–800 units/mL and >40–50 kg): 375 mg every 2 wk.
SUBQ (Adults and Children ≥1 yr, Pretreatment serum IgE >700–800 units/mL and >30–40 kg): 300 mg every 2 wk.
SUBQ (Adults and Children ≥1 yr, Pretreatment serum IgE >700–800 units/mL and >20–30 kg): 225 mg every 2 wk.
SUBQ (Adults and Children ≥1 yr, Pretreatment serum IgE >700–800 units/mL and ≥10–20 kg): 150 mg every 2 wk.
SUBQ (Adults and Children ≥1 yr, Pretreatment serum IgE >700–800 units/mL and ≥10–20 kg): 150 mg every 2 wk.
SUBQ (Adults and Children ≥1 yr, Pretreatment serum IgE >800–900 units/mL and >70–80 kg): 600 mg every 2 wk.
SUBQ (Adults and Children ≥1 yr, Pretreatment serum IgE >800–900 units/mL and >60–70 kg): 525 mg every 2 wk.
SUBQ (Adults and Children ≥1 yr, Pretreatment serum IgE >800–900 units/mL and >50–60 kg): 450 mg every 2 wk.
SUBQ (Adults and Children ≥1 yr, Pretreatment serum IgE >800–900 units/mL and >40–50 kg): 375 mg every 2 wk.
SUBQ (Adults and Children ≥1 yr, Pretreatment serum IgE >800–900 units/mL and >30–40 kg): 300 mg every 2 wk.
SUBQ (Adults and Children ≥1 yr, Pretreatment serum IgE >800–900 units/mL and >20–30 kg): 225 mg every 2 wk.
SUBQ (Adults and Children ≥1 yr, Pretreatment serum IgE >800–900 units/mL and ≥10–20 kg): 150 mg every 2 wk.
SUBQ (Adults and Children ≥1 yr, Pretreatment serum IgE >900–1000 units/mL and >60–70 kg): 600 mg every 2 wk.
SUBQ (Adults and Children ≥1 yr, Pretreatment serum IgE >900–1000 units/mL and >50–60 kg): 525 mg every 2 wk.
SUBQ (Adults and Children ≥1 yr, Pretreatment serum IgE >900–1000 units/mL and >40–50 kg): 450 mg every 2 wk.
SUBQ (Adults and Children ≥1 yr, Pretreatment serum IgE >900–1000 units/mL and >30–40 kg): 375 mg every 2 wk.
SUBQ (Adults and Children ≥1 yr, Pretreatment serum IgE >900–1000 units/mL and >25–30 kg): 300 mg every 2 wk.
SUBQ (Adults and Children ≥1 yr, Pretreatment serum IgE >900–1000 units/mL and >15–25 kg): 225 mg every 2 wk.
SUBQ (Adults and Children ≥1 yr, Pretreatment serum IgE >900–1000 units/mL and ≥10–15 kg): 150 mg every 2 wk.

SUBQ (Adults and Children ≥1 yr, Pretreatment serum IgE >1000–1100 units/mL and >50–60 kg): 600 mg every 2 wk.
SUBQ (Adults and Children ≥1 yr, Pretreatment serum IgE >1000–1100 units/mL and >40–50 kg): 450 mg every 2 wk.
SUBQ (Adults and Children ≥1 yr, Pretreatment serum IgE >1000–1100 units/mL and >30–40 kg): 375 mg every 2 wk.
SUBQ (Adults and Children ≥1 yr, Pretreatment serum IgE >1000–1100 units/mL and >25–30 kg): 300 mg every 2 wk.
SUBQ (Adults and Children ≥1 yr, Pretreatment serum IgE >1000–1100 units/mL and >15–25 kg): 225 mg every 2 wk.
SUBQ (Adults and Children ≥1 yr, Pretreatment serum IgE >1000–1100 units/mL and ≥10–15 kg): 150 mg every 2 wk.
SUBQ (Adults and Children ≥1 yr, Pretreatment serum IgE >1100–1200 units/mL and >50–60 kg): 600 mg every 2 wk.
SUBQ (Adults and Children ≥1 yr, Pretreatment serum IgE >1100–1200 units/mL and >40–50 kg): 525 mg every 2 wk.
SUBQ (Adults and Children ≥1 yr, Pretreatment serum IgE >1100–1200 units/mL and >30–40 kg): 450 mg every 2 wk.
SUBQ (Adults and Children ≥1 yr, Pretreatment serum IgE >1100–1200 units/mL and >20–30 kg): 300 mg every 2 wk.
SUBQ (Adults and Children ≥1 yr, Pretreatment serum IgE >1100–1200 units/mL and >15–20 kg): 225 mg every 2 wk.
SUBQ (Adults and Children ≥1 yr, Pretreatment serum IgE >1100–1200 units/mL and ≥10–15 kg): 150 mg every 2 wk.
SUBQ (Adults and Children ≥1 yr, Pretreatment serum IgE >1200–1300 units/mL and >40–50 kg): 525 mg every 2 wk.
SUBQ (Adults and Children ≥1 yr, Pretreatment serum IgE >1200–1300 units/mL and >30–40 kg): 450 mg every 2 wk.
SUBQ (Adults and Children ≥1 yr, Pretreatment serum IgE >1200–1300 units/mL and >25–30 kg): 375 mg every 2 wk.
SUBQ (Adults and Children ≥1 yr, Pretreatment serum IgE >1200–1300 units/mL and >20–25 kg): 300 mg every 2 wk.
SUBQ (Adults and Children ≥1 yr, Pretreatment serum IgE >1200–1300 units/mL and >12–20 kg): 225 mg every 2 wk.
SUBQ (Adults and Children ≥1 yr, Pretreatment serum IgE >1200–1300 units/mL and ≥10–12 kg): 150 mg every 2 wk.
SUBQ (Adults and Children ≥1 yr, Pretreatment serum IgE >1300–1500 units/mL and >40–50 kg): 600 mg every 2 wk.
SUBQ (Adults and Children ≥1 yr, Pretreatment serum IgE >1300–1500 units/mL and >30–40 kg): 525 mg every 2 wk.
SUBQ (Adults and Children ≥1 yr, Pretreatment serum IgE >1300–1500 units/mL and >25–30 kg): 375 mg every 2 wk.
SUBQ (Adults and Children ≥1 yr, Pretreatment serum IgE >1300–1500 units/mL and >15–25 kg): 300 mg every 2 wk.
SUBQ (Adults and Children ≥1 yr, Pretreatment serum IgE >1300–1500 units/mL and >12–15 kg): 225 mg every 2 wk.
SUBQ (Adults and Children ≥1 yr, Pretreatment serum IgE >1300–1500 units/mL and ≥10–12 kg): 150 mg every 2 wk.
SUBQ (Adults and Children ≥1 yr, Pretreatment serum IgE >1500–1850 units/mL and >30–40 kg): 600 mg every 2 wk.
SUBQ (Adults and Children ≥1 yr, Pretreatment serum IgE >1500–1850 units/mL and >25–30 kg): 450 mg every 2 wk.
SUBQ (Adults and Children ≥1 yr, Pretreatment serum IgE >1500–1850 units/mL and >20–25 kg): 375 mg every 2 wk.
SUBQ (Adults and Children ≥1 yr, Pretreatment serum IgE >1500–1850 units/mL and >15–20 kg): 300 mg every 2 wk.
SUBQ (Adults and Children ≥1 yr, Pretreatment serum IgE >1500–1850 units/mL and >12–15 kg): 225 mg every 2 wk.

Chronic Rhinosinusitis with Nasal Polyps

SUBQ (Adults Pretreatment serum IgE ≥30–100 units/mL and >90–150 kg): 300 mg every 4 wk.
SUBQ (Adults Pretreatment serum IgE ≥30–100 units/mL and >40–90 kg): 150 mg every 4 wk.
SUBQ (Adults Pretreatment serum IgE ≥30–100 units/mL and 30–40 kg): 75 mg every 4 wk.
SUBQ (Adults Pretreatment serum IgE >100–200 units/mL and >125–150 kg): 600 mg every 4 wk.
SUBQ (Adults Pretreatment serum IgE >100–200 units/mL and >90–125 kg): 450 mg every 4 wk.
SUBQ (Adults Pretreatment serum IgE >100–200 units/mL and >40–90 kg): 300 mg every 4 wk.
SUBQ (Adults Pretreatment serum IgE >100–200 units/mL and 30–40 kg): 150 mg every 4 wk.
SUBQ (Adults Pretreatment serum IgE >200–300 units/mL and >125–150 kg): 375 mg every 2 wk.
SUBQ (Adults Pretreatment serum IgE >200–300 units/mL and >90–125 kg): 600 mg every 4 wk.
SUBQ (Adults Pretreatment serum IgE >200–300 units/mL and >60–90 kg): 450 mg every 4 wk.

O

SUBQ (Adults Pretreatment serum IgE >200–300 units/mL and >40–60 kg): 300 mg every 4 wk.
SUBQ (Adults Pretreatment serum IgE >200–300 units/mL and 30–40 kg): 225 mg every 4 wk.
SUBQ (Adults Pretreatment serum IgE >300–400 units/mL and >125–150 kg): 525 mg every 2 wk.
SUBQ (Adults Pretreatment serum IgE >300–400 units/mL and >90–125 kg): 450 mg every 2 wk.
SUBQ (Adults Pretreatment serum IgE >300–400 units/mL and >70–90 kg): 600 mg every 4 wk.
SUBQ (Adults Pretreatment serum IgE >300–400 units/mL and >40–70 kg): 450 mg every 4 wk.
SUBQ (Adults Pretreatment serum IgE >300–400 units/mL and 30–40 kg): 300 mg every 4 wk.
SUBQ (Adults Pretreatment serum IgE >400–500 units/mL and >125–150 kg): 600 mg every 2 wk.
SUBQ (Adults Pretreatment serum IgE >400–500 units/mL and >90–125 kg): 525 mg every 2 wk.
SUBQ (Adults Pretreatment serum IgE >400–500 units/mL and >70–90 kg): 375 mg every 2 wk.
SUBQ (Adults Pretreatment serum IgE >400–500 units/mL and >50–70 kg): 600 mg every 4 wk.
SUBQ (Adults Pretreatment serum IgE >400–500 units/mL and 30–50 kg): 450 mg every 4 wk.
SUBQ (Adults Pretreatment serum IgE >500–600 units/mL and >90–125 kg): 600 mg every 2 wk.
SUBQ (Adults Pretreatment serum IgE >500–600 units/mL and >70–90 kg): 450 mg every 2 wk.
SUBQ (Adults Pretreatment serum IgE >500–600 units/mL and >60–70 kg): 375 mg every 2 wk.
SUBQ (Adults Pretreatment serum IgE >500–600 units/mL and >40–60 kg): 600 mg every 4 wk.
SUBQ (Adults Pretreatment serum IgE >500–600 units/mL and 30–40 kg): 450 mg every 4 wk.
SUBQ (Adults Pretreatment serum IgE >600–700 units/mL and >80–90 kg): 525 mg every 2 wk.
SUBQ (Adults Pretreatment serum IgE >600–700 units/mL and >60–80 kg): 450 mg every 2 wk.
SUBQ (Adults Pretreatment serum IgE >600–700 units/mL and >50–60 kg): 375 mg every 2 wk.
SUBQ (Adults Pretreatment serum IgE >600–700 units/mL and >40–50 kg): 600 mg every 4 wk.
SUBQ (Adults Pretreatment serum IgE >600–700 units/mL and 30–40 kg): 450 mg every 4 wk.
SUBQ (Adults Pretreatment serum IgE >700–800 units/mL and >80–90 kg): 600 mg every 2 wk.
SUBQ (Adults Pretreatment serum IgE >700–800 units/mL and >70–80 kg): 525 mg every 2 wk.
SUBQ (Adults Pretreatment serum IgE >700–800 units/mL and >50–70 kg): 450 mg every 2 wk.
SUBQ (Adults Pretreatment serum IgE >700–800 units/mL and >40–50 kg): 375 mg every 2 wk.
SUBQ (Adults Pretreatment serum IgE >700–800 units/mL and 30–40 kg): 300 mg every 2 wk.
SUBQ (Adults Pretreatment serum IgE >800–900 units/mL and >70–80 kg): 600 mg every 2 wk.
SUBQ (Adults Pretreatment serum IgE >800–900 units/mL and >60–70 kg): 525 mg every 2 wk.
SUBQ (Adults Pretreatment serum IgE >800–900 units/mL and >50–60 kg): 450 mg every 2 wk.
SUBQ (Adults Pretreatment serum IgE >800–900 units/mL and >40–50 kg): 375 mg every 2 wk.
SUBQ (Adults Pretreatment serum IgE >800–900 units/mL and 30–40 kg): 300 mg every 2 wk.
SUBQ (Adults Pretreatment serum IgE >900–1000 units/mL and >60–70 kg): 600 mg every 2 wk.
SUBQ (Adults Pretreatment serum IgE >900–1000 units/mL and >50–60 kg): 525 mg every 2 wk.
SUBQ (Adults Pretreatment serum IgE >900–1000 units/mL and >40–50 kg): 450 mg every 2 wk.
SUBQ (Adults Pretreatment serum IgE >900–1000 units/mL and 30–40 kg): 375 mg every 2 wk.
SUBQ (Adults Pretreatment serum IgE >1000–1100 units/mL and >50–60 kg): 600 mg every 2 wk.
SUBQ (Adults Pretreatment serum IgE >1000–1100 units/mL and >40–50 kg): 450 mg every 2 wk.
SUBQ (Adults Pretreatment serum IgE >1000–1100 units/mL and 30–40 kg): 375 mg every 2 wk.
SUBQ (Adults Pretreatment serum IgE >1100–1200 units/mL and >50–60 kg): 600 mg every 2 wk.
SUBQ (Adults Pretreatment serum IgE >1100–1200 units/mL and >40–50 kg): 525 mg every 2 wk.
SUBQ (Adults Pretreatment serum IgE >1100–1200 units/mL and 30–40 kg): 450 mg every 2 wk.
SUBQ (Adults Pretreatment serum IgE >1200–1300 units/mL and >40–50 kg): 525 mg every 2 wk.
SUBQ (Adults Pretreatment serum IgE >1200–1300 units/mL and 30–40 kg): 450 mg every 2 wk.
SUBQ (Adults Pretreatment serum IgE >1300–1500 units/mL and >40–50 kg): 600 mg every 2 wk.
SUBQ (Adults Pretreatment serum IgE >1300–1500 units/mL and 30–40 kg): 525 mg every 2 wk.

Availability

Lyophilized powder for injection: 150 mg/vial. **Solution for injection (prefilled syringes and autoinjectors):** 75 mg/0.5 mL, 150 mg/1 mL, 300 mg/2 mL.

NURSING IMPLICATIONS

Assessment

- Assess lung sounds and respiratory function before starting and periodically during therapy.
- Assess allergy symptoms (rhinitis, conjunctivitis, hives) before starting and periodically throughout therapy.
- Assess for allergic reactions (wheezing, shortness of breath, cough, chest tightness, trouble breathing, low BP, dizziness, fainting, rapid or weak heartbeat, anxiety, feeling of impending doom, flushing, itching, hives, feeling warm, swelling of the throat or tongue, throat tightness, hoarse voice, trouble swallowing) within 2 hr of injections; may occur beyond a year

after first dose. Observe patient for 2 hr after 1st 3 injections and then 30 min after subsequent injections. Epinephrine, diphenhydramine, and corticosteroids should be available in case of anaphylaxis.

- Monitor for injection site reactions (bruising, redness, warmth, burning, stinging, itching, hives, pain, induration, mass, inflammation). Usually occur within 1 hr of injection, last <8 days, and ↓ in frequency with subsequent dosing.

Lab Test Considerations

- **For Asthma and Nasal Polyps:** Measure serum IgE and body weight before starting therapy to determine dose. Adjust dose for significant changes in body weight during therapy. Serum IgE levels will ↑ following administration and ↑ may persist for up to 1 yr following discontinuation. Serum total IgE levels obtained <1 yr following discontinuation may not reflect steady state free IgE levels and should not be used to reassess the dosing regimen. If therapy is interrupted for ≥1 yr, retest total serum IgE levels to determine dose. A minimum of 3–6 mo of therapy is suggested to determine efficacy.
- **For Food Allergies:** Measure serum IgE and body weight before starting therapy to determine dose. Adjust dose for significant changes in body weight during therapy. Dosing should not be adjusted based on IgE levels taken during treatment or <1 yr following interruption of therapy. If therapy has been stopped for ≥1 yr, retest IgE levels to determine dose. Periodically reassess the need for continued therapy.

Implementation

- Doses of inhaled corticosteroids may be gradually ↓ with supervision of health care provider; do not discontinue abruptly.
- **SUBQ:** 1st 3 injections should be administered by a health care provider with no hypersensitivity reactions. Once therapy has been established, administration of prefilled syringe or autoinjector outside of a health care setting by a patient or a caregiver may be appropriate for selected patients. **Reconstitution:** To reconstitute, draw 1.4 mL of sterile water for injection into a 3-mL syringe with a 1-inch 18-gauge needle. With vial upright on a flat surface, inject sterile water into vial. Keep vial upright and gently swirl for approximately 1 min to evenly wet powder. Do not shake. Lyophilized omalizumab takes 15–20 min to dissolve. Gently swirl vial for 5–10 sec every 5 min to dissolve any remaining particles. Solution should be clear or slightly opalescent and may have small bubbles or foam around edge of vial. Do not use if particles are visible or if contents do not dissolve completely within 40 min. Invert vial for 15 seconds to allow solution to drain toward stopper. Solution may be somewhat viscous. In order to obtain full 1.2 mL dose, all of solution must be withdrawn from vial using a new 3-mL syringe with an 18-gauge needle before expelling any air or excess solution from syringe. Administer within 8 hr if refrigerated or within 4 hr if stored at room temperature. Discard unused solution.
- **For lyophilized powder in vials: Reconstitution:** To reconstitute, draw 1.4 mL of sterile water for injection into a 3-mL syringe with a 1-inch 18-gauge needle. With vial upright on a flat surface, inject sterile water into vial. Keep vial upright and gently swirl for approximately 1 min to evenly wet powder. Do not shake. Lyophilized omalizumab takes 15–20 min to dissolve. Gently swirl vial for 5–10 sec every 5 min to dissolve any remaining particles. Solution should be clear or slightly opalescent and may have small bubbles or foam around edge of vial. Do not use if particles are visible or if contents do not dissolve completely within 40 min. Invert vial for 15 seconds to allow solution to drain toward stopper. Solution may be somewhat viscous. In order to obtain full 1.2 mL dose, all of solution must be withdrawn from vial using a new 3-mL syringe with an 18-gauge needle before expelling any air or excess solution from syringe. Administer within 8 hr if refrigerated or within 4 hr if stored at room temperature. Discard unused solution.
- Replace 18-gauge needle with a 25-gauge needle for SUBQ injection. Inject into thigh, abdomen (avoiding 2 inches around naval), or upper arm if administered by caregiver or health care provider. Because solution is slightly viscous, injection may take 5–10 sec to administer. Divide doses >150 mg into 2 injection sites and inject at least 1 inch apart. If no hypersensitivity reactions occur, patient or caregiver may be taught injection technique for home use. Patient and caregiver must be able to recognize symptoms of anaphylaxis, treat anaphylaxis appropriately, and administer prefilled syringe using proper technique.

Patient/Family Teaching

- Explain purpose and side effects of medication. Advise patient to read *Patient Information* before starting therapy and with each injection in case of changes.
- Advise patient to notify health care provider of all Rx or OTC medications, vitamins, or herbal products being taken and to consult with health care provider before taking other medications.
- Instruct patients with asthma and nasal polyps not to discontinue or reduce other asthma medications, especially inhaled systematic corticosteroids, without consulting health care provider.

O

- Instruct patient and caregiver in correct preparation, injection technique, disposal of equipment, and monitoring for anaphylaxis.
- Advise patient to notify health care provider immediately if symptoms of an allergic reaction occurs and seek medical attention if needed.
- Rep: Advise women of reproductive potential to notify health care provider if pregnancy is planned or suspected or if breastfeeding.

Evaluation/Desired Outcomes
- Decreased incidence of exacerbations of asthma.
- Decreased severity of itching and quantity of hives.
- Decreased size of nasal polyps and decreased severity of nasal congestion.
- Reduction of type I allergic reactions, including anaphylaxis.

omega-3-acid ethyl esters
(oh-**me**-ga three **as**-id **eth**-il **es**-ters)

Lovaza

Classification

Therapeutic: lipid-lowering agents

Pharmacologic: fatty acids

Indications
Hypertriglyceridemia (triglycerides ≥500 mg/dL).

Action
Inhibits synthesis of triglycerides. **Therapeutic Effects:** Reduction of triglycerides.

Pharmacokinetics
Absorption: Well absorbed.
Distribution: Widely distributed to tissues.
Metabolism and Excretion: Incorporated into phospholipids.
Half-life: Unknown.

TIME/ACTION PROFILE (↓ triglycerides)

ROUTE	ONSET	PEAK	DURATION
PO	unknown	2 mo	unknown

Contraindications/Precautions
Contraindicated in: Hypersensitivity.
Use Cautiously in: Allergy/hypersensitivity to fish; OB: Safety not established in pregnancy; Lactation: Safety not established in breastfeeding; Pedi: Safety and effectiveness not established in children.

Adverse Reactions/Side Effects
Derm: rash. **GI:** ↑ liver enzymes, altered taste, eructation.

Interactions
Drug-Drug: May ↑ risk of bleeding with **aspirin** or **warfarin**.

Route/Dosage
PO (Adults): 4 g once daily *or* 2 g twice daily.

Availability (generic available)
Gelatin capsules (oil-filled): 1 g.

NURSING IMPLICATIONS
Assessment
- Obtain a diet history, especially with regard to fat consumption.

Lab Test Considerations
- Monitor serum triglyceride levels prior to and periodically during therapy.
- Monitor serum ALT periodically during therapy. May ↑ ALT.
- Monitor serum LDL-C levels periodically during therapy. May ↑ LDL-C.

Implementation
- Do not confuse Lovaza with lorazepam.
- An appropriate lipid-lowering diet should be followed before therapy and should continue during therapy.
- **PO:** May be taken as a single 4-g dose or as 2 g twice daily. May be administered with meals. ***DNC:*** Swallow capsules whole; do not break, dissolve, or chew. Do not puncture gelatin capsules.

Patient/Family Teaching
- Explain the purpose and side effects of omega-3-acid ethyl esters. Instruct patient to take medication as directed and not to skip doses or double up on missed doses. Encourage patient to take with meals. Take missed doses as soon as remembered, but if a day is missed, do not double doses the next day. Medication helps control but does not cure elevated serum triglyceride levels. Advise patient to read *Patient Information* before starting and with each Rx refill in case of changes.
- Emphasize the importance of follow-up exams to determine effectiveness.
- Advise patient that this medication should be used in conjunction with diet restrictions (fat, cholesterol, carbohydrates, alcohol), exercise, weight loss in overweight patients, and control of medical problems (such as diabetes mellitus and hypothyroidism) that may contribute to hypertriglyceridemia.
- Advise patient to notify health care provider of all Rx or OTC medications, vitamins, or herbal products being taken and to consult with health care provider before taking other medications.
- Rep: Advise women of reproductive potential to notify health care provider if pregnancy is planned or suspected or if breastfeeding.

Evaluation/Desired Outcomes
- Lowering of serum triglyceride levels. Patients who do not have an adequate response after 2 mo of treatment should be withdrawn from therapy.

BEERS

omeprazole (o-mep-ra-zole)

Losec, PriLOSEC, PriLOSEC OTC

Classification

Therapeutic: antiulcer agents

Pharmacologic: proton pump inhibitors

Indications

Symptomatic GERD. Erosive esophagitis due to acid-mediated GERD. Maintenance of healing of erosive esophagitis due to acid-mediated GERD. Duodenal ulcers (with or without anti-infectives for *Helicobacter pylori*). Short-term treatment of active benign gastric ulcer. Pathologic hypersecretory conditions, including Zollinger-Ellison syndrome. Reduction of risk of GI bleeding in critically ill patients. **OTC:** Heartburn occurring at least twice per week.

Action

Binds to an enzyme on gastric parietal cells in the presence of acidic gastric pH, preventing the final transport of hydrogen ions into the gastric lumen. **Therapeutic Effects:** Diminished accumulation of acid in the gastric lumen with lessened gastroesophageal reflux. Healing of duodenal ulcers.

Pharmacokinetics

Absorption: Rapidly absorbed following oral administration; immediate release formulation contains bicarbonate to prevent acid degradation.

Distribution: Good distribution into gastric parietal cells.

Protein Binding: 95%.

Metabolism and Excretion: Mostly metabolized by the liver via the CYP2C19 isoenzyme and to a lesser extent by the CYP3A4 isoenzyme; the CYP2C19 isoenzyme exhibits genetic polymorphism (15–20% of Asian patients and 3–5% of White and Black patients may be poor metabolizers and may have significantly ↑ omeprazole concentrations and an ↑ risk of adverse effects); inactive metabolites are excreted in urine (77%) and feces.

Half-life: 0.5–1 hr (↑ in hepatic impairment).

TIME/ACTION PROFILE (antisecretory effects)

ROUTE	ONSET	PEAK	DURATION
PO	within 1 hr	within 2 hr	72–96 hr

Contraindications/Precautions

Contraindicated in: Hypersensitivity to omeprazole or related drugs (benzimidazoles); Concurrent use of rilpivirine.

Use Cautiously in: Hepatic impairment (dose ↓ may be necessary); Patients using high doses for >1 yr (↑ risk of hip, wrist, or spine fractures; fundic gland polyps); Patients using therapy for >3 yr (↑ risk of vitamin B_{12} deficiency); Pre-existing risk of hypocalcemia; Lactation: Safety not established in breastfeeding; Pedi: Children <1 mo (safety and effectiveness not established); Geri: Appears on Beers list. ↑ risk of *Clostridioides difficile* infection, pneumonia, GI malignancies, bone loss, and fractures in older adults. Avoid scheduled use for >8 wk in older adults unless for high-risk patients (e.g., oral corticosteroid or chronic NSAID use) or patients with erosive esophagitis, Barrett esophagitis, pathological hypersecretory condition, or demonstrated need for maintenance therapy (e.g., failure of H_2 antagonist).

Adverse Reactions/Side Effects

CV: chest pain. **Derm:** ACUTE GENERALIZED EXANTHEMATOUS PUSTULOSIS, cutaneous lupus erythematosus, DRUG REACTION WITH EOSINOPHILIA AND SYSTEMIC SYMPTOMS (DRESS), itching, rash, STEVENS-JOHNSON SYNDROME, TOXIC EPIDERMAL NECROLYSIS. **F and E:** hypocalcemia (especially if treatment duration ≥3 mo), hypokalemia (especially if treatment duration ≥3 mo), hypomagnesemia (especially if treatment duration ≥3 mo). **GI:** abdominal pain, CLOSTRIDIOIDES DIFFICILE-ASSOCIATED DIARRHEA (CDAD), constipation, diarrhea, flatulence, fundic gland polyps, nausea, vomiting. **GU:** acute tubulointerstitial nephritis. **MS:** bone fracture. **Neuro:** dizziness, drowsiness, fatigue, headache, weakness. **Misc:** HYPERSENSITIVITY REACTIONS (INCLUDING ANAPHYLAXIS, ANGIOEDEMA, OR TUBULOINTERSTITIAL NEPHRITIS), systemic lupus erythematosus, vitamin B_{12} deficiency.

Interactions

Drug-Drug: May significantly ↓ levels and effectiveness of **rilpivirine**; concurrent use contraindicated. May ↑ levels and risk of toxicity of **antifungal agents**, **cilostazol**, **citalopram**, **diazepam**, **triazolam**, **cyclosporine**, **phenytoin**, **tacrolimus**, and **warfarin**; consider ↓ dose of cilostazol from 100 mg twice daily to 50 mg twice daily. May ↓ absorption and effectiveness of drugs requiring acidic pH, including **ketoconazole**, **itraconazole**, **iron salts**, **dasatinib**, **erlotinib**, **nilotinib**, **atazanavir**, **nelfinavir**, and **mycophenolate mofetil**; avoid concurrent use with **atazanavir** and **nelfinavir**. May ↑ levels and risk of toxicity of **digoxin** and **methotrexate**. **Voriconazole** may ↑ levels and risk of toxicity. May ↓ the antiplatelet effects of **clopidogrel**; avoid concurrent use. **Rifampin** may ↓ levels and effectiveness; avoid concurrent use. Hypomagnesemia and hypokalemia ↑ risk of **digoxin** toxicity.

Drug-Natural Products: **St. John's wort** may ↓ levels and effectiveness; avoid concurrent use.

O

Route/Dosage

Symptomatic GERD

PO (Adults): 20 mg once daily for up to 4 wk

PO (Children 1–16 yr and ≥20 kg): 20 mg once daily for up to 4 wk.

PO (Children 1–16 yr and 10–<20 kg): 10 mg once daily for up to 4 wk.

PO (Children 1–16 yr and 5–<10 kg): 5 mg once daily for up to 4 wk.

Erosive Esophagitis Due to Acid-Mediated GERD

PO (Adults): 20 mg once daily for 4–8 wk

PO (Children 1–16 yr and ≥20 kg): 20 mg once daily for 4–8 wk.

PO (Children 1–16 yr and 10–<20 kg): 10 mg once daily for 4–8 wk.

PO (Children 1–16 yr and 5–<10 kg): 5 mg once daily for 4–8 wk.

PO (Children 1 mo–<1 yr and ≥10 kg): 10 mg once daily for up to 6 wk.

PO (Children 1 mo–<1 yr and 5–<10 kg): 5 mg once daily for up to 6 wk.

PO (Children 1 mo–<1 yr and 3–<5 kg): 2.5 mg once daily for up to 6 wk.

Maintenance of Healing of Erosive Esophagitis Due to Acid-Mediated GERD

PO (Adults): 20 mg once daily for up to 12 mo.

PO (Children 1–16 yr and ≥20 kg): 20 mg once daily for up to 12 mo.

PO (Children 1–16 yr and 10–<20 kg): 10 mg once daily for up to 12 mo.

PO (Children 1–16 yr and 5–<10 kg): 5 mg once daily for up to 12 mo.

Duodenal Ulcers Associated With *Helicobacter pylori*

PO (Adults): 40 mg once daily in the morning with clarithromycin for 2 wk, then 20 mg once daily for 2 wk *or* 20 mg twice daily with clarithromycin 500 mg twice daily and amoxicillin 1000 mg twice daily for 10 days (if ulcer is present at beginning of therapy, continue omeprazole 20 mg daily for 18 more days); has also been used with clarithromycin and metronidazole.

Gastric Ulcer

PO (Adults): 40 mg once daily for 4–6 wk.

Gastric Hypersecretory Conditions

PO (Adults): 60 mg once daily initially; may ↑ up to 120 mg 3 times daily (doses >80 mg/day should be given in divided doses);

Reduction of Risk of GI Bleeding in Critically Ill Patients.

PO (Adults): 40 mg initially, then another 40 mg 6–8 hr later, followed by 40 mg once daily for up to 14 days.

Heartburn (OTC Use)

PO (Adults): 20 mg once daily for up to 14 days.

Availability (generic available)

Delayed-release tablets: 🍁 10 mg, 20 mg[OTC].
Delayed-release capsules: 10 mg, 20 mg, 40 mg.
Delayed-release powder for oral suspension (peach-mint flavor): 2.5 mg/packet, 10 mg/packet.
In combination with: metronidazole and clarithromycin in a compliance package (Losec 1-2-3 M); amoxicillin and clarithromycin in a compliance package (Losec 1-2-3-A) (both in Canada only); amoxicillin and rifabutin (Talicia); sodium bicarbonate (Konvomep, Zegerid [OTC]). See Appendix N.

NURSING IMPLICATIONS

Assessment

- Assess patient routinely for epigastric or abdominal pain and frank or occult blood in the stool, emesis, or gastric aspirate.
- Monitor bowel function. Report diarrhea, abdominal cramping, fever, and bloody stools to health care provider promptly as a sign of CDAD. May begin up to several weeks following cessation of therapy.
- Monitor for signs and symptoms of vitamin B_{12} deficiency with prolonged use (>1 yr) (pallor, fatigue, weakness, numbness or tingling in the hands and feet, difficulty with balance or coordination, confusion, glossitis [beefy tongue]). Consider screening for deficiency every 1–2 yr.

Lab Test Considerations

- Monitor CBC with differential periodically during therapy.
- May ↑ AST, ALT, alkaline phosphatase, and bilirubin.
- May ↑ serum gastrin concentrations during first 1–2 wk of therapy. Levels return to normal after discontinuation of omeprazole.
- Monitor INR and prothrombin time in patients taking warfarin.
- May cause hypomagnesemia. Monitor serum magnesium prior to and periodically during therapy.
- May cause false-positive results in diagnostic investigations for neuroendocrine tumors due to ↑ serum chromogranin A (CgA) levels secondary to drug-induced ↓ gastric acidity. Temporarily stop omeprazole ≥14 days before assessing CgA levels and consider repeating test if initial CgA levels are high.

Implementation

- Do not confuse Prilosec with Prozac or Pristiq. Do not confuse omeprazole with fomepizole.
- **PO:** Administer doses 30 min before meals, preferably in the morning. ***DNC:*** Swallow capsules and tablets whole; do not crush or chew. Capsules may be opened and sprinkled on cool applesauce; entire mixture should be ingested immediately and followed by a drink of water. Do not store for future use.

- *Powder for oral suspension:* Administer on empty stomach, ≥1 hr before a meal. Empty contents of 2.5-mg packet into 5 mL of water or contents of 10-mg packet into 15 mL of water. Stir. Leave 2–3 min to thicken. Stir and drink within 30 min. If material remains after drinking, add more water, stir, and drink immediately. For patients with nasogastric or enteral feeding, suspend feeding for 3 hr before and 1 hr after administration. Empty packet contents into a small cup containing 5 mL of water for 2.5-mg dose or 15 mL water for 10-mg dose using a catheter-tipped syringe. **Do not use other liquids or foods.** Immediately shake syringe and leave 2–3 min to thicken. Administer within 30 min. Refill the syringe with an equal amount of water. Shake and flush remaining contents from nasogastric or gastric tube into stomach.
- May be administered concurrently with antacids.

Patient/Family Teaching

- Explain the purpose and side effects of omeprazole. Instruct patient to take medication as directed before meals for the full course of therapy, even if feeling better. Take missed doses as soon as remembered but not if almost time for next dose. Do not double doses. Advise patient to read *Patient Information* before starting and with each Rx refill in case of changes.
- May cause occasional drowsiness or dizziness. Caution patient to avoid driving or other activities requiring alertness until response to medication is known.
- Instruct patient using multiple daily doses for longer than a year to report symptoms of osteoporosis-related fractures (hip, wrist, spine).
- Instruct patient to notify health care provider of all Rx or OTC medications, vitamins, or herbal products being taken and consult health care provider before taking any new medications, especially St. John's wort, clopidogrel, or rifampin.
- Advise patient to avoid alcohol, products containing aspirin or NSAIDs, and foods that may cause an increase in GI irritation.
- Advise patient to report onset of black, tarry stools; diarrhea; abdominal pain; or persistent headache to health care provider promptly.
- Instruct patient to notify health care provider of onset of black, tarry stools; diarrhea; abdominal pain; or persistent headache or if fever and diarrhea develop, especially if stool contains blood, pus, or mucus. Advise patient not to treat diarrhea without consulting health care provider.
- Rep: Advise women of reproductive potential to notify health care provider if pregnancy is planned or suspected or if breastfeeding.

Evaluation/Desired Outcomes

- Decrease in abdominal pain or prevention of gastric irritation and bleeding. Healing of duodenal ulcers can be seen on x-ray examination or endoscopy.
- Decrease in symptoms of GERD and erosive esophagitis. Therapy is continued for 4–8 wk after initial episode.

onabotulinumtoxinA
(**oh**-nuh-bot-yoo-**lye**-num **tox**-in aye)

Botox, Botox Cosmetic

Classification

Therapeutic: cosmetic agents

Pharmacologic: neurotoxins

Indications

Botox Cosmetic: Treatment of the following conditions: Temporary improvement in the appearance of moderate to severe glabellar lines (brow furrow) associated with corrugator and/or procerus muscle activity. Temporary improvement in the appearance of moderate to severe lateral canthal lines (crow's feet) associated with orbicularis oculi activity. Temporary improvement in the appearance of moderate to severe forehead lines associated with frontalis muscle activity (should be treated in conjunction with glabellar lines). Temporary improvement in the appearance of moderate to severe platysma bands associated with platysma band activity. **Botox:** Treatment of the following conditions: Spasticity, Cervical dystonia, Severe axillary hyperhidrosis that is refractory to topical agents, Blepharospasm associated with dystonia, Strabismus, Prevention of migraines in patients with chronic migraines (≥15 headaches/mo with headache lasting ≥4 hr/day), Urinary incontinence due to detrusor overactivity associated with a neurologic condition in adults who have an inadequate response to or are intolerant of an anticholinergic medication, Neurogenic detrusor overactivity in children ≥5 yr who have an inadequate response to or are intolerant of an anticholinergic medication, Overactive bladder with symptoms of urge urinary incontinence, urgency, and frequency in adults who have an inadequate response to or are intolerant of an anticholinergic medication.

Action

Produces partial chemical denervation by inhibiting the release of acetylcholine. Result is local decrease in muscle activity. **Therapeutic Effects:** Decreased brow furrow, crow's feet, forehead lines, and platysma bands with improved appearance. Decreased muscle tone in upper

O

and lower limbs. Decreased severity of abnormal head position and neck pain. Decreased sweating. Decreased blepharospasm. Decreased strabismus. Decreased frequency and duration of headaches. Reduced frequency of urinary incontinence episodes.

Pharmacokinetics

Absorption: Minimal systemic absorption; action is primarily local.
Distribution: Unknown.
Metabolism and Excretion: Unknown.
Half-life: Unknown.

TIME/ACTION PROFILE (improvement)

ROUTE	ONSET	PEAK	DURATION
IM†	1–2 days	unknown	3–4 mo
IM‡	3–4 days	unknown	3–4 mo
IM*	2 wk	unknown	3–4 mo
IM††	<2 wk	unknown	3–4 mo
IM**	1–2 days	unknown	2–6 wk
IM^	unknown	unknown	200 days
IM^^	unknown	unknown	3 mo

† Cosmetic; ‡ Blepharospasm; * Cervical dystonia; †† Spasticity; ** Strabismus; ^ Axillary hyperhidrosis; ^^Migraines.

Contraindications/Precautions

Contraindicated in: Hypersensitivity; Presence of infection at planned injection sites; Acute urinary tract infection and/or acute urinary retention (for urinary incontinence indication).
Use Cautiously in: Peripheral motor neuropathic diseases (e.g. amyotrophic lateral sclerosis, motor neuropathy) or neuromuscular junctional disorders (e.g. myasthenia gravis, Lambert-Eaton syndrome) (↑ risk of significant systemic effects such as dysphagia or respiratory compromise); Inflammation at planned injection site; Marked facial asymmetry, ptosis, excessive dermatochelasis, deep dermal scarring, thick sebaceous skin, or inability to lessen glabellar lines by physical spreading; Excessive weakness or atrophy in target muscles; Swallowing or breathing problems (for treatment of cervical dystonia; ↑ risk of dysphagia); Respiratory problems (for treatment of spasticity or detrusor overactivity associated with a neurologic condition; ↑ risk of pulmonary infection and worsening condition); OB: Safety not established in pregnancy; Lactation: Safety not established in breastfeeding; Pedi: Children <2 yr (safety and effectiveness not established); Geri: Use lowest effective dose in older adults.

Adverse Reactions/Side Effects

EENT: dry eye, eye irritation, photophobia, temporary eyelid droop, visual changes. **GI:** dysphagia, nausea. **GU:** urinary retention, urinary tract infection. **Local:** discomfort at injection sites. **MS:** arthralgia, local muscle weakness, myalgia. **Neuro:** fatigue, headache. **Resp:** upper respiratory tract infection, bronchitis, dyspnea. **Misc:** HYPERSENSITIVITY REACTIONS (INCLUDING ANAPHYLAXIS), SPREAD OF TOXIN EFFECT.

Interactions

Drug-Drug: Neuromuscular effects may be potentiated by **aminoglycosides**, **quinidine** and other **drugs that alter neuromuscular transmission**. Additive effects may occur with other forms of **botulinum toxin**.

Route/Dosage

Botox Cosmetic

Reduction of Glabellar Lines

IM (Adults): 0.1 mL (4 units) into each of five sites (two in each corrugator muscle and one in the procerus muscle; total dose of 20 units); not more frequently than every 3 mo.

Reduction of Lateral Canthal Lines

IM (Adults): 0.1 mL (4 units) into each of three sites per side in the lateral orbicularis oculi muscle (12 units per side; total dose of 24 units); not more frequently than every 3 mo.

Reduction of Forehead Lines

IM (Adults): 0.1 mL (4 units) into each of five sites in the frontalis muscle (total dose of 20 units); not more frequently than every 3 mo.

Reduction of Platysma Bands

IM (Adults): 0.05 mL (2 units) into each of four sites in upper segment of platysma muscle, below the jawline, and on each side, as well as 0.025 mL (1 unit) into each of five sites along each vertical neck band. Depending on platysma band severity, total dose may be 26 units (one band/side), 31 units (one band on one side, two bands on other side), or 36 units (two bands/side). Not to be administered more frequently than every 3 mo.

Botox

Upper Limb Spasticity

IM (Adults): *Biceps brachii:* 60–200 units divided in 2–4 sites; not more frequently than every 3 mo; *Brachioradialis:* 45–75 units divided in 1–2 sites; not more frequently than every 3 mo; *Brachialis:* 30–50 units divided in 1–2 sites; not more frequently than every 3 mo; *Pronator teres:* 15–25 units in one site; not more frequently than every 3 mo; *Pronator quadratus:* 10–50 units in one site; not more frequently than every 3 mo; *Flexor carpi radialis or flexor carpi ulnaris:* 12.5–50 units in one site; not more frequently than every 3 mo; *Flexor digitorum profundus or flexor digitorum sublimis:* 30–50 units in one site; not more frequently than every 3 mo; *Lumbricals/interossei:* 5–10 units in one site; not more frequently than every 3 mo; *Adductor pollicis or flexor pollicis longus:* 20 units in one site; not more frequently than every 3 mo; *Flexor pollicis brevis/opponens pollicis:* 5–25 units in one site; not more frequently than every 3 mo.
IM (Children ≥2 yr): 3–6 units/kg divided among affected muscles, with the following doses being used for

each muscle: *Biceps brachii:* 1.5–3 units/kg divided in 4 sites; not more frequently than every 3 mo; *Brachialis, flexor carpi radialis, or flexor carpi ulnaris:* 1–2 units/kg divided in 2 sites; not more frequently than every 3 mo; *Brachioradialis, flexor digitorum profundus, or flexor digitorum sublimis:* 0.5–1 units/kg divided in 2 sites; not more frequently than every 3 mo.

Lower Limb Spasticity

IM (Adults): *Gastrocnemius medial head, gastrocnemius lateral head, soleus, or tibialis posterior:* 75 units divided in 3 sites; not more frequently than every 3 mo; *Flexor hallucis longus or flexor digitorum longus:* 50 units divided in 2 sites; not more frequently than every 3 mo.
IM (Children ≥2 yr): 4–8 units/kg divided among affected muscles, with the following doses being used for each muscle: *Gastrocnemius, soleus, or tibialis posterior:* 1–2 units/kg divided in 2 sites; may be repeated after 3 mo, based on return of symptoms.

Cervical Dystonia

IM (Adults): Mean dose is 236 units divided among the affected muscles in patients previously treated with botulinum toxin; initial dose should be lower in previously untreated patients; subsequent dosing should be based on patient's head and neck position, localization of pain, muscle hypertrophy, patient response, and previous tolerability; total dose injected into sternocleidomastoid muscles should be ≤100 units (to ↓ incidence of dysphagia); not more frequently than every 3 mo.

Axillary Hyperhidrosis

IM (Adults): 50 units per axilla; may repeat when clinical effect diminishes.

Blepharospasm

IM (Adults and Children): 1.25–2.5 units into the medial and lateral pretarsal orbicularis oculi of the upper lid and into the lateral pretarsal orbicularis oculi of the lower lid; not more frequently than every 3 mo.

Strabismus

IM (Adults and Children ≥12 yr): *Vertical muscles and for horizontal strabismus <20 prism diopters:* 1.25–2.5 units in any one muscle; *Horizontal strabismus of 20–50 prism diopters:* 2.5–5 units in any one muscle; *Persistent VI nerve palsy of ≥1 mo:* 1.25–2.5 units in the medial rectus muscle.

Chronic Migraine

IM (Adults): 155 units divided among seven specific head/neck muscle areas (see prescribing information for dose to be injected into each area) every 12 wk.

Urinary Incontinence

IM (Adults): 200 units injected into the detrusor muscle; may repeat when clinical effect diminishes, but not more frequently than every 3 mo.

Overactive Bladder

IM (Adults): 100 units injected into the detrusor muscle; may repeat when clinical effect diminishes, but not more frequently than every 3 mo.

Pediatric Detrusor Overactivity associated with a Neurologic Condition

IM (Children ≥5 yr and ≥34 kg): 200 units injected into the detrusor muscle; may repeat when clinical effect diminishes, but not more frequently than every 3 mo.
IM (Children ≥5 yr and <34 kg): 6 units/kg injected into the detrusor muscle; may repeat when clinical effect diminishes, but not more frequently than every 3 mo.

Availability

Powder for injection (Botox Cosmetic): 50 units/vial, 100 units/vial. **Powder for injection (Botox):** 100 units/vial, 200 units/vial.

NURSING IMPLICATIONS

Assessment

- Assess for signs of anaphylaxis (dyspnea, rash, pruritus, laryngeal edema, wheezing) following administration. Keep epinephrine, an antihistamine, and resuscitation equipment close by during administration.
- Monitor for signs of the spread of toxin effects (asthenia, general muscle weakness, diplopia, ptosis, dysphagia, dysphonia, urinary incontinence, dyspnea). Pre-existing motor neuropathic or neuromuscular disorders ↑ risk of generalized muscle weakness. *If difficulties with swallowing, speech, or respiration occur,* immediately stop injections and provide appropriate medical care.

Implementation

- Clinicians administering botulinum toxin should understand neuromuscular anatomy of the area involved and potential alterations. Using *Botox* for unapproved uses may ↑ risk of adverse effects and fatality.
- Botulinum toxin products are not interchangeable. Determine appropriate product prior to administration.
- **Adults:** Inject no more frequently than every 3 mo, using lowest effective dose. Do not exceed 400 units/3 mo.
- **Children:** Total dose should not exceed the lower of 10 units/kg body weight or 340 units in a 3-mo interval. Total dose administered per treatment session in the upper limb should not exceed 6 units/kg or 200 units, whichever is lower. Total dose administered per treatment session in the lower limb should not exceed 8 units/kg or 300 units, whichever is lower.
- *Botox Cosmetic*: **Reconstitution:** Reconstitute 50 unit vial with 1.25 mL and 100 unit vial with

O

2.5 mL of 0.9% NaCl without preservatives. **Concentration:** 4 units/0.1 mL. Inject diluent slowly into vial at 45° angle. Discard vial if vacuum does not pull diluent into vial. Rotate vial gently, and record date and time of reconstitution on label. Solution should be clear, colorless, and particulate-free. Refrigerate solution and use within 24 hr of reconstitution; do not freeze. Discard unused solution. Unopened vials should be stored in refrigerator.

- **IM** Draw ≥0.5 mL of reconstituted solution into tuberculin syringe and expel any air bubbles from syringe barrel. Remove needle used for reconstitution and replace with a 30–33 gauge needle; ensure patency of needle. Inject each dose of 0.1 mL.
- *Botox*: **Reconstitution:** Slowly inject vial with proper amount of preservative free 0.9% NaCl, using proper syringe size (see package insert). **Concentration:** *For 100 unit vial*, use 1 mL of diluent for 10 units/0.1 mL; 2 mL of diluent for 5 units/0.1 mL; 4 mL of diluent for 2.5 units/0.1 mL; 8 mL of diluent for 1.25 units/0.1 mL; 10 mL of diluent for 1 unit/0.1 mL*For 200 unit vial*, use 1 mL of diluent for 20 units/0.1 mL; 2 mL of diluent for 10 units/0.1 mL; 4 mL of diluent for 5 units/0.1 mL; 8 mL of diluent for 2.5 units/0.1 mL; 10 mL of diluent for 2 units/0.1 mL. Discard vial if vacuum does not pull diluent into vial. Rotate vial gently, and record date and time of reconstitution on label. Solution should be clear, colorless, and free of particulates. Refrigerate solution and use within 24 hr of reconstitution; do not freeze. Discard unused solution. Unopened vials should be stored in refrigerator.
- **IM** Follow specific dose and administration recommendations for each indication.

Patient/Family Teaching

- Explain purpose of medication to patient. Review *Medication Guide* with patient prior to each administration.
- Inform patient that effects of onabotulinumtoxinA may spread beyond the site of local injection. Advise patient to notify health care provider immediately if problems swallowing, speaking, or breathing occur or if signs and symptoms of spread (asthenia, generalized muscle weakness, diplopia, blurred vision, ptosis, dysphagia, dysarthria, urinary incontinence, breathing difficulties) occur. May occur hours to weeks after injection.
- May cause loss of strength, muscle weakness, blurred vision, or drooping eyelids. Caution patient to avoid driving or other activities requiring alertness until response to medication is known.
- Rep: Advise women of reproductive potential to notify health care provider if pregnancy is planned or suspected or if breastfeeding.

Evaluation/Desired Outcomes

- Decreased brow furrow, crow's feet, forehead lines, and platysma bands with improved appearance.
- Reduction in forehead lines.
- Decreased muscle tone in upper and lower limbs.
- Decreased severity of abnormal head position and neck pain.
- Decreased sweating.
- Decreased blepharospasm.
- Decreased strabismus.
- Decreased frequency and duration of headaches.
- Decreased frequency of urinary incontinence episodes.

ondansetron (on-dan-se-tron)

🍁 Ondissolve ODF

Classification

Therapeutic: antiemetics

Pharmacologic: 5-HT_3 agonists

Indications

IV, PO: Prevention of nausea and vomiting associated with highly or moderately emetogenic chemotherapy. Prevention of postoperative nausea and vomiting.
PO: Prevention of nausea and vomiting associated with radiation therapy.

Action

Blocks the effects of serotonin at 5-HT_3 receptor sites (selective antagonist) located in vagal nerve terminals and the chemoreceptor trigger zone in the CNS. **Therapeutic Effects:** Decreased incidence and severity of nausea and vomiting following chemotherapy, radiation, or surgery.

Pharmacokinetics

Absorption: IV administration results in complete bioavailability; 100% absorbed following oral administration.
Distribution: Unknown.
Metabolism and Excretion: Extensively metabolized by the liver (primarily by CYP3A4); 5% excreted unchanged by the kidneys.
Half-life: *Adults:* 3.5–5.5 hr; *Children 5 mo–12 yr:* 2.9 hr.

TIME/ACTION PROFILE (antiemetic effect)

ROUTE	ONSET	PEAK	DURATION
PO, IV	rapid	15–30 min	4–8 hr
IM	rapid	40 min	unknown

Contraindications/Precautions

Contraindicated in: Hypersensitivity; Orally disintegrating tablets contain aspartame and should not be used in patients with phenylketonuria; Congenital long QT syndrome; Concurrent use of apomorphine.

Use Cautiously in: Hepatic impairment; Abdominal surgery (may mask ileus); Phenylketonuria (orally disintegrating tablets contain phenylalanine); OB: Use during pregnancy only if potential maternal benefit justifies potential fetal risk; Lactation: Safety of oral formulation not established in breastfeeding; IV formulation may be safe to use in breastfeeding; Pedi: Safety and effectiveness not established in children ≤3 yr (PO) or <1 mo (parenteral).

Adverse Reactions/Side Effects

CV: myocardial ischemia, QT interval prolongation, TORSADE DE POINTES. **Derm:** STEVENS-JOHNSON SYNDROME (SJS), TOXIC EPIDERMAL NECROLYSIS (TEN). **GI:** constipation, diarrhea, ↑ liver enzymes, abdominal pain, dry mouth. **Neuro:** headache, dizziness, drowsiness, extrapyramidal reactions, fatigue, weakness. **Misc:** SEROTONIN SYNDROME.

Interactions

Drug-Drug: **Apomorphine** ↑ risk of severe hypotension and loss of consciousness; concurrent use contraindicated. **Carbamazepine**, **phenytoin**, and **rifampin** may ↓ levels and effectiveness. Drugs that affect serotonergic neurotransmitter systems, including **SSRIs**, **SNRIs**, **tricyclic antidepressants**, **MAOIs**, **fentanyl**, **lithium**, **buspirone**, **tramadol**, **methylene blue**, and **triptans**, may ↑ risk of serotonin syndrome.

Route/Dosage

Prevention of Nausea/Vomiting Associated With Highly or Moderately Emetogenic Chemotherapy

PO (Adults): *Highly emetogenic chemotherapy:* 24 mg given 30 min before chemotherapy.
PO (Adults and Children >11 yr): *Moderately emetogenic chemotherapy:* 8 mg given 30 min before chemotherapy and repeated 8 hr later; 8 mg every 12 hr may be given for 1–2 days following chemotherapy.
PO (Children 4–11 yr): *Moderately emetogenic chemotherapy:* 4 mg given 30 min before chemotherapy and repeated 4 and 8 hr later; 4 mg every 8 hr may be given for 1–2 days following chemotherapy.
IV (Adults): 0.15 mg/kg (max dose = 16 mg) given 30 min before chemotherapy, repeated 4 and 8 hr later.
IV (Children 6 mo–18 yr): 0.15 mg/kg (max dose = 16 mg) given 30 min before chemotherapy, repeated 4 and 8 hr later.

Hepatic Impairment

PO, IM, IV (Adults): *Severe hepatic impairment:* Not to exceed 8 mg/day.

Prevention of Postoperative Nausea/Vomiting

PO (Adults): 16 mg given 1 hr before induction of anesthesia.
IM IV (Adults and Children >12 yr): 4 mg given before induction of anesthesia or postoperatively.
IV (Children 1 mo–12 yr and >40 kg): 4 mg given before induction of anesthesia or postoperatively.
IV (Children 1 mo–12 yr and ≤40 kg): 0.1 mg/kg given before induction of anesthesia or postoperatively.

Hepatic Impairment

PO, IM, IV (Adults): *Severe hepatic impairment:* Not to exceed 8 mg/day.

Prevention of Nausea/Vomiting Associated With Radiation Therapy

PO (Adults): 8 mg given 1–2 hr before radiation; may be repeated every 8 hr, depending on type, location, and extent of radiation.

Hepatic Impairment

PO, IM, IV (Adults): *Severe hepatic impairment:* Not to exceed 8 mg/day.

Availability (generic available)

Tablets: 4 mg, 8 mg, 24 mg. **Orally disintegrating tablets (contain aspartame) (strawberry flavor):** 4 mg, 8 mg. **Oral solution (strawberry flavor):** 4 mg/5 mL. **Solution for injection:** 2 mg/mL.

O

NURSING IMPLICATIONS

Assessment

- Assess for nausea, vomiting, abdominal distention, and bowel sounds before and following administration.
- Assess for extrapyramidal effects (involuntary movements, facial grimacing, rigidity, shuffling walk, trembling of hands) periodically during therapy.
- Monitor ECG in patients with hypokalemia, hypomagnesemia, HF, or bradyarrhythmias or those concurrently taking medications that prolong the QT interval.
- Assess for signs/symptoms of serotonin syndrome (confusion, delirium, agitation, coma, dilated pupils, tachycardia, hyperthermia, shivering, hyperreflexia, muscle rigidity, hypertension, vomiting, diarrhea, seizures). *If signs/symptoms of serotonin syndrome occur,* discontinue ondansetron.
- Assess for rash periodically during therapy. May cause SJS or TEN. *If severe rash occurs or if accompanied with fever, general malaise, fatigue, muscle or joint aches, blisters, oral lesions, conjunctivitis, hepatitis, or eosinophilia,* discontinue ondansetron.

Lab Test Considerations

- May transiently ↑ bilirubin, AST, and ALT.

Implementation

- 1st dose is administered prior to emetogenic event.

- **PO:** For orally disintegrating tablets, do not attempt to push through foil backing; with dry hands, peel back backing and remove tablet. Immediately place tablet on tongue; tablet will dissolve in seconds; then swallow with saliva. Administration of liquid is not necessary.

IV Administration

- **IV Push:** Administer undiluted (2 mg/mL) immediately before induction of anesthesia or postoperatively if nausea and vomiting occur shortly after surgery. **Rate:** Administer over ≥30 sec and preferably over 2–5 min.
- **Intermittent Infusion: Dilution:** Dilute doses for prevention of nausea and vomiting associated with chemotherapy in 50 mL of D5W, 0.9% NaCl, D5/0.9% NaCl, D5/0.45% NaCl for adults and in 10–50 mL D5W or 0.9% NaCl for children 6 mo–1 yr or < 10 kg. Solution is clear and colorless. Use within 24–48 hr after dilution. **Concentration:** 1 mg/mL. **Rate:** Administer each dose over 15 min.
- **Y-Site Compatibility:** acetaminophen, aldesleukin, alemtuzumab, amikacin, aminocaproic acid, amiodarone, anakinra, anidulafungin, argatroban, arsenic trioxide, ascorbic acid, atracurium, atropine, azithromycin, aztreonam, benztropine, bivalirudin, bleomycin, bumetanide, buprenorphine, busulfan, butorphanol, calcium chloride, calcium gluconate, carboplatin, carmustine, caspofungin, cefazolin, cefotaxime, cefoxitin, ceftaroline, ceftolozane/tazobactam, cefuroxime, chlorpromazine, ciprofloxacin, cisatracurium, cisplatin, cladribine, clindamycin, cyanocobalamin, cyclophosphamide, cyclosporine, cytarabine, dacarbazine, dactinomycin, daptomycin, daunorubicin, defibrotide, dexamethasone, dexmedetomidine, dexrazoxane, digoxin, diltiazem, diphenhydramine, dobutamine, docetaxel, dopamine, doxorubicin hydrochloride, doxorubicin liposomal, doxycycline, droperidol, enalaprilat, ephedrine, epinephrine, epirubicin, epoetin alfa, eptifibatide, erythromycin, esmolol, etoposide, etoposide phosphate, famotidine, fentanyl, filgrastim, floxuridine, fluconazole, fludarabine, folic acid, fosaprepitant, fosphenytoin, gemcitabine, gentamicin, glycopyrrolate, heparin, hydrocortisone, hydromorphone, idarubicin, ifosfamide, imipenem/cilastatin, imipenem/cilastatin/relebactam, irinotecan, isavuconazonium, isoproterenol, ketorolac, labetalol, leucovorin, levofloxacin, lidocaine, linezolid, magnesium sulfate, mannitol, melphalan, meperidine, mesna, methadone, methotrexate, metoclopramide, metoprolol, metronidazole, midazolam, mitomycin, mitoxantrone, morphine, moxifloxacin, multivitamins, mycophenolate, nafcillin, nalbuphine, naloxone, nicardipine, nitroglycerin, nitroprusside, norepinephrine, octreotide, oxacillin, oxaliplatin, oxytocin, paclitaxel, pamidronate, papaverine, penicillin G, pentamidine, pentostatin, phentolamine, phenylephrine, phytonadione, piperacillin/tazobactam, plazomicin, potassium acetate, potassium chloride, potassium phosphates, procainamide, prochlorperazine, promethazine, propranolol, protamine, pyridoxine, remifentanil, rocuronium, sodium acetate, sodium phosphates, succinylcholine, sufentanil, sulbactam/durlobactam, tacrolimus, tedizolid, telavancin, theophylline, thiotepa, tigecycline, tirofiban, tobramycin, topotecan, vancomycin, vasopressin, vecuronium, verapamil, vinblastine, vincristine, vinorelbine, voriconazole, zidovudine, zoledronic acid.
- **Y-Site Incompatibility:** acyclovir, allopurinol, aminophylline, amphotericin B deoxycholate, amphotericin B liposomal, ampicillin, ampicillin/sulbactam, azathioprine, blinatumomab, cefepime, chloramphenicol, dantrolene, diazoxide, ertapenem, foscarnet, furosemide, ganciclovir, gemtuzumab ozogamicin, indomethacin, letermovir, lorazepam, meropenem/vaborbactam, methohexital, micafungin, milrinone, pantoprazole, pemetrexed, pentobarbital, phenobarbital, phenytoin, rituximab, sargramostim, sodium bicarbonate, trastuzumab, trimethoprim/sulfamethoxazole.

Patient/Family Teaching

- Explain the purpose and side effects of ondansetron. Instruct patient to take as directed. Advise patient to read *Patient Information* before starting and with each Rx refill in case of changes.
- Advise patient to notify health care provider immediately if symptoms of irregular heartbeat; serotonin syndrome; or involuntary movement of eyes, face, or limbs occur.
- Advise patient to notify health care provider of all Rx or OTC medications, vitamins, or herbal products being taken and to consult with health care provider before taking other medications.
- Rep: Advise women of reproductive potential to notify health care provider if pregnancy is planned or suspected or if breastfeeding.

Evaluation/Desired Outcomes

- Prevention of nausea and vomiting associated with emetogenic cancer chemotherapy.
- Prevention of postoperative nausea and vomiting.
- Prevention of nausea and vomiting due to radiation therapy.

oritavancin (oh-rit-a-**van**-sin)

Kimyrsa, Orbactiv

Classification

Therapeutic: anti-infectives

Pharmacologic: lipoglycopeptides

Indications

Acute bacterial skin and skin structure infections caused by or suspected to be caused by susceptible designated gram-positive bacteria.

Action
Binds to bacterial cell wall, resulting in cell death. **Therapeutic Effects:** Bactericidal action against susceptible bacteria with resolution of infection. **Spectrum:** Active against *Staphylococcus aureus* (including methicillin-susceptible and resistant strains), *Streptococcus pyogenes*, *Streptococcus agalactiae*, *Streptococcus dysgalactiae*, *Streptococcus anginosus* (including *S. anginosus*, *S. intermidius*, and *S. constellatus*), and *Enterococcus faecalis* (vancomycin-susceptible strains only).

Pharmacokinetics
Absorption: IV administration results in complete bioavailability.
Distribution: Penetrates skin/skin structures.
Metabolism and Excretion: Slowly excreted unchanged in urine (5% in 2 wk) and feces (1% in 2 wk).
Half-life: 245 hr.

TIME/ACTION PROFILE (plasma concentrations)

ROUTE	ONSET	PEAK	DURATION
IV	rapid	end of infusion	≥2 wk

Contraindications/Precautions
Contraindicated in: Hypersensitivity (cross-sensitivity with other glycopeptides may occur); Heparin use for 120 hr (5 days) following administration of oritavancin (causes false ↑ aPTT); Confirmed/suspected osteomyelitis (alternate treatment required).
Use Cautiously in: Severe renal impairment; Severe hepatic impairment; OB: Safety not established in pregnancy; Lactation: Safety not established in breastfeeding; Pedi: Safety and effectiveness not established in children; Geri: Older adults may have ↑ sensitivity to drug effects.

Adverse Reactions/Side Effects
CV: tachycardia. **Derm:** limb/SUBQ abscess formation. **GI:** ↑ liver enzymes, CLOSTRIDIOIDES DIFFICILE ASSOCIATED DIARRHEA (CDAD), nausea, vomiting. **Local:** injection site reactions. **Neuro:** headache. **Misc:** HYPERSENSITIVITY REACTIONS (INCLUDING ANAPHYLAXIS), infusion reactions (including infusion-related reaction resembling vancomycin flushing syndrome).

Interactions
Drug-Drug: ↑ risk of bleeding with **warfarin**; avoid concurrent use, if possible. Affects the activities of several CYP450 enzymes; careful monitoring of other **drugs metabolized by the CYP450 system** that have narrow therapeutic indices to assess for toxicity or ineffectiveness is recommended.

Route/Dosage
IV (Adults): 1200 mg as a single dose.

Availability
Lyophilized powder for injection (Orbactiv): 400 mg/vial. **Lyophilized powder for injection (Kimyrsa):** 1200 mg/vial.

NURSING IMPLICATIONS
Assessment
- Assess signs and symptoms of infection at baseline and during therapy.
- Monitor for hypersensitivity reactions including anaphylaxis. *If acute reaction occurs,* immediately discontinue and initiate supportive measures.
- Monitor for diarrhea, abdominal pain, fever, and bloody stools. *If CDAD suspected,* discontinue oritavancin and treat as clinically indicated. May begin up to 2 mo following cessation of therapy.
- Monitor for infusion-related reaction (resembling vancomycin flushing syndrome: flushing of upper body, urticaria, pruritus, rash, chest pain, back pain, chills, rigor). *If symptoms occur,* consider stopping or slowing infusion until resolved.
- Monitor for signs/symptoms of osteomyelitis (fever, local erythema and pain, chills, diaphoresis, loss of range of motion). *If osteomyelitis is suspected or diagnosed,* discontinue oritavancin and institute alternate antibacterial therapy.

Lab Test Considerations
- Obtain specimens for culture and sensitivity before starting therapy. 1st dose may be given before receiving results.
- Monitor liver function tests. May ↑ ALT, AST, and bilirubin.
- May cause hyperuricemia and hypoglycemia.
- Causes falsely ↑ aPTT for 120 hr after infusion. Avoid heparin administration during this time. Use a nonphospholipid dependent coagulation test such as factor Xa assay if needed.
- Artificially prolongs PT and INR for up to 12 hr.

Implementation
- The two oritavancin products (*Orbactiv* and *Kimyrsa*) are different products. Directions for use are not interchangeable.

Orbactiv
- **Reconstitution:** Using three 400-mg vials, add 40 mL of sterile water for injection to each vial. Swirl gently to avoid foaming and ensure powder is completely dissolved. Solution is clear and colorless to pale yellow; do not administer if discolored or contains particulates. **Concentration:** 10 mg/mL. **Dilution:** Withdraw and discard 120 mL from 1000-mL bag of D5W. Withdraw

O

40 mL from each vial and add to D5W bag. Do not use 0.9% NaCl; may cause precipitation. **Concentration:** 1.2 mg/mL. Use within 6 hr at room temperature or 12 hr if refrigerated, including infusion time.

- **Rate:** Infuse over 3 hr. Flush line before and after infusion.

Kimyrsa

- **Reconstitution:** Add 40 mL sterile water for injection to 1200-mg vial. Swirl gently to avoid foaming. Solution is clear, colorless to pink; do not use if cloudy, discolored, or contains particulates. **Concentration:** 30 mg/mL. **Dilution:** Withdraw and discard 40 mL from a 250-mL IV bag of 0.9% NaCl or D5W. Withdraw 40 mL of reconstituted vial and add to IV bag of 0.9% NaCl or D5W to bring volume to 250 mL. **Concentration:** 4.8 mg/mL. Discard unused portion of reconstituted solution. Solution is stable for 4 hr at room temperature or 12 hr if refrigerated. Combined storage and infusion times should be within the stability times.
- **Rate:** Infuse over 1 hr.
- **Y-Site Compatibility:** (Applies to both oritavancin products) calcium gluconate, ciprofloxacin, dexmedetomidine, dobutamine, dopamine, epinephrine, famotidine, fentanyl, fluconazole, gentamicin, haloperidol, insulin, regular, lorazepam, midazolam, morphine, nitroglycerin, norepinephrine, phenylephrine, potassium chloride, tobramycin.
- **Y-Site Incompatibility:** (Applies to both oritavancin products) aminophylline, amphotericin B deoxycholate, aztreonam, bumetanide, clindamycin, furosemide, heparin, hydrocortisone, meropenem, nitroprusside, phenytoin, trimethoprim/sulfamethoxazole.

Patient/Family Teaching

- Explain purpose and side effects of medication. Advise patient to read *Patient Information* before starting therapy.
- Advise patient to notify health care provider of all Rx or OTC medications, vitamins, or herbal products being taken and to consult health care provider before taking other medications.
- Instruct patient to notify health care provider if signs and symptoms of hypersensitivity reactions (rash, hives, dyspnea, facial swelling) occur.
- Instruct patient to notify health care provider immediately if diarrhea, abdominal cramping, fever, or bloody stools occur and not to treat with antidiarrheals without consulting health care provider.
- Rep: Advise women of reproductive potential to notify health care provider if pregnancy is planned or suspected or if breastfeeding.

Evaluation/Desired Outcomes

- Resolution of the signs and symptoms of infection. Length of time for complete resolution depends on the organism and site of infection.

BEERS

orphenadrine
(or-**fenn**-a-dreen)

~~Norflex~~

Classification

Therapeutic: skeletal muscle relaxants (centrally acting)

Pharmacologic: diphenhydramine analogues

Indications

Muscle spasm associated with acute painful musculoskeletal conditions (as adjunct to rest and physical therapy).

Action

Skeletal muscle relaxation, probably due to CNS depression. **Therapeutic Effects:** Skeletal muscle relaxation, with decreased discomfort.

Pharmacokinetics

Absorption: Readily absorbed after oral and IM administration; IV administration results in complete bioavailability.

Distribution: Unknown.

Metabolism and Excretion: Mostly metabolized by the liver.

Half-life: 14 hr.

TIME/ACTION PROFILE (skeletal muscle effects)

ROUTE	ONSET	PEAK	DURATION
PO-ER	within 1 hr	6–8 hr	12 hr
IM	5 min	30 min	12 hr
IV	immediate	unknown	12 hr

Contraindications/Precautions

Contraindicated in: Hypersensitivity; Bladder-neck obstruction, prostatic hyperplasia, glaucoma, myasthenia gravis, peptic ulcer disease, or GI obstruction.

Use Cautiously in: Underlying cardiovascular disease; Renal impairment; OB: Safety not established in pregnancy; Lactation: Safety not established in breastfeeding; Pedi: Safety and effectiveness not established in children; Geri: Appears on Beers list. ↑ risk of anticholinergic adverse reactions, sedation, and fractures in older adults. Avoid use in older adults.

Adverse Reactions/Side Effects

CV: orthostatic hypotension, tachycardia. **EENT:** blurred vision, dry eyes. **GI:** constipation, dry mouth. **GU:** urinary retention. **Neuro:** CNS excitation, confusion, dizziness, drowsiness.

Interactions

Drug-Drug: Anticholinergics ↑ risk of anticholinergic side effects. ↑ risk of CNS depression with other **CNS depressants**, including **alcohol**, **antihistamines**,

antidepressants, **sedative/hypnotics**, or **opioid analgesics**.
Drug-Natural Products: Kava-kava, valerian, chamomile, or **hops** can ↑ risk of CNS depression.

Route/Dosage

PO (Adults): 100 mg twice daily.
IV, IM (Adults): 60 mg every 12 hr.

Availability (generic available)

Extended-release tablets: 100 mg. **Solution for injection:** 30 mg/mL.

NURSING IMPLICATIONS

Assessment

- Geri: Assess older adults for anticholinergic adverse effects (delirium, acute confusion, dizziness, dry mouth, blurred vision, urinary retention, constipation, tachycardia) and sedation.
- Assess for pain, muscle stiffness, and range of motion before and periodically throughout therapy.

Lab Test Considerations

- Monitor CBC and renal and hepatic function periodically during prolonged therapy.

Implementation

- Provide safety measures as indicated. Supervise ambulation and transfer of patients.
- **PO:** Administer without regard to food.
- *DNC:* Do not break, crush, or chew extended-release tablets.
- **IM** May be administered undiluted.

IV Administration

- **IV Push:** May be administered undiluted.
- **Y-Site Incompatibility:** Do not administer other drugs through same IV line.

Patient/Family Teaching

- Explain the purpose and side effects of orphenadrine. Advise patient to take medication as directed. Take missed doses within 1 hr; if not, return to regular dosing schedule. Do not double doses. Advise patient to read *Patient Information* before starting and with each Rx refill in case of changes.
- Encourage patient to comply with additional therapies prescribed for muscle spasm (rest, physical therapy, heat).
- Emphasize the importance of routine follow-up exams to monitor progress.
- Medication may cause dizziness, drowsiness, and blurred vision. Advise patient to avoid driving and other activities requiring alertness until response to drug is known.
- Instruct patient to make position changes slowly to minimize orthostatic hypotension.
- Advise patient to notify health care provider of all Rx or OTC medications, vitamins, or herbal products being taken and to consult with health care provider before taking other medications. Advise patient to avoid concurrent use of alcohol and other CNS depressants while taking this medication.
- Rep: Advise women of reproductive potential to notify health care provider if pregnancy is planned or suspected or if breastfeeding.

Evaluation/Desired Outcomes

- Decreased musculoskeletal pain and muscle spasticity.
- Increased range of motion.

oseltamivir (o-sel-**tam**-i-vir)
Tamiflu
Classification
Therapeutic: antivirals
Pharmacologic: neuraminidase inhibitors

Indications

Treatment of uncomplicated acute illness due to influenza infection in adults and children ≥2 wk who have had symptoms for ≤2 days. Prevention of influenza in patients ≥1 yr.

Action

Inhibits the enzyme neuraminidase, which may alter virus particle aggregation and release. **Therapeutic Effects:** Reduced duration or prevention of flu-related symptoms.

Pharmacokinetics

Absorption: Rapidly absorbed from the GI tract; 75% reaches systemic circulation as the active drug.
Distribution: Well distributed to tissues.
Metabolism and Excretion: Rapidly metabolized by the liver to oseltamivir carboxylate, the active drug. >99% excreted unchanged in urine.
Half-life: *Oseltamivir carboxylate:* 6–10 hr.

TIME/ACTION PROFILE (plasma concentrations)

ROUTE	ONSET	PEAK	DURATION
PO	unknown	unknown	12 hr

Contraindications/Precautions

Contraindicated in: Hypersensitivity; End-stage renal disease and not receiving dialysis.
Use Cautiously in: Renal impairment (↓ dose if CCr ≤60 mL/min); Hereditary fructose intolerance (75 mg of oral suspension contains 2 g of sorbitol); OB: Use during pregnancy only if potential maternal

O

benefit justifies potential fetal risk; Lactation: Use during breastfeeding only if potential maternal benefit justifies potential risk to infant; Pedi: Children <2 wk (safety and effectiveness not established for treatment); children <1 yr (safety and effectiveness not established for prevention). Oral suspension contains sodium benzoate; avoid use in neonates.

Adverse Reactions/Side Effects

Derm: ERYTHEMA MULTIFORME, STEVENS-JOHNSON SYNDROME (SJS), TOXIC EPIDERMAL NECROLYSIS (TEN). **GI:** nausea, vomiting. **Neuro:** abnormal behavior, agitation, confusion, delirium, hallucinations, insomnia, nightmares, SEIZURES, vertigo. **Resp:** bronchitis.

Interactions

Drug-Drug: May ↓ therapeutic effect of **influenza virus vaccine**; avoid use 2 days prior to and 2 wk after vaccine administration.

Route/Dosage

Treatment of Influenza

PO (Adults and Children ≥13 yr): 75 mg twice daily for 5 days.
PO (Children 1–12 yr and >40 kg): 75 mg twice daily for 5 days.
PO (Children 1–12 yr and 23.1–40 kg): 60 mg twice daily for 5 days.
PO (Children 1–12 yr and 15.1–23 kg): 45 mg twice daily for 5 days.
PO (Children 1–12 yr and ≤15 kg): 30 mg twice daily for 5 days.
PO (Infants 2 wk–<1 yr): 3 mg/kg/dose twice daily for 5 days.

Renal Impairment

PO (Adults): *CCr 30–60 mL/min:* 30 mg twice daily for 5 days; *CCr 10–30 mL/min:* 30 mg once daily for 5 days; *CCr ≥10 mL/min and on hemodialysis:* 30 mg after each hemodialysis session (not to exceed 5 days); *CCr ≥10 mL/min and on peritoneal dialysis:* 30-mg single dose immediately after a dialysis exchange; *CCr <10 mL/min and not on dialysis:* Not recommended.

Influenza Prevention

PO (Adults and Children ≥13 yr): 75 mg once daily for ≥10 days.
PO (Children 1–12 yr and >40 kg): 75 mg once daily for 10 days.
PO (Children 1–12 yr and 23.1–40 kg): 60 mg once daily for 10 days.
PO (Children 1–12 yr and 15.1–23 kg): 45 mg once daily for 10 days.
PO (Children 1–12 yr and ≤15 kg): 30 mg once daily for 10 days.

Renal Impairment

PO (Adults): *CCr 30–60 mL/min:* 30 mg once daily for ≥10 days; *CCr 10–30 mL/min:* 30 mg every other day for ≥10 days; *CCr ≥10 mL/min and on hemodialysis:* 30 mg after alternate hemodialysis sessions (treatment duration ≥10 days); *CCr ≥10 mL/min and on peritoneal dialysis:* 30 mg once weekly immediately after a dialysis exchange (treatment duration ≥10 days); *CCr <10 mL/min and not on dialysis:* Not recommended.

Availability (generic available)

Capsules: 30 mg, 45 mg, 75 mg. **Oral suspension (tutti-frutti flavor):** 6 mg/mL.

NURSING IMPLICATIONS

Assessment

- Monitor progression of influenza symptoms. Additional supportive treatment may be indicated.
- Monitor for signs of hypersensitivity reaction including anaphylaxis and serious skin reactions (TEN, SJS, erythema multiforme). *If symptoms occur,* discontinue oseltamivir and treat as indicated.

Implementation

- Begin therapy as soon as possible from the 1st sign of flu symptoms, within 2 days of exposure.
- **PO:** May be administered with food or milk to minimize GI irritation.
- Use correct oral dosing device for measuring oral solution. Dosing errors have occurred due to oseltamivir dosing in mg and solution in mL. Make sure units of measure on prescription instructions match dosing device provided with the drug.
- If oral suspension is not available, capsules may be opened and mixed with flavored foods (regular or sugar-free chocolate syrup, corn syrup, caramel topping, light brown sugar dissolved in water). If correct dose and oral suspension are not available, pharmacist may compound emergency supply of oral suspension from 75 mg capsules.

Patient/Family Teaching

- Explain purpose and side effects of medication. Advise patient to read *Patient Information* before starting therapy.
- Instruct patient to take oseltamivir as soon as influenza symptoms appear and to continue to take it as directed for the full course of therapy, even if feeling better. Take missed doses as soon as remembered unless within 2 hr of next dose. Do not double doses.
- Caution patient that oseltamivir should not be shared with anyone, even if they have the same symptoms.
- Advise patient that oseltamivir is not a substitute for an influenza vaccine. Patients should receive annual influenza vaccine according to immunization guidelines.
- Advise patients to report behavioral changes (hallucinations, delirium, abnormal behavior) to health care provider immediately.
- Advise patient to notify health care provider of all Rx or OTC medications, vitamins, or herbal products

being taken and to consult with health care provider before taking other medications.

- Rep: Advise women of reproductive potential to notify health care provider if pregnancy is planned or suspected or if breastfeeding.

Evaluation/Desired Outcomes

- Reduced duration or prevention of flu-related symptoms.

HIGH ALERT

osimertinib (oh-si-mer-ti-nib)

Tagrisso

Classification

Therapeutic: antineoplastics

Pharmacologic: epidermal growth factor receptor (EGFR) inhibitors

Indications

Metastatic epidermal growth factor receptor (EGFR) T790M mutation-positive non-small-cell lung cancer (NSCLC) in patients who have progressed on or after EGFR tyrosine kinase inhibitor therapy. First-line treatment of metastatic NSCLC in patients whose tumors have EGFR exon 19 deletions or exon 21 L858R mutations. First-line treatment of locally advanced or metastatic NSCLC in patients whose tumors have EGFR exon 19 deletions or exon 21 L858R mutations (in combination with pemetrexed and platinum-based chemotherapy). Adjuvant therapy after tumor resection of NSCLC in patients whose tumors have EGFR exon 19 deletions or exon 21 L858R mutations. Locally advanced, unresectable (stage III) NSCLC in patients whose disease has not progressed during or following concurrent or sequential platinum-based chemoradiation therapy and whose tumors have EGFR exon 19 deletions or exon 21 L858R mutations.

Action

Irreversibly binds to select mutant forms of EGFR (including T790M), resulting in inactivation of kinases that regulate proliferation and transformation; the T790M mutation is the most common mechanism of resistance to EGFR tyrosine kinase inhibitors. **Therapeutic Effects:** Improved progression-free survival.

Pharmacokinetics

Absorption: Well absorbed following oral administration.

Distribution: Extensively distributed to tissues.

Protein Binding: 95%.

Metabolism and Excretion: Mostly metabolized by the liver via the CYP3A4 isoenzyme to two active metabolites; 68% excreted in feces (2% as unchanged drug); 14% excreted in urine (2% as unchanged drug).

Half-life: 48 hr.

TIME/ACTION PROFILE (plasma concentrations)

ROUTE	ONSET	PEAK	DURATION
Oral	unknown	6 hr	24 hr

Contraindications/Precautions

Contraindicated in: OB: Pregnancy; Lactation: Lactation.

Use Cautiously in: Congenital long QT syndrome, HF, electrolyte abnormalities, or taking QT interval prolonging medications; End-stage renal disease (CCr <15 mL/min); Severe hepatic impairment; Rep: Women of reproductive potential and men with female partners of reproductive potential; Pedi: Safety and effectiveness not established in children.

Adverse Reactions/Side Effects

CV: cutaneous vasculitis, DEEP VEIN THROMBOSIS, HF, QT interval prolongation. **Derm:** dry skin, nail disorders, pruritus, rash, ERYTHEMA MULTIFORME (EM), STEVENS-JOHNSON SYNDROME (SJS), urticaria. **EENT:** ↑ lacrimation, blepharitis, blurred vision, cataracts, dry eye, eye pain, keratitis. **F and E:** hypermagnesemia, hyponatremia. **GI:** constipation, diarrhea, nausea, stomatitis. **Hemat:** anemia, lymphopenia, NEUTROPENIA, THROMBOCYTOPENIA, APLASTIC ANEMIA. **Metab:** ↓ appetite. **MS:** back pain. **Neuro:** fatigue, headache, STROKE. **Resp:** cough, INTERSTITIAL LUNG DISEASE (ILD)/PNEUMONITIS, PULMONARY EMBOLISM.

Interactions

Drug-Drug: Strong CYP3A4 inhibitors, including **itraconazole**, **nefazodone**, and **ritonavir**, may ↑ levels and risk of toxicity; avoid concurrent use. **Strong CYP3A4 inducers**, including **carbamazepine**, **rifampin**, and **phenytoin**, may ↓ levels and effectiveness; avoid concurrent use. May ↑ or ↓ **carbamazepine**, **cyclosporine**, **ergot derivatives**, **fentanyl**, **phenytoin**, or **quinidine**; avoid concurrent use. **QT interval prolonging drugs** may ↑ risk of torsades de pointes; avoid concurrent use. May ↑ levels and risk of toxicity of **P-glycoprotein substrates**, including **fexofenadine**. May ↑ levels and risk of toxicity of **breast cancer resistant protein substrates**, including **rosuvastatin**.

Drug-Natural Products: St. John's wort may ↓ levels and effectiveness; avoid concurrent use.

Route/Dosage

PO (Adults): 80 mg once daily. In patients with metastatic disease, continue until disease progression

O

or unacceptable toxicity. In adjuvant setting, continue until disease progression, unacceptable toxicity, or for up to 3 yr.

Availability

Tablets: 40 mg, 80 mg.

NURSING IMPLICATIONS

Assessment

- Assess for worsening respiratory symptoms (dyspnea, cough, hypoxia, fever) during therapy; may indicate ILD or pneumonitis. If signs and symptoms occur, hold medication. If ILD confirmed, permanently discontinue osimertinib. **Dosage adjustments for ILD/pneumonitis in patients who have not recently received platinum-based chemoradiation:** *Any Grade ILD/pneumonitis:* permanently discontinue osimertinib; **Dosage adjustments for ILD/pneumonitis in patients who have recently received platinum-based chemoradiation:** *Grade 1:* Hold therapy or continue as clinically appropriate; *Grade ≥2 ILD/pneumonitis:* Permanently discontinue osimertinib.
- Assess cardiac history and ECG at baseline. Monitor ECG periodically during therapy, especially in patients with congenital long QTc syndrome, HF, electrolyte abnormalities, or taking medications that prolong QTc interval. *If QTc interval >500 msec on ≥2 separate ECGs,* hold therapy until QTc interval <481 msec or recovery to baseline (if baseline QTc is ≥481 msec but <500 msec); then resume at 40-mg dose. *If QTc interval prolongation occurs with signs and symptoms of life-threatening arrhythmia,* permanently discontinue osimertinib.
- Assess for signs and symptoms of cardiomyopathy (HF, pulmonary edema, ↓ left ventricular ejection fraction [LVEF], stress cardiomyopathy) by echocardiogram and multigated acquisition scan prior to starting therapy and every 3 mo during therapy, especially in patients with cardiac risk factors. *If asymptomatic and absolute ↓ in LVEF of 10% from baseline and <50%,* withhold therapy for up to 4 wk. If improved to baseline, resume. If not improved to baseline, permanently discontinue osimertinib. *If symptomatic HF develops,* permanently discontinue osimertinib.
- Monitor for symptoms of keratitis (eye inflammation, lacrimation, light sensitivity, blurred vision, eye pain, red eye) during therapy. If symptoms occur, refer to an ophthalmologist.
- Assess for rash or signs and symptoms of SJS or EM periodically during therapy (fever, general malaise, fatigue, muscle or joint aches, red patches, blisters, oral lesions, conjunctivitis). *If SJS or EM suspected,* hold therapy. *If SJS or EM confirmed,* permanently discontinue osimertinib.
- Monitor for signs and symptoms of cutaneous (leukocytoclastic, urticarial vasculitis, IgA) vasculitis (multiple nonblancheable red papules on forearms, lower legs, or buttocks or large urticaria on trunk that do not go away within 24 hr and develop a bruised appearance). Interrupt therapy if suspected and evaluate; permanent discontinuation may be necessary.

Lab Test Considerations

- Verify negative pregnancy test before starting therapy.
  Patient selection is based on presence of EGFR exon mutations in tumor specimens. Confirm EGFR mutation by an FDA-approved test prior to treatment. Information on FDA-approved tests for the detection of EGFR mutations is available at http://www.fda.gov/companiondiagnostics.
- Monitor CBC with differential before starting and periodically during therapy. May cause lymphopenia, thrombocytopenia, anemia, and neutropenia. *If Grade ≥3 reaction occurs,* withhold osimertinib for up to 3 wk. *If improved to Grade ≤2,* resume at 80 mg or 40 mg daily. *If no improvement in 3 wk,* permanently discontinue osimertinib.
- Monitor electrolytes periodically during therapy. May cause hyponatremia and hypermagnesemia.

Implementation

- **PO:** Administer once daily without regard to food.
- For patients with difficulty swallowing, disperse tablet in 60 mL (2 oz) of only noncarbonated water. Stir until tablet is completely dispersed and swallow immediately; do not crush, heat, or ultrasonicate during preparation. Rinse container with 4–8 oz of water and drink or administer through nasogastric (NG) tube immediately. If administered via NG tube, disperse tablet in 15 mL of noncarbonated water; then use an additional 15 mL of water to transfer any residues in syringe. Administer 30 mL of solution via NG tube with 30 mL of water flushes.
- Geri: Higher incidence of Grade 3 or 4 adverse events have been reported, requiring more frequent dosage adjustments in older adults.

Patient/Family Teaching

- Explain purpose and side effects of osimertinib to patient. Instruct them to take medication as directed. Do not share medication with others, even if they have similar symptoms; may be harmful. Keep out of children's reach. Advise patient to read *Patient Information* prior to starting therapy and with each Rx dose refill in case of changes.
- Inform patient that side effects may include diarrhea, dry skin, stomatitis, fatigue, and ↓ appetite. Maintain adequate hydration and good oral hygiene.
- Advise patient to notify health care professional if signs and symptoms of lung problems (worsening lung symptoms, trouble breathing, shortness of breath, cough, fever), heart problems (pounding or racing heart, shortness of breath, swollen ankles or feet, light-headedness, fainting), eye symptoms,

rash (target lesions, severe blistering or peeling of skin), cutaneous vasculitis (multiple nonblanching red papules on forearms, lower legs, or buttocks or large hives on trunk that do not go away within 24 hr and develop a bruised appearance), and aplastic anemia (new or persistent fevers, bruising, bleeding, pallor) occur.

- Instruct patient to notify health care professional of all Rx or OTC medications, vitamins, or herbal products being taken and consult health care professional before taking any new medications.
- Rep: May cause fetal harm. Caution women of reproductive potential to use effective contraception during therapy and for 6 wk after final dose. Advise men with female partners of reproductive potential to use effective contraception during and for 4 mo after final dose. Advise patients to avoid breastfeeding during and for 2 wk after final dose. May impair fertility in women and men.

Evaluation/Desired Outcomes

- Improved progression-free survival.

ospemifene (os-pem-i-feen)

Osphena

Classification

Therapeutic: hormones

Pharmacologic: estrogen agonists/antagonists

Indications

Moderate to severe dyspareunia due to menopausal vulvar/vaginal atrophy. Moderate to severe vaginal dryness due to menopausal vulvar/vaginal atrophy.

Action

Has agonist (estrogen-like) effects on the endometrium of the uterus; effects are tissue-specific. **Therapeutic Effects:** Decreased dyspareunia. Decreased vaginal dryness.

Pharmacokinetics

Absorption: Well absorbed following oral administration; food enhances absorption 2–3-fold.

Distribution: Extensively distributed to tissues.

Protein Binding: >99%.

Metabolism and Excretion: Mostly metabolized by the liver via the CYP3A4 and CYP2C9 isoenzymes; 75% excreted in feces, 7% in urine as metabolites; minimal amounts excreted unchanged in urine.

Half-life: 26 hr.

TIME/ACTION PROFILE (improvement in symptoms)

ROUTE	ONSET	PEAK	DURATION
PO	within 12 wk	unknown	unknown

Contraindications/Precautions

Contraindicated in: Hypersensitivity; Undiagnosed abnormal genital bleeding; History/suspicion of estrogen-dependent cancer; History of/current thromboembolic disorder, including deep vein thrombosis (DVT), pulmonary embolism (PE), MI, or stroke; Known or suspected breast cancer; Severe hepatic impairment; OB: Pregnancy; Lactation: Lactation.

Use Cautiously in: Patients with risk factors for cardiovascular disease, arterial vascular disease, or venous thromboembolism (including hypertension, obesity, family history, tobacco use, diabetes mellitus, history of DVT/PE, or systemic lupus erythematosus); Long-term use (>4–5 yr); may ↑ risk of MI, stroke, invasive breast cancer, PE, DVT, and dementia in postmenopausal women; Women with a uterus (estrogen use without a progestin ↑ risk of endometrial cancer).

Adverse Reactions/Side Effects

CV: DVT, MI. **Derm:** ↑ sweating, hot flush. **GU:** genital/vaginal discharge. **MS:** muscle spasms. **Neuro:** STROKE. **Resp:** PE. **Misc:** HYPERSENSITIVITY REACTIONS (INCLUDING ANGIOEDEMA), MALIGNANCY (BREAST, ENDOMETRIAL).

Interactions

Drug-Drug: Fluconazole may ↑ levels and risk of toxicity; avoid concurrent use. **CYP3A4 or CYP2C9 inhibitors**, including **ketoconazole**, may ↑ levels and risk of toxicity. **Rifampin** may ↓ levels and effectiveness; avoid concurrent use. Avoid concurrent use of other **estrogens** or **estrogen agonist/antagonists** due to ↑ estrogen effects. May displace or be displaced by other **drugs that are highly protein bound**.

Route/Dosage

PO (Adults): 60 mg once daily.

Availability (generic available)

Tablets: 60 mg.

NURSING IMPLICATIONS

Assessment

- Assess amount of pain during intercourse and vaginal dryness prior to and periodically during therapy. Determine methods previously used to treat dyspareunia.
- Assess BP before and periodically during therapy.
- Monitor for hypersensitivity reactions (angioedema, urticaria, rash, pruritus). *If hypersensitivity reaction occurs,* discontinue ospemifene and provide supportive care.
- Inquire about breast health and date of last mammogram in postmenopausal women who have been on ospemifene long term (4–5 yr).

- Assess periodically for signs or symptoms of PE such as dyspnea, chest pain, cough, tachycardia, DVT such as lower extremity edema, erythema, pain with movements or walking, and dementia (changes in baseline cognition or mental status) in postmenopausal women who have been on ospemifene long term (4–5 yr). *If PE or DVT suspected,* permanently discontinue ospemifene.

Implementation

- **PO:** Administer once daily with food.

Patient/Family Teaching

- Explain purpose and side effects of ospemifene to patient. Instruct them to take medication as directed. Do not share medication with others, even if they have similar symptoms; may be harmful. Keep out of children's reach. Advise patient to read *Patient Information* sheet before starting therapy and with each Rx refill in case of changes.
- Advise patient to discuss dose and need for ospemifene every 3–6 mo as the shortest necessary duration of therapy is recommended.
- Advise women to perform monthly self breast exams and yearly breast exams by a health care provider. Mammograms should be scheduled based on patient age, risk factors, and prior mammogram results. Women should also follow yearly pelvic exams to monitor for uterine cancer.
- Advise patient to report unusual vaginal bleeding to health care provider immediately.
- Advise patient to report changes in vision or speech, sudden new severe headaches, severe pains in chest or legs with or without shortness of breath, weakness, or fatigue promptly to health care provider immediately.
- Inform patient that ospemifene may cause hot flashes, vaginal discharge, muscle spasm, and ↑ sweating.
- Patients who still have a uterus should discuss addition of progestin with health care provider.
- Instruct patient to notify health care provider of all Rx or OTC medications, vitamins, or herbal products being taken and consult health care provider before taking any new medications.
- Advise patient to notify health care provider of medication regimen before treatment or surgery.
- Caution patient that cigarette smoking, ↑ BP, high cholesterol, diabetes, and being overweight during estrogen therapy may ↑ risk of heart disease.
- Rep: May cause fetal harm. Advise women of reproductive potential to notify health care provider if pregnancy is planned or suspected and to avoid use during breastfeeding.

Evaluation/Desired Outcomes

- Decrease in pain during intercourse.
- Decreased vaginal dryness.

oxacillin, See PENICILLINS, PENICILLINASE RESISTANT.

HIGH ALERT

oxaliplatin (ox-a-li-pla-tin)

~~Eloxatin~~

Classification

Therapeutic: antineoplastics

Pharmacologic: alkylating agents

Indications

Adjuvant treatment of stage III colon cancer in patients who have undergone complete resection of the primary tumor (in combination with 5-fluorouracil and leucovorin). Advanced colorectal cancer (in combination with 5-fluorouracil and leucovorin). **Unlabeled Use:** Ovarian cancer that has progressed despite treatment with other agents.

Action

Inhibits DNA replication and transcription by incorporating platinum into normal cross-linking (cell-cycle nonspecific). **Therapeutic Effects:** Death of rapidly replicating cells, particularly malignant ones.

Pharmacokinetics

Absorption: IV administration results in complete bioavailability.

Distribution: Extensive tissue distribution.

Protein Binding: >90% (platinum).

Metabolism and Excretion: Undergoes rapid and extensive nonenzymatic biotransformation; excreted mostly by the kidneys.

Half-life: 391 hr.

TIME/ACTION PROFILE

ROUTE	ONSET	PEAK	DURATION
IV	unknown	unknown	unknown

Contraindications/Precautions

Contraindicated in: Hypersensitivity; Hypersensitivity to other platinum compounds; OB: Pregnancy; Lactation: Lactation.

Use Cautiously in: Renal impairment; HF, bradycardia, concurrent use of QT interval prolonging medications, hypokalemia, and hypomagnesemia; Rep: Women of reproductive potential and men with female partners of reproductive potential; Pedi: Safety and effectiveness not established in children; Geri: ↑ risk of adverse reactions in older adults.

Adverse Reactions/Side Effects

Adverse reactions are noted for the combination of oxaliplatin, 5-fluorouracil, and leucovorin.

CV: chest pain, edema, QT interval prolongation, thromboembolism, TORSADES DE POINTES. **EENT:** visual abnormalities. **F and E:** dehydration, hypokalemia. **GI:** diarrhea, nausea, vomiting, abdominal pain, anorexia, gastroesophageal reflux, stomatitis. **Hemat:** anemia, NEUTROPENIA, THROMBOCYTOPENIA, leukopenia. **Local:** injection site reactions. **MS:** RHABDOMYOLYSIS, back pain. **Neuro:** fatigue, neurotoxicity, POSTERIOR REVERSIBLE ENCEPHALOPATHY SYNDROME (PRES). **Resp:** cough, dyspnea, INTERSTITIAL LUNG DISEASE (ILD), PULMONARY FIBROSIS. **Misc:** HYPERSENSITIVITY REACTIONS (INCLUDING ANAPHYLAXIS), fever.

Interactions

Drug-Drug: Nephrotoxic agents may ↑ risk of nephrotoxicity. **QT interval prolonging medications**, including **Class Ia antiarrhythmics** and **Class III antiarrhythmics**, may ↑ risk of torsades de pointes.

Route/Dosage

IV (Adults): *Day 1:* 85 mg/m² with leucovorin 200 mg/m² at the same time over 2 hr, followed by 5-fluorouracil 400 mg/m² bolus over 2–4 min, then 5-fluorouracil 600 mg/m² as a 22-hr infusion. *Day 2:* Leucovorin 200 mg/m² over 2 hr, followed by 5-fluorouracil 400 mg/m² bolus over 2–4 min, then 5-fluorouracil 600 mg/m² as a 22-hr infusion. Cycle is repeated every 2 wk. Dosage ↓/alteration may be required for neurotoxicity or other serious adverse effects.

Renal Impairment

IV (Adults): *CCr <30 mL/min:* ↓ dose on Day 1 to 65 mg/m².

Availability (generic available)

Lyophilized powder for injection: 50 mg/vial, 100 mg/vial. **Solution for injection:** 5 mg/mL.

NURSING IMPLICATIONS

Assessment

- Assess for acute or delayed peripheral sensory neuropathy. *Acute onset* occurs within hr to 1–2 days of dosing, resolves within 14 days, and frequently recurs with further dosing (transient paresthesia, dysesthesia, and hypoesthesia of hands, feet, perioral area, or throat). Symptoms may be precipitated or exacerbated by exposure to cold or cold objects; avoid ice during symptoms. May also cause jaw spasm, abnormal tongue sensation, dysarthria, eye pain, and a feeling of chest pressure. *Persistent* (>14 days) causes paresthesias, dysesthesias, and hypoesthesias, but may also include deficits in proprioception that may interfere with daily activities (walking, writing, swallowing). Persistent neuropathy may occur without prior acute neuropathy and may improve upon discontinuation of oxaliplatin. **Adjuvant Therapy:** *For persistent Grade 2 neurosensory events that do not resolve,* ↓ dose to 75 mg/m². *For persistent Grade 3 neurosensory events,* consider discontinuing therapy. Do not alter 5-fluorouracil/leucovorin regimen. *For Grade 4 neuropathy,* discontinue oxaliplatin. **Advanced Colorectal Cancer:** *For persistent Grade 2 neurosensory events that do not resolve,* ↓ dose to 65 mg/m². *For persistent Grade 3 neurosensory events,* consider discontinuing therapy. Do not alter 5-fluorouracil/leucovorin regimen. *For Grade 4 neuropathy,* discontinue oxaliplatin.
- Monitor for signs/symptoms of anaphylaxis (rash, hives, swelling of lips or tongue, sudden cough). *If hypersensitivity reaction occurs,* permanently discontinue oxaliplatin and treat as indicated. Epinephrine, corticosteroids, and antihistamines should be readily available during therapy.
- Assess for signs/symptoms of pulmonary toxicity (nonproductive cough, dyspnea, crackles, radiological infiltrates). *If signs or symptoms occur,* hold and evaluate. *If pulmonary fibrosis or ILD confirmed,* permanently discontinue oxaliplatin.
- Monitor for signs/symptoms of PRES (headache, altered mental functioning, seizure, vision changes, with or without hypertension). *If PRES confirmed by MRI,* permanently discontinue oxaliplatin.
- Monitor ECG in patients with HF, bradyarrhythmias, and electrolyte abnormalities and in patients taking drugs known to prolong the QT interval.
- Monitor for signs/symptoms of rhabdomyolysis (muscle pain or weakness, dark, red-brown urine). *If rhabdomyolysis occurs,* permanently discontinue oxaliplatin.
- Monitor for signs/symptoms of GI adverse reactions (nausea, vomiting, diarrhea) during therapy. *If Grade 3 or 4 GI adverse reactions occur,* after recovery, ↓ oxaliplatin dose to 75 mg/m² and ↓ fluorouracil dose to 300 mg/m² as IV bolus and 500 mg/m² as 22-hr continuous infusion.

Lab Test Considerations

- Verify negative pregnancy test before starting therapy. Monitor WBC with differential, ALT, AST, bilirubin, and serum creatinine at baseline, before each oxaliplatin cycle and as indicated. **Adjuvant Therapy:** *For Grade 4 neutropenia or febrile neutropenia, or Grade 3 or 4 thrombocytopenia,* hold next dose until neutrophils ≥1.5 × 10⁹/L and platelets ≥75 × 10⁹/L; then ↓ oxaliplatin dose to 75 mg/m² and ↓ 5-fluorouracil dose to 300 mg/m² as IV bolus and 500 mg/m² as 22-hr infusion. **Advanced Colorectal Cancer:** *After recovery from grade 3–4 GI*

O

reactions (despite prophylactic treatment), grade 4 neutropenia, febrile neutropenia, or grade 3–4 thrombocytopenia: ↓ oxaliplatin dose to 65 mg/m² and ↓ 5-fluorouracil dose by 20% (300 mg/m² as IV bolus and 500 mg/m² as 22-hr infusion). Delay next dose until neutrophils ≥1.5 × 10⁹/L and platelets ≥75 × 10⁹/L. Monitor and correct electrolytes before starting therapy and periodically during therapy.

Implementation

- Correct hypokalemia and hypermagnesemia before starting therapy.
- Premedicate with antiemetic with or without dexamethasone. Prehydration is not required.

IV Administration

- **V** Oxaliplatin is a vesicant. If extravasation occurs, immediately stop infusion. Leave needle/cannula in place temporarily but do not flush the line. Gently aspirate extravasated solution; then remove needle/cannula. Elevate patient's extremity. Apply dry warm (if concerned for oxaliplatin-induced cold neuropathy) or dry cold compresses for 20 min 4 times day for 1–2 days. If extravasation of >40 mg of oxaliplatin occurs, consider high-dose oral dexamethasone to ↓ severity of resulting inflammatory reaction.
- **Reconstitution:** Reconstitute lyophilized powder with sterile water for injection or D5W by adding 10 mL to 50-mg vial or 20 mL to 100-mg vial. Gently swirl to dissolve. **Concentration:** 5 mg/mL. **Dilution:** Further dilute reconstituted solution in 250–500 mL of D5W. Diluted solution is stable for up to 6 hr at room temperature or up to 24 hr under refrigeration.
- **Intermittent Infusion:** Protect concentrated solution from light; do not freeze. **Dilution:** Must be further diluted with 250–500 mL of D5W. **Do not use 0.9% NaCl or any other chloride-containing solution for final solution.** Do not use aluminum needles or administration sets containing aluminum parts; aluminum may cause degradation of platinum compounds. May be stored in refrigerator for 24 hr or at room temperature for 6 hr. Diluted solution is not light-sensitive. Do not administer solutions that are discolored or contain particulates. **Concentration:** 0.2–0.6 mg/mL. **Rate:** Administer oxaliplatin simultaneously with leucovorin in separate bags via Y-line over 120 min. Prolonging infusion time to 6 hr may ↓ acute toxicities. Infusion times for fluorouracil and leucovorin do not need to change.
- Infusion line should be flushed with D5W prior to administration of other solutions or medications.
- **Y-Site Compatibility:** alemtuzumab, allopurinol, amikacin, aminocaproic acid, aminophylline, amiodarone, amphotericin B deoxycholate, amphotericin B liposomal, ampicillin, ampicillin/sulbactam, anidulafungin, argatroban, atracurium, azithromycin, aztreonam, bivalirudin, bleomycin, bumetanide, buprenorphine, butorphanol, calcium gluconate, carboplatin, caspofungin, cefazolin, cefotaxime, cefotetan, cefoxitin, ceftazidime, ceftriaxone, cefuroxime, chloramphenicol, chlorpromazine, ciprofloxacin, cisatracurium, cisplatin, clindamycin, cyclophosphamide, cyclosporine, cytarabine, dacarbazine, dactinomycin, daptomycin, daunorubicin, dexamethasone, dexmedetomidine, dexrazoxane, digoxin, diltiazem, diphenhydramine, dobutamine, docetaxel, dopamine, doxorubicin hydrochloride, doxorubicin liposomal, doxycycline, droperidol, enalaprilat, ephedrine, epinephrine, epirubicin, ertapenem, erythromycin, esmolol, etoposide, etoposide phosphate, famotidine, fentanyl, fluconazole, fludarabine, foscarnet, fosphenytoin, furosemide, gemcitabine, gemtuzumab ozogamicin, gentamicin, glycopyrrolate, granisetron, haloperidol, heparin, hetastarch, hydralazine, hydrocortisone, hydromorphone, idarubicin, ifosfamide, imipenem/cilastatin, insulin regular, irinotecan, isoproterenol, ketorolac, labetalol, leucovorin, levofloxacin, levoleucovorin calcium, lidocaine, linezolid, lorazepam, magnesium sulfate, mannitol, meperidine, meropenem, mesna, methadone, methylprednisolone, metoclopramide, metoprolol, metronidazole, midazolam, milrinone, minocycline, mitomycin, mitoxantrone, morphine, moxifloxacin, nafcillin, nalbuphine, naloxone, nicardipine, nitroglycerin, nitroprusside, norepinephrine, octreotide, ondansetron, paclitaxel, palonosetron, pemetrexed, pentamidine, phentolamine, phenylephrine, potassium acetate, potassium chloride, potassium phosphates, procainamide, prochlorperazine, promethazine, propranolol, rocuronium, sodium acetate, sodium bicarbonate, sodium phosphates, succinylcholine, sufentanil, tacrolimus, theophylline, thiotepa, tigecycline, tirofiban, tobramycin, topotecan, trimethoprim/sulfamethoxazole, vancomycin, vasopressin, vecuronium, verapamil, vinblastine, vincristine, vinorelbine, voriconazole, zidovudine, zoledronic acid.
- **Y-Site Incompatibility:** calcium chloride, cefepime, dantrolene, diazepam, sodium chloride.

Patient/Family Teaching

- Explain purpose and side effects of medication. Advise patient to read *Patient Information* before starting therapy.
- Inform patient of potential for peripheral neuropathy and potentiation by exposure to cold or cold objects. Advise patient to avoid cold drinks, use of ice in drinks or as ice packs, and to cover exposed skin prior to exposure to cold temperatures or cold objects. Caution patients to cover themselves with a blanket during infusion, avoid breathing deeply when exposed to cold air, wear warm clothing, cover mouth and nose with a scarf or pull-down ski cap to warm the air that goes to their lungs, avoid taking things from the freezer or refrigerator without

wearing gloves, drink fluids warm or at room temperature, always drink through a straw, avoid using ice chips for nausea, avoid running air conditioning at high levels in house or car, wash hands with warm water. Notify health care provider of response since last treatment before next infusion.

- Instruct patient to notify health care provider immediately if signs of allergic reactions occur.
- Instruct patient to notify health care provider immediately if signs of PRES, low blood cell counts (fever, persistent diarrhea, infection), persistent vomiting, signs of dehydration, cough or breathing difficulty, thirst, dry mouth, dizziness, ↓ urination, or signs of infection (fever, temperature of ≥100.5° F, cough that brings up mucus, chills or shivering, burning or pain on urination, pain on swallowing, sore throat, redness or swelling at IV site) occur.
- Rep: May cause fetal harm. Advise women of reproductive potential to use effective contraception during therapy and for ≥9 mo after final dose and to avoid breastfeeding during and for 3 mo after final dose. Advise men with female partners of reproductive potential to use effective contraception for 6 mo after final dose. May impair female and male fertility.

Evaluation/Desired Outcomes

- Decrease in size and spread of malignancies.

BEERS

oxazepam (ox-az-e-pam)

~~Serax~~

Classification

Therapeutic: antianxiety agents sedative/hypnotics

Pharmacologic: benzodiazepines

Schedule IV

Indications

Anxiety. Symptomatic treatment of alcohol withdrawal.

Action

Depresses the CNS, probably by potentiating GABA, an inhibitory neurotransmitter. **Therapeutic Effects:** Decreased anxiety. Diminished symptoms of alcohol withdrawal.

Pharmacokinetics

Absorption: Well absorbed following oral administration. Absorption is slower than with other benzodiazepines.

Distribution: Widely distributed. Crosses the blood-brain barrier.

Metabolism and Excretion: Metabolized by the liver to inactive compounds.

Protein Binding: 97%.

Half-life: 5–15 hr.

TIME/ACTION PROFILE (sedation)

ROUTE	ONSET	PEAK	DURATION
PO	45–90 min	unknown	6–12 hr

Contraindications/Precautions

Contraindicated in: Hypersensitivity; Cross-sensitivity with other benzodiazepines may exist; Comatose patients or those with pre-existing CNS depression; Uncontrolled severe pain; Angle-closure glaucoma; Some products contain tartrazine and should be avoided in patients with known intolerance.

Use Cautiously in: Hepatic impairment (may be preferred over some benzodiazepines due to short half-life); History of suicide attempt or substance use disorder; Severe chronic obstructive pulmonary disease; Myasthenia gravis; OB: Use late in pregnancy can result in sedation (respiratory depression, lethargy, hypotonia) and/or withdrawal symptoms (hyperreflexia, irritability, restlessness, tremors, inconsolable crying, feeding difficulties) in neonates; Lactation: Use while breastfeeding only if potential maternal benefit justifies potential risk to infant; Pedi: Children <6 yr (safety and effectiveness not established); Geri: Appears on Beers list. ↑ risk of cognitive impairment, delirium, falls, fractures, and motor vehicle accidents in older adults. If possible, avoid use in older adults.

Adverse Reactions/Side Effects

CV: tachycardia. **Derm:** rash. **EENT:** blurred vision. **GI:** constipation, diarrhea, drug-induced hepatitis, nausea, vomiting. **GU:** urinary problems. **Hemat:** leukopenia. **Neuro:** dizziness, drowsiness, confusion, depression, hangover, headache, impaired memory, paradoxical excitation, slurred speech. **Resp:** respiratory depression. **Misc:** physical dependence, psychological dependence, tolerance.

Interactions

Drug-Drug: Use with **opioids** or other **CNS depressants**, including other **benzodiazepines**, **nonbenzodiazepine sedative/hypnotics**, **anxiolytics**, **general anesthetics**, **muscle relaxants**, **antipsychotics**, and **alcohol** may cause profound sedation, respiratory depression, coma, and death; reserve concurrent use for when alternative treatment options are inadequate. May ↓ the therapeutic effectiveness of **levodopa**. **Hormonal contraceptives** or **phenytoin** may ↓ levels and effectiveness. **Theophylline** may ↓ sedative effects.

Drug-Natural Products: **Kava-kava**, **valerian**, **skullcap**, **chamomile**, or **hops** can ↑ risk of CNS depression.

O

Route/Dosage

PO (Adults): *Antianxiety agent:* 10–30 mg 3–4 times daily. *Sedative/hypnotic/management of alcohol withdrawal:* 15–30 mg 3–4 times daily.

PO (Geriatric Patients): 5 mg 1–2 times daily initially or 10 mg 3 times daily; may ↑ as needed.

Availability (generic available)

Capsules: 10 mg, 15 mg, 30 mg. **Tablets:** 🍁 10 mg, 🍁 15 mg, 🍁 30 mg.

NURSING IMPLICATIONS

Assessment

- Assess patient for anxiety and orientation, mood and behavior.
- Assess level of sedation (respiratory depression, ataxia, dizziness, slurred speech) periodically during therapy.
- Prolonged high-dose therapy may lead to psychological or physical dependence. Restrict the amount of drug available to patient. Assess regularly for continued need for treatment.
- Assess risk for addiction, abuse, or misuse prior to administration and periodically during therapy.
- Geri: Assess CNS effects and risk of falls. Institute falls prevention strategies.

Lab Test Considerations

- Monitor CBC and liver function tests periodically during prolonged therapy.
- May ↓ thyroidal uptake of ^{123}I and ^{131}I.

Implementation

- Medication should be tapered at completion of therapy (taper by 0.5 mg every 3 days). Sudden cessation of medication may lead to withdrawal (insomnia, irritability, nervousness, tremors).
- **PO:** Administer with food if GI irritation becomes a problem.

Patient/Family Teaching

- Explain purpose and side effects of medication. Advise patient to read *Patient Information* before starting therapy.
- Instruct patient to take missed doses within 1 hr; otherwise omit and resume regular schedule. Do not double or ↑ dose. If dose is less effective after a few weeks, notify health care provider.
- Caution patient not to stop taking oxazepam without consulting health care provider. Abrupt withdrawal may cause sweating, vomiting, muscle cramps, tremors, and seizures; may be life-threatening.
- Inform patient that oxazepam is usually prescribed for short-term use; do not take more than prescribed or for a longer period than prescribed.
- Advise patient that oxazepam is a drug with known abuse potential. Protect it from theft, and never give to anyone other than the individual for whom it was prescribed. Store out of sight and reach of children and in a location not accessible by others.
- Teach other methods to ↓ anxiety, such as exercise, support group, relaxation techniques.
- May cause drowsiness or dizziness. Caution patient to avoid driving or other activities requiring alertness until response to medication is known.
- Advise patient to notify health care provider of all Rx or OTC medications, vitamins, or herbal products being taken and to consult health care provider before taking other medications.
- Advise patient to avoid the use of alcohol or other CNS depressants, including opioids, concurrently with lorazepam; may cause respiratory depression and overdose. Instruct patient to consult health care provider before taking Rx, OTC, or herbal products concurrently with this medication.
- Geri: Instruct patient and family how to ↓ falls risk at home.
- Advise patient to notify health care provider of medication regimen prior to treatment or surgery.
- Emphasize the importance of follow-up exams to monitor effectiveness of medication.
- Rep: May cause fetal harm. Advise women of reproductive potential to use a nonhormonal method of contraception during use and to notify health care provider if pregnancy is planned or suspected or if breastfeeding. Monitor infants exposed to oxazepam during 2nd and 3rd trimester or immediately prior to or during childbirth for ↓ fetal movement and/or fetal heart rate variability, floppy infant syndrome, dependence, and symptoms of withdrawal (hypertonia, hyperreflexia, hypoventilation, irritability, tremors, diarrhea, vomiting); may occur shortly after delivery up to 3 wk after birth. Monitor breastfed infants for sedation and poor sucking. Encourage pregnant patients to enroll in the North American Antiepileptic Drug Pregnancy Registry by calling 1-888-233-2334; information is available at www.aedpregnancyregistry.org.

Evaluation/Desired Outcomes

- Decreased sense of anxiety.
- Increased ability to cope.
- Prevention or relief of acute agitation, tremor, and hallucinations during alcohol withdrawal.

BEERS

OXcarbazepine

(ox-kar-**baz**-e-peen)

Oxtellar XR, Trileptal

Classification

Therapeutic: anticonvulsants

Pharmacologic: carbamazepine analogues

Indications

Partial seizures (as monotherapy or adjunctive therapy). **Unlabeled Use:** Trigeminal neuralgia.

Action

Blocks sodium channels in neural membranes, stabilizing hyperexcitable states, inhibiting repetitive neuronal firing, and decreasing propagation of synaptic impulses. **Therapeutic Effects:** Decreased incidence of seizures.

Pharmacokinetics

Absorption: Rapidly absorbed after oral administration and rapidly converted to the active 10-hydroxy metabolite (MHD).
Distribution: Extensively distributed to tissues.
Metabolism and Excretion: Extensively converted to the active metabolite, MHD, which is then primarily excreted by the kidneys.
Half-life: *Oxcarbazepine:* 2 hr; *MHD:* 9 hr.

TIME/ACTION PROFILE (plasma concentrations)

ROUTE	ONSET	PEAK	DURATION
PO	PO	rapid	4.5 hr†

† Steady-state levels of MHD are reached after 2–3 days during twice-daily dosing.

Contraindications/Precautions

Contraindicated in: Hypersensitivity to oxcarbazepine, carbamazepine, or eslicarbazepine.
Use Cautiously in: All patients (may ↑ risk of suicidal thoughts/behaviors); Renal impairment (↓ dose if CCr <30 mL/min); Severe hepatic impairment; Rep: Women of reproductive potential; OB: May be teratogenic (associated with oral clefts and cardiac abnormalities); levels of active metabolites may gradually ↓ during pregnancy, which may ↑ seizure risk; use during pregnancy only if potential maternal benefit justifies potential fetal risk; Lactation: Use while breastfeeding only if potential maternal benefit justifies potential risk to infant; Pedi: Safety and effectiveness not established in children <2 yr (immediate release) or <6 yr (extended release); Geri: Appears on Beers list. May worsen or cause syndrome of inappropriate antidiuretic hormone (SIADH) secretion in older adults. Use with caution in older adults and closely monitor sodium concentrations when starting therapy or ↑ dose.
Exercise Extreme Caution in: Patients positive for HLA-B*1502 alleles (unless benefits clearly outweigh the risks) (↑ risk of serious skin reactions).

Adverse Reactions/Side Effects

Derm: acne, DRUG REACTION WITH EOSINOPHILIA AND SYSTEMIC SYMPTOMS (DRESS), rash, STEVENS-JOHNSON SYNDROME (SJS), TOXIC EPIDERMAL NECROLYSIS (TEN), urticaria. **EENT:** abnormal vision, diplopia, nystagmus. **Endo:** SIADH, hypothyroidism. **F and E:** ↑ thirst, hyponatremia. **GI:** abdominal pain, nausea, vomiting, dyspepsia. **Hemat:** lymphadenopathy. **Neuro:** ataxia, dizziness, drowsiness, gait disturbances, headache, tremor, vertigo, cognitive symptoms, SEIZURES, SUICIDAL THOUGHTS. **Misc:** hypersensitivity reactions.

Interactions

Drug-Drug: May ↑ levels and risk of toxicity of **CYP2C19 substrates**, including **phenytoin**, when used at doses greater than 1200 mg/day; may need to ↓ dose of phenytoin. May ↓ levels and effectiveness of **CYP3A4 substrates**, including **hormonal contraceptives**. **Carbamazepine**, **phenobarbital**, **phenytoin**, and **rifampin** may ↓ levels and effectiveness; monitor MHD levels during titration period; may need to adjust dose of oxcarbazepine.

Route/Dosage

Immediate-release tablets and oral suspension can be interchanged at equal doses.
PO (Adults): *Adjunctive therapy (immediate release):* 300 mg twice daily; may ↑ by up to 600 mg/day at weekly intervals up to 1200 mg/day (up to 2400 mg/day may be needed); *Conversion to monotherapy (immediate release):* 300 mg twice daily; may ↑ by 600 mg/day at weekly intervals, while other antiepileptic drugs are tapered over 3–6 wk; dose of oxcarbazepine should be ↑ up to 2400 mg/day over a period of 2–4 wk; *Initiation of monotherapy (immediate release):* 300 mg twice daily; ↑ by 300 mg/day every 3rd day, up to 1200 mg/day. Maximum maintenance dose should be achieved over 2–4 wk; *Adjunctive therapy or monotherapy (extended release):* 600 mg once daily for 1 wk; may ↑ by 600 mg/day at weekly intervals up to 1200–2400 mg once daily; *Concurrent use of strong CYP3A4 inducer (carbamazepine, phenobarbital, phenytoin, rifampin) (extended release):* Consider initiating therapy with 900 mg once daily.
PO (Children 2–16 yr): *Adjunctive therapy (immediate release):* 4–5 mg/kg twice daily (up to 600 mg/day); ↑ over 2 wk to achieve 900 mg/day in patients 20–29 kg, 1200 mg/day in patients 29.1–39 kg, and 1800 mg/day in patients >39 kg (range 6–51 mg/kg/day). In patients <20 kg, initial dose of 16–20 mg/kg/day may be used not to exceed 60 mg/kg/day. *Conversion to monotherapy (immediate release):* 8–10 mg/kg/day given twice daily; may ↑ by 10 mg/kg/day at weekly intervals, whereas other antiepileptic drugs are tapered over 3–6 wk; dose of oxcarbazepine should be ↑ up to 600–900 mg/day in patients ≤20 kg, 900–1200 mg/day in patients 25–30 kg, 900–1500 mg/day in patients 35–40 kg, 1200–1500 mg/day in patients 45 kg, 1200–1800 mg/day in patients 50–55 kg, 1200–2100 mg/day in patients 60–65 kg, and 1500–2100 mg/

O

day in patients 70 kg. Maximum maintenance dose should be achieved over 2–4 wk.

PO (Children 6–17 yr): *Adjunctive therapy or monotherapy (extended release):* 8–10 mg/kg once daily (up to 600 mg/day) for 1 wk; may ↑ by 8–10 mg/kg/day at weekly intervals over 2–3 wk to achieve 900 mg/day in patients 20–29 kg, 1200 mg/day in patients 29.1–39 kg, and 1800 mg/day in patients >39 kg; *Concurrent use of strong CYP3A4 inducer (carbamazepine, phenobarbital, phenytoin, rifampin) (extended release):* Consider initiating therapy with 12–15 mg/kg (max dose = 900 mg) once daily.

Renal Impairment

PO (Adults): *CCr<30 mL/min (immediate and extended release)*. Initiate therapy at 300 mg/day and ↑ slowly to achieve desired response.

Availability (generic available)

Immediate-release tablets: 150 mg, 300 mg, 600 mg. **Extended-release tablets:** 150 mg, 300 mg, 600 mg. **Oral suspension (lemon flavor):** 300 mg/5 mL.

NURSING IMPLICATIONS

Assessment

- Monitor closely for notable changes in behavior that could indicate the emergence or worsening of suicidal thoughts or behavior or depression.
- **Seizures:** Assess frequency, location, duration, and characteristics of seizure activity. Hyponatremia may ↑ frequency and severity of seizures. Implement seizure precautions as indicated.
- Monitor for CNS changes. May manifest as cognitive symptoms (psychomotor slowing, difficulty with concentration, speech or language problems), somnolence or fatigue, or coordination abnormalities (ataxia, gait disturbances).
- Monitor for skin reactions (rash, erythema, urticaria, pruritus, fever, blistering). Patients with HLA-B*1502 alleles are at ↑ risk for SJS and TEN. *If skin reactions occur,* discontinue oxcarbazepine.
- Monitor for signs/symptoms of DRESS (fever, rash, lymphadenopathy, facial swelling), associated with involvement of other organ systems (hepatitis, nephritis, hematologic abnormalities, myocarditis, myositis) during therapy. May resemble an acute viral infection. Eosinophilia is often present. *If signs/symptoms of DRESS occur,* discontinue oxcarbazepine.

Lab Test Considerations

- Monitor ECG and serum electrolytes before and periodically during therapy. May cause hyponatremia; usually occurs during the 1st 3 mo of therapy. May require dose ↓, fluid restriction, or discontinuation of therapy. Sodium levels return to normal within a few days of discontinuation.

Implementation

- Do not confuse oxcarbazepine with carbamazepine or oxaprozin.
- **PO:** Administer twice daily with or without food.
- Administer extended-release tablets on an empty stomach, >1 hr before or 2 hr after meals. ***DNC:*** Swallow extended-release tablets whole; do not crush, break, or chew.
- Shake oral suspension for ≥10 sec. Withdraw dose using oral dosing syringe supplied by manufacturer. May be mixed in a small glass of water just before administration or swallowed directly from syringe. Rinse syringe with warm water and allow to dry. Discard any unused portion after 7 wk of opening the bottle.

Patient/Family Teaching

- Explain purpose and side effects of medication. Advise patient to read *Patient Information* before starting therapy. Instruct patient to take oxcarbazepine in equally spaced doses as directed. Take missed doses as soon as possible but not just before next dose; do not double dose. Notify health care provider if >1 dose is missed. Medication should be gradually discontinued to prevent seizures.
- Instruct patient to notify health care provider of all Rx or OTC medications, vitamins, or herbal products being taken and to consult with health care provider before taking other medications. Advise patient not to take alcohol or other CNS depressants, including opioids, concurrently with this medication.
- May cause dizziness, drowsiness, or CNS changes. Advise patients to avoid driving or other activities requiring alertness until response to medication is known. Do not resume driving until health care provider gives clearance based on control of seizure disorder.
- Advise patient and caregiver to notify health care provider if thoughts about suicide or dying, attempts to commit suicide, new or worse depression, new or worse anxiety, feeling very agitated or restless, panic attacks, trouble sleeping, new or worse irritability, acting aggressive, being angry or violent, acting on dangerous impulses, an extreme ↑ in activity and talking, or other unusual changes in behavior or mood occur.
- Instruct patient to notify health care provider of medication regimen before treatment or surgery.
- Advise patient to carry identification describing disease and medication regimen at all times.
- Rep: Advise women of reproductive potential to use an additional nonhormonal method of contraception during therapy and until next menstrual period. Instruct patient to notify health care provider if pregnancy is planned or suspected. Encourage patients who become pregnant to

enroll in the North American Antiepileptic Drug Pregnancy Registry by calling 1-888-233-2334 or visiting www.aedpregnancyregistry.org. Enrollment must be done by patients themselves.

Evaluation/Desired Outcomes

- Decreased incidence of seizures.

oxiconazole, See ANTIFUNGALS (TOPICAL).

oxyBUTYnin (ox-i-byoo-ti-nin)

oxyBUTYnin (oral) ~~Ditropan, Ditropan XL~~

oxyBUTYnin (transdermal gel)
Gelnique

oxyBUTYnin (transdermal patch)
Oxytrol, Oxytrol for Women

Classification
Therapeutic: urinary tract antispasmodics
Pharmacologic: anticholinergics

Indications

Urinary symptoms that may be associated with neurogenic bladder, including: Frequent urination, Urgency, Nocturia, Urge incontinence. Overactive bladder with symptoms of urge incontinence, urgency, and frequency.

Action

Inhibits the action of acetylcholine at postganglionic receptors. Has direct spasmolytic action on smooth muscle, including smooth muscle lining the GU tract, without affecting vascular smooth muscle. **Therapeutic Effects:** Increased bladder capacity. Delayed desire to void. Decreased urge incontinence, urinary urgency, and frequency and decreased number of urinary accidents associated with overactive bladder.

Pharmacokinetics

Absorption: Rapidly absorbed following oral administration, but undergoes extensive first-pass metabolism. Transdermal absorption occurs by passive diffusion through intact skin and bypasses the first-pass effect.
Distribution: Highly bound (>99%) to plasma proteins. Widely distributed.
Metabolism and Excretion: Extensively metabolized by the liver via the CYP3A4 isoenzyme; one metabolite is pharmacologically active; metabolites are renally excreted with negligible (<0.1%) excretion of unchanged drug.
Half-life: 7–8 hr (oral and patch); 30–64 hr (gel).

TIME/ACTION PROFILE (urinary spasmolytic effect)

ROUTE	ONSET	PEAK	DURATION
PO	30–60 min	3–6 hr	6–10 hr (up to 24 hr with ER tablet)
TD-patch	within 24 hr	36 hr	3–4 days

Contraindications/Precautions

Contraindicated in: Hypersensitivity; Uncontrolled angle-closure glaucoma; Intestinal obstruction or atony; Urinary retention.
Use Cautiously in: Renal impairment; Hepatic impairment; Bladder outflow obstruction; Ulcerative colitis; Benign prostatic hyperplasia; Cardiovascular disease; Reflux esophagitis or gastrointestinal obstructive disorders; Patients with dementia receiving acetylcholinesterase inhibitors; Myasthenia gravis; Parkinson's disease (may worsen symptoms); Autonomic neuropathy (may worsen ↓ GI motility); OB: Safety not established in pregnancy; Lactation: Safety not established in breastfeeding; Pedi: Safety not established in children <18 yr (patch and gel) or <5 yr (oral); Geri: Poorly tolerated in older adults due to anticholinergic effects. Initiate treatment at lower doses.

Adverse Reactions/Side Effects

CV: chest pain, edema, tachycardia. **Derm:** ↓ sweating, *transdermal only:* application site reactions, hot flushes, pruritus. **EENT:** blurred vision, hoarseness. **GI:** <u>constipation</u>, <u>dry mouth</u>, <u>nausea</u>, abdominal pain, anorexia, diarrhea, dysphagia. **GU:** <u>urinary retention</u>. **Metab:** hyperthermia. **Neuro:** <u>dizziness</u>, <u>drowsiness</u>, agitation, confusion, hallucinations, headache. **Misc:** HYPERSENSITIVITY REACTIONS (INCLUDING ANAPHYLAXIS AND ANGIOEDEMA).

Interactions

Drug-Drug: ↑ anticholinergic effects with other **agents having anticholinergic properties**, including **amantadine**, **antidepressants**, **phenothiazines**, **disopyramide**, and **haloperidol**. Additive CNS depression with other **CNS depressants**, including **alcohol**, **antihistamines**, **antidepressants**, **opioids**, and **sedative/hypnotics**. **Ketoconazole**, **itraconazole**, **erythromycin**, and **clarithromycin** may ↑ levels and risk of toxicity. May ↓ the GI promotility effects of **metoclopramide**.

Route/Dosage

PO (Adults): *Immediate-release tablets:* 5 mg 2–3 times daily; not to exceed 5 mg 4 times daily; may start with 2.5 mg 2–3 times daily in older adults. *Extended-release tablets:* 5–10 mg once daily; may ↑ as needed (in 5-mg increments) up to maximum dose of 30 mg/day.

PO (Children >5 yr): *Immediate-release tablets:* 5 mg 2–3 times daily; not to exceed 15 mg/day. *Extended-release tablets (children ≥6 yr):* 5 mg once daily; may ↑ as needed (in 5-mg increments) up to maximum dose of 20 mg/day.
PO (Children 1–5 yr): 0.2 mg/kg/dose 2–3 times daily.
Transdermal (Adults): *Patch:* Apply one 3.9-mg system twice weekly (every 3–4 days); *Gel:* Apply contents of one sachet once daily.

Availability (generic available)

Immediate-release tablets: 2.5 mg, 5 mg.
Extended-release tablets: 5 mg, 10 mg, 15 mg.
Oral solution: 5 mg/5 mL. **Transdermal gel:** 10%.
Transdermal patch: 3.9 mg/24 hr[OTC].

NURSING IMPLICATIONS

Assessment

- Monitor voiding pattern, intake and output ratios, and for bladder distention prior to and periodically during therapy. Catheterization may be used to assess postvoid residual. Assess bladder function with cystometry prior to prescription of oxybutynin.
- Assess for CNS anticholinergic effects during therapy. *If symptoms (headache, dizziness, somnolence, confusion, hallucinations) occur,* consider discontinuation of oxybutynin.

Implementation

- Do not confuse oxybutynin with oxycodone, Oxycontin, or oxymorphone.
- **PO:** Immediate-release tabs should be administered on an empty stomach; ER tablets may be given with or without food. ***DNC:*** Extended-release tablets should be swallowed whole; do not break, crush, or chew.
- **Transdermal patch:** Apply patch to dry, intact skin on abdomen, hip, or buttock twice weekly (every 3 or 4 days). Application site should be rotated with each new patch to avoid reapplication to the same site within 7 days. Do not divide or cut the patch into pieces; do not use if damaged.
- **Transdermal gel:** Apply clear, colorless gel once daily to intact skin on abdomen (avoid area around navel), upper arms/shoulders, or thighs until dry. Rotate sites; do not use same site on consecutive days.

Patient/Family Teaching

- Instruct patient to take oxybutynin as directed. Take missed doses as soon as remembered unless almost time for next dose. Advise patient to read *Information for the Patient* prior to beginning therapy and with each Rx refill in case of new information.
- May cause drowsiness or blurred vision. Advise patient to avoid driving and other activities requiring alertness until response to medication is known.
- Advise patient to avoid concurrent use of alcohol and other CNS depressants while taking this medication.
- Instruct patient that frequent rinsing of mouth, good oral hygiene, and sugarless gum or candy may ↓ dry mouth. Notify health care professional if mouth dryness persists >2 wk.
- Advise patient to stop taking oxybutynin and notify health care professional immediately if signs of angioedema or anaphylaxis (swelling of face, tongue, or throat; rash; dyspnea) occur.
- Inform patient that oxybutynin ↓ the body's ability to perspire. Avoid strenuous activity in a warm environment because overheating may occur.
- Advise patient to notify health care professional if urinary retention occurs or if constipation persists. Discuss methods of preventing constipation, such as ↑ dietary fiber, water intake, and mobility.
- Advise patient to notify health care professional of all Rx or OTC medications, vitamins, or herbal products being taken and to consult with health care professional before taking other medications.
- Rep: Advise women of reproductive potential to notify health care professional if pregnancy is planned or suspected or if breastfeeding.
- Discuss need for continued medical follow-up. Periodic cystometry may be used to evaluate effectiveness. Ophthalmic exams should be performed periodically to detect glaucoma, especially in patients over 40 yr of age.
- **Transdermal patch:** Instruct patient on correct application and disposal of patch. Open pouch by tearing along arrows; apply immediately. Apply ½ patch to skin by removing ½ protective cover and applying to skin. Apply 2nd half by bending in half and rolling patch onto skin while removing protective liner. Press patch firmly in place.
- Remove slowly; fold in half, sticky sides together; and discard. Wash site with mild soap and water or a small amount of baby oil.
- Advise patient referred for MRI to remove patch prior to test and give directions for replacing patch.
- **Transdermal gel:** Instruct patient on correct application of oxybutynin gel. Do not apply to recently shaved skin; skin with rashes; or areas treated with lotions, oils, or powders. May be used with sunscreen. Wash area with mild soap and water and dry completely before applying. Tear packet open just before use and squeeze entire contents into hand or directly onto application site. Amount of gel will be size of a nickel. Gently rub into skin until dry. Wash hands immediately following application. Avoid application near open fire or when smoking; medication is flammable. Do not shower, bathe, swim, exercise, or immerse the application site in water for 1 hr after application. Cover application site with clothing if close skin-to-skin contact at application site is anticipated.

- Instruct patient to discontinue oxybutynin if skin sensitivity occurs.

Evaluation/Desired Outcomes

- Relief of bladder spasm and associated symptoms (frequency, urgency, nocturia, incontinence) in patients with a neurogenic or overactive bladder.

REMS HIGH ALERT

oxyCODONE (ox-i-koe-done)

OxyCONTIN, ✱ Oxy IR, ✱ OxyNEO, Roxicodone, Roxybond, ✱ Supeudol, Xtampza ER

Classification

Therapeutic: opioid analgesics

Pharmacologic: opioid agonists, opioid agonists/nonopioid analgesic combinations

Schedule II

Indications

Moderate to severe pain. Pain severe enough to require daily, around-the-clock long-term opioid treatment and for which alternative treatment options are inadequate (extended release [ER]) (children ≥11 yr should be tolerating a minimum opioid dose of ≥20 mg of oxycodone or equivalent for ≥5 days before initiating ER oxycodone therapy).

Action

Binds to opiate receptors in the CNS. Alters the perception of and response to painful stimuli, while producing generalized CNS depression. **Therapeutic Effects:** Decreased pain.

Pharmacokinetics

Absorption: Well absorbed from the GI tract.
Distribution: Widely distributed to tissues.
Protein Binding: 38–45%
Metabolism and Excretion: Mostly metabolized by the liver by the CYP3A4 isoenzyme and to a lesser extent by the CYP2D6 isoenzyme.
Half-life: 2–3 hr.

TIME/ACTION PROFILE (analgesic effects)

ROUTE	ONSET	PEAK	DURATION
PO	10–15 min	60–90 min	3–6 hr
PO-ER†	10–15 min	3 hr	12 hr

† Extended release.

Contraindications/Precautions

Contraindicated in: Hypersensitivity; Some products contain alcohol or bisulfites and should be avoided in patients with known intolerance or hypersensitivity; Significant respiratory depression; Paralytic ileus; Acute or severe bronchial asthma; Acute, mild, intermittent, or postoperative pain (extended release [ER])).
Use Cautiously in: Personal or family history of substance use disorder or mental illness; Head trauma; ↑ intracranial pressure; Severe renal impairment; Severe hepatic impairment; Hypothyroidism; Adrenal insufficiency; Seizure disorders; Undiagnosed abdominal pain; Prostatic hyperplasia; Difficulty swallowing or GI disorders that may predispose patient to obstruction (↑ risk for GI obstruction); OB: Avoid chronic use; prolonged use of opioids during pregnancy can result in neonatal opioid withdrawal syndrome; Lactation: Use while breastfeeding only if potential maternal benefit justifies potential risk to infant; Pedi: Children <11 yr (safety and effectiveness of ER products not established); Geri: ↑ risk of respiratory depression in older adults; initial dose ↓ recommended.

Adverse Reactions/Side Effects

CV: orthostatic hypotension. **Derm:** flushing, sweating. **EENT:** blurred vision, diplopia, miosis. **Endo:** adrenal insufficiency. **GI:** constipation, choking, dry mouth, GI obstruction, nausea, vomiting. **GU:** urinary retention. **Neuro:** confusion, sedation, dizziness, dysphoria, euphoria, floating feeling, hallucinations, headache, unusual dreams. **Resp:** RESPIRATORY DEPRESSION (INCLUDING CENTRAL SLEEP APNEA AND SLEEP-RELATED HYPOXEMIA). **Misc:** allodynia, opioid-induced hyperalgesia, physical dependence, psychological dependence, tolerance.

Interactions

Drug-Drug: Use with caution in patients receiving MAO inhibitors; may result in unpredictable reactions; ↓ initial dose of oxycodone to 25% of usual dose. Use with **benzodiazepines** or other **CNS depressants**, including other **opioids**, **nonbenzodiazepine sedative/hypnotics**, **anxiolytics**, **general anesthetics**, **muscle relaxants**, **antipsychotics**, and **alcohol**, may cause profound sedation, respiratory depression, coma, and death; reserve concurrent use for when alternative treatment options are inadequate. **Mixed agonist/antagonist analgesics**, including **nalbuphine** or **butorphanol**, and **partial agonist analgesics**, including **buprenorphine**, may ↓ oxycodone's analgesic effects and/or precipitate opioid withdrawal in physically dependent patients. **CYP3A4 inhibitors**, including **ritonavir**, **ketoconazole**, **itraconazole**, **fluconazole**, **clarithromycin**, **erythromycin**, **nefazodone**, **diltiazem**, **verapamil**, **nelfinavir**, and **fosamprenavir**, ↑ levels and risk of opioid toxicity; careful monitoring during initiation, dose changes, or discontinuation of the inhibitor is recommended. **CYP3A4 inducers**, including **carbamazepine**, **efavirenz**, **corticosteroids**, **modafinil**, **nevirapine**, **oxcarbazepine**, **phenobarbital**,

O

phenytoin, **rifabutin**, or **rifampin**, may ↓ levels and analgesia; if inducers are discontinued or dosage ↓, patients should be monitored for signs of opioid toxicity, and necessary dose adjustments should be made. **CYP2D6 inhibitors** may ↑ levels and risk of opioid toxicity. Drugs that affect serotonergic neurotransmitter systems, including **tricyclic antidepressants**, **SSRIs**, **SNRIs**, **MAO inhibitors**, **TCAs**, **tramadol**, **trazodone**, **mirtazapine**, **5-HT_3 receptor antagonists**, **linezolid**, **methylene blue**, and **triptans**, may ↑ risk of serotonin syndrome.

Route/Dosage

Larger doses may be required during chronic therapy. ER capsules are NOT bioequivalent to ER tablets.
PO (Adults ≥50 kg): *Opioid-naive patients:* 5–10 mg (immediate release [IR]) every 3–4 hr initially, as needed. Once optimal analgesia is obtained, patients with chronic pain may be converted to an equivalent 24-hr dose given in 2 divided doses as ER tablets every 12 hr.
PO (Adults <50 kg): *Opioid-naive patients:* 0.2 mg/kg (IR) every 3–4 hr initially, as needed. Once optimal analgesia is obtained, patients with chronic pain may be converted to an equivalent 24-hr dose given in 2 divided doses as ER tablets every 12 hr.
PO (Children ≥11 yr): 0.05–0.15 mg/kg (IR) every 4–6 hr as needed, as immediate-release product. Once optimal analgesia is obtained, patients with chronic pain may be converted to an equivalent 24-hr dose given in 2 divided doses as ER tablets every 12 hr.
Rect (Adults): 10–40 mg 3–4 times daily initially, as needed.

Hepatic Impairment

PO (Adults): ↓ initial dose by 50–66%.

Availability (generic available)

Immediate-release tablets (Roxicodone): 5 mg, 10 mg, 15 mg, 20 mg, 30 mg. **Immediate-release tablets (abuse deterrent) (Roxybond):** 5 mg, 15 mg, 30 mg. **Immediate-release capsules:** 5 mg. **Oral solution:** 5 mg/5 mL, 100 mg/5 mL (concentrated). **Extended-release tablets (abuse deterrent) (Oxycontin):** 10 mg, 15 mg, 20 mg, 30 mg, 40 mg, 60 mg, 80 mg. **Extended-release capsules (abuse deterrent) (Xtampza ER):** 9 mg, 13.5 mg, 18 mg, 27 mg, 36 mg.
Rectal suppositories: 🍁 10 mg, 🍁 20 mg. ***In combination with:*** aspirin (generic only), acetaminophen (Endocet, Nalocet, Percocet, Prolate); see Appendix N.

NURSING IMPLICATIONS

Assessment

- Assess type, location, and intensity of pain prior to and 1 hr (peak) after administration. When titrating opioid doses, ↑ of 25–50% should be administered until there is either a 50% ↓ in the patient's pain rating on a numerical or visual analog scale or the patient reports satisfactory pain relief. A repeat dose can be safely administered at the time of the peak if previous dose is ineffective and side effects are minimal.
- Patients taking ER tablets may also be given supplemental short-acting opioid doses for breakthrough pain.
- An equianalgesic chart (see Appendix I) should be used when changing routes or when changing from one opioid to another.
- Assess BP, HR, and respiratory rate before and periodically during administration. If respiratory rate <10/min, assess level of sedation. Physical stimulation may be sufficient to prevent significant hypoventilation. Dose may need to be ↓ by 25–50%. Initial drowsiness will ↓ with continued use. Monitor for respiratory depression, especially during initiation or following dose ↑; serious, life-threatening, or fatal respiratory depression may occur. May cause sleep-related breathing disorders (central sleep apnea, sleep-related hypoxemia).
- Geri: Pedi: Assess older adults and pediatric patients frequently; more sensitive to the effects of opioid analgesics and may experience side effects and respiratory complications more frequently.
- Prolonged use may lead to physical and psychological dependence and tolerance. This should not prevent patient from receiving adequate analgesia. Patients who receive oxycodone for pain rarely develop psychological dependence. Progressively higher doses may be required to relieve pain with long-term therapy; may ↑ risk of overdose. Prolonged use of opioids should be reserved for patients whose pain remains severe enough to require them and alternative treatment options continue to be inadequate. Many acute pain conditions treated in the outpatient setting require no more than a few days of an opioid pain medicine.
- Assess bowel function routinely. Prevention of constipation should be instituted with ↑ intake of fluids and bulk and laxatives to minimize constipating effects. Stimulant laxatives should be administered routinely if opioid use exceeds 2–3 days, unless contraindicated. Consider drugs for opioid induced constipation.
- Assess risk for opioid addiction, abuse, or misuse prior to administration. Abuse or misuse of extended-release preparations by crushing, chewing, snorting, or injecting dissolved product will result in uncontrolled delivery of oxycodone and can result in overdose and death. Abuse deterrent: *Xtampza ER* and *Oxycontin* are abuse deterrent formulations that are difficult to crush and if crushed result in a gel.

Lab Test Considerations

- May ↑ amylase and lipase.

Toxicity and Overdose

- If an opioid antagonist is required to reverse respiratory depression or coma, naloxone is the antidote. Dilute the 0.4-mg ampule of naloxone in 10 mL of 0.9% NaCl and administer 0.5 mL (0.02 mg) by IV push every 2 min. For children and patients weighing <40 kg, dilute 0.1 mg of naloxone in 10 mL of 0.9% NaCl for a concentration of 10 mcg/mL and administer 0.5 mcg/kg every 2 min. Titrate dose to avoid withdrawal, seizures, and severe pain.

Implementation

- ***High Alert:*** Accidental overdose of opioid analgesics has resulted in fatalities. Before administering, clarify all ambiguous orders. Pedi: Medication errors with opioid analgesics are common in pediatric patients; calculate doses carefully. Use appropriate measuring devices.
- Do not confuse short-acting oxycodone with long-acting Oxycontin. Do not confuse oxycodone with hydrocodone, oxybutynin, or oxymorphone. Do not confuse Oxycontin with MS Contin, oxybutynin, oxymorphone, or oxytocin.
- Explain therapeutic value of medication prior to administration to enhance the analgesic effect.
- Regularly administered doses may be more effective than as needed administration. Analgesic is more effective if given before pain becomes severe.
- Coadministration with nonopioid analgesics may have additive analgesic effects and may permit lower doses.
- When converting from IR to ER oxycodone, administer total daily oral oxycodone dose once daily; dose of ER product can be titrated every 3–4 days (see Appendix I). To convert from another opioid to ER oxycodone, convert to total daily dose of oxycodone and then administer 50% of this dose as ER oxycodone once daily; can then titrate dose every 3–4 days.
- Oxycodone should be discontinued gradually after long-term use to prevent withdrawal symptoms. For patients on long-acting agents who are physically opioid-dependent, initiate the taper by a small enough increment (no greater than 10–25% of total daily dose) to avoid withdrawal symptoms, and proceed with dose-lowering at an interval of every 2–4 wk. Patients who have been taking opioids for briefer periods of time may tolerate a more rapid taper. Monitor frequently to manage pain and withdrawal symptoms (restlessness; lacrimation; rhinorrhea; yawning; perspiration; chills; myalgia; mydriasis; irritability; anxiety; backache; joint pain; weakness; abdominal cramps; insomnia; nausea; anorexia; vomiting; diarrhea; ↑ BP, respiratory rate, or HR). If withdrawal symptoms occur, pause the taper for a period of time or ↑ the dose of opioid analgesic to the previous dose, and then proceed with a slower taper. Also, monitor patients for changes in mood, emergence of suicidal thoughts, or use of other substances. A multimodal approach to pain management may optimize the treatment of chronic pain, as well as assist with the successful tapering of the opioid analgesic.
- **PO:** May be administered with food or milk to minimize GI irritation.
- Administer solution with properly calibrated measuring device.
- **Extended Release:** ***DNC:*** Take one tablet at a time. Swallow ER tablet whole; do not crush, break, or chew. Taking broken, chewed, crushed, or dissolved ER tablets may lead to rapid release and absorption of a potentially fatal dose of oxycodone.
- Advise patients not to presoak, lick, or wet ER tablets prior to placing in the mouth. Take each tablet with enough water to ensure complete swallowing immediately after placing in mouth. Dose of ER preparations should be based on 24-hr opioid requirement determined with short-acting opioids then converted to extended-release form.
- ER oxycodone capsules (*Xtampza ER*) are not equivalent to ER oxycodone tablets (*Oxycontin*).
- ***REMS:*** FDA strongly encourages health care providers to complete a REMS-compliant education program that includes all the elements of the FDA Education *Blueprint for Health Care Providers Involved in the Management or Support of Patients with Pain,* available at www.fda.gov/OpioidAnalgesicREMSBlueprint. Information on programs can be found at 1-800-503-0784 or www.opioidanalgesicrems.com.
- Discuss availability of naloxone for emergency treatment of opioid overdose with the patient and caregiver and assess the potential need for access to naloxone, both when initiating and renewing therapy, especially if patient has household members (including children) or other close contacts at risk for accidental exposure or overdose. Consider prescribing naloxone, based on the patient's risk factors for overdose, such as concurrent use of CNS depressants, a history of opioid use disorder, or prior opioid overdose. However, the presence of risk factors for overdose should not prevent the proper management of pain in any patient.

Patient/Family Teaching

- Explain purpose and side effects of oxycodone to patient. Instruct them to take medication as directed and when to ask for pain medication. Do not share medication with others, even if they have similar

O

symptoms; may be harmful. Keep out of children's reach. Advise patient to read *Patient Information* before starting and with each Rx refill in case of changes.

- ***REMS:*** Instruct patient on how and when to ask for and take pain medication. Do not stop taking without discussing with health care provider; may cause withdrawal symptoms if discontinued abruptly after prolonged use. Do not ↑ doses without discussing with health care provider; may lead to overdose. Discuss safe use, risks, and proper storage and disposal of opioid analgesics with patients and caregivers with each Rx. The Patient Counseling Guide is available at www.fda.gov/OpioidAnalgesicREMSPCG.
- Advise patient that oxycodone is a drug with known abuse potential. Protect it from theft, and never give to anyone other than the individual for whom it was prescribed. Store out of sight and reach of children, and in a location not accessible by others.
- Educate patients and caregivers on how to recognize respiratory depression and emphasize the importance of calling 911 or getting emergency medical help right away in the event of a known or suspected overdose. Inform patients and caregivers about various ways to obtain naloxone as permitted by individual state naloxone dispensing and prescribing requirements or guidelines (Rx, direct from pharmacist, or state programs). OTC naloxone nasal spray is available at pharmacies nationwide for overdose or accidental ingestion.
- Advise patient to notify health care provider if pain control is not adequate or if severe or persistent side effects occur.
- Medication may cause drowsiness or dizziness. Advise patient to call for assistance when ambulating and to avoid driving or other activities that require alertness until response to the medication is known.
- Advise patients taking *Oxycontin* tablets that empty matrix tablets may appear in stool.
- Advise patient to make position changes slowly to minimize orthostatic hypotension.
- Emphasize the importance of aggressive prevention of constipation with the use of oxycodone.
- Advise patient to avoid concurrent use of alcohol or other CNS depressants with this medication; may cause overdose.
- Instruct patient to notify health care provider of all Rx or OTC medications, vitamins, or herbal products being taken and consult health care provider before taking any new medications.
- Encourage patient to turn, cough, and breathe deeply every 2 hr to prevent atelectasis.
- Advise patient that good oral hygiene, frequent mouth rinses, and sugarless gum or candy may decrease dry mouth.
- Rep: Advise patient to notify health care provider if pregnancy is planned or suspected or if breastfeeding. Inform patient of potential for neonatal opioid withdrawal syndrome with prolonged use during pregnancy. Monitor neonate for signs and symptoms of withdrawal symptoms (irritability, hyperactivity and abnormal sleep pattern, high-pitched cry, tremor, vomiting, diarrhea, failure to gain weight); usually occur the first days after birth. Monitor infants exposed to oxycodone through breast milk for excess sedation and respiratory depression. Doses <60 mg/day of the IR formulation are unlikely to result in clinically relevant exposure in breastfed infants. Chronic use may ↓ fertility in women and men.

Evaluation/Desired Outcomes

- Decrease in severity of pain without a significant alteration in level of consciousness or respiratory status.

HIGH ALERT

oxytocin (ox-i-toe-sin)

Pitocin

Classification

Therapeutic: hormones

Pharmacologic: oxytocics

Indications

IV: Induction of labor in patients with a medical indication for initiation of labor. **IV:** Facilitation of threatened abortion. **IV, IM:** Postpartum control of bleeding after expulsion of the placenta. NOT to be used for elective induction of labor.

Action

Stimulates uterine smooth muscle, producing uterine contractions similar to those in spontaneous labor. Has vasopressor and antidiuretic effects. **Therapeutic Effects:** Induction of labor. Control of postpartum bleeding.

Pharmacokinetics

Absorption: IV administration results in complete bioavailability.

Distribution: Widely distributed in extracellular fluid. Small amounts reach fetal circulation.

Metabolism and Excretion: Rapidly metabolized by liver and kidneys. Primarily excreted in urine as metabolites.

Half-life: 3–9 min.

TIME/ACTION PROFILE (↓ in uterine contractions)

ROUTE	ONSET	PEAK	DURATION
IV	immediate	unknown	1 hr
IM	3–5 min	unknown	30–60 min

Contraindications/Precautions

Contraindicated in: Hypersensitivity; Anticipated nonvaginal delivery.

Use Cautiously in: OB: 1st and 2nd stages of labor; slow infusion over 24 hr has caused water intoxication with seizure and coma or maternal death due to oxytocin's antidiuretic effect.

Adverse Reactions/Side Effects

Maternal adverse reactions are noted for IV use only

CV: maternal: hypotension**fetal:** arrhythmias. **F and E: maternal:** hypochloremia, hyponatremia, water intoxication. **GU: maternal:** ↑ uterine motility, painful contractions, abruptio placentae, ↓ uterine blood flow. **Neuro: maternal:** COMA, SEIZURES. **fetal:** INTRACRANIAL HEMORRHAGE. **Resp: fetal:** ASPHYXIA, hypoxia. **Misc:** hypersensitivity reactions.

Interactions

Drug-Drug: Severe hypertension may occur if oxytocin follows administration of **vasopressors**.

Route/Dosage

Induction/Stimulation of Labor

IV (Adults): 0.5–1 milliunits/min; ↑ by 1–2 milliunits/min every 30–60 min until desired contraction pattern established; dose may be ↓ after desired frequency of contractions is reached and labor has progressed to 5–6 cm dilation.

Postpartum Hemorrhage

IV (Adults): 10 units infused at 20–40 milliunits/min.
IM (Adults): 10 units after delivery of placenta.

Incomplete/Inevitable Abortion

IV (Adults): 10 units at a rate of 20–40 milliunits/min.

Availability (generic available)

Solution for injection: 10 units/mL.

NURSING IMPLICATIONS

Assessment

- Assess fetal maturity, presentation, and pelvic adequacy before administering oxytocin for induction of labor.
- Assess character, frequency, and duration of uterine contractions; resting uterine tone; and fetal HR frequently throughout administration. If contractions occur <2 min apart and are >50–65 mm Hg on monitor, if they last ≥60–90 sec, or if a significant change in fetal HR develops, stop infusion and turn patient onto the left side to prevent fetal anoxia. Notify health care provider immediately.
- Monitor maternal BP and HR frequently and fetal HR continuously throughout administration.
- Monitor for signs/symptoms of water intoxication (drowsiness, listlessness, confusion, headache, anuria).

Lab Test Considerations

- Monitor maternal electrolytes. Water retention may result in hypochloremia or hyponatremia.

Implementation

- Do not confuse oxytocin with Oxycontin.
- Do not administer oxytocin simultaneously by >1 route.
- **IM:** 10 units (1 mL) of oxytocin can be given after delivery of the placenta.

IV Administration

- **Continuous Infusion:** Rotate infusion container to ensure thorough mixing. Store solution in refrigerator, but do not freeze.
- Infuse via infusion pump for accurate dose. Oxytocin should be connected via Y-site injection to an IV of 0.9% NaCl for use during adverse reactions.
- Magnesium sulfate should be available if needed for relaxation of myometrium.
- Dose of oxytocin is determined by uterine response.
- **Induction of Labor: Dilution:** Dilute 1 mL (10 units) in 1000 mL of 0.9% NaCl, D5W, or LR. **Concentration:** 10 milliunits/mL. **Rate:** Begin infusion at 0.5–2 milliunits/min (0.05–0.2 mL); ↑ in increments of 1–2 milliunits/min at 15–30-min intervals until contractions simulate normal labor. Gradually ↑ dose at 30–60 min intervals in increments of 1–2 milliunits/min until the desired contraction pattern has been established. Once desired frequency of contractions has been reached and labor has progressed to 5–6 cm dilation, dose may be ↓ by similar increments.
- **Postpartum Bleeding: Dilution:** Dilute 1–4 mL (10–40 units) in 1000 mL of 0.9% NaCl, D5W, or LR. **Concentration:** 10–40 milliunits/mL. **Rate:** Begin infusion at 20–40 milliunits/min to control uterine atony. Adjust rate as indicated.
- **Incomplete or Inevitable Abortion: Dilution:** Dilute 1 mL (10 units) in 500 mL of 0.9% NaCl or D5W. **Concentration:** 20 milliunits/mL. **Rate:** Infuse 20–40 milliunits/min. Total dose should not exceed 30 units in a 12-hr period due to risk of water intoxication.
- **Y-Site Compatibility:** acetaminophen, acyclovir, allopurinol, amikacin, aminocaproic acid, aminophylline, amphotericin B liposomal, anidulafungin, argatroban, ascorbic acid, atracurium, atropine, azathioprine, azithromycin, aztreonam, benztropine, bivalirudin, bumetanide, buprenorphine, butorphanol, calcium chloride, calcium gluconate,

O

caspofungin, cefazolin, cefepime, cefotaxime, cefotetan, cefoxitin, ceftazidime, ceftriaxone, cefuroxime, chloramphenicol, chlorothiazide, ciprofloxacin, cisatracurium, clindamycin, cyclophosphamide, cyclosporine, daptomycin, dexamethasone, dexmedetomidine, digoxin, diltiazem, diphenhydramine, dobutamine, dopamine, doxycycline, droperidol, enalaprilat, ephedrine, epinephrine, epoetin alfa, eptifibatide, ertapenem, erythromycin, esmolol, famotidine, fentanyl, fluconazole, folic acid, foscarnet, fosphenytoin, furosemide, ganciclovir, gentamicin, glycopyrrolate, granisetron, heparin, hydrocortisone, hydromorphone, imipenem/cilastatin, isoproterenol, ketamine, ketorolac, labetalol, leucovorin, levofloxacin, lidocaine, linezolid, lorazepam, magnesium sulfate, mannitol, meperidine, meropenem, methadone, methylprednisolone, metoclopramide, metoprolol, metronidazole, midazolam, milrinone, minocycline, morphine, moxifloxacin, multivitamins, mycophenolate, nafcillin, nalbuphine, naloxone, nicardipine, nitroglycerin, nitroprusside, norepinephrine, ondansetron, oxacillin, palonosetron, pamidronate, papaverine, penicillin G, pentamidine, pentobarbital, phenobarbital, phentolamine, phenylephrine, phytonadione, piperacillin/tazobactam, potassium acetate, potassium chloride, potassium phosphates, procainamide, prochlorperazine, promethazine, propranolol, protamine, pyridoxine, sodium acetate, sodium bicarbonate, sodium phosphates, succinylcholine, sufentanil, tacrolimus, theophylline, thiamine, tigecycline, tirofiban, tobramycin, vancomycin, vasopressin, verapamil, voriconazole, zidovudine, zoledronic acid.

- **Y-Site Incompatibility:** dantrolene, diazepam, dimenhydrinate, indomethacin, methohexital, phenytoin, remifentanil, trimethoprim/sulfamethoxazole.

Patient/Family Teaching

- Explain purpose and side effects of medication. Advise patient to read *Patient Information* before starting therapy.
- Advise patient to notify health care provider of all Rx or OTC medications, vitamins, or herbal products being taken and to consult health care provider before taking other medications.
- Advise patient to expect contractions similar to menstrual cramps after administration has started.

Evaluation/Desired Outcomes

- Induction of labor.
- Control of postpartum bleeding.

HIGH ALERT

PACLitaxel (pak-li-tax-el)

~~Taxol~~

PACLitaxel protein-bound particles (albumin-bound)

Abraxane

Classification

Therapeutic: antineoplastics

Pharmacologic: taxoids

Indications

Paclitaxel: Advanced ovarian cancer (in combination with cisplatin). Non-small cell lung cancer (NSCLC) when potentially curative surgery and/or radiation therapy is not an option. Metastatic breast cancer unresponsive to other therapy. Node-positive breast cancer when administered sequentially to standard combination chemotherapy that includes doxorubicin. Treatment of AIDS-related Kaposi sarcoma. **Paclitaxel (albumin-bound):** Metastatic breast cancer after treatment failure or relapse where therapy included an anthracycline. Locally advanced or metastatic NSCLC when potentially curative surgery or radiation therapy is not an option (in combination with carboplatin). Metastatic pancreatic adenocarcinoma (in combination with gemcitabine).

Action

Interferes with the normal cellular microtubule function that is required for interphase and mitosis. **Therapeutic Effects:** Death of rapidly replicating cells, particularly malignant ones.

Pharmacokinetics

Absorption: IV administration results in complete bioavailability.

Distribution: Widely distributed to tissues.

Protein Binding: 89–98%.

Metabolism and Excretion: Highly metabolized by the liver primarily by the CYP2C8 and CYP3A4 isoenzymes; <10% excreted unchanged in urine.

Half-life: *Paclitaxel:* 13–52 hr; *Paclitaxel protein-bound particles (albumin-bound):* 27 hr.

TIME/ACTION PROFILE (effect on WBCs)

ROUTE	ONSET	PEAK	DURATION
IV	unknown	11 days	3 wk

Contraindications/Precautions

Contraindicated in: Hypersensitivity to paclitaxel, other taxanes, or castor oil (paclitaxel); Severe hypersensitivity to paclitaxel protein-bound particles (paclitaxel protein-bound particles); AST >10 times upper limit of normal (ULN) or total bilirubin >5 times ULN (paclitaxel protein-bound particles); Moderate or severe hepatic impairment (pancreatic adenocarcinoma only for paclitaxel protein-bound particles); Known alcohol intolerance; Neutrophil count ≤1500 cells/mm^3 (for patients with ovarian, lung, breast, or pancreatic cancer) or ≤1000 cells/mm^3 (for patients with AIDS-related Kaposi sarcoma); OB: Pregnancy; Lactation: Lactation.

Use Cautiously in: Moderate or severe hepatic impairment (↓ dose); Active infection; ↓ bone marrow reserve; Rep: Women of reproductive potential and men with female partners of reproductive potential; Pedi: Safety and effectiveness not established in children; Geri: Older adults may have ↑ risk of adverse reactions.

Adverse Reactions/Side Effects

CV: ECG changes, edema, hypotension, bradycardia. **Derm:** alopecia, STEVENS-JOHNSON SYNDROME (SJS), TOXIC EPIDERMAL NECROLYSIS (TEN). **GI:** ↑ liver enzymes, diarrhea, mucositis, nausea, vomiting, pancreatitis. **GU:** renal failure. **Hemat:** anemia, NEUTROPENIA, thrombocytopenia. **Local:** injection site reactions. **MS:** arthralgia, myalgia. **Neuro:** peripheral neuropathy, dizziness, headache, seizures. **Resp:** cough, dyspnea, interstitial pneumonia, PULMONARY EMBOLISM, PULMONARY FIBROSIS. **Misc:** HYPERSENSITIVITY REACTIONS (INCLUDING ANAPHYLAXIS), SEPSIS.

Interactions

Drug-Drug: CYP3A4 inhibitors, including **atazanavir**, **clarithromycin**, **itraconazole**, **ketoconazole**, **nefazodone**, **nelfinavir**, and **ritonavir**, may ↑ levels and risk of toxicity; concurrent use should be undertaken with caution. **CYP3A4 inducers**, including **carbamazepine**, **rifampin**, and **phenytoin**, may ↓ levels and effectiveness; concurrent use should be undertaken with caution. **Gemfibrozil** may ↑ levels and risk of toxicity; concurrent use should be undertaken with caution. ↑ risk of myelosuppression with other **antineoplastics** or **radiation therapy**. Myelosuppression ↑ when given after **cisplatin**. May ↑ levels and risk of toxicity of **doxorubicin**. May ↓ antibody response to and ↑ risk of adverse reactions from **live-virus vaccines**.

Route/Dosage

Paclitaxel

Ovarian Cancer

IV (Adults): *Previously untreated patients:* 175 mg/m^2 over 3 hr every 3 wk *or* 135 mg/m^2 over 24 hr every 3 wk, followed by cisplatin; *Previously treated patients:* 135 mg/m^2 *or* 175 mg/m^2 over 3 hr every 3 wk.

P

Hepatic Impairment

IV (Adults 24-hr infusion): *Transaminase levels <2 times ULN and bilirubin levels ≤1.5 mg/dL:* 135 mg/m² over 24 hr. *Transaminase levels 2–<10 times ULN and bilirubin levels ≤1.5 mg/dL:* 100 mg/m² over 24 hr. *Transaminase levels <10 times ULN and bilirubin levels 1.6–7.5 mg/dL:* 50 mg/m² over 24 hr. *Transaminase levels ≥10 times ULN or bilirubin levels >7.5 mg/dL:* Avoid use.

Hepatic Impairment

IV (Adults 3-hr infusion): *Transaminase levels <10 times ULN and bilirubin levels ≤1.25 times ULN:* 175 mg/m² over 3 hr. *Transaminase levels <10 times ULN and bilirubin levels 1.26–2 times ULN:* 135 mg/m² over 3 hr. *Transaminase levels <10 times ULN and bilirubin levels 2.01–5 times ULN:* 90 mg/m² over 3 hr. *Transaminase levels ≥10 times ULN or bilirubin levels >5 times ULN:* Avoid use.

Breast Cancer

IV (Adults): *Adjuvant treatment of node-positive breast cancer:* 175 mg/m² over 3 hr every 3 wk for 4 courses administered sequentially to doxorubicin-containing combination chemotherapy; *Failure of initial therapy for metastatic disease or relapse within 6 mo of adjuvant therapy:* 175 mg/m² over 3 hr every 3 wk.

Hepatic Impairment

IV (Adults 3-hr infusion): *Transaminase levels <10 times ULN and bilirubin levels ≤1.25 times ULN:* 175 mg/m² over 3 hr. *Transaminase levels <10 times ULN and bilirubin levels 1.26–2 times ULN:* 135 mg/m² over 3 hr. *Transaminase levels <10 times ULN and bilirubin levels 2.01–5 times ULN:* 90 mg/m² over 3 hr. *Transaminase levels ≥10 times ULN or bilirubin levels >5 times ULN:* Avoid use.

Non-Small Cell Lung Cancer

IV (Adults): 135 mg/m² over 24 hr every 3 wk, followed by cisplatin.

Hepatic Impairment

IV (Adults 24-hr infusion): *Transaminase levels <2 times ULN and bilirubin levels ≤1.5 mg/dL:* 135 mg/m² over 24 hr. *Transaminase levels 2–<10 times ULN and bilirubin levels ≤1.5 mg/dL:* 100 mg/m² over 24 hr. *Transaminase levels <10 times ULN and bilirubin levels 1.6–7.5 mg/dL:* 50 mg/m² over 24 hr. *Transaminase levels ≥10 times ULN or bilirubin levels >7.5 mg/dL:* Avoid use.

AIDS-Related Kaposi Sarcoma

IV (Adults): 135 mg/m² over 3 hr every 3 wk *or* 100 mg/m² over 3 hr every 2 wk (dose ↓/adjustment may be necessary in patients with advanced HIV infection).

Hepatic Impairment

IV (Adults 3-hr infusion): *Transaminase levels <10 times ULN and bilirubin levels ≤1.25 times ULN:* 175 mg/m² over 3 hr. *Transaminase levels <10 times ULN and bilirubin levels 1.26–2 times ULN:* 135 mg/m² over 3 hr. *Transaminase levels <10 times ULN and bilirubin levels 2.01–5 times ULN:* 90 mg/m² over 3 hr. *Transaminase levels ≥10 times ULN or bilirubin levels >5 times ULN:* Avoid use.

Paclitaxel Protein-Bound Particles (Albumin-Bound)

Breast Cancer

IV (Adults): 260 mg/m² over 30 min every 3 wk.

Hepatic Impairment

IV (Adults): *AST levels <10 times ULN and bilirubin levels 1.51–3 times ULN:* 200 mg/m² over 30 min every 3 wk; may ↑ to 260 mg/m² for the 3rd course based on individual tolerance; *AST levels <10 times ULN and bilirubin levels 3.01–5 times ULN:* 200 mg/m² over 30 min every 3 wk; may ↑ to 260 mg/m² for the 3rd course based on individual tolerance; *AST levels >10 times ULN or bilirubin levels >5 times ULN:* Avoid use.

Non-Small Cell Lung Cancer

IV (Adults): 100 mg/m² over 30 min on Days 1, 8, and 15 of each 21-day cycle.

Hepatic Impairment

IV (Adults): *AST levels <10 times ULN and bilirubin levels 1.51–3 times ULN:* 80 mg/m² over 30 min on Days 1, 8, and 15 of each 21-day cycle; may ↑ to 100 mg/m² for the 3rd course based on individual tolerance; *AST levels <10 times ULN and bilirubin levels 3.01–5 times ULN:* 80 mg/m² over 30 min on Days 1, 8, and 15 of each 21-day cycle; may ↑ to 100 mg/m² for the 3rd course based on individual tolerance; *AST levels >10 times ULN or bilirubin levels >5 times ULN:* Avoid use.

Pancreatic Adenocarcinoma

IV (Adults): 125 mg/m² over 30–40 min on Days 1, 8, and 15 of each 28-day cycle.

Hepatic Impairment

IV (Adults): *Moderate or severe hepatic impairment:* Avoid use.

Availability

Paclitaxel (generic available)

Solution for injection: 6 mg/mL.

Paclitaxel Protein-Bound Particles (Albumin-Bound)

Lyophilized powder for injection: 100 mg/vial.

NURSING IMPLICATIONS

Assessment

- Monitor vital signs frequently, especially during 1st hr of the infusion.
- Monitor cardiovascular status especially during 1st 3 hr of infusion. Hypotension and bradycardia are common but usually do not require treatment. Continuous ECG monitoring is recommended only for

patients with serious underlying conduction abnormalities or those concurrently taking doxorubicin.

- Monitor for bone marrow suppression. Assess for bleeding (bleeding gums; bruising; petechiae; guaiac stools, urine, or emesis) and avoid IM injections and taking rectal temperatures if platelet count is low. Apply pressure to venipuncture sites for 10 min. Assess for signs of infection during neutropenia. Anemia may occur. Monitor for dyspnea and orthostatic hypotension. Granulocyte-colony stimulating factor (G-CSF) may be used if necessary.
- Monitor intake and output, appetite, and nutritional intake. Paclitaxel causes nausea and vomiting in 50% of patients. Prophylactic antiemetics may be used. Adjust diet as tolerated to help maintain fluid and electrolyte balance and nutritional status.
- Assess for arthralgia and myalgia, which usually begin 2–3 days after therapy and resolve within 5 days. Pain is usually relieved by nonopioid analgesics but may be severe enough to require treatment with opioid analgesics.
- Assess for rash periodically during therapy. May cause SJS and TEN. *If rash severe or if accompanied with fever, general malaise, fatigue, muscle or joint aches, blisters, oral lesions, conjunctivitis, hepatitis, and/or eosinophilia,* discontinue paclitaxel.
- **Paclitaxel:** Monitor for hypersensitivity reactions continuously during the 1st 30 min and frequently thereafter. These occur frequently (19%), usually during the 1st 10 min of paclitaxel infusion, after the 1st or 2nd dose. Most common manifestations are dyspnea, flushing, tachycardia, rash, hypotension, and chest pain. If these occur, stop infusion and notify health care provider. Treatment may include bronchodilators, epinephrine, antihistamines, and corticosteroids. Keep these agents and resuscitative equipment close by in the event of an anaphylactic reaction. Other manifestations of hypersensitivity reactions include flushing and rash. Patients experiencing hypersensitivity reactions should not be rechallenged with paclitaxel.
- Assess for development of peripheral neuropathy. If severe symptoms occur, subsequent dose should be ↓ by 20%.
- **Paclitaxel Protein-Bound (Albumin-Bound):** Do not rechallenge patients who experience a severe hypersensitivity reaction.
- Sensory neuropathy is dose- and schedule-dependent. *If Grade ≥3 sensory neuropathy,* hold paclitaxel protein-bound (albumin-bound) until resolution to Grade <2 for metastatic breast cancer or until resolution to Grade ≤1 for NSCLC and pancreatic cancer followed by a dose ↓ for all subsequent courses of therapy.

Lab Test Considerations

- Verify negative pregnancy test before starting therapy.
- **Paclitaxel:** Monitor CBC and differential before and periodically during therapy. The nadir of leukopenia occurs in 11 days, with recovery by days 15–21. *If neutrophil counts <500/mm³ for ≥1 wk,* ↓ dose by 20% for subsequent courses.
- **Paclitaxel Protein-Bound Particles (Albumin-Bound):** Monitor CBC and differential frequently, including before starting therapy and prior to dosing on Day 1 (for breast cancer), 8, and 15 (for NSCLC and pancreatic cancer). **For Breast Cancer:** *If severe neutropenia (ANC <500 cells/mm³ for ≥7 days),* ↓ dose to 220 mg/m². *If recurrence of severe neutropenia,* ↓ dose to 180 mg/m². **For NSCLC:** *If neutropenic fever (ANC <500/mm³ with fever >38°C) OR delay of next cycle by >7 days for ANC <1500/mm³ OR ANC <500/mm³ for >7 days,* ↓ dose on 1st occurrence to 75 mg/m² and on 2nd occurrence, ↓ dose to 50 mg/m². For 3rd occurrence, discontinue therapy. *If severe neutropenia (ANC <500 cells/mm³ for ≥7 days),* ↓ dose in subsequent courses. *If platelet count <50,000/mm³,* for 1st occurrence, ↓ dose to 75 mg/m². Discontinue therapy at 2nd occurrence. **For Pancreatic Cancer:** *On Day 1, if ANC <1500 cells/mm³ OR platelet count <100,000 cells/mm³,* hold next dose until recovery. *On Day 8, if ANC 500–<1000 cells/mm³ OR platelet count 50,000–<75,000 cells/mm³,* ↓ dose one level; *on Day 8, if ANC <500 cells/mm³ OR <50,000 cells/mm³,* hold dose. *On Day 15, if Day 8 doses were ↓ or given without modification and ANC 500–<1000 cells/mm³ OR platelet count 50,000–<75,000 cells/mm³,* ↓ dose one level from Day 8. *On Day 15, if Day 8 doses were ↓ or given without modification and ANC <500 cells/mm³ OR platelet count <50,000 cells/mm³,* hold doses. *On Day 15, if Day 8 doses were held and ANC ≥1000 cells/mm³ OR platelet count ≥75,000 cells/mm³,* ↓ dose one level from Day 1. *On Day 15, if Day 8 doses were held and ANC 500–<1000 cells/mm³ OR platelet count 50,000–<75,000 cells/mm³,* ↓ dose two levels from Day 1. *On Day 15, if Day 8 doses were held and ANC <500 cells/mm³ OR platelet count <50,000 cells/mm³,* hold doses.
- Monitor AST, ALT, LDH, and bilirubin before and periodically during therapy.

P

Implementation

- Do not confuse paclitaxel with docetaxel or paclitaxel protein-bound particles.
- Paclitaxel should be administered under the supervision of a physician experienced in the use of cancer chemotherapeutic agents.

Paclitaxel

IV Administration

- Pretreatment is recommended for **all** patients and should include dexamethasone 20 mg PO (10 mg for patients with advanced HIV disease) 12 hr and 6 hr before paclitaxel, diphenhydramine 50 mg IV 30–60 min before paclitaxel, and famotidine 20 mg IV 30–60 min before paclitaxel.
- **V** Paclitaxel is a vesicant. If extravasation occurs, immediately stop infusion. Leave needle/cannula in place temporarily but do not flush the line. Gently aspirate extravasated solution; then remove needle/cannula. Elevate patient's extremity and apply dry cold compresses for 20 min 4 times day for 1–2 days. Initiate hyaluronidase antidote for refractory cases in addition to supportive management. For hyaluronidase, inject 1–6 mL (150 units/mL) into existing IV line; usual dose is 1 mL for each 1 mL of extravasated drug; if needle/cannula has been removed, inject SUBQ in a clockwise manner around area of extravasation; may repeat several times over the next 3–4 hr.
- **Intermittent Infusion: Dilution:** Dilute contents of 5 mL (30 mg) vials with 0.9% NaCl, D5W, D5/0.9% NaCl, or dextrose 5% in Ringer's solution. Although haziness in solution is normal, inspect for particulate matter or discoloration before use. Protect from light. Use an in-line filter of not >0.22-micron pore size. Solutions are stable for 27 hr at ambient temperature. Do not use PVC containers or administration sets. **Concentration:** 0.3–1.2 mg/mL. **Rate:** Dose for *breast cancer, ovarian cancer, or AIDS-related Kaposi sarcoma* is administered over 3 hr. Dose for *ovarian cancer* can also be administered as a 24 hr infusion.
- **Y-Site Compatibility:** acyclovir, alemtuzumab, allopurinol, amikacin, aminophylline, ampicillin, ampicillin/sulbactam, anidulafungin, argatroban, atracurium, azithromycin, aztreonam, bivalirudin, bleomycin, bumetanide, buprenorphine, busulfan, butorphanol, calcium chloride, calcium gluconate, carboplatin, carmustine, caspofungin, cefazolin, cefepime, cefotaxime, cefotetan, cefoxitin, ceftazidime, ceftriaxone, cefuroxime, chloramphenicol, ciprofloxacin, cisatracurium, cisplatin, cladribine, clindamycin, cyclophosphamide, cyclosporine, cytarabine, dacarbazine, dactinomycin, dantrolene, daptomycin, daunorubicin, dexamethasone, dexmedetomidine, dexrazoxane, diltiazem, diphenhydramine, dobutamine, dopamine, doxorubicin hydrochloride, doxycycline, droperidol, enalaprilat, ephedrine, epinephrine, epirubicin, ertapenem, erythromycin, esmolol, etoposide, etoposide phosphate, famotidine, fentanyl, floxuridine, fluconazole, fludarabine, fluorouracil, foscarnet, fosphenytoin, furosemide, ganciclovir, gemcitabine, gentamicin, glycopyrrolate, granisetron, haloperidol, heparin, hydralazine, hydrocortisone, hydromorphone, ifosfamide, imipenem/cilastatin, insulin regular, irinotecan, isoproterenol, ketorolac, leucovorin, levofloxacin, lidocaine, linezolid, lorazepam, magnesium sulfate, mannitol, meperidine, meropenem, mesna, methadone, methotrexate, metoclopramide, metoprolol, metronidazole, midazolam, milrinone, minocycline, mitomycin, morphine, moxifloxacin, nafcillin, nalbuphine, naloxone, nicardipine, nitroglycerin, nitroprusside, norepinephrine, octreotide, ondansetron, oxaliplatin, palonosetron, pamidronate, pantoprazole, pemetrexed, pentamidine, pentobarbital, pentostatin, phenobarbital, phentolamine, phenylephrine, piperacillin/tazobactam, potassium acetate, potassium chloride, potassium phosphates, procainamide, prochlorperazine, promethazine, propofol, remifentanil, rituximab, sodium acetate, sodium bicarbonate, sodium phosphates, succinylcholine, sufentanil, tacrolimus, theophylline, thiotepa, tigecycline, tirofiban, tobramycin, topotecan, trastuzumab, trimethoprim/sulfamethoxazole, vancomycin, vasopressin, vecuronium, verapamil, vinblastine, vincristine, vinorelbine, voriconazole, zidovudine, zoledronic acid.
- **Y-Site Incompatibility:** amiodarone, amphotericin B deoxycholate, amphotericin B liposomal, chlorpromazine, diazepam, digoxin, doxorubicin liposomal, gemtuzumab ozogamicin, idarubicin, indomethacin, labetalol, methylprednisolone, mitoxantrone, phenytoin, propranolol.

Paclitaxel Protein-Bound Particles (Albumin-Bound)

- Consider premedication in patients who have had prior hypersensitivity reactions to paclitaxel protein-bound (albumin-bound).
- **Dose Reduction for Pancreatic Cancer:** Full dose: 125 mm/m². 1st dose ↓: 100 mm/m². 2nd dose ↓: 75 mm/m². If additional dose ↓ required, discontinue therapy.

IV Administration

- Paclitaxel protein bound particles is an irritant. If extravasation occurs, immediately stop infusion. Leave needle/cannula in place temporarily but do not flush the line. Gently aspirate extravasated solution; then remove needle/cannula. Elevate patient's extremity and apply dry cold compresses for 20 min 4 times day for 1–2 days.

- **Intermittent Infusion: Reconstitution:** Reconstitute by slowly adding 20 mL to each vial over ≥1 min. Direct solution to inside wall of vial to prevent foaming. Allow vial to sit for >5 min to ensure proper wetting of cake/powder. Gently swirl or invert vial for ≥2 min until powder is completely dissolved; avoid foaming. If foaming or clumping occurs, allow vial to stand for 15 min until foaming dissolves. Suspension should be milky and homogenous without visible particles. If particles or settling are visible, gently invert vial to resuspend. **Concentration:** 5 mg/mL. Inject appropriate amount of reconstituted suspension into empty sterile PVC IV bag. Do not use an in-line filter during administration. Do not administer suspension that is discolored or contains particulate matter. Should be administered immediately but is stable for 8 hr if refrigerated. Discard unused portion. **Rate:** Administer over 30 min.
- **Y-Site Compatibility:** carboplatin, dexamethasone, gemcitabine, granisetron, palonosetron.

Patient/Family Teaching

- Explain purpose and side effects of medication. Advise patient to read *Patient Information* before starting therapy.
- Advise patient to notify health care provider of all Rx or OTC medications, vitamins, or herbal products being taken and to consult health care provider before taking other medications.
- Advise patient to notify health care provider immediately of rash, difficulty breathing, or symptoms of hypersensitivity reaction occurs.
- Instruct patient to notify health care provider promptly if fever; chills; cough; hoarseness; sore throat; signs of infection; lower back or side pain; painful or difficult urination; bleeding gums; bruising; petechiae; blood in stools, urine, or emesis; dyspnea; or orthostatic hypotension occurs. Caution patient to avoid crowds and persons with known infections. Instruct patient to use soft toothbrush and electric razor and to avoid falls. Caution patient not to drink alcoholic beverages or to take medication containing aspirin or NSAIDs; may precipitate gastric bleeding.
- May cause dizziness. Caution patient to avoid driving or other activities requiring alertness until response to medication is known.
- Instruct patient to notify health care provider if abdominal pain, yellow skin, weakness, paresthesia, gait disturbances, or joint or muscle aches occur.
- Instruct patient to inspect oral mucosa for redness and ulceration. If mouth sores occur, advise patient to use sponge brush and rinse mouth with water after eating and drinking. Stomatitis usually resolves in 5–7 days.
- Discuss with patient the possibility of hair loss. Complete hair loss usually occurs after 14–21 days and is reversible after discontinuation of therapy. Explore coping strategies.
- Instruct patient not to receive any vaccinations without advice of health care provider.
- Rep: Advise women of reproductive potential to use a nonhormonal method of contraception during therapy and for ≥6 mo after last dose of therapy and to avoid breastfeeding during therapy and for 2 wk after last dose. Advise men with female partners of reproductive potential to use effective contraception during therapy and for ≥3 mo after last dose. May impair fertility in women and men.

Evaluation/Desired Outcomes

- Death of rapidly replicating cells, particularly malignant ones.

HIGH ALERT

P

palbociclib (pal-bo-sye-klib)

Ibrance

Classification

Therapeutic: antineoplastics

Pharmacologic: kinase inhibitors

Indications

Advanced or metastatic hormone receptor (HR)-positive, human epidermal growth factor 2 (HER2)-negative breast cancer as initial endocrine-based therapy (in combination with an aromatase inhibitor). Advanced or metastatic HR-positive, HER2-negative breast cancer in patients with disease progression following endocrine therapy (in combination with fulvestrant). Locally advanced or metastatic, HR-positive, HER2-negative, endocrine-resistant, PIK3CA-mutated breast cancer following recurrence on or after completing adjuvant endocrine therapy (in combination with inavolisib and fulvestrant).

Action

Inhibits kinases (cyclin-dependent kinases 4 and 6) that are part of the signaling pathway for cell proliferation. **Therapeutic Effects:** Improved survival and decreased spread of breast cancer.

Pharmacokinetics

Absorption: 46% absorbed following oral administration.

Distribution: Unknown.

Metabolism and Excretion: Mostly metabolized (by CYP3A and sulfontransferase); 6.9% excreted unchanged in urine, 2.3% in feces.
Half-life: 29 hr.

TIME/ACTION PROFILE (improvement in progression-free survival)

ROUTE	ONSET	PEAK	DURATION
PO	within 4 mo	unknown	maintained throughout treatment

Contraindications/Precautions

Contraindicated in: OB: Pregnancy; Lactation: Lactation.
Use Cautiously in: Severe renal impairment; Severe hepatic impairment; Rep: Women of reproductive potential and men with female partners of reproductive potential; Pedi: Safety and effectiveness not established in children.

Adverse Reactions/Side Effects

CV: DEEP VEIN THROMBOSIS (DVT). **Derm:** alopecia. **EENT:** epistaxis. **GI:** ↓ appetite, stomatitis, vomiting, diarrhea, nausea. **GU:** ↓ fertility, ↑ serum creatinine. **Hemat:** anemia, leukopenia, NEUTROPENIA, thrombocytopenia. **Neuro:** peripheral neuropathy, weakness. **Resp:** INTERSTITIAL LUNG DISEASE (ILD), PULMONARY EMBOLISM (PE).

Interactions

Drug-Drug: CYP3A inhibitors, including **clarithromycin, itraconazole, ketoconazole, lopinavir/ritonavir, nefazodone, nelfinavir, posaconazole, ritonavir, verapamil**, and **voriconazole**, may ↑ levels and risk of toxicity; avoid concurrent use, if possible. If concurrent use necessary, ↓ palbociclib dose. **Strong CYP3A inducers**, including **carbamazepine, phenytoin**, and **rifampin**, may ↓ levels and effectiveness; avoid concurrent use. **Moderate CYP3A inducers**, including **bosentan, efavirenz, etravirine, modafinil**, and **nafcillin**, may ↓ levels and effectiveness; avoid concurrent use. May ↑ levels and risk of toxicity of **cyclosporine, dihydroergotamine, ergotamine, everolimus, fentanyl, midazolam, pimozide, quinidine, sirolimus**, and **tacrolimus**; if concurrent use necessary, dose ↓ may be necessary.
Drug-Natural Products: St. John's wort may ↓ levels and effectiveness; avoid concurrent use.
Drug-Food: Grapefruit/grapefruit juice may ↑ levels and risk of toxicity; avoid concurrent use.

Route/Dosage

PO (Adults): 125 mg once daily for 21 days, followed by 7 days off; *Concurrent use of strong CYP3A4 inhibitor:* 75 mg once daily for 21 days, followed by 7 days off.

Hepatic Impairment

PO (Adults): *Severe hepatic impairment:* 75 mg once daily for 21 days, followed by 7 days off.

Availability (generic available)

Capsules: 75 mg, 100 mg, 125 mg.

NURSING IMPLICATIONS

Assessment

- Monitor for signs/symptoms of infection (fever, chills, dizziness, shortness of breath, weakness) during therapy. Treat as medically appropriate. *For Grade ≥3 (if persisting despite medical treatment)*, withhold palbociclib until symptoms resolve to Grade ≤1. Resume at next ↓ dose.
- Monitor for signs/symptoms of venous thromboembolism such as PE (chest pain, dyspnea, tachycardia) or DVT (calf pain or tenderness, lower extremity edema, localized warmth or erythema). *If DVT or PE suspected*, discontinue palbociclib.
- Monitor for signs/symptoms of ILD (dyspnea, cough, hypoxia, fever). CT scan or chest x-ray can confirm. *If ILD suspected*, hold palbociclib. *If ILD confirmed*, permanently discontinue palbociclib.

Lab Test Considerations

- Verify negative pregnancy test before starting therapy.
- Monitor CBC with differential at baseline and beginning of each cycle, on Day 15 of 1st 2 cycles, and as clinically indicated. May ↓ neutrophils, lymphocytes, hemoglobin, and platelets. Median time to 1st episode of neutropenia is 15 days, and median duration of Grade ≥3 neutropenia is 7 days. May cause febrile neutropenia. *If Grade 3 hematologic toxicity occurs on Day 1 of cycle*, hold palbociclib and repeat CBC within 1 wk. When recovered to Grade ≤2, start next cycle at same dose. *If Grade 3 hematologic toxicity occurs on Day 15 of 1st 2 cycles*, continue palbociclib at current dose to complete cycle and repeat CBC on Day 22. *If Grade 4 hematologic toxicity occurs on Day 22*, hold palbociclib until recovery to Grade ≤2. Resume at next ↓ dose. Consider dose ↓ in cases of prolonged (>1 wk) recovery from Grade 3 neutropenia or recurrent Grade 3 neutropenia on Day 1 of subsequent cycles. *For Grade 3 ANC of 500–<1000/mm³ plus fever ≥38.5°C and/or infection*, hold palbociclib until recovery to Grade ≤2. Resume at next ↓ dose. *For Grade 4 hematologic toxicity*, hold palbociclib until recovery to Grade ≤2. Resume at next ↓ dose.
- May ↑ serum creatinine.

Implementation

- **PO:** Administer with food at the same time each day, for 21 consecutive days, followed by 7 days off treatment; combination with letrozole once daily given throughout 28-day cycle. ***DNC:*** Swallow capsules whole; do not open, crush, or chew; do not swallow capsules that are broken, cracked, or not intact.
- Pre/perimenopausal women treated with a combination of palbociclib + aromatase inhibitor or fulvestrant *or* palbociclib + inavolisib and fulvestrant

should also be treated with luteinizing hormone-releasing hormone (LHRH) agonist. Men treated with a combination of palbociclib + aromatase inhibitor *or* palbociclib + inavolisib and fulvestrant therapy should be considered for treatment with LHRH agonist.

- **Dose Reductions for Adverse Reactions:** Starting dose is 125 mg/day. 1st dose ↓ is to 100 mg/day; 2nd dose ↓ is to 75 mg/day; if further dose ↓ needed, discontinue therapy.

Patient/Family Teaching

- Explain the purpose and side effects of palbociclib. Instruct to take as directed. If a dose is vomited or missed, omit dose and take next dose at usual time; do not take an additional dose that day. Do not change dose or stop taking without consulting health care provider. Advise patient to read *Patient Information* before starting therapy and with each Rx refill in case of changes.
- Advise patient to avoid grapefruit or grapefruit products during therapy.
- Instruct patient to notify health care provider immediately and to seek medical care if fever or chills (even a low-grade fever can be serious) accompanied by weakness, tiredness, sore throat, mouth sores, rashes, flu-like symptoms, or respiratory illness occur; these could be associated with febrile neutropenia.
- Instruct patient to notify health care provider of all Rx or OTC medications, vitamins, or herbal products being taken and to consult with health care provider before taking other medications, especially St. John's wort.
- Rep: May cause fetal harm. Advise women of reproductive potential to notify health care provider if pregnancy is planned or suspected or if breastfeeding. Advise women of reproductive potential to use effective contraception and avoid breastfeeding during and for ≥3 wk after last dose. Advise men with female partners of reproductive potential to use effective contraception during and for ≥3 wk after last dose. Inform men that palbociclib may impair fertility.

Evaluation/Desired Outcomes

- Improved survival and decrease in the spread of breast cancer.

BEERS

paliperidone (pa-li-**per**-i-done)

Erzofri, Invega, Invega Hafyera, Invega Sustenna, Invega Trinza

Classification

Therapeutic: antipsychotics

Pharmacologic: benzisoxazoles

Indications

PO, IM Acute and maintenance treatment of schizophrenia (Erzofri, Invega, and Invega Sustenna). **IM:** Maintenance treatment of schizophrenia after patients have been adequately treated with Invega Sustenna for at least 4 mo (Invega Trinza). **IM:** Maintenance treatment of schizophrenia after patients have been adequately treated with either Invega Sustenna for at least 4 mo or Invega Trinza for at least one 3-mo cycle (Invega Hafyera). **PO, IM:** Acute treatment of schizoaffective disorder (as monotherapy or as adjunct to mood stabilizers and/or antidepressants) (Erzofri, Invega, and Invega Sustenna).

Action

May act by antagonizing dopamine and serotonin in the CNS. Paliperidone is the active metabolite of risperidone. **Therapeutic Effects:** Decreased manifestations of schizophrenia. Decreased manifestations of schizoaffective disorder.

Pharmacokinetics

Absorption: 28% absorbed following oral administration, food ↑ absorption; slowly absorbed after IM administration (concentrations higher and more rapidly achieved with administration into deltoid muscle).

Distribution: Unknown.

Metabolism and Excretion: 59% excreted unchanged in urine; 32% excreted in urine as metabolites.

Half-life: *PO:* 23 hr; *IM (Erzofri):* 27 days; *IM (Sustenna):* 25–49 days; *IM (Trinza):* 84–139 days; *IM (Hafyera):* 148–159 days.

TIME/ACTION PROFILE (plasma concentrations)

ROUTE	ONSET	PEAK	DURATION
PO	unknown	24 hr	24 hr
IM: Erzofri	unknown	16–28 days	1 mo
IM: Sustenna	unknown	13 days	1 mo
IM: Trinza	unknown	30–33 days	3 mo
IM: Hafyera	unknown	29–32 days	6 mo

Contraindications/Precautions

Contraindicated in: Hypersensitivity to paliperidone or risperidone; Concurrent use of drugs known to cause QT interval prolongation (including quinidine, procainamide, sotalol, amiodarone, chlorpromazine, thioridazine, moxifloxacin); History of congenital QTc prolongation or other cardiac arrhythmias; Bradycardia, hypokalemia, hypomagnesemia (↑ risk of QTc prolongation); Pre-existing severe GI narrowing (due to nature of tablet formulation); CCr <50 mL/min (for IM).

Use Cautiously in: Parkinson disease or dementia with Lewy bodies (↑ sensitivity to effects of antipsychotics); History of suicide attempt; History of HF, MI, conduction abnormalities, stroke, or TIA (↑ risk of orthostatic hypotension and syncope); Patients at risk for aspiration pneumonia or falls; History of seizures; Conditions that may ↑ body temperature (strenuous exercise, exposure to extreme heat, concurrent anticholinergics or risk of dehydration); ↓ GI transit time (may ↑ blood levels); May mask symptoms of some drug overdoses, intestinal obstruction, Reye syndrome, or brain tumor (due to antiemetic effect); Diabetes mellitus; Severe hepatic impairment; Renal impairment (↓ dose if CCr <80 mL/min); Low white blood cell count/absolute neutrophil count or history of drug-induced leukopenia/neutropenia (↑ risk of leukopenia/neutropenia); History of breast cancer; OB: Neonates at ↑ risk for extrapyramidal symptoms and withdrawal after delivery when exposed during the 3rd trimester; use only if maternal benefit outweighs fetal risk; Lactation: Use while breastfeeding only if potential maternal benefit justifies potential risk to infant; Pedi: Children <12 yr (safety and effectiveness not established); Geri: Appears on Beers list. ↑ risk of stroke, cognitive decline, and mortality in older adults with dementia. Avoid use in older adults, except for schizophrenia.

Adverse Reactions/Side Effects

CV: palpitations, tachycardia (dose related), bradycardia, orthostatic hypotension, QT interval prolongation. **EENT:** blurred vision. **Endo:** galactorrhea, gynecomastia, hyperglycemia, hyperprolactinemia. **GI:** abdominal pain, dry mouth, dyspepsia, nausea, swollen tongue. **GU:** ↓ fertility (women), amenorrhea, impotence, priapism. **Hemat:** AGRANULOCYTOSIS, leukopenia, neutropenia. **Metab:** dyslipidemia, weight gain. **MS:** back pain, dystonia (dose related). **Neuro:** drowsiness, extrapyramidal disorders (dose related), headache, insomnia, akathisia, anxiety, confusion, dizziness, dysarthria, fatigue, NEUROLEPTIC MALIGNANT SYNDROME, SEIZURES, syncope, tardive dyskinesia, tremor (dose related), weakness. **Resp:** dyspnea, cough. **Misc:** fever, HYPERSENSITIVITY REACTIONS (INCLUDING ANAPHYLAXIS AND ANGIOEDEMA).

Interactions

Drug-Drug: ↑ risk of CNS depression with other **CNS depressants**, including **alcohol**, **antihistamines**, **sedative/hypnotics**, or **opioid analgesics**. May antagonize the effects of **levodopa** or other **dopamine agonists**. ↑ risk of orthostatic hypotension with **antihypertensives**, **nitrates**, or other **agents that lower BP**. **Strong CYP3A4 inducers** or **strong P-glycoprotein inducers**, including **carbamazepine** or **rifampin**, may ↓ levels and effectiveness; avoid concurrent use with Invega Sustenna; if use of strong CYP3A4 or P-glycoprotein inducer necessary, consider using paliperidone tablets. **Valproic acid** may ↑ levels and risk of toxicity; may need to ↓ dose of paliperidone.
Drug-Natural Products: St. John's wort may ↓ levels and effectiveness; avoid concurrent use with Invega Sustenna.

Route/Dosage

Schizophrenia

PO (Adults): 6 mg once daily; may titrate by 3 mg/day at intervals of ≥5 days (range 3–12 mg/day).
PO (Children 12–17 yr): 3 mg once daily; may titrate by 3 mg/day at intervals of ≥5 days (not to exceed 6 mg if <51 kg or 12 mg if ≥51 kg).
IM (Adults): *Erzofri:* 351 mg initially, then 117 mg 4 wk later; continue with monthly maintenance dose of 117 mg (range of 39–234 mg based on efficacy and/or tolerability); *Invega Sustenna:* 234 mg initially, then 156 mg 1 wk later; continue with monthly maintenance dose of 117 mg (range of 39–234 mg based on efficacy and/or tolerability); *Invega Trinza:* Dose should be based on dose of previous 1-mo injection dose of Invega Sustenna. **If last dose of Invega Sustenna was 78 mg:** Administer 273 mg of Invega Trinza every 3 mo. **If last dose of Invega Sustenna was 117 mg:** Administer 410 mg of Invega Trinza every 3 mo. **If last dose of Invega Sustenna was 156 mg:** Administer 546 mg of Invega Trinza every 3 mo. **If last dose of Invega Sustenna was 234 mg:** Administer 819 mg of Invega Trinza every 3 mo. May adjust dose based on efficacy and/or tolerability (range: 273–819 mg). *Invega Hafyera:* Dose should be based on dose of previous 1-mo injection dose of Invega Sustenna or previous every 3-mo dose of Invega Trinza. **If last dose of Invega Sustenna was 156 mg:** Administer 1092 mg of Invega Hafyera every 6 mo. **If last dose of Invega Sustenna was 234 mg:** Administer 1560 mg of Invega Hafyera every 6 mo. **If last dose of Invega Trinza was 546 mg:** Administer 1092 mg of Invega Hafyera every 6 mo. **If last dose of Invega Trinza was 819 mg:** Administer 1560 mg of Invega Hafyera every 6 mo.

Renal Impairment

PO (Adults): *CCr 50–79 mL/min:* 3 mg/day initially; may ↑ to max of 6 mg/day; *CCr 10–<50 mL/min:* 1.5 mg/day initially; may ↑ to max of 3 mg/day.

Renal Impairment

IM (Adults): *CCr 50–79 mL/min: Erzofri:* 234 mg initially; then 78 mg 4 wk later; continue with monthly maintenance dose of 78 mg (range of 39–156 mg based on efficacy and/or tolerability); *Invega Sustenna:* 156 mg initially; then 117 mg 1 wk later; continue with monthly maintenance dose of 78 mg (range of 39–156 mg based on efficacy and/or tolerability); *Invega Trinza:* Once stabilized on Invega Sustenna, can then transition to appropriate dose of Invega Trinza (see above); *Invega Hafyera:* Once stabilized on Invega

Sustenna or Invega Trinza, can then transition to appropriate dose of Invega Hafyera (see above); *CCr <50 mL/min:* Use not recommended.

Schizoaffective Disorder

PO (Adults): 6 mg/day; may titrate by 3 mg/day at intervals of ≥4 days (range 3–12 mg/day).
IM (Adults): *Erzofri:* 351 mg initially; then 78–234 mg 4 wk later; continue with monthly maintenance dose of 78–234 mg (range based on efficacy and/or tolerability); *Invega Sustenna:* 234 mg initially; then 156 mg 1 wk later; continue with monthly maintenance dose of 78–234 mg (range based on efficacy and/or tolerability).

Renal Impairment

PO (Adults): *CCr 50–79 mL/min:* 3 mg/day initially; may ↑ to max of 6 mg/day; *CCr 10–<50 mL/min:* 1.5 mg/day initially; may ↑ to max of 3 mg/day.

Renal Impairment

IM (Adults): *CCr 50–79 mL/min: Erzofri:* 234 mg initially; then 78 mg 4 wk later; continue with monthly maintenance dose of 78 mg (range of 39–156 mg based on efficacy and/or tolerability); *Invega Sustenna:* 156 mg initially; then 117 mg 1 wk later; continue with monthly maintenance dose of 78 mg (range of 39–156 mg based on efficacy and/or tolerability); *CCr <50 mL/min:* Use not recommended.

Availability (generic available)

Extended-release tablets (Invega): 1.5 mg, 3 mg, 6 mg, 9 mg. **Extended-release intramuscular injection (Erzofri):** 39 mg/0.25 mL, 78 mg/0.5 mL, 117 mg/0.75 mL, 156 mg/mL, 234 mg/1.5 mL, 351 mg/2.25 mL. **Extended-release intramuscular injection (Invega Sustenna):** 39 mg/0.25 mL, ❋ 50 mg/0.5 mL , ❋ 75 mg/0.75 mL, 78 mg/0.5 mL, ❋ 100 mg/mL, 117 mg/0.75 mL, ❋ 150 mg/1.5 mL, 156 mg/mL, 234 mg/1.5 mL. **Extended-release intramuscular injection (Invega Trinza):** ❋ 175 mg/0.875 mL, ❋ 263 mg/1.315 mL, 273 mg/0.875 mL, ❋ 350 mg/1.75 mL, 410 mg/1.315 mL, ❋ 525 mg/2.625 mL, 546 mg/1.75 mL, 819 mg/2.625 mL. **Extended-release intramuscular injection (Invega Hafyera):** 1092 mg/3.5 mL, 1,560 mg/5 mL.

NURSING IMPLICATIONS

Assessment

- Monitor mental status (orientation, mood, behavior) before and periodically during therapy. Monitor closely for notable changes in behavior that could indicate the emergence or worsening of suicidal thoughts or behavior or depression, especially during early therapy. Restrict amount of drug available to patient.
- Assess weight and BMI initially and throughout therapy. Refer as appropriate for nutritional/weight and medical management.
- Obtain ECG at baseline. Monitor orthostatic BP (sitting, standing, lying down) and HR before and periodically during therapy. May cause prolonged QT interval, tachycardia, hypertension, and orthostatic hypotension. Protect patient from falls.
- Monitor for signs/symptoms of hyperglycemia (polydipsia, polyuria, polyphagia, nausea, weakness) during treatment.
- Monitor for onset of extrapyramidal side effects (*akathisia:* restlessness; *dystonia:* muscle spasms and twisting motions; *pseudoparkinsonism:* masklike face, rigidity, tremors, drooling, shuffling gait, dysphagia). Report these symptoms; ↓ of dose or discontinuation of medication may be necessary.
- Monitor for tardive dyskinesia (involuntary rhythmic movement of mouth, face, and extremities). Report immediately; may be irreversible.
- Monitor for development of neuroleptic malignant syndrome (fever, muscle rigidity, delirium, respiratory distress, tachycardia, seizures, diaphoresis, hypertension or hypotension, cardiac arrhythmia, pallor, tiredness). *If neuroleptic malignant syndrome suspected,* discontinue paliperidone.
- Monitor for signs/symptoms related to hyperprolactinemia (menstrual abnormalities, galactorrhea, sexual dysfunction, changes in libido, erectile or ejaculatory dysfunction).
- Assess for falls risk. Drowsiness, orthostatic hypotension, and motor and sensory instability ↑ risk. Institute prevention if indicated.

Lab Test Considerations

- Monitor fasting blood glucose at baseline, at wk 12, and annually in all patients; monitor more frequently for patients with risk factors for diabetes mellitus; patients with diabetes should be closely monitored for worsening glucose control.
- Monitor cholesterol levels at baseline, at wk 12, and every 5 yr thereafter.
- Monitor serum prolactin prior to and periodically during therapy. May ↑ serum prolactin levels.
- Monitor CBC frequently during initial months of therapy in patients with pre-existing or history of low WBC. May cause leukopenia, neutropenia, or agranulocytosis. *If leukopenia, neutropenia, or agranulocytosis occurs,* discontinue paliperidone.

Implementation

- ***High Alert:*** Do not confuse Invega Sustenna with Invega Trinza. Do no confuse Invega with Intuniv.

P

- **PO:** Administer once daily in the morning without regard to food. ***DNC:*** Tablets should be swallowed whole; do not crush, break, or chew. Observe patient when administering medication to ensure that medication is actually swallowed and not hoarded or cheeked.
- **IM:** *Erzofri:* Prior to administration, shake the prefilled syringe vigorously for ≥10 sec within 5 min prior to administration to ensure a homogeneous suspension. Administer as a single injection; do not administer as a divided injection; use only the needles provided within the dose kit. Administer initial and 2nd doses in deltoid using a 1½-inch 22-gauge needle for patients ≥90 kg (≥200 lb) or 1-inch 23-gauge needle for patients <90 kg (<200 lb). Monthly maintenance doses can be administered in either deltoid or gluteal sites. For gluteal injection, use 1½-inch 22-gauge needle regardless of patient weight. Monthly doses may be given up to 7 days before or after the monthly time point. *After 1st mo, if missed dose is within 4–6 wk of scheduled dose,* resume regular monthly dosing as soon as possible at the patient's previously stabilized dose, followed by return to normal monthly injections in either deltoid or gluteal muscle. *If >6 wk–6 mo since 1st injection,* resume at same dose the patient was previously stabilized on (unless patient was stabilized on a dose of 234 mg; then the 1st 2 injections should be 156 mg each). Administer a deltoid injection as soon as possible, administer a 2nd deltoid injection 1 wk later at the same dose, and thereafter resume previously stabilized dose 1 mo after the second injection in deltoid or gluteal sites. *If >6 mo since scheduled dose,* restart dosing with initial dose of 351 mg deltoid injection on day 1, and then resume previously stabilized dose 1 mo after the initial injection.
- **IM:** *Invega Sustenna:* Administer initial and 2nd doses in deltoid using a 1½-inch 22-gauge needle for patients ≥90 kg (≥200 lb) or 1-inch 23-gauge needle for patients <90 kg (<200 lb). Monthly maintenance doses can be administered in either deltoid or gluteal sites. For gluteal injection, use 1½-inch 22-gauge needle regardless of patient weight. To avoid missed dose, may give 2nd dose 4 days before or after the 1-wk time point. Monthly doses may be given up to 7 days before or after the monthly time point. *After 1st mo, if missed dose is within 4 wk of scheduled dose,* administer 2nd dose of 156 mg as soon as possible. Give 3rd dose of 117 mg in either deltoid or gluteal muscle 5 wk after 1st injection (regardless of timing of 2nd injection). Then return to normal monthly injections in either deltoid or gluteal muscle. *If >4 wk and <7 wk since 1st injection,* resume by administering 156 mg dose in deltoid as soon as possible, a 2nd 156 mg dose in deltoid in 1 wk, followed by monthly doses in deltoid or gluteal sites. *If >7 mo since scheduled dose,* administer using initial dosing schedule. During regular monthly dose schedule, *if <6 wk since last injection,* administer previously stabilized dose as soon as possible and then monthly. *If >6 wk since last injection,* resume dose previously stabilized on, unless stabilized on 234 mg (then 1st two injections should be 156 mg). Administer one dose in deltoid as soon as possible and then another deltoid injection of same dose 1 wk later; then resume regular monthly schedule. *If >6 mo since last injection,* administer using initial dosing schedule. Once stabilized on *Invega Sustenna*, can then transition to appropriate dose of *Invega Hafyera*.
- **IM:** *Invega Trinza:* Use only after ≥4 mo of monthly *Invega Sustenna* therapy. Prior to administration, shake the prefilled syringe vigorously for ≥15 sec within 5 min prior to administration to ensure a homogeneous suspension. *Deltoid injection:* For patients weighing <90 kg, use the 1-inch 22-gauge thin wall needle. For patients weighing ≥90 kg, use the 1½-inch 22-gauge thin wall needle. *Gluteal injection:* Regardless of patient weight, use 1½-inch 22-gauge thin wall needle. Initiate *Invega Trinza* when next 1-mo paliperidone dose is scheduled. *Avoid missed doses;* dose may be given 2 wk before or after 3 mo scheduled dose. *If more than 3½ mo (up to but <4 mo) since last dose,* administer previously administered dose as soon as possible; then continue with 3-mo injections. *If 4 mo up to and including 9 mo since last dose,* do NOT administer next dose. *If last dose was 273 mg,* administer 2 doses of 78 mg of *Invega Sustenna* one wk apart into deltoid muscle, then one dose of *Invega Trinza* 273 mg 1 mo after 2nd dose of *Invega Sustenna*. *If last dose was 410 mg,* administer 2 doses of 117 mg of *Invega Sustenna* 1 wk apart into deltoid muscle, then one dose of *Invega Trinza* 410 mg 1 mo after 2nd dose of *Invega Sustenna*. *If last dose was 819 mg,* administer 2 doses of 156 mg of *Invega Sustenna* 1 wk apart into deltoid muscle, then one dose of *Invega Trinza* 819 mg 1 mo after 2nd dose of *Invega Sustenna*. If >9 mo have elapsed since last injection of *Invega Trinza*, reinitiate treatment with *Invega Sustenna*. Then resume *Invega Trinza* after at least 4 mo of *Invega Sustenna*. Once stabilized on *Invega Trinza*, can then transition to appropriate dose of *Invega Hafyera*.
- **IM:** *Invega Hafyera* must be administered as a gluteal IM injection by a health care provider once every 6 mo. After shaking, solution is uniform, thick, and milky white; do not inject if discolored or contains particulate matter. Do not use needles from *Invega Sustenna* or *Invega Trinza*; may develop blockage. Begin *Invega Hafyera* only after therapy has been established with either once-a-month *Invega Sustenna* for ≥4 mo OR every-3-mo *Invega Trinza* for at least one 3-mo injection cycle. Begin

within 1 wk before or after next scheduled dose for *Invega Sustenna* or 2 wk before or after *Invega Trinza* dose. May give *Invega Hafyera* injection up to 2 wk before or 3 wk after the scheduled 6-mo dose to avoid a missed dose. **If >6 mo and 3 wk but <8 mo since last dose of *Invega Hafyera*,** restart with *Invega Sustenna. If last dose of Invega Hafyera was 1092 mg,* administer *Invega Sustenna* 156 mg into deltoid muscle on Day 1. Then 1 mo after Day 1, administer *Invega Hafyera* 1092 mg into gluteal muscle. *If last dose of Invega Hafyera was 1560 mg,* administer *Invega Sustenna* 234 mg into deltoid muscle on Day 1. Then 1 mo after Day 1, administer **Invega Hafyera** 1560 mg into gluteal muscle. **If 8 mo up to and including 11 mo since last dose of** *Invega Hafyera*, restart with *Invega Sustenna*. *If last dose of Invega Hafyera was 1092 mg,* administer *Invega Sustenna* 156 mg into deltoid muscle on Day 1 and 156 mg on Day 8. Then 1 mo after Day 8, administer *Invega Hafyera* 1092 mg into gluteal muscle. *If last dose of Invega Hafyera was 1560 mg,* administer *Invega Sustenna* 156 mg into deltoid muscle on Day 1 and 156 mg on Day 8. Then 1 mo after Day 1, administer *Invega Hafyera* 1560 mg into gluteal muscle. If >11 mo since the last dose of *Invega Hafyera,* restart therapy with *Invega Sustenna. Invega Hafyera* can be resumed after therapy with *Invega Sustenna* for at least 4 mo.

Patient/Family Teaching

- Explain purpose and side effects of paliperidone to patient. Instruct them to take medication as directed. Do not share medication with others, even if they have similar symptoms; may be harmful. Keep out of children's reach. Appearance of tablets in stool is normal and not of concern. Advise patient to read *Patient Information* before starting and with each Rx refill in case of changes.
- Emphasize the importance of routine follow-up exams and lab tests to monitor side effects and continued participation in psychotherapy to improve coping skills.
- Inform patient of the possibility of extrapyramidal symptoms, neuroleptic malignant syndrome, and tardive dyskinesia. Instruct patient to report these symptoms immediately to health care provider.
- Instruct patients with diabetes to monitor blood glucose more closely; advise patients without diabetes of symptoms of high blood glucose (↑ thirst, hunger, and urination).
- Advise patient to change positions slowly to minimize orthostatic hypotension. Protect from falls.
- May cause drowsiness and dizziness. Caution patient to avoid driving or other activities requiring alertness until response to medication is known.
- Advise patient and family to notify health care provider if thoughts about suicide or dying, attempts to commit suicide, new or worse depression, new or worse anxiety, feeling very agitated or restless, panic attacks, trouble sleeping, new or worse irritability, acting aggressive, being angry or violent, acting on dangerous impulses, an extreme ↑ in activity and talking, or other unusual changes in behavior or mood occur.
- Advise patient that extremes in temperature should also be avoided; this drug impairs body temperature regulation.
- Advise patient to notify health care provider of all Rx or OTC medications, vitamins, or herbal products being taken and to consult with health care provider before taking other medications, especially St. John's wort and alcohol.
- Advise patient to seek nutritional, weight, or medical management as needed for weight gain or cholesterol elevation.
- Instruct patient to notify health care provider promptly if sore throat, fever, unusual bleeding or bruising, rash, tremors, menstrual abnormalities, galactorrhea, or sexual dysfunction occur.
- Advise patient to notify health care provider of medication regimen before treatment or surgery.
- Rep: Advise women of reproductive potential to notify health care provider if pregnancy is planned or suspected or if breastfeeding. Encourage pregnant women to enroll in the National Pregnancy Registry for Atypical Antipsychotics by calling 1-866-961-2388 or visiting http://womensmentalhealth.org/clinical-and-research-programs/pregnancyregistry/. Monitor neonates for extrapyramidal and/or withdrawal symptoms (agitation, hypertonia, hypotonia, tremor, somnolence, respiratory distress, feeding disorder) and manage symptoms appropriately. Monitor infants exposed to paliperidone through breast milk for excess sedation, failure to thrive, jitteriness, and extrapyramidal symptoms (tremors and abnormal muscle movements). May temporarily cause female infertility.

Evaluation/Desired Outcomes

- Decrease in excited, manic behavior.
- Decrease in positive symptoms (delusions, hallucinations) of schizophrenia.
- Decrease in negative symptoms (social withdrawal; flat, blunted affect) of schizophrenia.

palonosetron
(pa-lone-**o**-se-tron)
~~Aloxi~~, Posfrea

Classification
Therapeutic: antiemetics
Pharmacologic: 5-HT_3 agonists

P

Indications
Prevention of acute and delayed nausea and vomiting caused by initial or repeat courses of moderately or highly emetogenic chemotherapy (moderately emetogenic chemotherapy for adults only). Prevention of postoperative nausea and vomiting for up to 24 hr after surgery.

Action
Blocks the effects of serotonin at receptor sites (selective antagonist) located in vagal nerve terminals and in the chemoreceptor trigger zones in the CNS. **Therapeutic Effects:** Decreased incidence and severity of nausea and vomiting following emetogenic chemotherapy or surgery.

Pharmacokinetics
Absorption: IV administration results in complete bioavailability.
Distribution: Well distributed to tissues.
Metabolism and Excretion: 50% metabolized by the liver via the CYP1A2, CYP2D6, and CYP3A4 isoenzymes to inactive metabolites; 40% excreted unchanged in urine.
Half-life: 40 hr.

TIME/ACTION PROFILE

ROUTE	ONSET	PEAK	DURATION
IV	within 30 min	unknown	7 days

Contraindications/Precautions
Contraindicated in: Hypersensitivity; cross-sensitivity with other 5-HT_3 antagonists may occur.
Use Cautiously in: OB: Safety not established in pregnancy; Lactation: Use while breastfeeding only if potential maternal benefit justifies potential risk to infant; Pedi: Neonates <1 mo (safety and effectiveness not established).

Adverse Reactions/Side Effects
GI: constipation, diarrhea. **Neuro:** dizziness, headache.

Interactions
Drug-Drug: Drugs that affect serotonergic neurotransmitter systems, including **SSRIs**, **SNRIs**, **tricyclic antidepressants**, **MAO inhibitors**, **fentanyl**, **lithium**, **buspirone**, **tramadol**, **methylene blue**, and **triptans**, may ↑ risk of serotonin syndrome

Route/Dosage
Prevention of Chemotherapy-Induced Nausea/Vomiting
IV (Adults): 0.25 mg given 30 min before start of chemotherapy.
IV (Children 1 mo–<17 yr): 20 mcg/kg (max dose = 1.5 mg) given 30 min before start of chemotherapy.

Prevention of Postoperative Nausea/Vomiting
IV (Adults): 0.075 mg given immediately before induction of anesthesia.

Availability (generic available)
Solution for injection: 0.05 mg/mL. ***In combination with:*** fosnetupitant (Akynzeo); netupitant (Akynzeo); see Appendix N.

NURSING IMPLICATIONS
Assessment
- Assess for nausea, vomiting, abdominal distention, and bowel sounds before and following administration.
- Assess for signs/symptoms of serotonin syndrome (confusion, delirium, agitation, coma, dilated pupils, tachycardia, hyperthermia, shivering, hyperreflexia, muscle rigidity, hypertension, vomiting, diarrhea, seizures). ↑ risk of serotonin syndrome with concurrent use of other serotonergic drugs (SSRIs, SNRIs, triptans). *If serotonin syndrome suspected,* discontinue palonosetron.

Lab Test Considerations
- May transiently ↑ bilirubin, AST, and ALT.

Implementation
- 1st dose is administered prior to emetogenic event.
- Repeated dose within a 7-day period is not recommended.

IV Administration
- **IV Push:** Administer dose undiluted 30 min before chemotherapy or immediately prior to the induction of anesthesia. Flush line before and after administration with 0.9% NaCl. Do not administer solutions that are discolored or contain particulate matter. **Rate:** In adults, administer over 30 sec 30 min before starting chemotherapy and over 10 sec for postoperative nausea and vomiting. In children, administer over 15 min 30 min before starting chemotherapy.
- **Y-Site Compatibility:** alemtuzumab, amikacin, aminocaproic acid, aminophylline, amiodarone, amphotericin B liposomal, ampicillin, ampicillin/sulbactam, anidulafungin, argatroban, atropine, azithromycin, aztreonam, bivalirudin, bleomycin, bumetanide, buprenorphine, busulfan, butorphanol, calcium acetate, calcium chloride, calcium gluconate, carboplatin, carmustine, caspofungin, cefazolin, cefepime, cefotaxime, cefotetan, cefoxitin, ceftazidime, ceftriaxone, cefuroxime, chloramphenicol, chlorpromazine, ciprofloxacin, cisatracurium, cisplatin, clindamycin, cyclophosphamide, cyclosporine, cytarabine, dacarbazine, dactinomycin, dantrolene, daptomycin, daunorubicin, dexamethasone, dexmedetomidine, dexrazoxane, digoxin, diltiazem, diphenhydramine, dobutamine, docetaxel, dopamine, doxorubicin hydrochloride, doxorubicin liposomal, droperidol, enalaprilat, ephedrine, epinephrine, epirubicin, eptifibatide, erythromycin, esmolol, etoposide, etoposide phosphate, famotidine, fentanyl, fluconazole, fludarabine, fluorouracil, fosaprepitant,

foscarnet, fosphenytoin, furosemide, gemcitabine, gentamicin, glycopyrrolate, haloperidol, heparin, hydralazine, hydrocortisone, hydromorphone, idarubicin, ifosfamide, insulin regular, irinotecan, isoproterenol, ketorolac, labetalol, leucovorin, levofloxacin, lidocaine, linezolid, lorazepam, magnesium sulfate, mannitol, melphalan, meperidine, meropenem, mesna, methadone, methotrexate, metoclopramide, metoprolol, metronidazole, midazolam, milrinone, mitomycin, mitoxantrone, morphine, moxifloxacin, nalbuphine, naloxone, neostigmine, nicardipine, nitroglycerin, nitroprusside, norepinephrine, octreotide, oxaliplatin, oxytocin, paclitaxel, paclitaxel protein bound, pamidronate, phenobarbital, phentolamine, phenylephrine, piperacillin/tazobactam, potassium acetate, potassium chloride, potassium phosphates, procainamide, prochlorperazine, promethazine, propofol, propranolol, remifentanil, rocuronium, sodium acetate, sodium bicarbonate, sodium phosphates, succinylcholine, sufentanil, tacrolimus, theophylline, thiotepa, tigecycline, tirofiban, tobramycin, topotecan, trimethoprim/sulfamethoxazole, vancomycin, vasopressin, vecuronium, verapamil, vinblastine, vincristine, vinorelbine, zidovudine.

- **Y-Site Incompatibility:** acyclovir, allopurinol, amphotericin B deoxycholate, diazepam, doxycycline, ganciclovir, gemtuzumab ozogamicin, imipenem/cilastatin, letermovir, methylprednisolone, minocycline, nafcillin, pantoprazole, pentamidine, pentobarbital, phenytoin.

Patient/Family Teaching

- Explain the purpose and side effects of palonosetron. Advise patient to read *Medication Guide* before starting and periodically during therapy in case of changes.
- Advise patient to notify health care provider if nausea or vomiting occur.
- Counsel patient to report symptoms of serotonin syndrome (confusion, sweating, fast heartbeat, fever, vomiting, hallucinations, muscle spasms, tremors, twitching).
- Rep: Advise women of reproductive potential to notify health care provider if pregnancy is planned or suspected or if breastfeeding.

Evaluation/Desired Outcomes

- Prevention of nausea and vomiting associated with initial and repeat courses of emetogenic cancer chemotherapy or surgery.

pamidronate (pa-**mid**-roe-nate)

Classification

Therapeutic: bone resorption inhibitors

Pharmacologic: bisphosphonates, hypocalcemics

Indications

Moderate to severe hypercalcemia associated with malignancy. Osteolytic bone lesions associated with multiple myeloma or breast cancer. Moderate to severe Paget disease.

Action

Inhibits resorption of bone. **Therapeutic Effects:** Decreased serum calcium. Decreased skeletal destruction in multiple myeloma or breast cancer. Decreased skeletal complications in Paget disease.

Pharmacokinetics

Absorption: IV administration results in complete bioavailability.

Distribution: Rapidly absorbed by bone. Reaches high concentrations in bone, liver, spleen, teeth, and tracheal cartilage. Approximately 50% of a dose is retained by bone and then slowly released.

Metabolism and Excretion: 50% excreted unchanged in the urine.

Half-life: Elimination half-life from plasma is biphasic: 1st phase 1.6 hr, 2nd phase 27.2 hr. Elimination half-life from bone is 300 days.

TIME/ACTION PROFILE (effect on serum calcium)

ROUTE	ONSET	PEAK	DURATION
IV	24 hr	7 days	unknown

Contraindications/Precautions

Contraindicated in: Hypersensitivity to pamidronate, other bisphosphonates, or mannitol; OB: Pregnancy; Lactation: Lactation.

Use Cautiously in: Underlying cardiovascular disease, especially HF (initiate saline hydration cautiously); Invasive dental procedures, cancer, receiving chemotherapy or corticosteroids, poor oral hygiene, periodontal disease, dental disease, anemia, coagulopathy, infection, or poorly fitting dentures (may ↑ risk of jaw osteonecrosis); History of thyroid surgery (may be at ↑ risk for hypocalcemia); Renal impairment (↓ dose); Pedi: Safety and effectiveness not established in children.

Adverse Reactions/Side Effects

CV: arrhythmias, hypertension, syncope, tachycardia. **EENT:** blurred vision, conjunctivitis, eye pain/inflammation, rhinitis. **Endo:** hypothyroidism. **F and E** hypocalcemia, hypokalemia, hypomagnesemia, hypophosphatemia, fluid overload. **GI:** nausea, abdominal pain, anorexia, constipation, vomiting. **GU:** nephrotoxicity. **Hemat:** leukopenia, anemia. **Local:** phlebitis. **MS:** muscle stiffness, pain, femur fractures, osteonecrosis (primarily of jaw). **Neuro:** fatigue. **Resp:** rales. **Misc:** fever.

Interactions

Drug-Drug: Hypokalemia and hypomagnesemia may ↑ risk of **digoxin** toxicity. **Calcium** and **vitamin D** will antagonize the beneficial effects of pamidronate. **Thalidomide** may ↑ risk of renal impairment.

Route/Dosage

Hypercalcemia of Malignancy

IV (Adults): *Moderate hypercalcemia (corrected serum calcium of 12–13.5 mg/dL):* 60–90 mg as single dose; may be repeated after 7 days. *Severe hypercalcemia (corrected serum calcium >13.5 mg/dL):* 90 mg as single dose; may be repeated after 7 days.

Osteolytic Lesions from Multiple Myeloma

IV (Adults): 90 mg once monthly.

Osteolytic Lesions from Metastatic Breast Cancer

IV (Adults): 90 mg every 3–4 wk.

Paget Disease

IV (Adults): 30 mg once daily for 3 days.

Availability (generic available)

Solution for injection: 3 mg/mL, 6 mg/mL, 9 mg/mL.

NURSING IMPLICATIONS

Assessment

- Monitor intake, output, and BP frequently during therapy. Assess for signs of fluid overload (edema, rales/crackles).
- Monitor signs/symptoms of hypercalcemia (nausea, vomiting, anorexia, weakness, constipation, thirst, cardiac arrhythmias).
- Observe for evidence of hypocalcemia (paresthesia, muscle twitching, laryngospasm, Chvostek or Trousseau sign). Protect symptomatic patients by elevating and padding side rails; keep bed in low position. Calcium and vitamin D supplementation recommended.
- Perform dental examination before initiation of treatment. Osteonecrosis of jaw more like to occur with dental extraction, periodontal disease, and poorly fitting dentures. Preventive dentistry recommended prior to treatment. Invasive dental procedures should be avoided if possible during treatment.
- Monitor IV site for phlebitis (pain, redness, swelling). Symptomatic treatment should be used if this occurs.
- Assess for bone pain. Treatment with nonopioid or opioid analgesics may be necessary.

Lab Test Considerations

- Verify pregnancy status when starting therapy and monitor regularly.
- Monitor serum electrolytes (including calcium, phosphate, potassium, and magnesium) closely. May cause hypokalemia, hypomagnesemia, hypophosphatemia, and hypocalcemia.
- Assess serum creatinine prior to each treatment. Monitor renal function periodically during therapy.
- Monitor CBC with differential during the 1st 2 wk of therapy.
- Monitor vitamin D levels.
- In Paget disease, monitor alkaline phosphatase and urinary hydroxyproline.
- In multiple myeloma, monitor urine albumin every 3–6 mo.

Implementation

- Initiate a vigorous saline hydration, maintaining a urine output of 2000 mL/24 hr, concurrently with pamidronate therapy. Patients should be adequately hydrated, but avoid overhydration. Use caution in patients with underlying cardiovascular disease, especially HF. Do not use diuretics prior to treatment of hypovolemia.
- Single doses of IV pamidronate should not exceed 90 mg due to the high risk of clinically significant deterioration in renal function, which may progress to renal failure.
- Use double gloves and a protective gown to prepare and administer. If possible, prepare in a biological safety cabinet or a compounding aseptic containment isolator; eye, face, and respiratory protection may be needed. Prepare and administer in a closed-system drug transfer device. During administration, if there is a potential that the substance could splash or if the patient may resist, use eye and face protection. Discard IV equipment in specially designated containers. Health care providers who are actively trying to conceive, who are pregnant or may become pregnant, and who are breastfeeding should avoid handling pamidronate.

IV Administration

- **Hypercalcemia: Dilution:** Dilute recommended dose in 1000 mL of 0.45% NaCl, 0.9% NaCl, or D5W. Solution is stable for 24 hr at room temperature. **Rate:** Administer over 2–24 hr (infuse over >2 hr in patients with renal impairment).
- **Multiple Myeloma: Dilution:** Dilute recommended dose in 500 mL of 0.45% NaCl, 0.9% NaCl, or D5W. **Rate:** Administer over 4 hr.
- **Breast Cancer: Dilution:** Dilute recommended dose in 250 mL of 0.45% NaCl, 0.9% NaCl, or D5W. **Rate:** Administer over 2 hr.
- **Paget Disease: Dilution:** Dilute recommended dose in 500 mL of 0.45% NaCl, 0.9% NaCl, or D5W. **Rate:** Administer over 4 hr.
- **Y-Site Compatibility:** acyclovir, alemtuzumab, allopurinol, amikacin, aminophylline, amphotericin B liposomal, ampicillin, ampicillin/sulbactam, anidulafungin, argatroban, arsenic, atracurium, azithromycin, aztreonam, bivalirudin, bleomycin, bumetanide, buprenorphine, butorphanol, carboplatin, carmustine, cefazolin, cefepime, cefotaxime, cefotetan, cefoxitin, ceftazidime, ceftriaxone, cefuroxime, chloramphenicol, chlorpromazine,

ciprofloxacin, cisatracurium, cisplatin, clindamycin, cyclophosphamide, cyclosporine, cytarabine, dacarbazine, daptomycin, dexamethasone, dexmedetomidine, dexrazoxane, digoxin, diltiazem, diphenhydramine, dobutamine, docetaxel, dopamine, doxorubicin hydrochloride, doxorubicin liposomal, doxycycline, droperidol, enalaprilat, ephedrine, epinephrine, epirubicin, ertapenem, erythromycin, esmolol, etoposide, etoposide phosphate, famotidine, fentanyl, fluconazole, fludarabine, fluorouracil, foscarnet, fosphenytoin, furosemide, ganciclovir, gemcitabine, gentamicin, glycopyrrolate, granisetron, haloperidol, heparin, hydralazine, hydrocortisone, hydromorphone, ifosfamide, imipenem/cilastatin, insulin regular, isoproterenol, ketorolac, labetalol, levofloxacin, lidocaine, linezolid, lorazepam, magnesium sulfate, mannitol, melphalan, meperidine, meropenem, mesna, methotrexate, methylprednisolone, metoclopramide, metoprolol, metronidazole, midazolam, milrinone, mitoxantrone, morphine, moxifloxacin, mycophenolate, nafcillin, nalbuphine, naloxone, nicardipine, nitroglycerin, nitroprusside, norepinephrine, octreotide, ondansetron, oxytocin, paclitaxel, palonosetron, pemetrexed, pentamidine, pentobarbital, phenobarbital, phentolamine, phenylephrine, piperacillin/tazobactam, potassium acetate, potassium chloride, potassium phosphates, procainamide, prochlorperazine, promethazine, propranolol, remifentanil, rocuronium, sodium acetate, sodium bicarbonate, sodium phosphates, succinylcholine, sufentanil, tacrolimus, theophylline, thiotepa, tigecycline, tirofiban, tobramycin, topotecan, trimethoprim/sulfamethoxazole, vancomycin, vasopressin, vecuronium, verapamil, vinblastine, vincristine, vinorelbine, voriconazole, zidovudine.

- **Y-Site Incompatibility:** amphotericin B deoxycholate, caspofungin, dantrolene, diazepam, gemtuzumab ozogamicin, leucovorin, phenytoin.

Patient/Family Teaching

- Explain the purpose and side effects of pamidronate. If an appointment is missed, contact health care provider as soon as possible to reschedule. Advise patient to read *Medication Guide* before starting and periodically during therapy in case of changes.
- Emphasize the need for keeping follow-up exams to monitor progress, even after medication is discontinued, to detect relapse.
- Advise patient to report signs of hypercalcemic relapse (bone pain, anorexia, nausea, vomiting, thirst, lethargy) or eye problems (pain, inflammation, blurred vision, conjunctivitis) to health care provider promptly.
- Advise patient to notify nurse of pain at the infusion site.
- Encourage patient to comply with dietary recommendations. Diet should contain adequate amounts of calcium and vitamin D.
- Advise patient to notify health care provider if bone pain is severe or persistent.
- Advise patient to maintain good oral hygiene and have regular dental examinations. Instruct patient to inform health care provider of pamidronate therapy prior to dental surgery. Tell patients with concurrent risk factors for osteonecrosis of the jaw to report signs/symptoms of this condition (gum loss; numbness; pain, swelling, or infection of jaw/gums).
- Advise patient to notify health care provider of all Rx or OTC medications, vitamins, or herbal products being taken and to consult with health care provider before taking other medications.
- Rep: May cause fetal harm. Advise women of reproductive potential to notify health care provider if pregnancy is planned or suspected and to avoid breastfeeding during therapy. May impair female and male fertility.

Evaluation/Desired Outcomes

- Lowered serum calcium levels.
- Decreased pain from lytic lesions.

P

pancrelipase (pan-kre-li-pase)

✱ Cotazym, Creon, ✱ Pancrease MT, Pancreaze, Pertzye, Viokace, Zenpep

Classification

Therapeutic: digestive agent

Pharmacologic: pancreatic enzymes

Indications

Pancreatic insufficiency associated with: Chronic pancreatitis, Pancreatectomy, Cystic fibrosis, GI bypass surgery, Ductal obstruction secondary to tumor.

Action

Contains lipolytic, amylolytic, and proteolytic activity. **Therapeutic Effects:** Increased digestion of fats, carbohydrates, and proteins in the GI tract.

Pharmacokinetics

Absorption: Unknown.
Distribution: Unknown.
Metabolism and Excretion: Unknown.
Half-life: Unknown.

TIME/ACTION PROFILE (digestant effects)

ROUTE	ONSET	PEAK	DURATION
PO	rapid	unknown	unknown

Contraindications/Precautions

Contraindicated in: Hypersensitivity to hog proteins.

Use Cautiously in: Gout, renal impairment, or hyperuricemia (may ↑ uric acid levels); OB: Systemic absorption during pregnancy expected to be minimal; significant fetal exposure not expected; Lactation: Systemic absorption expected to be minimal; significant exposure to breastfed infant not expected.

Adverse Reactions/Side Effects

Derm: hives, rash. **EENT:** nasal stuffiness. **GI:** abdominal pain (high doses only), diarrhea, nausea, stomach cramps, FIBROSING COLONOPATHY (HIGH DOSES ONLY), oral irritation. **GU:** hematuria. **Metab:** hyperuricemia. **Resp:** dyspnea, shortness of breath, wheezing. **Misc:** allergic reactions.

Interactions

Drug-Drug: Antacids (**calcium carbonate** or **magnesium hydroxide**) may ↓ effectiveness of pancrelipase. May ↓ the absorption of concurrently administered **iron supplements**.

Drug-Food: **Alkaline foods** destroy coating on enteric-coated products.

Route/Dosage

PO (Adults and Children ≥4 yr): Initiate with 500 lipase units/kg/meal; dose should be adjusted based on weight, clinical symptoms, and stool fat content; maximum dose = 2500 lipase units/kg/meal (or 10,000 lipase units/kg/day).

PO (Children >1 yr and <4 yr): Initiate with 1000 lipase units/kg/meal; dose should be adjusted based on weight, clinical symptoms, and stool fat content; maximum dose = 2500 lipase units/kg/meal (or 10,000 lipase units/kg/day).

PO (Children ≤1 yr): 2000–4000 lipase units per 120 mL of formula or breast milk.

Availability (generic available)

Tablets: 10,440 units lipase/39,150 units protease/39,150 units amylase, 20,880 units lipase/78,300 units protease/78,300 units amylase. **Delayed-release capsules:** 2600 units lipase/6200 units protease/10,850 units amylase, 3000 units lipase/9500 units protease/15,000 units amylase, 3000 units lipase/10,000 units protease/16,000 units amylase, 4000 units lipase/14,375 units protease/15,125 units amylase, 4200 units lipase/14,200 units protease/24,600 units amylase, 5000 units lipase/17,000 units protease/27,000 units amylase, 6000 units lipase/19,000 units protease/30,000 units amylase, 8000 units lipase/28,750 units protease/30,250 units amylase, 🍁 8000 units lipase/30,000 units protease/30,000 units amylase, 10,000 units lipase/34,000 units protease/55,000 units amylase, 10,500 units lipase/35,500 units protease/61,500 units amylase, 12,000 units lipase/38,000 units protease/60,000 units amylase, 13,800 units lipase/27,600 units protease/27,600 units amylase, 15,000 units lipase/51,000 units protease/82,000 units amylase, 16,000 units lipase/57,500 units protease/60,500 units amylase, 16,800 units lipase/56,800 units protease/98,400 units amylase, 🍁 20,000 units lipase/55,000 units protease/55,000 units amylase, 20,000 units lipase/68,000 units protease/109,000 units amylase, 20,700 units lipase/41,400 units protease/41,400 units amylase, 21,000 units lipase/54,700 units protease/83,900 units amylase, 23,000 units lipase/46,000 units protease/46,000 units amylase, 24,000 units lipase/76,000 units protease/120,000 units amylase, 25,000 units lipase/85,000 units protease/136,000 units amylase, 36,000 units lipase/114,000 units protease/180,000 units amylase, 40,000 units lipase/136,000 units protease/218,000 units amylase, 60,000 units lipase/189,600 units protease/252,600 units amylase.

NURSING IMPLICATIONS

Assessment

- Assess patient's nutritional status (height, weight, skin fold thickness, arm muscle circumference, lab values) prior to and periodically throughout therapy.
- Monitor stools for steatorrhea (foul smell, frothy).
- Assess patient for allergy to pork; sensitivity to pancrelipase may exist.

Lab Test Considerations

- May cause ↑ serum and urine uric acid concentrations. Consider monitoring in patients with gout, renal impairment, or hyperuricemia.

Implementation

- *Pancreaze* is not interchangeable with any other pancrelipase product.
- **PO:** Administer immediately before or with meals and snacks.
- ***DNC:*** Swallow tablets whole; do not crush, break, or chew.
- If unable to swallow whole, capsules may be opened and contents sprinkled on soft, acidic foods that can be swallowed without chewing (e.g., applesauce or Jell-O). Follow immediately with water or juice to ensure complete ingestion. Do not mix with alkaline foods prior to ingestion or coating will be destroyed.
- Half of the prescribed *Pancreaze* and *Pertzye* dose for an individualized full meal should be given with each snack. The total daily dose should reflect approximately three meals plus two or three snacks per day.
- Do not mix contents of *Pancreaze, Pertzye,* or *Creon* capsules directly into breast milk or formula. Capsule contents may be sprinkled on small amounts of acidic soft food with pH ≤4.5 (applesauce) and administered within 15 min. Contents of the capsule

may also be administered directly to the mouth, followed with breast milk or formula. Applesauce mixture of *Pertzye* can also be administered via a gastric tube.

- Do not mix *Zenpep* capsule contents directly into formula or breast milk prior to administration. Administer with applesauce, bananas, or pears (commercially prepared) and follow with breast milk or formula.

Patient/Family Teaching

- Encourage patients to comply with diet recommendations of health care professional (generally high calorie, high protein, low fat). Dose should be adjusted for fat content of diet. Usually 300 mg of pancrelipase is necessary to digest every 17 g of dietary fat. If a dose is missed, it should be omitted and next dose taken with next snack, as directed. Do not ↑ dose without consulting health care professional. Several days may be required to determine correct dose. Advise patient to read *Medication Guide* before starting therapy and with each Rx refill; information may be updated.
- Instruct patient not to chew tablets and to swallow them quickly with plenty of liquid to prevent mouth and throat irritation. Sit upright to enhance swallowing. Eating immediately after taking medication helps further ensure that the medication is swallowed and does not remain in contact with mouth and esophagus for a prolonged period. Patient should avoid sniffing powdered contents of capsules, as sensitization of nose and throat may occur (nasal stuffiness or respiratory distress).
- Advise patients and caregivers to notify health care professional if symptoms of fibrosing colonopathy (abdominal pain, distention, vomiting, constipation) occur. Symptoms occur more frequently with doses >6000 lipase units/kg of body weight per meal (10,000 lipase units/kg of body weight/day) and have been associated with colonic strictures in children <12 yr.
- Instruct patient to notify health care professional if joint pain, swelling of legs, gastric distress, or rash occurs.
- Instruct patient to notify health care professional immediately if difficulty breathing or hives occur.
- Rep: Advise female patients to notify health care professional if pregnancy is planned or suspected or if breastfeeding.

Evaluation/Desired Outcomes

- Improved nutritional status in patients with pancreatic insufficiency.
- Normalization of stools in patients with steatorrhea.

HIGH ALERT

panitumumab

(pan-i-**tu**-mu-mab)

Vectibix

Classification

Therapeutic: antineoplastics

Pharmacologic: kinase inhibitors

Indications

Wild-type RAS (wild type in KRAS and NRAS) metastatic colorectal cancer that has failed fluoropyrimidine-, oxaliplatin-, and irinotecan-containing chemotherapy (as monotherapy). Wild-type RAS (wild type in KRAS and NRAS) metastatic colorectal cancer (as first-line therapy with FOLFOX). KRAS G12C-mutated metastatic colorectal cancer in patients who have received prior treatment with fluoropyrimidine-, oxaliplatin-, and irinotecan-based chemotherapy (in combination with sotorasib).

Action

Binds to epidermal growth factor receptor, resulting in inactivation of kinases that regulate proliferation and transformation. **Therapeutic Effects:** Decreased progression of colorectal cancer.

Pharmacokinetics

Absorption: IV administration results in complete bioavailability.
Distribution: Unknown.
Metabolism and Excretion: Unknown.
Half-life: 7.5 days.

TIME/ACTION PROFILE (plasma concentrations)

ROUTE	ONSET	PEAK	DURATION
IV	unknown	end of infusion	unknown

Contraindications/Precautions

Contraindicated in: Concurrent use of leucovorin; RAS: mutant metastatic colorectal cancer or unknown RAS mutation status (↑ mortality and tumor progression); OB: Pregnancy; Lactation: Lactation.
Use Cautiously in: Rep: Women of reproductive potential; Pedi: Safety and effectiveness not established in children.

Adverse Reactions/Side Effects

CV: edema. **Derm:** acneiform dermatitis, dry skin, erythema, paronychia, pruritus, rash, skin exfoliation, skin fissures, abscesses, NECROTIZING FASCIITIS, photosensitivity. **EENT:** corneal perforation, eyelash growth, keratitis, ulcerative keratitis. **F and E** hypomagnesemia, hypocalcemia. **GI:** abdominal pain, constipation, diarrhea,

P

nausea, vomiting, stomatitis. **GU:** acute renal failure. **Neuro:** fatigue. **Resp:** cough, INTERSTITIAL LUNG DISEASE (ILD), PULMONARY FIBROSIS. **Misc:** INFUSION REACTIONS.

Interactions

Drug-Drug: None reported.

Route/Dosage

RAS Wild-Type Metastatic Colorectal Cancer

IV (Adults): 6 mg/kg every 14 days; continue until disease progression or unacceptable toxicity.

KRAS G12C: Mutated Metastatic Colorectal Cancer

IV (Adults): 6 mg/kg every 14 days; continue until disease progression, unacceptable toxicity, or until sotorasib is withheld or discontinued. Administer 1st sotorasib dose before 1st panitumumab infusion.

Availability

Solution for injection: 20 mg/mL.

NURSING IMPLICATIONS

Assessment

- Assess for dermatologic toxicity (dermatitis acneiform, pruritus, erythema, rash, skin exfoliation, paronychia, dry skin, skin fissures). If severe, may lead to infection (sepsis, septic death, abscesses requiring incision and drainage). *Upon 1st occurrence of Grade 3 dermatologic toxicity,* hold 1–2 doses; if skin improves to Grade <3, resume at original dose. *For 2nd occurrence of Grade 3 dermatologic toxicity,* hold 1–2 doses; if skin improves to Grade <3, resume at 80% of original dose. *For 3rd occurrence of Grade 3 dermatologic toxicity,* hold 1–2 doses; if skin improves to Grade <3, resume at 60% of original dose. *For Grade 4 dermatologic toxicity or 4th occurrence of a Grade 3 dermatologic toxicity,* permanently discontinue panitumumab.
- Monitor for signs/symptoms of infusion-related reactions (fever, chills, hypotension, dizziness, nausea, vomiting, urticaria, pruritus, shortness of breath, bronchospasm, angioedema) during and within 24 hr of infusion. *If mild to moderate infusion-related reaction occurs,* ↓ infusion rate by 50%. *If severe infusion-related reaction occurs,* stop panitumumab; may require permanent discontinuation.
- Monitor for signs/symptoms of ILD or pulmonary fibrosis (dyspnea, cough, hypoxia, fever). CT scan or chest x-ray can confirm. *If ILD or pulmonary fibrosis suspected,* hold therapy. *If ILD or pulmonary fibrosis confirmed,* permanently discontinue panitumumab.
- Monitor for diarrhea and dehydration during therapy. Provide supportive care including antiemetic or antidiarrheal as needed; hold panitumumab, if necessary.
- Monitor for evidence of keratitis, ulcerative keratitis, or corneal perforation. *If acute or worsening keratitis, ulcerative keratitis, or corneal perforation occur,* interrupt or discontinue panitumumab.

Lab Test Considerations

- Patient selection is based on RAS or KRAS G12C status. Prior to administration, assess RAS and KRAS G12C mutational status in colorectal tumors and confirm the absence of a RAS mutation in exons 2, 3, and 4. Information on FDA-approved tests for the detection of RAS and KRAS G12 Cmutations in patients with metastatic colorectal cancer is available at http://www.fda.gov/CompanionDiagnostics.
- Monitor electrolytes regularly during and for 8 wk after therapy. May cause hypomagnesemia, hypocalcemia, and hypokalemia. Replace electrolytes as needed.

Implementation

IV Administration

- **Intermittent Infusion: Dilution:** Dilute dose in 100 mL of 0.9% NaCl; dilute doses >1000 mg with 150 mL. **Concentration:** ≤10 mg/mL. Mix by inverting gently; do not shake. Solution is colorless and may contain a small amount of visible translucent to white, amorphous, proteinaceous particles. Do not administer solutions that are discolored or contain particulate matter. Store in refrigerator; do not freeze. Use diluted solution within 6 hr of preparation if stored at room temperature or within 24 hr if refrigerated.
- **Rate:** Administer over 60 min via infusion pump using a low-protein-binding 0.2-mcg or 0.22-mcg in-line filter. If 1st infusion is tolerated, subsequent infusions may be infused over 30–60 min. Administer doses >1000 mg over 90 min. Flush line before and after administration with 0.9% NaCl.
- **Y-Site Incompatibility:** Do not administer other drugs through same IV line.

Patient/Family Teaching

- Explain purpose and side effects of panitumumab. If an appointment is missed, reschedule as soon as possible. Advise patient to read *Patient Information* before starting and with each Rx refill in case of changes.
- Emphasize the importance of regular follow-ups and eye exams to monitor for side effects and periodic blood tests to monitor electrolyte levels.
- May cause photosensitivity. Caution patient to wear sunscreen and hats and to limit sun exposure. Advise patient to avoid tanning beds during treatment and for 2 mo following therapy, as sunlight may ↑ risk of dermatologic reactions.
- Instruct patient to report symptoms of hypomagnesemia, hypocalcemia, or hypokalemia (muscle twitches, spasms, weakness, or cramps; heart palpitations).

- Advise patient to notify health care provider if signs and symptoms of dermatologic toxicity, infusion reactions, pulmonary fibrosis, or ocular changes occur.
- Advise patient to notify health care provider of all Rx or OTC medications, vitamins, or herbal products being taken and to consult with health care provider before taking other medications.
- Rep: May cause fetal harm. Advise women of reproductive potential to notify health care provider if pregnancy is planned or suspected or if breastfeeding. Advise women of reproductive potential to use effective contraception and to avoid breastfeeding during therapy and for 2 mo after last dose. May impair fertility in women.

Evaluation/Desired Outcomes

- Decreased progression of colorectal cancer.

BEERS

☒ pantoprazole
(pan-**toe**-pra-zole)
✦ Pantoloc, Protonix, ✦ Tecta
Classification
Therapeutic: antiulcer agents
Pharmacologic: proton pump inhibitors

Indications

Erosive esophagitis associated with GERD. Maintenance of healing of erosive esophagitis. Pathologic hypersecretory conditions, including Zollinger-Ellison syndrome. **Unlabeled Use:** Adjunctive treatment of duodenal ulcers associated with *Helicobacter pylori*.

Action

Binds to an enzyme in the presence of acidic gastric pH, preventing the final transport of hydrogen ions into the gastric lumen. **Therapeutic Effects:** Diminished accumulation of acid in the gastric lumen, with lessened acid reflux. Healing of duodenal ulcers and esophagitis. Decreased acid secretion in hypersecretory conditions.

Pharmacokinetics

Absorption: Tablet is enteric-coated; absorption occurs only after tablet leaves the stomach.
Distribution: Unknown.
Protein Binding: 98%.
Metabolism and Excretion: Primarily metabolized by the CYP2C19 and CYP3A4 isoenzymes in the liver; ☒ the CYP2C19 isoenzyme exhibits genetic polymorphism (15–20% of Asian patients and 3–5% of White and Black patients may be poor metabolizers and may have significantly ↑ pantoprazole concentrations and an ↑ risk of adverse effects); inactive metabolites are excreted in urine (71%) and feces (18%).

Half-life: 1 hr.

TIME/ACTION PROFILE (effect on acid secretion)

ROUTE	ONSET†	PEAK	DURATION†
PO	2.5 hr	unknown	1 wk
IV	15–30 min	2 hr	unknown

† Onset = 51% inhibition; duration = return to normal following discontinuation.

Contraindications/Precautions

Contraindicated in: Hypersensitivity to pantoprazole or related drugs (benzimidazoles).
Use Cautiously in: Patients using high doses for >1 yr (↑ risk of hip, wrist, or spine fractures and fundic gland polyps); Patients using therapy for >3 yr (↑ risk of vitamin B$_{12}$ deficiency); Pre-existing risk of hypocalcemia; Risk of zinc deficiency (IV); OB: Use during pregnancy only if potential maternal benefit justifies potential fetal risk; Lactation: Use while breastfeeding only if potential maternal benefit justifies potential risk to infant; Pedi: Safety and effectiveness not established in children <18 yr (pathologic hypersecretory conditions), <5 yr (PO for erosive esophagitis associated with GERD), or <3 mo (IV for erosive esophagitis associated with GERD); Geri: Appears on Beers list. ↑ risk of *Clostridioides difficile* infection, pneumonia, GI malignancies, bone loss, and fractures in older adults. Avoid scheduled use for >8 wk in older adults unless for high-risk patients (e.g., oral corticosteroid or chronic NSAID use) or patients with erosive esophagitis, Barrett's esophagitis, pathological hypersecretory condition, or demonstrated need for maintenance therapy (e.g., failure of H$_2$ antagonist).

Adverse Reactions/Side Effects

Derm: ACUTE GENERALIZED EXANTHEMATOUS PUSTULOSIS, cutaneous lupus erythematosus, DRUG REACTION WITH EOSINOPHILIA AND SYSTEMIC SYMPTOMS (DRESS), STEVENS-JOHNSON SYNDROME, TOXIC EPIDERMAL NECROLYSIS. **Endo:** hyperglycemia. **F and E** hypocalcemia (especially if treatment duration ≥3 mo), hypokalemia (especially if treatment duration ≥3 mo), hypomagnesemia (especially if treatment duration ≥3 mo). **GI:** abdominal pain, CLOSTRIDIOIDES DIFFICILE-ASSOCIATED DIARRHEA (CDAD), diarrhea, eructation, flatulence, fundic gland polyps. **GU:** acute tubulointerstitial nephritis. **Hemat:** vitamin B$_{12}$ deficiency. **Local:** thrombophlebitis. **MS:** bone fracture. **Neuro:** headache. **Misc:** HYPERSENSITIVITY REACTIONS (INCLUDING ANAPHYLAXIS, ANGIOEDEMA, OR TUBULOINTERSTITIAL NEPHRITIS), systemic lupus erythematosis.

Interactions

Drug-Drug: May ↓ levels and effectiveness of **atazanavir** and **nelfinavir**; avoid concurrent use with either of these antiretrovirals. May ↓ absorption of drugs requiring acid pH, including **ketoconazole**, **itraconazole**, **ampicillin esters**, **iron salts**, **erlotinib**, and **mycophenolate mofetil**; concomitant use with **atazanavir** not recommended. May ↑ risk of bleeding with **warfarin** (monitor INR/PT). Hypomagnesemia and hypokalemia ↑ risk of **digoxin** toxicity. May ↑ **methotrexate** levels and risk of toxicity.

Route/Dosage

Erosive Esophagitis Associated With Gastroesophageal Reflux Disease

PO (Adults): *Short-term treatment:* 40 mg once daily for up to 8 wk; *Maintenance of healing:* 40 mg once daily.

PO (Children ≥5 yr): *15–39 kg:* 20 mg once daily for up to 8 wk; *≥40 kg:* 40 mg once daily for up to 8 wk.

IV (Adults): 40 mg once daily for up to 10 days.

IV (Children 1–17 yr and >40 kg): 40 mg once daily for up to days.

IV (Children 1–17 yr and >15–<40 kg): 20 mg once daily for up to days.

IV (Children 1–17 yr and ≤15 kg): 10 mg once daily for up to days.

IV (Children 3 mo–<1 yr and ≥12.5 kg): 10 mg once daily for up to days.

IV (Children 3 mo–<1 yr and <12.5 kg): 0.8 mg/kg once daily for up to days.

Pathologic Hypersecretory Conditions, Including Zollinger-Ellison Syndrome

PO (Adults): 40 mg twice daily, up to 120 mg twice daily.

IV (Adults): 80 mg every 12 hr (up to 240 mg/day).

Availability (generic available)

Delayed-release tablets: 20 mg, 40 mg. **Delayed-release oral suspension:** 40 mg/pkt. **Powder for injection:** 40 mg/vial. **Premixed infusion:** 40 mg/50 mL 0.9% NaCl, 40 mg/100 mL 0.9% NaCl, 80 mg/100 mL 0.9% NaCl.

NURSING IMPLICATIONS

Assessment

- Assess routinely for epigastric or abdominal pain and frank or occult blood in the stool, emesis, or gastric aspirate.
- Monitor bowel function. Diarrhea, abdominal cramping, fever, and bloody stools should be reported to health care professional promptly as a sign of CDAD. May begin up to several wk following cessation of therapy.
- Monitor injection site for thrombophlebitis. *If erythema or pain at the site occur,* remove catheter and provide appropriate medical care.
- Assess for hypersensitivity reactions, including severe cutaneous reactions. *If difficulty breathing, hives, or rash occur,* immediately discontinue therapy and provide appropriate medical evaluation and treatment.

Lab Test Considerations

- Monitor liver function tests. May ↑ AST, ALT, alkaline phosphatase, and bilirubin. Monitor serum magnesium and calcium before and periodically during therapy. May cause hypomagnesemia and hypocalcemia.
- May cause vitamin B_{12} deficiency with long-term use (>3 yr). IV formulation may cause zinc deficiency.

Implementation

- Do not confuse Protonix with Lotronex or protamine.
- Patients receiving IV should be converted to PO dosing as soon as possible, preferably within 7 days of starting.
- **PO:** Administer 30–60 min before meals. Best if taken before breakfast. If taking twice daily, take 1st dose before breakfast and 2nd dose before dinner. ***DNC:*** Swallow tables whole; do not break, crush, or chew.
- *Oral suspension:* Sprinkle granules on 1 teaspoon of applesauce or apple juice approximately 30 min before meals. Do not crush or chew granules. Take sips of water to make sure granules are washed down into the stomach. Granules may also be emptied into a small cup or spoon containing one teaspoon of apple juice. Stir for 5 sec (granules will not dissolve) and swallow immediately. To make sure that entire dose is taken, rinse container once or twice with apple juice to remove any remaining granules. Swallow immediately. Do not use with anything other than applesauce or apple juice. For *nasogastric tube or gastrostomy tube,* remove plunger from the barrel of a 60 mL catheter-tip syringe. Discard plunger. Connect catheter tip of syringe to a 16 French (or larger) tube. Hold syringe attached to tubing as high as possible while giving pantoprazole. Empty contents of packet into the barrel of the syringe. Add 10 mL (2 teaspoons) of apple juice and gently tap and/or shake the barrel of the syringe to help rinse the syringe and tube. Repeat at least twice more using the same amount of apple juice (10 mL or 2 teaspoons) each time. No granules should remain in the syringe.
- Antacids may be used concurrently.

IV Administration

- **IV Push: Reconstitution:** Reconstitute each vial with 10 mL of 0.9% NaCl. Reconstituted solution is stable for 6 hr at room temperature. Do not freeze. **Dilution:** Administer undiluted. **Concentration:** 4 mg/mL. **Rate:** Administer over >2 min.
- **Intermittent Infusion: Reconstitution:** Reconstitute each vial with 10 mL of 0.9% NaCl. Reconstituted

solution is stable for 6 hr at room temperature. Do not freeze. **Dilution:** Dilute further depending on age. *3 mo–< 1 yr:* Dilute with 21 mL 0.9% NaCl; *1–17 yr and adults:* Dilute with 100 mL 0.9% NaCl or 5% dextrose. Solution should be clear and free of particulates. **Concentration:** 1.3 mg/mL (3 mo–< 1 yr); 0.4–0.8 mg/mL (1–17 yr and adults). Diluted solution is stable for 24 hr at room temperature. **Rate:** Administer over 15 min through dedicated line or Y-site.

- **Y-Site Compatibility:** acetazolamide, allopurinol, alprostadil, aminocaproic acid, aminophylline, amphotericin B liposomal, ampicillin, ampicillin/sulbactam, anidulafungin, argatroban, arsenic trioxide, azithromycin, bleomycin, bumetanide, cangrelor, carboplatin, carmustine, ceftaroline, ceftolozane/tazobactam, ceftriaxone, cyclophosphamide, cytarabine, docetaxel, doxorubicin liposomal, doxycycline, eravacycline, ertapenem, fluorouracil, foscarnet, fosphenytoin, ganciclovir, granisetron, hetastarch, imipenem/cilastatin, irinotecan, isavuconazonium, meropenem/vaborbactam, mesna, methadone, methohexital, nafcillin, paclitaxel, penicillin G sodium, pentobarbital, phentolamine, phenylephrine, plazomicin, potassium chloride, procainamide, rifampin, succinylcholine, sufentanil, tedizolid, telavancin, theophylline, tigecycline, tirofiban, vasopressin, zidovudine, zoledronic acid.
- **Y-Site Incompatibility:** alemtuzumab, atropine, aztreonam, blinatumomab, buprenorphine, butorphanol, calcium chloride, cefepime, cefotaxime, cefotetan, chloramphenicol, chlorpromazine, ciprofloxacin, cisatracurium, cisplatin, dacarbazine, dactinomycin, dantrolene, daptomycin, daunorubicin, dexamethasone, dexmedetomidine, dexrazoxane, diazepam, diltiazem, diphenhydramine, dobutamine, doxorubicin hydrochloride, droperidol, ephedrine, epirubicin, esmolol, estrogens, conjugated, etoposide, etoposide phosphate, famotidine, fentanyl, fluconazole, fludarabine, gemcitabine, gemtuzumab ozogamicin, glycopyrrolate, haloperidol, hydralazine, hydroxyzine, idarubicin, ifosfamide, indomethacin, ketorolac, labetalol, leucovorin calcium, levofloxacin, lidocaine, linezolid, lorazepam, melphalan, meperidine, methotrexate, methylprednisolone, metoprolol, metronidazole, milrinone, mitomycin, mitoxantrone, moxifloxacin, multivitamins, mycophenolate, nalbuphine, naloxone, nicardipine, ondansetron, palonosetron, pemetrexed, pentamidine, phenytoin, posaconazole, potassium acetate, potassium phosphates, prochlorperazine, promethazine, propranolol, rocuronium, sodium acetate, sodium phosphate, thiotepa, topotecan, vecuronium, verapamil, vinblastine, vincristine, vinorelbine, voriconazole, solutions containing zinc.

Patient/Family Teaching

- Explain purpose and side effects of medication to patient. Advise patient to read *Patient Information* before starting therapy. Instruct patient to take medication as directed for the full course of therapy, even if feeling better.
- Instruct patient to notify health care professional of all Rx or OTC medications, vitamins, or herbal products being taken and consult health care professional before taking any new medications.
- Advise patient to avoid alcohol, products containing aspirin or NSAIDs, and foods that may cause an ↑ in GI irritation.
- Advise patient to report onset of black, tarry stools; diarrhea; or abdominal pain to health care professional promptly. Instruct patient to notify health care professional immediately if rash, diarrhea, abdominal cramping, fever, or bloody stools occur and not to treat with antidiarrheals without consulting health care professional.
- Rep: Advise women of reproductive potential to notify health care professional if pregnancy is planned or suspected or if breastfeeding.

P

Evaluation/Desired Outcomes

- Diminished accumulation of acid in the gastric lumen, with lessened acid reflux.
- Healing of duodenal ulcers and esophagitis.
- Decreased acid secretion in hypersecretory conditions.

paricalcitol, See VITAMIN D COMPOUNDS.

BEERS

PARoxetine

PARoxetine hydrochloride

(par-**ox**-e-teen)

Paxil, Paxil CR

PARoxetine mesylate

~~Brisdelle, Pexeva~~

Classification

Therapeutic: antianxiety agents, antidepressants

Pharmacologic: selective serotonin reuptake inhibitors (SSRIs)

Indications

Paxil, Paxil CR: Treatment of the following disorders: Major depressive disorder, Panic disorder, Social anxiety disorder. **Paxil:** Treatment of the following disorders:

Obsessive compulsive disorder (OCD), Generalized anxiety disorder, Post-traumatic stress disorder (PTSD). **Paxil CR:** Premenstrual dysphoric disorder. **Paroxetine mesylate (7.5-mg capsule):** Moderate to severe vasomotor symptoms associated with menopause.

Action

Inhibits neuronal reuptake of serotonin in the CNS, thus potentiating the activity of serotonin; has little effect on norepinephrine or dopamine; mechanism for benefit in treating vasomotor symptoms unknown. **Therapeutic Effects:** Antidepressant action. Decreased frequency of panic attacks, OCD, or anxiety. Improvement in manifestations of PTSD. Decreased dysphoria prior to menses. Decreased vasomotor symptoms in postmenopausal women.

Pharmacokinetics

Absorption: Completely absorbed following oral administration. Controlled-release tablets are enteric-coated and control medication release over 4–5 hr.
Distribution: Widely distributed throughout body fluids and tissues, including the CNS.
Protein Binding: 95%.
Metabolism and Excretion: Highly metabolized by the liver, primarily by the CYP2D6 isoenzyme; the CYP2D6 isoenzyme exhibits genetic polymorphism; ~7% of population may be poor metabolizers and may have significantly ↑ paroxetine concentrations and an ↑ risk of adverse effects. 2% excreted unchanged in urine.
Half-life: 21 hr.

TIME/ACTION PROFILE (antidepressant action)

ROUTE	ONSET	PEAK	DURATION
PO	1–4 wk	unknown	unknown

Contraindications/Precautions

Contraindicated in: Hypersensitivity; Concurrent use of MAO inhibitors or MAO-inhibitor-like drugs (linezolid or methylene blue); Concurrent use of thioridazine or pimozide; Lactation: Lactation.
Use Cautiously in: May ↑ risk of suicide attempt/ideation, especially during early treatment or dose adjustment; this risk appears to be greater in adolescents or children; History of mania; History of seizures; History of bipolar disorder; Angle-closure glaucoma; Severe renal impairment; Severe hepatic impairment; OB: Use during the 1st trimester may be associated with ↑ risk of cardiac malformations; consider fetal risk/maternal benefit; use during the 3rd trimester may result in neonatal serotonin syndrome requiring prolonged hospitalization, respiratory and nutritional support; Pedi: Safety and effectiveness not established in children; Geri: Appears on Beers list. May worsen or cause syndrome of inappropriate antidiuretic hormone (SIADH) secretion and/or hyponatremia in older adults. Use with caution in older adults and closely monitor sodium concentrations when starting therapy or ↑ dose.

Adverse Reactions/Side Effects

CV: chest pain, edema, hypertension, palpitations, postural hypotension, tachycardia, vasodilation. **Derm:** sweating, photosensitivity, pruritus, rash, STEVENS-JOHNSON SYNDROME (SJS). **EENT:** blurred vision, pharyngitis, rhinitis. **Endo:** SIADH. **F and E** hyponatremia. **GI:** constipation, diarrhea, dry mouth, nausea, ↓ appetite, abdominal pain, dyspepsia, flatulence, taste disturbances, vomiting, weight loss. **GU:** ↓ libido, delayed/absent orgasm, ejaculatory delay/failure, erectile dysfunction, genital disorders, infertility, urinary disorders, urinary frequency. **Hemat:** BLEEDING. **Metab:** ↑ appetite, weight gain. **MS:** back pain, bone fracture, myalgia, myopathy. **Neuro:** anxiety, dizziness, drowsiness, headache, insomnia, weakness, agitation, amnesia, confusion, depression, emotional lability, hangover, impaired concentration, malaise, NEUROLEPTIC MALIGNANT SYNDROME (NMS), paresthesia, SUICIDAL THOUGHTS/BEHAVIORS, syncope, tremor. **Resp:** cough. **Misc:** chills, fever, SEROTONIN SYNDROME, yawning.

Interactions

Drug-Drug: **MAO inhibitors** may result in serious, potentially fatal reactions; wait ≥2 wk after stopping MAO inhibitor before initiating paroxetine; wait ≥2 wk after stopping paroxetine before starting MAO inhibitors. **MAO-inhibitor-like drugs**, such as **linezolid** or **methylene blue**, may ↑ risk of serotonin syndrome; concurrent use contraindicated; do not start therapy in patients receiving **linezolid** or **methylene blue**; if **linezolid** or **methylene blue** need to be started in a patient receiving paroxetine, immediately discontinue paroxetine and monitor for signs/symptoms of serotonin syndrome for 2 wk or until 24 hr after last dose of linezolid or methylene blue, whichever comes first (may resume paroxetine therapy 24 hr after last dose of linezolid or methylene blue). **Pimozide** or **thioridazine** may ↑ risk of QT interval prolongation and torsades de pointes; concurrent use contraindicated. May ↑ levels and risk of toxicity of other **antidepressants**, **phenothiazines**, **class Ic antiarrhythmics**, **risperidone**, **atomoxetine**, **theophylline**, and **quinidine**; concurrent use should be undertaken with caution. **Cimetidine** may ↑ levels and risk of toxicity. **Phenobarbital** and **phenytoin** may ↓ levels and effectiveness. May ↓ the effectiveness of **digoxin** and **tamoxifen**. May ↑ risk of bleeding with **NSAIDs**, **aspirin**, **clopidogrel**, **prasugrel**, **ticagrelor**, **dabigatran**, **apixaban**, **edoxaban**, **rivaroxaban**, or **warfarin**. Drugs that affect serotonergic neurotransmitter systems, including **tricyclic antidepressants**, **SNRIs**, **fentanyl**, **lithium**, **buspirone**, **tramadol**,

meperidine, **methadone**, **amphetamines**, and **triptans**, may ↑ risk of serotonin syndrome
Drug-Natural Products: ↑ risk of serotonergic side effects including serotonin syndrome with **St. John's wort**, **SAMe**, and **tryptophan**.

Route/Dosage

Depression

PO (Adults): 20 mg as a single dose in the morning; may ↑ by 10 mg/day at weekly intervals (not to exceed 50 mg/day). *Controlled-release tablets:* 25 mg once daily initially. May ↑ at weekly intervals by 12.5 mg (not to exceed 62.5 mg/day).
PO (Geriatric Patients): 10 mg/day initially; may be slowly ↑ (not to exceed 40 mg/day). *Controlled-release tablets:* 12.5 mg once daily initially; may be slowly ↑ (not to exceed 50 mg/day).

Obsessive Compulsive Disorder

PO (Adults): 20 mg/day initially; ↑ by 10 mg/day at weekly intervals up to 40 mg (not to exceed 60 mg/day).

Panic Disorder

PO (Adults): 10 mg/day initially; ↑ by 10 mg/day at weekly intervals up to 40 mg (not to exceed 60 mg/day). *Controlled-release tablets:* 12.5 mg/day initially; ↑ by 12.5 mg/day at weekly intervals (not to exceed 75 mg/day).

Social Anxiety Disorder

PO (Adults): 20 mg/day. *Controlled-release tablets:* 12.5 mg/day initially; may ↑ by 12.5 mg/day weekly intervals (not to exceed 37.5 mg/day).

Generalized Anxiety Disorder

PO (Adults): 20 mg once daily initially; ↑ by 10 mg/day at weekly intervals (not to exceed 50 mg/day).

Post-Traumatic Stress Disorder

PO (Adults): 20 mg/day initially; may ↑ by 10 mg/day at weekly intervals (not to exceed 50 mg/day).

Premenstrual Dysphoric Disorder

PO (Adults): *Controlled-release tablets:* 12.5 mg once daily throughout menstrual cycle or during luteal phase of menstrual cycle only; may ↑ to 25 mg/day after 1 wk.

Menopausal Vasomotor Symptoms

PO (Adults): 7.5 mg once daily at bedtime.

Renal Impairment

PO (Adults): Paxil or Paxil CR:: *Severe renal impairment:* 10 mg/day initially; may slowly ↑ (not to exceed 40 mg/day). *Controlled-release tablets:* 12.5 mg once daily initially; may slowly ↑ (not to exceed 50 mg/day).

Hepatic Impairment

PO (Adults): Paxil or Paxil CR:: *Severe hepatic impairment:* 10 mg/day initially; may slowly ↑ (not to exceed 40 mg/day). *Controlled-release tablets:* 12.5 mg once daily initially; may slowly ↑ (not to exceed 50 mg/day).

Availability (generic available)

Paroxetine hydrochloride tablets: 10 mg, 20 mg, 30 mg, 40 mg. **Paroxetine hydrochloride controlled-release tablets:** 12.5 mg, 25 mg, 37.5 mg. **Paroxetine hydrochloride oral suspension (orange flavor):** 10 mg/5 mL. **Paroxetine mesylate capsules:** 7.5 mg.

NURSING IMPLICATIONS

Assessment

- Monitor appetite and nutritional intake. Weigh weekly. Notify health care provider of continued weight loss. Adjust diet as tolerated to support nutritional status.
- Assess for suicidal tendencies, especially during early therapy. Restrict amount of drug available to patient. Risk may be ↑ in adults ≤24 yr. After starting therapy, young adults should be seen by health care provider face-to-face at least weekly for 4 wk, then every other wk for next 4 wk, then at 12 wk, and then on advice of health care provider thereafter.
- Assess for signs and symptoms of serotonin syndrome (confusion, delirium, agitation, coma, dilated pupils, tachycardia, hyperthermia, shivering, hyperreflexia, muscle rigidity, hypertension, vomiting, diarrhea, seizures). ↑ risk of serotonin syndrome with concurrent use of other serotonergic drugs (SSRIs, SNRIs, triptans); discontinuation may be required.
- Monitor for signs and symptoms of NMS (hyperpyrexia, muscle rigidity, seizures, altered mental status, evidence of autonomic instability [irregular HR or BP, tachycardia, diaphoresis, cardiac arrhythmia]). *If signs/symptoms of NMS occur,* discontinue paroxetine.
- Assess for rash or signs/symptoms of SJS periodically during therapy (fever, general malaise, fatigue, muscle or joint aches, blisters, oral lesions, conjunctivitis). *If SJS suspected,* discontinue therapy and provide supportive care.
- Assess sexual function before starting paroxetine. Assess for changes in sexual function during treatment, including timing of onset; patient may not report.
- **Depression:** Monitor mental status (orientation, mood, behavior). Inform health care provider if patient demonstrates significant ↑ in anxiety, nervousness, or insomnia.
- **OCD:** Assess frequency of obsessive-compulsive behaviors. Note degree to which these thoughts and behaviors interfere with daily functioning.
- **Panic Attacks:** Assess frequency and severity of panic attacks.

P

- **Social Anxiety Disorder:** Assess frequency and severity of episodes of anxiety.
- **PTSD:** Assess manifestations periodically during therapy.
- **Premenstrual Dysphoria:** Assess symptoms of premenstrual distress before starting and during therapy.

Lab Test Considerations

- Verify negative pregnancy test before starting therapy.
- Assess sodium levels at baseline and then after 3–4 wk in high-risk patients (> 65 yr, previous history of antidepressant-induced hyponatremia, low body weight, concurrent use of thiazides or other hyponatremia-inducing agents).
- Monitor CBC and differential periodically during therapy. Report leukopenia or anemia.

Implementation

- Do not confuse paroxetine with fluoxetine, duloxetine, or piroxicam. Do not confuse Paxil with Doxil, Plavix, or Trexall.
- Paroxetine mesylate cannot be substituted with paroxetine (Paxil or Paxil CR) or generic paroxetine.
- Periodically reassess dose and continued need for therapy.
- During administration and when preparing tablets, wear double chemotherapy gloves, protective gown, and hair and shoe covers. Respiratory (N95) protection and eye/face protection are needed if there is risk of patient vomiting or spitting up. Single chemotherapy gloves are appropriate if handling and administering intact tablets from a unit-dose package. Health care providers who are actively trying to conceive, who are pregnant or may become pregnant, and who are breastfeeding should avoid handling paroxetine.
- **PO:** Administer as a single dose in the morning. May administer with food to minimize GI irritation.
- Swallow tablets whole. ***DNC:*** Do not crush, break, or chew. Shake suspension before administering.
- Taper to avoid potential withdrawal reactions.

Patient/Family Teaching

- Explain the purpose and side effects of paroxetine. Instruct patient to take as directed. Take missed doses as soon as possible and return to regular dosing schedule. Do not double doses. Caution patient to consult health care provider before discontinuing paroxetine. Daily doses should be decreased slowly. Abrupt withdrawal may cause dizziness, sensory disturbances, agitation, anxiety, nausea, and sweating. Advise patient to read *Medication Guide* before starting and with each Rx refill in case of changes.
- Emphasize the importance of follow-up exams to monitor progress. Encourage patient participation in psychotherapy to improve coping skills.
- May cause drowsiness or dizziness. Caution patient to avoid driving and other activities requiring alertness until response to the drug is known.
- Advise patient, family, and caregivers to look for suicidality, especially during early therapy or dose changes. Notify health care provider immediately if thoughts about suicide or dying, attempts to commit suicide, new or worse depression or anxiety, agitation or restlessness, panic attacks, insomnia, new or worse irritability, aggressiveness, acting on dangerous impulses, mania, or other changes in mood or behavior.
- Advise patient and caregivers to immediately notify health care provider if symptoms of serotonin syndrome occur.
- Instruct patient to notify health care provider of all Rx or OTC medications, vitamins, or herbal products being taken and consult health care provider before taking any new medications and to avoid alcohol or other CNS-depressant drugs, including opioids, during therapy.
- Inform patient that frequent mouth rinses, good oral hygiene, and sugarless gum or candy may minimize dry mouth. Saliva substitute may be used. Consult dentist if dry mouth persists for >2 wk.
- Advise patient to notify health care provider if headache, weakness, nausea, anorexia, anxiety, or insomnia persists.
- Inform patient that paroxetine may cause symptoms of sexual dysfunction. In men, ejaculatory delay or failure, ↓ libido, and erectile dysfunction may occur. In women, may result in ↓ libido and delayed or absent orgasm. Advise patient to notify health care provider if symptoms occur.
- Rep: Advise women of reproductive potential to notify health care provider immediately if pregnancy is planned or suspected and to avoid breastfeeding during therapy. Use in the month before delivery has been associated with an ↑ in the risk of postpartum hemorrhage. Infants exposed to paroxetine during 1st trimester have ↑ risk of congenital malformations, particularly cardiovascular malformations. If used during pregnancy, should be tapered during 3rd trimester to avoid neonatal serotonin syndrome. Monitor infants exposed to paroxetine for excess sedation, restlessness, agitation, poor feeding, poor weight gain, or respiratory distress; may ↑ risk of persistent pulmonary hypertension of the newborn. Inform patient of pregnancy exposure registry that monitors pregnancy outcomes in women exposed to antidepressants during pregnancy. Register patient by calling the National Pregnancy Registry for Antidepressants at 1-866-961-2388 or visiting online at https://womensmentalhealth.org/clinical-and-research programs/pregnancyregistry/antidepressants/.

Evaluation/Desired Outcomes

- Increased sense of well-being.
- Renewed interest in surroundings. May require 1–4 wk of therapy to obtain antidepressant effects.
- Decrease in obsessive-compulsive behaviors.
- Decrease in frequency and severity of panic attacks.

- Decrease in frequency and severity of episodes of anxiety.
- Improvement in manifestations of PTSD.
- Decreased dysphoria prior to menses.

patiromer (pa-tir-oh-mer)

Veltassa

Classification

Therapeutic: antidotes, electrolyte modifiers

Pharmacologic: cationic exchange resins

Indications

Mild to moderate hyperkalemia (if severe, more immediate measures such as calcium IV or insulin/glucose IV should be instituted).

Action

Contains calcium-sorbitol counterion and ↑ fecal potassium excretion through binding of potassium in the lumen of the GI tract. **Therapeutic Effects:** Reduced serum potassium concentrations.

Pharmacokinetics

Absorption: Not systemically absorbed.

Distribution: Not distributed.

Metabolism and Excretion: Eliminated in the feces.

Half-life: Unknown.

TIME/ACTION PROFILE)

ROUTE	ONSET	PEAK	DURATION
PO	7–12 hr	unknown	24 hr

Contraindications/Precautions

Contraindicated in: Hypersensitivity; History of bowel impaction, bowel obstruction, or severe constipation (may be ineffective and worsen condition).

Use Cautiously in: Pedi: Children <12 yr (safety and effectiveness not established).

Adverse Reactions/Side Effects

F and E hypokalemia, hypomagnesemia. **GI:** constipation, diarrhea, flatulence, nausea.

Interactions

Drug-Drug: May ↓ absorption and effectiveness of **bisoprolol**, **carvedilol**, **ciprofloxacin**, **levothyroxine**, **metformin**, **mycophenolate mofetil**, **nebivolol**, **quinidine**, **telmisartan**, and **thiamine**; administer ≥3 hr before or after patiromer.

Route/Dosage

PO (Adults): 8.4 g once daily; titrate dose at ≥1 wk intervals by 8.4 g once daily as needed to achieve desired serum potassium concentration (max = 25.2 g once daily).

PO (Children ≥12 yr): 4 g once daily; titrate dose at ≥1 wk intervals by 4 g once daily as needed to achieve desired serum potassium concentration (max = 25.2 g once daily).

Availability

Powder for oral suspension: 1 g/pkt, 8.4 g/pkt, 16.8 g/pkt, 25.2 g/pkt.

NURSING IMPLICATIONS

Assessment

- Monitor for bowel sounds and frequency and consistency of stools periodically during therapy. May cause constipation.

Lab Test Considerations

- Monitor serum potassium and magnesium periodically during therapy. May cause hypokalemia and hypomagnesemia. Consider magnesium supplements if hypomagnesemia occurs.

Implementation

- Due to delayed action, do not use patiromer as an emergency treatment of life-threatening hyperkalemia.
- **PO:** Administer immediately ≥3 hr before or 3 hr after other PO medications. Measure 1/3 cup of water. Pour half the water into a glass; then add patiromer and stir. Add the remaining half of the water and stir thoroughly. The powder will not dissolve and mixture will look cloudy. Add more water to the mixture as needed for desired consistency. Drink mixture immediately. If powder remains in the glass after drinking, add more water, stir, and drink immediately. Repeat as needed to ensure the entire dose is administered. May use other beverages or soft foods (applesauce, yogurt, pudding) instead of water to prepare mixture. Do not heat or add to heated foods or liquids. Do not take in dry form. Stable for 3 mo at room temperature or until the packet expiration date if refrigerated.

P

Patient/Family Teaching

- Instruct patient to take patiromer as directed and adhere to prescribed diet.
- Advise patient to take patiromer ≥3 hr before or 3 hr after other medications.
- Instruct patient to not heat suspension or add to heated foods or liquids. Do not take in dry form.
- Rep: Advise females of reproductive potential to notify health care professional if pregnancy is planned or suspected or if breastfeeding. Patiromer is not absorbed systemically, so it is not expected to harm fetus.

Evaluation/Desired Outcomes

- Reduced serum potassium concentrations.

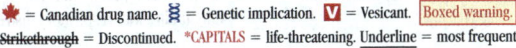

pegfilgrastim (peg-fil-**gra**-stim)
Fulphila, Fylnetra, ✦ Lapelga, Neulasta, Neulasta Onpro, Nyvepria, Stimufend, Udenyca, Ziextenzo

Classification
Therapeutic: colony-stimulating factors

Indications
To decrease the incidence of infection (febrile neutropenia) in patients with nonmyeloid malignancies receiving myelosuppressive antineoplastics associated with a high risk of febrile neutropenia. **Fylnetra, Neulasta, Stimufend, Udenyca, and Ziextenzo:** To increase survival in patients acutely exposed to myelosuppressive doses of radiation.

Action
Filgrastim is a glycoprotein that binds to and stimulates neutrophils to divide and differentiate. Also activates mature neutrophils. Binding to a polyethylene glycol molecule prolongs its effects. **Therapeutic Effects:** Decreased incidence of infection in patients who are neutropenic from chemotherapy. Improved survival in patients acutely exposed to myelosuppressive doses of radiation.

Pharmacokinetics
Absorption: Well absorbed following SUBQ administration.
Distribution: Unknown.
Metabolism and Excretion: Unknown.
Half-life: 15–80 hr.

TIME/ACTION PROFILE

ROUTE	ONSET	PEAK	DURATION
SUBQ	unknown	unknown	unknown

Contraindications/Precautions
Contraindicated in: Hypersensitivity to filgrastim or *Escherichia coli*–derived proteins.
Use Cautiously in: Patients with breast or lung cancer receiving chemotherapy and/or radiotherapy (↑ risk of myelodysplastic syndrome or acute myeloid leukemia); Patients with sickle cell disease (↑ risk of sickle cell crisis); Malignancy with myeloid characteristics; OB: Use during pregnancy only if potential maternal benefit justifies potential fetal risk; Lactation: Use while breastfeeding only if potential maternal benefit justifies potential risk to infant.

Adverse Reactions/Side Effects
CV: aortitis. **GI:** SPLENIC RUPTURE. **GU:** glomerulonephritis. **Hemat:** ACUTE MYELOID LEUKEMIA, leukocytosis, MYELODYSPLASTIC SYNDROME, SICKLE CELL CRISIS, thrombocytopenia. **MS:** medullary bone pain. **Resp:** ADULT RESPIRATORY DISTRESS SYNDROME (ARDS). **Misc:** CAPILLARY LEAK SYNDROME, HYPERSENSITIVITY REACTIONS (INCLUDING ANAPHYLAXIS).

Interactions
Drug-Drug: Simultaneous use with **antineoplastics** may have adverse effects on rapidly proliferating neutrophils; avoid use for 24 hr before and 24 hr following chemotherapy. **Lithium** may potentiate the release of neutrophils; concurrent use should be undertaken cautiously.

Route/Dosage
Patients with Cancer Receiving Myelosuppressive Chemotherapy
SUBQ (Adults and Children ≥45 kg): 6 mg per chemotherapy cycle.
SUBQ (Children 31–44 kg): 4 mg per chemotherapy cycle.
SUBQ (Children 21–30 kg): 2.5 mg per chemotherapy cycle.
SUBQ (Children 10–20 kg): 1.5 mg per chemotherapy cycle.
SUBQ (Children <10 kg): 0.1 mg/kg per chemotherapy cycle.

Patients Acutely Exposed to Myelosuppressive Doses of Radiation
SUBQ (Adults and Children ≥45 kg): *Fylnetra, Neulasta, Stimufend, Udenyca, or Ziextenzo:* 6 mg as soon as possible after suspected or confirmed exposure to radiation levels >2 gray (Gy), then 6 mg 1 wk later.
SUBQ (Children 31–44 kg): *Fylnetra, Neulasta, Stimufend, Udenyca, or Ziextenzo:* 4 mg as soon as possible after suspected or confirmed exposure to radiation levels >2 gray (Gy), then 4 mg 1 wk later.
SUBQ (Children 21–30 kg): *Fylnetra, Neulasta, Stimufend, Udenyca, or Ziextenzo:* 2.5 mg as soon as possible after suspected or confirmed exposure to radiation levels >2 gray (Gy), then 2.5 mg 1 wk later.
SUBQ (Children 10–20 kg): *Fylnetra, Neulasta, Stimufend, Udenyca, or Ziextenzo:* 1.5 mg as soon as possible after suspected or confirmed exposure to radiation levels >2 gray (Gy), then 1.5 mg 1 wk later.
SUBQ (Children <10 kg): *Fylnetra, Neulasta, Stimufend, Udenyca, or Ziextenzo:* 0.1 mg/kg as soon as possible after suspected or confirmed exposure to radiation levels >2 gray (Gy), then 0.1 mg/kg 1 wk later.

Availability
Solution for injection (prefilled syringes and autoinjectors): 6 mg/0.6 mL.

NURSING IMPLICATIONS
Assessment
- Assess patient for bone pain during therapy. Pain is usually mild to moderate and usually controllable with nonopioid analgesics, but may require opioid analgesics.
- Assess patient periodically for signs of ARDS (fever, lung infiltration, respiratory distress). *If ARDS*

occurs, treat condition and discontinue pegfilgrastim and/or withhold until symptoms resolve.

- Monitor for signs/symptoms of splenic rupture (left upper abdominal or shoulder pain) during therapy.
- Monitor for signs/symptoms of capillary leak syndrome (hypotension, hypoalbuminemia, edema, hemoconcentration). Treat symptomatically.
- Assess for signs/symptoms of aortitis (fever, abdominal pain, malaise, back pain, ↑ inflammatory markers [C-reactive protein, WBC]). *If aortitis suspected,* discontinue pegfilgrastim.
- May cause transient positive nuclear bone-imaging changes.

Lab Test Considerations

- Obtain baseline CBC. Monitor WBCs, hematocrit, and platelets regularly.
- May ↑ LDH, alkaline phosphatase, and uric acid.

Implementation

- Do not confuse Neulasta with Lunesta or Nuedexta.
- Pegfilgrastim should not be administered between 14 days before and 24 hr after administration of cytotoxic chemotherapy.
- Keep patients with sickle cell disease receiving pegfilgrastim well hydrated and monitor for sickle cell crisis. *If sickle cell crisis occurs,* discontinue pegfilgrastim.
- **SUBQ:** Administer SUBQ once per chemotherapy cycle. Do not administer solutions that are discolored or contain particulates. Do not shake. Store refrigerated; allow to reach room temperature for ≥30 min and maximum of 48 hr, but protect from light.
- **On-body Injector:** Small, one-time use, lightweight, battery-powered, and waterproof up to 8 feet for 1 hr. Filled by health care provider with a prefilled syringe before application. The prefilled syringe with *Neulasta* and the *On-body Injector* are part of *Neulasta Onpro kit*. The *On-body Injector* is applied directly to skin using a self-adhesive backing. The *On-body Injector* uses sounds and lights to inform its status. The prefilled syringe gray needle cap contains dry natural rubber, derived from latex; do not use if allergic to latex. Apply to intact, nonirritated skin on abdomen or back of arm. Back of arm may only be used if there is a caregiver available to monitor the status of the *On-body Injector*. Approximately 27 hr after the *On-body Injector* is applied, *Neulasta* will be delivered over approximately 45 min. Follow manufacturer's instructions for monitoring and removal. Instruct patients using the *On-body Injector* to notify health care provider immediately if they suspect the device may not have performed as intended in order to determine need for a replacement dose.

Patient/Family Teaching

- Instruct patient in technique for injection, care of medication, and disposal of equipment. Advise patient to read *Patient Information* before starting therapy and with each Rx refill in case of changes.
- Instruct patient on correct disposal technique for home administration. Caution patient not to reuse needle, syringe, or drug product. Provide a puncture-proof container for disposal of prefilled syringe.
- Emphasize the importance of adherence with therapy and regular monitoring of blood counts.
- Advise patient to notify health care provider immediately if signs of allergic reaction (shortness of breath, hives, rash, pruritus, laryngeal edema), ARDS (shortness of breath with or without a fever, trouble breathing, fast rate of breathing), kidney injury (swelling of face or ankles, blood in urine or dark-colored urine, urinating less than usual), capillary leak syndrome (swelling or puffiness, urinating less than usual, trouble breathing, swelling of abdomen, feeling of fullness, dizziness or feeling faint, general feeling of tiredness), myelodysplastic syndrome or acute myeloid leukemia (tiredness, fever, easy bruising or bleeding), inflammation of the aorta (fever, abdominal pain, feeling tired, back pain), or signs of splenic rupture (left upper abdominal or shoulder tip pain) occur.
- Advise patients with sickle cell disease to maintain hydration and to notify health care provider promptly if symptoms of sickle cell crisis occur.
- Advise patient to notify health care provider of all Rx or OTC medications, vitamins, or herbal products being taken and to consult with health care provider before taking other medications.
- Rep: Advise women of reproductive potential to notify health care provider if pregnancy is planned or suspected or if breastfeeding.

Evaluation/Desired Outcomes

- Decreased incidence of infection in patients who are neutropenic from chemotherapy.
- Improved survival in patients acutely exposed to myelosuppressive doses of radiation.

peginterferon beta-1a

(peg-in-ter-**feer**-on **bay**-ta)

Plegridy

Classification

Therapeutic: immune modifiers

Pharmacologic: interferons

Indications
Relapsing forms of multiple sclerosis (MS), including clinically isolated syndrome, relapsing-remitting disease, and active secondary progressive disease.

Action
Antiviral and immunoregulatory properties produced by interacting with specific receptor sites on cell surfaces may explain beneficial effects. Produced by recombinant DNA technology. Pegylation prolongs duration of action. **Therapeutic Effects:** Reduced incidence of relapse (neurologic dysfunction) and slowed physical disability.

Pharmacokinetics
Absorption: Extent of absorption following SUBQ or IM administration unknown.
Distribution: Widely distributed to tissues.
Metabolism and Excretion: Undergoes catabolism; excretion is mainly renal.
Half-life: 78 hr.

TIME/ACTION PROFILE (↓ relapse rates)

ROUTE	ONSET	PEAK	DURATION
SUBQ	within one mo	24–36 wk	unknown
IM	unknown	unknown	unknown

Contraindications/Precautions
Contraindicated in: Hypersensitivity to natural or recombinant interferon beta or peginterferon.
Use Cautiously in: History of depression or suicidal ideation; Latex allergy; History of seizures; Renal impairment; OB: Use during pregnancy only if potential maternal benefit justifies potential fetal risk; Lactation: Use while breastfeeding only if potential maternal benefit justifies potential risk to infant; Pedi: Safety and effectiveness not established in children; Geri: Safety and effectiveness not established in older adults.

Adverse Reactions/Side Effects
CV: HF. **Derm:** pruritus. **GI:** HEPATOTOXICITY, nausea, vomiting. **Hemat:** ↓ peripheral blood counts, HEMOLYTIC UREMIC SYNDROME, THROMBOTIC THROMBOCYTOPENIC PURPURA. **Local:** injection site reactions. **MS:** arthralgia, myalgia. **Neuro:** depression, headache, SEIZURES, SUICIDAL IDEATION, weakness. **Resp:** PULMONARY ARTERIAL HYPERTENSION (PAH). **Misc:** chills, fever, flu-like symptoms, AUTOIMMUNE DISORDERS, HYPERSENSITIVITY REACTIONS (INCLUDING ANAPHYLAXIS).

Interactions
Drug-Drug: ↑ myelosuppression may occur with other **myelosuppressive drugs**, including **antineoplastics**. **Hepatotoxic agents** may ↑ the risk of hepatotoxicity (↑ liver enzymes).
Drug-Natural Products: Astragalus, echinacea, and **melatonin** may ↑ risk of myelosuppression; avoid concurrent use.

Route/Dosage
IM, SUBQ (Adults): 63 mcg on Day 1, then 94 mcg on Day 15, and then 125 mcg every 14 days.

Availability
Solution for injection (prefilled pens and prefilled syringes): 63 mcg/0.5 mL, 94 mcg/0.5 mL, 125 mcg/0.5 mL.

NURSING IMPLICATIONS
Assessment
- Assess frequency of exacerbations of symptoms of MS periodically during therapy.
- Monitor for signs/symptoms of depression during therapy. *If depression occurs,* notify health care provider immediately.
- Monitor for signs/symptoms of hepatotoxicity (fatigue, nausea, upper abdominal pain, jaundice, scleral icterus, dark urine, clay-colored stools).
- Monitor for injection site reactions (erythema, pain, pruritus, edema, bruising, drainage, necrosis). Avoid injecting near area of reaction.
- Monitor patient with significant cardiac disease for worsening symptoms during initiation and periodically during therapy.
- Assess patients who develop unexplained symptoms (dyspnea, new or increasing fatigue) for PAH. *If other causes have been ruled out and a diagnosis of PAH is confirmed,* discontinue peginterferon beta-1a.

Lab Test Considerations
- Monitor AST, ALT, and bilirubin periodically during therapy.
- Monitor CBC with differential periodically during therapy. May cause anemia, ↓ lymphocytes, ↓ neutrophils, and ↓ platelets.

Implementation
- Administer prophylactic analgesics and/or antipyretics to prevent or minimize flu-like symptoms. Incidence of injection site reactions may be less with IM than with SUBQ dosing.
- Remove syringe from refrigerator and allow to warm to room temperature for 30 min before injection. Do not use warm water to warm. Solution is clear to slightly opalescent and colorless to slightly yellow. Do not administer solutions that are cloudy, discolored, or contain particulate matter.
- **SUBQ:** Inject SUBQ in abdomen, back of upper arm, or thigh every 14 days; rotate sites. Prefilled pens are for single dose; discard after use.
- For patients using SUBQ dosing for 1st time, titrate using the *Plegridy Starter Pack* for use with the prefilled syringe. Kit is supplied separately and contains two titration devices (*Dose 1 for Day 1:* 63 mcg, orange clip; *Dose 2 for Day 15:* 94 mcg, blue clip; *Dose 3 for Day 29 and every 14 days after:*

125 mcg, gray clip) to be used only with prefilled syringes for SUBQ use.

- **IM:** Rotate injection sites between left and right thighs.
- Protective cover of prefilled syringe for IM use contains latex. Avoid handling by latex-sensitive individuals. Monitor for allergic reactions.
- For patients using IM dosing for 1st time, titrate using the *Plegridy Titration Kit* for use with the prefilled syringe. Kit is supplied separately and contains two titration devices (*Dose 1 for Day 1:* 63 mcg, yellow clip; *Dose 2 for Day 15:* 94 mcg, purple clip; *Dose 3 for Day 29 and every 14 days after:* 125 mcg, no clip) to be used only with prefilled syringes for IM use.

Patient/Family Teaching

- Explain the purpose and side effects of peginterferon beta-1a. Instruct patient to take medication as directed; do not change dose or schedule without consulting health care provider. Advise patient to read *Medication Guide* prior to starting therapy and with each Rx refill in case of changes.
- Instruct patient in correct technique for injection and care and disposal of equipment. Avoid injecting into areas of skin irritation, redness, bruising, infection, or scarring. Check injection site 2 hr after injection for redness, swelling, and tenderness. Notify health care provider if skin reaction does not clear in a few days. Caution patient not to reuse needles or syringes and provide patient with a puncture-resistant container for disposal.
- Inform patient that flu-like symptoms (headache, fever, chills, myalgia, sweating, malaise, tiredness) may occur during therapy. Acetaminophen may be used for relief of fever and myalgias. Flu-like symptoms are not contagious.
- Advise patient to notify health care provider immediately if signs and symptoms of liver disease (yellowing of skin or whites of eyes, nausea, loss of appetite, tiredness, bleeding easily, confusion, sleepiness, dark-colored urine, pale stools), depression, suicidal thoughts, seizures, allergic reactions (itching; swelling of face, eyes, lips, tongue, or throat; trouble breathing; feeling faint; anxiousness; rash; hives), or autoimmune diseases (easy bleeding or bruising, thyroid gland problems, autoimmune hepatitis) occur.
- Instruct patient to notify health care provider of all Rx or OTC medications, vitamins, or herbal products being taken and to consult with health care provider before taking other medications.
- Rep: Advise women of reproductive potential to notify health care provider if pregnancy is planned or suspected or if breastfeeding.

Evaluation/Desired Outcomes

- Decrease in the frequency of relapse (neurologic dysfunction) in patients with relapsing-remitting MS.

pegloticase (peg-loe-ti-kase)

Krystexxa

Classification

Therapeutic: antigout agents

Pharmacologic: enzymes

Indications

Chronic gout in adults who have not responded to/cannot tolerate xanthine oxidase inhibitors, including allopurinol.

Action

Consists of recombinant uricase covalently bonded to monomethoxypoly(ethylene glycol); uricase catalyzes the oxidation of uric acid to allantoin, a water soluble by-product that is readily excreted in urine. **Therapeutic Effects:** ↓ serum uric acid levels with resultant ↓ in attacks of gout and its sequelae.

Pharmacokinetics

Absorption: IV administration results in complete bioavailability.

Distribution: Unknown.

Metabolism and Excretion: Unknown.

Half-life: Unknown.

TIME/ACTION PROFILE

ROUTE	ONSET	PEAK	DURATION
IV	rapid	within 24 hr	>300 hr

Contraindications/Precautions

Contraindicated in: Serious hypersensitivity, including anaphylaxis; Glucose-6-phosphate dehydrogenase (G6PD) deficiency (↑ risk of hemolysis and methemoglobinemia).

Use Cautiously in: HF (may ↑ risk of exacerbation); Retreatment after a drug-free interval (↑ risk of allergic reactions, monitor carefully); OB: Use during pregnancy only if clearly needed; Lactation: Use while breastfeeding only if potential maternal benefit justifies potential risk to infant; Pedi: Safety and effectiveness not established in children; Geri: Older adults may be more sensitive to drug effects.

Adverse Reactions/Side Effects

CV: chest pain. **Derm:** contusion/ecchymoses. **EENT:** nasopharyngitis. **GI:** nausea, constipation, vomiting. **Hemat:** HEMOLYSIS, METHEMOGLOBINEMIA. **Metab:** gout flare. **Misc:** INFUSION REACTIONS, HYPERSENSITIVITY REACTIONS (INCLUDING ANAPHYLAXIS).

Interactions

Drug-Drug: May interfere with the action of other **PEG-containing therapies.**

Route/Dosage

IV (Adults): 8 mg every 2 wk.

Availability

Solution for injection: 8 mg/mL.

NURSING IMPLICATIONS

Assessment

- Monitor for joint pain and swelling. Gout flares are expected to occur upon initiation of therapy. Administer prophylactic doses of colchicine or an NSAID ≥1 wk before and concurrently during the 1st 6 mo of therapy.
- Monitor for signs/symptoms of anaphylaxis (wheezing, perioral or lingual edema, hemodynamic instability, rash, urticaria) during and following infusion for ≥2 hr. Risk is higher in patients with uric acid level >6 mg/dL. *If anaphylaxis occurs,* immediately discontinue pegloticase and treat as indicated.
- Monitor for infusion reactions (rash, dyspnea, flushing, chest pain) during and for ≥1 hr after infusion. *If infusion reaction occurs,* slow or stop infusion; restart at slower rate.

Lab Test Considerations

- Screen patients at risk for G6PD deficiency before starting therapy. Patients of African, Mediterranean (including Southern European and Middle Eastern), and Southern Asian ancestry are at ↑ risk for G6PD deficiency. Do not administer pegloticase to patients with G6PD deficiency.
- Assess uric acid levels prior to infusions. *If uric acid level >6 mg/dL,* discontinue therapy. Risk of anaphylaxis and other infusion reactions is particularly high with two consecutive levels >6 mg/dL.

Implementation

- Premedicate with antihistamine and corticosteroid prior to infusion to ↓ risk of anaphylaxis and infusion reaction. Administer in a setting with professionals prepared to manage anaphylaxis and infusion reactions.
- Gout flare prophylaxis with either NSAIDs or colchicine can be started ≥1 wk before starting therapy and continued for ≥6 mo. Discontinue all oral urate-lowering medications before starting and during therapy.
- May be administered with methotrexate.

IV Administration

- **Intermittent Infusion:** Withdraw 1 mL of pegloticase from vial and inject into 250 mL bag of NaCl. Invert bag several times to mix; do not shake. Solution is clear and colorless; do not administer if discolored or contains precipitates. Solution is stable for 4 hr if refrigerated or at room temperature. Do not freeze. Protect from light. Bring solution to room temperature before administering. **Rate:** Infuse over 120 min. Do not administer via IV push or bolus.
- **Y-Site Incompatibility:** Do not administer other drugs through same IV line.

Patient/Family Teaching

- Explain purpose and side effects of medication. Advise patient to read *Patient Information* before starting therapy.
- Advise patient to notify health care provider immediately if signs of anaphylaxis or infusion reaction occur.
- Advise patient not to take pegloticase if they have G6PD deficiency.
- Inform patient that gout flares may initially ↑ during the 1st 3 mo of therapy. Advise patient to take concurrent colchicine or NSAIDs to ↓ flares.
- Advise patient to notify health care provider of all Rx or OTC medications, vitamins, or herbal products being taken and to consult with health care provider before taking other medications.
- Instruct patient not to take oral urate-lowering medications before or during therapy.
- Rep: Advise women of reproductive potential to notify health care provider if pregnancy is planned or suspected and to avoid breastfeeding during therapy.

Evaluation/Desired Outcomes

- ↓ in uric acid levels with resultant improvement in gout symptoms in patients with chronic gout.

HIGH ALERT

pembrolizumab

(pem-broe-li-zoo-mab)

Keytruda

Classification

Therapeutic: antineoplastics

Pharmacologic: monoclonal antibodies, programmed death-1 inhibitors

Indications

Unresectable or metastatic melanoma. Adjuvant treatment of Stage IIB, IIC, or III melanoma following complete resection. First-line treatment of patients with stage III non-small cell lung cancer (NSCLC), who are not candidates for surgical resection or definitive chemoradiation, or metastatic NSCLC and whose tumors express PD-L1 (tumor proportion score [TPS] ≥1%) and have no epidermal growth factor receptor (EGFR) or anaplastic lymphoma kinase (ALK) genomic tumor aberrations (as monotherapy). Metastatic NSCLC expressing PD-L1 (TPS ≥1%) that has progressed on or after platinum-containing chemotherapy (as monotherapy). Patients with EGFR or ALK genomic tumor aberrations should have disease progression on FDA-approved therapy for these aberrations prior to receiving pembrolizumab. Adjuvant treatment of Stage IB, II, or IIIA NSCLC following resection and platinum-based chemotherapy (as monotherapy). Resectable (tumors ≥4 cm or node positive) NSCLC (in combination with platinum-containing chemotherapy as neoadjuvant treatment, and then continued as a single agent as adjuvant treatment after surgery). 🧬 First-line treatment of metastatic nonsquamous NSCLC with no EGFR or ALK genomic tumor aberrations (in combination with pemetrexed and platinum chemotherapy). First-line treatment of unresectable advanced or metastatic malignant pleural mesothelioma (in combination with pemetrexed and platinum chemotherapy). First-line treatment of metastatic nonsquamous NSCLC (in combination with carboplatin and either paclitaxel or nab-paclitaxel [albumin-bound]). Recurrent or metastatic head and neck squamous cell carcinoma (HNSCC) that has progressed on or after platinum-containing chemotherapy. First-line treatment of metastatic or unresectable recurrent HNSCC (in combination with platinum and fluorouracil). 🧬 First-line treatment of metastatic or unresectable recurrent HNSCC expressing PD-L1 (combined positive score [CPS] ≥1). Resectable locally advanced HNSCC expressing PD-L1 (CPS ≥1) as a single agent as neoadjuvant treatment, continued as adjuvant treatment in combination with radiotherapy with or without cisplatin, and then as a single agent. Adults with relapsed or refractory classical Hodgkin lymphoma (cHL). Children with refractory cHL or cHL that has relapsed after ≥2 lines of therapy. Primary mediastinal large B-cell lymphoma that is refractory or that has relapsed after ≥2 prior lines of therapy (should not be used in patients who require urgent cytoreductive therapy). Locally advanced or metastatic urothelial carcinoma in patients who are not eligible for any platinum-containing chemotherapy. Locally advanced or metastatic urothelial carcinoma in patients who have disease progression during or following platinum-containing chemotherapy or within 12 mo of neoadjuvant or adjuvant treatment with platinum-containing chemotherapy. Locally advanced or metastatic urothelial carcinoma (in combination with enfortumab vedotin). Bacillus Calmette-Guerin (BCG)-unresponsive, high-risk, non-muscle-invasive bladder cancer with carcinoma in situ with or without papillary tumors in patients who are not eligible for or have elected not to undergo cystectomy. 🧬 Unresectable or metastatic microsatellite instability-high (MSI-H) or mismatch repair deficient (dMMR) solid tumors that have progressed following prior treatment and have no satisfactory alternative treatment options. 🧬 First-line treatment of unresectable or metastatic MSI-H or dMMR colorectal cancer. 🧬 First-line treatment of locally advanced unresectable or metastatic HER2-positive gastric or gastroesophageal junction adenocarcinoma (in combination with trastuzumab, fluoropyrimidine- and platinum-containing chemotherapy). First-line treatment of locally advanced unresectable or metastatic HER2-negative gastric or gastroesophageal junction adenocarcinoma in patients whose tumors express PD-L1 (CPS ≥1) (in combination with fluoropyrimidine- and platinum-containing chemotherapy). 🧬 Locally advanced or metastatic esophageal or gastroesophageal junction (tumors with epicenter 1–5 cm above the gastroesophageal junction) carcinoma that is not amenable to surgical resection or definitive chemoradiation either as monotherapy after ≥1 prior line of systemic therapy for patients with tumors of squamous cell histology that express PD-L1 (CPS ≥10) or in combination with platinum- and fluoropyrimidine-based chemotherapy in patients whose tumors that express PD-L1 (CPS ≥1). Locally advanced cervical cancer involving the lower third of the vagina, with or without extension to pelvic sidewall, or hydronephrosis/nonfunctioning kidney, or spread to adjacent pelvic organs (FIGO 2014 Stage III–IVA) (in combination with chemoradiotherapy). 🧬 Recurrent or metastatic cervical cancer expressing PD-L1 (CPS ≥1) that has progressed on or after chemotherapy. 🧬 Persistent, recurrent, or metastatic cervical cancer expressing PD-L1 (CPS ≥1) (in combination with chemotherapy, with or without bevacizumab). Hepatocellular carcinoma secondary to hepatitis B in patients who have received prior systemic therapy other than a PD-1/PD-L1-containing regimen. Locally advanced unresectable or metastatic biliary tract cancer (in combination with gemcitabine and cisplatin). Recurrent locally advanced or metastatic Merkel cell carcinoma. First-line treatment of advanced renal cell carcinoma (RCC) (in combination with axitinib or lenvatinib). Adjuvant treatment of RCC at intermediate-high or high risk of recurrence following nephrectomy, or following nephrectomy and resection of metastatic lesions. Primary advanced or recurrent endometrial carcinoma (in combination with carboplatin and paclitaxel, and then continued as a single agent). 🧬 Advanced endometrial carcinoma that is mismatch repair proficient (pMMR) or not MSI-H in patients who have disease progression following prior systemic therapy in any setting and are not candidates for curative surgery or radiation (in combination with lenvatinib). 🧬 Advanced endometrial carcinoma that is MSI-H or dMMR in patients who have disease progression following prior systemic therapy in any setting and are not candidates for curative surgery or radiation. 🧬 Unresectable or metastatic tumor mutational burden-high (TMB-H) [≥10 mutations/megabase] solid tumors that have progressed following prior treatment and have no satisfactory alternative treatment options. Recurrent or metastatic cutaneous squamous cell carcinoma that is

P

not curable by surgery or radiation. Locally recurrent unresectable or metastatic triple-negative breast cancer (TNBC) in patients whose tumors express PD-L1 (CPS ≥10) (in combination with chemotherapy). High-risk early-stage TNBC (in combination with chemotherapy as neoadjuvant treatment, and then continued as a single agent as adjuvant treatment after surgery).

Action

Programmed death receptor-1 (PD-1) blocking antibody (an IgG4 kappa immunoglobulin) that binds to PD-1 and blocks its interaction with its ligands, PD-L1 and PD-L2, resulting in activation of the immune system and decreased tumor growth. **Therapeutic Effects:** Decreased spread of melanoma, NSCLC, malignant pleural mesothelioma, HNSCC, cHL, urothelial carcinoma, MSI-H or dMMR solid tumors, MSI-H or dMMR colorectal cancer, gastric tumors, cervical cancer, endometrial cancer, esophageal cancer, primary mediastinal large B-cell lymphoma, hepatocellular carcinoma, biliary tract cancer, Merkel cell carcinoma, RCC, TMB-H solid tumors, cutaneous squamous cell carcinoma, and TNBC.

Pharmacokinetics

Absorption: IV administration results in complete bioavailability.
Distribution: Unknown.
Metabolism and Excretion: Unknown.
Half-life: 26 days.

TIME/ACTION PROFILE

ROUTE	ONSET	PEAK	DURATION
IV	within 3 mo	unknown	may persist for >8.8 mo

Contraindications/Precautions

Contraindicated in: OB: Pregnancy; Lactation: Lactation.
Use Cautiously in: Moderate or severe hepatic impairment; Solid organ transplant recipients (↑ risk of rejection); Allogeneic hematopoietic stem cell transplant recipients (↑ risk of transplantation complications); Rep: Women of reproductive potential; Pedi: Safety and effectiveness not established in children <2 yr (cHL, MSI-H cancer, primary mediastinal large B-cell lymphoma, and Merkel cell carcinoma) <12 yr (melanoma), or children <18 yr (all other indications).

Adverse Reactions/Side Effects

CV: MYOCARDITIS, pericarditis, vasculitis. **Derm:** pruritus, rash, DRUG REACTION WITH EOSINOPHILIA AND SYSTEMIC SYMPTOMS (DRESS), STEVENS-JOHNSON SYNDROME (SJS), TOXIC EPIDERMAL NECROLYSIS (TEN). **EENT:** iritis, uveitis. **Endo:** hyperglycemia, hyperthyroidism, hypoglycemia, hypothyroidism, ADRENAL INSUFFICIENCY, hypoparathyroidism, hypophysitis. **F and E** hypercalcemia, hyperkalemia, hypermagnesemia, hypocalcemia, hypokalemia, hypomagnesemia, hyponatremia, hypophosphatemia. **GI:** ↓ appetite, ↑ amylase, ↑ lipase, ↑ liver enzymes, constipation, diarrhea, nausea, COLITIS, gastritis, HEPATITIS, pancreatitis. **GU:** ↑ serum creatinine, nephritis. **Hemat:** ↑ activated partial thromboplastin time, ↑ INR, anemia, lymphopenia, neutropenia, thrombocytopenia, hemolytic anemia. **Metab:** hypercholesterolemia, hypertriglyceridemia, hypoalbuminemia. **MS:** ↑ CK, arthralgia, back pain, extremity pain, myalgia, myositis, RHABDOMYOLYSIS. **Neuro:** dizziness, fatigue, headache, insomnia, autoimmune neuropathy, ENCEPHALITIS, Guillain-Barré syndrome, MENINGITIS, myasthenic syndrome, myelitis. **Resp:** PNEUMONITIS. **Misc:** INFUSION-RELATED REACTIONS, SEPSIS.

Interactions

Drug-Drug: None reported.

Route/Dosage

Melanoma

IV (Adults): 200 mg every 3 wk until disease progression or unacceptable toxicity *or* 400 mg every 6 wk until disease progression or unacceptable toxicity.

Adjuvant Treatment of Melanoma

IV (Adults): 200 mg every 3 wk until disease recurrence, unacceptable toxicity, or up to 12 mo *or* 400 mg every 6 wk until disease recurrence, unacceptable toxicity, or up to 12 mo.
IV (Children≥12 yr): 2 mg/kg (max = 200 mg) every 3 wk until disease recurrence, unacceptable toxicity, or up to 12 mo.

Non-Small Cell Lung Cancer, Malignant Pleural Mesothelioma, Head and Neck Squamous Cell Carcinoma, Esophageal Cancer, Biliary Tract Cancer, or Locally Recurrent Unresectable or Metastatic Triple Negative Breast Cancer

IV (Adults): 200 mg every 3 wk until disease progression, unacceptable toxicity, or up to 24 mo *or* 400 mg every 6 wk until disease progression, unacceptable toxicity, or up to 24 mo. If being administered in combination with chemotherapy, should be administered prior to chemotherapy when given on the same day.

Locally Advanced Head and Neck Squamous Cell Carcinoma,

IV (Adults): 200 mg every 3 wk *or* 400 mg every 6 wk. As neoadjuvant therapy, administer as monotherapy for 6 wk or until disease progression that precludes definitive surgery or unacceptable toxicity. As adjuvant therapy, administer in combination with radiotherapy with or without cisplatin, and then continue as monotherapy. Continue until disease recurrence or unacceptable toxicity or up to 1 yr.

Adjuvant Treatment of Non-Small Cell Lung Cancer

IV (Adults): 200 mg every 3 wk until disease recurrence, unacceptable toxicity, or up to 12 mo *or* 400 mg every 6 wk until disease recurrence, unacceptable toxicity, or up to 12 mo.

Resectable Non-Small Cell Lung Cancer

IV (Adults): 200 mg every 3 wk. Neoadjuvant treatment in combination with platinum-containing chemotherapy for 12 wk or until disease progression that precludes definitive surgery, or unacceptable toxicity, followed by neoadjuvant treatment as monotherapy after surgery for 39 wk or until disease recurrence or unacceptable toxicity; *or* 400 mg every 6 wk. Neoadjuvant treatment in combination with platinum-containing chemotherapy for 12 wk or until disease progression that precludes definitive surgery, or unacceptable toxicity, followed by neoadjuvant treatment as monotherapy after surgery for 39 wk or until disease recurrence or unacceptable toxicity

Urothelial Carcinoma, Gastric Cancer, Cervical Cancer, Endometrial Carcinoma, Hepatocellular Carcinoma, Renal Cell Carcinoma, Cutaneous Squamous Cell Carcinoma, or Microsatellite Instability-High/Mismatch Repair Deficient Colorectal Cancer

IV (Adults): 200 mg every 3 wk until disease progression, unacceptable toxicity, or up to 24 mo *or* 400 mg every 6 wk until disease progression, unacceptable toxicity, or up to 24 mo. If being administered in combination with chemotherapy, chemoradiotherapy, bevacizumab, trastuzumab, paclitaxel, or carboplatin, should be administered prior to these therapies when given on the same day; if being administered in combination with enfortumab vedotin, should be administered after this medication when given on the same day.

Adjuvant Treatment of Renal Cell Carcinoma

IV (Adults): 200 mg every 3 wk until disease recurrence, unacceptable toxicity, or up to 12 mo *or* 400 mg every 6 wk until disease recurrence, unacceptable toxicity, or up to 12 mo.

Bacillus Calmette-Guerin-Unresponsive, High-Risk Non-Muscle-Invasive Bladder Cancer

IV (Adults): 200 mg every 3 wk until persistent or recurrent high-risk non-muscle invasive bladder cancer, disease progression, unacceptable toxicity, or up to 24 mo *or* 400 mg every 6 wk until persistent or recurrent high-risk non-muscle invasive bladder cancer, disease progression, unacceptable toxicity, or up to 24 mo.

Classical Hodgkin Lymphoma, Microsatellite Instability-High/Mismatch Repair Deficient Cancer, Primary Mediastinal Large B-Cell Lymphoma, Merkel Cell Carcinoma, or Tumor Mutational Burden-High Cancer

IV (Adults): 200 mg every 3 wk until disease progression, unacceptable toxicity, or up to 24 mo *or* 400 mg every 6 wk until disease progression, unacceptable toxicity, or up to 24 mo.

IV (Children≥2 yr): 2 mg/kg (max = 200 mg) every 3 wk until disease progression, unacceptable toxicity, or up to 24 mo.

High-Risk, Early-Stage Triple Negative Breast Cancer

IV (Adults): 200 mg every 3 wk for 24 wk (8 doses) (as neoadjuvant treatment in combination with chemotherapy) or until disease progression or unacceptable toxicity followed by 200 mg every 3 wk for up to 27 wk (9 doses) (as monotherapy as adjuvant treatment after surgery) *or* 400 mg every 6 wk for 24 wk (4 doses) (as neoadjuvant treatment in combination with chemotherapy) or until disease progression or unacceptable toxicity followed by 400 mg every 6 wk for up to 27 wk (5 doses) (as monotherapy as adjuvant treatment after surgery). If being administered in combination with chemotherapy, should be administered prior to chemotherapy when given on the same day.

Availability

Solution for injection: 25 mg/mL.

NURSING IMPLICATIONS

Assessment

- Monitor for signs/symptoms of immune-mediated pneumonitis (shortness of breath, chest pain, new or worse cough) periodically during therapy. Evaluate with x-ray. *If Grade ≥2 pneumonitis occurs,* treat with corticosteroids. *If Grade 2 pneumonitis occurs,* hold pembrolizumab. Resume therapy in patients with complete or partial resolution (Grade ≤1) after corticosteroid taper. *If Grades 3 or 4 or recurrent Grade 2 pneumonitis occurs,* permanently discontinue pembrolizumab.
- Monitor for immune-mediated nephritis (hematuria, ↑ BP, oliguria, edema, shortness of breath) during therapy. *If nephritis occurs with kidney dysfunction and treatment is interrupted or discontinued,* administer systemic corticosteroids (1–2 mg/kg/day prednisone or equivalent) until improvement to Grade ≤1; then follow corticosteroid taper.
- Monitor for signs/symptoms of immune-mediated colitis (diarrhea, abdominal pain, mucus or blood in stool, with or without fever). *If Grades 2 or 3 colitis occurs,* hold pembrolizumab. Resume therapy in patients with complete or partial resolution (Grades ≤1) after corticosteroid taper. Permanently discontinue pembrolizumab if no complete or partial response within 12 wk of initiating corticosteroids or

if unable to ↓ prednisone dose to ≤10 mg/day (or equivalent) within 12 wk of corticosteroid initiation. *If Grade 4 colitis occurs,* permanently discontinue pembrolizumab.

- Assess for signs/symptoms of immune-mediated hepatitis (yellowing of skin or whites of eyes, unusual darkening of urine, unusual tiredness, pain in right upper stomach) before each dose.
- Monitor for signs/symptoms of infusion-related reactions (rigors, chills, wheezing, pruritus, flushing, rash, hypotension, hypoxemia, fever). *If Grades 1 or 2 infusion-related reactions occur,* hold or slow rate of infusion. *If Grades 3 or 4 infusion-related reactions occur,* stop infusion and permanently discontinue pembrolizumab.
- Monitor for clinical signs/symptoms of hypophysitis (persistent or unusual headache, extreme weakness, dizziness or fainting, vision changes) during therapy. Other endocrinopathies to monitor for include Grade ≥2 adrenal insufficiency, type 1 diabetes, hyperthyroidism, thyroiditis, and hypothyroidism. *If Grade 3 or 4 endocrinopathies occur,* hold pembrolizumab until clinically stable.
- Assess for rash periodically during therapy. Topical emollients and/or topical corticosteroids may be adequate to treat mild to moderate nonexfoliative rashes. May cause SJS, TEN, and DRESS. *If rash, itching, blistering, or ulcers in mouth or other mucous membranes occur and SJS, TEN, or DRESS are suspected,* hold pembrolizumab and refer for assessment and treatment. *If SJS, TEN, or DRESS are confirmed,* permanently discontinue pembrolizumab.
- Monitor for signs/symptoms of encephalitis (headache, fever, tiredness or weakness, confusion, memory problems, sleepiness, hallucinations, seizures, stiff neck) periodically during therapy. *If Grade 2 neurological toxicities occur,* hold pembrolizumab; resume after complete or partial resolution (Grades 0–1) after corticosteroid taper. Permanently discontinue pembrolizumab if no complete or partial response (Grades 0–1) within 12 wk of initiating corticosteroids or if unable to ↓ prednisone dose to ≤10 mg/day (or equivalent) within 12 wk of corticosteroid initiation. *If Grade 3 or 4 neurological toxicities occur,* permanently discontinue pembrolizumab and administer corticosteroids at dose of 1–2 mg/kg/day prednisone or equivalent for immune-mediated encephalitis, followed by corticosteroid taper.
- Monitor for signs/symptoms of myocarditis (chest pain, dyspnea) during therapy. *If Grade 2, 3, or 4 myocarditis occurs,* permanently discontinue pembrolizumab.

Lab Test Considerations

- Verify negative pregnancy test prior to starting therapy.
- Patient selection is based on presence of positive PD-L1 expression in stage III NSCLC who are not candidates for surgical resection or definitive chemoradiation, metastatic NSCLC, first-line treatment of metastatic or unresectable recurrent HNSCC, metastatic gastric cancer (if PD-L1 expression is not detected in an archival gastric cancer specimen, evaluate feasibility of obtaining a tumor biopsy for PD-L1 testing), previously treated recurrent locally advanced or metastatic esophageal cancer, and recurrent or metastatic cervical cancer. For MSI-H/dMMR indications, select patients for pembrolizumab as a single agent based on MSI-H/dMMR status in tumor specimens. For TMB-H, select patients for pembrolizumab as a single agent based on TMB-H status in tumor specimens. For combination therapy for non-MSI-H/dMMR advanced endometrial carcinoma, select patients for pembrolizumab in combination with lenvatinib based on MSI or MMR status in tumor specimens. For use of pembrolizumab in combination with chemotherapy, select patients based on the presence of positive PD-L1 expression in locally recurrent unresectable or metastatic TNBC. Information on FDA-approved tests used for patient selection is available at http://www.fda.gov/CompanionDiagnostics.
- Monitor for ↑ serum creatinine before and periodically during therapy. *If Grade 2 or 3 ↑ in serum creatinine occur,* hold pembrolizumab. Resume in patients with complete or partial resolution (Grade ≤1) after corticosteroid taper. Permanently discontinue if no complete or partial resolution within 12 wk of last dose or inability to ↓ prednisone dose to ≤10 mg per day (or equivalent) within 12 wk of starting steroids. *If Grade 4 ↑ in blood creatinine occur,* permanently discontinue pembrolizumab.
- Monitor for liver function before and periodically during therapy. **For hepatitis with no tumor involvement:** *If AST/ALT >3 and ≤8 times upper limit of normal (ULN) or total bilirubin >1.5 and ≤3 times ULN,* hold pembrolizumab. Resume with complete or partial resolution (Grade ≤1) after corticosteroid taper. Permanently discontinue pembrolizumab if no complete or partial resolution within 12 wk of last dose or inability to ↓ prednisone dose to ≤10 mg per day (or equivalent) within 12 wk of starting steroids. *If AST or ALT >8 times ULN or total bilirubin >3 times ULN,* permanently discontinue pembrolizumab. **For hepatitis with tumor involvement of the liver:** *If baseline AST/ALT >1 and ≤3 times ULN and ↑ to >5 and ≤10 times ULN or baseline AST/ALT >3 and ≤5 times ULN and ↑ to >8 and ≤10 times ULN,* hold pembrolizumab. *If AST/ALT >10 times ULN or total bilirubin >3 times ULN,* permanently discontinue pembrolizumab.
- Monitor for changes in thyroid function at start of and periodically during therapy, and as indicated based

on clinical evaluation. Administer corticosteroids for Grade ≥3 hyperthyroidism; hold pembrolizumab for severe (Grade 3) hyperthyroidism and resume therapy when recovery to Grade ≤1. Permanently discontinue pembrolizumab for life-threatening (Grade 4) hyperthyroidism. Manage hypothyroidism with thyroid replacement without interruption of therapy or corticosteroids.

- Monitor serum blood glucose. May cause hyperglycemia or other signs and symptoms of diabetes.

Implementation

IV Administration

- **Intermittent Infusion: Dilution:** Withdraw required volume of pembrolizumab and transfer to IV bag of 0.9% NaCl or D5W. Mix using gently inversion. Solution is clear to slightly opalescent, colorless to slightly yellow; do not administer solution if discolored or contains particulate matter other than translucent to white proteinaceous particles. Solution is stable at room temperature for up to 6 hr including infusion time and 96 hr if refrigerated. **Concentration:** 1–10 mg/mL. **Rate:** Infuse through a sterile, nonpyrogenic, low-protein-binding 0.2–5-micron in-line or add-on filter over 30 min.
- **Y-Site Incompatibility:** Do not administer other drugs through same IV line.

Patient/Family Teaching

- Explain purpose and side effects of medication to patient. Advise patient to read *Patient Information* before starting therapy. Emphasize importance of keeping scheduled appointments for blood work or other laboratory tests.
- Instruct patient to notify health care provider of all Rx or OTC medications, vitamins, or herbal products being taken and to consult with health care provider before taking other medications.
- Advise patient to notify health care provider immediately if signs and symptoms of pneumonitis; colitis; hepatitis; kidney problems (change in amount or color of urine); hormone gland problems (rapid heartbeat, weight loss, ↑ sweating, weight gain, hair loss, feeling cold, constipation, deepening of voice, dizziness or fainting, persistent or unusual headache); change in taste; trouble sleeping; flu-like symptoms; or back, bone, joint, muscle, or neck pain occur.
- Rep: May cause fetal harm. Advise women of reproductive potential to use highly effective contraception and avoid breastfeeding during and for ≥4 mo after last dose.

Evaluation/Desired Outcomes

- Decreased spread of melanoma, NSCLC, malignant pleural mesothelioma, HNSCC, cHL, urothelial carcinoma, MSI-H or dMMR solid tumors, MSI-H or dMMR colorectal cancer, gastric tumors, cervical cancer, endometrial cancer, esophageal cancer, primary mediastinal large B-cell lymphoma, hepatocellular carcinoma, biliary tract cancer, Merkel cell carcinoma, RCC, TMB-H solid tumors, cutaneous squamous cell carcinoma, and TNBC.

HIGH ALERT

PEMEtrexed (pe-me-**trex**-ed)

Alimta, Axtle, Pemfexy, Pemrydi RTU

Classification

Therapeutic: antineoplastics

Pharmacologic: antimetabolites, folate antagonists

Indications

Malignant pleural mesothelioma as initial therapy when tumor is unresectable or patient is not a candidate for surgery (in combination with cisplatin). Metastatic nonsquamous non-small cell lung cancer (NSCLC) as initial therapy in patients without epidermal growth factor receptor or anaplastic lymphoma kinase genomic tumor aberrations (in combination with platinum-based therapy and pembrolizumab). Locally advanced or metastatic nonsquamous NSCLC as initial therapy (in combination with cisplatin). Locally advanced or metastatic nonsquamous NSCLC as maintenance treatment in patients whose disease has not progressed after 4 cycles of platinum-based first-line chemotherapy (as monotherapy). Recurrent metastatic nonsquamous NSCLC after previous chemotherapy (as monotherapy).

Action

Disrupts folate dependent metabolic processes involved in thymidine and purine synthesis. Converted intracellularly to polyglutamate form, which increases duration of action. **Therapeutic Effects:** Decreased growth and spread of mesothelioma. Improved survival in patients with nonsquamous NSCLC.

Pharmacokinetics

Absorption: IV administration results in complete bioavailability.

Distribution: Unknown.

Metabolism and Excretion: Minimal metabolism; 70–90% excreted unchanged in urine.

Half-life: 3.5 hr.

TIME/ACTION PROFILE (hematologic effects)

ROUTE	ONSET	PEAK	DURATION
IV	unknown	8–15 days	21 days

P

Contraindications/Precautions

Contraindicated in: Hypersensitivity; CCr <45 mL/min; OB: Pregnancy; Lactation: Lactation.

Use Cautiously in: Concurrent use of NSAIDs in patients with CCr 45–79 mL/min (avoid those with short half-lives); 3rd space fluid accumulation (ascites, pleural effusions); consider drainage prior to therapy; Hepatic impairment (dose alteration recommended); Rep: Women of reproductive potential and men with female partners of reproductive potential; Pedi: Safety and effectiveness not established in children.

Adverse Reactions/Side Effects

CV: chest pain. **Derm:** desquamation, rash, radiation recall, STEVENS-JOHNSON SYNDROME, TOXIC EPIDERMAL NECROLYSIS. **GI:** constipation, nausea, stomatitis, vomiting, anorexia, diarrhea, esophagitis, mouth pain. **GU:** ↓ fertility (men). **Hemat:** anemia, hemolytic anemia, leukopenia, thrombocytopenia. **Neuro:** neuropathy. **Resp:** pharyngitis, INTERSTITIAL PNEUMONITIS. **Misc:** fever, infection.

Interactions

Drug-Drug: NSAIDs, especially those with short half-lives, ↑ levels and risk of toxicity; avoid for 2 days before, day of, and 2 days after treatment. **Probenecid** ↑ levels. **Nephrotoxic agents** ↑ risk of nephrotoxicity.

Route/Dosage

Nonsquamous Non-Small Cell Lung Cancer

IV (Adults): *Initial therapy (with cisplatin):* 500 mg/m² on Day 1 of each 21-day cycle for up to 6 cycles (administer before cisplatin); *Initial therapy (with platinum-based therapy and pembrolizumab):* 500 mg/m² on Day 1 of each 21-day cycle for 4 cycles (administer before carboplatin or cisplatin and after pembrolizumab). Following completion of platinum-based therapy, pemetrexed may be administered as monotherapy or with pembrolizumab as maintenance therapy until disease progression or unacceptable toxicity; *Maintenance treatment (as monotherapy) or disease recurrence (as monotherapy):* 500 mg/m² on Day 1 of each 21-day cycle until disease progression or unacceptable toxicity.

Mesothelioma

IV (Adults): 500 mg/m² on Day 1 of each 21-day cycle until disease progression or unacceptable toxicity.

Availability (generic available)

Lyophilized powder for injection: 100 mg/vial, 500 mg/vial, 750 mg/vial, 1 g/vial. **Solution for injection:** 10 mg/mL, 25 mg/mL.

NURSING IMPLICATIONS

Assessment

- Monitor for blistering and exfoliative skin toxicity during therapy. *If severe skin toxicity occurs,* permanently discontinue pemetrexed.
- Monitor for signs/symptoms of interstitial pneumonitis (new onset dyspnea, cough, fever). *If signs/symptoms of interstitial pneumonitis occur and diagnosis confirmed,* permanently discontinue pemetrexed.
- Assess for radiation recall (rash, redness, swelling, pain, peeling skin) in patients who received radiation weeks to years before starting pemetrexed therapy. *If signs/symptoms of radiation recall occur,* permanently discontinue pemetrexed.
- Monitor for GI toxicities (mucositis, diarrhea). *If Grade 3 or 4 GI toxicities, except mucositis, or diarrhea requiring hospitalization occurs,* ↓ pemetrexed dose by 75%; delay initiation of next cycle until recovery to Grade ≤2. *If Grade 3 or 4 mucositis occurs,* ↓ pemetrexed dose by 50%; delay initiation of next cycle until recovery to Grade ≤2. *If recurrent Grade 3 or 4 GI toxicity occurs after two dose reductions,* permanently discontinue pemetrexed.
- Monitor for neurologic toxicities. *If Grade 3 or 4 neurologic toxicity occurs or after two dose reductions for any non-Grade 3 or 4 toxicity,* permanently discontinue pemetrexed.
- Monitor for bone marrow suppression. Assess for bleeding (bleeding gums; bruising; petechiae; guaiac stools, urine, and emesis) and avoid IM injections and taking rectal temperatures if platelet count is low. Apply pressure to venipuncture sites for 10 min. Assess for signs of infection during neutropenia. Anemia may occur. Monitor for dyspnea and orthostatic hypotension. Granulocyte-colony stimulating factor (G-CSF) may be used if necessary.

Lab Test Considerations

- Verify negative pregnancy test before initiation.
- Assess CCr before each dose and periodically as indicated. *If CCr <45 mL/min,* hold therapy until CCr recovers to ≥45 mL/min.
- Monitor CBC with differential before each dose and on Days 8 and 15 of each cycle and then as clinically indicated. May cause neutropenia, thrombocytopenia leukopenia, and anemia. Delay initiation of next cycle until ANC ≥1500 cells/mm³ and platelets ≥100,000 cells/mm³. *If ANC <500/mm³ and platelets ≥50,000/mm or platelets <50,000/mm³ without bleeding,* ↓ pemetrexed dose by 75%. *If platelets <50,000/mm³ with bleeding,* ↓ pemetrexed dose by 50%. *If Grade 3 or 4 myelosuppression occurs after two dose reductions,* discontinue premetrexed
- Monitor liver function tests periodically during therapy.

Implementation

- Do not confuse pemetrexed with pralatrexate.
- Administer 0.4–1 mg of folic acid once daily for 7 days preceding 1st dose of pemetrexed, and continue during therapy and for 21 days after last dose.

- Administer vitamin B_{12} 1 mg IM as a single dose during the week preceding 1st dose and every 3 cycles thereafter. Subsequent doses of vitamin B_{12} may be given on same day as pemetrexed. Do not substitute with oral vitamin B_{12}.
- Administer dexamethasone 4 mg twice daily on the day before, the day of, and the day after administration to ↓ risk of skin toxicity.

IV Administration

- Prepare solution in a biologic cabinet. Wear gloves, gown, and mask while handling medication.
- **Intermittent Infusion: Lyophilized powder for injection: Reconstitution:** Calculate number of vials needed for dose; vials contain excess to facilitate delivery. Reconstitute with preservative-free D5W injection; use 4.2 mL for each 100-mg vial or 20 mL for each 500-mg vial. **Concentration:** 25 mg/mL. Swirl gently until powder is completely dissolved. Solution is clear and colorless to yellow or green-yellow. Do not administer if discolored or contains particulates. **Dilution:** Further dilute with D5W for a total volume of 100 mL. May refrigerate reconstituted or diluted solution for up to 24 hr.
- **Solution for injection:** Determine volume needed for dose; withdraw calculated amount and transfer to empty IV bag. Do not dilute. Discard if solution is discolored or contains particulates. Immediately administer or store in bag at room temperature for up to 24 hr. **Rate:** Infuse over 10 min.
- **Y-Site Compatibility:** acyclovir, allopurinol, amikacin, aminocaproic acid, aminophylline, amiodarone, amphotericin B liposomal, ampicillin, ampicillin/sulbactam, atracurium, azithromycin, aztreonam, bivalirudin, bleomycin, bumetanide, buprenorphine, butorphanol, carboplatin, carmustine, ceftriaxone, cefuroxime, cisatracurium, cisplatin, clindamycin, cyclophosphamide, cyclosporine, cytarabine, dactinomycin, daptomycin, dexamethasone, dexmedetomidine, dexrazoxane, digoxin, diltiazem, diphenhydramine, docetaxel, dopamine, doxorubicin liposomal, enalaprilat, ephedrine, epinephrine, eptifibatide, ertapenem, esmolol, etoposide, etoposide phosphate, famotidine, fentanyl, fluconazole, fludarabine, fluorouracil, foscarnet, fosphenytoin, furosemide, ganciclovir, glycopyrrolate, granisetron, haloperidol, heparin, hydrocortisone, hydromorphone, ifosfamide, imipenem/cilastatin, insulin regular, isoproterenol, ketorolac, labetalol, leucovorin, levofloxacin, lidocaine, linezolid, lorazepam, magnesium sulfate, mannitol, meperidine, meropenem, mesna, methadone, methylprednisolone, metoclopramide, metoprolol, midazolam, milrinone, mitomycin, morphine, moxifloxacin, nafcillin, naloxone, nitroglycerin, norepinephrine, octreotide, oxaliplatin, paclitaxel, pamidronate, pentobarbital, phenobarbital, phentolamine, piperacillin/tazobactam, potassium acetate, potassium chloride, potassium phosphates, procainamide, promethazine, propranolol, remifentanil, rocuronium, sodium acetate, sodium bicarbonate, sodium phosphates, succinylcholine, sufentanil, tacrolimus, theophylline, thiotepa, tigecycline, tirofiban, trimethoprim/sulfamethoxazole, vancomycin, vecuronium, verapamil, vinblastine, vincristine, vinorelbine, zidovudine, zoledronic acid.
- **Y-Site Incompatibility:** anidulafungin, calcium chloride, calcium gluconate, caspofungin, cefazolin, cefepime, cefotaxime, cefotetan, cefoxitin, ceftazidime, chloramphenicol, chlorpromazine, ciprofloxacin, dacarbazine, dantrolene, daunorubicin, diazepam, dobutamine, doxorubicin hydrochloride, doxycycline, droperidol, epirubicin, erythromycin, gemcitabine, gentamicin, hydralazine, idarubicin, irinotecan, metronidazole, minocycline, mitoxantrone, nalbuphine, nicardipine, nitroprusside, ondansetron, pantoprazole, pentamidine, phenytoin, prochlorperazine, tobramycin, topotecan, vasopressin.

Patient/Family Teaching

- Explain purpose and side effects of medication. Advise patient to read *Patient Information* before starting therapy.
- Emphasize the importance of taking prophylactic folic acid and vitamin B_{12} to ↓ treatment-related hematologic and GI toxicity.
- Advise patient to notify health care provider immediately if signs and symptoms of infection (fever, sore throat), anemia, or neurotoxicity occur.
- Instruct patient to notify health care provider if persistent vomiting, diarrhea, or signs of dehydration occur.
- Instruct patient to notify health care provider of all Rx or OTC medications, vitamins, or herbal products being taken; to consult health care provider before taking any new medications, especially NSAIDs; and to avoid alcohol during therapy.
- Rep: May cause fetal harm. Advise women of reproductive potential to use effective contraception during therapy and for ≥6 mo after last dose and to avoid breastfeeding during therapy and for ≥1 wk after last dose. Advise men with female partners of reproductive potential to use effective contraception during therapy and for ≥3 mo after last dose. If pregnancy is planned or suspected, notify health care provider promptly. May impair fertility in men.

Evaluation/Desired Outcomes

- Decreased growth and spread of mesothelioma or NSCLC.

P

PENICILLINS (pen-i-sill-ins)

penicillin G aqueous
Pfizerpen
penicillin G benzathine
Bicillin L-A
penicillin V
Pen-VK

Classification
Therapeutic: anti-infectives
Pharmacologic: penicillins

Indications
Treatment of a wide variety of infections, including: Pneumococcal pneumonia, Streptococcal pharyngitis, Syphilis, Gonorrhea strains. Treatment of enterococcal infections (requires the addition of an aminoglycoside). Prevention of rheumatic fever. Should not be used as a single agent to treat anthrax. **Unlabeled Use:** Treatment of Lyme disease. Prevention of recurrent *Streptococcal pneumoniae* septicemia in children with sickle-cell disease.

Action
Inhibits bacterial cell wall synthesis. **Therapeutic Effects:** Bactericidal action against susceptible bacteria. **Spectrum:** Active against: Most gram-positive organisms, including many streptococci (*Streptococcus pneumoniae*, group A beta-hemolytic streptococci), staphylococci (non-penicillinase-producing strains), and *Bacillus anthracis*; Some gram-negative organisms, such as *Neisseria meningitidis* and *Neisseria gonorrhoeae* (only penicillin susceptible strains); Some anaerobic bacteria and spirochetes including *Borellia burgdorferi*.

Pharmacokinetics
Absorption: Variably absorbed from the GI tract. *Penicillin V:* resists acid degradation in the GI tract. *Benzathine penicillin:* IM absorption is delayed and prolonged and results in sustained therapeutic blood levels.
Distribution: Widely distributed, although CNS penetration is poor in the presence of uninflamed meninges.
Metabolism and Excretion: Minimally metabolized by the liver, excreted mainly unchanged by the kidneys.
Half-life: 30–60 min.

TIME/ACTION PROFILE (plasma concentrations)

ROUTE	ONSET	PEAK	DURATION
Penicillin V PO	rapid	0.5–1 hr	4–6 hr
Penicillin G IM	rapid	0.25–0.5 hr	4–6 hr
Penicillin G IV	rapid	end of infusion	4–6 hr
Benzathine penicillin IM	delayed	12–24 hr	3 wk

Contraindications/Precautions
Contraindicated in: Previous hypersensitivity to penicillins (cross-sensitivity may exist with cephalosporins and other beta-lactams); Hypersensitivity to benzathine (benzathine preparation only); Some products may contain tartrazine and should be avoided in patients with known hypersensitivity.
Use Cautiously in: Severe renal impairment (↓ dose); OB: Although safety not established in pregnancy, has been used safely; Lactation: Safety not established in breastfeeding; Geri: Consider ↓ body mass; age-related ↓ in renal, hepatic, and cardiac function; comorbidities; and concurrent drug therapy when prescribing and dosing.

Adverse Reactions/Side Effects
Derm: rash, ACUTE GENERALIZED EXANTHEMATOUS PUSTULOSIS, DRUG REACTION WITH EOSINOPHILIA AND SYSTEMIC SYMPTOMS (DRESS), STEVENS-JOHNSON SYNDROME (SJS), TOXIC EPIDERMAL NECROLYSIS (TEN), urticaria. **GI:** diarrhea, epigastric distress, nausea, vomiting, CLOSTRIDIOIDES DIFFICILE-ASSOCIATED DIARRHEA (CDAD). **GU:** interstitial nephritis. **Hemat:** eosinophilia, hemolytic anemia, leukopenia. **Local:** pain (at IM site), phlebitis. **Neuro:** SEIZURES. **Misc:** HYPERSENSITIVITY REACTIONS (INCLUDING ANAPHYLAXIS AND SERUM SICKNESS), superinfection.

Interactions
Drug-Drug: May ↓ effectiveness of **oral contraceptive agents**. **Probenecid** ↓ renal excretion and ↑ blood levels of penicillin (therapy may be combined for this purpose). **Neomycin** may ↓ absorption of penicillin V. May ↑ levels and risk of toxicity of **methotrexate**.

Route/Dosage
Penicillin G
IM, IV (Adults): *Most infections:* 1–5 million units every 4–6 hr.
IM, IV (Children): 8333–16,667 units/kg every 4 hr; 12,550–25,000 units/kg every 6 hr; up to 250,000 units/kg/day in divided doses, some infections may require up to 300,000 units/kg/day.
IV (Infants >7 days): 25,000 units/kg every 8 hr; *Meningitis:* 50,000–75,000 units/kg every 6 hr.
IV (Infants <7 days): 25,000 units/kg every 12 hr; *Streptococcus B meningitis:* 100,000–150,000 units/kg/day in divided doses.

Penicillin G Benzathine
IM (Adults): *Streptococcal infections/erysipeloid:* 1.2 million units as a single dose. *Primary, secondary, and early latent syphilis:* 2.4 million units as a single dose. *Tertiary and late latent syphilis (not neurosyphilis):* 2.4 million units once weekly for 3 wk. *Prevention of rheumatic fever:* 1.2 million units every 3–4 wk.
IM (Children >27 kg): *Streptococcal infections/erysipeloid:* 900,000–1.2 million units as a

single dose. *Primary, secondary, and early latent syphilis:* up to 2.4 million units as a single dose. *Late latent or latent syphilis of undetermined duration:* 50,000 units/kg once weekly for 3 wk. *Prevention of rheumatic fever:* 1.2 million units every 2–3 wk.

IM (Children <27 kg): *Streptococcal infections/erysipeloid:* 300,000–600,000 units as a single dose. *Primary, secondary, and early latent syphilis:* up to 2.4 million units as a single dose. *Late latent or latent syphilis of undetermined duration:* 50,000 units/kg once weekly for 3 wk. *Prevention of rheumatic fever:* 1.2 million units every 2–3 wk.

Penicillin V Potassium

PO (Adults and Children ≥12 yr): *Most infections:* 125–500 mg every 6–8 hr. *Rheumatic fever prevention:* 125–250 mg every 12 hr.

PO (Children <12 yr): *Lyme disease:* 12.5 mg/kg every 6 hr (unlabeled); prevention of *Streptococcus pneumoniae* sepsis in children with sickle cell disease: 125 mg twice daily.

Availability

Penicillin G Potassium Aqueous (generic available)

Powder for injection: 5 million units/vial, 20 million units/vial. **Premixed solution for injection:** 1 million units/50 mL, 2 million units/50 mL, 3 million units/50 mL.

Penicillin G Sodium Aqueous (generic available)

Powder for injection: 5 million units/vial.

Penicillin G Benzathine

Suspension for IM injection: 600,000 units/mL.

Penicillin V Potassium (generic available)

Oral solution: 125 mg/5 mL, 250 mg/5 mL. **Tablets:** 250 mg, 🍁 300 mg, 500 mg.

NURSING IMPLICATIONS

Assessment

- Assess for resolving infection (WBC and vital signs trends; appearance of wound, sputum, urine, and stool) during therapy.
- Obtain a history to determine previous use of and reactions to other beta-lactam antibiotics including cephalosporins. Persons with a negative history may still have an allergic response.
- Observe for signs/symptoms of hypersensitivity reactions (rash, urticaria, pruritus, flushing, dizziness, vomiting, abdominal pain) and angioedema (swelling of throat, lips, tongue, or face; dyspnea; wheezing; hoarseness). *If hypersensitivity reaction occurs,* discontinue drug immediately and provide supportive care. Keep epinephrine, an antihistamine, and resuscitation equipment close by in case of an anaphylactic reaction.
- Monitor for signs/symptoms of CDAD, including watery diarrhea with mucus, fever, abdominal pain or cramping, anorexia, nausea, and, in severe cases, dehydration, and blood or pus in the stool. May begin >2 mo after therapy. Report promptly to health care provider.
- Assess for rash or signs/symptoms of DRESS, TEN, or SJS frequently during therapy (fever, general malaise, fatigue, muscle or joint aches, blisters, oral lesions, conjunctivitis, hepatitis, eosinophilia). *If severe skin reaction occurs,* discontinue penicillin and provide supportive care; may be life-threatening. May recur once treatment is stopped.
- Monitor for seizure activity, particularly in patients with renal impairment. *If seizure occurs,* discontinue penicillin and treat as clinically indicated. Institute seizure precautions.
- Assess for signs/symptoms of superinfection such as oral thrush (white or yellow patches) or genital mycotic infections (pruritus and yeasty discharge). Treat infection promptly.

Lab Test Considerations

- Obtain specimens for culture and sensitivity before initiating therapy. 1st dose may be given before receiving results.
- Monitor renal function (including urinalysis), CBC with differential, and serum electrolytes before starting and routinely during *penicillin G* therapy.
- May cause positive direct Coombs test.
- Hyperkalemia may develop after large doses of *penicillin G potassium.*
- Monitor sodium concentrations in patient with hypertension or HF. Hypernatremia may develop after large doses of *penicillin G sodium.*
- May ↑ AST, ALT, LDH, and serum alkaline phosphatase. Monitor hepatic function with prolonged IV therapy with *penicillin G.*
- May cause leukopenia and neutropenia, especially with prolonged therapy or in hepatic impairment.

Implementation

- Do not confuse penicillin with penicillamine. Do not confuse penicillin G aqueous (potassium/sodium salts) with penicillin G benzathine.
- **PO:** May administer around the clock without regard to food, although *penicillin V* is best absorbed when taken with meals.
- Use calibrated measuring device for liquid preparations. Solution is stable for 14 days if refrigerated.

P

Penicillin G Potassium and Penicillin G Sodium

- **IM:** Inject *penicillin G* deep into a well-developed muscle mass at a slow, consistent rate to prevent blockage of the needle. Massage well. Accidental injury near or into a nerve can result in severe pain and dysfunction. Do not inject *penicillin G benzathine* in deltoid or anterolateral thigh.
- *Penicillin G potassium or sodium* may be diluted with lidocaine (without epinephrine) 1% or 2% to minimize pain from IM injection.
- Never give penicillin G benzathine suspension IV. May cause embolism or fatal reactions.

IV Administration

- V Penicillin G is a vesicant. If extravasation occurs, immediately stop infusion. Leave needle/cannula in place temporarily but do not flush the line. Gently aspirate extravasated solution; then remove needle/cannula. Elevate patient's extremity and apply dry cold compresses. Initiate hyaluronidase antidote for refractory cases in addition to supportive management. For hyaluronidase, inject a total of 1 mL (15 units/mL) intradermally or SUBQ as five separate 0.2-mL injections (using a tuberculin syringe) around the site of extravasation; if IV catheter remains in place, administer IV through the infiltrated catheter; may repeat in 30–60 min if no resolution.
- **IV:** Change IV sites every 48 hr to prevent phlebitis.
- Administer slowly and observe patient closely for signs of hypersensitivity; observe for hyperkalemia with *IV penicillin G potassium.*
- **Intermittent Infusion:** **Reconstitution:** Add 8.2 mL of sterile water for injection or 0.9% NaCl to the 5 million unit vial for a final concentration of 500,000 units *penicillin G*/mL; add 3.2 mL for a final concentration of 1 million units *penicillin G*/mL. Add 33 mL of sterile water for injection or 0.9% NaCl to the 20 million unit vial for a final concentration of 500,000 units *penicillin G*/mL; add 11.5 mL for a final concentration of 1 million units *penicillin G*/mL. Shake well before injection. **Dilution:** Doses of ≤ 3 million units should be diluted in ≥ 50 mL of D5W or 0.9% NaCl; doses of >3 million units should be diluted with 100 mL. **Concentration:** 100,000–500,000 units/mL (50,000 units/mL in neonates). **Rate:** Infuse over 1–2 hr (adults) or 15–30 min (children).
- **Continuous Infusion:** Doses of ≥ 10 million units may be diluted in 1 or 2 L. **Rate:** Infuse over 24 hr.

Penicillin G Potassium

- **Y-Site Compatibility:** acyclovir, amikacin, amiodarone, ascorbic acid, atropine, azathioprine, aztreonam, benztropine, bumetanide, buprenorphine, butorphanol, calcium chloride, calcium gluconate, cefazolin, cefotaxime, cefotetan, cefoxitin, ceftazidime, ceftolozane/tazobactam, ceftriaxone, cefuroxime, chloramphenicol, chlorothiazide, chlorpromazine, clindamycin, cyanocobalamin, cyclophosphamide, cyclosporine, dexamethasone, digoxin, diltiazem, diphenhydramine, dopamine, edetate calcium disodium, enalaprilat, ephedrine, epinephrine, epoetin alfa, esmolol, famotidine, fentanyl, fluconazole, folic acid, foscarnet, furosemide, gentamicin, glycopyrrolate, heparin, hydrocortisone, hydromorphone, imipenem/cilastatin, indomethacin, insulin, regular, isoproterenol, ketamine, ketorolac, lidocaine, magnesium sulfate, mannitol, meperidine, meropenem/vaborbactam, methylprednisolone, metoclopramide, metoprolol, midazolam, morphine, multivitamins, nafcillin, nalbuphine, naloxone, nicardipine, nitroglycerin, nitroprusside, norepinephrine, ondansetron, oxacillin, oxytocin, phenylephrine, phytonadione, potassium chloride, procainamide, prochlorperazine, propranolol, pyridoxine, sodium bicarbonate, sufentanil, sulbactam/durlobactam, tacrolimus, theophylline, thiamine, tobramycin, vancomycin, vasopressin, verapamil.
- **Y-Site Incompatibility:** amphotericin B deoxycholate, dantrolene, diazepam, diazoxide, dobutamine, doxycycline, ganciclovir, haloperidol, minocycline, papaverine, pentamidine, pentobarbital, phenytoin, protamine, tedizolid, tranexamic acid, trimethoprim/sulfamethoxazole.

Penicillin G Sodium

- **Y-Site Compatibility:** amikacin, ascorbic acid, atropine, azathioprine, aztreonam, benztropine, bumetanide, buprenorphine, butorphanol, calcium chloride, calcium gluconate, cefazolin, cefotaxime, cefotetan, cefoxitin, ceftazidime, ceftriaxone, cefuroxime, chloramphenicol, clindamycin, cyanocobalamin, cyclophosphamide, cyclosporine, dexamethasone, digoxin, dimenhydrinate, diphenhydramine, dopamine, edetate calcium disodium, enalaprilat, ephedrine, epinephrine, epoetin alfa, esmolol, famotidine, fentanyl, fluconazole, folic acid, furosemide, gentamicin, glycopyrrolate, heparin, hydrocortisone, imipenem/cilastatin, indomethacin, insulin, regular, isoproterenol, ketamine, ketorolac, levofloxacin, lidocaine, magnesium sulfate, mannitol, meperidine, meropenem, methylprednisolone, metoclopramide, metoprolol, midazolam, morphine, multivitamins, nafcillin, nalbuphine, naloxone, nitroglycerin, nitroprusside, norepinephrine, ondansetron, oxacillin, oxytocin, pantoprazole, penicillin G potassium, phenylephrine, phytonadione, plazomicin, potassium chloride, procainamide, prochlorperazine, propranolol, pyridoxine, sildenafil, sodium bicarbonate, sufentanil, theophylline, thiamine, tobramycin, vancomycin, vasopressin, verapamil.
- **Y-Site Incompatibility:** amphotericin B deoxycholate, dantrolene, diazepam, diazoxide, dobutamine, doxycycline, ganciclovir, haloperidol, labetalol, minocycline, morphine, papaverine, pentamidine, pentobarbital, phenobarbital, phenytoin, protamine, tranexamic acid, trimethoprim/sulfamethoxazole.

Patient/Family Teaching

- Explain the purpose and side effects of the medication. Instruct patient to take medication around the clock and to finish drug completely as directed, even if feeling better. Pedi: Instruct parents or caregivers to use calibrated measuring device with liquid preparations of *penicillin V*. Advise patient that sharing this medication may be dangerous. Advise patient to read *Patient Information* before starting therapy.
- Instruct patient to notify health care provider if symptoms do not improve.
- Advise patients and family to call 911 and seek urgent treatment for signs/symptoms of hypersensitivity reactions (difficulty breathing; chest tightness; hives; rash; feeling light-headed; itching; swelling of the face, lips, tongue, or throat).
- Advise patient to report signs/symptoms of superinfection (furry overgrowth on the tongue, white patches in mouth, vaginal itching or discharge, loose or foul-smelling stools).
- Instruct patient to notify health care provider if fever and diarrhea develop, especially if stool contains blood, pus, or mucus. Advise patient not to treat diarrhea without consulting health care provider.
- Patient with an allergy to penicillin should be instructed to always carry an identification card with this information.
- Advise patient to notify health care provider of all Rx or OTC medications, vitamins, or herbal products being taken and to consult with health care provider before taking other medications, especially probenecid.
- Rep: Advise women of reproductive potential to notify health care provider if pregnancy is planned or suspected or if breastfeeding. Advise patient taking oral contraceptives to use an additional nonhormonal method of contraception during therapy with penicillin and until next menstrual period.

Evaluation/Desired Outcomes

- Bactericidal action against susceptible bacteria.
- Resolution of signs and symptoms of infection. Length of time for complete resolution depends on the organism and site of infection.

V PENICILLINS, PENICILLINASE RESISTANT

dicloxacillin (dye-klox-a-**sill**-in)
nafcillin (naf-**sill**-in)
oxacillin (ox-a-**sill**-in)

Classification
Therapeutic: anti-infectives
Pharmacologic: penicillinase resistant penicillins

Indications

Treatment of the following infections due to penicillinase-producing staphylococci: Respiratory tract infections, Sinusitis, Skin and skin structure infections. **Dicloxacillin:** Osteomyelitis. **Nafcillin, oxacillin:** Are also used to treat: Bone and joint infections, Urinary tract infections, Endocarditis, Septicemia, Meningitis.

Action

Inhibits bacterial cell wall synthesis. Not inactivated by penicillinase enzymes. **Therapeutic Effects:** Bactericidal action. **Spectrum:** Active against most gram-positive aerobic cocci but less so than penicillin. Spectrum is notable for activity against: Penicillinase-producing strains of *Staphylococcus aureus*, *Staphylococcus epidermidis*. Not active against methicillin-resistant staphylococci.

Pharmacokinetics

Absorption: *Dicloxacillin:* Rapidly but incompletely (35–76%) absorbed from the GI tract following oral administration. *Nafcillin and oxacillin:* IV administration results in complete bioavailability; well absorbed from IM sites.
Distribution: Widely distributed; penetration into CSF is minimal, but sufficient in the presence of inflamed meninges.
Metabolism and Excretion: *Dicloxacillin:* Some metabolism by the liver (6–10%) and some renal excretion of unchanged drug (60%); small amounts eliminated in the feces via the bile. *Nafcillin, oxacillin:* Partially metabolized by the liver (nafcillin 60%, oxacillin 49%); partially excreted unchanged by the kidneys.
Half-life: *Dicloxacillin:* 0.5–1.1 hr (↑ in severe hepatic and renal impairment); *Nafcillin:* Neonates: 1–5 hr; Children 1 mo–14 yr: 0.75–1.9 hr; Adults: 0.5–1.5 hr (↑ in renal impairment); *Oxacillin:* Neonates: 1.6 hr; Children up to 2 yr: 0.9–1.8 hr; Adults: 0.3–0.8 hr (↑ in severe hepatic impairment).

TIME/ACTION PROFILE (plasma concentrations)

ROUTE	ONSET	PEAK	DURATION
Dicloxacillin (PO)	30 min	30–120 min	6 hr
Nafcillin (IM)	30 min	60–120 min	4–6 hr
Nafcillin (IV)	rapid	end of infusion	4–6 hr
Oxacillin (IM)	rapid	30 min	4–6 hr
Oxacillin (IV)	rapid	end of infusion	4–6 hr

Contraindications/Precautions

Contraindicated in: Hypersensitivity to penicillins (cross-sensitivity with cephalosporins may exist).
Use Cautiously in: Severe renal impairment; Severe hepatic impairment; Lactation: Use while breastfeeding

only if potential maternal benefit justifies potential risk to infant.

Adverse Reactions/Side Effects

Derm: rash, urticaria. **GI:** diarrhea, nausea, vomiting, ↑ liver enzymes, CLOSTRIDIOIDES DIFFICILE-ASSOCIATED DIARRHEA (CDAD). **GU:** acute kidney injury, hematuria, interstitial nephritis, proteinuria. **Hemat:** eosinophilia, leukopenia. **Local:** pain (at IM site), phlebitis. **Neuro:** SEIZURES (HIGH DOSES). **Misc:** HYPERSENSITIVITY REACTIONS (INCLUDING ANAPHYLAXIS AND SERUM SICKNESS), superinfection.

Interactions

Drug-Drug: Probenecid ↓ renal excretion and ↑ levels (treatment may be combined for this purpose). May ↓ effectiveness of **oral contraceptive agents**. May ↑ levels and risk of toxicity of **methotrexate**.

Route/Dosage

Dicloxacillin

PO (Adults and Children ≥40 kg): 125–250 mg every 6 hr (max dose = 2 g/day).

PO (Children <40 kg): 6.25–12.5 mg/kg every 6 hr; (up to 12.25 mg/kg every 6 hr has been used for osteomyelitis) (max dose = 2 g/day).

Nafcillin

IV (Adults): 500–2000 mg every 4–6 hr.

IM, (Adults): 500 mg every 4–6 hr.

IM, IV (Children): 50–200 mg/kg/day divided every 4–6 hr (max dose = 12 g/day).

IM, IV (Neonates >2 kg): 25 mg/kg every 8 hr for the 1st 7 days of life, then 25 mg/kg every 6 hr.

IM, IV (Neonates 1.2–2 kg): 25 mg/kg every 12 hr for the 1st 7 days of life, then 25 mg/kg every 8 hr.

IM, IV (Neonates 0–4 wk, <1.2 kg): 25 mg/kg every 12 hr.

Oxacillin

IM, IV (Adults and Children ≥40 kg): 250–2000 mg every 4–6 hr (max dose = 12 g/day).

IM, IV (Children <40 kg): 100–200 mg/kg/day divided every 4–6 hr (max dose = 12 g/day).

IM, IV (Neonates ≥2 kg): 25 mg/kg every 8 hr for the 1st 7 days of life, then 25 mg/kg every 6 hr.

IM, IV (Neonates 1.2–2 kg): 25 mg/kg every 12 hr for the 1st 7 days of life, then 25 mg/kg every 8 hr.

IM, IV (Neonates <1.2 kg): 25 mg/kg every 12 hr.

Availability

Dicloxacillin (generic available)

Capsules: 250 mg, 500 mg.

Nafcillin (generic available)

Powder for injection: 1 g/vial, 2 g/vial, 10 g/vial. **Premixed infusion:** 2 g/100 mL D5W.

Oxacillin (generic available)

Powder for injection: 1 g/vial, 2 g/vial, 10 g/vial. **Premixed infusion:** 2 g/50 mL D5W.

NURSING IMPLICATIONS

Assessment

- Assess patient for infection (vital signs; appearance of wound, sputum, urine, and stool; WBC) at beginning of and throughout therapy.
- Obtain a history before initiating therapy to determine previous use of and reactions to penicillins, cephalosporins, or other beta-lactam antibiotics. Persons with a negative history of penicillin sensitivity may still have an allergic response.
- Observe patient for signs/symptoms of hypersensitivity reactions, including anaphylaxis (rash, pruritus, laryngeal edema, wheezing, abdominal pain). *If hypersensitivity reaction occurs,* discontinue therapy and treat as indicated. Keep epinephrine, antihistamine, and resuscitation equipment close by.
- Assess for signs of phlebitis. Change IV site every 48 hr to prevent phlebitis.
- Monitor for diarrhea, abdominal pain, fever, and bloody stools. *If CDAD suspected,* discontinue therapy and treat as clinically indicated. May begin up to several weeks following cessation of therapy.

Lab Test Considerations

- Obtain specimens for culture and sensitivity prior to initiating therapy. 1st dose may be given before receiving results.
- May cause leukopenia and neutropenia, especially with prolonged therapy or hepatic impairment.
- May cause positive direct Coombs test result.
- May ↑ AST, ALT, LDH, and serum alkaline phosphatase.

Implementation

- **PO:** Administer around the clock on an empty stomach ≥1 hr before or 2 hr after food. Take with a full glass of water; acidic juices may ↓ absorption of penicillins.
- Use calibrated measuring device for liquid preparations. Shake well. Solution is stable for 14 days if refrigerated.

Nafcillin

IV Administration

- **V** Nafcillin is a vesicant. Monitor closely if administered through a peripheral IV administration. Can also be infused through a PICC. A central line should be used if continuous infusion administered. If extravasation occurs, immediately stop infusion. Leave needle/cannula in place temporarily but do not flush the line. Gently aspirate extravasated solution; then remove needle/cannula. Elevate patient's extremity and apply dry warm compresses. Initiate hyaluronidase antidote for refractory cases in addition to supportive management. For hyaluronidase, inject a total of 1 mL (15 units/mL) intradermally or SUBQ as five separate 0.2-mL injections (using a tuberculin syringe) around the site of extravasation; if IV catheter remains in place, administer IV through the infiltrated catheter; may repeat in 30–60 min if no resolution.

- **IV, IM: Reconstitution:** Add 3.4 mL to each 1-g vial or 6.8 mL to each 2-g vial, for a concentration of 250 mg/mL. Stable for 2–7 days if refrigerated.
- **IV Push: Dilution:** Dilute reconstituted solution with 15–30 mL sterile water, 0.45% NaCl, or 0.9% NaCl for injection. **Concentration:** 100 mg/mL. **Rate:** Administer over 5–10 min.
- **Intermittent Infusion: Dilution:** Dilute with sterile water for injection, 0.9% NaCl, D5W, D10W, D5/0.25% NaCl, D5/0.45% NaCl, D5/0.9% NaCl, D5/LR, Ringer's, or LR. Stable for 24 hr at room temperature, 96 hr if refrigerated. **Concentration:** 2–40 mg/mL. **Rate:** Infuse over ≥30–60 min to avoid irritation and phlebitis.
- **Y-Site Compatibility:** acyclovir, amikacin, aminophylline, amiodarone, ampicillin, anidulafungin, argatroban, arsenic trioxide, ascorbic acid, atracurium, atropine, aztreonam, benztropine, bivalirudin, bleomycin, bumetanide, buprenorphine, butorphanol, calcium chloride, calcium gluconate, carboplatin, carmustine, cefazolin, cefotaxime, cefotetan, cefoxitin, ceftazidime, ceftriaxone, cefuroxime, chlorpromazine, cisplatin, clindamycin, cyanocobalamin, cyclophosphamide, cyclosporine, dactinomycin, daptomycin, dexamethasone, digoxin, dobutamine, docetaxel, dopamine, doxorubicin liposomal, enalaprilat, ephedrine, epinephrine, epoetin alfa, erythromycin, etoposide, etoposide phosphate, famotidine, fentanyl, fluconazole, fludarabine, foscarnet, fosphenytoin, furosemide, ganciclovir, gemtuzumab ozogamicin, gentamicin, glycopyrrolate, granisetron, heparin, hydrocortisone, hydromorphone, imipenem/cilastatin, indomethacin, isoproterenol, ketorolac, leucovorin, lidocaine, linezolid, lorazepam, magnesium sulfate, mannitol, mesna, methadone, methylprednisolone, metoclopramide, metoprolol, metronidazole, milrinone, mitomycin, morphine, multivitamins, naloxone, nicardipine, nitroglycerin, nitroprusside, norepinephrine, octreotide, ondansetron, oxacillin, oxytocin, paclitaxel, pamidronate, pantoprazole, pemetrexed, penicillin G, pentobarbital, phenobarbital, phentolamine, phenylephrine, phytonadione, potassium acetate, potassium chloride, procainamide, prochlorperazine, propofol, propranolol, sodium bicarbonate, sufentanil, tacrolimus, theophylline, thiamine, thiotepa, tigecycline, tirofiban, tobramycin, vasopressin, vinblastine, voriconazole, zidovudine, zoledronic acid.
- **Y-Site Incompatibility:** alemtuzumab, amphotericin B, azathioprine, caspofungin, chloramphenicol, dacarbazine, dantrolene, daunorubicin, dexrazoxane, diazoxide, doxycycline, droperidol, epirubicin, fentanyl, folic acid, gemcitabine, haloperidol, hydralazine, idarubicin, irinotecan, meperidine, minocycline, mitoxantrone, mycophenolate, palonosetron, pentamidine, phenytoin, promethazine, protamine, pyridoxine, succinylcholine, topotecan, trimethoprim/sulfamethoxazole, vecuronium, vincristine, vinorelbine.

Oxacillin

IV Administration

- **IV, IM: Reconstitution:** Add 1.4 mL sterile water for injection to each 250-mg vial, 2.7 mL to each 500-mg vial, 5.7 mL to each 1-g vial, 11.5 mL to each 2-g vial, and 23 mL to each 4-g vial, for a concentration of 250 mg/1.5 mL. Stable for 3 days at room temperature or 7 days if refrigerated.
- **IV Push: Dilution:** Further dilute each reconstituted 250-mg or 500-mg vial with 5 mL sterile water or 0.9% NaCl for injection, 10 mL for each 1-g vial, 20 mL for each 2-g vial, and 40 mL for each 4-g vial. **Concentration:** 100 mg/mL. **Rate:** Administer slowly over 10 min.
- **Intermittent Infusion: Dilution:** Dilute with 0.9% NaCl, D5W, D5/0.9% NaCl, or LR. **Concentration:** 0.5–40 mg/mL. **Rate:** May be infused for up to 6 hr.
- **Y-Site Compatibility:** acyclovir, aminophylline, ascorbic acid, atracurium, atropine, aztreonam, benztropine, bumetanide, buprenorphine, butorphanol, cefazolin, cefotaxime, cefotetan, cefoxitin, ceftazidime, ceftriaxone, cefuroxime, chloramphenicol, chlorpromazine, clindamycin, cyanocobalamin, cyclophosphamide, cyclosporine, dexamethasone, digoxin, diltiazem, dopamine, doxapram, enalaprilat, ephedrine, epinephrine, epoetin alfa, erythromycin, famotidine, fentanyl, fluconazole, folic acid, foscarnet, furosemide, glycopyrrolate, heparin, hydrocortisone, hydromorphone, imipenem/cilastatin, insulin regular, isoproterenol, ketorolac, labetalol, levofloxacin, lidocaine, mannitol, methotrexate, metoclopramide, metoprolol, midazolam, milrinone, morphine, multivitamins, nafcillin, naloxone, nitroglycerin, nitroprusside, norepinephrine, ondansetron, oxytocin, papaverine, penicillin G, pentobarbital, phenobarbital, phenylephrine, phytonadione, potassium chloride, procainamide, prochlorperazine, propranolol, sufentanil, tacrolimus, theophylline, thiamine, vasopressin, zidovudine.
- **Y-Site Incompatibility:** amphotericin B deoxycholate, calcium chloride, calcium gluconate, dantrolene, diazepam, diazoxide, diphenhydramine, dobutamine, doxycycline, esmolol, gentamicin, haloperidol, hydralazine, minocycline, pentamidine, phenytoin, promethazine, protamine, pyridoxine,

P

succinylcholine, tobramycin, trimethoprim/sulfamethoxazole.

Patient/Family Teaching

- Explain purpose and side effects of medication. Advise patient to read *Patient Information* before starting therapy.
- Instruct patient to take medication around the clock and to finish the drug completely as directed, even if feeling better. Take missed dose as soon as remembered. Advise patient that sharing of this medication may be dangerous.
- Advise patient to notify health care provider of all Rx or OTC medications, vitamins, or herbal products being taken and to consult health care provider before taking other medications.
- Advise patient to report signs/symptoms of superinfection (black, furry overgrowth on the tongue; vaginal itching or discharge; loose or foul-smelling stools) and allergy.
- Instruct patient to notify health care provider if fever and diarrhea develop, especially if stool contains blood, pus, or mucus. Advise patient not to treat diarrhea without consulting health care provider.
- Instruct patient to notify health care provider if symptoms do not improve.
- Rep: Advise women of reproductive potential to notify health care provider if pregnancy is planned or suspected or if breastfeeding.

Evaluation/Desired Outcomes

- Resolution of the signs and symptoms of infection. Length of time for complete resolution depends on the organism and site of infection.

perindopril, See ANGIOTENSIN-CONVERTING ENZYME (ACE) INHIBITORS.

HIGH ALERT

pertuzumab

(per-**tue**-zue-mab)

Perjeta

Classification

Therapeutic: antineoplastics

Pharmacologic: HER2/neu receptor antagonists, monoclonal antibodies

Indications

HER2-positive metastatic breast cancer in patients who have not yet been treated with anti-HER2 agents or chemotherapy (in combination with docetaxel and trastuzumab [or trastuzumab hyaluronidase]). Neoadjuvant treatment of HER2-positive locally advanced, inflammatory, or early-stage breast cancer (either >2 cm in diameter or node-positive) (in combination with trastuzumab [or trastuzumab hyaluronidase] and chemotherapy). Adjuvant treatment of HER2-positive early breast cancer at high risk of recurrence (in combination with trastuzumab [or trastuzumab hyaluronidase] and chemotherapy).

Action

A monoclonal antibody that attaches to and blocks the human epidermal growth factor receptor 2 protein (HER2), resulting in cell growth arrest and apoptosis. **Therapeutic Effects:** Decreased spread of breast cancer.

Pharmacokinetics

Absorption: IV administration results in complete bioavailability.

Distribution: Minimally distributed to tissues.

Metabolism and Excretion: Unknown.

TIME/ACTION PROFILE

ROUTE	ONSET	PEAK	DURATION
IV	unknown	unknown	20 mo†

† Median duration of response.

Contraindications/Precautions

Contraindicated in: Hypersensitivity; OB: Pregnancy.

Use Cautiously in: Asian patients (↑ incidence of febrile neutropenia); Rep: Women of reproductive potential; Lactation: Safety not established in breastfeeding; Pedi: Safety and effectiveness not established in children.

Adverse Reactions/Side Effects

May reflect combination treatment with docetaxel and trastuzumab.

CV: peripheral edema, HF. **Derm:** alopecia, rash, dry skin, nail disorder. **EENT:** ↑ lacrimation. **GI:** ↓ appetite, diarrhea, nausea, vomiting. **Hemat:** ANEMIA, LEUKOPENIA, NEUTROPENIA. **MS:** arthralgia, myalgia. **Neuro:** dizziness, dysgeusia, fatigue, headache, insomnia, peripheral neuropathy, weakness. **Resp:** dyspnea. **Misc:** chills, fever, HYPERSENSITIVITY REACTIONS (INCLUDING ANAPHYLAXIS AND ANGIOEDEMA), INFUSION REACTIONS.

Interactions

Drug-Drug: ↑ risk of bone marrow depression/immunosuppression with other **bone marrow depressants/immunosuppressants** or **radiation therapy**.

Route/Dosage

Metastatic Breast Cancer

IV (Adults): 840 mg initially, then 420 mg every 3 wk.

Neoadjuvant Treatment of Breast Cancer

IV (Adults): 840 mg initially, then 420 mg every 3 wk for 3–6 cycles given preoperatively. Following surgery, administer 420 mg every 3 wk to complete 1 yr of treatment (up to 18 cycles).

Adjuvant Treatment of Breast Cancer

IV (Adults): 840 mg initially, then 420 mg every 3 wk for 1 yr (up to 18 cycles) or until disease recurrence or unacceptable toxicity.

Availability

Solution for injection: 30 mg/mL.

NURSING IMPLICATIONS

Assessment

- Assess left ventricular ejection fraction (LVEF) before starting pertuzumab and at regular intervals during therapy. **Metastatic Breast Cancer:** *If pretreatment LVEF ≥50%,* monitor prior to and about every 12 wk. *If LVEF ↓ to <40% or 40–45% with a ↓ of ≥10% points below pretreatment value,* hold pertuzumab and trastuzumab (or trastuzumab hyaluronidase) for ≥3 wk. *If after 3 wk, LVEF recovered to >45% or 40–45% with a ↓ of <10% points below pretreatment value,* resume pertuzumab and trastuzumab (or trastuzumab hyaluronidase). **Early Breast Cancer:** *If pretreatment LVEF ≥55%,* monitor prior to and about every 12 wk or once during neoadjuvant therapy. *If LVEF ↓ to <50% with a ↓ of ≥10% points below pretreatment value,* hold pertuzumab and trastuzumab (or trastuzumab hyaluronidase) for ≥3 wk. *If after 3 wk, LVEF recovered to >50% with a ↓ of <10% points below pretreatment value,* resume pertuzumab and trastuzumab (or trastuzumab hyaluronidase). For patients receiving anthracycline-based chemotherapy, a LVEF ≥50% is required after completion of anthracyclines before starting pertuzumab and trastuzumab.
- If trastuzumab is withheld or discontinued, withhold or discontinue pertuzumab. If docetaxel is discontinued, pertuzumab and trastuzumab therapy may continue. Dose ↓ are not recommended for pertuzumab.
- Assess patient closely for 60 min after initial infusion and 30 min after subsequent infusions for signs/symptoms of infusion-associated reaction (fever, chills, fatigue, headache, asthenia, hypersensitivity, vomiting). *If a significant infusion-associated reaction occurs,* slow or interrupt infusion and treat as indicated. Monitor until complete resolution of reaction. *If severe infusion reactions occur,* consider discontinuation of pertuzumab.
- Monitor patient for signs and symptoms of hypersensitivity reactions (rash, hives, itching, dyspnea, angioedema) occurs. *If hypersensitivity reaction occurs,* immediately discontinue pertuzumab. Keep medications and emergency equipment available for immediate use.

Lab Test Considerations

- Verify negative pregnancy status before starting therapy.
- Determine HER protein overexpression prior to therapy.
- Monitor CBC with differential periodically during therapy.

Implementation

IV Administration

- Administer pertuzumab, trastuzumab (or trastuzumab hyaluronidase), and taxane sequentially. Administer pertuzumab and trastuzumab (or trastuzumab hyaluronidase) in any order. Administer taxane after pertuzumab and trastuzumab (or trastuzumab hyaluronidase).
- Observe patient for 30–60 min after pertuzumab infusion and before any subsequent infusion of trastuzumab or taxane.
- **Intermittent Infusion: Dilution:** Withdraw appropriate volume of pertuzumab and dilute in 250 mL of 0.9% NaCl using a PVC or non-PVC polyolefin infusion bag. Gently invert to mix; do not shake. Administer immediately, or refrigerate for 24 hr; do not freeze. **Rate:** Infuse initial dose over 60 min and following doses over 30–60 min.
- For delayed or missed doses, if time between 2 sequential infusions is <6 wk, administer 420 mg dose of pertuzumab; do not wait until next planned dose. If time between 2 sequential infusions ≥6 wk, readminister initial 840 mg dose, followed every 3 wk by 420 mg dose.

Patient/Family Teaching

- Explain purpose and side effects of medication. Advise patient to read *Patient Information* before starting therapy.
- Advise patient to report signs/symptoms of infusion-associated and hypersensitivity reactions immediately.
- Advise patient to notify health care provider immediately if signs/symptoms of left ventricular dysfunction (new onset or worsening shortness of breath, cough, swelling of ankles/legs, swelling of face, palpitations, weight gain of >5 pounds in 24 hr, dizziness or loss of consciousness) occur.
- Instruct patient to notify health care provider promptly if fever; chills; cough; hoarseness; sore throat; signs of infection; lower back or side pain; painful or difficult urination; bleeding gums; bruising; petechiae; blood in stools, urine, or emesis; increased fatigue; or dyspnea occur. Caution patient to avoid crowds and persons with known infections. Instruct patient to use soft toothbrush and electric

P

razor and to avoid falls. Caution patient not to drink alcoholic beverages or take medication containing aspirin or NSAIDs; may precipitate gastric bleeding.
- Instruct patient to notify health care provider of all Rx or OTC medications, vitamins, or herbal products being taken and consult health care provider before taking any new medications.
- Rep: May cause fetal harm. Advise women of reproductive potential to notify health care provider immediately if pregnancy is planned or suspected or if breastfeeding. Caution patient to use effective contraception during therapy and for 7 mo following last dose. Inform patients who become pregnant while receiving pertuzumab of pregnancy pharmacovigilance program to monitor infant outcomes. Encourage patient to report exposure to Genentech Adverse Event Line: 1-888-835-2555. Monitor exposed pregnant patients for oligohydramnios.

Evaluation/Desired Outcomes
- Decreased spread of breast cancer.

pertuzumab/trastuzumab/hyaluronidase
(per-**tue**-zue-mab/traz-**too**-zoo-mab/hye-al-yoor-**on**-i-dase)

Phesgo

Classification

Therapeutic: antineoplastics

Pharmacologic: HER2/neu receptor antagonists, monoclonal antibodies

Indications
Neoadjuvant treatment of human epidermal growth factor receptor 2 protein (HER2)-positive locally advanced, inflammatory, or early-stage breast cancer (either >2 cm in diameter or node-positive) (in combination with chemotherapy). Adjuvant treatment of HER2-positive early breast cancer at high risk of recurrence (in combination with chemotherapy). HER2-positive metastatic breast cancer in patients who have not yet been treated with anti-HER2 agents or chemotherapy (in combination with docetaxel).

Action
Pertuzumab and trastuzumab: monoclonal antibody that binds to HER2 sites in breast cancer tissue and inhibits proliferation of cells that overexpress HER2; *Hyaluronidase:* Acts locally by depolymerizing hyaluronan, which increases permeability of the SUBQ tissue. **Therapeutic Effects:** Regression of breast cancer and metastases.

Pharmacokinetics
Pertuzumab

Absorption: 70% absorbed following SUBQ administration.

Distribution: Minimally distributed to tissues.

Metabolism and Excretion: Unknown.

Half-life: Unknown.

Trastuzumab

Absorption: 80% absorbed following SUBQ administration.

Distribution: Minimally distributed to tissues.

Metabolism and Excretion: Unknown.

Half-life: Unknown.

TIME/ACTION PROFILE (plasma concentrations)

ROUTE	ONSET	PEAK	DURATION
Pertuzumab (SUBQ)	unknown	4 days	unknown
Trastuzumab (SUBQ)	unknown	4 days	unknown

Contraindications/Precautions
Contraindicated in: Hypersensitivity; OB: Pregnancy.

Use Cautiously in: HF, uncontrolled hypertension, recent MI, arrhythmias, or prior anthracycline exposure (equivalent to >360 mg/m² of doxorubicin); Pulmonary disease or extensive tumor involvement of lungs (↑ risk of pulmonary toxicity); Dyspnea at rest (↑ risk of hypersensitivity reaction); Rep: Women of reproductive potential; Lactation: Use while breastfeeding only if potential maternal benefit justifies potential risk to infant; Pedi: Safety and effectiveness not established in children.

Adverse Reactions/Side Effects
CV: arrhythmias, HF, hypertension, peripheral edema. **Derm:** alopecia, dry skin, rash, dermatitis, erythema, nail discoloration, palmar-plantar erythrodysesthesia syndrome. **EENT:** epistaxis, ↑ lacrimation, dry eyes, rhinorrhea. **Endo:** hypoglycemia. **F and E:** hyperkalemia, hyponatremia, hypernatremia, hypokalemia. **GI:** ↓ appetite, ↑ liver enzymes, constipation, diarrhea, dyspepsia, hypoalbuminemia, nausea, stomatitis, vomiting, weight loss, abdominal pain, hemorrhoids, hyperbilirubinemia. **GU:** ↑ serum creatinine, urinary tract infection. **Hemat:** anemia, leukopenia, lymphocytopenia, neutropenia, thrombocytopenia. **Local:** injection site pain, injection site reaction. **MS:** arthralgia, myalgia, muscle spasm, pain. **Neuro:** dizziness, dysgeusia, fatigue, headache, insomnia, paresthesia, peripheral neuropathy. **Resp:** cough, dyspnea, upper respiratory tract infection, ACUTE RESPIRATORY DISTRESS SYNDROME, INTERSTITIAL PNEUMONITIS, pleural effusion, PULMONARY EDEMA, PULMONARY FIBROSIS. **Misc:** fever, HYPERSENSITIVITY REACTIONS (INCLUDING ANAPHYLAXIS AND ANGIOEDEMA).

Interactions
Drug-Drug: Use of an **anthracycline (daunorubicin, doxorubicin, or idarubicin)** following therapy may ↑ risk of cardiotoxicity; if possible, avoid anthracycline-based therapy for up to 7 mo following completion of therapy.

Route/Dosage

Do not substitute Phesgo with or for pertuzumab, trastuzumab, ado-trastuzumab emtansine, or fam-trastuzumab deruxtecan.

Neoadjuvant Treatment of Breast Cancer

SUBQ (Adults): *Initial dose:* Pertuzumab 1200 mg/trastuzumab 600 mg/hyaluronidase 10,000 units followed by maintenance dose in 3 wk; *Maintenance dose:* Pertuzumab 600 mg/trastuzumab 600 mg/hyaluronidase 20,000 units every 3 wk for 3–6 cycles as part of a treatment regimen for early breast cancer. Following surgery, continue pertuzumab/trastuzumab/hyaluronidase to complete 1 yr of treatment (up to 18 cycles) or until disease recurrence or unmanageable toxicity, whichever occurs 1st, as a part of a complete regimen for early breast cancer. In patients receiving an anthracycline-based regimen for early breast cancer, administer pertuzumab/trastuzumab/hyaluronidase following completion of the anthracycline. In patients receiving docetaxel or paclitaxel, administer docetaxel or paclitaxel after pertuzumab/trastuzumab/hyaluronidase.

Adjuvant Treatment of Breast Cancer

SUBQ (Adults): *Initial dose:* Pertuzumab 1200 mg/trastuzumab 600 mg/hyaluronidase 10,000 units followed by maintenance dose in 3 wk; *Maintenance dose:* Pertuzumab 600 mg/trastuzumab 600 mg/hyaluronidase 20,000 units every 3 wk for a total of 1 yr (up to 18 cycles) or until disease recurrence or unmanageable toxicity, whichever occurs 1st, as part of a complete regimen for early breast cancer. In patients receiving an anthracycline-based regimen for early breast cancer, administer pertuzumab/trastuzumab/hyaluronidase following completion of the anthracycline. In patients receiving docetaxel or paclitaxel, administer docetaxel or paclitaxel after pertuzumab/trastuzumab/hyaluronidase.

Metastatic Breast Cancer

SUBQ (Adults): *Initial dose:* Pertuzumab 1200 mg/trastuzumab 600 mg/hyaluronidase 10,000 units followed by maintenance dose in 3 wk; *Maintenance dose:* Pertuzumab 600 mg/trastuzumab 600 mg/hyaluronidase 20,000 units every 3 wk until disease recurrence or unmanageable toxicity. Administer docetaxel after pertuzumab/trastuzumab/hyaluronidase.

Availability

Solution for injection: pertuzumab 60 mg, trastuzumab 60 mg, and hyaluronidase 2000 units/mL, pertuzumab 80 mg, trastuzumab 40 mg, and hyaluronidase 2000 units/mL.

NURSING IMPLICATIONS

Assessment

- Conduct a cardiac assessment, including history, physical examination, and determination of left ventricular ejection fraction (LVEF) by echocardiogram or MUGA scan before starting therapy. Assess LVEF at regular intervals. May cause hypertension, arrhythmias, left ventricular dysfunction, HF, cardiomyopathy, and death. *For early breast cancer: with LVEF ≥55%,* monitor LVEF every 12 wk. Hold *Phesgo* for ≥3 wk for LVEF ↓ to <50% with a ↓ of ≥10% points below pretreatment value. Resume *Phesgo* after 3 wk if LVEF recovered to ≥50% or <10% points below pretreatment value. *For metastatic breast cancer with LVEF ≥50%,* monitor LVEF every 12 wk. Hold *Phesgo* for 3 wk for LVEF ↓ to either <40% or 40–45% with a ↓ of ≥10% points below pretreatment value. Resume *Phesgo* after 3 wk if LVEF has recovered to either >45% or 40–45% with a ↓ of <10% points below pretreatment value. After repeat assessment within 3 wk, if LVEF has not improved, has declined further, and/or patient is symptomatic, permanently discontinue *Phesgo*. After completion of therapy, continue to monitor for cardiomyopathy and assess LVEF measurements every 6 mo for ≥2 yr.
- Monitor for ≥30 min after initial dose and 15 min after each maintenance dose for signs of hypersensitivity or administration-related reactions. *If Grade 1 or 2 hypersensitivity reaction occurs,* premedicate with an analgesic, antipyretic, or antihistamine. *If anaphylaxis or severe injection-related reactions occur,* permanently discontinue *Phesgo*.
- Monitor for signs and symptoms of pulmonary toxicity (dyspnea, interstitial pneumonitis, pulmonary infiltrates, pleural effusions, noncardiogenic pulmonary edema, hypoxia, acute respiratory distress syndrome, pulmonary fibrosis) periodically during therapy.

Lab Test Considerations

- Obtain a negative pregnancy test before starting therapy.
- Patient selection is based on HER2 protein overexpression or HER2 gene amplification in tumor specimens using FDA-approved tests specific for breast cancer. Information on FDA-approved tests is available at http://www.fda.gov/CompanionDiagnostics.
- May exacerbate chemotherapy-induced neutropenia. May cause anemia, neutropenia, leukopenia, and febrile neutropenia.
- May ↑ serum creatinine, AST, ALT, and bilirubin and ↓ albumin.
- May ↓ potassium and glucose and ↑ sodium and potassium.

P

Implementation

- *Phesgo* has different dose and administration instructions than pertuzumab IV, trastuzumab IV, and SUBQ trastuzumab when administered alone. Do not use other drugs in place of *Phesgo*.
- *In patients receiving anthracycline-based regimen for early breast cancer,* administer *Phesgo* following completion of the anthracycline. *In patients receiving Phesgo for early breast cancer with a taxane,* administer taxane after *Phesgo*. *In patients receiving Phesgo for metastatic breast cancer with docetaxel,* administer docetaxel after *Phesgo*.
- **SUBQ:** Solution is clear to opalescent and colorless to slightly brownish; do not administer if cloudy, discolored, or contains particulates. Do not dilute; do not shake. Attach 25–27-gauge ⅜–⅝-inch needle to syringe just before injection. Solution is stable for up to 4 hr at room temperature or 24 hr if refrigerated. Inject into thigh only; alternate between right and left thigh with each dose. Inject initial dose of 15 mL over 8 min. Inject maintenance dose of 10 mL over 5 min. Inject at least 1 inch from previous site and avoid areas where skin is red, bruised, tender, or hard. Inject other SUBQ medications in different sites.

Patient/Family Teaching

- Explain purpose and side effects of medication to patient. Advise patient to read *Patient Information* before starting therapy.
- Advise patient to notify health care provider immediately if signs and symptoms of cardiomyopathy (new onset or worsening shortness of breath, cough, swelling of ankles or legs, swelling of face, palpitations, weight gain >5 pounds in 24 hr, dizziness, loss of consciousness) or pulmonary toxicity (shortness of breath or wheezing) occur.
- Advise patient to notify health care provider immediately if signs and symptoms of hypersensitivity and administration-related reactions (dizziness, nausea, chills, fever, vomiting, diarrhea, urticaria, swelling of face or neck, breathing problems, chest pain) occur.
- Advise patient to notify health care provider of all Rx or OTC medications, vitamins, or herbal products being taken and to consult with health care provider before taking other medications.
- Rep: May cause fetal harm. Advise women of reproductive potential to use effective contraception and to avoid breastfeeding for 7 mo after last dose. If *Phesgo* is administered during pregnancy or if a patient becomes pregnant while receiving *Phesgo* or within 7 mo following last dose of *Phesgo*, health care providers and patients should immediately report exposure to pharmacovigilance program at Genentech at 1-888-835-2555.

Evaluation/Desired Outcomes

- Regression of breast cancer and metastases.

phenazopyridine
(fen-az-oh-**peer**-i-deen)

Pyridium

Classification

Therapeutic: nonopioid analgesics

Pharmacologic: urinary tract analgesics

Indications

Provides relief from the following urinary tract symptoms, which may occur in association with infection or following urologic procedures:

Pain, Itching, Burning, Urgency, Frequency.

Action

Acts locally on the urinary tract mucosa to produce analgesic or local anesthetic effects. Has no antimicrobial activity. **Therapeutic Effects:** Diminished urinary tract discomfort.

Pharmacokinetics

Absorption: Well absorbed following oral administration.

Distribution: Unknown.

Metabolism and Excretion: Rapidly excreted unchanged in the urine.

Half-life: Unknown.

TIME/ACTION PROFILE (urinary analgesia)

ROUTE	ONSET	PEAK	DURATION
PO	unknown	5–6 hr	6–8 hr

Contraindications/Precautions

Contraindicated in: Hypersensitivity; Glomerulonephritis; Severe hepatitis, uremia, or renal failure; Renal impairment; Glucose-6-phosphate dehydrogenase deficiency.

Use Cautiously in: Hepatitis; OB: Safety not established in pregnancy; Lactation: Safety not established in breastfeeding.

Adverse Reactions/Side Effects

Derm: rash. **GI:** hepatotoxicity, nausea. **GU:** bright-orange urine, renal failure. **Hemat:** hemolytic anemia, methemoglobinemia. **Neuro:** headache, vertigo.

Interactions

Drug-Drug: None reported.

Route/Dosage

PO (Adults): 200 mg 3 times daily for 2 days.

PO (Children): 4 mg/kg 3 times daily for 2 days.

Availability (generic available)

Tablets: 95 mg[OTC], 100 mg, 🍁 200 mg[OTC], 🍁 200 mg[OTC], 200 mg.

NURSING IMPLICATIONS

Assessment

- Assess for urgency, frequency, and pain on urination before starting and during therapy.

Lab Test Considerations

- Culture and susceptibility studies should be sent. Phenazopyridine may mask symptoms of urinary tract infection and should not be used without evaluation and treatment of underlying cause of urinary pain.
- Renal function should be monitored periodically during therapy.
- Interferes with urine tests due to urine discoloration (glucose, ketones, bilirubin, steroids, protein).

Implementation

- ***High Alert:*** Do not confuse Pyridium with pyridoxine.
- Medication should be discontinued after pain or discomfort is relieved (usually 2 days for treatment of urinary tract infection). Concurrent antibiotic therapy should continue for full prescribed duration.
- **PO:** Administer without regard to food, or with food to ↓ GI irritation. ***DNC:*** Do not crush, break, or chew tablet.

Patient/Family Teaching

- Explain purpose and side effects of medication. Advise patient to read *Patient Information* before starting therapy.
- Inform patient that drug causes reddish-orange discoloration of urine that may stain clothing or bedding. May also cause staining of soft contact lenses.
- Instruct patient to notify health care provider if rash, skin discoloration, or unusual tiredness occurs.
- Rep: Advise women of reproductive potential to notify health care provider if pregnancy is planned or suspected or if breastfeeding.

Evaluation/Desired Outcomes

- Decrease in pain and burning on urination.

HIGH ALERT

phenelzine (fen-el-zeen)

Nardil

Classification

Therapeutic: antidepressants

Pharmacologic: monamine oxidase (MAO) inhibitors

Indications

Neurotic or atypical depression (usually reserved for patients who do not tolerate or respond to other modes of therapy [e.g., tricyclic antidepressants, SSRIs, SNRIs, electroconvulsive therapy]).

Action

Inhibits the enzyme monoamine oxidase, resulting in an accumulation of various neurotransmitters (dopamine, epinephrine, norepinephrine, and serotonin) in the body. **Therapeutic Effects:** Improved mood.

Pharmacokinetics

Absorption: Well absorbed from the GI tract.
Distribution: Unknown.
Metabolism and Excretion: Metabolized by the liver; excreted in urine as metabolites and unchanged drug.
Half-life: 12 hr.

TIME/ACTION PROFILE (antidepressant effect)

ROUTE	ONSET	PEAK	DURATION
PO	2–4 wk	3–6 wk	2 wk

Contraindications/Precautions

Contraindicated in: Hypersensitivity; Liver disease; Severe renal impairment; Pheochromocytoma; HF; Patients undergoing elective surgery requiring general anesthesia (should be discontinued ≥10 days before surgery); Excessive consumption of caffeine; Concurrent use of meperidine, SSRIs, SNRIs, tricyclic antidepressants, tetracyclic antidepressants, nefazodone, trazodone, procarbazine, selegiline, linezolid, carbamazepine, cyclobenzaprine, bupropion, buspirone, sympathomimetics, other MAO inhibitors, dextromethorphan, narcotics, alcohol, general anesthetics, diuretics, or tryptophan; Concurrent use of foods containing high concentrations of tyramine (see Appendix J).
Use Cautiously in: May ↑ risk of suicide attempt/ideation especially during early treatment or dose adjustment; this risk appears to be greater in adolescents or children; Schizophrenia; Bipolar disorder; Seizure disorders; Diabetes (↑ risk of hypoglycemia); OB: Safety not established in pregnancy; Lactation: Safety not established in breastfeeding; Pedi: Safety and effectiveness not established in children; Geri: ↑ risk of adverse reactions in older adults.

Adverse Reactions/Side Effects

CV: edema, orthostatic hypotension, HYPERTENSIVE CRISIS. **Derm:** pruritus, rash. **EENT:** blurred vision, glaucoma, nystagmus. **F and E** hypernatremia. **GI:** constipation, dry mouth, ↑ liver enzymes, abdominal pain, nausea, vomiting. **GU:** sexual dysfunction, urinary retention. **Metab:** weight gain. **Neuro:** dizziness, drowsiness, fatigue, headache, hyperreflexia, insomnia, tremor, twitching, weakness, euphoria, paresthesia, restlessness, SEIZURES, SUICIDAL THOUGHTS/BEHAVIORS.

Interactions

Drug-Drug: Serious, potentially fatal adverse reactions may occur with concurrent use of other **antidepressants (SSRIs, SNRIs, bupropion, tricyclics, tetracyclics, nefazodone, trazodone)**, **carbamazepine**, **cyclobenzaprine**, **procarbazine**, or **selegiline**. Avoid using within 2 wk of each other (wait 5 wk from end of **fluoxetine** therapy). Hypertensive crisis may occur with **amphetamines**, **levodopa**, **dopamine**, **epinephrine**, **norepinephrine**, **methylphenidate**, or **vasoconstrictors**. Hypertension or hypotension, coma, seizures, respiratory depression, and death may occur with **meperidine**; avoid using within 2–3 wk of MAO inhibitor therapy. **Dextromethorphan** may produce psychosis or bizarre behavior. Hypertension may occur with **buspirone**; avoid using within 2 wk of each other. Additive hypotension may occur with **antihypertensives**, **spinal anesthesia**, **opioids**, or **barbiturates**. Additive hypoglycemia may occur with **insulins** or **oral hypoglycemic agents**. Risk of seizures may be ↑ with **tramadol**.

Drug-Natural Products: Serious, potentially fatal adverse effects (serotonin syndrome) may occur with **St. John's wort** and **SAMe**. Hypertensive crises may occur with large amounts of **caffeine**-containing herbs (**cola nut**, **guarana**, or **malt**). Insomnia, headache, tremor, hypomania may occur with **ginseng**. Hypertensive crises, disorientation, and memory impairment may occur with **tryptophan** or supplements containing **tyrosine** or **phenylalanine**.

Drug-Food: Hypertensive crisis may occur with ingestion of foods containing high concentrations of **tyramine** (see Appendix J). Consumption of foods or beverages with high **caffeine** content ↑ the risk of hypertension and arrhythmias.

Route/Dosage

PO (Adults): 15 mg 3 times daily; ↑ to 60–90 mg/day in divided doses; after maximal benefit achieved, gradually ↓ to smallest effective dose (15 mg/day or every other day).

Availability

Tablets: 15 mg.

NURSING IMPLICATIONS

Assessment

- Assess mental status, mood changes, and anxiety level frequently.
- Monitor BP and HR before and frequently during therapy.
- Monitor intake and output and daily weight. Assess patient for peripheral edema and urinary retention.
- Assess for suicidal tendencies, especially during early therapy. Restrict amount of drug available to patient. Risk may be ↑ in adults ≤24 yr. After starting therapy, young adults should be seen by health care provider face-to-face at least weekly for 4 wk, then every other wk for next 4 wk, then at 12 wk, and then on advice of health care provider thereafter.

Lab Test Considerations

- Assess hepatic function periodically during prolonged or high-dose therapy.
- Monitor serum glucose closely in patients with diabetes; hypoglycemia may occur.

Toxicity and Overdose

- Concurrent ingestion of tyramine-rich foods and many medications may result in a life-threatening hypertensive crisis. Signs and symptoms of hypertensive crisis include chest pain, tachycardia or bradycardia, severe headache, nausea, vomiting, photosensitivity, neck stiffness, sweating, and enlarged pupils. Treatment includes IV phentolamine.
- Symptoms of overdose include anxiety, irritability, tachycardia, hypertension or hypotension, respiratory distress, dizziness, drowsiness, hallucinations, confusion, seizures, sluggish reflexes, fever, and diaphoresis. Treatment includes induction of vomiting or gastric lavage and supportive therapy as symptoms arise.

Implementation

- Do not administer these medications in the evening because the psychomotor stimulating effects may cause insomnia or other sleep disturbances.
- **PO:** Tablets may be crushed and mixed with food or fluids for patients with difficulty swallowing.

Patient/Family Teaching

- Instruct patient to take medication as directed. Take missed doses if remembered within 2 hr; otherwise, omit and return to regular dosage schedule. Do not discontinue abruptly as withdrawal symptoms (nausea, vomiting, malaise, nightmares, agitation, psychosis, seizures) may occur.
- Caution patient to avoid alcohol, CNS depressants, OTC drugs, and foods or beverages containing tyramine (see Appendix J) or excessive caffeine during and for ≥2 wk after therapy has been discontinued; they may precipitate a hypertensive crisis. Instruct patient to notify health care provider immediately if symptoms of hypertensive crisis (severe headache, palpitations, chest or throat tightness, sweating, dizziness, neck stiffness, nausea, vomiting) develop.
- Advise patient, family, and caregivers to look for suicidality, especially during early therapy or dose changes. Notify health care provider immediately if thoughts about suicide or dying, attempts to commit suicide, new or worse depression or anxiety, agitation or restlessness, panic attacks, insomnia, new or worse irritability, aggressiveness, acting on dangerous impulses, mania, or other changes in mood or behavior.
- May cause dizziness or drowsiness. Caution patient to avoid driving and other activities requiring alertness until response to medication is known.

- Caution patient to change positions slowly to minimize orthostatic hypotension. Older adults are at ↑ risk for this side effect.
- Instruct patient to consult with health care provider before taking any new prescription, OTC, or herbal product.
- Advise patient to notify health care provider if dry mouth, urinary retention, or constipation occurs. Frequent rinses, good oral hygiene, and sugarless candy or gum may ↓ dry mouth. An ↑ in fluid intake, fiber, and exercise may prevent constipation.
- Advise patient to notify health care provider of medication regimen before surgery. If possible, therapy should be discontinued at least 2 wk before surgery.
- Instruct patient to carry identification describing medication regimen at all times.
- Emphasize the importance of participation in psychotherapy if recommended by health care provider and follow-up exams to evaluate progress. Ophthalmologic testing should also be done periodically with long-term therapy.
- Rep: Advise women of reproductive potential to notify health care provider if pregnancy is planned or suspected or if breastfeeding.

Evaluation/Desired Outcomes

- Improved mood in depressed patients.
- Decreased anxiety.
- Increased appetite.
- Improved energy level.
- Improved sleep.
- Patients may require 3–6 wk of therapy before therapeutic effects of medication are seen.

BEERS

V PHENobarbital

(fee-noe-**bar**-bi-tal)

~~Luminal~~, Sezaby

Classification

Therapeutic: anticonvulsants, sedative/hypnotics

Pharmacologic: barbiturates

Schedule IV

Indications

Tonic-clonic (grand mal), partial, and febrile seizures in children. Preoperative sedative and in other situations in which sedation may be required. Hypnotic (short-term).

Action

Produces all levels of CNS depression. Depresses the sensory cortex, decreases motor activity, and alters cerebellar function. Inhibits transmission in the nervous system and raises the seizure threshold. Capable of inducing (speeding up) enzymes in the liver that metabolize drugs, bilirubin, and other compounds. **Therapeutic Effects:** Anticonvulsant activity. Sedation.

Pharmacokinetics

Absorption: Absorption is slow but relatively complete (70–90%).

Distribution: Unknown.

Metabolism and Excretion: 75% metabolized by the liver; 25% excreted unchanged by the kidneys.

Half-life: *Neonates:* 1.8–8.3 days; *Infants:* 0.8–5.5 days; *Children:* 1.5–3 days; *Adults:* 2–6 days.

TIME/ACTION PROFILE (sedation†)

ROUTE	ONSET	PEAK	DURATION
PO	30–60 min	unknown	>6 hr
IM, SUBQ	10–30 min	unknown	4–6 hr
IV	5 min	30 min	4–6 hr

† Full anticonvulsant effects occur after 2–3 wk of chronic dosing unless a loading dose has been used.

Contraindications/Precautions

Contraindicated in: Hypersensitivity; Comatose patients or those with pre-existing CNS depression; Severe respiratory disease with dyspnea or obstruction; Uncontrolled severe pain; Known alcohol intolerance (elixir only); Lactation: Lactation.

Use Cautiously in: Hepatic impairment; Severe renal impairment; History of suicide attempt or drug abuse; OB: Chronic use during pregnancy results in drug dependency in the infant; may result in coagulation defects and fetal malformation; acute use at term may result in respiratory depression in the newborn; Geri: Appears on Beers list. Older adults have ↑ risk of physical dependence and risk of toxicity at lower doses. If possible, avoid use in older adults.

P

Adverse Reactions/Side Effects

CV: IV: hypotension. **Derm:** DRUG REACTION WITH EOSINOPHILIA AND SYSTEMIC SYMPTOMS (DRESS), photosensitivity, rash, STEVENS-JOHNSON SYNDROME (SJS), TOXIC EPIDERMAL NECROLYSIS (TEN), urticaria. **GI:** constipation, diarrhea, nausea, vomiting. **Local:** phlebitis. **MS:** arthralgia, myalgia. **Neuro:** <u>hangover</u>, delirium, depression, drowsiness, excitation, lethargy, neuralgia, vertigo. **Resp:** respiratory depression**IV:** LARYNGOSPASM, bronchospasm. **Misc:** HYPERSENSITIVITY REACTIONS (INCLUDING ANGIOEDEMA AND SERUM SICKNESS), physical dependence, psychological dependence.

Interactions

Drug-Drug: Use with **opioid analgesics** may result in significant sedation, respiratory depression, coma, and death. Reserve concurrent use of these drugs for patients when alternative treatment options are inadequate; if concurrent use necessary, limit doses and durations to the minimum required.

Additive CNS depression with other **CNS depressants**, including **alcohol, antihistamines**, and other **sedative/hypnotics**. May ↓ levels and effectiveness of **hormonal contraceptives, warfarin, chloramphenicol, cyclosporine, dacarbazine, corticosteroids, tricyclic antidepressants, felodipine, clonazepam, carbamazepine, verapamil, theophylline, metronidazole**, and **quinidine**. May ↑ risk of hepatic toxicity of **acetaminophen. MAO inhibitors, valproic acid**, or **divalproex** may ↑ levels and risk of toxicity. **Rifampin** may ↓ levels and effectiveness. May ↑ risk of hematologic toxicity with **cyclophosphamide**.

Drug-Natural Products: Kava-kava, valerian, chamomile, or **hops** can ↑ risk of CNS depression. **St. John's wort** may ↓ levels and effectiveness.

Route/Dosage

Status Epilepticus

IV (Adults and Children >1 mo): 15–18 mg/kg in a single or divided dose (max loading dose = 20 mg/kg).

IV (Neonates): 15–20 mg/kg in a single dose. If clinically indicated, ≥15 min after completion of the initial loading dose, a 2nd loading dose may be administered over the subsequent 15 min as 20 mg/kg for term infants or 10–20 mg/kg for preterm infants.

Maintenance Anticonvulsant

IV, PO (Adults and Children >12 yr): 1–3 mg/kg/day in 1–2 divided doses.

IV, PO (Children >5 yr): 2–3 mg/kg/day in 1–2 divided doses.

IV, PO (Children ≤5 yr): 3–5 mg/kg/day in 1–2 divided doses.

Sedation

PO, IM (Adults): 30–120 mg/day in 2–3 divided doses. *Preoperative sedation:* 100–200 mg IM 1–1.5 hr before the procedure.

PO (Children): 2 mg/kg 3 times daily. *Preoperative sedation:* 1–3 mg/kg PO/IM/IV 1–1.5 hr before the procedure.

Hypnotic

PO, SUBQ, IV, IM (Adults): 100–320 mg at bedtime.

IV, IM, SUBQ (Children): 3–5 mg/kg at bedtime.

Hyperbilirubinemia

PO (Adults): 90–180 mg/day in 2–3 divided doses.

PO (Children <12 yr): 3–8 mg/kg/day in 2–3 divided doses; doses up to 12 mg/kg/day have been used.

Availability (generic available)

Tablets: 15 mg, 16.2 mg, 30 mg, 32.4 mg, 60 mg, 64.8 mg, 97.2 mg, 100 mg. **Elixir:** 20 mg/5 mL. **Lyophilized powder for injection:** 100 mg/vial. **Solution for injection:** 65 mg/mL, 130 mg/mL.

NURSING IMPLICATIONS

Assessment

- Monitor respiratory status, HR, and BP, and signs and symptoms of angioedema (swelling of lips, face, and throat; dyspnea) frequently in patients receiving IV therapy. Equipment for resuscitation and artificial ventilation should be readily available. Respiratory depression is dose-dependent.
- Monitor for infusion site reaction (pain, swelling, discoloration, temperature change in limb). *If signs/symptoms of infusion site reaction occur,* immediately discontinue injection.
- Assess for dermatologic toxicity. *At 1st sign of drug-related rash,* discontinue and do not resume therapy if symptoms suggest SJS or TEN.
- Monitor for signs and symptoms of multiorgan hypersensitivity reactions: DRESS (rash, fever, lymphadenopathy). May be associated with other organ involvement (hepatitis, hepatic failure, blood dyscrasias, acute multiorgan failure). If cause cannot be determined, discontinue phenobarbital immediately.
- Prolonged therapy may lead to psychological or physical dependence. Restrict amount of drug available to patient, especially if depressed, suicidal, or with a history of addiction.
- Geri: Older adults may react to phenobarbital with marked excitement, depression, and confusion. Monitor for these adverse reactions.
- **Seizures:** Assess location, duration, and characteristics of seizure activity.
- **Sedation:** Assess level of consciousness and anxiety when used as a preoperative sedative.
- Assess postoperative patients for pain with a pain scale. Phenobarbital may ↑ sensitivity to painful stimuli.

Lab Test Considerations

- Monitor hepatic and renal function and CBC periodically during prolonged therapy.
- Monitor serum folate concentrations periodically during therapy because of ↑ folate requirements of patients on long-term anticonvulsant therapy with phenobarbital.
- May ↓ bilirubin in neonates and in patients with congenital nonhemolytic unconjugated hyperbilirubinemia or seizure disorders.

Toxicity and Overdose

- Serum phenobarbital levels may be monitored when used as an anticonvulsant. Therapeutic blood levels are 10–40 mcg/mL. Symptoms of toxicity include confusion, drowsiness, dyspnea, slurred speech, and staggering.

Implementation

- Do not confuse phenobarbital with pentobarbital.
- Supervise ambulation and transfer of patients following administration. Two side rails should be raised

and call bell within reach at all times. Keep bed in low position. Institute seizure and fall precautions.

- When changing from phenobarbital to another anticonvulsant, gradually ↓ dose while concurrently ↑ dose of replacement anticonvulsant.
- **PO:** Tablets may be crushed and mixed with food or fluids. Oral solution may be taken undiluted or mixed with water, milk, or fruit juice. Use calibrated measuring device for accurate measurement of liquid dose.
- **IM:** Injections should be given deep into the gluteal muscle to minimize tissue irritation. Do not inject >5 mL into any one site, because of tissue irritation.

IV Administration

- V IV phenobarbital is a vesicant. Administer into a large vein. If extravasation occurs, immediately stop infusion. Leave needle/cannula in place temporarily but do not flush the line. Gently aspirate extravasated solution; then remove needle/cannula. Elevate patient's extremity and apply dry warm compresses. Initiate hyaluronidase antidote for refractory cases in addition to supportive management. For hyaluronidase, inject a total of 1 mL (15 units/mL) intradermally or SUBQ as five separate 0.2-mL injections (using a tuberculin syringe) around the site of extravasation; if IV catheter remains in place, administer IV through the infiltrated catheter; may repeat in 30–60 min if no resolution.
- **IV:** May require 15–30 min to reach peak concentrations in the brain. Administer minimal dose and wait for effectiveness before administering 2nd dose to prevent cumulative barbiturate-induced depression.
- **Intermittent Infusion: Lyophilized powder for injection:** **Reconstitution:** Reconstitute vial with 10 mL of 0.9% NaCl. **Concentration:** 10 mg/mL. Do not use solution that is not absolutely clear within 5 min after reconstitution or that contains a precipitate. Discard powder or solution that has been exposed to air for longer than 30 min. If not administered immediately, place vial in original carton to protect from light. Stable for 8 hr at room temperature or 24 hr if refrigerated. Administer solution undiluted. **Solution for injection:** Administer dose undiluted.
- **Rate:** Infuse over 15–30 min and no faster than 60 mg/min. Infuse large loading doses over 60 min. Titrate slowly for desired response. Rapid administration may result in respiratory depression.
- **Y-Site Compatibility:** acyclovir, amikacin, aminocaproic acid, aminophylline, amphotericin B liposomal, anidulafungin, argatroban, arsenic trioxide, ascorbic acid, atropine, azathioprine, azithromycin, aztreonam, benztropine, bivalirudin, bleomycin, bumetanide, butorphanol, caffeine citrate, calcium chloride, calcium gluconate, carboplatin, cefazolin, ceftazidime, ceftriaxone, chloramphenicol, chlorothiazide, cisplatin, clindamycin, cyanocobalamin, cyclophosphamide, cytarabine, dacarbazine, dactinomycin, daptomycin, dexamethasone, dexmedetomidine, dexrazoxane, digoxin, docetaxel, dopamine, doxapram, doxorubicin liposomal, edetate calcium disodium, enalaprilat, epoetin alfa, eptifibatide, ertapenem, etoposide, etoposide phosphate, famotidine, fentanyl, fluconazole, fludarabine, fluorouracil, folic acid, foscarnet, fosphenytoin, furosemide, ganciclovir, gemcitabine, gentamicin, glycopyrrolate, granisetron, heparin, hydrocortisone, ibuprofen lysine, ifosfamide, indomethacin, insulin regular, irinotecan, ketorolac, labetalol, leucovorin, linezolid, lorazepam, magnesium sulfate, mannitol, meropenem, mesna, methadone, methohexital, methotrexate, methylprednisolone, metoclopramide, metoprolol, metronidazole, milrinone, mitoxantrone, morphine, multivitamins, nafcillin, naloxone, nitroglycerin, nitroprusside, octreotide, oxacillin, oxytocin, paclitaxel, palonosetron, pamidronate, pemetrexed, pentobarbital, phenylephrine, phytonadione, piperacillin/tazobactam, potassium acetate, potassium chloride, procainamide, propofol, propranolol, rocuronium, sodium acetate, sodium bicarbonate, sufentanil, theophylline, thiotepa, tigecycline, tirofiban, tobramycin, vancomycin, vasopressin, vecuronium, vinblastine, vincristine, voriconazole, zoledronic acid.
- **Y-Site Incompatibility:** acetaminophen, alemtuzumab, amiodarone, amphotericin B deoxycholate, atracurium, buprenorphine, carmustine, caspofungin, cefotaxime, cefotetan, cefoxitin, cefuroxime, chlorpromazine, cyclosporine, dantrolene, daunorubicin, diazepam, diazoxide, diltiazem, diphenhydramine, dobutamine, doxorubicin hydrochloride, doxycycline, epinephrine, epirubicin, esmolol, gemtuzumab ozogamicin, haloperidol, idarubicin, meperidine, midazolam, minocycline, mitomycin, mycophenolate, nalbuphine, nicardipine, norepinephrine, ondansetron, papaverine, pentamidine, phenytoin, prochlorperazine, promethazine, protamine, pyridoxine, succinylcholine, thiamine, topotecan, trimethoprim/sulfamethoxazole, verapamil, vinorelbine.

Patient/Family Teaching

- Explain purpose and side effects of medication. Advise patient to read *Patient Information* before starting therapy.
- Advise patient to take medication as directed. Take missed dose as soon as remembered if not almost time for next dose; do not double doses.

P

- Advise patient on prolonged therapy not to discontinue medication without consulting health care provider. Abrupt withdrawal may precipitate seizures or status epilepticus.
- Medication may cause daytime drowsiness. Caution patient to avoid driving and other activities requiring alertness until response to medication is known. Do not resume driving until physician gives clearance based on control of seizure disorder.
- Caution patient to avoid taking alcohol or other CNS depressants, including opioids, concurrently with phenobarbital.
- Advise patient to notify health care provider if facial swelling, difficulty breathing, rash, skin peeling, fever, sore throat, mouth sores, unusual bleeding or bruising, nosebleeds, or petechiae occur.
- Teach sleep hygiene techniques (dark room, quiet, bedtime ritual, limit daytime napping, avoid nicotine and caffeine).
- Rep: Advise women of reproductive potential using oral contraceptives to use an additional nonhormonal contraceptive during therapy and until next menstrual period. Instruct patient to notify health care provider immediately if pregnancy is planned or suspected or if breastfeeding. Use during 3rd trimester of pregnancy may cause withdrawal symptoms (seizures, hyperirritability) in the neonate; symptoms of withdrawal may be delayed up to 14 days after birth. Monitor infant for respiratory depression if used during labor. A registry is available for women exposed to phenobarbital during pregnancy. Pregnant women may enroll themselves into the North American Antiepileptic Drug Pregnancy Registry (1-888-233-2334 or http://www.aedpregnancyregistry.org).
- Pedi: Advise parents or caregivers that child may experience irritability, hyperactivity, and/or sleep disturbances, which may diminish in a few days to a few weeks or may persist until drug is stopped. An alternative medication can be considered. Instruct parents to monitor for skin rash occurring 7–20 days after treatment begins and to contact a health care provider if rash occurs. Teach family about symptoms of toxicity (staggering, drowsiness, slurred speech).

Evaluation/Desired Outcomes

- Decrease or cessation of seizure activity without excessive sedation. Several wk may be required to achieve maximum anticonvulsant effects.
- Preoperative sedation.
- Improvement in sleep patterns.
- Decrease in serum bilirubin levels.

phentermine (fen-ter-meen)

~~Adipex-P~~, Lomaira

Classification

Therapeutic: weight control agents

Pharmacologic: appetite suppressants

Schedule IV

Indications

Short-term treatment of obesity in conjunction with other interventions (dietary restriction, exercise); used to produce and maintain weight loss in patients with a BMI ≥30 kg/m² or ≥27 kg/m² in the presence of other risk factors (diabetes, hypertension, hyperlipidemia).

Action

Decreases hunger by altering the chemical control of nerve impulse transmission in the appetite control center of the hypothalamus. **Therapeutic Effects:** Appetite suppression with resultant weight loss.

Pharmacokinetics

Absorption: Unknown.

Distribution: Unknown.

Metabolism and Excretion: Metabolized by the liver.

Half-life: 19–24 hr.

TIME/ACTION PROFILE (appetite suppression)

ROUTE	ONSET	PEAK	DURATION
PO	unknown	unknown	4 hr†

† For 8-mg tablets; ↑ to 12–14 hr for 30-mg capsules.

Contraindications/Precautions

Contraindicated in: Hypersensitivity or known intolerance to sympathomimetic amines or tartrazine; Cardiovascular disease; Hyperthyroidism; Uncontrolled hypertension; History of drug abuse; Agitation; Glaucoma; Concurrent or recent (within 14 days) MAO inhibitor therapy; Concurrent use of SSRI antidepressants; OB: Pregnancy; Lactation: Lactation.

Use Cautiously in: Diabetes mellitus; Pedi: Children ≤16 yr (safety and effectiveness not established).

Adverse Reactions/Side Effects

CV: hypertension, palpitations, tachycardia, VALVULAR ABNORMALITIES. **EENT:** blurred vision. **GI:** constipation, diarrhea, dry mouth, nausea, unpleasant taste, vomiting. **GU:** changes in libido, erectile dysfunction. **Neuro:** CNS stimulation, confusion, dizziness, dysphoria, euphoria, headache, insomnia, mental depression, restlessness. **Resp:** PULMONARY HYPERTENSION.

Interactions

Drug-Drug: **MAO inhibitors** may result in hypertensive crisis; concurrent use contraindicated; do not use within 14 days of MAO inhibitors. ↑ risk of adverse CNS events with **alcohol**. Concurrent use with **SSRI antidepressants** is not recommended. May ↓ **insulin** or **oral hypoglycemic** requirements in patients with diabetes. **Topiramate** may ↑ levels and risk of toxicity.

Route/Dosage

PO (Adults and Children >16 yr): *Capsules or orally disintegrating tablets:* 15–37.5 mg once daily; *Lomaira:* 8 mg 3 times daily.

Availability (generic available)

Tablets (Lomaira): 8 mg. **Orally disintegrating tablets:** 15 mg, 30 mg, 37.5 mg. **Capsules:** 15 mg, 30 mg, 37.5 mg. ***In combination with:*** topiramate (Qsymia). See Appendix N

NURSING IMPLICATIONS

Assessment

- Monitor weight and waist circumference every month for 1st 3 mo and then every 3 mo. Adjust concurrent medications (antihypertensives, antidiabetics, lipid-lowering agents) as needed.
- Monitor for CNS effects (delirium, mania, psychosis).
- Monitor BP and for pulmonary hypertension and valvular abnormalities (new-onset dyspnea, chest pain, syncope, lower extremity edema).
- Monitor for development of tolerance (no longer effective in suppressing appetite).

Implementation

- **PO:** Avoid administering at nighttime. Cut scored tablets for half dose if needed. Administer before or 1–2 hr after breakfast. Administer *Lomaira* 30 min before meals.
- **Orally disintegrating tablets:** Administer in morning with or without food. Gently remove tablet with dry hands from bottle and immediately place on top of tongue; then swallow with or without water.

Patient/Family Teaching

- Explain purpose and side effects of medication to patient. Advise patient to read *Patient Information* before starting therapy. Instruct patient to take medication as directed. Take missed dose as soon as remembered. Do not take two doses at the same time. Tolerance to anorectic effect usually develops within a few weeks. If this occurs, discontinue therapy. The recommended dose should not be exceeded. Medication may need to be discontinued gradually.
- Advise patient to notify health care provider of all Rx or OTC medications, vitamins, or herbal products being taken and to consult health care provider before taking other medications.
- Advise patient to adhere to a low-calorie diet and behavior modification counseling.
- May cause drowsiness. Advise patient to avoid driving or other activities requiring alertness until response to medication is known.
- Caution patient to avoid using alcohol or other CNS depressants with this medication.
- Advise patient to notify health care provider immediately if chest pain, ↓ exercise tolerance, fainting, or swelling of the feet or lower legs occurs.
- Caution patient not to use other weight loss products while taking phentermine.
- Rep: May cause fetal harm. Advise women of reproductive potential to use effective contraception and avoid breastfeeding during therapy. Advise women of reproductive potential to notify health care provider if pregnancy is planned or suspected.

Evaluation/Desired Outcomes

- Appetite suppression with resultant weight loss.

REMS

phentermine/topiramate

(**fen**-ter-meen/toe-**pyre**-a-mate)

Qsymia

Classification

Therapeutic: weight control agents

Pharmacologic: appetite suppressants

Schedule IV

Indications

Weight management as part of a program including caloric restriction and increased exercise in adults with obesity *or* with overweight with ≥1 weight-related comorbid condition. Weight management as part of a program including caloric restriction and increased exercise in children ≥12 yr old with obesity.

P

Action

Phentermine: Decreases appetite and food consumption; *Topiramate:* Decreases appetite and enhances satiety. **Therapeutic Effects:** Weight loss.

Pharmacokinetics

Phentermine

Absorption: Extent of absorption following oral administration unknown.

Distribution: Unknown.

Metabolism and Excretion: Metabolized by the liver.

Half-life: 19–24 hr.

Topiramate

Absorption: 80% absorbed following oral administration.

Distribution: Unknown

Metabolism and Excretion: Not extensively metabolized. 70% excreted unchanged in urine.

Half-life: 21 hr.

TIME/ACTION PROFILE (weight loss)

ROUTE	ONSET	PEAK	DURATION
PO	within 8 wk	16–32 wk	unknown

Contraindications/Precautions

Contraindicated in: Hypersensitivity/idiosyncracy to sympathomimetics (contains tartrazine); Glaucoma;

Hyperthyroidism; During/within 14 days of MAO inhibitors; End-stage renal disease on dialysis; Severe hepatic impairment; History of suicidal thought/active suicidal ideation; OB: Pregnancy; Lactation: Lactation.

Use Cautiously in: History of substance abuse; Ketogenic diet (↑ risk of kidney stones); Rep: Women of reproductive potential; Pedi: Children <12 yr (safety and effectiveness not established); may ↓ vertical growth; Geri: ↑ risk of adverse effects in older adults (consider age-related ↓ in cardiac, renal, and hepatic function; concurrent chronic disease states; and medications).

Adverse Reactions/Side Effects

CV: tachycardia, hypotension, palpitations. **Derm:** alopecia, ERYTHEMA MULTIFORME, oligohydrosis (↓ sweating), STEVENS-JOHNSON SYNDROME, TOXIC EPIDERMAL NECROLYSIS. **EENT:** acute myopia, blurred vision, eye pain, secondary angle closure glaucoma, visual field defects. **Endo:** hypoglycemia. **F and E** hypokalemia, metabolic acidosis. **GI:** altered taste, constipation, dry mouth, HEPATOTOXICITY. **GU:** ↑ serum creatinine, kidney stones. **Metab:** ↓ growth (children). **Neuro:** headache, insomnia, paresthesia, cognitive impairment, dizziness, mood disorders, SEIZURES (FOLLOWING ABRUPT DISCONTINUATION), SUICIDAL IDEATION. **Misc:** ALLERGIC REACTION, hyperthermia.

Interactions

Drug-Drug: ↑ risk of hypokalemia with **non-potassium-sparing diuretics**. ↑ risk of CNS depression with **other CNS depressants**, including **alcohol**, some **antihistamines**, **sedative/hypnotics**, **antipsychotics**, and **opioid analgesics**; avoid concurrent use of alcohol. Altered exposure to **oral contraceptives** may ↑ risk of irregular bleeding. **Carbamazepine** or **phenytoin** may ↓ levels and effectiveness. Concurrent use of topiramate with **valproic acid** may ↑ risk of hyperammonemia. Concurrent use of topiramate with **carbonic anhydrase inhibitors** may ↑ risk of metabolic acidosis and kidney stones. May ↓ levels and effectiveness of **pioglitazone**.

Route/Dosage

PO (Adults): Phentermine 3.75 mg/topiramate 23 mg once daily for 14 days; then ↑ to phentermine 7.5 mg/topiramate 46 mg once daily for 12 wk; then assess weight loss. If patient has not lost ≥3% of baseline body weight, ↑ to phentermine 11.25 mg/topiramate 69 mg once daily for 14 days; then ↑ to phentermine 15 mg/topiramate 92 mg once daily for 12 wk; then assess weight loss. If patient has not lost ≥5% of baseline body weight, discontinue therapy, as success is unlikely. Discontinuation should proceed by taking the phentermine 15 mg/topiramate 92 mg capsule every other day for 1 wk and then discontinue therapy.

PO (Children ≥12 yr): Phentermine 3.75 mg/topiramate 23 mg once daily for 14 days; then ↑ to phentermine 7.5 mg/topiramate 46 mg once daily for 12 wk; then assess BMI. If patient has not experienced a ↓ of ≥3% of baseline BMI, ↑ to phentermine 11.25 mg/topiramate 69 mg once daily for 14 days; then ↑ to phentermine 15 mg/topiramate 92 mg once daily for 12 wk; then assess BMI. If patient has not experienced a ↓ of ≥5% of baseline BMI, discontinue therapy, as success is unlikely. Discontinuation should proceed by taking the phentermine 15 mg/topiramate 92 mg capsule every other day for 1 wk and then discontinue therapy. If weight loss >2 lb/wk, consider ↓ dose.

Renal Impairment

PO (Adults and Children ≥12 yr): *CCr <50 mL/min:* Not to exceed phentermine 7.5 mg/topiramate 46 mg once daily.

Hepatic Impairment

PO (Adults and Children): *Moderate hepatic impairment:* Not to exceed phentermine 7.5 mg/topiramate 46 mg once daily.

Availability (generic available)

Capsules (contain tartrazine): phentermine 3.75 mg (immediate-release [IR])/topiramate 23 mg (extended-release [ER]) (for titration only), phentermine 7.5 mg (IR)/topiramate 46 mg (ER), phentermine 11.25 mg (IR)/topiramate 69 mg (ER) (for titration only), phentermine 15 mg (IR)/topiramate 92 mg (ER).

NURSING IMPLICATIONS

Assessment

- Monitor for weight loss and adjust concurrent medications (antihypertensives, antidiabetics, lipid-lowering agents) as needed. Evaluate weight loss after each 12 wk of therapy.
- Monitor closely for notable changes in behavior that could indicate the emergence or worsening of suicidal thoughts or behavior or depression. Discontinue therapy if these occur.
- Monitor BP and HR periodically during therapy; may cause ↑ in resting HR. May cause hypotension in patients treated with antihypertensives.

Lab Test Considerations

- Verify negative pregnancy test prior to starting therapy and monthly during therapy.
- Before starting and periodically during therapy, obtain a blood chemistry profile in all patients and blood glucose in patients with diabetes on antidiabetic medication.
- May cause hypoglycemia; monitor blood glucose closely in patients with diabetes.
- May cause metabolic acidosis; monitor serum bicarbonate before starting and periodically during therapy.
- May cause ↑ serum creatinine; peak ↑ observed after 4–8 wk of therapy. Monitor serum creatinine before and periodically during therapy; if persistent ↑ occur, ↓ dose or discontinue therapy.

- May cause hypokalemia; monitor serum potassium periodically during therapy.

Implementation

- ***REMS:*** Because of teratogenic risk, *Qsymia* is only available through certified pharmacies that are enrolled in the Qsymia certified pharmacy network. Information can be obtained at www.QsymiaREMS.com or by calling 1-888-998-4887.
- **PO:** Administer once daily in the morning without regard to food. Avoid dosing in the evening; may cause insomnia.

Patient/Family Teaching

- Explain purpose and side effects of medication to patient. Advise patient to read *Patient Information* before starting therapy. Instruct to take as directed. If dose is missed, take at next scheduled time. Do not take two doses at the same time or extra doses. Do not stop taking without consulting health care professional. Discontinue gradually, taking one dose every other day for ≥1 wk before stopping to prevent seizures. ***REMS:*** Explain *Qsymia* REMS requirements to patient.
- Instruct patient to notify health care professional of all Rx or OTC medications, vitamins, or herbal products being taken and consult health care professional before taking any new medications. Advise patient to avoid taking other CNS depressants, opioids, or alcohol.
- Advise patient to notify health care professional if sustained periods of heart pounding or racing while at rest; severe and persistent eye pain or significant changes in vision; changes in attention, concentration, memory, or difficulty finding words; or factors that can ↑ risk of acidosis (prolonged diarrhea, surgery, high-protein/low-carbohydrate diet, concomitant medications) occur.
- Inform patients and families of risk of suicidal thoughts and behavior (behavioral changes; emerging or worsening signs and symptoms of depression; unusual changes in mood; emergence of suicidal thoughts, behavior, or thoughts of self-harm). Advise that these should be reported to health care professional immediately.
- May cause changes in mental performance, motor performance, or vision. Caution patients to avoid driving and other activities requiring alertness until response to medication is known.
- Instruct patient to ↑ fluid intake to ↑ urinary output and ↓ risk of kidney stones.
- Advise patient to monitor for ↓ sweating and ↑ body temperature during physical activity, especially in hot weather.
- Rep: May cause fetal harm. Advise women of reproductive potential to use effective contraception and avoid breastfeeding during therapy. Advise patients to notify health care professional if pregnancy is planned or suspected. For patients taking combined oral contraceptives, may cause irregular bleeding and spotting;
  advise patient to continue oral contraceptive and notify health care professional if spotting is concerning.

Evaluation/Desired Outcomes

- Weight loss.

HIGH ALERT

V phenylephrine (fen-il-eff-rin)

Biorphen, Immphentiv, ✱ Neo-Synephrine, Vazculep

Classification

Therapeutic: vasopressors

Pharmacologic: adrenergics alpha adrenergic agonists, vasopressors

For ophthalmic use see Appendix B

Indications

Hypotension associated with shock that may persist after adequate fluid replacement. Hypotension associated with anesthesia. **Anesthesia adjunct:** Prolongation of the duration of spinal anesthesia. Localization of the effect of regional anesthesia.

Action

Constricts blood vessels by stimulating alpha-adrenergic receptors. **Therapeutic Effects:** Increased BP.

Pharmacokinetics

Absorption: Well absorbed from IM sites. IV administration results in complete bioavailability.
Distribution: Widely distributed to tissues.
Metabolism and Excretion: Metabolized by the liver into inactive metabolites.
Half-life: 2.5 hr.

TIME/ACTION PROFILE (vasopressor effects)

ROUTE	ONSET	PEAK	DURATION
IV	immediate	unknown	15–20 min
IM	10–15 min	unknown	0.5–2 hr
SUBQ	10–15 min	unknown	50–60 min

Contraindications/Precautions

Contraindicated in: Hypersensitivity to bisulfites.
Use Cautiously in: HF, coronary artery disease, or peripheral arterial disease; OB: Has been used safely during cesarean section procedure; safety of use during 1st or 2nd trimester of pregnancy not established; Lactation: Use while breastfeeding only if potential maternal

P

benefit justifies potential risk to infant; Pedi: Safety and effectiveness not established in children.

Adverse Reactions/Side Effects

CV: ARRHYTHMIAS, bradycardia, chest pain, hypertension, ischemia, tachycardia. **Derm:** pruritus. **GI:** epigastric pain, nausea, vomiting. **Local:** phlebitis, sloughing at IV site. **Neuro:** blurred vision, headache, insomnia, nervousness, tremor. **Resp:** dyspnea.

Interactions

Drug-Drug: General anesthetics may result in myocardial irritability; use with extreme caution. **MAO inhibitors**, **ergot alkaloids (methylergonovine)**, **oxytocics**, **tricyclic antidepressants**, **atropine**, **corticosteroids**, or **atomoxetine** result in severe hypertension. **Alpha-adrenergic blockers**, **PDE-5 inhibitors**, **calcium channel blockers**, **benzodiazepines**, **ACE inhibitors**, or **guanfacine** may antagonize vasopressor effects.

Route/Dosage

Hypotension

SUBQ IM (Adults): 2–5 mg.
SUBQ IM (Children): 0.1 mg/kg/dose every 1–2 hr as needed, maximum dose 5 mg.
IV (Adults): 0.2 mg (range 0.1–0.5 mg); may be repeated every 10–15 min *or* as an infusion at 100–180 mcg/min initially, 40–60 mcg/min maintenance.
IV (Children): 5–20 mcg/kg/dose every 10–15 min as needed or 0.1–0.5 mcg/kg/min infusion; titrate to effect.

Hypotension During Anesthesia

SUBQ, IM (Adults): 2–3 mg has been used 3–4 min before spinal anesthesia to prevent hypotension.
IM, SUBQ (Children): 0.5–1 mg/25 lb body weight.
IV (Adults): 40–100 mcg; may repeat every 1–2 min as needed (not to exceed total dose of 200 mcg); if BP remains low, initiate continuous infusion at 10–35 mcg/min (not to exceed 200 mcg/min).

Vasoconstrictor for Regional Anesthesia

Local: (Adults): Add 1 mg to every 20 mL of local anesthetic (yields a 1:20,000 solution).

Prolongation of Spinal Anesthesia

Spinal: (Adults): 2–5 mg added to anesthetic solution.

Availability (generic available)

Solution for injection: 0.1 mg/mL, 10 mg/mL.

NURSING IMPLICATIONS

Assessment

- Monitor BP every 2–3 min until stabilized and every 5 min thereafter during IV administration.
- Monitor ECG continuously for arrhythmias during IV administration.
- Assess IV site frequently throughout infusion.

Implementation

- ***High Alert:*** Patient harm and fatalities have occurred from medication errors with phenylephrine. Before administration, have 2nd practitioner independently check original order, dose calculations, concentration, route of administration, and infusion pump settings.

IV Administration

- V IV phenylephrine is a vesicant. Central line administration is preferred; extravasation may cause severe ischemic necrosis. If central line is not available, may administer for <72 hr through a peripheral IV catheter placed in a large vein at a proximal site (e.g., in or proximal to antecubital fossa). May also administer through a midline catheter. If extravasation occurs, immediately stop infusion. Leave needle/cannula in place temporarily but do not flush the line. Gently aspirate extravasated solution; then remove needle/cannula. Elevate patient's extremity and apply dry warm compresses. Initiate phentolamine antidote for refractory cases in addition to supportive management. For phentolamine, dilute 5–10 mg in 10 mL of 0.9% NaCl and administer SUBQ into extravasation site as soon as possible after extravasation; if IV catheter remains in place, administer initial dose IV through the infiltrated catheter. May repeat in 60 min if patient remains symptomatic. Nitroglycerin 2% topical ointment (1-inch strip applied to site of ischemia to cover affected area; may repeat every 8 hr as necessary) may be used as alternative to phentolamine.
- **IV:** Blood volume depletion should be corrected, if possible, before initiation of IV phenylephrine.
- **IV Push: Dilution:** Dilute each 1 mg with 9 mL of sterile water for injection or D5W. For *Biorphen*, the **0.1 mg/mL** solution must NOT be diluted prior to administration. **Rate:** Administer each single dose over 1 min.
- **Continuous Infusion: Dilution:** Dilute 10 mg in 250 or 500 mL of D5W or 0.9% NaCl. **Concentration:** 20 or 40 mcg/mL.
- **Rate:** Titrate rate according to patient response.
- **Y-Site Compatibility:** alemtuzumab, amikacin, aminophylline, amiodarone, amphotericin B liposomal, anidulafungin, argatroban, arsenic trioxide, ascorbic acid, atracurium, atropine, azithromycin, aztreonam, benztropine, bivalirudin, bleomycin, bumetanide, buprenorphine, butorphanol, calcium chloride, calcium gluconate, cangrelor, carboplatin, carmustine, caspofungin, cefazolin, cefotaxime, cefotetan, cefoxitin, ceftazidime, ceftazidime/avibactam, ceftolozane/tazobactam, ceftriaxone, cefuroxime, chloramphenicol, cisatracurium, cisplatin, clindamycin, cyanocobalamin, cyclophosphamide, cyclosporine, cytarabine, dacarbazine, dactinomycin, daptomycin, daunorubicin, dexamethasone, dexmedetomidine, dexrazoxane, digoxin, diltiazem, diphenhydramine, dobutamine, docetaxel, dopamine, doxorubicin hydrochloride,

doxycycline, enalaprilat, ephedrine, epinephrine, epirubicin, epoetin alfa, eptifibatide, eravacycline, ertapenem, erythromycin, esmolol, etomidate, etoposide, etoposide phosphate, famotidine, fentanyl, fluconazole, fludarabine, fluorouracil, folic acid, foscarnet, fosphenytoin, gentamicin, glycopyrrolate, granisetron, heparin, hydrocortisone, hydromorphone, idarubicin, ifosfamide, imipenem/cilastatin/relebactam, imipenem/cilastatin, irinotecan, isavuconazonium, isoproterenol, ketorolac, labetalol, leucovorin, levofloxacin, lidocaine, linezolid, lorazepam, magnesium sulfate, mannitol, meperidine, meropenem/vaborbactam, mesna, methadone, methotrexate, methylprednisolone, metoclopramide, metoprolol, metronidazole, micafungin, midazolam, milrinone, mitoxantrone, morphine, moxifloxacin, multivitamins, mycophenolate, nafcillin, nalbuphine, naloxone, nicardipine, nitroglycerin, nitroprusside, norepinephrine, octreotide, ondansetron, oritavancin, oxacillin, oxaliplatin, oxytocin, paclitaxel, palonosetron, pamidronate, pantoprazole, papaverine, penicillin G, pentobarbital, phenobarbital, phytonadione, piperacillin/tazobactam, plazomicin, potassium acetate, potassium chloride, procainamide, prochlorperazine, promethazine, propranolol, protamine, pyridoxine, remifentanil, rocuronium, sodium acetate, sodium bicarbonate, succinylcholine, sufentanil, sulbactam/durlobactam, tacrolimus, telavancin, theophylline, thiamine, thiotepa, tigecycline, tirofiban, tobramycin, topotecan, vancomycin, vasopressin, vecuronium, verapamil, vinblastine, vincristine, vinorelbine, voriconazole, zidovudine, zoledronic acid

- **Y-Site Incompatibility:** acyclovir, amphotericin B deoxycholate, azathioprine, dantrolene, diazepam, ganciclovir, indomethacin, insulin regular, minocycline, mitomycin, pentamidine, phenytoin, trimethoprim/sulfamethoxazole **Anesthesia:** Phenylephrine 2–5 mg may be added to spinal anesthetic solution to prolong anesthesia.
- Phenylephrine 1 mg may be added to each 20 mL of local anesthetic to produce vasoconstriction.

Patient/Family Teaching

- Explain purpose and side effects of phenylephrine to patient.
- Advise patient to notify health care provider of all Rx or OTC medications, vitamins, or herbal products being taken and to consult health care provider before taking other medications.
- **IV:** Instruct patient to report headache, dizziness, dyspnea, or pain at IV infusion site promptly.
- Rep: Advise women of reproductive potential to notify health care provider if pregnancy is planned or suspected or if breastfeeding.

Evaluation/Desired Outcomes

- Increased BP.

V phenytoin (fen-i-toyn)

Dilantin, Phenytek, ✱Tremytoine

Classification

Therapeutic: antiarrhythmics (group IB), anticonvulsants

Pharmacologic: hydantoins

Indications

Treatment/prevention of tonic-clonic (grand mal) seizures and complex partial seizures. **Unlabeled Use:** As an antiarrhythmic, particularly for ventricular arrhythmias associated with digoxin toxicity, prolonged QT interval, and surgical repair of congenital heart diseases in children. Neuropathic pain, including trigeminal neuralgia.

Action

Limits seizure propagation by altering ion transport. May also decrease synaptic transmission. Antiarrhythmic properties as a result of shortening the action potential and decreasing automaticity. **Therapeutic Effects:** Diminished seizure activity. Termination of ventricular arrhythmias.

Pharmacokinetics

Absorption: Absorbed slowly from the GI tract. Bioavailability differs among products; the Dilantin and Phenytek preparations are considered to be extended products. Other products are considered to be prompt release.

Distribution: Distributes into CSF and other body tissues and fluids. Preferentially distributes into fatty tissue.

Protein Binding: Adults 90–95%; ↓ protein binding in neonates (up to 20% free fraction available), infants (up to 15% free), and patients with hyperbilirubinemia, hypoalbuminemia, severe renal dysfunction, or uremia.

Metabolism and Excretion: Mostly metabolized by the liver via the CYP2C9 isoenzyme, and to a lesser extent by the CYP2C19 isoenzyme; the CYP2C9 isoenzyme exhibits genetic polymorphism (intermediate or poor metabolizers may have significantly ↑ phenytoin concentrations and an ↑ risk of adverse reactions); minimal amounts excreted in the urine.

Half-life: 22 hr (range 7–42 hr).

TIME/ACTION PROFILE (anticonvulsant effect)

ROUTE	ONSET	PEAK	DURATION
PO	2–24 hr (1 wk)*	1.5–3 hr	6–12 hr
PO-ER	2–24 hr (1 wk)	4–12 hr	12–36 hr
IV	0.5–1 hr (1 wk)	rapid	12–24 hr

* () = time required for onset of action without a loading dose.

P

Contraindications/Precautions

Contraindicated in: Hypersensitivity; Hypersensitivity to propylene glycol (phenytoin injection only); History of hepatotoxicity related to phenytoin; Alcohol intolerance (phenytoin injection and liquid only); Sinus bradycardia, sinoatrial block, 2nd- or 3rd-degree heart block, or Stokes-Adams syndrome (phenytoin injection only); OB: Pregnancy (↑ risk of congenital anomalies; ↑ risk of hemorrhage in newborn if used at term).

Use Cautiously in: All patients (may ↑ risk of suicidal thoughts/behaviors); Hepatic or renal disease (↑ risk of adverse reactions; dose reduction recommended for hepatic impairment); Severe cardiac or respiratory disease (use of IV phenytoin may result in an ↑ risk of serious adverse reactions); Cardiac disease (↑ risk of cardiac arrest or bradycardia); CYP2C9 intermediate or poor metabolizers (↑ risk of phenytoin toxicity); Lactation: Use while breastfeeding only if potential maternal benefit justifies potential harm to infant; Pedi: Suspension contains sodium benzoate, a metabolite of benzyl alcohol that can cause potentially fatal gasping syndrome in neonates; Geri: Use of IV phenytoin may result in an ↑ risk of serious adverse reactions in older adults.

Exercise Extreme Caution in: Patients positive for human leukocyte antigen (HLA) allele, HLA-B*1502 allele or carriers of CYP2C9*3 variant (unless benefits clearly outweigh the risks) (↑ risk of serious skin reactions).

Adverse Reactions/Side Effects

CV: hypotension (↑ with IV), bradycardia, CARDIAC ARREST, tachycardia. **Derm:** hypertrichosis, rash, ACUTE GENERALIZED EXANTHEMATOUS PUSTULOSIS, DRUG REACTION WITH EOSINOPHILIA AND SYSTEMIC SYMPTOMS (DRESS), exfoliative dermatitis, pruritus, purple glove syndrome, STEVENS-JOHNSON SYNDROME (SJS), TOXIC EPIDERMAL NECROLYSIS (TEN). **EENT:** diplopia, nystagmus. **GI:** gingival hyperplasia, nausea, constipation, drug-induced hepatitis, HEPATIC FAILURE, vomiting. **Hemat:** AGRANULOCYTOSIS, APLASTIC ANEMIA, leukopenia, lymphadenopathy, megaloblastic anemia, pure red cell aplasia, thrombocytopenia. **MS:** osteomalacia, osteoporosis. **Neuro:** ataxia, agitation, confusion, dizziness, drowsiness, dysarthria, dyskinesia, extrapyramidal syndrome, headache, insomnia, SUICIDAL THOUGHTS, vertigo, weakness. **Misc:** ANGIOEDEMA, fever.

Interactions

Drug-Drug: **Alcohol (acute ingestion), amiodarone, benzodiazepines, capecitabine, chloramphenicol, chlordiazepoxide, cimetidine, disulfiram, estrogens, ethosuximide, felbamate, fluconazole, fluorouracil, fluoxetine, fluvastatin, fluvoxamine, halothane, isoniazid, itraconazole, ketoconazole, methylphenidate, miconazole, oxcarbazepine, omeprazole, phenothiazines, salicylates, sertraline, sulfonamides, trazodone, voriconazole,** and **warfarin** may ↑ levels and risk of toxicity. **Alcohol (chronic ingestion), barbiturates, carbamazepine, diazepam, diazoxide, fosamprenavir, nelfinavir, rifampin, ritonavir, sucralfate, theophylline,** and **vigabatrin** may ↓ levels and effectiveness. May ↓ levels and effectiveness of **albendazole, amiodarone, apixaban, atorvastatin, benzodiazepines, carbamazepine, clozapine, cyclosporine, dabigatran, digoxin, edoxaban, efavirenz, estrogens, felbamate, fluvastatin, lacosamide, lamotrigine, lopinavir/ritonavir, methadone, mexiletine, nelfinavir, nifedipine, nimodipine, nisoldipine, oxcarbazepine, oral contraceptives, quetiapine, quinidine, rifampin, ritonavir, rivaroxaban, simvastatin, tacrolimus, theophylline, ticagrelor, topiramate, verapamil,** and **warfarin**. IV phenytoin and **dopamine** may cause additive hypotension. Additive CNS depression with other **CNS depressants**, including **alcohol, antihistamines, antidepressants, opioids,** and **sedative/hypnotics**. **Antacids** may ↓ absorption of orally administered phenytoin. ↑ systemic clearance of **methotrexate**, which has been associated with a worse event-free survival; phenytoin use is not recommended in children undergoing chemotherapy for acute lymphocytic leukemia. May ↑ risk of hyperammonemia when used with **valproate**.

Drug-Natural Products: St. John's wort may ↓ levels and effectiveness

Drug-Food: May ↓ absorption of **folic acid**. Concurrent administration of **enteral tube feedings** may ↓ absorption of oral phenytoin. **Folic acid** may ↓ levels and effectiveness.

Route/Dosage

IM administration is not recommended due to erratic absorption and pain on injection. Oral route should be used whenever possible.

Anticonvulsant

PO (Adults): Loading dose of 15–20 mg/kg as extended capsules in 3 divided doses given every 2–4 hr; maintenance dose 5–6 mg/kg/day given in 1–3 divided doses; usual dosing range = 200–1200 mg/day.

PO (Children 10–16 yr): 6–7 mg/kg/day in 2–3 divided doses.

PO (Children 7–9 yr): 7–8 mg/kg/day in 2–3 divided doses.

PO (Children 4–6 yr): 7.5–9 mg/kg/day in 2–3 divided doses.

PO (Children 0.5–3 yr): 8–10 mg/kg/day in 2–3 divided doses.

PO (Neonates up to 6 mo): 5–8 mg/kg/day in 2 divided doses; may require every-8-hr dosing.

IV (Adults): *Status epilepticus loading dose:* 15–20 mg/kg. Rate not to exceed 25–50 mg/min. *Maintenance dose:* Same as PO dosing above.

IV (Children): *Status epilepticus loading dose:* 15–20 mg/kg at 1–3 mg/kg/min. *Maintenance dose:* Same as PO dosing above.

Antiarrhythmic

IV (Adults): 50–100 mg every 10–15 min until arrhythmia is abolished, or a total of 15 mg/kg has been given, or toxicity occurs.
PO (Adults): Loading dose: 250 mg 4 times daily for 1 day, then 250 mg twice daily for 2 days, then maintenance at 300–400 mg/day in divided doses 1–4 times/day.
IV (Children): 1.25 mg/kg every 5 min; may repeat up to total loading dose of 15 mg/kg. *Maintenance dose:* 5–10 mg/kg/day in 2–3 divided doses IV or PO.

Availability (generic available)

Capsules: 30 mg, 100 mg, 200 mg, 300 mg. **Chewable tablets:** 50 mg. **Oral suspension:** 🍁 30 mg/5 mL, 125 mg/5 mL. **Solution for injection:** 50 mg/mL.

NURSING IMPLICATIONS

Assessment

- Assess mental status (orientation, mood, behavior) before starting and periodically during therapy. Monitor closely for notable changes in behavior that could indicate the emergence or worsening of suicidal thoughts or behavior or depression.
- Assess oral hygiene. Vigorous cleaning beginning within 10 days of initiation of therapy may help control gingival hyperplasia.
- Assess for phenytoin hypersensitivity syndrome (fever, skin rash, lymphadenopathy, angioedema). Rash usually occurs within the 1st 2 wk of therapy. Hypersensitivity syndrome usually occurs at 3–8 wk but may occur up to 12 wk after initiation of therapy. May lead to renal failure, rhabdomyolysis, or hepatic necrosis; may be fatal.
- Observe patient for development of rash. Discontinue phenytoin at the 1st sign of skin reactions. Serious adverse reactions such as exfoliative, purpuric, or bullous rashes or the development of lupus erythematosus, SJS, or TEN preclude further use of phenytoin or fosphenytoin. 🧬 SJS and TEN are significantly more common in patients with a particular HLA allele, HLA-B*1502 (occurs almost exclusively in patients with Asian ancestry, including Han Chinese, Filipinos, Malaysians, South Asian Indians, and Thais). Avoid using phenytoin as alternative to carbamazepine for patients who test positive. If less serious skin eruptions (measles-like or scarlatiniform) occur, phenytoin may be resumed after complete clearing of the rash. If rash reappears, further use of phenytoin should be avoided.
- Monitor for signs and symptoms of DRESS (fever, rash, lymphadenopathy, facial swelling), associated with involvement of other organ systems (hepatitis, nephritis, hematologic abnormalities, myocarditis, myositis) during therapy. May resemble an acute viral infection. Eosinophilia is often present. *If signs/symptoms of DRESS occur,* discontinue therapy.
- **Seizures:** Assess location, duration, frequency, and characteristics of seizure activity. EEG may be monitored periodically during therapy.
- Monitor BP, ECG, and respiratory function continuously during administration of IV phenytoin and throughout period when peak serum phenytoin levels occur (15–30 min after administration).
- **Arrhythmias:** Monitor ECG continuously during treatment of arrhythmias.

Lab Test Considerations

- Monitor CBC, serum calcium, albumin, and hepatic function prior to therapy, monthly for the 1st several months, and then periodically during therapy.
- May ↑ alkaline phosphatase, GGT, and glucose.
- Monitor serum folate concentrations periodically during prolonged therapy.

Toxicity and Overdose:

- Monitor serum phenytoin levels routinely. Therapeutic concentrations are 10–20 mcg/mL (8–15 mcg/mL in neonates) in patients with normal serum albumin and renal function. In patients with altered protein binding (neonates, patients with renal failure, hypoalbuminemia, acute trauma), free phenytoin serum concentrations should be monitored. Therapeutic serum free phenytoin concentrations are 1–2 mcg/mL.
- Progressive signs and symptoms of phenytoin toxicity include nystagmus, ataxia, confusion, nausea, slurred speech, and dizziness.

Implementation

- Implement seizure precautions.
- When transferring from phenytoin to another anticonvulsant, dose adjustments are made gradually over several wk.
- **PO:** Administer with or immediately after meals to minimize GI irritation. Shake liquid preparations well before pouring. Use a calibrated measuring device for accurate dose. Chewable tablets must be crushed or chewed well before swallowing. Capsules may be opened and mixed with food or fluids for patients with difficulty swallowing. To prevent direct contact of alkaline drug with mucosa, have patient swallow a liquid 1st, follow with mixture of medication, and then follow with 8 ounces of water, milk, or food.
- If patient is receiving enteral tube feedings, 2 hr should elapse between feeding and phenytoin administration. If phenytoin is administered via nasogastric

tube, flush tube with 2–4 ounces of water before and after administration.

- Do not interchange chewable phenytoin tablets with phenytoin sodium capsules; they are not bioequivalent.

IV Administration

- **IV:** Slight yellow color will not alter solution potency. If refrigerated, may form precipitate, which dissolves after warming to room temperature. Discard solution that is not clear.
- **V** IV phenytoin is a vesicant. Administer directly into a large peripheral or central vein through a large-gauge catheter. Following IV administration, 0.9% NaCl should be injected through the same needle or IV catheter to prevent irritation. Phenytoin is caustic to tissues; may lead to purple glove syndrome. If extravasation occurs, immediately stop infusion. Leave needle/cannula in place temporarily but do not flush the line. Gently aspirate extravasated solution; then remove needle/cannula. Elevate patient's extremity and apply dry warm compresses. Initiate hyaluronidase antidote for refractory cases in addition to supportive management. For hyaluronidase, inject a total of 1 mL (150 units/mL) intradermally or SUBQ as five separate 0.2-mL injections (using a tuberculin syringe) around the site of extravasation; if IV catheter remains in place, administer IV through the infiltrated catheter; may repeat in 30–60 min if no resolution.
- **IV Push:** Administer undiluted. **Rate:** Administer at a rate not to exceed 50 mg/min in adults or 1–3 mg/kg/min in children (or 50 mg/min, whichever is slower). Rapid administration may result in severe hypotension or arrhythmias.
- **Intermittent Infusion: Dilution:** Administer by mixing with no more than 50 mL of 0.9% NaCl. **Concentration:** 1–10 mg/mL. Administer immediately following admixture. Use tubing with a 0.45- to 0.22-micron in-line filter. **Rate:** Complete infusion within 1 hr at a rate not to exceed 50 mg/min. In patients who may develop hypotension, patients with cardiovascular disease, or older adults, do not exceed rate of 25 mg/min (may be as low as 5–10 mg/min). Maximum rate in neonates is 1–3 mg/kg/min. Monitor cardiac function and BP throughout infusion.
- **Y-Site Compatibility:** cisplatin.
- **Y-Site Incompatibility:** acetaminophen, acyclovir, alemtuzumab, amikacin, aminocaproic acid, aminophylline, amiodarone, amphotericin B deoxycholate, amphotericin B liposomal, ampicillin, ampicillin/sulbactam, anidulafungin, argatroban, arsenic trioxide, ascorbic acid, atropine, azathioprine, azithromycin, aztreonam, benztropine, bivalirudin, bleomycin, bumetanide, buprenorphine, butorphanol, calcium chloride, calcium gluconate, carboplatin, carmustine, caspofungin, cefazolin, cefepime, cefotaxime, cefotetan, cefoxitin, ceftazidime, ceftolozane/tazobactam, ceftriaxone, cefuroxime, chloramphenicol, chlorpromazine, ciprofloxacin, clindamycin, cyanocobalamin, cyclophosphamide, cyclosporine, cytarabine, dacarbazine, dactinomycin, dantrolene, daptomycin, daunorubicin, dexamethasone, dexmedetomidine, dexrazoxane, diazepam, digoxin, diltiazem, diphenhydramine, dobutamine, docetaxel, dopamine, doxorubicin hydrochloride, doxorubicin liposomal, doxycycline, enalaprilat, ephedrine, epinephrine, epirubicin, epoetin alfa, eptifibatide, ertapenem, erythromycin, etoposide, etoposide phosphate, fentanyl, fludarabine, fluorouracil, folic acid, fosphenytoin, furosemide, ganciclovir, gemcitabine, gemtuzumab ozogamicin, gentamicin, glycopyrrolate, granisetron, haloperidol, heparin, hydralazine, hydrocortisone, hydromorphone, idarubicin, ifosfamide, imipenem/cilastatin, imipenem/cilastatin/relebactam, indomethacin, insulin regular, irinotecan, isavuconazonium, isoproterenol, ketamine, ketorolac, labetalol, leucovorin, levofloxacin, lidocaine, linezolid, lorazepam, magnesium sulfate, mannitol, meperidine, meropenem, meropenem/vaborbactam, mesna, methadone, methotrexate, methylprednisolone, metoclopramide, metoprolol, metronidazole, micafungin, midazolam, milrinone, minocycline, mitoxantrone, morphine, moxifloxacin, multivitamins, mycophenolate, nafcillin, nalbuphine, naloxone, nicardipine, nitroglycerin, nitroprusside, norepinephrine, octreotide, ondansetron, oritavancin, oxacillin, oxytocin, paclitaxel, palonosetron, pamidronate, pantoprazole, papaverine, pemetrexed, penicillin G, pentamidine, pentobarbital, phenobarbital, phentolamine, phenylephrine, phytonadione, piperacillin/tazobactam, plazomicin, potassium acetate, potassium chloride, procainamide, prochlorperazine, promethazine, propofol, propranolol, protamine, pyridoxine, rocuronium, sodium acetate, sodium bicarbonate, succinylcholine, sufentanil, sulbactam/durlobactam, tacrolimus, tedizolid, theophylline, thiamine, thiotepa, tigecycline, tirofiban, tobramycin, topotecan, trimethoprim/sulfamethoxazole, vancomycin, vasopressin, vecuronium, verapamil, vinblastine, vincristine, vinorelbine, voriconazole, zoledronic acid

Patient/Family Teaching

- Explain purpose and side effects of medication. Advise patient to read *Patient Information* before starting therapy. Instruct patient to take as directed, at the same time each day. If a dose is missed from a once-a-day schedule, take as soon as possible and return to regular dosing schedule. If taking several doses a day, take missed dose as soon as possible within 4 hr of next scheduled dose; do not double doses. Consult health care provider if doses are missed for 2 consecutive days. Abrupt withdrawal may lead to status epilepticus.

- Advise patient to notify health care provider of all Rx or OTC medications, vitamins, or herbal products being taken and to consult health care provider before taking other medications.
- May cause drowsiness or dizziness. Caution patient to avoid driving or other activities requiring alertness until response to medication is known. Do not resume driving until health care provider gives clearance based on control of seizure disorder. Caution patient to avoid alcohol and CNS depressants.
- Instruct patient on importance of maintaining good dental hygiene and seeing dentist frequently for teeth cleaning to prevent tenderness, bleeding, and gingival hyperplasia. Starting oral hygiene program within 10 days of starting phenytoin therapy may minimize growth rate and severity of gingival enlargement. Patients <23 yr and those taking doses >500 mg/day are at ↑ risk for gingival hyperplasia.
- Advise patient that brands of phenytoin may not be equivalent. Check with health care provider if brand or dose form is changed.
- Advise patients with diabetes to monitor blood glucose carefully and to notify health care provider of significant changes.
- Instruct patient to notify health care provider of medication regimen prior to treatment or surgery.
- Advise patient not to take phenytoin within 2–3 hr of antacids.
- Advise patient to carry identification describing disease process and medication regimen at all times.
- Instruct patients that behavioral changes, skin rash, facial or perioral swelling, shortness of breath, fever, sore throat, mouth ulcers, easy bruising, petechiae, unusual bleeding, abdominal pain, chills, pale stools, dark urine, jaundice, severe nausea or vomiting, drowsiness, slurred speech, unsteady gait, swollen glands, or persistent headache should be reported to health care provider immediately. Advise patient and caregivers to notify health care provider if thoughts about suicide or dying, attempts to commit suicide, new or worse depression, new or worse anxiety, feeling very agitated or restless, panic attacks, trouble sleeping, new or worse irritability, acting aggressive, being angry or violent, acting on dangerous impulses, an extreme ↑ in activity and talking, or other unusual changes in behavior or mood occur.
- Rep: May cause fetal harm. Advise women of reproductive potential to use an additional nonhormonal method of contraception during therapy and until next menstrual period. Instruct women of reproductive potential to notify health care provider if pregnancy is planned or suspected or if breastfeeding. Encourage patients who become pregnant to enroll in the North American Antiepileptic Drug Pregnancy Registry that monitors outcomes in women exposed to antiepileptic drugs, such as phenytoin, by calling 1-888-233-2334 or visiting www.aedpregnancyregistry.org. Enrollment must be done by patients themselves. Monitor serum phenytoin concentrations periodically during pregnancy to determine need for dose adjustments. May cause depletion of vitamin K–dependent clotting factors in newborns. Administer vitamin K to mother before delivery and to neonate after birth to prevent bleeding related to ↓ levels of vitamin K–dependent clotting factors, which may occur in newborns exposed to phenytoin in utero.

Evaluation/Desired Outcomes

- Diminished seizure activity.
- Termination of ventricular arrhythmias.

phytonadione

(fye-toe-na-**dye**-one)

Classification

Therapeutic: antidotes, vitamins

Pharmacologic: fat-soluble vitamins

P

Indications

Prevention and treatment of hypoprothrombinemia, which may be associated with: Excessive doses of warfarin, Salicylates, Certain anti-infective agents, Nutritional deficiencies, Prolonged total parenteral nutrition. Prevention and treatment of vitamin K–deficiency bleeding in neonates.

Action

Acts as a vitamin K replacement. Required for hepatic synthesis of blood coagulation factors II (prothrombin), VII, IX, and X. **Therapeutic Effects:** Prevention of bleeding due to hypoprothrombinemia.

Pharmacokinetics

Absorption: Well absorbed following oral or SUBQ administration. Oral absorption requires presence of bile salts. Some vitamin K is produced by bacteria in the GI tract.

Distribution: Unknown.

Metabolism and Excretion: Rapidly metabolized by the liver.

TIME/ACTION PROFILE

ROUTE	ONSET	PEAK†	DURATION‡
PO	6–12 hr	unknown	unknown
SUBQ	1–2 hr	3–6 hr	12–14 hr
IV	1–2 hr	3–6 hr	12 hr

† Control of hemorrhage.

‡ Normal PT achieved.

Contraindications/Precautions

Contraindicated in: Hypersensitivity; Hypersensitivity or intolerance to benzyl alcohol (injection only).
Use Cautiously in: Hepatic impairment; Pedi: Use of injection formulations containing benzyl alcohol may lead to gasping syndrome in neonates and infants.
Exercise Extreme Caution in: Severe life-threatening reactions have occurred following IV administration; use other routes unless risk is justified.

Adverse Reactions/Side Effects

Derm: eczematous reactions, flushing, kernicterus, rash, scleroderma-like lesions, urticaria. **GI:** gastric upset, hyperbilirubinemia (large doses in very premature infants), unusual taste. **Hemat:** hemolytic anemia. **Local:** erythema, pain at injection site, swelling. **Misc:** HYPERSENSITIVITY REACTIONS.

Interactions

Drug-Drug: Large doses will counteract the effect of **warfarin**. Large doses of **salicylates** or broad-spectrum **anti-infectives** may ↑ vitamin K requirements. **Bile acid sequestrants, mineral oil,** and **sucralfate** may ↓ vitamin K absorption from the GI tract.

Route/Dosage

IV use of phytonadione should be reserved for patients with serious or life-threatening bleeding and elevated INR. Oral route is preferred in patients with elevated INRs and no serious or life-threatening bleeding. IM route should generally be avoided because of risk of hematoma formation.

Treatment of Hypoprothrombinemia Due to Vitamin K Deficiency (From Factors Other Than Warfarin)

SUBQ IV (Adults): 10 mg as single dose.
PO (Adults): 2.5–25 mg/day.
SUBQ IV (Children >1 mo): 1–2 mg as single dose.
PO (Children >1 mo): 2.5–5 mg/day.

Vitamin K Deficiency (Supratherapeutic INR) Secondary to Warfarin

PO (Adults): *INR ≥5 and <9 (no significant bleeding):* Hold warfarin and give 1–2.5 mg vitamin K; if more rapid reversal required, give ≤5 mg vitamin K; *INR >9 (no significant bleeding):* Hold warfarin and give 2.5–5 mg vitamin K.
IV (Adults): *Elevated INR with serious or life-threatening bleeding:* 10 mg slow infusion.

Prevention of Hypoprothrombinemia During Total Parenteral Nutrition

IV (Adults): 5–10 mg once weekly.
IV (Children): 2–5 mg once weekly.

Prevention of Vitamin K–Deficiency Bleeding in Neonates

IM (Neonates): 0.5–1 mg within 1 hr of birth; may repeat in 6–8 hr if needed. May be repeated in 2–3 wk if mother received previous anticonvulsant/anticoagulant/anti-infective/antitubercular therapy. 1–5 mg may be given IM to mother 12–24 hr before delivery.

Treatment of Vitamin K–Deficiency Bleeding in Neonates

IM, SUBQ (Neonates): 1–2 mg/day.

Availability (generic available)

Tablets: 5 mg. **Solution for injection:** 1 mg/0.5 mL, 10 mg/mL.

NURSING IMPLICATIONS

Assessment

- Monitor for signs and symptoms of occult bleeding (weakness, dizziness, pallor, petechiae, ecchymosis, guaiac stools, coffee ground emesis) or frank hemorrhage (epistaxis, bleeding gums, hematuria, rectal blood).
- Monitor HR and BP frequently; notify health care provider immediately if symptoms of internal bleeding or hypovolemic shock develop. Inform all personnel of patient's bleeding tendency to prevent further trauma. Apply pressure to all venipuncture sites for ≥5 min; avoid unnecessary IM injections.
- Monitor for signs/symptoms of hypersensitivity reactions (rash, urticaria, pruritus, flushing, dizziness, vomiting, abdominal pain) and angioedema (swelling of throat, lips, tongue, or face; dyspnea; wheezing; hoarseness). *If hypersensitivity reaction or angioedema occur,* discontinue phytonadione immediately and provide supportive care.
- Pedi: Monitor for side effects and adverse reactions. Children (especially neonates) may be especially sensitive to the effects and side effects of vitamin K.

Lab Test Considerations

- Monitor INR at baseline and during therapy to determine response and need for further therapy.

Implementation

- Administration of whole blood or plasma may also be required in severe bleeding because of the delayed onset of phytonadione.
- Phytonadione is an antidote for warfarin overdose but does not counteract the anticoagulant activity of heparin.
- **PO:** Administer without regard to food.
- PO is the recommended route, except when the clinical disorder prevents absorption. If parenteral administration is needed, SUBQ is the preferred route; IV and IM routes should be avoided whenever possible. Fatal hypersensitivity reactions, including anaphylaxis, have occurred during and immediately after IV and IM injection of phytonadione.
- **SUBQ:** Inject into the SUBQ tissue of the upper arms, outer side of upper thighs, or the abdomen (≥2 inches away from the umbilicus). Apply pressure for ≥ 5 min.
- **IM:** Inject into the anterolateral aspect of the thigh (neonates and infants). Apply pressure for ≥ 5 min.

IV Administration

- **Intermittent Infusion: Dilution:** Dilute in ≥ 50 mL of 0.9% NaCl, D5W, or D5/0.9% NaCl. **Rate:** Administer over 30–60 min. Rate should not exceed 1 mg/min.
- **Y-Site Compatibility:** amikacin, aminophylline, ascorbic acid, atracurium, atropine, azathioprine, aztreonam, benztropine, bumetanide, buprenorphine, butorphanol, calcium chloride, calcium gluconate, cefazolin, cefotaxime, cefotetan, cefoxitin, ceftazidime, ceftriaxone, cefuroxime, chloramphenicol, chlorpromazine, clindamycin, cyanocobalamin, cyclosporine, dexamethasone, digoxin, diphenhydramine, dopamine, doxycycline, enalaprilat, ephedrine, epinephrine, epoetin alfa, erythromycin, esmolol, famotidine, fentanyl, fluconazole, folic acid, furosemide, ganciclovir, gentamicin, glycopyrrolate, heparin, hydrocortisone, imipenem/cilastatin, insulin regular, isoproterenol, ketorolac, labetalol, lidocaine, mannitol, meperidine, metoclopramide, metoprolol, midazolam, minocycline, morphine, multivitamins, nafcillin, nalbuphine, naloxone, nitroglycerin, nitroprusside, norepinephrine, ondansetron, oxacillin, oxytocin, papaverine, penicillin G, pentamidine, pentobarbital, phenobarbital, phentolamine, phenylephrine, potassium chloride, procainamide, prochlorperazine, propranolol, pyridoxine, sodium bicarbonate, succinylcholine, sufentanil, theophylline, thiamine, tobramycin, vancomycin, vasopressin, verapamil.
- **Y-Site Incompatibility:** dantrolene, diazepam, magnesium sulfate, phenytoin, trimethoprim/sulfamethoxazole.

Patient/Family Teaching

- Explain the purpose and side effects of phytonadione. Instruct to take as directed. Take missed doses as soon as remembered unless almost time for next dose. Notify health care provider of missed doses. Advise patient to read *Patient Information* before starting and periodically during therapy in case of changes.
- Tell patient to report and seek treatment for signs and symptoms of bleeding (weakness; fast heartbeat; trouble breathing; dizziness; pale skin; tiredness; obvious bleeding in urine, stool, mouth, or nose; excessive menstrual flow).
- Cooking does not destroy substantial amounts of vitamin K. Patient should not drastically alter diet while taking vitamin K. See Appendix J for foods high in vitamin K.
- Caution patient to avoid IM injections and activities leading to injury. Use a soft toothbrush, do not floss, and shave with an electric razor until coagulation defect is corrected.
- Advise patient to notify health care provider of all Rx or OTC medications, vitamins, or herbal products being taken and to consult with health care provider before taking other medications and alcohol.
- Advise patient to inform health care provider of medication regimen prior to treatment or surgery.
- Advise patient to carry identification at all times describing disease process.
- Emphasize the importance of frequent lab tests to monitor coagulation factors.
- Rep: Advise women of reproductive potential to notify health care provider if pregnancy is planned or suspected or if breastfeeding.

Evaluation/Desired Outcomes

- Prevention or cessation of bleeding due to hypoprothrombinemia secondary to impaired intestinal absorption or oral anticoagulant, salicylate, or anti-infective therapy.
- Prevention of vitamin K–deficiency related hemorrhage in the neonate.

BEERS

pimavanserin
(pim-a-**van**-ser-in)

Nuplazid

Classification

Therapeutic: antipsychotics

Indications

Hallucinations and delusions associated with Parkinson disease psychosis.

Action

Exact mechanism is unknown. May work by acting as an inverse agonist and antagonist primarily at 5-HT^{2A} receptors and less at 5-HT^{2C} receptors. **Therapeutic Effects:** Reduced frequency and/or severity of hallucinations and delusions in patients with Parkinson disease psychosis.

Pharmacokinetics

Absorption: Unknown.

Distribution: Extensively distributed to tissues.

Protein Binding: 95%.

Metabolism and Excretion: Mostly metabolized by the liver (CYP3A4 and CYP3A5 isoenzymes) to an active metabolite. Primarily excreted in feces.

Half-life: 57 hr (pimavanserin); 200 hr (active metabolite).

TIME/ACTION PROFILE (plasma concentrations)

ROUTE	ONSET	PEAK	DURATION
PO	unknown	6 hr	unknown

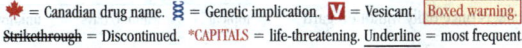

Contraindications/Precautions

Contraindicated in: Hypersensitivity; QT interval prolongation; Concurrent use of agents that prolong the QT interval (↑ risk of serious arrhythmias); History of arrhythmias, including bradycardia; Hypokalemia or hypomagnesemia (↑ risk of serious arrhythmias); Congenital long QT syndrome (↑ risk of serious arrhythmias); Severe renal impairment.

Use Cautiously in: OB: Safety not established in pregnancy; Lactation: Safety not established in breastfeeding; Pedi: Safety and effectiveness not established in children; Geri: Appears on Beers list. ↑ risk of stroke, cognitive decline, and mortality in older adults with dementia. Avoid use in older adults, except for psychosis in Parkinson disease.

Adverse Reactions/Side Effects

CV: peripheral edema, QT interval prolongation, TORSADES DE POINTES. **GI:** constipation, nausea. **Neuro:** confusion, gait disturbance, hallucinations. **Misc:** HYPERSENSITIVITY REACTIONS (INCLUDING ANGIOEDEMA).

Interactions

Drug-Drug: **Amiodarone**, **sotalol**, **quinidine**, **disopyramide**, **procainamide**, **thioridazine**, **chlorpromazine**, **moxifloxacin**, and **ziprasidone** may ↑ risk of serious ventricular arrhythmias; avoid concurrent use. **Strong CYP3A4 inhibitors**, including **clarithromycin**, **itraconazole**, and **ketoconazole**, may ↑ levels and risk of toxicity; ↓ pimavanserin dose. **Strong CYP3A4 inducers**, including **carbamazepine**, **phenytoin**, and **rifampin**, as well as **moderate CYP3A4 inducers**, including **efavirenz**, **modafinil**, **nafcillin**, and **thioridazine**, may ↓ levels and effectiveness; avoid concurrent use.

Drug-Natural Products: **St. John's wort** may ↓ levels and effectiveness; avoid concurrent use.

Drug-Food: **Grapefruit juice** may ↑ levels and risk of toxicity; avoid concurrent use.

Route/Dosage

PO (Adults): 34 mg once daily. *Concurrent use of strong CYP3A4 inhibitors:* 10 mg once daily.

Availability (generic available)

Capsules: 34 mg. **Tablets:** 10 mg.

NURSING IMPLICATIONS

Assessment

- Assess mental status (orientation, mood, behavior) before and periodically during therapy.
- Perform ECG if patient has a history of cardiac disease to monitor for prolong QT interval.
- Monitor for hypersensitivity reactions (rash, urticaria, symptoms consistent with angioedema [tongue swelling, circumoral edema, throat tightness, dyspnea]).

Implementation

- **PO:** Administer 2 tablets once daily without regard to food.
- Capsules can be taken whole or opened and entire contents sprinkled over a tablespoon (15 mL) of applesauce, yogurt, pudding, or a liquid nutritional supplement. Consume immediately without chewing; do not store for future use.

Patient/Family Teaching

- Explain purpose and side effects of medication. Advise patient to read *Patient Information* before starting therapy. Instruct patient to take pimavanserin as directed.
- Instruct patient to notify health care provider of all Rx or OTC medications, vitamins, or herbal products being taken and consult health care provider before taking any new medications, especially St. John's wort.
- Advise patient to notify health care provider of palpitations, chest pain, fatigue, or hypersensitivity reactions and to seek immediate medical attention if needed.
- Advise patient to avoid grapefruit or grapefruit juice.
- Rep: Advise women of reproductive potential to notify health care provider if pregnancy is planned or suspected or if breastfeeding.

Evaluation/Desired Outcomes

- Reduced frequency and/or severity of hallucinations and delusions in patients with Parkinson disease psychosis.

pimecrolimus
(pi-me-**cro**-li-mus)

Elidel

Classification

Therapeutic: immunosuppressants, (topical)

Indications

Short-term and intermittent long-term management of mild to moderate atopic dermatitis unresponsive to or in patients intolerant of conventional treatment.

Action

Inhibits T-cell and mast cell activation by interfering with production of inflammatory cytokines. **Therapeutic Effects:** Decreased severity of atopic dermatitis.

Pharmacokinetics

Absorption: Minimally absorbed through intact skin.

Distribution: Local distribution after topical administration.

Metabolism and Excretion: Systemic metabolism and excretion are negligible with local application.

Half-life: Not applicable.

TIME/ACTION PROFILE (improvement in symptoms)

ROUTE	ONSET	PEAK	DURATION
topical	within 6 days	unknown	unknown

Contraindications/Precautions

Contraindicated in: Hypersensitivity; Should not be applied to areas of active cutaneous viral infections (↑ risk of dissemination); Concurrent use of occlusive dressings; Malignant or premalignant skin conditions; Immunocompromised; Netherton syndrome (↑ absorption of pimecrolimus); Lactation: Lactation.

Use Cautiously in: Clinical infection at treatment site (infection should be treated/cleared prior to use); Skin papillomas (warts) (allow treatment/resolution prior to use); Natural/artificial sunlight (minimize exposure); OB: Use during pregnancy only if potential maternal benefit justifies potential fetal risk; Pedi: Children <2 yr (safety and effectiveness not established).

Adverse Reactions/Side Effects

Derm: SKIN CANCER. **Local:** burning. **Misc:** LYMPHOMA.

Interactions

Drug-Drug: None reported.

Route/Dosage

Topical (Adults and Children ≥2 yr): Apply thin film twice daily; rub in gently and completely.

Availability (generic available)

Cream: 1%.

NURSING IMPLICATIONS

Assessment

- Assess skin lesions before starting and periodically during therapy. Discontinue therapy after signs and symptoms of atopic dermatitis have resolved. Resume treatment at the 1st signs/symptoms of recurrence.

Implementation

- **Topical:** Apply a thin layer to affected area twice daily and rub in gently and completely. May be used on all skin areas including head, neck, and intertriginous areas. Do not use with occlusive dressings.
- Continuous long-term use of topical calcineurin inhibitors, including pimecrolimus, in any age group should be avoided, and application limited to areas of involvement with atopic dermatitis. Safety has not been established for noncontinuous use longer than 1 yr.

Patient/Family Teaching

- Explain purpose and side effects of medication. Advise patient to read *Patient Information* before starting therapy. Instruct patient on correct technique for application. Apply only as directed to external areas. Wash hands following application, unless hands are areas of application.
- Advise patient to notify health care provider of all Rx or OTC medications, vitamins, or herbal products being taken and to consult health care provider before taking other medications.
- Caution patient to avoid exposure to natural or artificial sunlight, including tanning beds, while using cream.
- Advise patient that pimecrolimus may cause skin burning. This occurs most commonly during 1st few days of application, is of mild to moderate severity, and improves within 5 days or as atopic dermatitis resolves.
- Advise patient to notify health care provider if no improvement is seen following 6 wk of treatment or at any time if condition worsens.
- Rep: Advise women of reproductive potential to notify health care provider if pregnancy is planned or suspected or if breastfeeding.

Evaluation/Desired Outcomes

- Decreased severity of atopic dermatitis.

pindolol, See BETA BLOCKERS (nonselective).

pioglitazone (pi-o-glit-a-zone)

Actos

Classification

Therapeutic: antidiabetics

Pharmacologic: thiazolidinediones

Indications

Type 2 diabetes mellitus.

Action

Improves sensitivity to insulin by acting as an agonist at receptor sites involved in insulin responsiveness and subsequent glucose production and utilization. Requires insulin for activity. **Therapeutic Effects:** Decreased insulin resistance, resulting in glycemic control without hypoglycemia.

Pharmacokinetics

Absorption: Well absorbed following oral administration.

Distribution: Well distributed to tissues.

Protein Binding: >99%. Active metabolites are also highly (>99%) bound.

Metabolism and Excretion: Extensively metabolized by the liver via the CYP2C8 isoenzyme; at least two metabolites have pharmacologic activity. Primarily excreted in feces and urine as metabolites.

Half-life: *Pioglitazone:* 3–7 hr; *total pioglitazone (pioglitazone plus metabolites):* 16–24 hr.

P

TIME/ACTION PROFILE (effects on blood glucose)

ROUTE	ONSET	PEAK	DURATION
PO	30 min	2–4 hr	24 hr

Contraindications/Precautions

Contraindicated in: Hypersensitivity; Type 1 diabetes; Diabetic ketoacidosis; Clinical evidence of active liver disease or ↑ ALT (>2.5 times upper limit of normal); Active bladder cancer; New York Heart Association (NYHA) Class III–IV HF; Pedi: Children.
Use Cautiously in: Edema; NYHA Class I–II HF; Hepatic impairment; History of bladder cancer; Women (may ↑ distal upper and lower limb fractures) Rep: Women of reproductive potential; OB: Safety not established in pregnancy; Lactation: Safety not established in breastfeeding.

Adverse Reactions/Side Effects

CV: edema, HF. **EENT:** macular edema. **GI:** ↑ liver enzymes, LIVER FAILURE. **GU:** BLADDER CANCER. **Hemat:** anemia. **MS:** fractures (arm, hand, foot) (women), RHABDOMYOLYSIS.

Interactions

Drug-Drug: May ↓ efficacy of **hormonal contraceptives**. **Strong CYP2C8 inhibitors**, including **gemfibrozil**, may ↑ levels and risk of toxicity. **Ketoconazole** may ↑ levels and risk of toxicity. **Insulin** may ↑ risk of fluid retention and worsening HF. **Topiramate** may ↓ levels and effectiveness.
Drug-Natural Products: Glucosamine may worsen blood glucose control. **Chromium** and **coenzyme Q-10** may ↑ risk of hypoglycemia.

Route/Dosage

PO (Adults): *No HF:* 15–30 mg once daily; may ↑ in increments of 15 mg/day to 45 mg/day if needed; *NYHA class I–II HF:* 15 mg once daily; may ↑ in increments of 15 mg/day to 45 mg/day if needed; *Concurrent use of gemfibrozil:* Do not exceed 15 mg once daily.

Availability (generic available)

Tablets: 15 mg, 30 mg, 45 mg. ***In combination with:*** metformin (Actoplus Met), glimepiride (Duetact), alogliptin; see Appendix N.

NURSING IMPLICATIONS

Assessment

- Monitor for signs/symptoms of hypoglycemia (nausea, tachycardia, sweating, hunger, weakness, dizziness, light-headedness, confusion, tremor, anxiety).
- Assess cardiac history and for signs and symptoms of HF (dyspnea, peripheral edema, rales/crackles, jugular venous distension) at initiation, during therapy, and with dose ↑.
- Monitor for signs/symptoms of hepatotoxicity (fatigue, nausea, upper abdominal pain, jaundice, scleral icterus, dark urine, clay-colored stools).
- Assess and monitor bone health. ↑ risk of fractures in female patients, especially in the distal upper limb (forearm, hand, wrist) or distal lower limb (foot, ankle, fibula, tibia).
- Screen for history of bladder cancer prior to initiation of therapy. Prolonged use >12 mo ↑ risk of bladder cancer.

Lab Test Considerations

- Monitor serum glucose periodically and A1c every 6 mo during therapy to evaluate effectiveness.
- Monitor CBC with differential periodically during therapy. May ↓ hemoglobin and hematocrit, usually during the 1st 4–12 wk of therapy; then levels stabilize.
- Monitor serum AST, ALT, alkaline phosphatase, and total bilirubin before starting therapy and periodically thereafter or if jaundice or symptoms of hepatic impairment occur. Patients with mild ALT ↑ should have more frequent monitoring. *If ALT ↑ to >3 times upper limit of normal (ULN),* recheck ALT promptly. Discontinue pioglitazone if ALT remains >3 times ULN.
- May cause transient ↑ in CK levels.

Implementation

- Do not confuse Actos with Actonel.
- Patients stabilized on a diabetic regimen who are exposed to stress, fever, trauma, infection, or surgery may require administration of insulin.
- **PO:** May be administered with or without meals.

Patient/Family Teaching

- Explain the purpose and side effects of pioglitazone. Instruct patient to take as directed. If dose for 1 day is missed, do not double dose the next day. Advise patient to read *Medication Guide* before starting therapy and with each Rx refill in case of changes.
- Explain need for continued medical follow-up to assess effectiveness and possible side effects of medication. Periodic lab tests may be needed.
- Explain to patient that this medication controls hyperglycemia but does not cure diabetes. Therapy is long term.
- Review signs of hypoglycemia and hyperglycemia with patient. If hypoglycemia occurs, advise patient to take a glass of orange juice or 2–3 teaspoons of sugar, honey, or corn syrup dissolved in water and notify health care provider.
- Advise patient to carry a form of sugar (sugar packets, candy) and identification describing disease process and medication regimen at all times.
- Encourage patient to follow prescribed diet, medication, and exercise regimen to prevent hypoglycemic or hyperglycemic episodes.

- Instruct patient in proper testing of serum glucose and ketones. These tests should be closely monitored during periods of stress or illness, and health care provider should be notified if significant changes occur.
- Advise patient to notify health care provider immediately if signs/symptoms of HF (trouble breathing, leg swelling, lung congestion, rapid weight gain) occur.
- Advise patient to notify health care provider immediately if signs of hepatic impairment (fatigue, nausea, upper abdominal pain, yellowing of skin or eyes, dark urine, light-colored stools) or bladder cancer (blood in urine, urinary pain or urgency) occur.
- Advise patient to inform health care provider of medication regimen before treatment or surgery.
- Rep: Insulin is the preferred method of controlling blood glucose during pregnancy. May cause ovulation in anovulatory women; counsel women of reproductive potential that higher doses of oral contraceptives or a form of contraception other than oral contraceptives may be required. Advise women of reproductive potential to notify health care provider promptly if pregnancy is planned or suspected or if breastfeeding.

Evaluation/Desired Outcomes

- Control of blood glucose levels.

piperacillin/tazobactam

(pi-**per**-a-sill-in/tay-zoe-**bak**-tam)

Zosyn

Classification

Therapeutic: anti-infectives

Pharmacologic: extended spectrum penicillins

Indications

Appendicitis and peritonitis. Skin and skin structure infections. Gynecologic infections. Community-acquired and nosocomial pneumonia.

Action

Piperacillin: Inhibits bacterial cell wall synthesis. Spectrum is extended compared with other penicillins. **Tazobactam:** Inhibits beta-lactamase, an enzyme that can destroy penicillins. **Therapeutic Effects:** Death of susceptible bacteria. **Spectrum:** Active against piperacillin-resistant beta-lactamase producing: *Bacteroides fragilis*, *E. coli*, *Acinetobacter baumanii*, *Klebsiella pneumoniae*, *Pseudomonas aeruginosa*, *Staphylococcus aureus*, *Haemophilus influenzae*.

Pharmacokinetics

Absorption: IV administration results in complete bioavailability.

Distribution: Widely distributed. Enters CSF well only when meninges are inflamed.

Metabolism and Excretion: Piperacillin (68%) and tazobactam (80%) are mostly excreted unchanged by the kidneys.

Half-life: *Adults:* 0.7–1.2 hr; *Children (6 mo–12 yr):* 0.7–0.9 hr; *Infants (2–5 mo):* 1.4 hr.

TIME/ACTION PROFILE (piperacillin plasma concentrations)

ROUTE	ONSET	PEAK	DURATION
IV	rapid	end of infusion	4–6 hr

Contraindications/Precautions

Contraindicated in: Hypersensitivity to penicillins, beta-lactams, cephalosporins, or tazobactam (cross-sensitivity may occur).

Use Cautiously in: Renal impairment (↑ risk of seizures) (↓ dose or ↑ interval recommended if CCr <40 mL/min); Seizure disorders; Sodium restriction; Critically ill patients (↑ risk of renal failure; use alternative antibiotic, if possible); OB: Safety not established in pregnancy; Lactation: Safety not established in breastfeeding; Pedi: Children <2 mo (safety and effectiveness not established).

Adverse Reactions/Side Effects

Derm: rash (↑ in patients with cystic fibrosis), ACUTE GENERALIZED EXANTHEMATOUS PUSTULOSIS, DRUG REACTION WITH EOSINOPHILIA AND SYSTEMIC SYMPTOMS (DRESS), STEVENS-JOHNSON SYNDROME (SJS), TOXIC EPIDERMAL NECROLYSIS (TEN), urticaria. **GI:** diarrhea, CLOSTRIDIOIDES DIFFICILE-ASSOCIATED DIARRHEA (CDAD), constipation, drug-induced hepatitis, nausea, vomiting. **GU:** interstitial nephritis, renal failure. **Hemat:** bleeding, leukopenia, neutropenia, thrombocytopenia. **Local:** pain, phlebitis. **MS:** RHABDOMYOLYSIS. **Neuro:** confusion, dizziness, headache, insomnia, lethargy, SEIZURES (HIGHER DOSES). **Misc:** fever (↑ in patients with cystic fibrosis), hemophagocytic lymphohistiocytosis, HYPERSENSITIVITY REACTIONS (INCLUDING ANAPHYLAXIS AND SERUM SICKNESS), superinfection.

Interactions

Drug-Drug: Probenecid ↓ renal excretion and ↑ levels. May alter excretion of **lithium**. **Potassium-losing diuretics**, **corticosteroids**, or **amphotericin B** may ↑ risk of hypokalemia. ↑ risk of hepatotoxicity with other **hepatotoxic agents**. May ↓ levels/effects of **aminoglycosides** in patients with renal impairment. May ↑ levels and risk of toxicity of **methotrexate**. **Vancomycin** may ↑ risk of acute kidney injury. May prolong the neuromuscular blockade associated with **vecuronium**.

P

Route/Dosage

Contains 2.84 mEq (65 mg) sodium/g of piperacillin; adult doses below expressed as combined piperacillin/tazobactam content.

Appendicitis/Peritonitis

IV (Adults and Children ≥2 mo and >40 kg): 3.375 g every 6 hr.
IV (Children ≥9 mo and ≤40 kg): 112.5 mg/kg every 8 hr.
IV (Infants 2–9 mo and ≤40 kg): 90 mg/kg every 8 hr.

Renal Impairment

IV (Adults): *CCr 20–40 mL/min:* 2.25 g every 6 hr; *CCr <20 mL/min:* 2.25 g every 8 hr; *Hemodialysis:* 2.25 g every 12 hr + 0.75 g following hemodialysis on hemodialysis days; *Continuous ambulatory peritoneal dialysis:* 2.25 g every 12 hr.

Nosocomial Pneumonia

IV (Adults and Children ≥2 mo and >40 kg): 4.5 g every 6 hr.
IV (Children ≥9 mo and ≤40 kg): 112.5 mg/kg every 6 hr.
IV (Infants 2–9 mo and ≤40 kg): 90 mg/kg every 6 hr.

Renal Impairment

IV (Adults): *CCr 20–40 mL/min:* 3.375 g every 6 hr; *CCr <20 mL/min:* 2.25 g every 6 hr; *Hemodialysis:* 2.25 g every 8 hr + 0.75 g following hemodialysis on hemodialysis days; *Continuous ambulatory peritoneal dialysis:* 2.25 g every 8 hr.

Skin and Skin Structure Infections, Gynecologic Infections, and Community-Acquired Pneumonia

IV (Adults): 3.375 g every 6 hr.

Renal Impairment

IV (Adults): *CCr 20–40 mL/min:* 2.25 g every 6 hr; *CCr <20 mL/min:* 2.25 g every 8 hr; *Hemodialysis:* 2.25 g every 12 hr + 0.75 g following hemodialysis on hemodialysis days; *Continuous ambulatory peritoneal dialysis:* 2.25 g every 12 hr.

Availability (generic available)

Powder for injection: 2.25 g (2 g piperacillin/0.25 g tazobactam)/vial, 3.375 g (3 g piperacillin/0.375 g tazobactam)/vial, 4.5 g (4 g piperacillin/0.5 g tazobactam)/vial, 13.5 g (12 g piperacillin/1.5 g tazobactam)/vial, 40.5 g (36 g piperacillin/4.5 g tazobactam)/vial. **Premixed infusion:** 2.25 g (2 g piperacillin/0.25 g tazobactam) in 50 mL of 0.45% NaCl, 3.375 g (3 g piperacillin/0.375 g tazobactam) in 50 mL of 0.3% NaCl, 4.5 g (4 g piperacillin/0.5 g tazobactam) in 100 mL of 0.45% NaCl.

NURSING IMPLICATIONS

Assessment

- Assess for resolving infection (WBC and vital signs trends; appearance of wound, sputum, urine, and stool) at beginning of and during therapy.
- Obtain a history before initiating therapy to determine previous use of and reactions to other beta-lactam antibiotics including cephalosporins. Persons with a negative history may still have an allergic response.
- Observe for signs/symptoms of anaphylaxis (rash, pruritus, laryngeal edema, wheezing). *If anaphylaxis occurs,* discontinue piperacillin/tazobactam. Keep epinephrine, an antihistamine, and resuscitation equipment close by in the event of an anaphylactic reaction.
- Monitor for signs/symptoms of CDAD, including watery diarrhea with mucus, fever, abdominal pain or cramping, anorexia, nausea, and, in severe cases, dehydration and blood or pus in the stool. May begin up to several weeks after therapy. Report promptly to health care provider.
- Assess for rash or signs and symptoms of skin reactions, including TEN or SJS, frequently during therapy (fever, general malaise, fatigue, muscle or joint aches, blisters, oral lesions, conjunctivitis, hepatitis, and/or eosinophilia). Discontinue at 1st sign of rash and provide supportive care; may be life-threatening. May recur once treatment is stopped.
- Monitor for signs and symptoms of DRESS (fever, rash, lymphadenopathy, and/or facial swelling), associated with involvement of other organ systems (hepatitis, nephritis, hematologic abnormalities, myocarditis, myositis) during therapy. May resemble an acute viral infection. Eosinophilia is often present. *If signs/symptoms of DRESS occur,* discontinue piperacillin/tazobactam.
- Monitor for signs and symptoms of rhabdomyolysis (malaise, myalgia, muscle cramps or weakness, dark or tea-colored urine).
- Monitor for seizure activity, particularly in patients with renal impairment; discontinue therapy if seizure occurs and treat as clinically indicated. Institute seizure precautions.
- Assess for signs and symptoms of superinfection such as oral thrush (white or yellow patches) or genital mycotic infections (pruritus and yeasty discharge). Treat infection promptly.
- Monitor for signs and symptoms of hemophagocytic lymphohistiocytosis (fever, rash, lymphadenopathy, hepatosplenomegaly, cytopenia); if these occur, discontinue piperacillin/tazobactam immediately and treat as needed.

Lab Test Considerations

- Evaluate renal and hepatic function, CBC with differential, and electrolytes prior to and routinely during therapy.
- Obtain specimens for culture and sensitivity prior to initiating therapy. 1st dose may be given before receiving results.
- May cause positive direct Coombs test.
- Monitor renal and hepatic function before starting and routinely during therapy. May ↑ BUN, serum creatinine, AST, ALT, serum bilirubin, alkaline phosphatase, and LDH.

- Monitor CBC with differential before starting and routinely during therapy. May cause leukopenia and neutropenia, especially with prolonged therapy or in hepatic impairment. May also cause ↓ hemoglobin and hematocrit, thrombocytopenia, and eosinophilia.
- May ↑ prothrombin and partial thromboplastin time.

Implementation

IV Administration

- If a dose of piperacillin/tazobactam is required that does not equal 2.25 g, 3.375 g, or 4.5 g, premixed infusion should not be used.
- **Intermittent Infusion: Reconstitution:** Reconstitute 2.25 g, 3.375 g, and 4.5 g single-dose vials with 10 mL, 15 mL, and 20 mL, respectively of 0.9% NaCl, sterile water for injection, or D5W. Swirl until dissolved. **Concentration:** 202.5 mg/mL (180 mg/mL of piperacillin and 22.5 mg/mL of tazobactam). **Dilution:** Dilute further in 50–150 mL of 0.9% NaCl, D5W, D5/0.9% NaCl, or LR. **Concentration:** 22.5–90 mg/mL of piperacillin/tazobactam (in children) Reconstituted vials stable for 24 hr at room temperature or 48 hr if refrigerated. Infusion stable for 24 hr at room temperature or 48 hr if refrigerated. Premixed bags are stable for 24 hr at room temperature or 14 days if refrigerated. **Rate:** Infuse over 30 min.
- **Y-Site Compatibility:** acetaminophen, allopurinol, amikacin, aminocaproic acid, aminophylline, amphotericin B liposomal, anidulafungin, argatroban, arsenic trioxide, aztreonam, bivalirudin, bleomycin, bumetanide, buprenorphine, busulfan, butorphanol, caffeine citrate, calcium chloride, calcium gluconate, cangrelor, carboplatin, carmustine, cefepime, ceftolozane/tazobactam, chloramphenicol, clindamycin, cyclophosphamide, cyclosporine, cytarabine, dactinomycin, daptomycin, dexamethasone, dexmedetomidine, dexrazoxane, diazepam, digoxin, dimenhydrinate, diphenhydramine, docetaxel, dopamine, enalaprilat, ephedrine, epinephrine, eptifibatide, eravacycline, erythromycin, esmolol, etoposide, etoposide phosphate, fentanyl, floxuridine, fluconazole, fludarabine, fluorouracil, foscarnet, fosphenytoin, furosemide, granisetron, heparin, hetastarch, hydrocortisone, hydromorphone, ifosfamide, isoproterenol, ketamine, ketorolac, leucovorin, lidocaine, linezolid, lorazepam, magnesium sulfate, mannitol, melphalan, meperidine, meropenem, meropenem/vaborbactam, mesna, methotrexate, methylprednisolone, metoclopramide, metoprolol, metronidazole, milrinone, morphine, naloxone, nitroglycerin, nitroprusside, norepinephrine, octreotide, ondansetron, oxytocin, paclitaxel, palonosetron, pamidronate, pemetrexed, pentobarbital, phenobarbital, phentolamine, phenylephrine, plazomicin, potassium acetate, potassium chloride, potassium phosphates, procainamide, remifentanil, rituximab, sargramostim, sildenafil, sodium acetate, sodium bicarbonate, sodium phosphates, succinylcholine, sufentanil, sulbactam/durlobactam, tacrolimus, tedizolid, telavancin, theophylline, thiotepa, tigecycline, tirofiban, trimethoprim/sulfamethoxazole, vasopressin, vinblastine, vincristine, voriconazole, zidovudine, zoledronic acid.
- **Y-Site Incompatibility:** acyclovir, alemtuzumab, amiodarone, amphotericin B deoxycholate, caspofungin, chlorpromazine, ciprofloxacin, cisplatin, dacarbazine, dantrolene, daunorubicin, diltiazem, dobutamine, doxorubicin hydrochloride, doxorubicin liposomal, doxycycline, droperidol, epirubicin, famotidine, ganciclovir, gemcitabine, gemtuzumab ozogamicin, glycopyrrolate, haloperidol, hydralazine, idarubicin, insulin regular, irinotecan, labetalol, levofloxacin, methadone, midazolam, minocycline, mitomycin, mitoxantrone, mycophenolate, nalbuphine, nicardipine, pentamidine, phenytoin, prochlorperazine, promethazine, propranolol, rocuronium, tobramycin, topotecan, tranexamic acid, trastuzumab, vecuronium, verapamil, vinorelbine.

Patient/Family Teaching

- Explain the purpose and side effects of piperacillin/tazobactam. Advise patient to read *Patient Information* before starting therapy.
- Instruct patient to notify health care provider if symptoms do not improve.
- Advise patients and family to call 911 and seek urgent treatment for signs and symptoms of hypersensitivity reactions (difficulty breathing; chest tightness; hives; rash; feeling light-headed; itching; swelling of the face, lips, tongue, or throat).
- Advise patient to report signs of superinfection (furry overgrowth on the tongue, white patches in mouth, vaginal itching or discharge, loose or foul-smelling stools).
- Caution patient to notify health care provider if fever and diarrhea occur, especially if stool contains blood, pus, or mucus. Advise patient not to treat diarrhea without consulting health care provider. May occur up to several weeks after discontinuation of medication.
- Advise patient to notify health care provider of all Rx or OTC medications, vitamins, or herbal products being taken and to consult with health care provider before taking other medications.
- Rep: Advise women of reproductive potential to notify health care provider if pregnancy is planned or suspected or if breastfeeding.

P

Evaluation/Desired Outcomes

- Bactericidal action against susceptible bacteria.
- Resolution of the signs and symptoms of infection. Length of time for complete resolution depends on the organism and site of infection.

pitavastatin See HMG-CoA REDUCTASE INHIBITORS (statins).

plecanatide (ple-kan-a-tide)

Trulance

Classification

Therapeutic: laxatives

Pharmacologic: guanylate cyclase-C agonists

Indications

Chronic idiopathic constipation. Irritable bowel syndrome with constipation.

Action

Locally ↑ cyclic guanosine monophosphate concentrations, which ↑ intestinal fluid and accelerates transit time. **Therapeutic Effects:** Increased frequency of complete spontaneous bowel movements.

Pharmacokinetics

Absorption: Minimally absorbed, action is primarily local.

Distribution: Stays within the GI tract with minimal distribution.

Metabolism and Excretion: Converted to its principal active metabolite within the GI tract. Plecanatide and active metabolite and then degrade in intestinal lumen to smaller peptides and amino acids. Excretion information unknown.

Half-life: Unknown.

TIME/ACTION PROFILE (improvement in symptoms)

ROUTE	ONSET	PEAK	DURATION
PO	1 wk	2–12 wk	2 wk†

† Following discontinuation.

Contraindications/Precautions

Contraindicated in: Known/suspected mechanical GI obstruction; Pedi: Children <6 yr (↑ risk of dehydration).

Use Cautiously in: OB: Safety not established in pregnancy; fetal exposure to plecanatide or its active metabolite unlikely; Lactation: Use while breastfeeding only if potential maternal benefit justifies potential risk to infant; Pedi: Children 6–18 yr (safety and effectiveness not established).

Adverse Reactions/Side Effects

GI: ↑ liver enzymes, abdominal distention, diarrhea, flatulence.

Interactions

Drug-Drug: None reported.

Route/Dosage

PO (Adults): 3 mg once daily.

Availability

Tablets: 3 mg.

NURSING IMPLICATIONS

Assessment

- Monitor bowel function (frequency, consistency) periodically during therapy. *If severe diarrhea occurs,* hold plecanatide and rehydrate patient.

Lab Test Considerations

- May ↑ ALT, and AST.

Implementation

- **PO:** Administer once daily without regard to food. Swallow tablet whole. Tablets can be crushed and mixed in room temperature applesauce or water. Do not mix with other foods or liquids. For administration with water, mix 30 mL of water into a cup with the tablet, swirl for ≥10 sec, and swallow entire amount immediately. Add an additional 30 mL of water if any part of the tablet remains; swirl again and swallow immediately.
- ***Administration through a gastric or nasogastric feeding tube:*** Mix about 30 mL of room temperature water into a cup with the crushed tablet and swirl for ≥15 sec. Flush the feeding tube with 30 mL water, draw up the mixture with a syringe, and administer mixture via the feeding tube immediately. Add an additional 30 mL of water to the cup if any part of the tablet remains, swirl for ≥15 sec, and use the same syringe to administer via the feeding tube. Flush the feeding tube with ≥10 mL of water after administration.

Patient/Family Teaching

- Explain the purpose and side effects of plecanatide. Instruct patient to take as directed. If a dose is missed, omit and take next dose at regular time; do not double doses. Advise patient to read *Patient Information* before starting and with each Rx refill in case of changes.
- Instruct patient to notify health care provider of all Rx or OTC medications, vitamins, or herbal products being taken and consult health care provider before taking any new medications.
- Rep: Advise women of reproductive potential to notify health care provider if pregnancy is planned or suspected or if breastfeeding.

Evaluation/Desired Outcomes

- Increased frequency of complete spontaneous bowel movements.

HIGH ALERT

polatuzumab vedotin
(pol-a-tooz-ue-mab ve-doe-tin)

Polivy

Classification

Therapeutic: antineoplastics

Pharmacologic: monoclonal antibodies

Indications
Previously untreated diffuse large B-cell lymphoma, not otherwise specified, or high-grade B-cell lymphoma in patients who have an International Prognostic Index score ≥2 (in combination with rituximab, cyclophosphamide, doxorubicin, and prednisone). Relapsed or refractory diffuse large B-cell lymphoma, not otherwise specified, after ≥2 prior therapies (in combination with bendamustine and rituximab).

Action
Binds to the CD79b antigen on the surface of B cells, releasing monomethylauristatin E (MMAE). MMAE binds to microtubules and kills dividing cells by inhibiting cell division and inducing apoptosis. **Therapeutic Effects:** Improved progression-free survival of previously untreated diffuse large B-cell lymphoma or high-grade B-cell lymphoma. Decreased progression of relapsed or refractory diffuse large B-cell lymphoma.

Pharmacokinetics
Absorption: IV administration results in complete bioavailability.

Distribution: Not widely distributed to tissues.

Metabolism and Excretion: Broken down into small peptides, amino acids, unconjugated MMAE, and unconjugated MMAE-related catabolites.

Half-life: *Antibody-conjugated MMAE:* 12 days; *Unconjugated MMAE:* 4 days.

TIME/ACTION PROFILE (plasma concentrations)

ROUTE	ONSET	PEAK	DURATION
IV	unknown	unknown	unknown

Contraindications/Precautions
Contraindicated in: Moderate or severe hepatic impairment; OB: Pregnancy; Lactation: Lactation.

Use Cautiously in: Peripheral neuropathy; Rep: Women of reproductive potential and men with female partners of reproductive potential; Pedi: Safety and effectiveness not established in children.

Adverse Reactions/Side Effects
F and E hypocalcemia, hypokalemia, hypophosphatemia. **GI:** ↓ appetite, ↑ amylase, ↑ lipase, ↑ liver enzymes, diarrhea, hypoalbuminemia, vomiting, weight loss, HEPATOTOXICITY, hyperbilirubinemia. **GU:** ↑ serum creatinine, ↓ fertility (men). **Hemat:** ANEMIA, lymphopenia, NEUTROPENIA, THROMBOCYTOPENIA. **MS:** arthralgia. **Neuro:** dizziness, fatigue, peripheral neuropathy, PROGRESSIVE MULTIFOCAL LEUKOENCEPHALOPATHY (PML). **Resp:** dyspnea. **Misc:** fever, INFECTION, infusion reactions, tumor lysis syndrome.

Interactions
Drug-Drug: Strong CYP3A inhibitors, including **ketoconazole**, may ↑ unconjugated MMAE levels and risk of toxicity. **Strong CYP3A inducers**, including **rifampin**, may ↓ unconjugated MMAE levels and effectiveness.

Route/Dosage
IV (Adults): 1.8 mg/kg every 21 days for 6 cycles.

Availability
Lyophilized powder for injection: 30 mg/vial, 140 mg/vial.

NURSING IMPLICATIONS
Assessment
- Monitor for signs/symptoms of peripheral neuropathy (hypoesthesia, hyperesthesia, paresthesia, dysesthesia, neuropathic pain, burning sensation, weakness, gait disturbance) during therapy. May occur as early as 1st cycle and effects are cumulative. **For patients receiving polatuzumab vedotin with rituximab, cyclophosphamide, doxorubicin, and prednisone:** *If Grade 2 peripheral sensory neuropathy occurs,* if recovered to Grade ≤1 before next dose, resume at same dose level. If Grade 2 continues at time of next dose, ↓ by one dose level. *If Grade 3 peripheral sensory neuropathy occurs,* hold polatuzumab vedotin until Grade ≤2 and ↓ by one dose level. *If Grade 4 peripheral neuropathy occurs,* permanently discontinue polatuzumab vedotin. *If Grade 2–3 peripheral motor neuropathy occurs,* hold polatuzumab vedotin until Grade ≤1 and ↓ by one dose level. *If Grade 4 peripheral motor neuropathy occurs,* permanently discontinue polatuzumab vedotin. **For patients receiving polatuzumab vedotin with bendamustine and rituximab:** *If Grade 2–3 peripheral neuropathy occurs,* hold polatuzumab vedotin until Grade ≤1. If recovered to Grade ≤1 before Day 14, restart next cycle at permanently ↓ dose of 1.4 mg/kg. If prior dose ↓ to 1.4 mg/kg already occurred, discontinue polatuzumab vedotin. If not recovered to Grade ≤1 before Day 14, discontinue polatuzumab

P

vedotin. *If Grade 4 peripheral neuropathy occurs,* discontinue polatuzumab vedotin.

- Monitor for signs/symptoms of infusion-related reactions (fever, chills, sweating, myalgia, headache, dizziness, nausea, vomiting, urticaria, pruritus, shortness of breath, wheezing) during and within 24 hr of infusion. *If Grade 1–3 infusion-related reactions occur,* hold infusion and give supportive treatment. For 1st instance of Grade 3 wheezing, bronchospasm, or generalized urticaria, permanently discontinue polatuzumab vedotin. For recurrent Grade 2 wheezing or urticaria or for recurrence of any Grade 3 symptoms, permanently discontinue polatuzumab vedotin. If symptoms completely resolve, resume infusion at 50% of rate achieved before interruption. If no infusion related symptoms occur, ↑ rate of infusion in increments of 50 mg/hr every 30 min. For next cycle, infuse over 90 min. If no infusion-related reaction occurs, infuse subsequent infusions over 30 min. Administer premedication for all cycles. *If Grade 4 infusion-related reactions occur,* immediately stop infusion. Give supportive treatment. Permanently discontinue polatuzumab vedotin.
- Monitor for signs/symptoms of infection (fever, chills, sore throat, cough, dyspnea, skin lesions) during therapy.
- Monitor for signs/symptoms of PML (new or worsening neurological, cognitive, or behavioral changes; progressive weakness; hemianopia; diplopia; other visual field defects; aphasia; loss of coordination), an opportunistic infection of the brain caused by the JC virus, which may be fatal. *If PML is suspected,* hold polatuzumab vedotin and any concurrent chemotherapy. *If PML diagnosis confirmed,* discontinue permanently polatuzumab vedotin.
- Assess for signs/symptoms of tumor lysis syndrome (malaise, tachycardia, hypotension, confusion, delirium, arthralgia, myalgia, muscle spasms or twitches, paresthesia, headache, dizziness, nausea, vomiting, dark urine, acute renal failure, hyperkalemia, hypocalcemia, hyperuricemia, hypophosphatemia) in patients with advanced stage disease and/or with ↑ tumor burden; may be fatal. Correct electrolyte abnormalities, monitor renal function and fluid balance, and administer supportive care, including dialysis, as indicated.
- Monitor for signs/symptoms of hepatotoxicity (fatigue, nausea, upper abdominal pain, jaundice, scleral icterus, dark urine, clay-colored stools).

Lab Test Considerations

- Verify negative pregnancy test before starting therapy.
- Monitor CBC during therapy. May cause neutropenia, thrombocytopenia, and anemia. Administer prophylactic granulocyte colony-stimulating factor (G-CSF) therapy for neutropenia in patients receiving polatuzumab vedotin with rituximab, cyclophosphamide, doxorubicin, and prednisone; consider prophylactic use of G-CSF therapy in patients receiving polatuzumab vedotin with bendamustine and rituximab. **For patients receiving polatuzumab ve dotin with rituximab, cyclophosphamide, doxorubicin, and prednisone:** *If Grade 3–4 neutropenia occurs,* hold all therapy until ANC recovers to >1000 cells/mcL. If ANC recovers to >1000 cells/mcL on or before Day 7, resume all therapy without dose ↓. Consider G-CSF prophylaxis for subsequent cycles, if not previously given. If ANC recovers to >1000 cells/mcL after Day 7, restart all therapy. Consider G-CSF prophylaxis for subsequent cycles, if not previously given. If prophylaxis was given, consider dose ↓ of polatuzumab vedotin. **For patients receiving polatuzumab vedotin with bendamustine and rituximab:** *If Grade 3–4 neutropenia occurs,* hold all therapy until ANC recovers to >1000 cells/mcL. If ANC recovers to >1000 cells/mcL on or before Day 7, resume all therapy without dose ↓. Consider G-CSF prophylaxis for subsequent cycles, if not previously given. If ANC recovers to >1000 cells/mcL after Day 7, restart all therapy. Consider G-CSF prophylaxis for subsequent cycles, if not previously given. If prophylaxis was given, consider dose ↓ of bendamustine. If dose ↓ of bendamustine has already occurred, consider dose ↓ of polatuzumab vedotin to 1.4 mg/kg.
- **For patients receiving polatuzumab vedotin with rituximab, cyclophosphamide, doxorubicin, and prednisone:** *If Grade 3–4 thrombocytopenia occurs,* hold all therapy until platelets recover to >75,000 cells/mcL. If platelets recover to >75,000 cells/mcL on or before Day 7, resume all therapy without dose ↓. If platelets recover to >75,000 cells/mcL after Day 7, restart all therapy, and consider dose ↓ of polatuzumab vedotin. **For patients receiving polatuzumab vedotin with bendamustine and rituximab:** *If Grade 3–4 thrombocytopenia occurs,* hold all therapy until platelets recover to >75,000 cells/mcL. If platelets recover to >75,000 cells/mcL on or before Day 7, resume all therapy without dose ↓. If platelets recover to >75,000 cells/mcL after Day 7, restart all therapy, with dose ↓ of bendamustine. If dose ↓ of bendamustine already occurred, consider dose ↓ of polatuzumab vedotin to 1.4 mg/kg.
- Monitor AST, ALT, and total bilirubin periodically during therapy.

Implementation

- **Dose reduction schedule** *Starting dose:* 1.8 mg/kg; *1st dose ↓:* 1.4 mg/kg; *2nd dose ↓:* 1 mg/kg; *Requirement for further dose ↓:* Discontinue polatuzumab vedotin.
- Administered with bendamustine and rituximab in any order.

- Premedicate with antihistamine and antipyretic 30–60 min prior to polatuzumab vedotin.
- Administer prophylaxis for *Pneumocystis jiroveci* pneumonia and herpesvirus during therapy.
- If a dose is missed, administer as soon as possible. Adjust schedule to maintain a 21-day interval between doses.

IV Administration

- ***High Alert:*** Fatalities have occurred with chemotherapeutic agents. Before administering, clarify all ambiguous orders; double-check single, daily, and course-of-therapy dose limits; have 2nd practitioner independently double-check original order, calculations, and infusion pump settings.
- **IV:** Use double gloves and a protective gown to prepare and administer. If possible, prepare in a biological safety cabinet; eye, face, and respiratory protection may be needed. Prepare and administer in a closed-system drug transfer device. During administration, if there is a potential that the substance could splash or if the patient may resist, use eye and face protection. Discard IV equipment in specially designated containers. If powder or solution comes in contact with skin or mucosa, wash thoroughly with soap and water.
- **Intermittent Infusion: Reconstitution:** Reconstitute each vial by slowly injecting 1.8 mL or 7.2 mL of sterile water for injection into 30-mg or 140-mg vial of polatuzumab respectively. Swirl gently; do not shake. Solution is colorless to slightly brown, clear to slightly opalescent; do not administer solutions that are cloudy, discolored, or contain particulate matter. Reconstituted solution is stable up to 48 hr if refrigerated or 8 hr at room temperature; do not freeze or expose to direct sunlight. **Concentration:** 20 mg/mL. **Dilution:** Dilute with ≥50 mL of 0.9% NaCl, 0.45% NaCl, or D5W. **Concentration:** 0.72–2.7 mg/mL. Gently invert to mix; do not shake. *If diluted with 0.9% NaCl,* solution is stable for up to 4 hr at room temperature or up to 24 hr if refrigerated. *If diluted with 0.45% NaCl,* solution is stable for up to 4 hr at room temperature or up to 18 hr if refrigerated. *If diluted with D5W,* solution is stable for up to 6 hr at room temperature or up to 36 hr if refrigerated. **Rate:** Infuse the initial dose over 90 min. Monitor patients for infusion-related reactions during the infusion and for ≥90 min following completion of the infusion. Infuse using a dedicated infusion line with a sterile, nonpyrogenic, low-protein-binding in-line or add-on filter (0.2- or 0.22-micron pore size) and catheter.
- **Y-Site Incompatibility:** Do not administer other drugs through same IV line.

Patient/Family Teaching

- Explain purpose and side effects of *Polivy*. Do not stop receiving drug without consulting health care provider. If an appointment is missed, contact health care provider as soon as possible to reschedule. Advise patient to read *Medication Guide* before starting and periodically during therapy in case of changes.
- Caution patient to notify health care provider immediately if signs and symptoms of bleeding, infection (≥fever of 38°C [100.4°F], chills, cough, pain on urination), PML (confusion, dizziness, loss of balance, difficulty talking or walking, changes in vision), tumor lysis syndrome (nausea, vomiting, diarrhea, lethargy), or hepatotoxicity (fatigue, nausea, upper abdominal pain, yellowing of skin or eyes, dark urine, light-colored stools) occur. Caution patient to avoid crowds and persons with known infections. Instruct patient to use soft toothbrush and electric razor and to avoid falls. Patient should also be cautioned not to drink alcoholic beverages or to take products containing aspirin or NSAIDs; may precipitate GI hemorrhage.
- Advise patient to notify health care provider if signs and symptoms of peripheral neuropathy (numbness or tingling of hands or feet, muscle weakness) or infusion-related reactions (fever, chills, rash, breathing problems within 24 hr of infusion) occur.
- Advise patient to notify health care provider of all Rx or OTC medications, vitamins, or herbal products being taken and to consult with health care provider before taking other medications.
- Rep: May cause fetal harm. Advise women of reproductive potential to use effective contraception during and for ≥3 mo after last dose and to avoid breastfeeding for ≥2 mo after last dose. Advise men with female partners of reproductive potential to use effective contraception during and for ≥5 mo after last dose. May impair male fertility.

Evaluation/Desired Outcomes

- Improved progression free survival of previously untreated diffuse large B-cell lymphoma or high-grade B-cell lymphoma.
- Decreased progression of relapsed or refractory diffuse large B-cell lymphoma.

polyethylene glycol 3350
(po-lee-**eth**-e-leen **glye**-kole)

🍁 ClearLax, 🍁 Comfilax, 🍁 Emolax, Gavilax, GlycoLax, 🍁 Hydralax, 🍁 Lax-a-Day, MiraLax, 🍁 PegaLax, 🍁 Relaxa, 🍁 RestoraLax

Classification
Therapeutic: laxatives
Pharmacologic: osmotics

P

Indications
Occasional constipation.

Action
Polyethylene glycol in solution acts as an osmotic agent, drawing water into the lumen of the GI tract. **Therapeutic Effects:** Evacuation of the GI tract without water or electrolyte imbalance.

Pharmacokinetics
Absorption: Nonabsorbable.
Distribution: Unknown.
Metabolism and Excretion: Excreted in fecal contents.
Half-life: Unknown.

TIME/ACTION PROFILE (bowel movement)

ROUTE	ONSET	PEAK	DURATION
PO	unknown	1–3 days	unknown

Contraindications/Precautions
Contraindicated in: GI obstruction; Gastric retention; Toxic colitis; Megacolon; Bowel perforation.
Use Cautiously in: Abdominal pain of uncertain cause, particularly if accompanied by fever; OB: Minimal systemic absorption; may be used during pregnancy when osmotic laxative needed; Lactation: Minimal systemic absorption; probably compatible with breastfeeding; Pedi: May be associated with metabolic acidosis and neuropsychiatric events in children.

Adverse Reactions/Side Effects
Derm: urticaria. **GI:** abdominal bloating, cramping, flatulence, nausea.

Interactions
Drug-Drug: None reported.

Route/Dosage
PO (Adults): 17 g (heaping tablespoon) in 8 ounces of water once daily; may be used for up to 2 wk.
PO (Children >6 mo): 0.2–0.8 g/kg once daily; titrate to effect (max = 17 g/day).

Availability (generic available)
Oral powder: 17 g/dose (in 14-ounce, 24-ounce, and 26-ounce containers).

NURSING IMPLICATIONS
Assessment
- Assess for abdominal distention, presence of bowel sounds, and usual pattern of bowel function.
- Assess color, consistency, and amount of stool produced.

Lab Test Considerations
- May cause electrolyte imbalances with diarrhea or use that is frequent or prolonged.

Implementation
- Do not confuse polyethylene glycol with propylene glycol.
- **PO:** Dissolve powder in 8 ounces of any beverage (hot or cold) prior to administration. Do not mix in starch-based thickeners used for patients with difficulty swallowing.

Patient/Family Teaching
- Explain the purpose and side effects of medication. Advise to take as directed. Advise patient to read *Patient Information* before starting therapy.
- Inform patient that 2–4 days may be required to produce a bowel movement; best results require 1–2 wk of use. Polyethylene glycol 3350 should not be used for >2 wk. Prolonged, frequent, or excessive use may result in electrolyte imbalance and laxative dependence.
- Advise patient to notify health care provider if nausea, vomiting or abdominal pain, unusual cramps, bloating, diarrhea or a sudden change in bowel habits for >2 wk occurs. Advise patient to discontinue use and consult health care provider if severe diarrhea, rectal bleeding, abdominal pain, bloating, cramping, or nausea gets worse or if they need to use for >1 wk.
- Advise patient to notify health care provider of all Rx or OTC medications, vitamins, or herbal products being taken and to consult with health care provider before taking other medications.
- Rep: Advise women of reproductive potential to notify health care provider if pregnancy is planned or suspected or if breastfeeding.

Evaluation/Desired Outcomes
- A soft, formed bowel movement.

REMS HIGH ALERT

pomalidomide
(pom-a-**lid**-oh-mide)
Pomalyst

Classification
Therapeutic: antineoplastics
Pharmacologic: immunomodulatory agents

Indications
Multiple myeloma in patients who have received ≥2 prior therapies including lenalidomide and a proteasome inhibitor and have progressed on or within 60 days of completion of previous treatment (with prednisone). AIDS-related Kaposi sarcoma after failure of highly active antiretroviral therapy. Kaposi sarcoma in patients who are HIV-negative.

Action
Inhibits proliferation and induced apoptosis of hematopoietic tumor cells. Proliferation of resistant multiple myeloma cell lines and may act synergistically with dexamethasone. Enhances T cell and natural killer cell-mediated immunity and inhibits production of proinflammatory cytokines. **Therapeutic Effects:** Decreased progression of multiple myeloma and Kaposi sarcoma.

Pharmacokinetics

Absorption: Well absorbed following oral administration.

Distribution: Enters semen.

Metabolism and Excretion: Primarily metabolized in the liver by CYP1A2 and CYP3A4 with some metabolism by CYP2C19 and CYP2D6. Metabolites excreted in urine and feces. Minimal amounts excreted unchanged in urine.

Half-life: *Normal subjects:* 9.5 hr; *Patients with myeloma:* 7.5 hr.

TIME/ACTION PROFILE

ROUTE	ONSET	PEAK	DURATION
PO	unknown	unknown	unknown

Contraindications/Precautions

Contraindicated in: Severe hypersensitivity; Blood should not be donated; Serum creatinine >3 mg/dL; Serum bilirubin >2 mg/dL and AST/ALT >3 times upper limit of normal; Concurrent use of pembrolizumab (↑ risk of mortality); OB: Pregnancy; Lactation: Lactation.

Use Cautiously in: Rep: Women of reproductive potential and men with female partners of reproductive potential; Pedi: Safety and effectiveness not established in children.

Adverse Reactions/Side Effects

CV: peripheral edema, DEEP VEIN THROMBOSIS (DVT), MI. **Derm:** dry skin, hyperhidrosis, night sweats, pruritus, rash, DRUG REACTION WITH EOSINOPHILIA AND SYSTEMIC SYMPTOMS (DRESS), skin exfoliation, STEVENS-JOHNSON SYNDROME (SJS), TOXIC EPIDERMAL NECROLYSIS (TEN). **Endo:** hyperglycemia. **F and E** hypercalcemia, hypocalcemia, hypokalemia, hyponatremia. **GI:** ↓ appetite, constipation, diarrhea, nausea, vomiting, HEPATOTOXICITY. **GU:** renal failure. **Hemat:** ANEMIA, leukopenia, lymphopenia, NEUTROPENIA, THROMBOCYTOPENIA. **MS:** arthralgia, back pain, bone pain, muscle spasms, muscle weakness, musculoskeletal pain, pain in extremity. **Neuro:** confusion, dizziness, insomnia, neuropathy, fatigue, STROKE, tremor, weakness. **Resp:** dyspnea, PULMONARY EMBOLISM (PE). **Misc:** fever, INFECTION, MALIGNANCY, chills, HYPERSENSITIVITY REACTIONS (INCLUDING ANAPHYLAXIS AND ANGIOEDEMA).

Interactions

Drug-Drug: CYP3A inhibitors, **CYP1A2 inhibitors**, or **P-glycoprotein (P-gp) inhibitors**, including **ketoconazole**, may ↑ levels and risk of toxicity; avoid concurrent use. **CYP3A inducers**, **CYP1A2 inducers**, or **P-gp inducers**, including **rifampin**, may ↓ levels and effectiveness; avoid concurrent use.

Route/Dosage

Multiple Myeloma

PO (Adults): 4 mg once daily on Days 1–21 of each 28-day cycle; continue until disease progression; *Concurrent use of strong CYP1A2 inhibitor:* 2 mg once daily on Days 1–21 of each 28-day cycle; continue until disease progression.

Renal Impairment

PO (Adults): *Hemodialysis:* 3 mg once daily (give dose after dialysis on hemodialysis days); continue until disease progression.

Hepatic Impairment

PO (Adults): *Mild or moderate hepatic impairment:* 3 mg once daily; continue until disease progression; *Severe hepatic impairment:* 2 mg once daily; continue until disease progression.

Kaposi Sarcoma

PO (Adults): 5 mg once daily on Days 1–21 of each 28-day cycle; continue until disease progression or unacceptable toxicity; *Concurrent use of strong CYP1A2 inhibitor:* 2 mg once daily on Days 1–21 of each 28-day cycle; continue until disease progression or unacceptable toxicity.

Renal Impairment

PO (Adults): *Hemodialysis:* 4 mg once daily on Days 1–21 of each 28-day cycle (give dose after dialysis on hemodialysis days); continue until disease progression or unacceptable toxicity.

Hepatic Impairment

PO (Adults): *Mild, moderate, or severe hepatic impairment:* 3 mg once daily on Days 1–21 of each 28-day cycle; continue until disease progression or unacceptable toxicity.

Availability (generic available)

Capsules: 1 mg, 2 mg, 3 mg, 4 mg.

NURSING IMPLICATIONS

Assessment

- Assess for signs of DVT and PE (dyspnea, chest pain, arm or leg swelling) periodically during therapy. Prophylactic anticoagulation is recommended.
- Monitor for signs and symptoms of SJS, TEN, and DRESS (rash, exfoliative dermatitis, eosinophilia, fever, lymphadenopathy, hepatitis, nephritis, pneumonitis, myocarditis, pericarditis) during therapy. May be fatal. *If Grade 2 or 3 skin rash occurs,* hold or discontinue pomalidomide. *If Grade 4 rash; exfoliative or bullous rash; or SJS, TEN, or DRESS occurs,* permanently discontinue pomalidomide.
- Monitor for hypersensitivity reactions (angioedema, skin exfoliation, bullae, severe dermatologic

P

reactions) during therapy. *If symptoms occur,* permanently discontinue pomalidomide.

Lab Test Considerations

- Verify two negative pregnancy tests before starting therapy. Pregnancy tests must be done within 10–14 days and within 24 hr of starting therapy. Once treatment has started, pregnancy tests should occur weekly during first 4 wk of use and then every 4 wk in women with a regular menstrual cycle and every 2 wk in women with an irregular cycle. Discontinue therapy if pregnancy is suspected or confirmed.
- Monitor liver function tests monthly. *If ↑ liver enzymes occurs,* hold pomalidomide. After return to baseline values, may consider resuming pomalidomide at ↓ dose.
- **Multiple Myeloma:** Monitor CBC with differential weekly for 1st 8 wk of therapy and at least monthly thereafter. May cause neutropenia. *If ANC <500 cells/mcL or febrile neutropenia (fever ≥38.5°C and ANC <1000 cells/mcL),* hold pomalidomide until ANC ≥500 cells/mcL and follow CBC weekly. If ANC returns to ≥500 cells/mcL, resume pomalidomide at 1 mg/day less than previous dose. *For each subsequent drop of ANC <500 cells/mcL,* hold pomalidomide and resume at 1 mg/day less than previous dose when ANC returns to ≥500 cells/mcL.
- May cause thrombocytopenia. *If platelets fall to <25,000 cells/mcL,* hold pomalidomide until platelets ≥50,000 cells/mcL and follow CBC weekly. When platelets return to >50,000 cells/mcL, resume pomalidomide at 1 mg/day less than previous dose. *For each subsequent drop of platelets <25,000 cells/mcL,* hold pomalidomide and resume at 1 mg/day less than previous dose when platelet count returns to ≥50,000 cells/mcL.
- Monitor liver function tests (AST, ALT, serum bilirubin) monthly during therapy. Hold pomalidomide if liver enzymes ↑. May restart therapy at a ↓ dose when levels return to normal. Permanently discontinue pomalidomide if unable to tolerate 1 mg once daily.
- **Kaposi sarcoma:** Monitor CBC every 2 wk for 1st 12 wk and monthly thereafter. May cause neutropenia. *If ANC 500–< 1000 cells/mcL,* for Day 1 of cycle, hold pomalidomide until ANC ≥1000 cells/mcL. Resume at same dose. During cycle, continue pomalidomide at same dose. *If ANC <500 cells/mcL,* hold pomalidomide until ANC ≥1000 cells/mcL. Resume at same dose.
- May cause febrile neutropenia. *If ANC <1000 cells/mcL and single temperature ≥38.3° C or ANC <1000 cells/mcL and sustained temperature ≥38° C for >1 hr,* hold pomalidomide until ANC ≥1000 cells/mcL. Resume at 1 mg/day less than previous dose.
- May cause thrombocytopenia. *If platelets 25,000–<50,000 cells/mcL,* for Day 1 of cycle, hold pomalidomide until platelets ≥50,000 cells/mcL. Resume at same dose. During cycle, continue at current dose. *If platelets <25,000 cells/mcL,* permanently discontinue pomalidomide. Permanently discontinue pomalidomide if unable to tolerate 1 mg once daily.
- May cause hyperglycemia, hyponatremia, hypokalemia, hypocalcamia, and hypercalcemia.

Implementation

- ***REMS:*** Pomalidomide is only available through PS-Pomalidomide REMS program. Prescribers and pharmacies must be certified. Patients must sign a patient-prescriber form and comply with REMS requirements. Women of reproductive potential who are not pregnant must comply with pregnancy testing and contraception requirements, and men must comply with contraception requirements.
- Thromboprophylaxis should be based on assessment of patient's underlying risk factors.
- **PO:** Administer with water on an empty stomach, without regard to food. ***DNC:*** Swallow capsule whole with water; do not open, break, or chew.

Patient/Family Teaching

- ***REMS:*** Instruct patient to comply with all aspects of the *PS-Pomalidomide REMS program*. Details available at www.PS-PomalidomideREMS.com.
- Explain purpose and side effects of medication to patient. Advise patient to read *Patient Information* before starting therapy. Instruct patient to take as directed daily at the same time each day. Missed doses may be taken up to 12 hr after the time it would be normally be taken. If >12 hr, skip dose and take regularly scheduled dose the next day; do not double doses.
- Advise patient to notify health care provider of all Rx or OTC medications, vitamins, or herbal products being taken and to consult with health care provider before taking other medications.
- Caution patient not to share pomalidomide with anyone, even someone who has similar symptoms.
- Instruct patient to avoid smoking during therapy; may ↓ efficacy of pomalidomide.
- Advise patient to notify health care provider if signs and symptoms of a blood clot (shortness of breath, chest pain, arm or leg swelling), heart attack (chest pain that may spread to arms, neck, jaw, back, or abdomen; feeling sweaty; shortness of breath; feeling sick or vomiting), or stroke (sudden numbness or weakness, especially on one side of body; severe headache or confusion; problems with vision, speech, or balance) occur.
- Advise patient to notify health care provider if signs and symptoms of liver problems (yellowing of skin or white part of eyes, dark or brown urine, pain on upper right side of abdomen, unusual bleeding or bruising, feeling tired), skin reactions (red, itchy skin rash; peeling of skin; blisters; severe itching; fever), or allergic reaction (swelling of lips, mouth, tongue, or throat; trouble breathing or swallowing; very fast heartbeat; feeling dizzy or faint; hives) occur.

- May cause dizziness and confusion. Caution patient to avoid driving and other activities requiring alertness until response to medication is known.
- Advise patient to avoid donating blood while taking pomalidomide and for 1 mo following therapy.
- Rep: May cause fetal harm. Inform women of reproductive potential that they must use one highly effective method (IUD, hormonal contraceptive, tubal ligation, partner's vasectomy) and one additional method (latex or synthetic condom, diaphragm, cervical cap) for 4 wk before, during therapy and interruptions of therapy, and for 4 wk after last dose and to avoid breastfeeding during therapy. May impair female fertility. Encourage pregnant women and pregnant female partners of men exposed to pomalidomide during pregnancy to enroll in the registry to monitor outcomes of pregnancy by calling 1-888-423-5436. Pomalidomide is present in semen. Male patients receiving pomalidomide must always use a latex or synthetic condom during any contact with women of reproductive potential and for 4 wk after last dose, even if they have undergone a successful vasectomy. Instruct men to avoid donating sperm while taking pomalidomide and for 1 mo after last dose.

Evaluation/Desired Outcomes

- Decrease progression of multiple myeloma and Kaposi sarcoma.

posaconazole

(po-sa-**kon**-a-zole)

Noxafil, ✱ Posanol

Classification

Therapeutic: antifungals

Pharmacologic: triazoles

Indications

PO, IV: Treatment of invasive aspergillosis (tablets and injection). **PO, IV:** Prevention of invasive *Aspergillus* and *Candida* infections in patients who are severely immunocompromised, such as hematopoietic stem cell transplant recipients with graft-versus-host disease or those with hematologic malignancies with prolonged neutropenia from chemotherapy (tablets, oral suspension, delayed-release oral suspension, and injection). **PO:** Treatment of oropharyngeal candidiasis (including candidiasis unresponsive to itraconazole or fluconazole) (oral suspension).

Action

Blocks ergosterol synthesis, a major component of fungal plasma membrane. **Therapeutic Effects:** Fungistatic/fungicidal action against susceptible fungi. **Spectrum:** *Aspergillus* spp., *Candida* spp.

Pharmacokinetics

Absorption: Well absorbed following oral administration; absorption is optimized by food; IV administration results in complete bioavailability.
Distribution: Extensive extravascular distribution and penetration into body tissues.
Protein Binding: >98%.
Metabolism and Excretion: Some metabolism via UDP glucuronidation; 66% eliminated unchanged in feces, 13% in urine (mostly as metabolites).
Half-life: 35 hr.

TIME/ACTION PROFILE (plasma concentrations)

ROUTE	ONSET	PEAK	DURATION
PO (suspension)	unknown	3–5 hr	8 hr
PO-ER	unknown	4–5 hr	24 hr
IV	unknown	2 hr	24 hr

Contraindications/Precautions

Contraindicated in: Hypersensitivity to posaconazole or other azole antifungals; Concurrent use of atorvastatin, ergot alkaloids, lovastatin, pimozide, quinidine, simvastatin, or sirolimus; Concurrent use of venetoclax at initiation and during the ramp-up phase; Hereditary fructose intolerance (for delayed-release oral suspension only).
Use Cautiously in: History of/predisposition to QTc interval prolongation including congenital QTc prolongation, concurrent medications that prolong the QTc interval, or electrolyte abnormalities (hypokalemia, hypomagnesemia); correct pre-existing abnormalities prior to administration; Moderate to severe renal impairment (CCr <50 mL/min); use only if justified by risk/benefit assessment (IV form should be avoided; use oral form only); Severe diarrhea, vomiting, or renal impairment (monitor for breakthrough fungal infections); OB: Use during pregnancy only if potential maternal benefit justifies potential fetal risk; Lactation: Use while breastfeeding only if potential maternal benefit justifies potential risk to infant; Pedi: Children <18 yr (IV) or <13 yr (oral) (safety and effectiveness not established).

Adverse Reactions/Side Effects

CV: QT interval prolongation, TORSADES DE POINTES. **Endo:** adrenal insufficiency, pseudoaldostonerism. **F and E** hypokalemia, hypomagnesemia, hypocalcemia. **GI:** diarrhea, nausea, vomiting, HEPATOCELLULAR DAMAGE, PANCREATITIS. **Neuro:** headache. **Resp:** cough. **Misc:** fever, HYPERSENSITIVITY REACTIONS.

Interactions

Drug-Drug: May ↑ **cyclosporine**, **sirolimus**, and **tacrolimus** levels and risk of toxicity; use with sirolimus contraindicated; for cyclosporine and tacrolimus, ↓ dose initially and monitor levels frequently. May ↑ **quinidine** and **pimozide** levels and the risk for arrhythmias; concurrent use contraindicated. May ↑ levels and risk of toxicity from **ergot alkaloids**, including **ergotamine** and **dihydroergotamine**; concurrent use contraindicated. May ↑ levels of **simvastatin**, **atorvastatin**, or **lovastatin** and the risk for rhabdomyolysis; concurrent use contraindicated. May ↑ risk of tumor lysis syndrome, neutropenia, and serious infection during initiation or the ramp-up phase of **venetoclax** in patients with chronic lymphocytic leukemia or small lymphocytic leukemia; concurrent use contraindicated. **Rifabutin**, **phenytoin**, **cimetidine**, and **efavirenz** may ↓ levels and effectiveness; avoid concurrent use. **Esomeprazole** and **metoclopramide** may ↓ levels and effectiveness. May ↑ **rifabutin** levels and risk of toxicity; avoid concurrent use. **QT interval prolonging drugs** may ↑ risk for QT interval prolongation and torsades de pointes; avoid concurrent use. May ↑ **digoxin** levels and risk of toxicity; monitor levels frequently. May ↑ **phenytoin**, **midazolam**, **ritonavir**, and **atazanavir** levels and risk of toxicity; monitor for excess clinical effect. May ↑ levels of and risk of neurotoxicity, syndrome of inappropriate antidiuretic hormone, and paralytic ileus with concurrent use of **vinca alkaloids**, including **vincristine** and **vinblastine**; consider using an alternative nonazole antifungal. May ↑ levels and risk of adverse cardiovascular reactions to **calcium channel blockers**; consider dosage reduction.

Route/Dosage

The oral suspension is NOT interchangeable with delayed-release tablets.

Treatment of Invasive Aspergillosis

May switch between use of IV and delayed-release tablets (another loading dose is not needed when switching between formulations).

PO (Adults and Children ≥13 yr): *Delayed-release tablets:* 300 mg twice daily on Day 1; then 300 mg once daily starting on Day 2 for a total of 6–12 wk.

IV (Adults and Children ≥13 yr): 300 mg twice daily on Day 1; then 300 mg once daily starting on Day 2 for a total of 6–12 wk.

Prophylaxis of Invasive *Aspergillus* and *Candida* Infections

PO (Adults and Children ≥13 yr): *Oral suspension:* 200 mg 3 times daily. Duration of therapy is based on recovery from neutropenia or immunosuppression.

PO (Adults and Children ≥2 yr and >40 kg): *Delayed-release tablets:* 300 mg twice daily on Day 1; then 300 mg once daily starting on Day 2. Duration of therapy is based on recovery from neutropenia or immunosuppression.

IV (Adults): 300 mg twice daily on Day 1; then 300 mg once daily starting on Day 2. Duration of therapy is based on recovery from neutropenia or immunosuppression.

IV (Children ≥2 yr): 6 mg/kg (max = 300 mg) twice daily on Day 1; then 6 mg/kg (max = 300 mg) once daily starting on Day 2. Duration of therapy is based on recovery from neutropenia or immunosuppression.

Treatment of Oropharyngeal Candidiasis

PO (Adults and Children ≥13 yr): *Oral suspension:* 100 mg twice daily on Day 1; then 100 mg once daily for the next 13 days. For refractory oropharyngeal candidiasis, give 400 mg twice daily; duration of therapy is based on the severity of the patient's underlying disease and clinical response.

Availability (generic available)

Delayed-release tablets: 100 mg. **Oral suspension (cherry flavor):** 40 mg/mL. **Solution for injection:** 18 mg/mL.

NURSING IMPLICATIONS

Assessment

- Assess for previous allergies to antifungal medicines (ketoconazole, fluconazole, itraconazole, voriconazole).
- Assess for signs and symptoms of fungal infection. If severe diarrhea or vomiting occurs, monitor closely for breakthrough fungal infection.
- Assess for hypersensitivity reactions (rash; hives; swelling of mouth, face, lips, tongue, or throat).
- Assess cardiac status. Obtain baseline ECG and periodically during therapy to monitor for arrhythmias and QT interval prolongation in high-risk patients.

Lab Test Considerations

- Monitor liver function tests before and periodically during therapy. May ↑ ALT, AST, alkaline phosphatase, and total bilirubin levels; generally reversible on discontinuation. *If clinical signs and symptoms of liver disease develop,* permanently discontinue posaconazole.
- May cause pseudoaldosteronism (new or exacerbation of hypertension and abnormal laboratory tests). Monitor for ↓ aldosterone, ↑ 11-deoxycortisol, ↓ potassium, and ↓ serum renin. If these occur, discontinue therapy, switch to another antifungal, or use of an aldosterone receptor antagonist may be necessary.
- Monitor electrolyte levels (may ↓ potassium, magnesium, and calcium) before starting and during therapy. Correct as necessary before and during therapy.

Implementation

- Delayed-release tablet and oral suspension are not interchangeable. Tablets are the preferred oral formulation for prophylaxis because they achieve higher plasma concentrations of drug.

- **PO:** Administer delayed-release tablets with food. *DNC:* Swallow tablets whole; do not divide, crush, or chew.
- Shake suspension well before use. Use spoon provided to ensure accurate dose. Administer during or within 20 min of a full meal, liquid nutritional supplement, or acidic carbonated beverage (e.g., ginger ale) to ↑ absorption. Rinse spoon for administration with water after each use. Alternative therapy or close monitoring for breakthrough fungal infections should be considered for patients unable to eat a full meal or tolerate a nutritional supplement.

IV Administration

- **Intermittent Infusion:** Allow solution to reach room temperature before administering. **Dilution:** Dilute in D5W, D5/0.45% NaCl, D5/0.9% NaCl, D5/20 mEq potassium, 0.45% NaCl, or 0.9% NaCl. **Concentration:** 1–2 mg/mL. Do not dilute with other solutions. Use immediately; stable for 24 hr if refrigerated. Discard unused solution. Solution is clear, colorless to yellow; do not administer solutions that are discolored or contain particulate matter. Administer through a 0.22-micron polyethersulfone or polyvinylidene difluoride filter via central venous line, including a central venous catheter or peripherally inserted central catheter line. If no central catheter available, may be administered through a peripheral venous catheter by slow intravenous infusion over 30 min only as a single dose in advance of central venous line placement or to bridge the period during which a central venous line is replaced or is in use for other intravenous treatment. **Rate:** Infuse slowly over 90 min. Do not give as a bolus.
- **Y-Site Compatibility:** amikacin, caspofungin, ciprofloxacin, daptomycin, dobutamine, famotidine, filgrastim, gentamicin, hydromorphone, levofloxacin, lorazepam, meropenem, micafungin, morphine, norepinephrine, potassium chloride, vancomycin.
- **Y-Site Incompatibility:** acetaminophen, acyclovir, cefepime, cefiderocol, furosemide, ganciclovir, imipenem/cilastatin/relebactam, insulin aspart, levetiracetam, methylprednisolone, metoclopramide, ondansetron, pantoprazole, piperacillin/tazobactam.

Patient/Family Teaching

- Explain purpose and side effects of medication to patient. Advise patient to read *Patient Information* before starting therapy. Instruct patient to take during or immediately (within 20 min) following a full meal or liquid nutritional supplement in order to enhance absorption. Take missed doses as soon as remembered.
- Instruct patient to notify health care professional of all Rx or OTC medications, vitamins, or herbal products being taken and consult health care professional before taking any new medications.
- Advise patient to notify health care professional if severe diarrhea or vomiting occurs (may ↓ posaconazole levels and allow breakthrough fungal infections) or if signs and symptoms of liver injury (itching, yellow eyes or skin, fatigue, flu-like symptoms) or change in HR or rhythm occur.
- Emphasize the need for routine laboratory and BP monitoring before and during therapy.
- Rep: May cause fetal harm. Advise women of reproductive potential to notify health care professional if pregnancy is planned or suspected and to avoid breastfeeding during therapy.

Evaluation/Desired Outcomes

- Fungistatic/fungicidal action against susceptible fungi.

potassium and sodium phosphates

(po-**tas**-e-um/**soe**-dee-um **foss**-fates)

K-Phos Neutral, K-Phos No. 2

Classification

Therapeutic: antiurolithics, mineral and electrolyte replacements/supplements

Indications

Treatment and prevention of phosphate depletion in patients who are unable to ingest adequate dietary phosphate. Adjunct therapy of urinary tract infections with methenamine. Prevention of calcium urinary stones. Phosphate salts of potassium may be used in hypokalemic patients with metabolic acidosis or coexisting phosphorus deficiency.

Action

Phosphate is present in bone and is involved in energy transfer and carbohydrate metabolism. Serves as a buffer for the excretion of hydrogen ions by the kidneys. Dibasic potassium phosphate is converted in renal tubule to monobasic salt, resulting in urinary acidification, which is required for methenamine hippurate or mandelate to be active as urinary anti-infectives. Acidification of urine increases solubility of calcium, decreasing calcium stone formation. **Therapeutic Effects:** Replacement of phosphorus in deficiency states. Urinary acidification. Increased efficacy of methenamine. Decreased formation of calcium urinary tract stones.

Pharmacokinetics

Absorption: Well absorbed following oral administration. Vitamin D promotes GI absorption of phosphates.

P

Distribution: Phosphates enter extracellular fluids and are then actively transported to sites of action.
Metabolism and Excretion: Excreted mainly (>90%) by the kidneys.
Half-life: Unknown.

TIME/ACTION PROFILE (effects on serum phosphate concentrations)

ROUTE	ONSET	PEAK	DURATION
PO	unknown	unknown	unknown

Contraindications/Precautions
Contraindicated in: Hyperkalemia (potassium salts); Hyperphosphatemia; Hypocalcemia; Severe renal impairment; Untreated Addison's disease (potassium salts).
Use Cautiously in: Hyperparathyroidism; Cardiac disease; Hypernatremia (sodium phosphate only); Hypertension (sodium phosphate only); Mild or moderate renal impairment.

Adverse Reactions/Side Effects
Related to hyperphosphatemia, unless otherwise indicated
CV: ARRHYTHMIAS, bradycardia, CARDIAC ARREST, ECG changes (absent P waves, widening of the QRS complex with biphasic curve, peaked T waves), edema. **GI:** diarrhea, abdominal pain, nausea, vomiting. **F and E** hyperkalemia, hypernatremia, hyperphosphatemia, hypocalcemia, hypomagnesemia. **MS: hypocalcemia, hyperkalemia:** muscle cramps. **Neuro:** confusion, dizziness, flaccid paralysis, headache, heaviness of legs, paresthesias, tremor, weakness.

Interactions
Drug-Drug: Potassium-sparing diuretics, ACE inhibitors, or **angiotensin II receptor blockers** may result in hyperkalemia. **Corticosteroids** may result in hypernatremia. **Calcium-, magnesium-**, or **aluminum-containing compounds** ↓ absorption of phosphates by formation of insoluble complexes. **Vitamin D** enhances the absorption of phosphates.
Drug-Food: Oxalates (in spinach and rhubarb) and **phytates** (in bran and whole grains) may ↓ absorption of phosphates by binding them in the GI tract.

Route/Dosage
Phosphorous Supplementation
PO (Adults and Children >4 yr): 250–500 mg (8–16 mmol) phosphorus (1–2 packets) 4 times daily.
PO (Children <4 yr): 250 mg (8 mmol) phosphorus (1 packet) 4 times daily.

Urinary Acidification
PO (Adults): 2 tablets 4 times/day.

Maintenance Phosphorus
PO (Adults): 50–150 mmol/day in divided doses.
PO (Children): 2–3 mmol/kg/day in divided doses.

Availability
Potassium and Sodium Phosphates
Tablets (K-Phos Neutral): elemental phosphorus 250 mg (8 mmol), sodium 298 mg (13 mEq), and potassium 45 mg (1.1 mEq). **Tablets (K-Phos No.2):** elemental phosphorus 250 mg (8 mmol), sodium 134 mg (5.8 mEq), and potassium 88 mg (2.3 mEq). **Powder for oral solution:** elemental phosphorus 250 mg (8 mmol), sodium 164 mg (7.1 mEq), and potassium 278 mg (7.1 mEq)/packet.

NURSING IMPLICATIONS
Assessment
- Assess patient for signs/symptoms of hypokalemia (weakness, fatigue, arrhythmias, presence of U waves on ECG, polyuria, polydipsia) and hypophosphatemia (anorexia, weakness, ↓ reflexes, bone pain, confusion, blood dyscrasias) throughout therapy.
- Monitor HR, BP, and ECG periodically during therapy in patients with cardiac disease.
- Assess volume status before and during therapy, including intake, output, and daily weight. Correct as indicated.

Lab Test Considerations
- Assess serum potassium before initiating therapy when correcting hypophosphatemia. *If potassium ≥4 mEq/L,* use alternate form of phosphorus.
- Monitor phosphate, potassium, sodium, magnesium, and calcium before starting and periodically during therapy. Normalize calcium level before initiating therapy.
- Monitor renal function studies before starting and periodically throughout therapy.
- Monitor urinary pH in patients receiving potassium and sodium phosphate as a urinary acidifier.

Implementation
- **PO:** Tablets should be dissolved in a full glass of water. Allow mixture to stand for 2–5 min to ensure it is fully dissolved. Solutions prepared by pharmacy should not be further diluted.
- Administer after meals to minimize GI irritation and laxative effect.
- Do not administer simultaneously with antacids containing aluminum, magnesium, or calcium.

Patient/Family Teaching
- Explain purpose and side effects of medication. Advise patient to read *Patient Information* before starting therapy.
- Instruct patient to take missed dose as soon as remembered unless within 1 or 2 hr of next dose. Explain that the tablets should not be swallowed whole and should be dissolved in water.
- Advise patient to notify health care provider of all Rx or OTC medications, vitamins, or herbal products

being taken and to consult health care provider before taking other medications.

- Instruct patients in low-sodium diet (see Appendix J).
- Advise patient of importance of maintaining a high fluid intake (drinking at least one 8-ounce glass of water each hour) to prevent kidney stones.
- Instruct the patient to notify health care provider if diarrhea, weakness, fatigue, muscle cramps, unexplained weight gain, swelling of lower extremities, shortness of breath, unusual thirst, or tremors occurs.
- Rep: Advise women of reproductive potential to notify health care provider if pregnancy is planned or suspected or if breastfeeding.

Evaluation/Desired Outcomes

- Prevention and correction of serum phosphate and potassium deficiencies.
- Maintenance of acidic urine.
- Decreased urine calcium, which prevents formation of renal calculi.

HIGH ALERT

V potassium chloride

(poe-**tass**-ee-um **klor**-ide)

Klor-Con, Klor-Con M10, Klor-Con M15, Klor-Con M20, ~~K-Tab,~~ ✱ Micro-K, Pokonza, ~~Slow-K~~

Classification

Therapeutic: mineral and electrolyte replacements/supplements

Indications

Treatment/prevention of potassium depletion.

Action

Maintain acid-base balance, isotonicity, and electrophysiologic balance of the cell. Activator in many enzymatic reactions; essential to transmission of nerve impulses; contraction of cardiac, skeletal, and smooth muscle; gastric secretion; renal function; tissue synthesis; and carbohydrate metabolism.
Therapeutic Effects: Replacement. Prevention of deficiency.

Pharmacokinetics

Absorption: Well absorbed following oral administration. IV administration results in complete availability.
Distribution: Enters extracellular fluid; then actively transported into cells.
Metabolism and Excretion: Excreted by the kidneys.
Half-life: Unknown.

TIME/ACTION PROFILE (↑ in serum potassium concentrations)

ROUTE	ONSET	PEAK	DURATION
PO	unknown	1–2 hr	unknown
IV	rapid	end of infusion	unknown

Contraindications/Precautions

Contraindicated in: Hyperkalemia; Severe renal impairment; Untreated Addison's disease; Some oral products may contain tartrazine (FDC yellow dye #5) or alcohol; avoid using in patients with known hypersensitivity or intolerance; Hyperkalemic familial periodic paralysis.
Use Cautiously in: Cardiac disease; Renal impairment; Diabetes mellitus (liquids may contain sugar); Hypomagnesemia (may make correction of hypokalemia more difficult); GI hypomotility including dysphagia or esophageal compression from left atrial enlargement (tablets, capsules).

Adverse Reactions/Side Effects

CV: ARRHYTHMIAS, ECG changes. **F and E** hyperchloremia, hyperkalemia. **GI:** abdominal pain, diarrhea, flatulence, nausea, vomiting **tablets, capsules only:** GI ulceration, stenotic lesions. **Local:** irritation at IV site. **Neuro:** confusion, paralysis, paresthesia, restlessness, weakness.

Interactions

Drug-Drug: Potassium-sparing diuretics, **ACE inhibitors**, or **angiotensin II receptor antagonists** may lead to hyperkalemia. **Anticholinergics** may ↑ GI mucosal lesions in patients taking wax-matrix potassium chloride preparations.

Route/Dosage

Expressed as mEq of potassium.

Normal Daily Requirements

PO (Adults): 40–80 mEq/day.
PO (Children): 2–3 mEq/kg/day.
PO (Neonates): 2–6 mEq/kg/day.

Prevention of Hypokalemia During Diuretic Therapy

PO (Adults): 20–40 mEq/day in 1–2 divided doses; single dose should not exceed 20 mEq.
PO (Neonates, Infants and Children): 1–2 mEq/kg/day in 1–2 divided doses.

Treatment of Hypokalemia

PO (Adults): 40–100 mEq/day in divided doses.
PO (Neonates, Infants and Children): 2–5 mEq/kg/day in divided doses.
IV (Adults): 10–20 mEq/dose (maximum: 40 mEq/dose) to infuse over 2–3 hr (maximum infusion rate: 40 mEq/hr).

P

IV (Neonates, Infants and Children): 0.5–1 mEq/kg/dose (maximum 30 mEq/dose) as an infusion to infuse at 0.3–0.5 mEq/kg/hr (maximum infusion rate 1 mEq/kg/hr).

Availability

Extended-release capsules: 8 mEq, 10 mEq. **Extended-release tablets:** 8 mEq, 10 mEq, 15 mEq, 20 mEq. **Oral solution:** 20 mEq/15 mL, 40 mEq/15 mL. **Powder for oral solution:** 20 mEq/pkt. **Concentrate for injection:** 0.1 mEq/mL, 0.2 mEq/mL, 0.3 mEq/mL, 0.4 mEq/mL, 1.5 mEq/mL, 2 mEq/mL, 3 mEq/mL. **Solution for IV infusion:** 10 mEq/L in various dextrose and saline solutions in 250-, 500-, and 100-mL containers, 20 mEq/L in dextrose/saline/LR in 250-, 500-, and 100-mL containers, 30 mEq/L in various dextrose and saline solutions in 250-, 500-, and 100-mL containers, 40 mEq/L in various dextrose and saline solutions in 250-, 500-, and 100-mL containers.

NURSING IMPLICATIONS

Assessment

- Assess for signs/symptoms of hypokalemia (weakness, fatigue, U wave on ECG, arrhythmias, polyuria, polydipsia) and hyperkalemia before and during therapy.
- Monitor HR, BP, and ECG periodically during IV therapy.
- Assess volume status before and during therapy, including intake, output, and daily weight. Correct as indicated.

Lab Test Considerations

- Monitor serum potassium before and periodically during therapy. *If serum potassium <2.5 mEq/L,* use IV potassium instead of oral to replenish. *If hypokalemia is refractory,* check serum magnesium and correct hypomagnesemia.
- Monitor renal function, bicarbonate, calcium, chloride, magnesium, phosphate, sodium, and acid/base balance periodically during therapy. Correct values as indicated.

Toxicity and Overdose

- Signs/symptoms of toxicity are those of hyperkalemia, including bradycardia, irregular HR, fatigue, weakness, paresthesia, confusion, dyspnea, chest pain, and ECG changes (peaked T waves, depressed ST segments, prolonged QT interval, widened QRS complex, loss of P wave, arrhythmias).
- Treatment includes discontinuation of potassium, administration of sodium bicarbonate to correct acidosis, dextrose and insulin to facilitate passage of potassium into cells, calcium salts to reverse ECG effects (in patients who are not receiving digoxin), sodium polystyrene used as an exchange resin, and/or dialysis for patient with impaired renal function.

Implementation

- ***High Alert:*** Medication errors involving too rapid infusion or bolus IV administration of potassium chloride have resulted in fatalities.
- Patients with renal tubular acidosis (hyperchloremic acidosis) may require other salts (potassium bicarbonate, potassium citrate, potassium gluconate).
- If hypokalemia is secondary to diuretic therapy, consider ↓ diuretic dose, unless there is a history of significant arrhythmia or concurrent digoxin therapy.
- **PO:** Administer with or after meals to ↓ GI irritation.
- Use of tablets and capsules should be reserved for patients who cannot tolerate liquid preparations. Capsules can be opened and sprinkled on soft food (pudding, applesauce) and swallowed immediately with a glass of water or juice. ***DNC:*** Do not chew or crush enteric-coated or extended-release tablets or capsules.
- Dissolve effervescent tablets in 3–8 ounces of cold water. Ensure that effervescent tablet is fully dissolved. Powders and solutions should be diluted in 4–8 ounces of cold water or juice. Instruct patient to drink slowly over 5–10 min.

IV Administration

- **IV:** ***High Alert:*** Never administer potassium IV push or bolus (may cause fatal cardiac arrest). Potassium must be diluted prior to IV administration. In general, the dose, concentration of infusion, and rate of administration may be dependent on patient condition/indication and specific institution policy.
- **V** Potassium chloride is a vesicant (at concentrations >0.1 mEq/mL). If extravasation occurs, immediately stop infusion. Leave needle/cannula in place temporarily but do not flush the line. Gently aspirate extravasated solution; then remove needle/cannula. Elevate patient's extremity and apply dry warm compresses. Initiate hyaluronidase antidote for refractory cases in addition to supportive management. For hyaluronidase, inject a total of 1 mL (150 units/mL) intradermally or SUBQ as five separate 0.2-mL injections (using a tuberculin syringe) around the site of extravasation; if IV catheter remains in place, administer IV through the infiltrated catheter; may repeat in 30–60 min if no resolution.
- **Continuous Infusion:** ***High Alert:*** Do not administer concentrations ≥1.5 mEq/mL undiluted; may cause cardiac arrest. Concentrated products have black caps on vials or black stripes above constriction on ampules and are labeled with a warning about dilution requirement. Each single dose must be diluted and thoroughly mixed in 100–1000 mL of IV solution. Usually limited to 80 mEq/L via peripheral line or 200 mEq/L via central line.
- Concentrations of 0.1 and 0.4 mEq/mL are intended for administration via calibrated infusion device and do not require dilution. **Rate:** ***High Alert:*** Infuse slowly, at a rate up to 10 mEq/hr in adults or 0.5 mEq/kg/hr in children in general care areas. Check hospital policy for maximum infusion rates (maximum rate in monitored setting is 40 mEq/hr in adults or 1 mEq/kg/hr in children in a peripheral line. May use higher concentrations via central line). Use an infusion pump.

- **Solution Compatibility:** May be diluted in D5W, D10W, D5/LR, D5/0.9% NaCl, D5/0.45% NaCl, 0.9% NaCl, 0.45% 0.9% NaCl, and LR. Available premixed with many of the above IV solutions.
- **Y-Site Compatibility:** acetaminophen, acyclovir, alemtuzumab, allopurinol, alprostadil, amikacin, aminocaproic acid, aminophylline, amphotericin B liposomal, anidulafungin, argatroban, arsenic trioxide, ascorbic acid, atracurium, atropine, azathioprine, aztreonam, benztropine, bivalirudin, bleomycin, bumetanide, buprenorphine, butorphanol, calcium gluconate, cangrelor, carboplatin, carmustine, caspofungin, cefazolin, cefiderocol, cefotaxime, cefotetan, cefoxitin, ceftaroline, ceftazidime, ceftazidime/avibactam, ceftobiprole, ceftolozane/tazobactam, ceftriaxone, cefuroxime, chlorothiazide, chlorpromazine, ciprofloxacin, cisatracurium, cisplatin, cladribine, clevidipine, clindamycin, cyanocobalamin, cyclophosphamide, cyclosporine, cytarabine, dacarbazine, dactinomycin, daptomycin, daunorubicin, dexamethasone, dexmedetomidine, dexrazoxane, digoxin, diltiazem, diphenhydramine, dobutamine, docetaxel, dopamine, doxorubicin hydrochloride, doxorubicin liposomal, doxycycline, edetate calcium disodium, enalaprilat, ephedrine, epinephrine, epirubicin, epoetin alfa, eptifibatide, ertapenem, erythromycin, esmolol, etoposide, etoposide phosphate, famotidine, fentanyl, filgrastim, fluconazole, fludarabine, folic acid, foscarnet, fosphenytoin, furosemide, ganciclovir, gemcitabine, gemtuzumab ozogamicin, gentamicin, glycopyrrolate, granisetron, heparin, hydrocortisone, hydromorphone, ibuprofen lysine, idarubicin, ifosfamide, imipenem/cilastatin, indomethacin, insulin aspart, insulin regular, irinotecan, isavuconazonium, isoproterenol, ketamine, ketorolac, labetalol, letermovir, leucovorin, levofloxacin, lidocaine, linezolid, lorazepam, magnesium sulfate, mannitol, melphalan, meperidine, meropenem, meropenem/vaborbactam, mesna, methadone, methohexital, methotrexate, methylprednisolone, metoclopramide, metoprolol, metronidazole, micafungin, midazolam, milrinone, mitomycin, mitoxantrone, morphine, moxifloxacin, multivitamin, mycophenolate, nafcillin, nalbuphine, naloxone, nicardipine, nitroglycerin, nitroprusside, norepinephrine, octreotide, omadacycline, ondansetron, oritavancin, oxacillin, oxaliplatin, oxytocin, paclitaxel, palonosetron, pamidronate, pantoprazole, papaverine, pemetrexed, penicillin G, pentobarbital, phenobarbital, phentolamine, phenylephrine, phytonadione, piperacillin/tazobactam, plazomicin, posaconazole, potassium acetate, procainamide, prochlorperazine, promethazine, propofol, propranolol, protamine, pyridoxine, remifentanil, rituximab, rocuronium, sargramostim, sodium acetate, sodium bicarbonate, succinylcholine, sufentanil, sulbactam/durlobactam, tacrolimus, tedizolid, telavancin, theophylline, thiamine, thiotepa, tigecycline, tirofiban, tobramycin, topotecan, trastuzumab, vancomycin, vasopressin, vecuronium, verapamil, vinblastine, vincristine, vinorelbine, voriconazole, zidovudine, zoledronic acid.
- **Y-Site Incompatibility:** amphotericin B deoxycholate, blinatumomab, dantrolene, diazepam, diazoxide, dimenhydrinate, haloperidol, pentamidine, phenytoin, trimethoprim/sulfamethoxazole.

Patient/Family Teaching

- Explain purpose and side effects of medication. Advise patient to read *Patient Information* before starting therapy.
- Explain that a missed dose should be taken as soon as remembered within 2 hr or omit and return to regular schedule. Do not double dose.
- Advise patient to notify health care provider of all Rx or OTC medications, vitamins, or herbal products being taken and to consult health care provider before taking other medications.
- Advise patient to notify health care provider if GI irritation or ulceration (nausea, vomiting, flatulence, abdominal pain, diarrhea) occurs.
- Advise patient to notify health care provider for signs and symptoms of hypokalemia (fatigue, constipation, palpitations, difficulty breathing) and hyperkalemia (abdominal pain, diarrhea, nausea, vomiting, chest pain, irregular heartbeat, extremity weakness or numbness).
- Caution patient to avoid salt substitutes or low-salt milk or food unless approved by health care provider. Patient should be advised to read all labels to prevent excess potassium intake.
- Advise patient regarding sources of dietary potassium (see Appendix J). Encourage compliance with recommended diet.
- Emphasize the importance of regular follow-up exams to monitor serum levels and progress.
- Rep: Advise women of reproductive potential to notify health care provider if pregnancy is planned or suspected or if breastfeeding.

Evaluation/Desired Outcomes

- Prevention and correction of serum potassium depletion.

pramipexole (pra-mi-pex-ole)

✱ Mirapex

Classification

Therapeutic: antiparkinson agents

Pharmacologic: dopamine agonists

Indications

Parkinson disease. Restless leg syndrome (immediate release only).

Action

Stimulates dopamine receptors in the striatum of the brain. **Therapeutic Effects:** Decreased tremor and rigidity in Parkinson disease. Decreased leg restlessness.

Pharmacokinetics

Absorption: >90% absorbed following oral administration.

Distribution: Widely distributed.

Metabolism and Excretion: 90% excreted unchanged in urine.

Half-life: 8 hr (↑ in older adults and patients with renal impairment).

TIME/ACTION PROFILE (plasma concentrations)

ROUTE	ONSET	PEAK	DURATION
PO	unknown	2 hr	8 hr
PO-ER	unknown	6 hr	24 hr

Contraindications/Precautions

Contraindicated in: Hypersensitivity; Major psychotic disorder; Impulsive control/compulsive behaviors.

Use Cautiously in: Renal impairment (↑ dosing interval if CCr <60 mL/min [immediate release] or CCr <50 mL/min [extended release]); OB: Safety not established in pregnancy; Lactation: Use while breastfeeding only if potential maternal benefit justifies potential risk to infant; may inhibit lactation; Pedi: Safety and effectiveness not established in children.

Adverse Reactions/Side Effects

CV: orthostatic hypotension. **Derm:** pruritus. **Endo:** syndrome of inappropriate antidiuretic hormone. **GI:** constipation, dry mouth, dyspepsia, nausea. **GU:** urinary frequency. **MS:** leg cramps, muscle pain, postural deformities, RHABDOMYOLYSIS. **Neuro:** amnesia, dizziness, drowsiness, hallucinations, weakness, abnormal dreams, aggression, agitation, confusion, delirium, delusions, disorientation, dyskinesia, extrapyramidal syndrome, headache, hypertonia, impulse control disorders (gambling, sexual, uncontrolled spending, binge/compulsive eating), insomnia, paranoid ideation, psychosis, SLEEP ATTACKS, unsteadiness/falling. **Misc:** tooth disease.

Interactions

Drug-Drug: Levodopa may ↑ risk of hallucinations and dyskinesia. **Cimetidine, diltiazem, triamterene, verapamil, quinidine, quinine,** and **cisplatin** may ↑ levels and risk of toxicity. **Dopamine antagonists,** including **butyrophenones, metoclopramide, phenothiazines,** or **thioxanthenes,** may ↓ effectiveness.

Route/Dosage

When switching from immediate-release to extended-release product, the same total daily dose can be used.

Parkinson Disease

PO (Adults): *Immediate release:* 0.125 mg 3 times daily initially; may ↑ every 5–7 days (range 1.5–4.5 mg/day in 3 divided doses); *Extended release:* 0.375 mg once daily; may ↑ to 0.75 mg once daily in 5–7 days, and then ↑ every 5–7 days by 0.75 mg/day (max dose = 4.5 mg/day).

Renal Impairment

PO (Adults Immediate release): *CCr 35–59 mL/min:* 0.125 mg twice daily initially; may ↑ every 5–7 days up to 1.5 mg twice daily; *CCr 15–34 mL/min:* 0.125 mg daily initially; may ↑ every 5–7 days up to 1.5 mg daily.

Renal Impairment

PO (Adults Extended release): *CCr 30–50 mL/min:* 0.375 mg every other day; may consider ↑ dose to 0.375 mg once daily after 1 wk based on response and tolerability; may ↑ in 0.375 mg increments after 1 wk (max dose = 2.25 mg/day).

Restless Leg Syndrome

PO (Adults): 0.125 mg daily 1–3 hr before bedtime. May be ↑ at 4–7 day intervals to 0.25 mg daily and then up to 0.5 mg daily.

Renal Impairment

PO (Adults Immediate release): *CCr 20–60 mL/min:* 0.125 mg daily 1–3 hr before bedtime. May ↑ at 14-day intervals to 0.25 mg daily and then up to 0.5 mg daily.

Availability (generic available)

Immediate-release tablets: 0.125 mg, 0.25 mg, 0.5 mg, 0.75 mg, 1 mg, 1.5 mg. **Extended-release tablets:** 0.375 mg, 0.75 mg, 1.5 mg, 2.25 mg, 3 mg, 3.75 mg, 4.5 mg.

NURSING IMPLICATIONS

Assessment

- Assess patient for signs/symptoms of psychosis (confusion, paranoid ideation, delusions, hallucinations, disorientation, aggression, agitation, delirium) and impulsive behavior. Risk of symptoms ↑ with age.
- Monitor ECG, BP, HR and for other signs of orthostatic hypotension frequently during dose adjustment and periodically during therapy.
- Assess patient for drowsiness, sleep disorders, and concurrent use of sedating medications or alcohol. *If significant daytime sleepiness or falling asleep during activities that require active participation occurs,* pramipexole may be discontinued.
- **Parkinson Disease:** Assess patient for signs/symptoms of Parkinson disease (tremor, muscle weakness and rigidity, ataxia) before and throughout therapy.
- **Restless Leg Syndrome:** Assess sleep patterns and frequency of restless leg disturbances.

Lab Test Considerations

- Assess renal function prior to initiation.

Implementation

- An attempt to ↓ dose of levodopa/carbidopa may be made cautiously during pramipexole therapy.
- Taper or discontinuation may cause withdrawal symptoms (apathy, anxiety, depression, fatigue, insomnia, sweating, pain); symptoms do not respond to levodopa. Consider readministration of pramipexole at lowest dose.
- **PO:** Administer with meals to minimize nausea; usually resolves with continued therapy. ***DNC:*** Swallow extended-release tablets whole; do not crush, break, or chew.

Patient/Family Teaching

- Explain purpose and side effects of medication. Advise patient to read *Patient Information* before starting therapy.
- Instruct patient to take missed dose or immediate-release product as soon as remembered if it is not almost time for next dose. If extended release tablet missed, skip dose and take next scheduled dose. Do not double doses. Consult health care provider before ↓ dose or discontinuing medication.
- May cause drowsiness and unexpected episodes of falling asleep. Caution patient to avoid driving or other activities requiring alertness until response to medication is known and to notify health care provider if episodes of falling asleep occur.
- Advise patient to notify health care provider if dyskinesia or postural deformities occur.
- Advise patient to notify health care provider if unexplained muscle pain, tenderness, weakness, or other signs of rhabdomyolysis occurs.
- Advise patient to change position slowly to minimize dizziness from orthostatic hypotension. May occur more frequently during initial therapy.
- Instruct patient to notify health care provider of all Rx or OTC medications, vitamins, or herbal products being taken and consult health care provider before taking any new medications.
- Advise patient to notify health care provider if new or ↑ gambling, sexual, or other intense urges or psychotic-like behaviors occur.
- Rep: Advise women of reproductive potential to notify health care provider if pregnancy is planned or suspected or if breastfeeding. Pramipexole may inhibit lactation.

Evaluation/Desired Outcomes

- Decreased tremor and rigidity in Parkinson disease.
- Decrease in restless legs and improved sleep.

prasterone (pras-ter-one)

Intrarosa

Classification

Therapeutic: none assigned

Pharmacologic: steroids

Indications

Moderate to severe dyspareunia due to menopause.

Action

Inactive steroid that is converted into active androgens and/or estrogens. Exact mechanism in treatment of vulvar and vaginal atrophy in menopausal women not fully established. **Therapeutic Effects:** Reduced severity of dyspareunia.

Pharmacokinetics

Absorption: Unknown.

Distribution: Unknown.

Metabolism and Excretion: Metabolized via dehydrogenase, reductase, and aromatase to estradiol and testosterone.

Half-life: Unknown.

TIME/ACTION PROFILE (↓ in severity of dyspareunia)

ROUTE	ONSET	PEAK	DURATION
Vag	unknown	12 wk	unknown

Contraindications/Precautions

Contraindicated in: Undiagnosed abnormal genital bleeding; Current or history of breast cancer.

Use Cautiously in: None reported.

Adverse Reactions/Side Effects

GU: vaginal discharge.

Interactions

Drug-Drug: None reported.

Route/Dosage

Vag (Adults): Insert one vaginal insert at bedtime.

Availability

Vaginal insert: 6.5 mg.

NURSING IMPLICATIONS

Assessment

- Assess for pain during intercourse periodically during therapy.
- Assess for current or history of breast cancer prior to use.

Implementation

- **Vag:** Insert vaginal insert at bedtime using applicator provided. Vaginal inserts can be stored at room temperature or refrigerated.

Patient/Family Teaching

- Explain purpose and side effects of medication. Advise patient to read *Patient Information* before starting therapy.

P

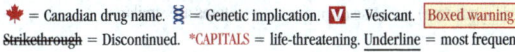

- Inform patient that vaginal discharge and abnormal PAP smear findings may occur with therapy.
- Advise patient to notify health care provider of all Rx or OTC medications, vitamins, or herbal products being taken and to consult with health care provider before taking other medications during therapy.

Evaluation/Desired Outcomes

- Decreased pain during intercourse.

pravastatin, See HMG-CoA REDUCTASE INHIBITORS (statins).

BEERS

prazosin (pra-zoe-sin)

~~Minipress~~

Classification

Therapeutic: antihypertensives

Pharmacologic: peripherally acting antiadrenergics

Indications

Mild to moderate hypertension. **Unlabeled Use:** Urinary outflow obstruction in patients with benign prostatic hyperplasia.

Action

Dilates both arteries and veins by blocking postsynaptic $alpha_1$-adrenergic receptors. Decreases contractions in smooth muscle of prostatic capsule. **Therapeutic Effects:** Lowering of BP. Decreased symptoms of prostatic hyperplasia (urinary urgency, urinary hesitancy, nocturia).

Pharmacokinetics

Absorption: 60% absorbed following oral administration.
Distribution: Widely distributed to tissues.
Protein Binding: 97%.
Metabolism and Excretion: Extensively metabolized by the liver. Minimal (5–10%) renal excretion of unchanged drug.
Half-life: 2–3 hr.

TIME/ACTION PROFILE (antihypertensive effects)

ROUTE	ONSET	PEAK	DURATION
PO	2 hr	2–4 hr†	10 hr

† Following single dose; maximal antihypertensive effects occur after 3–4 wk of chronic dosing.

Contraindications/Precautions

Contraindicated in: Hypersensitivity.
Use Cautiously in: Renal impairment (↑ sensitivity to effects; dose ↓ may be required); Angina; Patients undergoing cataract surgery (↑ risk of intraoperative floppy iris syndrome); OB: Use during pregnancy only if potential maternal benefit justifies potential fetal risk; other antihypertensives preferred in pregnancy; Lactation: Use while breastfeeding only if potential maternal benefit justifies potential risk to infant; Pedi: Safety and effectiveness not established in children; Geri: Appears on Beers list. ↑ risk of orthostatic hypotension in older adults. Avoid use for treatment of hypertension in older adults.

Adverse Reactions/Side Effects

CV: first-dose orthostatic hypotension, palpitations, angina, edema, syncope. **EENT:** blurred vision, intraoperative floppy iris syndrome. **GI:** abdominal cramps, diarrhea, dry mouth, nausea, vomiting. **GU:** erectile dysfunction, priapism. **Neuro:** dizziness, headache, weakness, depression, drowsiness.

Interactions

Drug-Drug: Additive hypotension with acute ingestion of **alcohol**, other **antihypertensives**, or **nitrates**. Antihypertensive effects may be ↓ by **NSAIDs**.

Route/Dosage

Hypertension

PO (Adults): 1 mg 2–3 times daily (give 1st dose at bedtime) for initial 3 days of therapy; then ↑ gradually to maintenance dose of 6–15 mg/day in 2–3 divided doses (not to exceed 20–40 mg/day).

Benign Prostatic Hyperplasia

PO (Adults): 1–5 mg twice daily.

Availability (generic available)

Capsules: 1 mg, 2 mg, 5 mg. **Tablets:** 🍁 1 mg, 🍁 2 mg, 🍁 5 mg.

NURSING IMPLICATIONS

Assessment

- Assess for first-dose orthostatic reaction (dizziness, weakness) and syncope. May occur 30 min–2 hr after initial dose and occasionally thereafter. Incidence may be dose related. Volume-depleted or sodium-restricted patients may be more sensitive. Observe patient closely during this period; take precautions to prevent injury. First dose may be given at bedtime to minimize this reaction.
- Monitor intake, output, and daily weight; assess for edema daily, especially at beginning of therapy.
- **Hypertension:** Monitor BP and HR frequently during initial dose adjustment and periodically during therapy. Report significant changes.
- **Benign Prostatic Hyperplasia:** Assess for symptoms of prostatic hyperplasia (urinary hesitancy, feeling of incomplete bladder emptying, interruption of urinary stream, impairment of size and force of urinary stream, terminal urinary dribbling, straining to start flow, dysuria, urgency) before and periodically during therapy.
- Rule out prostatic carcinoma before therapy; symptoms are similar.

Lab Test Considerations
- May ↑ BUN and creatinine.
- May ↓ sodium and potassium.

Implementation
- May be used in combination with diuretics or beta blockers to minimize sodium and water retention. If these are added to prazosin therapy, ↓ dose of prazosin initially and titrate to effect.
- **PO:** Administer daily dose at bedtime, without regards to meals, at the same time each day. If necessary, dose may be ↑ to twice daily.

Patient/Family Teaching
- Explain purpose and side effects of medication. Advise patient to read *Patient Information* before starting therapy. Instruct patient to take medication at the same time each day. Take missed doses as soon as remembered. If not remembered until next day, omit; do not double doses.
- Advise patient to notify health care provider of all Rx or OTC medications, vitamins, or herbal products being taken and to consult with health care provider before taking other medications, especially NSAIDs and cough, cold, or allergy remedies.
- Advise patient to weigh self twice weekly and assess feet and ankles for fluid retention.
- May cause dizziness or drowsiness. Advise patient to avoid driving or other activities requiring alertness until response to the medication is known.
- Caution patient to avoid sudden changes in position to ↓ orthostatic hypotension. Alcohol, CNS depressants, standing for long periods, hot showers, and exercising in hot weather should be avoided because of enhanced orthostatic effects.
- Instruct patient to notify health care provider of medication regimen before any surgery.
- Advise patient to notify health care provider immediately if erection lasts ≥4 hr or if frequent dizziness, fainting, or swelling of feet or lower legs occurs.
- Rep: Advise women of reproductive potential to notify health care provider if pregnancy is planned or suspected or if breastfeeding.
- **Hypertension:** Emphasize the importance of continuing to take this medication as directed, even if feeling well. Medication controls but does not cure hypertension.
- Encourage patient to comply with additional interventions for hypertension (weight reduction, low-sodium diet, smoking cessation, moderation of alcohol consumption, regular exercise, stress management).
- Instruct patient and caregivers on proper technique for BP monitoring. Advise them to check BP at least weekly and to report significant changes.

Evaluation/Desired Outcomes
- Lowering of BP.
- Decreased symptoms of prostatic hyperplasia (urinary urgency, urinary hesitancy, nocturia).

prednisoLONE, See CORTICOSTEROIDS (SYSTEMIC).

prednisONE, See CORTICOSTEROIDS (SYSTEMIC).

pregabalin (pre-gab-a-lin)
Lyrica, Lyrica CR

Classification
Therapeutic: analgesics, anticonvulsants
Pharmacologic: gamma aminobutyric acid (GABA) analogues, nonopioid analgesics

Schedule V

Indications
Immediate release and extended release: Treatment of the following conditions: Neuropathic pain associated with diabetic peripheral neuropathy, Postherpetic neuralgia. **Immediate release:** Treatment of the following conditions: Fibromyalgia, Neuropathic pain associated with spinal cord injury, Partial-onset seizures (adjunctive therapy).

Action
Binds to calcium channels in CNS tissues that regulate neurotransmitter release. Does not bind to opioid receptors. **Therapeutic Effects:** Decreased neuropathic or postherpetic pain. Decreased partial-onset seizures.

Pharmacokinetics
Absorption: Well absorbed (>90%) following oral administration.
Distribution: Well distributed to tissues; probably crosses the blood-brain barrier.
Metabolism and Excretion: Minimally metabolized; 90% excreted unchanged in urine.
Half-life: 6 hr.

TIME/ACTION PROFILE (↓ postherpetic pain)

ROUTE	ONSET	PEAK	DURATION
PO	unknown	2–4 wk	unknown

Contraindications/Precautions
Contraindicated in: Hypersensitivity; Known/suspected myopathy; Severe renal impairment (extended release only); Lactation: Lactation.

Use Cautiously in: All patients (may ↑ risk of suicidal thoughts/behaviors); Renal impairment (↓ dose if CCr <60 mL/min); HF; History of drug dependence/drug-seeking behavior; Respiratory impairment (↑ risk of respiratory depression); OB: Safety not established in pregnancy; Pedi: Children <1 mo (safety and effectiveness not established); Geri: Consider age-related ↓ in renal function when determining dose in older adults.

Adverse Reactions/Side Effects

CV: peripheral edema, PR interval prolongation. **Derm:** bullous pemphigoid, STEVENS-JOHNSON SYNDROME. **EENT:** blurred vision, double vision, vertigo. **GI:** dry mouth, abdominal pain, constipation, diarrhea, nausea, vomiting. **Hemat:** thrombocytopenia. **Metab:** ↑ appetite, weight gain. **MS:** ↑ CK. **Neuro:** dizziness, drowsiness, headache, impaired attention/concentration/thinking, SUICIDAL THOUGHTS/BEHAVIORS. **Resp:** RESPIRATORY DEPRESSION. **Misc:** fever, HYPERSENSITIVITY REACTIONS (INCLUDING ANGIOEDEMA).

Interactions

Drug-Drug: Pioglitazone may ↑ risk of fluid retention. ↑ risk of CNS and respiratory depression with other **CNS depressants**, including **opioids**, **alcohol**, **benzodiazepines**, or other **sedatives/hypnotics**.

Route/Dosage

Diabetic Neuropathic Pain

PO (Adults): *Immediate release:* 50 mg 3 times daily; ↑ over 7 days up to 100 mg 3 times daily. *Extended release:* 165 mg once daily after an evening meal; ↑ to 330 mg once daily after an evening meal within 1 wk.

Renal Impairment

PO (Adults): *CCr 30–60 mL/min:* Immediate release: 75–300 mg/day in 2–3 divided doses; Extended release: 82.5–330 mg once daily after an evening meal; *CCr 15–30 mL/min:* Immediate release: 25–150 mg/day in 1–2 divided doses; *CCr <15 mL/min:* Immediate release: 25–75 mg/day as a single daily dose.

Postherpetic Neuralgia

PO (Adults): *Immediate release:* 75 mg twice daily or 50 mg 3 times daily initially; may ↑ over 7 days to 300 mg/day in 2–3 divided doses; after 2–4 wk may ↑ to 600 mg/day in 2–3 divided doses. *Extended release:* 165 mg once daily after an evening meal; ↑ to 330 mg once daily after an evening meal within 1 wk; if pain is persistent after 2–4 wk, may then ↑ dose of up to 660 mg once daily after an evening meal.

Renal Impairment

PO (Adults): *CCr 30–60 mL/min:* Immediate release: 75–300 mg/day in 2–3 divided doses; Extended release: 82.5–330 mg once daily after an evening meal; *CCr 15–30 mL/min:* Immediate release: 25–150 mg/day in 1–2 divided doses; *CCr <15 mL/min:* Immediate release: 25–75 mg/day as a single daily dose.

Fibromyalgia

PO (Adults): *Immediate release:* 75 mg twice daily initially; may ↑ to 150 mg twice daily within 1 wk based on efficacy and tolerability. May ↑ to 225 twice daily.

Renal Impairment

PO (Adults): *CCr 30–60 mL/min:* Immediate release: 75–300 mg/day in 2–3 divided doses *CCr 15–30 mL/min:* Immediate release: 25–150 mg/day in 1–2 divided doses; *CCr <15 mL/min:* Immediate release: 25–75 mg/day as a single daily dose.

Spinal Cord Injury Neuropathic Pain

PO (Adults): *Immediate release:* 75 mg twice daily initially; may ↑ to 150 mg twice daily within 1 wk based on efficacy and tolerability; if insufficient pain relief after 2–3 wk, may ↑ to 300 twice daily.

Renal Impairment

PO (Adults): *CCr 30–60 mL/min:* Immediate release: 75–300 mg/day in 2–3 divided doses; *CCr 15–30 mL/min:* Immediate release: 25–150 mg/day in 1–2 divided doses; *CCr <15 mL/min:* Immediate release: 25–75 mg/day as a single daily dose.

Partial Onset Seizures

PO (Adults): *Immediate release:* 75 mg twice daily or 50 mg 3 times daily initially; may gradually ↑ on a weekly basis up to a max dose of 600 mg/day (in 2–3 divided doses).

PO (Children ≥1 mo and ≥30 kg): *Immediate release:* 2.5 mg/kg/day in 2–3 divided doses; may gradually ↑ on a weekly basis up to a max dose of 10 mg/kg/day in 2–3 divided doses (max = 600 mg/day).

PO (Children ≥1 mo and <30 kg): *Immediate release:* 3.5 mg/kg/day in 2–3 divided doses for patients ≥4 yr old or in 3 divided doses for patients 1 mo–<4 yr old; may gradually ↑ on a weekly basis up to a max dose of 14 mg/kg/day in 2–3 divided doses for patients ≥4 yr old or in 3 divided doses for patients 1 mo–<4 yr old.

Renal Impairment

PO (Adults): *CCr 30–60 mL/min:* Immediate release: 75–300 mg/day in 2–3 divided doses; *CCr 15–30 mL/min:* Immediate release: 25–150 mg/day in 1–2 divided doses; *CCr <15 mL/min:* Immediate release: 25–75 mg/day as a single daily dose.

Availability (generic available)

Immediate-release capsules: 25 mg, 50 mg, 75 mg, 100 mg, 150 mg, 200 mg, 225 mg, 300 mg. **Extended-release tablets:** 82.5 mg, 165 mg, 330 mg. **Oral solution:** 20 mg/mL.

NURSING IMPLICATIONS

Assessment

- Monitor closely for notable changes in behavior that could indicate the emergence or worsening of suicidal thoughts or behavior or depression.

- Monitor for hypersensitivity reactions (angioedema, hives, dyspnea, wheezing). Discontinue immediately and implement supportive measures if indicated.
- Monitor for respiratory depression (respiratory rate and oxygen saturation). Implement supportive measures if needed.
- **Diabetic Peripheral Neuropathy, Postherpetic Neuralgia, Fibromyalgia, and Spinal Cord Injury Pain:** Assess location, characteristics, and intensity of pain periodically during therapy.
- **Seizures:** Assess location, duration, and characteristics of seizure activity.

Lab Test Considerations

- May ↑ CK.
- May ↓ platelets.

Implementation

- Do not confuse Lyrica with Lopressor or Hydrea.
- Pregabalin should be discontinued gradually over ≥1 wk. Abrupt discontinuation may cause insomnia, nausea, headache, anxiety, sweating, and diarrhea when used for pain and may cause ↑ in seizure frequency when treating seizures.
- **PO:** May be administered without regard to meals. Oral solution may be stored at room temperature.

Patient/Family Teaching

- Explain purpose and side effects of medication. Advise patient to read *Patient Information* before starting therapy. Instruct patient to take medication as directed. Take missed doses as soon as remembered unless almost time for next dose; do not double doses. Do not discontinue abruptly.
- Advise patient to notify health care provider of all Rx or OTC medications, vitamins, or herbal products being taken and to consult with health care provider before taking other medications.
- May cause dizziness, drowsiness, and blurred vision. Caution patient to avoid driving or activities requiring alertness until response to medication is known. Advise patient to notify health care provider if changes in vision occur. Patients with seizures should not resume driving until health care provider gives clearance based on control of seizure disorder.
- Instruct patient to promptly report unexplained muscle pain, tenderness, or weakness, especially if accompanied by malaise or fever. Discontinue therapy if myopathy is diagnosed or suspected or if ↑ CK levels occur.
- Advise patient and caregiver to notify health care provider if thoughts about suicide or dying, attempts to commit suicide, new or worse depression, new or worse anxiety, feeling very agitated or restless, panic attacks, trouble sleeping, new or worse irritability, acting aggressive, being angry or violent, acting on dangerous impulses, an extreme ↑ in activity and talking, or other unusual changes in behavior or mood occur.
- Inform patient that pregabalin may cause edema and weight gain.
- Advise patient to notify health care provider if hypersensitivity reactions, respiratory depression, or rash occurs. Advise to seek immediate medical attention if needed.
- Caution patient to avoid alcohol or other CNS depressants, including opioids, with pregabalin; may cause respiratory depression and overdose.
- Instruct patient to notify health care provider of medication regimen before treatment or surgery.
- Advise patient to carry identification describing disease process and medication regimen at all times.
- Rep: Advise women of reproductive potential to notify health care provider if pregnancy is planned or suspected and to avoid breastfeeding during therapy. May impair male fertility. Encourage patients who become pregnant to enroll in the NAAED Pregnancy Registry by calling 1-800-233-2334 or visiting https://www.aedpregnancyregistry.org/.

Evaluation/Desired Outcomes

- Decreased neuropathic or postherpetic pain.
- Decreased partial-onset seizures.

P

prochlorperazine

(proe-klor-**pair**-a-zeen)

~~Compazine~~, Compro, ✱ Prochlorazine

Classification

Therapeutic: antiemetics, antipsychotics

Pharmacologic: phenothiazines

Indications

Nausea and vomiting.

Action

Alters the effects of dopamine in the CNS. Possesses significant anticholinergic and alpha-adrenergic blocking activity. Depresses the chemoreceptor trigger zone in the CNS. **Therapeutic Effects:** Diminished nausea and vomiting.

Pharmacokinetics

Absorption: Absorption from tablet is variable; may be better with oral liquid formulations. Well absorbed after IM administration.
Distribution: Widely distributed; high concentrations in the CNS.
Protein Binding: ≥90%.
Metabolism and Excretion: Highly metabolized by the liver and GI mucosa.
Half-life: Unknown.

TIME/ACTION PROFILE (antiemetic effect)

ROUTE	ONSET	PEAK	DURATION
PO	30–40 min	unknown	3–4 hr
Rect	60 min	unknown	3–4 hr
IM	10–20 min	10–30 min	3–4 hr
IV	rapid (min)	10–30 min	3–4 hr

Contraindications/Precautions

Contraindicated in: Hypersensitivity; Cross-sensitivity with other phenothiazines may exist; Angle-closure glaucoma; Bone marrow depression; Severe liver or cardiovascular disease; Hypersensitivity to bisulfites or benzyl alcohol (some parenteral products); Pedi: Children <2 yr or <9.1 kg.

Use Cautiously in: Diabetes mellitus; Respiratory disease; Prostatic hypertrophy; CNS tumors; Seizure disorder; Intestinal obstruction; At risk for falls; History of breast cancer; OB: Safety not established in pregnancy; Lactation: Safety not established in breastfeeding; Geri: Dose ↓ recommended; ↑ risk of mortality in older adults treated for dementia-related psychosis.

Adverse Reactions/Side Effects

CV: ECG changes, hypotension, tachycardia. **Derm:** photosensitivity, pigment changes, rash. **EENT:** blurred vision, dry eyes, lens opacities. **Endo:** galactorrhea, hyperprolactinemia. **GI:** constipation, dry mouth, anorexia, hepatitis, ileus. **GU:** pink or reddish-brown discoloration of urine, urinary retention. **Hemat:** AGRANULOCYTOSIS, leukopenia. **Metab:** hyperthermia. **Neuro:** extrapyramidal reactions, NEUROLEPTIC MALIGNANT SYNDROME, sedation, tardive dyskinesia. **Misc:** allergic reactions.

Interactions

Drug-Drug: Additive hypotension with **antihypertensives**, **nitrates**, or acute ingestion of **alcohol**. Additive CNS depression with other **CNS depressants**, including **alcohol**, **antidepressants**, **antihistamines**, **opioid analgesics**, **sedative/hypnotics**, or **general anesthetics**. Additive anticholinergic effects with other **drugs possessing anticholinergic properties**, including **antihistamines**, some **antidepressants**, **atropine**, **haloperidol**, and other **phenothiazines**. **Lithium** ↑ risk of extrapyramidal reactions. May mask early signs of **lithium** toxicity. ↑ risk of agranulocytosis with **antithyroid agents**. ↓ beneficial effects of **levodopa**. **Antacids** may ↓ absorption.

Drug-Natural Products: Kava-kava, **valerian**, **chamomile**, or **hops** can ↑ risk of CNS depression. ↑ anticholinergic effects with **angel's trumpet**, **jimson weed**, and **scopolia**.

Route/Dosage

Pediatric dose should not exceed 10 mg on the 1st day and then should not exceed 20 mg/day in children 2–5 yr or 25 mg/day in children 6–12 yr.

PO (Adults and Children ≥12 yr): 5–10 mg 3–4 times daily (not to exceed 40 mg/day).
PO (Children 18–39 kg): 2.5 mg 3 times daily *or* 5 mg twice daily (not to exceed 15 mg/day).
PO (Children 14–17 kg): 2.5 mg 2–3 times daily (not to exceed 10 mg/day).
PO (Children 9–13 kg): 2.5 mg 1–2 times daily (not to exceed 7.5 mg/day).
IM (Adults and Children ≥12 yr): 5–10 mg every 3–4 hr as needed. *Nausea/vomiting associated with surgery:* 5–10 mg; may be repeated once.
IM (Children 2–12 yr): 0.132 mg/kg; usually only one dose is required.
IV (Adults and Children ≥12 yr): 2.5–10 mg (not to exceed 40 mg/day). *Nausea/vomiting associated with surgery:* 5–10 mg; may be repeated once.
Rect (Adults): 25 mg twice daily.
Rect (Children 18–39 kg): 2.5 mg 3 times daily or 5 mg twice daily (not to exceed 15 mg/day).
Rect (Children 14–17 kg): 2.5 mg 2–3 times daily (not to exceed 10 mg/day).
Rect (Children 9–13 kg): 2.5 mg 1–2 times daily (not to exceed 7.5 mg/day).

Availability (generic available)

Tablets: 5 mg, 10 mg. **Solution for injection:** 5 mg/mL. **Suppositories:** 🍁 10 mg, 25 mg.

NURSING IMPLICATIONS

Assessment

- Monitor BP (sitting, standing, lying down), ECG, HR, and respiratory rate before and frequently during the period of dosage adjustment. May cause Q-wave and T-wave changes in ECG.
- Assess patient for level of sedation after administration.
- Monitor patient for onset of akathisia (restlessness or desire to keep moving) and extrapyramidal side effects (*parkinsonian:* difficulty speaking or swallowing, loss of balance control, pill rolling, masklike face, shuffling gait, rigidity, tremors; and *dystonic:* muscle spasms, twisting motions, twitching, inability to move eyes, weakness of arms or legs) every 2 mo during therapy and 8–12 wk after therapy has been discontinued. Report these symptoms; ↓ in dose or discontinuation may be necessary. Trihexyphenidyl or diphenhydramine may be used to control these symptoms.
- Monitor for tardive dyskinesia (uncontrolled rhythmic movement of mouth, face, and extremities; lip smacking or puckering; puffing of cheeks; uncontrolled chewing; rapid or worm-like movements of tongue). Report immediately; may be irreversible.
- Monitor for development of neuroleptic malignant syndrome (fever, respiratory distress, tachycardia, seizures, diaphoresis, hypertension or hypotension, pallor, tiredness, severe muscle stiffness, loss of

bladder control). Notify health care provider immediately if these symptoms occur.

- Assess for falls risk. Drowsiness, orthostatic hypotension, and motor and sensory instability ↑ risk. Institute prevention if indicated.
- **Antiemetic:** Assess patient for nausea and vomiting before and 30–60 min after administration.

Lab Test Considerations

- CBC and liver function tests should be evaluated periodically during therapy. May cause blood dyscrasias, especially between Wk 4 and 10 of therapy. Hepatotoxicity is more likely to occur between Wk 2 and 4 of therapy. May recur if medication is restarted. Liver function abnormalities may require discontinuation of therapy.
- May cause false-positive or false-negative pregnancy test results and false-positive urine bilirubin test results.
- May ↑ prolactin.

Implementation

- To prevent contact dermatitis, avoid getting solution on hands.
- Phenothiazines should be discontinued 48 hr before and not resumed for 24 hr after myelography; they ↓ seizure threshold.
- **PO:** Administer with food, milk, or a full glass of water to minimize gastric irritation.
- **IM:** Do not inject SUBQ. Inject slowly, deep into well-developed muscle. Keep patient recumbent for ≥30 min after injection to minimize hypotensive effects. Slight yellow color will not alter potency. Do not administer solution that is markedly discolored or that contains a precipitate.

IV Administration

- **IV Push:** Concentration: Dilute to a concentration of 1 mg/mL. Rate: Administer at a rate of 1 mg/min; not to exceed 5 mg/min.
- **Intermittent Infusion:** Dilution: Dilute 20 mg in up to 1 L dextrose, saline, Ringer's or LR, dextrose/saline, dextrose/Ringer's, or lactated Ringer's combinations.
- **Continuous Infusion:** Has been used as infusion with 20 mg/L of compatible solution.
- **Y-Site Compatibility:** acetaminophen, alemtuzumab, amikacin, amiodarone, anidulafungin, argatroban, arsenic trioxide, ascorbic acid, atracurium, atropine, azithromycin, benztropine, bleomycin, bumetanide, buprenorphine, butorphanol, carboplatin, carmustine, caspofungin, chlorpromazine, cisatracurium, cisplatin, cladribine, cyanocobalamin, cyclophosphamide, cyclosporine, cytarabine, dacarbazine, dactinomycin, daptomycin, daunorubicin, dexmedetomidine, dexrazoxane, digoxin, diltiazem, diphenhydramine, dobutamine, docetaxel, dopamine, doxorubicin hydrochloride, doxorubicin liposomal, doxycycline, enalaprilat, ephedrine, epinephrine, epirubicin, eptifibatide, erythromycin, esmolol, etoposide, famotidine, fentanyl, fluconazole, gentamicin, glycopyrrolate, granisetron, hetastarch, hydrocortisone, hydromorphone, idarubicin, ifosfamide, irinotecan, isoproterenol, labetalol, LR, leucovorin, lidocaine, linezolid, magnesium sulfate, mannitol, melphalan, meperidine, mesna, methadone, methotrexate, methylprednisolone, metoclopramide, metoprolol, metronidazole, milrinone, mitoxantrone, morphine, moxifloxacin, multivitamins, mycophenolate, nafcillin, nalbuphine, naloxone, nicardipine, nitroglycerin, norepinephrine, octreotide, ondansetron, oxacillin, oxaliplatin, oxytocin, paclitaxel, palonosetron, pamidronate, papaverine, penicillin G, phentolamine, phenylephrine, phytonadione, potassium acetate, potassium chloride, procainamide, promethazine, propofol, propranolol, protamine, pyridoxine, remifentanil, rituximab, rocuronium, sargramostim, sodium acetate, succinylcholine, sufentanil, tacrolimus, theophylline, thiamine, thiotepa, tigecycline, tirofiban, tobramycin, topotecan, trastuzumab, vancomycin, vasopressin, vecuronium, verapamil, vinblastine, vincristine, vinorelbine, zoledronic acid.
- **Y-Site Incompatibility:** acyclovir, aldesleukin, allopurinol, aminocaproic acid, aminophylline, amphotericin B deoxycholate, amphotericin B liposomal, ampicillin, ampicillin/sulbactam, azathioprine, aztreonam, bivalirudin, calcium chloride, cangrelor, cefazolin, cefepime, cefotaxime, cefotetan, cefoxitin, ceftazidime, ceftriaxone, cefuroxime, chloramphenicol, clindamycin, dantrolene, dexamethasone, diazepam, diazoxide, epoetin alfa, ertapenem, etoposide phosphate, filgrastim, fludarabine, fluorouracil, folic acid, foscarnet, fosphenytoin, furosemide, ganciclovir, gemcitabine, gemtuzumab ozogamicin, imipenem/cilastatin, indomethacin, insulin regular, ketorolac, levofloxacin, midazolam, minocycline, mitomycin, nitroprusside, pantoprazole, pemetrexed, pentamidine, pentobarbital, phenobarbital, phenytoin, piperacillin/tazobactam, sodium bicarbonate, trimethoprim/sulfamethoxazole

Patient/Family Teaching

- Instruct patient to take medication as directed and not to skip doses or double up on missed doses. Take missed doses as soon as remembered unless almost time for next dose. If >2 doses are scheduled

P

each day, missed dose should be taken within about 1 hr of the ordered time. Abrupt withdrawal may lead to gastritis, nausea, vomiting, dizziness, headache, tachycardia, and insomnia.

- Inform patient of possibility of extrapyramidal symptoms and tardive dyskinesia. Instruct patient to report these symptoms immediately to health care provider.
- Advise patient to change positions slowly to minimize orthostatic hypotension. Protect from falls.
- May cause drowsiness. Caution patient to avoid driving or other activities requiring alertness until response to medication is known.
- Caution patient to avoid alcohol and CNS depressants. Advise patient to notify health care provider of all Rx or OTC medications, vitamins, or herbal products being taken and to consult with health care provider before taking other medications and alcohol.
- Advise patient to use sunscreen and protective clothing when exposed to the sun to prevent photosensitivity reactions. Extremes in temperature should also be avoided, because this drug impairs body temperature regulation.
- Instruct patient to use frequent mouth rinses, good oral hygiene, and sugarless gum or candy to minimize dry mouth. Consult health care provider if dry mouth continues for >2 wk.
- Advise patient not to take prochlorperazine within 2 hr of antacids or antidiarrheal medication.
- Advise patient that increasing bulk and fluids in the diet and exercise may help minimize the constipating effects of this medication.
- Inform patient that this medication may turn urine pink to reddish-brown.
- Advise patient to notify health care provider of medication regimen before treatment or surgery.
- Instruct patient to notify health care provider promptly if sore throat, fever, unusual bleeding or bruising, skin rashes, weakness, tremors, visual disturbances, dark-colored urine, or clay-colored stools are noted.
- Rep: Advise women of reproductive potential to notify health care provider if pregnancy is planned or suspected or if breastfeeding. Maternal use of phenothiazines may cause jaundice or hyper- or hyporeflexia in newborn infants. Use during 3rd trimester may ↑ risk for abnormal muscle movements (extrapyramidal symptoms) and withdrawal symptoms in newborns following delivery; may include agitation, feeding disorder, hypertonia, hypotonia, respiratory distress, somnolence, and tremor; may be self-limiting or require hospitalization. Monitor infants breastfed by a mother taking prochlorperazine for drowsiness, skin reactions, and hypotension.
- Emphasize the importance of routine follow-up exams to monitor response to medication and detect side effects. Periodic ocular exams are indicated. Encourage continued participation in psychotherapy as ordered by health care provider.

Evaluation/Desired Outcomes

- Relief of nausea and vomiting.

progesterone (pro-**jess**-te-rone)

Crinone, Endometrin, Prometrium

Classification
Therapeutic: hormones
Pharmacologic: progestins

Indications

Crinone, Prometrium, and Oil for Injection: Secondary amenorrhea. **Oil for injection:** Abnormal uterine bleeding. **Prometrium:** Prevention of endometrial hyperplasia in postmenopausal women who have not had a hysterectomy (with estrogen). **Crinone and Endometrin:** Part of assisted reproductive technology in the management of infertility.

Action

Produces: Secretory changes in the endometrium, Increase in basal body temperature, Histologic changes in vaginal epithelium, Relaxation of uterine smooth muscle, Mammary alveolar tissue growth, Pituitary inhibition, Withdrawal bleeding in the presence of estrogen. **Therapeutic Effects:** Restoration of hormonal balance with control of uterine bleeding. Successful outcome in assisted reproduction.

Pharmacokinetics

Absorption: Micronization ↑ oral and vaginal absorption.
Distribution: Unknown.
Protein Binding: ≥90%.
Metabolism and Excretion: Metabolized by the liver; 50–60% eliminated by kidneys; 10% eliminated in feces.
Half-life: Several min.

TIME/ACTION PROFILE (plasma concentrations)

ROUTE	ONSET	PEAK	DURATION
PO	unknown	2–4 hr	unknown
Vaginal	unknown	34.8–55 hr	unknown
IM	unknown	19.6–28 hr	unknown

Contraindications/Precautions

Contraindicated in: Hypersensitivity; Hypersensitivity to parabens or sesame oil/seeds (IM suspension only); Hypersensitivity to peanuts (Prometrium only); Undiagnosed vaginal bleeding; Thromboembolic disease (e.g., deep vein thrombosis [DVT], pulmonary embolism [PE], MI, stroke); Protein C, protein S, or antithrombin deficiency or other thrombophilic disorder; Cerebrovascular disease; Severe hepatic impairment; Missed abortion; OB: Pregnancy.

Use Cautiously in: Long-term use (more than 4–5 yr); may ↑ risk of MI, stroke, invasive breast cancer, DVT, PE, and dementia in postmenopausal women; Breast cancer; Hepatic impairment; Cardiovascular disease; Depression; Lactation: Use while breastfeeding only if potential maternal benefit justifies potential risk to infant.

Adverse Reactions/Side Effects

CV: DVT, edema, MI, thrombophlebitis. **Derm:** chloasma, melasma, rash. **EENT:** retinal thrombosis. **Endo:** amenorrhea, breakthrough bleeding, breast tenderness, changes in menstrual flow, galactorrhea, spotting. **GI:** ↓ weight, constipation, hepatitis, nausea. **GU:** cervical erosions, pelvic pain, vaginal discharge. **Local:** irritation or pain at IM injection site. **Metab:** weight gain. **Neuro:** dementia, depression, headache, STROKE. **Resp:** PE. **Misc:** gingival bleeding, HYPERSENSITIVITY REACTIONS (INCLUDING ANAPHYLAXIS AND ANGIOEDEMA), MALIGNANCY (BREAST, ENDOMETRIAL, OVARIAN).

Interactions

Drug-Drug: May ↓ effectiveness of **bromocriptine** when used concurrently for galactorrhea and amenorrhea.

Route/Dosage

Secondary Amenorrhea

PO (Adults): 400 mg once daily in the evening for 10 days.
Vag (Adults): 45 mg (1 applicatorful of 4% gel) once every other day for up to 6 doses; may ↑ to 90 mg (1 applicatorful of 8% gel) once every other day for up to 6 doses.
IM (Adults): 100–150 mg (single dose) or 5–10 mg once daily for 6–8 days, given 8–10 days before expected menstrual period.

Abnormal Uterine Bleeding

IM (Adults): 5–10 mg once daily for 6 days.

Prevention of Endometrial Hyperplasia

PO (Adults): 200 mg once daily at bedtime for 12 days sequentially per 28-day cycle.

Assisted Reproductive Technology

Vag (Adults): *Patients who require progesterone supplementation:* 90 mg (1 applicatorful of 8% gel) once daily; if pregnancy occurs, may continue for up to 10–12 wk *or* 100 mg insert 2 or 3 times daily starting the day after oocyte retrieval and continuing for up to 10 wk total duration; *Patients with partial or complete ovarian failure who require progesterone replacement (intravaginal gel):* 90 mg (1 applicatorful of 8% gel) twice daily; if pregnancy occurs, may continue for up to 10–12 wk.

Availability (generic available)

Capsules (Prometrium): 100 mg, 200 mg. **Oil for intramuscular injection:** 50 mg/mL. **Vaginal gel (Crinone):** 4%, 8%. **Vaginal insert (Endometrin):** 100 mg. ***In combination with:*** estradiol (Bijuva). See Appendix N.

NURSING IMPLICATIONS

Assessment

- Monitor for signs and symptoms of venous thromboembolism, such as PE (chest pain, dyspnea, tachycardia) or DVT (calf pain or tenderness, lower extremity edema, localized warmth or erythema), or emerging cardiovascular disease, such as MI (chest pain, dyspnea, diaphoresis, dizziness, nausea) or stroke (weakness, slurred speech, confusion, dizziness); discontinue therapy in all patients if PE, DVT, stroke, or MI are suspected.
- Monitor BP periodically during therapy.
- Monitor intake and output and weekly weight. Report significant discrepancies or steady weight gain.
- Monitor for fluid retention; may exacerbate conditions such as HF or renal impairment.
- Monitor for breast tenderness, lumps, or discharge. Perform baseline mammogram before starting treatment.
- **Amenorrhea:** Assess patient's usual menstrual history. Administration of drug usually begins 8–10 days before anticipated menstruation. Withdrawal bleeding usually occurs 48–72 hr after course of therapy. Therapy should be discontinued if menses occur during injection series.
- **Dysfunctional Bleeding:** Monitor pattern and amount of vaginal bleeding (pad count). Bleeding should end by 6th day of therapy. Discontinue therapy if menses occur during injection series.

Lab Test Considerations

- Verify negative pregnancy test before starting therapy.
- Monitor hepatic function before and periodically during therapy. May ↑ alkaline phosphatase.
- May ↓ pregnanediol excretion concentrations.
- May ↑ low-density lipoprotein cholesterol and ↓ high-density lipoprotein cholesterol.
- May alter thyroid function test results.

Implementation

- Estrogen plus progestin therapy should not be used for the prevention of cardiovascular disease or dementia.
- Discontinuation of oral dose ≥4–6 wk prior to surgery associated with an ↑ risk of thromboembolism or prolonged immobilization is recommended.
- **PO:** Administer at bedtime. For patients who experience difficulty swallowing the capsules, take with a full glass of water while in the standing position.

P

- Handle intact tablets or capsules with single gloves; use double gloves, respiratory protection, and a protective gown in the preparation of tablets or capsules, including cutting, crushing, or manipulating, or handling uncoated tablets; optimally prepare in a ventilated control device.
- **IM:** Shake vial before preparing IM dose. Administer deep IM. Rotate sites.
- **Vag:** Vaginal gel and insert are administered with disposable applicator provided by manufacturer.
- Allow ≥6 hr after any other vaginal treatment before using vaginal gel.
- Vaginal insert is not recommended for use with other vaginal products.
- If dose ↑ is required from 4% gel to 8% gel, doubling the volume of the 4% gel will not accomplish dose ↑; changing to 8% gel is required.

Patient/Family Teaching

- Explain purpose and side effects of progesterone to patient. Instruct them to take medication as directed. Patient should not use tampons during therapy. Do not share medication with others, even if they have similar symptoms; may be harmful. Keep out of children's reach. Advise patient to read *Patient Information* sheet before starting therapy and with each Rx refill in case of changes.
- Inform postmenopausal women that long-term use may ↑ risk of MI, stroke, invasive breast cancer, PE, DVT, and dementia.
- Emphasize the importance of routine follow-up physical exams, including BP; breast, abdomen, and pelvic examinations; and Pap smears.
- Advise patient to report signs and symptoms of fluid retention (swelling of ankles and feet or weight gain) or hepatic impairment (yellowed skin or eyes, itchy skin, dark urine, light-colored stools).
- Advise patient to promptly report signs and symptoms of changes in vision or speech; sudden new, severe headaches; severe pains in chest or legs, with or without shortness of breath; weakness; or fatigue promptly to health care provider immediately.
- Instruct patient to notify health care provider if unusual vaginal bleeding, change in vaginal bleeding pattern, or spotting occurs.
- **Vag:** Instruct patient not to use vaginal gel concurrently with other vaginal agents. If these agents must be used concurrently, administer ≥6 hr before or after vaginal gel. Small white globules may appear as a vaginal discharge, possibly due to gel accumulation, even several days after use.
- Caution patient that cigarette smoking, high BP, high cholesterol, diabetes, and being overweight during progesterone therapy may ↑ risk of DVT or PE.
- Caution patient to use sunscreen and protective clothing to prevent photosensitivity reactions.
- Instruct patient to notify health care provider of all Rx or OTC medications, vitamins, or herbal products being taken and consult health care provider before taking any new medications or having surgery to avoid potential drug interactions.
- Rep: Advise women of reproductive potential to notify health care provider immediately if pregnancy is planned or suspected or if breastfeeding.

Evaluation/Desired Outcomes

- Reduction of uterine bleeding.
- Successful outcome in assisted reproduction.

BEERS HIGH ALERT

V promethazine

(proe-**meth**-a-zeen)

Phenergan, Promethegan

Classification

Therapeutic: antiemetics, antihistamines, sedative/hypnotics

Pharmacologic: phenothiazines

Indications

Various allergic conditions and motion sickness. Preoperative sedation. Treatment and prevention of nausea and vomiting. Adjunct to anesthesia and analgesia.

Action

Blocks the effects of histamine. Has inhibitory effect on the chemoreceptor trigger zone in the medulla, resulting in antiemetic properties. Alters the effects of dopamine in the CNS. Possesses significant anticholinergic activity. Produces CNS depression by indirectly decreased stimulation of the CNS reticular system. **Therapeutic Effects:** Relief of symptoms of histamine excess usually seen in allergic conditions. Diminished nausea or vomiting. Sedation.

Pharmacokinetics

Absorption: Well absorbed after oral (88%) and IM administration; rectal administration may be less reliable. IV administration results in complete bioavailability.
Distribution: Widely distributed to tissues.
Metabolism and Excretion: Metabolized by the liver.
Half-life: 9–16 hr.

TIME/ACTION PROFILE (noted as antihistaminic effects; sedative effects last 2–8 hr)

ROUTE	ONSET	PEAK	DURATION
PO, IM	20 min	unknown	4–12 hr
Rectal	20 min	unknown	4–12 hr
IV	3–5 min	unknown	4–12 hr

Contraindications/Precautions

Contraindicated in: Hypersensitivity; Comatose patients; Prostatic hypertrophy; Bladder-neck obstruction; Some products contain alcohol or bisulfites and should be avoided in patients with known intolerance; Angle-closure glaucoma; Pedi: Children <2 yr (may cause fatal respiratory depression).

Use Cautiously in: Hypertension; Cardiovascular disease; Hepatic impairment; Prostatic hypertrophy; Glaucoma; Asthma; Sleep apnea; Epilepsy; Underlying bone marrow depression; OB: Avoid chronic use during pregnancy; Lactation: Safety not established in breastfeeding; Pedi: Children >2 yr (use lowest effective dose and avoid concurrent respiratory depressants); Geri: Appears on Beers list. ↑ risk of anticholinergic adverse reactions in older adults, including falls, delirium, and dementia. Avoid use in older adults.

Adverse Reactions/Side Effects

CV: bradycardia, hypertension, hypotension, tachycardia. **Derm:** photosensitivity, rash, severe tissue necrosis upon infiltration at IV site. **EENT:** blurred vision, diplopia, tinnitus. **GI:** constipation, dry mouth, hepatitis. **Hemat:** blood dyscrasias. **Neuro:** confusion, disorientation, sedation, dizziness, extrapyramidal reactions, fatigue, insomnia, nervousness, NEUROLEPTIC MALIGNANT SYNDROME.

Interactions

Drug-Drug: Additive CNS depression with other **CNS depressants**, including **alcohol**, other **antihistamines**, **opioid analgesics**, and other **sedative/hypnotics**. Neuroleptic malignant syndrome can occur when used with **antipsychotics**. Additive anticholinergic effects with other **drugs possessing anticholinergic properties**, including other **antihistamines**, **antidepressants**, **atropine**, **haloperidol**, other **phenothiazines**, **quinidine**, and **disopyramide**. May precipitate seizures when used with **drugs that lower seizure threshold**. **MAO inhibitors** may ↑ risk of sedation and anticholinergic side effects.

Route/Dosage

Antihistamine

PO (Adults): 6.25–12.5 mg 3 times/day and 25 mg at bedtime.

PO (Children ≥2 yr): 0.1 mg/kg/dose (not to exceed 12.5 mg) every 6 hr during the day and 0.5 mg/kg/dose (not to exceed 25 mg) at bedtime.

IM, IV, Rect (Adults): 25 mg; may repeat in 2 hr.

Rect (Children ≥2 yr): 0.125 mg/kg every 4–6 hr *or* 0.5 mg/kg at bedtime.

Antivertigo (Motion Sickness)

PO (Adults): 25 mg 30–60 min before departure; may be repeated in 8–12 hr.

PO, Rect (Children ≥2 yr): 0.5 mg/kg (not to exceed 25 mg) 30–60 min before departure; may be given every 12 hr as needed.

Sedation

PO, Rect, IM, IV (Adults): 25–50 mg; may repeat every 4–6 hr if needed.

PO, Rect, IM (Children >2 yr): 0.5–1 mg/kg (not to exceed 50 mg) every 6 hr as needed.

Nausea/Vomiting

PO, Rect, IM, IV (Adults): 12.5–25 mg every 4 hr as needed; initial PO dose should be 25 mg.

PO, Rect, IM, IV (Children ≥2 yr): 0.25–1 mg/kg (not to exceed 25 mg) every 4–6 hr.

Availability (generic available)

Tablets: 12.5 mg, 25 mg, 50 mg. **Oral solution (cherry flavor):** 6.25 mg/5 mL. **Solution for injection:** 25 mg/mL, 50 mg/mL. **Suppositories:** 12.5 mg, 25 mg, 50 mg. ***In combination with:*** codeine, dextromethorphan, and/or phenylephrine in a variety of cough and cold preparations.

NURSING IMPLICATIONS

Assessment

- Monitor BP, HR, and respiratory rate frequently in patients receiving IV doses.
- Assess level of sedation after administration. Risk of sedation and respiratory depression are ↑ when administered concurrently with other drugs that cause CNS depression.
- Monitor patient for onset of extrapyramidal side effects (*akathisia:* restlessness; *dystonia:* muscle spasms and twisting motions; *pseudoparkinsonism:* masklike face, rigidity, tremors, drooling, shuffling gait, dysphagia). Notify health care provider if these symptoms occur.
- Monitor for development of neuroleptic malignant syndrome (fever, respiratory distress, tachycardia, seizures, diaphoresis, hypertension or hypotension, pallor, tiredness, severe muscle stiffness, loss of bladder control). Notify health care provider immediately if these symptoms occur.
- Assess for falls risk. Drowsiness, orthostatic hypotension, and motor and sensory instability ↑ risk. Institute prevention if indicated.
- Geri: Assess for adverse anticholinergic effects (delirium, acute confusion, dizziness, dry mouth, blurred vision, urinary retention, constipation, tachycardia).
- **Allergy:** Assess allergy symptoms (rhinitis, conjunctivitis, hives) before and periodically throughout course of therapy.
- **Antiemetic:** Assess for nausea and vomiting before and after administration.

Lab Test Considerations

- May cause false-positive or false-negative pregnancy test results.

P

- Evaluate CBC periodically during chronic therapy; blood dyscrasias may occur.
- May ↑ serum glucose.
- May cause false-negative results in skin tests using allergen extracts. Promethazine should be discontinued 72 hr before the test.

Implementation

- When administering promethazine concurrently with opioid analgesics, supervise ambulation closely to prevent injury from ↑ sedation.
- **PO:** Administer with food, water, or milk to minimize GI irritation. Tablets may be crushed and mixed with food or fluids for patients with difficulty swallowing.
- **IM:** Administer deep into well-developed muscle. SUBQ or inadvertent intra-arterial administration may cause severe tissue necrosis and is contraindicated.

IV Administration

- **IV:** ***High Alert:*** If administered IV, assess for burning and pain at IV site; may cause severe tissue injury. Avoid IV administration, if possible. Administer IV only if IM injection not possible. If pain occurs after IV administration, discontinue administration immediately and evaluate for possible arterial injection or perivascular extravasation, and initiate appropriate medical management.
- **V** IV promethazine is a vesicant. Dilution is required before administering IV. Administer into a large vein or preferably through a central venous catheter. If extravasation occurs, immediately stop infusion. Leave needle/cannula in place temporarily but do not flush the line. Gently aspirate extravasated solution; then remove needle/cannula. Elevate patient's extremity and apply dry warm or dry cold compresses. Initiate hyaluronidase antidote for refractory cases in addition to supportive management. For hyaluronidase, inject a total of 1 mL (15 units/mL) intradermally or SUBQ as five separate 0.2-mL injections (using a tuberculin syringe) around the site of extravasation; if IV catheter remains in place, administer IV through the infiltrated catheter; may repeat in 30–60 min if no resolution.
- **IV Push: Dilution:** Dilute with 0.9% NaCl or D5W. **Concentration:** ≤1 mg/mL. **Rate:** Administer each 25 mg slowly, over ≥10–15 min (max rate = 25 mg/min). Rapid administration may ↓ BP.
- **Y-Site Compatibility:** alemtuzumab, amikacin, aminocaproic acid, amiodarone, anidulafungin, argatroban, arsenic trioxide, ascorbic acid, atracurium, atropine, azithromycin, benztropine, bleomycin, bumetanide, buprenorphine, butorphanol, calcium chloride, calcium gluconate, carboplatin, caspofungin, ceftaroline, chlorpromazine, ciprofloxacin, cisatracurium, cisplatin, cladribine, cyanocobalamin, cyclophosphamide, cyclosporine, cytarabine, dacarbazine, dactinomycin, daptomycin, daunorubicin, dexmedetomidine, dexrazoxane, digoxin, diltiazem, diphenhydramine, dobutamine, docetaxel, dopamine, doxorubicin hydrochloride, doxycycline, edetate calcium disodium, enalaprilat, ephedrine, epinephrine, epirubicin, epoetin alfa, eptifibatide, ergonovine, erythromycin, esmolol, etoposide, etoposide phosphate, famotidine, fentanyl, filgrastim, fluconazole, fludarabine, gemcitabine, gentamicin, glycopyrrolate, granisetron, hydromorphone, idarubicin, ifosfamide, insulin, regular, irinotecan, isoproterenol, ketamine, labetalol, leucovorin, levofloxacin, lidocaine, linezolid, lorazepam, magnesium sulfate, mannitol, melphalan, meperidine, mesna, methadone, metoclopramide, metoprolol, metronidazole, midazolam, milrinone, mitoxantrone, morphine, moxifloxacin, mycophenolate, nalbuphine, naloxone, nicardipine, nitroglycerin, norepinephrine, octreotide, ondansetron, oxaliplatin, oxytocin, paclitaxel, palonosetron, pamidronate, pemetrexed, pentamidine, phentolamine, phenylephrine, potassium acetate, procainamide, prochlorperazine, propranolol, protamine, pyridoxine, remifentanil, rituximab, rocuronium, sargramostim, sodium acetate, succinylcholine, sufentanil, tacrolimus, theophylline, thiamine, thiotepa, tigecycline, tirofiban, tobramycin, topotecan, trastuzumab, vancomycin, vasopressin, vecuronium, verapamil, vinblastine, vincristine, vinorelbine, voriconazole, zoledronic acid.
- **Y-Site Incompatibility:** acyclovir, aldesleukin, allopurinol, aminophylline, amphotericin B deoxycholate, amphotericin B liposomal, ampicillin/sulbactam, azathioprine, cangrelor, carmustine, cefepime, cefotaxime, cefotetan, cefoxitin, ceftazidime, ceftobiprole, ceftriaxone, cefuroxime, chlorothiazide, clindamycin, dantrolene, diazepam, diazoxide, dimenhydrinate, doxorubicin liposomal, ertapenem, fluorouracil, folic acid, foscarnet, ganciclovir, gemtuzumab ozogamicin, indomethacin, ketorolac, methohexital, methylprednisolone, minocycline, mitomycin, morphine, nafcillin, nitroprusside, oxacillin, pantoprazole, pentobarbital, phenobarbital, phenytoin, piperacillin/tazobactam, sodium bicarbonate, trimethoprim/sulfamethoxazole.

Patient/Family Teaching

- Explain purpose and side effects of medication. Advise patient to read *Patient Information* before starting therapy. Review dose schedule with patient. If medication is ordered regularly and a dose is missed, take as soon as remembered unless time for next dose. Pedi: Caution caregivers to use only the measuring device accompanying the liquid medication and not to use household measuring devices.
- Advise patient to notify health care provider of all Rx or OTC medications, vitamins, or herbal products being taken and to consult with health care provider before taking other medications.
- May cause drowsiness. Caution patient to avoid driving or other activities requiring alertness until response to medication is known.

- Advise patient that frequent mouth rinses, good oral hygiene, and sugarless gum or candy may ↓ dry mouth. Health care provider should be notified if dry mouth persists >2 wk.
- Caution patient to use sunscreen and protective clothing to prevent photosensitivity reactions.
- Advise patient to change positions slowly to ↓ orthostatic hypotension. Protect from falls. Geri: Older adults are at ↑ risk.
- Caution patient to avoid concurrent use of alcohol and other CNS depressants with this medication.
- Instruct patient to notify health care provider if sore throat, fever, jaundice, or uncontrolled movements are noted.
- **Motion Sickness:** When used as prophylaxis for motion sickness, advise patient to take medication ≥30 min and preferably 1–2 hr before exposure to conditions that may cause motion sickness.
- Rep: Advise women of reproductive potential to notify health care provider if pregnancy is planned or suspected or if breastfeeding.

Evaluation/Desired Outcomes

- Relief of symptoms of histamine excess usually seen in allergic conditions.
- Diminished nausea or vomiting.
- Sedation.

HIGH ALERT

V propofol (proe-poe-fol)

Diprivan

Classification

Therapeutic: general anesthetics

Indications

Induction of general anesthesia. Maintenance of balanced anesthesia when used with other agents. Initiation and maintenance of monitored anesthesia care. Sedation of intubated, mechanically ventilated patients in intensive care units (ICUs).

Action

Short-acting hypnotic. Mechanism of action is unknown. Produces amnesia. Has no analgesic properties. **Therapeutic Effects:** Induction and maintenance of anesthesia.

Pharmacokinetics

Absorption: IV administration results in complete bioavailability.
Distribution: Rapidly and widely distributed. Crosses the blood-brain barrier well; rapidly redistributed to other tissues.
Protein Binding: 95–99%.
Metabolism and Excretion: Rapidly metabolized by the liver. Primarily excreted in urine as metabolites.
Half-life: 3–12 hr (blood-brain equilibration half-life 2.9 min).

TIME/ACTION PROFILE (loss of consciousness)

ROUTE	ONSET	PEAK	DURATION†
IV	40 sec	unknown	3–5 min

† Time to recovery is 8 min (up to 19 min if opioid analgesics have been used).

Contraindications/Precautions

Contraindicated in: Hypersensitivity to propofol, soybean oil, egg lecithin, or glycerol; OB: Crosses placenta; may cause neonatal depression; may affect child's brain development when used during 3rd trimester.
Use Cautiously in: Cardiovascular disease; Lipid disorders (emulsion may have detrimental effect); ↑ intracranial pressure; Cerebrovascular disorders; Hypovolemic patients (lower induction and maintenance dosage recommended); Lactation: Safety not established in breastfeeding; Pedi: Not recommended for induction of anesthesia in children <3 yr or for maintenance of anesthesia in infants <2 mo; not for ICU or preprocedure sedation; may affect brain development in children <3 yr; Geri: Lower induction and maintenance dose ↓ recommended in older adults.

P

Adverse Reactions/Side Effects

CV: bradycardia, hypotension, hypertension. **Derm:** flushing. **GI:** abdominal cramping, hiccups, nausea, vomiting. **GU:** discoloration of urine (green). **Local:** burning, pain, stinging, coldness, numbness, tingling at IV site. **MS:** involuntary muscle movements, perioperative myoclonia. **Neuro:** dizziness, headache. **Resp:** APNEA, cough. **Misc:** fever, PROPOFOL INFUSION SYNDROME.

Interactions

Drug-Drug: Additive CNS and respiratory depression with **alcohol**, **antihistamines**, **opioid analgesics**, and **sedative/hypnotics** (dose ↓ may be required). **Theophylline** may antagonize the CNS effects of propofol. Cardiorespiratory instability can occur when used with **acetazolamide**. **Fentanyl** may ↑ risk of serious bradycardia in children. ↑ risk of hypertriglyceridemia with **intravenous fat emulsion**.

Route/Dosage

General Anesthesia

IV (Adults <55 yr): *Induction:* 40 mg every 10 sec until induction achieved (2–2.5 mg/kg total). *Maintenance:* 100–200 mcg/kg/min. Rates of 150–200 mcg/kg/min are usually required during 1st 10–15 min after induction and then ↓ by 30–50% during 1st 30 min of maintenance. Rates of 50–100 mcg/kg/min are associated with optimal recovery time. May also be given intermittently in increments of 25–50 mg.

IV (Geriatric Patients, Cardiac Patients, Debilitated Patients, or Hypovolemic Patients): *Induction:* 20 mg every 10 sec until induction achieved (1–1.5 mg/kg total). *Maintenance:* 50–100 mcg/kg/min (dose in cardiac anesthesia ranges from 50–150 mcg/kg/min depending on concurrent use of opioid).

IV (Adults Undergoing Neurosurgical Procedures): *Induction:* 20 mg every 10 sec until induction achieved (1–2 mg/kg total). *Maintenance:* 100–200 mcg/kg/min.

IV (Children 3–16 yr): *Induction:* 2.5–3.5 mg/kg; use lower dose for children ASA III or IV.

IV (Children 2 mo–16 yr): *Maintenance:* 125–300 mcg/kg/min (following 1st 30 min of maintenance, rate should be ↓ if possible); younger children may require larger infusion rates compared to older children.

Monitored Anesthesia Care Sedation

IV (Adults <55 yr): *Initiation:* 100–150 mcg/kg/min infusion *or* 0.5 mg/kg as slow injection. *Maintenance:* 25–75 mcg/kg/min infusion or incremental boluses of 10–20 mg.

IV (Geriatric Patients, Debilitated Patients, or ASA III/IV Patients): *Initiation:* Use slower infusion or injection rates. *Maintenance:* 20% less than the usual adult infusion dose; rapid/repeated bolus dosing should be avoided.

ICU Sedation

IV (Adults): 5 mcg/kg/min for a minimum of 5 min. Additional increments of 5–10 mcg/kg/min over 5–10 min may be given until desired response is obtained. (Range 5–50 mcg/kg/min.) Dose should be reassessed every 24 hr.

Availability (generic available)

Lipid emulsion for injection: 10 mg/mL.

NURSING IMPLICATIONS

Assessment

- Assess respiratory status, HR, and BP continuously throughout propofol therapy. Frequently causes apnea lasting ≥60 sec. Maintain patent airway and adequate ventilation. Propofol should be used only by individuals experienced in endotracheal intubation, and equipment for this procedure should be readily available.
- Assess level of sedation and level of consciousness throughout and following administration.
- **ICU sedation:** Perform sedation vacation per institution protocol and assess neurological function daily during maintenance to determine minimum dose required for sedation. Maintain minimal level of sedation during these assessments; do not discontinue. Abrupt discontinuation may cause rapid awakening with anxiety, agitation, and resistance to mechanical ventilation.
- Monitor for propofol infusion syndrome (severe metabolic acidosis, hyperkalemia, lipemia, rhabdomyolysis, hepatomegaly, cardiac and renal failure). Most frequent with prolonged, high-dose infusions (>5 mg/kg/hr for >48 hr) but has also been reported following large-dose short-term infusions during surgical anesthesia. If prolonged sedation or ↑ dose is required or metabolic acidosis occurs, consider alternative method of sedation.

Lab Test Considerations

- Monitor LFTs, BUN, creatinine, and electrolytes (sodium, potassium, magnesium, calcium).
- Monitor triglycerides, CK, and lactic acid in extended use or high doses.

Toxicity and Overdose

- If overdose occurs, monitor BP, HR, and respiratory rates continuously. Maintain patent airway and assist ventilation as needed. If hypotension occurs, treatment includes IV fluids, repositioning, and vasopressors.

Implementation

- Do not confuse Diprivan with Diflucan.
- Dose is titrated to patient response.
- Propofol has no effect on the pain threshold. Adequate analgesia should *always* be used when propofol is used as an adjunct to surgical procedures.

IV Administration

- V Propofol is a vesicant. Administer into a large vein. If extravasation occurs, immediately stop infusion. Leave needle/cannula in place temporarily but do not flush the line. Gently aspirate extravasated solution; then remove needle/cannula. Elevate patient's extremity and apply dry cold compresses. Initiate hyaluronidase antidote for refractory cases in addition to supportive management. For hyaluronidase, inject a total of 1 mL (15 units/mL) intradermally or SUBQ as five separate 0.2-mL injections (using a tuberculin syringe) around the site of extravasation; if IV catheter remains in place, administer IV through the infiltrated catheter; may repeat in 30–60 min if no resolution. May also cause injection site pain; may be minimized if larger veins of the forearm or antecubital fossa are used, especially in pediatric patients. Pain may be ↓ by a prior injection of IV lidocaine (1 mL of a 1% solution).
- **IV Push: Dilution:** Usually administered undiluted. If dilution is necessary, use only D5W. Shake well before use. Solution is opaque, making detection of contaminants difficult. Do not use if separation of the emulsion is evident. Contains no preservatives; maintain sterile technique and administer immediately

after preparation. **Concentration:** Undiluted: 10 mg/mL. If dilution is necessary, dilute to concentration ≥2 mg/mL.

- Discard unused portions and IV lines at the end of anesthetic procedure or within 6 hr. *For ICU sedation,* discard after 12 hr if administered directly from vial or after 6 hr if transferred to a syringe or other container. Do not administer via filter <5-micron pore size.
- Aseptic technique is essential. Solution is capable of rapid growth of bacterial contaminants. Infections and subsequent deaths have been reported. **Rate:** Administer over 3–5 min. Titrate to desired level of sedation. Pedi: Induction doses may be administered over 20–30 sec.
- **Intermittent/Continuous Infusion: Dilution:** Administer undiluted. Allow 3–5 min between dose adjustments to allow for and assess the clinical effects. **Concentration:** 10 mg/mL.
- **Rate:** Based on patient's weight (see Route/Dosage section).
- **Y-Site Compatibility:** acyclovir, aminophylline, ampicillin, aztreonam, bumetanide, buprenorphine, butorphanol, calcium gluconate, cangrelor, carboplatin, cefazolin, cefepime, cefotaxime, cefotetan, cefoxitin, ceftaroline, ceftobiprole, cefuroxime, chlorpromazine, cisplatin, clevidipine, clindamycin, cyclophosphamide, cyclosporine, cytarabine, dexamethasone, dexmedetomidine, diphenhydramine, doxycycline, droperidol, enalaprilat, ephedrine, esmolol, famotidine, fentanyl, fluconazole, fluorouracil, furosemide, glycopyrrolate, granisetron, haloperidol, heparin, hydrocortisone, hydromorphone, ifosfamide, imipenem/cilastatin, insulin regular, isoproterenol, ketamine, labetalol, levetiracetam, lorazepam, mannitol, meperidine, milrinone, nafcillin, nalbuphine, naloxone, nitroprusside, norepinephrine, paclitaxel, palonosetron, pentobarbital, phenobarbital, potassium chloride, prochlorperazine, propranolol, sodium bicarbonate, sufentanil, tigecycline.
- **Y-Site Incompatibility:** acetaminophen, amikacin, calcium chloride, ceftolozane/tazobactam, ciprofloxacin, cisatracurium, diazepam, digoxin, doxorubicin hydrochloride, eravacycline, gentamicin, isavuconazonium, levofloxacin, methotrexate, methylprednisolone, metoclopramide, metronidazole, minocycline, mitoxantrone, phenytoin, plazomicin, sulbactam/durlobactam, tobramycin, verapamil.

Patient/Family Teaching

- Explain purpose and side effects of medication to patient or caregiver.
- Advise patient to notify health care provider of all Rx or OTC medications, vitamins, or herbal products being taken and to consult with health care provider before taking other medications.
- Inform patient that this medication will ↓ mental recall of the procedure.
- May cause drowsiness or dizziness. Advise patient to request assistance before ambulation and transfer and to avoid driving or other activities requiring alertness for 24 hr following administration.
- Advise patient to avoid alcohol, marijuana, other forms of cannabis, or prescriptions, including opioids, or OTC drugs that may slow CNS actions without the advice of a health care provider for 24 hr following administration.
- Rep: Advise women of reproductive potential to notify health care provider if pregnancy is planned or suspected or if breastfeeding. Monitor neonates for hypotonia and sedation following maternal exposure to propofol.

Evaluation/Desired Outcomes

- Induction and maintenance of anesthesia.

propranolol, See BETA BLOCKERS (nonselective).

protamine
(proe-ta-meen)

Classification
Therapeutic: antidotes
Pharmacologic: antiheparins

Indications

Acute management of severe heparin overdosage. Used to neutralize heparin received during dialysis, cardiopulmonary bypass, and other procedures. **Unlabeled Use:** Management of overdose of heparin-like compounds.

Action

A strong base that forms a complex with heparin (an acid). **Therapeutic Effects:** Inactivation of heparin.

Pharmacokinetics

Absorption: IV administration results in complete bioavailability.
Distribution: Unknown.
Metabolism and Excretion: Metabolic fate not known. Protamine-heparin complex eventually degrades.
Half-life: 7 min.

TIME/ACTION PROFILE (reversal of heparin effect)

ROUTE	ONSET	PEAK	DURATION
IV	30 sec–1 min	unknown	2 hr†

† Depends on body temperature.

P

Contraindications/Precautions

Contraindicated in: Hypersensitivity to protamine or fish.

Use Cautiously in: Patients who have received previous protamine-containing insulin or vasectomized men (↑ risk of hypersensitivity reactions); OB: Safety not established in pregnancy; use during pregnancy only if clearly needed; Lactation: Safety not established in breastfeeding; use while breastfeeding only if clearly needed.

Adverse Reactions/Side Effects

CV: bradycardia, hypertension, hypotension. **Derm:** flushing. **GI:** nausea, vomiting. **Hemat:** bleeding. **MS:** back pain. **Resp:** dyspnea, pulmonary edema, pulmonary hypertension. **Misc:** HYPERSENSITIVITY REACTIONS (INCLUDING ANAPHYLAXIS AND ANGIOEDEMA).

Interactions

Drug-Drug: None reported.

Route/Dosage

IV (Adults and Children): *Heparin overdose:* 1 mg of protamine/100 units of heparin. If given >30 min after heparin, give 0.5 mg of protamine/100 units of heparin (not to exceed 100 mg/2 hr). Further doses should be determined by coagulation tests. If heparin was administered subcutaneously, use 1–1.5 mg of protamine per 100 units of heparin (give 25–50 mg of the protamine dose slowly followed by a continuous infusion over 8–16 hr). *Enoxaparin overdose (unlabeled use):* 1 mg of protamine/1 mg of enoxaparin. *Dalteparin overdose (unlabeled use):* 1 mg of protamine/100 anti-Xa units of dalteparin. If required, a 2nd dose of 0.5 mg of protamine/100 anti-Xa units of dalteparin may be given 2–4 hr later if laboratory assessment indicates need.

Availability (generic available)

Solution for injection: 10 mg/mL.

NURSING IMPLICATIONS

Assessment

- Monitor for signs/symptoms of bleeding or hemorrhage during therapy (weakness, tachycardia, dyspnea, dizziness, pallor, fatigue, tarry stools, coffee ground emesis, obvious severe bleeding [bleeding gums, epistaxis, bleeding wounds]). Hemorrhage may recur 8–9 hr after therapy because of rebound effects of heparin. Rebound may occur as late as 18 hr after therapy in patients heparinized for cardiopulmonary bypass.
- BP should be monitored throughout therapy for immediate recognition of hypotensive reactions.
- Assess for allergy to fish (salmon) or previous reaction to or use of protamine insulin or protamine sulfate. Vasectomized men and individuals with severe left ventricular dysfunction or abnormal pulmonary hemodynamics also have higher risk of hypersensitivity reaction. Observe patient for signs and symptoms of hypersensitivity reaction (hives, edema, coughing, wheezing). Keep epinephrine, an antihistamine, and resuscitative equipment close by in the event of anaphylaxis.
- Assess for hypovolemia before initiation of therapy. Failure to correct hypovolemia may result in cardiovascular collapse from peripheral vasodilating effects of protamine sulfate.

Lab Test Considerations

- Monitor clotting factors, activated clotting time (ACT), aPTT, and thrombin time (TT) 5–15 min after therapy and again as necessary.

Implementation

- Do not confuse protamine with Protonix.
- Discontinue heparin infusion. In milder cases, overdose may be treated by heparin withdrawal alone.
- In severe cases, fresh frozen plasma or whole blood may also be required to control bleeding.
- Dose varies with type of heparin, route of heparin therapy, and amount of time elapsed since discontinuation of heparin.
- Do not administer >100 mg in 2 hr without rechecking clotting studies, as protamine sulfate has its own anticoagulant properties.

IV Administration

- **IV Push: Dilution:** May be administered undiluted. If further dilution is desired, D5W or 0.9% NaCl may be used. **Concentration:** 10 mg/mL. **Rate:** Administer by slow IV push over 1–3 min. Rapid infusion rate may result in hypotension, bradycardia, flushing, feeling of warmth, or anaphylaxis-like reaction. If these symptoms occur, stop infusion and notify health care provider. No more than 50 mg should be administered within a 10-min period.
- **Y-Site Compatibility:** acetaminophen, amikacin, aminophylline, ascorbic acid, atropine, azathioprine, aztreonam, benztropine, bumetanide, buprenorphine, butorphanol, calcium chloride, calcium gluconate, chlorpromazine, clindamycin, cyanocobalamin, cyclosporine, digoxin, diphenhydramine, dobutamine, dopamine, doxycycline, enalaprilat, ephedrine, epinephrine, epoetin alfa, erythromycin, esmolol, famotidine, fentanyl, fluconazole, ganciclovir, gentamicin, glycopyrrolate, imipenem/cilastatin, isoproterenol, labetalol, lidocaine, magnesium sulfate, mannitol, meperidine, metoclopramide, metoprolol, midazolam, morphine, multivitamins, nalbuphine, naloxone, nitroglycerin, nitroprusside, norepinephrine, ondansetron, oxytocin, papaverine, phentolamine, phenylephrine, phytonadione, potassium chloride, procainamide, prochlorperazine, promethazine, propranolol, pyridoxine, sodium bicarbonate, succinylcholine, sufentanil, theophylline,

thiamine, tobramycin, vancomycin, vasopressin, verapamil.

- **Y-Site Incompatibility:** amphotericin B deoxycholate, ampicillin, ampicillin/sulbactam, cefazolin, cefotaxime, cefotetan, cefoxitin, ceftazidime, ceftriaxone, cefuroxime, chloramphenicol, dantrolene, dexamethasone, diazepam, folic acid, furosemide, heparin, hydrocortisone, indomethacin, insulin regular, ketorolac, methylprednisolone, nafcillin, oxacillin, penicillin G, pentamidine, pentobarbital, phenobarbital, phenytoin, trimethoprim/sulfamethoxazole.

Patient/Family Teaching

- Explain purpose and side effects of protamine. Advise patient to read *Medication Guide* before starting and periodically during therapy in case of changes.
- Tell patient to report and seek treatment for signs and symptoms of bleeding (weakness; fast heartbeat; trouble breathing; dizziness; pale skin; tiredness; obvious bleeding in urine, stool, mouth, or nose).
- Advise patient to avoid activities that may result in bleeding (shaving, brushing teeth, receiving injections or rectal temperatures, ambulating) until risk of hemorrhage has passed.
- Advise patient to notify health care provider of all Rx or OTC medications, vitamins, or herbal products being taken and to consult with health care provider before taking other medications.
- Rep: Advise women of reproductive potential to notify health care provider if pregnancy is planned or suspected or if breastfeeding.

Evaluation/Desired Outcomes

- Control of bleeding.
- Normalization of clotting factors in heparinized patients.

pseudoephedrine

(soo-doe-e-**fed**-rin)

Silfedrine Children's, ~~Sudafed 12 Hour~~, Sudafed 24 Hour, Sudafed Children's, SudoGest, SudoGest 12 Hour

Classification

Therapeutic: allergy, cold and cough remedies, nasal drying agents/decongestants

Pharmacologic: adrenergics, alpha adrenergic agonists

Indications

Symptomatic management of nasal congestion associated with acute viral upper respiratory tract infections. Used in combination with antihistamines in the management of allergic conditions. Used to open obstructed eustachian tubes in chronic otic inflammation or infection.

Action

Stimulates alpha- and beta-adrenergic receptors. Produces vasoconstriction in the respiratory tract mucosa (alpha-adrenergic stimulation) and possibly bronchodilation ($beta_2$-adrenergic stimulation). **Therapeutic Effects:** Reduction of nasal congestion, hyperemia, and swelling in nasal passages.

Pharmacokinetics

Absorption: Well absorbed after oral administration.
Distribution: Appears to enter the CSF.
Metabolism and Excretion: Partially metabolized by the liver. 55–75% excreted unchanged by the kidneys (depends on urine pH).
Half-life: *Children:* 3.1 hr; *Adults:* 9–16 hr (depends on urine pH).

TIME/ACTION PROFILE (decongestant effects)

ROUTE	ONSET	PEAK	DURATION
PO	15–30 min	unknown	4–6 hr
PO-ER	60 min	unknown	12 hr

Contraindications/Precautions

Contraindicated in: Hypersensitivity to sympathomimetic amines; Hypertension or severe coronary artery disease; Concurrent MAO inhibitor therapy; Known alcohol intolerance (some liquid products); Pedi: Children <4 yr.
Use Cautiously in: Hyperthyroidism; Diabetes mellitus; Prostatic hyperplasia; Ischemic heart disease; Glaucoma; OB: May be associated with ↑ risk of congenital anomalies, especially in 1st trimester; Lactation: May lead to acute ↓ in milk production and irritability/agitation in infants.

Adverse Reactions/Side Effects

CV: palpitations, CARDIOVASCULAR COLLAPSE, hypertension, tachycardia. **Derm:** diaphoresis. **GI:** anorexia, dry mouth. **GU:** dysuria. **Neuro:** anxiety, nervousness, dizziness, drowsiness, excitability, fear, hallucinations, headache, insomnia, restlessness, SEIZURES, weakness. **Resp:** respiratory difficulty.

Interactions

Drug-Drug: **MAO inhibitors** may cause hypertensive crisis. Additive adrenergic effects with other **adrenergics**. **Beta blockers** may result in hypertension or bradycardia. **Drugs that acidify the urine** may ↓ effectiveness. **Phenothiazines** and **tricyclic antidepressants** potentiate pressor effects. **Drugs that alkalinize the urine (sodium bicarbonate, high-dose antacid therapy)** may ↑ risk of toxicity.
Drug-Food: **Foods that acidify the urine** may ↓ effectiveness. **Foods that alkalinize the urine** may ↑ risk of toxicity (see lists in Appendix J).

P

Route/Dosage

PO (Adults and Children >12 yr): *Immediate release:* 60 mg every 6 hr as needed (not to exceed 240 mg/day). *Extended release:* 120 mg every 12 hr *or* 240 mg every 24 hr.
PO (Children 6–12 yr): *Immediate release:* 30 mg every 6 hr as needed (not to exceed 120 mg/day).
PO (Children 4–5 yr): *Immediate release:* 15 mg every 6 hr (not to exceed 60 mg/day).

Availability (generic available)

Immediate-release tablets: 30 mg[OTC], 60 mg[OTC]. **Immediate-release capsules:** 🍁 60 mg[OTC]. **Extended-release tablets:** 120 mg[OTC], 240 mg[OTC]. **Extended-release capsules:** 🍁 240 mg[OTC]. **Liquid (grape and others):** 15 mg/5 mL[OTC], 30 mg/5 mL[OTC]. ***In combination with:*** antihistamines, acetaminophen, cough suppressants, and expectorants[OTC]. See Appendix N.

NURSING IMPLICATIONS

Assessment

- Assess congestion (nasal, sinus, eustachian tube) before and periodically during therapy.
- Monitor HR and BP before beginning therapy and periodically during therapy.
- Assess lung sounds and character of bronchial secretions. Maintain fluid intake of 1500–2000 mL/day to ↓ viscosity of secretions.

Implementation

- Do not confuse Sudafed with sotalol or Sudafed PE.
- Administer pseudoephedrine ≥2 hr before bedtime to minimize insomnia.
- **PO:** ***DNC:*** Extended-release tablets and capsules should be swallowed whole; do not crush, break, or chew. Contents of the capsule can be mixed with jam or jelly and swallowed without chewing for patients with difficulty swallowing.

Patient/Family Teaching

- Explain the purpose and side effects of pseudoephedrine. Instruct patient to take medication as directed and not to take more than recommended. Avoid taking at or near bedtime to prevent insomnia. Take missed doses within 1 hr; if remembered later, omit. Do not double doses. Keep out of children's reach. Caution parents to avoid OTC cough and cold products in children <4 yr. Advise patient to read *Medication Guide* before starting and periodically during therapy.
- Instruct patient to notify health care provider if nervousness, slow or fast HR, breathing difficulties, hallucinations, or seizures occur, because these symptoms may indicate overdose.
- Instruct patient to contact health care provider if symptoms do not improve within 7 days or if fever is present.
- Advise patient to notify health care provider of all Rx or OTC medications, vitamins, or herbal products being taken and to consult with health care provider before taking other medications. Instruct patient to avoid concurrent use with other OTC stimulants.
- Rep: May cause fetal harm. Avoid use during 1st trimester of pregnancy. Prolonged use later in pregnancy should also be avoided. Has been used for persistent idiopathic hyperlactation in patients who require medication therapy.

Evaluation/Desired Outcomes

- Decreased nasal, sinus, or eustachian tube congestion.

pyrazinamide

(peer-a-**zin**-a-mide)

Classification
Therapeutic: antituberculars

Indications

Active tuberculosis (TB) (in combination with other agents).

Action

Converted to pyrazinoic acid in susceptible strains of Mycobacterium, which lowers the pH of the environment. **Therapeutic Effects:** Bacteriostatic action against susceptible mycobacteria. **Spectrum:** Active against mycobacteria only.

Pharmacokinetics

Absorption: Well absorbed after oral administration.
Distribution: Widely distributed to tissues. Reaches high concentrations in the CNS (same as plasma).
Metabolism and Excretion: Mostly metabolized by the liver. Metabolite (pyrazinoic acid) has antimycobacterial activity; 3–4% excreted unchanged by the kidneys.
Half-life: *Pyrazinamide:* 9.5 hr. *Pyrazinoic acid:* 12 hr. Both are ↑ in renal impairment.

TIME/ACTION PROFILE (plasma concentrations)

ROUTE	ONSET	PEAK	DURATION
PO	unknown	1–2 hr (4–5 hr†)	24 hr

† For pyrazinoic acid.

Contraindications/Precautions

Contraindicated in: Hypersensitivity; Cross-sensitivity with ethionamide, isoniazid, niacin, or nicotinic acid may exist; Severe hepatic impairment.
Use Cautiously in: Gout; Renal failure; Diabetes mellitus; Acute intermittent porphyria; OB: Use during

pregnancy only if clearly needed; Lactation: Use while breastfeeding only if potential maternal benefit justifies potential risk to infant.

Adverse Reactions/Side Effects

Derm: acne, photosensitivity, rash. **GI:** anorexia, diarrhea, HEPATOTOXICITY, nausea, vomiting. **GU:** dysuria. **Hemat:** anemia, thrombocytopenia. **Metab:** hyperuricemia. **MS:** arthralgia, gouty arthritis.

Interactions

Drug-Drug: Rifampin may result in life-threatening hepatotoxicity; avoid concurrent use. May ↓ levels and effectiveness of **cyclosporine**. May ↓ effectiveness of **antigout agents**.

Route/Dosage

PO (Adults and Children): 15–30 mg/kg/day as a single dose. Up to 60 mg/kg/day has been used in isoniazid-resistant TB (not to exceed 2 g/day as a single dose or 3 g/day in divided doses). May also be given as 50–70 mg/kg 2–3 times weekly (not to exceed 2 g/dose on daily regimen, 3 g/dose for 3-times-weekly regimen, or 4 g/dose for twice-weekly regimen). *Patients with HIV:* 20–40 mg/kg/day for 1st 2 mo of therapy (maximum: 2 g/day); further dosing depends on regimen used.

Availability (generic available)

Tablets: 500 mg.

NURSING IMPLICATIONS

Assessment

- Perform mycobacterial studies and susceptibility tests before and periodically during therapy to detect possible resistance.
- Monitor for signs/symptoms of hepatotoxicity (fatigue, nausea, upper abdominal pain, jaundice, scleral icterus, dark urine, clay-colored stools), especially in patients with pre-existing liver disease or those at ↑ risk for hepatitis (alcoholism). Notify health care provider if suspected. Patients with hepatic impairment should receive pyrazinamide therapy only if crucial to treatment. *If severe hepatic damage occurs,* permanently discontinue pyrazinamide.

Lab Test Considerations

- Evaluate hepatic function before and every 2–4 wk during therapy. ↑ AST and ALT may not be predictive of clinical hepatitis and may return to normal levels during treatment.
- Monitor uric acid before and during therapy. May ↑ uric acid, resulting in precipitation of acute gout. *If hyperuricemia with acute gouty arthritis occurs,* permanently discontinue pyrazinamide.
- *Pulmonary TB with negative initial cultures:* Obtain sputum AFB smear and culture every month until 2 consecutive specimens are negative; perform chest x-rays after 2–3 mo of treatment and at the end of therapy.
- *Pulmonary TB with positive initial cultures:* Obtain sputum AFB smear and culture more frequently (every 2 wk) until 2 consecutive specimens are negative; repeat chest x-rays after 2 mo of treatment and at the end of therapy, if clinically indicated.
- May interfere with urine ketone determinations.

Implementation

- **PO:** May be given concurrently with isoniazid.

Patient/Family Teaching

- Explain the purpose and side effects of pyrazinamide. Advise patient to take medication as directed and not to skip doses or double up on missed doses. Take missed doses as soon as remembered unless almost time for next dose. Emphasize the importance of continuing therapy even after symptoms have subsided. Length of therapy depends on regimen being used and underlying disease states. Do not share medication with others, even if they have similar symptoms; may be harmful. Advise patient to read *Patient Information* before starting and with each Rx refill in case of changes.
- Explain need for continued medical follow-up to monitor progress and assess possible side effects of medication. Periodic lab tests will be needed. Advise patients to notify health care provider if no improvement is noticed after 2–3 wk of therapy.
- Inform patients with diabetes that pyrazinamide may interfere with urine ketone measurements.
- Advise patient to immediately report signs and symptoms of hepatotoxicity (fatigue, nausea, upper abdominal pain, yellowing of skin or eyes, dark urine, light-colored stools).
- Advise patient to immediately report signs and symptoms of gout (fever, pain, redness, swelling of the joints).
- Advise patients to use sunscreen and protective clothing to prevent photosensitivity reactions.
- Advise patient to notify health care provider of all Rx or OTC medications, vitamins, or herbal products being taken and to consult with health care provider before taking other medications.
- Rep: Advise women of reproductive potential to notify health care provider if pregnancy is planned or suspected or if breastfeeding. Monitor infants exposed to pyrazinamide via breast milk for jaundice.

P

Evaluation/Desired Outcomes

- Resolution of signs and symptoms of TB.
- Negative sputum cultures.

pyridoxine (vitamin B_6)

(peer-i-**dox**-een)

Classification

Therapeutic: vitamins

Pharmacologic: water soluble vitamins

Indications

Treatment and prevention of pyridoxine deficiency (may be associated with poor nutritional status or chronic debilitating illnesses). Treatment of pyridoxine-dependent seizures in infants. Treatment and prevention of neuropathy, which may develop from isoniazid, penicillamine, or hydralazine therapy. Treatment of isoniazid overdose >10 g.

Action

Required for amino acid, carbohydrate, and lipid metabolism. Used in the transport of amino acids, formation of neurotransmitters, and synthesis of heme. **Therapeutic Effects:** Prevention of pyridoxine deficiency. Prevention or reversal of neuropathy associated with hydralazine, penicillamine, or isoniazid therapy.

Pharmacokinetics

Absorption: Well absorbed from the GI tract.
Distribution: Stored in liver, muscle, and brain.
Metabolism and Excretion: Converted in RBCs to pyridoxal phosphate and another active metabolite. Amounts in excess of requirements are excreted unchanged by the kidneys.
Half-life: 15–20 days.

TIME/ACTION PROFILE

ROUTE	ONSET	PEAK	DURATION
PO, IM, IV	unknown	unknown	unknown

Contraindications/Precautions

Contraindicated in: Hypersensitivity to pyridoxine or any component.
Use Cautiously in: Parkinson disease (treatment with levodopa only); OB: Chronic ingestion of large doses may produce pyridoxine-dependency syndrome in newborn.

Adverse Reactions/Side Effects

Adverse reactions listed are seen with excessive doses only.

Neuro: sensory neuropathy, paresthesia. **Misc:** pyridoxine-dependency syndrome.

Interactions

Drug-Drug: Interferes with the therapeutic response to **levodopa** when used without carbidopa. Requirements are ↑ by **isoniazid, hydralazine, chloramphenicol, penicillamine, estrogens**, and **immunosuppressants**. May ↓ levels and effectiveness of **phenobarbital** and **phenytoin**.

Route/Dosage

Prevention of Deficiency (Recommended Daily Allowance)

PO (Adults and Children >14 yr): 1.2–1.7 mg/day (larger doses required with cycloserine, ethionamide, hydralazine, immunosuppressants, isoniazid, penicillamine, and estrogen-containing oral contraceptives).
PO (Children 9–13 yr): 1 mg/day (larger doses required with cycloserine, ethionamide, hydralazine, immunosuppressants, isoniazid, and penicillamine).
PO (Children 1–8 yr): 0.5–0.6 mg/day (larger doses required with cycloserine, ethionamide, hydralazine, immunosuppressants, isoniazid, and penicillamine).
PO (Infants 6–12 mo): 0.3 mg/day.
PO (Infants <6 mo): 0.1 mg/day.

Treatment of Deficiency

PO (Adults): 2.5–10 mg/day until clinical signs are corrected, then 2–5 mg/day.
PO (Children): 5–25 mg/day for 3 wk, then 1.5–2.5 mg/day.

Pyridoxine-Dependent Seizures

PO, IM, IV (Neonates and Infants): 10–100 mg initially, then 50–100 mg/day orally.

Drug-Induced Neuritis

PO: (Adults): *Treatment:* 100–300 mg/day; *Prophylaxis:* 25–100 mg/day.
PO (Children): *Treatment:* 10–50 mg/day; *Prophylaxis:* 1–2 mg/kg/day.

Isoniazid Overdose (>10 g)

IM, IV (Adults and Children): Amount in mg equal to amount of isoniazid ingested given as 1–4 g IV, then 1 g IM every 30 min.

Availability (generic available)

Tablets: 10 mg[OTC], 25 mg[OTC], 50 mg[OTC], 100 mg[OTC], 250 mg[OTC]. **Extended-release tablets:** 200 mg[OTC]. **Oral solution:** 12.5 mg/mL. **Solution for injection:** 100 mg/mL.

NURSING IMPLICATIONS

Assessment

- Assess signs/symptoms vitamin B_6 deficiency (anemia, dermatitis, cheilosis, irritability, seizures, nausea, vomiting) before and periodically throughout therapy. Institute seizure precautions in pyridoxine-dependent infants. Pyridoxine-dependent seizures should cease in 2–3 min after IV administration.
- Monitor respiratory rate, HR, and BP with large IV dose.

Lab Test Considerations

- May cause false elevations in urobilinogen concentrations.

Implementation

- Do not confuse pyridoxine with pralidoxime or Pyridium.
- Single B-vitamin deficiencies are infrequent; combination preparations are commonly administered.
- Administration of parenteral vitamin B_6 is indicated for patients who are NPO, have nausea and vomiting, or malabsorption syndromes.
- **PO:** *DNC:* Swallow extended-release capsules and tablets whole; do not crush, break, or chew. If unable to swallow capsule, the contents may be mixed with jam or jelly.
- **IM:** Rotate sites; burning or stinging at site may occur.
- **IV:** Administer by slow IV push or as infusion in standard IV solutions. Protect parenteral solution from light.
- **Rate:** Infusion rates of 15–30 min and up to 3 hr have been used.
- **Y-Site Compatibility:** amikacin, aminophylline, ascorbic acid, atracurium, atropine, aztreonam, benztropine, bumetanide, buprenorphine, butorphanol, calcium chloride, calcium gluconate, cefotaxime, cefotetan, cefoxitin, ceftazidime, ceftriaxone, cefuroxime, chlorpromazine, clindamycin, cyanocobalamin, cyclosporine, dexamethasone, digoxin, diphenhydramine, dobutamine, dopamine, doxycycline, enalaprilat, ephedrine, epinephrine, epoetin alfa, erythromycin, esmolol, famotidine, fentanyl, fluconazole, gentamicin, glycopyrrolate, heparin, insulin, regular, isoproterenol, labetalol, lidocaine, magnesium sulfate, mannitol, meperidine, metoclopramide, metoprolol, midazolam, minocycline, morphine, multivitamins, nalbuphine, naloxone, nitroglycerin, nitroprusside, norepinephrine, ondansetron, oxytocin, papaverine, penicillin G, pentamidine, phentolamine, phenylephrine, phytonadione, potassium chloride, procainamide, prochlorperazine, promethazine, propranolol, protamine, sodium bicarbonate, succinylcholine, sufentanil, theophylline, thiamine, tobramycin, vancomycin, vasopressin, verapamil.
- **Y-Site Incompatibility:** amphotericin B deoxycholate, azathioprine, cefazolin, chloramphenicol, dantrolene, diazepam, diazoxide, folic acid, furosemide, ganciclovir, hydrocortisone, imipenem/cilastatin, indomethacin, ketorolac, methylprednisolone, nafcillin, oxacillin, pentobarbital, phenobarbital, phenytoin, trimethoprim/sulfamethoxazole.

Patient/Family Teaching

- Explain purpose and side effects of medication. Advise patient to read *Patient Information* before starting therapy.
- Encourage patient to comply with diet recommended by health care provider. Explain that the best source of vitamins is a well-balanced diet. Foods high in vitamin B_6 include bananas, whole grains, potatoes, lima beans, and meats.
- Caution patient not to exceed RDA for pyridoxine. Large doses may cause unsteady gait, numbness in feet, and difficulty with hand coordination.
- Rep: Advise women of reproductive potential to notify health care provider if pregnancy is planned or suspected or if breastfeeding.

Evaluation/Desired Outcomes

- Decrease symptoms of vitamin B_6 deficiency.

P

BEERS

QUEtiapine (kwet-**eye**-a-peen)

SEROquel, SEROquel XR

Classification

Therapeutic: antipsychotics, mood stabilizers

Indications

Schizophrenia. Depressive episodes with bipolar disorder. Acute manic episodes associated with bipolar I disorder (as monotherapy [for adults or adolescents] or with lithium or divalproex [adults only]). Maintenance treatment of bipolar I disorder (with lithium or divalproex). Adjunctive treatment of depression.

Action

Probably acts by serving as an antagonist of dopamine and serotonin. Also antagonizes histamine H_1 receptors and alpha$_1$-adrenergic receptors. **Therapeutic Effects:** Decreased manifestations of psychoses, depression, or acute mania.

Pharmacokinetics

Absorption: Well absorbed after oral administration.
Distribution: Widely distributed.
Metabolism and Excretion: Extensively metabolized by the liver via the CYP3A4 isoenyzme to norquetiapine (active metabolite with anticholinergic properties); <1% excreted unchanged in the urine.
Half-life: 6 hr.

TIME/ACTION PROFILE (antipsychotic effects)

ROUTE	ONSET	PEAK	DURATION
PO	unknown	unknown	8–12 hr
PO-XR	unknown	unknown	unknown

Contraindications/Precautions

Contraindicated in: Hypersensitivity; Concurrent use of agents that prolong the QT interval (↑ risk of serious arrhythmias); History of arrhythmias, including bradycardia; Hypokalemia or hypomagnesemia (↑ risk of serious arrhythmias); Congenital long QT syndrome (↑ risk of serious arrhythmias).
Use Cautiously in: Cardiovascular disease, cerebrovascular disease, dehydration, or hypovolemia (↑ risk of hypotension); History of seizures or Alzheimer dementia; Diabetes (may ↑ risk of hyperglycemia); Patients at risk for aspiration pneumonia or falls; Hepatic impairment (dose ↓ may be necessary); Hypothyroidism (may be exacerbated); May ↑ risk of suicide attempt/ideation especially during early treatment or dose adjustment; this risk appears to be greater in adolescents or children; Low white blood cell count or history of drug-induced leukopenia/neutropenia (↑ risk of leukopenia/neutropenia); Urinary retention, prostatic hypertrophy, constipation, or ↑ intraocular pressure; History of breast cancer; OB: Neonates at ↑ risk for extrapyramidal symptoms and withdrawal after delivery when exposed during the 3rd trimester; use only if potential maternal benefit justifies potential fetal risk; Lactation: Use while breastfeeding only if potential maternal benefit justifies potential risk to infant; Pedi: Safety and effectiveness not established in children <18 yr (extended release) or <10 yr (immediate release); Geri: Appears on Beers list. ↑ risk of stroke, cognitive decline, and mortality in older adults with dementia. Avoid use in older adults, except for schizophrenia, bipolar disorder, adjunctive treatment of major depressive disorder, or psychosis in Parkinson disease.

Adverse Reactions/Side Effects

CV: ↑ BP (children), palpitations, peripheral edema, postural hypotension. **Derm:** ACUTE GENERALIZED EXANTHEMATOUS PUSTULOSIS, DRUG REACTION WITH EOSINOPHILIA AND SYSTEMIC SYMPTOMS (DRESS), STEVENS-JOHNSON SYNDROME (SJS), sweating. **EENT:** ear pain, pharyngitis, rhinitis. **Endo:** hyperglycemia, hyperprolactinemia, hypothyroidism. **GI:** anorexia, constipation, dry mouth, dyspepsia, GI OBSTRUCTION, PANCREATITIS. **GU:** ↓ fertility (women). **Hemat:** ↓ hemoglobin, AGRANULOCYTOSIS, leukopenia, neutropenia. **Metab:** weight gain, hyperlipidemia, hypertriglyceridemia. **MS:** rhabdomyolysis. **Neuro:** dizziness, cognitive impairment, extrapyramidal symptoms, NEUROLEPTIC MALIGNANT SYNDROME, sedation, SEIZURES, SUICIDAL THOUGHTS/BEHAVIORS, tardive dyskinesia. **Resp:** cough, dyspnea. **Misc:** flu-like syndrome.

Interactions

Drug-Drug: **QT interval prolonging medications**, including **macrolide antibiotics** (**erythromycin**, **clarithromycin**), **dofetilide**, **sotalol**, **quinidine**, **disopyramide**, **procainamide**, **thioridazine**, **chlorpromazine**, **droperidol**, **moxifloxacin**, **mefloquine**, **pentamidine**, **arsenic trioxide**, **citalopram**, **escitalopram**, **tacrolimus**, and **ziprasidone**, may ↑ risk of serious ventricular arrhythmias and should be avoided. ↑ CNS depression may occur with **alcohol**, **antihistamines**, **opioid analgesics**, and **sedative/hypnotics**. ↑ risk of hypotension with acute ingestion of **alcohol** or **antihypertensives**. **CYP3A inducers**, including **phenytoin**, **carbamazepine**, **barbiturates**, **rifampin**, or **corticosteroids**, may ↓ levels and effectiveness. **CYP3A inhibitors**, including **ketoconazole**, **itraconazole**, **fluconazole**, **protease inhibitors**, or **erythromycin**, may ↑ levels and risk of toxicity. Concurrent use of **anticholinergic medications** may ↑ risk of anticholinergic adverse reactions.

Route/Dosage

Schizophrenia

PO (Adults): *Immediate release:* 25 mg twice daily on Day 1; ↑ by 25–50 mg 2–3 times daily on Days 2 and 3, up to 300–400 mg/day in 2–3 divided doses by Day 4 (not to exceed 800 mg/day); *Extended release:* 300 mg once daily; ↑ by 300 mg/day (not to exceed 800 mg/day); older adults or patients with hepatic impairment should be started on immediate-release product and converted to extended-release product once effective dose is reached.

PO (Children 13–17 yr): *Immediate release:* 25 mg twice daily on Day 1; ↑ to 50 mg twice daily on Day 2; then ↑ to 100 mg twice daily on Day 3; then ↑ to 150 mg twice daily on Day 4; then ↑ to 200 mg twice daily on Day 5; may then ↑ by no more than 100 mg/day (not to exceed 800 mg/day).

Acute Manic Episodes Associated With Bipolar I Disorder

PO (Adults): *Immediate release:* 50 mg twice daily on Day 1; then ↑ to 100 mg twice daily on Day 2; then ↑ to 150 mg twice daily on Day 3; then ↑ to 200 mg twice daily on Day 4; may then ↑ by no more than 200 mg/day up to 400 mg twice daily on Day 6 if needed; *Extended release:* 300 mg once daily on Day 1, then 600 mg once daily on Day 2, then 400–800 mg once daily starting on Day 3.

PO (Children 10–17 yr): *Immediate release:* 25 mg twice daily on Day 1; then ↑ to 50 mg twice daily on Day 2; then ↑ to 100 mg twice daily on Day 3; then ↑ to 150 mg twice daily on Day 4; then ↑ to 200 mg twice daily on Day 5; may then ↑ by no more than 100 mg/day (not to exceed 600 mg/day).

Acute Depressive Episodes Associated With Bipolar Disorder

PO (Adults): *Immediate release or extended release:* 50 mg once daily at bedtime on Day 1; then ↑ to 100 mg daily at bedtime on Day 2; then ↑ to 200 mg daily at bedtime on Day 3; then ↑ to 300 mg daily at bedtime thereafter.

Maintenance Treatment of Bipolar I Disorder

PO (Adults): Continue at the dose required to maintain symptom remission (usual dosage: 400–800 mg/day given as once daily dose [extended release] or in two divided doses [immediate release]).

PO (Children 10–17 yr): Continue at the lowest dose required to maintain symptom remission.

Depression

PO (Adults): *Extended release:* 50 mg once daily on Days 1 and 2; then ↑ to 150 mg once daily starting on Day 3 (not to exceed 300 mg/day).

Availability (generic available)

Immediate-release tablets: 25 mg, 50 mg, 100 mg, 200 mg, 300 mg, 400 mg. **Extended-release tablets:** 50 mg, 150 mg, 200 mg, 300 mg, 400 mg.

NURSING IMPLICATIONS

Assessment

- Monitor mental status (mood, orientation, behavior) before and periodically during therapy.
- Assess for suicidal tendencies, especially during early therapy. Restrict amount of drug available to patient. Risk may be ↑ in children, adolescents, and adults ≤24 yr. After starting therapy, young adults should be seen by health care provider face-to-face at least weekly for 4 wk, then every other wk for next 4 wk, then at 12 wk, and then on advice of health care provider thereafter.
- Assess weight and BMI initially; then at Wk 4, Wk 8, and Wk 12; and then every 4 mo during therapy. Refer as appropriate for nutritional/weight management and medical management.
- Assess orthostatic vitals (HR and BP lying, sitting, standing) frequently during initial dosage adjustment and periodically throughout therapy. Titrate slowly and monitor closely; may cause orthostatic hypotension, bradycardia, and syncope. If hypotension occurs during dose titration, return to the previous dose.
- Observe patient carefully to ensure medication is swallowed and not hoarded or cheeked.
- Monitor for onset of akathisia (restlessness or desire to keep moving) and extrapyramidal side effects (*parkinsonian:* difficulty speaking or swallowing, loss of balance control, pill-rolling motion of hands, masklike face, shuffling gait, rigidity, tremors and dystonic muscle spasms, twisting motions, twitching, inability to move eyes, weakness of arms or legs) every 2 mo during therapy and 8–12 wk after therapy has been discontinued. Notify health care provider if these symptoms occur; ↓ in dose or discontinuation of medication may be necessary. Trihexyphenidyl or benztropine may be used to control these symptoms.
- Monitor for possible tardive dyskinesia (uncontrolled rhythmic movement of mouth, face, and extremities; lip smacking or puckering; puffing of cheeks; uncontrolled chewing; rapid or worm-like movements of tongue). Report these symptoms immediately; may be irreversible.
- Monitor frequency and consistency of bowel movements and assess for symptoms of hypomotility (nausea, vomiting, abdominal distension, abdominal pain). Symptoms range from constipation to paralytic ileus; ↑ risk with use of other anticholinergic

Q

medications. ↑ fiber and fluids in the diet and laxatives may help to minimize constipation. Prophylactic laxatives may be used for high-risk patients.

- Monitor for signs and symptoms of neuroleptic malignant syndrome (hyperpyrexia, muscle rigidity, seizures altered mental status, evidence of autonomic instability [irregular HR or BP, tachycardia, diaphoresis, cardiac arrhythmia]). Notify health care provider immediately if these symptoms occur.
- Assess for rash or signs and symptoms of SJS frequently during therapy (fever, general malaise, fatigue, muscle or joint aches, blisters, oral lesions, conjunctivitis, hepatitis, eosinophilia). Discontinue and provide supportive care; may be life-threatening.
- Monitor for signs of pancreatitis (nausea, vomiting, anorexia, persistent severe abdominal pain sometimes radiating to the back) during therapy.
- Quetiapine ↓ the seizure threshold. Institute seizure precautions for patients with history of seizure disorder.
- Monitor for symptoms related to hyperprolactinemia (menstrual abnormalities, galactorrhea, sexual dysfunction).
- Assess for falls risk. Drowsiness, orthostatic hypotension, and motor and sensory instability ↑ risk. Institute prevention if indicated.
- Monitor for signs and symptoms of DRESS (fever, rash, lymphadenopathy, facial swelling), associated with involvement of other organ systems (hepatitis, nephritis, hematologic abnormalities, myocarditis, myositis) during therapy. May resemble an acute viral infection. Eosinophilia is often present. Discontinue therapy if signs occur.

Lab Test Considerations

- May cause asymptomatic ↑ in AST and ALT.
- Assess fasting lipid profile at baseline, Wk 12, and every 5 yr thereafter. May ↑ total cholesterol and triglycerides.
- Monitor fasting blood glucose at baseline, Wk 12, and annually; patients with diabetes should be monitored more frequently.
- May cause anemia, thrombocytopenia, leukocytosis, and leukopenia.
- Monitor serum prolactin prior to and periodically during therapy. May ↑ serum prolactin levels.

Implementation

- Do not confuse quetiapine with olanzapine. Do not confuse Seroquel with Seroquel XR.
- If therapy is reinstituted after an interval of ≥1 wk off, follow initial titration schedule.
- **PO:** Administer without regard to food; however, extended-release tablets are best absorbed on an empty stomach. ***DNC:*** Extended-release tablets should be swallowed whole; do not break, crush, or chew.

Patient/Family Teaching

- Explain the purpose and side effects of quetiapine. Instruct patient to take as directed. Take missed doses as soon as remembered unless almost time for next dose; do not double doses. Consult health care provider prior to stopping; should be discontinued gradually. Stopping abruptly may cause insomnia, nausea, and vomiting. Advise patient of need for continued medical follow-up for psychotherapy, eye exams, and laboratory tests. Advise patient to read *Patient Information* before starting and with each Rx refill in case of changes.
- Instruct patient to notify health care provider of all Rx or OTC medications, vitamins, or herbal products being taken and to consult health care provider before taking any other medications. Caution patient to avoid concurrent use of alcohol and other CNS depressants.
- Inform patient of the possibility of extrapyramidal symptoms. Instruct patient to report symptoms immediately to health care provider.
- Advise patient to change positions slowly to minimize orthostatic hypotension. Protect from falls.
- May cause drowsiness. Caution patient to avoid driving or other activities requiring alertness until response to medication is known.
- Advise patient to avoid extremes in temperature; this drug impairs body temperature regulation.
- Advise patient, family, and caregivers to look for suicidality, especially during early therapy or dose changes. Notify health care provider immediately if thoughts about suicide or dying, attempts to commit suicide, new or worse depression or anxiety, agitation or restlessness, panic attacks, insomnia, new or worse irritability, aggressiveness, acting on dangerous impulses, mania, or other changes in mood or behavior.
- Refer patient for nutritional, weight, or medical management of dyslipidemia as indicated.
- Advise patient to notify health care provider of medication regimen before treatment or surgery.
- Instruct patient to notify health care provider promptly of sore throat, fever, unusual bleeding or bruising, constipation, or rash.
- Rep: Advise women of reproductive potential to notify health care provider if pregnancy is planned or suspected or if breastfeeding. May lead to temporary, reversible infertility in women. Consider early screening for gestational diabetes if used during pregnancy. Neonates

exposed to antipsychotic drugs during 3rd trimester are at risk for extrapyramidal and/or withdrawal symptoms following delivery. Monitor neonates for symptoms of agitation, hypertonia, hypotonia, tremor, somnolence, respiratory distress, excessive sedation, and feeding difficulties. Monitor infants exposed to quetiapine through breast milk for excessive sedation. There is a pregnancy exposure registry that monitors pregnancy outcomes in women exposed to atypical antipsychotics, during pregnancy. Health care providers are encouraged to advise patients to register by calling the National Pregnancy Registry for Atypical Antipsychotics at 1-866-961-2388 or visiting https://womensmentalhealth.org/clinical-and-research-programs/pregnancyregistry/.

Evaluation/Desired Outcomes

- Decrease in excited, manic behavior.
- Decrease in signs of depression in patients with bipolar disorder.
- Decrease in manic episodes in patients with bipolar I disorder.
- Decrease in positive symptoms (delusions, hallucinations) of schizophrenia.
- Decrease in negative symptoms (social withdrawal, flat, blunt affect) of schizophrenia.

quinapril, See ANGIOTENSIN-CONVERTING ENZYME (ACE) INHIBITORS.

BEERS

RABEprazole (ra-bep-ra-zole)

Aciphex, ~~Aciphex Sprinkle~~, Pariet

Classification
Therapeutic: antiulcer agents
Pharmacologic: proton-pump inhibitors

Indications

Gastroesophageal reflux disease (GERD). Duodenal ulcers (including combination therapy with clarithromycin and amoxicillin to eradicate *Helicobacter pylori* and prevent recurrence). Pathological hypersecretory conditions, including Zollinger-Ellison syndrome.

Action

Binds to an enzyme in the presence of acidic gastric pH, preventing the final transport of hydrogen ions into the gastric lumen. **Therapeutic Effects:** Diminished accumulation of acid in the gastric lumen, with lessened acid reflux. Healing of duodenal ulcers and esophagitis. Decreased acid secretion in hypersecretory conditions.

Pharmacokinetics

Absorption: Delayed-release tablet is designed to allow rabeprazole, which is not stable in gastric acid, to pass through the stomach intact. Subsequently 52% is absorbed after oral administration.
Distribution: Unknown.
Protein Binding: 96.3%.
Metabolism and Excretion: Mostly metabolized by the CYP3A4 and CYP2C19 isoenzymes in the liver; (the CYP2C19 enzyme system exhibits genetic polymorphism; 15–20% of Asian patients and 3–5% of White and Black patients may be poor metabolizers and may have significantly ↑ rabeprazole concentrations and an ↑ risk of adverse effects); 10% excreted in feces; remainder excreted in urine as inactive metabolites.
Half-life: 1–2 hr.

TIME/ACTION PROFILE (acid suppression)

ROUTE	ONSET	PEAK	DURATION
PO	within 1 hr	unknown	24 hr†

† Suppression continues to increase over the 1st wk of therapy.

Contraindications/Precautions

Contraindicated in: Hypersensitivity to rabeprazole or related drugs (benzimidazoles); Concurrent use of rilpivirine.
Use Cautiously in: Severe hepatic impairment (dose reduction may be necessary); Patients using high doses for >1 yr (↑ risk of hip, wrist, or spine fractures and fundic gland polyps); Patients using therapy for >3 yr (↑ risk of vitamin B_{12} deficiency); Pre-existing risk of hypocalcemia; OB: Safety not established in pregnancy; Lactation: Use while breastfeeding only if potential maternal benefit justifies potential risk to infant; Pedi: Children <12 yr (safety and effectiveness not established); Geri: Appears on Beers list. ↑ risk of *Clostridioides difficile* infection, pneumonia, GI malignancies, bone loss, and fractures in older adults. Avoid scheduled use for >8 wk in older adults unless for high-risk patients (e.g., oral corticosteroid or chronic NSAID use) or patients with erosive esophagitis, Barrett esophagitis, pathological hypersecretory condition, or demonstrated need for maintenance therapy (e.g., failure of H_2 antagonist).

Adverse Reactions/Side Effects

Derm: ACUTE GENERALIZED EXANTHEMATOUS PUSTULOSIS (AGEP), cutaneous lupus erythematosus, DRUG REACTION WITH EOSINOPHILIA AND SYSTEMIC SYMPTOMS (DRESS), photosensitivity, rash, STEVENS-JOHNSON SYNDROME (SJS), TOXIC EPIDERMAL NECROLYSIS (TEN). **F and E:** hypocalcemia (especially if treatment duration ≥3 mo), hypokalemia (especially if treatment duration ≥3 mo), hypomagnesemia (especially if treatment duration ≥3 mo). **GI:** abdominal pain, CLOSTRIDIOIDES DIFFICILE-ASSOCIATED DIARRHEA (CDAD), constipation, diarrhea, fundic gland polyps, nausea. **GU:** acute tubulointerstitial nephritis. **MS:** bone fracture, neck pain. **Neuro:** dizziness, headache, malaise. **Misc:** chills, fever, HYPERSENSITIVITY REACTIONS (INCLUDING ANAPHYLAXIS, ANGIOEDEMA, OR TUBULOINTERSTITIAL NEPHRITIS), systemic lupus erythematosus, vitamin B_{12} deficiency.

Interactions

Drug-Drug: May significantly ↓ levels and effectiveness of **rilpivirine**; concurrent use contraindicated. May ↓ absorption of drugs requiring acid pH, including **ketoconazole**, **itraconazole**, **atazanavir**, **iron salts**, **erlotinib**, **dasatinib**, **nelfinavir**, **nilotinib**, and **mycophenolate mofetil**; avoid concurrent use with **nelfinavir**. May ↑ levels and risk of toxicity of **digoxin**, **methotrexate**, and **tacrolimus**. Hypomagnesemia and hypokalemia may ↑ risk of **digoxin** toxicity. May ↑ risk of bleeding with **warfarin** (monitor INR).

Route/Dosage

Gastroesophageal Reflux Disease

PO (Adults): *Healing of erosive or ulcerative GERD:* 20 mg once daily for 4–8 wk; *Maintenance of healing of erosive or ulcerative GERD:* 20 mg once daily; *Symptomatic GERD:* 20 mg once daily for 4 wk (additional 4 wk may be considered for nonresponders).
PO (Children ≥12 yr): *Short-term treatment of symptomatic GERD:* 20 mg once daily for up to 8 wk.
PO (Children 1–11 yr): *≥15 kg:* 10 mg once daily for up to 12 wk (given as sprinkle); *<15 kg:* 5 mg once daily for up to 12 wk (given as sprinkle); may ↑ up to 10 mg once daily if inadequate response.

Duodenal Ulcers

PO (Adults): *Healing of duodenal ulcers:* 20 mg once daily for up to 4 wk.

H. pylori Eradication to Reduce the Risk of Duodenal Ulcer Recurrence (Triple Therapy)

PO (Adults): 20 mg twice daily for 7 days, with amoxicillin 1000 mg twice daily for 7 days and clarithromycin 500 mg twice daily for 7 days.

Pathological Hypersecretory Conditions, Including Zollinger-Ellison Syndrome

PO (Adults): 60 mg once daily initially; may be adjusted as needed and continued as necessary; doses up to 100 mg daily or 60 mg twice daily have been used.

Availability (generic available)

Delayed-release capsules (sprinkle): 10 mg.
Delayed-release tablets: ✱ 10 mg, 20 mg.

NURSING IMPLICATIONS

Assessment

- Assess routinely for epigastric or abdominal pain and frank or occult blood in the stool, emesis, or gastric aspirate.
- Monitor bowel function. Monitor for signs/symptoms of CDAD, including watery diarrhea with mucus, fever, abdominal pain or cramping, anorexia, nausea, and, in severe cases, dehydration, colitis, and blood or pus in the stool. Report to health care provider promptly. May begin up to several weeks following cessation of therapy.
- Monitor patients for development of severe cutaneous adverse reactions, including SJS, TEN, DRESS, and AGEP, including signs and symptoms of prodrome of fever, malaise, mucosal lesions, progressive skin rash, blisters, lymphadenopathy, conjunctivitis, myalgias, hepatitis, or eosinophilia. If a severe cutaneous adverse reaction is suspected, interrupt therapy until etiology of reaction is determined. Discontinue rabeprazole at the 1st sign of severe cutaneous adverse reactions.
- Monitor for signs and symptoms of acute tubulointerstitial nephritis (fever, rash, eosinophilia, flank pain, oliguria, hematuria), which can also initially appear as nonspecific symptoms of ↓ renal function (malaise, nausea, anorexia). Notify health care provider if suspected and discontinue use if confirmed.

Lab Test Considerations

- Monitor CBC with differential periodically during therapy.
- May cause hypomagnesemia, hypocalcemia, or hypokalemia. Monitor serum levels prior to and periodically during therapy.
- Vitamin B_{12} deficiency may occur with prolonged use >1–2 yr.

Implementation

- ***High Alert:*** Do not confuse rabeprazole with aripiprazole. Do not confuse Aciphex with Accupril or Aricept.
- **PO:** Administer without regard to food, preferably in the morning. ***DNC:*** Tablets should be swallowed whole; do not break, crush, or chew.
- For treatment of duodenal ulcers, take after a meal.
- For *Helicobacter pylori* eradication, take tablets with food.
- Capsules may be opened and sprinkled on a small amount of soft food (applesauce, fruit- or vegetable-based baby food, yogurt) or empty contents into small amount of liquid (infant formula, apple juice, pediatric electrolyte solution). Food or liquid should be at or below room temperature. Whole dose should be taken within 15 min of being sprinkled. Granules should not be chewed or crushed. Dose should be taken 30 min before a meal. Do not store mixture for future use.

Patient/Family Teaching

- Explain the purpose and side effects of rabeprazole. Instruct patient to take medication as directed for the full course of therapy, even if feeling better. Take missed doses as soon as remembered but not if almost time for next dose. Do not double doses. Advise patient to read *Patient Information* before starting and with each Rx refill in case of changes.
- May cause occasional drowsiness or dizziness. Caution patient to avoid driving or other activities requiring alertness until response to medication is known.
- Instruct patient to report symptoms of hypomagnesemia, hypocalcemia, or hypokalemia such as muscle twitches, spasms, weakness, or cramps, and heart palpitations.
- Advise patient to avoid alcohol, products containing aspirin or NSAIDs, and foods that may cause an ↑ in GI irritation.
- Caution patients to wear sunscreen and protective clothing to prevent photosensitivity reactions.
- Instruct patient to notify health care provider of onset of black, tarry stools; diarrhea; abdominal pain; or persistent headache or if fever and diarrhea develop, especially if stool contains blood, pus, or mucus. Advise patient not to treat diarrhea without consulting health care provider.
- Instruct patient to notify health care provider of all Rx or OTC medications, vitamins, or herbal products being taken and consult health care provider before taking any new medications.

R

- Rep: Advise women of reproductive potential to notify health care provider if pregnancy is planned or suspected or if breastfeeding.

Evaluation/Desired Outcomes

- Decrease in abdominal pain or prevention of gastric irritation and bleeding.
- Decrease in symptoms of GERD.
- Decreased acid secretion in hypersecretory conditions.

raloxifene (ra-lox-i-feen)

Evista

Classification

Therapeutic: bone resorption inhibitors

Pharmacologic: selective estrogen receptor modulators

Indications

Treatment and prevention of osteoporosis in postmenopausal women. Reduction in the risk of breast cancer in postmenopausal women with osteoporosis and those at high risk for invasive breast cancer.

Action

Binds to estrogen receptors, producing estrogen-like effects on bone, resulting in reduced resorption of bone and decreased bone turnover. **Therapeutic Effects:** Prevention of osteoporosis in patients at risk. Decreased risk of breast cancer.

Pharmacokinetics

Absorption: Although well absorbed (>60%), after oral administration, extensive first-pass metabolism results in 2% bioavailability.

Distribution: Extensively distributed to tissues.

Protein Binding: 95%.

Metabolism and Excretion: Extensively metabolized by the liver; undergoes enterohepatic cycling; excreted primarily in feces.

Half-life: 27.7 hr.

TIME/ACTION PROFILE (effects on bone turnover)

ROUTE	ONSET	PEAK	DURATION
PO	unknown	3 mo	unknown

Contraindications/Precautions

Contraindicated in: Hypersensitivity; History of thromboembolic events.

Use Cautiously in: Potential immobilization (↑ risk of thromboembolic events); History of stroke or transient ischemic attack; Atrial fibrillation; Hypertension; Cigarette smoking.

Adverse Reactions/Side Effects

CV: DEEP VEIN THROMBOSIS, MI. **Derm:** hot flush. **EENT:** retinal vein thrombosis. **MS:** leg cramps. **Neuro:** STROKE. **Resp:** PULMONARY EMBOLISM.

Interactions

Drug-Drug: Cholestyramine may ↓ absorption; avoid concurrent use. May alter effects of **warfarin** and other **highly protein-bound drugs.** Concurrent systemic **estrogen** therapy is not recommended.

Route/Dosage

PO (Adults): 60 mg once daily.

Availability (generic available)

Tablets: 60 mg.

NURSING IMPLICATIONS

Assessment

- Assess bone mineral density with x-ray, serum, and urine bone turnover markers (bone-specific alkaline phosphatase, osteocalcin, and collagen breakdown products) before and periodically during therapy.

Lab Test Considerations

- May ↑ triglycerides.
- May ↑ hormone-binding globulin (sex steroid-binding globulin, thyroxine-binding globulin, corticosteroid-binding globulin) with ↑ total hormone concentrations.
- May slightly ↓ in serum total calcium, inorganic phosphate, total protein, and albumin.
- May slightly ↓ in platelets.

Implementation

- **PO:** May be administered without regard to food.
- Calcium supplementation should be added to diet if daily intake is inadequate.

Patient/Family Teaching

- Explain purpose and side effects of medication. Advise patient to read *Patient Information* before starting therapy.
- Instruct patient on importance of adequate calcium and vitamin D intake or supplementation.
- Advise patient to discontinue alcohol consumption and smoking.
- Emphasize importance of regular weight-bearing exercise. Advise patient that raloxifene should be discontinued ≥72 hr before and during prolonged immobilization (recovery from surgery, prolonged bedrest). Instruct patient to avoid prolonged restrictions of movement during travel because of ↑ venous thrombosis risk.
- Advise patient that raloxifene will not ↓ hot flashes or flushes associated with estrogen deficiency and may cause hot flashes.
- Instruct patient to notify health care provider immediately if leg pain, redness, or ↑ warmth in lower leg; swelling of legs, hands, or feet; sudden chest pain; shortness of breath or coughing up blood; or sudden change in vision occur.

Evaluation/Desired Outcomes

- Prevention of osteoporosis in postmenopausal women.
- Reduced risk of breast cancer in postmenopausal women with osteoporosis and those at high risk for invasive breast cancer.

ramipril, See ANGIOTENSIN-CONVERTING ENZYME (ACE) INHIBITORS.

ranolazine (ra-**nole**-a-zeen)

✱ Corzyna, ~~Ranexa~~

Classification

Therapeutic: antianginals

Indications

Chronic angina pectoris.

Action

Does not ↓ BP or heart rate; remainder of mechanism is not known. **Therapeutic Effects:** Decreased frequency of angina.

Pharmacokinetics

Absorption: Highly variable.

Distribution: Unknown.

Metabolism and Excretion: Metabolized by the liver primarily by the CYP3A isoenzyme and to a lesser extent by the CYP2D6 isoenzyme; <5% excreted unchanged in urine and feces.

Half-life: 7 hr.

TIME/ACTION PROFILE (plasma concentrations)

ROUTE	ONSET	PEAK	DURATION
PO	unknown	2–5 hr	12 hr

Contraindications/Precautions

Contraindicated in: Hypersensitivity; Concurrent use of strong CYP3A inhibitors; Concurrent use of CYP3A inducers; Hepatic impairment; Lactation: Lactation.

Use Cautiously in: Renal impairment; OB: Use during pregnancy only if potential maternal benefit justifies potential fetal risk; Pedi: Safety and effectiveness not established in children; Geri: ↑ risk of adverse reactions in patients >75 yr.

Adverse Reactions/Side Effects

CV: palpitations, QT interval prolongation, TORSADES DE POINTES. **EENT:** tinnitus. **GI:** abdominal pain, constipation, dry mouth, nausea, vomiting. **GU:** acute renal failure. **Neuro:** dizziness, headache.

Interactions

Drug-Drug: Ketoconazole, itraconazole, clarithromycin, nefazodone, nelfinavir, and **ritonavir** significantly ↑ levels and risk of toxicity; concurrent use contraindicated. **Rifampin, rifabutin, rifapentin, phenobarbital, phenytoin,** and **carbamazepine** significantly ↓ levels and effectiveness; concurrent use contraindicated. **Verapamil, diltiazem, aprepitant, erythromycin,** and **fluconazole** may ↑ levels and risk of toxicity; do not exceed ranolazine dose of 500 mg twice daily. **Cyclosporine** and **paroxetine** may ↑ levels and risk of toxicity. May ↑ levels and risk of toxicity of **simvastatin, metoprolol, tricyclic antidepressants,** and **antipsychotics**. May ↑ **digoxin** levels and risk of toxicity; dose adjustment may be required.

Drug-Natural Products: St. John's wort significantly ↓ levels and effectiveness; concurrent use contraindicated.

Drug-Food: Grapefruit juice ↑ levels and risk of toxicity; do not exceed ranolazine dose of 500 mg twice daily.

Route/Dosage

PO (Adults): 500 mg twice daily initially; may ↑ to 1000 mg twice daily.

Availability (generic available)

Extended-release tablets: 500 mg, 1000 mg.

NURSING IMPLICATIONS

Assessment

- Assess location, duration, intensity, and precipitating factors of anginal pain.
- Monitor ECG at baseline and periodically during therapy to evaluate effects on QT interval.

Lab Test Considerations

- Monitor renal function after starting and periodically during therapy in patients with moderate to severe renal impairment (CCr <60 mL/min) for ↑ serum creatinine accompanied by ↑ BUN. Usually rapid onset, but does not progress and is reversible with discontinuation of ranolazine. *If acute renal failure occurs,* discontinue ranolazine.
- May cause transient eosinophilia.
- May ↓ hematocrit.

Implementation

- Ranolazine should be used in combination with calcium channel blockers, beta blockers, or nitrates.
- **PO:** May be administered without regard to food. ***DNC:*** Tablets should be swallowed whole; do not break, crush, or chew.

R

Patient/Family Teaching

- Explain purpose and side effects of medication to patient. Advise to read *Patient Information* before starting therapy.
- If dose is missed, instruct patient to take the usual dose at the next scheduled time; do not double doses. Explain that ranolazine is used for chronic therapy and will not help an acute angina episode.
- Advise patient to avoid grapefruit juice and grapefruit products when taking ranolazine.
- May cause dizziness and light-headedness. Caution patient to avoid driving and other activities requiring alertness until response to medication is known.
- Advise patient to notify health care professional if fainting occurs.
- Inform patient that ranolazine may cause changes in the ECG. Patient should inform health care professional if they have a personal or family history of QTc interval prolongation, congenital long QT syndrome, or proarrhythmic conditions such as hypokalemia.
- Instruct patient to notify health care professional of all Rx or OTC medications, vitamins, or herbal products being taken and consult health care professional before taking any new medications.
- Rep: Advise women of reproductive potential to notify health care professional if pregnancy is planned or suspected, or if breastfeeding.

Evaluation/Desired Outcomes

- Decrease in frequency of angina attacks.

rasagiline (ra-sa-ji-leen)

Azilect

Classification

Therapeutic: antiparkinson agents

Pharmacologic: monoamine oxidase type B inhibitors

Indications

Parkinson disease.

Action

Irreversibly inactivates monoamine oxidase (MAO) by binding to it at type B (brain sites); inactivation of MAO leads to increased amounts of dopamine available in the CNS. Differs from selegiline by its nonamphetamine characteristics. **Therapeutic Effects:** Improvement in symptoms of Parkinson disease, allowing increase in function.

Pharmacokinetics

Absorption: 36% absorbed following oral administration.

Distribution: Extensively distributed to tissues; readily crosses the blood-brain barrier.

Metabolism and Excretion: Extensively metabolized by the liver primarily by the CYP1A2 isoenzyme to an inactive metabolite; <1% excreted in urine.

Half-life: 1.3 hr; does not correlate with duration of MAO-B inhibition.

TIME/ACTION PROFILE

ROUTE	ONSET	PEAK	DURATION
PO	rapid	1 hr	40 days*

* Recovery of MAO-B function.

Contraindications/Precautions

Contraindicated in: Hypersensitivity; Concurrent use of meperidine, tramadol, methadone, or another MAO inhibitor; Moderate to severe hepatic impairment; Elective surgery requiring general anesthesia; Pheochromocytoma; Psychotic disorder.

Use Cautiously in: Mild hepatic impairment; OB: Safety not established in pregnancy; Lactation: Safety not established in breastfeeding; Pedi: Safety and effectiveness not established in children.

Adverse Reactions/Side Effects

CV: orthostatic hypotension (may ↑ levodopa-induced hypotension), ↑ BP, chest pain, syncope. **Derm:** alopecia, ecchymosis, MELANOMA, rash. **EENT:** conjunctivitis, rhinitis. **GI:** anorexia, dizziness, dyspepsia, gastroenteritis, vomiting. **GU:** ↓ libido, albuminuria. **Hemat:** leukopenia. **Metab:** weight loss. **MS:** arthralgia, arthritis, neck pain. **Neuro:** depression, dizziness, drowsiness, dyskinesia (may ↑ levodopa-induced dyskinesia), hallucinations, impulse control disorders (gambling, sexual), malaise, paresthesia, sleep driving, vertigo. **Resp:** asthma. **Misc:** fever, flu-like syndrome.

Interactions

Drug-Drug: **Meperidine**, **tramadol**, **methadone**, or other **MAO inhibitors** may ↑ risk of serotonin syndrome; concurrent use contraindicated. **CYP1A2 inhibitors**, including **ciprofloxacin**, may ↑ levels and risk of toxicity; dose adjustment recommended. **Dextromethorphan** may ↑ risk of psychosis/bizarre behavior; avoid concurrent use. ↑ risk of adverse reactions with **mirtazapine** and **cyclobenzapine**; avoid concurrent use. Hypertensive crisis may occur with **sympathomimetic amines**, including **amphetamines**, **pseudoephedrine**, **phenylephrine**, or **ephedrine**; avoid concurrent use. ↑ risk of serotonin syndrome with **tricyclic antidepressants**, **SSRIs**, and **SNRIs**; rasagiline should be discontinued ≥14 days prior to initiation of antidepressants (**fluoxetine** should be discontinued ≥5 wk prior to rasagiline therapy).

Drug-Natural Products: **St. John's wort** may ↑ risk of serotonin syndrome; avoid concurrent use.

Drug-Food: Ingestion of foods containing high amounts of **tyramine** (>150 mg) (e.g., cheese) may result in life-threatening hypertensive crisis.

Route/Dosage

PO (Adults): *Monotherapy or as adjunct therapy in patients not taking levodopa:* 1 mg once daily; *Concurrent levodopa therapy:* 0.5 mg once daily; may ↑ to 1 mg once daily; *Concurrent use of ciprofloxacin or other CYP1A2 inhibitors:* 0.5 mg once daily.

Hepatic Impairment

PO (Adults): *Mild hepatic impairment:* 0.5 mg once daily.

Availability (generic available)

Tablets: 0.5 mg, 1 mg.

NURSING IMPLICATIONS

Assessment

- Assess signs/symptoms of Parkinson disease (tremor, muscle weakness and rigidity, ataxic gait) before starting and periodically during therapy.
- Monitor for new onset or inadequately controlled hypertension periodically during therapy.
- Assess for serotonin syndrome (mental changes [agitation, hallucinations, coma], autonomic instability [tachycardia, labile BP, hyperthermia], neuromuscular aberrations [hyperreflexia, incoordination], or GI symptoms [nausea, vomiting, diarrhea]), especially in patients taking other serotonergic drugs (SSRIs, SNRIs, triptans).
- Assess patient for drowsiness, sleep disorders, and concurrent use of sedating medications or alcohol. *If significant daytime sleepiness or falling asleep during activities that require active participation occurs,* rasagiline may be discontinued.
- Assess for signs/symptoms of psychosis (confusion, paranoid ideation, delusions, hallucinations, disorientation, aggression, agitation, delirium) and ask specifically about impulsive and compulsive behaviors (gambling, binges, ↑ sexual urges). *If psychosis or inability to control urges occurs,* consider ↓ dose or discontinue therapy.

Lab Test Considerations

- May cause albuminuria, leukopenia, and abnormal liver function tests.

Implementation

- Do not confuse Azilect with Aricept. Do not confuse rasagiline with repaglinide.
- If used in combination with levodopa, a ↓ in levodopa dose may be considered based on individual results.
- **PO:** Administer once daily.

Patient/Family Teaching

- Explain purpose and side effects of medication. Advise patient to read *Patient Information* before starting therapy.
- Instruct patient to omit missed doses and take next dose as scheduled the following day. Do not double doses or discontinue abruptly; may cause ↑ temperature, muscular rigidity, altered consciousness, and autonomic instability.
- Caution patient to avoid alcohol, CNS depressants, and foods or beverages containing tyramine (see Appendix J) during and for ≥2 wk after therapy has been discontinued; they may precipitate a hypertensive crisis. Instruct patient to contact health care provider immediately if symptoms of hypertensive crisis (chest pain, tachycardia, bradycardia, severe headache, stiff/sore, nausea, vomiting, sweating, photosensitivity, enlarged pupils) or serotonin syndrome (mental changes [agitation, hallucinations, coma], autonomic instability, hyperreflexia, incoordination, nausea, vomiting, diarrhea) occur.
- Instruct patient to notify health care provider of all Rx or OTC medications, vitamins, or herbal products being taken and consult health care provider before taking any new medications. Caution patient to avoid use of St. John's wort and analgesics meperidine, tramadol, or methadone during therapy.
- Caution patient to avoid elective surgery requiring general anesthesia, cocaine, or local anesthesia containing sympathomimetic vasoconstrictors within 14 days of discontinuing rasagiline. If surgery is necessary sooner, benzodiazepines, rocuronium, fentanyl, morphine, and codeine may be used cautiously.
- Caution patient to change positions slowly to minimize orthostatic hypotension. Older adults are at ↑ risk.
- Caution patient to notify health care provider if new agitation; aggression; delirium; hallucinations; or new or ↑ gambling, sexual, or other intense urges occur.
- Inform patient that rasagiline may cause falling asleep while engaged in activities of daily living, including the operation of motor vehicles, conversations, and eating. Notify health care provider if periods of daytime sleepiness occur.
- Advise patient to notify health care provider immediately if severe headache, neck stiffness, heart racing, or palpitations occur.
- Rep: Advise women of reproductive potential to notify health care providers if pregnancy is planned or suspected or if breastfeeding.

Evaluation/Desired Outcomes

- Improvement in symptoms of Parkinson disease, allowing ↑ in function.

R

rasburicase

(ras-**byoor**-i-case)

Elitek, Fasturtec

Classification

Therapeutic: antigout agents, antihyperuricemics

Pharmacologic: enzymes

Indications

Initial management of increased uric acid levels in patients with leukemia, lymphoma, or other malignancies who are being treated with antineoplastics, which are expected to produce hyperuricemia.

Action

An enzyme that promotes the conversion of uric acid to allantoin, an inactive water-soluble compound. Produced by recombinant DNA technology. **Therapeutic Effects:** Decreased sequelae of hyperuricemia (nephropathy, arthropathy).

Pharmacokinetics

Absorption: IV administration results in complete bioavailability.

Distribution: Well distributed to tissues.

Metabolism and Excretion: Unknown.

Half-life: 18 hr.

TIME/ACTION PROFILE (↓ in uric acid)

ROUTE	ONSET	PEAK	DURATION
IV	rapid	unknown	4–24 hr

Contraindications/Precautions

Contraindicated in: Glucose-6-phosphate dehydrogenase (G6PD) deficiency (↑ risk of severe hemolysis); Previous allergic reaction, hemolysis, or methemoglobinemia from rasburicase; OB: Pregnancy; Lactation: Lactation.

Use Cautiously in: None reported.

Adverse Reactions/Side Effects

Derm: rash. **GI:** abdominal pain, constipation, diarrhea, mucositis, nausea, vomiting. **Hemat:** HEMOLYSIS, METHEMOGLOBINEMIA, neutropenia. **Neuro:** headache. **Resp:** respiratory distress. **Misc:** fever, HYPERSENSITIVITY REACTIONS (INCLUDING ANAPHYLAXIS), sepsis.

Interactions

Drug-Drug: None reported.

Route/Dosage

IV (Adults and Children): 0.2 mg/kg once daily for 5 days.

Availability

Lyophilized powder for injection: 1.5 mg/vial, 7.5 mg/vial.

NURSING IMPLICATIONS

Assessment

- Monitor for hypersensitivity reaction (chest pain, dyspnea, hypotension, urticaria). *If severe reaction occurs,* permanently discontinue rasburicase.

Lab Test Considerations

- Monitor patients for hemolysis. Screen patients at higher risk for G6PD deficiency (patients of African or Mediterranean ancestry) prior to therapy. *If hemolysis occurs,* permanently discontinue rasburicase.
- May cause methemoglobinemia. *If methemoglobinemia confirmed,* permanently discontinue rasburicase.
- May cause spuriously low uric acid levels in blood samples left at room temperature. Collect blood for uric acid levels in prechilled tubes containing heparin and immediately immerse and maintain in an ice water bath. Uric acid must be analyzed in plasma. Plasma samples must be assayed within 4 hr of collection.

Implementation

- Chemotherapy is initiated 4–24 hr after 1st dose of rasburicase.

IV Administration

- **Intermittent Infusion: Reconstitution:** Add 1 mL of diluent provided to each vial and mix by swirling gently. Do not shake or vortex. Reconstitute 7.5 mg vial with 5 mL of diluent. Solution should be clear and colorless. Do not use solution if discolored or contains particulates. **Dilution:** Remove dose from reconstituted vials and inject into infusion bag of 0.9% NaCl for a final total volume of 50 mL. Administer within 24 hr of reconstitution. Store reconstituted or diluted solution in refrigerator for up to 24 hr. **Rate:** Administer over 30 min. Do not administer as a bolus. Infuse through a separate line. Do not use a filter with infusion. If separate line is not possible, flush line with ≥15 mL of 0.9% NaCl prior to infusion.
- **Y-Site Incompatibility:** blinatumomab.

Patient/Family Teaching

- Explain purpose and side effects of medication. Advise patient to read *Patient Information* before starting therapy.
- Advise patient to notify health care provider of all Rx or OTC medications, vitamins, or herbal products being taken and to consult health care provider before taking other medications.
- Instruct patient to notify health care provider immediately if difficulty breathing, chest pain, or hives occur.
- Rep: May cause fetal harm. Advise women of reproductive potential to notify health care provider

if pregnancy is planned or suspected and to avoid breastfeeding during and for 2 wk after last dose.

Evaluation/Desired Outcomes

- Decreased sequelae of hyperuricemia. More than 1 course of therapy or administration beyond 5 days is not recommended.

REMS

ravulizumab

(rav-ue-liz-ue-mab)

Ultomiris

Classification

Therapeutic: hemostatic agents

Pharmacologic: complement inhibitors, monoclonal antibodies

Indications

Paroxysmal nocturnal hemoglobinuria. Atypical hemolytic uremic syndrome. Generalized myasthenia gravis in patients who are anti-acetylcholine receptor antibody-positive. Neuromyelitis optica spectrum disorder in patients who are anti-aquaporin-4 antibody positive.

Action

Binds to the complement protein C5 and inhibits its cleavage to C5a and C5b, preventing the production of the terminal complement complex, C5b-9, which is a necessary step in the initiation of hemolysis in paroxysmal noctural hemoglobinuria and development of thrombotic microangiopathy in atypical hemolytic uremic syndrome. Mechanism in generalized myasthenia gravis may be due to decreased deposition of C5b-9 complex at neuromuscular junction. Mechanism in neuromyelitis optica spectrum disorder may be due to inhibition of aquaporin-4 antibody-induced terminal complement C5b-9 deposition. **Therapeutic Effects:** Decreased hemolysis associated with paroxysmal noctural hemoglobinuria. Decreased complement-mediated thrombotic microangiopathy in atypical hemolytic uremic syndrome. Reduction in muscle weakness and improvement in ability to perform activities of daily living in generalized myasthenia gravis. Reduction in risk of relapse in neuromyelitis optica spectrum disorder.

Pharmacokinetics

Absorption: IV administration results in complete bioavailability.
Distribution: Distributed to tissues.
Metabolism and Excretion: Unknown.
Half-life: 50 days.

TIME/ACTION PROFILE (inhibition of serum free C5)

ROUTE	ONSET	PEAK	DURATION
IV	Rapid	End of infusion	8 wk

Contraindications/Precautions

Contraindicated in: Unresolved *Neisseria meningitidis* infection; Patients not vaccinated against *Neisseria meningitidis* (unless risk of delaying treatment outweighs risks of developing a meningococcal infection); Lactation: Lactation.
Use Cautiously in: OB: Use during pregnancy only if potential maternal benefit justifies potential fetal risk; Pedi: Children <1 mo (safety and effectiveness not established).

Adverse Reactions/Side Effects

GI: abdominal pain, diarrhea, nausea. **MS:** arthralgia. **Neuro:** headache, dizziness. **Resp:** upper respiratory tract infection. **Misc:** fever, HYPERSENSITIVITY REACTIONS (INCLUDING ANAPHYLAXIS), INFECTIONS (INCLUDING HAEMOPHILUS INFLUENZAE, NEISSERIA GONORRHOEAE, AND STREPTOCOCCUS PNEUMONIAE), infusion reactions, MENINGOCOCCAL INFECTIONS.

Interactions

Drug-Drug: None reported.

Route/Dosage

Paroxysmal Nocturnal Hemoglobinuria or Atypical Hemolytic Uremic Syndrome

IV (Adults and Children ≥1 mo and ≥100 kg): *Loading dose:* 3000 mg as a single dose (if switching from eculizumab, give loading dose 2 wk after last eculizumab dose); *Maintenance dose (initiated 2 wk after loading dose):* 3600 mg every 8 wk. Treatment should continue for ≥6 mo for atypical hemolytic uremic syndrome.
IV (Adults and Children ≥1 mo and 60–<100 kg): *Loading dose:* 2700 mg as a single dose (if switching from eculizumab, give loading dose 2 wk after last eculizumab dose); *Maintenance dose (initiated 2 wk after loading dose):* 3300 mg every 8 wk. Treatment should continue for ≥6 mo for atypical hemolytic uremic syndrome.
IV (Adults and Children ≥1 mo and 40–<60 kg): *Loading dose:* 2400 mg as a single dose (if switching from eculizumab, give loading dose 2 wk after last eculizumab dose); *Maintenance dose (initiated 2 wk after loading dose):* 3000 mg every 8 wk. Treatment should continue for ≥6 mo for atypical hemolytic syndrome.
IV (Adults and Children ≥1 mo and 30–<40 kg): *Loading dose:* 1200 mg as a single dose (if switching from eculizumab, give loading dose 2 wk after last eculizumab dose); *Maintenance dose (initiated 2 wk*

R

after loading dose): 2700 mg every 8 wk. Treatment should continue for ≥6 mo for atypical hemolytic uremic syndrome.
IV (Adults and Children ≥1 mo and 20–<30 kg): *Loading dose:* 900 mg as a single dose (if switching from eculizumab, give loading dose 2 wk after last eculizumab dose); *Maintenance dose (initiated 2 wk after loading dose)*: 2100 mg every 8 wk. Treatment should continue for ≥6 mo for atypical hemolytic uremic syndrome.
IV (Adults and Children ≥1 mo and 10–<20 kg): *Loading dose:* 600 mg as a single dose (if switching from eculizumab, give loading dose 2 wk after last eculizumab dose); *Maintenance dose (initiated 2 wk after loading dose)*: 600 mg every 4 wk. Treatment should continue for ≥6 mo for atypical hemolytic uremic syndrome.
IV (Adults and Children ≥1 mo and 5–<10 kg): *Loading dose:* 600 mg as a single dose (if switching from eculizumab, give loading dose 2 wk after last eculizumab dose); *Maintenance dose (initiated 2 wk after loading dose)*: 300 mg every 4 wk. Treatment should continue for ≥6 mo for atypical hemolytic uremic syndrome.

Generalized Myasthenia Gravis or Neuromyelitis Optica Spectrum Disorder

IV (Adults ≥100 kg): *Loading dose:* 3000 mg as a single dose (if switching from eculizumab, give loading dose 2 wk after last eculizumab dose); *Maintenance dose (initiated 2 wk after loading dose)*: 3600 mg every 8 wk.
IV (Adults 60–<100 kg): *Loading dose:* 2700 mg as a single dose (if switching from eculizumab, give loading dose 2 wk after last eculizumab dose); *Maintenance dose (initiated 2 wk after loading dose)*: 3300 mg every 8 wk.
IV (Adults 40–<60 kg): *Loading dose:* 2400 mg as a single dose (if switching from eculizumab, give loading dose 2 wk after last eculizumab dose); *Maintenance dose (initiated 2 wk after loading dose)*: 3000 mg every 8 wk.

Availability

Solution for injection: 10 mg/mL, 100 mg/mL.

NURSING IMPLICATIONS

Assessment

- Monitor for signs or symptoms of infusion reaction (lower back pain, ↓ or ↑ BP, infusion-related muscle pain or spasm, limb discomfort, rigors, dysgeusia) or drug hypersensitivity (allergic reaction) for ≥1 hr following completion of infusion. If signs of cardiovascular instability or respiratory compromise occur, interrupt infusion and institute supportive measures.
- Monitor for early signs and symptoms of meningococcal infections (headache with nausea or vomiting, headache and fever, headache with nuchal rigidity, stiff neck, stiff back, fever, fever and a rash, confusion, muscle aches with flu-like symptoms, eyes sensitive to light) during therapy. Evaluate immediately if infection is suspected. Consider discontinuation of therapy during treatment of serious meningococcal infections.
- **Paroxysmal Nocturnal Hemoglobinuria:** On discontinuation of therapy, monitor for signs and symptoms of hemolysis (↑ LDH, reappearance of fatigue, hemoglobinuria, abdominal pain, shortness of breath, major adverse vascular event, dysphagia, erectile dysfunction) for ≥16 wk. If signs and symptoms of hemolysis occur after discontinuation, including ↑ LDH, may require restarting ravulizumab.
- **Atypical Hemolytic Uremic Syndrome:** On discontinuation, monitor for signs and symptoms of complement-mediated thrombotic microangiopathy (changes in mental status, seizures, angina, dyspnea, thrombosis, ↑ BP) for ≥12 mo. In addition to clinical symptoms, monitor for ≥two concurrent lab values (↓ in platelet count ≥25% of baseline or peak platelet count during ravulizumab therapy; ↑ in serum creatinine ≥25% of baseline or to nadir during ravulizumab therapy; ↑ in serum LDH ≥25% of baseline or of nadir during ravulizumab therapy). If thrombotic microangiopathy complications occur on discontinuation, consider restarting ravulizumab.
- **Myasthenia Gravis:** Monitor for steady improvement in affected areas of muscle weakness. Signs of worsening or continued weakness include skeletal muscle weakness, eye and facial muscle weakness, drooping eyelids, blurred or double vision, difficulty swallowing, slurred speech, dyspnea, and being easily fatigued after periods of activity.
- **Neuromyelitis Optica Spectrum Disorder:** Monitor for symptoms in the eyes (pain, blurred vision, loss of vision in one or both eyes), muscles (weakness, spasms, pain, paresthesia, paralysis), bladder and bowel (incontinence), uncontrollable vomiting and hiccups, or confusion. In children, monitor for confusion, seizures, or coma.
- Pedi: Monitor children for signs of serious infections due to *Streptococcus pneumoniae* and *Haemophilus influenzae type b* such as pneumonia or bronchitis (tachypnea, cough, wheezing, fever), meningitis (severe headache, nausea and vomiting, fever, nuchal rigidity or stiff neck, Brudzinski or Kernig sign), ear infections, sinusitis, and conjunctivitis (inflammation, redness, drainage of the eye).

Lab Test Considerations

- Monitor LDH, serum creatinine, and platelet levels at baseline and for ≥12 mo after last dose; normalization or improvement in LDH and platelets, and ≥25%

improvement in serum creatinine from baseline indicates efficacy.

Implementation

- Vaccinate patients for meningococcal infection according to current Advisory Committee on Immunization Practices guidelines ≥2 wk before starting ravulizumab to ↓ risk of serious infection. May revaccinate patients considering duration of ravulizumab therapy. If ravulizumab is started immediately due to urgent need or vaccines are administered <2 wk before starting ravulizumab therapy, administer 2 wk of antibacterial prophylaxis. Administer vaccines as soon as possible if not prior to therapy initiation.
- Pedi: In children, may ↑ risk of developing serious infections due to *Streptococcus pneumoniae* and *Haemophilus influenzae type b*. Vaccinate for prevention of *Streptococcus pneumoniae* and *Haemophilus influenzae type b* infections according to Advisory Committee on Immunization Practices guidelines.
- ***REMS:*** Available only through *Ultomiris* and *Soliris REMS* program. Prescribers must enroll in program by accessing UltSolREMS.com or calling 1-888-765-4747 for more information.
- **Intermittent Infusion:** Solution is clear to translucent, slightly whitish; do not use solutions that are cloudy, discolored, or contain particulate matter. **Dilution:** Withdraw volume required and dilute with 0.9% NaCl. **Concentration:** Dilute to a final concentration of 5 mg/mL (for 10 mg/mL vials) or 50 mg/mL (for 100 mg/mL vials). Vials are single use only. Mix gently; do not shake. Do not mix 100 mg/mL and 10 mg/mL vials together. Protect from light; do not freeze. If not used immediately after preparation, store refrigerated for no longer than 24 hr, taking into account the expected infusion time. Once removed from refrigeration, administer within 6 hr if prepared with 10 mg/mL vials or within 4 hr if prepared with 100 mg/mL vials. Allow to warm to room temperature before infusing; do not heat in a microwave or with any heat source other than ambient air temperature. After administration, flush the entire line with 0.9% NaCl. **Rate:** Infuse through a 0.2- or 0.22-micron filter. Rate is based on body weight. See manufacturer's instructions for rate of loading dose and maintenance doses.
- **Y-Site Incompatibility:** Do not administer other drugs through same IV line.

Patient/Family Teaching

- Explain the purpose and side effects of ravulizumab to patient. Do not stop receiving drug without consulting health care provider. If an appointment is missed, contact health care provider as soon as possible to reschedule. Advise patient to read *Medication Guide* before starting and periodically during therapy in case of changes.
- Explain need for continued medical follow-up to assess effectiveness and possible side effects of medication. Periodic lab tests or exams may be needed.
- Caution patients about risk of meningococcal infection/sepsis. Advise patient to notify health care provider immediately if symptoms of meningitis or other infections occur. Inform patient of need for vaccination before starting therapy.
- Caution patients about risk of infections caused by *Streptococcus pneumoniae*, *Haemophilus influenzae type b*, and gonorrhea. Advise patient to consult health care provider if at risk for gonorrhea infection about gonorrhea prevention and regular testing.
- ***REMS:*** Inform patient of REMS program. Provide REMS educational materials and ensure patients are vaccinated with meningococcal vaccines. Enrollment in the *Ultomiris* and *Soliris REMS* and additional information are available by telephone: 1-888-765-4747 or at UltSolREMS.com.
- Instruct patient to carry *Ultomiris Patient Safety Card* that describes symptoms with them at all times and to immediately seek medical evaluation if symptoms occur during and for at least 8 mo after therapy.
- Advise patient to notify health care provider of all Rx or OTC medications, vitamins, or herbal products being taken and consult health care provider before taking any new medications.
- Rep: Advise women of reproductive potential to notify health care provider if pregnancy is planned or suspected and to avoid breastfeeding during therapy and for ≥8 mo after last dose. Patients or health care providers may call 1-833-793-0563 or go to UltomirisPregnancyStudy.com to enroll in or to obtain information about the pregnancy exposure registry that monitors pregnancy outcomes in women exposed to ravulizumab-cwvz.

Evaluation/Desired Outcomes

- Decreased hemolysis associated with paroxysmal nocturnal hemoglobinuria.
- Decreased complement-mediated thrombotic microangiopathy in atypical hemolytic uremic syndrome.
- Reduction in muscle weakness and improvement in ability to perform activities of daily living in generalized myasthenia gravis.
- Reduction in risk of relapse in neuromyelitis optica spectrum disorder.

R

relugolix/estradiol/norethindrone (rel-ue-goe-lix/es-tra-dye-ole/nor-eth-in-drone)

Myfembree

Classification

Therapeutic: hormones

Pharmacologic: GnRH antagonist, estrogens, progestins

Indications

Heavy menstrual bleeding associated with uterine fibroids in premenopausal women. Moderate to severe pain associated with endometriosis in premenopausal women.

Action

Relugolix: Reversibly binds to gonadotropin-releasing hormone (GnRH) receptors in the pituitary gland, causing a decrease in the release of luteinizing hormone and follicle-stimulating hormone, which subsequently leads to decreased serum concentrations of estradiol and progesterone; *Estradiol:* An estrogen that reduces the ↑ in bone resorption and resultant bone loss that can occur due to a ↓ in circulating estrogen concentrations from relugolix; *Norethindrone:* A progestin that protects the uterus from estrogen-induced endometrial hyperplasia. **Therapeutic Effects:** Reduction in menstrual blood loss in premenopausal women with uterine fibroids. Reduction in pain in premenopausal women with endometriosis.

Pharmacokinetics

Relugolix

Absorption: 12% absorbed following oral administration.

Distribution: Unknown.

Metabolism and Excretion: Primarily metabolized in the liver via the CYP3A4 isoenzyme (and to a lesser extent by CYP2C8). Primarily excreted in feces (81%; 4.2% as unchanged drug), with 4.1% excreted in urine (2.2% as unchanged drug).

Half-life: 61 hr.

Estradiol

Absorption: Well absorbed following oral administration.

Distribution: Widely distributed to tissues.

Metabolism and Excretion: Mostly metabolized by the liver and other tissues. Enterohepatic recirculation occurs; more absorption may occur from the GI tract.

Half-life: 16.6 hr.

Norethindrone

Absorption: Rapidly absorbed following oral administration.

Distribution: Widely distributed to tissues.

Metabolism and Excretion: Mostly metabolized by the liver. Metabolites primarily excreted in the urine (>50%), with 20–40% being excreted in feces.

Half-life: 8–9 hr.

TIME/ACTION PROFILE (plasma concentrations)

ROUTE	ONSET	PEAK	DURATION
PO (relugolix)	unknown	2 hr	unknown
PO (estradiol)	unknown	7 hr	unknown
PO (norethindrone)	unknown	1 hr	unknown

Contraindications/Precautions

Contraindicated in: Hypersensitivity; Women >35 yr who smoke; Current or history of deep vein thrombosis or pulmonary embolism; Cerebrovascular disease, cardiovascular disease, or peripheral vascular disease; Subacute bacterial endocarditis with valvular disease or atrial fibrillation; Inherited or acquired hypercoagulopathies; Uncontrolled hypertension; Headaches with focal neurological symptoms or migraine headaches with aura if >35 yr; Osteoporosis; Current or history of breast cancer or other hormone-sensitive malignancy; ↑ risk for hormone-sensitive malignancy; Hepatic impairment; Undiagnosed abnormal uterine bleeding; OB: Pregnancy.

Use Cautiously in: Underlying cardiovascular disease; Obesity; History of low trauma fracture or risk factors for osteoporosis or bone loss, including taking medications that may ↓ bone mineral density; History of suicidal ideation, depression, or anxiety; Submucosal uterine fibroids (↑ risk of prolapse or expulsion); Prediabetes or diabetes; Hypertriglyceridemia; Hypothyroidism or hypoadrenalism (may need to ↑ doses of thyroid hormone or cortisol replacement therapy); Lactation: Use while breastfeeding only if potential maternal benefit justifies potential risk to infant; Rep: Women of reproductive potential; Pedi: Safety and effectiveness not established in children.

Adverse Reactions/Side Effects

CV: DEEP VEIN THROMBOSIS, edema, hypertension, MI. **Derm:** hot flush, hyperhidrosis, night sweats, alopecia. **Endo:** hyperglycemia. **GI:** ↑ liver enzymes, cholecystitis, diarrhea, dyspepsia, nausea. **GU:** ↓ libido, amenorrhea, uterine bleeding, uterine fibroid expulsion/prolapse, vulvovaginal dryness. **Metab:** hypercholesterolemia, hypertriglyceridemia. **MS:** ↓ bone mineral density, arthralgia. **Neuro:** headache, anxiety, depression, dizziness, fatigue, irritability, STROKE, SUICIDAL THOUGHTS/BEHAVIORS. **Resp:** PULMONARY EMBOLISM. **Misc:** BREAST CANCER, HYPERSENSITIVITY REACTIONS (INCLUDING ANAPHYLAXIS AND ANGIOEDEMA).

Interactions

Drug-Drug: Corticosteroids, anticonvulsants, or **proton pump inhibitors** may ↑ risk of bone mineral density reduction and osteoporosis. **Hormonal contraceptives** may ↓ effectiveness of relugolix/estradiol/norethindrone and ↑ risk of thromboembolic events; avoid concurrent use. **P-glycoprotein (P-gp) inhibitors** may ↑ relugolix levels and risk of toxicity; avoid concurrent use. If concurrent use unavoidable, administer relugolix/estradiol/norethindrone 1st and then administer P-gp inhibitor ≥6 hr later. **Combined P-gp and strong CYP3A4 inducers** may ↓ relugolix/estradiol/norethindrone levels and effectiveness; avoid concurrent use.

Route/Dosage

PO (Adults): One tablet once daily. Start as early as possible after the onset of menses but no later than 7 days after menses has started. Duration of therapy not to exceed 24 mo.

Availability

Tablets: relugolix 40 mg/estradiol 1 mg/norethindrone 0.5 mg.

NURSING IMPLICATIONS

Assessment

- Monitor for signs and symptoms of thrombotic events (sudden unexplained partial or complete loss of vision, proptosis, diplopia, papilledema, retinal vascular lesions). *If arterial or venous thrombotic event occurs or is suspected,* immediately discontinue therapy. Risk is ↑ in women >35 yr who smoke and women with uncontrolled hypertension, dyslipidemia, vascular disease, or obesity. *For surgery associated with ↑ thromboembolism risk or prolonged immobilization,* discontinue therapy; ≥4–6 wk before surgery, if feasible.
- Assess bone mineral density by dual-energy x-ray absorptiometry (DXA) at baseline and periodically in women with heavy menstrual bleeding associated with uterine fibroids. In women with moderate to severe pain associated with endometriosis, annual DXA is recommended during therapy. Consider discontinuing therapy if risk associated with bone loss exceeds potential benefit of therapy. May add calcium and vitamin D supplement to ↑ bone mineral density.
- Assess for history of suicidal ideation, depression, and mood disorders before starting and just after initiating therapy to determine if risks of therapy outweigh benefits. Patients with new or worsening depression, anxiety, or other mood changes should be referred to a mental health provider. Advise patients to seek immediate medical attention for suicidal ideation and behavior. Re-evaluate the benefits and risks of continuing relugolix/estradiol/norethindrone if such events occur.
- Monitor for signs/symptoms of hypersensitivity reaction (anaphylaxis, urticaria, angioedema). *If hypersensitivity reaction occurs,* immediately discontinue relugolix/estradiol/norethindrone.

Lab Test Considerations

- Verify negative pregnancy test before starting therapy.
- May ↓ glucose tolerance and ↑ blood glucose.
- Monitor lipid levels. May ↑ cholesterol and triglycerides.
- May ↑ serum concentrations of binding proteins (thyroid-binding globulin, corticosteroid-binding globulin), which may ↓ free thyroid or corticosteroid hormone levels.

Implementation

- Begin therapy as soon as possible after menses onset and no later than 7 days after menses has started. If relugolix/estradiol/norethindrone is started later in the menstrual cycle, irregular and/or heavy bleeding may initially occur.
- Total duration of therapy is 24 mo.
- **PO:** Administer one tablet once daily at the same time, without regard to food.

Patient/Family Teaching

- Explain purpose and side effects of medication. Advise patient to read *Patient Information* before starting therapy.
- Instruct patient to take missed dose as soon as possible the same day and then resume regular scheduled dosing.
- Inform patient of the potential for bone loss and possible need for supplementation with calcium and vitamin D.
- Discuss with patient the possibility of hair loss. Explore methods of coping including discontinuing therapy.
- Instruct patient to notify health care provider of all Rx or OTC medications, vitamins, or herbal products being taken and consult health care provider before taking any new medications.
- Advise patient to notify health care provider immediately if signs and symptoms of thromboembolism (leg pain or swelling; sudden shortness of breath; double vision; bulging of eyes; sudden blindness; pain or pressure in chest, arm, or jaw; sudden, severe headache; weakness or numbness in arm or leg; trouble speaking) occur.
- Advise patient to notify health care provider immediately if suicidal thoughts or attempts, new or worse depression or anxiety, other changes in behavior or mood, or liver problems (jaundice, dark, amber-colored urine, feeling tired, nausea, vomiting, generalized swelling, right upper abdomen pain, bruising easily) occur.
- Rep: May cause early pregnancy loss if administered to pregnant women. Advise women of reproductive

R

potential to use effective nonhormonal contraception during therapy and for one wk after final dose. Avoid concurrent use of hormonal contraceptives containing estrogen during therapy; may ↑ risk of estrogen-associated adverse events and ↓ efficacy of relugolix/estradiol/norethindrone. Women who take relugolix/estradiol/norethindrone may experience amenorrhea or a ↓ in amount, intensity, or duration of menstrual bleeding, which may delay ability to recognize pregnancy. Inform patient of pregnancy exposure registry and call or encourage patient to call the Myfembree Pregnancy Exposure Registry at 1-855-428-0707.

Evaluation/Desired Outcomes

- Reduction in menstrual blood loss in premenopausal women with uterine fibroids.
- Moderate to severe pain associated with endometriosis in premenopausal women.

remdesivir (rem-de-si-vir)

Veklury

Classification

Therapeutic: antivirals

Pharmacologic: nucleoside analogues

Indications

Coronavirus 2019 (COVID-19) infection in patients who are hospitalized. COVID-19 infection in patients who are not hospitalized, have mild to moderate COVID-19, and are at high risk for progression to severe COVID-19, including hospitalization or death.

Action

As an adenosine nucleotide prodrug, remdesivir is metabolized to an active nucleoside triphosphate metabolite, after being distributed into cells. Remdesivir triphosphate acts as an adenosine triphosphate (ATP) analog and competes with ATP for incorporation into RNA chains by the SARS-CoV-2 RNA-dependent RNA polymerase, which results in delayed chain termination during viral RNA replication. **Therapeutic Effects:** Reduced time to recovery in hospitalized patients (hospital discharge, hospitalized but not requiring supplemental oxygen and no longer requiring ongoing care) from COVID-19 infection. Reduction in risk of hospitalization or all-cause mortality in nonhospitalized patients.

Pharmacokinetics

Absorption: IV administration results in complete bioavailability.

Distribution: Unknown.

Metabolism and Excretion: Remdesivir is a prodrug that is metabolized intracellularly to the active metabolite, remdesivir triphosphate. Primarily excreted in urine (74%, 10% as unchanged drug), with 18% of drug being excreted in feces.

Half-life: *Nucleoside triphosphate metabolite:* 20 hr.

TIME/ACTION PROFILE (median time to recovery)

ROUTE	ONSET	PEAK	DURATION
IV	unknown	11 days	unknown

Contraindications/Precautions

Contraindicated in: Hypersensitivity.

Use Cautiously in: OB: Safety not established in pregnancy; Lactation: Safety not established in breastfeeding.

Adverse Reactions/Side Effects

Endo: hyperglycemia. **GI:** nausea, ↑ liver enzymes, constipation. **GU:** acute kidney injury. **Hemat:** anemia. **Resp:** RESPIRATORY FAILURE. **Misc:** fever, HYPERSENSITIVITY REACTIONS (INCLUDING ANAPHYLAXIS AND ANGIOEDEMA), infusion reactions.

Interactions

Drug-Drug: Chloroquine or **hydroxychloroquine** may ↓ antiviral effects; avoid concurrent use.

Route/Dosage

IV (Adults and Children ≥40 kg): *Hospitalized patients:* 200 mg on Day 1, then 100 mg once daily starting on Day 2. Treatment duration = 10 days (patients requiring invasive mechanical ventilation and/or extracorporeal membrane oxygenation [ECMO]); 5 days (patients not requiring invasive mechanical ventilation and/or ECMO; if these patients are not improving after 5 days, treatment may be continued for another 5 days). *Nonhospitalized patients:* 200 mg on Day 1, then 100 mg once daily on Days 2 and 3.

IV (Children ≥28 days and 3–<40 kg): *Hospitalized patients:* 5 mg/kg on Day 1, then 2.5 mg/kg once daily starting on Day 2. Treatment duration = 10 days (patients requiring invasive mechanical ventilation and/or ECMO); 5 days (patients not requiring invasive mechanical ventilation and/or ECMO; if these patients are not improving after 5 days, treatment may be continued for another 5 days). *Nonhospitalized patients:* 5 mg/kg on Day 1, then 2.5 mg/kg once daily on Days 2 and 3.

IV (Children ≥28 days and 1.5–<3 kg): *Hospitalized patients:* 2.5 mg/kg on Day 1, then 1.25 mg/kg once daily starting on Day 2. Treatment duration = 10 days (patients requiring invasive mechanical ventilation and/or ECMO); 5 days (patients not requiring invasive mechanical ventilation and/or ECMO; if these patients are not improving after 5 days, treatment may be continued for another 5 days). *Nonhospitalized patients:* 2.5 mg/kg on Day 1, then 1.25 mg/kg once daily on Days 2 and 3.

IV (Children <28 days and ≥1.5 kg): *Hospitalized patients:* 2.5 mg/kg on Day 1, then 1.25 mg/kg once daily starting on Day 2. Treatment duration = 10 days (patients requiring invasive mechanical ventilation and/or ECMO); 5 days (patients not requiring invasive mechanical ventilation and/or ECMO; if these patients are not improving after 5 days, treatment may be continued for another 5 days). *Nonhospitalized patients:* 2.5 mg/kg on Day 1, then 1.25 mg/kg once daily on Days 2 and 3.

Availability

Lyophilized powder for injection: 100 mg/vial.

NURSING IMPLICATIONS

Assessment

- Monitor for signs/symptoms of COVID-19 infection (fever, cough, shortness of breath) before and periodically during therapy.
- Monitor for signs/symptoms of hypersensitivity reactions (hypotension, tachycardia, bradycardia, dyspnea, wheezing, angioedema, rash, nausea, vomiting, diaphoresis, shivering) during therapy and for ≥1 hr after infusion is complete. Slowing infusion rate to maximum time of 120 min may prevent reactions. *If clinically significant symptoms occur,* immediately discontinue infusion and begin symptomatic treatment.

Lab Test Considerations

- Monitor hepatic function before starting and during therapy as clinically appropriate. *If ALT ≥5 times upper limit of normal (ULN),* do not start remdesivir therapy. *If ALT ≥5 times ULN during therapy or ALT ↑ accompanied by signs/symptoms of liver inflammation or ↑ conjugated bilirubin, alkaline phosphatase, or INR,* hold remdesivir. Resume when ALT <5 times ULN.
- Monitor prothrombin time before starting and during therapy as clinically appropriate.

Implementation

- Administer remdesivir only in settings in which health care providers have immediate access to medications to treat a severe infusion or hypersensitivity reaction, such as anaphylaxis, and the ability to activate the emergency medical system.

IV Administration

- V Remdesivir is a vesicant. May be administered through a peripheral or central line. If extravasation occurs, immediately stop infusion. Leave needle/cannula in place temporarily but do not flush the line. Gently aspirate extravasated solution; then remove needle/cannula. Elevate patient's extremity and apply dry warm compresses.
- **Intermittent Infusion: Reconstitution:** Reconstitute vial with 19 mL of sterile water for injection. The powder for injection is the only approved formulation of remdesivir for patients weighing 1.5–<40 kg. Discard vial if vacuum does not pull sterile water for injection into vial. Shake vial for 30 sec. Allow contents to settle for 2–3 min for a clear solution. If contents not completely dissolved, shake for 30 sec and allow to settle for 2–3 min. Repeat until solution is clear. Reconstituted solution is stable for 4 hr at room temperature or 24 hr if refrigerated. **Concentration:** 5 mg/mL. **Dilution:** *For 100-mg dose,* withdraw and discard 20 mL from a 250-mL or 100-mL 0.9% NaCl infusion bag. Withdraw 20 mL of reconstituted solution and inject into infusion bag. *For 200-mg dose,* withdraw and discard 40 mL from a 250-mL or 100-mL 0.9% NaCl infusion bag. Withdraw 40 mL of reconstituted solution and inject into infusion bag. Gently invert bag 20 times to mix; do not shake. Solution is stable for 24 hr at room temperature or 48 hr if refrigerated. **Rate:** *Infuse 250 mL* over 30 min for rate of 8.33 mL/min, over 60 min for rate of 4.17 mL/min, or over 120 min for rate of 2.08 mL/min. *Infuse 100 mL* over 30 min for rate of 3.33 mL/min, over 60 min for rate of 1.67 mL/min, or over 120 min for rate of 0.83 mL/min.
- **Y-Site Compatibility:** fentanyl, furosemide, heparin, hydromorphone, morphine, octreotide.

Patient/Family Teaching

- Explain purpose of remdesivir to patient.
- Advise patient to notify health care provider immediately if signs and symptoms of hypersensitivity reactions (low blood pressure; changes in heartbeat; shortness of breath; wheezing; swelling of lips, face, or throat; rash; nausea; vomiting; sweating; shivering) occur.
- Instruct patient to notify health care provider of all Rx or OTC medications, vitamins, or herbal products being taken and to consult health care provider before taking other Rx, OTC, or herbal products, especially chloroquine or hydroxychloroquine.
- Rep: Advise women of reproductive potential to notify health care provider if pregnancy is planned or suspected or if breastfeeding during therapy.

Evaluation/Desired Outcomes

- Reduced time to recovery (hospital discharge, hospitalized but not requiring supplemental oxygen and no longer requiring ongoing care) from COVID-19 infection.

Rh_0(D) immune globulin IV, **See Rh_0(D) IMMUNE GLOBULIN.**

R

Rh_0(D) immune globulin microdose IM, IV, See Rh_0(D) IMMUNE GLOBULIN.

Rh_0(D) immune globulin microdose IM, See Rh_0(D) IMMUNE GLOBULIN.

Rh_0(D) immune globulin standard dose IM, See Rh_0(D) IMMUNE GLOBULIN.

Rh_0(D) IMMUNE GLOBULIN

(arr aych oh dee im-**yoon glob**-yoo-lin)

Rh_0(D) immune globulin standard dose IM

HyperRHO S/D Full Dose, RhoGAM

Rh_0(D) immune globulin microdose IM

HyperRHO S/D Mini-Dose, MICRhoGAM

Rh_0(D) immune globulin IV

WinRho SDF

Rh_0(D) immune globulin microdose IM, IV

Rhophylac

Classification

Therapeutic: vaccines/immunizing agents

Pharmacologic: immune globulins

Indications

IM, IV: Administered to Rh_0(D)-negative patients who have been exposed to Rh_0(D)-positive blood by: Pregnancy or delivery of a Rh_0(D)-positive infant; Abortion of a Rh_0(D)-positive fetus; Fetal-maternal hemorrhage due to amniocentesis, other obstetrical manipulative procedure, or intra-abdominal trauma while carrying a Rh_0(D)-positive fetus; Transfusion of Rh_0(D)-positive blood or blood products to a Rh_0(D)-negative patient. **IV:** Management of immune thrombocytopenic purpura (ITP).

Action

Prevent production of anti-Rh_0(D) antibodies in Rh_0(D)-negative patients who were exposed to Rh_0(D)-positive blood. Increase platelet counts in patients with ITP. **Therapeutic Effects:** Prevention of antibody response and hemolytic disease of the newborn (erythroblastosis fetalis) in future pregnancies of women who have conceived a Rh_0(D)-positive fetus. Prevention of Rh_0(D) sensitization following transfusion accident. Decreased bleeding in patients with ITP.

Pharmacokinetics

Absorption: IV administration results in complete bioavailability. Well absorbed from IM sites.

Distribution: Unknown.

Metabolism and Excretion: Unknown.

Half-life: 25–30 days.

TIME/ACTION PROFILE (plasma concentrations)

ROUTE	ONSET	PEAK	DURATION
IM	rapid	5–10 days	unknown
IV†	unknown	2 hr	unknown

† When given for ITP, platelet counts start to rise in 1–2 days, peak after 5–7 days, and last for 30 days.

Contraindications/Precautions

Contraindicated in: Prior hypersensitivity reaction to human immune globulin; Rh_0(D)- or Du-positive patients.

Use Cautiously in: ITP patients with pre-existing anemia (↓ dose if Hgb <10 g/dL). May also cause disseminated intravascular coagulation in ITP patients.

Adverse Reactions/Side Effects

CV: hypertension, hypotension. **Derm:** rash. **GI:** diarrhea, nausea, vomiting. **GU:** acute renal failure. **Hemat:** anemia. **ITP:** DISSEMINATED INTRAVASCULAR COAGULATION, INTRAVASCULAR HEMOLYSIS. **Local:** pain at injection site. **MS:** arthralgia, myalgia. **Neuro:** dizziness, headache. **Misc:** fever.

Interactions

Drug-Drug: May ↓ antibody response to some **live-virus vaccines (measles, mumps, rubella)**.

Route/Dosage

Rh_0(D) Immune Globulin (for IM use only)

Following Delivery

IM (Adults): *HyperRHO S/D Full Dose, RhoGAM:* 1 vial standard dose (300 mcg) within 72 hr of delivery.

Before Delivery

IM (Adults): *HyperRHO S/D Full Dose, RhoGAM:* 1 vial standard dose (300 mcg) at 26–28 wk.

Termination of Pregnancy (<13 wk Gestation)

IM (Adults): *HyperRHO S/D Mini-Dose, MICRhoGAM:* 1 vial of microdose (50 mcg) within 72 hr.

Termination of Pregnancy (>13 wk Gestation)

IM (Adults): *RhoGAM:* 1 vial standard dose (300 mcg) within 72 hr.

Large Fetal-Maternal Hemorrhage (>15 mL)

IM (Adults): *RhoGAM:* 20 mcg/mL of Rh_0(D)-positive fetal RBCs.

Transfusion Accident

IM (Adults): *HyperRHO S/D Full Dose, RhoGAM:* (Volume of Rh-positive blood administered × Hct of donor blood)/15 = number of vials of standard dose (300 mcg) preparation (round to next whole number of vials).

Rh_0(D) Immune Globulin IV (for IM or IV Use)

Following Delivery

IM, IV (Adults): *WinRho SDF:* 120 mcg within 72 hr of delivery. *Rhophylac:* 300 mcg within 72 hr of delivery.

Prior to Delivery

IM, IV (Adults): *WinRho SDF, Rhophylac:* 300 mcg at 28 wk; if initiated earlier in pregnancy, repeat every 12 wk.

Following Amniocentesis or Chorionic Villus Sampling

IM, IV (Adults): *WinRho SDF (before 34 wk gestation):* 300 mcg immediately; repeat every 12 wk during pregnancy. *Rhophylac:* 300 mcg within 72 hr of procedure.

Termination of Pregnancy, Amniocentesis, or Any Other Manipulation

IM, IV (Adults): *WinRho SDF:* 120 mcg within 72 hr after event.

Large Fetal-Maternal Hemorrhage/ Transfusion Accident

IM (Adults): *WinRho SDF:* 1200 mcg every 12 hr until total dose is given (total dose determined by amount of blood loss/hemorrhage).

IV (Adults): *WinRho SDF:* 600 mcg every 8 hr until total dose is given (total dose determined by amount of blood loss/hemorrhage).

Immune Thrombocytopenic Purpura

IV (Adults and Children): *WinRho SDF, Rhophylac:* 50 mcg/kg initially (if Hgb <10 g/dL, ↓ dose to 25–40 mcg/kg); further dosing/frequency determined by clinical response (range 25–60 mcg/kg). Each dose may be given as a single dose or in 2 divided doses on separate days.

Availability

Rh_0(D) Immune Globulin (for IM Use)

Solution for injection (prefilled syringes): 50 mcg (microdose: MICRhoGAM, HyperRHO S/D Mini-Dose), 300 mcg (standard dose: RhoGAM, HyperRHO S/D Full Dose).

Rh_0(D) Immune Globulin Intravenous (for IM or IV Use)

Injection: 300 mcg/vial, 500 mcg/vial, 3000 mcg/vial.
Prefilled syringes: 300 mcg/2 mL.

NURSING IMPLICATIONS

Assessment

- **IV:** Assess vital signs periodically during therapy in patients receiving IV Rh_0(D) immune globulin.
- **ITP:** Monitor for signs/symptoms of intravascular hemolysis (back pain, shaking chills, fever, hemoglobinuria), anemia, and renal impairment. If transfusions are required, use Rh_0(D)-negative packed red blood cells to prevent exacerbation of intravascular hemolysis.

Lab Test Considerations

- *Pregnancy:* Type and crossmatch of mother and newborn's cord blood must be performed to determine need for medication. Mother must be Rh_0(D)-negative and Du-negative. Infant must be Rh_0(D)-positive. If there is doubt regarding infant's blood type or if father is Rh_0(D)-positive, medication should be given.
- An infant born to a woman treated with Rh_0(D) immune globulin antepartum may have a weakly positive direct Coombs test result on cord or infant blood.
- *ITP:* Monitor platelets, RBCs, hemoglobin, and reticulocytes to determine effectiveness of therapy.

Implementation

- Do not give to infant, to Rh_0(D)-positive individual, or to Rh_0(D)-negative individual previously sensitized to the Rh_0(D) antigen. However, there is no more risk than when given to a woman who is not sensitized. When in doubt, administer Rh_0(D) immune globulin.
- Do not confuse IM and IV formulations. Rh immune globulin for IV administration is labeled "Rh Immune Globulin Intravenous." Rh Immune Globulin Intravenous may be given IM; however, Rh Immune Globulin (microdose and standard dose) is for IM use only and cannot be given IV.
- When using prefilled syringes, allow solution to reach room temperature before administration.
- **IM: Reconstitution:** Reconstitute Rh_0(D) immune globulin IV for IM use immediately before use with 1.25 mL of 0.9% NaCl. Inject diluent onto inside wall of vial and wet pellet by gently swirling until dissolved. Do not shake.
- Administer into the deltoid muscle. Dose should be given within 3 hr but may be given up to 72 hr after delivery, miscarriage, abortion, or transfusion.

IV Administration

- **IV Push: Reconstitution:** Reconstitute Rh_0(D) immune globulin IV for IV administration immediately before use with 2.5 mL of 0.9% NaCl. Inject diluent onto inside wall of vial and wet pellet by gently swirling until dissolved. Do not shake. **Rate:** Administer over 3–5 min.

R

Patient/Family Teaching

- **Pregnancy:** Explain to patient that the purpose of this medication is to protect future Rh_o (D)-positive infants.
- **ITP:** Explain purpose of medication to patient.
- Advise patient to notify health care provider if presence of dark urine, back pain, fever, chills, less urine passed, swelling, sudden weight gain, shortness of breath, rash, dizziness, or shaking. Symptoms can happen within 4–8 hr and up to 72 hr after dose.
- Advise patient to notify health care provider of all Rx or OTC medications, vitamins, or herbal products being taken and to consult with health care provider before taking other medications.

Evaluation/Desired Outcomes

- Prevention of antibody response and hemolytic disease of the newborn (erythroblastosis fetalis) in future pregnancies of women who have conceived a Rh_o (D)-positive fetus.
- Prevention of Rh_o (D) sensitization following transfusion accident.
- Decreased bleeding in patients with ITP.

HIGH ALERT

ribociclib (rye-boe-**sye**-klib)

Kisqali

Classification

Therapeutic: antineoplastics

Pharmacologic: kinase inhibitors

Indications

Adjuvant treatment of hormone receptor (HR)-positive, human epidermal growth factor receptor 2 (HER2)-negative stage II and III early breast cancer in patients at high risk of recurrence. Advanced or metastatic HR-positive, HER2-negative breast cancer (as initial endocrine-based therapy) (in combination with an aromatase inhibitor). Advanced or metastatic HR-positive, HER2-negative breast cancer (as initial endocrine-based therapy or following disease progression on endocrine therapy) (in combination with fulvestrant).

Action

Inhibits kinases (cyclin-dependent kinases 4 and 6) that are part of the signaling pathway for cell proliferation. **Therapeutic Effects:** Improved survival and decreased spread of breast cancer.

Pharmacokinetics

Absorption: 66% absorbed following oral administration.
Distribution: Extensively distributed to the tissues.
Metabolism and Excretion: Mostly metabolized in the liver by the CYP3A4 isoenzyme; 17% excreted unchanged in feces, 12% in urine.
Half-life: 32 hr.

TIME/ACTION PROFILE (plasma concentrations)

ROUTE	ONSET	PEAK	DURATION
PO	unknown	1–4 hr	unknown

Contraindications/Precautions

Contraindicated in: Congenital long QT syndrome; Uncorrected hypokalemia or hypomagnesemia; Recent MI, HF, unstable angina, bradycardia, uncontrolled hypertension, high degree atrioventricular block, severe aortic stenosis, or uncontrolled hypothyroidism; OB: Pregnancy; Lactation: Lactation.
Use Cautiously in: Severe renal impairment (↓ dose); Moderate or severe hepatic impairment (↓ dose); Rep: Women of reproductive potential; Pedi: Safety and effectiveness not established in children.

Adverse Reactions/Side Effects

CV: peripheral edema, QT interval prolongation, syncope. **Derm:** alopecia, pruritus, rash, DRUG REACTION WITH EOSINOPHILIA AND SYSTEMIC SYMPTOMS (DRESS), STEVENS-JOHNSON SYNDROME (SJS), TOXIC EPIDERMAL NECROLYSIS (TEN). **F and E:** hypokalemia, hypophosphatemia. **GI:** ↑ liver enzymes, abdominal pain, constipation, diarrhea, nausea, stomatitis, vomiting, HEPATOTOXICITY, hyperbilirubinemia. **GU:** ↑ serum creatinine, ↓ fertility (men). **Hemat:** anemia, NEUTROPENIA, THROMBOCYTOPENIA. **Metab:** ↓ appetite. **MS:** back pain. **Neuro:** fatigue, headache, insomnia. **Resp:** dyspnea, INTERSTITIAL LUNG DISEASE (ILD). **Misc:** fever.

Interactions

Drug-Drug: Strong CYP3A4 inhibitors, including **clarithromycin, itraconazole, ketoconazole, lopinavir/ritonavir, nefazodone, nelfinavir, posaconazole, ritonavir**, or **voriconazole**, may ↑ levels and the risk of toxicity; avoid concurrent use, if possible; if unavoidable, ↓ dose of ribociclib. **Strong CYP3A4 inducers**, including **carbamazepine, phenytoin**, or **rifampin**, can ↓ levels and effectiveness; avoid concurrent use. May ↑ levels and risk of toxicity of **cyclosporine, dihydroergotamine, ergotamine, everolimus, fentanyl, midazolam, pimozide, quinidine, sirolimus**, and **tacrolimus**; if concurrent use is required, dose ↓ may be necessary. **QT-interval-prolonging medications**, including **amiodarone, chloroquine, clarithromycin, disopyramide, haloperidol, methadone, moxifloxacin, ondansetron, pimozide, procainamide, quinidine, sotalol**, and **tamoxifen**, may ↑ risk of QT interval prolongation; avoid concurrent use.
Drug-Natural Products: St. John's wort may ↓ levels and effectiveness; avoid concurrent use.
Drug-Food: Grapefruit/grapefruit juice or **pomegranate/pomegranate juice** may ↑ levels and risk of toxicity; avoid ingestion.

Route/Dosage

Early Breast Cancer

PO (Adults): 400 mg once daily for 21 days, followed by 7 days off to complete a 28-day treatment cycle; continue treatment cycles for 3 yr or until disease progression or unacceptable toxicity. *Concurrent use of strong CYP3A4 inhibitor:* 200 mg once daily for 21 days, followed by 7 days off to complete a 28-day treatment cycle; continue treatment cycles for 3 yr or until disease progression or unacceptable toxicity.

Renal Impairment

PO (Adults): *Severe renal impairment:* 200 mg once daily for 21 days, followed by 7 days off to complete a 28-day treatment cycle; continue treatment cycles for 3 yr or until disease progression or unacceptable toxicity.

Advanced or Metastatic Breast Cancer

PO (Adults): 600 mg once daily for 21 days, followed by 7 days off to complete a 28-day treatment cycle; continue treatment cycles until disease progression or unacceptable toxicity. *Concurrent use of strong CYP3A4 inhibitor:* 400 mg once daily for 21 days, followed by 7 days off to complete a 28-day treatment cycle; continue treatment cycles until disease progression or unacceptable toxicity.

Renal Impairment

PO (Adults): *Severe renal impairment:* 200 mg once daily for 21 days, followed by 7 days off to complete a 28-day treatment cycle; continue treatment cycles until disease progression or unacceptable toxicity.

Hepatic Impairment

PO (Adults): *Moderate or severe hepatic impairment:* 400 mg once daily for 21 days, followed by 7 days off to complete a 28-day treatment cycle; continue treatment cycles until disease progression or unacceptable toxicity.

Availability

Tablets: 200 mg.

NURSING IMPLICATIONS

Assessment

- Monitor ECG prior to therapy. Avoid administering if QT interval >450 msec. Repeat ECG on Day 14 of first cycle, beginning of 2nd cycle, and as indicated. *If QT interval >480 msec,* suspend therapy. If QT interval prolongation resolves to <481 msec, resume therapy at same dose or next ↓ dose in advanced or metastatic breast cancer. *If QT interval ≥481 msec recurs,* interrupt dose until QT interval resolves to <481 msec; then resume ribociclib at next ↓ dose. *If QT interval >500 msec,* withhold therapy if >500 msec on ≥2 separate ECGs (within same visit). If QT interval prolongation resolves to <481 msec, resume therapy at next ↓ dose. *If QT interval prolongation is either >500 msec or >60 msec change from baseline AND associated with any of the following: torsades de pointes, polymorphic ventricular tachycardia, unexplained syncope, or signs and symptoms of serious arrhythmia; or if dose <200 mg/day is required,* permanently discontinue ribociclib.
- Monitor for signs and symptoms of ILD/pneumonitis (hypoxia, cough, dyspnea) during therapy. *If Grade 1 symptoms (asymptomatic) occur,* continue and treat symptomatically. *If Grade 2 symptoms occur,* hold therapy until ≤Grade 1.
  Resume at next ↓ dose. *If Grade 2 recurs,* permanently discontinue ribociclib. *If Grade 3 or Grade 4 symptoms (life-threatening) occur,* permanently discontinue ribociclib.
- Monitor for cutaneous reactions (rash, erythema, purpura) during therapy. *If Grade 1 (<10% body surface area [BSA] with active skin toxicity, no signs of systemic involvement) or Grade 2 (10–30% BSA with active skin toxicity, no signs of systemic involvement) occurs,* continue at same dose, initiate medical therapy, and monitor as clinically indicated. *If Grade 3 (severe rash not responsive to medical management; >30% BSA with active skin toxicity; signs of systemic involvement present; SJS) occurs,* hold ribociclib until the cause of has been determined. If the cause is SJS, TEN, or DRESS, permanently discontinue ribociclib. For other causes, hold dose until recovery to ≤Grade 1; then resume ribociclib at same dose level. If the cutaneous reaction recurs at Grade 3, resume ribociclib at the next ↓ dose. *If Grade 4 (any % BSA associated with extensive superinfection, with IV antibiotics indicated; life-threatening consequences; TEN) occurs,* permanently discontinue ribociclib.

Lab Test Considerations

- Verify negative pregnancy test prior to starting therapy.
- Monitor serum electrolytes (potassium, calcium, phosphorous, magnesium) prior to starting therapy, at beginning of 1st 6 cycles, and as indicated. Correct abnormalities before starting therapy.
- Monitor liver function before starting therapy, every 2 wk for 1st 2 cycles, at beginning of each subsequent 4 cycles, and as indicated. ***For AST and/or ALT ↑ from baseline, WITHOUT ↑ total bilirubin >2 times upper limit of normal (ULN): If Grade 1 (>ULN–3 times ULN),*** no dose adjustment. *If Grade 2 (>3–5 times ULN),* hold dose until recovery to ≤baseline grade; then resume at same dose. *If Grade 2 recurs,* resume ribociclib at next ↓ dose.

R

Do not interrupt dose for Grade 2 at baseline. *Grade 3 (>5–20 times ULN),* withhold dose until recovery to ≤baseline grade; then resume at next lower dose. *If Grade 3 recurs,* discontinue ribociclib. *If Grade 4 occurs (>20 times ULN),* discontinue ribociclib. ***Combined ↑ in AST and/or ALT WITH total bilirubin ↑, in absence of cholestasis:*** *If ALT and/or AST >3 times ULN along with total bilirubin >2 times ULN irrespective of baseline grade,* discontinue ribociclib.

- Monitor CBC before starting therapy, every 2 wk for 1st 2 cycles, at beginning of each subsequent 4 cycles, and as indicated. *If Grade 1 or 2 (ANC 1000/mm³ to <lower limit of normal) occurs,* no dose adjustment required. *If Grade 3 (ANC 500–1000/mm³) occurs,* interrupt dose until recovery to Grade ≤2. Resume therapy at same dose. *If toxicity recurs at Grade 3,* hold dose until recovery; then resume ribociclib at next ↓ dose. *If Grade 3 febrile neutropenia occurs,* suspend therapy until recovery of neutropenia to Grade ≤2. Resume therapy at next ↓ dose. *If Grade 4 (ANC <500/mm³) occurs,* withhold therapy until recovery to Grade ≤2. Resume ribociclib at next ↓ dose.

Implementation

- **Dose Reduction Schedule:** Starting dose: 600 mg/day. 1st dose reduction: 400 mg/day. 2nd dose reduction: 200 mg/day.
- **PO:** Administer once daily at the same time each day, preferably in the morning, without regard to food. *DNC:* Swallow tablets whole; do not crush, break, or chew. Do not administer tablets that are broken, cracked, or not intact.
- Pre/perimenopausal women or men taking ribociclib and an aromatase inhibitor or fulvestrant should be treated with a luteinizing hormone-releasing hormone agonist.

Patient/Family Teaching

- Instruct patient to take ribociclib as directed. If patient vomits after taking dose or misses dose, omit for that day. Take next dose at usual time the next day. Advise patient to read *Patient Information* prior to starting and with each Rx refill in case of changes.
- Advise patient to avoid eating pomegranate or grapefruit and to avoid drinking pomegranate or grapefruit juice during therapy.
- Advise patient to notify health care professional if signs and symptoms of heart rhythm problems (fast or irregular heart rate, dizziness, feeling faint), low white blood cell counts (fever and chills), liver problems (yellowing of skin or whites of eyes, jaundice, dark or brown tea-colored urine, feeling very tired, loss of appetite, pain on upper right side of abdomen, unusual bleeding or bruising), or skin reactions occur.
- Instruct patient to notify health care professional of all Rx or OTC medications, vitamins, or herbal products being taken and to consult with health care professional before taking other medications.
- Rep: May cause fetal harm. Advise women of reproductive potential to use effective contraception and to avoid breastfeeding during and for ≥3 wk after last dose of therapy. Inform male patients that ribociclib may impair fertility.

Evaluation/Desired Outcomes

- Improved survival and decreased spread of breast cancer.

rifabutin (riff-a-**byoo**-tin)

Mycobutin

Classification

Therapeutic: agents for atypical mycobacterium

Indications

Prevention of disseminated *Mycobacterium avium* complex disease in patients with advanced HIV infection.

Action

Appears to inhibit DNA-dependent RNA polymerase in susceptible organisms. **Therapeutic Effects:** Antimycobacterial action against susceptible organisms. **Spectrum:** Active against *M. avium* and most strains of *M. tuberculosis*.

Pharmacokinetics

Absorption: Well absorbed following oral administration (50–85%). Absorption ↓ in patients with HIV (20%).

Distribution: Widely distributed to body tissues and fluids.

Metabolism and Excretion: Mostly metabolized by the liver; <5% excreted unchanged by the kidneys.

Half-life: 45 hr.

TIME/ACTION PROFILE (plasma concentrations)

ROUTE	ONSET	PEAK	DURATION
PO	rapid	2–4 hr	24 hr

Contraindications/Precautions

Contraindicated in: Hypersensitivity. Cross-sensitivity with other rifamycins (rifampin) may occur; Active tuberculosis (TB); Concurrent use of cabotegravir/rilpivirine or voriconazole; Lactation: Lactation.

Use Cautiously in: OB: Use during pregnancy only if potential maternal benefit justifies potential fetal risk; Pedi: Safety and effectiveness not established in children.

Adverse Reactions/Side Effects

CV: chest pain, chest pressure. **Derm:** ACUTE GENERALIZED EXANTHEMATOUS PUSTULOSIS, DRUG REACTION WITH

EOSINOPHILIA AND SYSTEMIC SYMPTOMS (DRESS), rash, skin discoloration, STEVENS-JOHNSON SYNDROME (SJS), TOXIC EPIDERMAL NECROLYSIS (TEN). **EENT:** ocular disturbances. **GI:** altered taste, CLOSTRIDIOIDES DIFFICILE-ASSOCIATED DIARRHEA (CDAD), drug-induced hepatitis. **Hemat:** hemolysis, neutropenia, thrombocytopenia. **MS:** arthralgia, myositis. **Resp:** dyspnea. **Misc:** brown-orange discoloration of body fluids (urine, tears, saliva), flu-like syndrome.

Interactions

Drug-Drug: May significantly ↓ levels and effectiveness of **rilpivirine**; concurrent use with cabotegravir/rilpivirine contraindicated. **Voriconazole** may significantly ↑ levels and risk of toxicity of both rifabutin and voriconazole; concurrent use contraindicated. May ↓ levels and effectiveness of **estrogen-containing contraceptives**. May ↓ levels and effectiveness of **bictegravir** and **tenofovir alafenamide**; concurrent use with **bictegravir/emtricitabine/tenofovir alafenamide** is not recommended. May ↓ levels and effectiveness of **doravirine**; ↑ doravirine dose. May ↓ levels and effectiveness of **rilpivirine** and **tenofovir alafenamide**; concurrent use with **rilpivirine/tenofovir alafenamide/emtricitabine** not recommended. **Atazanavir/ritonavir**, **lopinavir/ritonavir**, and **tipranavir/ritonavir** may ↑ levels and risk of toxicity; ↓ rifabutin dose to 150 mg every other day or 150 mg 3 times weekly. May ↑ levels and risk of toxicity of **darunavir/ritonavir**; ↓ rifabutin dose to 150 mg every other day or 150 mg 3 times weekly. May ↓ levels and effectiveness of **elvitegravir**; concurrent use with elvitegravir/cobicistat not recommended. May ↓ levels and effectiveness of **etravirine**; concurrent use with etravirine with ritonavir or another protease inhibitor not recommended. **Nelfinavir** may ↑ levels and risk of toxicity; ↓ rifabutin dose to 150 mg once daily and ↓ nelfinavir dose. May ↓ levels and effectiveness of **sofosbuvir**; concurrent use not recommended. May ↑ levels and risk of toxicity of metabolite of **bedaquiline**; concurrent use not recommended. **Fluconazole** may ↑ levels and risk of toxicity. Concurrent use with **itraconazole** or **posaconazole** may ↑ levels and risk of toxicity of rifabutin and ↓ levels and effectiveness of itraconazole or posaconazole; avoid concurrent use. May ↓ levels and effectiveness of **dapsone** and **sulfamethoxazole/trimethoprim**. Concurrent use with **clarithromycin** may ↑ levels and risk of toxicity of rifabutin and ↓ levels and effectiveness of clarithromycin.

Route/Dosage

PO (Adults): 300 mg once daily. If GI upset occurs, may give as 150 mg twice daily with food.

Availability (generic available)

Capsules: 150 mg. ***In combination with:*** amoxicillin and omeprazole (Talicia). See Appendix N.

NURSING IMPLICATIONS

Assessment

- Monitor for signs of active TB (purified protein derivative [PPD], chest x-ray, sputum culture, blood culture, urine culture, biopsy of suspicious lymph nodes) prior to and during therapy. Rifabutin must not be administered to patients with active TB.
- Mycobacterial studies and susceptibility tests should be performed before and periodically during therapy to detect possible resistance. Perform chest x-ray after 2–3 mo and at end of treatment in patients with negative initial cultures.
- Assess lung sounds and character and amount of sputum periodically during therapy.
- Monitor for signs/symptoms of CDAD including watery diarrhea with mucus, fever, abdominal pain or cramping, anorexia, nausea, and, in severe cases, dehydration and blood or pus in the stool. May begin ≥2 mo after therapy. Report promptly to health care provider.
- Monitor patients for development of severe cutaneous adverse reactions, including DRESS, SJS, and TEN, including signs and symptoms of prodrome of fever, malaise, mucosal lesions, progressive skin rash, blisters, lymphadenopathy, conjunctivitis, myalgias, hepatitis, or eosinophilia. *If a severe cutaneous adverse reaction is suspected,* interrupt therapy until etiology of reaction is determined. Consultation with a dermatologist is recommended. *If a severe cutaneous adverse reaction is confirmed or for other Grade 4 skin reactions,* permanently discontinue rifabutin.
- Monitor for signs/symptoms of hypersensitivity reactions (hypotension, urticaria, angioedema, acute bronchospasm, conjunctivitis, thrombocytopenia, neutropenia) or flu-like syndrome (weakness, fatigue, muscle pain, nausea, vomiting, headache, fever, chills, aches, rash, itching, sweats, dizziness, shortness of breath, chest pain, cough, syncope, palpitations). *If hypersensitivity reaction occurs,* discontinue rifabutin.

Lab Test Considerations

- Monitor CBC periodically during therapy. May cause neutropenia and thrombocytopenia. Obtain acid-fast bacilli smear and culture from sputum monthly until two consecutive specimens are negative.

Implementation

- Do not confuse rifabutin with rifapentine.
- **PO:** Administer without regard to meals unless GI upset occurs on empty stomach. High-fat meals slow rate but do not ↓ absorption. May be mixed with foods such as applesauce.

R

Patient/Family Teaching

- Explain the purpose and side effects of rifabutin. Advise patient to take as directed. Do not skip doses or double up on missed doses. Emphasize the importance of continuing full course of therapy even if asymptomatic. Advise patient to read *Patient Information* before starting and with each Rx refill in case of changes.
- Emphasize the importance of regular follow-up exams to monitor progress and to check for side effects.
- Advise patient to notify health care provider promptly if signs and symptoms of neutropenia (sore throat, fever, signs of infection), thrombocytopenia (unusual bleeding or bruising), or hepatitis (yellow eyes and skin, nausea, vomiting, anorexia, unusual tiredness, weakness) occur.
- Advise patients and family to call 911 and seek urgent treatment for signs and symptoms of hypersensitivity reactions (difficulty breathing; chest tightness; hives; rash; feeling light-headed; itching; swelling of the face, lips, tongue, or throat).
- Caution patient to avoid the use of alcohol during this therapy, because this may ↑ the risk of hepatotoxicity.
- Instruct patient to notify health care provider immediately if diarrhea, abdominal cramping, fever, or bloody stools occur and not to treat with antidiarrheals without consulting health care providers.
- Instruct patient to report symptoms of myositis (myalgia, arthralgia) or uveitis (intraocular inflammation) to health care provider promptly.
- Inform patient that skin, saliva, sputum, sweat, tears, urine, and feces may become brown-orange and that soft contact lenses may become permanently discolored.
- Advise patient to notify health care provider of all Rx or OTC medications, vitamins, or herbal products being taken and to consult with health care provider before taking other medications.
- Rep: Advise women of reproductive potential to notify health care provider if pregnancy is planned or suspected and to avoid breastfeeding during therapy.

Evaluation/Desired Outcomes

- Antimycobacterial action against susceptible organisms.
- Prevention of disseminated MAC in patients with advanced HIV infection.

rifAMPin (rif-am-pin)

Rifadin, ~~Rimactane~~, ✦ Rofact

Classification

Therapeutic: antituberculars

Pharmacologic: rifamycins

Indications

Active tuberculosis (TB) (with other agents). Elimination of meningococcal carriers. **Unlabeled Use:** Prevention of disease caused by *Haemophilus influenzae* type B in close contacts. Synergy with other antimicrobial agents for *S. aureus* infections.

Action

- Inhibits RNA synthesis by blocking RNA transcription in susceptible organisms. **Therapeutic Effects:** Bactericidal action against susceptible organisms. **Spectrum:** Broad spectrum notable for activity against: *Mycobacterium* spp. *Staphylococcus aureus*, *H. influenzae*, *Legionella pneumophila*, *Neisseria meningitidis*.

Pharmacokinetics

Absorption: Well absorbed following oral administration.

Distribution: Widely distributed; enters CSF.

Protein Binding: 80%.

Metabolism and Excretion: Mostly metabolized by the liver; 60% eliminated in feces via biliary elimination.

Half-life: 3 hr.

TIME/ACTION PROFILE (plasma concentrations)

ROUTE	ONSET	PEAK	DURATION
PO	rapid	2–4 hr	12–24 hr
IV	rapid	end of infusion	12–24 hr

Contraindications/Precautions

Contraindicated in: Hypersensitivity; Concurrent use of atazanavir, darunavir, fosamprenavir, lurasidone, praziquantel, or tipranavir.

Use Cautiously in: History of liver disease (↑ risk of hepatotoxicity); Chronic liver disease, poor nutritional status, or prolonged use of antibacterial drugs or anticoagulants (↑ risk of vitamin K deficiency and subsequent coagulation disorders); Diabetes; Concurrent use of other hepatotoxic agents; OB: Safety not established in pregnancy; Lactation: Safety not established in breastfeeding.

Adverse Reactions/Side Effects

Derm: ACUTE GENERALIZED EXANTHEMATOUS PUSTULOSIS, DRUG REACTION WITH EOSINOPHILIA AND SYSTEMIC SYMPTOMS (DRESS), pruritus, rash, STEVENS-JOHNSON SYNDROME, TOXIC EPIDERMAL NECROLYSIS. **EENT:** red discoloration of tears. **GI:** abdominal pain, diarrhea, flatulence, heartburn, nausea, vomiting, HEPATOTOXICITY, red discoloration of saliva and teeth. **GU:** red discoloration of urine. **Hemat:** bleeding, hemolytic anemia, thrombocytopenia, THROMBOTIC MICROANGIOPATHY (INCLUDING THROMBOTIC THROMBOCYTOPENIC PURPURA AND HEMOLYTIC UREMIA SYNDROME). **MS:** arthralgia, muscle weakness, myalgia. **Neuro:** ataxia, confusion, drowsiness, fatigue, headache, weakness.

Resp: INTERSTITIAL LUNG DISEASE. **Misc:** flu-like syndrome, HYPERSENSITIVITY REACTIONS (INCLUDING ANGIOEDEMA).

Interactions

Drug-Drug: Significantly ↓ levels and effectiveness of **atazanavir**, **darunavir**, **fosamprenavir**, **lurasidone**, **praziquantel**, and **tipranavir**; concurrent use contraindicated. Significantly ↓ levels and effectiveness of **efavirenz**, **mifepristonequinine**, **sofosbuvir**, **ticagrelor**, and **zidovudine**; avoid concurrent use. Significantly ↓ levels and effectiveness of **hormonal contraceptives**; use nonhormonal birth control during rifampin therapy. May ↓ levels and effectiveness of numerous drugs, including **caspofungin**, **chloramphenicol**, **clarithromycin**, **cyclosporine**, **diazepam**, **diltiazem**, **disopyramide**, **doxycycline**, **fluconazole**, **glipizide**, **glyburide**, **haloperidol**, **ketoconazole**, **levothyroxine**, **losartan**, **lovastatin**, **metoprolol**, **mexiletine**, **morphine**, **moxifloxacin**, **nifedipine**, **nortriptyline**, **ondansetron**, **oxycodone**, **phenytoin**, **prednisolone**, **propafenone**, **propranolol**, **quinidine**, **simvastatin**, **tamoxifen**, **theophylline**, **toremifene**, **verapamil**, and **zolpidem**. May ↑ levels of active metabolite of **clopidogrel**, which may ↑ risk of bleeding; avoid concurrent use. May ↓ levels and effectiveness of **warfarin**; monitor INR regularly during concurrent therapy. May significantly ↓ levels and effectiveness of **itraconazole**; avoid use 2 wk before and during itraconazole therapy. May significantly ↓ levels and effectiveness of **irinotecan**; avoid use 2 wk before and during irinotecan therapy. May ↓ levels and effectiveness of **digoxin**; closely monitor serum digoxin concentrations and ↑ digoxin dose by 20–40% if needed. May significantly ↓ levels and effectiveness of **tacrolimus**; monitor tacrolimus whole blood concentrations regularly and ↑ tacrolimus dose as necessary. May ↓ levels and effectiveness of **methadone**, which may ↑ risk of withdrawal symptoms. Absorption may be ↓ by **antacids**; administer rifampin ≥1 hr prior to antacids. **Probenecid** and **trimethoprim/sulfamethoxazole** may ↑ levels and risk of toxicity. Concurrent use with **atovaquone** may ↓ atovaquone levels and effectiveness and ↑ levels and risk of toxicity of rifampin; avoid concurrent use. May ↓ levels and effectiveness of **dapsone**; may also ↑ levels and toxicity of the active metabolite of **dapsone**, which could ↑ the risk of methemoglobinemia.

Route/Dosage

Tuberculosis

PO, IV (Adults): 600 mg/day or 10 mg/kg/day (up to 600 mg/day) single dose; may also be given twice weekly.

PO, IV (Children and Infants): 10–20 mg/kg/day single dose or divided every 12 hr (not to exceed 600 mg/day); may also be given twice weekly.

Asymptomatic Carriers of Meningococcus

PO, IV (Adults): 600 mg every 12 hr for 2 days.

PO, IV (Children ≥1 mo): 10 mg/kg every 12 hr for 2 days (max: 600 mg/dose).

PO (Infants <1 mo): 5 mg/kg every 12 hr for 2 days.

H. influenzae Prophylaxis

PO (Adults): 600 mg/day for 4 days.

PO (Children): 20 mg/kg/day for 4 days (max: 600 mg/dose).

PO (Neonates): 10 mg/kg/day for 4 days.

Synergy for *S. aureus* Infections

PO (Adults): 300–600 mg twice daily.

PO (Children and Neonates): 5–20 mg/kg/day divided every 12 hr (max: 600 mg/dose).

Availability (generic available)

Capsules: 150 mg, 300 mg. **Powder for injection:** 600 mg/vial.

NURSING IMPLICATIONS

Assessment

- Perform mycobacterial studies and susceptibility tests prior to and periodically during therapy to detect possible resistance.
- Assess lung sounds and character and amount of sputum periodically during therapy.
- Monitor for signs and symptoms of interstitial lung disease. *If respiratory failure, pulmonary fibrosis, or acute respiratory distress syndrome occur,* discontinue rifampin immediately and initiate appropriate treatment.
- Monitor for signs and symptoms of DRESS (fever, rash, lymphadenopathy, facial swelling), associated with involvement of other organ systems (hepatitis, nephritis, hematologic abnormalities, myocarditis, myositis) during therapy. May resemble an acute viral infection. Eosinophilia is often present. Discontinue therapy if signs occur.
- Monitor for signs and symptoms of hypersensitivity reactions (fever, rash, urticaria, angioedema, hypotension, acute bronchospasm, conjunctivitis, thrombocytopenia, neutropenia, elevated liver transaminases), or flu-like syndrome (weakness, fatigue, muscle pain, nausea, vomiting, headache, chills, aches, itching, sweats, dizziness, shortness of breath, chest pain, cough, syncope, palpitations). Discontinue rifampin if symptoms occur.

Lab Test Considerations

- Evaluate renal function, CBC, and urinalysis periodically during therapy.
- Monitor hepatic function at least monthly during therapy. May ↑ AST, ALT, serum alkaline phosphatase, and bilirubin concentrations.
- May ↑ uric acid concentrations.

R

- May cause false-positive direct Coombs test results.
- May interfere with dexamethasone suppression test results; discontinue rifampin 15 days prior to test.
- May interfere with methods for determining serum folate and vitamin B levels and with urine tests based on color reaction.
- Monitor coagulation tests (PT, INR, aPTT) during therapy in patients at risk for vitamin K deficiency.

Implementation

- Do not confuse rifampin with rifaximin or Rifamate.
- May use vitamin K supplementation in patients at risk for vitamin K deficiency.
- **PO:** Administer medication on an empty stomach ≥1 hr before or 2 hr after meals with a full glass (240 mL) of water. If GI irritation becomes a problem, may be administered with food. Antacids may also be taken 1 hr prior to administration. Capsules may be opened and contents mixed with applesauce or jelly for patients with difficulty swallowing.
- Pharmacist can compound a syrup for patients unable to swallow capsules.

IV Administration

- Avoid extravasation; may cause local irritation and inflammation. If these occur, discontinue infusion and restart at another site.
- IV and oral doses are the same.
- **Intermittent Infusion: Reconstitution:** Inject 10 mL sterile water for injection into vial. Swirl gently to dissolve. Reconstituted solution is stable at room temperature ≤30 hr. **Concentration:** 60 mg/mL. Not to exceed 60 mg/mL. **Dilution:** Dilute further in 100 mL or 500 mL of D5W or 0.9% NaCl. Infusion is stable at room temperature for 8 hr (in D5W) or 6 hr (in 0.9% NaCl). **Rate:** Administer solutions diluted in 100 mL over 30 min and in those diluted in 500 mL over 3 hr.
- **Y-Site Compatibility:** amiodarone, bumetanide, caffeine citrate, ciprofloxacin, daptomycin, midazolam, pantoprazole, tigecycline, vancomycin.
- **Y-Site Incompatibility:** diltiazem.

Patient/Family Teaching

- Advise patient to take medication as directed, and not to skip doses or double missed doses. Emphasize importance of continuing therapy even after symptoms have subsided. Length of therapy for TB depends on regimen being used and underlying disease states. Patients on short-term prophylactic therapy should also be advised of the importance of compliance with therapy.
- Advise patient to notify health care professional promptly if signs and symptoms of hepatitis (yellow eyes and skin, nausea, vomiting, anorexia, unusual tiredness, weakness) or thrombocytopenia (unusual bleeding or bruising) occur.
- Advise patient to notify health care professional and stop rifampin immediately if signs and symptoms of severe cutaneous adverse reactions (rash, skin color changes or peeling, blisters, facial swelling, swollen lymph nodes, fever) occur.
- Caution patient to avoid the use of alcohol during this therapy; may ↑ risk of hepatotoxicity.
- Instruct patient to report the occurrence of flu-like symptoms (fever, chills, myalgia, headache) promptly.
- Advise patient to notify health care professional immediately if their symptoms of mycobacterial disease (cough, fever, tiredness, shortness of breath, malaise, headache, pain, night sweats, swollen lymph nodes, loss of appetite, weight loss, weakness, skin ulcers or lesions) worsen or recur.
- Rifampin may occasionally cause drowsiness. Caution patient to avoid driving or other activities requiring alertness until response to medication is known.
- Inform patient that saliva, sputum, teeth, sweat, tears, urine, and feces may become red-orange to red-brown and that soft contact lenses may become permanently discolored.
- Rep: Advise women of reproductive potential to notify health care professional if pregnancy is planned or suspected and to avoid breastfeeding during therapy. Rifampin may ↓ hormonal contraceptive efficacy. Alternate contraceptive should be used during therapy.
- Emphasize importance of regular follow-up exams to monitor progress and to check for side effects.

Evaluation/Desired Outcomes

- Bactericidal action against susceptible organisms.

rifAXIMin (ri-fax-i-min)

Xifaxan, ✱ Zaxine

Classification

Therapeutic: anti-infectives

Pharmacologic: rifamycins

Indications

Travelers' diarrhea due to noninvasive strains of *Escherichia coli*. Reduction in risk of overt hepatic encephalopathy recurrence. Irritable bowel syndrome with diarrhea.

Action

Inhibits bacterial RNA synthesis by binding to bacterial DNA-dependent RNA polymerase. **Therapeutic Effects:** Decreased severity of travelers' diarrhea. Decreased episodes of overt hepatic encephalopathy. Decreased signs/symptoms of irritable bowel syndrome with diarrhea. **Spectrum:** *Escherichia coli* (enterotoxigenic and enteroaggregative strains).

Pharmacokinetics

Absorption: Poorly absorbed (<0.4%); action is primarily in GI tract.
Distribution: 80–90% concentrated in gut.
Metabolism and Excretion: Almost exclusively excreted unchanged in feces.
Half-life: 6 hr.

ROUTE	ONSET	PEAK	DURATION
PO	unknown	unknown	unknown

Contraindications/Precautions

Contraindicated in: Hypersensitivity to rifaximin or other rifamycins; Diarrhea with fever or bloody stools; Diarrhea caused by other infectious agents; Lactation: Lactation.
Use Cautiously in: OB: Use during pregnancy only if potential maternal benefit justifies potential fetal risk; Pedi: Safety not established in children <18 yr (hepatic encephalopathy or irritable bowel syndrome with diarrhea) or <12 yr (travelers' diarrhea).

Adverse Reactions/Side Effects

CV: peripheral edema. **GI:** CLOSTRIDIOIDES DIFFICILE-ASSOCIATED DIARRHEA (CDAD). **Neuro:** dizziness.

Interactions

Drug-Drug: **P-glycoprotein inhibitors**, including **cyclosporine**, may ↑ levels and risk of toxicity. May cause fluctuations in INR when used with **warfarin**; closely monitor INR.

Route/Dosage

Travelers' Diarrhea

PO (Adults and Children ≥12 yr): 200 mg 3 times daily for 3 days.

Hepatic Encephalopathy

PO (Adults): 550 mg twice daily.

Irritable Bowel Syndrome With Diarrhea

PO (Adults): 550 mg 3 times daily for 14 days; if recurrence of symptoms, may treat up to an additional two times.

Availability

Tablets: 200 mg, 550 mg.

NURSING IMPLICATIONS

Assessment

- **Traveler's Diarrhea:** Assess frequency and consistency of stools and bowel sounds before and during therapy.
- Assess fluid and electrolyte balance and skin turgor for dehydration.
- **Hepatic Encephalopathy:** Assess mental status periodically during therapy.
- **Irritable Bowel Syndrome With Diarrhea:** Assess frequency and consistency of stools and other irritable bowel syndrome symptoms (bloating, cramping) daily.
- Monitor bowel function. Diarrhea, abdominal cramping, fever, and bloody stools should be reported to health care provider promptly as a sign of CDAD. May begin up to several weeks following cessation of therapy.

Lab Test Considerations

- May cause lymphocytosis, monocytosis, and neutropenia.

Implementation

- Do not confuse rifaximin with rifampin.
- **PO:** Administer with or without food.

Patient/Family Teaching

- Explain purpose and side effects of medication to patient. Advise patient to read *Patient Information* before starting therapy. Instruct patient to take as directed and to complete therapy, even if feeling better.
- Advise patient to notify health care provider of all Rx or OTC medications, vitamins, or herbal products being taken and to consult with health care provider before taking other medications.
- Advise patient to stop taking rifaximin if diarrhea symptoms get worse, persist >24–48 hr, or are accompanied by fever or blood in the stool. Consult health care provider if these occur. Advise patient not to treat diarrhea without consulting health care provider. May occur up to several weeks after discontinuation of medication.
- May cause dizziness. Caution patient to avoid driving and other activities requiring alertness until response to medication is known.
- Rep: Advise women of reproductive potential to notify health care provider if pregnancy is planned or suspected or if breastfeeding.

Evaluation/Desired Outcomes

- Decreased severity of travelers' diarrhea.
- Decreased episodes of overt hepatic encephalopathy.
- Decreased signs/symptoms of irritable bowel syndrome with diarrhea.

R

rilpivirine (ril-pi-vir-een)

Edurant, Edurant PED

Classification
Therapeutic: antiretrovirals
Pharmacologic: non-nucleoside reverse transcriptase inhibitors

Indications

Treatment-naive patients with HIV infection with HIV-1 RNA ≤100,000 copies/mL at start of therapy. Short-term treatment of HIV infection in patients with an HIV-1 RNA <50 copies/mL who are on a stable antiretroviral regimen with no history of treatment failure and with no known or suspected resistance to either cabotegravir or rilpivirine (in combination with cabotegravir) (to be used as either oral lead-in to assess the tolerability of rilpivirine prior to administration of cabotegravir/rilpivirine extended-release injection or oral therapy for patients who will miss planned injection dosing with cabotegravir/rilpivirine extended-release injection).

Action

Inhibits HIV-replication by noncompetitively inhibiting HIV reverse transcriptase. **Therapeutic Effects:** Slowed progression of HIV infection and decreased occurrence of sequelae. Increases CD4 cell counts and decreases viral load.

Pharmacokinetics

Absorption: Well absorbed following oral administration.
Distribution: Unknown.
Protein Binding: 99.7%.
Metabolism and Excretion: Mostly metabolized by the liver by the CYP3A isoenzyme; 25% excreted in feces unchanged, <1% excreted unchanged in urine.
Half-life: 50 hr.

TIME/ACTION PROFILE (plasma concentrations)

ROUTE	ONSET	PEAK	DURATION
PO	unknown	4–5 hr	24 hr

Contraindications/Precautions

Contraindicated in: Concurrent use of CYP3A inducers or proton pump inhibitors; Lactation: Breastfeeding not recommended in patients with HIV.
Use Cautiously in: Concurrent use of drugs that ↑ risk of torsades de pointes (may ↑ risk of arrhythmias); History of depression or suicide attempt; Hepatitis B or C; Pedi: Children <2 yr (safety and effectiveness not established).

Adverse Reactions/Side Effects

Derm: DRUG REACTION WITH EOSINOPHILIA AND SYSTEMIC SYMPTOMS (DRESS), rash. **Endo:** Grave's disease. **GI:** autoimmune hepatitis, hepatotoxicity. **MS:** polymyositis. **Neuro:** depression (↑ in children), dizziness, Guillain-Barré syndrome, headache, insomnia. **Misc:** immune reconstitution syndrome.

Interactions

Drug-Drug: **CYP3A inducers**, including **carbamazepine**, **dexamethasone** (more than a single dose), **oxcarbazepine**, **phenobarbital**, **phenytoin**, **rifampin**, or **rifapentine**, ↓ levels and effectiveness and promote virologic resistance; concurrent use contraindicated. **Proton pump inhibitors**, including **esomeprazole**, **lansoprazole**, **omeprazole**, **pantoprazole**, and **rabeprazole**, ↓ levels and effectiveness and may ↑ resistance; concurrent use contraindicated. Concurrent use with **antacids** may ↓ levels and effectiveness; use with caution; administer at least 2 hr before or 4 hr after rilpivirine. Concurrent use with **H_2 antagonists** may ↓ levels and effectiveness; use with caution; administer at least 12 hr before or 4 hr after rilpivirine. **Rifabutin** may ↓ levels; ↑ rilpivirine dose to 50 mg once daily during concurrent use. **Efavirenz**, **etravirine**, and **nevirapine** may ↓ levels; avoid concurrent use. **Darunavir/ritonavir**, **lopinavir/ritonavir**, **atazanavir/ritonavir**, **fosamprenavir/ritonavir**, **tipranavir/ritonavir**, **atazanavir**, **fosamprenavir**, and **nelfinavir** may ↑ levels. **Clarithromycin** or **erythromycin** may ↑ levels; consider using azithromycin. **Fluconazole**, **itraconazole**, **ketoconazole**, **posaconazole**, and **voriconazole** may ↑ levels; rilpivirine may ↓ **ketoconazole** levels. Concurrent use with **QT interval-prolonging drugs** may ↑ risk of serious arrhythmias. May ↓ levels of **methadone**; monitor clinical effects.
Drug-Natural Products: Concurrent use of **St. John's wort** ↓ blood levels and effectiveness and promote virologic resistance; concurrent use contraindicated.

Route/Dosage

Tablets and tablets for oral suspension are not interchangeable.

Treatment-Naive Patients With HIV Infection

PO (Adults and Children ≥2 yr and ≥25 kg): 25 mg once daily (tablets only); *Pregnant patients on stable rilpivirine regimen prior to pregnancy and virologically suppressed (HIV RNA <50 copies/mL):* 25 mg once daily; *Concurrent use of rifabutin:* 50 mg once daily (↓ to 25 mg once daily when rifabutin discontinued).
PO (Children ≥2 yr and 20–<25 kg): 15 mg once daily (tablets for oral suspension only).
PO (Children ≥2 yr and 14–<20 kg): 12.5 mg once daily (tablets for oral suspension only).

Combination Therapy With Cabotegravir for HIV Infection

PO (Adults and Children ≥12 yr and ≥35 kg): *Oral lead-in therapy to assess tolerability of rilpivirine:* 25 mg once daily (with oral cabotegravir 30 mg once daily) for ≥28 days; then switch to cabotegravir/rilpivirine extended-release injection. *To replace planned missed cabotegravir/rilpivirine extended-release injections for patients on monthly dosing schedule (if patient plans to miss scheduled monthly injection by >7 days):* 25 mg once daily (with oral cabotegravir

30 mg once daily) initiated at the same time as missed injection of cabotegravir/rilpivirine; then continued until day the cabotegravir/rilpivirine extended-release injection is restarted (oral replacement therapy can be continued for up to 2 mo). *To replace planned missed cabotegravir/rilpivirine extended-release injections for patients on every 2-mo dosing schedule (if patient plans to miss scheduled every 2-mo injection by >7 days):* 25 mg once daily (with oral cabotegravir 30 mg once daily) initiated the same time as missed injection of cabotegravir/rilpivirine; then continued until day the cabotegravir/rilpivirine extended-release injection is restarted (oral replacement therapy can be continued for up to 2 mo).

Availability

Tablets (Edurant): 25 mg. **Tablets for oral suspension (Edurant PED):** 2.5 mg. ***In combination with:*** cabotegravir (Cabenuva); dolutegravir (Juluca); emtricitabine and tenofovir alafenamide (Odefsey); emtricitabine and tenofovir disoproxil fumarate (Complera). See Appendix N.

NURSING IMPLICATIONS

Assessment

- Assess for change in severity of HIV symptoms and for symptoms of opportunistic infections during therapy.
- Monitor closely for notable changes in behavior that could indicate the emergence or worsening of suicidal thoughts or behavior or depression.
- Assess for rash periodically during therapy. May cause DRESS. Discontinue therapy if severe or if accompanied with fever, general malaise, fatigue, muscle or joint aches, blisters, oral lesions, conjunctivitis, hepatitis, or eosinophilia.

Lab Test Considerations

- Monitor viral load and CD4 cell count regularly during therapy.
- Monitor liver function tests before and periodically during therapy in patients with underlying liver disease, hepatitis B or C, or marked ↑ transaminases. May cause ↑ AST, ALT, and total bilirubin.
- May cause ↑ serum creatinine, total cholesterol, LDL cholesterol, and triglycerides.

Implementation

- **PO:** Administer tablets and tablets for oral suspension once daily with a meal in combination with other antiretrovirals.
- Place tablets for oral suspension in a cup; add 5 mL of room temperature water. Swirl the cup carefully for 1–2 min to disperse the tablets. The oral suspension can be further diluted with 5 mL of water, milk, orange juice, or applesauce. Discard any suspension not taken immediately. ***DNC:*** Do not crush the tablets for oral suspension.
- When administered with cabotegravir, administer rilpivirine with cabotegravir once daily at same time with a meal. Take last PO dose on same day as cabotegravir injection is started. If patient plans to miss a scheduled cabotegravir injection by >7 days, take daily PO therapy to replace up to 2 consecutive monthly injection visits. Take 1st PO dose 1 mo after last injection.

Patient/Family Teaching

- Emphasize the importance of taking rilpivirine as directed, at the same time each day. It must always be used in combination with other antiretroviral drugs. Do not take more than prescribed amount and do not stop taking without consulting health care professional. Take missed doses with a meal if remembered <12 hr of the time it is usually taken; then return to regular schedule. If > 12 hr from time dose is usually taken, omit dose and resume dosing schedule; do not double doses. Advise patient to read *Patient Information* prior to starting therapy and with each Rx refill in case of changes.
- Advise patient to take antacids 2 hr before or 4 hr after and H_2 antagonists 12 hr before or 4 hr after rilpivirine.
- Instruct patient that rilpivirine should not be shared with others.
- Inform patient that rilpivirine does not cure HIV or prevent associated or opportunistic infections. Rilpivirine may ↓ the risk of transmission of HIV to others through sexual contact or blood contamination. Caution patient to use a condom and to avoid sharing needles or donating blood to prevent spreading HIV to others. Advise patient that the long-term effects of rilpivirine are unknown at this time.
- Inform patients and families of risk of suicidal thoughts and behavior and advise that behavioral changes; emergency or worsening signs and symptoms of depression; unusual changes in mood; or emergence of suicidal thoughts, behavior, or thoughts of self-harm should be reported to health care professional immediately.
- Immune reconstitution syndrome may trigger opportunistic infections or autoimmune disorders. Notify health care professional if symptoms or rash occur.
- May cause dizziness. Caution patient to avoid driving or other activities requiring alertness until response to medication is known.
- Advise patient to notify health care professional of all Rx or OTC medications, vitamins, or herbal products being taken and to consult with health care professional before taking other medications, especially St. John's wort.
- Rep: Advise women of reproductive potential to use a nonhormonal method of birth control during

R

rilpivirine therapy. If pregnancy is suspected, notify health care professional promptly. Encourage health care professionals to enroll pregnant patients in the Antiretroviral Pregnancy Registry by calling 1-800-258-4263. Advise women of reproductive potential to avoid breastfeeding.

- Emphasize the importance of regular follow-up exams and blood counts to determine progress and monitor for side effects.

Evaluation/Desired Outcomes

- Delayed progression of HIV and decreased opportunistic infections in patients with HIV.
- Decrease in viral load and increase in CD4 cell counts.

rimegepant (ri-meg-je-pant)

Nurtec

Classification

Therapeutic: vascular headache suppressants

Pharmacologic: calcitonin gene-related peptide receptor antagonists

Indications

Acute treatment of migraine with or without aura. Preventive treatment of episodic migraines.

Action

Binds to and inhibits the calcitonin gene-related peptide (CGRP) receptor, which reduces the neuroinflammatory and vasodilatory effects of CGRP. **Therapeutic Effects:** Reduction in pain and other bothersome symptoms associated with migraine. Reduction in number of monthly migraine days.

Pharmacokinetics

Absorption: 64% absorbed following oral administration. High-fat foods may delay and ↓ extent of absorption.

Distribution: Extensively distributed to tissues.

Protein Binding: 96%.

Metabolism and Excretion: Primarily metabolized in liver via the CYP3A4 isoenzyme, and to a lesser extent by the CYP2C9 isoenzyme. Primarily excreted as unchanged drug in feces (42%) and urine (51%).

Half-life: 11 hr.

TIME/ACTION PROFILE (relief of migraine pain)

ROUTE	ONSET	PEAK	DURATION
PO	0.5 hr	2 hr	up to 48 hr

Contraindications/Precautions

Contraindicated in: Hypersensitivity; Severe hepatic impairment; End-stage renal disease (CCr <15 mL/min).

Use Cautiously in: OB: Safety not established in pregnancy; Lactation: Safety not established in breastfeeding; Pedi: Safety and effectiveness not established in children.

Adverse Reactions/Side Effects

GI: nausea. **Misc:** hypersensitivity reactions.

Interactions

Drug-Drug: Strong CYP3A4 inhibitors, including **itraconazole**, may significantly ↑ levels and risk of toxicity; avoid concurrent use. **Moderate CYP3A4 inhibitors** may ↑ levels and risk of toxicity; avoid another dose of rimegepant within 48 hr during concurrent use. **Strong CYP3A4 inducers**, including **rifampin**, or **moderate CYP3A4 inducers** may ↓ levels and effectiveness; avoid concurrent use. **P-glycoprotein inhibitors**, including **cyclosporine** or **quinidine**, may ↑ levels and risk of toxicity; avoid another dose of rimegepant within 48 hr during concurrent use.

Route/Dosage

Acute Migraine Treatment

PO (Adults): 75 mg as single dose (max dose = 75 mg/24 hr). Should not be used to treat >18 migraines in 30-day period.

Preventive Treatment of Episodic Migraines

PO (Adults): 75 mg every other day.

Availability

Orally disintegrating tablets (ODTs) (menthol flavor): 75 mg.

NURSING IMPLICATIONS

Assessment

- Assess pain location, character, intensity, duration, and associated symptoms (photophobia, phonophobia, nausea, vomiting) during migraine attack.
- Monitor frequency of migraine headaches in patients using rimegepant for prophylaxis.

Implementation

- Use dry hands when opening blister pack. Peel back foil covering of one blister and gently remove the ODT. Do not push ODT through foil. As soon as blister is opened, remove ODT and place on tongue; ODT may also be placed under tongue. ODT will disintegrate in saliva so that it can be swallowed without additional liquid. Take ODT immediately after opening blister pack. Do not store ODT outside the blister pack for future use.
- **PO: Treatment:** Administer ODT once daily as needed for migraine attacks. Limit dose to one ODT/day and no more than 18 doses in a 30-day period.
- **Prophylaxis:** Administer one ODT every other day for prevention of migraine headaches.

Patient/Family Teaching

- Explain purpose and side effects of medication to patient. Advise patient to read *Patient Information* before starting therapy. Instruct patient to take rimegepant as soon as symptoms of a migraine attack appear, but it may be administered any time during an attack. Do not take >75 mg in any 24-hr period.

- Advise patient to notify health care provider of all Rx or OTC medications, vitamins, or herbal products being taken and to consult with health care provider before taking other medications.
- Instruct patient using rimegepant for prevention to take as directed.
- Advise patient to avoid alcohol, which aggravates headaches, during rimegepant use.
- Advise patient that lying down in a darkened room following rimegepant administration may further help relieve headache.
- Inform patient of potential for hypersensitivity reactions and that these reactions can occur days after administration of rimegepant. Advise patient to notify health care provider immediately if signs or symptoms of hypersensitivity reactions (shortness of breath, rash) occur. Rimegepant should be discontinued if hypersensitivity reaction occurs.
- Rep: Advise women of reproductive potential to notify health care provider if pregnancy is planned or suspected or if breastfeeding. Inform patient of the pregnancy exposure registry that monitors outcomes in women exposed to *Nurtec* during pregnancy. For more information, health care providers or patients are encouraged to contact 1-877-366-0324, email nurtecpregnancyregistry@ppd.com, or visit nurtecpregnancyregistry.com.

Evaluation/Desired Outcomes

- Reduction in pain and other bothersome symptoms associated with migraine.
- Reduction in number of monthly migraine days.

risankizumab
(ris-an-kiz-ue-mab)

Skyrizi

Classification

Therapeutic: antipsoriatics

Pharmacologic: interleukin antagonists, monoclonal antibodies

Indications

Moderate to severe plaque psoriasis in patients who are candidates for phototherapy or systemic therapy. Active psoriatic arthritis (as monotherapy or in combination with non-biologic disease-modifying antirheumatic drugs [DMARDs]). Moderately to severely active Crohn disease. Moderately to severely active ulcerative colitis.

Action

Binds to the p19 protein subunit of the interleukin (IL)-23 cytokine to prevent its interaction with the IL-23 receptor. This cytokine is normally involved in inflammatory and immune responses. Binding to interleukins antagonizes their effects, inhibiting the release of proinflammatory cytokines and chemokines. **Therapeutic Effects:** Decrease in area and severity of psoriatic lesions. Improvement in clinical and symptomatic parameters of psoriatic arthritis. Improvement in clinical and endoscopic remission rates in Crohn disease. Improvement in clinical remission rates in ulcerative colitis.

Pharmacokinetics

Absorption: 89% absorbed following SUBQ administration. IV administration results in complete bioavailability.

Distribution: Well distributed to tissues.

Metabolism and Excretion: Broken down by catabolic processes into peptides and amino acids.

Half-life: *Plaque psoriasis:* 28 days; *Crohn disease:* 21 days.

TIME/ACTION PROFILE (plasma concentrations)

ROUTE	ONSET	PEAK	DURATION
SUBQ	unknown	3–14 days	12 wk
IV	unknown	unknown	unknown

Contraindications/Precautions

Contraindicated in: Hypersensitivity; Active, untreated infection.

Use Cautiously in: History of tuberculosis (TB) (possibility of reactivation); Cirrhosis (for Crohn disease only); OB: Use during pregnancy only if potential maternal benefit justifies potential fetal risk; Lactation: Safety not established in breastfeeding; Pedi: Safety and effectiveness not established in children.

Exercise Extreme Caution in: Chronic infection or history of recurrent infection.

Adverse Reactions/Side Effects

GI: hepatotoxicity (in Crohn disease and ulcerative colitis). **Local:** injection site reactions. **Neuro:** fatigue, headache. **Misc:** infection, HYPERSENSITIVITY REACTIONS (INCLUDING ANAPHYLAXIS).

Interactions

Drug-Drug: May ↓ antibody response to and ↑ risk of adverse reactions from **live vaccines**; avoid use during therapy.

Route/Dosage

Plaque Psoriasis and Psoriatic Arthritis

SUBQ (Adults): 150 mg initially and 4 wk later, then 150 mg every 12 wk.

Crohn Disease

IV (Adults): *Induction:* 600 mg initially and then at Wk 4 and Wk 8. At Wk 12, begin maintenance therapy (SUBQ) (see below).

SUBQ (Adults): *Maintenance:* 180 mg or 360 mg at Wk 12, and then every 8 wk.

Ulcerative Colitis

IV (Adults): *Induction:* 1200 mg initially and then at Wk 4 and Wk 8. At Wk 12, begin maintenance therapy (SUBQ) (see below).

SUBQ (Adults): *Maintenance:* 180 mg or 360 mg at Wk 12, and then every 8 wk.

Availability

Solution for SUBQ injection (prefilled pens): 150 mg/mL. **Solution for SUBQ injection (prefilled syringes):** 90 mg/mL, 150 mg/mL. **Solution for SUBQ injection (prefilled cartridge with on-body injector):** 150 mg/mL. **Solution for IV injection:** 60 mg/mL.

NURSING IMPLICATIONS

Assessment

- Assess patient for TB before starting, during, and after therapy. Do not administer risankizumab to patient with active TB. Consider anti-TB therapy before starting therapy in patients with a past history of latent or active TB in whom an adequate course of treatment cannot be confirmed.
- Assess skin lesions before and periodically during therapy.
- Monitor for signs/symptoms of infection (fever, chills, cough, dyspnea, skin infections) periodically during therapy.
- Monitor for signs/symptoms of hypersensitivity reactions (fainting; dizziness; feeling light-headed; chest tightness; swelling of face, eyelids, lips, mouth, tongue, or throat; skin rash; hives; trouble breathing or throat tightness; itching) during therapy.

Lab Test Considerations

- *For Crohn disease and ulcerative colitis:* Assess liver enzymes and bilirubin levels before starting therapy and periodically during induction for ≥12 wk.

Implementation

- Complete all age-appropriate vaccinations as recommended by current immunization guidelines before starting therapy.
- Before injecting, remove carton from refrigerator; without removing prefilled pen or prefilled syringe(s) from the carton, allow risankizumab to reach room temperature out of direct sunlight: 30–90 min for prefilled pen and 15–30 min for the prefilled syringe(s). Solution is colorless to slightly yellow and clear to slightly opalescent; may contain a few translucent to white particles. Do not use if solution is cloudy, discolored, or contains large particles. Do not freeze or shake.
- May use pen, prefilled syringe, or prefilled cartridge with supplied on-body injector for SUBQ injections. Follow manufacturer's *Instructions for Use* for each method.
- **SUBQ**: Inject into abdomen or thigh; may inject in upper outer arm if administered by health care provider or caregiver. Do not inject into areas where skin is tender, bruised, erythematous, indurated, or affected by psoriasis. If using 75 mg/0.83 mL syringes, 150-mg dose requires two syringes. Inject in different locations.

IV Administration

- **Intermittent Infusion: Dilution:** *For Crohn disease:* For a dose of 600 mg, add one vial (10 mL) to an IV bag or glass bottle containing 100 mL, 250 mL, or 500 mL of D5W or 0.9% NaCl; *For ulcerative colitis:* For a dose of 1200 mg, add two vials (20 mL) to an IV bag or glass bottle containing 250 mL or 500 mL of D5W or 0.9% NaCl. **Concentration:** 1.2–6 mg/mL. Discard any remaining solution in the vial. Do not shake vial or diluted solution. Allow diluted solution to warm to room temperature (if stored refrigerated) prior to administration. Complete infusion within 8 hr of dilution. Solution is stable for 8 hr at room temperature and up to 20 hr if refrigerated and protected from light. **Rate:** Infuse over ≥1 hr (600 mg dose) or ≥2 hr (1200 mg dose). At Wk 12, begin SUBQ maintenance therapy.

Patient/Family Teaching

- Explain purpose and side effects of medication to patient. Advise patient to read *Patient Information* before starting therapy. Instruct patient and/or caregiver about correct injection technique and disposal of equipment. Administer at Wk 0, Wk 4, and every 12 wk thereafter. If a dose is missed, administer as soon as possible; then resume dosing at the regular scheduled time.
- Instruct patient to notify health care provider of all Rx or OTC medications, vitamins, or herbal products being taken and to consult health care provider before taking other Rx, OTC, or herbal products.
- Advise patient to notify health care provider if signs and symptoms of infection (fever; sweats; chills; cough; shortness of breath; blood in mucus; muscle aches; warm, red, or painful skin or sores different from psoriasis; weight loss; diarrhea or stomach pain; burning on urination; urinating more often than usual) occur.
- Advise patient to avoid live vaccines during therapy.
- Rep: Advise women of reproductive potential to notify health care provider if pregnancy is planned or suspected or if breastfeeding. Delay live-virus immunizations in infants exposed in utero for ≥5 mo after birth. Inform pregnant patient of registry that monitors outcomes in women who become pregnant while treated with risankizumab. Encourage patient to enroll by calling 1877-302-2161.

Evaluation/Desired Outcomes

- Decrease in area and severity of psoriatic lesions.
- Improvement in clinical and symptomatic parameters of psoriatic arthritis.
- Improvement in clinical and endoscopic remission rates in Crohn disease.
- Improvement in clinical remission rates in ulcerative colitis.

risedronate (ris-ed-roe-nate)

Actonel, ✱ Actonel DR, Atelvia

Classification

Therapeutic: bone resorption inhibitors

Pharmacologic: bisphosphonates

Indications

Prevention and treatment of postmenopausal and corticosteroid-induced osteoporosis. Treatment of Paget disease in men and women. Treatment of osteoporosis in men.

Action

Inhibits bone resorption by binding to bone hydroxyapatite, which inhibits osteoclast activity. **Therapeutic Effects:** Reversal of the progression of osteoporosis with decreased fractures and other sequelae. Reduced bone turnover and resorption; normalization of serum alkaline phosphatase with reduced complications of Paget disease.

Pharmacokinetics

Absorption: Rapidly but poorly absorbed following oral administration (0.63% bioavailability).

Distribution: 60% of absorbed dose distributes to bone.

Metabolism and Excretion: 40% of absorbed dose is excreted unchanged by kidneys; unabsorbed drug is excreted in feces.

Half-life: *Initial:* 1.5 hr; *terminal:* 220 hr (reflects dissociation from bone).

TIME/ACTION PROFILE (effects on serum alkaline phosphatase)

ROUTE	ONSET	PEAK	DURATION
PO	within days	30 days	up to 16 mo

Contraindications/Precautions

Contraindicated in: Hypersensitivity; Severe renal impairment; Hypocalcemia; Abnormalities of the esophagus that delay esophageal emptying (e.g. strictures, achalasia); Inability to stand/sit upright for ≥30 min; OB: Pregnancy.

Use Cautiously in: History of upper GI disorders; Other disturbances of bone or mineral metabolism (correct abnormalities before initiating therapy); Dietary deficiencies (supplemental vitamin D and calcium may be required); Invasive dental procedures, cancer, receiving chemotherapy, corticosteroids, angiogenesis inhibitors, poor oral hygeine, periodontal disease, dental disease, anemia, coagulopathy, infection, or poorly fitting dentures (may ↑ risk of jaw osteonecrosis); Lactation: Use while breastfeeding only if potential maternal benefit justifies potential risk to infant.

Adverse Reactions/Side Effects

CV: chest pain, edema. **Derm:** rash, STEVENS-JOHNSON SYNDROME (SJS), TOXIC EPIDERMAL NECROLYSIS (TEN). **EENT:** amblyopia, conjunctivitis, dry eyes, eye pain/inflammation, tinnitus. **GI:** abdominal pain, diarrhea, belching, colitis, constipation, dysphagia, esophageal cancer, esophageal ulcer, esophagitis, gastric ulcer, nausea. **MS:** arthralgia, musculoskeletal pain, femur fractures, osteonecrosis (primarily of jaw). **Neuro:** weakness. **Resp:** asthma exacerbation. **Misc:** flu-like syndrome.

Interactions

Drug-Drug: NSAIDs or **aspirin** may ↑ risk of GI irritation. Absorption is ↓ by **calcium supplements** or **antacids**. **Proton pump inhibitors** and **H_2 antagonists** may cause a faster release of drug from the delayed-release product that can ↑ levels; concurrent use not recommended.

Drug-Food: Food ↓ absorption (administer ≥30 min before breakfast).

R

Route/Dosage

Prevention and Treatment of Postmenopausal Osteoporosis

PO (Adults): 5 mg once daily (immediate-release tablets) *or* 35 mg once weekly (immediate- or delayed-release tablets) *or* 75 mg taken on 2 consecutive days for a total of 2 tablets each mo (immediate-release tablets) *or* 150 mg once monthly (immediate-release tablets).

Prevention and Treatment of Glucocorticoid-Induced Osteoporosis

PO (Adults): 5 mg once daily (immediate-release tablets).

Treatment of Osteoporosis in Men

PO (Adults): 35 mg once weekly (immediate-release tablets).

Treatment of Paget Disease

PO (Adults): 30 mg once daily for 2 mo (immediate-release tablets); retreatment may be considered after 2 mo off therapy.

Availability (generic available)

Immediate-release tablets: 5 mg, 30 mg, 35 mg, 150 mg. **Delayed-release tablets (Atelvia):** 35 mg.

NURSING IMPLICATIONS

Assessment

- Perform a routine oral exam before starting therapy. Dental exam with appropriate preventative dentistry should be considered before therapy. Patients with history of tooth extraction, poor oral hygiene, gingival infections, diabetes, or use of a dental appliance or those taking immunosuppressive therapy, angiogenesis inhibitors, or systemic corticosteroids are at ↑ risk for osteonecrosis of the jaw.
- Assess for hypersensitivity reactions (angioedema, generalized rash, bullous skin reactions, SJS, TEN) and eye inflammation (iritis, uveitis).
- **Osteoporosis:** Assess patients via bone density study for low bone mass before and periodically during therapy.
- **Paget disease:** Assess for symptoms of Paget disease (bone pain, headache, ↓ visual and auditory acuity, ↑ skull size).

Lab Test Considerations

- *Osteoporosis:* Assess serum calcium before and periodically during therapy. Hypocalcemia and vitamin D deficiency should be treated before starting alendronate. May cause mild, transient ↑ of calcium and phosphate.
- *Paget disease:* Monitor alkaline phosphatase before and periodically during therapy to monitor effectiveness of therapy.

Implementation

- Do not confuse Actonel with Actos.
- **PO:** Administer *Actonel* 1st thing in the morning with 6–8 ounces of water, ≥30 min before other medications, beverages, or food. Waiting >30 min will improve absorption. Administer *Atelvia* right after breakfast with ≥4 ounces of water. ***DNC:*** Swallow tablet whole; do not crush, break, or chew.
- Calcium-, magnesium-, or aluminum-containing agents may interfere with absorption of risedronate and should be taken at a different time of day with food.
- Avoid administering delayed-release product with proton pump inhibitors or H_2 antagonists; may allow a faster release and ↑ drug level.

Patient/Family Teaching

- Explain purpose and side effects of medication to patient. Advise patient to read *Patient Information* before starting therapy.
- Advise patient to notify health care provider of all Rx or OTC medications, vitamins, or herbal products being taken and to consult with health care provider before taking other medications.
- Instruct patient on the importance of taking as directed. Risedronate should be taken with 6–8 ounces of water (mineral water, orange juice, coffee, and other beverages ↓ absorption). *If a dose of Actonel 35 mg is missed*, take one tablet the morning remembered; then return to the one tablet/week on the originally scheduled day; do not take two pills at once. *If one or both tablets of Actonel 75 mg are missed and the next month's scheduled doses are >7 days away*: If both Actonel 75-mg doses are missed, take one the morning remembered and one the next morning. If only one Actonel 75-mg tablet is missed, take the missed tablet on the morning of the day after remembered; then return to original schedule. Do not take more than two 75 mg tablets within 7 days. *If one or both tablets of Actonel 75 mg are missed and the next month's scheduled doses are within 7 days,* omit and return to schedule next month. *If one or both tablets of Actonel 150 mg are missed and the next month's scheduled doses are >7 days away,* take the missed tablet on the morning of the day after you remember; then return to original schedule. Do not take more than two 150-mg tablets within 7 days. *If one or both tablets of Actonel 75 mg are missed and the next month's scheduled doses are within 7 days,* omit and return to schedule next month.
- Caution patients to remain upright for ≥30 min following dose to facilitate passage to stomach and minimize risk of esophageal irritation.
- Advise patient to eat a balanced diet and consult health care provider about the need for supplemental calcium and vitamin D (see Appendix J).
- Inform patient that severe musculoskeletal pain may occur within days, months, or years after starting risedronate. Symptoms my resolve completely after discontinuation or slow or incomplete resolution may occur. Notify health care provider if severe pain occurs.
- Encourage patient to participate in regular exercise and to modify behaviors that ↑ the risk of osteoporosis (stop smoking, ↓ alcohol consumption).
- Advise patient to practice proper mouth care during therapy and to notify health care provider if signs and symptoms of osteonecrosis of the jaw (jaw pain, toothache, sores on gums) occur.
- Advise patient to inform health care provider of risedronate therapy before dental surgery.
- Rep: May cause fetal harm. Advise women of reproductive potential to notify health care provider if pregnancy is planned or suspected and to avoid breastfeeding during therapy. May impair female and male fertility.

Evaluation/Desired Outcomes

- Reversal of the progression of osteoporosis with decreased fractures and other sequelae.
- Reduced bone turnover and resorption; normalization of serum alkaline phosphatase with reduced complications of Paget disease.

BEERS

risperiDONE (riss-per-i-done)

RisperDAL, RisperDAL Consta, RisperDAL M-TAB, Rykindo, Uzedy

Classification

Therapeutic: antipsychotics, mood stabilizers

Pharmacologic: benzisoxazoles

Indications

PO, IM, SUBQ: Schizophrenia. **PO:** Acute manic or mixed episodes associated with bipolar I disorder (as monotherapy or in combination with lithium or valproate). **IM:** Maintenance treatment of bipolar I disorder (as monotherapy or in combination with lithium or valproate). **PO:** Irritability associated with autistic disorder.

Action

May act by antagonizing dopamine and serotonin in the CNS. **Therapeutic Effects:** Decreased symptoms of psychoses, bipolar mania, or autism.

Pharmacokinetics

Absorption: 70% after administration of tablets, solution, or orally disintegrating tablets. Following IM administration, small initial release of drug, followed by 3-wk lag; the rest of release starts at 3 wk and lasts 4–6 wk. Following SUBQ administration, initial release of drug occurs at 4–6 hr, with the rest of release occurring at 10–14 days after administration.

Distribution: Unknown.

Metabolism and Excretion: Primarily metabolized by the liver by the CYP2D6 isoenzyme to 9-hydroxyrisperidone (has similar pharmacological properties as risperidone). Risperidone and its active metabolite are renally eliminated.

Half-life: *Extensive metabolizers:* 3 hr for risperidone; 21 hr for 9-hydroxyrisperidone. *Poor metabolizers:* 20 hr for risperidone; 30 hr for 9-hydroxyrisperidone; *SUBQ:* 9–11 days.

TIME/ACTION PROFILE (clinical effects)

ROUTE	ONSET	PEAK	DURATION
PO	1–2 wk	unknown	up to 6 wk†
IM	3 wk	4–6 wk	up to 6 wk†
SUBQ	2 wk	6–8 wk	unknown

† After discontinuation.

Contraindications/Precautions

Contraindicated in: Hypersensitivity to risperidone or paliperidone; Lactation: Lactation.

Use Cautiously in: Renal or hepatic impairment (initial dose ↓ recommended); Underlying cardiovascular disease (↑ risk of arrhythmias and hypotension); History of seizures; History of drug abuse; Diabetes or risk factors for diabetes (may worsen glucose control); Patients at risk for aspiration or falls; History of breast cancer; Renal impairment; Hepatic impairment; OB: Neonates at ↑ risk for extrapyramidal symptoms and withdrawal after delivery when exposed during the 3rd trimester; use during pregnancy only if potential maternal benefit justifies potential fetal risk; Pedi: Safety and effectiveness not established in children <13 yr (schizophrenia), <10 yr (bipolar disorder), or <5 yr (autism); Geri: Appears on Beers list. ↑ risk of stroke, cognitive decline, and mortality in older adults with dementia. Avoid use in older adults, except for schizophrenia or bipolar disorder.

Adverse Reactions/Side Effects

CV: arrhythmias, orthostatic hypotension, syncope, tachycardia. **Derm:** itching/skin rash, ↑ pigmentation, dry skin, photosensitivity, seborrhea, STEVENS-JOHNSON SYNDROME, sweating, TOXIC EPIDERMAL NECROLYSIS. **EENT:** pharyngitis, rhinitis, visual disturbances. **Endo:** galactorrhea, hyperglycemia, hyperprolactinemia. **F and E:** polydipsia. **GI:** constipation, diarrhea, dry mouth, nausea, ↑ salivation, abdominal pain, anorexia, dyspepsia, dysphagia, vomiting, weight loss. **GU:** ↓ libido, dysmenorrhea/menorrhagia, ↓ fertility (women), amenorrhea, difficulty urinating, gynecomastia, impotence, polyuria, priapism. **Hemat:** AGRANULOCYTOSIS, leukopenia, neutropenia. **Metab:** weight gain, dyslipidemia. **MS:** arthralgia, back pain. **Neuro:** ↑ dreams, ↑ sleep duration, aggressive behavior, dizziness, extrapyramidal reactions, headache, insomnia, sedation, fatigue, impaired temperature regulation, nervousness, NEUROLEPTIC MALIGNANT SYNDROME, SEIZURES, tardive dyskinesia. **Resp:** cough, dyspnea. **Misc:** HYPERSENSITIVITY REACTIONS (INCLUDING ANAPHYLAXIS AND ANGIOEDEMA).

Interactions

Drug-Drug: May ↓ antiparkinsonian effects of **levodopa** or other **dopamine agonists**. **Strong CYP3A4 inducers**, including **carbamazepine**, **phenytoin**, **rifampin**, and **phenobarbital**, may ↓ levels and effectiveness; dose adjustments may be necessary. **Fluoxetine** and **paroxetine** may ↑ levels and risk of toxicity; dose adjustments may be necessary. **Clozapine**

R

may ↑ levels and risk of toxicity. ↑ CNS depression may occur with other **CNS depressants**, including **alcohol**, **antihistamines**, **sedative/hypnotics**, or **opioid analgesics**. **Methylphenidate** may ↑ risk of extrapyramidal symptoms.

Drug-Natural Products: Kava, **valerian**, or **chamomile** can ↑ CNS depression.

Route/Dosage

Schizophrenia

PO (Adults): 1 mg twice daily; ↑ by 1–2 mg/day no more frequently than every 24 hr to 4–8 mg daily.

PO (Children 13–17 yr): 0.5 mg once daily; ↑ by 0.5–1.0 mg no more frequently than every 24 hr to 3 mg daily. May administer half the daily dose twice daily if drowsiness persists.

IM (Adults): 25 mg every 2 wk; some patients may benefit from a higher dose of 37.5 or 50 mg every 2 wk.

IM (Geriatric Patients): 25 mg every 2 wk.

SUBQ (Adults): *Currently taking (switching from) 2 mg/day of oral risperidone:* Uzedy: 50 mg once monthly or 100 mg every 2 mo; *Currently taking (switching from) 3 mg/day of oral risperidone:* Uzedy: 75 mg once monthly or 150 mg every 2 mo; *Currently taking (switching from) 4 mg/day of oral risperidone:* Uzedy: 100 mg once monthly or 200 mg every 2 mo; *Currently taking (switching from) 5 mg/day of oral risperidone:* Uzedy: 125 mg once monthly or 250 mg every 2 mo; *Concurrent use of strong CYP2D6 inhibitor (e.g. fluoxetine or paroxetine):* Uzedy: When initiation of strong CYP2D6 inhibitor is expected, place patients on a lower dose of risperidone prior to the planned start of the strong CYP2D6 inhibitor. When a strong CYP2D6 inhibitor is initiated in patients already receiving the lowest risperidone dose (50 mg once monthly or 100 mg every 2 mo), continue treatment with these doses unless clinical judgment requires interruption of treatment. *Concurrent use of strong CYP3A4 inducer:* Uzedy: Upon initiation of therapy with a strong CYP3A4 inducer, closely monitor patients during the first 4–8 wk; the dose of Uzedy may need to be adjusted. A dose ↑ of Uzedy or additional oral risperidone may be considered.

Hepatic/Renal Impairment

PO (Adults): *Severe renal impairment (CCr <30 mL/min) or severe hepatic impairment:* Start with 0.5 mg twice daily; ↑ by 0.5 mg twice daily, up to 1.5 mg twice daily; then ↑ at weekly intervals if necessary.

Hepatic/Renal Impairment

IM (Adults): Start with 0.5 mg PO twice daily for 1st wk; then ↑ to 1 mg PO twice daily or 2 mg PO once daily during 2nd wk. If 2 mg/day PO dose is well tolerated, can initiate 12.5 mg or 25 mg IM every 2 wk.

Hepatic/Renal Impairment

SUBQ (Adults): *Uzedy:* Titrate patients up to at least 2 mg/day of oral risperidone before initiating Uzedy. If patient tolerates this dose of oral risperidone, consider SUBQ dose of 50 mg once monthly.

Acute Manic or Mixed Episodes Associated With Bipolar I Disorder

PO (Adults): 2–3 mg/day as a single daily dose; dose may be ↑ at 24-hr intervals by 1 mg (range 1–5 mg/day).

PO (Children 13–17 yr): 0.5 mg once daily; ↑ by 0.5–1 mg no more frequently than every 24 hr to 2.5 mg daily. May administer half the daily dose twice daily if drowsiness persists.

PO (Geriatric Patients): Start with 0.5 mg twice daily; ↑ by 0.5 mg twice daily, up to 1.5 mg twice daily; then ↑ at weekly intervals if necessary. May also be given as a single daily dose after initial titration.

Hepatic/Renal Impairment

PO (Adults): *Severe renal impairment (CCr <30 mL/min) or severe hepatic impairment:* Start with 0.5 mg twice daily; ↑ by 0.5 mg twice daily, up to 1.5 mg twice daily; then ↑ at weekly intervals if necessary.

Maintenance Treatment of Bipolar I Disorder

IM (Adults): 25 mg every 2 wk; some patients may benefit from a higher dose of 37.5 or 50 mg every 2 wk.

IM (Geriatric Patients): 25 mg every 2 wk.

Hepatic/Renal Impairment

IM (Adults): Start with 0.5 mg PO twice daily for 1st wk; then ↑ to 1 mg PO twice daily or 2 mg PO once daily during 2nd wk. If 2 mg/day PO dose is well tolerated, can initiate 12.5 mg or 25 mg IM every 2 wk.

Irritability Associated With Autistic Disorder

PO (Children 5–16 yr weighing <20 kg): 0.25 mg/day initially. After at least 4 days of therapy, may ↑ to 0.5 mg/day. Dose ↑ in increments of 0.25 mg/day may be considered at 2 wk or longer intervals. May be given as a single or divided dose.

PO (Children 5–16 yr weighing >20 kg): 0.5 mg/day initially. After at least 4 days of therapy, may ↑ to 1 mg/day. Dose ↑ in increments of 0.5 mg/day may be considered at 2 wk or longer intervals. May be given as a single or divided dose.

Hepatic/Renal Impairment

PO (Adults): *Severe renal impairment (CCr <30 mL/min) or severe hepatic impairment:* Start with 0.5 mg twice daily; ↑ by 0.5 mg twice daily, up to 1.5 mg twice daily; then ↑ at weekly intervals if necessary.

Availability (generic available)

Immediate-release tablets: 0.25 mg, 0.5 mg, 1 mg, 2 mg, 3 mg, 4 mg. **Orally disintegrating tablets (Risperdal M-Tabs):** 0.25 mg, 0.5 mg, 1 mg, 2 mg, 3 mg, 4 mg. **Oral solution:** 1 mg/mL. **Extended-release suspension for IM injection (Risperdal Consta, Rykindo):** 12.5 mg/vial kit, 25 mg/vial kit, 37.5 mg/vial kit, 50 mg/vial kit. **Extended-release suspension for SUBQ injection (Uzedy):** 50 mg/0.14 mL, 75 mg/0.14 mL, 100 mg/0.28 mL, 125 mg/0.35 mL, 150 mg/0.42 mL, 200 mg/0.56 mL, 250 mg/0.7 mL.

NURSING IMPLICATIONS

Assessment

- Monitor mental status (orientation, mood, behavior) and mood before and periodically during therapy. Monitor closely for notable changes in behavior that could indicate the emergence or worsening of suicidal thoughts or behavior or depression, especially during early therapy. Restrict amount of drug available to patient.
- Assess weight and BMI initially; at 4, 8, and 12 wk; and every 4 mo throughout therapy. Refer as appropriate for nutritional/weight and medical management. Pedi: May ↑ weight in children and adolescents.
- Monitor for symptoms of hyperglycemia (polydipsia, polyuria, polyphagia, weakness) periodically during therapy.
- Obtain ECG at baseline. Monitor BP (sitting, standing, lying down) and HR before and frequently during initial dose titration; repeat in 12 wk and then annually. May cause prolonged QT interval, tachycardia, and orthostatic hypotension. If hypotension occurs, dose may need to be ↓.
- Observe patient when administering medication to ensure medication is swallowed and not hoarded or cheeked.
- Monitor for onset of extrapyramidal side effects (*akathisia:* restlessness; *dystonia:* muscle spasms and twisting motions; *pseudoparkinsonism:* masklike face, rigidity, tremors, drooling, shuffling gait, dysphagia). Report these symptoms; ↓ of dose or discontinuation may be necessary. Trihexyphenidyl or benztropine may be used to control symptoms.
- Monitor for tardive dyskinesia (involuntary rhythmic movement of mouth, face, and extremities) every 6 mo. Report immediately; may be irreversible.
- Monitor for signs and symptoms of neuroleptic malignant syndrome (hyperpyrexia, muscle rigidity, seizures altered mental status, evidence of autonomic instability [irregular HR or BP, tachycardia, diaphoresis, cardiac arrhythmia]). *If neuroleptic malignant syndrome suspected,* discontinue risperidone.
- Monitor for signs/symptoms related to hyperprolactinemia (menstrual abnormalities, galactorrhea, sexual dysfunction, changes in libido, erectile or ejaculatory dysfunction).
- Assess for falls risk. Drowsiness, orthostatic hypotension, and motor and sensory instability ↑ risk. Institute prevention if indicated.
- Monitor for skin rash during therapy. May require discontinuation of therapy.

Lab Test Considerations

- May ↑ AST and ALT.
- May cause anemia, thrombocytopenia, leukocytosis, and leukopenia.
- Obtain fasting blood glucose at baseline, Wk 12, and annually thereafter.
- Monitor fasting lipid panel at baseline, Wk 12, and every 5 yr thereafter.
- Monitor CBC frequently during initial months of therapy in patients with pre-existing or history of ↓ WBC. May cause leukopenia, neutropenia, or agranulocytosis. *If ANC <1000 cells/mm³,* discontinue risperidone.
- Monitor serum prolactin before starting and periodically during therapy. May ↑ serum prolactin levels.

Implementation

- Do not confuse risperidone with ropinirole. Do not confuse Risperdal with Restoril or ropinirole.
- When switching from other antipsychotics, discontinue previous agents when starting risperidone and minimize the period of overlapping antipsychotic agents.
- If therapy is reinstituted after an interval off risperidone, follow initial titration schedule.
- For SUBQ use, give 1st injection on the day after the last dose of oral therapy.
- For IM use, establish tolerance with oral dosing before IM use and continue oral dosing for 3 wk following initial IM injection. *Risperdal Consta:* Take oral doses for 3 wk, starting with the 1st dose of risperidone. Then discontinue PO doses. *Rykindo:* Take oral doses for 7 days, starting with day of 1st dose of risperidone. After 7 days, discontinue PO doses. Do not ↑ dose more frequently than every 4 wk. When transitioning from *Risperdal Consta* (risperidone long-acting IM injection) to *Rykindo*, give 1st injection of same dosage 45 wk after last injection; oral supplementation is not recommended; do not ↑dose more frequently than every 4 wk.
- **PO:** Administer in the morning or evening.
- For *orally disintegrating tablets*, peel back foil to expose tablet; do not push tablet through foil. Use dry hands to remove tablet and immediately place entire tablet on tongue. Tablets disintegrate in mouth within sec or can be swallowed with or without liquid. Do not split or chew tablet. Unused tablets must be disposed of once removed.

R

- *Oral solution* can be administered directly from calibrated oral dosing syringe or mixed with water, coffee, orange juice, or low-fat milk; do not mix with cola or tea.
- **SUBQ**: Allow syringe to reach room temperature ≥30 min prior to administration. May be injected into abdomen or back of upper arm; avoid areas with nodules, lesions, excessive pigment, tattoos, irritation, redness, bruising, infection, stretch marks, or scarring. Rotate injection sites. Do not expel visible air bubble to ensure entire dose is given. Wait 23 sec before removing needle from tissue. Store dose pack in refrigerator.
- **IM** Allow the drug and diluent to reach room temperature ≥30 min prior to reconstitution. Reconstitute with 2 mL of diluent in dose pack. Shake well to mix suspension. Administer via deep deltoid (1-inch needle) or gluteal (2-inch needle) injection using enclosed safety needle; alternate arms or buttocks with each injection. *Rykindo* should only be administered via deep gluteal (2-inch needle) injection. Must be administered within 6 hr of reconstitution. Store dose pack in refrigerator.
- Do not combine dose strengths in a single injection.

Patient/Family Teaching

- Explain the purpose and side effects of risperidone. Instruct patient to take as directed. Keep out of children's reach. Do not stop receiving drug without consulting health care provider. If an appointment is missed, reschedule as soon as possible. Caution patient to consult health care provider before discontinuing. Pedi: Explain to parents the importance of using calibrated measuring device for accurate dosing. Advise patient to read *Medication Guide* before starting and with each Rx refill in case of changes.
- Emphasize the importance of routine follow-up exams to monitor side effects and continued participation in psychotherapy to improve coping skills.
- Inform patient of the possibility of extrapyramidal symptoms. Instruct patient to report these symptoms immediately to health care provider.
- Advise patient to change positions slowly to minimize orthostatic hypotension. Protect from falls.
- May cause drowsiness. Caution patient to avoid driving or other activities requiring alertness until response to medication is known.
- Advise patient and family to notify health care provider if thoughts about suicide or dying, attempts to commit suicide, new or worse depression, new or worse anxiety, feeling very agitated or restless, panic attacks, trouble sleeping, new or worse irritability, acting aggressive, being angry or violent, acting on dangerous impulses, an extreme ↑ in activity and talking, or other unusual changes in behavior or mood occur.
- Advise patient to use sunscreen and protective clothing when exposed to the sun to prevent photosensitivity reactions. Extremes in temperature should also be avoided; this drug impairs body temperature regulation.
- Instruct patient to notify health care provider of all Rx or OTC medications, vitamins, or herbal products being taken and consult health care provider before taking any new medications. Caution patient to avoid concurrent use of alcohol and other CNS depressants.
- Advise patient to notify health care provider of medication regimen before treatment or surgery.
- Instruct patient to notify health care provider promptly if sore throat, fever, unusual bleeding or bruising, rash, tremors, or symptoms of hyperglycemia occur.
- Rep: Advise women of reproductive potential to notify health care provider if pregnancy is planned or suspected and to avoid breastfeeding. Monitor neonates for extrapyramidal and/or withdrawal symptoms. Monitor infants exposed to risperidone through breast milk for excess sedation, failure to thrive, jitteriness, and extrapyramidal symptoms (tremors and abnormal muscle movements). Encourage women who become pregnant while taking risperidone to enroll in the National Pregnancy Registry for Atypical Antipsychotics at 1-866-961-2388 or visit http://womensmentalhealth.org/research/pregnancyregistry/. May impair fertility in women; usually reversible.

Evaluation/Desired Outcomes

- Decrease in excited, manic behavior.
- Decrease in positive symptoms (delusions, hallucinations) of schizophrenia.
- Decreased aggression toward others, deliberate self-injury, temper tantrums, and mood changes in children with autism.
- Decrease in negative symptoms (social withdrawal, flat, blunted affects) of schizophrenia.
- Decrease in autism symptoms.

ritlecitinib (rit-le-sye-ti-nib)

Litfulo

Classification

Therapeutic: none assigned

Pharmacologic: kinase inhibitors

Indications

Severe alopecia areata.

Action

Irreversibly inhibits Janus kinase 3 and the tyrosine kinase expressed in the hepatocellular carcinoma (TEC) kinase family by blocking the adenosine triphosphate binding site, both of which may inhibit T-cell activation. **Therapeutic Effects:** Reduction in scalp hair loss.

Pharmacokinetics

Absorption: 64% absorbed following oral administration.

Distribution: Unknown.

Metabolism and Excretion: Metabolized by multiple pathways, including glutathione S-transferase and several CYP450 enzymes (CYP3A, CYP2C8, CYP1A2, and CYP2C9). Primarily excreted as metabolites in the urine (66%), with 20% excreted in the feces.

Half-life: 1.3–2.3 hr.

TIME/ACTION PROFILE (↓ in scalp hair loss)

ROUTE	ONSET	PEAK	DURATION
PO	6–8 wk	unknown	≥24 wk

Contraindications/Precautions

Contraindicated in: Hypersensitivity; Active, serious infection; Severe hepatic impairment; Lactation: Lactation.

Use Cautiously in: Chronic, recurrent infection; Previous exposure to tuberculosis (TB); History of serious or opportunistic infection; Lived or traveled in areas of endemic TB or mycoses; Predisposed to infection; >50 yr old with ≥1 cardiovascular risk factor (may ↑ risk of all-cause mortality, cardiovascular death, MI, stroke, and thrombosis); Current or past history of smoking (↑ risk of malignancy, cardiovascular death, MI, or stroke); Known malignancy (other than a successfully treated nonmelanoma skin cancer or cervical cancer); OB: Safety not established in pregnancy; Pedi: Children <12 yr (safety and effectiveness not established); Geri: Infection risk may be ↑ in older adults.

Adverse Reactions/Side Effects

CV: ARTERIAL THROMBOSIS, CARDIOVASCULAR DEATH, DEEP VEIN THROMBOSIS (DVT), MI. **Derm:** acne, atopic dermatitis, folliculitis, rash, urticaria. **GI:** diarrhea, ↑ liver enzymes, stomatitis. **Hemat:** anemia, lymphopenia, thrombocytopenia. **MS:** ↑ CK. **Neuro:** headache, dizziness, STROKE. **Resp:** PULMONARY EMBOLISM (PE). **Misc:** fever, HYPERSENSITIVITY REACTIONS (INCLUDING ANAPHYLAXIS), INFECTION (INCLUDING TB, BACTERIAL, INVASIVE FUNGAL, VIRAL, AND OTHER INFECTIONS DUE TO OPPORTUNISTIC PATHOGENS), MALIGNANCY.

Interactions

Drug-Drug: May ↑ risk of adverse reactions and ↓ antibody response to **live vaccines**; avoid concurrent use. May ↑ levels and risk of toxicity of **CYP3A substrates**. May ↑ levels and risk of toxicity of **CYP1A2 substrates**. **Strong CYP3A inducers**, including **rifampin**, may ↓ levels and effectiveness; concurrent use not recommended.

Route/Dosage

PO (Adults): 50 mg once daily.

Availability

Capsules: 50 mg.

NURSING IMPLICATIONS

Assessment

- Assess scalp for hair regrowth periodically during therapy.
- Monitor for signs and symptoms of infection during and after therapy. *If a patient develops a serious or opportunistic infection,* interrupt ritlecitinib, promptly complete diagnostic testing appropriate for an immunocompromised patient, and start antimicrobial therapy. May resume ritlecitinib once the infection is controlled.
- Screen patient for latent TB before starting therapy. Do not administer ritlecitinib to patients with active TB. Start anti-TB therapy before starting ritlecitinib in patients with a new diagnosis of latent TB or previously untreated latent TB.
- May cause viral reactivation (herpes virus reactivation). If a patient develops herpes zoster, consider holding therapy until episode resolves.
- Monitor for signs and symptoms of a hypersensitivity reaction (dyspnea; feeling faint or dizzy; swelling of lips, tongue, or throat; urticaria; hives; rash) during therapy. *If hypersensitivity reaction occurs,* discontinue ritlecitinib.
- Monitor for thrombosis, including PE, DVT, and arterial thrombi. *If signs/symptoms of thrombosis occur,* permanently discontinue ritlecitinib.
- Perform periodic skin examination in ↑ risk patients of skin cancer.

Lab Test Considerations

- Monitor absolute lymphocyte counts (ALC) and platelet counts before starting therapy, at 4 wk after start of therapy, and then according to routine patient management. If ALC <500 cells/mm³ or platelet count <100,000 cells/mm³, hold ritlecitinib; may be restarted once levels return to above this value. If platelet count <50,000 cells/mm³, discontinue ritlecitinib.
- Screen for viral hepatitis at baseline. Initiation is not recommended in patients with hepatitis B or C.
- Monitor liver enzymes before starting and periodically during therapy. *If ↑ in ALT or AST are observed and drug-induced liver injury is suspected,* hold ritlecitinib until diagnosis determined.
- May ↑ CK.

Implementation

- Verify that all vaccinations, including prophylactic herpes zoster, are current before starting therapy. Avoid use of live-attenuated vaccines during treatment or shortly before starting therapy.

R

- **PO:** Administer once daily without regard to food. ***DNC:*** Swallow capsules whole; do not crush, split, or chew.

Patient/Family Teaching

- Explain the purpose and side effects of ritlecitinib. Instruct patient to take as directed. If a dose is missed, administer dose as soon as possible, unless it is <8 hr before next dose; then skip missed dose and resume dosing at the regular scheduled time. If therapy is held, a temporary interruption for <6 wk is not expected to result in significant loss of regrown scalp hair. Advise patient to read *Medication Information* before starting ritlecitinib and with each Rx refill in case of changes.
- Advise patients and family to call 911 and seek urgent treatment for signs and symptoms of hypersensitivity reactions (difficulty breathing; chest tightness; hives; rash; feeling light-headed; itching; swelling of the face, lips, tongue, or throat).
- Advise patients and family to call 911 and seek urgent treatment if signs and symptoms of MI or stroke (chest pain, dizziness, nausea, weakness, slurred speech, confusion, trouble breathing); or blood clots (swelling, pain, or tenderness in one or both legs; sudden, unexplained chest or upper back pain; shortness of breath or difficulty breathing; changes in vision, especially in one eye only) occur.
- Advise patient to notify health care provider if signs and symptoms of infections (fever; sweating; chills; muscle aches; cough or shortness of breath; blood in phlegm; weight loss; warm, red, or painful skin or sores on the body; diarrhea or stomach pain; burning on urination or urinating more often than usual; feeling very tired).
- Inform patient that ritlecitinib may ↑ risk of cancer (lymphoma, lung cancer). Advise patient to have periodic skin examinations and to tell health care provider if they have ever had any type of cancer.
- Instruct patient to notify health care provider of all Rx or OTC medications, vitamins, or herbal products being taken and consult health care provider before taking any new medications.
- Advise patient to avoid live attenuated vaccines during or shortly before starting therapy.
- Rep: Advise women of reproductive potential to notify health care provider if pregnancy is planned or suspected and to avoid breastfeeding during therapy and for 14 hr after last dose. If patient becomes pregnant while receiving ritlecitinib, health care provider should report pregnancy exposure to Pregnancy Exposure Registry by calling 1-877-390-2940.

Evaluation/Desired Outcomes

- Decrease in scalp hair loss.

ritonavir (ri-toe-na-veer)

Norvir

Classification

Therapeutic: antiretrovirals

Pharmacologic: protease inhibitors

Indications

HIV infection (in combination with other antiretrovirals).

Action

Inhibits the action of HIV protease and prevents the cleavage of viral polyproteins. **Therapeutic Effects:** Increased CD4 cell counts and decreased viral load with subsequent slowed progression of HIV infection and its sequelae.

Pharmacokinetics

Absorption: Appears to be well absorbed after oral administration.

Distribution: Poor CNS penetration.

Protein Binding: 98–99%.

Metabolism and Excretion: Primarily metabolized in the liver by the CYP3A4 and CYP2D6 isoenzymes; one metabolite has antiretroviral activity; 3.5% excreted unchanged in urine.

Half-life: 3–5 hr.

TIME/ACTION PROFILE (plasma concentrations)

ROUTE	ONSET	PEAK	DURATION
PO	rapid	4 hr*	12 hr

*Nonfasting.

Contraindications/Precautions

Contraindicated in: Hypersensitivity; Concurrent use of alfuzosin, amiodarone, apalutamide, colchicine, dihydroergotamine, dronedarone, ergotamine, flecainide, fluticasone, lomitapide, lovastatin, lurasidone, meperidine, methylergonovine, midazolam (PO), pimozide, propafenone, quinidine, ranolazine, simvastatin, sildenafil (Revatio), St. John's wort, triazolam, or voriconazole; Lactation: Breastfeeding not recommended in patients with HIV.

Use Cautiously in: Hepatic impairment or history of hepatitis; Diabetes mellitus; Hemophilia (↑ risk of bleeding); Structural heart disease, conduction abnormalities, ischemic heart disease, or HF (↑ risk of heart block); Pedi: Children <1 mo (safety and effectiveness not established).

Adverse Reactions/Side Effects

CV: heart block, orthostatic hypotension, PR interval prolongation, syncope. **Derm:** rash, skin eruptions, STEVENS-JOHNSON SYNDROME (SJS), sweating, TOXIC EPIDERMAL NECROLYSIS (TEN), urticaria. **EENT:** pharyngitis, throat irritation. **Endo:** hyperglycemia. **F and E:** dehydration. **GI:** abdominal pain, altered taste, anorexia, diarrhea, nausea, vomiting, constipation, dyspepsia, flatulence. **GU:** renal impairment. **Metab:** fat redistribution, hyperlipidemia. **MS:** ↑ CK, myalgia. **Neuro:** abnormal thinking, weakness, dizziness, headache, malaise, paresthesia, SEIZURES, somnolence. **Resp:** bronchospasm. **Misc:** fever, HYPERSENSITIVITY REACTIONS (INCLUDING ANAPHYLAXIS AND ANGIOEDEMA), immune reconstitution syndrome.

Interactions

Drug-Drug: May significantly ↑ levels and risk of toxicity from some **antiarrhythmics (amiodarone, dronedarone, flecainide, pimozide, propafenone, quinidine), ergot derivatives (dihydroergotamine, ergotamine, methylergonovine), fluticasone (inhalation), lomitapide, lurasidone, meperidine, ranolazine, sildenafil (Revatio), alfuzosin, lovastatin, simvastatin, voriconazole, midazolam (oral)**, and **triazolam**; concurrent use contraindicated. May significantly ↑ levels and risk of toxicity of **colchicine**; concurrent use in patients with renal or hepatic impairment contraindicated; ↓ colchicine dose in patients without renal or hepatic impairment. **Apalutamide** may ↓ levels and promote resistance; concurrent use contraindicated. May ↑ levels and risk of toxicity of **maraviroc**; ↓ maraviroc dose to 150 mg twice daily. May ↑ levels and risk of toxicity of **clarithromycin**; ↓ clarithromycin dose if CCr <60 mL/min. May ↑ levels and risk of toxicity of **rifabutin**; ↓ rifabutin dose to 150 mg every other day or 3 times weekly. May ↑ levels and risk of toxicity of certain **opioid analgesics (fentanyl, hydrocodone, oxycodone, tramadol)**; certain **NSAIDs (diclofenac, ibuprofen, indomethacin)**; certain **antiarrhythmics (disopyramide, lidocaine, mexiletine)**; certain **antidepressants (amitriptyline, clomipramine, desipramine, imipramine, nortriptyline, nefazodone, sertraline, trazodone, fluoxetine, paroxetine, venlafaxine)**; certain **antiemetics (dronabinol, ondansetron)**; certain **beta blockers (metoprolol, pindolol, propranolol, timolol)**; certain **calcium channel blockers (amlodipine, diltiazem, felodipine, isradipine, nicardipine, nifedipine, nimodipine, nisoldipine, verapamil)**; certain **immunosuppressants (cyclosporine, tacrolimus)**; certain **antipsychotics (chlorpromazine, haloperidol, perphenazine, risperidone, thioridazine)**; and also **atazanavir, darunavir, fosamprenavir, quinidine, tipranavir, bedaquiline, methamphetamine**, and **warfarin**; may need to ↓ dose. May ↑ levels and risk of toxicity of **vincristine** and **vinblastine**; consider holding or switching to another antiretroviral regimen that does not contain a CYP3A or P-glycoprotein inhibitor. May ↑ levels and risk of toxicity of **dasatinib** and **nilotinib**; may need to ↓ doses of dasatinib and nilotinib. May ↑ levels and risk of tumor lysis syndrome with **venetoclax** and **ibrutinib**; avoid concurrent use. May ↑ levels and risk of toxicity of **abemaciclib** and **neratinib**; avoid concurrent use. May ↑ levels and risk of toxicity of **glecaprevir/pibrentasvir, sofosbuvir/velpatasvir/voxilaprevir, ombitasvir**, and **paritaprevir**; avoid concurrent use. May ↑ levels and risk of toxicity of systemic, inhaled, nasal, or ophthalmic **corticosteroids (betamethasone, budesonide, ciclesonide, dexamethasone, fluticasone, methylprednisolone, mometasone, prednisone, triamcinolone)**; consider alternative corticosteroid such as beclomethasone or prednisolone. May ↓ levels and effectiveness of **hormonal contraceptives, zidovudine, bupropion**, and **theophylline**; dose alteration or alternative therapy may be necessary. **Clarithromycin** or **fluoxetine** may ↑ levels and risk of toxicity. ↑ risk of heart block with **beta blockers, verapamil, diltiazem, digoxin**, or **atazanavir**. May ↑ levels and risk of toxicity of phosphodiesterase type 5 inhibitors; ↓ starting doses not to exceed 25 mg within 48 hr for **sildenafil** (Viagra), 2.5 mg every 72 hr for **vardenafil**, and 10 mg every 72 hr for **tadalafil**. May ↑ risk of adverse effects with **salmeterol**; concurrent use not recommended. May ↑ risk of myopathy with **atorvastatin** or **rosuvastatin**; use lowest possible statin dose. May ↑ levels and risk of toxicity of **bosentan**; initiate bosentan at 62.5 mg once daily or every other day; if patient already receiving bosentan, discontinue bosentan ≥36 hr before initiation of ritonavir and then restart bosentan ≥10 days later at 62.5 mg once daily or every other day. May ↑ levels and risk of toxicity of **tadalafil (Adcirca)**; initiate tadalafil (Adcirca) at 20 mg once daily; if patient already receiving tadalafil (Adcirca), discontinue tadalafil (Adcirca) ≥24 hr before initiation of ritonavir and then restart tadalafil (Adcirca) ≥7 days later at 20 mg once daily. May ↑ levels and risk of toxicity of **quetiapine**; ↓ quetiapine dose to of current dose. **Dexamethasone** may ↓ levels and effectiveness; consider use of alternative corticosteroid, such as beclomethasone or prednisolone. **Encorafenib** and **ivosidenib** may ↑ risk of QT interval prolongation; avoid concurrent use, if possible. If concurrent use necessary, ↓ doses of encorafenib and ivosidenib. Concurrent use with **elagolix** may ↑ elagolix levels and ↓ ritonavir levels; do not use with elagolix 200 mg twice daily for >1 mo; do not use with elagolix 150 mg once daily for >6 mo. May ↑ levels and risk of toxicity of active metabolite of **fostamatinib**, which can ↑ risk of hepatotoxicity and neutropenia; may need to ↓ fostamatinib dose.

Drug-Natural Products: St. John's wort may ↓ levels and promote resistance; concurrent use contraindicated.

Drug-Food: Food ↑ absorption.

Route/Dosage

PO (Adults): 300 mg twice daily for 2–3 days, then 400 mg twice daily for 2–3 days, then 500 mg twice daily for 2–3 days, then 600 mg twice daily as maintenance.

PO (Children >1 mo): 250 mg/m^2 twice daily initially; ↑ by 50 mg/m^2 twice daily every 2–3 days up to 400 mg/m^2 twice daily (if unable to get up to 400 mg/m^2 twice daily, consider alternative antiretroviral therapy).

Availability (generic available)

Tablets: 100 mg. **Oral powder:** 100 mg/pkt.

NURSING IMPLICATIONS

Assessment

- Assess for change in severity of HIV symptoms and for signs/symptoms of opportunistic infections during therapy.
- Assess for rash (mild to moderate rash usually occurs in the 2nd wk of therapy and resolves within 1–2 wk of continued therapy). Monitor patients for development of severe cutaneous adverse reactions, such as SJS and TEN, including signs and symptoms of prodrome of fever, malaise, mucosal lesions, progressive skin rash, blisters, lymphadenopathy, conjunctivitis, myalgias, hepatitis, or eosinophilia. *If a severe cutaneous adverse reaction is suspected,* hold ritonavir until etiology of reaction is determined. Consultation with a dermatologist is recommended. *If a severe cutaneous adverse reaction is confirmed,* permanently discontinue ritonavir.
- Assess cardiac history and ECG at baseline; monitor for PR interval prolongation and 2nd- and 3rd-degree atrioventricular block.

Lab Test Considerations

- Monitor viral load at baseline and with modification of antiretroviral treatment, at 2–8 wk, then every 4–8 wk until values are below the limit of detection (<200 copies/mL), and then every 3–4 mo; if viral loads suppressed for >2 yr, monitoring may be extended to every 6 mo.
- Monitor CD4 cell counts at baseline and with modification of antiretroviral treatment and then every 3–6 mo during the 1st 2 yr of treatment and if the CD4 counts are <300 cells/mm^3 or viremia develops; if viral loads suppressed for >2 yr, monitoring may be extended to every 12 mo.
- Monitor CBC with differential at baseline then every 3–6 mo or when CD4 testing is done.
- Perform hepatitis B and C screening at baseline and with modification of antiretroviral treatment; may repeat screening every 12 mo in high-risk patients if results are negative at baseline.
- Monitor ALT, AST, GGT, and total bilirubin at baseline and with modification of antiretroviral treatment and then every 3–4 mo or more frequently if signs of hepatotoxicity develop. May ↑ AST, ALT, GGT, and total bilirubin.
- Monitor serum triglycerides and total cholesterol at baseline and then every 6–12 mo during therapy. May ↑ triglycerides.
- Monitor fasting blood glucose and A1c at baseline and with modification of antiretroviral treatment and then every 3–6 mo in patients with abnormal values or every 12 mo in patients with normal values. May cause hyperglycemia.
- Monitor basic chemistry, uric acid, and CK at baseline and with modification of antiretroviral treatment, at 2–8 wk, and then every 3–6 mo. May CK and uric acid.

Implementation

- Do not confuse ritonavir with Retrovir.
- **PO:** Administer with a meal or light snack. ***DNC:*** Swallow tablets whole; do not crush, break, or chew. Store tablets at room temperature.
- Oral powder may be mixed with applesauce, vanilla pudding, water, chocolate milk, or infant formula to ↓ the bitter flavor. Administer within 2 hr of preparation or discard.
- May be administered via feeding tubes compatible with ethanol and propylene glycol, such as silicone and polyvinyl chloride; do not use with polyurethane feeding tubes due to potential incompatibility.
- If nausea occurs on dose of 600 mg twice daily, may titrate by 300 mg twice daily for 1 day, then 400 mg twice daily for 2 days, then 500 mg twice daily for 1 day, and then 600 mg twice daily thereafter.
- Patients initiating concurrent therapy with nucleoside analogues may have less GI intolerance by initiating ritonavir for 2 wk and then adding the nucleoside analogue.

Patient/Family Teaching

- Explain the purpose and side effects of ritonavir. Emphasize the importance of taking as directed, at evenly spaced times during day. Do not take more than prescribed amount, and do not stop taking without consulting health care provider. Take missed doses as soon as remembered; do not double doses. Advise patient to read *Patient Information* before starting and with each Rx refill in case of changes.
- Emphasize the importance of regular follow-up exams and blood counts to determine progress and monitor for side effects.
- Because of potential for numerous drug interactions with ritonavir, advise patient to notify health care provider of all Rx or OTC medications, vitamins, or herbal products being taken and consult health care provider before taking any new medications, especially St. John's wort.
- Inform patient that ritonavir does not cure HIV or prevent associated or opportunistic infections. Ritonavir may ↓ the risk of transmission of HIV to others through sexual contact or blood contamination. Caution patient to use a condom during sexual

contact and to avoid sharing needles or donating blood to prevent spreading HIV to others.

- Inform patient that ritonavir may cause hyperglycemia. Advise patient to notify health care provider if ↑ thirst or hunger; unexplained weight loss; ↑ urination; fatigue; or dry, itchy skin occurs.
- Warn patient to report symptoms of arrhythmias and PR prolongation (fast heartbeat, skipped beats, palpitations, dizziness, light-headedness, trouble breathing, faintness).
- Instruct patient to notify health care provider immediately if rash occurs.
- Inform patient that redistribution and accumulation of body fat may occur, causing central obesity, dorsocervical fat enlargement (buffalo hump), peripheral wasting, breast enlargement, and cushingoid appearance. The cause and long-term effects are not known.
- Rep: Advise women of reproductive potential taking oral contraceptives to use a nonhormonal method of birth control during ritonavir therapy. If pregnancy is suspected, notify health care provider promptly. Encourage pregnant women to enroll in the Antiretroviral Pregnancy Registry by calling 1-800-258-4263. Advise women of reproductive potential to avoid breastfeeding during therapy.

Evaluation/Desired Outcomes

- Delayed progression of AIDS and decreased opportunistic infections in patients with HIV.
- Decrease in viral load and improvement in CD4 cell counts.

HIGH ALERT

riTUXimab (ri-tux-i-mab)

Riabni, Rituxan, ✦Riximyo, Ruxience, Truxima

Classification

Therapeutic: antineoplastics

Pharmacologic: monoclonal antibodies

Indications

Riabni, Rituxan, Ruxience, and Truxima: Treatment of the following conditions: Relapsed or refractory low-grade or follicular CD20-positive B-cell non-Hodgkin lymphoma (NHL) (as monotherapy); Previously untreated follicular CD20-positive B-cell NHL in combination with first-line chemotherapy and, in patients achieving a complete or partial response to rituximab in combination with chemotherapy, as single-agent maintenance therapy; Nonprogressing low-grade CD20-positive B-cell NHL following treatment with cyclophosphamide, vincristine, and prednisone (as monotherapy); Previously untreated diffuse large B-cell CD20-positive NHL (in combination with CHOP or another anthracycline-based chemotherapy regimen); CD-20 positive chronic lymphocytic leukemia (CLL) (in combination with fludarabine and cyclophosphamide); Moderately to severely active rheumatoid arthritis in patients who have had an inadequate response to ≥1 TNF antagonist therapies (with methotrexate); Granulomatosis with polyangiitis (Wegener granulomatosis) and microscopic polyangiitis (in combination with glucocorticoids); Moderate to severe pemphigus vulgaris. **Rituxan only:** Treatment of the following condition: Previously untreated advanced-stage CD20-positive diffuse large B-cell lymphoma, Burkitt lymphoma, Burkitt-like lymphoma, or mature B-cell acute leukemia (in combination with chemotherapy).

Action

Binds to the CD20 antigen on the surface of lymphoma cells, preventing the activation process for cell cycle initiation and differentiation. **Therapeutic Effects:** Death of lymphoma cells. Prolonged progression-free survival in CLL. Reduced signs and symptoms of rheumatoid arthritis. Achievement of complete remission in granulomatosis with polyangiitis, microscopic polyangiitis, and pemphigus vulgaris.

Pharmacokinetics

Absorption: IV administration results in complete bioavailability.

Distribution: Binds specifically to CD20 binding sites on lymphoma cells.

Metabolism and Excretion: Unknown.

Half-life: 59.8–174 hr (depending on tumor burden).

TIME/ACTION PROFILE (B-cell depletion)

ROUTE	ONSET	PEAK	DURATION
IV	within 14 days	3–4 wk	6–9 mo†

† Duration of depletion after 4 wk of treatment.

Contraindications/Precautions

Contraindicated in: Hypersensitivity to murine (mouse) proteins; OB: Can pass placental barrier potentially causing fetal B-cell depletion. Use during pregnancy only if clearly needed; Lactation: Lactation.

Use Cautiously in: Pre-existing bone marrow depression; Pre-existing cardiac or pulmonary conditions, history of rituximab-induced cardiopulmonary adverse reactions, or high numbers of circulating malignant cells (↑ risk of infusion-related reactions); Hepatitis B virus (HBV) infection (may reactivate infection during and for several mo after treatment); Systemic lupus erythematosus (may cause fatal progressive multifocal leukoencephalopathy

✦ = Canadian drug name. = Genetic implication. V = Vesicant. Boxed warning. ~~Strikethrough~~ = Discontinued. *CAPITALS = life-threatening. Underline = most frequent.

R

[PML]); HIV infection (may ↑ risk of HIV-associated lymphoma); Rep: Women of reproductive potential; Pedi: Safety and effectiveness not established for children <6 mo (mature B-cell lymphomas and B-cell acute leukemia), <2 yr (granulomatosis with polyangiitis and microscopic polyangiitis), and <18 yr (all other indications).

Adverse Reactions/Side Effects

CV: hypotension, ARRHYTHMIAS, peripheral edema. **Derm:** flushing, LICHENOID DERMATITIS, PARANEOPLASTIC PEMPHIGUS, STEVENS-JOHNSON SYNDROME (SJS), TOXIC EPIDERMAL NECROLYSIS (TEN), urticaria, VESICULOBULLOUS DERMATITIS. **Endo:** hyperglycemia. **F and E:** hypocalcemia. **GI:** abdominal pain, altered taste, dyspepsia, HBV REACTIVATION. **GU:** renal failure. **Hemat:** ANEMIA, NEUTROPENIA, THROMBOCYTOPENIA. **MS:** arthralgia, back pain. **Neuro:** headache, PML. **Resp:** bronchospasm, cough, dyspnea. **Misc:** infection, INFUSION-RELATED REACTIONS, TUMOR LYSIS SYNDROME.

Interactions

Drug-Drug: May ↓ antibody response to or ↑ risk of adverse reactions to **live vaccines**; avoid use during treatment; inactive vaccines should be administered ≥4 wk prior to start of therapy.

Route/Dosage

Relapsed or Refractory Low-Grade or Follicular CD20-Positive B-Cell Non-Hodgkin Lymphoma

IV (Adults): *Riabni, Rituxan, Ruxience, or Truxima:* 375 mg/m² once weekly for 4 or 8 doses; may retreat with 375 mg/m² once weekly for 4 doses.

Previously Untreated Follicular CD20-Positive B-Cell Non-Hodgkin Lymphoma

IV (Adults): *Riabni, Rituxan, Ruxience, or Truxima:* 375 mg/m² given on Day 1 of each cycle of chemotherapy with cyclophosphamide, vincristine, and prednisone for up to 8 doses; if patients experience complete or partial response, give 375 mg/m² (as monotherapy) every 8 wk for 12 doses (initiate this maintenance therapy 8 wk after completion of rituximab + cyclophosphamide/vincristine/prednisone regimen).

Nonprogressing Low-Grade CD20-Positive B-Cell Non-Hodgkin Lymphoma

IV (Adults): *Riabni, Rituxan, Ruxience, or Truxima:* For patients who have not progressed following 6–8 cycles of chemotherapy with cyclophosphamide, vincristine, and prednisone, 375 mg/m² given once weekly for 4 doses given every 6 mo for up to 16 doses.

Diffuse Large B-Cell Non-Hodgkin Lymphoma

IV (Adults): *Riabni, Rituxan, Ruxience, or Truxima:* 375 mg/m² given on Day 1 of each cycle of chemotherapy for up to 8 infusions.

Previously Untreated Mature B-Cell Lymphomas and B-Cell Acute Leukemia

IV (Children ≥6 mo): *Rituxan:* 375 mg/m²/dose in combination with systemic Lymphome Malin B chemotherapy regimen; administer 2 doses during each of the two induction courses (Day −2 and Day 1), and one dose during each of the two consolidation cycles (Day 1) (6 doses total).

Chronic Lymphocytic Leukemia

IV (Adults): *Riabni, Rituxan, Ruxience, or Truxima:* 375 mg/m² given on the day before initiating chemotherapy with fludarabine and cyclophosphamide, then 500 mg/m² on Day 1 of cycles 2–6 (every 28 days).

Rheumatoid Arthritis

IV (Adults): *Riabni, Rituxan, Ruxience, or Truxima:* 1000 mg every 2 wk for 2 doses; subsequent courses should be administered every 24 wk (not sooner than every 16 wk).

Granulomatosis With Polyangiitis and Microscopic Polyangiitis

IV (Adults): *Induction treatment:* Riabni, Rituxan, Ruxience, or Truxima: 375 mg/m² once weekly for 4 wk; *Follow-up treatment in patients who have achieved disease control with induction treatment:* Riabni, Rituxan, Ruxience, or Truxima: 500 mg every 2 wk for 2 doses (should be started 16–24 wk after last rituximab induction dose; if achieved disease control with another agent, start follow-up treatment within 4 wk after last induction dose of that agent), then 500 mg every 6 mo thereafter.

IV (Children ≥2 yr): *Induction treatment:* Riabni, Rituxan, Ruxience, or Truxima: 375 mg/m² once weekly for 4 wk; *Follow-up treatment in patients who have achieved disease control with induction treatment:* Riabni, Rituxan, Ruxience, or Truxima: 250 mg/m² every 2 wk for 2 doses (should be started 16–24 wk after last rituximab induction dose; if achieved disease control with another agent, start follow-up treatment within 4 wk after last induction dose of that agent), then 250 mg/m² every 6 mo thereafter.

Pemphigus Vulgaris

IV (Adults): *Riabni, Rituxan, Ruxience, or Truxima:* 1000 mg every 2 wk for 2 doses, then maintenance dose of 500 mg infusion at Month 12 and then every 6 mo thereafter. On relapse, administer 1000 mg.

Availability

Solution for injection: 10 mg/mL. ***In combination with:*** hyaluronidase (Rituxan Hycela). See Appendix N.

NURSING IMPLICATIONS

Assessment

- Monitor for signs/symptoms of infusion-related reactions (fever, chills/rigors, nausea, urticaria, fatigue, headache, pruritus, bronchospasm, dyspnea, sensation of tongue or throat swelling, rhinitis, vomiting, hypotension, flushing, pain at disease sites, pulmonary infiltrates, acute respiratory distress syndrome, MI, ventricular fibrillation, cardiogenic shock). Infusion-related events occur frequently within 30 min–2 hr of beginning 1st infusion and may resolve with slowing or discontinuing infusion. *If severe reactions occur,* immediately discontinue infusion and treat with glucocorticoids, epinephrine, bronchodilators, or oxygen, as needed. If decision is made to restart rituximab after symptoms resolve, resume infusion at ≥50% ↓ in rate. Incidence ↓ with subsequent infusions.

- Monitor for tumor lysis syndrome due to rapid ↓ in tumor volume (acute renal failure, hyperkalemia, hypocalcemia, hyperuricemia, hypophosphatemia), usually occurring 12–24 hr after 1st infusion. Risks are higher in patients with greater tumor burden; may be fatal. Correct electrolyte abnormalities, monitor renal function and fluid balance, and administer supportive care, including dialysis, as indicated.
- Monitor ECG during and immediately after infusion in patients with pre-existing cardiac conditions (arrhythmias, angina) or patients who have developed arrhythmias during previous infusions of rituximab. Life-threatening arrhythmias may occur.
- Assess for signs of PML (hemiparesis, apathy, confusion, cognitive deficiencies, ataxia) periodically during therapy.
- Assess for infection during and for 1 yr after therapy. Bacterial, fungal, and new or reactivated viral infections may occur. Screen patient for HBV infection prior to therapy. Discontinue rituximab and any concurrent chemotherapy in patients who develop viral hepatitis or other serious infections, and institute appropriate treatment.
- Assess for mucocutaneous reactions periodically during therapy. May cause SJS and TEN. Discontinue therapy if severe or if accompanied with fever, general malaise, fatigue, muscle or joint aches, blisters, oral lesions, conjunctivitis, hepatitis, or eosinophilia.

Lab Test Considerations

- Verify negative pregnancy status before starting therapy.
- Monitor CBC before starting and regularly during therapy and frequently in patients with blood dyscrasias. May cause anemia, thrombocytopenia, or neutropenia.
- Frequently causes B-cell depletion with an associated ↓ in serum immunoglobulins in a minority of patients; does not appear to cause an ↑ incidence of infection.
- Obtain HBsAg and anti-HBc to screen patient for HBV infection before initiating therapy. May cause reactivation of HBV up to 24 mo after therapy.

Implementation

- Do not confuse rituximab with infliximab. Do not confuse Rituxan with Rituxan Hycela.
- Transient hypotension may occur during infusion; antihypertensive medications may be held for 12 hr before infusion.
- **Rheumatoid Arthritis:** Administer 100 mg methylprednisolone IV or equivalent 30 min prior to each infusion to minimize infusion reactions.
- **Granulomatosis With Polyangiitis and Microscopic Polyangiitis:** Administer methylprednisolone 1000 mg IV per day for 1–3 days, followed by oral prednisone 1 mg/kg/day (not to exceed 80 mg/day and tapered per clinical need) to treat severe vasculitis symptoms. Begin regimen within 14 days prior to or with the initiation of rituximab; may continue during and after the 4-wk course of rituximab treatment.
- Prophylaxis against *Pneumocystis jiroveci* pneumonia and herpes virus recommended during treatment and for up to 12 mo following treatment as appropriate for patients with CLL, and during and for ≥6 mo following last rituximab infusion for patients with granulomatosis with polyangiitis and microscopic polyangiitis.

IV Administration

- **Intermittent Infusion: Dilution:** Dilute with 0.9% NaCl or D5W. **Concentration:** 1–4 mg/mL. Gently invert bag to mix. Solution is clear to slightly opalescent and colorless to slightly yellow; do not administer solutions that are cloudy, discolored, or contain particulate matter. Discard unused portion remaining in vial. Solution is stable for 12 hr at room temperature and for 24 hr if refrigerated. Unused portion of *Ruxience* diluted in 0.9% NaCl can be stored refrigerated for 16 days. **Rate:** Do not administer as an IV push or bolus.
- *1st infusion:* Administer at an initial rate of 50 mg/hr. If hypersensitivity or infusion-related events do not occur, rate may ↑ in 50-mg/hr increments every 30 min to a maximum of 400 mg/hr.
- *Subsequent infusions:* May administer at an initial rate of 100 mg/hr and ↑ in 100-mg/hr increments at 30-min intervals to a maximum of 400 mg/hr.
- For previously untreated NHL and B-cell NHL, if no Grade 3 or 4 infusion-related reactions occurred in Cycle 1, may administer via 90-min infusion using glucocorticoids. Begin at rate of 20% of dose over 30 min, with remaining 80% dose over 60 min. If tolerated, then can be used for remainder of therapy.
- **Y-Site Compatibility:** acyclovir, amikacin, aminophylline, ampicillin, ampicillin/sulbactam, aztreonam, bleomycin, bumetanide, buprenorphine,

R

busulfan, butorphanol, calcium gluconate, carboplatin, carmustine, cefazolin, cefotaxime, cefotetan, cefoxitin, ceftazidime, ceftriaxone, cefuroxime, chlorpromazine, cisplatin, clindamycin, cyclophosphamide, cytarabine, dactinomycin, daunorubicin, dexamethasone, dexrazoxane, digoxin, diphenhydramine, dobutamine, docetaxel, dopamine, doxorubicin liposomal, doxycycline, droperidol, enalaprilat, etoposide phosphate, famotidine, fentanyl, filgrastim, floxuridine, fluconazole, fludarabine, fluorouracil, ganciclovir, gemcitabine, gentamicin, granisetron, haloperidol, heparin, hydrocortisone, hydromorphone, idarubicin, ifosfamide, imipenem/cilastatin, irinotecan, leucovorin, lorazepam, magnesium sulfate, mannitol, meperidine, mesna, methotrexate, methylprednisolone, metoclopramide, metronidazole, mitomycin, mitoxantrone, morphine, nalbuphine, paclitaxel, pentamidine, piperacillin/tazobactam, potassium chloride, prochlorperazine, promethazine, sargramostim, theophylline, thiotepa, tobramycin, trimethoprim/sulfamethoxazole, vinblastine, vincristine, vinorelbine, zidovudine.

- **Y-Site Incompatibility:** aldesleukin, ciprofloxacin, cyclosporine, doxorubicin hydrochloride, furosemide, levofloxacin, minocycline, ondansetron, sodium bicarbonate, topotecan, vancomycin.

Patient/Family Teaching

- Explain purpose and side effects of medication to patient. Advise patient to read *Patient Information* before starting therapy.
- Advise patient to notify health care provider of all Rx or OTC medications, vitamins, or herbal products being taken and to consult health care provider before taking other medications.
- Advise patient to report signs/symptoms infusion-related reactions immediately.
- Instruct patient to notify health care provider promptly if painful ulcers or sores on skin, lips, or in mouth; blisters; peeling skin; rash; or pustule occur.
- Instruct patient to report signs/symptoms of hepatotoxicity (yellowing of the skin and eyes, unusual darkening of the urine, nausea, feeling tired or weak, vomiting) that persist over several days to health care provider immediately.
- Instruct patient to report signs/symptoms of PML (progressive weakness on one side of the body or clumsiness of limbs; disturbance of vision; changes in thinking, memory, and orientation leading to confusion and personality changes) that persist over several days to health care provider immediately.
- Instruct patient to notify health care provider promptly if fever; chills; cough; hoarseness; sore throat; signs of infection; lower back or side pain; painful or difficult urination; bleeding gums; bruising; petechiae; blood in stools, urine, or emesis; ↑ fatigue; dyspnea; or orthostatic hypotension occurs. Caution patient to avoid crowds and persons with known infections. Instruct patient to use soft toothbrush and electric razor and to avoid falls. Caution patient not to drink alcoholic beverages or take medication containing aspirin or NSAIDs; may precipitate gastric bleeding.
- Advise patient to consult health care provider prior to receiving any vaccinations.
- Rep: May cause fetal harm. Advise women of reproductive potential to use effective contraception during and for 12 mo following therapy and to avoid breastfeeding during therapy and for ≥6 mo after last dose. Observe newborns and infants of women taking rituximab during pregnancy for signs of infection.

Evaluation/Desired Outcomes

- Decrease in spread of malignancy.
- Prolonged progression-free survival in CLL.
- Reduced signs and symptoms of rheumatoid arthritis.
- Achievement of complete remission in granulomatosis with polyangiitis and microscopic polyangiitis.

BEERS HIGH ALERT

rivaroxaban (ri-va-**rox**-a-ban)

Xarelto

Classification

Therapeutic: anticoagulants

Pharmacologic: antithrombotics, factor Xa inhibitors

Indications

Prevention of deep vein thrombosis (DVT) that may lead to pulmonary embolism (PE) following knee or hip replacement surgery. Prevention of venous thromboembolism (VTE) and VTE-related death during hospitalization and following hospital discharge in patients admitted for an acute medical illness who are at risk for thromboembolic complications and not at high risk of bleeding. Treatment of DVT or PE. Reduction in risk of recurrence of DVT and/or PE in patients at continued risk for recurrent DVT or PE after completion of initial treatment for at least 6 mo. Reduction in risk of stroke/systemic embolism in patients with nonvalvular atrial fibrillation (AF). Reduction in risk of major cardiovascular events (cardiovascular death, MI, stroke) in patients with chronic coronary artery disease (in combination with aspirin). Reduction in risk of major thrombotic vascular events (MI, ischemic stroke, acute limb ischemia, major amputation of a vascular etiology) in patients with peripheral artery disease (PAD), including patients who have recently undergone a lower extremity revascularization procedure due to symptomatic PAD (in combination with aspirin). Treatment of VTE and the reduction in the risk of recurrent VTE in pediatric patients from birth to <18 yr after ≥5 days of initial parenteral anticoagulant treatment. Thromboprophylaxis in pediatric patients ≥2 yr with congenital heart disease who have undergone the Fontan procedure.

Action

Acts as selective factor X inhibitor that blocks the active site of factor Xa, inactivating the cascade of coagulation.
Therapeutic Effects: Treatment and prevention of thromboembolic events and major cardiovascular events.

Pharmacokinetics

Absorption: Well absorbed (80%) following oral administration; absorption occurs in the stomach and ↓ as it enters the small intestine.
Distribution: Unknown.
Metabolism and Excretion: 51% metabolized by the liver; 36% excreted unchanged in urine. Metabolites do not have anticoagulant activity.
Half-life: 5–9 hr.

TIME/ACTION PROFILE (anticoagulant effect)

ROUTE	ONSET	PEAK	DURATION
PO	unknown	2–4 hr†	24 hr

† Plasma concentrations.

Contraindications/Precautions

Contraindicated in: Hypersensitivity; Active major bleeding; Severe renal impairment (adults) (CCr <15 mL/min [DVT/PE treatment or prevention]); Prosthetic heart valves; Transcatheter aortic valve replacement (↑ risk of death and bleeding); Moderate to severe hepatic impairment or any liver pathology resulting in altered coagulation (adults); PE with hemodynamic instability or requiring thrombolysis or pulmonary embolectomy; Concurrent use of drugs that are combined P-glycoprotein (P-gp) inducers/strong CYP3A4 inducers or combined P-gp inhibitors/strong CYP3A4 inhibitors; Triple positive antiphospholipid syndrome (↑ risk of thrombosis); Lactation: Lactation; Pedi: Moderate or severe renal impairment (eGFR: <50 mL/min/1.73 m^2) (children ≥1 yr); serum creatinine above 97.5th percentile (children <1 yr); Pedi: Hepatic impairment in children; Pedi: Children <6 mo and any of the following (<37 wk of gestation at birth, <10 days of oral feeding, or <2.6 kg).
Use Cautiously in: Neuroaxial spinal anesthesia or spinal puncture, especially if concurrent with an indwelling epidural catheter, drugs affecting hemostasis, history of traumatic/repeated spinal puncture, or spinal deformity (↑ risk of spinal hematoma); CCr ≤50 mL/min (AF) (↓ dose); Use of feeding tube (proper placement of tube must be documented to ensure absorption); OB: Use during pregnancy only if potential maternal benefit justifies potential fetal risk; Rep: Women of reproductive potential with abnormal uterine bleeding (↑ risk of uterine bleeding); Geri: Appears on Beers list. ↑ risk of bleeding in older adults. Avoid use for long treatment of AF or VTE in favor of safer anticoagulant options.

Adverse Reactions/Side Effects

CV: syncope. **Derm:** blister, pruritus. **Hemat:** BLEEDING. **Local:** wound secretion. **MS:** extremity pain, muscle spasm.

Interactions

Drug-Drug: **Combined P-gp inhibitors/strong CYP3A4 inhibitors**, including **ketoconazole**, **itraconazole**, **lopinavir/ritonavir**, **ritonavir**, and **conivaptan**, may ↑ levels and risk of bleeding; avoid concurrent use. **Combined P-gp inducers/strong CYP3A4 inducers**, including **carbamazepine**, **phenytoin**, or **rifampin**, may ↓ levels and effectiveness; avoid concurrent use. **Combined P-gp inhibitors/moderate CYP3A4 inhibitors**, including **erythromycin**, in patients with renal impairment (CCr 15–79 mL/min) may ↑ levels and risk of bleeding; avoid concurrent use. ↑ risk of bleeding with other **anticoagulants**, **aspirin**, **clopidogrel**, **ticagrelor**, **prasugrel**, **fibrinolytics**, **NSAIDs**, **SNRIs**, or **SSRIs**.
Drug-Natural Products: **St. John's wort** may ↓ levels and effectiveness; avoid concurrent use.

Route/Dosage

Prevention of Deep Vein Thrombosis Following Knee or Hip Replacement Surgery

PO (Adults): 10 mg once daily, initiated 6–10 hr postoperatively (when hemostasis is achieved) and continued for 35 days after hip replacement or 12 days after knee replacement.

Prevention of Venous Thromboembolism in Acutely Ill Medical Patients at Risk for Thromboembolic Complications Not at High Risk of Bleeding

PO (Adults): 10 mg once daily while in the hospital and after hospital discharge for a total of 31–39 days.

Treatment of Deep Vein Thrombosis or Pulmonary Embolism

PO (Adults): 15 mg twice daily with food for 21 days, then 20 mg once daily with food for remainder of treatment period.

R

Reduction in Risk of Recurrent Deep Vein Thrombosis and/or Pulmonary Embolism in Patients at Continued Risk for Recurrent Deep Vein Thrombosis and/or Pulmonary Embolism

PO (Adults): 10 mg once daily to be initiated after ≥6 mo of standard anticoagulant treatment.

Reduction in Risk of Stroke/Systemic Embolism in Nonvalvular Atrial Fibrillation

PO (Adults): 20 mg once daily with evening meal.

Renal Impairment

PO (Adults): *CCr ≤50 mL/min:* 15 mg once daily with evening meal.

Reduction in Risk of Major Cardiovascular Events in Patients With Chronic Coronary Artery Disease or Reduction in Risk of Major Thrombotic Vascular Events in Peripheral Arterial Disease, Including Patients After Lower Extremity Revascularization Due to Symptomatic Peripheral Arterial Disease

PO (Adults): 2.5 mg twice daily.

Treatment of Venous Thromboembolism and Reduction in Risk of Recurrent Venous Thromboembolism in Pediatric Patients

PO (Children ≥50 kg): *Oral suspension or tablets:* 20 mg once daily with food to be initiated after ≥5 days of initial parenteral anticoagulation therapy. Continue therapy for ≥3 mo (unless <2 yr with catheter-related thrombosis).

PO (Children 30–49.9 kg): *Oral suspension or tablets:* 15 mg once daily with food to be initiated after ≥5 days of initial parenteral anticoagulation therapy. Continue therapy for ≥3 mo (unless <2 yr with catheter-related thrombosis).

PO (Children 12–29.9 kg): *Oral suspension:* 5 mg twice daily with feeding or food to be initiated after ≥5 days of initial parenteral anticoagulation therapy. Continue therapy for ≥3 mo (unless <2 yr with catheter-related thrombosis).

PO (Children 10–11.9 kg): *Oral suspension:* 3 mg three times daily with feeding or food to be initiated after ≥5 days of initial parenteral anticoagulation therapy. Continue therapy for ≥3 mo (unless <2 yr with catheter-related thrombosis).

PO (Children 9–9.9 kg): *Oral suspension:* 2.8 mg three times daily with feeding or food to be initiated after ≥5 days of initial parenteral anticoagulation therapy. Continue therapy for ≥3 mo (unless <2 yr with catheter-related thrombosis).

PO (Children 8–8.9 kg): *Oral suspension:* 2.4 mg three times daily with feeding or food to be initiated after ≥5 days of initial parenteral anticoagulation therapy. Continue therapy for ≥3 mo (up to 12 mo) unless <2 yr with catheter-related VTE in which duration should be 1 mo (up to 3 mo).

PO (Children 7–7.9 kg): *Oral suspension:* 1.8 mg three times daily with feeding or food to be initiated after ≥5 days of initial parenteral anticoagulation therapy. Continue therapy for ≥3 mo (up to 12 mo) unless <2 yr with catheter-related VTE in which duration should be 1 mo (up to 3 mo).

PO (Children 5–6.9 kg): *Oral suspension:* 1.6 mg three times daily with feeding or food to be initiated after ≥5 days of initial parenteral anticoagulation therapy. Continue therapy for ≥3 mo (up to 12 mo) unless <2 yr with catheter-related VTE in which duration should be 1 mo (up to 3 mo).

PO (Children 4–4.9 kg): *Oral suspension:* 1.4 mg three times daily with feeding or food to be initiated after ≥5 days of initial parenteral anticoagulation therapy. Continue therapy for ≥3 mo (up to 12 mo) unless <2 yr with catheter-related VTE in which duration should be 1 mo (up to 3 mo).

PO (Children 3–3.9 kg): *Oral suspension:* 0.9 mg three times daily with feeding or food to be initiated after ≥5 days of initial parenteral anticoagulation therapy. Continue therapy for ≥3 mo (up to 12 mo) unless <2 yr with catheter-related VTE in which duration should be 1 mo (up to 3 mo).

PO (Children 2.6–2.9 kg): *Oral suspension:* 0.8 mg three times daily with feeding or food to be initiated after ≥5 days of initial parenteral anticoagulation therapy. Continue therapy for ≥3 mo (up to 12 mo) unless <2 yr with catheter-related VTE in which duration should be 1 mo (up to 3 mo).

Thromboprophylaxis in Pediatric Patients With Congenital Heart Disease After Fontan Procedure

PO (Children ≥2 yr and ≥50 kg): *Oral suspension or tablets:* 10 mg once daily.

PO (Children ≥2 yr and 30–49.9 kg): *Oral suspension:* 7.5 mg once daily.

PO (Children ≥2 yr and 20–29.9 kg): *Oral suspension:* 2.5 mg twice daily.

PO (Children ≥2 yr and 12–19.9 kg): *Oral suspension:* 2 mg twice daily.

PO (Children ≥2 yr and 10–11.9 kg): *Oral suspension:* 1.7 mg twice daily.

PO (Children ≥2 yr and 8–9.9 kg): *Oral suspension:* 1.6 mg twice daily.

PO (Children ≥2 yr and 7–7.9 kg): *Oral suspension:* 1.1 mg twice daily.

Availability (generic available)

Tablets: 2.5 mg, 10 mg, 15 mg, 20 mg. **Oral suspension:** 1 mg/mL.

NURSING IMPLICATIONS

Assessment

- Monitor for bleeding (bleeding gums; nosebleed; unusual bruising; black, tarry stools; hematuria; fall in hematocrit or BP; guaiac-positive stools; bleeding from surgical site). Discontinue rivaroxaban if active bleeding occurs. Anticoagulant effects of rivaroxaban persist for about 24 hr after last dose. Anticoagulant effects cannot be reliably monitored with standard laboratory tests.
- Calculate a HAS-BLED score (hypertension, abnormal renal and liver function, stroke, bleeding, labile INRs, elderly, and drugs or alcohol) in high-risk patients at every follow-up to assess the risk of major bleeding during therapy.
- Monitor frequently for signs/symptoms of neurological impairment (numbness or weakness of legs, bowel or bladder dysfunction, back pain, tingling, muscle weakness); if noted, urgent treatment is required. Intrathecal or epidural catheter should not be removed earlier than 18 hr in young patients aged 20–45 yr and 26 hr in older adults aged 60–76 yr after last administration of rivaroxaban; next dose should be ≥ 6 hr after catheter removal.

Lab Test Considerations

- Assess renal function before starting therapy and periodically during treatment; frequency of monitoring depends on individual patient factors, including baseline renal function, concurrent drug therapy, comorbidities, and age. Monitor at least every 6 mo (every 3–6 mo in patients with renal impairment [CCr < 60 mL/min]) or during an acute illness that may worsen renal function.
- Monitor liver function at baseline and then yearly in healthy patients (every 3–6 mo in patients at risk of hepatic impairment or at-risk older adult patients [≥75 yr]). May ↑ AST, ALT, total bilirubin, and GGT.
- Assess CBC during initiation and at regular intervals (at least yearly) to assess trends in hemoglobin/hematocrit; assess more frequently if needed, especially in patients with active bleeding symptoms.

Toxicity and Overdose

- Antidote is andexanet alfa. May also consider prothrombin complex concentrate (PCC) or other procoagulant reversal agents such as activated prothrombin complex concentrate or recombinant factor VIIa for life-threatening bleeding. If PCC is used, monitoring anticoagulant effect of rivaroxaban using clotting test (PT, INR, or aPTT) or anti-FXa activity is not useful. Hemodialysis does not significantly contribute to rivaroxaban clearance. Protamine sulfate, vitamin K, and tranexamic acid do not reverse anticoagulant activity.

Implementation

- *When switching from warfarin to rivaroxaban,* discontinue warfarin and start rivaroxaban as soon as INR <3.0 in adults and <2.5 in pediatric patients to avoid periods of inadequate anticoagulation. *When switching from anticoagulants other than warfarin to rivaroxaban,* for adult or pediatric patients, start rivaroxaban 0–2 hr prior to next scheduled evening dose and omit dose of other anticoagulant. For continuous heparin, discontinue heparin and administer rivaroxaban at same time. *When switching from rivaroxaban to other anticoagulants with rapid onset,* for adult and pediatric patients currently taking rivaroxaban and transitioning to an anticoagulant with rapid onset, discontinue rivaroxaban and give 1st dose of the other anticoagulant (oral or parenteral) at the time that the next rivaroxaban dose was due. May discontinue rivaroxaban and begin both parenteral anticoagulant at time of next rivaroxaban dose. *When switching from rivaroxaban to warfarin,* overlap rivaroxaban with warfarin and measure INR just before next rivaroxaban dose; discontinue rivaroxaban when INR ≥2. Once rivaroxaban is discontinued, INR testing may be done reliably 24 hr after last dose.
- Discontinue ≥24 hr prior to surgery and other interventions. Restart as soon as hemostasis has been re-established.
- If rivaroxaban must be discontinued for reasons other than bleeding, consider replacing with another anticoagulant; discontinuation ↑ risk of thrombotic events.
- To ensure a therapeutic dose is maintained, monitor child's weight and review dose regularly, especially for children <12 kg.
- **PO:** *Prophylaxis of DVT following surgery:* Administer 1st dose 6–10 hr after surgery, once hemostasis has been established. To ↑ absorption, all doses should be taken with feeding or food. Do not break or split tablets.
- If unable to swallow tablet, 15 mg and 20 mg tablets may be crushed, mixed with applesauce, and administered immediately after mixing. Follow dose immediately with food.
- If administering crushed tablet via nasogastric or gastric feeding tube, check placement of tube. Rivaroxaban is absorbed from the stomach, not the small intestine. Suspend crushed tablet in 50 mL water and administer. Follow administration of 15-mg or 20-mg tablet immediately with food.
- Crushed tablets are stable in water or applesauce for up to 4 hr.

R

- Oral suspension may be given through nasogastric or gastric feeding tube. After administration, flush feeding tube with water.
- *Reduction in Risk of Stroke in Nonvalvular AF:* Administer with evening meal.
- *Treatment of DVT and/or PE:* Administer with food, at the same time each day.
- *Reduction in the Risk of Recurrence of DVT and/or PE in Patients at Continued Risk for DVT and/or PE, Prophylaxis of VTE in Acutely Ill Medical Patients at Risk for Thromboembolic Complications Not at High Risk of Bleeding, or Reduction of Risk of Major Cardiovascular Events (Cardiovascular Death, MI, and Stroke) in Chronic Coronary Artery Disease or PAD:* Administer without regard for food.

Patient/Family Teaching

- Explain purpose and side effects of rivaroxaban. Instruct patient to take as directed. *Adults:* Take missed doses as soon as remembered that day. If taking 2.5 mg twice daily, take a single 2.5 mg dose at next scheduled dose. If taking 15 mg twice daily, may take two 15-mg tablets to achieve 30 mg daily dose; then return to regular schedule. If taking 10 mg, 15 mg, or 20 mg once daily, take missed dose immediately; do not double dose. *Pediatric Patients:* If taking once a day, take missed dose as soon as possible once noticed, but only on the same day. If not possible, skip dose and continue with next dose as prescribed; do not take two doses to make up for a missed dose. If rivaroxaban is taken two times a day, take missed morning dose as soon as possible once it is noticed; a missed morning dose may be taken together with the evening dose. A missed evening dose can only be taken in the same evening. If rivaroxaban is taken three times a day, if a dose is missed, patient should skip missed dose and go back to the regular dosing schedule at the usual time without compensating for missed dose. If patient vomits or spits up dose within 30 min after receiving dose, give a new dose; if >30 min after dose is taken, do not readminister dose; take next dose as scheduled. If patient vomits or spits up dose repeatedly, contact child's doctor right away. Inform health care provider of missed doses at time of checkup or lab tests. Inform patients that anticoagulant effect may persist for 2–5 days following discontinuation. Advise patient to read the *Medication Guide* before starting therapy and with each Rx refill in case of changes.
- Caution patients not to discontinue medication early without consulting health care provider; may ↑ risk of stroke, DVT, or PE. If temporarily discontinued, restart as soon as possible.
- Inform patient having had neuraxial anesthesia or spinal puncture to watch for signs and symptoms of spinal or epidural hematoma (numbness or weakness of legs, bowel or bladder dysfunction). Notify health care provider immediately if symptoms occur.
- Advise patient to report any symptoms of unusual bleeding or bruising (bleeding gums; nosebleed; black, tarry stools; hematuria; excessive menstrual flow) and symptoms of spinal or epidural hematoma (tingling; numbness, especially in lower extremities; muscular weakness) to health care provider immediately.
- Instruct patient not to drink alcohol or take other Rx, OTC, or herbal products, especially those containing aspirin, NSAIDs, or St. John's wort, and not to start or stop any new medications during rivaroxaban therapy without advice of health care provider.
- Rep: Advise women of reproductive potential to notify health care provider if pregnancy is planned or suspected or if breastfeeding. Pregnant women are at ↑ risk of hemorrhage. Rivaroxaban should be used only if potential benefit justifies the potential risk to the mother and fetus. Monitor for bleeding in fetus and/or neonate of women taking rivaroxaban during pregnancy.

Evaluation/Desired Outcomes

- Prevention of blood clots and subsequent PE following knee/hip replacement surgery.
- Treatment of deep vein thrombosis DVT and pulmonary embolism PE.
- Treatment and prevention of thromboembolic events and major cardiovascular events.

rivastigmine (rye-va-stig-meen)

Exelon

Classification

Therapeutic: anti-Alzheimer's agents

Pharmacologic: cholinergics (cholinesterase inhibitors)

Indications

PO: Treatment of the following conditions: Mild to moderate dementia associated with Alzheimer disease. Mild to moderate dementia associated with Parkinson disease. **Transdermal:** Treatment of the following conditions: Mild, moderate, or severe dementia associated with Alzheimer disease. Mild to moderate dementia associated with Parkinson disease.

Action

Enhances cholinergic function by reversible inhibition of cholinesterase. **Therapeutic Effects:** Decreased dementia (temporary) associated with Alzheimer disease and Parkinson disease. Enhanced cognitive ability.

Pharmacokinetics

Absorption: Well absorbed following oral administration. Transdermal patch is slowly absorbed over 8 hr.
Distribution: Widely distributed to tissues.
Metabolism and Excretion: Rapidly and extensively metabolized by the liver; metabolites are excreted by the kidneys.
Half-life: *PO:* 1.5 hr; *Transdermal:* 24 hr.

TIME/ACTION PROFILE (improvement in dementia)

ROUTE	ONSET	PEAK	DURATION
PO	within 2 wk	up to 12 wk	unknown
Transdermal	unknown	unknown	unknown

Contraindications/Precautions

Contraindicated in: Hypersensitivity to rivastigmine or other carbamates; History of application site reactions with transdermal product suggestive of allergic contact dermatitis.
Use Cautiously in: History of asthma or obstructive pulmonary disease; History of GI bleeding; Sick sinus syndrome or other supraventricular cardiac conduction abnormalities; Moderate or severe renal impairment (dose ↓ may be needed); Mild or moderate hepatic impairment (dose ↓ may be needed); Patients weighing <50 kg (dose ↓ may be needed); OB: Safety not established in pregnancy; Lactation: Use during breastfeeding only if potential maternal benefit justifies potential risk to infant; Pedi: Safety and effectiveness not established in children.

Adverse Reactions/Side Effects

CV: edema, HF, hypotension. **Derm:** allergic dermatitis. **GI:** anorexia, diarrhea, nausea, vomiting, ↓ weight, abdominal pain, dyspepsia, flatulence. **Local:** application reactions (transdermal patch). **Neuro:** weakness, dizziness, drowsiness, headache, tremor. **Misc:** fever.

Interactions

Drug-Drug: Nicotine may ↓ levels and effectiveness.

Route/Dosage

PO (Adults): 1.5 mg twice daily initially; after ≥2 wk, may ↑ to 3 mg twice daily. Further increments may be made at 2-wk intervals up to 6 mg twice daily.
Transdermal (Adults): *Initial Dose:* 4.6 mg/24-hr transdermal patch initially; ↑ to 9.5 mg/24-hr transdermal patch after ≥4 wk; may ↑ to 13.3 mg/24-hr transdermal patch if needed (is recommended effective dose for patients with severe Alzheimer disease).

Hepatic Impairment

Transdermal (Adults): *Mild to moderate hepatic impairment:* Do not exceed dose of 4.6 mg/24 hr.

Availability (generic available)

Capsules: 1.5 mg, 3 mg, 4.5 mg, 6 mg. **Transdermal patch:** 4.6 mg/24 hr, 9.5 mg/24 hr, 13.3 mg/24 hr.

NURSING IMPLICATIONS

Assessment

- Assess cognitive function (memory, attention, reasoning, language, ability to perform simple tasks) periodically throughout therapy.
- Monitor for nausea, vomiting, anorexia, and weight loss.
- Monitor for hypersensitivity skin reactions; may occur after oral or transdermal administration. *If allergic contact dermatitis is suspected after transdermal use,* may switch to oral rivastigmine after negative allergy testing. *If disseminated hypersensitivity reaction of the skin occurs,* discontinue rivastigmine.

Implementation

- Patients switching from oral doses of <6 mg to transdermal doses should use 4.6 mg/24-hr patch. Patients taking oral doses of 6–12 mg may be converted directly to 9.5 mg/24-hr patch. Apply patch on the day following the last oral dose.
- **PO:** Administer in the morning and evening with food.
- **Transdermal:** Apply patch to clean, dry, hairless area that will not be rubbed by tight clothing. Upper or lower back is recommended; may also use upper arm or chest. Do not apply to red, irritated, or cut skin. Rotate sites to prevent irritation; do not use same site within 14 days. Remove adhesive liner and apply by pressing patch firmly until edges stick well. May be worn during bathing and hot weather. Every 24 hr, remove old patch and discard by folding in half and apply new patch to a new area.

R

Patient/Family Teaching

- **PO:** Explain the purpose and side effects of rivastigmine. Emphasize the importance of taking at regular intervals as directed. If a dose is missed for several days in a row, advise patient to contact health care provider, as drug may need to be restarted at a lower dose. Advise patient to read *Patient Information* before starting and with each Rx refill in case of changes.
- **Transdermal:** Instruct patient and caregiver on the correct application, rotation, and discarding of patch. Patch should be folded in half and discarded out of reach of children and pets; medication remains in discarded patch. Replace missed doses immediately and apply next patch at usual time. Advise patient and caregiver to avoid contact with eyes and to wash hands after applying patch. Avoid exposure to heat

sources (excessive sunlight, saunas, heating pads) for long periods.
- Advise patient and caregiver to notify health care provider if skin reactions occur.
- Advise patient referred for MRI test to discuss patch with referring health care provider and MRI facility to determine if removal of patch is necessary prior to test and for directions for replacing patch.
- Caution patient and caregiver that rivastigmine may cause dizziness. Caution patient to avoid driving or other activities requiring alertness until response to medication is known.
- Advise patient and caregiver to notify health care provider if nausea, vomiting, anorexia, or weight loss occur. If adverse effects become intolerable during treatment with *transdermal patch,* instruct patient to discontinue patches for several days and then restart at same or next lower dose level. If treatment is interrupted for more than several days, lowest dose level should be used when restarting and titrate according to Route and Dosage section.
- Advise patient and caregiver to notify health care provider of medication regimen prior to treatment or surgery.
- Inform patient and caregiver that improvement in cognitive functioning may take weeks to months and that the degenerative process is not reversed.
- Advise patient to notify health care provider of all Rx or OTC medications, vitamins, or herbal products being taken and to consult with health care provider before taking other medications.
- Rep: Advise women of reproductive potential to notify health care provider if pregnancy is planned or suspected or if breastfeeding.

Evaluation/Desired Outcomes
- Temporary improvement in cognitive function (memory, attention, reasoning, language, ability to perform simple tasks) in patients with Alzheimer disease.
- Improvement in cognitive function and overall functioning in patients with Parkinson disease.

rizatriptan (riz-a-**trip**-tan)
Maxalt, Maxalt-MLT

Classification
Therapeutic: vascular headache suppressants
Pharmacologic: 5-HT_1 agonists

Indications
Acute treatment of migraine with or without aura.

Action
Acts as an agonist at specific 5-HT_1 receptor sites in intracranial blood vessels and sensory trigeminal nerves. **Therapeutic Effects:** Cranial vessel vasoconstriction with associated decrease in release of neuropeptides and resultant decrease in migraine headache.

Pharmacokinetics
Absorption: Completely absorbed after oral administration, but first-pass metabolism results in 45% bioavailability.
Distribution: Unknown.
Metabolism and Excretion: Primarily metabolized by monoamine oxidase-A (MAO-A); minor conversion to an active compound; 14% excreted unchanged in urine.
Half-life: 2–3 hr.

TIME/ACTION PROFILE (plasma concentrations)

ROUTE	ONSET	PEAK	DURATION
PO	30 min	1–1.5 hr	unknown

Contraindications/Precautions
Contraindicated in: Hypersensitivity; Ischemic or vasospastic cardiovascular, cerebrovascular, or peripheral vascular syndromes; History of significant cardiovascular disease; Uncontrolled hypertension; Should not be used within 24 hr of other 5-HT_1 agonists or ergot-type compounds (dihydroergotamine); Basilar or hemiplegic migraine; Concurrent MAO-A inhibitor therapy or within 2 wk of discontinuing MAO-A inhibitor therapy; Phenylketonuria (orally disintegrating tablet contains aspartame).
Use Cautiously in: Severe renal impairment, especially in patients on dialysis; Moderate hepatic impairment; OB: Safety not established in pregnancy; Lactation: Safety not established in breastfeeding; Pedi: Safety and effectiveness not established in children <12 yr (oral films) or <6 yr (tablets and orally disintegrating tablets).
Exercise Extreme Caution in: Cardiovascular risk factors (hypertension, hypercholesterolemia, cigarette smoking, obesity, diabetes, strong family history, menopausal women or men >40 yr); use only if cardiovascular status has been evaluated and determined to be safe and 1st dose is administered under supervision.

Adverse Reactions/Side Effects
CV: chest pain, CORONARY ARTERY VASOSPASM, MI, myocardial ischemia, VENTRICULAR ARRHYTHMIAS. **Derm:** TOXIC EPIDERMAL NECROLYSIS. **GI:** dry mouth, nausea. **Neuro:** dizziness, drowsiness, weakness. **Misc:** HYPERSENSITIVITY REACTIONS (INCLUDING ANGIOEDEMA).

Interactions
Drug-Drug: Concurrent use with **MAO-A inhibitors** ↑ levels and adverse reactions (concurrent use or use within 2 wk of MAO inhibitor is contraindicated). Concurrent use with other **5-HT agonists** or

ergot-type compounds (dihydroergotamine) may result in ↑ vasoactive properties; avoid use within 24 hr of each other. **Propranolol** ↑ levels and risk of adverse reactions; ↓ dose of rizatriptan; rizatriptan not recommended in children <40 kg. ↑ risk of serotonin syndrome when used with **SSRIs** or **SNRIs**.
Drug-Natural Products: ↑ risk of serotonergic side effects including serotonin syndrome with **St. John's wort** and **SAMe**.

Route/Dosage

PO (Adults): 5–10 mg (use 5-mg dose in patients receiving propranolol); may be repeated in 2 hr; not to exceed 3 doses/24 hr.
PO (Children 6–17 yr and ≥40 kg): 10-mg single dose (use 5-mg dose in patients receiving propranolol).
PO (Children 6–17 yr and <40 kg): 5 mg single dose (do NOT use in patients receiving propranolol).

Availability (generic available)

Tablets: 5 mg, 10 mg. **Orally disintegrating tablets (Maxalt-MLT)(peppermint flavor):** 5 mg, 10 mg.

NURSING IMPLICATIONS

Assessment

- Assess pain location, character, intensity, and duration and associated symptoms (photophobia, phonophobia, nausea, vomiting) during migraine attack.
- Assess for serotonin syndrome (mental changes [agitation, hallucinations, coma], autonomic instability [tachycardia, labile BP, hyperthermia], neuromuscular aberrations [hyper-reflexia, incoordination], or GI symptoms [nausea, vomiting, diarrhea]), especially in patients taking other serotonergic drugs (SSRIs, SNRIs).
- Assess cardiovascular status in triptan-naive patients with multiple cardiovascular risk factors (↑ age, diabetes, hypertension, smoking, obesity, strong family history of coronary artery disease) before receiving rizatriptan. For patients with multiple cardiovascular risk factors who have a negative cardiovascular evaluation, consider administering the 1st dose of rizatriptan in a medically supervised setting and performing an ECG immediately following administration. Periodic cardiovascular evaluation in intermittent long-term users of rizatriptan may be used.

Implementation

- If migraine headache returns, a 2nd dose may be administered 2 hr after first dose. Maximum daily dose should not exceed 30 mg in any 24-hr period.
- **PO:** ***DNC:*** Tablets should be swallowed whole with liquid.
- Orally disintegrating tablets should be left in the package until use. Remove from the blister pouch. Do not push tablet through the blister; peel open the blister pack with dry hands and place tablet on tongue. Tablet will dissolve rapidly and be swallowed with saliva. No liquid is needed to take the orally disintegrating tablet.

Patient/Family Teaching

- Explain purpose and side effects of medication to patient. Advise patient to read *Patient Information* before starting therapy. Inform patient that rizatriptan should be used only during a migraine attack. It is meant to be used for relief of migraine attacks but not to prevent or reduce the number of attacks.
- Advise patient to notify health care professional of all Rx or OTC medications, vitamins, or herbal products being taken and to consult with health care professional before taking other medications.
- Instruct patient to administer rizatriptan as soon as symptoms of a migraine attack appear, but it may be administered at any time during an attack. If migraine symptoms return, a 2nd dose may be used. Allow ≥2 hr between doses, and do not use >30 mg in any 24-hr period.
- If patient has no response to 1st dose of rizatriptan, reconsider diagnosis of migraine before rizatriptan is administered to treat any subsequent attacks.
- Caution patient not to take rizatriptan within 24 hr of other vascular headache suppressants.
- Advise patient that lying down in a darkened room after rizatriptan administration may further help relieve headache.
- Advise patient that overuse (use >10 days/mo) may lead to exacerbation of headache (migraine-like daily headaches, or as a marked ↑ in frequency of migraine attacks). May require gradual withdrawal of rizatriptan and treatment of symptoms (transient worsening of headache).
- Advise patient to notify health care professional before next dose of rizatriptan if pain or tightness in the chest occurs during use. If pain is severe or does not subside, notify health care professional immediately. If feelings of tingling, heat, flushing, heaviness, pressure, drowsiness, dizziness, tiredness, or sickness develop, discuss with health care professional at next visit.
- May cause dizziness or drowsiness. Caution patient to avoid driving or other activities requiring alertness until response to medication is known.
- Caution patient to avoid alcohol, which aggravates headaches, during rizatriptan use.
- Advise patient to notify health care professional immediately if signs or symptoms of serotonin syndrome occur.

R

- Rep: Advise women of reproductive potential to notify health care professional if pregnancy is planned or suspected or if breastfeeding.

Evaluation/Desired Outcomes

- Decrease in migraine headache.

romosozumab

(**roe**-moe-**soz**-ue-mab)

Evenity

Classification

Therapeutic: bone resorption inhibitors

Pharmacologic: sclerostin inhibitors

Indications

Treatment of osteoporosis in postmenopausal women who are at high risk for a fracture or have failed or are intolerant to other medications used to treat osteoporosis.

Action

Inhibits sclerostin, which leads to increased bone formation and decreased bone resorption. **Therapeutic Effects:** Reduction in vertebral and nonvertebral fractures and improvement in bone mineral density.

Pharmacokinetics

Absorption: Unknown.

Distribution: Minimally distributed to tissues.

Metabolism and Excretion: Degraded into small peptides and amino acids; elimination pathway unknown.

Half-life: 12.8 days.

TIME/ACTION PROFILE (plasma concentrations)

ROUTE	ONSET	PEAK	DURATION
SUBQ	unknown	5 days	4 wk

Contraindications/Precautions

Contraindicated in: Hypersensitivity; Hypocalcemia (correct before administration); MI or stroke in past year (↑ risk of cardiovascular death, MI, or stroke).

Use Cautiously in: Risk factors for cardiovascular disease; Severe renal impairment or receiving dialysis (monitor serum calcium concentrations and calcium and vitamin D intake); Invasive dental procedures; cancer; receiving chemotherapy, corticosteroids, or angiogenesis inhibitors; poor oral hygiene; diabetes; gingival infections; periodontal disease; dental disease; anemia; coagulopathy; infection; or poorly fitting dentures (↑ risk of jaw osteonecrosis); Geri: Older adults may be more sensitive to drug effects.

Adverse Reactions/Side Effects

CV: CARDIOVASCULAR DEATH, MI, peripheral edema. **F and E:** hypocalcemia. **Local:** injection site reactions. **MS:** arthralgia, atypical femoral fracture, muscle spasm, osteonecrosis of the jaw. **Neuro:** headache, insomnia, paresthesia, STROKE. **Misc:** HYPERSENSITIVITY REACTIONS (INCLUDING ANAPHYLAXIS AND ANGIOEDEMA).

Interactions

Drug-Drug: None reported.

Route/Dosage

SUBQ (Adults): 210 mg once monthly for 12 mo.

Availability

Solution for injection (prefilled syringes): 105 mg/1.17 mL.

NURSING IMPLICATIONS

Assessment

- Assess bone density before and periodically during therapy.
- Monitor for new or unusual thigh, hip, or groin pain, which may indicate an incomplete femur fracture.
- Assess cardiac history. Avoid administration in patients who have had an MI or stroke within the preceding year. Monitor patients for signs and symptoms of emerging cardiovascular disease such as MI (chest pain, dyspnea, diaphoresis, dizziness, nausea) and stroke (unilateral weakness, slurred speech, confusion, dizziness). *If MI or stroke occurs, permanently discontinue romosozumab.*
- Monitor for signs/symptoms of hypocalcemia (muscle spasms, twitches, or cramps; peripheral or circumoral paresthesia) periodically during therapy. Correct hypocalcemia before initiating therapy.
- Perform a routine oral exam prior to initiation of therapy. Dental exam with appropriate preventative dentistry should be considered prior to therapy. Patients with history of tooth extraction, poor oral hygiene, gingival infections, diabetes, cancer, receiving radiation, anemia, coagulopathy, or use of a dental appliance or those taking immunosuppressive therapy, angiogenesis inhibitors, or systemic corticosteroids are at greater risk for osteonecrosis of the jaw.

Implementation

- Duration of therapy is limited to 1 yr due to ↓ effectiveness. If continued therapy is needed, continue therapy with an antiresorptive agent.
- Supplement patient with calcium and vitamin D during therapy.
- If a dose is missed, administer as soon as possible and reschedule monthly from date of last dose.
- **SUBQ:** Administer by a health care provider. Allow romosozumab to warm to room temperature for ≥30 min; do not warm in any other way. Solution is clear to opalescent, colorless to light yellow; do not administer solutions that are cloudy, discolored, or contain particulate matter. Do not shake. Dose requires two injections in separate sites: thigh,

abdomen, or outer area of upper arm. Do not inject into areas where the skin is tender, bruised, red, or hard. Avoid injecting into areas with scars or stretch marks. Refrigerate solution in original carton to protect from light; do not freeze. Stable for 30 days at room temperature.

Patient/Family Teaching

- Explain purpose and side effects of romosozumab to patient. Do not stop receiving drug without consulting health care provider. If an appointment is missed, contact health care provider as soon as possible to reschedule. Advise patient to read *Medication Guide* before starting and periodically during therapy in case of changes.
- Advise patients and family to call 911 and seek urgent treatment for signs and symptoms of hypersensitivity reactions (difficulty breathing; chest tightness; hives; rash; feeling light-headed; itching; swelling of the face, lips, tongue, or throat).
- Advise patients and family to call 911 and seek urgent treatment if signs and symptoms of MI or stroke (chest pain, dizziness, nausea, weakness, slurred speech, confusion, trouble breathing) occur.
- Advise patient to eat a balanced diet and consult health care provider about the need for supplemental calcium and vitamin D.
- Encourage patient to participate in regular exercise and to modify behaviors that ↑ risk of osteoporosis (stop smoking, ↓ alcohol consumption).
- Advise patient to notify health care provider if signs and symptoms if osteonecrosis of the jaw (pain, numbness, swelling of, or drainage from the jaw, mouth, or teeth); hypocalcemia (spasms, twitches, or cramps in muscles; numbness or tingling in fingers, toes, or around mouth); or thigh, hip, or groin pain occur.
- Advise parents to notify health care provider of all Rx or OTC medications, vitamins, or herbal products being taken and to consult with health care provider before taking other medications.
- Rep: Advise women of reproductive potential to notify health care provider if pregnancy is planned or suspected or if breastfeeding.

Evaluation/Desired Outcomes

- Reduction in vertebral and nonvertebral fractures and improvement in bone mineral density.

rOPINIRole (roe-pin-i-role)

~~Requip, Requip XL~~

Classification

Therapeutic: antiparkinson agents

Pharmacologic: dopamine agonists

Indications

Parkinson disease. Restless leg syndrome (immediate release only).

Action

Stimulates dopamine receptors in the brain. **Therapeutic Effects:** Decreased tremor and rigidity in Parkinson disease. Decreased leg restlessness.

Pharmacokinetics

Absorption: 55% absorbed following oral administration.

Distribution: Widely distributed to tissues.

Metabolism and Excretion: Extensively metabolized by the liver primarily by the CYP1A2 isoenzyme; <10% excreted unchanged in urine.

Half-life: 6 hr.

TIME/ACTION PROFILE

ROUTE	ONSET	PEAK	DURATION
PO	unknown	unknown	8 hr

Contraindications/Precautions

Contraindicated in: Hypersensitivity; Major psychotic disorder; Impulsive control/compulsive behaviors.

Use Cautiously in: Hepatic impairment (slower titration may be required); Severe cardiovascular disease; OB: Safety not established in pregnancy; Lactation: Use while breastfeeding only if potential maternal benefit justifies potential risk to infant; Pedi: Safety and effectiveness not established in children; Geri: ↑ risk of hallucinations in older adults.

Adverse Reactions/Side Effects

CV: <u>orthostatic hypotension</u>, hypertension, peripheral edema, syncope. **Derm:** sweating. **EENT:** abnormal vision. **GI:** constipation, dry mouth, dyspepsia, nausea, vomiting. **Neuro:** <u>dizziness</u>, <u>syncope</u>, aggression, agitation, confusion, delirium, delusions, disorientation, drowsiness, dyskinesia, fatigue, hallucinations, headache, impulse control disorders (gambling, sexual, uncontrolled spending, binge/compulsive eating), insomnia, paranoid ideation, psychosis, SLEEP ATTACKS, somnolence, weakness.

Interactions

Drug-Drug: CYP1A2 inhibitors, including **ciprofloxacin**, may ↑ levels and risk of toxicity. **CYP1A2 inducers**, including **cigarette smoke**, may ↓ levels and effectiveness. **Estrogens** may ↑ levels and risk of toxicity. **Phenothiazines, butyrophenones, thioxanthenes**, or **metoclopramide** may ↓ effectiveness. May ↑ effects of **levodopa**; consider ↓ dose of levodopa.

Route/Dosage

Parkinson Disease

PO (Adults): *Immediate release:* 0.25 mg 3 times daily for 1 wk, then 0.5 mg 3 times daily for 1 wk, then 0.75 mg 3 times daily for 1 wk, then 1 mg 3 times daily for 1 wk; then may ↑ by 1.5 mg/day every wk up to 9 mg/day; then may ↑ by up to 3 mg/day every wk up to 24 mg/day; *Extended release:* 2 mg once daily for 1–2 wk; may ↑ by 2 mg/day; do not exceed 8 mg/day in patients with advanced Parkinson disease or 12 mg/day in patients with early Parkinson disease.

Renal Impairment

PO (Adults): *Hemodialysis:* Immediate release: 0.25 mg 3 times daily; may ↑ dose as needed based on response and tolerability (not to exceed 18 mg/day).

Restless Leg Syndrome

PO (Adults): *Immediate release:* 0.25 mg once daily initially, 1–3 hr before bedtime. After 2 days, ↑ to 0.5 mg once daily and then to 1 mg once daily by the end of first wk of dosing; then ↑ by 0.5 mg weekly, up to 4 mg/day as needed/tolerated.

Renal Impairment

PO (Adults): *Hemodialysis:* Immediate release 0.25 mg once daily; may ↑ dose as needed based on response and tolerability (not to exceed 3 mg/day).

Availability (generic available)

Immediate-release tablets: 0.25 mg, 0.5 mg, 1 mg, 2 mg, 3 mg, 4 mg, 5 mg. **Extended-release tablets:** 2 mg, 4 mg, 6 mg, 8 mg, 12 mg.

NURSING IMPLICATIONS

Assessment

- Assess BP and HR periodically during therapy.
- Assess for drowsiness, sleep disorders, and concurrent use of sedating medications or alcohol. *If significant daytime sleepiness or falling asleep during activities that require active participation occurs,* ropinirole may be discontinued.
- Assess for signs/symptoms of psychosis (confusion, paranoid ideation, delusions, hallucinations, disorientation, aggression, agitation, delirium) and ask specifically about impulsive and compulsive behaviors (gambling, binges, ↑ sexual urges). *If psychosis or inability to control urges occurs,* consider ↓ dose or discontinue ropinirole.
- **Parkinson Disease:** Assess for signs/symptoms of Parkinson disease (tremor, muscle weakness and rigidity, ataxic gait) prior to and during therapy.
- **Restless Leg Syndrome:** Assess sleep patterns and frequency of restless leg events.
- Monitor for *augmentation* (earlier onset of symptoms in the evening or afternoon), ↑ in symptoms, spread of symptoms to other extremities, and *rebound* (new onset of symptoms in the early-morning hours). If signs/symptoms occur, consider dose adjustment or discontinuation of therapy.

Lab Test Considerations

- May ↑ BUN.

Implementation

- Do not confuse ropinirole with Risperdal or risperidone.
- **PO:** May be administered without regard to food. Administration with food may ↓ nausea. ***DNC:*** Swallow extended-release tablets whole; do not break, crush, or chew.
- Taper or discontinuation may cause withdrawal symptoms (apathy, anxiety, depression, fatigue, insomnia, sweating, pain); symptoms do not respond to levodopa. Trial readministration of ropinirole at lowest dose may be considered.

Patient/Family Teaching

- Explain purpose and side effects of medication. Advise patient to read *Patient Information* before starting therapy.
- Instruct patient to take missed doses as soon as possible; omit if almost time for next dose. Do not double doses or stop abruptly; may cause hyperpyrexia and confusion.
- Caution patient to change positions slowly to minimize symptoms of orthostatic hypotension and to notify health care provider if syncope related to bradycardia occurs. Older patients are at ↑ risk.
- Inform patient that ropinirole may cause falling asleep while engaged in activities of daily living, including the operation of motor vehicles, conversations, and eating. Notify health care provider if periods of daytime sleepiness occur.
- Advise patient to notify health care provider of all Rx or OTC medications, vitamins, or herbal products being taken and to consult health care provider before taking other medications, including alcohol and other CNS depressants.
- Advise patient that fluids, sugarless gum or candy, ice, or saliva substitutes may help minimize dry mouth. Consult health care provider if dry mouth continues for >2 wk.
- Advise patient to have periodic skin exams to check for lesions that may be melanoma.
- Advise patient to notify health care provider if new or ↑ gambling, sexual, or other impulse control disorders or psychotic-like behaviors occur.
- Rep: Advise women of reproductive potential to notify health care provider if pregnancy is planned or suspected or if breastfeeding. Advise patients that ropinirole could inhibit lactation.

Evaluation/Desired Outcomes

- Decreased tremor and rigidity in Parkinson disease.
- Decrease in restless legs and improved sleep.

rosuvastatin, See HMG-CoA REDUCTASE INHIBITORS (statins).

ruxolitinib (topical)

(rux-oh-li-ti-nib)

Opzelura

Classification

Therapeutic: none assigned

Pharmacologic: kinase inhibitors

Indications

Short-term and noncontinuous chronic treatment of mild to moderate atopic dermatitis in nonimmunocompromised patients whose disease is not adequately controlled with topical prescription therapies or when those therapies are not advisable. Nonsegmental vitiligo.

Action

Inhibits Janus kinase 1 and 2, which are normally involved in the signaling of hematopoiesis and immune processes. **Therapeutic Effects:** Decreased severity of atopic dermatitis. Reduction in depigmented areas in nonsegmental vitiligo.

Pharmacokinetics

Absorption: Systemic absorption occurs following topical administration and is dependent on dose and surface area of application.

Distribution: Unknown.

Protein Binding: 97%.

Metabolism and Excretion: Primarily metabolized in the liver via the CYP3A4 isoenzyme, with minor contribution from CYP2C9. Primarily excreted in the urine (74%), with 22% excreted in the feces. Less than 1% excreted as unchanged drug.

Half-life: 116 hr.

TIME/ACTION PROFILE (plasma concentrations)

ROUTE	ONSET	PEAK	DURATION
Topical	unknown	unknown	unknown

Contraindications/Precautions

Contraindicated in: Active, serious infection; Risk factor for thrombosis; Lactation: Lactation.

Use Cautiously in: Chronic or recurrent infection; History of a serious infection or opportunistic infection; Exposure to tuberculosis (TB); Resided or traveled in areas of endemic TB or endemic mycoses; >50 yr old with ≥1 cardiovascular risk factor (may ↑ risk of all-cause mortality, cardiovascular death, MI, stroke, and thrombosis); Known malignancy (other than a successfully treated nonmelanoma skin cancer or cervical cancer); Immunocompromised;OB: Other agents preferred for the topical treatment of atopic dermatitis and vitiligo in pregnancy; Pedi: Children <12 yr (safety and effectiveness not established).

Adverse Reactions/Side Effects

CV: ARTERIAL THROMBOSIS, CARDIOVASCULAR DEATH, DEEP VEIN THROMBOSIS. **Derm:** acne, erythema, folliculitis, NONMELANOMA SKIN CANCER, pruritus, urticaria. **EENT:** nasopharyngitis, rhinorrhea, tonsillitis. **GI:** diarrhea. **Hemat:** anemia, eosinophilia, neutropenia, thrombocytopenia. **Metab:** hyperlipidemia. **Neuro:** headache. **Resp:** PULMONARY EMBOLISM. **Misc:** fever, INFECTION (INCLUDING REACTIVATION TB AND OTHER OPPORTUNISTIC INFECTIONS DUE TO BACTERIAL, FUNGAL, VIRAL, AND MYCOBACTERIAL PATHOGENS), MALIGNANCY.

Interactions

Drug-Drug: Strong CYP3A4 inhibitors, including **ketoconazole**, may ↑ levels and risk of toxicity; avoid concurrent use.

Route/Dosage

Atopic Dermatitis

Topical: (Adults and Children ≥12 yr): Apply a thin layer twice daily to affected area(s) of up to 20% body surface area. Discontinue once signs/symptoms resolve. Reassess therapy if signs/symptoms have not resolved within 8 wk. Do not use more than one 60-g tube per wk or one 100-g tube per 2 wk.

Nonsegmental Vitiligo

Topical: (Adults and Children ≥12 yr): Apply a thin layer twice daily to affected area(s) of up to 10% body surface area. Reassess need for continued therapy if no meaningful improvement with repigmentation by 24 wk. Do not use more than one 60-g tube per wk or one 100-g tube per 2 wk.

Availability

Cream: 1.5%.

R

NURSING IMPLICATIONS

Assessment

- Assess area of skin affected before applying and periodically during therapy.
- Monitor signs and symptoms of infection during and after therapy. *If serious or opportunistic infection or sepsis occurs,* hold ruxolitinib; may resume when infection is controlled.
- Evaluate patients for latent and active TB infection before administration. Monitor for signs and symptoms of TB during therapy.
- Monitor for signs and symptoms of viral reactivation during therapy. *If herpes zoster occurs during therapy,* consider holding ruxolitinib until episode resolved.
- Assess for hepatitis B and C before starting therapy. Avoid therapy in patients with active hepatitis B or C.
- Perform periodic skin examination in ↑ risk patients of skin cancer.

Lab Test Considerations

- Monitor CBC periodically during therapy. May cause thrombocytopenia, anemia, and neutropenia. *If clinically significant cytopenias occur,* discontinue ruxolitinib. May ↑ total cholesterol, LDL-C, and triglycerides.

Implementation

- **Topical: Atopic dermatitis:** Apply a thin layer of ruxolitinib twice daily to affected areas of up to 20% body surface area. Stop using when signs/symptoms of atopic dermatitis (itch, rash, redness) resolve. If dermatitis does not improve within 8 wk, re-examine affected area.
- **Nonsegmental Vitiligo:** Apply a thin layer of ruxolitinib twice daily to affected areas of up to 10% body surface area; may require >24 wk. If no meaningful repigmentation occurs by 24 wk, re-evaluate affected area.

Patient/Family Teaching

- Explain purpose and side effects of medication. Advise patient to read *Patient Information* before starting therapy.
- Instruct patient to wash hands after applying, unless hands are being treated. Do not use in eyes, mouth, or vagina.
- Advise patient to notify health care provider if signs and symptoms of infections (fever; sweating; chills; muscle aches; cough or shortness of breath; blood in phlegm; weight loss; warm, red, or painful skin or sores on the body; diarrhea or stomach pain; burning on urination or urinating more often than usual; feeling very tired) occur.
- Advise patient to notify health care provider promptly if signs/symptoms of heart attack or stroke (pain or pressure in chest, throat, neck, jaw, stomach, arms, or back; shortness of breath; sweatiness; nausea; vomiting; dizziness; weakness in one part of body; slurred speech), blood clots (swelling, pain, or tenderness in one or both legs; sudden, unexplained chest or upper back pain; difficulty breathing; unusual bleeding, bruising, fever, or tiredness) occur.
- Inform patient that ruxolitinib may ↑ risk of cancer (lymphoma, lung cancer). Advise patient to have periodic skin examinations and to tell health care provider if they have ever had any type of cancer.
- Instruct patient to notify health care provider of all Rx or OTC medications, vitamins, or herbal products being taken and consult health care provider before taking any new medications during therapy.
- Rep: Advise women of reproductive potential to notify health care provider if pregnancy is planned or suspected and to avoid breastfeeding during therapy and for 4 wk after last dose. Encourage patients who are exposed to ruxolitinib during pregnancy to enroll in registry that monitors outcomes in pregnancy by calling 1-855-463-3463.

Evaluation/Desired Outcomes

- Decreased severity of atopic dermatitis.
- Reduction in depigmented areas in nonsegmental vitiligo.

sacubitril/valsartan

(sa-**ku**-bi-tril/val-**sar**-tan)

Entresto, Entresto Sprinkle

Classification

Therapeutic: vasodilators, heart failure agents

Pharmacologic: angiotensin II receptor antagonists, neprilysin inhibitors

Indications

Chronic HF in adults. Symptomatic HF in children ≥1 yr with systemic left ventricular systolic dysfunction.

Action

Sacubitril: A pro-drug converted to LBQ657, its active moiety. LBQ657 inhibits the enzyme neprilysin. Neprilysin degrades vasoactive peptides, including natriuretic peptides, bradykinin, and adrenomedullin, resulting in ↑ levels of these peptides, causing vasodilation and ↓ extracellular fluid volume via sodium excretion. *Valsartan:* Blocks vasoconstrictor and aldosterone-producing effects of angiotensin II at receptor sites, including vascular smooth muscle and the adrenal glands. **Therapeutic Effects:** Reduction in cardiovascular death and hospitalizations due to HF in adults. Reduction in NT-proBNP concentrations and improvement in cardiovascular outcomes in children.

Pharmacokinetics

Sacubitril

Absorption: ≥60% absorbed following oral administration.

Distribution: Widely distributed to tissues.

Protein Binding: 94–97%.

Metabolism and Excretion: Rapidly converted to LBQ657, its active form. LBQ657 is not significantly metabolized; 52–68% excreted in urine, primarily as LBQ657; 37–48% excreted in feces, primarily as LBQ657.

Half-life: *Sacubitril:* 1.4 hr. *LBQ657:* 11.5 hr.

Valsartan

Absorption: Absorption in combinations with sacubitril is more compared to oral administration of single-entity formulation.

Distribution: Widely distributed to tissues.

Protein Binding: 94–97%.

Metabolism and Excretion: Minimally metabolized by the liver; 13% excreted in urine; 86% in feces.

Half-life: 9.9 hr.

TIME/ACTION PROFILE (plasma concentrations)

ROUTE	ONSET	PEAK	DURATION
Sacubitril (PO)	unknown	0.5 hr	12 hr
Valsartan (PO)	unknown	1.5 hr	12 hr

Contraindications/Precautions

Contraindicated in: Hypersensitivity, hereditary angioedema, or history of angioedema from previous ACE inhibitors or ARBs; Concurrent use of ACE inhibitors during or for 36 hr before or after; Concurrent use with aliskiren in patients with diabetes or moderate to severe renal impairment (CCr <60 mL/min); Severe hepatic impairment; OB: Pregnancy; Lactation: Lactation.

Use Cautiously in: Volume- or salt-depleted patients or patients receiving high doses of diuretics (correct deficits before initiating therapy or initiate at lower doses); Black patients (may not be effective); Renal impairment due to primary renal disease or HF (may worsen renal function); Rep: Women of reproductive potential; Pedi: Children <1 yr (safety and effectiveness not established).

Adverse Reactions/Side Effects

CV: hypotension. **F and E:** hyperkalemia. **Neuro:** dizziness. **Resp:** cough. **Misc:** ANGIOEDEMA.

Interactions

Drug-Drug: NSAIDs and selective **COX-2 inhibitors** may ↑ the risk of renal impairment. ↑ risk of hypotension with other **antihypertensives** and **diuretics**. **Potassium-sparing diuretics**, **potassium-containing salt substitutes**, or **potassium supplements** may ↑ risk of hyperkalemia. ↑ risk of hyperkalemia, renal dysfunction, hypotension, and syncope with **ACE inhibitors** or **aliskiren**; avoid concurrent use with aliskiren in patients with diabetes or CCr <60 mL/min; avoid concurrent use with ACE inhibitors. May ↑ levels and risk of toxicity of **lithium**.

Route/Dosage

Tablets or Oral Suspension (suspension indicated where applicable)

PO (Adults): Sacubitril 49 mg/valsartan 51 mg twice daily initially; double dose in 2–4 wk to target dose of sacubitril 97 mg/valsartan 103 mg, as tolerated. *Patients not currently receiving ACE inhibitors or angiotensin II receptor blockers or receiving low doses of these agents:* Sacubitril 24 mg/valsartan 26 mg twice daily initially; double dose every 2–4 wk to target dose of sacubitril 97 mg/valsartan 103 mg, as tolerated.

PO (Children ≥1 yr and ≥50 kg): Sacubitril 49 mg/valsartan 51 mg twice daily initially; ↑ dose in 2 wk to sacubitril 72 mg/valsartan 78 mg twice daily, as tolerated; then ↑ dose again in 2 wk to target dose of sacubitril 97 mg/valsartan 103 mg twice daily, as tolerated. *Patients not currently receiving ACE inhibitors or angiotensin II receptor blockers or receiving low doses of these agents:* Sacubitril 24 mg/valsartan 26 mg twice daily initially; ↑ dose in 2 wk to sacubitril

S

49 mg/valsartan 51 mg twice daily, as tolerated; then ↑ dose again in 2 wk to sacubitril 72 mg/valsartan 78 mg twice daily, as tolerated; then ↑ dose again in 2 wk to target dose of sacubitril 97 mg/valsartan 103 mg twice daily, as tolerated.

PO (Children ≥1 yr and 40–<50 kg): Sacubitril 24 mg/valsartan 26 mg twice daily initially; ↑ dose in 2 wk to sacubitril 49 mg/valsartan 51 mg twice daily, as tolerated; then ↑ dose again in 2 wk to target dose of sacubitril 72 mg/valsartan 78 mg twice daily, as tolerated. *Patients not currently receiving ACE inhibitors or angiotensin II receptor blockers or receiving low doses of these agents:* 0.8 mg/kg (represents combined amount of sacubitril and valsartan) of oral suspension twice daily initially; ↑ dose in 2 wk to 1.6 mg/kg (represents combined amount of sacubitril and valsartan) of oral suspension twice daily, as tolerated; then ↑ dose in 2 wk to 2.3 mg/kg (represents combined amount of sacubitril and valsartan) of oral suspension twice daily, as tolerated; then ↑ dose again in 2 wk to target dose of 3.1 mg/kg (represents combined amount of sacubitril and valsartan) of oral suspension twice daily, as tolerated.

PO (Children ≥1 yr and <40 kg): 1.6 mg/kg (represents combined amount of sacubitril and valsartan) of oral suspension twice daily initially; then ↑ dose in 2 wk to 2.3 mg/kg (represents combined amount of sacubitril and valsartan) of oral suspension twice daily, as tolerated; then ↑ dose again in 2 wk to target dose of 3.1 mg/kg (represents combined amount of sacubitril and valsartan) of oral suspension twice daily, as tolerated. *Patients not currently receiving ACE inhibitors or angiotensin II receptor blockers or receiving low doses of these agents:* 0.8 mg/kg (represents combined amount of sacubitril and valsartan) of oral suspension twice daily initially; ↑ dose in 2 wk to 1.6 mg/kg (represents combined amount of sacubitril and valsartan) of oral suspension twice daily, as tolerated; then ↑ dose in 2 wk to 2.3 mg/kg (represents combined amount of sacubitril and valsartan) of oral suspension twice daily, as tolerated; then ↑ dose again in 2 wk to target dose of 3.1 mg/kg (represents combined amount of sacubitril and valsartan) of oral suspension twice daily, as tolerated.

Hepatic/Renal Impairment

PO (Adults): *Severe renal impairment (CCr <30 mL/min/1.73 m²) or moderate hepatic impairment:* Sacubitril 24 mg/valsartan 26 mg twice daily initially; double dose every 2–4 wk to target dose of sacubitril 97 mg/valsartan 103 mg, as tolerated.

Hepatic/Renal Impairment

PO (Children ≥1 yr and ≥50 kg): *Severe renal impairment (CCr <30 mL/min/1.73 m²) or moderate hepatic impairment:* Sacubitril 24 mg/valsartan 26 mg twice daily initially; ↑ dose in 2 wk to sacubitril 49 mg/valsartan 51 mg twice daily, as tolerated; then ↑ dose again in 2 wk to sacubitril 72 mg/valsartan 78 mg twice daily, as tolerated; then ↑ dose again in 2 wk to target dose of sacubitril 97 mg/valsartan 103 mg twice daily, as tolerated.

Hepatic/Renal Impairment

PO (Children ≥1 yr and 40–<50 kg): *Severe renal impairment (CCr <30 mL/min/1.73 m²) or moderate hepatic impairment:* 0.8 mg/kg (represents combined amount of sacubitril and valsartan) of oral suspension twice daily initially; ↑ dose in 2 wk to 1.6 mg/kg (represents combined amount of sacubitril and valsartan) of oral suspension twice daily, as tolerated; then ↑ dose in 2 wk to 2.3 mg/kg (represents combined amount of sacubitril and valsartan) of oral suspension twice daily, as tolerated; then ↑ dose again in 2 wk to target dose of 3.1 mg/kg (represents combined amount of sacubitril and valsartan) of oral suspension twice daily, as tolerated.

Hepatic/Renal Impairment

PO (Children ≥1 yr and <40 kg): *Severe renal impairment (CCr <30 mL/min/1.73 m²) or moderate hepatic impairment:* 0.8 mg/kg (represents combined amount of sacubitril and valsartan) of oral suspension twice daily initially; ↑ dose in 2 wk to 1.6 mg/kg (represents combined amount of sacubitril and valsartan) of oral suspension twice daily, as tolerated; then ↑ dose in 2 wk to 2.3 mg/kg (represents combined amount of sacubitril and valsartan) of oral suspension twice daily, as tolerated; then ↑ dose again in 2 wk to target dose of 3.1 mg/kg (represents combined amount of sacubitril and valsartan) of oral suspension twice daily, as tolerated.

Oral Pellets

PO (Children ≥1 yr and 34–<50 kg): Sacubitril 30 mg/valsartan 32 mg (using two sacubitril 15 mg/valsartan 16 mg capsules) twice daily initially; ↑ dose in 2 wk to sacubitril 45 mg/valsartan 48 mg (using three sacubitril 15 mg/valsartan 16 mg capsules) twice daily, as tolerated; then ↑ dose again in 2 wk to target dose of sacubitril 60 mg/valsartan 64 mg (using four sacubitril 15 mg/valsartan 16 mg capsules) twice daily, as tolerated. *Patients not currently receiving ACE inhibitors or angiotensin II receptor blockers or receiving low doses of these agents:* Use oral suspension (see above for dosing information).

PO (Children ≥1 yr and 26–<34 kg): Sacubitril 24 mg/valsartan 24 mg (using four sacubitril 6 mg/valsartan 6 mg capsules) twice daily initially; ↑ dose in 2 wk to sacubitril 30 mg/valsartan 32 mg (using two sacubitril 15 mg/valsartan 16 mg capsules) twice daily, as tolerated; then ↑ dose again in 2 wk to target dose of sacubitril 45 mg/valsartan 48 mg (using three sacubitril 15 mg/valsartan 16 mg capsules) twice daily, as

tolerated. *Patients not currently receiving ACE inhibitors or angiotensin II receptor blockers or receiving low doses of these agents:* Use oral suspension (see above for dosing information).
PO (Children ≥1 yr and 19–<26 kg): Sacubitril 18 mg/valsartan 18 mg (using three sacubitril 6 mg/valsartan 6 mg capsules) twice daily initially; ↑ dose in 2 wk to sacubitril 24 mg/valsartan 24 mg (using four sacubitril 6 mg/valsartan 6 mg capsules) twice daily, as tolerated; then ↑ dose again in 2 wk to target dose of sacubitril 30 mg/valsartan 32 mg (using two sacubitril 15 mg/valsartan 16 mg capsules) twice daily, as tolerated. *Patients not currently receiving ACE inhibitors or angiotensin II receptor blockers or receiving low doses of these agents:* Use oral suspension (see above for dosing information).
PO (Children ≥1 yr and 13–<19 kg): Sacubitril 12 mg/valsartan 12 mg (using two sacubitril 6 mg/valsartan 6 mg capsules) twice daily initially; ↑ dose in 2 wk to sacubitril 18 mg/valsartan 18 mg (using three sacubitril 6 mg/valsartan 6 mg capsules) twice daily, as tolerated; then ↑ dose again in 2 wk to target dose of sacubitril 24 mg/valsartan 24 mg (using four sacubitril 6 mg/valsartan 6 mg capsules) twice daily, as tolerated. *Patients not currently receiving ACE inhibitors or angiotensin II receptor blockers or receiving low doses of these agents:* Use oral suspension (see above for dosing information).
PO (Children ≥1 yr and <13 kg): Use oral suspension (see above for dosing information). *Patients not currently receiving ACE inhibitors or angiotensin II receptor blockers or receiving low doses of these agents:* Use oral suspension (see above for dosing information).

Availability (generic available)

Tablets: sacubitril 24 mg/valsartan 26 mg, sacubitril 49 mg/valsartan 51 mg, sacubitril 97 mg/valsartan 103 mg. **Oral pellets (sprinkle):** sacubitril 6 mg/valsartan 6 mg, sacubitril 15 mg/valsartan 16 mg.

NURSING IMPLICATIONS

Assessment

- Assess BP (lying, sitting, standing) and HR frequently during initial dose adjustment and periodically throughout therapy. Correct volume or salt depletion prior to administration of therapy. If hypotension occurs, consider ↓ dose of diuretics or concurrent antihypertensive agents. If hypotension persists, ↓ the dose or temporarily discontinue therapy. Permanent discontinuation of therapy is usually not required.
- Monitor daily weight and assess patient routinely for resolution of fluid overload (peripheral edema, rales/crackles, dyspnea, weight gain, jugular venous distention).
- Monitor for oliguria, progressive azotemia, and/or acute renal failure in patients with severe HF (renal function is dependent on the renin-angiotensin system).
- Assess patients for signs of angioedema (dyspnea, orofacial swelling); may occur more frequently in Black patients. If signs occur, discontinue therapy, provide supportive therapy, and monitor for airway compromise.

Lab Test Considerations

- Verify negative pregnancy test before starting therapy.
- Assess baseline hepatic function.
- Monitor renal function including BUN, serum creatinine, and eGFR. May ↑ BUN and serum creatinine. May require ↓ dose.
- May cause hyperkalemia. May require ↓ dose or temporary interruption of therapy.
- May ↓ hemoglobin and hematocrit.

Implementation

- **PO:** Administer twice daily without regard to food.
- If switching from an ACE inhibitor to sacubitril/valsartan, allow 36 hr between last ACE inhibitor dose and starting sacubitril/valsartan.
- *Entresto Sprinkle* can be substituted in patients unable to swallow tablets. Capsules should not be swallowed. ***DNC:*** Do not chew or crush the oral pellets. Open the capsule and sprinkle the contents onto 1–2 teaspoons of soft food. Consume food containing the oral pellets immediately after adding them. Empty capsule shells must be discarded after use. Use the entire contents of the capsules to achieve the dosage. Do not administer oral pellets via nasogastric, gastrostomy, or other enteral tubes because it may cause obstruction.

S

Patient/Family Teaching

- Explain the purpose and side effects of sacubitril/valsartan to patient. Instruct patient to take as directed, at the same time each day, even if feeling well. Take missed doses as soon as remembered if not almost time for next dose; do not double doses. Do not swallow *Entresto Sprinkle* capsules or crush the oral pellets. Open the capsule and sprinkle the entire contents onto 1–2 teaspoons of soft food. Consume food containing the oral pellets immediately after adding them. Empty capsule shells must be discarded after use. Warn patient not to discontinue therapy unless directed by health care provider. Advise patient to read *Patient Information* before starting therapy and with each Rx refill in case of changes.
- Emphasize the importance of follow-up exams to evaluate effectiveness of medication.
- Caution patient to avoid salt substitutes containing potassium or foods containing high levels of

potassium or sodium unless directed by health care provider. See Appendix J.

- Instruct patient to notify health care provider and immediately seek treatment if swelling of face, eyes, lips, or tongue or if difficulty swallowing or breathing occur.
- May cause dizziness. Caution patient to avoid driving or other activities requiring alertness until response to medication is known.
- Instruct patient to notify health care provider of all Rx or OTC medications, vitamins, or herbal products being taken and to avoid concurrent use of Rx, OTC, and herbal products, especially NSAIDs, potassium supplements, salt substitutes, ACE inhibitors, ARBs, lithium, or aliskiren, without consulting health care provider.
- Instruct patient to notify health care provider of medication regimen before treatment or surgery.
- Rep: May cause fetal harm. Advise women of reproductive potential to use contraception and avoid breastfeeding during therapy. Notify health care provider if pregnancy is planned or suspected. Sacubitril/valsartan should be discontinued as soon as possible when pregnancy is detected.

Evaluation/Desired Outcomes

- Decreased HF-related hospitalizations in adults with HF.
- Decreased NT-proBNP concentrations and improvement in cardiovascular outcomes in children with HF.

safinamide (sa-fin-a-mide)

✦ Onstryv, Xadago

Classification

Therapeutic: antiparkinson agents

Pharmacologic: monoamine oxidase type B inhibitors

Indications

Parkinson disease in patients who are experiencing "off" episodes (as adjunctive treatment to levodopa/carbidopa).

Action

Irreversibly inhibits monoamine oxidase B, which leads to ↑ dopamine levels in the CNS. **Therapeutic Effects:** Increased amount of "on" time without dyskinesia or with nontroublesome dyskinesia.

Pharmacokinetics

Absorption: 95% absorbed following oral administration.

Distribution: Extensively distributed to the tissues; readily crosses the blood-brain barrier.

Metabolism and Excretion: Extensively metabolized by hydrolytic oxidation or oxidative cleavage to inactive metabolites; 76% excreted in urine (primarily as inactive metabolites).

Half-life: 20–26 hr.

TIME/ACTION PROFILE (plasma concentrations)

ROUTE	ONSET	PEAK	DURATION
PO	unknown	2–3 hr	24 hr

Contraindications/Precautions

Contraindicated in: Hypersensitivity; Concurrent use of other MAO inhibitors; Concurrent use of opioids, SNRIs, TCAs, cyclobenzaprine, methylphenidate, amphetamine, or St. John's wort; Concurrent use of dextromethorphan; Severe hepatic impairment; Psychotic disorder; Lactation: Lactation.

Use Cautiously in: Retinal disease; Moderate hepatic impairment; OB: Use during pregnancy only if potential maternal benefit justifies potential fetal risk; Pedi: Safety and effectiveness not established in children.

Adverse Reactions/Side Effects

CV: hypertension, orthostatic hypotension. **EENT:** visual changes. **GI:** ↑ liver enzymes, nausea. **Neuro:** dyskinesia, ↑ fall risk, anxiety, drowsiness, hallucinations, impulse control disorders (gambling, sexual, binge eating), insomnia, paresthesia, psychosis, sleep attacks, sleep driving. **Resp:** cough. **Misc:** hypersensitivity reactions.

Interactions

Drug-Drug: **MAO inhibitors**, including **linezolid** and **isoniazid**, may ↑ risk of hypertensive crises; concurrent use contraindicated; separate administration by ≥14 days. **Meperidine**, **methadone**, **tramadol**, **SSRIs**, **SNRIs**, **TCAs**, **cyclobenzaprine**, **methylphenidate**, or **amphetamine** may ↑ risk of serotonin syndrome; concurrent use contraindicated; separate administration by ≥14 days; SSRIs may be used at the lowest dose possible. **Dextromethorphan** may result in psychosis/bizarre behavior; concurrent use contraindicated. Hypertensive crisis may occur with cough and cold products containing **sympathomimetic amines**, including **pseudoephedrine** and **phenylephrine**; monitor patient's BP closely. May ↑ levels and risk of toxicity of **imatinib**, **irinotecan**, **lapatinib**, **methotrexate**, **mitoxantrone**, **rosuvastatin**, **sulfasalazine**, and **topotecan**; monitor closely for adverse effects. **Dopamine antagonists**, including **antipsychotics** and **metoclopramide**, may ↓ effectiveness.

Drug-Natural Products: **St. John's wort** may ↑ risk of serotonin syndrome; concurrent use contraindicated.

Drug-Food: Ingestion of foods containing high amounts of **tyramine** (>150 mg) (e.g., cheese) may result in hypertensive crisis.

Route/Dosage

PO (Adults): 50 mg once daily; after 2 wk, may ↑ dose to 100 mg once daily.

Hepatic Impairment

PO (Adults): *Moderate hepatic impairment:* Do not exceed 50 mg/day; *Severe hepatic impairment:* Contraindicated.

Availability (generic available)

Tablets: 50 mg, 100 mg.

NURSING IMPLICATIONS

Assessment

- Assess signs/symptoms of Parkinson disease (tremor, muscle weakness and rigidity, ataxic gait) before starting and during therapy.
- Monitor for new-onset hypertension or hypertension not adequately controlled after starting safinamide. Sustained BP elevation may require dose ↓.
- Assess for serotonin syndrome (mental changes [agitation, hallucinations, coma], autonomic instability [tachycardia, labile BP, hyperthermia], neuromuscular aberrations [hyperreflexia, incoordination], and/or GI symptoms [nausea, vomiting, diarrhea]), especially in patients taking other serotonergic drugs (SSRIs, SNRIs, triptans).
- Assess for drowsiness, sleep disorders, and concurrent use of sedating medications or alcohol. *If significant daytime sleepiness or falling asleep during activities that require active participation occurs,* safinamide may be discontinued.
- Assess for signs/symptoms of psychosis (confusion, paranoid ideation, delusions, hallucinations, disorientation, aggression, agitation, delirium) and ask specifically about impulsive and compulsive behaviors (gambling, binges, ↑ sexual urges). *If psychosis or inability to control urges occurs,* consider ↓ dose or discontinue safinamide.

Lab Test Considerations

- May ↑ ALT or AST.

Implementation

- **PO:** Administer once daily, at the same time each day, without regard to food.

Patient/Family Teaching

- Explain purpose and side effects of medication. Advise patient to read *Patient Information* before starting therapy.
- Instruct patient to omit missed doses and to take next scheduled dose at usual time the following day. Do not double doses. Do not discontinue abruptly; may cause elevated temperature, muscular rigidity, altered consciousness, and autonomic instability.
- Caution patient to avoid alcohol, CNS depressants, and foods or beverages containing tyramine (see Appendix J) during and for ≥2 wk after therapy discontinued; they may precipitate a hypertensive crisis. Contact health care provider immediately if symptoms of hypertensive crisis or serotonin syndrome develop.
- Instruct patient to notify health care provider of all Rx or OTC medications, vitamins, or herbal products being taken and consult health care provider before taking any new medications, including St. John's wort, cough or cold products containing dextromethorphan, and the analgesics meperidine, tramadol, or methadone during therapy.
- Inform patient that safinamide may cause falling asleep while engaged in activities of daily living, including the operation of motor vehicles, conversations, and eating. Notify health care provider if periods of daytime sleepiness occur.
- Advise patient to notify health care provider if new or ↑ gambling, sexual, or other impulse control disorders or psychotic-like behaviors occur.
- Advise patient to have regular ophthalmic exams during therapy and to notify health care provider if visual changes occur.
- Rep: Advise women of reproductive potential to notify health care provider if pregnancy is planned or suspected or if breastfeeding.

Evaluation/Desired Outcomes

- Improvement in symptoms of Parkinson disease, allowing ↑ in function.

salmeterol (sal-me-te-role)

Serevent Diskus

Classification

Therapeutic: bronchodilators

Pharmacologic: adrenergics

S

Indications

As concurrent therapy for the treatment of asthma and the prevention of bronchospasm in patients who are currently taking but are inadequately controlled on an inhaled corticosteroid. Prevention of exercise-induced bronchospasm. Maintenance treatment to prevent bronchospasm in COPD.

Action

Produces accumulation of cyclic adenosine monophosphate at $beta_2$-adrenergic receptors. Relatively specific for $beta_2$ (pulmonary) receptors. **Therapeutic Effects:** Bronchodilation.

Pharmacokinetics

Absorption: Minimal systemic absorption follows inhalation.

Distribution: Action is primarily local.

Metabolism and Excretion: Metabolized in the liver via the CYP3A4 isoenzyme; 60% excreted in feces, 25% excreted in urine.
Half-life: 3–4 hr.

TIME/ACTION PROFILE (bronchodilation)

ROUTE	ONSET	PEAK	DURATION
Inhaln	10–25 min	3–4 hr	12 hr†

† 9 hr in adolescents.

Contraindications/Precautions

Contraindicated in: Hypersensitivity to salmeterol or milk proteins; Acute attack of asthma (onset of action is delayed); Patients not receiving an inhaled corticosteroid (↑ risk of asthma-related death); Patients whose asthma is currently controlled on low- or medium-dose inhaled corticosteroid therapy.
Use Cautiously in: Cardiovascular disease (including angina and hypertension); Seizure disorders; Diabetes; Glaucoma; Hyperthyroidism; Pheochromocytoma; Excessive use (may lead to tolerance and paradoxical bronchospasm); OB: Use during pregnancy only if potential maternal benefit justifies potential fetal risk; may inhibit contractions during labor; Lactation: Use while breastfeeding only if potential maternal benefit justifies potential risk to infant; Pedi: ↑ risk of asthma-related hospitalizations in children not receiving an inhaled corticosteroid; Pedi: Children <4 yr (safety and effectiveness not established).

Adverse Reactions/Side Effects

CV: palpitations, tachycardia. **GI:** abdominal pain, diarrhea, nausea. **MS:** muscle cramps/soreness. **Neuro:** headache, nervousness, tremor. **Resp:** cough, paradoxical bronchospasm.

Interactions

Drug-Drug: Beta blockers may ↓ therapeutic effects. **MAO inhibitors** and **tricyclic antidepressants** may potentiate cardiovascular effects. **Strong CYP3A4 inhibitors**, including **ketoconazole**, **itraconazole**, **ritonavir**, **atazanavir**, **clarithromycin**, **nefazodone**, or **nelfinavir**, may ↑ levels and risk of toxicity; concurrent use not recommended.
Drug-Natural Products: Use with caffeine-containing herbs (**cola nut**, **guarana**, **mate**, **tea**, **coffee**) ↑ stimulant effect.

Route/Dosage

Asthma

Inhaln (Adults and Children ≥4 yr): 50 mcg (1 inhalation) twice daily (approximately 12 hr apart).

Prevention of Exercise-Induced Bronchospasm

Inhaln (Adults and Children ≥4 yr): 50 mcg (1 inhalation) ≥30 min before exercise; additional doses should not be used for ≥12 hr.

COPD

Inhaln (Adults): 50 mcg (1 inhalation) twice daily (approximately 12 hr apart).

Availability

Powder for oral inhalation: 50 mcg/blister. ***In combination with:*** fluticasone (Advair Diskus, Advair HFA, Wixela Inhub). See Appendix N.

NURSING IMPLICATIONS

Assessment

- Assess lung sounds, BP, and HR before administration and periodically during therapy.
- Monitor pulmonary function tests before initiating therapy and periodically during therapy.
- Monitor for ↓ of asthma symptoms (wheezing, dyspnea, cough, orthopnea) during therapy.
- Observe for paradoxical bronchospasm (wheezing, dyspnea, tightness in chest, laryngeal spasm). Frequently occurs with 1st use of new canister or vial. *If paradoxical bronchospasm occurs,* discontinue salmeterol.
- Monitor for hypersensitivity reactions (anaphylaxis, urticaria, angioedema, rash). *If hypersensitivity reaction occurs,* discontinue salmeterol and initiate supportive treatment.

Lab Test Considerations

- May ↑ serum glucose concentrations; occurs rarely with recommended doses and is more pronounced with frequent use of high doses.
- May ↓ serum potassium concentrations, which are usually transient and dose related; rarely occurs at recommended doses and is more pronounced with frequent use of high doses.
- Monitor liver enzymes for any sign of hepatic disease prior to initiation of therapy.

Toxicity and Overdose

- Symptoms of overdose include persistent agitation, chest pain or discomfort, ↓ BP, dizziness, hyperglycemia, hypokalemia, seizures, tachyarrhythmias, persistent trembling, and vomiting.
- Treatment includes discontinuing salmeterol and other beta-adrenergic agonists and providing symptomatic, supportive therapy. Cardioselective beta blockers should be used cautiously because they may induce bronchospasm.

Implementation

- Salmeterol should be used along with an inhaled corticosteroid, not as monotherapy. Patients taking salmeterol twice daily should not use additional doses for exercise-induced bronchospasm. If symptoms arise between doses, administer a short-acting $beta_2$ agonist for immediate relief.
- **Inhaln:** Once removed from foil overwrap, discard diskus when every blister has been used or 6 wk have passed, whichever comes 1st.

Patient/Family Teaching

- Explain the purpose and side effects of salmeterol to patient. Teach proper technique of inhalation depending on the delivery device used and advise patient to take as directed. Do not use more than the prescribed dose. If a regularly scheduled dose is missed, use as soon as possible and resume regular schedule. Do not double doses. If symptoms occur before next dose is due, use a rapid-acting inhaled bronchodilator.
- Emphasize the importance of regular follow-up exams to determine progress during therapy.
- Instruct patient using *powder for inhalation* never to exhale into diskus device and always to hold device in a level horizontal position. Mouthpiece should be kept dry; never wash.
- Caution patient not to use salmeterol to treat acute symptoms. A rapid-acting inhaled beta-adrenergic bronchodilator should be used for relief of acute asthma attacks.
- Advise patients on chronic therapy not to use additional salmeterol to prevent exercise-induced bronchospasm. Patients using salmeterol for prevention of exercise-induced bronchospasm should not use additional doses of salmeterol for 12 hr after prophylactic administration.
- Advise patient to notify health care provider immediately if difficulty in breathing persists after use of salmeterol, if condition worsens, if more inhalations of rapid-acting bronchodilator than usual are needed to relieve an acute attack, or if using ≥4 inhalations of a rapid-acting bronchodilator for ≥2 consecutive days or more than one canister in an 8-wk period.
- Salmeterol should be used with inhaled corticosteroids and is not a substitute for corticosteroids or adrenergic bronchodilators. Advise patients using inhalation or systemic corticosteroids to consult health care provider before stopping or reducing therapy.
- Instruct patient to notify health care provider of all Rx or OTC medications, vitamins, or herbal products being taken and to avoid concurrent use of Rx, OTC, and herbal products without consulting health care provider.
- Rep: Advise women of reproductive potential to notify health care provider if pregnancy is planned or suspected or if breastfeeding.

Evaluation/Desired Outcomes

- Prevention of bronchospasm or reduction of frequency of acute asthma attacks in patients with chronic asthma. Improvement in asthma control can occur within 15 min of starting therapy, but full benefit may take ≥1 wk. Time to onset and degree of symptom relief will vary with individual.
- Prevention of exercise-induced asthma.
- Prevention of bronchospasm in COPD.

sarilumab (sar-il-ue-mab)

Kevzara

Classification

Therapeutic: antirheumatics, immunosuppressants,

Pharmacologic: interleukin antagonists

Indications

Moderately to severely active rheumatoid arthritis in patients who have not responded to ≥1 disease-modifying antirheumatic drugs (DMARD) (as monotherapy or in combination with methotrexate or other non-biologic DMARDs). Polymyalgia rheumatica in patients who had an inadequate response to corticosteroids or cannot tolerate a corticosteroid taper. Active polyarticular juvenile idiopathic arthritis (as monotherapy or in combination with non-biologic DMARDs).

Action

Acts as an inhibitor of interleukin-6 (IL-6) receptors by binding to them. IL-6 is a mediator of various inflammatory processes. **Therapeutic Effects:** Decreased pain and swelling with decreased rate of joint destruction in patients with rheumatoid arthritis and juvenile idiopathic arthritis. Sustained remission in polymyalgia rheumatica.

Pharmacokinetics

Absorption: Well absorbed via SUBQ injection.
Distribution: Well distributed to tissues.
Metabolism and Excretion: Metabolic pathway has not been defined. Elimination is predominantly through the linear, nonsaturable proteolytic pathway at high concentrations; at lower concentrations, elimination is predominately through nonlinear saturable target-mediated pathway.
Half-life: *200 mg every 2 wk dose:* up to 10 days; *150 mg every 2 wk dose:* up to 8 days.

TIME/ACTION PROFILE (plasma concentrations)

ROUTE	ONSET	PEAK	DURATION
SUBQ	unknown	2–4 days	28–43 days

Contraindications/Precautions

Contraindicated in: Hypersensitivity; Active infection; Hepatic impairment; ANC <2000/mm³ (<500/mm³ while on therapy) or platelet count <150,000/mm³ (<50,000/mm³ while on therapy); Concurrent use with biological DMARDs.
Use Cautiously in: Chronic or recurrent infection; History of serious or opportunistic infection; Exposure to tuberculosis (TB); Lived in or traveled to areas of endemic tuberculosis or endemic mycoses; Diverticulitis or concurrent use of NSAIDs or corticosteroids

S

(↑ risk for GI perforation); Severe renal impairment; OB: Use during pregnancy only if potential maternal benefit justifies potential fetal risk; Lactation: Use while breastfeeding only if potential maternal benefit justifies potential risk to infant; Pedi: Safety and effectiveness not established in children; Geri: ↑ risk of infections in older adults.

Adverse Reactions/Side Effects

GI: ↑ liver enzymes, GI PERFORATION. **Hemat:** NEUTROPENIA, THROMBOCYTOPENIA. **Local:** injection site reactions. **Metab:** dyslipidemia. **Misc:** INFECTION (INCLUDING TB, DISSEMINATED FUNGAL INFECTIONS, AND INFECTIONS WITH OPPORTUNISTIC PATHOGENS), hypersensitivity reactions, MALIGNANCY.

Interactions

Drug-Drug: May alter the activity of CYP450 enzymes; the effects of the following drugs should be monitored: **cyclosporine**, **theophylline**, **warfarin**, **hormonal contraceptives**, **atorvastatin**, and **lovastatin**. May ↓ antibody response to and ↑ risk of adverse reactions to **live-virus vaccines**; avoid concurrent use.

Route/Dosage

Rheumatoid Arthritis

SUBQ (Adults): 200 mg every 2 wk.

Polymyalgia Rheumatica

SUBQ (Adults): 200 mg every 2 wk (in combination with a corticosteroid taper). May be used as monotherapy once corticosteroid taper is completed.

Polyarticular Juvenile Idiopathic Arthritis

SUBQ (Adults and Children ≥63 kg): 200 mg every 2 wk.

Availability

Solution for SUBQ injection (prefilled syringes and pens): 150 mg/1.14 mL, 200 mg/1.14 mL.

NURSING IMPLICATIONS

Assessment

- Assess for signs of infection (fever, dyspnea, flu-like symptoms, diverticulitis symptoms, dysuria, cellulitis, wound infection) prior to injection. The most common are upper respiratory tract infections, bronchitis, and urinary tract infections. Signs and symptoms of inflammation may be lessened due to suppression from sarilumab. Infections may be fatal, especially in patients taking immunosuppressive therapy. *If patient develops a serious infection,* discontinue sarilumab until infection is controlled.
- Monitor patients for active and latent TB, and consider treating latent TB if positive prior to sarilumab initiation.
- Monitor for signs and symptoms of viral reactivation (herpes zoster [rash, blisters], hepatitis B [jaundice, dark urine, light-colored stools, fatigue, weakness, loss of appetite, nausea, vomiting, stomach pain]) during therapy.

Lab Test Considerations

- Verify negative pregnancy test prior to initiation.
- Assess lipid parameters approximately 4–8 wk after starting therapy and then every 6 mo. May ↑ LDL-C, HDL-C, and/or triglycerides.
- **Rheumatoid Arthritis:** Monitor neutrophil count prior to, at 4 and 8 wk after starting, and every 3 mo during therapy. Base dose modifications on measures from end of dosing interval. *If ANC >1000 cells/mm^3,* maintain current dose of sarilumab. *If ANC 500–1000 cells/mm^3,* withhold therapy until ANC >1000 cells/mm^3. Resume at 150 mg every 2 wk and ↑ to 200 mg every 2 wk as appropriate. *If ANC <500 cells/mm^3,* discontinue sarilumab.
- Monitor platelet count prior to, at 4 and 8 wk after starting, and every 3 mo during therapy. *If platelet count 50,000–100,000 cells/mm^3,* suspend therapy until platelets >100,000 cells/mm^3. Resume at 150 mg every 2 wk and ↑ to 200 mg every 2 wk as appropriate.
- Monitor AST and ALT prior to, at 4 and 8 wk after starting, and every 3 mo during therapy. *If ALT > upper limit of normal (ULN) to ≤3 times ULN,* consider modifying dose of concurrent DMARDs as clinically appropriate. *If ALT >3 times ULN to ≤5 times ULN,* hold therapy until ALT <3 times ULN. Resume at 150 mg every 2 wk and ↑ to 200 mg every 2 wk as appropriate. *If ALT >5 times ULN,* discontinue sarilumab.
- **Polymyalgia Rheumatica:** *If ANC <1000 cells/mm^3 at the end of the dosing interval, platelet count <100,000 cells/mm^3, or AST or ALT >3 times ULN,* discontinue sarilumab.
- **Polyarticular Juvenile Idiopathic Arthritis:** *If platelet count >50,000–100,000 cells/mm^3, ALT >3 times to ≤5 times ULN, or neutrophil count 500–<1000 cells/mm^3,* hold therapy. *If platelet count ≤50,000 cells/mm^3, ALT >5 times ULN, or neutrophil count <500 cells/mm^3,* discontinue sarilumab.

Implementation

- Update immunizations before starting therapy following current immunization guidelines for patients receiving immunosuppressive agents.
- Administer a tuberculin skin test prior to administration of sarilumab. Patients with latent TB should be treated for TB prior to therapy.
- Other DMARDs should be continued during sarilumab therapy.
- **SUBQ:** Refrigerate in original carton to protect from light; do not freeze. Only the prefilled syringe is approved for use in children. Allow dosage formulations to sit at room temperature for 30 min (prefilled syringe) or 60 min (prefilled pen) prior to administration; do not warm any other way. Do not shake. May be stored for up to 14 days in original carton at room temperature. Inject full amount in syringe.

Rotate injection sites; avoid areas where skin is tender, damaged, or has bruises or scars. Solution is clear and colorless to pale yellow; do not administer solutions that are discolored or contain particulate matter.

Patient/Family Teaching

- Explain the purpose and side effects of sarilumab to patient. Do not stop receiving drug without consulting health care provider. If an appointment or dose is missed, contact health care provider as soon as possible to reschedule. Instruct patient and caregiver in correct technique for SUBQ injections and care and disposal of equipment. Rotate injection sites. Do not inject where skin is tender, damaged, bruised, or scarred. Advise patient to read the *Medication Guide* before starting and with each Rx refill in case of changes.
- Caution patient to notify health care provider immediately if signs of infection (fever, sweating, chills, muscle aches, cough, shortness of breath, blood in phlegm, weight loss, warm, red or painful skin or sores, diarrhea or stomach pain that does not go away, burning on urination, urinary frequency, feeling tired) occur.
- Advise patient to immediately report and seek treatment for allergic reaction. Signs and symptoms of anaphylaxis might include swelling of face, lips, or tongue; hives; severe rash; shortness of breath; or chest pain.
- Advise patient to avoid receiving live vaccines during therapy.
- Instruct patient to notify health care provider of all Rx or OTC medications, vitamins, or herbal products being taken and consult health care provider before taking any new medications.
- Instruct patient to notify health care provider of medication regimen prior to treatment or surgery.
- Rep: Advise women of reproductive potential to notify health care provider if pregnancy is planned or suspected or if breastfeeding. Encourage women who become pregnant while taking sarilumab to participate in the pregnancy registry by going to https://mothertobaby.org/ongoing-study/kevzara/ or calling 1-877-311-8972.

Evaluation/Desired Outcomes

- Slowed progression of rheumatoid arthritis and polyarticular juvenile idiopathic arthritis.
- Sustained remission in polymyalgia rheumatica.

BEERS

scopolamine (scoe-pol-a-meen)

Transderm-Scop

Classification

Therapeutic: antiemetics

Pharmacologic: anticholinergics

Indications

Prevention of motion sickness. Prevention of postoperative nausea and vomiting.

Action

Inhibits the muscarinic activity of acetylcholine. Corrects the imbalance of acetylcholine and norepinephrine in the CNS, which may be responsible for motion sickness. **Therapeutic Effects:** Reduction of postoperative nausea and vomiting. Reduction of spasms.

Pharmacokinetics

Absorption: Well absorbed following transdermal administration.

Distribution: Crosses the blood-brain barrier.

Metabolism and Excretion: Mostly metabolized by the liver.

Half-life: 8 hr.

TIME/ACTION PROFILE (antiemetic, sedative properties)

ROUTE	ONSET	PEAK	DURATION
Transdermal	4 hr	unknown	72 hr

Contraindications/Precautions

Contraindicated in: Hypersensitivity; Angle-closure glaucoma; Acute hemorrhage; Tachycardia secondary to cardiac insufficiency or thyrotoxicosis; OB: Pregnant women with severe pre-eclampsia (may ↑ risk of seizures).

Use Cautiously in: Possible intestinal obstruction; Prostatic hyperplasia; Chronic renal, hepatic, pulmonary, or cardiac disease; Schizophrenia (may worsen condition); OB: Use during pregnancy only if potential maternal benefit justifies potential fetal risk; Lactation: Use while breastfeeding only if potential maternal benefit justifies potential risk to infant; Pedi: ↑ risk of adverse reactions in children due to anticholinergic effects; Geri: Appears on Beers list. ↑ risk of adverse reactions in older adults due to anticholinergic effects. Avoid use in older adults.

Adverse Reactions/Side Effects

CV: tachycardia, palpitations. **Derm:** ↓ sweating. **EENT:** blurred vision, mydriasis, photophobia. **GI:** dry mouth, constipation. **GU:** urinary hesitancy, urinary retention. **Neuro:** drowsiness, agitation, confusion, delusions, disorientation, hallucinations, paranoia, psychosis, speech disorder. **Misc:** HYPERTHERMIA.

Interactions

Drug-Drug: ↑ anticholinergic effects with **antihistamines**, **antidepressants**, **quinidine**, or **disopyramide**. ↑ CNS depression with **alcohol**, **antidepressants**, **antihistamines**, **opioid analgesics**, or **sedative/hypnotics**. May alter the absorption of other **orally administered drugs** by slowing motility of the

GI tract. May ↑ GI mucosal lesions in patients taking oral **wax-matrix potassium chloride preparations**. **Drug-Natural Products:** ↑ anticholinergic effects with **jimson weed** and **scopolia**.

Route/Dosage

Transdermal (Adults): *Motion sickness:* Apply 1 patch 4 hr prior to travel and then every 3 days (as needed); *Preoperative:* Apply 1 patch the evening before surgery (remove 24 hr after surgery).

Availability (generic available)

Transdermal system: 1.5 mg scopolamine/patch releases 0.5 mg scopolamine over 3 days.

NURSING IMPLICATIONS

Assessment

- Monitor for nausea and vomiting before and during therapy.
- Assess for signs/symptoms of urinary retention periodically during therapy; discontinue if difficulty urinating develops.
- Monitor for anticholinergic side effects such as ↓ in GI motility (constipation, obstruction), urinary retention, temporary dilation of pupils resulting in blurred vision, and ↑ intraocular pressure.
- Monitor for acute psychosis, agitation, speech disorder, hallucinations, paranoia, and delusions, especially in patients receiving other drugs concurrently that are associated with similar psychiatric effects; if condition occurs, discontinue scopolamine.
- Geri: Older adults may be more sensitive to neurological (drowsiness, disorientation, confusion) and psychiatric effects, as well as for risk of hyperthermia; consider more frequent monitoring.

Implementation

Transdermal: Apply ≥4 hr before exposure to travel to prevent motion sickness.

Patient/Family Teaching

- Educate patient on reason for scopolamine and side effects. Instruct them to use medication as directed. Take missed doses as soon as remembered. Do not double doses. Advise patient to read *Patient Information* before starting and with each Rx refill in case of changes.
- Advise patients if body temperature ↑ or if they are not sweating when exposed to warm conditions, to remove the transdermal patch and contact a health care provider.
- **Transdermal:** Instruct patient on application of transdermal patches. Apply ≥4 hr before exposure to travel to prevent motion sickness. Wash hands and dry thoroughly before and after application. Apply to hairless, clean, dry area behind ear; avoid areas with cuts or irritation. Apply pressure over system to ensure contact with skin. Once secured, avoid touching or applying pressure to system being worn. Do not cut the transdermal system; only one system should be worn at a time. System is effective for 3 days. If system becomes dislodged, replace with a new system on another site behind the ear. System is waterproof and not affected by bathing or showering.
- On removal, fold the used transdermal system in half with the sticky side together and discard in household trash in a manner that prevents accidental contact or ingestion by children, pets, or others. Wash hands thoroughly after removing system.
- Instruct patient to remove patch and notify health care provider immediately if symptoms of acute angle-closure glaucoma (pain or reddening of the eyes with pupil dilation) occur.
- Caution patients engaging in underwater sports of potentially distorting effects of scopolamine.
- Advise patient referred for MRI test to discuss patch with referring health care provider and MRI facility to determine if removal of patch is necessary prior to test and for directions for replacing patch.
- Rep: Advise women of reproductive potential to notify health care provider if pregnancy is planned or suspected or if breastfeeding. When the transdermal patch is used to prevent nausea and vomiting associated with surgery, dose adjustments are required prior to cesarean delivery. Avoid use of transdermal patches in pregnant patients with severe preeclampsia; may cause eclamptic seizures. Monitor for dry mouth, drowsiness, blurred vision, and dilation of the pupils in infant of a mother using transdermal scopolamine. May ↓ milk production.

Evaluation/Desired Outcomes

- Prevention of motion sickness.
- Prevention of postoperative nausea and vomiting.

secnidazole (sek-nid-a-zole)

Solosec

Classification

Therapeutic: anti-infectives

Pharmacologic: imidazoles

Indications

Bacterial vaginosis. Trichomoniasis.

Action

Disrupts DNA synthesis in susceptible organisms. **Therapeutic Effects:** Resolution of bacterial vaginosis. Resolution of trichomoniasis. **Spectrum:** Active against *Bacteroides spp., Gardnerella vaginalis, Prevotella spp., Mobiluncus spp.,* and *Trichomonas vaginalis.*

Pharmacokinetics

Absorption: Rapidly and completely absorbed following oral administration.

Distribution: Extensively distributed to tissues.

Metabolism and Excretion: Primarily metabolized by CYP450 system in liver; 15% excreted unchanged in urine.
Half-life: 17 hr.

TIME/ACTION PROFILE (plasma concentrations)

ROUTE	ONSET	PEAK	DURATION
PO	rapid	4 hr	unknown

Contraindications/Precautions
Contraindicated in: Hypersensitivity; cross-sensitivity with other imidazoles may occur; Cockayne syndrome (↑ risk of hepatotoxicity and death); Lactation: Lactation.
Use Cautiously in: OB: Safety not established in pregnancy; Pedi: Children <12 yr (safety and effectiveness not established).

Adverse Reactions/Side Effects
GI: abdominal pain, diarrhea, metallic taste, nausea, vomiting. **GU:** vulvovaginal candidiasis, vulvovaginal pruritus. **Neuro:** headache.

Interactions
Drug-Drug: Alcohol or preparations containing **ethanol** or **propylene glycol** may lead to nausea, vomiting, diarrhea, abdominal pain, dizziness, and headache. Avoid use during secnidazole therapy and for ≥2 days after completing therapy.

Route/Dosage
Bacterial Vaginosis
PO (Adults and Children ≥12 yr): 2 g as a single dose.

Trichomoniasis
PO (Adults and Children ≥12 yr): 2 g as a single dose. Any sexual partners should also be treated with a 2-g single dose.

Availability
Oral granules: 2 g/pkt.

NURSING IMPLICATIONS
Assessment
- Assess for signs/symptoms of bacterial vaginosis (thin white or gray vaginal discharge; pain, itching, or burning in the vagina; strong fishlike odor, especially after sex; burning on urination; itching around the outside of the vagina) before and periodically following secnidazole.
- Assess for signs/symptoms of trichomoniasis (foul-smelling vaginal discharge, genital itching, painful urination) before and periodically following secnidazole.

Lab Test Considerations
- Obtain specimen for culture and sensitivity before starting therapy.

Implementation
- **PO:** Administer packet once without regard to meals. Open packet and sprinkle entire contents onto applesauce, yogurt, or pudding. Granules will not dissolve. Consume all of the mixture within 30 min without chewing or crunching granules. May be followed with a 8 ounces of water to aid in swallowing. Granules are not intended to be dissolved in any liquid.

Patient/Family Teaching
- Explain purpose and side effects of medication. Advise patient to read *Patient Information* before starting therapy.
- Advise patient to notify health care provider of all Rx or OTC medications, vitamins, or herbal products being taken and to consult with health care provider before taking other medications during therapy.
- Advise patient to notify health care provider if signs and symptoms of vulvovaginal candidiasis (vaginal itching, white or yellowish discharge [discharge may be lumpy or look like cottage cheese]) occur. May require treatment with antifungal agents.
- Advise patient to avoid alcohol during and for 2 days after last dose of secnidazole. May cause nausea, vomiting, diarrhea, abdominal pain, dizziness, and headache when taken with alcohol.
- Rep: Advise women of reproductive potential to notify health care provider if pregnancy is planned or suspected. Advise female patient to avoid breastfeeding for ≥96 hr (4 days) following secnidazole dose.

Evaluation/Desired Outcomes
- Resolution of bacterial vaginosis.
- Resolution of trichomoniasis.

S

secukinumab
(sek-ue-**kin**-ue-mab)
Cosentyx

Classification
Therapeutic: antipsoriatics
Pharmacologic: interleukin antagonists, monoclonal antibodies

Indications
SUBQ: Treatment of the following conditions: Moderate to severe plaque psoriasis in patients who are candidates for systemic therapy or phototherapy; Active enthesitis-related arthritis; Moderate to severe hidradenitis suppurativa. **IV, SUBQ:** Treatment of the following conditions: Active psoriatic

arthritis (with or without methotrexate); Active ankylosing spondylitis; Active non-radiographic axial spondyloarthritis in patients with objective signs of inflammation.

Action

A monoclonal antibody that acts as an antagonist of interleukin (IL)-17A by selectively binding to it and preventing its interaction with the IL-17 receptor. Antagonism prevents the production of inflammatory cytokines and chemokines. **Therapeutic Effects:** Decreased plaque formation and spread in plaque psoriasis. Decreased progression of and decreased structural damage associated with psoriatic arthritis. Decreased signs and symptoms in ankylosing spondylitis. Decreased disease activity in non-radiographic axial spondyloarthritis. Decreased risk of disease flare in juvenile psoriatic arthritis and enthesitis-related arthritis. Reduction in abscesses and inflammatory nodules in hidradenitis suppurativa.

Pharmacokinetics

Absorption: Well absorbed following SUBQ administration. IV administration results in complete bioavailability.
Distribution: Levels in interstitial fluid of skin (lesional and nonlesional) are 27–40% those of serum.
Metabolism and Excretion: Catabolized into small peptides and amino acids.
Half-life: 22–31 days.

TIME/ACTION PROFILE (plasma concentrations)

ROUTE	ONSET	PEAK	DURATION
SUBQ	unknown	6 hr	unknown
IV	rapid	end of infusion	unknown

Contraindications/Precautions

Contraindicated in: Hypersensitivity; Acute viral hepatitis.
Use Cautiously in: Chronic infection/history recurrent infection (including tuberculosis [TB]); Inflammatory bowel disease (exacerbation may occur); OB: Use during pregnancy only if potential maternal benefit justifies potential fetal risk; Lactation: Use while breastfeeding only if potential maternal benefit justifies potential risk to infant; Pedi: Safety and effectiveness not established in children <18 yr (psoriatic arthritis, ankylosing spondylitis, non-radiographic axial spondyloarthritis, and hidradenitis suppurativa) or <6 yr (plaque psoriasis).

Adverse Reactions/Side Effects

Derm: eczematous eruptions. **GI:** diarrhea, inflammatory bowel disease. **Misc:** HYPERSENSITIVITY REACTIONS (INCLUDING ANAPHYLAXIS OR ANGIOEDEMA), INFECTION (INCLUDING HEPATITIS B VIRUS REACTIVATION).

Interactions

Drug-Drug: ↑ risk of adverse reactions with **live vaccines**; avoid concurrent use. Administration of **non-live vaccines** may not elicit antibody response sufficient to produce protection. May affect activity of CYP450 enzymes and may alter the effectiveness/toxicity of **CYP450 substrate**, including **warfarin** and **cyclosporine**; close monitoring is recommended and necessary dose modifications undertaken.

Route/Dosage

Plaque Psoriasis

SUBQ (Adults): 300 mg once weekly for 5 wk, then 300 mg every 4 wk; for select patients, a dose of 150 mg may be sufficient.
SUBQ (Children ≥6 yr and ≥50 kg): 150 mg once weekly for 5 wk, then 150 mg every 4 wk.
SUBQ (Children ≥6 yr and <50 kg): 75 mg once weekly for 5 wk, then 75 mg every 4 wk.

Psoriatic Arthritis

SUBQ (Adults): Initiate therapy with or without a loading dose. *With loading dose:* 150 mg once weekly for 5 wk; then 150 mg every 4 wk; if patient continues to have symptoms, may ↑ dose to 300 mg. *Without loading dose:* 150 mg every 4 wk; if patient continues to have symptoms, may ↑ dose to 300 mg.
IV (Adults): Initiate therapy with or without a loading dose. *With loading dose:* 6 mg/kg initially; then 1.75 mg/kg (max dose = 300 mg) every 4 wk. *Without loading dose:* 1.75 mg/kg (max dose = 300 mg) every 4 wk.
SUBQ (Children ≥2 yr and ≥50 kg): 150 mg once weekly for 5 wk; then 150 mg every 4 wk.
SUBQ (Children ≥2 yr and 15–<50 kg): 75 mg once weekly for 5 wk; then 150 mg every 4 wk.

Ankylosing Spondylitis

SUBQ (Adults): Initiate therapy with or without a loading dose. *With loading dose:* 150 mg once weekly for 5 wk; then 150 mg every 4 wk; if patient continues to have symptoms, may ↑ dose to 300 mg; *Without loading dose:* 150 mg every 4 wk; if patient continues to have symptoms, may ↑ dose to 300 mg.
IV (Adults): Initiate therapy with or without a loading dose. *With loading dose:* 6 mg/kg initially; then 1.75 mg/kg (max dose = 300 mg) every 4 wk. *Without loading dose:* 1.75 mg/kg (max dose = 300 mg) every 4 wk.

Non-radiographic Axial Spondyloarthritis

SUBQ (Adults): Initiate therapy with or without a loading dose. *With loading dose:* 150 mg once weekly for 5 wk; then 150 mg every 4 wk; *Without loading dose:* 150 mg every 4 wk.
IV (Adults): Initiate therapy with or without a loading dose. *With loading dose:* 6 mg/kg initially; then 1.75 mg/kg (max dose = 300 mg) every 4 wk. *Without loading dose:* 1.75 mg/kg (max dose = 300 mg) every 4 wk.

Enthesitis-Related Arthritis

SUBQ (Adults and Children ≥4 yr and ≥50 kg): 150 mg once weekly for 5 wk; then 150 mg every 4 wk.
SUBQ (Adults and Children ≥4 yr and 15–<50 kg): 75 mg once weekly for 5 wk; then 150 mg every 4 wk.

Hidradenitis Suppurativa

SUBQ (Adults): 300 mg once weekly for 5 wk; then 300 mg every 4 wk; if patient does not adequately respond, may ↑ dose to 300 mg every 2 wk.

Availability

Solution for SUBQ injection (caps contain latex) (prefilled syringes): 75 mg/0.5 mL, 150 mg/mL. **Solution for SUBQ injection (caps contain latex) (Sensoready pen):** 150 mg/mL. **Solution for SUBQ injection (UnoReady pen):** 150 mg/mL. **Solution for IV injection:** 25 mg/mL.

NURSING IMPLICATIONS

Assessment

- Assess skin lesions periodically during therapy for psoriasis.
- For patients with arthritis, assess pain, joint swelling and stiffness, and limitations of movement during therapy.
- For patients with hidradenitis suppurativa, assess armpits, groin, buttocks, and under breasts for new or worsening cysts or abscesses (including cellulitis) during therapy.
- Assess for signs/symptoms of infection (fever; dyspnea; sweats; chills; muscle aches; cough; blood in phlegm; weight loss; frequent or painful urination; warm, red, or painful skin or sores; diarrhea; stomach pain), including TB, prior to and periodically during therapy. New infections should be monitored closely; most common are upper respiratory tract infections, bronchitis, and urinary tract infections. Infections may be fatal, especially in patients taking immunosuppressive therapy.
- Assess for latex allergy. Needle cover of syringe contains latex and should not be handled by persons sensitive to latex.
- Monitor for signs/symptoms of anaphylaxis (urticaria, dyspnea, wheezing) and angioedema (facial or throat swelling, hoarseness) following injection. Provide necessary emergency care. Medications (antihistamines, corticosteroids, epinephrine) and equipment should be readily available in the event of a severe reaction. *If anaphylaxis or other severe allergic reaction occurs,* discontinue secukinumab.
- Assess for history of hepatitis B, which can be reactivated during therapy.
- Monitor patients with inflammatory bowel disease closely; may cause exacerbations.

Implementation

- Administer a tuberculin skin test prior to administration of secukinumab. Patients with active latent TB should be treated for TB prior to therapy.
- Immunizations should be current prior to initiating therapy. Patients on secukinumab may receive concurrent vaccinations, except for live vaccines.
- Administer initial injection under supervision of a health care provider.
- Vial is for institutional use only. With training, patient may use pen and prefilled syringes at home.
- Solution is clear to slightly opalescent and colorless to slightly yellow. Do not administer solutions that are cloudy, discolored, or contain particulate matter. Discard unused solution.
- **SUBQ:** Administer at a 45° angle in upper thighs or abdomen, avoiding the 2 inches around navel. Upper outer arm may be used if administered by caregiver. Put pressure on injection site for 10 sec; do not rub. Administer two injections at different sites for 300-mg dose. Rotate injection sites; avoid areas that are tender, bruised, hard, red, or affected by psoriasis. Refrigerate prefilled syringes and pens.

IV Administration

- **Intermittent Infusion: Dilution:** Withdraw and discard a volume of 0.9% NaCl from the infusion bag equal to the calculated volume of the solution required for the dose. *For a patient weighing ≤52 kg:* Use a 100-mL infusion bag for the loading dose and a 50-mL infusion bag for the maintenance dose; if a 50-mL bag is unavailable, use a 100-mL bag and withdraw and discard 50 mL using aseptic technique. *For a patient weighing >52 kg:* Use a 100-mL infusion bag for the loading dose and the maintenance dose. Withdraw the calculated volume of solution from the vial(s) and add slowly into the 0.9% NaCl infusion bag; gently invert to mix the bag to avoid foaming and do not shake. Administer as soon as possible. Store at room temperature for ≤4.5 hr or under refrigeration for ≤24 hr from the start of the time of the preparation (piercing the 1st vial) to the completion of infusion. Protect diluted solution from light when stored in refrigerator. Do not use if particulates or discoloration are noted prior to administration. **Rate:** Administer the infusion at a flow rate of about 3.3 mL/min for a 100-mL bag or 1.7 mL/min for a 50-mL bag with a total administration time of 30 min. On completion, flush the line with 0.9% NaCl to guarantee that all the solution for infusion in the line has been administered. Use only an infusion set with an in-line, sterile, nonpyrogenic, low-protein-binding filter with a pore size of 0.2 micrometer.

S

- **Y-Site Incompatibility:** Do not administer other drugs through same IV line.

Patient/Family Teaching

- Explain the purpose and side effects of secukinumab to patient. If an appointment is missed, contact health care provider as soon as possible to reschedule. Instruct patient on the correct technique for administering secukinumab. Review *Medication Guide*, preparation of dose, administration sites and technique, and disposal of equipment into a puncture-resistant container. Advise patient to review *Medication Guide* with each Rx in case of changes.
- Caution patient to notify health care provider immediately if signs of infection, severe rash, swollen face, or difficulty breathing occur while taking secukinumab.
- Advise patient to notify health care provider of all Rx or OTC medications, vitamins, or herbal products being taken and to consult with health care provider before taking other medications.
- Advise patient to avoid live vaccines during therapy.
- Instruct patient to notify health care provider of medication regimen prior to treatment or surgery.
- ***Sensoready Pen and UnoReady Pen*:** Adults may self-administer, if appropriate. Pediatric patients should not self-administer; a caregiver should inject pen. Use the UnoReady or Sensoready pen within 5 min of removing the cap. Allow refrigerated product to return to room temperature before administering. Clean area for injection with alcohol swab. Hold pen with cap pointing up. Check solution through window; if discolored, cloudy, or contains flakes, discard solution. Remove cap. Place pen, with window visible, against skin at a 90° angle and press button until 2 clicks are heard. 1st click indicates injection started; 2nd click indicates injection is almost complete. Hold pen in place until all solution is injected (10 sec) and green marker is visible in window and has filled window. Remove needle and press with a gauze pad or cotton ball for 10 sec. Do not rub injection site. Dispose of pen into a puncture-resistant container.
- Rep: Advise women of reproductive potential to notify health care provider if pregnancy is planned or suspected or if breastfeeding.

Evaluation/Desired Outcomes

- Reduced severity of plaques in patients with severe chronic plaque psoriasis.
- Reduction in abscesses and inflammatory nodules in hidradenitis suppurativa.
- Decreased progression of and decreased structural damage associated with psoriatic arthritis.
- Decreased risk of disease flare in juvenile psoriatic arthritis and enthesitis-related arthritis.
- Decreased signs and symptoms in ankylosing spondylitis.
- Decreased disease activity in non-radiographic axial spondyloarthritis.

selegiline (se-le-ji-leen)

~~Eldepryl~~, Emsam, Zelapar

Classification

Therapeutic: antiparkinson agents, antidepressants

Pharmacologic: monoamine oxidase type B inhibitors

Indications

PO: Parkinson disease in patients who fail to respond to levodopa/carbidopa alone (in combination with levodopa or levodopa/carbidopa). **Transdermal:** Major depressive disorder.

Action

Following conversion by MAO to its active form, selegiline inactivates MAO by irreversibly binding to it at type B (brain) sites; results in higher levels of monoamine neurotransmitters in the brain (dopamine, serotonin, norepinephrine). **Therapeutic Effects:** Increased response to levodopa/dopamine therapy in Parkinson disease. Decreased symptoms of depression.

Pharmacokinetics

Absorption: Well absorbed following oral administration. 25–30% of patch content is absorbed; levels are higher than those following oral administration because there is less first-pass hepatic metabolism.

Distribution: Widely distributed to tissues; crosses the blood-brain barrier.

Metabolism and Excretion: Mostly metabolized by the liver, primarily by the CYP2A6, CYP2C9, and CYP3A4/5 isoenzymes to N-desmethylselegiline, amphetamine, and methamphetamine as well as inactive metabolites. Primarily excreted in urine as metabolites.

Half-life: *Oral:* 10 hr; *Transdermal:* 20 hr.

TIME/ACTION PROFILE (beneficial effects in Parkinson disease)

ROUTE	ONSET	PEAK	DURATION
PO	2–3 days†	40–90 min†	unknown
Orally disintegrating	5 min†	10–15 min†	unknown
Transdermal	unknown	≥2 wk‡	unknown

† Beneficial effects in Parkinson disease;
‡ Antidepressant effects.

Contraindications/Precautions

Contraindicated in: Hypersensitivity; Pheochromocytoma; Major psychotic disorder; Concurrent use of opioids, other MAO inhibitors, St. John's wort, cyclobenzaprine, or dextromethorphan; Lactation: Lactation.

Use Cautiously in: History of peptic ulcer disease; Phenylketonuria (orally disintegrating tablets only); Elective surgery; May ↑ risk of suicide attempt/ideation, especially during early treatment or dose adjustment (transdermal only); History of mania (transdermal only); OB: Safety not established in pregnancy;

Pedi: Safety and effectiveness not established in children; Geri: ↑ risk of orthostatic hypotension in older adults.

Adverse Reactions/Side Effects

CV: orthostatic hypotension. **Derm: Transdermal:** application site reactions, acne, ecchymoses, pruritus, sweating. **GI:** nausea, abdominal pain, diarrhea, dry mouth. **Neuro:** aggression, agitation, confusion, delirium, delusions, disorientation, dizziness, fainting, hallucinations, headache, impulse control disorders(gambling, sexual, binge eating), insomnia, paranoia, psychosis, sedation, SEROTONIN SYNDROME, vivid dreams.

Interactions

Drug-Drug: Opioid analgesics (e.g., **meperidine**) or **cyclobenzaprine** may ↑ risk of serotonin syndrome; concurrent use contraindicated. Selegiline should be discontinued for ≥2 wk before initiating any of these medications. Other **MAO inhibitors**, including **linezolid**, may ↑ risk of hypertensive crises; concurrent use contraindicated. Selegiline should be discontinued for ≥2 wk before initiating any other medication with MAO inhibitor properties. Use with products containing **dextromethorphan** may lead to episodes of psychosis or bizarre behavior; concurrent use contraindicated. Drugs that affect serotonergic neurotransmitter systems, including **tricyclic antidepressants**, **SSRIs**, **SNRIs**, **fentanyl**, **buspirone**, **amphetamines**, and **triptans**, may ↑ risk of serotonin syndrome; avoid concurrent use with any antidepressant. Selegiline should be discontinued for ≥14 days before initiating any antidepressant. Fluoxetine should be discontinued for ≥5 wk before initiating selegiline. May initially ↑ risk of side effects (primarily dyskinesia) of **levodopa/carbidopa** (dose of levodopa/carbidopa may need to be ↓ by 10–30%). **Antipsychotics** and **metoclopramide** may ↓ effectiveness.
Drug-Natural Products: St. John's wort may ↑ risk of serotonin syndrome; concurrent use contraindicated.
Drug-Food: Doses >10 mg/day (tablets/capsules), >2.5 mg/day (orally disintegrating tablets), or >6 mg/24 hr (transdermal) may produce hypertensive reactions with **tyramine-containing foods** (see Appendix J).

Route/Dosage

Parkinson Disease

PO (Adults): *Capsules or tablets:* 5 mg twice daily with breakfast and lunch (some patients may require further dividing of doses: 2.5 mg 4 times daily). *Orally disintegrating tablets:* 1.25 mg once daily for ≥6 wk. After 6 wk, may ↑ to 2.5 mg once daily if effect not achieved and patient is tolerating medication.

Depression

Transdermal (Adults): Apply 6 mg/24-hr patch once daily initially; if necessary, may be ↑ at 2-wk intervals in increments of 3 mg/24-hr patch (max dose = 12 mg/24 hr).

Availability (generic available)

Capsules: 5 mg. **Tablets:** 5 mg. **Orally disintegrating tablets (contain phenylalanine) (Zelapar) (grapefruit flavor):** 1.25 mg. **Transdermal patch (Emsam):** 6 mg/24 hr, 9 mg/24 hr, 12 mg/24 hr.

NURSING IMPLICATIONS

Assessment

- Monitor BP and HR before and frequently during therapy for depression.
- **Parkinson Disease:** Assess for signs/symptoms of Parkinson disease (tremor, muscle weakness and rigidity, ataxic gait) before and during therapy.
- **Depression:** Assess mental status, mood changes, and anxiety level frequently. Assess for suicidal tendencies, agitation, irritability, and unusual changes in behavior, especially during early therapy. Assess for any personal or family history of bipolar disorder, mania, or hypomania before starting therapy.

Toxicity and Overdose

- Concurrent ingestion of tyramine-rich foods and many medications may result in a life-threatening hypertensive crisis. Signs and symptoms of hypertensive crisis include chest pain, tachycardia or bradycardia, severe headache, neck stiffness or soreness, nausea and vomiting, sweating, photosensitivity, and enlarged pupils. If hypertensive crisis occurs, discontinue selegiline and administer labetalol 20 mg slowly IV to control hypertension. Manage fever with external cooling. Monitor patient closely until symptoms have stabilized.

Implementation

- Do not confuse selegiline with Salagen. Do not confuse Zelapar with Zyprexa or Zydis.
- An attempt to ↓ the dose of levodopa/carbidopa by 10–30% may be made after 2–3 days of selegiline therapy.
- **PO:** Administer 5-mg tablet with breakfast and lunch.
- Administer *orally disintegrating tablets* in the morning, before breakfast and without liquid. Remove tablet gently from blister pack with clean, dry hands immediately before administering. Do not attempt to push tablet through backing. Tablet will disintegrate within sec when placed on tongue. Avoid food or liquid within 5 min of administering orally disintegrating tablets.

S

- **Transdermal:** Apply system to dry, intact skin on the upper torso such as chest, back, upper thigh, or outer surface of the upper arm once every 24 hr at the same time each day. Avoid areas that are hairy, oily, irritated, broken, scarred, or calloused. Wash area gently with soap and warm water; rinse thoroughly. Allow skin to dry completely before application. Apply immediately after removing from package. Do not alter the system (i.e., cut) in any way before application. Remove liner from adhesive layer and press firmly in place with palm of hand for 30 sec, especially around the edges, to make sure contact is complete. Remove used system and fold so that adhesive edges are together. Only one selegiline patch should be worn at a time. Dispose away from children and pets. Apply new system to a different site. Wash hands thoroughly with soap and water to remove any medicine that may have gotten on them.

Patient/Family Teaching

- Explain purpose and side effects of medication. Advise patient to read *Patient Information* before starting therapy. Instruct patient to take medication as directed. Take missed doses as soon as possible, but not if late afternoon or evening or almost time for next dose. Do not double doses. Caution patient that taking more than the prescribed dose may ↑ side effects and place patient at risk for hypertensive crisis if foods containing tyramine are consumed (see Appendix J).
- Advise patients taking selegiline ≥20 mg/day to avoid large amounts of tyramine-containing foods (see Appendix J), alcoholic beverages, large quantities of caffeine-containing beverages, or OTC or herbal cough or cold medications.
- Advise patient to notify health care provider of all Rx or OTC medications, vitamins, or herbal products being taken and to consult with health care provider before taking other medications. Caution patient to avoid use of St. John's wort and the analgesics meperidine, tramadol, and methadone during therapy.
- Caution patient and caregiver that selegiline may cause drowsiness and dizziness. Monitor and assist with ambulation and caution patient to avoid driving and other activities requiring alertness until response to medication is known.
- Inform patient and family of the signs and symptoms of MAO inhibitor–induced hypertensive crisis (severe headache, chest pain, nausea, vomiting, photosensitivity, enlarged pupils). Advise patient to notify health care provider immediately if severe headache or any other unusual symptoms occur. ≥14 days should elapse between discontinuation of selegiline and start of MAO inhibitor therapy.
- Caution patient to change positions slowly to minimize orthostatic hypotension.
- Advise patient to notify health care provider of signs and symptoms of serotonin syndrome (mental status changes [agitation, hallucinations, delirium, coma], autonomic instability [tachycardia, labile BP, dizziness, diaphoresis, flushing, hyperthermia], neuromuscular changes [tremor, rigidity, myoclonus, hyperreflexia, incoordination], seizures, GI symptoms [nausea, vomiting, diarrhea]).
- Advise patient to notify health care provider if agitation; aggression; delirium; hallucinations; or new or ↑ gambling, sexual, or other intense urges occur.
- Advise patient that ↑ fluids, sugarless gum or candy, ice, or saliva substitutes may help minimize dry mouth. Consult health care provider if dry mouth continues for >2 wk.
- Rep: Advise women of reproductive potential to notify health care provider if pregnancy is planned or suspected. Advise patient to avoid breastfeeding during and for 7 days after final dose.
- **Transdermal:** Instruct patient to apply patch as directed. Advise patients and caregivers to read the *Medication Guide about Using Antidepressants in Children and Teenagers*. Inform patient that improvement may be noticed after one to several weeks of therapy. Advise patient not to discontinue therapy without consulting health care provider.
- Caution patient to avoid alcohol and CNS depressants during and for ≥2 wk after therapy has been discontinued; they may precipitate a hypertensive crisis. Contact health care provider immediately if symptoms of hypertensive crisis develop. Patients taking 9 mg/24 hr or 12 mg/24 hr must avoid foods or beverages containing tyramine (see Appendix J) from the 1st day of the ↑ dose through 2 wk after discontinuation of selegiline transdermal therapy.
- Advise patient to avoid exposing application site to external sources of direct heat such as heating pads, electric blankets, heat lamps, saunas, hot tubs, heated water beds, and prolonged direct sunlight.
- Caution patient to change positions slowly to minimize orthostatic hypotension. Older adults are at ↑ risk for this side effect.
- Advise patient referred for MRI test to discuss patch with referring health care provider and MRI facility to determine if removal of patch is necessary before test and for directions for replacing patch.
- Advise patients and caregivers to notify health care provider if severe headache, neck stiffness, heart racing or palpitations, anxiety, agitation, panic attacks, insomnia, irritability, hostility, aggressiveness, impulsivity, akathisia, hypomania, mania, change in behavior, worsening of depression, or suicidal ideation occur, especially during initial therapy or during changes in dose.
- Advise patient to notify health care provider of medication regimen before treatment or surgery. If possible, therapy should be discontinued ≥2 wk before surgery.

Evaluation/Desired Outcomes

- Increased response to levodopa/dopamine therapy in Parkinson disease.
- Decreased symptoms of depression.

selexipag (se-lex-i-pag)
Uptravi
Classification
Therapeutic: vasodilators
Pharmacologic: prostacyclin receptor agonists

Indications

Pulmonary arterial hypertension (WHO Group I).

Action

Prostacyclin receptor (IP receptor) agonist that leads to dilation of the pulmonary and arterial vasculature. **Therapeutic Effects:** Delayed disease progression and reduced hospitalizations.

Pharmacokinetics

Absorption: 49% absorbed following oral administration; food delays and ↓ extent of absorption. IV administration results in complete bioavailability.
Distribution: Highly protein bound.
Protein Binding: 99%.
Metabolism and Excretion: Hydrolyzed by carboxylesterase-1 to form active metabolite, which contributes to pharmacologic activity. Also metabolized by CYP3A4 and CYP2C8 to form inactive metabolites. Primarily excreted in feces.
Half-life: 0.8–2.5 hr (selexipag); 6.2–13.5 hr (active metabolite).

TIME/ACTION PROFILE (plasma concentrations)

ROUTE	ONSET	PEAK	DURATION
PO	unknown	1–3 hr (selexipag); 3–4 hr (active metabolite)	unknown
IV	rapid	end of infusion	unknown

Contraindications/Precautions

Contraindicated in: Hypersensitivity; Concurrent use of strong CYP2C8 inhibitors; Severe hepatic impairment; Lactation: Lactation.
Use Cautiously in: Moderate hepatic impairment (↓ dose recommended); OB: Use during pregnancy only if potential maternal benefit justifies potential fetal risk; women with pulmonary hypertension are usually advised to avoid pregnancy; Pedi: Safety and effectiveness not established in children.

Adverse Reactions/Side Effects

Derm: flushing, rash. **GI:** diarrhea, jaw pain, nausea, vomiting, ↓ appetite. **Hemat:** anemia. **MS:** arthralgia, myalgia. **Neuro:** headache. **Resp:** PULMONARY EDEMA.

Interactions

Drug-Drug: Strong CYP2C8 inhibitors, including **gemfibrozil**, may significantly ↑ levels of selexipag and its active metabolite, which may ↑ risk of toxicity and effectiveness; concurrent use contraindicated. **Moderate CYP2C8 inhibitors**, including **clopidogrel**, **teriflunomide** and **deferasirox**, may ↑ levels of selexipag and its active metabolite; consider ↓ initial dose of selexipag to once daily. **CYP2C8 inducers**, including **rifampin**, may ↓ exposure to active metabolite; ↑ dose (up to twice the normal dose) of selexipag.

Route/Dosage

IV route should be used for patients who are temporarily unable to tolerate oral therapy.
PO (Adults): 200 mcg twice daily; ↑ dose by 200 mcg twice daily on weekly basis to highest tolerated dose (max = 1600 mcg twice daily); *Concurrent use of moderate CYP2C8 inhibitor:* 200 mcg once daily; ↑ dose by 200 mcg once daily on weekly basis as tolerated.
IV (Adults): IV dose should be based on patient's current dose of oral selexipag: *Previously taking selexipag 200 mcg PO twice daily:* 225 mcg IV twice daily; *Previously taking selexipag 400 mcg PO twice daily:* 450 mcg IV twice daily; *Previously taking selexipag 600 mcg PO twice daily:* 675 mcg IV twice daily; *Previously taking selexipag 800 mcg PO twice daily:* 900 mcg IV twice daily; *Previously taking selexipag 1000 mcg PO twice daily:* 1125 mcg IV twice daily; *Previously taking selexipag 1200 mcg PO twice daily:* 1350 mcg IV twice daily; *Previously taking selexipag 1400 mcg PO twice daily:* 1575 mcg IV twice daily; *Previously taking selexipag 1600 mcg PO twice daily:* 1800 mcg IV twice daily.

Hepatic Impairment

PO (Adults): *Moderate hepatic impairment:* 200 mcg once daily; ↑ dose by 200 mcg once daily on weekly basis as tolerated.

Availability (generic available)

Tablets: 200 mcg, 400 mcg, 600 mcg, 800 mcg, 1000 mcg, 1200 mcg, 1400 mcg, 1600 mcg. **Lyophilized powder for injection:** 1800 mcg/vial.

NURSING IMPLICATIONS

Assessment

- Monitor hemodynamic parameters and exercise tolerance prior to and periodically during therapy.

S

- Assess for pulmonary edema during therapy. *If associated pulmonary veno-occlusive disease confirmed,* discontinue selexipag.

Lab Test Considerations

- May cause hyperthyroidism.
- May cause ↓ hemoglobin.

Implementation

- **PO:** Administer twice daily; food may improve tolerability. ***DNC:*** Swallow tablets whole; do not break, crush, or chew. ↑ dose by 200 mcg weekly to highest dose tolerated up to 1600 mcg twice daily. If dose is not tolerated, ↓ to previous dose.

IV Administration

- **Intermittent Infusion: Reconstitution:** Bring selexipag injection to room temperature for 30–60 min. Protect vial from light at all times. Using a polypropylene syringe with 8.6 mL 0.9% NaCl and inject along vial wall. Gently invert vial; repeat until complete dissolution. Do not shake. Do not use if reconstituted solution appears cloudy, discolored, or contains particulates. **Concentration:** 225 mcg/mL. **Dilution:** Withdraw 100 mL 0.9% NaCl injection and transfer into an empty sterile glass container. Withdraw required volume of reconstituted solution with polypropylene syringe and dilute into glass container to obtain desired final dose. All remaining reconstituted solution must be discarded. Gently invert container five times. Wrap entire container with light-protective cover. Keep at room temperature and complete infusion within 4 hr of vial puncture. **Rate:** Infuse over 80 min using infusion set made of DEHP-free polyvinyl chloride, natural latex rubber-free microbore tubing protected from light. Do not use a filter. Once glass container is empty, continue infusion with 0.9% NaCl to infuse the remaining selexipag from the IV line.
- **Y-Site Incompatibility:** Do not administer other drugs through same IV line.

Patient/Family Teaching

- Instruct patient to take selexipag as directed. Take missed doses as soon as possible unless next dose is within 6 hr. If ≥3 days are missed, restart at lower dose and titrate. Do not stop selexipag without consulting health care professional.
- Advise patient to read *Patient Information* prior to starting therapy and with each Rx refill in case of changes.
- Advise patient to notify health care professional of difficulty breathing, cough, chest pain, or fatigue.
- Instruct patient to notify health care professional of all Rx or OTC medications, vitamins, or herbal products being taken and consult health care professional before taking any new medications.
- Rep: Advise females of reproductive potential to notify health care professional if pregnancy is planned or suspected and to avoid breastfeeding during therapy.

Evaluation/Desired Outcomes

- Slowed disease progression and reduced hospitalizations for pulmonary arterial hypertension.

semaglutide (sem-a-**gloo**-tide)

Ozempic, Rybelsus, Wegovy

Classification

Therapeutic: antidiabetics, weight control agents

Pharmacologic: glucagon-like peptide-1 (GLP-1) receptor agonists

Indications

Ozempic and Rybelsus: Type 2 diabetes mellitus (as adjunct to diet and exercise). **Ozempic:** To reduce the risk of major adverse cardiovascular events in patients with type 2 diabetes mellitus and established cardiovascular disease. **Ozempic:** To reduce the risk of sustained eGFR decline, end-stage kidney disease, and cardiovascular death in patients with type 2 diabetes mellitus and chronic kidney disease. **Wegovy:** Chronic weight management in: Adults who are obese (body mass index [BMI] ≥30 kg/m^2) *OR* are overweight (BMI ≥27 kg/m^2) with ≥1 weight-related comorbid condition (e.g., hypertension, dyslipidemia, type 2 diabetes) (as adjunct to reduced-calorie diet and ↑ physical activity). Pediatric patients ≥12 yr old who are obese (initial BMI ≥95th percentile standardized for age and sex) (as adjunct to reduced-calorie diet and ↑ physical activity). **Wegovy:** To reduce the risk of major adverse cardiovascular events (cardiovascular death, nonfatal MI, or nonfatal stroke) in adults with established cardiovascular disease and who are either obese or overweight.

Action

Acts as an acylated human glucagon-like peptide-1 (GLP-1, an incretin) receptor agonist; increases intracellular cyclic AMP (cAMP), leading to insulin release when glucose is elevated, which then subsides as blood glucose decreases toward euglycemia. Also decreases glucagon secretion and delays gastric emptying. Also helps to suppress appetite, leading to decreased caloric intake. **Therapeutic Effects:** Improved glycemic control. Reduction in risk of cardiovascular death, nonfatal MI, or nonfatal stroke patients with type 2 diabetes mellitus and established cardiovascular disease. Reduction in risk of sustained eGFR decline, end-stage kidney disease, and cardiovascular death in patients with type 2 diabetes mellitus and chronic kidney disease. Reduction in body weight.

Pharmacokinetics

Absorption: 89% absorbed following SUBQ injection; 0.4–1% absorbed following oral administration.
Distribution: Minimally distributed to tissues.

Protein Binding: >99%.
Metabolism and Excretion: Endogenously metabolized; eliminated in the urine (3% as unchanged drug) and feces.
Half-life: 1 wk.

TIME/ACTION PROFILE (plasma concentrations)

ROUTE	ONSET	PEAK	DURATION
SUBQ	unknown	1–3 days	unknown
PO	unknown	1 hr	unknown

Contraindications/Precautions

Contraindicated in: Hypersensitivity; Personal or family history of medullary thyroid carcinoma; Multiple endocrine neoplasia syndrome type 2; Type 1 diabetes; Diabetic ketoacidosis; Severe GI disease (including severe gastroparesis); Lactation: Avoid use of Rybelsus while breastfeeding.
Use Cautiously in: History of pancreatitis; Diabetic retinopathy (↑ risk of complications); History of angioedema or anaphylaxis to another GLP-1 receptor agonist; History of suicidal attempt or active suicidal ideations; Undergoing elective surgery or procedure requiring general anesthesia or deep sedation; OB: Use during pregnancy only if potential maternal benefit justifies potential fetal risk; insulin recommended for glucose management in pregnancy; Lactation: Use injectable formulations while breastfeeding only if potential maternal benefit justifies potential risk to infant; Rep: Women of reproductive potential; Pedi: Safety and effectiveness not established in children <12 yr (Wegovy) or <18 yr (Ozempic or Rybelsus).

Adverse Reactions/Side Effects

CV: ↑ heart rate. **Derm:** hair loss. **EENT:** retinopathy complications. **Endo:** hypoglycemia, MEDULLARY THYROID CARCINOMA. **GI:** abdominal pain, constipation, diarrhea, nausea, vomiting, ↓ appetite, ↑ amylase, ↑ lipase, abdominal distention, cholecystitis, cholelithiasis, dyspepsia, flatulence, PANCREATITIS, vomiting. **GU:** acute kidney injury. **Local:** injection site reactions. **Neuro:** fatigue, headache, dizziness, SUICIDAL BEHAVIOR/IDEATION (WEGOVY ONLY). **Resp:** aspiration. **Misc:** HYPERSENSITIVITY REACTIONS (INCLUDING ANAPHYLAXIS AND ANGIOEDEMA).

Interactions

Drug-Drug: Concurrent use with **agents that increase insulin secretion**, including **sulfonylureas** or **insulin**, may ↑ risk of serious hypoglycemia; use cautiously and consider dose ↓ of agent increasing insulin secretion. May alter absorption of concurrently administered **oral medications** due to delayed gastric emptying.

Route/Dosage

Type 2 Diabetes

Rybelsus formulations should not be substituted on a mg-per-mg basis. Only one formulation should be used at one time.
PO (Adults): *Rybelsus (formulation R1):* 3 mg once daily for 30 days, then 7 mg once daily; after 30 days, may ↑ to 14 mg once daily if additional glycemic control needed. *Rybelsus (formulation R2):* 1.5 mg once daily for 30 days, then 4 mg once daily; after 30 days, may ↑ to 9 mg once daily if additional glycemic control needed.
SUBQ (Adults): *Ozempic:* 0.25 mg once weekly initially for 4 wk, then 0.5 mg once weekly for 1 wk; may then ↑ dose after ≥4 wk, if additional glycemic control needed, to 1 mg once weekly; may then ↑ dose after ≥4 wk, if additional glycemic control needed, to 2 mg once weekly.

Reduction in Risk of Major Adverse Cardiovascular Events in Patients with Type 2 Diabetes Mellitus and Established Cardiovascular Disease

SUBQ (Adults): *Ozempic:* 0.25 mg once weekly initially for 4 wk, then 0.5 mg once weekly for 1 wk; may then ↑ dose after ≥4 wk, if additional glycemic control needed, to 1 mg once weekly; may then ↑ dose after ≥4 wk, if additional glycemic control needed, to 2 mg once weekly.

Reduction in Risk of Sustained eGFR Decline, End-Stage Kidney Disease, and Cardiovascular Death in Patients with Type 2 Diabetes Mellitus and Chronic Kidney Disease

SUBQ (Adults): *Ozempic:* 0.25 mg once weekly initially for 4 wk, then 0.5 mg once weekly for 1 wk; then ↑ dose after ≥4 wk to 1 mg once weekly.

Chronic Weight Management

SUBQ (Adults and Children ≥12 yr): *Wegovy:* 0.25 mg once weekly initially for 4 wk, then 0.5 mg once weekly for 4 wk, then 1 mg once weekly for 4 wk, then 1.7 mg once weekly for 4 wk, then 1.7 mg or 2.4 mg once weekly thereafter.

Reduction in Risk of Major Adverse Cardiovascular Events in Patients with Established Cardiovascular Disease Who Are Overweight or Obese

SUBQ (Adults): *Wegovy:* 0.25 mg once weekly initially for 4 wk, then 0.5 mg once weekly for 4 wk, then 1 mg once weekly for 4 wk, then 1.7 mg once weekly for 4 wk, then 1.7 mg or 2.4 mg once weekly thereafter.

S

Availability

Tablets (Rybelsus [formulation R1]): 3 mg, 7 mg, 14 mg. **Tablets (Rybelsus [formulation R2]):** 1.5 mg, 4 mg, 14 mg. **Solution for injection (Ozempic) (prefilled pens):** 2 mg/3 mL (delivers doses of 0.25 mg or 0.5 mg), 4 mg/3 mL (delivers dose of 1 mg), 8 mg/3 mL (delivers dose of 2 mg). **Solution for injection (Wegovy) (prefilled pens):** 0.25 mg/0.5 mL, 0.5 mg/0.5 mL, 1 mg/0.5 mL, 1.7 mg/0.75 mL, 2.4 mg/0.75 mL.

NURSING IMPLICATIONS

Assessment

- Observe patient taking concurrent insulin or medication that ↑ insulin secretion for signs/symptoms of hypoglycemia.
- Monitor for pancreatitis. *If pancreatitis suspected,* discontinue semaglutide. *If pancreatitis confirmed,* do not restart semaglutide.
- Monitor weight before and periodically during therapy.
- Monitor for signs/symptoms of hypersensitivity reactions (swelling of face, lips, tongue, or throat; problems breathing or swallowing; severe rash or itching; fainting or feeling dizzy; very rapid heartbeat) during therapy.
- Monitor HR regularly during therapy. *If sudden sustained ↑ in resting HR occurs,* discontinue semaglutide.

Lab Test Considerations

- Monitor A1c periodically during therapy to evaluate effectiveness.
- *Wegovy:* In patients with type 2 diabetes, monitor blood glucose prior to starting and during therapy.
- May ↑ lipase and amylase.
- Monitor renal function when initiating or escalating doses of semaglutide.

Implementation

- Patients stabilized on a diabetic regimen who are exposed to stress, fever, trauma, infection, or surgery may require administration of insulin.
- ***Switching between Rybelsus formulations:*** Do not switch between *Rybelsus* formulations during the initiation phase (Days 1–30); may switch between *Rybelsus* formulations after 30 days of treatment. When switching between formulations, initiate the other *Rybelsus* formulation the day after discontinuing the previous *Rybelsus* formulation. Patients treated with *Rybelsus (formulation R1)* 7 mg once daily can be switched to *Rybelsus (formulation R2)* 4 mg once daily. Patients treated with *Rybelsus (formulation R1)* 14 mg once daily can be switched to *Rybelsus (formulation R2)* 9 mg once daily.
- ***Switching from Ozempic to Rybelsus (formulation R1):*** One week after discontinuing *Ozempic* 0.5 mg SUBQ once weekly, start *Rybelsus (formulation R1)* 7 mg or 14 mg PO once daily.
- ***Switching from Ozempic to Rybelsus (formulation R2):*** One week after discontinuing *Ozempic* 0.5 mg SUBQ once weekly, start *Rybelsus (formulation R2)* 4 mg or 9 mg PO once daily.
- **PO:** Administer ≥30 min before 1st food, beverage, or other oral medications of the day with no more than 4 oz of plain water only. Waiting <30 min or taking *Rybelsus* with food, beverages (other than plain water), or other PO medications ↓ absorption and will lessen effects. Waiting >30 min to eat may ↑ absorption. ***DNC:*** Swallow tablets whole; do not split, crush, or chew.
- **SUBQ:** Administer once weekly on same day each wk, any time of day without regard to meals. May change day of injection as long as time between doses is >48 hr. Inject into abdomen, thigh, or upper arm, rotating sites each wk. Solution is clear and colorless; do not administer solutions that are cloudy, discolored, or contain particulate matter. Store pens in refrigerator in original box until administration to protect from light; do not freeze. *Wegovy:* Single-use pens are stable for up to 28 days. *Ozempic* multidose pens are stable if refrigerated without the needle for 56 days after 1st use. Use a new needle for each injection.
- *Wegovy:* If dose escalation is not tolerated, may delay dose escalation for 4 wk. If patients do not tolerate maintenance dose of 2.4 mg once weekly, dose can be temporarily ↓ to 1.7 mg once weekly, for a maximum of 4 wk. After 4 wk, ↑ to maintenance dose of 2.4 mg once weekly. Discontinue *Wegovy* if patient cannot tolerate 2.4-mg dose.

Patient/Family Teaching

- Instruct patient to take semaglutide as directed. If a PO dose is missed, omit dose and take next dose the following day. Instruct patient in correct technique for injection and disposal of materials. Follow manufacturer's instructions for pen use. Pen should never be shared between patients, even if needle is changed. Administer missed *Ozempic* doses as soon as remembered within 5 days of missed dose; if >5 days, skip dose and administer next dose on regular scheduled day. Administer missed *Wegovy* doses as soon as remembered. If one dose is missed and next scheduled dose is >2 days away (48 hr), administer *Wegovy* as soon as possible. If one dose is missed and the next scheduled dose is <2 days away (48 hr), omit dose and resume dosing on regularly scheduled day of wk. If >2 consecutive doses are missed, resume dosing as scheduled or restart *Wegovy* and follow dose escalation schedule; may ↓ occurrence of GI symptoms. Advise patient to read the *Medication Guide* before starting therapy and with each Rx refill in case of changes.

- Advise patient taking insulin to never mix insulin and semaglutide together. Give as two separate injections. Both injections may be given in the same body area but should not be given right next to each other.
- Explain to patient that this medication controls hyperglycemia but does not cure diabetes. Therapy is long term.
- Review signs/symptoms of hypoglycemia (sweating, hunger, dizziness, ↑ HR, irritability, confusion, seizures) and hyperglycemia (thirst, hunger, frequent urination, fatigue, blurred vision) with patient. Advise patient to carry a form of sugar and identification describing disease process and medication regimen at all times. *If hypoglycemia occurs,* advise patient to take a glass of orange juice or 2–3 teaspoons of sugar, honey, or corn syrup dissolved in water and notify health care provider.
- Encourage patient to follow prescribed diet, medication, and exercise regimen to prevent hypoglycemic or hyperglycemic episodes.
- Instruct patient in proper testing of serum glucose and ketones. These tests should be closely monitored during periods of stress or illness, and health care provider should be notified if significant changes occur.
- Advise patient to notify health care provider of all Rx or OTC medications, vitamins, or herbal products being taken and consult health care provider before taking any new medications.
- Advise patient to notify health care provider and discontinue semaglutide immediately if signs/symptoms of pancreatitis (nausea, vomiting, abdominal pain radiating to back), palpitations or ↑ HR while at rest, or hypersensitivity (swelling of face, lips, tongue, or throat; problems breathing or swallowing; severe rash or itching; fainting or feeling dizzy; very rapid heartbeat) occur.
- Inform patient of risk of benign and malignant thyroid C-cell tumors. Advise patient to notify health care provider if symptoms of thyroid tumors (lump in neck, hoarseness, trouble swallowing, shortness of breath) occur.
- Advise patient to inform health care provider of medication regimen before procedures or surgery due to ↑ risk of aspiration with general or deep sedation.
- Instruct patient with history of diabetic retinopathy to have ophthalmic monitoring for progression of disease throughout therapy.
- Rep: Insulin is the preferred method of controlling blood glucose during pregnancy. Advise women of reproductive potential and men with female partners of reproductive potential to discontinue semaglutide in women ≥2 mo before a planned pregnancy to allow for long washout period of semaglutide. Counsel women of reproductive potential to notify health care provider if pregnancy is planned or suspected or if breastfeeding. Encourage pregnant patients to enroll in registry that monitors outcomes in women exposed to semaglutide during pregnancy by calling 1-877-390-2760 or visiting www.wegovypregnancyregistry.com.

Evaluation/Desired Outcomes

- Improved glycemic control.
- Reduction in risk of cardiovascular death, nonfatal MI, or nonfatal stroke patients with type 2 diabetes mellitus and established cardiovascular disease.
- Reduction in risk of sustained eGFR decline, end-stage kidney disease, and cardiovascular death in patients with type 2 diabetes mellitus and chronic kidney disease.
- Reduction in body weight.

senna (sen-na)

Ex-Lax, Senokot

Classification

Therapeutic: laxatives

Pharmacologic: stimulant laxatives

Indications

Constipation, particularly when associated with: Slow transit time, Constipating drugs, Irritable or spastic bowel syndrome, Neurologic constipation.

Action

Active components of senna (sennosides) alter water and electrolyte transport in the large intestine, resulting in accumulation of water and increased peristalsis. **Therapeutic Effects:** Laxative action.

Pharmacokinetics

Absorption: Minimally absorbed following oral administration.

Distribution: Unknown.

Metabolism and Excretion: Unknown.

Half-life: Unknown.

TIME/ACTION PROFILE (laxative effect)

ROUTE	ONSET	PEAK	DURATION
PO	6–12 hr†	unknown	3–4 days

† May take as long as 24 hr.

Contraindications/Precautions

Contraindicated in: Hypersensitivity; Abdominal pain of unknown cause, especially if associated with fever; Rectal fissures; Ulcerated hemorrhoids; Known alcohol intolerance (some liquid products).

Use Cautiously in: Chronic use (may lead to laxative dependence); Possible intestinal obstruction; OB: Other agents recommended for treatment of constipation in pregnancy (↑ risk of electrolyte abnormalities).

S

Adverse Reactions/Side Effects

F and E: electrolyte abnormalities (chronic use or dependence). **GI:** cramping, diarrhea, nausea. **GU:** pink-red or brown-black discoloration of urine. **Misc:** laxative dependence.

Interactions

Drug-Drug: May ↓ absorption of other **orally administered drugs** because of ↓ transit time.

Route/Dosage

Larger doses have been used to treat/prevent opioid-induced constipation. Consult labeling of individual OTC products for more specific dosing information.

PO (Adults): 17.2–50 mg 1–2 times daily.

PO (Children 12–17 yr): 17.6–26.4 mg 1–2 times daily.

PO (Children 6–11 yr): 8.8–13.2 mg 1–2 times daily.

PO (Children 2–6 yr): 4.4–6.6 mg 1–2 times daily.

Availability (generic available)

Tablets: 8.6 mg[OTC], 15 mg [OTC], 17.2 mg[OTC], 25 mg[OTC]. **Syrup:** 8.8 mg/5 mL[OTC].

NURSING IMPLICATIONS

Assessment

- Assess for abdominal distention, presence of bowel sounds, and usual pattern of bowel function.
- Assess color, consistency, and amount of stool produced.

Implementation

- **PO:** Take with 8 ounces of water. Administer at bedtime for evacuation 6–12 hr later. Administer on an empty stomach for more rapid results.
- Shake oral solution well before administering.

Patient/Family Teaching

- Explain purpose and side effects of medication to patient. Advise patient to read *Patient Information* before starting therapy.
- Advise patient to notify health care provider of all Rx or OTC medications, vitamins, or herbal products being taken and to consult with health care provider before taking other medications.
- Advise patient that laxatives should be used only for short-term therapy. Long-term therapy may cause electrolyte imbalance and dependence.
- Encourage patient to use other forms of bowel regulation, such as ↑ fluid intake and fiber in the diet, and ↑ mobility. Normal bowel habits are individualized and may vary from 3 times/day to 3 times/wk.
- Inform patient that this medication may cause a change in urine color to pink, red, violet, yellow, or brown.
- Instruct patients with cardiac disease to avoid straining during bowel movements (Valsalva maneuver).
- Advise patient not to use laxatives when abdominal pain, nausea, vomiting, or fever is present.
- Rep: Advise women of reproductive potential to notify health care provider if pregnancy is planned or suspected or if breastfeeding.

Evaluation/Desired Outcomes

- Laxative action.

sertaconazole, See ANTIFUNGALS (TOPICAL).

BEERS

sertraline (ser-tra-leen)

Zoloft

Classification

Therapeutic: antidepressants

Pharmacologic: selective serotonin reuptake inhibitors (SSRIs)

Indications

Major depressive disorder. Panic disorder. Obsessive-compulsive disorder (OCD). Post-traumatic stress disorder (PTSD). Social anxiety disorder (social phobia). Premenstrual dysphoric disorder. **Unlabeled Use:** Generalized anxiety disorder.

Action

Inhibits neuronal uptake of serotonin in the CNS, thus potentiating the activity of serotonin. Has little effect on norepinephrine or dopamine. **Therapeutic Effects:** Antidepressant action. Decreased incidence of panic attacks. Decreased obsessive and compulsive behavior. Decreased feelings of intense fear, helplessness, or horror. Decreased social anxiety. Decrease in premenstrual dysphoria.

Pharmacokinetics

Absorption: Appears to be well absorbed after oral administration.

Distribution: Extensively distributed throughout body tissues.

Protein Binding: 98%.

Metabolism and Excretion: Extensively metabolized by the liver; one metabolite has some antidepressant activity; 14% excreted unchanged in feces.

Half-life: 24 hr.

TIME/ACTION PROFILE (antidepressant effect)

ROUTE	ONSET	PEAK	DURATION
PO	within 2–4 wk	unknown	unknown

Contraindications/Precautions

Contraindicated in: Hypersensitivity; Concurrent use of MAO inhibitors or MAO-inhibitor-like drugs (linezolid or methylene blue); Concurrent use of pimozide; Oral concentrate contains alcohol; avoid in patients with known intolerance.

Use Cautiously in: May ↑ risk of suicide attempt/ideation especially during early treatment or dose adjustment; this risk appears to be greater in adolescents or children; Severe renal impairment; Severe hepatic impairment; History of mania; Angle-closure glaucoma; OB: Use during 3rd trimester may result in neonatal serotonin syndrome requiring prolonged hospitalization and respiratory and nutritional support. Use during pregnancy only if potential maternal benefit justifies potential fetal risk; Pedi: Children <6 yr (safety and effectiveness not established); Geri: Appears on Beers list. May worsen or cause syndrome of inappropriate antidiuretic hormone (SIADH) secretion and/or hyponatremia in older adults. Use with caution in older adults and closely monitor sodium concentrations when starting therapy or ↑ dose.

Adverse Reactions/Side Effects

CV: chest pain, palpitations, QT interval prolongation, TORSADES DE POINTES. **Derm:** ↑ sweating, hot flashes, rash. **EENT:** pharyngitis, rhinitis, tinnitus, visual abnormalities. **Endo:** diabetes, SIADH. **F and E:** ↑ thirst, hyponatremia. **GI:** diarrhea, dry mouth, nausea, abdominal pain, altered taste, anorexia, constipation, dyspepsia, flatulence, vomiting. **GU:** ↓ libido, delayed/absent orgasm, ejaculatory delay/failure, erectile dysfunction, menstrual disorders, urinary disorders, urinary frequency. **Hemat:** BLEEDING. **Metab:** ↑ appetite. **MS:** back pain, myalgia. **Neuro:** dizziness, drowsiness, fatigue, headache, insomnia, tremor, agitation, anxiety, confusion, emotional lability, hypertonia, hypoesthesia, impaired concentration, manic reaction, nervousness, paresthesia, SUICIDAL THOUGHTS/BEHAVIORS, twitching, weakness, yawning. **Misc:** fever.

Interactions

Drug-Drug: Serious, potentially fatal reactions (hyperthermia; rigidity; myoclonus; autonomic instability, with fluctuating vital signs and extreme agitation, which may proceed to delirium and coma) may occur with **MAO inhibitors**. MAO inhibitors should be stopped ≥14 days before sertraline therapy. Sertraline should be stopped ≥14 days before MAO inhibitor therapy. **MAO-inhibitor-like drugs**, including **linezolid** or **methylene blue**, may ↑ risk of serotonin syndrome; concurrent use contraindicated; do not start therapy in patients receiving **linezolid** or **methylene blue**; if **linezolid** or **methylene blue** need to be started in a patient receiving sertraline, immediately discontinue sertraline and monitor for signs/symptoms of serotonin syndrome for 2 wk or until 24 hr after last dose of linezolid or methylene blue, whichever comes first (may resume sertraline therapy 24 hr after last dose of linezolid or methylene blue). May ↑ **pimozide** levels and risk of QT interval prolongation and ventricular arrhythmias; concurrent use contraindicated. Drugs that affect serotonergic neurotransmitter systems, including **tricyclic antidepressants**, **SNRIs**, **fentanyl**, **lithium**, **buspirone**, **tramadol**, **meperidine**, **methadone**, **amphetamines**, and **triptans**, may ↑ risk of serotonin syndrome. May ↑ sensitivity to **adrenergics** and ↑ the risk of serotonin syndrome. Concurrent use with **alcohol** is not recommended. May ↑ levels and risk of toxicity of **warfarin**, **phenytoin**, **tricyclic antidepressants**, some **benzodiazepines (alprazolam)**, or **clozapine**. ↑ risk of bleeding with **NSAIDs**, **aspirin**, **clopidogrel**, **prasugrel**, **ticagrelor**, **dabigatran**, **apixaban**, **edoxaban**, **rivaroxaban**, or **warfarin**. **Cimetidine** may ↑ levels and risk of toxicity. **QT interval prolonging medications** may ↑ risk of QT interval prolongation and torsades de pointes; avoid concurrent use.

Drug-Natural Products: ↑ risk of serotonergic side effects including serotonin syndrome with **St. John's wort** and **SAMe**.

Route/Dosage

Depression

PO (Adults): 50 mg once daily in the morning or evening initially; after several weeks, may ↑ at weekly intervals up to 200 mg/day, depending on response.

Obsessive Compulsive Disorder

PO (Adults): 50 mg once daily in the morning or evening initially; after several weeks, may ↑ at weekly intervals up to 200 mg/day, depending on response.

PO (Children 13–17 yr): 50 mg once daily.

PO (Children 6–12 yr): 25 mg once daily.

Panic Disorder

PO (Adults): 25 mg once daily initially; may ↑ after 1 wk to 50 mg once daily.

Post-Traumatic Stress Disorder

PO (Adults): 25 mg once daily for 7 days; then ↑ to 50 mg once daily; may then be ↑ if needed at intervals of at least 7 days (range 50–200 mg once daily).

Social Anxiety Disorder

PO (Adults): 25 mg once daily initially; then ↑ to 50 mg once daily; may be ↑ at weekly intervals up to 200 mg/day.

Premenstrual Dysphoric Disorder

PO (Adults): 50 mg/day initially either daily or daily during luteal phase of cycle. Daily dosing may be titrated upward in 50-mg increments at the beginning of a cycle. In luteal phase–only dosing, a 50-mg/day titration step for 3 days at the beginning of each luteal phase dosing period should be used (range 50–150 mg/day).

S

Availability (generic available)

Tablets: 25 mg, 50 mg, 100 mg. **Capsules:** ❋25 mg, ❋50 mg, ❋100 mg, 150 mg, 200 mg. **Oral solution (concentrated) (contains 12% alcohol):** 20 mg/mL.

NURSING IMPLICATIONS

Assessment

- Assess for suicidal tendencies, especially during early therapy. Restrict amount of drug available to patient. Risk may be ↑ in children, adolescents, and adults ≤24 yr. After starting therapy, children, adolescents, and young adults should be seen by health care provider at least weekly for 4 wk, every 3 wk for next 4 wk, and on advice of health care provider thereafter.
- Monitor appetite and nutritional intake. Weigh weekly. Notify health care provider of continued weight loss. Adjust diet as tolerated to support nutritional status.
- Assess for serotonin syndrome (mental changes [agitation, hallucinations, coma], autonomic instability [tachycardia, labile BP, hyperthermia], neuromuscular aberrations [hyperreflexia, incoordination], GI symptoms [nausea, vomiting, diarrhea]), especially in patients taking other serotonergic drugs (SSRIs, SNRIs, triptans). *If signs/symptoms of serotonin syndrome occur,* discontinue sertraline.
- Assess sexual function before starting sertraline. Assess for changes in sexual function during treatment, including timing of onset; patient may not report.
- **Depression:** Monitor mood changes. Inform health care provider if patient demonstrates significant ↑ in anxiety, nervousness, or insomnia.
- **OCD:** Assess for frequency of obsessive-compulsive behaviors. Note degree to which these thoughts and behaviors interfere with daily functioning.
- **Panic Attacks:** Assess frequency and severity of panic attacks.
- **PTSD:** Assess for feelings of fear, helplessness, and horror. Determine effect on social and occupational functioning.
- **Social Anxiety Disorder:** Assess for signs/symptoms of social anxiety disorder (blushing; sweating; trembling; tachycardia during interactions with new people, people in authority, or groups) periodically during therapy.
- **Premenstrual Dysphoric Disorder:** Assess for signs/symptoms of premenstrual dysphoric disorder (feeling angry, tense, or tired; crying easily; feeling sad or hopeless; arguing with family or friends for no reason; difficulty sleeping or paying attention; feeling out of control or unable to cope; having cramping, bloating, food craving, or breast tenderness) periodically during therapy.

Lab Test Considerations

- May cause false-positive urine screening tests for benzodiazepines.
- May cause hyperglycemia; monitor serum glucose if clinical symptoms occur.

Implementation

- Do not confuse sertraline with cetirizine or Soriatane.
- Periodically reassess dose and continued need for therapy.
- **PO:** Administer as a single dose in the morning or evening.
- For oral concentrate, use dropper provided to remove oral concentrate and mix with 4 ounces (½ cup) of water, ginger ale, lemon-lime soda, lemonade, or orange juice ONLY. Do not mix with other liquids. Take immediately after mixing. Do not mix in advance. Slight haze may appear after mixing; this is normal. Dropper dispenser contains dry natural rubber; advise patient with latex allergy.

Patient/Family Teaching

- Explain purpose and side effects of medication to patient. Advise patient to read *Patient Information* before starting therapy. Instruct to take as directed. Take missed doses as soon as possible and return to regular dosing schedule. Do not double doses. Do not stop abruptly; may cause dysphoric mood, irritability, agitation, dizziness, sensory disturbances (paresthesias such as electric shock sensations), anxiety, confusion, headache, lethargy, emotional lability, insomnia, and hypomania.
- Instruct patient to notify health care provider of all Rx or OTC medications, vitamins, or herbal products being taken and consult health care provider before taking any new medications, especially St. John's wort or SAMe.
- May cause drowsiness or dizziness. Caution patient to avoid driving and other activities requiring alertness until response to the drug is known.
- Advise patient, family, and caregivers to look for suicidality, especially during early therapy or dose changes. Notify health care provider immediately if thoughts about suicide or dying, attempts to commit suicide, new or worse depression or anxiety, agitation or restlessness, panic attacks, insomnia, new or worse irritability, aggressiveness, acting on dangerous impulses, mania, or other changes in mood or behavior occur.
- Advise patient and caregivers to immediately notify health care provider if signs/symptoms of serotonin syndrome occur.
- Advise patient to avoid alcohol or other CNS depressant drugs during therapy and to consult with health care provider before taking other medications and to avoid alcohol or other CNS depressant drugs, including opioids, during therapy.

- Inform patient that frequent mouth rinses, good oral hygiene, and sugarless gum or candy may minimize dry mouth. If dry mouth persists for >2 wk, consult health care provider regarding use of saliva substitute.
- Advise patient to wear sunscreen and protective clothing to prevent photosensitivity reactions.
- Advise patient to notify health care provider if headache, weakness, nausea, anorexia, anxiety, or insomnia persists or if bleeding (bruising, hematoma, epistaxis, petechiae) occurs.
- Inform patient that sertraline may cause symptoms of sexual dysfunction. In men, ejaculatory delay or failure, ↓ libido, and erectile dysfunction may occur. In women, may result in ↓ libido and delayed or absent orgasm. Advise patient to notify health care provider if symptoms occur.
- Emphasize the importance of follow-up exams to monitor progress. Encourage patient participation in psychotherapy to improve coping skills.
- Rep: Advise women of reproductive potential to notify health care provider immediately if pregnancy is planned or suspected or if breastfeeding. If used during pregnancy, should be tapered during 3rd trimester to avoid neonatal serotonin syndrome. Use in the month before delivery may ↑ risk of postpartum hemorrhage. Monitor infants exposed to sertraline for excess sedation, restlessness, agitation, poor feeding, poor weight gain, or respiratory distress; may ↑ risk of persistent pulmonary hypertension of the newborn. Inform patient of pregnancy exposure registry that monitors pregnancy outcomes in women exposed to antidepressants during pregnancy. Register patients by calling the National Pregnancy Registry for Antidepressants at 1-866-961-2388 or online at https://womensmentalhealth.org/research/pregnancyregistry/antidepressants.

Evaluation/Desired Outcomes

- Antidepressant action.
- Decreased incidence of panic attacks.
- Decreased obsessive and compulsive behavior.
- Decreased feelings of intense fear, helplessness, or horror.
- Decreased social anxiety.
- Decrease in premenstrual dysphoria.

sevelamer (se-vel-a-mer)

~~Renagel~~, Renvela

Classification

Therapeutic: electrolyte modifiers

Pharmacologic: phosphate binders

Indications

Hyperphosphatemia associated with end-stage renal disease.

Action

A polymer that binds phosphate in the GI tract, preventing its absorption. **Therapeutic Effects:** Decreased serum phosphate levels and reduction in the consequences of hyperphosphatemia (ectopic calcification, secondary hyperparathyroidism with osteitis fibrosa).

Pharmacokinetics

Absorption: Not absorbed; action is local (in GI tract).

Distribution: Unknown.

Metabolism and Excretion: Eliminated in feces.

Half-life: Unknown.

TIME/ACTION PROFILE (↓ in serum phosphate concentrations)

ROUTE	ONSET	PEAK	DURATION
PO	5 days	2 wk	unknown

Contraindications/Precautions

Contraindicated in: Hypersensitivity; Hypophosphatemia; Bowel obstruction.

Use Cautiously in: Dysphagia, swallowing disorders, severe GI motility disorders, or major GI tract surgery (avoid use of tablets); OB: Not systemically absorbed; no fetal exposure expected. May ↓ levels of folate and fat-soluble minerals; consider supplementation during pregnancy; Lactation: Not systemically absorbed; no expected presence in breast milk. May ↓ levels of folate and fat-soluble minerals; consider supplementation while breastfeeding; Pedi: Safety and effectiveness not established in children <18 yr (tablets) and children <6 yr (Renvela).

Adverse Reactions/Side Effects

GI: <u>diarrhea</u>, <u>dyspepsia</u>, <u>vomiting</u>, BLEEDING GI ULCER, BOWEL OBSTRUCTION/NECROSIS/PERFORATION, choking (tablet), colitis, constipation, dysphagia (tablet), ESOPHAGEAL OBSTRUCTION (TABLET), flatulence, nausea, ulceration.

Interactions

Drug-Drug: May ↓ absorption and effectiveness of other drugs, especially **drugs whose efficacy is dependent on tightly controlled blood levels**. ↓ absorption and effectiveness of **ciprofloxacin**.

Route/Dosage

PO (Adults): 800–1600 mg 3 times daily with meals; may titrate by 800 mg every 2 wk to achieve target serum phosphorus levels.

PO (Children ≥6 yr and BSA ≥1.2 m²): *Renvela:* 1600 mg 3 times daily with meals; may titrate by 800 mg every 2 wk to achieve target serum phosphorus levels.

S

PO (Children ≥6 yr and BSA 0.75–<1.2 m^2): *Renvela:* 800 mg 3 times daily with meals; may titrate by 400 mg every 2 wk to achieve target serum phosphorus levels.

Availability (generic available)

Powder for oral suspension: 800 mg/pkt, 2400 mg/pkt. **Tablets:** 400 mg, 800 mg.

NURSING IMPLICATIONS

Assessment

- Assess patient for GI side effects periodically during therapy.
- Monitor for signs/symptoms of ileus (abdominal distention, constipation, ↓ or absent bowel sounds) or GI perforation (nausea, abdominal pain, tarry stools, coffee ground emesis, pallor, anemia).

Lab Test Considerations

- Monitor phosphorous, calcium, bicarbonate, and chloride periodically during therapy. May ↓ folic acid and vitamins D, E, and K levels.

Implementation

- Doses of concurrent medications, especially antiarrhythmics, should be spaced ≥2 hr before or 3 hr after sevelamer. Ciprofloxacin dose must be extended to 6 hr after sevelamer.
- **PO:** Administer with meals. ***DNC:*** Do not break, chew, or crush tablets; contents expand in water.
- Use suspension for patients with swallowing disorders. Place contents of powder packet in a cup and mix thoroughly with ≥1 ounce of water for the 800-mg dose or 2 ounces of water for the 2400-mg dose packet. Stir mixture vigorously (it does not dissolve) and drink entire preparation within 30 min or resuspend the preparation right before drinking.

Patient/Family Teaching

- Explain the purpose and side effects of sevelamer. Instruct patient to take sevelamer with meals as directed and to adhere to prescribed diet. Advise patient to read *Patient Information* before starting and with each Rx refill in case of changes.
- Caution patient to space concurrent medications ≥1 hr before or 3 hr after sevelamer (6 hr for ciprofloxacin).
- Advise patient to notify health care provider if GI effects (worsening of existing constipation, bloody stools) occur.
- Advise patient to notify health care provider of all Rx or OTC medications, vitamins, or herbal products being taken and to consult with health care provider before taking other medications.
- Rep: Advise women of reproductive potential to notify health care provider if pregnancy is planned or suspected or if breastfeeding. Sevelamer is not systemically absorbed but may ↓ serum levels of fat-soluble vitamins and folic acid in pregnant and lactating women. May consider supplementation.

Evaluation/Desired Outcomes

- Decrease in serum phosphorous concentration to ≤5.5 mg/dL. Dose adjustment is based on serum phosphorous concentrations.

sildenafil (sil-den-a-fil)

Revatio, Viagra

Classification

Therapeutic: erectile dysfunction agents, vasodilators

Pharmacologic: phosphodiesterase type 5 inhibitors

Indications

Viagra: Erectile dysfunction (ED). **Revatio:** Pulmonary arterial hypertension (PAH) (WHO Group I).

Action

Viagra: Enhances effects of nitric oxide released during sexual stimulation. Nitric oxide activates guanylate cyclase, which produces increased levels of cyclic guanosine monophosphate (cGMP). cGMP produces smooth muscle relaxation of the corpus cavernosum, which promotes increased blood flow and subsequent erection. cGMP also leads to vasodilation of the pulmonary vasculature. Sildenafil inhibits the enzyme phosphodiesterase type 5 (PDE5); PDE5 inactivates cGMP. *Revatio:* Produces vasodilation of the pulmonary vascular bed. **Therapeutic Effects:** *Viagra:* Enhanced blood flow to the corpus cavernosum and erection sufficient to allow sexual intercourse. Requires sexual stimulation. *Revatio and Liqrev:* Improved exercise tolerance (or pulmonary hemodynamics) and delayed worsening of disease.

Pharmacokinetics

Absorption: Rapidly absorbed (41%) after oral administration; IV administration results in complete bioavailability.

Distribution: Widely distributed to tissues; negligible amount in semen.

Protein Binding: 96%.

Metabolism and Excretion: Primarily metabolized by the liver via the CYP3A4 isoenzyme; one metabolite is active and accounts for 20% or more of drug effect. Metabolites excreted mostly (80%) in feces; 13% excreted in urine.

Half-life: 4 hr (for sildenafil and active metabolite).

TIME/ACTION PROFILE (vasodilation, ability to produce erection)

ROUTE	ONSET	PEAK	DURATION
PO	within 1 hr	30–120 min	up to 4 hr

Contraindications/Precautions

Contraindicated in: Hypersensitivity; Concurrent use of nitrates or riociguat; Pulmonary veno-occlusive disease.

Use Cautiously in: Serious underlying cardiovascular disease (including history of MI, stroke, or serious arrhythmia within 6 mo), cardiac failure, or coronary artery disease with unstable angina; History of HF, coronary artery disease, uncontrolled hypertension (BP >170/110 mm Hg) or hypotension (BP <90/50 mm Hg), dehydration, autonomic dysfunction, or severe left ventricular outflow obstruction; Pulmonary hypertension secondary to sickle cell anemia (may ↑ risk of vaso-occlusive crises); Concurrent treatment with antihypertensives or glipizide; Renal impairment (CCr <30 mL/min, hepatic impairment; all result in ↑ blood levels; ↓ dose required with Viagra); Anatomic penile deformity (angulation, cavernosal fibrosis, Peyronie disease); Conditions associated with priapism (sickle cell anemia, multiple myeloma, leukemia); Bleeding disorders or active peptic ulceration; History of sudden severe vision loss or at risk for nonarteritic ischemic optic neuropathy (low cup-to-disc ratio in eye, age >50 yr, diabetes, hypertension, coronary artery disease, hyperlipidemia, smoking) (may ↑ risk of recurrence); Retinitis pigmentosa; Alpha adrenergic blockers (patients should be on stable dose of alpha blockers before starting sildenafil); OB: *Revatio and Liqrev:* Use during pregnancy only if potential maternal benefit justifies potential fetal risk; Lactation: *Revatio:* Safety not established; Pedi: *Revatio:* Safety and effectiveness not established in children <1 yr (Revatio); Geri: Older adults may have ↑ levels and may require lower doses.

Adverse Reactions/Side Effects

CV: hypotension, MI, SUDDEN DEATH, vaso-occlusive crises. **Derm:** flushing, rash. **EENT:** epistaxis, hearing loss, nasal congestion, vision loss. **GI:** dyspepsia, diarrhea. **GU:** priapism, urinary tract infection. **MS:** myalgia. **Neuro:** headache, dizziness, insomnia, paresthesia. **Misc:** HYPERSENSITIVITY REACTIONS (INCLUDING ANAPHYLAXIS).

Interactions

Drug-Drug: Concurrent use of **nitrates** may cause serious, life-threatening hypotension and is contraindicated. Concurrent use of **riociguat** may result in severe hypotension; concurrent use contraindicated. **CYP3A4 inhibitors**, including **cimetidine**, **erythromycin**, **tacrolimus**, **ketoconazole**, and **itraconazole**, and **protease inhibitor antiretrovirals**, including **nelfinavir** and **ritonavir**, may ↑ levels and the risk of toxicity, including hypotension (initial dose of sildenafil for ED should be ↓ to 25 mg); concurrent use of strong CYP3A inhibitors not recommended with oral Revatio. ↑ risk of hypotension with **alpha adrenergic blockers** and acute ingestion of **alcohol**. **CYP3A4 inducers**, including **rifampin**, **bosentan**, **barbiturates**, **carbamazepine**, **phenytoin**, **efavirenz**, **nevirapine**, **rifampin**, or **rifabutin**, may ↓ levels and effectiveness; dose adjustments may be necessary in the treatment of PAH. May ↑ levels and the risk of toxicity of **bosentan**. Use cautiously with **glipizide**. May ↑ the risk of bleeding with **warfarin**.

Route/Dosage

Erectile Dysfunction

PO (Adults): *Viagra:* 50 mg taken 1 hr before sexual activity (range 25–100 mg taken 30 min–4 hr before sexual activity); not more than once daily; *Concurrent use of Viagra with alpha-blocker antihypertensives:* Do not use 50–100 mg dose within 4 hr of alpha blocker; 25-mg dose may be taken anytime.

PO (Geriatric Patients ≥65 yr or with concurrent enzyme inhibitors): *Viagra:* 25 mg taken 1 hr before sexual activity (range 25–100 mg taken 30 min–4 hr before sexual activity); not more than once daily.

Hepatic/Renal Impairment

PO (Adults): *Viagra:* 25 mg taken 1 hr before sexual activity (range 25–100 mg taken 30 min–4 hr before sexual activity); not more than once daily.

Pulmonary Arterial Hypertension

IV therapy is indicated for patients unable to take PO therapy

PO (Adults): *Revatio:* 20 mg 3 times daily; may ↑ in 20-mg increments to 80 mg 3 times daily based on clinical response and tolerability.

PO (Children ≥1 yr and >45 kg): *Revatio:* 20 mg 3 times daily; may ↑ to 40 mg 3 times daily based on clinical response and tolerability.

PO (Children ≥1 yr and 21–45 kg): *Revatio:* 20 mg 3 times daily.

PO (Children ≥1 yr and ≤20 kg): *Revatio:* 10 mg 3 times daily.

IV (Adults): *Revatio:* 10 mg 3 times daily.

Availability (generic available)

Tablets (Revatio): 20 mg. **Tablets (Viagra):** 25 mg, 50 mg, 100 mg. **Oral suspension (grape flavor):** 10 mg/mL. **Solution for injection (Revatio):** 0.8 mg/mL.

NURSING IMPLICATIONS

Assessment

- Monitor BP and HR when used concurrently with medications that ↓ BP.
- Monitor for pulmonary edema (shortness of breath, swelling in hands or feet).

S

- **Viagra:** Determine the presence of ED before administration. Sildenafil has no effect in the absence of sexual stimulation.
- **Revatio:** Monitor hemodynamic parameters and exercise tolerance before and periodically during therapy.

Implementation

- Do not confuse Viagra with Allegra.
- **PO:** Dose for *ED* is administered 1 hr before sexual activity. May be administered 30 min–4 hr before sexual activity.
- Dose for *PAH* is administered 3 times daily without regard to food. Doses should be spaced 4–6 hr apart.
- Use syringe provided for accurate dosing of oral suspension. Shake well before using. Store in refrigerator if indicated. Oral suspension is stable for 60 days from date of reconstitution.

IV Administration

- **IV Push: Dilution:** Administer undiluted. Solution is clear and colorless; do not administer solutions that are cloudy, discolored, or contain a precipitate. **Rate:** Administer as a bolus three times daily.
- **Y-Site Incompatibility:** Do not administer other drugs through same IV line.

Patient/Family Teaching

- Explain purpose and side effects of medication to patient. Advise patient to read *Patient Information* before starting therapy. Instruct patient to take as directed. For *ED,* take approximately 1 hr before sexual activity and not more than once per day. For *PAH*, take missed doses as soon as remembered unless almost time for next dose; do not double doses.
- Advise patient to notify health care professional of all Rx or OTC medications, vitamins, or herbal products being taken and to consult health care professional before taking other medications. A review of all current medications and health problems is needed to make sure it is safe to take this drug.
- Advise patient that *Viagra* is not indicated for use in women.
- Caution patient not to take sildenafil concurrently with alpha-adrenergic blockers (unless on a stable dose) or nitrates. If chest pain occurs after taking sildenafil, instruct patient to seek immediate medical attention.
- Instruct patient to notify health care professional promptly if erection lasts >4 hr, or if experiencing sudden or ↓ vision loss in one or both eyes, ↓ or loss in hearing, ringing in the ears, or dizziness.
- Inform patient that sildenafil offers no protection against sexually transmitted diseases. Counsel patient that protection against sexually transmitted diseases and HIV infection should be considered.
- Rep: Advise women of reproductive potential to notify health care professional if pregnancy is planned or suspected or if breastfeeding.

Evaluation/Desired Outcomes

- *Viagra:* Enhanced blood flow to the corpus cavernosum and erection sufficient to allow sexual intercourse. Requires sexual stimulation.
- *Revatio:* Improved exercise tolerance (or pulmonary hemodynamics) and delayed worsening of disease.

silodosin (si-lo-do-sin)

~~Rapaflo~~

Classification

Therapeutic: benign prostatic hyperplasia (BPH) agents

Pharmacologic: alpha-adrenergic blockers

Indications

Benign prostatic hyperplasia (BPH).

Action

Blocks postsynaptic alpha$_1$-adrenergic receptors. Decreases contractions in the smooth muscle of the prostatic capsule. **Therapeutic Effects:** Decreased signs and symptoms of BPH (urinary urgency, hesitancy, nocturia).

Pharmacokinetics

Absorption: 32% absorbed following oral administration.

Distribution: Well distributed to tissues.

Protein Binding: 97%.

Metabolism and Excretion: Extensively metabolized by the liver by the CYP3A4 isoenzyme, UGT2B7, and other metabolic pathways; 33.5% excreted in urine and 54.9% in feces.

Half-life: 13.3 hr.

TIME/ACTION PROFILE (↓ in BPH symptoms)

ROUTE	ONSET	PEAK	DURATION
PO	rapid	24 hr	24 hr*

* Following discontinuation.

Contraindications/Precautions

Contraindicated in: Hypersensitivity; Concurrent use of strong CYP3A4 inhibitors. Severe renal impairment; Severe hepatic impairment;

Use Cautiously in: Cataract surgery (may cause intraoperative floppy iris syndrome); Moderate renal impairment (↓ dose); Geri: ↑ risk of orthostatic hypotension in older adults; Pedi: Safety and effectiveness not established in children.

Adverse Reactions/Side Effects

CV: orthostatic hypotension. **Derm:** pruritus, rash, urticaria. **GI:** diarrhea. **GU:** retrograde ejaculation. **Neuro:** dizziness, headache. **Misc:** allergic reactions.

Interactions

Drug-Drug: Strong CYP3A4 inhibitors, including **ketoconazole**, **clarithromycin**, **itraconazole**, and **ritonavir**, significantly ↑ levels and risk of toxicity; concurrent use contraindicated. **Moderate CYP3A4 inhibitors**, including **diltiazem**, **erythromycin**, and **verapamil**, may ↑ levels and risk of toxicity; use cautiously. Concurrent use with **antihypertensives** (including **calcium channel blockers** and **thiazide diuretics**), other **alpha blockers**, and **PDE-5 inhibitors** (including **sildenafil**, **tadalafil**, and **vardenafil**) ↑ the risk of dizziness and orthostatic hypotension. **P-glycoprotein inhibitors**, including **cyclosporine**, may ↑ levels and risk of toxicity; concurrent use not recommended.

Route/Dosage

PO (Adults): 8 mg once daily.

Renal Impairment

PO (Adults): *CCr 30–50 mL/min:* 4 mg once daily.

Availability (generic available)

Capsules: 4 mg, 8 mg.

NURSING IMPLICATIONS

Assessment

- Assess for signs/symptoms of BPH (urinary hesitancy, feeling of incomplete bladder emptying, interruption of urinary stream, impairment of size and force of urinary stream, terminal urinary dribbling, straining to start flow, dysuria, urgency) before and periodically during therapy.
- Assess for 1st-dose orthostatic hypotension and syncope. Monitor BP (lying and standing) during initial therapy and periodically thereafter. Observe patient closely during this period and take precautions to prevent injury.
- Monitor intake, output, and daily weight, and assess for edema daily, especially at beginning of therapy. Report weight gain or edema.
- Rectal exams before starting and periodically throughout therapy to assess prostate size are recommended.
- Rule out prostate cancer before initiating therapy; symptoms are similar.

Implementation

- ***High Alert:*** Do not confuse silodosin with sirolimus.
- **PO:** Administer with food at the same time each day.
- If unable to swallow capsule, may open capsule and sprinkle powder inside on a tablespoonful of applesauce. Swallow immediately, within 5 min, without chewing; follow with 8 ounces of cool water to ensure complete dose is swallowed. Use cool applesauce, soft enough to be swallowed without chewing. Do not store for future use or subdivide capsule contents.

Patient/Family Teaching

- Explain the purpose and side effects of silodosin. Instruct to take as directed with the same meal each day. Emphasize the importance of continuing to take this medication, even if feeling well. If a dose is missed, take as soon as remembered unless almost time for next dose. Do not double doses. Advise patient to read *Patient Information* before starting therapy and with each Rx refill in case of changes.
- Emphasize the importance of follow-up exams to evaluate effectiveness of medication.
- May cause dizziness. Caution patient to avoid driving or other activities requiring alertness until response to the medication is known.
- Caution patient to avoid sudden changes in position to ↓ orthostatic hypotension, especially patients with low BP or concurrently taking antihypertensives. Geri: Assess risk for falls; instruct patient and family in preventing falls at home.
- Instruct patient to notify health care provider of all Rx or OTC medications, vitamins, or herbal products being taken and consult health care provider before taking any new medications, especially cough, cold, or allergy remedies.
- Instruct patient to notify health care provider of medication regimen before any surgery. Patients planning cataract surgery should notify ophthalmologist of silodosin therapy prior to surgery.

Evaluation/Desired Outcomes

- Decreased symptoms of BPH (urinary urgency, hesitancy, nocturia).

S

simethicone (si-meth-i-kone)

Degas, Extra Strength Gas-X, Flatulex, ✱ Gas Relief, Gas-X, Genasyme, ✱ Infacol, Maximum Strength Mylanta Gas, Mylanta Gas, Mylicon, ✱ Ovol, ✱ Pediacol, Phazyme

Classification

Therapeutic: antiflatulent

Indications

Relief of painful symptoms of excess gas in the GI tract.

Action

Causes the coalescence of gas bubbles. Does not prevent the formation of gas. **Therapeutic Effects:** Passage of gas through the GI tract by belching or passing flatus.

Pharmacokinetics

Absorption: No systemic absorption occurs.
Distribution: Not systemically distributed.

Metabolism and Excretion: Excreted unchanged in the feces.
Half-life: Unknown.

TIME/ACTION PROFILE (antiflatulent effect)

ROUTE	ONSET	PEAK	DURATION
PO	immediate	unknown	3 hr

Contraindications/Precautions
Contraindicated in: Not recommended for infant colic.
Use Cautiously in: Abdominal pain of unknown cause, especially when accompanied by fever.

Adverse Reactions/Side Effects
None significant.

Interactions
Drug-Drug: None reported.

Route/Dosage
PO (Adults): 40–125 mg 4 times daily, after meals and at bedtime (up to 500 mg/day).
PO (Children 2–12 yr): 40 mg 4 times daily.
PO (Children <2 yr): 20 mg 4 times daily (up to 240 mg/day).

Availability (generic available)
Chewable tablets: 40 mg[OTC], 80 mg[OTC], 125 mg[OTC], 150 mg[OTC]. **Tablets:** 60 mg[OTC], 80 mg[OTC], 95 mg[OTC]. **Capsules:** 125 mg[OTC] 🍁 166 mg[OTC], 180 mg[OTC], 250 mg[OTC]. **Drops:** 40 mg/0.6 mL[OTC], 🍁 40 mg/mL[OTC], 🍁 95 mg/1.425 mL[OTC]. ***In combination with:*** antacids[OTC]. See Appendix N.

NURSING IMPLICATIONS
Assessment
- Assess for abdominal pain, distention, bowel sounds, and frequency of belching and flatus before starting and periodically throughout course of therapy.

Implementation
- **PO:** Administer after meals and at bedtime. Shake liquid preparation well before administration. Chewable tablets should be chewed thoroughly before swallowing for faster and more complete absorption.
- Drops can be mixed with 30 mL of cool water, infant formula, or other liquid as directed. Shake well before using.

Patient/Family Teaching
- Explain purpose and side effects of medication, and the importance of diet and exercise in gas prevention. Advise patient to read *Patient Information* before starting therapy.
- Advise patient to notify health care provider if symptoms persist.
- Advise patient to notify health care provider of all Rx or OTC medications, vitamins, or herbal products being taken and to consult health care provider before taking other medications.

Evaluation/Desired Outcomes
- Decrease in abdominal distention and discomfort.

---

simvastatin, See HMG-CoA REDUCTASE INHIBITORS (statins).

---

sirolimus (conventional)
(sir-**oh**-li-mus)
Rapamune

Classification
Therapeutic: immunosuppressants

Indications
Prevention of organ rejection in kidney transplantation (in combination with corticosteroids and cyclosporine). Lymphangioleiomyomatosis.

Action
Inhibits T-lymphocyte activation/proliferation, which occurs as a response to antigenic and cytokine stimulation; antibody production is also inhibited. **Therapeutic Effects:** Decreased incidence and severity of organ rejection. Improvement in pulmonary function in lymphangioleiomyomatosis.

Pharmacokinetics
Absorption: 14% absorbed following oral administration.
Distribution: Concentrates in erythrocytes; distributes to heart, intestines, kidneys, liver, lungs, muscle, spleen, and testes in high concentrations.
Protein Binding: 92%.
Metabolism and Excretion: Extensively metabolized in the liver via the CYP3A4 isoenzyme; 91% excreted in feces.
Half-life: 62 hr.

TIME/ACTION PROFILE (plasma concentrations)

ROUTE	ONSET	PEAK	DURATION
PO	rapid	1–2 hr	24 hr

Contraindications/Precautions
Contraindicated in: Hypersensitivity; Alcohol intolerance/sensitivity (solution contains ethanol); Liver or lung transplant patients; Severe hepatic impairment; OB: Pregnancy.
Use Cautiously in: Mild or moderate hepatic impairment; Lactation: Use while breastfeeding only if the potential maternal benefit justifies the potential risk to the infant; Rep: Women of reproductive potential; Pedi: Children <13 yr (safety and effectiveness not established).

Adverse Reactions/Side Effects

Reflects combined therapy with corticosteroids and cyclosporine

CV: edema, hypotension, pericardial effusion. **Derm:** acne, rash, ↓ wound healing, thrombocytopenic purpura. **Endo:** hyperglycemia. **F and E:** hypokalemia. **GI:** ascites, hepatotoxicity. **GU:** amenorrhea, infertility (men), menorrhagia, ovarian cysts, renal impairment. **Hemat:** leukopenia, thrombocytopenia, anemia. **Metab:** hypercholesterolemia, hypertriglyceridemia. **MS:** arthralgia. **Neuro:** insomnia, tremor, PROGRESSIVE MULTIFOCAL LEUKOENCEPHALOPATHY (PML). **Resp:** INTERSTITIAL LUNG DISEASE (ILD), PULMONARY HYPERTENSION. **Misc:** ANGIOEDEMA, INFECTION (INCLUDING ACTIVATION OF LATENT VIRAL INFECTIONS SUCH AS BK VIRUS–ASSOCIATED NEPHROPATHY AND CLOSTRIDIOIDES DIFFICILE-ASSOCIATED DIARRHEA), lymphocele, LYMPHOMA.

Interactions

Drug-Drug: Cyclosporine (modified) significantly ↑ levels and risk of toxicity; administer sirolimus 4 hr after cyclosporine. **Strong CYP3A4 inhibitors**, including **ketoconazole**, **voriconazole**, **itraconazole**, **clarithromycin**, and **erythromycin**, may ↑ levels and risk of toxicity; avoid concurrent use. **Diltiazem**, **verapamil**, **nicardipine**, **clotrimazole**, **fluconazole**, **metoclopramide**, **cimetidine**, **danazol**, **letermovir**, and **protease inhibitors** may ↑ levels and risk of toxicity; monitor sirolimus levels and adjust dose as necessary. **Strong CYP3A4 inducers**, including **rifampin** and **rifabutin**, may ↓ levels and effectiveness; avoid concurrent use. **Carbamazepine**, **phenobarbital**, **phenytoin**, and **rifapentine** may ↓ levels and effectiveness. Risk of renal impairment may be ↑ by concurrent use of other **nephrotoxic agents**. Concurrent use with **tacrolimus** and **corticosteroids** in lung transplantation may ↑ risk of anastomotic dehiscence; fatalities have been reported; not approved for this use. Concurrent use with **tacrolimus** and **corticosteroids** in liver transplantation may ↑ risk of hepatic artery thrombosis; fatalities have been reported; not approved for this use. **ACE inhibitors** may ↑ risk of angioedema. May ↓ antibody response to and ↑ risk of adverse reactions to **live-virus vaccines**; avoid vaccination. May ↑ levels and risk of toxicity of **verapamil**. **Cannabidiol** may ↑ levels and risk of toxicity; monitor sirolimus levels and adjust dose as necessary.

Drug-Natural Products: Echinacea and **melatonin** may interfere with immunosuppression. **St. John's wort** may ↓ levels and effectiveness.

Drug-Food: Grapefruit juice may ↑ levels and risk of toxicity; avoid concurrent ingestion.

Route/Dosage

Kidney Transplantation

PO (Adults and Children ≥13 yr and ≥40 kg): 6 mg loading dose, followed by 2 mg/day maintenance dose. *Dosing following cyclosporine withdrawal:* Patients at low to moderate risk for rejection after transplantation may be withdrawn from cyclosporine over 4–8 wk beginning 2–4 mo after transplant. Thereafter, sirolimus dose should be titrated upward to maintain a whole blood trough level of 12–14 ng/mL. Clinical assessment should also be used to gauge dose. Dose changes can be made at 7–14 day intervals. The following formula may also be used: sirolimus maintenance dose = current dose × (target concentration/current concentration). If a large ↑ is needed, a loading dose may be given and blood levels reassessed 3–4 days later. Loading dose may be calculated by the following formula: sirolimus loading dose = 3 × (new maintenance dose − current maintenance dose). Loading doses >40 mg should be spread over 2 days.

PO (Adults and Children ≥13 yr and <40 kg): 3 mg/m² loading dose, followed by 1 mg/m²/day maintenance dose. *Dosing following cyclosporine withdrawal:* Patients at low to moderate risk for rejection after transplantation may be withdrawn from cyclosporine over 4–8 wk beginning 2–4 mo after transplant. Thereafter, sirolimus dose should be titrated upward to maintain a whole blood trough level of 12–14 ng/mL. Clinical assessment should also be used to gauge dose. Dose changes can be made at 7–14 day intervals. The following formula may also be used: sirolimus maintenance dose = current dose × (target concentration/current concentration). If a large ↑ is needed, a loading dose may be given and blood levels reassessed 3–4 days later. Loading dose may be calculated by the following formula: sirolimus loading dose = 3 × (new maintenance dose − current maintenance dose). Loading doses >40 mg should be spread over 2 days.

Hepatic Impairment

PO (Adults and Children): *Mild or moderate hepatic impairment:* ↓ maintenance dose by 33%; loading dose is unchanged; *Severe hepatic impairment:* ↓ maintenance dose by 50%; loading dose is unchanged.

Lymphangioleiomyomatosis

PO (Adults): 2 mg once daily. Monitor whole blood trough level in 10–20 days and titrate dose to maintain level of 5–15 ng/mL. The following formula may also be used to adjust dose: sirolimus maintenance dose = current dose × (target concentration/current concentration). Further dose changes can be made at 7–14 day intervals. Once stable dose achieved, should monitor whole blood trough levels at least every 3 mo.

S

Hepatic Impairment

(Adults): *Mild or moderate hepatic impairment:* ↓ dose by 33%; *Severe hepatic impairment:* ↓ dose by 50%.

Availability (generic available)

Oral solution (contains alcohol): 1 mg/mL. **Tablet:** 0.5 mg, 1 mg, 2 mg.

NURSING IMPLICATIONS

Assessment

- Monitor BP closely during therapy. Hypertension is a common complication of sirolimus therapy and should be treated.
- Assess for any new neurological signs or symptoms that may be suggestive of PML. *If symptoms occur,* withhold dose and consult with neurologist. Consider ↓ amount of immunosuppression in patients.
- Monitor for signs and symptoms of lymphangioleiomyomatosis and ILD (wheezing; cough, which may be bloody; shortness of breath; chest pain; pneumothorax; pneumonitis) periodically during therapy.

Lab Test Considerations

- Monitor sirolimus blood levels when dose formulations are changed and in patients likely to have altered drug metabolism, patients ≥13 yr who weigh <40 kg, patients with hepatic impairment, and during concurrent administration of drugs that may interact with sirolimus. Trough concentrations ≥15 ng/mL are associated with an ↑ in adverse effects.
- Monitor lipid panel for hyperlipidemia. Provide appropriate medical intervention as indicated.
- May cause anemia, leukopenia, thrombocytopenia, and hypokalemia.
- May cause ↑ AST, ↑ ALT, hypophosphatemia, and hyperglycemia.
- Monitor renal function, including for proteinuria and serum creatinine, especially with coadministration of sirolimus and cyclosporine or other nephrotoxic medications. *If ↑ serum creatinine occurs,* consider discontinuing sirolimus or other nephrotoxic medications.

Implementation

- Do not confuse Rapamune with Rapaflo or sirolimus with silodosin.
- Only physicians experienced in immunosuppressive therapy and management of renal transplant patients should use sirolimus for prophylaxis of organ rejection in patients receiving renal transplants.
- Therapy with sirolimus should be started as soon as possible post-transplant. Concurrent therapy with cyclosporine and corticosteroids is recommended. Sirolimus should be taken 4 hr after cyclosporine.
- **PO:** Administer consistently with or without food. ***DNC:*** Swallow tablet whole; do not crush, break, or chew. Do not administer with or mix with grapefruit juice.
- For oral solution, use amber oral syringe to withdraw prescribed amount from bottle. Empty sirolimus from syringe into a glass or plastic container holding ≥2 ounces (60 mL) of water or orange juice; do not use other liquids. Stir vigorously and drink at once. Refill container with ≥4 ounces of additional liquid, stir vigorously, and drink at once.
- Store bottles in refrigerator. Protect from light. Solution may develop a slight haze when refrigerated; allow to stand at room temperature and shake gently until haze disappears. Sirolimus may remain in syringe at room temperature or refrigerated for up to 24 hr. Discard syringe after one use. Oral solution must be used within 1 mo of opening bottle.

Patient/Family Teaching

- Instruct patient to take sirolimus at the same time each day as directed. Do not skip or double up on missed doses. Do not discontinue medication without advice of health care provider.
- Advise patient to avoid grapefruit and grapefruit juice during therapy.
- Explain purpose and side effects of medication, reinforcing the need for lifelong therapy to prevent transplant rejection. Review symptoms of rejection for transplanted organ and stress need to notify health care provider immediately if they occur. Advise patient to read *Patient Information* before starting therapy.
- Advise patient to notify health care provider if swelling of face, eyes, or mouth; trouble breathing or wheezing; throat tightness; chest pain or tightness; dizziness; rash or peeling of skin; swelling of hands or feet; or symptoms of PML (hemiparesis, apathy, confusion, cognitive deficiencies, ataxia) occur.
- Advise patient to wear sunscreen and protective clothing and limit time in sunlight and UV light due to ↑ risk of skin cancer.
- Caution patient to notify health care provider if signs of infection or delayed wound healing occur.
- Advise patient to avoid vaccinations with a live virus during therapy; sirolimus may ↓ vaccine effectiveness.
- Rep: May cause fetal harm. Advise women of reproductive potential to notify health care provider if pregnancy is planned or suspected or if breastfeeding. Advise women of reproductive potential to use effective contraception prior to, during, and for 12 wk following therapy. May cause male and female infertility.
- Emphasize the importance of repeated lab tests during sirolimus therapy.

Evaluation/Desired Outcomes

- Prevention of transplanted kidney rejection.
- Reduction in symptoms of lymphangioleiomyomatosis.

SITagliptin (sit-a-glip-tin)

Brynovin, Januvia, Zituvio

Classification

Therapeutic: antidiabetics

Pharmacologic: enzyme inhibitors

Indications

Type 2 diabetes mellitus (as an adjunct to diet and exercise).

Action

Inhibits the enzyme dipeptidyl peptidase-4 (DPP-4), which slows the inactivation of incretin hormones, resulting in increased levels of active incretin hormones. These hormones are released by the intestine throughout the day and are involved in regulation of glucose homeostasis. Increased/prolonged incretin levels result in an increase in insulin release and decrease in glucagon levels. **Therapeutic Effects:** Improved control of blood glucose.

Pharmacokinetics

Absorption: 87% absorbed following oral administration.

Distribution: Extensively distributed to tissues.

Metabolism and Excretion: Undergoes minor metabolism by the liver via the CYP3A4 and CYP2C8 isoenzymes to inactive metabolites; 87% excreted in the urine (79% as unchanged drug), with 13% excreted in the feces.

Half-life: 12.4 hr.

TIME/ACTION PROFILE (plasma concentrations)

ROUTE	ONSET	PEAK	DURATION
PO	rapid	1–4 hr	24 hr

Contraindications/Precautions

Contraindicated in: Hypersensitivity; Type 1 diabetes mellitus.

Use Cautiously in: Renal impairment (↓ dose if CCr <45 mL/min); History of pancreatitis; History of angioedema to another DPP-4 inhibitor; History of HF or renal impairment (↑ risk of HF); OB: Safety not established in pregnancy; Lactation: Safety not established in breastfeeding; Pedi: Safety and effectiveness not established in children; Geri: Consider age-related ↓ in renal function when determining dose in older adults.

Adverse Reactions/Side Effects

CV: HF. **Derm:** bullous pemphigoid, rash, STEVENS-JOHNSON SYNDROME (SJS), urticaria. **EENT:** nasopharyngitis. **GI:** diarrhea, nausea, PANCREATITIS. **GU:** acute renal failure. **MS:** arthralgia, back pain, myalgia, RHABDOMYOLYSIS. **Neuro:** headache. **Resp:** upper respiratory tract infection. **Misc:** HYPERSENSITIVITY REACTIONS (INCLUDING ANAPHYLAXIS AND ANGIOEDEMA).

Interactions

Drug-Drug: May slightly ↑ levels of **digoxin**; monitoring recommended. ↑ risk of hypoglycemia when used with **insulin**, **glyburide**, **glipizide**, or **glimepiride**; may need to ↓ dose of insulin or sulfonylurea.

Route/Dosage

PO (Adults): 100 mg once daily.

Renal Impairment

PO (Adults): *CCr 30–<45 mL/min:* 50 mg once daily; *CCr <30 mL/min, hemodialysis, or peritoneal dialysis:* 25 mg once daily.

Availability (generic available)

Tablets: 25 mg, 50 mg, 100 mg. **Oral solution:** 25 mg/mL. ***In combination with:*** ertugliflozin (Steglujan); metformin (Janumet, Zituvimet); metformin XR (Janumet XR, Zituvimet XR). See Appendix N.

NURSING IMPLICATIONS

Assessment

- Observe for signs/symptoms of hypoglycemia (abdominal pain, sweating, hunger, weakness, dizziness, headache, tremor, tachycardia, anxiety).
- Monitor for signs/symptoms of pancreatitis (nausea; vomiting; anorexia; persistent, severe abdominal pain, sometimes radiating to the back) during therapy. *If pancreatitis occurs,* discontinue sitagliptin and monitor serum and urine amylase, amylase/CCr ratio, electrolytes, serum calcium, glucose, and lipase.
- Assess for rash periodically during therapy. May cause SJS. *If severe skin reaction occurs or if accompanied by fever, general malaise, fatigue, muscle or joint aches, blisters, oral lesions, conjunctivitis, hepatitis, or eosinophilia,* discontinue sitagliptin.

Lab Test Considerations

- Monitor A1c before starting and periodically during therapy.
- Monitor renal function before starting and periodically during therapy.

Implementation

- Do not confuse sitagliptin with saxagliptin or sumatriptan. Do not confuse Januvia with Jantoven or Janumet.
- Patients stabilized on a diabetic regimen who are exposed to stress, fever, trauma, infection, or surgery may require administration of insulin.
- **PO:** May be administered once daily without regard to food.

S

- For the oral solution, measure the dose using a calibrated oral syringe or oral dosing cup that is scored.

Patient/Family Teaching

- Instruct patient to take sitagliptin as directed. Take missed doses as soon as remembered, unless it is almost time for next dose; do not double doses. Advise patient to read the *Medication Guide* before starting and with each Rx refill in case of changes.
- Explain to patient that sitagliptin helps control hyperglycemia but does not cure diabetes. Therapy is usually long term.
- Encourage patient to follow prescribed diet, medication, and exercise regimen to prevent hyperglycemic or hypoglycemic episodes.
- Review signs/symptoms of hypoglycemia (sweating, hunger, dizziness, ↑ HR, irritability, confusion, seizures) and hyperglycemia (thirst, hunger, frequent urination, fatigue, blurred vision) with patient. Advise patient to carry a form of sugar and identification describing disease process and medication regimen at all times. *If hypoglycemia occurs,* advise patient to take a glass of orange juice or 2–3 teaspoons of sugar, honey, or corn syrup dissolved in water and notify health care provider.
- Instruct patient in proper testing of blood glucose and urine ketones. These tests should be monitored closely during periods of stress or illness, and health care provider notified if significant changes occur.
- Advise patient to stop taking sitagliptin and notify health care provider promptly if signs/symptoms of hypersensitivity reactions (rash; hives; swelling of face, lips, tongue, and throat; difficulty in breathing or swallowing), pancreatitis (nausea; vomiting; anorexia; persistent, severe abdominal pain, sometimes radiating to the back), or HF (fatigue, ↑ HR, difficulty breathing with exercise, swelling in legs and feet) occur.
- Instruct patient to notify health care provider if new or worsening arthritis, blisters, or erosions occur.
- Advise patient to notify health care provider of all Rx or OTC medications, vitamins, or herbal products being taken and to consult with health care provider before taking other medications.
- Advise women of reproductive potential to notify health care provider if pregnancy is planned or suspected or if breastfeeding.

Evaluation/Desired Outcomes

- Improved A1c, fasting plasma glucose, and 2-hr postprandial glucose levels.

V sodium bicarbonate

(**soe**-dee-um bye-**kar**-boe-nate)

Classification

Therapeutic: antiulcer agents

Pharmacologic: alkalinizing agents

Indications

PO, IV: Treatment of the following conditions: Metabolic acidosis. To alkalinize urine and promote excretion of certain drugs in overdose situations. **PO:** Antacid. **Unlabeled Use:** Stabilization of acid-base status in cardiac arrest and treatment of life-threatening hyperkalemia.

Action

Acts as an alkalinizing agent by releasing bicarbonate ions. Following oral administration, releases bicarbonate, which is capable of neutralizing gastric acid. **Therapeutic Effects:** Alkalinization. Neutralization of gastric acid.

Pharmacokinetics

Absorption: Following oral administration, excess bicarbonate is absorbed, resulting in metabolic alkalosis and alkaline urine. IV administration results in complete bioavailability.
Distribution: Widely distributed into extracellular fluid.
Metabolism and Excretion: Sodium and bicarbonate are excreted by the kidneys.
Half-life: Unknown.

TIME/ACTION PROFILE (PO = antacid effect; IV = alkalinization)

ROUTE	ONSET	PEAK	DURATION
PO	immediate	30 min	1–3 hr
IV	immediate	rapid	unknown

Contraindications/Precautions

Contraindicated in: Metabolic or respiratory alkalosis; Hypocalcemia; Hypernatremia; Excessive chloride loss; As an antidote following ingestion of strong mineral acids; Patients on sodium-restricted diets (oral use as an antacid only); Renal failure (oral use as an antacid only); Severe abdominal pain of unknown cause, especially if associated with fever (oral use as an antacid only).
Use Cautiously in: HF; Renal impairment; Concurrent corticosteroid therapy; Chronic use as an antacid (may cause metabolic alkalosis and possible sodium overload); Pedi: May ↑ risk of cerebral edema in children with diabetic ketoacidosis.

Adverse Reactions/Side Effects

CV: edema. **F and E:** metabolic alkalosis, hypernatremia, hypocalcemia, hypokalemia. **GI: PO:** flatulence, gastric distention. **Local:** irritation at IV site. **Neuro:** cerebral hemorrhage (with rapid injection in infants), tetany.

Interactions

Drug-Drug: Following oral administration, may ↓ absorption of **ketoconazole**. **Calcium-containing antacids** may lead to milk-alkali syndrome. Urinary alkalinization may result in ↓ **salicylate** or **barbiturate** levels; ↑ blood levels of **quinidine**, **mexiletine**,

flecainide, or **amphetamines**; ↑ risk of crystalluria from **fluoroquinolones**; ↓ effectiveness of **methenamine**. May negate the protective effects of **enteric-coated products**; do not administer within 1–2 hr of each other.

Route/Dosage

Contains 12 mEq of sodium/g.

Alkalinization of Urine

PO (Adults): 48 mEq (4 g) initially, then 12–24 mEq (1–2 g) every 4 hr (up to 48 mEq every 4 hr) or 1 teaspoon of powder every 4 hr as needed.
PO (Children): 1–10 mEq/kg/day (84–840 mg/kg/day) in divided doses.
IV (Adults and Children): 2–5 mEq/kg as a 4–8-hr infusion.

Antacid

PO (Adults): *Tablets/powder:* 325 mg–2 g 1–4 times daily or ½ teaspoon every 2 hr as needed. *Effervescent powder:* 3.9–10 g in water after meals; patients >60 yr should receive 1.9–3.9 g after meals.

Systemic Alkalinization/Cardiac Arrest

IV (Adults and Children and Infants): *Cardiac arrest/urgent situations:* 1 mEq/kg; may repeat 0.5 mEq/kg every 10 min. *Less urgent situations:* 2–5 mEq/kg as a 4–8-hr infusion.

Renal Tubular Acidosis

PO (Adults): 0.5–2 mEq/kg/day in 4–5 divided doses.
PO (Children): 2–3 mEq/kg/day in 3–4 divided doses.

Availability (generic available)

Oral powder: (20.9 mEq Na/ ½ teaspoon) in 120-, 240-, 480-, and 2400-g containers[OTC]. **Tablets:** 325 mg (3.9 mEq Na/tablet)[OTC], 🍁 500 mg (6.0 mEq Na/tablet[OTC], 650 mg (7.7 mEq Na/tablet)[OTC]. **Solution for injection:** 4.2% (0.5 mEq/mL), 8.4% (1 mEq/mL).

NURSING IMPLICATIONS

Assessment

- Assess fluid balance (intake, output, daily weight, edema, lung sounds) throughout therapy. Report symptoms of fluid overload (hypertension, edema, dyspnea, rales/crackles, frothy sputum) if they occur.
- Assess patient for signs of acidosis (disorientation, headache, weakness, dyspnea, hyperventilation), alkalosis (confusion, irritability, paresthesia, tetany, altered breathing pattern), hypernatremia (edema, weight gain, hypertension, tachycardia, fever, flushed skin, mental irritability), or hypokalemia (weakness, fatigue, U wave on ECG, arrhythmias, polyuria, polydipsia) throughout therapy.
- **Antacid:** Assess patient for epigastric or abdominal pain and frank or occult blood in the stool, emesis, or gastric aspirate.

Lab Test Considerations

- Monitor sodium, potassium, calcium, bicarbonate concentrations, serum osmolarity, acid-base balance, and renal function prior to and periodically throughout therapy.
- Obtain arterial blood gases frequently in emergency situations and during parenteral therapy.
- Monitor urine pH frequently when used for urinary alkalinization.
- Antagonizes effects of pentagastrin and histamine during gastric acid secretion test. Avoid administration during the 24 hr preceding the test.

Implementation

- May cause premature dissolution of enteric-coated tablets in the stomach.
- **PO:** Tablets must be taken with a full glass of water.
- When used in treatment of peptic ulcers, may be administered 1 and 3 hr after meals and at bedtime.

IV Administration

- **V** IV sodium bicarbonate at concentrations ≥4.2% is a vesicant. If extravasation occurs, immediately stop infusion. Leave needle/cannula in place temporarily but do not flush the line. Gently aspirate extravasated solution; then remove needle/cannula. Elevate patient's extremity and apply dry warm compresses. Initiate hyaluronidase antidote for refractory cases in addition to supportive management. For hyaluronidase, inject a total of 1 mL (150 units/mL) intradermally or SUBQ as five separate 0.2-mL injections (using a tuberculin syringe) around the site of extravasation; if IV catheter remains in place, administer IV through the infiltrated catheter; may repeat in 30–60 min if no resolution.
- **IV Push:** Used in cardiac arrest or urgent situations.
- **Dilution:** Use premeasured ampules or prefilled syringes to ensure accurate dose. **Rate:** Administer by rapid bolus. Flush IV line before and after administration to prevent incompatible medications used in arrest management from precipitating.
- **Continuous Infusion: Dilution:** May be diluted in dextrose, saline, and dextrose/saline combinations. Premixed infusions are already diluted and ready to use.
- **Rate:** May be administered over 4–8 hr.
- **Y-Site Compatibility:** acyclovir, alemtuzumab, amikacin, aminophylline, argatroban, arsenic trioxide, ascorbic acid, atropine, azithromycin, aztreonam, benztropine, bivalirudin, bleomycin, bumetanide, caffeine citrate, cangrelor, carboplatin, carmustine, cefazolin, cefepime, ceftaroline, ceftazidime, ceftobiprole, ceftolozane/tazobactam, ceftriaxone, chloramphenicol, cisplatin, cladribine, clindamycin, cyanocobalamin, cyclophosphamide, cyclosporine, cytarabine,

S

dacarbazine, daptomycin, daunorubicin, dexamethasone, dexmedetomidine, dexrazoxane, digoxin, docetaxel, enalaprilat, ephedrine, epoetin alfa, eptifibatide, ertapenem, erythromycin, esmolol, etoposide, etoposide phosphate, famotidine, fentanyl, filgrastim, fluconazole, fludarabine, fluorouracil, folic acid, foscarnet, fosphenytoin, furosemide, gemcitabine, gemtuzumab ozogamicin, gentamicin, glycopyrrolate, granisetron, heparin, hydrocortisone, ibuprofen lysine, ifosfamide, indomethacin, insulin regular, irinotecan, ketorolac, labetalol, levofloxacin, lidocaine, linezolid, lorazepam, magnesium sulfate, mannitol, melphalan, meropenem, meropenem/vaborbactam, mesna, methadone, methotrexate, methylprednisolone, metoclopramide, metoprolol, metronidazole, milrinone, mitomycin, mitoxantrone, morphine, moxifloxacin, multivitamins, nafcillin, naloxone, nitroglycerin, nitroprusside, octreotide, oxaliplatin, oxytocin, paclitaxel, palonosetron, pamidronate, pantoprazole, pemetrexed, penicillin G, pentobarbital, phenobarbital, phentolamine, phenylephrine, phytonadione, piperacillin/tazobactam, plazomicin, potassium acetate, potassium chloride, procainamide, propofol, propranolol, protamine, pyridoxine, remifentanil, rocuronium, sodium acetate, sufentanil, tacrolimus, thiotepa, tigecycline, tirofiban, tobramycin, trastuzumab, vancomycin, vasopressin, vecuronium, vinblastine, voriconazole, zoledronic acid.

- **Y-Site Incompatibility:** allopurinol, amiodarone, amphotericin B deoxycholate, amphotericin B liposomal, ampicillin, anidulafungin, atracurium, azathioprine, buprenorphine, butorphanol, calcium chloride, calcium gluconate, caspofungin, cefotaxime, cefotetan, cefoxitin, cefuroxime, chlorpromazine, dantrolene, diazepam, diazoxide, dimenhydrinate, diphenhydramine, dobutamine, dopamine, doxorubicin liposomal, doxycycline, epinephrine, epirubicin, eravacycline, ganciclovir, haloperidol, idarubicin, imipenem/cilastatin, isavuconazonium, isoproterenol, ketamine, leucovorin, meperidine, midazolam, mycophenolate, nalbuphine, nicardipine, norepinephrine, ondansetron, papaverine, pentamidine, phenytoin, prochlorperazine, promethazine, rituximab, sargramostim, succinylcholine, thiamine, topotecan, trimethoprim/sulfamethoxazole, verapamil, vincristine, vinorelbine.

Patient/Family Teaching

- Explain the purpose and side effects of sodium bicarbonate. Instruct patient to take medication as directed. Take missed doses as soon as remembered unless almost time for next dose. Advise patient to read *Medication Guide* before starting and periodically during therapy in case of changes.
- **Antacid:** Advise patient to avoid routine use of sodium bicarbonate for indigestion. Dyspepsia that persists >2 wk should be evaluated by a health care provider.
- Emphasize the importance of regular follow-up examinations to monitor serum electrolyte levels and acid-base balance and to monitor progress.
- Review symptoms of electrolyte imbalance with patients on chronic therapy; instruct patient to notify health care provider if these symptoms occur.
- Advise patient not to take milk products concurrently with this medication. Renal calculi or hypercalcemia (milk-alkali syndrome) may result.
- Advise patient on sodium-restricted diet to avoid use of baking soda as a home remedy for indigestion.
- Instruct patient to notify health care provider if indigestion is accompanied by chest pain, difficulty breathing, or diaphoresis or if stools become dark and tarry.
- Advise patient to notify health care provider of all Rx or OTC medications, vitamins, or herbal products being taken and to consult with health care provider before taking other medications.
- Rep: Advise women of reproductive potential to notify health care provider if pregnancy is planned or suspected or if breastfeeding. Frequent use of sodium bicarbonate as an antacid may result in metabolic alkalosis and fluid overload in both mother and fetus.

Evaluation/Desired Outcomes

- Increase in urinary pH.
- Clinical improvement of acidosis.
- Enhanced excretion of selected overdoses and poisonings.
- Decreased gastric discomfort.

sodium polystyrene sulfonate
(**soe**-dee-um po-lee-**stye**-reen **sul**-fon-ate)

Kayexalate, Kionex, SPS

Classification
Therapeutic: hypokalemic, electrolyte modifiers
Pharmacologic: cationic exchange resins

Indications

Mild to moderate hyperkalemia (if severe, more immediate measures such as sodium bicarbonate IV, calcium, or glucose/insulin infusion should be instituted).

Action

Exchanges sodium ions for potassium ions in the intestine (each 1 g is exchanged for 1 mEq potassium). **Therapeutic Effects:** Reduction of serum potassium concentrations.

Pharmacokinetics

Absorption: Distributed throughout the intestine but is nonabsorbable.
Distribution: Not distributed.
Metabolism and Excretion: Eliminated in the feces.
Half-life: Unknown.

TIME/ACTION PROFILE (↓ in serum potassium concentrations)

ROUTE	ONSET	PEAK	DURATION
PO	2–12 hr	unknown	6–24 hr
Rectal	2–12 hr	unknown	4–6 hr

Contraindications/Precautions

Contraindicated in: Life-threatening hyperkalemia (other, more immediate measures should be instituted); Hypersensitivity to saccharin or parabens (some products); Ileus; Abnormal bowel function (↑ risk for intestinal necrosis); Postoperative patients with no bowel movement (↑ risk for intestinal necrosis); History of impaction, chronic constipation, inflammatory bowel disease, ischemic colitis, vascular intestinal atherosclerosis, previous bowel resection, or bowel obstruction (↑ risk for intestinal necrosis); Known alcohol intolerance (suspension only).
Use Cautiously in: HF; Hypertension; Edema; Sodium restriction; Constipation.

Adverse Reactions/Side Effects

CV: edema. **F and E:** hypocalcemia, hypokalemia, hypomagnesemia. **GI:** constipation, fecal impaction, anorexia, gastric irritation, INTESTINAL NECROSIS, ischemic colitis, nausea, vomiting.

Interactions

Drug-Drug: May ↓ absorption of any other orally administered medication; administer sodium polystyrene sulfonate ≥3 hr before or after other oral medications (≥6 hr for patients with gastroparesis). Administration with **calcium** or **magnesium-containing antacids** may ↓ resin-exchanging ability and ↑ risk of systemic alkalosis. Hypokalemia may enhance **digoxin** toxicity. **Sorbitol** may ↑ risk of colonic necrosis; concurrent use not recommended.

Route/Dosage

4 level teaspoons = 15 g (4.1 mEq sodium/g).
PO (Adults): 15 g 1–4 times daily in water (up to 40 g 4 times daily).
Rect (Adults): 30–50 g as a retention enema; repeat as needed every 6 hr.
PO, Rect (Children): 1 g/kg/dose every 6 hr.

Availability (generic available)

Oral suspension: 15 g sodium polystyrene sulfonate with 20 g sorbitol/60 mL, 15 g sodium polystyrene sulfonate with 14.1 g sorbitol/60 mL. **Powder for suspension:** 15 g/bottle, 454 g/bottle.

NURSING IMPLICATIONS

Assessment

- Monitor for signs/symptoms of hyperkalemia (fatigue, muscle weakness, paresthesia, confusion, dyspnea, peaked T waves, depressed ST segments, prolonged QT segments, widened QRS complexes, loss of P waves, cardiac arrhythmias). Assess for development of hypokalemia (weakness, fatigue, arrhythmias, flat or inverted T waves, prominent U waves).
- Monitor intake, output, and daily weight. Assess for symptoms of fluid overload (dyspnea, rales/crackles, jugular venous distention, peripheral edema). Concurrent low-sodium diet may be ordered for patients with HF (see Appendix J).
- In patients receiving concurrent digoxin, assess for signs/symptoms of digoxin toxicity (anorexia, nausea, vomiting, visual disturbances, arrhythmias).
- Assess abdomen and note character and frequency of stools. Discontinue sodium polystyrene sulfonate if patient becomes constipated. Concurrent laxatives may be ordered to prevent constipation or impaction. Some products contain sorbitol to prevent constipation. Patient should ideally have 1–2 watery stools each day during therapy.

Lab Test Considerations

- Monitor potassium daily during therapy. Notify health care provider when potassium ↓ to 4–5 mEq/L.
- Monitor renal function and electrolytes (especially sodium, calcium, bicarbonate, and magnesium) before starting and periodically throughout therapy.

Implementation

- Consult health care provider regarding discontinuation of medications that may ↑ serum potassium (ACE inhibitors, angiotensin-receptor blockers, potassium-sparing diuretics, potassium supplements, salt substitutes).
- Administer oral doses ≥3 hr before or 3 hr after other medications (patients with gastroparesis may require a 6-hr separation).
- A laxative is often administered concurrently to prevent constipation.
- **PO:** For oral or nasogastric tube administration, shake suspension well before use. Solution is stable for 24 hr when refrigerated. When using powder, add prescribed amount to 3–4 mL water/g of powder. Shake well. Do not mix in orange juice or in any fruit juice known to contain potassium. Do not heat solution to enhance dissolution of powder; heating

S

impairs exchange resin properties. Chilling and adding syrup may improve palatability. May also be added to food. Resin cookie or candy recipes are available; discuss with pharmacist or dietitian.

- **Rect: Retention Enema:** Precede retention enema with cleansing enema. Administer solution via rectal tube or 28-French Foley catheter with 30-mL balloon. Insert tube at least 20 cm and tape in place.
- For retention enema, add powder to 100 mL of prescribed solution (usually sorbitol or 20% dextrose in water). Shake well to dissolve powder thoroughly; should be of liquid consistency. Position patient on left side and elevate hips on pillow if solution begins to leak. Follow administration of medication with additional 50–100 mL of diluent to ensure administration of complete dose. Encourage patient to retain enema as long as possible, ≥30–60 min.
- After retention period, irrigate colon with 1–2 L of non-sodium-containing solution. Y-connector with tubing may be attached to Foley or rectal tube; cleansing solution is administered through one port of the Y and allowed to drain by gravity through the other port.

Patient/Family Teaching

- Explain the purpose and side effects of sodium polystyrene sulfonate. Instruct on method of administration of medication to patient. Tell patient to separate dosing of other oral medications by ≥3 hr either before or after this drug. Advise patient to read *Medication Guide* before starting and periodically during therapy in case of changes.
- Advise patient to report GI symptoms, especially constipation.
- Advise patient to avoid taking antacids or laxatives during therapy, unless approved by health care provider; may cause systemic alkalosis.
- Instruct patient to report symptoms of hyperkalemia (fatigue, weakness, numbness, tingling, heart palpitations).
- Inform patient of need for frequent lab tests to monitor effectiveness.
- Advise patient to notify health care provider of all Rx or OTC medications, vitamins, or herbal products being taken and to consult with health care provider before taking other medications.

Evaluation/Desired Outcomes

- Normalization of serum potassium levels.

sofosbuvir/velpatasvir

(soe-**fos**-bue-vir/vel-**pat**-as-vir)

Epclusa

Classification

Therapeutic: antivirals

Pharmacologic: NS5B inhibitors, NS5A inhibitors

Indications

Chronic hepatitis C virus (HCV) genotype 1, 2, 3, 4, 5, or 6 infection in patients without cirrhosis or with compensated cirrhosis. Chronic HCV genotype 1, 2, 3, 4, 5, or 6 infection in patients with decompensated cirrhosis (in combination with ribavirin).

Action

Sofosbuvir: Inhibits the HCV NS5B RNA-dependent RNA polymerase, resulting in inhibition of viral replication. *Velpatasvir:* Inhibits the HCV NS5A protein, resulting in inhibition of viral replication. **Therapeutic Effects:** Decreased levels of HCV with sustained virologic response and lessened sequelae of chronic HCV infection.

Pharmacokinetics

Sofosbuvir

Absorption: Rapidly metabolized following absorption (extensive first-pass effect).

Distribution: Unknown.

Metabolism and Excretion: Extensively metabolized primarily to GS-461203, an active antiviral moiety, and then converted to GS-331007, which does not have antiviral activity. 80% excreted in urine mostly as GS-331007 (3.5% as unchanged drug); 14% excreted in feces; 2.5% excreted in expired air.

Half-life: *Sofosbuvir:* 0.4 hr; *GS-331007:* 25 hr.

Velpatasvir

Absorption: Well absorbed following oral administration.

Distribution: Unknown.

Protein Binding: >99.5%.

Metabolism and Excretion: Primarily metabolized in the liver via the CYP2B6, CYP2C8, and CYP3A4 isoenzymes. Primarily undergoes biliary excretion, with 94% excreted in feces and 0.4% eliminated in urine.

Half-life: 47 hr.

TIME/ACTION PROFILE (plasma concentrations)

ROUTE	ONSET	PEAK	DURATION
sofosbuvir (PO)	unknown	0.5–1 hr	24 hr
velpatasvir (PO)	unknown	3 hr	24 hr

Contraindications/Precautions

Contraindicated in: Situations when ribavirin is contraindicated (when ribavirin required); Concurrent use with other drugs/regimens containing sofosbuvir; Receiving immunosuppressant or chemotherapy medications (↑ risk of hepatitis B virus [HBV] reactivation); OB: Pregnant women or men whose partners are pregnant (when ribavirin is required; ribavirin may cause fetal harm); Lactation: Lactation (when ribavirin required).

Use Cautiously in: OB: Safety not established in pregnancy (when ribavirin not required); Lactation: Safety not established in breastfeeding (when ribavirin not required); Pedi: Children <3 yo (safety and effectiveness not established); Geri: Older adults may be more sensitive to drug's effects.

Adverse Reactions/Side Effects

Without Ribavirin

Derm: rash. **GI:** ↑ lipase, HBV REACTIVATION, nausea. **Neuro:** fatigue, headache, insomnia, irritability.

With Ribavirin

Derm: rash. **GI:** diarrhea, nausea, HBV REACTIVATION, ↑ lipase. **Hemat:** anemia. **Neuro:** fatigue, headache, insomnia.

Interactions

Drug-Drug: P-glycoprotein inducers may ↓ levels and effectiveness of sofosbuvir and velpatasvir; concurrent use not recommended. **Moderate or strong CYP2B6 inducers, moderate or strong CYP2C8 inducers**, or **moderate or strong CYP3A4 inducers** may ↓ levels and effectiveness of velpatasvir; concurrent use not recommended. **Amiodarone** may ↑ risk of symptomatic bradycardia when used with sofosbuvir-containing regimens; concurrent use not recommended; if amiodarone necessary, monitor patients in inpatient setting for 1st 48 hr of concurrent use and then monitor HR on outpatient basis for at least the 1st 2 wk of treatment; follow same monitoring procedure if discontinuing amiodarone immediately before initiation of sofosbuvir/velpatasvir. **Acid-reducing agents** may ↓ levels and effectiveness of velpatasvir; separate administration from **antacids**, including **magnesium hydroxide** and **aluminum hydroxide**, by 4 hr; administer **H_2-receptor antagonists** simultaneously or 12 hr apart from sofosbuvir/velpatasvir (dose of H_2 antagonist should not exceed famotidine 40 mg twice daily or equivalent); concurrent use with **proton pump inhibitors** not recommended (if proton pump inhibitor necessary, administer sofosbuvir/velpatasvir with food and take 4 hr before **omeprazole** 20 mg; use with other proton pump inhibitors not studied). May ↑ levels and risk of toxicity of **digoxin**; therapeutic monitoring of serum digoxin concentrations recommended. May ↑ levels and risk of toxicity of **topotecan**; concurrent use not recommended. **Carbamazepine, phenytoin, phenobarbital, oxcarbazepine, rifabutin**, and **rifampin** may ↓ levels and effectiveness of sofosbuvir and velpatasvir; concurrent use not recommended. **Efavirenz** may ↓ levels and effectiveness of velpatasvir; concurrent use not recommended. May ↑ levels and risk of toxicity of **tenofovir disoproxil fumarate**; monitor closely. **Tipranavir/ritonavir** may ↓ levels and effectiveness of sofosbuvir and velpatasvir; concurrent use not recommended. May ↑ levels and risk of toxicity of **rosuvastatin** and **atorvastatin**; rosuvastatin dose should not exceed 10 mg/day; monitor closely for atorvastatin-induced myopathy or rhabdomyolysis. May cause fluctuations in INR when used with **warfarin**; closely monitor INR. May ↑ risk of hypoglycemia when used with certain **antidiabetic agents**.

Drug-Natural Products: St. John's wort may ↓ levels and effectiveness of sofosbuvir and velpatasvir; concurrent use not recommended.

Route/Dosage

Dosing recommendations below may also be followed for patients coinfected with HIV.

PO (Adults): *Patients without cirrhosis or with compensated cirrhosis (including liver transplant recipients):* One 400-mg/100-mg tablet once daily for 12 wk; *Patients with decompensated cirrhosis:* One 400-mg/100-mg tablet once daily for 12 wk in combination with ribavirin.

PO (Children ≥3 yr or ≥30 kg): *Patients without cirrhosis or with compensated cirrhosis (including liver transplant recipients):* One 400-mg/100-mg tablet once daily for 12 wk *or* two 200-mg/50-mg tablets once daily for 12 wk *or* two 200-mg/50-mg pellet packets once daily for 12 wk; *Patients with decompensated cirrhosis:* One 400-mg/100-mg tablet once daily for 12 wk in combination with ribavirin *or* two 200-mg/50-mg tablets once daily for 12 wk in combination with ribavirin *or* two 200-mg/50-mg pellet packets once daily for 12 wk in combination with ribavirin.

PO (Children ≥3 yr or 17–<30 kg): *Patients without cirrhosis or with compensated cirrhosis (including liver transplant recipients):* one 200-mg/50-mg tablet once daily for 12 wk *or* one 200-mg/50-mg pellet packet once daily for 12 wk; *Patients with decompensated cirrhosis:* one 200-mg/50-mg tablet once daily for 12 wk in combination with ribavirin *or* one 200-mg/50-mg pellet packet once daily for 12 wk in combination with ribavirin.

PO (Children ≥3 yr or <17 kg): *Patients without cirrhosis or with compensated cirrhosis (including liver transplant recipients):* one 150-mg/37.5-mg pellet packet once daily for 12 wk; *Patients with decompensated cirrhosis:* one 150-mg/37.5-mg pellet packet once daily for 12 wk in combination with ribavirin.

Availability (generic available)

Tablets: sofosbuvir 200 mg/velpatasvir 50 mg, sofosbuvir 400 mg/velpatasvir 100 mg. **Oral pellets:** sofosbuvir 150 mg/velpatasvir 37.5 mg per pkt, sofosbuvir 200 mg/velpatasvir 50 mg per pkt.

NURSING IMPLICATIONS

Assessment

- Monitor for signs and symptoms of HBV reactivation (jaundice, dark urine, light-colored stools, fatigue, weakness, loss of appetite, nausea, vomiting, stomach pain) during therapy.

S

Lab Test Considerations

- Measure hepatitis B surface antigen (HBsAg) and hepatitis core antibody (anti-HBc) in all patients before starting HCV therapy. May cause HBV reactivation. Monitor for clinical and laboratory signs of hepatitis flare (↑ AST, ALT, and bilirubin; liver failure; death) or HBV reactivation (rapid ↑ in serum HBV DNA level) during HCV treatment and post-treatment follow-up.
- May cause ↑ serum lipase and amylase levels.
- May cause ↑ CK and indirect bilirubin levels.

Implementation

- **PO:** Administer one tablet daily without regard to food for 12 wk.
- Do not chew oral pellets; causes a bitter aftertaste. May be administered directly into mouth and swallowed whole or taken with food. In pediatric patients <6 yr, administer oral pellets with food to increase tolerability and palatability. Sprinkle oral pellets on one or more spoonfuls of nonacidic soft food (pudding, chocolate syrup, ice cream) at or below room temperature. Take oral pellets within 15 min of gently mixing with food and swallow entire contents without chewing.
- Administer antacids 4 hr apart from sofosbuvir/velpatasvir. May administer simultaneously or 12 hr apart with H_2-receptor antagonists at doses not to exceed famotidine 40 mg twice daily. Avoid administration with proton pump inhibitors; if medically necessary, administer sofosbuvir/velpatasvir with food and 4 hr before omeprazole 20 mg.

Patient/Family Teaching

- Explain the purpose and side effects of *Epclusa*. Instruct patient to take as directed. Do not skip or miss doses or stop medication without consulting health care provider. Advise patient to read *Patient Information* before starting and with each Rx refill in case of changes.
- Explain need for continued medical follow-up to assess effectiveness and possible side effects of medication. Periodic lab tests may be needed.
- Advise patient to notify health care provider if they have a history of HBV. May cause reactivation.
- Advise patient to report signs and symptoms of bradycardia (dizziness, light-headedness, faintness, weakness, slow heartbeat, heart palpitations).
- Instruct patient to notify health care provider of all Rx or OTC medications, vitamins, or herbal products being taken and consult health care provider before taking any new medications, especially St. John's wort or proton pump inhibitors.
- Rep: Advise patients to notify health care provider if pregnancy is planned or suspected or if breastfeeding. Advise women of reproductive potential who take *Epclusa* with ribavirin to use effective contraception during therapy and for 6 mo after therapy is completed. Notify health care provider immediately if pregnancy is suspected.

Evaluation/Desired Outcomes

- Decreased levels of HCV with sustained virologic response and lessened sequelae of chronic HCV infection.

solifenacin (so-li-**fen**-a-sin)

VESIcare

Classification

Therapeutic: urinary tract antispasmodics

Pharmacologic: anticholinergics

Indications

Overactive bladder with symptoms (urge incontinence, urgency, frequency) (tablets only).

Action

Acts as a muscarinic (cholinergic) receptor antagonist; antagonizes bladder smooth muscle contraction. **Therapeutic Effects:** Decreased symptoms of overactive bladder. Improved maximum cystometric capacity in neurogenic detrusor overactivity.

Pharmacokinetics

Absorption: 90% absorbed following oral administration.

Distribution: Extensively distributed to tissues.

Protein Binding: 98%.

Metabolism and Excretion: Extensively metabolized by liver via the CYP3A4 isoenzyme. 69% excreted in urine as metabolites, 22% in feces.

Half-life: *Tablets:* 45–68 hr.

TIME/ACTION PROFILE (plasma concentrations)

ROUTE	ONSET	PEAK	DURATION
Oral	unknown	3–8 hr	24 hr

Contraindications/Precautions

Contraindicated in: Hypersensitivity; Urinary retention; Gastric retention; Uncontrolled angle-closure glaucoma; Severe hepatic impairment; History of QT interval prolongation.

Use Cautiously in: Moderate hepatic impairment (lower dose recommended); Renal impairment; Bladder outflow obstruction; GI obstructive disorders, severe constipation, or ulcerative colitis; Myasthenia gravis; Angle-closure glaucoma; OB: Safety not established in pregnancy; Lactation: Safety not established in breastfeeding; Pedi: Safety and effectiveness not established in children.

Adverse Reactions/Side Effects

CV: palpitations, QT interval prolongation, tachycardia. **EENT:** blurred vision. **GI:** constipation, dry mouth, abdominal pain, dyspepsia, nausea. **GU:** urinary tract infection. **MS:** muscle weakness. **Neuro:** confusion, drowsiness, hallucinations, headache. **Misc:** HYPERSENSITIVITY REACTIONS (INCLUDING ANAPHYLAXIS AND ANGIOEDEMA).

Interactions

Drug-Drug: Strong CYP3A4 inhibitors, including **ketoconazole**, may significantly ↑ levels and risk of toxicity. **QT interval prolonging medications** may ↑ risk of QT interval prolongation; avoid concurrent use.

Route/Dosage

Overactive Bladder

PO (Adults): *Tablets:* 5 mg once daily; may ↑ to 10 mg once daily; *Concurrent use of strong CYP3A4 inhibitors:* Tablets: Not to exceed 5 mg once daily.

Renal Impairment

PO (Adults): *CCr <30 mL/min:* Tablets: Not to exceed 5 mg once daily.

Hepatic Impairment

PO (Adults): *Moderate hepatic impairment:* Tablets: Not to exceed 5 mg once daily.

Availability (generic available)

Tablets (Vesicare): 5 mg, 10 mg.

NURSING IMPLICATIONS

Assessment

- Monitor for signs/symptoms of hypersensitivity reaction (angioedema, anaphylaxis) after 1st and subsequent doses; may occur up to several hours afterward. *If swelling of the upper tongue, hypopharynx, or larynx occurs,* promptly discontinue solifenacin and provide therapy as indicated.
- **Overactive Bladder:** Monitor voiding pattern and assess symptoms of overactive bladder (urinary urgency, incontinence, frequency) before starting and periodically during therapy.

Implementation

- **PO:** Administer once daily without regard to food. ***DNC:*** Tablets must be swallowed whole; do not break, crush, or chew.

Patient/Family Teaching

- Explain purpose and side effects of medication. Advise patient to read *Patient Information* before starting therapy.
- *Overactive bladder:* if dose missed, omit and take next day; do not take 2 doses in same day.
- May cause dizziness and blurred vision. Caution patient to avoid driving and other activities that require alertness until response to medication is known.
- Advise patient to discontinue solifenacin and notify health care provider immediately if hives; rash; swelling of lips, face, tongue, or throat; or trouble breathing occurs.
- Inform patient of potential anticholinergic side effects (constipation, urinary retention, blurred vision, heat prostration in a hot environment) and to notify health care provider if symptoms persist.
- Instruct patient to notify health care provider of all Rx or OTC medications, vitamins, or herbal products being taken and consult health care provider before taking any new medications.
- Rep: Advise women of reproductive potential to notify health care provider if pregnancy is planned or suspected or if breastfeeding.

Evaluation/Desired Outcomes

- Decrease in symptoms of overactive bladder (urge urinary incontinence, urgency, frequency).

solriamfetol (sol-ri-am-fe-tol)

Sunosi

Classification

Therapeutic: central nervous system stimulants

Pharmacologic: dopamine norepinephrine reuptake inhibitors

Schedule IV

Indications

Excessive daytime sleepiness due to narcolepsy or obstructive sleep apnea.

Action

Selective dopamine and norepinephrine reuptake inhibitor. **Therapeutic Effects:** Improved wakefulness.

Pharmacokinetics

Absorption: 95% absorbed following oral administration; high-fat food delays absorption.
Distribution: Extensively distributed to tissues.
Metabolism and Excretion: Undergoes minimal metabolism; primarily excreted in urine as unchanged drug (95%).
Half-life: 7 hr.

TIME/ACTION PROFILE (plasma concentrations)

ROUTE	ONSET	PEAK	DURATION
PO	unknown	1.25–3 hr	unknown

Contraindications/Precautions

Contraindicated in: Concurrent use or use within 14 days of discontinuation of MAO inhibitors; End-stage renal disease.

Use Cautiously in: Cardiovascular disease, cerebrovascular disease, or hypertension; Moderate or severe renal impairment (↓ dose); Psychoses or bipolar disorder; History of drug (especially stimulants) or alcohol abuse; OB: Use during pregnancy only if potential maternal benefit justifies potential fetal risk; Lactation: Use while breastfeeding only if potential maternal benefit justifies potential risk to infant; Pedi: Safety and effectiveness not established in children; Geri: Because of reduced renal function, older adults may be at ↑ risk of adverse reactions.

Adverse Reactions/Side Effects

CV: ↑ BP, ↑ HR, palpitations. **Derm:** ↑ sweating. **GI:** ↓ appetite, abdominal pain, constipation, diarrhea, dry mouth, nausea. **Neuro:** headache, anxiety, dizziness, insomnia, irritability.

Interactions

Drug-Drug: Concurrent use with or within 14 days of discontinuation of **MAO inhibitors** may ↑ risk of hypertensive crises; concurrent use contraindicated. Use cautiously with other **drugs that ↑ BP or HR**. **Dopaminergic drugs** may have synergistic effects.

Route/Dosage

Narcolepsy

PO (Adults): 75 mg once daily; may ↑ to 150 mg once daily, if needed, after ≥3 days.

Renal Impairment

PO (Adults): *eGFR 30–59 mL/min/1.73 m²:* 37.5 mg once daily; may ↑ to 75 mg once daily after ≥7 days, if needed. *eGFR 15–29 mL/min/1.73 m²:* 37.5 mg once daily.

Obstructive Sleep Apnea

PO (Adults): 37.5 mg once daily; may double dose at intervals of at least every 3 days, if needed (max dose = 150 mg/day).

Renal Impairment

PO (Adults): *eGFR 30–59 mL/min/1.73 m²:* 37.5 mg once daily; may ↑ to 75 mg once daily after ≥7 days, if needed. *eGFR 15–29 mL/min/1.73 m²:* 37.5 mg once daily.

Availability

Tablets: 75 mg, 150 mg.

NURSING IMPLICATIONS

Assessment

- Observe and document frequency of narcoleptic episodes before starting and during therapy.
- Assess BP and HR; control hypertension before starting therapy. Monitor BP during therapy and treat new-onset hypertension and exacerbations of pre-existing hypertension. *If ↑ BP or HR that is not managed with dose ↓ or other intervention occurs,* consider discontinuing solriamfetol.
- Assess for emergence or exacerbation of psychiatric symptoms. *If symptoms occur,* consider dose ↓ or discontinuing solriamfetol.

Implementation

- **PO:** Administer upon waking without regard to food.

Patient/Family Teaching

- Explain purpose and side effects of medication. Advise patient to read *Patient Information* before starting therapy.
- Instruct patient to avoid taking medication within 9 hr of planned bedtime; may impair ability to fall asleep.
- Advise patient that sharing this medication with others is dangerous and illegal; Solriamfetol has abuse potential. Caution patient to protect it from theft and store out of sight and reach of children, in a location not accessible by others.
- Advise patient to notify health care provider if anxiety, insomnia, irritability, agitation, or signs of psychosis or bipolar disorders occur.
- Advise patient to notify health care provider of all Rx or OTC medications, vitamins, or herbal products being taken and to consult with health care provider before taking other medications. If alcohol is used during therapy, limit to moderate amounts.
- Rep: Advise women of reproductive potential to notify health care provider if pregnancy is planned or suspected or if breastfeeding. Monitor breastfed infants for agitation, insomnia, anorexia, and ↓ weight gain. Encourage pregnant patient to enroll in the registry to monitor outcomes for exposure to solriamfetol during pregnancy by calling 1-877-283-6220 or visiting www.SunosiPregnancyRegistry.com.

Evaluation/Desired Outcomes

- Improved ability to stay awake.

sotagliflozin

(soe-ta-gli-**floe**-zin)

Inpefa

Classification

Therapeutic: none assigned

Pharmacologic: sodium-glucose co-transporter 1 (SGLT1) inhibitors, sodium-glucose co-transporter 2 (SGLT2) inhibitors

Indications

To reduce the risk of cardiovascular death, hospitalization for HF, and urgent HF visits in patients with HF. To reduce the risk of cardiovascular death, hospitalization for HF, and urgent HF visits in patients with type 2 diabetes mellitus, chronic kidney disease, and other cardiovascular risk factors.

Action

Inhibits both sodium-glucose co-transporter 1 (SGLT1) and SGLT2. Inhibition of SGLT1 reduces intestinal absorption of glucose and sodium. Inhibition of SGLT2 reduces renal reabsorption of glucose and sodium, which reduces cardiac preload and afterload and sympathetic activity. Exact mechanism of cardiovascular benefit unknown. **Therapeutic Effects:** Reduction in the risk of cardiovascular death, hospitalization for HF and urgent HF visits.

Pharmacokinetics

Absorption: 25% absorbed following oral administration. High-caloric meals ↑ absorption.
Distribution: Extensively distributed to tissues.
Protein Binding: >93%.
Metabolism and Excretion: Primarily metabolized in the liver via UGT1A9 and to a lesser extent by the CYP3A4 isoenzyme. Primarily excreted in the urine (57%) with 37% excreted in the feces.
Half-life: 21–35 hr.

TIME/ACTION PROFILE (plasma concentrations)

ROUTE	ONSET	PEAK	DURATION
PO	unknown	1.25–3 hr	24 hr

Contraindications/Precautions

Contraindicated in: Hypersensitivity; Type 1 diabetes; Moderate or severe hepatic impairment; eGFR <15 mL/min/1.73 m² or hemodialysis; Rep: SGLT2 inhibitors are not recommended for the treatment of HF in women of reproductive potential; OB: 2nd and 3rd trimesters of pregnancy; SGLT2 inhibitors are not recommended for the treatment of HF during pregnancy; Lactation: Lactation.
Use Cautiously in: History of type 1 or 2 diabetes, pancreatitis, pancreatic surgery, acute febrile illness, reduced caloric intake due to illness or surgery, surgical procedures, volume depletion, or alcohol abuse (↑ risk of ketoacidosis); Hypovolemia, chronic kidney disease (eGFR <60 mL/min/1.73 m²), or concurrent use of loop diuretics (↑ risk of volume depletion or hypotension); History of genital mycotic infections; OB: Safety not established during 1st trimester of pregnancy; Pedi: Safety and effectiveness not established in children; Geri: Older adults may have ↑ risk of hypovolemia and hypotension.

Adverse Reactions/Side Effects

CV: hypotension. **Endo:** hypoglycemia (↑ with other medications). **F and E:** dehydration, KETOACIDOSIS. **GI:** diarrhea. **GU:** urinary tract infection (including pyelonephritis), acute kidney injury, genital mycotic infection, NECROTIZING FASCIITIS OF PERINEUM (FOURNIER GANGRENE). **Neuro:** dizziness.

Interactions

Drug-Drug: ↑ risk of hypoglycemia with **insulin** or **insulin secretagogues**; dose adjustments may be required. May ↑ levels and risk of toxicity of **digoxin**; closely monitor levels. **UGT inducers**, including **rifampin**, may ↓ levels and effectiveness. **May** ↓ **lithium** levels and effectiveness.

Route/Dosage

PO (Adults): 200 mg once daily; then after 2 wk, ↑ to 400 mg once daily.

Availability

Tablets: 200 mg, 400 mg.

NURSING IMPLICATIONS

Assessment

- Monitor fluid volume status at initiation and throughout therapy; correct volume status prior to therapy initiation, especially in patients with hypotension, renal impairment, or concurrently receiving diuretics.
- BP should be monitored throughout therapy; ↑ risk of symptomatic hypotension in older adults and those concurrently receiving diuretics.
- Monitor for signs and symptoms of hypoglycemia (nausea, tachycardia, sweating, hunger, dizziness, light-headedness, confusion, anxiety), especially if used concurrently with insulin and insulin secretagogues; dosage adjustment of insulin or insulin secretagogues may be necessary.
- Monitor for signs and symptoms of ketoacidosis regardless of blood glucose levels (weakness, fatigue, flushed face, nausea, vomiting, thirst, fruity breath, polyuria). Older adults and women at ↑ risk especially in 1st mo of therapy. Treat promptly and provide supportive care.
- Monitor for signs and symptoms of UTI (fever, dysuria, polyuria, hematuria, flank pain, suprapubic pain or pressure). Genital mycotic infections (genital pruritus, yeasty discharge) may occur, especially in patients with history of genital mycotic infections; women and uncircumcised men at higher risk. Treat infection promptly.
- Assess the lower limbs for signs and symptoms of infection, including osteomyelitis, new pain or tenderness, and sores or ulcers, especially in patients with a history of prior amputation, peripheral arterial disease, neuropathy, or diabetic foot ulcers.
- Assess for signs and symptoms of necrotizing fasciitis of the perineum (Fournier gangrene: tenderness, redness, or swelling of the genitals or perineum; fever; malaise; perineal skin discoloration or gangrenous appearance; drainage; sores; blisters; foul odor).

S

Lab Test Considerations

- Verify a negative pregnancy test before starting therapy.
- Assess renal function at baseline, regularly during therapy, and as clinically indicated. Can ↑ serum creatinine and ↓ eGFR.
- Check A1c twice yearly in patients who are meeting treatment goals, every 3 mo in patients whose therapy has changed or who are not meeting glycemic goals, and more frequently as clinically warranted.
- Monitor ketones in patients at risk for ketoacidosis.

Implementation

- Correct volume depletion prior to initiation, especially in older adults or those who are hypotensive, have renal impairment, or are concurrently receiving diuretics.
- **PO:** Administer once daily not >1 hr before the first meal of the day. ***DNC:*** Do not cut, crush, or chew tablets.
- If a dose is missed by >6 hr, take the next dose as prescribed the next day.
- Withhold sotagliflozin ≥3 days, if possible, prior to major surgery or procedures associated with prolonged fasting. Resume when the patient is clinically stable and resumed oral intake.

Patient/Family Teaching

- Explain purpose and side effects of medication to patient. Instruct patient to take medication as directed. If a dose is missed by >6 hr, take the next dose as prescribed the next day. Advise patient to read *Patient Information* before starting therapy.
- Teach the patient how and when to self-monitor blood glucose and how to treat hypoglycemia. Glucose tablets, glucose gel, cranberry juice, or hard candy should be kept at home for use in hypoglycemia emergency. Symptoms of hypoglycemia include nausea, rapid heartbeat, sweating, hunger, dizziness, light-headedness, confusion, and anxiety.
- Tell patient to maintain adequate hydration to prevent hypotension and report symptoms of hypotension (faintness, light-headedness, dizziness, palpitations, heart racing).
- Instruct patient to immediately seek treatment for and report symptoms of ketoacidosis (weakness, fatigue, flushed face, nausea, vomiting, thirst, fruity breath, frequent urination).
- Tell patient to immediately seek treatment for and report symptoms of necrotizing fasciitis of the perineum (Fournier gangrene: tenderness, redness, or swelling of the genitals or perineum; fever; malaise; perineal skin discoloration; sores; blisters; drainage; foul odor).
- Teach about the importance of and how to perform meticulous daily foot and lower leg care. Counsel patient to report new pain or tenderness, sores, ulcers, or infections involving the leg or foot.
- Advise patient to report symptoms of UTI (fever, frequent and painful urination, bloody urine, flank pain, pelvic pain or pressure) or genital mycotic infections (genital itchiness, yeasty discharge).
- Advise patient to notify health care professional of all Rx or OTC medications, vitamins, or herbal products being taken and to consult health care professional before taking other medications.
- Rep: Instruct women of reproductive potential to notify health care professional if pregnancy if planned or suspected and to avoid breastfeeding. Avoid use in 2nd and 3rd trimester of pregnancy and weigh risk vs. benefit of use during 1st trimester.

Evaluation/Desired Outcomes

- Reduction in the risk of cardiovascular death, hospitalization for HF and urgent HF visits.

BEERS

spironolactone
(speer-oh-no-**lak**-tone)

Aldactone, Carospir

Classification

Therapeutic: diuretics

Pharmacologic: potassium-sparing diuretics

Indications

New York Heart Association (NYHA) class II–IV HF. Hypertension. Edema associated with cirrhosis and nephrotic syndrome. Primary hyperaldosteronism (tablets only). **Unlabeled Use:** Acne. Hormone therapy for transgender females (male-to-female).

Action

Causes loss of sodium bicarbonate and calcium while saving potassium and hydrogen ions by antagonizing aldosterone. Directly inhibits testosterone secretion and androgen binding to the androgen receptor. **Therapeutic Effects:** Improved survival in patients with NYHA class II–IV HF. Weak diuretic and antihypertensive response when compared with other diuretics.

Pharmacokinetics

Absorption: >90% absorbed. Oral suspension results in 15–37% higher serum concentrations compared to tablets. Bioavailability ↑ with food.

Distribution: Crosses the placenta; enters breast milk.

Protein Binding: >90%.

Metabolism and Excretion: Converted by the liver to its active diuretic compound (canrenone). Primarily excreted in the urine.

Half-life: *Spironolactone:* 78–84 min; *Canrenone:* 13–24 hr.

TIME/ACTION PROFILE (diuretic effect)

ROUTE	ONSET	PEAK	DURATION
PO	unknown	1–3 hr	2–3 days†

† Multiple doses.

Contraindications/Precautions

Contraindicated in: Hypersensitivity; Severe renal impairment (CCr <30 mL/min); SCr >2.5 mg/dL (for patients with HF); Hyperkalemia; Addison's disease; Concurrent use of eplerenone; OB: Pregnancy.

Use Cautiously in: Hepatic impairment; Diabetes mellitus (↑ risk of hyperkalemia); Lactation: Use while breastfeeding only if potential maternal benefit justifies potential risk to infant; Pedi: Safety and effectiveness not established in children; Geri: ↑ risk of hyperkalemia in older adults.

Adverse Reactions/Side Effects

CV: arrhythmias. **Derm:** alopecia, DRUG RASH WITH EOSINOPHILIA AND SYSTEMIC SYMPTOMS (DRESS), pruritus, STEVENS-JOHNSON SYNDROME (SJS), TOXIC EPIDERMAL NECROLYSIS (TEN). **Endo:** amenorrhea, breast tenderness, deepening of voice, gynecomastia (in males), ↑ hair growth (in females), sexual dysfunction. **F and E:** hyperkalemia, hyponatremia, hyperchloremic metabolic acidosis. **GI:** GI irritation. **GU:** erectile dysfunction, dysuria. **Hemat:** agranulocytosis, thrombocytopenia. **MS:** muscle cramps. **Neuro:** dizziness, headache, sedation. **Misc:** HYPERSENSITIVITY REACTIONS (INCLUDING ANAPHYLAXIS).

Interactions

Drug-Drug: Use with **eplerenone** ↑ risk of hyperkalemia; concurrent use contraindicated. ↑ risk of hypotension with acute ingestion of **alcohol**, other **antihypertensive agents**, or **nitrates**. Use with **ACE inhibitors**, **NSAIDs**, **potassium supplements**, **angiotensin II receptor antagonists**, **potassium-sparing diuretics**, **angiotensin converting enzyme inhibitors**, or **cyclosporine** ↑ risk of hyperkalemia. ↓ **lithium** excretion. Antihypertensive and diuretic effectiveness may be ↓ by **NSAIDs**. May ↑ levels and risk of toxicity of **digoxin**; monitor levels closely. May ↑ levels and risk of toxicity of **CYP2C8 substrates**, including **repaglinide**. May ↑ levels and risk of toxicity of **CYP3A4/5 substrates**, including **midazolam**, **sirolimus**, or **tacrolimus**. ↓ hypoprothrombinemic effect of **oral anticoagulants**. **Cholestyramine** may ↑ risk of hyperkalemic metabolic acidosis. May ↑ prostate-specific antigen levels in patients receiving **abiraterone**; concurrent use not recommended.

Route/Dosage

Oral suspension is not therapeutically equivalents to tablets. If patient requires a dose >100 mg, use tablets, NOT suspension. Suspension doses >100 mg may result in higher than expected spironolactone concentrations.

Heart Failure

PO (Adults): *Serum potassium ≤5 mEq/L and eGFR>50 mL/min/1.73 m²:* Tablet: 25 mg once daily; may then ↑ to 50 mg once daily; if patient develops hyperkalemia with 25 mg once daily, ↓ dose to 25 mg every other day. Suspension: 20 mg once daily; may then ↑ to 37.5 mg once daily; if patient develops hyperkalemia with 20 mg once daily, ↓ dose to 20 mg every other day. *Serum potassium ≤5 mEq/L and eGFR 30–50 mL/min/1.73 m²:* Tablets: 25 mg every other day. Suspension: 10 mg once daily.

Hypertension

PO (Adults): Tablets: 25–100 mg/day as a single dose or 2 divided doses; may titrate dose every 2 wk (max dose = 100 mg/day). Suspension: 20–75 mg/day as a single dose or 2 divided doses; may titrate dose every 2 wk (max dose = 75 mg/day).

Edema

PO (Adults): Tablets: 25–200 mg/day as a single dose or 2 divided doses. Suspension: 75 mg/day as a single dose or 2 divided doses.

Primary Hyperaldosteronism

PO (Adults): 100–400 mg/day.

Acne (off-label use)

PO (Adults): 50–200 mg once daily.

Hormone Therapy for Transgender Females (off-label use)

PO (Adults): 25 mg once or twice daily in combination with other appropriate agents. Increase at 1-wk intervals based on serum testosterone levels and tolerability to a usual dose of 50–150 mg twice daily (max dose = 200 mg twice daily).

Availability (generic available)

Tablets: 25 mg, 50 mg, 100 mg. **Oral suspension (banana flavor):** 25 mg/5 mL. ***In combination with:*** hydrochlorothiazide.

NURSING IMPLICATIONS

Assessment

- Monitor intake and output ratios and daily weight during therapy.
- If medication is given as an adjunct to antihypertensive therapy, evaluate BP before administering and periodically during therapy.
- Assess patient frequently for development of hyperkalemia (fatigue, muscle weakness, paresthesia, confusion, dyspnea, cardiac arrhythmias). Patients who have diabetes mellitus or kidney disease and elderly patients are at increased risk of developing these symptoms.

S

- Periodic ECGs may be recommended in patients receiving prolonged therapy.
- Assess patient for skin rash frequently during therapy. Discontinue diuretic at first sign of rash; may be life-threatening. SJS or TEN may develop. Treat symptomatically; may recur once treatment is stopped.
- Monitor for signs and symptoms of DRESS (fever, rash, lymphadenopathy, facial swelling) periodically during therapy. Discontinue therapy if symptoms occur.

Lab Test Considerations

- Evaluate serum potassium levels prior to therapy, within 1 wk of starting therapy or dose increase, and routinely during therapy. If hyperkalemia occurs, decrease dose or discontinue therapy and treat hyperkalemia.
- Monitor BUN, serum creatinine, and electrolytes prior to and periodically during therapy. May cause ↑ serum magnesium, uric acid, BUN, creatinine, potassium, plasma renin activity, and urinary calcium excretion levels. May also cause ↓ sodium levels.
- Discontinue potassium-sparing diuretics 3 days prior to a glucose tolerance test because of risk of severe hyperkalemia.
- May cause false ↑ of plasma cortisol concentrations. Spironolactone should be withdrawn 4–7 days before test.

Implementation

- *Carospir* is not therapeutically equivalent to *Aldactone*; do not interchange.
- **PO:** Administer in AM to avoid interrupting sleep pattern.
- Administer with food or milk to minimize gastric irritation and to increase bioavailability.
- Oral suspension does not require dilution.

Patient/Family Teaching

- Emphasize the importance of continuing to take this medication, even if feeling well. Instruct patient to take medication at the same time each day. Take missed doses as soon as remembered unless almost time for next dose. Do not double doses.
- Caution patient to avoid salt substitutes and foods that contain high levels of potassium unless prescribed by health care professional.
- May cause dizziness. Caution patient to avoid driving or other activities requiring alertness until response to medication is known.
- Instruct patient to notify health care professional of all Rx or OTC medications, vitamins, or herbal products being taken and consult health care professional before taking any new medications, especially OTC decongestants, cough or cold preparations, or appetite suppressants due to potential for increased BP.
- Instruct patient to notify health care professional of medication regimen prior to treatment or surgery.
- Advise patient to notify health care professional if rash, muscle weakness or cramps, fatigue, or severe nausea, vomiting, or diarrhea occurs.
- Inform male patients that spironolactone may cause gynecomastia; may require dose decrease. Usually reversible.
- Rep: Advise females of reproductive potential to notify health care professional if pregnancy is planned or suspected or if breastfeeding.
- Emphasize the need for follow-up exams to monitor progress.
- **Hypertension:** Reinforce need to continue additional therapies for hypertension (weight loss, restricted sodium intake, stress reduction, moderation of alcohol intake, regular exercise, and cessation of smoking). Medication helps control but does not cure hypertension.
- Teach patient and family the correct technique for checking BP weekly.

Evaluation/Desired Outcomes

- Improved survival in patients with NYHA class II–IV HF.
- Increase in diuresis and decrease in edema while maintaining serum potassium level in an acceptable range.
- Decrease in BP.
- Prevention of hypokalemia in patients taking diuretics.
- Treatment of hyperaldosteronism.
- Reduced male characteristics in male-to-female transgender patients.

streptomycin, See AMINOGLYCOSIDES.

sucralfate (soo-kral-fate)

Carafate, Cytogard, Sulcrate, Sulcrate Plus

Classification

Therapeutic: antiulcer agents

Pharmacologic: GI protectants

Indications

Short-term management of duodenal ulcers. Maintenance (preventive) therapy of duodenal ulcers. **Unlabeled Use:** Management of gastric ulcer or gastroesophageal reflux. Prevention of gastric mucosal injury caused by high-dose aspirin or other NSAIDs in patients with rheumatoid arthritis or in high-stress situations (e.g., intensive care unit). **Suspension:** Mucositis/stomatitis/rectal or oral ulcerations from various etiologies.

Action

Aluminum salt of sulfated sucrose reacts with gastric acid to form a thick paste, which selectively adheres to the ulcer surface. **Therapeutic Effects:** Protection of ulcers, with subsequent healing.

Pharmacokinetics

Absorption: Systemic absorption is minimal (<5%).
Distribution: Unknown.
Metabolism and Excretion: >90% is eliminated in the feces.
Half-life: 6–20 hr.

TIME/ACTION PROFILE (mucosal protectant effect)

ROUTE	ONSET	PEAK	DURATION
PO	1–2 hr	unknown	6 hr

Contraindications/Precautions

Contraindicated in: Hypersensitivity.
Use Cautiously in: Renal failure (accumulation of aluminum can occur); Diabetes (↑ risk of hyperglycemia with suspension); Impaired swallowing (↑ risk of tablet aspiration).

Adverse Reactions/Side Effects

Derm: pruritus, rash. **Endo:** hyperglycemia (suspension). **GI:** constipation, diarrhea, dry mouth, gastric discomfort, indigestion, nausea. **Neuro:** dizziness, drowsiness. **Misc:** HYPERSENSITIVITY REACTIONS (INCLUDING ANAPHYLAXIS AND ANGIOEDEMA).

Interactions

Drug-Drug: May ↓ absorption of **phenytoin**, **fat-soluble vitamins**, or **tetracycline**. ↓ effectiveness when used with **antacids** or **cimetidine**. ↓ absorption of **fluoroquinolones**; separate administration by 2 hr.

Route/Dosage

Treatment of Ulcers

PO (Adults): 1 g 4 times daily, given 1 hr before meals and at bedtime; or 2 g twice daily, on waking and at bedtime.
PO (Adults): 1 g twice daily, given 1 hr before a meal.

Gastroesophageal Reflux

PO (Adults): 1 g 4 times daily, given 1 hr before meals and at bedtime.
PO (Children): 40–80 mg/kg/day divided every 6 hr, given 1 hr before meals and at bedtime.

Stomatitis

PO (Adults and Children): 5–10 mL of suspension; swish and spit or swish and swallow 4 times daily.

Proctitis

Rect (Adults): 2 g of suspension given as an enema once or twice daily.

Availability (generic available)

Oral suspension (cherry flavor): 1 g/10 mL, ✱ 200 mg/mL. **Tablets:** 1 g.

NURSING IMPLICATIONS

Assessment

- Assess for abdominal pain and frank or occult blood in the stool.

Lab Test Considerations

- Monitor blood glucose in patients with diabetes treated with oral suspension.

Implementation

- **PO:** Administer on an empty stomach, 1 hr before meals and at bedtime. Tablet may be broken or dissolved in water before ingestion.
- Oral suspension is only for oral use; do not administer IV. Shake well before use. Store at room temperature; do not freeze.
- If antacids are also required for pain, administer 30 min before or after sucralfate dose.

Patient/Family Teaching

- Explain purpose and side effects of medication. Advise patient to read *Patient Information* before starting therapy.
- Advise patient to continue with course of therapy for 4–8 wk, even if feeling better, to ensure ulcer healing. If a dose is missed, take as soon as remembered unless almost time for next dose; do not double doses.
- Advise patient to notify health care provider of all Rx or OTC medications, vitamins, or herbal products being taken and to consult health care provider before taking other medications.
- Advise patient that ↑ in fluid intake, dietary bulk, and exercise may prevent drug-induced constipation.
- Emphasize importance of routine examinations to monitor progress.

Evaluation/Desired Outcomes

- Decrease in abdominal pain.
- Prevention and healing of duodenal ulcers, seen by x-ray examination and endoscopy.

sugammadex

(soo-**gam**-ma-dex)
Bridion

Classification
Therapeutic: antidotes

Indications

Reversal of neuromuscular blockade induced by rocuronium or vecuronium in patients undergoing surgery.

Action

Forms a complex with rocuronium or vecuronium, reducing the amount of the neuromuscular blocker available to bind to nicotinic cholinergic receptors in the neuromuscular junction. **Therapeutic Effects:** Reversal of neuromuscular blocking effects.

Pharmacokinetics

Absorption: IV administration results in complete bioavailability.
Distribution: Well distributed.
Metabolism and Excretion: Primarily excreted unchanged in urine (95%); <1% excreted in feces.
Half-life: 2 hr (↑ in renal impairment).

TIME/ACTION PROFILE (reversal of neuromuscular blocking effects)

ROUTE	ONSET	PEAK	DURATION
IV	unknown	2–5 min	unknown

Contraindications/Precautions

Contraindicated in: Hypersensitivity; Severe renal impairment.
Use Cautiously in: Patients with coagulopathies or being treated with anticoagulants; OB: Safety not established in pregnancy; Lactation: Safety not established in breastfeeding; Rep: Women of reproductive potential (may ↓ efficacy of hormonal contraception).

Adverse Reactions/Side Effects

CV: bradycardia, hypotension. **GI:** nausea, vomiting. **Hemat:** ↑ aPTT, ↑ PT/INR. **Neuro:** headache. **Misc:** ANAPHYLAXIS.

Interactions

Drug-Drug: May ↓ levels and the effectiveness of **hormonal contraceptives**. Concurrent use with **unfractionated heparin, low molecular weight heparin, warfarin, dabigatran, edoxaban, rivaroxaban**, or **apixaban** may ↑ risk of bleeding.

Route/Dosage

Following sugammadex use, wait 24 hr before readministering rocuronium or vecuronium. If more immediate neuromuscular blockade is needed, a nonsteroidal neuromuscular-blocking agent (e.g., succinylcholine) may be required.

Routine Reversal of Rocuronium- or Vecuronium-Induced Blockade

IV (Adults and Children): *Deep block (if spontaneous recovery of twitch response has reached 1 to 2 post-tetanic counts and there are no twitch responses to train-of-four [TOF] stimulation):* 4 mg/kg (actual body weight) as a single dose; *Moderate block (if spontaneous recovery has reached the reappearance of the 2nd twitch [T2] in response to TOF stimulation):* 2 mg/kg (actual body weight) as a single dose.

Immediate Reversal of Rocuronium-Induced Blockade

IV (Adults): 16 mg/kg (actual body weight) as a single dose administered soon (3 min) after administration of a single dose of 1.2 mg/kg of rocuronium.

Availability (generic available)

Solution for injection: 100 mg/mL.

NURSING IMPLICATIONS

Assessment

- Monitor respiratory status from time of sugammadex injection until complete recovery of neuromuscular function to ensure adequate ventilation and maintenance of patent airway. Determine recovery through assessment of response to peripheral nerve stimulator, skeletal muscle tone, and respiratory measurements. To readminister rocuronium or vecuronium, minimum wait time is 5 min with 1.2 mg/kg of rocuronium or 4 hr for 0.6 mg/kg of rocuronium or 0.1 mg/kg of vecuronium; 24 hr is recommended.
- Monitor for signs and symptoms of anaphylaxis (urticaria, rash, erythema, flushing, skin eruption, hypotension, tachycardia, swelling of tongue, swelling of pharynx, bronchospasm, wheezing) following injection. May require vasopressors and ventilatory support.
- Monitor for bradycardia during and after injection. May require atropine if clinically significant.

Lab Test Considerations

- Monitor aPTT and PT/INR in patients with known coagulopathies, being treated with therapeutic anticoagulation, receiving thromboprophylaxis or drugs other than heparin and low molecular weight heparin, or receiving thromboprophylaxis drugs and who then receive a dose of 16 mg/kg sugammadex.

Implementation

IV Administration

- **IV Push (Adults):** Administer as a single undiluted bolus injection into an existing IV line with 0.9% NaCl, D5W, D2.5/0.45% NaCl, D5/0.9% NaCl, D5/isolyte P, LR, or Ringer's solution. Solution is clear and colorless to slightly yellow-brown; do not administer solutions that are discolored or contain particulate matter. **Rate:** Inject over 10 sec. Ensure line is flushed with 0.9% NaCl between sugammadex and other drugs.
- **IV Push (Children):** Administer as a single undiluted bolus injection (100 mg/mL) into an existing IV line with 0.9% NaCl, D5W, D2.5/0.45% NaCl, D5/0.9% NaCl, D5/isolyte P, LR, or Ringer's solution. To ↑ the accuracy of dosing in children, may be diluted by transferring entire contents of 2-mL vial of sugammadex to a bottle or IV bag containing 18 mL of 0.9% NaCl (resulting concentration 10 mg/mL).

Rate: Inject over 10 sec. Ensure line is flushed with 0.9% NaCl between sugammadex and other drugs.
- **Y-Site Incompatibility:** ondansetron, verapamil.

Patient/Family Teaching
- Rep: Advise women of reproductive potential to notify health care provider if pregnancy is planned or suspected or if breastfeeding. May ↓ effect of hormonal contraceptives for up to 7 days. Advise women to use an additional nonhormonal contraceptive method (e.g., condoms and spermicides) for next 7 days.

Evaluation/Desired Outcomes
- Reversal of neuromuscular blocking effects of rocuronium and vecuronium.

sulbactam/durlobactam
(sul-**bak**-tam/der-low-**bak**-tam)

Xacduro

Classification

Therapeutic: anti-infectives

Pharmacologic: beta-lactams, beta-lactamase inhibitors

Indications
Hospital-acquired bacterial pneumonia and ventilator-associated bacterial pneumonia caused by susceptible isolates of *Acinetobacter baumannii-calcoaceticus* complex.

Action
Sulbactam is a beta-lactam antibiotic and a beta-lactamase inhibitor that inhibits *Acinetobacter baumannii-calcoaceticus* complex penicillin-binding proteins. Durlobactam is a beta-lactamase inhibitor that protects sulbactam from being degraded by certain serine-beta-lactamases. **Therapeutic Effects:** Bactericidal action against susceptible bacteria. **Spectrum:** Active against the following gram-negative pathogen: *Acinetobacter baumannii-calcoaceticus* complex.

Pharmacokinetics
Absorption: IV administration results in complete bioavailability.

Distribution: Well distributed to tissues.

Metabolism and Excretion: Undergoes minimal metabolism. Primarily excreted by the kidneys, with 75–85% of sulbactam and 78% of durlobactam being excreted as unchanged drug.

Half-life: *Sulbactam:* 2–3 hr; *Durlobactam:* 2–3 hr.

TIME/ACTION PROFILE (plasma concentrations)

ROUTE	ONSET	PEAK	DURATION
IV	rapid	end of infusion	6 hr

Contraindications/Precautions
Contraindicated in: Hypersensitivity to sulbactam, durlobactam, or any beta-lactam antibiotic.

Use Cautiously in: Renal impairment (↓ dose if CCr <45 mL/min); CCr ≥130 mL/min; OB: Safety not established in pregnancy; Lactation: Safety not established in breastfeeding; Pedi: Safety and effectiveness not established in children; Geri: Consider age-related ↓ in renal function in determining dose in older adults.

Adverse Reactions/Side Effects
CV: arrhythmia. **F and E:** hypokalemia. **GI:** ↑ liver enzymes, diarrhea, CLOSTRIDIOIDES DIFFICILE-ASSOCIATED DIARRHEA (CDAD), constipation. **GU:** acute kidney injury. **Hemat:** anemia, thrombocytopenia. **Misc:** HYPERSENSITIVITY REACTIONS (INCLUDING ANAPHYLAXIS).

Interactions
Drug-Drug: Probenecid may ↓ renal excretion and ↑ levels of sulbactam; concurrent use not recommended.

Route/Dosage
IV (Adults): *CCr 45–129 mL/min:* Sulbactam 1 g/durlobactam 1 g every 6 hr for 7–14 days. *CCr ≥130 mL/min:* Sulbactam 1 g/durlobactam 1 g every 4 hr for 7–14 days.

Renal Impairment
IV (Adults): *CCr 30–44 mL/min:* Sulbactam 1 g/durlobactam 1 g every 8 hr for 7–14 days. *CCr 15–29 mL/min:* Sulbactam 1 g/durlobactam 1 g every 12 hr for 7–14 days. *CCr <15 mL/min (at baseline before initiating therapy):* Sulbactam 1 g/durlobactam 1 g every 12 hr for first 3 doses; then sulbactam 1 g/durlobactam 1 g every 24 hr to complete a total treatment course of 7–14 days. *CCr <15 mL/min (after initiating therapy):* Sulbactam 1 g/durlobactam 1 g every 24 hr for 7–14 days.

Availability
Lyophilized powder for injection: sulbactam 1 g/vial + durlobactam 0.5 g/vial (2 vials supplied).

NURSING IMPLICATIONS
Assessment
- Assess patient for infection (vital signs, wound appearance, sputum, urine, stool, WBCs) at beginning and throughout therapy.
- Obtain a history before initiating therapy to determine previous use of and reaction to carbapenems, penicillins, cephalosporins or other beta lactams.
- Monitor for signs/symptoms hypersensitivity reactions (rash, pruritus, laryngeal edema, anaphylaxis).

If symptoms occur, discontinue sulbactam/durlobactam and treat as indicated. Keep epinephrine, antihistamine, and resuscitation equipment close by.

- Monitor bowel function for diarrhea, abdominal cramping, fever, and bloody stools. *If CDAD suspected,* discontinue therapy and treat as clinically indicated. May begin up to several months following cessation of therapy.
- Monitor for rash; may lead to severe skin reactions.

Lab Test Considerations

- Obtain specimens for culture and sensitivity before therapy. 1st dose may be given before receiving results.
- May ↑ ALT and AST.
- May cause hypokalemia and thrombocytopenia.

Implementation

IV Administration

- **Intermittent Infusion:** *Xacduro* kit includes one clear single-dose vial of sulbactam 1 g and two amber single-dose vials of durlobactam 0.5 g as sterile powders. **Reconstitution:** Reconstitute *sulbactam* 1-g vial with 5 mL of sterile water for injection; gently shake to dissolve. Solution is clear, colorless to slightly yellow; do not use if cloudy, discolored, or contains particulates. Dilution must occur within 1 hr of reconstitution. Reconstitute each *durlobactam* 0.5-g vial with 2.5 mL of sterile water for injection; gently shake to dissolve. Solution is clear, light yellow to orange; do not use if cloudy, discolored, or contains particulates. Dilution must occur within 1 hr of reconstitution. **Dilution:** Withdraw 5 mL of reconstituted sulbactam and 5 mL (2.5 mL from each vial) of reconstituted durlobactam. Add total withdrawn volume of both sulbactam and durlobactam to a 100 mL bag of 0.9% NaCl. Discard unused portion. Store solution in refrigerator. Allow solution to reach room temperature over 15–30 min before administering; stable for 24 hr if refrigerated. **Rate:** Infuse over 3 hr.
- **Y-Site Compatibility:** amikacin, anidulafungin, azithromycin, aztreonam, bumetanide, calcium chloride, calcium gluconate, caspofungin, cefazolin, cefepime, cefiderocol, cefotetan, cefoxitin, ceftazidime, ceftolozane/tazobactam, ceftriaxone, cefuroxime, cisatracurium, dexamethasone, dexmedetomidine, digoxin, diltiazem, diphenhydramine, dobutamine, dopamine, doxycycline, epinephrine, eravacycline, ertapenem, esmolol, esomeprazole, famotidine, fentanyl, fluconazole, fosphenytoin, furosemide, gentamicin, heparin, hydrocortisone, hydromorphone, imipenem/cilastatin, imipenem/cilastatin/relebactam, insulin regular, isavuconazonium, labetalol, lidocaine, linezolid, lorazepam, magnesium sulfate, mannitol, meperidine, meropenem, meropenem/vaborbactam, mesna, methylprednisolone, metronidazole, micafungin, midazolam, milrinone, minocycline, morphine, naloxone, nicardipine, nitroglycerin, norepinephrine, octreotide, omadacycline, ondansetron, pantoprazole, penicillin G potassium, phenylephrine, piperacillin/tazobactam, plazomicin, potassium chloride, potassium phosphates, rocuronium, sodium bicarbonate, sodium phosphates, tigecycline, tobramycin, vancomycin, vasopressin.
- **Y-Site Incompatibility:** albumin, human, amiodarone, ceftaroline, ciprofloxacin, daptomycin, levofloxacin, phenytoin, propofol, vecuronium.

Patient/Family Teaching

- Explain purpose and side effects of medication. Advise patient to read *Patient Information* before starting therapy.
- Advise patient to report rash or signs of superinfection (furry overgrowth on the tongue, vaginal itching or discharge, loose or foul-smelling stools).
- Advise patient that serious allergic reaction may occur and to notify health care provider immediately if rash, swelling of face or airway, or difficulty breathing occur.
- Caution patient to notify health care provider if fever and diarrhea occur, especially if stool contains blood, pus, or mucus. Advise patient not to treat diarrhea without consulting health care provider. May occur up to several weeks after discontinuation of medication.
- Rep: Advise women of reproductive potential to notify health care provider if pregnancy is planned or suspected or if breastfeeding.

Evaluation/Desired Outcomes

- Resolution of signs and symptoms of infection. Length of time for complete resolution depends on the organism and site of infection.

sulconazole, See ANTIFUNGALS (TOPICAL).

sulfaSALAzine

(sul-fa-**sal**-a-zeen)

Azulfidine, Azulfidine EN-tabs, Salazopyrin

Classification

Therapeutic: antirheumatics (DMARD), gastrointestinal anti-inflammatories

Indications

Mild to moderate ulcerative colitis or as adjunctive therapy in severe ulcerative colitis. Rheumatoid arthritis unresponsive or intolerant to salicylates and/or NSAIDs.

Action

Locally acting anti-inflammatory action in the colon, where activity is probably a result of inhibition of prostaglandin synthesis. **Therapeutic Effects:** Reduction in the symptoms of ulcerative colitis or rheumatoid arthritis.

Pharmacokinetics

Absorption: 10–15% absorbed after oral administration.
Distribution: Widely distributed to tissues.
Protein Binding: 99%.
Metabolism and Excretion: Split by intestinal bacteria into sulfapyridine and 5-aminosalicylic acid. Some absorbed sulfasalazine is excreted by bile back into intestines; 15% excreted unchanged by the kidneys. Sulfapyridine also excreted mostly by the kidneys.
Half-life: 6 hr.

TIME/ACTION PROFILE (plasma concentrations)

ROUTE	ONSET	PEAK	DURATION
PO	1 hr	1.5–6 hr	6–12 hr

Contraindications/Precautions

Contraindicated in: Hypersensitivity reactions to sulfonamides, salicylates, or sulfasalazine; Cross-sensitivity with furosemide, sulfonylurea hypoglycemic agents, or carbonic anhydrase inhibitors may exist; Glucose-6-phosphate dehydrogenase deficiency (↑ risk of hemolysis); Hypersensitivity to bisulfites (mesalamine enema only); Urinary tract or intestinal obstruction; Porphyria.
Use Cautiously in: Severe renal impairment; Severe hepatic impairment; History of porphyria; Blood dyscrasias; OB: Neural tube defects have been reported; use during pregnancy only if potential maternal benefit justifies potential fetal risk; Lactation: May compete with bilirubin for binding sites on plasma proteins in the newborn and cause kernicterus; bloody stools or diarrhea reported in breastfed infants; Pedi: Children <2 yr (safety and effectiveness not established).

Adverse Reactions/Side Effects

Derm: rash, ACUTE GENERALIZED EXANTHEMATOUS PUSTULOSIS, DRUG REACTION WITH EOSINOPHILIA AND SYSTEMIC SYMPTOMS (DRESS), EXFOLIATIVE DERMATITIS, photosensitivity, STEVENS-JOHNSON SYNDROME (SJS), TOXIC EPIDERMAL NECROLYSIS (TEN), yellow discoloration. **GI:** anorexia, diarrhea, nausea, vomiting, drug-induced hepatitis. **GU:** crystalluria, infertility, oligospermia, orange-yellow discoloration of urine, renal impairment. **Hemat:** AGRANULOCYTOSIS, APLASTIC ANEMIA, blood dyscrasias, eosinophilia, hemolytic anemia, megaloblastic anemia, thrombocytopenia. **Neuro:** headache, peripheral neuropathy. **Resp:** pneumonitis. **Misc:** fever, HYPERSENSITIVITY REACTIONS (INCLUDING ANAPHYLAXIS AND ANGIOEDEMA).

Interactions

Drug-Drug: May ↑ risk of toxicity of **oral hypoglycemic agents**, **phenytoin**, **methotrexate**, **zidovudine**, or **warfarin**. ↑ risk of drug-induced hepatitis with other **hepatotoxic agents**. ↑ risk of crystalluria with **methenamine**. May ↑ levels and risk of toxicity of **mercaptopurine** or **thioguanine**.
Drug-Food: May ↓ **iron** and **folic acid** absorption.

Route/Dosage

Ulcerative Colitis

PO (Adults): 1 g every 6–8 hr (may start with 500 mg every 6–12 hr), followed by maintenance dose of 500 mg every 6 hr.
PO (Children >2 yr): *Initial:* 6.7–10 mg/kg every 4 hr *or* 10–15 mg/kg every 6 hr *or* 13.3–20 mg/kg every 8 hr. *Maintenance:* 7.5 mg/kg every 6 hr (not to exceed 2 g/day).

Rheumatoid Arthritis

PO (Adults): 500 mg–1 g/day (as delayed-release tablets) for 1 wk; then ↑ by 500 mg/day every week up to 2 g/day in 2 divided doses; if no benefit seen after 12 wk, ↑ to 3 g/day in 2 divided doses.
PO (Children ≥6 yr): 30–50 mg/kg/day in 2 divided doses (as delayed-release tablets); initiate therapy at 25% of planned maintenance dose and ↑ every 7 days until maintenance dose is reached (not to exceed 2 g/day).

Availability (generic available)

Tablets: 500 mg. **Delayed-release (enteric-coated) tablets (Azulfidine EN-tabs):** 500 mg.

S

NURSING IMPLICATIONS

Assessment

- Assess for allergies to sulfonamides and salicylates. Discontinue therapy if rash, difficulty breathing, swelling of face or lips, or fever occur.
- Monitor intake and output. Fluid intake should be sufficient to maintain a urine output of ≥1200–1500 mL/day to prevent crystalluria and stone formation.
- Assess for rash periodically during therapy. May cause SJS, TEN, and DRESS. Discontinue therapy if severe or if accompanied by fever, general malaise, fatigue, muscle or joint aches, blisters, oral lesions, conjunctivitis, hepatitis, or eosinophilia.
- **Ulcerative Colitis:** Assess abdominal pain and frequency, quantity, and consistency of stools at the beginning of and during therapy.
- **Rheumatoid Arthritis:** Assess range of motion and degree of swelling and pain in affected joints before and periodically during therapy.

Lab Test Considerations

- Monitor urinalysis, BUN, and serum creatinine before and periodically during therapy. May cause crystalluria and urinary cell calculi formation. *If renal function declines,* discontinue sulfasalazine.
- Monitor CBC with differential and liver function tests before and every 2 wk during 1st 3 mo of therapy, monthly during the 2nd 3 mo, and every 3 mo thereafter or as clinically indicated. *If blood dyscrasias occur,* discontinue sulfasalazine
- Higher than recommended doses can interfere with a variety of lab assays that use nicotinamide adenine dinucleotide or nicotinamide adenine dinucleotide phosphate (CK, AST/ALT, ammonia, thyroxine, glucose).

Implementation

- Do not confuse sulfasalazine with cefuroxime or sulfadiazine.
- Varying dosing regimens of sulfasalazine may be used to minimize GI side effects.
- **PO:** Administer after meals or with food to minimize GI irritation, with 8 ounces of water. ***DNC:*** Swallow enteric-coated tablets whole; do not crush or chew.

Patient/Family Teaching

- Explain purpose and side effects of medication. Advise patient to read *Patient Information* before starting therapy. Instruct patient on the correct method of administration. Advise patient to take medication as directed, even if feeling better. Take missed doses as soon as remembered unless almost time for next dose.
- Advise patient to notify health care provider of all Rx or OTC medications, vitamins, or herbal products being taken and to consult with health care provider before taking other medications.
- May cause dizziness. Caution patient to avoid driving or other activities that require alertness until response to medication is known.
- Advise patient to notify health care provider if skin rash, sore throat, fever, mouth sores, unusual bleeding or bruising, wheezing, fever, or hives occur.
- Caution patient to use sunscreen and protective clothing to prevent photosensitivity reactions.
- Inform patient that this medication may cause orange-yellow discoloration of urine and skin, which is not significant. May permanently stain contact lenses yellow.
- Instruct patient to notify health care provider if symptoms worsen or do not improve. If symptoms of acute intolerance (cramping, acute abdominal pain, bloody diarrhea, fever, headache, rash) occur, discontinue therapy and notify health care provider immediately.
- Instruct patient to notify health care provider if symptoms do not improve after 1–2 mo of therapy.
- Rep: May cause fetal harm. Advise women of reproductive potential to notify health care provider if pregnancy is planned or suspected and to avoid breastfeeding during therapy. Neural tube defects have been reported in infants of women taking sulfasalazine during pregnancy. Monitor newborns for kernicterus if mother taking sulfasalazine; monitor breastfed infants for bloody stool or diarrhea. Inform men that sulfasalazine may cause infertility; usually reversible.

Evaluation/Desired Outcomes

- Reduction in the symptoms of ulcerative colitis or rheumatoid arthritis.

HIGH ALERT

SULFONYLUREAS

glimepiride (glye-**me**-pye-ride)

~~Amaryl~~

glipiZIDE (**glip**-i-zide)

~~Glucotrol XL~~

glyBURIDE (**glye**-byoo-ride)

~~DiaBeta~~, Euglucon, ~~Glynase~~

Classification

Therapeutic: antidiabetics

Pharmacologic: sulfonylureas

Indications

Type 2 diabetes mellitus.

Action

Lower blood glucose by stimulating the release of insulin from the pancreas and increasing the sensitivity to insulin at receptor sites. May also decrease hepatic glucose production. **Therapeutic Effects:** Lowering of blood glucose in patients with diabetes.

Pharmacokinetics

Absorption: All agents are well absorbed after oral administration.

Distribution: *Glyburide:* Reaches high concentrations in bile and crosses the placenta.

Protein Binding: *Glimepiride:* 99.5%, *glipizide:* 99%, *glyburide:* 99%.

Metabolism and Excretion: All agents are mostly metabolized by the liver. *Glimepiride:* Converted to a metabolite with some hypoglycemic activity; *Glyburide:* Primarily metabolized by CYP2C9.

Half-life: *Glimepiride:* 5–9.2; *glipizide:* 2.1–2.6 hr; *glyburide:* 10 hr.

TIME/ACTION PROFILE (hypoglycemic activity)

ROUTE	ONSET	PEAK	DURATION
Glimepiride	unknown	2–3 hr	24 hr
Glipizide	15–30 min	1–2 hr	up to 24 hr
Glyburide	45–60 min	1.5–3 hr	24 hr

Contraindications/Precautions

Contraindicated in: Hypersensitivity; Hypersensitivity with sulfonamides (cross-sensitivity may occur); Type 1 diabetes; Diabetic coma or ketoacidosis; Concurrent use of bosentan (glyburide only).

Use Cautiously in: Glucose-6-phosphate dehydrogenase deficiency (↑ risk of hemolytic anemia); Renal or hepatic dysfunction (↑ risk of hypoglycemia); Infection, trauma, or surgery (may alter requirements for control of blood glucose); Impaired pituitary or adrenal function; Prolonged nausea or vomiting; Debilitated or malnourished patients (↑ risk of hypoglycemia); OB: Cross the placenta and ↑ risk of neonatal hypoglycemia; should be discontinued ≥2 wk before delivery; insulin recommended during pregnancy; Lactation: May ↑ risk of hypoglycemia in infant; use while breastfeeding only if benefit to patient outweighs potential risk to infant; Pedi: Safety and effectiveness not established; Geri: ↑ sensitivity; dose reduction may be required.

Adverse Reactions/Side Effects

Derm: ERYTHEMA MULTIFORME, photosensitivity, exfoliative dermatitis, rash. **Endo:** hypoglycemia. **F and E:** hyponatremia. **GI:** constipation, cramps, diarrhea, drug-induced hepatitis, heartburn, nausea, vomiting. **Hemat:** APLASTIC ANEMIA, agranulocytosis, hemolytic anemia, leukopenia, pancytopenia, thrombocytopenia. **Metab:** ↑ appetite, weight gain. **Neuro:** dizziness, drowsiness, headache, weakness.

Interactions

Drug-Drug: ↑ risk of elevated liver enzymes when **bosentan** used with glyburide (avoid concurrent use). Effectiveness may be ↓ by concurrent use of **diuretics**, **corticosteroids**, **atypical antipsychotics**, **danazol**, **phenothiazines**, **oral contraceptives**, **estrogens**, **progestins**, **glucagon**, **protease inhibitors**, **somatropin**, **thyroid preparations**, **phenytoin**, **niacin**, **sympathomimetics**, **calcium channel blockers**, and **isoniazid**. **Alcohol**, **ACE inhibitors**, **angiotensin II receptor blockers**, **chloramphenicol**, **fibric acid derivatives**, **fluoxetine**, **disopyramide**, **fluoroquinolones**, **MAO inhibitors**, **NSAIDs** (except diclofenac), **pentoxifylline**, **probenecid**, **salicylates**, **voriconazole**, **H_2 receptor antagonists**, **sulfonamides**, and **warfarin** may ↑ risk of hypoglycemia. Concurrent use with **warfarin** may alter the response to both agents (↑ effects of both initially, then ↓ activity); close monitoring recommended during any changes in dose. **Beta blockers** may mask the signs and symptoms of hypoglycemia. May ↑ **cyclosporine** levels. **Colesevelam** may ↓ effects; administer glyburide, glipizide, and glimepiride ≥4 hr before colesevelam. **Topiramate** may ↓ levels and effects of glyburide.

Route/Dosage

Glimepiride

PO (Adults): 1–2 mg once daily initially; may ↑ every 1–2 wk up to 8 mg/day (usual range 1–4 mg/day).

PO (Geriatric Patients): 1 mg once daily initially.

Glipizide

PO (Adults): 5 mg once daily initially; may ↑ by 2.5–5 mg/day at weekly intervals as needed (max dose = 40 mg/day immediate release; 20 mg/day extended release). Extended-release tablets are given once daily. Doses >15 mg/day of immediate-release tablets should be given as 2 divided doses.

PO (Geriatric Patients): 2.5 mg once daily initially.

Glyburide

PO (Adults): 2.5–5 mg once daily initially; may ↑ by 2.5–5 mg/day at weekly intervals (range 1.25–20 mg/day).

PO (Geriatric Patients): 1.25 mg once daily initially; may ↑ by 2.5 mg/day at weekly intervals.

Availability

Glimepiride (generic available)

Tablets: 1 mg, 2 mg, 4 mg. ***In combination with:*** pioglitazone (Duetact); rosiglitazone (Avandaryl); see Appendix N.

Glipizide (generic available)

Extended-release tablets: 2.5 mg, 5 mg, 10 mg. **Tablets:** 5 mg, 10 mg. ***In combination with:*** Metformin (Metaglip); see Appendix N.

Glyburide (generic available)

Tablets: 1.25 mg, 2.5 mg, 5 mg. ***In combination with:*** metformin (Glucovance); see Appendix N.

NURSING IMPLICATIONS

Assessment

- Monitor for signs/symptoms of hypoglycemia (sweating, hunger, weakness, dizziness, tremor, tachycardia, anxiety).
- Assess patient for allergy to sulfonamides.
- Assess skin and mucosal integrity for rapid spread of lesions or blistering.
- Patients on concurrent beta blocker therapy may have very subtle signs of hypoglycemia.

Lab Test Considerations

- Monitor serum glucose and A1c periodically during therapy to evaluate effectiveness of treatment.
- Monitor CBC periodically during therapy. Report ↓ in blood counts promptly.
- May ↑ AST, LDH, BUN, and serum creatinine.

Toxicity and Overdose

- Overdose is manifested by symptoms of hypoglycemia. Mild hypoglycemia may be treated with administration of oral glucose. Severe hypoglycemia should

S

be treated with IV D50W followed by continuous IV infusion of more dilute dextrose solution at a rate sufficient to keep serum glucose at approximately 100 mg/dL.

Implementation

- ***High Alert:*** Accidental administration of oral hypoglycemic agents to adults and children without type 2 diabetes has resulted in serious harm or death. Before administering, confirm that patient has type 2 diabetes.
- ***High Alert:*** Do not confuse glipizide with glyburide.
- Patients stabilized on a diabetic regimen who are exposed to stress, fever, trauma, infection, or surgery may require administration of insulin.
- To convert from other oral hypoglycemic agents, gradual conversion is not required. For insulin dose of <20 units/day, change to oral hypoglycemic agents can be made without gradual dose adjustment. Patients taking ≥20 units/day should convert gradually by receiving oral agent and ↓ insulin dose by 25–30% every day or every 2nd day with gradual insulin dose ↓ as tolerated. Monitor serum or urine glucose and ketones ≥3 times/day during conversion.
- **PO:** Administer once in the morning with breakfast or divided into 2 doses.
- Administer *glipizide* 30 min before a meal.

Patient/Family Teaching

- Explain purpose and side effects of medication to patient. Advise patient to read *Patient Information* before starting therapy. Advise patient to take at same time each day. Take missed doses as soon as remembered unless almost time for next dose. Do not take if unable to eat.
- Advise patient to notify health care provider of all Rx or OTC medications, vitamins, or herbal products being taken and to consult with health care provider before taking other medications.
- Explain to patient that this medication controls hyperglycemia but does not cure diabetes. Therapy is long term.
- Review signs of hypoglycemia and hyperglycemia with patient. If hypoglycemia occurs, advise patient to drink 4 ounces of orange juice or 2–3 teaspoons of sugar, honey, or corn syrup dissolved in water or an appropriate number of glucose tablets and notify health care provider.
- Encourage patient to follow prescribed diet, medication, and exercise regimen to prevent hypoglycemic or hyperglycemic episodes.
- Advise patient in proper testing of serum glucose and ketones. These tests should be closely monitored during periods of stress or illness and health care provider notified if significant changes occur.
- May occasionally cause dizziness or drowsiness. Advise patient to avoid driving or other activities requiring alertness until response to medication is known.
- Advise patient to avoid other medications, especially alcohol, while on this therapy without consulting health care provider. Concurrent use of alcohol may cause a disulfiram-like reaction (abdominal cramps, nausea, flushing, headaches, and hypoglycemia).
- Advise patient to use sunscreen and protective clothing to prevent photosensitivity reactions.
- Advise patient to inform health care provider of medication regimen before treatment or surgery.
- Advise patient to carry a form of sugar (sugar packets, candy) and identification describing disease process and medication regimen at all times.
- Advise patient to notify health care provider promptly if unusual weight gain, swelling of ankles, drowsiness, shortness of breath, muscle cramps, weakness, sore throat, rash, or unusual bleeding or bruising occurs.
- Rep: Insulin is the recommended method of controlling blood glucose during pregnancy. Advise women of reproductive potential to use a form of contraception other than oral contraceptives, to notify health care provider promptly if pregnancy is planned or suspected, and to avoid breastfeeding. If therapy continued during breastfeeding, monitor infant for hypoglycemia.

Evaluation/Desired Outcomes

- Lowering of blood glucose in patients with diabetes.

sulopenem etzadroxil/probenecid

(soo-loe-**pen**-em et-za-**drox**-il/ proe-**ben**-e-sid)

Orlynvah

Classification

Therapeutic: anti-infectives

Pharmacologic: uricosurics

Indications

Uncomplicated urinary tract infections in women who have limited or no alternative oral antibiotic treatment options.

Action

Sulopenem etzadroxil: Inhibits bacterial cell wall synthesis. *Probenecid:* Inhibits OAT3-mediated renal clearance of sulopenem, resulting in ↑ levels of sulopenem. **Therapeutic Effects:** Bactericidal action against susceptible bacteria. **Spectrum:** Active against the following gram-negative organisms: *Escherichia coli*, *Klebsiella pneumoniae*, *Proteus mirabilis*.

Pharmacokinetics

Sulopenem Etzadroxil

Absorption: 40% absorbed in fasting state; food ↑ absorption (64%).

Distribution: Well distributed to tissues.
Metabolism and Excretion: Prodrug that is hydrolyzed by esterases to the active drug, sulopenem, which then undergoes hydrolysis followed by dehydrogenation. 44% excreted in feces (27% as unchanged drug); 41% excreted in urine (3% as unchanged drug).
Half-life: 1.2 hr.

Probenecid
Absorption: Extent of absorption unknown.
Distribution: Minimally distributed to tissues.
Metabolism and Excretion: Routes of metabolism and excretion unknown.
Half-life: 3–4 hr.

TIME/ACTION PROFILE (plasma concentrations)

ROUTE	ONSET	PEAK	DURATION
PO	unknown	1–3 hr	12 hr

Contraindications/Precautions

Contraindicated in: Hypersensitivity; Serious hypersensitivity to other beta-lactams (cross-sensitivity may occur); Blood dyscrasias; Uric acid kidney stones; Concurrent use with ketorolac; CCr <15 mL/min or on hemodialysis.
Use Cautiously in: History of gout (↑ risk of nephrolithiasis); OB: Safety not established in pregnancy; Lactation: Safety not established in breastfeeding; Pedi: Safety and effectiveness not established in children.

Adverse Reactions/Side Effects

GI: diarrhea, abdominal pain, CLOSTRIDIOIDES DIFFICILE-ASSOCIATED DIARRHEA (CDAD), nausea, vomiting. **GU:** nephrolithiasis, vulvovaginal infection. **Metab:** gout, hyperuricemia. **Neuro:** headache. **Misc:** HYPERSENSITIVITY REACTIONS (INCLUDING ANAPHYLAXIS AND ANGIOEDEMA).

Interactions

Drug-Drug: May significantly ↑ levels and risk of toxicity of **ketorolac**; concurrent use contraindicated. May ↑ levels and risk of toxicity of **ketoprofen**; concurrent use not recommended. May ↑ levels and risk of toxicity of **indomethacin**, **lorazepam**, **naproxen**, **rifampin**, and **sulfonylureas**. May ↑ levels and risk of toxicity of **methotrexate**; avoid concurrent use. **OAT3 inhibitors** may ↑ levels and risk of toxicity.

Route/Dosage

PO (Adults): One tablet (sulopenem etzadroxil 500 mg/probenecid 500 mg) twice daily for 5 days.

Renal Impairment

PO (Adults): *CCr <15 mL/min or hemodialysis:* Use not recommended.

Availability

Tablets: sulopenem etzadroxil 500 mg/probenecid 500 mg.

NURSING IMPLICATIONS

Assessment

- Monitor for signs/symptoms of urinary tract infection (fever, dysuria, polyuria, hematuria, flank pain, suprapubic pain or pressure).
- Monitor for signs/symptoms of CDAD including watery diarrhea with mucus, fever, abdominal pain or cramping, anorexia, nausea, and in severe cases, dehydration, and blood or pus in the stool. May occur >2 mo after therapy.
- Monitor for signs/symptoms of hypersensitivity reactions (rash, urticaria, pruritus, flushing, dizziness, vomiting, abdominal pain) and angioedema (swelling of throat, lips, tongue, face, dyspnea, wheezing, hoarseness). *If hypersensitivity reaction occurs,* discontinue sulopenem etzadroxil/probenecid and provide supportive care.

Lab Test Considerations

- May cause hyperuricemia.

Implementation

- **PO:** Administer twice daily with food.

Patient/Family Teaching

- Explain purpose and side effects. Advise to take twice daily with food as directed. Take missed dose as soon as possible; do not double the dose. Do not share medication with others, even if they have similar symptoms; may be harmful. Advise patient to read *Patient Information* before starting therapy.
- Inform patient of the importance of receiving the full course of therapy even if feeling better. If urinary symptoms worsen or do not resolve, another appointment should be scheduled as soon as possible for re-evaluation.
- Instruct patient to notify health care professional immediately if diarrhea, abdominal cramping, fever, or bloody stools occur and not to treat with antidiarrheals without consulting health care professionals.
- Advise patients and family to call 911 and seek urgent treatment for signs and symptoms of hypersensitivity reactions such as difficulty breathing, chest tightness, hives, rash, feeling lightheaded, itching, swelling of the face, lips, tongue, or throat.
- Advise patient to notify health care professional of all Rx or OTC medications, vitamins, or herbal products being taken and to consult health care professional before taking other medications.
- Rep: Advise patient to notify health care professional if pregnancy is planned or suspected or if breastfeeding.

Evaluation/Desired Outcomes

- Bactericidal action against susceptible bacteria.

S

SUMAtriptan (soo-ma-**trip**-tan)

Imitrex, ✱ Imitrex DF, Imitrex STATdose, Onzetra Xsail, Tosymra, Zembrace SymTouch

Classification

Therapeutic: vascular headache suppressants

Pharmacologic: 5-HT_1 agonists

Indications

SUBQ PO Intranasal: Acute treatment of migraine attacks. **SUBQ:** Acute treatment of cluster headache episodes.

Action

Acts as a selective agonist of 5-HT_1 at specific vascular serotonin receptor sites, causing vasoconstriction in large intracranial arteries. **Therapeutic Effects:** Relief of acute attacks of migraine.

Pharmacokinetics

Absorption: Well absorbed (97%) after SUBQ administration. Absorption after oral administration is incomplete and significant amounts undergo substantial hepatic metabolism, resulting in poor bioavailability (14%). Well absorbed after intranasal administration.
Distribution: Well distributed to tissues.
Metabolism and Excretion: Mostly metabolized (80%) by the liver.
Half-life: 2 hr.

TIME/ACTION PROFILE (relief of migraine)

ROUTE	ONSET	PEAK	DURATION
PO	within 30 min	2–4 hr	up to 24 hr
SUBQ	30 min	up to 2 hr	up to 24 hr
Nasal	within 60 min	2 hr	unknown

Contraindications/Precautions

Contraindicated in: Hypersensitivity to sumatriptan or latex (needle shield of prefilled syringe contains rubber [latex derivative]); Ischemic heart disease or signs and symptoms of ischemic heart disease, Prinzmetal angina, or uncontrolled hypertension; Stroke or transient ischemic attack; Peripheral arterial disease (including but not limited to ischemic bowel disease); Hemiplegic or basilar migraine; Severe hepatic impairment.
Use Cautiously in: OB: Use during pregnancy only if potential maternal benefit justifies potential fetal risk; Lactation: Use while breastfeeding only if potential maternal benefit justifies potential risk to infant; Rep: Women of reproductive potential; Pedi: Safety and effectiveness not established in children; Geri: ↑ risk of cardiovascular complications in older adults.
Exercise Extreme Caution in: Cardiovascular risk factors (hypertension, hypercholesterolemia, smoking, obesity, diabetes, family history, menopausal women, men >40 yr); use only if cardiovascular status has been evaluated and determined to be safe and 1st dose is administered under supervision.

Adverse Reactions/Side Effects

CV: angina, chest pressure, chest tightness, coronary vasospasm, ECG changes, MI, transient hypertension. **Derm:** tingling, warm sensation, burning sensation, cool sensation, flushing. **EENT:** alterations in vision, nasal sinus discomfort, throat discomfort. **GI:** abdominal discomfort, dysphagia. **Local:** injection site reaction. **MS:** jaw discomfort, muscle cramps, myalgia, neck pain, neck stiffness. **Neuro:** dizziness, vertigo, anxiety, drowsiness, fatigue, feeling of heaviness, feeling of tightness, headache, malaise, numbness, tight feeling in head, weakness. **Misc:** HYPERSENSITIVITY REACTIONS (INCLUDING ANAPHYLAXIS AND ANGIOEDEMA).

Interactions

Drug-Drug: Risk of vasospastic reactions may be ↑ by concurrent use of **ergotamine** or **dihydroergotamine**; avoid use within 24 hr of each other. Avoid concurrent use with other **5HT_1 agonists**. **MAO inhibitors** may ↑ levels and risk of toxicity; do not use within 2 wk of discontinuing MAO inhibitor. ↑ risk of serotonin syndrome with **SSRIs**, **SNRIs**, **TCAs**, **meperidine**, **bupropion**, or **buspirone**; avoid concurrent use.
Drug-Natural Products: ↑ risk of serotonergic side effects, including serotonin syndrome, with **St. John's wort** and **SAMe**.

Route/Dosage

PO (Adults): 50–100 mg initially; if response is inadequate after ≥2 hr, may repeat dose (max = 100 mg/dose; 200 mg/24 hr).
SUBQ (Adults): 6 mg; may repeat after 1 hr (not to exceed 12 mg in 24 hr); *Zembrace SymTouch:* 3 mg; may repeat after 1 hr (not to exceed 12 mg/24 hr).
Intranasal (Adults): *Nasal spray (Imitrex):* Single dose of 5, 10, or 20 mg in 1 nostril; may be repeated in 2 hr (not to exceed 40 mg/24 hr or treatment of >5 episodes/mo); *Nasal spray (Tosymra):* Single dose of 10 mg in 1 nostril; may be repeated in 1 hr (not to exceed 30 mg/24 hr); *Nasal powder:* 11 mg in each nostril; may be repeated in 2 hr (not to exceed 44 mg/24 hr or treatment of >4 episodes/mo).

Hepatic Impairment

PO (Adults): Do not exceed single doses of 50 mg; if response is inadequate after ≥2 hr, may repeat dose (max = 200 mg/24 hr).

Availability (generic available)

Nasal powder capsules (Onzetra Xsail): 11 mg. **Nasal spray (Imitrex, Tosymra):** 5 mg/spray, 10 mg/spray, 20 mg/spray. **Solution for injection (auto-injectors):** 3 mg/0.5 mL, 4 mg/0.5 mL, 6 mg/0.5 mL. **Tablets:** 25 mg, 50 mg100 mg. ***In combination with:*** naproxen (Treximet); see Appendix N.

NURSING IMPLICATIONS

Assessment

- Assess pain location, intensity, duration, and associated symptoms (photophobia, phonophobia, nausea, vomiting) during migraine attack.
- Give initial SUBQ dose under observation to patients with potential for coronary artery disease, including postmenopausal women, men >40 yr, or patients with risk factors for coronary artery disease (hypertension, hypercholesterolemia, obesity, diabetes, smoking, or family history). Monitor BP before and for 1 hr after initial injection. If angina occurs, monitor ECG for ischemic changes.
- Monitor for serotonin syndrome in patients taking SSRIs or SNRIs concurrently with sumatriptan.

Implementation

- Do not confuse sumatriptan with sitagliptin or zolmitriptan.
- **PO:** Administer as soon as symptoms appear. ***DNC:*** Swallow tablets whole; do not crush, break, or chew. Tablets are film-coated to prevent contact with tablet contents, which have an unpleasant taste and may cause nausea and vomiting.
- **SUBQ:** Administer as a single injection. Solution is clear and colorless or pale yellow; do not use if dark-colored or cloudy or if beyond expiration date.
- **Intranasal:** Do not test the spray unit before use. Administer 10-mg dose as 2 sprays of 5 mg in one nostril or 1 spray in each nostril.
- **Nasal Powder:** Remove clear device cap from the reusable delivery device; then remove a disposable nosepiece from foil pouch and click nosepiece into device body. Press fully and promptly release white piercing button on device body to pierce capsule inside nosepiece. White piercing button should only be pressed once and released before administration to each nostril. Insert nosepiece into nostril making a tight seal. Rotate device to place mouthpiece into the mouth. Patient blows forcefully through mouthpiece to deliver the sumatriptan powder into nasal cavity. Vibration (e.g., a rattling noise) may occur, and indicates that patient is blowing forcefully, as directed. Once medication in the 1st nosepiece has been administered, remove and discard nosepiece.

Patient/Family Teaching

- Explain purpose and side effects of medication. Advise patient to read *Patient Information* before starting therapy.
- Advise patient to notify health care provider of all Rx or OTC medications, vitamins, or herbal products being taken and to consult with health care provider before taking other medications. Patients concurrently taking SSRI or SNRI antidepressants should notify health care provider promptly if signs of serotonin syndrome (mental status changes [agitation, hallucinations, coma], autonomic instability [tachycardia, labile BP, hyperthermia], neuromuscular aberrations [hyperreflexia, incoordination], gastrointestinal symptoms [nausea, vomiting, diarrhea]) occur.
- Inform patient that sumatriptan should be used only *during* a migraine attack. It is meant to be used for relief of migraine attacks but not to prevent or ↓ the number of attacks.
- Instruct patient to administer sumatriptan as soon as symptoms of a migraine attack appear, but it may be administered at any time during an attack.
- Advise patient that lying down in a darkened room after sumatriptan administration may further help relieve headache.
- Advise patient that overuse (>10 days/month) may lead to exacerbation of headache (migraine-like daily headaches or as a marked ↑ in frequency of migraine attacks). May require gradual withdrawal of sumatriptan and treatment of symptoms (transient worsening of headache).
- Advise patient to notify health care provider before next dose of sumatriptan if pain or tightness in chest occurs during use. If pain is severe or does not subside, notify health care provider immediately. If wheezing; heart throbbing; swelling of eyelids, face, or lips; skin rash; skin lumps; or hives occur, notify health care provider immediately, and do not take more sumatriptan without approval of health care provider. If usual dose fails to relieve three consecutive headaches or if frequency and/or severity ↑, notify health care provider. If feelings of tingling, heat, flushing, heaviness, pressure, drowsiness, dizziness, tiredness, or sickness develop, discuss with health care provider at next visit.
- Sumatriptan may cause dizziness or drowsiness. Caution patient to avoid driving or other activities requiring alertness until response to medication is known.
- Advise patient to avoid alcohol, which aggravates headaches, during sumatriptan use.
- **SUBQ:** Instruct patient on the proper technique for loading, administering, and discarding the *Imitrex STATdose pen* autoinjector. Patient information pamphlet is provided. Instructional video is available from the manufacturer. If migraine symptoms return after 1st injection, a 2nd injection may be used. Allow ≥1 hr between doses, and do not use >2 injections in any 24-hr period. Additional sumatriptan doses are not likely to be effective, and alternative medications

S

may be used. If no relief from 1st dose, unlikely 2nd dose will provide relief. Inform patient that pain or redness at the injection site usually lasts <1 hr.

- **Intranasal:** Instruct patient in proper technique for intranasal administration. Usual dose is a single spray in one nostril. If headache returns, a 2nd dose may be administered in ≥2 hr. Do not administer 2nd dose if no relief was provided by 1st dose without consulting health care provider.
- Rep: Advise women of reproductive potential to avoid using sumatriptan if pregnancy is planned or suspected or if breastfeeding. Adequate contraception should be used during therapy.

Evaluation/Desired Outcomes

- Relief of acute attacks of migraine.

suvorexant (soo-voe-**rex**-ant)

Belsomra

Classification

Therapeutic: sedative/hypnotics

Pharmacologic: orexin receptor antagonists

Schedule IV

Indications

Insomnia associated with difficulty in sleep onset and/or maintenance.

Action

Antagonizes the effects of orexins A and B, naturally occurring neuropeptides that promote wakefulness, by binding to their receptors. **Therapeutic Effects:** Improved sleep.

Pharmacokinetics

Absorption: 82% absorbed following oral administration; a high-fat meal will delay absorption and sleep onset. ↑ absorption in obese women.

Distribution: Well distributed to tissues.

Protein Binding: >99%.

Metabolism and Excretion: Extensively metabolized by the liver via the CYP3A isoenzyme and to a lesser extent by the CYP2C19 isoenzyme to inactive metabolites. 66% excreted in feces; 23% in urine, mostly as metabolites.

Half-life: 12 hr (↑ in hepatic impairment).

TIME/ACTION PROFILE (sleep)

ROUTE	ONSET	PEAK	DURATION
PO	30 min (delayed by food)	unknown	7 hr†

† Excess sedation may persist for several days after discontinuation.

Contraindications/Precautions

Contraindicated in: Narcolepsy; Severe hepatic impairment.

Use Cautiously in: History of substance abuse or drug dependence; Obese patients (↑ levels, especially in women; dose ↓ may be warranted); History of or concurrent psychiatric diagnoses; Underlying pulmonary disease; OB: Use during pregnancy only if potential maternal benefit justifies potential fetal risk; Lactation: Use while breastfeeding only if potential maternal benefit justifies potential risk to infant; Pedi: Safety and effectiveness not established in children; Geri: ↑ risk of falls in older adults.

Adverse Reactions/Side Effects

Adverse reactions, especially related to CNS depression are dose-related, especially at the 20-mg dose.

Neuro: drowsiness, cataplexy, complex sleep behaviors (including sleep driving, sleep walking, or engaging in other activities while sleeping), daytime drowsiness, hallucinations (during sleep), sleep paralysis, worsening of depression/suicidal ideation.

Interactions

Drug-Drug: Strong CYP3A inhibitors, including **clarithromycin, conivaptan, itraconazole, ketoconazole, nefazodone, nelfinavir, posaconazole,** and **ritonavir**, may ↑ risk of excessive sedation; avoid concurrent use. **Moderate CYP3A inhibitors**, including **aprepitant, atazanavir, ciprofloxacin, diltiazem, erythromycin, fluconazole, fosamprenavir, imatinib,** and **verapamil**, may result in ↑ sedation; ↓ suvorexant dose. Risk of CNS depression, next-day impairment, sleep-driving, and other complex behaviors while not fully awake ↑ with other **CNS depressants**, including **alcohol**, some **antihistamines, opioids**, other **sedative/hypnotics** (including **benzodiazepines**), and **tricyclic antidepressants**; dose adjustments may be necessary. **CYP3A inducers**, including **carbamazepine, phenytoin**, and **rifampin**, may ↓ levels and effectiveness. May alter **digoxin** levels; closely monitor serum digoxin concentrations.

Drug-Food: Grapefruit juice may ↑ levels and excess sedation; ↓ suvorexant dose.

Route/Dosage

PO (Adults): 10 mg within 30 min of going to bed; if well tolerated but not optimally effective, may ↑ dose the following night; not to exceed 20 mg (dose may not be repeated on a single night and should be when ≥7 hr of sleep time is anticipated before planned awakening). *Concurrent use of moderate CYP3A inhibitors:* 5 mg initially; may ↑ dose to 10 mg if lower dose is tolerated but not optimally effective. Lowest effective dose should be used.

Availability

Tablets: 5 mg, 10 mg, 15 mg, 20 mg.

NURSING IMPLICATIONS

Assessment

- Assess mental status, sleep patterns, and potential for abuse before administration. Prolonged use of >7–10 days may lead to physical and psychological dependence. Limit amount of drug available to the patient.
- Assess alertness at time of peak effect. Notify health care provider if desired sedation does not occur.

Implementation

- Before administering, ↓ external stimuli and provide comfort measures to ↑ effectiveness of medication.
- Protect patient from injury. Raise bed rails. Assist with ambulation. Remove potential safety hazards and items that may be harmful.
- Use lowest effective dose.
- **PO:** Administer no more than once/night and within 30 min of going to bed. Take only if ≥7 hr remaining before waking. ***DNC:*** Swallow tablets whole with 8 ounces of water. For faster onset of sleep, do not administer with or immediately after a meal.

Patient/Family Teaching

- Explain purpose and side effects of medication to patient. Advise patient to read *Patient Information* before starting therapy. Instruct patient to take as directed. Advise patient not to take suvorexant unless able to stay in bed for ≥7 hr before being active again. Do not take more than the amount prescribed because of the habit-forming potential. Not recommended for use >7–10 days.
- Advise patient to notify health care provider of all Rx or OTC medications, vitamins, or herbal products being taken and to consult with health care provider before taking other medications. Caution patient to avoid concurrent use of alcohol or other CNS depressants, including opioids.
- Because of rapid onset, advise patient to go to bed immediately after taking suvorexant.
- May cause daytime drowsiness or dizziness. Advise patient to avoid driving or other activities requiring alertness for ≥8 hr after dosing until response to this medication is known.
- Caution patient that complex sleep-related behaviors (sleep-driving) may occur while asleep. Inform caregivers of these behaviors and advise to notify health care provider if any occur.
- Advise patient to notify health care provider if depression worsens or suicidal thoughts occur.
- Advise patient to notify health care provider immediately if signs of anaphylaxis (swelling of the tongue or throat, trouble breathing, nausea, vomiting) occur.
- Rep: Advise women of reproductive potential to notify health care provider if pregnancy is planned or suspected or if breastfeeding.

Evaluation/Desired Outcomes

- Improved sleep.

suzetrigine (soo-se-tri-jeen)

Journavx

Classification

Therapeutic: nonopioid analgesics

Pharmacologic: sodium channel blockers

Indications

Moderate to severe acute pain.

Action

Acts as a selective blocker of the Na_v 1.8 voltage-gated sodium channel, which then inhibits transmission of pain signals from peripheral sensory neurons to the spinal cord and brain. **Therapeutic Effects:** Reduction in pain.

Pharmacokinetics

Absorption: Well absorbed following oral administration.

Distribution: Widely distributed to tissues.

Protein Binding: 99%.

Metabolism and Excretion: Primarily metabolized by the liver via the CYP3A isoenzyme to an active metabolite (M6–SUZ). 50% excreted in feces (primarily as metabolites), 44% excreted in urine (primarily as metabolites).

Half-life: *Suzetrigine:* 24 hr; *M6–SUZ:* 33 hr.

TIME/ACTION PROFILE (plasma concentrations)

ROUTE	ONSET	PEAK	DURATION
PO	unknown	3 hr	12 hr

Contraindications/Precautions

Contraindicated in: Concurrent use of strong CYP3A inhibitors. End-stage renal disease; Severe hepatic impairment.

Use Cautiously in: Moderate hepatic impairment (↓ dose); Rep: Women of reproductive potential; OB: Safety not established in pregnancy; Lactation: Safety not established in breastfeeding; Pedi: Safety and effectiveness not established in children.

S

Adverse Reactions/Side Effects

Derm: pruritus, rash. **GI:** nausea, vomiting. **GU:** renal impairment. **MS:** ↑ CK, muscle spasms.

Interactions

Drug-Drug: **Strong CYP3A inhibitors**, including **itraconazole**, may significantly ↑ levels and risk of toxicity; concurrent use contraindicated. **Moderate CYP3A inhibitors**, including **fluconazole**, may ↑ levels and risk of toxicity; ↓ suzetrigine dose. May ↓ levels and effectiveness of **CYP3A substrates**, including **midazolam**. **Strong CYP3A inducers**, including **rifampin**, and **moderate CYP3A inducers**, including **efavirenz**, may ↓ levels and effectiveness; avoid concurrent use. May ↓ levels and effectiveness of **hormonal contraceptives** containing progestins OTHER than levonorgestrel or norethindrone.
Drug-Natural Products: St. John's wort may ↓ levels and effectiveness; avoid concurrent use.
Drug-Food: Grapefruit juice may ↑ levels and risk of toxicity; avoid concurrent use.

Route/Dosage

PO (Adults): 100 mg initially, then 50 mg every 12 hr starting 12 hr after initial dose. Do not exceed treatment duration of 14 days. *Concurrent use of moderate CYP3A inhibitors:* 100 mg initially, then starting 12 hr after initial dose, give 50 mg every 12 hr for 3 doses, then 12 hr later, give 50 mg once daily. Do not exceed treatment duration of 14 days.

Hepatic Impairment

PO (Adults): 100 mg initially, then starting 12 hr after initial dose, give 50 mg every 12 hr for 3 doses, then 12 hr later, give 50 mg once daily. Do not exceed treatment duration of 14 days.

Availability

Tablets: 50 mg.

NURSING IMPLICATIONS

Assessment

- Assess pain level and location before and during therapy.
- Assess for pruritus, rash, and muscle spasms.

Lab Test Considerations

- May ↑ CK.
- May ↓ eGFR.
- Monitor liver function tests periodically during therapy.

Implementation

- Use for the shortest duration consistent with patient treatment goals; use >14 days has not been evaluated.
- **PO:** *DNC:* Swallow tablets whole. Do not chew or crush.
- Administer starting dose, 100 mg, on an empty stomach >1 hr before or 2 hr after food. Clear liquids may be consumed (water, apple juice, vegetable broth, tea, black coffee) during this time. Subsequent doses can be administered with or without food.

Patient/Family Teaching

- Explain purpose and side effects of medication to patient. Advise patient to read *Patient Information* before starting therapy. If a dose is missed, take the missed dose as soon as possible and then take the next scheduled dose at the recommended time. If >2 doses are missed, take 100 mg and then take the next scheduled dose at the recommended time.
- Advise patient to notify health care professional of all Rx or OTC medications, vitamins, or herbal products being taken and to consult health care professional before taking other medications.
- Advise patient to avoid foods or drinks containing grapefruit during therapy.
- Rep: Advise women of reproductive potential to notify health care professional if pregnancy is planned or suspected or if breastfeeding. Advise patient taking concurrent hormonal contraceptives containing progestins other than levonorgestrel and norethindrone to use additional nonhormonal contraceptives (condoms) or alternative contraceptives (a combined oral contraceptive containing ethinyl estradiol as the estrogen and levonorgestrel or norethindrone as the progestin or an intrauterine system) during treatment and for 28 days after final dose.

Evaluation/Desired Outcomes

- Reduction in pain.

TACROLIMUS
tacrolimus (oral, IV)
(ta-**kroe**-li-mus)
Advagraf, Astagraf XL,
Envarsus PA, Envarsus XR,
Prograf
tacrolimus (topical)
Protopic
Classification
Therapeutic: immunosuppressants

Indications
PO, IV: Prevention of organ rejection in patients who have undergone allogeneic liver, kidney, heart, or lung transplantation (in combination with other immunosuppressants) (extended release only indicated for kidney transplant). **Topical:** Moderate to severe atopic dermatitis in patients who do not respond to or cannot tolerate alternative conventional therapies.

Action
Inhibit T-lymphocyte activation. **Therapeutic Effects:** Prevention of transplanted organ rejection. Improvement in signs/symptoms of atopic dermatitis.

Pharmacokinetics
Absorption: Absorption following oral administration is erratic and incomplete (bioavailability ranges 5–67%); minimal amounts absorbed following topical use.
Distribution: Widely distributed to tissues.
Protein Binding: 99%.
Metabolism and Excretion: 99% metabolized by the liver; <1% excreted unchanged in the urine.
Half-life: *Liver transplant patients:* 11.7 hr; *healthy volunteers:* 21.2 hr.

TIME/ACTION PROFILE (immunosuppression)

ROUTE	ONSET	PEAK	DURATION
PO	rapid	1.3–3.2 hr*	12 hr
PO-ER	unknown	unknown	24 hr
IV	rapid	unknown	8–12 hr
Topical†	unknown	1–2 wk	unknown

* Blood level.
† Improvement in atopic dermatitis.

Contraindications/Precautions
Contraindicated in: Hypersensitivity to tacrolimus or to castor oil (a component in the injection); Concurrent use with cyclosporine (↑ risk of nephrotoxicity); Concurrent use of sirolimus (↑ risk of mortality and adverse reactions); Congenital long QT syndrome; Weakened/compromised immune system; Malignant or premalignant skin condition; Lactation: Lactation.
Use Cautiously in: Renal or hepatic impairment (dose ↓ may be required; if oliguria occurs, wait 48 hr before initiating tacrolimus); Severe infection, graft-versus-host disease, or human leukocyte antigen mismatch (↑ risk of thrombotic microangiopathy); Renal impairment (dose ↓ may be required; if oliguria occurs, wait 48 hr before initiating tacrolimus); Hepatic impairment (dose ↓ may be required); Exposure to sunlight/UV light (may ↑ risk of malignant skin changes); OB: Hyperkalemia and renal impairment may occur in the newborn; use during pregnancy only if potential maternal benefit justifies potential fetal risk; Pedi: Higher end of dosing range is required to maintain adequate blood levels in children.

Adverse Reactions/Side Effects
Noted primarily for PO and IV use.
CV: hypertension, peripheral edema, QT interval prolongation. **Derm:** pruritus, rash, alopecia, herpes simplex, hirsutism, impaired wound healing, photosensitivity, sweating. **EENT:** abnormal vision, amblyopia, sinusitis, tinnitus. **Endo:** hyperglycemia, hyperlipidemia. **F and E:** hyperkalemia, hypomagnesemia, hyperphosphatemia, hypocalcemia, hyponatremia, hypophosphatemia, metabolic acidosis, metabolic alkalosis. **GI:** ↑ liver enzymes, abdominal pain, anorexia, ascites, constipation, diarrhea, dyspepsia, nausea, vomiting, cholangitis, cholestatic jaundice, dysphagia, flatulence, GI BLEEDING, GI PERFORATION, oral thrush, peritonitis. **GU:** nephrotoxicity, urinary tract infection, ↓ fertility. **Hemat:** anemia, leukocytosis, leukopenia, thrombocytopenia, coagulation defects, pure red cell aplasia, thrombotic microangiopathy (including hemolytic uremic syndrome and thrombotic thrombocytopenia purpura). **Local: topical:** burning, stinging. **Metab:** ↑ appetite. **MS:** arthralgia, hypertonia, leg cramps, muscle spasm, myalgia, myasthenia, osteoporosis. **Neuro:** dizziness, headache, insomnia, paresthesia, tremor, abnormal dreams, agitation, anxiety, confusion, depression, emotional lability, hallucinations, neuropathy, POSTERIOR REVERSIBLE ENCEPHALOPATHY SYNDROME (PRES), psychoses, SEIZURES, somnolence. **Resp:** cough, pleural effusion, asthma, bronchitis, pharyngitis, pneumonia, pulmonary edema. **Misc:** generalized pain, chills, fever, HYPERSENSITIVITY REACTIONS (INCLUDING ANAPHYLAXIS), INFECTION (INCLUDING ACTIVATION OF LATENT VIRAL INFECTIONS SUCH AS BK VIRUS-ASSOCIATED NEPHROPATHY), MALIGNANCY (INCLUDING LYMPHOMA AND SKIN CANCER).

T

Interactions

Noted primarily for PO and IV use, but should be considered for topical use.

Drug-Drug: Aminoglycosides, **amphotericin B**, **cisplatin**, **nucleotide reverse transcriptase inhibitors**, **protease inhibitors**, or **cyclosporine** may ↑ risk of nephrotoxicity; allow 24 hr to pass after stopping cyclosporine before starting tacrolimus. **Potassium-sparing diuretics**, **ACE inhibitors**, or **angiotensin II receptor blockers** may ↑ risk of hyperkalemia. **Strong CYP3A4 inhibitors**, including **chloramphenicol**, **clarithromycin**, **cobicistat**, **itraconazole**, **ketoconazole**, **nefazodone**, **posaconazole**, **protease inhibitors**, and **voriconazole**, may significantly ↑ levels; ↓ tacrolimus dose by ⅔ when used with voriconazole or posaconazole; closely monitor tacrolimus whole blood trough concentrations. **Mild CYP3A4 inhibitors** and **moderate CYP3A4 inhibitors**, including **amiodarone**, **calcium channel blockers**, **cimetidine**, **clotrimazole**, **danazol**, **erythromycin**, **ethinyl estradiol**, **fluconazole**, **imatinib**, **isavuconazonium**, **lansoprazole**, **letermovir**, **nilotinib**, and **omeprazole**, may ↑ levels and risk of toxicity; closely monitor tacrolimus whole blood trough concentrations and adjust tacrolimus dose, if needed. **Magnesium/aluminum hydroxide** and **metoclopramide** may ↑ levels and risk of toxicity; closely monitor tacrolimus whole blood trough concentrations and adjust tacrolimus dose, if needed. **Strong CYP3A4 inducers**, including **carbamazepine**, **phenobarbital**, **phenytoin**, **rifabutin**, and **rifampin**, may ↓ levels and effectiveness; ↑ tacrolimus dose and closely monitor tacrolimus whole blood trough concentrations. **Mild CYP3A4 inducers** and **moderate CYP3A4 inducers**, including **methylprednisolone** or **prednisone**, may ↓ levels and effectiveness; closely monitor tacrolimus whole blood trough concentrations and adjust tacrolimus dose, if needed. **Vaccinations** may be less effective if given concurrently with tacrolimus (avoid use of live-virus vaccines). May ↑ levels and risk of toxicity of **mycophenolate mofetil** or **mycophenolic acid**. **Caspofungin** may ↓ levels and effectiveness; closely monitor tacrolimus whole blood trough concentrations and adjust tacrolimus dose, if needed. **Cannabidiol** may ↑ levels and risk of toxicity; monitor tacrolimus levels and adjust dose as necessary.

Drug-Natural Products: Astragalus, **echinacea**, and **melatonin** may interfere with immunosuppression. **St. John's wort** may ↓ levels and effectiveness; ↑ tacrolimus dose and closely monitor tacrolimus whole blood trough concentrations. **Schisandra sphenanthera** may significantly ↑ levels and risk of toxicity; closely monitor tacrolimus whole blood trough concentrations.

Drug-Food: Food ↓ the rate and extent of GI absorption. **Grapefruit juice** may ↑ levels and risk of toxicity; avoid concurrent use.

Route/Dosage

Because of the potential risk for anaphylaxis, the IV route of administration should be reserved for those patients unable to take the drug orally. Extended-release capsules are not interchangeable with immediate-release capsules/granules or other extended-release products. When converting between immediate-release capsules and granules, the total daily dose should remain the same. Black patients may require a higher dose to achieve desired tacrolimus trough concentrations. Patients with cystic fibrosis may also require a higher dose for lung transplantation due to ↓ bioavailability.

Kidney Transplantation

PO (Adults): *Immediate-release capsules (in combination with azathioprine):* 0.2 mg/kg/day in 2 divided doses initially; titrate to achieve recommended whole blood trough concentration; *Immediate-release capsules (in combination with mycophenolate mofetil and IL-2 antagonist):* 0.1 mg/kg/day in 2 divided doses initially; titrate to achieve recommended whole blood trough concentration; *Extended-release capsules (Astagraf XL) (in combination with basiliximab induction):* 0.15 mg/kg once daily (to be started either before or within 48 hr of completion of transplant); *Extended-release capsules (Astagraf XL) (without basiliximab induction):* 0.1 mg/kg given as single dose preoperatively within 12 hr prior to reperfusion, followed by 0.2 mg/kg once daily started postoperatively ≥4 hr after preoperative dose and within 12 hr after reperfusion; *Conversion from immediate-release capsules to extended-release capsules (Envarsus XR):* Initiate extended-release treatment with a once-daily dose that is 80% of the total daily dose of the immediate-release product (also appropriate for Black patients).

PO (Children): *Immediate-release capsules or suspension:* 0.3 mg/kg/day in 2 divided doses initially; titrate to achieve recommended whole blood trough concentration.

IV (Adults): 0.03–0.05 mg/kg/day as a continuous infusion initially; titrate to achieve recommended blood concentration.

Liver Transplantation

PO (Adults): *Immediate-release capsules:* 0.1–0.15 mg/kg/day in 2 divided doses initially; titrate to achieve recommended blood concentration.

PO (Children): *Immediate-release capsules:* 0.15–0.2 mg/kg/day in 2 divided doses initially; titrate to achieve recommended blood concentration. *Suspension:* 0.2 mg/kg/day in 2 divided doses initially; titrate to achieve recommended blood concentration.

IV (Adults): 0.03–0.05 mg/kg/day as a continuous infusion initially; titrate to achieve recommended blood concentration.

IV (Children): 0.03–0.05 mg/kg/day.

Heart Transplantation

PO (Adults): *Immediate-release capsules:* 0.075 mg/kg/day in 2 divided doses initially; titrate to achieve recommended blood concentration.

PO (Children): *Immediate-release capsules or suspension (without antibody induction treatment):* 0.3 mg/kg/day in 2 divided doses initially; titrate to achieve recommended whole blood trough concentration. *Immediate-release capsules or suspension (with antibody induction treatment):* 0.1 mg/kg/day in 2 divided doses initially; titrate to achieve recommended whole blood trough concentration.

IV (Adults): 0.01 mg/kg/day as a continuous infusion initially; titrate to achieve recommended blood concentration.

Lung Transplantation

PO (Adults): *Immediate-release capsules:* 0.075 mg/kg/day in 2 divided doses initially; titrate to achieve recommended blood concentration.

PO (Children): *Immediate-release capsules or suspension (without antibody induction treatment):* 0.3 mg/kg/day in 2 divided doses initially; titrate to achieve recommended whole blood trough concentration. *Immediate-release capsules or suspension (with antibody induction treatment):* 0.1 mg/kg/day in 2 divided doses initially; titrate to achieve recommended whole blood trough concentration.

IV (Adults): 0.01–0.03 mg/kg/day as a continuous infusion initially; titrate to achieve recommended blood concentration.

Atopic Dermatitis

Topical (Adults): Apply 0.03% or 0.1% ointment twice daily. Discontinue when signs/symptoms of atopic dermatitis resolve.

Topical (Children ≥2–15 yr): Apply 0.03% ointment twice daily. Discontinue when signs/symptoms of atopic dermatitis resolve.

Availability (generic available)

Capsules: 0.5 mg, 1 mg, 5 mg. **Extended-release capsules (Astagraf XL):** 0.5 mg, 1 mg, ✤ 3 mg, 5 mg. **Extended-release tablets (Envarsus XR):** 0.75 mg, 1 mg, 4 mg. **Granules for oral suspension:** 0.2 mg/pkt, 1 mg/pkt. **Solution for injection:** 5 mg/mL. **Topical ointment:** 0.03%, 0.1%.

NURSING IMPLICATIONS

Assessment

- Assess for signs/symptoms of PRES (headache, altered mental status, seizures, visual disturbances, hypertension) periodically during therapy. Confirm diagnosis by radiologic procedure. *If PRES is suspected or diagnosed,* maintain BP control and immediately ↓ immunosuppression. Symptoms are usually reversed on ↓ or discontinuation of immunosuppression.
- Monitor for signs/symptoms of opportunistic infection (persistent fever, malaise, sore throat, unusual bleeding or bruising).
- Monitor for signs/symptoms of neurotoxicity (headache, altered mental status, seizure, visual disturbance, delirium, coma).
- **Prevention of Organ Rejection:** Monitor BP closely during therapy. Hypertension is a common complication of tacrolimus therapy and should be treated.
- Observe patients receiving IV tacrolimus for the development of anaphylaxis (rash, pruritus, laryngeal edema, wheezing) for ≥30 min and frequently thereafter. *If signs/symptoms of anaphylaxis occur,* stop infusion and initiate treatment.
- **Atopic Dermatitis:** Assess skin lesions before and periodically during therapy.
- Use only for short time, not continuously, and in the minimum dose possible to ↓ risk of developing skin cancer.

Lab Test Considerations

- Tacrolimus blood level monitoring may be helpful in the evaluation of rejection and toxicity, dose adjustments, and assessment of compliance. *For kidney transplantation,* during the 1st 3 mo, most patients maintained tacrolimus whole blood concentrations of 7–20 ng/mL and then 5–15 ng/mL through 1 yr. *For de novo kidney transplantation,* during the 1st mo, most patients maintained tacrolimus whole blood concentrations of 6–11 ng/mL and then 4–11 ng/mL through mo 1. *For heart transplantation,* from wk 1 to 3 mo, most patients maintained tacrolimus trough whole blood concentrations of 8–20 ng/mL and then 6–18 ng/mL from 3–18 mo post-transplant.
- Monitor serum creatinine, potassium, and glucose closely. ↑ serum creatinine and ↓ urine output may indicate nephrotoxicity. May also cause insulin-dependent post-transplant diabetes mellitus (🧬 incidence is higher in Black and Hispanic patients).
- May also cause hyperuricemia, hypokalemia, hyperkalemia, hypomagnesemia, metabolic acidosis, metabolic alkalosis, hyperlipidemia, hyperphosphatemia, hypophosphatemia, hypocalcemia, and hyponatremia.
- Monitor CBC with differential. May cause anemia, leukocytosis, and thrombocytopenia.

Implementation

- Do not confuse Prograf with Prozac. Do not confuse tacrolimus with tamsulosin.
- Do not confuse immediate-release tacrolimus with extended-release tacrolimus.
- Should only be prescribed by health care providers experienced with immunosuppressive therapy and organ transplant patients.

T

- Begin therapy with tacrolimus no sooner than 6 hr post-transplantation. Concurrent therapy with corticosteroids is recommended in the early postoperative period.
- Tacrolimus should not be used concurrently with cyclosporine. Tacrolimus or cyclosporine should be discontinued ≥24 hr before starting the other.
- Oral therapy is preferred because of the risk of anaphylactic reactions with IV tacrolimus. IV therapy should be replaced with oral therapy as soon as possible.
- Adults should be started at the lower end of the dose range; children require higher doses to maintain blood trough concentrations similar to adults.
- Immediate and extended-release capsules are not interchangeable.
- **PO:** Initiate oral doses 8–12 hr after discontinuation of IV doses. Administer with or without food, but should be consistent, and at same time each day.
- *Extended-release capsules:* Administer at the same time each day, preferably in the morning, on an empty stomach ≥1 hr before or 2 hr after breakfast. ***DNC:*** Swallow capsules whole; do not chew, divide, or crush.
- **Topical:** Do not use continuously for a long time.
- **Topical:** Wash hands before applying. Apply a thin layer of ointment twice daily to affected skin. Use smallest amount of ointment needed to control signs and symptoms of eczema. Do not cover treated area with bandages, dressings, or wraps. If not treating areas on hands, wash hands with soap and water after applying to remove any ointment on hands.

IV Administration

- **Continuous Infusion: Dilution:** Dilute in 0.9% NaCl or D5W. May be stored in polyethylene or glass containers for 24 hr following dilution. Do not store in PVC containers. Do not administer solutions that are discolored or contain particulate matter. **Concentration:** 0.004–0.02 mg/mL. **Rate:** Infuse over 24 hr.
- **Y-Site Compatibility:** alemtuzumab, amikacin, aminocaproic acid, aminophylline, amiodarone, amphotericin B deoxycholate, amphotericin B liposomal, anidulafungin, argatroban, arsenic trioxide, atracurium, azithromycin, aztreonam, benztropine, bivalirudin, bleomycin, bumetanide, buprenorphine, busulfan, butorphanol, calcium chloride, calcium gluconate, carboplatin, carmustine, caspofungin, cefazolin, cefotaxime, cefotetan, cefoxitin, ceftazidime, ceftolozane/tazobactam, ceftriaxone, cefuroxime, chloramphenicol, chlorpromazine, ciprofloxacin, cisatracurium, cisplatin, clindamycin, cyclophosphamide, cyclosporine, cytarabine, dacarbazine, dactinomycin, daptomycin, daunorubicin, dexamethasone, dexmedetomidine, dexrazoxane, digoxin, diltiazem, diphenhydramine, dobutamine, docetaxel, dopamine, doxorubicin hydrochloride, doxorubicin liposomal, doxycycline, droperidol, enalaprilat, ephedrine, epinephrine, epirubicin, ertapenem, erythromycin, esmolol, etoposide, etoposide phosphate, famotidine, fentanyl, fluconazole, fludarabine, foscarnet, fosphenytoin, gemcitabine, gentamicin, glycopyrrolate, granisetron, haloperidol, heparin, hydralazine, hydrocortisone, hydromorphone, idarubicin, ifosfamide, imipenem/cilastatin, insulin regular, irinotecan, isavuconazonium, isoproterenol, ketorolac, labetalol, letermovir, leucovorin, levofloxacin, lidocaine, linezolid, lorazepam, magnesium sulfate, mannitol, meperidine, meropenem, mesna, methadone, methotrexate, methylprednisolone, metoclopramide, metoprolol, metronidazole, micafungin, midazolam, milrinone, minocycline, mitomycin, mitoxantrone, morphine, moxifloxacin, multivitamins, mycophenolate, nafcillin, nalbuphine, naloxone, nicardipine, nitroglycerin, nitroprusside, norepinephrine, octreotide, ondansetron, oxacillin, oxaliplatin, oxytocin, paclitaxel, palonosetron, pamidronate, pemetrexed, penicillin G potassium, pentamidine, phentolamine, phenylephrine, piperacillin/tazobactam, potassium acetate, potassium chloride, potassium phosphates, procainamide, prochlorperazine, promethazine, propranolol, remifentanil, rocuronium, sodium acetate, sodium bicarbonate, sodium phosphates, succinylcholine, sufentanil, tedizolid, theophylline, thiotepa, tigecycline, tirofiban, tobramycin, topotecan, vancomycin, vasopressin, vecuronium, verapamil, vinblastine, vincristine, vinorelbine, voriconazole, zidovudine, zoledronic acid.
- **Y-Site Incompatibility:** allopurinol, azathioprine, cefepime, dantrolene, diazepam, diazoxide, esomeprazole, folic acid, gemtuzumab ozogamicin, iron sucrose, levothyroxine, phenytoin.

Patient/Family Teaching

- Explain purpose and side effects of medication to patient. Advise patient to read *Patient Information* before starting therapy. Advise patient to take tacrolimus at the same time each day, with or without food, as directed. Do not skip or double up on missed doses. Do not discontinue medication without advice of health care provider. Take missed doses of extended-release capsule as soon as remembered unless >14 hr after scheduled dose; do not double doses.
- Advise patient to notify health care provider of all Rx or OTC medications, vitamins, or herbal products being taken and to consult with health care provider before taking other medications.
- Advise patient to inspect capsules with each new Rx, before taking. Contact health care provider if appearance of capsules or dose has changed.
- Advise patient to avoid grapefruit and grapefruit juice and alcohol during therapy.
- Reinforce the need for lifelong therapy to prevent transplant rejection. Review symptoms of rejection

for transplanted organ and stress need to notify health care provider immediately if they occur.
- Advise patient to avoid eating raw oysters or other shellfish; make sure they are fully cooked before eating.
- Instruct patient to notify health care provider if signs/symptoms of infection (fever; sweats; chills; cough or flu-like symptoms; muscle aches; warm, red, painful areas on skin) occur.
- Instruct patient to notify health care provider if signs/symptoms of diabetes mellitus (frequent urination, ↑ thirst or hunger), neurotoxicity (vision changes, deliriums, or tremors), or PRES occur.
- Advise patient to wear protective clothing and sunscreen to avoid photosensitivity reactions.
- Advise patient to avoid exposure to chickenpox, measles, mumps, and rubella. If exposed, see health care provider for prophylactic therapy.
- Instruct patient to notify health care provider of all Rx or OTC medications, vitamins, or herbal products being taken and consult health care provider before taking any new medications.
- Advise patient of the risk of lymphoma or skin cancer with tacrolimus therapy.
- **Topical:** Instruct patient to apply ointment as directed. Advise patient to read the *Medication Guide* prior to starting and with each Rx renewal; new information may be available.
- Advise patient not to bathe, shower, or swim right after applying; may wash off ointment. May use moisturizers with ointment. Instruct patient to check with health care provider first about products to use. If moisturizers are used, apply them after application of ointment.
- Advise patients to contact health care provider if their symptoms do not improve after 6 wk of therapy, if their symptoms worsen, or if they develop a skin infection.
- Instruct patient to use ointment only on areas of skin with atopic dermatitis.
- Advise patient to stop using the ointment when the signs/symptoms of atopic dermatitis go away.
- Advise patient to limit sun exposure during treatment.
- Advise patient of the risk of using topical tacrolimus during pregnancy.
- Inform patient of the risk of lymphoma or skin cancer with topical tacrolimus therapy.
- Rep: Advise women of reproductive potential to notify health care provider if pregnancy is planned or suspected, avoid breastfeeding during therapy, and discuss family planning with health care provider before starting therapy. May impair male and female fertility. Encourage female transplant recipients and women fathered by male transplant recipients to enroll in the Transplantation Pregnancy Registry International that monitors outcomes of women exposed to tacrolimus by calling 1-877-955-6877 or visiting https://www.transplantpregnancyregistry.org/.

Evaluation/Desired Outcomes

- Prevention of transplanted organ rejection.
- Improvement in signs/symptoms of atopic dermatitis.

tadalafil (ta-da-la-fil)

Adcirca, Alyq, Cialis, Tadliq

Classification

Therapeutic: erectile dysfunction agents, vasodilators

Pharmacologic: phosphodiesterase type 5 inhibitors

Indications

Cialis: Treatment of: Erectile dysfunction (ED), Benign prostatic hyperplasia (BPH). *Adcirca, Alyq, and Tadliq:* Pulmonary arterial hypertension (PAH).

Action

Increases cyclic guanosine monophosphate (cGMP) levels by inhibiting phosphodiesterase type 5, an enzyme responsible for the breakdown of cGMP. cGMP produces smooth muscle relaxation of the corpus cavernosum, which in turn promotes increased blood flow and subsequent erection. cGMP also leads to vasodilation of the pulmonary vasculature. **Therapeutic Effects:** *Cialis:* Enhanced blood flow to the corpus cavernosum and erection sufficient to allow sexual intercourse. Improved signs and symptoms of BPH. *Adcirca, Alyq, and Tadliq:* Improved exercise tolerance in PAH.

Pharmacokinetics

Absorption: Well absorbed following oral administration.

Distribution: Extensive tissue distribution; penetrates semen.

Protein Binding: 94%.

Metabolism and Excretion: Mostly metabolized by the liver via the CYP3A4 isoenzyme system; metabolites are excreted in feces (61%) and urine (36%).

Half-life: 17.5 hr.

TIME/ACTION PROFILE (vasodilation, improved erectile function)

ROUTE	ONSET	PEAK	DURATION
PO	rapid	0.5–6 hr	36

T

Contraindications/Precautions

Contraindicated in: Hypersensitivity; Concurrent use of nitrates or riociguat; Unstable angina, recent history of stroke, life-threatening HF within 6 mo, uncontrolled hypertension, arrhythmias, stroke within 6 mo, or MI within 90 days; Any other cardiovascular pathology precluding sexual activity; Known hereditary degenerative retinal disorders; Severe hepatic impairment; Severe renal impairment (Adcirca, Alyq, and Tadliq); Severe renal impairment (Cialis once-daily dosing); Pedi: Children or newborns.

Use Cautiously in: Left ventricular outflow obstruction; Penile deformity; Renal impairment; Underlying conditions predisposing to priapism, including sickle cell anemia, multiple myeloma, or leukemia; Bleeding disorders or active peptic ulcer disease; History of sudden severe vision loss or nonarteritic ischemic optic neuropathy; may ↑ risk of recurrence; Low cup-to-disk ratio, age >50 yr, diabetes, hypertension, coronary artery disease, hyperlipidemia, or smoking (↑ risk of nonarteritic ischemic optic neuropathy); Geri: ↑ risk of diarrhea in older adults.

Adverse Reactions/Side Effects

CV: hypotension, peripheral edema. **Derm:** flushing. **EENT:** hearing loss, nasal congestion, vision loss. **GI:** diarrhea, dyspepsia. **GU:** ↓ fertility, priapism. **MS:** back pain, limb pain, myalgia. **Neuro:** headache.

Interactions

Drug-Drug: Concurrent use of **nitrates** may cause serious, life-threatening hypotension and is contraindicated. Concurrent use of **riociguat** may result in severe hypotension; concurrent use contraindicated. ↑ risk of hypotension with **alpha-adrenergic blockers** and acute ingestion of **alcohol**; discontinue alpha-adrenergic blocker therapy ≥1 day before starting Cialis for BPH. **Strong CYP3A4 inhibitors**, including **ritonavir**, **ketoconazole**, and **itraconazole**, may ↑ levels and the risk of toxicity (dose adjustments recommended with Cialis; avoid concurrent use with Adcirca, Alyq, and Tadliq). **CYP3A4 inducers** may ↓ levels and its effectiveness; avoid concurrent use with Adcirca, Alyq, or Tadliq.

Route/Dosage

Cialis (for ED)

PO (Adults): 10 mg prior to sexual activity (range 5–20 mg; not to exceed one dose/24 hr) *or* 2.5 mg once daily (max: 5 mg/day); *Concurrent use of strong CYP3A4 inhibitors:* Single dose should not exceed 10 mg in any 72-hr period; for once-daily dose regimen, should not exceed 2.5 mg/day.

Renal Impairment

PO (Adults): *CCr 30–50 mL/min (as-needed dosing):* Initial dose should not exceed 5 mg/day; maximum dose should not exceed 10 mg in 48 hr; *CCr <30 mL/min (as-needed dosing):* Maximum dose should not exceed 5 mg in 72 hr; *CCr <30 mL/min (once-daily dosing):* Not recommended for use.

Hepatic Impairment

PO (Adults): *Mild or moderate hepatic impairment:* Daily dose should not exceed 10 mg (once-daily dose regimen not recommended); *Severe hepatic impairment:* Not recommended for use.

Cialis (for BPH or ED/BPH)

PO (Adults): 5 mg once daily; use for up to 26 wk when used concurrently with finasteride; *Concurrent use of strong CYP3A4 inhibitors:* Should not exceed 2.5 mg once daily.

Renal Impairment

PO (Adults): *CCr 30–50 mL/min:* Initial dose should not exceed 2.5 mg/day; maximum dose should not exceed 5 mg/day; *CCr <30 mL/min:* Not recommended for use.

Hepatic Impairment

PO (Adults): Not recommended for use.

Adcirca, Alyq, and Tadliq (for PAH)

PO (Adults): 40 mg once daily; *If receiving ritonavir for ≥1 wk:* start 20 mg once daily; may then ↑ to 40 mg once daily based on tolerability; *If initiating ritonavir while on Adcirca, Alyq, or Tadliq:* Stop Adcirca, Alyq, or Tadliq ≥24 hr before starting ritonavir; may reinitiate Adcirca, Alyq, or Tadliq at 20 mg once daily after ≥1 wk of therapy with ritonavir; may then ↑ to 40 mg once daily based on tolerability.

Renal Impairment

PO (Adults): *CCr 31–80 mL/min:* Start 20 mg once daily; may then ↑ to 40 mg once daily based on tolerability.

Hepatic Impairment

PO (Adults): *Mild or moderate hepatic impairment:* Start with 20 mg once daily.

Availability (generic available)

Tablets (Cialis): 2.5 mg, 5 mg, 10 mg, 20 mg. **Tablets (Adcirca or Alyq):** 20 mg. **Oral suspension (Tadliq) (peppermint flavor):** 20 mg/5 mL. ***In combination with:*** finasteride (Entadfi); macitentan (Opsynvi). See Appendix N.

NURSING IMPLICATIONS

Assessment

- ***Cialis for ED:*** Determine the presence of ED before administration. Tadalafil has no effect in the absence of sexual stimulation.
- ***Cialis for BPH:*** Assess for symptoms of BPH (urinary hesitancy, feeling of incomplete bladder emptying, interruption of urinary stream, impairment of size and force of urinary stream, terminal urinary dribbling, straining to start flow, dysuria, urgency) before and periodically during therapy.

- Digital rectal examinations should be performed before and periodically during therapy for BPH.
- ***Adcirca, Alyq, Tadliq*:** Monitor hemodynamic parameters and exercise tolerance prior to and periodically during therapy.

Implementation

- **PO:** For *ED:* Administer >30 min before sexual activity; effectiveness may continue for 36 hr.
- For *PAH, BPH, ED/BPH, or daily for ED:* Administer once daily at the same time each day.
- Administer without regard to food. ***DNC:*** Swallow tablets whole; do not crush, break, or chew.
- Shake suspension well for 30 sec before measuring dose.

Patient/Family Teaching

- Explain purpose and side effects of medication to patient. Advise patient to read *Patient Information* before starting therapy. Instruct patient to take as needed for ED >30 min before sexual activity and not more than once per day. Inform patient that sexual stimulation is required for an erection to occur after taking tadalafil. Instruct patient to take for PAH as directed.
- Advise patient to notify health care professional of all Rx or OTC medications, vitamins, or herbal products being taken and to consult with health care professional before taking other medications.
- Advise patient that tadalafil is not indicated for use in women.
- Caution patient not to take tadalafil concurrently with alpha-adrenergic blockers (unless on a stable dose) or nitrates. If chest pain occurs after taking tadalafil, instruct patient to seek immediate medical attention.
- Advise patient to avoid excess alcohol intake in combination with tadalafil; may ↑ risk of orthostatic hypotension, ↑ HR, ↓ standing BP, dizziness, and headache.
- Instruct patient to notify health care professional promptly if erection lasts >4 hr, they are not satisfied with their sexual performance, they develop unwanted side effects, or they experience sudden or ↓ vision loss in one or both eyes, ↓or loss in hearing, ringing in the ears, or dizziness.
- Inform patient that tadalafil offers no protection against sexually transmitted diseases. Counsel patient that protection against sexually transmitted diseases and HIV infection should be considered.
- Rep: Advise women of reproductive potential to notify health care professional if pregnancy is planned or suspected or if breastfeeding.

Evaluation/Desired Outcomes

- *Cialis:* Enhanced blood flow to the corpus cavernosum and erection sufficient to allow sexual intercourse and improve signs and symptoms of BPH.
- *Adcirca, Alyq, and Tadliq:* Improved exercise tolerance in PAH.

tafamidis (ta-fam-id-is)

Vyndamax, Vyndaqel

Classification

Therapeutic: none assigned

Pharmacologic: transthyretin stabilizers

Indications

Cardiomyopathy of wild type or hereditary transthyretin-mediated amyloidosis.

Action

Acts as a transthyretin (TTR) stabilizer by selectively binding to TTR at the thyroxine binding sites and stabilizing the tetramer of the TTR transport protein by slowing its dissociation into monomers, which is the rate-limiting step in the amyloidogenic process. **Therapeutic Effects:** Reduction in mortality and cardiovascular hospitalizations.

Pharmacokinetics

Absorption: Unknown.
Distribution: Well distributed to tissues.
Protein Binding: >99%.
Metabolism and Excretion: Metabolic pathway not fully known (may undergo glucuronidation). 59% excreted in feces (primarily as unchanged drug); 22% excreted in urine (primarily as metabolites).
Half-life: 49 hr.

TIME/ACTION PROFILE (plasma concentrations)

ROUTE	ONSET	PEAK	DURATION
PO	Unknown	4 hr	24 hr

Contraindications/Precautions

Contraindicated in: OB: Pregnancy; Lactation: Lactation.
Use Cautiously in: Rep: Women of reproductive potential; Pedi: Safety and effectiveness in children not established.

Adverse Reactions/Side Effects

No adverse reactions reported in prescribing information.

Interactions

Drug-Drug: May ↑ levels and risk of toxicity of **breast cancer-resistant protein substrates**, including **imatinib**, **methotrexate**, and **rosuvastatin**.

T

Route/Dosage

Vyndaqel

PO (Adults): 80 mg once daily.

Vyndamax

PO (Adults): 61 mg once daily.

Availability

Capsules (Vyndaqel): 20 mg. **Capsules (Vyndamax):** 61 mg.

NURSING IMPLICATIONS

Assessment

- Monitor cardiovascular status at baseline and as clinically indicated during therapy.

Lab Test Considerations

- Test for variant TTR genotype prior to initiation of therapy.

Implementation

- **PO:** Administer without regard to food. ***DNC:*** Swallow capsules whole. Do not crush, cut, or chew.

Patient/Family Teaching

- Explain purpose and side effects of medication. Advise patient to read *Patient Information* before starting therapy. If a dose is missed, instruct patient to take as soon as remembered or omit and take the next scheduled dose. Do not double doses.
- Advise patient to notify health care professional of all Rx or OTC medications, vitamins, or herbal products being taken and to consult health care professional before taking other medications.
- Rep: Advise women of reproductive potential of potential risk to fetus and to avoid breastfeeding during therapy. Notify health care professional if pregnancy is planned or suspected or if breastfeeding. Consider reporting pregnancy to Pfizer at 1-800-438-1985.

Evaluation/Desired Outcomes

- Reduction in mortality and cardiovascular hospitalizations.

HIGH ALERT

tamoxifen (ta-mox-i-fen)

Soltamox

Classification

Therapeutic: antineoplastics

Pharmacologic: antiestrogens

Indications

Estrogen-receptor positive metastatic breast cancer. Adjuvant treatment of early-stage estrogen-receptor positive breast cancer. To reduce the occurrence of contralateral breast cancer when used as adjuvant therapy for breast cancer. Prevention of breast cancer in high-risk patients. To reduce risk of invasive breast cancer in women with ductal carcinoma in situ following breast surgery and radiation.

Action

Competes with estrogen for binding sites in breast and other tissues. Reduces DNA synthesis and estrogen response. **Therapeutic Effects:** Suppression of tumor growth. Reduced incidence of breast cancer in high-risk patients.

Pharmacokinetics

Absorption: Well absorbed after oral administration.
Distribution: Widely distributed to tissues.
Metabolism and Excretion: Primarily metabolized by the liver via the CYP3A isoenzyme into N-desmethyltamoxifen and via the CYP2D6 isoenzyme into 4-hydroxytamoxifen. Both of these metabolites are further metabolized into endoxifen (N-desmethyltamoxifen via CYP2D6 and 4-hydroxytamoxifen via CYP3A). Both endoxifen and 4-hydroxytamoxifen are 30- to 100-fold more potent than tamoxifen in suppressing estrogen-dependent cell proliferation. The CYP2D6 enzyme system exhibits genetic polymorphism (~7% of population may be poor metabolizers and may have significantly ↓ endoxifen concentrations and ↓ effectiveness of tamoxifen). Slowly eliminated in the feces. Minimal amounts excreted in the urine.
Half-life: 7 days.

TIME/ACTION PROFILE (tumor response)

ROUTE	ONSET	PEAK	DURATION
PO	4–10 wk	several mo	several wk

Contraindications/Precautions

Contraindicated in: Hypersensitivity; Concurrent warfarin therapy with history of deep vein thrombosis (DVT) or pulmonary embolism (PE) (patients with ductal carcinoma in situ or at high risk for breast cancer only); OB: Pregnancy; Lactation: Lactation.
Use Cautiously in: ↓ bone marrow reserve; History of thromboembolic events; Rep: Women of reproductive potential.

Adverse Reactions/Side Effects

CV: DVT, edema. **Derm:** hot flashes. **EENT:** blurred vision. **F and E:** hypercalcemia. **GI:** nausea, vomiting. **GU:** UTERINE MALIGNANCIES, vaginal bleeding. **Hemat:** leukopenia, thrombocytopenia. **MS:** bone pain. **Neuro:** confusion, depression, headache, STROKE, weakness. **Resp:** PE. **Misc:** tumor flare.

Interactions

Drug-Drug: Estrogens may ↓ effectiveness. **Bromocriptine** may ↑ levels and risk of toxicity. May ↑ the anticoagulant effect of **warfarin**. Risk of thromboembolic events is ↑ by concurrent use of other **antineoplastics**.

Route/Dosage

Metastatic Breast Cancer

PO (Adults): 20 mg once daily *or* 20 mg twice daily.

Adjuvant Treatment of Breast Cancer

PO (Adults): 20 mg once daily for 5–10 yr.

Prevention of Breast Cancer in High-Risk Women or Ductal Carcinoma In Situ

PO (Adults): 20 mg once daily for 5 yr.

Availability (generic available)

Oral solution (licorice aniseed flavor): 10 mg/5 mL. **Tablets:** 10 mg, 20 mg.

NURSING IMPLICATIONS

Assessment

- Assess for an ↑ in bone or tumor pain. Confer with health care provider regarding analgesics. This transient pain usually resolves despite continued therapy.
- Monitor for signs and symptoms of venous thromboembolism such as PE (chest pain, dyspnea, tachycardia), DVT (calf pain or tenderness, lower extremity edema, localized warmth or erythema), or stroke (headache, facial numbness, unilateral weakness, aphasia, eye pain or swelling, vision changes). Discontinue therapy if suspected.
- Gynecologic examinations should be performed at initiation of therapy and annually to monitor for uterine malignancies; abnormal vaginal bleeding, menstrual irregularities, changes in vaginal discharge, or pelvic pain or pressure should be monitored; breast exam and mammogram should occur at baseline and periodically.
- Dual energy x-ray absorptiometry scans should be completed at baseline and every 1–2 yr. Evaluate osteoporosis and fracture risk in all patients. Risk of ↓ bone mineral density in premenopausal women.
- X-ray of thoracic and lumbar spine to rule out vertebral facture should be done in patients with kyphosis, height loss ≥6 cm, acute severe back pain, and in age ≥65 yr.
- Optical coherence tomography should be done at baseline and every 6 mo to detect tamoxifen maculopathy during treatment.

Lab Test Considerations

- Verify negative pregnancy test before starting therapy.
- An estrogen receptor assay should be assessed before initiation of therapy.
- Monitor CBC and platelets at baseline and periodically during therapy. May cause leukopenia and thrombocytopenia.
- Monitor serum cholesterol and triglyceride concentrations in patients with pre-existing hyperlipidemia. May cause ↑ concentrations.
- Bone mineral density panel (serum albumin, calcium and alkaline phosphatase, and phosphate and osteocalcin measurements) should be measured at baseline and periodically. May cause transient hypercalcemia in patients with metastases to the bone. If severe hypercalcemia develops, discontinue tamoxifen.
- Monitor hepatic function tests and thyroxine (T_4) periodically during therapy. May ↑ liver enzymes and thyroxine concentrations.

Implementation

- Handle intact tablets or capsules with single gloves; use double gloves, respiratory protection, and a protective gown in the preparation of tablets or capsules, including cutting, crushing, or manipulating, or the handling of uncoated tablets; optimally prepare in a ventilated control device. During administration, wear single gloves, and wear eye/face protection if the formulation is hard to swallow or if the patient may resist, vomit, or spit up.
- **PO:** Administer with food or fluids if GI irritation becomes a problem. Consult health care provider if patient vomits shortly after administration of medication to determine need for repeat dose.

Patient/Family Teaching

- Explain the purpose and side effects of tamoxifen. Instruct patient to take medication as directed. If a dose is missed, it should be omitted. Advise patient to read *Medication Guide* before starting therapy and with each Rx refill in case of changes.
- If skin lesions are present, inform patient that lesions may temporarily ↑ in size and number and may have ↑ erythema.
- Advise patient to report bone pain to health care provider promptly. This pain may be severe. Analgesics should be ordered to control pain. Inform patient that this may be an indication of the drug's effectiveness and will resolve over time.
- Instruct patient to monitor weight weekly. Weight gain or peripheral edema should be reported to health care provider.
- Advise patient that medication may cause hot flashes. Notify health care provider if these become bothersome.
- Instruct patient to notify health care provider promptly if pain or swelling of legs, shortness of breath, weakness, sleepiness, confusion, nausea, vomiting, weight gain, dizziness, headache, loss of appetite, or blurred vision occurs. Patient should also report menstrual irregularities, vaginal bleeding, or pelvic pain or pressure.
- Advise patient to notify health care provider of all Rx or OTC medications, vitamins, or herbal products being taken and to consult with health care provider before taking other medications.

T

- Rep: May cause fetal harm. Advise women of reproductive potential to use a nonhormonal method of contraception during therapy and for 2 mo after last dose and to avoid breastfeeding for 3 mo after last dose. May cause female infertility.

Evaluation/Desired Outcomes

- Decrease in the size or spread of breast cancer. Observable effects of therapy may not be seen for 4–10 wk after initiation.
- Reduced incidence of breast cancer in high-risk patients.

tamsulosin (tam-**soo**-loe-sin)

~~Flomax~~, Flomax CR

Classification
Therapeutic: benign prostatic hyperplasia (BPH) agents
Pharmacologic: alpha-adrenergic blockers

Indications

Benign prostatic hyperplasia (BPH).

Action

Decreases contractions in smooth muscle of the prostatic capsule by preferentially binding to alpha$_1$-adrenergic receptors. **Therapeutic Effects:** Decreased symptoms of BPH (urinary urgency, hesitancy, nocturia).

Pharmacokinetics

Absorption: >90% absorbed after oral administration.
Distribution: Widely distributed to tissues.
Protein Binding: 94–99%.
Metabolism and Excretion: Primarily metabolized by the liver via the CYP3A4 and CYP2D6 isoenzymes; the CYP2D6 enzyme system exhibits genetic polymorphism (~7% of population may be poor metabolizers and may have significantly ↑ tamsulosin concentrations and an ↑ risk of adverse effects). <10% excreted unchanged in urine.
Half-life: 14 hr.

TIME/ACTION PROFILE (↑ in urine flow)

ROUTE	ONSET	PEAK	DURATION
PO	unknown	2 wk	unknown

Contraindications/Precautions

Contraindicated in: Hypersensitivity.
Use Cautiously in: Patients at risk for prostate cancer (symptoms may be similar); Patients undergoing cataract surgery (↑ risk of intraoperative floppy iris syndrome); Sulfa allergy; CYP2D6 poor metabolizers (especially when using higher dose of 0.8 mg/day).

Adverse Reactions/Side Effects

CV: orthostatic hypotension. **EENT:** intraoperative floppy iris syndrome, rhinitis. **GU:** priapism, retrograde/diminished ejaculation. **Neuro:** dizziness, headache.

Interactions

Drug-Drug: Cimetidine may ↑ levels and the risk of toxicity. ↑ risk of hypotension with **doxazosin, prazosin,** and **terazosin**; concurrent use should be avoided. ↑ risk of hypotension with **sildenafil, tadalafil,** and **vardenafil**. Strong **CYP3A4 inhibitors** and **CYP2D6 inhibitors** may ↑ levels and the risk of toxicity; concurrent use should be avoided.

Route/Dosage

PO (Adults): 0.4 mg once daily after a meal; may ↑ after 2–4 wk to 0.8 mg/day.

Availability (generic available)

Capsules: 0.4 mg. ***In combination with:*** dutasteride (Jalyn); see Appendix N.

NURSING IMPLICATIONS

Assessment

- Assess patient for symptoms of BPH (urinary hesitancy, feeling of incomplete bladder emptying, interruption of urinary stream, impairment of size and force of urinary stream, terminal urinary dribbling, straining to start flow, dysuria, urgency) before and periodically during therapy.
- Assess patient for 1st-dose orthostatic hypotension and syncope. Incidence may be dose related. Observe patient closely during this period and take precautions to prevent injury. Monitor BP (lying and standing) and during initial therapy and periodically thereafter.
- Monitor intake and output ratios and daily weight, and assess for edema daily, especially at beginning of therapy. Report weight gain or edema.
- Rectal exams prior to and periodically throughout therapy to assess prostate size are recommended.
- Rule out prostate cancer before initiating therapy; symptoms are similar.

Implementation

- Do not confuse tamsulosin with tacrolimus.
- **PO:** Administer 30 min after the same meal each day. ***DNC:*** Swallow capsules whole; do not open, crush, or chew.
- If dose is interrupted for several days at either the 0.4-mg or 0.8-mg dose, restart therapy with the 0.4-mg/day dose.

Patient/Family Teaching

- Explain the purpose and side effects of tamsulosin. Instruct to take as directed with the same meal each day. Emphasize the importance of continuing to take this medication, even if feeling well. If a dose is missed, take as soon as remembered unless almost time for next dose. Do not double doses. Advise patient to read *Patient Information* before starting therapy and with each Rx refill in case of changes.

- Emphasize the importance of follow-up visits to determine effectiveness of therapy.
- May cause dizziness. Advise patient to avoid driving or other activities requiring alertness until response to medication is known.
- Caution patient to change positions slowly to minimize orthostatic hypotension, especially patients with low BP or concurrently taking antihypertensives. Geri: Assess risk for falls; instruct patient and family in preventing falls at home.
- Instruct patient to notify health care provider of all Rx or OTC medications, vitamins, or herbal products being taken and consult health care provider before taking any new medications, especially cough, cold, or allergy remedies.
- Rep: Tamsulosin is not indicated for use in women. Abnormal ejaculation, including ejaculation failure, retrograde ejaculation, and ↓ ejaculation have occurred with tamsulosin use in men. May impair male fertility. Symptoms are reversible when medication is discontinued.

Evaluation/Desired Outcomes

- Decreased symptoms of BPH (urinary urgency, hesitancy, nocturia).

REMS HIGH ALERT

tapentadol (ta-pen-ta-dol)

Nucynta, Nucynta ER, ✱ Nucynta IR

Classification

Therapeutic: analgesics (centrally acting), opioid analgesics

Pharmacologic: opioid agonists

Schedule II

Indications

Acute pain that is severe enough to require an opioid analgesic and for which alternative treatments are inadequate (immediate release only). Moderate to severe chronic pain in opioid-tolerant patients requiring use of daily, around-the-clock long-term opioid treatment and for which alternative treatment options are inadequate (extended release only). Pain associated with diabetic peripheral neuropathy in patients requiring around-the-clock opioid analgesia for an extended time (extended release only).

Action

Acts as a mu-opioid receptor agonist. Also inhibits the reuptake of norepinephrine. **Therapeutic Effects:** Decrease in pain severity.

Pharmacokinetics

Absorption: 32% absorbed following oral administration.

Distribution: Widely distributed.

Metabolism and Excretion: Undergoes extensive first-pass hepatic metabolism (97%); metabolites have no analgesic activity; metabolized drug is 99% renally excreted.

Half-life: 4 hr.

TIME/ACTION PROFILE (analgesic effect)

ROUTE	ONSET	PEAK	DURATION
PO	unknown	1 hr	4–6 hr

Contraindications/Precautions

Contraindicated in: Hypersensitivity; Significant respiratory depression in unmonitored settings or where resuscitative equipment is not readily available; Paralytic ileus; Severe renal impairment; Severe hepatic impairment; Concurrent use of MAO inhibitors or use of MAO inhibitors in the preceding 2 wk; Acute or severe bronchial asthma; Acute, mild, intermittent, or postoperative pain (extended release only); OB: Not recommended for use during labor and delivery; Pedi: Children ≥6 yr and ≥40 kg with renal or hepatic impairment.

Use Cautiously in: Personal or family history of substance use disorder or mental illness; Conditions associated with hypoxia, hypercapnea, or ↓ respiratory reserve, including asthma, chronic obstructive pulmonary disease, cor pulmonale, extreme obesity, sleep apnea syndrome, myxedema, kyphoscoliosis, CNS depression, use of other CNS depressants, or coma (↑ risk of further respiratory depression); use smallest effective dose; Seizure disorders; Moderate hepatic impairment; OB: Use during pregnancy only if potential maternal benefit justifies potential fetal risk. Chronic maternal treatment with opioids during pregnancy may result in neonatal opioid withdrawal syndrome; Lactation: Use while breastfeeding only if potential maternal benefit justifies potential risk to infant; Pedi: Safety and effectiveness not established in children <18 yr (extended release) or <6 yr and <40 kg (immediate release); Geri: ↑ risk of respiratory depression in older adults (dose ↓ suggested).

Adverse Reactions/Side Effects

CV: hypotension. **Endo:** adrenal insufficiency. **GI:** diarrhea, nausea, vomiting. **GU:** ↓ fertility. **Neuro:** allodynia, dizziness, headache, hyperalgesia, SEIZURES, somnolence. **Resp:** RESPIRATORY DEPRESSION (INCLUDING CENTRAL SLEEP APNEA AND SLEEP-RELATED HYPOXEMIA). **Misc:** allodynia, HYPERSENSITIVITY REACTIONS (INCLUDING

T

ANAPHYLAXIS AND ANGIOEDEMA), opioid-induced hyperalgesia, physical dependence, psychological dependence.

Interactions

Drug-Drug: **MAO inhibitors** or use of MAO inhibitors in the preceding 2 wk can result in potentially life-threatening adverse cardiovascular reactions due to additive effects on norepinephrine levels; concurrent use or use of MAO inhibitors in preceding 2 wk contraindicated. Use with **benzodiazepines** or other **CNS depressants**, including other **opioids**, **nonbenzodiazepine sedative/hypnotics**, **anxiolytics**, **general anesthetics**, **muscle relaxants**, **antipsychotics**, and **alcohol**, may cause profound sedation, respiratory depression, coma, and death; reserve concurrent use for when alternative treatment options are inadequate. **Alcohol** may ↑ levels and risk of toxicity. **Mixed agonist/antagonist analgesics**, including **nalbuphine** or **butorphanol**, and **partial agonist analgesics**, including **buprenorphine**, may ↓ tapentadol's analgesic effects and/or precipitate opioid withdrawal in physically dependent patients. Drugs that affect serotonergic neurotransmitter systems, including **tricyclic antidepressants**, **SSRIs**, **SNRIs**, **MAO inhibitors**, **TCAs**, **tramadol**, **trazodone**, **mirtazapine**, **5-HT$_3$ receptor antagonists**, **linezolid**, **methylene blue**, and **triptans**, may ↑ risk of serotonin syndrome.

Route/Dosage

When switching from immediate-release to extended-release product, the same total daily dose can be used.

PO (Adults): *Immediate release:* 50 mg, 75 mg, or 100 mg initially; then every 4–6 hr as needed and tolerated. If adequate analgesia is not achieved within first hr of first dose, additional dose may be given. Doses should not exceed 700 mg on the first day or 600 mg/day thereafter; *Extended release:* 50 mg twice daily; titrate dose up to 100–250 mg twice daily (not to exceed dose of 500 mg/day).

PO (Children ≥6 yr and ≥80 kg): *Immediate release:* 50 mg every 4 hr; may ↑ to 75 mg every 4 hr as needed and tolerated. If adequate analgesia still not achieved, may ↑ to 100 mg every 4 hr to maintain analgesia without intolerable side effects (not to exceed 7.5 mg/kg/day). Duration of treatment should not exceed 3 days.

PO (Children ≥6 yr and 60–79 kg): *Immediate release:* 50 mg every 4 hr; may ↑ to 75 mg every 4 hr as needed and tolerated (not to exceed 7.5 mg/kg/day). Duration of treatment should not exceed 3 days.

PO (Children ≥6 yr and 40–59 kg): *Immediate release:* 50 mg every 4 hr (not to exceed 7.5 mg/kg/day). Duration of treatment should not exceed 3 days.

Hepatic Impairment

PO (Adults): *Moderate hepatic impairment:* Immediate release: 50 mg every 8 hr initially; then titrate to maintain analgesia without intolerable side effects. Extended release: 50 mg once daily; may titrate up to maximum dose of 100 mg once daily if needed.

Availability

Immediate-release tablets: 50 mg, 75 mg, 100 mg. **Extended-release tablets:** 50 mg, 100 mg, 150 mg, 200 mg, 250 mg.

NURSING IMPLICATIONS

Assessment

- Assess type, location, and intensity of pain before and 1 hr (peak) after administration.
- Assess BP, HR, and respiratory rate before and periodically during administration. If respiratory rate <10/min, assess level of sedation. Dose may need to be ↓ by 25–50%. Respiratory depression does not ↑ in severity, only in duration, with ↑ dose. Monitor for respiratory depression, especially during initiation or following dose ↑; serious, life-threatening, or fatal respiratory depression may occur. May cause sleep-related breathing disorders (central sleep apnea, sleep-related hypoxemia).
- Geri/Pedi: Assess older adults and pediatric patients frequently; they are more sensitive to the effects of opioid analgesics and may experience side effects and respiratory complications more frequently.
- Patients taking extended-release tapentadol may require additional short-acting or rapid-onset opioid doses for breakthrough pain. Doses of short-acting opioids should be equivalent to 10–20% of 24 hr total and given every 2 hr as needed.
- Assess bowel function routinely. Prevention of constipation should be instituted with ↑ intake of fluids and bulk and with laxatives to minimize constipating effects. Administer stimulant laxatives routinely if opioid use exceeds 2–3 days, unless contraindicated. Consider drugs for opioid-induced constipation.
- Prolonged use may lead to physical and psychological dependence and tolerance, although these may be milder than with opioids. This should not prevent patient from receiving adequate analgesia. Patients who receive tapentadol for pain rarely develop psychological dependence.
- Monitor patient for seizures. May occur within recommended dose range. Risk is ↑ in patients with a history of seizures and in patients taking antidepressants (SSRIs, SNRIs, TCAs) or other drugs that ↓ the seizure threshold.
- Monitor for serotonin syndrome (mental-status changes [agitation, hallucinations, coma], autonomic instability [tachycardia, labile BP, hyperthermia], neuromuscular aberrations [hyperreflexia, incoordination], and/or GI symptoms [nausea, vomiting, diarrhea]) in patients taking SSRIs, SNRIs, triptans, TCAs, or MAO inhibitors concurrently with tapentadol.
- Assess risk for opioid addiction, abuse, or misuse prior to administration. Abuse or misuse of extended-release preparations by crushing, chewing, snorting, or injecting dissolved product will result in uncontrolled delivery of tapentadol and can result in overdose and death.

- Monitor for symptoms of opioid-induced hyperalgesia (↑ pain upon opioid dose ↑, ↓ pain upon opioid dose ↓, or pain from ordinarily nonpainful stimuli [allodynia]). If a patient is suspected to be experiencing opioid-induced hyperalgesia, consider appropriately ↓ the dose of the current opioid analgesic or using opioid rotation (safely switching patient to a different opioid moiety).

Toxicity and Overdose

- Overdose may cause respiratory depression. Naloxone may reverse some but not all of the symptoms of overdose. Treatment should be symptomatic and supportive. Maintain adequate respiratory exchange.

Implementation

- Explain therapeutic value of medication prior to administration to enhance the analgesic effect.
- Initial immediate-release dose of 50 mg, 75 mg, or 100 mg is individualized based on pain severity, previous experience with similar drugs, and ability to monitor patient. Second dose may be administered as soon as 1 hr after 1st dose if adequate pain relief is not obtained with 1st dose.
- Medication should be discontinued gradually after long-term use to prevent withdrawal symptoms. For patients on long-acting agents who are physically opioid dependent, initiate the taper by a small enough increment (e.g., no greater than 10%–25% of total daily dose) to avoid withdrawal symptoms, and proceed with dose-lowering at an interval of every 2–4 wk. Patients who have been taking opioids for briefer periods of time may tolerate a more rapid taper. Monitor frequently to manage pain and withdrawal symptoms (restlessness; lacrimation; rhinorrhea; yawning; perspiration; chills; myalgia; mydriasis; irritability; anxiety; backache; joint pain; weakness; abdominal cramps; insomnia; nausea; anorexia; vomiting; diarrhea; or ↑ BP, respiratory rate, or HR). If withdrawal symptoms occur, pause the taper for a period of time or ↑ the dose of opioid analgesic to the previous dose, and then proceed with a slower taper. Also, monitor patients for changes in mood, emergence of suicidal thoughts, or use of other substances. A multimodal approach to pain management may optimize the treatment of chronic pain and assist with the successful tapering of the opioid analgesic.
- **PO:** Tapentadol may be administered without regard to meals.
- Extended-release tapentadol must be taken one tablet at a time, with adequate water to ensure complete swallowing immediately after placement of the tablet in the mouth.
- ***DNC:*** Swallow extended-release tablets whole; do not crush, break, or chew.
- Use calibrated syringe to administer correct dose of oral solution.
- ***REMS:*** FDA strongly encourages health care providers to complete a REMS-compliant education program that includes all the elements of the FDA Education *Blueprint for Health Care Providers Involved in the Management or Support of Patients with Pain,* available at www.fda.gov/OpioidAnalgesicREMSBlueprint. Information on programs can be found at 1-800-503-0784 or www.opioidanalgesicrems.com.
- Discuss availability of naloxone for emergency treatment of opioid overdose with the patient and caregiver and assess the potential need for access to naloxone, both when initiating and renewing therapy, especially if patient has household members (including children) or other close contacts at risk for accidental exposure or overdose. Consider prescribing naloxone, based on the patient's risk factors for overdose, such as concurrent use of CNS depressants, a history of opioid use disorder, or prior opioid overdose. However, the presence of risk factors for overdose should not prevent the proper management of pain in any patient.

Patient/Family Teaching

- Explain purpose and side effects of tapentadol to patient.
- ***REMS:*** Instruct patient on how and when to ask for and take pain medication and to take tapentadol as directed; do not adjust dose without consulting health care provider. Report breakthrough pain and adverse reactions to health care provider. Do not take tapentadol if pain is mild or can be controlled with other pain medications, such as NSAIDs or acetaminophen. Do not stop abruptly; may cause withdrawal symptoms (anxiety, sweating, insomnia, rigors, pain, nausea, tremors, diarrhea, upper respiratory symptoms, hallucinations). ↓ dose gradually. Advise patient to read the *Medication Guide* prior to taking tapentadol and with each Rx refill in case of changes. Discuss safe use, risks, and proper storage and disposal of opioid analgesics with patients and caregivers with each Rx. The Patient Counseling Guide (PCG) is available at www.fda.gov/OpioidAnalgesicREMSPCG.
- Advise patient that tapentadol is a drug with known abuse potential. Protect it from theft, and never give to anyone other than the individual for whom it was prescribed; may be dangerous. Store out of sight and reach of children, and in a location not accessible by others.

- May cause dizziness and drowsiness. Caution patient to avoid driving or other activities requiring alertness until response to medication is known.
- Inform patient that tapentadol may cause seizures. Stop taking tapentadol and notify health care provider immediately if seizures occur.
- Advise patient to notify health care provider if signs of serotonin syndrome (agitation, restlessness, nausea and vomiting, abnormal eye movements, diarrhea, fast heartbeat, high BP, fever, loss of coordination, hallucinations) occur.
- Encourage patient to turn, cough, and breathe deeply every 2 hr to prevent atelectasis.
- Advise patient to change positions slowly to minimize orthostatic hypotension.
- Caution patient to avoid concurrent use of alcohol or other CNS depressants, including other opioids, with this medication.
- Emphasize the importance of aggressive prevention of constipation with the use of tapentadol.
- Educate patients and caregivers on how to recognize respiratory depression and emphasize the importance of calling 911 or getting emergency medical help right away in the event of a known or suspected overdose. Inform patients and caregivers about various ways to obtain naloxone as permitted by individual state naloxone dispensing and prescribing requirements or guidelines (Rx, direct from pharmacist, or state programs). OTC naloxone nasal spray is available at pharmacies nationwide for overdose or accidental ingestion.
- Instruct patient to notify health care provider of all Rx or OTC medications, vitamins, or herbal products being taken and consult health care provider before taking any new medications.
- Rep: Advise patient to notify health care provider if pregnancy is planned or suspected or if breastfeeding. Inform patient of potential for neonatal opioid withdrawal syndrome with prolonged use during pregnancy. Monitor neonate for signs and symptoms of withdrawal symptoms (irritability, hyperactivity and abnormal sleep pattern, high-pitched cry, tremor, vomiting, diarrhea, failure to gain weight); usually occur the first days after birth. Monitor infants exposed to tapentadol through breast milk for excess sedation and respiratory depression. Chronic use may ↓ fertility in women and men.

Evaluation/Desired Outcomes

- Decrease in severity of pain without a significant alteration in level of consciousness or respiratory status.

tavaborole, See ANTIFUNGALS (TOPICAL).

tedizolid (ted-eye-zoe-lid)

Sivextro

Classification

Therapeutic: anti-infectives

Pharmacologic: oxazolidinones

Indications

Acute bacterial skin and skin structure infections.

Action

Inhibits bacterial protein synthesis at the level of the 23S ribosome of the 50S subunit. **Therapeutic Effects:** Bacteriostatic action against enterococci, staphylococci, and streptococci, resulting in resolution of infection. **Spectrum:** Active against *Staphylococcus aureus*, including methicillin-resistant strains (MRSA), *Streptococcus pyogens*, *Streptococcus agalactiae*, *Streptococcus anginosus* group (including *Streptococcus anginosus*, *Streptococcus intermedius*, *Streptococcus constellatus*), and *Enterococcus faecalis*.

Pharmacokinetics

Absorption: IV administration results in complete bioavailability; well absorbed (91%) following oral administration.

Distribution: Well distributed to tissues.

Metabolism and Excretion: Rapidly converted by phosphatases to its active form; primarily excreted in feces (82%) and urine (18%) (<3% excreted unchanged in urine or feces).

Half-life: 12 hr.

TIME/ACTION PROFILE (plasma concentrations)

ROUTE	ONSET	PEAK	DURATION
PO	unknown	2.5 hr	24 hr
IV	rapid	end of infusion	24 hr

Contraindications/Precautions

Contraindicated in: Uncontrolled hypertension, pheochromocytoma, thyrotoxicosis, or concurrent use of sympathomimetic agents, vasopressors, or dopaminergic agents (↑ risk of hypertensive response); Carcinoid syndrome (↑ risk of serotonin syndrome); OB: Pregnancy.

Use Cautiously in: Neutropenia (safety and efficacy not established if WBC <1000 cells/mm³); Lactation: Use while breastfeeding only if potential maternal benefit justifies potential risk to infant.

Adverse Reactions/Side Effects

GI: CLOSTRIDIOIDES DIFFICILE-ASSOCIATED DIARRHEA (CDAD), diarrhea, nausea, vomiting. **Neuro:** dizziness, headache. **Misc:** infusion reactions.

Interactions

Drug-Drug: ↑ risk of hypertensive response with **MAO inhibitors, sympathomimetics** (e.g.,

pseudoephedrine), **vasopressors** (e.g., **epinephrine**, **norepinephrine**), and **dopaminergic agents** (e.g., **dopamine**, **dobutamine**); concurrent or recent use should be avoided. ↑ risk of serotonin syndrome with **SSRIs**, **TCAs**, **triptans**, **meperidine**, **bupropion**, or **buspirone**; avoid concurrent use. May ↑ levels and risk of toxicity of **methotrexate**, **topotecan**, or **rosuvastatin**; discontinue these medications temporarily during tedizolid treatment.

Route/Dosage

Tablets should NOT be used in children who weigh <35 kg.

PO, IV (Adults and Children ≥35 kg): 200 mg once daily for 6 days.
IV (Children ≥26 wk gestational age and 20–<35 kg): 60 mg twice daily for 6 days.
IV (Children ≥26 wk gestational age and 14–<20 kg): 40 mg twice daily for 6 days.
IV (Children ≥26 wk gestational age and 10–<14 kg): 30 mg twice daily for 6 days.
IV (Children ≥26 wk gestational age and 6–<10 kg): 20 mg twice daily for 6 days.
IV (Children ≥26 wk gestational age and 3–<6 kg): 12 mg twice daily for 6 days.
IV (Children ≥26 wk gestational age and 2–<3 kg): 6 mg twice daily for 6 days.
IV (Children ≥26 wk gestational age and 1–<2 kg): 3 mg/kg twice daily for 6 days.

Availability

Tablets: 200 mg. **Lyophilized powder for injection:** 200 mg/vial.

NURSING IMPLICATIONS

Assessment

- Assess for signs/symptoms of infection (vital signs; appearance of wound, sputum, urine, and stool; WBC) at beginning of and during therapy.
- Monitor for signs/symptoms of CDAD (diarrhea, abdominal cramping, fever, bloody stools). *If CDAD occurs, discontinue tedizolid and treat as indicated.* May begin up to several months following cessation of therapy.

Lab Test Considerations

- Obtain specimens for culture and sensitivity prior to initiating therapy. First dose may be given before receiving results.
- Consider alternate therapies in patients with neutrophil counts <1000 cells/mm^3.
- May cause anemia.

Implementation

- Dose adjustment is not necessary when switching from IV to oral formulation.
- **PO:** Administer without regard to food.

IV Administration

- **Intermittent Infusion: Reconstitution:** Reconstitute each vial with 4 mL of sterile water for injection. Gently swirl and let vial stand until completely dissolved; avoid shaking. **Concentration:** 50 mg/mL. **Dilution: For patients weighing ≥35 kg:** Slowly inject reconstituted solution into 250 mL bag of 0.9% NaCl or D5W. **For patients weighing <35 kg:** Prepare a stock solution by slowly injecting 1.6 mL of reconstituted solution into bag with 98.4 mL of 0.9% NaCl or D5W. Do not invert the vial during extraction. **Concentration:** 0.8 mg/mL. Next, add appropriate volume of stock solution to obtain dose to empty infusion bag or syringe. It may be necessary to round to the nearest graduation mark for smaller volumes. Gently invert bag to mix; avoid shaking to minimize foaming. Solution is clear and colorless to pale yellow; do not administer solution that is discolored or contains particulates. Must be infused within 24 hr after reconstitution at room temperature or under refrigeration. **Rate:** Infuse over 1 hr.
- **Y-Site Compatibility:** amikacin, amiodarone, ampicillin/sulbactam, anidulafungin, azithromycin, aztreonam, bumetanide, cefazolin, cefepime, cefiderocol, ceftazidime, ceftazidime/avibactam, ceftolozane/tazobactam, ceftriaxone, cefuroxime, ciprofloxacin, cisatracurium, daptomycin, dexamethasone, dexmedetomidine, digoxin, diltiazem, dopamine, epinephrine, eptifibatide, ertapenem, esomeprazole, famotidine, fentanyl, fosphenytoin, furosemide, heparin, hydrocortisone, hydromorphone, imipenem/cilastatin, insulin regular, labetalol, levofloxacin, lidocaine, lorazepam, mannitol, meperidine, meropenem, meropenem/vaborbactam, mesna, methylprednisolone, metoclopramide, metronidazole, micafungin, midazolam, milrinone, morphine, naloxone, nitroglycerin, norepinephrine, ondansetron, pantoprazole, penicillin G potassium, phenylephrine, piperacillin/tazobactam, plazomicin, potassium chloride, potassium phosphate, rocuronium, sodium bicarbonate, sodium phosphate, tacrolimus, tigecycline, vancomycin, vasopressin, vecuronium.
- **Y-Site Incompatibility:** albumin (human), calcium chloride, calcium gluconate, caspofungin, ceftaroline, cyclosporine, diphenhydramine, dobutamine, doxycycline, esmolol, gentamicin, isavuconazonium, magnesium sulfate, nicardipine, phenytoin, tobramycin.

Patient/Family Teaching

- Explain purpose and side effects of medication. Advise patient to read *Patient Information* before starting therapy.
- Advise patient to take full course of therapy, even if feeling better. Take missed doses as soon as

T

remembered unless <8 hr before next dose; then wait until next scheduled dose. Do not double dose.

- Advise patient to notify health care provider of all Rx or OTC medications, vitamins, or herbal products being taken and to consult with health care provider before taking other medications.
- Instruct patient to notify health care provider if changes in vision occur or immediately if diarrhea, abdominal cramping, fever, or bloody stools occur and not to treat with antidiarrheal without consulting health care provider.
- Rep: May cause fetal harm. Advise women of reproductive potential to notify health care provider if pregnancy is planned or suspected or if breastfeeding.

Evaluation/Desired Outcomes

- Resolution of signs and symptoms of infection. Length of time for complete resolution depends on organism and site of infection.

telavancin (tel-a-**van**-sin)

Vibativ

Classification

Therapeutic: anti-infectives

Pharmacologic: lipoglycopeptides

Indications

Complicated skin/skin structure infections caused by susceptible bacteria. Hospital-acquired and ventilator-associated bacterial pneumonia caused by *Staphylococcus aureus*.

Action

Inhibits bacterial cell wall synthesis by interfering with the polymerization and cross-linking of peptidoglycan. **Therapeutic Effects:** Bactericidal action against susceptible organisms. **Spectrum:** Active against *Staphylococcus aureus* (including methicillin-susceptible and -resistant strains), *Streptococcus pyogenes*, *Streptococcus agalactiae*, *Streptococcus anginosus* (including *S. anginosus*, *S. intermedius*, and *S. constellatus*), and *Enterococcus faecalis* (vancomycin-susceptible strains only).

Pharmacokinetics

Absorption: IV administration results in complete bioavailability.

Distribution: Minimal distribution to tissues.

Metabolism and Excretion: Metabolism is not known; 76% excreted unchanged in urine <1% in feces.

Half-life: 8 hr.

TIME/ACTION PROFILE (plasma concentrations)

ROUTE	ONSET	PEAK	DURATION
IV	unknown	end of infusion	24 hr

Contraindications/Precautions

Contraindicated in: Hypersensitivity; Congenital long QT syndrome, known prolongation of the QT interval, uncompensated HF, or severe left ventricular hypertrophy (↑ risk of fatal arrhythmias); Concurrent use of unfractionated heparin; OB: Pregnancy.

Use Cautiously in: Renal impairment (↓ dose if CCr ≤50 mL/min) (efficacy may be ↓ in patients with complicated skin/skin structure infections and CCr ≤50 mL/min) (↑ risk of mortality in patients with hospital-acquired or ventilator-associated pneumonia and CCr ≤50 mL/min; use only if benefit outweighs risk); Diabetes, HF, or hypertension (↑ risk of renal impairment); Lactation: Use while breastfeeding only if potential maternal benefit justifies potential risk to infant; Pedi: Safety and effectiveness not established in children (may be associated with poor outcomes in children <1 yr who have immature renal function); Geri: Consider age-related ↓ in renal function in older adults.

Adverse Reactions/Side Effects

CV: QT interval prolongation. **GI:** nausea, taste disturbance, vomiting, abdominal pain, CLOSTRIDIOIDES DIFFICILE-ASSOCIATED DIARRHEA (CDAD). **GU:** foamy urine, nephrotoxicity. **Neuro:** dizziness. **Misc:** ANAPHYLAXIS, infusion reactions.

Interactions

Drug-Drug: May artificially prolong activated partial thromboplastin time for up to 18 hr when used with **unfractionated heparin**; concurrent use contraindicated. **QT interval prolonging medications** may ↑ risk of arrhythmias. **NSAIDs, ACE inhibitors**, and **loop diuretics** may ↑ risk of nephrotoxicity.

Route/Dosage

Complicated Skin/Skin Structure Infections

IV (Adults): 10 mg/kg ever 24 hr for 7–14 days.

Renal Impairment

IV (Adults): *CCr 30–50 mL/min:* 7.5 mg/kg every 24 hr; *CCr 10–≤30 mL/min:* 10 mg/kg every 48 hr.

Hospital-Acquired/Ventilator-Associated Bacterial Pneumonia

IV (Adults): 10 mg/kg ever 24 hr for 7–21 days.

Renal Impairment

IV (Adults): *CCr 30–50 mL/min:* 7.5 mg/kg every 24 hr; *CCr 10–≤30 mL/min:* 10 mg/kg every 48 hr.

Availability

Lyophilized powder for injection: 750 mg/vial.

NURSING IMPLICATIONS

Assessment

- Assess for signs/symptoms of therapeutic response to treatment based on resolving infection (vital signs; appearance of wound, sputum, urine, and stool; WBC) throughout therapy.

- Assess cardiac history and ECG at baseline; avoid use in patients with long QT syndrome or cardiac arrhythmias associated with prolonged QT interval.
- Monitor for signs/symptoms of CDAD, including watery diarrhea with mucus, fever, abdominal pain or cramping, anorexia, nausea, and, in severe cases, dehydration, colitis, and blood or pus in the stool. May begin up to several weeks following cessation of therapy.
- Monitor for infusion-related reactions (resembling vancomycin flushing syndrome: flushing of upper body, urticaria, pruritus, rash). May resolve with stopping or slowing infusion.
- Observe patient for signs/symptoms of anaphylaxis (rash, pruritus, laryngeal edema, wheezing). Discontinue drug and notify health care provider immediately if symptoms occur. Keep epinephrine, an antihistamine, and resuscitation equipment close by in case of anaphylactic reaction.

Lab Test Considerations

- Verify negative pregnancy test before starting therapy.
- Obtain specimens for culture and sensitivity prior to therapy. First dose may be given before receiving results.
- Monitor CBC with differential.
- Monitor renal function (serum creatinine, CCr) prior to, every 48–72 hr during, and at the end of therapy. May cause nephrotoxicity. If ↓ renal function, reassess need for telavancin.
- May interfere with prothrombin time, INR, aPTT, activated clotting time, and coagulation-based factor Xa tests. Collect blood samples for these tests as close to next dose of telavancin as possible.
- Interferes with urine qualitative dipstick protein assays and quantitative dye methods; may use microalbumin assays.

Implementation

IV Administration

- **Intermittent Infusion:** Reconstitution: Reconstitute each vial with 45 mL of D5W, sterile water for injection, or 0.9% NaCl. Reconstitution time is usually <2 min but may require up to 20 min. Mix thoroughly with contents dissolved completely. Do not administer solution that is discolored or contains particulate matter. Discard vial if vacuum did not pull diluent into vial. Time in vial plus time in bag should not exceed 12 hr at room temperature or 7 days if refrigerated. Concentration: 15 mg/mL. Dilution: For doses of 150–800 mg, dilute further with 100–250 mL of D5W, 0.9% NaCl, or LR. Concentration: For doses <150 mg or >800 mg, dilute for a final concentration of 0.6–8 mg/mL. Rate: Administer over ≥60 min to minimize infusion reactions.
- **Y-Site Compatibility:** ampicillin/sulbactam, azithromycin, calcium gluconate, caspofungin, cefepime, ceftazidime, ceftriaxone, ciprofloxacin, dexamethasone, diltiazem, dobutamine, dopamine, doxycycline, ertapenem, famotidine, fluconazole, gentamicin, hydrocortisone, labetalol, letermovir, magnesium sulfate, mannitol, meropenem, metoclopramide, milrinone, norepinephrine, ondansetron, pantoprazole, phenylephrine, piperacillin/tazobactam, potassium chloride, potassium phosphates, sodium bicarbonate, sodium phosphates, tigecycline, tobramycin, vasopressin.
- **Y-Site Incompatibility:** amphotericin B deoxycholate, amphotericin B liposomal, digoxin, esomeprazole, furosemide, levofloxacin, micafungin.

Patient/Family Teaching

- Explain the purpose and side effects of telavancin. If an appointment is missed, contact health care provider as soon as possible to reschedule. Advise patient to read *Medication Guide* before starting and periodically during therapy in case of changes.
- Instruct the patient to notify health care provider if symptoms do not improve.
- Advise patient to report signs of superinfection (black, furry overgrowth on the tongue; vaginal itching or discharge; loose or foul-smelling stools).
- Instruct patient to notify health care provider if fever and diarrhea develop, especially if stool contains blood, pus, or mucus. Advise patient not to treat diarrhea without consulting health care provider.
- Inform patient that common side effects include taste disturbance, nausea, vomiting, headache, and foamy urine. Notify health care provider if difficulty breathing, chest pain, or palpitations occur.
- Advise patients and family to call 911 and seek urgent treatment for signs and symptoms of infusion-related reactions or anaphylaxis (flushing; difficulty breathing; chest tightness; hives; rash; feeling light-headed; itching; swelling of the face, lips, tongue, or throat).
- Instruct patient to notify health care provider of all Rx or OTC medications, vitamins, or herbal products being taken and consult health care provider before taking any new medications.
- Rep: May cause fetal harm. Advise women of reproductive potential to use effective contraception during therapy and for 2 days after last dose and to notify health care provider if pregnancy is suspected. Inform patient of pregnancy exposure registry that monitors pregnancy outcomes in women exposed to telavancin during pregnancy. Encourage pregnant patients to enroll in the VIBATIV pregnancy registry by calling 1-877-484-2700. May impair fertility in men.

T

Evaluation/Desired Outcomes

- Resolution of the signs and symptoms of infection. Length of time for complete resolution depends on the organism and site of infection.

telmisartan, See ANGIOTENSIN II RECEPTOR ANTAGONISTS.

BEERS

temazepam (tem-az-a-pam)

Restoril

Classification

Therapeutic: sedative/hypnotics

Pharmacologic: benzodiazepines

Schedule IV

Indications

Short-term management of insomnia (<4 wk).

Action

Acts at many levels in the CNS, producing generalized depression. Effects may be mediated by GABA, an inhibitory neurotransmitter. **Therapeutic Effects:** Relief of insomnia.

Pharmacokinetics

Absorption: Well absorbed after oral administration.
Distribution: Widely distributed; crosses blood-brain barrier. Accumulation of drug occurs with chronic dosing.
Protein Binding: 96%.
Metabolism and Excretion: Metabolized by the liver.
Half-life: 10–20 hr.

TIME/ACTION PROFILE (sedation)

ROUTE	ONSET	PEAK	DURATION
PO	30 min	2–3 hr	6–8 hr

Contraindications/Precautions

Contraindicated in: Hypersensitivity; Cross-sensitivity with other benzodiazepines may exist; Pre-existing CNS depression; Severe uncontrolled pain; Angle-closure glaucoma; Impaired respiratory function; Sleep apnea.
Use Cautiously in: Hepatic impairment; History of suicide attempt or drug addiction; OB: Use late in pregnancy can result in sedation (respiratory depression, lethargy, hypotonia) and/or withdrawal symptoms (hyperreflexia, irritability, restlessness, tremors, inconsolable crying, feeding difficulties) in neonates; Lactation: Use while breastfeeding only if potential maternal benefit justifies potential risk to infant; Pedi: Safety and effectiveness not established in children; Geri: Appears on Beers list. ↑ risk of cognitive impairment, delirium, falls, fractures, and motor vehicle accidents in older adults. If possible, avoid use in older adults.

Adverse Reactions/Side Effects

Derm: rash. **EENT:** blurred vision. **GI:** constipation, diarrhea, nausea, vomiting. **Neuro:** hangover, abnormal thinking, behavior changes, dizziness, drowsiness, hallucinations, lethargy, paradoxic excitation, sleep driving. **Misc:** physical dependence, psychological dependence.

Interactions

Drug-Drug: Use with **opioids** or other **CNS depressants**, including other **benzodiazepines**, **nonbenzodiazepine sedative/hypnotics**, **anxiolytics**, **general anesthetics**, **muscle relaxants**, **antipsychotics**, and **alcohol**, may cause profound sedation, respiratory depression, coma, and death; reserve concurrent use for when alternative treatment options are inadequate. May ↓ efficacy of **levodopa**. **Rifampin** or **smoking** may ↓ levels and effectiveness. **Probenecid** may prolong effects. Sedative effects may be ↓ by **theophylline**.
Drug-Natural Products: **Kava-kava, valerian, skullcap**, **chamomile**, or **hops** can ↑ risk of CNS depression.

Route/Dosage

PO (Adults): 15–30 mg at bedtime initially if needed; some patients may require only 7.5 mg.
PO (Geriatric Patients): 7.5 mg at bedtime.

Availability (generic available)

Capsules: 7.5 mg, 15 mg, 22.5 mg, 30 mg.

NURSING IMPLICATIONS

Assessment

- Assess mental status (orientation, mood, behavior) and potential for abuse prior to administering medication.
- Assess risk for addiction, abuse, or misuse prior to administration and periodically during therapy.
- Assess sleep patterns before and periodically throughout therapy.
- Prolonged high-dose therapy may lead to psychological or physical dependence. Restrict amount of drug available to patient, especially if patient is depressed or suicidal or has a history of addiction.
- Geri: Assess CNS effects and risk of falls. Institute falls prevention strategies.

Toxicity and Overdose

- If overdose occurs, flumazenil is the antidote. Do not use with patients with seizure disorder. May induce seizures.

Implementation

- Do not confuse Restoril with Risperdal.
- Supervise ambulation and transfer of patients after administration. Remove cigarettes. Side

rails should be raised and call bell within reach at all times.

- Gradually taper to discontinue or ↓ the dose to ↓ risk of withdrawal reactions, increased seizure frequency, and status epilepticus. If a patient develops withdrawal reactions, consider pausing taper or ↑ the dose to the previous tapered dose level. Subsequently ↓ the dose more slowly. Some patients may require longer tapering period (weeks–>12 mo).
- **PO:** Administer with food if GI irritation becomes a problem.

Patient/Family Teaching

- Instruct patient to take temazepam as directed. Teach sleep hygiene techniques (dark room, quiet, bedtime ritual, limit daytime napping, avoidance of nicotine and caffeine). If less effective after a few weeks, consult health care provider; do not ↑ dose. Advise patient to read *Medication Guide* before starting therapy and with each Rx refill in case of changes.
- Caution patient not to stop taking temazepam without consulting health care provider. Abrupt withdrawal may cause sweating, vomiting, muscle cramps, tremors, and seizures; may be life-threatening.
- Advise patient to take temazepam only if able to devote 8 hr to sleep.
- Advise patient that temazepam is a drug with known abuse potential. Protect it from theft, and never give to anyone other than the individual for whom it was prescribed. Store out of sight and reach of children and in a location not accessible by others.
- May cause daytime drowsiness or dizziness. Caution patient to avoid driving or other activities requiring alertness until response to medication is known. Geri: Instruct patient and family how to ↓ falls risk at home.
- Advise patient to avoid the use of alcohol and other CNS depressants and to consult health care provider before using OTC preparations that contain antihistamines or alcohol.
- Caution patient that complex sleep-related behaviors (sleep-driving, making phone calls, preparing and eating food, having sex, sleep walking) may occur while asleep. Inform patient to notify health care provider if sleep-related behaviors (may include sleep-driving: driving while not fully awake after ingestion of a sedative-hypnotic product, with no memory of the event) occur.
- Emphasize the importance of follow-up appointments to monitor progress.
- Rep: Advise women of reproductive potential to contact health care provider immediately if pregnancy is planned or suspected. Monitor infants exposed to temazepam during pregnancy or labor for several weeks or more prior to delivery for signs and symptoms of withdrawal (hypoactivity, hypotonia, hypothermia, respiratory depression, apnea, feeding problems, impaired metabolic response to cold stress). Monitor infants exposed to temazepam during breastfeeding for excessive sedation, poor feeding, and poor weight gain and advise family or caregiver to seek medical attention if they notice these signs. There is a pregnancy registry that monitors pregnancy outcomes in women exposed to psychiatric medications, including temazepam, during pregnancy. Health care providers are encouraged to register patients by calling the National Pregnancy Registry for Psychiatric Medications at 1-866-961-2388 or online at https://womensmentalhealth.org/pregnancyregistry/.

Evaluation/Desired Outcomes

- Improvement in sleep pattern with decreased number of nighttime awakenings, improved sleep onset, and increased total sleep time, which may not be noticeable until the 3rd day of therapy.

tenecteplase, See THROMBOLYTIC AGENTS.

tenofovir alafenamide

(te-**noe**-fo-veer al-a-**fen**-a-mide)

Vemlidy

Classification

Therapeutic: antiretrovirals

Pharmacologic: nucleoside reverse transcriptase inhibitors

T

Indications

Chronic hepatitis B virus (HBV) infection in patients with compensated liver disease.

Action

Converted by hydrolysis to tenofovir and subsequently phosphorylated to the active metabolite, tenofovir diphosphate, which inhibits replication of HBV through incorporation into viral DNA by the HBV reverse transcriptase, resulting in disruption of DNA synthesis. **Therapeutic Effects:** Decreased progression/sequelae of chronic HBV infection.

Pharmacokinetics

Absorption: Tenofovir alafenamide is a prodrug, which is hydrolyzed into tenofovir; absorption ↑ by high-fat meals.
Distribution: Unknown.

Metabolism and Excretion: Tenofovir is phosphorylated to tenofovir diphosphate (active metabolite); 32% excreted in feces, <1% in urine.
Half-life: 0.51 hr.

TIME/ACTION PROFILE (plasma concentrations)

ROUTE	ONSET	PEAK	DURATION
PO	unknown	0.5 hr	24 hr

Contraindications/Precautions

Contraindicated in: End-stage renal disease (CCr <15 mL/min) (not receiving hemodialysis); Decompensated hepatic impairment.
Use Cautiously in: Coinfection with HIV and chronic HBV; Renal impairment or receiving nephrotoxic medications (↑ risk of renal impairment); OB: Use during pregnancy only if potential maternal benefit justifies potential fetal risk; Lactation: Use while breastfeeding only if potential maternal benefit justifies potential risk to infant; Pedi: Children <6 yr (safety and effectiveness not established).

Adverse Reactions/Side Effects

GI: ↑ amylase, ↑ liver enzymes, abdominal pain, LACTIC ACIDOSIS/HEPATOMEGALY WITH STEATOSIS, nausea. **GU:** ACUTE RENAL FAILURE/FANCONI SYNDROME, glycosuria. **Metab:** hyperlipidemia. **MS:** ↑ CK, back pain. **Neuro:** fatigue, headache. **Resp:** cough.

Interactions

Drug-Drug: Nephrotoxic agents, including **NSAIDs**, ↑ risk of nephrotoxicity; avoid concurrent use. Medications that compete for active tubular secretion, including **acyclovir**, **cidofovir**, **ganciclovir**, **valacyclovir**, **valganciclovir**, or **aminoglycosides**, may ↑ levels and risk of toxicity; avoid concurrent use. **Carbamazepine**, **oxcarbazepine**, **phenobarbital**, **phenytoin**, **rifabutin**, **rifampin**, or **rifapentine** may ↓ levels and effectiveness; concurrent use with oxcarbazepine, phenobarbital, phenytoin, rifabutin, rifampin, or rifapentine not recommended; ↑ tenofovir alafenamide dose to 50 mg once daily when used with carbamazepine.
Drug-Natural Products: St. John's wort may ↓ levels and effectiveness; concurrent use not recommended.

Route/Dosage

PO (Adults and Children ≥6 yr and ≥25 kg): 25 mg once daily.

Renal Impairment

PO (Adults and Children ≥6 yr and ≥25 kg): *Hemodialysis:* Administer dose after dialysis session.

Availability (generic available)

Tablets: 25 mg. ***In combination with:*** bictegravir and emtricitabine (Biktarvy); darunavir, cobicistat, and emtricitabine (Symtuza); elvitegravir, cobicistat, and emtricitabine (Genvoya); emtricitabine (Descovy); emtricitabine and rilpivirine (Odefsey). See Appendix N.

NURSING IMPLICATIONS

Assessment

- Monitor for signs of hepatitis (jaundice, fatigue, anorexia, pruritus) during therapy. On discontinuation of therapy, monitor for clinical and laboratory signs of HBV exacerbation for at least several months after stopping therapy.

Lab Test Considerations

- Test patient for HIV-1 infection before starting therapy; tenofovir alafenamide should not be used alone in patient with HIV-1 infection.
- Monitor liver function tests and HBV levels during and following therapy. If therapy is discontinued, may cause severe exacerbation of HBV.
- Lactic acidosis may occur with hepatotoxicity causing hepatic steatosis; may be fatal, especially in women.
- May cause renal impairment. Monitor serum creatinine, estimated CCr, urine glucose, and urine protein before starting and periodically during therapy. Also assess serum phosphorous in patients with chronic kidney disease. Discontinue tenofovir alafenamide in patients who develop clinically significant ↓ in renal function or evidence of Fanconi syndrome.
- May ↑ ALT, AST, CK, amylase, and LDL cholesterol. May cause glycosuria.

Implementation

- **PO:** Administer once daily with food.

Patient/Family Teaching

- Instruct patient to take medication as directed. Avoid missing doses. Advise patient to read *Patient Information* before starting and with each Rx refill in case of changes.
- Advise patient to notify health care provider immediately if symptoms of lactic acidosis (weakness, fatigue, dizziness, muscle pain, trouble breathing, stomach pain with nausea or vomiting, cold extremities, fast or irregular heartbeat) or severe liver problems (yellow skin or whites of eyes, dark tea-colored urine, light-colored stool, loss of appetite, nausea, pain in right side of abdomen) occur.
- Instruct patient to notify health care provider of all Rx or OTC medications, vitamins, or herbal products being taken and consult health care provider before taking any new medications.
- Rep: Advise women of reproductive potential to notify health care provider if pregnancy is planned or suspected or if breastfeeding. Advise patient taking oral contraceptives to use a nonhormonal method of birth control during therapy. Inform patient of pregnancy exposure registry that monitors outcomes in women exposed to tenofovir alafenamide during pregnancy. Register patient in the Antiretroviral Pregnancy Registry by calling 1-800-258-4263.

Evaluation/Desired Outcomes

- Decreased progression/sequelae of chronic HBV infection.

teprotumumab

(tep-roe-toom-ue-mab)

Tepezza

Classification

Therapeutic: none assigned

Pharmacologic: insulin-like growth factor-1 receptor inhibitors, monoclonal antibodies

Indications

Thyroid eye disease (regardless of thyroid eye disease activity or duration).

Action

Exact mechanism in thyroid eye disease not fully characterized. Inhibits insulin-like growth factor-1 receptors. **Therapeutic Effects:** Reduction in proptosis (eyeball protrusion).

Pharmacokinetics

Absorption: IV administration results in complete bioavailability.

Distribution: Minimally distributed to extravascular tissues.

Metabolism and Excretion: Metabolized via proteolytic degradation. Excretion pathway not characterized.

Half-life: 20 days

TIME/ACTION PROFILE (plasma concentrations)

ROUTE	ONSET	PEAK	DURATION
IV	rapid	end of infusion	unknown

Contraindications/Precautions

Contraindicated in: OB: Pregnancy.

Use Cautiously in: Inflammatory bowel disease (IBD) (may cause exacerbation); Diabetes; Lactation: Safety not established in breastfeeding; Rep: Women of reproductive potential; Pedi: Safety and effectiveness not established in children.

Adverse Reactions/Side Effects

Derm: alopecia, dry skin. **EENT:** hearing impairment. **Endo:** hyperglycemia. **GI:** diarrhea, nausea. **MS:** muscle spasms. **Neuro:** fatigue, dysgeusia, headache. **Misc:** infusion reactions.

Interactions

Drug-Drug: None reported.

Route/Dosage

IV (Adults): 10 mg/kg initially; then 20 mg/kg every 3 wk for 7 additional doses.

Availability

Lyophilized powder for injection: 500 mg/vial.

NURSING IMPLICATIONS

Assessment

- Monitor for signs and symptoms of infusion reaction (transient increases in blood pressure, feeling hot, tachycardia, dyspnea, headache, muscular pain) during or within 90 min of infusion. Reactions are usually mild to moderate and can be managed with corticosteroids and antihistamines. If infusion reaction occurs, consider premedicating with an antihistamine, antipyretic, or corticosteroid and/or administering all subsequent infusions at a slower rate.
- Monitor patients with IBD for flare of disease. If IBD exacerbation is suspected, consider discontinuation of therapy.
- Assess patients' hearing before, during, and after treatment. If significant hearing loss occurs during therapy, consider discontinuation of therapy.

Lab Test Considerations

- Assess for elevated blood glucose and symptoms of hyperglycemia prior to infusion and continue to monitor during therapy. Ensure patients with hyperglycemia or pre-existing diabetes are under glycemic control before and during therapy.

Implementation

IV Administration

- **Intermittent Infusion: Reconstitution:** Reconstitute each vial with 10 mL of sterile water for injection. Powder has a cake-like appearance. Ensure stream of diluent is not directed onto the powder. Do not shake; gently swirl solution by rotating vial until powder is dissolved. **Concentration:** Final concentration is 47.6 mg/mL. **Dilution:** Further dilute in 0.9% NaCl. To maintain a constant volume in infusion bag, use a sterile syringe and needle to remove volume equivalent to amount of reconstituted solution to be placed into infusion bag. Withdraw required volume from reconstituted vial(s) based on the patient's weight (in kg) and transfer into an IV bag containing 0.9% NaCl for a total volume of 100 mL (for <1800 mg dose) or 250 mL (for ≥1800 mg and greater dose). Mix diluted solution by gentle inversion. Do not shake. Diluted solution is stable for 4 hr at room temperature or up to 48 hr if refrigerated and protected from light. If refrigerated prior to administration, allow diluted solution to reach room temperature prior to infusion. Solution is colorless or slightly brown, clear to opalescent; do not administer solutions that are cloudy, discolored, or contain particulate matter. **Rate:** Infuse over 90 min for first two infusions. If well

T

tolerated, may reduce subsequent infusions to 60 min. If not well tolerated, continue at 90 min. Do not administer as IV push or bolus.

- **Y-Site Incompatibility:** Do not infuse concomitantly with other agents.

Patient/Family Teaching

- Explain purpose of teprotumumab to patient.
- Advise patient to notify health care professional if symptoms of infusion reaction occur.
- Inform patient of risk of IBD. Instruct patient to notify health care professional immediately if diarrhea, with or without blood or rectal bleeding, associated with abdominal pain, or cramping/colic, urgency, tenesmus, or incontinence, occurs.
- May cause hyperglycemia. If diabetic, advise patient to discuss with health care professional need to adjust glycemic control measures, including medications as appropriate. Encourage compliance with glycemic control.
- Inform patient that hearing impairment may occur during therapy. Instruct patient to notify health care professional immediately if they experience any changes in hearing during therapy.
- Rep: May cause fetal harm. Advise females of reproductive potential to notify health care professional immediately if pregnancy is planned or suspected; discontinue teprotumumab if pregnancy occurs. Advise females of reproductive potential to use effective contraception during therapy and for 6 mo following last dose.

Evaluation/Desired Outcomes

- Reduction in proptosis (eyeball protrusion).

BEERS

terazosin (ter-ay-zoe-sin)

Hytrin

Classification

Therapeutic: antihypertensives

Pharmacologic: peripherally acting antiadrenergics

Indications

Mild to moderate hypertension (as monotherapy or in combination with other antihypertensives). Benign prostatic hyperplasia (BPH).

Action

Dilates both arteries and veins by blocking postsynaptic $alpha_1$-adrenergic receptors. Decreases contractions in smooth muscle of the prostatic capsule. **Therapeutic Effects:** Lowering of BP. Decreased symptoms of BPH (urinary urgency, hesitancy, nocturia).

Pharmacokinetics

Absorption: Well absorbed after oral administration.

Distribution: Unknown.

Metabolism and Excretion: 50% metabolized by the liver. 10% excreted unchanged by the kidneys. 20% excreted unchanged in feces. 40% eliminated in bile.

Half-life: 12 hr.

TIME/ACTION PROFILE

ROUTE	ONSET†	PEAK‡	DURATION†
PO-hypertension	15 min	6–8 wk	24 hr
PO-BPH	2–6 wk	unknown	unknown

† After single dose.

‡ After multiple oral dosing.

Contraindications/Precautions

Contraindicated in: Hypersensitivity.

Use Cautiously in: Dehydration, volume or sodium depletion (↑ risk of hypotension); Patients undergoing cataract surgery (↑ risk of intraoperative floppy iris syndrome); OB: Other antihypertensive agents preferred during pregnancy; Lactation: Safety not established in breastfeeding; Pedi: Safety and effectiveness not established in children; Geri: Appears on Beers list. ↑ risk of orthostatic hypotension in older adults. Avoid use for treatment of hypertension in older adults.

Adverse Reactions/Side Effects

CV: first-dose orthostatic hypotension, arrhythmias, chest pain, palpitations, peripheral edema, tachycardia. **Derm:** pruritus. **EENT:** nasal congestion, blurred vision, conjunctivitis, intraoperative floppy iris syndrome, sinusitis. **GI:** nausea, abdominal pain, diarrhea, dry mouth, vomiting. **GU:** erectile dysfunction, urinary frequency. **Metab:** weight gain. **MS:** arthralgia, back pain, extremity pain. **Neuro:** dizziness, headache, weakness, drowsiness, nervousness, paresthesia. **Resp:** dyspnea. **Misc:** fever.

Interactions

Drug-Drug: ↑ risk of hypotension with **sildenafil**, **tadalafil**, **vardenafil**, other **antihypertensives**, **nitrates**, or acute ingestion of **alcohol**. **NSAIDs**, **sympathomimetics**, or **estrogens** may ↓ effects of antihypertensive therapy.

Route/Dosage

Hypertension

PO (Adults): 1 mg initially; then slowly ↑ up to 5 mg/day (usual range 1–5 mg/day); may be given as single dose or in 2 divided doses (not to exceed 20 mg/day).

Benign Prostatic Hyperplasia

PO (Adults): 1 mg at bedtime; may be gradually ↑ up to 5–10 mg/day.

Availability (generic available)

Capsules: 1 mg, 2 mg, 5 mg, 10 mg.
Tablets: ✱ 1 mg, ✱ 2 mg, ✱ 5 mg, ✱ 10 mg.

NURSING IMPLICATIONS

Assessment

- Assess for first-dose orthostatic reaction (dizziness, weakness) and syncope. May occur 30 min–2 hr after initial dose and occasionally thereafter. Incidence may be dose related. Volume-depleted or sodium-restricted patients may be more sensitive. Observe patient closely during this period; take precautions to prevent injury. 1st dose may be given at bedtime to minimize this reaction. Geri: Older adults are at high risk of orthostatic hypotension.
- Monitor intake and output ratios and daily weight; assess for edema daily, especially at beginning of therapy.
- **Hypertension:** Monitor BP and HR frequently during initial dose adjustment and periodically during therapy. Report significant changes.
- **BPH:** Assess patient for symptoms of BPH (urinary hesitancy, feeling of incomplete bladder emptying, interruption of urinary stream, impairment of size and force of urinary stream, terminal urinary dribbling, straining to start flow, dysuria, urgency) before and periodically during therapy.
- Rule out prostatic carcinoma before therapy; symptoms are similar.

Implementation

- May be used in combination with diuretics or beta blockers to minimize sodium and water retention in treatment of hypertension. If these are added to terazosin therapy, ↓ dose of terazosin initially and titrate to effect.
- Restart use at the initial dose if therapy interrupted for several days or longer.
- If used with phosphodiesterase-5 inhibitor therapy, initiate at the lowest dose to avoid hypotension in patients taking terazosin.
- **PO:** Administer daily dose at bedtime. If necessary, dose may be ↑ to twice daily.

Patient/Family Teaching

- Explain the purpose and side effects of terazosin to patient. Instruct patient to take medication at the same time each day, preferably at bedtime to minimize side effects, especially the 1st dose. Take missed doses as soon as remembered. If not remembered until next day, omit; do not double doses. Advise patient against sudden discontinuation of drug, as this may cause rebound hypertension. Do not share medication with others, even if they have similar symptoms; may be harmful. Advise patient to read *Patient Information* before starting and with each Rx refill in case of changes.
- Advise patient to weigh self twice weekly and assess feet and ankles for fluid retention.
- May cause dizziness or drowsiness. Advise patient to avoid driving or other activities requiring alertness until response to the medication is known.
- Caution patient to avoid sudden changes in position to ↓ orthostatic hypotension. Alcohol, CNS depressants (including opioids), standing for long periods, hot showers, and exercising in hot weather should be avoided because of enhanced orthostatic effects.
- Advise patient to notify health care professional of all Rx or OTC medications, vitamins, or herbal products being taken and to consult with health care professional before taking other medications, especially NSAIDs or cough/cold/allergy remedies.
- Instruct patient to notify health care professional of medication regimen before any surgery.
- **Hypertension:** Emphasize the importance of continuing to take this medication as directed, even if feeling well. Medication controls but does not cure hypertension.
- Encourage patient to comply with additional interventions for hypertension (weight ↓, low-sodium diet, smoking cessation, moderation of alcohol consumption, regular exercise, stress management).
- Instruct patient and family on proper technique for BP monitoring. Advise them to check BP at least weekly and to report significant changes.
- Rep: Advise women of reproductive potential to notify health care professional if pregnancy is planned or suspected or if breastfeeding. Terazosin is not a preferred antihypertensive for use during pregnancy; consider transitioning to a preferred agent in patients planning to become pregnant.

Evaluation/Desired Outcomes

- Decrease in BP without appearance of side effects.
- Decreased symptoms of BPH. May require 2–6 wk of therapy before effects are noticeable.

terbinafine, See ANTIFUNGALS (TOPICAL).

terbutaline (ter-byoo-ta-leen)

Bricanyl Turbuhaler

Classification

Therapeutic: bronchodilators

Pharmacologic: adrenergics

Indications

Reversible airway disease due to asthma (SUBQ used for short-term control and oral agent as long-term control).

Unlabeled Use: Preterm labor (tocolytic) (terbutaline injection may only be used for short-term [≤72 hr] management of preterm labor to prolong pregnancy and allow for the administration of antenatal steroids).

Action

Results in the accumulation of cyclic adenosine monophosphate (cAMP) at beta-adrenergic receptors. Produces bronchodilation. Inhibits the release of mediators of immediate hypersensitivity reactions from mast cells. Relatively selective for $beta_2$ (pulmonary)-adrenergic receptor sites, with less effect on $beta_1$ (cardiac)-adrenergic receptors. **Therapeutic Effects:** Bronchodilation.

Pharmacokinetics

Absorption: 35–50% absorbed following oral administration but rapidly undergoes first-pass metabolism. Well absorbed following SUBQ administration.
Distribution: Unknown.
Metabolism and Excretion: Partially metabolized by the liver; 60% excreted unchanged by the kidneys.
Half-life: 5.7 hr.

TIME/ACTION PROFILE (bronchodilation)

ROUTE	ONSET	PEAK	DURATION
PO	within 60–120 min	within 2–3 hr	4–8 hr
SUBQ	within 15 min	within 0.5–1 hr	1.5–4 hr

Contraindications/Precautions

Contraindicated in: Hypersensitivity to adrenergic amines.
Use Cautiously in: Cardiac disease; Hypertension; Hyperthyroidism; Diabetes; Glaucoma; OB: Use for bronchodilation in pregnancy only if potential maternal benefit justifies potential fetal risk; Geri: Older adults are more susceptible to adverse reactions (may require dose ↓).

Adverse Reactions/Side Effects

CV: angina, arrhythmias, hypertension, myocardial ischemia, tachycardia. **Endo:** hyperglycemia. **F and E:** hypokalemia. **GI:** nausea, vomiting. **Neuro:** nervousness, restlessness, tremor, headache, insomnia. **Resp:** pulmonary edema.

Interactions

Drug-Drug: Concurrent use with other **adrenergics** (sympathomimetics) will have additive adrenergic side effects. **MAO inhibitors** may lead to hypertensive crisis. **Beta blockers** may negate its therapeutic effect.
Drug-Natural Products: Use with caffeine-containing herbs (**cola nut, guarana, mate, tea, coffee**) ↑ stimulant effect.

Route/Dosage

Asthma

PO (Adults and Children >15 yr): 2.5–5 mg 3 times daily (given every 6 hr) (not to exceed 15 mg/24 hr).
PO (Children 12–15 yr): 2.5 mg 3 times daily (given every 6 hr) (not to exceed 7.5 mg/24 hr).
PO (Children <12 yr): 0.05 mg/kg 3 times daily; may ↑ gradually (not to exceed 0.15 mg/kg 3–4 times daily or 5 mg/24 hr).
SUBQ (Adults and Children ≥12 yr): 250 mcg; may repeat in 15–30 min (not to exceed 500 mcg/4 hr).
SUBQ (Children <12 yr): 0.005–0.01 mg/kg; may repeat in 15–20 min.

Tocolysis (Off-Label)

IV (Adults): 2.5–10 mcg/min infusion; ↑ by 5 mcg/min every 10 min until contractions stop (not to exceed 30 mcg/min). After contractions have stopped for 30 min, ↓ infusion rate to lowest effective amount and maintain for 4–8 hr.

Availability (generic available)

Tablets: 2.5 mg, 5 mg. **Solution for injection:** 1 mg/mL.

NURSING IMPLICATIONS

Assessment

- Assess cardiac history and ECG at baseline.
- **Bronchodilator:** Assess lung sounds, respiratory pattern, BP, and HR before administration and during peak of medication. Monitor for symptomatic improvement of asthma attack. Note amount, color, and character of sputum produced, and notify health care provider of abnormal findings.
- Monitor pulmonary function tests before initiating therapy and periodically throughout therapy to determine effectiveness of medication.
- **Preterm Labor:** Monitor maternal BP and HR, frequency and duration of contractions, and fetal HR. Notify health care provider if contractions persist or ↑ in frequency or duration or if symptoms of maternal or fetal distress occur. Maternal side effects include tachycardia, palpitations, tremor, anxiety, and headache.
- Assess maternal respiratory status for symptoms of pulmonary edema (increased rate, dyspnea, rales/crackles, frothy sputum).
- Monitor mother and neonate for symptoms of hypoglycemia (anxiety; chills; cold sweats; confusion; cool, pale skin; difficulty in concentration; drowsiness; excessive hunger; headache; irritability; nausea; nervousness; rapid pulse; shakiness; unusual tiredness; weakness) and mother for hypokalemia (weakness, fatigue, U wave on ECG, arrhythmias).

Lab Test Considerations

- Monitor maternal serum glucose and electrolytes. May cause hypokalemia and hypoglycemia. Monitor neonate's serum glucose, because hypoglycemia may also occur in neonates.

Toxicity and Overdose

- Symptoms of overdose include persistent agitation, chest pain or discomfort, ↓ BP, dizziness, hyperglycemia, hypokalemia, seizures, tachyarrhythmias, persistent trembling, and vomiting.

- Treatment includes discontinuing beta-adrenergic agonists and symptomatic, supportive therapy. Cardioselective beta blockers are used cautiously because they may induce bronchospasm.

Implementation

- **PO:** Administer with meals to minimize gastric irritation.
- Tablet may be crushed and mixed with food or fluids for patients with difficulty swallowing.
- **SUBQ:** Administer SUBQ injections in lateral deltoid area. Do not use solution if discolored.

IV Administration

- **Continuous Infusion: Dilution:** May be diluted in D5W, 0.9% NaCl, or 0.45% NaCl. **Concentration:** 1 mg/mL (undiluted). **Rate:** Use infusion pump to ensure accurate dose. Begin infusion at 10 mcg/min. ↑ infusion rate by 5 mcg/min every 10 min until contractions cease. Maximum dose is 80 mcg/min. Begin to taper dose in 5 mcg/min decrements after a 30–60 min contraction-free period is attained. Switch to oral dose form after patient is contraction-free 4–8 hr on the lowest effective dose.
- **Y-Site Compatibility:** insulin regular.

Patient/Family Teaching

- Explain the purpose and side effects of terbutaline. Instruct patient to take medication as directed. If on a scheduled dosing regimen, take a missed dose as soon as possible; space remaining doses at regular intervals. Do not double doses. Caution patient not to exceed recommended dose; may cause adverse effects, paradoxical bronchospasm, or loss of effectiveness of medication. Do not share medication with others, even if they have similar symptoms; may be harmful. Keep out of children's reach. Advise patient to read *Patient Information* before starting and with each Rx refill in case of changes.
- Instruct patient to contact health care provider immediately if shortness of breath is not relieved by medication or is accompanied by diaphoresis, dizziness, palpitations, or chest pain.
- **Asthma:** Caution patient to avoid smoking and other respiratory irritants.
- Advise patient to notify health care provider of all Rx or OTC medications, vitamins, or herbal products being taken and to consult with health care provider before taking other medications. Advise patient there are multiple significant drug-drug interactions for this drug.
- **Preterm Labor:** Notify health care provider immediately if labor resumes or if significant side effects occur.
- Rep: Advise women of reproductive potential to notify health care provider if pregnancy is planned or suspected or if breastfeeding. Unintended tocolytic effects may occur. Serious adverse reactions, including death, have been reported after administration of terbutaline to pregnant women, including tachycardia, transient hyperglycemia, hypokalemia, arrhythmias, pulmonary edema, and myocardial ischemia. Transient fetal tachycardia or hypoglycemia may occur.

Evaluation/Desired Outcomes

- Prevention or relief of bronchospasm.
- Increase in ease of breathing.
- Control of preterm labor in a fetus of 20–36 wk gestational age.

terconazole, See ANTIFUNGALS (VAGINAL).

teriflunomide

(ter-i-**floo**-noe-mide)

Aubagio

Classification

Therapeutic: anti-multiple sclerosis agents

Pharmacologic: immune response modifiers, pyrimidine synthesis inhibitors

Indications

Relapsing forms of multiple sclerosis (MS), including clinically isolated syndrome, relapsing-remitting disease, and active secondary progressive disease.

Action

Inhibits an enzyme required for pyrimidine synthesis; has antiproliferative and anti-inflammatory effects.

Therapeutic Effects: ↓ incidence and severity of relapses in MS, with a decrease in disability progression.

Pharmacokinetics

Absorption: Well absorbed following oral administration.

Distribution: Well distributed to tissues.

Protein Binding: >99%.

Metabolism and Excretion: Metabolized via hydrolysis to inactive metabolites. 38% excreted in feces; 23% excreted in urine.

Half-life: 18–19 days.

TIME/ACTION PROFILE (↓ in disability progression)

ROUTE	ONSET	PEAK	DURATION
PO	3–6 mo	unknown	unknown

T

Contraindications/Precautions

Contraindicated in: Hypersensitivity to teriflunomide or leflunomide; Severe hepatic impairment; Concurrent use of leflunomide; Live-virus vaccinations; Active acute or chronic infection; Rep: Women of reproductive potential not using effective contraception; OB: Pregnancy; Lactation: Lactation.

Use Cautiously in: Mild or moderate hepatic impairment; Severe immunodeficiency, bone marrow disease, or severe uncontrolled infection; Concurrent use of neurotoxic medications or diabetes mellitus (↑ risk of peripheral neuropathy); Hypertension (control before therapy is initiated); Rep: Women of reproductive potential and men with female partners of reproductive potential; Pedi: Safety and effectiveness not established in children; Geri: ↑ risk of peripheral neuropathy in older adults.

Adverse Reactions/Side Effects

CV: hypertension. **Derm:** alopecia, DRUG REACTION WITH EOSINOPHILIA AND SYSTEMIC SYMPTOMS (DRESS), STEVENS-JOHNSON SYNDROME (SJS), TOXIC EPIDERMAL NECROLYSIS (TEN). **F and E:** hyperkalemia, hypophosphatemia. **GI:** ↑ liver enzymes, diarrhea, nausea, HEPATOTOXICITY. **GU:** acute renal failure (urate nephropathy). **Hemat:** leukopenia, neutropenia, thrombocytopenia. **Neuro:** paresthesia, peripheral neuropathy. **Misc:** HYPERSENSITIVITY REACTIONS (INCLUDING ANAPHYLAXIS, ANGIOEDEMA, AND URTICARIA), INFECTION (INCLUDING LATENT TUBERCULOSIS [TB] AND VIRAL INFECTIONS).

Interactions

Drug-Drug: May ↑ levels and risk of toxicity of **CYP2C8 substrates**, including **paclitaxel**, **pioglitazone**, and **repaglinide**. May ↓ levels and effectiveness of **CYP1A2 substrates**, including **alosetron**, **duloxetine**, **theophylline**, and **tizanidine**. May ↓ response to and ↑ risk of adverse reactions from **live vaccines**; avoid live vaccinations and consider long half-life of teriflunomide before administering. May ↑ levels and risk of toxicity of **ethinyl estradiol** and **levonorgestrel**. May ↑ risk of bleeding with **warfarin**. ↑ risk of additive immunosuppression with other **immunosuppressants** or **antineoplastics**; consider long half-life of teriflunomide. **Breast cancer resistant protein inhibitors**, including **cyclosporine**, **eltrombopag**, and **gefitinib**, may ↑ levels and risk of toxicity.

Route/Dosage

PO (Adults): 7 mg once daily *or* 14 mg once daily.

Availability (generic available)

Film-coated tablets: 7 mg, 14 mg.

NURSING IMPLICATIONS

Assessment

- Assess BP before starting and periodically during therapy. Treat hypertension as needed.
- Assess for rash periodically during therapy. May cause SJS or TEN. Discontinue teriflunomide if severe or if accompanied with fever, general malaise, fatigue, muscle or joint aches, blisters, oral lesions, conjunctivitis, hepatitis, or eosinophilia.
- Monitor for signs and symptoms of DRESS (fever; rash; lymphadenopathy and/or facial swelling; eosinophilia, in association with other organ system involvement, such as hepatitis, nephritis, hematologic abnormalities, myocarditis, or myositis, sometimes resembling an acute viral infection). Discontinue teriflunomide if DRESS is confirmed.

Lab Test Considerations

- Verify negative pregnancy test before starting therapy.
- Monitor liver function tests (transaminases, bilirubin) within 6 mo before starting therapy and monthly thereafter for at least the 1st 6 mo. Do not administer if ALT >2 times upper limit of normal (ULN). Consider discontinuing therapy if serum transaminases ↑ >3 times ULN.
- Monitor serum transaminases and bilirubin in patients with symptoms of liver dysfunction. If liver injury is suspected, discontinue teriflunomide, begin accelerated elimination procedure, and monitor liver function tests weekly until normal.
- Monitor CBC within 6 mo before starting and periodically during therapy based on signs and symptoms of infection. Mean ↓ in WBC occurs during 1st 6 wk and remains low during therapy.
- Monitor INR closely in patients taking warfarin.

Implementation

- Administer a tuberculin skin test prior to administration of teriflunomide. Patients with active latent TB should be treated for TB prior to therapy.
- **PO:** Administer once daily without regard to food.
- **Drug Elimination Procedure:** Women of reproductive potential who either wish to become pregnant or become pregnant during therapy and men who want to father a child must discontinue teriflunomide and go through one of the drug elimination procedures. Either of the following procedures is recommended to achieve nondetectable plasma levels <0.02 mg/L after stopping treatment with teriflunomide: (1) Administer cholestyramine 8 g every 8 hr for 11 days. If cholestyramine 8 g regimen is not well tolerated, cholestyramine 4 g every 8 hr can be used; *or* (2) Administer 50 g of oral activated charcoal powder every 12 hr for 11 days. Days do not need to be consecutive unless rapid lowering of levels is desired. Verify plasma levels <0.02 mg/L by two separate tests ≥14 days

apart. Plasma levels may take up to 2 yr to reach nondetectable levels without drug elimination procedure.

Patient/Family Teaching

- Instruct patient to take teriflunomide as directed. Advise patient to read *Medication Guide* before starting therapy and with each Rx refill in case of changes.
- Advise patient to notify health care provider promptly if symptoms of severe allergic reactions, liver problems (nausea, vomiting, stomach pain, ↓ appetite, tiredness, yellowing of skin or whites of eyes, dark urine), serious skin problems (redness or peeling), infection (fever, tiredness, body aches, chills, nausea, vomiting), or interstitial lung disease (cough, dyspnea, with or without fever) occur.
- Instruct patient to notify health care provider if symptoms of peripheral neuropathy (numbness and tingling in hands and feet different from symptoms of MS), kidney problems (flank pain), high potassium level (nausea or racing heartbeat), or high BP occur.
- Instruct patient to notify health care provider of all Rx or OTC medications, vitamins, or herbal products being taken and consult health care provider before taking any new medications.
- Instruct patient to avoid vaccinations with live vaccines during and following therapy without consulting health care provider.
- Discuss the possibility of hair loss with patient. Explore methods of coping.
- Rep: May cause fetal harm. Advise women of reproductive potential and male patients with female partners of reproductive potential to use effective birth control during therapy and until levels of teriflunomide <0.02 mg/L. If pregnancy is planned or suspected or if breastfeeding, notify health care provider immediately; an accelerated elimination procedure may be used to ↓ levels more rapidly. Women of reproductive potential are also recommended to undergo accelerated elimination procedure on discontinuation of therapy. Inform patient of pregnancy safety surveillance program that monitors pregnancy outcomes in women exposed to teriflunomide. Encourage to report pregnancy by calling 1-800-745-4447, option 2. Advise patient to avoid breastfeeding during therapy.

Evaluation/Desired Outcomes

- Decrease in the number of MS flares (relapses) and slowing of physical problems caused by MS.

BEERS REMS

TESTOSTERONE

(tess-**toss**-te-rone)

testosterone cypionate
Azmiro, Depo-Testosterone

testosterone enanthate
✱ Delatestryl, Xyosted

testosterone nasal gel
Natesto

testosterone pellets
Testopel

testosterone transdermal gel
Androgel, Testim, Vogelxo

testosterone transdermal solution
~~Axiron~~

testosterone undecanoate
Aveed, Jatenzo, Kyzatrex, Tlando

Classification
Therapeutic: hormones
Pharmacologic: androgens

Schedule III

Indications

Hypogonadism in men with low testosterone serum concentrations. Delayed puberty in men (enanthate and pellets). Androgen-responsive breast cancer in postmenopausal women (palliative) (enanthate). **Unlabeled Use:** Part of masculinizing hormone therapy in female-to-male (FtM) transgender patients.

Action

Responsible for the normal growth and development of male sex organs. Maintenance of male secondary sex characteristics: Growth and maturation of the prostate, seminal vesicles, penis, and scrotum; Development of male hair distribution; Vocal cord thickening; Alterations in body musculature and fat distribution. **Therapeutic Effects:** Correction of hormone deficiency in male hypogonadism: Initiation of male puberty. Suppression of tumor growth in some forms of breast cancer. Increased male characteristics in FtM transgender patients.

Pharmacokinetics

Absorption: Well absorbed from IM or SUBQ sites, through skin, or through nasal mucosa. Cypionate, enanthate, and undecanoate salts are absorbed slowly. Skin serves as reservoir for sustained release of testosterone into systemic circulation; 10% absorbed into systemic circulation during 24-hr period.

T

Distribution: Circulating testosterone is primarily bound in the serum to sex hormone-binding globulin and albumin.
Protein Binding: 98%.
Metabolism and Excretion: Metabolized by the liver. 90% eliminated in urine as metabolites.
Half-life: *Enanthate (IM), nasal gel, pellets, topical gel, topical solution, undecanoate:* 10–100 min; *cypionate:* 8 days; *enanthate (SUBQ):* Unknown.

TIME/ACTION PROFILE (androgenic effects†)

ROUTE	ONSET	PEAK	DURATION
IM—cypionate, enanthate	unknown	unknown	2–4 wk
IM—undecanoate	unknown	unknown	10 wk
SUBQ—enanthate	unknown	unknown	unknown
Nasal gel	unknown	unknown	3 mo
Oral	unknown	unknown	unknown
Pellets	unknown	unknown	3–6 mo
Transdermal (solution)	unknown	14 days	7–10 days
Transdermal (gel)	30 min	unknown	24 hr

† Response is highly variable among individuals; may take mo.

Contraindications/Precautions

Contraindicated in: Hypersensitivity; Men with breast or prostate cancer; Age-related hypogonadism (undecanoate [PO]); Some products contain benzyl alcohol and should be avoided in patients with known hypersensitivity; Women (pellets, nasal gel, tablets, topical gel, topical solution); OB: Pregnancy; Lactation: Lactation.
Use Cautiously in: Diabetes mellitus; Established cardiovascular disease or risk factors for cardiovascular disease; Hypertension; Renal or hepatic impairment; Benign prostatic hyperplasia; Hypercalcemia; Obesity or chronic lung disease (↑ risk of sleep apnea); Polycythemia; Nasal disorders, nasal/sinus surgery, nasal fracture in previous 6 mo, nasal fracture that caused deviated anterior nasal septum, mucosal inflammatory disorders (e.g. Sjögren syndrome), or sinus disorders (nasal gel); Pedi: Prepubertal males exposed to testosterone may experience premature development of secondary sexual characteristics, aggression, and other side effects; Geri: Appears on Beers list. ↑ risk of prostatic hyperplasia/carcinoma in older adults. Avoid use in older adults, except for confirmed hypogonadism with clinical symptoms.

Adverse Reactions/Side Effects

CV: edema, DEEP VEIN THROMBOSIS, ↑ BP, MI. **Derm:** male pattern baldness. **EENT:** deepening of voice- **nasal gel:** epistaxis, nasal scabbing, nasopharyngitis, rhinorrhea. **Endo: women:** change in libido, clitoral enlargement, ↓ breast size. **men:** acne, facial hair, gynecomastia, erectile dysfunction, oligospermia, priapism. **F and E:** hypercalcemia, hyperkalemia, hyperphosphatemia. **GI:** abdominal cramps, changes in appetite, HEPATOTOXICITY, nausea, vomiting. **buccal:** bitter taste, gingivitis, gum edema, gum tenderness. **GU:** ↓ fertility, ↓ sperm count, menstrual irregularities, nocturia, priapism, prostatic enlargement, urinary hesitancy, urinary incontinence. **Hemat:** ↑ hematocrit. **Local:** chronic skin irritation (transdermal), pain at injection/implantation site. **Metab:** hyperlipidemia. **Neuro:** anxiety, confusion, depression, fatigue, headache, STROKE, SUICIDAL THOUGHTS/BEHAVIOR, vertigo. **Resp:** PULMONARY EMBOLISM, PULMONARY OIL MICROEMBOLISM (WITH UNDECANOATE [IM]), sleep apnea. **Misc:** HYPERSENSITIVITY REACTIONS (INCLUDING ANAPHYLAXIS).

Interactions

Drug-Drug: May ↑ effects of **warfarin**, **oral hypoglycemic agents**, and **insulin**. **Corticosteroids** may ↑ risk of edema formation.

Route/Dosage

Replacement Therapy

IM (Adults): 50–400 mg every 2–4 wk (enanthate or cypionate); 750 mg initially, then at Wk 4, then every 10 wk (undecanoate).
SUBQ (Adults): 75 mg once weekly (enanthate).
Intranasal (Adults): One actuation (5.5 mg) in each nostril 3 times daily.
PO (Adults): *Jatenzo:* 158 mg twice daily; may titrate up to 396 mg twice daily based on serum testosterone concentrations. *Kyzatrex:* 200 mg twice daily; may titrate up to 400 mg twice daily based on serum testosterone concentrations. *Tlando:* 225 mg twice daily.
Transdermal (Adults): *Androgel 1% or Testim:* 5 g (contains 50 mg of testosterone; 5 mg systemically absorbed) applied once daily (morning preferable); if needed, may be ↑ to maximum of 10 g (contains 100 mg of testosterone; 10 mg systemically absorbed); *Androgel 1.62%:* 40.5 mg of testosterone (2 pump actuations) applied once daily (morning preferable); dose may be adjusted down to a minimum of 20.25 mg or up to a maximum of 81 mg of testosterone, if needed (dose based on serum testosterone concentrations); *Vogelxo:* 50 mg of testosterone (one tube, one packet, or 4 pump actuations) applied once daily; dose may be adjusted up to a maximum of 100 mg of testosterone, if needed (dose based on serum testosterone concentrations).
SUBQ (for implantation) (pellets): (Adults): 150–450 mg every 3–6 mo.
Topical (Adults): 60 mg (2 pump actuations) applied once daily; may be ↑ up to 120 mg (4 pump actuations) based on serum testosterone concentrations.

Delayed Male Puberty

IM (Children): 50–200 mg every 2–4 wk for up to 6 mo (enanthate).
SUBQ (for SUBQ implantation) (pellets): (Children): 150–450 mg every 3–6 mo.

Palliative Management of Breast Cancer

IM (Adults): 200–400 mg every 2–4 wk (enanthate).

Availability (generic available)

Capsules (Jatenzo): 158 mg, 198 mg, 237 mg. **Capsules (Kyzatrex):** 100 mg, 150 mg, 200 mg. **Capsules (Tlando):** 112.5 mg. **Nasal gel:** 5.5 mg/pump actuation. **Pellets:** 75 mg. **Solution for intramuscular injection (cypionate) (in oil):** 100 mg/mL, 200 mg/mL. **Solution for intramuscular injection (enanthate) (in oil):** 200 mg/mL. **Solution for intramuscular injection (undecanoate) (in oil) (Aveed):** 250 mg/mL. **Solution for SUBQ injection (enanthate) (autoinjector) (Xyosted):** 50 mg/0.5 mL, 75 mg/0.5 mL, 100 mg/0.5 mL. **Transdermal gel (Androgel):** 20.25 mg/packet (1.62%), 25 mg/packet (1%), 40.5 mg/packet (1.62%), 50 mg/packet (1%), 75-g metered dose pump (each pump dispenses 60 metered 12.5-mg doses [1%]), 88-g metered dose pump (each pump dispenses 60 metered 20.25-mg doses [1.62%]). **Transdermal gel (Testim):** 50 mg/unit–dose tube (1%). **Transdermal gel (Vogelxo):** 50 mg/packet or unit–dose tube (1%), 75-g metered dose pump (each pump dispenses 60 metered 12.5-mg doses [1%]). **Transdermal solution:** 30 mg/pump actuation.

NURSING IMPLICATIONS

Assessment

- Monitor intake and output, weigh patient twice weekly, and assess for edema. Report significant changes indicative of fluid retention.
- Assess cardiovascular risk and BP before and 6 wk after starting therapy. May ↑ BP. Treat new-onset and exacerbations of pre-existing hypertension with guideline-recommended medications. Regularly re-evaluate whether the benefits of testosterone therapy outweigh its risks in patients who have/develop cardiovascular risk factors or cardiovascular disease while receiving therapy.
- Assess for abuse using higher doses than prescribed and usually in conjunction with other anabolic androgenic steroids. May result in heart attack, HF, stroke, depression, hostility, aggression, liver toxicity, and infertility. Measure serum testosterone concentrations if abuse is suspected.
- **Men:** Monitor for precocious puberty in boys (acne, darkening of skin, development of male secondary sex characteristics: ↑ in penis size, frequent erections, growth of body hair). Bone age determinations should be measured every 6 mo to determine rate of bone maturation and effects on epiphyseal closure.
- Monitor for breast enlargement, persistent erections, and ↑ urge to urinate in men. Monitor for difficulty urinating in older men, because prostate enlargement may occur.
- In patients receiving injection of testosterone undecanoate, monitor in health care setting for 30 min after injection for signs of pulmonary oil microembolism (cough, dyspnea, throat tightening, chest pain, dizziness, syncope) or anaphylaxis.
- **Women:** Assess for virilism (deepening of voice, unusual hair growth or loss, clitoral enlargement, acne, menstrual irregularity).
- In women with metastatic breast cancer, monitor for signs/symptoms of hypercalcemia (nausea, vomiting, constipation, lethargy, loss of muscle tone, thirst, polyuria).

Lab Test Considerations

- Before therapy, measure serum testosterone concentrations in the morning on ≥2 separate days. Normal range (300–1050 ng/dL). Monitor serum testosterone concentrations 4–12 wk after starting therapy. Discontinue therapy if concentrations are consistently outside of normal range.
- Monitor hemoglobin and hematocrit periodically during therapy; may cause polycythemia.
- Monitor liver enzymes, prostate specific antigen, and serum cholesterol levels periodically during therapy. May ↑ AST, ALT, bilirubin, and cholesterol levels and suppress clotting factors II, V, VII, and X.
- Monitor serum and urine calcium levels and serum alkaline phosphatase concentrations in women with metastatic breast cancer.
- May ↑ sodium, chloride, potassium, and phosphate concentrations.
- Monitor blood glucose closely in patients with diabetes who are receiving oral hypoglycemic agents or insulin.
- *Transdermal Solution:* Measure serum testosterone concentrations after initiation of therapy to ensure desired concentrations (300–1050 ng/dL) are achieved. Adjust dose based on serum testosterone concentration from a single blood draw 2–8 hr after applying and ≥14 days after starting treatment or following dose adjustment. If concentration is <300 ng/dL, may ↑ daily dose from 60 mg (2 pump actuations) to 90 mg (3 pump actuations) or from 90 mg to 120 mg (4 pump actuations). If concentration >1050 ng/dL, ↓ daily testosterone dose from 60 mg (2 pump actuations) to 30 mg (1 pump actuation) as instructed by health care provider. If concentration consistently >1050 ng/dL at lowest daily dose of 30 mg (1 pump actuation), discontinue testosterone.
- *Nasal gel:* Monitor serum testosterone concentrations after 1 mo and periodically during therapy. If total testosterone concentrations consistently >1050 ng/dL, discontinue testosterone. If total testosterone concentrations are consistently <300 ng/dL, consider alternative therapy.

T

Implementation

- Range-of-motion exercises should be done with all bedridden patients to prevent mobilization of calcium from the bone.
- **PO:** Administer twice daily, in the morning and evening, with food.
- **IM:** Administer IM deep into gluteal muscle. Crystals may form when vials are stored at low temperatures; warming and shaking vial will redissolve crystals. Use of a wet syringe or needle may cause solution to become cloudy but will not affect its potency.
- ***REMS:*** Due to the risk of pulmonary oil microembolism, testosterone undecanoate injection may be prescribed only by prescribers registered in the *Aveed REMS* program. Required components of the *Aveed REMS* program include the following: prescribers must be certified with the *Aveed REMS* program by enrolling and complying with the REMS requirements; health care settings must be certified with the *Aveed REMS* program and have health care providers who are certified. Health care settings must have on-site access to equipment and personnel trained to manage serious pulmonary oil microembolism and anaphylaxis. Information about *Aveed* and the *Aveed REMS* program is available at www.aveedrems.com or by calling 1-855-755-0494.
- **SUBQ:** Pellets are to be implanted SUBQ by a health care provider.
- **Transdermal Solution:** Apply to axilla using applicator at the same time each morning, to clean, dry, intact skin. Do not apply to other parts of the body, including to the scrotum, penis, abdomen, shoulders, or upper arms. Prime pump when using for 1st time by depressing pump 3 times; discard any product dispensed directly into a basin, sink, or toilet; and then wash liquid away thoroughly. Prime only before 1st use of each pump. After priming, completely depress pump once with nozzle over applicator cup to dispense 30 mg of testosterone. Apply in 30 mg (1 pump actuation) increments. Place actuator into the axilla and wipe steadily down and up into the axilla. If solution drips or runs, wipe back up with applicator cup. Do not rub into skin with fingers or hand. Repeat process for each 30-mg dose needed. When repeat application to same axilla, allow axilla to dry completely before more is applied. Rinse applicator under room temperature running water and pat dry with a tissue. Allow axilla to dry completely before dressing. Solution has an alcohol base and is flammable until dry. Apply deodorant before application of testosterone solution. Avoid swimming or washing for 2 hr after application. Wash hands immediately with soap and water after application.
- **Transdermal Gel:** Apply gel once daily, preferably in the morning, to clean, dry, intact skin of shoulders and upper arms (*Androgel*, *Testim*, and *Vogelxo*), abdomen (Androgel only), or front or inner thighs (Fortesta). Gel should not be applied to scrotum (5–30 times more permeable than other sites). Refer to the chart on the pump label to determine how many full pump depressions are required for the daily prescribed dose.
- The dose of Fortesta should be titrated based on the serum testosterone concentration from a single blood draw 2 hr after applying Fortesta and at approximately 14 days and 35 days after starting treatment or following dose adjustment.
- **Intranasal:** Prime pump by inverting, depressing pump 10 times, discarding any amount dispensed directly into a sink, and washing gel away thoroughly with warm water. Wipe tip with a clean, dry tissue. If gel gets on hands, wash hands with warm water and soap. Priming should be done only before 1st use of each dispenser. Blow nose. Place right index finger on pump of actuator, and while in front of a mirror, slowly advance tip of actuator into left nostril upward until finger on the pump reaches the base of the nose. Tilt the actuator so that the opening on the tip of the actuator is in contact with the lateral wall of the nostril to ensure that the gel is applied to the nasal wall. Slowly depress the pump until it stops. Remove the actuator from the nose while wiping the tip along the inside of the lateral nostril wall to fully transfer the gel. Repeat with right nostril. Press on the nostrils at a point just below bridge of the nose and lightly massage. Refrain from blowing nose or sniffing for 1 hr after administration.

Patient/Family Teaching

- Explain purpose and side effects of medication to patient. Advise patient to read *Patient Information* before starting therapy. Advise patient to use as directed. Do not use higher than prescribed doses. Explain rationale for prohibiting use of testosterone for ↑ athletic performance. Testosterone is neither safe nor effective for this use and has a potential risk of serious side effects.
- Advise patient to notify health care provider of all Rx or OTC medications, vitamins, or herbal products being taken and to consult with health care provider before taking other medications.
- Advise patient to report the following signs and symptoms promptly: *in men,* priapism (sustained and often painful erections), difficulty urinating, or gynecomastia; *in women,* virilism (which may be reversible if medication is stopped as soon as changes are noticed) or hypercalcemia (nausea, vomiting, constipation, and weakness); *in men or women,* edema (unexpected weight gain, swelling of feet), hepatitis (yellowing of skin or eyes and abdominal pain), or unusual bleeding or bruising.
- Advise patients with diabetes to monitor blood closely for alterations in blood glucose concentrations.
- Emphasize the importance of regular follow-up physical exams, lab tests, and x-ray exams to monitor progress.

- Radiologic bone age determinations should be evaluated every 6 mo in prepubertal children to determine rate of bone maturation and effects on epiphyseal centers.
- **Transdermal Gel or Solution:** Explain application to patient.
- Advise patient that women and children should avoid contact with unclothed or unwashed application site. Virilization has been reported in children who were secondarily exposed to testosterone gel. Patients should cover the application site(s) with clothing (T-shirt) after solution has dried. For direct skin-to-skin contact, patient should wash application site thoroughly with soap and water to remove any testosterone residue. If unwashed or unclothed skin with testosterone solution comes in direct contact with skin of another person, wash area of contact with soap and water as soon as possible.
- **Intranasal:** Advise patient to notify health care provider if nasal signs or symptoms (nasopharyngitis, rhinorrhea, epistaxis, nasal discomfort, nasal scabbing) occur.
- Rep: May cause fetal harm. Advise women of reproductive potential to notify health care provider immediately if pregnancy is planned or suspected or if breastfeeding. May impair fertility.

Evaluation/Desired Outcomes

- Correction of hormone deficiency in male hypogonadism.
- Initiation of male puberty.
- Suppression of tumor growth in some forms of breast cancer.
- Increased male characteristics in FtM transgender patients.

REMS

thalidomide (tha-lid-oh-mide)

Thalomid

Classification

Therapeutic: antineoplastics, immunosuppressants

Indications

Cutaneous manifestations of moderate to severe erythema nodosum leprosum. Prevention (maintenance) and suppression of recurrent erythema nodosum leprosum. Newly diagnosed multiple myeloma (in combination with dexamethasone). **Unlabeled Use:** Behçet syndrome. HIV-associated wasting syndrome. Aphthous stomatitis (including HIV associated). Crohn disease.

Action

May suppress excess levels of tumor necrosis factor-alpha and alter leukocyte migration by altering characteristics of cell surfaces. **Therapeutic Effects:** Decreased skin lesions in erythema nodosum leprosum and prevention of recurrence. Slowed progression of multiple myeloma.

Pharmacokinetics

Absorption: 67–93% absorbed following oral administration.
Distribution: Well distributed to tissues.
Metabolism and Excretion: Hydrolyzed in plasma to multiple metabolites. Primarily excreted in the urine (92%; <4% as unchanged drug).
Half-life: 5–7 hr.

TIME/ACTION PROFILE (plasma concentrations)

ROUTE	ONSET	PEAK	DURATION
PO	unknown	2–5 hr	unknown

Contraindications/Precautions

Contraindicated in: Hypersensitivity; Seizure disorders; Concurrent use of pembrolizumab in patients with multiple myeloma (↑ risk of mortality); OB: Pregnancy; Lactation: Lactation.
Use Cautiously in: Rep: Women of reproductive potential and men with female sexual partners of reproductive potential; Pedi: Children <12 yr (safety and effectiveness not established).

Adverse Reactions/Side Effects

CV: bradycardia, edema, orthostatic hypotension, DEEP VEIN THROMBOSIS (DVT) (↑ RISK WITH DEXAMETHASONE IN MULTIPLE MYELOMA). **Derm:** DRUG REACTION WITH EOSINOPHILIA AND SYSTEMIC SYMPTOMS (DRESS), rash, STEVENS-JOHNSON SYNDROME (SJS), TOXIC EPIDERMAL NECROLYSIS (TEN), photosensitivity. **GI:** constipation. **Hemat:** neutropenia, thrombocytopenia. **Neuro:** dizziness, drowsiness, peripheral neuropathy, SEIZURES. **Resp:** PULMONARY EMBOLISM (PE) (↑ RISK WITH DEXAMETHASONE IN MULTIPLE MYELOMA). **Misc:** HYPERSENSITIVITY REACTIONS (INCLUDING ANAPHYLAXIS AND ANGIOEDEMA), TUMOR LYSIS SYNDROME.

Interactions

Drug-Drug: ↑ risk of CNS depression with **barbiturates, sedative/hypnotics, alcohol, chlorpromazine**, or other **CNS depressants**. **Agents that may cause peripheral neuropathy** may ↑ risk of peripheral neuropathy.
Drug-Natural Products: **Echinacea** and **melatonin** may interfere with immunosuppression.

Route/Dosage

Erythema Nodosum Leprosum

PO (Adults ≥50 kg): 100–300 mg once daily initially; up to 400 mg/day has been used, depending on previous

T

response. Every 3–6 mo, attempts should be made to taper and discontinue by 50 mg every 2–4 wk.
PO (Adults <50 kg): 100 mg once daily initially; up to 400 mg/day has been used, depending on previous response. Every 3–6 mo, attempts should be made to taper and discontinue by 50 mg every 2–4 wk.

Multiple Myeloma
PO (Adults): 200 mg once daily in 28-day treatment cycles.

Availability
Capsules: 50 mg, 100 mg, 150 mg, 200 mg.

NURSING IMPLICATIONS
Assessment
- Assess monthly for initial 3 mo and periodically during therapy to detect early signs of peripheral neuropathy (numbness, tingling, or pain in hands and feet). Commonly occurs with prolonged therapy, but has occurred following short-term use or following completion of therapy. May be severe and irreversible. Electrophysiologic testing may be done at baseline and every 6 mo to detect asymptomatic peripheral neuropathy. *If neuropathy symptoms occur,* discontinue thalidomide immediately to limit further damage. Reinstate therapy only if neuropathy returns to baseline.
- Monitor for signs/symptoms of hypersensitivity reaction (erythematous macular rash, fever, tachycardia, hypotension). May require discontinuation of therapy if severe. If reaction recurs when dosing is resumed, discontinue thalidomide.
- Monitor for signs/symptoms of bleeding (fatigue, dizziness, pallor, petechiae, epistaxis, tarry stools, coffee ground emesis) during therapy. May require dose interruption, reduction, or discontinuation.
- Monitor patients for development of severe cutaneous adverse reactions, including DRESS, SJS, and TEN, including signs/symptoms of prodrome of fever, malaise, mucosal lesions, progressive skin rash, blisters, lymphadenopathy, conjunctivitis, myalgias, hepatitis, or eosinophilia. *If a severe cutaneous adverse reaction is suspected,* hold thalidomide until etiology of reaction is determined. Consultation with a dermatologist is recommended. *If a severe cutaneous adverse reaction or Grade 3 or 4 skin rash is confirmed,* permanently discontinue thalidomide.
- Assess for signs/symptoms of tumor lysis syndrome (malaise, tachycardia, hypotension, confusion, delirium, arthralgia, myalgia, muscle spasms or twitches, paresthesia, headache, dizziness, nausea, vomiting, dark urine, acute renal failure, hyperkalemia, hypocalcemia, hyperuricemia, hypophosphatemia), especially in patients with high tumor burden. Supportive therapy may be necessary based on severity.
- **Multiple Myeloma:** Monitor for signs/symptoms of venous thromboembolism such as PE (chest pain, dyspnea, tachycardia) or DVT (calf pain or tenderness, lower extremity edema, localized warmth or erythema), especially in patients concurrently taking dexamethasone. Consider prophylaxis depending on patient risk factors.

Lab Test Considerations
- Verify negative pregnancy test before starting therapy with two negative tests. Pregnancy tests with a sensitivity of ≥50 mIU/mL must be done within 10–14 days and 24 hr prior to starting therapy. Once treatment has started, pregnancy tests should occur weekly during 1st 4 wk of use and then every 4 wk in women with a regular menstrual cycle and every 2 wk in women with an irregular cycle.
- Monitor WBC with differential during therapy. May ↓ WBC. If ANC ↓ to ≤750 cells/mm³ during therapy, re-evaluate medication regimen; if neutropenia persists, consider discontinuing therapy. May cause thrombocytopenia.
- Monitor viral load in HIV-seropositive patients after the 1st and 3rd mo of therapy and every 3 mo thereafter. May ↑ viral load levels.

Implementation
- Do not confuse Thalomid with thiamine.
- ***REMS:*** Due to teratogenic effects, thalidomide may be prescribed only by prescribers registered in the *Thalomid REMS* program. Required components of the *Thalomid REMS* program include the following: prescribers must be certified with the *Thalomid REMS* program by enrolling and complying with the REMS requirements; patients must sign a Patient-Physician Agreement Form and comply with the REMS requirements. Women of reproductive potential who are not pregnant must comply with the pregnancy testing and contraception requirements, and men must comply with contraception requirements. Pharmacies must be certified with the *Thalomid REMS* program, must only dispense to patients who are authorized to receive *Thalomid*, and must comply with REMS requirements. Information about *Thalomid* and the *Thalomid REMS* program is available at www.thalomidrems.com or by calling the REMS Call Center at 1-888-423-5436. Thalidomide is started within 24 hr of a negative pregnancy test with a sensitivity of at least 50 mIU/mL. Pregnancy testing must occur weekly during first month of therapy and then monthly thereafter in women with a regular menstrual cycle. For women with irregular menses, pregnancy testing should occur every 2 wk. If pregnancy occurs, thalidomide should be discontinued immediately. Any suspected fetal exposure must be reported to the FDA and the manufacturer, and patient should be referred to an obstetrician/gynecologist experienced in reproductive toxicity. Even

a single dose (1 capsule [regardless of strength]) taken by a pregnant woman during her pregnancy can cause severe birth defects.

- Handle intact tablets or capsules with single gloves; use double gloves, respiratory protection, and a protective gown in the preparation of tablets or capsules, including cutting, crushing, manipulating, or handling uncoated tablets. During administration, wear single gloves, and wear eye/face protection if the formulation is hard to swallow or if the patient may resist, vomit, or spit up. If powder from capsules comes into contact with the skin mucous membranes, wash thoroughly with soap and water.
- Corticosteroids may be used concurrently with thalidomide for patients with moderate to severe neuritis associated with a severe erythema nodosum leprosum reaction. Use of corticosteroids can be tapered and discontinued when neuritis resolves.
- **PO:** Administer once daily with water, preferably at bedtime and ≥1 hr after the evening meal. If divided doses are used, administer ≥1 hr after meals.

Patient/Family Teaching

- Explain the purpose and side effects of thalidomide. Instruct patient to take as directed. Tell patient to take drug at bedtime ≥1 hr after evening meal. Do not discontinue without notifying health care provider; dose should be tapered gradually. Explain *Thalomid REMS* program to patient. Keep out of children's reach. Advise patient to read *Patient Information* before starting and with each Rx refill in case of changes.
- Explain need for continued medical follow-up to assess effectiveness and possible side effects of medication. Periodic lab tests will be needed.
- Frequently causes drowsiness or dizziness. Caution patient to avoid driving or other activities requiring alertness until response to medication is known.
- Advise patient to immediately report signs/symptoms of thromboembolism (shortness of breath, chest pain, arm/leg swelling).
- Advise patient to immediately report signs/symptoms of SJS or TEN (flu-like symptoms, spreading red rash, skin/mucous membrane blistering).
- Advise patient to report signs/symptoms of infection, bleeding, or peripheral neuropathy (numbness, tingling, pain, or burning in hands/feet).
- Advise patient to change positions slowly to minimize orthostatic hypotension.
- Caution patient to use sunscreen and protective clothing to prevent photosensitivity reactions.
- Advise patient not to drink alcohol while taking drug.
- Instruct patient not to donate blood and male patients not to donate sperm while taking thalidomide and for 1 mo following discontinuation.
- Advise patient to notify health care provider of all Rx or OTC medications, vitamins, or herbal products being taken and to consult with health care provider before taking other medications.
- Rep: May cause fetal harm. Inform women of reproductive potential that they must use one highly effective method (IUD, hormonal contraceptive, tubal ligation, partner's vasectomy) and one additional method (latex condom, diaphragm, cervical cap) AT THE SAME TIME for ≥4 wk before, during therapy and interruptions of therapy, and for 4 wk following discontinuation of therapy, even with a history of infertility, unless due to a hysterectomy or patient has been postmenopausal naturally for 24 consecutive mo. Advise female patients to avoid breastfeeding during therapy. Men receiving thalidomide with female partners of reproductive potential must always use a latex condom during and for up to 4 wk following discontinuation, even if they have undergone a successful vasectomy. Thalidomide must be discontinued if pregnancy is suspected or confirmed. Suspected fetal exposure must be reported to FDA via MedWatch at 1-800-FDA-1088 and to manufacturer at 1-888-668-2528. Inform women of reproductive potential that there is a Pregnancy Exposure Registry that monitors pregnancy outcomes in women exposed to thalidomide during pregnancy and that they can contact the Pregnancy Exposure Registry by calling 1-888-423-5436. May impair male fertility.

Evaluation/Desired Outcomes

- Resolution of the signs and symptoms of active erythema nodosum leprosum reaction. Usually requires at least 2 wk of therapy; then taper medication in 50-mg decrements every 2–4 wk.
- Prevention of recurrent erythema nodosum leprosum. Tapering off medication should be attempted every 3–6 mo in decrements of 50 mg every 2–4 wk.
- Decrease in serum and urine paraprotein measurements in patients with multiple myeloma.

T

thiamine (vitamin B_1)

(**thye**-a-min)

Classification

Therapeutic: vitamins

Pharmacologic: water soluble vitamins

Indications

Treatment of thiamine deficiency (beriberi). Prevention of Wernicke encephalopathy. Dietary supplement in patients with GI disease, alcoholism, or cirrhosis.

Action

Required for carbohydrate metabolism. **Therapeutic Effects:** Replacement in deficiency states.

Pharmacokinetics

Absorption: Well absorbed from the GI tract by an active process. Excessive amounts are not absorbed completely. Also well absorbed from IM sites.
Distribution: Widely distributed to tissues.
Metabolism and Excretion: Metabolized by the liver. Excess amounts are excreted unchanged by the kidneys.
Half-life: Unknown.

TIME/ACTION PROFILE (time for symptoms of deficiency: edema and HF: to resolve†)

ROUTE	ONSET	PEAK	DURATION
PO, IM, IV	hr	days	days–wk

† Confusion and psychosis take longer to respond.

Contraindications/Precautions

Contraindicated in: Hypersensitivity; Known alcohol intolerance or bisulfite hypersensitivity (elixir only).
Use Cautiously in: Wernicke encephalopathy (condition may be worsened unless thiamine is administered before glucose).

Adverse Reactions/Side Effects

Adverse reactions and side effects are extremely rare and are usually associated with IV administration or extremely large doses.
CV: hypotension, VASCULAR COLLAPSE. **Derm:** cyanosis, pruritus, sweating, tingling, urticaria, warmth. **EENT:** tightness of the throat. **GI:** nausea. **Neuro:** restlessness, weakness. **Resp:** pulmonary edema, respiratory distress. **Misc:** ANGIOEDEMA.

Interactions

Drug-Drug: None reported.

Route/Dosage

Thiamine Deficiency (Beriberi)

PO (Adults): 5–10 mg 3 times daily.
PO (Children): 10–50 mg/day in divided doses.
IM, IV (Adults): 5–100 mg 3 times daily.
IM, IV (Children): 10–25 mg/day.

Dietary Supplement

PO (Adults): 1–1.6 mg/day.
PO (Children 4–10 yr): 0.9–1 mg/day.
PO (Children birth–3 yr): 0.3–0.7 mg/day.

Availability (generic available)

Tablets: 50 mg[OTC], 100 mg[OTC], 250 mg[OTC]. **Oral solution:** 25 mg/mL[OTC]. **Solution for injection:** 100 mg/mL.

NURSING IMPLICATIONS

Assessment

- Assess for signs/symptoms of thiamine deficiency (anorexia, GI distress, irritability, palpitations, tachycardia, edema, paresthesia, muscle weakness and pain, depression, memory loss, confusion, psychosis, visual disturbances, elevated serum pyruvic acid levels).
- Assess patient's nutritional status (diet, weight) before starting and during therapy.
- Monitor for signs/symptoms of anaphylaxis (wheezing, urticaria, edema) especially after repeat administration. *If hypersensitivity suspected,* administer one one-hundredth of the dose intradermally. If no reaction occurs after 30 min, administer full dose and observe for ≥30 min.

Lab Test Considerations

- May interfere with certain methods of testing serum theophylline, uric acid, and urobilinogen concentrations.

Implementation

- Do not confuse thiamine with Thalomid.
- **IM:** May cause tenderness and induration at injection site. Cool compresses may ↓ discomfort.

IV Administration

- **IV:** Sensitivity reactions and death have occurred from IV administration. An intradermal test dose is recommended in patients with suspected sensitivity.
- **IV Push: Concentration:** Administer undiluted at 100 mg/mL. **Rate:** Administer at a rate of 100 mg over 5 min.
- **Continuous Infusion: Dilution:** May be diluted in dextrose/Ringer's or LR combinations, dextrose/saline combinations, D5W, D10W, Ringer's and LR injection, 0.9% NaCl, or 0.45% NaCl.
- **Y-Site Compatibility:** amikacin, ascorbic acid, atracurium, atropine, aztreonam, benztropine, bumetanide, buprenorphine, butorphanol, calcium chloride, calcium gluconate, cefazolin, cefotaxime, cefotetan, cefoxitin, ceftriaxone, cefuroxime, chlorpromazine, clindamycin, cyanocobalamin, cyclosporine, dexamethasone, digoxin, diphenhydramine, dobutamine, dopamine, doxycycline, enalaprilat, ephedrine, epinephrine, erythromycin, esmolol, famotidine, fentanyl, gentamicin, glycopyrrolate, heparin, insulin regular, isoproterenol, labetalol, lidocaine, magnesium sulfate, mannitol, meperidine, metoclopramide, metoprolol, morphine, multivitamins, nafcillin, nalbuphine, naloxone, nitroglycerin, nitroprusside, norepinephrine, oxacillin, oxytocin, papaverine, penicillin G, pentamidine, phentolamine, phenylephrine, phytonadione, potassium chloride, procainamide, prochlorperazine, promethazine, propranolol, protamine, pyridoxine, succinylcholine, sufentanil, theophylline, tobramycin, vancomycin, vasopressin, verapamil.

- **Y-Site Incompatibility:** aminophylline, azathioprine, ceftazidime, chloramphenicol, dantrolene, diazepam, diazoxide, folic acid, furosemide, ganciclovir, hydrocortisone, imipenem/cilastatin, indomethacin, methylprednisolone, pentobarbital, phenobarbital, phenytoin, sodium bicarbonate, trimethoprim/sulfamethoxazole.

Patient/Family Teaching

- Explain purpose and side effects of medication. Advise patient to read *Patient Information* before starting therapy.
- Encourage patient to comply with dietary recommendations. Explain that the best source of vitamins is a well-balanced diet.
- Teach that foods high in thiamine include cereals (whole grain and enriched), meats (especially pork), and fresh vegetables.
- Caution patient not to exceed RDA for thiamine. Large doses may cause side effects.
- Advise patient to notify health care provider of all Rx or OTC medications, vitamins, or herbal products being taken and to consult health care provider before taking other medications.
- Rep: Thiamine requirements are ↑ during pregnancy, especially in women with prolonged nausea and vomiting. Advise women of reproductive potential to notify health care provider if pregnancy is planned or suspected or if breastfeeding. RDA for thiamine during lactation is 1.4 mg.

Evaluation/Desired Outcomes

- Prevention of or ↓ in signs and symptoms of vitamin B deficiency.
- Decrease in symptoms of neuritis, ocular signs, ataxia, edema, and heart failure may be seen within hr of administration and may disappear within a few days.
- Confusion and psychosis may take longer to respond and may persist if nerve damage has occurred.

HIGH ALERT

THROMBOLYTIC AGENTS

alteplase (al-te-plase)

Activase, ✦Activase rt-PA, Cathflo Activase

tenecteplase (te-nek-te-plase)

TNKase

Classification

Therapeutic: thrombolytics

Pharmacologic: plasminogen activators

Indications

Alteplase, tenecteplase: Acute MI. Acute ischemic stroke. **Alteplase:** Acute massive pulmonary emboli (PE). **Alteplase:** Occluded central venous access devices.

Action

Directly activate plasminogen, converting it to plasmin, which is then able to degrade fibrin present in clots. **Therapeutic Effects:** Lysis of thrombi in coronary arteries, with preservation of ventricular function or improvement of ventricular function (and ↓ risk of HF or death). Lysis of PE. Lysis of thrombi causing ischemic stroke, reducing risk of neurologic sequelae. Restoration of cannula or catheter patency and function.

Pharmacokinetics

Absorption: IV administration results in complete bioavailability. Intracoronary administration or administration into occluded catheters or cannulae has a more localized effect.
Distribution: Minimally distributed to tissues.
Metabolism and Excretion: *Alteplase, tenecteplase:* Rapidly metabolized by the liver.
Half-life: *Alteplase:* 35 min; *tenecteplase:* 20–24 min (initial phase), 90–130 min (terminal phase).

TIME/ACTION PROFILE (fibrinolysis)

ROUTE	ONSET	PEAK	DURATION
Alteplase IV	30 min	60 min	unknown
Tenecteplase IV	rapid	unknown	unknown

Contraindications/Precautions

Contraindicated in: Active internal bleeding; History of cerebrovascular accident; Recent (within 2 mo) intracranial or intraspinal injury or trauma; Intracranial neoplasm, AV malformation, or aneurysm; Severe uncontrolled hypertension; Known bleeding tendencies; Hypersensitivity; cross-sensitivity with other thrombolytics may occur.
Use Cautiously in: Recent (within 10 days) major surgery, trauma, GI, or GU bleeding; Left heart thrombus; Severe renal impairment; Severe hepatic impairment; Hemorrhagic ophthalmic conditions; Septic phlebitis; Previous puncture of a noncompressible vessel; Subacute bacterial endocarditis or acute pericarditis; OB: Safety not established in pregnancy; Lactation: Safety not established in breastfeeding; Pedi: Safety not established in children; Geri: ↑ risk of intracranial bleeding in patients >75 yr.
Exercise Extreme Caution in: Concurrent use of anticoagulant therapy (↑ risk of intracranial bleeding).

Adverse Reactions/Side Effects

CV: hypotension, reperfusion arrhythmias. **Derm:** ecchymoses, flushing, urticaria. **EENT:** epistaxis, gingival bleeding. **GI:** nausea, vomiting. **Hemat:** BLEEDING. **Local:** hemorrhage at injection site, phlebitis. **MS:** musculoskeletal pain. **Neuro:** INTRACRANIAL

T

HEMORRHAGE. **Resp:** bronchospasm, hemoptysis. **Misc:** fever, HYPERSENSITIVITY REACTIONS (INCLUDING ANAPHYLAXIS).

Interactions

Drug-Drug: Aspirin, other **NSAIDs**, **warfarin**, **heparin**, **low molecular weight heparins**, **direct thrombin inhibitors**, **eptifibatide**, **tirofiban**, **clopidogrel**, **ticagrelor**, **prasugrel**, or **dipyridamole** may ↑ risk of bleeding, although these agents are frequently used together or in sequence. **Antifibrinolytic agents**, including **aminocaproic acid** or **tranexamic acid**, may ↓ effectiveness.

Drug-Natural Products: Anise, **arnica**, **chamomile**, **clove**, **dong quai**, **fenugreek**, **feverfew**, **garlic**, **ginger**, **ginkgo**, **Panax ginseng**, or **licorice** may ↑ risk of bleeding.

Route/Dosage

Alteplase

Myocardial Infarction (Accelerated or Front-Loading Infusion)

IV (Adults): 15 mg bolus, then 0.75 mg/kg (up to 50 mg) over 30 min, then 0.5 mg/kg (up to 35 mg) over next 60 min; usually accompanied by heparin therapy.

Myocardial Infarction (3-Hr Infusion)

IV (Adults >65 kg): 60 mg over 1st hr (6–10 mg given as a bolus over first 1–2 min), 20 mg over the 2nd hr, and 20 mg over the 3rd hr for a total dose of 100 mg.

IV (Adults <65 kg): 0.75 mg/kg over 1st hr (0.075–0.125 mg/kg given as a bolus over first 1–2 min), 0.25 mg/kg over the 2nd hr, and 0.25 mg/kg over the 3rd hr for a total dose of 1.25 mg/kg (not to exceed 100 mg total).

Pulmonary Embolism

IV (Adults): 100 mg over 2 hr; follow with heparin.

Acute Ischemic Stroke

IV (Adults): 0.9 mg/kg (not to exceed 90 mg), given as an infusion over 1 hr, with 10% of the dose given as a bolus over the 1st min.

Occluded Venous Access Devices

IV (Adults and Children >30 kg): 2 mg/2 mL instilled into occluded catheter; if unsuccessful, may repeat once after 2 hr.

IV (Adults and Children <30 kg): 110% of the lumen volume (not to exceed 2 mg in 2 mL) instilled into occluded catheter; if unsuccessful, may repeat once after 2 hr.

Tenecteplase

Myocardial Infarction

IV (Adults <60 kg): 30 mg as a single dose.

IV (Adults ≥60 kg and <70 kg): 35 mg as a single dose.

IV (Adults ≥70 kg and <80 kg): 40 mg as a single dose.

IV (Adults ≥80 kg and <90 kg): 45 mg as a single dose.

IV (Adults ≥90 kg): 50 mg as a single dose.

Acute Ischemic Stroke

IV (Adults ≥90 kg): 25 mg as a single dose.

IV (Adults ≥80 kg and <90 kg): 22.5 mg as a single dose.

IV (Adults ≥70 kg and <80 kg): 20 mg as a single dose.

IV (Adults ≥60 kg and <70 kg): 17.5 mg as a single dose.

IV (Adults <60 kg): 15 mg as a single dose.

Availability

Alteplase

Powder for injection: 2 mg/vial, 50 mg/vial, 100 mg/vial.

Tenecteplase

Powder for injection: 25 mg/vial, 50 mg/vial.

NURSING IMPLICATIONS

Assessment

- Begin therapy as soon as possible after the onset of symptoms.
- Monitor vital signs, including temperature, continuously for coronary thrombosis and at least every 4 hr during therapy for other indications. Do not use lower extremities to monitor BP. Notify health care provider if systolic BP >180 mm Hg or diastolic BP >110 mm Hg. Should not be given if hypertension is uncontrolled. Inform health care provider if hypotension occurs. Hypotension may result from the drug, hemorrhage, or cardiogenic shock.
- Assess carefully for bleeding every 15 min during the 1st hr of therapy, every 15–30 min during the next 8 hr, and at least every 4 hr for the duration of therapy. Frank bleeding may occur from sites of invasive procedures or from body orifices. Internal bleeding may also occur (↓ neurologic status; abdominal pain with coffee grounds emesis or black, tarry stools; hematuria; joint pain). If uncontrolled bleeding occurs, stop medication and notify health care provider immediately.
- Assess neurologic status during therapy. Altered sensorium or neurologic changes may be indicative of intracranial bleeding.
- Assess for hypersensitivity reactions (anaphylaxis). *If hypersensitivity reaction occurs,* discontinue therapy and implement supportive measures (epinephrine) as indicated.
- **MI:** Monitor ECG continuously. Notify health care provider if significant arrhythmias occur. Monitor cardiac enzymes. Radionuclide myocardial scanning and/or coronary angiography may be ordered 7–10 days after therapy to monitor effectiveness of therapy.
- Assess intensity, character, location, and radiation of chest pain. Note presence of associated symptoms

(nausea, vomiting, diaphoresis). Notify health care provider if chest pain is unrelieved or recurs.

- Monitor heart sounds and breath sounds frequently. Inform health care provider if signs/symptoms of HF occur (rales/crackles, dyspnea, S_3 heart sound, jugular venous distention).
- **Acute Ischemic Stroke:** Assess neurologic status. Determine time of onset of stroke symptoms. Alteplase must be administered within 3–4.5 hr of onset (within 3 hr in patients >80 yr, those taking oral anticoagulants, those with a baseline National Institutes of Health Stroke Scale score of 25, or those with both a history of stroke and diabetes).
- **PE:** Monitor HR, BP, hemodynamics, and respiratory status (rate, degree of dyspnea, arterial blood gases).
- **Cannula/Catheter Occlusion:** Monitor ability to aspirate blood as indicator of patency. Ensure that patient exhales and holds breath when connecting and disconnecting IV syringe to prevent air embolism.

Lab Test Considerations

- Hematocrit, hemoglobin, platelet count, fibrin/fibrin degradation product titer, fibrinogen concentration, PT, thrombin time, and aPTT may be evaluated before and frequently during therapy. Bleeding time may be assessed before therapy if patient has received platelet inhibitors.
- Obtain type and crossmatch and have blood available at all times in case of hemorrhage.
- Stools should be tested for occult blood loss and urine for hematuria periodically during therapy.

Toxicity and Overdose

- ***High Alert:*** If local bleeding occurs, apply pressure to site. If severe or internal bleeding occurs, discontinue infusion. Clotting factors and/or blood volume may be restored through infusions of whole blood, packed RBCs, fresh frozen plasma, or cryoprecipitate. Do not administer dextran; it has antiplatelet activity. Aminocaproic acid may be used as an antidote.

Implementation

- ***High Alert:*** Overdose and underdose of thrombolytic medications have resulted in patient harm or death. Have second practitioner independently check original order, dose calculations, and infusion pump settings.
- Do not confuse Activase with Cathflo Activase or TNKase. Do not confuse TNKase with t-PA.
- Thrombolytic agents should be used only in settings in which hematologic function and clinical response can be adequately monitored.
- Insert 2 IV lines before therapy; one for the thrombolytic agent, the other for any additional infusions.
- Avoid invasive procedures, such as IM injections or arterial punctures, with this therapy. If such procedures must be performed, apply pressure to all arterial and venous puncture sites for ≥30 min. Avoid venipunctures at noncompressible sites (jugular vein, subclavian site).
- Acetaminophen may be ordered to control fever.

Alteplase

IV Administration

- **Intermittent Infusion: Activase: Reconstitution:** Use sterile water for injection as diluent (do not use bacteriostatic water). Reconstitute 20-mg vials with 20 mL and 50-mg vials with 50 mL using an 18-gauge needle. Avoid excess agitation during dilution; swirl or invert gently to mix. Solution may foam upon reconstitution. Bubbles will resolve upon standing a few minutes. Solution will be clear to pale yellow. Stable for 8 hr at room temperature. **Dilution:** May be further diluted immediately before use in an equal amount of 0.9% NaCl or D5W. **Concentration:** 1 mg/mL. **Rate:** See Route and Dosage section for specific rates. Flush line with 20–30 mL of saline at completion of infusion to ensure entire dose is received.
- **Y-Site Compatibility:** eptifibatide, lidocaine, metoprolol, propranolol, tobramycin, vancomycin.
- **Y-Site Incompatibility:** bivalirudin, cangrelor, dobutamine, dopamine, heparin, nitroglycerin.
- **IV Push: Cathflo Activase: Reconstitution:** Reconstitute by withdrawing 2.2 mL of sterile water for injection (provided) and injecting into vial, directing diluent into powder. Allow slight foaming to dissipate by letting vial stand undisturbed. Do not use bacteriostatic water. Mix by gently swirling to dissolve; complete dissolution should occur within 3 min. Do not shake. Solution should be colorless to pale yellow. Use solution within 8 hr. **Concentration:** 1 mg/mL. **Rate:** Withdraw 2 mL of reconstituted solution and instill into occluded catheter. After 30 min dwell time, attempt to aspirate blood. If catheter remains occluded, allow 120 min dwell time. If catheter function is not restored after one dose, 2nd dose may be instilled. If catheter function is restored, aspirate 4–5 mL of blood to remove *Cathflo Activase* and residual clot. Gently irrigate catheter with 0.9% NaCl.

Tenecteplase

IV Administration

- **IV Push: Reconstitution:** Reconstitute vial with 10 mL of sterile water for injection (do not use bacteriostatic water), directing the stream into the powder. Slight foaming may occur; large bubbles will dissipate if left standing undisturbed for several min. Swirl gently until contents are completely dissolved;

T

do not shake. Solution is clear and colorless to pale yellow. Withdraw dose from reconstituted vial with the syringe and discard unused portion. Once dose is in syringe, stand the shield assembly vertically on a flat surface (with green side down) and passively recap the red hub cannula. Remove the entire shield assembly, including the red hub cannula, by twisting counterclockwise. Shield assembly also contains the clear-ended blunt plastic cannula; retain for split septum IV access. Solution may be refrigerated and administered within 8 hr. **Concentration:** 5 mg/mL. **Rate:** Administer over 5 sec. Flush line with saline-containing solution before and following administration of tenecteplase. Precipitate forms in line when administered with dextrose-containing solutions.

- **Y-Site Incompatibility:** Do not administer other drugs through same IV line.

Patient/Family Teaching

- Explain purpose and side effects of medication to patient. Advise patient to read *Patient Information* before starting therapy.
- Advise patient to notify health care provider of all Rx or OTC medications, vitamins, or herbal products being taken and to consult with health care provider before taking other medications.
- Advise patient to report hypersensitivity reactions (rash, dyspnea) and bleeding or bruising.
- Explain need for bedrest and minimal handling during therapy to avoid injury. Avoid all unnecessary procedures such as shaving and vigorous tooth brushing.
- Rep: Advise women of reproductive potential to notify health care provider if pregnancy is planned or suspected or if breastfeeding.

Evaluation/Desired Outcomes

- Lysis of thrombi in coronary arteries, with preservation of ventricular function or improvement of ventricular function (and ↓ risk of HF or death).
- Lysis of PE.
- Lysis of thrombi causing ischemic stroke, reducing risk of neurologic sequelae.
- Restoration of cannula or catheter patency and function.

BEERS

ticagrelor (tye-ka-grel-or)

Brilinta

Classification

Therapeutic: antiplatelet agents

Pharmacologic: platelet aggregation inhibitors

Indications

To reduce the risk of cardiovascular death, MI, and stroke in patients with acute coronary syndrome (ACS) or a history of MI. Also reduces the risk of stent thrombosis in patients who have received an intracoronary stent for ACS (in combination with aspirin). To reduce the risk of first MI or stroke in patients with coronary artery disease who are at high risk for such events (in combination with aspirin). To reduce the risk of stroke in patients with acute ischemic stroke (NIH Stroke Scale score ≤5) or high-risk transient ischemic attack (TIA) (in combination with aspirin).

Action

Both parent drug and its active metabolite inhibit platelet aggregation by reversibly interacting with platelet $P2Y_{12}$ ADP-receptors, preventing signal transduction and platelet activation. **Therapeutic Effects:** Reduction in risk of cardiovascular death, MI, and stroke associated with ACS. Reduction in stent thrombosis. Reduction in risk of first MI or stroke in high-risk patients with coronary artery disease. Reduction in risk of stroke in patients with acute ischemic stroke or TIA.

Pharmacokinetics

Absorption: 36% absorbed following oral administration.

Distribution: Well distributed to tissues.

Protein Binding: 99%.

Metabolism and Excretion: Mostly metabolized in the liver by the CYP3A4 isoenzyme, with some metabolism by the CYP3A5 isoenzyme, with conversion to an active metabolite (AR-C124910XX); excretion primarily via biliary secretion; <1% excreted unchanged or as active metabolite in urine.

Half-life: *Ticagrelor:* 7 hr; *Active metabolite:* 9 hr.

TIME/ACTION PROFILE (inhibition of platelet aggregation)

ROUTE	ONSET	PEAK	DURATION
PO	within 30 min	4 hr	5 days†

† Following discontinuation.

Contraindications/Precautions

Contraindicated in: Hypersensitivity; Active bleeding; History of intracranial bleeding; Impending coronary artery bypass graft surgery or other surgery (discontinue 5 days prior); Severe hepatic impairment (↑ risk of bleeding); Use of thrombolytics for treatment of acute ischemic stroke; Lactation: Lactation.

Use Cautiously in: Moderate hepatic impairment; History of sick sinus syndrome, 2nd- or 3rd-degree heart block, or bradycardia-related syncope in the absence of a pacemaker; Hypotension following recent coronary artery bypass graft surgery or percutaneous coronary intervention in patients receiving ticagrelor (consider bleeding as a cause); OB: Use during pregnancy only if potential maternal benefit justifies potential fetal risk; Pedi: Safety and effectiveness not established in children; Geri: Appears on Beers list. ↑ risk of major bleeding compared to clopidogrel, especially in patients ≥75 yr old. Use with caution in older adults, especially in patients ≥75 yr old.

Adverse Reactions/Side Effects

CV: bradycardia, heart block. **Endo:** gynecomastia. **Hemat:** BLEEDING. **Resp:** dyspnea, central sleep apnea, Cheyne-Stokes respiration. **Misc:** HYPERSENSITIVITY REACTIONS (INCLUDING ANGIOEDEMA).

Interactions

Drug-Drug: Strong CYP3A4/5 inhibitors, including **atazanavir**, **clarithromycin**, **itraconazole**, **ketoconazole**, **nefazodone**, **nelfinavir**, **ritonavir**, and **voriconazole**, may ↑ levels and risk of bleeding; avoid concurrent use. **Strong CYP3A inducers**, including **carbamazepine**, **dexamethasone**, **phenobarbital**, **phenytoin**, and **rifampin**, may ↓ levels and effectiveness; avoid concurrent use. **P-glycoprotein inhibitors**, including **cyclosporine**, may ↑ levels and risk of bleeding. May ↑ levels and risk of toxicity of **lovastatin**, **simvastatin**, and **rosuvastatin**; avoid use of lovastatin and simvastatin doses >40 mg/day. Effectiveness is ↓ by **aspirin** >100 mg/day (maintain aspirin at 75–100 mg/day). May alter **digoxin** levels; monitoring recommended. Risk of bleeding ↑ by **anticoagulants**, **fibrinolytics**, and chronic **NSAIDs**. **Opioids** may ↓ absorption of ticagrelor and its active metabolite and ↓ antiplatelet effects; consider using parenteral antiplatelet in patients with ACS if concurrent use of opioids needed.

Route/Dosage

Acute Coronary Syndrome or History of Myocardial Infarction

PO (Adults): *Loading dose:* 180 mg; followed by *maintenance dose:* 90 mg twice daily for 1 yr; then 60 mg twice daily.

Coronary Artery Disease Without a History of Myocardial Infarction or Stroke

PO (Adults): 60 mg twice daily.

Acute Ischemic Stroke or Transient Ischemic Attack

PO (Adults): *Loading dose:* 180 mg; followed by *maintenance dose:* 90 mg twice daily for up to 30 days.

Availability (generic available)

Tablets: 60 mg, 90 mg.

NURSING IMPLICATIONS

Assessment

- Assess for signs/symptoms of stroke, peripheral vascular disease, or MI periodically during therapy.
- Monitor for signs/symptoms of bleeding (pallor of skin and conjunctiva, fatigue, weakness, easy bruising, nosebleeds, bleeding gums, hematuria), including GI bleeding (hematochezia, melena, coffee ground emesis). If bleeding occurs, manage without discontinuing ticagrelor as prematurely stopping this medication can ↑ risk of cardiovascular events.
- Observe for signs/symptoms of hypersensitivity reactions (rash, facial swelling, pruritus, laryngeal edema, wheezing). *If hypersensitivity reaction occurs,* discontinue ticagrelor. Keep epinephrine, an antihistamine, and resuscitation equipment close by in case of anaphylactic reaction.

Lab Test Considerations

- May ↑ uric acid and serum creatinine.
- May cause false negative results in heparin-induced platelet aggregation assay for patients with heparin-induced thrombocytopenia.

Implementation

- Do not confuse Brilinta with Briviact.
- **PO:** Administer without regard to food.
- For patients unable to swallow, tablets can be crushed and mixed with water. Mixture can also be administered via a nasogastric tube.
- For patients with history of ACS, MI, acute ischemic stroke, or TIA, administer the 1st maintenance dose of ticagrelor 6–12 hr after loading dose.
- Patients who have received a loading dose of clopidogrel may be started on ticagrelor.
- For ACS or history of MI, initiate ticagrelor with a daily maintenance dose of aspirin 75–100 mg daily. *If patient has undergone percutaneous coronary intervention,* consider single antiplatelet therapy per evolving risk for thrombotic versus bleeding events.
- For acute ischemic stroke or TIA, administer a loading dose of aspirin (300–325 mg) and a daily maintenance dose of aspirin (75–100 mg) with ticagrelor.
- Discontinue ticagrelor 5 days before planned surgical procedures with a major risk of bleeding. If ticagrelor must be temporarily discontinued, restart as soon as possible. Premature discontinuation of therapy may ↑ risk of MI, stent thrombosis, and death.

Patient/Family Teaching

- Instruct patient to take ticagrelor exactly as directed. Take missed doses as soon as possible unless almost time for next dose; do not double doses. Do not discontinue ticagrelor without consulting health care provider; may ↑ risk of cardiovascular events. Advise patient to read the *Medication Guide* before starting therapy and with each Rx refill in case of changes.

T

- Advise patient that daily aspirin should not exceed 100 mg and to avoid taking other medications that contain aspirin.
- Inform patient that they will bleed and bruise more easily and it will take longer to stop bleeding. Advise patient to notify health care provider promptly if unusual, prolonged, or excessive bleeding or blood in stool or urine occurs.
- Inform patient that ticagrelor may cause shortness of breath, which usually resolves during therapy. Advise patient to notify health care provider if unexpected or severe shortness of breath or symptoms of hypersensitivity reactions occur.
- Advise patient to notify health care provider of medication regimen prior to treatment or surgery or dental procedure. Prescriber should be consulted before stopping ticagrelor.
- Instruct patient to notify health care provider of all Rx or OTC medications, vitamins, or herbal products being taken and consult health care provider before taking any new medications, especially aspirin or NSAIDs.
- Rep: Advise women of reproductive potential to notify health care provider if pregnancy is planned or suspected and to avoid breastfeeding during therapy.

Evaluation/Desired Outcomes

- Decreased thrombotic cardiovascular events in patients with ACS.
- Reduction in risk of first MI or stroke in high-risk patients with coronary artery disease.
- Reduction in risk of stroke in patients with acute ischemic stroke or TIA.

tigecycline (tye-gi-**sye**-kleen)

Tygacil

Classification

Therapeutic: anti-infectives

Pharmacologic: glycylcyclines

Indications

Complicated skin/skin structure infections, complicated intra-abdominal infections, or community-acquired bacterial pneumonia caused by susceptible bacteria (should only be used when alternative treatments are not suitable; should NOT be used for diabetic foot infections).

Action

Inhibits bacterial protein synthesis by binding to the 30S ribosomal subunit. **Therapeutic Effects:** Resolution of infection. **Spectrum:** Active against the following gram-positive bacteria: *Enterococcus faecalis* (vancomycin-susceptible strains only), *Staphylococcus aureus* (methicillin-sensitive and methicillin-resistant strains), *Streptococcus agalactiae*, *Streptococcus anginosus*, *Streptococcus pneumoniae* (penicillin-susceptible isolates), and *Streptococcus pyogenes*. Also active against these gram-negative organisms: *Citrobacter freundii*, *Enterobacter cloacae*, *Escherichia coli*, *Haemophilus influenzae*, *Legionella pneumophila*, *Klebsiella oxytoca*, and *Klebsiella pneumoniae*. Additionally active against the following anaerobes: *Bacteroides fragilis*, *Bacteroides thetaiotaomicron*, *Bacteroides uniformis*, *Bacteroides vulgatus*, *Clostridium perfringens*, and *Peptostreptococcus micros*.

Pharmacokinetics

Absorption: IV administration results in complete bioavailability.

Distribution: Widely distributed with good penetration into gall bladder, lung, and colon.

Metabolism and Excretion: Minimal metabolism; primary route of elimination is biliary/fecal excretion of unchanged drug and metabolites (59%), 33% renal (22% unchanged).

Half-life: 27.1 hr (after 1 dose); 42.4 hr after multiple doses.

TIME/ACTION PROFILE (plasma concentrations)

ROUTE	ONSET	PEAK	DURATION
IV	rapid	end of infusion	12 hr

Contraindications/Precautions

Contraindicated in: Hypersensitivity; Diabetic foot infections; Hospital-acquired or ventilator-associated pneumonia (↑ risk of mortality and ↓ effectiveness); Pedi: Children.

Use Cautiously in: Complicated intra-abdominal infections due to perforation; Severe hepatic impairment (↓ maintenance dose); OB: Use during pregnancy only if potential maternal benefit outweighs potential fetal risk; may cause permanent teeth discoloration and suppress bone growth in fetus, especially when used during 2nd or 3rd trimester; Lactation: Use while breastfeeding only if potential maternal benefit justifies potential risk to infant; Geri: Older adults may be more sensitive to adverse effects.

Adverse Reactions/Side Effects

Derm: photosensitivity, rash, STEVENS-JOHNSON SYNDROME (SJS). **Endo:** hyperglycemia, hypoglycemia. **F and E:** hypocalcemia, hyponatremia. **GI:** nausea, vomiting, ↑ liver enzymes, anorexia, CLOSTRIDIOIDES DIFFICILE-ASSOCIATED DIARRHEA (CDAD), dry mouth, jaundice, PANCREATITIS. **GU:** ↑ serum creatinine. **Hemat:** hypofibrinogenemia. **Local:** injection site reactions. **Neuro:** dysgeusia, intracranial hypertension, somnolence. **Resp:** pneumonia. **Misc:** DEATH, HYPERSENSITIVITY REACTIONS (INCLUDING ANAPHYLAXIS).

Interactions

Drug-Drug: May ↓ effectiveness of **hormonal contraceptives**. Effects on **warfarin** are unknown; monitoring recommended. May ↑ trough levels and risk of toxicity of **calcineurin inhibitors**, including **cyclosporine** and **tacrolimus**.

Route/Dosage

IV (Adults): 100 mg initially, then 50 mg every 12 hr for 5–14 days (skin/skin structure infections and intra-abdominal infections) or 7–14 days (pneumonia).

Hepatic Impairment

IV (Adults): *Severe hepatic impairment:* 100 mg initially, then 25 mg every 12 hr.

Availability (generic available)

Lyophilized powder for injection: 50 mg/vial.

NURSING IMPLICATIONS

Assessment

- Assess for infection (vital signs; appearance of wound, sputum, urine, and stool; WBC) at beginning of and during therapy.
- Before initiating therapy, obtain a history of tetracycline hypersensitivity; may be cross-reactive and should be avoided with known hypersensitivity to tetracyclines.
- Monitor for signs/symptoms of hypersensitivity reaction. *If symptoms occur,* immediately discontinue tigecycline and treat as indicated. Keep emergency medication and equipment nearby during therapy.
- Monitor for signs/symptoms of CDAD (diarrhea, abdominal cramping, fever, bloody stools). *If CDAD occurs,* discontinue tigecycline and treat as indicated. May begin up to several weeks following cessation of therapy.
- Assess for signs/symptoms of pancreatitis (nausea, vomiting, abdominal pain, ↑ serum lipase or amylase) periodically during therapy. *If pancreatitis suspected,* consider discontinuation of tigecycline.
- Monitor patients for development of severe cutaneous adverse reactions, including SJS. Assess for rash, fever, general malaise, fatigue, muscle or joint pain, blisters, oral lesions, and conjunctivitis periodically during therapy. *If signs/symptoms of SJS occur,* discontinue tigecycline.

Lab Test Considerations

- Obtain specimens for culture and sensitivity before initiating therapy. 1st dose may be given before receiving results.
- Monitor CBC with differential.
- Monitor blood coagulation parameters, including fibrinogen, before and regularly during therapy.
- May ↑ alkaline phosphatase, amylase, bilirubin, LDH, AST, and ALT. *If hepatic dysfunction occurs,* monitor progression and evaluate risk and benefit of continuing therapy. Hepatic dysfunction may occur after discontinuation of therapy.
- May cause ↑ BUN, azotemia, acidosis, and hyperphosphatemia. *If any of these abnormalities occur,* discontinue tigecycline.
- May cause hyperglycemia, hypokalemia, hypoproteinemia, hypocalcemia, or hyponatremia.

Implementation

- May cause yellow-brown discoloration and softening of teeth and bones if administered prenatally, during lactation, or early childhood through 8 yr.

IV Administration

- **Intermittent Infusion:** Reconstitute each vial with 5.3 mL of 0.9% NaCl or D5W. Reconstituted solution should be yellow to orange in color. Do not administer if discolored or contains particulates. **Concentration:** 10 mg/mL. **Dilution:** Dilute further in 100 mL of D5W, LR, or 0.9% NaCl. Reconstituted solution should be yellow to orange in color. Do not administer if discolored or contains particulates. Infusion is stable for up to 24 hr at room temperature or for up to 48 hr if refrigerated. **Concentration:** ≤1 mg/mL. **Rate:** Infuse over 30–60 min.
- **Y-Site Compatibility:** acetylcysteine, acyclovir, allopurinol, amikacin, aminocaproic acid, aminophylline, amphotericin B liposomal, ampicillin, ampicillin/sulbactam, argatroban, arsenic trioxide, atracurium, azithromycin, aztreonam, bivalirudin, bumetanide, buprenorphine, busulfan, butorphanol, calcium chloride, calcium gluconate, cangrelor, carboplatin, carmustine, caspofungin, cefazolin, cefepime, cefiderocol, cefotaxime, cefotetan, cefoxitin, ceftazidime, ceftazidime/avibactam, ceftolozane/tazobactam, ceftriaxone, cefuroxime, ciprofloxacin, cisatracurium, cisplatin, clindamycin, cyclophosphamide, cyclosporine, cytarabine, dacarbazine, dactinomycin, daptomycin, daunorubicin, dexamethasone, dexmedetomidine, dexrazoxane, digoxin, diltiazem, diphenhydramine, dobutamine, docetaxel, dopamine, doxorubicin hydrochloride, doxorubicin liposomal, droperidol, enalaprilat, ephedrine, epinephrine, eptifibatide, ertapenem, erythromycin, esmolol, etoposide, etoposide phosphate, famotidine, fentanyl, fluconazole, fludarabine, fluorouracil, foscarnet, fosphenytoin, furosemide, ganciclovir, gemcitabine, gentamicin, glycopyrrolate, granisetron, haloperidol, heparin, hydrocortisone, hydromorphone, ifosfamide, imipenem/cilastatin, insulin regular, irinotecan, isavuconazonium, isoproterenol, ketorolac, labetalol, letermovir, leucovorin, levofloxacin, lidocaine, linezolid, lorazepam, magnesium sulfate, mannitol,

T

melphalan, meperidine, meropenem, meropenem/vaborbactam, mesna, methohexital, methotrexate, metoclopramide, metoprolol, metronidazole, midazolam, milrinone, mitomycin, mitoxantrone, morphine, moxifloxacin, mycophenolate, nafcillin, nalbuphine, naloxone, nitroglycerin, nitroprusside, norepinephrine, octreotide, ondansetron, oxaliplatin, oxytocin, paclitaxel, palonosetron, pamidronate, pantoprazole, pemetrexed, pentamidine, pentobarbital, phenobarbital, phenylephrine, piperacillin/tazobactam, plazomicin, potassium acetate, potassium chloride, potassium phosphates, procainamide, prochlorperazine, promethazine, propofol, propranolol, remifentanil, rocuronium, sodium acetate, sodium bicarbonate, sodium phosphates, succinylcholine, sufentanil, sulbactam/durlobactam, tacrolimus, tedizolid, telavancin, theophylline, thiotepa, tirofiban, tobramycin, topotecan, trimethoprim/sulfamethoxazole, vancomycin, vasopressin, vecuronium, vinblastine, vincristine, vinorelbine, zidovudine, zoledronic acid.

- **Y-Site Incompatibility:** amiodarone, amphotericin B deoxycholate, bleomycin, chloramphenicol, chlorpromazine, dantrolene, diazepam, epirubicin, esomeprazole, hydralazine, idarubicin, nicardipine, phenytoin, verapamil.

Patient/Family Teaching

- Explain purpose and side effects of medication. Advise patient to read *Patient Information* before starting therapy.
- Advise patient to take full course of therapy, even if feeling better. Skipping doses or not completing full course may result in ↓ effectiveness and ↑ risk of bacterial resistance.
- Instruct patient to notify health care provider if fever and diarrhea develop, especially if stool contains blood, pus, or mucus. Advise patient not to treat diarrhea without consulting health care provider.
- Advise patient to notify health care provider if superinfection (black, furry overgrowth on the tongue; vaginal itching or discharge; loose or foul-smelling stools), rash, pruritus, or urticaria occur.
- Pedi: Caution parent that tigecycline use during infancy through 8 yr may cause permanent discoloration of the teeth and reversible bone growth inhibition.
- Rep: Advise women of reproductive potential to notify health care provider if pregnancy is planned or suspected. Advise women of reproductive potential to use a nonhormonal method of contraception while taking tigecycline and until next menstrual period. Use during the 2nd and 3rd trimesters may cause permanent yellow-gray-brown discoloration of the teeth and reversible inhibition of bone growth in the fetus. Advise patient to avoid breastfeeding during and for 9 days after last dose.

Evaluation/Desired Outcomes

- Resolution of signs and symptoms of infection.

tildrakizumab

(til-dra-**kiz**-ue-mab)

Ilumya

Classification

Therapeutic: antipsoriatics

Pharmacologic: interleukin antagonists, monoclonal antibodies

Indications

Moderate to severe plaque psoriasis in patients who are candidates for phototherapy or systemic therapy.

Action

Binds to the p19 protein subunit of the interleukin (IL)-23 cytokine to prevent its interaction with the IL-23 receptor. This cytokine is normally involved in inflammatory and immune responses. Binding to interleukins antagonizes their effects, inhibiting the release of proinflammatory cytokines and chemokines. **Therapeutic Effects:** Decrease in area and severity of psoriatic lesions.

Pharmacokinetics

Absorption: 73–80% absorbed following SUBQ administration.

Distribution: Well distributed to tissues.

Metabolism and Excretion: Broken down by catabolic processes into peptides and amino acids.

Half-life: 23 days.

TIME/ACTION PROFILE (plasma concentrations)

ROUTE	ONSET	PEAK	DURATION
SUBQ	unknown	6 days	12 wk

Contraindications/Precautions

Contraindicated in: Hypersensitivity; Active, untreated infection.

Use Cautiously in: History of tuberculosis (TB) (possibility of reactivation); OB: Use during pregnancy only if potential maternal benefit justifies potential fetal risk; Lactation: Use while breastfeeding only if potential maternal benefit justifies potential risk to infant; Pedi: Safety and effectiveness not established in children.

Exercise Extreme Caution in: Chronic infection or history of recurrent infection.

Adverse Reactions/Side Effects

GI: diarrhea. **Local:** injection site reactions. **Misc:** infection, HYPERSENSITIVITY REACTIONS (INCLUDING ANGIOEDEMA AND URTICARIA).

Interactions

Drug-Drug: May ↓ antibody response to and ↑ risk of adverse reactions from **live vaccines**; avoid use during therapy.

Route/Dosage

SUBQ (Adults): 100 mg initially and 4 wk later, then 100 mg every 12 wk.

Availability

Solution for injection (prefilled syringes): 100 mg/mL.

NURSING IMPLICATIONS

Assessment

- Assess affected area(s) prior to and periodically during therapy.
- Monitor for hypersensitivity reaction (angioedema, urticaria). *If hypersensitivity reaction occurs,* discontinue tildrakizumab immediately and initiate treatment as indicated.
- Assess for latent TB with a tuberculin skin test prior to initiation of therapy. Treatment of latent TB should be started before initiating therapy with tildrakizumab. Monitor for signs/symptoms of active TB during and after therapy.
- Assess for signs/symptoms of infection (fever, dyspnea, flu-like symptoms, frequent or painful urination, redness or swelling at the site of a wound), including tuberculosis, prior to injection. Monitor new infections (respiratory, urinary) closely. *If a clinically important or serious infection occurs, or if infection is unresponsive to treatment,* monitor closely and consider discontinuing tildrakizumab until infection resolves.

Implementation

- Do not confuse Ilumya with Ilaris.
- Injection should be administered by a health care professional.
- Update all age appropriate immunizations before initiating therapy.
- **SUBQ:** Allow prefilled syringe to sit in carton at room temperature for 30 min prior to injection. Solution is clear to slightly opalescent, colorless to slightly yellow; do not administer if cloudy, discolored, or contains particulates. Air bubbles in solution do not need removal; do not shake. Inject into abdomen, thigh, or upper arm. Do not inject within 2 inches of umbilicus, or into skin that is tender, bruised, erythematous, indurated, affected by psoriasis or into scars, stretch marks, or blood vessels. Follow manufacturer's directions for retractable needle syringe. Store in refrigerator in original carton until time of use; do not freeze. May store at room temperature in original carton for up to 30 days.

Patient/Family Teaching

- Explain purpose and side effects of medication. Advise patient to read *Patient Information* before starting therapy.
- Explain that if a dose is missed, administer as soon as possible, then resume at regularly scheduled interval.
- Advise patient to notify health care professional if signs/symptoms of hypersensitivity reaction (feel faint; swelling of face, eyelids, lips, mouth, tongue or throat; skin rash, trouble breathing, or chest tightness occur.
- Instruct patient to notify health care professional if signs or symptoms of chronic or acute infection occur.
- Instruct patient to avoid receiving live vaccines during therapy.
- Advise patient to notify health care professional of all Rx or OTC medications, vitamins, or herbal products being taken and to consult health care professional before taking other medications.
- Rep: Advise women of reproductive potential to notify health care professional if pregnancy is planned or suspected or if breastfeeding.

Evaluation/Desired Outcomes

- Decrease in extent and severity of psoriatic lesions.

---

timolol, **See BETA BLOCKERS (nonselective).**

---

tioconazole, **See ANTIFUNGALS (VAGINAL).**

---

tiotropium (tye-o-**trope**-ee-yum)

✱ Spiriva, Spiriva Handihaler, Spiriva Respimat

Classification
Therapeutic: bronchodilators
Pharmacologic: anticholinergics

Indications

Long-term maintenance treatment of bronchospasm due to COPD. Reduction of exacerbations in patients with COPD. Long-term maintenance treatment of asthma.

Action

Acts as anticholinergic by selectively and reversibly inhibiting M_3 receptors in smooth muscle of airways.
Therapeutic Effects: Decreased incidence and severity of bronchospasm in COPD and asthma.

Pharmacokinetics

Absorption: *Handihaler:* 19% absorbed following inhalation; *Respimat:* 33% absorbed following inhalation.

Distribution: Extensive tissue distribution; due to route of administration, ↑ concentrations occur in lung.
Metabolism and Excretion: 74% excreted unchanged in urine; 25% of absorbed drug is metabolized.
Half-life: 5–6 days.

TIME/ACTION PROFILE (bronchodilation)

ROUTE	ONSET	PEAK	DURATION
Inhaln	rapid	5 min	24 hr

Contraindications/Precautions

Contraindicated in: Hypersensitivity to tiotropium or ipratropium.
Use Cautiously in: Hypersensitivity to atropine or milk proteins; Narrow-angle glaucoma, prostatic hyperplasia, or bladder-neck obstruction (may worsen condition); CCr ≤60 mL/min (monitor closely); OB: Safety not established in pregnancy; Lactation: Safety not established in breastfeeding; Pedi: Children <6 yr (safety and effectiveness not established).

Adverse Reactions/Side Effects

CV: tachycardia. **Derm:** rash. **EENT:** glaucoma. **GI:** dry mouth, constipation. **GU:** urinary difficulty, urinary retention. **Resp:** paradoxical bronchospasm. **Misc:** HYPERSENSITIVITY REACTIONS (INCLUDING ANGIOEDEMA).

Interactions

Drug-Drug: Should not be used concurrently with **ipratropium** due to risk of additive anticholinergic effects.

Route/Dosage

COPD

Inhaln (Adults): *Handihaler:* 18 mcg once daily; *Respimat:* 2 inhalations of 2.5 mcg once daily.

Asthma

Inhaln (Adults and Children ≥6 yr): *Respimat:* 2 inhalations of 1.25 mcg once daily.

Availability (generic available)

Dry powder capsules for inhalation (Handihaler): 18 mcg. **Inhalation solution (Respimat):** 1.25 mcg/inhalation in cartridge (delivers 28 or 60 metered inhalations), 2.5 mcg/inhalation in cartridge (delivers 28 or 60 metered inhalations).

NURSING IMPLICATIONS

Assessment

- Assess respiratory status (rate, breath sounds, degree of dyspnea) and HR before administration and at peak of medication effect.
- Assess for paradoxical bronchospasm (wheezing). If occurs, hold medication and notify health care provider immediately. Treatment should consist of an inhaled short-acting beta$_2$-agonist (albuterol).
- Monitor for hypersensitivity reactions (urticaria, angioedema, rash, bronchospasm, anaphylaxis, itching). Implement supportive care as indicated.

Implementation

- Do not confuse Spiriva with Apidra or Inspra.
- Capsules are for inhalation only and must not be swallowed.
- **Inhaln:** See Appendix C for administration of inhalation medications.

Patient/Family Teaching

- Explain purpose and side effects of medication to patient. Advise to read *Patient Information* before starting therapy. Instruct to take exactly as directed. Take missed doses as soon as remembered unless almost time for the next dose; space remaining doses evenly during day. Do not double doses.
- Advise patient to notify health care provider of all Rx or OTC medications, vitamins, or herbal products being taken and to consult health care provider before taking other medications, including eye drops.
- Advise patient that tiotropium is not to be used for acute bronchospasm attacks but may be continued during an acute exacerbation.
- Advise patient to notify health care provider immediately if signs and symptoms of angioedema (swelling of the lips, tongue, or throat; itching; rash) or signs of glaucoma (eye pain or discomfort, blurred vision, visual halos or colored images in association with red eyes from conjunctival congestion and corneal edema) occur.
- Caution patient to avoid spraying medication in eyes; may cause blurring of vision and pupil dilation.
- Advise patient that rinsing mouth after using inhaler, good oral hygiene, and sugarless gum or candy may minimize dry mouth; usually resolves with continued treatment.
- **Handihaler:** Instruct patient in proper use and cleaning of the Handihaler inhaler. Review the *Patient's Instructions for Use* guide with patient. Capsules should be stored in sealed blisters; remove immediately before use or effectiveness of capsules is reduced. Tear blister strip carefully to expose only one capsule at a time. Discard capsules that are inadvertently exposed to air. *Spiriva* should be administered only via the Handihaler, and the Handihaler should not be used with other medications. When disposing of capsule, tiny amount of powder left in capsule is normal.
- **Respimat:** Advise patient to prime inhaler by actuating inhaler toward the ground until an aerosol cloud is visible; then repeat process 3 more times. If not used for >3 days, actuate inhaler once to prepare inhaler for use. If not used for >21 days, actuate inhaler until an aerosol cloud is visible; then repeat 3 more times to prepare inhaler for use. Discard 3 mo from 1st use.

- Rep: Advise women of reproductive potential to inform health care provider if pregnancy is planned or suspected or if breastfeeding.

Evaluation/Desired Outcomes

- Decreased incidence and severity of bronchospasm in COPD and asthma.

tirzepatide (tir-zep-a-tide)

Mounjaro, Zepbound

Classification

Therapeutic: antidiabetics

Pharmacologic: glucagon-like peptide-1 (GLP-1) receptor agonists, glucose-dependent insulinotropic polypeptide (GIP) receptor agonists

Indications

Mounjaro: Type 2 diabetes mellitus (as adjunct to diet and exercise). **Zepbound:** Treatment of the following conditions: Chronic weight management in patients who are obese (body mass index [BMI] ≥30 kg/m^2) *OR* are overweight (BMI ≥27 kg/m^2) with ≥1 weight-related comorbid condition (e.g. hypertension, dyslipidemia, type 2 diabetes, obstructive sleep apnea, or cardiovascular disease) (in combination with reduced-calorie diet and increased physical activity). Moderate to severe obstructive sleep apnea in patients with obesity.

Action

Acts as a glucose-dependent insulinotropic polypeptide receptor and glucagon-like peptide-1 (GLP-1) receptor agonist; increases insulin secretion and reduces glucagon secretion, both in a glucose-dependent manner. Also slows gastric emptying. Also helps to suppress appetite, leading to decreased caloric intake. **Therapeutic Effects:** Improved glycemic control. Reduction in body weight. Reduction in apneic/hypoapneic episodes per hour.

Pharmacokinetics

Absorption: 80% absorbed following subcutaneous administration.

Distribution: Minimally distributed to tissues.

Protein Binding: 99%.

Metabolism and Excretion: Metabolized by proteolytic cleavage, beta oxidation, and amide hydrolysis. Excreted in the urine and feces, with very little being eliminated as unchanged drug.

Half-life: 5 days.

TIME/ACTION PROFILE (plasma concentrations)

ROUTE	ONSET	PEAK	DURATION
SUBQ	unknown	8–72 hr	unknown

Contraindications/Precautions

Contraindicated in: Hypersensitivity; Personal or family history of medullary thyroid carcinoma; Multiple endocrine neoplasia syndrome type 2; Type 1 diabetes; Severe GI disease (including severe gastroparesis).

Use Cautiously in: History of pancreatitis; Diabetic retinopathy (↑ risk of complications); History of angioedema or anaphylaxis to another GLP-1 receptor agonist; History of suicide or active suicidal ideation; Undergoing elective surgery or procedure requiring general anesthesia or deep sedation; Rep: Women of reproductive potential; OB: Use during pregnancy only if potential maternal benefit justifies potential fetal risk; insulin recommended for glucose management in pregnancy; Lactation: Use while breastfeeding only if potential maternal benefit justifies potential risk to infant; Pedi: Safety and effectiveness not established in children.

Adverse Reactions/Side Effects

CV: ↑ HR, hypotension. **Derm:** hair loss. **EENT:** retinopathy complications. **Endo:** hypoglycemia, MEDULLARY THYROID CARCINOMA. **GI:** ↓ appetite, constipation, diarrhea, nausea, vomiting, ↑ amylase, ↑ lipase, abdominal distension, abdominal pain, cholecystitis, cholelithiasis, dyspepsia, flatulence, gastroesophageal reflux disease, PANCREATITIS. **GU:** acute kidney injury. **Local:** injection site reactions. **Neuro:** dizziness, dysesthesia, dysgeusia, fatigue, SUICIDAL THOUGHTS/BEHAVIOR. **Resp:** aspiration. **Misc:** HYPERSENSITIVITY REACTIONS (INCLUDING ANAPHYLAXIS AND ANGIOEDEMA).

Interactions

Drug-Drug: Concurrent use with **agents that increase insulin secretion**, including **sulfonylureas** or **insulin**, may ↑ the risk of serious hypoglycemia; use cautiously and consider dose ↓ of agent increasing insulin secretion. May alter absorption of concurrently administered **oral medications**, including **oral hormonal contraceptives**, due to delayed gastric emptying; advise patients taking oral hormonal contraceptive to switch to a nonoral contraceptive method or add a barrier contraceptive method for 4 wk after initiating therapy and for 4 wk after each dose escalation of tirzepatide.

Route/Dosage

Type 2 Diabetes

SUBQ (Adults): *Mounjaro:* 2.5 mg once weekly initially for 4 wk; then ↑ to 5 mg once weekly; may then ↑ dose in 2.5 mg/wk increments every 4 wk, if needed, to achieve glycemic goals (max weekly dose = 15 mg/wk).

T

Chronic Weight Management

SUBQ (Adults): *Zepbound:* 2.5 mg once weekly initially for 4 wk; then ↑ to 5 mg once weekly; may then ↑ dose in 2.5 mg/wk increments every 4 wk, if needed, to achieve weight loss goals. Recommended maintenance dose is 5 mg/wk, 10 mg/wk, or 15 mg/wk.

Obstructive Sleep Apnea

SUBQ (Adults): *Zepbound:* 2.5 mg once weekly initially for 4 wk; then ↑ to 5 mg once weekly; then ↑ dose in 2.5 mg/wk increments every 4 wk to achieve recommended maintenance dose of 10 mg/wk or 15 mg/wk.

Availability

Solution for injection (prefilled pens and single-dose vials): 2.5 mg/0.5 mL, 5 mg/0.5 mL, 7.5 mg/0.5 mL, 10 mg/0.5 mL, 12.5 mg/0.5 mL, 15 mg/0.5 mL.

NURSING IMPLICATIONS

Assessment

- Observe patient taking concurrent insulin for signs/symptoms of hypoglycemic reactions (sweating, hunger, weakness, dizziness, tremor, tachycardia, anxiety, headache, blurred vision, slurred speech, irritability).
- If thyroid nodules or ↑ serum calcitonin are noted, patient should be referred to an endocrinologist.
- Monitor for signs/symptoms of pancreatitis (persistent severe abdominal pain, sometimes radiating to the back, with or without vomiting). *If pancreatitis suspected,* discontinue tirzepatide. *If pancreatitis confirmed,* do not restart tirzepatide.
- Monitor for signs/symptoms of hypersensitivity reactions (anaphylaxis, angioedema) during therapy.
- Monitor for new or worsening depression, suicidal thoughts or behaviors, or any unusual changes in mood or behavior. *If patient experiences suicidal thoughts or behaviors,* discontinue tirzepatide.
- Monitor weight before and periodically during therapy.

Lab Test Considerations

- Monitor A1c twice yearly in patients who have stable glycemic control and are meeting treatment goals. Monitor quarterly in patients in whom treatment goals have not been met or with therapy change.
- *Zepbound:* In patients with type 2 diabetes, monitor blood glucose prior to starting and during therapy.
- May ↑ lipase and amylase.

Implementation

- Patients stabilized on a diabetic regimen who are exposed to stress, fever, trauma, infection, or surgery may require administration of insulin.
- **SUBQ:** Administer once weekly at any time of the day, without regard to food. Day of week may be changed as long as ≥72 hr before next dose. The pen is a single-dose device that does not require priming before injection. Inject into abdomen, thigh, or upper arm. Rotate injection sites with each dose. Solution is clear and colorless to slightly yellow; do not administer solutions that are cloudy, discolored, or contain particulate matter. Store pens in refrigerator; can also be stored at room temperature for up to 21 days; do not freeze. Store in the original carton to protect from light.
- When using with insulin, administer as separate injections; never mix. If injecting tirzepatide and insulin in same body region, injections should not be close to each other.

Patient/Family Teaching

- Explain purpose and side effects of medication to patient. Advise patient to read *Patient Information* before starting therapy. Instruct patient on use of pen and to use as directed. Advise patient to rotate injection sites with each dose. Follow manufacturer's instructions for pen use. Pen should never be shared between patients, even if needle is changed. Store pen in refrigerator; do not freeze. After initial use, pen may be stored at room temperature for up to 21 days. Emphasize the importance of routine follow-up exams.
- Advise patient to notify health care provider of all Rx or OTC medications, vitamins, or herbal products being taken and consult health care provider before taking any new medications.
- Take missed dose as soon as remembered within 4 days after the missed dose. If >4 days have passed, skip the missed dose and administer the next dose on the regularly scheduled day.
- Advise patient taking insulin and tirzepatide to never mix insulin and tirzepatide together. Give as 2 separate injections. Both injections may be given in the same body area, but should not be given right next to each other.
- Explain to patient that this medication controls hyperglycemia but does not cure diabetes. Therapy is long term.
- Review signs/symptoms of hypoglycemia and hyperglycemia with patient. If hypoglycemia occurs, advise patient to take a glass of orange juice or 2–3 teaspoons of sugar, honey, or corn syrup dissolved in water and notify health care provider.
- Encourage patient to follow prescribed diet, medication, and exercise regimen to prevent hypoglycemic or hyperglycemic episodes.
- Instruct patient in proper testing of serum glucose and ketones. These tests should be closely monitored during periods of stress or illness, and health care provider should be notified if significant changes occur.
- Advise patient to notify health care provider if changes in vision occur during therapy.

- Advise patient to notify health care provider immediately if signs/symptoms of pancreatitis (nausea, vomiting, abdominal pain) or hypersensitivity (swelling of face, lips, tongue, or throat; problems breathing or swallowing; severe rash or itching; fainting or feeling dizzy; very rapid heartbeat) occur.
- Inform patient of risk of benign and malignant thyroid tumors. Advise patient to notify health care provider if signs/symptoms of thyroid tumors (lump in neck, hoarseness, trouble swallowing, shortness of breath) occur.
- Advise patient to inform health care provider of medication regimen before procedures or surgery due to ↑ risk of aspiration with general or deep sedation.
- Advise patient to carry a form of sugar (sugar packets, candy) and identification describing disease process and medication regimen at all times.
- Rep: Insulin is the preferred method of controlling blood glucose during pregnancy. Counsel women of reproductive potential to notify health care provider if pregnancy is planned or suspected or if breastfeeding. Advise patients using oral hormonal contraceptives to switch to a nonoral contraceptive method or add a barrier method of contraception for 4 wk after initiation and for 4 wk after each dose escalation.

Evaluation/Desired Outcomes

- Improved glycemic control.
- Reduction in body weight.
- Reduction in apneic/hypoapneic episodes per hour.

tiZANidine (tye-zan-i-deen)

Zanaflex

Classification

Therapeutic: antispasticity agents (centrally acting)

Pharmacologic: adrenergics

Indications

Spasticity.

Action

Acts as an agonist at central alpha-adrenergic receptor sites. Reduces spasticity by increasing presynaptic inhibition of motor neurons. **Therapeutic Effects:** Decreased spasticity, allowing better function.

Pharmacokinetics

Absorption: Completely absorbed after oral administration but rapidly metabolized, resulting in 40% bioavailability.

Distribution: Widely distributed.

Metabolism and Excretion: 95% metabolized by the liver.

Half-life: 2.5 hr.

TIME/ACTION PROFILE (reduced muscle tone)

ROUTE	ONSET	PEAK	DURATION
PO	unknown	1–2 hr	3–6 hr

Contraindications/Precautions

Contraindicated in: Hypersensitivity; Concurrent use of strong CYP1A2 inhibitors.

Use Cautiously in: Severe renal impairment; Hepatic impairment; Concurrent antihypertensive therapy; OB: Safety not established in pregnancy; Lactation: Safety not established in breastfeeding; Pedi: Safety and effectiveness not established in children; Geri: Dose ↓ may be necessary in older adults due to ↓ clearance.

Adverse Reactions/Side Effects

CV: hypotension, bradycardia. **Derm:** rash, skin ulcers, sweating. **EENT:** blurred vision, pharyngitis, rhinitis. **GI:** abdominal pain, diarrhea, dry mouth, dyspepsia, constipation, ↑ liver enzymes, vomiting. **GU:** urinary frequency. **MS:** back pain, myasthenia. **Neuro:** anxiety, depression, dizziness, paresthesia, sedation, weakness, dyskinesia, hallucinations, nervousness, speech disorder. **Misc:** fever, HYPERSENSITIVITY REACTIONS (INCLUDING ANAPHYLAXIS AND ANGIOEDEMA).

Interactions

Drug-Drug: **Strong CYP1A2 inhibitors**, including **ciprofloxacin** and **fluvoxamine**, may significantly ↑ levels and risk of hypotension and sedation; concurrent use contraindicated. **Moderate CYP1A2 inhibitors** or **weak CYP1A2 inhibitors**, including **acyclovir**, **amiodarone**, **cimetidine**, **mexiletine**, **propafenone**, and **zileuton**, may ↑ levels and risk of toxicity; avoid concurrent use. **Hormonal contraceptives** may ↑ levels and risk of toxicity; avoid concurrent use. ↑ risk of hypotension with **antihypertensives**, especially **alpha$_2$-adrenergic agonist antihypertensives**; avoid concurrent use with alpha$_2$-adrenergic agonists. ↑ CNS depression may occur with **alcohol** or other **CNS depressants**, including some **antidepressants**, **sedative/hypnotics**, **antihistamines**, and **opioid analgesics**.

Route/Dosage

Tablets are not interchangeable with capsules

PO (Adults): 2 mg every 6–8 hr initially (no more than 3 doses/24 hr); ↑ by 2–4 mg/dose every 1–4 days up to 16 mg/dose or 36 mg/day.

Renal Impairment

PO (Adults): *CCr <25 mL/min:* 2 mg every 6–8 hr initially (no more than 3 doses/24 hr); ↑ by 2 mg/dose every 1–4 days up to 16 mg/dose or 36 mg/day.

Hepatic Impairment

PO (Adults): 2 mg every 6–8 hr initially (no more than 3 doses/24 hr); ↑ by 2 mg/dose every 1–4 days up to 16 mg/dose or 36 mg/day.

Availability (generic available)

Tablets: 2 mg, 4 mg. **Capsules:** 2 mg, 4 mg, 6 mg. **Oral solution:** 2 mg/5 mL.

NURSING IMPLICATIONS

Assessment

- Assess muscle spasticity before and periodically during therapy.
- Monitor BP and HR, especially during dose titration. May cause orthostatic hypotension, bradycardia, dizziness, and, rarely, syncope. Effects are usually dose related.
- Observe patient for drowsiness, dizziness, and asthenia. *If symptoms occur,* consider ↓ dose.

Lab Test Considerations

- Monitor AST/ALT at baseline and 1 mo after maximum dose achieved.
- May ↑ glucose, alkaline phosphatase, AST, and ALT.

Implementation

- Do not confuse tizanidine with nizatidine or tiagabine.
- Dose should be titrated carefully to prevent side effects. When discontinuing tizanidine, especially in patient on high dose for long period or with concurrent opioid use, ↓ dose by 2–4 mg/day to minimize withdrawal.
- **PO:** Take consistently with or without food to ↓ variability in plasma concentration.

Patient/Family Teaching

- Explain purpose and side effects of medication. Advise patient to read *Patient Information* before starting therapy.
- Advise patient to avoid stopping tizanidine. Tizanidine needs to be discontinued gradually under guidance of health provider.
- May cause dizziness and drowsiness. Advise patient to avoid driving or other activities requiring alertness until response to drug is known.
- Instruct patient to change positions slowly to minimize orthostatic hypotension.
- Advise patient to notify health care provider immediately if difficulty breathing; urticaria; or swelling of face, throat, or tongue occur.
- Advise patient to notify health care provider if hallucinations occur.
- Advise patient to notify health care provider of all Rx or OTC medications, vitamins, or herbal products being taken and to consult health care provider before taking other medications. Caution patient to avoid alcohol or other CNS depressants.
- Inform patient that frequent rinses, good oral hygiene, and sugarless candy or gum may diminish dry mouth. An ↑ in fluid intake, fiber, and exercise may ↓ constipation risk.
- Rep: Advise women of reproductive potential to notify health care provider if pregnancy is planned or suspected or if breastfeeding.

Evaluation/Desired Outcomes

- Decrease in muscle spasticity with ↑ ability to perform activities of daily living.

tobramycin, See AMINOGLYCOSIDES.

tocilizumab (toe-si-liz-oo-mab)

Actemra, Actemra ACTPen, Avtozma, Tofidence, Tyenne

Classification

Therapeutic: antirheumatics, immunosuppressants

Pharmacologic: interleukin antagonists

Indications

Actemra, Avtozma, Tofidence, and Tyenne: Management of the following disorders: Moderately to severely active rheumatoid arthritis in patients who have not responded to ≥1 disease-modifying antirheumatic drug (DMARD) (as monotherapy or in combination with methotrexate or other non-biologic DMARDs); Active systemic juvenile idiopathic arthritis (as monotherapy or in combination with methotrexate); Active polyarticular juvenile idiopathic arthritis (as monotherapy or in combination with methotrexate); Giant cell arteritis. **Actemra, Avtozma, and Tofidence:** Coronavirus disease 2019 (COVID-19) in hospitalized patients who are receiving systemic corticosteroids and require supplemental oxygen, noninvasive or invasive mechanical ventilation, or extracorporeal membrane oxygenation. **Actemra only:** Management of the following disorders: Chimeric antigen receptor T cell–induced severe or life-threatening cytokine release syndrome; Systemic sclerosis-associated interstitial lung disease (ILD).

Action

Acts as an inhibitor of interleukin-6 (IL-6) receptors by binding to them. IL-6 is a mediator of various inflammatory processes. **Therapeutic Effects:** Slowed progression of rheumatoid arthritis, systemic/polyarticular juvenile idiopathic arthritis, giant cell arteritis. Resolution of cytokine release syndrome. Slowing in rate of decline in pulmonary function in systemic sclerosis-associated ILD. Reduced mortality and prolonged time to mechanical ventilation in COVID-19.

Pharmacokinetics

Absorption: IV administration results in complete bioavailability; 80% absorbed following SUBQ administration.

Distribution: Minimally distributed to tissues.

Metabolism and Excretion: Unknown.

Half-life: *4 mg/kg dose:* up to 11 days; *8 mg/kg:* up to 13 days.

TIME/ACTION PROFILE (improvement)

ROUTE	ONSET	PEAK	DURATION
IV	within 1 mo	4 mo	unknown
SUBQ	unknown	unknown	unknown

Contraindications/Precautions

Contraindicated in: Hypersensitivity; Active infection (for all indications other than COVID-19); Active hepatic disease/impairment; ANC <2000/mm³ (<500/mm³ while on therapy) or platelet count below 100,000/mm³ (<50,000/mm³ while on therapy) (for rheumatoid arthritis, giant cell arteritis, systemic sclerosis-associated ILD, polyarticular juvenile idiopathic arthritis, and systemic juvenile idiopathic arthritis); ANC <1000/mm³ or platelet count below 50,000/mm³ (for COVID-19); Lactation: Lactation.

Use Cautiously in: Patients at risk for GI perforation, including patients with diverticulitis; Renal impairment; Hepatic impairment; Patients with risk factors for tuberculosis (TB); OB: Use during pregnancy only if potential maternal benefit justifies potential fetal risk; Pedi: Children <2 yr (safety and effectiveness not established); Geri: ↑ risk of adverse reactions in older adults.

Adverse Reactions/Side Effects

CV: hypertension. **Derm:** DRUG REACTION WITH EOSINOPHILIA AND SYSTEMIC SYMPTOMS (DRESS), rash, STEVENS-JOHNSON SYNDROME. **EENT:** nasopharyngitis. **GI:** ↑ liver enzymes, GI PERFORATION, HEPATOTOXICITY. **Hemat:** NEUTROPENIA, THROMBOCYTOPENIA. **Metab:** hyperlipidemia. **Neuro:** headache, dizziness. **Misc:** INFECTION (INCLUDING TB, DISSEMINATED FUNGAL INFECTIONS AND INFECTIONS WITH OPPORTUNISTIC PATHOGENS), HYPERSENSITIVITY REACTIONS (INCLUDING ANAPHYLAXIS), infusion reactions.

Interactions

Drug-Drug: May alter the activity of CYP450 enzymes; the effects of the following drugs should be monitored: **cyclosporine**, **theophylline**, **warfarin**, **hormonal contraceptives**, **atorvastatin**, and **lovastatin**. Concurrent use of other hepatotoxic medications, including **methotrexate**, may ↑ risk of hepatotoxicity. May ↓ antibody response to and ↑ risk of adverse reactions to **live-virus vaccines**; do not administer concurrently.

Route/Dosage

Rheumatoid Arthritis

IV (Adults): *Actemra, Avtozma, Tofidence, or Tyenne:* 4 mg/kg every 4 wk; may ↑ to 8 mg/kg every 4 wk based on clinical response.

SUBQ (Adults ≥100 kg): *Actemra, Avtozma, or Tyenne:* 162 mg once weekly.

SUBQ (Adults <100 kg): *Actemra, Avtozma, or Tyenne:* 162 mg every 2 wk; may ↑ to every wk based on clinical response.

Systemic Juvenile Idiopathic Arthritis

IV (Children ≥2 yr and ≥30 kg): *Actemra, Avtozma, Tofidence, or Tyenne:* 8 mg/kg every 2 wk.

IV (Children ≥2 yr and <30 kg): *Actemra, Avtozma, Tofidence, or Tyenne:* 12 mg/kg every 2 wk.

SUBQ (Children ≥2 yr and ≥30 kg): *Actemra, Avtozma, or Tyenne:* 162 mg once weekly.

SUBQ (Children ≥2 yr and <30 kg): *Actemra, Avtozma, or Tyenne:* 162 mg every 2 wk.

Polyarticular Juvenile Idiopathic Arthritis

IV (Children ≥2 yr and ≥30 kg): *Actemra, Avtozma, Tofidence, or Tyenne:* 8 mg/kg every 4 wk.

IV (Children ≥2 yr and <30 kg): *Actemra, Avtozma, Tofidence, or Tyenne:* 10 mg/kg every 4 wk.

SUBQ (Children ≥2 yr and ≥30 kg): *Actemra, Avtozma, or Tyenne:* 162 mg every 2 wk.

SUBQ (Children ≥2 yr and <30 kg): *Actemra, Avtozma, or Tyenne:* 162 mg every 3 wk.

Giant Cell Arteritis

IV (Adults): *Actemra, Avtozma, Tofidence, or Tyenne:* 6 mg/kg (max = 600 mg/dose) every 4 wk (with a tapering course of corticosteroids).

SUBQ (Adults): *Actemra, Avtozma, or Tyenne:* 162 mg once weekly (with a tapering course of corticosteroids); may also consider giving 162 mg every 2 wk (with a tapering course of corticosteroids) based on clinical response.

Cytokine Release Syndrome

IV (Adults and Children ≥2 yr and ≥30 kg): *Actemra only:* 8 mg/kg (max = 800 mg/dose) initially; if patient does not clinically improve after initial dose, up to 3 additional doses may be administered every 8 hr.

IV (Adults and Children ≥2 yr and <30 kg): *Actemra only:* 12 mg/kg initially; if patient does not clinically improve after initial dose, up to 3 additional doses may be administered every 8 hr.

Systemic Sclerosis-Associated Interstitial Lung Disease

SUBQ (Adults): *Actemra only:* 162 mg once weekly.

T

COVID-19

IV (Adults): *Actemra, Avtozma, or Tofidence:* 8 mg/kg (max = 800 mg) as single dose; if clinical signs/symptoms worsen or do not improve, may administer another 8 mg/kg (max = 800 mg) dose ≥8 hr after initial dose.

Availability

Solution for IV injection: 20 mg/mL. **Solution for SUBQ injection (autoinjectors or prefilled syringes):** 162 mg/0.9 mL.

NURSING IMPLICATIONS

Assessment

- Assess pain and range of motion before and periodically during therapy.
- Assess for signs of infection (fever, dyspnea, flu-like symptoms, frequent or painful urination, redness or swelling at the site of a wound), including TB, prior to injection. Monitor new infections closely; most common are upper respiratory tract infections, bronchitis, and urinary tract infections. Signs and symptoms of inflammation may be lessened due to suppression from tocilizumab. Infections may be fatal, especially in patients taking immunosuppressive therapy. If patient develops a serious infection, discontinue tocilizumab until infection is controlled.
- Monitor for injection site reactions (redness and/or itching, rash, hemorrhage, bruising, pain, swelling). Rash will usually disappear within a few days. Application of a towel soaked in cold water may relieve pain or swelling.
- Assess for hypersensitivity reactions and signs of anaphylaxis (urticaria, dyspnea, facial edema) following injection. Medications (antihistamines, corticosteroids, epinephrine) and equipment should be readily available in the event of a severe reaction. Discontinue tocilizumab immediately if anaphylaxis or other severe allergic reaction occurs.
- In patients with COVID-19, monitor for signs and symptoms of new infections during and after therapy. Evaluate patients for risk factors for TB. In patients with COVID-19, it is not necessary to test for latent TB infection before starting therapy. For all other indications, assess patient for latent TB with a tuberculin skin test prior to initiation of therapy. Treatment of latent TB should be started before therapy with tocilizumab.
- Assess for signs and symptoms of systemic fungal infections (fever, malaise, weight loss, sweating, cough, dyspnea, pulmonary infiltrates, serious systemic illness with or without concurrent shock). Ascertain if patient lives in or has traveled to areas of endemic mycoses. Consider empiric antifungal treatment for patients at risk of histoplasmosis and other invasive fungal infections until the pathogens are identified. Consult with an infectious diseases specialist. Consider stopping tocilizumab until the infection has been diagnosed and adequately treated.

Lab Test Considerations

- Assess CBC before starting and after 4–8 wk and then every 3 mo during therapy.
- *If ANC >1000 cells/mm³*, maintain dose. *If ANC 500–1000 cells/mm³*, hold IV tocilizumab until ANC >1000 cells/mm³; then resume at 4 mg/kg and ↑ to 8 mg/kg as clinically appropriate or ↓ SUBQ tocilizumab to every other week, and then ↑ frequency to every week as clinically appropriate. *If ANC <500 cells/mm³*, discontinue tocilizumab.
- *If platelet count 50,000–100,000 cells/mm³*, hold tocilizumab until platelet count >100,000/mm³; then resume IV dosing at 4 mg/kg and ↑ to 8 mg/kg as clinically appropriate or ↓ SUBQ tocilizumab to every other week and then ↑ frequency to every week as clinically appropriate. *If platelet count <50,000 cells/mm³*, discontinue tocilizumab.
- **For rheumatoid arthritis and ILD,** obtain liver enzymes (ALT, AST, alkaline phosphatase, and total bilirubin) before starting, every 4–8 wk after start of therapy for 1st 6 mo, and every 3 mo thereafter. *If liver enzymes persistently ↑ >1–3 times upper limit of normal (ULN)*, ↓ IV tocilizumab dose to 4 mg/kg and ↓ SUBQ injection to every other week or hold tocilizumab until AST/ALT have normalized. *If liver enzymes >3–5 times ULN (confirmed by repeat testing)*, hold tocilizumab until liver enzymes <3 times ULN and then follow recommendations for liver enzymes ↑ >1–3 times ULN. *If liver enzymes >5 times ULN or persistent ↑ >3 times ULN*, discontinue tocilizumab. **For giant cell arteritis,** monitor liver enzymes before starting therapy, every 4–8 wk after start of therapy for 1st 6 mo, and every 3 mo thereafter. *If liver enzymes persistently ↑ >1–3 times ULN*, hold tocilizumab until AST/ALT have normalized and ↓ SUBQ injection to every other week or hold tocilizumab until AST/ALT have normalized. *If liver enzymes >3–5 times ULN (confirmed by repeat testing)*, hold tocilizumab until liver enzymes <3 times ULN and then follow recommendations for liver enzymes ↑ >1–3 times ULN. *If liver enzymes >5 times ULN or persistent ↑ >3 times ULN*, discontinue tocilizumab. **For systemic juvenile idiopathic arthritis and polyarticular juvenile idiopathic arthritis,** monitor liver enzymes at the time of 2nd administration and thereafter every 4–8 wk for polyarticular juvenile idiopathic arthritis and every 2–4 wk for systemic juvenile idiopathic arthritis.
- Monitor lipid levels after 4–8 wk of therapy; then follow clinical guidelines for management of hyperlipidemia. May ↑ total cholesterol, triglycerides, LDL-C, or HDL-C.

Implementation

- Administer a tuberculin skin test before administration of tocilizumab (for all indications other than COVID-19). Patients with latent TB should be treated for TB prior to therapy.
- Immunizations should be current before starting therapy. Patients on tocilizumab may receive concurrent vaccinations, except for live vaccines.
- Other DMARDs should be continued during tocilizumab therapy.
- When transitioning from IV to SUBQ administration, administer 1st SUBQ dose instead of next scheduled IV dose.
- Pedi: Do not change dose based on single visit weight; weight fluctuates.
- **SUBQ:** Solution is clear and colorless to pale yellow; do not administer solutions that are discolored or contain particulate matter. Discard unused solution. Rotate injection sites; avoid sites with moles, scars, and areas where skin is tender, bruised, red, hard, or not intact.

IV Administration

- **Intermittent Infusion:** Dilution: Withdraw volume of 0.9% NaCl or 0.45% NaCl from a 100-mL bag (50-mL bag for children <30 kg) equal to volume of solution required for patient's dose. Slowly add tocilizumab from each vial to infusion bag. Invert slowly to mix; avoid foaming. Do not infuse solutions that are discolored or contain particulate matter. Diluted solution is stable for 24 hr if refrigerated or at room temperature; protect from light. Allow solution to reach room temperature before infusing. Rate: Infuse over 60 min. Do not administer via IV push or bolus.
- **Y-Site Incompatibility:** Do not administer other drugs through same IV line.

Patient/Family Teaching

- Explain purpose and side effects of medication to patient. Advise patient to read *Patient Information* before starting therapy. If a dose is missed, contact health care provider to schedule next infusion. Instruct patient and caregiver in correct technique for SUBQ injections and care and disposal of equipment.
- Instruct patient to notify health care provider of all Rx or OTC medications, vitamins, or herbal products being taken and consult health care provider before taking any new medications.
- Caution patient to notify health care provider immediately if signs of infection (fever; sweating; chills; muscle aches; cough; shortness of breath; blood in phlegm; weight loss; warm, red, or painful skin or sores; diarrhea or stomach pain; burning on urination; urinary frequency; feeling tired), fever and stomach-area pain that does not go away, change in bowel habits, severe rash, swollen face, or difficulty breathing occurs. If signs/symptoms of anaphylaxis occur, discontinue injections and notify health care provider immediately.
- Instruct patient to notify health care provider of medication regimen prior to treatment or surgery.
- Rep: Advise women of reproductive potential to notify health care provider if pregnancy is planned or suspected or if breastfeeding. Inform patient of pregnancy exposure registry that monitors outcomes in women exposed to tocilizumab. Register patient by calling 1-877-311-8972; health care provider or patient can call to register.

Evaluation/Desired Outcomes

- Slow progression of rheumatoid arthritis, systemic/polyarticular juvenile idiopathic arthritis, and giant cell arteritis.
- Resolution of cytokine release syndrome.
- Slowing in rate of decline in pulmonary function in systemic sclerosis-associated ILD.
- Reduced mortality and prolonged time to mechanical ventilation in COVID-19.

tofacitinib (toe-fa-**sye**-ti-nib)

Xeljanz, Xeljanz XR

Classification

Therapeutic: antirheumatics

Pharmacologic: kinase inhibitors

T

Indications

Moderately to severely active rheumatoid arthritis in patients who have had an inadequate response/intolerance to ≥1 tumor necrosis factor (TNF) blocker (as monotherapy or in combination with nonbiologic disease-modifying antirheumatic drugs [DMARDs]) (not to be used with biologic DMARDs or potent immunosuppressants, including azathioprine and cyclosporine) (immediate-release and extended-release tablets only). Active psoriatic arthritis in patients who have had an inadequate response/intolerance to ≥1 TNF blocker (in combination with other nonbiologic DMARDs) (not to be used with biologic DMARDs or potent immunosuppressants, including azathioprine and cyclosporine) (immediate-release and extended-release tablets only). Active ankylosing spondylitis in patients who have had an inadequate response/intolerance to ≥1 TNF blocker (not to be used with biologic DMARDs or potent immunosuppressants, including azathioprine and cyclosporine) (immediate-release and extended-release tablets only). Moderately to severely active ulcerative colitis in patients who have had an inadequate response/intolerance to ≥1 TNF blocker (not to be used with biologic therapies or potent immunosuppressants, including azathioprine and cyclosporine) (immediate-release and extended-release tablets only). Active polyarticular course juvenile idiopathic arthritis in patients who have had an inadequate response/intolerance to ≥1 TNF blocker (not to be used with biologic DMARDs or potent immunosuppressants, including azathioprine and cyclosporine) (immediate-release tablets and oral solution only).

Action

Acts as a Janus kinase inhibitor. Some results of inhibition include decreased hematopoiesis and immune cell function. Decreases circulating killer cells, increases B cell count, and decreases serum C-reactive protein.
Therapeutic Effects: Improvement in clinical and symptomatic parameters of rheumatoid arthritis, psoriatic arthritis, ankylosing spondylitis, ulcerative colitis, and polyarticular course juvenile idiopathic arthritis.

Pharmacokinetics

Absorption: 74% absorbed following oral administration.
Distribution: Well distributed to tissues.
Metabolism and Excretion: Primarily metabolized by the liver via the CYP3A4 isoenzyme, with some contribution from the CYP2C19 isoenzyme. 30% renal excretion of the parent drug.
Half-life: 3 hr.

TIME/ACTION PROFILE (clinical improvement)

ROUTE	ONSET	PEAK	DURATION
PO	within 2 wk	3 mo	unknown
PO-ER	unknown	unknown	unknown

Contraindications/Precautions

Contraindicated in: Active infection; ↑ risk for thrombosis; History of MI or stroke; Lymphocyte count <500 cells/mm³, ANC <1000 cells/mm³, or Hgb <9 g/dL; Severe hepatic impairment; Lactation: Lactation.
Use Cautiously in: Patients with rheumatoid arthritis who are >50 yr old and have ≥1 cardiovascular risk factor (↑ risk of all-cause mortality, cardiovascular death, MI, stroke, and thrombosis); Current or past history of smoking (↑ risk of malignancy, cardiovascular death, MI, or stroke); Chronic or recurrent infection; Known malignancy; Risk of GI perforation; Chronic lung disease (↑ risk of infection); Japanese patients (↑ risk of herpes zoster); OB: Use during pregnancy only if potential maternal benefit justifies potential fetal risk; Pedi: Safety and effectiveness not established in children <18 yr (rheumatoid arthritis, psoriatic arthritis, ulcerative colitis) or <2 yr (active polyarticular course juvenile idiopathic arthritis); Geri: Infection risk may be ↑ in older adults.

Adverse Reactions/Side Effects

CV: ARTERIAL THROMBOSIS, CARDIOVASCULAR DEATH, DEEP VEIN THROMBOSIS (DVT), MI, peripheral edema. **Derm:** erythema, pruritus, rash. **F and E:** dehydration. **GI:** ↑ liver enzymes, abdominal pain, diarrhea, dyspepsia, gastritis, GI PERFORATION, vomiting. **GU:** ↑ serum creatinine. **Hemat:** anemia, neutropenia. **Metab:** hyperlipidemia. **MS:** arthralgia, joint swelling, musculoskeletal pain, tendonitis. **Neuro:** fatigue, headache, insomnia, paresthesia, STROKE. **Resp:** PULMONARY EMBOLISM (PE). **Misc:** DEATH, fever, HYPERSENSITIVITY REACTIONS (INCLUDING ANGIOEDEMA AND URTICARIA), INFECTION (INCLUDING TUBERCULOSIS [TB], BACTERIAL, INVASIVE FUNGAL INFECTIONS, VIRAL, AND OTHER INFECTIONS DUE TO OPPORTUNISTIC PATHOGENS), MALIGNANCY.

Interactions

Drug-Drug: May ↑ risk of adverse reactions and ↓ antibody response to **live vaccines**; avoid concurrent use. **Strong CYP3A4 inhibitors**, including **ketoconazole**, or **moderate CYP3A4 inhibitors/strong CYP2C19 inhibitors**, including **fluconazole**, may ↑ levels and risk of toxicity; dose ↓ recommended. **Strong CYP3A4 inducers**, including **rifampin**, may ↓ levels and effectiveness; avoid concurrent use. ↑ risk of immunosuppression when used concurrently with other potent **immunosuppressants**, including **azathioprine, cyclosporine, tacrolimus, antineoplastics**, or **radiation therapy**.

Route/Dosage

Rheumatoid Arthritis, Psoriatic Arthritis, and Ankylosing Spondylitis

PO (Adults): *Immediate-release tablets:* 5 mg twice daily; *Extended-release tablets:* 11 mg once daily; *Concurrent use of strong CYP3A4 inhibitors or concurrent use of moderate CYP3A4 inhibitor with a strong CYP2C19 inhibitor:* 5 mg once daily (immediate-release tablets); if taking 11 mg once daily (extended-release tablets), then switch to 5 mg once daily (immediate-release tablets).

Renal Impairment

PO (Adults): *Moderate or severe renal impairment:* 5 mg once daily (immediate-release tablets); if taking 11 mg once daily (extended-release tablets), then switch to 5 mg once daily (immediate-release tablets). For patients undergoing hemodialysis, administer dose after dialysis session.

Hepatic Impairment

PO (Adults): *Moderate hepatic impairment:* 5 mg once daily (immediate-release tablets); if taking 11 mg once daily (extended-release tablets), then switch to 5 mg once daily (immediate-release tablets).

Ulcerative Colitis

PO (Adults): *Immediate-release tablets:* Induction: 10 mg twice daily for ≥8 wk; based on therapeutic response, may transition to maintenance dose or continue 10 mg twice daily for an additional 8 wk. Discontinue therapy if inadequate response achieved after 16 wk using 10 mg twice daily. Maintenance: 5 mg twice daily; if patient experiences loss of response on 5 mg twice daily, then use 10 mg twice daily after assessing the benefits and risks and use for the shortest duration; use lowest effective dose to maintain response; *Extended-release tablets:* Induction: 22 mg once daily for ≥8 wk; based on therapeutic response, may transition to maintenance dose or continue 22 mg once daily for an additional 8 wk. Discontinue therapy if inadequate response achieved after 16 wk using 22 mg once daily. Maintenance: 11 mg once daily; if patient experiences loss of response on 11 mg once daily, then use 22 mg once daily after assessing the benefits and risks and use for the shortest duration; use lowest effective dose to maintain response; *Concurrent use of strong CYP3A4 inhibitors or concurrent use of moderate CYP3A4 inhibitor with a strong CYP2C19 inhibitor:* If taking 10 mg twice daily (immediate-release tablets), ↓ to 5 mg twice daily (immediate-release tablets); if taking 5 mg twice daily (immediate-release tablets), ↓ to 5 mg once daily (immediate-release tablets). If taking 22 mg once daily (extended-release tablets), then ↓ to 11 mg once daily (extended-release tablets); if taking 11 mg once daily (extended-release tablets), then switch to 5 mg once daily (immediate-release tablets).

Renal Impairment

PO (Adults): *Moderate or severe renal impairment:* If taking 10 mg twice daily (immediate-release tablets), ↓ to 5 mg twice daily (immediate-release tablets); if taking 5 mg twice daily (immediate-release tablets), ↓ to 5 mg once daily (immediate-release tablets). If taking 22 mg once daily (extended-release tablets), then ↓ to 11 mg once daily (extended-release tablets); if taking 11 mg once daily (extended-release tablets), then switch to 5 mg once daily (immediate-release tablets). For patients undergoing hemodialysis, administer dose after dialysis session.

Hepatic Impairment

PO (Adults): *Moderate hepatic impairment:* If taking 10 mg twice daily (immediate-release tablets), ↓ to 5 mg twice daily (immediate-release tablets); if taking 5 mg twice daily (immediate-release tablets), ↓ to 5 mg once daily (immediate-release tablets). If taking 22 mg once daily (extended-release tablets), then ↓ to 11 mg once daily (extended-release tablets); if taking 11 mg once daily (extended-release tablets), then switch to 5 mg once daily (immediate-release).

Active Polyarticular Course Juvenile Idiopathic Arthritis

PO (Children ≥2 yr and ≥40 kg): *Immediate-release tablets or oral solution:* 5 mg twice daily. *Concurrent use of strong CYP3A4 inhibitors or concurrent use of moderate CYP3A4 inhibitor with a strong CYP2C19 inhibitor:* 5 mg once daily (immediate-release tablets or oral solution).

PO (Children ≥2 yr and 20–<40 kg): *Oral solution:* 4 mg twice daily. *Concurrent use of strong CYP3A4 inhibitors or concurrent use of moderate CYP3A4 inhibitor with a strong CYP2C19 inhibitor:* 4 mg once daily (oral solution).

PO (Children ≥2 yr and 10–<20 kg): *Oral solution:* 3.2 mg twice daily. *Concurrent use of strong CYP3A4 inhibitors or concurrent use of moderate CYP3A4 inhibitor with a strong CYP2C19 inhibitor:* 3.2 mg once daily (oral solution).

Renal Impairment

PO (Children ≥2 yr and ≥40 kg): *Moderate or severe renal impairment:* Immediate-release tablets or oral solution: 5 mg once daily. For patients undergoing hemodialysis, administer dose after dialysis session.

Renal Impairment

PO (Children ≥2 yr and 20–<40 kg): *Moderate or severe renal impairment:* Oral solution: 4 mg once daily. For patients undergoing hemodialysis, administer dose after dialysis session.

Renal Impairment

PO (Children ≥2 yr and 10–<20 kg): *Moderate or severe renal impairment:* Oral solution: 3.2 mg once daily. For patients undergoing hemodialysis, administer dose after dialysis session.

Hepatic Impairment

PO (Children ≥2 yr and ≥40 kg): *Moderate hepatic impairment:* Immediate-release tablets or oral solution: 5 mg once daily.

Hepatic Impairment

PO (Children ≥2 yr and 20–<40 kg): *Moderate hepatic impairment:* Oral solution: 4 mg once daily.

Hepatic Impairment

PO (Children ≥2 yr and 10–<20 kg): *Moderate hepatic impairment:* Oral solution: 3.2 mg once daily.

Availability (generic available)

Immediate-release tablets: 5 mg, 10 mg. **Extended-release tablets:** 11 mg, 22 mg. **Oral solution (grape flavor):** 1 mg/mL.

T

NURSING IMPLICATIONS

Assessment

- Assess pain and range of motion before and periodically during therapy.
- Assess for signs and symptoms of infection, including opportunistic infections and TB, prior to and periodically during therapy. *If sepsis or serious infection occurs,* interrupt therapy and provide appropriate diagnostic testing, antimicrobial therapy, and close monitoring. Most common are pneumonia, cellulitis, herpes zoster, urinary tract infection, diverticulitis, and appendicitis. Infections may be fatal, especially in patients taking immunosuppressive therapy.
- Assess for signs and symptoms of systemic fungal infections (fever, malaise, weight loss, sweats, cough, dypsnea, pulmonary infiltrates, serious systemic illness with or without concurrent shock). Ascertain if patient lives in or has traveled to areas of endemic mycoses. Consider empiric antifungal treatment for patients at risk of histoplasmosis and other invasive fungal infections until pathogen identified. Consult with infectious diseases specialist. Consider stopping tofacitinib until the infection has been diagnosed and adequately treated.
- Monitor for thrombosis, including PE, DVT, and arterial thrombi. *If symptoms of thrombosis occur,* permanently discontinue tofacitinib.

Lab Test Considerations

- Monitor CBC with differential prior to and periodically during therapy. Do not initiate tofacitinib in patients with lymphocyte count <500 cells/mm^3, ANC <1000 cells/mm^3, or Hgb <9 g/dL.
- Monitor lymphocyte count at baseline and every 3 mo thereafter. *If lymphocyte count ≥500 cells/mm^3,* maintain dose. *If lymphocyte count <500 cells/mm^3 and confirmed by repeat testing,* permanently discontinue tofacitinib.
- Monitor neutrophil count at baseline, after 4–8 wk of therapy, and every 3 mo thereafter. *If ANC >1000 cells/mm^3,* maintain dose. *If ANC 500–1000 cells/mm^3,* interrupt dosing until ANC >1000 cells/mm^3. *If ANC <500 cells/mm^3 and confirmed by repeat testing,* permanently discontinue tofacitinib.
- Monitor Hgb at baseline, after 4–8 wk of therapy, and every 3 mo thereafter. *If ↓ in Hgb ≤2 g/dL and Hgb ≥9.0 g/dL and confirmed by repeat testing,* maintain dose. *If ↓ in Hgb >2 dL and Hgb <8.0 g/dL,* interrupt administration of tofacitinib until Hgb values have normalized.
- Monitor liver enzymes prior to and periodically during therapy.
- Monitor total cholesterol, LDL-C, and HDL-C for 4–8 wk following initiation of therapy.
- Complete tuberculin skin test prior to initiation of therapy. Treatment of latent TB should be started before therapy with tofacitinib.

Implementation

- Immunizations should be current prior to initiating therapy. Patients on tofacitinib should not receive live vaccines.
- Screen patient for viral hepatitis before starting therapy.
- Extended-release tablets are not interchangeable with oral solution.
- *To switch from immediate release to extended release,* patients treated with *Xeljanz* 5 mg twice daily may be switched to *Xeljanz XR* 11 mg once daily the day following the last dose of *Xeljanz* 5 mg.
- **PO:** Administer twice daily without regard to food. *DNC:* Swallow extended-release tablets whole; do not crush, break, or chew.
- Oral solution is clear and colorless. Administer oral solution using the included press-in bottle adapter and oral dosing syringe.

Patient/Family Teaching

- Instruct patient to take tofacitinib as directed. Advise patient to read *Medication Guide* before starting and with each Rx refill in case of changes.
- Advise patient to notify health care provider immediately if signs of infection (fever; sweating; chills; muscle aches; cough; shortness of breath; blood in phlegm; weight loss; warm, red, or painful skin or sores; diarrhea or stomach pain; burning on urination or urinating more often than normal; feeling very tired) occur.
- Advise patient to notify health care provider immediately if signs hypersensitivity (facial swelling, hives) or stomach or intestinal perforation (fever, stomach-area pain that does not go away, change in bowel habits) occur.
- Inform patient ≥50 yr of age with ≥1 cardiovascular risk factor that risk of death from all causes is ↑ with tofacitinib use. They should discontinue therapy if they experience heart attack or stroke.
- Inform patient that risk of malignancy and lymphoproliferative disorders is ↑ with tofacitinib use and periodic cancer screens, including skin assessments, are recommended.
- Advise patient to notify health care provider of all Rx or OTC medications, vitamins, or herbal products being taken and to consult with health care provider before taking other medications.
- Instruct patient to notify health care provider of medication regimen prior to treatment or surgery.
- Rep: Advise women of reproductive potential to notify health care provider if pregnancy is planned or suspected. Advise women to avoid breastfeeding during therapy and for ≥18 hr after the last dose of oral solution or 36 hr after the last dose of extended-release tablets. May impair female fertility.
- Emphasize importance of follow-up lab tests to monitor for adverse reactions.

Evaluation/Desired Outcomes

- Decreased pain and swelling with improved physical functioning and ↓ rate of joint destruction in patients with rheumatoid arthritis, psoriatic arthritis, ankylosing spondylitis, and polyarticular course juvenile idiopathic arthritis.
- Decrease in diarrhea and abdominal pain in patients with ulcerative colitis.

tolnaftate, See ANTIFUNGALS (TOPICAL).

tolterodine (tol-ter-oh-deen)

~~Detrol, Detrol LA~~

Classification

Therapeutic: urinary tract antispasmodics

Pharmacologic: anticholinergics

Indications

Overactive bladder with symptoms of urinary frequency, urgency, or urge incontinence.

Action

Acts as a competitive muscarinic receptor antagonist, resulting in inhibition of cholinergically mediated bladder contraction. **Therapeutic Effects:** Decreased urinary frequency, urgency, and urge incontinence.

Pharmacokinetics

Absorption: Well absorbed (77%) following oral administration.

Distribution: Extensively distributed to tissues.

Protein Binding: 96.3%.

Metabolism and Excretion: Extensively metabolized by the liver, via the CYP2D6 isoenzyme; (the CYP2D6 enzyme system exhibits genetic polymorphism; 7% of population may be poor metabolizers and may have significantly ↑ tolterodine concentrations and an ↑ risk of adverse effects); one metabolite (5-hydroxymethyltolterodine) is active; other metabolites are excreted in urine.

Half-life: *Tolterodine:* 1.9–3.7 hr; *5-hydroxymethyltolterodine:* 2.9–3.1 hr.

TIME/ACTION PROFILE (effects on bladder function)

ROUTE	ONSET	PEAK	DURATION
PO	unknown	unknown	12 hr

Contraindications/Precautions

Contraindicated in: Hypersensitivity to tolterodine or fesoterodine; Urinary retention; Gastric retention; Severe hepatic impairment; End-stage renal disease; Uncontrolled angle-closure glaucoma; Lactation: Lactation.

Use Cautiously in: GI obstructive disorders, including pyloric stenosis (↑ risk of gastric retention); Significant bladder outflow obstruction (↑ risk of urinary retention); Controlled angle-closure glaucoma; Myasthenia gravis; Mild to moderate hepatic impairment (↓ dose); Severe renal impairment (↓ dose); OB: Use during pregnancy only if potential maternal benefit justifies potential fetal risk; Pedi: Safety and effectiveness not established in children.

Adverse Reactions/Side Effects

EENT: blurred vision, dry eyes. **GI:** <u>dry mouth</u>, constipation, dyspepsia. **Neuro:** <u>dizziness</u>, <u>headache</u>, sedation. **Misc:** HYPERSENSITIVITY REACTIONS (INCLUDING ANAPHYLAXIS AND ANGIOEDEMA).

Interactions

Drug-Drug: Strong CYP3A4 inhibitors, including **erythromycin**, **clarithromycin**, **cyclosporine**, **itraconazole**, **ketoconazole**, and **vinblastine**, may ↑ levels and risk of toxicity.

Route/Dosage

Immediate-Release Tablets

PO (Adults): 2 mg twice daily; may be lowered depending on response; *Concurrent use of strong CYP3A4 inhibitors:* 1 mg twice daily.

Hepatic/Renal Impairment

PO (Adults): *Mild to moderate hepatic impairment or CCr 10–30 mL/min:* 1 mg twice daily.

Extended-Release Capsules

PO (Adults): 4 mg once daily; may be lowered depending on response; *Concurrent use of strong CYP3A4 inhibitors:* 2 mg once daily.

Hepatic/Renal Impairment

PO (Adults): *Mild to moderate hepatic impairment or (CCr 10–30 mL/min):* 2 mg once daily.

Availability (generic available)

Extended-release capsules: 2 mg, 4 mg. **Tablets:** 1 mg, 2 mg.

NURSING IMPLICATIONS

Assessment

- Assess for urinary urgency, frequency, urge incontinence, and GI obstruction at baseline and periodically during therapy.
- Monitor for signs/symptoms of anaphylaxis and angioedema (difficulty breathing, upper airway obstruction, ↓ BP, rash, swelling of face or neck). *If symptoms occur,* discontinue tolterodine and treat as indicated. Keep emergency medication and equipment nearby when given in hospital.

T

- Monitor for anticholinergic CNS effects (dizziness, somnolence) especially after starting therapy or ↑ dose.

Implementation
- **PO:** Administer without regard to food.
- ***DNC:*** Extended-release capsules should be swallowed whole; do not open, crush, dissolve, or chew.

Patient/Family Teaching
- Explain purpose and side effects of medication. Advise patient to read *Patient Information* before starting therapy.
- May cause dizziness and blurred vision. Caution patient to avoid driving or other activities requiring alertness until response to medication is known.
- Instruct patient to notify health care provider immediately if rash or signs/symptoms of anaphylaxis or angioedema occur.
- Inform patient that frequent rinses, good oral hygiene, and sugarless candy or gum may diminish dry mouth. An ↑ in fluid intake, fiber, and exercise may ↓ constipation risk.
- Rep: Advise women of reproductive potential to notify health care provider if pregnancy is planned or suspected or if breastfeeding.

Evaluation/Desired Outcomes
- Decreased urinary frequency, urgency, and urge incontinence.

REMS

tolvaptan (tol-vap-tan)

Jinarc, Jynarque, Samsca

Classification

Therapeutic: electrolyte modifiers

Pharmacologic: vasopressin antagonists

Indications
Samsca: Significant hypervolemic and euvolemic hyponatremia (serum sodium <125 mEq/L or less marked symptomatic hyponatremia that has resisted correction by fluid restriction), including patients with HF and syndrome of inappropriate antidiuretic hormone. **Jynarque:** Patients at risk of rapidly progressing autosomal dominant polycystic kidney disease.

Action
Acts as a selective vasopressin V2-receptor antagonist, resulting in increased renal water excretion and increased serum sodium. **Therapeutic Effects:** Correction of hyponatremia (Samsca). Slowed deterioration of renal function (Jynarque).

Pharmacokinetics
Absorption: 40% absorbed following oral administration.

Distribution: Well distributed to tissues.

Protein Binding: >99%.

Metabolism and Excretion: Extensively metabolized in the liver via the CYP3A4 isoenzyme; 59% excreted in the feces (19% as unchanged drug), with 40% excreted in the urine (<1% as unchanged drug).

Half-life: 12 hr.

TIME/ACTION PROFILE

ROUTE	ONSET	PEAK	DURATION
PO	within 8 hr	2–4 hr†	7 days

† Plasma concentrations.

Contraindications/Precautions
Contraindicated in: Hypersensitivity; Hepatic impairment; Urgent need to acutely raise serum sodium (Samsca); Patients who cannot appropriately sense/respond to thirst; Hypovolemia; Uncorrected abnormal serum sodium concentrations (Jynarque); Anuria; Uncorrected urinary outflow obstruction; Lactation: Lactation.

Use Cautiously in: Severe malnutrition, alcoholism, or advanced liver disease (↑ risk of osmotic demyelination; correct electrolyte abnormalities at a slower rates); Cirrhosis (↑ risk of GI bleeding; use only when the need to treat outweighs risk); OB: Use during pregnancy only if potential maternal benefit justifies potential fetal risk; Pedi: Safety and effectiveness not established in children; Geri: Older adults may have ↑ sensitivity to effects.

Adverse Reactions/Side Effects
CV: palpitations. **Derm:** dry skin, rash. **Endo:** hyperglycemia. **F and E:** thirst, hypernatremia, hypovolemia. **GI:** constipation, diarrhea, dry mouth, ↓ appetite, dyspepsia, HEPATOTOXICITY. **GU:** polyuria. **Metab:** hyperuricemia. **Neuro:** dizziness, weakness, osmotic demyelination. **Misc:** HYPERSENSITIVITY REACTIONS (INCLUDING ANAPHYLAXIS).

Interactions
Drug-Drug: Strong CYP3A inhibitors, including **ketoconazole, clarithromycin, itraconazole, nelfinavir, ritonavir**, and **nefazodone**, as well as **moderate CYP3A inhibitors**, including **erythromycin, fluconazole, aprepitant, diltiazem**, and **verapamil**, may ↑ levels and risk of toxicity; avoid concurrent use. **CYP3A inducers**, including **rifampin**, may ↓ levels and effectiveness; avoid concurrent use with Jynarque; dosage adjustments may be necessary with Samsca. **P-glycoprotein inhibitors**, including **cyclosporine**, may ↑ levels and risk of toxicity; dosage adjustments may be necessary. May ↑ risk of hyperkalemia with **angiotensin II receptor blockers, ACE inhibitors**, and **potassium-sparing diuretics**. **Diuretics** may ↑ risk of too rapidly correcting serum sodium

concentrations. May inhibit effects of **desmopressin**; avoid concurrent use.
Drug-Food: Grapefruit juice may ↑ levels and the risk of toxicity; avoid concurrent use.

Route/Dosage

Samsca and Jynarque should not be used interchangeably.

Hyponatremia (Samsca)

PO (Adults): 15 mg once daily initially; may ↑ at intervals of ≥1 day to 30 mg once daily, up to a maximum of 60 mg once daily. Do not use for longer than 30 days.

Autosomal Dominant Polycystic Kidney Disease (Jynarque and Jinarc)

PO (Adults): 60 mg/day initially (taken as 45 mg upon wakening and then 15 mg 8 hr later); may be ↑ after at least 1 wk to 90 mg/day (taken as 60 mg upon wakening and then 30 mg 8 hr later); may then be ↑ after at least 1 wk to 120 mg/day (taken as 90 mg upon wakening and then 30 mg 8 hr later); *Concurrent use of moderate CYP3A inhibitors:* 30 mg/day initially (taken as 15 mg upon wakening and then 15 mg 8 hr later); may be ↑ after at least 1 wk to 45 mg/day (taken as 30 mg upon wakening and then 15 mg 8 hr later); may then be ↑ after at least 1 wk to 60 mg/day (taken as 45 mg upon wakening and then 15 mg 8 hr later).

Availability (generic available)

Tablets (Jynarque): 15 mg, 30 mg, 45 mg, 60 mg, 90 mg. **Tablets (Samsca):** 15 mg, 30 mg.

NURSING IMPLICATIONS

Assessment

- **Samsca:** Monitor neurologic status and assess for signs and symptoms of osmotic demyelination syndrome (trouble speaking, dysphagia, drowsiness, confusion, mood changes, involuntary movements, weakness, seizures), especially during initiation and after titration. If a rapid ↑ in sodium or symptoms occur, discontinue *Samsca* and consider administration of hypotonic fluid.
- **Jynarque:** Monitor for signs and symptoms of liver injury (fatigue, anorexia, right upper abdominal discomfort, dark urine, jaundice) periodically during therapy. If symptoms occur, discontinue *Jynarque*.
- Monitor fluid balance. If hypovolemia occurs interrupt or discontinue tolvaptan and provide supportive care (monitor vital signs, balance fluid and electrolytes).

Lab Test Considerations

- Monitor serum sodium frequently during initiation and dose titration and periodically during therapy. Too rapid correction of hyponatremia (>12 mEq/L/24 hr) can cause osmotic demyelination syndrome.
- Monitor serum potassium in patients with serum potassium >5 mEq/L or taking medication known to ↑ potassium.
- **Jynarque:** Monitor ALT, AST, and bilirubin 2 wk and 4 wk after starting therapy, then monthly for 1st 18 mo, and every 3 mo thereafter. If ALT, AST, or bilirubin ↑ to >2 times upper limit of normal (ULN), immediately discontinue *Jynarque*; repeat tests as soon as possible (within 48–72 hr). If levels stabilize or resolve, *Jynarque* may be reinitiated with ↑ frequency of monitoring as long as ALT and AST remain below 3 times ULN. Do not restart in patients with signs or symptoms of hepatic injury or whose ALT or AST is ever >3 times ULN during therapy with tolvaptan, unless another explanation for liver injury exists and the injury has resolved. In patients with a stable, low baseline AST or ALT, an ↑ >2 times baseline, even if <2 times ULN, may indicate early liver injury. Suspend and promptly (48–72 hr) re-evaluate liver enzymes before reinitiating therapy with more frequent monitoring.

Implementation

- ***REMS:*** REMS requirements are for *Jynarque* product.
- Initiate and reinitiate *Samsca* in a hospital where serum sodium can be closely monitored.
- Avoid fluid restriction during first 24 hr of therapy.
- **PO:** Administer once daily without regard to meals.

Patient/Family Teaching

- Instruct patient to take tolvaptan as directed. Avoid drinking grapefruit juice during therapy; may cause ↑ levels. Take missed doses as soon as remembered, but not if just before next dose; do not double doses. Do not stop and restart therapy. Restarting therapy may require hospitalization.
- ***REMS:*** Explain requirements of *Tolvaptan for ADPKD Shared System REMS* program (providers must be certified and inform patients of risk of hepatotoxicity; patient must enroll, comply with ongoing monitoring requirements, and get *Jynarque* from pharmacies participating in REMS program).
- Inform patients they can continue fluid ingestion in response to thirst during therapy and should have water available to drink at all times during therapy. Following discontinuation of therapy, resume fluid restriction.
- Advise patient to notify health care provider immediately if signs and symptoms of hepatotoxicity (feeling tired, fever, loss of appetite, rash, nausea, itching, right upper abdomen pain or tenderness, yellowing of skin and white part of eye, vomiting, dark urine) occur.

- Advise patient to notify health care provider of all Rx or OTC medications, vitamins, or herbal products being taken and to consult with health care provider before taking other medications.
- Advise patient to notify health care provider if signs of dehydration (vomiting, diarrhea, inability to drink normally, dizziness, feeling faint) or bleeding (vomiting bright red blood, dark blood clots, or coffee-ground-like material; black, tarry stools; bloody stools).
- Rep: Advise women of reproductive potential to notify health care provider if pregnancy is planned or suspected and to avoid breastfeeding.

Evaluation/Desired Outcomes

- Normalization of serum sodium levels. Therapy should be limited to 30 days (Samsca).
- Slowed deterioration of renal function (Jynarque).

topiramate (toe-**peer**-a-mate)

Eprontia, Qudexy XR, Topamax, Topamax Sprinkle, Trokendi XR

Classification

Therapeutic: anticonvulsants, mood stabilizers

Indications

Partial-onset seizures (as monotherapy or adjunctive therapy). Primary generalized tonic-clonic seizures (as monotherapy or adjunctive therapy). Seizures due to Lennox-Gastaut syndrome (as adjunctive therapy). Prevention of migraine headache. **Unlabeled Use:** Adjunct in treatment of bipolar disorder. Infantile spasms.

Action

Action may be due to: Blockade of sodium channels in neurons; Enhancement of gamma-aminobutyrate, an inhibitory neurotransmitter; Prevention of activation of excitatory receptors. **Therapeutic Effects:** Decreased incidence of seizures. Decreased incidence/severity of migraine headache.

Pharmacokinetics

Absorption: 80% absorbed following oral administration.
Distribution: Minimally distributed to tissues.
Metabolism and Excretion: Not extensively metabolized. 70% excreted unchanged in urine.
Half-life: *Immediate release:* 21 hr; *Extended release:* 31 hr.

TIME/ACTION PROFILE (plasma concentrations†)

ROUTE	ONSET	PEAK	DURATION
PO	unknown	2 hr	12 hr
PO-ER	unknown	24 hr	unknown

† After single dose.

Contraindications/Precautions

Contraindicated in: Hypersensitivity; Recent alcohol use (within 6 hr before and after use of extended-release product); Metabolic acidosis (on metformin) (with extended-release product only).
Use Cautiously in: All patients (may ↑ risk of suicidal thoughts/behaviors); Dehydration; Patients predisposed to metabolic acidosis; Sulfa allergy; Renal impairment (↓ dose if CCr <70 mL/min/1.73 m²); Hepatic impairment; Rep: Women of reproductive potential; OB: Use during pregnancy only if potential maternal benefit justifies potential fetal risk; Lactation: Use while breastfeeding only if potential maternal benefit justifies potential risk to infant; Pedi: Safety and effectiveness not established in children <2 yr (immediate release) and <6 yr (extended release); children are more prone to oligohydrosis, hyperthermia, metabolic acidosis, ↓ bone mineral density, and ↓ growth; Geri: Consider age-related ↓ in renal/hepatic impairment, concurrent disease states, and drug therapy in older adults.

Adverse Reactions/Side Effects

Derm: oligohydrosis (↑ in children), STEVENS-JOHNSON SYNDROME, TOXIC EPIDERMAL NECROLYSIS. **EENT:** abnormal vision, diplopia, nystagmus, ↑ intraocular pressure, acute myopia/secondary angle closure glaucoma, mydriasis, ocular pain, ocular redness, retinal detachment, visual field defects. **Endo:** ↓ growth (children). **F and E:** hyperchloremic metabolic acidosis. **GI:** nausea, weight loss, abdominal pain, anorexia, constipation, dry mouth, hyperammonemia. **GU:** kidney stones. **Hemat:** BLEEDING, leukopenia. **Metab:** hyperthermia (↑ in children). **MS:** ↓ bone mineral density (↑ in children). **Neuro:** ataxia, cognitive disorders, dizziness, drowsiness, fatigue, impaired concentration/memory, nervousness, paresthesia, psychomotor slowing, sedation, speech problems, aggression, agitation, anxiety, confusion, depression, encephalopathy, malaise, mood problems, SEIZURES, SUICIDAL THOUGHTS/BEHAVIORS, tremor. **Misc:** fever.

Interactions

Drug-Drug: Alcohol use within 6 hr before or after use of Trokendi XR may significantly alter topiramate levels; use during this time frame contraindicated. **Phenytoin**, **carbamazepine**, or **valproic acid** may ↓ levels and effectiveness. May ↑ levels and risk of toxicity of **phenytoin**, **amitriptyline**, or **lithium**. May ↓ levels and effectiveness of **hormonal contraceptives**, **risperidone**, or **valproic acid**. ↑ risk of CNS depression with **alcohol** or other **CNS depressants**. **Carbonic anhydrase inhibitors** (e.g., **acetazolamide** or **zonisamide**) may ↑ risk of metabolic acidosis and kidney stones. **Valproic acid** may ↑ risk of hyperammonemia, encephalopathy, and hypothermia. ↑ risk of bleeding with **aspirin**, **clopidogrel**, **ticagrelor**,

prasugrel, **warfarin**, **dabigatran**, **rivaroxaban**, **apixaban**, **edoxaban**, **NSAIDs**, or **SSRIs**.

Route/Dosage

Epilepsy (monotherapy)

PO (Adults and Children ≥10 yr): *Immediate release:* 25 mg twice daily initially; gradually ↑ at weekly intervals to 200 mg twice daily over a 6-wk period; *Extended release (Qudexy XR or Trokendi XR):* 50 mg once daily initially; gradually ↑ at weekly intervals to 400 mg once daily over a 6-wk period.

PO (Children 2–<10 yr [6–<10 yr for Trokendi XR] and >38 kg): *Immediate release:* 25 mg once daily in the evening initially, gradually ↑ at weekly intervals to 125 mg twice daily over a 5–7-wk period; if needed may continue to titrate dose on a weekly basis up to 200 mg twice daily; *Extended release (Qudexy XR or Trokendi XR):* 25 mg once daily for 1 wk; then ↑ to 50 mg once daily for 1 wk; then ↑ by 25–50 mg/day at weekly intervals over a 5–7-wk period to target dose of 250–400 mg once daily.

PO (Children 2–<10 yr [6–<10 yr for Trokendi XR] and 32–38 kg): *Immediate release:* 25 mg once daily in the evening initially; gradually ↑ at weekly intervals to 125 mg twice daily over a 5–7-wk period; if needed, may continue to titrate dose on a weekly basis up to 175 mg twice daily; *Extended release (Qudexy XR or Trokendi XR):* 25 mg once daily for 1 wk; then ↑ to 50 mg once daily for 1 wk; then ↑ by 25–50 mg/day at weekly intervals over a 5–7-wk period to target dose of 250–350 mg once daily.

PO (Children 2–<10 yr [6–<10 yr for Trokendi XR] and 23–31 kg): *Immediate release:* 25 mg once daily in the evening initially; gradually ↑ at weekly intervals to 100 mg twice daily over a 5–7-wk period; if needed, may continue to titrate dose on a weekly basis up to 175 mg twice daily; *Extended release (Qudexy XR or Trokendi XR):* 25 mg once daily for 1 wk; then ↑ to 50 mg once daily for 1 wk; then ↑ by 25–50 mg/day at weekly intervals over a 5–7-wk period to target dose of 200–350 mg once daily.

PO (Children 2–<10 yr [6–<10 yr for Trokendi XR] and 12–22 kg): *Immediate release:* 25 mg once daily in the evening initially; gradually ↑ at weekly intervals to 100 mg twice daily over a 5–7-wk period; if needed, may continue to titrate dose on a weekly basis up to 150 mg twice daily; *Extended release (Qudexy XR or Trokendi XR):* 25 mg once daily for 1 wk; then ↑ to 50 mg once daily for 1 wk; then ↑ by 25–50 mg/day at weekly intervals over a 5–7-wk period to target dose of 200–300 mg once daily.

PO (Children 2–<10 yr [6–<10 yr for Trokendi XR] and ≤11 kg): *Immediate release:* 25 mg once daily in the evening initially; gradually ↑ at weekly intervals to 75 mg twice daily over a 5–7-wk period; if needed, may continue to titrate dose on a weekly basis up to 125 mg twice daily; *Extended release (Qudexy XR or Trokendi XR):* 25 mg once daily for 1 wk; then ↑ to 50 mg once daily for 1 wk; then ↑ by 25–50 mg/day at weekly intervals over a 5–7-wk period to target dose of 150–250 mg once daily.

Renal Impairment

PO (Adults): *CCr <70 mL/min:* ↓ dose by 50%.

Epilepsy (adjunctive therapy)

PO (Adults and Children ≥17 yr): *Immediate release:* 25–50 mg/day initially; ↑ by 25–50 mg/day at weekly intervals up to 200–400 mg/day in 2 divided doses (200–400 mg/day in 2 divided doses for partial seizures or Lennox-Gastaut syndrome and 400 mg/day in 2 divided doses for primary generalized tonic-clonic seizures); *Extended release (Qudexy XR or Trokendi XR):* 25–50 mg once daily initially; ↑ by 25–50 mg/day at weekly intervals up to 200–400 mg once daily (for partial seizures or Lennox-Gastaut syndrome) and 400 mg once daily (for primary generalized tonic-clonic seizures).

PO (Children 2–16 yr): *Immediate release and extended release (Qudexy XR):* 25 mg once daily at night initially for first wk; ↑ at 1–2 wk intervals by 1–3 mg/kg/day up to 5–9 mg/kg/day in 2 divided doses.

PO (Children 6–16 yr): *Extended release (Trokendi XR):* 25 mg once daily at night initially for first wk; ↑ at 1–2 wk intervals by 1–3 mg/kg/day up to 5–9 mg/kg/day given once daily at night.

Renal Impairment

PO (Adults): *CCr <70 mL/min:* ↓ dose by 50%.

Migraine Prevention

PO (Adults and Children ≥12 yr): *Immediate release:* 25 mg at night initially; ↑ by 25 mg/day at weekly intervals up to target dose of 100 mg/day in 2 divided doses; *Extended release (Qudexy XR):* 25 mg once daily initially; ↑ by 25 mg/day at weekly intervals up to target dose of 100 mg once daily.

Renal Impairment

PO (Adults): *CCr <70 mL/min:* ↓ dose by 50%.

Availability (generic available)

Immediate-release tablets: 25 mg, 50 mg, 100 mg, 200 mg. **Extended-release capsules (Qudexy XR):** 25 mg, 50 mg, 100 mg, 150 mg, 200 mg. **Extended-release capsules (Trokendi XR):** 25 mg, 50 mg, 100 mg, 200 mg. **Oral solution (Eprontia) (mixed berry flavor):** 25 mg/mL. **Sprinkle capsules:** 15 mg, 25 mg. ***In combination with:*** phentermine (Qsymia). See Appendix N.

T

NURSING IMPLICATIONS

Assessment

- Monitor closely for notable changes in behavior that could indicate the emergence or worsening of suicidal thoughts or behavior or depression.
- Pedi: Monitor growth rate (height and weight) in children; may have negative effects on height and weight.
- **Seizures:** Assess location, duration, and characteristics of seizure activity. Implement seizure precautions if indicated.
- **Migraines:** Assess pain location, intensity, duration, and associated symptoms (photophobia, phonophobia, nausea, vomiting) during migraine attack. Monitor frequency and intensity of pain on pain scale.
- **Bipolar Disorder:** Assess mental status (mood, orientation, behavior) and cognitive abilities before and periodically during therapy.

Lab Test Considerations

- Monitor CBC with differential before starting and periodically during therapy. Frequently causes anemia.
- May ↑ AST and ALT. Monitor periodically during therapy.
- Evaluate serum bicarbonate before starting and periodically during therapy. Monitor for signs/symptoms of metabolic acidosis (hyperventilation, fatigue, anorexia, cardiac arrhythmias, stupor). If metabolic acidosis occurs, dosing taper or discontinuation may be necessary.

Implementation

- Do not confuse Topamax with Toprol XL.
- **PO:** Administer with or without food.
- ***DNC:*** Do not break/crush tablets because of bitter taste.
- Contents of the sprinkle capsules can be sprinkled on a small amount (5 mL) of soft food, such as applesauce, custard, ice cream, oatmeal, pudding, or yogurt. To open, hold the capsule upright so the word "TOP" is visible and readable. Carefully twist off the clear portion of the capsule. Can be opened over the small portion of the food. Sprinkle the entire contents of the capsule onto the food. Be sure the patient swallows the entire spoonful of the sprinkle/food mixture immediately without chewing. Follow with fluids immediately to make sure all of the mixture is swallowed. Never store a sprinkle/food mixture for use at another time.
- ***DNC:*** Swallow extended-release capsules *(Trokendi XR)* whole; do not sprinkle on food, break, crush, dissolve, or chew.
- ***DNC:*** Swallow extended-release capsules *(Qudexy XR)* whole; may be opened and sprinkled on soft food; do not crush or chew. Swallow immediately; do not save for later.

Patient/Family Teaching

- Explain purpose and side effects of medication to patient. Advise to read *Patient Information* before starting therapy. Instruct to take exactly as directed. Take missed doses as soon as possible but not just before next dose; do not double doses. Notify health care provider if >1 dose is missed. Medication should be gradually discontinued to prevent seizures and status epilepticus.
- Advise patient to notify health care provider of all Rx or OTC medications, vitamins, or herbal products being taken and to consult health care provider before taking other medications.
- May ↓ sweating and ↑ body temperature. Advise patient, especially caregivers/parents, to provide adequate hydration and monitoring, especially during hot weather.
- May cause dizziness, drowsiness, confusion, and difficulty concentrating. Caution patients to avoid driving or other activities requiring alertness until response to medication is known.
- Advise patient to maintain a fluid intake of 2000–3000 mL/day to prevent the formation of kidney stones.
- Instruct patient to notify health care provider immediately if periorbital pain or blurred vision occur. Medication should be discontinued if ocular symptoms occur. May lead to permanent loss of vision.
- Advise patient and caregivers/family to notify health care provider if thoughts about suicide or dying, attempts to commit suicide, new or worse depression, new or worse anxiety, feeling very agitated or restless, panic attacks, trouble sleeping, new or worse irritability, acting aggressive, being angry or violent, acting on dangerous impulses, an extreme increase in activity and talking, other unusual changes in behavior or mood, or rash occur.
- Inform patient that topiramate may cause encephalopathy. If signs/symptoms (unexplained lethargy, vomiting, changes in mental status) occur, notify health care provider.
- Caution patient to make position changes slowly to minimize orthostatic hypotension.
- Advise patient not to take alcohol or other CNS depressants concurrently with this medication. Avoid alcohol 6 hr before and after taking *Trokendi XR*.
- Instruct patient to notify health care provider of medication regimen before treatment or surgery.
- Advise patient to use sunscreen and wear protective clothing to prevent photosensitivity reactions.
- Advise patient to carry identification describing disease and medication regimen at all times.
- Rep: May cause fetal harm. Infants exposed to topiramate during pregnancy are at ↑ risk for cleft lip and/or cleft palate and for being small for gestational age. Advise women of reproductive potential to use a nonhormonal form of contraception while taking

topiramate; may make hormonal contraceptives less effective. Advise women of reproductive potential to notify health care provider if pregnancy is planned or suspected or if breastfeeding. If pregnancy occurs, encourage patient to enroll in the North American Drug Pregnancy Registry by calling 1-888-233-2334 or visiting https://www.aedpregnancyregistry.org/.

Evaluation/Desired Outcomes

- Decreased incidence of seizures.
- Decreased incidence/severity of migraine headache.

HIGH ALERT

topotecan (toe-poe-**tee**-kan)

Hycamtin

Classification

Therapeutic: antineoplastics

Pharmacologic: enzyme inhibitors

Indications

IV: Metastatic ovarian cancer that has not responded to previous chemotherapy. Small cell lung cancer unresponsive to first line therapy. Stage IV-B persistent or recurrent cervical cancer not amenable to treatment with surgery or radiation (with cisplatin). **PO:** Relapsed small cell lung cancer in patients with a complete or partial prior response and who are ≥45 days from the end of first-line chemotherapy.

Action

Interferes with DNA synthesis by inhibiting the enzyme topoisomerase. **Therapeutic Effects:** Death of rapidly replicating cells, particularly malignant ones.

Pharmacokinetics

Absorption: IV administration results in complete bioavailability. 40% absorbed following oral administration.

Distribution: Well distributed to tissues.

Metabolism and Excretion: Small amounts metabolized by the liver. 18–33% excreted in feces; 20–50% excreted in urine (primarily as metabolites).

Half-life: *PO:* 3–6 hr; *IV:* 2–3 hr.

TIME/ACTION PROFILE (effects on WBCs)

ROUTE	ONSET	PEAK	DURATION
PO	unknown	1–2 hr	24 hr
IV	within days	11 days	7 days

Contraindications/Precautions

Contraindicated in: Hypersensitivity; OB: Pregnancy; Lactation: Lactation.

Use Cautiously in: Renal impairment (↓ dose if CCr <40 mL/min); Platelet count <25,000 cells/mm³ (↓ dose); History of interstitial lung disease (ILD), pulmonary fibrosis, lung cancer, thoracic radiation, or use of pneumotoxic drugs or colony stimulating factors; Rep: Women of reproductive potential; Geri: Older adults may require dose ↓ due to age-related ↓ in renal function.

Adverse Reactions/Side Effects

Derm: alopecia. **GI:** abdominal pain, diarrhea, nausea, vomiting, ↑ liver enzymes, anorexia, constipation, stomatitis. **Hemat:** ANEMIA, NEUTROPENIA, THROMBOCYTOPENIA. **MS:** arthralgia. **Neuro:** headache, fatigue, weakness. **Resp:** dyspnea, ILD.

Interactions

Drug-Drug: P-glycoprotein inhibitors, including **amiodarone**, **azithromycin**, **captopril**, **carvedilol**, **clarithromycin**, **conivaptan**, **cyclosporine**, **diltiazem**, **dronedarone**, **erythromycin**, **felodipine**, **itraconazole**, **ketoconazole**, **lopinavir**, **ritonavir**, **quinidine**, **ranolazine**, **ticagrelor**, or **verapamil**, may ↑ levels and risk of toxicity; avoid concurrent use. Neutropenia is prolonged by concurrent use of **filgrastim**; do not use filgrastim until day 6, 24 hr following completion of topotecan. ↑ myelosuppression with other **antineoplastics** (especially **cisplatin**) or **radiation therapy**. May ↓ antibody response to and ↑ risk of adverse reactions from **live-virus vaccines**.

Route/Dosage

PO (Adults): 2.3 mg/m²/day for 5 days starting on Day 1 of a 21-day course (round calculated oral dose to nearest 0.25 mg and prescribe the minimum number of 1 mg and 0.25 mg capsules with the same number of capsules prescribed for each of the 5 days).

IV (Adults): *Ovarian and Small Cell Lung Cancer:* 1.5 mg/m²/day for 5 days starting on Day 1 of a 21-day course; *Cervical Cancer:* 75 mg/m² on Days 1, 2, and 3 followed by cisplatin on Day 1 and repeated every 21 days.

Renal Impairment

PO (Adults): *CCr 30–49 mL/min:* 1.5 mg/m²/day for 5 days starting on Day 1 of a 21-day course; may ↑ dose after 1st course by 0.4 mg/m²/day if no severe hematologic or GI toxicities occur; *CCr <30 mL/min:* 0.6 mg/m²/day for 5 days starting on Day 1 of a 21-day course; may ↑ dose after 1st course by 0.4 mg/m²/day if no severe hematologic or GI toxicities occur.

Renal Impairment

IV (Adults): *CCr 20–39 mL/min:* 0.75 mg/m²/day for 5 days starting on Day 1 of a 21-day course; *Cervical Cancer:* Administer at standard doses only if serum creatinine ≤1.5 mg/dL; do not administer if serum creatinine >1.5 mg/dL.

Availability (generic available)

Capsules: 0.25 mg, 1 mg. **Powder for injection:** 4 mg/vial. **Solution for injection:** 1 mg/mL.

NURSING IMPLICATIONS

Assessment

- Monitor vital signs frequently during administration.
- Monitor for bone marrow depression. Assess for bleeding (bleeding gums; bruising; petechiae; guaiac stools, urine, and emesis) and avoid IM injections and taking rectal temperatures if platelet count is low. Apply pressure to venipuncture sites for 10 min. Assess for signs of infection during neutropenia. Anemia may occur. Monitor for ↑ fatigue, dyspnea, and orthostatic hypotension.
- Nausea and vomiting are common. Pretreatment with antiemetics should be considered.
- Monitor for signs/symptoms of ILD (cough, fever, dyspnea, hypoxia). *If ILD confirmed,* discontinue topotecan.

Lab Test Considerations

- Verify negative pregnancy test before starting therapy.
- Monitor CBC with differential and platelet count before administration and frequently during therapy. Baseline neutrophil count ≥1500 cells/mm³ and platelet count ≥100,000 cells/mm³ are required before 1st dose. The nadir of neutropenia occurs in 11 days, with a duration of 7 days. The nadir of thrombocytopenia occurs in 15 days, with a duration of 5 days. The nadir of anemia occurs in 15 days. Subsequent doses should not be administered until neutrophils recover to >1000 cells/mm³, platelets recover to >100,000 cells/mm³, and hemoglobin levels recover to 9 g/dL. ***Topotecan monotherapy:*** *If neutrophils <500 cells/mm³ or platelets <25,000 cells/mm³,* ↓ dose to 1.25 mg/m² or administer granulocyte-colony stimulating factor (G-CSF) starting no sooner than 24 hr following the last dose (specifically for neutropenia). ***When topotecan used with cisplatin:*** *If febrile neutropenia (neutrophils <1000 cells/mm³ with temperature of ≥100.4°F or platelets <25,000 cells/mm³,* ↓ dose to 0.6 mg/m² (and to 0.45 mg/m² if necessary) or administer G-CSF starting no sooner than 24 hr following the last dose (specifically for neutropenia).
- Monitor liver function. May ↑ AST, ALT, and bilirubin.

Implementation

- ***High Alert:*** Check dose carefully before administration.
- **PO:** Administer with or without food. ***DNC:*** Swallow capsules whole; do not open, crush, or chew. If vomiting occurs after taking dose, do not replace dose.
- Do not administer capsules to patients with Grade 3 or 4 diarrhea. When recovered to Grade ≤1, resume with dose ↓ by 0.4 mg/m²/day for subsequent courses.

IV Administration

- Wear gloves, gown, and mask while handling IV medication. Discard IV equipment in specially designated containers.
- Topotecan is an irritant. If extravasation occurs, immediately stop infusion. Leave needle/cannula in place temporarily but do not flush the line. Gently aspirate extravasated solution; then remove needle/cannula. Elevate patient's extremity and apply dry cold compresses for 20 min 4 times day for 1–2 days.
- **Intermittent Infusion: Reconstitution:** Reconstitute each vial with 4 mL of sterile water for injection. **Dilution:** Dilute further in D5W or 0.9% NaCl. Infusion is stable for 24 hr at room temperature or up to 7 days if refrigerated. Solution is yellow to yellow-green. **Concentration:** 10–50 mcg/mL. **Rate:** Infuse over 30 min.
- **Y-Site Compatibility:** alemtuzumab, amikacin, amiodarone, anidulafungin, argatroban, aztreonam, bivalirudin, buprenorphine, butorphanol, calcium chloride, carboplatin, caspofungin, cefazolin, cefotaxime, cefotetan, cefoxitin, ceftriaxone, cefuroxime, chloramphenicol, chlorpromazine, ciprofloxacin, cisatracurium, cisplatin, cyclophosphamide, cyclosporine, dacarbazine, dactinomycin, daptomycin, daunorubicin, dexmedetomidine, dexrazoxane, diltiazem, diphenhydramine, dobutamine, docetaxel, dopamine, doxorubicin hydrochloride, doxorubicin liposomal, doxycycline, droperidol, enalaprilat, ephedrine, epinephrine, erythromycin, esmolol, etoposide, etoposide phosphate, famotidine, fentanyl, fluconazole, fludarabine, furosemide, gemcitabine, gemtuzumab ozogamicin, gentamicin, glycopyrrolate, granisetron, haloperidol, heparin, hetastarch, hydralazine, hydrocortisone, hydromorphone, idarubicin, ifosfamide, insulin regular, isoproterenol, labetalol, leucovorin, levofloxacin, lidocaine, linezolid, lorazepam, magnesium sulfate, mannitol, meperidine, mesna, methadone, methylprednisolone, metoclopramide, metoprolol, metronidazole, midazolam, milrinone, minocycline, mitoxantrone, morphine, moxifloxacin, nalbuphine, naloxone, nitroglycerin, nitroprusside, norepinephrine, octreotide, ondansetron, oxaliplatin, paclitaxel, palonosetron, pamidronate, pentamidine, phenylephrine, potassium chloride, procainamide, prochlorperazine, promethazine, propranolol, remifentanil, succinylcholine, sufentanil, tacrolimus, theophylline, thiotepa, tigecycline, tirofiban, tobramycin, vancomycin, vasopressin, vecuronium, verapamil, vinblastine,

vincristine, vinorelbine, voriconazole, zidovudine, zoledronic acid.
- **Y-Site Incompatibility:** acyclovir, allopurinol, aminophylline, amphotericin B deoxycholate, ampicillin, ampicillin/sulbactam, bumetanide, calcium gluconate, cefepime, ceftazidime, clindamycin, dantrolene, dexamethasone, diazepam, digoxin, ertapenem, fluorouracil, foscarnet, fosphenytoin, ganciclovir, hydrocortisone, imipenem/cilastatin, ketorolac, meropenem, methohexital, mitomycin, nafcillin, pantoprazole, pemetrexed, pentobarbital, phenobarbital, phenytoin, piperacillin/tazobactam, potassium acetate, potassium phosphates, rituximab, sodium bicarbonate, sodium phosphates, trastuzumab, trimethoprim/sulfamethoxazole.

Patient/Family Teaching
- Explain purpose and side effects of medication to patient. Advise to read *Patient Information* before starting therapy. Instruct patient to take as directed. If vomiting occurs after taking, do not replace dose; notify health care provider. Do not take missed doses; take next scheduled dose and notify health care provider. If any capsules are broken or leaking, do not touch with bare hands; dispose of capsules and wash hands with soap and water.
- Advise patient to notify health care provider of all Rx or OTC medications, vitamins, or herbal products being taken and to consult health care provider before taking other medications.
- May cause drowsiness or sleepiness during and for several days after therapy. Caution patient to avoid driving and other activities requiring alertness until response to medication is known.
- Advise patient to notify health care provider if fever; chills; sore throat; signs of infection; bleeding gums; bruising; petechiae; blood in urine, stool, or emesis; or signs and symptoms of interstitial lung disease occur. Caution patient to avoid crowds and persons with known infections. Instruct patient to use soft toothbrush and electric razor. Patient should be cautioned not to drink alcoholic beverages or take products containing aspirin or NSAIDs.
- May cause diarrhea. Advise patient to notify health care provider if diarrhea with fever, stomach pain, or cramps or for diarrhea that occurs >3 times/day.
- Discuss with patient the possibility of hair loss. Explore methods of coping.
- Instruct patient not to receive any vaccinations without advice of health care provider.
- Rep: May cause fetal harm. Advise women of reproductive potential to use effective contraception during therapy and for 6 mo after last

dose and to avoid breastfeeding during therapy and for 1 wk after last dose. Advise men with female partners of reproductive potential to use effective contraception during therapy and for 3 mo after last dose. May impair fertility in men and women.

Evaluation/Desired Outcomes
- Death of rapidly replicating cells, particularly malignant ones.

torsemide, See DIURETICS (LOOP).

| | BEERS | REMS | HIGH ALERT |

☒ **traMADol** (tra-ma-dol)
ConZip, ✦ Durela, ✦ Ralivia, ✦ Tridural, ~~Ultram, Ultram ER,~~ ✦ Zytram XL
Classification
Therapeutic: analgesics (centrally acting), opioid analgesics
Pharmacologic: opioid agonists

Schedule IV

Indications
Moderate to moderately severe pain (extended-release formulations indicated for patients who require around-the-clock pain management).

Action
Acts as a mu-opioid receptor agonist. Inhibits reuptake of serotonin and norepinephrine in the CNS. **Therapeutic Effects:** Decreased pain.

Pharmacokinetics
Absorption: *Immediate release:* 75% absorbed after oral administration; *Extended release:* 85–90% (compared with immediate release).
Distribution: Widely distributed to tissues.
Metabolism and Excretion: ☒ Mostly metabolized by the liver (primarily by the CYP2D6 and CYP3A4 isoenzymes); primarily metabolized by the CYP2D6 isoenzyme to active metabolite with analgesic activity (M1); CYP2D6 enzyme system exhibits genetic polymorphism; 7% of population may be poor metabolizers and may have significantly ↑ concentrations of tramadol and ↓ concentrations of M1 metabolite. 1–10% of White patients, 3–4% of Black patients, and 1–2% of East Asian patients may be CYP2D6 ultra-rapid metabolizers and have significantly ↑ concentrations of M1 metabolite. 30% eliminated unchanged in the urine.

Half-life: *Tramadol (immediate release):* 6–8 hr, *Extended release:* 7.9 hr; *Active metabolite:* 7–9 hr; both are ↑ in renal or hepatic impairment.

TIME/ACTION PROFILE (analgesia)

ROUTE	ONSET	PEAK	DURATION
PO–immediate release	1 hr	2–3 hr	4–6 hr
PO–extended release	unknown	12 hr	24 hr

Contraindications/Precautions

Contraindicated in: Hypersensitivity; Cross-sensitivity with opioids may occur; Significant respiratory depression; Acute or severe bronchial asthma (in unmonitored setting or in absence of resuscitative equipment); Known or suspected GI obstruction (including paralytic ileus); Concurrent use of MAO inhibitors (or use within the past 14 days); Patients who are acutely intoxicated with alcohol, sedatives/hypnotics, centrally acting analgesics, opioid analgesics, or psychotropic agents; Patients who are physically dependent on opioid analgesics (may precipitate withdrawal); Ultra-rapid metabolizers of CYP2D6 (↑ risk of respiratory depression and death); Severe renal impairment (extended release); Hepatic impairment (extended release). Lactation: Lactation; Pedi: Children <12 yr, children <18 yr following tonsillectomy and/or adenoidectomy, and children 12–18 yr who are postoperative; have obstructive sleep apnea, obesity, severe pulmonary disease, or neuromuscular disease; or are taking other medications that cause respiratory depression (↑ risk of respiratory depression and death).

Use Cautiously in: Personal or family history of substance use disorder or mental illness; History of epilepsy or risk factors for seizures; Diabetes mellitus (↑ risk of hypoglycemia); Severe renal impairment (immediate release) (↑ dosing interval); Hepatic impairment (immediate release) (↑ dosing interval in patients with cirrhosis); Suicidal or prone to addiction (↑ risk of suicide); Excessive use of alcohol (↑ risk of suicide); ↑ intracranial pressure or head trauma; OB: Use during pregnancy only if potential maternal benefit justifies potential fetal risk. Chronic maternal treatment with opioids during pregnancy may result in neonatal opioid withdrawal syndrome; Geri: Appears on Beers list. May worsen or cause hyponatremia in older adults. Use with caution in older adults and monitor sodium concentrations closely when initiating therapy or ↑ the dose. Use extended-release formulation with extreme caution in patients >75 yr.

Adverse Reactions/Side Effects

Derm: pruritus, sweating. **EENT:** visual disturbances. **Endo:** hypoglycemia. **F and E:** hyponatremia. **GI:** constipation, nausea, abdominal pain, anorexia, diarrhea, dry mouth, dyspepsia, flatulence, vomiting. **GU:** ↓ fertility, menopausal symptoms, urinary retention/frequency. **Neuro:** dizziness, headache, somnolence, anxiety, confusion, coordination disturbance, euphoria, hypertonia, malaise, nervousness, SEIZURES, sleep disorder, stimulation, weakness. **Resp:** RESPIRATORY DEPRESSION (INCLUDING CENTRAL SLEEP APNEA AND SLEEP-RELATED HYPOXEMIA). **Misc:** allodynia, opioid-induced hyperalgesia, physical dependence, psychological dependence, tolerance.

Interactions

Drug-Drug: **MAO inhibitors** ↑ risk of adverse reactions; concurrent use or use within previous 14 days contraindicated. Use with **benzodiazepines** or other **CNS depressants**, including other **opioids**, **nonbenzodiazepine sedative/hypnotics**, **anxiolytics**, **general anesthetics**, **muscle relaxants**, **antipsychotics**, and **alcohol**, may cause profound sedation, respiratory depression, coma, and death; reserve concurrent use for when alternative treatment options are inadequate. **Mixed agonist/antagonist analgesics**, including **nalbuphine** or **butorphanol**, and **partial agonist analgesics**, including **buprenorphine**, may ↓ tramadol's analgesic effects and/or precipitate opioid withdrawal in physically dependent patients. ↑ risk of seizures with high doses of **penicillins**, **cephalosporins**, **phenothiazines**, **opioid analgesics**, or **antidepressants**. **CYP2D6 inhibitors**, including **quinidine**, **fluoxetine**, **paroxetine**, and **bupropion**, may ↓ levels of active metabolite (M1) and lead to ↓ analgesic effects. **CYP3A4 inhibitors**, including **erythromycin**, **clarithromycin**, **ketoconazole**, **itraconazole**, and **protease inhibitors**, may allow for a greater degree of metabolism via CYP2D6 and ↑ levels of the active metabolite (M1), leading to respiratory depression. **CYP3A4 inducers** may ↓ levels and effectiveness. Drugs that affect serotonergic neurotransmitter systems, including **SSRIs**, **SNRIs**, **MAO inhibitors**, **TCAs**, **trazodone**, **mirtazapine**, **5-HT$_3$ receptor antagonists**, **linezolid**, **methylene blue**, and **triptans**, may ↑ risk of serotonin syndrome.

Drug-Natural Products: **Kava-kava**, **valerian**, or **chamomile** can ↑ risk of CNS depression. ↑ risk of serotonin syndrome with **St. John's wort**.

Route/Dosage

Immediate Release

PO (Adults ≥18 yr): *Rapid titration:* 50–100 mg every 4–6 hr (not to exceed 400 mg/day [300 mg in patients >75 yr]). *Gradual titration:* 25 mg/day initially; ↑ by 25 mg/day every 3 days to reach dose of 25 mg 4 times daily; then ↑ by 50 mg/day every 3 days to reach dose of 50 mg 4 times daily; may then use 50–100 mg every 4–6 hr (maximum dose = 400 mg/day).

Renal Impairment

PO (Adults): *CCr <30 mL/min:* ↑ dosing interval to every 12 hr (not to exceed 200 mg/day).

Hepatic Impairment

PO (Adults): *Severe hepatic impairment:* 50 mg every 12 hr.

Extended Release

PO (Adults): *Not currently receiving immediate release:* 100 mg once daily initially; may then titrate every 5 days up to 300 mg/day; *Currently receiving immediate release:* Calculate 24-hr total dose of immediate-release product and give same dose (rounded down to next lowest 100-mg increment) of ER once daily (maximum dose = 300 mg/day).

Availability (generic available)

Immediate-release tablets: 25 mg, 50 mg, 100 mg. **Extended-release capsules (Conzip):** 100 mg, 200 mg, 300 mg. **Extended-release tablets:** ✱ 75 mg, 100 mg ✱ 150 mg, 200 mg, 300 mg ✱ 400 mg. **Oral solution (grape flavor):** 5 mg/mL. ***In combination with:*** acetaminophen (generic only).

NURSING IMPLICATIONS

Assessment

- Assess type, location, and intensity of pain before and 2–3 hr (peak) after administration.
- Monitor BP at start of and periodically during therapy; hypotension can occur in patients with compromised ability to maintain BP.
- Assess respiratory rate and level of consciousness before and periodically during administration. Observe closely for signs of sedation and respiratory depression, especially when converting from immediate-release to extended-release formulations.
- Assess bowel function routinely. Prevention of constipation should be instituted with ↑ intake of fluids and bulk and with laxatives to minimize constipating effects. Administer stimulant laxatives routinely if opioid use exceeds 2–3 days, unless contraindicated. Consider drugs for opioid-induced constipation.
- Prolonged use may lead to physical and psychological dependence and tolerance, although these may be milder than with other opioids. This should not prevent patient from receiving adequate analgesia. Patients who receive tramadol for pain rarely develop psychological dependence. If tolerance develops, changing to an opioid agonist may be required to relieve pain. Prolonged use of opioids should be reserved for patients whose pain remains severe enough to require them and for whom alternative treatment options continue to be inadequate. Many acute pain conditions treated in the outpatient setting require no more than a few days of an opioid pain medicine.
- Monitor for signs/symptoms of hyponatremia (confusion, disorientation) during therapy, especially during early therapy and with older adults. *If signs and symptoms of hyponatremia occur,* begin treatment (fluid restriction) and discontinue tramadol.
- Monitor patient for seizures. May occur within recommended dose range. Risk is ↑ with higher doses and in patients taking antidepressants (SSRIs, SNRIs, TCAs, MAO inhibitors), opioid analgesics, or other drugs that ↓ the seizure threshold. Also monitor for serotonin syndrome (mental status changes [agitation, hallucinations, coma], autonomic instability [tachycardia, labile BP, hyperthermia], neuromuscular aberrations [hyperreflexia, incoordination], GI symptoms [nausea, vomiting, diarrhea]) in patients taking these drugs concurrently.
- Assess risk for opioid addiction, abuse, or misuse prior to administration. Abuse or misuse of extended-release preparations by crushing, chewing, snorting, or injecting dissolved product will result in uncontrolled delivery of tramadol and can result in overdose and death.

Lab Test Considerations

- May cause ↑ serum creatinine, ↑ liver enzymes, ↓ hemoglobin, and proteinuria.
- May cause hypoglycemia. Monitor blood glucose in patients with predisposing risk factors, including diabetes or renal impairment.
- May cause hyponatremia. Geri: Monitor sodium levels regularly when initiating therapy, ↑ the dose, or using extended-release formulation with older adults, especially >75 yr.

Toxicity and Overdose

- Overdose may cause respiratory depression and seizures. Naloxone may reverse some but not all of the symptoms of overdose. Treatment should be symptomatic and supportive. Maintain adequate respiratory exchange. Hemodialysis is not helpful because it removes only a small portion of administered dose. Seizures may be managed with barbiturates or benzodiazepines; naloxone ↑ risk of seizures.

Implementation

- ***High Alert:*** Do not confuse tramadol with trazodone.
- Tramadol is considered to provide more analgesia than codeine 60 mg but less than combined aspirin 650 mg/codeine 60 mg for acute postoperative pain.
- For chronic pain, daily doses of 250 mg of tramadol provide pain relief similar to that of 5 doses/day of acetaminophen 300 mg/codeine 30 mg, 5 doses/day

T

of aspirin 325 mg/codeine 30 mg, or 2–3 doses/day of acetaminophen 500 mg/oxycodone 5 mg.

- Explain therapeutic value of medication before administration to enhance the analgesic effect.
- Regularly administered doses may be more effective than as-needed administration. Analgesic is more effective if given before pain becomes severe.
- Initiate treatment at the lowest dose necessary to achieve adequate analgesia. Titrate the dose based upon the individual patient's response.
- Extended release: If converting from other opioids, discontinue all other around-the-clock opioid drugs; no established conversion ratios are defined. It is safer to underestimate a patient's 24-hr tramadol requirements and provide rescue medication (e.g., immediate-release opioid) than to overestimate the 24-hr tramadol dosage and manage an adverse reaction due to an overdose.
- Tramadol should be discontinued gradually after long-term use to prevent withdrawal symptoms. For patients on long-acting agents who are physically opioid-dependent, initiate the taper by a small enough increment (no greater than 10–25% of total daily dose) to avoid withdrawal symptoms, and proceed with dose-lowering at an interval of every 2–4 wk. Patients who have been taking opioids for briefer periods of time may tolerate a more rapid taper. Monitor frequently to manage pain and withdrawal symptoms (restlessness; lacrimation; rhinorrhea; yawning; perspiration; chills; myalgia; mydriasis; irritability; anxiety; backache; joint pain; weakness; abdominal cramps; insomnia; nausea; anorexia; vomiting; diarrhea; ↑ BP, respiratory rate, or HR). If withdrawal symptoms occur, pause the taper for a period of time or ↑ the dose of opioid analgesic to the previous dose, and then proceed with a slower taper. Also, monitor patients for changes in mood, emergence of suicidal thoughts, or use of other substances. A multimodal approach to pain management may optimize the treatment of chronic pain and assist with the successful tapering of the opioid analgesic.
- **PO:** Tramadol may be administered without regard to meals. ***DNC:*** Swallow extended-release tablets and capsules whole; do not crush, break, dissolve, or chew. When administering oral solution, use a calibrated oral syringe or other dosing device with metric units of measurements to correctly measure the prescribed amount of medication.
- ***REMS:*** FDA strongly encourages health care providers to complete a REMS-compliant education program that includes all the elements of the FDA Education *Blueprint for Health Care Providers Involved in the Management or Support of Patients with Pain,* available at www.fda.gov/OpioidAnalgesicREMSBlueprint. Information on programs can be found at 1-800-503-0784 or www.opioidanalgesicrems.com.
- Discuss availability of naloxone for emergency treatment of opioid overdose with the patient and caregiver and assess the potential need for access to naloxone, both when initiating and renewing therapy, especially if patient has household members (including children) or other close contacts at risk for accidental exposure or overdose. Consider prescribing naloxone, based on the patient's risk factors for overdose, such as concurrent use of CNS depressants, a history of opioid use disorder, or prior opioid overdose. However, the presence of risk factors for overdose should not prevent the proper management of pain in any patient.

Patient/Family Teaching

- ***REMS:*** Explain purpose and side effects of tramadol to patient. Instruct them to take medication as directed and when to ask for pain medication. Never use household teaspoons or tablespoons to measure dose for oral solution; always use a calibrated measuring device. Do not share medication with others, even if they have similar symptoms; may be harmful. Do not stop taking without discussing with health care provider; may cause withdrawal symptoms if discontinued abruptly after prolonged use. Do not ↑ doses without discussing with health care provider; may lead to overdose. Discuss safe use, risks, and proper storage and disposal of opioid analgesics with patients and caregivers with each Rx. The Patient Counseling Guide is available at https://opioidanalgesicrems.com/patientCounselingGuide.html Advise patient to read *Patient Information* before starting and with each Rx refill in case of changes.
- May cause dizziness and drowsiness. Caution patient to avoid driving or other activities requiring alertness until response to medication is known.
- Emphasize the importance of aggressive prevention of constipation with the use of tramadol.
- Advise patient that tramadol is a drug with known abuse potential. Protect it from theft, and never give to anyone other than the individual for whom it was prescribed. Store out of sight and reach of children and in a location not accessible by others.
- Educate patients and caregivers on how to recognize respiratory depression and emphasize the importance of calling 911 or getting emergency medical help right away in the event of a known or suspected overdose. Inform patients and caregivers about various ways to obtain naloxone as permitted by individual state naloxone dispensing and prescribing requirements or guidelines (Rx, direct from pharmacist, or state programs). OTC nasal spray is available at pharmacies nationwide for overdose or accidental ingestion.

- Advise patient to change positions slowly to minimize orthostatic hypotension.
- Caution patient to avoid concurrent use of alcohol or other CNS depressants, including other opioids, with this medication. Advise patient to notify health care provider before taking other RX, OTC, or herbal products concurrently.
- Advise patient to notify health care provider if seizures or if symptoms of serotonin syndrome (agitation, confusion, fever, elevated BP, rapid heartbeat, sweating, nausea, vomiting, loss of coordination) occur.
- Encourage patient to turn, cough, and breathe deeply every 2 hr to prevent atelectasis.
- Rep: Advise women of reproductive potential to notify health care provider if pregnancy is planned or suspected and to avoid breastfeeding during therapy. Inform patient of potential for neonatal opioid withdrawal syndrome with prolonged use during pregnancy. Monitor neonate for signs and symptoms of withdrawal symptoms (irritability, hyperactivity and abnormal sleep pattern, high-pitched cry, tremor, vomiting, diarrhea, failure to gain weight); usually occur the 1st days after birth. Monitor infants exposed to tramadol through breast milk for excess sedation and respiratory depression. Neonatal seizures, fetal death, and stillbirth have been reported with tramadol immediate-release products. Chronic use may ↓ fertility in men and women.

Evaluation/Desired Outcomes

- Decrease in severity of pain without a significant alteration in level of consciousness or respiratory status.

HIGH ALERT

trametinib (tra-me-ti-nib)

Mekinist

Classification

Therapeutic: antineoplastics

Pharmacologic: kinase inhibitors

Indications

Metastatic or unresectable melanoma with the BRAF V600E or V600K mutation (as monotherapy in patients who are BRAF-inhibitor treatment-naive or in combination with dabrafenib). Adjuvant treatment of melanoma with the BRAF V600E or V600K mutation (in combination with dabrafenib). Metastatic non-small cell lung cancer (NSCLC) with the BRAF V600E mutation (in combination with dabrafenib). Locally advanced or metastatic anaplastic thyroid cancer in patients with the BRAF V600E mutation who have no satisfactory locoregional treatment options (in combination with dabrafenib). Metastatic or unresectable solid tumors with the BRAF V600E mutation in patients who have progressed following prior treatment and have no satisfactory alternative treatment options (in combination with dabrafenib). Low-grade glioma with the BRAF V600E mutation in patients who require systemic therapy (in combination with dabrafenib).

Action

Inhibits the activity of kinases, enzymes that promote cellular proliferation. **Therapeutic Effects:** Improved progression-free survival and overall survival in melanoma. Decreased progression of NSCLC, anaplastic thyroid cancer, and solid tumors. Decreased progression of and improved progression-free survival in low-grade glioma.

Pharmacokinetics

Absorption: Well absorbed following oral administration.

Distribution: Unknown.

Protein Binding: 97.4%.

Metabolism and Excretion: 50% metabolized, 80% eliminated in feces (metabolites and parent compound), 20% excreted in urine (mostly as metabolites).

Half-life: 3.9–4.8 days.

TIME/ACTION PROFILE (response)

ROUTE	ONSET	PEAK	DURATION
PO	1 mo	2 mo	5–7 mo

Contraindications/Precautions

Contraindicated in: OB: Pregnancy; Lactation: Lactation.

Use Cautiously in: Severe renal impairment; Moderate or severe hepatic impairment; Rep: Women of reproductive potential and men with female partners of reproductive potential; Pedi: Safety and effectiveness not established in children <18 yr (melanoma, NSCLC, anaplastic thyroid cancer) or <1 yr (solid tumors or glioma).

Adverse Reactions/Side Effects

CV: CARDIOMYOPATHY, hypertension, DEEP VEIN THROMBOSIS (DVT). **Derm:** acneiform dermatitis, rash, cellulitis, DRUG REACTION WITH EOSINOPHILIA AND SYSTEMIC SYMPTOMS (DRESS), dry skin, erythema, folliculitis, palmar-plantar erythrodysesthesia syndrome, paronychia, photosensitivity, pruritus, STEVENS-JOHNSON SYNDROME. **EENT:** blurred vision, dry eye, retinal pigment epithelial detachment (RPED), retinal vein occlusion. **Endo:** hyperglycemia. **GI:** abdominal pain, diarrhea, ↑ liver enzymes, stomatitis, COLITIS, GI PERFORATION. **GU:** ↓ fertility (women). **Hemat:** BLEEDING, hemophagocytic lymphohistiocytosis. **MS:** rhabdomyolysis. **Neuro:** dizziness, dysgeusia, Guillain-Barré syndrome, INTRACRANIAL HEMORRHAGE, peripheral neuropathy. **Resp:**

T

INTERSTITIAL LUNG DISEASE (ILD), PULMONARY EMBOLISM (PE). **Misc:** fever (including serious febrile reactions), lymphedema, MALIGNANCY.

Interactions

Drug-Drug: None reported.

Route/Dosage

Unresectable/Metastatic Melanoma, Non-Small Cell Lung Cancer, or Anaplastic Thyroid Cancer

PO (Adults): 2 mg once daily; continue until disease progression or unacceptable toxicity.

Adjuvant Treatment of Unresectable/Metastatic Melanoma

PO (Adults): 2 mg once daily; continue until disease recurrence or unacceptable toxicity for up to 1 yr.

Unresectable/Metastatic Solid Tumors

PO (Adults): 2 mg once daily; continue until disease progression or unacceptable toxicity.

PO (Children ≥1 yr and ≥51 kg): 2 mg once daily; continue until disease progression or unacceptable toxicity.

PO (Children ≥1 yr and 38–50 kg): 1.5 mg once daily; continue until disease progression or unacceptable toxicity.

PO (Children ≥1 yr and 26–37 kg): 1 mg once daily; continue until disease progression or unacceptable toxicity.

Low-Grade Glioma

Oral Tablets

PO (Children ≥1 yr and ≥51 kg): 2 mg once daily; continue until disease progression or unacceptable toxicity.

PO (Children ≥1 yr and 38–50 kg): 1.5 mg once daily; continue until disease progression or unacceptable toxicity.

PO (Children ≥1 yr and 26–37 kg): 1 mg once daily; continue until disease progression or unacceptable toxicity.

Oral Solution

PO (Children ≥1 yr and ≥51 kg): 2 mg once daily; continue until disease progression or unacceptable toxicity.

PO (Children ≥1 yr and 46–50 kg): 1.6 mg once daily; continue until disease progression or unacceptable toxicity.

PO (Children ≥1 yr and 42–45 kg): 1.4 mg once daily; continue until disease progression or unacceptable toxicity.

PO (Children ≥1 yr and 38–41 kg): 1.25 mg once daily; continue until disease progression or unacceptable toxicity.

PO (Children ≥1 yr and 34–47 kg): 1.15 mg once daily; continue until disease progression or unacceptable toxicity.

PO (Children ≥1 yr and 30–33 kg): 1 mg once daily; continue until disease progression or unacceptable toxicity.

PO (Children ≥1 yr and 26–29 kg): 0.9 mg once daily; continue until disease progression or unacceptable toxicity.

PO (Children ≥1 yr and 22–25 kg): 0.85 mg once daily; continue until disease progression or unacceptable toxicity.

PO (Children ≥1 yr and 18–21 kg): 0.7 mg once daily; continue until disease progression or unacceptable toxicity.

PO (Children ≥1 yr and 14–17 kg): 0.55 mg once daily; continue until disease progression or unacceptable toxicity.

PO (Children ≥1 yr and 12–13 kg): 0.45 mg once daily; continue until disease progression or unacceptable toxicity.

PO (Children ≥1 yr and 11 kg): 0.4 mg once daily; continue until disease progression or unacceptable toxicity.

PO (Children ≥1 yr and 9–10 kg): 0.35 mg once daily; continue until disease progression or unacceptable toxicity.

PO (Children ≥1 yr and 8 kg): 0.3 mg once daily; continue until disease progression or unacceptable toxicity.

Availability (generic available)

Tablets: 0.5 mg, 2 mg. **Oral solution (strawberry flavor):** 0.05 mg/mL.

NURSING IMPLICATIONS

Assessment

- Assess left ventricular ejection fraction (LVEF) by echocardiogram or multigated acquisition scan before starting, after 1 mo, and then every 2–3 mo during therapy. *If asymptomatic and absolute ↓ LVEF of ≥10% from baseline and below institutional lower limits of normal from pretreatment value,* hold trametinib for up to 4 wk. *If LVEF improves to normal within 4 wk,* resume trametinib at lower dose. *If not improved to normal LVEF value after 4 wk,* permanently discontinue trametinib. *If symptomatic cardiomyopathy or absolute ↓ LVEF >20% of baseline that is below institutional lower limits of normal,* permanently discontinue trametinib.
- Perform ophthalmic exam at baseline. *If patient reports visual disturbance,* within 24 hr, perform comparative exam. *If RPED occurs,* hold trametinib. *If RPED improves within 3 wk,* resume trametinib at same or ↓ dose. *If no RPED improvement within 3 wk,* resume trametinib at ↓ dose or permanently discontinue. *If retinal vein occlusion occurs,* permanently discontinue trametinib.

- Assess for signs and symptoms of ILD (cough, dyspnea, hypoxia, pleural effusion, infiltrates). *If ILD or pneumonitis occur,* permanently discontinue trametinib.
- Monitor for serious or worsening skin reactions every 2 mo during and for 6 mo following therapy. *If severe cutaneous adverse reactions occur,* permanently discontinue trametinib. *If intolerable Grade 2 or Grade 3 or 4 skin toxicity occurs,* hold trametinib for up to 3 wk. *If intolerable Grade 2 or Grade 3 or 4 skin toxicity improved within 3 wk,* resume trametinib at ↓ dose. *If intolerable Grade 2 or if Grade 3 or 4 skin toxicity not improved despite interruption of therapy for 3 wk,* permanently discontinue trametinib.
- Monitor BP periodically during therapy. May cause hypertension.
- Monitor temperature during therapy. Also monitor for signs/symptoms of infection and renal impairment during and following severe pyrexia. May cause serious febrile reactions. *If fever of 100.4°–104°F or 1st symptoms in case of recurrence,* hold trametinib as monotherapy or both trametinib and dabrafenib until fever resolves; resume at same or ↓ dose, administering antipyretics as secondary prophylaxis. *If fever >104°F or complicated by rigors, hypotension, dehydration, or renal failure,* hold trametinib as monotherapy or both trametinib and dabrafenib until fever resolves for ≥24 hr; resume at same or ↓ dose, administering antipyretics as secondary prophylaxis, or permanently discontinue trametinib.
- Monitor for signs/symptoms of venous thromboembolism (shortness of breath, chest pain, arm or leg swelling). *If uncomplicated DVT or PE occurs,* hold trametinib for up to 3 wk. If improved to Grade ≤1, resume trametinib at ↓ dose. *If uncomplicated DVT or PE improved within 3 wk or if life-threatening PE occurs,* permanently discontinue trametinib.
- Monitor for signs/symptoms of hemorrhage. *If Grade 3 hemorrhage occurs,* hold trametinib until hemorrhage improved; then resume at ↓ dose. *If Grade 3 hemorrhage does not improve or Grade 4 hemorrhage occurs,* permanently discontinue trametinib.
- Monitor for signs/symptoms of colitis and GI perforation.
- Perform dermatologic exam prior to initiation of combination therapy with trametinib and dabrafenib, every 2 mo during therapy, and for up to 6 mo following discontinuation.
- Monitor patients receiving combination therapy with trametinib and dabrafenib closely for signs/symptoms of noncutaneous malignancies and hemophagocytic lymphohistiocytosis. *If hemophagocytic lymphohistiocytosis occurs,* discontinue trametinib and provide appropriate treatment.

Lab Test Considerations

- Verify negative pregnancy before starting therapy.
- Confirm presence of BRAF V600E or V600K mutation in tumor specimens prior to starting therapy with trametinib. Information on FDA-approved tests for the detection of BRAF V600E mutations is available at http://www.fda.gov/CompanionDiagnostics. May ↑ AST, ALT, and alkaline phosphatase.
- May cause hypoalbuminemia.
- May cause cytopenia, neutropenia, lymphopenia, and anemia.
- May cause hyperglycemia. Monitor blood sugar at baseline and periodically during therapy when administered with dabrafenib.

Implementation

- **Recommended Dose Reductions:** *1st dose ↓ (for tablets):* ↓ by 0.5 mg/day. *2nd dose ↓ (for tablets):* ↓ by 0.5 mg/day. *If unable to tolerate a maximum of two ↓ (for tablets):* Permanently discontinue trametinib. Refer to drug label for oral solution dose ↓ when adverse reactions occur.
- **PO:** Administer tablets on an empty stomach ≥1 hr before or 2 hr after a meal approximately 24 hr apart. Administer oral solution with low-fat meal or on an empty stomach. If infant is unable to tolerate fasting conditions, may give breast milk or formula on demand. ***DNC:*** Swallow tablets whole; do not crush or break.
- **Oral solution:** Add 90 mL distilled or purified water to the bottle. Reattach lid and gently shake until powder has dissolved into clear solution. Insert dosing adapter into bottle neck and store at room temperature. Do not freeze. Once reconstituted, oral solution can be used for 35 days. Administer from oral dosing syringe or feeding tube.

Patient/Family Teaching

- Instruct patient to take trametinib as directed ≥1 hr before or 2 hr after meals approximately 24 hr apart. Take missed doses as soon as remembered unless within 12 hr of next dose; then omit and take regularly scheduled dose. If vomiting occurs after administration, do not take an additional dose; take the next dose at its scheduled time. Store in refrigerator in original bottle with desiccant; do not place in pill boxes. Oral solution is intended to be prepared and administered by a caregiver. Advise patient to read *Patient Information* before starting therapy and with each Rx refill in case of changes.
- Inform patient of potential side effects. Advise patient to notify health care provider if signs/symptoms of HF (pounding or racing heart, shortness of

T

breath, swelling of feet or ankles, dizziness), visual disturbances (blurred vision, loss of vision, seeing colored dots, seeing a blurred outline or halo around objects, other visual changes), dyspnea, progressive or intolerable rash (acne; redness, swelling, peeling, or tenderness of hands or feet), hypertension (severe headache, blurry vision, dizziness), hemorrhage (headache, dizziness, weakness, coughing or vomiting blood [or coffee-ground texture], red or black tarry stools, easy bruising), skin changes (new wart, sore or reddish bump that bleeds or does not heal, change in size or color of a mole), hyperglycemia (↑ thirst, urinating more often than normal, ↑ amount of urine), or severe diarrhea occur.

- Advise patient to notify health care provider of all Rx or OTC medications, vitamins, or herbal products being taken and to consult with health care provider before taking other medications.
- Rep: Advise women of reproductive potential and men with female partners of reproductive potential to use a highly effective form of contraception during and for ≥4 mo after last dose. Use a nonhormonal form of contraception; trametinib may ↓ effectiveness of hormonal contraceptives. Advise women of reproductive potential to notify health care provider if pregnancy is suspected and to avoid breastfeeding during and for 4 mo after last dose. May impair fertility in women.

Evaluation/Desired Outcomes

- Improved progression-free survival and overall survival in melanoma.
- Decreased progression of NSCLC, anaplastic thyroid cancer, and solid tumors.
- Decreased progression of and improved progression-free survival in low-grade glioma.

trandolapril, See ANGIOTENSIN-CONVERTING ENZYME (ACE) INHIBITORS.

HIGH ALERT

tranexamic acid

(tran-ex-**am**-ikas-id)

Cyklokapron, Lysteda

Classification

Therapeutic: hemostatic agents

Pharmacologic: antifibrinolytics, plasminogen inactivators

Indications

IV: Prevention or reduction of hemorrhage during and following dental surgery in hemophiliacs. **PO:** Cyclic heavy menstrual bleeding.

Action

Inhibits activation of plasminogen, thereby preventing the conversion of plasminogen to plasmin. **Therapeutic Effects:** Decreased bleeding following dental surgery in hemophiliacs. Reduced need for replacement therapy. Reduced menstrual blood loss.

Pharmacokinetics

Absorption: IV administration results in complete bioavailability; 45% absorbed following oral administration.

Distribution: Penetrates readily into joint fluid and synovial membranes.

Metabolism and Excretion: 95% excreted unchanged in urine.

Half-life: *IV:* 2 hr (↑ in renal impairment); *Oral:* 11 hr.

TIME/ACTION PROFILE (plasma concentrations)

ROUTE	ONSET	PEAK	DURATION
IV	unknown	unknown	7–8 hr
PO	unknown	2.5 hr	unknown

Contraindications/Precautions

Contraindicated in: Hypersensitivity; Thromboembolic disorders (current, history of, or at risk for); Acquired defective color vision (IV); Subarachnoid hemorrhage; Concurrent use of combination hormonal contraception (PO).

Use Cautiously in: Renal impairment (↑ dosing interval); Hematuria originating in the upper urinary tract; Conditions associated with ↑ thrombus formation; OB: Use during pregnancy only if potential maternal benefit justifies potential fetal risk; Lactation: Use while breastfeeding only if potential maternal benefit justifies potential risk to infant.

Adverse Reactions/Side Effects

CV: hypotension, thromboembolism. **EENT:** visual abnormalities. **GI:** diarrhea, nausea, vomiting. **MS:** pain. **Neuro:** headache, dizziness, SEIZURES. **Misc: PO:** ANAPHYLAXIS.

Interactions

Drug-Drug: Concurrent use of **hormonal contraceptives** with oral tranexamic acid may ↑ risk of thrombosis; concurrent use contraindicated. Concurrent use of **clotting factor complexes** may ↑ the risk of thrombotic complications (give tranexamic acid 8 hr following clotting factor replacement therapy). May ↑ the procoagulant effects of **all-trans retinoic acid.** ↓ effectiveness with **thrombolytic agents.**

Route/Dosage

IV (Adults and Children): 10 mg/kg just prior to surgery with appropriate replacement therapy; then 10 mg/kg 3–4 times daily for 2–8 days.

Renal Impairment

IV (Adults and Children): *SCr 1.36–2.83 mg/dL:* 10 mg/kg twice daily; *SCr 2.83–5.66 mg/dL:* 10 mg/kg daily; *SCr >5.66 mg/dL:* 10 mg/kg every 48 hr or 5 mg/kg once daily.

PO (Adults): 1300 mg 3 times daily for a maximum of 5 days during menstruation.

Renal Impairment

PO (Adults): *SCr 1.41–2.8 mg/dL:* 1300 mg twice daily for a maximum of 5 days during menstruation; *SCr 2.81–5.7 mg/dL:* 1300 mg daily for a maximum of 5 days during menstruation; *SCr >5.7 mg/dL:* 650 mg daily for a maximum of 5 days during menstruation.

Availability (generic available)

Premixed infusion: 1 g/100 mL 0.7% NaCl. **Solution for injection:** 100 mg/mL. **Tablets:** ✱ 500 mg, 650 mg.

NURSING IMPLICATIONS

Assessment

- **Prevention of postsurgical hemorrhage:** Observe site of surgery for excessive bleeding.
- **Heavy menstrual bleeding:** Monitor menstrual flow prior to and during therapy.
- Patients taking tranexamic acid for more than several days should have ophthalmologic examinations to detect visual abnormalities prior to and at regular intervals during and after therapy. Discontinue therapy if visual changes occur.

Implementation

- ***High Alert:*** Serious adverse reactions, including seizures and arrhythmias, have occurred when administering tranexamic acid incorrectly via the intrathecal route instead of through the IV route. Confirm the correct route of administration for tranexamic acid, and avoid confusion with other injectable solutions that might be administered at the same time.
- **PO:** Administer 3 times daily without regard to food. Swallow tablets whole; do not crush, break, or chew.

IV Administration

- **Intermittent Infusion: Dilution:** May be diluted with most solutions, such as electrolyte, carbohydrate, amino acid, and dextran solutions. Prepare mixture on day of infusion. **Rate:** Infuse at a rate not to exceed 100 mg (1 mL)/min. More rapid administration has resulted in hypotension.
- **Y-Site Compatibility:** clevidipine, defibrotide, heparin.
- **Y-Site Incompatibility:** ampicillin, ampicillin/sulbactam, blinatumomab, penicillin G, piperacillin/tazobactam.

Patient/Family Teaching

- Instruct patient to take medication as directed; do not take more than 6 tablets/day, for longer that 5 days in any menstrual cycle, or when not menstruating. Take missed doses as soon as remembered; then take next dose as least 6 hr later; do not double doses. Advise patient to read *Patient Information* before starting and with each Rx refill in case of changes.
- Advise patient to stop medication and inform health care professional of any changes in vision. Inform patients on prolonged therapy of the importance of regular ophthalmologic follow-up.
- Instruct patient to notify health care professional of all Rx or OTC medications, vitamins, or herbal products being taken and consult health care professional before taking any new medications. Caution patient to avoid taking hormonal contraceptives and products containing aspirin or NSAIDs without consulting health care professional.
- Instruct patient to notify health care professional if signs and symptoms of thrombosis (severe, sudden headache; pains in chest, groin, or legs, especially calves; sudden loss of coordination; sudden and unexplained shortness of breath; slurred speech; visual changes; weakness or numbness in arm or leg) or anaphylaxis (shortness of breath, throat tightness, rash) occur.
- Instruct patient to notify health care professional if heavy menstrual bleeding persists or worsens or if bleeding does not lessen after 2 cycles or tranexamic acid seems to stop working.
- Rep: Advise females of reproductive potential to notify health care professional if pregnancy is planned or suspected or if breastfeeding.

Evaluation/Desired Outcomes

- Prevention of hemorrhage during and following dental surgery in hemophiliacs.
- Reduced menstrual blood loss.

HIGH ALERT

trastuzumab

(traz-**too**-zoo-mab)

Herceptin, Hercessi, Herzuma, Kanjinti, Ogivri, Ontruzant, Trazimera

Classification

Therapeutic: antineoplastics

Pharmacologic: monoclonal antibodies

Indications

HER2-overexpressing metastatic gastric or gastroesophageal adenocarcinoma in patients who have not received prior treatment for metastatic disease (in combination with cisplatin and capecitabine or 5-fluorouracil). HER2-overexpressing node-positive or node-negative breast cancer (as part of one of the following regimens: doxorubicin, cyclophosphamide, and either paclitaxel or docetaxel; or docetaxel and carboplatin) (as adjuvant therapy). HER2-overexpressing node-positive or node-negative breast cancer (to be used alone after multimodality anthracycline-based therapy) (as adjuvant therapy). HER2-overexpressing metastatic breast cancer (as first-line therapy) (in combination with paclitaxel). HER2-overexpressing metastatic breast cancer in patients who have already received ≥1 other chemotherapy regimens for metastatic disease (as monotherapy).

Action

A monoclonal antibody that binds to HER2 sites in breast cancer tissue and inhibits proliferation of cells that overexpress HER2 protein. **Therapeutic Effects:** Regression of breast, gastric, or gastroesophageal cancer and metastases.

Pharmacokinetics

Absorption: IV administration results in complete bioavailability.
Distribution: Unknown.
Metabolism and Excretion: Unknown.
Half-life: Unknown.

TIME/ACTION PROFILE (plasma concentrations)

ROUTE	ONSET	PEAK	DURATION
IV	unknown	unknown	unknown

Contraindications/Precautions

Contraindicated in: OB: Pregnancy; Lactation: Lactation.
Use Cautiously in: Pre-existing pulmonary conditions; Hypersensitivity to trastuzumab, Chinese hamster ovary cell proteins, or other components of the product; Hypersensitivity to benzyl alcohol (use sterile water for injection instead of bacteriostatic water, which accompanies the vial); Rep: Women of reproductive potential; Pedi: Safety not established in children; Geri: Older adults may have ↑ risk of cardiotoxicity.
Exercise Extreme Caution in: Pre-existing cardiac dysfunction.

Adverse Reactions/Side Effects

CV: ARRHYTHMIAS, edema, HF, hypertension, tachycardia. **Derm:** rash, acne, herpes simplex. **EENT:** pharyngitis, rhinitis, sinusitis. **GI:** abdominal pain, anorexia, diarrhea, nausea, vomiting. **Hemat:** anemia, leukopenia. **MS:** pain, arthralgia, bone pain. **Neuro:** depression, dizziness, headache, insomnia, neuropathy, paresthesia, peripheral neuritis, weakness. **Resp:** ACUTE RESPIRATORY DISTRESS SYNDROME, cough, dyspnea, INTERSTITIAL PNEUMONITIS, PULMONARY EDEMA, PULMONARY FIBROSIS. **Misc:** chills, fever, INFECTION, flu-like syndrome, INFUSION REACTIONS (INCLUDING ANAPHYLAXIS AND ANGIOEDEMA).

Interactions

Drug-Drug: **Anthracyclines**, including **daunorubicin**, **doxorubicin**, or **idarubicin**, may ↑ risk of cardiotoxicity; if possible, avoid anthracycline-based therapy for up to 7 mo after stopping trastuzumab. **Paclitaxel** may ↑ levels and risk of toxicity.

Route/Dosage

Adjuvant Treatment of Breast Cancer

IV (Adults): *During and following paclitaxel, docetaxel, or docetaxel/carboplatin:* 4 mg/kg initially; then 2 mg/kg once weekly during chemotherapy for the 1st 12 wk (paclitaxel or docetaxel) or 18 wk (docetaxel/carboplatin); 1 wk after the last weekly dose, give 6 mg/kg every 3 wk. Do not exceed treatment duration of 1 yr. *As single agent within 3 wk following completion of multimodality, anthracycline-based chemotherapy regimens:* 8 mg/kg initially; then 6 mg/kg every 3 wk. Do not exceed treatment duration of 1 yr.

Metastatic Breast Cancer

IV (Adults): 4 mg/kg initially; then 2 mg/kg once weekly until disease progression.

Metastatic Gastric Cancer

IV (Adults): 8 mg/kg initially; then 6 mg/kg every 3 wk until disease progression.

Availability

Lyophilized powder for injection: 150 mg/vial, 420 mg/vial. ***In combination with:*** hyaluronidase (Herceptin Hylecta). See Appendix N.

NURSING IMPLICATIONS

Assessment

- Assess for infusion-related symptoms (chills, fever, nausea, vomiting, pain [in some cases at tumor sites], headache, dizziness, dyspnea, hypotension, rash, asthenia) following initial infusion. Severe reactions (bronchospasm, anaphylaxis, angioedema, hypoxia, severe hypotension) may occur during or immediately following the initial infusion. May be treated with epinephrine, corticosteroids, diphenhydramine, bronchodilators, and oxygen. *If dyspnea or severe hypotension occurs,* interrupt infusion. *If severe reaction occurs,* permanently discontinue trastuzumab.

- Assess for signs and symptoms of HF (dyspnea, ↑ cough, paroxysmal nocturnal dyspnea, peripheral edema, S_3 gallop, ↓ left ventricular ejection fraction [LVEF]) prior to and frequently during therapy. Perform baseline assessment of cardiac history, physical exam, and LVEF with ECG or multiple gated acquisition (MUGA) scan. Monitor LVEF every 3 mo, at completion of therapy, and then every 6 mo for ≥2 yr. *If ≥16% absolute ↓ in LVEF from pretreatment values or an LVEF value below institutional limits of normal and ≥10% absolute ↓ in LVEF from pretreatment values occurs,* hold trastuzumab. Repeat LVEF measures every 4 wk if dose is held for significant left ventricular dysfunction.
- Monitor patient for signs of pulmonary hypersensitivity reactions (dyspnea, pulmonary infiltrates, pleural effusion, noncardiogenic pulmonary edema, hypoxia, acute respiratory distress syndrome). Patients with symptomatic pulmonary disease or extensive lung tumor involvement are at ↑ risk. *If severe symptoms occur,* discontinue trastuzumab.

Lab Test Considerations

- Verify negative pregnancy test before starting therapy.
  HER2 protein overexpression is used to determine whether treatment with trastuzumab is indicated. HER2 protein overexpression is detected by HercepTest (IHC assay) and PathVysion (FISH assay).
- May cause anemia and leukopenia.

Implementation

- ***High Alert:*** Do not confuse trastuzumab with ado-trastuzumab.
- ***High Alert:*** Fatalities have occurred with chemotherapeutic agents. Before administering, clarify all ambiguous orders; double-check single, daily, and course-of-therapy dose limits; have second practitioner independently double-check original order, dose calculations, and infusion pump settings.
- May be administered in the outpatient setting.
- *If a dose is missed by ≤1 wk,* administer usual maintenance dose as soon as possible. Do not wait until next planned cycle. Administer subsequent maintenance doses 7 days or 21 days later according to the weekly or three-weekly schedules, respectively. *If a dose is missed by >1 wk,* administer a reloading dose as soon as possible. Administer subsequent maintenance doses 7 days or 21 days later according to weekly or three-weekly schedules, respectively.

IV Administration

- **Intermittent Infusion: Reconstitution:** Reconstitute each vial with 7.4 mL of sterile water for injection, directing the stream of diluent into lyophilized cake of trastuzumab. Swirl the vial gently; do not shake. May foam slightly; allow the vial to stand undisturbed for 5 min. Solution should be clear to slightly opalescent and colorless to pale yellow, without particulate matter. Stable for 24 hr if refrigerated. **Concentration:** 21 mg/mL. **Dilution:** Add calculated dose to 250 mL bag of 0.9% NaCl. Invert bag gently to mix. Infusion is stable for up to 24 hr if refrigerated. **Rate:** Infuse the 4 mg/kg loading dose over 90 min and the weekly 2 mg/kg dose over 30 min or 6 mg/kg dose over 30–90 min every 3 wk, or 8 mg/kg dose over 90 min if the loading dose was well tolerated. Do not administer as an IV push or bolus.
- **Y-Site Compatibility:** acyclovir, aminophylline, ampicillin, ampicillin/sulbactam, bleomycin, bumetanide, buprenorphine, busulfan, butorphanol, calcium gluconate, carboplatin, carmustine, cefazolin, ceftazidime, ceftriaxone, cefuroxime, ciprofloxacin, cisplatin, cyclophosphamide, cytarabine, dactinomycin, daunorubicin, dexamethasone, digoxin, diphenhydramine, dobutamine, docetaxel, dopamine, doxorubicin hydrochloride, doxorubicin liposomal, doxycycline, droperidol, enalaprilat, etoposide phosphate, famotidine, fentanyl, filgrastim, fluconazole, fluorouracil, ganciclovir, gemcitabine, gentamicin, granisetron, haloperidol, heparin, hydrocortisone, hydromorphone, ifosfamide, imipenem/cilastatin, leucovorin, lorazepam, magnesium sulfate, mannitol, meperidine, mesna, methotrexate, methylprednisolone, metoclopramide, metronidazole, minocycline, mitomycin, mitoxantrone, paclitaxel, pentamidine, potassium chloride, prochlorperazine, promethazine, remifentanil, sargramostim, sodium bicarbonate, theophylline, thiotepa, tobramycin, trimethoprim/sulfamethoxazole, vancomycin, vinblastine, vincristine, vinorelbine, zidovudine.
- **Y-Site Incompatibility:** aldesleukin, amikacin, amphotericin B deoxycholate, aztreonam, cefotaxime, cefotetan, cefoxitin, chlorpromazine, clindamycin, cyclosporine, fludarabine, furosemide, idarubicin, irinotecan, levofloxacin, morphine, nalbuphine, ondansetron, piperacillin/tazobactam, topotecan.

Patient/Family Teaching

- Explain purpose and side effects of medication to patient. Advise patient to read *Patient Information* before starting therapy.

T

- Advise patient to notify health care provider of all Rx or OTC medications, vitamins, or herbal products being taken and to consult health care provider before taking other medications.
- Advise patients to contact a health care provider immediately if signs and symptoms of HF (new onset or worsening shortness of breath, cough, swelling of the ankles/legs, swelling of face, palpitations, weight gain >5 pounds in 24 hr, dizziness, loss of consciousness) or hypersensitivity reactions (dizziness, nausea, chills, fever, vomiting, diarrhea, urticaria, angioedema, breathing problems, chest pain) occur.
- Caution patient to avoid crowds and persons with known infections.
- Advise patient not to receive any vaccinations without advice of health care provider.
- Rep: May cause fetal harm. Advise women of reproductive potential to notify health care provider immediately if pregnancy is planned or suspected and to avoid breastfeeding. Caution patient to use effective contraception during therapy and for 7 mo following last dose. Monitor infants exposed to trastuzumab for oligohydramnios, pulmonary hypoplasia, skeletal abnormalities, and neonatal death. Encourage women who may be exposed during pregnancy to report exposure to the Genentech Adverse Event Line at 1-888-835-2555.

Evaluation/Desired Outcomes

- Regression of breast, gastric, or gastroesophageal cancer and metastases.

traZODone (traz-oh-done)

~~Desyrel~~, Raldesy

Classification

Therapeutic: antidepressants

Indications

Major depression. **Unlabeled Use:** Insomnia.

Action

Alters the effects of serotonin in the CNS. **Therapeutic Effects:** Antidepressant action, which may develop only over several wk.

Pharmacokinetics

Absorption: Well absorbed after oral administration.
Distribution: Widely distributed to tissues.
Protein Binding: 89–95%.
Metabolism and Excretion: Extensively metabolized by the liver via the CYP3A4 isoenzyme; minimal excretion of unchanged drug by the kidneys.
Half-life: 5–9 hr.

TIME/ACTION PROFILE (antidepressant effect)

ROUTE	ONSET	PEAK	DURATION
PO	1–2 wk	2–4 wk	wk

Contraindications/Precautions

Contraindicated in: Hypersensitivity; Recovery period after MI; Concurrent electroconvulsive therapy; Concurrent use of MAO inhibitors or MAO-inhibitor-like drugs (linezolid or methylene blue); Angle-closure glaucoma; Lactation: Lactation.
Use Cautiously in: May ↑ risk of suicide attempt/ideation especially during early treatment or dose adjustment; this risk appears to be greater in adolescents or children; Cardiovascular disease; Hypovolemia or dehydration (↑ risk of syndrome of inappropriate antidiuretic hormone secretion [SIADH]); Severe renal impairment (↓ dose); Severe hepatic impairment (↓ dose); OB: Other agents preferred for treatment of depression or insomnia in pregnancy; Pedi: Safety and effectiveness not established in children; Geri: ↑ risk of SIADH in older adults. Initial dose ↓ recommended in older adults.

Adverse Reactions/Side Effects

CV: hypotension, arrhythmias, chest pain, hypertension, palpitations, QT interval prolongation, tachycardia. **Derm:** rash. **EENT:** blurred vision, tinnitus. **F and E:** hyponatremia, SIADH. **GI:** dry mouth, constipation, diarrhea, excess salivation, flatulence, nausea, vomiting. **GU:** erectile dysfunction, hematuria, priapism, urinary frequency. **Hemat:** anemia, leukopenia. **MS:** myalgia. **Neuro:** drowsiness, confusion, dizziness, dysgeusia, fatigue, hallucinations, headache, insomnia, nightmares, slurred speech, SUICIDAL THOUGHTS/BEHAVIORS, syncope, tremor, weakness.

Interactions

Drug-Drug: Serious, potentially fatal reactions (hyperthermia, rigidity, myoclonus, autonomic instability, with fluctuating vital signs and extreme agitation, which may proceed to delirium and coma) may occur with concurrent **MAO inhibitors**. MAO inhibitors should be stopped ≥14 days before trazodone therapy. Trazodone should be stopped ≥14 days before MAO inhibitor therapy. **MAO-inhibitor-like drugs**, such as **linezolid** or **methylene blue**, may ↑ risk of serotonin syndrome; concurrent use contraindicated; do not start therapy in patients receiving **linezolid** or **methylene blue**; if **linezolid** or **methylene blue** need to be started in a patient receiving trazodone, immediately discontinue trazodone and monitor for signs/symptoms of serotonin syndrome for

2 wk or until 24 hr after last dose of linezolid or methylene blue, whichever comes first (may resume trazodone therapy 24 hr after last dose of linezolid or methylene blue). May ↑ **digoxin** or **phenytoin** levels and the risk of toxicity. ↑ CNS depression with other **CNS depressants**, including **alcohol**, **opioid analgesics**, and **sedative/hypnotics**. ↑ risk of hypotension with **antihypertensives**, acute ingestion of **alcohol**, or **nitrates**. **Fluoxetine** may ↑ levels and risk of toxicity. **CYP3A4 inhibitors**, including **ritonavir** and **ketoconazole**, may ↑ levels and risk of toxicity. **CYP3A4 inducers**, including **carbamazepine**, may ↓ levels and effectiveness. Drugs that affect serotonergic neurotransmitter systems, including **tricyclic antidepressants**, **fentanyl**, **buspirone**, **tramadol** and **triptans**, may ↑ the risk of serotonin syndrome. ↑ risk of bleeding with **NSAIDs**, **aspirin**, **clopidogrel**, **prasugrel**, **ticagrelor**, or **warfarin**. **Diuretics** may ↑ risk of SIADH.

Drug-Natural Products: Kava-kava, **valerian**, or **chamomile** can ↑ CNS depression. ↑ risk of serotonergic side effects including serotonin syndrome with **St. John's wort** and **SAMe**.

Route/Dosage

Depression

PO (Adults): 150 mg/day in 3 divided doses; ↑ by 50 mg/day every 3–4 days until desired response (not to exceed 400 mg/day in outpatients or 600 mg/day in hospitalized patients).

PO (Geriatric Patients): 75 mg/day in divided doses initially; may be ↑ every 3–4 days.

Insomnia

PO (Adults): 25–100 mg at bedtime.

Availability (generic available)

Tablets: 50 mg, 100 mg, 150 mg, 300 mg. **Oral solution:** 10 mg/mL.

NURSING IMPLICATIONS

Assessment

- Monitor BP and HR before and during initial therapy. Monitor ECGs in patients with pre-existing cardiac disease before and periodically during therapy to detect arrhythmias.
- Assess for possible sexual dysfunction.
- Assess for serotonin syndrome (mental changes [agitation, hallucinations, coma], autonomic instability [tachycardia, labile BP, hyperthermia], neuromuscular aberrations [hyperreflexia, incoordination], GI symptoms [nausea, vomiting, diarrhea]), especially in patients taking other serotonergic drugs (SSRIs, SNRIs, triptans).
- **Depression:** Assess mental status (orientation, mood, and behavior) frequently.
- Assess for suicidal tendencies, especially during early therapy. Restrict amount of drug available to patient. Risk may be ↑ in patients ≤24 yr. After starting therapy, young adults should be seen by health care provider at least weekly for 4 wk, every 3 wk for next 4 wk, and on advice of health care provider thereafter.

Lab Test Considerations

- Assess CBC and renal and hepatic function before starting and periodically during therapy. Slight, clinically insignificant ↓ in leukocyte and neutrophil counts may occur.
- May cause hyponatremia, especially in older adults, those on diuretics, and those who are hypovolemic. *If symptomatic hyponatremia occurs,* discontinue trazodone and treat as indicated.

Implementation

- Do not confuse trazodone with tramadol.
- **PO:** Administer with or immediately after meals to minimize side effects (nausea, dizziness) and allow maximum absorption. A larger portion of the total daily dose may be given at bedtime to ↓ daytime drowsiness and dizziness.

Patient/Family Teaching

- Explain purpose and side effects of medication. Advise patient to read *Patient Information* before starting therapy.
- Instruct patient to take missed dose as soon as remembered. Do not take if within 4 hr of next scheduled dose; do not double dose.
- Advise patient to consult health care provider before discontinuing medication; gradual dose reduction is necessary to prevent discontinuation syndrome.
- May cause drowsiness and blurred vision. Caution patient to avoid driving and other activities requiring alertness until response to drug is known.
- Caution patient to change positions slowly to minimize orthostatic hypotension.
- Advise patient to avoid concurrent use of alcohol or other CNS depressant drugs.
- Advise patient family, and caregivers to look for suicidality, especially during early therapy or dose changes. Notify health care provider immediately if thoughts about suicide or dying, attempts to commit suicide, new or worse depression or anxiety, agitation or restlessness, panic attacks, insomnia, new or worse irritability, aggressiveness, acting on dangerous impulses, mania, or other changes in mood or behavior occur.
- Advise patient and caregivers to immediately notify health care provider if symptoms of serotonin

T

syndrome (mental changes [agitation, hallucinations, coma], autonomic instability [tachycardia, labile BP, hyperthermia], neuromuscular aberrations [hyperreflexia, incoordination], GI symptoms [nausea, vomiting, diarrhea]) occur.

- Advise patient to notify health care provider of all Rx or OTC medications, vitamins, or herbal products being taken and to consult with health care provider before taking other medications, especially aspirin and NSAIDs.
- Inform patient that frequent rinses, good oral hygiene, and sugarless candy or gum may diminish dry mouth. Health care provider should be notified if this persists >2 wk. An ↑ in fluid intake, fiber, and exercise may prevent constipation.
- Advise patient to notify health care provider of medication regimen before treatment or surgery.
- Instruct patient to notify health care provider if priapism, irregular heartbeat, fainting, confusion, skin rash, or tremors occur or if dry mouth, nausea and vomiting, dizziness, headache, muscle aches, constipation, or diarrhea becomes pronounced.
- Rep: Advise women of reproductive potential to notify health care provider if pregnancy is planned and to avoid breastfeeding during therapy.

Evaluation/Desired Outcomes

- Resolution of depression.
- Increased sense of well-being.
- Renewed interest in surroundings.
- Increased appetite.
- Improved energy level.
- Improved sleep.

treprostinil (tre-pross-ti-nil)

Orenitram, Remodulin, Tyvaso, Tyvaso DPI, Yutrepia

Classification

Therapeutic: vasodilators

Pharmacologic: prostacyclins

Indications

IV SUBQ: Treatment of the following disorders: Pulmonary arterial hypertension (WHO Group 1); Pulmonary arterial hypertension in patients requiring transition from epoprostenol. **Inhaln PO:** Pulmonary arterial hypertension (WHO Group 1). **Inhaln:** Pulmonary hypertension associated with interstitial lung disease (WHO Group 3).

Action

Treprostinil is a prostacyclin that produces direct vasodilation of pulmonary and systemic arterial vascular beds. Also inhibits platelet aggregation. **Therapeutic Effects:** Decreased exercise-associated symptoms and delayed disease progression.

Pharmacokinetics

Absorption: IV administration results in complete bioavailability. Rapidly and completely (near 100%) absorbed following SUBQ administration; 64–72% absorbed after oral inhalation; 17% absorbed after oral administration.

Distribution: Well distributed to extravascular tissues.

Protein Binding: 91%.

Metabolism and Excretion: Primarily metabolized by the liver via the CYP2C8 isoenzyme; metabolites are renally excreted; minimal excretion of unchanged drug in urine.

Half-life: *SUBQ:* 4 hr *Dry powder inhalation:* 27–50 min.

TIME/ACTION PROFILE (clinical improvement)

ROUTE	ONSET	PEAK	DURATION
SUBQ/IV	unknown	1 wk	unknown
Inhaln (soln)	unknown	unknown	unknown
Inhaln (dry powder)	unknown	unknown	unknown
PO	unknown	unknown	unknown

Contraindications/Precautions

Contraindicated in: Known hypersensitivity; Moderate or severe hepatic impairment (PO only).

Use Cautiously in: Renal impairment; Hepatic impairment (dose ↓ recommended in mild to moderate hepatic impairment [for parenteral] and mild hepatic impairment [PO]); Pulmonary disease (inhalation only); Diverticulosis (PO only) (tablet shell does not dissolve); OB: Use during pregnancy only if potential maternal benefit justifies potential fetal risk; Lactation: Safety not established in breastfeeding; Pedi: Safety and effectiveness not established in children ≤16 yr (parenteral) or children <18 yr (inhalation and PO).

Adverse Reactions/Side Effects

CV: edema, hypotension. **Derm:** rash, pruritus, flushing. **F and E:** hypokalemia. **GI:** diarrhea, nausea. **Hemat:** bleeding. **Local:** infusion site pain/reaction. **MS:** jaw pain. **Neuro:** headache, dizziness. **Resp:** cough (inhalation only), bronchospasm (inhalation only), dyspnea (inhalation only).

Interactions

Drug-Drug: ↑ risk of hypotension with **antihypertensives, diuretics,** or **vasodilators. CYP2C8 inhibitors**, including **gemfibrozil**, may ↑ levels and risk of toxicity. **CYP2C8 inducers**, including **rifampin**, may ↓ levels and effectiveness. Risk of bleeding may be ↑ by concurrent use of **anticoagulants**.

Route/Dosage

SUBQ, IV (Adults): *Naive to prostacyclin therapy:* 1.25 ng/kg/min; may ↓ to 0.625 ng/kg/min if intolerance occurs. Increments of no more than 1.25 ng/kg/min may be made weekly for the 1st 4 wk and then no more than 2.5 ng/kg/min weekly for the remainder of therapy. Avoid abrupt discontinuation or rapid ↓ in dosing; *Patients requiring transition from epoprostenol:* Initiate at 10% of current epoprostenol dose; ↑ dose as epoprostenol dose is ↓.

PO (Adults): 0.25 mg every 12 hr with food; may ↑ by 0.25–0.5 mg every 12 hr every 3–4 days to achieve optimal clinical response (max dose = 21 mg every 12 hr); *Concurrent gemfibrozil therapy:* ↓ initial dose to 0.125 mg every 12 hr; may ↑ by 0.125 mg every 12 hr every 3–4 days to achieve optimal clinical response.

Inhaln (Adults): *Solution for oral inhalation (Tyvaso):* 3 breaths (18 mcg) 4 times daily (administered every 4 hr while awake); may ↑ by 3 breaths/treatment every 1–2 wk until target dose of 9 breaths (54 mcg) 4 times daily (administered every 4 hr while awake) is achieved. *Dry powder inhaler (Tyvaso DPI):* 16 mcg 4 times daily (administered every 4 hr while awake); ↑ by 16 mcg/treatment every 1–2 wk until target dose of 48–64 mcg 4 times daily (administered every 4 hr while awake) is achieved. *Powder for oral inhalation (for patients who are treprostinil naive) (Yutrepia):* 26.5 mcg (in two breaths) 3–5 times/day; ↑ by 26.5 mcg/treatment every week until target dose of 79.5–106 mcg 4 times daily is achieved. *Powder for oral inhalation (for patients transitioning from treprostinil solution for oral inhalation) (Yutrepia):* Current Tyvaso dose of ≤5 breaths: 26.5 mcg (in two breaths) 3–5 times/day; ↑ by 26.5 mcg/treatment every week until target dose of 79.5–106 mcg 4 times daily is achieved. Current Tyvaso dose of 6–8 breaths: 53 mcg (in two breaths) 3–5 times/day; ↑ by 26.5 mcg/treatment every week until target dose of 79.5–106 mcg 4 times daily is achieved. Current Tyvaso dose of 9–11 breaths: 79.5 mcg (in two breaths) 3–5 times/day; ↑ by 26.5 mcg/treatment every week until target dose of 79.5–106 mcg 4 times daily is achieved. Current Tyvaso dose of 12–14 breaths: 106 mcg (in two breaths) 3–5 times/day. Current Tyvaso dose of 15–17 breaths: 132.5 mcg (in two breaths) 3–5 times/day. Current Tyvaso dose of ≥18 breaths: 159 mcg (in two breaths) 3–5 times/day.

Hepatic Impairment

SUBQ, IV (Adults): *Mild or moderate hepatic impairment:* ↓ initial dose to 0.625 ng/kg/min (using ideal body weight).

Hepatic Impairment

PO (Adults): *Mild hepatic impairment:* ↓ in initial dose to 0.125 mg every 12 hr; may ↑ by 0.125 mg every 12 hr every 3–4 days to achieve optimal clinical response.

Availability (generic available)

Extended-release tablets (Orenitram): 0.125 mg, 0.25 mg, 1 mg, 2.5 mg, 5 mg. **Solution for injection (Remodulin):** 1 mg/mL, 2.5 mg/mL, 5 mg/mL, 10 mg/mL. **Powder for oral inhalation (Yutrepia):** 26.5 mcg, 53 mcg, 79.5 mcg, 106 mcg. **Solution for oral inhalation (Tyvaso):** 0.6 mg/mL. **Dry powder for inhalation (Tyvaso DPI):** 16 mcg/cartridge, 32 mcg/cartridge, 48 mcg/cartridge, 64 mcg/cartridge.

NURSING IMPLICATIONS

Assessment

- Monitor for signs/symptoms of improvement in pulmonary arterial hypertension (↓ dyspnea, ↑ exercise tolerance) periodically during therapy.
- Monitor for signs/symptoms of excessive bleeding.
- **IV:** Assess for infusion site reaction (pain, erythema, induration, rash) during therapy.
- **Inhaln:** Monitor BP during therapy.
- Monitor for bronchospasm, especially in patients with history of hyperreactive airway.

Implementation

- Treprostinil should be used only by clinicians experienced in the treatment of pulmonary arterial hypertension. Initiation of therapy should be in a setting with equipment and personnel for monitoring and emergency treatment.
- Assess patient's ability to accept and administer treprostinil and to insert and care for infusion system prior to initiating therapy.
- Dose should be ↑ for lack of improvement or worsening in symptoms or ↓ for excessive side effects or infusion site reactions.
- SUBQ route is preferred to ↓ risk of blood stream infections. IV route may be used if SUBQ route is not tolerated due to severe site pain or reaction.
- Avoid abrupt withdrawal or large dose ↓; may result in worsening of symptoms of pulmonary arterial hypertension.
- **Transitioning from SUBQ or IV Route to PO:** ↓ SUBQ or IV dose up to 30 ng/kg/min per day while simultaneously ↑ PO dose up to 6 mg per day (2 mg, 3 times daily) if tolerated.
- **PO:** Administer with food every 12 hr for twice-daily dosing and every 8 hr for three-time daily dosing. *DNC:* Swallow tablets whole; do not crush, break, or chew. Do not take a tablet that is damaged or broken.
- If PO therapy must be interrupted, consider temporary SUBQ or IV infusion. May use implantable IV infusion pump using same dose as external infusion pump.

T

- **SUBQ:** Administer without diluting solution via a self-inserted SUBQ catheter and an infusion pump designed for SUBQ drug delivery. During use, a single syringe can be administered up to 72 hr. A single vial should be used for up to 14 days after initial introduction into vial. Do not administer solution if discolored or contains particulates. Refer to manufacturer's instructions. **Rate:** SUBQ infusion rate (using undiluted treprostinil) may be calculated with the following formula: **Undiluted SUBQ infusion rate** (mL/hr) = **[Dose** (ng/kg/min) × **weight** (kg) × **0.00006]/treprostinil vial strength** (mg/mL).

IV Administration

- **Continuous Infusion:** Administer via a surgically placed indwelling central venous catheter, using an infusion pump designed for intravenous drug delivery or implantable infusion pump. If clinically necessary, a temporary peripheral intravenous cannula, preferably placed in a large vein, may be used for short-term administration. Use of a peripheral IV infusion for more than a few hours ↑ risk of thrombophlebitis. **Dilution:** 50–100 mL of sterile water for injection, 0.9% NaCl, Sterile Diluent for Remodulin, Sterile Diluent for Flolan, or Sterile Diluent for Epoprostenol Sodium. Do not administer solution if discolored or contains particulates. **Concentration:** Amount of diluent and concentration are calculated based on dose needed, patient weight, and volume of reservoir. Diluted solutions are stable for up to 48 hr in concentrations as low as 0.004 mg/mL at room temperature.
- **Rate:** Administer via infusion set with in-line 0.22- or 0.2-micron pore size filter. IV infusion rate (using undiluted treprostinil) may be calculated with the following formula: **Undiluted IV infusion rate** (mL/hr) = **[Dose** (ng/kg/min) × **weight** (kg) × **0.00006]/treprostinil vial strength** (mg/mL).
- **Inhaln:** Use **solution for oral inhalation** only with *Tyvaso Inhalation System*. Administer as supplied. Solution is clear and colorless to slightly yellow; do not use if discolored or contains particulates. Do not mix with other medications. Twist top off ampule and squeeze entire contents into medicine cup. Cap device and store upright for remaining sessions/day. Discard medicine cup and any remaining medication at end of each day and clean device according to instructions. A single inhalation delivers approximately 6 mcg of treprostinil. Administer in 4 separate treatments each day approximately 4 hr apart, during waking hours. If initial 3 breaths are not tolerated, may ↓ to 1 or 2 breaths. One ampule of *Tyvaso* contains a sufficient volume of medication for all four treatment sessions in a single day.
- **Inhaln:** Use **dry powder inhaler** *(Tyvaso DPI)* only with *Tyvaso DPI Inhaler*. A single inhalation is administered per cartridge. Administer in 4 separate treatments each day approximately 4 hr apart, during waking hours. Use **capsules for oral powder inhalation** only with *Yutrepia Inhaler*. Capsules come in various strengths depending on dose. Inhale within 5 min of opening and always inhale each capsule twice for full dose. Protect blister pack from moisture and light.

Patient/Family Teaching

- Explain purpose and side effects of medication. Advise patient to read *Patient Information* before starting therapy.
- **For PO and inhalation self-administration,** instruct patient on device preparation, dosing, administration, cleaning, and maintenance, as indicated; keep backup device on hand to avoid interruption of therapy. If dose is missed, take as soon as possible. If ≥2 are missed, must restart titration at lowest dose. Advise patient that empty shell of oral tablet may appear in stool and is not concerning. **For IV or SUBQ administration,** instruct patient on catheter insertion and use of pump. Advise patient to have immediate access to backup pump and infusion set so infusion is not interrupted. Do not stop therapy abruptly; may result in worsening of symptoms.
- Advise patient to inform health care provider if headache, nausea, vomiting, restlessness, anxiety, or infusion site reaction occurs.
- Inform patient and family that therapy may be required for years to control disease.
- Instruct patient to notify health care provider of all Rx or OTC medications, vitamins, or herbal products being taken and consult health care provider before taking any new medications.
- **Rep:** Advise women of reproductive potential to notify health care provider if pregnancy is planned or suspected or if planning to breastfeed.

Evaluation/Desired Outcomes

- Improved exercise tolerance in patients with pulmonary arterial hypertension.

triamcinolone, See CORTICOSTEROIDS (NASAL).

triamcinolone, See CORTICOSTEROIDS (SYSTEMIC).

triamcinolone, See CORTICOSTEROIDS (TOPICAL).

BEERS

trimethoprim/sulfamethoxazole

(trye-**meth**-oh-prim/sul-fa-meth-**ox**-a-zole)

Bactrim, Bactrim DS, Septra, Sulfatrim, Sulfatrim DS, Sulfatrim Pediatric

Classification

Therapeutic: anti-infectives, antiprotozoals

Pharmacologic: folate antagonists, sulfonamides

Indications

Treatment of: Bronchitis, *Shigella* enteritis, Otitis media, *Pneumocystis jirovecii* pneumonia (PJP), Urinary tract infections, Traveler's diarrhea. Prevention of PJP in patients with HIV. **Unlabeled Use:** Biliary tract infections, osteomyelitis, burn and wound infections, chlamydial infections, endocarditis, gonorrhea, intra-abdominal infections, nocardiosis, rheumatic fever prophylaxis, sinusitis, eradication of meningococcal carriers, prophylaxis of urinary tract infections, and an alternative agent in the treatment of chancroid. Prevention of bacterial infections in immunosuppressed patients.

Action

Combination inhibits the metabolism of folic acid in bacteria at two different points. **Therapeutic Effects:** Bactericidal action against susceptible bacteria. **Spectrum:** Active against many strains of gram-positive aerobic pathogens, including: *Streptococcus pneumoniae*, *Staphylococcus aureus*. Has activity against many aerobic gram-negative pathogens, such as: *Enterobacter*, *Klebsiella*, *Morganella morganii*, *Escherichia coli*, *Proteus mirabilis*, *Proteus vulgaris*, *Shigella*, *Haemophilus influenzae*, *Pneumocystis jirovecii*. Not active against *Pseudomonas aeruginosa*.

Pharmacokinetics

Absorption: Well absorbed from the GI tract.

Distribution: Widely distributed to tissues. Crosses the blood-brain barrier.

Metabolism and Excretion: Some metabolism by the liver (20%); remainder excreted unchanged by the kidneys.

Half-life: *Trimethoprim:* 6–11 hr; *sulfamethoxazole:* 9–12 hr, both prolonged in renal failure.

TIME/ACTION PROFILE (plasma concentrations)

ROUTE	ONSET	PEAK	DURATION
PO	rapid	2–4 hr	6–12 hr
IV	rapid	end of infusion	6–12 hr

Contraindications/Precautions

Contraindicated in: Hypersensitivity to sulfonamides or trimethoprim; History of drug-induced immune thrombocytopenia due to sulfonamides or trimethoprim; Megaloblastic anemia secondary to folate deficiency; Severe renal impairment; Severe hepatic impairment; Concurrent use with dofetilide; Lactation: Avoid breastfeeding in infants who have glucose-6-phosphate dehydrogenase (G6PD) deficiency or hyperbilirubinemia; Pedi: Children <2 mo (can cause kernicterus).

Use Cautiously in: Mild or moderate renal impairment (↓ dose if CCr <30 mL/min); Mild or moderate hepatic impairment; G6PD deficiency (↑ risk hemolysis); HIV (↑ risk of adverse reactions); Concurrent use with other products containing propylene glycol (IV only) (↑ risk of lactic acidosis); OB: ↑ risk of neural tube defects, cardiovascular malformations, urinary tract defects, oral clefts, and club foot in fetus when used during pregnancy; use during pregnancy only if potential maternal benefit justifies potential fetal risk; Lactation: Use while breastfeeding only if potential maternal benefit justifies potential risk to infant; Geri: Appears on Beers list. Use with caution in older adults taking an angiotensin-converting enzyme inhibitor, angiotensin II receptor blocker, or angiotensin receptor/neprilysin inhibitor and in those with a ↓ CCr because of ↑ risk of hyperkalemia.

Adverse Reactions/Side Effects

CV: hypotension. **Derm:** rash, ACUTE FEBRILE NEUTROPHILIC DERMATOSIS, ACUTE GENERALIZED EXANTHEMATOUS PUSTULOSIS (AGEP), DRUG REACTION WITH EOSINOPHILIA AND SYSTEMIC SYMPTOMS (DRESS), ERYTHEMA MULTIFORME (EM), FEBRILE NEUTROPHILIC DERMATOSIS, photosensitivity, STEVENS-JOHNSON SYNDROME (SJS), TOXIC EPIDERMAL NECROLYSIS (TEN). **Endo:** hypoglycemia. **F and E:** hyperkalemia, hyponatremia. **GI:** nausea, vomiting, cholestatic jaundice, CLOSTRIDIOIDES DIFFICILE-ASSOCIATED DIARRHEA (CDAD), diarrhea, HEPATIC NECROSIS, hepatitis, pancreatitis, stomatitis. **GU:** crystalluria. **Hemat:** AGRANULOCYTOSIS, APLASTIC ANEMIA, HEMOPHAGOCYTIC LYMPHOHISTIOCYTOSIS, hemolytic anemia, leukopenia, megaloblastic anemia, thrombocytopenia. **Local:** phlebitis. **Neuro:** depression, fatigue, hallucinations, headache, insomnia, kernicterus (neonates). **Misc:** fever, HYPERSENSITIVITY REACTIONS (INCLUDING ANAPHYLAXIS AND RESPIRATORY FAILURE).

Interactions

Drug-Drug: May ↑ **dofetilide** levels and the risk of QT interval prolongation with arrhythmias; concurrent use contraindicated. May ↑ levels and risk of toxicity of **phenytoin**; closely monitor phenytoin levels. May ↑ levels of and risk of bleeding from **warfarin**; closely monitor INR. May ↑ hypoglycemic effects

T

of **sulfonylureas, pioglitazone, repaglinide,** and **metformin**. May ↑ levels and risk of toxicity of **methotrexate**; avoid concurrent use. May ↑ risk of thrombocytopenia from **thiazide diuretics**, especially in older adults. May ↑ risk of nephrotoxicity associated with **cyclosporine**; avoid concurrent use. May ↑ levels and risk of toxicity of **digoxin**, especially in older adults; closely monitor digoxin levels. **Indomethacin** may ↑ levels and risk of toxicity; avoid concurrent use. **ACE inhibitors** and **angiotensin receptor blockers** may ↑ risk of hyperkalemia; avoid concurrent use. May ↓ the effectiveness of **tricyclic antidepressants**. May ↑ risk of myelosuppression with **zidovudine**. May ↑ **procainamide** levels and risk of QT interval prolongation with arrhythmias; closely monitor procainamide levels.

Route/Dosage

Dosing based on trimethoprim content.

Bacterial Infections

PO, IV (Adults and Children >2 mo): *Mild to moderate infections:* 6–12 mg of trimethoprim/kg/day divided every 12 hr; *Serious infection/PJP:* 15–20 mg of trimethoprim/kg/day divided every 6–8 hr.

PO (Adults): *Urinary tract infection/chronic bronchitis:* 1 double-strength tablet (160 mg trimethoprim/800 mg sulfamethoxazole) every 12 hr for 10–14 days.

Urinary Tract Infection Prophylaxis

PO, IV (Adults and Children >2 mo): 2 mg of trimethoprim/kg/dose once daily or 5 mg of trimethoprim/kg/dose twice weekly.

P. jirovecii Pneumonia Prevention

PO (Adults): 1 double-strength tablet (160 mg trimethoprim/800 mg sulfamethoxazole) once daily (may also be given 3 times weekly).

PO (Children >1 mo): 150 mg of trimethoprim/m^2/day divided every 12 hr or given as a single dose on 3 consecutive days/wk (not to exceed 320 mg trimethoprim/1600 mg sulfamethoxazole per day).

Availability (generic available)

Tablets: 🍁 20 mg trimethoprim/100 mg sulfamethoxazole, 80 mg trimethoprim/400 mg sulfamethoxazole, 160 mg trimethoprim/800 mg sulfamethoxazole (double-strength). **Oral suspension (cherry, grape flavors):** 40 mg trimethoprim/200 mg sulfamethoxazole per 5 mL. **Solution for injection:** 16 mg trimethoprim/80 mg sulfamethoxazole per mL (contains 40% propylene glycol).

NURSING IMPLICATIONS

Assessment

- Assess for sulfonamide allergy prior to initiation.
- Assess for infection (vital signs; appearance of wound, sputum, urine, and stool; WBC) at beginning of and during therapy.
- Inspect IV site frequently for infusion reaction, including phlebitis.
- Monitor for signs/symptoms of hypersensitivity reaction and anaphylaxis. *If symptoms occur,* immediately discontinue therapy and treat as indicated. Keep emergency medication and equipment nearby during therapy.
- Assess for signs/symptoms of hemophagocytic lymphohistiocytosis (fever, hepatosplenomegaly, rash, lymphadenopathy, neurologic symptoms, cytopenias, ↑ ferritin, hypertriglyceridemia, liver enzyme and coagulation abnormalities). *If hemophagocytic lymphohistiocytosis suspected,* discontinue trimethoprim/sulfamethoxazole immediately and treat as indicated.
- Monitor intake and output. Fluid intake should be sufficient to maintain a urine output of ≥1200–1500 mL daily to prevent crystalluria and stone formation.
- Monitor for signs/ symptoms of CDAD (diarrhea, abdominal cramping, fever, bloody stools). *If CDAD occurs,* discontinue trimethoprim/sulfamethoxazole and treat as indicated. May begin up to several weeks following cessation of therapy.
- Assess for rash periodically during therapy. May cause SJS, TEN, EM, and AGEP. *If severe skin reaction occurs or if accompanied with fever, general malaise, fatigue, muscle or joint aches, blisters, oral lesions, conjunctivitis, hepatitis, or eosinophilia,* discontinue trimethoprim/sulfamethoxazole.

Lab Test Considerations

- Obtain specimens for culture and sensitivity before initiating therapy. 1st dose may be given before receiving results.
- Monitor CBC, including platelets, and urinalysis periodically during therapy.
- May ↑ serum bilirubin, potassium, serum creatinine, and alkaline phosphatase.
- May cause hypoglycemia.

Implementation

- Do not confuse DS (double-strength) formulations with single-strength formulations.
- Do not administer medication IM.
- **PO:** Administer around the clock with a full glass of water. Use calibrated measuring device for liquid preparations.

IV Administration

- **Intermittent Infusion: Dilution:** Dilute each 5 mL of trimethoprim/sulfamethoxazole with 125 mL of D5W (stable for 24 hr at room temperature). May also dilute each 5 mL of drug with 75 mL of D5W if fluid restriction is required (stable for 6 hr at room temperature). Do not refrigerate. **Concentration:** ≤1.06 mg/mL. **Rate:** Infuse over 60–90 min.

- **Y-Site Compatibility:** acyclovir, aldesleukin, alemtuzumab, allopurinol, aminocaproic acid, amphotericin B liposomal, anidulafungin, argatroban, arsenic trioxide, azithromycin, bivalirudin, bleomycin, cangrelor, carboplatin, carmustine, cefepime, cefiderocol, ceftaroline, ceftobiprole, cisplatin, cyclophosphamide, cytarabine, dactinomycin, daptomycin, defibrotide, dexmedetomidine, diltiazem, dimenhydrinate, docetaxel, doxorubicin liposomal, edetate disodium, eptifibatide, ertapenem, etoposide, etoposide phosphate, filgrastim, fludarabine, fluorouracil, fosphenytoin, gemcitabine, gemtuzumab ozogamicin, granisetron, hydromorphone, ifosfamide, irinotecan, leucovorin, levofloxacin, linezolid, lorazepam, melphalan, meropenem, mesna, methotrexate, metronidazole, milrinone, mitomycin, mitoxantrone, octreotide, oxaliplatin, paclitaxel, palonosetron, pamidronate, pemetrexed, piperacillin/tazobactam, potassium acetate, remifentanil, rituximab, sargramostim, sodium acetate, thiotepa, tigecycline, tirofiban, trastuzumab, vecuronium, vinblastine, vincristine, voriconazole, zidovudine, zoledronic acid.
- **Y-Site Incompatibility:** amikacin, aminophylline, amphotericin B deoxycholate, ampicillin, ampicillin/sulbactam, ascorbic acid, atropine, azathioprine, benztropine, blinatumomab, bumetanide, buprenorphine, butorphanol, calcium chloride, calcium gluconate, caspofungin, cefazolin, cefotaxime, cefotetan, cefoxitin, ceftazidime, ceftriaxone, cefuroxime, chloramphenicol, chlorpromazine, clindamycin, cyanocobalamin, cyclosporine, dacarbazine, dantrolene, daunorubicin, dexamethasone, dexrazoxane, diazepam, diazoxide, digoxin, diphenhydramine, dobutamine, dopamine, doxorubicin hydrochloride, doxycycline, ephedrine, epinephrine, epirubicin, epoetin alfa, erythromycin, famotidine, fentanyl, fluconazole, folic acid, furosemide, ganciclovir, gentamicin, glycopyrrolate, haloperidol, hydralazine, hydrocortisone, idarubicin, imipenem/cilastatin, indomethacin, insulin regular, isoproterenol, ketamine, ketorolac, lidocaine, mannitol, methadone, methylprednisolone, metoclopramide, metoprolol, midazolam, minocycline, multivitamins, mycophenolate, nafcillin, nalbuphine, naloxone, nitroglycerin, nitroprusside, norepinephrine, ondansetron, oritavancin, oxacillin, oxytocin, papaverine, penicillin G, pentamidine, pentobarbital, phenobarbital, phentolamine, phenylephrine, phenytoin, phytonadione, potassium chloride, procainamide, prochlorperazine, promethazine, propranolol, protamine, pyridoxine, sodium bicarbonate, succinylcholine, sufentanil, theophylline, thiamine, tobramycin, topotecan, vancomycin, verapamil, vinorelbine.

Patient/Family Teaching

- Explain purpose and side effects of medication. Advise patient to read *Patient Information* before starting therapy.
- Advise patient to take full course of therapy, even if feeling better, and to take missed dose as soon as remembered unless almost time for next dose. Skipping doses or not completing full course may result in ↓ effectiveness and ↑ risk of bacterial resistance.
- Instruct patient to notify health care provider if rash or fever and diarrhea develop, especially if diarrhea contains blood, mucus, or pus. Advise patient not to treat diarrhea without consulting health care provider.
- Emphasize importance of regular follow-up exams to monitor blood counts in patients on prolonged therapy.
- Caution patient to use sunscreen and protective clothing to prevent photosensitivity reaction.
- Advise patient to notify health care provider if rash, sore throat, fever, mouth sores, or unusual bleeding or bruising occurs.
- Advise patient to notify health care provider of all Rx or OTC medications, vitamins, or herbal products being taken and to consult with health care provider before taking other medications.
- Instruct patient to notify health care provider if signs/symptoms of infection do not improve within a few days.
- Rep: May cause fetal harm. Advise women of reproductive potential to notify health care provider if pregnancy is planned or suspected or if breast-feeding. Fetal exposure during pregnancy may lead to congenital malformations, neural tube defects, cardiovascular malformations, urinary tract defects, oral clefts, and club foot.

Evaluation/Desired Outcomes

- Resolution of the signs and symptoms of infection. Length of time for complete resolution depends on organism and site of infection.
- Resolution of symptoms of traveler's diarrhea.
- Prevention of PJP pneumonia in patients with HIV.

T

ubrogepant (ue-broe-je-pant)

Ubrelvy

Classification

Therapeutic: vascular headache suppressants

Pharmacologic: calcitonin gene-related peptide receptor antagonists

Indications

Acute treatment of migraine with or without aura.

Action

Binds to and antagonizes the calcitonin gene-related peptide (CGRP) receptor, which reduces the neuroinflammatory and vasodilatory effects of CGRP.
Therapeutic Effects: Relief of pain associated with acute migraine attacks.

Pharmacokinetics

Absorption: Rapidly absorbed. Absorption delayed by high-fat food.
Distribution: Widely distributed to tissues.
Metabolism and Excretion: Primarily metabolized by the liver via the CYP3A4 isoenzyme to inactive metabolites. Eliminated in bile/feces (42% as unchanged drugs) and urine (6% as unchanged drug).
Half-life: 5–7 hr.

TIME/ACTION PROFILE (pain relief)

ROUTE	ONSET	PEAK	DURATION
PO	30–60 min	2 hr	24 hr

Contraindications/Precautions

Contraindicated in: Hypersensitivity; Concurrent use of strong CYP3A4 inhibitors; End-stage renal disease.
Use Cautiously in: Hypertension; Raynaud phenomenon; Severe renal impairment (↓ dose); Severe hepatic impairment (↓ dose); OB: Safety not established in pregnancy; Lactation: Use while breastfeeding only if potential maternal benefit justifies potential risk to infant; Pedi: Safety and effectiveness not established in children.

Adverse Reactions/Side Effects

CV: hypertension, Raynaud phenomenon. **GI:** dry mouth, nausea. **Neuro:** drowsiness. **Misc:** HYPERSENSITIVITY REACTIONS (INCLUDING ANAPHYLAXIS AND FACIAL/THROAT EDEMA).

Interactions

Drug-Drug: Strong CYP3A4 inhibitors, including **clarithromycin**, **itraconazole**, or **ketoconazole**, may significantly ↑ levels and risk of toxicity; concurrent use contraindicated. **Moderate CYP3A4 inhibitors** and **weak CYP3A4 inhibitors**, including **ciprofloxacin**, **cyclosporine**, **fluconazole**, **fluvoxamine**, or **verapamil**, may ↑ levels and risk of toxicity; ↓ ubrogepant dose. **Strong CYP3A4 inducers**, including **phenobarbital**, **phenytoin**, or **rifampin**, may significantly ↓ levels and effectiveness; avoid concurrent use. **Moderate CYP3A4 inducers** or **weak CYP3A4 inducers** may ↓ levels and effectiveness; ↑ ubrogepant dose. **P-glycoprotein (P-gp) inhibitors** and **breast cancer resistant protein (BCRP) inhibitors**, including **carvedilol**, **eltrombopag**, or **quinidine**, may ↑ levels and risk of toxicity; ↓ ubrogepant dose.
Drug-Natural Products: St. John's wort may ↓ levels and effectiveness; avoid concurrent use.
Drug-Food: Grapefruit juice may ↑ levels and risk of toxicity; ↓ ubrogepant dose.

Route/Dosage

PO (Adults): 50 mg or 100 mg initially; if response is inadequate at 2 hr, may repeat dose (not to exceed 200 mg/24 hr). *Concurrent use of moderate CYP3A4 inhibitors:* 50 mg initially (not to exceed 50 mg/24 hr). *Concurrent use of weak CYP3A4 inhibitors:* 50 mg initially; if response is inadequate at 2 hr, may repeat dose (not to exceed 100 mg/24 hr). *Concurrent use of weak or moderate CYP3A4 inducers:* 100 mg initially; if response is inadequate at 2 hr, may repeat dose (not to exceed 200 mg/24 hr). *Concurrent use of P-gp or BCRP inhibitors:* 50 mg initially; if response is inadequate at 2 hr, may repeat dose (not to exceed 100 mg/24 hr).

Renal Impairment

PO (Adults): *CCr 15–29 mL/min:* 50 mg initially; if response is inadequate at 2 hr, may repeat dose (not to exceed 100 mg/24 hr).

Hepatic Impairment

PO (Adults): *Severe hepatic impairment:* 50 mg initially; if response is inadequate at 2 hr, may repeat dose (not to exceed 100 mg/24 hr).

Availability

Tablets: 50 mg, 100 mg.

NURSING IMPLICATIONS

Assessment

- Assess pain location, character, intensity, and duration and associated symptoms (photophobia, phonophobia, nausea, vomiting) during migraine.
- Monitor for hypersensitivity reaction, including anaphylaxis, minutes to days after administration. *If reaction occurs,* immediately discontinue ubrogepant and treat as indicated.
- Monitor for new-onset or worsening hypertension. *If either occur,* consider discontinuing ubrogepant if no alternate etiology found or BP is inadequately controlled.

- Assess for signs/symptoms of recurrent, worsening or new-onset Raynaud phenomenon. *If signs/symptoms occur,* discontinue ubrogepant.

Implementation

- **PO:** Administer without regard to food. If needed, a 2nd dose may be taken ≥2 hr after initial dose.

Patient/Family Teaching

- Explain purpose and side effects of medication. Advise patient to read *Patient Information* before starting therapy.
- Instruct patient to take ubrogepant as soon as symptoms of a migraine occur, but it may be administered any time during an attack. If migraine symptoms return, a 2nd dose may be used; allow ≥2 hr between doses, and do not use more than 100 mg in any 24-hr period.
- Inform patient that ubrogepant should only be used during a migraine. It is meant to be used for relief of migraine but not to prevent or ↓ the number of events.
- Advise patient to avoid grapefruit and grapefruit juice during therapy. Instruct patient not take a 2nd tablet within 24 hr if grapefruit or grapefruit juice was consumed.
- May cause dizziness or drowsiness. Caution patient to avoid driving or other activities requiring alertness until response to medication is known.
- Advise patient to avoid alcohol, which aggravates headaches, during therapy.
- Advise patient that lying down in a darkened room following ubrogepant administration may further help relieve headache.
- Advise patient to notify health care provider of all Rx or OTC medications, vitamins, or herbal products being taken and to consult with health care provider before taking other medications, especially St. John's wort.
- Advise patient to notify health care provider immediately if signs and symptoms of hypersensitivity reaction (anaphylaxis, dyspnea, facial or throat swelling, rash, hives, itching) occur.
- Rep: Advise women of reproductive potential to notify health care provider if pregnancy is planned or suspected or if breastfeeding. Encourage patient to enroll in registry that monitors outcomes in patients who become pregnant while taking ubrogepant by calling 1-833-277-0206 or visiting http://empresspregnancyregistry.com.

Evaluation/Desired Outcomes

- Relief of migraine attack.

ulipristal, See CONTRACEPTIVES, HORMONAL.

upadacitinib (ue-pad-a-sye-ti-nib)

Rinvoq, Rinvoq LQ

Classification

Therapeutic: antirheumatics

Pharmacologic: kinase inhibitors

Indications

Rinvoq: Treatment of the following disorders: Moderately to severely active rheumatoid arthritis in patients who have had an inadequate response/intolerance to ≥1 tumor necrosis factor (TNF) blocker (not to be used with other Janus kinase [JAK] inhibitors, biologic disease-modifying antirheumatic drugs [DMARDs] or potent immunosuppressants [including azathioprine or cyclosporine]); Refractory, moderate to severe atopic dermatitis in patients whose disease is not adequately controlled with other systemic drug products, including biologics, or when use of those therapies are not recommended (not to be used with other JAK inhibitors, biologic immunomodulators, or other immunosuppressants); Moderately to severely active ulcerative colitis in patients who have had an inadequate response/intolerance to ≥1 TNF blocker (not to be used with other JAK inhibitors, biological therapies, or potent immunosuppressants [including azathioprine or cyclosporine]); Moderately to severely active Crohn disease in patients who have had an inadequate response/intolerance to ≥1 TNF blocker (not to be used with other JAK inhibitors, biological therapies, or potent immunosuppressants [including azathioprine or cyclosporine]); Active ankylosing spondylitis in patients who have had an inadequate response/intolerance to ≥1 TNF blocker (not to be used with other JAK inhibitors, biologic DMARDs, or potent immunosuppressants [including azathioprine or cyclosporine]); Active non-radiographic axial spondyloarthritis in patients with objective signs of inflammation who have had an inadequate response or intolerance to TNF blocker therapy (not to be used with other JAK inhibitors, biologic DMARDs, or potent immunosuppressants [including azathioprine or cyclosporine]). Giant cell arteritis (not to be used with other JAK inhibitors, biological therapies, or potent immunosuppressants [including azathioprine or cyclosporine]). **Rinvoq and Rinvoq LQ:** Treatment of the following disorders: Active psoriatic arthritis in patients who have had an inadequate response/intolerance to ≥1 TNF blocker (not to be used with other JAK inhibitors, biologic DMARDs or potent immunosuppressants [including azathioprine or cyclosporine]); Active polyarticular

U

juvenile idiopathic arthritis in patients who have had an inadequate response or intolerance to ≥1 TNF blocker (not to be used with other JAK inhibitors, biologic DMARDs, or potent immunosuppressants [including azathioprine or cyclosporine]).

Action

Inhibits JAK enzymes, which prevents the activation of signal transducers, and activators of transcription, which ultimately results in decreased hematopoiesis and immune cell function. **Therapeutic Effects:** Improvement in clinical and symptomatic parameters of rheumatoid arthritis, psoriatic arthritis, atopic dermatitis, ulcerative colitis, Crohn disease, ankylosing spondylitis, non-radiographic axial spondyloarthritis, polyarticular juvenile idiopathic arthritis, and giant cell arteritis.

Pharmacokinetics

Absorption: Well absorbed following oral administration.
Distribution: Unknown.
Metabolism and Excretion: Primarily metabolized by the liver via the CYP3A4 isoenzyme and to a lesser extent by the CYP2D6 isoenzyme; 38% excreted in feces and 24% excreted in urine as unchanged drug.
Half-life: 8–14 hr.

TIME/ACTION PROFILE (clinical improvement)

ROUTE	ONSET	PEAK	DURATION
PO	within 2 wk	3 mo	unknown

Contraindications/Precautions

Contraindicated in: Hypersensitivity; Active infection; Lymphocyte count <500 cells/mm³, ANC <1000 cells/mm³, or hemoglobin <8 g/dL; ↑ risk for thrombosis; History of MI or stroke; End-stage renal disease (CCr <15 mL/min) (atopic dermatitis and ulcerative colitis only); Severe hepatic impairment; OB: Pregnancy; Lactation: Lactation.
Use Cautiously in: Patients who are >50 yr old and have ≥1 cardiovascular risk factor (↑ risk of all-cause mortality, cardiovascular death, MI, stroke, and thrombosis); Current or past history of smoking (↑ risk of malignancy, cardiovascular death, MI, or stroke); Known malignancy; Previously exposed to tuberculosis (TB); History of serious or opportunistic infection; Resided or traveled in areas of endemic TB or endemic mycoses; Underlying conditions that predispose to infection; History of diverticulitis or use of NSAIDs (↑ risk of GI perforation); End-stage renal disease (rheumatoid arthritis, psoriatic arthritis, Crohn disease, ankylosing spondylitis, non-radiographic axial spondyloarthritis, giant cell arteritis, polyarticular juvenile idiopathic arthritis); Rep: Women of reproductive potential; Pedi: Safety and effectiveness not established in children <18 yr (rheumatoid arthritis and ulcerative colitis), <12 yr (atopic dermatitis), or <2 yr (psoriatic arthritis and polyarticular juvenile idiopathic arthritis).

Adverse Reactions/Side Effects

CV: ARTERIAL THROMBOSIS, CARDIOVASCULAR DEATH, DEEP VEIN THROMBOSIS, MI. **GI:** ↑ liver enzymes, GI PERFORATION, nausea. **Hemat:** anemia, lymphopenia, NEUTROPENIA. **Metab:** dyslipidemia. **MS:** ↑ CK. **Neuro:** STROKE. **Resp:** cough, PULMONARY EMBOLISM. **Misc:** DEATH, fever, HYPERSENSITIVITY REACTIONS (INCLUDING ANAPHYLAXIS AND ANGIOEDEMA), INFECTION (INCLUDING TB, BACTERIAL, INVASIVE FUNGAL, VIRAL, OR OPPORTUNISTIC INFECTIONS), MALIGNANCY.

Interactions

Drug-Drug: May ↑ risk of adverse reactions and ↓ antibody response to **live vaccines**; avoid concurrent use. **Strong CYP3A4 inhibitors**, including **ketoconazole** or **clarithromycin**, may ↑ levels and risk of toxicity; avoid concurrent use. **Strong CYP3A4 inducers**, including **rifampin**, may ↓ levels and effectiveness; concurrent use not recommended. **NSAIDs** may ↑ risk of GI perforation; concurrent use requires careful monitoring. ↑ risk of immunosuppression when used with other potent **immunosuppressants**, including **azathioprine**, **cyclosporine**, **tacrolimus**, **antineoplastics**, or **radiation therapy**.
Drug-Food: **Grapefruit** or **grapefruit juice** may ↑ levels and risk of toxicity; avoid concurrent use.

Route/Dosage

Rinvoq extended-release tablets are not interchangeable with Rinvoq LQ oral solution.

Rheumatoid Arthritis, Ankylosing Spondylitis, or Non-Radiographic Axial Spondyloarthritis

PO (Adults): *Rinvoq:* 15 mg once daily.

Psoriatic Arthritis

PO (Adults): *Rinvoq:* 15 mg once daily.
PO (Children ≥2 yr and ≥30 kg): *Rinvoq:* 15 mg once daily *or Rinvoq LQ:* 6 mg twice daily.
PO (Children ≥2 yr and 20–<30 kg): *Rinvoq LQ:* 4 mg twice daily.
PO (Children ≥2 yr and 10–<20 kg): *Rinvoq LQ:* 3 mg twice daily.

Atopic Dermatitis

PO (Geriatric Patients ≥65 yr): *Rinvoq:* 15 mg once daily.
PO (Adults and Children 12–64 and ≥40 kg): *Rinvoq:* 15 mg once daily. If adequate response not achieved, may ↑ to 30 mg once daily. If adequate response not achieved with 30 mg once daily, discontinue therapy. *Concurrent use of strong CYP3A4 inhibitors:* Rinvoq: 15 mg once daily.

Renal Impairment

(Adults and Children ≥12 yr and ≥40 kg): *CCr 15–<30 mL/min:* Rinvoq: 15 mg once daily. *CCr <15 mL/min:* Rinvoq: Not recommended.

Ulcerative Colitis

PO (Adults): *Induction therapy:* Rinvoq: 45 mg once daily for 8 wk. *Maintenance therapy:* Rinvoq: 15 mg once daily; may ↑ to 30 mg once daily if patients have refractory, severe, or extensive disease. If adequate response not achieved with 30 mg once daily, discontinue therapy. *Concurrent use of strong CYP3A4 inhibitors:* Induction therapy (Rinvoq): 30 mg once daily for 8 wk. Maintenance therapy (Rinvoq): 15 mg once daily.

Renal Impairment

PO (Adults): *CCr 15–<30 mL/min:* Induction therapy (Rinvoq): 30 mg once daily for 8 wk. Maintenance therapy (Rinvoq): 15 mg once daily. *CCr <15 mL/min:* Rinvoq: Not recommended.

Hepatic Impairment

PO (Adults): *Mild or moderate hepatic impairment:* Induction therapy (Rinvoq): 30 mg once daily for 8 wk. Maintenance therapy (Rinvoq): 15 mg once daily.

Crohn Disease

PO (Adults): *Induction therapy:* Rinvoq: 45 mg once daily for 12 wk. *Maintenance therapy:* Rinvoq: 15 mg once daily; may ↑ to 30 mg once daily if patients have refractory, severe, or extensive disease. If adequate response not achieved with 30 mg once daily, discontinue therapy. *Concurrent use of strong CYP3A4 inhibitors:* Induction therapy (Rinvoq): 30 mg once daily for 12 wk. Maintenance therapy (Rinvoq): 15 mg once daily.

Renal Impairment

PO (Adults): *CCr 15–<30 mL/min:* Induction therapy (Rinvoq): 30 mg once daily for 12 wk. Maintenance therapy (Rinvoq): 15 mg once daily. *CCr <15 mL/min:* Rinvoq: Not recommended.

Hepatic Impairment

PO (Adults): *Mild or moderate hepatic impairment:* Induction therapy (Rinvoq): 30 mg once daily for 12 wk. Maintenance therapy (Rinvoq): 15 mg once daily.

Polyarticular Juvenile Idiopathic Arthritis

PO (Children ≥2 yr and ≥30 kg): *Rinvoq:* 15 mg once daily *or Rinvoq LQ:* 6 mg twice daily.
PO (Children ≥2 yr and 20–<30 kg): *Rinvoq LQ:* 4 mg twice daily.
PO (Children ≥2 yr and 10–<20 kg): *Rinvoq LQ:* 3 mg twice daily.

Giant Cell Arteritis

PO (Adults): 15 mg once daily (in combination with a corticosteroid taper), then 15 mg once daily following discontinuation of corticosteroids.

Availability

Extended-release tablets (Rinvoq): 15 mg, 30 mg, 45 mg. **Oral solution (Rinvoq LQ):** 1 mg/mL.

NURSING IMPLICATIONS

Assessment

- Assess pain and range of motion before and periodically during therapy.
- Assess for signs/symptoms of infection (fever, dyspnea, flu-like symptoms, frequent or painful urination, redness or swelling at the site of a wound), including TB and hepatitis B virus, prior to and periodically during therapy. Monitor new infections closely; most common are upper respiratory tract infections, bronchitis, and urinary tract infections. Infections may be fatal, especially in patients taking immunosuppressive therapy. If patient develops a serious infection, including serious opportunistic infection, interrupt therapy until infection is controlled.
- Assess for latent TB with a tuberculin skin test prior to initiation of therapy. Treatment of latent TB should be started before therapy with upadacitinib.
- Screen for hepatitis B virus infection before starting therapy.
- Assess skin for new lesions periodically during therapy; ↑ risk of skin cancer.
- Monitor for signs/symptoms of thrombosis (swelling, pain, or tenderness in the leg; sudden unexplained chest pain; shortness of breath) during therapy.
- Monitor patients at risk for GI perforation (patients with a history of diverticulitis and those taking concurrent medications, including NSAIDs or corticosteroids). Evaluate promptly patients presenting with new-onset abdominal pain for early identification of GI perforation.

Lab Test Considerations

- Verify negative pregnancy test before starting therapy.
- Monitor neutrophil count at baseline and periodically during therapy. *If ANC <1000 cells/mm³*, hold upadacitinib; restart once ANC returns above this value.
- Monitor lymphocyte count at baseline and periodically during therapy. *If absolute lymphocyte count <500 cells/mm³*, hold upadacitinib; restart once absolute lymphocyte count returns above this value.
- May cause anemia. Monitor hemoglobin at baseline and periodically during therapy. *If hemoglobin <8 g/dL*, hold upadacitinib.

U

- May ↑ total cholesterol, LDL-C, and HDL-C. Monitor levels 12 wk after starting therapy and periodically thereafter for hyperlipidemia.
- Monitor liver enzymes at baseline and periodically thereafter. *If AST or ALT are ↑ and drug-induced liver injury is suspected,* hold upadacitinib.

Implementation
- Immunizations, including prophylactic zoster vaccinations, should be current before starting therapy. Patients on upadacitinib may receive concurrent vaccinations, except for live vaccines.
- **PO:** *Extended-release tablets:* Administer once daily without regard to food. ***DNC:*** Swallow tablets whole; do not split, crush, or chew. *Oral solution:* Administer twice daily without regard to food using the provided press-in bottle adapter and oral dosing syringe.

Patient/Family Teaching
- Explain the purpose and side effects of upadacitinib to patient. Instruct patient to take upadacitinib as directed. Do not stop receiving drug without consulting health care provider. Advise patient to read *Patient Information* before starting therapy and with each Rx refill in case of changes.
- Emphasize the importance of regular lab tests to monitor for adverse drug reactions.
- Caution patient to avoid grapefruit or grapefruit juice during therapy.
- Advise patient to avoid live vaccines during therapy.
- Caution patient to notify health care provider immediately if signs of infection (fever; sweating; chills; muscle aches; cough; shortness of breath; blood in phlegm; weight loss; warm, red, or painful skin or sores; diarrhea or stomach pain; burning on urination or urinating more often than normal; feeling very tired), heart attack (chest pain, trouble breathing, sweating, dizziness, nausea), stroke (weakness, slurred speech, confusion, dizziness), or blood clots occur.
- Caution patient to notify health care provider immediately if signs/symptoms of stomach or intestinal perforation (fever, stomach-area pain that does not go away, change in bowel habits) occur.
- Advise patient to notify health care provider of all Rx or OTC medications, vitamins, or herbal products being taken and to consult with health care provider before taking other medications.
- Instruct patient to notify health care provider of medication regimen prior to treatment or surgery.
- Inform patient of ↑ risk of lymphoma and other cancers. Advise patient to have periodic skin exams for new lesions of skin cancer.
- Instruct patients to contact their health care provider if medication residue is observed repeatedly in stool or ostomy output.
- Rep: May cause fetal harm. Advise women of reproductive potential to use effective contraception during and for 4 wk after last dose and to avoid breastfeeding during therapy and for 6 days after last dose. Advise women of reproductive potential to notify health care provider if pregnancy is planned or suspected. If pregnancy occurs during therapy, report to the AbbVie Inc.'s Adverse Event reporting line at 1-800-633-9110, or FDA at 1-800-FDA-1088 or www.fda.gov/medwatch.

Evaluation/Desired Outcomes
- Improved symptoms, physical function, and decreased fatigue in patients with rheumatoid arthritis, psoriatic arthritis, atopic dermatitis, ulcerative colitis, Crohn disease, ankylosing spondylitis, non-radiographic axial spondyloarthritis, polyarticular juvenile idiopathic arthritis, and giant cell arteritis.

ustekinumab
(uss-te-**kin**-oo-mab)

Imuldosa, ✱ Jamteki, Otulfi, Pyzchiva, Selarsdi, Starjemza, Stelara, Steqeyma, Wezlana, Yesintek

Classification

Therapeutic: antipsoriatics

Pharmacologic: interleukin antagonists, monoclonal antibodies

Indications
Moderate to severe plaque psoriasis in patients who are candidates for phototherapy or systemic therapy. Active psoriatic arthritis (as monotherapy or with methotrexate). Moderately to severely active Crohn disease. Moderately to severely active ulcerative colitis.

Action
Binds to the p40 protein subunit used by both the interleukin (IL) 12 and IL-23 cytokines. These cytokines are involved in inflammatory and immune responses, including natural killer cell activation and CD4+ T-cell differentiation and activation. Binding to interleukins antagonizes their effects, disrupting IL-12 and IL-23 mediated signaling and cytokine cascades. **Therapeutic Effects:** Decrease in area and severity of psoriatic lesions. Decreased progression of psoriatic arthritis. Reduced signs and symptoms and maintenance of clinical remission of Crohn disease and ulcerative colitis.

Pharmacokinetics
Absorption: Well absorbed following SUBQ administration. IV administration results in complete bioavailability.

Distribution: Minimally distributed to tissues.
Metabolism and Excretion: Broken down by catabolic processes into peptides and amino acids.
Half-life: *Psoriasis:* 15–46 days; *Crohn disease:* 19 days.

TIME/ACTION PROFILE (plasma concentrations)

ROUTE	ONSET	PEAK	DURATION
45 mg SUBQ	unknown	13.5 days	12 wk
90 mg SUBQ	unknown	7 days	12 wk
IV	unknown	unknown	unknown

Contraindications/Precautions

Contraindicated in: Hypersensitivity; Active untreated infection.
Use Cautiously in: History of known malignancy or tuberculosis (TB) (possibility of reactivation); >60 yr, history of prolonged immunosuppressant therapy, or history of PUVA treatment (↑ risk of skin cancer); OB: Use during pregnancy only if potential maternal benefit justifies potential fetal risk; Lactation: Use while breastfeeding only if potential maternal benefit justifies potential risk to infant; Pedi: Safety and effectiveness not established in children <18 yr (Crohn disease) or <6 yr (psoriasis or psoriatic arthritis).
Exercise Extreme Caution in: Chronic infection or history of recurrent infection.

Adverse Reactions/Side Effects

Local: erythema. **Neuro:** fatigue, headache, POSTERIOR REVERSIBLE ENCEPHALOPATHY SYNDROME (PRES). **Resp:** eosinophilic pneumonia, interstitial pneumonia, RESPIRATORY FAILURE. **Misc:** HYPERSENSITIVITY REACTIONS (INCLUDING ANAPHYLAXIS AND ANGIOEDEMA), INFECTION, MALIGNANCY.

Interactions

Drug-Drug: May ↓ antibody response to and ↑ risk of adverse reactions from **live vaccines**. May ↓ desired antibody response to **non-live vaccines**. May affect the activity of CYP450 drug-metabolizing enzymes; when treatment is started during concurrent **CYP450 substrates**, especially those with a narrow therapeutic indices, including **warfarin** and **cyclosporine**; appropriate monitoring and dose adjustment should be carried out.

Route/Dosage

Plaque Psoriasis

SUBQ (Adults and Children ≥6 yr and >100 kg): 90 mg initially and 4 wk later, then 90 mg every 12 wk.
SUBQ (Adults ≤100 kg): 45 mg initially and 4 wk later, then 45 mg every 12 wk.
SUBQ (Children ≥6 yr and 60–100 kg): 45 mg initially and 4 wk later, then 45 mg every 12 wk.
SUBQ (Children ≥6 yr and <60 kg): *Otulfi, Selarsdi, Starjemza, Stelara, Steqeyma, Wezlana, and Yesintek:* 0.75 mg/kg initially and 4 wk later, then 0.75 mg/kg every 12 wk.

Psoriatic Arthritis

SUBQ (Adults): 45 mg initially and 4 wk later, then 45 mg every 12 wk.
SUBQ (Adults and Children ≥6 yr and >100 kg and with coexistent moderate to severe plaque psoriasis): 90 mg initially and 4 wk later, then 90 mg every 12 wk.
SUBQ (Children ≥6 yr and ≥60 kg): 45 mg initially and 4 wk later, then 45 mg every 12 wk.
SUBQ (Children ≥6 yr and <60 kg): *Otulfi, Selarsdi, Starjemza, Stelara, Steqeyma, Wezlana, and Yesintek:* 0.75 mg/kg initially and 4 wk later, then 0.75 mg/kg every 12 wk.

Crohn Disease and Ulcerative Colitis

IV, SUBQ (Adults >85 kg): 520 mg IV infusion, then 90 mg SUBQ 8 wk later, then 90 mg every 8 wk.
IV, SUBQ (Adults 56–85 kg): 390 mg IV infusion, then 90 mg SUBQ 8 wk later, then 90 mg every 8 wk.
IV, SUBQ (Adults ≤55 kg): 260 mg IV infusion, then 90 mg SUBQ 8 wk later, then 90 mg every 8 wk.

Availability

Solution for IV injection: 5 mg/mL. **Solution for SUBQ injection:** 45 mg/0.45 mL (vials and prefilled syringes), 90 mg/1 mL (prefilled syringes).

NURSING IMPLICATIONS

Assessment

- Assess for signs of infection (fever, dyspnea, flu-like symptoms, frequent or painful urination, redness or swelling at the site of a wound) prior to injection. *If existing or new infection occurs,* monitor closely; infections can be fatal while on immunosuppressive therapy. Patients genetically deficient in IL-12/IL-23 are particularly vulnerable to disseminated infections; consider diagnostic testing.
- Assess patient for latent TB with a tuberculin skin test prior to initiation of therapy. Treatment of latent TB should be started before therapy with ustekinumab.
- Monitor for signs and symptoms of PRES (visual disturbance, seizure, headache, altered mentation). *If PRES suspected,* discontinue ustekinumab.
- Monitor for signs/symptoms of hypersensitivity reaction (rash; urticaria; chest tightness; wheezing; feeling faint; dyspnea; throat tightness; swelling of face, eyelids, tongue, or throat) during therapy. *If*

symptoms occur, immediately discontinue ustekinumab and treat as indicated.

- **Crohn Disease:** Evaluate symptomatic response between 6 and 10 wk to determine need to modify therapy.
- **Psoriasis:** Assess affected area(s) prior to and periodically during therapy; improvement in psoriatic lesions is indicative of efficacy.
- **Psoriatic Arthritis:** Assess swollen or tender joints; ↓ in joint pain or number of joints affected is indicative of efficacy.

Implementation

- Immunizations should be current prior to initiating therapy. Patients on ustekinumab may receive concurrent vaccinations, except for live vaccines.
- **SUBQ**: Should be administered by health care provider unless patient or caregiver has been trained to administer injection. Administer using a 1-mL syringe with 27-gauge, ½-inch needle in upper arm, gluteal region, thigh, or abdomen; rotate site. Do not administer in areas that are tender, bruised, erythematous, or indurated. Solution is colorless to light yellow and may contain a few small translucent or white particles; do not administer if discolored, cloudy, or contains other particulates. Do not shake. Store solution in refrigerator; do not freeze.
- For prefilled syringe, inject full contents of syringe; maintain pressure on plunger head and remove from skin; slowly allow empty syringe to move up to cover needle with needle guard. Needle cover contains latex.

IV Administration

- **Intermittent Infusion:** Calculate the dose and the number of vials needed based on patient weight. Withdraw equal volume as dose from 250-mL bag of 0.9% NaCl or 0.45% NaCl. Withdraw 26 mL from each vial of ustekinumab needed and add to 250-mL bag; mix gently. Solution is clear and colorless to light yellow; do not administer if discolored or contains particulates. Solution is stable for 7 hr at room temperature. Discard remaining solution. **Rate:** Infuse over ≥1 hr through a 0.2-micrometer in-line, sterile, nonpyrogenic, low-protein-binding filter.
- **Y-Site Incompatibility:** Do not administer other drugs through same IV line.

Patient/Family Teaching

- Explain purpose and side effects of medication. Advise patient to read *Patient Information* before starting therapy.
- Instruct patient on the appropriate steps for measuring accurate dose, administration technique, and disposal of equipment, if self-administering. Notify patient that the needle cover on the prefilled syringe contains latex.
- Advise patient to not stop receiving drug without consulting health care provider.
- Explain need for continued medical follow-up to assess effectiveness and possible side effects of medication. If an appointment is missed, reschedule as soon as possible.
- Inform patient of ↑ risk for infection and to notify health care provider immediately if signs of anaphylaxis or infection (fever; sweats; chills; muscle aches; cough; shortness of breath; blood in phlegm; weight loss; warm, red, or painful sores; diarrhea or stomach pain; burning or urination or urinary frequency; tiredness) occur.
- Inform patient that ustekinumab may ↑ risk for cancer and to obtain preventive screening.
- Advise patient to notify health care provider if signs/symptoms of PRES (headache, seizures, confusion, visual problems) occur.
- Advise patient not to receive live vaccinations during therapy.
- Instruct patient to notify health care provider of all Rx or OTC medications, vitamins, or herbal products being taken and consult health care provider before taking any new medications.
- Instruct patient to notify health care provider of medication regimen prior to treatment or surgery.
- **Rep:** Advise women of reproductive potential to notify health care provider if pregnancy is planned or suspected or if breastfeeding. Delay live-virus immunizations in infants exposed in utero for ≥6 mo after birth.

Evaluation/Desired Outcomes

- Decrease in extent and severity of psoriatic lesions.
- Decreased progression of psoriatic arthritis.
- Reduced signs and symptoms and maintenance of clinical remission of Crohn disease or ulcerative colitis.

valACYclovir

(val-ay-**sye**-kloe-veer)

Valtrex

Classification

Therapeutic: antivirals

Indications

Treatment of herpes zoster (shingles). Treatment/suppression of genital herpes. Reduction of transmission of genital herpes. Treatment of chickenpox. Treatment of herpes labialis (cold sores).

Action

Rapidly converted to acyclovir. Acyclovir interferes with viral DNA synthesis. **Therapeutic Effects:** Inhibited viral replication, decreased viral shedding, and reduced time to healing of lesions. Reduced transmission of genital herpes.

Pharmacokinetics

Absorption: 54% bioavailable as acyclovir after oral administration of valacyclovir.

Distribution: CSF concentrations of acyclovir are 50% of plasma concentrations.

Metabolism and Excretion: Rapidly converted to acyclovir via intestinal/hepatic metabolism. Primarily excreted in the urine as acyclovir.

Half-life: 2.5–3.3 hr; up to 14 hr in renal impairment (acyclovir).

TIME/ACTION PROFILE (plasma concentrations†)

ROUTE	ONSET	PEAK	DURATION
PO	unknown	1.5–2.5 hr	8–24 hr

† Acyclovir.

Contraindications/Precautions

Contraindicated in: Hypersensitivity to valacyclovir or acyclovir.

Use Cautiously in: Renal impairment (↓ dose/↑ dosing interval if CCr <50 mL/min); Pedi: Safety and effectiveness not established in children <18 yr (herpes zoster or genital herpes), <12 yr (herpes labialis), or <2 yr (chickenpox); Geri: Dose ↓ may be necessary in older adults due to ↑ risk of acute renal failure and CNS side effects.

Adverse Reactions/Side Effects

GI: nausea, abdominal pain, anorexia, constipation, diarrhea. **GU:** crystalluria, RENAL FAILURE. **Hemat:** THROMBOTIC THROMBOCYTOPENIC PURPURA/HEMOLYTIC UREMIC SYNDROME (WITH USE OF HIGH DOSES IN IMMUNOSUPPRESSED PATIENTS). **Neuro:** headache, agitation, confusion, delirium, dizziness, encephalopathy, hallucinations, SEIZURES, weakness.

Interactions

Drug-Drug: Probenecid and **cimetidine** may ↑ levels and risk of toxicity, especially in patients with renal impairment. Concurrent use of other **nephrotoxic drugs** ↑ risk of adverse renal effects.

Route/Dosage

Herpes Zoster

PO (Adults): 1 g 3 times daily for 7 days.

Renal Impairment

PO (Adults): *CCr 30–49 mL/min:* 1 g every 12 hr. *CCr 10–29 mL/min:* 1 g every 24 hr. *CCr <10 mL/min:* 500 mg every 24 hr.

Genital Herpes

PO (Adults): *Initial treatment:* 1 g twice daily for 10 days. *Recurrence:* 500 mg twice daily for 3 days. *Suppression of recurrence:* 1 g once daily or 500 mg once daily in patients experiencing <10 recurrences/yr. *Suppression of recurrence in patients with HIV:* 500 mg every 12 hr. *Reduction of transmission:* 500 mg once daily for source partner.

Renal Impairment

PO (Adults): *CCr 10–29 mL/min:* 1 g every 24 hr for initial treatment of genital herpes, 500 mg every 24 hr for treatment of recurrent episodes of genital herpes, 500 mg every 48 hr for suppression of genital herpes in patients with <10 recurrences/yr, 500 mg every 24 hr for suppression of genital herpes in patients with ≥10 recurrences/yr or patients with HIV. *CCr <10 mL/min:* 500 mg every 24 hr for initial treatment of genital herpes, 500 mg every 24 hr for treatment of recurrent episodes of genital herpes, 500 mg every 48 hr for suppression of genital herpes in patients with <10 recurrences/yr, 500 mg every 24 hr for suppression of genital herpes in patients with ≥10 recurrences/yr or patients with HIV.

Herpes Labialis

PO (Adults and Children ≥12 yr): 2 g initially, then 2 g 12 hr later.

Renal Impairment

PO (Adults): *CCr 30–49 mL/min:* 1 g initially, then 1 g 12 hr later. *CCr 10–29 mL/min:* 500 mg initially, then 500 mg 12 hr later. *CCr <10 mL/min:* 500 mg as a single dose.

Chickenpox

PO (Children ≥2 yr): 20 mg/kg 3 times daily for 5 days (not to exceed 1 g 3 times daily).

Availability (generic available)

Tablets: 500 mg, 1 g.

V

NURSING IMPLICATIONS

Assessment

- Assess lesions for type, location, and severity before and daily during therapy.
- Monitor for signs/symptoms of thrombotic thrombocytopenic purpura/hemolytic uremic syndrome (thrombocytopenia, microangiopathic hemolytic anemia, neurologic findings, renal impairment, fever). Requires prompt treatment; may be fatal.

Lab Test Considerations

- Monitor BUN and serum creatinine.

Implementation

- ***High Alert:*** Do not confuse valacyclovir with valganciclovir. Do not confuse Valtrex with Valcyte.
- **PO:** Administer with or without food.
- **Herpes Zoster:** Implement valacyclovir therapy as soon as possible after the onset of signs/symptoms of herpes zoster; most effective if started within 48 hr of the onset of zoster rash. Efficacy of treatment started >72 hr after rash onset is unknown.
- **Genital Herpes and Herpes Labialis:** Implement treatment for genital herpes as soon as possible after onset of symptoms (tingling, itching, burning).
- **Chickenpox:** Initiate therapy at the earliest sign or symptom; preferably within 24 hr of onset of rash.

Patient/Family Teaching

- Explain purpose and side effects of medication. Advise patient to read *Patient Information* before starting therapy. Instruct to take exactly as directed for the full course of therapy. Take missed doses as soon as remembered if not just before next dose; do not double doses.
- Advise patient to notify health care provider of all Rx or OTC medications, vitamins, or herbal products being taken and to consult health care provider before taking other medications.
- Advise patient to maintain adequate hydration during therapy.
- Advise patient to notify health care provider promptly if CNS signs/symptoms (aggressive behavior, unsteady movement, shaky movements, confusion, speech problems, hallucinations, seizures, coma) occur.
- Advise patient to notify health care provider of signs or symptoms of extreme fatigue, bruising or bleeding, dark urine or yellow skin or eyes, pale skin, change in the amount of urine passed, change in eyesight, or fever.
- **Herpes Zoster:** Advise patient that valacyclovir does not prevent the spread of infection to others. Precautions should be taken around others who have not had chickenpox or varicella vaccine or are immunosuppressed until all lesions have crusted.
- **Genital Herpes and Herpes Labialis:** Advise patient that valacyclovir does not prevent the spread of herpes labialis to others. Advise patient to avoid contact with others while lesions or symptoms are present. Valacyclovir ↓ transmission of genital herpes to others. Advise patient to practice safe sex (avoid sexual intercourse when lesions are present and wear a condom made of latex or polyurethane during sexual contact).
- Rep: Advise women of reproductive potential to notify health care provider if pregnancy is planned or suspected or if breastfeeding.

Evaluation/Desired Outcomes

- Inhibited viral replication, decreased viral shedding, and reduced time to healing of lesions.
- Reduced transmission of genital herpes.

valbenazine (val-ben-a-zeen)

Ingrezza, Ingrezza Sprinkle

Classification

Therapeutic: none assigned

Pharmacologic: reversible monoamine depleters

Indications

Tardive dyskinesia. Chorea associated with Huntington disease.

Action

Acts as a reversible inhibitor of the vesicular monoamine transporter 2, which inhibits the reuptake of serotonin, norepinephrine, and dopamine into vesicles in presynaptic neurons. **Therapeutic Effects:** Reduced severity of tardive dyskinesia. Reduction in chorea.

Pharmacokinetics

Absorption: 49% absorbed following oral administration.

Distribution: Well distributed to tissues.

Protein Binding: >99%.

Metabolism and Excretion: Rapidly and extensively metabolized by the liver via hydrolysis to the active metabolite, α-dihydrotetrabenazine (α-HTBZ); also metabolized via the CYP3A4 isoenzyme to form other minor metabolites. α-HTBZ is further metabolized, in part, via the CYP2D6 isoenzyme. The CYP2D6 isoenzyme exhibits genetic polymorphism; 7% of population may be poor metabolizers and may have significantly ↑ concentrations and an ↑ risk of adverse effects. 60% eliminated in urine (<2% as unchanged drug); 30% eliminated in feces (<2% as unchanged drug).

Half-life: 15–22 hr (valbenazine and α-HTBZ).

TIME/ACTION PROFILE (plasma concentrations)

ROUTE	ONSET	PEAK	DURATION
PO	unknown	0.5–1 hr	unknown

Contraindications/Precautions

Contraindicated in: Hypersensitivity; Congenital long QT syndrome or history of torsades de pointes; Lactation: Lactation.

Use Cautiously in: Patients with Huntington disease with history of depression or suicidal thoughts/attempts; Poor CYP2D6 metabolizers or taking strong CYP2D6 inhibitor (may need to ↓ valbenazine dose); Moderate or severe hepatic impairment (↓ dose); OB: Safety not established in pregnancy; Pedi: Safety and effectiveness not established in children.

Adverse Reactions/Side Effects

EENT: blurred vision. **GI:** constipation, nausea, vomiting, xerostomia. **GU:** urinary retention. **MS:** arthralgia, bradykinesia. **Neuro:** fatigue, sedation/somnolence, akathisia, balance difficulty, DEPRESSION, dizziness, gait disturbances, headache, NEUROLEPTIC MALIGNANT SYNDROME (NMS), parkinsonism, restlessness, SUICIDAL THOUGHTS/BEHAVIORS, tremor, unsteady gait. **Misc:** HYPERSENSITIVITY REACTIONS (INCLUDING ANGIOEDEMA).

Interactions

Drug-Drug: MAO inhibitors may ↑ risk of serotonin syndrome and/or ↓ the effectiveness of valbenazine; avoid concurrent use. **Strong CYP3A4 inhibitors**, including **itraconazole**, **ketoconazole**, or **clarithromycin**, may ↑ levels of valbenazine and its active metabolite (α-HTBZ) and the risk of toxicity; ↓ valbenazine dose. **Strong CYP2D6 inhibitors**, including **fluoxetine**, **paroxetine**, or **quinidine**, may ↑ levels of the active metabolite (α-HTBZ) and the risk of toxicity; may need to ↓ valbenazine dose. **Strong CYP3A4 inducers**, including **rifampin**, **carbamazepine**, or **phenytoin**, may ↓ levels and effectiveness; concurrent use not recommended. May ↑ levels and risk of toxicity of **digoxin**.

Drug-Natural Products: St. John's wort may ↓ levels and effectiveness; concurrent use not recommended.

Route/Dosage

Tardive Dyskinesia

PO (Adults): 40 mg once daily; after 1 wk, ↑ to 80 mg once daily. *Known CYP2D6 poor metabolizer:* 40 mg once daily (with no additional titration). *Concurrent use of strong CYP3A4 inhibitors or strong CYP2D6 inhibitors:* 40 mg once daily (with no additional titration).

Hepatic Impairment

PO (Adults): *Moderate or severe hepatic impairment:* 40 mg once daily (with no additional titration).

Chorea Associated with Huntington Disease

PO (Adults): 40 mg once daily; ↑ by 20 mg/day every 2 wk until achieve recommended dose of 80 mg once daily. *Known CYP2D6 poor metabolizer:* 40 mg once daily (with no additional titration). *Concurrent use of strong CYP3A4 inhibitors or strong CYP2D6 inhibitors:* 40 mg once daily (with no additional titration).

Hepatic Impairment

PO (Adults): *Moderate or severe hepatic impairment:* 40 mg once daily (with no additional titration).

Availability (generic available)

Capsules: 40 mg, 60 mg, 80 mg. **Sprinkle capsules:** 40 mg, 60 mg, 80 mg.

NURSING IMPLICATIONS

Assessment

- Monitor for changes in signs and symptoms of tardive dyskinesia (uncontrolled rhythmic movement of mouth, face, and extremities; lip smacking or puckering; puffing of cheeks; uncontrolled chewing; rapid or worm-like movements of tongue; excessive eye blinking) periodically during therapy.
- Assess cardiac history and ECG at baseline; avoid use in patients with long QT syndrome or torsade de pointes.
- Monitor patients with Huntington disease for new or worsening depression and suicidal ideation or behaviors. If these reactions occur and do not resolve, consider discontinuing valbenazine.
- Monitor for signs and symptoms of hypersensitivity (angioedema involving the larynx, glottis, lips, and eyelids). *If signs and symptoms of hypersensitivity occur,* discontinue valbenazine.
- Monitor for signs and symptoms of NMS (hyperpyrexia, muscle rigidity, altered mental status, evidence of autonomic instability [irregular HR or BP, tachycardia, diaphoresis, cardiac arrhythmia]). *If symptoms of NMS occur,* immediately discontinue valbenazine. Recurrence of NMS has been reported with resumption of therapy. If therapy with valbenazine is needed after recovery from NMS, patients should be monitored for signs of recurrence.

Implementation

- **PO:** Administer once daily without regard to food.
- Open and sprinkle the entire contents of the sprinkle capsule over a bowl containing a small amount (1 tablespoonful) of soft food such as applesauce, yogurt, or pudding. Do not sprinkle the contents of the capsule into milk or drinking water. Stir the contents of the capsule into the soft food with the tablespoon and swallow the drug/food mixture

V

immediately. Mixture can be stored for up to 2 hr at room temperature. Discard any unused portion after 2 hr. Following administration of the drug/food mixture, drink a glass (e.g., 240 mL) of water. Do not administer via nasogastric, gastrostomy, or other enteral tubes because it may cause obstruction.

Patient/Family Teaching

- Explain the purpose and side effects of valbenazine to patient. Instruct patient to take valbenazine as directed. Do not stop taking valbenazine without consulting health care provider. Advise patient to read *Patient Information* before starting and with each Rx refill in case of changes.
- Advise patient and family to monitor for changes, especially sudden changes, in mood, behaviors, thoughts, or feelings. If new or worse feelings of sadness or crying spells; lack of interest in friends or activities; sleeping a lot more or less; feelings of unimportance, guilt, hopelessness, or helplessness; irritability or aggression; feeling more or less hungry; having difficulty paying attention; or thoughts of hurting self or ending life occur, notify health care provider promptly.
- Explain need for continued medical follow-up to assess effectiveness and possible side effects of medication.
- May cause drowsiness. Caution patient to avoid driving and other activities requiring alertness until response to medication is known.
- Advise patient to notify health care provider if symptoms of NMS or heart rhythm problems (fast, slow, or irregular heartbeat; shortness of breath; fever; dizziness; fainting; severe muscle rigidity) occur.
- Instruct patient to notify health care provider of all Rx or OTC medications, vitamins, or herbal products being taken and consult health care provider before taking any new medications.
- Rep: Advise women of reproductive potential to notify health care provider if pregnancy is planned or suspected and to avoid breastfeeding during therapy and for 5 days after last dose.

Evaluation/Desired Outcomes

- Decrease in severity of uncontrolled movements.
- Reduction in chorea.

valGANciclovir

(val-gan-**sye**-kloe-veer)

Valcyte

Classification

Therapeutic: antivirals

Indications

Treatment of cytomegalovirus (CMV) retinitis in patients with AIDS. Prevention of CMV disease in kidney, kidney/pancreas, and heart transplant patients at risk.

Action

Valganciclovir is a prodrug, which is rapidly converted to ganciclovir by intestinal and hepatic enzymes. CMV virus converts ganciclovir to its active form (ganciclovir phosphate) inside host cell, where it inhibits viral DNA polymerase. **Therapeutic Effects:** Antiviral effect directed preferentially against CMV-infected cells.

Pharmacokinetics

Absorption: 59% absorbed following oral administration, rapidly converted to ganciclovir.
Distribution: Widely distributed to tissues, including CSF.
Metabolism and Excretion: Rapidly converted to ganciclovir; ganciclovir is mostly excreted by the kidneys.
Half-life: 4.1 hr (intracellular half-life of ganciclovir phosphate is 18 hr).

TIME/ACTION PROFILE (ganciclovir plasma concentrations)

ROUTE	ONSET	PEAK	DURATION
PO	rapid	2 hr	12–24 hr

Contraindications/Precautions

Contraindicated in: Hypersensitivity to valganciclovir or ganciclovir; Hemodialysis; Undergoing liver transplantation; OB: Pregnancy; Lactation: Lactation.
Use Cautiously in: Renal impairment (↓ dose if CCr <60 mL/min); Pre-existing bone marrow depression; Previous or concurrent myelosuppressive drug therapy or radiation therapy; Rep: Women of reproductive potential and men with female partners of reproductive potential; Pedi: Children <4 mo (safety and effectiveness not established); Geri: Age-related ↓ in renal function requires dosage ↓ in older adults.

Adverse Reactions/Side Effects

GI: abdominal pain, diarrhea, nausea, vomiting. **GU:** ↓ fertility, renal impairment. **Hemat:** ANEMIA, APLASTIC ANEMIA, NEUTROPENIA, PANCYTOPENIA, THROMBOCYTOPENIA. **Neuro:** headache, insomnia, agitation, ataxia, confusion, dizziness, hallucinations, paresthesia, peripheral neuropathy, psychosis, sedation, SEIZURES. **Misc:** fever, HYPERSENSITIVITY REACTIONS (INCLUDING ANAPHYLAXIS), INFECTION, MALIGNANCY.

Interactions

Drug-Drug: ↑ risk of hematologic toxicity with **zidovudine**. **Probenecid** may ↑ levels and risk of toxicity. Patients with renal impairment may experience accumulation of metabolites of **mycophenolate**.
Drug-Food: Food ↑ absorption.

Route/Dosage

Treatment of CMV Disease

PO (Adults): *Induction:* 900 mg twice daily for 21 days; *Maintenance treatment or patients with inactive CMV retinitis:* 900 mg once daily.

Renal Impairment

(Adults): *CCr 40–59 mL/min:* Induction: 450 mg twice daily for 21 days. Maintenance treatment or patients with inactive CMV retinitis: 450 mg once daily. *CCr 25–39 mL/min:* Induction: 450 mg once daily for 21 days. Maintenance treatment or patients with inactive CMV retinitis: 450 mg every 2 days. *CCr 10–24 mL/min:* Induction: 450 mg every 2 days for 21 days. Maintenance treatment or patients with inactive CMV retinitis: 450 mg twice weekly.

Prevention of CMV Disease in Transplant Patients

PO (Adults): *Kidney/pancreas or heart transplant:* 900 mg once daily, starting 10 days prior to transplant and continued for 100 days after; *Kidney transplant:* 900 mg once daily, starting 10 days prior to transplant and continued for 200 days after.
PO (Children 4 mo–16 yr): *Kidney transplant:* Dose is based on body surface area (BSA) and CCr. Dose = 7 × BSA × CCr (see prescribing information for equations used for BSA and CCr); all calculated doses should be rounded to nearest 25 mg (max = 900 mg) and administered as oral solution; should be started 10 days prior to transplant and continued for 200 days after.
PO (Children 4 mo–16 yr): *Heart transplant:* Dose is based on BSA and CCr. Dose = 7 × BSA × CCr (see prescribing information for equations used for BSA and CCr); all calculated doses should be rounded to nearest 25 mg (max = 900 mg) and administered as oral solution; should be started 10 days prior to transplant and continued for 100 days after.

Renal Impairment

PO (Adults): *CCr 40–59 mL/min:* 450 mg once daily; *CCr 25–39 mL/min:* 450 mg every 2 days; *CCr 12–24 mL/min:* 450 mg twice weekly.

Availability (generic available)

Tablets: 450 mg. **Oral solution (tutti-frutti flavor):** 50 mg/mL.

NURSING IMPLICATIONS

Assessment

- Culture for CMV (urine, blood, throat) may be taken prior to administration. However, a negative CMV culture does not rule out CMV retinitis. Diagnosis of CMV retinitis should be determined by ophthalmoscopy prior to treatment with valganciclovir. If symptoms do not respond after several weeks, resistance to valganciclovir may have occurred. Ophthalmologic exams should be performed weekly during induction and every 2 wk during maintenance or more frequently if the macula or optic nerve is threatened. Progression of CMV retinitis may occur during or following valganciclovir treatment.
- Assess for signs/symptoms of infection (fever, chills, flu-like symptoms, cough, hoarseness, lower back or side pain, sore throat, dysuria, hematuria, cellulitis, erythematous nonhealing wound). Notify health care provider if these symptoms occur.
- Assess for bleeding (bleeding gums, bruising, petechiae, weakness, tachycardia, dyspnea, dizziness, pallor, fatigue, tarry stools, coffee ground emesis). Avoid IM injections and taking rectal temperatures. Apply pressure to venipuncture sites for 10 min.

Lab Test Considerations

- Verify negative pregnancy test before starting therapy.
- May cause neutropenia, anemia, and thrombocytopenia. Monitor CBC with differential closely during therapy. Do not administer if ANC <500 cells/mm^3, platelet count <25,000 cells/mm^3, or hemoglobin <8 g/dL. Recovery begins within 3–7 days of discontinuation of therapy. Consider hematopoietic growth factor treatment in patients with severe leukopenia, neutropenia, anemia, or thrombocytopenia.
- Monitor BUN and serum creatinine at least once every 2 wk during therapy. May ↑ serum creatinine. Monitor renal function in children using a modified Schwartz formula for calculations of CrCl and consider changes in height and body weight.

Implementation

- Do not confuse valganciclovir with valacyclovir. Do not confuse Valcyte with Valtrex.
- During administration and when preparing or handling tablets, wear double chemotherapy gloves, protective gown, and hair and shoe covers; optimally prepare in a ventilated control device. Respiratory (N95) protection and eye/face protection is needed if there is risk of patient vomiting or spitting up. Single chemotherapy gloves are appropriate if handling and administering intact tablets from a unit-dose package. Health care providers who are actively trying to conceive, who are pregnant or may become pregnant, and who are breastfeeding should avoid handling valganciclovir.
- **PO:** Administer tablets and oral solution with food. Adults should take tablets, not oral solution. Handle valganciclovir tablets carefully. ***DNC:*** Do not break or crush. Avoid direct contact with broken or crushed tablets. If contact with the skin or mucous membranes occurs, wash thoroughly with soap and water and rinse eyes thoroughly with plain water.
- For oral solution, shake well prior to use. Use oral dispenser provided for accurate dose. Store oral solution in refrigerator for no longer than 49 days.

V

Patient/Family Teaching

- Explain the purpose and side effects of valganciclovir. Instruct patient to take with food, as directed. Take missed doses as soon as remembered, unless almost time for next dose; do not double doses. Advise patient to read *Patient Information* before starting therapy and with each Rx refill in case of changes.
- Instruct patient on proper handling and to avoid direct contact of skin or mucous membranes with any broken or crushed tablet, powder for oral solution, or reconstituted oral solution. Keep valganciclovir out of children's reach.
- Advise patient to maintain adequate hydration to avoid renal toxicity.
- Explain need for continued medical follow-up to assess effectiveness and possible side effects of medication. Regular blood counts and eye exams will be needed.
- Inform patient that valganciclovir is not a cure for CMV retinitis. Progression of retinitis may continue in immunocompromised patients during and following therapy. Advise patients to have regular ophthalmic exams at least every 4–6 wk. Duration of therapy for CMV prevention is based on the duration and degree of immunosuppression.
- May cause seizures, sedation, dizziness, ataxia, and/or confusion. Caution patient not to drive or do other activities requiring alertness until response to medication is known.
- Advise patient to promptly report unexplained weight loss, persistent weakness and fatigue, swollen lymph nodes, abnormal bleeding, unusual pain or bruising, or new lumps to health care provider.
- Advise patient to notify health care provider if fever; chills; sore throat; other signs of infection; bleeding gums; bruising; petechiae; or blood in urine, stool, or emesis occurs. Caution patient to avoid crowds and persons with known infections. Instruct patient to use soft toothbrush and electric razor. Patient should be cautioned not to drink alcoholic beverages or take products containing aspirin or NSAIDs.
- Caution patient to use sunscreen and protective clothing to prevent photosensitivity reactions.
- Advise patient to notify health care provider of all Rx or OTC medications, vitamins, or herbal products being taken and to consult with health care provider before taking other medications.
- Rep: May cause fetal harm. Advise women of reproductive potential to use effective contraception during and for ≥30 days following therapy and to avoid breastfeeding. Advise men with female partners of reproductive potential to use a barrier method of contraception during and for ≥90 days following therapy. Advise patient to notify health care provider immediately if pregnancy is suspected. May cause temporary or permanent infertility in men and women.

Evaluation/Desired Outcomes

- Management of the symptoms of CMV retinitis in patients with AIDS.
- Prevention of CMV disease in kidney, kidney/pancreas, and heart transplant patients at risk.

valproate sodium, See VALPROATES.

VALPROATES

divalproex sodium
(dye-val-**proe**-ex **soe**-dee-um)
Depakote, Depakote ER, Depakote Sprinkle, Epival

valproate sodium
(val-**proe**-ate **soe**-dee-um)
~~Depacon~~

valproic acid (val-**proe**-ik **as**-id)
~~Depakene~~

Classification
Therapeutic: anticonvulsants, vascular headache suppressants

Indications

Monotherapy and adjunctive therapy for simple and complex absence seizures. Monotherapy and adjunctive therapy for complex partial seizures. Adjunctive therapy for patients with multiple seizure types, including absence seizures. **Divalproex sodium only:** Manic episodes associated with bipolar disorder. Prevention of migraine headache.

Action

Increase levels of GABA, an inhibitory neurotransmitter in the CNS. **Therapeutic Effects:** Suppression of seizure activity. Decreased manic episodes. Decreased frequency of migraine headaches.

Pharmacokinetics

Absorption: Well absorbed following oral administration; divalproex is enteric-coated, and absorption is delayed. Extended-release form produces lower blood levels. IV administration results in complete bioavailability.
Distribution: Rapidly distributed into plasma and extracellular water. Cross blood-brain barrier.
Protein Binding: 80–90% (↓ in neonates, older adults, renal impairment, or chronic hepatic impairment).
Metabolism and Excretion: Mostly metabolized by the liver; minimal amounts excreted unchanged in urine.
Half-life: Adults: 9–16 hr.

TIME/ACTION PROFILE (onset = anticonvulsant effect; peak = blood levels)

ROUTE	ONSET	PEAK	DURATION
PO–liquid	2–4 days	15–120 min	6–24 hr
PO–capsules	2–4 days	1–4 hr	6–24 hr
PO–delayed-release products	2–4 days	3–5 hr	12–24 hr
PO–extended-release products	2–4 days	7–14 hr	24 hr
IV	2–4 days	end of infusion	6–24 hr

Contraindications/Precautions

Contraindicated in: Hypersensitivity; Hepatic impairment; Known/suspected urea cycle disorders (may result in fatal hyperammonemic encephalopathy); Mitochondrial disorders caused by mutations in mitochondrial DNA polymerase gamma (↑ risk for potentially fatal hepatotoxicity); Rep: Women of reproductive potential not using effective contraception (for migraine prophylaxis only); OB: Pregnancy (for migraine prophylaxis only); Lactation: Lactation; Pedi: Children <2 yr with suspected mitochondrial disorder caused by mutations in mitochondrial DNA polymerase gamma (↑ risk for potentially fatal hepatotoxicity).

Use Cautiously in: All patients (may ↑ risk of suicidal thoughts/behaviors); Bleeding disorders; Renal impairment; Hepatic impairment; Organic brain disease; Bone marrow depression; Rep: Women of reproductive potential (use for seizure disorders or bipolar disorders only if other medications are ineffective, poorly tolerated, or inappropriate); OB: Pregnancy (may cause fetal harm, including ↓ IQ, neurodevelopmental disorders [including autism spectrum disorders and attention-deficit hyperactivity disorder], neural tube defects, hearing impairment/loss, and other major congenital malformations); use for seizure disorders or bipolar disorders only if other medications are ineffective, poorly tolerated, or inappropriate; Geri: ↑ risk of adverse effects in older adults.

Adverse Reactions/Side Effects

CV: peripheral edema. **Derm:** ACUTE GENERALIZED EXANTHEMATOUS PUSTULOSIS, alopecia, DRUG REACTION WITH EOSINOPHILIA AND SYSTEMIC SYMPTOMS (DRESS), ERYTHEMA MULTIFORME, rash, STEVENS JOHNSON SYNDROME, TOXIC EPIDERMAL NECROLYSIS. **EENT:** visual disturbances. **GI:** abdominal pain, anorexia, diarrhea, indigestion, nausea, vomiting, constipation, HEPATOTOXICITY, PANCREATITIS. **Hemat:** thrombocytopenia, leukopenia. **Metab:** ↑ appetite, HYPERAMMONEMIA, weight gain. **Neuro:** agitation, dizziness, headache, insomnia, sedation, tremor, ataxia, confusion, depression, HYPOTHERMIA, SUICIDAL THOUGHTS. **Misc:** HYPERSENSITIVITY REACTIONS (INCLUDING ANGIOEDEMA).

Interactions

Drug-Drug: ↑ risk of bleeding with **warfarin**. **Aspirin**, **carbamazepine**, **chlorpromazine**, **cimetidine**, **erythromycin**, or **felbamate** may ↑ levels and the risk of toxicity. ↑ risk of CNS depression with other **CNS depressants**, including **alcohol**, **antihistamines**, **antidepressants**, **opioid analgesics**, **MAO inhibitors**, and **sedative/hypnotics**. **MAO inhibitors** and other **antidepressants** may ↓ seizure threshold and ↓ effectiveness. **Carbamazepine**, **ertapenem**, **imipenem**, **meropenem**, **methotrexate**, **phenobarbital**, **phenytoin**, **estrogen-containing contraceptives**, or **rifampin** may ↓ levels and effectiveness. May ↑ levels and risk of toxicity of **carbamazepine**, **diazepam**, **amitriptyline**, **nortriptyline**, **ethosuximide**, **lamotrigine**, **phenobarbital**, **phenytoin**, **rufinamide**, **topiramate**, or **zidovudine**; dosage adjustments of these medications may be necessary. May ↑ levels and risk of toxicity of **propofol**; ↓ propofol dose. **Topiramate** may ↑ risk of hypothermia and hyperammonemia, with or without encephalopathy. **Cholestyramine** may ↓ levels and effectiveness; separate administration by 3 hr. **Cannabidiol** may ↑ risk of liver enzyme elevation; monitor liver enzymes closely during concurrent therapy.

Route/Dosage

Regular-release and delayed-release formulations usually given in 2–4 divided doses daily; extended-release formulation (Depakote ER) usually given once daily.

Seizure Disorders

PO (Adults and Children >10 yr): *Single-agent therapy (complex partial seizures):* Initial dose of 10–15 mg/kg/day in 1–4 divided doses; ↑ by 5–10 mg/kg/day weekly until therapeutic response achieved (not to exceed 60 mg/kg/day); when daily dose exceeds 250 mg, give in divided doses. *Polytherapy (complex partial seizures):* Initial dose of 10–15 mg/kg/day; ↑ by 5–10 mg/kg/day weekly until therapeutic response achieved (not to exceed 60 mg/kg/day); when daily dosage exceeds 250 mg, give in divided doses.

PO (Adults and Children >2 yr [>10 yr for Depakote ER]): *Simple and complex absence seizures:* Initial dose of 15 mg/kg/day in 1–4 divided doses; ↑ by 5–10 mg/kg/day weekly until therapeutic response achieved (not to exceed 60 mg/kg/day); when daily dose exceeds 250 mg, give in divided doses.

IV (Adults and Children): Give same daily dose and at same frequency as was given orally; switch to oral formulation as soon as possible.

Rect (Adults and Children): Dilute syrup 1:1 with water for use as a retention enema. Give 17–20 mg/kg load, maintenance 10–15 mg/kg/dose every 8 hr.

V

Bipolar Disorder

PO (Adults): *Depakote:* Initial dose of 750 mg/day in divided doses initially; titrated rapidly to desired clinical effect or trough plasma levels of 50–125 mcg/mL (not to exceed 60 mg/kg/day). *Depakote ER:* Initial dose of 25 mg/kg once daily; titrated rapidly to desired clinical effect of trough plasma levels of 85–125 mcg/mL (not to exceed 60 mg/kg/day).

Migraine Prevention

PO (Adults and Children ≥16 yr): *Depakote:* 250 mg twice daily (up to 1000 mg/day). *Depakote ER:* 500 mg once daily for 1 wk; then ↑ to 1000 mg once daily.

Availability

Valproic Acid (generic available)

Capsules: 250 mg. **Oral solution:** 250 mg/5 mL.

Valproate Sodium (generic available)

Solution for injection: 100 mg/mL.

Divalproex Sodium (generic available)

Delayed-release tablets (Depakote): 125 mg, 250 mg, 500 mg. **Extended-release tablets (Depakote ER):** 250 mg, 500 mg. **Sprinkle capsules:** 125 mg.

NURSING IMPLICATIONS

Assessment

- **Seizures:** Assess location, duration, frequency, and characteristics of seizure activity. Institute seizure precautions.
- **Bipolar Disorder:** Assess mood, ideation, and behavior frequently.
- **Migraine Prophylaxis:** Monitor frequency and intensity of migraine headaches.
- Geri: Assess older adults for excessive somnolence.
- Assess for suicidal tendencies, especially during early therapy. Restrict amount of drug available to patient. Risk may be ↑ in children, adolescents, and adults ≤24 yr.
- Monitor for signs/symptoms of hepatotoxicity (malaise, weakness, lethargy, facial edema, vomiting, anorexia). *If hepatotoxicity occurs,* discontinue therapy and initiate alternate therapy.
- Monitor for signs/symptoms of pancreatitis (abdominal pain, nausea, vomiting, anorexia). *If pancreatitis occurs,* discontinue therapy and initiate alternate therapy initiated.
- Monitor for signs/symptoms of DRESS (fever, rash, lymphadenopathy, hepatitis, nephritis, hematological abnormalities, myocarditis, myositis, eosinophilia). *If signs/symptoms occur and DRESS is confirmed,* discontinue valproate; do not restart.

Lab Test Considerations

- Monitor CBC and bleeding time before and periodically during therapy. May cause leukopenia and thrombocytopenia.
- Monitor hepatic function (LDH, AST, ALT, and bilirubin) and serum ammonia before starting and periodically during therapy. May cause hepatotoxicity; monitor closely, especially during initial 6 mo of therapy; fatalities have occurred. *If hyperammonemia occurs,* discontinue therapy.
- May interfere with accuracy of thyroid function tests.
- May cause false-positive results in urine ketone tests.

Toxicity and Overdose

- Therapeutic serum levels range from 50–100 mcg/mL (50–125 mcg/mL for mania). Doses are gradually ↑ until a predose serum concentration ≥50 mcg/mL is reached. However, a good correlation among daily dose, serum level, and therapeutic effects has not been established. Monitor patients receiving near the maximum recommended dose of 60 mg/kg/day for toxicity.

Implementation

- Do not confuse *Depakote ER* and regular dose forms.
- *Depakote ER* produces lower blood levels than *Depakote* dosing forms. If switching from *Depakote* to *Depakote ER*, ↑ dose by 8–20%.
- Single daily doses are usually administered at bedtime because of sedation.
- **PO:** Administer with or immediately after meals to minimize GI irritation. ***DNC:*** Swallow extended-release and delayed-release tablets and capsules whole; do not open, break, or chew; will cause mouth or throat irritation and destroy extended release mechanism. Do not administer tablets with milk or carbonated beverages (may cause premature dissolution). Delayed-release divalproex sodium may cause less GI irritation than valproic acid capsules.
- Geri: ↓ starting dose in older adults. ↑ doses more slowly and with regular monitoring for fluid and nutritional intake, dehydration, somnolence, and other adverse reactions.
- Shake liquid preparations well before pouring. Use calibrated measuring device to ensure accurate dose. Oral solution may be mixed with food or other liquids to improve taste.
- Sprinkle capsules may be swallowed whole or opened and entire capsule contents sprinkled on a teaspoonful of soft, cool food (applesauce, pudding). Do not chew mixture. Administer immediately; do not store for future use.
- To convert from valproic acid to divalproex sodium, initiate divalproex sodium at same total daily dose and dosing schedule as valproic acid. Once patient is stabilized on divalproex sodium, attempt administration 2–3 times daily.
- **Rect** Dilute syrup 1:1 with water for use as a retention enema.

IV Administration

- **Intermittent Infusion: Dilution:** May be diluted in ≥50 mL of D5W, 0.9% NaCl, or LR. Solution is stable for 24 hr at room temperature. Concentration: 2 mg/mL. Rate: Infuse over 60 min (≤20 mg/min). Rapid infusion may cause ↑ side effects. Has been given as an infusion of ≤15 mg/kg over 5–10 min (1.5–3 mg/kg/min). Rapid loading doses of 20 to 40 mg/kg have been administered over 1 to 5 min. In pediatric patients, an infusion rate of 1.5 to 3 mg/kg/min has been recommended.

- **Y-Site Compatibility:** cefepime, ceftazidime, dobutamine, dopamine, meropenem, naloxone.
- **Y-Site Incompatibility:** vancomycin.

Patient/Family Teaching

- Explain purpose and side effects of medication to patient. Advise patient to read *Patient Information* before starting therapy. Advise to take as directed. If a dose is missed on a once-a-day schedule, take as soon as remembered that day. If on a multiple-dose schedule, take it within 6 hr of the scheduled time; then space remaining doses throughout the remainder of the day. Abrupt withdrawal may lead to status epilepticus.
- Advise patient to notify health care provider of all Rx or OTC medications, vitamins, or herbal products being taken and to consult with health care provider before taking other medications, especially CNS depressants or opioids. Caution patient to avoid alcohol during therapy.
- May cause drowsiness or dizziness. Advise patient to avoid driving or other activities requiring alertness until effects of medication are known. Explain to patient not to resume driving until physician gives clearance based on control of seizure disorder.
- Advise patient and family/caregiver to notify health care provider if thoughts about suicide or dying, attempts to commit suicide, new or worse depression, new or worse anxiety, feeling very agitated or restless, panic attacks, trouble sleeping, new or worse irritability, acting aggressive, being angry or violent, acting on dangerous impulses, an extreme ↑ in activity and talking, or other unusual changes in behavior or mood occur.
- Instruct patient to notify health care provider of medication regimen prior to treatment or surgery.
- Advise patient to notify health care provider if anorexia, abdominal pain, severe nausea and vomiting, yellow skin or eyes, fever, sore throat, malaise, weakness, facial edema, lethargy, unusual bleeding or bruising, pregnancy, or loss of seizure control occurs. Children <2 yr of age are especially at risk for fatal hepatotoxicity.
- Advise patient to carry identification at all times describing medication regimen.
- Emphasize the importance of routine exams to monitor progress.
- Rep: May cause fetal harm. Advise women of reproductive potential to use effective contraception during therapy and to notify health care provider immediately if pregnancy is planned or suspected or if breastfeeding. Dietary folic acid supplementation prior to conception and during 1st trimester of pregnancy ↓ the risk for congenital neural tube defects in the general population. May cause abnormal clotting and hepatic failure in pregnant woman and neonate. May cause adverse effects on neurodevelopment, including ↑ in autism spectrum disorders and attention-deficit hyperactivity disorder, ↓ IQ, neural tube defects, and hearing impairment/loss. Advise pregnant patients taking valproates to enroll in the North American Anti Epileptic Drug Pregnancy Registry to monitor outcomes by calling 1-888-233-2334 or visiting www.aedpregnancyregistry.org; patient must enroll themselves. May cause male infertility. Monitor breastfed infant for signs of liver damage, including jaundice and unusual bruising or bleeding.

Evaluation/Desired Outcomes

- Suppression of seizure activity.
- Decreased manic episodes.
- Decreased frequency of migraine headaches.

valproic acid, See VALPROATES.

valsartan, See ANGIOTENSIN II RECEPTOR ANTAGONISTS.

V vancomycin

(van-koe-**mye**-sin)

Firvanq, Vancocin

Classification

Therapeutic: anti-infectives

Indications

IV: Potentially life-threatening infections when less toxic anti-infectives are contraindicated. Particularly useful in staphylococcal infections, including: endocarditis, meningitis, osteomyelitis, pneumonia, septicemia, soft-tissue infections in patients who have allergies to penicillin or its derivatives or when sensitivity testing demonstrates resistance to methicillin. **PO:** Staphylococcal enterocolitis or diarrhea due to *Clostridioides difficile*.

Action

Binds to bacterial cell wall, resulting in cell death. **Therapeutic Effects:** Bactericidal action against susceptible organisms. **Spectrum:** Active against gram-positive pathogens, including: Staphylococci (including methicillin-resistant strains of *Staphylococcus aureus*), Group A beta-hemolytic streptococci, *Streptococcus pneumoniae*, *Corynebacterium*, *Clostridioides difficile*, *Enterococcus faecalis*, *Enterococcus faecium*.

Pharmacokinetics

Absorption: Poorly absorbed from the GI tract.
Distribution: Widely distributed to tissues. Some penetration (20–30%) of CSF.
Metabolism and Excretion: Oral doses excreted primarily in the feces; IV vancomycin eliminated almost entirely by the kidneys.
Half-life: *Neonates:* 6–10 hr; *Children 3 mo–3 yr:* 4 hr; *Children >3 yr:* 2–2.3 hr; *Adults:* 5–8 hr (↑ in renal impairment).

TIME/ACTION PROFILE (plasma concentrations)

ROUTE	ONSET	PEAK	DURATION
IV	rapid	end of infusion	12–24 hr

Contraindications/Precautions

Contraindicated in: Hypersensitivity.
Use Cautiously in: Renal impairment (↓ dose if CCr ≤80 mL/min); Hearing impairment; Intestinal obstruction or inflammation (↑ systemic absorption when given orally); OB: Pharmacokinetics of IV vancomycin may be altered in pregnancy (volume of distribution may be ↑); systemic absorption of PO vancomycin expected to be minimal; Lactation: Use while breastfeeding only if potential maternal benefit justifies potential risk to infant.

Adverse Reactions/Side Effects

CV: hypotension. **Derm:** ACUTE GENERALIZED EXANTHEMATOUS PUSTULOSIS, DRUG REACTION WITH EOSINOPHILIA AND SYSTEMIC SYMPTOMS (DRESS), LINEAR IGA BULLOUS DERMATOSIS, rash, STEVENS-JOHNSON SYNDROME (SJS), TOXIC EPIDERMAL NECROLYSIS (TEN). **EENT:** ototoxicity. **GI:** nausea, vomiting. **GU:** nephrotoxicity. **Hemat:** eosinophilia, leukopenia. **Local:** phlebitis. **MS:** back and neck pain. **Misc:** chills, fever, HYPERSENSITIVITY REACTIONS (INCLUDING ANAPHYLAXIS), vancomycin flushing syndrome (with rapid infusion).

Interactions

Drug-Drug: May cause additive ototoxicity and nephrotoxicity with other **ototoxic** and **nephrotoxic drugs**, including **aspirin**, **aminoglycosides**, **cyclosporine**, **cisplatin**, and **loop diuretics**. May enhance neuromuscular blockade from **nondepolarizing neuromuscular blocking agents**. ↑ risk of histamine flush when used with **general anesthetics** in children.

Route/Dosage

Serious Systemic Infections

IV (Adults): 500 mg every 6 hr *or* 1 g every 12 hr (up to 4 g/day).
IV (Children >1 mo): 40 mg/kg/day divided every 6–8 hr. *Staphylococcal CNS infection:* 60 mg/kg/day divided every 6 hr; maximum dose: 1 g/dose.
IV (Neonates 1 wk–1 mo and >2000 g): 15–20 mg/kg every 8 hr.
IV (Neonates 1 wk–1 mo and 1200–2000 g): 10–15 mg/kg every 8–12 hr.
IV (Neonates 1 wk–1 mo and <1200 g): 15 mg/kg every 24 hr.
IV (Neonates <1 wk and >2000 g): 10–15 mg/kg every 8–12 hr.
IV (Neonates <1 wk and 1200–2000 g): 10–15 mg/kg every 12–18 hr.
IV (Neonates <1 wk and <1200 g): 15 mg/kg every 24 hr.
IT (Adults): 20 mg/day.
IT (Children): 5–20 mg/day.
IT (Neonates): 5–10 mg/day.

Renal Impairment

IV (Adults): An initial loading dose of 750 mg–1 g (not less than 15 mg/kg); serum level monitoring is optimal for choosing maintenance dose in patients with renal impairment; these guidelines may be helpful. *CCr 50–80 mL/min:* 1 g every 1–3 days; *CCr 10–50 mL/min:* 1 g every 3–7 days; *CCr <10 mL/min:* 1 g every 7–14 days.

Endocarditis Prophylaxis in Penicillin-Allergic Patients

IV (Adults and Adolescents): 1 g single dose 1 hr preprocedure.
IV (Children): 20 mg/kg single dose 1 hr preprocedure.

Diarrhea Due to *C. difficile*

PO (Adults): 125 mg every 6 hr for 10 days.
PO (Children): 40 mg/kg/day divided into 3 or 4 doses for 7–10 days (not to exceed 2 g/day).

Staphylococcal Enterocolitis

PO (Adults): 500–2000 mg/day in 3–4 divided doses for 7–10 days.
PO (Children): 40 mg/kg/day in 3–4 divided doses for 7–10 days (not to exceed 2 g/day).

Availability (generic available)

Capsules: 125 mg, 250 mg. **Powder for oral solution (grape flavor):** 3.75 g/bottle, 7.5 g/bottle, 15 g/bottle. **Premixed infusion:** 500 mg/100 mL D5W, 750 mg/150 mL D5W, 1000 mg/200 mL D5W or 0.9% NaCl, 1250 mg/200 mL D5W, 1500 mg/300 mL D5W, 1750 mg/350 mL D5W, 2000 mg/400 mL D5W.

Solution for injection: 250 mg/vial, 500 mg/vial, 750 mg/vial, 1 g/vial, 1.5 g/vial, 5 g/vial, 10 g/vial, 100 g/vial.

NURSING IMPLICATIONS

Assessment

- Assess patient for infection (vital signs; appearance of wound, sputum, urine, and stool; WBC) at beginning of and throughout therapy.
- Monitor IV site for phlebitis and other administration reactions; rotate infusion sites. *If symptoms occur,* immediately stop infusion and treat as indicated.
- Monitor for signs/symptoms of anaphylaxis and vancomycin flushing syndrome (hypotension; pruritus; flushing of face, neck, or upper body; pain and muscle spasm of chest and back). *If symptoms occur,* stop infusion immediately and treat as indicated. Keep emergency medication and equipment close by during therapy.
- Monitor for severe dermatologic reactions such as TEN, SJS, and DRESS. *At 1st sign of rash, mucosal lesions, or blisters,* immediately discontinue vancomycin and treat as indicated.
- Evaluate 8th cranial nerve function by audiometry and serum vancomycin concentrations prior to and throughout therapy in patients with borderline renal function or those >60 yr of age. Prompt recognition and intervention are essential in preventing permanent damage.
- Monitor intake, output, and daily weight. Cloudy or pink urine may be a sign of nephrotoxicity.
- Assess for signs of superinfection (black, furry overgrowth on tongue; vaginal itching or discharge; loose or foul-smelling stools).
- Monitor for signs/symptoms of CDAD (diarrhea, abdominal cramping, fever, bloody stools). *If CDAD occurs,* discontinue vancomycin and treat as indicated. May begin up to several weeks following cessation of therapy.

Lab Test Considerations

- Obtain specimens for culture and sensitivity prior to initiating therapy. 1st dose may be given before receiving results.
- Monitor CBC, renal function, and urinalysis for casts, albumin, or cells in the urine periodically during therapy. *If acute kidney injury occurs,* discontinue vancomycin or ↓ dose.
- Monitor vancomycin concentrations, periodically during therapy. *If acute kidney injury occurs,* discontinue vancomycin or ↓ dose.

Toxicity and Overdose

- Trough concentrations should not exceed 10 mcg/mL (mild to moderate infection) or 15–20 mcg/mL (severe infection).

Implementation

- Vancomycin must be given orally for treatment of staphylococcal enterocolitis and *C. difficile*-associated diarrhea. Orally administered vancomycin is not effective for other types of infections.
- **PO:** Use calibrated measuring device for liquid preparations. Shake well before use. Oral solution is stable for 14 days if refrigerated.

IV Administration

- V IV vancomycin is a vesicant. Monitor closely if administered through a peripheral IV. Can also be infused through a midline catheter or PICC. If extravasation occurs, immediately stop infusion. Leave needle/cannula in place temporarily but do not flush the line. Gently aspirate extravasated solution; then remove needle/cannula. Elevate patient's extremity and apply dry cold compresses. Initiate hyaluronidase antidote for refractory cases in addition to supportive management. For hyaluronidase, inject a total of 1 mL (15 units/mL) intradermally or SUBQ as five separate 0.2-mL injections (using a tuberculin syringe) around the site of extravasation; if IV catheter remains in place, administer IV through the infiltrated catheter; may repeat in 30–60 min if no resolution.
- **Intermittent Infusion: Reconstitution:** Add 10 mL or 20 mL of sterile water for injection to 500-mg or 1-g vials, respectively. Solution stable for 14 days if refrigerated. **Concentration:** 50 mg/mL. **Dilution:** Dilute further with ≥100 mL of 0.9% NaCl, D5W, D5/0.9% NaCl, or LR for every 500 mg of vancomycin being administered. Infusion is stable for 96 hr if refrigerated. **Concentration:** ≤5 mg/mL. **Rate:** Infuse over ≥60 min (90 min for doses >1 g). Do not administer rapidly or as a bolus, to minimize risk of thrombophlebitis, hypotension, and vancomycin flushing syndrome. May need to slow infusion further to 1.5–2 hr if flushing syndrome occurs.
- **IT: Dilution:** Dilute with preservative-free 0.9% NaCl. **Concentration:** 1–5 mg/mL. **Rate:** Directly instill into ventricular cerebrospinal fluid.
- **Y-Site Compatibility:** acetaminophen, acetylcysteine, acyclovir, aldesleukin, alemtuzumab, allopurinol, alprostadil, alteplase, amikacin, aminocaproic acid, amiodarone, anidulafungin, argatroban, arsenic trioxide, ascorbic acid, atracurium, atropine, azithromycin, benztropine, bleomycin, bumetanide, buprenorphine, butorphanol, caffeine citrate, calcium chloride, calcium gluconate, cangrelor, carboplatin, carmustine, caspofungin, ceftazidime, chlorpromazine, ciprofloxacin, cisatracurium, cisplatin, clindamycin, cyanocobalamin, cyclophosphamide, cyclosporine, cytarabine, dacarbazine, dactinomycin, daunorubicin, dexamethasone,

V

dexmedetomidine, dexrazoxane, digoxin, diltiazem, diphenhydramine, dobutamine, docetaxel, dopamine, doxapram, doxorubicin hydrochloride, doxorubicin liposomal, doxycycline, enalaprilat, ephedrine, epinephrine, epirubicin, eptifibatide, eravacycline, ertapenem, erythromycin, esmolol, etoposide, etoposide phosphate, famotidine, fentanyl, filgrastim, fluconazole, fludarabine, folic acid, fosphenytoin, gemcitabine, gentamicin, glycopyrrolate, granisetron, hydromorphone, ifosfamide, imipenem/cilastatin/relebactam, insulin aspart, insulin, regular, irinotecan, isavuconazonium, isoproterenol, ketamine, labetalol, levetiracetam, levofloxacin, lidocaine, linezolid, lorazepam, magnesium sulfate, mannitol, melphalan, meperidine, meropenem, meropenem/vaborbactam, mesna, methadone, metoclopramide, metoprolol, metronidazole, midazolam, milrinone, minocycline, mitoxantrone, morphine, multivitamins, mycophenolate, nalbuphine, naloxone, nicardipine, nitroglycerin, nitroprusside, norepinephrine, octreotide, ondansetron, oxaliplatin, oxytocin, paclitaxel, palonosetron, pamidronate, pantoprazole, papaverine, pemetrexed, penicillin G, pentamidine, pentobarbital, phenobarbital, phentolamine, phenylephrine, phytonadione, plazomicin, posaconazole, potassium acetate, potassium chloride, procainamide, prochlorperazine, promethazine, propranolol, protamine, pyridoxine, remifentanil, rifampin, sildenafil, sodium acetate, sodium bicarbonate, succinylcholine, sufentanil, sulbactam/durlobactam, tacrolimus, tedizolid, thiamine, thiotepa, tigecycline, tirofiban, tobramycin, topotecan, trastuzumab, vasopressin, vecuronium, verapamil, vinblastine, vincristine, vinorelbine, voriconazole, zidovudine, zoledronic acid.

- **Y-Site Incompatibility:** albumin, human, aminophylline, amphotericin B deoxycholate, amphotericin lipid complex, amphotericin B liposomal, azathioprine, bivalirudin, blinatumomab, cefiderocol, chloramphenicol, dantrolene, daptomycin, defibrotide, diazepam, diazoxide, dimenhydrinate, epoetin alfa, fluorouracil, furosemide, ganciclovir, gemtuzumab ozogamicin, ibuprofen lysine, idarubicin, indomethacin, ketorolac, leucovorin, methylprednisolone, mitomycin, moxifloxacin, phenytoin, rituximab, trimethoprim/sulfamethoxazole, valproate sodium.

Patient/Family Teaching

- Explain purpose and side effects of medication. Advise patient to read *Patient Information* before starting therapy.
- Advise patient to take missed oral dose as soon as remembered unless almost time for next dose; do not double dose.
- Instruct patient to notify health care provider if signs of hypersensitivity, tinnitus, vertigo, or hearing loss occur.
- Advise patient to notify health care provider if no improvement of infection is seen in a few days.
- Patients with a history of rheumatic heart disease or valve replacement need to be taught importance of using antimicrobial prophylaxis prior to invasive dental or medical procedures.
- Rep: Advise women of reproductive potential to notify health care provider if pregnancy is planned or suspected or if breastfeeding.

Evaluation/Desired Outcomes

- Resolution of signs and symptoms of infection. Length of time for complete resolution depends on organism and site of infection.
- Endocarditis prophylaxis.

vardenafil (var-**den**-a-fil)

Classification

Therapeutic: erectile dysfunction agents

Pharmacologic: phosphodiesterase type 5 inhibitors

Indications

Erectile dysfunction (ED).

Action

Increases cyclic guanosine monophosphate (cGMP) levels by inhibiting phosphodiesterase type 5, an enzyme responsible for the breakdown of cGMP. cGMP produces smooth muscle relaxation of the corpus cavernosum, which in turn promotes increased blood flow and subsequent erection. **Therapeutic Effects:** Enhanced blood flow to the corpus cavernosum and erection sufficient to allow sexual intercourse. Requires sexual stimulation.

Pharmacokinetics

Absorption: 15% absorbed following oral administration; absorption is rapid.

Distribution: Extensive tissue distribution; penetrates semen.

Protein Binding: 95%.

Metabolism and Excretion: Mostly metabolized by the liver via the CYP3A4 isoenzyme and to a lesser extent by the CYP2C isoenzyme. M1 metabolite has anti-ED activity. Parent drug and metabolites are mostly excreted in feces. 2–6% renally eliminated.

Half-life: 4–6 hr.

TIME/ACTION PROFILE

ROUTE	ONSET	PEAK	DURATION
PO	rapid	0.5–2 hr	4 hr

Contraindications/Precautions

Contraindicated in: Hypersensitivity; Concurrent use of nitrates or riociguat; Unstable angina, recent history of stroke, life-threatening arrhythmias, or HF or MI within 6 mo; Known hereditary degenerative retinal disorders; Congenital or acquired QT prolongation or concurrent use of Class IA or III antiarrhythmics; End-stage renal disease requiring dialysis; Moderate hepatic impairment (orally disintegrating tablets only); Severe hepatic impairment.

Use Cautiously in: Other serious underlying cardiovascular disease or left ventricular outflow obstruction; Penile deformity; Underlying conditions predisposing to priapism, including sickle cell anemia, multiple myeloma, or leukemia; Bleeding disorders or active peptic ulcer diseases; History of sudden severe vision loss or nonarteritic ischemic optic neuropathy (NAION); may ↑ risk of recurrence; Low cup-to-disk ratio, age >50 yr, diabetes, hypertension, coronary artery disease, hyperlipidemia, or smoking (↑ risk of NAION); Geri: Older adults may have ↑ levels; ↓ dose required.

Adverse Reactions/Side Effects

Derm: flushing. **EENT:** HEARING LOSS, rhinitis, sinusitis, VISION LOSS. **GI:** dyspepsia, nausea. **GU:** priapism. **Neuro:** headache, amnesia, dizziness. **Misc:** flu syndrome.

Interactions

Drug-Drug: **Nitrates** may cause serious, life-threatening hypotension; concurrent use contraindicated. **Riociguat** may result in severe hypotension; concurrent use contraindicated. **Class IA antiarrhythmics**, including **quinidine** or **procainamide**, or **Class III antiarrhythmics**, including **amiodarone** or **sotalol**, may ↑ risk of serious arrhythmias; avoid concurrent use. **Strong CYP3A4 inhibitors**, including **atazanavir**, **clarithromycin**, **cobicistat**, **itraconazole**, **ketoconazole**, and **ritonavir**, and **moderate CYP3A4 inhibitors**, including **erythromycin**, may ↑ levels and risk of toxicity; avoid concurrent use with orally disintegrating tablets; ↓ dose of tablets. ↑ risk of hypotension with **alpha-adrenergic blockers** and acute ingestion of **alcohol**; patients should be on stable dose of alpha blockers before starting vardenafil (should start therapy with tablets [orally disintegrating tablets should not be used]).

Route/Dosage

The tablets and orally disintegrating tablets are not interchangeable; the orally disintegrating tablets provide a higher level of systemic exposure compared to the tablets.

Tablets

PO (Adults): 10 mg taken 1 hr prior to sexual activity (range 5–20 mg; not to exceed one dose/24 hr); *Concurrent use of cobicistat or ritonavir:* Single dose should not exceed 2.5 mg in any 72-hr period; *Concurrent use of atazanavir, clarithromycin, ketoconazole 400 mg daily, or itraconazole 400 mg daily:* Single dose should not exceed 2.5 mg/24 hr; *Concurrent use of ketoconazole 200 mg daily, itraconazole 200 mg daily, or erythromycin:* Single dose should not exceed 5 mg/24 hr; *Concurrent use of stable alpha-blocker therapy (not on potent CYP3A4 inhibitor):* 5 mg initial dose; titrate as tolerated; *Concurrent use of stable alpha-blocker and potent CYP3A4 inhibitor therapy:* 2.5 mg initial dose; titrate as tolerated.

PO (Geriatric Patients ≥65 yr): 5 mg initial dose; titrate as tolerated.

Hepatic Impairment

PO (Adults): *Moderate hepatic impairment:* May start with 5 mg dose (not to exceed 10 mg).

Orally Disintegrating Tablets

PO (Adults): 10 mg taken 1 hr prior to sexual activity (not to exceed one dose/24 hr).

Availability (generic available)

Tablets: 2.5 mg, 5 mg, 10 mg, 20 mg. **Orally disintegrating tablets (peppermint flavor):** 10 mg.

NURSING IMPLICATIONS

Assessment

- Assess for the presence of ED before administration. Vardenafil has no effect in the absence of sexual stimulation.
- Assess cardiac history, BP, and ECG at baseline.

Implementation

- *Tablets* and *orally disintegrating tablets* are not interchangeable.
- **PO:** *Tablets* are usually administered 1 hr before sexual activity. May be administered 30 min to 4 hr before sexual activity.
- Administer *orally disintegrating tablets* 1 hr before sexual activity. These tablets should be left in the package until use. Remove from the blister pouch. Do not push tablet through the blister; peel open the blister pack with dry hands and place tablet on tongue. Tablet will dissolve rapidly and be swallowed with saliva. No liquid is needed to take the orally disintegrating tablet.
- May be administered without regard to food.

Patient/Family Teaching

- Explain the purpose and side effects of vardenafil. Instruct patient to take approximately 30 min–1 hr before sexual activity and not more than once per day. Inform patient that sexual stimulation is required for an erection to occur after taking vardenafil. Do not share medication with others, even if they have similar symptoms; may be harmful. Advise patient to

V

read *Patient Information* before starting and with each Rx refill in case of changes.

- Advise patient that vardenafil is not indicated for use in women.
- Caution patient not to take vardenafil concurrently with alpha-adrenergic blockers (unless on a stable dose) or nitrates. If chest pain occurs after taking vardenafil, instruct patient to seek immediate medical attention.
- Instruct patient to notify health care provider promptly if erection lasts >4 hr or if sudden or ↓ vision loss in one or both eyes, loss or ↓ in hearing, ringing in the ears, or dizziness occurs.
- Instruct patient to notify health care provider of all Rx or OTC medications, vitamins, or herbal products being taken and consult health care provider before taking any new medications.
- Inform patient that vardenafil offers no protection against sexually transmitted diseases. Counsel patient that protection against sexually transmitted diseases and HIV infection should be considered.

Evaluation/Desired Outcomes

- Male erection sufficient to allow intercourse.

varenicline (systemic)

(var-**en**-i-kleen)

Champix, ~~Chantix~~

Classification

Therapeutic: smoking deterrents

Pharmacologic: nicotine agonists

Indications

Smoking cessation (in combination with nonpharmacologic support).

Action

Selectively binds to alpha$_4$, beta$_2$ nicotinic acetylcholine receptors, acting as a nicotine agonist; prevents the binding of nicotine to receptors. **Therapeutic Effects:** Decreased desire to smoke.

Pharmacokinetics

Absorption: 100% absorbed following oral administration.

Distribution: Unknown.

Metabolism and Excretion: Minimally metabolized; 92% excreted in urine unchanged.

Half-life: 24 hr.

TIME/ACTION PROFILE

ROUTE	ONSET	PEAK	DURATION
PO	unknown	3–4 hr	24 hr

Contraindications/Precautions

Contraindicated in: Hypersensitivity; Lactation: Lactation.

Use Cautiously in: Severe renal impairment (↓ dose if CCr <30 mL/min); Stable cardiovascular disease (may ↑ risk of cardiovascular events); Psychiatric illness; Seizure disorders; OB: Use during pregnancy only if potential maternal benefit outweighs potential fetal risk; Pedi: Safety not established in children; Geri: Consider age-related ↓ in renal function in older adults.

Adverse Reactions/Side Effects

CV: MI, syncope. **Derm:** flushing, hyperhidrosis, acne, dermatitis, dry skin, STEVENS-JOHNSON SYNDROME (SJS). **EENT:** blurred vision, visual disturbances. **GI:** diarrhea, gingivitis, nausea, ↑ liver enzymes, constipation, dyspepsia, dysphagia, enterocolitis, eructation, flatulence, gallbladder disorder, GI bleeding, vomiting. **Hemat:** anemia. **Metab:** ↑ appetite. **MS:** arthralgia, back pain, musculoskeletal pain, muscle cramps, myalgia, restless legs. **Neuro:** ↓ attention span, depression, dizziness, insomnia, irritability, restlessness, abnormal dreams, aggression, agitation, amnesia, anxiety, delusions, disorientation, dissociation, hallucinations, HOMICIDAL THOUGHTS/BEHAVIOR, hostility, mania, migraine, mood changes, panic, paranoia, psychosis, SEIZURES, sleepwalking, STROKE, SUICIDAL THOUGHTS/BEHAVIOR. **Misc:** accidental injury, chills, fever, HYPERSENSITIVITY REACTIONS (INCLUDING ANGIOEDEMA), mild physical dependence.

Interactions

Drug-Drug: Smoking cessation may ↑ levels and risk of toxicity of **theophylline**, **warfarin**, and **insulin**. Risk of adverse reactions (nausea, vomiting, dizziness, fatigue, headache) may be ↑ with **nicotine** replacement therapy (nicotine transdermal patches). **Alcohol** may ↑ risk of worsening neuropsychiatric events.

Route/Dosage

PO (Adults): Treatment is started 1 wk prior to planned smoking cessation (may also begin dosing and then quit smoking between days 8 and 35 of treatment); 0.5 mg once daily on the 1st 3 days, then 0.5 mg twice daily for the next 4 days, then 1 mg twice daily.

Renal Impairment

PO (Adults): *CCr <30 mL/min:* 0.5 mg daily; may ↑ to 0.5 mg twice daily.

Availability (generic available)

Tablets: 0.5 mg, 1 mg.

NURSING IMPLICATIONS

Assessment

- Assess for desire to stop smoking and monitor for therapeutic response such as ↓ or elimination of cigarette smoking.
- Monitor for nausea. Usually dose-dependent. May require dose reduction.

- Assess and monitor mental status, mood changes, and affect, especially during initial few months of therapy and during dose changes. Assess for suicidal tendencies. Risk may be ↑ in children, adolescents, and adults ≤24 yr. Inform health care provider if patient demonstrates significant ↑ in signs of depression (depressed mood, loss of interest in usual activities, significant change in weight and/or appetite, insomnia or hypersomnia, ↑ fatigue, feelings of worthlessness, slowed thinking or impaired concentration, suicide attempt or suicidal/homicidal ideation). If so, restrict amount of drug available to patient.
- Assess for rash periodically during therapy. May cause SJS. *If severe skin reaction occurs or if accompanied with fever, general malaise, fatigue, muscle or joint aches, blisters, oral lesions, conjunctivitis, hepatitis, or eosinophilia,* discontinue varenicline.

Lab Test Considerations

- May cause anemia.
- Monitor renal function in older adults.

Implementation

- **PO:** Administer after eating with a full glass of water.

Patient/Family Teaching

- Explain the purpose and side effects of varenicline. Instruct patient to take as directed after eating and with a full glass of water. Set a date to stop smoking. Start taking varenicline 1 wk before quit date. Patient may also begin varenicline and then quit smoking between days 8 and 35 of therapy. Begin with 0.5 mg/day for the 1st 3 days; then for the next 4 days, take one 0.5-mg tablet in the morning and in the evening. After 1st 7 days, ↑ to 1-mg tablet in the morning and evening. Advise patient to read *Medication Guide* before starting therapy and with each Rx refill in case of changes.
- Encourage patient to attempt to quit, even if they had early lapses after quit day. Provide patient with educational materials and counseling to support attempts to quit smoking.
- Caution patient not to share varenicline with others. May be harmful.
- Advise patient to stop taking varenicline and contact health care provider promptly if agitation; depressed mood; any changes in behavior that are not typical of nicotine withdrawal; suicidal thoughts or behavior; rash with mucosal lesions or skin reaction; or chest pain, pressure, or dyspnea occur. Encourage patient to reduce amount of alcohol consumed until effects of medication are known.
- May cause blurred vision, dizziness, and disturbance in attention. Caution patient to avoid driving and other activities requiring alertness until response to medication is known.
- Inform patient that nausea; insomnia; and vivid, unusual, or strange dreams may occur and are usually transient. Advise patient to notify health care provider if these symptoms are persistent and bothersome; dose reduction may be considered.
- Instruct patient to notify health care provider of all Rx or OTC medications, vitamins, or herbal products being taken and consult health care provider before taking any new medications. Inform patient that some medications may require dose adjustments after quitting smoking.
- Rep: Advise women of reproductive potential to notify health care provider if pregnancy is planned or suspected or if breastfeeding. Monitor breastfed infants for seizures and excessive vomiting.

Evaluation/Desired Outcomes

- Smoking cessation. Patients who have successfully stopped smoking at the end of 12 wk should take an additional 12-wk course to increase the likelihood of long-term abstinence. Patients who do not succeed in stopping smoking during 12 wk of initial therapy or who relapse after treatment should be encouraged to make another attempt once factors contributing to the failed attempt have been identified and addressed.

HIGH ALERT

V vasopressin

(vay-soe-**press**-in)

~~Pitressin~~, Vasostrict

Classification

Therapeutic: hormones

Pharmacologic: antidiuretic hormones, vasopressors

Indications

Central diabetes insipidus due to deficient antidiuretic hormone. Vasodilatory shock. **Unlabeled Use:** Gastrointestinal hemorrhage.

Action

Alters the permeability of the renal collecting ducts, allowing reabsorption of water. Directly stimulates musculature of GI tract. In high doses, acts as a nonadrenergic peripheral vasoconstrictor. **Therapeutic Effects:** Decreased urine output and increased urine osmolality in diabetes insipidus. Increased BP.

Pharmacokinetics

Absorption: IM absorption may be unpredictable. IV administration results in complete bioavailability.

V

Distribution: Well distributed to tissues.
Metabolism and Excretion: Rapidly degraded by the liver and kidneys; <5% excreted unchanged by the kidneys.
Half-life: <10 min.

TIME/ACTION PROFILE (antidiuretic effect)

ROUTE	ONSET	PEAK	DURATION
IM, SUBQ	unknown	unknown	2–8 hr
IV	unknown	unknown	30–60 min

Contraindications/Precautions

Contraindicated in: Hypersensitivity to 8-L arginine vasopressin or chlorobutanol (only in multidose vial); Chronic renal failure.
Use Cautiously in: Perioperative polyuria (↑ sensitivity to vasopressin effects); Comatose patients; Seizures; Migraine headaches; Asthma; HF; Cardiovascular disease; Renal impairment; OB: Higher doses (0.07 units/min) for vasodilatory shock may be needed in 2nd and 3rd trimesters; Lactation: Safety not established in breastfeeding; Geri: Older adults may have ↑ sensitivity to effects.

Adverse Reactions/Side Effects

CV: angina, chest pain, MI. **Derm:** ↑ sweating, paleness, perioral blanching. **Endo:** diabetes insipidus. **F and E** water intoxication (higher doses). **GI:** abdominal cramps, belching, diarrhea, flatulence, heartburn, nausea, vomiting. **Neuro:** "pounding" sensation in head, dizziness, trembling. **Misc:** allergic reactions, fever.

Interactions

Drug-Drug: Antidiuretic effect may be ↓ by concurrent administration of **clozapine**, **lithium**, **demeclocycline**, and **foscarnet**. Antidiuretic effect may be ↑ by concurrent administration of **cyclophosphamide**, **enalapril**, **felbamate**, **haloperidol**, **ifosfamide**, **pentamidine**, **tricyclic antidepressants**, **SSRIs**, or **vincristine**. Vasopressor effect may be ↑ by concurrent administration of **ganglionic blocking agents**, **indomethacin**, or **catecholamines**. **Furosemide** ↑ urine flow.

Route/Dosage

Diabetes Insipidus

IM, SUBQ (Adults): 5–10 units 2–4 times daily.
IM, SUBQ (Children): 2.5–10 units 2–4 times daily.
IV (Adults and Children): 0.0005 units/kg/hr; double dose every 30 min as needed to a maximum of 0.01 units/kg/hr.

Vasodilatory Shock

IV (Adults): 0.01 units/min; titrate by 0.005 units/min every 10–15 min until target BP achieved (max dose = 0.07 units/min).
IV (Infants and Children): 0.0003–0.002 units/kg/min, titrate to effect.

GI Hemorrhage

IV (Adults): 0.2–0.4 units/min; then titrate to maximum dose of 0.9 units/min; if bleeding stops, continue same dose for 12 hr; then taper off over 24–48 hr.
IV (Children): 0.002–0.005 units/kg/min then titrate to maximum dose of 0.01 units/kg/min; if bleeding stops, continue same dose for 12 hr; then taper off over 24–48 hr.

Availability (generic available)

Premixed infusion: 20 units/100 mL D5W or 0.9% NaCl, 40 units/100 mL D5W or 0.9% NaCl. **Solution for injection:** 20 units/mL.

NURSING IMPLICATIONS

Assessment

- Monitor BP, HR, and ECG periodically throughout therapy.
- **Diabetes Insipidus:** Monitor urine osmolality and urine volume frequently to determine effects of medication. Assess patient for symptoms of dehydration (excessive thirst, dry skin and mucous membranes, tachycardia, poor skin turgor). Weigh patient daily, monitor intake and output, and assess for edema.

Lab Test Considerations

- Monitor urine specific gravity during therapy.
- Monitor serum electrolyte concentrations periodically during therapy.

Toxicity and Overdose

- Signs and symptoms of water intoxication include confusion, drowsiness, headache, weight gain, difficulty urinating, seizures, and coma.
- Treatment of overdose includes water restriction and temporary discontinuation of vasopressin until polyuria occurs. If symptoms are severe, administration of mannitol, hypertonic dextrose, urea, and/or furosemide may be used.

Implementation

- Do not confuse vasopressin with desmopressin.
- Aqueous vasopressin injection may be administered SUBQ or IM for diabetes insipidus.
- Administer 1–2 glasses of water at the time of administration to minimize side effects (blanching of skin, abdominal cramps, nausea).

IV Administration

- V Vasopressin is a vesicant. Central line administration is preferred. If extravasation occurs, immediately stop infusion. Leave needle/cannula in place temporarily but do not flush the line. Gently aspirate extravasated solution; then remove needle/cannula. Elevate patient's extremity and apply dry warm compresses. Initiate nitroglycerin topical ointment antidote for refractory cases in addition to supportive management. For nitroglycerin, apply 1-inch strip of 2% topical ointment to site of ischemia to cover affected area; may repeat every 8 hr as necessary. Phentolamine or terbutaline may be used as alternatives to topical nitroglycerin. For phentolamine, dilute 5–10 mg in 10 mL of 0.9% NaCl and administer SUBQ into extravasation site as soon as possible after extravasation; if IV catheter remains in place, administer initial dose IV through the infiltrated catheter. May repeat in 60 min if patient remains symptomatic. For terbutaline, for large areas of extravasation, dilute 1 mg in 10 mL of 0.9% NaCl and administer SUBQ into extravasation site; may repeat in 15 min if necessary; for small areas of extravasation, dilute 1 mg in 1 mL of 0.9% NaCl and administer 0.5 mg (0.5 mL) SUBQ into extravasation site; may repeat in 15 min if necessary.

- **Continuous Infusion: Dilution:** Dilute 2.5 mg (no fluid restriction) or 5 mg (fluid restriction) of vasopressin in 500 mL or 100 mL, respectively, of 0.9% NaCl or D5W. Solution is clear and colorless; do not administer solutions that are cloudy, discolored, or contain particulates. **Concentration:** 0.1 units/mL or 1 unit/mL. Solution is stable for 18 hr at room temperature or 24 hr if refrigerated. Rate: See Route/Dosage section.
- **Y-Site Compatibility:** acyclovir, alemtuzumab, allopurinol, amikacin, aminocaproic acid, aminophylline, amiodarone, amphotericin B liposomal, anidulafungin, argatroban, arsenic trioxide, ascorbic acid, atracurium, atropine, azathioprine, azithromycin, aztreonam, benztropine, bivalirudin, bleomycin, bumetanide, buprenorphine, busulfan, butorphanol, calcium chloride, calcium gluconate, carboplatin, carmustine, caspofungin, cefazolin, cefepime, cefotaxime, cefotetan, cefoxitin, ceftaroline, ceftazidime, ceftazidime/avibactam, ceftolozane/tazobactam, ceftriaxone, cefuroxime, chloramphenicol, chlorpromazine, ciprofloxacin, cisatracurium, cisplatin, clindamycin, cyanocobalamin, cyclophosphamide, cyclosporine, cytarabine, dacarbazine, dactinomycin, daptomycin, dexamethasone, dexmedetomidine, dexrazoxane, digoxin, diltiazem, diphenhydramine, dobutamine, docetaxel, dopamine, doxorubicin hydrochloride, doxorubicin liposomal, doxycycline, droperidol, enalaprilat, ephedrine, epinephrine, epirubicin, epoetin alfa, eravacycline, ertapenem, erythromycin, esmolol, etoposide, etoposide phosphate, famotidine, fentanyl, fluconazole, fludarabine, fluorouracil, folic acid, foscarnet, fosphenytoin, ganciclovir, gemcitabine, gentamicin, glycopyrrolate, granisetron, heparin, hetastarch, hydrocortisone, hydromorphone, hydroxyzine, idarubicin, ifosfamide, imipenem/cilastatin, insulin, aspart, irinotecan, isavuconazonium, isoproterenol, ketorolac, labetalol, LR, leucovorin, levetiracetam, levofloxacin, lidocaine, linezolid, lorazepam, magnesium sulfate, mannitol, melphalan, meperidine, meropenem, meropenem/vaborbactam, mesna, methadone, methohexital, methotrexate, methylprednisolone, metoclopramide, metoprolol, metronidazole, micafungin, midazolam, milrinone, mitomycin, mitoxantrone, morphine, moxifloxacin, multivitamin, mycophenolate, nafcillin, nalbuphine, naloxone, nicardipine, nitroglycerin, nitroprusside, norepinephrine, octreotide, ondansetron, oxacillin, oxaliplatin, oxytocin, paclitaxel, palonosetron, pamidronate, pantoprazole, papaverine, penicillin G, pentamidine, pentobarbital, phenobarbital, phentolamine, phenylephrine, phytonadione, piperacillin/tazobactam, plazomicin, potassium acetate, potassium chloride, potassium phosphates, procainamide, prochlorperazine, promethazine, propranolol, protamine, pyridoxine, remifentanil, rocuronium, sildenafil, sodium acetate, sodium bicarbonate, sodium phosphates, succinylcholine, sufentanil, sulbactam/durlobactam, tacrolimus, tedizolid, telavancin, theophylline, thiamine, thiotepa, tigecycline, tirofiban, tobramycin, topotecan, vancomycin, vecuronium, verapamil, vinblastine, vincristine, vinorelbine, voriconazole, zidovudine, zoledronic acid.
- **Y-Site Incompatibility:** dantrolene, diazepam, diazoxide, gemtuzumab ozogamicin, indomethacin, pemetrexed, phenytoin

Patient/Family Teaching

- Explain purpose of vasopressin to patient.
- Advise patient of rationale for drinking water at time of administration to minimize side effects. Inform patient that these side effects are not serious and usually disappear quickly.
- Caution patient to avoid concurrent use of alcohol while taking vasopressin.
- Rep: Advise women of reproductive potential to notify health care provider if pregnancy is planned or suspected or if breastfeeding. Due to ↑ clearance of vasopressin in the 2nd and 3rd trimester, the dose of vasopressin may need to be ↑. May produce tonic uterine contractions that could threaten the continuation of pregnancy.
- Patients with diabetes insipidus should carry identification at all times describing disease process and medication regimen.

Evaluation/Desired Outcomes

- ↓ urine volume.
- Relief of polydipsia.
- ↑ urine osmolality in patients with central diabetes insipidus.
- ↑BP.

V

vedolizumab
(ve-doe-**liz**-yoo-mab)
Entyvio

Classification
Therapeutic: gastrointestinal anti-inflammatories
Pharmacologic: monoclonal antibodies, integrin receptor antagonists

Indications
Moderately to severely active ulcerative colitis. Moderately to severely active Crohn's disease.

Action
A monoclonal antibody that binds to certain integrins, blocking their interaction with substances involved in mucosal cell adhesion, also inhibits migration of memory T-lymphocytes across endothelium into inflamed GI tissue. **Therapeutic Effects:** Decreased chronic GI inflammation and symptomatology associated with ulcerative colitis and Crohn's disease.

Pharmacokinetics
Absorption: IV administration results in complete bioavailability.
Distribution: Minimally distributed to tissues.
Metabolism and Excretion: Unknown.
Half-life: 25 days.

TIME/ACTION PROFILE (clinical improvement)

ROUTE	ONSET	PEAK	DURATION
IV	within 6 wk	unknown	up to 8 wk

Contraindications/Precautions
Contraindicated in: Hypersensitivity; Active severe infection.
Use Cautiously in: OB: Use during pregnancy only if potential maternal benefits justify potential fetal risk; Lactation: Use while breastfeeding only if potential maternal benefit justifies potential risk to infant; Pedi: Safety and effectiveness not established in children.

Adverse Reactions/Side Effects
Derm: pruritus, rash. **GI:** ↑ liver enzymes, oropharyngeal pain. **MS:** arthralgia, back pain, extremity pain. **Neuro:** headache, fatigue, PROGRESSIVE MULTIFOCAL LEUKOENCEPHALOPATHY (PML). **Resp:** cough. **Misc:** fever, HYPERSENSITIVITY REACTIONS (INCLUDING ANAPHYLAXIS), INFECTION, INFUSION REACTIONS.

Interactions
Drug-Drug: May ↓ antibody response to and ↑ risk of adverse reactions from **live-virus vaccines**; complete immunizations prior to treatment. Concurrent use with **natalizumab** may ↑ risk of infections and PML; avoid concurrent use. Concurrent use with **TNF blockers** may ↑ risk of infections; avoid concurrent use. May affect activity of CYP450 enzymes and may alter the effectiveness/toxicity of **CYP450 substrate**.

Route/Dosage
IV (Adults): 300 mg initially, then 2 and 6 wk later, then every 8 wk; treatment may be continued if beneficial response is obtained by wk 14.
SUBQ (Adults): 108 mg every 2 wk (beginning after ≥2 IV doses [at Week 0 and Week 2]); treatment may be continued if beneficial response is obtained by Week 14.

Availability
Lyophilized powder for IV injection: 300 mg/vial. **Solution for SUBQ injection (prefilled syringes or pens):** 108 mg/0.68 mL.

NURSING IMPLICATIONS
Assessment
- Assess abdominal pain and frequency, quantity, and consistency of stools at beginning and during therapy.
- Assess for signs of hypersensitivity or infusion-related reactions (dyspnea; bronchospasm; urticaria; flushing; rash; swelling of lips, tongue, throat, or face; wheezing; hypertension; tachycardia). *If anaphylaxis or serious allergic reactions occur,* discontinue vedolizumab and treat symptoms.
- Monitor for new signs or symptoms suggestive of PML, a life threatening, opportunistic CNS infection, during and for ≥6 mo after therapy. Signs and symptoms are diverse and progressive over wks to mo. *If PML suspected,* stop therapy and consult neurologist; if diagnosis confirmed, permanently discontinue vedolizumab.

Lab Test Considerations
- May ↑ serum AST, ALT, and bilirubin. Discontinue vedolizumab if jaundice or other evidence of liver injury occur.

Implementation
- Perform test for latent tuberculosis (TB). If positive, begin treatment for TB prior to starting vedolizumab therapy. Monitor for TB throughout therapy, even if latent TB test is negative.
- Ensure patient is up to date according to current immunization guidelines before starting therapy.
- Following the first two IV doses administered at Week 0 and Week 2, may be switched to SUBQ injection at Week 6. Discontinue therapy in patients who show no evidence of therapeutic benefit by Week 14. May be switched from IV infusion to SUBQ injection for patients in clinical response or remission beyond Week 6. To switch patients to SUBQ injection, administer first SUBQ dose in place of the next scheduled IV infusion and every 2 wk thereafter. Inspect the solution visually for particulates and discoloration prior to administration. Solution in *Entyvio* prefilled syringe or *Entyvio Pen* is clear to moderately

opalescent, colorless to slightly yellow solution; do not use with visible particulates or discoloration.

- **SUBQ:** Administer each SUBQ injection at a different anatomic location (thigh, any quadrant of abdomen, or upper arm) from the previous injection. Do not inject into moles, scars, bruises, or areas where the skin is tender, erythematous, or indurated.

IV Administration

- **Intermittent Infusion: Reconstitution:** Reconstitute with 4.8 mL sterile water for injection, 0.9% NaCl, or LR using 21- to 25-gauge needle. Direct stream to wall of vial to prevent excessive foaming. Gently swirl vial for ≥15 sec to dissolve; do not invert or shake vigorously. Allow to sit for up to 20 min at room temperature for reconstitution and settling of foam. If not fully dissolved after 20 min, allow another 10 min. Do not use vial if not dissolved within 30 min. Solution is clear or opalescent, colorless to light brownish-yellow; do not administer solutions that are cloudy, discolored, or contain particulates. Swirl gently and invert vial three times prior to withdrawing dose. Use immediately after reconstitution. Reconstituted solution is stable for 8 hr if refrigerated. **Dilution:** Add 5 mL of reconstituted solution to 250 mL 0.9% NaCl or LR. Gently mix bag. Use as soon as possible. Use solutions diluted with LR immediately or store in refrigerator for up to 6 hr. Solutions diluted with 0.9% NaCl are stable for up to 12 hr at room temperature or 24 hr if refrigerated; do not freeze. **Rate:** Infuse over 30 min; do not administer as IV push or bolus. Flush line with 30 mL of 0.9% NaCl or LR after infusion.
- **Y-Site Incompatibility:** Do not administer other drugs through same IV line.

Patient/Family Teaching

- Explain purpose of vedolizumab to patient. Advise patient to read *Medication Guide* prior to therapy.
- Instruct patient and/or caregiver in proper technique to administer SUBQ injection. If SUBQ injection is interrupted or if a scheduled dose(s) of SUBQ *Entyvio* is missed, inject next SUBQ dose as soon as possible and then every 2 wk thereafter. In the event of incomplete dose administration (patient attempts administration of dose with *Entyvio Pen* but is uncertain if a full dose was administered), instruct the patient to call their pharmacy or health care professional.
- Instruct patient to report symptoms of PML (progressive unilateral weakness; changes in vision, memory, orientation, and personality), hypersensitivity reactions, hepatotoxicity (yellowing of the skin and eyes, unusual darkening of the urine, anorexia, nausea, feeling tired or weak, vomiting, right upper abdominal pain) to health care professional immediately.
- Inform patient of risk of infection. Advise patient to notify health care professional if symptoms of infection (fever, chills, muscle aches, shortness of breath, runny nose, cough, sore throat, red or painful skin, open cuts or sores, tiredness, pain during urination) occur.
- Advise patient to avoid live and oral vaccines during therapy.
- Advise patient to notify health care professional of all Rx or OTC medications, vitamins, or herbal products being taken and to consult with health care professional before taking other medications.
- Rep: Advise women of reproductive potential to notify health care professional if pregnancy is planned or suspected or if breastfeeding.

Evaluation/Desired Outcomes

- Decreased chronic GI inflammation and symptomatology associated with ulcerative colitis and Crohn's disease. Discontinue therapy if no improvement by Week 14.

BEERS

venlafaxine (ven-la-fax-een)

~~Effexor~~, Effexor XR

Classification

Therapeutic: antidepressants, antianxiety agents

Pharmacologic: selective serotonin/norepinephrine reuptake inhibitors

Indications

Major depressive disorder. Generalized anxiety disorder (Effexor XR only). Social anxiety disorder (extended release only). Panic disorder (extended release only). **Unlabeled Use:** Premenstrual dysphoric disorder.

Action

Inhibits serotonin and norepinephrine reuptake in the CNS. **Therapeutic Effects:** Decrease in depressive symptomatology, with fewer relapses/recurrences. Decreased anxiety. Decrease in panic attacks.

Pharmacokinetics

Absorption: 92–100% absorbed after oral administration.

Distribution: Extensive distribution into body tissues.

Metabolism and Excretion: Extensively metabolized on first pass through the liver (primarily through the CYP2D6 isoenzyme); the CYP2D6 isoenzyme exhibits genetic polymorphism (~7% of population

V

may be poor metabolizers and may have significantly ↑ venlafaxine concentrations and an ↑ risk of adverse effects). One metabolite, O-desmethylvenlafaxine (ODV), has antidepressant activity. 5% of venlafaxine is excreted unchanged in urine; 30% of the active metabolite is excreted in urine.

Half-life: *Venlafaxine:* 3–5 hr; *ODV:* 9–11 hr (both are ↑ in hepatic/renal impairment).

TIME/ACTION PROFILE (antidepressant action)

ROUTE	ONSET	PEAK	DURATION
PO	within 2 wk	2–4 wk	unknown

Contraindications/Precautions

Contraindicated in: Hypersensitivity; Concurrent use of MAO inhibitors or MAO-inhibitor-like drugs (linezolid or methylene blue); Lactation: Lactation.

Use Cautiously in: May ↑ risk of suicide attempt/ideation, especially during early treatment or dose adjustment; this risk appears to be greater in adolescents or children; Cardiovascular disease, including hypertension; Renal impairment (↓ dose); Hepatic impairment (↓ dose); Seizures or neurologic impairment; Mania; History of drug abuse; Angle-closure glaucoma; OB: Use during pregnancy only if potential maternal benefit justifies potential fetal risk (potential for discontinuation syndrome or toxicity in the neonate when venlafaxine is taken during the 3rd trimester); Pedi: Safety and effectiveness not established in children; Geri: Appears on Beers list. May worsen or cause syndrome of inappropriate antidiuretic hormone (SIADH) secretion and/or hyponatremia in older adults. Use with caution in older adults and closely monitor sodium concentrations when starting therapy or ↑ dose.

Adverse Reactions/Side Effects

CV: chest pain, hypertension, palpitations, tachycardia. **Derm:** ecchymoses, itching, photosensitivity, rash. **EENT:** rhinitis, visual disturbances, epistaxis, tinnitus. **Endo:** SIADH. **GI:** abdominal pain, altered taste, anorexia, constipation, diarrhea, dry mouth, dyspepsia, nausea, vomiting, weight loss. **GU:** ↓ libido, delayed/absent orgasm, ejaculatory delay/failure, erectile dysfunction, urinary frequency, urinary retention. **Hemat:** BLEEDING. **Neuro:** abnormal dreams, anxiety, dizziness, headache, insomnia, nervousness, paresthesia, weakness, abnormal thinking, agitation, confusion, depersonalization, drowsiness, emotional lability, NEUROLEPTIC MALIGNANT SYNDROME, SEIZURES, SUICIDAL THOUGHTS/BEHAVIORS, twitching, worsening depression. **Misc:** chills, discontinuation syndrome, SEROTONIN SYNDROME, yawning.

Interactions

Drug-Drug: Concurrent use with **MAO inhibitors** may result in serious, potentially fatal reactions; wait ≥2 wk after stopping MAO inhibitor before initiating venlafaxine; wait ≥1 wk after stopping venlafaxine before starting MAO inhibitor. **MAO-inhibitor-like drugs**, including **linezolid** or **methylene blue**, may ↑ risk of serotonin syndrome; concurrent use contraindicated; do not start therapy in patients receiving **linezolid** or **methylene blue**; if **linezolid** or **methylene blue** need to be started in a patient receiving venlafaxine, immediately discontinue venlafaxine and monitor for signs/symptoms of serotonin syndrome for 2 wk or until 24 hr after last dose of linezolid or methylene blue, whichever comes first (may resume venlafaxine therapy 24 hr after last dose of linezolid or methylene blue). Drugs that affect serotonergic neurotransmitter systems, including **tricyclic antidepressants**, **SNRIs**, **fentanyl**, **lithium**, **buspirone**, **tramadol**, **meperidine**, **methadone**, **amphetamines**, and **triptans**, may ↑ risk of serotonin syndrome. May ↑ levels and risk of toxicity of **desipramine** and **haloperidol**. **Cimetidine** may ↑ levels and risk of toxicity; may be more pronounced in older adults, those with hepatic or renal impairment, or those with pre-existing hypertension. **Ketoconazole** may ↑ levels and risk of toxicity. ↑ risk of bleeding with **NSAIDs**, **aspirin**, **clopidogrel**, **prasugrel**, **ticagrelor**, **dabigatran**, **apixaban**, **edoxaban**, **rivaroxaban**, or **warfarin**.

Drug-Natural Products: **Kava-kava**, **valerian**, **chamomile**, or **hops** can ↑ risk of CNS depression. ↑ risk of serotonergic side effects, including serotonin syndrome, with **St. John's wort** and **SAMe**.

Route/Dosage

Major Depressive Disorder

PO (Adults): *Tablets:* 75 mg/day in 2–3 divided doses; may ↑ by up to 75 mg/day every 4 days, up to 225 mg/day (not to exceed 375 mg/day in 3 divided doses); *Extended-release capsules:* 75 mg once daily (some patients may be started at 37.5 mg once daily) for 4–7 days; may ↑ by up to 75 mg/day at intervals of not less than 4 days (not to exceed 225 mg/day).

Renal Impairment

PO (Adults): *CCr 10–70 mL/min:* ↓ daily dose by 25% (immediate release); *CCr 30–89 mL/min:* ↓ daily dose by 25–50% (extended release); *CCr <30 mL/min:* ↓ daily dose by ≥50% (extended release); *Hemodialysis:* ↓ daily dose by ≥50%.

Hepatic Impairment

PO (Adults): *Mild, moderate, or severe hepatic impairment:* ↓ daily dose by 50%.

General Anxiety Disorder

PO (Adults): *Extended-release capsules:* 75 mg once daily (some patients may be started at 37.5 mg once daily) for 4–7 days; may ↑ by up to 75 mg/day at intervals of not less than 4 days (not to exceed 225 mg/day).

Renal Impairment
PO (Adults): *CCr 10–70 mL/min:* ↓ daily dose by 25% (immediate release); *CCr 30–89 mL/min:* ↓ daily dose by 25–50% (extended release); *CCr <30 mL/min:* ↓ daily dose by ≥50% (extended release); *Hemodialysis:* ↓ daily dose by ≥50%.

Hepatic Impairment
PO (Adults): *Mild, moderate, or severe hepatic impairment:* ↓ daily dose by 50%.

Social Anxiety Disorder
PO (Adults): *Extended-release capsules:* 75 mg once daily.

Renal Impairment
PO (Adults): *CCr 10–70 mL/min:* ↓ daily dose by 25% (immediate release); *CCr 30–89 mL/min:* ↓ daily dose by 25–50% (extended release); *CCr <30 mL/min:* ↓ daily dose by ≥50% (extended release); *Hemodialysis:* ↓ daily dose by ≥50%.

Hepatic Impairment
PO (Adults): *Mild, moderate, or severe hepatic impairment:* ↓ daily dose by 50%.

Panic Disorder
PO (Adults): *Extended-release capsules:* 37.5 mg once daily for 7 days; may then ↑ to 75 mg once daily; may then ↑ by 75 mg/day every 7 days (not to exceed 225 mg/day).

Hepatic Impairment
PO (Adults): *Mild, moderate, or severe hepatic impairment:* ↓ daily dose by 50%.

Renal Impairment
PO (Adults): *CCr 10–70 mL/min:* ↓ daily dose by 25% (immediate release); *CCr 30–89 mL/min:* ↓ daily dose by 25–50% (extended release); *CCr <30 mL/min:* ↓ daily dose by ≥50% (extended release); *Hemodialysis:* ↓ daily dose by ≥50%.

Availability (generic available)
Immediate-release tablets: 25 mg, 37.5 mg, 50 mg, 75 mg, 100 mg. **Extended-release tablets:** 37.5 mg, 75 mg, 112.5 mg, 150 mg, 225 mg. **Extended-release capsules:** 37.5 mg, 75 mg, 150 mg.

NURSING IMPLICATIONS
Assessment
- Screen patients for a personal or family history of bipolar disorder, mania, or hypomania before starting therapy.
- Assess mental status and mood changes. Inform health care provider if patient demonstrates significant ↑ in anxiety, nervousness, or insomnia.
- Assess for suicidal tendencies, especially during early therapy. Restrict amount of drug available to patient. Risk may be ↑ in adults ≤24 yr. After starting therapy, young adults should be seen by health care provider at least weekly for 4 wk, every 3 wk for next 4 wk, and on advice of health care provider thereafter.
- Monitor BP before and periodically during therapy. Sustained hypertension may be dose-related; ↓ dose or discontinue therapy if this occurs.
- Monitor appetite and nutritional intake. Weigh weekly. Report continued weight loss. Adjust diet as tolerated to support nutritional status.
- Assess for serotonin syndrome (mental changes [agitation, hallucinations, coma], autonomic instability [tachycardia, labile BP, hyperthermia], neuromuscular aberrations [hyperreflexia, incoordination], GI symptoms [nausea, vomiting, diarrhea]), especially in patients taking other serotonergic drugs (SSRIs, SNRIs, triptans). *If serotonin syndrome occurs,* discontinue venlafaxine and any other serotonergic agents; initiate appropriate medical interventions.
- Assess sexual function before starting and during therapy, including timing of onset.

Lab Test Considerations
- Monitor CBC with differential periodically during therapy. May cause anemia, leukocytosis, leukopenia, thrombocytopenia, basophilia, and eosinophilia.
- May ↑ alkaline phosphatase, bilirubin, AST, ALT, BUN, and serum creatinine.
- May ↑ cholesterol.
- May cause hyperglycemia, hypoglycemia, hyperkalemia, hypokalemia, hyperuricemia, hyperphosphatemia, hypophosphatemia, and hyponatremia.
- May cause false-positive immunoassay screening tests for phencyclidine and amphetamine.

Implementation
- Do not confuse Effexor XR with Enablex.
- **PO:** Administer venlafaxine with food.
- ***DNC:*** Swallow extended-release capsules and tablets whole; do not crush, break, or chew.
- Extended-release capsules may be opened and contents sprinkled on a spoonful of applesauce. Take immediately and follow with a glass of water. Do not store mixture for later use.

Patient/Family Teaching
- Instruct patient to take venlafaxine as directed at the same time each day. Take missed doses as soon as possible unless almost time for next dose. Do not double doses or discontinue abruptly. Patients taking venlafaxine for >6 wk should have dose gradually ↓ before discontinuation to prevent dizziness, nausea, headache, irritability, insomnia, diarrhea, anxiety, fatigue, abnormal dreams, and hyperhidrosis; discontinuation may take several months.

V

- Advise patient, family, and caregivers to look for suicidality, especially during early therapy or dose changes. Notify health care provider immediately if thoughts about suicide or dying, attempts to commit suicide, new or worse depression or anxiety, agitation or restlessness, panic attacks, insomnia, new or worse irritability, aggressiveness, acting on dangerous impulses, mania, or other changes in mood or behavior occur.
- Advise patient to notify health care provider immediately if symptoms of serotonin syndrome (agitation, hallucinations, ↑ HR, hyperthermia, hyperreflexia, incoordination) occur.
- May cause drowsiness or dizziness. Caution patient to avoid driving or other activities requiring alertness until response to the drug is known.
- Instruct patient to notify health care provider of all Rx or OTC medications, vitamins, or herbal products being taken and consult health care provider before taking any new medications. Caution patient to avoid taking alcohol or other CNS-depressant drugs, including opioids, during therapy.
- Instruct patient to notify health care provider if signs of allergy (rash, hives) occur.
- Inform patient that venlafaxine may cause symptoms of sexual dysfunction. In men, ejaculatory delay or failure, ↓ libido, and erectile dysfunction may occur. In women, may result in ↓ libido and delayed or absent orgasm. Advise patient to notify health care provider if symptoms occur.
- Rep: Advise women of reproductive potential to notify health care provider immediately if pregnancy is planned or suspected or if breastfeeding. Use during last month of pregnancy ↑ risk of postpartum hemorrhage. If used during pregnancy, should be tapered during 3rd trimester to avoid neonatal serotonin syndrome. Monitor infants exposed to venlafaxine for excess sedation, restlessness, agitation, poor feeding, poor weight gain, and respiratory distress; may ↑ risk of persistent pulmonary hypertension of the newborn. Inform patient of pregnancy exposure registry that monitors pregnancy outcomes in women exposed to antidepressants during pregnancy. Register patients by calling the National Pregnancy Registry for Antidepressants at 1-844-405-6185 or visiting online at https://womensmentalhealth.org/research/pregnancyregistry/antidepressants/.
- Emphasize the importance of follow-up exams to monitor progress.

Evaluation/Desired Outcomes

- Increased sense of well-being.
- Renewed interest in surroundings. Need for therapy should be periodically reassessed.
- ↓ anxiety.

verapamil, See CALCIUM CHANNEL BLOCKERS.

BEERS

vilazodone (vil-az-oh-done)

Viibryd

Classification

Therapeutic: antidepressants

Pharmacologic: selective serotonin reuptake inhibitors (SSRIs), benzofurans

Indications

Major depressive disorder.

Action

Increases serotonin activity in the CNS by inhibiting serotonin reuptake. Also binds selectively with high affinity to 5-HT_{1A} receptors and is a 5-HT_{1A} receptor partial agonist.

Therapeutic Effects: Improvement in symptoms of depression.

Pharmacokinetics

Absorption: 72% absorbed following oral administration with food.

Distribution: Unknown.

Protein Binding: 96–99%.

Metabolism and Excretion: Mostly metabolized by the liver, primarily by the CYP3A4 isoenzyme; 1% excreted unchanged in urine.

Half-life: 25 hr.

TIME/ACTION PROFILE (plasma concentrations)

ROUTE	ONSET	PEAK	DURATION
PO	unknown	4–5 hr	unknown

Contraindications/Precautions

Contraindicated in: Concurrent use of MAO inhibitors or MAO-inhibitor-like drugs (linezolid or methylene blue).

Use Cautiously in: May ↑ risk of suicide attempt/ideation especially during early treatment or dose adjustment; this risk appears to be greater in adolescents or children; Bipolar disorder (may ↑ risk of mania/hypomania); Angle-closure glaucoma; OB: Use during pregnancy only if potential maternal benefit justifies potential fetal risk; Lactation: Use while breastfeeding only if potential maternal benefit justifies potential risk to infant; Pedi: Safety and effectiveness not established in children; Geri: Appears on Beers list. May worsen or cause syndrome of inappropriate antidiuretic hormone (SIADH) secretion and/or hyponatremia in older adults. Use with caution in older adults and closely monitor sodium concentrations when starting therapy or ↑ dose.

Adverse Reactions/Side Effects

Endo: SIADH. **F and E:** hyponatremia. **GI:** diarrhea, nausea, dry mouth, PANCREATITIS, vomiting. **GU:** ↓ libido, delayed/absent orgasm, ejaculatory delay/failure, erectile dysfunction. **Hemat:** BLEEDING. **Neuro:** insomnia, abnormal dreams, dizziness, NEUROLEPTIC MALIGNANT-LIKE SYNDROME, restlessness, SEIZURES, sleep paralysis, SUICIDAL THOUGHTS/BEHAVIORS. **Misc:** SEROTONIN SYNDROME.

Interactions

Drug-Drug: Concurrent use with, or use within 14 days of starting or stopping, **MAO inhibitors** may ↑ risk of neuroleptic malignant syndrome or serotonin syndrome and should be avoided. **MAO-inhibitor-like drugs**, such as **linezolid** or **methylene blue**, may ↑ risk of serotonin syndrome; concurrent use contraindicated; do not start therapy in patients receiving **linezolid** or **methylene blue**; if **linezolid** or **methylene blue** need to be started in a patient receiving vilazodone, immediately discontinue vilazodone and monitor for signs/symptoms of serotonin syndrome for 2 wk or until 24 hr after last dose of linezolid or methylene blue, whichever comes first (may resume vilazodone therapy 24 hr after last dose of linezolid or methylene blue). Drugs that affect serotonergic neurotransmitter systems, including **tricyclic antidepressants**, **SNRIs**, **fentanyl**, **lithium**, **buspirone**, **tramadol**, **meperidine**, **methadone**, **amphetamines**, and **triptans**, may ↑ risk of serotonin syndrome. ↑ risk of bleeding with **NSAIDs**, **aspirin**, **clopidogrel**, **prasugrel**, **ticagrelor**, **dabigatran**, **apixaban**, **edoxaban**, **rivaroxaban**, or **warfarin**. **Strong CYP3A4 inhibitors**, including **ketoconazole**, may ↑ levels and risk of toxicity. **Moderate CYP3A4 inhibitors**, including **erythromycin**, may ↑ levels and risk of toxicity; ↓ dose. **Strong CYP3A4 inducers**, including **carbamazepine**, may ↓ levels and effectiveness.

Drug-Natural Products: ↑ risk of serotonin syndrome with **St. John's wort**.

Route/Dosage

PO (Adults): 10 mg once daily for one wk; then 20 mg once daily for one wk; dose may be ↑ to 40 mg once daily (recommended dose = 20–40 mg/day). *Concurrent use of strong CYP3A4 inhibitors:* Not to exceed 20 mg/day; *Concurrent use of strong CYP3A4 inducers (if used for >14 days):* May need to ↑ dose up to twofold (daily dose should not exceed 80 mg).

Availability (generic available)

Tablets: 10 mg, 20 mg, 40 mg.

NURSING IMPLICATIONS

Assessment

- Assess mental status and mood changes. Inform health care provider if patient demonstrates significant ↑ in anxiety, nervousness, or insomnia.
- Before starting therapy, screen patient for bipolar disorder (detailed psychiatric history, including family/personal history of suicide, bipolar disorder, or depression). Use cautiously in patients with a positive history.
- Assess for suicidal tendencies, especially during early therapy. Restrict amount of drug available to patient. Risk may be ↑ in adults ≤24 yr. After starting therapy, young adults should be seen by health care provider at least weekly for 4 wk, every 3 wk for next 4 wk, and on advice of health care provider thereafter.
- Assess for signs and symptoms of hyponatremia (headache, difficulty concentrating, memory impairment, confusion, weakness, unsteadiness). May require discontinuation of therapy.
- Assess for serotonin syndrome (mental changes [agitation, hallucinations, coma], autonomic instability [tachycardia, labile BP, hyperthermia], neuromuscular aberrations [hyperreflexia, incoordination], GI symptoms [nausea, vomiting, diarrhea]), especially in patients taking other serotonergic drugs (SSRIs, SNRIs, triptans).
- Monitor for development of neuroleptic malignant syndrome (fever, muscle rigidity, altered mental status, respiratory distress, tachycardia, seizures, diaphoresis, hypertension or hypotension, pallor, tiredness, loss of bladder control). Discontinue vilazodone and notify health care provider immediately if these symptoms occur.
- Assess baseline sexual function before starting vilazodone. Assess for changes in sexual function during treatment, including timing of onset.

Lab Test Considerations

- Monitor serum sodium concentrations periodically during therapy. May cause hyponatremia potentially as a result of SIADH.
- May alter anticoagulant effects. Monitor patients receiving warfarin, NSAIDs, or aspirin concurrently.

Implementation

- **PO:** Administer vilazodone with food; administration without food can result in inadequate drug concentrations and may ↓ effectiveness.
- *When discontinuing therapy after prolonged treatment (>3 wk)*, ↓ dose gradually. If taking 40 mg once daily, ↓ to 20 mg once daily for 4 days, followed by 10 mg once daily for 3 days. If taking

V

20 mg once daily, ↓ to 10 mg once daily for 7 days. *When discontinuing therapy after brief treatment (2–3 wk),* taper over 1–2 wk; <2 wk treatment generally does not need taper. Patients with a history of antidepressant withdrawal symptoms or on a high dose may require a slower taper (>4 wk). *If intolerable withdrawal symptoms occur during taper,* resume the previously prescribed dose and/or ↓ dose at a more gradual rate. Patients with a history of discontinuation syndrome on long-term treatment (>6 mo) may benefit from tapering over >3 mo.

Patient/Family Teaching

- Explain purpose and side effects of medication to patient. Advise patient to read *Patient Information* before starting therapy. Instruct patient to take as directed at the same time each day. Take missed doses as soon as possible unless almost time for next dose. Do not double doses or discontinue abruptly. Gradually ↓ dose before discontinuation. Emphasize the importance of follow-up exams to monitor progress, and encourage patient participation in psychotherapy.
- Instruct patient to notify health care provider of all Rx or OTC medications, vitamins, or herbal products being taken and to avoid concurrent use of Rx, OTC, and herbal products, especially NSAIDs, aspirin, and warfarin, without consulting health care provider.
- Advise patient, family, and caregivers to look for suicidality, especially during early therapy or dose changes. Notify health care provider immediately if thoughts about suicide or dying, attempts to commit suicide, new or worse depression or anxiety, agitation or restlessness, panic attacks, insomnia, new or worse irritability, aggressiveness, acting on dangerous impulses, mania, or other changes in mood or behavior occur.
- Advise patient and caregivers to notify health care provider immediately if symptoms of serotonin syndrome occur.
- Caution patient of the risk of serotonin syndrome and neuroleptic malignant syndrome, especially when taking triptans, tramadol, tryptophan supplements, and other serotonergic or antipsychotic agents.
- May cause dizziness. Caution patient to avoid driving or other activities requiring alertness until response to the drug is known.
- Caution patient to avoid taking alcohol or other CNS-depressant drugs, including opioids, during therapy.
- Inform patient that symptoms of sexual dysfunction can occur. Advise men that ejaculatory delay or failure, ↓ libido, and erectile dysfunction may occur. Advise women that ↓ libido and delayed or absent orgasm may occur. Advise patient to notify health care provider if symptoms occur.
- Rep: Advise women of reproductive potential to notify health care provider immediately if pregnancy is planned or suspected or if breastfeeding. Use during last month of pregnancy ↑ risk of postpartum hemorrhage. If used during pregnancy, should be tapered during 3rd trimester to avoid neonatal serotonin syndrome. Monitor infants exposed to vilazodone for excess sedation, restlessness, agitation, poor feeding, poor weight gain, or respiratory distress; may ↑ risk of persistent pulmonary hypertension of the newborn. Encourage pregnant patients to enroll in pregnancy exposure registry that monitors outcomes of women exposed to antidepressants during pregnancy by contacting National Pregnancy Registry for Antidepressants at 1-866-961-2388 or visiting online at https://womensmentalhealth.org/research/pregnancyregistry/antidepressants/.

Evaluation/Desired Outcomes

- Improve symptoms of depression.
- ↓ anxiety.

HIGH ALERT

vinBLAStine (vin-**blass**-teen)

Classification

Therapeutic: antineoplastics

Pharmacologic: vinca alkaloids

Indications

Palliative treatment of the following: Hodgkin lymphoma, Lymphocytic lymphoma, Histiocytic lymphoma, Advanced mycosis fungoides, Testicular carcinoma, Kaposi sarcoma, Breast cancer.

Action

Binds to proteins of mitotic spindle, causing metaphase arrest. Cell replication is stopped as a result (cell cycle specific for M phase). **Therapeutic Effects:** Death of rapidly replicating cells, particularly malignant ones.

Pharmacokinetics

Absorption: IV administration results in complete bioavailability.

Distribution: Does not cross the blood-brain barrier well.

Metabolism and Excretion: Converted by the liver to an active antineoplastic compound; excreted in the feces via biliary excretion, with some renal elimination.

Half-life: 24 hr.

TIME/ACTION PROFILE (effects on WBC counts)

ROUTE	ONSET	PEAK	DURATION
IV	5–7 days	10 days	7–14 days

Contraindications/Precautions

Contraindicated in: Hypersensitivity; OB: Pregnancy; Lactation: Lactation.

Use Cautiously in: Infection; ↓ bone marrow reserve; Hepatic impairment (↓ dose by 50% if serum bilirubin >3 mg/dL); Rep: Women of reproductive potential.

Adverse Reactions/Side Effects

Derm: alopecia, dermatitis, vesiculation. **Endo:** syndrome of inappropriate antidiuretic hormone (SIADH). **GI:** nausea, vomiting, anorexia, constipation, diarrhea, stomatitis. **GU:** gonadal suppression. **Hemat:** anemia, leukopenia, thrombocytopenia. **Local:** phlebitis. **Metab:** hyperuricemia. **Neuro:** depression, neuritis, paresthesia, peripheral neuropathy, SEIZURES, weakness. **Resp:** BRONCHOSPASM.

Interactions

Drug-Drug: Additive bone marrow depression with other **antineoplastics** or **radiation therapy**. Bronchospasm may occur in patients who have been previously treated with **mitomycin**. May ↓ antibody response to **live-virus vaccines** and ↑ risk of adverse reactions. May ↓ levels and effectiveness of **phenytoin**.

Route/Dosage

IV (Adults): *Initial:* 3.7 mg/m² (100 mcg/kg) as a single dose; ↑ weekly as tolerated by 1.8 mg/m² (50 mcg/kg) to maximum of 18.5 mg/m² (usual dose is 5.5–7.4 mg/m²). *Maintenance:* 10 mg 1–2 times/mo or one increment less than last dose every 7–14 days.

IV (Children): *Initial:* 2.5 mg/m² as a single dose; ↑ weekly as tolerated by 1.25 mg/m² to maximum of 7.5 mg/m². *Maintenance:* one increment less than last dose every 7 days.

Availability (generic available)

Solution for injection: 1 mg/mL.

NURSING IMPLICATIONS

Assessment

- Monitor BP, HR, and respiratory rate during therapy. Bronchospasm and acute or progressive dyspnea can be life-threatening and may occur at time of infusion or several hours to weeks later.
- May cause nausea and vomiting. Monitor intake, output, appetite, and nutritional intake. Prophylactic antiemetics may be used. Adjust diet as tolerated.
- Monitor for signs/symptoms of myelosuppression, consisting of anemia (weakness, fatigue, dizziness, pallor of skin and sclera), neutropenia (malaise, fatigue, fever, chills, sore throat, lymphadenopathy, infections), or thrombocytopenia (petechiae, purpura, epistaxis, bleeding). Assess for signs of infection during neutropenia.
- Assess for bleeding (bleeding gums, bruising, petechiae, weakness, tachycardia, dyspnea, dizziness, pallor, fatigue, tarry stools, coffee ground emesis) and avoid IM injections and taking rectal temperatures if platelet count is low. Apply pressure to venipuncture sites for 10 min.
- Monitor for signs/symptoms of neuropathy or neurotoxicity (blurred or double vision, difficulty in walking, drooping eyelids, headache, fingers, toe or jaw pain, paresthesia in the fingers and toes, constipation, abdominal pain, urinary retention, postural hypotension, loss of deep tendon reflexes).
- Monitor for signs/symptoms of gout (↑ uric acid, joint pain, edema). Encourage patient to drink ≥2 L of fluid per day. Allopurinol or alkalinization of urine may be used to ↓ uric acid levels.

Lab Test Considerations

- Monitor CBC with differential prior to and routinely throughout therapy. If WBC <2000 cells/mm³, hold subsequent doses until WBC ≥4000 cells/mm³. The nadir of leukopenia occurs in 5–10 days and recovery usually occurs 7–14 days later. Thrombocytopenia may also occur in patients who have received radiation or other chemotherapy agents.
- Monitor liver function (AST, ALT, LDH, bilirubin) and renal function (BUN, serum creatinine) before starting and periodically throughout therapy.
- May ↑ uric acid. Monitor periodically during therapy.
- Monitor serum sodium periodically, especially if SIADH suspected.

Implementation

- ***High Alert:*** Fatalities have occurred with chemotherapeutic agents. Before administering, clarify all ambiguous orders; double-check single, daily, and course-of-therapy dose limits; have second practitioner independently double-check original order, dose calculations, and infusion pump settings. Do not administer SUBQ, IM, or intrathecally (IT). IT administration is fatal. Vinblastine must be dispensed in an overwrap stating, "For IV use only." Overwrap should remain in place until immediately before administration.
- ***High Alert:*** Do not confuse vinblastine with vincristine.
- When preparing from a vial or ampule, wear double chemotherapy gloves, protective gown, respiratory (N95) protection, and hair and shoe covers; optimally prepare in a ventilated control device. When administering, add eye/face protection if there is a potential that the substance could splash. Severe irritation or corneal ulceration may occur if splashed into eye. Use a closed-system drug transfer device when dosage form allows. Prepare in a minibag, not a syringe. Single chemotherapy gloves are appropriate

if administering from prefilled bag. Discard IV equipment in specially designated containers.

- Do not inject into extremities with impaired circulation; may cause thrombophlebitis.

IV Administration

- **V** Vinblastine is a vesicant. If extravasation occurs, immediately stop infusion. Leave needle/cannula in place temporarily but do not flush the line. Gently aspirate extravasated solution; then remove needle/cannula. Elevate patient's extremity and apply dry warm compresses for 20 min 4 times day for 1–2 days. Initiate hyaluronidase antidote by injecting 1–6 mL (150 units/mL) into existing IV line; usual dose is 1 mL for each 1 mL of extravasated drug. If needle/cannula has been removed, inject SUBQ in a clockwise manner around area of extravasation or administer 1 mL as five separate 0.2 mL injections SUBQ into extravasation site; may repeat several times over next 3–4 hr.
- **IV Push: Dilution:** Dilute each 10 mg with 10 mL of 0.9% NaCl for injection with phenol or benzyl alcohol. Solution is clear. Reconstituted medication is stable for 28 days if refrigerated. **Concentration:** 1 mg/mL. **Rate:** Administer each single dose over 1 min through Y-site injection of a free-flowing infusion of 0.9% NaCl or D5W.
- **Intermittent Infusion: Dilution:** Dilute in 25 to 50 mL of 0.9% NaCl, D5W, or LR. Dilution in large volumes (100–250 mL) or prolonged infusion (≥30 min) ↑ chance of vein irritation and extravasation.
- **Y-Site Compatibility:** acyclovir, alemtuzumab, allopurinol, amikacin, aminophylline, amiodarone, ampicillin, ampicillin/sulbactam, anidulafungin, argatroban, arsenic trioxide, atracurium, aztreonam, bivalirudin, bleomycin, bumetanide, buprenorphine, busulfan, butorphanol, calcium chloride, calcium gluconate, carboplatin, carmustine, caspofungin, cefazolin, cefotaxime, cefotetan, cefoxitin, ceftazidime, ceftriaxone, cefuroxime, chloramphenicol, chlorpromazine, ciprofloxacin, cisatracurium, cisplatin, clindamycin, cyclophosphamide, cyclosporine, dacarbazine, dactinomycin, daptomycin, daunorubicin, dexamethasone, dexmedetomidine, dexrazoxane, digoxin, diltiazem, diphenhydramine, dobutamine, docetaxel, dopamine, doxorubicin hydrochloride, doxorubicin liposomal, doxycycline, droperidol, enalaprilat, ephedrine, epinephrine, epirubicin, ertapenem, erythromycin, esmolol, etoposide, etoposide phosphate, famotidine, fentanyl, filgrastim, fluconazole, fludarabine, fluorouracil, foscarnet, fosphenytoin, ganciclovir, gemcitabine, gentamicin, glycopyrrolate, granisetron, haloperidol, heparin, hetastarch, hydralazine, hydrocortisone, hydromorphone, idarubicin, ifosfamide, imipenem/cilastatin, insulin regular, irinotecan, isoproterenol, ketorolac, labetalol, leucovorin, levofloxacin, lidocaine, linezolid, lorazepam, magnesium sulfate, mannitol, melphalan, meperidine, meropenem, mesna, methadone, methohexital, methotrexate, metoclopramide, metoprolol, metronidazole, midazolam, milrinone, mitomycin, mitoxantrone, morphine, moxifloxacin, nafcillin, nalbuphine, naloxone, nitroglycerin, nitroprusside, norepinephrine, octreotide, ondansetron, oxaliplatin, paclitaxel, palonosetron, pamidronate, pemetrexed, pentamidine, pentobarbital, phenobarbital, phentolamine, phenylephrine, piperacillin/tazobactam, potassium acetate, potassium chloride, potassium phosphates, procainamide, prochlorperazine, promethazine, propranolol, remifentanil, rituximab, sargramostim, sodium acetate, sodium bicarbonate, sodium phosphates, succinylcholine, sufentanil, tacrolimus, theophylline, thiotepa, tigecycline, tirofiban, tobramycin, topotecan, trastuzumab, trimethoprim/sulfamethoxazole, vancomycin, vasopressin, vecuronium, verapamil, vincristine, vinorelbine, voriconazole, zidovudine, zoledronic acid.
- **Y-Site Incompatibility:** amphotericin B deoxycholate, amphotericin B liposomal, cefepime, dantrolene, diazepam, furosemide, gemtuzumab ozogamicin, pantoprazole, phenytoin.

Patient/Family Teaching

- Explain the purpose and side effects of vinblastine. Do not stop receiving without consulting health care provider. If an appointment is missed, contact health care provider as soon as possible to reschedule. Advise patient to read *Medication Guide* before starting and periodically during therapy in case of changes.
- Explain need for continued medical follow-up to assess effectiveness and possible side effects of medication. Periodic lab tests will be needed.
- Advise patient to notify health care provider if fever, chills, sore throat, or signs of infection occur. Caution patient to avoid crowds and persons with known infections.
- Tell patient to report and seek treatment for signs and symptoms of bleeding (weakness; fast heartbeat; trouble breathing; dizziness; pale skin; tiredness; obvious bleeding in urine, stool, mouth, or nose). Instruct patient to use soft toothbrush and electric razor. Caution patient not to drink alcoholic beverages or take products containing aspirin or NSAIDs.
- Instruct patient to inspect oral mucosa for redness and ulceration. Advise patient that if ulceration occurs, to avoid spicy foods, use sponge brush, and rinse mouth with water after eating and drinking. Topical agents may be used if mouth pain interferes

with eating. Stomatitis pain may require treatment with opioid analgesics.

- Instruct patient to report symptoms of neurotoxicity (paresthesia, pain, difficulty walking, persistent constipation).
- Advise patient that jaw pain, pain in organs containing tumor tissue, nausea, and vomiting may occur. Avoid constipation and report other adverse reactions.
- Discuss with patient the possibility of hair loss. Explore coping strategies.
- Instruct patient not to receive any vaccinations without advice of health care provider.
- Advise patient to notify health care provider of all Rx or OTC medications, vitamins, or herbal products being taken and to consult with health care provider before taking other medications.
- Rep: May cause fetal harm. Advise women of reproductive potential to notify health care provider if pregnancy is planned or suspected and to avoid breastfeeding during therapy. Adverse effects to a fetus may be caused by both men or women receiving treatment with vinblastine. Contraception should be used during therapy and for ≥2 mo after last dose. If need to use during pregnancy, avoid during 1st trimester, leave a 3-wk time period between the last chemotherapy dose and anticipated delivery, and do not administer chemotherapy beyond week 33 of gestation. If treatment cannot be deferred until after delivery in patients with early stage Hodgkin lymphoma, may be administered safely and effectively in the latter phase of pregnancy. Encourage patient to enroll in the pregnancy registry for all cancers diagnosed during pregnancy at Cooper University Health (1-856-757-7876). May cause infertility in men.

Evaluation/Desired Outcomes

- Regression of malignancy without the appearance of detrimental side effects.

HIGH ALERT

V vinCRIStine (vin-kriss-teen)

~~Vincasar PFS~~

Classification

Therapeutic: antineoplastics

Pharmacologic: vinca alkaloids

Indications

Used alone and in combination with other treatment modalities (antineoplastics, surgery, or radiation therapy) in treatment of: Hodgkin disease, Leukemias, Neuroblastoma, Malignant lymphomas, Rhabdomyosarcoma, Wilms tumor, Other tumors.

Action

Binds to proteins of mitotic spindle, causing metaphase arrest. Cell replication is stopped as a result (cell cycle specific for M phase). Has little or no effect on bone marrow. **Therapeutic Effects:** Death of rapidly replicating cells, particularly malignant ones.

Pharmacokinetics

Absorption: IV administration results in complete bioavailability.

Distribution: Rapidly and widely distributed; extensively bound to tissues.

Metabolism and Excretion: Metabolized by the liver and eliminated in the feces via biliary excretion.

Half-life: 10.5–37.5 hr.

TIME/ACTION PROFILE (effects on blood counts†)

ROUTE	ONSET	PEAK	DURATION
IV	unknown	4 days	7 days

† Usually mild.

Contraindications/Precautions

Contraindicated in: Hypersensitivity; OB: Pregnancy; Lactation: Lactation.

Use Cautiously in: Infection; ↓ bone marrow reserve; Hepatic impairment (↓ dose if serum bilirubin >3 mg/dL); Rep: Women of reproductive potential.

Adverse Reactions/Side Effects

Derm: <u>alopecia</u>. **EENT:** cortical blindness, diplopia. **Endo:** syndrome of inappropriate antidiuretic hormone (SIADH). **GI:** <u>nausea</u>, <u>vomiting</u>, abdominal cramps, anorexia, constipation, ileus, stomatitis. **GU:** gonadal suppression, nocturia, oliguria, urinary retention. **Hemat:** anemia, leukopenia, thrombocytopenia (mild and brief). **Local:** <u>phlebitis</u>, tissue necrosis (from extravasation). **Metab:** hyperuricemia. **Neuro:** <u>ascending peripheral neuropathy</u>, agitation, depression, insomnia, mental status changes. **Resp:** bronchospasm.

Interactions

Drug-Drug: Bronchospasm may occur in patients who have been previously treated with **mitomycin**. **l-asparaginase** may ↑ levels and risk of toxicity; give vincristine 12–24 hr before asparaginase. May ↓ antibody response to **live-virus vaccines** and ↑ risk of adverse reactions.

Route/Dosage

IV (Adults): 10–30 mcg/kg (0.4–1.4 mg/m²) as a single dose; may repeat weekly (not to exceed 2 mg/dose).

V

IV (Children >10 kg): 1.5–2 mg/m² as a single dose; may repeat weekly.
IV (Children <10 kg): 50 mcg/kg as a single dose; may repeat weekly.

Availability (generic available)

Solution for injection: 1 mg/mL.

NURSING IMPLICATIONS

Assessment

- Monitor BP, HR, and respiratory rate during therapy.
- Monitor for hypersensitivity reaction (rash, edema, anaphylaxis) during infusion. *If symptoms occur,* immediately discontinue vincristine and treat as indicated.
- Monitor neurologic status. Assess for paresthesia (numbness, tingling, pain), loss of deep tendon reflexes (Achilles reflex is usually first involved), weakness (wrist drop or footdrop, gait disturbances), cranial nerve palsies (jaw pain, hoarseness, ptosis, visual changes), autonomic dysfunction (ileus, difficulty voiding, orthostatic hypotension, impaired sweating), and CNS dysfunction (↓ level of consciousness, agitation, hallucinations).
- Monitor intake, output, and daily weight. *If ↓ urine output with hyponatremia occurs,* it may indicate SIADH and usually responds to fluid restriction.
- Assess nutritional status. *If nausea or vomiting occurs,* use an antiemetic to minimize symptoms.
- Monitor for signs/symptoms of gout (↑ uric acid, joint pain, edema). Encourage patient to drink ≥2 liters of fluid per day. Allopurinol or alkalinization of urine may be used to ↓ uric acid levels.

Lab Test Considerations

- Monitor CBC with differential before starting and periodically throughout therapy. May cause slight leukopenia 4 days after therapy, which resolves within 7 days. Platelet count may ↑ or ↓.
- Monitor liver function (AST, ALT, LDH, bilirubin) and renal function (BUN, serum creatinine) before starting and periodically throughout therapy.
- May ↑ uric acid. Monitor periodically during therapy.

Implementation

- ***High Alert:*** Fatalities have occurred with chemotherapeutic agents. Before administering, clarify all ambiguous orders; double-check single, daily, and course-of-therapy dose limits; have second practitioner independently double-check original order, dose calculations, and infusion pump settings. Do not administer SUBQ, IM, or intrathecally (IT). IT administration is fatal. Vincristine must be dispensed in an overwrap stating "For IV use only." Overwrap should remain in place until immediately before administration.
- ***High Alert:*** Do not confuse vincristine with vinblastine.
- Should be administered by individuals experienced in the administration of this medication.
- Solution should be prepared in a biologic cabinet. Wear gloves, gown, and mask while handling medication. Discard IV equipment in specially designated containers.

IV Administration

- V Vincristine is a vesicant. If extravasation occurs, immediately stop infusion. Leave needle/cannula in place temporarily but do not flush the line. Gently aspirate extravasated solution; then remove needle/cannula. Elevate patient's extremity and apply dry warm compresses for 20 min 4 times day for 1–2 days. Initiate hyaluronidase antidote by injecting 1–6 mL (150 units/mL) into existing IV line; usual dose is 1 mL for each 1 mL of extravasated drug. If needle/cannula has been removed, inject SUBQ in a clockwise manner around area of extravasation or administer 1 mL as five separate 0.2-mL injections SUBQ into extravasation site; may repeat several times over next 3–4 hr.
- **IV Push: Concentration:** Administer undiluted at 1 mg/mL. **Rate:** Administer each dose over 1 min through Y-site injection of a free-flowing infusion of 0.9% NaCl or D5W.
- **Y-Site Compatibility:** acyclovir, alemtuzumab, allopurinol, amikacin, aminocaproic acid, aminophylline, amiodarone, amphotericin B liposomal, ampicillin, ampicillin/sulbactam, anidulafungin, argatroban, arsenic trioxide, atracurium, azithromycin, aztreonam, bivalirudin, bleomycin, bumetanide, buprenorphine, butorphanol, calcium chloride, calcium gluconate, carboplatin, carmustine, caspofungin, cefazolin, cefotetan, cefoxitin, ceftazidime, ceftriaxone, cefuroxime, chlorpromazine, ciprofloxacin, cisatracurium, cladribine, cisplatin, cladribine, clindamycin, cyclophosphamide, cyclosporine, cytarabine, dacarbazine, dactinomycin, daptomycin, daunorubicin, dexamethasone, dexmedetomidine, dexrazoxane, digoxin, diltiazem, diphenhydramine, dobutamine, docetaxel, dopamine, doxorubicin hydrochloride, doxorubicin liposomal, doxycycline, droperidol, enalaprilat, ephedrine, epinephrine, epirubicin, ertapenem, erythromycin, esmolol, etoposide, etoposide phosphate, famotidine, fentanyl, filgrastim, fluconazole, fludarabine, fluorouracil, foscarnet, fosphenytoin, fosphenytoin, ganciclovir, gemcitabine, gentamicin, granisetron, haloperidol, heparin, hetastarch, hydrocortisone, hydromorphone, ifosfamide, imipenem/cilastatin, insulin regular, isoproterenol, ketorolac, labetalol, leucovorin, levofloxacin, lidocaine, linezolid, lorazepam, magnesium sulfate, mannitol, melphalan, meperidine, meropenem, mesna, methadone, methohexital, methotrexate,

methylprednisolone, metoclopramide, metoprolol, metronidazole, midazolam, milrinone, minocycline, mitomycin, mitoxantrone, morphine, moxifloxacin, nalbuphine, naloxone, nicardipine, nitroglycerin, nitroprusside, norepinephrine, octreotide, ondansetron, oxaliplatin, paclitaxel, palonosetron, pamidronate, pemetrexed, pentamidine, pentobarbital, phenobarbital, phenylephrine, piperacillin/tazobactam, potassium acetate, potassium chloride, potassium phosphates, procainamide, prochlorperazine, promethazine, propranolol, remifentanil, rituximab, rocuronium, sargramostim, sodium acetate, sodium phosphates, succinylcholine, sufentanil, tacrolimus, theophylline, thiotepa, tigecycline, tirofiban, tobramycin, topotecan, trastuzumab, trimethoprim/sulfamethoxazole, vancomycin, vasopressin, vecuronium, verapamil, vinblastine, vinorelbine, voriconazole, zidovudine, zoledronic acid.

- **Y-Site Incompatibility:** amphotericin B deoxycholate, cefepime, diazepam, gemtuzumab ozogamicin, idarubicin, nafcillin, pantoprazole, phenytoin.

Patient/Family Teaching

- Explain purpose and side effects of medication. Advise patient to read *Patient Information* before starting therapy.
- Emphasize need for periodic lab tests to monitor for side effects.
- Instruct patient to notify health care provider immediately if redness, swelling, or pain at injection site occurs.
- Instruct patient to report symptoms of neurotoxicity (numbness and tingling, pain, difficulty walking, persistent or severe constipation, abdominal pain). Advise patient to ↑ fluid intake, dietary fiber, and exercise to minimize constipation; stool softeners or laxatives may be used.
- Advise patient to notify health care provider of signs and symptoms of urinary retention (difficulty urinating, weak stream, abdominal pain).
- Advise patient to notify health care provider of fever; chills; sore throat; signs of infection; bleeding gums; bruising; petechiae; blood in urine, stool, or emesis; or mouth sores. Caution patient to avoid crowds and persons with known infections.
- Discuss the possibility of hair loss. Explore coping strategies.
- Instruct patient not to receive any vaccinations without advice of health care provider.
- Rep: May cause fetal harm. Advise women of reproductive potential to notify health care provider if pregnancy is planned or suspected and to avoid breastfeeding during therapy. Contraception should be used during therapy and ≥2 mo after last dose.

Evaluation/Desired Outcomes

- Regression of malignancy without the appearance of detrimental side effects.

HIGH ALERT

V vinorelbine

(vine-oh-**rel**-been)

~~Navelbine~~

Classification

Therapeutic: antineoplastics

Pharmacologic: vinca alkaloids

Indications

Inoperable non-small cell lung cancer (as monotherapy or in combination with cisplatin).

Action

Binds to a protein (tubulin) of cellular microtubules, where it interferes with microtubule assembly. Cell replication is stopped as a result (cell cycle-specific for M phase). **Therapeutic Effects:** Death of rapidly replicating cells, particularly malignant ones.

Pharmacokinetics

Absorption: IV administration results in complete bioavailability.

Distribution: Highly bound to platelets and lymphocytes.

Metabolism and Excretion: Mostly metabolized by the liver. ≥1 metabolite is active. Large amounts eliminated in feces; 11% excreted unchanged by the kidneys.

Half-life: 28–44 hr.

TIME/ACTION PROFILE (effect on WBCs)

ROUTE	ONSET	PEAK	DURATION
IV	unknown	7–10 days	7–15 days

Contraindications/Precautions

Contraindicated in: Hypersensitivity; Active infection; ↓ bone marrow reserve; OB: Pregnancy; Lactation: Lactation.

Use Cautiously in: Hepatic impairment (↓ dose if total bilirubin >2 mg/dL); Debilitated patients (↑ risk of hyponatremia); Granulocytopenia (temporarily discontinue or ↓ dose); Rep: Women of reproductive potential; Pedi: Safety and effectiveness not established in children.

Adverse Reactions/Side Effects

CV: chest pain. **Derm:** alopecia, rash. **F and E:** hyponatremia. **GI:** constipation, nausea, ↑ liver enzymes, abdominal pain, anorexia, diarrhea, vomiting. **Hemat:** ANEMIA, NEUTROPENIA,

V

THROMBOCYTOPENIA. **Local:** irritation (at IV site), phlebitis. **MS:** arthralgia, back pain, jaw pain, myalgia. **Neuro:** fatigue, neurotoxicity. **Resp:** shortness of breath.

Interactions

Drug-Drug: ↑ bone marrow depression with other **antineoplastics** or **radiation therapy**. **Cisplatin** ↑ risk and severity of bone marrow depression. **Mitomycin** or **chest radiation** ↑ risk of pulmonary reactions.

Route/Dosage

IV (Adults): 30 mg/m² once weekly.

Hepatic Impairment

IV (Adults): *Total bilirubin 2.1–3 mg/dL:* 15 mg/m² once weekly; *Total bilirubin ≥3 mg/dL:* 7.5 mg/m² once weekly.

Availability (generic available)

Solution for injection: 10 mg/mL.

NURSING IMPLICATIONS

Assessment

- Monitor BP, HR, and respiratory rate during therapy. *If acute shortness of breath and severe bronchospasm occur,* treat with corticosteroid, bronchodilator, and supplemental oxygen as clinically indicated.
- Assess frequently for signs of infection (sore throat, temperature, cough, mental status changes), especially when nadir of granulocytopenia is expected.
- Monitor neurologic status. Assess for paresthesia (numbness, tingling, pain), loss of deep tendon reflexes (Achilles reflex is usually first involved), weakness (wrist drop or footdrop, gait disturbances), cranial nerve palsies (jaw pain, hoarseness, ptosis, visual changes), autonomic dysfunction (constipation, ileus, difficulty voiding, orthostatic hypotension, impaired sweating), and CNS dysfunction (↓ level of consciousness, agitation, hallucinations). The incidence of neurotoxicity associated with vinorelbine is less than that of other vinca alkaloids.
- Monitor intake and output and daily weight for significant discrepancies. *If ↓ urine output with hyponatremia occurs,* it may indicate SIADH and usually responds to fluid restriction.
- Assess nutritional status. *If nausea or vomiting occurs,* use an antiemetic to minimize symptoms.
- Monitor for signs/symptoms of gout (↑ uric acid, joint pain, edema). Encourage patient to drink ≥2 liters of fluid per day. Allopurinol or alkalinization of urine may be used to ↓ uric acid levels.

Lab Test Considerations

- Monitor CBC prior to each dose and routinely during therapy. The nadir of granulocytopenia usually occurs 7–10 days after vinorelbine administration, and recovery usually follows within 7–15 days. *If granulocytes <1500 cells/mm³,* ↓ dose or hold vinorelbine. *If repeated fevers and/or sepsis occur during granulocytopenia,* modify future dose of vinorelbine. May also cause mild to moderate anemia. Thrombocytopenia rarely occurs.
- Monitor liver function (AST, ALT, LDH, bilirubin) and renal function (BUN, serum creatinine) before starting and periodically during therapy. May ↑ uric acid; monitor periodically during therapy.

Implementation

- ***High Alert:*** Fatalities have occurred with chemotherapeutic agents. Before administering, clarify all ambiguous orders; double-check single, daily, and course-of-therapy dose limits; have second practitioner independently double-check original order, dose calculations, and infusion pump settings.
- Solution should be prepared in a biologic cabinet. Wear gloves, gown, and mask while handling medication. Discard IV equipment in specially designated containers.

IV Administration

- V Vinorelbine is a vesicant. If extravasation occurs, immediately stop infusion. Leave needle/cannula in place temporarily but do not flush the line. Gently aspirate extravasated solution; then remove needle/cannula. Elevate patient's extremity and apply dry warm compresses for 20 min 4 times day for 1–2 days. Initiate hyaluronidase antidote by injecting 1–6 mL (150 units/mL) into existing IV line; usual dose is 1 mL for each 1 mL of extravasated drug. If needle/cannula has been removed, inject SUBQ in a clockwise manner around area of extravasation, or administer 1 mL as five separate 0.2-mL injections SUBQ into extravasation site; may repeat several times over next 3–4 hr.
- **IV Push: Dilution:** Dilute vinorelbine with 0.9% NaCl or D5W. **Concentration:** 1.5–3 mg/mL. **Rate:** Infuse over 6–10 min into Y-site closest to bag of a free-flowing IV or into a central line.
- Flush vein with ≥75–125 mL of 0.9% NaCl or D5W administered over ≥10 min following vinorelbine infusion.
- **Intermittent Infusion: Dilution:** Dilute vinorelbine with 0.9% NaCl, D5W, 0.45% NaCl, D5/0.45% NaCl, Ringer's, or lactated Ringer's injection. Solution should be colorless to pale yellow. Do not administer if discolored or contains particulates. Diluted solution is stable for 24 hr at room temperature. **Concentration:** 0.5–2 mg/mL. **Rate:** Infuse over 6–10 min (up to 30 min) into Y-site closest to bag of a free-flowing IV or into a central line.
- Flush vein with ≥75–125 mL of 0.9% NaCl or D5W administered over ≥10 min following vinorelbine infusion.
- **Y-Site Compatibility:** amikacin, amiodarone, anidulafungin, argatroban, arsenic trioxide,

atracurium, aztreonam, bleomycin, bumetanide, buprenorphine, butorphanol, calcium chloride, calcium gluconate, carboplatin, carmustine, caspofungin, cefotaxime, ceftazidime, chlorpromazine, ciprofloxacin, cisatracurium, cisplatin, clindamycin, cyclophosphamide, cyclosporine, cytarabine, dacarbazine, dactinomycin, daptomycin, daunorubicin hydrochloride, dexamethasone, dexmedetomidine, dexrazoxane, digoxin, diltiazem, diphenhydramine, dobutamine, docetaxel, dopamine, doxorubicin hydrochloride, doxorubicin liposomal, doxycycline, droperidol, enalaprilat, ephedrine, epinephrine, epirubicin, ertapenem, erythromycin, etoposide, etoposide phosphate, famotidine, fentanyl, filgrastim, floxuridine, fluconazole, fludarabine, fosphenytoin, gemcitabine, gentamicin, glycopyrrolate, granisetron, haloperidol, hydralazine, hydrocortisone, hydromorphone, idarubicin, ifosfamide, imipenem/cilastatin, insulin, regular, irinotecan, isoproterenol, labetalol, leucovorin, levofloxacin, lidocaine, linezolid, lorazepam, magnesium sulfate, mannitol, melphalan, meperidine, meropenem, mesna, methadone, methotrexate, metoclopramide, metoprolol, metronidazole, midazolam, milrinone, mitoxantrone, morphine, moxifloxacin, nalbuphine, naloxone, nitroglycerin, norepinephrine, octreotide, ondansetron, oxaliplatin, paclitaxel, palonosetron, pamidronate, pemetrexed, pentamidine, phentolamine, phenylephrine, plicamycin, potassium acetate, potassium chloride, potassium phosphates, procainamide, prochlorperazine, promethazine, propranolol, rituximab, sodium acetate, sodium phosphates, succinylcholine, sufentanil, tacrolimus, theophylline, tigecycline, tirofiban, tobramycin, topotecan, trastuzumab, vancomycin, vasopressin, vecuronium, verapamil, vinblastine, vincristine, voriconazole, zidovudine, zoledronic acid.

- **Y-Site Incompatibility:** acyclovir, allopurinol, aminophylline, amphotericin B deoxycholate, amphotericin B liposomal, ampicillin, cefazolin, cefepime, cefotetan, cefoxitin, ceftriaxone, cefuroxime, dantrolene, diazepam, fluorouracil, foscarnet, furosemide, ganciclovir, ketorolac, methohexital, methylprednisolone, mitomycin, nafcillin, nitroprusside, pantoprazole, phenobarbital, phenytoin, piperacillin/tazobactam, sodium bicarbonate, trimethoprim/sulfamethoxazole.

Patient/Family Teaching

- Explain purpose and side effects of medication. Advise patient to read *Patient Information* before starting therapy.
- Instruct patient to notify health care provider immediately if redness, swelling, or pain at injection site occurs.
- Instruct patient to report symptoms of neurotoxicity (numbness and tingling, pain, difficulty walking, persistent or severe constipation, abdominal pain). Advise patient to ↑ fluid intake, dietary fiber, and exercise to minimize constipation; stool softeners or laxatives may be used.
- Advise patient to notify health care provider of signs and symptoms of urinary retention (difficulty urinating, weak stream, abdominal pain).
- Advise patient to notify health care provider of fever; chills; sore throat; signs of infection; bleeding gums; bruising; petechiae; blood in urine, stool, or emesis; or mouth sores. Caution patient to avoid crowds and persons with known infections.
- Discuss with patient the possibility of hair loss and explore coping strategies.
- Emphasize the need for periodic lab tests to monitor for side effects.
- Instruct patient not to receive any vaccinations without advice of health care provider.
- Rep: May cause fetal harm. Advise women of reproductive potential to use effective contraception during therapy and ≥2 mo after last dose and to avoid breastfeeding during and for 9 days after last dose.

Evaluation/Desired Outcomes

- Decrease in size or spread of malignancy without detrimental side effects.

VITAMIN D COMPOUNDS

calcifediol (kal-si-fe-**dye**-ol)
Rayaldee

calcitriol (kal-si-**trye**-ole)
Rocaltrol

cholecalciferol
(kol-e-kal-**sif**-e-role)
Delta-D3, ✱ Euro D

doxercalciferol
(**dox**-er-kal-**sif**-e-role)
~~Hectorol~~

ergocalciferol
(**er**-goe-kal-**sif**-e-role)
Drisdol

paricalcitol (par-i-**kal**-si-tole)
Zemplar

Classification
Therapeutic: vitamins
Pharmacologic: fat-soluble vitamins

Indications

Cholecalciferol: Secondary hyperparathyroidism in patients with stage 3 or 4 chronic kidney disease and serum total 25-hydroxyvitamin D levels <30 ng/mL. **Calcitriol:** Treatment of the following conditions: Hypocalcemia in chronic renal dialysis; Hypocalcemia in patients with hypoparathyroidism or pseudohypoparathyroidism; Secondary hyperparathyroidism and resulting metabolic bone disease in predialysis patients with moderate to severe renal insufficiency. **Cholecalciferol:** Treatment or prevention of vitamin D deficiency. **Doxercalciferol:** Treatment of the following conditions: Secondary hyperparathyroidism in patients undergoing chronic renal dialysis (IV and PO); Secondary hyperparathyroidism in patients with Stage 3 or 4 chronic kidney disease (PO only). **Ergocalciferol:** Treatment of the following conditions: Familial hypophosphatemia; Hypoparathyroidism; Vitamin D–resistant rickets. **Paricalcitol:** Prevention and treatment of secondary hyperparathyroidism in patients with Stage 3 or 4 (PO) or Stage 5 (PO and IV) chronic kidney disease.

Action

Calcifediol is a prohormone of the active form of vitamin D_3, calcitriol. Cholecalciferol requires activation in the liver and kidneys to create the active form of vitamin D_3 (calcitriol). Doxercalciferol and ergocalciferol require activation in the liver to create the active form of vitamin D_2. Paricalcitol is a synthetic analogue of calcitriol. Vitamin D promotes the absorption of calcium and ↓ parathyroid hormone concentration. **Therapeutic Effects:** Treatment and prevention of deficiency states, particularly bone manifestations. Improved calcium and phosphorous homeostasis in patients with chronic kidney disease.

Pharmacokinetics

Absorption: *Calcifediol, calcitriol, doxercalciferol, ergocalciferol, paricalcitol:* Well absorbed following oral administration. *Doxercalciferol, paricalcitol:* IV administration results in complete bioavailability.

Distribution: Unknown.

Protein Binding: *Calcifediol:* >98%; *Calcitriol and paricalcitol:* 99.9%.

Metabolism and Excretion: *Calcifediol:* Converted to calcitriol by the 1-alpha-hydroxylase enzyme, CYP27B1, in kidney; also metabolized by CYP24A1 to inactive metabolites; primarily excreted in feces. *Calcitriol:* Undergoes enterohepatic recycling and is excreted mostly in bile. *Cholecalciferol:* Converted by the liver and kidneys to calcitriol (active form of vitamin D_3). *Ergocalciferol:* Converted to active form of vitamin D_2 by sunlight, the liver, and the kidneys. *Doxercalciferol:* Converted by the liver to the active form of vitamin D_2. *Paricalcitol:* Mostly metabolized by the liver and excreted via hepatobiliary elimination.

Half-life: *Calcifediol:* 25 days. *Calcitriol:* 5–8 hr. *Cholecalciferol:* 14 hr. *Doxercalciferol:* 32–37 hr (up to 96 hr). *Paricalcitol:* 14–20 hr.

TIME/ACTION PROFILE (effects on serum calcium)

ROUTE	ONSET	PEAK	DURATION
Calcifediol-PO	2 wk	20 wk	unknown
Calcitriol-PO	2–6 hr	2–6 hr	3–5 days
Cholecalciferol-PO	unknown	unknown	unknown
Doxercalciferol PO	unknown	8 wk	1 wk
Doxercalciferol-IV	unknown	8 wk	1 wk
Ergocalciferol-PO	12–24 hr	unknown	up to 6 mo
Paricalcitol-PO	unknown	2–4 wk	unknown
Paricalcitol IV	unknown	up to 2 wk	unknown

Contraindications/Precautions

Contraindicated in: Hypersensitivity; Hypercalcemia; Vitamin D toxicity; Concurrent use of magnesium-containing antacids or other vitamin D supplements; Known intolerance to tartrazine (ergocalciferol); Malabsorption problems (cholecalciferol and ergocalciferol).

Use Cautiously in: OB: Safety not established in pregnancy; Lactation: Use while breastfeeding only if potential maternal benefit outweighs potential risk to infant; Pedi: Safety and effectiveness of calcifediol and doxercalciferol not established in children.

Adverse Reactions/Side Effects

Seen primarily as manifestations of toxicity (hypercalcemia).

CV: calcifediol: arrhythmias, edema, HF, hypertension. **doxercalciferol:** bradycardia. **paricalcitol:** palpitations. **Derm:** pruritus. **EENT:** conjunctivitis, photophobia, rhinorrhea. **F and E:** HYPERCALCEMIA **calcifediol:** hyperkalemia, hyperphosphatemia, polydipsia. **GI:** ↓ appetite, ↑ liver enzymes, abdominal pain, anorexia, constipation, dry mouth, nausea, PANCREATITIS, polydipsia, vomiting, weight loss. **GU:** ↓ libido, albuminuria, azotemia, nocturia, polyuria. **Hemat: calcifediol:** anemia. **Local:** pain at injection site. **Metab:** hyperthermia. **MS:** bone pain, muscle pain. **doxercalciferol:** arthralgia. **paricalcitol:** metastatic calcification. **Neuro: calcifediol:** dysgeusia, headache, SEIZURES, somnolence, weakness. **calcifediol:** confusion. **doxercalciferol:** dizziness, malaise. **Resp: doxercalciferol and ergocalciferol:** dyspnea. **Misc: calcitriol:** allergic reactions, chills, fever. **doxercalciferol:** HYPERSENSITIVITY REACTIONS (INCLUDING ANAPHYLAXIS, ANGIOEDEMA, HYPOTENSION, DYSPNEA, AND CARDIAC ARREST).

Interactions

Drug-Drug: Cholestyramine, colestipol, or **mineral oil** may ↓ absorption. **Calcium-containing drugs, thiazide diuretics**, and other **vitamin D analogs** may ↑ risk of hypercalcemia. **Corticosteroids** may ↓ effectiveness. Using calcifediol, calcitriol, doxercalciferol, or paricalcitol with **digoxin** may ↑ risk of arrhythmias. Vitamin

D requirements ↓ by **phenytoin**, **fosphenytoin**, **sucralfate**, **barbiturates**, and **primidone**. **Magnesium-containing drugs** may lead to hypermagnesemia. **Calcium-containing drugs** may ↑ risk of hypercalcemia. **Phenobarbital**, **rifampin**, **atazanavir**, **clarithromycin**, **erythromycin**, **itraconazole**, **ketoconazole**, **nefazodone**, **nelfinavir**, **ritonavir**, **verapamil**, and **voriconazole** may alter requirements for calcifediol, doxercalciferol, and paricalcitol; monitoring of calcium and phosphorus recommended.
Drug-Food: Ingestion of **foods high in calcium content** (see Appendix J) may lead to hypercalcemia.

Route/Dosage

Calcifediol

PO (Adults): 30 mcg once daily at bedtime; if desired intact PTH level (iPTH) remains ↑ after 3 mo, ↑ to 60 mcg once daily at bedtime. Maintenance dose should target total 25-hydroxyvitamin D levels of 30–100 ng/mL, iPTH levels within desired therapeutic range, serum calcium <9.8 mg/dL, and serum phosphorus ≤5.5 mg/dL.

Calcitriol

PO (Adults): *Hypocalcemia during dialysis:* 0.25 mcg once daily or every other day; if needed, may ↑ by 0.25 mcg/day at 4–8-wk intervals (typical dosage = 0.5–1 mcg/day). *Hypoparathyroidism:* 0.25 mcg once daily initially; if needed, may ↑ by 0.25 mcg/day at 2–4-wk intervals (typical dosage = 0.5–2 mcg/day). *Predialysis patients:* 0.25 mcg once daily (up to 0.5 mcg/day).
PO (Children): *Hypocalcemia during dialysis:* 0.25–2 mcg once daily. *Hypoparathyroidism (children ≥6 yr):* 0.25 mcg once daily initially; if needed, may ↑ by 0.25 mcg/day at 2–4-wk intervals (typical dosage = 0.5–2 mcg/day). *Hypoparathyroidism (children 1–5 yr):* 0.25–0.75 mcg once daily. *Hypoparathyroidism (children <1 yr):* 0.04–0.08 mcg/kg/day. *Predialysis patients (children ≥3 yr):* 0.25 mcg once daily (up to 0.5 mcg/day). *Predialysis patients (children <3 yr):* 10–15 ng/kg/day.
IV (Adults): *Hypocalcemia during dialysis:* 0.5 mcg (0.01 mcg/kg) 3 times weekly. May ↑ by 0.25–0.5 mcg/dose at 2–4-wk intervals (typical maintenance dose = 0.5–3.0 mcg 3 times weekly [0.01–0.05 mcg/kg 3 times weekly]).
IV (Children): *Hypocalcemia during dialysis:* 0.01–0.05 mcg/kg 3 times weekly.

Cholecalciferol

PO (Adults): 400–1000 units once daily.
PO (Infants): *Exclusively or partially breastfed:* 400 units once daily.

Doxercalciferol

PO (Adults): *Dialysis patients:* 10 mcg 3 times weekly (at dialysis); dose may be adjusted by 2.5 mcg at 8-wk intervals based on iPTH concentrations (maximum dose = 20 mcg 3 times weekly). *Nondialysis patients:* 1 mcg once daily; dose may be adjusted by 0.5 mcg at 2-wk intervals based on iPTH concentrations (maximum dose = 3.5 mcg/day).
IV (Adults): 4 mcg 3 times weekly at the end of dialysis; dose may be adjusted by 1–2 mcg at 8-wk intervals based on iPTH concentrations (maximum dose = 6 mcg 3 times weekly).

Ergocalciferol

PO (Adults): *Vitamin D–resistant rickets:* 12,000–500,000 units/day (to be used with phosphate supplement). *Familial hypophosphatemia:* 10,000–80,000 units/day (with phosphorus 1–2 g/day). *Hypoparathyroidism:* 50,000–200,000 units/day (to be used with calcium supplement).
PO (Children): *Vitamin D–resistant rickets:* 40,000–80,000 units/day (to be used with phosphate supplement). *Familial hypophosphatemia:* 10,000–80,000 units/day (with phosphorus 1–2 g/day). *Hypoparathyroidism:* 50,000–200,000 units/day (to be used with calcium supplement).
PO (Infants): *Exclusively or partially breastfed:* 400 units once daily.

Paricalcitol

Stage 3 or 4 Chronic Kidney Disease

PO (Adults): *Baseline iPTH concentration ≤500 pg/mL:* Initiate with 1 mcg once daily or 2 mcg 3 times weekly; dose can be adjusted at 2–4-wk intervals based on iPTH, calcium, and phosphate concentrations. *Baseline iPTH concentration >500 pg/mL:* Initiate with 2 mcg once daily or 4 mcg 3 times weekly; dose can be adjusted at 2–4-wk intervals based on iPTH, calcium, and phosphate concentrations.

Stage 5 Chronic Kidney Disease

PO (Adults): Initial dose (in mcg) is based on following equation: baseline iPTH concentration (pg/mL)/80; dose should be given 3 times weekly; dose can be adjusted at 2–4-wk intervals based on iPTH, calcium, and phosphate concentrations.
IV (Adults and Children ≥5 yr): 0.04–0.1 mcg/kg 3 times weekly during dialysis; dose can be adjusted by 2–4 mcg at 2–4-wk intervals based on iPTH, calcium, and phosphate concentrations (doses up to 0.24 mcg/kg have been used).

Availability

Calcifediol

Extended-release capsules: 30 mcg.

V

Calcitriol (generic available)
Capsules: 0.25 mcg, 0.5 mcg. **Oral solution:** 1 mcg/mL.

Cholecalciferol (generic available)
Capsules: 1000 units^OTC, 2000 units^OTC, 5000 units^OTC, 10,000 units^OTC, 25,000 units^OTC, 50,000 units^OTC. **Chewable tablets:** 400 units^OTC. **Oral solution:** 400 units/mL^OTC, 5000 units/mL^OTC. **Tablets:** 400 units^OTC, 1000 units^OTC, 2000 units^OTC, 3000 units^OTC, 5000 units^OTC, 50,000 units^OTC. ***In combination with:*** alendronate (Fosamax Plus D), see Appendix N.

Doxercalciferol (generic available)
Capsules: 0.5 mcg, 1 mcg, 2.5 mcg. **Solution for injection:** 2 mcg/mL.

Ergocalciferol (generic available)
Capsules: 50,000 units. **Oral solution:** 8000 units/mL^Rx, OTC. **Tablets:** 400 units, 2000 units.

Paricalcitol (generic available)
Capsules: 1 mcg, 2 mcg, 4 mcg. **Solution for injection:** 2 mcg/mL, 5 mcg/mL.

NURSING IMPLICATIONS

Assessment

- Assess for signs/symptoms of vitamin D deficiency (fatigue, depression, weakness, bone or muscle pain) before starting and periodically during therapy.
- Monitor for signs/symptoms of hypercalcemia (feeling tired, difficulty thinking clearly, loss of appetite, nausea, vomiting, constipation, ↑ thirst, ↑ urination, weight loss) during therapy. *If hypercalcemia occurs,* consider dose adjustment and monitor closely.
- Observe patient carefully for evidence of hypocalcemia (paresthesia, muscle twitching, laryngospasm, colic, cardiac arrhythmias, Chvostek or Trousseau sign).
- **Calcifediol:** Monitor for signs/symptoms of adynamic bone disease (fractures) during therapy. May develop if iPTH concentrations are abnormally low due to suppression.
- Pedi: Monitor height and weight; growth arrest may occur in prolonged high-dose therapy.
- **Rickets/Osteomalacia:** Assess for bone pain and weakness before starting and during therapy.

Lab Test Considerations

- Ensure serum calcium <9.8 mg/dL before starting *calcifediol* therapy. For *calcifediol,* monitor calcium, phosphorus, total 25-hydroxyvitamin D, and iPTH at least every 3 mo after starting therapy or dose adjustment and then at least every 6–12 mo. For *calcitriol,* monitor calcium and phosphate twice weekly initially; then monitor calcium, magnesium, alkaline phosphatase, and iPTH at least monthly. For *cholecalciferol,* monitor calcium, phosphate, and alkaline phosphatase periodically. For *doxercalciferol,* monitor ionized calcium, phosphate, and iPTH before starting therapy, then weekly during the 1st 12 wk, and then periodically. Also monitor alkaline phosphatase periodically. For *ergocalciferol,* monitor calcium and phosphate every 2 wk. For oral *paricalcitol,* monitor calcium, phosphate, and iPTH at least every 2 wk for the 1st 3 mo or after dose adjustment, then monthly for 3 mo, and then every 3 mo. For IV *paricalcitol,* monitor calcium and phosphate twice weekly until dose stabilized and then at least monthly. Monitor iPTH every 3 mo.
- The serum calcium × phosphate product (Ca × P) should not exceed 70 mg^2/dL^2 (55 mg^2/dL^2 for doxercalciferol).
- Calcitriol may falsely ↑ cholesterol levels.

Toxicity and Overdose

- Toxicity is manifested as hypercalcemia, hypercalciuria, and hyperphosphatemia. Assess patient for appearance of nausea, vomiting, anorexia, weakness, constipation, headache, bone pain, and metallic taste. Later symptoms include polyuria, polydipsia, photophobia, rhinorrhea, pruritus, and cardiac arrhythmias. Treatment usually consists of discontinuation of calcitriol, a low-calcium diet, use of low-calcium dialysate in peritoneal dialysis patients, and administration of a laxative. IV hydration and loop diuretics may be ordered to ↑ urinary excretion of calcium. Hemodialysis may also be used.

Implementation

- **PO:** May be administered without regard to meals. Measure solution accurately with calibrated dropper provided by manufacturer. May be mixed with juice, cereal, or food or dropped directly into mouth. Calcitriol capsules or solution should be protected from light and swallowed whole.
- **Calcifediol**: ***DNC:*** Administer at bedtime; swallow capsules whole, do not open, crush, or chew.

IV Administration

- **IV Push:** Administer *doxercalciferol* and *paricalcitol* undiluted by rapid injection through the catheter at the end of a hemodialysis period.
- **Y-Site Incompatibility:** Do not administer other drugs through same IV line.

Patient/Family Teaching

- Explain purpose and side effects of medication. Advise patient to read *Patient Information* before starting therapy.
- Advise patient to take missed dose as soon as remembered that day, unless almost time for next dose; do not double dose. If *calcifediol* is missed, omit and take next dose at regularly scheduled time; do not double dose.
- Review diet modifications with patient. See Appendix J for foods high in calcium and vitamin D. Renal

patients must still consider renal failure diet in food selection. Health care provider may order concurrent calcium supplement.

- Encourage patient to comply with dietary recommendations of health care provider. Explain that the best source of vitamins is a well-balanced diet and the importance of sunlight exposure. See Appendix J for foods high in vitamin D.
- Caution patient not to exceed RDA for vitamin supplementation.
- Advise patient to notify health care provider of all Rx or OTC medications, vitamins, or herbal products being taken and to consult health care provider before taking other medications.
- Advise patient to avoid concurrent use of antacids containing magnesium.
- Review symptoms of overdose and instruct patient to report these promptly to health care provider.
- Emphasize the importance of follow-up exams to evaluate therapy effectiveness.
- Rep: Advise women of reproductive potential to notify health care provider if pregnancy is planned or suspected or if breastfeeding. Monitor infants exposed to calcifediol through breast milk for signs/symptoms of hypercalcemia (seizures, vomiting, constipation, weight loss) and serum calcium concentrations.

Evaluation/Desired Outcomes

- Normalization of serum calcium and parathyroid hormone levels.
- Resolution or prevention of vitamin D deficiency.
- Improvement in symptoms of vitamin D–resistant rickets.
- **Calcifediol:** Serum total hydroxyvitamin D levels between 30 and 100 ng/mL, iPTH levels within therapeutic range, serum calcium (corrected for low albumin) within normal range, and serum phosphorus <5.5 mg/dL.

vonoprazan (von-oh-pra-zan)

Voquezna

Classification

Therapeutic: antiulcer agents

Pharmacologic: potassium-competitive acid blockers

Indications

Erosive esophagitis and relief of heartburn associated with erosive esophagitis. Maintenance of healed erosive esophagitis and relief of heartburn associated with erosive esophagitis. Relief of heartburn associated with nonerosive gastroesophageal reflux disease. *Helicobacter pylori* infection (in combination with amoxicillin or with amoxicillin and clarithromycin).

Action

Acts as a potassium-competitive acid blocker that suppresses basal and stimulated gastric acid secretion at the secretory surface of the gastric parietal cell through inhibition of the H^+, K^+-ATPase enzyme system in a potassium competitive manner. **Therapeutic Effects:** Healing and maintenance of healing of erosive esophagitis. Relief of heartburn associated with erosive esophagitis and nonerosive gastroesophageal reflux disease. Resolution of *Helicobacter pylori* infection.

Pharmacokinetics

Absorption: Extent of absorption following oral administration unknown.

Distribution: Extensively distributed to extravascular tissues.

Metabolism and Excretion: Metabolized in the liver to inactive compounds via the CYP2B6, CYP2C9, CYP2C19, CYP2D6, and CYP3A4/5 isoenzymes as well as sulfo- and glucuronosyl-transferases. Primarily excreted in the urine (67%; 8% as unchanged drug), with 31% excreted in the feces (<2% as unchanged drug).

Half-life: 6.8–7.9 hr.

TIME/ACTION PROFILE (antisecretory effects)

ROUTE	ONSET	PEAK	DURATION
PO	2–3 hr	unknown	24 hr

Contraindications/Precautions

Contraindicated in: Hypersensitivity; Concurrent use of rilpivirine-containing products; Severe renal impairment (for treatment of *Helicobacter pylori* infection); Moderate or severe hepatic impairment (for treatment of *Helicobacter pylori* infection); Lactation: Lactation.

Use Cautiously in: Patients using high doses for >1 yr (↑ risk of hip, wrist, or spine fractures and fundic gland polyps); Severe renal impairment (↓ dose recommended for treatment of erosive esophagitis); Moderate or severe hepatic impairment (↓ dose recommended for treatment of erosive esophagitis); OB: Safety not established in pregnancy; Pedi: Safety and effectiveness not established in children.

Adverse Reactions/Side Effects

CV: hypertension. **Derm:** STEVENS-JOHNSON SYNDROME (SJS), TOXIC EPIDERMAL NECROLYSIS (TEN). **F and E:** hypocalcemia (especially if treatment duration ≥3 mo), hypokalemia (especially if treatment duration

V

≥3 mo), hypomagnesemia (especially if treatment duration ≥3 mo). **GI:** abdominal distension, abdominal pain, CLOSTRIDIOIDES DIFFICILE-ASSOCIATED DIARRHEA (CDAD), diarrhea, dyspepsia, fundic gland polyps, gastritis, nausea. **GU:** acute tubulointerstitial nephritis, urinary tract infection. **Hemat:** vitamin B_{12} deficiency. **MS:** bone fracture. **Misc:** HYPERSENSITIVITY REACTIONS (INCLUDING ANAPHYLAXIS).

Interactions

Drug-Drug: May ↓ **rilpivirine** levels and ↑ risk of resistance; concurrent use contraindicated. May ↓ absorption of drugs requiring acid pH, including **ketoconazole**, **itraconazole**, **atazanavir**, **nelfinavir**, **iron salts**, **dasatinib**, **erlotinib**, **nilotinib**, and **mycophenolate mofetil**; avoid concurrent use with **atazanavir** and **nelfinavir**. Hypomagnesemia and hypokalemia ↑ risk of **digoxin** toxicity. **Diuretics** may ↑ risk of hypomagnesemia and hypokalemia. May ↑ levels and risk of toxicity of **CYP3A substrates**, including **midazolam**. May ↓ antiplatelet effects of **clopidogrel**; avoid concurrent use. May ↑ levels and risk of toxicity of **CYP2C19 substrates**, including **citalopram** and **cilostazol**. **Strong CYP3A inducers**, including **rifampin**, and **moderate CYP3A inducers**, including **efavirenz**, may ↓ levels and effectiveness; avoid concurrent use.

Route/Dosage

Erosive Esophagitis and Relief of Heartburn Associated with Erosive Esophagitis

PO (Adults): 20 mg once daily for 8 wk.

Renal Impairment

PO (Adults): *CCr <30 mL/min:* 10 mg once daily for 8 wk.

Hepatic Impairment

PO (Adults): *Moderate or severe hepatic impairment:* 10 mg once daily for 8 wk.

Maintenance of Healed Erosive Esophagitis and Relief of Heartburn Associated with Erosive Esophagitis

PO (Adults): 10 mg once daily for up to 6 mo.

Relief of Heartburn Associated with Non-Erosive Gastroesophageal Reflux Disease

PO (Adults): 10 mg once daily for 4 wk.

Helicobacter pylori Infection

PO (Adults): *In combination with amoxicillin (dual therapy) or amoxicillin and clarithromycin (triple therapy):* 20 mg twice daily for 14 days.

Renal Impairment

PO (Adults): *CCr <30 mL/min:* Not recommended.

Hepatic Impairment

PO (Adults): *Moderate or severe hepatic impairment:* Not recommended.

Availability

Tablets: 10 mg, 20 mg. ***In combination with:*** amoxicillin (Voquezna Dual Pak); amoxicillin and clarithromycin (Voquezna Triple Pak). See Appendix N.

NURSING IMPLICATIONS

Assessment

- Endoscopic evaluation should be done initially in older patients and for those who have a suboptimal response or an early symptomatic relapse after completing treatment.
- Monitor for signs/symptoms of severe cutaneous adverse reactions including SJS and TEN (prodrome of fever, flu-like symptoms, mucosal lesions, progressive skin rash, lymphadenopathy). *If SJS or TEN confirmed,* permanently discontinue vonoprazan.
- Monitor for signs/symptoms of CDAD including watery diarrhea with mucus, fever, abdominal pain or cramping, anorexia, nausea, and in severe cases, dehydration, colitis, and blood or pus in the stool. Use shortest treatment duration as possible.
- Monitor for signs/symptoms of hypersensitivity reactions (rash, urticaria, pruritus, flushing, dizziness, vomiting, abdominal pain). *If hypersensitivity reaction occurs,* discontinue vonoprazan and provide supportive care.
- Evaluate patients with suspected acute tubulointerstitial nephritis for allergic reaction vs. infection; Allergic signs/symptoms from tubulointerstitial nephritis may include fever, polyuria, rash, and eosinophilia with normal urinalysis while urinary tract infection signs/symptoms may include fever, polyuria, dysuria, flank pain, WBCs in urine, and leukocyte esterase in urine.

Lab Test Considerations

- Assess magnesium and calcium levels prior to initiation and monitor periodically. May cause hypomagnesemia, leading to hypocalcemia and/or hypokalemia. May exacerbate underlying hypocalcemia in patients with preexisting risk of hypocalcemia (i.e., hypoparathyroidism).
- May ↓ vitamin B12 levels.

Implementation

- **PO:** Administer with or without food.
- ***DNC:*** Swallow tablets whole; do not crush or chew.

Patient/Family Teaching

- Explain purpose and side effects of vonoprazan. Advise to take as directed with food and swallow tablets whole; do not crush or chew. *Missed dose for H pylori infection:* take the next dose if missed

≤4 hr. If >4 hr have passed, skip the missed dose and take the next dose at the regularly scheduled time. *Missed dose for healed erosive esophagitis or nonerosive gastroesophageal reflux disease:* take the next dose if missed ≤12 hr. If >12 hr have passed, skip the missed dose and take the next dose at the regularly scheduled time. Advise patient to read *Patient Information* before starting therapy and with each Rx refill in case of changes.

- Advise patient to report and immediately seek treatment for any unusual progressive rashes, fever, flu-like symptoms, mouth sores, or swollen lymph nodes.
- Instruct patient to report signs/symptoms of hypomagnesemia, hypocalcemia, or hypokalemia such as muscle cramps and spasms, twitching, numbness and tingling in the hands and feet, palpitations, or weakness.
- Advise patient to report persistent diarrhea especially if watery diarrhea with mucus or blood, fever, abdominal pain or cramping, nausea; urinary symptoms such as frequent urination, urinary pain, or flank pain.
- Advise patient to notify health care professional of all Rx or OTC medications, vitamins, or herbal products being taken and to consult health care professional before taking other medications. Avoid use with St. John's Wort or rifampin.
- Rep: Advise patient to notify health care professional if pregnancy is planned or suspected, and to avoid breastfeeding during therapy. Report pregnancies to the Phathom Pharmaceutical, Inc Adverse Event reporting line at 1-888-775-7428.

Evaluation/Desired Outcomes

- Healing and maintenance of healing of erosive esophagitis.
- Relief of heartburn associated with erosive esophagitis and nonerosive gastroesophageal reflux disease.
- Resolution of *Helicobacter pylori* infection.

voriconazole

(vor-i-**kon**-a-zole)

Vfend

Classification

Therapeutic: antifungals

Pharmacologic: azoles

Indications

Invasive aspergillosis. Candidemia (in patients without neutropenia) and serious *Candida* infections in skin, bladder, abdomen, kidney, and wounds. Esophageal candidiasis. Scedosporiosis and fusariosis in patients intolerant of or refractory to other therapies.

Action

Inhibits fungal ergosterol synthesis leading to production of abnormal fungal plasma membrane. **Therapeutic Effects:** Antifungal activity. **Spectrum:** Spectrum is notable for activity against: *Aspergillus* spp., *Candida* spp., *Scedosporium apiospermum*, *Fusarium* spp.

Pharmacokinetics

Absorption: 96% absorbed following oral administration; IV administration results in complete bioavailability.

Distribution: Widely distributed to tissues.

Metabolism and Excretion: Primarily metabolized by liver via the CYP2C19, CYP2C9, and CYP3A4 isoenzymes; <2% excreted unchanged in urine. The CYP2C19 isoenzyme exhibits genetic polymorphism; 15–20% of Asian patients and 3–5% of White and Black patients may be poor metabolizers and may have significantly ↑ voriconazole concentrations and an ↑ risk of adverse effects.

Half-life: Dose-dependent (adults: 6–9 hr); ↑ in hepatic impairment.

TIME/ACTION PROFILE (plasma concentrations)

ROUTE	ONSET	PEAK	DURATION
PO	rapid	1–2 hr	12 hr
IV	rapid	end of infusion	12 hr

Contraindications/Precautions

Contraindicated in: Concurrent use of dihydroergotamine, carbamazepine, efavirenz (≥400 mg/day), ergotamine, finerenone, ivabradine, lurasidone, naloxegol, phenobarbital, pimozide, rifabutin, rifampin, ritonavir (400 mg every 12 hr), quinidine, sirolimus, St. John's wort, tolvaptan, and venetoclax; Tablets contain lactose and should be avoided in patients with galactose intolerance, Lapp lactase deficiency, or glucose-galactose malabsorption; Severe hepatic impairment; OB: Pregnancy.

Use Cautiously in: Mild to moderate hepatic impairment (↓ IV and PO maintenance doses); Renal impairment (CCr <50 mL/min) (vehicle in IV formulation can accumulate resulting in toxicity; avoid use of IV unless potential benefit greatly outweighs potential risk, use oral form only); Congenital/acquired QT interval prolongation, HF, sinus bradycardia, hypokalemia, hypomagnesemia, or symptomatic arrhythmias; Hematologic malignancy (↑ risk of hepatotoxicity); Rep: Women of reproductive potential; Lactation: Use while breastfeeding only if potential maternal benefit justifies potential risk to infant; Pedi: Children <2 yr (safety and effectiveness not established); suspension contains benzyl alcohol, which may cause potentially

V

fatal gasping syndrome in neonates; ↑ risk of photosensitivity reactions in children.

Adverse Reactions/Side Effects

CV: changes in BP, edema, QT interval prolongation, tachycardia. **Derm:** DRUG REACTION WITH EOSINOPHILIA AND SYSTEMIC SYMPTOMS (DRESS), MELANOMA, photosensitivity, rash, SQUAMOUS CELL CARCINOMA, STEVENS-JOHNSON SYNDROME (SJS), TOXIC EPIDERMAL NECROLYSIS. **EENT:** visual disturbances, eye hemorrhage. **Endo:** ADRENAL INSUFFICIENCY, hyperglycemia. **F and E:** hypokalemia, hypomagnesemia. **GI:** abdominal pain, diarrhea, HEPATOTOXICITY, nausea, pancreatitis, vomiting. **MS:** fluorosis, periostitis. **Neuro:** dizziness, hallucinations, headache. **Misc:** chills, fever, infusion reactions.

Interactions

Drug-Drug: **Carbamazepine**, **phenobarbital**, and **rifampin** may significantly ↓ levels and effectiveness; concurrent use contraindicated. May significantly ↑ levels of **ivabradine**, **pimozide**, and **quinidine**, which can ↑ the risk of QT interval prolongation and torsades de pointes; concurrent use contraindicated. May significantly ↑ levels and risk of toxicity of **dihydroergotamine**, **ergotamine**, **lurasidone**, **sirolimus**, and **tolvaptan**; concurrent use contraindicated. May ↑ levels of **naloxegol**, which could precipitate symptoms of opioid withdrawal; concurrent use contraindicated. Concurrent use with **efavirenz** at dose of ≥400 mg every 24 hr is contraindicated, as it may significantly ↑ efavirenz levels and significantly ↓ voriconazole levels; if used together, ↑ oral maintenance dose of voriconazole to 400 mg every 12 hr and ↓ dose of efavirenz to 300 mg daily. Concurrent use with **ritonavir** at dose of 400 mg every 12 hr is contraindicated, as ritonavir may significantly ↓ voriconazole levels; use with ritonavir at dose of 100 mg every 12 hr; should be avoided if possible. Concurrent use with **rifabutin** may significantly ↑ rifabutin levels and significantly ↓ voriconazole levels; concurrent use contraindicated; if used together, ↑ oral maintenance dose of voriconazole to 400 mg every 12 hr and ↓ dose of efavirenz to 300 mg daily. Concurrent use with **venetoclax** at initiation and during ramp-up phase in patients with chronic lymphocytic leukemia or small lymphocytic leukemia is contraindicated because may ↑ risk of tumor lysis syndrome. May significantly ↑ levels of **finerenone**, which could ↑ risk of hyperkalemia; concurrent use contraindicated. **Fluconazole** may ↑ levels and risk of toxicity; avoid concurrent use. May ↑ levels and risk of toxicity of **cyclosporine**; ↓ cyclosporine dose by 50%. May ↑ levels and risk of toxicity of **tacrolimus**; ↓ tacrolimus dose to 1/3 of the starting dose. May ↑ levels and risk of toxicity of **glasdegib**; avoid concurrent use. May ↑ levels and risk of toxicity of tyrosine kinase inhibitors, including **axitinib**, **bosutinib**, **cabozantinib**, **ceritinib**, **cobimetinib**, **dabrafenib**, **dasatinib**, **ibrutinib**, **nilotinib**, **ribociclib**, and **sunitinib**; if concurrent use cannot be avoided, ↓ tyrosine kinase inhibitor dose. May ↑ levels and risk of toxicity of **eszopiclone**; ↓ eszopiclone dose. May ↑ levels and risk of toxicity of **tretinoin**; closely monitor patient for signs/symptoms of pseudotumor cerebri or hypercalcemia. May ↑ levels and risk of toxicity of **HMG-CoA reductase inhibitors**, some **benzodiazepines (alprazolam, midazolam, triazolam)**, **fentanyl**, **oxycodone**, **NSAIDs (ibuprofen, diclofenac)**, some **calcium channel blockers**, **sulfonylureas (glipizide, glyburide)**, **phenytoin**, **warfarin**, and **vinca alkaloids (vincristine, vinblastine)**; dose ↓ may be needed and careful monitoring required during concurrent use. May ↑ **methadone** levels and risk of QT interval prolongation. May ↑ levels of **corticosteroids** and risk of adrenal suppression. May ↑ levels and risk of toxicity of **ivacaftor**; ↓ ivacaftor dose. Concurrent use with **hormonal contraceptives** containing **ethinyl estradiol** and **norethindrone** may ↑ voriconazole, ethinyl estradiol, and norethindrone levels. May ↑ levels and risk of toxicity of **everolimus**; concurrent use not recommended. May ↑ levels and risk of toxicity of **omeprazole**; if patient receiving ≥40 mg/day of omeprazole, ↓ omeprazole dose by 50%. Similar effects may occur with other **proton pump inhibitors**. May ↑ levels and risk of toxicity of **protease inhibitors** and **non-nucleoside reverse transcriptase inhibitors**; frequent monitoring recommended. **Non-nucleoside reverse transcriptase inhibitors** may induce or inhibit the metabolism of voriconazole; frequent monitoring recommended. **Letermovir** may ↓ levels and effectiveness; avoid concurrent use. Use with **methotrexate** may ↑ risk of photosensitivity reactions.
Drug-Natural Products: **St. John's wort** may significantly ↓ levels and effectiveness; concurrent use contraindicated.

Route/Dosage

Invasive Aspergillosis, Scedosporiosis, or Fusariosis

IV, PO (Adults ≥40 kg): *Loading dose (IV):* 6 mg/kg IV every 12 hr for 2 doses, followed by *maintenance dose (IV)* of 4 mg/kg IV every 12 hr (use 5 mg/kg IV every 12 hr if concurrently using with phenytoin). Continue IV therapy for ≥7 days; then switch to oral maintenance dose once patient has clinically improved and can tolerate oral medications. *Maintenance dose (PO):* 200 mg PO every 12 hr (use 400 mg PO every 12 hr if concurrently using with phenytoin or efavirenz); if response inadequate, may ↑ to 300 mg every 12 hr. Total duration of therapy: ≥6–12 wk.
IV, PO (Adults <40 kg): *Loading dose (IV):* 6 mg/kg IV every 12 hr for 2 doses, followed by *maintenance dose (IV)* of 4 mg/kg IV every 12 hr (use 5 mg/kg IV every 12 hr if concurrently using with phenytoin). Continue IV therapy for ≥7 days; then switch to oral maintenance dose once patient has clinically improved and can tolerate oral medications. *Maintenance dose*

(PO): 100 mg PO every 12 hr (use 200 mg PO every 12 hr if concurrently using with phenytoin; use 400 mg PO every 12 hr if concurrently using with efavirenz); if response inadequate, may ↑ to 150 mg every 12 hr. Total duration of therapy: ≥6–12 wk.
IV, PO (Children ≥15 yr): *Loading dose (IV):* 6 mg/kg IV every 12 hr for 2 doses, followed by *maintenance dose (IV)* of 4 mg/kg IV every 12 hr. Continue IV therapy for ≥7 days; then switch to oral maintenance dose once patient has clinically improved and can tolerate oral medications.
Maintenance dose (PO): 200 mg every 12 hr; if response inadequate, may ↑ to 300 mg every 12 hr. Total duration of therapy: ≥6–12 wk.
IV, PO (Children 12–14 yr and ≥50 kg): *Loading dose (IV):* 6 mg/kg IV every 12 hr for 2 doses, followed by *maintenance dose (IV)* of 4 mg/kg IV every 12 hr. Continue IV therapy for ≥7 days; then switch to oral maintenance dose once patient has clinically improved and can tolerate oral medications. *Maintenance dose (PO):* 200 mg every 12 hr; if response inadequate, may ↑ to 300 mg every 12 hr. Total duration of therapy: ≥6–12 wk.
IV, PO (Children 12–14 yr and <50 kg): *Loading dose (IV):* 9 mg/kg IV every 12 hr for 2 doses, followed by *maintenance dose (IV)* of 8 mg/kg IV every 12 hr; if response inadequate, may ↑ maintenance dose by 1 mg/kg. Continue IV therapy for ≥7 days; then switch to oral maintenance dose once patient has clinically improved and can tolerate oral medications. *Maintenance dose (PO):* 9 mg/kg every 12 hr (not to exceed 350 mg every 12 hr); if response inadequate, may ↑ by 1 mg/kg or 50 mg (not to exceed 350 mg every 12 hr). Total duration of therapy: ≥6–12 wk.
IV, PO (Children 2–11 yr): *Loading dose (IV):* 9 mg/kg IV every 12 hr for 2 doses, followed by *maintenance dose (IV)* of 8 mg/kg IV every 12 hr; if response inadequate, may ↑ maintenance dose by 1 mg/kg. Continue IV therapy for ≥7 days; then switch to oral maintenance dose once patient has clinically improved and can tolerate oral medications. *Maintenance dose (PO):* 9 mg/kg every 12 hr (not to exceed 350 mg every 12 hr); if response inadequate, may ↑ by 1 mg/kg or 50 mg (not to exceed 350 mg every 12 hr). Total duration of therapy: ≥6–12 wk.

Hepatic Impairment

IV, PO (Adults): *Mild or moderate hepatic impairment:* Use standard IV loading dose; ↓ maintenance doses (IV or PO) by 50%; *Severe hepatic impairment:* Not recommended.

Candidemia in Non-Neutropenic Patients or Other Deep Tissue *Candida* Infections

IV, PO (Adults ≥40 kg): *Loading dose (IV):* 6 mg/kg IV every 12 hr for 2 doses, followed by *maintenance dose (IV)* of 3–4 mg/kg IV every 12 hr (use 5 mg/kg IV every 12 hr if concurrently using with phenytoin). Switch to oral dosing once patient has clinically improved and can tolerate oral medications. *Maintenance dose (PO):* 200 mg PO every 12 hr (use 400 mg PO every 12 hr if concurrently using with phenytoin or efavirenz); if response inadequate, may ↑ to 300 mg every 12 hr. Total duration of therapy: ≥14 days following resolution of symptoms or following last positive culture, whichever is longer.
IV, PO (Adults <40 kg): *Loading dose (IV):* 6 mg/kg IV every 12 hr for 2 doses, followed by *maintenance dose (IV)* of 3–4 mg/kg IV every 12 hr (use 5 mg/kg IV every 12 hr if concurrently using with phenytoin). Switch to oral dosing once patient has clinically improved and can tolerate oral medications. *Maintenance dose (PO):* 100 mg PO every 12 hr (use 200 mg PO every 12 hr if concurrently using with phenytoin; use 400 mg PO every 12 hr if using concurrently with efavirenz); if response inadequate, may ↑ to 150 mg every 12 hr. Total duration of therapy: ≥14 days following resolution of symptoms or following last positive culture, whichever is longer.
IV, PO (Children ≥15 yr): *Loading dose (IV):* 6 mg/kg IV every 12 hr for 2 doses, followed by *maintenance dose (IV)* of 3–4 mg/kg IV every 12 hr. Switch to oral dosing once patient has clinically improved and can tolerate oral medications. *Maintenance dose (PO):* 200 mg every 12 hr; if response inadequate, may ↑ to 300 mg every 12 hr. Total duration of therapy: ≥14 days following resolution of symptoms or following last positive culture, whichever is longer.
IV, PO (Children 12–14 yr and ≥50 kg): *Loading dose (IV):* 6 mg/kg IV every 12 hr for 2 doses, followed by *maintenance dose (IV)* of 3–4 mg/kg IV every 12 hr. Switch to oral dosing once patient has clinically improved and can tolerate oral medications. *Maintenance dose (PO):* 200 mg every 12 hr; if response inadequate, may ↑ to 300 mg every 12 hr. Total duration of therapy: ≥14 days following resolution of symptoms or following last positive culture, whichever is longer.
IV, PO (Children 12–14 yr and <50 kg): *Loading dose (IV):* 9 mg/kg IV every 12 hr for 2 doses, followed by *maintenance dose (IV)* of 8 mg/kg IV every 12 hr; if response inadequate, may ↑ maintenance dose by 1 mg/kg. Switch to oral dosing once patient has clinically improved and can tolerate oral medications. *Maintenance dose (PO):* 9 mg/kg every 12 hr (not to exceed 350 mg every 12 hr); if response inadequate, may ↑ by 1 mg/kg or 50 mg (not to exceed 350 mg every 12 hr). Total duration of therapy: ≥14 days following resolution of symptoms or following last positive culture, whichever is longer.

IV, PO (Children 2–11 yr): *Loading dose (IV):* 9 mg/kg IV every 12 hr for 2 doses, followed by *maintenance dose (IV)* of 8 mg/kg IV every 12 hr; if response inadequate, may ↑ maintenance dose by 1 mg/kg. Switch to oral dosing once patient has clinically improved and can tolerate oral medications. *Maintenance dose (PO):* 9 mg/kg every 12 hr (not to exceed 350 mg every 12 hr); if response inadequate, may ↑ by 1 mg/kg or 50 mg (not to exceed 350 mg every 12 hr). Total duration of therapy: ≥14 days following resolution of symptoms or following last positive culture, whichever is longer.

Hepatic Impairment

IV, PO (Adults): *Mild or moderate hepatic impairment:* Use standard IV loading dose; ↓ maintenance doses (IV or PO) by 50%; *Severe hepatic impairment:* Not recommended.

Esophageal Candidiasis

PO (Adults ≥40 kg): 200 mg every 12 hr (use 400 mg every 12 hr if concurrently using with phenytoin or efavirenz); if response inadequate, may ↑ to 300 mg every 12 hr. Duration of therapy: ≥14 days and for ≥7 days following resolution of symptoms.

PO (Adults <40 kg): 100 mg every 12 hr (use 200 mg every 12 hr if concurrently using with phenytoin; use 400 mg every 12 hr if using concurrently with efavirenz); if response inadequate, may ↑ to 150 mg every 12 hr. Duration of therapy: ≥14 days and for ≥7 days following resolution of symptoms.

PO (Children ≥15 yr): 200 mg every 12 hr; if response inadequate, may ↑ to 300 mg every 12 hr. Duration of therapy: ≥14 days and for ≥7 days following resolution of symptoms.

PO (Children 12–14 yr and ≥50 kg): 200 mg every 12 hr; if response inadequate, may ↑ to 300 mg every 12 hr. Duration of therapy: ≥14 days and for ≥7 days following resolution of symptoms.

IV, PO (Children 12–14 yr and <50 kg): Initiate therapy with *maintenance dose (IV)* of 4 mg/kg IV every 12 hr; if response inadequate, may ↑ maintenance dose by 1 mg/kg. Switch to oral dosing once patient has clinically improved and can tolerate oral medications. *Maintenance dose (PO):* 9 mg/kg every 12 hr (not to exceed 350 mg every 12 hr); if response inadequate, may ↑ by 1 mg/kg or 50 mg (not to exceed 350 mg every 12 hr). Total duration of therapy: ≥14 days and for ≥7 days following resolution of symptoms.

IV, PO (Children 2–11 yr): Initiate therapy with *maintenance dose (IV)* of 4 mg/kg IV every 12 hr; if response inadequate, may ↑ maintenance dose by 1 mg/kg. Switch to oral dosing once patient has clinically improved and can tolerate oral medications. *Maintenance dose (PO):* 9 mg/kg every 12 hr (not to exceed 350 mg every 12 hr); if response inadequate, may ↑ by 1 mg/kg or 50 mg (not to exceed 350 mg every 12 hr). Total duration of therapy: ≥14 days and for ≥7 days following resolution of symptoms.

Hepatic Impairment

IV, PO (Adults): *Mild or moderate hepatic impairment:* Use standard IV loading dose; ↓ maintenance doses (IV or PO) by 50%; *Severe hepatic impairment:* Not recommended.

Availability (generic available)

Tablets: 50 mg, 200 mg. **Oral suspension (orange flavor):** 40 mg/mL. **Powder for injection:** 200 mg/vial.

NURSING IMPLICATIONS

Assessment

- Monitor for signs/symptoms of fungal infections before and during therapy.
- Monitor ECG and QT interval before and periodically during therapy.
- Monitor visual function, including visual acuity, visual field, and color perception, in patients receiving >28 days of therapy. Vision usually returns to normal within 14 days after discontinuation of therapy.
- Monitor for allergic reactions (flushing, fever, sweating, tachycardia, chest tightness, dyspnea, faintness, nausea, pruritus, rash) during infusions. Symptoms occur immediately upon start of infusion. May require discontinuation of voriconazole.
- Monitor patients with risk factors for acute pancreatitis (recent chemotherapy, hematopoietic stem cell transplantation) for signs/symptoms of pancreatitis (abdominal pain, ↑ serum amylase and lipase).
- Assess for rash periodically during therapy. May cause SJS. *If severe skin reaction occurs or if accompanied with fever, general malaise, fatigue, muscle or joint aches, blisters, oral lesions, conjunctivitis, hepatitis, or eosinophilia,* discontinue voriconazole.

Lab Test Considerations

- Obtain specimens for culture and histopathology before therapy to isolate and identify organism. Therapy may be started before results are received.
- Monitor liver function tests (AST, ALT, and bilirubin) before starting, weekly during 1st mo, and monthly during therapy. If abnormal liver function tests occur, monitor for development of severe hepatic injury. *If liver enzymes markedly ↑ or clinical signs and symptoms of liver disease develops,* discontinue voriconazole.
- Monitor renal function during therapy.

Implementation

- Do not confuse Vfend with Venofer, or Vimpat.
- Once patient can tolerate oral medication, PO voriconazole may be used.

- Correct electrolyte disturbances (hypokalemia, hypomagnesemia, hypocalcemia) before starting and during therapy.
- **PO:** Administer >1 hr before or after a meal.
- Shake suspension well (approximately 10 sec) before measuring suspension. Use oral dispenser provided to ensure accurate dose. Do not mix suspension with other medicine, flavored liquid, or syrup. Store suspension at room temperature up to 14 days; then discard.

IV Administration

- Do not administer voriconazole with blood products or concentrated electrolytes, even in separate lines. Nonconcentrated electrolytes can be infused at same time, but separate lines must be used. TPN can be administered simultaneously but must be via separate line or via a different port in a multilumen catheter.
- **Intermittent Infusion: Reconstitution:** Reconstitute each 200-mg vial with 19 mL of sterile water for injection. **Concentration:** 10 mg/mL. **Dilution:** Withdraw and discard equal volume of diluent from infusion bag or bottle to be used. Withdraw required volume of voriconazole solution from vial(s) and add to appropriate volume of 0.9% NaCl, LR, D5/LR, D5/0.45% NaCl, D5W, 0.45% NaCl, or D5/0.9% NaCl. Reconstituted solution stable for 24 hr if refrigerated. Discard partially used vials. **Concentration:** 0.5–5 mg/mL. **Rate:** Infuse over 1–3 hr at a rate not to exceed 3 mg/kg/hr.
- **Y-Site Compatibility:** acyclovir, alemtuzumab, allopurinol, amikacin, aminocaproic acid, aminophylline, amiodarone, amphotericin B liposomal, ampicillin, ampicillin/sulbactam, anidulafungin, argatroban, arsenic trioxide, azithromycin, aztreonam, bivalirudin, bleomycin, buprenorphine, butorphanol, bumetanide, calcium acetate, calcium chloride, calcium gluconate, cangrelor, carboplatin, carmustine, caspofungin, cefazolin, cefiderocol, cefotaxime, cefotetan, cefoxitin, ceftaroline, ceftazidime, ceftobiprole, ceftriaxone, chloramphenicol, chlorpromazine, ciprofloxacin, cisatracurium, cisplatin, clindamycin, cyclophosphamide, cytarabine, dacarbazine, dactinomycin, daptomycin, daunorubicin, dexamethasone, dexmedetomidine, dexrazoxane, digoxin, diltiazem, diphenhydramine, dobutamine, docetaxel, dopamine, doxycycline, droperidol, enalaprilat, ephedrine, epinephrine, epirubicin, ertapenem, erythromycin, esmolol, etoposide, etoposide phosphate, famotidine, fentanyl, fluconazole, fludarabine, fluorouracil, foscarnet, fosphenytoin, furosemide, ganciclovir, gemcitabine, gentamicin, glycopyrrolate, granisetron, haloperidol, heparin, hydralazine, hydrocortisone, ifosfamide, imipenem/cilastatin, imipenem/cilastatin/relebactam, insulin regular, irinotecan, isoproterenol, ketorolac, labetalol, leucovorin, levofloxacin, lidocaine, linezolid, lorazepam, magnesium sulfate, mannitol, melphalan, meperidine, meropenem, mesna, methadone, methohexital, methotrexate, methylprednisolone, metoclopramide, metoprolol, metronidazole, midazolam, milrinone, minocycline, mitomycin, morphine, mycophenolate, nafcillin, nalbuphine, naloxone, nicardipine, nitroglycerin, norepinephrine, octreotide, ondansetron, oxaliplatin, oxytocin, paclitaxel, pamidronate, pentamidine, pentobarbital, phenobarbital, phenylephrine, piperacillin/tazobactam, potassium acetate, potassium chloride, potassium phosphates, procainamide, promethazine, propranolol, remifentanil, rocuronium, sodium acetate, sodium bicarbonate, sodium phosphates, succinylcholine, sufentanil, tacrolimus, theophylline, thiotepa, tirofiban, tobramycin, topotecan, trimethoprim/sulfamethoxazole, vancomycin, vasopressin, vecuronium, verapamil, vinblastine, vincristine, vinorelbine, zidovudine, zoledronic acid.
- **Y-Site Incompatibility:** amphotericin B deoxycholate, busulfan, cefepime, cyclosporine, dantrolene, diazepam, doxorubicin hydrochloride, gemtuzumab ozogamicin, idarubicin, mitoxantrone, moxifloxacin, nitroprusside, pantoprazole, phenytoin.

Patient/Family Teaching

- Explain purpose and side effects of medication to patient. Advise patient to read *Patient Information* before starting therapy. Advise patient to take as directed, on an empty stomach.
- Instruct patient to notify health care provider of all Rx or OTC medications, vitamins, or herbal products being taken and consult health care provider before taking any new medications.
- May cause blurred vision, photophobia, and dizziness. Caution patient to avoid driving and other activities requiring alertness until response to medication is known. Also advise patient to avoid driving at night.
- Advise patient to avoid direct sunlight, sunlamps, and tanning beds. Use sunscreen and protective clothing to prevent severe sunburn. Advise patient to have dermatologic evaluation on a regular basis to allow early detection and management of premalignant lesions; squamous cell carcinoma of the skin and melanoma have been reported during long-term therapy.
- Advise patient to notify health care provider if rash or signs and symptoms of allergic reaction occur.
- Rep: May cause fetal harm. Advise women of reproductive potential to use effective contraception and notify health care provider if pregnancy is planned

V

or suspected or if breastfeeding. Monitor for adverse reactions if voriconazole is administered concurrently with oral contraceptives.

Evaluation/Desired Outcomes

- Resolution of fungal infections.

BEERS

vortioxetine

(vor-tye-**ox**-e-teen)

Trintellix

Classification

Therapeutic: antidepressants

Pharmacologic: selective serotonin reuptake inhibitors (SSRIs)

Indications

Major depressive disorder.

Action

Selectively inhibits the reuptake of serotonin in the CNS. May also act as a 5-HT_{1A} agonist and as a 5-HT_3 antagonist. **Therapeutic Effects:** Antidepressant action.

Pharmacokinetics

Absorption: Well absorbed (75%) following oral administration.

Distribution: Extensive extravascular distribution.

Protein Binding: 98%.

Metabolism and Excretion: Primarily metabolized by the liver via the CYP2D6 isoenzyme; the CYP2D6 enzyme system exhibits genetic polymorphism (~7% of population may be poor metabolizers and may have significantly ↑ vortioxetine concentrations and an ↑ risk of adverse effects). 59% excreted in urine as metabolites, 26% in feces as metabolites, minimal renal excretion of unchanged drug.

Half-life: 66 hr.

TIME/ACTION PROFILE (antidepressant effect)

ROUTE	ONSET	PEAK	DURATION
PO	1–2 wk	4–8 wk	unknown

Contraindications/Precautions

Contraindicated in: Hypersensitivity; Concurrent use of MAO inhibitors or MAO-inhibitor-like drugs (linezolid or methylene blue); OB: Pregnancy.

Use Cautiously in: May ↑ risk of suicide attempt/ideation especially during early treatment or dose adjustment; this risk appears to be greater in adolescents or children; History of bipolar disorder (may activate mania/hypomania); CYP2D6 poor metabolizers; Angle-closure glaucoma; Lactation: Use while breastfeeding only if potential maternal benefit justifies potential risk to infant; Pedi: Safety and effectiveness not established in children; Geri: Appears on Beers list. May worsen or cause syndrome of inappropriate antidiuretic hormone (SIADH) secretion and/or hyponatremia in older adults. Use with caution in older adults and closely monitor sodium concentrations when starting therapy or ↑ dose.

Adverse Reactions/Side Effects

Endo: SIADH. **F and E:** hyponatremia . **GI:** constipation, nausea. **GU:** ↓ libido, delayed/absent orgasm, ejaculatory delay/failure, erectile dysfunction. **Hemat:** bleeding. **Neuro:** SUICIDAL THOUGHTS/BEHAVIORS. **Misc:** HYPERSENSITIVITY REACTIONS (INCLUDING ANAPHYLAXIS AND ANGIOEDEMA), SEROTONIN SYNDROME.

Interactions

Drug-Drug: Concurrent use of **MAO inhibitors** for psychiatric conditions or within 21 days of discontinuing vortioxetine is contraindicated; do not use vorioxetine within 14 days of discontinuing MAOIs used for psychiatric conditions, nor should vorioxetine be started in patients receiving **linezolid** or **intravenous methylene blue** due to risk of serious adverse reactions, including serotonin syndrome. Drugs that affect serotonergic neurotransmitter systems, including **tricyclic antidepressants, SNRIs, fentanyl, lithium, buspirone, tramadol, meperidine, methadone, amphetamines**, and **triptans**, ↑ risk of serotonin syndrome. **Strong CYP2D6 inhibitors**, including **bupropion, fluoxetine, paroxetine**, or **quinidine**, may ↑ levels and risk of toxicity. **Strong CYP2D6 inducers**, including **carbamazepine, phenytoin**, or **rifampin**, may ↓ levels and effectiveness. ↑ risk of bleeding with **aspirin, NSAIDs, anticoagulants, thrombolytics, antiplatelet agents**, and other **drugs affecting coagulation.**

Drug-Natural Products: ↑ risk of serotonin syndrome with **St. John's wort**.

Route/Dosage

PO: (Adults): 10 mg once daily initially; may ↑ to 20 mg once daily; some patients may only tolerate daily doses of 5 mg; *CYP2D6 poor metabolizers:* Daily dose should not exceed 10 mg; *Concurrent use of CYP2D6 inhibitors:* ↓ dose by 50%; *Concurrent use of strong CYP2D6 inducers for >14 days:* Consider ↑ dose (not to exceed three times the original dose). If daily dose 15–20 mg/day, do not discontinue abruptly; taper to 10 mg/day for 1 wk before discontinuing.

Availability (generic available)

Tablets: 5 mg, 10 mg, 20 mg.

NURSING IMPLICATIONS

Assessment

- Monitor mood changes. Inform health care provider if patient demonstrates significant increase in anxiety, nervousness, or insomnia.
- Screen patients for personal or family history of bipolar disorder, mania, or hypomania prior to starting therapy.
- Assess for suicidal tendencies, especially during early therapy. Restrict amount of drug available to patient. Risk may be ↑ in adults ≤24 yr. After starting therapy, young adults should be seen by health care provider at least weekly for 4 wk, every 3 wk for next 4 wk, and on advice of health care provider thereafter.
- Monitor for signs and symptoms of hypersensitivity reactions (rash, hives, swelling, difficulty breathing). Stop vortioxetine and treat symptomatically.
- Assess for sexual side effects (erectile dysfunction; ↓ libido).
- Monitor for serotonin syndrome (mental changes [agitation, hallucinations, coma], autonomic instability [tachycardia, labile BP, hyperthermia], neuromuscular aberrations [hyperreflexia, incoordination], GI symptoms [nausea, vomiting, diarrhea]), especially in patients taking other serotonergic drugs (SSRIs, SNRIs, triptans).

Lab Test Considerations

- May cause hyponatremia.

Implementation

- **PO:** Administer once daily at the same time each day without regard to meals.

Patient/Family Teaching

- Instruct patient to take vortioxetine at the same time each day as directed. Advise patient taking 15 mg/day or 20 mg/day of vortioxetine not to stop abruptly; may cause headache, muscle tension, mood swings, sudden outbursts of anger, dizziness, and runny nose. Instruct patient to read *Medication Guide* before starting therapy and with each Rx refill in case of changes.
- Inform patient that nausea is common in 1st wk of therapy and is dose related. Usually ↓ in frequency after 1st wk, but may persist.
- Caution patient to report signs and symptoms of hyponatremia (headache, difficulty concentrating, memory impairment, confusion, weakness, unsteadiness; these may worsen to hallucinations, syncope, seizures, coma, respiratory arrest, death) to health care provider promptly.
- Advise patient, family, and caregivers to look for suicidality, especially during early therapy or dose changes. Notify health care provider immediately if thoughts about suicide or dying, attempts to commit suicide, new or worse depression or anxiety, agitation or restlessness, panic attacks, insomnia, new or worse irritability, aggressiveness, acting on dangerous impulses, mania, or other changes in mood or behavior occur.
- Caution patient and caregiver to look for signs of activation of mania/hypomania (greatly ↑ energy, severe sleeping problems, racing thoughts, reckless behavior, unusually grand ideas, excessive happiness or irritability, talking more or faster than usual), especially in patients with a history or family history of bipolar disorder, mania, or hypomania.
- Instruct patient to notify health care provider of all Rx or OTC medications, vitamins, or herbal products being taken and consult health care provider before taking any new medications, especially St. John's wort. Advise patient to avoid taking other CNS depressants or alcohol. Also, taking aspirin, NSAIDs, warfarin, or other anticoagulants may increase risk of bleeding.
- Inform patient that medication may cause ↓ libido.
- Advise patient to notify health care provider if symptoms of hypersensitivity reaction or serotonin syndrome occur or if nausea persists.
- Rep: Advise women of reproductive potential to notify health care provider if pregnancy is planned or suspected or if breastfeeding. Use during last month of pregnancy ↑ risk of postpartum hemorrhage. If taken during the 3rd trimester, may ↑ risk of neonatal complications requiring prolonged hospitalization. Newborn may have toxicity or withdrawal symptoms resulting in breathing difficulty (respiratory distress, cyanosis, apnea, seizures, temperature instability feeding difficulties, behavioral issues) and may ↑ risk of persistent pulmonary hypertension of the newborn. Consider benefits of breastfeeding, mother's need for vortioxetine, and potential adverse effects on child before breastfeeding.
- Emphasize the importance of follow-up exams to monitor progress.

Evaluation/Desired Outcomes

- Increased sense of well-being.
- Renewed interest in surroundings. May require 1–4 wk of therapy to obtain antidepressant effects.

V

BEERS HIGH ALERT

warfarin (war-fa-rin)

~~Coumadin~~, Jantoven

Classification

Therapeutic: anticoagulants

Pharmacologic: coumarins

Indications

Prophylaxis and treatment of: Deep vein thrombosis, Pulmonary embolism, Thromboembolism associated with atrial fibrillation. Management of MI. Prevention of thrombus formation and embolization after prosthetic valve placement.

Action

Interferes with hepatic synthesis of vitamin K–dependent clotting factors (II, VII, IX, and X). **Therapeutic Effects:** Prevention of thromboembolic events.

Pharmacokinetics

Absorption: Well absorbed from the GI tract after oral administration.

Distribution: Minimally distributed to tissues.

Protein Binding: 99%.

Metabolism and Excretion: Primarily metabolized by the liver via the CYP2C9 isoenzyme, with some metabolism via the CYP3A4 isoenzyme; the CYP2C9 isoenzyme exhibits genetic polymorphism (intermediate or poor metabolizers may have significantly ↑ (S)-warfarin concentrations and an ↑ risk of adverse reactions).

Half-life: 42 hr.

TIME/ACTION PROFILE (effects on coagulation tests)

ROUTE	ONSET	PEAK	DURATION
PO	36–72 hr	5–7 days†	2–5 days‡

† At a constant dose

‡ After discontinuation

Contraindications/Precautions

Contraindicated in: Uncontrolled bleeding; Open wounds; Active ulcer disease; Recent brain, eye, or spinal cord injury or surgery; Severe hepatic impairment; Uncontrolled hypertension; OB: Pregnancy.

Use Cautiously in: Malignancy; History of ulcer, liver disease, or acute kidney injury; History of poor compliance; Asian patients or those who carry the CYP2C9*2 allele and/or the CYP2C9*3 allele, or with the VKORC1 AA genotype (↑ risk of bleeding with standard dosing; lower initial doses should be considered); Rep: Women of reproductive potential; Pedi: Has been used safely in children, but may require more frequent INR assessments; Geri: Appears on Beers list. ↑ risk of major bleeding when compared to direct acting oral anticoagulants (DOACs) in older adults. Avoid starting as initial therapy for treatment of nonvalvular atrial fibrillation or venous thromboembolism unless alternative options (DOACs) are contraindicated or there are significant barriers to their use. If already using warfarin, it may be reasonable to continue treatment, especially if INR is well controlled (i.e., >70% time in therapeutic range) and no adverse effects.

Adverse Reactions/Side Effects

Derm: dermal necrosis. **GI:** cramps, nausea. **GU:** CALCIPHYLAXIS. **Hemat:** BLEEDING. **Misc:** fever.

Interactions

Drug-Drug: Androgens, capecitabine, cefotetan, chloramphenicol, clopidogrel, disulfiram, fluconazole, fluoroquinolones, itraconazole, metronidazole (including vaginal use), **thrombolytics, eptifibatide, tirofiban, sulfonamides, quinidine, quinine, NSAIDs, valproates,** and **aspirin** may ↑ risk of bleeding. Chronic use of **acetaminophen** may ↑ risk of bleeding. Chronic **alcohol** ingestion may ↓ effectiveness; if chronic **alcohol** abuse results in significant liver damage, may ↑ risk of bleeding due to ↓ production of clotting factors. Acute **alcohol** ingestion may ↑ risk of bleeding. **Barbiturates, carbamazepine, rifampin,** and **hormonal contraceptives containing estrogen** may ↓ levels and effectiveness.

Drug-Natural Products: St. John's wort may ↓ levels and effectiveness. ↑ bleeding risk with **anise, arnica, chamomile, clove, dong quai, fenugreek, feverfew, garlic, ginger, ginkgo, Panax ginseng,** and **licorice.**

Drug-Food: Ingestion of large quantities of **foods high in vitamin K content** (see list in Appendix J) may antagonize the anticoagulant effect of warfarin.

Route/Dosage

PO (Adults): 2–5 mg/day for 2–4 days; then adjust daily dose by results of INR. Initiate therapy with lower doses in older adults or in Asian patients or those with CYP2C9*2 and/or CYP2C9*3 alleles or VKORC1 AA genotype.

PO (Children >1 mo): *Initial loading dose:* 0.2 mg/kg (maximum dose: 10 mg) for 2–4 days; then adjust daily dose by results of INR. Use 0.1 mg/kg if hepatic impairment is present. *Maintenance dose range:* 0.05–0.34 mg/kg/day.

Availability (generic available)

Tablets: 1 mg, 2 mg, 2.5 mg, 3 mg, 4 mg, 5 mg, 6 mg, 7.5 mg, 10 mg.

NURSING IMPLICATIONS

Assessment

- Assess for signs of bleeding and hemorrhage (bleeding gums; nosebleed; unusual bruising; tarry, black stools; hematuria; fall in hematocrit or BP; guaiac-positive stools, urine, or nasogastric aspirate).
- Assess for additional or ↑ thrombosis.

Lab Test Considerations

- Monitor PT, INR, and other clotting factors frequently during therapy and more frequently in patients with renal impairment. In general, an INR of 2–3 is recommended for most patients receiving warfarin.
- Asian patients and those who carry the CYP2C9*2 allele and/or the CYP2C9*3 allele, or those with VKORC1 AA genotype may require more frequent monitoring and lower doses.
- Geri: Patients >60 yr exhibit greater than expected PT/INR response. Monitor for side effects at lower therapeutic ranges.
- Pedi: May be more difficult to achieve and maintain therapeutic PT/INR ranges in children. Assess PT/INR levels more frequently.
- Monitor hepatic function and CBC before starting and periodically throughout therapy.
- Monitor stool and urine for occult blood before and periodically during therapy.

Toxicity and Overdose

- Withholding one or more doses of warfarin is usually sufficient if INR is excessively elevated or if minor bleeding occurs. If overdose occurs or anticoagulation needs to be immediately reversed, the antidote is vitamin K (phytonadione). Administration of whole blood or plasma also may be required in severe bleeding because of the delayed onset of vitamin K.

Implementation

- ***High Alert:*** Do not confuse Jantoven with Janumet or Januvia.
- Because of the large number of medications capable of significantly altering warfarin's effects, careful monitoring is recommended when new agents are started or other agents are discontinued. Interactive potential should be evaluated for all new medications (Rx, OTC, herbal).
- **PO:** Administer medication at same time each day; requires 3–5 days to reach effective levels; usually begun while patient is still on heparin.
- Do not interchange brands; potencies may not be equivalent.

Patient/Family Teaching

- Explain purpose and side effects of medication. Advise patient to read *Patient Information* before starting therapy.
- Instruct patient to take missed doses as soon as remembered that day; do not double doses. Inform health care provider of missed doses at time of checkup or lab tests. Inform patients that anticoagulant effect may persist for 2–5 days following discontinuation.
- Instruct patient to carry identification describing medication regimen at all times and to inform all health care personnel caring for patient on anticoagulant therapy before lab tests, treatment, or surgery.
- Emphasize the importance of frequent lab tests to monitor coagulation factors.
- Review foods high in vitamin K (see Appendix J). Patient should have consistent limited intake of these foods, as vitamin K is the antidote for warfarin, and alternating intake of these foods will cause coagulation to fluctuate. Advise patient to avoid cranberry juice or products during therapy.
- Caution patient to avoid IM injections and activities leading to injury. Instruct patient to use a soft toothbrush, not to floss, and to shave with an electric razor during warfarin therapy. Advise patient that venipunctures and injection sites require application of pressure to prevent bleeding or hematoma formation.
- Advise patient to notify health care provider of unusual bleeding or bruising (bleeding gums; nosebleed; black, tarry stools; hematuria; excessive menstrual flow) and pain, color, or temperature change to any area of the body. Notify patient with deficiency in protein C and/or S mediated anticoagulant response that they may be at ↑ risk for tissue necrosis.
- Advise patient to notify health care provider of all Rx or OTC medications, vitamins, or herbal products being taken and to consult health care provider before taking other medications, especially alcohol, aspirin or other NSAIDs.
- Rep: May cause fetal harm. Advise women of reproductive potential to use effective contraception during and for 1 mo after last dose. Advise patient to notify health care provider if pregnancy is planned or suspected or if breastfeeding.

Evaluation/Desired Outcomes

- Prevention of thromboembolic events.

W

xanomelene/trospium

(zan-**oh**-me-leen/**trose**-pee-um)

Cobenfy

Classification

Therapeutic: antipsychotics

Pharmacologic: cholinergics, anticholinergics

Indications

Schizophrenia.

Action

Xanomelene: Acts as an agonist at M1 and M4 muscarinic acetylcholine receptors in the CNS. *Trospium:* Acts as a muscarinic antagonist. The mechanism of both xanomelene and trospium in treatment of schizophrenia is unclear. **Therapeutic Effects:** Decreased manifestations of schizophrenia.

Pharmacokinetics

Xanomelene

Absorption: High-fat meals ↑ absorption by 30%.

Distribution: Extensively distributed to tissues.

Metabolism and Excretion: Primarily metabolized in the liver via the CYP1A2, CYP2C9, CYP2C19, CYP2D6, and CYP2B6 isoenzymes. 78% excreted in urine; 12% excreted in feces.

Half-life: 5 hr.

Trospium

Absorption: Low- or high-fat meals ↓ absorption by 85–90%.

Distribution: Well distributed to tissues.

Metabolism and Excretion: Primarily metabolized via ester hydrolysis and glucuronic acid conjugation. Primarily excreted in urine (85–90% as unchanged drug).

Half-life: 6 hr.

TIME/ACTION PROFILE

ROUTE	ONSET	PEAK	DURATION
PO	unknown	1–2 hr	12 hr

Contraindications/Precautions

Contraindicated in: Hypersensitivity; Urinary retention; Moderate to severe renal impairment; Hepatic impairment; Active biliary disease (including symptomatic gallstones); Gastric retention; Untreated, narrow-angle glaucoma.

Use Cautiously in: GI obstructive disorders; Ulcerative colitis, intestinal atony, or myasthenia gravis; OB: Safety not established in pregnancy; Lactation: Safety not established in breastfeeding; Pedi: Safety and effectiveness not established in children; Geri: Older adults may be at ↑ risk of adverse reactions.

Adverse Reactions/Side Effects

CV: hypertension, orthostatic hypotension, tachycardia. **EENT:** blurred vision. **GI:** constipation, dyspepsia, nausea, vomiting, ↑ liver enzymes, ↑ salivation, abdominal pain, diarrhea, dry mouth, gastroesophageal reflux disease. **GU:** dysuria, urinary hesitancy, urinary retention, urinary tract infection. **Neuro:** confusion, dizziness, hallucinations, sedation. **Resp:** cough. **Misc:** HYPERSENSITIVITY REACTIONS (INCLUDING ANGIOEDEMA).

Interactions

Drug-Drug: Strong CYP2D6 inhibitors may ↑ xanomelene levels and risk of toxicity. Drugs eliminated by active tubular secretion may ↑ trospium levels and risk of toxicity. May ↑ levels and risk of toxicity of **CYP3A4 substrates** or **P-glycoprotein substrates**. May ↑ risk of anticholinergic effects when used with other **anticholinergic drugs**. May alter absorption of concurrently administered drugs.

Route/Dosage

PO (Adults): One xanomelene 50 mg/trospium 20 mg capsule twice daily for ≥2 days, then ↑ to one xanomelene 100 mg/trospium 20 mg capsule twice daily for ≥5 days, then ↑ to one xanomelene 125 mg/trospium 30 mg capsule twice daily.

PO (Geriatric Patients): Start with one xanomelene 50 mg/trospium 20 mg capsule twice daily. Consider slower titration process. Max dose = one xanomelene 100 mg/trospium 20 mg twice daily.

Availability

Capsules: xanomelene 50 mg/trospium 20 mg, xanomelene 100 mg/trospium 20 mg, xanomelene 125 mg/trospium 30 mg.

NURSING IMPLICATIONS

Assessment

- Assess HR at baseline and as clinically indicated during therapy.
- Monitor for signs/symptoms of urinary retention. *If urinary retention occurs,* consider discontinuing xanomelene/trospium, ↓ dose, and/or referring for urologic evaluation.
- Monitor for signs/symptoms of anticholinergic CNS effects upon initiation and dose ↑. *If CNS effects occur,* consider ↓ dose or discontinuing xanomelene/trospium.

Lab Test Considerations

- Assess liver enzymes and bilirubin at baseline and as clinically indicated during therapy. *If clinical signs of liver injury, or ALT levels >5 times upper limit of normal or baseline values occur,* discontinue xanomelene/trospium.

Implementation

- **PO:** Administer 1 hr before or ≥2 hr after food. Do not open capsules.

Patient/Family Teaching

- Explain purpose and side effects of medication. Advise patient to read *Patient Information* before starting therapy.
- Advise patient to notify health care professional of all Rx or OTC medications, vitamins, or herbal products being taken and to consult health care professional before taking other medications.
- Instruct patients to notify health care professional for symptoms of urinary retention (urinary hesitancy, weak stream, incomplete bladder emptying, painful urination).
- Advise patient to immediately notify health care professional for signs/symptoms of angioedema (swelling of face, lips, tongue, larynx).
- Advise patient to notify health care professional for signs/symptoms of ↓ GI motility or hepatic injury (dyspepsia, nausea, vomiting, upper abdominal pain, jaundice, itching), or anticholinergic CNS effects (dizziness, confusion, hallucinations, somnolence).
- Advise patient not to drive or operate heavy machinery until they know how therapy affects them.
- Rep: Advise women of reproductive potential to notify health care professional if pregnancy is planned or suspected, or if breastfeeding. Encourage pregnant patient to enroll in registry that monitors outcomes in patients who become pregnant while taking xanomelene/trospium by calling 1-866-961-2388 or visiting https://womensmentalhealth.org/research/pregnancyregistry/atypicalantipsychotic/.

Evaluation/Desired Outcomes

- Decreased manifestations of schizophrenia.

BEERS

zaleplon (za-lep-lon)

~~Sonata~~

Classification

Therapeutic: sedative/hypnotics

Schedule IV

Indications

Short-term management of insomnia in patients unable to get ≥4 hr of sleep; especially useful in sleep initiation disorders.

Action

Produces CNS depression by binding to GABA receptors in the CNS. Has no analgesic properties.
Therapeutic Effects: Induction of sleep.

Pharmacokinetics

Absorption: Rapidly absorbed following oral administration.
Distribution: Well distributed to tissues.
Metabolism and Excretion: Extensively metabolized in the liver (mostly by aldehyde oxidase and some by the CYP3A4 isoenzyme).
Half-life: 1 hr.

TIME/ACTION PROFILE

ROUTE	ONSET	PEAK	DURATION
PO	within min	unknown	3–4 hr

Contraindications/Precautions

Contraindicated in: Hypersensitivity; History of experiencing complex sleep behaviors with zaleplon; Severe hepatic impairment; OB: Pregnancy; Lactation: Lactation.
Use Cautiously in: Mild or moderate hepatic impairment or weight ≤50 kg (initiate therapy at lowest dose); Impaired respiratory function; History of suicide attempt; Pedi: Safety and effectiveness not established in children; Geri: Appears on Beers list. ↑ risk of cognitive impairment, delirium, falls, fractures, and motor vehicle accidents in older adults. Avoid use in older adults.

Adverse Reactions/Side Effects

CV: peripheral edema. **Derm:** photosensitivity. **EENT:** abnormal vision, altered sense of smell, ear pain, epistaxis, hearing sensitivity, ocular pain. **GI:** abdominal pain, anorexia, colitis, dyspepsia, nausea. **GU:** dysmenorrhea. **Neuro:** abnormal thinking, amnesia, anxiety, behavior changes, COMPLEX SLEEP BEHAVIORS (INCLUDING SLEEP DRIVING, SLEEP WALKING, OR ENGAGING IN OTHER ACTIVITIES WHILE SLEEPING), depersonalization, dizziness, drowsiness, hallucinations, headache, hyperesthesia, impaired memory (briefly following dose), impaired psychomotor function (briefly following dose), malaise, nightmares, paresthesia, tremor, vertigo, weakness. **Misc:** fever.

Interactions

Drug-Drug: Cimetidine may ↑ levels and risk of toxicity; initiate therapy at a lower dose. Additive CNS depression with other **CNS depressants**, including **alcohol**, **antihistamines**, **opioid analgesics**, other **sedative/hypnotics**, **phenothiazines**, and **tricyclic antidepressants**. **CYP3A4 inducers**, including **rifampin**, **phenytoin**, **carbamazepine**, and **phenobarbital**, may ↓ levels and effectiveness.
Drug-Natural Products: Kava-kava, **valerian**, **chamomile**, or **hops** can ↑ risk of CNS depression.
Drug-Food: Concurrent ingestion of a **high-fat meal** slows the rate of absorption.

Route/Dosage

PO (Adults <65 yr): 10 mg (range 5–20 mg) at bedtime.

Hepatic Impairment

PO (Adults): Initiate therapy at 5 mg at bedtime (not to exceed 10 mg at bedtime).

Availability (generic available)

Capsules: 5 mg, 10 mg.

NURSING IMPLICATIONS

Assessment

- Assess mental status, sleep patterns, and potential for abuse prior to administering this medication. Zaleplon is used to treat short-term difficulty in falling asleep; ↓ time to sleep onset. May not ↑ total sleep time or ↓ number of wakenings after falling asleep. Prolonged use of >7–10 days may lead to physical and psychological dependence. Limit amount of drug available to the patient.
- Assess patient for pain and medicate as needed. Untreated pain ↓ sedative effect.
- Assess for complex sleep behaviors (sleep-walking, sleep-driving, or engaging in activities while not fully awake). May cause serious injuries and even death; if these behaviors occur, discontinue immediately if identified.

Implementation

- Do not confuse Sonata with Soriatane.
- Before administering, reduce external stimuli and provide comfort measures to ↑ effectiveness.
- Protect patient from injury. Supervise ambulation and transfer of patient after administration. Remove any cigarettes. Side rails should be raised and call bell within reach at all times.
- **PO:** ***DNC:*** Tablets should be swallowed whole with full glass of water immediately before bedtime or after going to bed and experiencing difficulty falling asleep. Do not administer with or immediately after a high-fat or heavy meal.

Patient/Family Teaching

- Explain purpose and side effects of medication. Advise patient to read *Patient Information* before starting therapy.
- Instruct patient not to take more than the amount prescribed because of the habit-forming potential. Not recommended for use longer than 7–10 days. Rebound insomnia (1–2 nights) may occur when stopped. If used for ≥2 wk, abrupt withdrawal may result in dysphoria, insomnia, abdominal or muscle cramps, vomiting, sweating, tremors, and seizures.
- Because of rapid onset, advise patient to go to bed immediately after taking zaleplon.
- May cause daytime drowsiness or dizziness. Advise patient to avoid driving or other activities requiring alertness until response to this medication is known.
- Inform patient that amnesia may occur, but can be avoided if only taken when they can get >4 hr sleep.
- Caution patient that complex sleep-related behaviors (sleep-driving, making phone calls, preparing and eating food, having sex, sleep walking) may occur while asleep. Inform patient to notify health care provider if sleep-related behaviors (may include sleep-driving: driving while not fully awake after ingestion of a sedative-hypnotic product, with no memory of the event) occur.
- Advise patient to notify health care provider of all Rx or OTC medications, vitamins, or herbal products being taken and to consult health care provider before taking other medications.
- Caution patient to avoid concurrent use of alcohol or other CNS depressants, including opioids.
- Rep: May cause fetal harm. Use is not recommended during pregnancy or breastfeeding. Advise women of reproductive potential to notify health care provider if pregnancy is planned or suspected or if breastfeeding.

Evaluation/Desired Outcomes

- Improved ability to fall asleep; ↓ time to sleep onset.

zavegepant (za-ve-je-pant)

Zavzpret

Classification

Therapeutic: vascular headache suppressants

Pharmacologic: calcitonin gene-related peptide receptor antagonists

Indications

Acute treatment of migraine with or without aura.

Action

Binds to and inhibits the calcitonin gene-related peptide (CGRP) receptor, which reduces the neuroinflammatory and vasodilatory effects of CGRP. **Therapeutic Effects:** Reduction in pain and other bothersome symptoms associated with migraine.

Pharmacokinetics

Absorption: 5% absorbed following intranasal administration.

Distribution: Extensively distributed to tissues.

Protein Binding: 90%.

Metabolism and Excretion: Primarily metabolized in liver via the CYP3A4 isoenzyme and to a lesser extent by the CYP2D6 isoenzyme. Primarily excreted as unchanged drug in feces (80%) and urine (11%).

Half-life: 6.55 hr.

TIME/ACTION PROFILE (relief of migraine pain)

ROUTE	ONSET	PEAK	DURATION
IN	0.5 hr	2 hr	up to 48 hr

Contraindications/Precautions

Contraindicated in: Hypersensitivity; Severe renal impairment; Severe hepatic impairment.

Use Cautiously in: Hypertension; Raynaud phenomenon; OB: Safety not established in pregnancy; Lactation: Safety not established in breastfeeding; Pedi: Safety and effectiveness not established in children.

Adverse Reactions/Side Effects

CV: hypertension, Raynaud phenomenon. **EENT:** nasal discomfort. **GI:** taste disorders, nausea, vomiting. **Misc:** hypersensitivity reactions.

Interactions

Drug-Drug: Organic anion transporting polypeptide 1B3 (OATP1B3) inhibitors or **sodium taurocholate cotransporting polypeptide (NTCP) transporter inhibitors**, including **rifampin**, may ↑ levels and risk of toxicity; avoid concurrent use. **Organic anion transporting polypeptide 1B3 (OATP1B3) inducers** or **sodium taurocholate cotransporting polypeptide (NTCP) transporter inducers** may ↓ levels and effectiveness; avoid concurrent use. **Intranasal decongestants** may ↓ absorption of zavegepant; avoid concurrent use. If concurrent use unavoidable, administer intranasal decongestant ≥1 hr after zavegepant.

Route/Dosage

Intranasal (Adults): Single dose of 10 mg in one nostril.

Z

Availability

Nasal spray: 10 mg/spray.

NURSING IMPLICATIONS

Assessment

- Assess pain location, character, intensity, duration, and associated symptoms (photophobia, phonophobia, nausea, vomiting) of migraine pain.
- Monitor frequency of migraine headaches.
- Monitor BP periodically and more frequently in patients with pre-existing HTN.
- Monitor for signs and symptoms of hypersensitivity reactions (anaphylaxis, dyspnea, rash, pruritus, urticaria, facial edema). *If hypersensitivity reaction occurs,* discontinue zavegepant and treat appropriately.

Implementation

- **Intranasal:** Administer a single 10 mg spray in one nostril, as needed. Do not administer more than one spray in each 24 hr period.

Patient/Family Teaching

- Instruct patient to administer zavegepant as directed. Do not test or prime the nasal spray before use. Advise patient to read the *Patient Information* before starting therapy and with each Rx refill in case of changes.
- Advise patient to avoid using intranasal decongestants with zavegepant; may ↓ absorption of zavegepant. If concurrent use is unavoidable, administer intranasal decongestants ≥1 hr after zavegepant administration.
- Advise patient to notify health care provider immediately if signs or symptoms of hypersensitivity reactions (shortness of breath; rash; swelling of the face, mouth, tongue, or throat) occur.
- Advise patient to report symptoms of ↑ BP or worsening pre-existing hypertension.
- Advise patient to notify health care provider of all Rx or OTC medications, vitamins, or herbal products being taken and to consult with health care provider before taking other medications.
- Rep: Advise women of reproductive potential to notify health care provider if pregnancy is planned or suspected or if breastfeeding.

Evaluation/Desired Outcomes

- Decrease in pain and symptoms associated with migraine headaches.

zidovudine (zye-doe-vue-deen)

Retrovir

Classification

Therapeutic: antiretrovirals

Pharmacologic: nucleoside reverse transcriptase inhibitors

Indications

HIV infection (in combination with other antiretrovirals). Reduction of maternal/fetal transmission of HIV. **Unlabeled Use:** Chemoprophylaxis after occupational exposure to HIV.

Action

Following intracellular conversion to its active form, inhibits viral RNA synthesis by inhibiting the enzyme DNA polymerase (reverse transcriptase). Prevents viral replication. **Therapeutic Effects:** Virustatic action against selected retroviruses. Slowed progression and decreased sequelae of HIV infection. Decreased viral load and improved CD4 cell counts. Decreased transmission of HIV to infants born to HIV-infected mothers.

Pharmacokinetics

Absorption: Well absorbed following oral administration.

Distribution: Widely distributed; enters the CNS.

Metabolism and Excretion: Mostly (75%) metabolized by the liver; 15–20% excreted unchanged by the kidneys.

Half-life: 1 hr.

TIME/ACTION PROFILE (plasma concentrations)

ROUTE	ONSET	PEAK	DURATION
PO	unknown	0.5–1.5 hr	4 hr
IV	rapid	end of infusion	4 hr

Contraindications/Precautions

Contraindicated in: Hypersensitivity; Lactation: Breastfeeding not recommended in mothers with HIV.

Use Cautiously in: ↓ bone marrow reserve (↓ dose for anemia or granulocytopenia); Women and obese patients (↑ risk of lactic acidosis and severe hepatomegaly); Latex allergy (IV only); Severe renal impairment; Severe hepatic impairment; Geri: Select dose carefully due to potential for age-related ↓ in hepatic, renal, or cardiac function in older adults.

Adverse Reactions/Side Effects

Derm: nail pigmentation. **Endo:** gynecomastia. **F and E:** LACTIC ACIDOSIS. **GI:** abdominal pain, diarrhea, nausea, anorexia, dyspepsia, HEPATOMEGALY (WITH STEATOSIS), oral mucosa pigmentation, PANCREATITIS, vomiting. **Hemat:** ANEMIA, NEUTROPENIA, pure red-cell aplasia, thrombocytosis. **Metab:** lipoatrophy. **MS:** back pain, MYOPATHY. **Neuro:** headache, weakness, ↓ mental acuity, anxiety, confusion, depression, dizziness, insomnia, restlessness, SEIZURES, syncope, tremor. **Misc:** immune reconstitution syndrome.

Interactions

Drug-Drug: ↑ bone marrow depression with other **agents having bone marrow–depressing**

properties, **antineoplastics**, **radiation therapy**, or **ganciclovir**. ↑ risk of neurotoxicity with **acyclovir**. Toxicity may be ↑ by concurrent administration of **probenecid** or **fluconazole**. **Clarithromycin** may ↓ levels and effectiveness.

Route/Dosage

HIV

PO (Adults): 100 mg every 4 hr while awake or 200 mg 3 times daily or 300 mg twice daily (depends on combination and clinical situation).
PO (Children ≥4 wk and ≥30 kg): 300 mg twice daily or 200 mg 3 times daily.
PO (Children ≥4 wk and 9–29.9 kg): 9 mg/kg twice daily or 6 mg/kg 3 times daily.
PO (Children ≥4 wk and 4–8.9 kg): 12 mg/kg twice daily or 8 mg/kg 3 times daily.
IV (Adults and Children >12 yr): 1 mg/kg every 4 hr. Change to oral therapy as soon as possible.
IV (Children): 120 mg/m² every 6 hr (not to exceed 160 mg/dose) or 20 mg/m²/hr as a continuous infusion.

Prevention of Maternal/Fetal Transmission of HIV Infection

PO (Adults >14 wk Pregnant): 100 mg 5 times daily until onset of labor.
IV (Adults during Labor and Delivery): 2 mg/kg over 1 hr; then continuous infusion of 1 mg/kg/hr until umbilical cord is clamped.
PO (Neonates): 2 mg/kg every 6 hr until 6 wk of age.
IV (Neonates): 1.5 mg/kg every 6 hr until 6 wk of age.

Availability (generic available)

Tablets: 300 mg. **Capsules:** 100 mg. **Oral solution:** 50 mg/5 mL. **Solution for injection:** 10 mg/mL. ***In combination with:*** lamivudine (Combivir); abacavir and lamivudine; see Appendix N.

NURSING IMPLICATIONS

Assessment

- Assess patient for change in severity of symptoms of HIV and for signs/symptoms of opportunistic infections during therapy.
- Assess for inflammatory response related to immune reconstitution syndrome (residual opportunistic infection, autoimmune disorder). *If signs of immune reconstitution syndrome occur,* evaluate and treat as indicated.

Lab Test Considerations

- Monitor viral load and CD4 counts prior to and periodically during therapy.
- Monitor CBC every 2 wk during the first 8 wk of therapy, then every 4 wk after the 1st 2 mo if well tolerated, or monthly during the 1st 3 mo and every 3 mo thereafter unless indicated in patients who are asymptomatic or have early symptoms. Commonly causes granulocytopenia and anemia. Anemia may occur 2–4 wk after initiation of therapy and may respond to epoetin therapy. Granulocytopenia usually occurs after 6–8 wk of therapy. *If hemoglobin <7.5 g/dL or ↓ of >25% from baseline and/or granulocyte count <750 cells/mm³ or ↓ of >50% from baseline occurs,* consider ↓ dose, discontinuing zidovudine, or transfusing blood. May gradually resume when bone marrow recovered.
- May ↑ AST, ALT, and alkaline phosphatase. *If lactic acidosis or severe hepatotoxicity occurs,* hold zidovudine; may be fatal, especially in women.
- Monitor serum amylase, lipase, and triglycerides periodically during therapy. Elevated serum levels may indicate pancreatitis and require discontinuation.

Implementation

- Do not confuse Retrovir with ritonavir.
- **PO:** Administer doses around the clock.
- Pedi: For neonates, use an oral syringe with 0.1-mL graduations to ensure accurate dosing of oral solution.
- **IV:** Patient should receive the IV infusion only until oral therapy can be administered.

IV Administration

- **Intermittent Infusion:** Vial stoppers contain latex; may cause allergic reaction in latex-sensitive individuals. **Dilution:** Remove calculated dose from the vial and dilute with D5W or 0.9% NaCl. Do not use discolored solution. Stable for 24 hr at room temperature or 48 hr if refrigerated. **Concentration:** ≤4 mg/mL. **Rate:** Infuse at a constant rate over 1 hr in adults or over 30 min in neonates. Avoid rapid infusion or bolus injection.
- **Continuous Infusion:** Has also been administered via continuous infusion.
- **Y-Site Compatibility:** acyclovir, alemtuzumab, allopurinol, amikacin, aminocaproic acid, amiodarone, amphotericin B deoxycholate, amphotericin B liposomal, anidulafungin, argatroban, arsenic trioxide, azithromycin, aztreonam, bivalirudin, bleomycin, carboplatin, carmustine, caspofungin, cefepime, ceftazidime, ceftriaxone, cisatracurium, cisplatin, clindamycin, cyclophosphamide, cytarabine, dacarbazine, dactinomycin, daptomycin, daunorubicin, dexamethasone, dexmedetomidine, diltiazem, dobutamine, docetaxel, dopamine, doxorubicin hydrochloride, doxorubicin liposomal, epirubicin, eptifibatide, ertapenem, erythromycin, etoposide, etoposide phosphate, filgrastim, fluconazole, fludarabine, fluorouracil,

Z

foscarnet, fosphenytoin, gemcitabine, gentamicin, granisetron, heparin, hetastarch, hydromorphone, idarubicin, ifosfamide, imipenem/cilastatin, irinotecan, leucovorin, levofloxacin, linezolid, lorazepam, melphalan, meperidine, meropenem, mesna, methadone, methotrexate, metoclopramide, metronidazole, milrinone, mitomycin, mitoxantrone, morphine, mycophenolate, nafcillin, nicardipine, octreotide, ondansetron, oxacillin, oxaliplatin, oxytocin, paclitaxel, palonosetron, pamidronate, pantoprazole, pemetrexed, pentamidine, phenylephrine, piperacillin/tazobactam, potassium acetate, potassium chloride, remifentanil, rituximab, rocuronium, sargramostim, sodium acetate, tacrolimus, thiotepa, tigecycline, tirofiban, tobramycin, topotecan, trastuzumab, trimethoprim/sulfamethoxazole, vancomycin, vasopressin, vecuronium, vinblastine, vincristine, vinorelbine, voriconazole, zoledronic acid.

- **Y-Site Incompatibility:** dexrazoxane, gemtuzumab ozogamicin.

Patient/Family Teaching

- Explain purpose and side effects of medication. Advise patient to read *Patient Information* before starting therapy.
- Instruct patient to take around the clock, even if sleep is interrupted. Emphasize the importance of compliance with therapy, not taking more than prescribed amount, and not discontinuing without consulting health care provider. Advise patient to take missed dose as soon as remembered unless almost time for next dose; do not double dose.
- Zidovudine may cause dizziness or fainting. Caution patient to avoid driving or other activities requiring alertness until response to medication is known.
- Inform patient that zidovudine does not cure HIV and may ↓ risk of transmission of HIV to others through sexual contact or blood contamination. Caution patient to use a condom during sexual contact and avoid sharing needles or donating blood to prevent spreading HIV to others.
- Instruct patient to notify health care provider promptly if signs of lactic acidosis (feel very weak or tired; feel cold, especially in arms and legs; unusual muscle pain; feel dizzy or light-headed; trouble breathing; fast or irregular heartbeat; stomach pain with nausea and vomiting) or liver problems (yellowing of skin or white part of eyes; loss of appetite; nausea; dark or tea-colored urine; pain, aching, or tenderness on right side of abdomen; light-colored stools) occur.
- Instruct patient to notify health care provider promptly if signs of pancreatitis (nausea, vomiting, abdominal pain) or immune reconstitution syndrome (signs and symptoms of an infection or autoimmune disorder) occur.
- Instruct patient to notify health care provider promptly if fever, sore throat, signs of infection, muscle weakness, or shortness of breath occurs. Caution patient to avoid crowds and persons with known infections. Instruct patient to use soft toothbrush, to use caution when using toothpicks or dental floss, and to have dental work done prior to therapy or deferred until blood counts return to normal.
- Advise patient to notify health care provider of all Rx or OTC medications, vitamins, or herbal products being taken and to consult with health care provider before taking other medications.
- Inform patient that redistribution and accumulation of body fat may occur, causing central obesity, dorsocervical fat enlargement (buffalo hump), peripheral muscle wasting, breast enlargement, and cushingoid appearance.
- Rep: Advise women of reproductive potential to notify health care provider if pregnancy is planned or suspected and to avoid breastfeeding. Advise patient taking oral contraceptives to use a nonhormonal method of birth control during therapy. Inform patient of pregnancy exposure registry that monitors outcomes in women exposed to zidovudine during. Enroll patients in the Antiretroviral Pregnancy Registry by calling 1-800-258-4263.
- Emphasize importance of regular follow-up exams and blood counts to determine progress and monitor for side effects.

Evaluation/Desired Outcomes

- Decrease in viral load and ↑ in CD4 counts in patients with HIV.
- Delayed progression of AIDS and ↓ opportunistic infections in patients with HIV.
- Reduction of maternal/fetal transmission of HIV.

BEERS

ziprasidone (zi-pra-si-done)

Geodon, Zeldox

Classification

Therapeutic: antipsychotics, mood stabilizers

Pharmacologic: piperazine derivatives

Indications

Schizophrenia; IM form is reserved for control of acutely agitated patients. Acute manic or mixed episodes associated with bipolar I disorder (oral only). Maintenance treatment of bipolar I disorder (as adjunct to lithium or valproate) (oral only).

Action

Effects probably mediated by antagonism of dopamine type 2 (D2) and serotonin type 2 ($5\text{-}HT_2$). Also antagonizes α_2 adrenergic receptors. **Therapeutic Effects:** Diminished schizophrenic behavior. Reduced symptoms of mania.

Pharmacokinetics

Absorption: 60% absorbed following oral administration; 100% absorbed from IM sites.
Distribution: Well distributed to tissues.
Protein Binding: 99%.
Metabolism and Excretion: 99% metabolized by the liver; <1% excreted unchanged in urine.
Half-life: *PO:* 7 hr; *IM:* 2–5 hr.

TIME/ACTION PROFILE (plasma concentrations)

ROUTE	ONSET	PEAK	DURATION
PO	within hrs	1–3 days†	unknown
IM	rapid	60 min	unknown

† Steady state achieved following continuous use.

Contraindications/Precautions

Contraindicated in: Hypersensitivity; History of QT interval prolongation (persistent QTc interval >500 msec), arrhythmias, recent MI or uncompensated HF; Concurrent use of MAO inhibitors or MAO-inhibitor-like drugs (linezolid or methylene blue); Concurrent use of other drugs known to prolong the QT interval, including quinidine, dofetilide, sotalol, other class Ia and III antiarrhythmics, pimozide, sotalol, thioridazine, chlorpromazine, pentamidine, arsenic trioxide, mefloquine, tacrolimus, droperidol, and moxifloxacin; Hypokalemia or hypomagnesemia.
Use Cautiously in: Concurrent diuretic therapy or diarrhea (may ↑ the risk of hypotension, hypokalemia, or hypomagnesemia); Hepatic impairment; History of cardiovascular or cerebrovascular disease; Hypotension, concurrent antihypertensive therapy, dehydration, or hypovolemia (may ↑ risk of orthostatic hypotension); At risk for aspiration pneumonia or falls; History of suicide attempt; History of breast cancer; OB: Neonates at ↑ risk for extrapyramidal symptoms and withdrawal after delivery when exposed during the 3rd trimester; use during pregnancy only if potential maternal benefit justifies potential fetal risk; Lactation: Use while breastfeeding only if potential maternal benefit justifies potential risk to infant; Pedi: Safety and effectiveness not established in children; Geri: Appears on Beers list. ↑ risk of stroke, cognitive decline, and mortality in older adults with dementia. Avoid use in older adults, except for schizophrenia or bipolar disorder.

Adverse Reactions/Side Effects

CV: orthostatic hypotension, QT interval prolongation. **Derm:** DRUG REACTION WITH EOSINOPHILIA AND SYSTEMIC SYMPTOMS (DRESS), rash, STEVENS-JOHNSON SYNDROME (SJS), urticaria. **EENT:** rhinorrhea. **Endo:** galactorrhea, hyperglycemia, hyperprolactinemia. **GI:** constipation, diarrhea, nausea, dysphagia. **GU:** amenorrhea, impotence. **Hemat:** AGRANULOCYTOSIS, leukopenia, neutropenia. **Metab:** hyperlipidemia, weight gain. **Neuro:** dizziness, drowsiness, restlessness, extrapyramidal reactions, NEUROLEPTIC MALIGNANT SYNDROME, seizures, syncope, tardive dyskinesia. **Resp:** cough.

Interactions

Drug-Drug: **MAO inhibitors** and **MAO-inhibitor-like drugs**, such as **linezolid** or **methylene blue**, may ↑ risk of serotonin syndrome. MAO inhibitors should be stopped ≥14 days before starting ziprasidone. Ziprasidone should be stopped ≥3 days before starting an MAO inhibitor. Concurrent use of **quinidine**, **dofetilide**, **other class Ia and III antiarrhythmics**, **pimozide**, **sotalol**, **thioridazine**, **chlorpromazine**, **pentamidine**, **arsenic trioxide**, **mefloquine**, **tacrolimus**, **droperidol**, **moxifloxacin**, or other agents that prolong the QT interval may result in potentially life-threatening adverse drug reactions; concurrent use contraindicated. Additive CNS depression may occur with **alcohol**, **antidepressants**, **antihistamines**, **opioid analgesics**, or **sedative/hypnotics**. Levels and effectiveness may be ↓ by **carbamazepine**. Levels and effects may be ↑ by **ketoconazole**. Drugs that affect serotonergic neurotransmitter systems, including **tricyclic antidepressants**, **SSRIs**, **SNRIs**, **fentanyl**, **lithium**, **buspirone**, **tramadol**, **meperidine**, **methadone**, **amphetamines**, and **triptans**, may ↑ risk of serotonin syndrome.
Drug-Natural Products: ↑ risk of serotonergic side effects, including serotonin syndrome, with **St. John's wort**.

Route/Dosage

Schizophrenia

PO (Adults): 20 mg twice daily initially; dose increments may be made at 2-day intervals up to 80 mg twice daily.
IM (Adults): 10–20 mg as needed up to 40 mg/day; may be given as 10 mg every 2 hr or 20 mg every 4 hr.

Acute Manic or Mixed Episodes Associated with Bipolar I Disorder

PO (Adults): 40 mg twice on 1st day, then 60 or 80 mg twice daily on 2nd day, then 40–80 mg twice daily.

Maintenance Treatment of Bipolar I Disorder (As Adjunct to Lithium or Valproate)

PO (Adults): Continue same dose on which patient was initially stabilized (range: 40–80 mg twice daily).

Z

Availability (generic available)

Capsules: 20 mg, 40 mg, 60 mg, 80 mg. **Lyophilized powder for injection:** 20 mg/vial.

NURSING IMPLICATIONS

Assessment

- Monitor mental status (orientation, mood, behavior) before starting and periodically during therapy.
- Assess weight and BMI initially and periodically during therapy.
- Monitor BP (sitting, standing, lying) and HR before starting and frequently during initial dose titration. *If QTc interval persistently >500 msec,* discontinue ziprasidone. Patients who experience dizziness, palpitations, or syncope may require further evaluation (e.g., Holter monitoring).
- Assess for rash during therapy. May be treated with antihistamines or corticosteroids. Usually resolves upon discontinuation of ziprasidone. Medication should be discontinued if no alternative etiology for rash is found. May cause SJS or DRESS. *If severe skin reaction occurs or if accompanied with fever, general malaise, fatigue, muscle or joint aches, blisters, oral lesions, conjunctivitis, hepatitis, or eosinophilia,* discontinue ziprasidone.
- Observe carefully when administering medication to ensure medication is actually taken and not hoarded or cheeked.
- Monitor for onset of akathisia (restlessness or desire to keep moving) and extrapyramidal side effects (*parkinsonian:* difficulty speaking or swallowing, loss of balance control, pill rolling of hands, masklike face, shuffling gait, rigidity, tremors and dystonic muscle spasms, twisting motions, twitching, inability to move eyes, weakness of arms or legs) every 2 mo during therapy and 8–12 wk after therapy has been discontinued. Notify health care provider if these symptoms occur, as reduction in dose or discontinuation of medication may be necessary. Trihexyphenidyl or benztropine may be used to control these symptoms.
- Although not yet reported for ziprasidone, monitor for possible tardive dyskinesia (uncontrolled rhythmic movement of mouth, face, and extremities; lip smacking or puckering; puffing of cheeks; uncontrolled chewing; rapid or worm-like movements of tongue). Report these symptoms immediately; may be irreversible.
- Monitor frequency and consistency of bowel movements. ↑ bulk and fluids in the diet may help to minimize constipation.
- Ziprasidone lowers the seizure threshold. Institute seizure precautions for patients with history of seizure disorder.
- Monitor for signs/symptoms of neuroleptic malignant syndrome (fever, respiratory distress, tachycardia, seizures, diaphoresis, hypertension or hypotension, pallor, tiredness). Notify health care provider immediately if these symptoms occur.
- Monitor for signs/symptoms related to hyperprolactinemia (menstrual abnormalities, galactorrhea, sexual dysfunction).
- Assess for falls risk. Drowsiness, orthostatic hypotension, and motor and sensory instability ↑ risk. Institute prevention if indicated.

Lab Test Considerations

- Monitor serum potassium and magnesium before starting and periodically during therapy. Patients with low potassium or magnesium should have levels treated and checked prior to resuming therapy. Obtain fasting blood glucose and cholesterol levels initially and periodically during therapy.
- Monitor CBC frequently during initial months of therapy in patients with pre-existing or history of low WBC. May cause leukopenia, neutropenia, or agranulocytosis. *If leukopenia, neutropenia, or agranulocytosis occurs,* discontinue ziprasidone.
- Monitor serum prolactin before starting and periodically during therapy. May ↑ serum prolactin levels.

Implementation

- Dose adjustments should be made at intervals of no less than 2 days. Usually patients should be observed for several wk before dose titration.
- Patients on parenteral therapy should be converted to oral doses as soon as possible.
- **PO:** Administer capsules with food or milk to ↓ gastric irritation. ***DNC:*** Swallow capsules whole; do not open, crush, or chew.
- **IM: Reconstitution:** Add 1.2 mL of sterile water for injection to the vial; shake vigorously until all drug is dissolved for a concentration of 20 mg/mL. Discard unused portion. Do not mix with other products or solutions. Do not administer solutions that are discolored or contain particulate matter.

Patient/Family Teaching

- Instruct patient to take medication as directed, at the same time each day. Do not discontinue medication without discussing with health care provider, even if feeling well. Patients on long-term therapy may need to discontinue gradually.
- Advise patient of need for continued medical follow-up for psychotherapy, eye exams, and laboratory tests.
- Inform patient of possibility of extrapyramidal symptoms. Instruct patient to report these symptoms immediately.
- Advise patient to change positions slowly to minimize orthostatic hypotension. Protect from falls.
- May cause seizures and drowsiness. Caution patient to avoid driving or other activities requiring alertness until response to medication is known.

- Advise patient to notify health care provider of all Rx or OTC medications, vitamins, or herbal products being taken and to consult with health care provider before taking other medications. Caution patient to avoid concurrent use of alcohol and other CNS depressants, including opioids.
- Advise patient to notify health care provider of medication regimen prior to treatment or surgery.
- Instruct patient to notify health care provider promptly if dizziness, loss of consciousness, palpitations, menstrual abnormalities, galactorrhea, or sexual dysfunction occur.
- Rep: Advise women of reproductive potential to notify health care provider if pregnancy is planned or suspected and to avoid breastfeeding during therapy. Monitor neonates exposed to ziprasidone during 3rd trimester for extrapyramidal and/or withdrawal symptoms. Some neonates recovered within hours or days without specific treatment; others required prolonged hospitalization. Monitor infants exposed through breast milk for excess sedation, irritability, poor feeding, and extrapyramidal symptoms (tremors and abnormal muscle movements). May impair fertility in women. Inform pregnant patients of registry that monitors outcomes in pregnant women exposed to atypical antipsychotics. Register patients by contacting the National Pregnancy Registry for Atypical Antipsychotics at 1-866-961-2388 or visiting http://womensmentalhealth.org/research/pregnancyregistry/.

Evaluation/Desired Outcomes

- Decrease in acute excited, manic behavior.
- Decrease in positive (delusions, hallucinations) and negative symptoms (social withdrawal, flat, blunted affect) of schizophrenia.
- Management of signs and symptoms of bipolar I disorder.

zoledronic acid

(zoe-led-**dron**-ic **as**-id)

✱ Aclasta, Reclast, ✱ Zometa

Classification

Therapeutic: bone resorption inhibitors, electrolyte modifiers, hypocalcemics

Pharmacologic: bisphosphonates

Indications

Hypercalcemia of malignancy. Multiple myeloma and metastatic bone lesions from solid tumors. Paget disease. Treatment of osteoporosis in men. Treatment and prevention of osteoporosis in postmenopausal women. Treatment and prevention of glucocorticoid-induced osteoporosis in patients expected to be on glucocorticoids for ≥12 mo.

Action

Inhibits bone resorption. Inhibits increased osteoclast activity and skeletal calcium release induced by tumors. **Therapeutic Effects:** Decreased serum calcium. Decreased serum alkaline phosphatase. Decreased fractures, radiation/surgery to bone, or spinal cord compression in patients with multiple myeloma or metastatic bone lesions. Decreased hip, vertebral, or nonvertebral osteoporosis-related fractures in postmenopausal women. Increased bone mass in men, postmenopausal women, and patients on prolonged corticosteroid therapy.

Pharmacokinetics

Absorption: IV administration results in complete bioavailability.

Distribution: Concentrated in and binds to bone.

Metabolism and Excretion: Mostly excreted unchanged by the kidneys.

Half-life: 167 hr.

TIME/ACTION PROFILE (effect on serum calcium)

ROUTE	ONSET	PEAK	DURATION
IV	within 4 days	4–7 days	30 days

Contraindications/Precautions

Contraindicated in: Hypersensitivity to zoledronic acid or other bisphosphonates; Severe renal impairment (CCr <35 mL/min) or acute renal failure; Hypocalcemia (correct before administering); adequate supplemental calcium and vitamin D required; OB: Pregnancy.

Use Cautiously in: History of aspirin-induced asthma; Chronic renal impairment, concurrent use of diuretics or nephrotoxic drugs, or dehydration (↑ risk of renal impairment; correct deficits prior to use); Concurrent use of nephrotoxic drugs; Invasive dental procedures; cancer; receiving chemotherapy, corticosteroids, or angiogenesis inhibitors; undergoing radiation; poor oral hygiene; periodontal disease; dental disease; anemia; coagulopathy; infection; or poorly fitting dentures (may ↑ risk of osteonecrosis of the jaw); Lactation: Use while breastfeeding only if potential maternal benefit justifies potential risk to infant; Pedi: Potential for long-term retention in bone in children; use in children only if potential benefit outweighs potential risk; Geri: ↑ risk of renal impairment in older adults.

Adverse Reactions/Side Effects

CV: <u>hypotension</u>, chest pain, leg edema. **Derm:** pruritus, rash, STEVENS-JOHNSON SYNDROME, TOXIC

Z

EPIDERMAL NECROLYSIS. **EENT:** conjunctivitis. **F and E:** hypophosphatemia, hypocalcemia, hypokalemia, hypomagnesemia. **GI:** abdominal pain, constipation, diarrhea, nausea, vomiting, dysphagia. **GU:** ↓ fertility (women), renal impairment/failure. **Hemat:** anemia. **MS:** musculoskeletal pain, femur fractures, osteonecrosis (primarily of the jaw). **Neuro:** agitation, anxiety, confusion, insomnia. **Resp:** asthma exacerbation. **Misc:** fever, flu-like syndrome.

Interactions

Drug-Drug: Loop diuretics, calcitonin, or **aminoglycosides** may ↑ risk of hypocalcemia. **NSAIDs** may ↑ risk of nephrotoxicity.

Route/Dosage

Paget Disease

IV (Adults): 5 mg as a single dose (information regarding retreatment unknown).

Treatment of Osteoporosis in Men or Postmenopausal Women or Treatment/Prevention of Glucocorticoid-Induced Osteoporosis

IV (Adults): 5 mg once yearly.

Prevention of Osteoporosis in Postmenopausal Women

IV (Adults): 5 mg every 2 yr.

Hypercalcemia of Malignancy

IV (Adults): 4 mg; may be repeated after 7 days.

Multiple Myeloma or Bone Metastases from Solid Tumors

IV (Adults): 4 mg every 3–4 wk (has been used for up to 15 mo).

Availability (generic available)

Premixed infusion: 4 mg/100 mL, 5 mg/100 mL. **Solution for injection:** 0.8 mg/mL.

NURSING IMPLICATIONS

Assessment

- Monitor intake and output. Initiate a vigorous saline hydration promptly and maintain a urine output of 2 L/day during therapy. Patients should be adequately hydrated, but avoid overhydration. Do not use diuretics before treatment of hypovolemia.
- Assess for acute-phase reaction (fever, myalgia, flu-like symptoms, headache, arthralgia). Usually occur within 3 days of dose and resolve within 3 days of onset, but may take 7–14 days to resolve; incidence ↓ with repeat dosing.
- Perform a routine oral exam before starting therapy. Dental exam with appropriate preventative dentistry should be considered before therapy. Patients with history of tooth extraction; poor oral hygiene; gingival infections; diabetes, cancer; receiving radiation; anemia; coagulopathy; use of a dental appliance; or taking immunosuppressive therapy, angiogenesis inhibitors, or systemic corticosteroids are at ↑ risk for jaw osteonecrosis.
- **Hypercalcemia:** Monitor signs/symptoms of hypercalcemia (nausea, vomiting, anorexia, weakness, constipation, thirst, cardiac arrhythmias).
- Assess for hypocalcemia (paresthesia, muscle twitching, laryngospasm, Chvostek or Trousseau sign).
- **Paget Disease:** Assess for signs/symptoms of Paget disease (bone pain, headache, ↓ visual and auditory acuity, ↑ skull size) periodically during therapy.
- **Osteoporosis:** Assess patient via bone density study for ↓ bone mass before and periodically during therapy.

Lab Test Considerations

- Verify negative pregnancy test before starting therapy.
- Monitor CCr, calculated based on actual body weight using the Cockcroft-Gault formula, before each treatment. Patients with a normal serum creatinine before treatment who develop an ↑ of 0.5 mg/dL within 2 wk of next dose should have next dose withheld until serum creatinine is within 10% of baseline value. Patients with an abnormal serum creatinine before treatment and with an ↑ of 1 mg/dL within 2 wk of next dose should have next dose withheld until serum creatinine is within 10% of baseline value.
- Assess serum calcium, phosphate, and magnesium before and periodically during therapy. If hypocalcemia, hypophosphatemia, or hypomagnesemia occur, temporary supplementation may be required. Hypocalcemia and vitamin D deficiency should be treated before initiating zoledronic acid therapy.
- Monitor CBC with differential and hemoglobin and hematocrit closely during therapy.
- *Paget Disease:* Monitor serum alkaline phosphatase before and periodically during therapy to monitor effectiveness.

Implementation

- Vigorous saline hydration alone may be sufficient to treat mild, asymptomatic hypercalcemia. Adequate rehydration is required before administration.
- Patients treated for Paget disease should take 1500 mg of calcium and 800 units of vitamin D each day, particularly during the 2 wk after dosing. Patients with osteoporosis should take 1200 mg of calcium and 800–1000 units of vitamin D each day. Patients with multiple myeloma and bone metastasis of solid tumors should take 500 mg of calcium and 400 units of vitamin D each day.
- Administration of acetaminophen or ibuprofen following administration may ↓ the incidence of acute-phase reaction symptoms.

IV Administration

- **Intermittent Infusion:**
- **Dilution:** Dilute 4 mg in 100 mL of 0.9% NaCl or D5W. If not used immediately, may be refrigerated for up to 24 hr. *Reclast* comes ready to use 5 mg in 100 mL solution. If refrigerated, allow solution to reach room temperature before administration. Do not administer solution that is discolored or contains particulate matter. **Concentration:** 0.04–0.05 mg/mL. **Rate:** Administer infusion over >15 min. Rapid infusions ↑ risk of renal deterioration and renal failure.
- **Y-Site Compatibility:** acyclovir, allopurinol, amikacin, aminocaproic acid, aminophylline, amiodarone, amphotericin B liposomal, ampicillin, ampicillin/sulbactam, anidulafungin, argatroban, arsenic trioxide, azithromycin, aztreonam, bivalirudin, bleomycin, bumetanide, buprenorphine, busulfan, butorphanol, carboplatin, carmustine, caspofungin, cefazolin, cefepime, cefotaxime, cefotetan, cefoxitin, ceftazidime, ceftriaxone, cefuroxime, chloramphenicol, chlorpromazine, ciprofloxacin, cisatracurium, cisplatin, clindamycin, cyclophosphamide, cyclosporine, cytarabine, dacarbazine, dactinomycin, daptomycin, daunorubicin, dexamethasone, dexmedetomidine, dexrazoxane, digoxin, diltiazem, diphenhydramine, dobutamine, docetaxel, dopamine, doxorubicin, doxorubicin liposomal, doxycycline, droperidol, enalaprilat, ephedrine, epinephrine, epirubicin, eptifibatide, ertapenem, erythromycin, esmolol, etoposide, etoposide phosphate, famotidine, fentanyl, fluconazole, fludarabine, fluorouracil, foscarnet, fosphenytoin, furosemide, ganciclovir, gemcitabine, gentamicin, glycopyrrolate, granisetron, haloperidol, heparin, hydralazine, hydrocortisone, hydromorphone, idarubicin, ifosfamide, imipenem/cilastatin, insulin regular, irinotecan, isoproterenol, ketorolac, labetalol, levofloxacin, lidocaine, linezolid, lorazepam, magnesium sulfate, mannitol, melphalan, meperidine, meropenem, mesna, methadone, methotrexate, methylprednisolone, metoclopramide, metoprolol, metronidazole, midazolam, milrinone, mitomycin, mitoxantrone, morphine, moxifloxacin, mycophenolate, nafcillin, nalbuphine, naloxone, nicardipine, nitroglycerin, nitroprusside, norepinephrine, octreotide, ondansetron, oxaliplatin, oxytocin, paclitaxel, pantoprazole, pemetrexed, pentamidine, pentobarbital, phenobarbital, phenylephrine, piperacillin/tazobactam, potassium acetate, potassium chloride, potassium phosphates, procainamide, prochlorperazine, promethazine, propranolol, remifentanil, rocuronium, sodium acetate, sodium bicarbonate, sodium phosphates, succinylcholine, sufentanil, tacrolimus, theophylline, thiotepa, tigecycline, tirofiban, tobramycin, topotecan, trimethoprim/sulfamethoxazole, vancomycin, vecuronium, verapamil, vinblastine, vincristine, vinorelbine, voriconazole, zidovudine.
- **Y-Site Incompatibility:** alemtuzumab, dantrolene, diazepam, gemtuzumab ozogamicin, phenytoin..

Patient/Family Teaching

- Explain purpose and side effects of medication to patient. Advise patient to read *Patient Information* before starting therapy. Emphasize the importance of lab tests to monitor progress.
- Advise patient to notify health care provider of all Rx or OTC medications, vitamins, or herbal products being taken and to consult with health care provider before taking other medications.
- Advise patient of the importance of adequate hydration. Patient should be instructed to drink ≥2 glasses of water before receiving dose.
- Advise patient to eat a balanced diet and consult health care provider about the need for supplemental calcium and vitamin D.
- Inform patient that severe musculoskeletal pain may occur within days, months, or years after starting zoledronic acid. Symptoms may resolve completely after discontinuation or slow or incomplete resolution may occur. Notify health care provider if severe pain occurs.
- Encourage patient to participate in regular exercise and to modify behaviors that ↑ the risk of osteoporosis (smoking cessation, ↓ alcohol consumption).
- Advise patient to notify health care provider if signs and symptoms of jaw osteonecrosis (pain, numbness, swelling of, or drainage from the jaw, mouth, or teeth) or hypocalcemia (spasms, twitches, or cramps in muscles; numbness or tingling in fingers, toes, or around mouth) or thigh, hip, or groin pain occur.
- Advise patient to inform health care provider of zoledronic acid therapy before dental surgery.
- Rep: May cause fetal harm. Advise women of reproductive potential to use effective contraception and avoid breastfeeding during and after therapy. May impair fertility in women.

Evaluation/Desired Outcomes

- Decreased serum calcium.
- Decreased serum alkaline phosphatase.
- Decreased fractures, radiation/surgery to bone, or spinal cord compression in patients with multiple myeloma or metastatic bone lesions.

Z

- Decreased hip, vertebral, or nonvertebral osteoporosis-related fractures in postmenopausal women.
- Increased bone mass in men, postmenopausal women, and patients on prolonged corticosteroid therapy.

ZOLMitriptan (zole-mi-trip-tan)

Zomig, Zomig Rapimelt, ~~Zomig-ZMT~~

Classification

Therapeutic: vascular headache suppressants

Pharmacologic: 5-HT_1 agonists

Indications

Acute treatment of migraine headache.

Action

Acts as an agonist at specific 5-HT_1 receptor sites in intracranial blood vessels and sensory trigeminal nerves. **Therapeutic Effects:** Relief of acute attacks of migraine.

Pharmacokinetics

Absorption: Well absorbed (40%) following oral and intranasal administration.

Distribution: Unknown.

Metabolism and Excretion: Mostly metabolized by the liver; some conversion to metabolites that are more active than zolmitriptan. 8% excreted unchanged in urine.

Half-life: 3 hr (for zolmitriptan and active metabolite).

TIME/ACTION PROFILE (relief of headache)

ROUTE	ONSET	PEAK	DURATION
PO	unknown	1.5 hr*	unknown
Intranasal	unknown	3 hr	unknown

* 3 hr for orally disintegrating tablets.

Contraindications/Precautions

Contraindicated in: Hypersensitivity; Significant underlying heart disease (including ischemic heart disease, history of MI, coronary artery vasospasm, uncontrolled hypertension); Stroke or transient ischemic attack; Peripheral vascular disease (including but not limited to ischemic bowel disease); Concurrent (or within 24 hr) use of other 5-HT agonists, ergotamine, or ergot-type medications; Hemiplegic or basilar migraine; Symptomatic Wolff-Parkinson-White syndrome or other arrhythmias; Moderate to severe hepatic impairment (nasal spray only).

Use Cautiously in: Cardiovascular risk factors (hypertension, hypercholesterolemia, cigarette smoking, obesity, diabetes, strong family history, menopausal women, men>40 yr [use only if cardiovascular status has been evaluated and determined to be safe and 1st dose is administered under supervision]); Hepatic impairment (use lower doses of oral); **OB:** Safety not established in pregnancy; **Lactation:** Use while breastfeeding only if potential maternal benefit justifies potential risk to infant; **Pedi:** Safety and effectiveness not established in children <18 yr (oral); children <12 yr (intranasal).

Adverse Reactions/Side Effects

CV: angina, chest pain/pressure/tightness/heaviness, hypertension, MI, palpitations. **Derm:** sweating, warm/cold sensation. **EENT:** throat pain/tightness/pressure. **GI:** dry mouth, dyspepsia, dysphagia, nausea. **MS:** myalgia, myasthenia. **Neuro:** dizziness, drowsiness, hypoesthesia, paresthesia, vertigo, weakness.

Interactions

Drug-Drug: Because of ↑ risk of cerebral vasospasm, avoid concurrent use of other **5-HT agonists (naratriptan, sumatriptan, rizatriptan)** and/or **ergot-type preparations (dihydroergotamine)**. **MAO inhibitors** ↑ levels and risk of toxicity; avoid use within 2 wk of MAO inhibitors. **Hormonal contraceptives** may ↑ levels and risk of toxicity. **Cimetidine** ↑ levels and risk of toxicity. ↑ risk of serotonin syndrome with **SSRIs**, **SNRIs**, **TCAs**, **triptans**, **meperidine**, **bupropion**, or **buspirone**; avoid concurrent use.

Drug-Natural Products: ↑ risk of serotonergic side effects including serotonin syndrome with **St. John's wort** and **SAMe**.

Route/Dosage

PO (Adults): 1.25–2.5 mg initially; if headache returns, dose may be repeated after 2 hr (not to exceed 10 mg/24 hr); *Concurrent use of cimetidine:* Single dose not to exceed 2.5 mg (not to exceed 5 mg/24 hr).

Hepatic Impairment

PO (Adults): *Moderate to severe hepatic impairment (oral tablets only):* 1.25 mg initially; if headache returns, dose may be repeated after 2 hr (not to exceed 5 mg/24 hr).

Intranasal (Adults and Children ≥12 yr): Single 2.5 mg initially (maximum single dose = 5 mg); may be repeated after 2 hr (not to exceed 10 mg/24 hr); *Concurrent use of cimetidine:* Single dose not to exceed 2.5 mg (not to exceed 5 mg/24 hr).

Availability (generic available)

Tablets: 2.5 mg, 5 mg. **Orally disintegrating tablets:** 2.5 mg, 5 mg. **Nasal spray:** 2.5 mg/100 mcL unit-dose spray device (package of 6), 5 mg/100 mcL unit-dose spray device (package of 6).

NURSING IMPLICATIONS

Assessment

- Assess pain location, intensity, duration, and associated symptoms (photophobia, phonophobia, nausea, vomiting) during migraine attack.

- Monitor for serotonin syndrome in patients taking SSRIs or SNRIs concurrently with zolmitriptan.

Implementation

- Do not confuse zolmitriptan with sumatriptan.
- **PO:** Initial dose is 2.5 mg. Lower doses can be achieved by breaking 2.5-mg tablet.
- *Orally disintegrating tablets* should be left in the package until use. Remove from the blister pouch. Do not push tablet through the blister; peel open the blister pack with dry hands and place tablet on tongue. Do not break orally disintegrating tablet. Tablet will dissolve rapidly and be swallowed with saliva. No liquid is needed to take the orally disintegrating tablet.
- **Intranasal:** Remove cap from nasal spray. Hold upright and block 1 nostril. Tilt head slightly back, insert devicc into opposite nostril, and depress plunger. May repeat in 2 hr.

Patient/Family Teaching

- Explain purpose and side effects of medication to patient. Advise patient to read *Patient Information* before starting therapy.
- Advise patient to notify health care provider of all Rx or OTC medications, vitamins, or herbal products being taken and to consult with health care provider before taking other medications.
- Advise patient that zolmitriptan should be used only during a migraine attack. It is meant to be used to relieve migraine attack, not to prevent or ↓ the number of attacks.
- Advise patient to administer zolmitriptan as soon as symptoms appear, but it may be administered any time during an attack. If migraine symptoms return, a 2nd dose may be used. Allow ≥2 hr between doses, and do not use >10 mg in any 24-hr period.
- If dose does not relieve headache, additional zolmitriptan doses are not likely to be effective; notify health care provider.
- Advise patient that lying down in a darkened room following zolmitriptan administration may further help relieve headache.
- May cause dizziness or drowsiness. Caution patient to avoid driving or other activities requiring alertness until response to medication is known.
- Advise patient to notify health care provider before next dose of zolmitriptan if pain or tightness in the chest occurs during use. If pain is severe or does not subside, notify health care provider immediately. If wheezing; heart throbbing; swelling of eyelids, face, or lips; skin rash; skin lumps; or hives occur, notify health care provider immediately and do not take more zolmitriptan without approval of health care provider. If feelings of tingling, heat, flushing, heaviness, pressure, drowsiness, dizziness, tiredness, or sickness develop, discuss with health care provider at next visit.
- Advise patient to avoid alcohol, which aggravates headaches, during zolmitriptan use.
- Advise patient that overuse (>10 days/mo) may lead to exacerbation of headache (migraine-like daily headaches or as a marked ↑ in frequency of migraine attacks). May require gradual withdrawal of zolmitriptan and treatment of symptoms (transient worsening of headache).
- Advise patient taking SSRI or SNRI antidepressants to notify health care provider if signs/symptoms of serotonin syndrome (mental status changes [agitation, hallucinations, coma], autonomic instability [tachycardia, labile BP, hyperthermia], neuromuscular aberrations [hyperreflexia, incoordination], gastrointestinal symptoms [nausea, vomiting, diarrhea]) occur.
- Rep: Advise women of reproductive potential to notify health care provider if pregnancy is planned or suspected or if breastfeeding. Holding breastfeeding for 24 hr after the maternal dose will minimize infant exposure via breast milk.

Evaluation/Desired Outcomes

- Relief of acute attacks of migraine.

BEERS

zolpidem (zole-pi-dem)

Ambien, Ambien CR, Edluar,
🍁 Sublinox

Classification

Therapeutic: sedative/hypnotics

Schedule IV

Indications

Insomnia with difficulties in sleep initiation (generic sublingual tablets are indicated for insomnia when a middle-of-the-night awakening is followed by difficulty returning to sleep).

Action

Produces CNS depression by binding to GABA receptors. Has no analgesic properties. **Therapeutic Effects:** Sedation and induction of sleep.

Pharmacokinetics

Absorption: Rapidly absorbed following oral administration. Controlled-release formulation releases 10 mg immediately, then another 2.5 mg later.

Distribution: Unknown.

Z

Metabolism and Excretion: Converted to inactive metabolites, which are excreted by the kidneys; clearance of sublingual tablet lower in women than in men.
Half-life: 2.5–3 hr (↑ in older adults and patients with hepatic impairment).

TIME/ACTION PROFILE (sedation)

ROUTE	ONSET	PEAK*	DURATION
PO	rapid	30 min–2 hr	6–8 hr
PO-ER	rapid	2–4 hr	6–8 hr
SL	rapid	unknown	unknown

* Food delays peak levels and effects.

Contraindications/Precautions

Contraindicated in: Hypersensitivity; History of experiencing complex sleep behaviors with zolpidem; Severe hepatic impairment (↑ risk of hepatic encephalopathy).
Use Cautiously in: History of previous psychiatric illness, suicide attempt, or drug or alcohol abuse; Pulmonary disease; Sleep apnea; Myasthenia gravis; Mild or moderate hepatic impairment (↑ risk of hepatic encephalopathy; ↓ initial dose); OB: May ↑ risk of respiratory depression in neonates after birth; Lactation: Use while breastfeeding only if potential maternal benefit justifies potential risk in infants; Pedi: Safety and effectiveness not established in children; Geri: Appears on Beers list. ↑ risk of cognitive impairment, delirium, falls, fractures, and motor vehicle accidents in older adults. Avoid use in older adults.

Adverse Reactions/Side Effects

EENT: blurred vision, double vision. **GI:** diarrhea, nausea, vomiting. **Neuro:** daytime drowsiness, dizziness, abnormal thinking, agitation, amnesia, behavior changes, COMPLEX SLEEP BEHAVIORS (INCLUDING SLEEP-DRIVING, SLEEP-WALKING, OR ENGAGING IN OTHER ACTIVITIES WHILE SLEEPING), delirium, hallucinations, prolonged reaction time. **Resp:** respiratory depression. **Misc:** HYPERSENSITIVITY REACTIONS (INCLUDING ANAPHYLAXIS), physical dependence, psychological dependence, tolerance.

Interactions

Drug-Drug: ↑ risk of CNS and respiratory depression with **sedatives/hypnotics**, **alcohol**, **phenothiazines**, **tricyclic antidepressants**, **opioids**, or **antihistamines**. **CYP3A4 inducers**, including **rifampin**, may ↓ levels and effectiveness. **CYP3A4 inhibitors**, including **ketoconazole**, may ↑ levels and risk of toxicity; consider ↓ zolpidem dose.
Drug-Natural Products: Kava-kava, **valerian**, or **chamomile** can ↑ risk of CNS depression. **St. John's wort** may ↓ levels and effectiveness; avoid concurrent use.
Drug-Food: Food ↓ and delays absorption.

Route/Dosage

PO, SL (Adults): *Tablets or SL tablets (Edluar):* 5 mg (for women) and 5–10 mg (for men) at bedtime; may ↑ to 10 mg at bedtime if 5-mg dose not effective; *SL tablets (generic):* 1.75 mg (for women) or 3.5 mg (for men) once upon awakening in the middle of the night; *Extended-release tablets:* 6.25 mg (for women) and 6.25–12.5 mg (for men) at bedtime; may ↑ to 12.5 mg at bedtime if 6.25-mg dose not effective.
PO, SL (Geriatric Patients, Debilitated Patients, or Patients with Mild/Moderate Hepatic Impairment): *Tablets or SL tablets (Edluar):* Do not exceed dose of 5 mg at bedtime; *Extended-release tablets:* Do not exceed dose of 6.25 mg at bedtime.
SL (Geriatric Patients, Patients Taking Concurrent CNS Depressants, or Patients with Mild/Moderate Hepatic Impairment): *SL tablets (generic):* Do not exceed dose of 1.75 mg at bedtime (in either men or women).

Availability (generic available)

Immediate-release tablets: 5 mg, 10 mg. **Immediate-release capsules:** 7.5 mg. **Extended-release tablets:** 6.25 mg, 12.5 mg. **Sublingual tablets (Edluar):** 5 mg, 10 mg. **Sublingual tablets:** 1.75 mg, 3.5 mg.

NURSING IMPLICATIONS

Assessment

- Assess mental status, sleep patterns, and potential for abuse prior to administration. Prolonged use for >7–10 days may lead to physical and psychological dependence. Limit amount of drug available to the patient.
- Assess alertness at time of peak effect. Notify health care provider if desired sedation does not occur.
- Assess for pain. Medicate as needed. Untreated pain ↓ sedative effects.
- Monitor respiratory status; ↑ risk of respiratory depression should be considered before prescribing zolpidem in patients with respiratory impairment, including sleep apnea and myasthenia gravis, or with concurrent opioid use.
- Assess for complex sleep behaviors (sleep-walking, sleep-driving, or engaging in activities while not fully awake). May cause serious injuries and even death; if these behaviors occur, discontinue immediately if identified.

Implementation

- ***High Alert:*** Do not confuse Ambien with ambrisentan. Do not confuse zolpidem with Zyloprim.
- Before administering, ↓ external stimuli and provide comfort measures to ↑ effectiveness of medication.

- Implement safety measures to protect patient from injury.
- Use lowest effective dose.
- **PO:** Swallow tablets whole with full glass of water. For faster onset of sleep, do not administer with or immediately after a meal.
- *DNC:* Swallow extended-release tablets whole; do not crush, break, or chew.
- **SL:** To open the blister pack, separate the individual blisters at the perforations. Peel off top layer of paper and push tablet through foil. Place the tablet under the tongue; allow to disintegrate; do not swallow or take with water.
- Only take if ≥4 hr left before awakening.

Patient/Family Teaching

- Explain purpose and side effects of medication to patient. Advise patient to read *Patient Information* before starting therapy. Instruct patient to take as directed. Take as a single dose and do not readminister during the same night. Advise patient not to take zolpidem unless able to stay in bed a full night (7–8 hr) before being active again. Do not take more than the amount prescribed because of the habit-forming potential. Not recommended for use >7–10 days. If used for >2 wk, abrupt withdrawal may result in fatigue, nausea, flushing, light-headedness, uncontrolled crying, vomiting, GI upset, panic attack, or nervousness.
- Advise patient to notify health care provider of all Rx or OTC medications, vitamins, or herbal products being taken and to consult health care provider before taking other medications.
- Because of rapid onset, advise patient to go to bed immediately after taking zolpidem.
- May cause daytime drowsiness or dizziness. Advise patient to avoid driving or other activities requiring alertness until response to this medication is known.
- Caution patient that complex sleep-related behaviors (sleep-driving, making phone calls, preparing and eating food, having sex, sleep walking) may occur while asleep. Inform patient to notify health care provider if sleep-related behaviors occur.
- Advise patient to notify health care provider immediately if signs/symptoms of anaphylaxis (swelling of the tongue or throat, trouble breathing, nausea, vomiting) occur.
- Caution patient to avoid concurrent use of alcohol or other CNS depressants, including opioids.
- Rep: Advise women of reproductive potential to notify health care provider if pregnancy is planned or suspected or if breastfeeding. Monitor neonates exposed to zolpidem during pregnancy and breastfeeding for signs of excess sedation, hypotonia, and respiratory depression.

Evaluation/Desired Outcomes

- Sedation and induction of sleep.

zuranolone (zoo-ran-oh-lone)

Zurzuvae

Classification

Therapeutic: antidepressants

Pharmacologic: corticosteroids, gamma aminobutyric acid (GABA) enhancers

Schedule IV

Indications

Postpartum depression.

Action

Although not fully understood, thought to be related to positive allosteric modulation of GABA-A receptors. **Therapeutic Effects:** Reduction in depressive symptoms.

Pharmacokinetics

Absorption: Extent of absorption following oral administration unknown. Absorption ↑ with fat-containing foods.

Distribution: Extensively distributed to tissues.

Metabolism and Excretion: Extensively metabolized in the liver via the CYP3A4 isoenzyme to inactive metabolites. 45% excreted in urine; 41% excreted in feces primarily as metabolites.

Half-life: 19.7–24.6 hr.

TIME/ACTION PROFILE (↓ in depressive symptoms)

ROUTE	ONSET	PEAK	DURATION
PO	3 days	unknown	at least 45 days

Contraindications/Precautions

Contraindicated in: OB: Pregnancy.

Use Cautiously in: History of substance use disorder or drug abuse; Moderate or severe renal impairment; Severe hepatic impairment; Rep: Women of reproductive potential; Lactation: Use while breastfeeding only if potential maternal benefit justifies potential risk to infant; Pedi: Safety and effectiveness not established in children.

Adverse Reactions/Side Effects

Derm: rash. **EENT:** nasopharyngitis, sinus congestion. **GI:** abdominal pain, diarrhea, dry mouth. **GU:** urinary tract infection. **MS:** muscle twitching, myalgia. **Neuro:** dizziness, sedation, anxiety, confusion, fatigue, gait disturbances, memory impairment, SUICIDAL THOUGHTS/BEHAVIORS, tremor. **Misc:** physical dependence.

Interactions

Drug-Drug: Use with **benzodiazepines** or other **CNS depressants**, including **opioids**, **nonbenzodiazepine sedative/hypnotics**, **anxiolytics**, **muscle relaxants**, and **alcohol**, may cause profound sedation, loss of consciousness, or respiratory depression; avoid concurrent use; if concurrent use unavoidable, ↓ zuranolone dose. **Strong CYP3A4 inhibitors**, including **itraconazole**, may ↑ levels and risk of toxicity; ↓ zuranolone dose. **Strong CYP3A4 inducers**, including **rifampin**, may ↓ levels and effectiveness; avoid concurrent use.

Route/Dosage

PO (Adults): 50 mg once daily in the evening for 14 days. If patients experience CNS adverse effects within the 14-day period, consider ↓ dose to 40 mg once daily in the evening within the 14-day period. *Concurrent use of strong CYP3A4 inhibitors:* 30 mg once daily in the evening for 14 days.

Renal Impairment

PO (Adults): *eGFR <60 mL/min/1.73 m²:* 30 mg once daily in the evening for 14 days.

Hepatic Impairment

PO (Adults): *Severe hepatic impairment:* 30 mg once daily in the evening for 14 days.

Availability

Capsules: 20 mg, 25 mg, 30 mg.

NURSING IMPLICATIONS

Assessment

- Monitor for mood changes (new or worsening depression or anxiety, agitation or restlessness, panic attacks, insomnia, new or worsening irritability, aggression, acting on dangerous impulses, mania).
- Assess for suicidal thoughts and behaviors, especially in patients ≤24 yr.
- Assess for potential risks of misuse, abuse, and addition due to potential physical dependence.

Implementation

- Administer once daily in the evening for 14 days with fat-containing food (400–1000 calories, 25–50% fat).

Patient/Family Teaching

- Explain purpose and side effects of medication to patient. Advise patient to read *Patient Information* before starting therapy. Instruct patient to take as directed. If an evening dose is missed, take next dose at the regular time the following evening. Do not take extra capsules on the same day to make up for the missed dose. Continue taking once daily until remainder of 14-day treatment course is completed.
- Instruct patient to notify health care provider of all Rx or OTC medications, vitamins, or herbal products being taken and consult health care provider before taking any new medications. Advise patient to avoid taking other CNS depressants, including alcohol, benzodiazepines, opioids, and tricyclic antidepressants; may cause falls, somnolence, cognitive impairment, and respiratory depression.
- Inform patients that zuranolone causes driving impairment due to CNS depressant effects. Caution patient to avoid driving and other activities requiring alertness until >12 hr after zuranolone administration for the duration of the 14-day treatment course. Inform patients that they may not be able to assess their own driving competence or the degree of driving impairment caused by zuranolone.
- Advise patient, family, and caregivers to look for suicidality, especially during early therapy or dose changes. Notify health care provider immediately if thoughts about suicide or dying, attempts to commit suicide, new or worsening depression or anxiety, agitation or restlessness, panic attacks, insomnia, new or worsening irritability, aggression, acting on dangerous impulses, mania, or other changes in mood or behavior occur.
- Advise patient about potential risks of misuse, abuse, and substance use disorder (addiction).
- Rep: May cause fetal harm. Advise women of reproductive potential to use effective contraception during treatment with zuranolone and for 1 wk after the final dose. Advise pregnant patients of the potential risk of infant exposed to zuranolone in utero. Advise women with reproductive potential to notify health care provider if pregnancy is planned or suspected or if breastfeeding. There is a pregnancy exposure registry that monitors pregnancy outcomes in patients exposed to antidepressants, including zuranolone, during pregnancy. Health care providers are encouraged to register patients by calling the National Pregnancy Registry for Antidepressants at 1-866-961-2388 or visiting online at https://womensmentalhealth.org/research/pregnancyregistry/antidepressants/.

Evaluation/Desired Outcomes

- Reduction in depressive symptoms.

Drugs Approved in Canada

These monographs describe medications approved for use in Canada by the Therapeutic Products Directorate, a division of Health Canada's Health Products and Food Branch. The medications are not approved by the United States Food and Drug Administration.

alfacalcidol (al-fa-kal-si-dol)

One-Alpha

Classification
Therapeutic: vitamins
Pharmacologic: vitamin D analogues

Indications

Hypocalcemia, secondary hyperparathyroidism, and osteodystrophy associated with chronic renal failure.

Action

Stimulates intestinal absorption of calcium and phosphorus, reabsorption of calcium from bone, and renal reabsorption of calcium. Does not require renal activation. **Therapeutic Effects:** Improved calcium and phosphorus homeostasis in patients with chronic kidney disease.

Pharmacokinetics

Absorption: Completely absorbed following oral administration.
Distribution: Unknown.
Protein Binding: Extensively to vitamin D–binding protein.
Metabolism and Excretion: Following absorption, 50% is rapidly converted by liver to active metabolite (1,25–$(OH)_2D_3$; 13% renally excreted.
Half-life: 3 hr.

TIME/ACTION PROFILE (plasma concentrations of active metabolite)

ROUTE	ONSET†	PEAK	DURATION‡
PO	6 hr	12 hr	few days–1 wk
IV	unknown	4 hr	few days–1 wk

† Effect on intestinal calcium absorption, bone pain, and muscle weakness improve within 2 wk–3 mo.
‡ Effect on serum calcium concentrations following discontinuation.

Contraindications/Precautions

Contraindicated in: Hypersensitivity, Lactation: Lactation.
Use Cautiously in: OB: Use during pregnancy only if potential maternal benefit justifies potential fetal risk; Pedi: Safety and effectiveness not established in children.

Adverse Reactions/Side Effects

CV: ARRHYTHMIAS, hypertension. **Derm:** pruritus, rash. **EENT:** conjunctivitis, photophobia. **F and E:** ↑ thirst, HYPERCALCEMIA, hyperphosphatemia, hyperthermia, polydipsia. **GI:** constipation, nausea, anorexia, dry mouth, PANCREATITIS, vomiting. **GU:** ↓ libido, albuminuria, hypercalciuria, nocturia, polyuria. **Metab:** hypercholesterolemia, hyperthermia. **MS:** arthralgia, myalgia. **Neuro:** headache, drowsiness, dysgeusia, weakness.

Interactions

Drug-Drug: Hypercalcemia ↑ risk of toxicity from **digoxin**. ↑ risk of toxicity with other **vitamin D analogs**. **Bile acid sequestrants**, including **cholestyramine**, or **mineral oil** may ↓ absorption and effectiveness. **Barbiturates** and other **anticonvulsants** may ↓ levels and effectiveness; larger doses of alfacalcidol may be required.

Route/Dosage

PO (Adults): *Predialysis patients:* 0.25 mcg/day for 2 mo initially; if necessary, ↑ dose by 0.25 mcg/day every 2 mo (usual range 0.5–1 mcg/day); *Dialysis patients:* 1 mcg/day; if necessary, ↑ dose by 0.5 mcg/day every 2–4 wk (usual range 1–2 mcg/day; max = 3 mcg/day). When normalization occurs, ↓ dose to minimum amount required to maintain normal serum calcium concentrations.
IV (Adults): *Dialysis patients:* 1 mcg during each dialysis session (2–3 times weekly); if necessary, ↑ dose weekly by 1 mcg per dialysis session up to 12 mcg/wk (range 1.5–12 mcg/wk). When normalization occurs, ↓ dose to minimum amount required to maintain normal serum calcium concentrations.

Availability

Soft gel capsules: 0.25 mcg, 1 mcg. **Oral drops:** 2 mcg/mL. **Solution for injection (contains ethanol and propylene glycol):** 2 mcg/mL.

NURSING IMPLICATIONS

Assessment

- Assess for signs of vitamin D deficiency before and during treatment.
- Assess for bone pain and weakness during therapy; usually ↓ within 2 wk to 3 mo.

Lab Test Considerations

- *For predialysis patients:* Monitor serum calcium and phosphate concentrations monthly and electrolytes periodically during treatment. *For dialysis patients:* Monitor serum calcium at least twice weekly during dose titration. If hypercalcemia occurs, ↓ dose of alfacalcidol by 50% and stop all calcium supplements until calcium concentrations return to normal. May ↑ plasma phosphorous concentrations. Maintain serum phosphate concentrations <2 mmol/L. Monitor inorganic phosphorus, magnesium, alkaline phosphatase, serum creatinine, BUN, 24-hr urinary calcium, and protein as needed.

Toxicity and Overdose

- Toxicity is manifested as hypercalcemia, hypercalciuria, and hyperphosphatemia. Assess for appearance of nausea, vomiting, anorexia, weakness, constipation, headache, bone pain, and metallic taste. Later symptoms include polyuria, polydipsia, photophobia, rhinorrhea, pruritus, and cardiac arrhythmias. Notify health care provider immediately if these signs/symptoms of hypervitaminosis D occur. Treatment usually consists of discontinuation of alfacalcidol, a low-calcium diet, and stopping calcium supplements. Persistent or markedly ↑ serum calcium concentrations in dialysis patients may be corrected by dialysis against a calcium-free dialysate.

Implementation

- **PO:** Administer with food. Swallow capsules whole; do not divide. Use calibrated dropper with oral solution for accurate dose. Oral solution may be mixed with water or milk.
- **IV:** Administer IV during hemodialysis. Shake well before use. Keep refrigerated. Single use vials; discard unused portion.

Patient/Family Teaching

- Explain purpose and side effects of medication to patient. Advise patient to read *Patient Information* before starting therapy. Advise patient to take medication as directed. Do not stop taking without consulting with health care provider. If dose is missed, take missed dose as soon as possible. If it is almost time for the next dose, skip dose and administer on regular schedule. Do not double the dose.
- Advise patient to notify health care provider of all Rx or OTC medications, vitamins, or herbal products being taken and to consult with health care provider before taking other medications.
- Advise patient and family/caregiver to notify health care provider if signs/symptoms of hypercalcemia occur.
- Review diet modifications with patient. See Appendix J for foods high in calcium and vitamin D. Patients with kidney disease must still consider renal failure diet in food selection. Health care provider may order concurrent calcium supplement.
- Encourage patient to comply with dietary recommendations. Explain that best source of vitamins is a well-balanced diet with foods from all four basic food groups and sunlight exposure for vitamin D.
- Advise patient to avoid concurrent use of antacids containing magnesium during therapy.
- Rep: Advise women of reproductive potential to notify health care provider if pregnancy is planned or suspected or if breastfeeding.

Evaluation/Desired Outcomes

- Improved calcium and phosphorous concentrations in patients with kidney disease.

bezafibrate (bezz-uh-fibe-rate)

Bezalip SR

Classification

Therapeutic: lipid-lowering agents

Pharmacologic: fibric acid derivatives

Indications

Use in conjunction with diet and other modalities in the treatment of hypercholesterolemia (type IIa and IIb mixed hyperlipidemia, to ↓ serum TG, LDL-C, and apolipoprotein B and ↑ HDL-C and apolipoprotein A). Hypertriglyceridemia (type IV and V hyperlipidemias) in patients at risk of pancreatitis and other sequelae.

Action

Inhibits TG synthesis. **Therapeutic Effects:** Lowered cholesterol and TGs, ↑ HDL-C, with ↓ risk of pancreatitis and other sequelae.

Pharmacokinetics

Absorption: Well absorbed (100%) following oral administration.

Distribution: Unknown.

Metabolism and Excretion: 50% metabolized. 50% excreted unchanged in urine; 3% excreted in feces.

Half-life: 1–2 hr.

TIME/ACTION PROFILE (plasma concentrations)

ROUTE	ONSET	PEAK	DURATION
PO	unknown	3–4 hr	24 hr

Contraindications/Precautions

Contraindicated in: Hypersensitivity/photosensitivity to bezafibrate or other fibric acid or fibrate derivatives; Severe hepatic or renal impairment (CCr <60 mL/min), primary biliary cirrhosis, gallstone or gallbladder disease, or hypoalbuminemia; OB: Pregnancy; Lactation: Lactation.

Use Cautiously in: History of liver disease; Geri: Consider age-related ↓ in renal function; avoid in patients >70 yr; Pedi: Limited experience in children at a dose of 10–20 mg/kg/day.

Adverse Reactions/Side Effects

Derm: alopecia, photosensitivity, pruritus, rash, urticaria. **GI:** dyspepsia, flatulence, gastritis, ↓ appetite, abdominal distension, abdominal pain, cholestasis, constipation, diarrhea, nausea. **GU:** erectile dysfunction, renal failure. **MS:** muscle cramps, muscle weakness, myalgia, RHABDOMYOLYSIS. **Neuro:** dizziness, headache. **Misc:** HYPERSENSITIVITY REACTIONS (INCLUDING ANAPHYLAXIS).

Interactions

Drug-Drug: ↑ risk of bleeding with **oral anticoagulants**; ↓ anticoagulant dose by 50% with frequent monitoring. **Cyclosporine** may ↑ risk of severe myositis/rhabdomyolysis. **Immunosuppressants** may ↑ risk of reversible renal impairment. ↑ risk of myopathy with **HMG CoA reductase inhibitors (statins)**; combination therapy should be undertaken with extreme caution; must be discontinued at the 1st signs of myopathy and should not be undertaken in the presence of predisposing factors including impaired renal function, severe infection, trauma, surgery, hormonal/electrolyte imbalance or ↑ alcohol intake. ↑ risk of serious hypoglycemia with **insulin** or **sulfonylureas**. **MAO inhibitors** may ↑ risk of hepatotoxicity. **Cholestyramine** and other **bile-acid sequestrants** may ↓ absorption and effectiveness; separate administration by ≥2 hr. Effectiveness may be ↓ by **estrogen**.

Route/Dosage

PO (Adults): 400 mg once daily.

Availability

Sustained-release tablet: 400 mg.

NURSING IMPLICATIONS

Assessment

- Obtain a diet history with regard to fat consumption. Before starting bezafibrate, every attempt should be made to obtain a normal TG concentration with diet, exercise, and weight loss.
- Assess for cholelithiasis (epigastric pain after meals, pain that radiates to right shoulder or back). If gallbladder studies are indicated and gallstones confirmed, discontinue therapy.
- Assess for hypersensitivity reactions (anaphylaxis). *If hypersensitivity reaction occurs,* discontinue bezafibrate immediately and implement supportive measures (epinephrine) as indicated.

Lab Test Considerations

- Monitor serum lipids before and periodically during therapy.
- May ↑ AST and ALT. Monitor liver enzymes periodically during therapy. Baseline tests are recommended after 3–6 mo and at least yearly thereafter. Discontinue bezafibrate if AST or ALT levels ↑ >3 times upper limit of normal.
- If muscle tenderness develops during therapy, monitor CK. If CK is >10 times the upper limit of normal or if myopathy occurs, discontinue bezafibrate.

Implementation

- **PO:** Administer without regard to meals. ***DNC:*** Swallow sustained-release tablets whole; do not crush, break, or chew.

Patient/Family Teaching

- Explain purpose and side effects of medication to patient. Advise patient to read *Patient Information* before starting therapy. Advise patient to take the medication as directed. Missed doses should be taken as soon as remembered; do not double dose. Advise patient that medication helps control but does not cure ↑ serum TG concentrations.
- Advise patient to notify health care provider of all Rx or OTC medications, vitamins, or herbal products being taken and to consult with health care provider before taking other medications.
- Advise patient that medication should be taken in conjunction with diet restrictions of fat, cholesterol, carbohydrates, and alcohol, as well as an exercise regimen and smoking cessation.
- Advise patient to notify health care provider of unexplained muscle pain or weakness, tiredness, fever, nausea, vomiting, or abdominal pain. If hypersensitivity reactions (anaphylaxis) occurs, advise patient to seek immediate medical attention.
- Rep: Advise women of reproductive potential to immediately notify health care provider if pregnancy is planned or suspected, and advise to use strict birth control measures. If pregnancy occurs despite birth control, discontinue bezafibrate. If planning a pregnancy, bezafibrate should discontinued several months before conception.

Evaluation/Desired Outcomes

- Lowered cholesterol and TGs, increased HDL-C, with decreased risk of pancreatitis and other sequelae.

buserelin (bue-se-**rel**-in)

Suprefact

Classification

Therapeutic: antineoplastics, hormones

Pharmacologic: luteinizing hormone-releasing hormone (LHRH) analogues

Indications

SUBQ: Initial and maintenance palliative treatment of advanced hormone-dependent prostate cancer (usually in combination with an antiandrogen).

Intranasal: Maintenance palliative treatment of advanced hormone-dependent prostate cancer (usually in combination with an antiandrogen). Nonsurgical treatment of endometriosis.

Action

Acts as a synthetic analog of endogenous gonadotropin-releasing hormone (GnRH/LHRH). Chronic use results in inhibited secretion of gonadotropin release and gonadal steroid production. The overall effect is due to downregulation of pituitary LHRH receptors. In men, testosterone synthesis and release are ↓. In women, secretion of estrogen is ↓. **Therapeutic Effects:** Decreased spread of advanced prostate cancer. Decreased sequelae of endometriosis (pain, dysmenorrhea).

Pharmacokinetics

Absorption: *SUBQ:* 70%; *intranasal:* 1–3%; *implant:* drug is slowly absorbed over 2–3 mo.
Distribution: Accumulates in liver, kidneys and anterior pituitary lobe.
Metabolism and Excretion: Metabolized in liver and kidneys and by enzymes on membranes in the pituitary gland.
Half-life: *SUBQ:* 80 min; *intranasal:* 1–2 hr; *implant:* 20–30 days.

TIME/ACTION PROFILE

ROUTE	ONSET	PEAK	DURATION
prostate cancer†	7 days	4 mo	until discontinuation
endometriosis‡ (intranasal)	unknown	unknown	duration of treatment

† ↓ in testosterone concentrations.
‡ Symptom improvement.

Contraindications/Precautions

Contraindicated in: Hypersensitivity; Nonhormonal-dependent prostate cancer or previous orchiectomy; Women with undiagnosed vaginal bleeding; OB: Pregnancy; Lactation: Lactation.
Use Cautiously in: Prostate cancer with urinary tract obstruction or spinal lesions; Pedi: Safety and effectiveness not established in children (injection contains benzyl alcohol).

Adverse Reactions/Side Effects

CV: edema, hypertension. **Derm:** hot flashes, acne. **EENT:** nasal irritation (nasal spray). **Endo:** glucose intolerance, gynecomastia, testosterone flare. **GI:** constipation, nausea. **GU:** ↓ libido, menorrhagia, vaginal dryness, impotence, suppression of ovulation. **Hemat:** anemia. **Unlabeled Use:** injection site reactions. **MS:** bone pain, osteoporosis. **Neuro:** headache (nasal spray), insomnia, weakness, depression, dizziness. **Misc:** transient exacerbation of metastatic prostate cancer or endometriosis.

Interactions

Drug-Drug: Risk of serious arrhythmias may be ↑ by **amiodarone, disopyramide, dofetilide, flecainide ibutilide, propafenone quinidine, sotalol, antipsychotics, antidepressants** (including **amitriptyline** and **nortriptyline**), **methadone, macrolides, fluoroquinolones, azole antifungals, 5-HT3 antagonists, beta-2 receptor agonists, pentamidine,** and **quinine**.

Route/Dosage

Prostate cancer

SUBQ (Adults): *Initial treatment:* 500 mcg every 8 hr for 7 days; *Maintenance treatment:* 200 mcg once daily.
Intranasal (Adults): *Maintenance treatment:* 400 mcg (200 mcg in each nostril) 3 times daily.

Endometriosis

Intranasal (Adults): 400 mcg (200 mcg in each nostril) 3 times daily. Treatment is usually continued for 6 mo; not to exceed 9 mo.

Availability

Solution for SUBQ injection (contains benzyl alcohol): 1000 mcg/mL. **Intranasal solution:** 1000 mcg/mL (delivers 100 mcg/actuation).

NURSING IMPLICATIONS

Assessment

- **Cancer:** Monitor patients with vertebral metastases for ↑ back pain and ↓ sensory/motor function.
- Monitor intake and output and assess for bladder distention in patients with urinary tract obstruction during initiation of therapy.
- **Endometriosis:** Assess for signs/symptoms of endometriosis before and periodically during therapy. Amenorrhea usually occurs within 8 wk of initial administration and menses usually resume 8 wk after completion.

Lab Test Considerations

- Verify negative pregnancy test before starting therapy.
- Monitor serum testosterone concentrations every 3 mo during treatment in men. When treatment begins, testosterone concentrations can temporarily markedly ↑, and patients may need another medication to ↓ concentrations.
- Monitor blood glucose in patients with diabetes frequently; may affect blood glucose.

Implementation

Prostate Cancer

- **SUBQ:** Only use syringes that come with kit for accurate dose. Inject into fatty tissue of abdomen, arm, or leg 3 times/day for 7 days; then once daily during maintenance.
- **Intranasal:** When used as maintenance, begin nasal spray in each nostril 3 times daily. If patient also receives decongestant nasal spray, wait 30 min to give buserelin spray before or after the decongestant.

Endometriosis

- **Intranasal:** Administer one spray in each nostril 3 times daily for 6–9 mo.

Patient/Family Teaching

- Explain purpose and side effects of medication to patient. Advise patient to read *Patient Information* before starting therapy.
- Advise patient to notify health care provider of all Rx or OTC medications, vitamins, or herbal products being taken and to consult with health care provider before taking other medications.
- Advise men that they may experience breast swelling and tenderness, ↓ libido, hot flashes and sweats, impotence, and weight gain. Notify health care provider if these symptoms occur.
- Advise women that they may experience ↓ libido, constipation, painful sexual intercourse, menopausal symptoms, and changes in hair growth. Notify health care provider if these symptoms occur.
- **SUBQ:** Advise patient in proper technique for self-injection and care and disposal of equipment. Use only syringes included in kit. Instruct patients that syringes may only be used once and then discarded.
- **Intranasal:** Advise patient on proper nasal spray technique. Prime pump before use.
- Advise patient that the nasal spray can cause nose bleeds and may change smell and taste senses.
- Rep: May cause fetal harm. Advise women of reproductive potential to notify health care provider if pregnancy is planned or suspected or breastfeeding. Oral contraceptives should be discontinued before starting therapy; patients should employ a nonhormonal method of contraception during therapy. Advise men and women to use contraception while taking this drug.

Evaluation/Desired Outcomes

- Decreased spread of advanced prostate cancer.
- Decreased sequelae of endometriosis (pain, dysmenorrhea).

cannabidiol (ka-**na**-bi-dye-ole) **delta-9–tetrahydrocannabinol (THC)**
(**del**-ta nine tet-re-hye-dro-ka-**na**-bi-nole)

🍁 Sativex

Classification

Therapeutic: analgesic adjuncts, antispasticity agents

Pharmacologic: cannabinoids

Indications

Adjunct treatment of spasticity in adults with multiple sclerosis (MS) who have not responded to other therapies. Analgesic adjunct in the management of neuropathic pain in patients with MS or advanced cancer who have not responded to opioids or other analgesics for severe pain.

Action

Acts on cannabinoid receptors located in pain pathways in the brain, spinal cord, and peripheral nerve terminals. Has analgesic and muscle relaxant properties. **Therapeutic Effects:** Decreased pain and spasticity.

Pharmacokinetics

Absorption: Buccal absorption is slower than inhalation.

Distribution: Highly lipid soluble; distributes and accumulates in fatty tissues.

Metabolism and Excretion: Some first-pass hepatic metabolism occurs; highly metabolized by the CYP450 enzyme system. Metabolites can be stored in fatty tissues and rereleased over time (up to weeks); one metabolite of THC is pharmacologically active (11-hydroxy-THC). Further metabolism occurs in renal and biliary systems.

Half-life: Biexponential half-lives with short initial phases of *Cannabidiol:* 1.4–1.8 hr; *THC:* 1.3–1.7 hr; *11-hydroxy-THC:* 1.9–2.1 hr; terminal elimination half-life of *cannabinoids:* 24–26 hr or more.

TIME/ACTION PROFILE (analgesic and antispasticity effects)

ROUTE	ONSET	PEAK†	DURATION
cannabidiol	unknown	1.6–2.8 hr	up to 12 hr
THC	unknown	1.6–2.4 hr	up to 12 hr

† Plasma concentrations peak more quickly when administered under the tongue.

Contraindications/Precautions

Contraindicated in: Hypersensitivity to cannabinoids, propylene glycol, or peppermint oil; Serious cardiovascular disease, including ischemic heart disease, arrhythmias, poorly controlled hypertension, or severe HF; History of schizophrenia/psychoses; Sore/inflamed mucosa (may alter absorption); OB: Pregnancy; Lactation: Lactation; Pedi: Safety and effectiveness not established in children.

Use Cautiously in: Epilepsy/recurrent seizures; Substance use; Perioperative state (consider possible changes in cardiovascular status); History of depression/suicide attempt or ideation; Severe renal impairment; Cancer patients with urinary tract pathology (↑ risk of urinary tract adverse reactions); Severe hepatic impairment; Rep: Women of reproductive potential; Geri: Use cautiously in older adults.

Adverse Reactions/Side Effects

CV: hypertension, palpitations, postural hypotension, tachycardia. **GI:** appetite change, constipation, dry mouth, mucosal/teeth discoloration, nausea(↑ in cancer patients), stomatitis. **GU:** urinary retention (↑ in cancer patients). **Local:** application site irritation. **Neuro:** dizziness, fatigue, confusion, depression, disorientation, drowsiness, dysgeusia, euphoria, hallucinations, psychotic reactions, SUICIDAL THOUGHTS/BEHAVIORS, weakness. **Misc:** physical dependence, psychological dependence.

Interactions

Drug-Drug: ↑ risk of CNS depression with other **CNS depressants**, including **alcohol**, some **antidepressants**, some **antihistamines**, **benzodiazepines**, **GABA inhibitors**, **sedative/hypnotics**, **opioids**, and **psychotropics/antipsychotics**. Cannabidiol may ↑ levels and risk of toxicity of **amitriptyline**, **fentanyl**, and **sufentanil**.
Drug-Natural Products: ↑ risk of intoxication with other forms of **cannabis**.

Route/Dosage

Buccal: (Adults): *Day 1:* One spray in the morning and one in the evening; may ↑ by 1 spray/day on subsequent days. Time between sprays should be ≥15 min. If unacceptable effects occur, temporarily discontinue and restart at a lower number of sprays/day or use longer intervals between sprays. Titrate to optimal maintenance dose (usual range 4–8 sprays/day, usually not >12 sprays/day; higher doses have been used/tolerated). Adjust dose to changes in patient condition.

Availability

Buccal spray contains ethanol (50% v/v), propylene glycol, and peppermint oil: Each mL contains *Cannabidiol:* 25 mg and *THC:* 27 mg/mL. Delivers 100 microliters/spray; each spray provides cannabidiol 2.5 mg and THC 2.7 mg.

NURSING IMPLICATIONS

Assessment

- Assess spasticity, pain levels, sleep quality, and functional improvement during therapy.
- Assess neurological status, gait, and coordination before and during therapy.
- Monitor for mood changes and suicidal thoughts or behaviors, especially in those with history of psychiatric illness.
- Assess mucosal integrity for stomatitis and mouth ulcers.

Lab Test Considerations

- Monitor liver function tests periodically during therapy.

Implementation

- Prime pump before 1st use. Shake vial gently and remove protective cap. Hold vial in an upright position and press firmly and quickly on the actuator 2 or 3 times, until a fine spray appears. Point spray into a tissue, away from patient.
- **Buccal:** Administer one spray 2 times/day, in morning and in evening, on 1st day. Administer under tongue or in buccal area. Rotate sites in mouth to avoid irritation. Effects should be noticed in about 30 min. Do not spray the back of throat or into nose. After 1st day, ↑ dose by 1 spray every 24 hr, spacing doses evenly. No more than 12 doses should be used over a 24-hr period. Space each spray by ≥15 min.

Patient/Family Teaching

- Explain purpose and side effects of medication to patient. Advise patient to read *Patient Information* before starting therapy. Advise to take as directed.
- Advise patient to notify health care provider of all Rx or OTC medications, vitamins, or herbal products being taken and to consult with health care provider before taking other medications.
- Advise patient and caregiver if any suicidal thoughts or behaviors occur to notify health care provider immediately.
- Educate patient on correct spray technique. Advise patient to rotate sites in the mouth between the tongue and buccal locations.
- Advise patient to store unopened bottles in refrigerator. Do not freeze. Keep away from sources of heat such as direct sunlight or flames (product is flammable). Opened bottles may be stored at room temperature. Keep out of reach of children.
- Advise patient that any unused contents should be discarded after 28 days. Do not dispose of medications in wastewater (e.g., down the sink or in the toilet) or in household garbage. Consult pharmacist how to dispose of expired or unneeded medication.
- Advise patient about the potential for dependency. Tolerance as well as psychological and physical dependence may occur with prolonged use. Use cautiously with a history of drug or alcohol abuse and advise patient to avoid alcohol and other drugs while taking cannabidiol.
- Advise patient of impairment to physical or mental abilities and to avoid activities that require mental alertness until response to medication is known.
- Rep: Advise women of reproductive potential to notify health care provider if pregnancy is planned or suspected or if breastfeeding.

Evaluation/Desired Outcomes

- Decreased pain and spasticity.

cilazapril (sye-**lay**-za-pril)
Inhibace

Classification
Therapeutic: antihypertensives
Pharmacologic: ACE inhibitors

Indications
Hypertension (as monotherapy or in combination with other antihypertensives). HF.

Action
ACE inhibitors block the conversion of angiotensin I to the vasoconstrictor angiotensin II. ACE inhibitors also prevent the degradation of bradykinin and other vasodilatory prostaglandins. ACE inhibitors also ↑ plasma renin concentrations and ↓ aldosterone concentrations. Net result is systemic vasodilation. **Therapeutic Effects:** Lowering of BP in hypertensive patients. Improved symptoms in patients with HF.

Pharmacokinetics
Absorption: Well absorbed following oral administration; rapidly converted to active metabolite, cilazaprilat (57% bioavailability for cilazaprilat).
Distribution: Unknown.
Metabolism and Excretion: Cilazaprilat is eliminated unchanged by the kidneys (91%).
Half-life: *Early elimination phase:* 0.9 hr; *terminal elimination phase (enzyme-bound cilazaprilat):* 36–49 hr.

TIME/ACTION PROFILE (effects on hemodynamics)

ROUTE	ONSET	PEAK	DURATION
PO (hypertension)	within 1 hr	3–7 hr	12–24 hr
PO (HF)	1–2 hr	2–4 hr	24 hr

Contraindications/Precautions
Contraindicated in: Hypersensitivity; History of angioedema with previous use of ACE inhibitors; Concurrent use with aliskiren in patients with diabetes or moderate to severe renal impairment (CCr <60 mL/min); OB: Pregnancy; Lactation: Lactation.
Use Cautiously in: Renal impairment, hepatic impairment, hypovolemia, hyponatremia, or concurrent diuretic therapy; Black patients with hypertension (monotherapy less effective and may require additional therapy; ↑ risk of angioedema); Surgery/anesthesia (hypotension may be exaggerated); Rep: Women of reproductive potential; Geri: Initial dose ↓ recommended in older adults due to age-related ↓ in renal function; Pedi: Safety and effectiveness not established in children.
Exercise Extreme Caution in: Family history of angioedema.

Adverse Reactions/Side Effects
CV: hypotension, chest pain, edema, tachycardia. **Derm:** flushing, pruritus, rash. **F and E:** hyperkalemia. **GI:** abdominal pain, anorexia, constipation, diarrhea, nausea, vomiting. **GU:** erectile dysfunction, proteinuria, renal impairment. **Hemat:** AGRANULOCYTOSIS. **Metab:** hyperuricemia. **MS:** back pain, myalgia. **Neuro:** dysgeusia, dizziness, drowsiness, fatigue, headache, insomnia, vertigo, weakness. **Resp:** cough, dyspnea. **Misc:** ANGIOEDEMA, fever.

Interactions
Drug-Drug: Excessive hypotension may occur with **diuretics**, other **antihypertensives**, or **alcohol**. ↑ risk of hyperkalemia with **potassium supplements**, **potassium-sparing diuretics**, or **potassium-containing salt substitutes**. ↑ risk of hyperkalemia, renal impairment, hypotension, and syncope with **angiotensin II receptor antagonists** or **aliskiren**; avoid concurrent use with aliskiren in patients with diabetes or CCr <60 mL/min. **NSAIDs** and selective **COX-2 inhibitors** may blunt the antihypertensive effect and ↑ the risk of renal impairment. May ↑ levels and risk of toxicity of **lithium**.

Route/Dosage
Hypertension
PO (Adults ≤65 yr): *As monotherapy:* 2.5 mg once daily initially; may ↑ every 2 wk by 2.5 mg/day; usual dose 2.5–5 mg once daily; max = 10 mg/day. Twice-daily administration may be necessary in some patients; *With diuretics:* 0.5 mg once daily initially; titrate carefully.
PO (Adults >65 yr): *As monotherapy:* 1.25 mg once daily initially; titrate carefully.

Renal Impairment
PO (Adults): *CCr >40 mL/min:* 1 mg once daily initially; titrate carefully (max dose = 5 mg/day); *CCr 10–40 mL/min:* 0.5 mg once daily initially; titrate carefully (max dose = 2.5 mg/day); *CCr <10 mL/min:* 0.25–0.5 mg once or twice weekly according to BP response.

Hepatic Impairment
PO (Adults): 0.5 mg once daily or less.

Heart Failure
PO (Adults): 0.5 mg/day with careful monitoring; after 5 days, dose may ↑ to 1 mg/day; dose may then be carefully titrated as needed/tolerated up to 2.5 mg/day; rarely patients may require 5 mg/day.

Renal Impairment

PO (Adults): *CCr >40 mL/min:* 0.5 mg once daily (max dose = 2.5 mg/day); *CCr 10–40 mL/min:* 0.25–0.5 mg once daily (max dose = 2.5 mg/day); *CCr <10 mL/min:* 0.25–0.5 mg once or twice weekly according to BP response.

Availability

Tablets: 1 mg, 2.5 mg, 5 mg. ***In combination with:*** hydrochlorothiazide (Inhibace Plus)

NURSING IMPLICATIONS

Assessment

- Assess for signs/symptoms of angioedema (dyspnea, facial swelling, stridor). Implement emergent supportive measures as needed.
- **Hypertension:** Monitor BP and HR frequently during initial dose adjustment and periodically during therapy.
- **Heart Failure:** Monitor daily weight and assess frequently for fluid overload (dyspnea, rales/crackles, weight gain, jugular venous distention).

Lab Test Considerations

- Monitor BUN, serum creatinine, and electrolytes periodically during therapy.
- Monitor CBC periodically. May cause agranulocytosis.
- May ↑ AST, ALT, alkaline phosphatase, bilirubin, uric acid, and glucose.

Implementation

- **PO:** Administer with or without food.

Patient/Family Teaching

- Explain purpose and side effects of medication to patient. Advise patient to read *Patient Information* before starting therapy. Advise to take as directed. Take missed dose as soon as remembered. If not until the following day, skip missed dose. Do not double doses.
- Advise patient to notify health care provider of all Rx or OTC medications, vitamins, or herbal products being taken and to consult with health care provider before taking other medications.
- Advise patient to change positions slowly to minimize hypotension. Use of alcohol, standing for long periods, exercising, and hot weather may ↑ risk of orthostatic hypotension.
- May cause dizziness. Advise patient to avoid driving and other activities requiring alertness until response to medication is known.
- Educate patient on proper technique for monitoring BP. Advise patient to check BP and weight weekly and record and report results to health care provider.
- Provide patient with additional interventions for hypertension control (weight ↓, low-sodium diet, smoking cessation, exercise regimen, stress management, moderation of alcohol consumption). Medication controls but does not cure hypertension.
- Advise patient that cilazapril may cause a dry, hacking nonproductive cough that usually occurs within the 1st few months of treatment and generally resolves within 1–4 wk after discontinuation. Advise to notify health care provider is cough becomes bothersome.
- Rep: Advise women of reproductive potential to use contraception and to notify health care provider if pregnancy is planned or suspected or if breastfeeding. Discontinue medication immediately if pregnancy is confirmed.

Evaluation/Desired Outcomes

- Lowering of BP in hypertensive patients.
- Improved symptoms in patients with HF.

cloxacillin (klox-a-**sill**-in)

Classification

Therapeutic: anti-infectives

Pharmacologic: penicillinase resistant penicillins

Indications

Treatment of the following infections due to penicillinase-producing staphylococci: Respiratory tract infections, Sinusitis, Septicemia, Endocarditis, Osteomyelitis, Skin and skin structure infections.

Action

Bind to bacterial cell wall, leading to cell death. Not inactivated by penicillinase enzymes. **Therapeutic Effects:** Bactericidal action. **Spectrum:** Active against most gram-positive aerobic cocci. Spectrum is notable for activity against: Penicillinase-producing strains of *Staphylococcus aureus* and *Staphylococcus epidermidis*. Not active against methicillin-resistant *Staphylococcus aureus*.

Pharmacokinetics

Absorption: IV administration results in complete bioavailability. Moderately absorbed (50%) following oral administration.

Distribution: Widely distributed; penetration into CSF is minimal but sufficient in the presence of inflamed meninges.

Metabolism and Excretion: Some metabolism by the liver (9–22%) and some renal excretion of unchanged drug (20%).

Half-life: 0.5–1.1 hr (↑ in severe hepatic impairment, renal impairment, and neonates).

TIME/ACTION PROFILE

ROUTE	ONSET	PEAK	DURATION
PO	30 min	30–120 min	6 hr
IM	unknown	unknown	6 hr
IV	rapid	end of injection/infusion	6 hr

Contraindications/Precautions

Contraindicated in: Previous hypersensitivity to penicillin (cross-sensitivity exists with cephalosporins and other beta-lactam antibiotics).

Use Cautiously in: Severe renal impairment; Severe hepatic impairment; OB: Safety and effectiveness not established in pregnancy; Lactation: Safety and effectiveness not established in breastfeeding; Pedi: Safety and effectiveness not established in premature and newborn infants.

Adverse Reactions/Side Effects

Derm: rash, urticaria. **GI:** diarrhea, epigastric distress, nausea, vomiting, CLOSTRIDIOIDES DIFFICILE-ASSOCIATED DIARRHEA (CDAD). **GU:** interstitial nephritis. **Hemat:** eosinophilia, leukopenia. **Neuro:** SEIZURES. **Misc:** HYPERSENSITIVITY REACTIONS (INCLUDING ANAPHYLAXIS AND SERUM SICKNESS), superinfection.

Interactions

Drug-Drug: May ↓ effectiveness of **oral contraceptive agents**. **Probenecid** ↓ renal excretion and ↑ levels (therapy may be combined for this purpose). May ↑ levels and risk of toxicity of **methotrexate**.

Drug-Food: Food ↓ oral absorption by 50%.

Route/Dosage

PO (Adults): 250–500 mg every 6 hr.

PO (Children ≥40 kg): 250–500 mg every 6 hr (max dose = 6 g/day).

PO (Children 5–<40 kg): 50 mg/kg/day divided every 6 hr (max dose = 4 g/day).

IM, IV (Adults): 1–2 g every 4–6 hr.

IM, IV (Children): 100–200 mg/kg/day in divided doses every 6 hr (max = 2 g/dose).

Availability

Capsules: 250 mg, 500 mg. **Oral solution:** 125 mg/5 mL. **Lyophilized powder for injection:** 250 mg/vial, 500 mg/vial, 1 g/vial, 2 g/vial.

NURSING IMPLICATIONS

Assessment

- Assess for infection (vital signs; appearance of wound, sputum, urine, and stool) initially and during therapy.
- Obtain a history before initiating therapy to determine previous use of and reactions to cephalosporins or other beta-lactam antibiotics. Patients with no history of penicillin sensitivity may still have an allergic response.
- Assess for hypersensitivity reactions (anaphylaxis, rash, pruritus, laryngeal edema, wheezing, abdominal pain). *If hypersensitivity reaction occurs,* discontinue cloxacillin and notify health care provider immediately. Implement emergent supportive measures (epinephrine) as indicated.
- Monitor bowel function and assess for CDAD (diarrhea, abdominal cramping, fever, bloody stools). Notify health care provider promptly. May begin up to several weeks following cessation of therapy.

Lab Test Considerations

- Obtain specimens for culture and sensitivity before initiating therapy. 1st dose may be given before receiving results.
- May cause leukopenia and neutropenia, especially with prolonged therapy or hepatic impairment.
- May cause positive direct Coombs test result.
- May ↑ AST, ALT, LDH, and alkaline phosphatase.

Implementation

- **PO:** Administer around the clock on an empty stomach ≥1 hr before or 2 hr after meals. Take with 8 ounces of water. Acidic juices may ↓ absorption of penicillins. ***DNC:*** Swallow whole. Do not crush, chew, or open capsules.
- Use calibrated measuring device for liquid preparations. Shake well. Solution is stable for 14 days if refrigerated.
- **IM Reconstitution:** Reconstitute 250-mg and 500-mg vials with 1.9 mL and 1.7 mL, respectively, of sterile water for injection. Shake well to dissolve. Stable for 24 hr at room temperature or 48 hr if refrigerated. **Concentration:**125 mg/mL (250-mg vial) and 250 mg/mL (500-mg vial).

IV Administration

- **IV Push: Reconstitution:** Reconstitute 250-mg, 500-mg, and 1-g vials with 4.9 mL, 4.8 mL, and 9.6 mL, respectively, of sterile water for injection. Shake well. Use reconstituted solution immediately. **Concentration:** 50–100 mg/mL. **Rate:** Administer over 2–4 min.
- **Intermittent Infusion: Reconstitution:** Reconstitute 1-g and 2-g vials with 3.4 mL and 6.8 mL, respectively, of sterile water for injection. Add to an appropriate infusion fluid in amount calculated to give desired dose. Shake well to dissolve. Use solution immediately. **Concentration:** 250 mg/mL. **Rate:** Infuse over 30–40 min.
- **Y-Site Compatibility:** acetylcysteine, acyclovir, aminophylline, amiodarone, amphotericin B liposomal, atropine, benztropine, caffeine citrate, calcium chloride, calcium gluconate, caspofungin, cefazolin, ceftazidime, ceftriaxone, cefotaxime, cefoxitin, cefuroxime, chloramphenicol, chlorothiazide, clindamycin, cyclophosphamide, cyclosporine, dexamethasone, digoxin, dopamine, epinephrine, edetate calcium disodium, esmolol, fentanyl, fluconazole, furosemide, heparin,

hydrocortisone, insulin regular, isoproterenol, ketamine, levofloxacin, lidocaine, magnesium sulfate, mannitol, meropenem, methohexital, methylprednisolone, metoclopramide, metronidazole, milrinone, naloxone, nitroprusside, norepinephrine, ondansetron, oxytocin, penicillin G, phenobarbital, phentolamine, piperacillin/tazobactam, potassium chloride, procainamide, prochlorperazine, propranolol, sildenafil, sodium bicarbonate, succinylcholine, sufentanil, voriconazole.

- **Y-Site Incompatibility:** amikacin, azithromycin, blinatumomab, chlorpromazine, ciprofloxacin, diazepam, diphenhydramine, dobutamine, droperidol, labetalol, lorazepam, midazolam, morphine, nitroglycerin, phenytoin, potassium phosphates, rocuronium, trimethoprim/sulfamethoxazole, tobramycin.

Patient/Family Teaching

- Explain purpose and side effects of medication to patient. Advise patient to read *Patient Information* before starting therapy. Advise patient to take medication around the clock and to finish the drug completely as directed, even if feeling better. Missed doses should be taken as soon as remembered. Advise patient that sharing of this medication may be dangerous.
- Advise patient to notify health care provider of all Rx or OTC medications, vitamins, or herbal products being taken and to consult with health care provider before taking other medications.
- Advise patient to report signs of superinfection (black, furry overgrowth on the tongue; vaginal itching or discharge; loose or foul-smelling stools) and allergy.
- Advise patient to notify health care provider if fever and diarrhea develop, especially if stool contains blood, pus, or mucus. Advise patient not to treat diarrhea without consulting health care provider.
- Advise patient to notify health care provider if symptoms do not improve.
- Rep: Advise women of reproductive potential to notify health care provider if pregnancy is planned or suspected or if breastfeeding. Advise patient taking oral contraceptives to use an additional nonhormonal method of contraception during therapy with penicillin and until next menstrual period.

Evaluation/Desired Outcomes

- Bactericidal action.

cyproterone (sy-proe-te-rone)

Androcur

Classification

Therapeutic: antineoplastics, hormones

Pharmacologic: antiandrogens

Indications

Palliative treatment of advanced prostate cancer.

Action

Has antiandrogenic and progestogenic/antigonadotropic properties, resulting in blocked binding of the active metabolite of testosterone on the surface of prostatic cancer cells and ↓ production of testicular testosterone. **Therapeutic Effects:** Decreased spread of prostate cancer.

Pharmacokinetics

Absorption: *PO:* Completely absorbed. *IM:* delayed and prolonged absorption after depot injection.

Distribution: Unknown.

Metabolism and Excretion: Metabolized by the CYP3A isoenzyme; excreted in feces (60%) and urine (33%) as unchanged drug and metabolites.

Half-life: *PO:* 38 hr; *IM:* 4 days.

TIME/ACTION PROFILE (plasma concentrations)

ROUTE	ONSET	PEAK	DURATION
PO	unknown	3–4 hr	8–12 hr
IM (depot)	unknown	3–4 days	1–2 wk

Contraindications/Precautions

Contraindicated in: Hypersensitivity; Liver disease/hepatic impairment/liver tumors (not due to prostate cancer); Dubin-Johnson syndrome; Rotor syndrome; History of meningioma; Wasting diseases (not related to prostate cancer); Severe depression; Thromboembolism.

Use Cautiously in: Cardiovascular disease; Renal impairment.

Adverse Reactions/Side Effects

CV: edema, HF, hypotension, MI, syncope, tachycardia, THROMBOEMBOLISM, vasovagal reactions. **Derm:** ↑ sweating, dry skin, hot flashes, patchy hair loss. **Endo:** adrenal suppression, antiandrogen withdrawal syndrome, glucose intolerance, gynecomastia. **F and E:** hypercalcemia. **GI:** anorexia, constipation, diarrhea, HEPATOTOXICITY, LIVER TUMORS, nausea, vomiting. **GU:** impotence, infertility. **Hemat:** anemia, thrombocytopenia. **Metab:** hyperlipidemia. **MS:** osteoporosis. **Neuro:** fatigue, weakness, depression, MENINGIOMAS. **Resp:** cough, dyspnea, pulmonary microembolism. **Misc:** allergic reactions.

Interactions

Drug-Drug: Antiandrogenic effect may be ↓ by **alcohol**. Effectiveness/long-term survival may be ↓ by concurrent **GnRH agonist** treatment. ↑ risk of myopathy with **HMG CoA reductase inhibitors (statins)**. **Strong CYP3A4 inhibitors**, including **clotrimazole**, **itraconazole**, **ketoconazole** and **ritonavir**, may ↑ levels and risk of toxicity. **Strong CYP3A4 inducers**, including **phenytoin** and **rifampin**, may ↓ levels and effectiveness.

Drug-Natural Products: St. John's wort may ↓ levels and effectiveness.

Route/Dosage

PO (Adults): 200–300 mg/day in 2–3 divided doses (max dose = 300 mg/day); *After orchiectomy:* 100–200 mg/day.

IM (Adults): 300 mg once weekly; *After orchiectomy:* 300 mg every 2 wk.

Availability

Oil for IM depot injection: 100 mg/mL. **Tablets:** 50 mg. **In combination with:** ethinyl estradiol (Diane-35, Cyestra-35, Cleo-35).

NURSING IMPLICATIONS

Assessment

- Assess for signs/symptoms of thromboembolism (chest pain, dyspnea, vital signs, level of consciousness). *If thromboembolism occurs,* discontinue cyproterone.
- Monitor mood changes, especially during 1st 6–8 wk. Note degree to which these thoughts and behaviors interfere with daily functioning. Inform health care provider if patient demonstrates significant ↑ in anxiety, nervousness, or insomnia.

Lab Test Considerations

- Monitor PSA during therapy. May ↑ PSA. Discontinue cyproterone if PSA ↑ occurs and monitor for 6–8 wk for withdrawal response before decision to proceed with other prostate cancer therapy.
- May impair carbohydrate metabolism. Monitor fasting blood glucose and glucose tolerance tests periodically during therapy, especially in patients with diabetes. May require dose changes in insulin or other antidiabetic agents.
- Monitor CBC periodically during therapy.
- Monitor liver function tests before and periodically during therapy and if symptoms of hepatotoxicity occur. Elevated liver enzymes may develop several weeks to months after therapy starts. *If hepatotoxicity occurs,* discontinue cyproterone.
- Monitor adrenocortical function tests by serum cortisol assay periodically during therapy.

Implementation

- **PO:** Administer at the same time each day, after meals and with liquids. Dose is usually lower after orchiectomy.
- **IM:** Administer slowly and avoid IV injection, which can lead to pulmonary microembolism.

Patient/Family Teaching

- Explain purpose and side effects of medication to patient. Advise patient to read *Patient Information* before starting therapy. Advise to take as directed. Take missed doses as soon as remembered, unless almost time for next dose; then skip missed dose and resume usual dosing schedule. Do not double dose.
- Advise patient to notify health care provider of all Rx or OTC medications, vitamins, or herbal products being taken and to consult with health care provider before taking other medications.
- Advise patient that benign breast lumps may occur; they generally subside 1–3 mo after discontinuation of therapy and/or after dose ↓. Dose ↓ should be weighed against the risk of inadequate tumor control.
- Advise patient to avoid alcohol during therapy.
- May cause fatigue and lassitude during 1st few weeks of therapy; then diminishes. Caution patient to avoid driving and other activities requiring alertness until response to medication is known.
- Advise patient that sperm count and volume of ejaculate ↓ with therapy. Infertility is common but reversible when therapy is discontinued (usually within 3–5 mo but may take up to 20 mo).
- Discuss with patient potential for patchy hair loss. Explore methods of coping.

Evaluation/Desired Outcomes

- Decreased spread of prostate cancer.

danaparoid (da-**nap**-a-roid)

✱ Orgaran

Classification

Therapeutic: anticoagulants

Pharmacologic: heparins (low molecular weight)

Indications

Prevention of thromboembolic phenomena, including deep vein thrombosis (DVT) and pulmonary emboli (PE) after surgical procedures known to ↑ the risk of such complications (knee/hip replacement, abdominal surgery). Treatment of nonhemorrhagic stroke. Treatment/prevention of thromboembolic phenomena in patients with a history of heparin-induced thrombocytopenia (HIT).

Action

Potentiates the inhibitory effect of antithrombin on factor Xa and thrombin. Danaparoid sodium is a heparinoid. **Therapeutic Effects:** Prevention of thrombus formation.

Pharmacokinetics

Absorption: 100% absorbed after SUBQ administration; IV administration results in complete bioavailability.

Distribution: Unknown.

Metabolism and Excretion: Excreted mostly by the kidneys.

Half-life: 25 hr.

TIME/ACTION PROFILE (anticoagulant effect)

ROUTE	ONSET	PEAK	DURATION
SUBQ	unknown	4–5 hr	12 hr

Contraindications/Precautions

Contraindicated in: Hypersensitivity to danaparoid sodium, pork products, or sulfites; Uncontrolled bleeding; Lactation: Lactation.

Use Cautiously in: Severe renal impairment (↓ dose); Severe hepatic impairment; Retinopathy (hypertensive or diabetic); Untreated hypertension; Recent history of ulcer disease; Spinal/epidural anesthesia; History of congenital or acquired bleeding disorder; Malignancy; OB: Safety and effectiveness not established in pregnancy; Pedi: Safety and effectiveness not established in children; Geri: Dose ↓ may be necessary in older adults with severe renal impairment.

Exercise Extreme Caution in: Severe uncontrolled hypertension; Bacterial endocarditis; Recent CNS or ophthalmologic surgery.

Adverse Reactions/Side Effects

CV: edema. **Derm:** ecchymoses, pruritus, rash, urticaria. **GI:** ↑ liver enzymes, constipation, nausea, vomiting. **GU:** urinary retention. **Hemat:** anemia, BLEEDING, thrombocytopenia. **Local:** erythema/irritation/pain at injection site, hematoma. **Neuro:** dizziness, headache, insomnia. **Misc:** fever.

Interactions

Drug-Drug: Risk of bleeding may be ↑ by **anticoagulants**, including **warfarin**, **dabigatran**, **rivaroxaban**, **apixaban**, or **edoxaban**, or **drugs that affect platelet function**, including **aspirin**, **NSAIDs**, **dipyridamole**, some **penicillins**, **clopidogrel**, **ticagrelor**, or **prasugrel**.

Route/Dosage

Prophylaxis of DVT/PE (non-HIT patients)

SUBQ (Adults): 750 anti-Xa units every 12 hr starting 1–4 hr preoperatively and ≥2 hr postoperatively for 7–10 days or until ambulatory (up to 14 days). *Following orthopedic, major abdominal surgery, and thoracic surgery:* 750 anti-Xa units, twice daily up to 14 days; initiate 1–4 hr preoperatively.

IV, SUBQ (Adults): *Nonhemorrhagic stroke:* Up to 1000 anti-Xa units IV, followed by 750 anti-Xa units SUBQ twice daily for 7–14 days.

HIT

IV: SUBQ (Adults): *DVT/PE prophylaxis, current HIT, >90 kg:* 1250 anti-Xa units SUBQ 2–3 times daily for 7–10 days (initial bolus of 1250 anti-Xa units IV may be used); *DVT/PE prophylaxis, current HIT, ≤90 kg:* 750 anti-Xa units SUBQ 2–3 times daily for 7–10 days (initial bolus of 1250 anti-Xa units IV may be used); *DVT/PE prophylaxis, past (>3 mo) HIT, >90 kg:* 750 anti-Xa units SUBQ 3 times daily *OR* 1250 anti-Xa units SUBQ twice daily for 7–10 days; *DVT/PE prophylaxis, past (>3 mo) HIT, ≤90 kg:* 750 anti-Xa units SUBQ 2–3 times daily for 7–10 days; *DVT/PE treatment, thrombus <5 days, >90 kg:* 3750 anti-Xa units IV bolus, then 400 anti-Xa units/hr for 4 hr, then 300 anti-Xa units/hr for 4 hr, then 150–200 anti-Xa units/hr for 5–7 days *OR* 1750 anti-Xa units SUBQ twice daily for 4–7 days; *DVT/PE treatment, thrombus <5 days, 55–90 kg:* 2250–2500 anti-Xa units IV bolus, then 400 anti-Xa units/hr for 4 hr, then 300 anti-Xa units/hr for 4 hr, then 150–200 anti-Xa units/hr for 5–7 days *OR* 2000 anti-Xa units SUBQ twice daily for 4–7 days; *DVT/PE treatment, thrombus <5 days, ≤55 kg:* 1250–1500 anti-Xa units IV bolus, then 400 anti-Xa units/hr for 4 hr, then 300 anti-Xa units/hr for 4 hr, then 150–200 anti-Xa units/hr for 5–7 days *OR* 1500 anti-Xa units SUBQ twice daily for 4–7 days; *DVT/PE treatment, thrombus ≥5 days, >90 kg:* 1250 anti-Xa units IV bolus, then 750 anti-Xa units SUBQ 3 times daily *OR* 1250 anti-Xa units SUBQ 2–3 times daily; *DVT/PE treatment, thrombus ≥5 days, ≤90 kg:* 1250 anti-Xa units IV bolus, then 750 anti-Xa units SUBQ 2–3 times daily; *Surgical prophylaxis, nonvascular surgery, >90 kg:* 750 anti-Xa units SUBQ 1–4 hr before procedure; repeat ≥6 hr after procedure; then 1250 anti-Xa units SUBQ twice daily *OR* 750 anti-Xa units SUBQ 3 times daily for 7–10 days; *Surgical prophylaxis, nonvascular surgery, ≤90 kg:* 750 anti-Xa units SUBQ 1–4 hr before procedure; repeat ≥6 hr after procedure; then 750 anti-Xa units SUBQ twice daily for 7–10 days; *Surgical prophylaxis, embolectomy, >90 kg:* 2250–2500 anti-Xa units IV bolus before procedure, then 150–200 anti-Xa units/hr starting ≥6 hr after procedure for 5–7 days *OR* 750 anti-Xa units SUBQ 2–3 times daily or change to oral anticoagulant after several days; *Surgical prophylaxis, embolectomy, 55–90 kg:* 2250–2500 anti-Xa units IV bolus before procedure, then 1250 anti-Xa units SUBQ twice daily starting ≥6 hr after procedure, then 750 anti-Xa units SUBQ 2–3 times daily or change to oral anticoagulant after several days; *Cardiac catheterization, >90 kg:* 3750 anti-Xa units IV bolus before procedure; *Cardiac catheterization, <90 kg:* 2500 anti-Xa units IV bolus before procedure; *Percutaneous transluminal coronary angioplasty:* 2500 anti-Xa units IV bolus before procedure, then 150–200 anti-Xa units/hr for 1–2 days after procedure; may receive 750 anti-Xa units SUBQ 2–3 times daily or oral anticoagulant after several days of IV therapy; *Intra-aortic balloon pump catheterization, >90 kg:* 3750 anti-Xa units IV bolus before procedure, then 150–200 anti-Xa units/hr or a 2nd bolus of 1250 anti-Xa units IV *OR* 750 anti-Xa units SUBQ 2–3 times daily *OR* 1250 anti-Xa units SUBQ twice daily; *Intra-aortic balloon pump catheterization, <90 kg:* 2500 anti-Xa units IV bolus before procedure, then 150–200 anti-Xa units/hr or a 2nd bolus of 1250 anti-Xa units IV *OR* 750 anti-Xa units SUBQ 2–3 times daily *OR* 1250 anti-Xa units SUBQ twice daily; *Peripheral vascular bypass:* 2250–2500 anti-Xa units IV bolus before procedure, then 150–200 anti-Xa units/hr started ≥6 hr after procedure for 5–7 days *OR* 750 anti-Xa units SUBQ 2–3 times daily or change to oral anticoagulant; *Cardiopulmonary bypass:* 125 anti-Xa units/kg IV bolus after thoracotomy, then 3 anti-Xa units/mL as priming fluid, then 7 anti-Xa units/kg/hr (started at bypass hookup and stopped 45 min before expected end of bypass), then 1250 anti-Xa units SUBQ twice daily or 750 anti-Xa units 3 times daily or 150–200 anti-Xa units/hr IV started 6 hr after procedure. *Hemodialysis, every other day or less frequently:* 3750 anti-Xa units IV bolus before 1st 2 hemodialysis, then 3000 anti-Xa units IV bolus (if plasma antifactor Xa level <300 units/L) or 2500 anti-Xa units IV (if plasma antifactory Xa levels 300–350) or 2000 anti-Xa units IV (if plasma antifactor Xa levels 350–400); *Hemodialysis, every other day or less frequently, <55 kg:* 2500 anti-Xa units IV bolus before 1st 2 hemodialysis, then 2000 anti-Xa units IV bolus (if plasma antifactory Xa level <300 units/L), or 1500 anti-Xa units IV (if plasma antifactory Xa levels 300–400); *Hemodialysis, daily:* 3750 anti-Xa units IV before 1st dialysis, then 2500 before 2nd dialysis; *Hemodialysis, daily, <55 kg:* 2500 anti-Xa units IV before 1st dialysis, then 2000 before 2nd dialysis; *Hemofiltration, 55–90 kg:* 2500 anti-Xa units IV bolus, then 600 anti-Xa units/hr for 4 hr, then 400 anti-Xa units/hr for 4 hr, then 200–600 anti-Xa units/hr to maintain plasma anti-Xa concentrations of 500–1000 units/L; *Hemofiltration, <55 kg:* 2000 anti-Xa units IV bolus, then 400 anti-Xa units/hr for 4 hr, then 150–400 anti-Xa units/hr to maintain anti-Xa concentrations of 500–1000 units/L.

Availability

Solution for injection (contains sulfites): 750 anti-Xa units/0.6 mL ampule.

NURSING IMPLICATIONS

Assessment

- Assess for signs/symptoms of bleeding (bleeding gums; nosebleed; unusual bruising; black, tarry stools; hematuria; ↓ in hematocrit or BP; guaiac-positive stools; bleeding from surgical site). Notify health care provider if these occur.
- Assess for evidence of additional or ↑ thrombosis. Symptoms will depend on area of involvement. Monitor neurological status frequently for signs of neurological impairment. May require urgent treatment.
- Assess for hypersensitivity reactions (chills, fever, urticaria).
- Monitor patients with epidural catheters frequently for signs/symptoms of neurologic impairment. **SUBQ:** Observe injection sites for hematomas, ecchymosis, or inflammation.

Lab Test Considerations

- Monitor CBC and stools for occult blood periodically during therapy. Monitor platelet count every other day for 1st wk, twice weekly for next 2 wk, and weekly thereafter. If thrombocytopenia occurs, monitor closely. If hematocrit ↓ unexpectedly, assess patient for potential bleeding sites.
- Special monitoring of clotting times (aPTT) is not necessary.
- May ↑ AST, ALT, and alkaline phosphatase.

Toxicity and Overdose

- Danaparoid sodium is not reversed with protamine sulfate. If overdose occurs, discontinue danaparoid sodium. Transfusion with fresh frozen plasma and plasmapheresis has been used if bleeding is uncontrollable.

Implementation

- Cannot be used interchangeably (unit for unit) with unfractionated heparin or other low-molecular-weight heparins.
- Conversion to oral anticoagulant therapy (unless it is contraindicated) should not be started until adequate antithrombotic control with parenteral danaparoid sodium has been achieved; conversion may take up to 5 days.
- **SUBQ:** Administer deep into SUBQ tissue. Alternate injection sites daily between the left and right anterolateral and left and right posterolateral abdominal wall. Inject entire length of needle at a 45° or 90° angle into a skin fold held between thumb and forefinger; hold skin fold throughout injection. Do not aspirate or massage. Rotate sites frequently. Do not administer IM because of danger of hematoma formation. Solution should be clear; do not inject solution containing particulate matter.
- If excessive bruising occurs, ice cube massage of site before injection may lessen bruising.

IV Administration

- **IV Push:** SUBQ is preferred route. **Dilution:** If administered IV, give as a bolus. May dilute with 0.9% NaCl, D5/0.9% NaCl, Ringer's, LR, or mannitol. Stable for up to 48 hr at room temperature. **Rate:** Push rapidly.

- **Y-Site Incompatibility:** Do not administer other drugs through same IV line.

Patient/Family Teaching

- Explain purpose and side effects of medication to patient. Advise patient to read *Patient Information* before starting therapy. Advise patient in correct technique for self-injection and care and disposal of equipment.
- Advise patient to notify health care provider of all Rx or OTC medications, vitamins, or herbal products being taken and to consult with health care provider before taking other medications.
- Advise patient to report any symptoms of unusual bleeding or bruising, dizziness, itching, rash, fever, swelling, or difficulty breathing to health care provider immediately.
- Advise patient not to take aspirin, naproxen, or ibuprofen without consulting health care provider while on danaparoid sodium therapy.
- Rep: Advise women of reproductive potential to notify health care provider if pregnancy is planned or suspected or if breastfeeding.

Evaluation/Desired Outcomes

- Prevention of thrombus formation.

domperidone (dom-per-i-done)

Classification
Therapeutic: gastric stimulant
Pharmacologic: butyrophenones dopamine antagonists

Indications

Symptoms associated with GI motility disorders, including subacute/chronic gastritis and diabetic gastroparesis. Nausea/vomiting associated with dopamine agonist antiparkinson therapy. **Unlabeled Use:** To stimulate lactation.

Action

Acts as a peripheral dopamine receptor blocker. ↑ GI motility, peristalsis, and ↓ esophageal sphincter pressure. Facilitates gastric emptying and ↓ small bowel transit time. ↑ prolactin levels. **Therapeutic Effects:** Improved GI motility. Decreased nausea/vomiting associated with dopamine agonist antiparkinson therapy.

Pharmacokinetics

Absorption: Well absorbed following oral administration.
Distribution: Does not cross the blood-brain barrier.
Protein Binding: 93%.
Metabolism and Excretion: Undergoes extensive first-pass hepatic metabolism, much via the CYP3A4 isoenzyme. 31% excreted in urine; 66% excreted in feces.
Half-life: 7 hr.

TIME/ACTION PROFILE (plasma concentrations)

ROUTE	ONSET	PEAK	DURATION
PO	unknown	30 min	6–8 hr

Contraindications/Precautions

Contraindicated in: Hypersensitivity/intolerance; Concurrent use of ketoconazole; Prolactinoma; Conditions where GI stimulation is dangerous, including GI hemorrhage/mechanical obstruction/perforation; Lactation: Lactation.
Use Cautiously in: History of breast cancer; Severe renal impairment (dose adjustment may be necessary during chronic therapy); Hepatic impairment; OB: Use during pregnancy only if potential maternal benefit justifies potential fetal harm; Pedi: Safety and effectiveness not established in children.

Adverse Reactions/Side Effects

Derm: hot flashes, rash. **GI:** dry mouth. **GU:** amenorrhea, impotence. **Endo:** galactorrhea, gynecomastia, hyperprolactinemia. **Neuro:** headache, insomnia.

Interactions

Drug-Drug: **Ketoconazole** may ↑ levels and risk of cardiovascular toxicity; concurrent use contraindicated; other **azole antifungals**, **macrolide anti-infectives**, and **protease inhibitors** may have similar effects. **QT interval prolonging medications** may ↑ risk of QT interval prolongation. Effectiveness may be ↓ by **anticholingeric medications**. Due to effects on gastric motility, absorption of drugs from the small intestine may be accelerated, while absorption of drugs from the stomach may be slowed, especially **sustained-release** or **enteric-coated** formulations.
Drug-Food: Grapefruit juice may ↑ levels and risk of toxicity.

Route/Dosage

Upper Gastrointestinal Motility Disorders

PO (Adults): 10 mg 3 times daily (max = 30 mg/day).

Renal Impairment

PO (Adults): Depending on degree of impairment, dosing during chronic therapy should be ↓ to once or twice daily.

Nausea/Vomiting Due to Dopamine Agonists

PO (Adults): 10 mg 3 times daily; higher doses may be required during dose titration (max = 30 mg/day).

Renal Impairment

PO (Adults): Depending on degree of impairment, dosing during chronic therapy should be ↓ to once or twice daily.

Availability
Tablets: 10 mg.

NURSING IMPLICATIONS
Assessment
- Assess for nausea, vomiting, abdominal distention, and bowel sounds before and after administration.
- Monitor BP (sitting, standing, lying down) and HR before and periodically during therapy. May cause prolonged QT interval, tachycardia, and orthostatic hypotension, especially in patients >60 yr or taking >30 mg/day.
- Monitor for signs/symptoms related to hyperprolactinemia (menstrual abnormalities, galactorrhea, sexual dysfunction).

Lab Test Considerations
- May ↑ ALT, AST, and cholesterol.
- Monitor serum prolactin before and periodically during therapy. May ↑ prolactin.

Implementation
- **PO:** Administer 15–30 min before meals and at bedtime.

Patient/Family Teaching
- Explain purpose and side effects of medication to patient. Advise patient to read *Patient Information* before starting therapy. Advise to take as directed.
- Advise patient to notify health care provider of all Rx or OTC medications, vitamins, or herbal products being taken and to consult with health care provider before taking other medications.
- Advise patient to avoid grapefruit juice during therapy.
- Advise patient to notify health care provider if galactorrhea (excessive or spontaneous flow of breast milk), gynecomastia (excessive development of male mammary gland), menstrual irregularities (spotting or delayed periods), palpitations, irregular heartbeat (arrhythmia), dizziness, or fainting occur.
- Rep: Advise women of reproductive potential to notify health care provider if pregnancy is planned or suspected or if breastfeeding.

Evaluation/Desired Outcomes
- Improved GI motility.
- Decreased nausea/vomiting associated with dopamine agonist antiparkinson therapy.

flupentixol (floo-pen-tiks-ol)
🍁 Fluanxol, 🍁 Fluanxol Depot

Classification
Therapeutic: antipsychotics
Pharmacologic: thioxanthenes

Indications
Maintenance treatment of schizophrenia in patients whose symptomatology does not include excitement, agitation, or hyperactivity.

Action
Alters the effects of dopamine in the CNS. Has some anticholinergic and alpha-adrenergic blocking activity.
Therapeutic Effects: Diminished signs and symptoms of schizophrenia.

Pharmacokinetics
Absorption: *Flupentixol dihydrochloride:* 40% absorbed following oral administration; *Flupentixol decanoate:* Slowly released from IM injection sites.
Distribution: Distributes to lungs, liver, and spleen; enter CNS; extensive tissue distribution.
Protein Binding: 99%.
Metabolism and Excretion: Mostly metabolized; metabolites do not have antipsychotic activity.
Most metabolites are excreted in feces; some renal elimination.
Half-life: *Flupentixol dihydrochloride:* 35 hr; *Flupentixol decanoate:* 3 wk.

TIME/ACTION PROFILE (antipsychotic effect)

ROUTE	ONSET	PEAK	DURATION
PO	within 2–3 days	3–8 hr (blood level)	8 hr
IM (depot)	24–72 hr	4–7 days (blood level)	2–4 wk

Contraindications/Precautions
Contraindicated in: Hypersensitivity to flupentixol or other thioxanthines (cross-sensitivity with phenothiazines may occur); CNS depression due to any cause, including comatose states, cortical brain damage (known or suspected), or circulatory collapse; Opiate, alcohol, or barbiturate intoxication; Hepatic impairment, cerebrovascular insufficiency, or severe cardiovascular pathology.
Use Cautiously in: Brain tumors or intestinal obstruction (may mask symptoms); Patients exposed to extreme heat or organophosphorous insecticides; Risk factors for/history of stroke; Any risk factors for QT prolongation, including hypokalemia, hypomagnesemia, genetic predisposition, cardiovascular disease history (including bradycardia), recent MI, HF, or arrhythmias; Known/suspected glaucoma; History of seizures (may ↓ seizure threshold); Parkinson disease (may worsen symptoms); OB: Use during pregnancy only if potential maternal benefit justifies potential fetal risk; Lactation: Safety and effectiveness not established in breastfeeding; Pedi: Safety and effectiveness not

established in children; Geri: ↑ risk of stroke, cognitive decline, and mortality in older adults with dementia.

Adverse Reactions/Side Effects

CV: tachycardia, hypotension, QT interval prolongation, THROMBOEMBOLISM. **Derm:** photosensitivity, rash, sweating. **EENT:** blurred vision. **Endo:** glucose intolerance, hyperprolactinemia. **GI:** constipation, dry mouth, excess salivation, hepatotoxicity. **GU:** ↓ libido, menstrual irregularities, urinary retention. **Hemat:** agranulocytosis, granulocytopenia, neutropenia. **Metab:** weight gain. **MS:** osteoporosis. **Neuro:** dizziness, extrapyramidal symptoms, NEUROLEPTIC MALIGNANT SYNDROME, sedation, tardive dyskinesia.

Interactions

Drug-Drug: ↑ CNS depression with other **CNS depressants**, including **alcohol**, some **antidepressants**, some **antihistamines**, **anxiolytics**, **benzodiazepines**, and **sedative/hypnotics**. ↑ risk of QT prolongation and serious arrhythmias with **class Ia and III antiarrhythmics**, some **antipsychotics** (including **thioridazine**), **macrolides**, and **fluoroquinolones**; avoid concurrent use. **Diuretics** and other **drugs affecting electrolytes** may ↑ risk of QT interval prolongation and serious arrhythmias. **Anticholinergic medications** may ↑ risk of anticholinergic adverse reactions, including paralytic ileus. May ↑ levels and risk of toxicity of **tricyclic antidepressants**. ↑ risk of extrapyramidal symptoms with **metoclopramide**. May ↓ effectiveness of **levodopa** and **dopamine agonists**.

Route/Dosage

PO (Adults): 1 mg 3 times daily initially; ↑ by 1 mg every 2–3 days until desired response; usual effective dose is 3–6 mg/day in divided doses (up to 12 mg/day has been used); if insomnia occurs, ↓ evening dose.

IM (Adults): Initiate with a 5–20 mg test dose (use 5-mg dose in older adults) of the 2% injection. Patients previously treated with long-acting neuroleptic injections may tolerate initial doses of 20 mg. A 2nd 20-mg dose may be given 4–10 days later and then 20–40 mg every 2–3 wk depending on response. Oral flupentixol should be continued, but gradually ↓ in the 1st wk following depot injection. Guidelines for conversion from oral to depot IM injection: daily oral dose (mg) × 4 = dose of depot IM injection (mg) given every 2 wk *or* daily oral dose (mg) × 8 = depot IM injection (mg) given every 4 wk.

Availability

Tablets (flupentixol dihydrochloride): 0.5 mg, 3 mg, 5 mg. **Solution for depot IM injection (flupentixol decanoate: contains medium-chain triglycerides [coconut oil]):** 20 mg/mL (2%), 100 mg/mL (10%).

NURSING IMPLICATIONS

Assessment

- Assess mental status (orientation, mood, behavior) before and periodically during therapy.
- Monitor BP (sitting, standing, lying), HR, ECG, and respiratory rate before and frequently during the period of dose adjustment. May cause QT interval prolongation.
- Observe carefully when administering oral medication to ensure that medication is actually taken and not hoarded.
- Assess weight and BMI initially and during therapy.
- Assess fluid intake and bowel function. ↑ fiber and fluids in the diet help minimize constipation.
- Monitor for onset of akathisia (restlessness or desire to keep moving) and extrapyramidal side effects (*parkinsonian:* difficulty speaking or swallowing, loss of balance control, pill rolling, masklike face, shuffling gait, rigidity, tremors; *dystonic:* muscle spasms, twisting motions, twitching, inability to move eyes, weakness of arms or legs) every 2 mo during therapy and 8–12 wk after therapy has been discontinued. ↓ in dose or discontinuation of medication may be necessary. Benztropine or diphenhydramine may be used to control these symptoms.
- Monitor for tardive dyskinesia (uncontrolled rhythmic movement of mouth, face, and extremities; lip smacking or puckering; puffing of cheeks; uncontrolled chewing; rapid or worm-like movements of tongue). Report immediately; may be irreversible.
- Monitor for development of neuroleptic malignant syndrome (fever, respiratory distress, tachycardia, seizures, diaphoresis, arrhythmias, hypertension or hypotension, pallor, tiredness, severe muscle stiffness, loss of bladder control). Report immediately.
- Monitor for signs/symptoms related to hyperprolactinemia (menstrual abnormalities, galactorrhea, sexual dysfunction).

Lab Test Considerations

- Monitor CBC and liver function tests periodically during treatment. May ↑ AST, ALT, and alkaline phosphatase.
- Monitor blood glucose before and periodically during therapy. May cause hyperglycemia.
- Monitor serum prolactin before and periodically during therapy. May ↑ prolactin.
- May cause false-positive pregnancy tests.

Implementation

- **PO:** Initially, take tablets 3 times daily, without regard to food. Dose will ↑ for 1st few days until desired results. Maintenance dose is usually taken in morning.
- When converting to IM doses, PO dose is usually continued in ↓doses for 1st wk.

- **IM:** Inject deep IM preferably into gluteus maximus. Solution is a yellow viscous oil; aspirate before injection to ensure dose is not injected IV. Do not administer solutions that are discolored, hazy, or contain particulate matter. Doses >2 mL should be administered as divided doses between two injection sites.
- For large doses or pain with large volume, flupentixol decanoate 10% (100 mg/mL) solution may be used instead of the 2% (20 mg/mL) solution.

Patient/Family Teaching

- Explain purpose and side effects of medication to patient. Advise patient to read *Patient Information* before starting therapy. Advise to take as directed. If a dose is missed, omit and take next dose as scheduled. Discontinuation should be gradual; abrupt discontinuation may cause withdrawal symptoms (nausea, vomiting, anorexia, diarrhea, rhinorrhea, sweating, myalgias, paresthesias, insomnia, restlessness, anxiety, agitation, vertigo, feelings of warmth and coldness, tremor). Symptoms begin within 1–4 days of withdrawal and abate within 7–14 days.
- Advise patient to notify health care provider of all Rx or OTC medications, vitamins, or herbal products being taken and to consult with health care provider before taking other medications.
- Advise patient of possibility of extrapyramidal symptoms and tardive dyskinesia. Caution patient to report these symptoms immediately to health care provider.
- Advise patient to change positions slowly to minimize orthostatic hypotension.
- Medication may cause drowsiness. Advise patient to avoid driving or other activities requiring alertness until response to medication is known.
- Advise patient to avoid concurrent use of alcohol and other CNS depressants.
- Advise patient to notify health care provider promptly if sore throat, fever, unusual bleeding or bruising, rash, weakness, tremors, visual disturbances, dark-colored urine, or clay-colored stools occur.
- Advise patient to avoid sun exposure and to wear protective clothing and sunscreen when outdoors.
- Advise patient to notify health care provider of medication regimen before treatment or surgery.
- Rep: Advise women of reproductive potential to notify health care provider if pregnancy is planned or suspected or if breastfeeding.

Evaluation/Desired Outcomes

- Diminished signs and symptoms of schizophrenia.

fusidic acid (fyoo-**sid**-ik **as**-id)

✦ Fucidin, ✦ Fucithalmic

Classification
Therapeutic: anti-infectives

Indications

Topical: Primary and secondary bacterial skin infections, including impetigo contagiosa, erythrasma, and secondary skin infections such as infected wounds/burns. **Ophth:** Superficial eye infections.

Action

Inhibits bacterial protein synthesis. **Therapeutic Effects:** Resolution of localized bacterial infections. **Spectrum:** Greatest activity against gram-positive organisms, including: *Staphylococcus aureus, Streptococcus pyogenes. Corynebacterium spp.*

Pharmacokinetics

Absorption: Unknown.
Distribution: Unknown.
Metabolism and Excretion: Absorbed drug is extensively metabolized.
Half-life: 5–6 hr.

TIME/ACTION PROFILE

ROUTE	ONSET	PEAK	DURATION
Top	unknown	unknown	6–8 hr
Ophth	unknown	unknown	12 hr

Contraindications/Precautions

Contraindicated in: Hypersensitivity to fusidic acid or other components of the formulation (topical ointment contains lanolin).
Use Cautiously in: OB: Use during pregnancy only if potential maternal benefit justifies potential fetal risk; Lactation: Safety and effectiveness not established in breastfeeding; Pedi: Ophthalmic formulation not indicated for use in neonatal conjunctivitis.

Adverse Reactions/Side Effects

Derm: mild local irritation.

Interactions

Drug-Drug: None reported.

Route/Dosage

Topical: (Adults and Children): Apply to affected area 3–4 times daily.
Ophth (Adults and Children): One drop into conjunctival sac of both eyes every 12 hr for 7 days.

Availability

Topical cream: 2%. **Topical ointment (contains lanolin):** 2%. **Ophthalmic viscous drops (microcrystalline suspension):** 1%. ***In combination with:*** hydrocortisone (Fucidin H)

NURSING IMPLICATIONS

Assessment

- Assess involved areas of skin and mucous membranes before and frequently during therapy. ↑ skin irritation may indicate need to discontinue medication.

Implementation

- Do not confuse topical product with ophthalmic product.
- **Topical:** Consult health care provider for proper cleansing technique before applying medication. Apply small amount to cover affected area completely. Avoid the use of occlusive wrappings or dressings unless directed by health care provider.
- **Ophth:** Contact lenses should not be worn during treatment. Administer 1 drop into conjunctival sac of both eyes every 12 hr for 7 days. See Appendix C for instructions.

Patient/Family Teaching

- Explain purpose and side effects of medication to patient. Advise patient to read *Patient Information* before starting therapy. Advise to apply medication as directed for full course of therapy, even if feeling better.
- Advise patient to notify health care provider of all Rx or OTC medications, vitamins, or herbal products being taken and to consult with health care provider before taking other medications.
- Advise patient to report ↑ skin irritation or lack of response to therapy to health care provider.
- Rep: Advise women of reproductive potential to notify health care provider if pregnancy is planned or suspected or if breastfeeding.

Evaluation/Desired Outcomes

- Resolution of localized bacterial infections.

methotrimeprazine

(meth-oh-try-**mep**-ra-zeen)

Methoprazine, Nozinan

Classification

Therapeutic: antipsychotics, nonopioid analgesics

Pharmacologic: phenothiazines

Indications

Psychotic disturbances. As an analgesic and adjunct in pain due to cancer, trigeminal neuralgia, intercostal neuralgia, phantom limb pain, and muscular discomforts. Nausea/vomiting. Insomnia.

Action

Antagonizes dopamine receptors; also antagonizes alpha-1, alpha-2, serotonin, and muscarinic receptors. **Therapeutic Effects:** Decreased manifestations of psychotic disturbances. Reduction in severity of pain. Reduction in nausea/vomiting.

Pharmacokinetics

Absorption: Well absorbed after oral and IM administration. IV administration results in complete bioavailability.

Distribution: Enters CSF.

Metabolism and Excretion: Mostly metabolized by the liver. Some metabolites are active; 1% excreted unchanged by the kidneys.

Half-life: 15–30 hr.

TIME/ACTION PROFILE

ROUTE	ONSET	PEAK	DURATION
PO (plasma concentrations)	unknown	2.7–2.9 hr	8–12 hr
IM (analgesia)	unknown	20–40 min	8 hr (up to 24 hr in children)

Contraindications/Precautions

Contraindicated in: Hypersensitivity to methotrimeprazine, phenothiazines, or sulfites; Blood dyscrasias; Hepatic impairment; Patients in coma or those who have overdosed on CNS depressants, including alcohol, analgesics, opioids, or sedative/hypnotics; OB: Pregnancy.

Use Cautiously in: History of seizures; History of glaucoma or prostatic hypertrophy (↑ risk of anticholinergic adverse reactions); Bradycardia, electrolyte abnormalities, congenital/acquired prolonged QT interval, or concurrent use of drugs that may prolong QT interval (↑ risk of serious arrhythmias); Underlying cardiovascular disease, including stroke, arteriosclerosis, or thromboembolism (↑ risk of adverse cardiovascular effects); Lactation: Safety and effectiveness not established in breastfeeding; Geri: ↑ risk of stroke, cognitive decline, and mortality in older adults with dementia.

Adverse Reactions/Side Effects

CV: orthostatic hypotension, bradycardia, palpitations, tachycardia. **EENT:** nasal congestion. **Endo:** hyperglycemia, hyperprolactinemia. **GI:** constipation, abdominal discomfort, dry mouth, nausea, vomiting. **GU:** difficulty in urination. **Hemat:** blood dyscrasias. **Local:** pain at injection site. **Neuro:** amnesia, drowsiness, sedation, disorientation, euphoria, extrapyramidal reactions, headache, NEUROLEPTIC MALIGNANT SYNDROME (NMS), SEIZURES, slurred speech, tardive dyskinesia, weakness. **Misc:** chills.

Interactions

Drug-Drug: ↑ CNS depression with other **CNS depressants**, including **alcohol**, **antihistamines**, **antidepressants**, **opioids**, or **sedative/hypnotics**; ↓ dose of these agents by 50% initially. ↑ anticholinergic effects with **antihistamines**, **antidepressants**, **phenothiazines**, **quinidine**, **disopyramide**, **atropine**, or **scopolamine**; ↓ doses of atropine or scopolamine. Reverses vasopressor effects of

epinephrine; avoid concurrent use; if vasopressor required, use phenylephrine or norepinephrine. ↑ risk of hypotension with acute ingestion of **alcohol**, **nitrates**, **MAO inhibitors**, or **antihypertensives**. **Succinylcholine** may result in tachycardia, hypotension, CNS stimulation, delirium, and ↑ extrapyramidal symptoms.
Drug-Natural Products: Kava, **valerian**, **skullcap**, **chamomile**, or **hops** may ↑ risk of CNS depression.

Route/Dosage

PO (Adults): *Minor conditions:* 6–25 mg/day in 3 divided doses (if sedation occurs, use smaller daytime doses and a larger dose at bedtime); *Nighttime sedative:* 10–25 mg as a single bedtime dose; *Psychoses/intense pain:* 50–75 mg/day in 2–3 divided doses; may ↑ dose to desired effect (doses of ≥1 g/day have been used; if dose exceeds 100–200 mg/day, administer in divided doses and keep patient on bedrest).
PO (Children): 0.25 mg/kg/day in 2–3 divided doses (not to exceed 40 mg/day in children <12 yr).
IM (Adults): *Postoperative analgesic adjunct:* 10–25 mg every 8 hr; if given with opioids, ↓ opioid dose by 50%.
IM (Children): *Analgesia:* 62.5–125 mcg (0.0625–0.125 mg)/kg/day single dose or divided doses; change to oral medication as soon as possible.
IV (Children): *Palliative care setting:* 62.5 mcg (0.0625 mg)/kg/day as a slow infusion.

Availability

Tablets: 2 mg, 5 mg, 25 mg, 50 mg. **Solution for injection:** 25 mg/mL.

NURSING IMPLICATIONS

Assessment

- Assess type, location, and intensity of pain before and 30 min after administration.
- Monitor BP frequently after injection. Orthostatic hypotension, fainting, syncope, and weakness frequently occur 10 min–12 hr after administration. Patient should remain supine for 6–12 hr after injection.
- Assess weight and BMI initially and throughout therapy.
- Observe patient carefully for extrapyramidal side effects (*parkinsonian:* difficulty speaking or swallowing, loss of balance control, pill rolling, masklike face, shuffling gait, rigidity, tremors; *dystonic:* muscle spasms, twisting motions, twitching, inability to move eyes, weakness of arms or legs). Usually occur only after prolonged or high-dose therapy. Usually resolve with dose ↓ or administration of antiparkinsonian agent.
- Monitor for tardive dyskinesia (involuntary rhythmic movement of mouth, face, and extremities). Report immediately and discontinue therapy; may be irreversible.
- Monitor for development of NMS (fever, respiratory distress, tachycardia, seizures, diaphoresis, hypertension or hypotension, pallor, tiredness). *If signs/symptoms of NMS occur,* discontinue methotrimeprazine immediately.
- Methotrimeprazine potentiates the action of other CNS depressants but can be given in conjunction with modified doses of opioid analgesics for management of severe pain. This medication does not significantly depress respiratory status and can be useful where pulmonary reserve is low.
- Monitor for signs/symptoms of hyperprolactinemia (menstrual abnormalities, galactorrhea, sexual dysfunction).

Lab Test Considerations

- Monitor CBC before and periodically during therapy.
- Monitor liver function tests periodically throughout long-term (>30 days) therapy.
- Monitor blood glucose before and periodically during therapy. May cause hyperglycemia.
- Monitor serum prolactin before and periodically during therapy. May ↑ prolactin.

Implementation

- **PO:** Administer during day or only at night depending on indication.
- **IM:** Do not inject SUBQ. Inject slowly into deep, well-developed muscle. Rotate injection sites.

IV Administration

- **Intermittent Infusion:** For patients on palliative care, may be infused as 0.0625 mg/kg/day in 250 mL of D5W. **Rate:** Infuse slowly, at 20–40 drops/min.
- **Y-Site Compatibility:** fentanyl, hydromorphone, methadone, morphine, sufentanil.
- **Y-Site Incompatibility:** heparin.

Patient/Family Teaching

- Explain purpose and side effects of medication to patient. Advise patient to read *Patient Information* before starting therapy. Advise to take medication as directed. Take missed doses as soon as remembered unless almost time for next dose; do not double dose.
- Advise patient to notify health care provider of all Rx or OTC medications, vitamins, or herbal products being taken and to consult with health care provider before taking other medications.

- Advise patient on how and when to ask for pain medication.
- Advise patients to make position changes slowly and to remain recumbent for 6–12 hr after administration to minimize orthostatic hypotension.
- May cause drowsiness. Caution patient to request assistance with ambulation and transfer and to avoid driving or other activities requiring alertness until response to the medication is known.
- Advise patient to avoid taking alcohol or other CNS depressants concurrently with this medication.
- Advise patient to use sunscreen and protective clothing when exposed to the sun. Extremes of temperature should also be avoided because this drug impairs body temperature regulation.
- Advise patient to use frequent mouth rinses, good oral hygiene, and sugarless gum or candy to minimize dry mouth.
- Advise patient to notify health care provider promptly if sore throat, fever, unusual bleeding or bruising, rash, weakness, tremors, dark-colored urine, clay-colored stools, or signs of blood clots (swelling, pain, and redness in an arm or leg that can be warm to touch; sudden chest pain; difficulty breathing; heart palpitations) occur.
- Rep: Advise women of reproductive potential to notify health care provider if pregnancy is planned or suspected or if breastfeeding. Use should be avoided during 3rd trimester because of ↑ risk of agitation, hypotonia, tremor, somnolence, respiratory distress, and feeding disturbances in newborn.

Evaluation/Desired Outcomes

- Decreased manifestations of psychotic disturbances.
- Reduction in severity of pain.
- Reduction in nausea/vomiting.

moclobemide

(moe-**kloe**-be-mide)

Manerix

Classification

Therapeutic: antidepressants

Pharmacologic: monamine oxidase (MAO) inhibitors, benzamides

Indications

Depression.

Action

Short-acting, reversible inhibitor of monoamine oxidase type A. Increases concentrations of serotonin, norepinephrine, and dopamine. **Therapeutic Effects:** Decreased symptoms of depression, with improved mood and quality of life.

Pharmacokinetics

Absorption: 98% absorbed following oral administration, but undergoes first-pass hepatic metabolism, resulting in 90% bioavailability.

Distribution: Unknown.

Metabolism and Excretion: Extensively metabolized (partially by CYP2C19 and CYP2D6); very small amounts are pharmacologically active; <1% excreted unchanged in urine.

Half-life: 1.5 hr (↑ with dose).

TIME/ACTION PROFILE

ROUTE	ONSET	PEAK	DURATION
PO	days–several wk (antidepressant effect)	0.5–3.5 hr (plasma concentrations)	24 hr (MAO-A inhibition)

Contraindications/Precautions

Contraindicated in: Hypersensitivity; Acute confusional states; Concurrent use of tricyclic antidepressants; Concurrent use of SSRIs or other MAO inhibitors; **Use Cautiously in:** History of suicide attempt or ideation; History of thyrotoxicosis or pheochromocytoma (possible risk of hypertensive reaction); Renal impairment; Severe hepatic impairment (↓ dose); OB: Safety and effectiveness not established in pregnancy; Lactation: Safety and effectiveness not established in breastfeeding; Pedi: Safety and effectiveness not established in children.

Adverse Reactions/Side Effects

CV: hypotension. **Neuro:** agitation, insomnia, restlessness, SUICIDAL THOUGHTS/BEHAVIORS, tremor.

Interactions

Drug-Drug: Selegiline greatly ↑ sensitivity to tyramine; concurrent use contraindicated. **Tricyclic antidepressants** may result in severe adverse reactions; concurrent use contraindicated. Should not be used with **SSRIs** or other **MAO inhibitors**; when making a switch, allow 4–5 half-lives of previous drug; for **fluoxetine**, wait ≥5 wk. May ↑ levels of and risk of QT prolongation with **thioridazine**; avoid concurrent use. Excessive **alcohol** should be avoided. **Cimetidine** may ↑ levels and risk of toxicity; ↓ moclobemide dose by 50%. Because of the potential for interactions with **anesthetics**, especially local anesthetics containing **epinephrine**, moclobemide should be discontinued ≥2 days before procedures. Concurrent use with **opioids** should be avoided; dosage adjustments may be necessary. **Sympathomimetics**, including **ephedrine** and **amphetamines**, may ↑ BP; avoid concurrent use. **Dextromethorphan** may ↑ risk of vertigo, tremor, nausea, and vomiting; avoid concurrent use. **Antihypertensives** may ↑ risk of hypotension.

Drug-Food: Ingestion of large amounts of **tyramine-containing foods**, including some cheeses and **Marmite yeast extract**, may result in hypertension and arrhythmias.

Route/Dosage

PO (Adults): 150 mg twice daily initially; may ↑ gradually after one wk, as needed/tolerated (max = 600 mg/day).

Hepatic Impairment

PO (Adults): *Severe hepatic impairment or concurrent use of cimetidine:* ↓ daily dose to ⅓–½ of standard dose.

Availability

Tablets: 100 mg, 150 mg, 300 mg.

NURSING IMPLICATIONS

Assessment

- Monitor BP and HR before and frequently during therapy. Report significant changes promptly.
- Monitor mood changes. Assess for suicidal tendencies, especially during early therapy. Restrict amount of drug available to patient.
- Monitor intake and output and daily weight. Assess for peripheral edema and urinary retention.

Lab Test Considerations

- Monitor liver and kidney function periodically during treatment.
- Monitor serum glucose closely in patients with diabetes; hypoglycemia may occur.

Toxicity and Overdose

- Concurrent ingestion of tyramine-rich foods and many medications may result in a life-threatening hypertensive crisis. Signs/symptoms of hypertensive crisis include chest pain, tachycardia, severe headache, nausea and vomiting, photosensitivity, and enlarged pupils. Treatment includes IV phentolamine.
- Symptoms of overdose include anxiety, irritability, tachycardia, hypertension or hypotension, respiratory distress, dizziness, drowsiness, hallucinations, confusion, seizures, fever, and diaphoresis. Treatment includes induction of vomiting or gastric lavage and supportive therapy as symptoms arise.

Implementation

- **PO:** Administer after meals. ***DNC:*** Swallow tablet whole. Do not crush, break, or chew. Dose may be adjusted gradually during the 1st wk of therapy.

Patient/Family Teaching

- Explain purpose and side effects of medication to patient. Advise patient to read *Patient Information* before starting therapy. Advise to take as directed. Take missed doses if remembered unless almost time for next dose; do not double doses. Do not discontinue abruptly; withdrawal symptoms (nausea, vomiting, malaise, nightmares, agitation, psychosis, seizures) may occur.
- Advise patient to notify health care provider of all Rx or OTC medications, vitamins, or herbal products being taken and to consult with health care provider before taking other medications.
- Advise patient to avoid alcohol, CNS depressants, OTC drugs, and foods or beverages containing tyramine (see Appendix J) during and for ≥2 wk after therapy has been discontinued; they may precipitate a hypertensive crisis. Contact health care provider immediately if symptoms of hypertensive crisis develop.
- Advise patient to notify health care provider if neck stiffness, changes in vision, diarrhea, constipation, rapid/pounding heartbeat, sudden and severe headache, stiff neck, confusion, disorientation, slurred speech, behavioral changes, or seizures occur.
- Advise patient, family, and caregivers to notify health care provider if thoughts about suicide or dying, attempts to commit suicide, new or worse depression, new or worse anxiety, feeling very agitated or restless, panic attacks, trouble sleeping, new or worse irritability, acting aggressive, being angry or violent, acting on dangerous impulses, an extreme ↑ in activity and talking, or other unusual changes in behavior or mood occur.
- Advise patient to carry identification describing medication regimen.
- Rep: Advise women of reproductive potential to notify health care provider if pregnancy is planned or suspected or if breastfeeding.

Evaluation/Desired Outcomes

- Decreased symptoms of depression, with improved mood and quality of life.

pinaverium (pin-ah-veer-ee-um)

🍁 Dicetel

Classification

Therapeutic: anti-irritable bowel syndrome agents

Pharmacologic: calcium channel blockers

Indications

Management of symptoms of irritable bowel syndrome (IBS), including abdominal pain, bowel disturbances, and discomfort. Treatment of symptoms related to biliary tract disorders.

Action

Acts as a calcium channel blocker with specific selectivity for intestinal smooth muscle. Relaxes GI (mainly colon) and biliary tracts; inhibits colonic motor response to food/pharmacologic stimulation.
Therapeutic Effects: Decreased symptoms of IBS.

Pharmacokinetics

Absorption: Poorly absorbed (1–10%).
Distribution: Distributes selectively to digestive tract.
Protein Binding: 97%.
Metabolism and Excretion: Minimal enterohepatic cycling; eliminated almost entirely in feces. Some metabolism.
Half-life: 1.5 hr.

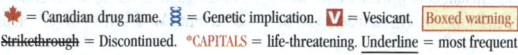

TIME/ACTION PROFILE (plasma concentrations)

ROUTE	ONSET	PEAK	DURATION
PO	unknown	1 hr	unknown

Contraindications/Precautions

Contraindicated in: Hypersensitivity; Galactose intolerance/Lapp lactase deficiency/glucose-galactose malabsorption; Lactation: Lactation.

Use Cautiously in: Pre-existing esophageal lesions/hiatal hernia; OB: Safety and effectiveness not established in pregnancy; Pedi: Safety and effectiveness not established in children.

Adverse Reactions/Side Effects

GI: constipation, diarrhea, distention, dry mouth, epigastric pain/fullness, esophageal irritation, nausea. **Derm:** rash. **Neuro:** drowsiness, headache, vertigo.

Interactions

Drug-Drug: Anticholinergic medications may ↑ spasmolytic effects.

Route/Dosage

PO (Adults): 50 mg 3 times daily; may ↑ as needed/tolerated up to 100 mg 3 times daily.

Availability

Tablets (contain lactose): 50 mg, 100 mg.

NURSING IMPLICATIONS

Assessment

- Assess for signs/symptoms of IBS (abdominal pain or discomfort, bloating, constipation).
- Assess for lactose intolerance; product contains lactose.

Implementation

- **PO:** Administer tablet with 8 ounces of water and food. ***DNC:*** Swallow tablet whole; do not crush, chew, or suck. If >3 tablets/day prescribed, take additional tablets with 8 ounces of water and a snack. May be irritating to esophagus. Do not take the tablet while lying down or just before bedtime.

Patient/Family Teaching

- Explain purpose and side effects of medication to patient. Advise patient to read *Patient Information* before starting therapy. Advise patient to take as directed. Take missed doses as soon as remembered unless almost time for next dose; do not double doses.
- Advise patient to notify health care provider of all Rx or OTC medications, vitamins, or herbal products being taken and to consult with health care provider before taking other medications.
- Advise patient to notify health care provider if the following side effects persist or worsen: stomach pain or fullness, nausea, constipation or diarrhea, heartburn, headache, dry mouth, dizziness, skin rash.
- Instruct patient to avoid alcohol intake while taking this medication.
- Rep: Advise women of reproductive potential to notify health care provider if pregnancy is planned or suspected or if breastfeeding.

Evaluation/Desired Outcomes

- Decreased symptoms of IBS.

propiverine (pro-**piv**-e-reen)

Mictoryl, Mictoryl Pediatric

Classification

Therapeutic: antispasmodics

Pharmacologic: anticholinergics

Indications

Urinary incontinence and/or increased urinary frequency and urgency associated with overactive bladder.

Action

Exhibits anticholinergic and calcium-modulating properties. The efferent connection of the pelvic nerve is inhibited due to anticholinergic action, resulting in relaxation of bladder smooth muscle. Inhibits the calcium influx and modulates the intracellular calcium in urinary bladder smooth muscle cells, causing musculotropic spasmolysis. **Therapeutic Effects:** Reduced urinary incontinence, frequency, and urgency.

Pharmacokinetics

Absorption: 50–60% absorbed following oral administration (↑ with high-fat meal).

Distribution: Extensively distributed to tissues.

Protein Binding: 90–95%.

Metabolism and Excretion: Primarily metabolized by the liver; 60% excreted in urine (<1% as unchanged drug); 21% excreted in feces.

Half-life: 14–20 hr.

TIME/ACTION PROFILE (plasma concentrations)

ROUTE	ONSET	PEAK	DURATION
PO	30 min–1 hr	2–10 hr	24 hr

Contraindications/Precautions

Contraindicated in: Hypersensitivity; Bladder outflow obstruction with urinary retention; Bowel obstruction; Fructose intolerance or sucrase-isomaltase insufficiency; Galactose intolerance/Lapp lactase deficiency/glucose-galactose malabsorption; Intestinal atony; Myasthenia gravis; Severe ulcerative colitis; Toxic megacolon; Uncontrolled angle-closure glaucoma; Moderate or severe hepatic impairment.

Use Cautiously in: Autonomic neuropathy; Arrhythmia; Hiatus hernia with reflux esophagitis; Prostatic enlargement; Class IV HF; Tachycardia; Renal impairment; Mild hepatic impairment; OB: Safety and effectiveness not established in pregnancy; Lactation: Safety and effectiveness not established in breastfeeding; Pedi: Children <5 yr (safety and effectiveness not established).

Adverse Reactions/Side Effects

CV: hypotension, palpitations, tachycardia. **Derm:** pruritus, rash. **EENT:** dry mouth. **GI:** abdominal pain, constipation, dyspepsia. **GU:** bladder and urethral symptoms, urinary retention. **Neuro:** blurred vision, confusion, dizziness, fatigue, headache, restlessness, sedation, tremor.

Interactions

Drug-Drug: Tricyclic antidepressants, **benzodiazepines**, and **anticholinergics** may ↑ risk of toxicity. May ↑ effects of **amantadine**, **phenothiazines**, and **beta agonists**. **Cholinergics** may ↓ effectiveness. **Isoniazid** may ↑ risk of hypotension. May ↓ effectiveness of **metoclopramide**.

Route/Dosage

PO (Adults): *Extended-release capsules:* 30 mg once daily; may ↑ to a max of 45 mg once daily.
PO (Children ≥35 kg): 15 mg twice daily (max = 30 mg/day).
PO (Children <35 kg): *Immediate-release tablets:* 0.8 mg/kg/day in 2 divided doses; alternatively, the following body weight adjusted dosing may be used. *29–34 kg:* 10 mg in morning and 15 mg in evening. *23–28 kg:* 10 mg 2 times daily. *17–22 kg:* 5 mg in morning and 10 mg in evening. *12–16 kg:* 5 mg twice daily.

Renal Impairment

PO (Adults): *CCr <30 mL/min:* Max dose = 30 mg/day.

Availability

Immediate-release tablets: 5 mg. **Extended-release capsules:** 30 mg, 45 mg.

NURSING IMPLICATIONS

Assessment

- Before starting therapy, rule out alternative causes of pollakiuria and nocturia (organic bladder disease such as UTI or malignancy, HF).
- Assess urinary frequency, urgency, incontinence, and bladder spasms before and periodically during therapy.
- Monitor for urinary retention. Measure postvoid residual if needed.
- Monitor for ECG changes (tachycardia, arrhythmias, and prolonged QT interval) during therapy.

Lab Test Considerations

- Monitor hepatic function. *If liver enzymes and/or bilirubin ↑ above normal values,* discontinue propiverine.

Implementation

- **PO:** Administer with or without food. ***DNC:*** Swallow extended-release capsules whole. Do not crush, break, or chew.
- Immediate-release tablets should be taken ≥1 hr before meals.

Patient/Family Teaching

- Explain purpose and side effects of medication to patient. Advise patient to read *Patient Information* before starting therapy. Advise patient it may take several days to notice improvement in symptoms. Advise if dose is missed, the next dose should be taken as planned. Do not double dose. The prescribed dosing schedule should be continued.
- Advise patient to notify health care provider of all Rx or OTC medications, vitamins, or herbal products being taken and to consult with health care provider before taking other medications.
- Advise patient to notify health care provider if signs and symptoms of glaucoma (blurred vision, eye pain, headache, side vision loss) and worsening neuropathy occur.
- Caution patient to avoid driving or other activities requiring alertness until response to medication is known.
- Advise patient to perform good oral hygiene and sugarless gum or candy for dry mouth.
- Advise patient about adequate fluid intake and fiber-rich diet to prevent constipation.
- Rep: Advise women of reproductive potential to notify health care provider if pregnancy is planned or suspected or if breastfeeding.

Evaluation/Desired Outcomes

- Reduced urinary incontinence, frequency, and urgency.

trimebutine (try-**meh**-boo-teen)
Classification
Therapeutic: lower gastrointestinal tract motility, spasmolytics

Indications

Symptomatic treatment of irritable bowel syndrome (IBS). Postoperative paralytic ileus.

Action

Acts as a spasmolytic. **Therapeutic Effects:** Decreased symptoms of IBS. Resumption of intestinal transit following abdominal surgical procedures.

Pharmacokinetics

Absorption: Rapidly absorbed following oral administration.
Distribution: Unknown.
Metabolism and Excretion: Extensively metabolized; <2.4% excreted unchanged in urine.
Half-life: 2.7–3.1 hr.

TIME/ACTION PROFILE (symptom relief)

ROUTE	ONSET	PEAK	DURATION
PO	within 3 days–2 wk	1 hr (plasma concentrations)	>1 wk (following discontinuation)

Contraindications/Precautions

Contraindicated in: Hypersensitivity.
Use Cautiously in: OB: Safety and effectiveness not established in pregnancy; Lactation: Safety and effectiveness not established in breastfeeding; Pedi: Children <12 yr (safety and effectiveness not established).

Adverse Reactions/Side Effects

GI: diarrhea, dry mouth, dyspepsia, epigastric pain, nausea. **Derm:** hot/cold sensation, rash. **Neuro:** dizziness, drowsiness, dysgeusia, fatigue, headache.

Interactions

Drug-Drug: None reported.

Route/Dosage

PO (Adults): 200 mg 3 times daily.

Availability

Tablets: 100 mg, 200 mg.

NURSING IMPLICATIONS

Assessment

- Assess for symptoms of IBS (cramping, constipation, and diarrhea; mucus in stools).
- Assess for abdominal distention and assess bowel sounds.
- Monitor intake and output.

Implementation

- **PO:** Administer as prescribed before meals.

Patient/Family Teaching

- Explain purpose and side effects of medication to patient. Advise patient to read *Patient Information* before starting therapy. Advise to take as directed.
- Advise patient to notify health care provider of all Rx or OTC medications, vitamins, or herbal products being taken and to consult with health care provider before taking other medications.
- Advise patient to avoid driving or operating heavy machinery until response to medication is known.
- Advise patient to avoid alcohol use during therapy.
- Advise patient to notify health care provider of persistent or worsening symptoms.
- Rep: Advise women of reproductive potential to notify health care provider if pregnancy is planned or suspected or if breastfeeding.

Evaluation/Desired Outcomes

- Decreased symptoms of IBS.
- Resumption of intestinal transit following abdominal surgical procedures.

vernakalant (ver-nak-a-lant)

Brinavess

Classification

Therapeutic: antiarrhythmics (class III)

Indications

Rapid conversion of recent onset atrial fibrillation to sinus rhythm for nonsurgical (≤7 days) and post–cardiac surgery patients (≤3 days).

Action

Prolongs atrial refractoriness without significantly affecting ventricular refractoriness by blocking specific potassium channels. Slows impulse conduction in atria by blocking sodium channels in concentration, voltage, and frequency-dependent manner.
Therapeutic Effects: Conversion of atrial fibrillation to sinus rhythm.

Pharmacokinetics

Absorption: IV administration results in complete bioavailability.
Distribution: Widely distributed to tissues.
Metabolism and Excretion: Mostly metabolized by the liver via the CYP2D6 isoenzyme; the CYP2D6 isoenzyme exhibits genetic polymorphism; ~7% of population may be poor metabolizers and may have significantly ↑ vernakalant concentrations and an ↑ risk of adverse effects.
Half-life: 3–5.5 hr

TIME/ACTION PROFILE

ROUTE	ONSET	PEAK	DURATION
IV	8–14 min	immediately	2–4 hr

Contraindications/Precautions

Contraindicated in: Hypersensitivity; Hypotension (systolic BP <100 mm Hg); Severe aortic stenosis; New York Heart Association Class III or IV HF; QT interval >440 msec; Congenital or acquired long QT syndrome; Severe bradycardia; Sinus node dysfunction or 2nd-/3rd-degree AV heart block, in the absence of a pacemaker; Acute coronary syndrome or acute decompensated HF within the last 30 days.
Use Cautiously in: Hepatic impairment; OB: Safety and effectiveness not established in pregnancy; Lactation: Safety and effectiveness not established in breastfeeding; Pedi: Safety and effectiveness not established in children.

Adverse Reactions/Side Effects

CV: atrial fibrillation, atrial flutter, bradycardia, heart block, hypertension, hypotension, VENTRICULAR TACHYCARDIA. **Derm:** ↑ sweating, hot flushing, pruritus. **EENT:** nasal discomfort. **F and E:** hypokalemia. **GI:** diarrhea, nausea, vomiting. **Local:** infusion site pain. **Neuro:** dizziness, dysgeusia, fatigue, headache, paresthesia. **Resp:** cough, dyspnea.

Interactions

Drug-Drug: None reported.

Route/Dosage

IV (Adults): 3 mg/kg infused over 10 min (for patients weighing ≥113 kg, max initial dose = 339 mg). If conversion to sinus rhythm does not occur within 15 min after the end of the initial infusion and the patient remains hemodynamically stable, a 2nd infusion of 2 mg/kg may be administered over 10 min (for patients weighing ≥113 kg, max dose of 2nd infusion = 226 mg). Cumulative doses >5 mg/kg should not be administered within 24 hr.

Availability

Solution for injection: 20 mg/mL (each vial contains 3.5 mmol [80 mg] of sodium).

NURSING IMPLICATIONS

Assessment

- Ensure patient is adequately hydrated and anticoagulated in accordance with treatment guidelines.
- Monitor vital signs and provide continuous cardiac rhythm monitoring before, during, and after administration. Assess for signs/symptoms of sudden ↓ in BP or HR, and significant QT interval prolongation during 1st infusion and >15 min after completion of infusion. Assess vital signs and provide continuous cardiac rhythm monitoring for >2 hr after completion of 2nd infusion.
- Monitor for sinus arrest or clinically significant bradycardia after converting to sinus rhythm. Resuscitation equipment and the capability to place a temporary pacemaker should be readily available.

Lab Test Considerations

- Monitor potassium before and during treatment. May cause hypokalemia.
- May ↑ AST, GGT, BUN, and serum creatinine.
- May ↓ hemoglobin.

Implementation

IV Administration

- Before administration, confirm patient eligibility for treatment by completing the supplied Pre-Infusion Checklist. The checklist is provided with the medication or is available at https://www.cipherpharma.com/wp-content/uploads/2019/10/Brinavess-English-Checklist-ENFR.pdf.
- Verify amiodarone, procainamide, flecainide, or ibutilide have not been administered within 4 hr before treatment.
- Do not administer via IV push or bolus.
- In case of accidental overdose or excessive infusion flow rate of injection, discontinue infusion immediately.
- **Intermittent Infusion: Dilution:** *If ≤100 kg:* Add 25 mL of vernakalant to 100 mL of 0.9% NaCl, LR, or D5W. *If >100 kg:* Add 30 mL of vernakalant to 120 mL of 0.9% NaCl, LR, or D5W. Diluted sterile solution should be clear, colorless to pale yellow. **Concentration:** 4 mg/mL. **Rate:** Infuse over 10 min.
- **Y-Site Incompatibility:** Do not administer other drugs through same IV line.

Patient/Family Teaching

- Explain purpose and side effects of treatment to patient.
- Advise patient to notify health care provider of all Rx or OTC medications, vitamins, or herbal products being taken and to consult with health care provider before taking other medications.
- Advise patient that treatment will be in a hospital or emergency room setting. Explain that the 1st infusion is to be administered for 10 min. A 2nd dose may be needed if the HR has not returned to normal within 15 min after 1st dose.
- Rep: Advise women of reproductive potential to notify health care provider if pregnancy is planned or suspected or if breastfeeding.

Evaluation/Desired Outcomes

- Suppression of irregular heart rhythm.

zopiclone (zoe-pi-clone)

✱ Imovane

Classification

Therapeutic: sedative/hypnotics

Pharmacologic: cyclopyrrolones

Indications

Short-term treatment of insomnia characterized by difficulty falling asleep and frequent/early awakenings.

Action

Interacts with GABA-receptor complexes; not a benzodiazepine. **Therapeutic Effects:** Improved sleep with decreased latency and increased maintenance of sleep.

Pharmacokinetics

Absorption: Rapidly absorbed (75%) following oral administration.

Distribution: Rapidly distributed from extravascular compartment.
Metabolism and Excretion: Primarily metabolized by the liver via the CYP3A4 isoenzyme; metabolites have minimal sedative/hypnotic activity; 4–5% excreted unchanged in urine.
Half-life: 5 hr.

TIME/ACTION PROFILE

ROUTE	ONSET	PEAK	DURATION
PO	rapid	2 hr	6 hr

Contraindications/Precautions

Contraindicated in: Hypersensitivity; Myasthenia gravis; Severe hepatic impairment; Severe respiratory impairment (including sleep apnea); Galactose intolerance (5 mg tablet contains lactose); OB: Pregnancy; Lactation: Lactation.
Use Cautiously in: Renal, hepatic, or pulmonary impairment (dosage ↓ may be recommended); Past history of paradoxical reactions to sedative/hypnotics or alcohol or violent behavior; History of depression or suicidal ideation; Geri: May ↑ risk of falls, confusion, or anterograde amnesia in older adults (use lowest effective dose); Pedi: Safety and effectiveness not established in children.
Exercise Extreme Caution in: History of substance/alcohol abuse.

Adverse Reactions/Side Effects

GI: bitter taste, anorexia, constipation, dry mouth, dyspepsia. **Neuro:** abnormal thinking, behavioral changes, sleep-driving. **Misc:** HYPERSENSITIVITY REACTIONS (INCLUDING ANAPHYLAXIS AND ANGIOEDEMA).

Interactions

Drug-Drug: ↑ risk of CNS depression with other **CNS depressants**, including **antihistamines**, **antidepressants**, **opioids**, **sedative/hypnotics**, and **antipsychotics**. ↑ levels and risk of CNS depression with **CYP3A4 inhibitors**, including **erythromycin ketoconazole**, **itraconazole**, **clarithromycin**, **nefazodone**, **ritonavir**, and **nelfinavir**; ↓ dose may be necessary. **CYP3A4 inducers**, including **carbamazepine**, **phenobarbital**, **phenytoin**, **rifampicin**, and **rifampin**, may ↓ levels and effectiveness; dose ↑ may be necessary.

Route/Dosage

PO (Adults): 3.75–7.5 mg taken immediately before bedtime; not to exceed 7.5 mg or 7–10 days use. Geri: 3.75 mg initially taken immediately before bedtime; may ↑ up to 7.5 mg if needed.

Hepatic/Renal Impairment

PO (Adults): 3.75 mg initially taken immediately before bedtime; may ↑ up to 7.5 mg if needed.

Availability

Tablets: 5 mg, 7.5 mg.

NURSING IMPLICATIONS

Assessment

- Assess mental status, sleep patterns, and previous use of sedative/hypnotics. Prolonged use of >7–10 days may lead to physical and psychological dependence.
- Assess alertness at time of peak of drug. Notify health care provider if desired sedation does not occur.
- Assess level of pain and medicate as needed. Untreated pain ↓ sedative effects.

Implementation

- Before administering, ↓ external stimuli and provide comfort measures to ↑ effectiveness of medication.
- Promote a safe environment.
- Use lowest effective dose.
- **PO:** Administer immediately before bedtime on an empty stomach.

Patient/Family Teaching

- Explain purpose and side effects of medication to patient. Advise patient to read *Patient Information* before starting therapy.
- Advise patient to notify health care provider of all Rx or OTC medications, vitamins, or herbal products being taken and to consult with health care provider before taking other medications.
- Advise patient to take as directed. Advise patient not to take zopiclone unless able to stay in bed a full night (7–8 hr) before being active again. Do not take more than the amount prescribed because of the habit-forming potential. Not recommended for use >7–10 days. If used for >2 wk, abrupt withdrawal may result in fatigue, nausea, flushing, light-headedness, uncontrolled crying, vomiting, GI upset, panic attack, or nervousness.
- Because of rapid onset, advise patient to go to bed immediately after taking zopiclone.
- May cause daytime drowsiness or dizziness. Advise patient to avoid driving or other activities requiring alertness until response to this medication is known.
- Advise patient that complex sleep-related behaviors (sleep-driving) may occur while asleep.
- Advise patient to notify health care provider immediately if signs/symptoms of anaphylaxis (swelling of the tongue or throat, trouble breathing, nausea, vomiting) occur.
- Advise patient to avoid concurrent use of alcohol or other CNS depressants.
- Rep: Advise women of reproductive potential to notify health care provider if pregnancy is planned or suspected or if breastfeeding.

Evaluation/Desired Outcomes

- Relief of insomnia by improved falling asleep and decreased frequency of nocturnal and early morning awakenings.

zuclopenthixol

(zoo-kloe-pen-**thix**-ole)

✦ Clopixol, ✦ Clopixol-Acuphase, ✦ Clopixol Depot

Classification

Therapeutic: antipsychotics

Pharmacologic: thioxanthenes

Indications

Schizophrenia.

Action

Exhibits high affinity for dopamine D_1 and D_2 receptors and α_1-adrenergic and 5-HT_2 receptors. Dopaminergic blockade produces neuroleptic activity. **Therapeutic Effects:** Decreases psychoses due to schizophrenia.

Pharmacokinetics

Absorption: Well absorbed following oral administration; slowly absorbed from IM sites.
Distribution: Widely distributed to tissues.
Metabolism and Excretion: Primarily metabolized by the liver via the CYP2D6 isoenzyme; the CYP2D6 isoenzyme exhibits genetic polymorphism; ~7% of population may be poor metabolizers and may have significantly ↑ metoprolol concentrations and an ↑ risk of adverse effects; metabolites do not have antipsychotic activity; minimal amounts excreted unchanged in urine.
Half-life: *PO:* 20 hr.

TIME/ACTION PROFILE (antipsychotic effect)

ROUTE	ONSET	PEAK	DURATION
PO	within hours	4 hr (plasma concentrations)	8–24 hr
IM (acuphase)	2–4 hr	8 hr (sedation)	2–3 days
IM (depot)	within 3 days	3–7 days (plasma concentrations)	2–4 wk

Contraindications/Precautions

Contraindicated in: Narrow-angle glaucoma.
Use Cautiously in: Electrolyte abnormalities, concurrent use of diuretics or drugs affecting QT interval, or history of cardiovascular disease (↑ risk of serious arrhythmias); Intestinal pathology or brain lesions (antiemetic effect may mask symptoms); History of seizures (may ↓ seizure threshold); Parkinson disease (may cause deterioration); Risk factors/history of stroke; Renal impairment; Hepatic impairment; OB: Use during pregnancy only if potential maternal benefit justifies potential fetal risk; Lactation: Safety and effectiveness not established in breastfeeding; Pedi: Safety and effectiveness not established in children; Geri: ↑ risk of stroke, cognitive decline, and mortality in older adults with dementia.

Adverse Reactions/Side Effects

CV: arrhythmias, hypotension, tachycardia, THROMBOEMBOLISM. **Derm:** ↑ sweating, photosensitivity. **EENT:** abnormal vision accommodation. **Endo:** hyperprolactinemia, hyperglycemia. **F and E:** ↑ thirst. **GI:** constipation, dry mouth, diarrhea, vomiting. **GU:** ↓ libido, abnormal urination. **Hemat:** anemia, granulocytopenia. **Metab:** weight gain. **MS:** myalgia. **Neuro:** dizziness, extrapyramidal symptoms, fatigue, sedation, NEUROLEPTIC MALIGNANT SYNDROME, tardive dyskinesia, syncope, weakness.

Interactions

Drug-Drug: ↑ risk of CNS depression with other **CNS depressants**, including **alcohol**, some **antihistamines**, some **antidepressants**, **anxiolytics**, **barbiturates**, **benzodiazepines**, and **sedative/hypnotics**. **CYP2D6 inhibitors** may ↑ levels and risk of toxicity. **Diuretics**, **lithium**, **class Ia and III antiarrhythmics**, some **antipsychotics** (including **thioridazine**), **macrolides**, and **fluoroquinolones** ↑ risk of QT interval prolongation and serious arrhythmias; avoid concurrent use. ↑ risk of anticholinergic adverse reactions with other **anticholingeric drugs**. ↑ risk of hypotension with **antihypertensives** and **diuretics**. Concurrent use with **tricyclic antidepressants** may result in altered metabolism and effects of both. ↑ risk of extrapyramidal symptoms with **metoclopramide**. May ↓ effectiveness of **levodopa** and **dopamine agonists**.

Route/Dosage

PO (Adults): *Acute psychoses:* 10–50 mg/day in 2–3 divided doses initially; may ↑ by 10–20 mg/day every 2–3 days; titrate according to response. Usual dose range is 20–60 mg/day; doses >100 mg/day are not recommended. Dose should be ↓ to lowest dose needed to control symptoms (20–40 mg/day). After maintenance dose is established, give as a single daily dose.
IM (Adults): *Acuphase:* 50–150 mg; may be repeated every 2–3 days if necessary; some patients may need an additional dose 1–2 days after 1st injection only; care must be taken to avoid overmedicating due to delay in absorption and antipsychotic effects. Max dose = 400 mg or 4 injections. Acuphase is not meant for long-term use; duration should not >2 wk. If dose >2 mL, divide dose and give in 2 different sites. If PO maintenance is needed, initiate 2–3 days

following the last dose of Acuphase. If depot is used for maintenance, may be given concurrently with the last injection of Acuphase. *Suggested transfer regimen to PO dosing:* If Acuphase dose was 50 mg, then oral dose could be 20 mg/day; if Acuphase dose was 100 mg, then oral dose could be 40 mg/day; if Acuphase dose was 150 mg, then oral dose could be 60 mg/day. *Suggested transfer regimen to depot dosing:* If Acuphase dose was 50 mg, then depot dose could be 100 mg IM every 2 wk. If Acuphase dose was 100 mg, then depot dose could be 200 mg IM every 2 wk. If Acuphase dose was 150 mg, then depot dose could be 300 mg IM every 2 wk.

IM (Adults): *Depot:* Usual maintenance dose is 150–300 mg every 2–4 wk; regimens should be individualized according to response; care must be taken not to overmedicate due to delayed/prolonged absorption and effects. If dose >2 mL, divide dose and give in 2 different sites.

Availability

Tablets (contain castor oil): 10 mg, 25 mg. **Zuclopenthixol acetate injection (Acuphase) (contains medium-chain triglycerides):** 50 mg/mL. **Zuclopenthixol decanoate injection (Depot) (contains medium-chain triglycerides):** 200 mg/mL.

NURSING IMPLICATIONS

Assessment

- Assess mental status (orientation, mood, behavior) before and periodically during therapy.
- Observe carefully when administering oral medication to ensure that medication is actually taken and not hoarded.
- Assess weight and BMI initially and during therapy.
- Assess fluid intake and bowel function. ↑ fiber and fluids in the diet help minimize constipation.
- Monitor for onset of akathisia (restlessness or desire to keep moving) and extrapyramidal side effects (*parkinsonian:* difficulty speaking or swallowing, loss of balance control, pill rolling, masklike face, shuffling gait, rigidity, tremors; *dystonic:* muscle spasms, twisting motions, twitching, inability to move eyes, weakness of arms or legs) every 2 mo during therapy and 8–12 wk after therapy has been discontinued. ↓ in dose or discontinuation of medication may be necessary. Benztropine or diphenhydramine may be used to control these symptoms.
- Monitor for tardive dyskinesia (uncontrolled rhythmic movement of mouth, face, and extremities; lip smacking or puckering; puffing of cheeks; uncontrolled chewing; rapid or worm-like movements of tongue). Report immediately; may be irreversible.
- Monitor for development of neuroleptic malignant syndrome (fever, respiratory distress, tachycardia, seizures, diaphoresis, arrhythmias, hypertension or hypotension, pallor, tiredness, severe muscle stiffness, loss of bladder control). Report immediately.
- Monitor for symptoms related to hyperprolactinemia (menstrual abnormalities, galactorrhea, sexual dysfunction).

Lab Test Considerations

- Monitor CBC and liver function tests every 6 mo and periodically as needed during treatment. May ↑ AST, ALT, and alkaline phosphatase.
- Monitor blood glucose before and periodically during therapy. May cause hyperglycemia.
- Monitor serum prolactin before and periodically during therapy. May ↑ prolactin.

Implementation

- **PO:** Administer before or after meals.
- **IM:** Administer deep in large muscle. A test dose may be ordered for 1st administration.

Patient/Family Teaching

- Explain purpose and side effects of medication to patient. Advise patient to read *Patient Information* before starting therapy. Advise to take as directed. If a dose is missed, omit and take next dose as scheduled. Discontinuation should be gradual.
- Advise patient to notify health care provider of all Rx or OTC medications, vitamins, or herbal products being taken and to consult with health care provider before taking other medications.
- Advise patient of possibility of extrapyramidal symptoms and tardive dyskinesia. Caution patient to report these symptoms immediately to health care provider.
- Advise patient to change positions slowly to minimize orthostatic hypotension.
- Medication may cause drowsiness. Caution patient to avoid driving or other activities requiring alertness until response to medication is known.
- Advise patient to notify health care provider promptly if sore throat, fever, unusual bleeding or bruising, rash, weakness, tremors, visual disturbances, dark-colored urine, or clay-colored stools occur.
- Advise patient to avoid sun exposure and to wear protective clothing and sunscreen when outdoors.
- Advise patient to notify health care provider of medication regimen before treatment or surgery.
- Rep: Advise women of reproductive potential to notify health care provider if pregnancy is planned or suspected or if breastfeeding or planning to breastfeed. Infants exposed in the 3rd trimester may exhibit extrapyramidal and withdrawal reactions, including agitation, hypertonia, hypotonia, tremor, somnolence, respiratory distress, and feeding disorders.

Evaluation/Desired Outcomes

- Decreased symptoms of schizophrenia (delusions; hallucinations; social withdrawal; flat, blunt affect).

BEERS CRITERIA

The Beers criteria for potentially inappropriate medication use in adults 65 and older in the United States is a compilation of drugs and drug classes found to increase the risk of adverse events in older adults. Frequently, older adults are more sensitive to the medications or their side effects. These adverse events have significant economic and quality of life costs for society and individuals and can result in more frequent hospitalizations, permanent injury, or death. Often, the potential for adverse events can be minimized by prescribing safer alternatives or prescribing at the lowest effective dose.

ALPRAZolam (avoid use) (Xanax, Xanax XR)

amiodarone (avoid use as first-line therapy for atrial fibrillation unless heart failure or significant left ventricular hypertrophy present) (Nexterone, Pacerone)

amitriptyline (avoid use) (Elavil)

amoxapine (avoid use)

ARIPiprazole (avoid use, except in schizophrenia, bipolar disorder, or adjunctive treatment of major depressive disorder) (Abilify, Abilify Asimtufii, Abilify Maintena, Aristada, Aristada Initio, Opipza)

asenapine (avoid use, except in schizophrenia or bipolar disorder) (Saphris, Secuado)

aspirin (avoid use for primary prevention of cardiovascular disease; avoid chronic use for pain [at doses >325 mg/day] unless other alternatives are not effective and the patient can take a gastroprotective agent; avoid short-term use for pain [at doses >325 mg/day] in combination with oral or parenteral corticosteroids, anticoagulants, or antiplatelet agents unless other alternatives are not effective and the patient can take a gastroprotective agent)

atropine (avoid use of all formulations except for ophthalmic formulations) (Atropen)

benztropine (avoid use of oral formulation)

brexpiprazole (avoid use, except in schizophrenia, adjunctive treatment of major depressive disorder, or agitation associated with dementia due to Alzheimer's disease) (Rexulti)

bumetanide (use with caution) (Burinex)

butalbital (avoid use)

canagliflozin (use with caution) Invokana

carBAMazepine (use with caution) (Carbatrol, Epitol, Equetro, TEGretol, TEGretol CR, TEGretol XR)

cariprazine (avoid use, except in schizophrenia, bipolar disorder, or adjunctive treatment of major depressive disorder) (Vraylar)

carisoprodol (avoid use) (Soma)

chlordiazePOXIDE (avoid use)

chlordiazePOXIDE-amitriptyline (avoid use)

chlorothiazide (use with caution) (Diuril)

chlorpheniramine (avoid use) (Chlor-Trimeton, Chlor-Trimeton Allergy, Ed Chlorphed Jr)

chlorproMAZINE (avoid use, except in schizophrenia, bipolar disorder, or for short-term use as an antiemetic)

chlorthalidone (use with caution) (Hemiclor, Thalitone)

chlorzoxazone (avoid use)

citalopram (use with caution) (CeleXA)

clidinium-chlordiazepoxide (avoid use) (Librax)

cloBAZam (avoid use) (Onfi, Sympazan)

clomiPRAMINE (avoid use) (Anafranil)

clonazePAM (avoid use) (KlonoPIN, Rivotril)

cloNIDine (avoid use for first-line treatment of hypertension) (Catapres-TTS, Duraclon, Nexiclon XR, Onyda XR)

clorazepate (avoid use)

cloZAPine (avoid use, except in schizophrenia, bipolar disorder, or psychosis in Parkinson disease) (Clozaril, Versacloz)

cyclobenzaprine (avoid use) (Amrix, Fexmid)

cyproheptadine (avoid use)

dabigatran (use caution in selecting over apixaban for long-term treatment of nonvalvular atrial fibrillation or venous thromboembolism) (Pradaxa)

dapagliflozin (use with caution) (Farxiga, Forxiga)

desipramine (avoid use) (Norpramin)

desmopressin (avoid use for treatment of nocturia or nocturnal polyuria) (Bipazen, DDAVP, DDAVP Melt, Octostim)

dessicated thyroid (avoid use) (Adthyza, Armour Thyroid)

desvenlafaxine (use with caution) (Pristiq)

dexlansoprazole (avoid scheduled use for >8 wk unless for high-risk patients [e.g., oral corticosteroid or chronic NSAID use] or patients with erosive esophagitis, Barrett's esophagitis, pathological hypersecretory condition, or demonstrated need for maintenance treatment [e.g., failure of H_2 antagonist]) (Dexilant)

dextromethorphan-quinidine (use with caution) (Nuedexta)

diazePAM (avoid use) (Diastat, Libervant, Valium, Valtoco)

diclofenac (avoid chronic use unless other alternatives are not effective and the patient can take a gastroprotective agent; avoid short-term use in combination with oral or parenteral corticosteroids, anticoagulants, or antiplatelet agents unless other alternatives are not effective and the patient can take a gastroprotective agent) (Cambia, Flector, Lofena, Pennsaid, Voltaren, Zipsor)

dicyclomine (avoid use)

diflunisal (avoid chronic use unless other alternatives are not effective and the patient can take a gastroprotective agent; avoid short-term use in combination with oral or parenteral corticosteroids, anticoagulants, or antiplatelet agents unless other alternatives are not effective and the patient can take a gastroprotective agent) (Dolobid)

digoxin (avoid use for first-line treatment of atrial fibrillation or heart failure; if used, avoid using dose >0.125 mg/day) (Lanoxin)

dimenhyDRINATE (avoid use) (Dramamine, Driminate, Gravol)

BEERS CRITERIA continued

diphenhydrAMINE (avoid use of oral formulations) (Benadryl)

dipyridamole (avoid use of short-acting formulation) (Persantine)

doxazosin (avoid use for treatment of hypertension) (Cardura, Cardura XL)

doxepin (avoid use of dose >6 mg/day) (Silenor Sinequan)

doxylamine (avoid use)

dronedarone (avoid use in patients with permanent atrial fibrillation or HF) (Multaq)

DULoxetine (use with caution) (Drizalma Sprinkle)

empagliflozin (use with caution) (Jardiance)

ertugliflozin (use with caution) (Steglatro)

escitalopram (use with caution) (Cipralex, Lexapro)

esomeprazole (avoid scheduled use for >8 wk unless for high-risk patients [e.g., oral corticosteroid or chronic NSAID use], or patients with erosive esophagitis, Barrett's esophagitis, pathological hypersecretory condition, or demonstrated need for maintenance treatment [e.g., failure of H_2 antagonist]) (NexIUM, NexIUM 24HR)

estazolam (avoid use)

estrogens (with or without progestins) (avoid use of systemic estrogens; intravaginal formulations acceptable to use for treatment of dyspareunia, recurrent lower urinary tract infections, and other vaginal symptoms)

eszopiclone (avoid use) (Lunesta)

etodolac (avoid chronic use unless other alternatives are not effective and the patient can take a gastroprotective agent; avoid short-term use in combination with oral or parenteral corticosteroids, anticoagulants, or antiplatelet agents unless other alternatives are not effective and the patient can take a gastroprotective agent)

FLUoxetine (use with caution) (PROzac)

fluPHENAZine (avoid use, except in schizophrenia)

flurbiprofen (avoid chronic use unless other alternatives are not effective and the patient can take a gastroprotective agent; avoid short-term use in combination with oral or parenteral corticosteroids, anticoagulants, or antiplatelet agents unless other alternatives are not effective and the patient can take a gastroprotective agent) (Lurbiro)

fluvoxaMINE (use with caution) (Luvox)

furosemide (use with caution) (Furoscix, Lasix)

glimepiride (avoid use as first- or second-line monotherapy or as add-on treatment unless there are significant barriers to the use of safer and more effective agents; if a sulfonylurea is used, glipizide is preferred)

glipiZIDE (avoid use as first- or second-line monotherapy or as add-on treatment unless there are significant barriers to the use of safer and more effective agents; if a sulfonylurea is used, this is the preferred agent) (Glucotrol XL)

glyBURIDE (avoid use as first- or second-line monotherapy or as add-on treatment unless there are significant barriers to the use of safer and more effective agents; if a sulfonylurea is used, glipizide is preferred)

growth hormone (avoid use, except for confirmed growth hormone deficiency due to an established etiology)

guanFACINE (avoid use for treatment of hypertension) (Intuniv, Intuniv XR)

haloperidol (avoid use, except in schizophrenia, bipolar disorder, or for short-term use as antiemetic) (Haldol Decanoate)

hydroCHLOROthiazide (use with caution) (Inzirqo)

hydrOXYzine (avoid use) Atarax, Vistaril

hyoscyamine (avoid use) (Hyosyne, Levbid, Levsin, Nulev, Oscimin)

ibuprofen (avoid chronic use unless other alternatives are not effective and the patient can take a gastroprotective agent; avoid short-term use in combination with oral or parenteral corticosteroids, anticoagulants, or antiplatelet agents unless other alternatives are not effective and the patient can take a gastroprotective agent) (Advil, Motrin)

iloperidone (avoid use, except in schizophrenia) (Fanapt)

imipramine (avoid use)

indomethacin (avoid chronic use unless other alternatives are not effective and the patient can take a gastroprotective agent; avoid short-term use in combination with oral or parenteral corticosteroids, anticoagulants, or antiplatelet agents unless other alternatives are not effective and the patient can take a gastroprotective agent) (Indocin)

insulin (avoid use of regimens containing only short- or rapid-acting insulin without concurrent use of basal or long-acting insulin)

ketorolac (avoid chronic use unless other alternatives are not effective and the patient can take a gastroprotective agent; avoid short-term use in combination with oral or parenteral corticosteroids, anticoagulants, or antiplatelet agents unless other alternatives are not effective and the patient can take a gastroprotective agent) (Sprix, Toradol)

lansoprazole (avoid scheduled use for >8 wk unless for high-risk patients [e.g., oral corticosteroid or chronic NSAID use], or patients with erosive esophagitis, Barrett's esophagitis, pathological hypersecretory condition, or demonstrated need for maintenance treatment [e.g., failure of H_2 antagonist]) (Prevacid, Prevacid 24HR, Prevacid SoluTab)

levomilnacipran (use with caution) (Fetzima)

LORazepam (avoid use) (Ativan, Loreev XR)

lumateperone (avoid use, except in schizophrenia or bipolar disorder) (Caplyta)

lurasidone (avoid use, except in schizophrenia or bipolar disorder) (Latuda)

meclizine (avoid use) (Bonine)

megestrol (avoid use)

meloxicam (avoid chronic use unless other alternatives are not effective and the patient can take a gastroprotective agent; avoid short-term use in combination with oral or parenteral corticosteroids, anticoagulants, or antiplatelet agents unless other alternatives are not effective and the patient can take a gastroprotective agent) (Xifyrm)

meperidine (avoid use) (Demerol)

BEERS CRITERIA continued

meprobamate (avoid use)

metaxalone (avoid use)

methocarbamol (avoid use) (Robaxin, Tanlor)

methylTESTOSTERone (avoid use, except for confirmed hypogonadism with clinical symptoms) (Methitest)

metoclopramide (avoid use, except in gastroparesis [use should generally not exceed 12 wk]) (Gimoti, Reglan)

midazolam (avoid use) (Nayzilam, Seizalam)

milnacipran (use with caution) (Savella)

mineral oil (avoid oral use) (Fleet Oil)

mirtazapine (use with caution) (🍁 Remeron, Remeron RD, Remeron SolTab)

nabumetone (avoid chronic use unless other alternatives are not effective and the patient can take a gastroprotective agent; avoid short-term use in combination with oral or parenteral corticosteroids, anticoagulants, or antiplatelet agents unless other alternatives are not effective and the patient can take a gastroprotective agent) (Relafen DS)

naproxen (avoid chronic use unless other alternatives are not effective and the patient can take a gastroprotective agent; avoid short-term use in combination with oral or parenteral corticosteroids, anticoagulants, or antiplatelet agents unless other alternatives are not effective and the patient can take a gastroprotective agent) (Aleve, 🍁 Anaprox, Anaprox DS, 🍁 Maxidol, Naprelan, Naprosyn)

NIFEdipine (avoid use of immediate-release formulation) (🍁 Adalat XL, Procardia XL)

nitrofurantoin (avoid use if CCr <30 mL/min or for long-term suppression of urinary tract infections) (Macrobid, Microdantin)

nortriptyline (avoid use) (🍁 Aventyl, Pamelor)

OLANZapine (avoid use, except in schizophrenia, bipolar disorder, or for short-term use as antiemetic) (ZyPREXA, ZyPREXA Relprevv, ZyPREXA Zydis)

olanzapine-fluoxetine (avoid use, except in bipolar disorder or treatment-resistant depression) (Symbyax)

olanzapine-samidorphan (avoid use, except in schizophrenia or bipolar disorder) (Lybalvi)

omeprazole (avoid scheduled use for >8 wk unless for high-risk patients [e.g., oral corticosteroid or chronic NSAID use], or patients with erosive esophagitis, Barrett's esophagitis, pathological hypersecretory condition, or demonstrated need for maintenance treatment [e.g., failure of H_2 antagonist]) (🍁 Losec, PriLOSEC, PriLOSEC OTC)

orphenadrine (avoid use)

oxaprozin (avoid chronic use unless other alternatives are not effective and the patient can take a gastroprotective agent; avoid short-term use in combination with oral or parenteral corticosteroids, anticoagulants, or antiplatelet agents unless other alternatives are not effective and the patient can take a gastroprotective agent) (Coxanto, Daypro)

oxazepam (avoid use)

OXcarbazepine (use with caution) (Oxtellar XR, Trileptal)

paliperidone (avoid use, except in schizophrenia) (Erzofri, Invega, Invega Hafyera, Invega Sustenna, Invega Trinza)

pantoprazole (avoid scheduled use for >8 wk unless for high-risk patients [e.g., oral corticosteroid or chronic NSAID use], or patients with erosive esophagitis, Barrett's esophagitis, pathological hypersecretory condition, or demonstrated need for maintenance treatment [e.g., failure of H_2 antagonist]) (🍁 Pantoloc, Protonix, 🍁 Tecta)

PARoxetine (avoid use) (Paxil, Paxil CR)

perphenazine (avoid use, except in schizophrenia or for short-term use as antiemetic)

perphenazine-amitriptyline (avoid use, except in schizophrenia or major depressive disorder with anxiety/agitation)

PHENobarbital (avoid use) (Sezaby)

pimavanserin (avoid use, except in psychosis in Parkinson disease) (Nuplazid)

piroxicam (avoid chronic use unless other alternatives are not effective and the patient can take a gastroprotective agent; avoid short-term use in combination with oral or parenteral corticosteroids, anticoagulants, or antiplatelet agents unless other alternatives are not effective and the patient can take a gastroprotective agent)

prasugrel (use with caution, especially in patients ≥75 years old; if used in patients ≥75 years old, consider using a lower dose [5 mg]) (Effient)

prazosin (avoid use for treatment of hypertension)

primidone (avoid use) (Mysoline)

promethazine (avoid use) (🍁 Histanil, Phenergan, Promethegan)

QUEtiapine (avoid use, except in schizophrenia, bipolar disorder, adjunctive treatment of major depressive disorder, or psychosis in Parkinson disease) (SEROquel, SEROquel XR)

RABEprazole (avoid scheduled use for >8 wk unless for high-risk patients [e.g., oral corticosteroid or chronic NSAID use], or patients with erosive esophagitis, Barrett esophagitis, or pathological hypersecretory condition, or demonstrated need for maintenance treatment [e.g., failure of H_2 antagonist]) (Aciphex, 🍁 Pariet)

risperiDONE (avoid use, except in schizophrenia or bipolar disorder) (Perseris, RisperDAL, RisperDAL Consta, Rykindo, Uzedy)

rivaroxaban (avoid use for long-term treatment of atrial fibrillation or venous thromboembolism in favor of safer anticoagulant options) (Xarelto)

scopolamine (avoid use) (Transderm-Scop)

sertraline (use with caution) (Zoloft)

sulindac (avoid chronic use unless other alternatives are not effective and the patient can take a gastroprotective agent; avoid short-term use in combination with oral or parenteral corticosteroids, anticoagulants, or antiplatelet agents unless other alternatives are not effective and the patient can take a gastroprotective agent)

temazepam (avoid use) (Restoril)

BEERS CRITERIA continued
terazosin (avoid use for treatment of hypertension) (Tezruly)
testosterone (avoid use, except for confirmed hypogonadism with clinical symptoms) (Androgel, Aveed, Azmiro, 🍁 Delatestryl, Depo-Testosterone, Jatenzo, Kyzatrex, Natesto, Testim, Testopel, Tlando, Undecatrex, Vogelxo, Xyosted)
thioridazine (avoid use, except in schizophrenia)
thiothixene (avoid use, except in schizophrenia)
ticagrelor (use with caution, especially in patients ≥75 years old) (Brillinta)
torsemide (use with caution) Soaanz
traMADol (use with caution) (ConZip, 🍁 Durela, 🍁 Ralivia, 🍁 Tridural, 🍁 Zytram XL)
triazolam (avoid use) (Halcion)
trihexyphenidyl (avoid use)
trimethoprim-sulfamethoxazole (use with caution in patients taking an angiotensin-converting enzyme inhibitor, angiotensin receptor blocker, or angiotensin receptor/neprilysin inhibitor, and in those with a reduced CCr) (Bactrim, Bactrim DS, 🍁 Septra, 🍁 Sulfatrim, 🍁 Sulfatrim DS, Sulfatrim Pediatric)
venlafaxine (use with caution) (Effexor XR)
vilazodone (use with caution) (Viibryd)
vortioxetine (use with caution) (Trintellix)
warfarin (avoid starting as initial therapy for treatment of nonvalvular atrial fibrillation or venous thromboembolism unless alternative options [direct oral anticoagulants] are contraindicated or there are significant barriers to their use; if already using, may be reasonable to continue treatment, especially if INR is well controlled [i.e. >70% time in therapeutic range] and no adverse effects) (Jantoven)
zaleplon (avoid use)
ziprasidone (avoid use, except in schizophrenia or bipolar disorder) (Geodon, 🍁 Zeldox)
zolpidem (avoid use) (Ambien, Ambien CR, Edluar, 🍁 Sublinox)

The 2023 American Geriatrics Society Beers Criteria® Update Expert Panel. (2023). American Geriatrics Society 2023 updated AGS Beers Criteria® for potentially inappropriate medication use in older adults. *Journal of the American Geriatrics Society*, *71*(7), 2052–2081. https://doi.org/10.1111/jgs.18372

DRUGS ASSOCIATED WITH INCREASED RISK OF FALLS IN OLDER ADULTS

Many factors are associated with falls in older adults, including frailty, disease, vision, polypharmacy, and certain medications. Below is a list of drugs associated with falls. Assess older adults on these medications for fall risk and implement fall reduction strategies.

ACE Inhibitors
benazepril (Lotensin)
captopril
enalapril (Epaned, Vasotec)
fosinopril
lisinopril (Qbrelis, Zestril)
moexipril
perindopril
quinapril (Accupril)
ramipril (Altace)
trandolapril

Angiotensin II Receptor Antagonists
azilsartan (Edarbi)
candesartan (Atacand)
irbesartan (Avapro)
losartan (Arbli, Cozaar)
olmesartan (Benicar)
telmisartan (Micardis)
valsartan (Diovan)

Antiarrhythmics
digoxin (Lanoxin)
disopyramide (Norpace, Norpace CR)

Anticonvulsants
carbamazepine (Carbatrol, Epitol, Equetro, Tegretol, Tegretol XR)
ethosuximide (Zarontin)
felbamate (Felbatol)
gabapentin (Gabarone, Gralise, Neurontin)
lamotrigine (Lamictal, Lamictal ODT, Lamictal XR, Subvenite)
levetiracetam (Elepsia XR, Keppra, Keppra XR, Roweepra, Spritam)
methsuximide (Celontin)
phenobarbital (Sezaby)
phenytoin (Dilantin, Phenytek)
pregabalin (Lyrica, Lyrica CR)
primidone (Mysoline)
tiagabine
topiramate (Eprontia, Qudexy XR, Topamax, Topamax Sprinkle, Trokendi XR)
valproate (Depakote, Depakote ER, Depakote Sprinkles)
zonisamide (Zonegran, Zonisade)

Antidepressants
amitriptyline
amoxapine
bupropion (Aplenzin, Forfivo XL, Wellbutrin SR, Wellbutrin XL)
citalopram (Celexa)
clomipramine (Anafranil)
desipramine (Norpramin)
doxepin (Silenor)
duloxetine (Drizalma Sprinkle)
escitalopram (Lexapro)
fluoxetine (Prozac)
fluvoxamine
imipramine
isocarboxazid (Marplan)
mirtazapine (Remeron, Remeron SolTab)
nefazodone
paroxetine (Paxil, Paxil CR)
phenelzine (Nardil)
protriptyline
sertraline (Zoloft)
tranylcypromine (Parnate)
trazodone (Raldesy)
trimipramine
venlafaxine (Effexor XR)

Antihistamines/Antinauseants
dimenhydrinate (Dramamine, Driminate)
diphenhydramine (Benadryl)
hydroxyzine (Vistaril)
meclizine (Bonine)
metoclopramide (Gimoti, Reglan)
prochlorperazine (Compro)
promethazine (Phenergan, Promethegan)
scopolamine patch (Transderm Scop)

Antiparkinsonian Agents
amantadine (Gocovri)
bromocriptine (Cycloset, Parlodel)
entacapone (Comtan)
levodopa/carbidopa (Crexont, Dhivy, Duopa, Rytary, Sinemet)
pramipexole
selegiline (Emsam, Zelapar)

Antipsychotics (Atypical)
aripiprazole (Abilify, Abilify Asimtufii, Abilify Maintena, Opipza, Aristada, Aristada Initio)
clozapine (Clozaril, Versacloz)
olanzapine (Zyprexa, Zyprexa Relprevv, Zyprexa Zydis)
paliperidone (Erzofri, Invega, Invega Hafyera, Invega Sustenna, Invega Trinza)
quetiapine (Seroquel, Seroquel XR)
risperidone (Perseris, Risperdal, Risperdal Consta, Rykindo, Uzedy)
ziprasidone (Geodon)

Antipsychotics (Typical)
chlorpromazine
fluphenazine
haloperidol (Haldol Decanoate)
loxapine (Adasuve)
perphenazine
pimozide
thioridazine
thiothixene
trifluoperazine

Anxiolytics
buspirone (Bucapsol)
meprobamate

Benzodiazepines (Long-Acting)
chlordiazepoxide
clonazepam (Klonopin)
clorazepate
diazepam (Libervant, Valium, Valtoco)
flurazepam

Benzodiazepines (Intermediate-Acting)
alprazolam (Xanax, Xanax XR)
estazolam
lorazepam (Ativan, Loreev XR)
oxazepam
temazepam (Restoril)

Benzodiazepines (Short-Acting)
triazolam (Halcion)

Beta Blockers
acebutolol
atenolol (Tenormin)
bisoprolol
carvedilol (Coreg, Coreg CR)
labetalol
metoprolol (Kaspargo Sprinkle, Lopressor, Toprol XL)
propranolol (Hemangeol, Inderal LA, Inderal XL, InnoPran XL)
timolol

Calcium Channel Blockers
amlodipine (Katerzia, Norliqva, Norvasc)
diltiazem (Cardizem, Cardizem CD, Cardizem LA, Cartia XT, Matzim LA, Tiadylt ER, Tiazac)
felodipine
isradipine
nicardipine (Cardene IV)
nifedipine (Procardia XL)
nisoldipine (Sular)
verapamil (Verelan PM)

Diuretics
amiloride/hydrochlorothiazide
bumetanide (Bumex)
furosemide (Furoscix, Lasix)
hydrochlorothiazide (Inzirqo)
triamterene/hydrochlorothiazide

Opioid Analgesics
codeine
fentanyl
hydrocodone (Hysingla ER)
hydromorphone (Dilaudid)
levorphanol
meperidine (Demerol)
methadone (Methadose)
morphine (Duramorph, Infumorph, Mitigo, MS Contin)
oxycodone (Oxaydo, OxyContin, Roxicodone, Roxybond, Xtampza ER)
oxymorphone

Skeletal Muscle Relaxants
baclofen (Baclofen, Fleqsuvy, Gablofen, Lioresal, Ozobax DS)

Vasodilators
doxazosin (Cardura, Cardura XL)
hydralazine
isosorbide dinitrate/mononitrate (Isordil Titradose)
nitroglycerin (Minitran, Nitro-Bid, Nitro-Dur, Nitro-Time, Nitrolingual, Nitrostat, Rectiv)
prazosin
terazosin (Tezruly)

American Geriatrics Society, British Geriatrics Society, and American Academy of Orthopedic Surgeons Panel on Falls Prevention. (2001). Guideline for the prevention of falls in older persons. *Journal of the American Geriatrics Society*, *49*(5), 664–672.
Hoel, R.W., Giddings Connolly, R.M., & Takahashi, P.Y. (2021). Polypharmacy management in older patients. *Mayo Clinic Proceedings*, *96*(1), 242–256. https://doi.org/10.1016/j.mayocp.2020.06.012

DO NOT CRUSH!

Do not crush any oral medication that is labeled as:

Antineoplastic **(AN)**
Buccal **(BU)**
Delayed Release **(DR)**
Enteric Coated **(EC)**
Extended Release **(ER)**
Effervescent Tablet **(EVT)**
Film coated **(FC)**
Mucous Membrane Irritant **(MMI)**
Orally Disintegrating Tablets **(ODT)**
Sublingual **(SL)**

Do not crush any oral medication that ends in the following letters:

CD CR ER LA SR XL XR XT

MEDICATIONS THAT SHOULD NOT BE CRUSHED:

Abirtega Tablet **(EN)**
Absorica Capsule **(MMI)**
Acamprosate Tablet **(DR)**
Accrufer Capsule **(MMI)**
Acetazolamide ER Capsule **(ER)**
Aciphex Tablet **(DR)**
Actonel Tablet **(FC, MMI)**
Adderall XR Capsule **(ER)**—see code "C"
Adzenys XR-ODT Tablet **(ER, ODT)**—see codes "A," "E"
Afinitor Tablet **(AN, MMI)**—see codes "F," H"
Akeega Tablet **(AN)**
Alecensa Capsule **(AN)**
Alkindi Sprinkle—see codes "A," "C"
Allegra-D 12-Hour or 24-Hour Tablet **(ER)**
Altoprev Tablet **(ER)**
Alunbrig Tablet **(AN, FC)**
Alvaiz Tablet **(FC)**—see code "A"
Ambien CR Tablet **(ER, FC)**
Amitiza Capsule **(gelatin coated)**
Amnesteem Capsule **(MMI)**
Amoxicillin/Clavulanate ER Tablet **(ER)**—see codes "A," "B"
Ampyra Capsule **(ER, FC)**
Amrix Capsule **(ER)**—see code "C"
Aplenzin Tablet **(ER)**
Apriso Capsule **(ER)**
Aptensio XR Capsule **(ER)**—see codes "A," "C"
Aptivus Capsule **(oil emulsion within spheres) (crushing, breaking, or chewing can leave bitter taste)**
Arakoda Tablet **(FC)**
Aricept 23-mg Tablet **(crushing may ↑ rate of absorption)**
Arthrotec Tablet **(DR, MMI)**—see code "F"
Aspirin/Dipyridamole ER Capsule **(ER)**
Aspruzyo Sprinkle **(FC)**
Astagraf XL Capsule **(ER)**—see code "A"
Atelvia Tablet **(DR, MMI)**
Atomoxetine Capsule **(contents can cause ocular irritation)**
Attruby Tablet **(FC)**
Augtyro Capsule **(AN)**
Austedo XR Tablet **(ER, FC)**
Avodart Capsule **(liquid filled, MMI)**—see codes "F," "H"
Azulfidine EN Tablet **(DR)**
Bafiertam Capsule **(DR)**
Balsalazide Capsule—see code "C"
Balversa Tablet **(AN, FC)**
Bayer Low-Dose Aspirin Tablet **(EC)**
Belbuca Buccal Film **(BU) (chewing or swallowing may ↓ bioavailability)**—see code "E"
Belsomra Tablet **(FC)**
Benzonatate Capsule **(chewing or crushing may cause local anesthesia of mucous membranes, which could lead to choking)**
Biltricide Tablet **(crushing, breaking, or chewing can leave bitter taste)**—see code "B"
Binosto Tablet **(EVT)**—see codes "A," "G"
Bonjesta Tablet **(ER)**
Bosulif Tablet **(AN, FC)**—see code "F"
Brenzavvy Tablet **(FC)**
Briviact Tablet **(FC) (crushing, breaking, or chewing can leave bitter taste)**—see code "A"
Brukinsa Capsule **(AN)**
Budesonide DR Capsule **(DR)**—see code "C"
Cabometyx Tablet **(AN)**—see code "F"
Calquence Tablet **(AN)**
Camzyos Capsule
Caprelsa Tablet **(AN, FC, MMI) (may be dissolved in water)**
Carbaglu Tablet **(dissolve in water)**
Carbatrol Capsule **(ER)**—see codes "A," "C"
Carbidopa/Levodopa ER Tablet **(ER)**—see code "B"
Cardizem CD/LA Capsule **(ER)**
Cardizem Tablet **(FC)**
Cardura XL Tablet **(ER)**
Cartia XT Capsule **(ER)**
Cefaclor ER Tablet **(ER, FC)**—see code "A"
Cefuroxime Tablet **(crushing, breaking, or chewing can leave bitter taste)**
Cellcept Capsule/Tablet **(FC, MMI)**—see codes "A," "H"
Cerdelga Capsule
Chlorpheniramine ER Tablet **(ER)**
Cholbam Capsule—see code "C"
Cibinqo Tablet **(FC)**
Claravis Capsule **(liquid filled, MMI)**
Clarinex-D 12-Hour Tablet **(ER)**
Clarithromycin ER Tablet **(ER, FC)**—see code "A"
Claritin-D 12-Hour/24-Hour Tablet **(ER)**
Cobenfy Capsule **(ER)**
Colestid Tablet—see code "A"
Cometriq Capsule **(AN)**—see code "F"
Concerta Tablet **(ER)**—see code "A"
Contrave Tablet **(ER)**
Conzip Capsule **(ER) (crushing, chewing, or dissolving can leave bitter taste)**—see code "A"
Copiktra Capsule **(AN)**
Coreg CR Capsule **(ER)**—see code "C" Cotellic Tablet **(AN, FC)**
Cotempla XR-ODT Tablet **(ER, ODT)**—see codes "A," "E"
Crenessity Capsule—see code "A"
Creon Capsule **(DR, MMI)**—see code "C"
Cresemba Capsule **(opening the capsule may ↓ absorption)**
Crexont Capsule **(ER)**—see code "C"
Cuvrior Tablet **(FC)**
Cyclophosphamide Capsule/Tablet **(AN)**—see codes "F," "H"
Dantizen Tablet **(AN)**
Darifenacin ER Tablet **(ER)**
Daurismo Tablet **(AN, FC)**
Depakote Tablet **(DR)**—see code "A"
Depakote ER Tablet **(ER)**—see code "A"
Depakote Sprinkle Capsule—see code "C"
Detrol LA Capsule **(ER)**
Dexedrine Capsule **(ER)**—see code "A"
Dexilant Capsule **(DR)**—see code "C"
Diacomit Capsule—see code "A"
Diclegis Tablet **(DR)**
Diclofenac ER Tablet **(ER, MMI)**—see code "A"
Diflunisal Tablet **(FC, MMI)**
Doryx MPC Tablet **(DR)**—see code "A"
Drisdol Capsule **(liquid filled)**—see code "A"
Droxia Capsule—see codes "A," "F," "H"
Duavee Tablet **(FC)**—see code "H"
Duexis Tablet **(FC, MMI)**
Dulcolax Tablet **(EC)**—see code "D"
Duloxetine DR Capsule **(DR)**
Dyanavel XR Tablet **(ER)**—see code "A"
EC-Naprosyn Tablet **(DR, EC)**—see codes "A," "D"
Ecotrin Tablet **(EC, MMI)**
Edluar SL Tablet **(SL)**—see code "E"
Edurant Tablet **(FC)**
E.E.S. Tablet **(crushing, chewing, or dissolving can leave bitter taste)**
Effer-K Tablet **(EVT)**—see code "G"
Effexor XR Capsule **(ER)**—see code "C"
Elepsia XR Tablet **(ER)**—see code "A"
Emend Capsule—see code "A"
Emrosi Capsule **(ER)**
Ensacove Capsule **(AN)**
Entresto Sprinkle **(MMI)**
Envarsus XR Tablet **(ER)**—see code "A"
Equetro Capsule **(ER)**—see codes "A," "C"
Ergomar SL Tablet **(SL)**—see code "E"
Erivedge Capsule **(AN)**—see code "F"

MEDICATIONS THAT SHOULD NOT BE CRUSHED:

Erleada Tablet **(AN, FC) (may dissolve in water)**
Ery-Tab Tablet **(DR)**—see code **"A"**
Erythromycin DR Capsule **(DR)**—see codes **"A," "C"**
Etodolac ER Tablet **(ER)**
Exjade Tablet **(dissolve in water, orange juice, or apple juice)**
Ezallor Sprinkle—see code **"C"**
Fabhalta Capsule
Felodipine Tablet **(ER)**
Fenofibric Acid DR Capsule **(DR)**
Ferrous Gluconate Tablet **(MMI)**
Ferrous Sulfate Tablet **(EC, MMI)**—see code **"A"**
Fetzima Capsule **(ER)**
Flomax Capsule—see code **"C"**
Fluoxetine DR Capsule **(DR)**—see code **"A"**
Fluvoxamine ER Capsule **(ER)**
Focalin XR Capsule **(ER)**—see code **"C"**
Forfivo XL Tablet **(FC)**
Fosamax Tablet **(MMI)**
Fosamax Plus D Tablet **(MMI)**
Fotivda Capsule **(AN)**
Fruzaqla Capsule **(AN)**
Galafold Capsule
Galantamine ER Capsule **(ER)**—see code **"A"**
Geodon Capsule
Gleevec Tablet **(MMI) (may dissolve in water or apple juice)**—see codes **"A," "F," "H"**
Gleostine Capsule **(AN, gelatin coated)**—see code **"H"**
Glucotrol XL Tablet **(ER)**
Glumetza Tablet **(ER)**—see code **"A"**
Gocovri Capsule **(ER)**—see codes **"A," "C"**
Gralise Tablet **(ER, FC)**—see code **"A"**
Hetlioz Capsule—see code **"A"**
Horizant Tablet **(ER)**—see code **"A"**
Hycamtin Capsule **(AN) (can make oral solution with solution for injection)**
Hydrea Capsule **(AN)**—see codes **"A," "F," "H"**
Hydromorphone ER Tablet **(ER) (crushing, chewing or dissolving may ↑ risk of fatal overdose)**—see code **"A"**
Hysingla ER Tablet **(ER) (crushing, chewing or dissolving may ↑ risk of fatal overdose)**
Ibandronate Tablet **(MMI)**
Ibrance Capsule/Tablet **(AN, FC)**
Iclusig Tablet **(AN, FC)**
Idhifa Tablet **(AN, FC)**
Imbruvica Capsule/Tablet **(AN, FC)**—see code **"A"**
Impavido Capsule—see code **"F"**
Inderal LA Capsule **(ER)**—see code **"A"**
Indomethacin ER Capsule **(ER)**—see codes **"A," "C"**
Inlyta Tablet **(AN, FC) (can make oral suspension)**
Innopran XL Capsule **(ER)**—see code **"A"**
Inpefa Tablet **(FC)**
Inqovi Tablet **(AN, FC)**
Intelence Tablet **(may dissolve in water)**
Intuniv Tablet **(ER)**
Invega Tablet **(ER)**
Invokamet XR Tablet **(ER, FC)**
Isentress Tablet **(FC)**—see code **"A"**
Isentress HD Tablet **(FC)**—see code **"A"**
Isosorbide Mononitrate ER Tablet **(ER)**—see code **"B"**
Itovebi Tablet **(AN)**
Jalyn Capsule **(MMI)**—see codes **"F," "H"**
Janumet XR Tablet **(ER, FC)**
Jaypirca Tablet **(AN, FC)**—see code **"F"**
Jentadueto XR Tablet **(ER, FC)**
Jornay PM Capsule **(ER)**—see codes **"A," "C"**
Journavx Tablet **(FC)**
Juxtapid Capsule
Kaletra Tablet **(FC)**—see code **"A"**
Kalydeco Tablet **(FC)**—see code **"A"**
Kapspargo Capsule **(ER)**—see code **"A"**
Kazano Tablet **(FC)**
Keppra Tablet **(FC) (crushing, breaking, or chewing can leave bitter taste)**—see code **"A"**
Keppra XR Tablet **(ER, FC)**—see code **"A"**
Ketoprofen ER Capsule **(ER, MMI)**
Kisqali Tablet **(AN, FC)**
Klor-Con Tablet **(ER, FC)**—see code **"A"**
Klor-Con M Tablet **(ER)**—see codes **"A," "B"**
Korlym Tablet
Koselugo Capsule **(AN)**
Krazati Tablet **(AN, FC)**
Krintafel Tablet **(FC)**
Lagevrio Capsule—see code **"C"**
Lamictal XR Tablet **(ER, FC)**
Lazcluze Tablet **(AN, FC)**
Lenvima Capsule **(AN) (may dissolve in water or apple juice)**
Lescol XL Tablet **(ER)**
Letairis Tablet **(FC)**—see code **"F"**
Levbid Tablet **(ER)**—see codes **"A," "B"**
Lialda Tablet **(DR)**
Linzess Capsule **(gelatin coated)**—see code **"C"**
Lipofen Capsule
Litfulo Capsule
Lithobid Tablet **(ER, FC)**—see code **"A"**
Lonsurf Tablet **(AN, FC)**
Lorbrena Tablet **(AN, FC)**—see code **"H"**
Loreev XR Capsule—see codes **"A," "C"**
Lovaza Capsule **(liquid filled)**
Lumakras Tablet **(AN, FC) (may dissolve in water)**
Lunesta Tablet **(FC) (crushing, breaking, or chewing can leave bitter taste)**
Lupkynis Capsule
Lybalvi Tablet **(FC)**
Lynparza Tablet **(AN, FC)**—see code **"H"**
Lyrica CR Tablet **(ER, FC)**—see code **"A"**
Lysodren Tablet **(AN)**
Lytgobi Tablet **(AN)**
Macrobid Capsule
Matzim LA Tablet **(ER)**
Mavenclad Tablet **(AN)**—see code **"H"**
Mavyret Pellets **(mix with food, not liquid)**
Mayzent Tablet **(FC)**
Meclizine Tablet
Mekinist Tablet **(AN, FC)**—see code **"A"**
Mesalamine DR Capsule **(DR)**—see code **"C"**
Mestinon Tablet **(ER)**—see code **"A"**
Metadate CD Capsule **(ER)**—see codes **"A," "C"**
Minocycline DR Tablet **(ER)**—see code **"B"**
Motpoly XR Capsule **(ER)**—see code **"A"**
Motrin Tablet **(crushing, breaking, or chewing can leave bitter taste)**—see code **"A"**
MS Contin Tablet **(ER) (crushing, chewing, or dissolving may ↑ risk of fatal overdose)**—see code **"A"**
Mucinex Tablet **(ER)**—see code **"A"**
Mucinex D Tablet **(ER)**—see codes **"A," "B"**
Mucinex DM Tablet **(ER)**—see code **"A"**
Mycapssa Capsule **(DR)**
Mydayis Capsule **(ER)**—see code **"C"**
Myfortic Tablet **(DR)**—see codes **"A," "H"**
Myrbetriq Tablet **(ER, FC)**—see code **"A"**
Mytesi Tablet **(DR, FC)**
Namenda XR Capsule **(ER)**—see codes **"A," "C"**
Namzaric Capsule **(ER)**—see code **"C"**
Naprelan Tablet **(ER, FC)**—see code **"A"**
Nerlynx Tablet **(AN)**
Neurontin Capsule/Tablet **(FC)**—see codes **"A," "B," "C"**
Nevirapine ER Tablet **(ER)**—see code **"A"**
Nexavar Tablet **(AN, FC)**
Nexiclon XR Tablet **(ER)**—see code **"B"**
Nexium Capsule **(DR)**—see codes **"A," "C"**
Nexium 24HR Capsule/Tablet **(DR)**—see codes **"A," "C"**
Niacin ER Tablet **(ER)**
Nicorette Lozenge—see code **"E"**
Ninlaro Capsule **(AN)**

DO NOT CRUSH! continued

MEDICATIONS THAT SHOULD NOT BE CRUSHED:

Nitro-Time Capsule **(ER)**
Nitrostat SL Tablet **(SL)**—see code "**E**"
Norpace CR Capsule **(ER)**
Northera Capsule
Norvir Tablet **(FC)**—see code "**A**"
Noxafil Tablet **(DR, FC)**—see code "**A**"
Nubeqa Tablet **(AN, FC)**
Nucynta ER Tablet **(ER, FC) (crushing, chewing or dissolving may ↑ risk of fatal overdose)**
Ofev Capsule **(crushing or chewing can leave bitter taste)**
Ogsiveo Tablet **(AN, FC)**
Ojjaara Tablet **(AN)**
Onglyza Tablet **(FC)**
Onureg Tablet **(AN, FC)**
Opfolda Capsule—see code "**C**"
Opsumit Tablet **(FC)**
Oravig Buccal Tablet **(BU)**
Orenitram Tablet **(ER)**
Orgovyx Tablet **(FC)**
Orphenadrine Citrate ER Tablet **(ER)**
Orserdu Tablet **(AN, FC)**
Oseni Tablet **(FC)**
Otezla Tablet **(FC)**
Oxaydo Tablet **(may obstruct feeding tubes if crushed)**—see code "**A**"
Oxtellar XR Tablet **(ER)**—see code "**A**"
Oxybutynin ER Tablet **(ER)**—see code "**A**"
OxyContin Tablet **(ER, FC) (crushing, chewing or dissolving may ↑ risk of fatal overdose)**—see code "**A**"
Oxymorphone ER Tablet **(ER, FC) (crushing, chewing or dissolving may ↑ risk of fatal overdose)**
Pancreaze Capsule **(DR, MMI)**—see code "**C**"
Paxil Tablet **(FC)**—see codes "**A**," "**B**"
Paxil CR Tablet **(ER, FC)**—see codes "**A**," "**F**"
Paxlovid Tablet **(FC)**
Pemazyre Tablet **(AN)**
Pentasa Capsule **(ER)**—see code "**C**"
Pentoxifylline ER Tablet **(ER)**
Pertzye Capsule **(DR, MMI)**—see code "**C**"
Piqray Tablet **(FC)**
Piroxicam Capsule **(MMI)**
Pomalyst Capsule **(AN)**
Pradaxa Capsule **(breaking, chewing, or emptying may ↑ bioavailability)**—see code "A"
Pramipexole ER Tablet **(ER)**
Prevacid Capsule **(DR)**—see code "**C**"
Prevacid 24HR Capsule **(DR)**
Prevacid SoluTab Tablet **(ODT) (may dissolve in water to administer via nasogastric tube)**
Prevymis Tablet **(FC)**—see code "**A**"
Prilosec OTC Tablet **(DR)**—see code "**A**"
Pristiq Tablet **(ER)**
Procardia XL Tablet **(ER, FC)**
Procysbi Capsule **(DR)**—see codes "**A**," "**C**"
Promacta Tablet **(FC)**—see code "**A**"
Propafenone ER Capsule **(ER)**
Propecia Tablet **(FC)**—see code "**F**"
Proscar Tablet **(FC)**—see code "**F**"
Protonix Tablet **(DR)**—see code "**A**"
Pylera Capsule **(MMI)**
Pyrukynd Tablet **(FC)**
Qelbree Capsule **(ER)**—see code "**C**"
Qinlock Tablet **(AN)**
Qudexy XR Capsule **(ER)**—see codes "**A**," "**C**"
Quinidine Gluconate ER Tablet **(ER)**
Ranolazine ER Tablet **(ER, FC)**—see code "**A**"
Rapamune Tablet **(FC)**—see code "**A**"
Rayaldee Capsule **(ER)**
Rayos Tablet **(DR)**—see code "**A**"
Relexxii Tablet **(ER)**
Retevmo Tablet **(AN)**
Revlimid Capsule—see code "**F**"
Reyataz Capsule **(gelatin coated)**—see code "**A**"
Rezlidhia Capsule **(AN)**
Rezurock Tablet **(FC)**
Ribavirin Capsule
Rinvoq Tablet **(ER)**—see code "**A**"
Ritalin LA Capsule **(ER)**—see codes "**A**," "**C**"
Ropinirole ER Tablet **(ER, FC)**
Roweepra Tablet **(crushing or chewing can leave bitter taste)**—see code "**A**"
Rozlytrek Capsule **(AN)**—see code "**A**"
Rukobia Tablet **(ER, FC)**
Rybelsus Tablet
Rydapt Capsule **(AN, liquid filled)**
Rytary Capsule **(ER)**—see code "**C**"
Saphris SL Tablet **(SL)**—see code "**E**"
Saxagliptin/Metformin ER Tablet **(ER, FC)**
Scemblix Tablet **(AN, FC)**—see code "**B**"
Sensipar Tablet **(FC) (cutting tablets may cause variable dosing accuracy)**
Seroquel XR Tablet **(ER)**
Sevelamer Tablet **(FC) (expands in liquid when crushed or broken)**—see code "**A**"
Siklos Tablet **(FC) (may dissolve in water)**—see codes "**A**," "**F**," "**H**"
Sotyktu Tablet **(FC)**
Sporanox Capsule—see code "**A**"
Spritam ODT **(ODT)**—see codes "**A**," "**E**"
Sprycel Tablet **(AN)**—see code "**F**"
Stalevo Tablet **(FC)**
Stivarga Tablet **(AN, FC)**—see code "**F**"
Suboxone SL Film **(SL)**—see code "**E**"
Sudafed 12-Hour/24-Hour Tablet **(ER)**—see code "**A**"
Sular Tablet **(ER, FC)**
Symdeko Tablet **(FC)**
Synjardy XR Tablet **(SR)**
Syprine Capsule
Tabrecta Tablet **(AN, FC)**
Tafinlar Capsule **(AN)**
Tafinlar Tablet for Suspension **(AN) (dissolve in water)**
Tagrisso Tablet **(AN, FC) (may dissolve in water)**
Talzenna Capsule **(AN)**
Targretin Capsule **(AN, liquid filled)**
Tarpeyo Capsule **(DR)**
Tasigna Capsule **(AN)**—see code "**C**"
Tavneos Capsule
Tazverik Tablet **(AN, FC)**
Tecfidera Capsule **(DR)**
Tegretol XR Tablet **(ER)**—see code "**A**"
Temodar Capsule **(AN, MMI)**—see codes "**F**," "**H**"
Tepmetko Tablet **(AN) (may dissolve in water)**
Theo-24 Capsule **(ER)**—see codes "**A**," "**C**"
Tiadylt ER Capsule **(ER)**—see code "**C**"
Tiazac Capsule **(ER)**—see code "**C**"
Tibsovo Tablet **(AN, FC)**
Tivicay PD Tablet **(may dissolve in water)**
Tolsura Capsule **(gelatin coated)**—see code "**A**"
Topamax Capsule, Tablet **(FC) (crushing, breaking, or chewing can leave bitter taste)**—see codes "**A**," "**C**"
Toprol XL Tablet **(ER)**—see codes "**A**," "**B**"
Torpenz Tablet **(AN, MMI)**—see code "**H**"
Toviaz Tablet **(ER, FC)**
Trazodone Tablet **(crushing or chewing can leave bitter taste)**—see codes "**A**," "**B**"
Tretinoin Capsule **(AN)**—see code "**C**"
Treximet Tablet **(FC) (crushing, chewing, or breaking may cause rapid absorption)**
Trikafta Tablet **(FC)**
Triumeq PD Tablet **(dissolve in water)**
Trokendi XR Capsule **(ER)**—see code "**A**"
Truqap Tablet **(AN, FC)**
Tukysa Tablet **(AN)**
Turalio Capsule **(AN)**
Tylenol 8-Hour Arthritis Pain Tablet **(ER)**—see code "**A**"
Uceris Tablet **(ER)**
Uptravi Tablet **(FC)**
Urocit-K Tablet **(ER)**
Uroxatral Tablet **(ER)**
Vafseo Tablet **(FC)**
Valcyte Tablet **(FC, MMI)**—see codes "**A**," "**F**," "**H**"

DO NOT CRUSH! continued

MEDICATIONS THAT SHOULD NOT BE CRUSHED:

Valproic Acid Capsule **(MMI)**—see code **"A"**
Vanflyta Tablet **(AN, FC)**
Vascepa Capsule
Venclexta Tablet **(AN, FC)**
Veozah Tablet **(FC)**
Verapamil ER Tablet **(ER)**
Verelan Capsule **(DR)**—see code **"C"**
Verelan PM Capsule **(ER)**—see code **"C"**
Verzenio Tablet **(AN)**
Vesicare Tablet **(FC) (crushing, breaking, or chewing can leave bitter taste)**—see code **"A"**
Vijoice Tablet **(AN) (may dissolve in water)**—see code **"A"**
Vimovo Tablet **(DR)**
Vimpat Tablet **(FC)**—see code **"A"**
Viokace Tablet **(MMI)**
Vitrakvi Capsule **(AN)**—see code **"A"**
Vonjo Capsule **(AN)**
Voranigo Tablet **(AN, FC)**
Votrient Tablet **(AN, FC) (crushing may ↑ bioavailability)**—see code **"F"**
Vumerity Capsule **(DR)**
Vyndamax Capsule **(liquid filled)**
Vyndaqel Capsule **(liquid filled)**
Welireg Tablet **(AN, FC)**
Wellbutrin SR/XL Tablet **(ER, FC)**
Xalcori Capsule **(AN) (may dissolve in water)**
Xanax XR Tablet **(ER)**—see code **"A"**
Xeljanz XR Tablet **(ER)**—see code **"A"**
Xeloda Tablet **(AN, FC)**
Xenleta Tablet **(FC)**
Xigduo XR Tablet **(ER, FC)**
Xospata Tablet **(AN)**
Xpovio Tablet **(AN, FC)**
Xtampza ER Capsule **(ER)**—see code **"C"**
Xtandi Capsule/Tablet **(AN)**—see code **"F"**
Yargesa Capsule—see code **"C"**
Zegerid Capsule—see code **"A"**
Zejula Tablet **(AN, FC)**
Zelboraf Tablet **(AN, FC)**
Zenatane Capsule **(gelatin coated, MMI)**
Zenpep Capsule **(DR, MMI)**—see code **"C"**
Zeposia Capsule
Zileuton ER Tablet **(ER)**
Zituvimet XR Tablet **(ER, FC)**
Zokinvy Capsule —see code **"C"**
Zolinza Capsule **(AN, MMI)**
Zortress Tablet **(AN, MMI)**—see codes **"F," "H"**
Zubsolv SL Tablet **(SL)**—see code **"E"**
Zydelig Tablet **(AN, FC)**
Zytiga Tablet **(AN, FC)**
Yonsa Tablet **(AN)**
Zavesca Capsule—see code **"C"**

CODES:

A: Liquid forms are available.
B: Tablets that are scored may be broken in half.
C: Capsule can be opened—contents may be used/sprinkled on certain foods or liquids as recommended by the manufacturer.
D: Do not take with antacids or milk products.
E: Disintegrates on or under the tongue—do not chew.
F: Women of reproductive potential should not handle crushed or broken tablets or the contents of opened capsules.
G: Effervescent tablets must be dissolved in the volume of diluent recommended by the manufacturer.
H: Avoid direct contact with skin, as may enhance tumor development.

Pharmacist's Letter. (2025, April). *Meds That Should Not Be Crushed.* Therapeutic Research Center. https://pharmacist.therapeuticresearch.com/en/Content/Segments/PRL/2014/Aug/Meds-That-Should-Not-Be-Crushed-7309

LIST OF CONFUSED DRUG NAMES

Drug Name	Confused Drug Name
Accupril	Aciphex
acetaminophen	acetaZOLAMIDE
acetaZOLAMIDE	acetaminophen
acetic acid for irrigation	glacial acetic acid
Aciphex	Accupril
Aciphex	Aricept
Activase	Cathflo Activase
Activase	TNKase
Actonel	Actos
Actos	Actonel
Adacel (Tdap)	Daptacel (DTaP)
Adderall	Adderall XR
Adderall XR	Adderall
ado-trastuzumab emtansine	trastuzumab
Afrin (oxymetazoline)	Afrin (saline)
Afrin (saline)	Afrin (oxymetazoline)
Aggrastat	argatroban
Allegra	Viagra
ALPRAZolam	clonazePAM
ALPRAZolam	LORazepam
amantadine	amiodarone
Ambien	ambrisentan
Ambisome	amphotericin B
ambrisentan	Ambien
aMILoride	amLODIPine
amiodarone	amantadine
amLODIPine	aMILoride
amphotericin B	Ambisome
amphotericin B	amphotericin B liposomal
amphotericin B liposomal	amphotericin B
antacid	Atacand
anticoagulant citrate dextrose solution formula A	anticoagulant sodium citrate solution
anticoagulant sodium citrate solution	anticoagulant citrate dextrose solution formula A
Apidra	Spiriva
apixaban	axitinib
argatroban	Aggrastat
Aricept	Aciphex
Aricept	Azilect
ARIPiprazole	proton pump inhibitors
ARIPiprazole	RABEprazole
Arista AH (absorbable hemostatic agent)	Arixtra
Arixtra	Arista AH (absorbable hemostatic agent)
Atacand	antacid
atomoxetine	atorvastatin
atorvastatin	atomoxetine
axitinib	apixaban
azaCITIDine	azaTHIOprine
azaTHIOprine	azaCITIDine
Azilect	Aricept
BabyBIG	HBIG (hepatitis B immune globulin)
Benadryl	benazepril
benazepril	Benadryl
Betadine (with povidone-iodine)	Betadine (without povidone-iodine)
Betadine (without povidone-iodine)	Betadine (with povidone-iodine)
betaine (anhydrous form)	betaine HCl

Drug Name	Confused Drug Name
betaine HCl	betaine (anhydrous form)
Bicillin C-R	Bicillin L-A
Bicillin L-A	Bicillin C-R
Blisovi 24 Fe	Blisovi Fe 1/20
Blisovi Fe 1/20	Blisovi 24 Fe
Brevibloc	Brevital
Brevital	Brevibloc
Brilinta	Briviact
Briviact	Brilinta
BUPivacaine	ROPivacaine
buprenorphine	HYDROmorphone
buPROPion	busPIRone
busPIRone	buPROPion
Cabenuva	cabotegravir
cabotegravir	Cabenuva
captopril	carvedilol
carBAMazepine	OXcarbazepine
CARBOplatin	CISplatin
Cardene	Cardizem
Cardizem	Cardene
carvedilol	captopril
Cathflo Activase	Activase
ceFAZolin	cefoTEtan
ceFAZolin	cefOXitin
ceFAZolin	cefTAZidime
ceFAZolin	cefTRIAXone
cefoTEtan	ceFAZolin
cefoTEtan	cefOXitin
cefoTEtan	cefTAZidime
cefoTEtan	cefTRIAXone
cefOXitin	ceFAZolin
cefOXitin	cefoTEtan
cefOXitin	cefTAZidime
cefOXitin	cefTRIAXone
cefTAZidime	ceFAZolin
cefTAZidime	cefoTEtan
cefTAZidime	cefOXitin
cefTAZidime	cefTRIAXone
cefTRIAXone	ceFAZolin
cefTRIAXone	cefoTEtan
cefTRIAXone	cefOXitin
ceftriaxone	cefTAZidime
cefuroxime	sulfaSALAzine
CeleBREX	CeleXA
CeleBREX	Cerebyx
CeleXA	CeleBREX
CeleXA	Cerebyx
CeleXA	ZyPREXA
Cerebyx	CeleBREX
Cerebyx	CeleXA
cetirizine	sertraline
chlordiazePOXIDE	chlorproMAZINE
chlorproMAZINE	chlordiazePOXIDE
CISplatin	CARBOplatin
citalopram	escitalopram
Claritin-D	Claritin-D 24
Claritin-D 24	Claritin-D
cloBAZam	clonazePAM
clomiPHENE	clomiPRAMINE
clomiPRAMINE	clomiPHENE
clonazePAM	ALPRAZolam
clonazePAM	cloBAZam
clonazePAM	cloNIDine

Brand names always start with an uppercase letter. Some brand names incorporate tall man letters in initial characters and may not be readily recognized as brand names. Brand name products appear in black; generic/other products appear in red.

LIST OF CONFUSED DRUG NAMES continued

Drug Name	Confused Drug Name
clonazePAM	cloZAPine
clonazePAM	LORazepam
cloNIDine	clonazePAM
cloNIDine	cloZAPine
cloNIDine	KlonoPIN
cloZAPine	clonazePAM
cloZAPine	cloNIDine
Clozaril	Colazal
coagulation factor IX (recombinant)	factor IX complex, vapor heated
coenzyme Q10	Cometriq
Colace	Cozaar
Colazal	Clozaril
colchicine	Cortrosyn
Cometriq	coenzyme Q10
Cortrosyn	colchicine
Cozaar	Colace
Cozaar	Zocor
cycloPHOSphamide	cycloSERINE
cycloPHOSphamide	cycloSPORINE
cycloSERINE	cycloPHOSphamide
cycloSERINE	cycloSPORINE
cycloSPORINE	cycloPHOSphamide
cycloSPORINE	cycloSERINE
cycloSPORINE	cycloSPORINE modified
cycloSPORINE modified	cycloSPORINE
Cymbalta	Symbyax
dabigatran	vigabatrin
DACTINomycin	DAPTOmycin
Daptacel (DTaP)	Adacel (Tdap)
DAPTOmycin	DACTINomycin
DAUNOrubicin	DOXOrubicin
DAUNOrubicin	IDArubicin
Depakote	Depakote ER
Depakote ER	Depakote
DEPO-Medrol	SOLU-Medrol
Depo-Provera	Depo-subQ provera 104
Depo-subQ provera 104	Depo-Provera
desipramine	disopyramide
desmopressin	vasopressin
dexAMETHasone	dexmedeTOMIDine
Dexilant	DULoxetine
dexmedeTOMIDine	dexAMETHasone
dexmethylphenidate	methadone
diazePAM	dilTIAZem
Diflucan	Diprivan
dilTIAZem	diazePAM
dimenhyDRINATE	diphenhydrAMINE
diphenhydrAMINE	dimenhyDRINATE
Diprivan	Diflucan
disopyramide	desipramine
DOBUTamine	DOPamine
DOCEtaxel	PACLitaxel
DOPamine	DOBUTamine
Doxil	Paxil
DOXOrubicin	DAUNOrubicin
DOXOrubicin	DOXOrubicin liposomal
DOXOrubicin	IDArubicin
DOXOrubicin liposomal	DOXOrubicin
Dramamine (dimenhyDRINATE)	Dramamine (ginger root)
Dramamine (dimenhyDRINATE)	Dramamine (meclizine)
Dramamine (ginger root)	Dramamine (dimenhyDRINATE)
Dramamine (ginger root)	Dramamine (meclizine)
Dramamine (meclizine)	Dramamine (dimenhyDRINATE)
Dramamine (meclizine)	Dramamine (ginger root)
droNABinol	droPERidol
droPERidol	droNABinol
Dulcolax (bisacodyl)	Dulcolax (docusate sodium)
Dulcolax (docusate sodium)	Dulcolax (bisacodyl)
DULoxetine	Dexilant
DULoxetine	FLUoxetine
DULoxetine	PARoxetine
edetate calcium disodium	edetate disodium
edetate disodium	edetate calcium disodium
elvitegravir, cobicistat, emtricitabine, and tenofovir alafenamide	elvitegravir, cobicistat, emtricitabine, and tenofovir disoproxil fumarate
elvitegravir, cobicistat, emtricitabine, and tenofovir disoproxil fumarate	elvitegravir, cobicistat, emtricitabine, and tenofovir alafenamide
Enbrel	Levbid
Engerix-B adult	Engerix-B pediatric/adolescent
Engerix-B pediatric/adolescent	Engerix-B adult
ePHEDrine	EPINEPHrine
EPINEPHrine	ePHEDrine
epiRUBicin	eriBULin
eriBULin	epiRUBicin
escitalopram	citalopram
factor IX complex, vapor heated	coagulation factor IX (recombinant)
Fanapt	Xanax
Farxiga	Fetzima
fentaNYL	SUFentanil
Fetzima	Farxiga
flavoxATE	fluvoxaMINE
Flonase	Flovent
Flovent	Flonase
flumazenil	influenza virus vaccine
FLUoxetine	DULoxetine
FLUoxetine	PARoxetine
fluPHENAZine	fluvoxaMINE
fluvoxaMINE	flavoxATE
fluvoxaMINE	fluPHENAZine
Fluzone High-Dose Quadrivalent	Fluzone Quadrivalent
Fluzone Quadrivalent	Fluzone High-Dose Quadrivalent
fomepizole	omeprazole
gabapentin	gemfibrozil
gemfibrozil	gabapentin
gentamicin	gentian violet
gentian violet	gentamicin
glacial acetic acid	acetic acid for irrigation
glipiZIDE	glyBURIDE
glyBURIDE	glipiZIDE

Brand names always start with an uppercase letter. Some brand names incorporate tall man letters in initial characters and may not be readily recognized as brand names. Brand name products appear in black; generic/other products appear in red.

MEDICATION SAFETY TOOLS | List of Confused Drug Names

LIST OF CONFUSED DRUG NAMES continued

Drug Name	Confused Drug Name
guaiFENesin	guanFACINE
guanFACINE	guaiFENesin
HBIG (hepatitis B immune globulin)	BabyBIG
Healon	Hyalgan
HMG-CoA reductase inhibitors ("statins")	nystatin
HumaLOG	HumuLIN
HumaLOG	NovoLOG
HumaLOG Mix 75/25	HumuLIN 70/30
HumuLIN	HumaLOG
HumuLIN	NovoLIN
HumuLIN 70/30	HumaLOG Mix 75/25
HumuLIN R U-100	HumuLIN R U-500
HumuLIN R U-500	HumuLIN R U-100
Hyalgan	Healon
hydrALAZINE	hydroCHLOROthiazide
hydrALAZINE	HYDROmorphone
hydrALAZINE	hydrOXYzine
Hydrea	Lyrica
hydroCHLOROthiazide	hydrALAZINE
hydroCHLOROthiazide	hydroxychloroquine
hydroCHLOROthiazide	hydrOXYzine
HYDROcodone	oxyCODONE
HYDROmorphone	buprenorphine
HYDROmorphone	hydrALAZINE
HYDROmorphone	hydrOXYzine
HYDROmorphone	morphine
HYDROmorphone	oxyMORphone
hydroxychloroquine	hydroCHLOROthiazide
hydroxychloroquine	hydroxyurea
hydroxyurea	hydroxychloroquine
hydroxyurea	hydrOXYzine
hydroxyurea	Ure-Na (palatable form of oral urea)
hydrOXYzine	hydrALAZINE
hydrOXYzine	hydroCHLOROthiazide
hydrOXYzine	HYDROmorphone
hydrOXYzine	hydroxyurea
IDArubicin	DAUNOrubicin
IDArubicin	DOXOrubicin
IDArubicin	idaruCIZUmab
idaruCIZUmab	IDArubicin
Ilaris	Ilumya
Ilumya	Ilaris
inFLIXimab	riTUXimab
influenza virus vaccine	flumazenil
influenza virus vaccine	perflutren lipid microspheres
influenza virus vaccine	tuberculin purified protein derivative (PPD)
Inspra	Spiriva
Intuniv	Invega
Invega	Intuniv
ISOtretinoin	tretinoin
Jantoven	Janumet
Jantoven	Januvia
Janumet	Jantoven
Janumet	Januvia
Janumet	Sinemet
Januvia	Jantoven
Januvia	Janumet
Kaletra	Keppra

Drug Name	Confused Drug Name
Keppra	Kaletra
Ketalar	ketorolac
ketamine	ketorolac
ketorolac	Ketalar
ketorolac	ketamine
ketorolac	methadone
KlonoPIN	cloNIDine
labetalol	LaMICtal
labetalol	lamoTRIgine
LaMICtal	labetalol
LaMICtal	LamISIL
LamISIL	LaMICtal
lamiVUDine	lamoTRIgine
lamoTRIgine	labetalol
lamoTRIgine	lamiVUDine
lamoTRIgine	levETIRAcetam
lamoTRIgine	levothyroxine
Lanoxin	levothyroxine
Lanoxin	naloxone
lanthanum carbonate	lithium carbonate
Lantus	Latuda
Lasix	Wakix
Latuda	Lantus
leucovorin calcium	Leukeran
leucovorin calcium	LEVOleucovorin
Leukeran	leucovorin calcium
Leukeran	Myleran
Levbid	Enbrel
levETIRAcetam	lamoTRIgine
levETIRAcetam	levOCARNitine
levETIRAcetam	levoFLOXacin
levOCARNitine	levETIRAcetam
levoFLOXacin	levETIRAcetam
LEVOleucovorin	leucovorin calcium
levothyroxine	lamoTRIgine
levothyroxine	Lanoxin
levothyroxine	liothyronine
linaCLOtide	linaGLIPtin
linaGLIPtin	linaCLOtide
liothyronine	levothyroxine
Lipitor	ZyrTEC
lithium carbonate	lanthanum carbonate
Lopressor	Lyrica
LORazepam	ALPRAZolam
LORazepam	clonazePAM
LORazepam	Lovaza
Lotronex	Protonix
Lovaza	LORazepam
Lunesta	Neulasta
Lupron Depot-3 Month	Lupron Depot-Ped
Lupron Depot-Ped	Lupron Depot-3 Month
Lyrica	Hydrea
Lyrica	Lopressor
Malarone	mefloquine
medroxy-PROGESTERone	methylPREDNISolone
medroxy-PROGESTERone	methylTESTOSTERone
mefloquine	Malarone
memantine	methadone
metFORMIN	metroNIDAZOLE
methadone	dexmethylphenidate
methadone	ketorolac

Brand names always start with an uppercase letter. Some brand names incorporate tall man letters in initial characters and may not be readily recognized as brand names. Brand name products appear in black; generic/other products appear in red.

LIST OF CONFUSED DRUG NAMES continued

Drug Name	Confused Drug Name
methadone	memantine
methadone	methylphenidate
methadone	metOLazone
methazolAMIDE	methIMAzole
methazolAMIDE	metOLazone
methIMAzole	methazolAMIDE
methIMAzole	metOLazone
methotrexate	metOLazone
methylphenidate	methadone
methylPREDNISolone	medroxyPROGESTERone
methylPREDNISolone	methylTESTOSTERone
methylTESTOSTERone	medroxyPROGESTERone
methylTESTOSTERone	methylPREDNISolone
metOLazone	methadone
metOLazone	methazolAMIDE
metOLazone	methIMAzole
metOLazone	methotrexate
metoprolol succinate	metoprolol tartrate
metoprolol tartrate	metoprolol succinate
metroNIDAZOLE	metFORMIN
metyraPONE	metyroSINE
metyroSINE	metyraPONE
miFEPRIStone	miSOPROStol
migALAstat	migLUstat
migLUstat	migALAstat
miSOPROStol	miFEPRIStone
mitoMYcin	mitoXANTRONE
mitoXANTRONE	mitoMYcin
morphine	HYDROmorphone
morphine - non-concentrated oral liquid	morphine - oral liquid concentrate
morphine - oral liquid concentrate	morphine - non-concentrated oral liquid
Motrin	Neurontin
MS Contin	OxyCONTIN
Mucinex D	Mucinex DM
Mucinex DM	Mucinex D
Myleran	Leukeran
nalbuphine	naloxone
naloxone	Lanoxin
naloxone	nalbuphine
Neo-Synephrine (phenylephrine)	neostigmine
neostigmine	Neo-Synephrine (phenylephrine)
neratinib	nilotinib
neratinib	niraparib
Neulasta	Lunesta
Neulasta	Nuedexta
Neurontin	Motrin
NexAVAR	NexIUM
NexIUM	NexAVAR
niCARdipine	NIFEdipine
niCARdipine	niMODipine
NIFEdipine	niCARdipine
NIFEdipine	niMODipine
nilotinib	neratinib
nilotinib	niraparib
niMODipine	niCARdipine
niMODipine	NIFEdipine
niraparib	neratinib
niraparib	nilotinib
nizatidine	tiZANidine
NovoLIN	HumuLIN
NovoLIN	NovoLOG
NovoLIN 70/30	NovoLOG Mix 70/30
NovoLOG	HumaLOG
NovoLOG	NovoLIN
NovoLOG Flexpen	NovoLOG Mix 70/30 Flexpen
NovoLOG Mix 70/30	NovoLIN 70/30
NovoLOG Mix 70/30 Flexpen	NovoLOG Flexpen
Nuedexta	Neulasta
nystatin	HMG-CoA reductase inhibitors ("statins")
OLANZapine	QUEtiapine
omeprazole	fomepizole
Oracea	Orencia
Orencia	Oracea
oxaprozin	OXcarbazepine
OXcarbazepine	carBAMazepine
OXcarbazepine	oxaprozin
oxyBUTYnin	oxyCODONE
oxyBUTYnin	OxyCONTIN
oxyBUTYnin	oxyMORphone
oxyCODONE	HYDROcodone
oxyCODONE	oxyBUTYnin
oxyCODONE	OxyCONTIN
oxyCODONE	oxyMORphone
OxyCONTIN	MS Contin
OxyCONTIN	oxyBUTYnin
OxyCONTIN	oxyCODONE
OxyCONTIN	oxyMORphone
OxyCONTIN	oxytocin
oxyMORphone	HYDROmorphone
oxyMORphone	oxyBUTYnin
oxyMORphone	oxyCODONE
oxyMORphone	OxyCONTIN
oxytocin	OxyCONTIN
PACLitaxel	DOCEtaxel
PACLitaxel	PACLitaxel protein-bound particles
PACLitaxel protein-bound particles	PACLitaxel
PARoxetine	DULoxetine
PARoxetine	FLUoxetine
PARoxetine	piroxicam
Paxil	Doxil
Paxil	Plavix
Paxil	Trexall
PAZOPanib	PONATinib
PEMEtrexed	PRALAtrexate
penicillAMINE	penicillin
penicillin	penicillAMINE
PENTobarbital	PHENobarbital
perflutren lipid microspheres	influenza virus vaccine
PHENobarbital	PENTobarbital
piroxicam	PARoxetine
Plavix	Paxil
Plavix	Pradaxa
polyethylene glycol	propylene glycol
PONATinib	PAZOPanib

Brand names always start with an uppercase letter. Some brand names incorporate tall man letters in initial characters and may not be readily recognized as brand names. Brand name products appear in black; generic/other products appear in red.

LIST OF CONFUSED DRUG NAMES continued

Drug Name	Confused Drug Name
potassium acetate	sodium acetate
Pradaxa	Plavix
PRALAtrexate	PEMEtrexed
pralidoxime	pyridoxine
prednisoLONE	predniSONE
predniSONE	prednisoLONE
PriLOSEC	Pristiq
PriLOSEC	PROzac
Pristiq	PriLOSEC
Prograf	Proscar
Prograf	PROzac
propylene glycol	polyethylene glycol
Proscar	Prograf
Proscar	Provera
protamine	Protonix
proton pump inhibitors	ARIPiprazole
Protonix	Lotronex
Protonix	protamine
Provera	Proscar
Provera	PROzac
PROzac	PriLOSEC
PROzac	Prograf
PROzac	Provera
Pyridium	pyridoxine
pyRIDostigmine	pyridoxine
pyridoxine	pralidixime
pyridoxine	Pyridium
pyridoxine	pyRIDostigmine
QUEtiapine	OLANZapine
quiNIDine	quiNINE
quiNINE	quiNIDine
RABEprazole	ARIPiprazole
Rapaflo	Rapamune
Rapamune	Rapaflo
rasagiline	repaglinide
Remeron	Rozerem
repaglinide	rasagiline
Restoril	RisperDAL
Retrovir	ritonavir
ribavirin	riboflavin
riboflavin	ribavirin
rifabutin	rifapentine
rifAMPin	rifAXIMin
rifapentine	rifabutin
rifAXIMin	rifAMPin
RisperDAL	Restoril
RisperDAL	rOPINIRole
risperiDONE	rOPINIRole
ritonavir	Retrovir
Rituxan	Rituxan Hycela
Rituxan Hycela	Rituxan
riTUXimab	inFLIXimab
romiDEPsin	romiPLOStim
romiPLOStim	romiDEPsin
rOPINIRole	RisperDAL
rOPINIRole	risperiDONE
ROPivacaine	BUPivacaine
Rozerem	Remeron
Salagen	selegiline
SandIMMUNE	SandoSTATIN
SandoSTATIN	SandIMMUNE
SAXagliptin	SITagliptin
selegiline	Salagen
SEROquel	SEROquel XR
SEROquel XR	SEROquel
sertraline	cetirizine
silodosin	sirolimus
Sinemet	Janumet
sirolimus	silodosin
SITagliptin	SAXagliptin
SITagliptin	SUMAtriptan
Slynd	Syeda
sodium acetate	potassium acetate
Solu-CORTEF	SOLU-Medrol
SOLU-Medrol	DEPO-Medrol
SOLU-Medrol	Solu-CORTEF
SORAfenib	SUNItinib
sotalol	Sudafed
Spiriva	Apidra
Spiriva	Inspra
Spravato	Steglatro
Steglatro	Spravato
Sudafed	sotalol
Sudafed	Sudafed PE
Sudafed 12 Hour	Sudafed 12 Hour Pressure + Pain
Sudafed 12 Hour Pressure + Pain	Sudafed 12 Hour
Sudafed PE	Sudafed
SUFentanil	fentaNYL
sulfADIAZINE	sulfaSALAzine
sulfaSALAzine	cefuroxime
sulfaSALAzine	sulfADIAZINE
SUMAtriptan	SITagliptin
SUMAtriptan	ZOLMitriptan
SUNItinib	SORAfenib
Syeda	Slynd
Symbyax	Cymbalta
tacrolimus	tamsulosin
talquetamab	teclistamab
Talvey	Tecvayli
tamsulosin	tacrolimus
Tarceva	Tresiba
teclistamab	talquetamab
Tecvayli	Talvey
TEGretol	TEGretol XR
TEGretol XR	TEGretol
terbinafine	terbutaline
terbutaline	terbinafine
tetanus diphtheria toxoid (Td)	tuberculin purified protein derivative (PPD)
Thalomid	thiamine
thiamine	Thalomid
Thrombate III	thrombin topical (recombinant)
thrombin topical (recombinant)	Thrombate III
tiaGABine	tiZANidine
tiZANidine	nizatidine
tiZANidine	tiaGABine
TNKase	Activase
TNKase	t-PA
Tobradex	Tobrex
Tobrex	Tobradex
Topamax	Toprol-XL
Toprol-XL	Topamax

Brand names always start with an uppercase letter. Some brand names incorporate tall man letters in initial characters and may not be readily recognized as brand names. Brand name products appear in black; generic/other products appear in red.

LIST OF CONFUSED DRUG NAMES continued

Drug Name	Confused Drug Name
Toujeo	Tradjenta
Toujeo	Tresiba
Toujeo	Trulicity
t-PA	TNKase
Tracleer	Tricor
Tradjenta	Toujeo
Tradjenta	Tresiba
Tradjenta	Trulicity
tra**MAD**ol	tra**ZOD**one
trastuzumab	ado-trastuzumab emtansine
tra**ZOD**one	tra**MAD**ol
Tresiba	Tarceva
Tresiba	Toujeo
Tresiba	Tradjenta
Tresiba	Trulicity
tretinoin	**ISO**tretinoin
Trexall	Paxil
Tricor	Tracleer
tromethamine	Trophamine
Trophamine	tromethamine
Trulicity	Toujeo
Trulicity	Tradjenta
Trulicity	Tresiba
tuberculin purified protein derivative (PPD)	influenza virus vaccine
tuberculin purified protein derivative (PPD)	tetanus diphtheria toxoid (Td)
Tylenol	Tylenol PM
Tylenol PM	Tylenol
Ure-Na (palatable form of oral urea)	hydroxyurea
val**ACY**clovir	val**GAN**ciclovir
Valcyte	Valtrex
val**GAN**ciclovir	val**ACY**clovir
Valtrex	Valcyte
Varivax	VZIG (varicella-zoster immune globulin)
vasopressin	desmopressin
Venofer	Vfend
Venofer	Vimpat

Drug Name	Confused Drug Name
Vfend	Venofer
Vfend	Vimpat
Viagra	Allegra
vigabatrin	dabigatran
Vimpat	Venofer
Vimpat	Vfend
vin**BLAS**tine	vin**CRIS**tine
vin**CRIS**tine	vin**BLAS**tine
Viracept	Viramune
Viramune	Viracept
VZIG (varicella-zoster immune globulin)	Varivax
Wakix	Lasix
Wellbutrin SR	Wellbutrin XL
Wellbutrin XL	Wellbutrin SR
Xanax	Fanapt
Xeloda	Xenical
Xenical	Xeloda
Yasmin	Yaz
Yaz	Yasmin
Zegerid	Zestril
Zelapar	Zy**PREXA**Zydis
Zestril	Zegerid
Zestril	Zetia
Zestril	Zy**PREXA**
Zetia	Zestril
Zocor	Cozaar
Zocor	Zyr**TEC**
ZOLMitriptan	**SUMA**triptan
Zovirax	Zyvox
Zy**PREXA**	Cele**XA**
Zy**PREXA**	Zestril
Zy**PREXA**	Zyr**TEC**
Zy**PREXA** Zydis	Zelapar
Zyr**TEC**	Lipitor
Zyr**TEC**	Zocor
Zyr**TEC**	Zy**PREXA**
Zyr**TEC**	Zyr**TEC**-D
Zyr**TEC**-D	Zyr**TEC**
Zyvox	Zovirax

Brand names always start with an uppercase letter. Some brand names incorporate tall man letters in initial characters and may not be readily recognized as brand names. Brand name products appear in black; generic/other products appear in red.

Institute of Safe Medication Practices. (2024). ISMP lists of confused drug names. https://online.ecri.org/hubfs/ISMP/Resources/ISMP_ConfusedDrugNames.pdf

FDA-APPROVED LIST OF GENERIC DRUG NAMES WITH TALL MAN (MIXED CASE) LETTERS

Drug Name with Tall Man (Mixed Case) Letters	Confused with	Drug Name with Tall Man (Mixed Case) Letters	Confused with
bu**PROP**ion	bus**PIR**one	hydr**OXY**zine	hydr**ALAZINE**—**HYDRO**morphone
bus**PIR**one	bu**PROP**ion	medroxy**PROGES-TER**one	methyl**PREDNIS**olone—methyl**TESTOSTER**one
clomi**PHENE**	clomi**PRAMINE**		
clomi**PRAMINE**	clomi**PHENE**	methyl**PREDNIS**olone	medroxy**PROGESTER**one—methyl**TESTOSTER**one
cyclo**SERINE**	cyclo**SPORINE**		
cyclo**SPORINE**	cyclo**SERINE**	methyl**TESTOSTER**one	medroxy**PROGESTER**one—methyl**PREDNIS**olone
DAUNOrubicin	**DOXO**rubicin		
dimenhy**DRINATE**	diphenhydr**AMINE**	mito**XANTRONE**	Not specified
diphenhydr**AMINE**	dimenhy**DRINATE**	ni**CAR**dipine	**NIFE**dipine
DOBUTamine	**DOP**amine	**NIFE**dipine	ni**CAR**dipine
DOPamine	**DOBUT**amine	predniso**LONE**	predni**SONE**
DOXOrubicin	**DAUNO**rubicin	predni**SONE**	predniso**LONE**
glipi**ZIDE**	gly**BURIDE**	risperi**DONE**	r**OPINIR**ole
gly**BURIDE**	glipi**ZIDE**	r**OPINIR**ole	risperi**DONE**
hydr**ALAZINE**	hydr**OXY**zine—**HYDRO**morphone	vin**BLAS**tine	vin**CRIS**tine
HYDROmorphone	hydr**OXY**zine—hydr**ALAZINE**	vin**CRIS**tine	vin**BLAS**tine

US food and Drug Administration (FDA) and Institute of Safe Medication Practices (ISMP). (2023). *FDA and ISMP lists of look-alike drug names with recommended tall man (mixed case letters)*. https://online.ecri.org/hubfs/ISMP/Resources/ISMP_Look-Alike_Tallman_Letters.pdf

ISMP LIST OF ADDITIONAL DRUG NAMES WITH TALL MAN (MIXED CASE) LETTERS

Drug Name with Tall Man (Mixed Case) Letters	Confused with	Drug Name with Tall Man (Mixed Case) Letters	Confused with
ALPRAZolam	**LOR**azepam—clonaze**PAM**	cef**TRIAX**one	ce**FAZ**olin—cefo**TE**tan—cef**OX**itin—cef**TAZ**idime
a**MIL**oride	am**LODIP**ine		
am**LODIP**ine	a**MIL**oride	Cele**BREX***	Cele**XA***
ARIPiprazole	**RABE**prazole	Cele**XA***	Cele**BREX***
aza**CITID**ine	aza**THIO**prine	chlordiaze**POXIDE**	chlorpro**MAZINE**
aza**THIO**prine	aza**CITID**ine	chlorpro**MAZINE**	chlordiaze**POXIDE**
BUPivacaine	**ROP**ivacaine	**CIS**platin	**CARBO**platin
car**BAM**azepine	**OX**carbazepine	clo**BAZ**am	clonaze**PAM**
CARBOplatin	**CIS**platin	clonaze**PAM**	**ALPRAZ**olam—clo**BAZ**am—clo**NID**ine—clo**ZAP**ine—**LOR**azepam
ce**FAZ**olin	cefo**TE**tan—cef**OX**itin—cef**TAZ**idime—cef**TRIAX**one		
		clo**NID**ine	clonaze**PAM**—clo**ZAP**ine—Klono**PIN***
cefo**TE**tan	ce**FAZ**olin—cef**OX**itin—cef**TAZ**idime—cef**TRIAX**one	clo**ZAP**ine	clonaze**PAM**—clo**NID**ine
		cyclo**PHOS**phamide	cyclo**SERINE**—cyclo**SPORINE**
cef**OX**itin	ce**FAZ**olin—cefo**TE**tan—cef**TAZ**idime—cef**TRIAX**one		
		cyclo**SERINE**	cyclo**PHOS**phamide—cyclo**SPORINE**
cef**TAZ**idime	ce**FAZ**olin—cefo**TE**tan—cef**OX**itin—cef**TRIAX**one	cyclo**SPORINE**	cyclo**PHOS**phamide—cyclo**SERINE**

*Brand names always start with an uppercase letter. Some brand names incorporate tall man letters in initial characters and may not be readily recognized as brand names. An asterisk follows all brand names in ISMP List of Additional Drug Names with Tall Man Letters.

© **ISMP 2023**. Permission is granted to reproduce material for internal newsletters or communications with proper attribution. Other reproduction is prohibited without written permission from ISMP. Report actual and potential medication errors to the Medication Errors Reporting Program (MERP) online at www.ismp.org or by calling 1-800-FAIL-SAF(E).

US food and Drug Administartion (FDA) and Institute of Safe Medication Practices (ISMP). (2023). *FDA and ISMP lists of look-alike drug names with recommended tall man (mixed case letters)*. https://online.ecri.org/hubfs/ISMP/Resources/ISMP_Look-Alike_Tallman_Letters.pdf

ISMP LIST OF ADDITIONAL DRUG NAMES WITH TALL MAN (MIXED CASE) LETTERS continued

Drug Name with Tall Man (Mixed Case) Letters	Confused with
DACTINomycin	**DAPTO**mycin
DAPTOmycin	**DACTIN**omycin
DEPO-Medrol*	**SOLU**-Medrol*
dex**AMETH**asone	dexmede**TOMID**ine
dexmede**TOMID**ine	dex**AMETH**asone
diaze**PAM**	dil**TIAZ**em
dil**TIAZ**em	diaze**PAM**
DOCEtaxel	**PACL**itaxel
DOXOrubicin	**IDA**rubicin
dro**NAB**inol	dro**PER**idol
dro**PER**idol	dro**NAB**inol
DULoxetine	**FLU**oxetine – **PAR**oxetine
e**PHED**rine	**EPINEPH**rine
EPINEPHrine	e**PHED**rine
epi**RUB**icin	eri**BUL**in
eri**BUL**in	epi**RUB**icin
fenta**NYL**	**SUF**entanil
flavox**ATE**	fluvoxa**MINE**
FLUoxetine	**DUL**oxetine – **PAR**oxetine
flu**PHENAZ**ine	fluvoxa**MINE**
fluvoxa**MINE**	flavox**ATE** – flu**PHENAZ**ine
guai**FEN**esin	guan**FACINE**
guan**FACINE**	guai**FEN**esin
Huma**LOG***	Humu**LIN***
Humu**LIN***	Huma**LOG***
hydr**ALAZINE**	hydro**CHLORO**thiazide – hydr**OXY**zine
hydro**CHLORO**thiazide	hydr**ALAZINE** – hydr**OXY**zine
HYDROcodone	oxy**CODONE**
HYDROmorphone	morphine – oxy**MOR**phone
hydr**OXY**zine	hydr**ALAZINE** – hydro**CHLORO**thiazide
IDArubicin	DOXOrubicin – idaru**CIZU**mab
idaru**CIZU**mab	**IDA**rubicin
in**FLIX**imab	ri**TUX**imab
ISOtretinoin	tretinoin
Klono**PIN***	clo**NID**ine
La**MIC**tal*	Lam**ISIL***
Lam**ISIL***	La**MIC**tal*
lami**VUD**ine	lamo**TRI**gine
lamo**TRI**gine	lami**VUD**ine
lev**ETIRA**cetam	lev**OCARN**itine – levo**FLOX**acin
lev**OCARN**itine	lev**ETIRA**cetam
levo**FLOX**acin	lev**ETIRA**cetam
LEVOleucovorin	leucovorin
LORazepam	**ALPRAZ**olam – clonaze**PAM**
met**FORMIN**	metro**NIDAZOLE**
methazol**AMIDE**	methi**MAZOLE** – met**OL**azone
methi**MAZOLE**	methazol**AMIDE** – met**OL**azone
met**OL**azone	methazol**AMIDE** – methi**MAZOLE**
metro**NIDAZOLE**	met**FORMIN**
metyra**PONE**	metyro**SINE**
metyro**SINE**	metyra**PONE**
mi**FEPRIS**tone	mi**SOPROS**tol
mig**ALA**stat	mig**LU**stat
mig**LU**stat	mig**ALA**stat
mi**SOPROS**tol	mi**FEPRIS**tone
mito**MY**cin	mito**XANTRONE**
mito**XANTRONE**	mito**MY**cin
Nex**AVAR***	Nex**IUM***
Nex**IUM***	Nex**AVAR***
ni**CAR**dipine	**NIFE**dipine – ni**MOD**ipine
NIFEdipine	ni**CAR**dipine – ni**MOD**ipine
ni**MOD**ipine	ni**CAR**dipine – **NIFE**dipine
Novo**LIN***	Novo**LOG***
Novo**LOG***	Novo**LIN***
OLANZapine	**QUE**tiapine
OXcarbazepine	car**BAM**azepine
oxy**BUTY**nin	oxy**CODONE** – Oxy**CONTIN*** – oxy**MOR**phone
oxy**CODONE**	**HYDRO**codone – oxy**BUTY**nin – Oxy**CONTIN*** – oxy**MOR**phone
Oxy**CONTIN***	oxy**BUTY**nin – oxy**CODONE** – oxy**MOR**phone
oxy**MOR**phone	**HYDRO**morphone – oxy**BUTY**nin – oxy**CODONE** – Oxy**CONTIN***
PACLitaxel	**DOCE**taxel
PARoxetine	**DUL**oxetine – **FLU**oxetine
PAZOPanib	**PONAT**inib
PEMEtrexed	**PRALA**trexate
penicill**AMINE**	penicillin
PENTobarbital	**PHEN**obarbital

*Brand names always start with an uppercase letter. Some brand names incorporate tall man letters in initial characters and may not be readily recognized as brand names. An asterisk follows all brand names in ISMP List of Additional Drug Names with Tall Man Letters.

US food and Drug Administration (FDA) and Institute of Safe Medication Practices (ISMP). (2023). *FDA and ISMP lists of look-alike drug names with recommended tall man (mixed case letters)*. https://online.ecri.org/hubfs/ISMP/Resources/ISMP_Look-Alike_Tallman_Letters.pdf

ISMP LIST OF ADDITIONAL DRUG NAMES WITH TALL MAN (MIXED CASE) LETTERS continued

Drug Name with Tall Man (Mixed Case) Letters	Confused with
PHENobarbital	**PENT**obarbital
PONATinib	**PAZOP**anib
PRALAtrexate	**PEME**trexed
Pri**LOSEC***	**PRO**zac*
PROzac*	Pri**LOSEC***
QUEtiapine	**OLANZ**apine
qui**NID**ine	qui**NINE**
qui**NINE**	qui**NID**ine
RABEprazole	**ARIP**iprazole
rif**AMP**in	rif**AXIM**in
rif**AXIM**in	rif**AMP**in
Risper**DAL***	r**OPINIR**ole
risperi**DONE**	r**OPINIR**ole
ri**TUX**imab	in**FLIX**imab
romi**DEP**sin	romi**PLOS**tim
romi**PLOS**tim	romi**DEP**sin
r**OPINIR**ole	Risper**DAL***– risperi**DONE**
Sand**IMMUNE***	Sando**STATIN***
Sando**STATIN***	Sand**IMMUNE***
SAXagliptin	**SIT**agliptin
SITagliptin	**SAX**agliptin–**SUMA**triptan
Solu–**CORTEF***	**SOLU**–**M**edrol*
SOLU–**M**edrol*	Solu–**CORTEF***– **DEPO**Medrol*
SORAfenib	**SUNI**tinib
SUFentanil	fenta**NYL**
sulf**ADIAZINE**	sulfa**SALA**zine
sulfa**SALA**zine	sulf**ADIAZINE**
SUMAtriptan	**SIT**agliptin–**ZOLM**itriptan
SUNItinib	**SORA**fenib
tia**GAB**ine	ti**ZAN**idine
ti**ZAN**idine	tia**GAB**ine
tra**MAD**ol	tra**ZOD**one
tra**ZOD**one	tra**MAD**ol
val**ACY**clovir	val**GAN**ciclovir
val**GAN**ciclovir	val**ACY**clovir
ZOLMitriptan	**SUMA**triptan
Zy**PREXA***	Zyr**TEC***
Zyr**TEC***	Zy**PREXA***

*Brand names always start with an uppercase letter. Some brand names incorporate tall man letters in initial characters and may not be readily recognized as brand names. An asterisk follows all brand names in ISMP List of Additional Drug Names with Tall Man Letters.

US food and Drug Administration (FDA) and Institute of Safe Medication Practices (ISMP). (2023). *FDA and ISMP lists of look-alike drug names with recommended tall man (mixed case letters)*. https://online.ecri.org/hubfs/ISMP/Resources/ISMP_Look-Alike_Tallman_Letters.pdf

PEDIATRIC INTRAVENOUS MEDICATION QUICK REFERENCE CHART

Risk of fluid overload in infants and children is always a consideration when administering IV medications. The following table provides maximum concentrations—the smallest amount of fluid necessary for diluting specific medications—and the maximum rate at which the medications be given.

Drug	Maximum Concentration	Maximum Rate
acetaminophen	10 mg/mL	Infuse over 15 min
acetazolamide	100 mg/mL	500 mg/min
acyclovir	7 mg/mL	Infuse over ≥1 hr
adenosine	3 mg/mL	Give over 1–2 sec
allopurinol	6 mg/mL	Infuse over ≥30 min
amikacin	10 mg/mL	Infuse over 30–60 min
aminocaproic acid	20 mg/mL	Infuse over 10–60 min
aminophylline	25 mg/mL (IV push) 1 mg/mL (intermittent infusion)	Infuse over 15–30 min
amphotericin B deoxycholate	0.1 mg/mL (peripherally) 0.25 mg/mL (centrally)	Infuse over 2–6 hr (peripherally or centrally)
amphotericin B liposomal	2 mg/mL	Infuse over 2 hr
ampicillin	100 mg/mL	IV push: Dose ≤500 mg: Give over 3–5 min; Dose >500 mg: Give over 10–15 min Intermittent infusion: Infuse over ≥20 min (neonates) or 10–15 min (infants, children, and adolescents)
ampicillin/sulbactam	30 mg/mL (ampicillin)	IV push: Give over 10–15 min Intermittent infusion: Infuse over 15–30 min
anidulafungin	0.77 mg/mL	≤1.1 mg/min
atropine	1 mg/mL	Give over 1 min
azathioprine	10 mg/mL (IV push) <10 mg/mL (intermittent infusion)	IV push: Give over 5 min Intermittent infusion: Infuse over 30–60 min
azithromycin	2 mg/mL	Infuse over 1 hr
aztreonam	20 mg/mL	IV push: Give over 3–5 min Intermittent infusion: Infuse over 20–60 min
belimumab	4 mg/mL	Infuse over 1 hr
bezlotoxumab	10 mg/mL	Infuse over 1 hr
brivaracetam	10 mg/mL	Give over 2–15 min
bumetanide	0.25 mg/mL (IV push) 0.04 mg/mL (intermittent infusion)	Give over 1–2 min
caffeine citrate	20 mg/mL	Infuse over 10–20 min
calcium chloride	20 mg/mL	100 mg/min
calcium gluconate	50 mg/mL	100 mg/min
caspofungin	0.5 mg/mL	Infuse over 1 hr
cefazolin	138 mg/mL (IV push) 20 mg/mL (intermittent infusion)	IV push: Give over 3–5 min Intermittent infusion: Infuse over 10–60 min
cefepime	160 mg/mL	Intermittent infusion: Infuse over 30 min Extended infusion: Infuse over 3–4 hr
cefotaxime	200 mg/mL (IV push) 60 mg/mL (intermittent infusion)	IV push: Give over 3–5 min Intermittent infusion: Infuse over 15–30 min
cefoxitin	180 mg/mL (IV push) 125 mg/mL (intermittent infusion)	IV push: Give over 3–5 min Intermittent infusion: Infuse over 15–60 min
ceftaroline	12 mg/mL	Neonates and infants <2 mo: Infuse over 30–60 min; Infants ≥2 mo, children, and adolescents: Infuse over 5–60 min
ceftazidime	180 mg/mL (IV push) 40 mg/mL (intermittent infusion) 30 mg/mL (continuous infusion)	IV push: Give over 3–5 min Intermittent infusion: Infuse over 15–30 min
ceftazidime/avibactam	Ceftazidime 40 mg/mL and avibactam 10 mg/mL	Infuse over 2 hr
ceftobiprole	5.33 mg/mL (≥3 mo–<12 yr) 2.67 mg/mL (≥12 yr)	Infuse over 2 hr

PEDIATRIC INTRAVENOUS MEDICATION QUICK REFERENCE CHART continued

Drug	Maximum Concentration	Maximum Rate
ceftolozane/tazobactam	Ceftolozane 16.3 mg/mL and tazobactam 8.1 mg/mL	Ceftolozane dose <2 g: Infuse over 1 hr; Ceftolozane dose of 2 g: Infuse over 3 hr
ceftriaxone	40 mg/mL	IV push: Give over 2–5 min Intermittent infusion: Infuse over 1 hr (neonates) or 30 min (infants, children, and adolescents)
cefuroxime	100 mg/mL (IV push) 137 mg/mL (intermittent infusion)	IV push: Give over 3–5 min Intermittent infusion: Infuse over 15–30 min
cetirizine	10 mg/mL	Give over 1–2 min
chlorothiazide	28 mg/mL	IV push: Give over 3–5 min Intermittent infusion: Infuse over 30 min
chlorpromazine	1 mg/mL	0.5 mg/min
ciprofloxacin	2 mg/mL	Infuse over 60 min
clindamycin	18 mg/mL	30 mg/min
cyclosporine	2.5 mg/mL	Infuse over 2–6 hr
dalbavancin	5 mg/mL	Infuse over 30 min
dexamethasone	10 mg/mL	Dose ≤10 mg: Give over 1–4 min Dose >10 mg: Infuse over 15–30 min
dexmedetomidine	4 mcg/mL	Infuse loading dose over 10–20 min
diazepam	5 mg/mL	1–2 mg/min
digoxin	100 mcg/mL	Infuse over 5–10 min
diphenhydramine	50 mg/mL	IV push: ≤25 mg min Intermittent infusion: Infuse over 10–15 min
enalaprilat	1.25 mg/mL	Give over 5 min
ertapenem	20 mg/mL	Infuse over 30 min
erythromycin	5 mg/mL	Infuse over 20–120 min
esomeprazole	0.8 mg/mL	Infuse over 10–30 min
ethacrynic acid	2 mg/mL	Infuse over 5–30 min
famotidine	4 mg/mL (IV push) 0.2 mg/mL (intermittent infusion)	IV push: Give over ≥2 min Intermittent infusion: Infuse over 15–30 min
fentanyl	50 mcg/mL	Give over 3–5 min; infuse larger doses (>5 mcg/kg) over 5–10 min
fluconazole	2 mg/mL	Infuse over 1–2 hr
flumazenil	0.1 mg/mL	0.2 mg/min
fosaprepitant	1 mg/mL	Infants ≥6 mo and children <12 yr: Infuse over 60 min; Children 12–17 yr: Infuse over 30 min
foscarnet	12 mg/mL (peripherally) 24 mg/mL (centrally)	60 mg/kg/hr
fosphenytoin	25 mg/mL	2 mg/kg/min
furosemide	10 mg/mL	0.5 mg/kg/min
ganciclovir	10 mg/mL	Infuse over 1 hr
gentamicin	10 mg/mL	Infuse over 30–120 min
glycopyrrolate	0.2 mg/mL	Give over 1–2 min
granisetron	1 mg/mL (IV push) 50 mcg/mL (intermittent infusion)	IV push: Give over 30 sec Intermittent infusion: Infuse over 30–60 min
hydralazine	20 mg/mL	Give over 1–2 min
hydrocortisone	50 mg/mL (IV push) 5 mg/mL (intermittent infusion)	IV push: Give over 30 sec Intermittent infusion: Infuse over 20–30 min
hydromorphone	4 mg/mL	Give over 2–3 min
ibuprofen	4 mg/mL	Infuse over ≥10 min
ibuprofen lysine	5 mg/mL	Infuse over 15 min
imipenem/cilastatin	5 mg/mL	Dose ≤500 mg: Infuse over 20–30 min; Dose >500 mg: Infuse over 40–60 min

PEDIATRIC INTRAVENOUS MEDICATION QUICK REFERENCE CHART continued

Drug	Maximum Concentration	Maximum Rate
indomethacin	1 mg/mL	Infuse over 20–30 min
infliximab	4 mg/mL	Infuse over 2 hr
isavuconazonium	1.5 mg/mL	Infuse over 1 hr
ketamine	50 mg/mL (IV push) 2 mg/mL (continuous infusion)	IV push: 0.5 mg/kg/min
ketorolac	30 mg/mL	Give over 1–5 min
labetalol	5 mg/mL (IV push) 1 mg/mL (continuous infusion)	IV push: 10 mg/min
lacosamide	10 mg/mL	Infuse over 30–60 min
levetiracetam	20 mg/mL (neonates) 50 mg/mL (infants, children, and adolescents)	Neonates: Concentration ≤15 mg/mL: Infuse over 10–15 min; Concentration of 20 mg/mL: 1 mg/kg/min Infants, children, and adolescents: Concentration ≤15 mg/mL: Infuse over 15 min; Concentration of 50 mg/mL: Infuse over 5–10 min
levocarnitine	8 mg/mL	Give over 2–3 min
levothyroxine	100 mcg/mL	Give over 2–3 min
linezolid	2 mg/mL	Infuse over 30–120 min
lorazepam	2 mg/mL	2 mg/min or 0.05 mg/kg over 2–5 min
magnesium sulfate	200 mg/mL	Infuse over 10–20 min
meperidine	10 mg/mL	Give over 5 min
meropenem	50 mg/mL (IV push) 20 mg/mL (intermittent or extended infusion)	IV push: Give over 3–5 min Intermittent infusion: Infuse over 15–30 min Extended infusion: Infuse over 3–4 hr
methylprednisolone	125 mg/mL (IV push) 2.5 mg/mL (intermittent infusion)	IV push: Give over 1–5 min Intermittent infusion: Infuse over 15–60 min
metoclopramide	5 mg/mL (IV push) 0.4 mg/mL (intermittent infusion)	IV push: Dose ≤10 mg: Give over 1–2 min Intermittent infusion: Dose >10 mg: Infuse over ≥15 min
metronidazole	5 mg/mL	Infuse over 30–60 min
micafungin	1.5 mg/mL	Infuse over 1 hr
midazolam	5 mg/mL	Give over 20–30 sec (5 min in neonates)
milrinone	200 mcg/mL	Loading dose: Give over 10 min
morphine	5 mg/mL (IV push or intermittent infusion) 1 mg/mL (continuous infusion)	IV push: Give over 4–5 min Intermittent infusion: Infuse over 15–30 min
mycophenolate	6 mg/mL	Infuse over 2 hr
nafcillin	125 mg/mL	IV push: Give over 5–10 min Intermittent infusion: Infuse over 30–60 min
naloxone	0.04 mg/mL (IV push) 400 mcg/mL (continuous infusion)	Give over 30 sec
ondansetron	2 mg/mL (IV push) 1 mg/mL (intermittent infusion)	IV push: Give over 2–5 min Intermittent infusion: Infuse over 15–30 min
oxacillin	100 mg/mL (IV push) 40 mg/mL (intermittent infusion)	IV push: Give over 10 min Intermittent infusion: Infuse over 15–30 min
palonosetron	30 mcg/mL	Prevention of chemotherapy-induced nausea/vomiting: Infuse over 15 min Prevention of postoperative nausea/vomiting: Give over 10 sec
pantoprazole	4 mg/mL (IV push) 0.8 mg/mL (intermittent infusion)	IV push: Give over 2 min Intermittent infusion: Infuse over 15 min
penicillin G	150,000 units/mL	Infuse over 15–30 min
pentamidine	6 mg/mL	Infuse over 1–2 hr
pentobarbital	50 mg/mL	50 mg/min

PEDIATRIC INTRAVENOUS MEDICATION QUICK REFERENCE CHART continued

Drug	Maximum Concentration	Maximum Rate
phenobarbital	65 mg/mL	30 mg/min
phenytoin	10 mg/mL	Neonates: 1 mg/kg/min; Infants, children, and adolescents: 3 mg/kg/min
phytonadione	10 mg/mL	1 mg/min
piperacillin/tazobactam	Piperacillin 80 mg/mL and tazobactam 10 mg/mL	Intermittent infusion: Infuse over 30 min Extended infusion: Neonates: Infuse over 3 hr; Infants, children, and adolescents: Infuse over 4 hr
posaconazole	2 mg/mL	Infuse over 90 min
potassium chloride	80 mEq/L (peripherally) 300 mEq/L (centrally)	≤0.5 mEq/kg/hr
propranolol	1 mg/mL	Infuse over 10 min
protamine	10 mg/mL	5 mg/min
remdesivir	1.25 mg/mL	Infuse over 30–120 min
rifampin	6 mg/mL	Infuse over 30–270 min
rocuronium	10 mg/mL	Give over 10 sec
tacrolimus	0.02 mg/mL	Infuse over 2–24 hr
tedizolid	0.8 mg/mL	Infuse over 1 hr
tobramycin	10 mg/mL	Infuse over 20–60 min
trimethoprim/sulfamethoxazole	1 mL drug per 15 mL diluent	Infuse over 60–90 min
valproate sodium	50 mg/mL	3 mg/kg/min
vancomycin	10 mg/mL	Infuse over 60 min
verapamil	2.5 mg/mL	Give over 2–3 min
voriconazole	5 mg/mL	3 mg/kg/hr
zidovudine	4 mg/mL	Infuse over 30–60 min

† UpToDate Lexidrug, via UpToDate Inc. Accessed August 15, 2025.

APPENDICES

APPENDIX A

Recent Drug Approvals

Highlighted below are select drugs recently approved by the FDA. To access other newly released drugs online, print purchasers can use their free trial to Davis Nursing Consult. See the inside front cover for access details.

HIGH ALERT

datopotamab deruxtecan (da-toe-poe-tah-mab der-ux-tee-kan)

Datroway

Classification

Therapeutic: antineoplastics

Pharmacologic: monoclonal antibodies, enzyme inhibitors

Indications

Unresectable or metastatic, hormone receptor positive, human epidermal growth factor receptor 2 (HER2)-negative (IHC 0, IHC 1+ or IHC 2+/ISH-) breast cancer in patients who have received prior endocrine-based therapy and chemotherapy for unresectable or metastatic disease.

Contraindications/Precautions

Contraindicated in: OB: Pregnancy; Lactation: Lactation.

Use Cautiously in: Mild or moderate renal impairment (CCr 30–<90 mL/min) (↑ risk of interstitial lung disease (ILD)/pneumonitis); Moderate hepatic impairment (total bilirubin >1.5–3 times upper limit of normal and any AST); Rep: Women of reproductive potential and men with female partners of reproductive potential; Pedi: Safety and effectiveness not established in children.

Adverse Reactions/Side Effects

Derm: alopecia, rash, dry skin, hyperpigmentation, pruritus. **EENT:** dry eye, keratitis, ↑ lacrimation, blepharitis, blurred vision, conjunctivitis, meibomian gland dysfunction, photophobia, visual impairment. **F and E:** hypocalcemia. **GI:** ↓ appetite, ↑ liver enzymes, abdominal pain, constipation, diarrhea, nausea, stomatitis, vomiting, dry mouth. **GU:** ↓ fertility. **Hemat:** anemia, leukopenia, lymphopenia, neutropenia. **Neuro:** cough, fatigue, headache. **Resp:** ILD/PNEUMONITIS. **Misc:** infusion-related reactions.

Route/Dosage

IV (Adults ≥90 kg): 540 mg every 3 wk; continue until disease progression or unacceptable toxicity.

IV (Adults <90 kg): 6 mg/kg every 3 wk; continue until disease progression or unacceptable toxicity.

delgocitinib (del-goe-sye-ti-nib)

Anzupgo

Classification

Therapeutic: none assigned

Pharmacologic: kinase inhibitors

Indications

Moderate to severe chronic hand eczema that is not adequately controlled with topical corticosteroids or when those therapies are not advisable.

Contraindications/Precautions

Contraindicated in: Active, serious infection.

Use Cautiously in: Chronic or recurrent infection; Exposure to tuberculosis; History of a serious infection or opportunistic infection; Underlying condition that predisposes to infection; >50 yr old with ≥1 cardiovascular risk factor (may ↑ risk of all-cause mortality, cardiovascular death, MI, stroke, and thrombosis); OB: Safety not established in pregnancy; Lactation: Safety not established in breastfeeding; Pedi: Safety and effectiveness not established in children.

Adverse Reactions/Side Effects

Derm: bacterial skin infection, erythema, NONMELANOMA SKIN CANCER, pruritus. **Hemat:** leukopenia, neutropenia. **Local:** application site pain. **Neuro:** paresthesia. **Misc:** infection (including viral reactivation).

Route/Dosage

Topical **(Adults):** Apply a thin layer twice daily to affected areas only on the hands and wrists. Do not use more than one 30-g tube per 2 wk or one 60-g tube per mo.

HIGH ALERT

landiolol (lan-dye-oh-lol)

Rapiblyk

Classification

Therapeutic: antiarrhythmics

Pharmacologic: beta-blockers

Indications

Short-term reduction of ventricular rate in patients with supraventricular tachycardia including atrial fibrillation and atrial flutter.

Contraindications/Precautions

Contraindicated in: Hypersensitivity; Severe sinus bradycardia, sick sinus syndrome, or >1st-degree heart block; Decompensated HF; Cardiogenic shock; Pulmonary hypertension; Moderate or severe hepatic impairment.

Use Cautiously in: Hypovolemia (↑ risk of hypotension); 1st-degree heart block, sinus node dysfunction, or conduction disorders (↑ risk of bradycardia and heart block); Reactive airway disease; Diabetes mellitus (may ↑ risk mask signs of hypoglycemia); Prinzmetal angina (↑ risk of angina); Untreated pheochromocytoma (initiate only after alpha blocker therapy started); Raynaud disease or peripheral vascular disease; Renal impairment (↑ risk of hyperkalemia); Mild hepatic impairment; Metabolic acidosis (↑ risk of hyperkalemia renal tubular acidosis); Hyperthyroidism (may mask symptoms); History of severe allergic reactions (intensity of reactions may be ↑); OB: Safety not established in pregnancy; Lactation: Safety not established in breastfeeding; Pedi: Safety and effectiveness not established in children; Geri: Older adults may have ↑ sensitivity to beta blockers; initial dose ↓ recommended.

Adverse Reactions/Side Effects

CV: bradycardia, HF, hypotension. **Endo:** hypoglycemia. **F and E:** hyperkalemia. **Local:** infusion site reactions. **Misc:** HYPERSENSITIVITY REACTIONS (INCLUDING ANAPHYLAXIS).

Route/Dosage

IV (Adults): *Normal cardiac function:* 9 mcg/kg/min infusion initially; then ↑ by 9 mcg/kg/min every 10 min to achieve adequate ventricular rate control (max dose = 36 mcg/kg/min). *Impaired cardiac function:* 1 mcg/kg/min infusion initially; then ↑ by 1 mcg/kg/min every 15 min to achieve adequate ventricular rate control (max dose = 36 mcg/kg/min).

lebrikizumab (leb-ri-kiz-ue-mab)

Ebglyss

Classification

Therapeutic: anti-inflammatories

Pharmacologic: interleukin antagonists, monoclonal antibodies

Indications

Moderate to severe atopic dermatitis in patients whose disease is not adequately controlled with topical prescription therapies or when those therapies are not advisable (can be used with or without topical corticosteroids; topical calcineurin inhibitor use should be reserved for sensitive areas only, including face, neck, and intertriginous and genital areas).

Contraindications/Precautions

Contraindicated in: Hypersensitivity.

Use Cautiously in: Pre-existing helminth infections; OB: Safety not established in pregnancy; Lactation: Safety not established in breastfeeding; Pedi: Children <12 yr (safety and effectiveness not established).

Adverse Reactions/Side Effects

EENT: conjunctivitis, keratitis. **Hemat:** eosinophilia. **Local:** injection site reactions. **Misc:** HYPERSENSITIVITY REACTIONS (INCLUDING ANGIOEDEMA).

Route/Dosage

Subcut (Adults and Children ≥12 yr and ≥40 kg): 500 mg (given as two 250-mg injections) initially; then 500 mg (given as two 250-mg injections) in 2 wk; then 250 mg every 2 wk. In patients who achieve clear or almost clear skin after 16 wk of therapy, may ↓ dose to 250 mg every 4 wk.

ocrelizumab/hyaluronidase (ok-re-liz-ue-mab/hye-al-yoor-on-i-dase)

Ocrevus Zunovo

Classification

Therapeutic: anti-multiple sclerosis agents

Pharmacologic: monoclonal antibodies

Indications

Relapsing forms of multiple sclerosis (MS), including clinically isolated syndrome, relapsing-remitting disease, and active secondary progressive disease. Primary progressive MS.

Contraindications/Precautions

Contraindicated in: Hypersensitivity to ocrelizumab or hyaluronidase; Active hepatitis B virus (HBV) infection (may reactivate infection during and for several months after treatment); Active infection; History of life-threatening reaction to ocrelizumab.

Use Cautiously in: Patients who are immunocompromised or receiving other immunosuppressants; Rep: Women of reproductive potential; OB: Safety not established in pregnancy (may cause fetal B-cell depletion); Lactation: Safety not established in breastfeeding; Pedi: Safety and effectiveness not established in children.

Adverse Reactions/Side Effects

CV: peripheral edema. **GI:** diarrhea, HBV REACTIVATION, IMMUNE-MEDIATED COLITIS. **Hemat:** neutropenia. **Local:** injection reactions. **MS:** back pain. **Neuro:** depression, PROGRESSIVE MULTIFOCAL LEUKOENCEPHALOPATHY

(PML). **Resp:** cough. **Misc:** INFECTION, MALIGNANCY (PRIMARILY BREAST CANCER).

Route/Dosage

Subcut (Adults): Ocrelizumab 920 mg/hyaluronidase 23,000 units every 6 mo.

pivmecillinam (piv-meh-**sil**-li-nam)

Pivya

Classification

Therapeutic: anti-infectives

Pharmacologic: penicillins

Indications

Uncomplicated urinary tract infections in female patients.

Contraindications/Precautions

Contraindicated in: Serious hypersensitivity to penicillins or cephalosporins; Primary or secondary carnitine deficiency resulting from inherited disorders of mitochondrial fatty acid oxidation and carnitine metabolism, and other inborn errors of metabolism; Porphyria.

Use Cautiously in: OB: May cause a false-positive test for isovaleric acidemia during newborn screening if administered shortly before delivery; Lactation: Use while breastfeeding only if potential maternal benefit justifies potential risk to infant; Pedi: Safety and effectiveness not established in children.

Adverse Reactions/Side Effects

Derm: ACUTE GENERALIZED EXANTHEMATOUS PUSTULOSIS (AGEP), DRUG REACTIONS WITH EOSINOPHILIA AND SYSTEMIC SYMPTOMS (DRESS), STEVENS-JOHNSON SYNDROME (SJS), TOXIC EPIDERMAL NECROLYSIS (TEN). **GI:** CLOSTRIDIOIDES DIFFICILE-ASSOCIATED DIARRHEA (CDAD), diarrhea, nausea. **GU:** genital pruritus, vulvovaginal candidiasis. **Neuro:** headache. **Misc:** carnitine deficiency, HYPERSENSITIVITY REACTIONS (INCLUDING ANAPHYLAXIS), porphyria.

Route/Dosage

PO (Adults): 185 mg 3 times daily for 3–7 days.

resmetirom (res-me-**tir**-om)

Rezdiffra

Classification

Therapeutic: none assigned

Pharmacologic: thyroid hormone receptor agonists

Indications

Noncirrhotic nonalcoholic steatohepatitis with moderate to advanced liver fibrosis (in combination with diet and exercise).

Contraindications/Precautions

Contraindicated in: Moderate to severe hepatic impairment.

Use Cautiously in: Severe renal impairment; OB: Safety not established in pregnancy; Lactation: Safety not established in breastfeeding; Pedi: Safety and effectiveness not established in children.

Adverse Reactions/Side Effects

CV: arrhythmias, palpitations. **Derm:** pruritus, erythema. **Endo:** hypoglycemia. **GI:** ↓ appetite, ↑ liver enzymes, diarrhea, nausea, abdominal pain, abnormal feces, cholecystitis, cholelithiasis, constipation, flatulence, obstructive pancreatitis, vomiting. **GU:** uterine bleeding. **MS:** tendinopathy. **Neuro:** depression, dizziness, dysgeusia, vertigo. **Misc:** hypersensitivity reactions.

Route/Dosage

PO (Adults ≥100 kg): 100 mg once daily. *Concurrent use of moderate CYP2C8 inhibitor:* 80 mg once daily.
PO (Adults <100 kg): 80 mg once daily. *Concurrent use of moderate CYP2C8 inhibitor:* 60 mg once daily.

rilzabrutinib (ril-za-**broo**-ti-nib)

Wayrilz

Classification

Therapeutic: none assigned

Pharmacologic: kinase inhibitors

Indications

Persistent or chronic immune thrombocytopenia in patients who have had an insufficient response to a previous treatment.

Contraindications/Precautions

Contraindicated in: Severe renal impairment; Moderate or severe hepatic impairment; OB: Pregnancy; Lactation: Lactation.

Use Cautiously in: Rep: Women of reproductive potential; Pedi: Safety and effectiveness not established in children.

Adverse Reactions/Side Effects

EENT: nasopharyngitis. **GI:** abdominal pain, diarrhea, nausea, HEPATOTOXICITY, dyspepsia, vomiting. **Hemat:** neutropenia. **MS:** arthralgia. **Neuro:** headache, dizziness. **Resp:** cough. **Misc:** INFECTION.

Route/Dosage

PO: (Adults): 400 mg twice daily.

vadadustat (vad-a-doo-stat)

Vafseo

Classification

Therapeutic: antianemics

Pharmacologic: hypoxia-inducible factor prolyl hydroxylase inhibitors

Indications

Anemia due to chronic kidney disease in patients who have been receiving dialysis for ≥3 mo.

Contraindications/Precautions

Contraindicated in: Hypersensitivity; Uncontrolled hypertension; Acute coronary syndrome, stroke, or TIA within past 3 mo; Active, acute liver disease or cirrhosis; Active malignancy; Lactation: Lactation.

Use Cautiously in: Cardiovascular or cerebrovascular disease; History of GI erosion, peptic ulcer disease, concurrent use of medications that ↑ risk of GI erosion, and current tobacco smokers and alcohol drinkers; OB: Safety not established in pregnancy; Pedi: Safety and effectiveness not established in children.

Adverse Reactions/Side Effects

CV: hypertension, abdominal pain, DEEP VEIN THROMBOSIS (DVT) (ESPECIALLY WITH HGB >11 G/DL), MI (ESPECIALLY WITH HGB >11 G/DL), VASCULAR ACCESS THROMBOSIS (ESPECIALLY WITH HGB >11 G/DL). **GI:** diarrhea, ↑ liver enzymes, dyspepsia, gastroesophageal erosion, HEPATOTOXICITY, nausea, vomiting. **Neuro:** dizziness, fatigue, headache, PULMONARY EMBOLISM (PE) (ESPECIALLY WITH HGB >11 G/DL), SEIZURES, STROKE (ESPECIALLY WITH HGB >11 G/DL). **Misc:** DEATH (ESPECIALLY WITH HGB >11 G/DL), MALIGNANCY.

Route/Dosage

Not Being Treated With Erythropoietin-Stimulating Agent (ESA)

PO (Adults): 300 mg once daily.

Being Switched From ESA

PO (Adults): 300 mg once daily. During transition phase, if Hgb ↓ to <9 g/dL or if Hgb response is unacceptable, may consider RBC transfusions or ESA treatment. *If patient receives RBC transfusions,* continue vadadustat treatment. *If patient receives ESA rescue treatment,* hold vadadustat treatment until Hgb ≥10 g/dL. Hold vadadustat until 2 days after last epoetin dose, 7 days after last darbepoetin dose, or 14 days after last methoxy polyethylene glycol-epoetin beta dose. When reinitiating vadadustat, resume at previous dose or ↑ previous dose by 150 mg.

vanzacaftor/tezacaftor/deutivacaftor (van-zah-kaf-tor/tez-a-kaf-tor/due-tiv-a-kaf-tor)

Alyftrek

Classification

Therapeutic: cystic fibrosis therapy adjuncts

Pharmacologic: transmembrane conductance regulator potentiators

Indications

Cystic fibrosis (CF) in patients who have ≥1 F508del mutation or another responsive mutation in the cystic fibrosis transmembrane conductance regulator (CFTR) gene.

Contraindications/Precautions

Contraindicated in: Severe hepatic impairment.

Use Cautiously in: Severe renal impairment or end-stage renal disease; Moderate hepatic impairment (not recommended; if necessary, use only if benefit outweighs risk); OB: Safety not established in pregnancy; Lactation: Safety not established in breastfeeding; Pedi: Children <6 yr (safety and effectiveness not established).

Adverse Reactions/Side Effects

CV: ↑ BP. **Derm:** rash. **EENT:** nasopharyngitis, oropharyngeal pain, cataracts, rhinorrhea, sinus congestion, sinusitis. **GI:** abdominal pain, constipation, diarrhea, HEPATOTOXICITY, nausea, vomiting. **MS:** ↑ CK, arthralgia, back pain. **Neuro:** fatigue, headache. **Resp:** cough, upper respiratory tract infection, dyspnea, hemoptysis. **Misc:** fever, HYPERSENSITIVITY REACTIONS (INCLUDING ANAPHYLAXIS), influenza.

Route/Dosage

PO (Adults and Children ≥12 yr): Two tablets of vanzacaftor 10 mg/tezacaftor 50 mg/deutivacaftor 125 mg once daily. *Concurrent use of strong CYP3A inhibitor:* One tablet of vanzacaftor 10 mg/tezacaftor 50 mg/deutivacaftor 125 mg once weekly. *Concurrent use of moderate CYP3A inhibitor:* One tablet of vanzacaftor 10 mg/tezacaftor 50 mg/deutivacaftor 125 mg every other day.

PO (Children 6–12 yr and ≥40 kg): Two tablets of vanzacaftor 10 mg/tezacaftor 50 mg/deutivacaftor 125 mg once daily. *Concurrent use of strong CYP3A inhibitor:* One tablet of vanzacaftor 10 mg/tezacaftor 50 mg/deutivacaftor 125 mg once weekly. *Concurrent use of moderate CYP3A inhibitor:* One tablet of vanzacaftor 10 mg/tezacaftor 50 mg/deutivacaftor 125 mg every other day.

PO (Children 6–12 yr and <40 kg): Three tablets of vanzacaftor 4 mg/tezacaftor 20 mg/deutivacaftor 50 mg once daily. *Concurrent use of strong CYP3A*

inhibitor: Two tablets of vanzacaftor 4 mg/tezacaftor 20 mg/deutivacaftor 50 mg once weekly. *Concurrent use of moderate CYP3A inhibitor:* Two tablets of vanzacaftor 4 mg/tezacaftor 20 mg/deutivacaftor 50 mg every other day.

DISCONTINUED DRUGS

Generic Name (Brand Name)	Reason for Discontinuation
abciximab (ReoPro)	Discontinued by manufacturer
amifostine (Ethyol)	Discontinued by manufacturer
amobarbital (Amytal)	Discontinued by manufacturer
belantamab mafodotin (Blenrep)	Discontinued by manufacturer
bezlotoxumab (Zinplava)	Discontinued by manufacturer
brexanolone (Zulresso)	Discontinued by manufacturer
brompheniramine	Discontinued by manufacturer
cascara sagrada	Discontinued by manufacturer
celecoxib/tramadol (Seglentis)	Discontinued by manufacturer
cortisone (🍁 Cortone)	Discontinued by manufacturer
daprodustat (Jesduvroq)	Discontinued by manufacturer
dexamethasone (topical) (Aeroseb-Dex)	Discontinued by manufacturer
dimercaprol (British anti-lewisite)	Discontinued by manufacturer
dolasetron (Anzemet)	Discontinued by manufacturer
enfuvirtide (Fuzeon)	Discontinued by manufacturer
estramustine (Emcyt)	Discontinued by manufacturer
exenatide (Bydureon BCise)	Discontinued by manufacturer
fentaNYL (buccal tablet) (Fentora)	Discontinued by manufacturer
fentaNYL (oral transmucosal lozenge) (Actiq)	Discontinued by manufacturer
finasteride/tadalafil (Entadfi)	Discontinued by manufacturer
gepirone (Exxua)	Discontinued by manufacturer
ingenol (Picato)	Discontinued by manufacturer
inotersen (Tegsedi)	Discontinued by manufacturer
levamlodipine (Conjupri)	Discontinued by manufacturer
obeticholic acid (Ocaliva)	Discontinued by manufacturer
oliceridine (Olinvyk)	Discontinued by manufacturer
ozenoxacin (Xepi)	Discontinued by manufacturer
palivizumab (Synagis)	Discontinued by manufacturer
piperacillin	Discontinued by manufacturer
retapamulin (Altabax)	Discontinued by manufacturer
reteplase (Retavase)	Discontinued by manufacturer
rifamycin (Aemcolo)	Discontinued by manufacturer
sodium phenylbutyrate/taurursodiol (Relyvrio)	Discontinued by manufacturer

DISCONTINUED DRUGS (continued)

Generic Name (Brand Name)	Reason for Discontinuation
somatropin (recombinant) (Humatrope)	Discontinued by manufacturer
somatropin (recombinant) (Nutropin AQ NuSpin)	Discontinued by manufacturer
streptozocin (Zanosar)	Discontinued by manufacturer
vorapaxar (Zontivity)	Discontinued by manufacturer
voxelotor (Oxbryta)	Discontinued by manufacturer
zalcitabine (ddC)	Discontinued by manufacturer

APPENDIX B
Ophthalmic Medications

General Info: See Appendix C for administration techniques for ophthalmic agents.
Consult health care provider regarding:
- Concurrent use of contact lenses (medication or additives may be absorbed by the lens).
- Concurrent administration of other ophthalmic agents (order and spacing may be important).

ADRs = adverse reactions.

DRUG NAME	DOSE	NOTES
Alpha-1 Blocker		
Uses: Treatment of pharmacologically induced mydriasis produced by adrenergic agonists (e.g., phenylephrine) or parasympatholytic (e.g., tropicamide) agents. **CAUTIONS:** Avoid use in presence of active ocular inflammation.		
phentolamine (Ryzumvi)	**Adults and children ≥12 yr:** 1–2 drops of 0.75% solution. **Children 3–11 yr:** 1 drop of 0.75% solution.	• ADRs: irritation, conjunctival hyperemia
Alpha-2 Agonists		
Uses: Open-angle glaucoma and other forms of intraocular hypertension (↓ formation of aqueous humor); brimonidine also available as over-the-counter product to ↓ ocular redness. **CAUTIONS:** Systemic absorption may result in adverse cardiovascular and CNS reactions (especially in patients with cardiovascular disease); avoid use in patients predisposed to acute angle-closure glaucoma.		
apraclonidine (Iopidine)	**Adults:** *Open-angle glaucoma:* 1–2 drops of 0.5% solution 3 times daily; *Postoperative ↓ of intraocular pressure:* 1 drop of 1% solution 1 hr before surgery and upon completion of surgery.	• A selective alpha-adrenergic agonist • Monitor BP and HR • Avoid concurrent use with MAO inhibitors • ADRs: *ophthalmic:* irritation, mydriasis; *systemic:* allergic reactions, arrhythmias, bradycardia, drowsiness, dry nose, fainting, headache, nervousness, weakness
brimonidine (Alphagan P, Lumify [OTC], Lumify Preservative Free [OTC])	**Adults and children ≥2 yr:** *Glaucoma:* 1 drop of 0.1–0.2% solution 3 times daily (8 hr apart). **Adults and children ≥5 yr:** *Ocular redness (Lumify):* 1 drop of 0.025% solution every 6–8 hr as needed (up to 4 times daily).	• A selective alpha-adrenergic agonist • Avoid concurrent use with MAO inhibitors • Tricyclic antidepressants may ↓ effectiveness; additive CNS depression may occur with other CNS depressants, additive adverse cardiovascular effects with other cardiovascular agents • ADRs: *ophthalmic:* irritation; *systemic:* drowsiness, dizziness, dry mouth, headache, weakness, muscular pain
Anesthetics		
Uses: Provide brief local anesthesia to allow measurement of intraocular pressure, removal of foreign bodies, or other superficial procedures. **CAUTIONS:** Repeated use may result in ↑ risk of CNS and cardiovascular toxicity; cross-sensitivity with some local anesthetics may occur.		
chloroprocaine (Iheezo)	**Adults:** 3 drops of 3% gel (single dose).	• ADRs: conjunctival hyperemia, mydriasis, irritation
lidocaine (Akten)	**Adults and children:** 2 drops of 3.5% gel (single dose).	• Does not interact with ophthalmic cholinesterase inhibitors • ADRs: *ophthalmic:* irritation; *systemic:* irregular heartbeat, CNS depression

DRUG NAME	DOSE	NOTES
proparacaine (Alcaine)	**Adults and children:** 1–2 drops of 0.5% solution (single dose).	• Does not interact with ophthalmic cholinesterase inhibitors • ADRs: *ophthalmic:* irritation; *systemic:* irregular heartbeat, CNS depression
tetracaine (Altacaine)	**Adults:** 1–2 drops of 0.5% solution (single dose).	• May interact with ophthalmic cholinesterase inhibitors, resulting in ↑ duration of action and risk of toxicity • ADRs: *ophthalmic:* irritation; *systemic:* irregular heartbeat, CNS depression

Antibacterials

Uses: Localized superficial ophthalmic infections (e.g., bacterial conjunctivitis).
CAUTIONS: Small amounts may be absorbed and result in hypersensitivity reactions.

DRUG NAME	DOSE	NOTES
azithromycin (AzaSite)	**Adults and children ≥1 yr:** 1 drop of 1% solution twice daily (given 8–12 hr apart) for 2 days, then once daily for 5 more days.	• When used to treat ocular chlamydial infections, concurrent systemic therapy is required • ADRs: eye irritation
bacitracin	**Adults and children:** ¼–½-inch ointment strip every 3–4 hr for acute infections or 2–3 times daily for mild to moderate infections.	• ADRs: eye irritation
besifloxacin (Besivance)	**Adults and children ≥1 yr:** 1 drop of 0.6% suspension 3 times daily (given 4–12 hr apart) for 7 days.	• ADRs: headache, eye irritation
ciprofloxacin (Ciloxan)	**Adults and children of all ages (solution) or ≥2 yr (ointment):** *Bacterial conjunctivitis:* Solution: 1–2 drops of 0.3% solution every 2 hr while awake for 2 days, then every 4 hr while awake for 5 more days; Ointment: ½-inch strip 3 times daily for 2 days, then twice daily for 5 more days; *Corneal ulcers:* Solution: 2 drops of 0.3% solution every 15 min for 6 hr, then every 30 min while awake for rest of day, then every hr while awake for next 24 hr, then every 4 hr while awake for next 12 days or longer if re-epithelialization does not occur.	• May cause harmless white crystalline precipitate that resolves over time • ADRs: altered taste, systemic allergic reactions, photophobia, discomfort
erythromycin	**Adults and children:** *Treatment of infections:* ½-inch ointment strip 2–6 times daily. **Infants:** *Prophylaxis of ophthalmia neonatorum:* ½-inch ointment strip in each eye as a single dose.	• ADRs: irritation
gatifloxacin (Zymaxid)	**Adults and children ≥1 yr:** 1 drop of 0.5% solution every 2 hr while awake (up to 8 times/day) for 1 day, then 2–4 times daily while awake for 6 more days.	• ADRs: irritation, headache, ↓ visual acuity, taste disturbance
gentamicin	**Adults and children:** *Solution:* 1–2 drops of 0.3% solution every 2–4 hr.	• ADRs: irritation, burning, stinging

DRUG NAME	DOSE	NOTES
levofloxacin	**Adults and children ≥6 yr:** *Bacterial conjunctivitis:* 1–2 drops of 0.5% solution every 2 hr while awake for 2 days (up to 8 times/day); then every 4 hr while awake for 5 more days (up to 4 times/day). *Corneal ulcers:* 1–2 drops of 1.5% solution every 30 min—2 hr while awake and 4–6 hr after going to bed for 3 days; then every 1–4 hr while awake until completion of therapy.	• ADRs: altered taste, systemic allergic reactions, photophobia
moxifloxacin (Vigamox)	**Adults and children:** 1 drop of 0.5% solution 3 times daily for 7 days.	• ADRs: irritation, ↓ visual acuity
ofloxacin (Ocuflox)	**Adults and children ≥1 yr:** *Bacterial conjunctivitis:* 1–2 drops of 0.3% solution every 2–4 hr while awake for 2 days, then 4 times daily for 5 more days; *Corneal ulcer:* 1–2 drops of 0.3% solution every 30 min while awake and every 4–6 hr while sleeping for 2 days, then every hr while awake for 4–6 more days, then 4 times daily until cured.	• ADRs: altered taste, systemic allergic reactions, photophobia
sulfacetamide	**Adults and children ≥2 mo:** *Solution:* 1–2 drops of 10% solution every 2–3 hr while awake (less frequently at night) for 7–10 days; *Ointment:* ½-inch strip every 3–4 hr and at bedtime for 7–10 days.	• Cross-sensitivity with other sulfonamides (including thiazides) may occur • ADRs: local irritation
tobramycin (Tobrex)	**Adults and children ≥2 mo:** *Solution:* 1–2 drops of 0.3% solution every 2–4 hr depending on severity of infection; *Ointment:* ½-inch strip every 8–12 hr.	• Ointment may impair corneal wound healing • ADRs: irritation, burning, stinging, blurred vision (ointment)

Anticholinergics

Uses: Preparation for cycloplegic refraction; induction of mydriasis; uveitis.

CAUTIONS: Use cautiously in patients with a history of glaucoma; systemic absorption may cause anticholinergic effects such as confusion, unusual behavior, flushing, hallucinations, slurred speech, drowsiness, swollen stomach (infants), tachycardia, or dry mouth.

atropine (Isopto Atropine)	**Adults and children ≥3 mo:** *Cycloplegia/mydriasis:* Solution: 1–2 drops of 1% solution 40 min before procedure; Ointment: 0.3–0.5 cm strip 1–2 times daily.	• Effects on accommodation may last 6 days; mydriasis may last 12 days • ADRs: irritation, blurred vision, photophobia
cyclopentolate (Cyclogyl)	**Adults:** 1–2 drops of 0.5–2% solution; may repeat in 5–10 min. **Children:** 1 drop of 0.5–2% solution; may be followed 5–10 min later by 1 drop of 0.5–1% solution.	• Peak of cycloplegia is within 25–75 min and lasts 6–24 hr • Peak of mydriasis is within 30–60 min and may last several days • 2% solution used for heavily pigmented iris • ADRs: irritation, blurred vision, photophobia

DRUG NAME	DOSE	NOTES
homatropine	**Adults and children ≥3 mo:** *Cycloplegic refraction:* 1–2 drops of 5% solution; may repeat in 5–10 min for 2 more doses; *Uveitis:* 1–2 drops of 5% solution 2–3 times daily (up to every 4 hr).	• Cycloplegia and mydriasis may last for 24–72 hr • ADRs: irritation, blurred vision, photophobia
tropicamide (Mydriacyl)	**Adults and children:** 1–2 drops of 0.5–1% solution (single dose).	• Stronger solution/repeated dosing may be required in patients with dark irises • Peak effect occurs in 20–40 min • Cycloplegia lasts 2–6 hr; mydriasis lasts up to 7 hr • ADRs: irritation, blurred vision, photophobia

Antifungal
Uses: Fungal blepharitis, conjunctivitis, and keratitis.
CAUTIONS: Small amounts may be absorbed and result in hypersensitivity reactions.

natamycin (Natacyn)	**Adults:** *Fungal keratitis:* 1 drop of 5% suspension every 1–2 hr for 3–4 days, then 6–8 times/day for 2–3 wk; *Fungal blepharitis or conjunctivitis:* 1 drop of 5% suspension every 4–6 hr for 2–3 wk.	• ADRs: irritation, swelling

Antihistamines
Uses: Various forms of allergic conjunctivitis.

alcaftadine (Lastacaft [OTC])	**Adults and children ≥2 yr:** 1 drop of 0.25% solution once daily.	• ADRs: transient burning/stinging, headache
azelastine	**Adults and children ≥3 yr:** 1 drop of 0.05% solution twice daily.	• ADRs: transient burning/stinging, headache, bitter taste
bepotastine (Bepreve)	**Adults and children ≥2 yr:** 1 drop of 1.5% solution twice daily.	• ADRs: taste disturbance, headache, local irritation
cetirizine (Zerviate)	**Adults and children ≥2 yr:** 1 drop of 0.24% solution twice daily (given 8 hr apart).	• ADRs: transient burning/stinging, ↓ visual acuity
epinastine	**Adults and children ≥2 yr:** 1 drop of 0.05% solution twice daily.	• ADRs: headache, local irritation
ketotifen (Alaway [OTC], Zaditor)	**Adults and children ≥3 yr:** 1 drop of 0.025% solution twice daily (given 8–12 hr apart).	• ADRs: local irritation
olopatadine (Pataday [OTC])	**Adults and children ≥2 yr:** *0.1% solution:* 1 drop twice daily (given 6–8 hr apart); *0.2% solution:* 1 drop once daily; *0.7% solution:* 1 drop once daily.	• ADRs: headache, conjunctival irritation

Antiparasitic
Uses: Demodex blepharitis.

lotilaner (Xdemvy)	**Adults:** 1 drop of 0.25% solution every 12 hr for 6 wk.	• ADRs: burning, stinging

DRUG NAME	DOSE	NOTES
Antivirals		
Uses: Herpetic conjunctivitis and keratitis. **CAUTIONS:** Small amounts may be absorbed and result in hypersensitivity reactions.		
ganciclovir (Zirgan)	**Adults and children ≥2 yr:** 1 drop of 0.15% gel 5 times daily (every 3 hr while awake) until corneal ulcer heals, then 3 times daily for 7 days.	• ADRs: blurred vision, irritation, keratopathy
trifluridine	**Adults and children ≥6 yr:** 1 drop of 1% solution every 2 hr while awake (up to 9 drops/day) until re-epithelialization occurs, then every 4 hr while awake for 7 more days (not to exceed 21 days).	• ADRs: burning, stinging, keratopathy
Artificial Tears/Ocular Lubricants (sterile buffered isotonic solutions/ointments)		
Uses: Artificial tears: Keep the eyes moist with isotonic solutions and wetting agents in the management of dry eyes due to lack of tears; also provide lubrication for artificial eyes. Ocular lubricants: Provide lubrication and protection in a variety of conditions including exposure keratitis, ↓ corneal sensitivity, corneal erosions, keratitis sicca, during/following ocular surgery or removal of a foreign body.		
Artificial tears (Bion Tears, Genteal Tears, HypoTears, LiquiTears, Murine Tears, Nature's Tears, Soothe, Systane, 🍁 Teardrops, Tears Naturale, Viva-Drops)	**Adults and children:** *Artificial tears:* Solution: 1–2 drops 3–4 times daily; Insert: 1 insert 1–2 times daily; *Ocular lubricants:* small amount instilled into conjunctiva several times daily.	• May alter effects of other concurrently administered ophthalmic medications • ADRs: photophobia, lid edema stinging (insert only), transient blurred vision, eye discomfort
Beta Blockers		
Uses: Open-angle glaucoma and other forms of ocular hypertension (↓ formation of aqueous humor). **CAUTIONS:** Systemic absorption is minimal but may occur. Systemic absorption may result in additive adverse cardiovascular effects (bradycardia, hypotension), especially when used with other cardiovascular agents (antihypertensives, antiarrhythmics). Other systemic adverse reactions may occur, including bronchospasm or delirium (older adults). Concurrent use with ophthalmic epinephrine may ↓ effectiveness.		
betaxolol (Betoptic S)	**Adults and children:** 1 drop of 0.25% suspension or solution twice daily.	• ADRs: conjunctivitis, ↓ visual acuity, ocular burning, rash (may be less likely than others to cause bronchospasm if systemically absorbed)
carteolol	**Adults:** 1 drop of 1% solution twice daily.	• ADRs: ocular burning, ↓ visual acuity
levobunolol	**Adults:** 1–2 drops of 0.5% solution once daily.	• ADRs: conjunctivitis, ↓ visual acuity, ocular burning, rash
timolol (Betimol, Istalol, Timoptic, Timoptic Ocudose, Timoptic-XE)	**Adults:** *Solution:* 1 drop of 0.25–0.5% solution 1–2 times daily; *Gel-forming solution:* 1 drop of 0.25–0.5% solution once daily. **Children:** *Solution:* 1 drop of 0.25–0.5% solution twice daily; *Gel-forming solution:* 1 drop of 0.25–0.5% solution once daily.	• ADRs: conjunctivitis, ↓ visual acuity, ocular burning, rash
Carbonic Anhydrase Inhibitors		
Uses: Open-angle glaucoma and other forms of ocular hypertension (↓ formation of aqueous humor). **CAUTIONS:** May exacerbate kidney stones; should not be used in patients with CCr <30 mL/min; may have cross-sensitivity with sulfonamides.		
brinzolamide (Azopt)	**Adults:** 1 drop of 1% suspension 3 times daily.	• ADRs: burning, stinging, unusual taste
dorzolamide	**Adults and children:** 1 drop of 2% solution 3 times daily.	• ADRs: bitter taste, ocular irritation, or allergy

DRUG NAME	DOSE	NOTES

Cholinergics (direct-acting)

Uses: Open-angle glaucoma (facilitates the outflow of aqueous humor); also used to facilitate miosis after ophthalmic surgery or before examination (to counteract mydriatics). Pilocarpine (Vuity) used for presbyopia.
CAUTIONS: Conditions in which pupillary constriction occurs should be avoided. If significant systemic absorption occurs, bronchospasm, sweating, and ↑ urination and salivation may occur.

acetylcholine (Miochol-E)	**Adults:** 0.5–2 mL instilled into anterior chamber before or after securing one or more sutures.	● ADRs: corneal edema, corneal clouding
carbachol (Miostat)	**Adults:** 0.5 mL instilled into anterior chamber before or after securing sutures.	● ADRs: blurred vision, altered vision, stinging, eye pain
pilocarpine (Qlosi, Vuity)	**Adults:** *Presbyopia:* Vuity: 1 drop of 1.25% solution once daily. An additional drop (in each eye) may be administered 3–6 hr after 1st dose; Qlosi: 1 drop of 0.4% solution once daily, or as needed, up to twice daily. An additional drop (in each eye) may be administered 2–3 hr after 1st dose. **Adults and children ≥2 yr:** *Glaucoma:* 1 drop of 1–4% solution up to 4 times daily; *Counteracting mydriatic sympathomimetics:* 1 drop of 1–4% solution (may be repeated prior to surgery). **Children <2 yr:** *Glaucoma:* 1 drop of 1% solution 3 times daily.	● ADRs: blurred vision, altered vision, stinging, eye pain, headache

Cholinergic (cholinesterase inhibitor)

Uses: Open-angle glaucoma not controlled with short-acting miotics or other agents; also used in varying doses for accommodative esotropia (diagnosis and treatment).
CAUTIONS: Enhances neuromuscular blockade from succinylcholine; intensifies the actions of cocaine and some other local anesthetics; additive toxicity with antimyasthenics, anticholinergics, and cholinesterase inhibitors (including some pesticides). Use cautiously in patients with history or risk of retinal detachment.

echothiophate (Phospholine Iodide)	**Adults:** 1 drop of 0.125% solution 1–2 times daily.	● Irreversible cholinesterase inhibitor ● May cause hyperactivity in patients with Down syndrome ● ADRs: blurred vision, change in vision, brow ache, miosis, eyelid twitching, watering eyes

Corticosteroids

Uses: Inflammatory eye conditions including allergic conjunctivitis, nonspecific superficial keratitis, anterior endogenous uveitis; infectious conjunctivitis (with anti-infectives); corneal injury; suppression of graft rejection following keratoplasty; postoperative inflammation; dry eye disease; macular edema.
CAUTIONS: Use cautiously in patients with infectious ocular processes (avoid in herpes simplex keratitis), especially fungal and viral ocular infections (may mask symptoms); diabetes, glaucoma, or epithelial compromise.

dexamethasone (Dextenza, Dexycu, Maxidex, Ozurdex)	**Adults and children:** *Solution:* 1–2 drops of 0.1% solution every hr during the day and every 2 hr during the night; gradually ↓ the dose to 1 drop every 4 hr, then to 3–4 times daily; *Suspension:* 1–2 drops of 0.1% suspension up to 4–6 times daily; *Implant:* one 0.7-mg implant injected into affected eye; *Insert:* one 0.4-mg insert (releases 0.4 mg dose for up to 30 days); *Suspension for injection:* 0.005 mL of 9% suspension injected into posterior chamber at end of ocular surgery.	● As condition improves, ↓ frequency of administration of ophthalmic solution/suspension ● ADRs: corneal thinning, ↑ intraocular pressure, irritation

DRUG NAME	DOSE	NOTES
difluprednate (Durezol)	**Adults and children:** *Postoperative inflammation:* 1 drop of 0.05% emulsion 4 times daily beginning 24 hr after surgery and continued for 2 wk, then 2 times daily for 1 wk; then taper; *Uveitis:* 1 drop of 0.05% emulsion 4 times daily for 14 days; then taper.	• As condition improves, ↓ frequency of administration • ADRs: blepharitis, photophobia, ↓ visual acuity
fluorometholone (Flarex, FML, FML Forte)	**Adults and children ≥2 yr:** *Suspension:* 1–2 drops of 0.1% suspension 4 times daily (up to 2 drops every 2 hr during initial 24–48 hr) or 1 drop of 0.25% suspension 2–4 times daily (up to 1 drop every 4 hr during initial 24–48 hr).	• As condition improves, ↓ frequency of administration • ADRs: corneal thinning, ↑ intraocular pressure, irritation
loteprednol (Alrex, Eysuvis, Inveltys, Lotemax, Lotemax SM)	**Adults:** *Allergic conjunctivitis:* Alrex: 1 drop of 0.2% suspension 4 times daily; *Dry eye disease:* Eysuvis: 1–2 drops of 0.25% suspension 4 times daily for up to 2 wk; *Inflammatory conditions:* Lotemax: 1–2 drops of 0.5% suspension 4 times daily (up to 1 drop every hr may be used in first wk); *Postoperative inflammation/pain:* Lotemax gel/suspension: 1–2 drops of 0.5% gel/suspension 4 times daily beginning 24 hr after surgery and continued for 2 wk or 1 drop of 0.38% gel 3 times daily beginning 24 hr after surgery and continued for 2 wk; Lotemax ointment: ½-inch strip 4 times daily beginning 24 hr after surgery and continued for 2 wk; Inveltys: 1–2 drops of 1% suspension 2 times daily beginning 24 hr after surgery and continued for 2 wk. **Children:** *Postoperative inflammation/pain:* Lotemax gel: 1–2 drops of 0.5% gel 4 times daily beginning 24 hr after surgery and continued for 2 wk.	• ADRs: corneal thinning, ↑ intraocular pressure, irritation
prednisolone (Pred Forte, Pred Mild)	**Adults and children:** 1–2 drops of 0.12–1% solution/suspension 2–4 times daily.	• As condition improves, ↓ frequency of administration • ADRs: corneal thinning, ↑ intraocular pressure, irritation

DRUG NAME	DOSE	NOTES
Immunomodulators		
Uses: Keratoconjunctivitis sicca and vernal keratoconjunctivitis. **CAUTIONS:** Tear production is not ↑ during concurrent use of ophthalmic NSAIDs or punctal plugs.		
cyclosporine (Cequa, Restasis, Verkazia, Vevye)	**Adults and children ≥16 yr:** *Keratoconjunctivitis sicca:* Restasis: 1 drop of 0.05% emulsion every 12 hr. **Adults:** *Keratoconjunctivitis sicca:* Cequa: 1 drop of 0.09% solution every 12 hr; Vevye: 1 drop of 0.1% solution every 12 hr. **Adults and children ≥4 yr:** *Vernal keratoconjunctivitis:* Verkazia: 1 drop of 0.1% emulsion 4 times daily until signs/symptoms resolve.	• Emulsion should be inverted to obtain uniform opaque appearance prior to use. • ADRs: irritation, blurred vision, conjunctival hyperemia
lifitegrast (Xiidra)	**Adults:** 1 drop of 5% solution every 12 hr.	• Emulsion should be inverted to obtain uniform opaque appearance prior to use. • ADRs: headache, irritation, blurred vision, metallic taste
Mast Cell Stabilizers		
Uses: Vernal keratoconjunctivitis and allergic conjunctivitis. **CAUTIONS:** Require several days of treatment before effects are seen.		
cromolyn	**Adults and children ≥4 yr:** 1–2 drops of 4% solution 4–6 times daily.	• ADRs: irritation
nedocromil (Alocril)	**Adults and children ≥3 yr:** 1–2 drops of 2% solution twice daily throughout period of exposure to allergen.	• ADRs: headache, ocular burning, unpleasant taste, nasal congestion
Nonsteroidal Anti-inflammatory Drugs		
Uses: Pain/inflammation following surgery (bromfenac, diclofenac, ketorolac, nepafenac); allergic conjunctivitis (ketorolac); inhibition of perioperative miosis (flurbiprofen). **CAUTIONS:** Cross-sensitivity with systemic NSAIDs may occur; concurrent use of anticoagulants, other NSAIDs, thrombolytics, some cephalosporins, and valproates may ↑ the risk of bleeding. May slow/delay healing. Avoid contact lens use.		
bromfenac (Bromsite, Prolensa)	**Adults:** *Generic:* 1 drop of 0.09% solution once daily starting 1 day before surgery and continued on day of surgery and for 2 wk after surgery; *Bromsite:* 1 drop of 0.075% solution twice daily starting 1 day before surgery and continued on day of surgery and for 2 wk after surgery; *Prolensa:* 1 drop of 0.07% solution once daily starting 1 day before surgery and continued on day of surgery and for 2 wk after surgery.	• Contains sulfites • ADRs: irritation, headache
diclofenac	**Adults:** *Cataract surgery:* 1 drop of 0.1% solution 4 times daily starting 24 hr after surgery and for 2 wk after surgery; *Corneal refractive surgery:* 1–2 drops of 0.1% solution within hour before surgery and within 15 min after surgery; then continue 4 times daily for up to 3 days.	• ADRs: irritation, allergic reactions

DRUG NAME	DOSE	NOTES
flurbiprofen	**Adults:** 1 drop of 0.03% solution every 30 min, beginning 2 hr prior to surgery (4 drops total in each eye).	● ADRs: irritation, allergic reactions
ketorolac (Acular, Acular LS, Acuvail)	**Adults and children ≥2 yr:** *Allergic conjunctivitis:* Acular: 1 drop of 0.5% solution 4 times daily; *Postoperative pain/inflammation:* Acular: 1 drop of 0.5% solution 4 times daily starting 24 hr after cataract surgery and for 2 wk after surgery; Acular LS: 1 drop of 0.4% solution 4 times daily for up to 4 days after corneal refractive surgery; Acuvail: 1 drop of 0.45% solution twice daily starting 1 day before cataract surgery and continued for 2 wk after surgery.	● ADRs: irritation, allergic reactions
nepafenac (Ilevro, Nevanac)	**Adults and children ≥10 yr:** *Ilevro:* 1 drop of 0.3% suspension once daily starting one day before cataract surgery and continued for 2 wk after surgery; instill 1 additional drop 30–120 min before surgery; *Nevanac:* 1 drop of 0.1% suspension 3 times daily starting one day before cataract surgery and continued for 2 wk after surgery.	● ADRs: irritation, photophobia, headache, hypertension, nausea/vomiting

Ocular Decongestants/Vasoconstrictors

Uses: ↓ ocular congestion due to irritation by vasoconstricting conjunctival blood vessels; stronger solutions have mydriatic effects. Oxymetazoline (Upneeq) used for acquired blepharoptosis.

CAUTIONS: Systemic absorption may result in adverse cardiovascular effects; excessive/prolonged use may produce rebound hyperemia; use caution in patients at risk for acute angle-closure glaucoma; cardiovascular effects may be exaggerated by MAO inhibitors and dose adjustment may be required within 21 days of MAO inhibitors; ↑ risk of arrhythmias with inhalation anesthetics.

naphazoline	**Adults:** 1–2 drops of 0.012% solution up to 4 times daily (for up to 3 days) or 1–2 drops of 0.1% solution every 3–4 hr as needed.	● ADRs: *ophthalmic:* rebound hyperemia; *systemic:* dizziness, headache, nausea, sweating, weakness
oxymetazoline (Upneeq)	**Adults:** 1 drop of 0.1% solution once daily.	● ADRs: *ophthalmic:* rebound hyperemia; *systemic:* headache, insomnia, nervousness, tachycardia
phenylephrine	**Adults and children:** *Mydriasis:* 1 drop of 2.5–10% solution; may repeat in 3–5 min as needed (max = 3 drops/eye).	● ADRs: *ophthalmic:* blurred vision, irritation; *systemic:* dizziness, tachycardia, hypertension, paleness, sweating, trembling
tetrahydrozoline (Visine [OTC])	**Adults:** 1–2 drops of 0.05% solution 2–4 times daily.	● ADRs: *ophthalmic:* irritation; *systemic:* tachycardia, hypertension

Prostaglandin Agonists

Uses: Open-angle glaucoma (↑ outflow of aqueous humor).

CAUTIONS: May change eye color to brown; will form precipitate with thimerosal-containing products; can be used with other agents to ↓ intraocular pressure.

bimatoprost (Durysta, Lumigan)	**Adults and children ≥16 yr:** 1 drop of 0.01–0.03% solution once daily in the evening. **Adults:** One implant in anterior chamber of affected eye.	● ADRs: local irritation, foreign body sensation, ↑ eyelash growth, ↑ brown pigmentation in iris

DRUG NAME	DOSE	NOTES
latanoprost (Iyuzeh, Xalatan, Xelpros)	**Adults:** 1 drop of 0.005% solution/ emulsion once daily in the evening.	• ADRs: local irritation, foreign body sensation, ↑ eyelash growth, ↑ brown pigmentation in iris
latanoprostene (Vyzulta)	**Adults and children >16 yr:** 1 drop of 0.024% solution once daily in the evening.	• ADRs: conjunctival hyperemia, local irritation, eye pain, ↑ eyelash growth, ↑ brown pigmentation in iris
omidenepag isopropyl (Omlonti)	**Adults:** 1 drop of 0.002% solution once daily in the evening.	• ADRs: conjunctival hyperemia, photophobia, blurred vision, dry eye, eye pain, headache, ↑ eyelash growth, ↑ brown pigmentation in iris
tafluprost (Zioptan)	**Adults:** 1 drop of 0.0015% solution once daily in the evening.	• ADRs: local irritation, foreign body sensation, ↑ eyelash growth, ↑ brown pigmentation in iris
travoprost (iDose TR, Travatan Z)	**Adults and children ≥16 yr:** *Solution:* 1 drop of 0.004% solution once daily in the evening. *Implant:* one 75 mcg implant injected into affected eye.	• ADRs: local irritation, foreign body sensation, ↑ eyelash growth, ↑ brown pigmentation in iris

Rho Kinase Inhibitor

Uses: Open-angle glaucoma or ocular hypertension (↑ outflow of aqueous humor).
CAUTIONS: Can be used with other agents to ↓ intraocular pressure.

netarsudil (Rhopressa)	**Adults:** 1 drop of 0.02% solution once daily in the evening.	• ADRs: conjunctival hyperemia, corneal verticillata, conjunctival hemorrhage eye pain, epithelial corneal edema, bacterial keratitis

Semifluorinated Alkane

Uses: Dry eye disease.

perfluorohexyloctane (Miebo)	**Adults:** 1 drop of 100% solution 4 times daily.	• ADRs: blurred vision

Transient Receptor Potential Melastatin 8 Agonist

Uses: Dry eye disease.

acoltremon (Tryptyr)	**Adults:** 1 drop of 0.003% solution twice daily.	• ADRs: eye pain

APPENDIX C

Medication Administration Techniques

Subcutaneous Injection Sites

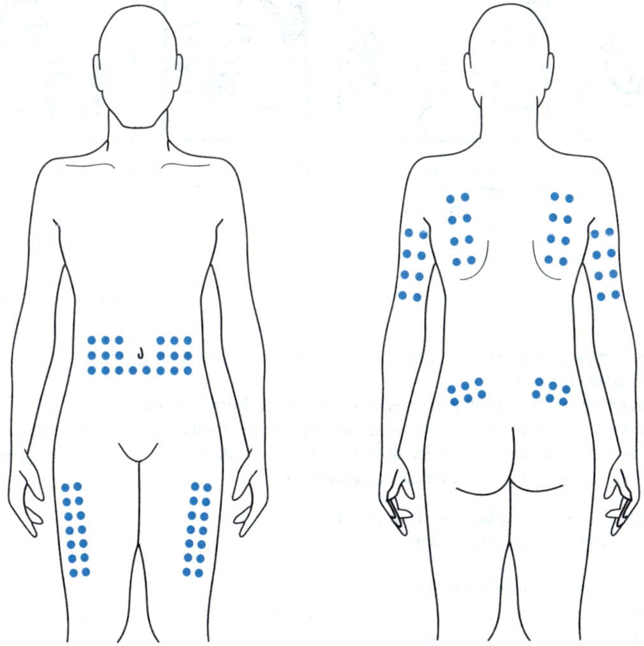

Administration of Ophthalmic Medications

For instillation of ophthalmic solutions, instruct patient to lie down or tilt head back and look at ceiling. Pull down on lower lid, creating a small pocket, and instill solution into pocket. With systemically acting drugs, apply pressure to the inner canthus for 1–2 min to minimize systemic absorption. Instruct patient to gently close eye. Wait 5 min before instilling 2nd drop or any other ophthalmic solutions.

For instillation of ophthalmic ointment, instruct patient to hold tube in hand for several minutes to warm. Squeeze a small amount of ointment (¼–½ in.) inside lower lid. Instruct patient to close eye gently and roll eyeball around in all directions with eye closed. Wait 10 min before instilling any other ophthalmic ointments.

Do not touch cap or tip of container to eye, fingers, or any surface.

Administration of Medications with Metered-Dose Inhalers

Instruct patient on the proper use of the metered-dose inhaler. There are 3 methods of using a metered-dose inhaler. Shake inhaler well. (1) Take a drink of water to moisten the throat; place the inhaler mouthpiece 2 finger-widths away from mouth; tilt head back slightly. While activating the inhaler, take a slow, deep breath for 3–5 sec; hold the breath for 10 sec; and breathe out slowly. (2) Exhale and close lips firmly around mouthpiece. Administer during second half of inhalation, and hold breath for as long as possible to ensure deep instillation of medication. (3) Use of spacer. Consult health care professional to determine method desired prior to instruction. Allow 1–2 min between inhalations. Rinse mouth with water or mouthwash after each use to minimize dry mouth and hoarseness. Wash inhalation assembly at least daily in warm running water.

For use of dry powder inhalers, turn head away from inhaler and exhale (do not blow into inhaler). Do not shake. Close mouth tightly around the mouthpiece of the inhaler and inhale rapidly.

Steps for Using Your Inhaler

1. Remove the cap and hold inhaler upright.
2. Shake the inhaler.
3. Tilt your head back slightly and breathe out slowly.
4. Position the inhaler in one of the following ways (A or B is optimal, but C is acceptable for those who have difficulty with A or B. C is required for breath-activated inhalers):

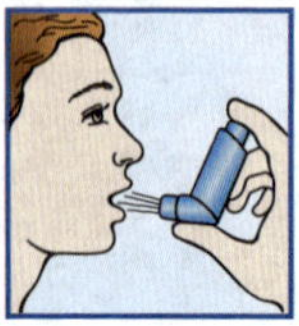

A. Open mouth with inhaler 1 to 2 inches away.

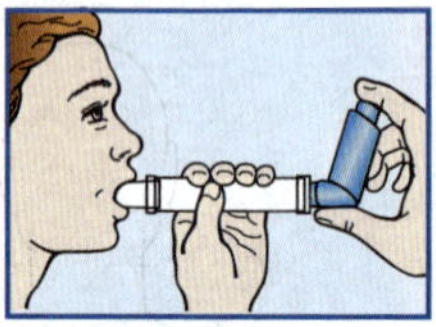

B. Use space/holding chamber (this is recommended especially for young children and for people using corticosteroids).

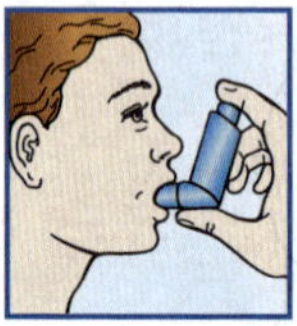

C. In the mouth. Do not use for corticosteroids.

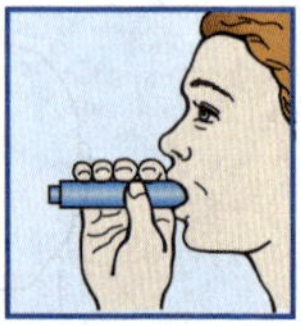

D. NOTE: Inhaled dry powder capsules require a different inhalation technique. To use a dry powder inhaler, it is important to close the mouth tightly around the mouthpiece of the inhaler and to inhale rapidly.

5. Press down on the inhaler to release medication as you start to breathe in slowly.
6. Breathe in slowly (3–5 sec).
7. Hold your breath for 10 sec to allow the medicine to reach deeply into your lungs.
8. Repeat puff as directed. Waiting 1 min between puffs may permit second puff to penetrate your lungs better.
9. Spacers/holding chambers are useful for all patients. They are particularly recommended for young children and older adults and for use with **inhaled corticosteroids**.

Avoid common inhaler mistakes. Follow these inhaler tips:

- Breathe out before pressing your inhaler.
- Inhale slowly.
- Breathe in through your mouth, not your nose.
- Press down on your inhaler at the start of inhalation (or within the first sec of inhalation).
- Keep inhaling as you press down on inhaler.
- Press your inhaler only once while you are inhaling (one breath for each puff).
- Make sure you breathe in evenly and deeply.
- If you are using a short-acting bronchodilator inhaler and a corticosteroid inhaler, use the bronchodilator 1st, and allow 5 min to elapse before using the corticosteroid.

Other inhalers have become available in addition to the one illustrated here. Different types of inhalers may require different techniques.

Administration of Medications by Nebulizer

Administer in a location where patient can sit comfortably for 10–15 min. Plug in compressor. Mix medication as directed, or empty unit-dose vials into nebulizer. Do not mix different types of medications without checking with health care professional. Assemble mask or mouthpiece and connect tubing to port on compressor. Have patient sit in a comfortable upright position. Make sure that mask fits properly over nose and mouth and that mist does not flow into eyes, or put mouthpiece into mouth. Turn on compressor. Instruct patient to take slow deep breaths. If possible, patient should hold breath for 10 sec before slowly exhaling. Continue this process until medication chamber is empty. Wash mask in hot soapy water; rinse well and allow to air dry before next use.

Administration of Nasal Sprays

Clear nasal passages of secretions prior to use. If nasal passages are blocked, use a decongestant immediately prior to use to ensure adequate penetration of the spray. Keep head upright. Breathe in through nose during administration. Sniff hard for a few minutes after administration.

Intramuscular Injection Sites

Deltoid site

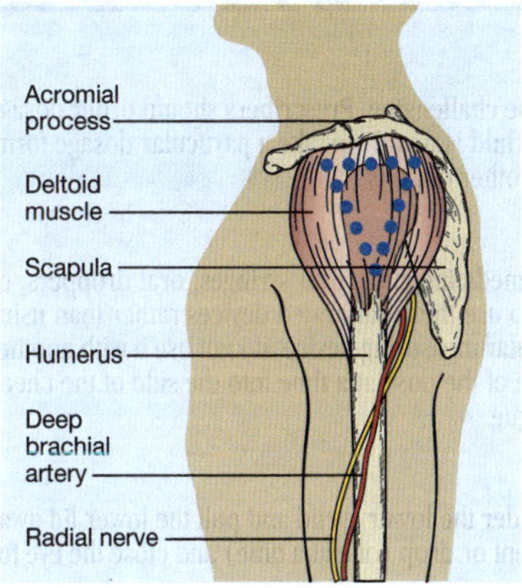

Ventrogluteal site

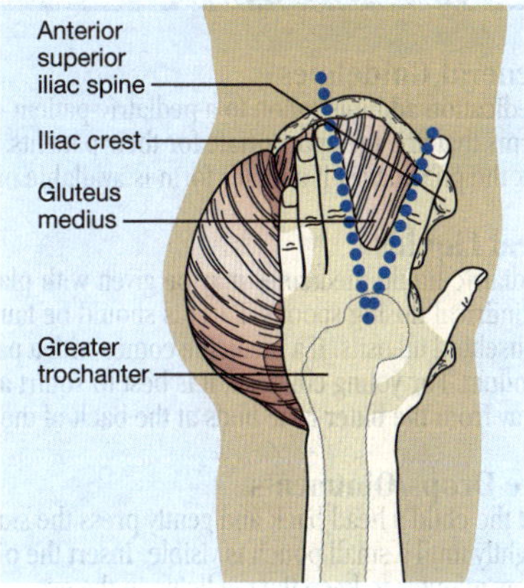

Vastus lateralis site

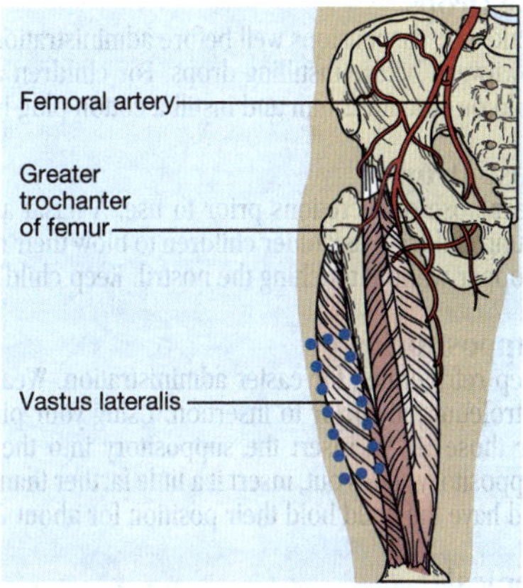

The deltoid and ventrogluteal sites are the preferred sites for adults; the vastus lateralis site is preferred in children under 2 yr of age.

APPENDIX D

Administering Medications to Children

General Guidelines

Medication administration to a pediatric patient can be challenging. Prescribers should order dosage forms that are age appropriate for their patients. If a child is unable to take a particular dosage form, ask the pharmacist if another form is available or for other options.

Oral Liquids

Pediatric liquid medicines may be given with plastic medicine cups, oral syringes, oral droppers, or cylindrical dosing spoons. Parents should be taught to use these calibrated devices rather than using household utensils. If a medicine comes with a particular measuring device, do not use it with another product. For young children, it is best to squirt a little of the dose at a time into the side of the cheek away from the bitter taste buds at the back of the tongue.

Eye Drops/Ointments

Tilt the child's head back and gently press the skin under the lower eyelid and pull the lower lid away slightly until a small pouch is visible. Insert the ointment or drop (one at a time) and close the eye for a few minutes to keep the medicine in the eye.

Ear Drops

Shake otic suspensions well before administration. For children <3 yr, pull the outer ear outward and downward before instilling drops. For children ≥3 yr, pull the outer ear outward and upward. Keep child on side for 2 min and instill a cotton plug into ear.

Nose Drops

Clear nose of secretions prior to use. A nasal aspirator (bulb syringe) may be used in infants and young children. Ask older children to blow their nose. Tilt child's head back over a pillow and squeeze dropper without touching the nostril. Keep child's head back for 2 min.

Suppositories

Keep refrigerated for easier administration. Wearing gloves, moisten the rounded end with water or petroleum jelly prior to insertion. Using your pinky finger for children <3 yr and your index finger for those ≥3 yr, insert the suppository into the rectum about 1 inch beyond the sphincter. If the suppository slides out, insert it a little farther than before. Hold the buttocks together for a few minutes and have the child hold their position for about 20 min, if possible.

Topicals

Clean affected area and dry well prior to application. Apply a thin layer to the skin and rub in gently. Do not apply coverings over the area unless instructed to do so by the prescriber.

Metered-Dose Inhalers

Generally the same principles apply in children as in adults, except the use of spacers is recommended for young children (see Appendix C).

APPENDIX E

Formulas Helpful for Calculating Doses

Ratio and Proportion

A ratio is the same as a fraction and can be expressed as a fraction (½) or in the algebraic form (1:2). This relationship is stated as *one is to two*.

A proportion is an equation of equal fractions or ratios.

$$\frac{1}{2}=\frac{4}{8}$$

To calculate doses, begin each proportion with the two known values, for example 15 grains = 1 gram (known equivalent) or 10 milligrams = 2 milliliters (dose available) on one side of the equation. Next, make certain that the units of measure on the opposite side of the equation are the same as the units of the known values and are placed on the same level of the equation.

Problem A: $$\frac{15\text{ gr}}{1\text{ g}}=\frac{10\text{ gr}}{x\text{ g}}$$

Problem B: $$\frac{10\text{ mg}}{2\text{ mL}}=\frac{5\text{ mg}}{x\text{ mL}}$$

Once the proportion is set up correctly, cross-multiply the opposing values of the proportion.

Problem A: $$\frac{15\text{ gr}}{1\text{ g}}\times\frac{10\text{ gr}}{x\text{ g}}$$

$$15x=10$$

Problem B: $$\frac{10\text{ mg}}{2\text{ mL}}\times\frac{5\text{ mg}}{x\text{ mL}}$$

$$10x=10$$

Next, divide each side of the equation by the number with the x to determine the answer. Then, add the unit of measure corresponding to x in the original equation.

Problem A: $$\frac{15x}{15}=\frac{10}{15}$$

$$x=\frac{2}{3}\text{ or } 0.6\text{ g}$$

Problem B: $$\frac{10x}{10}=\frac{10}{10}$$

$$x=1\text{ mL}$$

Calculation of IV Drip Rate

To calculate the drip rate for an intravenous infusion, 3 values are needed:

I. The amount of solution and corresponding time for infusion. May be ordered as:

1000 mL over 8 hr

or

125 mL/hr

II. The equivalent in time to convert hr to min.

1 hr = 60 min

III. The drop factor or number of drops that equal 1 mL of fluid. (This information can be found on the IV tubing box.)

10 gtt = 1 mL

Set up the problem by placing each of the 3 values in a proportion.

$$\frac{125\text{ mL}}{1\text{ hr}} \times \frac{1\text{ hr}}{60\text{ min}} \times \frac{10\text{ gtt}}{1\text{ mL}}$$

Units of measure can be canceled out from the upper and lower levels of the equation. The units cancel, leaving:

$$\frac{125}{1} \times \frac{1}{60\text{ min}} \times \frac{10\text{ gtt}}{1}$$

Next, multiply each level across and divide the numerator by the denominator for the answer.

$$\frac{125}{1} \times \frac{1}{6\text{ min}} \times \frac{1\text{ gtt}}{1}$$

125/6 = 20.8 or 21 gtt/min

Calculation of Creatinine Clearance (CCr) in Adults from Serum Creatinine

$$\text{Men: CCr} = \frac{\text{ideal body weight (kg)} \times (140 - \text{age})}{72 \times \text{serum creatinine (mg/dL)}}$$

Women: CCr = 0.85 × calculation for men

Calculation of Body Surface Area (BSA) in Adults and Children

Dubois method:

$$\text{SA (cm}^2) = \text{wt (kg)}^{0.425} \times 71.84$$

$$\text{SA (m}^2) = \text{K} \times \sqrt[3]{\text{wt}^2\text{ (kg)}}$$ (common K value 0.1 for toddlers, 0.103 for neonates)

Simplified method:

$$\text{BSA (m}^2) = \sqrt{\frac{\text{ht (cm)} \times \text{wt (kg)}}{3600}}$$

Body Mass Index

$$\text{BMI} = \text{wt (kg)/ht (m}^2)$$

APPENDIX F

Pediatric Dosage Calculations

Most drugs in children are dosed according to body weight (mg/kg) or body surface area (BSA) (mg/m^2). Care must be taken to properly convert body weight from pounds to kilograms (1 kg = 2.2 lb) before calculating doses based on body weight. Doses are often expressed as mg/kg/day or mg/kg/dose; therefore, orders written "mg/kg/d," which is confusing, *require further clarification from the prescriber.*

Chemotherapeutic drugs are commonly dosed according to body surface area, which requires an extra verification step (BSA calculation) prior to dosing. Medications are available in multiple concentrations; therefore, *orders written in "mL" rather than "mg" are not acceptable and require further clarification.*

Dosing also varies by indication; therefore, diagnostic information is helpful when calculating doses. The following examples are typically encountered when dosing medication in children.

Example 1.

Amoxicillin oral suspension will be given to a 1-yr-old child weighing 22 lb for otitis media at a dose of 40 mg/kg/day in 2 divided doses. The suspension is available at a concentration of 400 mg/5 mL. How many milliliters should be administered to the child for each dose?

Step 1. Convert pounds to kg:	22 lb × 1 kg/2.2 lb = 10 kg
Step 2. Calculate the dose in mg:	10 kg × 40 mg/kg/day = 400 mg/day
Step 3. Divide the dose by the frequency:	400 mg/day ÷ 2 = 200 mg/dose
Step 4. Convert the mg dose to mL:	200 mg/dose ÷ 400 mg/5 mL = **2.5 mL**

Example 2.

Ceftriaxone is being prescribed for a 5-yr-old child weighing 18 kg for meningitis at a dose of 100 mg/kg IV once daily. After reconstitution, the concentration of ceftriaxone solution in the vial is 40 mg/mL. How many milliliters of the solution should be administered to this child for each dose?

Step 1. Calculate the dose in mg:	18 kg × 100 mg/kg/day = 1800 mg/day
Step 2. Divide the dose by the frequency:	1800 mg/day ÷ 1 (daily) = 1800 mg/dose
Step 3. Convert the mg dose to mL:	1800 mg/dose ÷ 40 mg/mL = **45 mL**

Example 3.

Vincristine is being administered to a 4-yr-old child (height 97 cm; weight 37 lb) with leukemia at a dose of 2 mg/m^2. Vincristine is available in a vial at a concentration of 1 mg/mL. How many milliliters should be administered to this child for each dose?

Step 1. Convert pounds to kg:	37 lb × 1 kg/2.2 lb = 16.8 kg
Step 2. Calculate BSA:	$\sqrt{16.8 \text{ kg} \times 97 \text{ cm}/3600} = 0.67 \text{ m}^2$
Step 3. Calculate the dose in mg:	2 mg/m^2 × 0.67 m^2 = 1.34 mg
Step 4. Calculate the dose in mL:	1.34 mg ÷ 1 mg/mL = **1.34 mL**

APPENDIX G

Normal Values of Common Laboratory Tests

SERUM TESTS

HEMATOLOGIC	MEN	WOMEN
Hemoglobin	14–17.3 g/dL	11.7–15.5 g/dL
Hematocrit	42–52%	36–48%
Red blood cells (RBC)	4.51–6.01 million/mm³	4.01–5.51 million/mm³
Mean corpuscular volume (MCV)	77–97 (micrometer)³	78–102 (micrometer)³
Mean corpuscular hemoglobin (MCH)	27–35 picogram	27–35 picogram
Mean corpuscular hemoglobin concentration (MCHC)	32–36 g/dL	32–36 g/dL
Erythrocyte sedimentation rate (ESR)	≤20 mm/hr	≤30 mm/hr
Leukocytes (WBC)	4500–11,100/mm³	4500–11,100/mm³
Neutrophils	40–75% (2700–6500/mm³)	40–75% (2700–6500/mm³)
Bands	3–8% (150–700/mm³)	3–8% (150–700/mm³)
Eosinophils	0–5.5% (50–400/mm³)	0–5.5% (50–500/mm³)
Basophils	0–1% (0–100/mm³)	0–1% (0–100/mm³)
Monocytes	4–9% (200–400/mm³)	4–9% (200–400/mm³)
Lymphocytes	14–44% (1500–3700/mm³)	14–44% (1500–3700/mm³)
T lymphocytes	60–80% of lymphocytes	60–80% of lymphocytes
B lymphocytes	10–20% of lymphocytes	10–20% of lymphocytes
Platelets	150,000–450,000/mm³	150,000–450,000/mm³
Prothrombin time (PT)	10–13 sec	10–13 sec
Activated partial thromboplastin time (aPTT)	30–45 sec	30–45 sec

CHEMISTRY	MEN	WOMEN
Sodium	135–145 mEq/L	135–145 mEq/L
Potassium	3.5–5.3 mEq/L	3.5–5.3 mEq/L
Chloride	97–107 mEq/L	97–107 mEq/L
Bicarbonate (HCO3)	19–25 mEq/L	19–25 mEq/L
Total calcium	8.4–10.2 mg/dL or 4.5–5.5 mEq/L	8.4–10.2 mg/dL or 4.5–5.5 mEq/L
Ionized calcium	4.64–5.52 mg/dL or 2.1–2.6 mEq/L	4.64–5.52 mg/dL or 2.1–2.6 mEq/L
Phosphorus/phosphate	2.5–4.5 mg/dL	2.5–4.5 mg/dL
Magnesium	1.6–2.2 mg/dL or 1.5–2.5 mEq/L	1.6–2.2 mg/dL or 1.5–2.5 mEq/L
Glucose	65–99 mg/dL	65–99 mg/dL
Osmolality	275–295 mOsm/kg	275–295 mOsm/kg
Ammonia (NH3)	10–80 mcg/dL	10–80 mcg/dL
Amylase	100–300 U/L	100–300 U/L
Creatine kinase total (CK)	50–204 U/L	36–160 U/L
Creatine kinase isoenzymes, MB fraction	0–4% in MI	0–4% in MI
Lactic dehydrogenase (LDH)	90–156 U/L	90–156 U/L
Protein, total	6–8 g/d	6–8 g/d
Albumin	3.7–5.1 g/dL	3.7–5.1 g/dL

HEPATIC	MEN	WOMEN
AST	20–40 U/L	15–30 U/L
ALT	19–36 IU/mL	24–36 IU/mL
Total bilirubin	0.3–1.2 mg/dL	0.3–1.2 mg/dL
Conjugated bilirubin	0.0–0.3 mg/dL	0.0–0.3 mg/dL
Unconjugated (indirect) bilirubin	0.2–1.1 mg/dL	0.2–1.1 mg/dL
Alkaline phosphatase	35–142 U/L	25–125 U/L

RENAL	MEN	WOMEN
BUN	8–21 mg/dL	8–21 mg/dL
Creatinine	0.61–1.21 mg/dL	0.51–1.11 mg/dL
Uric acid	4.0–8.2 mg/dL	2.5–7.3 mg/dL

ARTERIAL BLOOD GASES	MEN	WOMEN
pH	7.35–7.45	7.35–7.45
Po^2	80–95 mm Hg	80–95 mm Hg
Pco^2	35–45 mm Hg	35–45 mm Hg
O^2 saturation	95–99%	95–99%
Base excess	+3–(−2)	+3–(−2)
Bicarbonate (HCO^{3-})	22–26 mEq/L	22–26 mEq/L

URINE TESTS

URINE	MEN	WOMEN
pH	4.5–8.0	4.5–8.0
Specific gravity	1.005–1.03	1.005–1.03

APPENDIX H

Controlled Substances Schedules

General

A controlled substance is any type of drug that the federal government has categorized as having significant potential for abuse or addiction. While controlled substances are regulated in both the United States (U.S.) and Canada, differences exist between the two countries with respect to scheduling and enforcement.

IN THE U.S.:

The Drug Enforcement Agency (DEA), an arm of the U.S. Justice Department, classifies controlled substances according to five schedules, based on whether they have a currently accepted medical use in treatment in the U.S., the potential for abuse and dependence liability (physical and psychological) of the medication, and likelihood of causing dependence when abused. Some states may have stricter prescription regulations. Physicians, dentists, podiatrists, and veterinarians may prescribe controlled substances. Nurse practitioners and physician assistants may also prescribe controlled substances with limitations that vary from state to state.

Schedule I (C-I):

Potential for abuse is so high as to be unacceptable. Have no currently accepted medical use in the United States. May be used for research with appropriate limitations. Examples are marijuana, LSD, and heroin.

Schedule II (C-II):

High potential for abuse that may lead to severe physical and psychological dependence (amphetamines, opioid analgesics, certain barbiturates). Outpatient prescriptions must be in writing. In emergencies, telephone orders may be acceptable if a written prescription is provided within 72 hr. No refills are allowed.

Schedule III (C-III):

Substances in this schedule have a potential for abuse less than substances in Schedules I or II, and abuse may lead to moderate or low physical dependence or high psychological dependence (certain nonbarbiturate sedatives, certain nonamphetamine CNS stimulants, certain opioid analgesics). Outpatient prescriptions can be refilled 5 times within 6 mo from date of issue if authorized by prescriber. Telephone orders are acceptable.

Schedule IV (C-IV):

Less abuse potential than Schedule III with minimal liability for physical or psychological dependence (certain sedatives/hypnotics, certain antianxiety agents, certain nonamphetamine CNS stimulants, some barbiturates, benzodiazepines). Outpatient prescriptions can be refilled 6 times within 6 mo from date of issue if authorized by prescriber. Telephone orders are acceptable.

Schedule V (C-V):

Minimal abuse potential. Number of outpatient refills determined by prescriber. Some products (cough suppressants with small amounts of codeine, antidiarrheals containing paregoric, pregabalin) may be available without prescription to patients >18 yr of age.

IN CANADA:

The federal ***Controlled Drugs and Substances Act (CDSA)*** along with the ***Narcotic Control Regulations***, Part G of the ***Food and Drug Regulations***, and the ***Benzodiazepines and Other Targeted Substances Regulations***, regulate narcotics, controlled drugs, and targeted substances.

The CDSA classifies controlled substances according to eight schedules and three classes of precursors. While a few examples are listed below, a complete list of drugs scheduled in Canada's Controlled Drugs and Substances act can be accessed at: https://laws-lois.justice.gc.ca/eng/acts/C%2D38.8/

Schedule I

—Opioids and derivatives and related drugs (e.g., morphine, oxycodone, heroin).

Schedule II
—Cannabis (marijuana) and derivatives.

Schedule III
—Amphetamines and related drugs and substances (e.g., methylphenidate, LSD).

Schedule IV
—Barbiturates and derivatives, anabolic steroids and related drugs, and benzodiazepines (e.g., diazepam).

Schedule VI
—Precursors Class A (e.g., pseudoephedrine and salts).
—Precursors Class B (e.g., acetone, toluene).
—Precursors Class C (mixtures of the above).

Schedules VII & VIII
—Cannabis and its resins in varying amounts.
(Note: In Canada marijuana may be used for medical purposes. It is regulated by the Access to Cannabis for Medical Purposes Regulations, which can be accessed at: https://www.laws-lois.justice.gc.ca/eng/regulations/SOR-2016-230/page-1.html)

The CDSA federally regulates conditions of sale, distribution, and accountability relating to controlled substances. Provincial legislation complements how patients access controlled substances from regulated health professionals. As such, it is imperative for an individual to become familiar with legislation pertaining to the specific province they are working in. Some federal regulations are as follows:

Narcotic drug—Two subcategories of prescription narcotics—"Straight" Narcotics and Verbal Prescription Narcotics

(e.g., codeine, morphine, fentanyl, oxycodone)

Straight Narcotics
- All single active ingredient products containing a narcotic, along with all narcotics for parenteral use and narcotic compounds containing >1 narcotic entity or <2 non-narcotic ingredients.
- Prescription can be written, faxed, or generated electronically in an authorized provincial electronic health record and must be signed and dated by prescriber.
- Refills are not permitted, but a prescription may be dispensed in divided portions. Prescription transfers from one pharmacist to another are not permitted.

Verbal Prescription Narcotic
(e.g., Tylenol No. 2 and Tylenol No. 3)
- Refers to oral combination products containing only one narcotic and ≥2 non-narcotic ingredients in a therapeutic dose. (Excluding diacetylmorphine, oxycodone, hydrocodone, methadone, or pentazocine. This means that an oral combination product that contains these drugs cannot be classified as a Verbal Prescription Narcotic.)
- Similar rules as above but prescriptions may also be verbal.

Exempted Codeine Preparations
(e.g., Tylenol No. 1)
- Under federal regulations, products containing codeine (meaning codeine phosphate or its equivalent) may be purchased over the counter, without a prescription, provided they have two other medicinal ingredients and a **maximum** of 8 mg of codeine per solid oral dose unit or 20 mg per 30 mL of liquid.
- The product may not be supplied if there are reasonable grounds to suspect the product will be used for other than recognized medical or dental purposes.

Controlled Drugs—Part 1
(e.g., Dexedrine, Ritalin, pentobarbital, secobarbital)
- Refers to drugs listed in Part I of the Schedule to Part G of the Food and Drug Regulations.

- Prescription may be written or verbal; no refills allowed if prescription is verbal.
- Refills are permitted if the number of repeats and the frequency or interval between refills is specified. Prescription transfers are not permitted.

Controlled Drugs—Parts 2 and 3

(e.g., other barbiturates and anabolic steroids)

- Refers to drugs listed in Parts II and III of the Schedule to Part G of the Food and Drug Regulations.
- Prescription may be written or verbal.
- Refills are permitted if prescribed in writing or verbally and the number of repeats and frequency or interval between refills is specified. Prescription transfers are not permitted.

Benzodiazepines and Other Targeted Substances

(e.g., lorazepam, diazepam)

- Refers to all benzodiazepines except flunitrazepam, which is listed in Schedule III of the Act as an illicit substance.
- Prescriptions may be written or verbal. Refills are permitted if the prescription is less than 1 yr old and the prescriber specifies the number of times it can be refilled. If the prescriber indicated the interval between refills, the pharmacist cannot refill the prescription if that interval has expired. Prescription transfers are permitted, but only once.

Resources:

1 Minister of Justice. (2023). *Controlled Drugs and Substances Act*. https://laws-lois.justice.gc.ca/PDF/C-38.8.pdf
2 National Association of Pharmacy Regulatory Authorities. (2025). https://www.napra.org
3 U.S. Department of Justice, Drug Enforcement Administration. (2025). *Controlled Substance Schedules*. https://www.dea.gov/drug-information/drug-scheduling

APPENDIX I

Equianalgesic Dosing Guidelines

OPIOID ANALGESICS STARTING ORAL DOSE COMMONLY USED FOR SEVERE PAIN

	EQUIANALGESIC DOSE		STARTING ORAL DOSE			
NAME	**ORAL***	**PARENTERAL†**	**ADULTS**	**CHILDREN**	**COMMENTS**	**PRECAUTIONS AND CONTRAINDICATIONS**
Morphine-like agonists (mu agonists)						
morphine	30 mg	10 mg	15–30 mg	0.3 mg/kg	Standard of comparison for opioid analgesics. Sustained release preparations (MS Contin) release over 8–12 hr. Other formulations (MS Contin) last 12–24 hr. Generic sustained release morphine preparations are now available.	For all opioids, caution in patients with impaired ventilation, bronchial asthma, ↑ intracranial pressure, liver failure.
hydromorphone (Dilaudid)	7.5 mg	1.5 mg	Opioid nave: 4–8 mg	0.06 mg/kg	Slightly shorter duration than morphine. Sustained release preparations release over 24 hr.	
fentanyl	—	0.1 mg	—	—		
oxycodone	20 mg	—	10–20 mg	0.2 mg/kg		
methadone	10 mg	5 mg	5–10 mg	0.2 mg/kg	Good oral potency, long plasma half-life (24–36 hr).	Accumulates with repeated dosing, requiring decreases in dose size and frequency, especially on days 2–5. Use with caution in older adults.

NAME	EQUIANALGESIC DOSE ORAL*	PARENTERAL†	STARTING ORAL DOSE ADULTS	CHILDREN	COMMENTS	PRECAUTIONS AND CONTRAINDICATIONS
levorphanol	2 mg (acute), 1 mg (chronic)	—	2–4 mg	0.04 mg/kg	Long plasma half-life (12–16 hr, but may be as long as 90–120 hr after one wk of dosing).	Accumulates on days 2 and 3. Use with caution in older adults.
oxymorphone (Opana)	10 mg	—	—	—	—	
meperidine (Demerol)	300 mg	100 mg	Not Recommended	—	Slightly shorter acting than morphine; accumulates with repetitive dosing causing CNS excitation; avoid in children with impaired renal function or who are receiving monoamine oxidase inhibitors.	Use with caution. Normeperidine (toxic metabolite) accumulates with repetitive dosing causing CNS excitation and a high risk of seizure. Avoid in children, renal impairment, and patients on monoamine oxidase inhibitors.
Centrally acting mu agonists						
tramadol (Ultram, ConZip)	120 mg	—	50–100 mg every 4–6 hr	—	Prodrug; significant serotonin reuptake inhibition. Maximum dose: IR 400 mg/day; ER 300 mg/day.	Caution with pre-existing seizure disorder, concurrent use of medications that ↓ seizure threshold, or medications that ↑ risk of serotonin syndrome.
tapentadol (Nucynta)	100 mg	—	50–100 mg every 4–6 hr	—	Sustained release preparation (Nucynta ER) releases over 12 hr. Blocks reuptake of norepinephrine > serotonin.	Caution with pre-existing seizure disorder or concurrent use of medications that ↓ seizure threshold.

	EQUIANALGESIC DOSE		STARTING ORAL DOSE			
NAME	**ORAL**	**PARENTERAL†**	**ADULTS**	**CHILDREN**	**COMMENTS**	**PRECAUTIONS AND CONTRAINDICATIONS**
Mixed agonists–antagonists (kappa agonists)						
nalbuphine	—	10 mg	10 mg every 3–6 hr	0.1–0.2 mg/kg every 3–4 hr	Not available orally; not scheduled under Controlled Substances Act. Kappa agonist, partial mu antagonist.	Incidence of psychotomimetic effects lower than with pentazocine; may precipitate withdrawal in opioid-dependent patients.
butorphanol	—	2 mg	1–4 mg every 3–4 hr (IM); 0.5–2 mg every 3–4 hr (IV)	—	Kappa agonist, partial mu antagonist. Also available in nasal spray.	Likenalbuphine.
Partial agonist						
buprenorphine	—	0.4 mg	0.3 mg every 6–8 hr (IM/IV)	2–12 yr: 0.2–0.6 mg every 4–6 hr (IM/IV)	Sublingual tablets now available both plain and with naloxone for opioid-dependent patient management for specially certified physicians. These tablets are not approved as analgesics. Also available as a long-acting transdermal patch (Butrans), and buccal film (Belbuca).	May precipitate withdrawal in opioid-dependent patients; not readily reversed by naloxone; avoid in labor.

* Starting dose should be lower for older adults.

† These are standard parenteral doses for acute pain in adults and can also be used to convert doses for IV infusions and repeated small IV boluses. For single IV boluses, use half the IM dose. IV doses for children >6 mo. = parenteral equianalgesic dose times weight (kg)/100.

‡ Irritating to tissues with repeated IM injections.

Kishner, S. (2022). Opioid equivalents and conversions. Medscape. https://emedicine.medscape.com/article/2138678-overview?form;eqfpf

GUIDELINES FOR PATIENT-CONTROLLED INTRAVENOUS OPIOID ADMINISTRATION FOR ADULTS WITH ACUTE PAIN

DRUG*	USUAL STARTING DOSE AFTER LOADING	USUAL DOSE RANGE	USUAL LOCKOUT (MIN)	USUAL LOCKOUT RANGE (MIN)
Morphine (1 mg/mL)	1 mg	0.5–2.5 mg	8	5–10
Hydromorphone (0.2 mg/mL)	0.2 mg	0.05–0.4 mg	8	5–10
Fentanyl (50 mcg/mL)	20 mcg	10–50 mcg	6	5–8

* Standard concentrations for most PCA machines are listed in parentheses.

Modified from *American Pain Society, Principles of Analgesic Use in the Treatment of Acute Pain and Cancer Pain*, 7th ed., American Pain Society, 2016.

FENTANYL TRANSDERMAL DOSE BASED ON DAILY MORPHINE DOSE*

ORAL 24-HR MORPHINE (mg/day)	TRANSDERMAL FENTANYL (mg/day)	FENTANYL TRANSDERMAL (mcg/hr)
30–90	0.6	25
91–150	1.2	50
151–210	1.8	75
211–270	2.4	100
271–330	3.0	125
331–390	3.6	150
391–450	4.2	175
451–510	4.8	200
511–570	5.4	225
571–630	6.0	250
631–690	6.6	275
691–750	7.2	300
For each additional 60 mg/day	+0.6	+25

* A 10-mg IM or 60-mg oral dose of morphine every 4 hr for 24 hr (total of 60 mg/day IM or 360 mg/day oral) was considered approximately equivalent to fentanyl transdermal 100 mcg/hr.

APPENDIX J

Food Sources for Specific Nutrients

Potassium-Rich Foods

artichoke
avocado
bananas
beet greens
bok choy
breadfruit
cantaloupe
cassava
coconut water
dried fruits
durian
grapefruit
honeydew
jackfruit
kiwi
kohlrabi
lima beans
mango
meats
milk
dried peas and beans
nuts
oranges/orange juice
papaya
peach
pear
plantains
pomegranate fruit and juice
pomelo
potatoes (white and sweet)
prunes/prune juice
pumpkin
rutabaga
salt substitute
spinach
sunflower seeds
Swiss chard
tomatoes/tomato juice
vegetable juice
winter squash (acorn, butternut, hubbard)

Sodium-Rich Foods

baking mixes (pancakes, muffins)
barbecue sauce
buttermilk
salted butter/margarine
canned chili
canned seafood
canned soups
canned spaghetti sauce
cured meats
dry onion soup mix
fast foods
frozen dinners
macaroni and cheese
microwave dinners
Parmesan cheese
pickles
salad dressings (prepared)
salt
salted pretzels, potato chips
sauerkraut
tomato ketchup

Calcium-Rich Foods

almond (milk/nuts)
calcium-fortified foods
canned salmon/sardines
cheese
cream soups (with milk)
greens: collard/mustard/turnip
kale
milk
soy (beans/milk)
spinach
tofu
yogurt

Vitamin K–Rich Foods

asparagus
beet greens
broccoli
brussels sprouts
cabbage
collard greens
dandelion leaves
garden cress
green tea leaves
kale
mustard greens
parsley
spinach
Swiss chard
turnip greens

Low-Sodium Foods

canned pumpkin
egg yolk
fresh vegetables
fruit
grits (not instant)
honey
jams and jellies
low-calorie mayonnaise
macaroons
puffed wheat and rice
dried peas and beans
sherbet
unsalted nuts
whiskey

Foods That Acidify Urine

cheeses
corn
cranberries
eggs
fish
grains (breads and cereals)
lentils
meats
nuts (Brazil, filberts, walnuts)
pasta
plums
poultry
prunes
rice

Foods That Alkalinize Urine

all fruits except cranberries, prunes, plums
all vegetables (except corn)
milk
nuts (almonds, chestnuts)

Foods Containing Tyramine

aged cheeses (blue, Boursault, brick, Brie, Camembert, cheddar, Emmentaler, Gruyère, mozzarella, Parmesan, Romano, Roquefort, Stilton, Swiss)
American processed cheese
avocados (especially overripe)
bananas
bean curd
beer and ale
caffeine-containing beverages (coffee, tea, colas)
caviar
chocolate
distilled spirits
fermented sausage (bologna, salami, pepperoni, summer sausage)
liver
meats prepared with tenderizer
miso soup
overripe fruit
peanuts
raisins
raspberries
red wine (especially Chianti)
sauerkraut
sherry
shrimp paste
smoked or pickled fish
soy sauce
vermouth
yeasts
yogurt

Iron-Rich Foods

cereals
clams
dried beans and peas
dried fruit
leafy green vegetables
lean red meats
molasses (blackstrap)
organ meats

Vitamin D–Rich Foods

canned salmon, sardines, tuna
cereals
fish
fish liver oils
fortified milk
nonfat dry milk

Foods That Interact With/Inhibit the CYP3A4 Isoenzyme

grapefruit
grapefruit juice
Seville oranges
tangelos

APPENDIX K

Insulins and Insulin Therapy

The goal of insulin therapy for patients with diabetes is to provide coverage that most closely resembles endogenous insulin production and results in the best glycemic control without hypoglycemia. Although daytime control of hyperglycemia may be accomplished with bolus doses of rapid-acting insulin analogs, elevations in fasting glucose may remain a problem. If fasting blood glucose levels remain elevated, the basal insulin dose (intermediate or long-acting) may have to be adjusted.

Most insulins used today are recombinant DNA human insulins. Produced through genetic engineering, synthetic human insulin is "manufactured" by yeast or nonpathogenic *E. coli*. In recent years, pharmaceutical companies have developed several new types and formulations of insulin.

Different insulins are distinguished by how quickly they are absorbed, the time and length of peak activity, and overall duration of action. Onset, peak, and duration of action times are approximate and vary according to individual factors such as injection site, blood supply, concurrent illnesses, lifestyle, and exercise level. These factors can vary from patient to patient and can vary in any patient from day to day.

There are 5 kinds of insulins: rapid-acting, short-acting, intermediate-acting, long-acting, and combination insulins.

Rapid-Acting Insulins

Rapid-acting insulins are analogs of regular insulin. An analog is a chemical structure very similar to another but differing in one component. Admelog/Humalog/Lyumjev (lispro), Apidra (glulisine), and Fiasp/Kirsty/Merilog/Novolog (aspart) are rapid-acting insulin analogs. The amino acid sequences of these analogs are nearly identical to human insulin. They differ in the positioning of certain proteins, which allows them to enter the bloodstream rapidly—within 15 min of subcutaneous injection. This closely mimics the body's own insulin response and allows greater flexibility in eating schedules for diabetic patients. Also, because these insulins leave the bloodstream quickly, the risk of hypoglycemic episodes several hours after the meal is lessened. The peak time for rapid-acting insulins is 1–2 hr, and the duration is 3–4 hr. Rapid-acting insulin solutions are clear. Insulin aspart, insulin glulisine, and insulin lispro (100 units/mL only) can be given IV in selected situations under medical supervision.

Short-Acting Insulins

Regular insulin is a short-acting insulin and is available commercially as Humulin R or Novolin R. The onset of regular insulin is 0.5–1 hr; its peak activity occurs 2–4 hr after subcutaneous injection and its duration of action is 5–7 hr. This time/action profile makes rigid meal scheduling necessary, as the patient must estimate that a meal will occur within 45 min of injection. Short-acting insulin solutions are clear. Regular insulin (100 units/mL only) can be given IV.

Intermediate-Acting Insulins

Intermediate-acting insulin contains protamine, which delays onset, peak, and duration of action to provide basal insulin coverage. Basal insulins are given to control blood glucose levels throughout the day when not eating. Commercially, intermediate-acting insulins are available as Humulin N or Novolin N. (The "N" stands for NPH.) Action starts between 2 and 4 hr after injecting. Peak activity occurs between 4 and 10 hr. Duration of action lasts 10–16 hr. The addition of protamine causes the cloudy appearance of intermediate-acting insulins and results in the formulation being a suspension rather than a solution. This is why these insulins must be gently mixed before administering. Intermediate-acting insulins can be mixed with short- or rapid-acting insulins to provide both basal and bolus coverage. Intermediate-acting insulins should not be administered IV.

Long-Acting Insulins

Long-acting insulins have the most delayed onset and the longest duration of all insulins. Products include Basaglar/Lantus/Rezvoglar/Semglee/Toujeo (glargine) and Tresiba (degludec). Peaks are not as prominent in long-acting insulins. In fact, insulin glargine has no real peak action because it forms slowly dissolving crystals in the subcutaneous tissue. The onset of action of insulin glargine is 3–4 hr and for insulin degludec is within 2 hr after SUBQ injection. Full activity occurs within 4–5 hr and remains constant for 24 hr. Even though these insulins are clear solutions, they cannot be diluted or mixed with any other insulin or solution. Mixing these insulins with other insulin products can alter the onset of action and time to peak effect. If bolus insulin is to be given at the same time as insulin glargine or insulin degludec, two separate syringes and injection sites must be used. Long-acting insulins should not be administered IV.

Combination Insulins

Various combinations of premixed insulins are available, containing fixed proportions of two different insulins, usually a short- and an intermediate-acting insulin. Typically, the intermediate-acting insulin makes up 70–75% of the mixture, with rapid- or short-acting insulin making up the remainder. Onset, peak, and duration vary according to each specific product. Brand names of these products include Humulin 70/30 (70% NPH, 30% regular), Humalog Mix 75/25 (75% insulin lispro protamine suspension and 25% insulin lispro), Humalog Mix 50/50 (50% insulin lispro protamine suspension and 50% insulin lispro), and Novolin 70/30 (70% NPH, 30% regular), or Novolog Mix 70/30 (70% insulin aspart protamine suspension and 30% insulin aspart).

BRAND NAME	GENERIC NAME	TYPE OF INSULIN	ONSET/PEAK/DURATION
Humalog Mix 75/25 Humalog Mix 50/50	insulin lispro protamine suspension and insulin lispro injection mixtures	Combination	15–30 min/2.8 hr/24 hr
Novolog Mix 70/30	insulin aspart protamine suspension and insulin aspart injection mixtures	Combination	15 min/1–4 hr/18–24 hr
Humulin 70/30	NPH/regular insulin mixture	Combination	30 min/2–12 hr/24 hr
Novolin 70/30	NPH/regular insulin mixture	Combination	30 min/2–12 hr/24 hr
Apidra	insulin glulisine	Rapid-Acting	Within 15 min/1–2 hr/3–4 hr
Admelog, Humalog, or Lyumjev	insulin lispro	Rapid-Acting	Within 15 min/1–2 hr/3–4 hr
Fiasp, Kirsty, Merilog, or Novolog	insulin aspart	Rapid-Acting	Within 15 min/1–2 hr/3–4 hr
Humulin R	regular insulin (SUBQ)	Short-Acting	½–1 hr/2–4 hr/5–7 hr
Novolin R	regular insulin (SUBQ)	Short-Acting	½–1 hr/2–4 hr/5–7 hr
Humulin R	regular insulin (IV)	Short-Acting	10–30 min/15–30 min/30–60 min
Novolin R	regular insulin (IV)	Short-Acting	10–30 min/15–30 min/30–60 min
Humulin N	NPH	Intermediate-Acting	2–4 hr/4–10 hr/10–16 hr
Novolin N	NPH	Intermediate-Acting	2–4 hr/4–10 hr/10–16 hr
Basaglar, Lantus, Rezvoglar, Semglee, or Toujeo	insulin glargine	Long-Acting	3–4 hr/No Peak/24 hr
Tresiba	insulin degludec	Long-Acting	Within 2 hr/12 hr/up to 42 hr

APPENDIX L

Differences in U.S. and Canadian Pharmaceutical Practices

In the U.S. and Canada, most drugs are prescribed and used similarly. However, certain processes and actions of the U.S. and Canadian pharmaceutical industries differ in significant ways, affecting both consumers and health care providers. Safety, marketing, and availability are three of these issues.

Safety

Controversy related to the importation of medications from Canada by U.S. consumers has sometimes raised concerns about the safety of these drugs. These fears are unfounded; in fact, the Canadian approval and manufacturing processes are very similar to U.S. processes. Both countries have pharmaceutical-related standards, laws, and policies to ensure that chemical entities marketed for human diseases and conditions are safe and effective. The process of taking a new drug from the laboratory to the pharmacy shelves includes:

Scientific development. The process begins with research. Scientists develop a new molecular entity targeted at a specific disease, symptom, or condition.

Patenting. A manufacturer applies for a patent, which prevents other drug companies from manufacturing a chemically identical drug. Patent protection lasts 20 years in the U.S. and Canada. After a patent expires, any manufacturer can make generic versions of the chemical; generic drugs typically cost much less than the brand-name drugs.

Preclinical testing. Before a drug is taken by human subjects, preclinical testing of the chemical is performed first on animals. Testing helps identify drug action, toxicity effects, side effects, adverse reactions, dose amounts and routes, and administration procedures. This phase can last anywhere from 3 to 5 years.

Permission to begin clinical testing. Once a drug is found to have demonstrable positive health effects and is safe for animal consumption, a manufacturer seeks permission to begin clinical studies with human subjects. In the U.S., this process is called New Drug Application and is administered by the Food and Drug Administration (FDA). In Canada, the process is referred to as a Clinical Trial Application and is administered by Health Canada.

Clinical trials. Clinical trials are initiated to establish the potential benefits and risks for humans. Several subphases are required in the clinical trials phase whereby increasingly larger sample sizes are necessary.

Phase 0: A new designation for first-in-human trials, which are designed to assess whether the drug affects humans in a manner that is expected.

Phase 1: Between 20 and 80 healthy volunteers are recruited to assess safety, tolerance, dose ranges, pharmacokinetics, and pharmacodynamics.

Phase 2: Up to 300 patient volunteers with the drug-targeted disease are enrolled to assess efficacy and toxicity. Variables from Phase I trials may also be assessed.

Phase 3: Between 1000 and 3000 patient volunteers are entered into a randomized, double-blinded study designed to confirm drug effectiveness, comparability with existing treatments, and further exploration of potential and real side effects.

Ongoing surveillance of a drug for rare or long-term effects, or Phase 4 in Canada, continues after approval is received and marketing begun.

Approval. The results of the clinical studies are reviewed by Health Canada in Canada and by the FDA in the U.S. These regulatory bodies assess all aspects of a drug, including the labeling. The approval process is often deemed excessively long by physicians and patients who are anxious to try new remedies for refractory or terminal diseases. Efforts are ongoing to shorten the process in both countries. For example, Health Canada is collaborating with the FDA to develop a harmonized system for new drug submissions. The Common Electronic Submissions Gateway between Health Canada and the U.S. FDA allows submissions to be sent to both countries in a common platform.

Marketing. Once a drug has been approved, it can be prescribed to consumers or, if it does not require a prescription, purchased by them.

Postmarketing surveillance. More clinical data become available when a drug is marketed and used by many people for longer periods of time. "Pharmacovigilance" is the term used to refer to the process of ongoing assessment of a drug's safety and effectiveness during this phase. In Canada, this includes Adverse Drug Reaction reporting by consumers and health professionals as described in "Detecting and Managing Adverse Drug Reactions."

Differences Between Canadian and U.S. Drug Pricing and Marketing

One major difference between Canadian and U.S. drug regulatory processes is pricing. In Canada, the Patented Medicine Prices Review Board regulates the prices that manufacturers can charge for prescription and nonprescription medicines. This is to ensure that prices are not excessive. No such control exists in the U.S., with postrebate prices for medications in the U.S. being approximately 10–15% higher than in Canada.[1]

Another difference is in advertising. In the U.S., manufacturers can market drugs directly, and forcefully, to consumers, a controversial privilege that has resulted in consumers requesting specific medications despite not necessarily understanding all of the risks and benefits. In Canada, such advertising is limited and subject to the approval of the Advertising Standards Canada agency and the Pharmaceutical Advertising Advisory Board. The Institute of Medicine had recommended a two-year moratorium on direct-to-consumer advertising for new drugs to better monitor safety; however, this proposal was never enacted as regulation. Instead, in May 2024, the FDA introduced a new requirement that all television and radio advertisements communicate risks more clearly.[2]

Natural Health Products

In Canada, Natural Health Products (NHPs) are regulated by Health Canada under the Natural Health Products Regulations. All NHPs must have a product license, and the Canadian sites that manufacture, package, label, and import these products must have a site license. A Natural Product Number or Homeopathic Medicine Number is issued for the product only after it has been reviewed by Health Canada for its safety and efficacy. The term "Natural Product" refers to vitamins and mineral supplements, herbal remedies, traditional and homeopathic medicines, probiotics, and other products, such as amino acids, enzymes, essential fatty acids, protein supplements, or personal care items for consumption that contain natural ingredients.

In the U.S., the FDA classifies natural products as food products under the Dietary Supplements Health Education Act, so claims about the ability of a supplement to diagnose, prevent, treat, or cure a disease are prohibited. It is not necessary, however, for natural products to undergo review or approval or for testing to be done for identity and purity of active ingredients.

Drug Schedule, Availability, and Pregnancy Category Differences

In Canada, drug schedules are used to classify medication according to accessibility. The Canadian drug schedules as defined by the National Pharmacy Regulatory Authorities are:

- **Schedule I:** Available only by prescription and provided by a pharmacist.
- **Schedule II:** Available only from a pharmacist; does not require a prescription; must be kept in an area with no public access (i.e., behind-the-counter).
- **Schedule III:** Available via open access in a pharmacy only (i.e. over-the-counter) to guarantee access to a pharmacist; does not require a prescription.
- **Unscheduled:** Can be sold in any store without professional supervision.

Each province and territory in Canada decides where to schedule each individual drug (except opioids and controlled substances), frequently changing schedules as new evidence is obtained. (Note: The province of Québec has not adopted this national model.)
The U.S. in contrast, categorizes medications according to two general classes:

- **Prescription Only:** Available only by prescription and provided by a pharmacist.
- **Over-the-Counter (OTC):** Available via open access in the pharmacy.

As a result of these differences in accessibility, some potentially dangerous drugs (such as insulin and codeine-containing cough medicines) are available only with a prescription in the U.S. and available without a prescription but in consultation with a pharmacist in Canada. Similarly, some Canadian drugs are available in combinations not found in the U.S. (see Appendix N for new Canadian combination drugs). There can also be significant variation within Canada due to each province and territory independently scheduling drugs, with the exception of narcotics and controlled substances. Other differences also exist with respect to drug availability between the two countries.

REFERENCES

SOURCES CITED

1 Jenei, K. Prasad, V., & Lythgoe, M.P. (2022). High US drug prices have global implications. *BMJ*, *376*(o693). https://doi.org/10.1136/bmj.o693

2 Johns, L., & Mezuk, B. (2025). Patient as consumers: Reflections on the FDA's new rule on direct-to consumer advertising. *American Journal of Preventive Medicine*, *68*(1), 210–214. https://doi.org/10.1016/j.amepre.2024.08.013

ADDITIONAL RESOURCES

Government of Canada. (2025, August 10). *Common electronic submissions gateway*. https://www.canada.ca/en/health-canada/services/drugs-health-products/drug-products/applications-submissions/guidance-documents/common-electronic-submissions-gateway.html

Government of Canada. (2025, August 10). *Health Canada*. https://www.canada.ca/en/health-canada.html

Government of Canada. (2025, August 10). *Natural health product regulation in Canada: Overview*. https://www.canada.ca/en/health-canada/services/drugs-health-products/natural-non-prescription/regulation.html

U.S. Food and Drug Administration. (2025, August 10). https://www.fda.gov

Comprehensive Index*

*Entries for **generic** names appear in **boldface type.** Trade names appear in regular type, with Canadian names preceded by a maple leaf icon (🍁). **CLASSIFICATIONS** appear in **BOLDFACE SMALL CAPS**. *Combination Drugs* appear in *italics* and can be accessed in Appendix N online at fadavis.com, herbal products are preceded by a yin-yang icon (☯) and can be accessed in Appendix M online at fadavis.com, and drugs with genetic implications are preceded by a double-helix icon (🧬). Immunizations can be accessed in Appendix O online at fadavis.com.

*Entries for **generic** names appear in **boldface type.** Trade names appear in regular type, with Canadian names preceded by a maple leaf icon (). **CLASSIFICATIONS** appear in **BOLDFACE SMALL CAPS**. *Combination Drugs* appear in *italics* and can be accessed in Appendix N online at fadavis.com, herbal products are preceded by a yin-yang icon () and can be accessed in Appendix M online at fadavis.com, and drugs with genetic implications are preceded by a double-helix icon (). Immunizations can be accessed in Appendix O online at fadavis.com.

*Entries for **generic** names appear in **boldface type.** Trade names appear in regular type, with Canadian names preceded by a maple leaf icon (🍁). **CLASSIFICATIONS** appear in **BOLDFACE SMALL CAPS**. *Combination Drugs* appear in *italics* and can be accessed in Appendix N online at fadavis.com, herbal products are preceded by a yin-yang icon (☯) and can be accessed in Appendix M online at fadavis.com, and drugs with genetic implications are preceded by a double-helix icon. Immunizations can be accessed in Appendix O online at fadavis.com.

*Entries for **generic** names appear in **boldface type.** Trade names appear in regular type, with Canadian names preceded by a maple leaf icon (🍁). **CLASSIFICATIONS** appear in **BOLDFACE SMALL CAPS**. *Combination Drugs* appear in *italics* and can be accessed in Appendix N online at fadavis.com, herbal products are preceded by a yin-yang icon (☯) and can be accessed in Appendix M online at fadavis.com, and drugs with genetic implications are preceded by a double-helix icon (🧬). Immunizations can be accessed in Appendix O online at fadavis.com.

*Entries for **generic** names appear in **boldface type.** Trade names appear in regular type, with Canadian names preceded by a maple leaf icon (🍁). CLASSIFICATIONS appear in BOLDFACE SMALL CAPS. *Combination Drugs* appear in *italics* and can be accessed in Appendix N online at fadavis.com, herbal products are preceded by a yin-yang icon (☯) and can be accessed in Appendix M online at fadavis.com, and drugs with genetic implications are preceded by a double-helix icon (🧬). Immunizations can be accessed in Appendix O online at fadavis.com.

*Entries for **generic** names appear in **boldface type.** Trade names appear in regular type, with Canadian names preceded by a maple leaf icon (🍁). **CLASSIFICATIONS** appear in **BOLDFACE SMALL CAPS.** *Combination Drugs* appear in *italics* and can be accessed in Appendix N online at fadavis.com, herbal products are preceded by a yin-yang icon (☯) and can be accessed in Appendix M online at fadavis.com, and drugs with genetic implications are preceded by a double-helix icon (🧬). Immunizations can be accessed in Appendix O online at fadavis.com.

*Entries for **generic** names appear in **boldface type.** Trade names appear in regular type, with Canadian names preceded by a maple leaf icon (🍁). **CLASSIFICATIONS** appear in **BOLDFACE SMALL CAPS**. *Combination Drugs* appear in *italics* and can be accessed in Appendix N online at fadavis.com, herbal products are preceded by a yin-yang icon (☯) and can be accessed in Appendix M online at fadavis.com, and drugs with genetic implications are preceded by a double-helix icon (🧬). Immunizations can be accessed in Appendix O online at fadavis.com.

*Entries for **generic** names appear in **boldface type.** Trade names appear in regular type, with Canadian names preceded by a maple leaf icon (🍁). **CLASSIFICATIONS** appear in **BOLDFACE SMALL CAPS**. *Combination Drugs* appear in *italics* and can be accessed in Appendix N online at fadavis.com, herbal products are preceded by a yin-yang icon (☯) and can be accessed in Appendix M online at fadavis.com, and drugs with genetic implications are preceded by a double-helix icon (🧬). Immunizations can be accessed in Appendix O online at fadavis.com.

D

*Entries for **generic** names appear in **boldface type.** Trade names appear in regular type, with Canadian names preceded by a maple leaf icon (🍁). **CLASSIFICATIONS** appear in **BOLDFACE SMALL CAPS.** *Combination Drugs* appear in *italics* and can be accessed in Appendix N online at fadavis.com, herbal products are preceded by a yin-yang icon (☯) and can be accessed in Appendix M online at fadavis.com, and drugs with genetic implications are preceded by a double-helix icon (🧬). Immunizations can be accessed in Appendix O online at fadavis.com.

*Entries for **generic** names appear in **boldface type.** Trade names appear in regular type, with Canadian names preceded by a maple leaf icon (🍁). CLASSIFICATIONS appear in BOLDFACE SMALL CAPS. *Combination Drugs* appear in *italics* and can be accessed in Appendix N online at fadavis.com, herbal products are preceded by a yin-yang icon (☯) and can be accessed in Appendix M online at fadavis.com, and drugs with genetic implications are preceded by a double-helix icon. Immunizations can be accessed in Appendix O online at fadavis.com.

*Entries for **generic** names appear in **boldface type.** Trade names appear in regular type, with Canadian names preceded by a maple leaf icon (🍁). **CLASSIFICATIONS** appear in **BOLDFACE SMALL CAPS.** *Combination Drugs* appear in *italics* and can be accessed in Appendix N online at fadavis.com, herbal products are preceded by a yin-yang icon (☯) and can be accessed in Appendix M online at fadavis.com, and drugs with genetic implications are preceded by a double-helix icon (🧬). Immunizations can be accessed in Appendix O online at fadavis.com.

*Entries for **generic** names appear in **boldface type.** Trade names appear in regular type, with Canadian names preceded by a maple leaf icon. **CLASSIFICATIONS** appear in **BOLDFACE SMALL CAPS**. *Combination Drugs* appear in *italics* and can be accessed in Appendix N online at fadavis.com, herbal products are preceded by a yin-yang icon and can be accessed in Appendix M online at fadavis.com, and drugs with genetic implications are preceded by a double-helix icon. Immunizations can be accessed in Appendix O online at fadavis.com.

COMPREHENSIVE INDEX

*Entries for **generic** names appear in **boldface type.** Trade names appear in regular type, with Canadian names preceded by a maple leaf icon (🍁). **CLASSIFICATIONS** appear in **BOLDFACE SMALL CAPS**. *Combination Drugs* appear in *italics* and can be accessed in Appendix N online at fadavis.com, herbal products are preceded by a yin-yang icon (☯) and can be accessed in Appendix M online at fadavis.com, and drugs with genetic implications are preceded by a double-helix icon (🧬). Immunizations can be accessed in Appendix O online at fadavis.com.

I

*Entries for **generic** names appear in **boldface type.** Trade names appear in regular type, with Canadian names preceded by a maple leaf icon (🍁). **CLASSIFICATIONS** appear in **BOLDFACE SMALL CAPS**. *Combination Drugs* appear in *italics* and can be accessed in Appendix N online at fadavis.com, herbal products are preceded by a yin-yang icon (☯) and can be accessed in Appendix M online at fadavis.com, and drugs with genetic implications are preceded by a double-helix icon (🧬). Immunizations can be accessed in Appendix O online at fadavis.com.

*Entries for **generic** names appear in **boldface type.** Trade names appear in regular type, with Canadian names preceded by a maple leaf icon. **CLASSIFICATIONS** appear in **BOLDFACE SMALL CAPS**. *Combination Drugs* appear in *italics* and can be accessed in Appendix N online at fadavis.com, herbal products are preceded by a yin-yang icon and can be accessed in Appendix M online at fadavis.com, and drugs with genetic implications are preceded by a double-helix icon. Immunizations can be accessed in Appendix O online at fadavis.com.

*Entries for **generic** names appear in **boldface type.** Trade names appear in regular type, with Canadian names preceded by a maple leaf icon ( ). **CLASSIFICATIONS** appear in **BOLDFACE SMALL CAPS.** *Combination Drugs* appear in *italics* and can be accessed in Appendix N online at fadavis.com, herbal products are preceded by a yin-yang icon ( ) and can be accessed in Appendix M online at fadavis.com, and drugs with genetic implications are preceded by a double-helix icon ( ). Immunizations can be accessed in Appendix O online at fadavis.com.

*Entries for **generic** names appear in **boldface type.** Trade names appear in regular type, with Canadian names preceded by a maple leaf icon (🍁). **CLASSIFICATIONS** appear in **BOLDFACE SMALL CAPS**. *Combination Drugs* appear in *italics* and can be accessed in Appendix N online at fadavis.com, herbal products are preceded by a yin-yang icon (☯) and can be accessed in Appendix M online at fadavis.com, and drugs with genetic implications are preceded by a double-helix icon. Immunizations can be accessed in Appendix O online at fadavis.com.

*Entries for **generic** names appear in **boldface type.** Trade names appear in regular type, with Canadian names preceded by a maple leaf icon (🍁). **CLASSIFICATIONS** appear in **BOLDFACE SMALL CAPS**. *Combination Drugs* appear in *italics* and can be accessed in Appendix N online at fadavis.com, herbal products are preceded by a yin-yang icon (☯) and can be accessed in Appendix M online at fadavis.com, and drugs with genetic implications are preceded by a double-helix icon (🧬). Immunizations can be accessed in Appendix O online at fadavis.com.

*Entries for **generic** names appear in **boldface type.** Trade names appear in regular type, with Canadian names preceded by a maple leaf icon (🍁). **CLASSIFICATIONS** appear in **BOLDFACE SMALL CAPS**. *Combination Drugs* appear in *italics* and can be accessed in Appendix N online at fadavis.com, herbal products are preceded by a yin-yang icon (☯) and can be accessed in Appendix M online at fadavis.com, and drugs with genetic implications are preceded by a double-helix icon (🧬). Immunizations can be accessed in Appendix O online at fadavis.com.

*Entries for **generic** names appear in **boldface type.** Trade names appear in regular type, with Canadian names preceded by a maple leaf icon (). **CLASSIFICATIONS** appear in **BOLDFACE SMALL CAPS**. *Combination Drugs* appear in *italics* and can be accessed in Appendix N online at fadavis.com, herbal products are preceded by a yin-yang icon () and can be accessed in Appendix M online at fadavis.com, and drugs with genetic implications are preceded by a double-helix icon (). Immunizations can be accessed in Appendix O online at fadavis.com.

*Entries for **generic** names appear in **boldface type.** Trade names appear in regular type, with Canadian names preceded by a maple leaf icon (🍁). **CLASSIFICATIONS** appear in **BOLDFACE SMALL CAPS**. *Combination Drugs* appear in *italics* and can be accessed in Appendix N online at fadavis.com, herbal products are preceded by a yin-yang icon (☯) and can be accessed in Appendix M online at fadavis.com, and drugs with genetic implications are preceded by a double-helix icon. Immunizations can be accessed in Appendix O online at fadavis.com.

COMPREHENSIVE INDEX

*Entries for **generic** names appear in **boldface type.** Trade names appear in regular type, with Canadian names preceded by a maple leaf icon (🍁). **CLASSIFICATIONS** appear in **BOLDFACE SMALL CAPS**. *Combination Drugs* appear in *italics* and can be accessed in Appendix N online at fadavis.com, herbal products are preceded by a yin-yang icon (☯) and can be accessed in Appendix M online at fadavis.com, and drugs with genetic implications are preceded by a double-helix icon (🧬). Immunizations can be accessed in Appendix O online at fadavis.com.

*Entries for **generic** names appear in **boldface type.** Trade names appear in regular type, with Canadian names preceded by a maple leaf icon (🍁). **CLASSIFICATIONS** appear in **BOLDFACE SMALL CAPS**. *Combination Drugs* appear in *italics* and can be accessed in Appendix N online at fadavis.com, herbal products are preceded by a yin-yang icon (☯) and can be accessed in Appendix M online at fadavis.com, and drugs with genetic implications are preceded by a double-helix icon (🧬). Immunizations can be accessed in Appendix O online at fadavis.com.

*Entries for **generic** names appear in **boldface type.** Trade names appear in regular type, with Canadian names preceded by a maple leaf icon (🍁). **CLASSIFICATIONS** appear in **BOLDFACE SMALL CAPS**. *Combination Drugs* appear in *italics* and can be accessed in Appendix N online at fadavis.com, herbal products are preceded by a yin-yang icon (☯) and can be accessed in Appendix M online at fadavis.com, and drugs with genetic implications are preceded by a double-helix icon (🧬). Immunizations can be accessed in Appendix O online at fadavis.com.

COMPREHENSIVE INDEX

*Entries for **generic** names appear in **boldface type.** Trade names appear in regular type, with Canadian names preceded by a maple leaf icon (🍁). **CLASSIFICATIONS** appear in **BOLDFACE SMALL CAPS**. *Combination Drugs* appear in *italics* and can be accessed in Appendix N online at fadavis.com, herbal products are preceded by a yin-yang icon (☯) and can be accessed in Appendix M online at fadavis.com, and drugs with genetic implications are preceded by a double-helix icon (🧬). Immunizations can be accessed in Appendix O online at fadavis.com.

*Entries for **generic** names appear in **boldface type.** Trade names appear in regular type, with Canadian names preceded by a maple leaf icon (🍁). **CLASSIFICATIONS** appear in **BOLDFACE SMALL CAPS**. *Combination Drugs* appear in *italics* and can be accessed in Appendix N online at fadavis.com, herbal products are preceded by a yin-yang icon (☯) and can be accessed in Appendix M online at fadavis.com, and drugs with genetic implications are preceded by a double-helix icon (🧬). Immunizations can be accessed in Appendix O online at fadavis.com.

*Entries for **generic** names appear in **boldface type.** Trade names appear in regular type, with Canadian names preceded by a maple leaf icon (🍁). **CLASSIFICATIONS** appear in **BOLDFACE SMALL CAPS**. *Combination Drugs* appear in *italics* and can be accessed in Appendix N online at fadavis.com, herbal products are preceded by a yin-yang icon (☯) and can be accessed in Appendix M online at fadavis.com, and drugs with genetic implications are preceded by a double-helix icon (🧬). Immunizations can be accessed in Appendix O online at fadavis.com.

Measurement Conversion Table

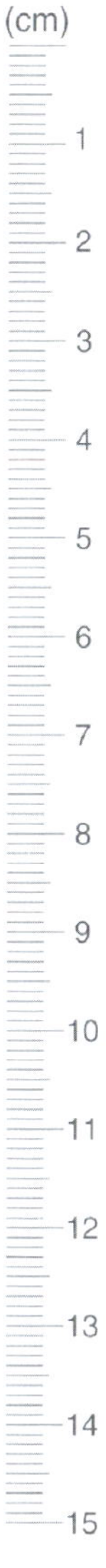

Metric System Equivalents

1 gram (g) = 1000 milligrams (mg)
1000 grams = 1 kilogram (kg)
0.001 milligram = 1 microgram (mcg)
1 liter (L) = 1000 milliliters (ml)
1 milliliter = 1 cubic centimeter (cc)
1 meter = 100 centimeters (cm)
1 meter = 1000 millimeters (mm)

Conversion Equivalents

Volume

1 milliliter = 15 minims (M) = 15 drops (gtt)

5 milliliters = 1 fluidram = 1 teaspoon (tsp)

15 milliliters = 4 fluidrams = 1 tablespoon (T)

30 milliliters = 1 ounce (oz) = 2 tablespoons

480 milliliters = 1 pint (pt)

960 milliliters = 1 quart (qt)

Weight

1 kilogram = 2.2 pounds (lb)
1 gram (g) = 1000 milligrams
0.6 gram = 600 milligrams
0.5 gram = 500 milligrams
0.325 gram = 325 milligrams = 5 grains (gr)
0.065 gram = 65 milligrams = 1 grain

Length

2.5 centimeters = 1 inch

Centigrade/Fahrenheit Conversions

$C = (F - 32) \times {}^{5}/_{9}$
$F = (C \times {}^{9}/_{5}) + 32$

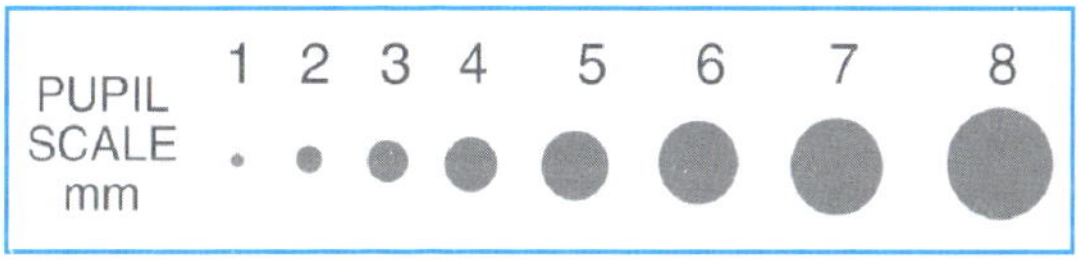

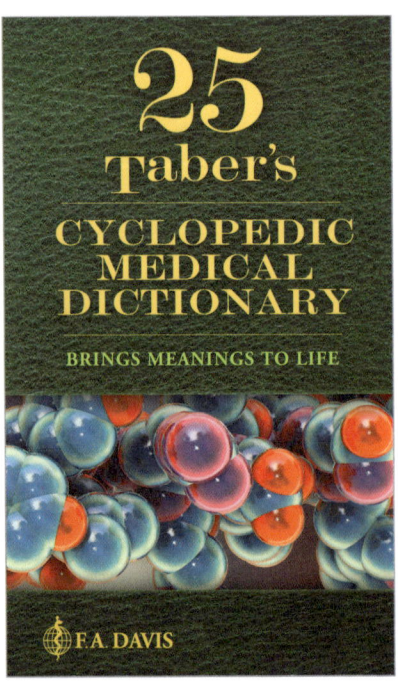

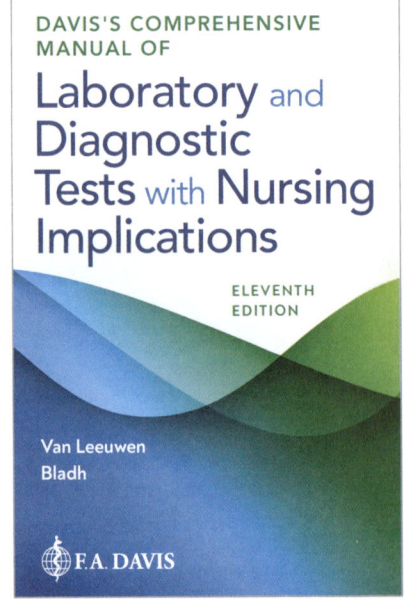

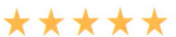